Debbie J. O'Hare.

To Veo,

A second-hand book for a first class career,

All my love,

Debbie

xxx

Essential Surgical Practice

Essential Surgical Practice

Edited by

A. Cuschieri MD ChM FRCS(Eng) FRCS(Edin)

Professor and Head of Department of Surgery, University of Dundee, Ninewells Hospital, Dundee

G. R. Giles MD FRCS

Professor and Head of Department of Surgery, St James's University Hospital, Leeds

A. R. Moossa MD FRCS(Eng) FRCS(Edin) FACS

Professor of Surgery, and Chairman of the Department of Surgery, University of California, San Diego; Surgeon-in-Chief, University of California Medical Center, San Diego, California

Second edition

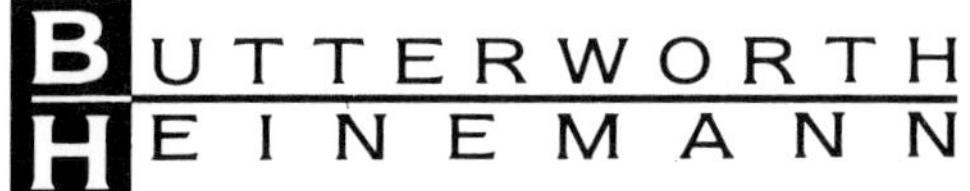

Butterworth-Heinemann Ltd
Linacre House, Jordan Hill, Oxford OX2 8DP

 PART OF REED INTERNATIONAL BOOKS

OXFORD LONDON BOSTON
MUNICH NEW DELHI SINGAPORE SYDNEY
TOKYO TORONTO WELLINGTON

First published 1982
Reprinted 1986
Second edition 1988
Reprinted 1992

British Library Cataloguing in Publication Data
Essential surgical practice
1. Surgery
I. Cuschieri, A. II. Giles, G. R.
III. Moossa, A. R.
617 RD31

ISBN 0 7506 0791 2
ISBN 0 7506 0886 2 International Edition

Printed and bound in Great Britain by
BPCC Hazells Ltd
Member of BPCC Ltd

Preface to the Second Edition

Our principal original aim in producing *Essential Surgical Practice* was to provide a comprehensive textbook of general surgery and allied specialties for the postgraduate student in surgical training. Inevitably since the first edition there have been changes in surgical practice which have necessitated extensive modifications and revision of the text. Furthermore, the first edition contained some imbalances of emphasis and other omissions which we felt required correction. Our approach to this second edition has been to improve and to update almost all of the chapters and in some instances to replace them entirely. However, the basic format remains as in the first edition with an early section on general aspects of surgery designed to provide a scientific base for the subsequent material. Although we deliberately do not include orthopaedic surgery in our remit, an entirely new section concerned with trauma has been added. This is written by American surgeons with a special interest in trauma, for this area of surgery has as yet to develop fully within the United Kingdom. It is our belief that the management and surgical treatment of the injured patient will require much more formalised training over the next 10 years and for this reason we believe that the new section will be more than justified. Following the same reasoning we have moved the section on transplant surgery into the general section as this is an area of surgical practice which has come of age and should no longer be considered to be on the fringe of a surgeon's interest. This chapter has been linked with the chapter on vascular access procedures which are required in a number of areas of practice outwith renal failure support.

This second edition is not intended as a reference book for the fully trained surgeon, and even for the surgical trainee there will still be the need to read detailed reviews of specialist areas of surgery. We do believe, however, that the second edition of *Essential Surgical Practice* provides an organized up-to-date account of modern surgical practice which covers the core material for those surgeons preparing for their postgraduate examinations.

We are grateful to our Publishers for their assistance in preparing the second edition and are indebted in particular to Dr G. Smaldon, whose tireless efforts and constant cajoling were instrumental in the completion of the second edition. Finally, we would like to thank our secretaries Mrs D. Bickerdike, Mrs I. Poole and Mrs J. Mackenzie for their invaluable secretarial assistance.

A. Cuschieri
G. R. Giles
A. R. Moossa

Preface to the First Edition

While we must admit to some self-doubt about the need for yet another textbook of surgery, we are conscious that there has been a distinct change in surgical practice over the past two to three decades. Whereas formerly there were surgical conditions requiring surgical procedures with defined results, risks, morbidity and success rates, the present-day surgical patient is often suffering from a variety of conditions requiring medical control or therapy. Thus the surgeon can no longer isolate himself from the advances which have occurred in our knowledge of surgical pathophysiology and from modern therapeutics. This basic need is reflected in our construction of this book which has a large section concerned with general aspects of management and a careful presentation at the beginning of each chapter of the basic anatomical and physiological principles which govern the natural function and disorders of each system.

We believe that we have produced a book in which the basic principles of practice are outlined and explained comprehensively but we have chosen not to include the practice of orthopaedics. Our reasons for doing so have been greatly influenced by the ready availability of excellent textbooks of orthopaedic surgery and the fact that this specialty has moved considerably from the practice of the general surgeon. Furthermore, we have not included detailed technique of operative procedures. We believe that cryptic descriptions of surgical operations in standard textbooks of clinical surgery are often misleading. The trainee surgeon ought to learn his operative surgery via the apprentice system offered by his senior peers and by reference to manuals of operative surgery.

It has not been our intention to produce a comprehensive reference textbook. Instead we hope to have compiled a manual of core surgical knowledge which is pertinent to the needs of the postgraduate surgical trainees in general surgery and its attendant specialties, particularly during the formative parts of their careers. Where it seemed appropriate we have asked our authors to indicate the likely future developments in their field and to provide a brief bibliography of good review articles or monographs so that the more discerning student may delve deeper into that subject. In order to restrict the size of the book an extensive bibliography has been omitted.

We are indebted to our authors who have attempted to maintain a uniform style and for their tolerance in allowing us to alter their scripts in minor details in order to avoid overlap of subject matter and to bring the style closer together.

We are indebted to the publishers for their guidance, useful advice, practical suggestions and for endeavouring to implement our views on presentation and layout of the text wherever possible. Their unfailing co-operation has been much appreciated. Finally, our special thanks go to our secretaries, Mrs J. Mackenzie, Mrs M. Kill, Mrs M. E. Cullingworth, Mrs I. Poole and Mrs J. Smith who between them bore the brunt of typing the main drafts of each chapter.

A. Cuschieri
G. R. Giles
A. R. Moossa

Contributors

C. E. Anagnostopoulos MD
Professor and Head, Cardiothoracic Surgery, State University of New York at Stony Brook, USA; Formerly Professor of Surgery, University of Chicago, San Diego

Andrew G. Batchelor BSc(Hons) MB BS FRCS(Eng) FRCS(Plastic Surgery)
Consultant Plastic Surgeon, St James's University Hospital, Leeds

Peter R. F. Bell MB ChB FRCS MD
Professor of Surgery, University of Leicester

Ian A. D. Bouchier MD ChB MD FRCP FRCP(Edin) FRSE
Professor and Head of Department of Medicine, Edinburgh Royal Infirmary

Paul F. Bradley MB BS FDS RCS(Eng) FRD RCS(Edin) BDS MRCS
Professor of Oral and Maxillofacial Surgery, University of Edinburgh and Honorary Consultant to Edinburgh Royal Infirmary

K. C. Calman MD PhD FRCP FRCS(Glas) FRSE
Dean of Postgraduate Medicine and Professor of Postgraduate Medical Education, University of Glasgow; Consultant in Clinical Oncology, Victoria Informary, Glasgow

John Chamberlain MB ChB FRCS(Edin)
Consultant Vascular Surgeon, Freeman Hospital, Newcastle upon Tyne; Honorary Clinical Lecturer in Surgery, University of Newcastle upon Tyne

D. Charlesworth DSc MD FRCS
Reader in Surgery, Victoria University of Manchester; Honorary Consultant Surgeon, University Hospital of South Manchester

R. A. Clark MB FRCP(Edin)
Consultant Physician and Head of Department of Respiratory Diseases, King's Cross Hospital, Dundee; Honorary Senior Lecturer, Department of Medicine, University of Dundee

H. Alan Crockard FRCS(Eng) FRCS(Edin)
Consultant Neurosurgeon, National Hospitals for Nervous Diseases, University College Hospital and The Middlesex Hospital, London

P. O. Daily MD FACS FACC FACCP
Clinical Professor of Surgery, and Head, Division of Cardiothoracic Surgery, University of California, San Diego; Director, Cardiovascular Surgery, Donald N. Sharp Memorial Hospital and Children's Hospital and Health Center, San Diego, California

R. F. Deane MB ChB FRCS(Edin) FRCS(Glas)
Consultant Urologist, Department of Urology, Western Infirmary, Glasgow

Peter H. Dickinson MS(Illinois) FRCS(Eng) FRCS(Edin)
Honorary Consultant Surgeon, Royal Victoria Infirmary, Newcastle upon Tyne; Honorary Lecturer in Surgery, University of Newcastle upon Tyne

William Duncan FRCP(Edin) FRCP(C) FRCS(Eng) FRCR(Lond) FACR(Hon)
Chief, Department of Radiation Oncology, Ontario Cancer Institute, Princess Margaret Hospital, Toronto; Professor, University of Toronto, Canada

J. C. Forrester ChM FRCS(Glas, Edin and Eng)
Consultant Surgeon, Ninewells Hospital, Dundee; Senior Lecturer in Surgery, University of Dundee

W. Frain-Bell MD FRCP
Physician-in-Charge, Department of Dermatology, Ninewells Hospital, Dundee; Senior Consultant in Dermatology, Tayside Health Board

Neill V. Freeman MB FRCS(Edin) FRCS
Consultant Paediatric and Neonatal Surgeon, Wessex Regional Centre for Paediatric Surgery, Southampton General Hospital; Senior Lecturer, Department of Surgery, University of Southampton

H. M. Gilles MD DSc FRCP FFCM DTM & H
Emeritus Professor of Tropical Medicine, University of Liverpool

P. J. Guillou BSc MD FRCS(Eng)
Senior Lecturer in Surgery and Consultant Surgeon, University Department of Surgery, St James's University Hospital, Leeds. Professor of Surgery (Elect) St Marys Hospital, London

Andrew Gunn RD MB ChB FRCS(Edin)
Consultant Surgeon, Ninewells Hospital and Medical School; Honorary Senior Lecturer in Surgery, University of Dundee.

T. B. Hargreave MS FRCS(Eng) FRCS(Edin)
Senior Lecturer, Department of Surgery, Edinburgh University; Honorary Consultant Urological and Renal Transplant Surgeon, Western General Hospital, Edinburgh

Graham L. Hill MD ChM FRCS(Eng) FRACS FALS
Professor and Chairman, University Department of Surgery, Auckland Hospital, Auckland, New Zealand

Jeffrey S. Hillman FRCS(Edin)
Consultant Ophthalmic Surgeon, St James's University Hospital, Leeds; Senior Clinical Lecturer in Ophthalmology, University of Leeds

Julian Hoff MD
Professor and Head, Section of Neurosurgery, University of Michigan, Ann Arbor, Michigan

David B. Hoyt MD
Assistant Professor of Surgery, Associate Director, Trauma Service, University of California, San Diego

C. S. Humphrey MD FRCS
Consultant Surgeon and Gastroenterologist, the Rochdale Hospitals, Rochdale, Lancashire

V. V. Kakkar MB BS FRCS FRCS(Edin)
Professor of Surgical Science, Director of Thrombosis Research Unit, King's College School of Medicine and Dentistry, University of London; Honorary Consultant Surgeon, King's College Hospital Group, London

M. R. B. Keighley MS FRCS
Professor of Surgery, The General Hospital, Birmingham

James Levett MD
Assistant Professor of Surgery, University of Chicago, Chicago, Illinois

M. S. McCormick MB ChB FRCS(Eng)
Consultant Otorhinolaryngologist to The Royal Liverpool Hospital and Arrowe Park District General Hospital, Wirral; Honorary Senior Lecturer, Department of Otorhinolaryngology, University of Liverpool

H. N. MacDonald PhD FRCOG
Consultant Obstetrician and Gynaecologist, St James's University Hospital, Leeds

John C. McGregor MB BSc(Hons) FRCS(Eng) FRCS(Edin)
Consultant Plastic and Reconstructive Surgeon; Honorary Senior Lecturer in Orthopaedics, University of Edinburgh

Robert C. Mackersie MD
Assistant Clinical Professor of Surgery, University of California, San Diego

A. G. D. Maran MD FRCS FACS
Head of Department of Otolaryngology, University of Edinburgh

Adrian Marston MA DM MCh(Oxon) FRCS(Eng) MD(Hon)
Consultant Surgeon, The Middlesex and University College Hospitals, London; Senior Lecturer in Surgery, University of London

A. J. Mearns MB FRCS(Eng) FRCS(Edin)
Cardiothoracic Surgeon, Bradford Royal Infirmary; Senior Visiting Research Fellow in Control Engineering, University of Bradford

Mark M. Mitchell MS MD
Associate Clinical Professor, Department of Anesthesiology, University of California, San Diego

William Y. Moores MD FACS
Associate Clinical Professor of Surgery, University of California, San Diego; Chief, Cardiothoracic Surgery Service, San Diego Veterans Administration Medical Center, San Diego

J. E. Newsam MB FRCS(Edin)
Consultant Urological Surgeon and Honorary Senior Lecturer, Western General Hospital, Edinburgh

Robert W. Parsons MD
Professor in Surgery and Pediatrics, University of Chicago Pritzker School of Medicine, Chicago, Illinois

Michael Powell FRCS(Eng)
Consultant Neurosurgeon, National Hospitals for Nervous Diseases, London

P. E. Preece MD(Wales) FRCS(Edin) FRCS(Eng)
Senior Lecturer and Honorary Consultant Surgeon, Ninewells Hospital and Medical School, Dundee

Alastair W. S. Ritchie MD FRCS(Edin)
Senior Registrar in Urology, Western General Hospital, Edinburgh

Martin C. Robson MD
Professor and Chairman, Division of Plastic and Reconstructive Surgery, Wayne State University School of Medicine, Detroit, Michigan

Marc M. Sedwitz MD
Assistant Professor of Surgery, University of California, San Diego

Steven R. Shackford MD FACS
Associate Professor of Surgery; Chief, Division of Trauma; Director, Regional Trauma Center, University of California, San Diego

A. J. Shearer MB ChB FFARCS
Consultant and Honorary Senior Lecturer in Anaesthesia, Ninewells Hospital and Medical School, Dundee

P. Sheridan MB FRCP(Eng)
Consultant Physician, Seacroft Hospital, Leeds

Bruce E. Stabile MD FACS
Associate Professor of Surgery, University of California at San Diego School of Medicine; Chief, Surgical Service, Veterans Administration Medical Center, San Diego

P. M. Stell ChM FRCS
Professor and Head of Department, Department of Otorhinolaryngology, University of Liverpool, Royal Liverpool Hospital

E. B. Stinson MD
Thelma and Henry Doelger Professor of Cardiovascular Surgery, Stanford Medical Center, Stanford, California

D. G. T. Thomas MA BCh FRCP(Glas) FRCS(Edin)
Consultant Neurosurgeon, The National Hospitals for Nervous Diseases and Senior Lecturer, Institute of Neurology, London

Kenneth Till MA MB BChir(Cantab) FRCS(Eng)
Honorary Consulting Neurological Surgeon, The Hospital for Sick Children, Great Ormond Street and University College Hospital, London

J. Tinker BSc FRCS(Glas) FRCP(Lond)
Director of the Intensive Therapy Unit, The Middlesex Hospital, London

M. G. Walker ChM FRCS(Edin)
Consultant Vascular Surgeon, Royal Infirmary, Manchester.

R. A. B. Wood MRCP(Lond) FRCS(Eng) FRCS(Edin)
Senior Lecturer in Surgery, University of Dundee; Honorary Consultant Surgeon, Tayside Health Board

Douglas R. Zusman MD
Assistant Clinical Professor of Surgery, University of California, San Diego; Co-Director, Heart Transplantation, Sharp Memorial Hospital, San Diego, California

Contents

Section 1

General Surgical Aspects

1 Wounds and their Management

J. C. Forrester

The life of an organism depends principally upon the preservation of its internal environment and this is based on its capacity to maintain and restore the integrity of its tissues. This inherent tendency to heal is so marked that its study is neglected by comparison with 'high technology' matters, such as organ transplantation and intensive care.

In earlier times the wound was assessed somewhat indirectly by studies of breaking strength and collagen content. Today we are able to look beyond these parameters to the behaviour of the individual cells in the wound. They are the prime movers in the healing process. When they function well the wound heals uneventfully.

THE ELEMENTS OF HEALING

Three distinct elements contribute to the process of wound repair.

1. Epithelization

This is the process by which surface covering of the wound is restored by a combination of cell migration and multiplication. The stimulus for epithelial repair is unknown. The loss of contact between cells undoubtedly plays a part. When an area is denuded of epithelium the marginal cells divide and migrate across the bare area. The activity ceases when epithelial contact is re-established with adjacent epithelial cells. There is also evidence that the loss of epithelial cover is associated with a fall in the level of a local inhibitory hormone or chalone which is synthesized by the epithelial cells. Epithelization proceeds most rapidly in a moist, highly oxygenated environment.

2. Contraction

This is the process by which the edges of an open wound gradually close together. It is a form of tissue migration that involves the entire thickness of the skin and subcutaneous tissues. It, therefore, proceeds most readily in areas where the skin is loose, such as the buttocks and the back of the neck. It is due to forces exerted by specialized fibroblasts in the wound. These cells have contractile elements in their cytoplasm and are named myofibroblasts. The process of contraction is physiological and must be distinguished from the pathological process of scar contracture or cicatrization which causes distortion and limitation of movement.

3. Connective Tissue Formation

This is the process by which the main body of the wound is united. It plays a fundamental role in all but the most superficial injuries and the strength of a wound following surgery is dependent on it. This is the most important element of the three and many studies of wound healing are simply examinations of this component in isolation.

TYPES OF HEALING

Although the elements of tissue repair are the same, open and closed wounds heal rather differently. When an incision is closed with sutures and heals without complication it is said to heal by first intention. Union takes place by a combination of epithelization and connective tissue formation. When an open wound is allowed to close naturally, union is accomplished by a combination of all three—wound contraction, connective tissue formation and epithelization. This is known as healing by second intention or by granulation.

Prior to the development of granulation tissue, the closed wound is much more susceptible to infection than the open wound. For this reason a heavily contaminated wound is often only partially closed. The deeper layers are secured but the subcutaneous tissues and skin are left open. Once healing is established and granulation tissue has formed the wound may be closed without fear of invasive infection developing. This technique is called delayed primary closure or secondary suture and this type of healing is known as healing by third intention.

PHASES OF HEALING

In deeper wounds, strength recovery is often an important attribute. Studies in the 1920s showed that this occurred in the phasic manner typical of many biological processes. In the first few days the wound has no recordable strength. Following this, strength increases rapidly. Finally, after a few weeks, the process slows up and further increases in strength occur much more slowly. These features of strength recovery correlate well with observed changes in the wound and healing is often considered as a three phase event.

In the first few days when the wound has no strength, little seems to be happening and this is called the *lag* phase. However, there is intense enzymic and leucocytic activity with breakdown and removal of devitalized tissue. A better term is the *preparation* phase, for the foundations for repair are being laid. During the next few weeks the scene is dominated by the proliferation of cells and capillaries. Neutrophils and macrophages are prominent and fibroblasts lay down collagen in increasing amounts. In an open wound this fibrocellular tissue is recognized as granulation tissue. This is the phase of *proliferation* or *fibroplasia*. After a variable number of weeks, these wound activities slow down. Fibroblasts and capillaries are less in evidence but strength progressively increases. This third phase is the one of *maturation* or *differentiation* which lasts many months.

THE ORGAN OF REPAIR

During the phase of proliferation the new tissue in the wound can be thought of as a repair organ (*Fig.* 1.1); its delicate stroma and extensive capillary network provide both physical and nutritional support for its component cells. The function of this organ is connective tissue formation. The fibroblast is the key cell synthesizing collagen and intercellular ground substance. Its activities together with those of the supporting macrophages are dependent on a readily available supply of oxygen. As a result cells and capillaries develop together as a unit and grow until the wound is filled. This new vascular connective tissue—granulation tissue—is most obvious in open wounds but it is also present between the edges of a healing incised wound. As time passes the fibroblasts and capillaries become much less prominent and a mature fibrous scar remains.

Wound Strength

The recovery of strength has obvious clinical significance and has proved to be one of the most useful indications of the progress of repair. Early studies of wound-breaking strength showed that the apparently well healed wound was still remarkably weak. These results, although criticized by bioengineers, have now been confirmed using approved bioengineering techniques. Skin and scar are complex visco-elastic materials which cannot be fully characterized unless tensile strength and extension (stretch) are recorded synchronously. Plotted together they describe a curve (load–extension) which reflects the ability of the scar to resist rupture (energy absorption) (*Fig.* 1.2). Studies of this sort show that, if anything, the wound is weaker than believed (*Fig.* 1.3). The findings are remarkably uniform demonstrating only a 50–70% recovery of strength by the end of 6 months. It appears that total recovery is rarely achieved. Such low recordings need not cause alarm for the absolute values are more than enough to meet the stresses imposed by every day life. These observations in animal wounds are confirmed in studies of excised human skin wounds (*Fig.* 1.4).

Wound Histology

Light microscope studies show a characteristic sequence of events (*Fig.* 1.5). As time elapses after wounding, specific cell populations appear on the scene. Neutrophils predominate in the first day or two and monocytes (macrophages) peak about 24 hours later. By 5 or 6 days fibroblasts are found in large numbers and their presence is paralleled by the development of a microcirculation. Collagen is readily identified in increasing amounts after the fourth day.

A characteristic sequence of enzyme changes is also seen

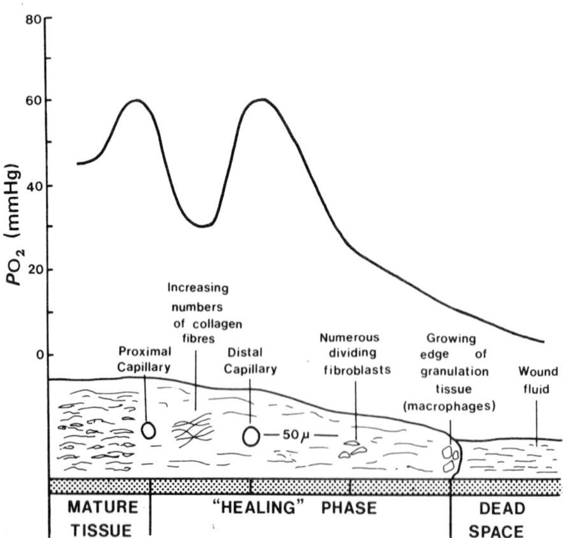

Fig. 1.1 Profile of a healing wound. It is a delicate system of cells and capillaries. New tissue grows from the 'vital' edge towards the central dead space. Direct measurements of Po_2 in this granulation tissue show a steady fall from the normal mature tissue level of around 45 mmHg to anoxic levels in the centre of the wound. Macrophages have a lower oxygen requirement than fibroblasts and are found at the free edge of the growing tissue. (After Silver I. A. 1980.)

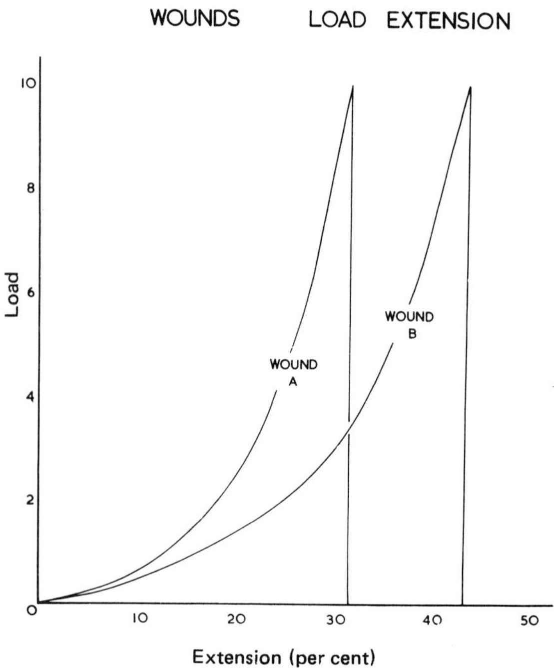

Fig. 1.2 Load–extension curves for wounds which break under the same load but differ in their degree of extension. Wound A is less pliable than wound B and is therefore more easily ruptured. The ability to resist rupture (energy absorption) is measured by the area under the curve.

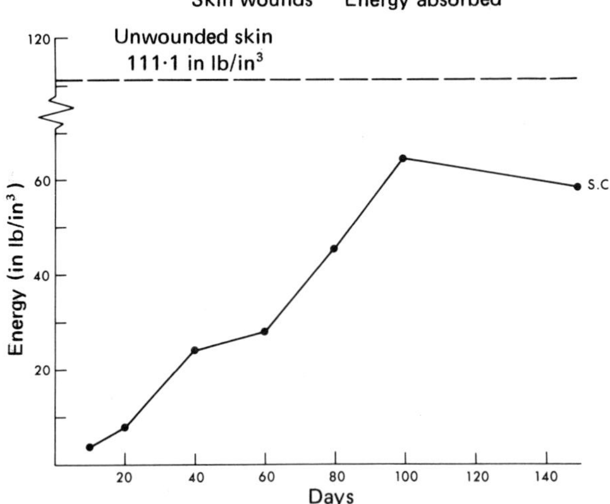

Fig. 1.3 The ability of a wound to resist rupture expressed as its energy absorption. There is only a 50% recovery by 150 days. (Reproduced by permission from Forrester J. C. et al. (1969) *J. Surg. Res.* **9**, 207–212.)

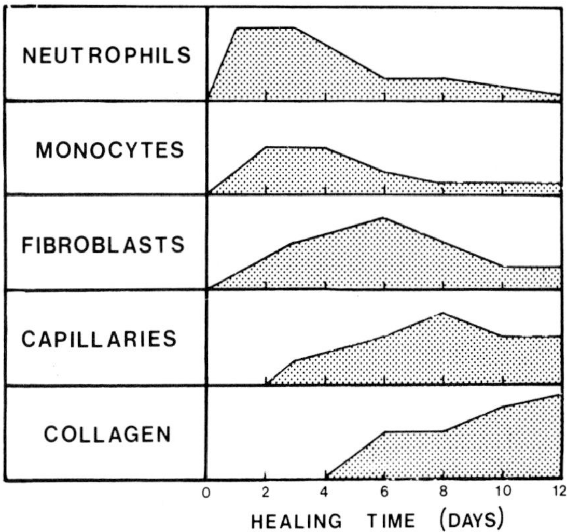

Fig. 1.5 The characteristic sequence of events in the first few days of wound healing. Neutrophils and monocytes appear first. Collagen appears following development of a functioning fibroblast-capillary system.

(*Fig.* 1.6). When identified histochemically these can be used to calculate the age of the wound in hours.

Collagen is responsible for most of the strength of the wound and the observed scar weakness is associated with physical changes in the collagen. When the wound is examined by polarized light normal collagen stands out as a clearly birefringent material. However, the wound scar does not exhibit this property during the first 6 months of healing. This lack of birefringence indicates a failure of organization at the molecular or small fibril level. Physical factors, such as fibre shape and weave, are important in determining the mechanical properties of skin and scar. These are best displayed by scanning electron microscope examination. In unwounded skin the collagen fibrils lie in well organized bundles (*Fig.* 1.7). In sutured wounds, the collagen fibrils lie in a relatively haphazard manner (*Fig.* 1.8). As time passes, the collagen fibrils in the wound coalesce to form large irregular masses (*Fig.* 1.9). Remodelling is minimal. As yet there is no evidence that the normal architectural network is ever restored.

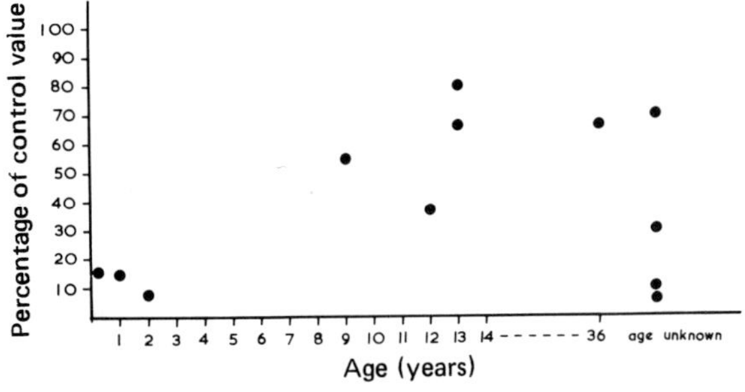

Fig. 1.4 The tensile strength of human skin wounds expressed as a percentage of intact skin. In the first 2-year period skin wounds are less than 20% of control value and even at 13 years there is still quite a marked weakness. (Reproduced by permission from Douglas D. M. et al. (1969) *Br. J. Surg.* **56**, 219–222.)

Wound Biochemistry

Of all the soft-tissue components that make up the body, only collagen has sufficient strength of its own to be responsible for the observed mechanical properties of unwounded tissue and firmly healed scar. The total amount of collagen rises very rapidly in a healing wound and normal levels are usually attained within a few weeks. However, strength continues to increase long after the collagen content has returned to normal. Clearly the quality of the collagen in the wound alters as time goes by.

Recent studies using radioactive tracer techniques have clarified the situation (*Fig.* 1.10). The total amount of collagen in the wound stabilizes after a few weeks but the rate of collagen synthesis and lysis remains high for considerably longer. This dynamic state may continue indefinitely for active collagenase has been isolated from healing wounds after 30 years. This balanced state of synthesis and lysis may explain several healing defects. In keloid and hypertrophic scars, over-production of collagen seems to be due to a relatively low rate of lysis. In scurvy it is the synthesis of collagen which fails and the wound weakens under the continued lytic process.

Collagen forms 30% of the total protein content of most animals. The collagen molecule is a rigid rod 300 nm long and 1·5 nm wide. Each molecule is composed of three polypeptide chains bound in a left-handed helix. The molecule itself is twisted the opposite way into a right-handed super-helix. The polypeptide chains of collagen are themselves remarkable. Over half the molecule is composed of the three amino acids glycine, proline and hydroxyproline. Both the carboxyl end and the amino terminal of the molecule are non-helical and the entire structure is held together by hydrogen bonds. These are relatively weak and the bulk of the strength of mature collagen is attributable to strong intermolecular and intramolecular covalent bonds. The individual amino acids are assembled in the endoplasmic reticulum of the fibroblast (*Fig.* 1.11), beginning at the amino

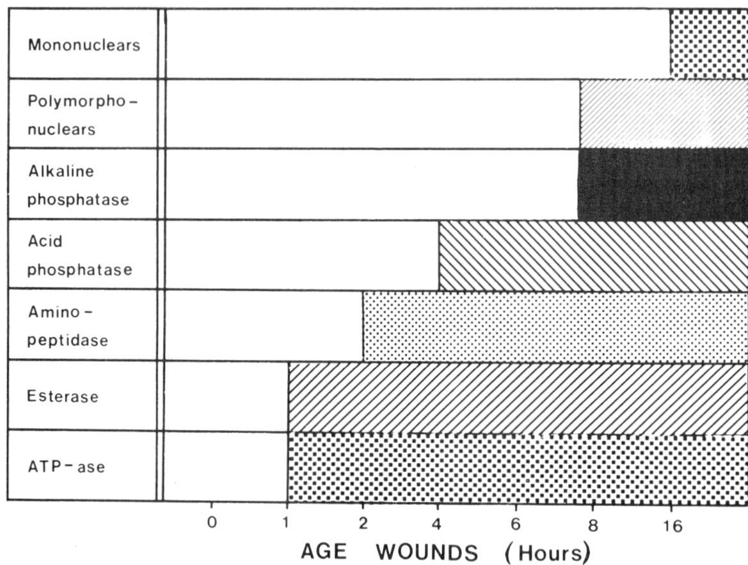

Fig. 1.6 Schematic diagram showing the histochemical estimation of the age of antemortem skin wounds. (Reproduced by permission from Raekallio J. (1972) *Forensic Sci.* **1**, 3–16.)

terminal and proceeding towards the carboxyl end. A unique feature in synthesis is that neither hydroxyproline nor hydroxylysine is incorporated directly into the collagen molecule. Instead a proline-rich collagen precursor (protocollagen) is formed. Hydroxylation then proceeds under the influence of protocollagen hydroxylase. Requirements of this enzyme are oxygen, alpha-ketoglutarate, ferrous iron and ascorbic acid. Each of these may interfere with collagen metabolism in experimental studies but the only one of practical importance is ascorbic acid, deficiency of which delays collagen synthesis. The incompletely synthesized collagen cannot be excreted from the fibroblasts and distends their endoplasmic reticulum in a characteristic way (*Fig.* 1.12).

It has recently become apparent that several different genes direct collagen synthesis. Five distinct types of collagen have been identified in vertebrate tissues. Type I characterizes mature bone and skin. Type II is found in hyaline cartilage, Type III features in cardiovascular structures, infant skin, and the granulation tissue of healing skin wounds. Types IV and V are associated with basement membranes. The significance of these different collagens is not yet clear but their presence does help explain why cutaneous scar tissue behaves differently from the surrounding dermis. Scar collagen contains both Types I and III and differs in its degree of hydroxylation of lysine and glycosylation of hydroxylysine. The cross-linking pattern is also different.

All connective tissues contain varying amounts of ground

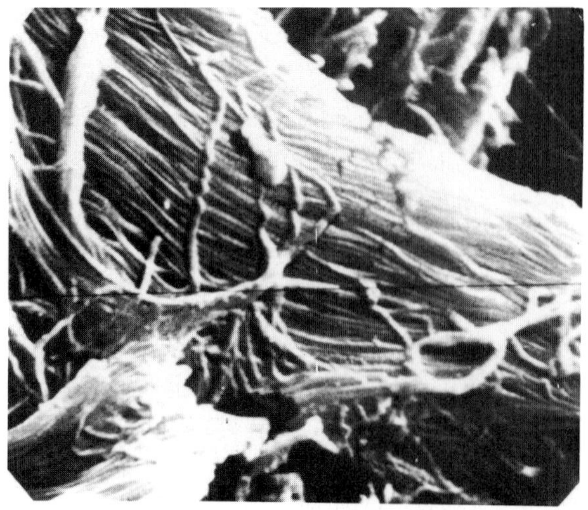

Fig. 1.7 Scanning electron micrograph of part of a normal collagen fibre showing that it is made up of bundles of cross-banded fibrils (×9000). (Reproduced by permission from Forrester J. C. et al. (1969) *Nature* **221**, 373–374.)

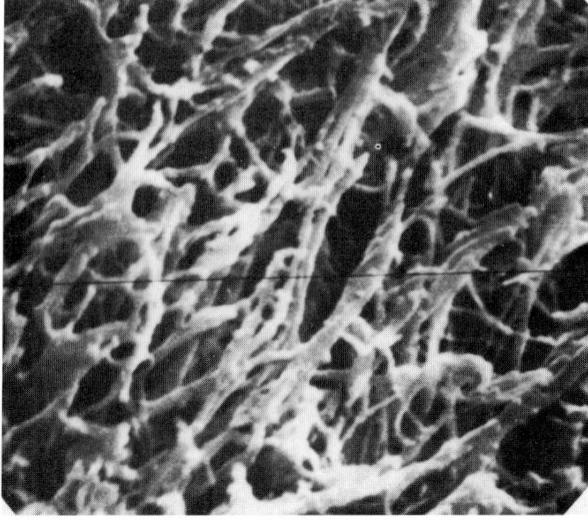

Fig. 1.8 Scanning electron micrograph of a 10-day sutured wound showing the randomly orientated collagen fibrils. They show little tendency to aggregate. Cross-banding is not apparent (×9000). (Reproduced by permission from Forrester J. C. et al. (1969) *Nature* **221**, 373–374.)

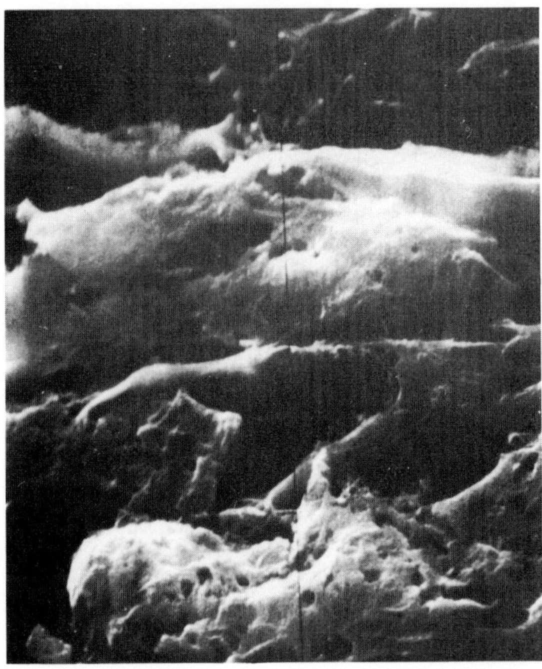

Fig. 1.9 Scanning electron micrograph of a representative portion of a 100-day wound. The collagen fibrils have aggregated to form large collagen masses but normal fibre architecture has not been restored (×3150). (Reproduced by permission from Forrester J. C. et al. (1969) *Nature* **221**, 373–374.)

substance. This amorphous matrix between the cells and fibres contains protein–glycosaminoglycan complexes called proteoglycans. The fibroblast synthesizes collagen, glycosaminoglycans and fibronectin. This latter component of the matrix is a large glycoprotein with important influences on both intercellular adhesion and cell to matrix adhesion.

The functions of the proteoglycans and fibronectin are incompletely understood but appear to play a part in the organization and precipitation of collagen fibres. The ground substance has, in addition, important effects on the mechanical properties of the mature tissue. The wound is a fibre–gel–fluid system and the mechanical properties of this complex material differ significantly from those of the fibrous tissue alone.

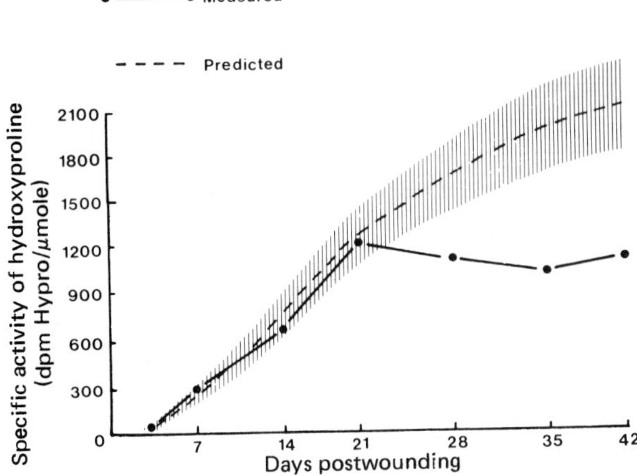

Fig. 1.10 Comparison of scar collagen accumulation predicted from its rate of synthesis with that actually measured. Total collagen does not increase after 3 weeks even though it continues to be synthesized and deposited at a rapid rate. Collagen is now being removed as quickly as it is formed (collagenolysis). The difference between the curves represents scar collagen turnover. (Reproduced by permission from Madden J. W. and Peacock E. E. jun. (1971) *Ann. Surg.* **174**, 511–520.)

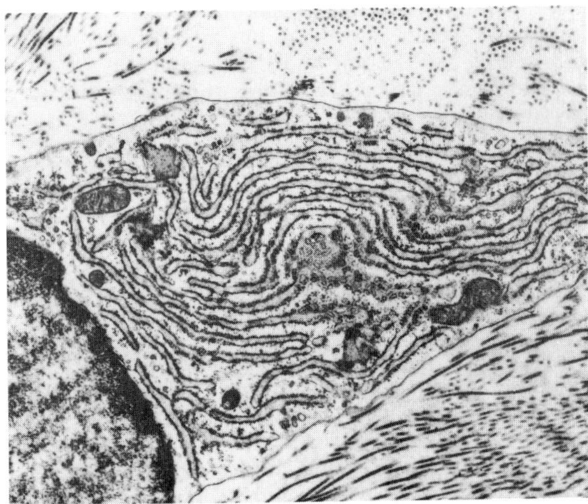

Fig. 1.11 Electron micrograph of part of a normal fibroblast. Note the characteristic well-developed endoplasmic reticulum. The lining ribosomes, which are responsible for its 'rough' appearance, are the active site of collagen synthesis. New collagen fibrils are rapidly excreted and are seen here surrounding the cell. Electron micrograph (×9000). (By courtesy of Professor Russell Ross, Seattle.)

FACTORS AFFECTING HEALING

A large number of factors influence the rate of healing. One or two of these have a clear but somewhat unpredictable

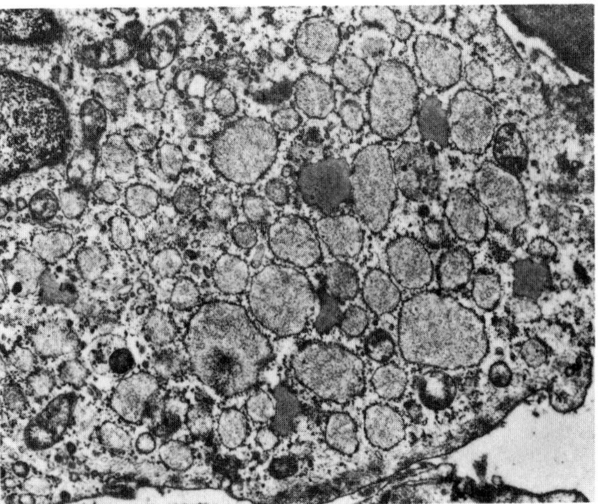

Fig. 1.12 Electron micrograph of part of a scorbutic fibroblast. Note the typical distended endoplasmic reticulum. There is no sign of collagen but it will appear within 24 hours of providing ascorbic acid. Electron micrograph (×9000). (By courtesy of Professor Russell Ross, Seattle.)

effect. For example, jaundice and uraemia adversely affect healing in experimental studies but in clinical work often seem to have little bearing on the end result. Several, however, do regularly affect the process of healing and deserve special mention.

Age

Healing proceeds more rapidly in the young, provided they are well nourished. The increased vigour of repair may explain why hypertrophic scars and keloids are more common in early life.

Nutrition

Clinical evidence suggests that wounds do not heal well in the debilitated or malnourished. However, recent work underlines the biological priority of the wound. Patients have to be severely protein depleted before healing is affected. Ascorbic acid is required for the synthesis and maintenance of collagen. Following injury, body stores are rapidly depleted and a scorbutic state may be induced. When this happens, collagen synthesis is impaired and healing is delayed. In older wounds where collagen turnover is still active, scars have been known to re-open. In countries where zinc is deficient, healing may be delayed. This is exceedingly rare in Great Britain.

Vascularity

Wounds heal well in areas like the face where the blood supply is good. The converse is found where blood flow is poor. The most striking examples are found in ischaemic vascular disease of the lower limb. Recent clinical studies have shown that both wound healing and the overall metabolic response to trauma are optimal when the environmental temperature is raised to 30°C. The combination of increased blood flow and warmth following sympathectomy has been shown to improve healing in patients with peripheral vascular disease.

A minimal inflammatory stimulus is required for healing to progress normally. If anti-inflammatory drugs, such as cortisone, are administered in the first few days after wounding, healing is likely to be delayed. Once healing is established cortisone does not appear to interfere with it. In practice wounds do heal in patients receiving long-term steroid therapy. However, the process is slow and more susceptible to complications.

Sepsis

Local infection is perhaps the most important cause of delayed wound healing and dehiscence. Collagen synthesis is depressed and collagenolysis is increased. This adversely affects the strength of repair and makes the cutting out of sutures more likely.

Oxygen

During the last two decades it has become clear that oxygen is the most important wound nutrient. A wound can only heal if its cells are functioning in a healthy vigorous fashion. Direct examination of the granulation tissue growing into a wound chamber shows a number of regular features (*see Fig.* 1.1). Po_2 levels fall steadily from the normal mature tissue level of around 45 mmHg (6·0 kPa) to levels close to zero in the centre of the wound. Fibroblast activity is maximal up to 50–80 µm away from the nearest normally perfused capillary. At this point Po_2 levels of between 10 and 20 mmHg

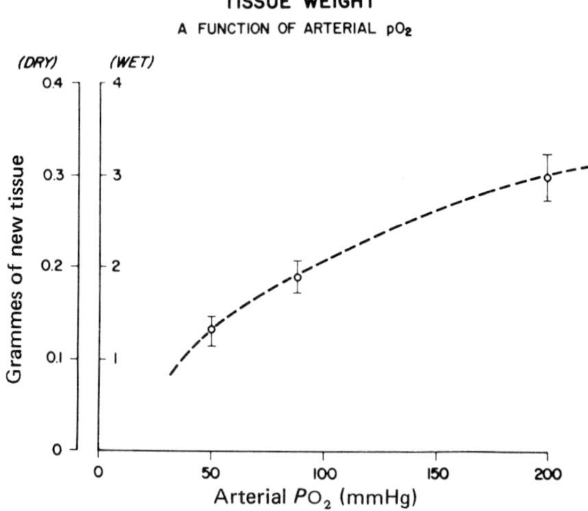

Fig. 1.13 The amount of new tissue formed in a wound is considerably greater when arterial PO_2 is increased by changing the ambient oxygen from 14 to 20 to 45% for 25 days. (Reproduced by permission from Hunt T. K. (1970) *J. Trauma* **10**, 1001–1009.)

(1·3–2·6 kPa) are regularly recorded. Macrophages have a lower oxygen requirement than fibroblasts and are found at the free edge of the growing granulation tissue. Even in these areas of very low oxygen tension they are still able to ingest bacteria but there is uncertainty about their ability to kill the ingested organisms. Increased oxygen uptake is invariably associated with the killing mechanism since the process is mediated by the peroxidase system. The delivery of nutrient oxygen to the wound is impaired by a number of local factors, such as tissue trauma and tight suturing techniques. More serious problems arise when wound capillary perfusion is impaired by systemic disorders. By far the most serious of these is the capillary shut-down associated with decreases in circulating blood volume. The wound, together with the splanchnic and cutaneous circulation, is the first to shut down in an attempt to maintain circulation to vital centres. Similar effects are observed in states of increased blood viscosity and cardiopulmonary decompensation. Finally, there is clear evidence that increasing the oxygen supply to a wound induces greater collagen production (*Fig.* 1.13) although it does not appear to affect the overall rate of healing. It must be borne in mind that collagen synthesis is only one of the many components that contribute to wound healing.

Wound Dressings

The undisturbed wound heals best and dressings may therefore impair the healing of open wounds by damaging the delicate new cells and capillaries on the wound surface.

Two recently developed materials largely overcome this problem. One is a wet polyacrilamide gel (Geliperm). This non-adherent sheet maintains a moist, well-oxygenated environment without encouraging bacterial growth. The second material is ideal for dressing deeper wounds. It is a Silastic foam which is poured into the wound and quickly sets to provide an exact fit. It, too, is inert and non-adherent. These two synthetic materials optimize the healing of an open wound by providing gentle inert support and cover.

WOUND FAILURE

Most wounds heal uneventfully, but failures do occur from time to time. These are the matters that cause surgeons most concern in everyday practice since they not only prolong the patient's stay in the ward but also may endanger life. Although healing is a unified response to injury, failures tend to present in three quite distinct ways. Acute failures are wound infection and wound dehiscence. Both of these problems may have repercussions later but there is one problem associated primarily with older wounds. This chronic failure is the condition of pathological fibrosis due to the overproduction of scar tissue.

Wound Fibrosis

This abnormally contracting state is often a late sequela of injury or inflammatory disease and features a whole range of chronic fibrotic processes from simple adhesions in peritoneum and tendon sheath to interstitial pulmonary fibrosis. Other troublesome examples are benign oesophageal stricture, mitral stenosis, hepatic cirrhosis and the post-traumatic cerebral scar. Attempts are now being made to control this pathological fibrosis by specific antifibrotic treatment of the scar and non-specific methods aimed at diminishing the inflammatory process that precedes fibroblast activation.

Drugs that affect collagen metabolism have more striking effects in the wound than elsewhere because of its high rate of turnover. Collagen synthesis can be prevented by interfering with hydroxylation of protocollagen within the fibroblast. This may be accomplished by removing cofactors, such as iron and ascorbic acid, or disturbing the configuration of the un-hydroxylated molecule with proline analogues. These techniques work *in vitro* but are disappointing in practice. Perhaps the most effective approach is to delay the maturation of the wound by preventing polymerization of tropocollagen. Simple accumulation of un-cross-linked collagen does not interfere with function. It is the rigid cross-linked collagen that causes fibrosis and deforming contractures. The abnormal physical behaviour appears to be associated with failure of soft-tissue remodelling following the irretrievable fixation of collagen fibril patterns by rapid intermolecular cross-linking when collagen is deposited in the young wound. When physical forces are applied to the wound before polymerization is complete the fibrils are aligned and mechanical properties enhanced. More useful effects follow when polymerization is arrested using β-aminopropionitrile. This drug works by blocking aldehyde formation and cross-linking. Penicillamine has similar effects. It chelates newly formed aldehydes before they take part in bond formation. The un-cross-linked collagen is free to organize in more physiological patterns and these are maintained when cross-linking is allowed to proceed. Since these new molecular patterns are reflected in the shape and weave of the collagen fibres themselves, the physical properties of the scar should be nearer normal.

Non-specific methods are aimed at controlling fibrosis by limiting the inflammatory process that precedes fibroblast activation. Anti-inflammatory drugs of steroid and non-steroid type have proved useful here and it seems likely that more specific agents will follow when the tissue activators of fibroblasts are properly identified. When tissue is injured lysosomal enzymes are released and damage the macrophages. The damaged macrophages stimulate fibroblasts to increase collagen production. In this way trauma creates necrosis and fibrosis results. If necrosis is reduced fibrosis is less. Studies in silicotic lung disease suggest that zinc may be useful here. It stabilizes lysosomes and protects macrophages from damage by silica. There is a considerable reduction in necrosis and fibrosis.

The present methods of managing fibrosis are imprecise, relying on surgical excision and judicious use of corticosteroids. The need for effective antifibrotic therapy is obvious. Until it is available the serious health hazard of excessive scar formation remains.

Wound Infection

This is the commonest and most troublesome disorder of wound healing. In the first studies attention was quite naturally directed towards the aerial contamination of wounds by bacteria. Since wound infection is rarely observed before the third or fourth postoperative day, it was widely believed that contamination was mainly a postoperative problem and that attention to ward design and dressing care would solve the problem. Yet there has been good evidence to the contrary since the early 1930s (*Fig.* 1.14). A primarily closed wound has no resistance at all to bacteria swabbed on its surface during the first 6 hours. After that time it becomes increasingly difficult to infect the wound until at 5 days it is as resistant as the surrounding skin. In practice, a wound is not subjected to such a severe challenge and clinical studies have shown that although an occlusive dressing would seem indicated for the first few days, it can in fact be left exposed with safety provided it is dry and not close to an obvious source of contamination, such as a colostomy.

Recent work suggests that so far as general surgery is concerned the main source of contaminating organisms is endogenous. Several studies of aerial bacteria in the operating theatre show significant variations in levels associated with the levels of activity of theatre personnel (*Fig.* 1.15). Although these levels may fluctuate quite widely the infection rate remains remarkably constant (*Fig.* 1.16). Also, if airborne infection was important it would be expected that operations of similar magnitude and duration would be equally likely to be followed by infection. However, this is not the case. In general surgical procedures the main source

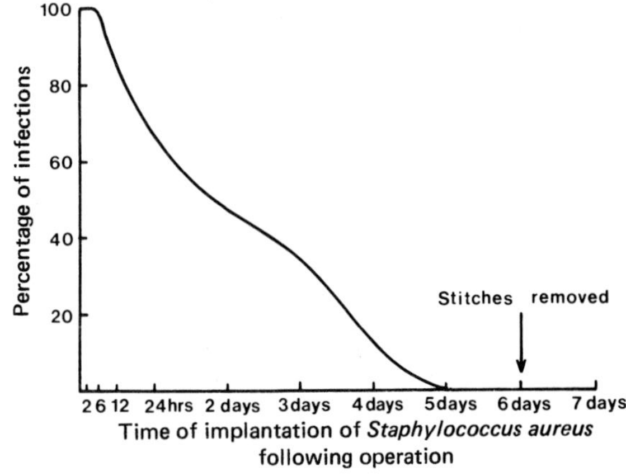

Fig. 1.14 The vulnerability of a healing incised wound to surface contamination with micro-organisms. During the first 6 hours it has no resistance. Thereafter it becomes increasingly resistant to invasion, and by 5 days it is as resistant as normal skin. (After DuMortier (1933) *Surg. Gynecol. Obstet.* **56**, 762–766.)

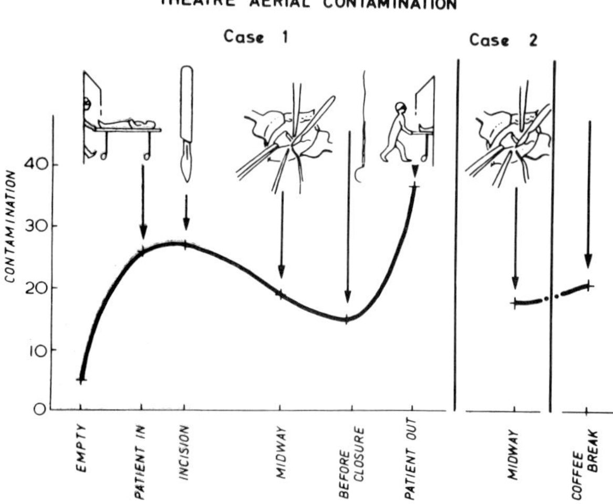

Fig. 1.15 Aerial contamination assessed during operations using a slit-sampler. Bacterial counts rise during operation and peak levels correspond with the increased movements of personnel at the beginning and the end of the procedure. (Reproduced by permission from Doig C. M. (1969) Aspects of Bacterial Carriage and Dissemination in a General Hospital. ChM Thesis, University of Dundee.)

of contaminating bacteria is the patient's own tissues. Airborne bacteria are responsible for only about 5% of infections.

Four different categories of wounds are recognized. Each has its own predictable rate of infection. A *clean wound* is an aseptic wound for an operation that does not transect the gastrointestinal, genito-urinary or tracheobronchial system. Familiar examples are lumbar sympathectomy and mastectomy. Reported infection rates here are usually between 1 and 4%. The *clean-contaminated* wound is one in which the gastrointestinal or respiratory tract is entered without significant spillage. A clean operation with a minor

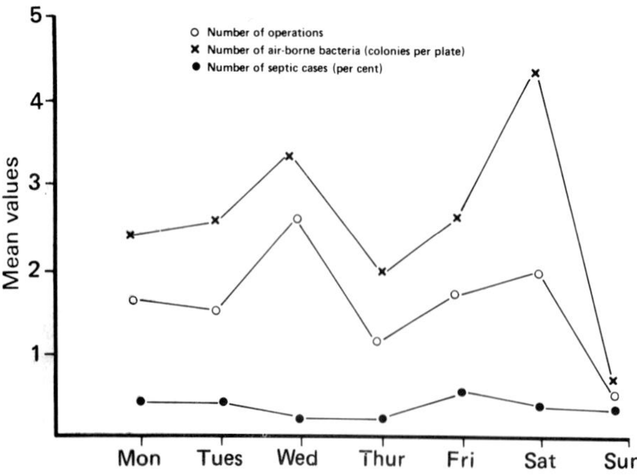

Fig. 1.16 Effect of theatre activity on aerial bacteria and wound sepsis. During the week, staff activity is stable and bacteria levels correlate with the number of operations performed. On Saturday, staff changes lead to increased activity of personnel and significantly higher bacterial counts. Despite these variations wound sepsis rates are unchanged. (Reproduced by permission from Burke J. F. (1964) *Monogr. Surg. Sci.* **1**, 301–345.)

break in sterile technique also comes into this category. The reported infection rates here are between 5 and 15%. The *contaminated* wound is one in which there has been gross spillage from gastrointestinal tract or, in the case of urinary and biliary procedures there is clear infection present. A clean wound with a major break in sterile technique may come into this category. The reported infection rates here are between 15 and 25% (when prophylactic antibiotics or antiseptics are not used). The fourth category is the *dirty* wound. In these cases the wound surfaces are directly contaminated by purulent material or continuing discharges from hollow viscera. Infection rates are unpredictable but usually greater than 25%.

In theory, the greater the number of organisms implanted in a wound the higher is the chance of infection developing. Just as infection cannot develop in the absence of bacteria, their simple presence is not enough. It has been repeatedly shown that organisms can be cultivated from most clean wounds at the end of an operation yet few become infected. The bacterial factors relate to the numbers and virulence of the organisms. In practice these are remarkably predictable. Host factors include general disorders such as inborn defects of resistance and immunity and more specific problems like chronic granulomatous disease and disease states associated with phagocyte malfunction. Wound factors are given less attention than is their due, perhaps because they relate in large measure to matters of individual surgical technique.

Local trauma from excessive retraction, over-zealous diathermy haemostasis or imprecise suture ligation will vitiate the most painstaking attention to the aseptic aspects of an operation. By contrast only 5% of a large series of emergency thoracotomy incisions became infected despite a complete absence of aseptic technique. In this series trauma was negligible and retraction forces were supported by the ribs rather than the soft tissues. Injuries elsewhere in the body also affect the incidence of wound infection but here the problem appears to be associated with factors such as hypovolaemia, increased blood viscosity and poor wound perfusion. The presence of extraneous material in a wound increases the chance of infection developing. The presence of a single piece of sterile silk suture material has been shown to enhance the infectivity of staphylococci by some ten thousand times. The presence of a tied silk suture has been shown to double the chance of a contaminated wound becoming infected. When tissue is devitalized by ligature the enhancement is even more marked (*Fig.* 1.17).

When wound perfusion is poor the availability of oxygen is decreased. The lowered levels of tissue P_{O_2} impair the function of the phagocytic cells at the wound surface. Bacteria are able to multiply in a relatively unimpeded manner and infection results. Increasing tissue oxygenation lowers the infection rate in strictly controlled experimental studies but does not have a useful application in clinical practice.

The usefulness of prophylactic antibiotics is now beyond doubt. Since bacteria multiply quickly the appropriate antibiotic must be administered as soon as possible. Antibiotics are most effective when given immediately and completely ineffective when administered more than 3 hours after bacterial inoculation (*Fig.* 1.18).

When indicated, prophylactic antibiotics should be administered routinely. In clean wounds where the natural infection rate is low, there is rarely any indication for their use. The exception is where any infection would be potentially catastrophic. This is mainly in vascular procedures where every measure is undertaken to avoid local infection

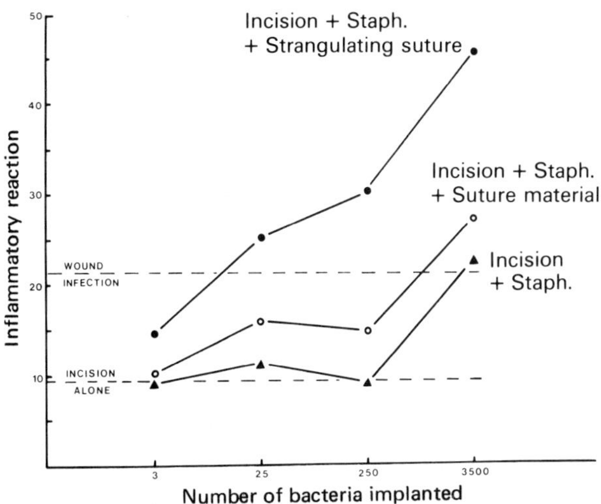

Fig. 1.17 The presence of extraneous material in a wound enhances the likelihood of infection developing. The presence of one tied silk suture doubles the chance of a contaminated wound becoming infected. (After Howe G. (1966) *Surg. Gynecol. Obstet.* **123**, 507–514.)

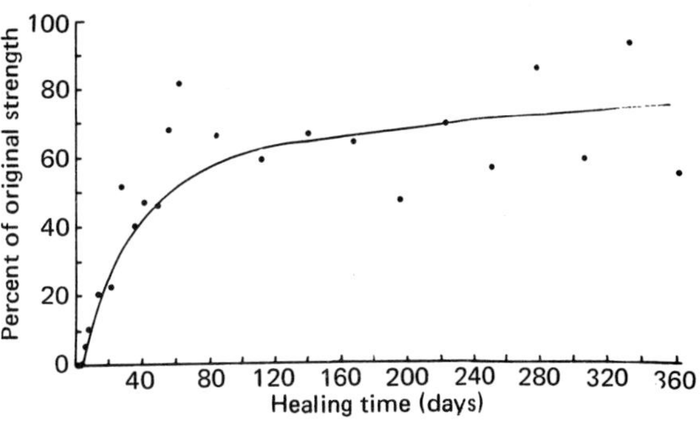

Fig. 1.19 Breaking strength of healing aponeurotic wounds. Strength increases rapidly for several weeks but then slows. There is only 70% recovery by the end of a year. (After Douglas D. M. (1952) *Br. J. Surg.* **40**, 79–84.)

with the attendant graft failure. In dirty wounds the bacterial contamination is so high that antibiotic medication is unlikely to reduce their numbers significantly. The main application of prophylactic antibiotics therefore lies in the moderately contaminated wound. Since the bacteria are unidentified at this stage a broad-spectrum antibiotic, such as cefuroxime, is selected. Metronidazole may be added. A single intraoperative dose appears to be sufficient and this routine minimizes possible toxic effects and the breeding out of resistant strains. Although topical application can be as effective the systemic administration of antibiotics is generally more certain. Antiseptics do not require matching to the contaminating organisms. Topical applications of iodine preparations prove highly effective. The reduced infection rate is comparable with that obtained with antibiotics.

Dehiscence

It is always a catastrophe when the edges of a healing wound break asunder. At its least the patient requires a second operation and hospital stay is prolonged. In other situations, particularly cardiac or vascular, it may be immediately fatal. In a high proportion of cases wound infection precedes and determines the result. However, even the apparently well healed wound exhibits biological features that make it less than completely secure.

Although collagen is rapidly synthesized in the wound, strength is recovered quite slowly (*Fig.* 1.19). It takes almost 3 months for aponeurosis to recover 70% of its original strength. By the end of a year it is a little stronger but the defect appears to be permanent. This weakness has particular relevance to healing in tissues of great natural strength, such as tendon or aponeurosis.

The second normal biological feature of repair is the softening of the tissues in the wound edge by collagenase activity (*Fig.* 1.20). The edges of a wound may appear firm and strong at the time the wound is repaired. However, this is far from the case a few days later. Collagenase is released when the wound is made and it diffuses into the tissues a few mm on either side. As a result the tissues at the wound edge become softened and are less able to hold any suture inserted at that point.

While strength of a wound is recovering, collagen synthesis and collagen lysis are delicately balanced. Wound strength is therefore adversely affected by any factor delaying collagen synthesis or increasing collagen lysis. Synthesis is impaired when there has been preoperative starvation sufficient to lower the body weight by about 20%. Impaired collagen synthesis is also found in patients on long-term steroid therapy. Radiation injury, uraemia, jaundice and diabetes have similar effects on fibroblast function.

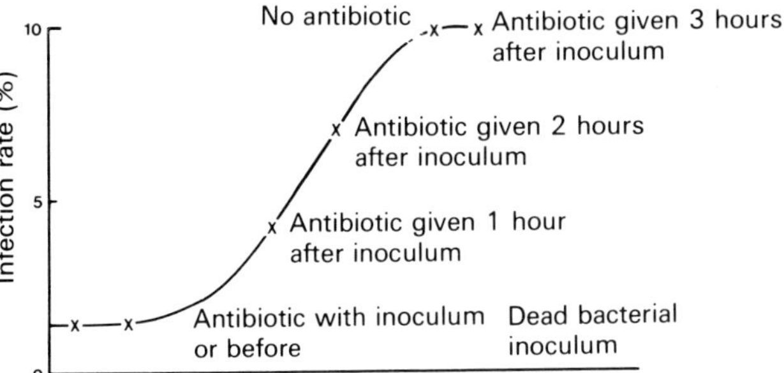

Fig. 1.18 Effect of systemic antibiotic on a contaminated wound. Prophylactic antibiotics are really only effective if given immediately. When they are administered more than 3 hours after bacterial inoculation they do not influence the incidence of infection. (After Burke J. F. (1961) *Surgery* **50**, 161–168.)

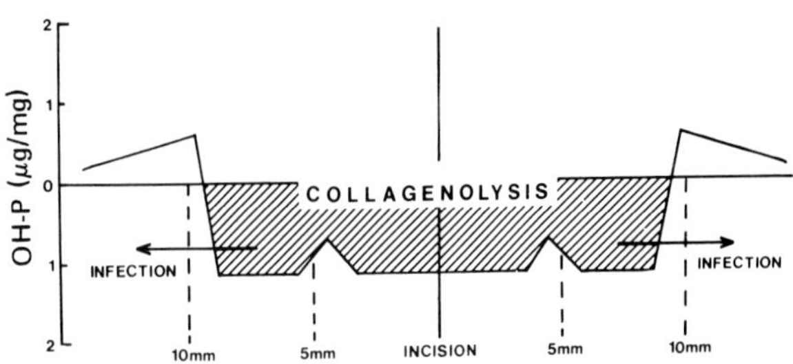

Fig. 1.20 The chemically active zone of an incised wound extends for at least 5 mm on either side of it. Collagen lysis is prominent in the first weak and is even more marked when infection is present. (After Adamsons R. J. et al. (1966) *Surg. Gynecol. Obstet.* **123**, 515–521.) The zero line is the concentration in normal abdominal wall.

These same factors may be present during operation but far more serious disturbances of collagen formation are associated with procedures in which a period of hypovolaemia occurs. Experimental work shows that even brief episodes of hypovolaemia without noticeable falls in blood pressure are associated with impaired wound perfusion and quite marked anoxia. Collagen synthesis and wound strength often take 4 or 5 days to get back to normal levels. Tissue trauma is the other major intraoperative factor associated with poor fibroblast function and impaired recovery of strength.

In the postoperative period a day or two's starvation is commonplace and this is unlikely to affect wound healing, provided the preoperative nutritional state of the patient was adequate. A variety of drugs, such as steroids, actinomycin, 5-fluorouracil and methotrexate, delay collagen synthesis by, in effect, paralysing the fibroblasts. Hypovolaemia with its associated wound hypoxia is still the most important source of trouble. Collagen lysis is encouraged by almost every agent that is associated with impaired collagen production. However, local trauma and infection are by far the most important stimulators of collagenolytic activity.

Wound dehiscence is therefore minimized by ensuring that the wound tissue is well nourished and oxygenated. This is achieved by a combination of gentle surgical technique and rapid restoration of circulating blood volume when it is reduced. An important aspect of surgical technique is suture use and selection. This activity requires considerable skill and judgement since a compromise situation has to be reached in every case. Sutures are required until the wound has sufficient strength to be self-supporting. On the other hand, sutures are foreign bodies and as such increase the likelihood of infection developing. This in turn is an important cause of delayed healing due to impaired collagen synthesis and increased collagen lysis.

Sutures are foreign bodies with inherent tissue-irritating propensities. The first essential is to use the finest sutures at all times. Materials with high tensile strength are, therefore, best (*Fig.* 1.21). The metallic sutures are the strongest and the natural sutures such as silk and catgut are the weakest. Synthetic materials, whether absorbable or non-absorbable, have an intermediate position. Since the metals usually cause more technical problems, the synthetic materials are usually the ideal choice. The bulk of foreign material is also

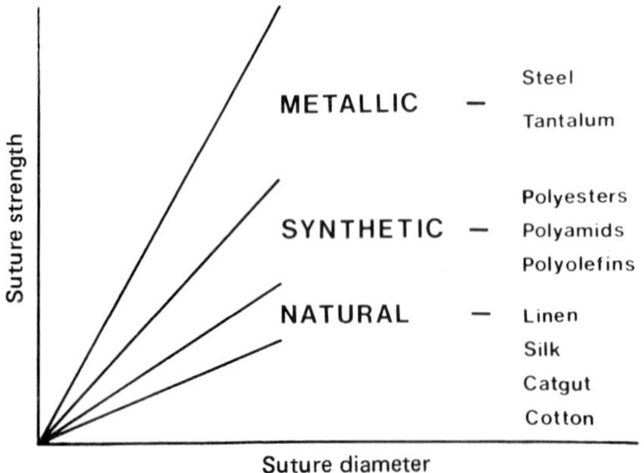

Fig. 1.21 The strength of a suture determines the size which is used. Natural fibres are the weakest and metallic ones are the strongest. The synthetics lie between and provide a fine suture of high strength. When they are used, less foreign material is implanted in the wound.

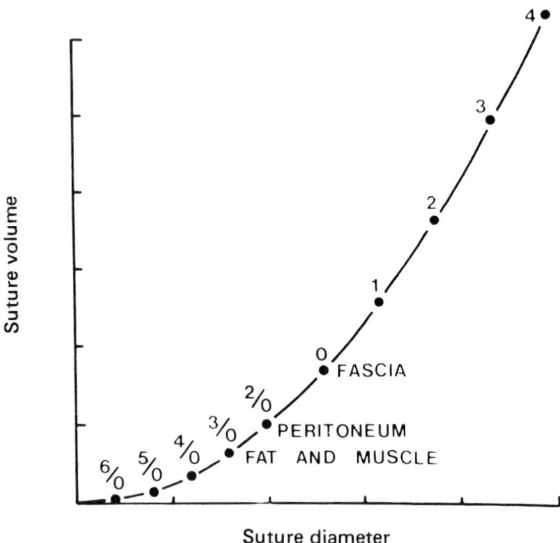

Fig. 1.22 The volume of implanted material goes up with the square of the diameter and selection of a suture one size heavier than necessary results in significantly more material being left behind in the wound.

minimized by selecting sutures at the finer end of the range. The volume of implanted material goes up with the square of the diameter and selection of a suture one size heavier than necessary results in significantly more material being left behind in the wound (*Fig.* 1.22). In any case it makes little sense to use a suture whose strength is much above the tissues it is holding together. Most tissues in the body are remarkably weak and it is only in the condensed collagen layers that holding power approaches that of 1/0 chromic catgut. In other tissues a much finer suture will suffice.

The next point is the lack of relationship between absorbability and suture strength (*Fig.* 1.23). Absorbable sutures lose strength rapidly and provide little effective support after a month. Despite this the suture may persist, apparently intact, for 90 days or more. In these cases it acts as a foreign body without helping support the wound.

The next consideration is the extent to which the particular suture irritates the tissues. All sutures do this to some degree (*Fig.* 1.24). In general, the natural materials are the most irritating and the synthetic monofilaments the least; the braided synthetics have an intermediate position. This inflammatory response to suture insertion delays healing and

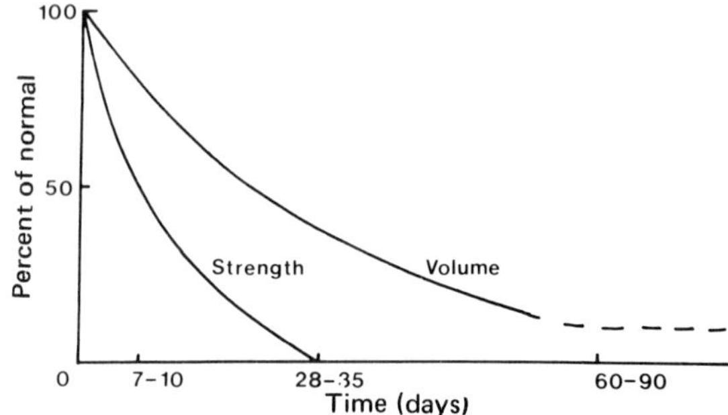

Fig. 1.23 Absorbable sutures lose strength much more quickly than non-absorbable. After one month they provide little if any support although continuing to act as a foreign body.

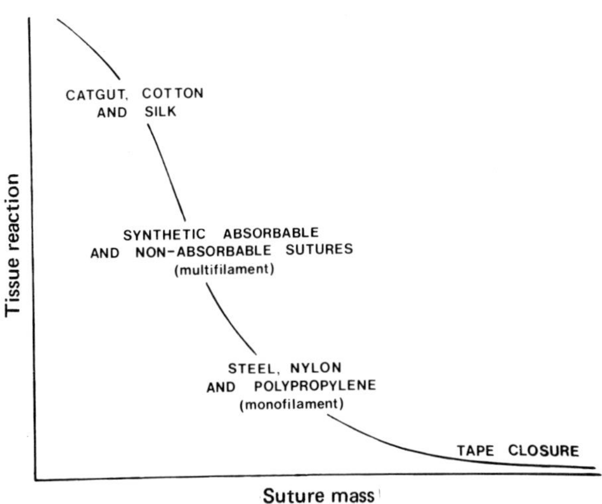

Fig. 1.24 Tissue reaction and suture material. The degree of tissue irritation elicited by a suture is an important determinant of wound infection. In general the natural materials are the most irritating and the synthetic monofilaments the least.

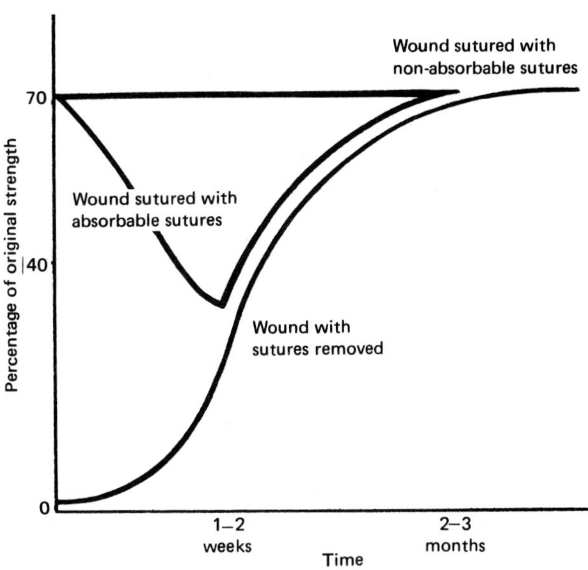

Fig. 1.25 Suture material and fascial healing. The unsutured fascial wound takes about 3 months to recover its strength. The sutured wound has this strength immediately. However, if the suture is absorbable its support steadily diminishes and wound strength falls to that of the unsutured tissue before it starts to recover. The critical point is between the first and second weeks and wound dehiscence is particularly common then.

enhances the infectivity of pathogens. Although this effect is minimized by using bland monofilaments it is not entirely eliminated and the ideal closure would be one in which sutures were dispensed with as in the tape closure of skin.

PRACTICAL APPLICATIONS IN WOUND REPAIR

Effective wound repair minimizes both infection and dehiscence. The selection of sutures is facilitated by picturing the wound as a delicate fibrocellular tissue with high oxygen requirements. Strength recovers slowly and the wound edges soften postoperatively as a result of collagenase released by local trauma and potentiated by infection.

The Fascial Wound

Few tissues hold sutures well but condensed collagen layers, such as fascia, do have significant holding power. However, they heal slowly, and, if strength is the desired feature of repair, the continued support of a non-absorbable suture is necessary. As soon as the wound is sutured it has considerable strength (*Fig.* 1.25). This is entirely due to the suture support. The wound itself has little strength until approximately 3 months have passed. It requires suture support until then and this can only be provided with certainty by non-absorbable materials. The use of absorbable sutures is by no means always associated with dehiscence but their progressive loss in strength means that there is a critical zone around the end of 2 weeks. It is no coincidence that, in earlier days, this was the time at which wound dehiscence commonly occurred.

The midline incision provides quick and easy access to the abdomen and dehiscence can virtually be eliminated when the particular characteristics of wound and suture are borne in mind. The aim is gentle prolonged support with a minimum amount of non-irritating suture material. A synthetic monofilament fits these requirements and insertion about 1 cm to the side of the wound ensures that it is safely outside the lytic zone. A continuous suturing technique is useful here since the stitch is to some extent self-adjusting and may accommodate to the patient's movement without unduly cutting into the wound tissue and causing local anoxia with all that entails. This technique is open to the criticism that a single break in the suture is likely to be catastrophic. This is not borne out in practice. In a series of over 500 consecutive midline closures, wound failures were a rarity and on every occasion the problem was 'cutting out' of the suture following prolonged local wound infection. In no case did the suture break.

Skin Closure

When fascial closure is secure skin repair need not be particularly strong and management is directed towards preventing wound infection and leaving a cosmetically acceptable scar. Wound infection is primarily a subcutaneous problem since this tissue offers little resistance to infection and pus accumulation. When bacterial contamination is severe it is best to treat the wound by delayed primary closure or perhaps simply to allow it to heal by second intention. When contamination is less severe it is sufficient to avoid percutaneous suture and use surgical tape to approximate the wound edges. In cases of technical difficulty a continuous subcuticular stitch usefully approximates the skin edges. It can be readily removed if infection supervenes otherwise it is left in place until the patient is about to be discharged. The end result is cosmetically good and the marked diminution in wound pain is particularly beneficial. Patients move around readily and the usual problems associated with immobility are notable by their absence.

When skin is approximated with conventional percutaneous sutures a small but significant zone of the wound is immediately fixed within rigid confines (*Fig.* 1.26). The normal inflammatory response of healing is associated with local swelling and the suture now cuts into the tissue. Local pain discourages movement but more serious is the locally impaired oxygenation. Even relatively small anoxic areas

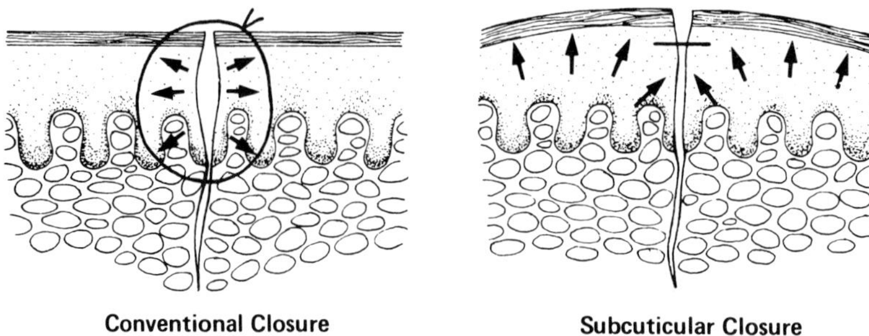

Fig. 1.26 Postoperative wound oedema is confined by percutaneous sutures. The suture cuts into the tissues causing pain and ischaemia. If the wound is contaminated infection is potentiated. When a subcuticular closure is used the tissues ride up over the oedema and discomfort is minimized. The microcirculation is maintained and infection is not enhanced.

may be sufficient to impair neutrophil function and as a result contaminating bacteria increase in number to the point where wound infection becomes inevitable. A simple way to overcome this is to use a continuous subcuticular stitch or surgical tape closure. Both these techniques allow the dispersion of tissue tension and encourage good capillary perfusion and wound oxygenation at all times.

The Contaminated Wound

The least favourable environment for bacteria is the open wound. If the cutaneous layers of a heavily contaminated wound are left open, invasive infection does not develop and once the newly forming granulation tissue has developed the wound may be secondarily closed without undue fuss. The other helpful measures are avoidance of non-irritating suture material or better still surgical tape closure of the skin edges. The question of prophylactic antibiotic administration has been referred to earlier and has a quite precise role to play here.

Repair of Special Tissues

The healing reactions of incised and open wounds are characteristic of the body's envelope of skin and fascia. Visceral healing shows some differences, perhaps because strength recovery is not usually so important.

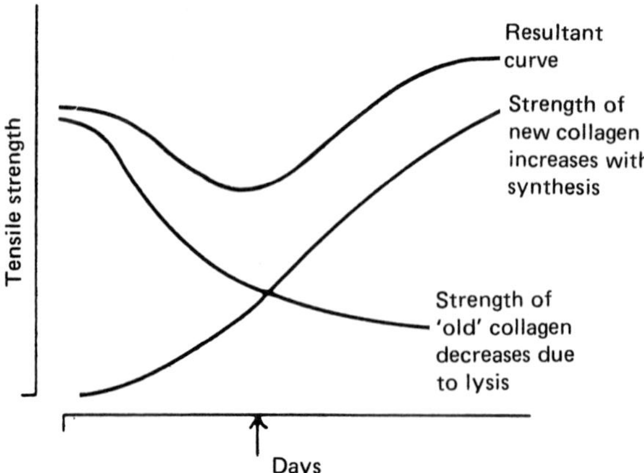

Fig. 1.27 The strength of colonic anastomoses is dependent on the balance between collagen lysis and synthesis. Since both these activities are marked the strength of colonic wounds is readily upset by factors interfering with collagen metabolism. (Reproduced by permission from Hunt T. K. and Hawley P. R. (1969) *Dis. Colon Rectum* **12**, 167–171.)

Bowel does not have great strength. Following anastomosis healing is very rapid and normal strength is recovered within 3 weeks. However, anastomotic leakage can be a problem, particularly in the colon and oesophagus. This is surprising when healing seems to be so rapid. However, it is this very rapidity which is often to blame. Collagen has an unusually high turnover rate in healing anastomoses. During the first 4–6 days up to 40% of the pre-existing collagen in the anastomosis is lost due to the very high levels of local collagenase activity (*Fig.* 1.27). Normally, strength is maintained by rapid synthesis of new collagen. However, with such high rates of synthesis and lysis the balance is easily upset. Local factors, such as trauma, foreign material and bacterial contamination all have adverse effects. The mechanical effects of food and faeces compound the problem. Where an anastomotic leakage is thought likely, tension-relieving sutures are always useful.

In the urinary tract healing is remarkably rapid. Quite large mucosal losses are rapidly covered by normal urothelium. Distensibility is the most valuable property of the bladder and tensile strength is always low in normal tissue. It is, therefore, not surprising to find that collagen synthesis in bladder wounds is maximal at 5 days and tensile strength is fully recovered by 3 weeks. Since prolonged suture strength is not required absorbable sutures suffice.

In blood vessels the connective tissue response is limited. Because of this, continued suture support is usually required for months. Accurate apposition is essential to ensure smooth healing and to avoid turbulent flow with local thrombosis. In prosthetic grafts a pseudo-intima rapidly develops but longitudinal ingrowth of fibrous tissue is limited to a few centimetres at either end. This new graft lining is relatively unstable and may come loose and occlude the vessel lower down. A more physiological graft material is the double-velour. This open meshwork material is pre-clotted with the patient's own blood and following establishment of flow is healed through the wall by the activities of fibroblasts and macrophages. Small capillary blood vessels are also seen. Artificial heart valves require particularly secure support. It should be remembered that they have to bear the brunt of around 40 million beats per year.

SUMMARY

Wound healing is a complex phenomenon affected by many factors. In concept however, it is relatively simple. The healing organ is a delicate capillary cell system (fibroblasts and macrophages). The basic functioning of this healing unit is adversely affected by anything from a heavy-handed approach at operation to factors affecting wound perfusion. Good tissue oxygenation enhances resistance to bacterial invasion and improves collagen synthesis.

Healing is slow and incomplete. Where strength recovery is important the continued support of non-absorbable sutures is required. Collagen turnover in the wound is relatively high and often prolonged. The deposition and removal of collagen is delicately balanced and readily upset by sepsis, shock and trauma as well as the presence of foreign material.

Most wounds heal well but failures of healing such as infection and dehiscence are particularly troublesome. In general surgery the source of infecting organisms is mainly the gastrointestinal tract. Micro-organisms can be cultured from most wounds but few become septic. The wound has an innate ability to resist infection provided it is kept healthy, and this basically means it is well nourished and supplied with as much oxygen as it requires. When prophylactic antibiotics are required they must be given as close to the time of bacterial seeding as possible.

Dehiscence or wound breakdown is found when sutures fail before the wound has fully recovered its strength. Commonly the stitches cut out because they are too near the wound edge.

Wound repair is the technical exercise whereby the wound is closed at the end of an operation. The prime consideration is gentle technique with the aim of minimally disturbing the delicate capillary blood supply and wound oxygenation. So far as *fascial closure* is concerned the suture of choice is a synthetic monofilament such as nylon or polypropylene. These provide permanent non-irritating support with the added advantage of not requiring removal should sepsis supervene. Since collagenase activity is marked and the wound edges unpredictably soft the sutures should be inserted well back from the wound edge to provide secure and even support. In this way the wound is supported from without rather than having the edges pulled together by fine stitches at the wound edge. In skin, the situation is different. Tape closure or subcuticular monofilament closure is associated with the lowest incidence of infection in contaminated wounds. However, where infection seems likely, the best routine is still delayed primary closure.

Further Reading

Adamsons R. J., Musco F. and Enquist I. F. (1966) The chemical dimensions of a healing incision. *Surg. Gynecol. Obstet.* **123**, 515–521.

Altemeier W. A., Burke J. F., Pruit B. A. et al. (ed.) (1984) *Manual on Control of Infection in Surgical Patients*, 2nd ed. Philadelphia, Lippincott.

Bornstein P. and Sage H. (1980) Structurally distinct collagen types. *Ann. Rev. Biochem.* **49**, 957–1003.

Chvapil M. (1975) Pharmacology of fibrosis: definitions, limits and perspectives. *Life Sci.* **16**, 1345–1362.

Douglas D. M., Forrester J. C. and Ogilvie R. R. (1969) Physical characteristics of collagen in the later stages of wound healing. *Br. J. Surg.* **56**, 219–222.

Forrester J. C. (1972) Suture materials and their use. *Br. J. Hosp. Med.* **8**, 578–592.

Forrester J. C. (1976) Surgical wound biology. *J. R. Coll. Surg. Edinb.* **21**, 239–249.

Forrester J. C., Zederfeldt B. H. and Hunt T. K. (1969) A bioengineering approach to the healing wound. *J. Surg. Res.* **9**, 207–212.

Gabbiani G. (1981) The myofibroblast: a key cell for wound healing and fibrocontractive diseases. *Prog. Clin. Biol. Res.* **54**, 183–194.

Hares M. M., Hegarty M. A., Warlow J. et al. (1981) A controlled trial to compare systemic and intra-incisional cefuroxime prophylaxis in high risk gastric surgery. *Br. J. Surg.* **68**, 276–280.

Hohn D. C. (1977) Leukocyte phagocytic function and dysfunction. *Surg. Gynecol. Obstet.* **144**, 99–104.

Mosher D. R. (1980) Fibronectin. *Prog. Hemost. Thromb.* **5**, 111–151.

Myers J. A. (1983) Geliperm: a non-textile wound dressing. *Pharm. J.* **230**, 263–264.

Niinikoski J., Hunt T. K. and Dunphy J. E. (1972) Oxygen supply in healing tissue. *Am. J. Surg.* **123**, 247–252.

Peacock E. E. (1981) Pharmacologic control of surface scarring in human beings. *Ann. Surg.* **193**, 592–597.

Polk H. C. and Lopez-Mayor J. F. (1969) Postoperative wound infection: a prospective study of determinant factors and prevention. *Surgery* **66**, 97–103.

Postlethwaite A. E., Keski-Oja J., Balian G. et al. (1981) Induction of fibroblast chemotaxis by fibronectin. *J. Exp. Med.* **153**, 494–499.

Prockop D. J., Kivirikko K. I., Tuderman L. et al. (1979) The biosynthesis of collagen and its disorders. *N. Engl. J. Med.* **302**, 13–23 and 77–85.

Rudolph R. (1979) Location of the force of wound contraction. *Surg. Gynecol. Obstet.* **148**, 547–551.

Silver I. A. (1977) Local factors in tissue oxygenation. *J. Clin. Pathol.* **30**, Suppl. 11, 7–13.

Silver I. A. (1980) The physiology of wound healing. In: Hunt T. K. (ed.) *Wound Healing and Wound Infection*. New York, Appleton-Century-Crofts, pp. 11–28.

Stone H. H., Haney B. B., Kolb L. D. et al. (1979) Prophylactic and preventive antibiotic therapy. *Ann. Surg.* **189**, 691–699.

Wood R. A. B., Williams R. H. P. and Hughes L. E. (1977) Foam elastomer dressings in the management of open granulating wounds. *Br. J. Surg.* **64**, 554–557.

2 *Ulcers, Abscesses, Sinuses, Fistulas and Foreign Body Reactions*

R. A. B. Wood and A. Cuschieri

Many of the conditions covered in this chapter have a common and close association with granulation tissue. The word comes from the 'grainy' appearance of the wound surface which derives from the numerous capillary loops and buds growing within it and giving it its red appearance. Following tissue injury, bleeding and then coagulation within a primitive fibrin clot stimulate an inflammatory response. The blood vessels in the area of the wound dilate, circulation slows and the white cells congregate on the walls of the dilated vessels. The capillaries near the wound become more permeable to inflammatory exudate containing plasma, white cells and some red cells. These early cells mainly undergo lysis releasing their contents. Monocytes from the blood and macrophages from the tissue increase in number and assume phagocytic activity throughout the inflammatory phase of wound healing. The macrophages also attract fibroblasts which start to proliferate. Fibroblasts produce collagen, fibronectin and polyglycans (ground substance). The macrophages synthesize many proteins including interferons, lipid enzymes and lysosomes. This inflammatory phase lasts 3–5 days and then recedes. The reconstructive or reparative phase is characterized by an increasing number of macrophages and fibroblasts at the expense of neutrophils which become progressively scanty. The fibroblasts produce a collagen-rich tissue cross-linked with fibronectin. This tissue contracts and the randomly distributed collagen is subsequently remodelled and replaced with new fibres laid down along stress lines. This process continues for a long time until the gain in the strength of the wound approximates to that of normal tissue, but it never completely reaches it.

Education concerning the management of granulating wounds is often inadequate. The poor management of these wounds prolongs the inflammatory phase of wound healing with consequent delay in the patient's recovery. At best this amounts to a failure of healing or early recurrence of the condition. The commonest mistake is the inadequate surgical drainage of an abscess or a granulating wound, the case being usually done by an unsupervised trainee at the end of a busy operating list. The after-care, designed to ensure correct dressing and drainage of the wound, is often neglected in the outpatient department with monthly or even longer appointments. Scanty follow-up notes reveal 'almost healed' repeated time and again. The reliance on prolonged antibiotics to control residual discharge which is assumed to be infection, is misplaced. The situation can only be remedied by adequate surgical intervention to ensure free drainage and thus end the inflammatory phase of healing so that the repair phase can begin.

The management of these conditions requires a planned approach with attention to detail and an exact diagnosis which sometimes requires radiological and other imaging tests. A misdiagnosis or inappropriate management may convert a simple treatable condition into one of a more serious nature, e.g., a high-level rectal fistula may be produced from a low-level one by inappropriate forcible probing of the wound.

ULCERS

An ulcer is a break in the continuity of an epithelial surface usually with an inflamed and granulating base. A clinical history of the ulcer and an assessment of the general medical condition of the patient precedes the accurate description of the ulcer site, size and shape. The ulcer edge and base, with a description of the state of the neighbouring skin or epithelial surface and draining lymph nodes are also important in the differential diagnosis. A rolled edge suggests a neoplastic lesion (*Fig.* 2.1), whereas a traumatic ulcer exhibits neoepithelial ingrowth from the sides of the ulcer. The base of an ulcer will contain granulation tissue which will be seen as either clean, red healthy granular tissue or necrotic slough which may obscure deep extensions or tracts. Whenever present, these result in continued slough formation within the ulcer crater by failure of correct drainage. Some ulcers occur in particular sites and can be diagnosed by the history and the examination. Others may need biopsy of the edge of the ulcer to determine their exact nature.

State of the Ulcer

An appreciation of the overall state of an ulcer is an important guide to the clinical management. An ulcer may be acutely inflamed with a surrounding area of cellulitis which may require appropriate antibiotic therapy. More often, it is chronically inflamed with adherent slough due to inadequate drainage from deep extensions or secondary tracts. Weak ulcers are covered with poor quality granulation tissue (pale and atrophic) and exhibit delayed epithelial healing. They may be due to specific infections, such as syphilis or tuberculosis (Chapter 5) but are more commonly ischaemic in origin due to peripheral vascular disease predominantly in

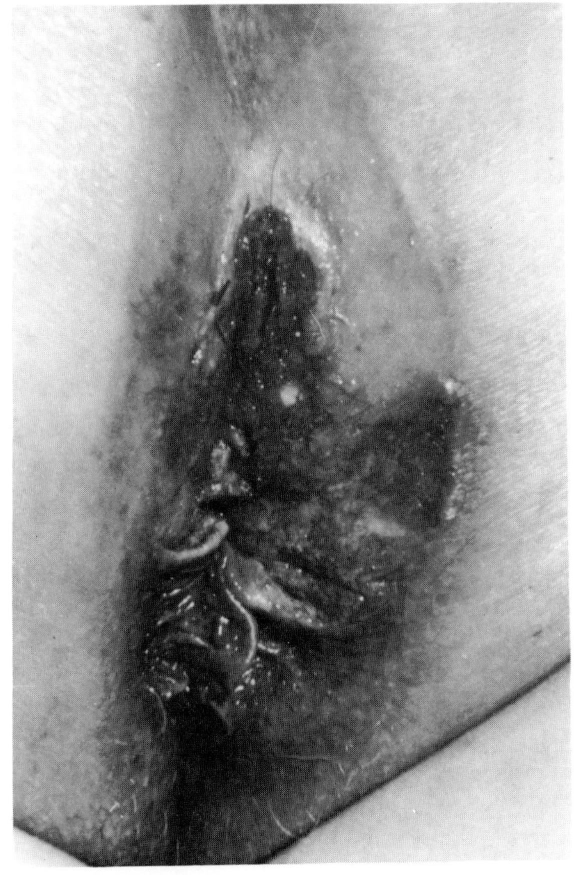

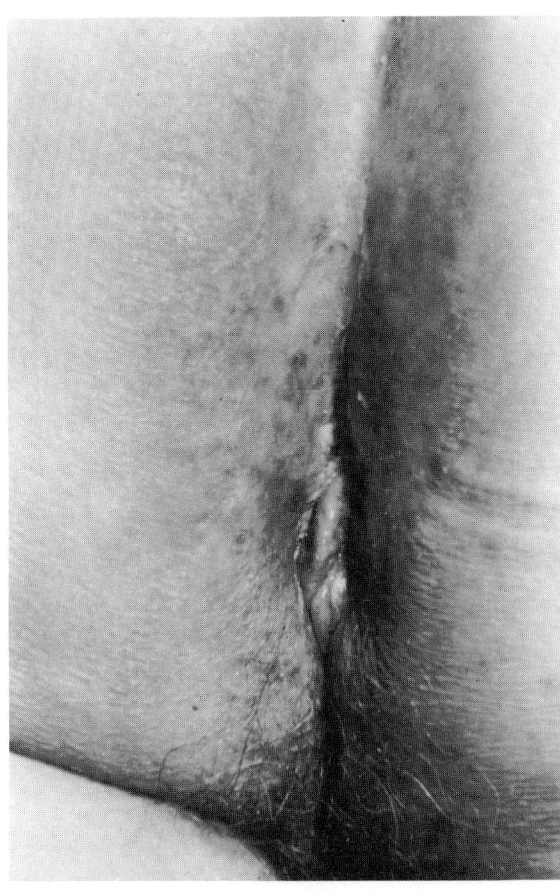

a b

Fig. 2.1 a, Squamous-cell carcinoma of the anal region. The lesion presented as an ulcer with a rolled edge and a granulating base. The patient was successfully treated by radiotherapy. b, Appearance of the perianal region of the same patient two years later.

the lower limbs. Indurated or callous ulcers which have a densely fibrotic surrounding and a deep perforating base with sharply cut edges with little or no tendency to healing are typified by the neuropathic (neurogenic, trophic) ulcers.

Types of Ulcers

The common types of ulcerating lesions encountered in surgical practice include:

1. Malignant ulcers of the skin (Chapter 14) and of the gastrointestinal tract (Chapters 67 and 74).
2. Peptic ulceration of the stomach and duodenum (Chapter 67).
3. Pressure sores or decubitus ulcers and ischaemic ulcers.
4. Gravitational ulcers.
5. Secondary infective ulcers due to drainage of abscesses and infection of an operative wound.
6. Traumatic ulcers, extensive ulcers of this kind are often encountered in patients on long-term systemic steroid therapy, where because of dermal atrophy, even minor trauma may result in full thickness skin loss (*Fig.* 2.2).
7. Ulcers associated with specific dermatological or systemic disease (Chapter 14).
8. Neuropathic ulcers (*Fig.* 2.3) arise from repeated trauma to an insensitive area of skin, as in a diabetic neuropathy or disseminated sclerosis. There may also be an associated ischaemic process.
9. Specific infective ulcers: acute viral, i.e. herpes simplex ulcers (encountered in surgical patients after critical illness, chest infection or in the immunosuppressed patient), spirochaetal ulcers due to *Treponema pallidum*, tuberculous and fungal ulcers.
10. Aphthous ulceration. This common ailment is of unknown aetiology and causes recurrent very painful ulcers usually on the floor of the mouth.
11. Iatrogenic ulcers may result from extravasation of an irritant fluid during intravenous drug administration (*Fig.* 2.4).
12. Ulcers artefacta: these are self-inflicted by the patient.

Principles of Ulcer Treatment

1. The determination of the exact aetiology of the ulcer is essential to successful therapy. Often, the diagnosis is obvious because of the site and local characteristics of the lesion. In every instance, however, a thorough physical examination is necessary and the clinical findings often provide essential clues to the underlying disorder (e.g. arterial disease, neuropathy). Where doubt remains as to the exact nature of the ulcer, a biopsy of its edge should be performed. There is no evidence that this procedure alters the prognosis of an ulcer even if it is malignant, as long as the correct management of that ulcer is undertaken soon afterwards. In the case of ulcers adjacent to bony surfaces,

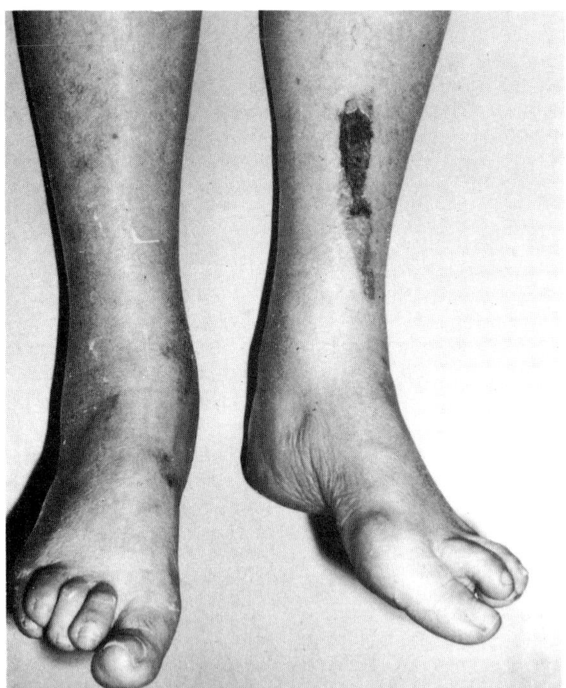

Fig. 2.2 Avulsion of the skin of the left shin in a patient on systemic steroid therapy. The injury was sustained in a minor fall.

an underlying osteomyelitis or osteonecrosis (*Fig.* 2.5) should be excluded by appropriate radiological examination of the affected part. The haemoglobin level should be estimated in all patients with ulcers. Other investigations will vary with the exact details of the individual patient.

2. A clean ulcer with healthy granulation tissue exudes a serous discharge and should be dressed twice daily or more often if the discharge is copious, as it often is, during the early stages of healing. The standard dressing is a cotton gauze roll soaked in a mild antiseptic (sodium hypochlorite) packed lightly into all parts of the ulcer base. Sodium

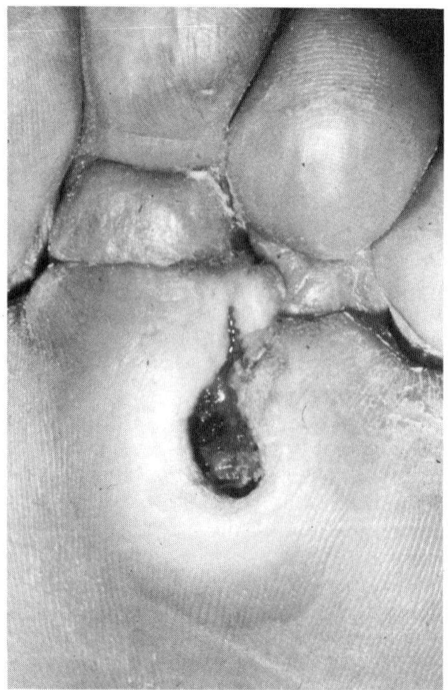

Fig. 2.3 Neuropathic ulcer in a patient with diabetes mellitus.

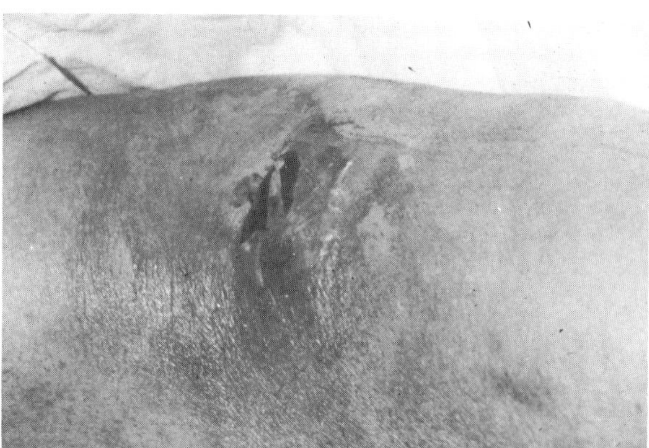

Fig. 2.4 Extravasation of doxorubicin (adriamycin) causing tissue necrosis and an ulcer in the antecubital fossa.

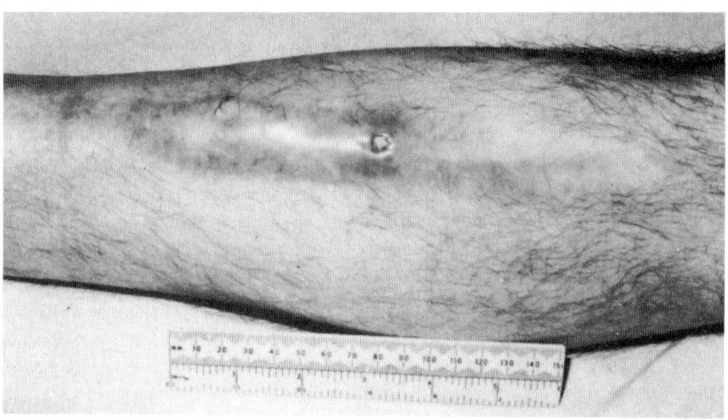

a

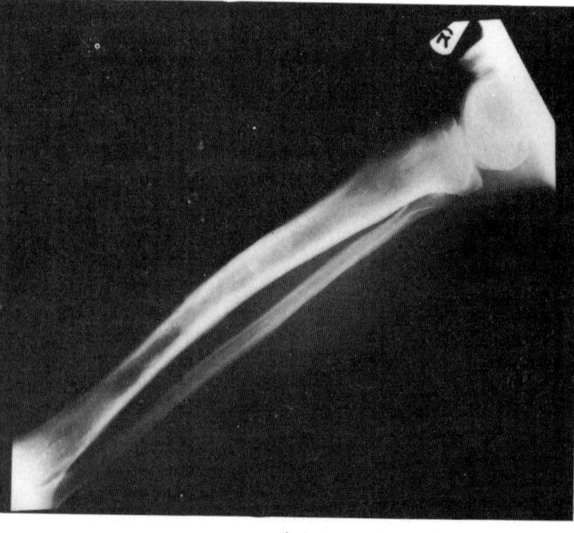

b

Fig. 2.5 *a*, Chronic osteomyelitis of the right tibia with discharging ulcer on the skin containing obvious sequestrum in its base. *b*, Radiograph of the region showing chronic osteomyelitis with sclerosis.

hypochlorite has been shown to impair capillary circulation and is toxic to granulation tissue. Sodium chloride 0·9% should be used instead but this must be changed regularly and not be allowed to dry out. Chlorhexidine 0·05% in water causes only slight disturbance of the capillary flow. Discomfort from this type of packing occurs more often nowadays as the cotton dressings contain variable amounts of cellulose especially within the warp. This absorbs liquid more rapidly than cotton and therefore expands into a hard mass which causes discomfort to the patient earlier by a pressure effect. As woven dressings shed a few fibres, pure cellulose dressings should not be used as they may delay healing of the granulation tissue by the incorporation of particles of cellulose deep in the granulation tissue (*Fig.* 2.6). All macroscopically visible fibre particles should be removed between each dressing change. Dressings often cause discomfort when removed from the ulcer edge especially at points of contact with nerve endings. They often become adherent to the granulation tissue, the superficial layer of which is avulsed on removal of the dressing, resulting in some bleeding from the capillary loops. This occurs more extensively when the wound/dressing combination is allowed to become dry.

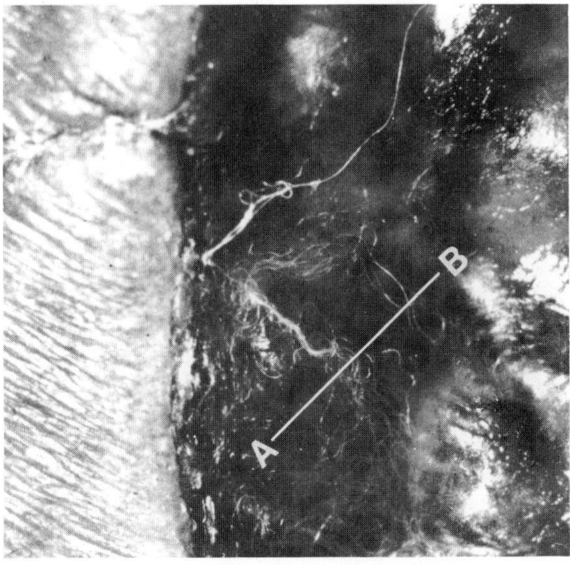

a

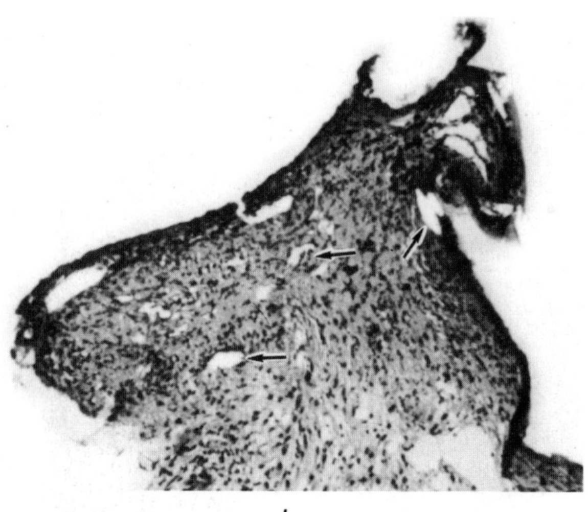

b

Fig. 2.6 *a*, Edge of granulating perineal wound showing cellulose filaments on the surface of the wound. Some filaments are embedded within the granulation tissue. (Reproduced by permission from the British Medical Journal.) *b*, Histological section of the above wound taken from A–B region showing birefringent cellulose particles (arrows) within the granulation tissue.

The ideal dressing for granulation tissue is one which is soft, absorbent, non-adherent and non-allergenic. Such a dressing does not exist but a near compromise is silicone foam elastomer which forms a tailor-made soft, comfortable and non-adherent spongy dressing which is taken out by the patient, washed and reinserted without any significant discomfort or the need for nursing assistance. Silicone foam elastomer can only be used effectively if drainage from the ulcer or abscess is adequate, the cavity is unilocular and its walls have mature healthy granulation tissue without any significant slough formation (*Fig.* 2.7*a–f*). As a result of their inert nature, silicones cause less stimulation of granulation tissue formation than gauze dressing which should be used for the first three days of the wound packing.

There are other groups of dressings for ulcers; microporous polyurethane films are suitable for relatively shallow wounds. They can be left in place for several days. They are permeable to gases and water vapour but prevent large molecules and bacteria from entering the wound. They are suitable for skin graft donor sites and have been shown to reduce epithelial healing times compared with traditional gauze dressings. They should not be used where there is excess exudate or in the presence of established infection. Hydrocolloid gels which may have a polyurethane base provide good wound protection. This hydrophilic compound forms a gel when it comes in contact with fluid and thus it is reputed to provide a good environment for healing and acts as a bacteriological barrier. Unfortunately the gel is not permeable to oxygen. Although these hydrocolloid dressings reduce pain, especially from ulcer edges, they are unsuitable for deep granulating wounds. Polysaccharide dextranomers are powder or bead-like dressings consisting of polysaccharide microspheres. They absorb exudate and mop up bacteria and slough. They need to be changed at least twice day, otherwise they encourage bacterial growth within them.

3. Adequate drainage and desloughing of the base of an ulcer is essential for healing. Many agents are advocated for the softening and separation of slough. Often the cheapest and most effective method is removal by excision of the dead tissue (*Fig.* 2.8). This may expose secondary extensions of the main ulcer cavity or bridging of the wound (*Fig.* 2.9) which will require opening up to ensure adequate drainage.

4. In general, antibiotics are unwarranted in granulating wounds since healthy granulation tissue forms a very effective natural barrier against bacterial invasion and is virtually impermeable to both topical and systemic antibiotics. The indications for antibiotic therapy in the management of ulcers are limited to patients with infected ulcers surrounded by a cellulitis and ulcers of specific bacterial origin such as syphilis or tuberculosis (Chapter 5). The situation regarding antibiotics may change as evidence accumulates of the importance of bacteria in some specific sites such as hidradenitis suppurativa, duct ectasia and pilonidal sinus. Thus delayed healing of granulating wounds has been described in patients in association with mixed bacterial colonization of the wound with aerobes and anaerobes.

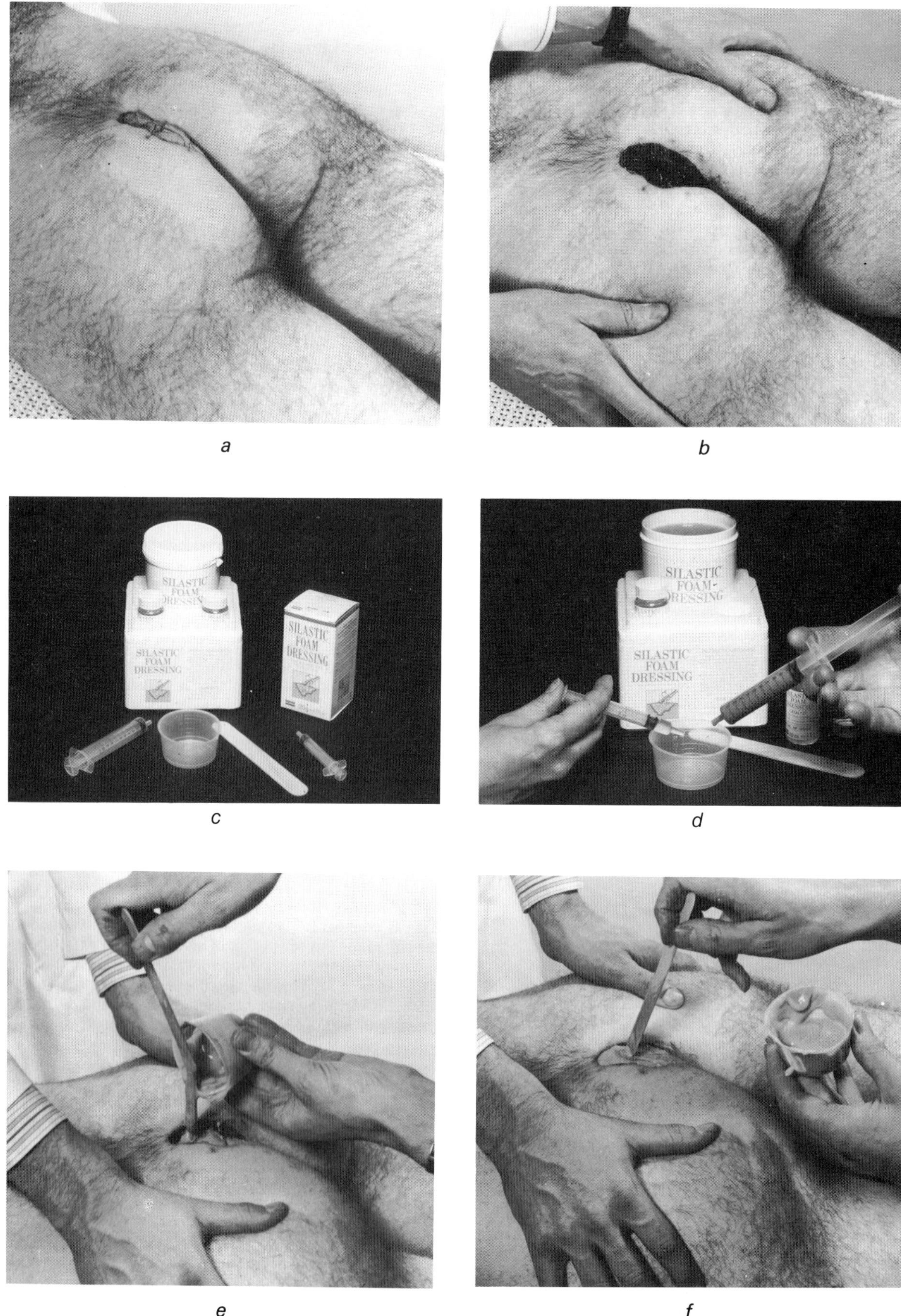
a
b
SILASTIC FOAM DRESSING
SILASTIC FOAM DRESSING
SILASTIC FOAM DRESSING
c
SILASTIC FOAM-DRESSING
SILASTIC FOAM DRESSING
d
e
f

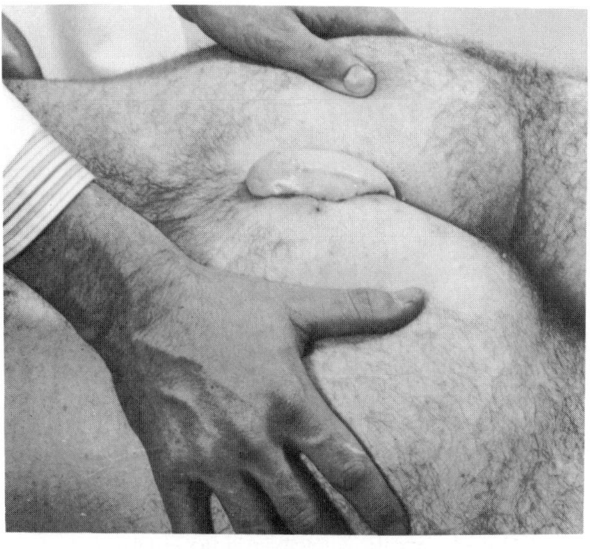

g

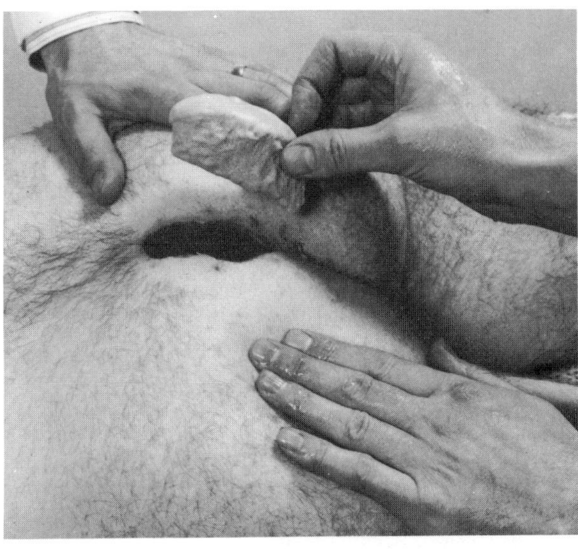

h

Fig. 2.7 Silicone foam elastomer dressing for open granulating wounds. *a*, Wound resulting from excision of pilonidal sinus, initially packed with acriflavine gauze stitched to the edges of the wound. The gauze pack is removed 3–4 days later. *b*, A clean granulating wound with mature and firm walls is seen when the pack is removed. A close inspection is necessary to exclude any pocketing, bridging and adherent slough. *c*, Materials and equipment necessary for the application of silicone foam elastomer dressing. *d*, The foam elastomer and catalyst (17:1 parts) are mixed together and stirred vigorously in a plastic container. *e*, With the edges of the wound held widely apart, the solution is poured into the wound. *f*, The foam expands as it sets within a few minutes. The wooden spatula is used to mould the surface of the dressing and to remove overspill at the edges. *g*, The complete foam dressing in situ. *h*, The tailor-made dressing can be removed quite painlessly and rinsed in clean water or mild antiseptic solution and reintroduced by the patient himself. As the cavity contracts and healing progresses, the original foam dressing rides up and needs to be replaced by a new silicone foam elastomer dressing weekly.

5. The formation of weak granulation tissue may result from a systemic disorder (myxoedema), malnutrition, long-term therapy with steroids, local ischaemia or specific infections (tuberculosis). Apart from the correction of specific abnormalities, zinc-containing lotions (red lotion, scarlet red) which stimulate granulation tissue formation, have a long established usage in these situations and some clinical trials have indicated possible benefit from this treatment.

6. Surgical treatment, apart from routine desloughing, is often necessary to deal with certain types of ulcers. The procedures include excision of chronic (callous) ulcers, skin grafting and the use of rotational skin flaps (Chapter 22).

Decubitus Ulcer (Pressure Sore)

These occur over the sacral area, the backs of the heels, elbows and back. They may be painless or painful at some time during their development or healing. Many of the afflicted patients are unconscious or unable to communicate

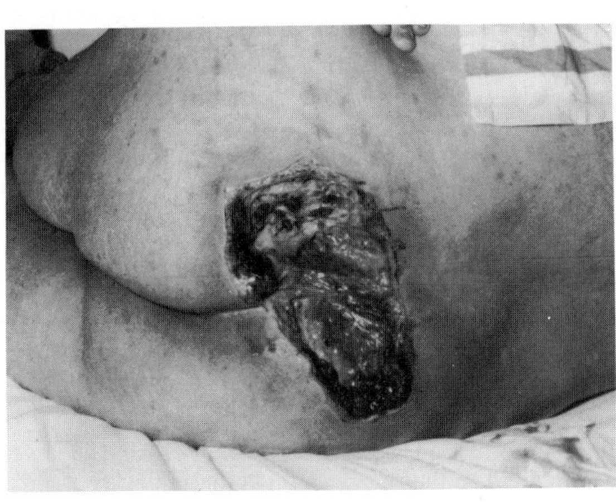

a

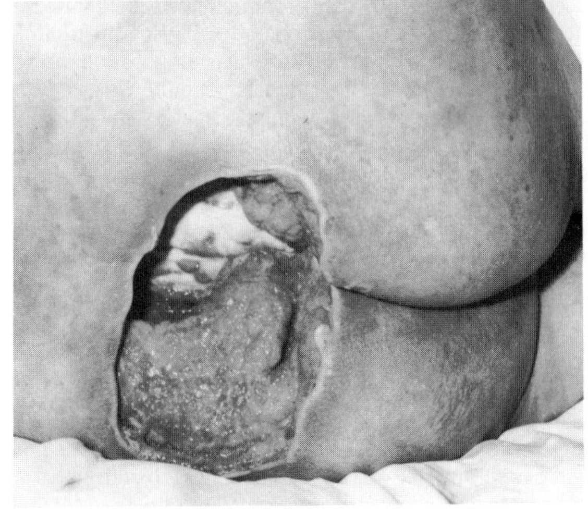

b

Fig. 2.8 Ulcer before (*a*) and after (*b*) desloughing.

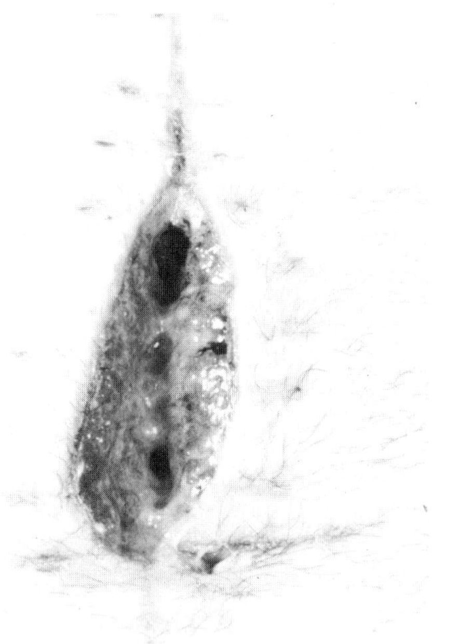

Fig. 2.9 Lower part of a midline epigastric wound healing by granulation but there is bridging of tissue impairing drainage from the depths of the wound.

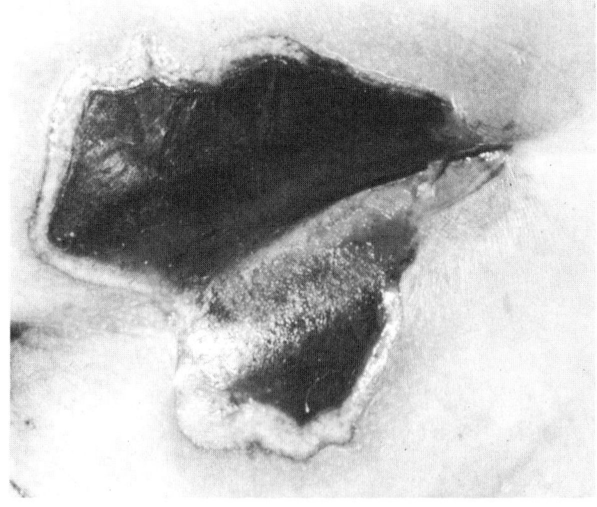

Fig. 2.10 Extensive decubitus ulcer in the sacral region. Thick adherent slough covers most of the ulcer which is surrounded by an area of cellulitis denoting the necessity for antibiotic therapy in addition to desloughing.

any discomfort. Impaired mobility, old age and neurological disease, such as disseminated sclerosis, often accompanied by incontinence of urine and faeces due to sphincter disturbances, make this one of the commonest complications of the chronic invalid or the critically ill. The pathophysiology is that of localized constant pressure over a contact area, causing ischaemia with eventual necrosis, first of the underlying subcutaneous fat, and subsequently of the skin, which remains sensitive to pain only at the edge of the ischaemic area, where cell death is incomplete.

The gangrenous skin eventually separates, leaving necrotic subcutaneous tissue and fat, which overlies the developing granulation tissue (*Fig.* 2.10). The ulcer may extend to and involve, tendon and bone. This destructive process is accentuated by the presence of an increased metabolic rate, such as pyrexia from a postoperative chest infection. No hospital ward is immune from this complication of prolonged recumbency. The emphasis should always be on prevention as this is much more satisfactory than the long drawn-out healing process of the established disease. Patients who are unable to move by themselves must be turned at least 2-hourly, day and night. Many aids are available to distribute the patient's weight, e.g. sheepskin blankets, ripple air beds, etc. Although these can help the individual patient, the main preventive measures are 2-hourly turning of the patient, skin hygiene and frequent massage after the application of talcum powder. The latter should be avoided in the presence of broken skin.

The investigation of a patient with a pressure sore should include full blood count and film. Any anaemia is corrected after serum folate, B_{12}, and iron samples have been taken where appropriate. Plasma electrolytes, blood urea and fasting glucose should be performed routinely. Metabolic and endocrine abnormalities should be corrected as uraemia, diabetes and hypothyroidism delay the formation of granulation tissue. The area around the ulcer should be radiographed in two planes to exclude osteomyelitis of the underlying bone. This needs to be eradicated, usually by surgical drainage of the abscess and removal of sequestra before healing of the ulcer can occur.

Many decubitus ulcers are in a poor surgical condition from inadequate drainage. Slough and dead tissue should be removed until capillary loop bleeding is just encountered. It is at this point that the patient will feel a little pain. The undermined skin edges should be excised to produce an ulcer from which serous discharge can drain adequately at all times and in all positions of the patient. The commonest reason for failure of decubitus ulcer to heal is continued pressure on the ulcerated area. Slough may reform early in the treatment and this should be repeatedly excised until healthy granulation tissue has formed over the whole of the ulcer crater. The formation of an abscess in an undermined area can cause bacterial septicaemia. Antibiotic therapy against Gram-negative organisms is indicated until drainage has been carried out.

When used in the management of pressure sores, silicone foam elastomer is allowed to flow over the edge of the ulcer resulting in a large cushion which helps to spread the weight of a patient over a larger surface area of the body (*Fig.* 2.11). In most cases, the above management will lead to healing of the ulcer which accelerates as soon as the patient becomes ambulant. The patient who is confined to bed may have an ulcer which is very resistant to treatment by postural drainage and dressings. The use of rotation skin flaps of the buttocks over the sacral area and split skin grafts for the heels may be necessary.

Gravitational Ulcers (Venous, Varicose, Stasis Ulcers)

These are the commonest ulcers encountered in general surgical practice. Gravitational ulcers are chronic, tend to recur after healing and cause considerable morbidity. Their typical location is on the medial side above the malleolus but are also found on the lateral aspect of the ankle. Occasionally extensive ulcers may form circumferential lesions around the lower leg. Gravitational ulcers have a typical appearance and are usually associated with the signs of chronic venous

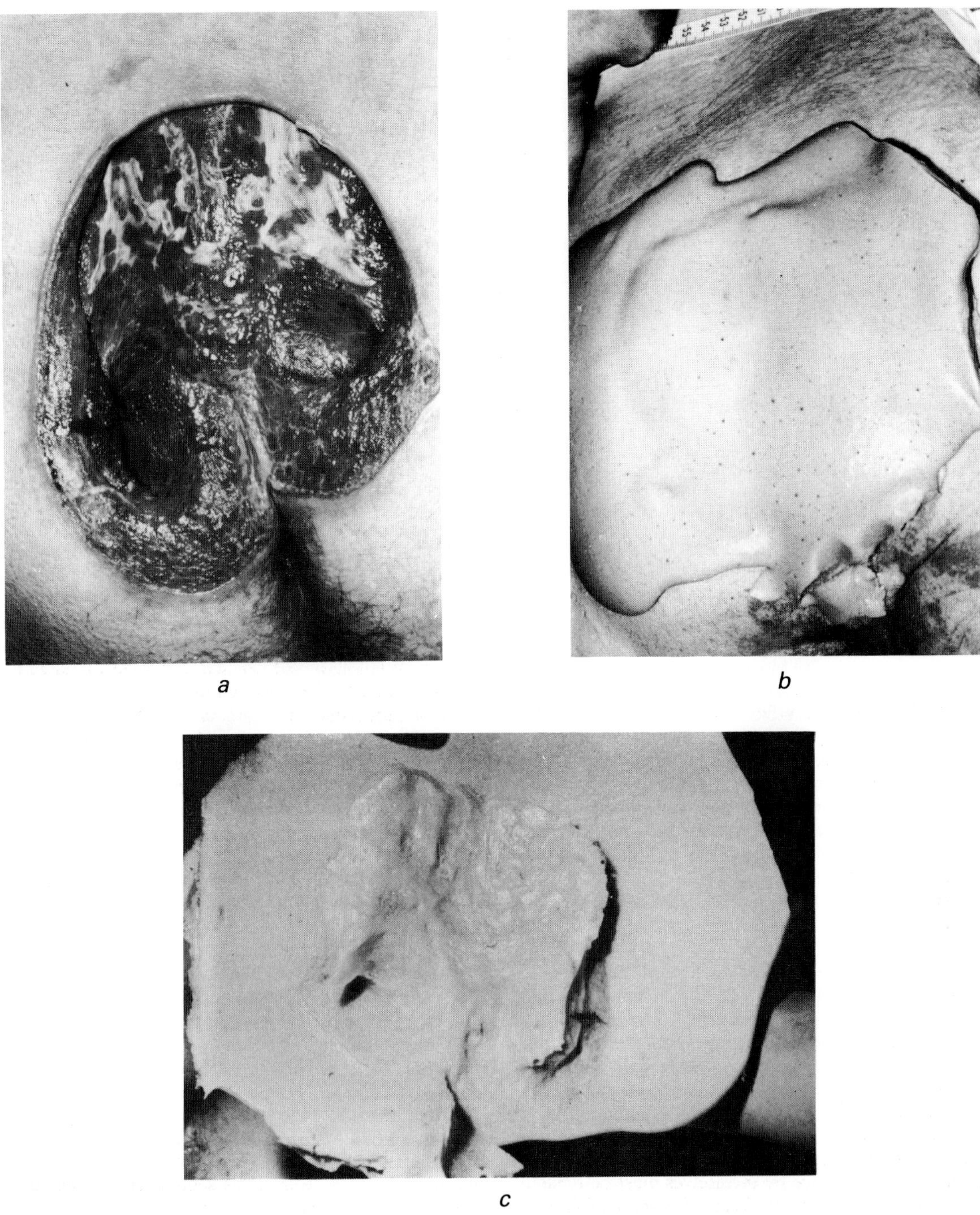

Fig. 2.11 Large silicone foam elastomer cushion for a large decubitus ulcer: *a*, Clean ulcer, *b*, Silicone foam elastomer cushion in situ. *c*, Silicone foam elastomer showing central plug and surrounding cushion.

insufficiency. Dermatitis is often present with surrounding brown discoloration, thickening of the skin and oedema of the limb. The ulcer itself may contain areas covered with slough, or fresh red granulation tissue which is surrounded by a thin pink zone. This is skin that is either breaking down or starting to heal (*Fig.* 2.12). The ulcer may extend deeply to involve the bone. Pain is felt from the edge of the ulcer and at various times during the repeated healing/breakdown cycles from the base of the ulcer as it involves nerve endings.

The pathophysiology is not fully understood. It is more commonly seen in patients with varicose veins and a past history of venous thrombosis. There is usually perforator vein incompetence between the deep and superficial veins which may occur as a separate entity or in conjunction with saphenofemoral incompetence. During activity the contractions of the muscles of the calf pump blood in a cephalad direction in the deep system. The resulting high venous pressure is transmitted to the superficial venous system in

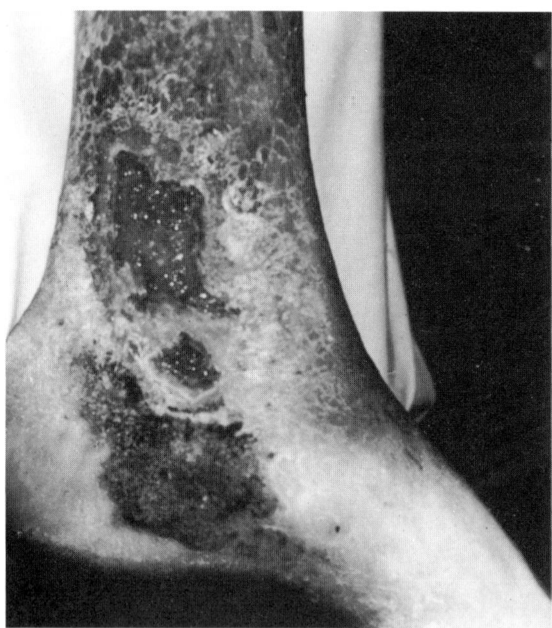

Fig. 2.12 Gravitational ulcer.

the presence of perforator valve incompetence and leads to extravasation of plasma and blood cells. As the oedematous legs of patients in cardiac failure do not commonly develop ulcers, other factors which adversely affect tissue metabolism are involved in the development of venous ulcers in addition to the high venous pressure in the superficial system. Fibrin deposition around the small vessels with impairment of tissue oxygenation and nutrition has been held responsible for the local necrosis and ulcer formation in these patients. In time, the subcutaneous tissue becomes firm with a fibrous/leathery feel (liposclerosis).

There is often a family history of varicose veins and a personal history of deep vein thrombosis during an acute illness or pregnancy. It is important in the differential diagnosis to exclude an ischaemic ulcer of the limb by checking the peripheral pulses. If these cannot be felt because of oedema, a convenient method is to use the Doppler ultrasound system. The ultrasound probe can also be used to detect perforator vein incompetence and also popliteal vein incompetence. Any suspicion of malignancy which may rarely occur in a very chronic granulating ulcer (Marjolin ulcer) must be excluded by biopsy.

The Trendelenburg test is performed with the patient in the supine position with the limb elevated. After the blood has been massaged out of the varicose veins, a rubber tourniquet is placed around the upper thigh to occlude the long saphenous vein and the patient is then asked to stand up. Immediate filling of the veins of the lower limb suggests incompetence of the perforator veins between the deep and superficial calf veins. Slow filling of these veins at first with rapid filling when the tourniquet is released indicates that both saphenofemoral incompetence and deep perforator incompetence are present. If filling of the varicose veins is only witnessed after the tourniquet is released incompetence is predominantly at the saphenofemoral junction.

If a Doppler ultrasound is not available and doubt about the state of the deep system patency exists, bilateral phlebograms should be performed. A past history of deep vein thrombosis should indicate the distinct possibility that the varicose veins are secondary to a blocked deep venous system. These patients always require a phlebogram and if the diagnosis is confirmed, obliteration of the superficial varicose veins is contraindicated as it will considerably aggravate the chronic venous insufficiency of the limb.

The mainstay of treatment for gravitational ulcers is the reduction of the venous pressure in the superficial veins. In mild cases where breakdown of skin is only just occurring, correctly fitting supportive stockings/tights, may be used. However, if oedema is present, bandaging of the legs from behind the toes to the mid-thigh after the ulcer has been dressed with a pure cotton or Jelonet dressing is required. As the bandages rapidly become stretched and loose, they should be reapplied by the patient every 4 h. The leg should be kept elevated whenever the patient is sedentary. Walking should be encouraged and obese patients should be made to lose weight by a low calorie diet. There are many proprietary preparations for varicose ulcers but none have shown any particular proven advantage in randomized trials. Dressings incorporating topical antibiotics should not be used as these will eventually produce an allergic reaction of the skin (*Fig.* 2.13). A dressing which is non-adherent when wet is ideal. Many of the severe ulcers persist for several years and are designated as resistant. More often than not, however, these apparent failures can be attributed to inadequate conservative management. Moderate-sized ulcers which respond to pressure dressings may be treated by sclerotherapy to the varicose veins using the Fegan technique with sodium tetradecyl sulphate (STD). After 1·5 ml of the STD are injected into the vein, a small dressing pad is placed over the injection site as the needle is withdrawn and further compression pads are placed over the vein. The leg is bandaged with 4 in (10 cm) crêpe to the lower leg and 6 in (15 cm) crêpe above the knee. A 4-in (10 cm) elastoplast is then put on top of the crêpe bandaging and the patient then wears elastic support stockings over the whole dressing. The patient is instructed to walk away from the clinic as this prevents the accumulation of the sclerosant fluid within the deep vein and ensures limitation of thrombosis to the superficial veins and the incompetent perforators. The patient must walk 3–4 miles per day and be active all day. After 2 weeks, the bandages and foam pads are removed and the legs re-dressed for a further 4 weeks. Sclerotherapy is not recommended for patients with obese legs or patients on oral contraceptives.

Reduction of venous pressure can be undertaken by surgical treatment. The Trendelenburg high ligation of the saphenous vein and its tributaries is performed if saphenofemoral incompetence is present. Stripping of the veins from the ankle to thigh is not recommended as this may remove the long saphenous nerve with a loss of sensation between the first and second toes. Other patients may complain of pain and tenderness at the ankle wound. A Linton subfascial ligation of the calf vein perforators, which is performed through a longitudinal medial incision, is indicated if perforator incompetence is demonstrated. However, this operation requires careful patient selection. In the presence of extensive destruction of the valves of the deep venous system, even the combined Trendelenburg ligation and Linton procedure may not achieve ulcer healing and these patients require to wear knee-length elastic compression stockings indefinitely to keep the ulcer healed. Whenever possible, healing of the ulcer by bed rest and elevation should precede surgical intervention for incompetent perforator veins.

Skin grafting of varicose ulcers can allow skin cover at an early stage but the results of both partial- and full-thickness

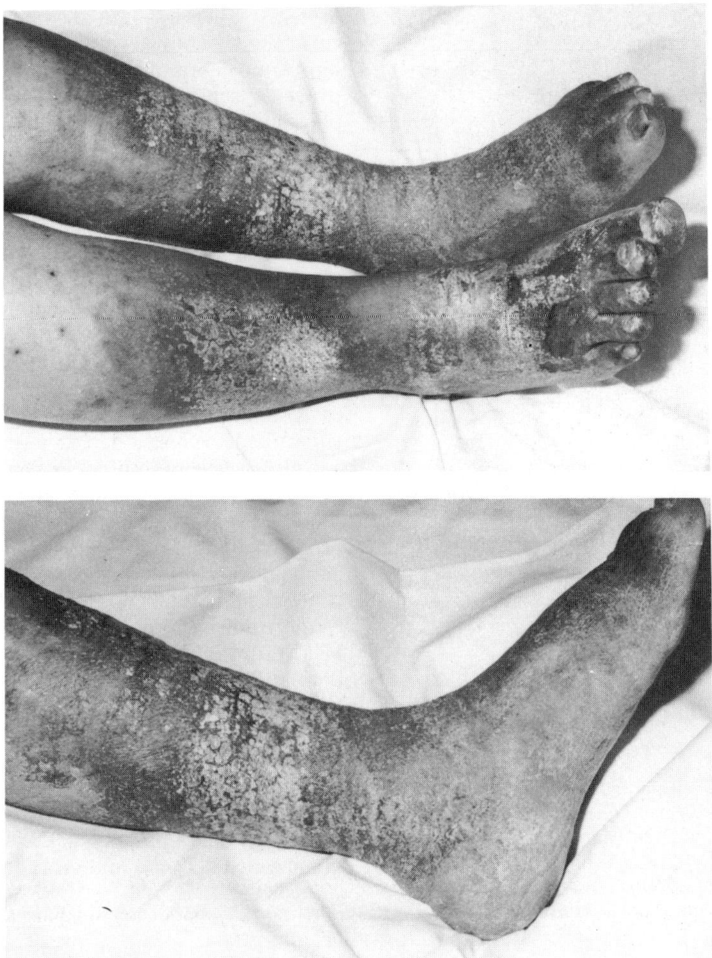

Fig. 2.13 Allergic dermatitis resulting from long-term application of antibiotic cream for gravitational ulceration.

grafting are by no means certain and bed rest to ensure an adequate take may need to be prolonged. Recently, a clinical trial has shown that autologous pinch grafts achieve ulcer healing in about 65% of patients and are more effective than porcine dermis. Skin grafting does not alter the pathophysiology of the condition so that recurrence of venous stasis ulceration can occur.

Ischaemic Ulcer

The ischaemic (vascular) ulcer is usually initiated by minor trauma to an ischaemic limb. Thus the anterior tibial region above the ankle is the commonest site for these ulcers (*Fig.* 2.14). A history of trauma or constant pressure by some object with symptoms of intermittent claudication or rest pain and previous trouble with healing of skin should lead one to suspect this condition. Ischaemic ulcers may also be associated with other medical conditions such as rheumatoid arthritis, especially with the Felty's syndrome and erythema induratum (Bazin).

The skin is atrophic and the ulcer is shallow with poor quality granulation tissue and absent or impaired epithelial healing. The whole area has a poor blood supply, the limb feeling cold, hairless, with deformed nails and frequently associated chronic paronychia. Evidence of peripheral vascular disease will be found on clinical examination and non-invasive investigations (Doppler, thermography). Occasionally, because of cutaneous warmth and hyperaemia caused by superadded infection, especially in the diabetic patient, one may be misled into thinking that the leg is less ischaemic than it really is. Examination of cardiovascular and respiratory systems should also be undertaken. Investigation must include ECG, chest radiography, full blood count, electrolytes and urea, blood glucose and tests for rheumatoid or connective tissue disorders. The affected limb should be radiographed. Thermography is an excellent non-invasive method of assessing the upper limit of limb ischaemia except in the presence of superadded infection usually in the diabetic.

Management depends on the presence or absence of a surgically correctable arterial lesion. This usually entails arteriography to outline the extent of an arterial block, the state of collateral circulation and the distal run-off. Digital vascular imaging (DVI) is proving successful for imaging larger vessel disease, but is less useful for vessels below the popliteal fossa. Patients with ischaemic ulcers usually have small vessel involvement which is not delineated by this technique. Correction of a block in a major vessel may give a dramatic improvement in leg perfusion and in ulcer healing. Femoropopliteal bypass surgery, whilst successful, is generally regarded as a holding procedure of limb salvage. This is

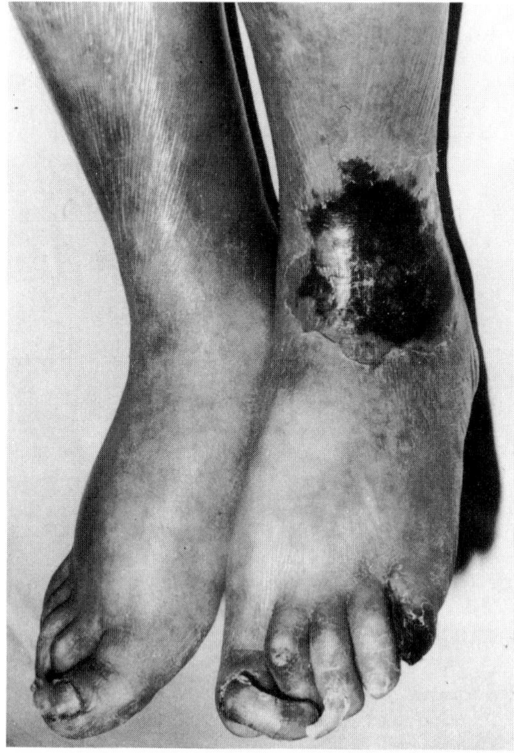

Fig. 2.14 Ischaemic ulcer following injury sustained after a fall whilst under the influence of alcohol. The patient had extensive peripheral vascular disease with absent femoral pulses.

even more the case when femoroposterior tibial bypass is undertaken. Percutaneous transfemoral balloon dilatation (Gunzig angioplasty) is usually not suitable for ischaemic ulcer patients because of the diffuse nature of the arterial disease which involves the small vessels. Lumbar sympathectomy increases the blood flow to the respective extremity largely by opening arteriovenous anastomoses. Enhancement of the skin's nutritional blood flow is demonstrated in only 60% of patients. Sympathectomy is unlikely to impart any benefit and may indeed be harmful if the ankle pressure is below 30 mmHg, in the presence of established neuropathy and ischaemia of the forefoot, and after direct arterial surgery. Sympathectomy is usually considered if arteriography precludes direct arterial surgery. Skin grafting of ischaemic ulcers is considered in Chapter 22.

Chronic Infective Ulcers

Chronic infections which can cause ulceration of the skin are uncommon in the UK. Tuberculous ulcers most commonly on the leg and perianal region are seen from time to time in immigrant members of the community. Other skin lesions associated with specific infections are dealt with elsewhere in this book (Chapters 5 and 14).

Malignant Ulcers of the Skin

These are considered in Chapter 14.

ABSCESSES

An abscess starts as a focal accumulation of neutrophils in an area of liquefactive necrosis around a large inoculum of bacteria. When established, it constitutes a fluctuant localized collection of pus within a pyogenic membrane. Pus is a semiliquid debris of necrotic leucocytes and tissue cells. The pyogenic membrane is composed of an inner layer of neutrophils and an outer zone of vascular granulation tissue.

The neutrophils are attracted to the focus of infection by chemotaxis and release proteolytic enzymes as they undergo necrosis in the pus. At the periphery of the necrotic tissue and neutrophils, some haemorrhage occurs from the damaged blood vessels. Activated platelets stimulate fibroblasts and together with the blood vessels and viable polymorphs and monocytes form granulation tissue (pyogenic membrane). More neutrophils and macrophages are drawn into the cavity as it expands. This expansion is favoured by the proteolytic breakdown of large molecules within the abscess cavity to form more osmotically active particles. The granulation tissue acts as a barrier to bacteria, but also prevents adequate levels of antibiotics penetrating the cavity. Most antibiotics are inactivated by a number of different factors in the pus, the exact mechanism varying with the specific mode of action of the particular antibiotic. This inactivation of antibiotic activity by pus is well established especially with gentamicin. Although pus contains the highest bacterial count within an abscess, the bacteria within pus appear to be in a resting phase and are not metabolically active. This dormant phase reduces the uptake of antibiotics by the bacteria and contributes to the inefficacy of antibiotic treatment in the presence of established pus formation.

In time, numerous macrophages appear within the fibroblastic zone and these cells come to be in close proximity to areas of active necrosis. With healing, the macrophages replace the neutrophil population within the pyogenic membrane which becomes less vascular and finally contracts into a residual scar.

Abscesses may form anywhere in the body and the nature of the infecting organisms varies with the particular site of abscess formation. Thus subcutaneous abscesses are mainly caused by *Staphylococcus aureus.* Internally, the situation is more complex and intra-abdominal abscesses are caused by a variety of disease processes: appendicitis, diverticular disease with pericolic abscess or perforation, perforated peptic ulcer or malignant disease of the bowel. Some are the result of a leaking surgical anastomosis and these incur a considerable morbidity and mortality, sepsis from this cause being one of the common causes of death in surgical wards. In many instances, the infection is polymicrobial and derived from enteric organisms: coliform organisms, *Streptococcus faecalis*, clostridial organisms and bacteroides. Less commonly, sepsis may develop from external inoculation of dirt and bacteria during trauma from car accidents, stabbing, gunshot wounds and extensive crush injuries. The risk of infection with clostridial organisms is high in these patients especially in the presence of dead or crushed/devitalized tissue which, for this reason, always requires prompt surgical removal. Bloodborne intra-abdominal infection is rare, but occasionally *Mycobacterium tuberculosis*, gonococcus, streptococcal and pneumococcal organisms may cause primary peritonitis.

The patients most at risk of intra-abdominal abscess formation are those who have large inoculum of bacteria from a perforated colon or oesophagus. The risk of severe sepsis is substantially less with perforation of the stomach, duodenum and small bowel as the normal resident bacterial count is low in these organs. However, bacterial overgrowth occurs in the small intestine when this becomes obstructed and in the stomach when acid secretion is reduced or absent.

Increasing patient age, obesity, malnutrition, shock and a decreased immunocompetence increase the risk of sepsis and abscess formation even after minor contamination. Surgical treatment for intra-abdominal abscesses undertaken on these high-risk patients is accompanied by a substantial mortality with reported rates of up to 30%. Thus, antibiotic therapy should be started preoperatively in all infected and contaminated acute intra-abdominal conditions. The choice of antibiotic regimen is based on the best guess against the organisms likely to be present. It usually includes metronidazole to provide cover against anaerobes particularly *Bacteroides fragilis*.

Except for minor superficial skin abscesses, there is usually a systemic reaction with toxicity and intermittent pyrexia. Tenderness and pain may be present and later this may become severe and throbbing in quality, especially when the pus is under tension. Some abscesses may be silent, even when large, with no localizing signs on physical examination but the patient develops signs of toxicity and a hypercatabolic state which may progress to multisystem organ failure. With all abscesses, there is the ever-present risk of bacterial invasion of the bloodstream and septicaemia. Rupture of an intra-abdominal abscess results in widespread peritonitis.

Some abscesses may resolve as a result of prompt and appropriate systemic antibiotic therapy. The abscess contents become liquefied by proteolytic digestion and the watery debris is gradually reabsorbed. The residual scar/cavity may eventually calcify (*Fig.* 2.15). If the abscess is near the surface, it may drain spontaneously and thereafter resolve.

The circulation around an expanding abscess may become compromised by a pressure effect and result in thrombosis and cell death. This process accounts for the tracking of large abscesses usually along specified fascial compartments. The drainage of an abscess releases the pressure within the abscess cavity. Aside from the evacuation of pus and reduction of the bacterial load, this has the effect of altering the environment and immediately improves the penetration of antibiotics into the abscess cavity. There is also some evidence that following drainage of an abscess, the bacteria may resume replication and thus become more sensitive to antibiotics.

Treatment of Abscesses

An abscess may be secondary to a serious underlying disease (carcinoma of the lung, caecal carcinoma, diverticular disease of the colon, etc.) and the appropriate treatment of the underlying condition then assumes priority when or shortly after the acute situation has settled with fluid replacement and antibiotics.

The onset of shock, rigors, a rising pulse rate and pyrexia should be an indication for blood cultures, systemic antibiotic therapy, and fluid replacement. Evacuation of pus should not be delayed. A biopsy of the wall of the abscess should be sent in all cases if a malignancy is not to be missed. Tissue and a large quantity of pus should be sent for bacteriological culture. A swab is much less effective in obtaining an accurate bacteriological culture unless sent to the laboratory in an appropriate transport medium.

The diagnosis of an abscess site, especially within the abdomen may be obvious from the history and localizing signs. Plain radiographs of the abdomen may reveal a localized ileus, soft-tissue swelling or sympathetic chest effusion if the abscess is situated in the subphrenic region. Contrast radiology may show displacement or discontinuity or leak from an abdominal hollow viscus. Some patients may not exhibit any localizing signs especially if they have received preoperative antibiotics. Ultrasound examination by modern equipment is useful in delineating the abscess in 60–80% of patients (*Fig.* 2.16). Radionuclide scintiscanning with

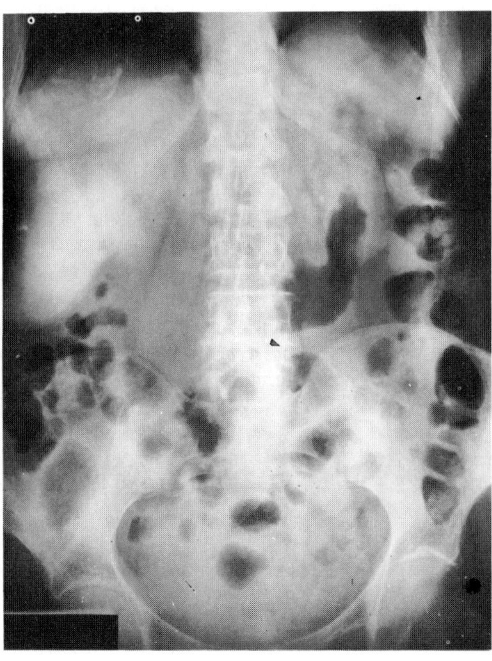

a

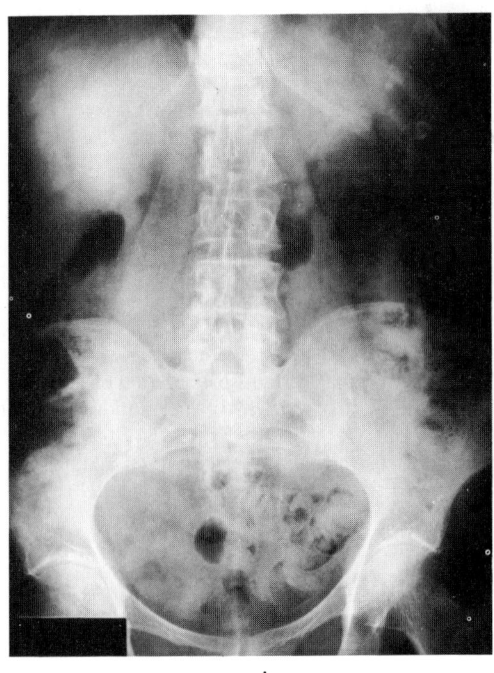

b

Fig. 2.15 *a*, Calcified liver abscess demonstrated in a plain abdominal film in 1980. *b*, This was not present on a previous abdominal film of the same patient obtained in 1975.

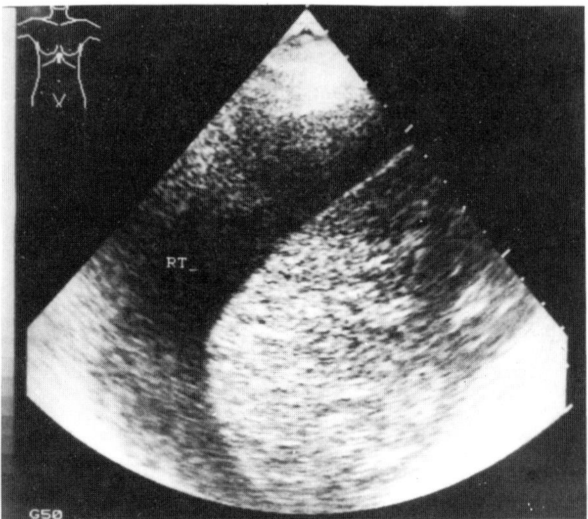

Fig. 2.16 Longitudinal ultrasound scan of the right lobe of the liver showing a large subhepatic abscess.

^{111}Indium labelled-autologous leucocytes is also used to localize pus (*Fig.* 2.17). Although this is more accurate than gallium scanning, it does not distinguish between inflammation and abscess formation. CT scanning is the most accurate method for the detection of intra-abdominal abscesses, rates of over 95% accuracy being reported.

Treatment may be undertaken using aspiration and/or percutaneous drainage of the abscess under ultrasound or CT guidance, where radiological expertise is available. Catheters are left in the abscess cavity and soon after the drainage has begun, the nature of the drainage fluid from the abscess cavity becomes more liquid. Percutaneous drainage of abscesses is effective and has replaced surgical drainage in some hospitals. Multilocular abscess cavities require the guided insertion of several drainage catheters.

Formal surgical drainage is still the method of choice in many institutions. The drainage of intra-abdominal abscesses should be planned and done by a senior surgeon as the morbidity and mortality in this high-risk group is considerable. Any doubts as to a firm fibrous area being an abscess cavity within the abdomen should be tested by aspiration with a needle and syringe. After the abscess cavity has been evacuated and an adequate specimen of pus sent for bacteriological culture, all the loculi are broken down and a silicone drain, with gutter or side holes, placed in a dependent position. The drain should be connected to a closed external collecting system. With large abscesses, sump suction drains are used and attached to a low pressure suction pump (Robert Shaw). Subsequent progress of an abscess cavity is monitored by radiology after injection of a contrast medium through a fine tube placed inside the drain (*Fig.* 2.18). There may be more than one site of an abscess and failure of clinical improvement requires a second look inside the abdomen to search for residual pus. As a pancreatic abscess resulting from pancreatic necrosis, is often accompanied by recurrent intra-abdominal sepsis, the entire abdominal wound is left open with proflavine packing of the pancreatic bed. This is renewed every 24–48 h under intravenous sedation until the wound heals by granulation.

Skin and Subcutaneous Abscesses

These are the most common type of abscesses encountered in surgical practice and occur at particular sites in various age groups. The staphylococcal abscess or boil on the neck or buttock in the young adolescent can occur from infected sweat glands blocked by debris or comedones. These abscesses often discharge and resolve spontaneously but some continue to enlarge and require surgical drainage. A carbuncle can be regarded as a confluence of several boils and results in extensive destruction of the skin and subcutaneous

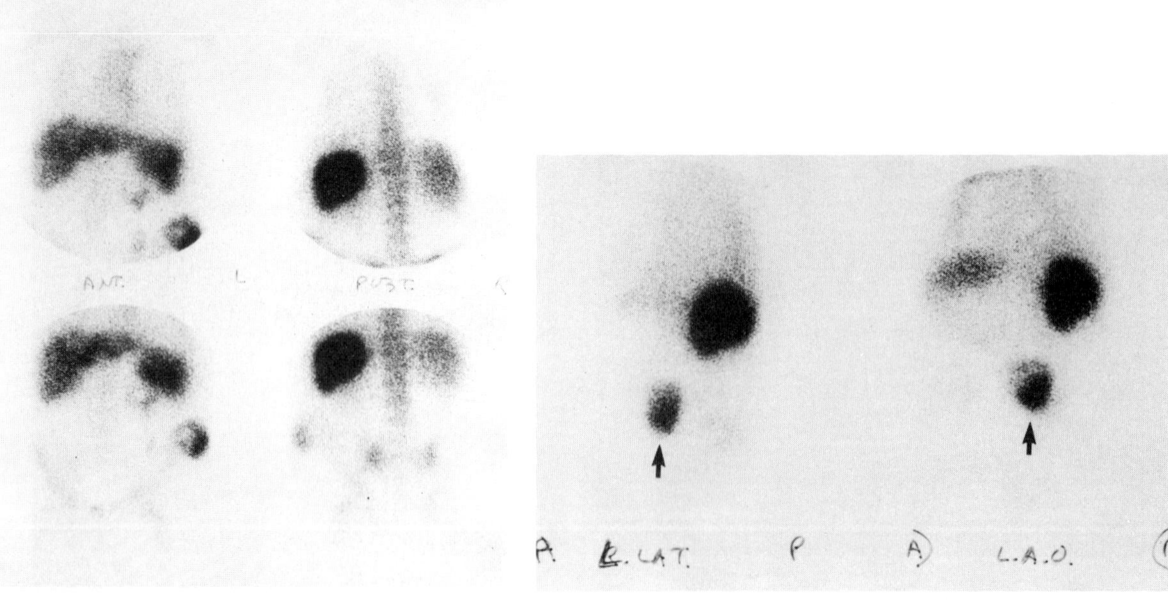

Fig. 2.17 ^{111}Indium-labelled autologous white cell scan in a patient who developed abdominal tenderness and septic shock 7 days after a left colon resection. *a*, The anterior and posterior views of the abdomen show hot areas over the liver, spleen and the left iliac fossa. *b*, The lateral views demonstrate the collection anterior to the colonic anastomosis (arrow).

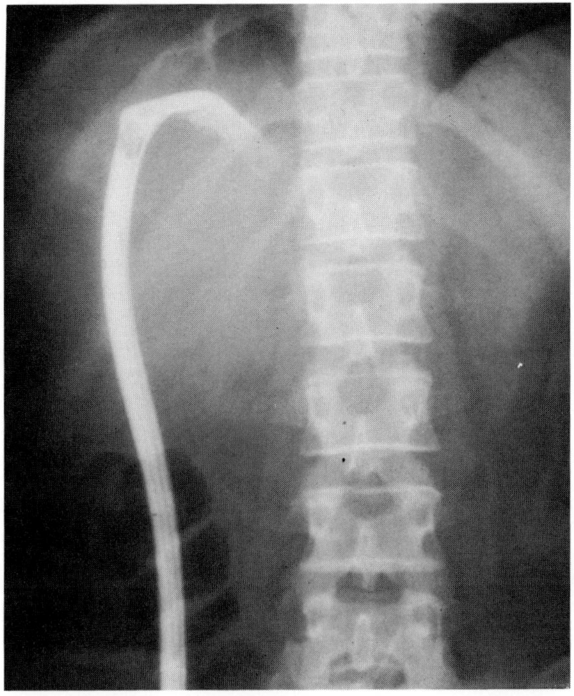

Fig. 2.18 This 70-year-old lady had undergone drainage of a central hepatic abscess. The radiograph shows the drainage tube within the liver. A fine catheter has been inserted inside the drainage tube for the injection of contrast material. As no residual cavity is demonstrated, the drainage tube can be removed.

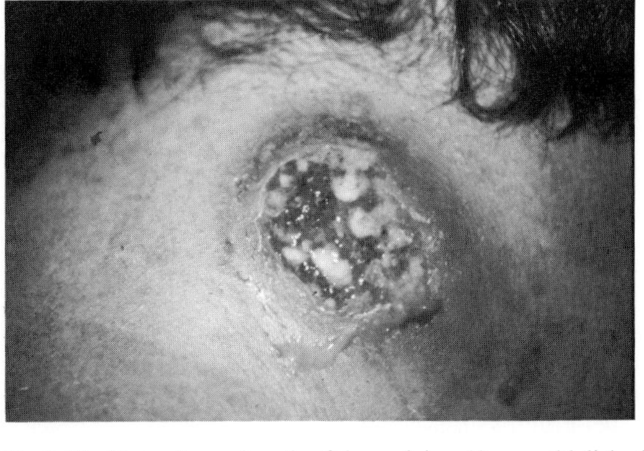

Fig. 2.19 Extensive carbuncle of the neck in a 40-year-old diabetic patient.

fat (*Fig.* 2.19). They are less commonly encountered nowadays except in the debilitated and diabetic patient.

Other common abscesses are perianal and ischiorectal abscesses. Bacteriological examination of the pus may indicate to the surgeon the likely source of infection: skin or bowel. These abscesses always require drainage. A significant proportion of abscesses in this region occur in association with perianal fistula (*Fig.* 2.20). At operation only very gentle probing of these abscess cavities is permissible to avoid the risk of secondary tract formation and conversion of a low to a high rectal fistula.

Breast Abscesses

These are encountered predominantly in the female during

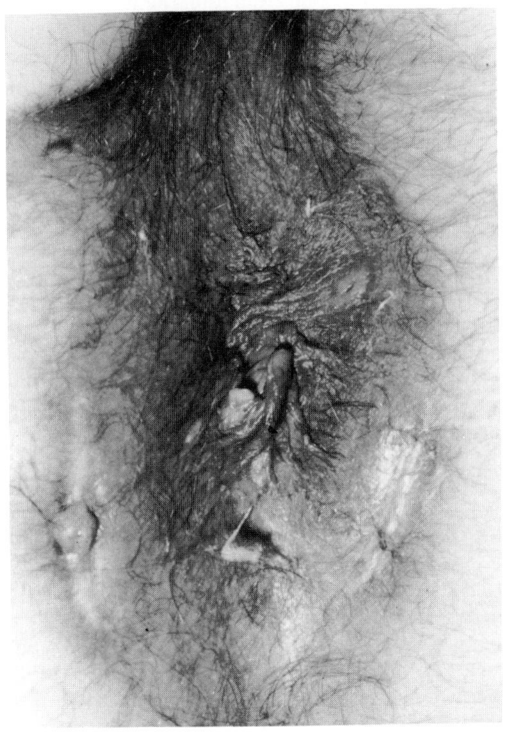

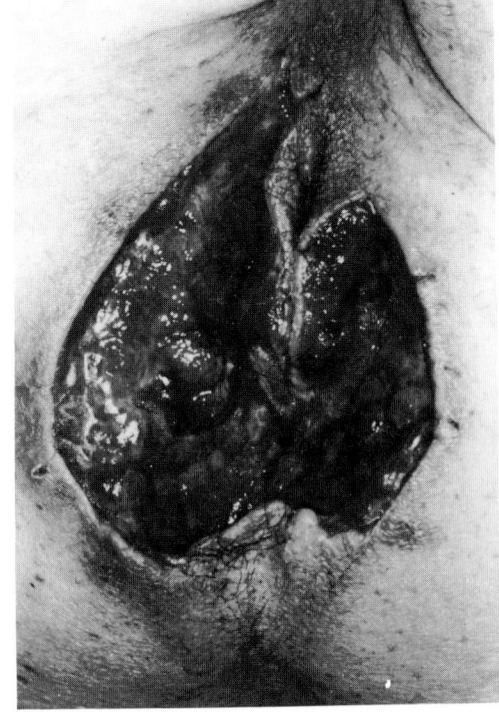

a

b

Fig. 2.20 *a*, Recurrent perianal fistula with two external orifices posterolateral to the anal margin. The fistula was of the horseshoe variety. *b*, Wound resulting from excision of the fistulous tracts.

the child-bearing age, most commonly in the puerperium and during breast feeding, but may occur at other times and in different age groups. Puerperal mastitis develops as a complication of milk engorgement, the breast parenchyma becoming secondarily infected with skin organisms. *Staphylococcus aureus* infections are the most common. The diffuse mastitis soon matures into multiloculated abscess with pain, oedema, induration and fluctuation. Early treatment with antibiotics and expression of milk may cause a resolution in some cases. If no decrease in the area of redness has occurred within 24 h, then referral for a surgical opinion is advisable. A breast abscess which remains undrained on antibiotics may result in the so-called antibioma which forms a hard mass consisting of dense fibrotic chronically inflamed breast tissue. Prompt surgical drainage of breast abscesses is necessary to avoid extensive destruction of breast parenchyma and permanent deformity (*Fig.* 2.21).

Breast abscess formation is also a feature of mammary duct ectasia. In this condition the lactiferous ducts just deep to the nipple become blocked with dead epithelial cells. The ducts dilate distally and become filled with necrotic cellular debris. There is a surrounding area of inflammatory cellular infiltrate containing giant cells and plasma cells (plasma cell mastitis). The increasing numbers of reports in the literature of bacteria being isolated in patients with this condition has led to the suggestion that duct ectasia may have a primary infective aetiology. Discharge of the abscess through the skin of the areola may result in mammary duct fistula (*Fig.* 2.22).

Breast abscesses are best drained through circumareolar or circumferential incisions. The loculi are broken down with the finger and the cavity packed or the skin sutured after the insertion of a dependent drain. Others introduce and tie a large nylon stitch around the abscess to occlude the cavity (closed method of treatment). Manual evacuation of milk from the affected breast should be encouraged as soon as the acute pain and tenderness have settled following drainage. Abscess formation due to duct ectasia requires subsequent removal of the associated dilated ducts to prevent recurrence (Urban operation). This is carried out through an inferior or medial circumareolar incision and a wedge of breast tissue containing the dilated ducts and associated inflamed breast parenchyma is removed.

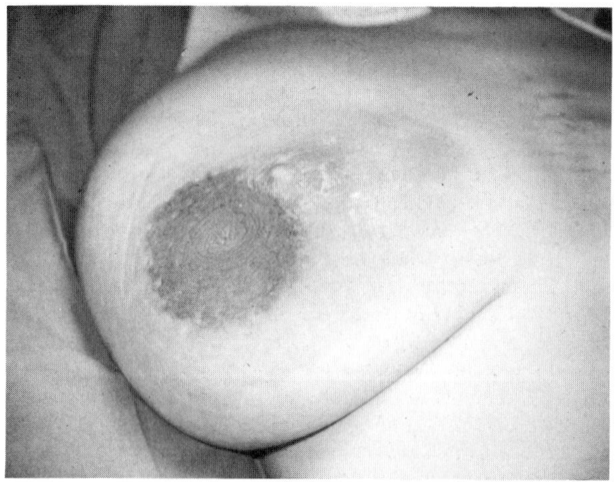

Fig. 2.21 A large breast abscess pointing to the areola in a postpartum female. The cavity was the size of a grapefruit with considerable destruction of the breast tissue.

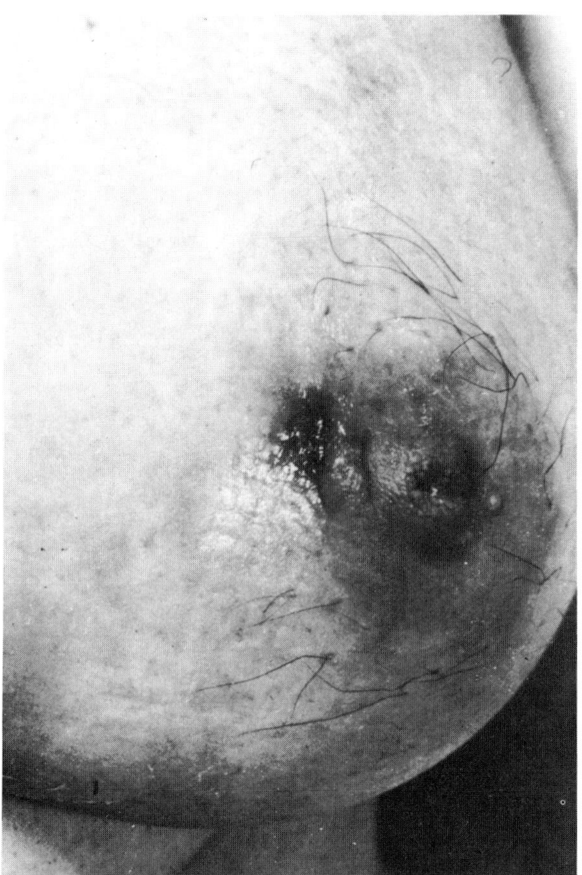

Fig. 2.22 Periductal mastitis with fistula formation.

It is important to stress that inflammatory breast cancer (mastitis carcinosa) may mimic septic mastitis and breast abscess (*Fig.* 2.23). If this suspicion is raised, xerography and a needle aspiration of Tru-cut biopsy should be performed initially as incision of these neoplastic breasts leads to disastrous fungation of the tumour.

Appendix Abscess

This arises as a result of a missed or delayed diagnosis of acute appendicitis, and the onset of a localized perforation of the inflamed appendix usually in the right iliac fossa. It may occur at any age, but is more common in the very young and elderly. The presenting symptoms include pain, abdominal distension and vomiting, due to intestinal obstruction, or pyrexia and toxicity. Examination may reveal a fixed tender mass in the right iliac fossa, or the suprapubic region. There may be inflammatory oedema of the overlying skin. An intermittent pyrexia, tachycardia and leucocytosis are usually present. A straight radiograph of the abdomen may show localized ileus with fluid levels and a soft-tissue mass. Differential diagnosis in the adult and elderly is from a caecal carcinoma (which may indeed co-exist with an appendix abscess), Crohn's disease and other ileocaecal granulomas, and perforation of a solitary caecal diverticulum. Initial management is with intravenous fluids, nil by mouth and systemic antibiotics. Nasogastric suction is instituted if abdominal distension is present. Increase in the size of the mass, cellulitis, pain, tenderness and toxicity or a rising pulse rate indicate failure of resolution and the need for

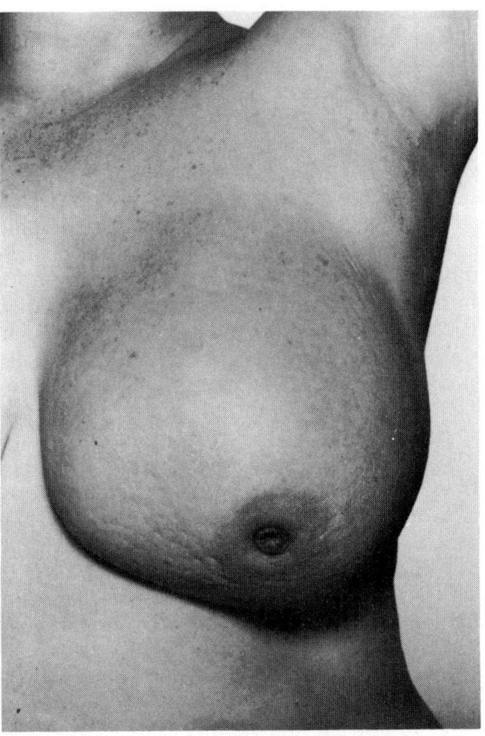

Fig. 2.23 This patient presented 5 months postpartum because of inability to breast feed from the left side. Mastitis carcinoma was confirmed by needle biopsy. The patient died 6 months later of disseminated disease.

prompt surgical intervention. Urgent drainage of an appendix mass may allow appendicectomy at the same time as drainage if the patient is fit and the appendix can be easily seen. More often, however, an interval appendicectomy is performed a few months later. In the meantime a barium enema should be performed in all adult and elderly patients. Doubts as to the presence of a carcinoma and/or caecal diverticulum, which can cause great difficulty even at operation, should be resolved by a right hemicolectomy with primary anastomosis if the area is free from faecal contamination. If there is obstruction of the small bowel with dilated bowel and contamination, it is safer to perform a double-barrelled ileostomy which is closed some 3–4 weeks later.

Pelvic Abscess

This may complicate acute appendicitis and pelvic infection or be secondary to peritonitis caused by perforation of a hollow viscus, e.g. perforated appendicitis. Perforated sigmoid diverticulitis or a slow localized leak from carcinoma of the sigmoid colon may present as a pelvic abscess. Symptoms of any type of particular illness may not have been noticed by the stoical patient and he may present eventually with toxicity and diarrhoea. The diarrhoea is intense and is accompanied by tenesmus, passage of liquid faeces and a great deal of mucus. Even in the young adult patient, faecal incontinence may occur. Examination of the patient's abdomen may reveal a suprapubic mass if the abscess is large. In the early stages of pelvic abscess formation, rectal examination reveals an oedematous and boggy mucosa. Subsequently, a tender mass is felt anteriorly but the posterior rectal wall feels normal. In the female patient, vulval oedema and tenderness on moving the cervix may be present. Leucocytosis is invariable but there are usually no radiological abnormalities on the straight abdominal films.

Oral fluid intake by the patient is encouraged, intravenous fluid therapy being instituted if the patient is toxic or dehydrated. Daily rectal examination is performed to assess the progress of the mass. The majority of pelvic abscesses drain spontaneously either into the rectum, especially if an anastomosis has previously been made, or the vaginal vault in the female, especially in a patient with previous hysterectomy. Antibiotic therapy is started if there is evidence of systemic sepsis after blood cultures have been taken. Continued severe symptoms of diarrhoea and toxicity with an enlarging fluctuant mass require surgical drainage. The patient is catheterized and in the lithotomy position, an operating proctoscope is passed into the rectum. The area of maximum fluctuation is then needled. As soon as pus is aspirated, a long handled knife is passed over the needle and a small incision made. A specimen of pus is sent for bacteriological examination and a finger is then introduced into the abscess cavity. The loculi are broken down gently but no attempt at curettage of the abscess walls is made because of the risk of damage to adherent bowel loops. Suprapubic exploration is occasionally warranted if the abscess is massive. Following successful treatment of a pelvic abscess, the appropriate radiological and endoscopic investigations are performed to determine the primary cause if this was not apparent at the time of presentation. When gastrointestinal disease is excluded, a gynaecological opinion should be sought in all female patients.

Intra-loop Abscesses

The diagnosis of these abscesses which are often multiple, can be very difficult. The condition may be suspected after a particularly contaminated and lengthy laparotomy for a generalized peritonitis due to a perforated hollow viscus. An intra-loop abscess may also result from a silent perforation, trauma to intra-abdominal organs, acute pancreatitis or leakage from an anastomotic suture line. Toxicity is often initially absent and the condition is usually heralded by abdominal distension and paralytic ileus with effortless vomiting of bile-stained fluid which subsequently becomes 'coffee-ground' in appearance and ultimately faeculent. The patient becomes obviously catabolic with a low serum albumin and hypokalaemia. Other electrolyte deficiencies resulting from prolonged ileus include hypocalcaemia and hypomagnesaemia which may cause confusion and delirium. Plain abdominal radiographs may show fluid levels, dilated loops of bowel and on auscultation, an absence of bowel sounds. Occasionally, a soft-tissue mass with a gas/fluid interface may be demonstrated. Abdominal ultrasound examination may indicate the presence of loop abscesses, but abdominal distension, oedematous skin and intestinal gas often preclude reliable interpretation of this investigation. Scintiscanning with indium-labelled autologous white cells may be helpful (*Fig.* 2.17). CT scanning is the most reliable method for the detection of intra-abdominal abscesses. Often the diagnosis remains a clinical one and a decision on surgical intervention is made because of continued weight loss, despite adequate parenteral feeding and evidence of intra-abdominal sepsis with fever, prolonged ileus, persistent leucocytosis and anaemia. Adequate surgical exposure is essential as the entire peritoneal cavity, including the lesser sac and abdominal contents, must be examined. All pus is evacuated, fibrinous deposits carefully removed and a full saline wash-out of the peritoneal cavity is performed. Tetracycline peritoneal lavage has been shown in an uncontrolled trial to reduce the recurrence of intra-abdominal loop abscesses. This report requires confirmation, as on theoretical grounds, the activity of the tetracycline in this situation is questionable. Any leaking anastomosis is best treated by exteriorization which is also indicated if intestinal resection is required because of necrosis of bowel or doubtful viability.

SINUSES

A sinus is a discharging blind-ended tract which opens on to an epithelial surface and often leads to an abscess cavity. However, a sinus cannot always be easily differentiated from a fistula as the internal opening of the latter may be difficult to demonstrate. The key to the correct treatment of a sinus is the detection of any associated deep abscess cavity or complex deep extensions of the sinus tract (*Fig.* 2.24). Failure to do this will result in a recurrence of the sinus at the same site or adjacent location.

The discharge from a sinus should always be submitted for bacteriological examination. Most of the pathogens isolated will be skin organisms or gut commensals, but occasionally specific infections, such as tuberculosis, actinomycosis or fungosis may be found, the last being encountered usually as secondary infection of a chronic abscess cavity. Examination of the sinus requires more than a cursory inspection of the external discharging opening. Very gentle probing with a fine malleable probe is used to assess the depth, direction and multiplicity of tracts, and may suggest further investigation of the condition with the aid of a sinogram. If the sinus has a narrow exit, a fine radio-opaque polythene catheter can be gently introduced until its progress is halted. A water/based contrast medium such as Angiographin 45%, is then injected through the catheter under image intensification. When the cavity or deep sinus has been demonstrated, appropriate radiographs are obtained in two planes for a permanent record. A larger skin opening such as a perineal sinus requires the exit tract to be obstructed with a Foley balloon catheter. Contrast is then injected into the sinus cavity until leakage occurs around the balloon at the skin level. This contrast study may reveal that the sinus is in fact a fistulous communication (*Fig.* 2.25).

In the management of any sinus, after the appropriate evaluation has been carried out as detailed above, the wound is laid open or excised and a biopsy of the tissue from the wall of the sinus is sent for histological examination. The vast majority of these biopsies will show granulation tissue only but if routine pathological examination is omitted, sooner or later a metastatic growth will be missed or some specific inflammatory disease will remain undiagnosed with persistence of the sinus or early recurrence.

Cervical sinuses due to tuberculous infection of the lymph glands in the neck are being encountered in many large towns within the UK, especially among the immigrant population. The collar-stud shape of the related abscess cavity is due to penetration of the investing layer of deep cervical fascia by the tuberculous abscess before bursting through the skin to form the sinus. The condition is discussed further in Chapter 23.

Osteomyelitis may uncommonly present as a discharging sinus, which indicates longstanding chronic osseous infection with sequestrum formation. The occurrence of a sinus after surgical treatment of osteomyelitis indicates inadequate removal of necrotic bone. If untreated, the area may become secondarily infected by fungal organisms or rarely by actinomycosis.

Pilonidal Sinus

The term pilonidal is of Greek derivation and means 'nest of hairs'. It is one of the commonest types of sinus seen in general surgical practice and is usually found in the natal

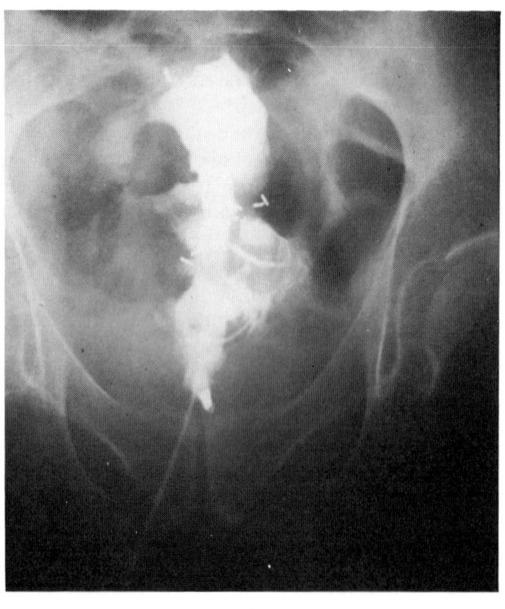

a

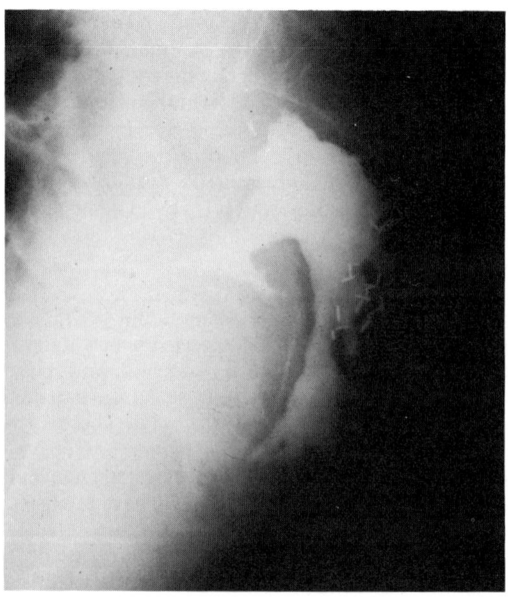

b

Fig. 2.24 Postero-anterior (*a*) and lateral (*b*) radiographs obtained after injecting contrast material through a fine catheter inserted into a chronic discharging sinus in the lower anterior abdominal wall. The patient had undergone a panproctocolectomy and ileostomy for Crohn's disease 4 years previously. The sinograms demonstrate a large abscess cavity extending to the pelvic floor.

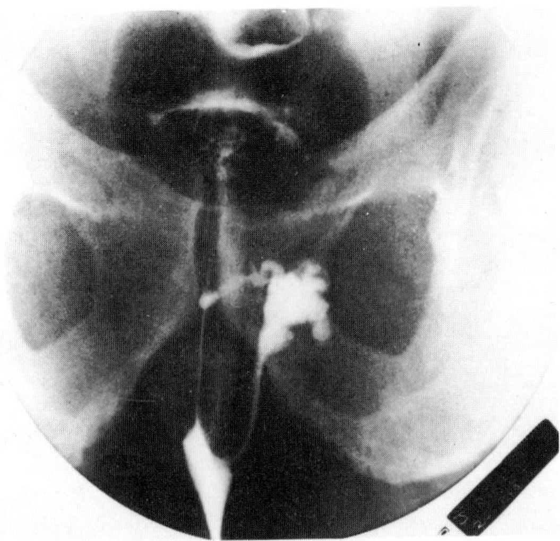

Fig. 2.25 Sinogram showing abscess cavity and a high-level fistulous communication with the rectum. The catheter is seen entering the abscess cavity. Contrast reaches and outlines the rectum before flowing down into the anal canal.

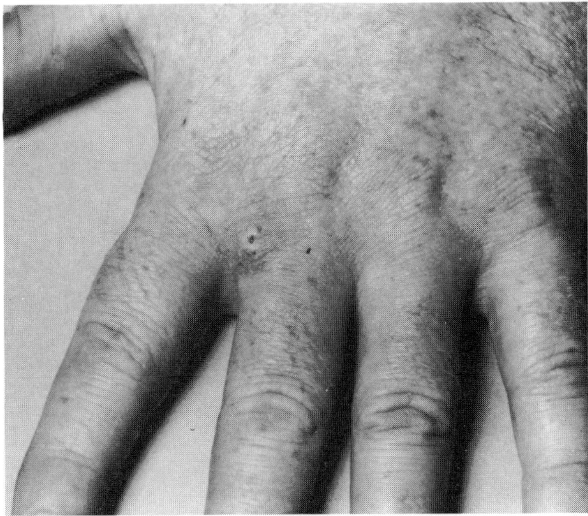

Fig. 2.26 Pilonidal sinus in the digital cleft between index and the middle finger in a barber.

cleft. Pilonidal sinus is an acquired condition and is thought to arise from loose hair shafts which are continuously shed from the body and migrate root first to the natal cleft during walking and thereafter are forced into the enlarging sweat glands by the gluteal contractions. Previously held theories of an embryological nature attributed the origin of a pilonidal sinus variously to a sequestratian dermoid, a traction dermoid and to persistence of the medullary canal defect.

Initially and in some patients indefinitely, pilonidal sinuses cause minimal reaction and symptoms but with the onset of secondary infection with skin commensals and blockage of sinus exit, recurring pain, swelling, discharge and occasionally bleeding are experienced by the patient. Untreated, the abscess discharges but often this is followed by recurrence and progressive extension with multiple sinus tracts and openings. The commonest sites other than the natal cleft, are between the toes and fingers, especially in barbers (*Fig.* 2.26). The now almost equal sex incidence of pilonidal sinus is probably related to the modern female fashion of tight fitting clothes. The condition was commonly encountered in servicemen during the Second World War (jeep disease).

A pilonidal sinus which has not been infected should be left untreated. Many forms of treatment are advocated by experts in a particular technique (phenol injection, incision, excision with primary closure) but they are all accompanied by recurrence rates of 16–40% and none has proved superior to adequate excision of the sinus. Both the acute abscess and the chronically discharging sinus can be treated in the same manner with excision of about half a centimetre of skin on either side of the sinus tract (*Fig.* 2.27). This will allow full drainage and formation of healthy granulation tissue, resulting in healing from the depths of the cavity. The wound edges are kept apart by flavine emulsion gauze roll which is sutured with a few laterally placed sutures and left in situ for 3–4 days. The patient may take baths during this time. When this dressing is removed, a clean granulating wound with stiff walls is observed. This allows healing from the base by contraction of the wound and by the newly formed collagenous tissue. The skin edges must, however, be kept apart until healing is almost complete with either daily packing with a gauze roll done by a district nurse or more conveniently and with less discomfort by the patient if the cavity is packed with silicone foam elastomer dressing. These methods will help to prevent bridging of the granulating wound until epithelial healing can finally seal the shallow granulating wound.

Hidradenitis Suppurativa

Another condition characterized by recurrent abscess/sinus formation is hidradenitis suppurativa. This is thought to be an abnormality of the apocrine sweat glands of the body which are found mainly in the axillae, groins, perineum and around the nipples. In affected individuals, the glands form recurrent abscesses after puberty with repeated attacks of pain and inflammation which may be very troublesome to the patient. These abscesses may resolve or burst spontaneously forming chronic discharging sinuses. The condition may be improved by low dose tetracycline therapy which is thought to reduce the apocrine secretion, but if very troublesome with repeated abscess formation, complete excision of the area containing the apocrine glands is required. The excision must be radical if recurrence at the edges is to be avoided. As the affected areas are difficult to graft, the wounds are left open to heal by granulation tissue with a surprisingly good cosmetic result (*Fig.* 2.28).

Sinus Formation following Surgery on the Gastrointestinal Tract

A wound sinus may form subsequent to initial healing of a surgical abdominal wound. A commonly encountered variety is the *stitch* sinus which is the result of non-absorbable suture material acting as a focus to a small infection within the wound. These sinuses are more commonly encountered after closure of a dirty or potentially contaminated wound than after clean operations. They tend to persist over many months and produce an inconvenient seropurulent discharge (*Fig.* 2.29). The incidence of stitch sinuses is diminished by ensuring that knots are tied and buried away from the subcutaneous plane. Healing of a persistent sinus requires the removal of the suture. This is usually done with sinus

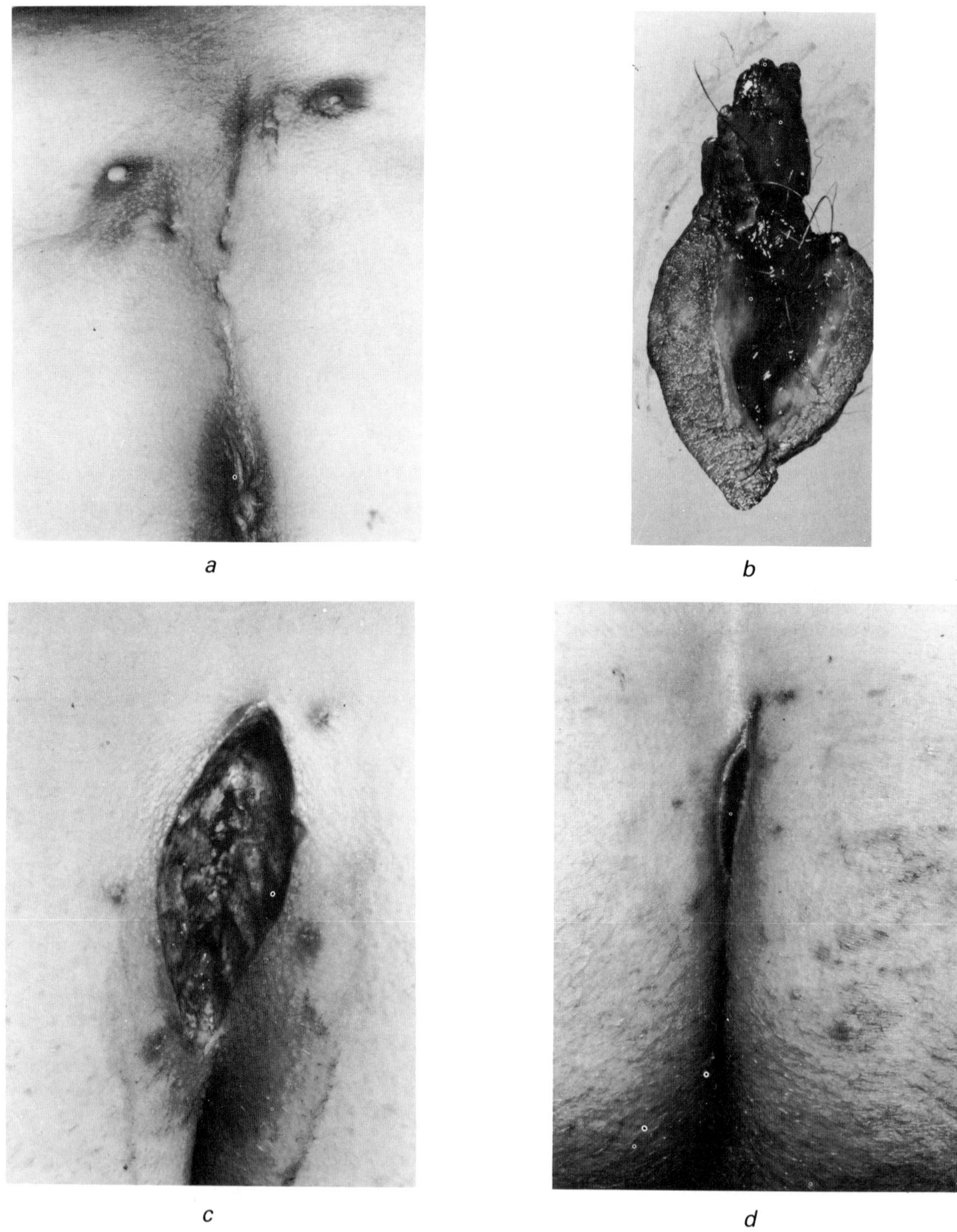

Fig. 2.27 *a*, Recurrent pilonidal sinus with three discharging tracts and a central pit. Note scars from previous incisions. *b*, Excised sinus showing the nest of hairs. *c*, Resulting cavity after removal of gauze pack 4 days after excision of sinus. *d*, Appearance of the wound on the 18th postoperative day.

forceps after the skin has been injected with local anaesthetic. In patients with contaminated wounds, e.g. emergency operations for acute abdominal conditions, the skin and subcutaneous tissues are left open to heal by granulation tissue or a delayed skin closure performed a few days later. As granulation tissue grows over and buries non-absorbable sutures, sinus formation is not a problem after healing of an abdominal wound by granulation (*Fig.* 2.30).

Larger sinuses, sometimes unrelated to the abdominal wound, are commonly encountered after operations for Crohn's disease. They may result from contamination at operation or occur in association with a small intra-loop abscess or a leak from a diseased bowel or anastomosis. The localized abscess may discharge through the abdominal wall (*Fig.* 2.31) or wound forming a fistula if the abscess cavity still connects with the bowel lumen. The internal orifice may

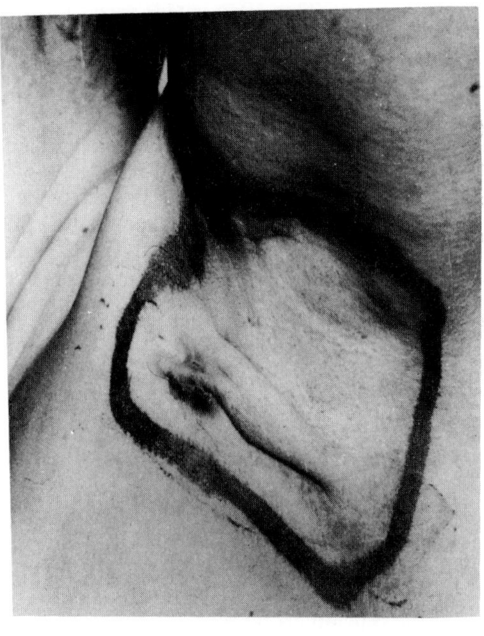

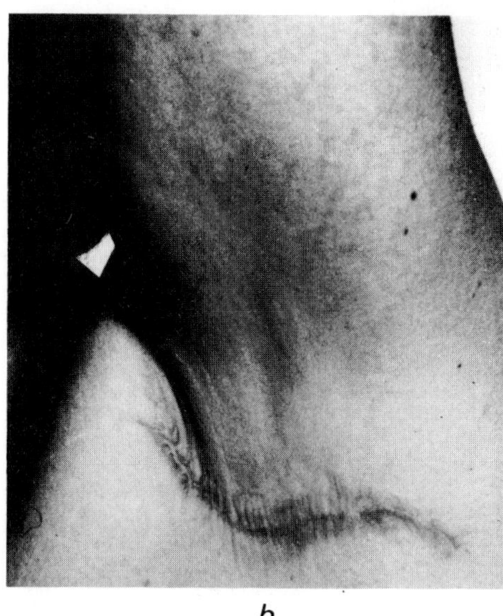

Fig. 2.28 *a*, Hidradenitis suppurativa of the axilla. *b*, End result after surgical excision and healing by granulation.

have healed in which case a chronic discharging sinus will be seen which cannot drain adequately because of the associated intra-abdominal abscess cavity. Longstanding discharge from this type of sinus may eventually lead to secondary amyloidosis and death from cardiac, renal and adrenal failure.

The pathological evolution of a sinus is well exemplified by the perineal sinus occurring after a panproctocolectomy for inflammatory bowel disease (*Fig.* 2.32), and less commonly after abdominoperineal resection for carcinoma of the rectum. Faecal contamination at operation increases the incidence of this complication. A perineal sinus is most commonly encountered after resection for Crohn's disease and there is some evidence that the granulation tissue in this disease may not contract or heal normally as non-caseating granulomas are sometimes demonstrable in the granulation tissue of these patients. Primary closure of a wound at

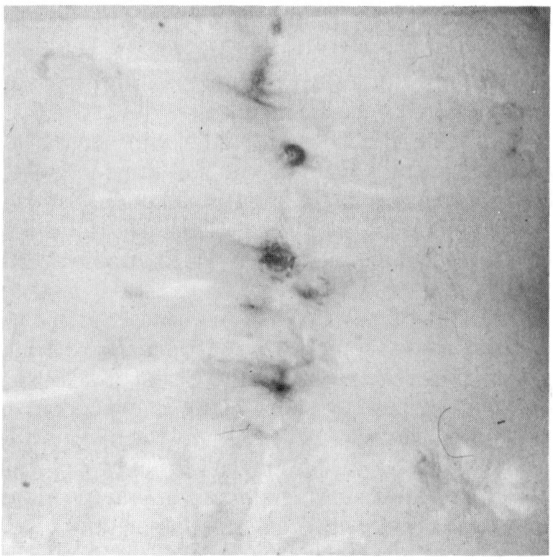

Fig. 2.29 Stitch sinus in a patient after resection and primary anastomosis of the sigmoid colon for perforated diverticular disease. The sinus persisted until the non-absorbable prolene suture was removed.

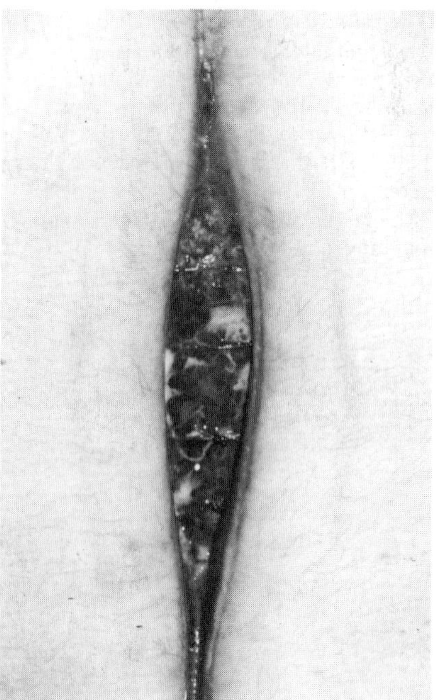

Fig. 2.30 In this patient who underwent an emergency operation for generalized peritonitis, the skin and subcutaneous tissues were left open. Interrupted nylon sutures can be seen within the granulation tissue which grew over the sutures allowing complete healing without sinus formation.

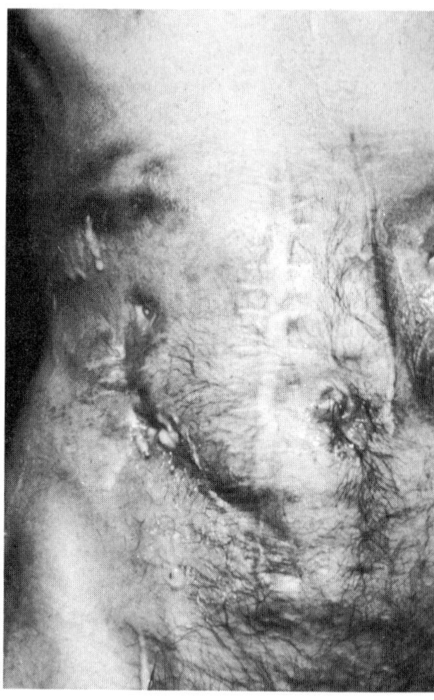

Fig. 2.31 Multiple discharging sinuses in the right abdominal wall in a patient suffering from Crohn's disease. The sinuses are connected with multiple intra-abdominal abscesses.

operation with drains inserted into the curve of the sacrum may well appear to achieve primary healing for several days. Often, however, the wound becomes inflamed and the patient may become toxic with a pyrexia and raised white count. Opening the perineal wound releases the pus of the acute abscess but is followed by persistent discharge over prolonged periods since the deeper loculus of the dumb-bell shaped cavity (situated above the levator muscles) cannot drain properly. A Foley catheter sinogram will show a narrowing at the level of the coccyx and levator ani muscles, fibres of which sweep back around the area of excised rectum. Thus the disharge from the pelvic space in front of the sacral concavity drains inadequately especially when the patient is supine. Treatment after evaluation by sinography, requires opening and wide excision to form a unilocular well-draining cavity. This often entails excision of the coccyx, granulation tissue and some muscle of the levator ani to remove the area of constriction. Many surgeons do not close the pelvic peritoneum and this allows small bowel and omentum to fill the pelvis. This probably helps to prevent a large space occurring below the pelvic peritoneum in which infection can develop. To prevent bowel dropping out through the pelvic floor, omentum has been advocated as a living package material. As granulation tissue contracts, healing can be checked with repeated sinograms but relaxation of weekly follow-up in the outpatient department cannot be allowed until the deep sacral wound has healed to the level of levator ani.

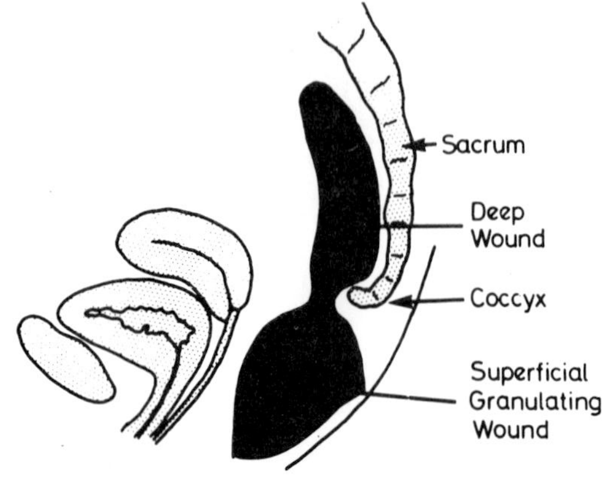

Fig. 2.32 Diagrammatic representation of the shape of a perineal sinus after panproctocolectomy. The coccyx and fibres of the pubococcygeus result in an hour-glass narrowing.

FISTULAS

A fistula is a communication betwen two epithelial or endothelial surfaces. It is usually an acquired condition when it is lined by granulation tissue, but may have some epithelium growing down the ends of the tract. It can be a congenital and life-threatening condition (e.g. oesophageal atresia with a fistulous communication with the trachea). External fistulas involve the skin (enterocutaneous) whereas internal fistulas can affect adjacent organs contiguously or more commonly through an intervening abscess cavity (entero-enteric, enterocolic, vesicocolic, etc.). Arteriovenous fistulas are considered in the vascular section.

The majority of internal abdominal fistulas result from an underlying gastrointestinal disease (colonic diverticular disease, Crohn's disease, colonic carcinoma, radiation enteritis, intestinal tuberculosis, chronic cholecystitis etc.). External abdominal fistulas arise as a complication of surgery on or trauma to the intra-abdominal organs such as anastomotic leakage, accidental or unrecognized injury during operation (*Fig.* 2.33). Other external fistulas are due to primary abscess formation which involves bowel and the skin and these are best exemplified by the perianal fistulas (*Fig.* 2.34).

The secondary effects of internal abdominal fistulas depend on the exact site and pathology of the condition causing it. Malabsorption and steatorrhoea may result from bacterial overgrowth with bile salt deconjugation and diminished bile salt pool. This may occur with entero-enteric and enterocolic fistulas. Cholangitis may follow bilio-enteric fistula. Severe cystitis with pneumaturia may be caused by the presence of vesicocolic fistula etc.

Constitutional effects are minimal with external colonic fistulas. By contrast, malnutrition and fluid and electrolyte depletion accompany high output small bowel fistulas. Skin excoriation and digestion of the abdominal wall is a serious feature of pancreatic, duodenal and high small bowel fistulas (*Fig.* 2.35).

Internal abdominal, perianal and anorectal fistulas seldom, if ever, close spontaneously. Healing of external abdominal fistulas can be expected if there is no distal obstruction to the involved bowel. This healing is dependent on the adequate drainage of any abscesses and the maintenance of a good nutritional state. Prophylaxis should be instituted against abdominal wall excoriation by attention to local skin care. This may be obtained by use of Stomadhesive as a seal to the skin through which drainage of the fistula may be undertaken with the aid of adequate sump suction drain. A fistula through a diseased segment of bowel is much less likely to heal, but this will depend to a certain extent on the pathology present.

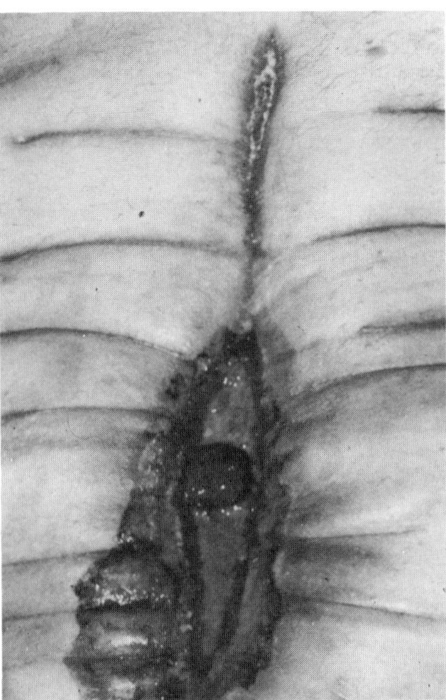

Fig. 2.33 A small-bowel fistula in the base of a granulating abdominal wound. This followed a difficult abdominal exploration for colonic diverticular disease.

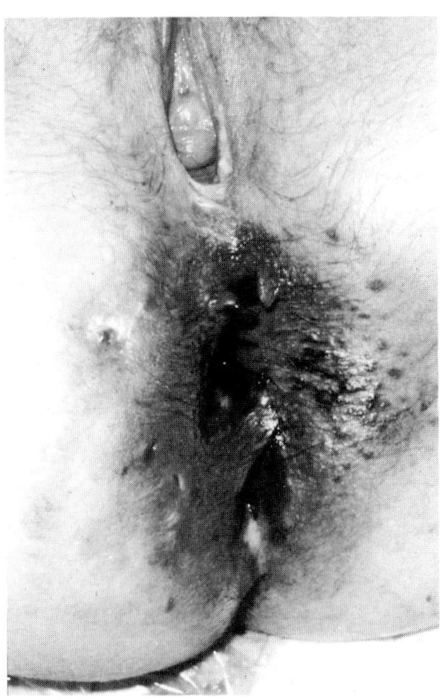

Fig. 2.34 Multiple perineal fistulas in a patient with extensive Crohn's disease of the rectum.

Management is, therefore, complex and requires definition of the exact underlying pathological anatomy by appropriate contrast radiology with a sinogram and/or barium enema, barium meal follow-through. Surgical intervention is required for internal fistulas and for external abdominal fistulas associated with distal obstruction, or where contrast radiology has shown discontinuity of the bowel, and in the presence of underlying neoplastic intestinal disease, or when conservative medical management with parenteral nutrition has failed to produce healing.

Mammary Duct Fistula

This occurs most commonly in patients with mammary duct ectasia, but may complicate other breast disorders. The patients present with recurrent attacks of non-cyclical breast pain and local areas of inflammation (periductal mastitis) which can proceed to abscess formation. These were thought to be sterile, but bacteria have now been demonstrated in some of the biopsies from patients with this condition. These periductal abscesses may resolve spontaneously, however, without the need for antibiotic therapy. If aerobes and anaerobes are, however, isolated in a patient who has required biopsy, then appropriate antibiotics may be necessary to prevent recurrence. There is often a history of creamy coloured nipple discharge in between attacks. Incision of an abscess or its spontaneous discharge, usually through the areolar skin may then be followed by the

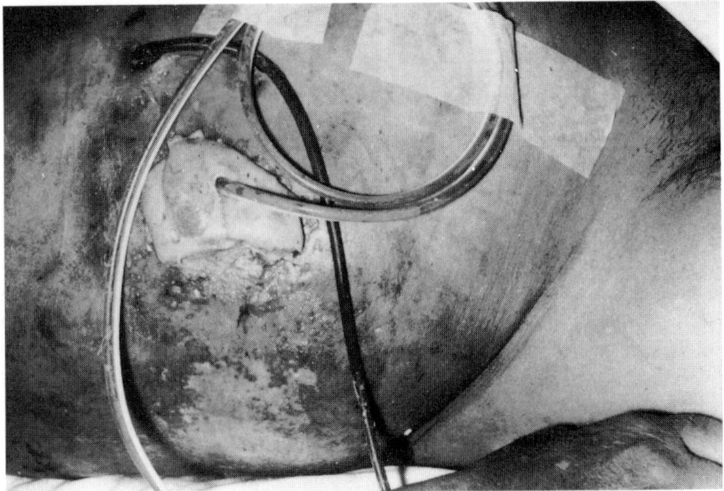

Fig. 2.35 High small-bowel fistula following surgical excision for Crohn's disease. There is extensive excoriation of the skin of the abdominal wall.

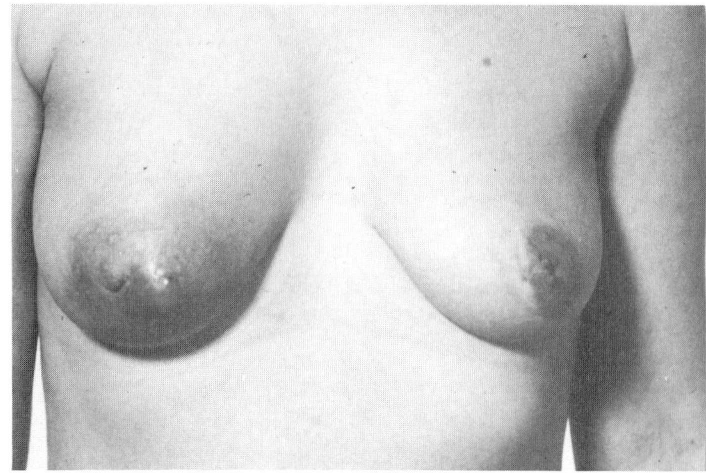

Fig. 2.36 Duct ectasia in a patient with previous surgery to the left breast which has an indrawn nipple and a scarred areola. On the right side, there is a discharging abscess and a mammary duct fistula.

development of a mammary duct fistula which continues to discharge small amounts of clear or creamy fluid. Persistence of a fistula is due to the blocked lactiferous duct at the nipple. If skin closure occurs, there is a further build-up of secretion and pain followed by pointing and discharge, resulting in an intermittent fistula. Examination may reveal bilateral nipple retraction and scars from previous surgical biopsy or abscess drainage (*Fig.* 2.36). The condition may be bilateral at the time of presentation or recur on the contralateral side at a later date. The breasts may be tender or feel normal, depending on the state of inflammation at the particular time of examination.

Treatment of a mammary duct fistula entails excision of the fistula, together with a wedge of breast tissue. If duct ectasia is present, a subareolar excision of all the nipple duct tissue is required.

Biliary Fistulas

These are classified as external which are secondary to bile duct trauma or leakage from accessory bile ducts and gallbladder bed, and internal which are classified into three types: bilio-enteric; broncho-biliary and bilio-pleural; bilio-biliary.

Most commonly, trauma to the biliary tract is iatrogenic and sustained during cholecystectomy. Leakage of bile may occur from damaged common hepatic or common bile duct, cut accessory bile ducts or cystic duct stump due to slipped ligature. Leakage of bile from the drain site is noticed in the early postoperative period. There is no skin excoriation and the bile leakage is collected in a Hollister type bag. Fluid and electrolyte replacement is necessary and definitive treatment of any bile duct damage is undertaken after appropriate radiological investigations. Management of bile duct injuries is discussed in Chapter 69. If drainage is inadequate, the patient becomes toxic from the accumulated infected bile usually in the subphrenic spaces and lesser sac, and may go on to develop frank biliary peritonitis. External biliary fistula may also arise as a complication of hepatic trauma or liver resection.

Bilio-enteric Fistulas

Spontaneous fistulas of this type are commonly caused by cholelithiasis (Chapter 69) and less commonly carcinoma of the hepatic flexure or extrahepatic bile ducts. The most common variety is the cholecystoduodenal fistula which may present acutely with cholangitis or gallstone ileus. The patients are usually elderly and treatment is by surgical intervention.

Iatrogenic choledochoduodenal fistula may result following the inadvisable and rough use of rigid probes (e.g. Bâke's dilators). As these metal sounds are forced through the Vaterian segment of the common bile duct, a false passage or fistula may be created during operations on the biliary tract. The onset of symptoms is usually delayed. Recurrent pain is the predominant symptom and is usually diagnosed as postcholecystectomy sydrome. Some patients, however, present with cholangitis. Endoscopic retrograde cholangiography usually outlines the fistula. Treatment is by choledochojejunostomy.

Broncho-biliary and Bilio-pleural Fistulas

These are secondary to subphrenic abscess formation resulting from bile duct or liver injuries. Treatment consists of adequate drainage of the subphrenic space and correction of biliary obstruction. Pulmonary lobectomy is not indicated as the fistulas invariably heal with this management.

Bilio-biliary Fistulas

These are rare and consist of a communication between the gallbladder or cystic duct and the common bile duct or common hepatic duct usually in patients with gallstones (Mirizzi's syndrome). The presenting symptoms are jaundice and pain. Treatment is surgical and indeed the exact pathological anatomy is usually first defined at laparotomy. Operative findings include dense adhesions in the subphrenic region with the gallbladder adherent to the extrahepatic bile duct system. In this eventuality the initial cholangiogram should be performed through the gallbladder. A partial cholecystectomy down to the fistula zone is carried out leaving a cuff of the gallbladder next to the fistula, no attempt being made to take the fistula down. A silicone T-tube is placed in the common bile duct through the fistula and the residual cuff of gallbladder wall sutured around the

T-tube which is left in situ for 6–8 weeks, depending on the radiological assessment by T-tube cholangiography.

Pancreatic Fistula

Pancreatic fistulas may be internal or external and carry a substantial morbidity from sepsis, haemorrhage and persistent pancreatitis.

An external fistula may be secondary to a pancreatic abscess complicating acute pancreatitis, but may also follow abdominal trauma and operative intervention. Pancreatic fistulas may result from pancreatic resections or iatrogenic trauma, e.g. damage to the tail of the pancreas during splenectomy or following pancreatic biopsy. However, the incidence of this complication following biopsy of the pancreas has been grossly exaggerated and biopsy is indicated before radical pancreatic resection for suspected pancreatic cancer. Wedge biopsy is safer and more accurate than Tru-cut needle biopsy, except for periampullary lesions, where a transduodenal needle biopsy is the procedure of choice. Fine needle aspiration cytology is both accurate and safe and is replacing other forms of biopsy in a number of centres.

The consequences of an external pancreatic fistula are similar to those of a high small bowel/duodenal fistula. Although the output tends to be lower, skin digestion is marked. Management is essentially similar to that of a high small bowel fistula. Endoscopic retrograde cholangiopancreatography is invaluable to outline associated lesions, e.g. abscesses, pseudocysts, duct stenoses, etc. and in defining the nature of the surgical treatment required if the fistula persists with conservative treatment.

An internal pancreatic fistula is almost always due to a pancreatic abscess which complicates acute pancreatitis in 1–5% of patients. The signs and symptoms include the disappearance of a previously palpable tender abdominal mass and the onset of gastrointestinal bleeding in a patient with prolonged pancreatitis. The most common fistulous communication is with the transverse colon, but stomach, duodenum, small intestinal and pleural cavity may be implicated. Bleeding occurs either from the fistula margin in the intestine or the abscess cavity and if this involves the splenic artery, it may be massive. Treatment of internal pancreatic fistula consists of drainage of the abscess cavity and this often results in spontaneous healing of the fistula. Pancreaticocolic fistula usually requires a colostomy and resection of the affected part of the colon may be necessary if the fistula persists. Bleeding from a pancreatic fistula is treated by embolization ligature of the bleeding point, the exact localization of which may be achieved by selective coeliac axis arteriography if the condition of the patient will allow this investigative procedure.

Gastrocutaneous Fistulas

These are usually iatrogenic following unrecognized operative injuries during splenectomy or vagotomy. Partial necrosis of the lesser curve to duodenum anastomosis after a Billroth 1 gastrectomy may also result in a gastric leak and fistula. Some apparently arise as a result of erosion by drains. A small percentage are caused by benign gastric ulcer, pancreatic abscess and pancreatic carcinoma. The diagnosis is usually delayed until 2–3 weeks after surgical intervention. There is considerable skin irritation and a high incidence of sepsis with subphrenic abscess formation. The loss of gastric juice may lead to an alkalosis and electrolyte depletion. Diagnosis may be quickly established by the administration of methylene blue but a contrast fistulogram or a barium swallow/meal should be done to delineate the exact pathological anatomy and any associated gastric disease.

Treatment is conservative and consists of nasogastric suction, correction of fluid and electrolyte abnormalities, nutritional support, parenteral cimetidine (to cut down the volume and acidity of the fistulous loss) and control of sepsis.

Nutrition is maintained either by the parenteral route or by means of a fine catheter feeding jejunostomy (Chapter 8). The majority of gastrocutaneous fistulas are not associated with carcinoma and heal with the above supportive treatment.

Gastrojejunocolic Fistula

This severe complication is usually found in association with inoperable carcinoma of the stomach or transverse colon. It is less frequently encountered as a result of recurrent ulcer at a gastrojejunal anastomosis largely due to the overall improvement in the results of ulcer management and surgical treatment. Some patients in the peptic ulcer group are subsequently found to be suffering from the Zollinger–Ellison syndrome.

The symptoms are profound with vomiting of foul-smelling material, diarrhoea, weight loss and inanition. There is a gross bacterial overgrowth of the small bowel contents leading to severe malabsorption with hypoproteinaemia and anaemia. In addition, there is irritation of the colonic mucosa by the dehydroxylated and deconjugated bile acids aggravating the diarrhoea and leading to a hypokalaemia. Chronic bleeding from the fistula is common and contributes to the anaemia. Examination reveals evidence of weight loss and an abdominal mass or scars from previous ulcer surgery. The diagnosis is strongly suspected at gastroscopy from the stench and residue found in the stomach, and is confirmed by a barium meal (*Fig.* 2.37) or enema. Initial management consists of correction of fluid and electrolyte abnormalities and anaemia, together with parenteral nutrition. Surgical treatment depends on the exact causation. Triple resection with a temporary proximal colostomy is required for ulcer cases. This includes a total gastrectomy in patients with the Zollinger–Ellison syndrome. Palliative resection may be possible in cancer cases but often the emphasis is on comfortable terminal care.

Small-bowel Fistulas

The outlook with these fistulas has been significantly improved over the past decade with the advent of effective nutritional support, better skin stoma management and the avoidance of early surgical intervention wherever possible as this is attended by a substantial mortality.

The majority (80–90%) of small-bowel fistulas follow operations on the intestinal tract either from anastomotic leakage or iatrogenic injury (*see Figs.* 2.33 and 2.35). Often the anastomotic dehiscence is attributed to the presence of underlying small bowel disorder, Crohn's disease being the most common, but radiation enteritis and intestinal tuberculosis featuring often in several published series. Apart from small-bowel disease, risk factors include old age, systemic or local bowel hypoxia, hypoproteinaemia, diabetes mellitus, and hepatic cirrhosis. A small-bowel fistula may also complicate both blunt and penetrating abdominal trauma.

Modern conservative management results in spontaneous closure of 70–80% of small-bowel fistulas and carries an

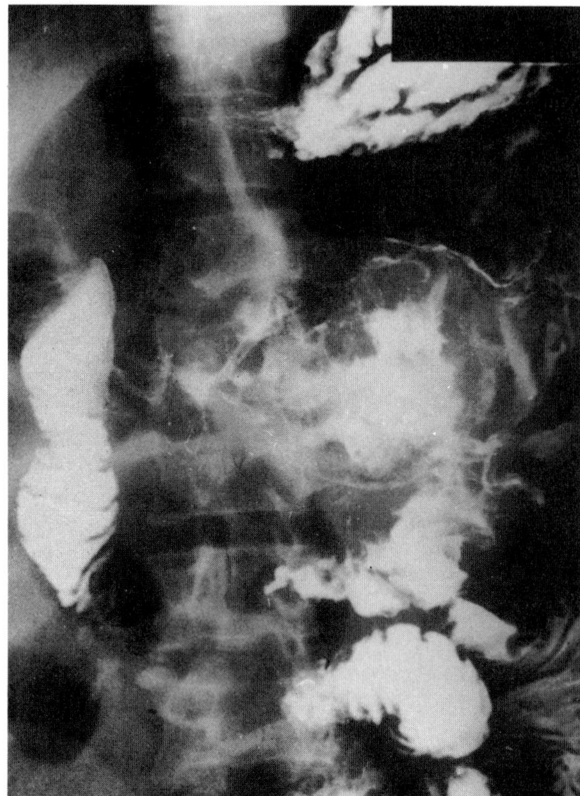

Fig. 2.37 Barium meal showing a gastrojejunocolic fistula due to gastric carcinoma.

average mortality of 6–10%. Surgical intervention performed when conservative management has failed has a reported mortality of 20%. The favourable prognostic factors include:

Distal (ileal) fistula
Output less than 500 ml per 24 h (low-output fistulas)
Late occurrence (after 14th postoperative day)
Absence of associated fistulas
No wound dehiscence.

The diagnosis is always obvious. Investigations are required to outline the exact pathological anatomy. The useful radiological investigations are a small-bowel enema with barium sulphate and a fistulogram obtained after insertion of a Foley catheter through the external orifice of the fistula

Treatment

Conservative

The mainstays of medical management are:
Nutritional support
Meticulous collection of fistulous discharge
Skin-stoma care
Control of sepsis

NUTRITIONAL SUPPORT. Initially this is by the parenteral route with the use of a subclavian line. The objective is to provide a daily intake of 2500 calories in the feed, consisting of dextrose, lipid and amino acid solution with some vitamins and trace elements. Attention to the electrolyte requirements with particular emphasis on K^+, Ca^{++}, Mg^{++} and phosphate is essential in all patients on prolonged parenteral nutrition. If loss is prolonged, estimation of trace elements is needed and deficiencies encountered corrected in order to obtain recovery from the prolonged small-bowel ileus. A separate intravenous line may be needed to maintain fluid and electrolyte balance. Elemental diets are used when the patient has been weaned off nasogastric suction, the fistula is distal and its output is low. They should be administered in an iso-osmolar state since hypertonic solution are poorly tolerated by the patient, cause abdominal discomfort and distension and enhance secretion by the intestinal mucosa and thus losses through the fistula.

COLLECTION OF FISTULOUS DISCHARGE. Nasogastric suction is used in patients with ileus and to minimize the fistula output when this is high. The collection of the fistulous discharge is best achieved by sump suction drainage. If collection bags are used meticulous fitting is required to avoid soiling and digestion of the peristomal skin.

SKIN-STOMA CARE. Silicone barrier cream may be used initially but Stomadhesive is best for long-term care. Karaya gum powder may be useful in irregular defects around the stoma before the application of Stomadhesive. In difficult cases, where the above methods prove inadequate, lactic acid irrigation of the fistula is effective in preventing autodigestion of the abdominal wall.

Surgical

The absolute indications for operative intervention are:

Intestinal distal obstruction
Peritonitis
Abscess formation
Bowel discontinuity
Presence of malignant disease
Persistent inflammatory bowel disease

In the absence of the above indications, medical treatment is continued but if a significant output remains after 4–5 weeks, operative intervention is necessary. Surgical treatment entails complete mobilization of the small bowel with resection of the involved segment. If the bowel ends appear healthy an end-to-end anastomosis is performed, otherwise, and in all cases of doubt, the two ends should be exteriorized. Exclusion of the involved loop is satisfactory when the rest of the small bowel is healthy. The results of this procedure are generally inferior to those of resection, except in patients with radiation enteritis.

External Colonic Fistulas

These most commonly follow colonic surgery, including colostomy closure. Trauma accounts for some cases as does perforated colonic diverticular disease and cancer. The patient may complain of a slight feeling of nausea or loss of appetite. Eventually, faeculent fluid appears from a drain site, the wound or both. If the patient is passing flatus and some faeces per rectum, the fistula usually closes spontaneously, but this may take a period of several weeks or months during which time the patient will need to wear a colostomy-type appliance if the output is greater than can be managed by two dressing changes per day. A limited barium enema and/or a fistulogram is necessary if the faecal discharge is copious, to determine continuity of the bowel or the presence of stricture formation causing distal obstruction. Either radiological procedure is terminated if an abscess cavity is outlined. Colonic fistulas tend to form

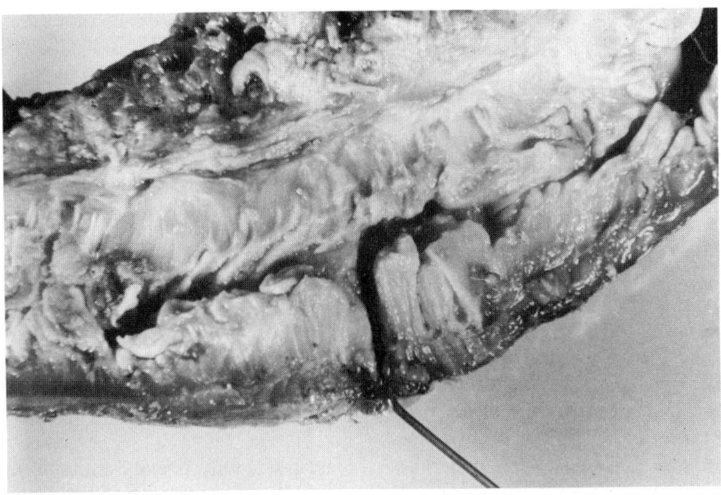

Fig. 2.38 Colovesical fistula due to diverticular disease: resected portion of sigmoid colon showing the fistulous tract, narrowed colon with sacculation of the wall and pericolic inflammatory thickening of fat.

granulating tracts earlier than small-bowel fistulas. The nutritional consequences of external colonic fistulas are minor and skin excoriation is not encountered unless diarrhoea is present.

Operative treatment is indicated for abscess formation, substantial bowel discontinuity or distal stricture and when the fistula persists. It consists of mobilization of the colon on either side of the fistula, excision of the affected area and end-to-end anastomosis using interrupted non-absorbable sutures. A double-barrel exteriorization is performed in the presence of significant sepsis and large abscesses.

Colovesical and Colovaginal Fistulas

The former is one of the commonest forms of internal abdominal fistulas. Both are usually encountered in association with diverticular disease and a pericolic abscess which perforates into the bladder or vagina, especially in females after hysterectomy, as this allows the diseased bowel to lie directly onto the bladder or the vaginal vault (*Fig.* 2.38). Less commonly these fistulas may be due to cervical or rectal carcinoma. Crohn's disease of the large and small bowel may be complicated by the development of entero/colovesical fistula. Radiotherapy for malignant disease of the pelvis accounts for the majority of rectovaginal/vesical fistulas.

The patient with a colovesical fistula presents with severe and intractable urinary tract infection. The urine is foul-smelling and cloudy and later may become faeculent. Gas may be passed through the urethra as pneumaturia, giving a sensation of slight stopping and starting of the urinary stream. The patient may present with toxicity due to ascending urinary infection and septicaemia. Blood cultures are taken and urine submitted for microscopy and culture. A demonstration of the fistulous tract by contrast radiology is necessary and this usually requires a high pressure system, such as barium enema or a micturating cystogram, but even then the fistula may not be demonstrated. Cystoscopy reveals a severe cystitis with reddened oedematous mucosa occasionally through which gas may be seen to pass into the bladder on suprapubic pressure.

Faecal discharge from the vagina is diagnostic of a colo- or rectovaginal fistula. This is best demonstrated by a barium enema. It is often difficult to visualize the actual fistulous tract on speculum inspection of the vagina, the most common finding being an area of raised, intensely inflamed vaginal lining and local tenderness.

Treatment of colovesical fistula is surgical with resection of the bowel and closure of the bladder wall in two layers with absorbable sutures. If the fistula is due to diverticular disease, adequate resection well back to normal bowel is necessary. This often entails full mobilization of left colon and splenic flexure with anastomosis between transverse colon and rectum and a proximal defunctioning colostomy. If the condition of the patient is precarious, initial surgical treatment is by a proximal defunctioning colostomy with resection and closure as a staged procedure when the patient's condition improves.

A rectovaginal fistula that has resulted from radiotherapy for gynaecological malignancy may require treatment by separation of two connecting organs by surgery and a living omental patch between them to obtain healing.

BIOLOGICAL REACTIONS TO FOREIGN BODIES AND IMPLANT MATERIALS

The effects of retained foreign bodies and intentional implants are dominated by the local connective-tissue response and in the case of implants within the vascular tree by complex phenomena connected with foreign-surface induced thrombogenesis and mechanical haemolysis. However, systemic effects resulting from the release of breakdown products of material are possible and may affect organ function distant from the implant site although in clinical practice, this systemic response to implants has not been a significant problem.

Although neoplastic change following implantation of foreign body material in the human has not been reported, tumours have been produced in animals after injection of metallic powder and salts (cobalt powder, metallic nickel, lead salts, etc.) or insertion of polymeric materials (cellophane, phenolformaldehyde films and discs). On the basis of the experimental data available, the induction of tumour formation in man would have to exceed 20 years and, therefore, the malignant potential of the various polymeric implants in clinical use may not yet have been realized. The majority of the experimental neoplasms produced in this way have been fibrosarcomas.

Local Response to Implanted Materials and Foreign Bodies

The initial response is an acute inflammatory reaction of varying severity with the accumulation of polymorphs and subsequently macrophages in the vicinity of the implant. If the material is chemically and physically inert, the connective-tissue response may differ little from the normal postoperative fibrosis, the end result being the formation of a fibrous tissue capsule around the implant so that the material becomes isolated and virtually extracorporeal.

A granulomatous reaction with the formation of granulation tissue containing macrophages and multinucleate giant cells of the foreign body type is evoked by more irritant implants and foreign bodies (wood, silicates, retained gauze swabs). This often proceeds to abscess formation, sterile or otherwise, and will persist until either the material is extruded or is slowly degraded by proteolytic enzymes released into the abscess cavity which may eventually calcify.

Finally, necrosis of the adjacent tissue is the response evoked by implants or foreign bodies which are chemically, mechanically or thermally active.

The factors which affect the tissue response to implants, apart from their chemical and physical characteristics, include mechanical instability of the implant and infection. Relative movement between the implant and adjacent tissue causes repeated trauma and determines the disposition of the fibrous tissue formation. Infection is the most important complication in clinical implant surgery. It may be difficult to dissociate the effects of low-grade infection from those due to the prosthetic material itself. Whilst there is good evidence that the pathogenicity of bacteria is increased by the presence of a foreign body, and overt infections, e.g. grafts and around metal prostheses are extremely difficult to eradicate and often necessitate removal of the implant, there is insufficient evidence for the commonly held view that wounds containing non-living foreign bodies are more susceptible to infection. Certainly, skin sutures used for the approximation of skin edges appear to carry a higher risk of infection than sutureless closure and this effect is related more to the material characteristics than the physical structure of the suture itself. Moreover, certain implant procedures are attended by a higher risk of sepsis, e.g. total hip replacement, prosthetic mitral valve replacement and silicone lined shunt in the treatment of hydrocephalus, etc. However, special factors such as old age, poor general condition or diminished resistance to infection may contribute to the infection rate in these patients.

In general, metal and alloys are more reactive than polymer-based materials because of the induction of electrochemical processes. Corrosion causes a slow solution of the material. Metal corrosion which affects stainless steel results in the formation of corrosive products. Both processes result in the intracellular and extracellular accumulation of steel particles, fibrous reaction and a chronic inflammatory cell infiltrate.

Silicone-based implant materials can elicit four types of tissue response: toxic, degradable, 'inert' and bioactive responses. Bioactive silicates elicit a specific prolonged response by means of a controlled surface reaction. These can be used to bond to soft tissues, collagen and bone. So far limitation of their usefulness has been due to their poor mechanical strength which does not withstand weight bearing. They are, however, already available as middle ear devices, dental root replacements and for faciomaxillary augmentation.

The physical form of an implant influences the intensity of the reaction. For every material that has been studied, the tissue reaction has been reported to be more pronounced when the material was implanted in a particulate form, probably because this results in a vast increase in the surface of the material. Within normal limits the quality of surface finish has little effect on the tissue reaction but the response is modified by the porosity of the implant surface.

Polymeric Materials

The tissue reaction to polymeric materials is complex and difficult to evaluate, as apart from the chemical formulation, it is affected by the associated impurities (residual monomer, additives, catalysts) and the physical form (liquid, solid, porous and particulate) of the implant and the site of implantation. In addition, there are significant species differences, and, therefore, the results of animal experimentation are not invariably applicable to man.

The available literature on the biocompatability of various polymeric metals is both extensive and difficult to interpret. Only those compounds which are in current established clinical usage will be discussed in this chapter.

The *polyamides* are better known by the generic name Nylon. All these polymers are susceptible to *in vivo* degradation by slow hydrolysis and for this reason are no longer used for long-term implantation. They excite a moderate to severe fibroblastic reaction with giant-cell formation. Monofilament nylon is still popular with many surgeons for closure of operative wounds and repair of hernias.

Polypropylene, which is a member of the polyolefins, is not biodegradable and is relatively inert. When implanted it becomes encapsulated by mature fibrous tissue without any chronic round-cell infiltrates and giant cells. It is used for prosthetic heart valves, arthroplasties and as a suture material, especially in vascular surgery, where its low coefficient of friction allows it to glide through the tissue with minimum trauma.

Ivalon (polyvinyl alcohol) sponge excites a very severe vascular fibroblastic reaction with giant-cell formation and leads to intense fibrosis and calcification. The material is used surgically in repair of rectal prolapse to achieve fixation of the mobilized rectum to the sacral concavity.

Teflon (Dacron, Fluon) is polytetrafluoroethylene (PTFE). In its expanded form it is also marketed as Goretex. This polymer is regarded as one of the most tissue-compatible of all the biomaterials currently available for implantation purposes. PTFE does not absorb water and is not biodegradable. It is the standard material used in the knitted, woven and velour forms for synthetic vascular prostheses. Although PTFE has a low coefficient of friction, it wears badly when subjected to repeated physical stress and undergoes particulate fragmentation, thus leading to a pronounced tissue reaction which is not encountered with the solid material. For this reason it is no longer used in joint replacement surgery. The initial response to implanted PTFE consists of a minimal chronic round-cell infiltrate. This is followed by a smooth tough encapsulation.

The changes following the insertion of a vascular prosthesis commence with the deposition of fibrin on the inner lining and interstices of the graft. A layer of fibroblasts subsequently covers the inner surface following absorption of the fibrin coating. In its turn the fibroblastic layer becomes covered by new endothelium (neo-intima). In the human a cellular layer of fibrin persists deep to the fibroblastic zone. There is evidence that the cells which accumulate in the graft are derived from three sources: lateral spread from the cut vessel ends, ingrowth from surrounding tissue and deposition from the circulating blood. This neo-intima still has a predisposition to a platelet adhesion and blood clot formation within the vascular prosthesis, necessitating in some patients long-term anticoagulation. Recent attempts to overcome this involve seeding the graft with endothelial cells grown in culture.

Polymethylmethacrylate (PMMA) is used extensively as an acrylic cement in joint replacement surgery. There is an exothermic reaction of polymerization and hardening of the cement which may damage adjacent tissues. Most damage occurs immediately. This can involve fat embolism, but late damage can occur from fibrous tissue reaction producing constriction and damage to organs and fibrous contraction around nervous tissue. At late follow-up methacrylate cement is frequently found covered with an amorphous and caseous looking debris when examined under the microscope. Although the cement is forced to go between the irregularities of the bone, it is this amorphous caseous debris which may allow a movement of the cemented object, eventually causing prosthetic loosening.

Medical grade *polymethylsiloxane* (silicone) is one of the most inert implantable materials when used in its polymerized solid state. It is encapsulated by a thin fibrous sheet which contains a few fibroblasts, a few myofibroblasts and occasional giant cells. The material has been used very extensively in medical practice for implantable tubes (shunts and stents) and space-occupying prostheses (mammary implants and skin expanders). Systemic dispersion of silicone particles is known to occur from aortic ball valves made of the material and from silicone tubing used in the roller pumps during dialysis for renal failure and during cardiopulmonary bypass perfusion. This can be minimized by correct roller pump setting. Long-term contamination may result in granuloma formation within the liver and silicone-containing lymphadenopathy has been reported draining from areas containing silicone finger joints. Substitution of the silicone products with plastic material does not appear to be a promising approach, as similar but more intensive macrophage uptake has been seen with these materials. A more intensive reaction is however elicited by the polydimethylsiloxane fluid which was at one time injected into the chest wall to give mammary enlargement. This resulted in intense fibrosis, round-cell infiltrate and cyst formation. This reaction was also associated with atrophy of fat, suggesting a possible chemical interaction with the adipose tissue cells. Modern mammary prostheses are composed of an inner silicone gel covered with a thin layer of the polymerized silicone elastomer to minimize the tissue reaction. However, encapsulation of these implants still can be a significant problem necessitating in some patients closed capsular disruption or open division of the capsule surrounding the implant. This problem may be reduced with the newer silicone elastomer envelopes which are being manufactured with very low bleed characteristics. This retains the much more active gel in the capsule even after capsular puncture. It is this leakage of the gel which is thought to be a potent source of the fibrous tissue formation and contraction.

Further Reading

Brennan S. S. and Leaper D. J. (1985) The effects of antiseptics on the healing wound: a study using the rabbit ear chamber. *Br. J. Surg.* **72,** 780–782.

Bundred N. J., Dixon J. M. J., Lumsden A. B. et al. (1985) Are the lesions of duct ectasia sterile? *Br. J. Surg.* **72,** 844–845.

Gerzof S. G. and Johnson W.C. (1984) Radiologic aspects of diagnosis and treatment of abdominal abscesses. *Surg. Clin. North Am.* **64,** 53–65.

Hendri L. L. and Wilson J. (1986) Biocompatiblity of silicones for medical use. In: Evered D. and O'Connor M. (ed.) *Silicone Biochemistry* (Ciba Foundation Symposium). Chichester, Wiley.

Negus D. (1985) Prevention and treatment of venous ulceration. *Ann. R. Coll. Surg. Engl.* **67**, 144–148.

Turner T. D., Schmidt R. J. and Harding K. G. (ed.) (1986) *Advances in Wound Management.* Chichester, Wiley Media Medica Publications.

Williams D. F. and Roaf R. (1973) *Implants in Surgery.* London, Saunders.

3 The Investigation and Treatment of Surgical Infections

M. R. B. Keighley and G. R. Giles

INTRODUCTION

The biological state of man is not a germ-free environment. Quite the contrary, it is a delicately precisioned symbiotic relationship between man, his systemic and local protective mechanisms, and his microbial flora. If any alteration occurs in this normal equilibrium between the resident microbes and the host, the bacteria's pathogenic potential is enhanced and an infection is frequently the end-result.

The surgeon has a special interest in microbiological science and its practical applications. Too often only scant attention is paid to the requirements of this area of medical science which is illogical when one considers that many surgical problems and failures are the result of infection and an inability to control this process. Diagnostic medical microbiology is especially important and is concerned with: (i) the isolation and identification of infectious agents; (ii) the demonstration of immune responses, e.g. antibody levels; and (iii) the rational selection of antimicrobials for treatment.

It is equally important to know when and how to take specimens, which laboratory investigations to request and how to interpret the results. It is not always recognized that the result of the laboratory tests depends upon the quality of the specimen, the care with which it is obtained, the timing and, of course, the skills of the laboratory. Not uncommonly the laboratory has little chance of performing satisfactory work because the clinician has not given due care when obtaining the specimen. Furthermore, in order to involve the laboratory staff directly, they should be informed in some detail of the clinical setting and the working diagnosis.

As already indicated, considerable discipline is required in the selection, timing and collection of specimens (*vide infra*), especially as many bacteria are susceptible to physical changes or contamination by chemicals. The methods used, must favour the survival of the micro-organism.

The most significant tests are obtained by study of sites normally sterile, e.g. blood, CSF, synovial and pleural cavities. However, much of the body has a normal flora and the investigation of a site for potential pathogens must take account of this normal flora of each particular site.

The type of specimen will depend upon the clinical problem and if a particular organ system seems to be involved, repeated specimens are taken from that source. In the absence of any clue, repeated samples of blood and urine are obtained and the other systems sequentially examined. In any case, certain points in the acquisition of the samples are paramount:

1. The sample should be relatively pure, i.e. sputum not saliva, from the depth of wound, not from the surface;
2. Sufficient quantity is needed;
3. Avoidance of contamination of the specimen;
4. Specimens obtained before starting antibiotics;
5. Once obtained, the specimens require immediate attention in the laboratory.

These points apply particularly to specimens aimed to culture bacteria and fungi, but viral specimens do not need to come from the main anatomical site involved in the infection. Viral specimens should be obtained as soon as possible after the onset of the illness and, if necessary, repeat nasopharyngeal washings or stool specimens can be obtained. Specimens for possible chlamydial infections need to be taken from the infection site. For both viral and chlamydial infections, the samples should be placed in antibiotic-containing transport media. Unlike bacterial specimens, it is possible to store these specimens in a refrigerator for 24 hours or even frozen at −70 °C.

ISOLATION OF THE INFECTIVE AGENTS

Specimen Staining

The demonstration of an infective agent normally requires that the infected material is both stained and cultured. Microscopic examination of both stained and unstained material is straightforward, quick and cost effective. It is less effective when the numbers of organisms are small and 10^5 organisms/ml are required if the organisms are to be demonstrated on a smear. Materials with 10^2–10^3 organisms/ml will culture on solid media but materials with fewer organisms require liquid media.

Gram staining is perhaps the most useful diagnostic test, for the Gram reaction not only indicates Gram-positive and negative organisms but also demonstrates morphology, e.g. cocci, rods, etc. Although no true diagnoses can be made, certain assumptions may be made if it is clinically imperative, e.g. clusters of Gram-positive cocci may well be staphylococci where Gram-positive chains of cocci are more likely to be streptococci.

Probably all specimens should be stained for mycobacteria by Ziehl–Neelsen stain or by the more sensitive auramine-rhodamine fluorescent stain. Monoclonal antibodies labelled with fluorescein and ELISA antigen recognition techniques are likely to be increasingly used and permit more specific identification especially with difficult organisms, e.g. *Bordetella pertussis* and *Legionella pneumonophila*. Special stains, e.g. methenamine silver nitrate and periodic acid–Schiff (PAS) are required for protozoa such as *Pneumocystis carinii* or for fungi. Where fungal infection is a real possibility, it may be better to examine unstained specimens or after treatment with 10% potassium hydroxide which lyses tissue around the hyphae and makes them more visible.

Culture of Specimens

The isolation and culture of clinical specimens requires conditions for aerobic, facultative anaerobic and anaerobic organisms and several culture media are used. Most aerobic and facultative anaerobes will grow on blood agar although organisms such as Neisseria and Haemophilus grow better on chocolate agar. Enteric organisms grow best on MacConkey agar or EMB agar. As many surgical infections result from intestinal contamination, it is particularly relevant to culture for true anaerobes in these patients. In addition to the media described above, an improved yield follows the use of high supplemented agar with haemin and vitamin K and other media containing antibiotics which inhibit the growth of enteric Gram-negative rods and facultative anaerobic or aerobic Gram-positive cocci. Broth cultures are commonly used to examine tissues with a low bacterial content and may give positive results when the solid media are negative. Many yeasts will grow on the media used to culture bacteria but most fungi grow better on specific media, e.g. Sabouraud's dextrose agar with antibiotics. Cultures for fungi are separately incubated at 25–30 °C and 37 °C.

Viruses are grown in cell culture systems depending upon the provisional diagnosis.

COLLECTION OF SPECIMENS

Wounds, Abscesses and Tissue Biopsies

Pus in closed and previously undrained soft-tissue abscesses frequently only contain one organism as the causative agent. Most commonly this will be a Staphyloccocus, Streptococcus or a coliform organism. However, when there are multiple abscesses, particularly in the abdominal cavity and when the abscesses are open to mucosal surfaces, there are usually multiple micro-organisms, of which it is impossible to know which are the more significant ones. There may be similar difficulties in complex abscesses in which the more superficial pus is cultured but deeper parts contain different bacteria and may have a different antibiotic specificity. In these deep lesions it is necessary to culture by both aerobic and anaerobic methods.

Fluids from the peritoneal cavity, the pleura or synovial spaces need to be collected with meticulous technique in order to avoid infection from the surrounding tissues. Considerable information may be obtained by microscopic smears and where fluid has been aspirated from a body cavity, this may be centrifuged to concentrate the organisms. Cell counts of fluid removed under these circumstances may be considered to be infected if the protein content exceeds 3 g/dl and the cell count exceeds 500–1000 cells/μl. A predominance of polymorph leucocytes in these fluids suggests an untreated pyogenic infection whereas if lymphocytes or monocytes predominate then some form of chronic infective agent should be suspected.

Gastrointestinal Tract Specimens

It is an established fact that many patients admitted as 'acute abdomens' to a surgical ward, are in fact suffering from acute infectious episodes. Faeces or rectal swabs must be cultured as they are the most readily available specimens, but inspection of the stool may reveal the presence of blood, mucus or parasites and microscopical examination may show the ova of parasites, protozoa or helminths. Specimens are suspended in both broth and on solid media. The laboratory will make special attempts to demonstrate Salmonella and Shigella infections on specific media. Campylobacter are best isolated on Campi-BAP or Skirrow's medium, cultured at a higher temperature of 40–42 °C. Many viruses are the cause of gastrointestinal illness, but it is often difficult to assign a particular significance to a viral agent cultured from the stool in view of the large numbers that are normally present.

Respiratory Secretions

Although most sore throats are due to viral infections, a small proportion in adults and a slightly larger proportion in children are associated with bacterial invasion of which the beta-haemolytic streptococcus, diphtheria and Candida are the most common. Throat swabs are taken from the tonsillar fossae and a separate one from the posterior pharyngeal wall. There is an abundance of normal flora and thus there is little advantage in performing microscopical examination of smears on the throat swabs. It is difficult to obtain specimens from the nasopharynx, which are not contaminated with normal flora. The middle ear is relatively inaccessible, although the ear drum may be punctured and allow aspiration of fluid. In half the cases of otitis media the fluid appears bacteriologically sterile.

The lower respiratory tract is studied by examining the sputum but there is almost inevitable contamination by the saliva and normal mouth flora. Thus it is important to obtain sputum which has truly been expectorated from the lower respiratory tract. This collection may be induced by the inhalation of saline aerosols or, alternatively, by tracheal intubation; bronchoscopic examination or even open lung biopsy is occasionally necessary in the diagnosis of *Pneumocystis carinii* infections or that due to the Legionella organisms. Culture media should be suitable for the growth of pneumococci, Klebsiella, fungi and mycobacteria. Most upper respiratory tract infections are the result of viruses and the diagnosis of a viral infection will depend largely on the rise of specific antibody titres occurring 2–3 weeks later rather than by a demonstration in culture of the infecting organism.

Urine

It is always worthwhile investigating the urine of patients with pyrexia of unknown origin or when there are specific symptoms relating to the genitourinary tract. The urine secreted by the kidney is sterile unless contamination has occurred. This is also true for bladder urine; however, the urethra does have a normal flora. Satisfactory specimens can be obtained from the male by the collection of a midstream specimen but careful precautions are necessary in the female if this technique is to be used and there is always liable to be contamination from the surrounding skin and labia. Occasionally it is necessary to catheterize the bladder for satisfactory specimens and still further the ureters may be cannulated separately in order to obtain separate specimens from right and left kidneys. Because the many micro-organisms multiply in the urine at room or body temperature, it is necessary that urine specimens are delivered to the laboratory very quickly. There is particular value in the examination by microscopy which may reveal the presence of leucocytes or epithelial cells and this is particularly relevant when the bacterial concentrations are greater than 10^5 organisms/ml. A Gram stain will commonly show that Gram-negative rods are present. Pus cells may be present without bacteria and may suggest that genitourinary tuberculosis is present. Urine is normally cultured on solid media although there are simplified methods available to estimate the number of bacteria in the urine, e.g. Agar-coated pipettes, dip-slide and Agar spoons. The presence of more than 10^5 bacteria/ml of the same type in two consecutive specimens establishes the diagnosis of active urinary tract infection in almost 100% of cases. If fewer than 10^4 colonies are present, this suggests that the organisms result from contamination. Intermediate counts indicate the need for further specimens.

Blood

This investigation is done too infrequently and should be performed repeatedly in all patients with pyrexia of unknown origin or high pyrexias in the postoperative state. It is an invaluable aid in determining the identity of organisms because it is rare for more than one organism to be cultured. Furthermore, the sensitivity of the identified organism to antibiotics should enable the most appropriate therapy to be given. It is vital that the technique for blood collection is rigidly disciplined and includes the most careful use of sterile equipment with aseptic techniques, the use of strict antiseptics on the skin which should not be touched except with sterile gloves and the collection of sufficient blood to add to both aerobic and anaerobic culture bottles. It is important that the bottles be taken to the laboratory promptly. Blood culture bottles are examined two to three times a day for the first two days and thereafter daily. Normally the cultures are kept and examined for one week. Most of the laboratories routinely Gram stain and subculture after the first 24 hours of incubation. In severe infections, particularly those taken from patients with shock, it is appropriate to culture two blood specimens taken 30 minutes apart obtained from different anatomical sites.

Micro-organisms growing in blood specimens do not necessarily reflect a septicaemic state and it is important to differentiate true positives from contaminated specimens. The growth of the same organism in repeated cultures is strongly indicative of a true finding whereas the growth of different organisms suggests contamination, though this is possible in rare instances following aortic replacement when an enterovascular fistula has developed. The growth of normal skin flora, e.g. *Staphylococcus epidermidis* or diphtheroids also suggests contamination, although this is still a significant finding in a patient with a vascular prosthesis. One common sense point is that the organism which is finally cultured should bear some clinical relevance to the suspected site, e.g. patients with intra-abdominal sepsis are more likely to have a Gram-negative organism circulating in the blood.

NORMAL HUMAN MICROBIOLOGICAL FLORA

The resident flora of the skin and mucous membranes is relatively consistent for the age of the host and always tends to re-establish, whereas transient flora consists of both pathogenic and non-pathogenic organisms which are resident only for a period of time (hours, days, weeks) but rarely gain significance while the normal residual flora is present. There are not normally resident viral populations.

The resident flora, whilst not essential, can aid the host, e.g. by synthesizing vitamin K in the gut. More importantly, the resident flora prevents the colonization of pathogenic bacteria, presumably by competition for nutrients, toxic or inhibitory products or competition for cellular receptors. When the normal flora is suppressed, the potential exists for the pathogenic bacteria to expand.

Normal flora can become pathogenic under certain circumstances, e.g. movement into a new environment: respiratory tract to bloodstream (*Streptococcus viridans*); intestinal tract to peritoneal cavity (Bacteroides sp.).

Skin

The resident flora of the skin is of particular interest to the practising surgeon. The predominant organisms are aerobic and non-aerobic Staphylococci, α-haemolytic Streptococci, Corynebacterium, Propionibacterium, enterococci, e.g. *Streptococcus faecalis,* fungi and yeasts in skin folds.

Upper Respiratory Tract

In the oropharynx, *Streptococcus viridans* is the dominant organism, together with diphtheroids and Staphylococci, but once the teeth erupt, bacteroides, anaerobic Vibrios, Fusobacterium and lactobacilli establish and yeasts and Actinomyces can be found on tonsillar tissue.

The predominant flora of the nose consists of corynebacteria, streptococci, *Staphylococcus aureus* and *Staphylococcus epidermidis.* The main organisms in the upper respiratory tract include: Haemophilus; pneumococci and haemolytic streptococci; Staphylococci, Neisseria, Mycoplasma and Bacteroides.

Gastrointestinal Tract

Although sterile at birth, the gastrointestinal tract becomes colonized with the effect of feeding. In breast-fed children, there is a predominance of lactobacilli but bottle-fed babies have a mixed flora. In the normal adult the acidity of the stomach reduces the bacterial content to 10^3–10^5 micro-organisms/gram of content and affords considerable protection against pathogens. As the pH of intestinal content increases, 10^5–10^8 bacteria/gram of content are found in the jejunum and 10^8–10^{10} bacteria/gram of colonic content. In the upper small bowel, lactobacilli and enterococci predominate but from the lower ileum onwards, the flora is faecal. By the sigmoid colon 10^{11} bacteria/gram of content are found and form 10–30% of the faecal weight. In the adult colon 95%+ are anaerobes (*Bacteroides fragilis*), Clostridia and anaerobic streptococci. The remaining fraction consists of Proteus, Pseudomonas, Lactobacilli and Candida.

Urogenital Tract

The vagina at birth is colonized by lactobacilli (Döderlein's bacilli) but a mixed flora takes over until puberty when the lactobacilli reappear in large numbers and contribute to the maintenance of an acid pH. If the lactobacilli are suppressed, yeasts and various bacteria are able to produce inflammation. After the menopause, the lactobacilli disappear and a mixed flora of Bacteroides sp., Clostridia, *Gardnerella vaginalis, Ureaplasma urealyticum.* The cervical mucus contains a lysozyme and has some antibacterial action. However, in many women, the vaginal introitus supports the flora of the perineum and perianal area and may lead to repeated attacks of cystitis.

The anterior urethra of both sexes may be contaminated by organisms similar to those found in the perineum. These organisms can be regularly cultured in the voided urine in numbers of 10^2–10^3/ml.

The Relevance of Normal Microbiological Flora

The culture of certain organisms such as Brucella, *Mycobacterium tuberculosis* and *Salmonella typhi* are always pathogenic. However, many infections are the result of action by micro-organisms normally present in the host. If the type of organism found in a body fluid is unusual, e.g. Gram-negative rods in sputum of a patient with pneumonia, then it may be assumed that this organism is responsible even though it may be represented elsewhere as normal flora. Conversely, in the culture of intra-abdominal abscesses, quite often multiple organisms are found and although these are consistent with normal flora and are reported as such, they are acting as pathogens.

Yeasts are often found in cultures of normal flora and are not usually relevant unless the patient is immunosuppressed or receiving parenteral nutritional therapy.

ANTIMICROBIAL THERAPY

The development of the modern era of antimicrobial therapy began with discovery of the sulphonamides and the discovery of penicillin made by Fleming in 1929 but applied practically by Chain and Florey in 1940. Initially, the antimicrobial agents were isolated from the media upon which moulds, e.g. streptomycin, had grown but many have since been synthesized.

Mechanisms of Action

Four areas of action are recognized:

1. Inhibition of Cell Wall Synthesis

The cell wall of a bacterium is a semirigid casing which permits a high internal osmotic pressure. Gram-positive micro-organisms have 3–5 times the osmotic pressure of Gram-negative bacteria. All penicillins and cephalosporins have a selective action on cell wall synthesis. These drugs are bound to receptors on the cell wall and lead to cell elongation or perforation. It is probable that the inhibitors of autolytic enzymes are inactivated and cell lysis results in isotonic environment. The lack of host toxicity of penicillins and cephalosporin is due to the absence of a cell wall with peptidoglycans in animals.

The resistance of a bacteria to penicillins and cephalosporins is partly dependent upon the organism's production of β-lactamases which open the β-lactam ring of these drugs. Other penicillins, e.g. cloxacillin, have an ability to bind these lactamases and protects the action of other penicillins, e.g. ampicillin, from destruction. Some bacteria have antibiotic resistance because of an absence of penicillin receptors or due to a failure of β-lactam to activate the autolytic enzymes.

Bacitracin, vancomycin and novobiocin act by interfering with the formation of the cell wall.

2. Inhibition of Protein Synthesis

The aminoglycosides (streptomycin, gentamicin, tobramycin, amikacin, kanamycin) probably bind to a specific receptor protein of the bacterial ribosome. In some manner this blocks the initiation of peptide formation and results in the break-up of the polysomes to monosomes incapable of protein synthesis.

The tetracyclines inhibit protein synthesis by blocking the introduction of amino acids into peptide chains. The action is inhibitory and reversible upon removal of the drug. Chloramphenicol attaches to a different point on the ribosome but also prevents peptide chain formation by inhibiting peptidyl transferase. Both tetracyclines and chloramphenicol are bacteriostatic. Erythromycin, lincomycin and clindamycin have the same basic action although at different molecular sites.

3. Inhibition of Nucleic Acid Synthesis

Some agents are effective inhibitors of DNA synthesis or act by binding to RNA polymerase, e.g. rifampicin. For many bacteria para-aminobenzoic acid (PABA) is an essential metabolite in the synthesis of folic acid. Sulphonamides can substitute for PABA and ultimately the failure of folic acid synthesis leads to a cessation of cell growth. Tubercle bacilli are not inhibited by sulphonamides but para-aminosalicylic acid is effective. Trimethoprim inhibits dihydrofolic acid reductase which normally produces tetrahydrofolate and ultimately DNA synthesis. It is thought that when trimethoprim and sulphonamides are used in combination, there is sequential inhibition of DNA production. Nalidixic acid, also inhibits DNA production.

4. Inhibition of Cell Membrane Function

If the functional integrity of the cell wall is disrupted, intracellular protein molecules are leaked and cell damage results. Polymyxins are the most active agents against the bacterial cell wall and polyene (amphotericin B) against fungi. Imidazoles act against fungi by inhibiting the synthesis of membrane lipids.

Laboratory Selection of Antimicrobial Agents

The selection of an antimicrobial agent can be sensibly made initially on the basis of the clinical site of infection. However, in hospitals, many bacteria show drug resistance which makes it imperative to measure antimicrobial sensitivity. Two principal methods are used:

1. Diffusion method. A filter paper disc containing measured quantities of drug is placed on a suitable medium heavily seeded with the micro-organism under investigation. After incubation, the diameter of the zone of inhibition is taken as evidence of drug action. The use of a disc for each antibiotic requires careful standardization of the test but permits a report of 'resistant' or 'susceptible'.
2. Dilution method. Graded concentrations of the antimicrobial agent are incorporated into fluid or solid culture media and these are subsequently inoculated with the test organism. Although this approach allows for a quantitative result to be reported, in terms of the concentrations required for inhibition, the scheme is very time consuming.

Clinical Selection of Antibiotics

In many situations, the relationship between the clinical syndrome and the aetiological organism is sufficiently constant to allow an intuitive selection of an antimicrobial agent while waiting for laboratory results. The best guess of the aetiological organism will depend upon the age of the patient, the site of infection, the place where the infection developed, e.g. home or hospital, and predisposing factors, e.g. concomitant steroids, immune deficiency. Once the organism is identified, an appropriate therapeutic regimen is more easily planned but because of bacterial resistance, adjustments may be required once the sensitivity is known.

There are indications for employing more than one antibiotic simultaneously. In the seriously ill patient, e.g. with Gram-negative septicaemia or bacterial meningitis in children, two or three organisms may be responsible. The use of two drugs may stop the emergence of resistant organisms, particularly in the treatment of tuberculosis. It may also be possible to achieve synergism of action between certain agents or to reduce individual doses and prevent toxicity, e.g. penicillins enhance the uptake of aminoglycosides by enterococci. One drug may affect the bacterial cell wall and allow the entry of the second drug, e.g. trimethoprim and polymyxins against *Serratia marcescens*. Alternatively, inactivation of one antimicrobial agent can be prevented by another, e.g. clavulanic acid can protect amoxycillin from β-lactamase inactivation.

A summary of some of the many available choices for antibiotic selection is summarized in *Table* 3.1. There is a constant development of new agents but many of the original drugs are still very effective, particularly when the infection has been acquired outside a hospital.

Estimation of Antimicrobial Concentration

The estimation of antibiotic concentrations in serum or other body fluids is required when using drugs of known toxicity, when the drug complications are dose-related and when a drug has a narrow therapeutic range. Occasionally, as in the treatment of bacterial endocarditis, drug levels are estimated at the peak levels and back-titrated against the involved organism to ensure a sufficiently bactericidal level.

The aminoglycosides and gentamicin, in particular, require careful assay for trough levels. Where renal impairment is present, the interval between doses must be lengthened. The therapeutic range of gentamicin is 2–10 μg/ml but it is likely that the peak concentrations are not responsible for the nephrotoxic and ototoxic side-effects; more likely it is the 'area under the curve' following the injection. A trough level of 2·5 μg/ml indicates the need for dose reduction; conversely, a peak level of less than 5 μg/ml and undetectable trough level suggests the need to increase the dose. Because of these difficulties, it is more convenient to use a normogram which utilizes the sex-related serum creatinine level for the patient's age and relates this to body weight to provide the initial loading dose and subsequent maintenance dose. These normograms are not applicable to patients in renal failure or children where repeated assays are required. Most assays titrate the antibiotic-containing fluid against known sensitive organisms in which the zone of inhibition is measured against a logarithmic graph of antibiotic standards.

Interaction of Antibiotics

Antimicrobial synergy may result from potentiation at a biochemical level, assistance to cellular penetration or protection. The most obvious biochemical synergy is shown by the combination of trimethoprim and sulphonamides or mecillinam and cephalexin. Antibiotics which act at the cell wall level (β-lactam) may interfere with the bacteria's ability to resist another drug's penetration, e.g. penicillin and aminoglycosides against *Streptococcus faecalis*. The protection against antibiotic degradation by β-lactamases has been attempted somewhat unsuccessfully by combining doxacillin and ampicillin against Gram-negative bacilli. More recently, broad-spectrum enzyme inhibitors have been developed e.g. clavulanic acid in combination with amoxycillin.

There are occasions when two antibiotics can interfere with each other's activity (*Table* 3.2). This phenomenon has been known for many years whereby a bacteriostatic agent such as tetracycline or chloramphenicol blocks the action of the β-lactam antibiotics whose affect depends upon cell growth. Occasionally two drugs interact chemically, e.g. carbenicillin and gentamicin in which the β-lactam ring of the penicillins and amino groups of the gentamicins combine so that both drugs are inactivated. Although this inactivation is unlikely to occur at therapeutic concentrations it does mean that the drugs should not be mixed in intravenous solutions.

Table 3.1 Choice of antimicrobial agents

	First choice	*Alternatives*
1. Aerobes		
a. Gram-positive		
Staphylococcus aureus	Cloxacillin	Cefamandole Cefazolin
Streptococcus pyogenes	Penicillin	Clindamycin Erythromycin
Streptococcus faecalis	Ampicillin	Co-trimoxazole Vancomycin
Streptococcus pneumoniae	Ampicillin	Co-trimoxazole
b. Gram-negative		
Escherichia coli	Gentamicin	Cefazolin Ampicillin
Proteus sp.	Gentamicin	Cefazolin Ticarcillin
Klebsiella sp.	Gentamicin	Cefazolin
Pseudomonas sp.	Tobramycin	Cefazolin Carbenicillin
Enterobacter sp.	Gentamicin	Cefazolin Amiracin
Acinetobacter sp.	Gentamicin	Cefazolin
Haemophilus influenzae	Ampicillin	Cefuroxime Tetracycline
2. Anaerobes		
a. Gram-positive		
Peptostreptococcus sp.	Penicillin Metronidazole	Cefamandole Clindamycin
Peptococcus sp.	Metronidazole	Clindamycin
Clostridium sp.	Penicillin	Metronidazole
b. Gram-negative		
Bacteroides fragilis	Metronidazole	Chloramphenicol Clindamycin
Bacteroides melaninogenicus	Penicillin	Cefamandole Metronidazole
Bifidobacterium sp.	Metronidazole	Clindamycin
Fusobacterium sp.	Penicillin	Tetracycline

Table 3.2 Antimicrobial incompatibilities

Main drug	*Incompatible drugs*
Penicillin	Tetracycline, vancomycin, amphotericin B
Chloramphenicol	Tetracycline, vancomycin, vitamin B complex, hydrocortisone
Gentamicin	Carbenicillin
Methicillin	Tetracyclines
Cephalothin	Erythromycin, tetracyclines

Side-effects of Antimicrobial Therapy

Approximately 5% of patients have an adverse reaction to antibiotic therapy, although most are of minor significance. Local irritation and phlebitis are common after intravenous infusion, and gastrointestinal disturbances found after oral administration. Many antibiotic doses contain large amounts of sodium and can result in congestive cardiac failure, particularly where renal function is poor. Both hepatic and renal dysfunction may permit accumulation of the antibiotics or their metabolites with toxic side-effects. Tetracyclines produce staining of immature bone and teeth and all these agents should be avoided under 8 years of age. Finally, some antibiotics induce hepatic enzyme activity, e.g. rifampicin and result in increased degradation of other agents to diminish their activity, e.g. contraceptive pills.

The β-lactam agents are most likely to produce hypersensitivity reactions. Structural similarities between different penicillins and also to the cephalosporins result in a degree of cross-sensitivity reactions between the two antibiotic groups. These hypersensitivity reactions can occur immediately after exposure with nausea, vomiting, urticaria or anaphylaxis. More commonly the reactions are delayed particularly after ampicillin and cephalosporins. Skin rashes may be of all types and are often of a generalized maculopapular type and associated with fever particularly after viral infections, e.g. cytomegalovirus, glandular fever. The sulphonamides, clindamycin and co-trimoxazole are commonly associated with skin eruptions which in its most severe form constitutes the Stevens–Johnson syndrome. Skin rashes after antimicrobial therapy are particularly common in patients with a history of eczema or asthma.

The suppression of normal gut flora can give rise to superinfection from candidiasis usually in the upper gastrointestinal tract but occasionally throughout the gut. Alternatively, an overgrowth of *Staphylococcus aureus* leads to severe enterocolitis, although this complication is rare in current practice. More recently, patients who develop diarrhoea after broad-spectrum antibiotics, are recognized to be suffering from toxins released by *Clostridium difficile*. Vancomycin is an appropriate agent once the toxins have been assayed in the faeces.

Neurotoxicity is commonly exhibited, after the poorly controlled administration of aminoglycosides, by diminished high-frequency hearing and vestibular damage demonstrated by an unsteady gait and nystagmus (*Table* 3.3). More serious encephalitic reactions are occasionally seen after high doses of penicillins, cephalosporins and nalixidic acid. Peripheral neuropathy may follow the use of isoniazid, chloramphenicol, metronidazole and nitrofurantoin. Aminoglycosides produce neuromuscular blockade by an anticholinesterase effect and by competing with calcium.

Table 3.3 Adverse interactions between antimicrobials and other drugs

Antibiotic	*Interfering drug*	*Result*
Cephaloridine	Diuretics	Nephrotoxicity
Gentamicin Tobramycin	Cephaloridine Diuretics	Nephrotoxicity
Chloramphenicol Sulphonamides	Phenytoin	Phenytoin toxicity
Griseofulvin	Warfarin	Decreased anticoagulation
Sulphonamides Chloramphenicol	Anticoagulants	Increased anticoagulation

Marrow toxicity is a well-known complication of sulphonamides and co-trimoxazole can induce megaloblastic damage. Chloramphenicol is notorious for producing occasional cases of aplastic anaemia (mortality rate 50%) or less serious cases of progressive anaemia, neutropenia and thrombocytopenia. Penicillins may occasionally produce (Coombs positive) haemolytic anaemia and selective white cell depression may be found with ampicillin, methicillin and carbenicillin, particularly where immunosuppressive drugs are also in use.

THERAPEUTIC AGENTS

Various forms of therapy may exert a profound influence on a patient's susceptibility to infection. Long- and short-term steroid therapy causes a depression of the inflammatory response. Immunosuppressive agents and cytotoxic drugs depress phagocytosis, impair the reticuloendothelial system and the bone marrow. Radiotherapy has a similar effect. In addition, by causing epithelial ulceration, it enhances the likelihood of bacterial invasion. Antimicrobial agents which suppress the normal bacterial flora may allow overgrowth of other organisms. This phenomenon is extremely dangerous in hospital if the common resident flora are susceptible and favours the selection of multiresistant bacteria which are often difficult to treat.

Additionally, there are several antimicrobial agents which not only affect the invading organism but can be detrimental to the host. Gentamicin, tetracycline, and sulphadiazine inhibit C_3 conversion, thus preventing bacteriolysis via the alternate pathway. Low-dose therapy with chloramphenicol can suppress the primary humoral immune response.

Antimicrobial Agents

Antimicrobial agents can be classified as antiseptics or antibiotics.

Antiseptics

Antiseptics are chemicals which are capable of killing free-living, commensal or pathogenic micro-organisms. They may be of natural, semi-synthetic or synthetic origin. Only a few chemicals, such as formaldehyde or halogens, are sporicidal and some agents, such as the mercury salts, are almost entirely bacteriostatic. Most antiseptics require a long exposure to be effective. Many antiseptics also have corrosive and staining properties.

The common antiseptics include heavy metals (mercury and silver salts), the halogens (hypochlorite and iodine compounds), oxidizing agents (hydrogen peroxide), ether, alcohols and dyes (aniline and acridine compounds). Also included in the antiseptics are the quaternary ammonium salts (of which cetrimide is the most important) together with phenols and cresols (which include hexachlorophene). The most important antiseptic in surgical practice is chlorhexidine, which is used extensively for sterilizing instruments and surgical skin preparation. The actions of various antiseptics are shown in *Table* 3.4.

Although antiseptics play an important part in skin preparation and in the management of burn patients, their value in established infection and as prophylaxis has been questioned.

Antibiotics (*Table* 3.1)

An antibiotic describes a chemical substance produced by one organism that in low concentrations is capable of inhibiting the growth of another micro-organism.

Table 3.4 Properties of commonly used antiseptics (antimicrobial agents) (from Gilmore et al., 1978)

Antiseptic	*Anti-bacterial spectrum*	*Sporicidal*	*Bactericidal*	*Acquired bacterial resistance*
Alcohols	Wide	No	Yes	No
Dyes	G+>G−	No	Slowly	Yes
Halogens	Complete	Yes	Yes	No
Formaldehyde	Complete	Yes	Yes	No
Metallic salts	G+>G−	No	Slowly	Yes
Phenols	Complete	No	In high conc.	Yes
Ammonium compounds	G+>G−	No	Yes	Yes
Chlorhexidine	G+>G−	No	Yes	Yes

G+ = Gram positive.
G− = Gram negative.

Penicillins

Penicillin is produced naturally by the mould penicillium. Many variants have been prepared by chemical modification of the penicillin nucleus resulting in a different spectrum of activity and susceptibility to penicillinase. Penicillinase is an enzyme which is produced by many micro-organisms, which destroys the β-lactam ring and abolishes the activity of the antibiotic. All penicillins have an allergic potential, causing skin rashes, urticaria and anaphylaxis. Benzylpenicillin is useful against streptococci, clostridia and oral anaerobes; most staphylococci are resistant to penicillin. Cloxacillin is useful for infections caused by *S. aureus*. Ampicillin is the antibiotic of choice for infections caused by *S. faecalis* but it has now become of little value in hospital practice against Gram-negative organisms because of a high incidence of resistance. Carbenicillin is similar to ampicillin but is much more active against *Pseudomonas aeruginosa*. All of the penicillins mentioned, apart from cloxacillin, are susceptible to β-lactamase and therefore have limited clinical value apart from streptococcal sepsis.

Cephalosporins

All cephalosporins except cefoxitin are semi-synthetic and are bactericidal. There are a large variety of different cephalosporins which differ in their antibacterial and pharmacokinetic properties. Most are effective against *S. aureus* and aerobic Gram-negative bacteria. Cefoxitin at high concentration is also effective against *Bacteroides fragilis*. Allergy is common to all compounds but nephrotoxicity is an important complication of cephaloridine, especially in patients receiving diuretics.

Aminoglycosides

The aminoglycosides include streptomycin, kanamycin, neomycin, tobramycin, gentamicin and amikacin. Streptomycin is rarely used other than for treatment of tuberculosis. Neomycin can only be taken by mouth and although it has been widely used in the past for bowel preparation this form of prophylaxis should be discontinued in favour of short-term systemic agents. Of the remaining compounds, gentamicin remains the treatment of choice for most aerobic Gram-negative infections with the exception of tobramycin which is more effective against *Pseudomonas aeruginosa*. Amikacin should be reserved for gentamicin-resistant Gram-negative bacilli.

Tetracyclines

These are only bacteriostatic and although they have a wide range of activity most tetracyclines are now unsuitable for prophylaxis and therapy because of the high frequency of bacterial resistance. Large doses of tetracycline can produce fatal hepatic disease which is often seen in late pregnancy or in other individuals receiving in excess of 3 g/day.

Clindamycin

Clindamycin is a synthetic derivative of lincomycin and is extremely effective against staphylococci, streptococci and bacteroides. However, in view of the high incidence of pseudomembranous colitis following the use of this agent in gastrointestinal surgery its routine use can no longer be recommended.

Metronidazole

This trichomonacide has now become the drug of choice for anaerobic infection. Metronidazole is effective for treatment and prevention of large bowel and gynaecological sepsis. Metronidazole is also a radio-sensitizing agent. Toxicity is rare but side-effects, such as rashes and nausea, may occur.

Co-trimoxazole

This antibiotic is a mixture of trimethoprim and sulphamethoxazole. It is effective against a wide range of aerobic and anaerobic species and is valuable for treatment of urinary infections. Toxicity includes rashes and neutropenia.

Chloramphenicol

This antibiotic is valuable when other antibiotics have failed. Resistance of Gram-negative bacteria is low because the drug is rarely used on account of the occasional reports of fatal bone marrow depression.

Antiviral Therapy

The significance of viral infections in the surgical patient is underestimated. Unexplained pyrexial illnesses, postoperative atypical pneumonias, herpes labialis and shingles are all common clinical manifestations. Improved diagnoses may be made by checking body fluids for virus and looking in the serum for a raised or rising titre of antibodies against common viruses: Herpes species, cytomegalic, influenza, etc. As yet there are only a limited number of antiviral agents available but many others will be developed over the next years. *Table* 3.5 summarizes the indications for use and it should be stressed that these agents are especially valuable in the immunocompromised patient.

Table 3.5 Antiviral agents

Drug	*Indication*
Idoxuridine (topic)	Herpetic skin lesions
Vidarabine (Ara-C)	Herpetic skin lesion Herpes zoster Herpes encephalitis
Acyclovir	Herpetic skin lesions Herpes encephalitis Herpes zoster
Amantidine	Influenza A Prophylaxis and treatment

ESTABLISHED INFECTION

Principles of Surgical Therapy

Treatment of established infection relies upon attention to surgical principles combined with intelligent use of antimicrobial therapy. The principles of surgical management are drainage of pus and débridement with secondary suture of heavily contaminated wounds. Antimicrobial agents cannot be expected to succeed alone if there is dead tissue and a collection of pus within a walled-off cavity. By contrast, surgical drainage is rarely necessary if infection is not associated with pus, as in leucopenic patients, in patients with superficial cellulitis or in patients with an inflamed segment of acute diverticular disease without abscess.

Examples of Established Infection

Staphylococcal Sepsis

S. aureus is responsible for a variety of clinical syndromes including furuncle, carbuncle, acute infections of the hand, such as paronychia, infected web space, and suppurative tenosynovitis. *S. aureus* remains the most frequent isolate from subcutaneous abscess and acute osteomyelitis. In most cases the source of organism is haematogenous but localization may be related to local trauma or a penetrating wound. The principles of treatment are drainage of pus and early antibiotic therapy. Cloxacillin is the antibiotic of choice for most of these syndromes, but the antibiotic may have to be changed, as in osteomyelitis, or if another organism such as streptococcus is isolated. Early antibiotic therapy for osteomyelitis and superficial infections may render surgical drainage unnecessary. If the infection has proceeded to formation of pus, drainage is mandatory. There is evidence to support the concept of early drainage and immediate primary skin closure, if the patient has already received high doses of an appropriate antimicrobial.

Streptococcal Sepsis

It is remarkable how the incidence of acute streptococcal infection has declined. The most important syndromes are cellulitis and erysipelas. Both conditions are due to a spreading subcutaneous infection associated with rapid lymphangitis and septicaemia in the absence of pus formation. Localization by natural defences is inefficient and is dependent upon anatomical tissue planes. There is a rapidly expanding, diffuse, red swelling. Special examples include orbital cellulitis, Ludwig's angina and pelvic cellulitis. There may be localized complications due to expanding tissue planes or venous thrombosis. Unlike staphylococcal sepsis, drainage is rarely necessary provided high doses of penicillin are used.

Sepsis in Open Wounds

Open wounds are invariably colonized by bacteria and infection is common if there is extensive necrosis of muscle following road accidents or agricultural injury. Occasionally subcutaneous infection in wounds may be complicated by gas gangrene or tetanus. The principal infecting organisms are *S. aureus* and those that comprise the coliforms. The management of traumatic wounds involves complete excision of all devitalized tissues and delayed skin closure. These principles have had to be relearned during the early years of almost all armed combat. Wounds must be thoroughly cleaned and fasciotomy may also be required. Primary wound closure should never be performed in the presence of foreign material or devitalized tissues.

However, investigators have found through the technique of bacterial quantification that successful wound closure can be achieved more rapidly when the bacterial level in the wound is 10^5 or fewer organisms/gram of tissue. Experimentally the optimal time for closure has been shown to be on or after the fourth post-wounding day. However, when acute traumatic wounds are closed primarily within the first 3 hours post-injury one can expect 0% infection rate. It has been documented that these wounds have bacterial counts between $\leqslant 10^2$ and $\leqslant 10^5$. Wounds received after 5 hours had bacterial counts $>10^5$, all presenting with post-traumatic wound infections if closed primarily. Therefore the 'golden period' can be equated to the time it takes for the bacteria to reach a level of 10^5/gram of tissue. Appropriate antibacterial therapy is recommended when it is especially effective against the aetiological agent of the infection. When traumatic wounds are properly managed and all surface contamination eliminated, the causative agent of infection will be, in all probability, a single species.

Tetanus

Tetanus is a potentially lethal complication of infected dirty wounds. It is caused by the neurotoxin of *Clostridium tetani* which acts upon the nerve cells of the cerebrospinal axis and also paralyses the cholinergic motor fibres to the eye. Most susceptible are the nerves of the medulla oblongata. A more in-depth discussion of this disease can be found in Chapter 5.

Gas Gangrene

The term 'gas gangrene' implies synergistic gangrene from gas-forming bacteria. However, most clinicians associate the term specifically with *Clostridium perfringens* (*welchii*) infection. Although *Cl. perfringens* is an important cause of synergistic gangrene, it is by no means the only bacterium responsible. Other species include certain gas-forming coliforms: peptostreptococci, fusobacteria, bifidobacteria, bacteroides and other clostridia. Gas gangrene and the anaerobic infections are discussed in Chapter 5.

Urinary Tract Sepsis

Repeated urinary infections, particularly in the male subject, usually indicate an anatomical or physiological abnormality in the urinary tract. Stenosis at the pelvi-ureteric junction, at the ureteric orifice, the bladder neck or the urethra are the most common abnormalities and often require surgical correction. Vesico-ureteric reflux or neuro-muscular abnormalities at the pelvi-ureteric junction account for physiological stasis with bacterial overgrowth. The most frequent pathogens are *E. coli*, Klebsiella sp., *Streptococcus faecalis*, *Staphylococcus aureus*, Proteus sp., and *Pseudomonas aeruginosa*. If the urinary infection is associated with pyelonephritis, an antibiotic which provides high blood levels, such as co-trimoxazole, ampicillin, or one of the cephalosporins would be advised. For bacteriuria it would be more advisable to use a urinary antiseptic, such as nalidixic acid or nitrofurantoin.

Pelvic Inflammatory Disease

Pelvic sepsis usually presents as an unexplained fever, abdominal pain, urinary frequency and/or vaginal discharge. There is an expanding cellulitis in the parametrium which may later form a tubo-ovarian pelvic abscess. The condition is often secondary to salpingitis and may be complicated by septic thrombophlebitis and septicaemia. The organisms usually responsible are: coliforms and anaerobic species or *Neisseria gonorrhoeae*. Treatment should be by antimicrobials using metronidazole and a cephalosporin. Operation is usually only required for drainage of pus. The subject is further discussed in Chapter 79.

Abdominal Sepsis

Many aspects of abdominal sepsis, such as acute cholecystitis, acute appendicitis, acute diverticular disease and the complications of granulomatous bowel disease, will be dealt with elsewhere in this book. Abdominal sepsis may also present with unexplained septicaemia or pyrexia of unknown origin. Careful clinical and radiological investigation will then be necessary to exclude a pelvic abscess, and infected abdominal viscus or intra-abdominal abscess. The latter include subhepatic and subphrenic abscesses which may complicate a silent perforation of an abdominal viscus, psoas abscess as a complication of colonic carcinoma or ileocaecal Crohn's disease and pericolic abscess resulting from diverticular disease or carcinoma. The abscess will require surgical drainage and concurrent or subsequent intestinal resection under appropriate antibiotic cover in patients with inflammatory bowel disease or carcinoma.

Septicaemic Shock

Profound circulatory collapse, oliguria, acidosis, fever and rigors are some of the common clinical manifestations of septicaemic shock. This clinical picture may be due to circulating endotoxins which are the breakdown products of Gram-negative bacterial cell wall. The presence of circulating endotoxin may be detected by the limulus lysate test, but there are difficulties in standardizing this investigation. Endotoxaemia implies the rapid destruction of bacteria by the body's own immune defence mechanisms.

The value of steroids for treatment of septic shock is doubtful. Special attention should be paid to the correction of fluid and electrolyte balance, renal function and some patients will also require assisted ventilation. High doses of a bactericidal antibiotic effective against the likely infecting organisms should be given immediately. However, caution should be exercised when dealing with Gram-negative organisms since rapid destruction of these agents could result in endotoxic shock and death.

Septicaemia, not attended by acidosis or circulatory changes, implies the rapid proliferation of bacteria in the circulation, whereas bacteraemia is the mere presence of bacteria in the circulation not exceeding counts greater than 10^3/ml of blood. An interesting note is that the incidence of septicaemia increases as the quantitative bacteriology of the wound increases. In both of these conditions it is important to try to identify the source of sepsis by careful clinical, radiological and biochemical study. Blood cultures should be performed before antibiotics are started. If clinical examination suggests a respiratory or urinary tract infection, antibiotics should be started and then changed according to sputum or urine cultures. If the patient has obstructive jaundice, early biliary decompression under antibiotic cover may be necessary if the current chemotherapy alone has failed. When there is localized intra-abdominal sepsis this will require antibiotics and drainage. If the patient has a limp or complains of bone pain, an acute septic arthritis or osteomyelitis should be suspected and treated accordingly.

ACQUIRED INFECTION

Principles of Surgical Therapy

Under no circumstances should antimicrobial prophylaxis be considered a substitute for good surgical technique. There is an increased risk of surgical sepsis following prolonged operations, if there has been inadequate haemostasis, if non-degradable materials, such as sutures, are left in the wound, if operation has compromised blood supply to an organ and whenever open drains are used. Whenever a hollow viscus containing bacteria, such as the colon, is opened, there is greater risk of infection. Under these circumstances the operation site should be isolated from the rest of the abdominal cavity with packs, the bowel should have been cleared of all visible intracolonic faecal material by efficient preoperative bowel preparation and wound closure should only be performed after changing into new gloves and gowns. Whenever possible closed suction drains should be used. If open drains are necessary they must be brought out through a separate incision. There is no evidence that wound protection reduces the incidence of postoperative sepsis. Antimicrobial irrigation may be beneficial in this instance. If there is obvious operative contamination of an abdominal wound, the skin and subcutaneous tissue should be left opened and allowed to heal by secondary intention.

Principles of Hospital Routine

Audit is an important means of maintaining a low incidence of postsurgical infection. Audit will improve surgical discipline and also provide early recognition of an outbreak of sepsis. If there is an epidemic of staphylococcal sepsis, elective operations should be stopped. Nasal swabs should be obtained from patients and staff to detect carriers. Carriers should be treated and not allowed to return for duty until this organism has been eliminated. Patients with sepsis should also be isolated and discharged as soon as possible.

Hygiene in the ward and in theatre is also important. Hand washing will reduce the risk of cross-infection in the ward. Severely infected cases should be isolated and barrier nursed. The patient should be adequately prepared for operation and shaving is best avoided where possible. Skin preparation should be with solutions of 0·5% chlorhexidine in 70% alcohol or 1% povidone-iodine. Surgeons should scrub with detergent solutions of chlorhexidine or iodine. Hats and masks should be worn to reduce dispersal of organisms but more important are measures to minimize the amount of movement and talking in theatre. The theatres should be equipped with a properly filtered air supply using 2 μm filters and the pressure should be greater than surrounding parts. The ventilation should achieve 300 changes of air per hour and a laminar air flow has been advised for orthopaedic implant surgery. Adequacy of instrument sterilization by autoclave, antiseptics or ethylene oxide should be checked periodically.

Principles of Antimicrobial Prophylaxis

The principle of antimicrobial prophylaxis is that a high dose of the antibiotic should be present in the tissues and circulation at the time at which the bacteria will be inoculated into the operation site. The antibiotic should be bactericidal and can be given in very large doses, preferably by the intravenous route. The first dose should be given 2–4 hours before the operation. A second and third dose should then be given at intervals after the operation. It is quite unnecessary to prolong the antibiotic therapy. Systemic administration provides predictable serum levels and should be used in preference to topical or oral agents. Furthermore, systemic prophylaxis will minimize the risk of bacterial resistance, superinfection and antibiotic-associated colitis.

However, the route and sequence of administration should be examined, so that adequate antimicrobial levels can be achieved both in the circulation and in the involved tissue. Experimental studies have shown that an intravenous push of ampicillin achieves levels four times greater than with intravenous infusion. Yet wound fluid levels were higher when the drug was given intramuscularly even after 6 hours. Wound fluid levels of gentamicin were equal when administered either by intramuscular injection or intravenous push.

Prevention of Hospital Acquired Infection (*Table* 3.6)

Burn Wound Sepsis

A more in-depth discussion of this subject is found in Chapter 21. All local cutaneous defences against bacterial invasion are virtually destroyed in this type of injury. Coupled with the destruction of the first line of defence to bacterial invasion are modifications in the systemic response such as hypovolaemia and an altered immune mechanism. Hence septicaemia and infection of the burned area are potentially lethal complications of even partial thickness burns. Sepsis is also frequently responsible for delayed healing and unsuccessful skin grafting.

β-haemolytic streptococcus is the most common transient flora and is the initial threat to the burns patient. Therefore penicillin is used prophylactically for 72 hours. A decrease in cross-contamination can be achieved by the use of single bedded units, plenum ventilation, barrier nursing, early excision and grafting and topical antiseptic agents. Autocontamination remains difficult to control. Rates of 14% are in evidence after 2 weeks and are as high as 76% after 4 weeks due to endogenous organisms.

Topical antimicrobials are used extensively to control burn wound sepsis. Some of these include: silver sulfadiazine, silver nitrate, mafenide acetate, povidone-iodine ointment and gentamicin sulphate cream. Polyvalent pseudomonas vaccine is also effective in reducing mortality from burn sepsis.

Intravenous Catheter Sepsis

Septic complications of intravenous therapy include superficial thrombophlebitis and septicaemia. Septicaemia is most frequent in patients with centrally placed catheters used for nutritional therapy or manometry. Staphylococci and occasionally coliforms are the predominant bacteria isolated from septicaemic patients and fungi are also of clinical importance. Intravenous catheter sepsis may be due to exogenous bacteria introduced into the intravenous solution, the giving set or the skin puncture site, because of breaks in aseptic techniques. However, it most likely occurs from the latter as a direct result of the endogenous (resident or transient) microflora being introduced during catheter insertion. Occasionally, a contamination may be due to episodes of bacteraemia from a distant site, such as an intra-abdominal abscess. Prevention of catheter sepsis is achieved by avoiding the intravenous route whenever nutrition can be administered into the intestinal tract. When parenteral nutrition is necessary it should be performed by a team of medical, nursing and pharmacy personnel. Electrolytes, vitamins and drugs should never be added to solutions outside the sterile environment of a laminar flow hood in the pharmacy department. Skin dressings and giving sets should be changed regularly. There is no place for antibiotic prophylaxis and prolonged exposure to antimicrobials increases the risk of fungal septicaemia.

Table 3.6 Policy of short-term antibiotic prophylaxis

Burns	Penicillin initial 72 hours
Intravenous catheter	None
Implant surgery	Cloxacillin
Urinary catheter	None
Gastrointestinal	
Gastric*	Cephazolin for carcinoma and reconstructive gastric surgery and bleeding
Biliary*	Cephazolin for acute biliary surgery, choledocholithiasis and repeat operations
Appendicectomy	Metronidazole
Colorectal	Metronidazole and gentamicin
Gynaecology*	Cephalosporin or metronidazole for hysterectomy only

*=Selective.

Infected Implants

The incidence of infection after inserting prosthetic implants at operation is low but the consequences are disastrous. Infection of prosthetic heart valves carries a mortality rate of over 60%; there is a high mortality and amputation rate if a Dacron graft becomes infected after peripheral vascular surgery. Chronic osteomyelitis may occur following prosthetic joint replacement and meningitis or ventriculitis is also a hazard of neurosurgical shunts. In all of these circumstances, the principal pathogen is *Staphylococcus aureus*. Prevention should rely upon reducing airborne contamination at operation by facilities to achieve ultraclean air, use of impervious clothing and skin preparation. In view of the consequences of postoperative sepsis, short-term antibiotic prophylaxis would also be advised.

Urinary Catheter Sepsis

Catheter-acquired infections are common; bacteriuria is almost universal in patients with prolonged bladder drainage. The common urinary isolates are *E. coli*, *S. faecalis*, and Pseudomonas sp. There is no justification for using antibiotics to prevent urinary infection in catheterized patients. Prevention should rely upon a strict aseptic technique for the introduction and care of catheters, use of a closed system of drainage and avoidance of clot retention in postoperative patients by encouraging a rapid diuresis.

Gynaecological Sepsis

In gynaecological surgery pelvic sepsis and wound infection are only a problem after vaginal or abdominal hysterectomy and under these circumstances short-term cephalosporins and metronidazole have been shown to reduce morbidity. The aetiological agents responsible for sepsis are *E. coli*, *Bacteroides fragilis* and Peptostreptococcus sp.

Postoperative Respiratory Infections

Respiratory complications occur frequently after upper abdominal or thoracic procedures but pathogenic bacteria are isolated from less than a third of patients with productive cough, fever and radiological signs of infection. The principal bacteria are haemophilus sp., *S. pneumoniae*, *Klebsiella pneumoniae* and occasionally *Pseudomonas aeruginosa*. Patients who are particularly at risk are those with chronic airways disease, the smokers and the obese. There is little, if any, evidence that prophylactic antibiotics prevent chest infection and their use should be reserved for patients with severe respiratory disease or patients with infected sputum.

On the other hand, it is much more desirable to cancel elective operations in patients with respiratory infection and to insist on vigorous physiotherapy and adequate postoperative analgesia in the remainder rather than rely on prophylactic antibiotics.

Abdominal Sepsis

Infection in the wound, septicaemia and abdominal or pelvic abscess are frequent complications of gastrointestinal operations. These complications usually occur as a result of bacteria being inoculated into the operation site from the intestinal tract during the surgical procedure (primary sepsis). Sepsis may also result from intestinal contamination following anastomotic dehiscence (secondary sepsis). Primary sepsis may be prevented by prophylactic antibiotics, whereas secondary sepsis complicating anastomotic breakdown represents inadequate surgical technique for which antibiotic prophylaxis is unlikely to be of value. The organisms responsible for infection vary with the site of operation and the pathology.

Gastric Surgery

In gastric surgery endogenous sepsis is common following operations for gastric carcinoma, reconstructions for bile vomiting and emergency surgery for bleeding, whereas sepsis is uncommon in patients requiring operation for duodenal ulcer, particularly if the intestinal tract has not been opened as in highly selective vagotomy. The bacterial colonization of the stomach is dependent upon pH and the most frequent pathogens are streptococci, *E. coli*, staphylococci as well as *Bacteroides oralis* and Peptostreptococcus sp. A policy of selective antimicrobial prophylaxis with a cephalosporin can be based upon the pH of gastric aspirates. Under these circumstances, antibiotics would be advised only if the pH is greater than 4·0. Alternatively, gastric contents can be aspirated at preoperative endoscopy so that the choice of antibiotic as well as their need can be defined.

Biliary Surgery

Sepsis in biliary surgery is most common following emergency operation for acute cholecystitis and surgery for common bile duct stones or strictures. The most frequent pathogens are *E. coli* and Klebsiella sp. However, in one study, using quantitative bacteriological techniques, culturing both the gallbladder bile and the gallbladder wall, *S. aureus* was the most frequent organism isolated. *E. coli*, Klebsiella-enterobacter group and β-haemolytic streptococcus were isolated less frequently. Selective prophylactic antibiosis with a cephalosporin can be based upon clinical criteria or by the use of Gram-stained films of bile aspirated from the gallbladder at the very beginning of the operation. Cephalosporins are also advised to cover procedures like endoscopic retrograde cholangiopancreatography (ERCP) and percutaneous transhepatic cholangiography (PTC) where septicaemia is a recognized hazard.

Appendicectomy

Most patients requiring an appendicectomy have established infection in the abdomen before operation and under these circumstances the term prophylaxis is inappropriate. However, the risk of sepsis following appendicectomy is sufficiently high to justify a single dose of metronidazole per rectum for all patients and particularly when appendicectomy is performed in conjunction with biliary or gynaecological procedures.

Colorectal Surgery

The greatest risk of endogenous abdominal sepsis is amongst patients having emergency or elective colorectal operations. The principal pathogens are *Bacteroides fragilis* and *E. coli*. These bacteria are increased in number within the small bowel of patients with intestinal obstruction and Crohn's disease. However, if cultures are taken periodically throughout the surgical procedure one would find that after 2 hours, the isolation of anaerobes will be reduced from 95% to 5% due to the exposure of the bowel to atmospheric oxygen. Infection rate due to anaerobes in this type of surgical procedure is between 10 and 15%. On account of the high incidence of infection in patients with inflammatory bowel disease and colorectal carcinoma, prophylaxis would be advised irrespective of anatomical site of operation. There are three possible routes of antibiotic administration in colorectal surgery. Topical agents may be instilled into the wound but they are unlikely to prevent septicaemia or intra-abdominal abscess. Oral agents, such as metronidazole and neomycin, may be used with bowel preparation in an attempt to reduce the bacterial flora of the colon; however, they are ineffective in the presence of obstruction, they encourage bacterial resistance and are more likely to cause pseudomembranous colitis. For this reason short-term systemic antimicrobials should be advised, using metronidazole and an aminoglycoside in all patients requiring colorectal operations (*Table* 3.6).

Further Reading

Ad Hoc Committee of the Committee on Trauma, Division of Medical Sciences (1964) National Research Council Report: Postoperative wound infections: The influence of ultraviolet irradiation of the operating room and the influence of various other factors. *Ann. Surg.* 160 (Suppl. 1), 1–192.

Keighley M. R. B. and Burdon B. (1979) *Antimicrobial Prophylaxis in Surgery*. Tunbridge Wells, Pitman Medical.

Robson M. C., Krizek T. J. and Heggers J. P. (1973) Biology of surgical infection. In: *Current Problems in Surgery*, Chicago, Year Book Medical Publishers.

4 Parasitic Infestations of Surgical Importance

H. M. Gilles and A. Cuschieri

HYDATID DISEASE

This disease can be caused by any one of three species of the genus *Echinococcus—E. granulosus, E. multilocularis* and *E. oligaettas*. Since the epidemiological and pathological features of these three tapeworms are very similar, a detailed description of *E. granulosus* only is given here. Hydatid disease which is caused by the larval form of *E. granulosus*, has a cosmopolitan distribution, being particularly prevalent in the sheep- and cattle-raising areas of the world.

Parasitology

The adult echinococcus is a small tapeworm which inhabits chiefly the upper part of the small intestines of canines, especially dogs and wolves. When the ova, which are passed in the faeces, are swallowed by man or other intermediate hosts (e.g. sheep, cattle, horses, etc.) the enclosed embryo is liberated in the duodenum. It penetrates the intestinal mucosa, reaches the portal circulation, and is usually held up in the liver within 12 h to develop into a hydatid cyst. If the embryo passes the liver filter, it enters the general circulation, and thus reaches the lungs and other parts of the body. Two main varieties of cyst occur: the unilocular and the multilocular. The unilocular hydatid cyst (*Fig.* 4.1) develops a wall with two layers: an outer thick, laminated layer, and an inner (germinal) layer which is composed of a protoplasmic matrix containing many nuclei. Around the cyst there is a connective-tissue capsule formed by the tissues of the host. Bulb-like processes known as brood capsules arise from the germinal layer. The brood capsules undergo localized proliferation and invagination of their walls to form scolices (tapeworm heads). Each scolex is borne on a pedicle and has suckers and hooklets. Some of the brood capsules separate from the walls and settle to the bottom of the cyst as a fine granular sediment, 'hydatid sand'. As the hydatid cyst enlarges, invaginations of the wall may give rise to daughter cysts and from them grand-daughter cysts may arise in a similar manner. In some cases in which no effective encapsulation occurs, the daughter cysts develop as a result of evaginations of the cyst wall producing the multilocular or alveolar hydatid cyst. This variety of cyst is caused by *E. multilocularis*.

When the hydatid is eaten by definitive hosts (dogs, foxes, wolves etc.) the numerous larvae develop into sexually mature worms in a few weeks.

Dogs are usually affected when they eat the infected viscera of sheep or cattle (*Fig.* 4.2). Infected ova may live for weeks in shady environments but are quickly destroyed by sunlight and high temperatures. Man acquires hydatid disease when he swallows infected ova as a result of his close association with dogs. Although infection is usually acquired in childhood, clinical symptoms do not appear until adult life. The dog faeces contaminating fleeces of sheep can also be an indirect source of human infection. It has been shown that in Kenya hydatid cysts are present in more than 30% of cattle, sheep and goats, though the disease in man occurs

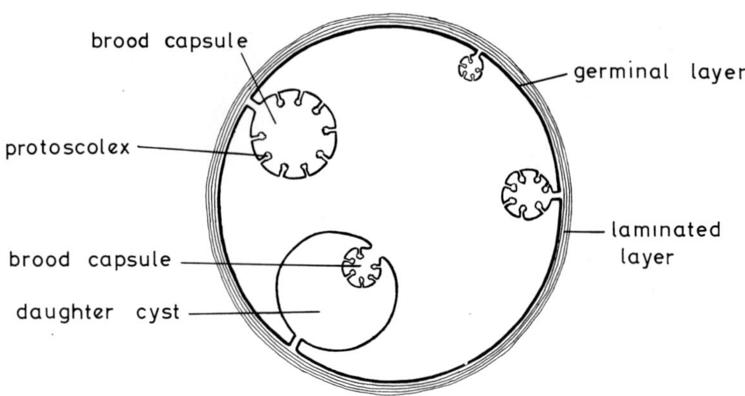

Fig. 4.1 Composition of a unilocular hydatid cyst.

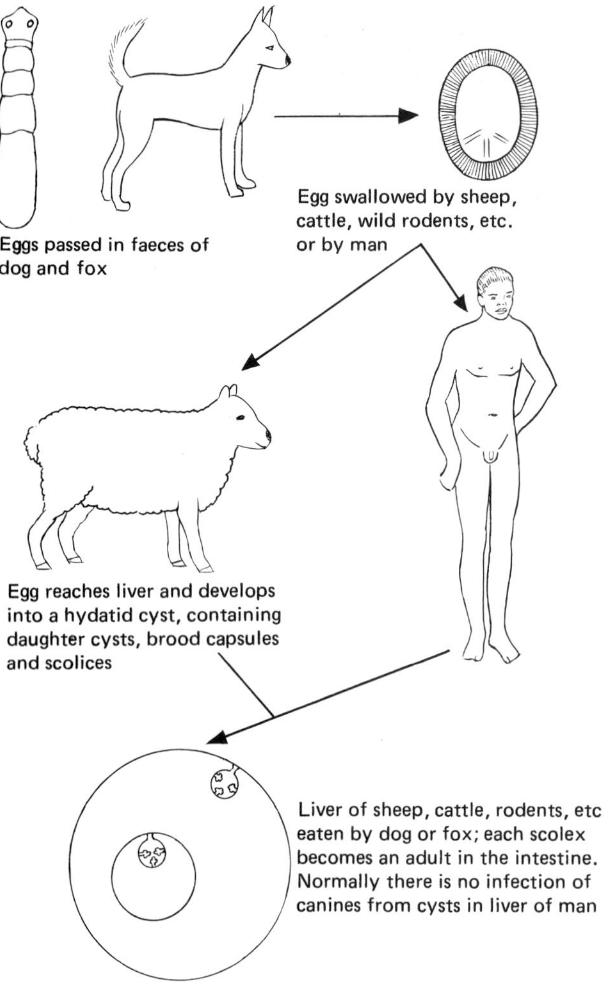

Eggs passed in faeces of dog and fox
Egg swallowed by sheep, cattle, wild rodents, etc. or by man
Egg reaches liver and develops into a hydatid cyst, containing daughter cysts, brood capsules and scolices
Liver of sheep, cattle, rodents, etc. eaten by dog or fox; each scolex becomes an adult in the intestine. Normally there is no infection of canines from cysts in liver of man

Fig. 4.2 Life cycle of *Echinococcus granulosus.*

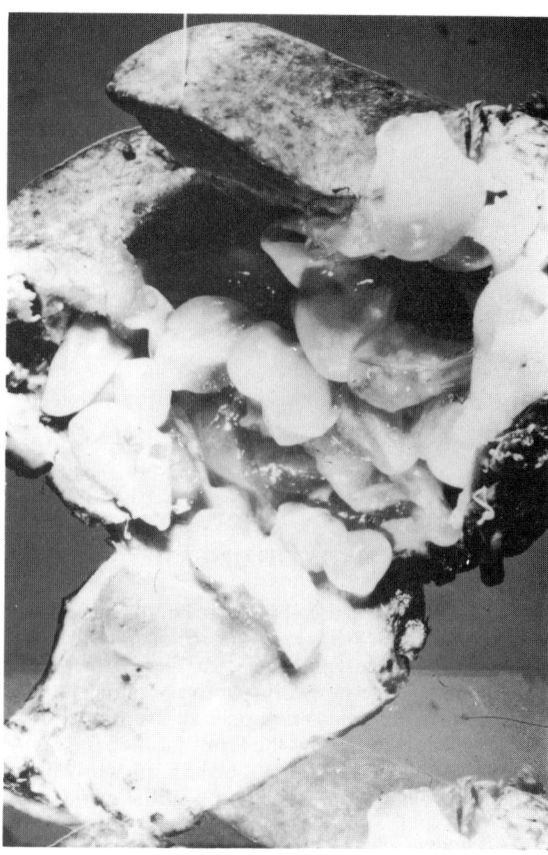

Fig. 4.3 Hydatid disease of the liver.

infrequently except in the areas of Turkana where canines are heavily infected. Turkana tribesmen are the most heavily infected people in Kenya because of the intimate contact between children and canines—here dogs are used to clean the face and anal regions of babies.

Pathology

When the ingested ovum reaches the duodenum, the hexacanth embryo is released and penetrates the intestinal wall to enter the portal circulation and thus reach the liver, most commonly the right lobe. Cysts are usually single but may be multiple and involve the left lobe. Larvae may pass through the liver to infect other organs in addition: lungs (71%), muscle (5%), brain (5%), spleen (2·5%), kidneys (2%), other abdominal organs (5%), bone (0·5%) and rarely the heart, thyroid and other organs. During the stage of migration, there may be a mild reaction with fever and urticarial skin rashes. There is an eosinophilic reaction to the larva itself which subsides as the host's fibrous tissue capsule thickens. In man the hydatid cyst may be (*a*) the classic unilocular, (*b*) the osseous, or (*c*) the alveolar.

The alveolar multiloculated cyst is usually found in the liver and has a sponge-like appearance (*Fig.* 4.3). In the brain it resembles a bunch of grapes (*Fig.* 4.4). The small cysts are usually sterile, consisting of an external laminated

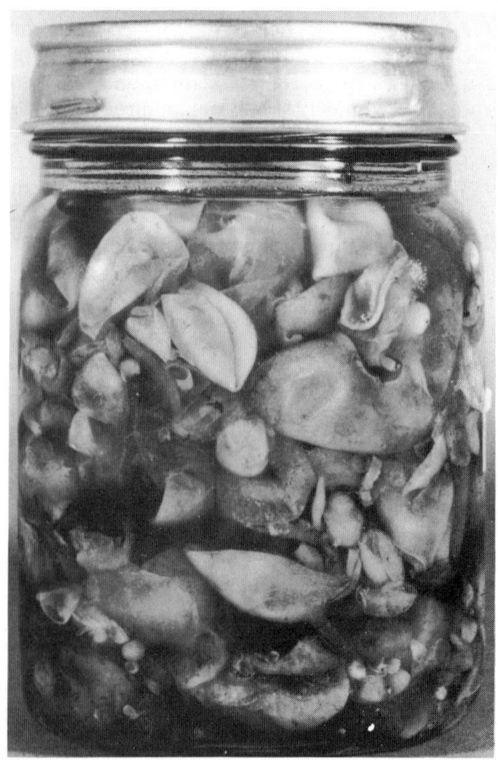

Fig. 4.4 Hydatid cysts.

membrane enclosing glairy greenish fluid. They are separated from each other by the connective tissue of the host in which areas of necrosis and calcification are found. A number of the cysts must, however, be fertile as metastases are the rule.

The classic unilocular hydatid may be sterile but is usually fertile and surrounded by fibrosis produced by the host following a granulomatous reaction. Rupture of fertile cysts, depending on their site, causes dissemination of daughter cysts and scolices with the formation of secondary metastatic hydatids. The escape of the cyst fluid and 'hydatid sand' may cause a severe allergic reaction with urticarial lesions, pruritus, fever, abdominal pain, dyspnoea, cyanosis, delirium and syncope. In addition, there is a marked eosinophilia.

In bone the usual fibrous capsule of the host is not formed and instead of being round, the cyst assumes an irregular branching shape as it penetrates the bony canals. Erosion of bone occurs and the medullary cavity is eventually invaded, when the cyst assumes its normal spherical form. The more highly vascularized areas, the epiphyses of long bones and the centres of the vertebral bodies, ilium and ribs, are the most frequently affected sites. Radiologically they appear as rounded areas of rarefaction. Spontaneous fractures may occur.

Clinical Features

The liver and lungs are the organs involved by the disease in over 90% of cases and hepatic hydatid accounts for three-quarters of these. Although the infection is usually contracted in childhood, a hydatid cyst of the liver may not produce symptoms until adult life, and an interval of over 30 years has been known to exist between primary infection and manifestation of symptoms. Most commonly the cyst is situated in the right lobe and measures 7 cm in diameter. Macroscopically it is surrounded by a greyish-white fibrous coat and compressed liver substance. It contains a glairy fluid and may harbour daughter cysts. Exogenous cysts communicate with the biliary tree and contain bile-stained fluid (*Fig.* 4.5). Secondary infection may occur (*Salmonellae* and pyogenic organisms). Rupture of the cyst may result from secondary infection, trauma or operative intervention. The possible severe allergic manifestations consequent on rupture have already been described and constitute a grave complication of abdominal echinococcosis. Rupture may also occur into the gallbladder, biliary tree, pleural cavity or hepatic veins with secondary metastases in the lungs. Coincident hydatid disease and primary liver cell carcinoma is well documented but no causal relationship between the two has been established.

The alveolar cyst may occur in the liver but is most frequently found in the lung in children. Rupture may be caused by coughing, infection or muscular strain. A chronic pulmonary abscess may result if infection is present. When the cyst ruptures into a bronchus, scolices may be present in the sputum. Rupture may also occur into the mediastinum or pleural cavity with secondary dissemination. Pneumo- and haemothorax are other possible complications.

In the brain, the cysts are usually single and present as a space-occupying lesion. Rupture may disseminate the lesions to the subarachnoid space of the cord. The spinal cord may also be affected by extension of a hydatid from the vertebrae or paravertebral tissues. Scolices may occasionally be seen in the CSF. The hydatids are usually fertile. Cerebral embolic secondaries have been reported from primary hydatid cysts in the lungs, liver and heart.

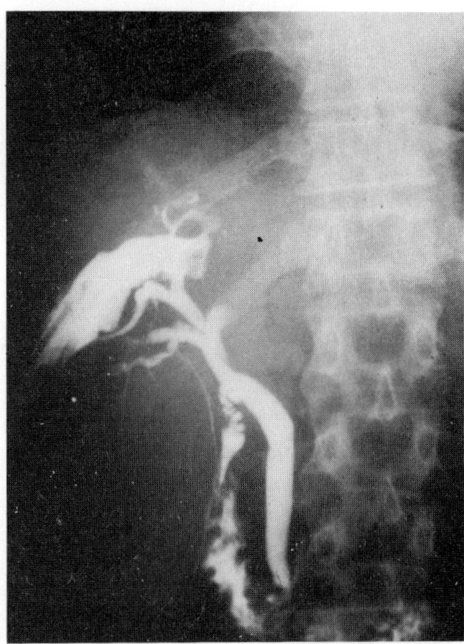

Fig. 4.5 Hydatid cyst of the liver communicating with the dorsocranial branch of the right hepatic duct.

Hydatid disease of the heart may be first discovered at autopsy. During life the cysts may rupture into the pericardium or into the chambers of the heart with consequent pulmonary metastases or systemic embolization causing thrombosis, infarction, or aneurysm formation. Constrictive pericarditis may follow rupture of a cyst into the pericardium.

The cysts are usually single in the spleen and kidneys where they may rupture into the renal pelvis producing renal colic and dysuria with the passage of hydatid material in the urine. Echinococcus may rarely involve other sites: orbit, ovaries, broad ligament and uterus.

Investigations

If the hydatid cysts rupture, the contents—hooklets, scolices, etc.—may be found in the faeces, sputum or urine. Moderate eosinophilia is present (300–2000/mm^3) and the immunoglobulin level may be raised. Radiological examination will often reveal the presence and location of the hydatid cysts (*Fig.* 4.6). Ultrasound examination has proved

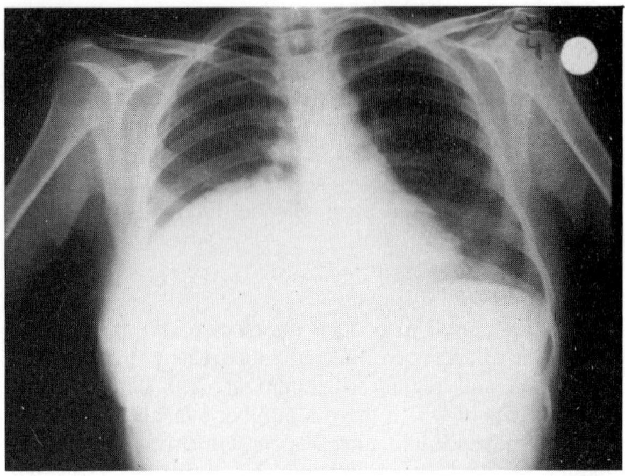

Fig. 4.6 Plain radiograph outlining a large liver with marked elevation of the right hemidiaphragm caused by a hydatid cyst in the right lobe.

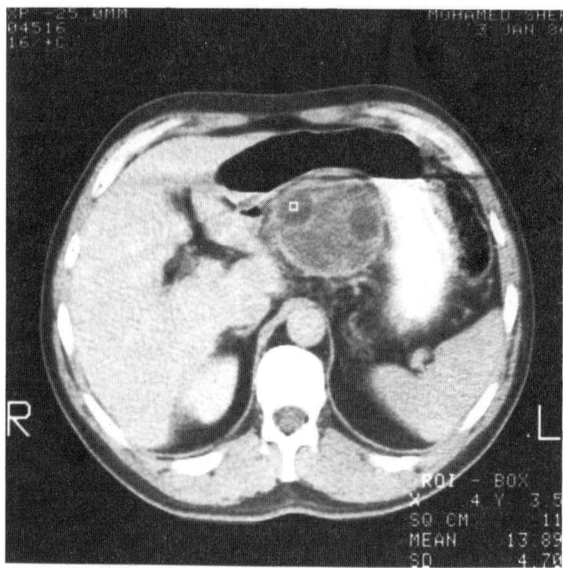

Fig. 4.7 CT scan showing a large hydatid cyst of the pancreas containing daughter cysts. The pancreas is a rare site of involvement by hydatid disease. (By courtesy of Dr Moh'd Saad FRCS, Chairman of Surgical Dept, Adan Hospital, Kuwait.)

very useful particularly when applied to the liver and other abdominal viscera. CT scanning can give valuable information on the cyst contents, its size and precise location (*Fig.* 4.7). It is the best method for establishing the diagnosis of intracranial hydatid disease. Selective angiography is less commonly used for the detection of hepatic hydatid since the advent of ultrasound scanning.

The sensitivity of the Casoni test varies from 57 to 100% in patients with known hydatid disease. A positive test may persist for several years after excision of the cyst. It appears, therefore, that the crude sterile hydatid fluid used in the Casoni test does not give specific results. An intradermal test antigen made up from an extract of lyophilized cyst material of *E. multilocularis* from experimental infections in gerbils is preferable. The complement-fixation test is positive in 70% of patients and may remain so for 2 years after the elimination of the infection. The indirect haemagglutination test is positive in 90% of cases and only 2% of control sera give measurable titres. Other serological tests used are the bentonite flocculation test (71% sensitive), the latex flocculation test, precipitin tests and conglutination tests.

The detection of circulating scolex antigen by countercurrent immunoelectrophoresis (CIE) or the enzyme-linked immunosorbent assay (ELISA) appears to give the most reliable results at present. The detection of the circulating antigen may be positive even when antibody tests are negative.

Medical Treatment

The methods used to control the disease are aimed at the prevention of access to infected carcasses by dogs and the registration and regular treatment of dogs with effective anthelmintics of which there a number available for veterinary use: mebendazole, nitroscanate, bunamidine and praziquantel. Any of these given at 3-monthly intervals will eliminate echinococcus together with other cestodes, such as *Taenic multiceps* and *T. ovis* whose larval forms cause disease and economic loss in sheep.

Although operation remains the definitive therapy for hydatid disease, several reports have shown that the use of mebendazole often results in death and shrinkage of the cyst, thereby avoiding the need for surgical intervention. Research suggests that serum levels greater than 1100 ng/ml 1–3 h after an oral dose may be required to kill the parasite. To achieve this, a dose of 200 mg/kg/day of mebendazole in three divided doses is required for about 16 weeks. Albendazole, an absorbable relative of mebendazole shows even greater promise. A dose of 10 mg/kg/day in two divided doses for 7–60 days has been followed by regression of the cyst in many cases.

Surgical Treatment of Hydatid Disease of the Liver

See Chapter 68.

Pulmonary Hydatid Disease

This is considered in Chapter 39.

AMOEBIASIS

The only amoeba pathogenic in the gut is *Entamoeba histolytica.* The parasite lives in the large intestine causing ulceration of the mucosa with consequent diarrhoea. Secondary lesions may occur, most commonly in the liver but other tissues can be affected, e.g. lungs, brain, genital organs and skin. Amoebiasis has a worldwide distribution but clinical disease occurs most frequently in tropical and subtropical latitudes. It is found in countries where standards of personal and environmental sanitation are low.

Parasitology

The amoeba multiplies by binary fission. It lives in the lumen of the large intestine where under suitable conditions, it invades the mucous membrane and submucosa and ingests red blood cells. When diarrhoea occurs, amoebae are expelled and can be detected in the freshly passed fluid stools. Amoebae are very sensitive to environmental changes and are thus short-lived outside the body. When there is no diarrhoea and other conditions are favourable for encystation, the amoebae cease feeding, become spherical, secrete a cyst wall and the nucleus divides twice to form the characteristic mature 4-nucleate cyst. This is the infective form and when ingested, the cyst hatches in the lower part of the small intestine/proximal colon and a 4-nucleate amoeba emerges from the cyst. After a series of nuclear and cytoplasmic divisions, each multinucleate amoeba gives rise to 8 uninucleate amoebae which establish themselves and multiply in the large intestine.

In most populations where *E. histolytica* is endemic, prevalence remains stable and the incidence and morbidity rates are low. Individual infections are often of long duration and reinfection is common. The disease is spread by cyst passers who may be classified into two main groups: *(a)* convalescents who have recovered from an acute attack, and *(b)*, individuals who can recall no clinical evidence of infection. The latter are probably the more common source of infection, even in countries with high standards of hygiene. Bad sanitation is more important than climate in the predominance of overt infection in the tropics. Carrier rates of *E. histolytica* among symptomless subjects have varied from 20 to 80% in some communities. The parasite can be transmitted by direct contact through the contaminated hands of cyst carriers, e.g. in institutions; it is also transmitted indirectly by means of contaminated food, such as raw vegetables fertilized with fresh human faeces, and through the intermediary of food handlers and flies.

Pathology

The large intestine is usually the primary site of infection and in order of frequency the regions affected are the caecum, flexures, descending colon and rectum. The appendix is sometimes involved and rarely the ileum. Macroscopically the large intestine may be studded with discrete ulcers with overhanging edges, the intervening mucosa being relatively normal. These vertical deep ulcers are in contrast to the superficial shallow spreading ulcers seen in bacillary dysentery. The ulcers spread laterally in the submucosa and become confluent. Large areas of mucosa are thus lost and greenish, shaggy sloughs may involve the muscle coat and extend even to the serosa in severe cases. In patients in whom the host–parasite balance has been altered either by drugs, concurrent disease or pregnancy, the entire mucosa may be sloughed and the underlying amoebic infection may be difficult to detect. The wall of the bowel is thickened and friable (*Fig.* 4.8).

Penetration of the basement membrane and the muscularis is usual in lesions seen at necropsy. The amoebae spread laterally beneath the muscularis and the intestinal epithelium forming large 'flask-shaped' or 'water-bottle' ulcers. These ulcers have overhanging edges and consist of a zone of necrosis surrounded by a low-grade inflammatory reaction with a predominance of lymphocytes and macrophages. A variable fibroblastic reaction is present. Amoebae are found at the periphery of the lesion in the submucosa and the muscle layers. They may also be seen in the necrotic tissue itself (*Fig.* 4.9).

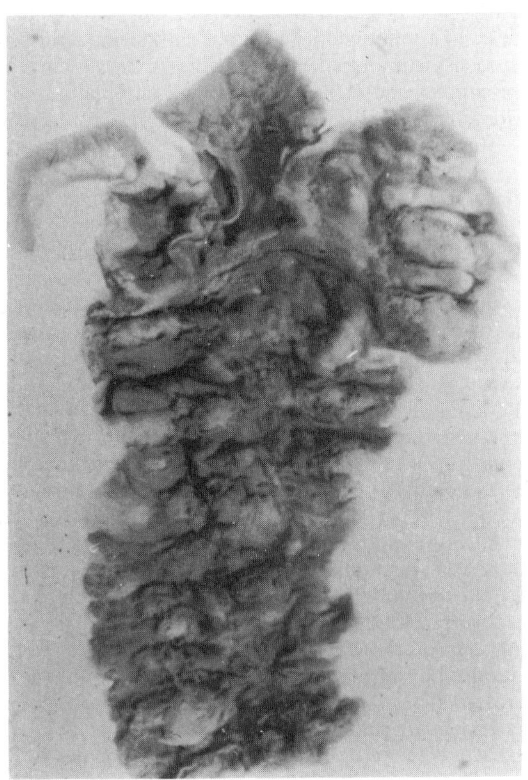

Fig. 4.8 Fulminating amoebic colitis resulting from the use of steroids given for a mistaken diagnosis of ulcerative colitis.

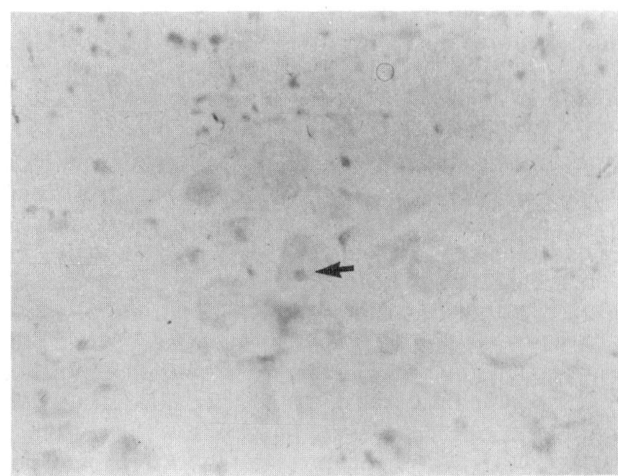

Fig. 4.9 Amoebic colitis section of colon. Note the *E. histolytica* trophozoites.

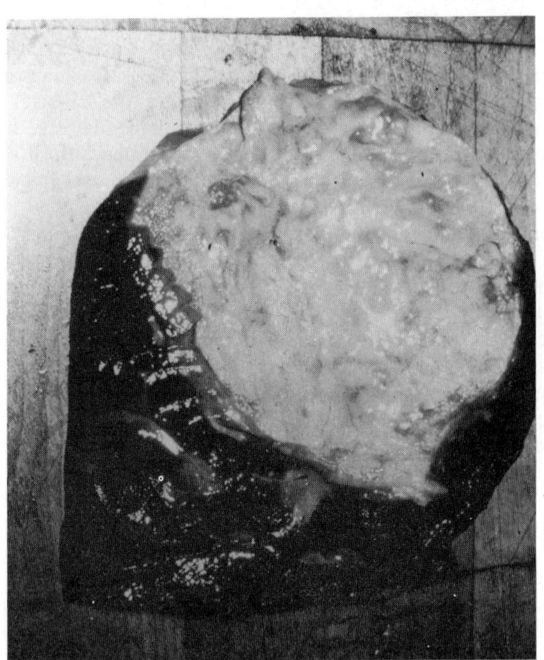

Fig. 4.10 Large single amoebic abscess of the liver.

Liver abscess (*Fig.* 4.10) is the most common extra-intestinal complication. The abscess is usually single but multiple abscesses are not uncommon. The right lobe of the liver is the most frequently affected, especially the posterior portion of the dome. Involvement of the left lobe only is, however, well documented. Bile would appear to destroy the amoebae as the gallbladder is never affected. In over 50% of patients with amoebic liver abscess, there is no evidence of amoebic infection on stool examination. The amoebae cause lysis of the liver parenchyma primarily in the periportal region. An expanding area of necrosis ensues and the abscess cavity may reach a diameter of 12 cm. The cavity contains sterile, chocolate-coloured fluid (the result of lysis of liver cells), granular debris and a few inflammatory cells. Amoebae may or may not be present in the pus. Histologically, the wall of the abscess consists of necrotic tissue and compressed liver parenchyma containing a variable infiltrate of monocytes, plasma cells, lymphocytes and fibroblasts.

Amoebae may be encountered in the area of coagulative necrosis or in the least affected compressed liver tissue.

Clinical Features

The classic picture produced by invasive intestinal amoebiasis is amoebic dysentery, the symptoms of which appear within a week or two of infection or may be delayed for months to years. The onset is usually gradual, with some looseness for a few days followed by evacuation of 6–12 mucoid bloodstained motions per day. Colic and tenesmus are unusual unless there is a lesion immediately inside the anus when tenesmus may be marked. Physical examination may be negative. Occasionally, and especially during more severe attacks, there is palpable thickening of the caecum or left colon with tenderness on pressure. Pyrexia is absent and there is little prostration. The duration of an attack of average severity may be a few days but it may linger on for some weeks. The attack usually subsides spontaneously. There follows a period of remission varying from a few days to several months, even years. During remission, the patient is often constipated. Another attack of dysentery then follows. This sequence of relapses and remissions may continue for several years and is typical of the disease. At any time complications, e.g. amoebic liver abscess, may develop. Complications are encountered in one-fifth of neglected cases. In malnourished individuals or in patients with coincident debilitating disorders, the attacks may be prolonged and very severe, even fatal. Fulminating amoebiasis is also encountered in patients on steroids and other immunosuppressive therapy. The fulminating disease has a sudden onset with swinging fever, chills, sweating and very severe dysentery with rapid dehydration and prostration. In such cases the stools are liquid with flecks of faecal matter and variable amounts of blood and mucus. There may be severe intestinal haemorrhage or perforation, followed by amoebic peritonitis. The mortality in untreated cases is high.

The direct complications of an intestinal infection are haemorrhage from erosion of a large vessel in the bowel wall, transmural extension of the infection with the formation of amoebic granulomas (amoebomas) and frank perforation. In addition to sudden perforation of an amoebic ulcer with the development of an acute surgical abdomen, a form of slow leakage through an extensively diseased bowel may result in peritonitis. The onset is not dramatic but peritonitis must be suspected in patients whose condition deteriorates and in whom there is increased abdominal distension or signs of ileus. Plain radiology reveals free gas in the peritoneal cavity. Other local complications include amoebic strictures which may occur in any part of the colon and intussusception which is rare. All complications are unusual in the common attacks of average severity.

The clinical features of amoeboma include a palpable mass usually in the right iliac fossa, low-grade fever, tenderness and symptoms and signs of intestinal obstruction. Clinically such a lesion may be indistinguishable from a neoplasm, ileocaecal tuberculosis, an appendix mass or a mycetoma.

In the early stages of an amoebic abscess, the patient complains of discomfort and fullness in the liver region. The liver enlarges and becomes tender. Moderate fever develops, at first intermittent and subsequently remittent. Sweating is severe especially at night. The patient becomes anorexic and loses weight. The liver tenderness is maximal over the site of the abscess usually in the right intercostal region laterally over the lower rib cage. The enlarged liver may cause obvious bulging of the chest wall and upper abdomen.

Chest wall movement is restricted on the affected side. The patient finds deep breathing painful and thus develops a shallow tachypnoea. The liver dullness is increased upwards and radiology reveals a raised immobile diaphragm on the affected side. The liver edge is usually palpable well away from the abscess area and often projects 2–3 fingers below the costal margin; it is firm and tender. Jaundice is uncommon but may occur. Most cases have a moderate polymorphonuclear leucocytosis ranging from 12 000 to 15 000/mm^3. The ESR is raised.

Signs of pulmonary involvement (collapse and pleural effusion) are usually limited to the base of the right lung above the raised immobile diaphragm. When the hepatic abscess ruptures through the diaphragm into the lung, the abscess contents discharge into the bronchial tree and the patient develops a cough with expectoration of the classic 'anchovy sauce' sputum which usually contains amoebae and lysed liver tissue. Untreated, the abscess may involve other regions: the pericardial sac (especially when situated in the left lobe), peritoneal cavity with involvement of adjacent intra-abdominal organs, and through the chest/abdominal wall to the exterior.

Embolic spread may result in abscess formation in other organs including the brain. It is probable that most abscesses in other organs are derived from metastatic spread from an initial liver abscess. However, primary brain and pulmonary lesions have been reported; in the latter case the sputum is creamy white and not anchovy.

The diagnosis of amoebiasis is established by the identification of *E. histolytica.* During an acute attack of dysentery microscopical examination of the bloodstained loose motions or of specimens removed at sigmoidoscopy will reveal the presence of motile amoebae, some with engorged red cells. In asymptomatic infections and during remissions, the stool is semiformed and contains *E. histolytica* cysts. These contain one or more bar-shaped chromatoid bodies and staining with iodine reveals 1–4 nuclei and a glycogen mass. Repeated stool examinations (6–10) should be made before absence of infection can be assumed. Concentration techniques for cysts are available, and cultural methods may assist diagnosis in scanty infections.

A sigmoidoscopic examination often yields useful information. The appearances consist of small yellow ulcers with surrounding hyperaemia, and a normal mucous membrane in between the ulcers. In chronic cases, amoebic lesions may appear as 'pinpoint craters' which are irregularly disposed.

The diagnosis of extra-intestinal amoebiasis can be difficult as concomitant dysentery is only present in 5–10% of patients. Chest radiographs show abnormalities in 75% of cases: elevated diaphragm with diminished movement on screening, basal collapse, patchy opacities and pleural effusion. Ultrasound examination is invaluable both in the diagnosis and aspiration of amoebic liver abscess. Serial ultrasound scanning is used to assess healing of an amoebic liver abscess. Radio-isotope and CT scanning are other useful and reliable diagnostic modalities for the detection and localization of hepatic amoebic abscesses.

Serological tests are useful in suspected cases of amoeboma and in those patients diagnosed as ulcerative colitis who have been to the tropics. The serodiagnostic tests include direct immunofluorescence, gel diffusion, countercurrent immunoelectrophoresis and enzyme-linked immunosorbent assay. An iso-enzyme electrophoretic technique is now available which differentiates the invasive from the non-invasive form of *E. histolytica*.

Treatment

Metronidazole (Flagyl) continues to give good results in both amoebic dysentery and liver abscess. Tinidazole is also effective. Asymptomatic intestinal amoebiasis can be treated by either diloxanide furoate (Furamide), 500 mg orally t.d.s. for 10 days, or di-iodohydroxyquinoline (Diodoquin) 600 mg t.d.s. for 21 days.

Attacks of acute amoebic dysentery are treated by metronidazole 400 mg orally t.d.s. for 5 days. Alternative regimens include emetine hydrochloride, 1 mg/kg (not exceeding 65 mg/day) intramuscularly or subcutaneously in two divided doses each day for 4–10 days; or dehydroemetine 1·5 mg/kg daily (not exceeding 90 mg/day). Neither of these drugs should be given to patients with cardiac disease. They are best avoided during pregnancy and in the aged. Therapy with these drugs must be supervised and the patient should be confined to bed. The emetine injections are stopped once the acute signs have subsided and treatment of the intestinal infection is continued with tetracycline and diloxanide furoate or Diodoquin.

For amoebic abscess of the liver, metronidazole 800 mg t.d.s. for 10 days is usually adequate. This regimen will also clear any contiguous complication or intestinal infection. A supplementary course of diodoquin or furamide will ensure that all cysts are cleared. Aspiration is needed for all large abscesses causing a grossly elevated immobilized hemidiaphragm (*Fig.* 4.11), if chemotherapy does not bring relief, or if there is a mass with very localized tenderness, or if the abscess appears to be pointing. Percutaneous aspiration of amoebic liver abscess is best performed under ultrasound guidance.

Surgical Management

Surgical intervention may be necessary in: (i) Fulminating amoebic colitis; (ii) Amoebic perforations of the intestine; (iii) Amoebic liver abscess.

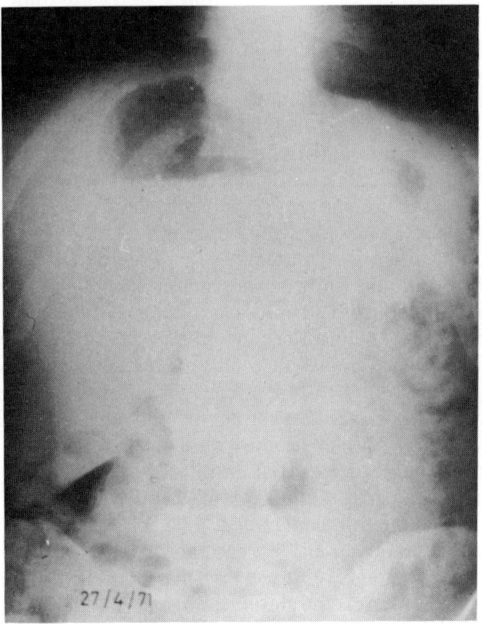

Fig. 4.11 Radiological appearance of large amoebic abscess. Note elevation of the diaphragm from the underlying abscess.

FULMINATING AMOEBIC COLITIS. Surgical treatment is indicated when the patient continues to deteriorate despite medical therapy (severe diarrhoea, toxicity, abdominal tenderness), in the presence of radiological evidence of toxic colonic dilatation, and the onset of an acute episode such as perforation/severe bleeding. Undoubtedly, the best operative treatment is primary resection with exteriorization of the bowel ends. The mortality from the condition, which in the past approximated to 100% has been reduced to about 50% with improved medical treatment and early and aggressive surgical intervention.

AMOEBIC BOWEL PERFORATION. This occurs in 1–2% of patients hospitalized for the disease. Although any segment of the small and large intestine may be involved, the most commonly affected sites are the caecum, ascending and sigmoid colon. Multiple localized or diffuse perforations are encountered in 25% of cases coming to surgery.

Three types of perforation are recognized: extraperitoneal, perforation of a granuloma or ulcer without acute dysentery, and perforation associated with the fulminant disease. Anti-amoebic drug therapy is the primary treatment for all localized extraperitoneal perforations. Surgery is indicated only if the patient's condition deteriorates and rupture appears imminent. Diversion of the faecal stream by an ileocolostomy beyond any colonic involvement and local drainage is the recommended treatment, except in perforations associated with gangrene in cases of fulminant amoebic colitis.

AMOEBIC LIVER ABSCESS. The majority of amoebic liver abscesses respond to medical treatment with or without percutaneous aspiration. Surgical treatment is reserved for when medical treatment has failed to produce complete resolution and for certain specific indications which include: (i) Frank or impending rupture; (ii) Onset of complications such as secondary infection or haemorrhage; (iii) Abscess in the left lobe because of the difficulties of aspiration in this area and the risk of rupture of the abscess into the pericardial sac.

In general, patients requiring surgical drainage have advanced disease and the overall mortality of this group is high (30–40%). A period of anti-amoebic therapy lasting a minimum of 4 days before surgical intervention has been shown to reduce the mortality significantly. Transbronchial rupture is usually well tolerated and curative, although rarely it may cause fatal pneumonitis or lung abscess. Rupture into the pleural cavity is accompanied by shock, respiratory distress and empyema. This situation requires urgent intervention to drain the abscess and the empyema, and to ensure early re-expansion of the collapsed lung. Intraperitoneal rupture requires adequate peritoneal toilet in addition to drainage of the abscess cavity.

COMPLICATIONS FOLLOWING SURGICAL DRAINAGE. Apart from respiratory complications and shock, the commonly encountered postoperative sequelae are liver failure and biliary peritonitis or fistulas. Massive haemorrhage is rare and ameobiasis of the skin is unusual if adequate anti-amoebic drug therapy is started before surgery.

SCHISTOSOMIASIS

The three common species infecting man are *Schistosoma haematobium*, *S. mansoni*, and *S. japonicum*. It has been estimated that a total of about 200 million persons are affected in various parts of the world. *S. haematobium* occurs in many parts of Africa, parts of the Middle East and a few foci in Southern Europe (Portugal). *S. mansoni* is found in the Nile delta, Africa, South America and the Caribbean. *S. japonicum* occurs in China, Japan, the Philippines and other foci in the Far East. Other schistosomes which infect man include *S. bovis*, *S. matthei* and *S. intercalatum*.

Parasitology

These worms are trematodes with the peculiar morphological feature whereby the male is folded to form a gynaecophoric canal in which the female is carried. The adult worms are found in the veins: *S. haematobium* predominantly in the vesical plexus, *S. mansoni* in the inferior mesenteric vein, and *S. japonicum* most commonly in the superior mesenteric vein.

The female lays eggs which pass through the bladder or bowel into urine and faeces respectively. A proportion of the eggs are retained in the tissues and some are carried to the liver, lungs and other organs. If an excreted egg lands in water, it hatches and produces a free-living form, the miracidium, which swims about by ciliary activity. It next invades an intermediate host, a snail of the appropriate species. Within the snail, it undergoes a process of asexual multiplication, passing through intermediate stages of redia and sporocyst to become the mature cercaria. This is the infective larval stage for man. It emerges from the snail and swims, being propelled by its forked tail. On contact with man, the cercaria penetrates the skin, sheds its tail and becomes a schistosomule. The latter migrates to the usual site for mature adults of the species. Various species of snails act as the intermediate hosts of schistosomes. The respective life cycles are shown in *Figs.* 4.12, 4.13, 4.14.

Man is the reservoir of *S. haematobium* but naturally acquired infection with *S. mansoni* has been found in various animals, including primates. *S. japonicum* is widely distributed in various animals—cats, dogs, cattle, pigs and rats—and these constitute a significant part of the reservoir. Man acquires the infection by wading, swimming, bathing or washing clothes and utensils in polluted waters. Certain occupational groups, e.g. farmers and fishermen, are at high risk. The age and sex distribution of schistosomiasis varies from area to area. One fairly common pattern is of high prevalence rates of active infection in children who excrete large quantities of eggs, and a lower prevalence rate of active infection among adults; the latter exhibit late manifestations and sequelae of the infection. Epidemiological studies indicate that the load of infection is an important factor in determining the severity of pathological lesions and clinical manifestations.

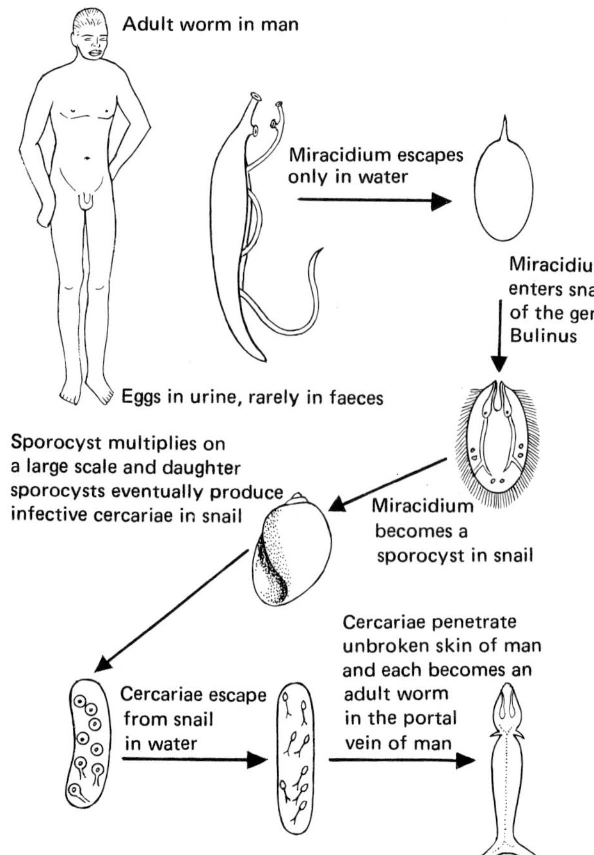
Adult worm in man
Miracidium escapes only in water
Miracidiun enters snai of the gen Bulinus
Eggs in urine, rarely in faeces
Sporocyst multiplies on a large scale and daughter sporocysts eventually produce infective cercariae in snail
Miracidium becomes a sporocyst in snail
Cercariae penetrate unbroken skin of man and each becomes an adult worm in the portal vein of man
Cercariae escape from snail in water

Fig. 4.12 Life cycle of *S. haematobium*.

Pathology

S. haematobium

This affects mainly the urinary tract. The lesions produced in the bladder are various. They include acute and polypoid lesions, fibrous plaques, 'ground-glass' lesions, sandy patches, ulceration, stricture, leucoplakia and cystitis glandularis, fibrosis and calcification of the bladder wall, and bladder-neck obstruction. None the less the bladder may appear normal macroscopically even in fairly severe infections and mucosal biopsies and press preparations are necessary if *S. haematobium* infection is suspected.

In the acute stage the bladder may only be hyperaemic, with or without petechial haemorrhages. Ova retained in the vesical tissues, most commonly in the subepithelial layer, result in the formation of pseudotubercles when the bladder becomes studded with small yellow seed-like bodies surrounded by a zone of hyperaemia, later resembling white sago grains. They are most frequently situated in the trigone, with the base and lateral walls next most commonly affected. Adult schistosomes are often present in the neighbouring vesical veins. Nodules or polyps may be formed by coalescence of these tubercles, hyperplasia of the mucosa, and early fibrosis and hypertrophy of muscle. These proliferating papillomatous or granulomatous lesions are initially hyperaemic and are responsible for the vesical filling defects seen radiologically in the early stages (*Fig.* 4.15). These proliferative mulberry-like lesions subsequently shrink to become white fibrous plaques as the ova become calcified, the mucosa atrophies and fibrosis of the connective tissue ensues. The bladder mucosa may eventually present a flat ground-glass appearance due to widespread atrophy of the epithelium and diffuse underlying fibrosis. A fibrocalcific type of polyp is also commonly encountered. This is a small, usually solitary lesion with a raised surface resembling the sandy patch. Its central core consists of dense fibrous tissue surrounding dilated capillaries and calcified ova. The epithelium is denuded. The third variety of polyp is villous in nature and is less common. It exhibits thickened club-shaped fronds covered by hyperplastic epithelium. These polyps rarely resemble the usual bladder papilloma with its delicate fronds covered by transitional epithelium.

The most common lesion encountered in vesical schistosomiasis is the 'sandy patch'. This late lesion is most often

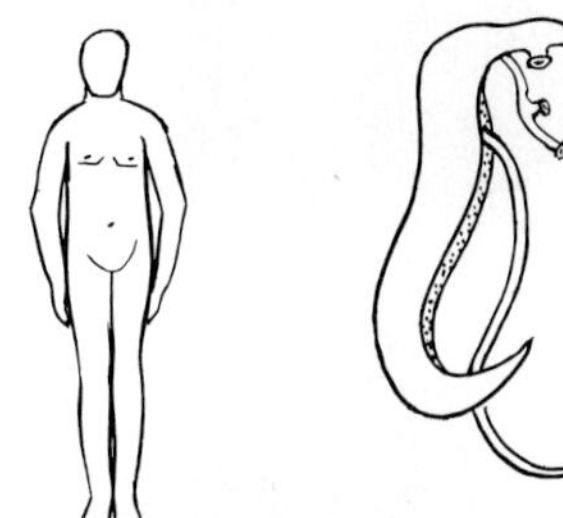
Adult worm in man
Eggs in faeces, rarely in urine

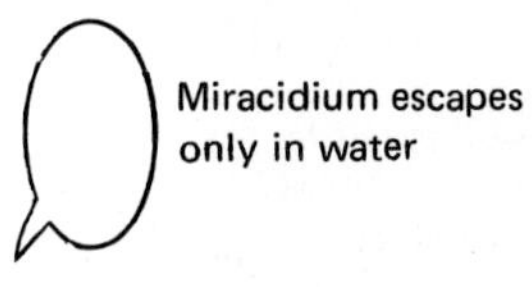
Miracidium escapes
only in water

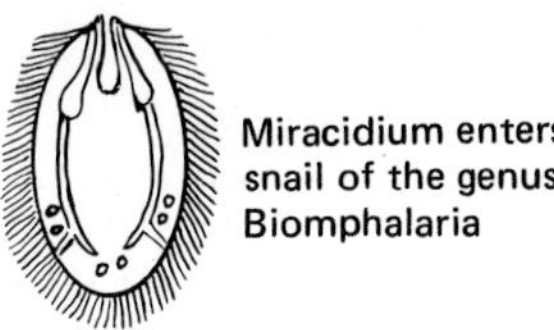
Miracidium enters
snail of the genus
Biomphalaria

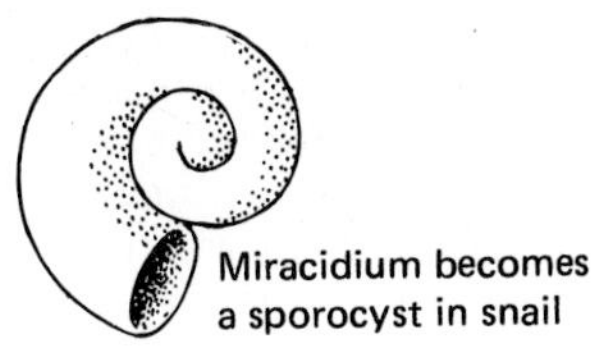
Miracidium becomes
a sporocyst in snail

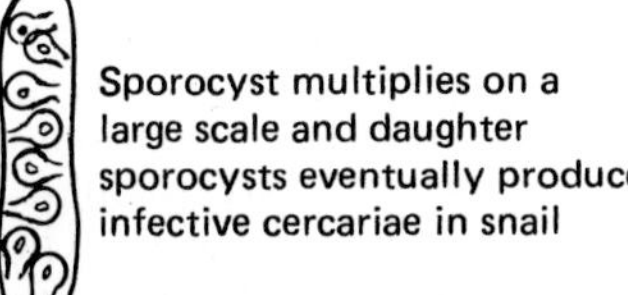
Sporocyst multiplies on a
large scale and daughter
sporocysts eventually produce
infective cercariae in snail

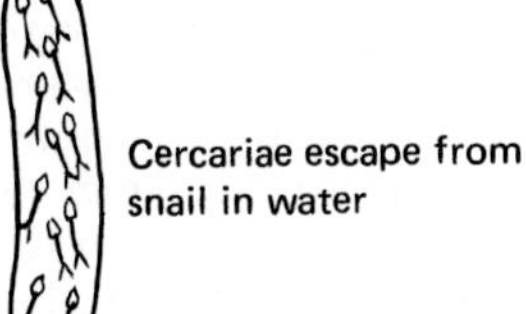
Cercariae escape from
snail in water

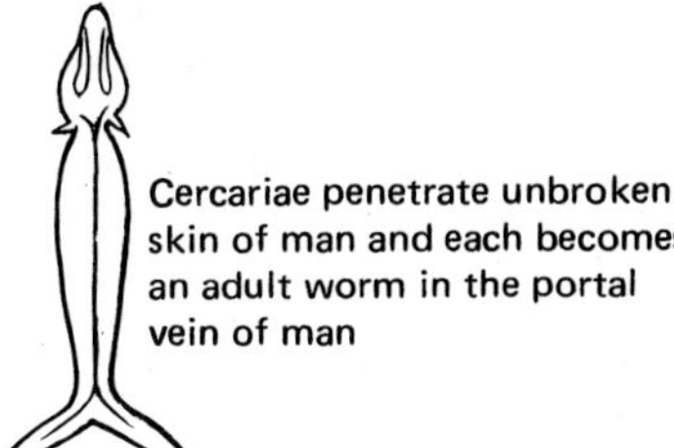
Cercariae penetrate unbroken
skin of man and each becomes
an adult worm in the portal
vein of man

Fig. 4.13 Life cycle of *S. mansoni*.

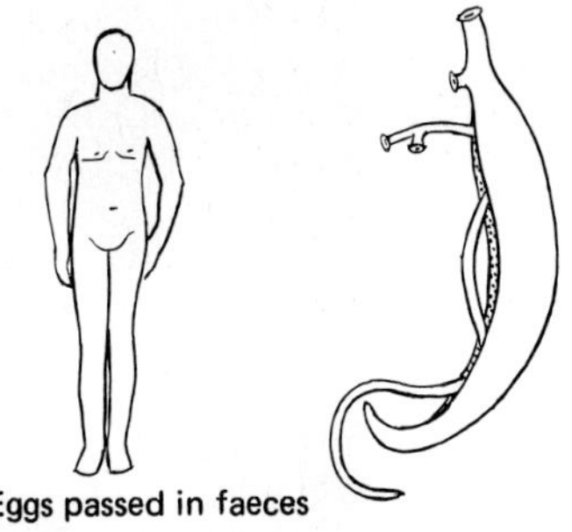
Adult worm in man, horses, cattle, etc.
Eggs passed in faeces

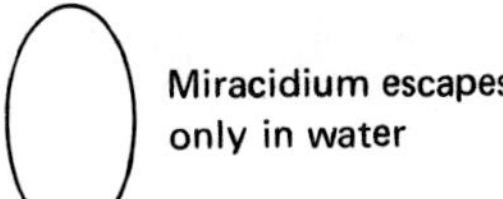
Miracidium escapes
only in water

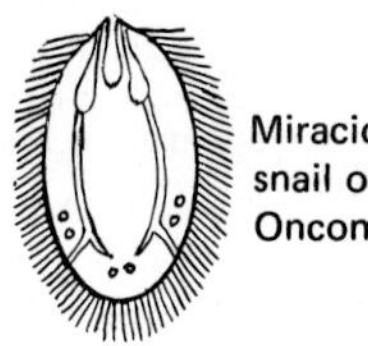
Miracidium enters
snail of the genus
Oncomelania

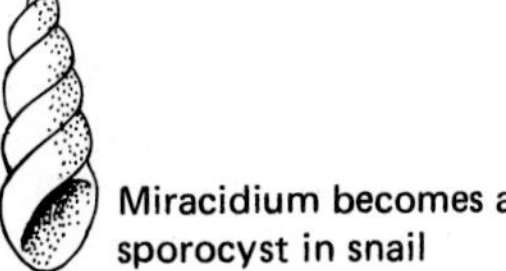
Miracidium becomes a
sporocyst in snail

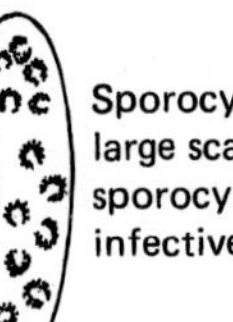
Sporocyst multiplies on a
large scale and daughter
sporocysts eventually produce
infective cercariae in snail

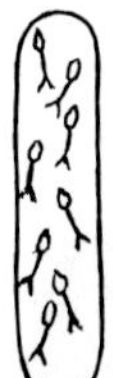
Cercariae escape from
snail in water

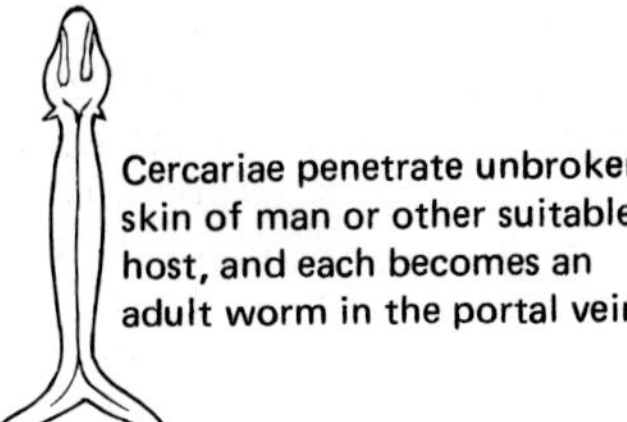
Cercariae penetrate unbroken
skin of man or other suitable
host, and each becomes an
adult worm in the portal vein

Fig. 4.14 Life cycle of *S. japonicum*.

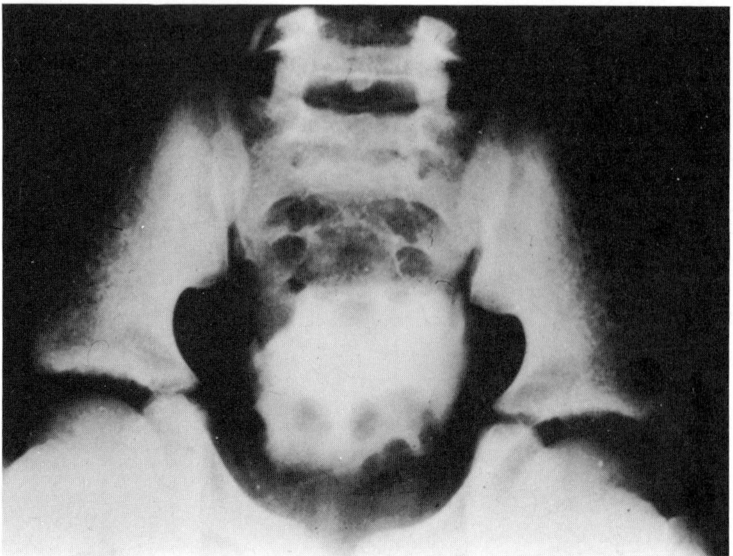

Fig. 4.15 Granulomatous lesions in *S. haematobium* infection seen radiologically as bladder filling defects.

seen in the trigone where the mucosa appears roughened, raised and greyish golden brown in colour (*Fig.* 4.16). The overlying epithelium may be irregularly thickened or atrophic with areas of metaplasia. In the submucosa and muscularis, pseudotubercles and foreign body granulomas may be seen surrounding ova in various stages of disintegration or calcification, but the predominant feature is dense fibrosis. At this stage, the cellular reaction is usually absent or scanty with occasional lymphocytes and plasma cells. Less commonly, there may be a fairly heavy lymphocytic infiltration, and the presence of lymph follicles has been described.

The bladder epithelium may undergo atrophy or become markedly hyperplastic. Foci of leucoplakia may be present. The mucosa at the edge of the nodules/polyps becomes folded, forming shallow pits or pseudoglands, the lumina of which may become occluded by the hypertrophied epithelium with the formation of broad epithelial pegs which may become detached, resulting in the appearance of isolated islets of epithelium in the submucosa—the so-called Brunn's nests. These epithelial downgrowths may become vesicular and lined by tall columnar cells (cystitis glandularis) and in the presence of lymphocyte infiltration, may resemble cystitis cystica. These changes are non-specific and are seen in other chronic bladder infections with obstruction or stone formation. Squamous metaplasia may supervene in these lesions.

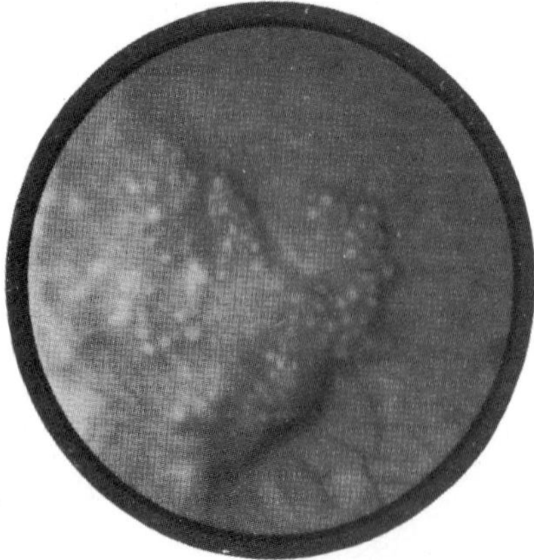

Fig. 4.16 Sandy patches of the bladder in *S. haematobium* infection. (By courtesy of Georg Thieme Verlag, publishers of *Atlas der Urologischen Endoskopie* by H. J. Reuter.)

The incidence of intractable ulceration of the mucosa and bladder wall varies in different endemic areas, being common in Egypt and rare in Zimbabwe and West Africa. It leads to bacterial infection which may spread rapidly to involve the ureters, kidneys, peritoneum and periurethral regions, and adjacent bowel with the development of multiple abscesses, septicaemia and death. The urethra may be directly involved, with consequent stricture formation, and, less commonly, an elephantoid condition of the penis.

In vesical schistosomiasis all types of bladder lesions may be seen in one bladder and all areas of the bladder wall may be involved. In the most severe cases, the whole thickness of the bladder wall may become fibrotic and calcified; in others, focal muscular hypertrophy and diverticula may be found. Bladder neck obstruction from fibrosis is a late complication which is seen frequently in Egypt and leads to urinary retention often in association with multiple sinuses in the scrotum and perineum.

Varying degrees of ureteric involvement are encountered in 70% of patients and are commoner in males. The lower thirds of the ureters are often involved as they share a common blood supply with the bladder. In addition, there may be secondary changes in the ureters induced by the bladder lesions. In endemic areas vesico-ureteric reflux with or without hydronephrosis is observed in up to 20% during the acute stages of infection in children. These changes are likely to be the result of oedema and congestion following pseudotubercle formation in the region of the intramural part of the ureters with consequent distortion. All the lesions and their consequences previously described in the bladder are also encountered in the ureters. Either stricture and/or dilatation of the ureters eventually result (*Fig.* 4.17).

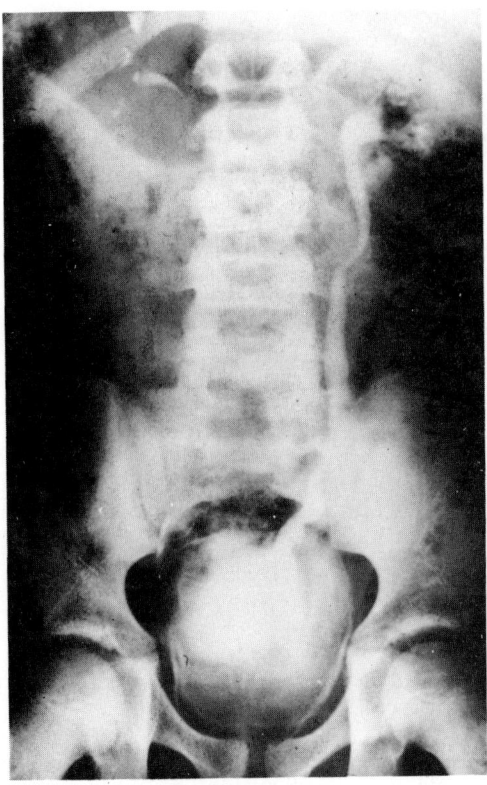

Fig. 4.17 Gross dilatation and tortuosity of the ureter in *S. haematobium* infection. Note also calcification of the bladder.

Fibrosis of the bladder may lead to stenosis of the ureteric orifices. Linear calcification in the ureteric wall, usually at the lower end, is pathognomonic. At other times, the calcification is punctate (ureteritis calcinosa), arising in the contents of ureteritis cystica. Calcification may also occur in a ureteral polyp. Any of these lesions may lead to obstruction with a dilated tortuous ureter and hydronephrosis, and progressive renal impairment. Obstructive renal failure is a well-known entity in this condition and even anuria can occur. Secondary infection of the obstructed kidney results in pyonephrosis.

Renal lesions directly due to the parasite are rare, but occasionally ova are found in the renal parenchyma or in the submucosa of the pelvicalyceal system. Interstitial nephritis has also been described. Rarely, adult worms may enter the interlobular veins and after their death cause an acute eosinophilic necrotizing lesion. Calcification of the renal capsule without renal parenchymal involvement has been reported.

S. mansoni and S. japonicum

Ova are discharged from the mesenteric veins through the mucosa into the intestinal lumen. Some of the ova are, however, retained in the tissues and excite an eosinophilic reaction with the formation of multiple eosinophilic abscesses. In the large intestine, the mucosa is reddened and granular with pin-point yellowish elevations surrounded by a hyperaemic zone. Shallow ulcers may form. These are more extensive in *S. japonicum* than in *S. mansoni* infection. The inflammatory reaction in the submucosa causes epithelial hyperplasia with the formation of sessile or pedunculated polyps. Polypoid lesions of the colon occur in 17–20% of Egyptian patients with schistosomiasis. The muscular layer and the serosa are frequently involved and the pseudotubercles may be associated with a focal exudative peritonitis and intestinal adhesions. Inflammatory masses may be produced in the intestinal wall—'bilharzioma'. With progressive fibrosis, the intestinal wall becomes rigid and the lumen stenosed. The mesentery is thickened and thrombosis of its veins may occur. Granulomatous lesions may be present in the mesenteric and retroperitoneal lymph nodes. These form masses which may stimulate a neoplasm—the pseudotumour. Caecocolic intussusception, intestinal obstruction, and rectal prolapse may supervene. With secondary infection, ischiorectal and anorectal abscesses and fistulas may form, and fibroepithelial polyps are not uncommon in the anal region. It has been suggested that the colitis seen in *S. japonicum* infections may be a premalignant condition.

Pyloric obstruction has been described in *S. japonicum* infection, and lesions may be found in the stomach, peritoneum and pancreas. Infection of the appendix is common and rarely the small intestine may be more affected than the colon.

As the ova in these infections are released in the portal venous system, the liver is invariably affected, the degree of involvement depending on the intensity of the infection. The liver is involved earlier and more severely in *S. japonicum* due to the larger number of ova produced by this schistosome. The liver may be contracted, enlarged or of normal size and its capsule shows a fine to coarse nodularity. The liver consistency is firm and the cut surface exhibits white 'clay-pipe stems' coarsing through the parenchyma which appears otherwise normal. The clay-pipe stem fibrotic areas are the result of terminal fibrosis originally caused by ova in and around the portal venous radicles (*Fig.* 4.18). Some of the intrahepatic portal venules may be dilated, others obliterated. Focal nodular hyperplasia may be seen in the subcapsular region and a fine periportal fibrosis has been described in Egypt.

The ova are trapped in the intrahepatic portal venules and only occasionally reach the sinusoids. The surrounding reaction varies from acute eosinophilic to the dense collagenous. Large acute abscesses may form in *S. japonicum* infections. Affected veins may be completely occluded by the granulomatous reaction with destruction of the elastic and muscle layers. Sclerosis, endarteritis and thrombophlebitis involve the portal vein branches, particularly in the portal tracts. Thin-walled vascular channels form in the fibrosed portal tracts. These are referred to as 'angiomatoids' and result either from recanalization of thrombosed veins or as adaptive communications between the portal and hepatic circulations. An increase in the number and size of the intrahepatic branches of the hepatic artery explains the maintenance of a normal liver blood flow in many patients with the disease. None the less changes are also seen in the arterioles, some of which exhibit hypertrophy and intimal proliferation. Hypertrophied nerve trunks and bile ducts may be seen in the distorted portal tracts.

The parenchymal cells of the liver are usually unaffected and overall the liver function remains good despite established portal hypertension. Parenchymal cell damage may arise from widespread vascular occlusion and anoxic episodes. Focal atrophy, fatty change and haemorrhage have been described, probably accounting for the nodular hyperplasia which may be seen in the subcapsular region. Acute liver cell necrosis may be precipitated by massive variceal haemorrhage or portal vein thrombosis.

Although ova are more frequently found in the lungs in *S.*

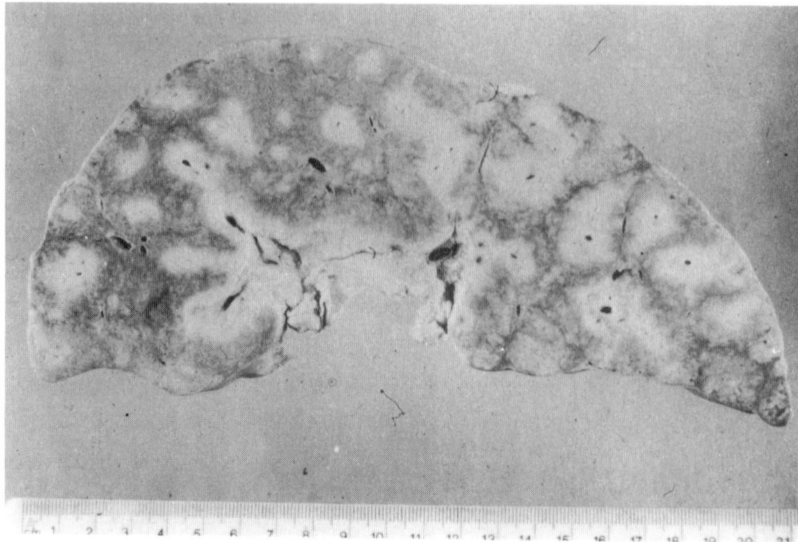

Fig. 4.18 Gross appearance of the cut liver surface in *S. japonicum* infestation. This type of fibrosis also occurs in *S. mansoni* infection.

haematobium infections, the more severe pathological effects are observed in the late stages of *S. japonicum* and *S. mansoni* infections with the development of portal hypertension and portosystemic venous collaterals. The pulmonary changes may be widespread and produce a clinical picture of cor pulmonale or chronic respiratory failure with cyanosis.

Cerebral involvement is more common in *S. japonicum* infection and spinal cord disease in *S. mansoni.* Small tubercles are found in the meninges and in the white and grey matter of the brain and cord. The lesions usually contain large numbers of ova in necrotic material surrounded by eosinophils, polymorphs and multinucleated giant cells with an outer layer of epithelioid cells and lymphocytes.

Clinical Features

During the stage of invasion and maturation of the worm which lasts about 12 weeks, the patient may develop a generalized illness with fever, malaise, exhaustion and sometimes diarrhoea and abdominal discomfort. Urticaria may develop and eosinophilia is nearly always present. This initial illness is known as the 'Katoyama syndrome' and is thought to result from a temporary state of antigen excess which exists until the host's antibody production is mobilized. The illness is usually seen in those who become infected for the first time and is more frequently encountered in immigrants than in natives of the endemic areas. It may on occasions be very severe and even fatal. This stage of initial illness occurs in all the three schistosomal infections.

S. haematobium

The stage of established infection occurs 10–12 weeks after cercarial penetration and is manifested by frank haematuria and egg extrusion. The haematuria is intermittent and often transitory. Episodes of haematuria continue to be experienced by untreated patients though these attacks become less severe with time. Microscopic examination of the urine reveals the presence of RBCs between attacks. The blood lost in the urine is rarely sufficient to cause anaemia and averages 6 ml/day in moderately severe infections. The excretion of the ova in the urine diminishes over the years. Proteinuria and amino aciduria have been reported but they do not contribute to the protein malnutrition except in extreme cases.

BLADDER. Initially the patient complains of dysuria, frequency and urgency of micturition. When schistosomal ulceration occurs, it is accompanied by suprapubic or perineal pain. Two clinicopathological entities have been described: (i) Sloughing of polypoid patches in early active disease; and (ii) Chronic ulceration at sites of heavy egg deposition. Polypoid lesions of the bladder may persist as polyps into the later inactive stages of the disease if the initial active infection is heavy.

Vesical fibrosis with contraction of the bladder and calcification occur in chronic infections. The calcification occurs in the dead ova rather than in the bladder tissues and is common in children and young adults. Radiological evidence of bladder calcification thus indicates that the patient had an initial heavy bilharzial infection. The calcified ova can be demonstrated beneath the urothelium and in some instances breaking through it. The significance of this is that a patient could have a 'calcified' bladder but, in time, as the calcified ova are discharged, the bladder wall returns to relative normality. Occasionally the bladder is large and atonic. This is thought to result from a reduced blood supply but may also be due to bladder neck obstruction.

URETERS. Ureteric involvement is common and usually bilateral. When unilateral, the left ureter is more often affected. Severe infections produce sandy patches, polyps, ureteritis cystica or glandularis, and ulcers. Stenosis of the ureter is a common occurrence. It usually affects the intramural segment, less often the lower third and, rarely, the upper half of the ureter. Proximal to the stricture, the ureter becomes dilated (hydroureter), lengthened and tortuous. Hydroureter may develop in the absence of stenosis from functional incoordination or aperistalsis. Proximal bacterial infection and stone formation are the sequelae of ureteric obstruction.

KIDNEYS. Hydronephrosis and pyonephrosis are the result of the obstructive uropathy. Pyelonephritis occurs frequently in these patients. An association between *S. haematobium* and the nephrotic syndrome has been suggested but remains unproven. Systemic hypertension has been reported in some areas (South Africa and Gambia) but no clear-cut relationship has been established.

Bacteriuria is often present in hospital patients. The 'pus' cells in the urine of these patients have been shown to be eosinophils derived from the inflammatory lesions around the ova in the bladder wall, and their numbers correlate with amounts of eggs excreted in the urine and are not related to the bacterial colony counts. *S. haematobium* infection in Egypt predisposes the patient to the development of a carrier state for *Salmonella typhi* and *S. paratyphi.* It has been suggested that the main site of salmonella infection in these patients is the urinary tract and their symptoms resemble those of the other urinary tract infections.

CALCULI. These are common in Egypt where they occur in 25% of infected individuals but are rare in most other parts of Africa. They occur in the bladder, ureters, kidneys and urethra. They consist of a central core of oxalate surrounded by an outer coat of urate often incorporating schistosome ova. Urinary stasis consequent on granuloma/stricture formation is the most important contributory factor. Disappearance of some of these calculi following successful medical therapy with resolution of the granuloma and associated obstructive uropathy has been documented. This is most likely to happen in young patients in whom fibrosis and irreversible stenosis has not had time to develop.

ASSOCIATION WITH VESICAL CANCER. There is evidence for an association between *S. haematobium* infestation and the development of bladder cancer. Thus in endemic areas, vesical cancer occurs at a younger age than in Europe and North America, there is no male preponderance, and the most common type of tumour is the squamous-cell carcinoma (40–75%) in contrast to the transitional-cell variety encountered in the Western hemisphere. Schistosomal bladder cancer arises commonly from the anterior and posterior walls, rarely from the trigone and superior apical regions, and is diffuse (multicentric) in one-third of cases. Various theories have been suggested to account for the pathogenesis: chronic irritation, miracidial toxin, beta-glucuronidase activity in the urine. Chronic irritation of the bladder mucosa by a persistently alkaline urine has been postulated following secondary infection of schistosomal cystitis by urea-splitting organisms. Irritation has also been ascribed to the continued rubbing of the mucosa against the calcified eggs in the submucosa.

The enzyme beta-glucuronidase is excreted in the urine of patients with active *S. haematobium* infection. This enzyme has been shown to be present in the miracidia, cercaria and the adult worm. In the presence of dietary and other exogenous carcinogenic compounds, the increased urinary beta-glucuronidase may hydrolyse inactive carcinogenic glucuronides, releasing the active carcinogen. There is good evidence for this hypothesis. Thus in Egypt raised levels of urinary metabolites of tryptophan, serotonin and the carcinogen 3-hydroxyanthranilic acid have been demonstrated in the urine of infected patients and very high levels (eight times the normal values) were observed in cases with bladder cancer. In an area of Uganda where plantains form the basic diet, high urinary levels of serotonin metabolites and particularly 5-hydroxyindole acetic acid were found. Bladder cancer is not uncommon in this area although *S. haematobium* is not widespread. Differences in the indoles excreted by *S. haematobium* patients in Maputo and Johannesburg have also been reported and considered to be due to dietary factors.

S. mansoni and S. japonicum

The onset of egg laying in a first infection is accompanied by bloody diarrhoea. The lesions in the colon are variable; there may be segmental roughening of the mucosa with congestion, small ulcers and, in the late stages, 'sandy patches' resembling those described in the bladder in *S. haematobium.* The mucosa may be thrown up into folds and polyps may develop especially in *S. mansoni* infection. Polyposis is due to a high localized egg burden damaging the muscularis mucosa. The polyps are therefore inflammatory in nature with little or no adenomatous hyperplasia, and are reversible with medical treatment. In some cases, severe dysentery associated with frank ulceration and massive haemorrhage occurs and is often fatal.

Perforation and stricture of the colon occur but are uncommon. Prolapse of the rectum has been described in association with polyps. Pseudotumour is a rare complication and may mimic carcinoma. It represents an exuberant connective-tissue reaction to a conglomeration of schistosomal granulomas and may be palpable, and situated inside or outside the intestinal lumen. It may cause stenosis.

Hepatosplenic schistosomiasis occurs in individuals with a heavy worm load about 5–15 years after infection. It has, however, been described in children. Ova are deposited in the terminal radicles of the portal vein with granuloma formation and fibrosis of the portal tracts. The ensuing portal hypertension is associated with splenomegaly (often massive), oesophageal varices and ascites. A higher seropositive incidence of the hepatitis B antigen status has been noted in individuals suffering from hepatosplenic schistosomiasis when compared with other patients and blood donors. *S. mansoni* infection may be associated with chronic *Salmonella* septicaemia and the nephrotic syndrome. Treatment of the schistosome infection may lead to the resolution of the associated disease.

Diagnosis can only be established by the demonstration of living schistosome eggs in the urine, stool or biopsy material. Dead eggs only signify past infection; they may remain in the tissues or be voided in the excreta for years after death of the adult worms. Eggs of *S. mansoni* and *S. japonicum* are sought in the stool; those of *S. haematobium* in mid-day urine specimens. Biopsy of the rectal mucosa is helpful, as is cystoscopy in *S. haematobium.* Serodiagnostic tests are of little clinical use.

Medical Treatment

The drugs of choice for the treatment of *S. haematobium* infection are metriphonate (Bilarcil) 7·5 mg/kg orally for 3 doses, each given at 15-day intervals, or Praziquantel (Biltricide) in a single oral dose of 20 mg/kg. *S. mansoni* infections are treated with oxamniquine 20–30 mg/kg/day for 3 days, or praziquantel in a single oral dose of 20 mg/kg after meals. Praziquantel is the drug of choice for *S. japonicum* and is administered in a single dose of 30 mg/kg.

Surgical Aspects

The need for surgical intervention in schistosomiasis may arise from the development of complications of the disease, e.g. portal hypertension, bilharzial granuloma of the gastro-intestinal tract and obstructive uropathy.

Portal Hypertension

Schistosomiasis causes a parenchymal block usually without significant hepatocellular dysfunction or reduction of the hepatic blood flow. Minor degrees of portal hypertension and hypersplenism may be reversed with specific anthelmintic therapy. Treatment is required for oesophageal varices only if bleeding has occurred. Increasingly, many of these patients are being managed with repeated sclerotherapy through the flexible endoscope. Surgical intervention is indicated if bleeding cannot be controlled in this way, or recurs, as it often does, after a full course of sclerotherapy. The general consensus of opinion is against the use of portocaval shunts in patients who have bled from their oesophageal varices as the majority are prone to develop severe encephalopathy after this procedure. Reports on the use of selective decompression by distal trans-splenic decompression (Warren shunt) have been favourable. Overall the best results in the management of these patients have been obtained by the use of splenectomy with porto-azygos disconnection or the more extensive devascularization procedure of Sugiura.

Bilharzial Granuloma of the Gastrointestinal Tract

This complication predominantly affects the large bowel, although small intestinal and appendiceal lesions have been reported. Small bowel granuloma usually presents with acute small bowel obstruction or, more rarely, with mesenteric infarction.

The clinical features of large bowel bilharzial granuloma are varied. The patient may have chronic symptoms—vague abdominal pain, palpable mass in the lower abdomen, passage of blood and mucus, anaemia and rectal prolapse—when the diagnosis is usually made by sigmoidoscopy and biopsy. The sigmoidoscopic and radiological appearances may, however, be difficult to differentiate from polyposis coli. Occasionally the patient presents with a large bowel obstruction and at operation a sigmoid lesion is found which is macroscopically indistinguishable from carcinoma. In the majority of cases, the colonic granulomatous lesion occurs in the descending colon, sigmoid and rectum.

In the elective situation after adequate bowel preparation, resection beyond the diseased mucosa with primary anastomosis is usually advocated. In patients with obstructive disease or when emergency surgery is needed, resection with exteriorization (Paul–Mikulicz) is indicated.

Obstructive Uropathy

There has been an increasing criticism of the use of cystoscopy in urinary schistosomiasis because of the real hazard of introducing secondary infection. The use of this endoscopic investigation should be selective as in diagnostic problem cases (e.g. exclusion of neoplasia). In any event, cystoscopy should not be undertaken except under conditions of strict surgical asepsis and in the presence of facilities for biopsy and radiological investigations.

The surgical treatment of obstructed ureters remains controversial. An accurate assessment of the extent of the ureteric disease and the state of the bladder is essential to a successful outcome. Adequate excision of the obstructed diseased segment with direct re-implantation or by means of ileal conduits with vesico-ileal anastomosis have given the best results. The most common cause of failure is inadequate excision. The operation of ileocaeco-urethroplasty is a difficult and hazardous procedure which should only be attempted in specialized units.

MALARIA

Malaria is still the most widely spread communicable disease in the tropics. An annual number of 250 million clinical cases are reported, and with an estimated overall mortality of 1%, 2·5 million persons die directly from malaria in the Indian subcontinent with 10 million cases reported from India and 7 million from Pakistan in 1977. The two most common parasites are *Plasmodium vivax* and *P. falciparum*.

Parasitology

The complete life cycle of the human malaria parasite embraces a period of development within the mosquito, and a period of infection in man (*Fig.* 4.19). After ingestion of infected human blood, a period of development lasting 10–14 days occurs in the mosquito resulting in the production of sporozoites. A bite infects the human host with these forms, which remain in the circulating blood for 30 min, then enter tissue cells notably in the liver. During the next 7–9 days, the sporozoites develop in the parenchymal cells of the liver. This stage of development is known as the pre-erythrocytic cycle. The cryptozoic schizonts so formed rupture and release numerous merozoites, most of which enter the circulation to invade the erythrocytes, thus starting the erythrocytic cycle. As in the short sporozoite phase, no symptoms of malaria are experienced during the pre-erythrocytic cycle. The plasmodium first appears in red cells as a small speck of chromatin surrounded by scanty cytoplasm, and soon becomes a ring-shaped trophozoite. As the parasite develops, pigment particles appear in the cytoplasm, and the chromatin becomes more prominent. Chromatin division then proceeds and, when complete, there is formed the mature schizont containing daughter merozoites. The parasitized red blood cells now rupture, releasing merozoites, the majority of which re-enter erythrocytes to re-initiate erythrocytic schizogony. In *P. falciparum* infection the erythrocytic cycle takes 36–48 h (subtertian); in *P. vivax* and *P. ovale* infection 48 h (tertian), and in *P. malariae* 74 h (quartan). The powers of invasion of the species of plasmodia differ considerably. *P. vivax* develops most easily in the youngest erythrocytes, so that at any time not more than 2% of red cells are invaded. *P. malariae* develops chiefly in the older red cells, the infection rate seldom exceeding 2%. In *P. falciparum* infection rates of up to 15% of red cells have been noted, and preference for young erythrocytes has been demonstrated.

In response to an unknown stimulus a number of the merozoites released after erythrocytic schizogony develop into male and female forms known as gametocytes which are inert in the human. Gametocytes provide the reservoir of infection, enabling mosquitoes to perpetuate the malaria cycle, and remain within the red cell for the duration of their survival (up to 120 days). A certain proportion of merozoites liberated in the pre-erythrocytic phase do not enter the bloodstream. Instead they re-enter the liver cells to produce the secondary or metacryptozoic schizonts which are responsible for the persistence of the exo-erythrocytic (EE) cycle. The reappearance of malaria after clinical cure results from the parasite's ability to persist in the tissues in this EE form. The eventual discharge of merozoites from these EE forms into the bloodstream initiates a relapse. The EE cycle occurs in *P. vivax*, *P. ovale* and *P. malariae* infections.

P. vivax can usually produce relapses up to three years after infection; while *P. malariae* has occasionally relapsed 10–30 years after a primary infection. Patients suffering from *P. ovale* malaria have been recently documented in

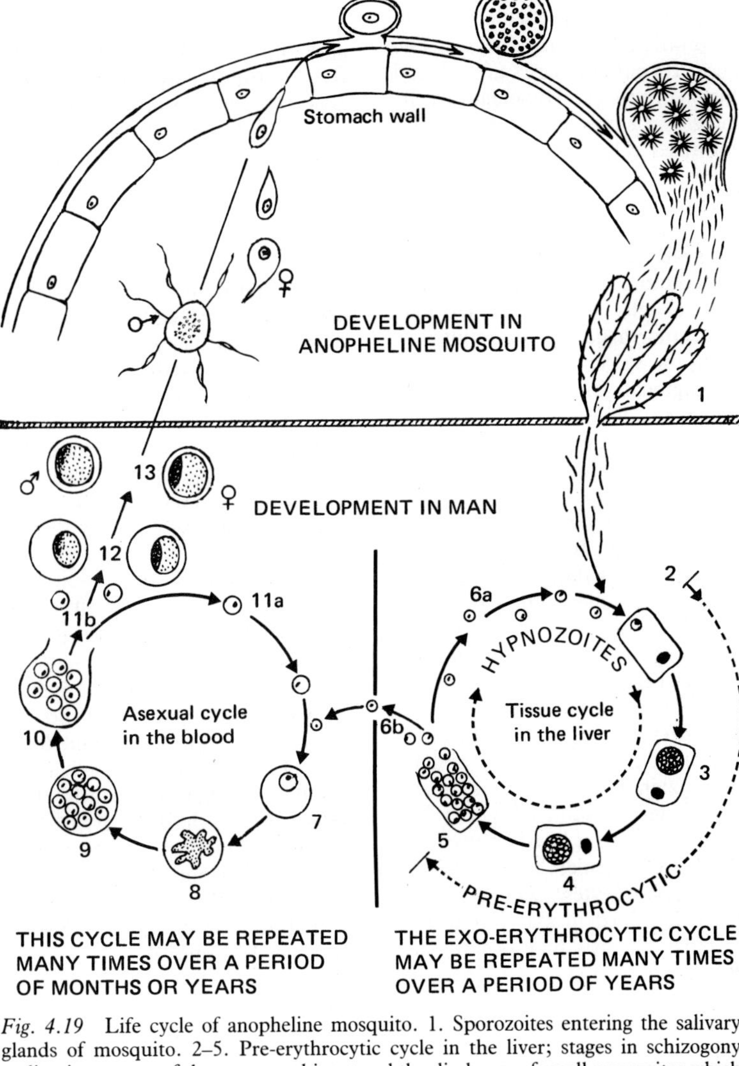

Fig. 4.19 Life cycle of anopheline mosquito. 1. Sporozoites entering the salivary glands of mosquito. 2–5. Pre-erythrocytic cycle in the liver; stages in schizogony ending in rupture of the mature schizont and the discharge of small merozoites which enter the bloodstream. 6*a*. Hypnozoites in liver responsible for initial invasion of erythrocytes and for subsequent relapses. *6*b*–11*a*. Erythrocytic schizogony. 7. Ring form. 8. Trophozoite. 9. Mature schizont. 10. Merozoites discharged on rupture of schizont. 11*a*. Merozoites about to enter the red blood cells to recommence erythrocytic schizogony. 11*b*. Immature gametocyte about to enter red blood corpuscle. 12. Immature male and female gametocytes. 13. Mature gametocytes awaiting ingestion by anopheline mosquito.

*No hypnozoites occur in *P. falciparum*.

Europe and the USA. All the infections were contracted in West Africa and a relatively long latent period was noticed. The infections were of considerable severity but spontaneous recovery was the rule. As the liver phase does not persist in *P. falciparum* infection, relapses do not occur after adequate medical treatment.

Malaria is transmitted by various species of anopheles mosquitoes. Transmission can also occur through transfusion of blood and blood products, and by syringe passage amongst drug addicts. In non-endemic areas, air travel is mostly responsible for the cases seen. It has been shown that Duffy blood groups are involved in the racial immunity of West African Negroes to *P. vivax* infection, while haemoglobin S heterozygotes (AS), and heterozygote females deficient in G–6–PD (Gd^{A-}/Gd^{B}) are protected against the lethal effects of *P. falciparum* malaria.

Pathology

The only type of malaria which is directly fatal is that caused by *P. falciparum.* The pathology of malaria in the various organs refers mainly to the changes seen in this infection. The most severe lesions in the CNS occur in cerebral malaria. The meninges are grossly congested, the small vessels of which are packed with parasitized cells. The haemolytic anaemia is often severe. The bone marrow becomes hyperaemic and extends into the shafts of the long bones. In the acute stage its vessels are full of parasitized erythrocytes, and haemozin is present in the reticuloendothelial cells and monocytes. There is a marked normoblastic hyperplasia even in the absence of a reticulocytosis in the peripheral blood, and a proliferation of myelocytes. The spleen is enlarged and tense. Its cut surface is greyish red with prominent Malpighian corpuscles. Histologically its blood vessels, Billroth cords and sinusoids are filled with parasitized red cells. Parasitized cells and haemozoin are seen in the pulp histiocytes and sinusoidal lining cells. Pigment may be found lying free in the pulp and sinusoids, and in our experience it is also found in the germinal follicles. A splenic smear reveals developing forms of parasites and haemozoin lying free and contained in monocytes. Degeneration of the endothelial cells of splenic vessels may occur causing thrombosis, haemorrhage and infarction.

With increasing immunity the spleen becomes jet black due to excess deposition of pigment. Gradually as the congestion decreases and the pigment disappears and the parasitized cells become scanty, the spleen diminishes in size. Its capsule becomes greyish, fibrotic and wrinkled with perisplenitis and fibrosis in the splenic pulp.

The pathological changes in the liver vary according to the immunological status of the individual. In cerebral malaria, the liver is enlarged and tense, and is dark red to grey in colour. If, however, the anaemia has been gross the liver, though enlarged, is pale. Histologically, the striking feature in the acute stage is the gross congestion of the sinusoids and centrilobular veins by parasitized erythrocytes. The Kupffer cells are hypertrophied and contain parasitized and unparasitized cells, remnants of parasites, haemozoin masses and at times haemosiderin. The parenchymal cells may contain haemosiderin but never haemozoin. One of the striking and constant histological features is degeneration and necrosis in the centrilobular regions in the absence of heart failure. The renal vessels, particularly the glomerular capillaries, are congested with parasitized erythrocytes. Acute diffuse glomerulonephritis has been described in association with *P. falciparum* malaria. Tubular necrosis may occasionally occur. Changes in the adrenals are variable. Degenerative and necrotic changes may affect the inner zone of the cortex with loss of lipid. The more usual finding, however, is gross congestion and haemorrhage.

In patients who die of pulmonary oedema, the lungs at postmortem are congested and oedematous, and exhibit hyaline membrane formation, thickened alveolar septa and areas of alveolar haemorrhage. The basic lesion appears to be injury to the capillaries of the lung with congestion and leakage of oedema fluid. No parasitized erythrocytes are encountered in the lungs in these patients.

Clinical Features

The clinical presentation of *P. vivax* and *P. falciparum* are as follows:

P. vivax

Fever is the most constant sign. After a brief period of remittent pyrexia, the pattern of intermittent, regularly recurring fever every second day is established. The classic features of the attack—cold stage, hot stage, sweating stage—are unusual in infants and children. General symptoms similar to those described for *P. falciparum* infection may occur but are usually milder. The spleen enlarges early in the disease, some degree of anaemia may be present, and there is often mild leucopenia. When the fever is high, convulsions may occur in children. *P. vivax* malaria is rarely fatal.

P. falciparum

There is little that is typical about this type, and its many and various symptoms can be very misleading. A common misconception concerns the periodicity of the fever which, especially in first attacks, is irregular and of daily occurrence. Headache, malaise, nausea, vomiting, and generalized joint pains may be the only additional presenting symptoms of an uncomplicated attack. On physical examination, there may be hepatosplenomegaly and a variable degree of anaemia. This rather undramatic clinical picture can deteriorate suddenly into one with severe manifestations and a fatal outcome. Abdominal presentations resembling appendicitis and acute abdomen have been described.

Among the pernicious manifestations, the following are commonly recognized: cerebral malaria, renal insufficiency/failure, gastrointestinal malaria, algid malaria, malarial anaemia, hyperpyrexia, pulmonary oedema and malarial haemoglobinuria. Patients are also usually dehydrated and may have herpes labialis. Jaundice with or without hepatic failure is a manifestation that is frequently misdiagnosed as infective hepatitis.

P. malariae

The only important clinical manifestation of this malaria is the production of the nephrotic syndrome in children with longstanding untreated infections.

A conclusive diagnosis of malaria can only be made by the detection of the parasite in the blood. Thick blood films are preferable to thin smears for this purpose especially in light infections. When the parasitaemia is gross, an attempt should be made to quantify the infection. Careful daily monitoring of the intensity of the parasitaemia is vital when assessing the effect of treatment as well as predicting prognosis. It is important to stress that complete parasite clearance often takes 72 h, and that the concomitant use of corticosteroids or any other anti-inflammatory drug may prolong this interval.

Treatment

It is important to emphasize that treatment comprises two equally important components: antiparasitic and supportive, i.e. the conventional management of the various manifestations associated with severe *P. falciparum* infection, such as renal failure, coma, convulsions, hepatic failure, dehydration, etc. The routine use of anticoagulants in malaria is to be avoided.

Antiparasitic Treatment

P. FALCIPARUM. Two basic decisions must be made before the start of antiparasitic treatment. First, has the patient acquired his infection in an area where *P. falciparum* is sensitive or resistant to chloroquine? Secondly, is the patient ill enough to require parenteral therapy or will oral treatment be sufficient?

Chloroquine-resistant Malaria: Of all the human parasites, only *P. falciparum* has become resistant to chloroquine. The areas where chloroquine-resistant malaria has been proven are South America, East Asia, the Indian subcontinent, and East and Central Africa. It is probably wise to treat all very severe cases of falciparum malaria initially with parenteral quinine, irrespective of their geographical source of origin. There are three degrees of chloroquine resistance—the patient's fever and parasitaemia respond to chloroquine but parasitaemia reappears within 28 days; the patient's fever responds to treatment but parasitaemia persists from the outset; and neither the fever nor the parasitaemia respond to treatment.

The dose schedules for the oral treatment of *P. falciparum* malaria are shown in *Table* 4.1.

P. VIVAX. The treatment of vivax malaria is a combination of the 3-day course of oral chloroquine (*Table* 4.1) together with a course of oral primaquine in a dose of 7·5 mg twice daily for 14–21 days. Patients should be screened for G–6–PD deficiency before primaquine therapy.

Table 4.1 Dose schedules for the oral treatment of *P. falciparum* malaria

A. Chloroquine-sensitive areas	
Day 1	Chloroquine or Amodiaquine 600 mg (base) Chloroquine or Amodiaquine 300 mg (base) 8 h later
Day 2	Chloroquine or Amodiaquine 300 mg (base)
Day 3	Chloroquine or Amodiaquine 300 mg (base)
Day 4	Chloroquine or Amodiaquine 300 mg (base)
B. Areas resistant to 4-aminoquinolines but sensitive to Fansidar	
Day 6	Quinine (or Quinidine) 600 mg every 8 h for 5 days A single dose of sulphadoxine or sulphalene 1500 mg and pyrimethamine 75 mg (i.e. 3 tablets of Fansidar or Metakelfin)
C. Areas with resistance to both 4-aminoquinolines and Fansidar	
	Quinine (or Quinoline) 600 mg every 8 h for 7 days together with Tetracycline 250 mg every 6 h or (500 mg twice daily) for 7 days

N.B. If parenteral therapy is indicated, expert advice should be sought.

Table 4.2 Chemoprophylaxis of malaria

A. For areas where there is no chloroquine resistance

i. Chloroquine 300 mg (base) once weekly

or

ii. Proguanil 200 mg once daily

B. For areas where chloroquine-resistance occurs

i. Chloroquine 300 mg (base) once weekly, together with Proguanil 200 mg daily

or

ii. Mefloquine 250 mg once weekly

Chemoprophylaxis of Malaria

The details of the regimens are shown in *Table* 4.2. The prophylactic treatment should be started 1 week before departure and continued for 4 weeks after returning from the endemic area.

FILARIASIS

The more common of the several species of filarial parasites transmitted by various arthropod vectors include *Wuchereria bancrofti, Onchocerca volvulus, Brugia malayi* and *Loa loa.* Some of these essentially tropical and subtropical diseases produce elephantiasis of the lower limbs and genitalia due to the occlusion and sclerosis of the lymphatics by the adult worms resulting in gross lymphoedema. Many infestations remain subclinical.

The life history of the various parasites which infest man follow a common pattern although details vary from species to species. The adult male and female worms of an infested person reproduce in the deep tissues. The long, thin larvae are known as microfilariae. These enter the peripheral bloodstream at specific hours depending on the filarial species and the feeding habits of the associated arthropod vector. In the insect (mosquitoes, blackflies, midges, etc.), the microfilariae mature and migrate to the biting structures of the arthropod and thus enter the bloodstream of the next victim of the insect bite. Further maturation occurs in the human where the adult worms congregate into masses causing granulomatous painful swellings, the site of which depends on the species. *Wuchereria bancrofti* is the main cause of elephantiasis and hydrocoele.

Treatment

Chemotherapy with Hetrazan results in destruction of the worms. Prevention includes elimination of sources of the arthropod vectors, the use of screening and insect repellents, and periodic treatment with diethylcarbamazine.

NON-FILARIAL ELEPHANTIASIS

Elephantiasis of the lower limbs has been consistently reported in certain areas of East Africa and Ethiopia where there is no filariasis. Recent studies have shown that these cases of non-filarial elephantiasis of the lower limbs are the result of an obstructive lymphopathy of the peripheral lymphatics caused by aluminosilicate and silica absorbed from the soil through the skin of the feet.

Further Reading

Bell D. R. (1985) *Lecture Notes in Tropical Medicine.* 2nd ed. Oxford, Blackwell.

Gilles H. M. (1984) *Recent Advances in Tropical Medicine.* Edinburgh, Churchill Livingstone.

Jordan P. and Webbe G. (1982) *Schistosomiasis. Epidemiology, Treatment and Control.* London, Heinemann.

Peters W. and Gilles H. M. (1981) *A Colour Atlas of Tropical Medicine and Parasitology.* 8th ed. London, Wolfe Medical Publications.

Saidi F. (1976) *Surgery of Hydatid Disease.* London, Saunders.

Simjee A. E. (1984) Amoebiasis. Infection and tropical disease. *Med. Int.* **4**, p. 137.

5 Specific Infections of Surgical Importance

A. Cuschieri and H. M. Gilles

GAS GANGRENE AND RELATED ANAEROBIC INFECTIONS

Gas Gangrene

Despite the widespread distribution of clostridial spores, gas gangrene is extremely rare in civilian practice (0·1/100 000/annum). Contamination of wounds, which must be a common occurrence, is therefore not usually followed by infection. The essential factor required for spore germination and production of the illness is reduced oxygen tension. This may result from severe contusion and lacerations with necrotic tissue, devitalization of a wound by compression, impaired blood supply, foreign bodies implanted in the depths of a punctured wound such as shrapnel or pieces of clothing (which may cause pressure necrosis and promote pyogenic infection), and soil. This induces tissue necrosis by virtue of its high content of ionizable calcium salts and silicic acid. The oxygen tension of a wound may be further lowered by coexisting infection with pyogenic organisms. Gas gangrene has been reported following injection of adrenaline into the buttocks where the skin is often contaminated by clostridial spores from the patient's own gastrointestinal tract.

Bacteriology

Gas gangrene is a mixed clostridial infection by saccharolytic (pathogenic) and proteolytic (saprophytic) organisms. The true pathogens are *Clostridium perfringens* (*Cl. welchii*), *Cl. novyi* (*Cl. oedematiens*) and *Cl. septicum*. Type A *Cl. perfringens* is the most important human pathogen. It produces the α-toxin which is a lecithinase and breaks down the phospholipid constituents of red cells with the production of severe haemolysis. Other exotoxins produced by some strains of *Cl. perfringens* include haemolysin (θ-toxin), collagenase (κ-toxin), hyaluronidase (μ-toxin) and deoxyribonuclease (ν-toxin).

The exotoxins produce a cellulitis and a progressive myonecrosis. They ferment the muscle carbohydrate with the production of lactic acid and gas (H_2, CO_2). The discharge from the wound is initially odourless. Spread of the necrosis occurs as a result of the exotoxin release and ischaemia from pressure by gas and exudate within tight muscle compartments. The affected area becomes tense, oedematous and crepitant. At first, the dead muscle is odourless and brick-red in colour. Progressive putrefaction by saprophytic clostridia (*Cl. sporogenes*, *Cl. histolyticum*) of the dead muscle mass completes the pathological process with the production of the characteristic 'fishy' odour and the greenish-black appearance of the affected area.

The profound toxaemia is due to the circulating exotoxins which may result in shock, haemolytic anaemia, renal failure and jaundice. The organisms themselves do not invade the bloodstream except as an agonal event and this accounts for the foamy liver and gas bubbles found in other organs in some cases at necropsy.

Clinical Features

The majority of gas gangrene infections are exogenous and result from contamination of large wounds as obtains in agricultural tractor injuries, severe comminuted compound fractures sustained in road traffic accidents and battle casualties. An appreciable number of cases in civilian practice are, however, endogenous in origin and are due to contamination by bowel organisms. In the Western Hemisphere, gas gangrene is most commonly encountered following amputation for peripheral vascular disease. Risk factors in this group include incontinence and diabetes. Other instances of endogenous gas gangrene include criminal abortion and infections following intestinal and less commonly biliary surgery.

The incubation period between the initiating incident and the onset of the clostridial infection varies from 1 day to 4 weeks, and its duration carries an inverse relationship to the severity of the illness and the mortality. The clinical differentiation of clostridial cellulitis from the more severe clostridial myonecrosis has become increasingly inappropriate with earlier diagnosis and the frequent difficulties in distinguishing one from the other on clinical grounds alone. Furthermore, the demonstration of gas by the elicitation of crepitus or by radiography (*Fig.* 5.1) is not essential for the diagnosis as non-gas-forming clostridial infections of wounds are well documented. Indeed the most acceptable and useful clinical classification is into *gas-forming* and *non-gas-forming* clostridial infections. The most important factor which determines whether the infection remains localized and non-crepitant, or becomes invasive with the production of severe toxaemia and gas formation is the presence of dead muscle. Thus the majority of cases following amputation for peripheral vascular disease fall into the gas-forming group, whereas other operations tend to result in wound infection with little if any gas formation.

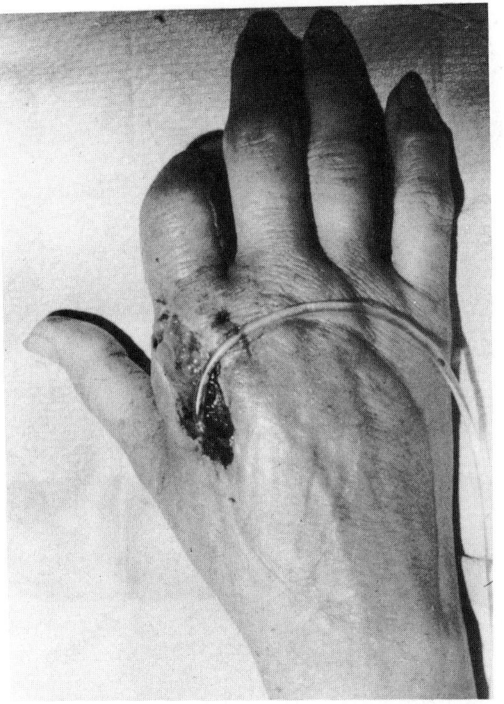

a

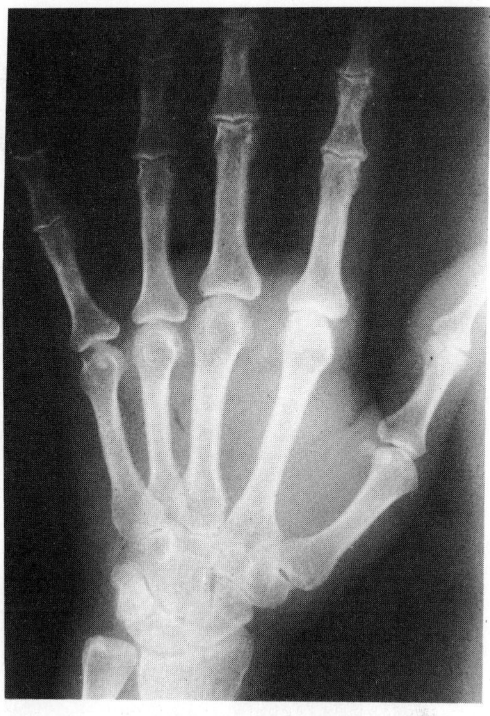

b

Fig. 5.1 *a*, Gas gangrene of the hand. *b*, Radiograph of *the same hand* showing gas in the soft tissues.

Non-gas-forming Infections

The disease is mild and apart from pyrexia, there is minimal, if any, toxicity. The wound is oedematous and erythematous, and may develop a brownish discoloration. Crepitus is absent; pain and tenderness are not severe. The mortality directly attributable to the clostridial infection is negligible.

Gas-forming Infections

The incubation period is usually under three days and the onset is acute. The condition declares itself by severe pain in the region of the wound and the rapid development of toxaemia, drowsiness, fever and tachycardia. The affected area becomes swollen, tense, oedematous and extremely tender. The discharge may be serous or bloodstained. It is variable in amount and is initially odourless but subsequently becomes sweet to foul smelling. Gas is detected by crepitus and by radiological examination. The overlying skin goes through a series of changes from intense white to inflammatory erythema with ecchymosis, bullae formation and frank greenish black gangrene (*Fig.* 5.2). In severe cases jaundice, haemolysis and renal failure develop and often contribute to the death of the patient. The overall mortality

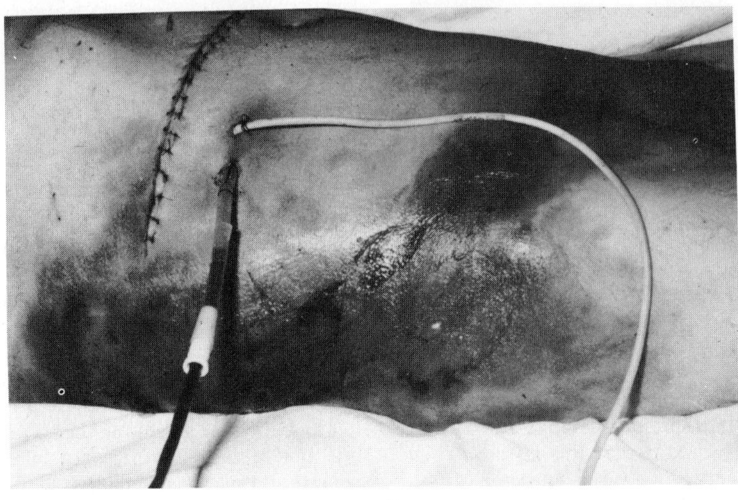

a

Fig. 5.2 *a*, Gas gangrene of the abdominal wall in a patient following exploration of the common bile duct for calculous disease. *(continued over)*

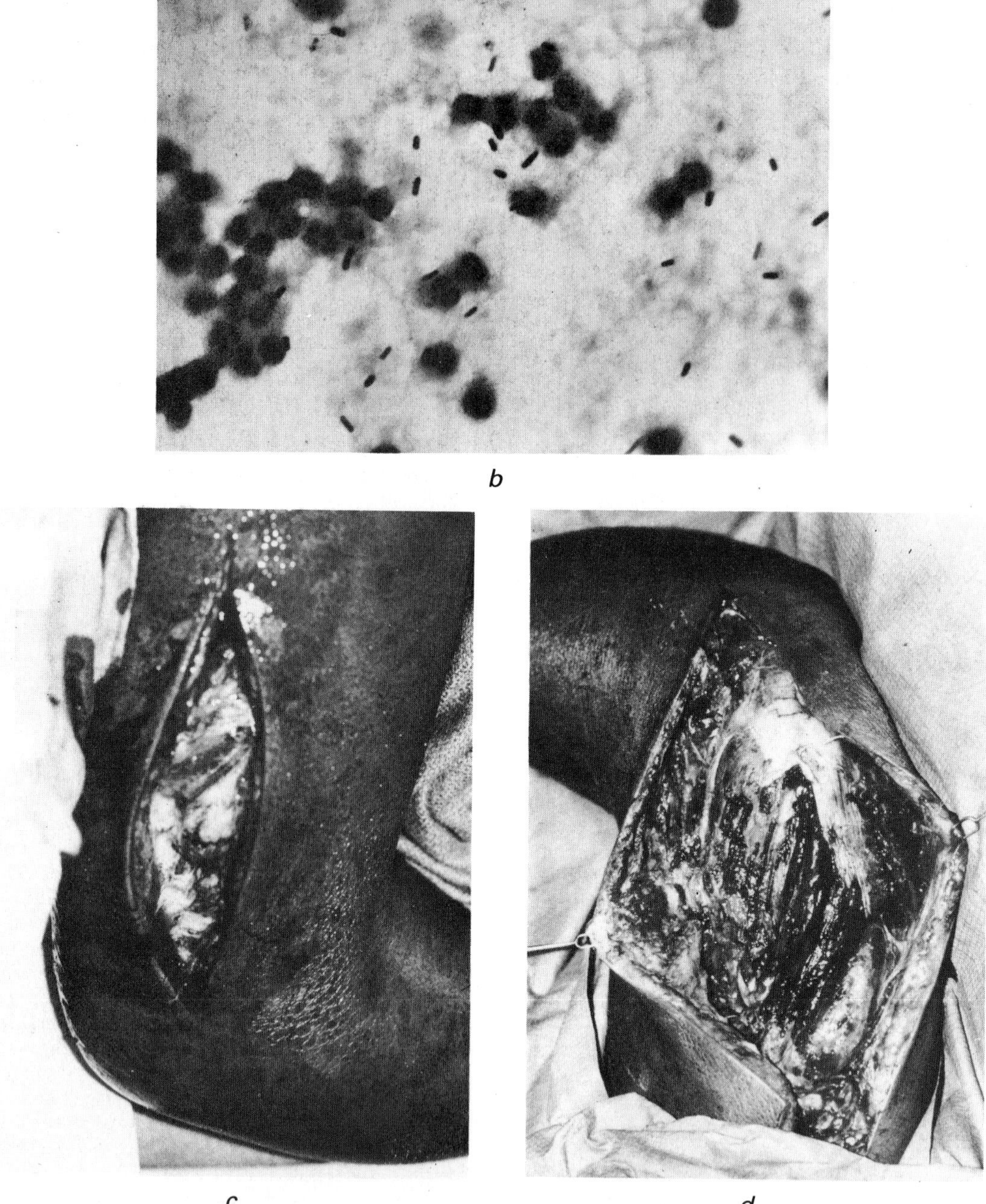

(*Fig. 5.2 continued*) *b*, Microscopy of the needle aspirate from the same patient showing clostridial organisms which were also isolated from the T-tube bile. *c*, Gas gangrene of the upper arm. Note bulging of the oedematous crepitant tissues after incision of the skin. *d*, Same patient as in *c*. Extensive necrosis of the upper arm muscles.

is 40% but the mortality directly due to overwhelming clostridial infection is 11–15%.

Treatment

The treatment of gas gangrene consists of general resuscitative measures for shock and specific therapy: antibiotics, antitoxin, surgical treatment and hyperbaric oxygen (when available).

Antibiotic Therapy

There is now both clinical and experimental evidence to indicate the value of antibiotic therapy in the prophylaxis against gas gangrene both in civilian practice, e.g. amputation for peripheral vascular disease, and in battle casualties. The prophylactic antibiotic therapy must be started before the operation or soon after the injury, and should be continued until healing is complete if the risk is high.

The benefit of antibiotic therapy in established clostridial infection remains doubtful largely because of poor antibiotic penetration into ischaemic tissue. Nevertheless, it still constitutes standard orthodox treatment in these potentially lethal infections, and is certainly beneficial in mixed infections. Initially parenteral benzyl penicillin is administered in large doses (1–2 mega units 4–6-hourly) to all patients except those with a known history of penicillin sensitivity where metronidazole, or clindamycin, or vancomycin, or chloramphenicol are used instead. Tetracycline and erythromycin have moderate activity against most clostridial species but are considered lesser alternatives because of the development of drug resistance. The treatment is continued for a minimum of 7 days and the regimen may have to be altered to suit the bacteriology and sensitivity tests of the individual case.

Surgical Treatment

Surgical treatment should be carried out immediately after resuscitation and is delayed only if facilities for hyperbaric oxygen therapy are availabe (*vide infra*), when operative intervention is postponed until completion of the first hyperbaric treatment. The aim of surgical treatment is the adequate excision of all necrotic tissue regardless of any anatomical defects thus produced. Pus is evacuated and the excised wound is thoroughly irrigated with hydrogen peroxide solution. The aggressive excision of all dead and infected tissue at the first operation is crucial to the survival of the patient. In limb infections, this may necessitate an amputation. No attempt is made to provide primary skin cover, and the wound is packed with gauze soaked in dilute hypochlorite solution. The patient is returned to the operating theatre 24–48 h later for a dressing change under general anaesthesia. Any residual necrotic areas are excised down to bleeding tissues, after which the wound is dressed as before. Reconstructive surgery/skin grating is delayed until the infection has been totally eradicated.

Hyperbaric Oxygen Therapy

Despite the continued controversy there is now sufficient evidence to indicate that hyperbaric oxygen therapy does benefit patients with pure clostridial infections, and may result in rapid improvement in the clinical condition and in limb salvage. Hyperbaric oxygen therapy is started soon after the initial resuscitation and before surgical intervention. It consists of repeated treatments of 1½–2 h at a pressure of 250 h kPa (2·5 atm).

Clostridial Enterocolitis

This results from the ingestion of improperly cooked food contaminated by *Cl. perfringens*. The disease is usually self-limiting and causes severe colicky abdominal pain and diarrhoea. The organism is present in the stool in high counts and can be demonstrated by a Gram-stained smear. Occasionally, the condition is more severe and leads to widespread necrosis of the bowel (primarily the small intestine) and is then referred to as enteritis necrotica. In addition to severe abdominal pain, vomiting and diarrhoea, the patient exhibits signs of peritonitis with profound toxaemia and shock. The condition carries a very high mortality.

NON-CLOSTRIDIAL INFECTIVE GANGRENE

Various clinical syndromes have been described as infective non-clostridial gangrene. The most common causative organisms are anaerobic streptococci but necrotizing infections with *E. coli* and bacteroides are well documented. The most common member of the bacteroides species responsible for infective gangrene is *Fusiformis fusiformis* which is often accompanied by *Borrelia vincentii* although it is doubtful if the latter plays any part in the disease process. These gangrenous conditions usually arise on a background of debility, atherosclerosis and diabetes mellitus. The causative anaerobes often act in association with *Streptococcus pyogenes*, staphylococci and coliform bacilli. However, in some well-documented cases of infective cutaneous and subcutaneous gangrene, a causative organism has not been isolated, despite repeated attempts at culture. In some cases a precipitating factor, e.g. trauma, operation or viral infection, initiates the condition; in others, particularly in diabetic patients, the morbid process arises spontaneously.

A commonly used pathological classification is into *cutaneous* and *subcutaneous* gangrene. In cutaneous gangrene which is also referred to as *progressive bacterial gangrene*, the necrosis is limited to the skin only and systemic signs are minimal or absent. Subcutaneous gangrene is also known as *necrotizing fasciitis*. The necrotic process primarily involves the subcutaneous fat and the deep fascia sparing the underlying muscle layer. Necrosis of the skin is secondary to the development of thrombosis of the perforating vessels as they course through the necrotic infected deeper layers. Subcutaneous gangrene is a serious rapidly spreading condition which is accompanied by toxaemia and may be fatal.

Although the above classification is now well established, it is important to stress that there is a wide spectrum of allied infections, some of which cannot be readily put into either of these two categories. A more embracing and clinically useful classification is shown in *Table 5.1*.

Table 5.1 Non-clostridial gangrene

Cutaneous gangrene (progressive bacterial gangrene)
Subcutaneous gangrene (necrotizing fasciitis)
Meleney's undermining ulcer
Cancrum oris and noma vulva—protein calorie malnutrition
Infected vascular gangrene
Streptococcal myositis
Human bite infection

Meleney's Postoperative Synergistic Gangrene

This is now referred to as progressive bacterial grangrene or synergistic necrotizing cellulitis. It is a cutaneous gangrene due to a synergistic infection with a microaerophilic non-haemophilic streptococcus and *S. aureus* but other synergistic combinations have been reported. It usually follows operative drainage of abscesses although cases unrelated to sepsis have been documented recently, particularly in patients with diabetes mellitus or severe atherosclerosis. The condition consists of a painful, slowly spreading infection of the skin which initially assumes a bright red coloration, subsequently changing to purple and black with the development of gangrene (*Fig.* 5.3). Systemic illness is mild or absent. Treatment is with antibiotics and surgical excision. The most favoured antibiotic combination is benzyl penicillin, metronidazole and gentamicin. Bacteriological specimens (discharge and tissue specimens) should be plated immediately. Surgical treatment should not be delayed and consists of wide excision with delayed skin cover.

Meleney's Chronic Undermining Ulcer

This infection is caused by a haemolytic microaerophilic streptococcus and usually develops after surgery on the intestinal or genital tracts. The infection and necrosis start in the subcutaneous tissues (*Fig.* 5.4) but the disease progressively affects the deeper tissues to involve the pelvis.

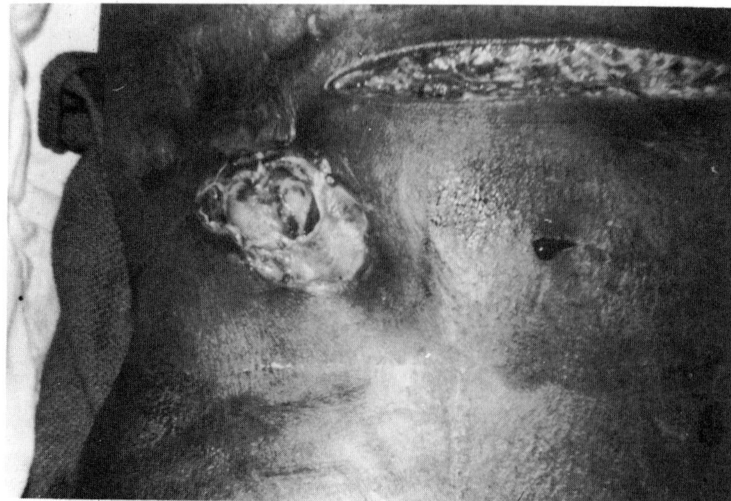

Fig. 5.3 Meleney's postoperative synergistic gangrene. Culture revealed the presence of a *S. aureus* and a microaerophilic non-haemolytic streptococcus.

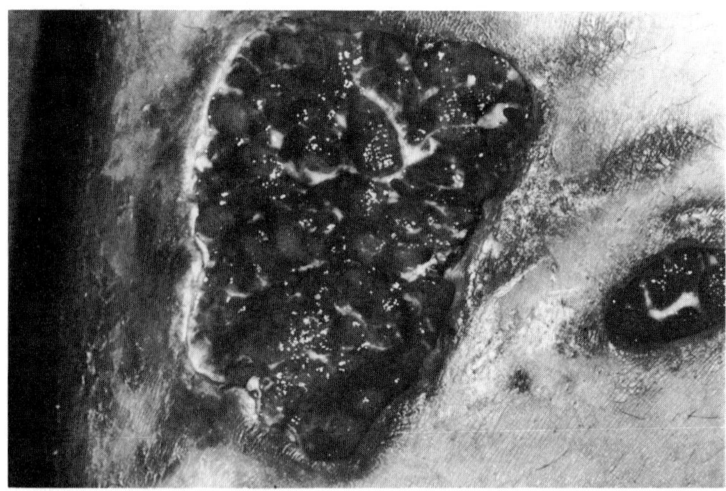

Fig. 5.4 Meleney's chronic undermining ulcers in the right iliac fossa in a renal transplant patient.

Treatment is with a combination of benzyl penicillin and metronidazole together with surgical excision and delayed skin cover.

Cancrum Oris and Noma Vulva

These are instances of mucocutaneous gangrene affecting the mouth (cancrum oris) or the vulva (noma vulva). They arise on a background of malnutrition in children, and are usually preceded by an infectious illness, such as measles. The infection is often a mixed one, but the protagonists are either anaerobic streptococci or members of the bacteroides species. The disease results in a slow but relentless necrosis of the perioral (or vulval tissues), and death may result from inhalation pneumonia. In addition to the appropriate antibiotic treatment, correction of the underlying malnutrition is essential. Surgical excision of the necrotic tissue is necessary. Skin cover and plastic reconstruction are delayed until the infection has been cleared and the patient's nutritional status is improved.

Necrotizing Fasciitis

This subcutaneous gangrene is also known as haemolytic streptococcal gangrene, hospital gangrene and gangrenous erysipelas. It includes such conditions as perineal phlegmon (*Fig.* 5.5) and Fournier's scrotal gangrene (*Fig.* 5.6). It is caused by haemolytic streptococci and less commonly by haemolytic staphylococci. Various other organisms have been identified in some of these infections including coliforms, bacteroides, diphtheroids and pseudomonas. Most commonly, the condition arises following surgery or trauma. Spontaneous cases have been described although in some of these patients, the preceding trauma may have been so slight as to be ignored or forgotten by the patient. The most commonly affected sites are the extremities, followed by the lower trunk including the external genitalia and perineum.

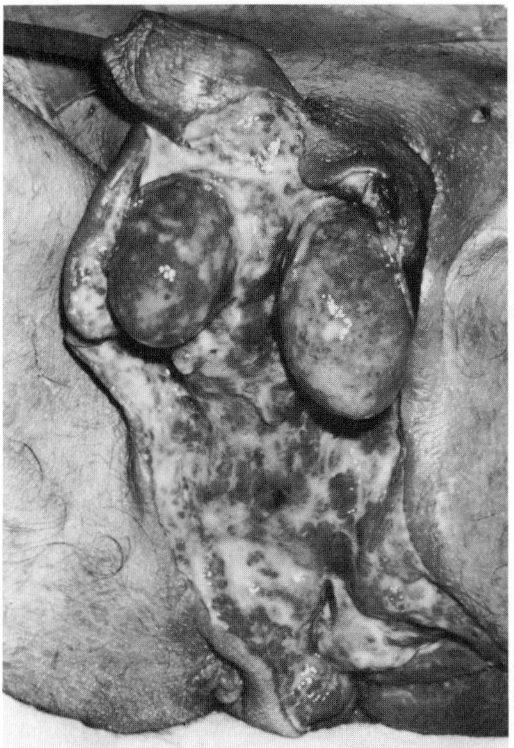

Fig. 5.5 Extensive perineal phlegmon involving the skin of the scrotum and proximal part of the penile shaft.

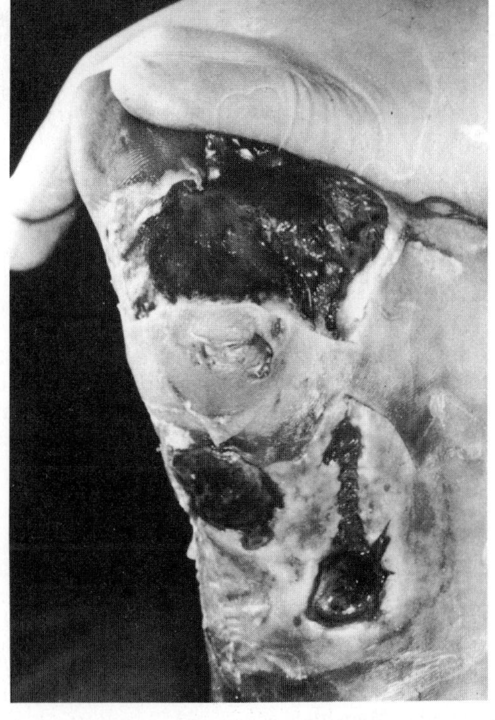

Fig. 5.7 Necrotizing fasciitis of the sole of the foot.

The exact mechanism for the subcutaneous necrosis is unknown but appears to be related to the binding of the mucopeptide fraction of the bacterial cell wall with dermal collagen. The necrosis never involves the muscle layer and skin involvement is secondary to thrombosis of the perforating vessels coursing through the infected necrotic area.

The disease is always serious and carries a definite mortality. The affected part is initially very painful but then becomes numb due to involvement of the sensory nerve fibres. The process spreads rapidly through the subcutaneous fatty/fascial plane with reddish discoloration, inflammatory oedema (sometimes bullous), necrosis, and eventual sloughing of the underlying skin (*Fig.* 5.7). Systemic manifestations are often present and the toxaemia may be severe with pyrexia, tachycardia and shock. Blood cultures should always be taken in these patients.

Treatment includes resuscitation with intravenous crystalloid solutions/plasma expanders/blood, antibiotic therapy

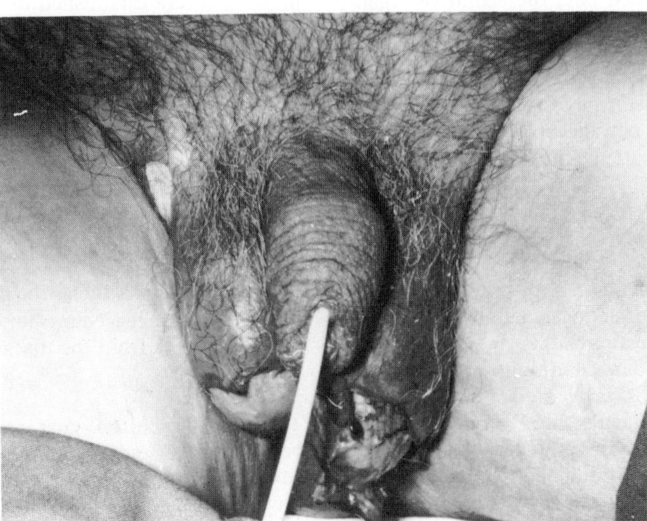

Fig. 5.6 Fournier's gangrene (necrotizing fasciitis) with partial necrosis of the scrotal skin.

using a triple regimen (benzyl penicillin, metronidazole and an aminoglycoside), and early wide surgical excision/drainage along the lines described in the gas gangrene section of this chapter.

OTHER NON-CLOSTRIDIAL ANAEROBIC INFECTIONS

These may arise spontaneously or follow amputations for peripheral vascular disease, trauma or intestinal surgery. They include *infected vascular gangrene,* and *streptococcal myositis.* A significant percentage of the reported cases have occurred in diabetic patients. The majority are serious infections with profound toxaemia and extensive gangrene with gas formation. The overall reported mortality is 30–35%. No benefit has been reported from hyperbaric oxygen in anaerobic non-clostridial wound infections and the mainstays of treatment are general resuscitative measures, antibiotics and early surgical excision with delayed skin cover.

Infected Vascular Gangrene

This has a gradual onset. The affected part (usually foot) becomes painful, swollen, black and foul smelling. Radiographs show extensive gas formation in the tissues of the involved foot. The infection is a mixed one with faecal organisms, most commonly *B. fragilis* and *Peptostreptococcus.* Toxaemia is usually mild.

Streptococcal Myositis

The onset may be subacute or insidious. Once established, the infection is always severe with profound toxaemia. There is marked swelling and severe pain in the affected part. The skin often assumes a copper tinge. The discharge is profuse and seropurulent. Gas formation, though present, is slight and the inflamed part has a slight sour smell. The muscle layers become oedematous but necrosis is not a significant feature.

HUMAN BITE INFECTIONS

The anaerobic infections caused by human bites can be particularly virulent and cause marked tissue destruction. The infection is usually a mixed one, the causative organisms being a combination of two or more of the following: *B. melaninogenicus, Fusobacterium spp.*, anaerobic cocci and spirochetes. The antibiotic of choice is penicillin which is administered in high dosage. It is rare for amputation of the affected digit to be necessary nowadays. The importance of tetanus prophylaxis in these patients must not be forgotten.

TETANUS

In the vast majority of cases tetanus is an exogenous infection, although rare instances of endogenous infections have been reported after septic abortion and surgical operations on the gastrointestinal tract. The conditions governing the germination of the spores of *Cl. tetani* are identical to those of gas gangrene and necessitate the local production of a reduced oxygen tension. The most common portal of entry worldwide is the umbilical stump following the application of dung to this region in newborn babies which is practised in some developing countries. Elsewhere the lower limbs constitute the commonest site of entry. Usually the wound is a minor one but is always penetrating in nature. In some 25% of cases in the West, the portal of entry is not evident at the time of diagnosis. Other sources of infection include piercing of the ear lobes, tattooing, burns, parenteral injections including vaccination, skin lesions, especially leg ulcers and those which lead to scratching, nasal foreign bodies and ear infections. The disease is well recognized in drug addicts.

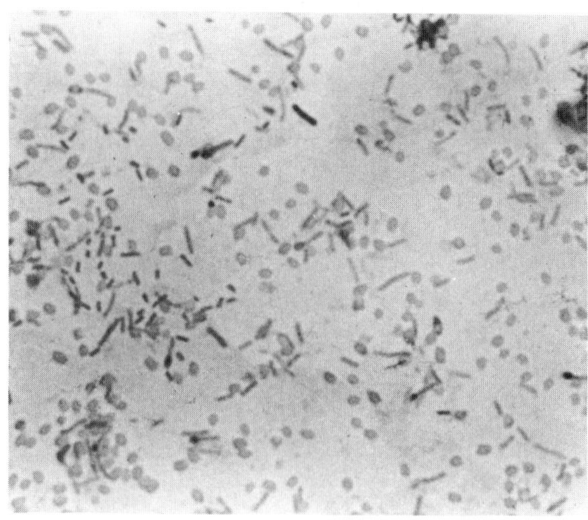

Fig. 5.8 Clostridium tetani organisms.

Cl. tetani (Fig. 5.8) produces two exotoxins. The most important is a neurotoxin called tetanospasmin which is responsible for the disease. A haemolytic toxin called tetanolysin has been separated from tetanospasmin. The second toxin acts on the peripheral neuromuscular junctions but does not play a significant role in the production of tetanus. Tetanospasmin reaches the central nervous system along the axons of motor nerve trunks, probably in the tissue spaces between the nerve fibres, and acts by blocking the inhibitory impulses at motor synapses. This results in two forms of contractions of striated smooth muscle: tonic (spasm) characteristic of early disease and clonic (convulsions) which indicate severe established disease.

The overall mortality of tetanus is 10–15%. Adverse factors include extremes of age, short incubation period, type of injury and severity of the illness. Thus, whereas mild to moderate tetanus carries a small mortality, death from the disease occurs in 30–40% of patients with severe tetanus. Death usually results from asphyxia from involvement of the muscles of respiration and cardiovascular complications resulting from sympathetic overactivity.

Clinical Features

Neonatal tetanus is by far the commonest type in developing countries where it accounts for 70% of cases. It is best considered separately from the disease in children and adults.

Neonatal Tetanus

The clinical picture is characteristic and the disease usually becomes manifest on the eighth day, hence the popular name 'eight-day disease'. It starts with a failure to suckle on the 3rd day. This is followed quickly by spasm of the facial muscles (risus sardonicus) and masseter (lock jaw) and progression to generalized clonic spasms with flexion of the arms, clenched fists, extension of the lower limbs and plantar flexion of the toes.

Children and Adults

The majority of patients (95%) who develop tetanus have not previously been immunized. The incubation period ranges from 4 to 10 days, the shorter the interval the more severe the disease. The progress of the disease (the time from the first symptom to the onset of tetanus) varies according to the severity of the disease but the full blown picture is reached by the 3rd day in 70% of cases.

The condition declares itself by stiffness, twitching and cramps limited to the same spinal segment as the area of infection (local tetanus). Other early symptoms and signs include muscle pains, headaches, irritability and restlessness, constipation, sweating and tachycardia. This is followed by the development of spasm of the masseter muscles, facial musculature and the muscles of deglutition (dysphagia). In the full blown picture, there are generalized clonic convulsions which may be triggered by mild external stimuli (sound, movement of personnel etc.). As the extensor muscles are more powerful than the flexor muscles, the patient classically assumes a position of opisthotonos. It is characteristic of tetanus that the muscles do not relax between convulsive attacks, and this distinguishes tetanic convulsions from those caused by strychnine poisoning.

Tetanus is nowadays classified into mild (no dysphagia or respiratory distress), moderate (presence of dysphagia and respiratory distress) and severe which is accompanied by gross spasticity and major spasms.

Treatment

Prophylaxis

The best method of preventing the disease is by active immunization with tetanus toxoid (a formolized preparation of the exotoxin adsorbed on to aluminium hydroxide or phosphate). Three injections are administered, with the second injection 6 weeks after the first, and the third injection 6–12 months after the second. A booster injection is given at 10-year intervals and at times of wounding. Booster toxoid injections are not necessary if a patient sustains a wound within 5 years of completion of an active immunization course or booster dose. However, if the period since the last toxoid injection exceeds 5 years, but is less than 10 years, a booster should be administered. In the absence of a history of active immunization, or if the period since the last toxoid injection exceeds 10 years, passive immunization with human tetanus immunoglobulin (tetanus immune globulin, TIG) in a dose of 250 u intramuscularly is indicated. This single dose provides adequate immunity for about 4 weeks. If the wound is not healed by this time, a second injection is administered. Active immunization with toxoid should be started at the same time using a different limb in those not previously immunized, or a single booster dose of toxoid is administered to those patients who had allowed their active immunity to lapse for more than 10 years. The use of equine antitetanic serum (ATS) is no longer justified because of its questionable value and the risks of serum sickness and anaphylactic reactions.

Treatment of the Established Disease

Specific measures include surgical attention to the wound (if present) with excision and open packing with antibiotic and hydrogen peroxide. Benzyl penicillin is administered in a dose of 1 mega unit every 4 h for 7 days, and human tetanus immunoglobulin is given in a dose of 2000–4000 u intramuscularly. In a recent study metronidazole (500 mg orally 6-hourly or 1 g rectally by suppository 8-hourly) was found to be more effective than procaine penicillin. In neonatal tetanus good results have been obtained with intrathecal TIG and prednisolone. For mild tetanus, the patient only requires sedation with diazepam. Tracheostomy and sedation is necessary for patients with moderate tetanus. In severe disease, the patient is curarized and kept on carefully monitored intermittent positive-pressure ventilation. The very severe cases with sympathetic overactivity and cardiovascular complications (tachycardia, labile hypertension, vasoconstriction, myocardial instability) require anaesthesia, mechanical ventilation and adrenergic blockade.

CHRONIC BACTERIAL INFECTIONS

These are produced by the species of the order *Actinomycetales*, so named because the bacterial cells may branch to form hyphae. With some species (*Actinomyces israelii*) this branching tendency is marked and simulates the appearances of a fungal growth (*actino* = radial, *myces* = fungus). The composition of the order *Actinomycetales* is shown in *Table 5.2*.

Streptomycetaceae are not pathogenic to man. The genus *Streptomyces* is, however, of medical importance as it contains numerous species valuable for the production of antibiotics (streptomycin, tetramycin, etc.). Most species of *Nocardia* are harmless and live on decaying organic matter in the soil. A few species, e.g. *Nocardia asteroides* can cause an infection of the lung which is often fatal and may be mistaken for tuberculosis. Other species (*N. madurae*, *N. brasiliensis*) are known to produce a chronic disease of hands or feet similar to actinomycosis.

Tuberculosis

In conjunction with all the mycobacteria, the tubercle bacilli are non-sporing, immobile, aerobic and Gram positive. Differential staining methods are used to identify the mycobacteria as after heat staining with carbol fuchsin, these bacteria, with the exception of some *Nocardia* species, are unique in resisting decolorization after treatment with strong acids and alcohol (acid fast).

There are several strains of non-pathogenic saprophytes in the soil and on plants (e.g. *M. phlei*) and on the human skin (*M. smegmatis*). The pathogenic status of several other species is still not fully clarified but some are often found in tuberculosis-like pulmonary disorders or in association with established tuberculosis. They are referred to variously as

Table 5.2 The actinomycetales

Order	*Family*	*Genus*	*Species (pathogenic)*
Actinomycetales	Mycobacteriaceae	Mycobacterium	M. tuberculosis M. leprae
	Actinomycetaceae	Actinomyces Nocardia	A. israelii N. asteroides N. madurae
	Streptomycetaceae	Streptomyces	—

atypical, environmental, anonymous, or MOTT (Mycobacteria Other than Typical Tubercle) to differentiate them from the established pathogens, e.g. *M. tuberculosis* and *M. bovis*.

The precise differentiation of the various mycobacteria is obviously important. Culture is usually performed on the Löwenstein–Jensen medium and requires 6 weeks although faster growth can be obtained in Dubos medium. No single test is said to be reliable in the identification of *M. tuberculosis* and *M. bovis*, although tests for virulence in guinea pigs (*M. tuberculosis*) and rabbits (*M. bovis*) are amongst the most reliable of the diagnostic tests. *M. tuberculosis* is the only species known to produce niacin on culture.

Following the eradication of tuberculous herds and the introduction of pasteurization of milk, bovine tuberculosis is rarely encountered in the Western Hemisphere and most of the reported fatal cases are pulmonary infections. The vast majority of cases in these countries are caused by *M. tuberculosis*, usually as a result of inhalation of organisms present in fresh droplets or dust contaminated with dried sputum by a patient with open pulmonary tuberculosis. Both bovine and human infections are still common in economically deprived areas, such as parts of the African continent, Latin America and India.

Pathology

It has been estimated that 90% of all tuberculous infections involve the lungs, but the infection may affect practically any organ or tissue. The commonly recognized extrapulmonary infections include tuberculosis of the skin, lymph nodes, bones and joints, genito-urinary system, abdomen and intestines, and CNS.

Tuberculous lesions assume one of two forms: the proliferative and the exudative. The more common proliferative lesion which is usually encountered in the lungs and solid organs is the tubercle follicle. This consists of an area of coagulative necrosis (caseation) due primarily to hypersensitivity to the tuberculoprotein, surrounded by epithelioid and Langhans giant cells (both derived from macrophages), and an outer zone of small round cells consisting mainly of lymphocytes and fibroblasts.

The exudative form of tuberculosis is typically encountered in infections of serous cavities, e.g. tuberculous pleurisy/peritonitis, and epithelial surfaces (sterile pyuria in renal tuberculosis). It results in the formation of a cellular exudate rich in fibrin together with a dense infiltration of the tissue with lymphocytes.

Childhood tuberculosis is characterized by marked involvement of the regional lymph nodes, as exemplified by the primary complex (Ghon focus at the periphery of the lung midzone and hilar lymphadenopathy), and tabes mesenterica where a small focus in the intestine is associated with marked enlargement of the mesenteric lymph nodes which at times rupture causing tuberculous peritonitis. By contrast in the adult, lymph-node enlargement is not marked and the disease either heals by fibrosis or extends locally by caseation, liquefaction and cavitation, with little tendency to bloodstream dissemination. This altered tissue response in the adult is no longer thought to be due to previous exposure to the tubercle bacillus, and appears to be the result of tissue maturation.

Softening and liquefaction of the caseous material underlies the development of tuberculous 'cold abscess'. The liquefied debris may track along fascial planes as in the psoas abscess originating from spinal tuberculosis (*Fig.* 5.9), or point to the surface with the eventual formation of tuberculous sinuses, e.g. collar-stud abscess in the neck from tuberculous lymphadenitis, and scrotal sinuses from tuberculous epididymitis.

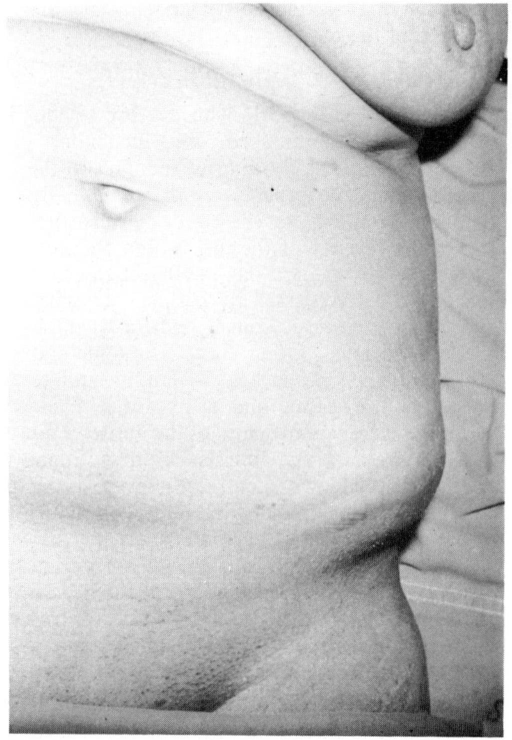

a

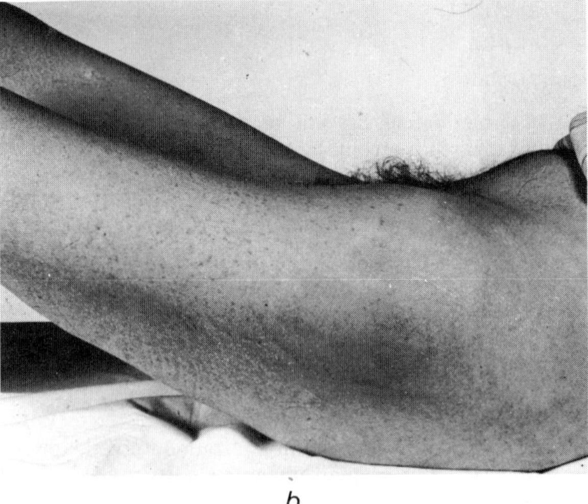

b

Fig. 5.9 *a*, Tuberculous abscess in the left iliac fossa. *b*, Tuberculous abscess due to spinal disease extending behind the inguinal ligament into the femoral triangle.

Involvement of a pulmonary vein by a tuberculous focus in the lung may lead to bloodstream dissemination and miliary tuberculosis, especially if resistance is lowered by poor nutrition, debility, old age, disease and immunosuppressive drugs such as steroids. If the bloodstream inoculum is small, the bacilli may be destroyed by the cells of the reticuloendothelial system. Failing this, they may either produce metastatic disease immediately or remain quiescent with reactivation some years later. These lesions are referred to as 'local metastatic tuberculosis' and account for the majority of tuberculous infections encountered in surgical practice.

Clinical Features

The general symptoms of active tuberculous infections include malaise, asthenia, weight loss, mild fever and night sweats. The symptomatology is, however, extremely varied and the disease can simulate many other disorders.

Tuberculosis is a disease of malnutrition and overcrowding. Other predisposing factors include poor general health, chronic disease, silicosis, and diabetes. Certain ethnic groups such as the Australian aborigines, black Africans and the American Indians, are particularly susceptible.

Allergy (Hypersensitivity) and Acquired Immunity

Tuberculous infection, subclinical or otherwise, results in the development of a cell-mediated allergy (delayed hypersensitivity) to tuberculoprotein which causes caseation and an accelerated macrophage response. This hypersensitivity which indicates present or past infection, can be determined by the tuberculin skin reaction which consists of the intracutaneous injection of Purified Protein Derivative (PPD) which is derived from and has replaced Koch's Old Tuberculin (OT). The delayed hypersensitivity, although closely related to, is not the mechanism of the acquired immunity to tuberculosis. This immunity which is only partial, is cell mediated by sensitized lymphocytes. Active immunization with BCG (Bacille Calmette–Guérin) is generally recommended for tuberculin-negative individuals. Complications of BCG inoculations are rare and include local abscess formation, regional lymphadenitis and, rarely, systemic infection with progressive pulmonary disease. The latter has been reported following attempts at immunotherapy with BCG in patients with malignant disease.

Treatment

Effective modern chemotherapy is followed by an almost universal cure rate without the necessity for long-term follow-up. It has eliminated the need for sanatorium management. The drugs available include streptomycin, para-aminosalicylic acid (PAS), isoniazid, rifampicin, pyrazinamide and ethambutol (Chapter 39).

Leprosy

It is estimated that 15 million people in the world have leprosy. Leprosy is common throughout most of Africa, Southern Asia, the Far East, and South and Central America. There are about 400 active cases registered in the UK. However, no case of indigenously contracted leprosy has been reported in Britain.

M. leprae, the causative organism, is a slender and acid-fast rod, occurring either singly or in clusters (globi) in the reticuloendothelial cells. This slowly multiplying organism has been grown in the foot pads of mice and the armadillo, but not in an artificial culture medium. The infectivity of leprosy is a function of the concentration of leprosy bacilli in the body of the patient, and the chances of viable bacilli emerging and remaining viable and pathogenic to susceptible contacts. Leprosy is not a very contagious disease. The disease is frequently contracted in childhood or adolescence, revealing itself in symptoms and signs some years later. This silent period is commonly 2–5 years, and often longer. Bacilli-laden nasal discharge is probably the main source of infection, but bacilliferous ulcerations, sweaty, hairy skin and maternal milk may contain viable bacilli. Infection may be acquired by inhalation or through abrasions in the skin.

Pathology

The pathological lesions depend on the type and extent of the immune response. If cell-mediated immunity is strong, *tuberculoid* lesions form. The reaction consists of a non-specific accumulation of giant cells, epthelioid cells, histiocytes and lymphocytes. Lymphocytic infiltrations are observed around and within nerve bundles. Bacilli are scanty and the lepromin test is positive.

When cell-mediated immunity is depressed, *lepromatous* leprosy results. The whole dermis is replaced by highly bacilliferous tissue that invades the adnexa and eventually destroys superficial nerves, pigment-forming cells, sweat and sebaceous glands and hair follicles. The target tissues are the Schwann cells, endothelial cells and muscle cells. Bacilli may be also found in the liver, bone marrow, spleen, kidneys and lungs.

Acute vasculitis, caused by immune complexes, may give rise to erythema nodosum leprosum, or other manifestations such as iritis, neuritis, orchitis, lymphadenitis and myositis. Longstanding untreated lepromatous leprosy can result in chronic nephritis and amyloidosis.

Clinical Features

Leprosy encompasses a whole spectrum of disease in between the two main types: lepromatous and tuberculoid. The earliest manifestation which is qualified as indeterminate, consists of a small, hypopigmented macule (2–5 cm) appearing anywhere in the body and often healing spontaneously. Determinate lesions that progress to clinical disease may arise out of indeterminate ones or *de novo*. Their subsequent features will depend on whether the disease is predominantly tuberculoid or lepromatous in nature.

Tuberculoid Leprosy

In this type (*Fig.* 5.10), there are a few or solitary skin lesions measuring 2–5 cm in diameter, often with a raised edge. The lesions are dry, hairless and anaesthetic. They are hypopigmented in dark-skinned and coppery in white-skinned individuals. Local or distant cutaneous nerve thickening occurs. The commonest sites of nerve involvement are the ulnar nerve at the elbow, the median at the wrist, the common peroneal in the popliteal fossa, the posterior tibial around the medial malleolus, and the greater auricular over the sternomastoid muscle. Sensory, motor and autonomic nerve trunks are affected. Nerve damage occurs early in tuberculoid leprosy.

Lepromatous Leprosy

This presents as a widespread symmetrical macular rash, slightly hypopigmented or erythematous, affecting the face, extensor surface of the limbs and the upper trunk. The midline of the back, the axillae, groins and scalp are usually spared. There is congestion of and discharge from the nose, the mucosa of which is thickened and yellow. Iritis may occur.

As the disease progresses, the skin, especially of the face, becomes thickened and nodular with thinning or loss of the eyebrows (*Fig.* 5.11). Symmetrical enlargements of the peripheral nerves occurs, with widespread peripheral anaesthesia and muscular weakness. Painless neuropathic ulceration, absorption of the extremities of the digits, wrist drop, foot drop and claw hand occur (*Fig.* 5.12). Nerve damage is

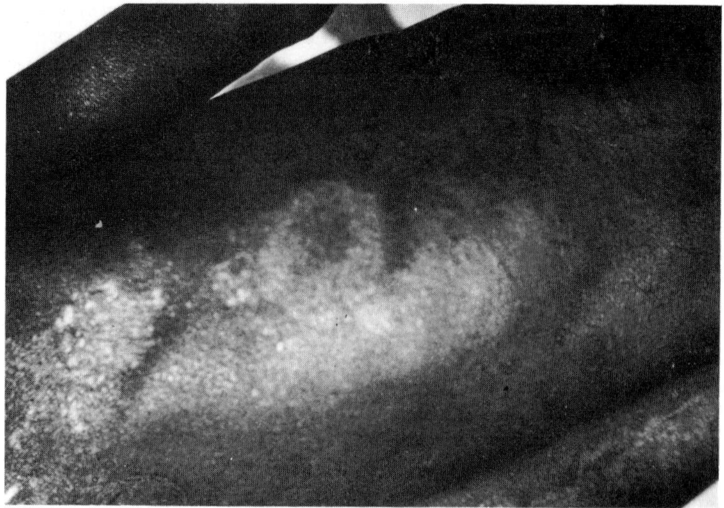

Fig. 5.10 Tuberculoid leprosy.

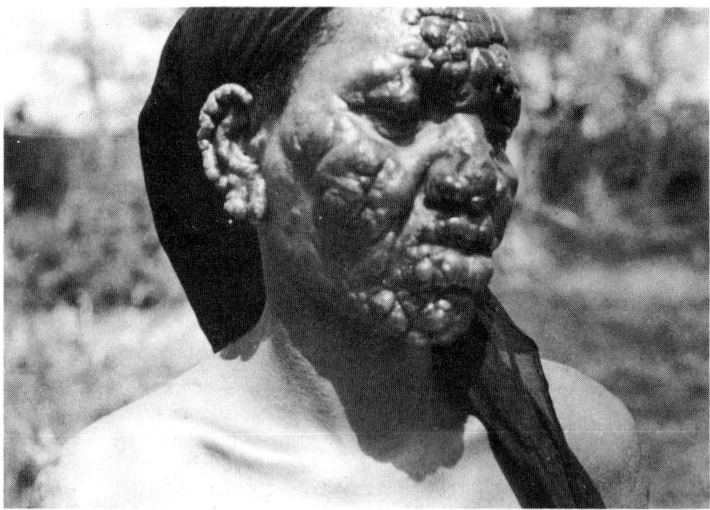

Fig. 5.11 Lepromatous leprosy.

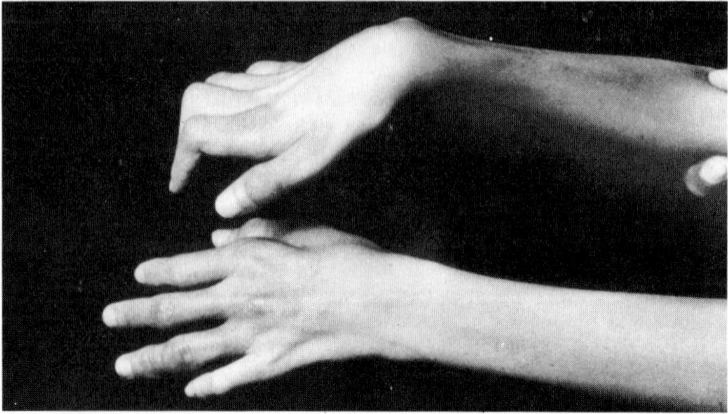

Fig. 5.12 Claw hand in advanced tuberculoid leprosy. With early treatment this lesion should never be seen.

observed late in lepromatous leprosy. Although acute exacerbations are found in all kinds of leprosy, they are most serious in the lepromatous type. An acute relapse is often heralded by an attack of erythema nodosum leprosum, and manifests widespread sensitivity phenomena in the skin, uveal tract, nerves, lymph nodes and joints.

Borderline Leprosy

The presenting features are not typical of either the tuberculoid or lepromatous disease. The disease may be arrested at this stage or progress in either direction. In *borderline tuberculoid leprosy* the lesions are more numerous and varied than in the pure tuberculoid disease. The peripheral nerves are thickened and sensation is impaired. It is a common presentation in Africans. Asian and European patients usually present with *borderline lepromatous leprosy*. Symmetry of the skin lesions is less constant while the nodules are often discrete, red and fleshy. Early nerve damage is found.

The possibility of leprosy should always be remembered when an individual who resided for some time in an endemic area, or comes from the tropics/subtropics, complains of a chronic non-itching patch in the skin that does not respond to treatment. The presence of diminished cutaneous sensation within an area of hypopigmentation makes the diagnosis more likely. Similarly, if the patient presents with an ulcer on the sole of the foot, or complains either of neurological symptoms which do not fit into a well-organized pattern, or of signs of damage to a peripheral nerve, particularly the ulnar or the posterior tibial, accompanied by a skin rash; then leprosy must be seriously considered as a diagnosis.

Examination of dermal material obtained by the slit-scrape method reveals numerous bacilli in lepromatous or borderline lepromatous leprosy, while in paucibacillary disease (tuberculoid and borderline tuberculoid) bacteria are scanty and difficult to demonstrate. The smear is made by pinching the skin firmly, e.g. of the ear lobe or suspected lesion, then making a small stab incision into the dermis, and scraping it with the turned blade. Tissue juice, free of blood, is placed on a slide, dried and stained with a modified Ziehl–Neelsen's method. Bacilli are also often found in the nasal discharge. Histological examination confirms the diagnosis.

Treatment

Time, sympathy and reassurance to the patient and his relatives are important. There is still a good deal of unjustified stigma associated with the diagnosis of leprosy.

Multibacillary Disease

The treatment of lepromatous and borderline lepromatous leprosy entails the administration of three drugs to minimize the development of dapsone resistance which is becoming increasingly common. The regimen consists of: (i) Rifampicin 600 mg once monthly, supervised with (ii) Dapsone 100 mg daily, self-administered, and (iii) Clofazimine 50 mg daily, self-administered together with 300 mg monthly, supervised. Where clofazimine is unacceptable because of its effects on skin colour, it should be replaced with ethionamide 250 mg self-administered. This triple drug combination should be given for a minimum of 2 years, and whenever possible until each patient with multibacillary disease has achieved skin smear negativity.

Paucibacillary Disease

Tuberculoid and borderline tuberculoid leprosy are treated with: (i) Rifampicin 600 mg once monthly, supervised for 6 months, and (ii) Dapsone 100 mg daily, self-administered for 6 months.

The education of the patient who has some degree of motor or sensory deficit will help to prevent much of the damage that results from unappreciated trauma. Judicious physiotherapy will help to maintain muscle tone and power, and preserve useful function. The services of a chiropodist will reduce the likelihood of ulceration developing in an anaesthetic foot. Surgical correction may be necessary for established deformities of the hands, feet or face. Patients suffering from lepromatous or borderline lepromatous leprosy are liable to develop serious eye complications, particularly iridocyclitis which has an insidious and painless onset. Regular checks by an ophthalmologist are therefore advisable.

Acute exacerbations in multibacillary disease require hospitalization with complete physical and mental rest. If symptoms are not relieved by aspirin 0·6 g three times daily, chlorpromazine is adminstered for 5 days. Patients with severe symptoms or those who develop new erythema nodosum leprosum lesions require treatment with corticosteroids or clofazimine or thalidomide:

1. Prednisolone. This is administered in a dose of 30 mg daily until the acute manifestations are controlled. Thereafter the dose is reduced rapidly and then stopped usually within 4 weeks of the start of the treatment. An alternative regimen involves commencing with a daily dose of 5 mg, increasing by 5 mg/day until the manifestations are completely controlled. This dose is then maintained for 7 days, and then gradually reduced. If new lesions appear during this process, the prednisolone dose is increased just sufficiently to control the symptoms, and then maintained at this level for a further week before slow reduction is resumed.

2. Clofazimine. When this drug is used in the treatment of multibacillary disease, the risks of acute exacerbation developing are considerably reduced. In the treatment of the established reactional episode, clofazimine is given in a daily dose of 100 mg, rising to 200 or even 300 mg/day until the acute signs and symptoms are controlled. Then the dose is gradually reduced until 100 mg every other day is being administered. Prednisolone and clofazimine may be given together in severe cases. A dose of 300 mg of clofazimine cannot be extended beyond 4 weeks.

3. Thalidomide. This is an extremely useful drug where its use is legally permitted. A dose of 400 mg/day will control even severe symptoms.

Ideally those who have been exposed to a patient suffering from leprosy, especially the multibacillary variety, and in particular where the source case has been untreated for some time or inadequately treated, should be examined every 3 months for several years; this applies particularly to children and to adults who share the same sleeping quarters as the parents. The evidence at present suggests that BCG vaccination will enhance any existing innate resistance to leprosy challenge. BCG should therefore be offered to any child and young adult who are not strongly tuberculin positive and who have been in close contact with a patient suffering from leprosy.

Dapsone given prophylactically for a lengthy period to individuals who were in close contact with a case of infectious leprosy will confer some protection against the development of the disease. Hence prophylactic dapsone should be recommended to those who have been in prolonged and intimate contact with a previously undiagnosed patient. The oral prophylactic dose of dapsone is as follows:

Up to 4 years, 25 mg/week; 4–7 years, 50 mg/week; 7–12 years, 75 mg/week; 12–15 years, 100 mg/week; and over 15 years, 200 mg/week.

Actinomycosis

This is a rare chronic infection caused by *Actinomyces israelii*, most commonly in the region of the lower jaw (cervicofacial). The disease is characterized by the formation of loculated abscesses with marked induration and sinus formation (*Fig.* 5.13).

Pathogenesis

Actinomyces israelii occurs as a normal commensal in the human mouth. The organism is anaerobic and Gram positive but not acid fast. Although the precise conditions governing the development of this endogenous infection are not known, the disease often follows trauma, such as extraction of a carious tooth. The traumatic implantation of the organism appears necessary for the genesis of the disease and cases following human bites or penetrating hand injuries resulting from violent contact with human teeth (punch actinomycosis) are well documented. The disease starts as an area of acute suppurative inflammation which persists as a chronic process with the formation of multiple loculated abscess cavities surrounded with dense fibrosis. Colonies of the organism occur in the pus as small, greyish-yellow granules (sulphur granules), and consist of a densely felted mass of filaments surrounded by radially disposed club shaped excrescences (*Fig.* 5.14). These clubs are not formed during artificial culture.

The disease spreads mainly by direct contact with considerable destruction of tissue and multiple sinus formation. Bloodborne spread is important as exemplified by the spread of ileocaecal actinomycosis via the portal vein to the liver, with the development of multiple intercommunicating loculated liver abscesses (honeycomb liver). Pulmonary infection may also disseminate via the bloodstream to other organs such as bones, kidneys and CNS.

In most instances, actinomycosis starts in the cervicofacial region (70%). In other instances, the primary infection

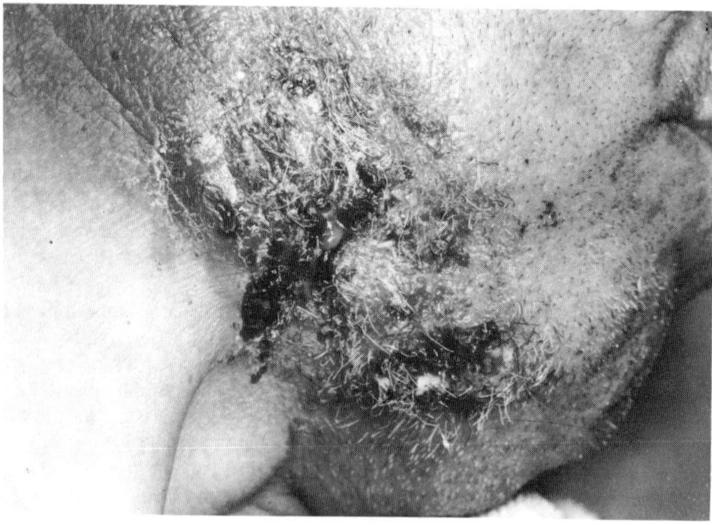

Fig. 5.13 Cervicofacial actinomycosis.

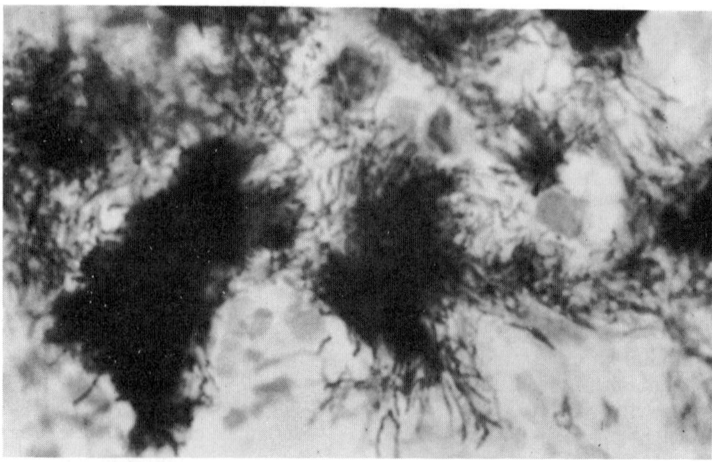

Fig. 5.14 Microscopy of the sulphur granules from a patient with cervicofacial actinomycosis.

occurs in the ileocaecal region (20%), or lungs (10%). Ileocaecal actinomycosis is discussed in Chapter 72 and pulmonary actinomycosis in Chapter 39.

Treatment

The organism has a wide spectrum of sensitivity to commonly used antibiotics, such a penicillin and lincomycin. Prognosis is good following prolonged antibiotic treatment, particularly in cervicofacial disease.

SYPHILIS

This venereal disease is caused by *Treponema pallidum* and is transmitted by direct intimate contact in the presence of moisture. Both hetero- and homosexual intercourse with an infected partner account for the vast majority of infections. The most common portal of entry is the genital region followed by the mouth or lips. Transmission by fomites is rare since the organisms are destroyed by rapid drying but rare such instances have been documented including 'second hand chewing gum'. Placental transmission of *T. pallidum* is well documented. In addition, infants may be infected prenatally, or rarely acquire extragenital infection during delivery from a mother with acute syphilis. The infants with congenital syphilis have lesions at birth or acquire them soon after.

T. pallidum is a delicate spiral filament which can be demonstrated by dark field illumination or flourescent antibody techniques in exudates from primary and secondary lesions of the disease.

Pathology and Clinical Course

Following penetration of the skin or mucous membrane, the organism spreads along the lymphatics and lymph nodes to reach the bloodstream within hours of exposure. The primary lesion which appears some 2–4 weeks later, is known as the *chancre*, and is found most often in the genitalia, mouth and lips. It consists of a painless indurated papule which breaks down to form a typically flat, hard ulcer (*Fig.* 5.15), and heals completely even without treatment. The associated regional lymphadenopathy is also painless.

The disease becomes generalized (secondary syphilis) within 2–3 months of infection. A widespread skin eruption (papular, vesicular or bullous) develops predominantly on the face, palms and soles. In addition, other lesions such as condylomata lata, mucous patches and serpiginous ulcers occur, usually at mucocutaneous junctions. Constitutional symptoms include low-grade fever, sore throat, headaches, joint and muscle pain, generalized lymphadenopathy, iridoyclitis and anaemia. The disease remains highly infective during this stage. All the secondary lesions heal spontaneously.

Tertiary syphilis is characterized by destructive lesions of a localized or diffuse nature which probably result from hypersensitivity to the spirochaetal antigens. The classical localized lesion is the gumma which consists of an area of coagulative necrosis surrounded by a zone of lymphocytes, plasma cells and macrophages. Both giant and epithelioid cells are much less frequent than in the tuberculous lesion. Adjacent arteries exhibit marked endarteritis obliterans. The most common sites of gumma include the testes, the liver and bones (nose, palate, skull, clavicle, ulna and tibia). The bony lesions account for the deformities of tertiary syphilis, e.g. saddle nose (*Fig.* 5.16).

The diffuse tertiary lesions of syphilis include syphilitic aortitis and vasculitis, cerebral syphilis (meningovascular and parenchymatous), and diffuse syphilitic osteitis. The vascular lesions lead to weakening of the media with aneurysm formation and, in the case of the ascending aorta, aortic regurgitation.

Meningovascular syphilis is characterized by focal meningitis, vascular episodes due to endarteritis and isolated cranial nerve palsies. Parenchymatous neurosyphilis comprises tabes dorsalis and generalized paralysis of the insane. In the former there is degenerative demyelination and gliosis affecting the posterior columns of the spinal cord and the posterior spinal nerve roots resulting in the characteristic high stepping gait. General paralysis of the insane is a chronic syphilitic meningo-encephalitis. The disease affects the frontal lobes most severely.

Diffuse syphilitic inflammation of the bones in tertiary syphilis is exemplified by the sabre tibia (*Fig.* 5.17) where the apparent bowing is due to deposition of new periosteal

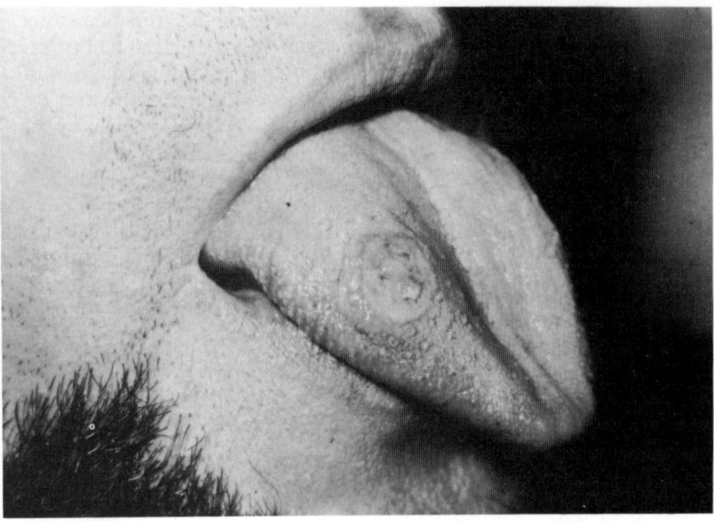

Fig. 5.15 Syphilitic ulcer of the tongue (primary lesion).

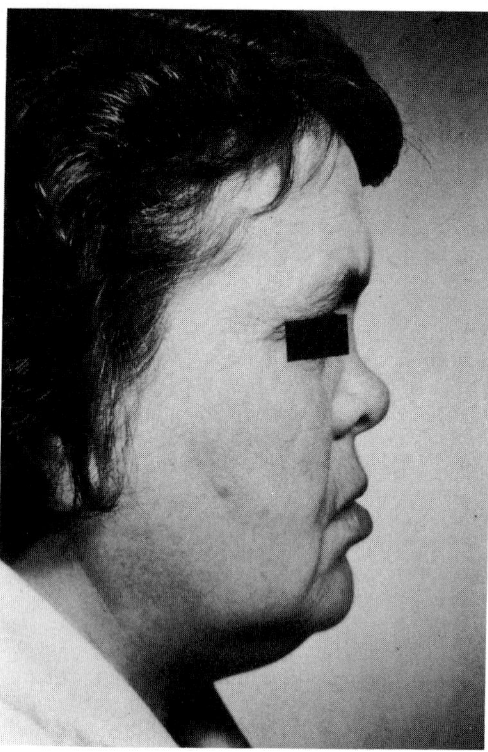

Fig. 5.16 Saddle nose deformity in tertiary syphilis.

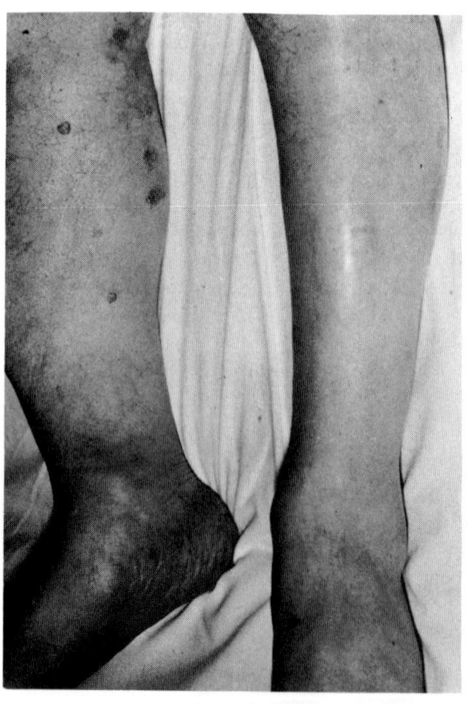

Fig. 5.17 Diffuse syphilitic osteitis resulting in a sabre tibia.

bone, and the worm-eaten appearance of the skull which results from the combined effects of destruction and new bone formation.

Diagnostic Tests

T. pallidum cannot be grown on culture. However, it can be easily identified from the exudate of primary and secondary lesions by dark-ground illumination or fluorescent antibody staining. Serological tests become positive 10–20 days after the acquisition of the infection, and are based on either the Wassermann or the treponemal antibody. The Wassermann antibody reacts with an alcoholic extract of beef heart (cardiolipin), the active component of which is diphosphatidylglycerol. This antigen was extracted at the Venereal Disease Research Laboratory (VDRL) and is used in the complement-fixation and the more sensitive flocculation test (Kahn and the VDRL tests). As the Wassermann antigen is not specific to *T. pallidum*, false positive reactions are encountered in a variety of conditions. These include other treponemal infections, leprosy, malaria, trypanosomiasis, infectious mononucleosis, collagen disease, pregnancy, Coxsackie B virus infection and autoimmune haemolytic anaemia.

The serological tests using the treponemal antibody are more specific (fewer false positive reactions) but still do not distinguish between syphilis and yaws. They include the Reiter protein complement-fixation test, the treponema pallidum immobilization test (TPI), and the flourescent treponemal antibody test (FTA).

Treatment

Both primary and secondary syphilis respond readily to adequate treatment which is usually by intramuscular penicillin.

NON-VENEREAL TREPONEMATOSES

These comprise a group of endemic infections caused by treponemes which are morphologically indistinguishable from *T. pallidum* and give positive reactions with the serological tests for syphilis. They are, however, non-venereal in origin, are usually acquired in childhood, and are characterized by cutaneous manifestations. They include yaws, pinta and endemic or non-venereal syphilis.

Yaws

This is also known as framboesia and is the most widespread of the endemic treponematoses. It is most commonly encountered in tropical and subtropical regions, and is caused by *T. pertenue*. Transmission is by non-venereal personal or household contact directly, or by termites and flies. The incubation period lasts 3–5 weeks. The disease begins with a primary lesion (mother yaw) which is accompanied by a mild systemic upset. The characteristic secondary raspberry-like lesions (framboise) develop several weeks to months later, and affect the whole body. The lesions on the soles of the feet are particularly painful and crippling. Crops of new lesions appear from time to time as old ones heal, but there are often latent periods. The disease causes a marked progressive destruction of skin, cartilage and bone, producing severe disfigurement not dissimilar from leprosy with which yaw used to be mistaken. A single injection of slow-release penicillin is curative.

Pinta

This skin disease is endemic in the tropical regions of the Americas and is caused by *T. carateum*. Contrary to other treponemal infections, it does not cause ulceration or tissue destruction. The skin lesions are initially flat and erythematous. These change to hyperpigmented spots (blue spotting) during the intermediate or secondary stage and finally to areas of depigmentation (white spotting). The possibility of vector transmission has been raised as the disease is common in rural areas where it may involve all the residents. However, personal non-venereal contact 'herd infection' is generally held to be responsible for the transmission of the disease.

Endemic Syphilis

Endemic or non-venereal syphilis is recognized in various countries where it is known by different popular names: skerljevo in Bosnia (Yugoslavia), bejel amongst the Bedouins in the Sahara desert, and dichuchwa in Botswana. It is caused by *T. pallidum* which is apparently identical to that responsible for venereal syphilis. Transmission is thought to be by direct contact and fomites including infected drinking water and flies. Affected individuals do not develop a primary lesion (chancre). The manifestations include generalized papular or circinate rash, condylomas, ulceration in the mouth and pharynx and lymphadenitis. Late lesions similar to venereal syphilis are encountered, such as gumma, destruction of the nasal septum, periostitis, etc.

GONORRHOEA

This is one of the most common diseases in the Western hemisphere. The incidence in the UK is 118 per 100000 and is higher in Scandinavian countries and the USA. It is caused by *Neisseria gonorrhoeae*, and in the vast majority of cases transmission is by sexual intercourse.

Clinical Features

In the female, the disease causes an acute purulent inflammation of the vulva, cervix, uterus and adnexa. Presentation with acute pelvic peritonitis and tubo-ovarian abscess formation is not unusual. Secondary involvement of the rectum (proctitis) is found in 50% of females. Rarely the rectum is the primary site of infection.

In adult life, the vagina is relatively resistant to gonococcal infection. This is not so in prepubertal girls probably because of the immature and unkeratinized vaginal epithelium. Thus, gonococcal vaginitis and vulvovaginitis may occur in this age group. However, most cases of vulvovaginitis in prepubertal girls are not venereal in origin but result from endogenous infection with neisseria from the upper respiratory tract, the organisms being introduced into the vagina by dirty hands, towels, clothing, etc. The respiratory bacteria responsible for most of these infections include *Neisseria sicca*, *N. flava*, *N. catarrhalis* and *N. meningitidis*. Vulvovaginitis in both children and adults can be caused by *Candida albicans* and *Trichomonas vaginalis*.

In the male, infection with *N. gonorrhoeae* results in inflammation of the urethra which often involves the epididymis, seminal vesicles, bladder and prostate. The untreated urethral inflammation may lead to stricture formation of the bulbar or spongy urethra.

In both sexes gonococcal inflammation may result in infertility due to stricture of the fallopian tubes in the female and vas deferens in the male. One of the disastrous consequences of gonococcal infection in the female used to be infection of the eyeballs of the neonate during delivery. Gonococcal ophthalmia neonatorum used to be the most frequent cause of blindness in infancy but is rarely encountered nowdays since the advent of effective chemotherapy and the introduction of instillations of silver nitrate or other antiseptic into the eye of the newborn.

Treatment

Gonococcal infections are usually sensitive to penicillin which is the first-choice antibiotic. Tetracyclines are used for resistant infections which account for 25% of cases.

OTHER VENEREAL DISEASES

These include venereal granulomatoses (lymphogranuloma venereum and granuloma inguinale), chancroid, genitourinary trichomoniasis, venereal herpes simplex infection, AIDS and genital warts (condylomata acuminata).

Lymphogranuloma Venereum

Lymphogranuloma venereum (LGV), also known as tropical bubo, is caused by *Chlamydia trachomatis*. Chlamydiae are obligate intracellular parasites and for this reason used to be considered as viruses and referred to as Bedsonia or Miyagawanella. They, however, contain all the characteristics of bacteria, including a complex cell wall, but lack the metabolic enzymes necessary for an independent existence. *Chlamydia trachomatis* is subdivided into strains which cause LGV (three serotypes), and others that are responsible for oculogenital infections.

LGV is common in tropical countries and is contracted by sexual intercourse, the reservoir of infection being the cervix in the asymptomatic female and the rectal mucosa in the asymptomatic homosexual male. It produces a papular, ulcerative or bullous lesion in the genital region which is not often painful and which heals spontaneously. This is followed within 1–6 weeks by gross lymphadenopathy (buboes). The enlarged lymph nodes in the ilio-inguinal regions suppurate, and subsequently ulcerate, discharging seropurulent material. The disease may involve the pelvic organs and rectum in the female. It often becomes chronic with extensive scarring leading to elephantiasis and fibrous strictures of the rectum, vagina and urethra. Sulphonamide therapy (5 g daily for 7 days) gives good results in early cases. Tetracyclines are indicated when sulphonamides have failed. Surgical treatment should only be undertaken after an adequate course of antibiotic therapy. Abscesses should be aspirated and incision avoided.

Granuloma Inguinale

This is found in certain tropical countries and the Southern United States. It is an infection with Donovan bodies (*Donovania granulomatosis*). Although infection is generally regarded to be acquired by sexual intercourse, extragenital inoculation may occur. The primary lesion is a papule which subsequently ulcerates. In the male, it is usually found on the penis but other sites are well documented in both sexes. However, the majority of the primary lesions occur in the genital, perineal, perianal or pubic regions. A 5-day course of streptomycin (4 g daily) is curative in most instances. Aureomycin, tetracycline and chloramphenicol are also effective.

Chancroid

Chancroid (soft chancre) is caused by *Haemophilus ducreyi* and is transmitted by sexual contact. The infection is commoner and more severe in males. The disease starts as a soft macule usually in the foreskin 3–10 days after exposure. The

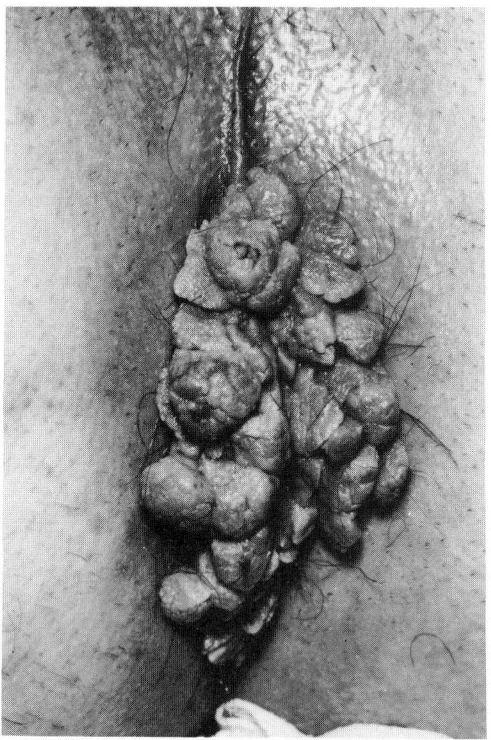

Fig. 5.18 Condylomata acuminata of the perianal region.

lesion subsequently becomes necrotic and produces a ragged ulcer which may result in substantial penile destruction. The ulcers may be multiple and vary considerably in size. In the female ulcerative lesions are found on the vulva and vagina. The inguinal lymph nodes become enlarged, painful and may suppurate. Treatment is by sulphonamides and tetracycline in the first instances. Resistant cases respond to cephalothin.

Condylomata Acuminata

The term 'condylomata acuminata' (genital warts) is used to differentiate these pointed warts from the flat condylomata lata of syphilis. Genital warts result from infection with a papovavirus and occur in the genital, perineal and perianal regions (*Fig.* 5.18), and may be followed by the appearance of similar warts elsewhere in the body. Treatment is by the application of 10% podophyllin or diathermy excision.

HERPETOVIRIDAE INFECTIONS

The family of herpesviruses—*Herpetoviridae*—comprises a large number of viruses but only four are pathogenic to man. These include the herpes simplex virus (HVS), the varicella zoster virus (VZV), cytomegalovirus (CMV) and the Epstein–Barr virus (EBV). They are important because of their common and ubiquitous occurrence and because of the association in some instances with the development of certain neoplastic conditions. Moreover, they can cause serious and often fatal infections in debilitated and immunocompromised patients.

These viral infections cause an initial, often mild and inconsequential, primary infection, following which the virus remains dormant in a non–infectious state (latent) at certain sites, e.g. sensory ganglia in HSV and probably in VZV. From time to time, reactivation of the virus with occurrence of clinical manifestations, such as cold sore, shingles, etc. may follow a febrile illness, operation, menstruation, radiotherapy, etc. The latency site for the EBV genome is thought to be the B-lymphocytes whereas the CMV genome appears to persist in the renal tubules, leucocytes (particularly polymorphs), parotid gland and cervix.

Herpes Simplex Infections

There are two recognized strains: HSV1 which is responsible for the majority of non-genital infections, and HSV2 which accounts for most of the ocular and genital infections. Infection with the HSV is widespread and prevalence ranges from 50 to 100% depending on the socio-economic status. The infection is acquired in the first instance by close personal contact and genital herpes is now one of the well-recognized venereal diseases in the West with a rising incidence such that in Great Britain genital herpes is twice as common as syphilis.

Labial Herpes

This is the commonest type of infection caused by HSV1. The portal of entry is the mouth and the vesicular lesions occur most commonly on the lips ('cold sore') but may be severe especially in the neonate, debilitated and the immunocompromised where they may cause extensive gingivostomatitis with intraoral/pharyngeal ulceration, fever and cervical lymphadenopathy. Rarely the infection may disseminate to the brain, liver and adrenals and is then usually fatal.

Labial herpes is the commonest recurrent type. Precipitating factors include fever, exposure to sunlight and menstruation. Each crop of labial vesicles is preceded by a burning sensation in the skin of the affected site.

Cutaneous Herpes

Although HSV does not penetrate intact healthy skin, infections may occur in patients with skin disorders and in the presence of burns and lacerations leading to an extensive vesicular eruption (eczema herpeticum). In burn patients, the infection may become widely disseminated and lead to severe and often fatal pneumonia.

Ocular Herpes

Most of these infections are due to HSV1 except those acquired in the neonatal period from an infected mother. The eye lesions include follicular conjunctivitis which may progress to corneal involvement with the formation of dendritic ulcers and corneal opacities. Corticosteroids enhance the eye damage caused by the virus and should be avoided in these infections.

CNS Infections

HSV infections may cause encephalitis, radiculitis, myelitis and meningitis. The encephalitis is usually the result of reactivation of latent infection.

Genital Herpes

Although the majority of genital herpes are due to HSV2, some are undoubtedly caused by HSV1. The disease which is sexually transmitted has an incubation period of 2–20 days with an average of 6 days. The primary infection is followed by recurrent attacks which are usually less severe with intervening periods of latency during which the patient feels well and has no clinical manifestations of the disease. The risk of transmission of the disease is highest during an acute attack but asymptomatic individuals may pass on the disease to their sexual partners. There is strong circumstantial evidence linking herpes simplex infection of the cervix with the development of cervical cancer, and there is a fourfold increased risk of cancer of the cervix in women with genital herpes. More recently an association between cancer of the vulva and genital herpes has been suggested though the evidence linking the two conditions is inconclusive at present.

A primary attack is heralded by systemic symptoms due to the viraemia: malaise, fever and myalgia. The lesions are found on the penis and perianal region in the male and the labia, clitoris, vagina, cervix, perineum and perianal region in the female. They consist of painful vesicles which ulcerate, then crust and heal spontaneously. Neuralgia is often present.

The severe pain during an acute attack may precipitate acute retention of urine.

Treatment of Herpes Virus Infections

As the virus is metabolically inactive during a latency period, treatment is futile at this stage. Effective therapy with the new antiviral agent acyclovir is now possible provided it is started early during a first or recurrent attack. There is a preferential uptake of the drug by infected (virally colonized) cells where it is activated by a virus-specific thymidine kinase forming acyclovir triphosphate which inhibits the viral DNA polymerase.

Varicella Zoster Virus Infections

The painful clinical condition known as zoster (formerly herpes zoster) is always the result of a reactivation of the same virus which causes chickenpox. Although in some instances no apparent cause for this activation is clinically obvious, in others a state of depressed cell-mediated immunity is present due to trauma, malignancy and immunosuppressive drugs, particularly in patients undergoing organ transplantation.

In the severely immunocompromised patient, the infection may be systemic with the development of pneumonia and involvement of other organs such as liver, CNS, adrenals and pancreas, and then carries an appreciable mortality.

In the more usual condition an exanthematous rash develops over a dermatome supplied by a specific dorsal nerve root and extramedullary nerve ganglion. The dermatomes supplied by the third dorsal to the second lumbar segment of the spinal cord are the ones most commonly affected, followed by that supplied by the fifth cranial nerve. Pain and paraesthesiae often predate the development of the vesicular rash. The most distressing feature of the disease is the development of a severe neuralgia (St Anthony's fire) which may persist for several weeks and require specialist treatment.

Cytomegalovirus Infections

The pattern of infection with CMV varies with the socio-economic state of the country. In poor developing countries with overcrowding and poor sanitation, the disease is acquired early in life and by the age of 5 years, the vast majority of children become seropositive for the virus. In the West, neonatal infection is rare and most primary infections are acquired in adolescence mainly from kissing and sexual intercourse such that the prevalence of seropositive individuals rises to 60–70% by the age of 60 years. The disease can be transmitted by the transfusion of blood products (particularly fresh blood and pooled platelet donations), and organ and bone marrow transplantation. It is thus a real hazard in transplant patients and in patients with leukaemia, since transmission of the virus may be followed by serious infection consequent on the immunosuppressed state of the patient leading to pneumonia, hepatitis, haemolytic anaemia, leucopenia and thrombocytopenia. The average reported mortality of this generalized disease is 2% but figures as high as 15–20% have been reported especially in bone marrow transplant recipients.

The infection may be transmitted to the fetus across the placenta. This may result in intrauterine death and spontaneous abortion. The vast majority of congenitally infected babies appear normal at birth but 10–30% of them will suffer brain damage (microcephaly) and mental retardation. A few babies show the classic cytomegalic inclusion disease, the features of which are similar to those of the generalized disease encountered in the immunosuppressed adult.

Infection in a normal adolescent may be asymptomatic or the individual may develop fever, sore throat, lymphadenopathy and hepatosplenomegaly. The clinical picture is very similar to that of glandular fever but the Paul–Bunnell test is negative. The blood may contain the characteristic intranuclear inclusions (owl eye) within atypical mononuclear cells. Anti-CMV antibodies can be demonstrated following the primary infection. In susceptible immunocompromised patients, the risk of CMV infection can be reduced by using blood and organs from CMV-negative donors, transfusion of leucocyte-free blood, and the administration of high titre anti-CMV immunoglobulin to the recipients.

Epstein–Barr Virus Infections

Aside from causing glandular fever (infectious mononucleosis), infection with the EBV leads to the development of African Burkitt's lymphoma and nasopharyngeal carcinoma. Infectious mononucleosis is a disease of the West with a peak incidence in adolescence and young adult life. It is transmitted in the saliva by kissing and is often referred to as the 'kissing disease'. The incubation period varies from 4 to 7 weeks, and is followed by the development of malaise, fever, asthenia, sore throat, lymphadenopathy and splenomegaly. The blood picture shows a lymphocytosis with more than 10% atypical monocytes. The Paul–Bunnell test which detects the presence of heterophile antibodies to sheep red blood cells, is positive. The liver function tests are often deranged during the first week of the illness which usually lasts 3–4 weeks. However, prolonged asthenia and debility for several months after the acute illness is quite common.

Human Immunodeficiency Virus—AIDS

This is discussed in Chapter 10.

FUNGAL INFECTIONS (MYCOSES)

From the clinical standpoint, fungal infections are best divided into cutaneous, subcutaneous and deep. Risk factors include prolonged antibiotic therapy which encourages the growth and establishment of commensal fungal organisms such as candida, leucopenia and T-lymphocyte depression which are associated with invasive and potentially fatal fungal disease.

The *cutaneous* (superficial) mycoses have a worldwide distribution and include dermatophytosis (ringworm), superficial candidosis (thrush), pityriasis versicolor, etc.

The *subcutaneous* fungal infections are largely restricted to the tropical and subtropical regions and often arise by direct implantation of soil fungal organisms through the skin of the soles of the feet, e.g. mycetoma and sporotrichosis.

A number of conditions result from *deep*-seated fungal infections which may be difficult to treat and prove fatal, particularly when the patient is immunosuppressed and debilitated. These include some fungal infections that have similar clinical characteristics: histoplasmosis, cryptococcosis, coccidiomycosis and blastomycosis. They are all caused by inhalation of infected soil dust, and the primary lesion is pulmonary. Although usually self-limiting, the disease may spread via the bloodstream to involve other organs causing serious and times fatal illness. Many of the histological features encountered in these deep-seated fungal infections are similar to those found in tuberculosis. These infections are discussed in Chapter 39.

Finally, *systemic* mycoses may arise from superficial and deep-seated fungal infections when the patient's immune response is depressed by disease, such as leukaemia, and immunosuppressive drugs including cytotoxic agents.

Candidosis

The candida species of fungi occur as commensals in the mouth, alimentary tract and the vagina. Infection with *Candida albicans* has been increasingly encountered in clinical practice, and is now one of the common fungal diseases arising as an opportunistic (nosocomial) infection in the debilitated, seriously ill patients, the immunosuppressed, individuals with primary immunological deficiency disorders affecting the T-lymphocytes, and finally as a superinfection in patients on broad-spectrum antibiotic therapy.

The infection is encountered in several clinical forms. Oral candidosis (thrush) and the vaginal and perianal (*Fig.* 5.19) infection are common and occur most commonly after antibiotic therapy. Vaginal candidosis is also common in conditions which result in a low pH of the vaginal contents from excess of glycogen in the vaginal cells, such as pregnancy, diabetes and women on the contraceptive pill. Cutaneous circumoral infection (*perlèche*) and chronic paronychia may also occur in these patients.

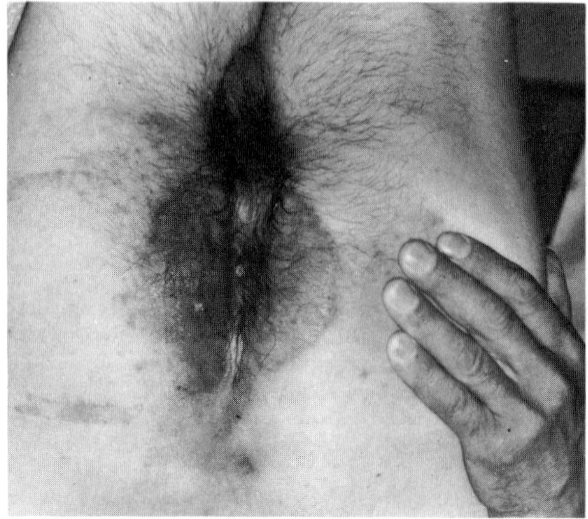

Fig. 5.19 Perianal candidosis.

Alimentary and Pulmonary Candidosis

The oral infection may extend to involve the gastrointestinal tract, particularly the oesophagus, following prolonged therapy with broad-spectrum antibiotics. Both alimentary and pulmonary candidosis may arise as opportunistic infections in the presence of impaired cell-mediated immunity, e.g. immunosuppressed individuals, lymphoreticulosis, cytotoxic therapy.

Generalized (Systematic) Candidosis

This is the most serious form and is characterized by bloodstream spread to any organ but most commonly to the kidneys and the endocardium. This serious systemic nosocomial infection is encountered during parenteral nutrition, in patients with prosthetic devices and grafts, in transplant patients, and immunological deficiency disorders characterized by a T-lymphocyte depression. The general clinical features of systemic candidosis include high fever, hypotension, rigors and renal impairment. The reported overall survival following appropriate systemic antifungal treatment is 65–70%.

Several types of primary immunological diseases affecting T-lymphocyte function are associated with the widespread development of chronic mucocutaneous candidosis. The immunological deficit varies from patient to patient.

Pulmonary candidosis is dealt with in Chapter 39.

Mycetoma

This is a localized infection of the skin and subcutaneous tissues of the extremities, usually the feet and less frequently the hand. It is found in developing countries. The infection is caused by organisms normally resident in the soil which are implanted by thorn and similar injuries in individuals who walk barefooted. Bacterial mycetoma is due to infection with species of nocardia or actinomyces (actinomycetoma). Fungal mycetoma (eumycetoma, maduromycoses) is endemic in certain countries such as India, and is caused by various fungi, including *Madurella mycetomi*, *Allescheria boydii* and *Aspergillus nidulans*. The disease results in chronic suppuration with severe tissue destruction and multiple discharging sinuses (*Fig.* 5.20). In both bacterial and fungal mycetoma, osteomyelitis of the bones of the foot may develop and adversely affect the prognosis.

In bacterial mycetoma, treatment with the appropriate antibacterial agent together with surgical drainage and débridement may prove effective. The fungal mycetomas, by contrast, seldom respond to antifungal chemotherapy as the organisms acquire a protective cement sheath or develop thickened cell walls which limit the efficacy of the drugs *in vivo*. None the less a trial of treatment with an antifungal agent, such as griseofulvin, flucytosine or ketoconazole, may be effective in patients with early and limited disease and without bone involvement. In most instances, however, amputation is necessary to achieve eradication of the disease.

Treatment of Systemic Fungal Infections

General considerations are important since antifungal therapy alone may be insufficient. Thus, infected prosthetic implants need to be removed or replaced, e.g. heart valves. Whenever possible, the immune depression is reversed at least partially by reduction of the dose of the immunosuppressive agents. Variable and conflicting results have been obtained by the administration of transfer factor and transfusion of leucocytes.

Intravenous amphotericin B remains the mainstay of ther-

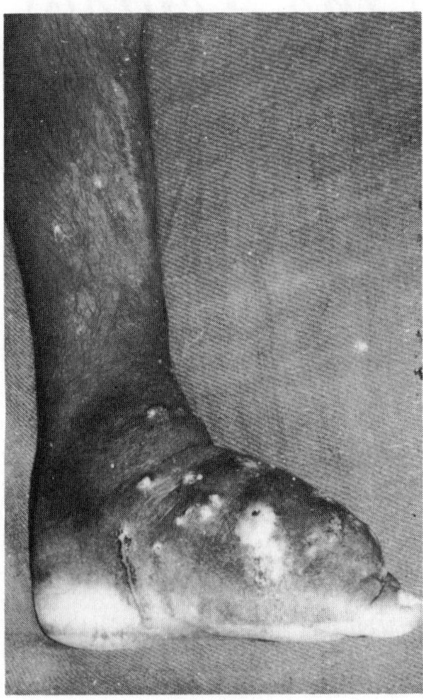

a

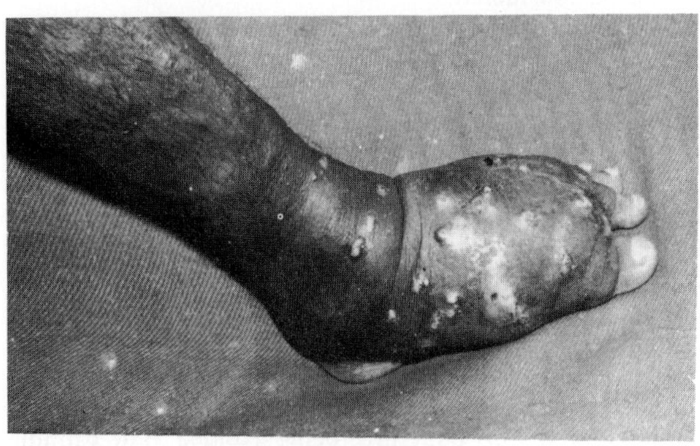

b

Fig. 5.20 a, b, Fungal mycetoma of the foot showing swelling, chronic induration with multiple sinuses and fungal granules. The nature of the infective agent is determined by paraffin sections of the granules stained with haematoxylin and eosin. Gram, Ziehl–Neelsen, periodic acid–Schiff, and Gomori's methanamine silver technique. (By courtesy of Dr M. G. Muthukumarasamy, Kilpauk Medical College, India.)

apy for systemic fungal infections. It is administered in 5% dextrose, initially in a dose of 0·25 mg/kg/24 h and increasing gradually over a period of 4–6 days to 1·0 mg/kg/day. The daily dose is administered over a period of 3–4 h. Since it deteriorates rapidly in solution on exposure to sunlight, the intravenous solution must be shielded. Treatment is monitored by blood levels which should be kept in the 1–3 μg/ml range. The main disadvantage of amphotericin B is its toxicity: rigors, hypotension, phlebitis, hepatic damage, renal damage, anaemia, leucopenia and hypokalaemia. The prior intravenous administration of either hydocortisone (50–100 mg) or chlorpheniramine (10 mg) is stated to reduce some of the early side-effects. In order to minimize toxicity, amphotericin B is often administered in a reduced dose in combination with other drugs. Various combinations are used including amphotericin B + flucytosine for cryptococcosis, rifampicin + amphotericin B for candidosis and blastomycosis. Altering the rate of infusion and alternate day treatment may help to reduce the incidence and severity of the side-effects. Other measures that have been recommended to reduce toxicity include heparin infusion against phlebitis, and mannitol and bicarbonate to minimize renal damage.

5-Flucytosine is a synthetic antifungal agent which can be administered orally or intravenously. It is active mainly against *Candida* and *Cryptococcus*. Apart from its side-effects (diarrhoea, rashes, leucopenia and hepatitis), its main disadvantage is the rapid emergence of resistance.

A number of imidazoles have significant antifungal activity. The two most often used are ketoconazole which is administered orally (200–600 mg), and miconazole which is given intravenously since it is poorly absorbed after oral administration. Ketoconazole has less side-effects than miconazole which may cause rashes, phlebitis, ventricular tachycardia and anaphylaxis. Drug resistance to the use of imidazoles is rare, and they have a broad spectrum of activity against many fungi (except aspergilli) and some Gram-positive bacteria. All the other imidazoles (clotrimazole, econazole, tioconazole) are mainly used as topical antifungal agents. Oral ketoconazole is advocated as a prophylactic measure in transplant patients.

Treatment of Cutaneous Fungal Infections

Topical polyenes (natamycin, nystatin, candicidin) are used as 1–2% creams or ointments, as suspensions or tablets (oral/vaginal). The topical imidazole preparations are also effective. In cases of chronic mucocutaneous candidosis associated with T-lymphocyte immune defects, treatment with transfer factor gives varying results.

Further Reading

Ahmadsyah I. and Salim A. (1985) Treatment of tetanus: an open study to compare the efficacy of procaine penicillin and metronidazole. *Br. Med. J.* **291**, 648-650.

Evans A. S. and Feldman H. A. (1982) *Bacterial Infections of Humans. Epidemiology and Contol.* New York, Plenum Medical Book Company.

Figegold S. M. (1977) *Anaerobic Bacteria in Human Disease.* New York, Academic Press.

Speller D. C. E. (1980) *Antifungal Chemotherapy.* Chichester, John Wiley.

Waters M. (1984) Leprosy. In: *Recent Advances in Tropical Medicine.* Edinburgh, Churchill Livingstone.

Wilcocks C. and Manson-Bahr P. E. C. (1986) *Manson's Tropical Diseases*, 18th ed. London, Baillière Tindall.

6 Management of the Acutely Injured and Seriously Ill Patient

Jack Tinker

INTRODUCTION

The acutely injured or critically ill surgical patient presents or develops failure of one or more of the major physiological systems. The assessment and management of the disturbed physiology that this incurs reflects the practice of intensive care and is the theme of this chapter.

The separate systems failure are considered individually for matters of convenience. They often coexist and are always interrelated, patients dying on an intensive care unit frequently develop what is now called 'multiple organ system failure' (MOSF). Management in these cases is dictated by a balance of priorities. The development of systemic or localized (even occult) infection is a crucial step for the progression from single to multiple organ system failure and greatly decreases the prognosis for survival. Prevention and prompt effective treatment of infection is a vital aspect of intensive care.

MONITORING THE CRITICALLY ILL PATIENT

Critical illness, whatever its cause, is characterized by severity, multisystem affliction and rapidity of change. Its management has, therefore, to be founded on the frequent or continuous measurement of many physiological variables.

As the number of physiological variables that are measured has increased through the advance of technology, so has it become important to select those that are relevant to the particular physiological derangement(s) present. Consequently, it is helpful to consider the variables systematically. It is also prudent to consider whether the measurements taken will aid in management, as all interventional techniques carry with them some degree of morbidity or even mortality.

Cardiovascular System

Electrocardiogram

The ECG provides continuous information concerning heart rate and rhythm and facilitates the rapid detection of various cardiac arrhythmias.

Arterial Blood Pressure (ABP)

The arterial blood pressure is a cornerstone of haemodynamic monitoring, for both hypo- and hypertension are frequently encountered. Unfortunately, there are still some misconceptions of its value. Its level is determined by the product of blood flow and the resistance to this flow; it is not, therefore, synonymous with arterial flow and hypotension is not the *sine qua non* of shock. When considering the level of arterial pressure the adequacy of perfusion should be considered.

The use of indwelling arterial cannulas to measure ABP has distinct advantages for the care of the critically ill patient. First, it gives a continuous and accurate reading of systolic, diastolic and mean pressures, along with a simultaneous display of the pressure waveform. The latter may give an indication of the state of contractility of the myocardium along with a visual impression of stroke volume and total peripheral resistance. Also, pressure waveform display will demonstrate the effect of cardiac arrhythmias on the pumping mechanism of the heart. Secondly, intra-arterial cannulas are convenient sampling points in those patients who require frequent blood gas estimations and repeated blood tests; the discomfort and complications of repeated arterial and venous punctures being avoided. The cannula should be inserted under local anaesthesia into the radial or brachial artery. It should be remembered that the accuracy of this and other direct measuring systems mentioned below depends upon accurate calibration and technical problems should always be considered in the case of spurious or grossly abnormal readings which seem out of keeping with the patient's general state before any rapid interventional measures are taken. In particular the attachment of ECG electrodes and the positioning of transducers in pressure monitoring systems should be given close attention.

Central Venous Pressure (CVP)

The CVP is, by definition, the pressure in the right atrium. It is a complex variable, being influenced by the venous return to the right atrium, the functional state of the right ventricle, the degree of venous tone, the intrapericardial pressure and the intrathoracic pressure. If the tricuspid valve is functioning normally then the CVP equates to the end-diastolic pressure in the right ventricle and is a measure of the preload to this chamber.

Measurement

A radio-opaque catheter may be passed from a subclavian, internal jugular or antecubital vein into the right atrium. This should be performed under full aseptic technique using a guide wire. Use of a femoral vein is not recommended because of the increased risk of sepsis and the possibility of inferior vena caval thrombosis. The patient should be placed in a head-down position to minimize the risk of air embolism and to increase venous return which will also aid puncture of the central veins. After insertion of the catheter no fluid should be infused through it unless blood can be easily withdrawn; the position of the tip must always be checked on a chest radiograph for not infrequently catheters double back, pass into veins of the neck or enter the right ventricle. Ideally, the tip should be located at the lower border of the superior vena cava or in the upper third of the right atrium away from the tricuspid valve (*Fig.* 6.1). Catheters introduced from subclavian or internal jugular veins are notoriously liable to migrate and require firm fixation to the skin with a suture after insertion. Measurements of CVP inferred from catheters located in an external jugular vein are inaccurate and should not be used.

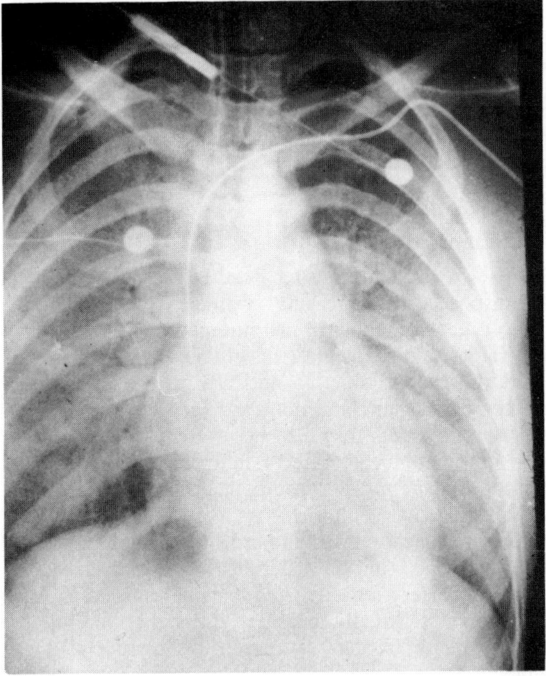

Fig. 6.1 A portable chest radiograph; the central venous catheter is correctly positioned in the right atrium.

From the catheter CVP should preferably be measured continuously using a pressure transducer, or if such facilities are not available, intermittently using a fluid manometer. A constant and carefully located zero-reference level is essential for accurate measurement, for small changes in the value of the CVP can reflect significant changes in cardiovascular function. Either the midaxillary line in the fourth intercostal space or the sternal angle can be used as zero levels; the former is often preferred since it is at the anatomical level of the right atrium. CVP varies with the phases of respiration and all readings should be documented at the end of expiration.

Normal Values

Measured from the midaxillary line the normal range is 3–7 mmHg (0·4–1·0 kPa) and from the sternal angle it is 0–3 mmHg (0–0·4 kPa).

Complications of Central Venous Cannulation

The literature abounds with reports of complications and their possible occurrence highlights the need for care during the insertion of catheters and for the highest standards of care once they are in place. Complication rates are minimal with skilled operators and it is a sensible policy in a hospital for a limited number of doctors to assume responsibility for carrying out all central venous cannulation.

1. DAMAGE TO ADJACENT STRUCTURES applies particularly to the use of the subclavian vein. Damage to the pleura can result in a pneumothorax and haemothorax may arise from damage to the subclavian artery, and on the left side damage of the thoracic duct can produce a chylothorax. These may occur singularly or together. Lacerations of the brachial artery or subclavian vein may also be produced. In patients with impaired haemostasis access via the subclavian and to some extent the internal jugular veins is particularly hazardous. The clotting defect should be reversed if possible prior to insertion. If this is not possible a peripheral approach via the antecubital fossa should be used.

2. SEPTICAEMIA, due to the introduction of infecting organisms through the catheter, is a constant threat. The development of multiple-lumen catheters now means that drugs and, in the short term, parenteral nutrition, may be infused through a CVP cannula. For long-term parenteral nutrition a separate feeding line should be inserted and tunnelled subcutaneously proximal to the insertion.

If an unexplained fever develops blood cultures should be taken through the distal lumen of the cannula and from a peripheral vein, the catheter should then be removed and the tip sent for bacteriological culture.

3. PENETRATION OF THE HEART OR GREAT VESSELS from erosion by the catheter tip is an infrequent but dangerous complication. Penetration of the right atrium will result in a pericardial effusion and tamponade whilst erosion through the superior vena cava results in a haemomediastinum or a haemothorax.

4. SHEARING of the catheter and possible embolism of the distal fragment is most likely to occur when catheters are introduced through a needle or with simultaneous multiple insertion at the same site. CVP catheters should never be withdrawn through an introducer needle, and when inserting more than one at the same site care should be taken not to 'skewer' any catheters already inserted with a subsequent needle approach.

5. THROMBOPHLEBITIS results from chemical and physical irritation of the vein and does not necessarily imply the presence of infection. Recent work suggests that some degree of thrombophlebitis often occurs following central vein cannulation though it is rarely of clinical significance. The incidence of thrombophlebitis is increased following repeated cannulation of the vein and increases with the length of time the catheter is left in situ. CVP cannulas should be removed and resited if necessary after 4–7 days.

6. AIR EMBOLISM is a constant danger with CVP cannulation and the measuring and infusion systems should be well sealed and carefully examined frequently.

7. SPINAL CORD INFARCTION due to irritation and spasm of one of the arteries of the costocervical plexus has been reported.

Because it is a composite variable the interpretation of CVP requires a great deal of prudence. Changes or trends over a period of time are more meaningful than a single isolated reading and on every occasion its values must be construed with those of other haemodynamic variables.

A low CVP implies reduction in the circulating blood volume and a consequent reduction in right ventricular preload. This might be the result of an absolute hypovolaemia, a reduction in venous tone (relative hypovolaemia) or a combination of both of these. An increase in venous tone can, likewise, give a normal CVP in the presence of hypovolaemia and during fluid replacement its value may rise above the normal level before the volume deficit has been corrected since venous relaxation is relatively slow.

A higher than normal CVP can be due to an increase in circulating blood volume, right ventricular failure or right ventricular constriction, as in pericardial tamponade. Tricuspid incompetence will produce high CVPs, though the alteration in waveform is diagnostic.

Apart from being a qualification of the volaemic state of the patient as described, the CVP is used as a guide to myocardial dysfunction as reflected in raised ventricular end diastolic pressures and raised atrial pressures. The CVP is a guide to events on the right side of the heart, using right-sided pressures to infer left-sided function depends on parallel functioning ventricles. In pure right ventricular failure (secondary to pulmonary hypertension, right ventricular outflow tract obstruction and pure right ventricular infarction) there will be a gross disturbance in the balance of function, which is also often present in acute cardiorespiratory disease. Reliance solely on CVP measurement in such circumstances may be erroneous and great care is needed in interpreting results. In the case of primary right ventricular dysfunction higher than normal right-sided filling pressures may be needed to facilitate adequate filling to the left side of the heart. Conversely, where left-sided function is affected more than the right a normal right-sided pressure may result in greatly raised left-sided filling pressures with the risk of causing cardiogenic pulmonary oedema. In clinical practice, in spite of these problems, measurement of the CVP, if correctly interpreted, is a valuable aid to patient management.

Pulmonary Artery Wedge Pressure (PAWP)—Pulmonary Artery Occlusion Pressure (PAOP)

The insertion of pulmonary artery catheters has now become relatively common on intensive care units. Occluding a small branch of the PA with a balloon-tipped catheter leads to a free communication between the tip and the pulmonary venous system. Pulmonary capillary pressure equates with left atrial pressure and thus in the absence of mitral valve disease gives an accurate estimate of left ventricular end-diastolic pressure (LVEDP) (and therefore preload). Thus one may produce a quantitative estimation of the functional state of the left ventricle.

The value of PAOP and hence LAP depends on the state of the left ventricle and the magnitude of pulmonary venous return. Low levels would tend to indicate hypovolaemia (relative or absolute) and high levels hypervolaemia or a failing left ventricle (if no mitral valve disease is present). Recent refinements in technology have increased the number of parameters that can be measured using the catheters.

Measurement

The catheters are inserted in the manner described for CVP measurement. Having advanced into a large intrathoracic vein the balloon is inflated and the catheter guided by the display of the pressure waveform until it occludes a small branch of the pulmonary artery. This pressure is the PAOP. The balloon is then deflated and the PA trace should reappear. The catheter may be left in situ for up to 72 hours. Should occlusion be technically impossible pulmonary artery diastolic pressure may be used as an alternative.

Complications of PA Catheterization

These include pulmonary artery thrombosis, knotting and coiling of the catheter, rupture of a pulmonary artery, PA haemorrhage, atrial and ventricular arrhythmias and bacterial endocarditis. Studies of morbidity and mortality have reported figures of 25–53% and 0–2% respectively. The technique is, therefore, not without risk and the potential benefits must be clearly defined before insertion. The main complication is pulmonary infarction which is likely to occur if the catheter occludes a vessel for long periods (this may be with or without the balloon inflated since the catheter can migrate). For this reason it is safer to continuously monitor the pressure waveform.

The Value of PAOP

The use of pulmonary artery catheters is becoming more circumspect with increasing awareness of their attendant risks. In general, though, measurement of PAOP may provide valuable physiological insight in patients with dissociated ventricular function and also in the differentiation between cardiogenic and non-cardiogenic pulmonary oedema. Measurements may also be of great value in the diagnosis of 'anatomical' defects following acute myocardial infarction; acute mitral incompetence and acute perforation of the ventricular septum.

Advances in catheter and microchip technology mean that various signals can now be measured or derived using pulmonary artery catheters and bedside computers. Cardiac output may be directly measured using thermodilution and mixed venous oxygen saturation by oximetry. Derived values include pulmonary vascular resistance, peripheral resistance, shunt fraction, oxygen consumption, content and delivery and various haemodynamic indices such as stroke volume and stroke work. Whilst these values may be of interest, the major use remains the measurement of PAOP.

Cardiac Output

This is most accurately measured directly by the thermodilution technique. Indirect methods using transthoracic impedence reflect trends in cardiac output but do not give absolute values. Ultrasonographic methods measuring thoracic aortic blood flow remain experimental. A simple and commonly used method is core and peripheral temperature difference measured using rectal or oesophageal probes and a thermistor probe on the big toe. With low cardiac output (or poor peripheral perfusion as following cardiopulmonary bypass) the difference may be of the order of 10 °C (normal value 2 °C).

Respiratory System

Respiratory Rate and Rhythm

These are usually measured and recorded by the nursing staff.

Tidal and Minute Volumes

These are easily measured with a Wright's respirometer and have great importance during mechanical ventilation. The expiratory peak flow can similarly be measured with a peak flow meter and is helpful in the management of patients with airway obstruction. Airway pressure—peak, mean and continuous—may be measured on most ventilators.

Arterial Blood Gases and Acid–base Measurements

Blood gas profiles provide values for partial pressures of oxygen and carbon dioxide (Po_2 and Pco_2), pH, standard bicarbonate, base deficit and saturation for both arterial and venous samples. Arterial samples should be assayed immediately or kept chilled to avoid falls in Po_2 and pH and rises in Pco_2 which occur as metabolic processes continue after the sample has been taken. Devices now exist for cutaneous measurement of Po_2 and arterial oxygen saturation. The former has been shown to be less accurate in adults than in neonates, especially where skin blood flow is reduced.

Renal and Metabolic Function

Urine Output

Urine output should be measured hourly using a urinary catheter and urinometer. Regular urine samples should be measured for electrolytes and osmolarity and 24-hour timed collections for the determination of creatinine clearance. Nitrogen balance should be calculated in catabolic patients particularly being managed with total parenteral nutrition.

Regular plasma urea and electrolytes should be measured in all critically ill patients along with appropriate assays pertinent to the patient's state.

Serial measures or urine and plasma osmolality also provide additional information concerning renal function. The plasma colloid osmotic pressure can be readily measured using a membrane osmometer and knowledge of its value may be helpful in various oedematous states.

SHOCK

Classification of Shock

A low cardiac output with reduced organ blood flow and inadequate or inappropriate delivery of oxygen to the tissues is central to the problem of acute circulatory failure, commonly known as shock. It is caused by a reduction in blood volume, a deterioration in cardiac function or a combination of both. Clinical evidence of hypoperfusion usually appears as the cardiac index falls to below 2L/m^2 and if uncorrected will lead to global derangement of body function. The eventual breakdown of cellular metabolism and microcirculatory homeostasis leads to irreversible cardiovascular collapse.

1. Hypovolaemic Shock

This is due to a fall in circulating blood volume from haemorrhage, plasma loss, as occurs in severe burns, or loss of extracellular fluid, as occurs in fistulas, vomiting or diarrhoea. Where capillary integrity is damaged, as in septicaemia, fluid may be lost into the extravascular compartment, in severe ileus or volvulus, hypovolaemia may result because of fluid sequestered in the bowel.

2. Cardiogenic Shock (Pump Failure)

This is the most commonly seen following acute myocardial infarction (>45% of the left ventricle needs to be involved) but will also occur after cardiac surgery, as a result of tamponade or following massive pulmonary embolus.

3. Septicaemic Shock

This may occur in any infection and is thought to be due to the release of foreign polysaccharides or proteins. It has increased in incidence dramatically in recent years. *Table* 6.1 shows some of the predisposing factors.

Table 6.1 Predisposing factors for the development of septicaemic shock

Immunosuppressive drugs	—cancer therapy —transplantation
Corticosteroids	
Broad-spectrum antibiotics	
Diabetes mellitus	
Long-term indwelling catheters	
Prolonged survival following severe injury	
Abdominal surgery (especially biliary)	
Pelvic surgery	

In surgical practice septicaemic shock usually complicates Gram-negative rod infections with organisms such as *E. coli*, *Klebsiella pneumoniae*, Proteus sp., and *Pseudomonas aeruginosa* in that order of precedence. All these species have been shown to produce endotoxin. The most commonly implicated Gram-positive causes of septicaemic shock are *Staph. aureus* and *Strep. pneumoniae*. Other causative infections include those due to Gram-negative anaerobes, Gram-positive aerobes, rickettsiae, fungi and viruses. The latter two show a particular prevalence in the patient who is immunosuppressed. Septicaemic shock may occur with or without signs of infection such as chills, rigors or pyrexia, but such features will often be absent in the immunosuppressed. Septicaemic shock often presents with an increased cardiac output and a reduced vascular resistance. However, as the condition progresses, cardiac output gradually falls with a rising peripheral resistance.

The division of shock into three types is helpful although it conceals the fact that there are many features common to all forms, and in the later stages all three types merge as distinguishing features are lost. Septicaemic shock is a combination of myocardial depression and hypovolaemia from loss of capillary integrity; endotoxaemia develops in the late stages of hypovolaemic shock when mucosal resistance breaks down and particularly when gut ischaemia occurs.

The Pathophysiology of Shock

In order to maintain an adequate circulation to vital structures, a number of neural and hormonal mechanisms are reflexly activated in response to the reduced cardiac output. There is a marked increase of sympatho-adrenal activity with an outpouring of adrenaline and noradrenaline from the adrenal medullas. The main actions of these hormones are mediated via cellular cyclic adenosine monophosphate (cyclic AMP), stimulating adenyl cyclase they increase the levels of cyclic AMP. In addition, they accelerate the breakdown of glycogen in cardiac muscle and this may provide some energy for the failing heart.

The autonomic response increases heart rate and myocardial contractility and constricts arterioles and venules, especially those in the cutaneous and visceral circulations. Cardiac output rises and together with the increased peripheral resistance elevates the arterial pressure. The venoconstriction, by decreasing the capacity of the venous vascular bed, promotes venous return to the heart and also helps sustain the cardiac output. Some degree of circulatory autoregulation may help to protect the renal, coronary and cerebral circulations. If sustained, this autonomic response will lead to impaired oxygen delivery to peripheral tissues and to the development of tissue acidosis.

The effects of the catecholamines are augmented by the release of cortisol and glucagon and by the actions of aldosterone and antidiuretic hormone in conserving sodium and water. A reduced blood volume also stimulates renin release and the formation of the potent vasopressor, angiotensin II.

Nevertheless, despite circulatory adjustments, tissue blood flow and therefore oxygen delivery becomes inadequate. In the face of sustained hypoxia there is global development of the 'sick cell syndrome'. Pyruvic acid is unable to pursue its pathway in the Krebs cycle and is therefore reduced to lactic acid with a fall in ATP production. This lactic acidosis becomes manifest initially intracellularly and then systemically. Such events will also be occurring in the myocardial cell where acidosis will lead to an impaired response to catecholamine stimulation and myocardial depression due to impaired excitation/contraction coupling. Lactic acidosis alters vascular reactivity and permeability and fluid leaks from the circulation into the interstitial spaces. This process is exacerbated by the presence of histamine, kinins and prostaglandins. The continuing loss of plasma increases the viscosity of the blood and therefore its resistance to flow. Cardiac output eventually begins to decline irreversibly.

Tissue hypoxia leads to the release of a number of vasoactive substances including 'myocardial depressants'. A specific 'myocardial depressant factor' has been identified that is mainly released from the ischaemic pancreas. This substance causes direct myocardial depression and further vasoconstriction in the splanchnic bed. In septicaemic shock the complex sequence of events is initiated by the action of bacterial endotoxins which primarily affect the microcirculation and do not themselves have a direct effect on the myocardium. Endotoxins cause endothelial damage, release of vasoactive substances and further toxins and produce gross disturbances in the microcirculation. They are also inherently cytotoxic.

Severe sustainment of all types of shock may also be complicated by the development of disseminated intravascular coagulation with further organ damage and a haemorrhagic diathesis.

The Clinical Features of Shock

The causative factors may be obvious and add to the features that are directly attributable to the low cardiac output and increased sympathoadrenal activity. The skin is pale, cold and clammy and there may be a tachycardia or arrhythmias. The blood pressure may be low or normal. In hypovolaemic shock the venous pressure is low, whilst in cardiogenic shock it will tend to be high. Reduced renal blood flow will lead to oliguria and, if not reversed, the development of acute renal failure. Reduced cerebral blood flow along with abnormalities in cerebral microcirculation may lead to development of an encephalopathy with confusion and deterioration in the level of consciousness.

Tachycardia, hypotension and a rise in venous pressure are features of pericardial tamponade and thus must be excluded if its presence is a possibility. This is especially important in the postoperative cardiac surgical patient and in cases of chest injury where myocardial contusion may be an additional complicating factor.

Assessment of the Shocked Patient

Cardiac output is the product of stroke volume and heart rate and it is therefore important to assess both variables.

1. Heart Rate

ECG monitoring usually shows a sinus tachycardia but various tachyarrhythmias may occur which can further depress cardiac output. Bradycardia is usually associated with cardiogenic shock and may reflect atrioventricular block.

2. Stroke Volume

Stroke volume is influenced by three variables: ventricular preload, myocardial contractility and ventricular afterload (total peripheral resistance).

Preload equates to the ventricular end diastolic volume which up to a certain level is proportional to the force of contraction of the heart muscle (Starling relationship). Its level may be estimated from the CVP, however, when there is imbalance of ventricular function the PAOP gives an estimate of the LV preload.

Contractility is a measure of the heart muscle's ability to alter its force of contraction independent of muscle fibre length. It has been described in many ways but is most easily considered in terms of the Starling Ventricular Function Curve where preload (CVP or PAOP) is plotted on the abscissa and stroke volume on the ordinate (*Fig.* 6.2). The

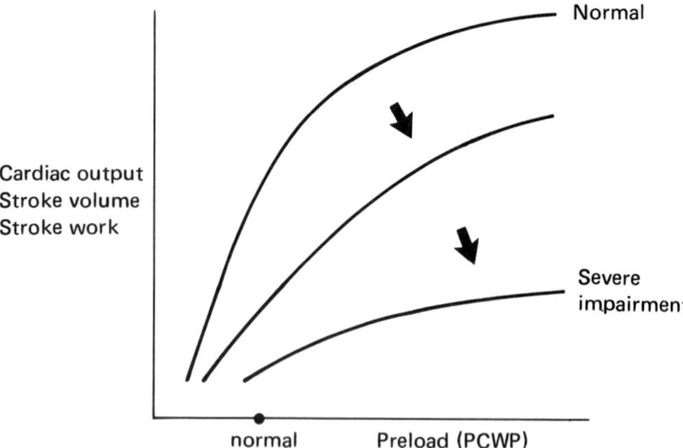

Fig. 6.2 Ventricular function curves.

slope and position of the resulting curve reflects the prevailing contractile state. The normal curve has an initial steep rate of rise where small alterations in preload produce large changes in stroke volume. At higher levels the proportional change in stroke volume for a given change in preload decreases. Impaired contractility (e.g. myocardial ischaemia, sepsis, acidosis) 'moves' the curve down and to the right. Conversely, improved contractility (inotropic support, correction of hypoxia and acidosis, revascularization) will effectively move the curve upwards and to the left.

Afterload is an expression of the resistance to ventricular muscle shortening during systole; the degree of shortening and hence the stroke volume varying inversely with the afterload. It is dominated by the total peripheral resistance (TPR) and may be inferred clinically from the degree of vasoconstriction, estimated from the arterial pressure waveform or calculated if cardiac output is measured.

Blood gas estimation should be performed regularly along with urea and electrolytes.

Sequential determination of the haematocrit gives information of the trend of red cell to plasma ratios.

The Treatment of Shock

Any precipitating factors need to be treated where possible; surgical intervention should be integrated into the overall plan of treatment with patients being resuscitated prior to surgery whenever possible. Irrespective of the nature of the shock there are two prime therapeutic objectives, increasing cardiac output and restoring regional blood flow and both can be achieved by manipulating the determinants of cardiac output, correcting metabolic disturbances and correcting disturbances of heart rate and rhythm.

1. Cardiac Output

a. Optimizing Ventricular Preload

INCREASE. Pure hypovolaemia in the absence of myocardial depression reduces preload and thus stroke volume. Administration of fluids will increase the preload and restore cardiac output. This would normally be monitored using CVP measurement. If contractility is normal the response will be rapid and fluids may be given relatively quickly (e.g. by administering rapid boluses with concomitant measurement of CVP, BP and urine output). If, however, there is myocardial depression or imbalanced ventricular function fluid administration should be cautious as overzealous correction can precipitate pulmonary oedema. Similarly in hypoalbuminaemic states care should be taken since in the presence of low plasma oncotic pressures normal or relatively low left ventricular end diastolic pressures may be sufficient to precipitate pulmonary oedema.

The question as to which type of fluid to use is contentious and teaching varies. It is generally accepted that at packed cell volumes of less than 30% the administration of blood (whole or packed red cells) is indicated. The choice of fluid replacement, other than that to optimize oxygen carrying capacity of blood, lies between crystalloid and colloid solutions. Larger volumes of crystalloid than colloid are needed for the same haemodynamic effect as a proportion is quickly lost from the intravascular compartment. Approximately three times the volume of blood lost has to be given as crystalloid to restore pressures to normal. Large volumes of crystalloid may produce osmotic abnormalities and have been implicated in the pathogenesis of ARDS. Colloid solutions are, however, more expensive and all have been shown to have side-effects, albeit of low incidence, associated with their use. In cases of water and sodium depletion and when only small volumes of blood/plasma are lost then replacement with colloids seems to be more logical. The choice of colloid solution used depends to some extent on availability but the principle is to keep plasma oncotic and hydrostatic pressures normal. In the healthy well nourished adult large stores of albumin are available to be mobilized within 24 hours to replenish that lost; albumin administration in such individuals is unwarranted. If patients are hypoalbuminaemic then albumin administration should be considered as well as synthetic substitutes.

COLLOID SOLUTIONS FOR VOLUME EXPANSION. Human Albumin Solution 4·0–4·5%: Available from pooled human plasma. It remains the 'gold standard' for volume replacement when blood is not indicated. It contains 2·3 mmol K and 140 mmol Na. There is no risk of infection and no deleterious effect on the reticuloendothelial system. It is, however, expensive and in relatively short supply in some areas and indiscriminate use is unjustifiable. Some degree of fibrinolysis occurs due to a pre-kallikrein activating effect and there is an incidence of severe anaphylactoid reaction of 0·004%.

Synthetic Plasma Substitutes: An ideal plasma substitute should have an osmotic pressure comparable to that of plasma, remain in the circulation long enough to effect its function and then be completely dispersed by metabolism or excretion.

Three types are currently available; dextrans, gelatins and hydroxyethylstarches. All can produce anaphylactoid reactions ranging in clinical severity from skin eruptions to anaphylactic shock. They are, however, rare, the overall combined incidence for minor and major reactions being 0·3% and 0·033% respectively.

Dextrans. The use of these has declined principally because of the fear of anaphylaxis (highest incidence of all synthetic substitutes) and renal failure due to the increased viscosity of the urine. They impair coagulation being fibrinoplastic and inhibit platelet function; sometimes in large volumes they produce an acquired form of von Willebrand's disease. The plasma half-lives ranges from 2 to 4 hours for dextran 40 to 24 hours for dextran 70. Dextran 40 is hypertonic, producing a volume effect equal to twice that infused; dextran 70 is isotonic.

Gelatins. These are the most commonly used plasma expanders. They are isotonic and have an average plasma half-life of 4·5 hours. They have no appreciable effect on haemostasis but have been implicated as causing reticulo-endothelial impaired function. Infusion of large volumes is thought by some to increase the incidence of ARDS and acute renal failure but this is certainly not proven.

Hydroxyethylstarches. The newest of the synthetic substitutes, these have the lowest risk of anaphylaxis, produce no deleterious effects on renal function and have long plasma half-lives (48 hours) with approximately 5% being in the circulation 2 weeks after infusion. There is some suggestion that high volumes may depress reticuloendothelial function by blocking uptake (as with gelatins) and infusion of large volumes may produce an acquired von Willebrand-like syndrome. The use of synthetic solutions with oxygen carrying capacity still remains experimental and some are not yet appropriate for clinical use.

THE PROBLEMS OF MASSIVE BLOOD TRANSFUSION. Massive blood transfusion has been defined as greater than 8 units over 4 hours or greater than 15 units in 24 hours (85% of blood now issued is in the form of packed cells rather than whole blood). Transfusions of these amounts of stored blood produce a number of problems.

1. Haemostasis. Blood stored for more than 24 hours contains no functioning platelets, 10% of Factors V and VIII and 20% of Factor XI. Significant dilutional thrombocytopenia may develop along with clotting factor deficiency. Clinical bleeding will require correction with fresh frozen plasma.

2. Microaggregates. Dead white cells along with fibrin and platelet aggregates are found in stored blood and have been implicated in the pathogenesis of ARDS and acute renal failure. Filters of varying pore size (20–40 μm) have been used in an effort to prevent these complications but they have inherent complications of their own such as

removal of viable platelets, if present, embolism from the filter and blockage. Their use remains controversial.

3. Citrate toxicity. Citrate present in stored blood may produce toxic effects as increased levels reduce the serum ionized calcium. If citrate metabolism is impaired, as in liver disease or low cardiac output states, muscle tremors and ECG changes of hypocalcaemia may ensue; 5–10 ml calcium gluconate with alternate units of blood during massive transfusion is believed to prevent this. Recent alternative formulations of blood have decreased this effect and its clinical significance is somewhat disputed.

4. Hypothermia. Stored blood is kept at 4 °C and in massive transfusion hypothermia may develop. Blood warmers should be used if possible.

5. Other problems include:

Hyperkalaemia
Metabolic acidosis
Impaired oxygen delivery to tissues because of low levels of 2,3-DPG in the red cells and the transmission of infection

DECREASE OF VENTRICULAR PRELOAD. Hypervolaemia or left ventricular failure will raise the preload and if pulmonary artery pressure rises pulmonary oedema may develop. PA pressure may be reduced by decreasing circulating volume, dilating pulmonary arteries or by decreasing venous return to the heart by the use of venodilators.

Venesection now has little use in the reduction of circulating volume except in an emergency where other means are now available. Loop diuretics such as frusemide increase sodium and water clearance by the kidneys though in acute pulmonary oedema frusemide causes venodilatation and this may be its principal mode of action in this circumstance. In acute heart failure associated with renal impairment, haemofiltration may enable the excess fluid to be effectively removed in a controlled fashion. Venodilatation using nitrates to decrease venous return will also decrease preload in addition to improving coronary artery blood flow. Sodium nitroprusside (an arteriolar dilator) also produces PA dilation and may be employed. The hypotensive effects of these drugs (especially nitroprusside) may prohibit their use.

b. Improving Myocardial Contractility

When preload has been optimized and cardiac output is still insufficient, myocardial contractility may be improved by the use of positive inotropic drugs. It should be remembered that correction of metabolic abnormalities, such as acidosis, and optimizing oxygenation can play as important a role as inotropic drugs in this respect.

Many drugs have positive inotropic properties although those used in critical care are primarily catecholamines. With the exception of dopamine, which may be used to dilate renal arteries, the catecholamines are used for their beta-1 receptor mediated increase in contractility of the myocardium. Other circulatory effects are due to stimulation of alpha and beta-2 receptors, adrenergic neurone stimulation, dopaminergic receptor stimulation and beta-1 mediated effects on heart rate and conduction (*Table* 6.2). All have short half-lives and need to be given by continuous infusion for a sustained effect.

Selection of an individual agent is dependent on matching its activcity to the underlying physiological disturbance, remembering that the distribution of blood flow may be as important as its increase.

The ideal inotropic agent should increase contractility with a negligible effect on heart rate (tachycardia increases myocardial oxygen consumption). It may be advantageous to have some beta-2 activity, although any vasodilatation-induced hypotension produced in this fashion should be offset at least in part by the increased contractility. Dopaminergic activity may be of benefit. An inotrope should not be arrhythmogenic, not stimulate adrenergic neurones nor produce excessive vasoconstriction.

All catecholamines increase cardiac work and may extend the size of a myocardial infarction. Any increase in oxygen demand should be matched by oxygen delivery.

Dobutamine in many respects satisfies a number of these conditions and is regarded by some as the inotrope of first choice. It does not seem to have the same inotropic efficacy as dopamine but has less unwanted effects. It combines inotropic activity with beta-2 mediated vasodilatation and has limited chronotropic activity and tendency to provoke arrhythmias. It has been shown to improve myocardial blood flow and its use in patients following myocardial infarction does not increase infarct size and may even limit extension. The dose range is 2–40 μg/kg/min.

Dopamine is the most widely used inotropic agent. It combines good beta-1 effects with the additional benefit of dopaminergically mediated renal vasodilatation. In high doses the alpha-mediated vasoconstrictor effects predominate and unwanted tachycardia and arrhythmias may then limit its use. Dose range is 1–30 μg/kg/min.

The combination of dopamine and dobutamine in the shocked patient with renal hypoperfusion has been used to good effect.

Isoprenaline increases cardiac output but distribution of any increase is primarily to skeletal muscle as a result of beta-2 mediated vasodilatation. It may produce arrhythmias and can cause excessive tachycardia. Hypotension may result from vasodilatation and the coronary circulation can be compromised which if combined with excessive rate may lead to a severe imbalance between oxygen supply and demand. Dose range is 0·02–0·18 μg/kg/min.

Table 6.2 Spectrum of activity of catecholamines

	Vascular		*Cardiac*			*Adrenergic*	*Dopaminergic*
	α Vasoconstriction	β_2 Vasodilatation	d*p*/d*t*	β_1 Conduction	Rate		
Dopamine	0 – + + + +	0 – +	+ + + +	+ +	+ +	+ + + +	+ +
Dobutamine	0 – +	0 – + +	+ + + +	+	+	0	0
Noradrenaline	+ + + +	0	+ + + +	+ + + +	+ + + +	+ + + +	0
Isoprenaline	0	+ + + +	+ + + +	+ + + +	+ + + +	0	0
Adrenaline	+ + +	+	+ + + +	+ + + +	+ + + +	+ +	0

Adrenaline will produce an increase in cardiac output though its spectrum of action distributes blood to skeletal muscles rather than to vital organs. Diastolic blood pressure falls and this may compromise coronary oxygen delivery. There is a marked increase in cardiac work and oxygen consumption and a high incidence of arrhythmias. Whilst its side-effects prohibit its routine use it remains the agent of choice in cardiac arrest (asystole) as it is the most potent drug available for that use. Dose range is 0·06–0·18 μg/kg/min.

Noradrenaline is only used in extreme circumstances because of its excessive vasoconstrictor activity. Dose range is 0·01–0·07 μg/kg/min.

c. Reducing Ventricular Afterload

If contractility and preload have been optimized but cardiac output still remains inadequate then reduction of ventricular afterload may be of benefit. Afterload as described above may be equated to total peripheral resistance and is reduced using vasodilators of one form or another. All vasodilators may produce hypotension and adequate preload must be ensured prior to their administration. In practice their use is normally confined to those patients with a systolic blood pressure of 90 mmHg (12·0 kPa) or above. The theoretical reason for their being of benefit is that with a lower peripheral resistance the left ventricle will be able to empty more at the end of each beat and therefore the cardiac output will improve.

There are a number of indications for the use of vasodilators:

1. Malignant hypertension and hypertensive crises (particularly hypertension following cardiac surgery);
2. Poor peripheral perfusion associated with high peripheral resistance;
3. Acute left ventricular failure with or without clinical pulmonary oedema;
4. Acute pulmonary oedema associated with acute mitral incompetence;
5. Severe resistant angina;
6. Myocardial infarction with low cardiac output.

Vasodilators may be divided into directly or indirectly acting.

DIRECT. The most commonly used in intensive care practice are sodium nitroprusside and nitrates such as nitroglycerin or isosorbide dinitrate.

Sodium nitroprusside is a rapidly acting potent vasodilator primarily acting directly on arterioles though having some action on venules. It produces a fall in peripheral resistance and venous return, thus reducing ventricular preload as well as afterload and as a consequence it may produce profound hypotension. Direct arterial pressure monitoring is advised when using this drug.

Nitroglycerine and other intravenous nitrates act directly and are predominantly venous dilators. The resultant fall in venous return produces a fall in preload; afterload is also reduced because it also relaxes arteriolar smooth muscle. Myocardial oxygen delivery is increased as coronary artery dilatation occurs. Pulmonary vascular resistance falls dropping afterload to the right ventricle. As a group they are less potent than nitroprusside.

Hydralazine given by i.v. boluses of 10–20 mg may be used to reduce afterload; it acts directly on arteriolar smooth muscle.

Nifedipine may be given orally; its calcium channel blocking activity causing arteriolar dilatation. Dose is 10–20 mg.

Prostacyclin (PGI_2) is a recently developed directly acting vasodilator acting on the pulmonary and systemic circulation. It is an arachidonic acid metabolite and has anticoagulant properties.

INDIRECT. Alpha-blocking drugs, phentolamine and chlorpromazine, reduce afterload as do beta-2 agonists such as salbutamol. The former are now rarely used as their effect may be prolonged and shorter acting, more easily controlled drugs are available. Salbutamol often causes excessive tachycardia.

2. Heart Rate and Rhythm

Attention should always be given to the heart rate whilst manipulating cardiac output. Sinus tachycardia rarely requires control, tachy- and bradyarrhythmias which affect haemodynamic performance should be promptly treated. If arrhythmias arise attention should be given to the adequacy of oxygenation and to the level of potassium.

3. Oxygenation

The arterial P_{O_2} should be kept between 9·3–13·3 kPa; hyperoxygenation should be avoided. Resorting to IPPV should be a last resort in the shocked patient and the use of facemask CPAP or PEEP systems should be considered.

4. Metabolic Acidosis

In the absence of ketosis or renal failure lactic acidosis secondary to impaired tissue perfusion is the most common cause in the critically ill.

Metabolic acidosis will impair cardiac function due to a fall in intracellular pH and this impairs myocardial response to catecholamines. Acidosis increases sympathetic tone, stimulating endogenous catecholamine release, and also enhances conversion of dopamine to noradrenaline with further, perhaps inappropriate, vasoconstriction.

Restoration of cardiac output and tissue perfusion will lead to correction of the acidosis. However, should the pH fall to less than 7·1 alkalinization should be commenced with small amounts of sodium bicarbonate (25–50 mmol) until the pH rises to 7·1.

5. Mechanical Support of the Circulation

If pharmacological support fails mechanical support may be of use in certain cases. Those currently available include intra-aortic balloon counterpulsation pumps (IABC), ventricular assist devices and a variety of other systems. IABC is the most commonly used.

The IABC catheter is balloon tipped. This is positioned in the thoracic aorta distal to the left subclavian artery. It is inserted through an introducer into the femoral artery or positioned during surgery under direct vision. The balloon is filled with CO_2 or helium and is inflated by an external pump.

The balloon is set to inflate and deflate by synchronization with the patient's ECG. Thus during systole deflation decreases afterload and in diastole inflation augments aortic diastolic pressure and enhances coronary blood flow.

Indications

1. Postcardiac surgical cardiogenic shock and inability to wean from cardiopulmonary bypass.
2. In acute myocardial infarction where circulatory support is needed during investigations prior to planned surgical intervention.

3. In patients with recurrent myocardial ischaemic episodes for pain relief and support during coronary arteriography.

4. In selected cases of septicaemic shock where myocardial depression is profound but the control of sepsis is judged to be possible.

Complications of Shock

Continuing hypoperfusion leads to eventual multiple organ system failure. Endothelial integrity is lost and infection and septicaemia may occur. Respiratory, hepatic and renal failure may all develop. Disseminated intravascular coagulation is common in severe circulatory failure and may potentiate the various organ failures.

Prognosis

Shock resulting from pure hypovolaemia carries an excellent prognosis if the causative lesions can be rapidly corrected. Mortality now arises after the initial resuscitation due to respiratory and renal failure. Acute renal failure occurring in this context still has a mortality of 50% and ARDS mortality remains at around 60%. The most ominous complication following shock is the development of septicaemia and multiple organ system failure. Cardiogenic shock following myocardial infarction still has a grave prognosis of up to 70%.

Cardiac Arrest

Cardiac arrest implies the sudden cessation of effective heart function usually because of ventricular fibrillation or ventricular asystole although the two are not mutually exclusive.

Aetiology

There are many possible causes which may occur separately or together in the surgical patient.

1. Myocardial ischaemia can often precipitate cardiac arrest and this most often occurs following myocardial infarction or acute coronary insufficiency. Patients with coronary artery disease are particularly at risk.

2. Hypotension from whatever cause may precipitate cardiac arrest especially in the presence of coronary artery disease or hypoxia.

3. Hypokalaemia may lead to the development of ventricular ectopics which in turn may cause spontaneous cardiac arrest.

4. Hyperkalaemia which may result from renal failure, metabolic acidosis or inadvertent rapid or excessive administration of potassium-containing solutions can cause cardiac arrest.

5. Hypoxia is a common cause and may occur in respiratory failure or as a result of patient disconnection from ventilator or oxygen supply, or under anaesthesia.

6. Hypothermia, a body temperature below 30 °C, predisposes to the development of ventricular fibrillation. During cardiac surgery the patient may be cooled to as low as 15 °C when asystole develops.

7. Increase in vagal tone due to drugs (e.g. suxamethonium) or to stimulation during surgery may precipitate asystole. The latter particularly occurs during surgery on the brain, middle ear, biliary tract, pelvic organs and the jaw.

8. Drug overdose particularly with catecholamines (incorrect dilution), digitalis and tricyclic antidepressants may cause arrest as can normal doses when there is abnormal sensitivity to their action, e.g. hypokalaemia, hypoxia and acidosis.

9. Physical irritation of the myocardium as may occur during cardiothoracic surgery, the passage of intracardiac catheters and guide wires for central venous cannulation can also provoke cardiac arrest.

Clinical Features

Syncope and impalpable major pulses (femoral/carotid) in the previously awake patients or loss of arterial pressure waveform and ECG changes in the unconscious patient are the hallmarks of the condition.

Survival depends on rapid diagnosis and intervention. Irreversible brain damage occurs after 3–4 minutes of cessation of circulation and prolonged cardiovascular standstill diminishes the chance of restoring effective cardiac function.

Management

Management may be divided into initial cardiopulmonary resuscitation (CPR), secondary treatment of any underlying rhythm disturbance and finally the aftercare following the arrest.

a. Initial Resuscitation

1. An initial precordial thump may be tried by giving a vigorous blow to the lower sternum (precordial thump). This should only be considered immediately after arrest has occurred otherwise it is a fruitless and time-wasting exercise.

2. Begin external cardiac massage (ECM). This should be at a rate of 60–80 per minute and should depress the sternum approximately 4 cm. ECM if performed correctly can sustain the circulation for long periods. Internal massage should be considered in postcardiac surgical patients, patients with severe chest injuries, in the presence of tamponade or haemothorax, or in patients with an otherwise good prognosis where ECM is ineffective.

3. The airway should be cleared and ventilation commenced with 100% oxygen using initially an oral airway and mask. Unless trained personnel are immediately at hand, face mask ventilation should be performed, before any attempt is made at endotracheal intubation, to ensure some immediate oxygenation. Intubation should then be performed and ventilation commenced. The ratio of compressions to breaths varies from protocol to protocol and may be 5 : 1, 10 : 2, 1 : 1 in 'new CPR'.

Whilst the above measures are instituted the following should ideally be performed by another person. If little help is available then ventilation and ECM must take priority.

4. Good venous access should be gained. In the author's opinion an internal jugular cannula should be inserted in all patients following cardiac arrest. Wide-bore cannulas in large arm veins are an acceptable second best.

5. ECG monitoring should be commenced.

6. Insertion of a radial artery cannula for repeated blood gas estimations.

b. Definitive Treatment

1. VENTRICULAR FIBRILLATION. A D.C. shock should be given as soon as possible. Some authorities would advocate this even without ECG monitoring if any delay in setting up occurs. The initial charge should be 100 J, increased to 400 J in steps if unsuccessful. CPR should be continued between shocks.

If fine fibrillation is present, 5–10 ml 1 : 10 000 i.v. adrenaline should be given to 'coarsen' it prior to defibrillation. Calcium chloride (5 ml of 10%) may also be given to facilitate this action.

Should these measures fail, lignocaine 1–1·5 mg/kg as an i.v. bolus should be given followed, if successful, by an infusion at an initial rate of 4 mg/hour. If lignocaine fails then bretylium tosylate (5–10 mg/kg) or mexiletine (100–250 mg at 25 mg/min) has been successful.

Disopyramide, amiodarone and flecainide have all been used to treat intractable or resistant ventricular fibrillation, specialist opinion being sought prior to their use.

2. VENTRICULAR ASYSTOLE. This is more difficult to treat that ventricular fibrillation and it usually signifies more severe myocardial pathology. The treatment remains empirical and the following drugs are used;

Adenaline 1–5 mg
Atropine 1–2 mg
Isoprenaline 1–3 mg followed by an infusion of 4–8 μg/min
Noradrenaline 1–5 mg
Calcium chloride 10% 5–10 ml

Cardiac pacing should be attempted should facilities exist if pharmacological measures fail. Recent advances in technology include transcutaneous pacing electrodes, pacing pulmonary artery catheters and oesophageal electrodes.

Abnormalities of arterial pH, oxygenation and potassium levels will impair resuscitative efforts and levels should be frequently monitored during prolonged resuscitation.

3. METABOLIC ACIDOSIS. Acidosis, if present, should be treated as outlined above. There is no place for excessive administration of bicarbonate at the beginning of resuscitation in the manner that is often practised. Excessive bicarbonate administration may lead to metabolic alkalosis (pH >7·55) which has been shown to be associated with an increased mortality rate. It has also been postulated that bicarbonate administration may lead to a fall in intracellular pH as CO_2 is formed and diffuses across cell membranes more rapidly than the negatively charged bicarbonate.

4. POTASSIUM HAEMOSTASIS. Hypokalaemia should be treated with i.v. potassium chloride, diluted and given over 5–10 minutes.

Hyperkalaemia may be the precipitating factor, occurring in renal failure, acidosis and as a result of overzealous administration. Treatment is described in the section on renal failure.

5. CEREBRAL PROTECTION. No firm evidence for the protective effect of any drug given during cardiac arrest for this has been documented. There is some evidence that calcium channel blockers (verapamil and nifedipine) may be of benefit.

c. Abandoning Resuscitation

There are no firm rules on this and decisions should be tailored to the individual circumstances, paying particular attention to the aetiology, duration of the arrest and the patient's underlying condition.

In general terms efforts are normally abandoned after 30–45 minutes if there is no electrical activity or persistent electromechanical dissociation. Prolonged efforts may be fully justified in young patients and particularly where hypothermia is present at the time of arrest. The assessment of neurological damage is notoriously difficult immediately after resuscitation and should be deferred.

d. Aftercare

This varies from patient to patient and the degree of support given will depend upon the individual circumstances. Treatment generally centres around:

1. Treatment of cardiogenic shock and pulmonary oedema
2. Monitoring and preservation of renal function
3. Preservation of brain function.

If consciousness is not recovered some degree of ischaemic brain damage can be assumed to have occurred if no other cause is apparent. An aggressive approach to this should be taken if full support is indicated. Review of neurological function should take place every 24 hours. This aim of treatment is to prevent any brain oedema occurring and to limit any oedema already present. Management includes:

a. Avoiding hypo- or hypertensive episodes, keeping cerebral perfusion pressure at adequate levels.

b. Maintaining arterial P_{O_2} within normal limits.

c. Hyperventilation, when IPPV is required, to a Pa_{CO_2} of 25–30 mmHg (3·3–4·0 kPa).

d. Paralysis and sedation to prevent incoordinate action between ventilator and patient or coughing which raises venous pressure and therefore ICP.

e. Monitoring and stabilizing blood sugar, electrolytes and plasma osmolarity.

f. Treating seizures as they develop. This may require the use of EEG monitoring in paralysed patients.

g. Dexamethasone is often given in an attempt to decrease brain oedema in doses 4 mg 6-hourly but is of no proven value in global cerebral oedema.

h. Routine insertion of ICP monitoring probes has been advocated by some authorities.

ACUTE RESPIRATORY FAILURE (ARF)

Patients requiring intensive care frequently develop arterial hypoxaemia as a consequence of respiratory insufficiency. It may follow a wide variety of insults traditionally divided into two groups—those with direct mechanisms of lung damage (contusion, pneumonitis from noxious gases or vapours or aspiration) and those in which the lung damage is a consequence of some distant but systemic process (sepsis, pancreatitis, DIC). The severity of pulmonary dysfunction is, however, extremely variable.

The critically ill patient may develop ARF from any number of precipitating factors though only a small number of the hypoxaemic population—resistant to oxygen enrichment or continuous positive airway pressure by facemask—require endotracheal intubation and ventilation. Similarly, only a small number of these patients will develop the classic features of the Adult Respiratory Distress Syndrome (ARDS) and it is to the management of this syndrome that this section is primarily directed, though the correction of any precipitating factor and hypoxaemia is the basis for the treatment of any variety of respiratory failure.

Pathology

The pathological changes seen in the lung can be divided into three phases: an initial exudative phase followed by a proliferative phase and, if survival occurs, a final regenerative phase of varying degree. Macroscopically the lungs become engorged and may weigh as much as 2000 g (normal 300 g). Microscopically, protein-rich and fibrinous exudates are followed by hyaline membrane deposition and interstitial fibrosis. Survival is characterized by regression of fibrotic changes in 70% of lung after 18 months. Intra-alveolar haemorrhage may occur in some cases. Oedema occurs in ARDS as a result of the breakdown of endothelial integrity and is thus protein rich and non-cardiogenic in origin. Left atrial pressure and therefore PAOP should be normal though in the later stages cardiac failure will exacerbate the problem. If hypoalbuminaemia develops low plasma oncotic pressure will facilitate the movement of water into the interstitium.

Pathophysiology

The pathological changes described above lead to characteristic abnormalities in pulmonary function:

1. Severe hypoxaemia develops as there is increasing ventilation/perfusion V/Q mismatch and falling functional residual capacity.
2. Falling compliance produces an increased work of breathing.
3. Pulmonary artery pressure increases.
4. $P\text{aco}_2$ is initially low as hypoxaemia and stiffened lungs stimulate ventilatory drive. In the later stages however $P\text{aco}_2$ rises as its clearance becomes inadequate.

Clinical Features

The clinical diagnosis of ARDS has changed little since it was first described. Typically, patients present with respiratory distress characterized by tachypnoea and dyspnoea. This may occur at the same time as any precipitating factor or may be delayed in onset. Classically the chest X-ray shows bilateral diffuse pulmonary infiltrates, however these may be absent in patients receiving continuous positive airways pressure (CPAP) or positive end-expiratory pressure (PEEP).

In non-survivors there is an almost inevitable development of multiple organ system failure, frequently complicated by sepsis, the overall mortality rate is of the order of 60%.

Treatment

There does not exist any specific form of therapy for ARDS and management is essentially based on correcting hypoxaemia and general supportive therapy. Of vital importance is the prompt diagnosis and treatment of infection as sepsis in these patients carries with it a grave prognosis.

Correction of Hypoxaemia

When treating hypoxaemia it is important to remember that oxygen delivery to tissues depends both on arterial oxygen content and cardiac output. $P\text{ao}_2$ should be measured in combination with values for haemoglobin and % saturation if possible. $P\text{ao}_2$ values above 8·0 kPa show little incremental increase in content for increases in partial pressure and striving to obtain values greater than this is of little benefit. However, below this value small decrements in tension produce significant decreases in content. At levels below 4·0 kPa oxygen transport from capillaries to cells becomes inadequate.

Hypoxaemia may be corrected in two ways, by increasing inspired concentration (FIO_2), and by increasing mean airway pressure which leads to an increase in functional residual capacity (FRC) and prevention of collapse of alveoli (and therefore improves arterial oxygenation). Oxygenation may be improved by extracorporeal means but this remains experimental.

1. Increasing Inspired Concentration

This may be used in combination with increased mean airway pressures or on its own in the first instance. Patients who can breathe without assistance can wear masks or nasal spectacles which will increase the inspired concentration by a variable amount depending on make. Venturi masks provide concentrations between 24 and 60%, Hudson masks are less accurate and provide concentrations up to 60%. Nasal spectacles provide between 20 and 45%. (It should be remembered that in the presence of a severe pulmonary shunt increasing FIO_2 will not be effective.)

All oxygen-enriched air should be adequately humidified and delivered to the patient at a temperature of 37 °C. Oxygen in high concentrations has been shown to produce similar morphological changes in the lungs as those seen in ARDS. It has also been demonstrated to produce a fall in vital capacity and FRC due to absorption atelectasis. Inspired concentrations greater than 60% should therefore be avoided whenever possible.

2. Increasing Airway Pressures—CPAP/PEEP

Where maximum inspired concentrations of O_2 are failing to provide adequate $P\text{ao}_2$ oxygenation may be improved by preventing collapse of small airways and increasing the FRC. It is now possible to do this in spontaneously breathing patients by administering PEEP or CPAP with a facemask.

a. PEEP/CPAP. These improve oxygenation by increasing FRC and by preventing collapse of small alveoli. At a given FIO_2 CPAP/PEEP administration will improve $P\text{ao}_2$. Increasing airway pressures will decrease cardiac output (by restricting venous return), increase the risk of barotrauma, increase dead space ventilation and stimulate the release of ADH. In the spontaneously breathing patient the work of breathing (and therefore O_2 consumption) will also be increased.

The criteria for instituting these measures varies in different centres but generally if the $P\text{ao}_2$ is less than 8·0 kPa on an FIO_2 >50% it would be appropriate. Normal levels range from 5 to 15 cmH_2O though higher levels have been used. Spontaneously breathing patients do not tolerate levels of greater than 10 cmH_2O. When measures such as these fail to improve oxygenation or patient tolerance becomes a problem artificial ventilation should be instituted.

b. INTERMITTENT POSITIVE-PRESSURE VENTILATION. In surgical patients there may be many different reasons for instituting IPPV; in the case of ARDS the decision is usually based on deteriorating respiratory function or a desire to decrease oxygen consumption. The following factors should be taken into account when deciding to institute IPPV:

1. Exhaustion
2. Rising respiratory rate
3. Falling $P\text{ao}_2$
4. $P\text{ao}_2 < 8·0$ kPa with FIO_2 60%
5. Decreasing lung volumes
6. Inadequate CO_2 clearance
7. O_2 demand higher than the ability to supply (the diaphragm may consume up to 20% of available oxygen in respiratory distress).

IPPV benefits the patient in these circumstances due to its facility to;

1. Improve ventilation–perfusion imbalance due to re-

cruitment of closed alveoli and improved overall gas distribution

2. Increase the FRC
3. Decrease the work of breathing
4. Facilitate increased minute volumes.

IPPV does, however, have attendant complications and the most serious in cases of ARDS is the increased risk of nosocomial respiratory infection which gravely influences the prognosis, otherwise the complications are the same as described for PEEP and CPAP with the additional risks associated with endotracheal intubation or tracheostomy. As with PEEP/CPAP impairment of cardiac output due to a decreased venous return may occur and an adequate circulating volume as judged by CVP or PAOP measurement should be maintained.

Endotracheal tubes and tracheostomies require meticulous nursing to prevent infection and local damage. With care endotracheal tubes may be left in place for up to 10 days before changing or converting to a tracheostomy.

Along with IPPV most ventilators allow for addition of CPAP/PEEP into the circuit. Ideally in these cases the ventilator should be volume preset with sufficient monitoring facilities to ensure that airway pressures do not rise too high and that a desired minute ventilation is achieved.

WEANING FROM IPPV. Weaning is a complex process which differs in each individual patient. There are no set criteria or time limits and management is essentially clinical. Generally speaking, other systems should be relatively stable (though on occasion cessation of IPPV produces dramatic improvement in cardiovascular function). Some suggested respiratory criteria for the institution of weaning are:

Vital capacity	$\geqslant$ 5·0 l
Inspiratory force	$\geqslant$ 10·0 cmH_2O
Minute volume	$\geqslant$ 18·0 l
Respiratory rate	< 45 per min
pH	> 7·3
Pa_{O_2} (FIO_2 0·4)	> 8·0 kPa

Other Measures

Care should be taken of the patient's general condition, in particular to the overall state of nutrition and, if necessary, parenteral or enteral nutrition should be instituted. Renal failure is a common sequelae of ARDS and urinary function should be meticulously observed. Patients often become anaemic and should be transfused when the haemoglobin falls below 9·0 g/L.

Fluid Balance

Fluid balance is complex in cases of ARDS and the CVP should be routinely measured. The syndrome is characterized by the loss of capillary integrity and at the time of diagnosis a great deal of plasma may already have been lost into the interstitium. Plasma should be replaced with human albumin fraction and the plasma oncotic pressure should be kept within normal limits. PAOP should be measured when interpretation of the CVP is in doubt.

Prognosis

Acute respiratory failure is a complex problem, a critically ill patient may develop lethal respiratory complications or may become critically ill because of acute respiratory failure. Although we possess considerable information of the physiological derangements little is known of the exact mechanisms of acute lung injury. Not surprisingly, therefore, treatment is still primarily directed to the correction of hypoxia rather than the underlying pathology.

The mortality of acute respiratory failure remains high; in the absence of specialized care it can be as great as 70% but many intensive care units have reduced this figure to between 20 and 40% (*see also* Chapter 9).

ACUTE RENAL FAILURE

In acute renal failure (ARF) there is a sudden and significant decrease in the glomerular filtration rate (GFR) with loss of the renal control of internal homeostasis. The low GFR is the direct consequence of a reduction in renal blood flow which in ARF falls to 30–40% of normal levels. There is also a diversion of intrarenal blood flow away from the cortex which further reduces the GFR. Afferent renal arteriolar constriction, probably due to high renal renin levels, and ischaemic cortical cell swelling add to the vascular insufficiency.

Clinically these changes become manifest as oliguria which is a hallmark of ARF.

Oliguria is variously quoted in terms of urine outputs that range from 400 to 700 ml/24 hours. In critically ill patients, however, urine output must be measured each hour and oliguria is defined as a urine flow of less than 20 ml/h.

ARF may complicate many forms of 'surgical' illness usually as an aftermath of any form of shock. In these cases renal function may be further impaired by Gram-negative endotoxaemia, disseminated intravascular coagulation (DIC), myoglobinuria, haemoglobinuria, various nephrotoxins and the presence of jaundice. Primary intrinsic renal disease, such as glomerulonephritis and pyelonephritis, is uncommon in surgical patients whilst the causes and problems of urinary tract obstruction are of specialist interest.

A Classification of ARF

With such a diverse aetiology it is helpful, practically, to group the causes of ARF into three categories; prerenal, renal and postrenal.

Prerenal failure is related to the reduction in renal blood flow and will resolve if this is quickly restored. If, however, the state of diminished perfusion persists structural changes occur in the kidney and the disorder is no longer immediately reversible. This state is often described as acute tubular necrosis (ATN) and represents the most common form of established ARF that is encountered in critically ill patients. Necrosis of renal tubules is, however, a very variable feature and there is a feeling in some quarters that the term should be abandoned in favour of either 'vasomotor nephropathy' or 'acute reversible intrinsic renal failure'. Renal cortical necrosis is a more significant diagnosis because of its irreversibility and can only be made on biopsy or the subsequent clinical course.

Postrenal failure is a possible result of any form of urinary tract obstruction and the occurrence of anuria, rather than oliguria, is always suggestive of such a cause. Its possible presence must always be considered in the differential diagnosis of ARF and if there is any doubt about the patency of the urinary tract, it must be investigated using high dose intravenous pyelography, ultrasound imaging or isotope excretion studies. Further consideration of obstructive uropathy is outside the scope of this chapter.

Diagnosis of ARF

When a postrenal cause is not implicated, the differential diagnosis of oliguria rests between prerenal failure and ATN, which in practical terms is the difference between an immediately correctable condition and one that has become established.

In prerenal failure, once the cardiac output has been restored, the urine volume should increase although in some cases there may be a delay of a few hours before this is noted. If inotopric support is required to increase the cardiac output, dopamine, because it increases renal blood flow and tubular sodium excretion, is the agent of first choice.

If oliguria persists after the renal circulation has been restored then ATN may have developed and any temptation to give more fluid to 'flush out the kidneys' must be resisted for this will only promote the development of the various syndromes of fluid overload. At this stage the measurement of urine and plasma osmolality and urine sodium concentration may give some guidance. A urine osmolality in excess of 500 mmol/L or a urine–plasma osmolality ratio greater than 1·5 suggests a prerenal disturbance. Similarly, a urine sodium concentration of less than 10 mmol/L indicates that the renal tubules are still able to absorb sodium in response to a reduced blood volume. Conversely a urine osmolality equal to that of plasma and a urine sodium concentration greater than 50 mmol/L are indicative of ATN.

The Course of Acute Tubular Necrosis

There is still debate concerning the influence of diuretics, mannitol and frusemide in particular, on the course of established ATN.

Mannitol is a relatively non-toxic polyhydric alcohol that is filtered by the glomeruli, it reduces water reabsorption and increases tubular excretion of electrolytes. Prophylactic administration of mannitol to high-risk patients undergoing abdominal surgery has some protective effect against the development of ARF, but its value when given after the insult is less certain. Current opinion suggests that it might be tried in a single dose of 25 g that should not be repeated if the urine volume is not increased. Mannitol is not metabolized and if it is retained it can produce a hyperosmolar syndrome and expansion of the extracellular fluid volume which might precipitate pulmonary oedema.

Frusemide, a potent loop diuretic, is probably the drug that is given most frequently in an endeavour to influence the course of ARF. It increases renal cortical blood flow transiently and its diuretic action may relieve any element of tubular obstruction. However, in spite of these possible benefits, clincial trials have failed to provide any convincing evidence that frusemide prevents or reverses the progression of ARF, whereas there is some evidence to show that it may increase the nephrotoxicity of various antibiotics. Certainly the use of frusemide to treat postoperative oliguria cannot be too strongly condemned. The majority of these patients require additional fluid replacement, and if diuretics are given they will produce a greater degree of hypovolaemia and may actually precipitate ARF. Frusemide should be restricted to those patients who remain oliguric after adequate fluid replacement. Then, if given as an infusion of 1 g over a period of 4 hours, it might produce an increase in urine volume but will probably not influence the overall course of the ARF. In certain situations this increased volume may be of great practical significance, for instance, to allow increased quantities of high calorie intravenous fluids to be given.

Biochemical Disturbances in ARF

These reflect the kidneys' impaired excretory function, the catabolic nature of critical illness and the sometimes inappropriate water and electrolyte replacement.

1. Water and Sodium

Hyponatraemia is very common and is almost always dilutional, the total body content of sodium is not significantly reduced. The plasma sodium concentration will increase with fluid restriction. Only in those situations where the underlying disease is associated with large losses of sodium is hyponatraemia likely to be truly depletional.

2. Potassium

Potassium is primarily an intracellular cation but the relatively small extracellular component has a profound effect on cardiac and skeletal muscle excitability. In ARF the major route of potassium excretion is reduced and its concentration in the plasma increases. The magnitude and rate of this rise are increased by release of potassium from damaged tissue, by an increased rate of catabolism and as a consequence of haemolysis or an extracellular acidosis. High plasma levels can develop with alarming rapidity. Above 6 mmol/L various cardiac arrhythmias may occur and if the increase continues, these are followed by conduction disturbances, peaking of the T waves and eventually, usually with levels above 7 mmol/L, cardiac arrest.

Hypokalaemia is relatively rare, only developing when there are large extrarenal losses of potassium.

3. Hydrogen Ions

Failure to excrete hydrogen ions leads to a metabolic acidosis. Initially, hyperventilation may restore the pH to within normal limits and the excess hydrogen ions can be buffered by the plasma bicarbonate. When the limits of compensation are exceeded the pH falls; this will occur more rapidly in catabolic patients, in those with an associated lactic acidosis and in the presence of ventilatory failure.

The increase in intracellular hydrogen ion concentration leads to an exchange of these ions for potassium ions across cell membranes and the plasma potassium increases.

4. Nitrogenous Products

In uncomplicated cases the blood urea usually increases at a rate of 6 mmol/L each 24 hours. In highly catabolic patients the rate of rise is in excess of this, sometimes as great as 40 mmol/L. An increase in serum creatinine is, except in the presence of severe muscle damage, more directly related to the disturbed renal function and in hypercatabolic states the urea–creatinine ratio increases.

5. Calcium

A moderate degree of hypocalcaemia is common in ARF. Tetany is, however, uncommon because the level of ionized calcium is increased by the metabolic acidosis and hypermagnesaemia may also be present.

Clinical Manifestations of ARF

These reflect the effects of the various fluid and electrolyte disturbances on the different systems.

Respiratory

Surgical patients suffering from the effects of trauma, infection or fluid overload may have severe respiratory failure requiring IPPV. In patients with ARF the presence or development of dyspnoea may be the consequence of pulmonary oedema, metabolic acidosis, pulmonary infection occurring singly or in combination.

Cardiovascular

Pulmonary and systemic oedema are usually the result of fluid overload although left ventricular failure might be present after cardiac surgery, in septicaemia, following chest trauma or for reasons not related to the primary illness. Oedema formation is facilitated by hypoalbuminaemia and abnormal capillary permeability.

Hypertension is again associated with overhydration and pericarditis only develops with high levels of blood urea. Various arrhythmias may occur and are usually related to changes in the plasma potassium level.

Gastrointestinal

Non-specific symptoms of anorexia, nausea and vomiting are common and may be due to water overload. Hiccups occur in the later stages and diarrhoea not infrequently follows nasogastric feeding with hyperosmolar solutions. Gastrointestinal bleeding from gastric erosions, stress ulcers, oesophagitis or, more rarely, severe colitis is a constant threat; the accumulation of blood in the gastrointestinal tract following such a haemorrhage increases the quantities of nitrogenous substances absorbed and the blood urea rises rapidly.

Neurological

Drowsiness, confusion and coma are in part related to the development of cerebral oedema and also to the numerous metabolic disturbances. The EEG in such situations usually shows non-specific changes compatible with a 'metabolic encephalopathy'.

Haemopoietic

A normocytic, normochromic anaemia due to suppression of erythropoiesis develops as ARF progresses. Coagulation disturbances are frequent and vary in severity. Platelet function is impaired by high levels of blood urea and varying degrees of DIC are common.

Infection

Phagocytic function and immune mechanisms are impaired in uraemia and infection is now recognized as the commonest cause of death in ARF. Open wounds and peritoneal contamination can lead to septicaemia and there is a serious risk of secondary infection through central venous, dialysis and urinary catheters. The prolonged use of broad-spectrum antibiotics may lead to the emergence of resistant organisms and colonization of the upper respiratory and urinary tracts. Prophylactic use of antibiotics in ARF is therefore not indicated and might have dangerous consequences.

Management of ARF

The early restoration of cardiac output and renal blood flow is essential if ATN is to be avoided. However, once it is established the goal of the initial treatment is to prevent or control the deviations of fluid and electrolyte balance. If this cannot be achieved then dialysis becomes necessary.

The measures include:

1. Restriction of water intake to 400 ml/day plus the volume of fluid lost from any other sources. Sodium is given only to replace measured losses either in the urine or more usually from the gastrointestinal tract. It is deceptively easy to overhydrate a patient in ARF and it has to be remembered that endogenous water production is of the order of 400–500 ml/day and that insensible loss from the respiratory tract must be ignored if the patient is receiving humidified air and oxygen.

2. Curtailment of potassium intake unless there are large extrarenal losses; these must be measured and replaced accordingly to avoid hypokalaemia. Sudden elevation of plasma potassium may be controlled temporarily by the administration of intravenous glucose and insulin (100 ml of 50% glucose plus 25 units of soluble insulin), sodium bicarbonate (100 ml of an 8·4% solution) or calcium gluconate (100 ml of a 10% solution) aided by the use of ion exchange resins in the calcium phase (30–60 g q.i.d. orally or rectally).

3. Provision of a high caloric intake within the limits imposed by fluid intake. Oral feeding is rarely possible and nasogastric feeding, even using fine bore tubes, often provokes diarrhoea which poses difficult nursing problems. The calories are therefore best provided intravenously in the form of 50% dextrose given through a central venous catheter. Additional insulin will almost certainly be required to prevent the development of hyperglycaemia. Insulin resistance is a feature of critical illness and consequently large quantities of insulin may be required and are best administered from a constant infusion pump.

Fat solutions are possible alternatives to dextrose if there is no abnormality of liver function, although their clearance is also delayed in uraemic patients.

Nitrogen should not be given at this stage and only later if the calorie intake is sufficiently high to control catabolism. Anabolic steroids are sometimes given in an effort to promote anabolism but they are of doubtful value.

4. *Control of Metabolic Acidosis.* The arterial pH should not fall below 7·1. Sodium bicarbonate will increase the pH if necessary but its use incurs a very high sodium intake.

5. *Treatment of Infection.* Proven infection requires early and vigorous treatment. Blood cultures must always be taken before starting antibiotics and in ARF the dosage of several antibiotics requires adjustment.

6. *Modification of Drug Treatment.* Many drugs are excreted via the kidneys and others may be nephrotoxic. Very careful monitoring and regulation of dosage is therefore essential. Those most likely to cause further renal damage are the aminoglycosides, amphotericin, cephaloridine (especially if given with diuretics) and low molecular weight dextrans.

Gentamicin is widely used for the treatment of Gram-negative infections and its dosage must be reduced in ARF and then controlled according to measured plasma levels. Digoxin is, likewise, a drug that is commonly used in seriously ill patients and in ARF it may be hazardous because sensitivity to its action is greatly affected by changes in plasma potassium, calcium and magnesium and toxic manifestations may appear at blood levels usually regarded as safe.

Dialysis

In the critically ill surgical patient with ARF the measures described are only likely to be of a temporary holding nature prior to dialysis. Whilst there are numerous clinical and biochemical criteria given as indications for dialysis (*Table* 6.3) these should be anticipated rather than awaited for they reflect severe disturbances of function. Dialysis should therefore be carried out at an early stage rather than at the time the complications have developed.

Table 6.3 Indications for dialysis

Clinical deterioration especially when associated with overhydration	
Bood urea	Above 35 mmol/L
Serum creatinine	Above 900 μmol/L
Hyperkalaemia	Serum potassium above 6·5 mmol/L and not responsive to other measures
Severe metabolic acidosis	pH lower than 7·1

Whether peritoneal or haemodialysis is chosen depends upon a number of factors.

Peritoneal dialysis is a relatively simple technique and if the abdominal wall and peritoneum are intact can be very effective. Fluid exchanges of 1–2 L are used, usually at a rate of 2 L/h or proportionately smaller volumes in children. There is no need to leave fluid 'dwelling' in the peritoneal cavity and a continuous flow in and out enables a satisfactory exchange rate to be maintained and minimizes the risks of catheter blockage. There are three strengths of peritoneal dialysis fluid currently available but only two are commonly used; an approximately isotonic fluid with 1·36% glucose and a hypertonic solution containing 6·36% glucose. The latter is formulated for the rapid removal of water in severely overhydrated patients, it is highly irritant to the peritoneum and should only be used for a limited period.

No potassium is added to the first few fluid exchanges but once the plasma potassium falls to below 4 mmol/L additions will be required.

There are a number of possible difficulties and complications of peritoneal dialysis. Pain may be troublesome, especially with hypertonic solutions, and can be reduced by the addition of 50 mg lignocaine to each litre of dialysate. Drainage of fluid from the peritoneal cavity may be inadequate and may require frequent turning of the patient or repositioning of the catheter; occasionally fluid extravasates into the abdominal wall.

During its insertion the catheter may perforate a loop of bowel and cause a bacterial peritonitis. This is heralded by the appearance of a cloudy drainage fluid. Dialysis should be continued with an appropriate antibiotic, usually gentamicin, added to the dialysate. Surgical repair is urgently required.

Haemodialysis is more efficient than peritoneal dialysis, the clearance of urea being some four times greater. It is also more comfortable for the patient and does not cause protein loss. It does, however, require extra equipment and access to the circulation via an arteriovenous shunt. The dialysis membrane is usually either cellophane or cuprophane arranged in plates, coils or hollow tubes to provide a large surface area for exchange. Peritoneal dialysis relies on an osmotic gradient whereas haemodialysis requires a pressure difference across the membrane leading to ultrafiltration of plasma; this cannot be achieved if the patient is hypotensive.

In hospital or unit where haemodialysis is common practice it will be the preferred method. Where this is not the case peritoneal dialysis, if feasible, is a satisfactory and simpler alternative.

Haemofiltration

This technique has gained increasing popularity in the management of acute renal failure in the Intensive Therapy Unit. The process imitates glomerular filtration and the haemofilter may be connected into an arteriovenous or venovenous circuit. Blood is anticoagulated with heparin or prostacyclin and large volumes of filtrate can be removed (1 L/h). When continuous filtration is used the biochemical abnormalities associated with ARF can be relatively easily corrected. The technique causes minimal haemodynamic changes and is an acceptable alternative to dialysis.

Renal biopsy. The oliguric period of ATN usually lasts between 7 and 20 days. Should it persist beyond 4 weeks then a renal biopsy should be considered to establish a definitive diagnosis. If this show the features of ATN, dialysis is continued; if, however, acute cortical necrosis is present the patient should, if appropriate, be transferred to a chronic dialysis programme.

The Diuretic Phase of ARF follows from the oliguric phase and may last for a similar period. Large volumes of unconcentrated urine are passed and there is still a significant degree of renal impairment. The blood urea may continue to rise and significant losses of sodium and potassium may occur. Very careful fluid and electrolyte control is still required.

Prognosis of ARF

ARF still carries a high mortality which, in surgical patients, may be as high as 50%, particularly in patients over 50 years of age. Infection is the commonest cause of death for reasons that are not always obvious but may be related to the presence of impaired cellular and humoral immunity in ARF.

ACUTE HEPATIC FAILURE (AHF)

This develops either as a consequence of massive necrosis of liver cells in a previously normal liver or from lesser degrees of necrosis in a chronically diseased liver. Most cases of acute liver failure are due to viral hepatitis (A, B, non-A non-B) or drug overdose (paracetamol). Rare causes include mushroom poisoning and shock. In surgical patients it is the result of reduced hepatic blood flow as might occur in any form of shock; septicaemia and right ventricular failure with high portal venous pressures intensify the effects of the ischaemia. Virus B hepatitis may follow blood transfusion and if it is of the fulminant type it will lead to liver failure. Repeated anaesthesia with halothane or exposure to hepatotoxic drugs are other possible causes.

Because of the central physiological role of the liver any major disturbance of its function produces a varied and complex clinical picture. Deepening coma, as a result of an hepatic encephalopathy, is often the first feature to develop but in patients who are also suffering from other disorders that affect the level of consciousness, it may be difficult to detect. Increasing jaundice and the occurrence of a haemorrhagic tendency are commonly associated.

Metabolic Disturbances in Liver Failure

Encephalopathy

Encephalopathy is due to the retention of 'toxic' metabolites, a number of which have still to be identified. Ammonia and mercaptans have been incriminated and also a number of false neurotransmitters, such as octopamine and beta-phenyl ethylalanine. These interfere with cerebral function by displacing the normal transmitters, dopamine and noradrenaline, from their sites of action. Many of the 'toxic' substances are derived from the bacterial breakdown of protein in the gut and their effects on cerebral function are increased by the presence of other metabolic disturbances, notably hypoxia, hypoglycaemia and hyponatraemia.

Coagulation Disorders

Normal blood coagulation is affected by an impaired synthesis of Factors II, V, VII, IX, X and fibrinogen, the occurrence of disseminated intravascular coagulation and the development of thrombocytopenia.

Bleeding may arise from acute erosions in the stomach or from areas of oesophagitis in the lower third of the oesophagus. Nasopharyngeal or tracheal suction may also be sufficient to cause bleeding into the airways.

Hypoglycaemia

Hypoglycaemia is a common feature; the liver glycogen stores are depleted and the hepatic uptake of glucose, necessary for the further synthesis of glycogen, is impaired. Gluconeogenesis is also reduced and increased blood levels of insulin have been reported in some cases.

Electrolyte and Acid–base Disorders

Hypokalaemia and hyponatraemia are common. The latter is probably due to a redistribution of sodium into the intracellular compartment; hypernatraemia is almost always the result of over-zealous sodium replacement. Hyperventilation is a feature of the earlier stages of hepatic encephalopathy and results in a respiratory alkalosis. A metabolic acidosis is a late feature due to tissue hypoperfusion and reduced hepatic clearance of lactic acid.

Renal Failure

Renal failure has a significant association with acute hepatic failure. Hypotension, endotoxaemia and altered vascular reactivity may all contribute.

Respiratory Failure

In the deeper stages of coma there is loss of the protective airway reflexes and pulmonary aspiration becomes an increasing risk. Irregularities of respiration also develop and may culminate in sudden respiratory arrest; they are probably the consequence of an increasing intracranial pressure due to cerebral oedema.

Hypoxaemia, in acute hepatic failure, can arise from infection or pulmonary oedema; arteriovenous anastomoses have also been described. The occurrence of pulmonary oedema is facilitated by a low plasma osmotic pressure and an increased alveolar–capillary permeability.

Cardiovascular Problems

Hypotension in association with a low peripheral vascular resistance is a common feature of acute hepatic failure. The vasodilatation is partly due to the accumulation of false neurotransmitters at sympathetic nerve endings. Arrhythmias are commonly due to hypokalaemia and a fall in cardiac output may result from haemorrhage or septicaemia.

Cerebral Oedema, often with cerebral herniation, is found in a high percentage of patients who have died from acute hepatic failure. Its presence in life is related to the encephalopathy and its rapid progress leads to sudden, often life-threatening, neurological deterioration.

Diagnosis

Diagnosis of AHF is based on the clinical features in combination with biochemical evidence of disordered liver function. The transaminase enzymes are usually very high at the onset and may fall rapidly afterwards. The bilirubin and alkaline phosphate also increase whilst serum albumin falls. Studies of blood coagulation will show varying degrees of impairment.

Management

The management of AHF is largely supportive in an attempt to provide sufficient time for surviving liver cells to regenerate. When it develops as a secondary consequence of cardiovascular failure the prognosis is usually governed by the nature of circulatory disorder. If it arises as a primary event then mortality relates to the depth of the coma, and is between 80 and 90% for patients with Grade IV encephalopathy.

Encephalopathy

All protein is withdrawn from the diet and oral neomycin is given to reduce the bacterial flora of the gut. Some caution is necessary in the presence of renal failure because significant amounts of neomycin are absorbed and toxic levels may accumulate. The bowel contents are reduced by the use of magnesium sulphate enemas and oral lactulose; apart from promoting diarrhoea, lactulose is also thought 'to trap' ammonia in the bowel by lowering the pH of the colonic contents.

All forms of sedation must be withheld if at all practically possible. Agitations and confusion may, however, make the patient unmanageable and then small doses of diazepam should be given.

Correction of all the metabolic disturbances is also an integral part of the treatment of acute hepatic encephalopathy. Up to the present time none of the more aggressive methods that have been used for treating severe encephalopathy such as exchange transfusion, cross-circulation and charcoal perfusion have proved to be of value. Currently the use of haemodialysis with a polyacrylonitrile membrane is being investigated. Animal experiments suggest that the removal of compounds with molecular weights ranging from 1500 to 5000 improves the level of coma.

Coagulation Disturbances

Clotting factors can be replaced as necessary using fresh frozen plasma; if a large number of units are required a very large sodium load is given and problems might arise in the presence of renal and cardiac failure.

DIC in AHF rarely requires the use of heparin and those patients with a thrombocytopenia of less than 20 000 should be given a transfusion of platelets.

Cimetidine, an H_2 receptor antagonist, should be given routinely in an i.v. dose of 200–400 mg 4–6-hourly. It has proved to be an effective prophylaxis against gastric bleeding in AHF. It is recommended that the pH of the gastric aspirate be kept above 5.

Hypoglycaemia

A continuous infusion of 10, 20 and 50% dextrose may be needed to combat the inevitable tendency to hypoglycaemia. A central venous catheter is required for this infusion and merits meticulous attention because patients with AHF are very prone to develop septicaemia. If measurement of central venous pressure is also required then a second central catheter should be inserted. If the subclavian vein is used for cannulation the state of coagulation should be corrected before a catheter is inserted.

Electrolyte and Acid–base Disturbances

Careful monitoring of water and electrolyte balance is essential. Hyponatraemia is usually due to dilution rather than true sodium depletion and is not an indication for the infusion of normal saline. Hypokalaemia may be marked and should be vigorously corrected using intravenous potassium chloride. Hypomagnesaemia and hypophosphataemia may also require treatment.

The respiratory alkalosis does not require treatment but its presence will aggravate the hypokalaemia and move the haemoglobin dissociation curve leftwards, possibly interfering with oxygen delivery to the tissues.

Metabolic acidosis usually signifies a reduced cardiac output and treatment in the first instance should be aimed at improving this; sodium bicarbonate should be reserved for resistant cases. If the acidosis is related to renal failure then some form of dialysis will be required.

Renal Failure

Renal failure, if established, should be managed on the lines indicated in the previous section. In AHF the urine output should be maintained above 1 ml/min if possible. Infusion of dopamine in low dosages (2–5 μg/kg/min) is of value in maintaining glomerular filtration and hence urine output. In this situation it is preferable to frusemide and mannitol.

Respiratory Failure

In the deeply comatose the airway must be protected with an endotracheal tube. IPPV may be required for either hypoxaemic or ventilatory failure.

Cerebral Oedema

High levels of intracranial pressure have been recorded in AHF. These have not been prevented by prophylactic dexamethasone treatment and were only partially responsive to mannitol therapy. It appears that more details of the pathogenesis of this form of cerebral oedema are required before more effective means of reversing it can be defined.

Prognosis

Despite improvements in conservative therapy and continuing developments in haemodialysis the mortality of severe AHF remains high (75–80%).

Further Reading

Berk J. L., Sampliner J. E., Artz J. S. et al. (1976) *Handbook of Critical Care.* Boston, Little Brown.

Ledingham I. McA. (ed.) (1977) *Recent Advances in Intensive Therapy.* London, Churchill Livingstone.

Siegel J. H. (1987) *Trauma.* London, Churchill Livingstone.

Tinker J. and Rapin M. (1983) *Care of the Critically Ill Patient.* Berlin, Springer-Verlag.

7 Fluid and Electrolyte Therapy and Disorders of Acid–base Balance

Graham L. Hill

INTRODUCTION

Most surgical illness and operative intervention profoundly alter the balance and distribution of body fluids and electrolytes. A good understanding of the metabolism of salt, water and electrolytes is therefore essential to the care of surgical patients. In this chapter, some basic concepts of body composition and surgical physiology will firstly be outlined before discussing the changes in body fluids that occur in surgical illness and how each of them may be treated.

BASIC CONCEPTS OF BODY COMPOSITION AND SURGICAL PHYSIOLOGY

Body Composition

Body Mass, Body Fat and the Fat-free Body Mass

The body mass may be thought of as being composed of two broad subdivisions, Body Fat and the Fat-free Body Mass.

Body Fat

This is largely neutral storage fat and therefore does not contain water. It is the major energy store of the body.

Fat-free Body Mass

Composed of water, protein, minerals and glycogen. In healthy subjects 72% of the fat-free body mass is water (this may increase to over 80% in very ill surgical patients) and this is subdivided into intracellular water and extracellular water. About 55% of the protein in the body is enclosed inside cells, the remainder being solute protein (mainly plasma protein) and extracellular connective-tissue protein and skeletal protein. By weight most of the minerals in the body are in the skeleton. Although the rest of the minerals in the body weigh less than half a kilogram, they are of crucial importance in determining water distribution. Glycogen weighs less than half a kilogram and provides an energy source in emergency situations.

In clinical practice it is usual to prescribe fluid, electrolyte, energy and protein requirements according to body mass. Since fluid and electrolyte exchanges in the body occur in its fat-free portion, considerable errors may occur if no cognizance is taken of the varying proportion of body mass due to *fat* that occurs from patient to patient. Not only does body fat comprise a greater proportion of body weight in women but it increases in both sexes with increasing age (*Fig.* 7.1). It is important also to remember that not all the fat in the body is in subcutaneous tissue. Nearly half of it is in less visible sites, particularly the abdominal cavity. A good clinical guide is the axiom: *the more fat, the less lean. In other words, for two patients of equal weight the fatter patient has less fluid, electrolyte and metabolic requirements.*

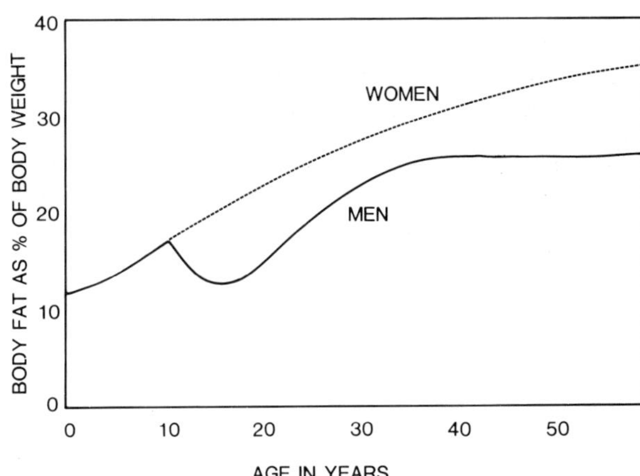

Fig. 7.1 This diagram shows that an increasing proportion of body weight is composed of fat as age increases. Note that after puberty the proportion of weight that is fat is always greater in females, i.e. if a female is the same weight as her male counterpart of the same age her metabolic, fluid and electrolyte requirements will be less.

Body Water Content and Distribution

The total body water may be divided into two major compartments, the extracellular water (ECW) and the intracellular water (ICW) which are separated by the cell membranes. The ICW is the site of all the metabolic processes of the body and the ECW is the compartment which provides a constant external environment for the cells. Edelman has classified ECW into five phases (*Fig.* 7.2) namely: (i) Plasma; (ii) Interstitial fluid—lymph; (iii) Connective tissues and cartilage water; (iv) Bone water; and (v) Transcellular fluid. Except for transcellular fluid each of these water phases corresponds to a well-defined anatomical space. Transcellular fluid is that fraction of the ECW which is formed by the

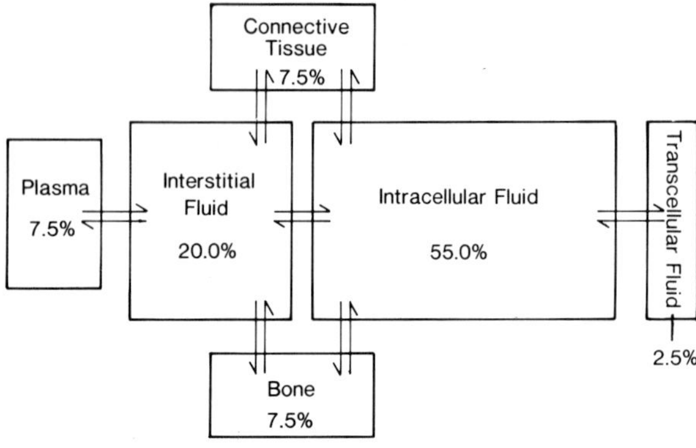

Fig. 7.2 Schematic diagram of the distribution of body water in a healthy young man. If labelled water is injected into the plasma of a patient it is distributed throughout these compartments within 2–4 h. (After Edelman I. S. and Leibman J. 1959, *Am. J. Med.* 27, 261.)

activity of the secretory cells but is not a transudate of plasma or lymph. The major component of the transcellular fluid is the intraluminal gastrointestinal water. Other transcellular fluids are found in the exocrine glands, liver, biliary tree, kidneys, eyes and the cerebrospinal fluid.

The emphasis from *Fig.* 7.2 of body water helps understanding of fluid shifts that may occur in surgical patients. The most familiar example is that of the patient with distal intestinal obstruction in whom the total transcellular fluid content of the intestine may be five or ten times that of normal and this is at the expense of other ECW. Invasive sepsis or extensive burns are other clinical examples in which large fluid translocations occur. In soft-tissue injuries or after extensive dissection from a major surgical procedure extracellular fluid accumulates around the area of injury.

Almost all illness results in a redistribution of body water. ECW tends to be maintained as wasting proceeds. The ECW, including plasma and interstitial water, maintains volume while cell mass shrinks. The practical implication of this is that very wasted surgical patients who are not clinically sodium and water depleted are intolerant of excessive salt and water loads; there is a tendency to oedema, hypoproteinaemia and hypotonicity.

Body Sodium Content and Distribution

Fig. 7.3 shows the distribution of body sodium in the average normal adult male. It gives a picture of how administered sodium will diffuse readily into the different compartments of extracellular water. When radio-labelled sodium is administered it is found that there is a sizeable pool of rapidly exchangeable sodium, a slowly exchangeable pool of sodium and probably a non-exchangeable pool of sodium in bone. Bone contains up to 40% of the total body content of sodium; thus exchangeable sodium is significantly less than the total body quantity. All the non-bone sodium is in exchange equilibrium with radio-labelled sodium in about 24 h.

Body Potassium Content and Distribution

Total body potassium content can be measured in a whole body counter and it can be demonstrated that almost all the potassium in the body is exchangeable in about 48 h when the whole body counting method is compared with the radio-potassium dilution technique. Almost all the potassium in the body is inside cells. Extracellular potassium is

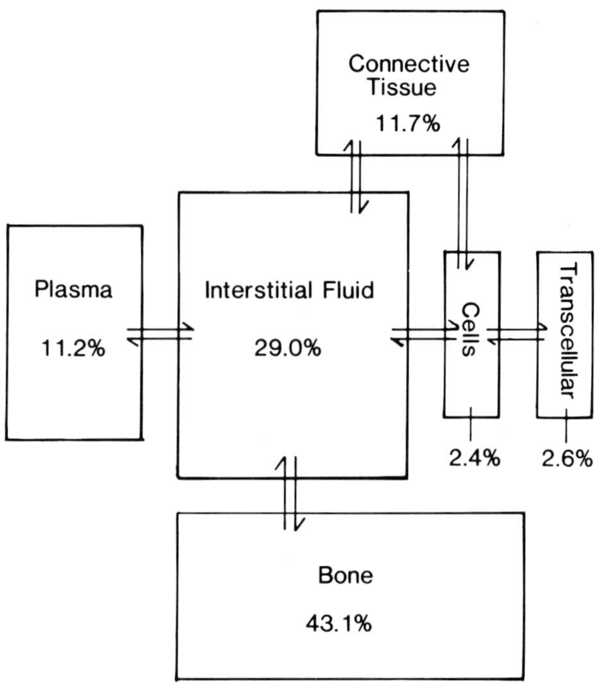

Fig. 7.3 Schematic diagram of the distribution of body sodium in a normal young adult man. (After Edelman I. S. and Leibman J. 1959, *Am. J. Med.* 27, 266.)

but a tiny fraction of the total body content. In a fit young male with 17 L of extracellular water only 65 mmol (out of a total body content of 3500 mmol), is effectively outside cells. The total plasma potassium may vary from as little as 7 mmol in a small woman to 21 mmol in a large man.

It is thought that most cells contain a constant concentration of potassium (150 mmol/L of ICW). Hence the total cell mass of the body (body cell mass) in healthy man can be calculated from measurements of total body potassium. Unfortunately in some surgical illness and during recovery the concentration of intracellular potassium may vary considerably and in these situations body cell mass cannot then be estimated reliably. Body potassium depletion may occur when there is loss of cell substance but may also occur as a true intracellular depletion. Isolated pH changes invoke a change in the distribution of potassium between ICW and ECW. A certain amount of intracellular potassium (about 100–200 mmol) is associated with glycogen storage in liver and muscle cells. It can be rapidly lost or gained in early starvation or carbohydrate refeeding.

Body Chloride Content and Distribution

The 'ideal' 70-kg man contains about 2300 mmol of chloride. Seventy per cent of this is in plasma, interstitial fluid and lymph. It is thus predominantly an extracellular ion though some is present in intracellular fluid and specific chloride-secreting cells such as the testes, ovary, intestinal and gastric mucosa and skin, and a significant part is localized in connective tissue. In clinical practice it is thought that since chloride is sufficiently restricted to the plasma and interstitial fluid it can be regarded as an index of extracellular fluid volume. Probably almost all the body chloride is exchangeable. Total plasma chloride content may change under pathophysiological circumstances independent of changes of plasma volume since hyperchloraemia may appear in some varieties of metabolic acidosis and hypochloraemia often is present in patients with metabolic alkalosis.

Other Ions of Clinical Importance

Magnesium

The total body content of magnesium in the average adult is about 1000 mmol, about half of which is incorporated in bone and is only slowly exchangeable. The distribution of magnesium is similar to that of potassium, the major proportion being intracellular. Plasma magnesium concentration normally ranges between 0·8–1·2 mmol/L. The kidneys show remarkable ability to conserve magnesium and this ion is essential for the function of most enzyme systems and depletion is characterized by neuromuscular and central nervous system hyperactivity. The normal daily intake of magnesium is about 10 mmol/day.

Calcium

Approximately 99% of the 1–1·2 kg of calcium in the body is concentrated in the skeleton. Thus a relatively small but profoundly important fraction of the total body calcium is in soft tissues and extracellular fluid.

Calcium is an important mediator of neuromuscular function. The usual dietary intake of calcium is about 3 g/day, and most of this is excreted unabsorbed in the faeces. The normal serum calcium concentration is maintained by vitamin D, parathormone and calcitonin. Acidosis increases and alkalosis decreases the serum calcium concentration. Approximately half the serum calcium is bound to plasma proteins, mainly albumin, but it is the remaining ionized calcium (i.e. about 40% of the total serum calcium) which is the fraction responsible for the biological effect.

Surgical Physiology

Osmolality and Tonicity of the Body Fluids

The chemical composition of the plasma, the interstitial fluid-lymph compartment and the intracellular fluid compartment of the body is shown in *Table* 7.1. It can be seen that the extracellular fluid has sodium as the principal cation and chloride and bicarbonate as the principal anions. There are minor differences in ionic composition between the plasma and interstitial fluid occasioned by the difference in protein concentration but for clinical purposes they may be considered equal.

The difference in ionic composition between the intracellular and extracellular fluid compartments is due to the selective permeability of the cell wall. Although water freely diffuses through this semipermeable membrane, the passage of sodium and its salts into cells is restricted, while that of potassium and its salts is promoted. This ability of water to diffuse freely across the cell membrane means that the total solute concentration (osmolality) of all body fluid compartments is identical.

Apart from calcium, zinc, magnesium and other trace metals, nearly all the osmotically active cations in the body are represented by the exchangeable sodium and exchangeable potassium. In normal subjects it has been found that there is a high correlation between the sum of these cations and the total content of water in the body, demonstrating clearly the osmotic homogeneity of the body. In 1958, Edelman and his colleagues found in a variety of normal and pathological subjects that there was a close relationship between the serum sodium concentration and the concentration of the total exchangeable cations in total body water (*Fig.* 7.4). Most clinical abnormalities of the serum sodium concentration can be explained if this concept is understood.

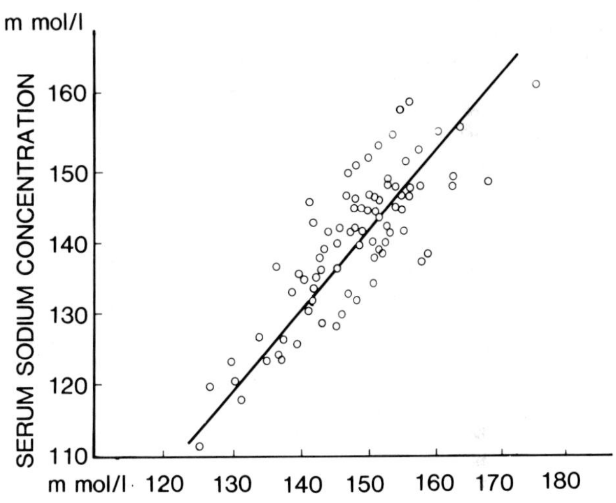

Fig. 7.4 This diagram redrawn from the classic paper of Edelman I. S. et al. 1958, *J. Clin. Invest.* **37**, 1236, shows the close relationship between serum sodium concentration and the concentration of the exchangeable cation ($NA_E + K_E$) in total body water for a wide variety of normal and sick subjects. F. D. Moore pointed out that this relationship is an expression of the osmotic homogeneity of the body and most clinical abnormalities of the serum sodium concentration can be explained by reference to it.

In surgical illness any condition that alters the effective osmotic pressure between the extracellular and intracellular compartments will result in redistribution of water between the compartments. In surgical practice hypotonicity occurs quite commonly and is reflected by a low serum sodium concentration. The decrease in effective osmotic pressure in ECW will result in a transfer of water from the extracellular to the intracellular fluid compartments. It is important to understand that depletion or increase of the extracellular fluid compartment without a change in the concentration of ions (osmolality) will not result in transfer of water from the intracellular space. The intracellular fluid shares in losses or gains that involve a change in concentration or composition

Table 7.1 Electrolyte concentration of body fluids (mmol/L)

Electrolyte concentration	*Plasma*	*Interstitial fluid*	*Intracellular fluid*
Cations			
Na^+	142	144	10
K^+	4	4	150
Ca^{++}	2·5	1·5	2
Mg^{++}	1·5	0·5	20
Anions			
Cl^-	103	114	10
HCO_3^-	27	30	10
SO_4^{--}	1·5	1·5	70
PO_4^{---}	1	1	45

of the extracelluiar fluid but does not share in changes involving loss of isotonic volume only.

It can be seen then that the distribution of water in the body is controlled by the osmolality of its fluid compartments. Dr F. D. Moore who wrote the classic *Metabolic Care of the Surgical Patient* teaches that the body as a whole acts as an osmometer in that an osmolality observed in any one part of the body must be present throughout the whole body.

In plasma about 98% of the osmolality consists of electrolyte; one-half of this is sodium, i.e. the total plasma osmolality is numerically twice the sodium concentration in mmol/L plus a small increment (about 8 mosm/kg due to other particles). Clinically any plasma osmolality beyond 'twice the sodium' may be assumed to be due to abnormal accumulations of osmotically active particles, including glucose, urea, lactate, mannitol, alcohol and others in renal failure.

Water Gain and Losses

Table 7.2 shows a water balance constructed for a normal 70-kg man living in a temperate climate. The normal subject drinks about 1500 ml of water/day and the rest of his water intake comes from water contained in solid food and from the food as it is oxidized in the body. Water is lost from the stool, urine, and also as insensible loss. Insensible losses are from the skin and the lungs and these increase when the patient is hypermetabolic, is over-breathing or is febrile. Shown in this table are the minimal amounts of water that can be lost, together with the maximum amounts that may be lost in extremes of surgical illness and stress.

Salt Gain and Losses

Normal man takes in about 100 mmol of sodium and 100 mmol of chloride per day. Balance is maintained primarily by the kidneys which excrete salt that is taken in in excess of need. Under conditions of reduced intake or extrarenal losses of sodium the normal kidney can reduce sodium excretion to less than 1 mmol/day and sodium may disappear from the faeces and the sweat (*Table* 7.3). In clinical practice 1 mmol of sodium per kg body weight per day is a useful guideline for maintenance requirements.

Potassium Gain and Losses

The normal subject takes in about 100 mmol of potassium per day and excretes about 60 mmol in his urine and the remainder in his faeces. Fluid from the small intestine contains much less potassium than that which is found in faeces. When potassium depletion occurs in patients with losses of small bowel content (e.g. enterocutaneous fistulas) it is because there has been renal conservation of sodium at the expense of potassium with consequent high output of urinary potassium.

Composition of Gastrointestinal Secretions

To construct a proper balance sheet in a surgical patient who has abnormal losses from the gastrointestinal tract it is important to have a working knowledge of the volume and composition of the different types of gastrointestinal fluids (*Table* 7.4). Gastrointestinal losses are usually isotonic or slightly hypotonic although there are considerable variations in their composition. In a patient with normal kidneys, though, these matter little. In clinical practice gastrointestinal losses are replaced by an isotonic salt solution. If the loss is from the stomach it is replaced litre for litre with 'normal saline' (0·9% saline) to which 15 mmol of K^+ have been added. Other losses from the gastrointestinal tract, including that fluid which accumulates in the lumen of the intestine when it is obstructed, can be replaced litre for litre with Ringer-lactate solution (Hartmann's). Villous tumours of the colon or rectum may secrete fluid with a high potassium concentration and clinical manifestations of hypokalaemia may be observed.

Acid–base Fundamentals

The Meaning of pH

The pH notation is a useful means of expressing H^+ concentrations of the body, because the H^+ concentrations happen to be low, relative to those of other cations. Thus, the

Table 7.2 24-hour average intake and output of water in an adult

Intake		*Output*	
Oral liquids	1300 ml (0–1500 ml/h)	Urine	1500 ml (300 ml–1400 ml/h)
Water in food	900 ml (0–1500 ml)	Stool	200 ml (0–2500 ml/h)
Water of oxidation	300 ml (125–800 ml)	Insensible:	
		Lungs	300 ml (200 ml–1500 ml)
		Skin	500 ml (200 ml–1000 ml/h)
Totals	2500 ml		2500 ml

Table 7.3 Intake and output of sodium in an adult subject (shown are average values together with minimal and maximal values that are possible in sickness and health)

Intake	*Output*	
Diet 50–100 mmol/day (0–100 mmol/h)	Urine	10–100 mmol/day (0–200 mmol/L)
	Stool	0–20 mmol/day (0–300 mmol/h)
	Skin	10–60 mmol/day (0–300 mmol/h)

Table 7.4 Composition of gastrointestinal secretions

Intestinal Tract Locality	*Volume (ml)*	*Na^+ (mmol/L)*	*K^+ (mmol/L)*	*Cl^- (mmol/L)*	*HCO_3^- (mmol/L)*
Saliva	1500	10	25	10	30
Gastric juice (fasting)	1500	60	15	90	15
Pancreatic fistula	700	140	5	75	120
Biliary fistula	500	145	5	100	40
Jejunostomy	2000–3000	110	5	100	30
Ileostomy	500	115	8	45	30
Proximal colostomy	300	80	20	45	30
Diarrhoeal stools	500–15000	120	25	90	45

normal Na^+ concentration of arterial plasma that has been equilibrated with red blood cells is 145 mmol/L, whereas the H^+ concentration is 0·00004 mmol/L. The pH (that is the negative logarithm of 0·00004) is therefore 7·4. The enormous range encompassed by the logarithmic pH scale can be understood if it is thought of in linear terms. Thus there is about twice as much H^+ in a solution of pH 7·1 (H^+ concentration is 0·000079 mmol/L) as there is at pH 7·4 (H^+ concentration is 0·000039 mmol/L). Body cells can function normally between pH 7·2 and pH 7·5, a range of 400% alteration in H^+ concentration.

The Disposal of Acid in the Body

A variety of organic acids is produced during the metabolism of carbohydrate, fat and proteins. The body is constantly working to prevent a metabolic acidosis due to these metabolic processes and surgical illness may upset this balance. Appreciable quantities of lactic acid, pyruvic acid and other acids sometimes accumulate in the blood in surgical patients. Oxidation of sulphur-containing amino acids generates H^+ and SO_4^{--} and metabolism of phosphorus containing substances such as nucleoproteins generate H^+ and PO_4^{---}. The H^+ formed by metabolism in the tissues is in large part hydrated to H_2CO_3 and the total H^+ load from this source is over 12 500 mmol/day. Most of the CO_2 is excreted in the lungs, and only small amounts of the H^+ ions from this source are excreted by the kidneys. Common sources of excessive acid loads are strenuous exercise (lactic acid) and diabetic ketosis. Failure of diseased kidneys to excrete a normal acid load is also a cause of acidosis.

Alkalosis is less of a problem than acidosis but the body has a much more limited power of compensation. In surgery the most common cause of alkalosis is loss of acid from the body due to vomiting of gastric juice. This is, of course, equivalent to adding alkali to the body.

The Henderson–Hasselbalch Equation

The principal buffers in the extracellular fluid are haemoglobin, protein and carbonic acid (H_2CO_3). As a buffer, the position of H_2CO_3 is unique because it is converted to H_2O and CO_2, and the CO_2 is then excreted in the lungs.

The function of this principal buffer system is expressed in the Henderson–Hasselbalch equation, which defines the pH in terms of the ratio of the salt and acid:

$$pH = pK + \log \frac{[HCO_3^-]}{[H_2CO_3]}.$$

The equation shows that the pH of the extracellular fluid is determined primarily by the ratio of base bicarbonate (mainly sodium bicarbonate) to the amount of carbonic acid (related to the CO_2 content of alveolar air) present in the blood. The symbol $[H_2CO_3]$ stands for the concentration of carbonic acid plus dissolved CO_2. In normal subjects the ratio $\frac{HCO_3^-}{H_2CO_3}$ is 20:1 and the pK 6·1.

Thus pH = 6·1 + log $[20_{10}]$ = 7·4.

The amount of carbonic acid and dissolved CO_2 is proportional to the P_{CO_2}. The plasma HCO_3^- (which cannot be measured directly) is the total measurable CO_2 of plasma minus the dissolved CO_2, the carbonic acid and the carbamino – CO_2. Constants have been derived experimentally such that the Henderson–Hasselbalch equation for the bicarbonate system in plasma can be written in the following form:

$$pH = 6{\cdot}1 + \log \left| \frac{HCO_3^-}{0{\cdot}03\,Pa\,CO_2} \right|$$

(0·03 is the solubility coefficient of CO_2).

This is the clinically applicable form of the equation, because HCO_3^- cannot be measured directly but pH and P_{CO_2} can be measured with suitable accuracy using pH and P_{CO_2} glass electrodes and HCO_3^- can then be calculated.

Four Types of Acid–base Disorder

When acid is added to the buffer system just described (metabolic acidosis), the concentration of bicarbonate (the numerator in the Henderson–Hasselbalch equation) will decrease. Ventilation will immediately increase to eliminate larger quantities of CO_2 with a subsequent decrease in the carbonic acid (the denominator in the Henderson–Hasselbalch equation) until the 20:1 ratio is re-established. Slower more complete compensation is effected by the kidneys with increased excretion of acid salts and retention of bicarbonate. The reverse will occur if *an alkali is added to the system (metabolic alkalosis). Respiratory acidosis and alkalosis* are produced by disturbances of ventilation with an increase or decrease in the denominator and the resultant change of the 20:1 ratio. Compensation is primarily renal, with a retention of bicarbonate and increased excretion of acid salts in respiratory acidosis and the reverse process in respiratory alkalosis. The four distinct types of acid–base disturbances are shown in *Table* 7.5. From this table it can be seen that the pH and P_{CO_2} from a freshly drawn arterial blood sample are necessary for diagnosis. *Thus measurements of pH and P_{CO_2} and calculation of bicarbonate concentration are required for a complete understanding of the acid–base status of a patient.*

Anion Gap

In the body, electrical neutrality is maintained by balancing the total number of cations with the total number of anions. This principle can be utilized clinically in patients with

Table 7.5 Four basic types of acid–base disorders—before and after partial compensation

	METABOLIC				RESPIRATORY			
	Acidosis		*Alkalosis*		*Acidosis*		*Alkalosis*	
	uncompensated	compensated	uncompensated	compensated	uncompensated	compensated	uncompensated	compensated
pH	↓↓	↓	↑↑	↑	↓↓	↓	↑↑	↑
P_{CO_2}	N	↓	N	↑	↑↑	↑↑	↓↓	↓↓
Plasma HCO_3^-	↓↓	↓	↑↑	↑	N	↑	N	↓

suspected acid–base disorders by measuring the serum sodium, chloride and bicarbonate concentrations. Normally the extracellular concentration of the cations (mainly sodium) equals the sum of the extracellular concentrations of the anions (chloride and bicarbonate) plus a constant. This constant equals about 8 mmol/L. If the sum of the concentrations of these two anions plus 8 is less than the serum sodium concentration, an anion gap is said to exist. Determination of the anion gap may prove quite helpful in assessing the cause of metabolic acidosis. Metabolic acidosis (resulting in an anion gap) may occur in patients with renal insufficiency in which phosphate and sulphate as well as organic acid anions are retained, or in ketoacidosis in which keto acids accumulate in the blood, or lactic acidosis, as arises in hypoxia.

Endocrine and Metabolic Response to Injury

It is important to understand the characteristic physiological changes which follow sepsis, surgical operation or accidental trauma, for these are the sum of the effects of a complex neuroendocrine reflex. The reflex is initiated by fear, pain, hypovolaemia, hypoxia, tissue injury and/or sepsis (afferent limb) and serves the body by means of metabolic and circulatory adjustments (efferent limbs) which lead to correction of the initial disturbance. The sum of all these effects needs to be appreciated in order to manage patients with problems of volume, concentration or composition of body fluids.

Reflex Responses to Injury or Sepsis

Sepsis, surgical operation, or other forms of trauma cause a series of physiological derangements which activate a number of different *efferent pathways* which are shown in *Fig.* 7.5. The early response to trauma can be blocked by section of the nerves to the area being traumatized although conscious perception of pain is not necessary for the neuroendocrine response. Although perception of pain at the site of injury and efferent impulses related to changes in effective circulating blood volume play the over-riding roles in the early neuroendocrine response to trauma, as injury progresses, other stimuli such as acidosis, hypoxia, hypercapnia, changes in body temperature as well as the release of local factors from injured tissues may all come into play.

Efferent Limb

The efferent arc of the reflex response to injury arises in basically two locations: the pituitary and the brainstem. The output of the *pituitary* is a set of hormones that act either directly on effector organs or via the release of mediating hormones. The efferent fibres of the parasympathetic nervous system and sympathetic nervous system carry the outflow of the *brainstem* to the periphery either directly, or indirectly by affecting the release of peripheral hormones.

Pituitary hormones involved in the metabolic response to trauma include ACTH, vasopressin, endorphins and enkephalins, growth hormone and prolactin.

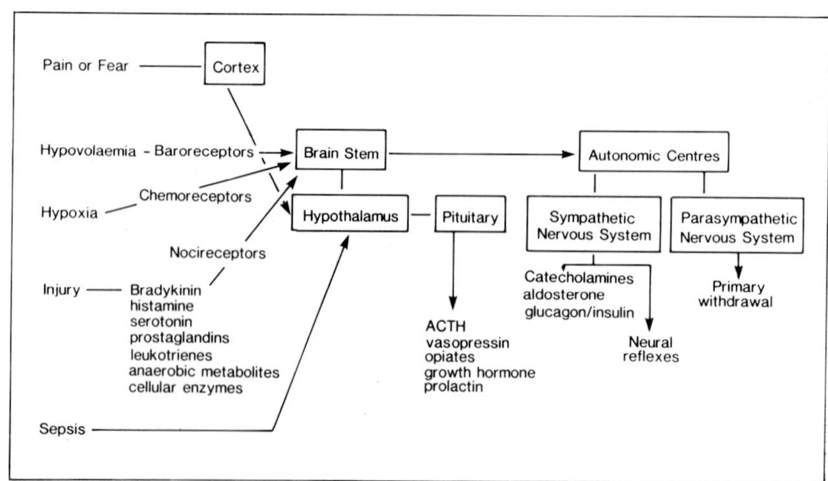

Fig. 7.5 Schema shows a simplified overview of the reflex response to pain, hypovolaemia, hypoxia, injury and sepsis. (Adapted from Gann & Lilly. 1984, *Prog. Crit. Care Med.* **1**, 17.)

Corticotropin-releasing factor is secreted from the median eminence. This compound is carried by the vessels of the hypothalamo–hypophyseal portal system into the anterior pituitary, where it acts upon the chromophobe cells to release ACTH. *ACTH* acts on the cells of the zona fasciculata in the adrenal leading to the biosynthesis of cortisol. *Cortisol* is required for the complete restitution of blood volume after haemorrhage. It appears to be involved in a shift of fluid from the intracellular compartment into the interstitial space. Cortisol also has wide ranging metabolic actions including inhibition of glycogenolysis and increase in gluconeogenesis from muscle amino acids. It inhibits the action of insulin and may affect the immune system.

The prime stimuli that lead to secretion of *vasopressin* are increased osmolality of the plasma and reduction of effective blood volume. In the early response to injury *blood volume changes* take precedence over tonicity. Vasopressin has several major areas of activity, the most important of which is to control renal free water handling. It increases permeability of the collecting system and this is the prime determinant of renal free water clearance.

There are two main groups of *opiate peptides* that are released from the pituitary in injured patients—endorphin and the enkephalins. They probably inhibit sympathetic tone and modulate sympathetic activity at the spinal level.

Increased circulating *growth hormone* occurs in response to the stress of surgery and trauma. The effects of this increase are either directly or through the action of *somatomedins*, a family of hormones which possess insulin-like activity. The important actions of growth hormone in the post-traumatic patient are metabolic rather than on fluid and electrolyte metabolism. Growth hormone inhibits the action of insulin in muscle, thereby decreasing net glucose uptake. *Prolactin*, like growth hormone has mainly metabolic effects in injured patients.

Thyroid hormones and thyroid-stimulating hormones are unaffected by injury or surgery. *Luteinizing hormone and follicle-stimulating hormone* are suppressed after surgery.

There are also *hormones under autonomic control* which are released as a response to injury or sepsis. There is an increase in *catecholamines, renin, aldosterone* and alteration in the *glucagon–insulin* ratio in septic and injured surgical patients. Catecholamines affect tissues through interaction with specific cell surface receptors and affect heart rate and blood pressure.

Catecholamines also act in a wide variety of tissues, through stimulation of other hormones; renin is increased and hence renal handling of water and sodium, and insulin and glucagon secretion are also altered by catecholamines. There is an increase in circulating glucagon and a relative decrease in insulin secretion. In haemorrhage and particularly when there is hypovolemia, *renin* and hence angiotensin are released. The latter is a potent vasoconstrictor and also has direct chronotropic and inotropic effects on the myocardium. It also acts on the median eminence and pituitary to increase secretion of vasopressin and ACTH. Angiotensin 2 is a major stimulus to secretion of aldosterone by the cells of the adrenal zona glomerulosa. Aldosterone acts on the renal tubule, the colon, terminal ileum, salivary glands and sweat glands to retain sodium.

Following trauma the effects of *autonomic nervous activity* and increased circulating catecholamines on the pancreas result in the release of glucagon and all inhibition of insulin secretion. There is a relative hypoinsulinaemia with respect to the circulating glucose concentrations. The ratio of insulin to glucagon, which is presented to the liver, is the critical determinant of the balance of hepatic anabolism and catabolism. Glucagon has a profound effect at the periphery in septic and injured patients and probably accounts for the increased muscle catabolism with the consequent loss of nitrogen and potassium in the urine. At the same time the suppression of the action of insulin in muscle by catecholamines, growth hormone and cortisol, limits substrate utilization.

The Net Effect of the Endocrine and Metabolic Response to Injury

From the point of view of fluid and electrolyte balance, these neuroendocrine responses to injury are of course essential to the immediate short-term survival of the patient. Nevertheless these changes possess a number of detrimental attributes as well: persistent water and sodium retention, inadequate clearance of metabolic byproducts and tissue factors, which leads to acidosis, poor substrate utilization and increased protein catabolism.

CLASSIFICATION OF BODY FLUID CHANGES

Shires has evolved the clinically useful concept that body fluid and electrolyte disorders can be classified into *volume changes, concentration changes and compositional changes.*

Volume Changes

Volume Deficit

By far the commonest fluid and electrolyte disorder encountered in surgical practice is a deficit of extracellular fluid. Intestinal obstruction, vomiting, excessive diarrhoea, severe trauma, major surgery associated with an extensive dissection, fluid loss from an enterocutaneous fistula, extensive burns, sepsis and shock, all result in a *net loss of extracellular fluid*. This, in the acute phase, cannot be diagnosed from laboratory information, for plasma sodium (and total body osmolality) have not been altered. Over a longer period of time, laboratory tests will show a rising blood urea and plasma creatinine, due to reduced glomerular filtration. The signs and symptoms of extracellular fluid volume deficit are set out in *Table* 7.6. Clinically it is quite useful to know that these symptoms and signs roughly equate to the size of the deficit sustained by the patient. Body composition studies in patients with deficits of extracellular fluid suggest that the deficit can be mild (1–2 L of ECF) moderate (2–4 L of ECF) or severe (5 or more litres of ECF).

Table 7.6 Signs and symptoms of extracellular fluid deficit

Deficit	*Mild (1–2 L ECF)**	*Moderate (2–4 L ECF)**	*Severe (5–9 L ECF)**
Symptoms	Gives history of recent loss of ECF	Apathy, anorexia Tachycardia Collapsed veins	Stupor or coma Ileus Pale, hypotensive Cold extremities Absent pulses
Signs	Usually no signs	↓ Tissue turgor Dry tongue	↓ Tissue turgor Sunken eyes

* Calculated for 70-kg subject with normal body fat stores.

Volume Excess

Apart from that which is associated with pulmonary oedema due to heart failure, extracellular fluid volume excess is caused either by the administration of large quantities of sodium-containing fluids (which is sometimes necessary to preserve renal function in septic patients) or is secondary to renal or hepatic failure. The plasma volume, or the interstitial volume, or both, are increased. The sign of interstitial volume overload is oedema and the signs of plasma volume overload are hypertension, tachycardia and increased venous pressure. It is important to stress that very depleted patients who ordinarily have a large extracellular water volume are not tolerant to excesses of sodium-containing fluids and may readily become overloaded. The surgeon will find such patients who have excessive amounts of extracellular fluid administered prior to surgery, have oedema of the walls of the stomach, colon and small bowel. This makes suturing more difficult, increasing the likelihood of anastomotic disruption.

Concentration Changes

Tonicity of the body fluids is a reflection of the plasma sodium concentration. Hyponatraemia or hypernatraemia in their early stages are not recognizable clinically. Nevertheless abnormal concentrations of plasma sodium should be noted and appropriate corrections made before clinical signs are seen.

Hyponatraemia

Most patients with hyponatraemia are hypotonic due to overhydration plus antidiuresis. Overhydration is due to excessive water administered orally or parenterally (e.g. 5% dextrose in water), and oxidation of fat or protein with production of free water. Vasopressin, as discussed above, is increased in patients suffering from acute surgical illness, immediately after surgical operation or tissue injury, and in chronic wasting disease. In surgical practice hyponatraemia is not uncommonly caused by the replacement of salt-rich losses with salt-poor fluids, i.e. there is a sodium lack with a 'relative' water retention.

Hyponatraemia, defined as serum sodium <130 mmol/L is clinically characterized by signs which reflect excessive intracellular water. When severe, the patient may have signs of central nervous system dysfunction including confusion, areflexia and later convulsions. Many hyponatraemic states are asymptomatic until the serum sodium level falls below 120 mmol/L. Following closed head injury, mild hyponatraemia is more serious because increased intracellular water adds to the problem caused by an increase of intracranial pressure. Most hyponatraemic states are dealt with by withholding water but when severe and associated with symptoms hypertonic salt solutions should be given cautiously, perhaps with frusemide or mannitol to promote water loss.

Hypernatraemia

The patient with hypernatraemia usually presents with dry, sticky mucous membranes, a red, swollen tongue and flushed skin. The common clinical cause is water deficit. This is true dehydration whereas 'surgical dehydration' is most often extracellular fluid depletion. The treatment of hypernatraemia is to encourage water drinking or to add free water intravenously as dextrose in water. It is important not to correct a hyperosmolar state too rapidly as this may lead to brain oedema.

Compositional Changes

Compositional abnormalities, which are clinically important, include changes in *acid–base balance* and concentration changes of *potassium, magnesium and calcium.*

Acid–base Changes

In *Table* 7.5 a broad outline of each of the four main types of acid–base disorder before and after partial compensation was shown. The clinical manifestations and the treatment of these compositional disorders will now be discussed.

Respiratory Acidosis

This condition is due to alveolar hypoventilation leading to retention of CO_2. There may be depression of the respiratory centre from drugs, injury and some forms of chronic pulmonary disease. In such patients the P_{CO_2} is chronically elevated and the bicarbonate concentration rises to compensate for this. Such patients need special management in the operative and postoperative period. Atelectasis, pneumonia and hypoventilation due to pain from the abdominal incision may exacerbate respiratory acidosis. At operation infiltration of the incision site with local anaesthetic agents and transverse incisions are used by some surgeons to lessen wound pain. Postoperative management includes measures to ensure adequate ventilation: analgesia (via 'pain pump') bronchodilators, physiotherapy and incentive spirometry. The management of patients with very large upper abdominal incisions may be helped by the use of epidural anaesthesia, although intensive care with mechanical ventilation may be required.

Respiratory Alkalosis

Respiratory alkalosis is due to hyperventilation and is sometimes seen on surgical wards and in intensive care units. Apprehension, pain, hypoxia and acidosis are the usual causes. Deliberate mechanical hyperventilation is used in the management of patients with severe head injury. In other intensive care patients who have respiratory alkalosis, this may be due to the improper use of the mechanical ventilator. There is a depression of the arterial P_{CO_2} and an elevation of the pH. The bicarbonate falls to compensate if the condition persists.

The dangers of severe respiratory alkalosis are those due to impaired oxygen delivery and hypokalaemia such as ventricular arrhythmias. Hypokalaemia occurs because potassium ions enter cells in exchange for hydrogen ions and there is an excessive urinary potassium loss in exchange for sodium. Treatment is primarily directed towards preventing the condition by the proper use of mechanical ventilators and correcting any pre-existing potassium deficits.

Metabolic Acidosis

This may result from the retention of acid (diabetic acidosis, lactic acidosis) or the loss of bicarbonate as occurs in diarrhoea, the short-gut syndrome, pancreatic fistulas or high output enterocutaneous fistulas. There is a low arterial pH and bicarbonate concentration. The initial compensation is an increase in rate and depth of breathing and reduction of the arterial P_{CO_2}.

A common cause of severe metabolic acidosis in surgical patients is acute circulatory failure causing tissue hypoxia and accumulation of lactic acid. Acute haemorrhagic shock may result in a rapid and profound drop in the arterial pH. Another cause of metabolic acidosis in surgery is the replacement of chloride ion in excess of that which has been lost.

The use of large volumes of 'normal saline' (154 mmol of chloride ion/L) to replace extracellular fluid deficits or losses from the small intestine may provide excessive chloride. The treatment of metabolic acidosis should be towards correction of the underlying disorder when possible. In hypovolaemic patients, the use of Ringer–lactate solution (Hartmann's) and blood to restore tissue perfusion results in a rapid reversal of the problem. It is recommended that bicarbonate therapy should be reserved for the treatment of severe metabolic acidosis, particularly when associated with circulatory impairment, e.g. following cardiac arrest when partial correction of the pH may be essential to restore myocardial function. The initial dose of bicarbonate should be 1 mmol/kg of body weight of HCO_3 as $NaHCO_3$ and that the decision for additional bicarbonate should be based on measurements of pH and P_{CO_2}.

Metabolic Alkalosis

Metabolic alkalosis results from the loss of acid or the gain of bicarbonate. Both the pH and plasma bicarbonate concentration are elevated. Compensation for metabolic alkalosis is primarily by renal mechanisms, since respiratory compensation is very small. The majority of patients with metabolic alkalosis have some degree of hypokalaemia resulting from an entry of potassium into cells in exchange for H^+ and an excessive urinary potassium loss in exchange for sodium.

The commonest cause of metabolic alkalosis in surgical patients is loss of gastric juice from persistent vomiting or gastric suction. It is also an accompaniment of untreated pyloric stenosis. There is loss of fluid with a high chloride and hydrogen ion concentration. Initial compensation is by the loss of sodium and bicarbonate in the urine but as extracellular fluid is lost there is an attempt to conserve sodium by the kidney and potassium and hydrogen ions are excreted into the urine in increasing quantities, resulting in an uncompensated alkalosis and profound hypokalaemia. The initially alkaline urine therefore becomes acid after a period of time, due to hydrogen ion excretion. Management includes replacement of the extracellular fluid volume deficit with 0·9% sodium chloride solution ('N' saline), in addition to replacement of potassium. It is important to remember that potassium should never be given to patients until volume repletion has been obtained and a good urine output has been established. The vast majority of patients with metabolic alkalosis and normal renal function can be treated with 0·9% saline and potassium alone. A very small number of patients with severe hypochloraemia and excessive nasogastric drainage may be refractory to even large amounts of 0·9% saline and potassium. In the past ammonium chloride was recommended in such circumstances but more recently 0·1 N–0·2 N hydrochloric acid has been shown to be safe and effective therapy for correction of very severe metabolic alkalosis. A solution of 150 ml of 1 N hydrochloric acid added to 1 L of sterile water gives an isotonic solution containing 300 mmol of hydrogen ion and chloride ion. The solution is administered over a 12-h period with frequent measurements of pH and P_{CO_2}. Usually 1 or 2 L are sufficient to correct the immediate problem and this gives the surgeon time to correct the underlying cause.

Clinical Steps for Evaluating a Patient with a Suspected Acid–base Disorder

A properly taken *history* should give a fairly clear idea of the type of acid–base disorder that might be encountered. Evaluation of the *clinical signs* may be useful, for example, tetany may be a manifestation of alkalosis; cyanosis may reflect respiratory failure. The *routine laboratory data*, i.e. venous blood electrolytes and bicarbonate should be evaluated before an arterial puncture is decided upon. First the serum *bicarbonate* concentration should be looked at. An elevation represents either a metabolic alkalosis or a metabolic compensation for a respiratory acidosis and a depression signifies either a metabolic acidosis or a metabolic compensation for respiratory alkalosis. Next the concentration of serum potassium is noted. If high, there may be acidosis; if low, there maybe alkalosis. If plasma chloride has been measured a high level suggests hyperchloraemic metabolic acidosis and a low level suggests metabolic alkalosis.

The *anion* gap may then be calculated. If the sum of the concentration of serum chloride and serum bicarbonate +8 is less than the serum sodium concentration, then an anion gap is present. This suggests a metabolic acidosis.

Frequently, adequate assessment of a patient's acid–base status can be made in this way from the history, physical examination and an analysis of the data from a venous blood sample. The decision to determine *arterial* blood pH and P_{CO_2} depends on the need to confirm the clinical impression; in very sick patients, the determination is essential. Measurement of pH and P_{CO_2} are also necessary to document a mixed disturbance of acid–base balance and determine the extent of acidosis or alkalosis upon which the need for treatment should be based.

Compositional Changes due to Abnormal Concentrations of Potassium, Magnesium and Calcium

Hyperkalaemia

Significant quantities of intracellular potassium are released into the extracellular space in response to severe injury, surgical stress or acidosis. In these situations dangerous hyperkalaemia (greater than 6 mmol/L) is rarely encountered if renal function is normal. The patient may suffer from nausea and vomiting, small bowel colic and diarrhoea. The electrocardiogram may show high peaked T waves, widened QRS complex and depressed ST segments. Heart block and asystolic cardiac arrest may develop with increasing concentrations of serum potassium.

Treatment of hyperkalaemia consists of immediate measures to reduce the serum potassium level, withholding of all administered potassium and correction of the underlying cause, if possible. If the plasma level is very high, e.g. >7 mmol/L and there is ECG or clinical evidence of cardiac malfunction, treatment should include the administration of glucose and insulin (100 ml 50% dextrose + 10 units of insulin), calcium (10 ml of 10% calcium gluconate by slow intravenous infusion) and if there is acidosis 1 ml/kg of $NaHCO_3$. Such patients may require urgent haemodialysis. Lesser degrees of hyperkalaemia can usually be managed by K^+ restriction, glucose and insulin and cation-exchange resins, administered either orally or by rectum in doses of 15–30 g every 12 h.

Hypokalaemia

Patients presenting for surgery may have been taking diuretics for long periods and have low levels of plasma as a consequence. More commonly, hypokalaemia occurs in surgical patients with alkalosis, after massive isotonic sodium replacement and when there have been large losses of gastrointestinal fluids. Increased renal loss of potassium occurs with both respiratory and metabolic alkalosis. Potassium is in competition with hydrogen ion for renal tubular excretion in exchange for sodium ion. Renal tubular excretion of potassium is increased when large amounts of sodium are infused and when there is renal tubular dysfunction. The development of hypokalaemia in patients with high losses of intestinal fluid is caused by renal loss of potassium occurring secondary to sodium retention which occurs in response to the loss of sodium from the gut.

The signs of potassium deficit are related to failure of normal contractility of skeletal muscle, smooth muscle and cardiac muscle. They include weakness that may progress to flaccid paralysis, diminished or absent tendon reflexes and paralytic ileus. Sensitivity to digitalis with atrial tachyarrhythmias and ventricular premature beats may occur. In addition, the ECG may show flattening of T waves, the development of U waves and depression of ST segments. The treatment of hypokalaemia involves intravenous administration of K^+ at a rate of administration which should not exceed 20 mmol/h. *Fig.* 7.6 shows that when

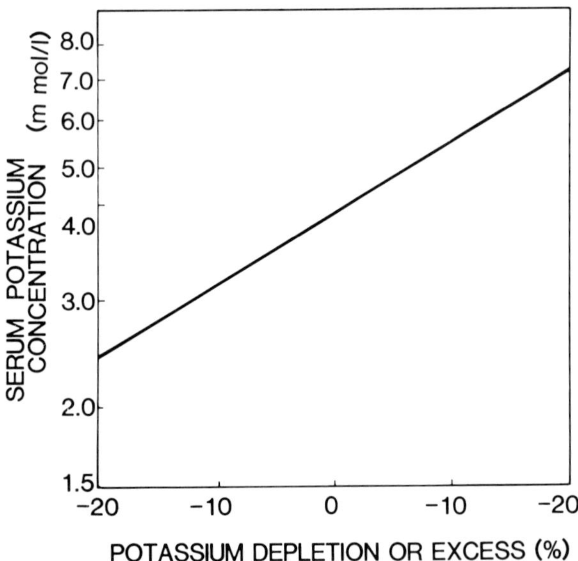

Fig. 7.6 The relationship of the serum potassium concentration to the total body content of potassium when the pH is within normal limits. With excessive external losses of potassium the serum K^+ falls: a loss of 10% of total body K^+ (i.e. about 350 mmol in a young man of normal build) drops the serum K^+ concentration from 4–3 mmol/L at normal pH.

acid–base disturbances are not present, serum potassium concentration is related to the degree of depletion of the total body potassium. It can be seen that a loss of 10% of total body potassium drops the serum potassium from 4 to 3 mmol at normal pH. This can be a useful guide to deciding on the initial rate of replenishment of a patient with hypokalaemia, although the situation should be reassessed every 6 h.

Magnesium Deficiency

Alcoholic patients, or those with high output ileostomies, enterocutaneous fistulas or severe diarrhoea may suffer from magnesium deficiency. The signs and symptoms of magnesium deficiency are clinically the same as calcium deficiency, including hyperactive tendon reflexes, muscle tremors and tetany. Hypocalcaemia is usually noted particularly in those patients who have symptoms of tetany. The diagnosis may be missed if the clinician is not aware that neuromuscular symptoms occurring in patients with high intestinal losses is more likely to be due to magnesium deficiency than calcium deficiency. Plasma magnesium levels are usually low, but they are not wholly reliable. Treatment of magnesium deficiency is by the parenteral administration of magnesium sulphate or magnesium chloride solutions. If renal function is normal and there is a severe depletion, as much as 20–30 mmol can be administered in a 24-h period. When large doses are given, the heart rate, blood pressure, respiration and electrocardiogram should be monitored closely.

Magnesium Excess

Symptomatic hypermagnesaemia is rare, but is occasionally seen in patients with renal failure.

Hypocalcaemia

Hypocalcaemia occurs in hypoparathyroidism, severe pancreatitis, renal failure, severe trauma, massive blood transfusion and overwhelming sepsis. Except in patients with hypoparathyroidism it is not treated, for the condition is most often self-limiting. Intravenous calcium, as calcium gluconate, or calcium chloride may be needed for acute symptoms as after parathyroidectomy. More chronic problems are dealt with by giving oral vitamin D supplements and calcium.

Hypercalcaemia

In surgical patients hypercalcaemia is most frequently caused by cancer with bony metastasis, hyperparathyroidism, ectopic production of parathormone, hyperthyroidism, prolonged immobilization and Paget's disease of bone. Hypercalcaemia may impair renal concentrating mechanisms resulting in polyuria. Severe hypercalcaemia can cause coma and death. The treatment of severe hypercalcaemia is to expand the extracellular fluid with isotonic saline and enhance calcium excretion by diuretics. Mithramycin is used when hypercalcaemia is associated with metastatic cancer.

FLUID AND ELECTROLYTE THERAPY

Parenteral Solutions

The composition of various intravenous fluids which are commonly used, is shown in *Table* 7.7.

A good isotonic salt solution for replacing gastrointestinal losses and repairing pre-existing volume deficits in the absence of gross abnormalities of concentration and composition, is *Ringer-lactate* or Hartmann's solution. This solution contains 130 mmol of sodium, balanced by 109 mmol of chloride and 28 mmol of lactate and has minimal effect on normal body fluid composition and pH even when infused and in large quantities. The chief disadvantage of Ringer-lactate solution is that its sodium concentration is lower than that of plasma. This rarely presents a clinical problem, provided it is remembered in extreme situations that the solution furnishes approximately 100 ml of free water for each litre administered. The remainder of the solutions shown in *Table* 7.7 are used to correct specific deficits. Choice of a particular fluid depends on the volume state of the patient and the type of concentration or compositional abnormality present.

Isotonic sodium chloride (0·9% of saline or 'N' saline) which contains 154 mmol of sodium and 154 mmol of chloride per litre, may under some circumstances provide excessive

Table 7.7 Composition of commonly used parenteral fluids (electrolyte content mmol/L)

	Cations				*Anions*			Energy
	Na	K	Ca	Mg	Cl	HCO_3^-	HPO_4^-	Kcal
ECF	142	4	2·5	1·5	103	27	3	—
Ringer-lactate (Hartmann's solution)	130	4	3		109	28	—	—
0·9% Sodium chloride	154	—	—	—	154	—	—	—
5% Dextrose	—	—	—	—	—	—	—	200/L
Hypotonic (1/5 'N' saline) (0·18% saline + 4·2% dextrose)	30	—	—	—	—	—	—	168/L
Potassium chloride (20% KCl)	—	25 mmol K^+ in 10 ml of 20% solution			25 mmol Cl^- in 10 ml of 20% solution			—

chloride ion and metabolic acidosis may develop. This solution is ideal, however, for the initial correction of an extracellular fluid volume deficit in the presence of hyponatraemia, hypochloraemia, and metabolic alkalosis. Water and sugar can be supplied as 5% *dextrose in water* or hypotonic sodium solution with sugar which is usually given as so called '*fifth-normal saline*' (0·18% saline, 4·2% dextrose).

Maintenance, Replacement and Repair

All good fluid therapy requires attention to three areas:

1. Maintenance of daily requirements of fluid and electrolyte.
2. Replacement of ongoing losses.
3. Repair of deficits of volume, concentration or composition.

Maintenance of Daily Requirements of Fluid and Electrolyte

In *Tables* 7.2 and 7.3, the normal daily exchange of water and sodium are shown. In temperate climates the daily maintenance requirement of an adult patient for water is 2500 ml. Different populations vary in their salt intake, but a good rule of thumb is that normal patients require 1 mmol of sodium/kg body weight/24 h. Looking at the available solutions, these daily requirements can be usefully provided in one of two ways.

500 ml of 'N' saline (0·9% saline), plus 2 L of 5% dextrose

or

2500 ml of one-fifth 'N' saline (0·18% saline + 4·2% dextrose).

To each of these regimens K^+ is added at the rate of 1 mmol/kg of body weight/24 h.

Two notes of caution must be observed when supplying maintenance needs after a surgical operation.

1. Potassium is usually unnecessary and may prove dangerous if given during the first 24 h following surgery. The obligatory breakdown of cells releases potassium after surgery, flooding the extracellular fluid and providing sufficient quantity during the early postoperative period.

2. The stress of operation stimulates the release of aldosterone and vasopressin with the accompanying retention of sodium and water, which may prove harmful to the patient with compromised renal or cardiac reserve, if restriction of fluid administration is not made. Recent evidence suggests that adequate intraoperative maintenance of extracellular fluid volume will overcome this postoperative need for fluid restriction, but nevertheless the surgeon should be ready to restrict intravenous fluids for the first 24 h or so. This is especially important in patients who are nutritionally depleted.

Replacement of Ongoing Losses

In surgical patients the commonest losses are from the gastrointestinal tract. Vomiting, biliary or pancreatic fistulas, enterocutaneous fistulas or severe diarrhoea, all necessitate replacement of fluid over and above maintenance requirements. From *Table* 7.4 it can be seen that the majority of gastrointestinal secretions can be replaced by an isotonic saline solution. If the losses are from vomiting then replacement is best litre for litre with 0·9% saline to which 15 mmol of potassium chloride have been added. Losses from other sites lower in the gastrointestinal tract can be usefully replaced by Ringer-lactate solution, litre for litre.

If losses from the gastrointestinal tract are greater than a litre each day for several days, these should be pooled and sent to the laboratory for more specific electrolyte analysis of sodium, chloride and potassium so that appropriate adjustments can be made to ensure more precise replacement.

Abnormal losses can also occur in two other situations:

1. Evaporation

From evaporation from the skin and respiratory tract. The patient with a high fever, or respiratory rate of 35 respirations or more, may lose an additional 500 ml or more of water each day. Thus in writing fluid orders an extra 500 ml of 5% dextrose in water will be necessary for patients of this type.

2. Sequestration

A number of surgical conditions lead to sequestration of extracellular fluid such that it is unavailable for normal exchange. When the *intestine is obstructed* the bidirectional movement of sodium and water across the intestinal mucosa is altered such that there is a net secretion of fluid (which resembles extracellular fluid) into the lumen of the intestine. In prolonged obstruction this may amount to a loss of extracellular fluid equivalent to 5–10 L of the body weight. This is best replaced by Ringer-lactate solution.

Sequestration of extracellular fluid also occurs at the site of operative trauma. It thus depends on the degree and magnitude of the surgery. Only several hundred millilitres of fluid are lost in an inguinal hernia repair and this is of no importance physiologically. On the other hand, extracellular fluid sequestered after a complex operation involving lysis of extensive adhesions, or a total gastrectomy or proctocolectomy may be substantial. It has been shown that when lactated Ringer's solution is given at a rate of about 500 ml/h during major abdominal surgery of this type, the problem of postoperative renal failure is almost entirely eliminated. Thus in major abdominal surgery it is recommended that Ringer-lactate solution should be continually administered at this rate throughout the operative procedure and an additional 500 ml of Ringer-lactate solution should be provided each day to the maintenance needs in the early postoperative period. The response to this treatment is judged according to the urine output which should be around 50 ml/h.

In patients with obvious malnutrition extracellular fluid is already expanded and such a regimen must be administered with considerable caution. We have already seen that such patients may be intolerant of extra sodium.

Repair of Volume Deficits

The most common volume change, indeed the most common fluid and electrolyte problem encountered in surgical patients is extracellular fluid deficit. Depletion of the extracellular fluid compartment without changes in concentration or composition is a problem found in many acutely ill surgical patients. For instance, in patients with complete small bowel obstruction, there may be a massive shift of extracellular fluid volume into the lumen of the intestine. The patient with massive ascites, burns or crush injuries, or peritonitis has a translocation of extracellular fluid into a so-called *'third space'*. This fluid is non-functional because it is no longer able to participate in the normal functions of the extracellular fluid and it may just as well have been lost externally. It is helpful to be able roughly to estimate extracellular fluid deficits to give confidence in replenishment and in this context the signs and symptoms in relation to these deficits as shown in *Fig.* 7.6 are a good starting point.

It must be stressed that plasma volume should be restored rapidly to improve oxygen delivery but interstitial fluid replacement should be repleted at a slower rate. Patients with strangulating bowel obstruction, peritonitis from a perforated diverticulum, or a perforated duodenal ulcer may need more urgent replenishment of interstitial fluid volume. In these circumstances rapid replacement of fluid deficit with good urine flow may be accomplished in one to three hours, following which laparotomy is performed.

The rate of repletion in other patients depends to some extent on the rate of the development of the deficit. Also an elderly patient adapts more slowly. Reassessment of the clinical situation is mandatory before giving more fluid. An especially helpful guide to fluid balance is the hourly measurement of urine volume. In the absence of diuretics or glycosuria, an adult patient who excretes 50 ml of urine per hour is in satisfactory equilibrium.

The type of fluid replaced will depend in most cases on how it has been lost and the serum electrolyte profile. If electrolytes are relatively normal in the face of obvious volume depletion, losses can be assumed to have been isosmotic with plasma and should be replaced with Ringer-lactate solution. In contrast, if chloride losses exceed sodium losses, as occurs with vomiting, isotonic saline is generally preferred as replacement fluid. Potassium should not be added to any of these fluids until adequate urine output of 50 ml/h is obtained.

Correction of Concentration and Compositional Deficits

The treatment of hyponatraemia, hypernatraemia and alterations in acid–base balance has been discussed above.

Establishing Fluid Balance

So-called fluid balance is potentially one of the most abused techniques in surgical practice. Extensive analytical facilities and a complete metabolic balance study are usually quite unnecessary in ordinary clinical practice. What is necessary is a concept of the broad principles of water and electrolyte balance and the ability to correlate this with the patient's symptoms and signs.

Using established data for the electrolyte content of different gastrointestinal fluids, it is possible to carry the management along on a daily basis with the patient in reasonable water and sodium balance and acid–base regulation. A simple record is kept of intake and output by all routes, using approximations where daily analysis would not be justified. An accurate record of the volume and nature of the 24-h oral and i.v. intake is made and the 24-h outputs from nasal, gastric tube or other losses from drains or fistulas and volume of urine excreted are measured. In order to put such management into effect, some sort of record or chart of the gains and losses should be kept. The exact form of this chart is immaterial. As part of the clinical balance procedure the patient's weight should be followed closely. In patients suffering from acute disease or injury any rapid gain in weight may be assumed to be due to the addition of water and salt to the body. Only under the circumstances of treating serious sepsis or major trauma, established dehydration, desalting water loss, or interstitial sequestration oedema does one expect weight gain to occur.

By the same token, excessive or sudden losses of weight indicate loss of salt and water from the body; sudden loss of weight in the region of 500–1000 g or more in a 24-h period, means quite serious under-administration of fluid; on the other hand, the brisk diuresis and natriuresis that occur during recovery from serious surgical illness results in a rapid weight loss that heralds a return to normal function.

Further Reading

Beck L. H. (ed.) (1981) Symposium on Body Fluid and Electrolyte Disorders. *Med. Clin. North Am.* **65**, 148.
Edelman I. S. and Leibman J. (1959) Anatomy of body water and electrolytes. *Am. J. Med.* **27**, 256.
Thoren L. (ed.) (1983) Symposium on Fluid and Electrolyte Problems in Surgery. *World J. Surg.* **7**, 565.

8 Nutrition in Surgical Practice

Graham L. Hill

MALNUTRITION IN SURGICAL PATIENTS—CLINICAL SYNDROMES

There is a growing awareness that malnutrition is common in many surgical patients. In children, where the problem has been more thoroughly studied, protein energy malnutrition is a spectrum of severe malnutrition in which three types are discernible: marasmus, kwashiorkor and marasmic kwashiokor.

Marasmus is the outcome of a diet which is properly balanced but there is not enough available; *kwashiorkor* results from a diet which is inadequate but contains relatively more calories than protein. The child with marasmus is underweight with gross wasting of muscle and subcutaneous tissues; he is a walking skeleton. Plasma albumin is usually normal and oedema is not present. The child with kwashiorkor has profound hypoalbuminaemia and he is oedematous. There is marked muscle wasting although this must be carefully looked for because of the relatively well-preserved subcutaneous tissue and oedema.

There are striking similarities between these childhood syndromes and the types of malnutrition seen in adult

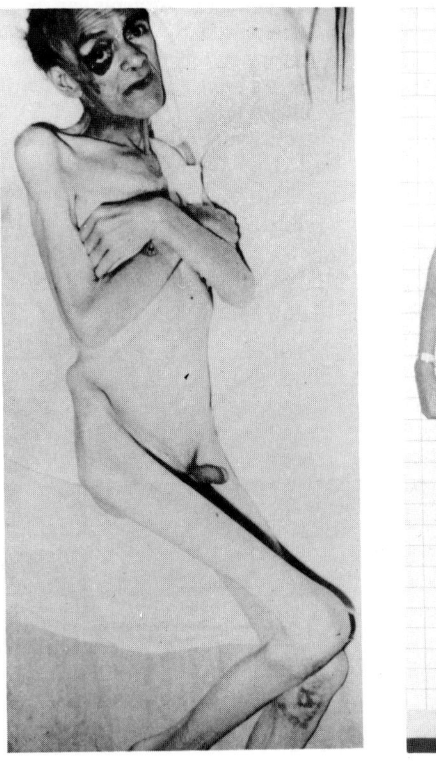

a

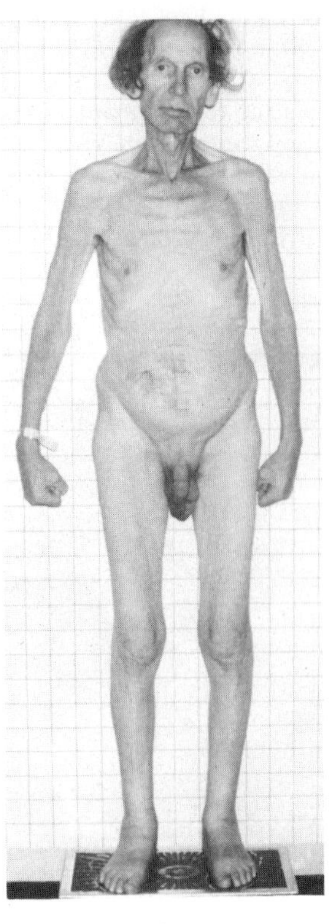

b

Fig. 8.1 a, This patient has marked wasting of fat and muscle and the skeleton is prominent. Plasma albumin level was 39 g/l. He resembles a child with *marasmus*. b, This patient has muscle wasting but this is partly obscured by the relatively well preserved subcutaneous tissue and by oedema. Plasma albumin level was 28 g/l. This condition resembles that of the child with *kwashiorkor*.

surgical patients suffering from protein energy malnutrition (*Fig.* 8.1). The *cachectic patient*, with profound wasting of both subcutaneous fat and muscle looks like a walking skeleton and his disordered metabolism is similar to that of the child with *marasmus*. On the other hand *patients with trauma and sepsis* have increased metabolic requirements and much of these are derived from catabolism of body protein. In addition, they may also lose additional protein from inflammatory exudates and the combined effect is wasted muscles, hypoalbuminaemia and low plasma concentrations of some of the proteins which are secreted by the liver and gastrointestinal tract such as transferrin, prealbumin and retinol-binding protein. Clearly this adult clinical syndrome which is seen in severe trauma and sepsis is not unlike that seen in children with *kwashiorkor*.

In children it has been established that protein energy malnutrition (PEM) is associated with immuno-incompetence, impaired phagocytic function, poor inflammatory response, delayed wound healing and even mental depression and apathy. There is now no doubt that similar problems occur in severely malnourished surgical patients too, although the same degree of starvation, trauma or sepsis does not always cause the same degree of impairment in different patients. This depends on the energy and protein stores of the patient before his illness, the degree of the energy deficit and his adaptation to it. In clinical practice it means that the surgeon should not be so concerned about how much the patient has lost, although that is important, he should focus his attention on what is left in terms of body fat, body protein and immune function.

PATHOGENESIS OF PROTEIN ENERGY MALNUTRITION IN SURGICAL PATIENTS

In a patient in energy balance the total amount of energy which is taken in by the body either orally or by the intravenous route equals that which is put out as heat and work. If the patient cannot eat and no nutrition is given intravenously there is negative energy balance, the body stores of fat and protein are utilized and the patient loses weight. If the output of heat rises (e.g. raised metabolic expenditure after major trauma) or the output of work increases (e.g. increased work of breathing in respiratory distress) there is also negative energy balance, the body stores of fat and protein are utilized and the patient loses weight.

The *total metabolic expenditure* is not increased even after major operations such as gastrectomy or colectomy. The *resting* metabolic expenditure is increased about 10% after such operations but the energy expended by physical activity (*active* metabolic expenditure) is reduced by a similar amount so that the total metabolic expenditure is unchanged. The weight loss after elective surgery is almost entirely due therefore to lack of energy intake and indeed the metabolic changes occurring after this sort of surgery can be shown to be very similar to those that occur after simple starvation and the rate of weight loss is almost identical.

In very major surgery, multiple trauma and invasive sepsis the resting metabolic expenditure is raised 20–40% and in extensive burns it may be raised 100%. In such patients the metabolic assault is then much greater for not only is energy intake usually reduced or absent, the energy output is raised as well. In these circumstances the rate of weight loss is more rapid than in simple starvation. This is due not only to the profound energy imbalance but also to increased amounts of protein being burned as fuel. For every 1 g of protein burned, 5 g of lean tissue are lost. In starvation, on the other hand, when relatively anhydrous fat is utilized for fuel, only about 1 g of weight is lost for every 1 g of fat burned.

Before the surgeon can properly understand the altered metabolism of patients with severe catabolic illness it is necessary for him to understand something of the physiology of *simple acute starvation*. Cahill's well known schema illustrates this well (*Fig.* 8.2). It can be seen that there are two primary fuel sources: muscle protein and fat. Glycogen in liver and muscle makes a very small contribution in comparison with these stores. Glucose is derived from

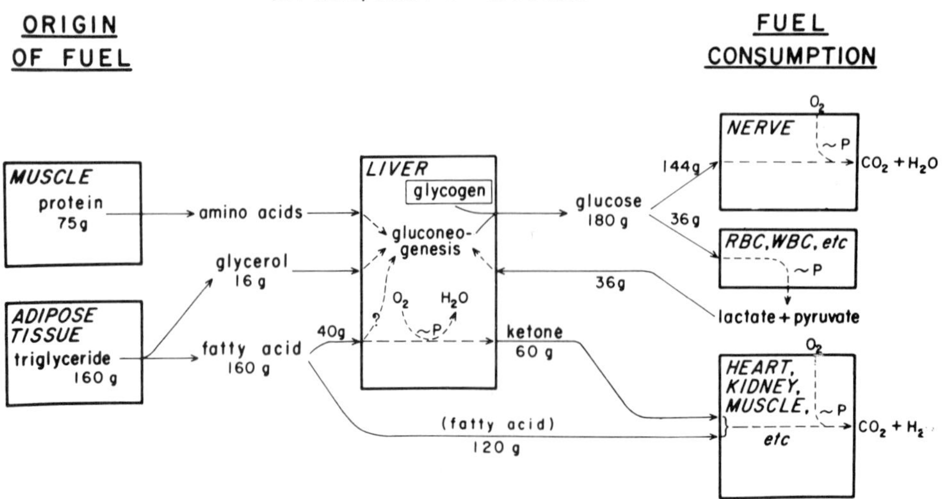

Fig. 8.2 Fuel metabolism in a normal man fasted for 24 h. Muscle and adipose tissue are the primary fuel sources and the fuel for the brain is glucose. (From Cahill G. F. (1970) *N. Engl. J. Med.* **282**, 668.)

gluconeogenesis. The new glucose formed in this way comes in part from muscle amino acids and in part from glycerol, which comes from fat. In early fasting about 180 g of glucose are made and most of this is utilized as a fuel by the brain, but some is also used by red and white blood cells, bone marrow and renal medulla. The rest of the body derives its energy from fat.

If *fasting is prolonged* marked changes in metabolism occur. The body cannot continue to supply the brain's energy need from muscle amino acids for erosion of body protein would be considerable and survival would be threatened. The body adapts to reduce the need of the brain for glucose by substituting its fuel supply and in prolonged fasting the brain utilizes ketone bodies, derived from fat for its energy needs (*Fig.* 8.3).

In severe injury, very major surgery, extensive burns and invasive sepsis profound metabolic changes occur, mainly as a result of the neuroendocrine responses described in the previous chapter. There is increased protein catabolism, a decrease in protein anabolism and an alteration in glucose

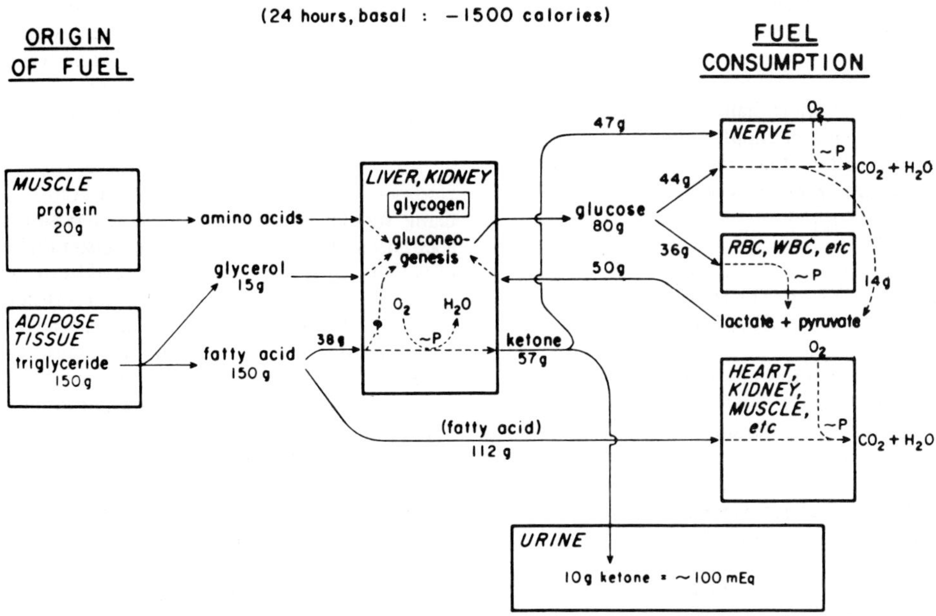

Fig. 8.3 Fuel metabolism in prolonged fasting. The patient has adapted by burning less muscle protein. The brain is now using ketones as fuel. (From Cahill G. F. (1970) *N. Engl. J. Med.* **282**, 668.)

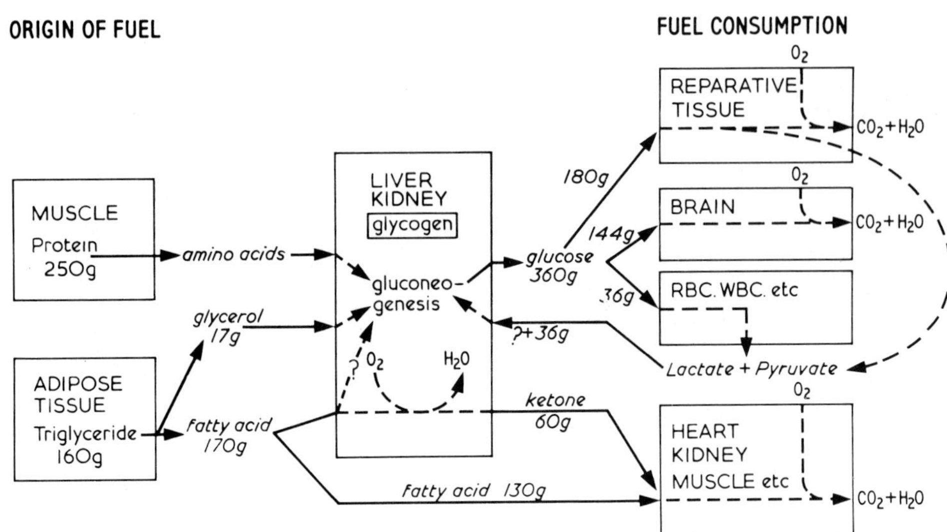

Fig. 8.4 Fuel metabolism in a patient with severe trauma. Reparative tissue is using glucose as fuel. This comes from gluconeogenesis from amino acids of muscle. (From Cahill G. F. et al. (1970). In: Fox C. L. and Nahas G. G. (ed.) *Body Fluid Replacement in the Surgical Patient*, p. 286, New York, Grune & Stratton.)

metabolism. The major alteration in energy metabolism is an increased gluconeogenesis to provide glucose for reparative tissues. *Fig.* 8.4 shows that while fat continues to be the main energy source, polymorphonuclear leucocytes, particularly when exhibiting phagocytosis, utilize glucose avidly and fibroblasts receive their energy in this way as well. In rapidly healing tissues the metabolism of glucose to lactate probably provides the main energy source. In this way the traumatized or septic patient has a special need for extra glucose and this is provided by catabolism of muscle protein.

It is not difficult then to understand how the marasmic starving surgical patient—who is not septic or severely injured—has wasting of both muscle and fat (*see Fig.* 8.1). The septic or severely injured patient, on the other hand, is quite different. He has a disproportionate wasting from body protein stores. Muscle bellies are shrunken, and plasma albumin and the short half-life plasma proteins, transferrin, prealbumin and retinol-binding protein fall to low levels. The clinical picture then is more that of kwashiorkor or marasmic kwashiorkor than marasmus (*see Fig.* 8.1).

INCIDENCE OF PROTEIN ENERGY MALNUTRITION IN SURGICAL PATIENTS

There have been several studies of the prevalence of malnutrition in surgical patients. In one large American tertiary care hospital, more than 50% of the surgical patients showed evidence of protein energy malnutrition. Another survey in a major teaching hospital in Great Britain where the type of surgery undertaken was of the major elective type showed that malnutrition was less common than stated by the American workers but it was nevertheless common (about 50%) in patients who had suffered some complication after a major operation. Evidence from prospective studies suggests that only about 5% of patients coming to hospital for elective major surgery have clinically important protein energy malnutrition. It should be stressed that patients with marginal malnutrition before a major operation can develop severe postoperative malnutrition if food intake is delayed for more than a few days.

DIAGNOSIS OF MALNUTRITION IN SURGICAL PATIENTS

There are now a great number of tests being advised for nutritional assessment (*Table* 8.1) but a good history and physical examination and a small number of laboratory tests are all that are usually required.

The purpose of the history and *physical examination* is to determine the extent of body fat and protein depletion and to gain some idea of how this effects physiological function. When taking the *history* the surgeon should ask specifically about energy intake (food and drinks) and energy output (fever, vomiting and diarrhoea). A useful check is to remember that if intake from meals has been half that of normal over the past month, then it might be expected that the patient will have lost 5 kg of bodyweight.

The next important question in the patient's history is 'how much weight has been lost?' This is best discovered by asking the patient what his weight was when he was well and then to measure his present weight. Asking the patient directly in this way has been shown to be more accurate than

Table 8.1 Some tests currently used by research workers to assess nutritional status

Clinical history	Calcium metabolism
Social history	Phosphorus metabolism
Physical examination	Magnesium metabolism
GI function tests	Zinc balance
CNS function tests	Copper balance
Calorimetry	Selenium balance
Plasma proteins	Anthropometry
Plasma amino acids	Computer aided tomography
Muscle amino acids	Xeroradiography
Tests of carbohydrate metabolism	Multiple isotope dilution tests
Tests of lipid metabolism	K^{40} counting
Tests of endocrine function	Neutron activation analysis
Water-soluble vitamins	Non-specific immunocompetence
Fat-soluble vitamins	Specific immunocompetence

using standard weight tables but even so considerable inaccuracies can occur. It is for this reason that other evidence of weight loss (e.g. loose-fitting clothes or comments from family members) should be sought for. Although there is no absolute amount of weight loss that can be considered to be of prognostic importance there is evidence that loss of 15–20% of body weight is likely to be associated with impairment of a number of important bodily functions.

Lastly, specific enquiry is made about recent alterations in physiological function. Abnormal tiredness, loss of endurance, breathlessness and failure to heal minor wounds all suggest that protein deficiency is sufficient to interfere with recovery.

Physical examination should be directly concerned with determining body stores of fat and protein. Although sophisticated anthropomorphic indices are sometimes recommended, careful palpation of the subcutaneous tissue over biceps and triceps (for fat stores) and the muscle bellies of the arms and legs (for protein stores) will usually reveal clinically significant depletion of these body stores. Inspection of the temporalis, spinatus and interosseous muscles are also good indications of muscle wasting. In patients with severe trauma or sepsis it is important to remember that fat folds may still be preserved even though considerable muscle wasting has occurred. *Table* 8.2 shows some other physical signs which are indicative of malnutrition and can be helpful in deciding when marginal malnutrition is present.

Plasma proteins are usually normal in the marasmic type of patient but when trauma and sepsis are present low levels of plasma albumin are frequently seen. When the level is below 32 g/L then severe malnutrition is usually present and many other markers of malnutrition will be found to be low. Low

Table 8.2 Some physical signs of malnutrition

Hair	Easy pluckability
Skin	Petechial, purpura, extreme thinness
Face	Nasolabial seborrhoea
Lips	Cheilosis, angular fissures
Tongue	Atrophy of papillae
Glands	Enlargement of salivary glands
Extremities	Dependent oedema

levels of plasma transferrin, plasma prealbumin and retinol-binding protein have been shown to be associated with an increased incidence of sepsis. Very severe malnutrition is associated with immuno-incompetence and recently some workers have suggested that delayed hypersensitivity skin testing should be used to determine if clinically significant malnutrition is present in surgical patients. It is now generally agreed, however, that patients whose immune state is depressed because of malnutrition can usually be picked out by the clinical methods which have already been mentioned.

It is a lot easier to *follow* the nutritional state of a patient than to assess it for the first time. Nutritional progress can be followed by regular measurements of body weight and plasma albumin as well as clinical assessment of physiological function. For patients receiving nutritional therapy it is frequently recommended that studies of nitrogen balance be made. Such studies are of great value to physicians who have a special interest in this sort of work and where the nursing staff are trained in the meticulous techniques required. In most routine hospital practice the inaccuracies of these techniques may make them unreliable. If errors occur they suggest that more nitrogen retention has occurred than has really happened in fact and this may lead to false optimism about the progress of the patient.

INDICATIONS FOR NUTRITIONAL THERAPY BEFORE MAJOR SURGERY

Studley showed many years ago that patients with peptic ulcer disease had a postoperative mortality of 33% when their preoperative weight loss was more than 20%. In contrast, in patients who had lost less body weight than this, the mortality rate was 3·5%. This, together with animal experiments which showed that profound hypoproteinaemia was associated with delayed wound healing and increased sepsis, has led some surgeons to prescribe preoperative nutritional therapy to many patients before undertaking major surgery.

Unfortunately, recent prospective studies have failed to confirm these findings and it is now realized that weight loss unaccompanied by impairment of physiological function does not increase the likelihood of nutrition associated postoperative complications. As a general guidline, body weight loss of 15–20% below well weight accompanied by clinical evidence of muscle weakness (respiratory and limb) and reduced physical endurance should alert the clinician to the possibility of increased risk of nutrition associated complications. If the plasma albumin level is less than 32 g/L it is likely that sepsis is present or has been in the recent past, and that postoperative septic complications and impaired wound healing are a possiblity. In such circumstances and particularly when the anticipated surgical procedure is a large one it is reasonable to consider 1–2 weeks of nutritional repletion before undertaking surgery.

INDICATIONS FOR NUTRITIONAL THERAPY AFTER MAJOR SURGERY

It is even more difficult to decide on the indications for nutritional therapy after major surgery. There is no question that nutritional therapy is required in the *hypercatabolic septic patient* who is losing weight and few would disagree that the patient who develops an *enterocutaneous fistula* in the postoperative period needs nutritional support as well as complete rest of the gastrointestinal tract. However, the correct time to give nutritional therapy to patients who do not have these complications after surgery is not known. Several studies have demonstrated that there is little or no advantage in the routine administration of calories and nitrogen after elective major surgery, although there is some evidence that very malnourished patients or those in whom very large granulating wounds are present may benefit from such treatment. A useful rule is that nutritional therapy should be considered if the patient has lost more than 15–20% of the weight when he was well and there is no immediate prospect of his eating normally. This is based on studies of starving volunteers who showed prolonged return to physical fitness when more than 20% of their body weight was lost.

NUTRITIONAL MANAGEMENT

Once it has been determined that nutritional supplementation is needed then the best method of delivering this sort of therapy must be decided upon. Over the past 15 years a number of techniques have been developed which have achieved the proper management of most nutritional problems that will be encountered in surgical practice. These are *oral sip feeding*, *tube feeding* and, if the gastrointestinal tract is non-functional, *parenteral feeding*.

For each of these methods to be successful a knowledge of basic patient requirements is necessary (*Table* 8.3).

Table 8.3 Basic patient nutritional requirements

	Daily requirement/ kg body weight
Water	30–50 ml
Calories	30–50 kcal
Nitrogen	0·20–0·35 g
Sodium	0·9–1·2 mmol
potassium	0·7–0·9 mmol

Magnesium, calcium, chloride and phosphate together with trace elements and vitamins should always be included.

Sip Feeding

Some patients who can eat but require extra calories and protein can be helped by sip feeding.

With suitable palatable liquid feeds, such as Complan, Thrive or Sustagen considerable extra energy and protein can be obtained by a patient who sips small volumes hour by hour throughout the day. About half of such patients are unable to do this satisfactorily complaining of bloating and abdominal cramps but the remainder find the effort demanded not too great and up to 2000 kcal and 50 g of extra protein can be given in this way. Ensure, Isocal and Osmolite contain balanced proportions of protein, carbohydrate and fat with electrolytes and provide a complete and balanced diet and are used when the patient is unable to take solid food.

Tube Feeding

For many patients requiring nutritional support the gastrointestinal tract is functional and therefore the easiest way of giving them nutrients. In the past a gastrostomy was the 'tube feeding' route most favoured but nasogastric tube

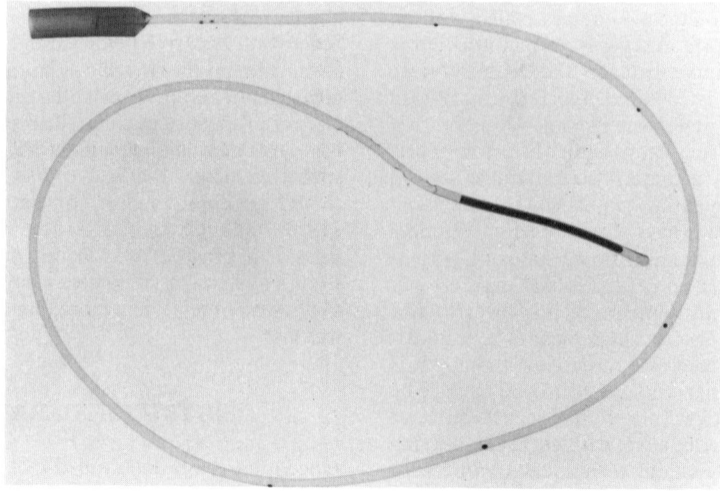

Fig. 8.5 Nasogastric tube feeding. The tube is made of silicone rubber (No. 7 F gauge) and has a tiny mercury weight at its tip. The patient can be fed using this tube for many days without discomfort.

feeding and jejunostomy feeding have practically superseded it.

Nasogastric Feeding

The recent introduction of fine bore, soft nasogastric tubes is a major advance in clinical nutrition and has enabled many patients to be fed by the enteral route who formerly might have been fed parenterally. The simplest tube to use is a fine bore silicone rubber tube with a tiny mercury weight at its tip. This is simply slipped through the nose and down the oesophagus but it is wise to confirm its placement in the stomach by radiography. Most patients find these tubes quite comfortable even over long periods (*Fig.* 8.5) and only rarely can they not be tolerated.

Although it is often stated that an ordinary diet carefully 'blenderized' can be used with these tubes, intermittent blockage can be an annoying and time-consuming problem. It is a lot easier in practice to use one of the defined formula diets (Clinifeed, Isocal or Ensure) for this purpose. Whenever dietary preparations are administered into the gastrointestinal tract via tubes it is best to employ constant infusion pumps to ensure a constant rate of delivery over the day. The disadvantage of nasogastric feeding is its poor tolerance by some patients because of delayed gastric emptying. The use of pumps decreases the incidence of abdominal cramps, vomiting and diarrhoea.

It is sometimes said that chemically defined bulk-free elemental diets should be used for nasogastric feeding. This is not always so. They are indicated when there is some deficiency of digestive enzymes or a very short gut but the cheaper and less complicated defined formula liquid feeds are probably better absorbed when the intestine is normal.

The patient on enteral feeding should be monitored closely. Daily measurements of body weight and fluid balance should be done, fractional urine sugars should be measured throughout the day. Twice weekly measurements of plasma electrolytes and albumin should also be performed. The sort of surgical patients in whom nasogastric tube feeding may be applicable include *short gut syndrome* (2–3 months after operation), *Crohn's disease*, *low enterocutaneous fistulas* (distal ileum or colon, *burns*, *trauma* and some patients with a *malabsorption syndrome*.

Jejunosotomy Feeding

Some clinical circumstances prohibit the use of nasogastric feeding. When there is a blockage, a fistula or a recent anastomosis in the oesophagogastric, gastric or duodenal regions, jejunosotomy is particularly useful. Recently the technique of fine catheter needle jejunostomy has been introduced (*Fig.* 8.6). A submucosal tunnel about 10 cm long is created in a loop of jejunum about 30 cm from the duodenal jejunal flexure using a stainless-steel needle. A fine plastic catheter 40 cm long with an internal diameter of 1·0 mm is threaded through the needle into the jejunum. The needle is withdrawn over the catheter and a purse string suture inserted in the jejunal wall around the the catheter. Using the same needle the catheter is threaded through the anterior abdominal wall; finally the loop of jejunum is attached to the peritoneum and the catheter fixed to the skin. Before feeding, radio-opaque material is injected through the catheter to confirm its position in the bowel lumen.

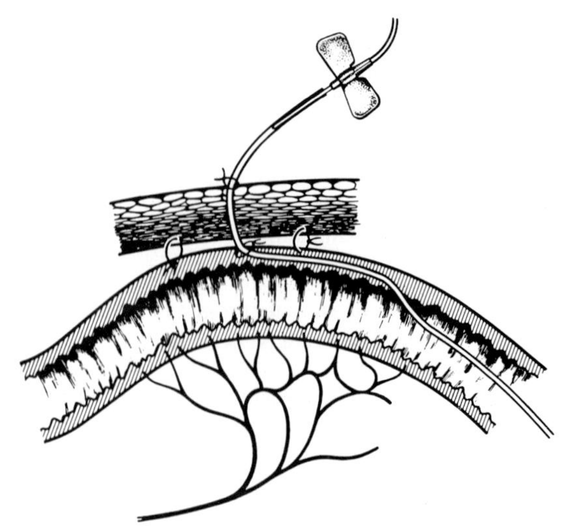

Fig. 8.6 Fine needle catheter jejunostomy.

A liquid diet (either elemental or defined formula) is infused constantly through the catheter beginning with half strength for the first day or two. If this is tolerated the volume and strength are increased until patient requirements are met.

This type of feeding is particularly valuable after oesophageal surgery where a prolonged period without oral intake is anticipated, especially in a patient who is already malnourished.

Parenteral Nutrition

Over the past 15 years or so the safe administration of nutrients by vein has become a practical form of therapy which can be given in most hospitals. Complete nutritional needs can be supplied safely over weeks, months or even years, provided there is a clear understanding of the principles involved. The nutrient solutions which contain amino acids, dextrose, minerals and vitamins are unstable if stored for extended periods of time and these separate ingredients must be mixed together in the hospital pharmacy under very strict aseptic techniques shortly before they are administered. The ratio of calories to nitrogen must be adequate (at least 150 kcal/g nitrogen) and they both must be administered simultaneously. The nutrients must be given in quantities considerably greater than the basic calorie and nitrogen requirements and it has been found that about 40 kcal/kg body weight per day and 0·3 g N/kg/day are needed to achieve gains of body protein.

Indications for the Use of Intravenous Nutrition

The principal indications for intravenous nutrition are found in seriously ill patients suffering from protein calorie malnutrition, intra-abdominal sepsis and severe trauma where the use of the gastrointestinal tract for feeding is not possible. Because the treatment itself is associated with a lot of complications and can be quite dangerous there must be very clear indications for its use. A useful reminder is that parenteral feeding will be the nutritional therapy of choice when the gastrointestinal tract is *blocked*, *short*, *fistulated*, *inflamed* or *cannot cope with demands*.

1. Gastrointestinal Tract is Blocked

Feeding by the intravenous route is required to avoid or correct malnutrition when the oesophagus, stomach or duodenum are blocked by stricture, neoplasm or an extrinsic mass. The very cachectic patient with gastric outlet obstruction is a good example. Blockages in the small or large bowel are usually dealt with directly by surgery although parenteral feeding may be required in the postoperative stage.

2. Gastrointestinal Tract is Short

Patients with the short gut syndrome usually require parenteral nutrition for the first 2 months or so postoperatively. Diarrhoea which is usually present in profuse amounts after massive enterectomy results from increased secretions encouraged by the osmotic stimulation of salt and water secretion that follows malabsorption of luminal content. Initially, this should be controlled by giving the patient nothing by mouth to reduce any osmotic stimuli. There may also be substantial losses secondary to gastric hypersecretion and malabsorption of endogenous secretions. For these reasons the patient is commenced on parenteral nutrition. Water, energy, protein and appropriate amounts of sodium, potassium, magnesium and trace metals are administered together with an H_2-blocking drug in a single container. Losses should be measured and replaced accordingly. The length of time the patient with the short gut syndrome remains on parenteral nutrition receiving nothing by mouth varies from 3 weeks to 2–3 months before stool volume reaches a plateau and electrolyte losses become predictable. Because enteral nutrition is necessary for optimal small bowel adaptation, oral feeding should be initiated as soon as feacal output and electrolyte losses reach a plateau. In some patients, usually with less than one metre of remaining intestine home parenteral feeding will be necessary, possibly on a permanent basis. There are several hundred patients receiving home total parenteral nutrition throughout the world and a number have been treated in this way for several years.

3. Gastrointestinal Tract is Fistulated

Patients with enterocutaneous fistulas proximal to the distal ileum should receive nothing by mouth and be given parenteral nutrition. Ileal and colonic fistulas may be treated with tube feeding provided the ouput from them is low (<100 ml/day). About 50% of fistulas from the small intestine will close spontaneously with this treatment. Certain types of fistulas will not close and will require surgery—in particular, when the fistula arises in an area of Crohn's disease or in an area of irradiated bowel. Any fistula that shows no sign of closing after 6 weeks of total gut rest should be investigated to determine the cause of non-closure and surgery should be undertaken when appropriate.

4. Gastrointestinal Tract is Inflamed

There is a lot of debate over the value of total gut rest and intravenous nutrition for patients with inflammatory bowel disease when it is used as a primary therapy. There is no doubt, however, that a lot of patients with partial obstruction of the small intestine secondary to Crohn's disease undergo spontaneous remission with total gut rest, steroids and total parenteral nutrition. Many malnourished patients, requiring surgery for inflammatory bowel disease will require parenteral feeding both before and after operation. Patients with inflammation inside the abdominal cavity but outside the gastrointestinal tract (e.g. intra-abdominal abscesses or pancreatitis) often require periods of total gut rest and nutritional support.

5. Gastrointestinal Tract cannot Cope

Often, in severe trauma or other hypercatabolic states sufficient calories and nitrogen cannot be supplied via the gastrointestinal tract. In such cases parenteral nutrition is required.

Lastly, parenteral nutrition has been advocated for patients in *acute renal failure* and also in some patients with *hepatic failure*.

The Nutrient Solution

For short periods such as the few weeks required by most surgical patients, a simple solution of 8·5% synthetic amino acids and 50% dextrose has been found to be uncomplicated in use and beneficial to the patient. One litre of this solution (500 ml 8·5% amino acids + 500 ml 50% dextrose) provides 1000 kcal and 6·8 g of nitrogen. To this solution is added albumin, sodium, potassium, magnesium, phosphorus, calcium, acetate, chloride, trace elements and vitamins as required from day to day.

Severe hypoalbuminaemia, i.e. 30 g/l, must be treated at the commencement of the course of parenteral nutrition. From 25 to 50 g/day of salt-poor albumin given during the first few days may restore the colloid osmotic pressure while supplementing protein nutrition. In the patient with severe diarrhoea and considerable faecal protein loss, or a large abscess cavity, albumin may be required throughout the course of treatment. Sodium requirements in the average adult patient are 50 mmol for each litre of nutrient solution. Both sodium and potassium are supplied as the acetate, chloride or acid phosphate as salt depending on the day-to-day requirements of these salts.

It is important to remember that the need for potassium and phosphorus may be very high in the severely debilitated patient. In order to achieve positive nitrogen balance and tissue synthesis, not only must adequate calories and sufficient nitrogen be provided but also potassium and phosphorus must be supplied in sufficient quantities to support cellular growth without causing hypokalaemia or hypophosphataemia. It is recommended that the usual daily dose of potassium be approximately 40 mmol for each 1000 calories administered. The need for potassium may prove to be greater than this, but the exact requirement can be controlled according to daily plasma levels. The normal daily requirement of phosphorus is met by adding 20 mEq to each 1000 calories, but decreased plasma levels may demand up to twice or even three times this amount in patients whose weight gain is maximal. From 2 to 4 mmol of magnesium sulphate are added to each litre of solution, although in patients suffering from severe malnutrition in which magnesium loss has occurred, 8 mmol should be added to each litre until the deficiency is corrected. Hypomagnesaemia will often occur within a week of intravenous hyperalimentation if magnesium is not added, and for this reason the need to add this element must be emphasized.

It is recommended that 3 mmol of calcium be added to each litre of hyperalimentation fluid but only one ampoule of the intravenous vitamin preparation MVI or Multibionta is given each day. These vitamin preparations are used because they contain both fat-soluble and water-soluble vitamins. Folic acid, vitamin K and vitamin B_{12} are administered separately as needed. Usually 10 mg of vitamin K and 15 mg of folate are given i.m. at least once weekly and vitamin B_{12} is given initially and again every 2 weeks.

Many surgical patients with malnutrition are severely anaemic, and the normal red cell volume is restored by the administration of whole blood or packed cells. The trace elements such as zinc (4 mg), copper (1·5 mg), manganese (0·5 mg), chromium (20 mg), iodine (100 mg) and selenium (50 mg) are added to the nutrient solution daily but additional zinc is required to achieve protein gain, particularly in patients with gastrointestinal losses. If there is less than 300 g/day of stool or small intestinal drainage zinc balance can be achieved by supplementation with 3·0 mg of elemental zinc/day. If there are fistula losses of 2 litres or so zinc balance can be achieved only if 30 mg of elemental zinc/day are given.

Administration via Subclavian Catheter

The hypertonic nature of the solutions used for intravenous feeding requires their delivery into a large central vein to avoid sepsis and thrombosis. The safest and most reliable technique for long-term intravenous therapy in adults is via percutaneous catheterization of the superior vena cava by way of the subclavian vein.

There is a widespread fear that intravenous nutrition is associated with a high rate of catheter tip sepsis with consequent septicaemia. It has now been shown that catheter-related sepsis is an avoidable complication if strict adherence to time-honoured principles of aseptic technique is adopted. The principles are simple enough. No additions are made to the litre bottles of nutrient solutions once they leave the pharmacy. A specified person, usually a nurse highly motivated to avoid complications, must change the catheterization site dressings and the intravenous administration tubing every second day. In practice, a simple regimen of changing the dressing every Monday, Wednesday, and Friday works well in with the weekly hospital routine. Each dressing is aseptically removed. The skin surrounding the catheter entrance site is prepared with a povidone-iodine solution for 3 min. Antimicrobial ointment is applied to the skin entrance catheter site, and a sterile water repellent dressing (e.g. Opsite) is reapplied. It is vital to maintain the integrity of the delivery tubing. Blood and blood products may not be administered or withdrawn via the catheter, and CVP must not be monitored through the hyperalimentation catheter. It is permissible when other venous sites are not easily obtainable to administer water and electrolytes and an intermittent bolus of antibiotics through the side arm of the intravenous drip tubing. This tubing is considered an integral part of the hyperalimentation delivery system and is changed three times weekly by the nurse in charge of hyperalimentation. Infection is thought to be catheter related and, therefore, the catheter is removed in the following circumstances: a positive blood culture which is unassociated with a known site of infection and an occult fever which does not subside after replacement of the delivery tubing and nutrient solution.

Catheter Placement

This is the most important step in the practical execution of a successful hyperalimentation course. The technique shown in *Figs.* 8.7 to 8.10 has gained wide acceptance and is associated with the least amount of problems. With practice, there is almost no occasion on which this route cannot be used. The catheter must be radio-opaque and preferably made of silicone. A 20 cm (8 in) long 16 gauge radio-opaque catheter passed through a 5 cm (2 in) long 14 gauge needle under scrupulous aseptic conditions is a well proven and safe system.

The patient is placed on his back with the foot of the bed elevated 15°. A small pad is placed between the shoulder blades to allow the shoulders to drop backwards. The skin is scrubbed with an antiseptic solution and drapes are carefully placed and scrupulous aseptic precautions are observed. Local anaesthetic is infiltrated into the skin, subcutaneous tissue and periosteum at the inferior border just lateral to the midpoint of the clavicle. The needle, attached to a small syringe, is advanced towards the tip of the finger placed into the suprasternal notch (*Fig.* 8.7). The needle should be very close to the inferior surface of the clavicle and penetration of the subclavian vein is signalled by a rush of blood into the syringe. The needle is advanced a few millimetres more to ensure that it is entirely within the vein. The patient is then asked to perform a Valsalva manoeuvre, the thumb is held over the needle hub as the syringe is removed. The radio-opaque catheter is then introduced through the needle and threaded into the superior vena cava (*Fig.* 8.8). The needle is then withdrawn from the patient and a small plastic cuff is fitted over the junction of the catheter and needle tip. The catheter is then connected to an intravenous administration set and a slow infusion of normal saline is begun while the catheter is sewn to the skin ((*Fig.* 8.9). Povidone-iodine ointment is applied around the entrance of the catheter into the skin and a dressing is applied over it including the

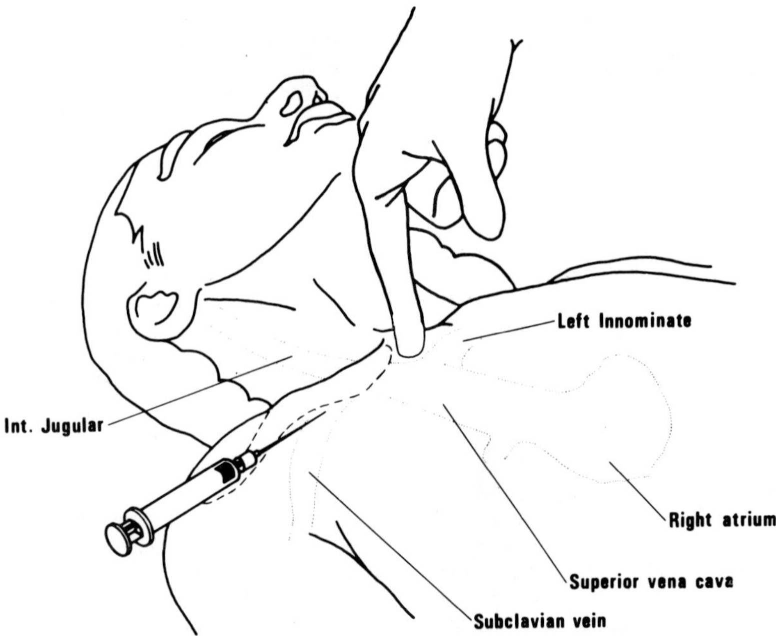

Fig. 8.7 A 14 gauge needle is inserted just lateral to the mid part of the clavicle and directed forward by a finger tip that is pressed firmly into the suprasternal notch. Puncture of the subclavian vein is indicated by a flush of blood into the syringe. (From Dudrick S. J. and Copeland E. M. (1973) Parenteral hyperalimentation. In: Nyhus L. M. (ed.), *Surgery Annual.* New York, Appleton-Century-Crofts.)

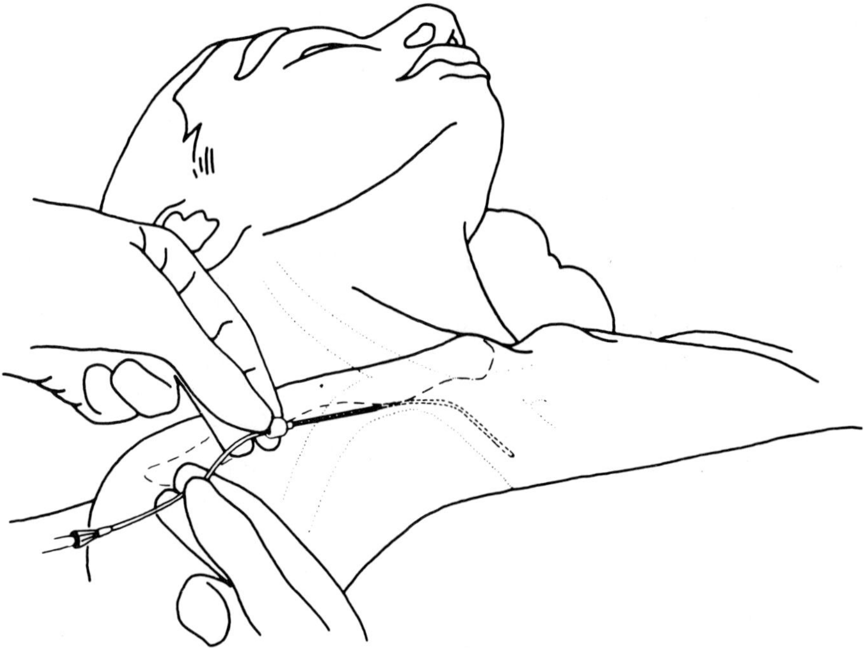

Fig. 8.8 The 16 gauge catheter is advanced into the vein to lie in the superior vena cava. (From Dudrick S. J. and Copeland E. M. (1973) Parenteral hyperalimentation. In: Nyhus L. M. (ed.), *Surgery Annual.* New York, Appleton-Century-Crofts.)

junction of the intravenous tubing and the hub of the catheter (*Fig.* 8.10).

For long-term parenteral feeding, radio-opaque silicone catheters (Broviac or Hickman) are used. These feeding lines are inserted using a similar surgical approach and then tunnelled subcutaneously over a long distance from the entrance of the catheter into the subclavian vein. This subcutaneous tunnelling reduces the risk of catheter sepsis.

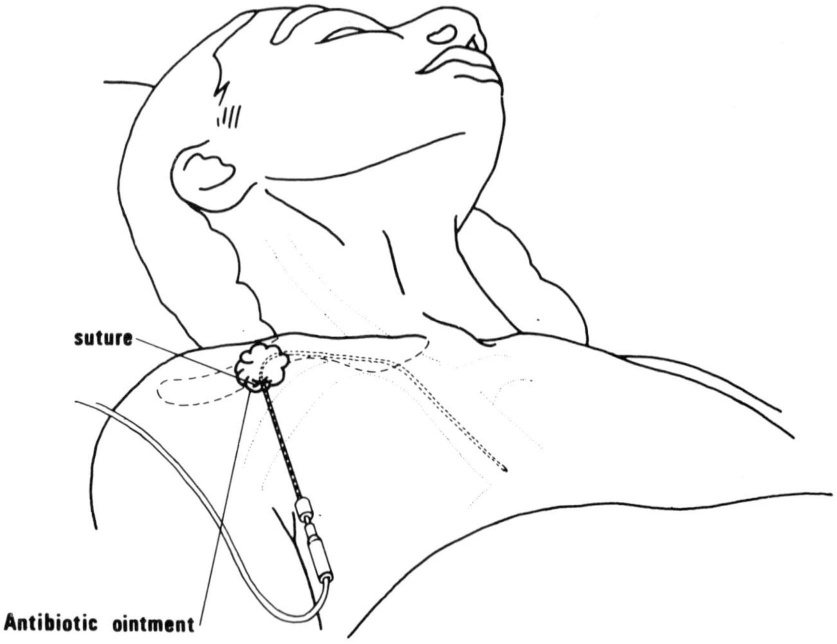

Fig. 8.9 The catheter is sutured to the skin and antiseptic ointment is placed around the catheter at the skin entrance site. (From Dudrick S. J. and Copeland E. M. (1973) Parenteral hyperalimentation. In: Nyhus L. M. (ed.), *Surgery Annual*. New York, Appleton-Century-Crofts.)

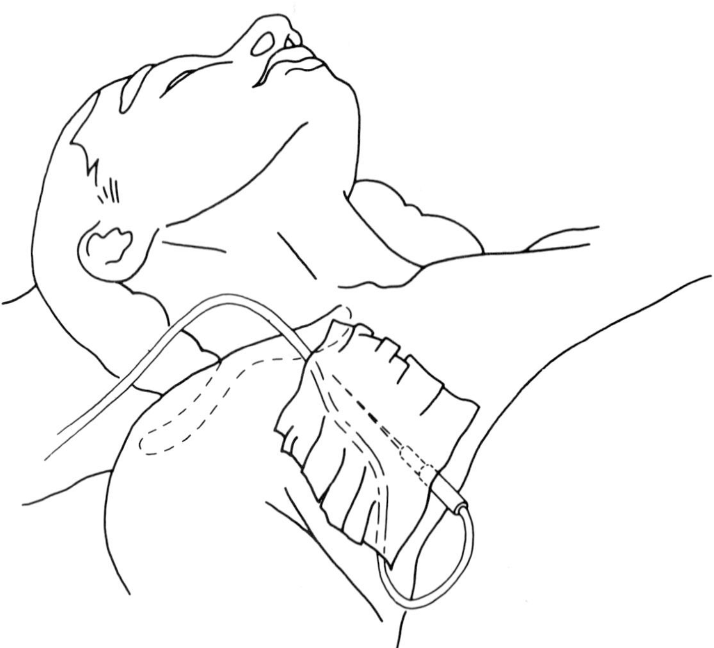

Fig. 8.10 Sterile dressing secures the catheter and tubing in place. The site is cleansed every second day and the infusion tubing is changed. (From Dudrick S. J. and Copeland E. M. (1973) Parenteral hyperalimentation. In: Nyhus L. M. (ed.), *Surgery Annual*. New York, Appleton-Century-Crofts.)

More recently, the Port-A-Cath system has been introduced (*see* Chapter 72) and would appear to be ideal for patients requiring home parenteral nutrition indefinitely.

A chest radiograph is taken immediately after insertion to confirm the position of the catheter in the vena cava and to check for possible pneumothorax. With close attention to these details of insertion complications are minimal, the most common problem being an occasional pneumothorax, particularly in a very emaciated patient where puncture of the apical pleura is more likely.

Administration of Nutrient Solution

The hypertonic solution (1800-2400 mosmol) *must* be delivered at a constant rate during each 24-h period. Usually 1–1·5 litre (1000 cal + 6·8 g nitrogen) is given in the first 24-h period followed by the administration of 1000 ml every 12 h for the next 48-h period. Supplemental water, sodium and potassium are given separately as indicated from the plasma levels. This careful administration by moderate increments avoids hyperosmolarity problems and gives the pancreas time to adapt with increased insulin output in response to the glucose load. Within 3 or 4 days most patients cope well with 3 litre (3000 cal) per day. After this plateau is reached (i.e. no spillage of sugar in the urine), it is sometimes necessary to increase the intake to 3500 ml to get positive nitrogen balance and effective weight gain. Throughout the course of intravenous feeding plasma levels of sodium, potassium, chloride, phosphate, sugar, urea and albumin are measured. Accurate daily weighings are also essential, and the maximum sustained weight gain is never much more than 0·3 kg/day. Gains greater than this most often indicate retention of water. In a very sick patient where fluid overload could be life-threatening it is safer to be content with maintaining body weight than with positive weight gain. Fractional urine sugars are checked every 6 hours not only to monitor possible hyperglycaemia and consequent osmotic diuresis but also to monitor the uniform rate of delivery of the nutrient solution. If a patient, during a specified nursing shift, is constantly showing a 3+ to 4+ urine sugar, it is not hard to pinpoint the problem, but if constant glycosuria is noted in a non-diabetic patient, the rate of delivery must be slowed until the excess sugar disappears. Sometimes, especially in septic patients, a constant glycosuria will appear even before maximum calories for weight gain are reached. This situation is remedied by the cautious administration of soluble insulin (about 20–50 units/l) in each bottle of the nutrient solution.

Administration during the Operative Period

Although it is permissible to continue to administer the nutrient solution during the operative period, it is safer and less complex to decrease the quantity to 2 litre the day before surgery, and during the operative period, administer through the central venous catheter 5% dextrose solution at the rate of 1 litre every 8 h. Abrupt cessation of the intravenous hyperalimentation may lead to 'rebound' insulin shock because insulin secretion continues for a day or so after the high glucose load is discontinued.

The Use of Fat Emulsions

Ten or twenty per cent soybean oil emulsions (Intralipid) are available as energy sources for intravenous nutrition. Although there are other energy sources available, dextrose and lipid are the only satisfactory ones. Lipid emulsions are expensive and in most surgical patients on short courses of parenteral nutrition (< 3 weeks) they are really not necessary. For periods longer than this lipid emulsion (1 litre of 10% solution 2 times each week) should be given to prevent fatty acid deficiencies. Some surgeons use lipid emulsions routinely for the non-protein calorie source in patients being fed i.v. and current evidence suggests that the procedure is less complicated and the patient is more easily managed when half the energy source is provided as lipid and half as dextrose. In very stressed patients a combination of glucose and fat is the best non-protein energy source providing triglyceride intolerance is absent.

THE WAY AHEAD

A number of controlled trials are in progress or are being planned which should help to solve the problem of who should be fed before and after major surgery. Trials are being conducted on cancer patients to decide if nutritional therapy will improve the outcome of patients receiving either surgical; chemotherapeutic or radiotherapeutic regimens.

In the future it may be possible to prescribe specific amino acid solutions for specific conditions. Already there are special formulations for renal failure and hepatic failure and it is hoped that advances will enable such solutions to be developed for patients with severe trauma, sepsis and advanced neoplasia.

There will be improvements in catheter technology and better pumps for accurate delivery of nutrient solutions. Although more hospitals will be able to administer parenteral nutrition safely and exposure to this type of treatment will be part of all surgeons' training it is likely that very complicated patients will continue to be treated by centres with a special interest in this type of work.

Further Reading

Clowes G. H. A. et al. (1983) Muscle proteolysis induced by a circulating peptide in patients with sepsis or trauma. *N. Engl. J. Med.* **308**, 545.

Dudrick S. J. et al. (1984) 100 patient years of ambulatory home total parenteral nutrition. *Ann. Surg.* **199**, 770.

Editorial (1983) Why the protein loss in sepsis and trauma? *Lancet* **1**, 858.

Editorial (1986) Indicators of surgical risk. *Lancet* **1**, 1422.

Hackett A. F. et al. (1979) Eating patterns in patients recovering from major surgery: A study of voluntary food intake and energy balance. *Br. J. Surg.* **66**, 415.

Hill G. L. (1983) Operative strategy in the treatment of enterocutaneous fistulas. *World J. Surg.* **7**, 495.

Hill G. L. (1985) Massive enterectomy: indications and management. *World J. Surg.* **9**, 833.

Hill G. L. and Church J. M. (1984) Energy and protein requirements of general surgical patient requiring intravenous nutrition. *Br. J. Surg.* **71**, 1.

Streat S. J. and Hill G. L. (1987) Nutritional support in the management of critically ill patients in surgical intensive care. *World J. Surg.* **11**, 194–201.

9 Medical Therapy in Surgical Practice

A. Cuschieri

ADVERSE DRUG REACTIONS AND INTERACTIONS

Adverse drug reactions in clinical practice are an ever-increasing problem and account for a sizeable morbidity and mortality which, though inevitable in view of the complexity of the modern therapeutic armamentarium, nevertheless can be minimized by the careful selection of drug therapy and constant vigilance. A frequent and necessary exercise in modern surgical practice involves the identification of various drug preparations. A substantial majority of middle-aged and elderly patients requiring surgical care arrive in hospital with a variety of medicaments the nature of which is usually unknown to the patient. On ascertaining the exact nature of the drugs, it often transpires that some are unnecessary and others may be detrimental, particularly hypnotics, which tend to cause confusion in the aged. The exact chemical formulation must be ascertained as some of the drugs may interact with specific therapy started during the hospital stay. Rarely, specific bizarre surgical syndromes may follow drug treatment.

Adverse Drug Reactions

In 1969 the Committee of the World Health Organization defined an adverse drug reaction as 'one which is noxious, unintended and occurs at doses normally used in man for prophylaxis, diagnosis and therapy'. This definition therefore, excludes the effects of both intentional and accidental overdose. Drug reactions fall into four broad categories:

Dose-related
Non-dose-related
Long-term
Teratogenic.

Dose-related Adverse Reactions

These may be produced by virtue of an excessive therapeutic effect (e.g. bleeding from recent surgical wounds due to use of anticoagulants, hypoglycaemia from excessive insulin, etc.) or by the development of side-effects which may be pharmacological (e.g. blurred vision following propantheline administration) or toxic such as vestibular damage by gentamicin, especially in patients suffering from renal failure, marrow depression from cytotoxic chemotherapy, etc. Other dose-related adverse reactions may be caused by secondary effects, e.g. superinfection of the gastrointestinal tract following the administration of broad-spectrum antibiotics or the reactivation of tuberculosis in immunosuppressed patients. The difference between the dose required to produce a therapeutic effect by a drug and the dose which produces toxic effects is referred to as the *therapeutic ratio*. This is obviously an important determining factor in the development of toxic side-effects.

Non-dose-related Adverse Reactions

These include idiosyncrasy to a particular drug. This is usually genetically determined and predisposes the individual to an abnormal reaction following the administration of certain drugs. Examples of this type of response include the haemolysis caused by sulphonamides or aspirin in patients with G-6-PD deficiency. Drug allergy is also not related to dose and although sensitization to a drug may be produced by any route of administration, it is most commonly encountered after topical applications.

Long-term Reactions

Long-term effects may be produced as a result of prolonged treatment, e.g. chronic interstitial nephritis and papillary necrosis may follow the long-term administration of analgesic mixtures containing phenacetin, aspirin or amidopyrone. They may also be delayed, the adverse effects occurring months or years after the cessation of treatment, e.g. the hypothyroidism which follows ^{131}I therapy or lymphoma and leukaemia which may develop some time after immunosuppressive or cytotoxic therapy.

Teratogenic Reactions

Thalidomide, apart from causing incalculable human suffering, created formidable surgical problems. All new drugs must now undergo a rigorous testing for teratogenicity in animals before being tested in humans in phase one studies.

Risk Factors for Adverse Drug Reactions

The risk is greater with the following:

Administration of drugs with a narrow therapeutic ratio, e.g. digoxin, warfarin, antihypertensive drugs.
Elderly patients.
Patients with hepatic and renal disease.
Multiple prescriptions

The risk increases with the number of drugs prescribed to the patient. Often, proprietary (trade) names are used without the clinician being fully aware of the exact chemical formulation. This is especially hazardous as many of these contain more than one drug.

Drug Interactions

These may result in *antagonism* causing a loss of the therapeutic effect of a particular drug, *potentiation* leading to an excessive therapeutic effect, *increased toxicity* or the development of an *unusual reaction* which does not occur with either drug alone.

Chemical and physical interactions between drugs may result in their *inactivation* when they are used in combination. Adding drugs to intravenous fluids is commonly contraindicated. Thus, heparin is completely inactivated and frusemide is precipitated by dextrose solutions, and calcium salts precipitate in sodium bicarbonate. Dextrose–saline/saline affects the stability of many antibiotics which results in a substantial loss of their activity. Examples include benzylpenicillin, ampicillin, methicillin and gentamicin. Certain antibiotic combinations are manifestly incompatible when added to intravenous fluids. The Na^+ and K^+ salts of benzylpenicillin and the semisynthetic penicillins inactivate gentamicin and precipitate the tetracyclines; carbenicillin inactivates colistin and gentamicin is itself inactivated by kanamycin. Many other drug incompatabilities in intravenous fluids have been documented and therefore, in general, one should avoid mixing drugs in intravenous fluids whenever possible.

The mechanisms involved in *in vivo* drug interactions include effects on transport to the site of action due to changes in absorption and/or protein binding. Thus phenylbutazone displaces warfarin from the binding sites and thereby potentiates its anticoagulant effect. Intracellular transport may also be altered. For example, the antihypertensive effect of guanethidine is inhibited by the concomitant administration of tricyclic antidepressants and sympathomimetic amines, both of which block the active transport mechanism necessary for guanethidine to enter the cell.

Drug interaction may also cause alterations in the renal excretion of certain agents, e.g. phenylbutazone interferes with the excretion of chlorpropamide causing hypoglycaemia. Drug metabolism may also be altered due either to enzyme induction, as occurs when warfarin metabolism is stimulated by barbiturates, or by enzyme inhibition, e.g. anticholinesterase drugs which potentiate the action of suxamethonium and may cause prolonged apnoea. Monoamine oxidase inhibitors potentiate the actions of sympathomimetic amines.

Drug interaction may result from competition at specific receptor sites or from an additive physiological effect. Thus, sedatives, tranquillizers, anaesthetic agents, alcohol, narcotic analgesics and antidepressants may induce severe hypotension in patients on antihypertensive drugs. Potentiation of tubocurarine may be produced by drugs with neuromuscular blocking activity such as the aminoglycosides.

Electrolyte abnormalities induced by drugs may be of sufficient magnitude to cause significant side-effects. Thus, carbenoxolone or steroid therapy may induce hypokalaemia and enhance digitalis toxicity, and hyponatraemia caused by the excessive administration of diuretics increases the hypotensive effects of sedatives and tranquillizers.

The mechanisms of many types of drug interactions are not fully understood and the clinician should take this factor into consideration when an unexplained or unexpected deterioration in the condition of the patient occurs.

DRUG-INDUCED DISORDERS

The disorder may develop during the drug treatment or some time (months to years) after its withdrawal. The changes may or may not be reversible and often result in a significant morbidity and mortality. Several categories are recognized and many are important in surgical practice. Disorders caused by antibiotic therapy are discussed in Chapter 3.

Fibrotic Disorders

These are outlined in *Table* 9.1. Some are now of historical interest as the precipitant drug has been withdrawn from clinical practice.

Table 9.1 Drug-induced fibrotic disorders

Disorder	*Drug responsible*
Dupuytren's contracture	Phenobarbitone
Myocardial fibrosis and constrictive pericarditis	Methysergide
Pulmonary fibrosis	Bleomycin, busulphan, melphalan, cyclophosphamide, methotrexate, nitroso-ureas, amiodarone, nitrofurantoin, methysergide
Oculomucocutaneous syndrome	Practolol
Retroperitoneal fibrosis	Methysergide, phenacetin, methyldopa
Carpal tunnel syndrome	Oral contraceptives, high-dose progesterone, thalidomide, disulfiram

Oculomucocutaneous Syndrome

This consisted of a sclerosing peritonitis and pathological changes in other sites (eyes, skin, ears, pleura and pericardium) and was induced by the beta-blocker practolol which was introduced in 1970. Shortly after its introduction, side-effects were recognized. At first, these appeared to be restricted to the skin, the eyes and the ears. A large variety of skin lesions were described and the eye lesions resulted in the development of the dry-eye syndrome with keratinization, symblepharon, corneal thinning, opacification and ulceration. Deafness and tinnitus occurred from involvement of the auditory nerve. A sclerosing peritonitis was later described. This is different from retroperitoneal fibrosis and occurred after 2–3 years' treatment with normal doses of practolol. The condition presented as one of acute or acute-on-chronic small bowel obstruction. At laparotomy, the visceral and parietal peritoneal surfaces were found to be covered by a greyish-white pseudomembrane which invested the small intestine like a capsule or cocoon. In some patients the anterior and lateral parietal peritoneum was also involved resulting in complete obliteration of the peritoneal cavity. The pseudomembrane was avascular and could be peeled from the underlying bowel without excessive bleeding. Histological examination of the membrane showed a mesothelial lining below which were prominent lamellar layers of collagen with a collection of lymphocytes and macrophages separating the deeper aspect from the serosa of the bowel. Although other beta-blockers (propranolol, oxprenolol, timolol, metoprolol, atenolol) have been suggested to rarely induce a similar condition, there is no firm evidence to link these with the development of sclerosing peritonitis since this condition may occur, albeit rarely, spontaneously.

Retroperitoneal Fibrosis

Usually, this condition is idiopathic. In addition to the retroperitoneal fibrosis which often causes an obstructive uropathy, there may be involvement of the mediastinum, aorta, myocardium/pericardium/heart valves (fibrosis, valve regurgitation, constrictive pericarditis), thyroid gland, orbit and the gallbladder. The disorder presents with weight loss, anorexia, abdominal and back pain radiating to the thighs and testes, and a raised ESR. Continuous long-term administration of methysergide may induce the condition. Other drugs have also been implicated (phenacetin, methyldopa, etc.) but without confirmation.

Pulmonary Fibrosis

This is most commonly the result of cytotoxic therapy especially with bleomycin and busulphan. The condition is usually irreversible and often fatal, although prednisolone therapy has been reported to be effective in reversing the signs of pulmonary toxicity in some cases. The pathological picture consists of fibrosing alveolitis, interstitial fibrosis, alveolar squamous metaplasia and hyalinization. The onset is variable, from days to several months after the initiation of therapy. The clinical manifestations of the disorder include fever, cough and dyspnoea.

Carpal Tunnel Syndrome

Although included in the fibrotic category, drug-induced carpal tunnel syndrome is more often the result of either oedema (oral contraceptives, high-dose progesterone therapy), a neuropathy (thalidomide, disulfiram), or synovitis induced by injecting diazepam intravenously on the anterolateral aspect of the wrist.

Gastrointestinal and Hepatobiliary Disorders

Some of the common drug-induced disorders are shown in *Table* 9.2. Drug-induced cholestatic jaundice and hepatitis are discussed in Chapter 69.

Table 9.2 Drug-induced gastrointestinal and hepatobiliary disorders

Disorder	*Drug*
Ulcers and haemorrhage	Aspirin and NANSAIDs
Strictures	Potassium chloride
Pseudo-obstruction	Tricyclic antidepressants, MAOI, narcotic analgesics, excess purgation
Cholestatic jaundice and hepatitis	*See* Chapter 69
Peliosis hepatitis	Androgens, oestrogens, methotrexate
Focal nodular hyperplasia and hepatic adenomas	Oral contraceptives, androgens
Hepatocellular carcinomas	Androgens, oral contraceptives
Reye's syndrome	Aspirin in children
Acute cholecystitis	Diuretics, ? parenteral nutrition

Gastrointestinal Bleeding and Ulceration

The association between regular heavy aspirin ingestion and gastric ulceration is well established. An increasing problem in the past decade has been the significant increase in gastrointestinal ulceration (gastric and duodenal) presenting with bleeding or perforation in patients above the age of 60 years who have taken non-aspirin, non-steroidal anti-inflammatory drugs (NANSAIDs) for osteo- or rheumatoid arthritis. These drugs are known to produce gastric erosions and microbleeding and in a recent case-controlled study, a high proportion of patients admitted with perforated and bleeding peptic ulcers were noted to be regular users of NANSAIDs, the most common of which were indomethacin, piroxicam, naproxen and ibuprofen. It has been estimated that in the UK NANSAID ingestion accounts for 2000 cases of bleeding each year with an estimated 10% mortality.

The thiazide diuretics induce a hypokalaemia which is particularly dangerous because it intensifies the action of digoxin on the myocardium. To obviate this sequence, a combined entero-coated tablet containing the diuretic and a core of potassium chloride was introduced. The use of this formulation led to the development of ulceration in the small bowel. This presented with haemorrhage, perforation or intestinal obstruction due to stricture formation. This complication was caused by the rapid release of potassium chloride over a short segment of small intestine. The high concentration of potassium chloride produced a focal mucosal necrosis with a varying degree of submucosal erosion and an acute-on-chronic inflammatory reaction. Since then, the formulation of the tablet has been altered such that the solubility of the potassium chloride was lowered by coating the crystals with an inert wax-sugar combination. This resulted in a much slower release of potassium over a period of several hours.

Liver Tumours

The vast majority of both benign and malignant liver tumours are not the consequence of drug administration. However, a definite association between the development of both liver-cell adenoma and hepatocellular carcinoma and oral contraceptive use and androgen intake has been established. The association between oral contraception and focal nodular hyperplasia is less certain and disputed by some.

Focal nodular hyperplasia is an entirely benign condition which resembles the regenerative nodules of cirrhosis on histological examination. It is difficult to diagnose on needle biopsies of the liver and often requires an excision biopsy for confirmation.

Liver-cell adenoma complicating oral contraception and androgen administration is very rare. The lesion usually measures 10 cm or more at the time of diagnosis. The tumour, though benign, is very vascular and presents acutely with rupture and bleeding in some 30% of cases. The progression to a hepatocellular carcinoma is debatable. Regression of the tumour may occur on withdrawal of oral contraception and androgen treatment.

There are some notable differences between the hepatocellular carcinomas which complicate oral contraception and androgen administration and those arising spontaneously. In the first instances, the steroid-associated tumours are more vascular and exhibit no vessel encasement on hepatic arteriography. This accounts for their common presentation with bleeding and rupture which occur in 55% of cases. Furthermore, these malignant tumours are not accompanied by an elevation of the serum alphafetoprotein level.

Cholecystitis

The administration of thiazide diuretics predisposes to the development of acute cholecystitis in patients who harbour gallstones. An association between prolonged parenteral nutrition and the development of both gallstones and acute acalculous cholecystitis has been reported but this requires confirmation. It is as yet unclear whether the prolonged fasting or the underlying illness rather than the parenteral nutrition is responsible for the development of acute acalculous cholecystitis in these patients.

Reye's Syndrome

This frequently fatal condition consisting of encephalopathy and liver failure due to yellow atrophy, occurs in children who are given aspirin usually for chickenpox. There is some evidence that the condition results from the release of the 'tumour necrosis factor' from macrophages brought about by the aspirin.

Endocrine and Metabolic Disorders

Drug-induced endocrine disorders are common and cover a wide spectrum (*Table* 9.3). Both hyper- and hypoactivity may be induced by medication usually over long periods.

Table 9.3 Drug-induced endocrine and metabolic disorders

Disorder	*Drug*
Hyperprolactinaemia	Phenothiazines, benzodiazepines, monoamine oxidase inhibitors, metoclopramide, butyrophenones
Growth retardation	Corticosteroids, androgens
Hyperthyroidism	Iodide preparations, amiodarone, lithium
Hypothyroidism	Sulphonylureas, phenylbutazone, aminoglutethimide, amiodarone, pentazocine, cyclophosphamide, ethionamide, lithium
Adrenal insufficiency	Steroids, metyrapone, aminoglutethimide, trilostane, ketoconazole, etomidate, oral anticoagulants
Gonadal dysfunction	Combination chemotherapy
Gynaecomastia	Oestrogens, spironolactone, digitalis, cimetidine, isoniazid, ethionamide, griseofulvin
Dilutional hyponatraemia	Chlorpropamide, carbamazepine, vincristine, cyclophosphamide, cisplatin
Partial nephrogenic diabetes insipidus	Lithium, demeclocycline
Osteoporosis	Steroids

Hyperprolactinaemia

The manifestations of hyperprolactinaemia include galactorrhoea, oligomenorrhoea/amenorrhoea, loss of libido and infertility in females, and impotence, gynaecomastia and decreased libido in males. It is produced by drugs which either deplete the hypothalamic stores of catecholamines or which block dopamine receptors, as prolactin secretion is normally under the inhibitory control of hypothalamic dopamine. Examples of drugs which cause this abnormality include phenothiazines, butyrophenones, monoamine oxidase inhibitors, metoclopramide, tricyclic antidepressants and cimetidine.

Growth Retardation

This is encountered in prepubertal children following long-term administration of corticosteroids which reduce the release of growth hormone and delay bone maturation. Androgens cause premature fusion of the epiphyses and thereby stunt growth despite an early temporary acceleration of linear growth. Drug-induced hypothyroidism may also be a cause of retardation of growth in children.

Thyroid Dysfunction

Both hyper- and hypothyroidism may be encountered. The most common cause of drug-induced hyperthyroidism is the administration of iodide-containing preparations in areas of endemic iodine deficiency. Rarely, hyperthyroidism may be caused by other drugs including lithium and the anti-arrhythmic agent, amiodarone.

Drug-induced hypothyroidism is commoner than hyperactivity. It may follow prolonged iodide administration. The precipitant drugs either interfere with the trapping of iodine or block its organification (aminoglutethimide, phenylbutazone, sulphonylureas, etc.). The exact mechanisms responsible for the hypothyroidism encountered with other drugs (lithium, amiodarone) are not known.

Adrenal Insufficiency

Suppression of the hypothalamic–pituitary–adrenal axis results from the continued administration of cortisone (and synthetic glucocorticoids) in a dose exceeding daily physiological requirements (20–30 mg hydrocortisone or equivalent/day). This suppression of corticotrophin secretion may persist for several months after slow withdrawal of therapy and may even be permanent. These patients therefore require replacement steroid during stress periods, including surgical operations. Adrenal insufficiency due to suppression of corticotrophin release can also occur as a complication of prolonged therapy with cyproterone acetate (an anti-androgen) which is often used in the treatment of hirsutism.

Gonadal Dysfunction

This is frequently encountered in patients undergoing systemic chemotherapy especially in males who often develop permanent azoospermia following combination chemotherapy. In most young females recovery of ovarian function is usual after cessation of chemotherapy although permanent ovarian failure is often encountered in older women.

Metabolic Abnormalities

These are wide-ranging and constitute one of the most common side-effects of drug medication. A dilutional hyponatraemia is caused by a variety of drugs which reduce the excretion of free water as a result of increased release of vasopressin from the neurohypophysis in addition to a direct antidiuretic action on the renal tubule, e.g. chlorpropamide, carbamazepine, etc., and certain cytotoxic agents (vincristine, cisplatin, cyclophosphamide) which cause an inappropriate antidiuresis. The recognition of this dilutional hyponatraemia is important as excessive saline administration may precipitate circulatory overload in these patients.

One of the most important consequences of long-term high-dose steroid therapy is osteoporosis which leads to considerable disability from back pain and pathological fractures.

Genito-urinary Disorders

A large variety of drugs are nephrotoxic. Some of the most commonly implicated ones are outlined in *Table* 9.4. Whenever possible, nephrotoxic drugs should be avoided in patients with known renal impairment. In addition, drugs which are excreted by the kidneys should be administered in a reduced dosage and blood levels obtained to ensure against toxic levels.

The most common drugs responsible for precipitating retention of urine in surgical practice are narcotic analgesics, anticholinergics and loop diuretics. Recently, epididymitis has been reported as a complication of the anti-arrhythmic drug, amiodarone.

Haematological Disorders

The important drug-induced haematological disorders in surgical practice are myelosuppression varying from a neutropenia to complete agranulocytosis and bleeding disorders which most commonly arise as a result of drug interactions during warfarin therapy, particularly in patients who require long-term oral anticoagulation.

In surgical practice, myelosuppression is usually due to cytotoxic therapy which requires regular monitoring by full blood counts to detect onset of this complication. Reduction of the dosage or complete withdrawal, depending on the severity of the blood picture, is indicated. This often results in haematological improvement. In patients with severe bone marrow depression, blood transfusions and cell component therapy (e.g. platelets) may be required as supportive measures in addition to treatment with corticosteroids or anabolic steroids (oxymetholone).

Potentiation of warfarin is the result of a reduction in its metabolism by concomitantly administered drugs, some of which are shown in *Table* 9.5. It is important to realize that some drugs have the opposite effect. They reduce the anticoagulant effect of warfarin, usually by enzyme induction, e.g. barbiturates, rifampicin, dischloralphenazone.

Neuromuscular Disorders

The surgically important disorders in this category are shown in *Table* 9.6. Neuromuscular blockade can result from:

Presynaptic inhibition.
Postsynaptic blockade of the acetylcholine receptors.
Combined pre- and postsynaptic effect.
Inhibition of ionic conductances across the muscle membrane such that an end-plate potential cannot be generated.

Postoperative peripheral respiratory depression is due either to drug interactions leading to potentiation of the effects and duration of muscle relaxants (*Table* 9.6), or to the occurrence of suxamethonium apnoea. This is usually an inherited disorder which is characterized by an abnormal pseudocholinesterase which is incapable of inactivating suxamethonium. An acquired form may be the result of hepatic disease or drug interaction (*Table* 9.6).

Certain drugs can aggravate or unmask latent myasthenia gravis. This is distinguished from the drug-induced myasthenic syndrome by the demonstration of antibodies to acetylcholine receptors in the plasma (AChR-ab). The drug-induced syndrome is very rare. It is encountered in elderly patients and individuals with renal impairment if the blood levels of the precipitant drugs are high and hypocalcaemia or hyperkalaemia is present.

Table 9.4 Drug-induced genito-urinary disorders

Disorder	*Drug*
Papillary necrosis	Phenacetin, amidopyrine, etc.
Renal failure	Neomycin, cephaloridine, cephalothin, colistin, vancomycin, amphotericin, cisplatin, penicillamine, cyclosporin, anti-inflammatory drugs, etc.
Retention of urine	Anticholinergic drugs, narcotic analgesics, diuretics
Epididymitis	Amiodarone

Table 9.5 Drug-induced haematological disorders

Disorder	*Drug*
Myelosuppression	Cytotoxic agents, carbimazole, sulphonamides, etc.
Bleeding tendency—potentiation of warfarin	NSAIDs, co-trimoxazole, metronidazole, latamoxef, cephamandole, erythromycin, neomycin, ketoconazole, miconazole, alcohol, danazol, clofibrate, cimetidine, anabolic steroids, etc.
Haemolysis	Salazopyrine, sulphonamides, aspirin, etc.
Thrombosis	Oral contraceptives

Table 9.6 Drug-induced neuromuscular disorders

Disorder	*Drug*
Postoperative respiratory depression	Aminoglycosides, polymyxins, tetracyclines, lincomycin, clindamycin, chloroquine
Suxamethonium apnoea	Phenelzine, ecothiopate, aprotinin, ketamine, procaine, promazine, lignocaine, clindamycin, lincomycin, lithium
Aggravation of myasthenia gravis	Aminoglycosides, procainamide, beta-blockers, chloroquine, phenytoin, lithium etc.
Myasthenic syndrome	Aminoglycosides, polymyxins, anticonvulsants, beta-blockers

Psychiatric Disorders

These are the commonest drug-induced disorders encountered in the West nowadays. They are most often encountered in the elderly. The causal relation with a particular drug may be difficult to establish. A complete check of the patient's recent medication is essential. Withdrawal of the suspected precipitant drug(s) is followed by an improvement in the mental state and thus confirms the diagnosis. The

Table 9.7. Drug-induced psychiatric syndromes

Disorder	*Drug*
Delirium	Hypnotics, alcohol, most antidepressants, neuroleptics, antihistamines, hyoscine, atropine, beta-blockers, digoxin, cimetidine
Psychotic states	Phenylephrine, salbutamol, propranolol, levodopa, bromocriptine, pentazocine, dihydrocodeine, indomethacin
Mania	Tricyclics, MAOIs, corticosteroids, aminophylline, levodopa
Depression	Methyldopa, clonidine, propranolol, phenobarbitone, corticosteroids, indomethacin, fenfluramine, oral contraceptives, chloroquine, cycloserine

various psychiatric disorders which may be induced by commonly prescribed drugs are shown in *Table* 9.7.

DRUGS COMMONLY USED IN SURGICAL PRACTICE

These are antibiotics, analgesics, cytotoxic agents, anticoagulants and related drugs, diuretics, steroids and inotropic agents. Antibiotics, cytotoxic agents and analgesics are considered elswhere in the book (Chapters 3, 11, 13).

Anticoagulants and Related Drugs

Heparin

This produces immediate anticoagulation and is given parenterally as it is inactivated by mouth. Heparin is believed to act by enhancing the effects of antithrombin III, thereby inactivating several clotting factors including Factor X (Xa). It also potentiates the naturally-occurring inhibitors of Factor X (Xa). For therapeutic purposes, heparin is administered intravenously, preferably by continuous pump infusion as its action is short lived. For this reason, when heparin is given by intermittent intravenous injection, the time interval between doses should not exceed 6 hours. Usually, oral anticoagulation is started at the same time and heparin is withdrawn on the third day. If oral anticoagulants cannot be administered, anticoagulation is continued with heparin when the dose is adjusted by the estimation of the partial thromboplastin time. In the prophylaxis against deep vein thrombosis, low-dose heparin is administered subcutaneously.

Haemorrhage as a result of heparin administration usually subsides soon after withdrawal of the drug. If rapid reversal is required, this is achieved by protamine sulphate which is given as a slow intravenous infusion. One mg of protamine sulphate inhibits 100 u of heparin. The maximum permissible dose of protamine sulphate is 50 mg and large doses have an anticoagulant effect. The other complication of heparin is hypersensitivity which is manifested by fever, lacrimation, urticaria and conjunctival itching.

Ancrod (Arvin)

This is an effective parenteral anticoagulant. It acts by producing controlled therapeutic defibrination. It is used mainly in the treatment of established thrombo-embolic disease where it is administered intravenously and in its prophylaxis especially for orthopaedic procedures in the elderly, e.g. fractures of the femur, hip joint replacement. The main advantage of ancrod in the treatment of thrombo-embolic disease is the absence of a rebound hypercoagulability when treatment is stopped. Haemorrhage may occur during therapy. This can be managed either with reconstituted freeze-dried fibrinogen or the administration of ancrod antivenom. The other complication is anaphylaxis which is treated with adrenaline and hydrocortisone.

Oral Anticoagulants

These consist of dicoumarol and warfarin which have an identical mode of action. In the UK, warfarin is preferred in view of its more rapid action and the smaller doses required. Oral anticoagulants are used for both short- and long-term therapy. They antagonize vitamin K and therefore act by inhibiting the synthesis of Factors II, VII, IX and X. The anticoagulant effect is not achieved until 36–48 h after initiation of therapy which is monitored by the estimation of the prothrombin time. Bleeding during therapy with oral anticoagulants requires immediate cessation of the drug, estimation of the prothrombin time, administration of phytomenadione (vitamin K_1) and fresh frozen plasma, together with investigation of the cause which is usually either overdosage or potentiation by other drugs.

Patients who are kept on long-term anticoagulant therapy (e.g. prosthetic heart valves) require to carry anticoagulant cards.

Antiplatelet Drugs

These agents reduce platelet adhesiveness and thereby inhibit thrombus formation on the arterial side of the circulation. They are ineffective in the treatment of venous thrombosis. They include aspirin, dipyridamole (Persantin), and sulphinpyrazone (Anturan). Antiplatelet agents are used in conjunction with oral anticoagulants in patients with prosthetic heart valves. Other indications include coronary arterial disease, after cardiac transplanatation, transient cerebral ischaemic attacks and diabetic retinopathy.

Fibrinolytic Agents

Fibrinolytic agents are used to activate the plasmin system responsible for fibrinolysis in order to lyse intravascular thrombi and embolized clots, e.g. major deep-vein thrombosis, pulmonary embolism, rethrombosis after arterial surgery, clotting of A–V shunts, myocardial infarction, etc. Treatment must be started soon after the onset of the intravascular clotting and ideally within 1–2 h. More recently their use has been extended to the treatment of empyema where they are instilled into the pleural cavity.

Two agents are available: streptokinase and urokinase. The former is of bacterial origin and is therefore strongly antigenic, whereas urokinase is extracted from human male urine and is non-antigenic. Their mode of action differs. Urokinase acts by activating plasminogen to plasmin directly in contrast to streptokinase which activates the proactivator to form the activator of plasminogen.

Streptokinase is the agent which has been used for the treatment of thrombo-embolic venous disease and acute arterial thrombosis. It is infused intravenously in isotonic saline, 5% dextrose or haemaccel (100 000 units in 100 ml) in a loading dose of 250 000–500 000 units over 30–60 min. This neutralizes antibodies to streptokinase commonly found in humans due to prior exposure to streptococci.

Maintenance dose consists of 100 000 u/h for 72 h for deep vein thrombosis and 24 h for pulmonary embolism. In arterial thrombosis, the duration of treatment varies from 24 to 72 h. Therapy which is monitored by the thrombin time, results in a decrease in the plasminogen and fibrinogen level with an increase in the level of fibrin degradation products. Herparin therapy, as a constant infusion, is started 3–4 h after the end of the streptokinase infusion, when the thrombin time has decreased to less than twice the control value, to prevent recurrence of the thrombosis. In view of its marked antigenicity, streptokinase therapy should be covered routinely with intravenous hydrocortisone (100 mg) which is given prior to the loading injection. The other important complication is haemorrhage. This requires immediate cessation of therapy and the administration of an antifibrinolytic agent (tranexamic acid, 10 mg/kg). Because of the inevitable rise in the antistreptokinase titre, repeated therapy is contraindicated within 3–6 months.

In surgical practice, use of urokinase has been restricted to recanalization of clotted A–V shunts when 5000–25 000 u in 2–3 ml are instilled into the affected shunt which is then clamped off for 2–4 h.

Diuretics

The commonly used diuretics in surgical practice are:

Thiazide—chlorothiazide, bendrofluazide
Loop—frusemide, ethacrynic acid
Osmotic—mannitol
Potassium-sparing diuretics—triamterene
Aldosterone antagonist—spironolactone.

The thiazide diuretics are usually administered as chronic medications in patients with oedema due to heart disease. They act directly on the kidney tubules and increase the excretion of sodium, chloride, bicarbonate and potassium. As the excretion of chloride is proportionately greater than bicarbonate, prolonged therapy may be followed by hypochloraemic alkalosis in addition to hypokalaemia. They should, thus, be used with extreme caution in patients with liver disease as they can precipitate encephalopathy.

The loop diuretics are more powerful and are often used in surgical practice in oliguric patients after expansion of the blood volume has been achieved. They act primarily on the ascending limb of Henle and on both the proximal and distal tubules, inhibiting the reabsorption of sodium and chloride through the entire length of the renal tubule. They act within 15 min of an intravenous injection. Usually frusemide in a dose of 40 mg is administered, but some advocate much larger doses (100–200 mg) in oliguric patients although the validity and enhanced efficacy of these larger doses are suspect. Loop diuretics cause hypokalemia and may lead to encephalopathy in patients with chronic liver disease.

Mannitol is extensively used in surgical practice and common indications include:

Renal shut down (oliguria) following hypovolaemia and subsequent to volume replacement.
To reduce intracranial pressure in neurosurgery.
As a prophylaxis against renal failure in jaundiced patients undergoing surgical intervention.

Mannitol is a sugar which is only marginally metabolized by the liver. It therefore expands the plasma volume and exerts its diuretic action by increasing the osmotic pressure of the glomerular filtrate. This results in impaired reabsorption of water and solutes (sodium, chloride, potassium, calcium, phosphorus, magnesium, urea, etc.). Aside from electrolyte disturbances, pulmonary oedema and congestive heart failure may be induced by mannitol therapy especially in patients with severe renal disease and diminished cardiac reserve. It is thus contraindicated in anuric patients and in individuals with known cardiac disease or pre-existing pulmonary congestion. It is administered as a 20% solution in a dose of 1·5–2 g/kg over a period of 30–60 min. It is important to stress that any hypovolaemia must be corrected before mannitol infusion is considered.

Spironolactone inhibits the aldosterone-mediated reabsorption of sodium and is used in patients with ascites due to chronic liver disease either alone or in combination with a loop diuretic. It does not cause hypokalaemia which is an important consideration in cirrhotic patients. It is active by mouth. The initial dose is 25 mg t.d.s. but this may be increased to 200–300 mg daily, if necessary, to obtain a diuresis.

Inotropic Drugs

Inotropic drugs are cardiac stimulants and include the cardiac glycosides, β_1-adrenoreceptor drugs and methylxanthines.

Cardiac Glycosides

The positive inotropic activity of digoxin and other cardiac glycosides is mediated via an action on the Na^+ and K^+-ATPase. The principal indication for their use is congestive cardiac failure associated with atrial fibrillation. They are no longer used as chronic medication in mild heart failure especially in the elderly. As potassium and digoxin share the same myocardial binding sites, hypokalaemia exaggerates the toxic effects of the cardiac glycosides which are cardiac and extracardiac. The cardiac side-effects precede the extracardiac ones and include ventricular bigeminy, multifocal ventricular extrasystoles, ventricular tachycardia and heart block.

β_1-Adrenoreceptor Drugs

The β_1-receptors are situated in the myocardial muscle fibres and their stimulation by these drugs results in an increased activity of the adenylate cyclase system and enhanced Ca^{++} uptake by the sarcoplasmic reticulum of the myocardium. They also stimulate the peripheral alpha or β_2-receptors to a varying extent. The resulting peripheral vasoconstriction or the oxygen-wasting tachycardia is undesirable in patients with cardiac decompensation (adrenaline, noradrenaline, isoprenaline).

The most widely used drug of this category in intensive surgical care is dopamine (Intropin) which exerts its beneficial effects by acting on different receptors at various dose ranges as follows:

In small doses (1–5 μg/kg/min), dopamine dilates the renal and mesenteric vascular beds by its unique action on 'dopaminergic' receptors. The effect on the kidneys results in an increase in the renal blood flow, glomerular filtration rate, sodium excretion and urine output.

At a higher dose range (5–20 μg/kg/min), dopamine has a direct inotropic action on the myocardium by its action on the β_1-receptors, causing a dose-related increase in the cardiac output with a minimal increase in the heart rate. The blood pressure rises as a consequence of the enhanced cardiac output.

In high doses (20 μg/kg/min and above), dopamine, in addition to increasing the cardiac output further, stimulates the alpha receptors on the peripheral blood vessels causing a systemic vasoconstriction and a further rise in the blood pressure. Despite this, the renal blood flow is maintained at a high level.

The most frequent reported reactions to dopamine are ectopic beats, tachycardia, anginal pain, palpitations, dyspnoea, nausea and vomiting. Dopamine is contraindicated in uncorrected tachyarrhythmias and in patients with phaeochromocytomas.

Dobutamine is also a selective stimulant of the β_1-receptors of the myocardium. It is also used in cardiogenic shock but has no advantages over dopamine and no selective action on the renal bood flow.

Steroids

As treatment with steroid hormones and their synthetic analogues is both complex and attended by a significant morbidity, it should never be undertaken lightly.

Corticosteroids

These include a wide range of substances synthesized by the adrenal cortex with a 21-carbon steroid nucleus. The basic physiological actions which are shared to a varying extent by all the adrenal corticosteroid hormones are:

Retention of sodium by the kidney and its excretion of osmotically free water.
Deposition of glycogen in the liver.
Increased protein breakdown.
Stabilization of cell membranes and an anti-inflammatory effect.
Mobilization of fat in response to adrenaline.

Adrenal corticosteroids, such as cortisol and cortisone, with a predominant effect on carbohydrate metabolism and usually with an associated anti-inflammatory action, are referred to as glucocorticoids; whereas, aldosterone which has a marked action on sodium retention and potassium excretion, is known as the mineralocorticoid.

The synthetic analogues may possess either action (*Table* 9.8). The selective action of these synthetic derivatives allows a more favourable therapeutic ratio than the naturally-occurring hormones. Cortisone is no longer used for replacement therapy. Prednisolone is the glucocorticoid most commonly used by mouth for long-term therapy. Prednisone is only active after conversion to prednisolone in the body.

Table 9.8 Relative potencies of some corticosteroids using hydrocortisone as the reference compound

Steroid	*Anti-inflammatory effect*	*Relative Na^+ retaining action*
Hydrocortisone	1·0	1·0
Cortisone	0·8	0·8
Prednisone	4·0	0·8
Prednisolone	4·0	0·8
Methyl prednisolone	5·0	0·5
Fludrocortisone	10·0	125·0
Triamcinolone	5·0	0
Betamethasone	25·0	0
Dexamethasone	25·0	0

Therapeutic Uses

Topical Application

These drugs are often used as topical ointments for a variety of skin disorders (*see* Chapter 22) and for mild distal inflammatory bowel disease as prednisolone suppositories and enemas (Chapter 74).

Topical steroid applications are often attended with side-effects. Secondary infection is common, including folliculitis, boils and fungal infections due to a local suppression of the inflammatory response. Allergy, causing a contact eczema, occurs very frequently following the topical application of steroids, particularly when these are combined with antibiotics. Prolonged topical steroid applications lead to atrophy of the skin due to loss of dermal collagen. Absorption through the skin into the bloodstream with suppression of the pituitary–adrenal axis occurs to a significant extent in children with the more potent corticosteroid applications and in adults if more than 30 g daily are used. Topical steroids should not be used in:

The presence of cutaneous infection.
When a definite diagnosis has not been made.
In gravitational ulcers in which they cause delayed healing due to inhibition of collagen formation.

Systemic Steroid Therapy

Systemic corticosteroid replacement therapy may be essential as in Addison's disease and hypopituitarism. More commonly, systemic corticosteroids are used in emergency life-threatening states and for long-term suppression of inflammation and the immune response.

EMERGENCY USE. There is still considerable controversy regarding the benefit of high-dose corticosteroid therapy during various acute illnesses and practice varies from centre to centre. There is, however, agreement that such treatment is valuable in the following situations:

Acute adrenal insufficiency.
Organ transplantation.
Severe acute exacerbation of inflammatory bowel disease.
Acute exacerbations of connective-tissue disorders and vasculitides.
Raised intracranial pressure from cerebral oedema caused by tumours and infarcts.
Status asthmaticus.
Pulmonary aspiration.
Adult respiratory distress syndrome.
Anaphylactic reactions.
Blood transfusion reactions.

Disagreement still exists on the value of high-dose steroid therapy in septic shock because although there is experimental evidence for their benefit, the few clinical trials which have been conducted have produced equivocal results. In practice, a short course consisting of 50 mg hydrocortisone/kg/24 h (or equivalent) in divided doses is administered by those in favour of this treatment in septic shock with a view to achieving systemic vasodilatation, maintaining the integrity of cell membranes and neutralizing the endotoxin.

Systemic corticosteroids, such as dexamethasone, are ineffective in the cerebral oedema which complicates liver failure and are contraindicated in acute pancreatitis. Whereas corticosteroids do not impart any benefit in fulminant (acute) hepatic failure, they significantly improve survival in subacute hepatic necrosis, chronic active hepatitis, alcoholic hepatitis and non-alcoholic cirrhosis in the female.

SUPPRESSION OF THE INFLAMMATORY RESPONSE. Systemic corticosteroids are now used less frequently and more selectively for this purpose. The principles of long-term suppression with steroids include a short period (1–2 weeks) during which high doses are administered to achieve a maximal response, followed by a gradual reduction until either the drug, usually prednisolone, is withdrawn or a small maintenance dose is continued. Rapid steroid withdrawal is harmful because, apart from increasing the risk of a 'flare up', it may also precipitate acute adrenal insufficiency. If the maintenance dose necessary to suppress the disease is greater than 20 mg of prednisolone or its equivalent, serious complications will develop within 12 months. The disorders for which systemic corticosteroids may be used in selected cases include:

Rheumatoid arthritis.
Rheumatic carditis.
The nephrotic syndrome in childhood.
Connective-tissue disorders and vasculitides.
Malignant conditions, e.g. advanced breast cancer, acute lymphocytic leukaemia, etc.
Autoimmune haemolytic anaemias.
Ulcerative colitis and Crohn's disease.
Neurological disorders, e.g. multiple sclerosis, Bell's palsy, etc.
Bronchial asthma of the severe chronic non-allergic type.
Certain skin disorders, e.g. pemphigus, etc.
Sarcoidosis.

All patients on long-term corticosteroid therapy should carry steroid cards.

The therapeutic effects of ACTH are not identical to those of corticosteroids and there is no predictable response by the adrenal to a given dose of ACTH. This polypeptide hormone and its synthetic analogue, corticosyn, have extra-adrenal effects which include a melanophore-stimulating action which causes hyperpigmentation. The main advantage of ACTH therapy is the maintenance of the functional integrity of the adrenal cortex. However, because of the unpredictable steroid response and because ACTH must be given by intramuscular injection, oral corticosteroids are used in preference to ACTH therapy except in children in whom prolonged steroid therapy may result in growth inhibition. A number of disorders seem to respond more readily to ACTH than systemic corticosteroids. These include multiple sclerosis and some acute allergic conditions. The main indications for the administration of ACTH in clinical practice are in the diagnosis of adrenal cortical function and its reserve capacity, and for adrenal suppression consequent on steroid withdrawal. The contraindications to systemic corticosteroid and ACTH therapy are:

Tuberculosis.
Local or systemic infections (unless controlled).
Congestive cardiac failure.
Hypertension.
Active peptic ulceration.
Psychosis.
Renal dysfunction.
Diabetes mellitus.
Glaucoma.
Myasthenia gravis.
Thrombo-embolic disease.
Pregnancy.

ADVERSE REACTIONS TO SYSTEMIC CORTICOSTEROIDS. A number of side-effects are inevitable after prolonged use of these agents. These include increased protein breakdown which is associated with atrophy of dermal collagen, striae, bruising, muscle wasting; myopathy and osteoporosis, the latter often leading to pathological fractures; the development of hirsutism and the cushingoid habitus with the typical moon face, buffalo hump, supraclavicular fat pads, central obesity and acne; fluid and electrolyte disturbances, e.g. hypokalaemic alkalosis and oedema; hyperglycaemia and glycosuria; diminished resistance to both acute and chronic bacterial infections; adrenal suppression and inability to respond to stress, including surgical intervention; immunosuppression and elevation of the blood urea. Other sporadic complications, some of which may be life-threatening, include peptic ulcer perforation and bleeding, cardiac failure, psychoses and behavioural changes, precipitation/aggravation of diabetes mellitus, hypertension, growth stunting in children, posterior subcapsular cataracts and amenorrhoea.

The adverse reactions that may develop on withdrawal of steroid therapy include:

Reactivation of the disease.
A withdrawal syndrome consisting of fever, myalgia, arthralgia and malaise.
Adrenal insufficiency.
Peripheral neuropathy.

Androgens and Anabolic Steroids

The most powerful naturally-occurring androgenic hormone is testosterone. Derivatives of testosterone with a pronounced anabolic and reduced androgenic effect include ethyloestrenol (taken orally), stanozolol (oral and intramuscular), nandrolone and nandrolone phenylpropionate, the last two being administered as depot intramuscular injection. None of the currently available steroids are entirely free of androgenic effects. In general, anabolic steroids have proved disappointing in those conditions characterized by muscle and tissue wasting, e.g. osteoporosis, chronic debilitating conditions and protein breakdown after major surgery, trauma or sepsis. They are used in the treatment of some aplastic anaemias and in advanced breast cancer.

The only indications for androgen treatment nowadays are hypogonadism and hypopituitarism (in conjunction with chorionic gonadotrophin and menotrophin). Neither androgens nor anabolic steroids should be administered for delayed puberty and allied growth disorders for despite an initial acceleration of linear growth, they lead to premature fusion of the epiphyses and result in short stature. Androgens and some of the anabolic steroids are known to cause hepatic tumours in humans after prolonged therapy. The other adverse reactions to anabolic steroids and androgens are cholestatic jaundice, fluid and salt retention, hirsutism and masculinization in some females.

Oestrogens

The primary oestrogens produced by the ovaries are oestrone and oestradiol-17β. Oestriol which is a metabolite of oestradiol is much less potent than either oestrone or oestradiol. Several synthetic oestrogens are available. The most commonly used non-steroidal synthetic oestrogen is stilboestrol, whereas the most powerful synthetic steroidal derivative is ethinyloestradiol. Oestrogens are used in the treatment of some patients with prostatic cancer. Their use in advanced or recurrent breast cancer has been largely replaced by the anti-oestrogen tamoxifen.

The important adverse responses to oestrogens are the stimulation of the breast parenchyma, cervical and uterine cancers and thrombo-embolic disease, especially in post-operative patients, in individuals suffering from varicose veins and in obese and diabetic women. Older females also complain of dyspepsia and withdrawal vaginal bleeding.

Progestogens

These compounds act on tissues which are sensitized by oestrogens. Progestogens fall into two categories: nortestosterone analogues (e.g. ethisterone, norethisterone) and progesterone and its derivatives (allyloestrenol, dydrogesterone, hydroxyprogesterone, medroxyprogesterone). The nortestosterone analogues are partially metabolized to potent oestrogens in the body and, therefore, have oestrogenic as well as progesterone-like effects. The progestogens are used for oral contraception in conjunction with oestrogens and in certain gynaecological disorders. They can also be effective in endometrial, renal and breast cancer. The progestogens which are used in malignancy are norethisterone, hydroxyprogesterone, medroxyprogesterone and megestrol. In advanced breast cancer, they are administered in high dosage in patients who relapse after a remission obtained with tamoxifen. Overall, a 30% objective response rate is obtained in these patients. Progestogens do not have any serious side-effects.

SPECIFIC MEDICAL DISORDERS COMMONLY ENCOUNTERED IN SURGICAL PRACTICE

Hypertension

The presence of *severe* hypertension undoubtedly increases the risk of surgery and its control by medical therapy reduces the incidence of all its serious complications: strokes, coronary heart disease, congestive cardiac failure, retinopathy and renal impairment. There is, however, controversy on the effect of medical treatment in reducing the incidence of these complications in patients with mild to moderate hypertension. Surgical intervention is not attended by a significant increase in morbidity/mortality in this group. In surgical practice hypertension is encountered in three circumstances:

High blood pressure is discovered during routine physical examination for a surgical disorder.
Patients on medical treatment for essential hypertension may develop a surgical condition which requires medical treatment.
Surgical treatment is required for a disorder causing secondary hypertension.

Previously Undiagnosed Hypertension

The first step is the confirmation of the presence of hypertension and its severity, since one elevated reading may be misleading and result from apprehension which may be induced by the surgical consultation. The blood pressure measurement must be repeated preferably over a period of a few weeks if the surgical condition permits. Severe hypertension is diagnosed if the systolic blood pressure is above 170 mmHg or the diastolic pressure exceeds 110 mmHg. On confirmation of the hypertension, elective surgery should be postponed, especially if the hypertension is severe. All patients require the following investigations:

Urinalysis
Full blood count and ESR
Serum electrolytes
Blood urea/creatinine
ECG
Chest radiography

In young patients where the possibility of secondary hypertension is distinctly greater, some of the following additional tests are necessary: intravenous pyelogram, renal scan, renal and adrenal angiography, differential renal function studies, skull radiograph, EEG and brain scan, plasma renin activity and catecholamine excretion rate. The majority of patients turn out to have essential hypertension. Medical treatment is then started and surgical intervention is performed once the hypertension has been controlled.

Patients on Medical Therapy for Hypertension requiring Operative Intervention

The medical treatment of hypertension entails the use of cardioselective beta-blockers which do not penetrate the blood–brain barrier (Atenolol, acebutolol) and thiazide diuretics. When beta-blockers are contraindicated (e.g. in bronchial asthma), a vasodilator (prazosin, nifedipine, verapamil) is added if control of the hypertension is not achieved by the diuretic. Central agents (methyldopa) are used when the above regimens have not been successful or are contraindicated. Captopril, an orally active potent vasodilator which is an inhibitor of angiotensin-I converting enzyme, is reserved for resistant or renal hypertension in view of its toxicity (neutropenia and renal damage).

The medical treatment is continued until the operation but exact details of the drug regimen and dosage must be known to the anaesthetist because of possible interaction with anaesthetic drugs. Diuretic-induced hypokalaemia, if present, must be corrected. In addition, the cardiac and renal reserve must be assessed in these patients by a blood urea and creatinine, exercise ECG and chest radiography.

Patients Referred for Surgical Treatment of Secondary Hypertension

Hypertension may be secondary to cerebral, endocrine, renal and vascular disease (*Table* 9.9). Some of these are amenable to surgical treatment. Management of the endocrine group is discussed in Chapter 63. The most difficult in terms of haemodynamic changes in the peri-operative period, is phaeochromocytoma. This requires a period of alpha- and beta-blockade before the operation, as removal of the tumour would otherwise be followed by catastrophic hypotension.

The management of renal artery stenosis remains problematic in that the results of surgery can be disappointing although control of the hypertension can be achieved by surgery in carefully selected cases. Percutaneous balloon angioplasty is practised in some centres in preference to surgical intervention in the first instance.

Cardiac Disease

The functional status of patients with heart disease varies and is currently categorized into four classes (*Table* 9.10). Patients in class I and II will have few symptoms and surgical intervention carried out with the necessary precautions, monitoring, and with available cardiologist's advice carries a minimal risk.

Patients with class I and II disease have a diminished cardiac reserve and overt cardiac failure can be precipitated

Table 9.9 Types and aetiology of secondary hypertension

CEREBRAL	Brain tumour*
ENDOCRINE	Primary aldosteronism (Conn's syndrome)*
	Phaeochromocytoma*
	Cushing's syndrome*
	Hyperparathyroidism*
RENAL	Renal artery stenosis*
	Acute/chronic glomerulonephritis
	Pyelonephritis
	Polycystic kidneys
	Diabetes mellitus
	Polyarteritis nodosa
VASCULAR	Coarctation of the aorta*
	Porphyria
	Polycythaemia rubra vera

*Surgical treatment necessary or considered.

Table 9.10 New York Heart Association: functional status of patients with heart disease

Class	*Description*
I	No limitation of ordinary physical activity
II	Dyspnoea after ordinary physical activity, e.g. walking
III	Marked limitation such that less than ordinary activity causes dyspnoea, e.g. unable to walk on the level without disability
IV	Dyspnoea at rest

by:

Drugs: beta-blockers and anti-arrhythmic agents.
Infection.
Intravenous fluids and especially blood transfusion.
Anaemia.

Surgical treatment is contraindicated in patients with class IV and should be postponed in class III patients until cardiac compensation is obtained by medical treatment. Surgery should also be postponed, whenever possible, for at least 3 months after myocardial infarction because of the risks of severe arrhythmia and a further possible fatal episode of myocardial infarction in the perioperative period. It is essential to administer prophylactic antibiotics (amoxycillin) in any patient with compensated valvular heart disease who is to undergo surgical intervention and endoscopy because of the risks of endocarditis.

The cardiac disorders with which the general surgeon should be familiar are cardiac failure, myocardial infarction, cardiogenic shock, dysrhythmias and cardiac arrest.

Cardiac Failure

Cardiac failure is defined as a state in which the heart fails to maintain an adequate circulation for the needs of the body despite satisfactory venous filling. It is classified into left, right and congestive (combined left and right failure). The causes of cardiac failure can be grouped under four headings:

1. PRESSURE OVERLOAD. Induced by aortic stenosis, hypertension, hypertrophic cardiomyopathy causing left ventricular failure, and pulmonary stenosis or pulmonary hypertension resulting in right ventricular failure.
2. VOLUME OVERLOAD (PRELOAD). Follows aortic/mitral valve regurgitation and arteriovenous fistula (left heart failure) and atrial/ventricular septal defects and pulmonary/tricuspid valve regurgitation causing right heart failure.
3. IMPAIRMENT OF CARDIAC MUSCLE. Most commonly due to coronary heart disease and less frequently to various types of cardiomyopathy and myocarditis.
4. HIGH OUTPUT CARDIAC FAILURE. Results from pulmonary emphysema, hyperthyroidism, Paget's disease and beriberi.

Left Ventricular Failure

The manifestations include dyspnoea, exertional fatigue and weakness and pulmonary oedema. The latter results from rapid pulmonary venous and capillary hypertension which induces a marked transudation of fluid into the alveoli and bronchial mucosa. The patient becomes acutely distressed with severe dyspnoea and hypoxia. On auscultation, moist fine crepitations are present especially at the lung bases in addition to rhonchi caused by the oedematous narrowing of the bronchi (cardiac asthma). The patient is pale or cyanosed and sweaty. A tachycardia is present. The blood pressure is usually elevated.

Right Heart Failure

Right heart failure is commonly secondary to left heart failure but it can be caused by lung disease (chronic cor pulomale), and primary cardiac disease, e.g. pulmonary or mitral valve stenosis, tricuspid regurgitation and congenital heart disease. It is accompanied by an elevated pulmonary artery pressure which results in systemic venous congestion, peripheral oedema, ascites and hepatomegaly. The jugular venous pressure is elevated. In addition, there is a loud pulmonary second sound. Acute right ventricular failure is caused by pulmonary embolism.

Treatment of Heart Failure

The cause of the cardiac failure must be identified, after which treatment consists of correcting the precipitating factors and bed rest during which passive and active leg exercises should be encouraged. Oxygen is administered by mask or nasal catheters. In left ventricular failure, morphine sulphate, 5–10 mg, is administered intravenously to reduce the tachypnoea and anxiety. Aminophylline may be given in a dose of 0·5 mg by slow intravenous injection to relieve bronchospasm and diminish the venous pressure.

The specific treatment of cardiac failure entails the administration of diuretics intravenously to increase water and electrolyte excretion by the kidneys, the use of inotropic drugs to enhance myocardial contractility and vasodilator drugs to relieve pressure and volume overload particularly in patients with severe heart failure.

For moderate to severe heart failure, the loop diuretics (frusemide, ethacrynic acid) are indicated in view of their potency and immediate action. The thiazide diuretics are used in patients with mild cardiac failure and for chronic therapy when potassium supplements are added or spironolactone is administered instead.

The most commonly used inotropic drugs are the cardiac glycosides (digoxin, digitoxin). They are indicated in patients with congestive failure with associated atrial fibrillation where their main beneficial effect is to slow the heart rate. Other inotropic drugs such as dopamine are restricted to patients with severe cardiac failure due to diminished myocardial contractility and in partients with cardiogenic shock.

Vasodilator therapy (nitrates, nitroprusside, prazosin, captopril) are restricted to patients with severe cardiac failure. Intravenous nitroprusside is particularly beneficial in cardiac failure due to myocardial infarction.

Myocardial Ischaemia

Myocardial ischaemia is due to coronary atheromatous disease and can present as:

Angina pectoris
Myocardial infarction
Sudden death from ventricular fibrillation
Arrhythmias

The established risk factors for ischaemic heart disease include: age, male sex, smoking, race (Caucasian), country, serum cholesterol level, hypertension, obesity, diabetes, diet (high dietary saturated fatty acids and cholesterol), and personality type (aggressive, competitive, ambitious). The highest incidence of deaths from myocardial infarction in men is found in Finland, Netherlands, Scotland, Northern Ireland and USA. The lowest incidence in an industrialized country is reported in Japan.

With the advent of coronary bypass surgery to revascularize the myocardium, investigations are now routinely performed in patients with manifestations of ischaemic heart disease. These include coronary angiograms in all patients with angina <40 years. In older patients, treadmill exercise with 12-lead ECG is performed initially and angiography carried out if the test is positive. Coronary angiography is also performed in patients after a myocardial infarction.

Angina Pectoris

The cardiac pain of angina pectoris is usually described by patients as an ache or a tightness, often accompanied by breathlessness. It is situated in the retrosternal region and may be accompanied by a choking sensation which may simulate the discomfort of oesophageal disease. The pain radiates to the root of the neck and along the lower border of the axilla and down the medial border of the arm, usually the left. It is often precipitated by exercise, emotion, large meal and a change of temperature, and is relieved by rest and sublingual nitrates. Pain occurring at rest indicates more severe disease: unstable angina (acute coronary insufficiency, preinfarction angina) or myocardial infarction. Unstable angina can be differentiated from myocardial infarction—the pain is relieved by sublingual nitrates and the cardiac enzymes are not elevated. Some 15% of patients with unstable angina go on to develop a myocardial infarction. It is therefore considered to be a medical emergency which requires hospitalization and full investigation as treatment, including coronary bypass surgery, may prevent the occurrence of myocardial infarction.

Myocardial Infarction

The pain of myocardial infarction is more severe than in angina and is at times vice-like. It lasts in excess of 30 min and is accompanied by pallor, perspiration, nausea and sometimes, vomiting. However, when it occurs in the postoperative period, myocardial infarction is often painless (silent infarct).

In addition to the pain, the manifestations of myocardial infarction are: an anxious patient, tachycardia and irregular pulse (atrial fibrillation, extrasystoles). The blood pressure is normal at first but may fall subsequently. Hypotension is a bad prognostic sign especially if unaccompanied by arrhythmias. Bradycardia, when it occurs, signifies heart block. On auscultation a third heart sound and basal crepitations (heart failure) are heard. Other findings include a harsh systolic apical murmur (ruptured mitral valve) or rarely, a harsh systolic murmur along left sternal edge which is due to rupture of the ventricular septum. Both conditions are accompanied by severe heart failure. The ECG tracing is initially normal. Then S–T segment elevation with peaked T-waves and Q-waves are observed within hours. The T-wave inversion reverts to normal during the subsequent few days and S–T segment, within weeks. The cardiac enzymes which are monitored are creatine kinase (CK), its myocardial specific isoenzyme CK-MB, AST and LDH. The first three reach peak elevation within 24–48 h. LDH is useful in detecting myocardial infarction which occurred a few days previously since it remains elevated for 7 days and reaches its peak at 3 days. Chest radiography is performed to detect pulmonary oedema (heart failure). The CK-MB isoenzyme is particularly helpful in postoperative patients when elevation of the other enzymes in the absence of myocardial infarction is common.

Arrhythmias

The important ones to the surgeon are atrial fibrillation, heart block and ventricular fibrillation. In addition to primary heart disease, atrial fibrillation is common in the elderly (11%). The incidence of complete heart block in healthy patients aged 75 years and over is 1%.

Atrial Fibrillation

This may be paroxysmal (intermittent) or chronic. Paroxysmal atrial fibrillation is the commonest cause of left ventricular failure in the elderly. It is treated with the anti-arrhythmic drug amiodarone. The drug treatment of patients with chronic fibrillation is digoxin. Dislodgement of the atrial clots may lead to the development of embolic disease such as mesenteric vascular occlusion. Elective surgery should be postponed until correction of the arrhythmia has been achieved.

Heart Block

Complete heart block is treated with the implantation of a permanent demand pacemaker before surgical intervention is carried out.

Ventricular Fibrillation

This requires immediate defibrillation and other cardiac arrest support measures.

Diabetes Mellitus

Diabetes mellitus is a common endocrine disorder which affects approximately 1% of the population in the Western hemisphere. Its essential biochemical feature is a persistent elevation of the blood glucose above the normal range: fasting blood glucose >6 mmol/L (100 mg/100 ml) and random glucose >9 mmol/L (162 mg/ml). The diabetic state is usually permanent although a transient carbohydrate intolerance may occasionally be found during the course of some acute illnesses and certain endocrine disorders.

The disease is of interest to the surgeon largely because of its complications. It causes an individual to be more sensitive to protein depletion, disturbances of carbohydrate intake and to water and electrolyte changes associated with surgical intervention. The main metabolic danger of undiagnosed or poorly controlled diabetes is the development of a severe ketoacidosis during the course of an acute illness. Furthermore, diabetic ketoacidosis may be a cause of severe abdominal pain, thus mimicking an acute abdomen.

Whilst a well-controlled young diabetic patient is in no greater danger of infection than a normal individual, uncontrolled diabetes is accompanied by a greater incidence of infection. Although a normal polymorphonuclear leucocytosis occurs in a diabetic in the presence of infection, the phagocytic activity of the leucocytes is impaired. There is also a tendency for an overgrowth of micro-organisms in uncontrolled diabetes, resulting in an increased incidence of non-clostridial gas-forming wound infections. In diabetic ketoacidosis precipitated by a surgical infection, granulocyte mobilization is impaired in addition to the reduced phagocytic activity. Furthermore, antibody formation is depressed.

Small vessel disease in the form of non-specific thickening of the basement membrane occurs in the ageing diabetic in addition to the ordinary changes of atherosclerosis in the major vessels. The resulting peripheral ischaemia and neuropathy lead to an increased frequency of infection by both anaerobic and microaerophilic organisms and trophic ulcers of the feet follow repeated minor trauma. Diabetic nephropathy in the form of glomerulosclerosis, usually accompanied by retinopathy, complicates the disease in 15% of patients who have been diabetic for 20 years or more. Whereas coronary heart disease is commoner in the diabetic than in the general population and is the single most common cause of death in these patients, there is no firm evidence for an increased incidence of cerebrovascular accidents in diabetic individuals.

Neuropathy is related to the duration rather than the severity of the diabetes and is, therefore, encountered usually in the elderly. The commonest type is a chronic sensory loss associated with paraesthesia in the legs and feet and absent ankle jerks. The development of a Charcot's type of arthropathy and trophic ulceration is common in this condition. Other types of neuropathy encountered in the diabetic include mixed subacute sensory and motor neuropathy causing impotence, diarrhoea and an atonic bladder.

The severity of the diabetic state is determined by the degree of insulin deficiency caused by the beta-cell hypofunction. Insulin consists of two chains (A, B) linked by disulphide bonds and like all other polypeptide hormones, it interacts with highly specific receptors (glycoproteins) located in the cell membranes of the target tissues. The combination between insulin and its receptors is an essential first step in the *in vivo* activity of this hormone, the effects of which can be conveniently described as rapid and long-term. The rapid actions of insulin are increased glucose uptake and metabolism by muscle and adipose tissue, increased glycogen formation within the liver, an increased synthesis of proteins especially in the muscles and a decreased release of fatty acids from the adipose tissue stores. The long-term actions are enhancement of the activity of some enzymes concerned with glucose metabolism and a depression of the activity of enzymes involved in gluconeogenesis.

Insulin release is chiefly governed by elevations in the blood glucose but certain amino acids, such as arginine, also promote insulin release. Thus a protein-rich meal raises the blood levels of insulin. The sulphonylurea drugs are used therapeutically in some cases of maturity-onset diabetes to promote release of the hormone by the endocrine cells of the pancreas.

Hormones which antagonize the actions of insulin include glucagon, adrenaline, growth hormone, adrenal steroids and ACTH. A specific insulin antagonist has been identified and suggested as a cause of diabetes but its exact role, if any, in the pathophysiology of the disease remains uncertain.

Two main types of diabetes are recognized: the insulin-dependent (juvenile-onset, ketosis-prone) and the non-insulin-dependent diabetes (maturity-onset, ketosis non-prone). It should be appreciated, however, that many patients fall in between the two main categories. Insulin-dependent and maturity-onset diabetes are aetiologically different. The inherited tendency is stronger in the maturity-onset variety which has been estimated to be three times greater in the children of diabetic parents than in the offspring of non-diabetic individuals. In the juvenile insulin-dependent type, a genetic predisposition is associated with certain HLA types, such as B_8, B_{15} and B_{12}, but the action of a non-genetic agent, e.g. a pancreotropic viral infection, is required in order to promote the disease. The region of the sixth human chromosome where the HLA loci are located is in close proximity to the D locus which is concerned with the immune response. The hypothesis currently in favour is that insulin-dependent diabetes is consequent on an immune disorder which results either in failure to eradicate a pancreotropic virus or in autoimmune reaction against the islet tissue. Both a seasonal incidence of juvenile-onset diabetes and high titres of antibodies to Coxsackie virus have been reported in these patients. Furthermore, islet-cell antibodies are found in 60–80% of newly diagnosed insulin-dependent diabetes.

Non-genetic disorders may also be responsible for the development of diabetes. The glucose tolerance test is often abnormal in acute pancreatitis but the impairment of the carbohydrate metabolism in this condition is usually temporary except in those patients who develop acute pancreatic necrosis. Acute pancreatitis in an established diabetic leads to a greatly increased insulin requirement and may precipitate ketoacidosis. Diabetes may occur in chronic pancreatitis due to the progressive destruction of the gland but this complication is less common than steatorrhoea. Haemochromatosis, otherwise known as bronze diabetes, is associated with the development of diabetes mellitus in 75% of cases. This disorder which is much commoner in males than females, is characterized by pigmentation, hepatosplenomegaly (cirrhosis), absence of body hair, chondrocalcinosis and arthritis. It is due to an accumulation of iron in the tissues from excessive absorption. Total pancreatectomy is invariably followed by diabetes which may be difficult to control. These patients have a particular tendency to hypoglycaemia because the pancreatectomy also results in the loss of the alpha cells and therefore glucagon production which normally antagonizes the action of insulin.

Carbohydrate intolerance (hormone-induced diabetes) is commonly found in Cushing's syndrome, in individuals suffering from phaeochromocytoma, and the rare glucagonoma syndrome. Drug-induced diabetes is encountered in patients on glucocorticoid or ACTH therapy and has been reported during treatment with benzothiazide diuretics and thyroxine.

Clinical Features of Diabetes Mellitus

The classic symptoms of diabetes mellitus include thirst, polyuria, tiredness and weight loss. The clinical differences between the insulin-dependent and the non-insulin-dependent diabetes are shown in *Table* 9.11. The diagnosis is confirmed by the finding of a glycosuria accompanied by a persistently raised blood glucose. More elaborate tests such as the glucose tolerance test (GTT) are required in borderline cases. A glucose tolerance test requires the performance

Table 9.11 Clinical types of diabetes mellitus

Clinical features	*Insulin-dependent*	*Non-insulin-dependent*
Sex ratio	Males=females	Females >males
Age	Children and adolescents	Middle age and elderly
Onset	Usually acute	Gradual
Weight loss	Often marked	Usually absent, often obese
Ketoacidosis	Common	Rare and mild
Plasma insulin level	Low or absent	Normal or reduced
Response to insulin	Sensitive	Relatively insensitive
Effects of hypoglycaemic agents	None	Responsive

of a fasting blood sugar followed by the administration of 50–100 g of glucose after which the blood glucose is estimated at 30, 60, 90 and 120 min. Modifications of the GTT include the intravenous test where the glucose load is administered intravenously and the results expressed in terms of the rate of fall of the blood glucose values after injection, and the augmented GTT when 100 g of cortisone are administered prior to the ingestion of the glucose load (steroid test). These modifications and the measurement of plasma insulin levels are rarely necessary in routine clinical practice. The C-peptide assay provides an indirect assessment of the blood insulin concentration since it is formed in equimolar amounts to insulin from proinsulin. The tolbutamide tolerance test is not used in the diagnosis of diabetes mellitus. This test is useful in the biochemical detection of an insulinoma in which condition it stimulates an excessive release of insulin causing a profound and prolonged hypoglycaemia.

Treatment

Insulin-dependent Diabetes

These patients require replacement therapy. Until recently, the insulins which were available for human use in diabetic patients were extracted from ox and beef pancreas. Porcine insulin differs from human insulin in the C-terminal amino acid of the B-chain (B30) which consists of alanine in the pig as opposed to threonine in the human. In addition to this, bovine insulin has two other different amino acids to the sequence found in human insulin, alanine instead of threonine in position A8 and valine instead of isoleucine in position A10. These animal species insulins are therefore antigenic and produce both high and low affinity antibodies. The antibodies which develop are, however, largely due to contaminants such as proinsulin and pancreatic peptides. These insulin antibodies are the cause of the lipoatrophy at the site of insulin injection and account for the development of insulin resistance. They also delay the appearance of insulin into the circulation following subcutaneous administration and prolong the intravenous half-life of injected insulin. Other suggested adverse effects of these antibodies include effect on the fetus of diabetic women from transplacental passage causing neonatal hypoglycaemia, macrosomia and microangiopathy, and the development of diabetic autonomic neuropathy as the antibodies cross-react with the nerve growth factor.

The development of monocomponent (single peak) neutral insulins of porcine origin was an important practical advance in reducing the antibody problem associated with insulin administration. The term 'monocomponent' implies that after purification by chromatography and electrophoresis, only one component remains in these highly purified insulins. The semisynthetic enzyme-modified porcine (emp) insulin was developed as a further safeguard against the development of insulin antibodies. It has the human amino acid sequence. This is achieved by replacing the B30 alanine residue of porcine insulin with a threonine residue by enzymatic means, thus converting it to human insulin. Human insulin synthesized by recombinant DNA technology using bacteria containing the genetically engineered plasmids, has now been evaluated clinically. It is designated by the prefix 'crb'—chain, recombinant DNA, bacteria. Biosynthetic human insulin was the first product produced by genetic engineering administered to humans. Its activity is similar to that of highly purified monocomponent insulin but it is absorbed more quickly after subcutaneous injection and its duration of action is shorter. Human insulin is now administered to newly-diagnosed diabetics, to diabetic pregnant mothers and those individuals needing short-term or intermittent treatment. At the moment, there is no good reason for converting established diabetic patients from pork to human insulin.

Soluble, crystalline insulin starts to act within 1 hour, has a maximal effect for 2–3 h and a total duration of action of about 8 h. In order to prolong its action, various complexes and combinations have been developed (*Table* 9.12). All insulin preparations are of 40 or 80 u/ml, strength. The

Table 9.12 Insulin preparations

SHORT-ACTING	Soluble insulin: highly purified (hp) pork or beef, single peak (sp) pork or beef, human-emp and human-crb.
INTERMEDIATE-ACTING	Isophane suspensions, 30/70 amorphous/crystalline suspensions.
LONG-ACTING	Protamine zinc suspensions.
MIXTURES OF SHORT- AND INTERMEDIATE-ACTING INSULINS	

standard insulin syringe BS 1619 is available in two sizes (1·0 ml, 2·0 ml) but there are now several different types of disposable insulin syringes.

Non-insulin-dependent Diabetes

In the first instance, management depends on whether the patient is overweight or not. Initially, diabetic patients who are not overweight are treated by carbohydrate restriction alone. A sulphonylurea drug, such as glibenclamide or chlopropamide, is added if control is not achieved by carbohydrate restriction alone. The sulphonylureas act by promoting the release of endogenous insulin and by decreasing hepatic glucose output. The biguanide, metformin, is used if persistent hyperglycaemia cannot be prevented by one of the sulphonylurea drugs. The action of biguanides is not dependent on the presence of functional islet tissue. They increase the glucose uptake by peripheral tissues and enhance the insulin sensitivity. They are incapable of producing hypoglycaemia. Phenformin, also a biguanide, has been abandoned because of the risk of lactic acidosis, a complication that occurs very rarely with metformin.

If the diabetic patient is overweight, a weight-reducing diet is started and drug therapy along the lines described above, is introduced only if diet fails to control the disease.

Insulin therapy is only considered in maturity-onset diabetes when therapy with diet and oral hypoglycaemic agents has not resulted in adequate control of the diabetic state.

Diabetic Coma

This is commonly due to diabetic ketoacidosis but coma may occur in the absence of ketosis (aketotic diabetic coma, hyperosmolar coma).

Diabetic Ketoacidosis

This results from an insulin lack and is characterized by hyperglycaemia and ketosis. The precipitating causes include the omission of insulin and acute infections. Not infrequently, diabetic ketoacidosis may be the presenting feature of a previously undiagnosed diabetic. The resulting glycosuria and osmotic diuresis cause dehydration from loss of water and electrolytes with the development of haemoconcentration and shock. The ketosis is caused by the increased breakdown of fat and results in acidosis, hyperventilation and vomiting, the latter aggravating the dehydration. The vomiting is frequently followed by generalized abdominal pain. If no treatment is given, the patient becomes increasingly drowsy, unconscious and finally dies in deep coma. Apart from signs of dehydration, shock and mental confusion or coma, the face is flushed and the breath has a characteristically sweet smell due to the acetone content. The abdominal signs which may occur include guarding, distension, reduced or absent bowel sounds and a succusion splash due to a paralytic ileus which is thought to be due to intracellular hypokalaemia.

The biochemical changes associated with diabetic ketoacidosis include hyperglycaemia and ketonuria. The level of blood glucose is not, however, a reliable guide to the severity of the illness. The pH is low and the bicarbonate level of the blood is greatly reduced. The serum electrolytes are commonly normal although the K^+ concentration may be raised. The blood urea is elevated and is a good guide to the prognosis. Leucocytosis is common even in the absence of infection.

TREATMENT. The treatment of diabetic ketoacidosis involves:

i. The administration of soluble insulin together with replacement of the fluid and electrolyte losses. In an adult, soluble insulin is administered by intravenous infusion at a rate of 5 u/h, preferably by means of a constant infusion pump. In children under the age of 10 years, the dose is reduced to 2–3 u/h. Insulin therapy is maintained until a satisfactory and consistent response is obtained which usually takes place between 4 and 8 hours after commencing treatment, and is monitored by blood glucose and electrolyte estimations performed 2-hourly until such control is achieved.

ii. The intravenous fluid therapy consists of the rapid administration of isotonic saline initially at the rate of 1 L/h reducing to 1 L 3-hourly as the dehydration and overbreathing improve. As the blood glucose falls in response to treatment, K^+ re-enters the cell. If at any stage, the serum K^+ falls below 4·0 mmol/L, 1–2 g KCl (13–26 mmol) are administered hourly via the saline drip throughout the duration of the insulin therapy. $NaHCO_3$ may be necessary to correct the acidosis, the exact requirements being calculated from the base deficit.

iii. In addition to the above measurements, nasogastric suction is instituted and a broad-spectrum antibiotic administered if there is any evidence of infection. Oxygen therapy has been advocated to correct the hypoxaemia and to prevent the development of cardiac arrhythmias.

Aketotic Diabetic Coma

This condition differs from diabetic ketoacidosis in that the dehydration is not accompanied by overt signs of ketosis and hyperventilation is absent. This complication is more frequently found in previously undiagnosed diabetics and appears to be more common amongst certain ethnic groups such as the West Indian immigrants to the UK. It is characterized by a marked elevation of the blood glucose level and plasma osmolality. Although the level of ketones in the plasma is elevated, acidosis is not marked and the plasma bicarbonate level is only slightly reduced. The condition carries a significant mortality of between 10 and 20%, and because of the severe hyperosmolar state, arterial thrombotic episodes are common.

TREATMENT. Because these patients are usually rather sensitive to insulin, only 3 u/h of soluble insulin should be administered intravenously via the constant infusion pump system.

Fluid therapy consists of large amounts of isotonic or 0·45% saline, depending on the plasma osmolality. Intravenous K^+ supplements are required during insulin therapy and, lastly, heparin is administered either intravenously or subcutaneously in view of the considerable risk of thrombosis. In other respects, the management is similar to that of diabetic ketoacidosis.

Management of Diabetes before and after Surgical Intervention

This depends on the magnitude of the operation and the severity of the diabetes:

i. No special preopoerative treatment is required for operations performed under local anaesthesia.

ii. A diabetic not receiving insulin, undergoing an operation under general anaesthesia, can be managed without special care but requires close postoperative observation. The clinical state should be monitored together with the blood sugar level and the presence or absence of both glycosuria and ketonuria noted. Soluble insulin by 4-hourly injections or low-dose continuous infusion giving 1–3 u/h is administered if there is significant loss of control of the diabetes.

iii. The insulin-treated diabetic patient undergoing a major operation requires special pre- and postoperative care. This consists of:

An intravenous 5% dextrose drip is set up in all these patients.

If the patient is on a single daily injection of insulin, this is converted to two injections (morning and evening) of soluble insulin, each consisting of half the daily requirement.

The morning injection is omitted if surgery is undertaken early in the day, and is administered 4–5 h before the operation if this is to be performed in the afternoon. This dose of insulin should be covered by the usual breakfast carbohydrate given as 50% dextrose.

In all these patients, the blood glucose requires to be estimated before the patient leaves the ward and at 2-hourly intervals thereafter.

The insulin requirements are best administered as a low-dose pump infusion at 1–2 u/h.

Postoperatively, 3 L of 5% dextrose or dextrose-saline are administered daily by intravenous infusion until oral feeding commences. The blood glucose and electrolyte levels should be monitored and the presence of any glycosuria or ketonuria noted when the necessary adjustment to the insulin regimen is made. This monitoring is continued until the patient is back on his usual preoperative regimen of insulin.

Hypoglycaemia

This is the commonest complication of insulin therapy and must be distinguished from spontaneous hypoglycaemia which may rarely be caused by islet-cell tumours and more commonly is reactive (functional) in origin when it results from an exaggerated insulin response to a rise in the blood glucose and is commonly encountered after gastric surgery for peptic ulceration.

The time of onset of exogenous insulin-induced hypoglycaemia depends upon the time of the injection and the type of insulin used. Patients with moderate to high concentrations of insulin antibodies show a delay in the recovery from exogenous insulin-induced hypoglycaemia. Hypoglycaemia may also complicate therapy with the sulphonylurea compounds but not with the biguanide drugs.

Symptoms and Signs

These are produced when the blood glucose falls below 2 mmol/L and include hunger, sweating, palpitations, tremor, tingling sensations and mental changes such as slow cerebration, fainting, aggressive behaviour, epileptiform convulsions and coma.

The patient is observed to be pale with tachycardia although the blood pressure and respiratory rate remain normal. Signs in the central nervous system include mono- or hemiplegia, incoordination of the eye movements and extensor plantar responses. The mental state varies from drowsiness to aggressive behaviour or coma.

Treatment

Hypoglycaemic attacks are best prevented by ensuring adequate buffer carbohydrate feeds at suitable time intervals depending on the nature of the hypoglycaemic agents used. These attacks are especially likely to occur in patients after total pancreatectomy and may be fatal in these patients. Diabetic patients should carry cards in addition to carbohydrate foods such as sweets, sugar lumps etc. These are taken if the patient starts to experience symptoms of hypoglycaemia. The treatment of established hypoglycaemia consists of the administration of glucose by mouth or intravenously depending on the clinical state of the patient.

Artificial Pancreas

This consists of circuits incorporating blood chemistry sensors and microchip-controlled pump delivery systems which monitor the blood glucose, insulin and electrolyte levels continuously and deliver the necessary amount of dextrose and insulin at an appropriate rate via an intravenous line. They are as yet not routinely used in the management of diabetes and ketoacidosis. They have been useful in the assessment of the insulin requirements of an unstable diabetic who proves difficult to control by conventional means. A period of attachment to the machine will measure accurately the average insulin and glucose requirements. They have also been used during operations for the removal of insulinomas not only for maintaining normal glucose levels during surgery, but also for ensuring that all the secreting neoplastic tissue has been removed.

Haemorrhagic Disorders

The congenital hereditary disorders within this category which are of surgical interest are haemophilia A, Factor IX deficiency (Christmas disease, haemophilia B) and von Willebrand's disease. Congenital deficiencies of Factors V and VII are easily corrected with an infusion of fresh frozen plasma. The important acquired haemorrhagic disorders are disseminated intravascular coagulation, the bleeding diathesis associated with liver disease and thrombotic thrombocytopenic purpura. The last is considered in Chapter 71.

Haemophilia

The condition is a sex-linked recessive disorder, the male exhibiting the disease and the female acting as a carrier, although approximately one-third of all cases occur without any family history, suggesting that spontaneous mutation may occur.

The underlying pathological feature is a deficiency of the procoagulant activity of the Factor VIII complex, a low molecular weight globulin known as anti-haemophiliac globulin/fraction (AHG, AHF). The other components of the Factor VIII complex, Factor VIII antigen and von Willebrand's cofactor (Factor VIIIvw) are present in normal amounts. Haemophilia A is rare and occurs in about 6 per 100 000 of the population being distinctly commoner in Caucasians.

The clinical severity of haemophilia A is determined by the reduced Factor VIII (AHG) activity. If any members of the family are involved, the severity of the defect appears to be the same in all those affected. The unit of measurement used to assess the disease is the international unit of Factor VIII. One international unit is based on the activity of 1·0 ml of average fresh normal plasma, also described as having 100% activity. In a normal individual, Factor VIII activity varies between 60 and 100%. Individuals with levels between 26 and 40% are, in practice, unlikely to bleed unless subjected to major surgery or trauma; a level of 6–25% indicates mild haemophilia with a tendency to bleed only if injured. If, however, the level reaches between 1 and 5%, bleeding will follow minor trauma and haemarthroses are likely. Below this level, the disease is particularly severe and spontaneous bleeding (gums, intramuscular, haematuria, haemarthrosis) can be expected.

Diagnosis

The diagnosis of haemophilia A should always be suspected in a patient with a bleeding tendency and a classic family history in whom a normal platelet count is found together with a normal bleeding and prothrombin time. Further investigation shows that the kaolin–cephalin time is prolonged and accompanied by a normal prothrombin time and reduced levels of Factors VIII (AHG) and IX.

Treatment

The indications for surgical intervention in the haemophiliac are precisely the same as a normal individual except for those patients in whom antibodies to Factor VIII have developed due to previous treatment. Basically, should the haemophiliac develop a major bleed or require surgery, then the low level of AHG should be made good by replacement therapy so that the level exceeds 30%. Plasma is insufficient to correct the disorder, cryoprecipitate or preferably AHG concentrates (Factorate, Kryobulin) are needed.

Cryoprecipitate was developed following the observation that a cold precipitate of plasma was rich in AHG. Fresh plasma is snap frozen and then thawed at 4°C when a string precipitate, the cryoprecipitate, is left in the plasma. This contains approximately 50% of the AHG of the original material. The supernatant plasma is removed and the cryoprecipitate is then frozen.

AHG (AHF) concentrates in a lyophilized state are used nowadays for the treatment of active bleeding and to cover surgical intervention and dental extractions. The concentrates are prepared from pooled human plasma obtained from donors found negative for HBsAg by the radioimmunoassay method. The concentrates come in vials containing 250 or 500 u. They are stored at 4 °C and keep their potency at this temperature for 2 years. They are reconstituted before use in 20–40 ml of sterile water. The High Potency Factorate is a purified preparation with lower levels of fibrinogen and other non-AHG protein per international unit than intermediate purity AHG preparations.

The formula for the amount of Factor VIII to be administered is:

$$\text{Requirements of Factor VIII} = \frac{\text{Wt in kg} \times \text{the desired Factor VIII rise (\%)}}{k(1\cdot5)}$$

The dose required and the frequency with which it should be given are determined by the type of bleeding (minor, major), the weight of the patient and by the fact that the half-life of Factor VIII is about 12 h. In a surgical setting, the initial level of Factor VIII should first be assayed so that required dose can be determined. The assay should be repeated at intervals throughout the course of treatment. The aim of treatment, particularly if the patient is to undergo major surgery, is to obtain an initial plasma level of about 0·8 u/ml (80% of normal) and then maintain the level above 40% for some 7–10 days by repeated intravenous administration of AHG concentrate at 12-hourly intervals.

Complications of Therapy

These are: hepatitis due to HBV, transmission of the AIDS virus with the development of acquired immune deficiency syndrome, development of inhibitors to AHG which neutralize its activity, and allergic reactions.

The presence of inhibitors should be suspected when an apparently adequate dose of Factor VIII raises the plasma level only slightly, transiently, or not at all. The incidence of inhibitory antibodies increases with repeated treatments and overall estimates vary from 5 to 21%; the development of these inhibitors makes treatment exceedingly complicated, if not impossible. Animal concentrates (bovine and porcine) have been used in patients with resistance to human AHG concentrates. Early reports with immunosuppression using cyclophosphamide have been encouraging but require confirmation. Activated Factor IX concentrates are of considerable value when high concentrations of inhibitor antibodies preclude the use of AHG. The basis of such therapy is that these concentrates contain certain activated factors which may bypass the point of action of Factor VIII in the haemostatic process and thus circumvent the problem created by the anti-AHG antibodies.

Allergic reactions are relatively rare. The reaction usually occurs during or within 1–2 h. The symptoms may consist of headaches, backache, urticaria, rigor, fever and tightness in the chest (bronchospasm) and, rarely, pulmonary oedema. Minor reactions may be treated with antihistamines and major ones require subcutaneous adrenaline and intravenous hydrocortisone.

Haemophilia B (Christmas Disease)

This inherited disorder due to deficiency of Factor IX, is clinically indistinguishable from haemophilia A and was recognized as a separate entity in 1952. It is a much less common condition than Factor VIII deficiency and affects only 1 per 1 000 000 of the population. Like haemophilia A, Christmas disease is also inherited as a sex-linked recessive characteristic. It mimics haemophilia A so closely that it can be differentiated only by a direct assay of Factor IX.

Replacement therapy is with Factor IX concentrates which are available in most haemophiliac centres.

Von Willebrand's Disease

This condition was first described by von Willebrand in the inhabitants of the Åland Islands in the Baltic sea. The disease is inherited as an autosomal dominant trait and, therefore, appears in consecutive generations affecting both males and females equally and is associated with bleeding from mucous membranes, haemarthrosis and postoperative haemorrhage. The basic abnormality is a deficiency of the Factor VIII antigen and Factor VIIIvw which is essential for platelet adhesiveness and for aggregation of platelets by the antibiotic ristocetin. The haematological tests show a prolonged bleeding time with a normal clotting time, reduced platelet adhesiveness and absent platelet aggregation with a normal platelet count. Fresh plasma contains both the missing factors and is used as the replacement therapy. Alternatively, cryoprecipitate may be used. The AHG factor concentrates lack the von Willebrand cofactor (VIIIvw) and are therefore ineffective in this condition.

Disseminated Intravascular Coagulation

This syndrome arises from the intravascular activation of procoagulant factors, chiefly thrombin, and platelet aggregation/adhesion leading to widespread thrombosis of the microcirculation of several organs, a consumptive coagulopathy and a secondary activation of plasminogen to plasmin causing a concurrent fibrinolysis. The net result is multiple organ damage/failure (adult respiratory distress syndrome, acute renal failure, hepatic insufficiency and CNS changes) and a generalized bleeding tendency manifested as petechiae/ecchymosis and bleeding from the mucous membranes (gastrointestinal haemorrhage, haematuria, epistaxis, etc.).

The important causes are shown in *Table* 9.13, the commonest in surgical practice being sepsis.

Haematological Findings

The consumptive coagulopathy leads to a multifactorial deficiency with prolongation of the prothrombin, thrombin and kaolin–cephalin time. The fibrin split products are elevated and thrombocytopenia is present and may be severe (<50 000). The level of antithrombin III is reduced as it is also consumed by the excessive thrombin and clot formation. The level of antithrombin III is a good guide to prognosis and to recovery from the disease.

Table 9.13 Causes of disseminated intravascular coagulation

SEPSIS	Toxin-induced endothelial damage and platelet aggregation
HAEMOLYSIS	ADP and RBC membrane phospholipids activate the procoagulants and induce platelet aggregation
TISSUE TRAUMA	Crush injuries, burns
IMMUNE REACTIONS	Antigen–antibody complex and complement-mediated intravascular coagulation.
PERITONEOVENOUS SHUNTING FOR ASCITES	Cellular debris, endotoxin or procoagulant in the ascitic fluid
OBSTETRIC COMPLICATIONS	Abruptio placentae, amniotic fluid embolism, etc.
ADVANCED CANCER	Predominantly thrombotic manifestations.

Treatment

In the first instance the initiating cause must be treated vigorously. This is particularly important in relation to sepsis. Hypovolaemia is corrected by fresh blood collected in heparin. The bleeding tendency is reversed by the use of fresh frozen plasma and cryoprecipitate. Some advocate the use of intravenous heparin early on in the disease to reduce the thrombotic tendency and augment antithrombin III activity. Heparin is, however, contraindicated in the presence of open wounds and overt active bleeding. More recently, the administration of concentrates of antithrombin III has given very favourable results. This normal inhibitor of Factor Xa and thrombin reduces both the abnormal intravascular clotting and the exaggerated fibrinolysis. The current consensus of opinion is against the use of antifibrinolytic agents in this condition, since the abnormal fibrinolytic state is secondary and may indeed be beneficial in preventing widespread thrombosis and organ failure. Platelet transfusions are administered if the patient is actively bleeding and has a significant thrombocytopenia.

Bleeding Associated with Liver Disease

The bleeding associated with liver disease may be due to a depletion of the clotting factors, to an enhanced fibrinolysis and a low platelet count with defective platelet function. All the clotting factors with the exception of Factors VIII and XII are synthesized by the liver. The vitamin K-dependent factors are reduced in cholestatic jaundice because of the malabsorption of vitamin K. This results in a prolongation of the prothrombin time which is reversed by parenteral phytomenadione. In advanced liver disease such as end-stage cirrhosis, the multifactorial deficiency is more severe and is characterized by prolongation of both the prothrombin and the kaolin–cephalin time which do not respond to parenteral vitamin K analogues. The clotting deficiency results from a synthetic failure due to hepatocyte decompensation and can only be temporarily corrected by replacement therapy using fresh frozen plasma and cryoprecipitate. In addition to the thrombocytopenia, platelet function is abnormal. This is thought to be secondary to the excess fibrin degradation products (from the exaggerated fibrinolysis) and to the elevated serum bilirubin.

Further Reading

Breckenridge A. (1983) *Hypertension* (Seminar). London, Update.

British National Formulary, No. 10, 1985. A joint publication of the British Medical Association and the Pharmaceutical Society of Great Britain.

Edmondson H. A., Henderson B. and Benton B. (1976) Liver-cell adenomas associated with use of oral contraceptives. *N. Engl. J. Med.* **294**, 470–472.

Karam J. H. and Etzwiler D. D. (ed.) (1983) International Symposium on Human Insulin. *Diabetes Care*, 6 (suppl 2): 1–68.

Lui K., Cedres L. B. et al. (1982) Relationship of education to major risk factors and death from coronary heart disease, cardiovascular disease and all causes. *Circulation* **66**, 1308–1314.

Smiddy F. C. (1981) *Medical Management of the Surgical Patient* 2nd ed. London, Arnold.

Somerville K., Faulkner G. and Langman M. (1986) Non-steroidal anti-inflammatory drugs and bleeding peptic ulcer. *Lancet* **1**, 462–464.

10 Preoperative, Operative and Postoperative Care

A. Cuschieri

The care of the patient undergoing surgical treatment is designed to achieve four objectives:

1. Reduction in the mortality and morbidity from surgery and general anaesthesia.
2. Safety of patients and staff during the conduct of the operation.
3. Pain relief.
4. Smooth convalescence and early rehabilitation.

PREOPERATIVE CARE

The assessment of the operative risks and fitness for general anaesthesia are the major issues at this stage. Adequate preoperative care, however, entails the consideration of other important factors, such as establishment of an adequate rapport with the patient, the general preparation of the patient for surgery and the institution of prophylactic measures against the onset of specific complications. Preoperative care therefore includes:

1. Assessment of operative risks—selection of patients.
2. Assessment of the fitness for general anaesthesia and surgery.
3. Adequate explanation to the patient of the nature of the operative procedure.
4. Correction of nutritional, blood volume, fluid and electrolyte deficiencies.
5. Institution of prophylactic measures against common postoperative complications.
6. General preparation of the patient for surgery.
7. Reasoned estimate of the amount of blood required to cover the operation (blood tariff).
8. Assessment of the likely postoperative course and the probable need for intensive care after the operation.

Assessment of Operative Risks

There is some truth in the statement that the beneficial effects of a surgical operation are inversely proportional to the magnitude of the surgical procedure. This consideration emphasizes the need for *careful patient selection which involves an exercise of clinical judgement whereby the relative benefits from a given surgical procedure is balanced against the known risks and complications of that treatment.* This decision is taken against the background knowledge regarding the natural history of the untreated disease from which the patient is suffering. Whereas this decision to operate may be straightforward, as in the emergency treatment of life-threatening disorders, it is often more difficult for planned elective procedures incurring a definite mortality. Nowhere is this decision more difficult than in the use of prophylactic operations for symptomless disease.

Extreme attitudes are always wrong, and such statements as the 'patient has to earn the operation' or 'the best place for a gastric ulcer is in the bucket' are expressions of rigid views borne of an unaudited experience and testify to an inadequate appreciation of human suffering. Moreover, the careful selection of patients for surgery does not entail the rejection of patients for surgical treatment because of the presence of risk factors which could adversely affect the overall results of a given personal experience. The prime consideration is always the welfare of the patient, and *patient selection is exclusively concerned with the decision regarding the best form of treatment for a particular patient in the light of individual and personal circumstances* (age, intercurrent disease, mental attitude and overall risks), including the patient's own expressed wishes.

Good selection of patients for surgery also entails an *early decision that medical/conservative management has failed,* as other risk factors being equal, the overall operative mortality commensurate with magnitude of the operation concerned, is lowest for those procedures undertaken under elective conditions. Thus, for example, the mortality following colectomy for ulcerative colitis is highest when this is performed as an emergency because of colonic perforation, intermediate when undertaken urgently for toxic megacolon and lowest when the procedure is performed electively because of failure of medical treatment.

Another aspect of patient selection is *referral for specialized treatment.* This concerns both inter- and intra-specialty tertiary referrals. The latter include patients with iatrogenic injuries (e.g. bile duct strictures), major hepatic surgery, patients with severe and persistent symptoms after gastric surgery, bleeding oesophageal varices and major reconstructive procedures on the gastrointestinal tract. These are situations which require special expertise and back-up facilities. As the optimal results of remedial surgery are obtained at the first attempt at correction, the situation where a surgeon who has not the necessary experience, is prepared 'to have a go' should not arise.

Fitness for Surgery and General Anaesthesia

Assuming surgical competence, every patient is fit for

Table 10.1 Physical status scale: American Society of Anesthesiologists (ASA)

Class	*Physical status*
1	A normally healthy individual: no organic, physiological, biochemical, or psychiatric disturbance
2	A patient with mild to moderate systemic disease: this may or may not be related to the disorder requiring surgical treatment, e.g. diabetes mellitus, hypertension
3	A patient with severe systemic disease which is not incapacitating, e.g. heart disease with limited exercise tolerance, uncontrolled hypertension or diabetes, etc.
4	A patient with incapacitating systemic disease that is a constant threat to life with or without surgery, e.g. congestive cardiac failure, severe and persistent angina
5	A moribund patient who is not expected to live and where surgery is performed as a last resort, e.g. ruptured aortic aneurysm
E	A patient who requires an emergency operation

surgery. Neither is the term 'fitness for general anaesthesia' strictly accurate as the condition of many seriously ill patients is actually improved during anaesthesia. What one is really assessing is the chances of survival of the patient beyond the postoperative period notwithstanding the secondary effects of surgery and anaesthesia. In the majority of cases *postoperative death is due to a combination of factors which include intercurrent disease, surgical complications and the adverse pulmonary effects of anaesthesia.* The preoperative assessment of risk is therefore difficult and imprecise but is influenced by the preoperative condition of the patient. The American Society of Anesthesiologists' grading scale of the preoperative 'physical status' of the patient is outlined in *Table* 10.1. Initially the system was introduced to describe and select patients for clinical trials but is now being increasingly adopted for routine clinical use. Although the preoperative assessment of risk has become the domain of anaesthetists, a joint consultation between the surgeon and his anaesthetist is preferable. The use of outpatient assessment clinics to examine patients awaiting elective surgery is gaining popularity. The patients are seen by the anaesthetist 1–2 weeks before admission. This practice results in fewer patients arriving unfit for surgery.

The evaluation of the patient entails:

I. History

Respiratory disease and smoking

Cardiac and vascular disease including deep vein thrombosis

Other medical disorders—bleeding diathesis, hypertension, diabetes etc.

Previous anaesthetic experience—intractable vomiting, volatile agents used, specific anaesthetic complications e.g. suxamethonium apnoea, malignant hyperpyrexia, etc.

Drugs and alcohol intake

II. Physical Examination

Nutrition

Mental state

Dentures

Abnormalities of jaw and neck

Respiratory system

Cardiovascular system

III. Investigations

a. Routine: Blood grouping and antibody screen. Hb, chest radiography only in patients with cardiorespiratory disease/symptoms, in the elderly, and in smokers, patients with possible metastases, recent immigrants from countries where tuberculosis is still endemic; ward examination of urine. An ECG should be carried out in all patients over 50 years and those with cardiac cardiac disease and hypertension. Urea and electrolyte estimation are performed in all patients undergoing major surgery, in patients on diuretics, suspected renal impairment or patients on i.v. fluid therapy

b. Special: Pulmonary function tests, sputum culture and blood gas analysis in patients with respiratory disease or when respiratory problems are anticipated. Forced expiratory volume in one second (FEV_1) and forced vital capacity are good indicators of obstructive and restrictive airways disease and are easily carried out with a Vitallograph

Clotting factor studies in all patients with haemorrhagic disease or jaundice

Screening for sickle cells in the appropriate ethnic groups

Elderly Patients

Patients over 60 years of age incur an enhanced risk which is largely the result of limited mobility, frequent presence of intercurrent disease and diminished reserve of cardiac/renal function which restricts the ability to cope with a prolonged period of illness in the event of postoperative complications. This enhanced risk is dependent more on the physiological state than the chronological age and no patient should be denied an operation on the basis of age alone. Elderly patients require an intensive preoperative evaluation to assess their respiratory, cardiac and renal reserves. Both intravenous fluids and blood transfusion have to be administered cautiously and with adequate monitoring as elderly patients are prone to develop circulatory overload. Aged patients require smaller doses of narcotic agents. They are likewise sensitive to sedative and hypnotic drugs which often precipitate restlessness and mental confusion in this age group.

Respiratory Disease and Smoking

The incidence of respiratory disease in surgical patients varies with the population (urban/rural, occupation, social class, etc.) and in Western Countries ranges from 25 to 50%. Obstructive lung disease is followed by a higher incidence of postoperative pulmonary complications than restrictive airways disease. Whenever possible, surgery on patients with acute respiratory infections should be postponed until 2 weeks after resolution of the infection. The timing of elective surgery in patients with chronic respiratory disease should coincide with a remission and after a period of intensive physiotherapy, breathing exercises and appropriate medical treatment with antibiotics and bronchodilators.

All patients with respiratory disease and smokers require pulmonary function tests to determine the type of respiratory disease (obstructive/restrictive), assess the respiratory reserve and the need for ventilatory support after surgery. Postoperative problems (chest infections, segmental/lobar collapse) are exceedingly common in patients with chronic bronchitis and in heavy smokers.

Smoking increases the risk of surgery and anaesthesia by virtue of its adverse effects on the cardiovascular and respiratory systems. Carbon monoxide and nicotine are responsible for the immediate cardiovascular effects. Consequent on the formation of carboxyhaemoglobin, carbon monoxide reduces the amount of haemoglobin available for combination with oxygen and alters the oxygen dissociation curve such that the affinity of haemoglobin for oxygen is enhanced. It also has a weak negative inotropic action on the heart.

Nicotine causes an increase in heart rate and blood pressure. Thus it enhances the demand of the myocardium for oxygen while carbon monoxide decreases the supply. Elimination of both carbon monoxide and nicotine with improvement in the cardiovascular fitness is complete following a 12–24 h abstention from smoking. There is a sixfold increase in the postoperative respiratory morbidity in patients who smoke more than 10 cigarettes/day. The responsible factors include small airways disease, hypersecretion of a thick, viscid mucus (secretional airway obstruction) and impairment of tracheobronchial clearance. A 2–3 months' abstinence from smoking is necessary before any beneficial influence on postoperative respiratory morbidity is witnessed. Smoking also depresses the immune response. It induces a reduction in the immunoglobulin levels, natural killer cell activity, neutrophil chemotaxis and pulmonary alveolar macrophage activity. Full recovery of the immune function requires a 6–8 weeks' period of abstinence from smoking. The only benefit from smoking appears to be that of a reduced incidence of isotopically detected postoperative deep vein thrombosis when compared to non-smokers. However, there is no evidence that smokers who abstain for several weeks before elective surgery incur an enhanced risk of deep vein thrombosis.

There is therefore sufficient information to allow sound advice to be given to smokers before elective surgery. A 6–8 weeks' abstinence will result in an improvement in the pulmonary function, a reduction in the postoperative respiratory morbidity and a return towards a normal immune response. Those patients who find it impossible to stop smoking for this period (or indefinitely), will derive some benefit in terms of improved cardiovascular function from a short period of abstinence (12–24 h) before their operation. This applies particularly to patients with ischaemic heart disease.

Cardiovascular Disease

The important risk factors relating to life-threatening complications are shown in *Table* 10.2. Whenever possible, surgical intervention should be delayed for a minimum of 3, and preferably 6, months following myocardial infarction. It is inadvisable to stop antihypertensive therapy before surgery because of the resulting cardiovascular instability and the enhanced risk of cardiovascular accidents. The exact details of any antihypertensive therapy is required by the anaesthetist to avoid adverse drug interaction and hypotensive episodes. Patients with Stokes–Adams attacks have a great risk of developing complete heart block during anaesthesia.

Table 10.2 Risk factors for life-threatening cardiac complications

Cardiac	Infarction within 6 months
	Dysrhythmias
	Atrial or ventricular extrasystoles
	Non-sinus rhythm or failure
	Third heart sound
	Jugular venous distension
	Significant valvular aortic stenosis
Others	Poor general/medical condition
	Old age (>70 years)
	Major intraperitoneal/thoracic operation
	Emergency operation

These patients and those with heart rates <40/min in the presence of a normal or increased supraventricular rate, should have a pacemaker inserted preoperatively, even as an emergency.

The correction of anaemia, as opposed to the need to replace blood volume deficits, has been overstated. There is no evidence that the correction of mild anaemia is necessary or indeed desirable before surgical intervention. Most patients in this category have adjusted to the reduced haemoglobin load and the associated haemodilution may indeed be beneficial in ensuring adequate tissue perfusion in the perioperative period. Indeed, the practice of controlled haemodilution down to a PCV of 30–35% has been reported to reduce morbidity and the need for autologous blood, as the patient's own blood is administered at the end of the operative procedure. If anaemic patients are to be transfused, this should be undertaken slowly and 7–10 days prior to the surgical procedure to allow for haemodynamic stabilization. In situations where the transfusion may result in heart failure, the slow administration of whole blood together with a loop diuretic, such as frusemide, is considered preferable to the transfusion of packed cells because of viscosity problems.

Drug Therapy

A substantial number of patients coming to surgical intervention are on drug therapy. There are some drugs which should be continued up to the time of the operation. These include antihypertensive agents and steroids. Other drugs must be discontinued two weeks before general anaesthesia. These are *monoamine oxidase inhibitors* (MAOI) which cause an accumulation of noradrenaline in the nerve terminals (when severe hypertension, pyrexia and convulsions can occur with vasopressors and narcotics), *tricyclic antidepressants* which block the re-uptake of noradrenaline into nerve terminals and have anticholinergic properties (potentiate the actions of noradrenaline and atropine-like drugs), *fenfluramine* which interacts with halogenated anaesthetics inducing dysrhythmias, *lithium* which prolongs the action of neuromuscular blocking agents, and *phenothiazines* which may induce tremor and restlessness during intravenous induction with barbiturates.

Oral Contraceptives

The risk of postoperative deep vein thrombosis in women on the combined (oestrogen + progesterone) pill is double that of non-users. This is related to a reduction in the activity of antithrombin III induced by the additive effect of the combined pill and general anaesthesia. This enhanced risk is not seen with the progestogen-only pill which need not be stopped over the time of elective surgery, however major. The recommendations in the British National Formulary are as follows: oestrogen-containing contraceptives should be discontinued 4 weeks before major elective surgery and alternative contraceptive arrangements made (e.g. Depo-Provera). In the emergency situation or when the patient, by oversight, is admitted on an oestrogen-containing pill, prophylactic low-dose heparin should be administered. Cessation of combined oral contraceptive therapy is not necessary in patients undergoing minor surgery with early ambulation and in patients taking the progestogen-only pill.

Obese Patients

These patients have an increased risk of respiratory complications, deep vein thrombosis, wound infection and dehiscence. In addition, they have a higher incidence of intercurrent disease and have a restricted mobility. The technical difficulty of the operative procedure is also enhanced. This may increase the risk of iatrogenic injury and jeopardize a successful outcome. Whenever possible, controlled weight reduction is recommended before elective surgical treatment.

Diabetic Patients

These patients require special management which is discussed in Chapter 9. The importance of avoiding dehydration in the diabetic patient undergoing surgery cannot be overstressed.

Prophylactic Measures

Certain general principles are so self-evident that they are infrequently reiterated and remembered only in sad retrospection following the occurrence of avoidable tragedies. Good nursing care, safe prescription and administration of drugs, error-proof methods of patient identification, reassurance of the patient and an adequate explanation of the intended treatment to relieve anxiety, marking of the operation site, the maintenance of essential replacement therapy, etc., whenever abused or misused may directly or indirectly lead to disastrous consequences. *The ultimate prophylactic measure in surgical practice is an obsession to check and double check.*

Specific Prophylaxis

There are a number of specific prophylactic measures which are indicated not routinely but selectively in some patients owing to the presence of risk factors which predispose to certain complications.

Prevention of Infective Endocarditis

The findings of the survey conducted by the British Cardiac Society has shown that 43% of patients who developed infective endocarditis, either had normal hearts or a previously unrecognized cardiac abnormality before the onset of the disease, stressing the fact that the valves of normal hearts can be infected and destroyed in severe septicaemic episodes. In this respect, the patients at risk include the elderly patients, diabetics, alcoholics, the immunosuppressed and drug addicts. Streptococci are the most common responsible organisms for infective endocarditis (viridans in 48%, other streptococci in 15%), followed by staphylococci (19%), enteric bacteria (14%), and a wide variety of organisms. Aside from dental work, the invasive procedures which may result in bacteraemic episodes include all common gastrointestinal and genitourinary operations, endoscopic procedures, liver biopsy and percutaneous transhepatic cholangiography, blood donation, phlebography, haemodialysis, fractures and cardiac catheterization. In a recent study, bacteraemia was reported in 17–20% of patients after nasotracheal intubation.

The recommendations of the British Society for Antimicrobial Chemotherapy for patients at risk because of cardiac lesions are: *amoxycillin for dental procedures; erythromycin for those allergic to penicillin; and a combination of amoxycillin and gentamicin against bowel organisms.* The provision of antibiotic cover in the elderly patients with apparently normal hearts is unsettled but the consensus view is that such a policy is not without risk in view of the large number of patients above the age of 60 undergoing surgical, investigative and dental procedures.

Chemoprophylaxis against Surgical Infections

In the UK National Survey of Hospital Infections performed in 1981, a total of 19% of patients were found to have infections. In 9%, the infection was acquired in hospital and wound infections accounted for 20% of these. Antibiotic prophylaxis is not an alternative to good surgical practice including a strict aseptic technique and is only used when the risk of infection is high and the results of infection (if it occurs) are serious. The situations in surgical practice where chemoprophylaxis is indicated because of proven benefit are shown in *Table* 10.3. The principles governing safe and effective antibiotic prophylaxis in surgical practice are well established and include:

Table 10.3 Chemoprophylaxis against surgical infections

Clinical condition/situation	*Antibiotic regimen*
Colorectal surgery	Systemic aminoglycoside (or cephalosporin) + metronidazole
Gastro-oesophageal surgery	Systemic cephalosporin or beta-lactam antibiotics or acetylureido-penicillins
Acute appendicitis	Intrarectal metronidazole
Biliary surgery	Systemic cephalosporin or co-trimoxazole
Prosthetic surgery (includes vascular grafts)	Flucloxacillin or cephalosporin

1. Therapeutic tissue concentrations of the antibiotic must be present at the time of the skin incision and maintained throughout the operation. In any event the antibiotic should not be administered more than 12 h prior to the operation.

2. The antibiotic should, whenever possible, be bactericidal in nature so that it need never be given for more than 48 h.

3. The choice of agent(s) depend(s) on the pathogens most likely to be encountered in a given situation.

4. Topical antibiotics are less effective and do not provide protection against intra-abdominal abscesses and septicaemia.

With the newer cephalosporins a single dose is administered either intramuscularly 2 h before the operation or intravenously at the time of induction. Some consider the single-dose regimen to be as effective and safer than the three-dose regimen, when the initial dose is repeated at 12 and 24 h after operation. Antibiotic prophylaxis should not be used in clean operations. There is no evidence that it prevents postoperative chest infections even in patients with tracheostomies or endotracheal tubes.

Prophylaxis against Deep Vein Thrombosis

The risk of venous thromboembolic disease in patients undergoing surgical treatment is influenced by a number of factors, the most important of which are: age, nature and extent of the procedure, presence of varicose veins, malignant disease, obesity, cardiac disease, and a history of previous deep vein thrombosis/pulmonary embolism. It is useful to divide patients into three categories depending on their risk of developing this potentially lethal complication (*Table* 10.4), since this influences the decision for specific prophylaxis against deep vein thrombosis and indicates the appropriate method which should be used. The available methods for the prevention of deep vein thrombosis are:

SUBCUTANEOUS LOW-DOSE HEPARIN. Heparin is administered in a dose of 5000 u 2 h before the operation and then either 8- or 12-hourly for the duration of the risk period, that is until the patient is fully ambulant. The 8-hourly regimen is associated with a significant increase in the incidence of wound haematoma. Low-dose subcutaneous heparin is the treatment of choice in general surgical patients within the moderate risk category. It is now clear that it does not provide adequate protection in general surgical patients falling within the high-risk category, particularly in those patients with a history of recent venous thrombosis. Prophylaxis in this group is best achieved by a combined regimen (low-dose heparin + dihydroergotamine or low-dose heparin + external pneumatic compression), or oral anticoagulation with intermittent external pneumatic compression or continuous intravenous heparin. The latter is administered by a calibrated infusion pump. The heparin infusion is started before surgery and adjusted to maintain the heparin level in the blood to 0·1 u/ml. This is gradually increased to 0·2 u/ml in the postoperative period.

All anticoagulant methods of prophylaxis are contraindicated in neurosurgical patients because of the risk of postoperative intracranial haemorrhage. Subcutaneous low-dose heparin is not routinely used in genitourinary practice because of the risk of bleeding, except in patients undergoing extensive pelvic surgery for invasive carcinoma of the pelvic organs where it is usually combined with external pneumatic compression.

ORAL ANTICOAGULANTS. These are administered in doses that result in a prolongation of the prothrombin time to between one and a half and twice the control value. The major disadvantage of this regimen is increased perioperative bleeding. A modified approach whereby the treatment is commenced 2–3 days after the operation reduces the risk of bleeding to acceptable levels.

DEXTRAN 70/40. Prophylaxis with dextran 70 or 40 is as effective as low-dose heparin in the prevention of fatal pulmonary embolism after general surgical operations. The dextran solution is administered in a volume of 500 ml at the time of surgery and repeated once daily for the first 2–5 days. Its disadvantages include hypersensitivity reactions, circulatory overload in the elderly and a slight risk of bleeding when commenced at the time of surgery. Dextran prophylaxis has become the treatment of choice in patients undergoing elective hip surgery.

EXTERNAL PNEUMATIC COMPRESSION (EPC) AND GRADUATED COMPRESSION STOCKINGS. EPC is an effective method of prophylaxis against deep vein thrombosis in general

Table 10.4a Risk groups for venous thromboembolic disease

Low risk	*Moderate risk*	*High risk*
<40 years Minor surgical procedures lasting <30 min No immobilization	>40 years Upper abdominal/thoracic procedures lasting >30 min	Recent venous thromboembolism Extensive abdominal/pelvic surgery for malignant disease

Table 10.4b Risk groups for venous thromboembolic disease and their prophylaxis

Category	*Incidence of* Ileofemoral vein thrombosis	*Incidence of* Fatal pulmonary embolism	*Recommended regimen*
Low risk	<1·0%	<0·01%	GCS with early ambulation
Moderate risk	2–8%	0·1–0·7%	Low-dose heparin or dextran or EPC
High risk	6–12%	1·0–2·0%	Combined regimens or i.v. heparin

GCS = graduated compression stockings.
EPC = external pneumatic compression.

surgical, urological and neurosurgical patients provided the device is worn throughout the postoperative period. It is often used in combination with other methods of prophylaxis such as anticoagulants or dextran. Similar results are achieved by the use of graduated compression stockings which are cheaper and more comfortable than the pneumatic appliances.

Prevention of Renal Failure

The cause of renal failure in the postoperative period is often multifactorial. Damage may result from hypoxia, hypotension, the accumulation or presence of endogenous nephrotoxic substances (such as free haemoglobin, myoglobin, endotoxin and excess bilirubin) or drug-induced nephrotoxicity. The high-risk groups include patients undergoing cardiopulmonary bypass and aortic surgery, jaundiced patients and those with significant hypovolaemia from blood loss or severe fluid and electrolyte deficits. Apart from avoiding known precipitating factors, effective prophylaxis is based on the maintenance of an adequate renal perfusion and oxygenation. Specific prophylaxis of renal failure in these high-risk groups is based on the proven observation that if sodium reabsorption is inhibited, the hypoxic damage due to a fall in the renal blood flow is greatly reduced. This natriuresis is achieved by a loop diuretic (frusemide) or an osmotic diuretic (mannitol). The resulting diuresis requires fluid replacement. In patients with jaundice due to large bile duct obstruction, the preoperative oral administration of bile salts (Na^+ cholate) reduces the incidence and morbidity from renal failure by blocking the absorption of endotoxin produced by the gut microflora. In a more recent clinical trial, lactulose (30 ml t.d.s. b.m.) was found to protect against renal failure in patients with obstructive jaundice.

General Preparation of the Patient for Surgery

Nursing Procedures

Routine measures include bathing the patient, application of identification bracelets, removal of dentures and other items such as jewellery, prosthesis, etc., administration of the premedication at the specified time, and total starvation for 4–6 h before surgery. Whole body disinfection by means of 4% chlorhexidine gluconate soap showers on the preoperative day, the preoperative evening and the morning of the operative day, has been shown to reduce dramatically the incidence of wound infections after elective surgery and is widely practised in Sweden.

The patient should be requested to empty his bladder on the morning of the operation. Although still widely used, shaving enhances the incidence of wound infection especially if performed several hours before the operation. It causes a myriad of tiny wounds in the skin which encourage bacterial growth. The use of depilatory creams is preferable in this respect, although repeated application may result in toxic skin reactions.

Gastrointestinal Preparation

There is little doubt that adequate preparation reduces both the morbidity and mortality following surgery on the gastrointestinal tract. In the emergency situation, the insertion of a nasogastric tube to evacuate gastric contents is mandatory and its routine use has reduced the incidence of aspiration during induction.

Patients with pyloric stenosis may require frequent gastric washes via the nasogastric tube with isotonic saline, and the procedure repeated until the effluent is reasonably clear and free of food debris. However, the routine insertion of a nasogastric tube in patients undergoing elective abdominal surgery is inappropriate, causes unnecessary discomfort to most patients and incurs a certain morbidity with a higher incidence of chest infections, oesophagitis and sore throat. The only indication for nasogastric suction in elective surgical practice is after total oesophagectomy when the stomach is mobilized to the neck for anastomosis to the cervical oesophagus. These patients are at risk of aspiration particularly if the recurrent laryngeal nerves have been damaged. In this situation, the ordinary Ryle's tube is inadequate and a Salem sump tube attached to a suction machine is necessary to ensure that the stomach is kept empty.

Adequate bowel preparation is necessary for procedures on the intestinal tract and is particularly relevant to colonic surgery. Both mechanical preparation and bowel sterilization are important as they reduce infection and leakage rates. Traditional mechanical cleansing of the colon entails a liquid low-residue diet, purgation and colonic washouts with tap water. The use of the Varipaque enema has greatly facilitated mechanical preparation of the colon and is being increasingly used in favour of the traditional methods. Other methods of bowel preparation include the use of elemental diets, oral mannitol and saline infusion of the gastrointestinal tract. Mannitol (10–20%) is given orally as an orange-flavoured solution (300 ml) on two occasions with a 12–24-h interval. It is very simple to administer and works by inducing a drastic osmotic purgation which may cause some dehydration. It also leads to the production of methane by the colonic organisms. Diathermy should not be used to open the bowel in patients whose colon was mechanically prepared by mannitol because of the danger of explosion. An alternative orally-administered solution is Golytely. This consists of a balanced crystalloid solution of PEG. About 2 litres of the orange-flavoured solution achieves very satisfactory mechanical cleansing of the bowel. The irrigation technique involves the rapid infusion of 3–4 litres of isotonic saline via a nasogastric tube. The infusion is continued until the intestinal tract is cleared of faecal matter. The technique is poorly tolerated by some patients, particularly the elderly, and induces distressing colic in patients with stenotic lesions.

Irrespective of the technique used, mechanical preparation of the colon is often incomplete in the presence of a distal stenosing lesion and the proximal colon may have to be cleared of faecal matter at the time of surgery. There are two techniques for achieving this safely. The first method (retrograde) uses a special tube (Muir) which is introduced via a colotomy proximal to the stenosing lesion. The second technique (prograde) involves an appendicectomy with insertion of a DePezzer/Malecot catheter through the appendix stump into the caecum. Alternatively, the tube is inserted through a small stab incision in the terminal ileum through the ileocaecal valve into the caecum (*Fig.* 10.1).

Mechanical bowel preparation has no effect on the bacterial counts in the colon. Effective reduction of the colonic bacterial population is achieved by the oral administration of neomycin and erythromycin or neomycin and metronidazole on the day prior to operation. Some surgeons have abandoned bowel sterilization and rely on systemic antibiotic cover (cephalosporin + metronidazole) using the three-dose regimen.

Catheterization

The bladder should be catheterized in all patients undergoing pelvic operations, in patients at risk from renal failure and those who require prolonged intravenous fluid therapy.

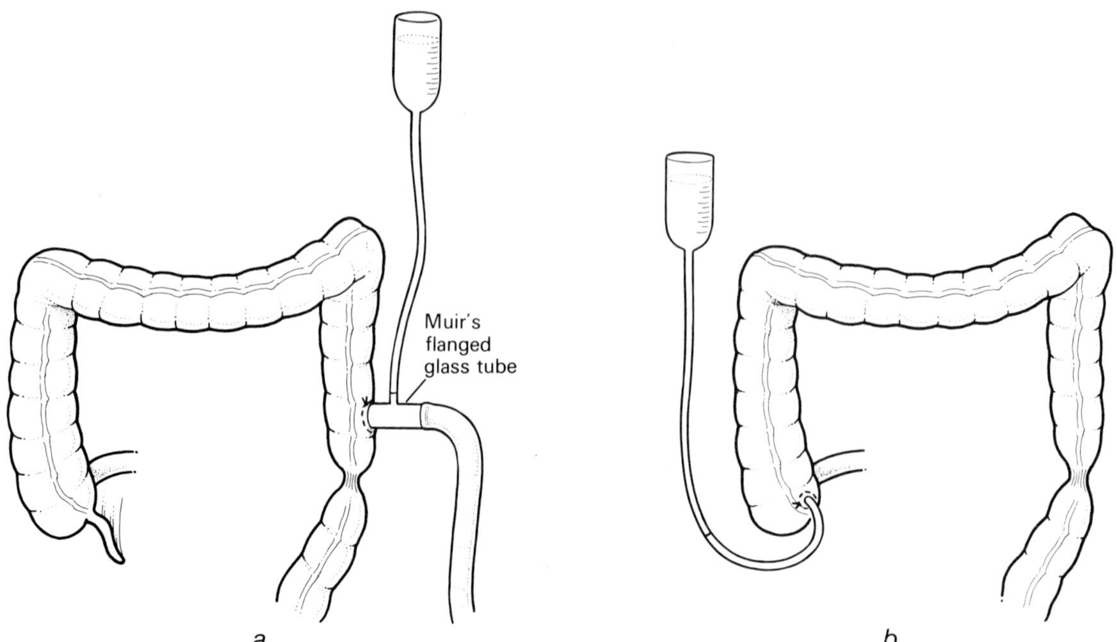

Fig. 10.1 *a*, Diagrammatic representation of the use of Muir's technique for cleaning the colon of faecal matter proximal to a stenosing lesion at operation (retrograde technique). The Muir's tube is introduced into the colon proximal to the lesion and held in place by a tight purse-string suture. The Paul's tubing attached to the exit end of the Muir's tube is clamped and 1–1·5 L of detergent solution is run into the colon which is then kneaded to break down the faecal concretions. On release of the clamp, the colonic contents are discharged via the Paul's tubing into a bucket containing antiseptic solution. *b*, Prograde method of dealing with faecal impaction of the colon proximal to a stenotic lesion at operation. An appendicectomy is performed and a Malecot or DePezzer catheter (size 24–26) is introduced into the caecum and held in place by a purse-string suture. The detergent solution is then run into the colon and the catheter is clamped. The colon is massaged to break down the faecal concretions. Thereafter, the tubing is unclamped and the colonic contents siphoned off. Alternatively, the catheter is introduced into the caecum via a stab wound in the terminal ileum.

Parenteral Nutrition

This is discussed in Chapter 8. A period of parenteral nutrition may be needed in patients with carcinoma of the stomach and the oesophagus who often have clinical and biochemical evidence of malnutrition. The decision should not be taken lightly since the overall benefit may be marginal. If considered necessary, parenteral nutrition should be maintained for a minimum of 10–14 days to impart any real benefit. The central venous line (Broviac or Hickman) should be inserted in theatre with full aseptic precautions.

Consent for Operation

The onus of this rests with the surgeon or one of his junior staff. Consent for surgery should be obtained at least one day before planned surgical intervention and should be prefaced by a clear explanation of the nature of the intended operation.

Premedication

In the past the scope of premedication was to ensure the smooth induction and maintenance of anaesthesia by reducing salivation and secretions, raising the threshold of pain and producing euphoria. Since the advent of intravenous induction, the primary goal has been to relieve anxiety which is present in the majority of patients before surgery. Often the patients cannot explain why they are anxious although some may have had previous unfortunate experiences with inhalational anaesthesia and surgical complications. Children who have had repeated operations are often frightened.

Drug premedication does not absolve the surgeon and anaesthetist from reassuring the patient and providing him with an adequate explanation of the intended operation. *Narcotics* (opiates) have become less popular as premedicating agents. In the first instance, timing of the injection is crucial since their effects wear off after 1 h. This becomes an important consideration when the operation is delayed. Secondly, they have undesirable side-effects, e.g. nausea, vomiting and cardiorespiratory depression. *Barbiturates* are seldom used nowadays. *Phenothiazines* produce sedation and antiemesis at the expense of increased restlessness, tachycardia and hypotension. However, promethazine + pethidine is popular with some anaesthetists as the promethazine enhances the sedative effect of pethidine and reduces its emetic effect.

The *benzodiazepines* are the most popular premedicating agents nowadays. They have anxiolytic and hypnotic effects and act on receptors in the cerebral cortex and limbic system in addition to facilitating GABA (gamma-aminobutyric acid) transmission. Their main advantages include minimal cardiorespiratory depression and high blood levels after oral administration. They are effective within 1 h of oral administration and their actions last for 2–4 h. The amnesia produced by the benzodiazepines is particularly helpful in patients undergoing endoscopy and operations under local anaesthesia. Some of the commonly used benzodiazepines are shown in *Table* 10.5.

Anticholinergic drugs are only used for the reduction of salivation in oral surgery and in the prevention of bradycardia in response to surgical stimulation (oculocardiac reflex, carotid bifurcation surgery, etc.). The agents most

Table 10.5 Benzodiazepines used for sedation

Drug	*Mean elimination half-life* (hours)	*Dose and route of administration*
Diazepam	33	0·1 mg/kg i.v.
	32	10 mg b.m.
Lorazepam	13	5 mg i.v.
	14	5 mg b.m.
Oxazepam	8	45 mg b.m.
Nitrazepam	30	5 mg b.m.
Temazepam	8	20 mg b.m.
Triazolam	4	0·25 mg b.m.

commonly used are atropine and hyoscine although glycopyrronium bromide has a more powerful antisialogogue action and cardiovascular stability than atropine.

OPERATIVE CARE

Good operative care militates against the occurrence of accidental hazards to the patient and attending staff. Furthermore it ensures the safe execution and completion of the surgical treatment. The design of modern operating theatres, although conducive towards the attainment of these goals, in no way absolves the staff from the strict observation of fundamental surgical principles governing the safe execution of surgical procedures: strict aseptic ritual, reduction of human traffic to the bare minimum possible, exclusion of infected individuals from the theatre suite and a relaxed atmosphere.

Operating Theatre

The following are the basic characteristics of modern operating theatre suites:

1. A well-designed layout to facilitate traffic and communication with essential services such as the Theatre Service Sterile Supply Unit, Blood Transfusion, Pathology and Microbiology Departments.
2. Positive-pressure filtered air ventilation with frequent air changes (20/min) to reduce bacterial airborne infection.
3. Piped services for anaesthetic oxygen and other gases, electric power cables for electrocautery, suction and monitoring purposes.
4. Ducting of escaped anaesthetic gases.
5. Monitoring and radiological imaging equipment.
6. Safety features designed to prevent electrical mishaps and discharges from static electricity—waterproof sockets, careful siting of electrical switches well above floor level, antistatic floors and footwear.

Skin Preparation

The skin bacteria comprise a resident and transient group of organisms (*Table* 10.6). The resident flora may change particularly in patients who have been hospitalized for long periods. As it is not possible to sterilize the skin, the term 'preparation' is used. The aim of this is to reduce the resident flora by the application of antiseptic solutions. The various preparations in common usage are shown in *Table* 10.7. In general, their efficacy in terms of reduction of the skin sample counts of viable bacteria is improved by repeated use. All the available antiseptics have limitations. Thus chlorhexidine is not sporicidal.

Table 10.6 Skin bacterial flora

Resident Flora	*Staph. aureus* (some patients)
	Staphylococcus spp.
	Diphtheroids
	Micrococci
	Gram-negative bacilli
Transient Flora	*Staph. aureus*
	Pseudomonas spp.
	Other Gram-negative organisms
	Clostridial spores

The use of intra-abdominal packs soaked in antiseptic solution is used by some surgeons during gastrointestinal surgery. If this practice is adopted, the antiseptic used must not be toxic locally and after absorption into the bloodstream. A fire hazard is well documented when electrocautery is used close to packs soaked in an alcohol-based antiseptic.

Wound Protectors

As the vast majority of wound infections are endogenous in origin, protection of the operative wound from gross contamination is practised by some, either with plastic drapes or

Table 10.7 Antiseptic solutions used for the preoperative preparation of the skin

Preparation	*Mean % reduction in skin-viable bacterial count*	
	After 1 treatment	After 6 treatments
Chlorhexidine, 4%	86·7	99·2
Povidone-iodine, 10%	68	99·7
Hexachlorophane, 3%	46·3	91·9
Irgasan DP 300, 2%	11·2	95·8
Chlorhexidine, 0·5%, in 95% ethanol	97·9	99·7
Phenolic, 0·1%, in 95% ethanol	91·8	99·5
Chlorhexidine, 0·5%, in water	65·1	91·8

Modified from Lowbury E. J. L. (1982) Special problems in hospital antiseptics. In: Russell A. O. (ed). *Principles and Practice of Disinfection, Preservation and Sterilization.* Oxford, Blackwell Scientific Publications. pp. 262–284.

with antiseptic-soaked swabs (chlorhexidine). The disadvantage of plastic drapes is that their removal cannot be achieved without some contamination of the wound. To date, there has not been any firm evidence that the use of wound protectors significantly reduces the incidence of postoperative wound infection.

Infectivity of Surgical Procedures

The majority of infections complicating surgical procedures are endogenous from the patient's own resident organisms. With good modern theatre practice, the risk of airborne infection is low and can be ignored except in prosthetic implant surgery and in the immunocompromised patient. The use of micro-environment modules and biological isolators is an established practice in joint replacement surgery and in patients at risk from opportunistic infections.

It is customary to classify surgical procedures into three categories depending on their infectivity risk. *Clean* operations do not involve bowel and are conducted in the absence of sepsis. Ideally these procedures should carry a negligible infection rate. *Potentially infected* procedures include all elective operations on hollow viscera which usually or on occasions harbour pathogenic organisms, e.g. biliary tract, gastrointestinal tract. The postoperative infection rate of this group is due largely to endogenous infection and can be substantially minimized by appropriate antibiotic prophylaxis and careful surgery designed to avoid spillage of the intraluminal contents into the peritoneal cavity. Procedures carried out for or in the presence of sepsis are referred to as *infected* operations. The surgical principles governing the management of infected cases include treatment of the underlying pathology, efficient peritoneal toilet which entails complete evacuation of pus, detritus and fibrin plaques, and culture of infected material. In addition, there is clear evidence for the value of two procedures in the management of severe intra-abdominal sepsis:

1. Peritoneal lavage with antibiotic–isotonic saline solutions (tetracycline, second-generation cephalosporin).
2. Delayed closure of the abdominal wall. This usually refers to delayed closure of the skin and subcutaneous tissue layers on the premise that wound infection is likely. The muscle layer is closed with non-absorbable monofilament material and the wound is then packed with gauze soaked in proflavine emulsion. In situations where gross sepsis is encountered and recurrent abscess formation is considered likely, the entire wound is left unsutured and the infected region of the peritoneal cavity and the wound are packed. Evisceration is prevented either by the application of an Opsite dressing (*Fig.* 10.2) or by a Marlex mesh (fitted with a zip) which is stitched to the edges of the skin wound. The packing is renewed under intravenous sedation and analgesia at intervals of 1–2 days when the wound and the affected region are inspected and any necessary toilet carried out (*Fig.* 10.3). In these severely septic abdominal cases, the antibiotic regimen must be based on the results of the bacteriological culture and sensitivity tests. Often the infection is a mixed one with both Gram-negative aerobes and anaerobes. Extra precautions are instituted in the operating theatre during and immediately after the completion of infected cases to prevent spread of infection. The theatre is thoroughly cleaned and the floor mopped with antiseptic solution before its further use.

Clean operations should precede potentially infected procedures in elective surgical lists. Infected cases are performed last or preferably in a separate theatre reserved for this purpose.

Prevention of Mishaps and Injuries to the Patient

These avoidable tragedies include: operating on the wrong patient and site, drug abuse, damage to the venous intima, compression or traction injuries, electrocautery burns, and retention of swabs and instruments. These accidents are preventable by attention to detail and by a practice involving inbuilt safety checks designed to approximate as near as possible to the ideal foolproof situation.

Patient Identification

This process starts with the salutory practice of the surgeon having a brief chat with the patient before induction. Apart

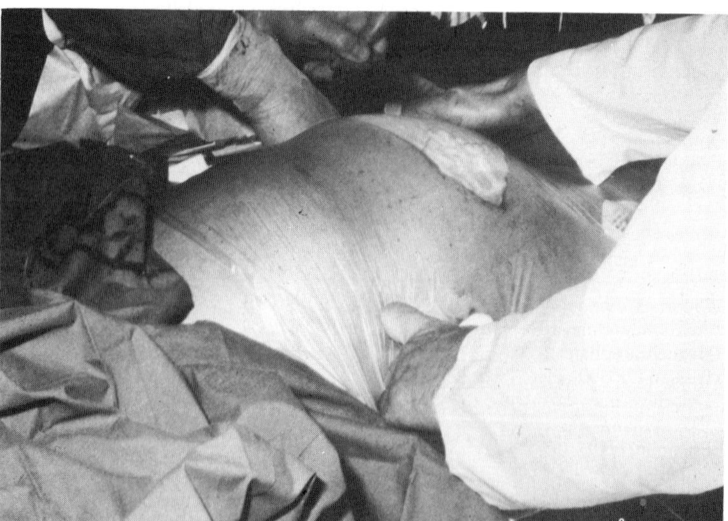

Fig. 10.2 Non-closure of the abdominal wall in severe sepsis (anterior coeliotomy, marsupuliazation). The patient had pancreatic necrosis with peripancreatic abscess formation. After resection of the pancreatic sequestrum, evacuation of the abscess and saline lavage, the space between the transverse colon and the stomach extending between the pancreatic bed and the parietes is packed with proflavine emulsion gauze. Evisceration is prevented by the application of an Opsite dressing.

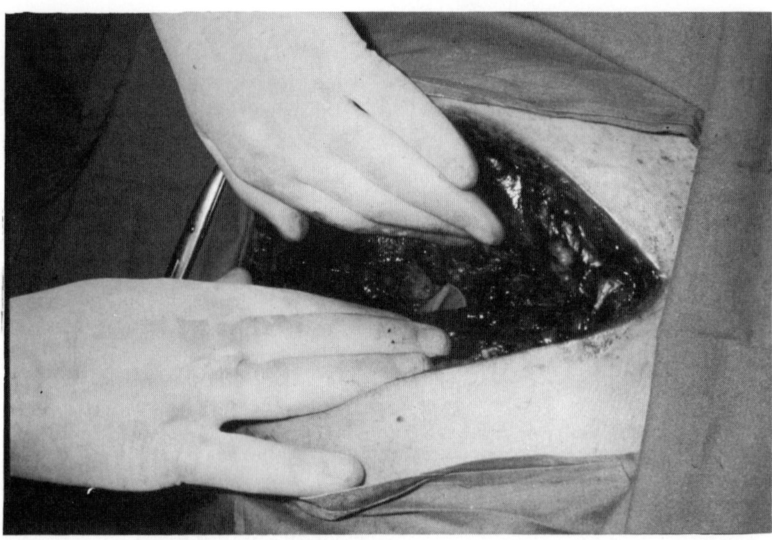

Fig. 10.3 Renewal of the pack and toilet of the cavity is performed every 24–48 h under intravenous sedation in the operating theatre until sepsis is eliminated and healing is well under progress.

from being a source of reassurance to the patient, this occasion provides an opportunity for a final check on the identification of the patient with cross reference to the identification bracelets, case notes, marked operation site and relevant radiographs which should always be put up on the viewing box.

Drug Abuse

This is largely the responsibility of the anaesthetist and covers not only the parenteral administration of drugs during the surgical procedure but also the safe induction and maintenance of general anaesthesia with adequate muscle relaxation. Adverse drug interaction, abnormal reaction to drugs and anaesthetic agents can be avoided or envisaged by adequate preoperative assessment, including detailed drug and anaesthetic histories of the patient.

Damage to the Venous Intima

The use of soft rubber mattresses and careful positioning of the patient minimizes but does not abolish prolonged calf vein compression during prolonged surgical procedures. The use of external pneumatic compression reduces the incidence of deep vein thrombosis. Alternatively, electrical calf-muscle stimulation or graduated compression stockings may be used.

Nerve Injuries

These neuropraxic injuries though recoverable, are a source of temporary anxiety and disability to the patient. They arise from faulty positioning of the patient and are due to compression or traction of nerve trunks. The most common positions of the patient which predispose to these injuries include the Trendelenburg tilt, the left or right lateral thoracic positions, hyperabduction of the arm, and lithotomy. The nerves most commonly injured are the popliteal, brachial plexus, radial and ulnar nerves. Adequate positioning and the use of padding to protect bony prominences are essential safeguards.

Electrocautery Hazards

All diathermy generators (transistorized or valve oscillators) operate within the radiofrequency range of 0·5–3 MHz. In the conventional earthing system, the return pathway of the current is through the patient and the indifferent electrode back to the machine. Faulty equipment and use may cause a number of complications, including thermoelectrical burns to the patient and surgeon, conflagration on the skin surface, electrocution and explosion. The common cause of these mishaps, apart from faulty equipment and inadvertent activation of the diathermy generator, is faulty application of the indifferent electrode (*Fig.* 10.4). In this eventuality, the conventional generator can still work by virtue of its monopolar effect, in which case the current returns through the patient, table, floor and back to the earth terminal of the machine. Any contact of the patient with metallic objects (arm rests, edge of table, stirrups, etc.) which provide earthing will result in a localized current of an intensity high enough to induce a thermoelectrical burn at the point of contact.

Burns and electrical shocks sustained by the surgeon are usually due to an unrecognized hole in the glove which will cause a substantial reduction of the dielectric between a non-insulated dissecting forceps and the surgeon's fingers. The use of insulated diathermy forceps obviates this eventuality.

The modern diathermy generators have earth-free isolated circuits and were developed specifically to prevent the return of electrical current through the earth back to the machine in the event of faulty application of the indifferent electrode. With these modern earth-free generators, the diathermy will not function unless the indifferent electrode is correctly applied to the patient. There is little doubt that the new generation of earth-free electrocautery machines has resulted in a substantial reduction of diathermy accidents. None the less they are not entirely safe and the earth-free circuit can still cause thermoelectrical burns under certain circumstances which include poor insulation of the generator, current leakage and contact of the indifferent electrode with the pedestal of the table.

Retained Swabs and Instruments

It is universal practice nowadays to have three counts, the first two being taken before closure, and the final count

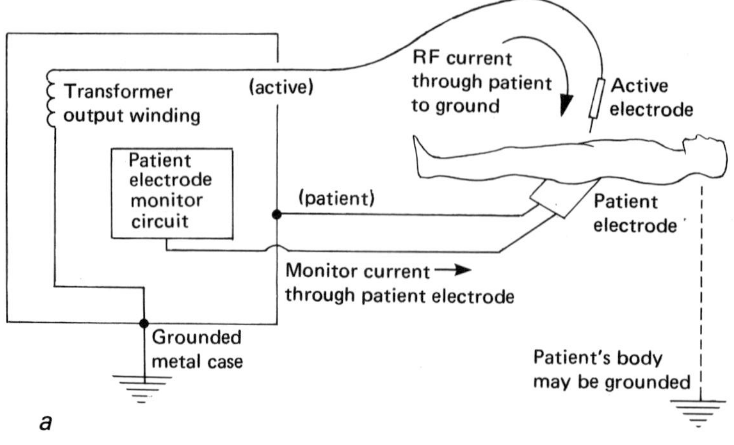

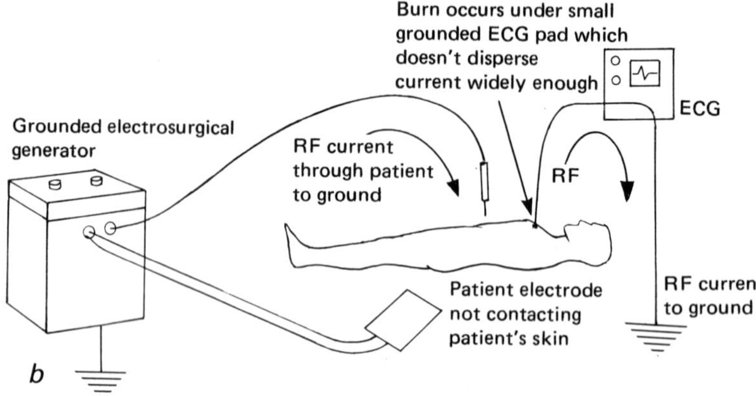

Fig. 10.4 Sequence of events leading to a thermoelectric burn of the patient following faulty application of the indifferent electrode of a diathermy generator using the conventional earthing system. (*a*) Correct application of the indifferent (patient's) electrode. (*b*) Faulty application of the patient's electrode.

before the patient is reversed. The most frequent cause for concern nowadays is a small needle usually from an atraumatic suture. A radiograph of the area is undertaken if after a thorough search and recount the item is still missing.

Use of Surgical Drains

There are few more controversial issues in surgical practice than the use of drains. Some surgeons insert drains routinely, others selectively and an increasing cohort, only when they have to, as in the drainage of abscess cavities. Drains come in various shapes and sizes and are referred to by a confusing array of eponymous names. The major factor which determines the performance of drains is the tissue reaction to the material composition of the drain. *Latex rubber* is soft but excites a profound inflammatory reaction within 24 h which encases the drain, rendering it totally ineffective. *PVC* is much less reactive and therefore more efficient. It is, however, firm and unyielding and tends to harden and split with prolonged use, especially when in contact with bile. The best drain material is *silicone* which is the least reactive, most pliable and shows no tendency to harden with prolonged use.

Drainage Systems

Various systems are used and they are best discussed separately.

Open (Static) Drainage

The drain (Penrose, multitubular, corrugated, Ragnall) is exteriorized either through the operation wound or via a separate stab wound stitched to the skin or held in place by a safety pin and covered with a gauze pad. This type of drainage contributes in a substantial way to wound infection and to the general dissemination of bacteria in surgical wards.

Closed Syphon Drainage

In this system, tube drains of PVC or silicone are connected to drainage bags equipped with a one-way valve at the entrance to the bag and a drainage tap at the opposite end. This allows daily emptying without disruption of the connection between the drain and the collecting bag. Some systems incorporate bacteriological filters as an added precaution against infection via the drain path.

Closed Suction Drainage

Firm polyethylene tubes with multiple perforations are connected to portable suction devices. Some utilize a low pressure vacuum (−100 to −150 mmHg) such as the Portovac and the Reliavac systems. Others employ a higher negative pressure (−300 to −500 mmHg), e.g. Redivac and Sterimed. Closed suction drains are of proven efficacy particularly in the drainage of the parietes. There is little to choose between the various types in terms of efficiency.

Sump Suction Drainage

This is the most efficient system of drainage and is particularly suited to the collection of irritant discharges or those which contain activated digestive enzymes (high small bowel and pancreatic fistulas). The drain has a parallel air vent which prevents the adjacent soft tissues from being sucked into the lumen of the drain when the negative pressure is applied. Some of the available sump suction drains incorporate a bacteriological filter inside the air vent to prevent contamination of the cavity with airborne bacteria. Most are made of PVC but silicone sump suction drains are now available.

Underwater Seal Drainage

This is essential for drainage of the pleural space. The drains are straight or angulated near the tip and are constructed of PVC or silicone.

Indications

The present position regarding the use of drains can best be summarized as follows:

Conditions in which the Use of Drains is a Life-saving Measure

The only disorder that comes into this category is tension pneumothorax where the rapid insertion of an apical drain is the sole factor affecting the immediate survival of the patient. There is an increased incidence of tension pneumothorax in patients on positive-pressure ventilation and prophylactic use of chest drains in these patients has been advocated although this policy is not widely practised.

Conditions in which Drainage Imparts Undoubted Therapeutic Benefit or Constitutes a Safe Prophylactic Measure

These include:

1. Chest drainage—Haemo/pneumothorax, empyema.
2. Thoracotomy, cardiothoracic procedures, oesophageal resections and perforations.
3. Drainage of abscesses and infected cysts.
4. Sump suction drainage for gastrointestinal, biliary and pancreatic fistulas.
5. Closed suction drainage after extensive dissections and elevation of skin flaps.
6. After operations for injuries to solid organs and partial/subtotal excision of vascular organs.

Conditions where Drainage is Generally Advocated but its Value Remains Unproven

Either routine or selective drainage is carried out in the following:

1. Cholecystectomy and exploration of the common bile duct.
2. Duodenal stump after Polya gastrectomy and gastroduodenal anastomosis.
3. Anterior resection, particularly after the low variety.
4. Pancreatic resections.

Conditions where Drainage is Counterproductive

There is good evidence both from retrospective reports and clinical trials that drainage can be harmful either by introducing infection within the peritoneal cavity or by increasing the incidence of wound infection. In one trial it appeared to nullify the beneficial effects of antibiotics on wound infection.

The conditions where drainage is not recommended are:

1. Peritonitis due to perforation of a hollow viscus—the use of drains is certainly no substitute for adequate peritoneal toilet and lavage.
2. Acute appendicitis.
3. Acute pancreatitis.

There is no doubt that drainage is essential after certain surgical procedures. Often, however, there is no reason for its use other than habit. The use of drains must be selective and should be tempered with the realization that drains cause a definite morbidity which includes pain, increased incidence of wound infection, impaired healing, pressure necrosis of oedematous hollow organs, restricted mobility and delayed convalescence.

PREVENTION OF VIRAL DISEASE

Surgeons and their theatre staff are at risk of contracting certain serious and potentially fatal viral disorders. The most important are viral hepatitis, cytomegalovirus infections and acquired immune deficiency syndrome (AIDS). Special procedures are necessary to avoid virus transmission to other patients and the attendant staff. In addition, a clearly laid out protocol should be established for immediate use in the event of accidental exposure. Effective immunization is now possible against hepatitis B infection. In the case of hepatitis A and B, the infectivity of the patient can be ascertained from the serum markers.

Viral Hepatitis

Viral hepatitis is the most common liver disease in the world today. It can result in death during the acute phase from fulminant liver failure due to massive liver cell necrosis, or lead to chronic active hepatitis and cirrhosis, a carrier state, and in the case of the hepatitis B virus (HBV), to the development of primary liver cell cancer. Three types are recognized: Hepatitis A which is caused by the Hepatitis A Virus (HAV), Hepatitis B resulting from infection by the Hepatitis B Virus (HBV), and the non-A non-B variety (also referred to as NANB hepatitis) which has no markers for either the HAV or the HBV or indeed for any other known hepatotropic virus.

Hepatitis A

This was formerly called infectious hepatitis and is caused by an enteric virus (HAV) which is present in the faeces of patients before the development of jaundice. The antibody to the virus is known as anti-HAV. It is present in high titres in the serum early on during the acute infection when it belongs to the IgM class. The IgG antibody indicates past infection and is present in 40–50% of the urban population in Britain.

Hepatitis B

It has been estimated that the HBV is carried by 5% of the world's population. The infection is largely blood borne with an incubation period of 12 weeks. The condition was formerly known as serum or post-transfusion hepatitis. HBV has been fully characterized. The whole virus (viron) is known as the Dane particle and consists of a core covered by surface antigen (HBsAg). The latter is formed in excess as separate tubules and spheres. The core of the virus contains a core antigen (HBcAg) which is never found in the circulating blood, the 'e' antigen (HBeAg), double-stranded DNA, and a DNA polymerase. Antibodies are formed to the

Table 10.8 Guide to the interpretation of serum markers of hepatitis B

HBsA	*HBeAg*	*Anti-HBe*	*Anti-HBc*	*Anti-HBs*	*Interpretation*
+	+	–	–	–	Incubation period or early acute hepatitis B
+	+	–	+	–	Acute hepatitis B or persistent carrier
+	–	+	+	–	Late acute hepatitis B or persistent carrier
+	–	–	+	–	Late acute hepatitis B or persistent carrier
–	–	+	+	+	Convalescent acute hepatitis B
–	–	–	+	+	Past infection

various antigens and can be detected in the peripheral blood (anti-HBs, anti-HBc, anti-HBe). The Dane particle is found in the peripheral blood at some time in all patients during the acute infection and in some carriers. HBsAg is also present in the peripheral blood during the acute stage of the disease and is used to define long-term carriers. The HBeAg is present early on during the course of the acute infection and is usually associated with high titres of HBsAg and the presence of Dane particles (HBV). It is the best marker of probable infectivity and usually converts to anti-HBe soon after jaundice develops. The HBeAg is also found in 15% of carriers. Anti-HBs denotes recovery in acute infection and denotes immunity. Anti-HBc is detected in the peripheral blood early on during the acute infection. It is not protective and is present in all carriers. Anti-HBe is present in convalescent patients and in the majority of carriers. It is associated with a low probability of infectivity. The interpretation of the various serum markers of hepatitis B is outlined in *Table* 10.8.

Hepatitis B is frequently followed by the development of chronic active hepatitis and subsequently, cirrhosis of the liver. The viral genome (DNA) of HBV becomes incorporated in the host DNA and this integration has been shown to be a necessary step in the development of primary liver carcinoma. The role of HBV in the pathogenesis of this tumour is probably greater than has hitherto been realized.

The risk to the surgeon during a 40-year career of contracting hepatitis B has been estimated at 30–40%. The risk of developing fulminant liver failure as a result of the infection is 0·1% and that of a chronic carrier state, 4%. The risk to patients from an infectious surgeon is not known but appears to be remote as only two such occurrences have been reported in the literature and both were cardiothoracic surgeons. Vaccination against hepatitis B is now considered advisable for all surgeons.

NANB Hepatitis

This is diagnosed by exclusion of HAV, HBV, cytomegalovirus and other hepatotropic viruses. It is probably caused by more than one virus but these have not been identified as yet. With the advent of screening of blood donations for the HBsAg, NANB accounts for over 90% of all transfusion-related hepatitis and approximately 7–10% of transfused patients acquire the infection. The disease is also transmitted by Factor VIII and Factor IX concentrates and one report suggests that haemophiliacs develop NANB hepatitis following their first exposure to these concentrates. Outbreaks following intravenous administration of immunoglobulin have been reported. The incubation period varies widely but averages 8 weeks and the disease is clinically indistinguishable from hepatitis A or B. Approximately 40% of patients who contract the NANB infection go on to develop chronic hepatitis.

Hepatitis B Vaccine

There are several effective vaccines against hepatitis B. Most are prepared from fully purified, formalin-inactivated B surface antigen (HBsAg). More recently a recombinant hepatitis B vaccine has been developed and shown to be as active in terms of anti-HBs response as the plasma-derived vaccine. Of the latter, the one most widely used is the vaccine prepared at the Merck Institute of Therapeutic Research. The vaccination programme with the Merck vaccine consists of three 40 mg doses administered at zero time, 2 months and a booster at 6 months. This regimen is effective in preventing the development of hepatitis B if administration is started within a few weeks of exposure, that is after an interval which is less than the incubation period of the disease. It is being used increasingly as a prophylaxis in medical and nursing staff who are accidentally inoculated with HBV by contaminated instruments, e.g. needle pricks and scalpel wounds, either alone or in combination with hyperimmune globulin.

Cytomegalovirus Infections

These are a major cause of morbidity and mortality in immunosuppressed patients. Solid organ transplant patients acquire the infection from the transplanted viscus whereas individuals receiving bone marrow grafts and leukaemic patients are infected by the transfused blood products. Cytomegalovirus (CMV) infections are considered in Chapter 5.

Acquired Immune Deficiency Syndrome

The responsible agent is a retrovirus which is generally known as the Human Immunodeficiency Virus (HIV), formerly known as Human T-cell Lymphotropic Virus type 3 (HTLV3). The virus can persist in the blood for long periods in the presence of antibody (anti-HIV) and has been isolated from blood, semen and saliva. A distinction must be made between HIV infection, AIDS, and persistent generalized lymphadenopathy (PGL). The available information indicates that about 30% of HIV infections result in the development of AIDS and the same proportion result in PGL. AIDS is defined as 'a reliably diagnosed disease which is indicative of an underlying cellular immune deficiency occurring in an individual with no other cause for the immune deficiency or any other defined cause for reduced resistance to the disease'. The 'reliably diagnosed disease' consists of one or more of the following: *Pneumocystis carinii* pneumonia and other opportunistic infections, Kaposi's sarcoma in a patient less than 60 years of age and cerebral lymphoma. Kaposi's sarcoma is a multifocal metastasizing malignant reticulosis consisting of spindle pleomorphic cells separated by spaces without endothelium but containing RBCs. The condition affects predominantly the skin although visceral (liver, spleen and lymph nodes, stomach, colon, heart, lungs) and osseous involvement is not uncommon. The other opportunistic infections are protozoal and helminthic infections (cryptosporidosis, strongyloidosis, toxoplasmosis), fungal infections (aspergillosis, candidiasis, cryptococcosis), bacterial infections (atypical mycobacteriosis), and viral infections (cytomegalovirus, herpes simplex virus and progressive multifocal leukoencephalopathy).

PGL is also known as the AIDS-related complex and is defined as 'the presence of two or more symptoms or signs of specific chronic unexplained conditions for three months or longer, together with two or more abnormal laboratory signs'. The symptoms and signs include non-inguinal lymphadenopathy, weight loss, fever, diarrhoea, fatigue/malaise and night sweats. In addition, two or more of the following laboratory findings must be present: decreased T-helper cells, decreased T-helper/T-suppressor ratio, anaemia or leucopenia or thrombocytopenia, elevated serum globulins, decreased blastogenic response of lymphocytes to mitogens, cutaneous anergy to multiple skin test antigens, and increased levels of circulating immune complexes.

AIDS is largely confined to homosexual and bisexual males (90%) although heterosexual contacts of infected homosexual males may contract the infection which has also been documented in infants born to infected mothers. Drug addicts/users sharing syringes and needles are also at risk. The vast majority of patients with haemophilia A who have received imported Factor VIII have become infected (positive for anti-HIV). To date about one-third have gone on to develop PGL or AIDS and a few have already died of the disease. Some of the sexual partners of seropositive patients with haemophilia A have become positive for anti-HIV. Current evidence indicates that HIV is transmitted by blood and semen. There is no firm evidence for transmission by any other route.

MEASURES DESIGNED TO PREVENT SPREAD OF VIRAL INFECTIONS AMONGST MEDICAL AND NURSING STAFF

Transmission of viral disease to members of staff may occur as a result of:

1. Direct percutaneous inoculation of infected blood, e.g. accidental needle pricks or scalpel wounds.
2. Spillage of infected blood on the skin may introduce infection through minute skin wounds/abrasions.
3. Contamination of mucosal surfaces by infected blood, e.g. accidental splashing of eyes.
4. Transfer of infected material via fomites, e.g. blood-contaminated equipment.

The established procedures designed to minimize transmission of viral disease in hospital practice are:

1. Identification of Patient's Infectivity

By the appropriate serological tests.

2. Special Arrangements for Admission and Ward Care of Infected Patients

These patients should be admitted and kept in single room accommodation (preferably with en suite toilet facilities) and barrier nursing. All staff involved with the patient or handling specimens obtained from him should be aware of the diagnosis. Long-sleeved gowns and masks should be worn by all staff. Additional isolation techniques are necessary when invasive procedures are undertaken, e.g. gloves, plastic aprons and eye protection. Room cleaning should include daily floor mopping and damp dusting with hypochlorite (Chloros diluted 1 in 100 giving 1000 ppm available chlorine).

3. Treatment of Used Disposable Items and Clinical Waste Material

Soft disposables should be double bagged and incinerated. Disposable instruments including needles are placed in an impervious container of metal or thick cardboard before incineration.

4. Treatment of Used Non-disposable Equipment

Whenever possible, these should be sterilized by heat; otherwise chemical disinfection is carried out by soaking for at least one hour either in 2% glutaraldehyde or a 10% dilution of formaldehyde solution BP. However, chemical sterilization is less satisfactory than autoclaving.

5. Additional Precautions by the Operating Team

All the members of the operating team should wear disposable plastic aprons beneath disposable gowns, double gloves and eye goggles. Extra special care is taken to prevent accidental injuries, blood spurting and spillage. All the external surfaces of equipment, trolleys, etc. within the theatre and the floor are wiped with Chloros or glutaraldehyde at the end of the procedure.

6. Disposal of the Deceased

In the event of death, the corpse is inserted in a polythene cadaver bag before coffining and the undertakers should be informed.

POSTOPERATIVE CARE

Following surgery, reversal and extubation, the patient is either transferred to the recovery ward within the operating theatre suite or, in the case of major surgery, directly to the Intensive Care Unit. Detailed postoperative instructions are written down and the drug therapy prescribed in the hospital prescription sheet. The operation notes should be dictated soon after the operation when details are still fresh in the surgeon's mind, meantime a brief note is entered in the case notes on the essential findings and the nature of the surgical procedure. At the end of a period of observation in the recovery ward, if the patient's condition is considered stable, transfer to the ward takes place. Alternatively, the patient's condition may warrant admission to the Intensive Care Unit. The advantages of a recovery ward include:

1. Close observation can be kept on the patient during the early recovery period by fully qualified nurses under supervision by an anaesthetist. This, together with monitoring of the vital signs, allows the early recognition of physiological derangements.
2. The recovery ward is fully equipped with essential services and emergency equipment necessary to deal with the onset of life-threatening complications, e.g. acute hypoxia and cardiac arrest.
3. Immediate access to the operating theatre in the event of a complication, such as haemorrhage, necessitating further surgical intervention.

Pain Relief

This is dealt with in Chapter 13. Satisfactory pain relief is essential for adequate respiratory exchange, effective coughing and early mobilization. Yet despite agreement on these issues, some two-thirds of all surgical patients are allowed to experience pain which is often inadequately treated by inexperienced staff using the standard PRN regimen of postoperative medication with narcotic analgesics. In practice this often means that the availability of the treatment depends on how demanding the patient is and on the attitude of the nursing staff.

Basic Nursing Care and Instructions

Many modern surgical wards are designed on the principle of progressive nursing care whereby the patients are grouped on the extent of observation, care and attention they require from the nursing staff. The postoperative orders on the nature and frequency of observation of the vital signs, treatment, fluid balance and special instructions such as the care of drains, wounds, etc. should be clearly written down on the appropriate charts.

Wound dressings are carried out in the treatment room. The overall management of wounds is outlined in Chapter 1. Whilst therapeutic nasogastric suction is of unquestionable value in the decompression of acute gastric dilatation and established ileus, its routine prophylactic use after abdominal surgery is not recommended as there is no evidence that it imparts any benefit. It increases the discomfort of the patient, limits the efficacy of coughing in clearing bronchial secretions and therefore predisposes to postoperative chest infection.

Certain minor ailments, such as vomiting, nausea, hiccups and minor degrees of abdominal distension and discomfort, are common after surgery and are initially managed with simple conservative measures but when persistent they may indicate the onset of serious complications and the situation then calls for a careful reappraisal.

Postoperative Complications

In general the incidence of postoperative complications is related directly to the preoperative condition of the patient and the magnitude of the surgical procedure, and inversely to the extent of the preoperative preparation and care. The general complications following planned surgical intervention are often the result of intercurrent disease and can usually be anticipated. Complications specific to the operation are a reflection of surgical expertise, surgical judgement and operative decision-making, and the nature and site of the disease for which surgery was performed. Other things being equal, the incidence of postoperative complications is highest for emergency procedures, intermediate for urgent operations and lowest for elective or planned intervention. The important postoperative complications are shown in *Table* 10.9 which also lists the various relevant chapters. The incidence of all these complications can be minimized with good preoperative care and early ambulation, together with the use of specific prophylactic measures whenever indicated. Complications specific to a particular operation are reduced as a result of careful surgical technique and experience.

Table 10.9 Postoperative complications

Complication	*Relevant chapters*
Respiratory: collapse, infection, aspiration, pulmonary insufficiency	9, 10, 13, 38
Cardiovascular complications	6, 10, 55
Thromboembolic disease	9, 57
Postoperative haemorrhage	6
Sepsis	3, 6
Gastrointestinal derangements: paralytic ileus acute gastric dilatation, anastomotic failure	67, 75
Postoperative retention of urine	82
Postoperative renal failure	6, 81
Postoperative jaundice, hepatic insufficiency	69
Wound infection and dehiscence	1, 3, 76
Postoperative confusion and neuropsychiatric disturbances. Cerebrovascular accidents	
Others: acute parotitis, acalculous cholecystitis, etc.	24, 69

Postoperative Pulmonary Complications

Respiratory Changes Consequent on Anaesthesia and Surgery

During the administration of general anaesthesia, there is an increase in the right-to-left shunting of the pulmonary blood flow and a depression in the ciliary activity of the bronchial mucosa. These changes are temporary and pulmonary function has usually returned to normal within one hour of surgery and general anaesthesia. None the less, hypoxaemia is extremely common during the first two postoperative days. The hypoxaemia is the result of diaphragmatic elevation which causes a reduction in the functional residual capacity (FRC) and underventilation of the lung bases to which the greater proportion of the pulmonary blood flow is distributed. Elevation and tenting of the diaphragm is due to an increase in the abdominal pressure usually from gastrointestinal distension and to pain, particularly from upper abdominal vertical wounds, which induces reflex contraction of the abdominal musculature. The rise in the intra-abdominal pressure after surgery is especially pronounced after reduction and repair of large ventral hernias and in the morbidly obese.

An increased bronchorrhoea is encountered in habitual smokers and in patients with chronic bronchitis. The impaired ciliary activity in these two groups further aggravates the bronchiolar and bronchial obstruction by viscid mucus plugs. The categories of patients at risk of respiratory complications are shown in *Table* 10.10. Thoracic operations are not accompanied by an increased risk of postoperative pulmonary complications. The important postoperative pulmonary complications are: pulmonary collapse and consolidation, aspiration, pulmonary embolism and respiratory insufficiency.

Pulmonary Collapse and Consolidation

Although the terms atelectasis and collapse are often used synonymously, atelectasis refers to lung parenchyma which has never been expanded. The correct term for the postoperative condition is therefore pulmonary collapse. This arises from impaired ventilation of the lung bases and accumulation of bronchial secretions. It may be patchy and segmental or more extensive with unilateral or bilateral lobar collapse. Oxygenation is impaired and hypoxaemia of varying severity ensues. Infection with consolidation often supervenes in the collapsed lobe or segment, the most common organisms responsible being *Haemophilus influenzae* and *Streptococcus pneumoniae*, although coliform infections are not uncommon after abdominal operations. The clinical picture is extremely varied. On the one hand, the patient may experience little inconvenience. Others develop

Table 10.10 Patients at risk of postoperative pulmonary complications

Condition	*Mechanism*
Obesity	Reduced functional residual capacity
Chronic obstructive airways disease	Secretional airway obstruction from bronchorrhoea and absence of ciliary activity
Chronic smokers	Secretional airway obstruction from bronchorrhoea, diminished ciliary activity, carboxyhaemoglobinaemia
Restrictive airways disease	Diminished vital capacity
Elderly and enfeebled	Aspiration
Cystic fibrosis	Bronchial obstruction by viscid secretions, pneumothorax
Operation damage to recurrent laryngeal nerve(s)	Ineffective cough, aspiration. Respiratory obstruction if bilateral

a mild pyrexia and a productive cough and are rapidly improved with physiotherapy aimed at encouraging deep breathing and expectoration of bronchial secretions. In the elderly, obese, chronic smokers or patients with pre-existing pulmonary disease, the condition is more severe with tachypnoea, cyanosis, dullness to percussion over the lower lobe(s) and bronchial breathing. These patients require antibiotic treatment, oxygen administered with a controlled oxygen therapy mask giving an inspired O_2 concentration of 30–40%, humidification and vigorous physiotherapy. Co-trimoxazole is the first-line antibiotic most commonly used in postoperative chest infections until the results of the sputum culture and sensitivity tests become available. If the chest radiograph shows extensive collapse—lobar or pulmonary, urgent fibreoptic bronchoscopy and clearing of the bronchial secretions by powerful suction is necessary. However, some rely initially on nasally-introduced endobronchial catheters for this purpose and proceed to bronchoscopy if this method, in association with physiotherapy, proves unsuccessful. Vigorous physiotherapy is maintained to prevent further collapse and the situation is monitored by daily postero-anterior chest radiographs. All patients with serious chest infections and lung collapse should have repeated blood gas estimations and the arterial Po_2 should not be allowed to fall below 10 kPA (75 mmHg). In a few patients, the secretional airway obstruction continues despite energetic therapy. These patients require endotracheal intubation and assisted ventilation. Some may, however, be considerably improved by the use of the minitracheostomy (*Fig.* 10.5). This disposable device which permits the insertion of a fine catheter into the tracheal lumen through the cricothyroid membrane is very effective in clearing the bronchial secretions in patients who are unable to expectorate effectively despite adequate physiotherapy (*see also* p. 631).

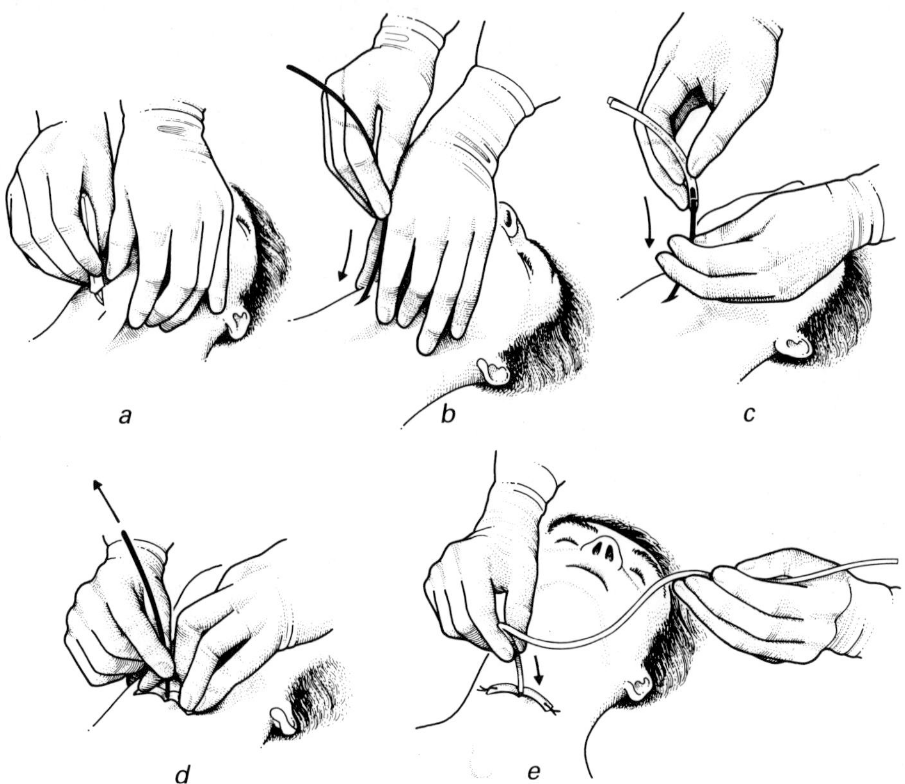

Fig. 10.5 The Mini-Trach (disposable minitracheostomy kit). This consists of a 4·0 mm PVC cannula (*c*) which is introduced over a plastic curved introducer (*b*) through a small stab incision in the skin (*a*) and cricothyroid membrane after the application of local anaesthetic solution. The end of the cannula is split into two wings which are stitched to the skin (*d*). The correct positioning of the cannula which has a radio-opaque marker, is checked by radiology to ensure that the tip is in the trachea and not down the right or left bronchus. The cannula is wide enough to admit the insertion of endobronchial suction catheters (*e*). The technique is invaluable in patients with persistent secretional airway obstruction despite vigorous physiotherapy and obviates the need of formal tracheostomy in many of these patients.

Two other options are used routinely in high-risk cases in some centres. The use of the disposable incentive spirometer (*Fig.* 10.6) greatly improves deep breathing and is of undoubted benefit if the patient is well motivated and uses it. Alternatively, others prefer the Entonox apparatus which is premixed with 50% nitrous oxide in oxygen to achieve the same objective and administer additional analgesia. More recently the use of the respiratory stimulant doxapram as an intravenous infusion (1·0–1·5 mg/kg) during the first two hours of the postoperative period, has been reported to improve arterial oxygen during the first two postoperative days. However, this drug is contraindicated in patients with ischaemic heart disease as it is a powerful myocardial stimulant and may cause severe arrhythmias.

Aspiration

Massive aspiration of the gastric contents into the bronchopulmonary tree is a serious complication which may proceed to cardiorespiratory failure and continues to carry a high mortality. Minor degrees of pulmonary aspiration are common and manifest themselves clinically as postoperative pneumonia and pulmonary abscess. The presence of a cuffed endotracheal tube is not a complete safeguard against minor degrees of aspiration which is also well documented in patients with a tracheostomy. In this respect, large-volume low-pressure cuff tubes are said to be more protective than the standard variety although recent evidence casts doubts on this assumption. Prophylactic nasogastric intubation after elective abdominal surgery increases the risk of aspiration.

Massive aspiration occurs either during induction and endotracheal intubation or during recovery from general anaesthesia, particularly in the elderly and enfeebled. Later on during the postoperative period, the condition may complicate acute gastric dilatation and paralytic ileus. In the emergency situation, a full stomach is a well-recognized hazard and underlies the importance of aspiration of the stomach contents prior to induction of general anaesthesia.

Massive aspiration of gastric contents induces severe bronchospasm and a chemical pneumonitis which is associated with significant fluid shifts from the circulating blood to the pulmonary parenchyma and circulatory collapse. In addition, the patient becomes markedly cyanosed and tachypnoeic. Moist rales and diminished air entry, particularly over the lung bases, are found on auscultation. The condition may progress to the adult respiratory distress syndrome with myocardial failure requiring inotropic support. The treatment entails vigorous suction toilet of the bronchial tree, administration of pure oxygen by intermittent positive-pressure ventilation, bronchodilators, methylprednisolone and antibiotics.

Other Pulmonary Complications

These include pneumothorax and pleural effusion. The most common cause of pneumothorax in the postoperative period is insertion of a central venous or feeding line and a chest radiograph is necessary after this procedure to exclude this potential complication. There is also an enhanced risk of pneumothorax in patients on positive-pressure ventilation presumably from rupture of pre-existing bullae. The insertion of an underwater seal drain is usually followed by rapid expansion of the lung. Negative suction is applied to the system if the expansion of the lung is delayed or becomes static after initial improvement. Intrapleural tetracycline is administered to promote pleural adhesions and fixation of the lung to the chest wall in resistant or recurrent cases.

Pleural effusions may be secondary to other pulmonary pathology such as collapse/consolidation, pulmonary infarction and secondary deposits. They may also result from congestive cardiac failure. A pleural effusion following oesophageal resection indicates leakage from the anastomosis and precedes the development of a frank empyema. As air, in addition to fluid, leaks into the pleural space from the oesophageal lumen, the chest radiograph shows a distinct fluid level (*Fig.* 10.7). A unilateral pleural effusion occurring late in the postoperative period usually signifies subdiaphragmatic infection.

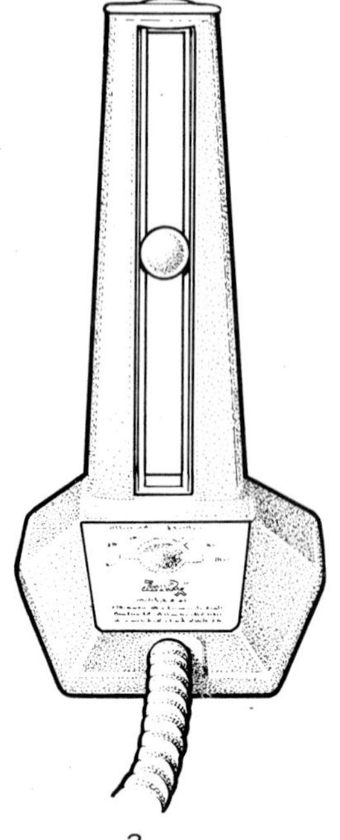

a

DIAL SETTING

1800	1800	3600	5400	7200	9000	10,800	12,600	14,400	16,200	18,000
1440	1440	2880	4320	5760	7200	8640	10,080	11,520	12,960	14,400
1095	1095	2190	3285	4380	5475	6570	7665	8760	9855	10,950
765	765	1530	2295	3060	3825	4590	5355	6120	6885	7650
505	505	1010	1515	2020	2525	3030	3535	4040	4545	5050
285	285	570	855	1140	1425	1710	1995	2280	2565	2850
145	145	290	435	580	725	870	1015	1160	1305	1450
	1	2	3	4	5	6	7	8	9	10

SECONDS PATIENT HOLDS BALL AT THE TOP

Figures represent minimum volume in cubic centimetres.

b

Fig. 10.6 Incentive spirometer: *a*, The calibrated dial of this disposable instrument indicates the minimum flow (ml/sec) at the various dial settings which are required to be generated by the patient's inspiratory effort to raise the ball to the top of the flow chamber. *b*, The chart shows the minimum volume obtained for efforts up to 10 seconds in length at the various settings.

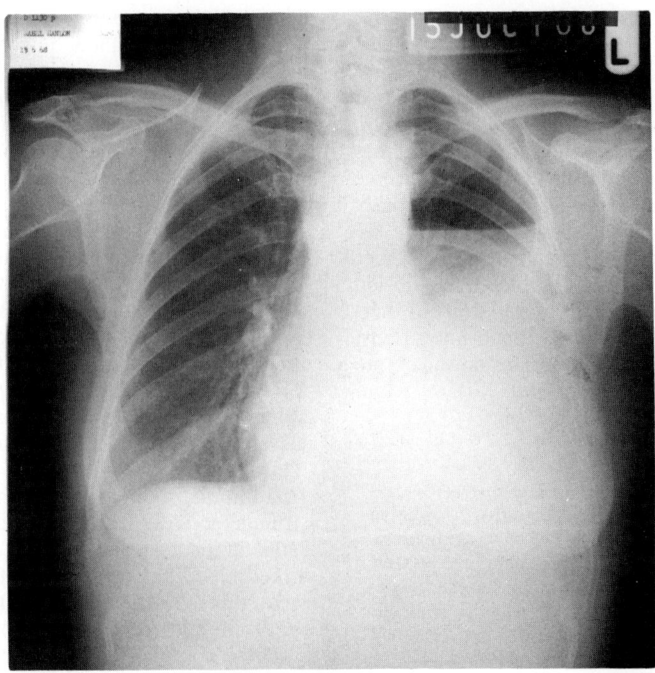

Fig. 10.7 Postero-anterior chest radiograph depicting a fluid level after dilatation of an oesophageal stricture indicating escape of fluid and air from the oesophageal lumen.

Postoperative Cerebral Complications

These include cerebrovascular accidents and various neuropsychiatric disturbances, some of which can be predicted and their severity, if not incidence, reduced by careful preoperative management.

Cerebrovascular Accidents

These are often precipitated by sudden hypotension during or after surgery in elderly hypertensive patients with severe atherosclerosis. Postoperative strokes are also a well-documented hazard after carotid endarterectomy and occur in 1–3% of these operations. They may arise from emboli released at or after surgery, ischaemia during the period of carotid clamping, and postoperative thrombosis of the internal carotid artery. Cerebrovascular accidents may also complicate open cardiac surgery although this is less common nowadays as a result of the increased safety and efficiency of modern extracorporeal perfusion systems.

Neuropsychiatric Disturbances

These are frequent and cover a wide spectrum of disorders. The commonest is *mental confusion* with agitation and disorientation in the elderly. This may arise on a background of senile dementia due to cerebral atrophy but is often precipitated or worsened by the injudicious administration of sedative and hypnotic drugs. A metabolic cause should be excluded in all cases, irrespective of age. Mental confusion, altered sleep rhythm and increasing somnolence may be the result of hepatic encephalopathy in patients with chronic liver disease. *Anxiety* and *depression* are common in cancer patients and often require medication with anxiolytics in addition to reassurance, especially when the surgical treatment is considered to be potentially curative. *Acute toxic confusional state* is a well-recognized acute psychiatric disorder which occurs in some patients during a serious illness or after a major surgical intervention. It must be differentiated from relapses of previous psychiatric disorders, such as schizophrenia, and requires expert management by a psychiatrist and constant observation by a special nurse.

There is a syndrome which affects patients who are recovering from a major illness or operation in Intensive Care Units. It is variously referred to as the ICU syndrome, silent psychosis, and postcardiotomy delirium when it follows open heart surgery. The patient's perception and memory are impaired and is unable to think and hold a conversation. He may become restless or apathetic or confused and in severe cases, delirious. The condition is thought to result from sleep deprivation, pain, prolonged drug administration, anxiety and fear. Full recovery is the norm but this may take several weeks to months.

Delirium Tremens (Acute Alcohol Withdrawal Syndrome)

This can be predicted in most instances from a detailed medical and drinking history. Prodromal symptoms include anxiety and tremors. The fully developed condition is characterized by extreme agitation and overactivity, visual hallucinations, total confusion, pyrexia and, less commonly, convulsions. It leads to rapid dehydration and often to abdominal wound dehiscence. Chlormethiazole 0·8% (Heminevrin) is administered as an intravenous infusion of 30–50 ml. The solution is run quickly at 60 drops/min (4 ml/min) until the patient becomes drowsy. Thereafter the drip rate is decreased to 10–15 drops/min and frequent checks on the level of consciousness are maintained. Oral therapy with chlormethiazole capsules is commenced as soon as possible. Chlormethiazole is contraindicated in acute pulmonary insufficiency. Adequate rehydration and the correction of metabolic alkalosis are important features of the management of these patients. Prevention of delirium tremens in susceptible patients can be achieved by the administration of intravenous alcohol (5% ethanol in 5% dextrose, 150 ml/h) to maintain the blood alcohol level at 2–10 mg/100 ml.

BLOOD TRANSFUSION

There can be little doubt that the major advances in operative surgery were made possible by the availability of blood transfusion. The beneficial impact of blood transfusion on survival which spanned right across the surgical disciplines was not, however, achieved without certain mishaps, some of which have only been realized recently. Other previously unrecognized hazards primarily of an infective nature are likely to emerge in the future. This cumulative experience has resulted in a change of attitude to blood transfusion which is nowadays regarded as a form of replacement therapy to be used only for certain clearly defined indications. The blood products available to the clinicians nowadays are shown in *Table* 10.11.

Table 10.11 Blood products

I. Whole blood	Anticoagulant/preservative solution most commonly used is acid-citrate-dextrose (ACD). Other preservative solutions used are citrate-phosphate-dextrose (CPD) which maintains higher red cell levels of 2,3-DPG, and ACD-adenine which increases the storage time permissible (35–42 days).
II. Blood components	i. Red cells ii. Platelets iii. Granulocytes iv. Whole plasma (fresh frozen, reconstituted v. Cryoprecipitate (Factor VIII)
III. Plasma fractions	i. Clotting factor concentrates ii. Immunoglobulin preparations: human normal immunoglobulin (HNI) and human specific immunoglobulin (HSI) iii. Saline albumin solution (also known as plasma protein fraction) iv. Salt-poor albumin

There are three indications for the transfusion of blood and blood products:

1. Hypovolaemia.
2. Diminished red cell mass.
3. Specific blood component deficiencies—component replacement therapy (Factor VIII, platelets, etc.).

Volume Replacement

The need to replace a depleted blood volume may arise as a result of haemorrhage or burns. It is also required by those surgical procedures involving the use of an extracorporeal circulation. Blood transfusion is not required for moderate blood loss (up to 1·0 L). In this situation the blood volume should be replaced by plasma protein fraction (PPF) or an artificial plasma expander (Dextran, Hemaccel). PPF is nowadays used in preference to dried reconstituted human plasma because of the following advantages: availability, less risk of disease transmission and a more balanced electrolyte content.

Blood transfusion is, however, necessary for massive haemorrhage. Restoration of the blood volume is started with a rapid transfusion of PPF or whatever is available (plasma expanders, electrolyte solutions). As the loss of the red cell mass is substantial, the replacement by blood transfusion at an early stage in severe haemorrhage is necessary. The recently introduced rapid low ionic strength compatibility techniques allow provision of fully crossmatched blood as promptly as former emergency procedures, i.e. within 30 min. Thus the use of unmatched group O Rh-negative blood is rarely justified in modern hospital practice.

A transfusion which is equivalent to the patient's own blood volume within 12 h is defined as a massive blood transfusion. This is attended by certain metabolic, haemodynamic and respiratory complications especially when the transfusion requirements are carried out entirely with stored (ACD) blood. On storage at 4 °C, the red cells lose their 2,3-diphosphoglycerate activity (2,3-DPG) resulting in an increased affinity for oxygen. Stored blood has few functioning platelets and is deficient in clotting factors (V, VIII). Both the pH and the K^+ content are increased with storage and these may impair myocardial function. The elevated citrate level after massive blood transfusion leads to a lowering of the ionized Ca^{++} level of the patient's blood. In addition, significant hypothermia may be induced in a patient receiving large quantities of stored blood. The presence of platelet and leucocyte aggregates (50–200 μm) in stored blood has been implicated as one of the aetiological factors in the development of the adult respiratory distress syndrome (postperfusion lung).

These complications can be largely prevented or minimized by the adoption of certain measures. These include the administration of 1 unit of fresh blood for every 5–10 units of stored blood, and intravenous 10% calcium gluconate, 10 ml for every litre of transfused citrated blood. Warming of the blood prior to transfusion is necessary when the infusion rate exceeds 50 ml/min, during massive transfusions, in exchange transfusion in the neonate and in patients with strong cold agglutinins. The use of micro-aggregate blood filters is generally recommended during massive transfusion and is thought to diminish the incidence of the adult respiratory distress syndrome. However, their benefit has never been established by clinical trials and their use leads to a further loss of platelets and coagulation factors, and incurs a theoretical risk of disseminated intravascular coagulation by the generation of thromboplastin.

Blood Transfusion Requirements for Surgical Procedures

Recurrent shortages of blood are becoming increasingly common in hospital practice. To some extent this is the result of wastage of red cell units through outdating which is consequent on the widespread practice of ordering more blood to cover operations than is actually needed. Several audit surveys in the UK and USA have shown an excessively high ratio of blood crossmatched to that transfused. Wastage is enhanced when, as often happens, the Blood Transfusion Department is not informed soon enough that some or all of the blood has not been used. Recrossmatching of the blood which has not been transfused is therefore delayed often to the extent that it cannot be used for other patients. This unnecessary crossmatching of blood has led a number of Regional Transfusion Centres to formulate 'Tariffs' (maximum blood order schedules) which indicate the appropriate amounts of blood to be crossmatched for the various operations (*Table* 10.12). The use of these tariffs is combined with a policy of performing only the blood grouping and antibody screening in those patients undergoing operations which do not usually require blood. The tariff for any given operation may be increased by virtue of certain clinical considerations, such as anaemia, anticipated finding of malignancy, previous radiotherapy, reoperation, etc. The tariff practice has been validated by a number of studies which have demon-

Table 10.12 Maximum surgical blood order tariff

Operation	*Blood requirements*		
	Routine tariff group and screening procedure (G+S) or units crossmatched	Increased tariff due to clinical considerations	Indication leading to increased tariff
General Surgery			
Abdominoperineal resection	4		
Bowel resection	3		
Breast biopsy/lumpectomy	G + S		
Cholecystectomy	G + S		
Partial gastrectomy	G + S		
Total gastrectomy	3	4	Thoracotomy
Haemorrhoidectomy	G + S		
Hernia repair	G + S		
Ileostomy	G + S		
Laparotomy	G + S	2	Malignancy
Liver biopsy	G + S		
Radical mastectomy	2		
Simple mastectomy	G + S		
Splenectomy (elective)	2		
Thyroidectomy	G + S		
Vagotomy (Truncal, HSV)	G + S		
Varicose vein operations	G + S		
Urology			
Partial cystectomy	2		
Total cystectomy	4		
Transurethral resection of bladder lesions	G + S	2	Larger tumours
Nephrectomy	2		
Nephrolithotomy	2		
Prostatectomy	2		
Thoracic Surgery			
Oesophagogastrectomy	4		
Hiatus hernia	G + S		
Pneumothorax	G + S		
Thoracotomy for pulmonary resection	3	4	Reoperation
Mediastinoscopy	2		
Arterial Surgery			
Aortic aneurysm	6	10–12	Ruptured
Femoropopliteal bypass	3		

(After Napier J. A. F. et al. (1985) *Br. Med. J.* **291**, 799–801, by courtesy of the Editor.)

strated its safety and efficiency in terms of a substantial reduction in the amount of unused and wasted blood.

Anaemia

As the anaemic patient is more liable to haemodynamic complications, especially circulatory overload, blood transfusion should be avoided in the anaemic patient whenever possible. Furthermore, a firm diagnosis of the morphological type and therefore the likely cause of the anaemia should be made before blood is transfused. The indications for blood transfusion of the anaemic patient are:

1. The presence of a critically low haemoglobin level.
2. An impending surgical operation.
3. Refractory anaemia—blood dyscrasias, chronic renal disease, etc.

All patients with a haemoglobin level of 7·0 g/l or less require a blood transfusion. If this is administered as red-cell concentrates, the rate should not exceed 250 ml in 4 h. This amount raises the haemoglobin level by 1–1·5 g/l. Alternatively, whole blood may be administered at a rate of 500 ml every 6 h, preferably covered with a loop diuretic (frusemide) to remove the excess fluid. In any event all anaemic patients should be transfused only during the day and observed closely for signs of circulatory overload.

Whenever possible, preoperative anaemia which is usually of the iron deficiency type, should be treated by haematinics (oral iron) and blood transfusion avoided. If the operation is urgent, the management depends on the severity of the anaemia and the nature of the intended operation, together with a realistic estimate (tariff) of the likely blood loss during surgery. Thus patients with a haemoglobin of 10·0 g or more do not require a preoperative blood transfusion but the requirement for crossmatched blood is increased by an extra 2–3 units above the usual tariff for the operation. If blood transfusion is considered necessary before an operation (Hb $<$ 10·0 g), it is advisable for this to be carried out at least two days before the operation to allow for haemodynamic adjustment and the recovery of function of the transfused red cells.

Transfusion of Fresh Blood

The indications for the use of fresh blood are fortunately

infrequent. They include disseminated intravascular coagulation, massive haemorrhage, major liver trauma and bleeding associated with liver disease. The transfusion of fresh blood for haemorrhagic disorders has been largely replaced by fresh frozen plasma, blood component and clotting factor(s) therapy.

Platelet Transfusions

Transfusion of platelet concentrates ($0{\cdot}8 \times 10^{11}$ platelets/unit) may be necessary in the presence of bleeding due to severe thrombocytopenia. Serious bleeding is unlikely if the platelet count exceeds 40 000/μl. In surgical practice, the need for platelet transfusion may arise after massive blood replacement, open heart surgery, hepatic transplantation and in patients with bleeding oesophageal varices. Estimates of the platelet transfusion requirements are based on the patient's platelet count and his surface area. The factors which adversely effect platelet survival in the circulation include active bleeding, splenomegaly, platelet antibodies, drugs, fever and disseminated intravascular coagulation. A decline in the haemostatic efficacy is observed with repeated platelet transfusions. Platelet concentrates must be administered using a specially designed platelet infusion set which incorporates a filter to remove any platelet aggregates which, if infused, become trapped in the pulmonary capillaries and cause pulmonary oedema.

Frozen Red Cell Bank

With the use of cryoprotective agents (glycerol, hydroxyethyl starch), satisfactory storage of red cells at −80° to −196 °C (mechanical deep freezing or liquid nitrogen storage) for long periods up to 10 years has been achieved. This method of storage removes leucocytes, platelets and any viral particles, thereby reducing the incidence of both transmission of viral diseases and immunization to tissue antigens. Red cells recovered from a frozen bank are consequently of particular value to patients on a renal dialysis programme and are being increasingly used in transplant surgery including hepatic transplantation.

Blood Transfusion Reactions

It is important to appreciate that the hazards of blood transfusion are not limited to the recipient but also affect the donor, and it is well for the clinician to be aware of this, especially in a society where blood is donated by unpaid volunteers, as though extremely rare, deaths from myocardial infarction and cerebral thrombosis have been reported in donors of blood. The usual minor complications encountered in blood donors are bruising, local reaction to antiseptics/dressings and vasovagal attacks.

The complications of transfusion of blood and blood components in the recipient are shown in *Table* 10.13.

Table 10.13 Complications of blood transfusion in the recipient

I. Febrile reactions	
II. Bacterial contamination	
III. Immune reactions	
IV. Physical complications	i. Circulatory overload ii. Air embolism iii. Pulmonary embolism iv. Thrombophlebitis v. ARDS
V. Metabolic complications	i. Hyperkalaemia ii. Citrate toxicity and hypocalcaemia iii. Release of vasoactive peptides iv. Release of plasticizers from PVC-phthalates
VI. Transmission of disease	i. Hepatitis: B, NANB, less commonly A, cytomegalovirus (CMV), and Epstein–Barr virus (EBV) ii. AIDS (Factor VIII) iii. Syphilis iv. Brucellosis v. Toxoplasmosis vi. Malaria vii. American trypanosomiasis (Chagas' disease)
VII. Haemorrhagic reactions	i. After massive transfusion of stored blood ii. Disseminated intravascular coagulation
VIII. Haemosiderosis	After repeated transfusion in patients with haematological disease

Febrile Reactions

The routine establishment of quality control in the manufacture of both intravenous fluids and disposable giving sets has virtually eliminated pyrogenic reactions. Pyrexia following blood transfusion is nowadays usually due to leucocyte incompatibility. These reactions are usually encountered after multiple transfusions and their occurrence indicates the need for leucocyte antibody testing in these patients should further transfusion be required, in which case leucocyte-poor blood should be used.

Transfusion of Contaminated Blood

A number of bacterial species, such as pseudomonas and coliforms, multiply in stored blood at 4 °C. These psychrophilic bacteria metabolize the citrate and produce endotoxins. The effect of transfusion of such contaminated blood is catastrophic and often fatal. Fortunately the complication is rare. Although gross contamination may be obvious by the presence of marked haemolysis resulting in black discoloration of the blood, not infrequently there is no discernible change in the macroscopic appearance of the blood even on close inspection. The clinical picture is dominated by profound circulatory collapse, dyspnoea, vomiting and diarrhoea within minutes of the start of the transfusion, and the development of disseminated intravascular coagulation. Treatment entails the immediate cessation of the transfusion, institution of antibiotic therapy active against coliforms and pseudomonas, together with the necessary supportive measures to combat the endotoxic shock. Treatment with monoclonal antibody to endotoxin has been shown to reduce the mortality in septicaemic patients and it seems likely that this form of treatment will become a useful adjunct in the management of these patients. The blood should be returned to the laboratory for culture and emergency investigation of centrifuged specimens for organisms and free haemoglobin.

Physical Complications

These include heart failure, air embolism and pulmonary thromboembolic disease. Air embolism has been virtually abolished with the introduction of plastic packs. Pulmonary embolism of aggregates of leucocytes and platelets may arise during massive transfusion of stored blood and lead to adult respiratory distress syndrome.

Immune Reactions

These are classified as haemolytic and non-haemolytic reactions. The classic haemolytic reaction results from the transfusion of ABO incompatible blood. Despite accurate red-cell grouping tests and sensitive matching methods, this complication is still encountered, largely from wrong donations since the administration to a patient of the wrong blood carries a 1 in 3 chance of ABO incompatibility. The patient experiences severe back pain, marked dyspnoea and develops profound shock soon after the start of the transfusion. Urticaria is frequent. The urine becomes dark red (haemoglobinuria) and the urine output falls often with the development of renal failure. The condition may also be further complicated by the development of disseminated intravascular coagulation. Treatment consists of cessation of the blood transfusion, careful monitoring of the patient and supportive management of the complications (renal failure, DIC).

Non-haemolytic reactions include severe immediate hypersensitivity reactions and mild allergic or anaphylactoid reactions. Both are reactions to transfused immunoglobulins (IgA) as a result of anti-IgA in the patient's plasma. The reaction results in the release of vasoactive peptides and activation of complement. The severe anaphylactic reaction is accompanied by profound hypotension, dyspnoea and cutaneous flushing. It is fortunately rare (1 in 20 000 transfusions) and responds to the termination of the transfusion, intravenous hydrocortisone and subcutaneous adrenaline. Antihistamines are used in the prophylaxis and active treatment of non-allergic reactions accompanied by urticaria.

Repeated transfusions as in patients with refractory anaemias and renal dialysis patients often result in alloimmunization to leucocyte and platelet antigens. This is the commonest cause of severe febrile reactions in these patients. In these situations the administration of red cells from which most of the other formed elements have been removed (leucocytes, platelets, soluble histocompatibility antigens) is used. This leucocyte-poor blood may be prepared in several ways: inverted centrifugation, dextran sedimentation, nylon filtration, saline washing and recovery of red cells from the frozen bank.

Transmission of Disease

Bacterial, protozoal and viral disorders can be transmitted by blood transfusion (*Table* 10.13). With the establishment of the screening of donors for evidence of present or past infection with the HBV, hepatitis B is now a rare complication of blood transfusion, and most instances of post-transfusion hepatitis are due to non-A non-B disease (NANB). The development of AIDS in haemophilia patients who received Factor VIII has been a most unfortunate experience and points to other as yet unknown hazards of blood transfusion which should never be undertaken lightly.

Effect of Blood Transfusion on Survival of Renal Allografts

There is now good evidence that the transfusions of autologous compatible blood prior to renal transplantation improve the overall survival of renal grafts. The exact reason(s) for this beneficial effect is unknown but two hypotheses have been put forward. The first is based on the premise that transfusions hyperimmunize the patient. Thus when high-dose immunosuppression is given at the time of transplantation, the clones of reactive cells are killed or inactivated. By contrast, in the non-transfused patients, the high dose immunosuppression administered at the time of transplantation does not coincide with the period of maximal immune stimulation and activity which occurs with the onset of rejection. The second hypothesis postulates that after repeated blood transfusions and the consequent development of HLA antibodies, it is difficult to match the patient, but should a match be found, the chances of graft survival will be enhanced.

Effect of Blood Transfusion on Survival after Surgery for Cancer

Several studies, all of which have been retrospective, have shown that patients with cancer, especially colorectal, survive longer if they do not receive blood transfusions at the time of their surgical treatment. In addition, tumour recurrence rate is four times higher in patients who are transfused in the perioperative period when compared with those who do not receive blood. Although they have not been confirmed by prospective controlled clinical studies, these findings are worrying and stress the importance of avoiding perioperative blood transfusion in patients undergoing colonic resection for carcinoma. The measures which help to achieve this objective include: treatment of preoperative anaemia by oral iron supplements, use of controlled preoperative haemodilution with autotransfusion and prevention of surgical bleeding.

Further Reading

Cheadle W. G., Vitale G. C., Mackie C. R. et al. (1985) Prophylactic postoperative nasogastric decompression: A prospective study of its requirement and the influence of cimetidine in 200 patients. *Ann. Surg.* **202,** 361–366.

Chodoff P., Margand P. M. S. and Knowles C. L. (1975) Short term abstinence from smoking: its place in preoperative preparation. *Crit. Care Med.* **31,** 131–133.

Dudrick S. J., Baue A. E., Eiseman B. et al. (ed.) (1983) *Manual of Preoperative and Postoperative Care.* American College of Surgeons Philadelphia, Saunders.

Evans H. J. R., Torrealba V., Hudd C. et al. (1984) The effect of preoperative bile salt administration on postoperative renal function in patients with obstructive jaundice. *Br. J. Surg.* **69,** 706–708.

Fowkes F. G. R., Evans K. T., Hartley G. et al. (1986) Multicentre trial of four strategies to reduce use of a radiological test. *Lancet* **1,** 367–370.

Jones R. M. (1985) Preoperative care. Smoking before surgery: the case for stopping. *Br. Med. J.* **290,** 1763–1764.

Lowbury E. J. L. (1982) Special problems in hospital antiseptics. In: Russell A. O., Hugo W. B. and Ayliffe G. A. A. (ed.) *Principles and Practice of Disinfection, Preservation and Sterilization.* Oxford, Blackwell Scientific Publications, pp. 262–284.

Meers P. D., Ayliffe G. A. J., Emmerson A. M. et al. (1981) Report on the national survey of infection in hospitals. *J. Hosp. Infect.* **2,** Suppl. 1–15.

Napier J. A. F., Biffin A. H., Lay D. (1985) Efficiency of use of blood for surgery in south and mid Wales. *Br. Med. J.* **291**, 799–801.

Pettigrew R. A. and Hill G. L. (1986) Indicators of surgical risks and clinical judgement. *Br. J. Surg.* **73**, 47–51.

Simmons N. A., Cawson R. A., Clarke C. et al. (1982) The antibiotic prophylaxis of infective endocarditis. Report of the working party of the British Society for Antimicrobial Chemotherapy. *Lancet,* **2**, 1323–1326.

11 Principles of Clinical Oncology

K. C. Calman and G. R. Giles

INTRODUCTION

Oncology as a clinical and scientific discipline has developed considerably in the past decade. The word itself comes from the Greek, oncos = mass. Oncology is concerned with the study of tumours, both benign and malignant. The difference between benign and malignant neoplastic disease is an important one. Benign tumours tend to resemble the parent tissue, are well differentiated, may have a capsule and do not spread. Their problems relate either to local pressure effects, or to the secretion of specific chemicals, such as hormones. Malignant tumours, on the other hand, may not resemble the parent tissue closely, are often poorly differentiated, and spread and invade both locally and widely throughout the body. It is this latter characteristic which is the distinguishing mark of the malignant tumour. This difference is in most instances fairly clear at a clinical level. However, there are a number of situations in which this distinction still requires clarification. The first relates to a number of rare tumours (e.g. the teratomas) in which it may be extremely difficult, at a histological level, to differentiate between the two. Similarly, the definition of 'carcinoma-in-situ' implies the characteristics of invasion without its being evident histologically. Finally, there is the difficult area of premalignant disease, and the recognition of the change from benign to malignant.

Cancer, in cellular terms, can be defined as an abnormal mass of tissue, the growth of which exceeds and is uncoordinated with that of normal tissues and persists in the same excessive manner after cessation of the stimuli which evoked the change.

A more useful clinical definition, however, is that cancer is not one disease, but a group of related diseases which share certain characteristics. This implies that the aetiology, natural history, prognosis and treatment may be different for each type of cancer, and indeed for each pathological variant at specific sites.

CARCINOGENESIS

As described above, cancer is a disorder of growth. The process by which this change in growth pattern occurs, the change from benign to malignant, is known as carcinogenesis. Individual agents, chemical, physical and biological which induce this change are known as carcinogens.

Molecular Basis of Carcinogenesis Oncogenes

The last few years have seen tremendous changes in our understanding of carcinogenesis. It is now clear that in human cancer, the molecular event which sets in motion the transformation from benign to malignant, is the activation of a series of genes, known as oncogenes. Such genes have now been mapped on human chromosomes, and the hypothesis is that the activation is triggered by a variety of carcinogens. When activated these genes produce gene-products, some of which have now been characterized. It is the gene products which are responsible for some of the characteristics of malignancy, such as invasion, metastasis and metabolic alterations in the cancer cell.

The greater understanding of oncogenes and their role in carcinogenesis has dramatically changed the direction of cancer research towards finding ways of controlling oncogene function or modifying the effects of gene products. These facts should be borne in mind in relation to the following description of individual agents which may cause cancer.

In therapeutic terms the discovery of human oncogenes has been of importance in the interpretation of the effects of currently available therapies, and in the search for new approaches to cancer management.

Historically, one of the first clinical observations made in this field was by a surgeon, Percival Pott, who recognized the high incidence of scrotal cancer in chimney sweeps, and related this to soot and dirt. He also demonstrated the real value of identifying a carcinogen in that by its removal, in this case by the prevention of chimney sweeping by young boys, cancer of this type could almost be eliminated. The power of prevention was thus demonstrated. It has been variously estimated that between 70 and 80% of all cancers are environmentally determined. This figure is based on several assumptions which require confirmation but is a useful working hypothesis.

Many factors have been associated with the aetiology of cancer and they are briefly summarized here.

Chemical Carcinogenesis

Since Percival Potts' discovery of the high incidence of scrotal cancer in chimney sweeps, evidence has mounted on the effect of chemicals in the induction of cancer. A very large number of chemicals, organic and inorganic, are known to be associated with increased risk (*Table* 11.1). Where these have been identified in industrial processes it is

Table 11.1 Chemicals and foods recognized as carcinogens in the human

CHEMICAL

Carcinogens	*Targets in the human*
2-Naphthylamine Benzidine 4-aminobiphenyl 4-nitrobiphenyl N,N-bis(2-chloroethyl)-2-naphthylamine	Urinary bladder
bis(2-chlorethyl) sulphide Chromium compounds Chloromethyl methyl ether	Lungs
Cigarette smoke	Lungs, pancreas and other tissues
Certain soots, tars, oils, arsenic compounds	Lungs and skin
Asbestos	Lungs and pleura
Nickel compounds	Lungs and nasal sinuses
Betel nuts	Buccal mucosa
Vinyl chloride	Liver
Diethylstilboestrol	Vagina

FOOD

I *Carcinogens from green plants*
- Cycasin
- Nitrosamines and nitrosamides
- Pyrrolizidine alkaloids
- Allyl and propenyl benzine derivatives
- Bracken, fern
- Polycyclic hydrocarbons

II *Carcinogens elaborated by fungi*
- Aflatoxins
- Sterigmatocystin
- Yellow rice toxins
- Griseofulvin

III *Carcinogens produced by actinomycetes and bacteria*
- Streptomyces products
  - Actinomycin D
  - Mitomycin C
  - Streptozocin
- Ethionine
- Nitrosamines

IV *Carcinogens from animal meat—fat*

V *Industrial carcinogens and pesticides*

usually possible to eliminate them and institute preventive measures.

Physical Carcinogenesis

Radiation in various forms is known to be associated with increased carcinogenic risk. Ultraviolet radiation may also be important in the induction of skin cancer, including melanoma. Chronic irritation of the skin may lead to malignant change, e.g. Marjolin's ulcer.

Biological Agents

A variety of biological agents, notably viruses and parasites, are known to be associated with cancer.

Viruses

For many years a search has gone on for viruses which would induce cancer in man. It has recently been possible to identify a number of viruses which fit into this category, including the Epstein–Barr virus (EBV) and Burkitt's lymphoma, hepatitis B virus and hepatocellular carcinoma, human papilloma virus and carcinoma of the cervix and human immunodeficiency virus (HIV) and the Kaposi's sarcoma associated with AIDS. In addition, some rarer forms of human leukaemia have a viral aetiology.

Parasites

Several parasitic infections are known to be associated with a higher incidence of cancer, notably schistosomiasis and bladder cancer and, in some instances, colonic cancer.

Personal Habits

There seems little doubt that life style and personal habits do have an influence on the incidence of cancer. Cigarette smoking is perhaps the most obvious of these and this can be correlated with an increased incidence of lung, bladder and pancreatic cancer. Diet may also be of considerable importance and the debate in relation to the role of dietary fibre and fat in the induction of cancer of the colon has not been fully resolved. Diet may also be important in the development of breast cancer. Food additives are a potential source of carcinogens, e.g. nitrites, cyclamates, etc.

Hormones and Drugs

Although essentially an extension of chemical carcinogenesis the cancers associated with these substances can also be classified as iatrogenic. Thus the relationship between oestrogens and endometrial cancer and the use of the contraceptive pill and hepatic lesions have been documented. Many of the alkylating agents used in the treatment of human cancer are also carcinogenic. It is likely that others remain to be fully documented. A particular problem is that of transplacental carcinogenesis and the classic example of this is the use of stilboestrol in early pregnancy and the subsequent development of vaginal cancer in the female offspring.

Methods of Detecting Carcinogenesis

The majority of discoveries relating to carcinogens have come from clinical or epidemiological studies. Their major drawback is that they rely on serendipity and may require decades of observation before the link between carcinogen and the cancer are finally established. The testing of new compounds can be done using experimental animal models though this can be expensive and the results may not be directly relevant to man. Newer approaches to this problem use bacterial or cellular models. These methods are promising and may allow more efficient screening of large numbers of compounds.

GENETIC ASPECTS OF ONCOLOGY

It is not possible to show genetic influences on cancer development in the clear manner which is evident in some other clinical syndromes. Neoplastic cells may show metabolic evidence forming new products, e.g. ectopic hormones and embryonic antigen production, that fundamental changes have occurred which involve both mutational and regulatory change in the genetic material. However, more probably genetic influence acts by determining the host susceptibility to carcinogen exposure and cancer progression. It is clear that some foci of malignant cells remain dormant for prolonged periods of time. This period of quiescence may be disturbed by alterations in the hormonal environment or by the response to trauma in which a background of cell repair, cell proliferation and replication

Table 11.2 Cancers associated with clinical syndromes

Disease	*Mode of transfer*	*Tumour susceptibility*
Neurofibromatosis	AD	Glioma, meningioma, phaeochromocytoma, sarcoma
Tuberous sclerosis	AD	Glioma, neurofibroma, astrocytoma
Porphyria cutaneous tarda	AD	BCC, Hepatocellular carcinoma
Albinism	AR	BCC, SCC
Tyrosinaemia	AR	Hepatocellular carcinoma
Polyposis coli	AD	Carcinoma colon
Gardner's syndrome	AD	Carcinoma colon, endocrine carcinoma
Peutz–Jeghers syndrome	AD	Ovarian, carcinoma duodenum and small bowel
Ataxia telangiectasia	AR	Leukaemia, reticuloses
IgA deficiency	Not clear	Lymphoreticular also carcinoma stomach, bladder, breast
IgM deficiency	Not clear	Lymphoreticular, neuro-blastoma

AD = autosomal dominant. AR = autosomal recessive

develop, e.g. colonic polyposis and ulcerative colitis. There is also evidence that with genetically transmitted diseases in which immunocompetence is lowered, there is an increased risk of malignancy, e.g. agammaglobulinaemia, Wiskott–Aldridge syndrome and ataxia telangiectasia. *Table* 11.2 lists the recognized genetically transmitted disorders and higher risk of malignancy.

There is little evidence that a general susceptibility to cancer can be inherited although there are families which appear to have large numbers of cancers. It has to be admitted that there may be many reasons for the cancers to be clustered in families, e.g. exposures to common carcinogens, diet, occupations or transmission of viruses. There has been a tendency to play down the genetic influences in such situations and look only for external influences. However, studies of relatives of women with breast cancer reveal that the age-adjusted frequency is 17% of first-degree relatives of premenopausal patients with bilateral disease compared with 3% of control cases. Less obvious changes in incidence are seen in the families of patients suffering cancers of the lung, prostate, bladder, uterus and ovary. With some rarer tumours such as retinoblastoma, phaeochromocytoma and melanoma it looks as though two types of tumour exist, one genetically determined and the other is a non-genetic form. The genetic form seems to occur at an earlier age, have male predominance and a somewhat improved prognosis. In fact it is improbable that the two forms exist separately but rather that they express the two extremes of genetic influence. It is thought that future research will reveal genetic markers or viral oncogenes on peripheral cells which will enable the identification of these susceptible individuals at an early age and permit effective screening for early neoplastic change in target organs.

Preneoplasia

There are several instances in which this state may be said to occur: (i) conditions which are not neoplastic or proliferative but appear to carry an increased risk of cancer. Examples in this category include chronic inflammatory processes although the role played by inflammation is uncertain, e.g. chronic atrophic gastritis and pernicious anaemia with gastric carcinoma, ulcerative colitis with colonic carcinoma. Another type of example relates to chromosomal abnormalities: Down's syndrome and increased risk of leukaemia; (ii) proliferative disorders in which the neoplasms are not always derived from the proliferating tissue, e.g. von Recklinghausen's disease and increased risk of glioma and mesangioma tuberous sclerosis with increased retinal, renal and myocardial tumours; (iii) true preneoplastic lesions are those conditions which are more liable to develop infiltrative lesions of the affected tissue, although not invariably. Carcinoma-in-situ is an example of this type where there are cytological appearances of neoplastic change but the lesion remains bounded by a basement membrane, e.g. carcinoma of cervix, carcinoma of colon in familial colonic polyposis. It is quite probable that the incidence of preinvasive cancer or carcinoma-in-situ is greater than invasive cancer. This suggests that many preinvasive cancers are controlled at that level, possibly by immunological means.

Epidemiological Studies

Epidemiology is an important tool in the study of malignant disease. It is useful in several ways:

1. To define the causes of the disease.
2. To define the size of the problem.
3. To identify high risk groups.
4. To identify bad prognostic groups.
5. To define associated diseases which might affect prognosis.

The extent of a cancer in community terms is described by frequency studies. The development of new cases of a cancer type defines the *incidence* of the disease whereas the *prevalence* constitutes the number of cases, both new and old, within the community. By an analysis of cancer frequencies within communities, it may be possible to define high-risk groups in whom special measures are required. This type of analysis can be directed to determine whether particular age groups or ethnic communities are especially prone to individual cancers. Alternatively, unusually increased frequences may suggest aetiological factors.

Thus epidemiological and demographic data should allow the surgeon (i) to define the size of problem relating to a particular cancer site of interest; (ii) to know which groups of patients are at high risk; (iii) to identify those characteristics of the patient or tumour which will determine the behaviour of the cancer. In planning a management approach to a particular form of cancer, these variables should be identified whenever possible.

SCREENING

The methods to be used to screen for individual tumours will be discussed in the relevant sections of the book. However, it is useful to discuss the basic philosophy of screening at this stage. Any method of early detection of cancer applied to a large population assumes:

1. That the test is reliable and indicates the presence of cancer.
2. That there are few false positives and false negatives.
3. That the test is easy to apply and interpret.

4. That the test is inexpensive.
5. That it does not incur a significant hazard to the population screened.
6. That early diagnosis, and subsequent treatment will significantly alter the natural history of the disease.

It is this last aspect which is most specifically related to a knowledge of the biology and natural history of the disease. This is illustrated in *Fig.* 11.1. If early intervention simply means earlier treatment without altering the growth pattern of the disease, then it is possibly of little value. However, if treatment shifts the curve (*Fig.* 11.2) indicating not only an increase in the survival time but also an increase in the quality of life, then it will be worthwhile.

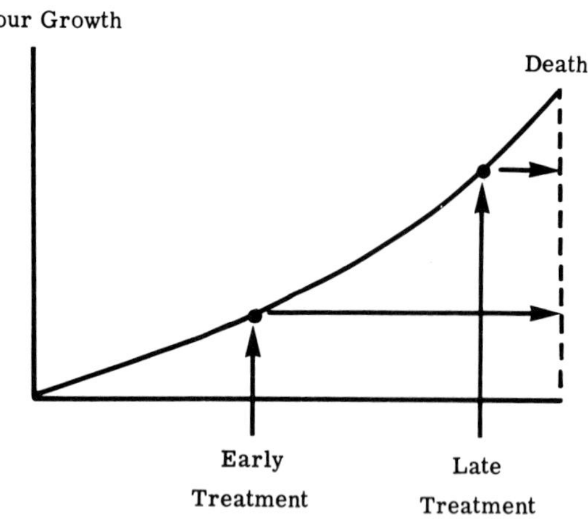

Fig. 11.1 Effect of early or late treatment on survival. In this figure although early treatment is associated with a longer overall survival there has been no change in the natural history by early treatment.

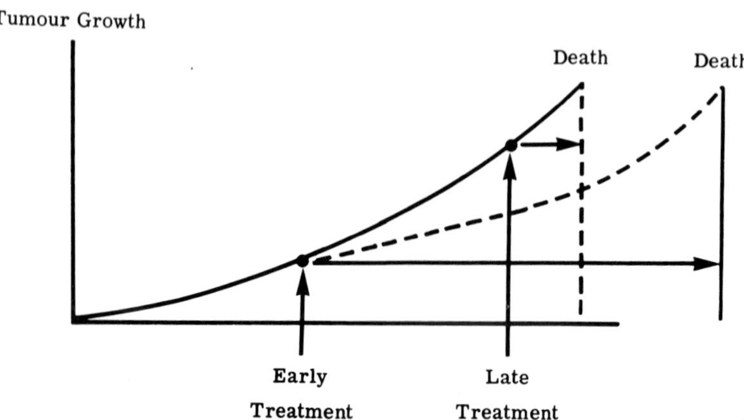

Fig. 11.2 Effect of early or late treatment on survival. In this figure early treatment is associated with a change in the survival curve and represents a real survival benefit from treatment.

Early Detection of Cancer

It would seem that there can be little controversy about the concept that if a cancer is detected earlier in its time course, then improved survival is to be expected. There are two points of methodological error in handling data of this type. The point of 'onset error' arises from the fact that if early detection advances the time of diagnosis of a disease then the period from diagnosis to death will lengthen (improved 5-year survival rate), irrespective of whether treatment has altered the natural history of the disease. It is possible to adjust for this factor if the extent of the lead time can be assessed. The second type of error results from the effect of the screening agent on the earlier diagnosis of cases which would normally be subclinically prevalent. The probability is that a slow growing tumour will be detected more readily than a fast growing cancer. Thus the survival of patients detected by screening programmes may well prove better than control cases but is not due to early diagnosis alone. It is possible to overcome this problem by grouping patients in different treatment schedules according to pathological staging, but even this approach can be misleading (*see below*).

It should be clear, therefore, that in those tumours which metastasize at an early stage, there is less chance of altering the natural history. The converse is also true. The concept of 'early diagnosis' is not relevant to a number of human malignant tumours at the present time, and the term 'earlier diagnosis' is more appropriate. It is important to point out, however, that the earlier the diagnosis is made, the greater the chance of detecting a lesion which is amenable to potentially curative treatment. Prevention and earlier diagnosis are perhaps the two most powerful weapons we have in the control of the cancer problem.

TUMOUR BIOLOGY

From the previous discussion it should be evident that a knowledge of tumour biology is essential for the management of the cancer patient. Solid tumours are composed of masses of cells which have different growth potentials and biological characteristics.

In the first instance it is important to note that the tumour mass is not solely composed of cancer cells. Indeed in some experimental tumours up to 50% of the tumour mass may be composed of non-cancer cells. These include the fibrous tissue stroma, blood vessels and host cells of various types, including lymphocytes, macrophages, leucocytes, mast cells, etc. Some of these cell types may be critical to the growth of the tumour. Blood vessels are derived from host tissue and are essential for the nourishment of the cancer. The role of macrophages and lymphocytes may be very important in determining the pattern of tumour growth.

Not only are the cells of a tumour composed of a variety of cell types, but the cancer cells themselves may differ. Indeed they may change with the evolution of the cancer. It is conventional to divide the cancer cells into three compartments (*Fig.* 11.3). The first of these is the growth fraction of the tumour. The cells in this compartment are actively dividing and are responsible for the growth of the tumour. The second compartment is the non-proliferating compartment composed of cells, not in active division, but capable of doing so if appropriately stimulated. This compartment, also known as the clonogenic fraction, is of considerable importance. If the growth fraction is eliminated then it is the cells in this compartment which are stimulated to divide and are recruited into the growing compartment. These residual, quiescent cells therefore have the capacity to repopulate a tumour or to set up a secondary tumour when stimulated. The third compartment, also a non-proliferating compartment is composed of dead cells or cells with only a limited capacity for cell division.

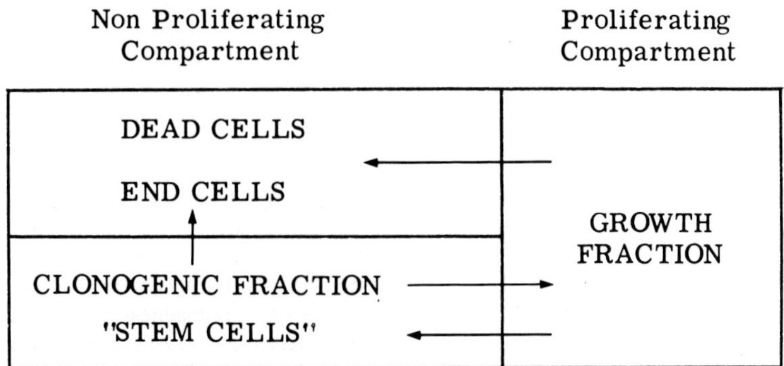

Fig. 11.3 Tumour kinetics. The tumour may be divided into several compartments depending on whether or not the cells are growing (growth fraction), have the capacity to grow (clonogenic fraction) or are end cells.

Growth control in normal tissues is a balance between cell division and cell loss. For many solid tumours the rate of cell division and the doubling time may be less than the normal tissue counterpart. The growth of the tumour therefore is likely to be related to a decrease in cell loss rather than an increase in the rate of cell division. The fact that cancer cells may divide more slowly than normal cells is of considerable practical importance if cytotoxic drugs are to be used.

The growth of a neoplastic tumour does not occur in a linear fashion, but is Gompertzian, that is to say that small tumours grow rapidly and logarithmically, and, as the tumour becomes larger, the growth rate slows down. This is related to many factors including a decreased blood supply, tumour necrosis, pressure effects and nutrition. Thus, small tumours tend to grow fast and large tumours more slowly. These growth kinetics are described as Gompertzian (*Fig.* 11.4). In addition, small tumours tend to have a large growth fraction (indicating that they would be more susceptible to cytotoxic drugs and radiotherapy), while large tumours have a small growth fraction (suggesting the contrary). Theoretically if part of a tumour is surgically removed, the growth characteristics of the remaining cancer cells, including secondary lesions, may change.

A tumour which is 1 cm^3 is normally considered to be at the limit of clinical detectability. Even so this tumour is likely to contain 10^9 cells. Even if the tumour could be detected at 1 mm^3 size, then it would contain approximately 10^6 cells. The possibility, therefore, that invasion and spread will have occurred even at this stage must be considered real indeed.

During the process of cell division the cell goes through several distinct phases. These are known as the cell cycle.

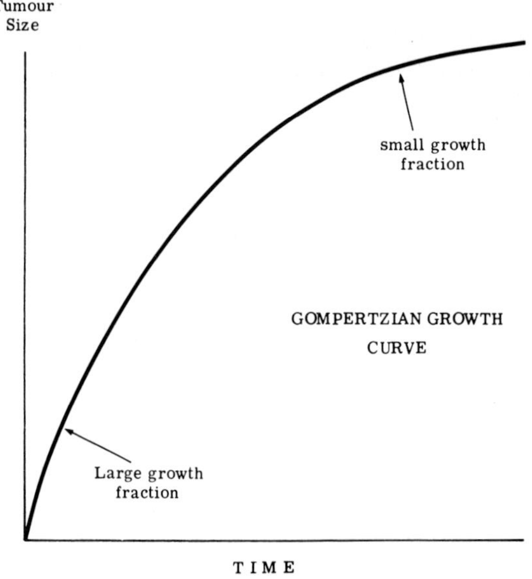

Fig. 11.4 Growth kinetics of tumours. As tumours increase in size their growth rate slows. Initially the tumour has a large growth fraction, but as the tumour volume increases, this is reduced.

Following mitosis the cell can either become an end cell, become a resting (clonogenic) cell or enter the cell cycle again (*Fig.* 11.5). The first phase of the cycle is known as the G_1 phase (first gap) where the cell synthesizes normal tissue proteins and performs the usual work of the cell. This then progresses to the S phase (synthetic phase) where DNA synthesis occurs. Following this there is a second gap (G_2) and then the cell goes again into mitosis. The cell cycle is of considerable importance in relation to chemotherapy and will be referred to later. Those resting or clonogenic cells are

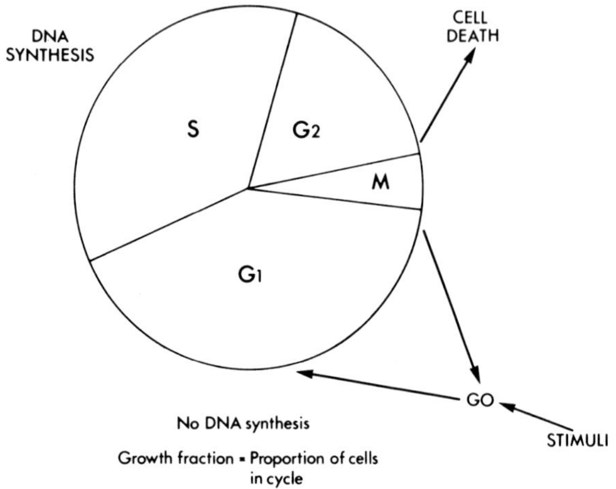

Fig. 11.5 The cell cycle. This describes the changes which take place during the time before and after cell division. M = mitosis, G_1 = first gap, S = synthetic phase, G_2 = second gap, G_0 = quiescent phase.

also referred to as cells in G_0, an important concept in relation to the growth of the tumour.

As well as being different in terms of growth, cancer cells also differ morphologically in their relation to the parent organ. The degree of differentiation of the tumour is an important prognostic factor in many tumour types. Poorly differentiated tumours are associated with a poorer prognosis than well-differentiated lesions. The degree of differentiation (or anaplasia) is also known as grading, and, though often subjective, the histological grading of the tumour is of real practical significance. Another feature of pathological importance is the histogenesis of the tumour, that is the cell type of origin. In many instances this is simple enough to define and has little therapeutic or biological significance. In some tumour types, however, the cell of origin may be very important indeed. In the leukaemias, the lymphomas and testicular and ovarian cancers, the histogenesis will determine the prognosis and possibly the treatment.

INVASION AND METASTASIS

Invasion

As has been previously mentioned one of the main characteristics of malignant neoplasia is invasion. The mechanisms by which direct invasion can occur are not entirely clear and several have been postulated. Thus direct extension due to pressure as the tumour increases in size, pushing cells between tissue planes, may be one such factor. There is some evidence that cancer cells are more mobile than normal cells, though it is just as likely that the mobility is related to lack of cohesiveness.

Most of our knowledge of this particular characteristic of malignant disease is derived from experimental studies of which the early work by Abercrombie and colleagues is fundamental. It is known that two cultures of fibroblasts will move in opposite directions (Contact Inhibition of Movement phenomenon). However, in a mixed culture of sarcoma and fibroblasts, the neoplastic cells freely infiltrate the fibroblast layer. This ability to infiltrate fibroblast cultures increases with the dedifferentiation of the tumour and the phenomenon is also shown with human cell lines of carcinoma of cervix and breast. Not all malignant cells have this ability and it is suggested that certain 'sentinel cells' are present in the malignant cell population which are able to 'blaze a trail' for the remainder. Monolayer cultures of vascular endothelium are more capable of resisting infiltration than other tissues. There is also the hypothesis that cancer cells release into the intercellular matrix, enzymes or 'toxins' which break down connective tissue barriers so assisting the local spread of the cancer cell.

Conversely, it is thought that the inflammatory process and stromal proliferation will facilitate malignant invasion. It is quite probable that tumours are capable of releasing substances capable of stimulating growth of normal tissues such as vascular tissue and have particular importance in establishment of metastases, e.g. angiogenesis factor.

All tumours, both benign and malignant have a background stroma of connective tissue and blood vessels which provides a matrix for metabolic exchanges. In anaplastic tumours collagen is somewhat scant and conversely is abundant in scirrhous cancers. Tumour growth is always associated with angiogenesis even though the new blood vessels show a grossly abnormal structure. New capillary growth can affect the subsequent growth rate of tumours. If angiogenesis can be inhibited, this would be a potent method of inhibiting tumour growth, particularly of metastases.

Metastasis

The natural history of a malignant tissue can be represented by the analogue diagram of *Fig.* 11.6.

The ability to metastasize is suggested by histological features of the tissue and is usually more common with dedifferentiated lesions, the exceptions being gliomas, chondrosarcomas and basal cell tumours. Conversely, extremely well differentiated cancers of the thyroid and adrenal glands readily metastasize. Some cancers tend to lose isoantigen identity as the metastasizing potential develops. Other strong factors include kinetic characteristics. Tumours with a naturally high degree of lymphocytic infiltration, e.g. seminomas, malignant melanomas and choriocarcinomas have a better prognosis than suggested by morphological appearances.

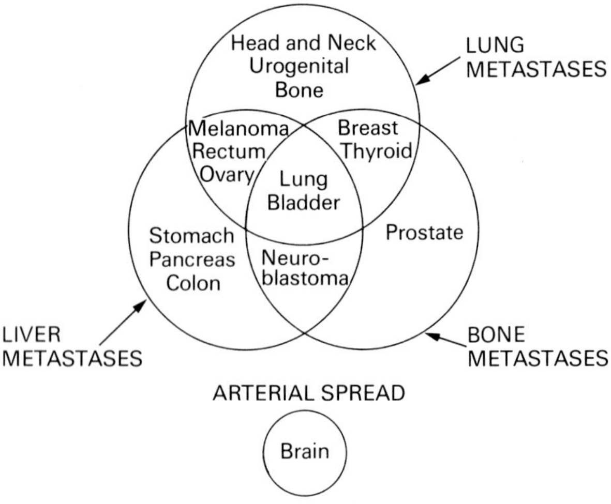

Fig. 11.6 Predominant sites of tumours leading to lung, liver and bone metastatic disease.

The process of metastasis is a complicated one and has only recently been studied in some detail. Perhaps the first point to make is that not every cancer cell appears capable of metastasizing. From animal experiments it has become clear that only a proportion of cancer cells are able to spread widely. The second point is that there appears to be some specificity in the site of spread of particular tumours. This is, of course, partly related to the site of the primary tumour and local anatomical factors, but, in addition, experimental studies have demonstrated site specificity of metastasizing cells. The third point which is perhaps self-evident is that metastases themselves can spread. This is relevant when the primary tumour is excised leaving small metastases behind.

The dissemination of malignant cells follows invasion of lymphatic and blood vessels. The lodgement of neoplastic cells within a lymph node is not invariably followed by a metastatic deposit and this event is partly determined by characteristics of the malignant cells, e.g. carcinomas frequently produce lymph node deposits, sarcomas do so infrequently. The presence of tumour cells in the bloodstream has been extensively investigated and is more commonly found in advanced disease. It is quite likely that many circulating tumour cells have little capacity to produce metastatic disease, although clearly the presence of vascular invasion is a sign of poor prognosis. Malignant cells arrested in the capillary circulation may or may not become surrounded by a fibrin thrombosis but seem to show migration between endothelial cells. These extravasated cells may die from metabolic causes in the interstitium but surviving cells develop a fibrovascular stroma which permits more rapid growth (*Fig.* 11.7). Products released by tumour cells may enable growth of metastases in selected sites, e.g. parathormone and osteo-activating factor appear to promote bone secondaries.

One reason for discussing the mechanism of metastasis in some detail is that it highlights several ways in which the process could be interrupted. First, the cell could be stopped from leaving the primary tumour; secondly the cell could be killed in the bloodstream or prevented from adhering to the vessel wall; thirdly the cell could be inhibited from penetrating the blood vessel and growing into a secondary tumour.

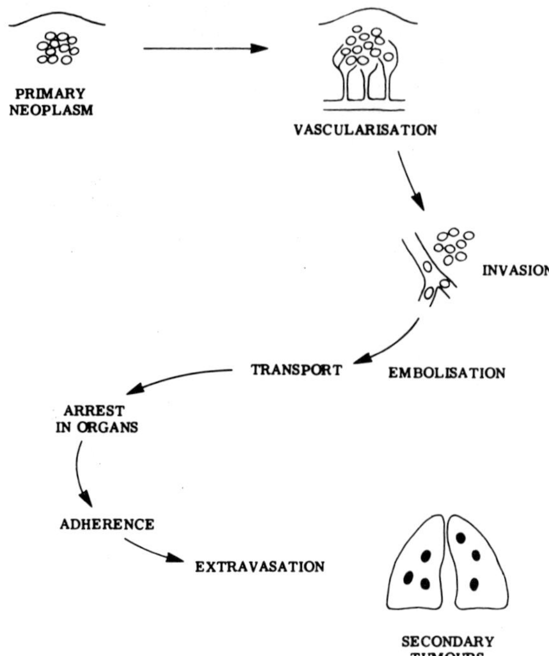

Fig. 11.7 Pathways of invasion and metastases. The primary neoplasms become vascularized, tumour cells invade and spread setting up secondary tumours.

The pattern of development of metastatic spread is largely explicable in both anatomical and mechanical forms, e.g. blood and bone metastases are trapped commonly in liver and lungs respectively, direct invasion of paravertebral venous plexuses leads to spinal deposits. The occurrence of metastases in the brain, skin and adrenal show that the arterial circulation may be involved although the fact that certain organs are uncommon sites, e.g. spleen, skeletal and cardiac muscle suggests a degree of selectivity in the 'soil into which the seeds are planted'. Experimentally there are many extraneous insults which when applied to an organ seem to make it more susceptible to metastatic disease. Matters are not so clear in the clinical field although it appears that previous local irradiation may be such a factor. This area of clinical research may be a fruitful one for experimentally it can be shown that the administration of high lipid diet, dextrans and reticuloendothelial blockade all enhance hepatic metastases.

Staging

It is a common observation that localized cancer gives a better prognosis than disseminated disease and this has led to the concept of 'early' and 'late' cases. This is not necessarily an accurate view because the state of advancement of the neoplasm depends upon the rate of growth, type of cancer, length of symptoms before diagnosis and treatment, and host immune response. It is more appropriate to document accurately the extent of the cancer by defined terms. The objectives in favour of clinicopathological staging are:

1. To assist in the evaluation of clinical care.
2. To give an indication of prognosis.
3. To aid treatment planning.
4. To allow comparative trials using patients in different centres.

The TNM system helps meet these requirements by providing an objective assessment of the anatomical extent of the disease.

This system is based on the assessment of:

1. The extent of the primary tumour —T
2. The condition of the regional lymph nodes —N
3. The absence or presence of distant metastases —M

Some tumours are more easily fitted into this scheme than others and it is particularly suitable for cancers that are accessible. Each category is subdivided, e.g. T1, T2, T3, T4 indicating an increasing extent of the primary tumour and may be judged in terms of measured size or degree of penetration through the organ. The additional subdivisions include T0—where the main organ shows no clinical evidence of primary tumour but metastases in nodes or elsewhere indicate than an occult tumour does exist and Tx where it proves to be impossible to assess the extent of the primary tumour. TIS indicates carcinoma-in-situ.

Nodal status is described as N1, N2, N3 and indicates the involvement of more distant lymph glands. Each primary tumour will have specific and appropriate grades of lymph node drainage.

The use of M0 indicates no metastases can be detected clinically. M1 is used to indicate the presence of metastases other than in lymph nodes. MX is used when the presence of metastases cannot be assessed clinically.

Following operation it is usually possible to add pathological data into the staging procedure. P1–4 grades the degree of penetration of the primary tumour within the organ of origin. G1–3 indicates increasing degrees of histological malignancy.

This complex scheme of clinical and pathological information can be drawn together for each type of cancer and can lead to broad clinical stages which allow meaningful comparisons.

Assessment of Metastatic Spread

With the improvement in imaging techniques, the extent of tumour spread may also be assessed by physical means. However, this may not always be worthwhile particularly in those tumours which are rapidly metastasizing, e.g. lung cancer. It is also debatable whether the detection of metastatic spread in the asymptomatic patient offers any clinical benefit.

Brain

Nuclide brain scans produce an extremely low yield in the neurologically normal patient. Conversely, solitary scan abnormalities may indicate benign disorders, e.g. meningiomas, even if metastatic disease is clinically obvious elsewhere. CT scans do detect smaller cerebral metastases than those seen on nuclide scans. However, a false negative rate of 40% has been found. CT scans produce more accurate morphological information particularly of benign conditions.

Lung

The most effective screening procedure for pulmonary metastases is a carefully taken PA and lateral chest radiograph. Tomograms rarely detect metastatic nodules not seen on the chest radiograph, however, CT of the chest will definitely reveal more metastases particularly those less than 6 mm. The extra sensitivity of the technique produces a false positive rate of 50% for these small nodules and the information cannot, therefore, be relied upon to change clinical decisions. One particular situation in which CT scans are especially helpful is in deciding whether to excise what seems to be a solitary metastasis. If metastases are found at some distance from the resection, then surgery would be contraindicated.

Liver

Isotope scans performed in patients without hepatomegaly and undisturbed liver function tests are not worthwhile. If these clinical tests are negative, only 5–10% show lesions on static scans and an equal incidence of false positives. This is particularly high in patients with fatty infiltration or alcoholic liver disease. Benign disorders may also produce filling defects which may be interpreted as metastatic disease. Surprisingly, CT scans are no more sensitive than nuclide investigations but are more specific. A CT scan may be indicated if a therapeutic decision will be based on the result. The position of ultrasound is so operator-dependent that it is difficult to evaluate its role. It does not seem sufficiently dependable to base clinical decisions on this technique alone.

Bone

Nuclide bone scans are very non-specific and careful attention to other clinical aspects are required when solitary non-articular bone lesions are found (33% are due to benign causes). Normally, scanning is only indicated for the symptom of bone pain and a raised alkaline phosphatase. However, clinical judgements may still be influenced in breast and prostatic cancer even though the patient is asymptomatic in bone. Skeletal radiographs are required to confirm the scan findings and to exclude benign disease.

By staging procedures it has become possible to define more accurately which patients will benefit from aggressive therapy and which patients require only localized treatment. Having established the importance of staging in Hodgkin's disease, and, having defined its natural history more fully, treatment programmes have been rationalized although the value of aggressive staging is now being questioned. The same is true in breast cancer. Multiple investigations of the patient, associated with adequate follow-up have not only allowed a greater understanding of the biology of the disease, but have begun to show which investigations are really necessary.

Cancer Markers

Staging, or the definition of the extent of disease, would be greatly improved if a simple test was available which would allow quantitation of the tumour mass and the search for appropriate biological markers (hormones, oncofetal antigens, enzymes and other products of cellular metabolism) has been one of the most fascinating in cancer research. The simplest markers are hormones, either secreted by a tumour of endocrine origin or by an ectopic hormone-producing cancer. The complete removal or destruction of the lesion should result in the disappearance of excess amounts of hormone and the level of hormone which can be used to predict response to therapy. Perhaps the most useful of all hormone markers is the secretion of chorionic gonadotrophin by choriocarcinoma, the amount of hormone secreted being directly related to the tumour mass.

Unfortunately, it seems that such biological markers are available for the rarer forms of cancer and do not seem to apply to the more common and often less easily treated neoplasms. One of the first markers which became available was carcino-embryonic antigen (CEA). Initially it was considered that this marker was specifically associated with the presence of colonic cancer. It has subsequently been shown, however, that the presence of CEA in the blood is not specific for colonic cancer and indeed its level may be elevated in patients who have benign disease (cirrhosis of liver, viral hepatitis, cigarette smoking, etc.). CEA is therefore of little use as a screening test, though it may be of value in the detection of recurrent colonic cancer.

CEA is one of a group of glycoproteins known as the oncofetal proteins, because of their presence in fetal tissues. Alpha-fetoprotein (AFP) is another such compound and may be elevated in the blood of patients who have primary liver cancer. Although AFP may be encountered in benign disorders, high levels are always associated with primary hepatic malignancy. Another useful tumour associated antigen for gastrointestinal and pancreatic malignancy is Ca 9-19.

In testicular teratoma the serial monitoring of the AFP level is of considerable value in determining the response of the tumour to therapy (*Fig.* 11.8). Other markers that have been used in monitoring recurrence and disease activity include urinary hydroxyproline, serum immune complexes, γ-glutamyltranspeptidase, alkaline phosphatase, serum amyloid protein, prolyl-hydroxylase, polyamines (spermine, spermidine) etc. Many of these are not in routine use.

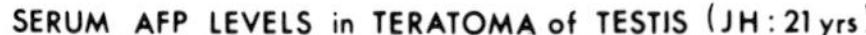

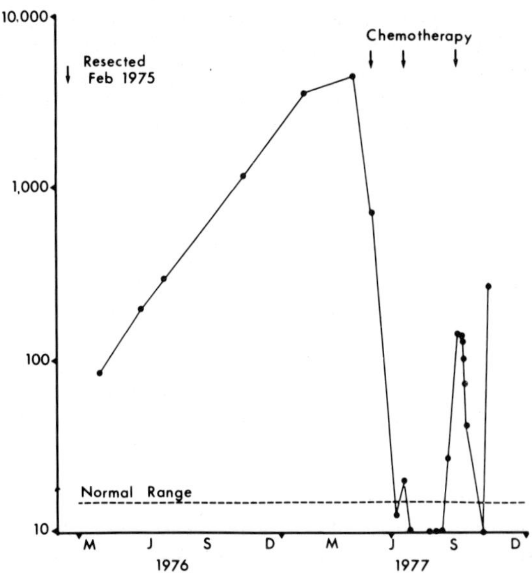

Fig. 11.8 Use of serum markers to follow response to treatment. The serum AFP (alphafetoprotein) is used to monitor response to therapy, the fall in levels being related to tumour cell death.

CLINICAL PROBLEMS ASSOCIATED WITH CANCER

These may be divided into three broad groups:

1. Clinical syndromes associated with the primary lesion or its spread, e.g. ectopic hormones, bone marrow involvement, etc.
2. Clinical syndromes associated with the treatment given to the patient, e.g. effects of surgical procedures on the gastrointestinal tract, induction of haematological toxicity or infection secondary to the use of drugs or radiotherapy.
3. Clinical syndromes not associated with either.

In each of these types of syndromes the concept of 'support' has been built up. Thus nutritional support, haematological support, support during infection are all part of the management of the cancer patient. The concept of 'support' is, however, broader than this, and should include emotional, psychological and spiritual help. The patient must be treated as a whole.

Clinical Syndromes Associated with Cancer

The important ones include the following:

Nutritional and Metabolic

Patients with solid tumours frequently suffer from malnutrition and disordered metabolism. This may not only affect the patient's overall prognosis and sense of well being but may directly affect the management plan. Thus surgical procedures may be more hazardous in this type of patient and there are indications that the response to chemotherapy and radiotherapy may also be related to the nutritional status.

The metabolic consequences of neoplasia are multiple and include the problems associated with hepatic and renal damage in cancer patients. Hyperuricaemia may occur in patients with cancer either because of rapid growth rate of the tumour, or because of increased cell death due to treatment. The prophylactic value of uricosuric agents in these cases is well known. Other metabolic problems include those related to the secretion of hormones, either ectopically produced or from tumours of endocrine glands. These effects may be the initial presenting feature of the patient and this is especially the case in lung cancer. Inappropriate ADH and ACTH secretion are relatively common, and the others such as the secretion of parathormone-like hormones, erythropoietin etc., are less frequently encountered.

Hypercalcaemia is a special problem frequently associated with patients with advanced cancer. The mechanism of hypercalcaemia relates especially to bone destruction or to the secretion of a parathormone-like hormone. This may be compounded by immobilization and renal insufficiency. Hypercalcaemia is associated with a multiplicity of symptoms including anorexia, weight loss, nausea and vomiting, constipation, psychological and neurological disturbances, polyuria and polydipsia.

Neurological Problems Associated with Cancer

In addition to direct invasion of the CNS or peripheral nerves with cancer cells giving rise to a wide variety of clinical signs and symptoms, other clinical syndromes also occur which seem more likely to be associated with the distant effects of the cancer. Commonly, these include myopathies, neuropathies, cord lesions and progressive multifocal leuco-encephalopathy—the latter two examples being extremely rare.

Haematological Problems

These are usually related to blood loss, nutritional problems or the effects of marrow involvement. Anaemia is common and is multifactorial. Where no obvious blood loss is suspected then it is likely that it is related to the 'anaemia of chronic diseases', a non-specific anaemia. Nutritional aspects should be considered, especially if the patient has anorexia or has had a surgical procedure involving the gastrointestinal tract. Marrow involvement usually manifests itself by anaemia, leucopenia and thrombocytopenia or a leuco-erythroblastic picture. Any of these may be the major clinical problem. Where bleeding is apparent the patient may require active haematological support (transfusion of fresh blood, clotting factors). Where possible, however, effective therapy is directed towards the neoplastic process, e.g. cytotoxic therapy for leukaemia; this approach may not be relevant for solid tumours.

Infection

This may be associated directly with the tumour, e.g. bladder involvement and cystitis, infection and atelectasis in lung cancer, or due to leucopenia and marrow involvement.

Dermatological Manifestations

These are discussed in Chapter 14.

The intensive care of the patient with cancer using nutritional, haematological or infection support, raises ethical questions and the clinician involved must be quite clear as to the aims of treatment and the overall prognosis and management plan for the patient. As treatment becomes more aggressive and as results of treatment improve, so the need for such support is likely to increase. As previously mentioned, the emotional and psychological support of the patient should not be overlooked.

Clinical Problems not Associated with Cancer or its Treatment

It is easy to assume that all symptoms and signs which the cancer patient has are associated with local extension or spread of the tumour. Yet cancer patients can develop other diseases and these sinister symptoms may be related to simple disorders. Infection is perhaps the most commonly confused clinical problem. Chest infections, in particular, may be assumed to be related to metastases and potentially treatable disease, e.g. tuberculosis, may be missed.

Other effects of cancer relate directly to their spread to involve vital organs, such as the lungs, respiratory tract or cardiovascular system.

Clinical Syndromes Associated with Treatment

The clinician should be fully aware, at all times, of the morbidity and mortality which he may induce by treatment. Surgical treatment has a definite morbidity and in each case the consequences of this should be borne in mind. As far as radiotherapy and chemotherapy are concerned there is little doubt that the complications which can be induced have been responsible for a great deal of suffering. The side-effects which can result may be divided into minor effects which are non-life-threatening and these include nausea, vomiting, diarrhoea, alopecia and local effects of treatment. Though these may be described as minor, they are of considerable importance to the patient. The life-threatening side-effects include haemorrhage, leucopenia, severe infection and second malignancies.

This latter consequence is of special significance in those patients who have early and potentially curable cancers who are then given adjuvant radiotherapy or chemotherapy following surgery.

THE CONTROL OF CANCER

There are potentially three ways by which cancer control can be achieved. First of all the particular cancer could be prevented. This, unfortunately, is only applicable to a limited number of cancers at present, but is potentially an extremely powerful method.

The second method for cancer control involves diagnosing the lesion before it has spread. In this instance early treatment, by removing the entire lesion would be curative. Once again, however, there are real limitations in the number of cancers which can be detected early, or in which screening is a viable proposition. It seems unlikely that in the next few years more refined methods of diagnosis will be available.

The final method of cancer control is concerned with the treatment of the patient whose disease has advanced locally or in whom distant spread has already occurred. This comprises the largest group of patients who present with cancer and for whom treatment is to be administered. Viewed in this way, the management of the cancer patient, by treatment, is seen as a logical extension of the concept of cancer control. It is the area of most concern to clinicians, and in which recent advances in treatment have contributed a great deal towards the control of individual cancers.

THE MANAGEMENT OF THE PATIENT WITH CANCER

Before discussing in detail the types of management which are available it is useful to consider certain general principles. In the first of these the clinician must decide on the aim of treatment:

1. To eradicate the disease and cure the patient.
2. To control the disease for a period of time.
3. To improve the quality of life.

While these aims are not mutually exclusive the approach to the patient will be different depending on the aim of treatment. In the first case the treatment is likely to be aggressive, prolonged and perhaps toxic. In the latter case treatment becomes less important as preservation of quality of life becomes more so. As the treatment of one type of cancer becomes better, so the aims of treatment may change. If current therapy is generally ineffective for long-term control, then the most important aspect for the patient is likely to be quality of life. If, however, there is a dramatic improvement in prognosis because of a new treatment, then the aim may change correspondingly. Such a change has been achieved in the testicular teratomas.

The second important concept in management is the consideration of the patient as a whole or complete individual, with a family, home, friends, work and leisure; as an individual who has thoughts, feelings and emotions. While often difficult to quantitate, these aspects of care are just as important as the diagnosis, investigation and treatment.

When faced with a patient who has, or may have had cancer, it is useful to have a flow chart which will outline the management plan (*Fig.* 11.9). In the first instance the whole patient is considered as are his reactions to his illness. The diagnosis is established and, with rare exceptions, this must be based on histological examination. With the diagnosis made, the clinician then considers prognostic factors related to the tumour and to the host. On the basis of this information treatment is then considered, first by defining the aims of treatment and the potential modalities or types of treatment available. At this point the decision must be made either to treat or not to treat the patient. This is not an irrevocable decision and can obviously be modified depending on the prognosis of the patient. In addition a decision not to treat a *tumour* does *not* mean that the *patient* should

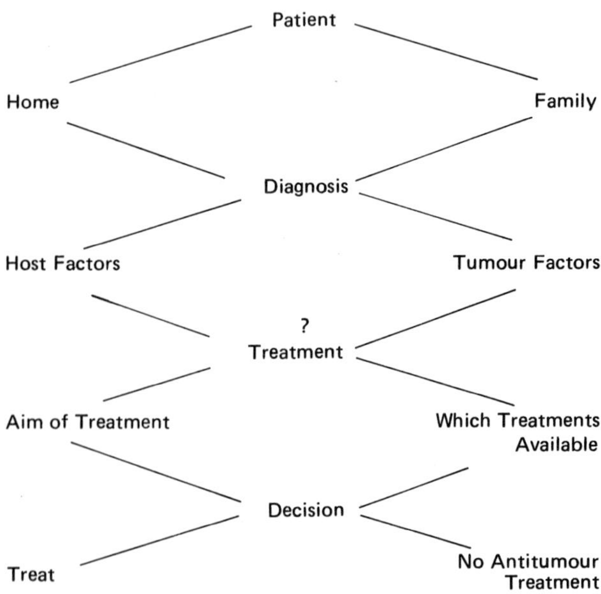

Fig. 11.9 Flow chart of decision making in relation to cancer treatment.

not be treated, as many methods may still be available to improve quality of life.

Throughout the treatment period the clinician must be constantly aware of the psychological morbidity which can be induced by simply making the diagnosis of cancer and then compounding this with treatment which may be mutilating or toxic. The treatment of cancer by radiotherapy, surgery or chemotherapy is associated with significant side-effects in almost all instances, and this must be taken into account when planning treatment.

The recognition of these problems does raise the question of communication between the patient and the doctor, and indeed between the patient and the cancer care team. This is an area in which personal judgement is critical, together with a knowledge of the patient's personality and those of his immediate family. In general it would be correct to say that more patients are now aware of their diagnosis and, in general, expect more communication from their medical advisers.

Principles of Treatment

One of the most important aspects of modern cancer management is the emphasis on the combination of different forms (or modalities) of therapy. Thus, combined modality therapy has been responsible for the improved survival rates in a number of different forms of cancer. The surgeon should therefore see himself as part of a team of specialists involved in the integrated management of the patient. It is essential, therefore, that he is familiar with other forms of treatment of cancer and can actively participate and lead in the development of newer therapeutic methods.

Surgery in the Management of the Patient

Surgery remains the mainstay of treatment in the majority of solid tumours. Surgical techniques are usually necessary for establishing the diagnosis, and the initial procedure on the primary tumour is often surgical. However, as a knowledge of the natural history of cancer increases and improvements in other forms of cancer treatment become established, so the role of surgical management may change. This may simply involve a change in timing of the surgical procedures, other modalities being used first, or a change in outlook, less or more radical procedures being required.

In the treatment of the primary lesion the surgical concept has been to remove the tumour in its entirety, wherever possible, and without excessive damage to normal adjacent tissues. In some instances this procedure is combined with simultaneous *en bloc* dissection of the regional lymph nodes. The arguments for these procedures were based on the fact that cancer was thought to spread centrifugally, first regional, then distant lymph nodes being involved with eventual blood-borne spread. This concept has been challenged, as it is now clear that in some forms of cancer blood-borne spread can occur without node involvement. Nevertheless the excision of regional lymph nodes remains an important part of the surgical treatment of some forms of cancer.

The above procedures are used where the aim of treatment is to remove as much as possible of the tumour bulk in the hope of completely eradicating the cancer. This may not be possible and in many cases a knowledge of the natural history or staging will make it clear that curative surgery is not possible. It is in this situation that other modalities of treatment are added.

Surgical treatment, however, has a much wider role than biopsy, and removal of the primary tumour. A great deal can often be done to improve the quality of life of the patient by using palliative procedures such as bypass operations and local resections. Surgical treatment is being increasingly used in the excision of secondary tumours which may be present within the abdominal cavity, the liver, the thorax and the brain. Such procedures often result in prolongation and improved quality of life, and an ability to introduce other forms of treatment after bulk removal of the tumour. Reduction of tumour burden has become an important principle in cancer management.

The surgeon's role has also increased in the field of diagnosis and staging. This has been particularly the case in the lymphomas where staging laparotomies have become part of the management plan. More recently surgical staging procedures have become important in other forms of cancer, particularly in the testicular teratomas. As other methods of cancer treatment become more aggressive so there will be an increasing need to define the extent of cancer spread. In conjunction with new investigative techniques, surgical procedures will continue to be part of this process.

A further area of particular concern to surgeons are reconstruction procedures following, or in association with primary surgery. Although this has focused particularly on breast cancer surgery, the concept is certainly applicable to other sites. Once again a concern to improve the quality of life for the patient is paramount.

Surgical methods are also of importance in the hormonal treatment of cancer. Oophorectomy, orchidectomy, adrenalectomy and hypophysectomy all have their place. As drug therapy becomes more effective, however, especially in the field of hormone antagonists so this area of the surgeon's work may change.

Radiotherapy

This area is fully covered in Chapter 12. Suffice it to say that radiotherapy is an integral part of the management of the cancer patient and a knowledge of its role in the management of particular forms of cancer is essential for the practising surgeon.

Chemotherapy

Over the past 20 years there have been major changes in the role of drug therapy in the treatment of cancer. This is partly because of the development of new drugs but also because of the introduction of combination chemotherapy in which several active drugs are used in treatment. The ideal drug, or drug combination, has not yet been found, yet the improvements made in the treatment of some forms of cancer make it necessary to consider the integration of chemotherapy into the management of many of the cancers regularly seen by surgeons.

At the present time there are over 40 active drugs which have been shown to have activity against forms of cancer. If two or three drug combinations are considered then the number of potential interactions is enormous. Many of the active drugs have been discovered by chance though it has been possible to design some of these using the basic principles of biochemical pharmacology. The screening for new drugs is a costly and time-consuming exercise, yet necessary to identify new agents of clinical value.

Once a potentially useful drug has been identified its introduction into clinical practice is in three phases. The phase I study is carried out to investigate the toxicity of the drug and to establish its clinical pharmacology. When this has been completed a phase II study is then performed using the drug in the most appropriate way based on the phase I study. The aim of the phase II investigation is to establish the clinical activity of the drug based on its effect on a variety of different forms of cancer. If the phase II study shows the drug has activity then a phase III study is performed which investigates, in greater detail, the effects of the drug in particular tumour types before introducing it into combinations.

The mechanism of action of chemotherapeutic agents can be described in many ways, and be linked to chemical structure, biochemical function, or site of action on the cell cycle. Each method of classification has its own advantages and disadvantages. A limitation of all methods of classification, however, is that they focus attention on one method or mode of action, while the drug itself may have several. One classification commonly used is that based on the mechanism of action on the biochemical pathways leading to DNA synthesis or replication. Drugs may therefore be classified as follows.

Alkylating Agents

These drugs (e.g. cyclophosphamide, nitrogen mustard, chlorambucil, melphalan, etc.) are highly reactive agents which are able to bind to important biological molecules such as proteins or DNA. By binding to these molecules they inhibit or restrict their function.

Antimetabolites

These drugs (e.g. 5-fluorouracil, methotrexate, cytosine arabinoside, 6-mercaptopurine, etc.) act by inhibiting specific metabolic pathways, usually those of DNA synthesis, thus preventing cell replication and inducing cell death.

Vinca Alkaloids

These drugs (vincristine, vinblastine, vindesine) act specifically by inhibiting or arresting cells in mitosis, thus functioning as spindle poisons.

Antibiotics

A wide range of such compounds are now available and include adriamycin, bleomycin, streptozocin, actinomycin D and mitomycin C. Their mechanism of action is complex but it is likely that they interact with the double-stranded DNA molecule preventing its replication.

Miscellaneous Agents

It is naturally impossible to classify all cytotoxic drugs in the ways described above. Indeed several of these drugs may act in more than one way to produce their cytotoxic effect. For some drugs, however, the mechanism of action is by no means clear.

Mechanism of Action in Relation to the Cell Cycle

As previously described, the cell cycle may be divided into a number of phases and it is possible to classify chemotherapeutic agents on the basis of their site of action on the cell cycle. In general most drugs have no effect if the cell is not in cycle.

Using animal models drugs can be divided into:

1. Cycle non-specific. These drugs are active at all phases of the cell cycle and include cyclophosphamide, the nitrosoureas, and adriamycin.
2. Cycle specific or phase specific. These drugs act only at certain parts of the cycle, e.g. mitosis—vincristine, bleomycin; s-phase—cytosine arabinoside, hydroxyurea, methotrexate.

A knowledge of the kinetics of drug action may be useful in the design of drug combinations.

Mechanisms of Selectivity and Drug Resistance

The problems of selectivity and resistance are central to an understanding of the use of drugs in clinical practice. All cytotoxic drugs are effective against cancer cells if given in large enough doses. However, the therapeutic ratio of most of the drugs used (that is the ratio of the maximum tolerated dose to the minimum effective dose) is often very small. This means that toxicity and effectiveness are closely related. Thus no matter how effective the drug may be, it may not be able to be used in an appropriate combination because of toxicity. Great care must therefore be exercised in the use of these drugs.

Resistance to Cytotoxic Agents

It may be useful to distinguish between intrinsic resistance to drug action and acquired resistance which arises after several exposures of the drug. Acquired resistance may result from the selection of resistant mutant cells by destruction of the sensitive cell population or by a biochemical modification of the initially sensitive cells. These modifications may include:

1. Altered cell kinetics.
2. Inaccessibility of the cells to drug action, e.g. fibrosis.
3. Altered immune responses to cancer cell antigens.
4. Impaired transport through cell membrane.
5. Undetermined biochemical changes, e.g. increased level of drug catabolizing enzymes, decreased levels of activating enzymes, deletion of specific cell-binding proteins necessary for cytostatic activity of drug, repair of damaged DNA and RNA.

In an attempt to overcome drug resistance cytotoxic drugs are administered in combination in order to delay the emergence of drug resistance. However, it seems that many tumours are still able to overcome the impact of separated metabolic insults. It is likely that insufficient attention has been paid in the past to the effect of combination therapy on the immune response and altered antigenicity which permits emergence of the resistant strain.

Effect of Drugs on the Growth Kinetics of the Tumour

As was described earlier, tumours are composed of different growth compartments and in general chemotherapeutic agents act only on the growth fraction. Even with a very effective agent which would reduce the growth fraction almost completely, there would still be recruitment of cells from the non-dividing clonogenic compartment. This is one of the major reasons for giving chemotherapeutic agents over a prolonged period of time.

It is usual nowadays to administer drugs intermittently. In this way side-effects can often be minimized and efficacy improved. From a kinetic point of view it may also explain why in some instances a drug is effective and in others it is not. In *Fig.* 11.10 drug treatment is given with reduction in tumour size, but at the same time marrow toxicity occurs and the drug has been discontinued. Thus, although the cancer was sensitive to the drug, host toxicity has prevented repeated drug administration. This is in contrast to *Fig.* 11.11 where the cancer is responsive to the agent and where the host tissues have been able to recover more rapidly than the tumour, allowing selectivity of cytotoxicity. Tumour resistance may also result in tumour growth (*Fig.* 11.12).

Combination Chemotherapy

One of the most important advances in the use of drug therapy in the treatment of cancer was the introduction of

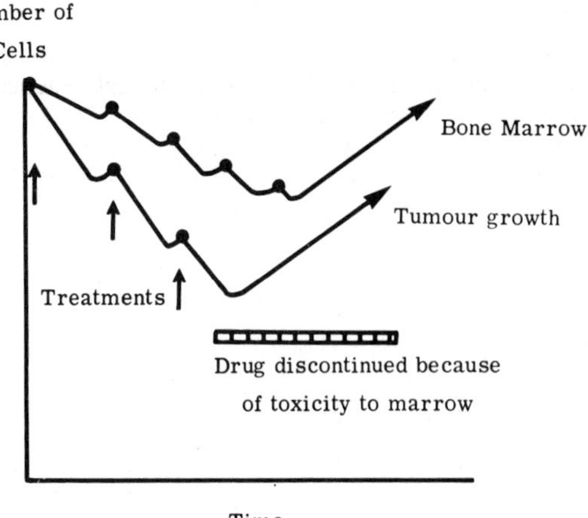

Fig. 11.10 Effect of marrow toxicity on drug response. Repeated treatments have resulted in bone marrow toxicity. The drug has been discontinued and the tumour regrows.

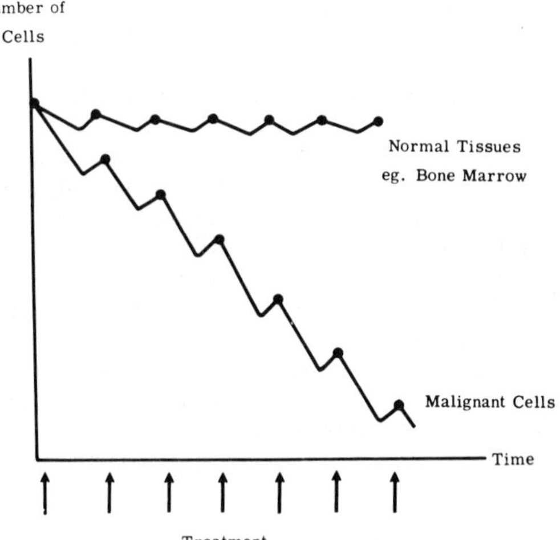

Fig. 11.11 Differential effect of treatment on normal and malignant cells. The drug is administered and the bone marrow is not damaged and a tumour response occurs.

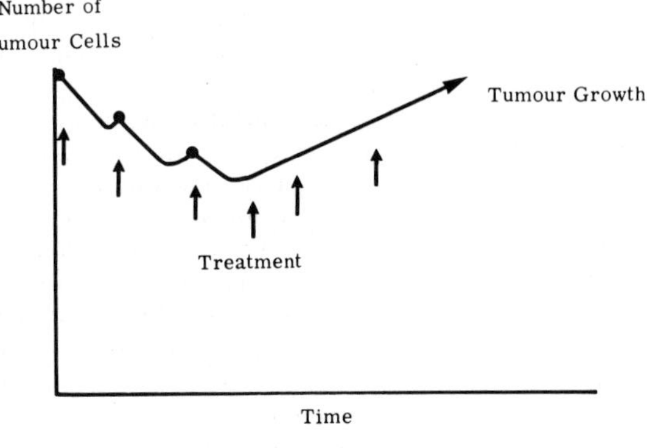

Fig. 11.12 Effect of drug resistance on tumour growth. Although drug treatment is initially effective in reducing the size of the tumour, resistance develops and the tumour grows in spite of repeated drug administration.

drug combinations. In almost all types of cancer, with some important exceptions, combinations of drugs are superior to single agents.

Combinations of drugs have been designed in a variety of ways though some of the most effective combinations have been discovered by chance. Combinations may be based on known biochemical synergisms or kinetic differences. The principles of combination chemotherapy are usually stated as follows:

1. Drugs used should be active as single agents against the particular cancer to be treated.
2. Drugs having similar toxicities should be avoided.
3. Drugs having different mechanisms of action or different sites of action should be used together.
4. Drugs used in combination should be used in doses as near as possible to their maximum doses when used as single agents.

Design of Combination Chemotherapy for Clinical Use

As with the overall management of the patient with cancer it is useful to have a plan for the selection of use of *drug combinations* (*Fig.* 11.13).

As before, the patient must be considered as an individual and prior to the commencement of chemotherapy the aims of treatment and possible side-effects should be reviewed. The choice of chemotherapy will depend on the diagnosis, and site and histology of the tumour and the condition of the patient. The individual drugs are then considered in the light of their effect as single agents, possible combinations and kinetic parameters. On the basis of this information a tentative treatment protocol is drawn up. The administration of this protocol is then considered in two ways. First,

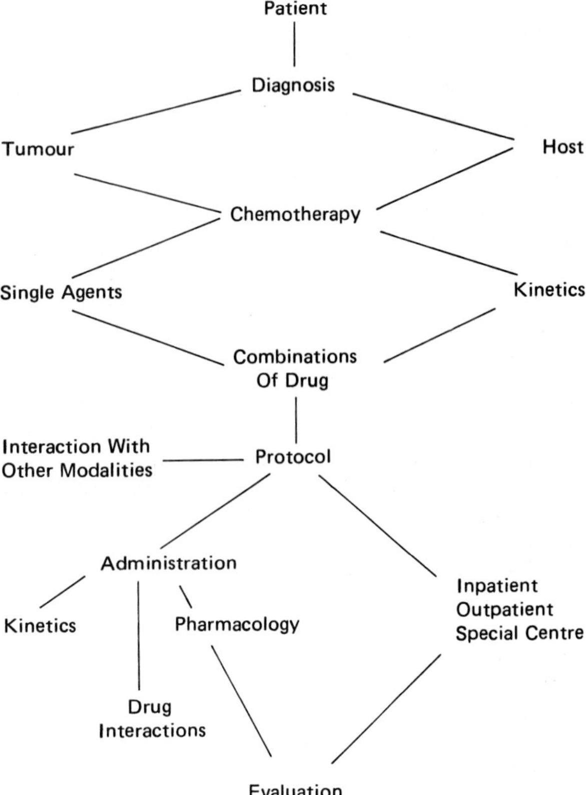

Fig. 11.13 Treatment plan for cancer patients.

the relationship to other forms of treatment, possible drug interactions, the pharmacology of the drugs and their kinetics. The second relates to where, and by whom, the drugs are to be administered. This will vary from protocol to protocol but it is essential that this is considered at an early stage.

Finally, it is paramount that the treatment protocol is evaluated and its results accurately recorded and reported. In most instances these drugs will be given as part of a clinical trial and the importance of such trials in the future management of the cancer patient cannot be overstressed.

The Role of Chemotherapy in the Treatment of Cancer

Although the most successful use of cytotoxic agents has occurred in the management of leukaemia and lymphoma, there is the ever present hope that it will ultimately prove possible to combine the modalities of surgery, radiotherapy and chemotherapy in therapeutic programmes capable of altering the natural history of common solid tumours. In fact, such developments have either been established, e.g. certain childhood embryonal cancers and carcinoma, or are nearly evaluated, e.g. testicular cancer, soft-tissue sarcomas. Other tumours such as breast and ovarian cancer are often responsive to cytotoxic treatment and this can play a significant role if applied at the correct time in the patient's course.

Surprisingly it looks as though some tumours are more sensitive than normal tissues to the action of drugs, although this is not usually the case. Furthermore it is known that some normal tissues affected by cytotoxic drugs are usually capable of proliferating more rapidly than neoplastic tissue and repair drug-induced damage before tumour cells can do so. Despite these encouraging observations, cytotoxic drug therapy has not yet significantly assisted cancer control of most solid tumours.

Table 11.3 Cancer chemotherapy

Cancers in which drugs have been responsible for some patients achieving a normal life span	
Acute leukaemia in children	Ewing's sarcoma
Hodgkin's disease	Wilms' tumour
Histiocytic lymphoma	Burkitt's lymphoma
Skin cancer	Retinoblastoma
Testicular carcinoma	Choriocarcinoma
Embryonal rhabdomyosarcoma	
Cancers in which responders to chemotherapy have had demonstrated improvement in survival	
Ovarian carcinoma	Lymphocytic lymphomas
Breast carcinoma	Neuroblastoma
Adult acute leukaemias	Oat-cell lung cancer
Multiple myeloma	Malignant insulinoma
Endometrial carcinoma	Gastrointestinal cancer
Prostatic cancer	Osteogenic sarcomas
Cancers responsive to drugs for which clinically useful improvement in survival of responders has not been clearly demonstrated	
Head and neck cancers	Malignant carcinoid tumours
Central nervous system cancer	
Endocrine gland tumours	Soft-tissue sarcomas
Cancers only marginally responsive or unresponsive to chemotherapeutic agents	
Hypernephroma	Pancreatic carcinoma
Bladder carcinoma	Hepatocellular carcinoma
Cancer of the oesophagus	Thyroid carcinoma
Epidermoid carcinoma of the lung	Malignant melanoma

Local Infusion Chemotherapy

There has been a revival of interest in this approach to cytotoxic drug delivery, largely because of new developments in implantable or miniaturized external pumps; rather than a breakthrough in drug design. As malignant tissue develops a neo-circulation drawn from the local arterial supply, it is possible to deliver high concentrations of drug in small volumes to the tumour provided that a single arterial supply is present. Because total drug doses are lower and spill-over into the general circulation is reduced, there may be less systemic toxicity. Furthermore, it is quite often possible to provide continuous delivery of the drug which is useful when administering cell cycle active agents such as fluorouracil and floxuridine. Implantation of catheters into the common hepatic artery are currently of great interest. A response rate of 50% is normally achieved but the median survival of patients with metastatic disease is still only one year and it has not yet been demonstrated that improved survival occurs over matched controls. It remains to be shown that arterial infusion of cytotoxic drugs is advantageous but with the availability of totally implantable, refillable and rechargeable pumps there is an added stimulus to investigate new drug schedules and means of increasing the potency of established drugs.

The use of drugs in the management of cancer is a rapidly changing field. It is possible therefore only to give an overall view of its role, recognizing that this might change at any time. The following summarizes the current place of chemotherapy in individual cancers (*Table* 11.3). Chemotherapy is now an established part of cancer management and its role is likely to develop in the future.

Complications of Chemotherapy

As has been mentioned the therapeutic index for anticancer drugs is small. Toxicity is therefore a major problem and in some cases can be severe enough to be life threatening. If they are used properly then the side-effects can be minimized, but there is need to exercise great care in their use, and, in some instances, administration should be restricted to special centres.

A wide variety of non-specific complications are associated with chemotherapeutic agents. These include nausea, vomiting and mucositis. This latter problem, affecting mainly the mouth, throat and gastrointestinal tract, can be especially difficult to deal with, particularly if complicated by superinfection. Alopecia occurs fairly frequently, particularly if certain drugs, such as adriamycin, are used. Haematological problems, leucopenia, thrombocytopenia do occur, and may be an accepted part of management if treatment is aggressive. Active haematological support must be given in this instance, with the use of prophylactic antibiotics to prevent infection together with leucocyte and platelet support. If the patient is severely immunosuppressed reverse barrier nursing or the use of protected environments may be required. Where indicated white cell transfusions may be necessary, though this is rare. Wherever possible the drugs used should be administered in doses which do not cause severe leucopenia. It should be remembered that this risk is compounded by previous or concurrent radiotherapy.

Chemotherapeutic agents induce a variety of hormonal changes and affect endocrine organ function. Of particular importance is the effect on testicular and ovarian activity. In the premenopausal woman menstruation may cease and following termination of therapy infertility may occur. This is also found in relation to testicular function, though in this instance sperm banking may be used, prior to treatment, in case infertility occurs. There is no evidence that the offspring of individuals who have had chemotherapy have any greater chance of developing birth defects or genetic abnormalities.

On the other hand, it would appear that the incidence of second tumours arising in patients who have had chemotherapy is higher than would be expected. Although the risk is not great it is certainly real, and must constantly be remembered, particularly when drugs are being used in an adjuvant setting, in fit patients, and over a long period of time.

In addition to the non-specific toxicities described above certain specific complications are known. These include the cardiotoxicity associated with the use of adriamycin and daunomycin, the lung toxicity with bleomycin and busulphan, the renal toxicity with methotrexate and cis-platinum, and the bladder toxicity with cyclophosphamide. These side-effects may become so severe as to be life threatening. However, with careful pretreatment assessment and attention to detail these can be avoided in most instances.

Adjuvant Chemotherapy

Originally the use of chemotherapy was restricted to patients with advanced cancer. With increasing safety, it has been applied to patients identified as being at high risk of developing recurrent cancer after attempts at curative surgery. The concept involved makes the assumption that small volumes of occult secondary cancer are more sensitive to chemotherapy than advanced cancer. There is little evidence as yet to support this view but it would seem that both pre- and postmenopausal patients with breast cancer and involved axillary nodes show marginal gains in disease-free survival after combination chemotherapy. Although colorectal cancer patients have been exhaustively evaluated after adjuvant 5-fluorouracil, there is no evidence that this agent is active enough to improve survival patterns.

Hormones in the Treatment of Cancer

Hormonal methods of treatment have an important part to play in the management of cancer, not only as therapeutic modalities, in their own right, but as methods for symptom control and general support of the patient.

Mechanism of Action of Hormones

It has been known for some time that only a proportion of patients with breast cancer respond to hormone therapy, as evidenced by tumour regression. Methods of predicting such response have been tried over the years but it is only recently that techniques have been developed which allow such a prediction to be of real clinical value.

With tumours which are responsive to steroid hormones it is known (*Fig.* 11.14) that the hormone is taken into the cell and binds to a specific receptor. This receptor then moves into the cell nucleus and the hormone interacts with cellular DNA to produce the biochemical effect of the hormone. By estimating for the presence or absence of such receptors in tumour tissue it has been possible to correlate this with response. Thus, if receptors are present within a specific cancer, it is probable that the patient will respond to hormonal therapy. If these are not present then the chances of response are very small. This measurement of receptor status has real clinical value.

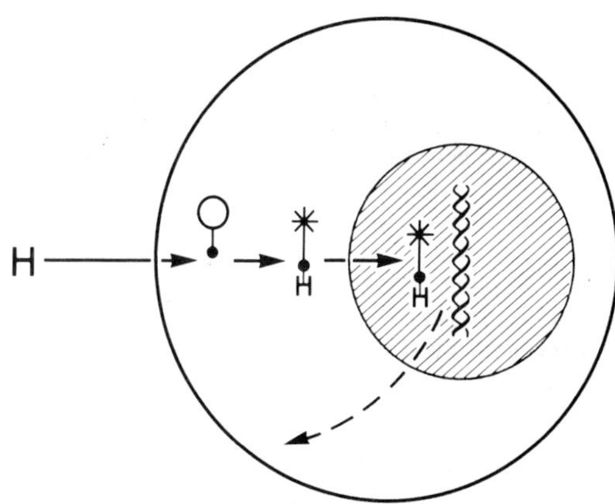

Fig. 11.14 Mechanism of action of steroid hormones on cell receptors. The hormone enters the cell, binds specifically to a receptor which is then translated into the nucleus where it interacts with the genome.

Use of Hormones in the Treatment of Cancer

Hormonal procedures can be employed in a number of different forms of cancer and are usually used in the following ways:

1. Ablative procedures—oophorectomy, adrenalectomy, etc. In this instance a source of hormone secretion is removed.
2. Added hormones—e.g. prednisolone, progestogens, oestrogens, androgens, etc. These compounds are used to produce specific antitumour effects.
3. Hormone antagonists, e.g. tamoxifen.
4. Drugs which interfere with hormone synthesis or release, e.g. aminoglutethimide.

Hormonal procedures have been used to treat male and female breast cancer, prostatic cancer and endometrial cancer. They have also been used in renal cancer, where the effect of the compounds (usually progestogens) is not clear cut. Corticosteroids are used in the treatment of leukaemias, lymphomas and myelomas.

Other Uses of Steroid Hormones

The corticosteroids in particular do have a place in the management of other aspects of cancer care. Thus, anorexia may respond to small doses of prednisolone and as part of the overall management of hypercalcaemia the corticosteroids may be of benefit. The value of dexamethasone in the management of raised intracranial pressure is well known. The use of androgens in the treatment of marrow complications has also been of some value.

IMMUNOTHERAPY

Although many virally and clinically induced cancers will induce a strong rejection response, there are many others in which the immune response is minimal. The lack of an immune response may be due to lack of tumour cell antigenicity or lack of host immune responsiveness. It is in this latter area which there may be host genetic influence via Ir genes (Immune Response genes). Reseach has identified a major Ir complex close to the MHC complex (*see* Chapter 77 but there are likely to be many others not so easily located. The function of the Ir gene is not known but it may act to recognize antigens by T cells and B cell antibody formation. This influence may be an all or none effect on the immune response, other genes appear to control the timing or the magnitude of the response (modifying genes). Presumably these genes exact a crucial influence in the host response to a proliferating neoplastic target. Experimentally it is known that some animals are resistant to certain oncogeneic viruses, presumably Ir genes restrict viral replication. In humans, it may be that the Epstein–Barr virus is controlled by Ir genes.

The mechanism of the effector system in cancer immunology remains uncertain. The evaulation of cell-mediated reactions against tumour associated antigens is relatively new, although there is hard data that both T- and non-T-cell effectors are involved. The contribution of the various antibody classes is quite uncertain. Although the attention of the researcher, both experimentally and clinically, naturally turns towards cancer cell killing, it is important also to consider the cytostatic effects of the immune system. It is quite likely that the latency of dominant cancer cells are the most important phenomenon of tumour immunology. There has, perhaps, been far too much attention directed along the investigative lines so successful in the analysis of organ transplantation, which may not be appropriate for tumour immunology.

In the same manner, more investigation is required of the effect of blocking serum factors. From transplantation research it is known that transplantation antigen antibodies (e.g. anti-H_2 antibodies) are capable of inhibiting sensitized lymphocytes. The antigen may also be inhibitory particularly for non-T cells and may be more important than antibody. It is known that serum blocking factors commonly disappear after removal of a primary tumour. This suggests that the tumour contributes to the blocking activity, e.g. release of membrane antigen. Different tumours and different cells within the same tumour vary in their ability to shed cell membrane antigen. Potentially the release of these blocking factors is capable of influencing the metastasizing capability of tumours.

The basic mechanisms of the immune response are described elsewhere (Chapter 77). This section will concentrate on the potential use of immunotherapy in cancer management.

There is a certain amount of evidence from animals and clinical studies that tumours may be susceptible to control by immunological means. This evidence, in humans, is by no means conclusive and has been challenged. The use of immunotherapy as a therapeutic modality is based on the assumption that modulation of the immune response would allow the control of tumour growth and that the effector arms of the response would destroy cancer cells.

To modify the immune response either active or passive immunotherapy may be used (*Table* 11.4) and this may be either specific or non-specific. Most of the clinical studies which have been reported have used active, non-specific methods such as the use of BCG, *Corynebacterium parvum* or levamisole. In some instances this has been combined with the use of autologous irradiated tumour cells in an attempt at making the response more specific.

Table 11.4 Traditional immunotherapy methods

	Active	*Passive*
Specific	Tumour cell extracts	Sensitized cells
	Tumour vaccines	Serum
Non-specific	BCG	White cell transfusions
	C. parvum	Serum factors
	Levamisole	

There are other antitumour phenomena which can be shown at least experimentally to be of use in cancer control. A revival of interest in the interferons has shown that α interferon is clinically effective against hairy cell leukaemia, but few other tumour systems. However, when recombinant interferon is combined with dacarbazine against melanoma and adriamycin against solid tumours, e.g. pancreatic, then a synergistic effect is obtained. It is becoming clear that interferons are best used in relatively low dosage for there is evidence that clinical disease may be accelerated by high doses and this may be due to an impairment of cellular responses. It is probable that a use of low-dose interferon will be made in the postoperative period when cellular responses to cancer (natural killer cell activity) are at their lowest. Non-cellular by-products of immune cells are now identifiable as lymphokines and these substances can be produced in quantity by molecular engineering. These substances, particularly interleukin 2 (IL2), are capable of stimulating and maturing cytotoxic T-lymphocytes and experimentally this has been effective against a number of murine tumours. There is considerable toxicity from IL2 when given systemically but it may be equally effective when given into tumour. IL2 can be used to stimulate autologous lymphocytes *ex vivo*, and the activated cells returned to the patient. Initial results are encouraging and clinical trials are in progress. Finally, two other products of macrophagic and lymphocyte metabolism have been identified: tumour neurosis factor and lymphotoxin. These agents appear to control the mobilization of energy sources at a cellular level and could be responsible for cancer cachexia as well as being capable of producing tumour neurosis.

Results of the Use of Immunotherapy

It would be fair to say that in general the results of immunotherapy in the treatment of cancer have been disappointing. In only a few instances has any real benefit been shown. There are several reasons for this. The first is that the techniques used, e.g. non-specific stimulation, may be far too crude to show any effects. Secondly, immunotherapy has often been used in patients with very advanced disease in whom other treatments have already failed. Under these circumstances it is perhaps not surprising that treatment is ineffective. Finally, adequate evaluation of treatment has often been lacking and interpretation and analysis of the data before sufficient patients have been studied has given a false impression of its value.

REHABILITATION AND TERMINAL CARE

Reference has already been made to the importance of the quality of life. Nowhere is this more important than in the patient who requires terminal care or rehabilitation following surgery or other forms of cancer therapy. Both terminal care and rehabilitation must be seen as active processes requiring the same high standards of care, investigation and treatment as in other aspects of cancer care. The team approach is invaluable and the role of the nurse, health visitor, physiotherapist, occupational therapist, etc. is not difficult to envisage.

At the stage of terminal care communication is of tremendous importance. The correct approach to the patient, together with a concern for care, can mean an enormous amount to the patient and the family.

At an earlier stage rehabilitation is also an area which should be pursued actively and all available expertise harnessed for the benefit of the patient. This applies to the patient who has just had a mastectomy, a colostomy, or a procedure on the head and neck, where the known psychological morbidity is high. Effective communication, help and advice, at this stage can improve the quality of life.

12 Ionizing Radiation and Radiotherapy

W. Duncan

The use of ionizing radiations in medicine began within a year of the discovery of X-rays in 1897. However, the philosophy and practice of modern radiotherapy are based on physical and biological principles, together with technical innovations introduced in the early 1950s. To a large extent these developments arose out of research conducted during and immediately following the Second World War, particularly concerning the peaceful uses of atomic energy. Two additions to our therapeutic armamentarium which led dramatically to the increasing application of radiotherapy and to its greater effectiveness in the field of cancer management require special mention (*Table* 12.1). The first was the manufacture of linear accelerators and telecobalt therapy machines which provided sources of high energy (megavoltage) X- and γ-rays which permitted the more effective treatment of deep-seated tumours with complete skin sparing. Secondly, the artificial production of radionuclides for medical purposes added significantly to the scope of sophisticated radiotherapy techniques (*Table* 12.2).

Table 12.1 Ionizing radiations in medical use

Electromagnetic radiations	X- and γ rays
Corpuscular or particulate radiations	Electrons or beta rays
	Protons
	Neutrons
	Pions
	Helium nuclei
	Other light atomic nuclei
	Carbon
	Neon
	Argon

Table 12.2 Radionuclides used in clinical oncology

Element	*Radio-nuclide*	*Emission*	*Half-life*
Phosphorus	^{32}P	Beta	14 days
Strontium	^{90}Sr	Beta	28 years
Yttrium	^{90}Yt	Beta	2·54 days
Iodine	^{125}I	Gamma	60 days
Iodine	^{131}I	Beta and gamma	8 days
Iridium	^{192}Ir	Gamma	74 days
Gold	^{198}Au	Beta and gamma	2·7 days
Cobalt	^{60}Co	Gamma	5·3 years
Caesium	^{137}Cs	Gamma	33 years
Radium	^{226}Ra	Beta and gamma	1300 years
Californium	^{252}Cf	Neutron and gamma	2·6 years

THE PHYSICAL INTERACTION OF RADIATION WITH MATTER

Ionizing radiations are absorbed to a varying degree in different tissues by a number of specific interactions. The processes by which the energy from radiation is transferred to tissues are complex and are known as attenuation. As a result of attenuation radiations may be scattered or absorbed, giving rise to other particles and radiations. X- and γ-rays, protons and electrons interact with the orbital electrons of atoms, while neutrons, pions and heavy charged particles react with atomic nuclei. The nature of these processes and their relative importance depend on the type of radiation, its energy and the atomic composition of the tissue responsible for its attenuation.

With most X- and γ-rays two processes are important—scattering and the photoelectric effect. When very high energy X-rays (mainly over 20 MV) interact with tissues the photon may be absorbed by the electrons with the production of 'positive' and 'negative' electrons—so-called pair production. Routine radiotherapy is usually given with megavoltage X-rays (photons) of between 4 and 20 MV peak energy, with occasional accelerators providing X-ray beams up to 35 MV.

Alternatively, electrons which have similar biological properties to photons are preferred in some centres for the treatment of superficial tumours.

Some explanation should be given at this point about the importance of megavoltage X-rays and their advantages in clinical practice. Their principal advantages are four-fold. The penetration of the beam is so good that excellent dose distribution at depth may be obtained that readily allow the treatment of deep-seated tumours. No tumour can be considered inaccessible to well-planned radiotherapy. Secondly, the energy of megavoltage X-ray beams is such that the secondary electrons produced when they interact with the skin are scattered predominantly in a forward direction. This results in the maximum dose of radiation building up under the surface affording significant sparing of the overlying skin. Severe skin reactions may therefore be avoided. Since most of the energy transfer from the beam to the tissues is by a form of 'elastic' scattering, which is relatively independent of the atomic composition of tissues, there is very similar absorption of radiation dose in all tissues (for example in bone and muscle). By comparison, using 250 kV X-rays, almost three times as much energy would be absorbed in the bone as in soft tissues. This relatively high dose absorbed in bone was responsible for high incidence radiation osteitis when tolerance dose levels were delivered. The introduction of megavoltage radiation has led to a great reduction in this particular complication.

The actual measurement of absorbed dose of radiation is obviously of importance. In 1954 the unit of absorbed dose was agreed for the first time and became known as the 'rad', being equal to the absorption of 100 erg/gram of tissue. The international community has now adopted a unit of absorbed dose in terms of the SI units. The new standard is equivalent to 1 joule/kg and is known as the 'gray'. One gray (Gy) is equal to 100 rad.

PHYSICOCHEMICAL EFFECTS OF RADIATION

When ionizing radiations interact with the biologically important targets they may do so either by 'direct' or 'indirect' action *'Direct' action* describes the primary ionization of important macromolecular structures in the biological target. *'Indirect' action* describes the effect of reactive species produced in water in the biological system which secondarily ionize the sensitive biological targets. Indirect action concerns therefore the radiolysis of water. For our purposes the breakdown of water by radiation releases five important species—$OH^{\cdot}$, ^{e}aq, $H^{\cdot}$, H_2O_2 and $H_2^{\cdot}$.

These highly reactive products of radiolysis then react with the biological targets in the cell, leading to disruption and perhaps irreversible damage of macromolecular structures. The most important product is the hydroxyl radical ($OH^{\cdot}$) which is an oxidizing agent. The aqueous electron (^{e}aq), which is a free electron surrounded by a cage of water molecules, is another highly reactive species which is a powerful reducing agent. In general, oxidative reactions are the more important in that they are more likely to produce irreversible damage in the cell, damage is 'fixed' by the oxidative processes.

The biological effects of radiation may therefore be primarily modified in two ways. Either the intrinsic sensitivity of the biological target may be altered, or the reactivity of the species produced by the radiolysis of water may be modified.

One method of altering the sensitivity of the target is to introduce thymidine analogues into the structure of DNA. The halogenated pyrimidines 5-BUdR and 5-IUdR, bromo- and iodo-desoxyuridine, to the extent that they are incorporated in DNA, will increase the sensitivity of mammalian cells to X-rays. The treatment of cells by heating at 40 °C or above (hyperthermia) before or after irradiation also introduces stresses and eventually damage the DNA which will lead to an increase in the lethal effects of radiation. Other techniques involve influencing the reactive species produced in water. Such manipulations form the basis of chemical radioprotection and also provide the basis of several methods of radiosensitization employed in clinical practice. An important point in these reactions is that the protective or sensitizing chemical agents must be present at the time of irradiation for they are interacting in physicochemical processes that are extremely fast.

One of the most powerful radiosensitizing agents is oxygen. It is thought that oxygen molecules would react principally with the hydrogen radical $H^{\cdot}$ to give $HO_2^{\cdot}$, the hydroperoxy radical, which would increase the oxidative effect. This however, is unlikely to be the complete explanation. It is suggested that following the formation of superoxide ions ($O_2^{\cdot}$) an enzyme, superoxide dismutase, may catalyse the reactions to form hydrogen peroxide and molecular oxygen. Biochemical damage would then be fixed as a result of powerful oxidative reactions. It may also be the case that certain types of physicochemical damage are oxygen-dependent while other types of fixed damage are not. The exact mechanisms involved are obviously complex and are not yet completely understood, but examination of the 'oxygen effect' has had a greater influence on recent developments in radiotherapy than any other radiobiological phenomena. The converse of course holds true that hypoxia produces a radioprotective influence on biological systems. Many animal tumours have been shown to contain a proportion (10–20%) of hypoxic cells and it is thought that some human cancers may also have a hypoxic yet clonogenic population of cells that are relatively radioresistant and may be the source of recurrent disease after unsuccessful radiotherapy.

In 1954 techniques became available which allowed the culture of mammalian cells to be undertaken consistently *in vitro*. By exploiting this technique the response of mammalian cells to different doses of radiation could be measured, and provided the basis of modern quantitative radiobiology on which so much of our present understanding depends.

Fig. 12.1 illustrates a typical mammalian cell survival curve in which the dose is plotted in a linear manner and the surviving fraction of cells on a logarithmic scale. It is seen that the response of mammalian cells at first is described by a very shallow initial slope or shoulder region. In this region cells appear to be able to absorb a certain dose of radiation, called the quasi-threshold dose (Dq), before reaching a point where depopulation is proportional to the absorbed dose of radiation. There is no actual threshold dose for mammalian cells. Most survival curves have an initial slope, the value of which depends on the size of dose fraction. In the proportional or exponential portion of the survival curve equal increments of dose produce similar levels of depopulation.

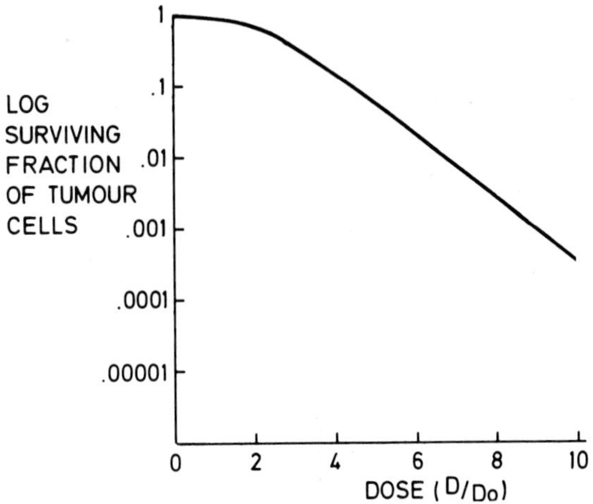

Fig. 12.1 Typical cell survival curve following X-irradiation.

The steepness of this exponential slope is measured by 1/Do where Do is known as the mean lethal dose (on average producing one lethal hit per cell). By definition and for reasons consistent with a mathematical description of the target theory of the nature of lethal radiation damage, the Do value is defined as the dose of radiation that will reduce the population to 37% (0·37 being 1/e and for exponential survival curves and surviving fraction SF = $e^{-D/Do}$). Since small dose fractions are usually given during a course of radiotherapy much more interest is now given to the Do of the initial slope of the curve.

It was of considerable interest and importance to find that there is only a small range of Do values for mammalian cells (range 100–400 cGy). In fact, most mammalian cell lines in culture have Do values in the range of 150–250 cGy.

Another finding of direct clinical relevance is that the mean lethal doses (Do) of normal and tumour cells from the same tissue of origin are similar. There is no consistent difference in the radiosensitivity of normal and tumour cells. Differences in intrinsic radiosensitivity cannot alone explain the ability of radiotherapy to eradicate tumours while its related surrounding normal tissues are preserved.

The 'shoulder' region of mammalian survival curves is the source of even greater interest. It is recognized that the size of the shoulder (Dq value) is a measure of the capacity of mammalian cells to recover from sublethal radiation damage. It is a manifestation of the ability of mammalian cells to protect the genome which may be demonstrated after many types of noxious insults. Following irradiation this capacity to recover has been shown to vary greatly between different types of cell. The values of Dq range from 50 to 500 cGy *in vitro* and the values tend to be much higher when measured *in vivo*. In a sense this quasi-threshold dose may be regarded as a measure of wasted radiation, in terms of cell killing, with each radiation exposure, and it is principally this effect which requires the dose of radiation when given in fractionated treatments to be increased in order to achieve the same biological effect.

Other techniques that have been used since 1976 have indicated that the response to radiation of mammalian tissues *in vivo* is perhaps better described by a continuously bending cell survival curve. The mathematical relationships of cell survival to dose are represented by what is known as the linear-quadratic model. The initial slope of the survival curve is determined by a function (α) which is proportional to the dose and the final slope by a function (β) is proportional to the square of the dose. Experimental studies have shown that tumours and actively responding normal tissues have a more steep initial slope than late responding tissues. There is as yet little firm data about the response of normal tissues or tumours to very small doses per fraction. However, it is thought that the differential killing of cancer cells compared with normal cells may be significantly increased by using very small dose fractions. It is possible that by giving doses per fraction of less than about 1·4 Gy, the probability of tumour control may be increased without any increase in the late normal tissue morbidity. It is necessary to give two or more of these small dose fractions each day to avoid the problem of tumour repopulation that would be likely if the overall treatment time were increased to allow the desired total dose to be given. Regimes of 'hyperfractionation' and accelerated fractionation are now being evaluated in clinical trials.

Another important biological factor determining the response of mammalian cells to radiation is the cell 'age' or its position in the mitotic cycle. Cells in mitosis are most susceptible to the lethal effects of irradiation while cells in late S, when the nuclear material has been duplicated, are most resistant. In any normal tissue or in a tumour population there will be varying numbers of cells in each phase of the cell cycle, the numbers being on average proportional to the time spent in each phase. Since the difference in mean lethal dose (Do) between M cells and late S phase cells is a factor of about 3, the degree of cell killing in a mixed population will depend greatly on its cell age distribution. Ideally, for maximum effect the tumour should be exposed to radiation when the majority of cells are in mitosis, but attempts at sychnronization have not been successful. Indeed it has to be acknowledged that perhaps only 50% of the tumour cell population is in cycle, the remainder being in resting or Go phase which is even more resistant to radiation.

The response of tissues to fractionated irradiation must also take repopulation into account. Human tumours have a wide range of doubling times, but most normal epithelial tissues will grow much faster—particularly following injury. It is therefore considered advantageous to divide a course of radiotherapy into many daily fractions, usually between 15 and 30, which allows some differential repopulation of normal tissues that have to be included within the treatment volume and the tumour itself. Radiotherapy attempts to optimize the selective depopulation of the tumour while minimizing the cell loss in normal tissues by the technique of fractionation. Fractionation will also allow for reoxygenation of hypoxic tumours, which should increase their radiocurability.

The parameters of the cell survival curve will change throughout a course of treatment as a result of changes in the intrinisic radiosensitivity of the population, the amount of recovery of sublethal damage, differential repopulation and with the redistribution of cell age in the irradiated tissues and tumour. It is by exploiting these subtle biological factors that radiotherapy can often produce an excellent therapeutic ratio, i.e. a high probability of local tumour control associated with low incidence of normal tissue morbidity.

These concepts may be demonstrated by examining the relationship of the cell survival curve to local tumour control and morbidity. It is generally accepted that in order to sterilize a tumour by irradiation, every cell has to be killed by the irradiation. There is little evidence to invoke concepts of immunological cytotoxicity, or necrosis secondary to vascular damage, to account for tumour cell destruction. One may then see from the cell survival curve that the probability of local tumour control (*Fig.* 12.2) depends essentially on the number of clonogenic cells it contains and on its radiosensitivity measured by the mean lethal dose. For fractionated radiotherapy the effective value would be measured from the appropriate portion of the initial slope of the survival curve.

The surviving fraction of cells may then be obtained since SF = $e^{-D/Do}$, where D is the total delivered. If the number of clonogenic cells in the tumour ('N') is known then the probability of cure is given by $e^{-(SF \times N)}$. It has been explained that normal cells have very similar cell survival characteristics to tumour cells, and so the dose-response curves for local tumour control and for normal tissue morbidity are not dissimilar (*Fig.* 12.3). Their relationship may be further illustrated by comparing the changing therapeutic ratio with increasing doses of radiation (*Fig.* 12.4).

It may be recognized that in most clinical applications there is initially a rapid increase in tumour control probability while there is small increase in the probability of normal tissue morbidity. A point (or dose) will be reached beyond which the rate of increase in morbidity greatly exceeds that of the increase in probability of local tumour control. That point may be called the 'optimum' dose. The radiation oncologist has to know the optimum dose levels for the different histological types of tumour and for different sizes of tumours which they wish to treat. In some clinical sites, such as larynx, it may be considered advisable to accept, say, a 10% morbidity in the larynx. These complications which are remediable by laryngectomy may be preferred to an increase in tumour recurrences associated with a lower radiation dose.

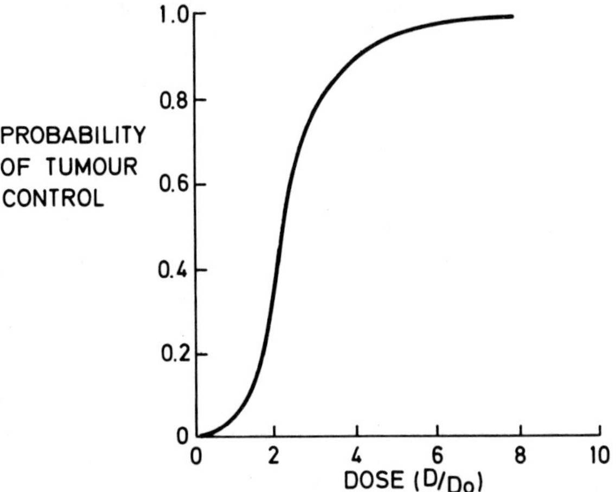

Fig. 12.2 Relationship of tumour control probability to radiation dose.

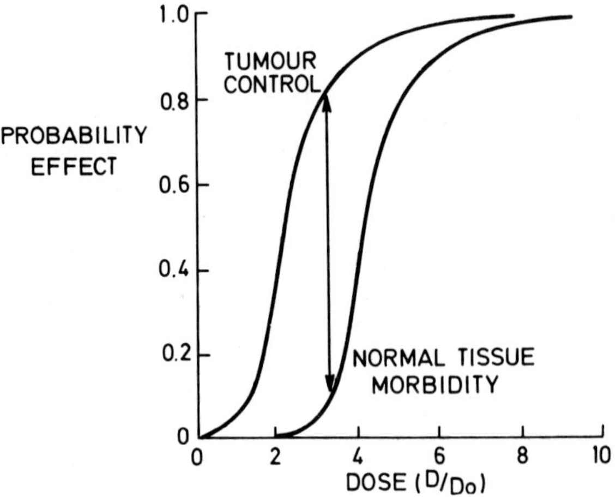

Fig. 12.3 Dose response curves for tumour and normal tissues indicating the therapeutic ratio.

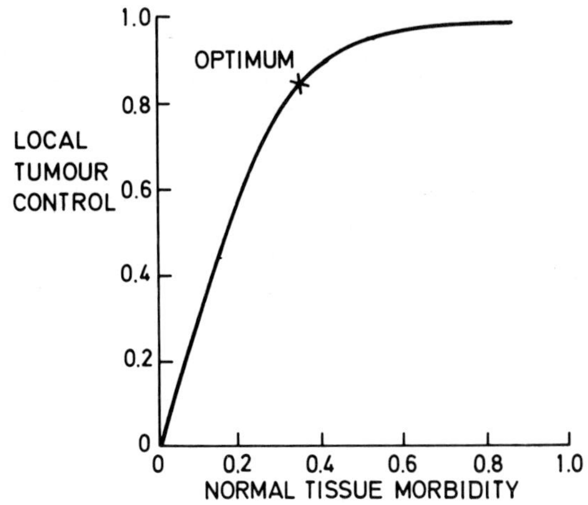

Fig. 12.4 The concept of optimum dose.

Although there is only a small range of variation in the 'intrinsic' radiosensitivity of mammalian cells they will, with a few notable exceptions such as the lymphocyte, show evidence of the lethal effects of radiation only when they enter mitosis. The rate at which tumours and normal tissues therefore show their response to radiation damage depends essentially on the cell turnover, the population kinetics of irradiated tissues. The intestinal villi have a very rapid turnover and within hours of irradiation damage will be obvious. In the brain only a few types of cells are capable of replication and their turnover rate is very low; damage therefore will be manifest relatively late compared with gut. In tumours, likewise, time is required after completion of radiotherapy to allow for the maximum effect of radiation to be manifest. It should be noted that some cancers such as the cystic basal-cell carcinoma in the skin may, although quite small, take up to 6 months to regress after effective radiotherapy.

The dose level which produces the acceptable level of late morbidity in normal tissues following radical or definitive radiotherapy is known as the 'tolerance' dose. In clinical practice when the objective is cure, normal tissue tolerance doses are usually prescribed. The probability of local tumour control, therefore, for any given type of tumour, will then depend on its size; the larger the tumour the lower the probability of it being sterilized by the radiation dose that may safely be given to the normal tissues. Some radiotherapists may in these circumstances be prepared to advise that the morbidity rate should be increased in order to increase tumour control. It is not considered that such an approach regularly be adopted and alternative forms of management should be considered in these circumstances.

DEFINITIVE OR RADICAL RADIOTHERAPY

The detailed assessment of patients with cancer is essential before a definitive opinion can be given about optimal management and the factors to be taken into account are given in *Table* 12.3. Their consideration often demands the experience and skill of several specialists in determining the best therapeutic approach for each patient. In cancers where there is no evidence of widespread dissemination the choice of management will normally be between surgery and

Table 12.3 Features of importance in the choice of treatment

1. Site of tumour
2. Histology of tumour
3. Stage of advancement
4. Biological characteristics of tumour
5. Biological characteristics of host
6. Age and general condition
7. Specific intercurrent disease or disability
8. Emotional status

radiotherapy. Associated with that choice, the decision must also be taken as to whether treatment is to be definitive (i.e. potentially curative) or palliative. In radiotherapy practice it is commonly accepted that there should be at least a 10% chance of complete local control and long-term survival before radical treatment is undertaken. It is implied in such a decision that patients with advanced cancer should not be required to endure the rigours of definitive management if they have little chance of cure. The total burden of physical and emotional stress which results from aggressive management must not be excessive in relation to the proportion of patients who may be successfully treated.

The indications for radical radiotherapy are given in *Table* 12.4, listed in a way which also gives some indication of the principles of radical or definitive radiotherapy.

Table 12.4 Indications for radical radiotherapy

I. *Primary Elective Management*	
Operable Lesions	*a*. Optimum control rates
	b. Preservation of form and function
Inoperable Lesions	*a*. Local extension
	b. General unfitness for surgery
II. *Primary Combined Management*	
Adjuvant to Surgery	*a*. Local residual disease
	b. Lymph node metastases
	c. (Other metastases)
Adjuvant to Chemotherapy	*a*. Local residual disease
	b. Protected organs (sanctuary sites)
III. *Secondary Management*	
After Elective Surgery	*a*. Local recurrence
	b. Lymph node metastases

PRIMARY ELECTIVE MANAGEMENT

Primary elective management by radiotherapy is accepted now for many types of primary tumours. These are tumours such as squamous carcinoma of the tongue which have been shown to be best managed by radiotherapy rather than surgery. Another example is the more advanced stages of carcinoma of the uterine cervix for which radiotherapy has for long been established as the treatment of choice. Many patients with localized lymphoreticular neoplasms, of which Hodgkin's disease is a good example, are also best treated by irradiation.

A very important advantage of radiotherapy is that often successful treatment may be carried out while retaining the function of some vital or important organ. Tumours of the brain are of course in this category, but cancer of the bladder is another very good example. Cancers of the larynx and pharynx may also be treated by primary irradiation with results similar to that achieved by radical surgery, but with the great advantage of retaining the voice and the ability to swallow normally.

It must be remembered that some forms of cancer which are inoperable may well be within the scope of radical radiotherapy. Cancer of the thyroid frequently presents with a large, fixed gland often associated with metastatic regional lymph node involvement. Radiotherapy is often able to eradicate the disease locally. Cancer of the prostate is often inoperable when the diagnosis is made, and yet large numbers of patients with this disease will have prolonged disease-free survival after radical radiotherapy.

It must also be acknowledged that many patients who may be unfit for surgery because of their age or general unfitness, or perhaps because of some specific intercurrent disease may well be able to complete a course of definitive radiotherapy. At times, too, patients may refuse elective surgery for their cancer while radiotherapy may be acceptable to them and which may offer an equally good probability of success.

PRIMARY COMBINED MANAGEMENT

Primary combined management by radiotherapy and surgery is becoming increasingly employed in times when patients are often seen and assessed by a multidisciplinary group of clinicians before decisions on management are taken. It is possible in these circumstances to plan a joint management programme which may offer improved chances of eradicating the tumour, sometimes with less morbidity than would have been associated with either treatment alone. The planned approach may involve radiation being given preoperatively or postoperatively.

The value of preoperative radiotherapy has not yet been firmly established in clinical trials, but important principles are involved in its use.

The objectives are to reduce the probability of local recurrence and perhaps also minimize the risk of distant dissemination. It is, however, generally recognized that distant spread has usually occurred before the presentation of the primary cancer and is not determined by surgical manipulation. Seldom is an 'inoperable' cancer made 'operable' by giving preoperative radiotherapy.

Preoperative radiotherapy may be given as a course of treatment delivering a dose of radiation two-thirds to three-quarters that of radical treatment. Usually a course of 'high-dose' preoperative radiotherapy would be given over 4–6 weeks. Thereafter a delay of further 4–6 weeks is allowed for the immediate radiation reaction to resolve, and then definitive excision is performed. The administration of such high radiation doses may contribute in small measure to an increase in postoperative morbidity. Preoperative radiotherapy has been shown to improve the 5-year survival of patients with stage T3 transitional-cell carcinoma of the bladder, and patients with operable breast cancer have also been demonstrated in a randomly controlled clinical trial to have a better survival following preoperative radiotherapy.

An alternative approach is to give a relatively low dose of radiation before operation. This technique minimizes the delay before definitive removal of the tumour and should not influence the operative procedure or the operative morbidity. A single dose of 500 cGy X-irradiation should reduce the tumour cell population by about two orders of magnitude (10^{-2}). Such a reduction in the number of viable tumour cells at the time of the operation should reduce the probability of local implantation and of disseminating viable clonogenic cells into the circulation.

A 'low-dose' preoperative regime of 500 cGy has been shown (in one trial, but not another) to improve survival in patients with Dukes' C stage rectal cancer after abdominoperineal resection. Also in patients with rectal cancer undergoing abdominoperineal resection a slightly higher dose, 2000 cGY given in ten daily fractions, has been shown not only to improve survival in patients with advanced disease (Dukes' C), but also to have reduced the incidence of local recurrence and of metastatic disease. In cancer of the bladder, too, this 'low-dose' level of radiation has been considered to be effective although this has not been demonstrated by a proper trial. Preoperative radiotherapy, and especially low-dose preoperative radiotherapy, requires further evaluation at other sites. There is evidence that the results of oesophagectomy may be improved by preoperative irradiation, although no controlled study has been reported. When further trials are reported the real improvement that has been demonstrated in patients with advanced bladder and rectal tumours may well be reflected in results of preoperative irradiation at other sites.

Postoperative radiotherapy has had much more general appeal to surgeons, particularly when given to selected patients with recognized residual disease at the time of operation. There are a number of tumours with which this policy of selective postoperative radiotherapy has been shown to be of benefit. Tumours of the thyroid and parotid glands, the ovary, and of the body of the uterus come into this category. There are other tumours such as Wilms's tumour where postoperative radiotherapy should be given, except in children under the age of 2 years, even when an encapsulated tumour has been completely removed. The other application of postoperative radiotherapy concerns the treatment of regional lymph nodes following excision of the primary tumour.

A clear example of this type of combined management is simple mastectomy without axillary lymph node dissection, followed by radical radiotherapy for breast cancer. However, new policies of surgical management have been introduced since the importance of histological evidence of axillary node involvement in determining further management has been documented.

The role of postoperative radiotherapy in the control of regional (and juxta regional) lymph nodes in germ-cell tumours of the testis is presently under review. There is no doubt that irradiation will control metastases from seminoma of the testis. Some controversy exists about the management of involved retroperitoneal nodes from teratoma of the testis, although the only controlled trial to investigate the relative effectiveness of primary elective irradiation and lymphadenectomy has shown no significant difference in the survival rates. The use of effective regimes of cytotoxic chemotherapy now plays an important role in the management of patients with metastatic germ cell tumours. As a result, both surgery and irradiation are less frequently employed than in the past to control lymph node and other metastases in these patients.

In the management of certain lymphoreticular neoplasms and acute lymphatic leukaemia in children, radiotherapy is regularly given as part of a combined management. Patients with Stage III Hodgkin's disease commonly have regions of bulky lymph nodes so large that resolution is incomplete after intensive chemotherapy. Radiotherapy to these sites of bulky disease considerably improves their prognosis. In leukaemia a high proportion of patients in apparent complete remission will relapse in the brain and testes, organs within which the tumour cells are protected from the effects of cytotoxic drugs. Prophylactic irradiation of the brain is part of routine management of many children with acute lymphoblastic leukaemia, and the high probability of later developing testicular disease may lead to testicular irradiation also being advised in these children.

SECONDARY MANAGEMENT BY RADIOTHERAPY

Secondary management by radiotherapy after failed surgery has never produced encouraging results. On many occasions the development of local recurrence or of regional lymph node heralds metastates, the presentation of generalized disease. These patients, for example with breast cancer, do have a very unfavourable prognosis. Exceptionally, in some sites such as the bladder, recurrence of a T2 tumour after endoscopic resection does justify a course of radical radiotherapy which carries a high probability of local control of the tumour.

A SYNOPSIS OF CURRENT PRACTICE

The principles involved in radical treatment have been described in some detail. There follows a brief account of the role of radiotherapy in current clinical practice. It should be recognized that the management of most forms of cancer is changing as new techniques are tried and confirmed to be of value. Steady progress is being recorded and it is impossible to provide a synopsis of radiotherapy which will fully reflect current thoughts on the indications for its use and the steadily improving results that are being reported.

Breast Cancer

In patients with apparently localized disease, the most important factors in deciding the management are the stage of the primary tumour and the degree of regional lymph node involvement. Secondarily the menopausal status of the patient may influence the choice of systemic medication. In the last few years there has been increasing attention paid to determining the minimum effective local management, together with concentration on the need for systemic management in most patients with breast cancer.

Patients with operable cancers are normally treated primarily by simple mastectomy and axillary node sampling. If the axillary nodes are found histologically not to be involved with tumour, postoperative radiotherapy would not be advised. If the axillary nodes are found to contain tumour metastases, radiotherapy to the chest wall (which has an increased risk of local recurrence in these patients) and regional lymph nodes should normally be given. Many of these patients may also be given several courses of cytotoxic chemotherapy if premenopausal or endocrine therapy, such as tamoxifen, if postmenopausal or a combination of both. If systemic treatment is being given many oncologists would withhold radiotherapy until there is evidence of local recurrence. Some surgeons may continue to advise a Halsted-type radical mastectomy. There is no indication routinely to give these patients postoperative radiotherapy, unless there is evidence of gross residual disease.

Patients with breast cancer under 3·0 cm in diameter, with or without mobile axillary nodes, are increasingly being managed without mastectomy. It would seem that excellent cosmetic results can be obtained, with good long-term survival rates, by local excision and radiotherapy to the breast. Irradiation may be by radionuclide implantation of the breast using ^{192}Iridium wire, or by electron or X-ray beams. External beam therapy may be added to the regional lymph nodes if axillary node biopsy demonstrates nodal involvement. Alternatively, some surgeons may rely on axillary-node dissection to control lymph node metastases.

Patients with more advanced inoperable disease in the breast also should benefit from radical irradiation. Many techniques are employed, but all include the breast, axillary and supraclavicular nodes, together with the ipsilateral internal mammary lymph node chain in the fields of irradiation. Local control of the breast tumour should be achieved in at least 75% of these patients. Simple mastectomy may occasionally be advised in some patients with local recurrence in the breast, and may contribute to long-term survival. Overall the survival rates of these patients (without involved supraclavicular nodes) should be about 40% at 5 years and with 15% surviving 10 years or more.

Lung Cancer

Lung cancer remains a special challenge not only because of the high incidence of the disease, but also in that most patients present with such advanced disease that they are unsuitable for radical treatment. Squamous carcinoma of the lung, if operable, is best managed by surgery, and anaplastic carcinomas are equally well managed by surgery or radiotherapy. The indiscriminate use of radical radiotherapy techniques in patients with advanced bronchial carcinoma is ill-advised. A simple palliative approach is often highly effective and is described later. Occasionally a fit patient with a small (<2·0 cm diameter) tumour with no evidence of metastatic disease, but who is not suitable for surgery, may be given radical radiotherapy. However, results are poor, with a 5-year survival rate of no more than 10%. Systemic cytotoxic chemotherapy is now regularly given to patients with small cell carcinomas and, although survival rates are improved, the margin of benefit is small.

Brain Tumours

Brain tumours in the adult are usually supratentorial gliomas, often poorly differentiated lesions with a poor prognosis. Radiotherapy is therefore usually palliative, providing a mean survival of 12 months or so. Medulloblastoma, however, although a highly aggressive tumour, is highly responsive to radiotherapy, and radical radiotherapy would always be advised. The posterior cranial fossa, the site of the primary tumour, and the whole cerebrospinal axis require to be included in the fields of irradiation because of the propensity of this tumour to spread by this route. With modern techniques about half of the children treated in this way will be long-term survivors.

Urological Cancer

The three most common tumours of the kidney are the renal-cell carcinoma, carcinoma of the renal pelvis and Wilms's tumour, the embryonal adenomyosarcoma of childhood. Only in the management of Wilms's tumour does radiation play an essential role.

Wilms's tumour, although rare, represents about 20% of children's cancer. The diagnosis can usually be made with a high degree of certainty by clinical examination and intravenous excretory urography. The standard practice is then to proceed to laparotomy and nephrectomy at which time the tumour is staged. If the tumour is very large preoperative radiotherapy may be given. The tumour is dramatically radiosensitive and regression quickly follows, so that operation need not be delayed for long. Further treatment then depends on the age of the child and the stage of the tumour.

It is now accepted that children under 2 years of age with tumours completely resected and shown to be confined to the kidney do not require postoperative irradiation. They will simply go on actinomycin D for one year. All other children, and those with more advanced disease, require postoperative abdominal irradiation and chemotherapy using actinomycin D and vincristine. There is debate about whether the whole abdomen or the renal bed and para-aortic lymph nodes need be irradiated. Results indicate little difference between the two techniques. The addition of cytotoxic chemotherapy with radiotherapy has almost doubled survival in these patients.

The treatment of choice for renal-cell carcinoma is nephrectomy, and radiotherapy may be of some value when given postoperatively for obvious residual disease. Preoperative radiotherapy has been evaluated and shown to be of no benefit even in locally advanced tumours.

The decision about the best management for patients with localized bladder cancer depends essentially on the stage of disease and the histological type and grading of the tumour. Superficial tumours and those with superficial muscle invasion (except Grade III lesions) are best dealt with by transurethral resection. All other tumours may be considered for treatment primarily by radiotherapy. Recurrent tumours following a course of transurethral resections may also be considered for irradiation. Optimum results seem to be obtained by small field irradiation of the bladder which would include only the perivesical and internal iliac nodes within the fields of treatment. It should be possible to control the bladder tumour in almost two-thirds of patients. Cystectomy should be advised for those patients with recurrent tumour after radiotherapy without evidence of spread of disease and who are fit for the operation.

Patients with carcinoma of the prostate with no evidence of lymph node or haematogenous metastases should be considered for radical radiotherapy. The radiation technique and dosage recommended is similar to that for bladder cancer. Excellent results have been obtained with 80% 5-year disease-free survival for Stage A disease, 70% for Stage B and 55% for Stage C. It has been demonstrated in controlled trials that there is no advantage in the simultaneous administration of oestrogens in these patients. Excellent results have also been reported following the permanent implantation of the prostate with ^{125}Iodine seeds in patients with small cancers. This technique may preserve potency better than external beam radiotherapy.

Gynaecological Cancer

Radical radiotherapy is a highly effective method of managing cancer of the uterine cervix and is the primary treatment in many centres throughout the world. Most centres use techniques which combine external beam megavoltage irradiation with intracavitary irradiation, employing radium, caesium-137 or cobalt-60. Some clinicians can claim that equally good results may be obtained in patients with the cancer confined to the cervix following Wertheim's hysterectomy. In patients with expansile disease in the cervix producing a barrel-shaped lesion, it is generally agreed that hysterectomy may give better results than radiotherapy. Often the distribution of radiation dose from the intracavitary sources is less than ideal in these patients. When the cancer has spread beyond the cervix radiotherapy is the treatment of choice. The results of treatment depend primarily of course on the clinical stage of the disease and the following survival rates should normally be obtained.

Stage	*5-year survival rate*
I	85%
IIa	75%
IIb	65%
IIIa	45%
IIIb	35%

Treatment of carcinoma of the body of the uterus remains primarily surgical, although preoperative radiotherapy probably improves the probability of local control and long-term survival in the more advanced cases. Preoperative radiotherapy is usually given in the form of intracavitary irradiation including the body of the uterus and the vaginal vault (the site of most recurrences). There may be some advantage in employing external beam radiotherapy to cover the whole pelvis and vagina, although the relative merits of these two techniques have not been properly evaluated. It must be remembered that in patients unfit for radical surgery or with inoperable disease, definitive radiotherapy may still be indicated. It has been suggested that the results of 'operable' disease by irradiation may be very similar to those following surgery. About 25% of patients with locally inoperable cancer in the body uterus may be expected to survive 5 years after radical radiotherapy.

The role of radiotherapy in the management of patients with ovarian cancer is less well established. Certainly it seems there is no advantage in giving postoperative irradiation following complete surgery for early cancer. However, when the disease is more advanced there is now some evidence that it is advisable to give megavoltage irradiation and that the whole abdomen should be included in the treatment. Particular attention has to be paid to treating the subdiaphragmatic areas which have been shown to be a common site of recurrent disease in the abdomen. It is clear, too, that when ovarian cancers are found not to be completely resectable, survival following radiotherapy is improved when surgery has removed as much as possible of the primary tumour.

Gastrointestinal Cancer

Cancers of the gastrointestinal tract have been considered wrongly to be completely radioresistant tumours. Experience is limited in the use of radiotherapy in their management, except in sites such as the oesophagus and anus. The prognosis of patients with carcinoma of the oesophagus is poor even in patients with relatively small tumours less than 7·0 cm in length and with no evidence of extrathoracic spread. Radical radiotherapy for patients with these small tumours will provide a 5-year survival rate of about 10%, probably similar to that following surgery. It is interesting that women with this disease have a survival rate almost twice that of men in series managed by radical radiotherapy.

Carcinoma of the stomach commonly presents so late that curative treatment either by excision or irradiation is seldom feasible. There is no evidence at present that definitive radiotherapy has a role, but it is claimed that preoperative radiotherapy may have a contribution to make as part of combined primary management. Intraoperative radiotherapy is being evaluated.

The value of preoperative radiotherapy has been demonstrated in patients with carcinoma of the rectum. Patients with Dukes' C stage cancers who had abdominoperineal resections have been shown to have improved 5-year survival rates (47%) when given low dose preoperative radiotherapy. Superficial (mucosal) carcinomas of the rectum respond well to radiotherapy and over 75% will be controlled at five years. This success rate may be no better than that expected after surgery, but obviously radiotherapy should be considered for patients who are unfit for surgery. There is an interest in treating deeply invasive carcinoma of the rectum primarily by irradiation, particularly tumours situated inferiorly to the peritoneal reflection. Again patients treated in this way have generally been those considered to be unsuitable for surgery because of their general condition. However, 5-year survival rates as high as 25% have been reported for patients with inoperable rectal carcinoma following radical radiotherapy. Postoperative radiotherapy (with or without adjuvant chemotherapy) has also been demonstrated to be advantageous to patients with Dukes' Stages B and C cancer of the rectum after curative resection. Significant improvement in both local tumour control and survival has been reported.

'Head and Neck' Cancer

The treatment of choice for many patients with cancer of the mouth is radiotherapy. Surgery, however, now has an equally important role. In many sites not only are control rates better than following surgery, but the cosmetic and functional results are better. Small lesions in the mouth may be very readily treated by surgery and advanced cancers involving the medulla or maxilla are best excised if possible.

The most common lesion in the mouth is squamous carcinoma arising on the lateral border of the middle third of the tongue. When the tumour is no greater than 2·5 cm in diameter and minimally infiltrating the substance of the tongue, a single plane radionuclide implant remains the treatment of choice. About 70% of these cancers will be locally controlled by radiotherapy alone. Similar lesions in the cheek or on the palate may also be considered for implantation using radium caesium needles, iridium wire or gold grains. Larger lesions require external beam therapy using megavoltage equipment or surgical excision. Mouth cancer is commonly associated with metastatic lymph nodes in the neck and, when mobile, are normally best dealt with by block dissection. When the involved node or nodes may be included in the radiation treatment volume *en bloc* with the primary cancer, it may be advantageous to adopt this treatment policy.

Cancers of the larynx and pharynx are often treated electively by irradiation with very good results. Small cancers of the glottis respond very well indeed and about 80% of patients can be cured, many with an excellent voice, following radiotherapy. It would seem that only in the very large infiltrating tumours in the larynx and pharynx, particularly if there is airway obstruction, would surgery be advised and offer a better chance of survival than after radiotherapy. Metastatic lymph nodes developing after treatment of the primary tumour are best managed by radical dissection. However, there is still considerable controversy regarding the management of these tumours, surgical excision being preferred in some centres.

Lymphoreticular Diseases

Lymphoreticular diseases are conveniently classified as Hodgkin's disease and non-Hodgkin's lymphomas. Several subclassifications exist for each of these and are recognized to be of clinical importance in indicating the natural history of the disease.

Hodgkin's disease predominantly occurs in lymph nodes, particularly in the cervical region, and normally spreads by involvement of contiguous lymph nodes. Later the liver and spleen, bone marrow and other organs may be involved. For patients with localized Hodgkin's disease involving one or two contiguous groups of lymph nodes radiotherapy is the treatment of choice. About 75% of patients will have complete remission of the disease with minimal side-effects of treatment.

Laparotomy with splenectomy and liver and lymph node biopsy is considered by many to be advantageous in most patients with apparently early disease. This adds to the accuracy of clinical staging of the disease and contributes in an important way to management if the spleen is involved.

When the disease involves nodes on both sides of the diaphragm radiotherapy in the form of total nodal irradiation gives excellent results. Cytotoxic chemotherapy is to be advised if there are constitutional symptoms of disease present, with radiotherapy being given afterwards to sites of gross lymph node involvement. When the disease is generalized and involving liver, bone marrow and other organs, chemotherapy is the treatment of choice.

Non-Hodgkin's lymphomas are a much less well-defined group of diseases. They involve often extranodal sites, the pharynx, gastrointestinal tract, thyroid gland, bone, testes and ovary. Their natural history is much less uniform than Hodgkin's disease and the pattern of spread much more capricious and unpredictable. The histological type of the tumour, degree of differentiation and stromal reaction are of great importance in determining their behaviour. Patients with diffuse, poorly differentiated tumours respond badly to all forms of management. Chemotherapy is normally to be advised but in some local radiotherapy may be highly effective and should be considered especially in older patients. In patients with non-Hodgkin's lymphomas showing nodular histology, especially with well-differentiated tumours, local radiotherapy, e.g. to the thyroid or nasopharynx, gives excellent results. In most patients, however, cytotoxic chemotherapy would normally be the treatment of choice, with the addition of radiotherapy to the primary site of disease if complete resolution has not been quickly obtained.

Soft-tissue and Bone Sarcomas

In most of these tumours the treatment of choice is excision combined with postoperative irradiation. When soft-tissue sarcomas are so large that surgery is not considered feasible, or would result in severe functional or cosmetic disability, then subradical ('debulking') resection is to be advised followed by radical radiotherapy to the residual tumours. It is not sufficiently well recognized that this form of combined primary management will achieve local control of the disease in over 85% of patients, often with remarkably little morbidity. Of course a problem remains in dealing with disseminated disease which commonly occurs in these patients, particularly associated with the poorly differentiated tumours.

A similar approach is now being evaluated in managing bone sarcomas in the limbs. Local excision of the tumour is being undertaken with insertion of a prosthesis, followed by radical radiotherapy. These patients are in many centres given systemic cytotoxic chemotherapy to attempt to control latent metastatic disease, but the efficacy of the regimes being used at present has yet to be confirmed.

Skin Cancer

Basal-cell carcinoma is the commonest form of invasive skin cancer and in 80% of patients arises on the face. These cancers are characteristically slow growing with a history of many months' duration, and commonly are small superficial lesions on presentation. Results of treatment by superficial X-rays or surgery are equally good. Radiotherapy is often the preferred treatment because of its simplicity. In tropical climates, however, surgery may be the treatment of choice because of the greater risk of late radiation necrosis in treated areas exposed to strong sunlight. Lesions on the trunk also may be better managed by excision as the radiation reactions are often more troublesome in these areas.

Squamous-cell carcinoma also arises commonly on exposed areas, particularly on the ear, lip and dorsum of the hand. The results of X-ray therapy again are excellent but in some circumstances, e.g. if the cartilage in the ear is involved, surgery may be performed. The risk of lymph node metastases has to be recognized with squamous-cell cancer, and surgery is to be advised when this complication presents.

Malignant melanoma is best managed by radical surgical excision. The response of melanoma to X-ray therapy is unpredictable and, although new techniques of radiotherapy are being explored at present, it cannot be advised as part of definitive management for patients with operable malignant melanoma.

PALLIATIVE RADIOTHERAPY

Many patients still present with cancer so advanced that cure is impossible. In these circumstances great clinical judgement must be exercised to consider how best the distressing features of the disease may be alleviated. Certain important principles of management are to be commended, and are equally applicable to the indications for surgery, cytotoxic chemotherapy or radiotherapy. Palliative treatment should always be directed to the alleviation of specific symptoms or signs of cancer. The treatment should be simple, short, effective and free of any lasting complications. It may be found that such treatment may be of emotional benefit, but relief of physical signs or symptoms of disease should always be the objective of palliative management. There is no case of radiotherapy to be used as a 'placebo'. Indeed it is seldom possible to guarantee that radiotherapy will be entirely free of side-effects. It should be recognized that frequently the administration of analgesic, narcotic and other symptomatic medication may be the best management of patients with advanced cancer rather than treatment of specific features of the disease by radiotherapy. In addition, the timely use of pain-relieving surgical procedures must be kept in mind, particularly in the patient with slowly progressive disease and who is otherwise quite fit.

Radiotherapy is often highly effective in controlling the distressing local symptoms and signs of cancer which are now considered in some detail (*Table* 12.5).

Table 12.5 Indications for palliative radiotherapy

1. Relief of pain
2. Healing of ulceration
3. Control of haemorrhage
4. Relief of obstruction
5. Suppression of effusions
6. Relief of neurological complications
7. Control of systemic symptoms and signs

Relief of pain is a most important consideration in the treatment of cancer for its control may greatly enhance the quality of the remainder of the patient's life. Metastatic tumour in bone is the most common cause of pain, and breast cancer is the most frequent form of cancer producing this distressing complication. In breast cancer systemic management with hormones or cytotoxic chemotherapy may be indicated, or an endocrine ablative procedure. However, often local irradiation is quickly effective and may be used alone or at times in addition to systemic management. Rapid and usually complete pain relief should be obtained in 85% of patients.

Bony metastases from other cancers such as bronchial, prostate, colon, bladder and kidney may also respond well to simple palliative X-ray therapy. It should also be recognized that pain from primary bone tumours, including osteosarcoma, can usually be relieved by local X-ray therapy, as well as the highly radioresponsive tumours such as myeloma and Ewing's sarcoma.

Tumour metastases in the pleura and those involving the capsule of the liver, may also give rise to severe pain, and local radiotherapy may be found to be much more effective than systemic chemotherapy.

Special attention should be paid to the prevention of fractures by irradiating weight-bearing regions of the skeleton found to be the site of metastatic disease—even in the absence of local symptoms. Irradiation may often result in tumour resolution and reconstruction and consolidation of the bone so that weight-bearing may safely continue. If a fracture does occur in a long bone internal fixation is usually necessary, and is combined with local irradiation if full activity is to be restored.

Healing of ulceration may also be promoted by radiotherapy. Ulcerated cancers may commonly be the cause of concern and distress from bleeding, discharge or the effects of secondary infection. There may be associated pain or discomfort. In patients with advanced tumours it may be possible to obtain only partial healing of the ulcerated lesion, but this may be effective in alleviating most of the associated symptoms. A very significant contribution may be made by radiotherapy to ulcerated recurrent or primary cancers of the breast. Recurrences in the perineal scar following abdominoperineal resection for rectal cancer may also respond to palliative radiotherapy. Inoperable rectal cancer may also produce distressing symptoms and pain, bleeding and mucoid discharge from its ulcerated surface can be alleviated in about 75% of patients.

Control of haemorrhage, which may be one of the greatest sources of anxiety to patients and relatives, is commonly achieved by radiotherapy. Severe haemorrhage may often be a serious problem in patients with advanced cancers of the uterine cervix, uterine body and bladder. Occasionally it may complicate cancers of the mouth, pharynx and bronchus. Radiotherapy can usually decrease and often arrest bleeding and palliation for this reason is usually indicated. Bleeding from renal-cell carcinoma responds slowly and uncertainly following palliative radiotherapy, and other techniques such as arterial embolization are rather to be advised.

Great care has of course to be taken not to prolong the act of dying, with the possibility of developing still further complications of advancing malignant disease, by inappropriate efforts to control haemorrhage.

Relief of symptoms of obstruction can be dramatic following well-considered radiotherapy. Superior mediastinal compression is usually the result of direct invasion of the superior vena cava by anaplastic cancer of the bronchus. It is an extremely distressing complication which is quickly relieved by a short course of X-ray therapy. In patients with severe congestion of the head and neck it is advisable to give corticosteroids before beginning in an attempt to minimize the increase in oedema which may follow the first dose of X-rays. Other tumours, such as thyroid cancer and, rarely, malignant lymphomas, may also cause superior mediastinal compression and may respond well to radiotherapy.

Obstruction produced by oesophageal cancer may be relieved in about 50% of patients, and will remain controlled for the short remaining life-span of these patients. Equally effective palliation may be achieved by the insertion of an oesophageal tube in selected patients. This technique, if applicable, has the advantage of being immediately effective, whereas some weeks will normally elapse before the obstructive lesion resolves after radiotherapy. Obstruction of the ureters in advanced cancer of the bladder or uterine cervix is seldom relieved by radiotherapy and is not considered an indication for palliative radiotherapy. Bilateral ureteric obstruction is always a sign of very advanced, locally infiltrative cancer, and progressive renal failure is perhaps the least uncomfortable complication of incurable malignant disease in the pelvis.

Neurological complications are relatively uncommon but may be a cause of great concern. Retrobulbar metastases may produce distressing disfigurement and interference with vision. The primary tumour, such as leukaemia, one of the lymphomas or a neuroblastoma, may be highly radiosensitive and dramatic palliation may quickly and easily be achieved. Retinal metastases may at times arise from breast cancer when timely irradiation may restore vision and considerably improve the patient's morale.

The clinical features of progressive intracranial metastases can be an enormous problem for patients, relatives and for medical and nursing staff. It is often beneficial to irradiate the brain which may alleviate the most distressing symptoms. Dexamethasone may be added which should help provide early symptomatic improvement and usually can be discontinued after completion of radiotherapy. It should be noted that in the case of bronchial carcinoma in particular, irradiation of cerebral metastases is regularly found to be of value and also may be associated with surprisingly long survival.

Symptoms and signs of pressure on the spinal cord are normally best dealt with by oral dexamethasone and radiotherapy to the site of obstruction. Occasionally surgical decompression may be advisable. This management gives as good a chance of restoration of full neurological function as surgical decompression, regardless of the type of cancer. When a primary tumour, such as a malignant lymphoma or neuroblastoma, is highly radiosensitive, radiotherapy alone can often successfully be employed or at times combined with cytotoxic chemotherapy.

An advanced primary cancer or metastatic deposit may produce distressing local features which may be alleviated by palliative radiotherapy, even if only partial tumour resolution is obtained. One site of special importance is the oral cavity, where radiotherapy is normally beneficial even in the most advanced stages of the disease. Death from mouth cancer, that is often slowly progressive, results from inanition. It is important to control as best one can the complications of slowly progressive local disease, such as difficulty in eating and swallowing, pain, excessive salivation, bleeding and perhaps fistula formation. Almost all of these patients will benefit from palliative radiotherapy.

Another palliative role of radiotherapy in the management of large, slow growing tumours is a technique to achieve 'growth restraint'. A dose of radiation, 300–500 cGy is given weekly for 2 or 3 months usually to a large inoperable carcinoma or sarcoma. The aim of this is to prevent further extension of tumour and perhaps avoid further local complications, although sometimes considerable resolution may be obtained.

Systemic effects of cancer, caused not by metastatic

lesions but by the production of hormones or biologically active polypeptides or similar substances, can occasionally cause the most distressing complications of various types of cancer. These effects may be seen in about 15% of patients with advanced cancer, but it is estimated that as many again have subclinical abnormalities.

The most common metabolic feature of advanced malignant disease is cachexia, a single cause for which has not as yet been identified. In many of the lymphomas and anaplastic carcinomas a feeling of well-being and weight increase may follow a course of palliative radiotherapy to the primary tumour. Other features, such as anorexia, episodic fever and pruritus, may also be relieved by radiotherapy in patients with advanced lymphomas.

A large number of metabolic consequences of ectopic hormone production may occur, and some of the more common but still extremely rare syndromes are described.

ACTH secretion, usually by an oat-cell carcinoma of the bronchus, results in adrenal hyperplasia and the continuous secretion of cortisol. This may not give rise to the features of classic Cushing's syndrome which takes time to develop, but the effects of renal loss of potassium may be most severe, although the other metabolic effects are also seen. Management of this syndrome with aminoglutethimide, alone or in combination with metyrapone, is difficult and usually unsuccessful. If an oat-cell carcinoma of the bronchus is the cause (and not for example medullary cancer of the thyroid) palliative radiotherapy of the primary lesion may give prompt symptomatic relief.

Some trophoblastic tumours such as chorion carcinoma and undifferentiated or trophoblastic tumours of the testis may secrete a thyroid-stimulating hormone giving rise to many of the disabling features of hyperthyroidism. Palliative radiotherapy of the metastatic lesions may help to control the troublesome symptoms, although cytotoxic chemotherapy may be preferred and antithyroid drugs are effective if needed.

Hypercalcaemia may be produced by a parathyroid-like hormone secreted by a squamous-cell carcinoma of the bronchus or renal-cell carcinoma. This syndrome has to be distinguished from hypercalcaemia due to widespread bone metastases but which is usually associated with breast cancer. Prednisolone 10 mg t.d.s. initially will usually reduce the serum levels of calcium, but radiotherapy should always be considered as well in patients with bronchial or renal carcinoma.

Spontaneous hypoglycaemia may occur as a feature of islet-cell tumours of the pancreas, but may also be a troublesome symptom of large mesenchymal tumours, particularly fibrosarcoma. A number of insulin-like substances have been identified. The hypoglycaemia seldom responds to treatment with glucagon, but diazoxide (Eudemine) and streptozotocin may be helpful. These tumours may be very slow growing and radiotherapy can help to bring the features of flushing, sweating, drowsiness and eventually coma and fits under better control.

Serious hyponatraemia can result from the ectopic production of ADH (antidiuretic hormone) produced by tumours, most commonly by an oat-cell carcinoma of the bronchus. In this case palliative radiotherapy to the primary cancer is advised and possibly avoids the need for water restriction and the administration of fludrocortisone and potassium supplements.

Myasthenia gravis may be associated with tumours of the thymus, but may be a feature of lung cancer—usually oat-cell carcinoma. The myasthenia responds poorly to prostigmine and to edrophonium chloride (Tensilon), and the muscle weakness may respond to guanidine, but irradiation of the primary tumour will usually produce marked neurological improvement.

Hypertrophic pulmonary osteoarthropathy is found in association with bronchial and mediastinal tumours and with pulmonary Hodgkin's disease, but rarely with secondary lung tumours. The involved joints can be extremely painful and disabling but the manifestations will disappear with successful treatment of the primary tumour which is best often achieved by radiation.

Carcinomatous neuropathies and myopathies are a strange group of non-metastatic complications of cancer usually arising most commonly in the lung, stomach and ovary. Their causation is puzzling because they are three times more common in treated patients than those untreated, and also in that they are more common in patients without metastases. It has been said that irradiation of the primary can be effective in improving carcinomatous myasthenia. It is very doubtful if palliative radiotherapy to the primary tumour improves the features of the other types of neuromyopathies, and certainly in peripheral neuropathy recovery is rare.

The management of the patient with incurable cancer will often involve the collaborative efforts of several specialists. It is important that each should be knowledgeable about what the others can contribute. The radiation oncologist has a duty to decide in the light of experience whether or not to treat, just as the surgeon will decide for or against operation. It must be recognized that no one, patients or the profession, benefits by the indiscriminate use of specialist techniques when responsible restraint may be the kindest and most appropriate advice. At that time the administration of analgesics, narcotic drugs or other symptomatic medication, skilled nursing and emotional support may be what is required.

RADIOTHERAPY FOR BENIGN CONDITIONS

Radiotherapy is now employed in the management of benign conditions only when certain clear indications exist. The techniques and dose of irradiation must minimize the risks of damage to normal tissues, and particularly the risks of inducing leukaemia or other malignant change. For these reasons radiotherapy is normally reserved for the management of benign conditions when other methods have failed or are absolutely contraindicated.

There are two endocrine conditions for which radiotherapy is still primarily indicated with excellent results. Hyperthyroidism in patients over the age of 40 years may be safely and effectively treated with ^{131}Iodine. In patients with a large goitre thyroidectomy may be preferred. Radio-iodine is also an effective method of treatment of recurrence after thyroidectomy and when thyrotoxicosis is complicated by other serious illnesses. A problem of radio-iodine therapy is the increasing incidence of hypothyroidism with time, and systematic follow-up of these patients must be undertaken.

Acromegaly associated with visual field impairment is best managed by hypophysectomy. If, after operation, the stimulated growth hormone remains elevated, small field beam directed radiotherapy to the pituitary fossa is indicated. In the absence of visual field defects pituitary irradiation should be given. Relatively low doses (3000 cGy in 10 fractions over 2 weeks) are normally advised, although this may produce normal growth hormone levels in about half the patients. However, improvement may be seen over several years. Prolactinomas may also respond to similar treatment. Chromophobe adenomas, by far the most common of the pituitary adenomas, may be very satisfactorily managed in this way. Higher doses of radiation may be given to the pituitary either by 90 yttrium rod implantation or, in highly specialized centres, proton irradiation has been employed which can localize the distribution of dose within the fossa. These techniques which certainly more effectively ablate the pituitary also carry much greater risks of complications, such as damage to the optic chiasma or adjacent structures.

Keloid formation may require treatment, and irradiation can help to avoid a recurrence of the problem. If symptoms demand, excision is to be advised, and immediate postoperative irradiation of the incision (single exposure of 1000 cGy) will usually prevent further recurrence. Irradiation does little to influence the mature keloid.

Excessive bone formation may occur after artificial hip replacement or other orthopaedic operations. The effects may be seriously disabling (particularly in association with DISH syndrome) and postoperative radiotherapy has been found to be effective in preventing recurrence of this problem.

Corneal vascularization after grafting may be a problem and the application of ^{90}Sr plaque, a beta-ray emitter, to the eye (500 cGy single exposure) is often effective. If necessary, this application may be repeated.

The artificial induction of the menopause may be beneficial in managing menorrhagia when surgery is not advised. For example, in a patient with severe cirrhosis or disabling multiple sclerosis the simple application of a short course of X-ray therapy may greatly improve the patient's morale and well-being and help further management.

Finally, the symptoms of ankylosing spondylitis may be dramatically relieved by radiotherapy. The well-documented risk of developing leukaemia or other tumours has led to radiation being used in selected patients only if they have been shown to be refractory to or intolerant of drug therapy. Accordingly, very few patients are now considered for X-ray therapy which is given only to the focal areas of active disease when indicated in the face of persistent pain and disability. Doses of 1500 cGy in 10 fractions over 2 weeks are adequate. It should be noted also that radiotherapy is most likely to be effective in relieving the granulomatous phase of the disease, usually within 5 years of presentation of the typical form of ankylosing spondylitis. Atypical syndromes will respond less well to irradiation which will normally give excellent lasting relief to well-selected patients

NEW TECHNIQUES IN RADIOTHERAPY

There is much effort and expensive investment at present made to improve the effectiveness of radiotherapy. Radiation techniques, like surgery, are forms of local management which too often are unsuccessful in controlling primary tumours. It is of the greatest importance that every effort be made to enhance the effectiveness of local management, while at the same time techniques of systemic management for metastatic disease continue to be developed. It has been estimated that about one-third of patients with cancer die of uncontrolled primary disease without evidence of dissemination. It has to be recognized also that too many patients with cancer present with so advanced disease that curative therapy is impossible. With our present knowledge and techniques twice as many patients with cancer could be cured if they had only sought earlier advice.

The techniques that are at present being evaluated are given in *Table* 12.6. The major effort in radiotherapy in the past ten years has been directed to the evaluation of the 'oxygen effect' in radiotherapy, and in the development of new techniques to reduce its importance. It has been well established that the relative resistance of hypoxic cells is reduced by almost 50% by the application of densely ionizing (or high LET) radiations suitable for treating deep-seated cancers. Fast neutron radiation has been studied most and although early reports were encouraging, when results were compared with those of X-ray therapy, subsequent trials have failed to confirm the substantial improvements that were claimed previously. It has been suggested that some types of tumour regarded as resistant to X-ray therapy for reasons other than hypoxia may be more responsive to fast neutron irradiation. Soft-tissue sarcomas, salivary gland tumours and gastric cancers are among the tumours that may be more effectively treated by fast neutrons, but randomly controlled trials have not yet been completed. Negative pi-mesons (pions) are tiny subatomic particles which produce high LET radiations following interaction with tissues. Their production requires very expensive high energy particle accelerators and only two facilities of this kind are available at Vancouver, Canada and at Villigen, Switzerland. Pions have the additional advantage of providing an extremely well-defined volume of high dose densely ionizing radiation at the end of their tracks. These features may allow better sparing of surrounding normal tissues, and also more effective treatment of the cancer.

Table 12.6 New techniques in radiotherapy

Physical
High LET radiations
Other particulate radiations
Hyperthermia
Chemical
Radiation sensitizers
Potentiating agents
Additive agents
Biological
Fractionation (hyperfractionation)
Kinetic analysis
Cell synchronization

At present only preliminary results have been reported, but they do not indicate that there will be major improvements in cancer control.

High energy atomic nuclei of carbon, nitrogen, argon and neon also have the dual advantage of providing high LET radiations (with low oxygen dependence) and excellent dose distribution. The only centre with the facility to examine the possible clinical advantages of these radiations is at the Bevalac particle accelerator in California.

Irradiation with protons or helium ions may be modulated to provide well-circumscribed volumes of high dose while sparing surrounding normal tissues. They are not, however, densely ionizing radiations, and in that respect would not be expected to have any biological advantage over megavoltage X-ray therapy. Eight centres in the world are at present engaged in their evaluation. Excellent results have been reported of the treatment by protons of ocular melanomas, and other intracranial lesions. The treatment of cancer of the prostate with these particles is also giving encouraging results

There is great interest in the killing of mammalian cells by heating and its application in cancer therapy. It is also known that there is a synergistic action of hyperthermia on the effects of X-irradiation. The evidence is that the lethal action of heating is associated with the denaturization of proteins, although the exact target has not been identified. In respect of the interaction of heating and irradiation short exposures of high temperatures (about 45 °C), which itself kills cells, results principally in a loss of the ability to recover from sublethal radiation damage (reduced Dq value). Longer exposure to temperature elevation of about 40–42 °C, which produces little cell killing, will result in an enhanced sensitivity to irradiation (reduced Do value). A criticial point in these differences is found at 43 °C. Hypoxic cells seem to be slightly more sensitive to high temperature (above 45 °C) exposure than well-oxygenated tissues. The cell age sensitivity of cells to hyperthermia is quite different from that to X-rays in that S phase cells are the most responsive to heating. These differences and the potential advantages of their interaction are being explored in a number of clinical studies designed to measure the effectiveness of combined hyperthermia and X-irradiation in cancer therapy.

Clinical radiation sensitization has always held the possibility of improving the effectiveness of radiotherapy. The problem has been to develop agents which will selectively sensitize tumour cells, while the normal cell response remains unchanged. The electron-affinic group of drugs of which misonidazole (a close relative of metronidazole) is an early example, is now undergoing clinical trials. Their application has been limited by neurotoxicity, but several new drugs (which are both safer and more effective) are now the subject of clinical trials. These drugs selectively sensitize hypoxic cells which are known to occur in tumours, and laboratory research suggests that may be an effective way of reducing the 'oxygen effect'. The best documented radiation sensitizer is oxygen. Patients may be treated in hyperbaric oxygen (3 atmospheres) so that it is carried in the plasma to hypoxic tumours at the time of irradiation. Randomly controlled trials have demonstrated the advantage of this technique, but its routine use is complex and time consuming and not without considerable hazard, and it has failed to gain general acceptance.

Other chemical agents, such as actinomycin D, 5-fluorouracil, bleomycin, cis-platinum and puromycin, may potentiate the effects of irradiation. Clinical studies have as yet failed to provide convincing evidence of improvement of the therapeutic ratio by combining these agents with X-ray therapy. Interest at present is directed to the additive effects of drugs, such as methotrexate and cyclophosphamide, that by reducing the number of viable cells in the cancer before X-ray therapy is given may increase the probability of local tumour control.

Regimes of fractionation have been developed empirically over many years and there is no rational basis for their use. Tumour cells, such as malignant melanoma, which are thought to have a large shoulder region (Dq value) on a survival curve, may be much more effectively treated by relatively fewer but larger fractions of dose. Clinical studies have demonstrated that this is so, although further trials are required to confirm these early reports.

It is now recognized that the radiotherapy of most common cancers may be improved by giving an increased number of very small dose fractions. This technique, known as hyperfractionation, requires that two or three fractions are given each day. These small dose fractions are thought to be relatively more effective in killing cancer cells, which are rapidly growing, than normal cells the depletion of which determines late radiation-related morbidity. Substantial gains in the therapeutic ratio could follow the introduction of this technique for the treatment of some cancers. Randomized trials comparing hyperfractionation with conventional treatment are in progress.

Detailed information on the tumour cell population kinetics might also be used to advantage in designing better treatment regimes. Tumours with a high growth fraction and short cell cycle time (such as Burkitt's lymphoma) are better treated by irradiation two or three times each day rather than by daily exposures. New techniques make it possible to analyse the kinetic parameters of tumours which may in turn help develop a more rational basis of dose fractionation. We are aware that there is almost a three-fold difference in the sensitivity of mammalian cells to irradiation throughout the cell cycle. Exploitation of techniques that would allow either tumour or normal cells to be synchronized could have a major influence on the effectiveness of radiotherapy. It may also be advantageous to shorten the overall treatment time for some cancers.

These new techniques are the subject of much laboratory and clinical research, and it can be expected that many of these developments will eventually contribute to the steady improvement in cancer management in the next decade.

Further Reading

Fajardo L. F. (1982) *Pathology of Radiation Injury*. New York, Masson.

Fletcher G. H. (1980) *Textbook of Radiotherapy*, 3rd ed. Philadelphia, Lea & Febiger.

Meredith W. J. and Massey J. B. (1977) *Fundamental Physics of Radiology*, 3rd ed. Bristol, Wright.

Potten C. S. and Hendry J. H. (ed.) (1983) *Cytotoxic Insult and Tissue*. London, Churchill Livingstone.

Steel G. G., Adams G. E. and Peckham M. J. (ed.) (1983) *The Biological Basis of Radiotherapy*. Amsterdam, Elsevier.

13 *The Principles of Anaesthesia*

Alfred J. Shearer

A knowledge of the principles of anaesthesia is necessary to the practice of surgery. The two specialties function in close collaboration and each requires a basic understanding of the other. There are often conflicting priorities and balanced judgement is required. In deciding when to operate, for example, the urgency of the procedure and the benefits to the health of the patient must be weighed against the risks and the need for preoperative treatment. Surgery, like anaesthesia, has many adverse effects on physiological homeostasis intraoperatively and the surgical insult plays a greater part in the aetiology of some postoperative complications than is often realized. For major procedures, especially in the thorax and abdomen, fitness for surgery becomes a more important consideration than the ability to withstand anaesthesia. The principles and the skills involved in the management of the patient under anaesthesia have a much wider application in the total care of the surgical patient. This may be most obvious when intensive care or resuscitation is required, but the treatment of any unstable patient and the provision of analgesia are equally important examples.

PREOPERATIVE CARE

Preoperative assessment involves a screening process to identify factors which may increase the morbidity or mortality associated with the intended procedure. Such factors may include coexisting disease, treatment with certain drugs, susceptibility to specific anaesthetic problems or the pathological consequences of the surgical condition itself. These must be fully assessed so that the risks involved can be evaluated. The perioperative therapy, anaesthetic technique, surgical procedure and postoperative requirements can then be considered with a view to avoiding or minimizing the risk to the patient. Because present-day practice is usually to carry out this assessment after the patient has been admitted for elective surgery, full investigation and treatment may sometimes dictate that the planned operation date be postponed. At the other extreme, when the surgical condition demands immediate intervention, only a very brief assessment and essential resuscitation may be all that is possible. The increasing number of minor and intermediate procedures now being done on a day-case basis is of benefit to the patient and the health service. This requires careful selection of patients and an efficient system of preoperative assessment. Written consent is required for surgery and anaesthesia but it must be informed consent. Adequate explanation of the proposed procedures is not only a legal requirement but necessary in reassuring the patient. The prospect of an operation can be very frightening and a sympathetic ear can go a long way to reducing the degree of sedation that may be required for premedication. Strict protocol is necessary in the routine preparation of patients for theatre as mishaps arising from oversight or error can be disastrous and are unforgivable.

Assessment

Full preoperative assessment includes a comprehensive history and examination, a search of existing medical records and investigation as appropriate. The objective is first to define any problems and risk factors. Relevant features must then be fully evaluated in the context of the proposed surgery.

A full medical history is required and must include details of the presenting and other current symptoms, drug therapy, adverse reactions or allergies, family history, life style and social circumstances. It is important to elucidate any problems related to anaesthesia which the patient or any relative may have had in the past. Systematic enquiry and examination must be comprehensive but with special emphasis on the respiratory and cardiovascular systems. Only limited investigation is required for screening purposes. *Table* 13.1 shows the commonest indications for preoperative tests. Beyond this, a test is only justified if there is clinical evidence for the presence of coexisting disease.

Intercurrent Disease

Chronic Respiratory Disease

Patients with pre-existing respiratory disease have a high incidence of intraoperative and postoperative respiratory complications. Problems arise because of airway irritability, excessive sputum production and reduced pulmonary reserve. Airway irritability causes coughing, breath holding, excessive secretions, bronchospasm, laryngeal spasm and vomiting during general anaesthesia. Excessive sputum production increases the incidence of pulmonary collapse and bronchopneumonia, particularly if the sputum is infected preoperatively. This is a greater problem after thoracic or abdominal surgery which makes effective coughing and

Table 13.1 Common indications for preoperative tests

Preoperative test	*Common indications*
Urinalysis	All in-patients
Haemoglobin	Major surgery
Urea and electrolytes	>70 years Impaired gastrointestinal intake Significant gastrointestinal losses Renal disease Diabetes Diuretic, digoxin or steroid therapy
ECG	Cardiorespiratory disease >40 years
Chest radiography	Acute respiratory symptoms Possible metastasis Cardiorespiratory disease, Tuberculosis risk } if no radiograph in previous 12 months >50 years for major abdominal surgery
Blood glucose	Diabetes Corticosteroid therapy
Prothrombin time and partial thromboplastin time	Hepatobiliary disease (repeat after parenteral vitamin K) Bleeding disorder Anticoagulant therapy
Platelet count and bleeding time	Bleeding disorder

expectoration more difficult. High airways resistance, poor pulmonary compliance and air trapping may exacerbate this problem of postoperative sputum retention. Patients with impaired respiratory function can tolerate less respiratory insult before respiratory failure supervenes. Impaired respiratory function results from excessive work of breathing and less efficient gaseous exchange. High airways resistance and low lung compliance both increase the work of breathing, while factors such as loss of lung tissue and air trapping reduce the efficiency of gas exchange due to ventilation and perfusion mismatching. Severe cases may also have a loss of ventilatory sensitivity to carbon dioxide or right heart failure. Anaesthesia and surgery, particularly abdominal or thoracic surgery, can both adversely affect pulmonary function and cause respiratory failure in these cases.

Preoperative assessment is geared towards determining the degree of chronic impairment and the presence of the reversible elements of infection and bronchospasm. These reversible features should be treated before embarking on elective non-urgent surgery. Assessment of the chronic state is necessary before deciding on fitness for surgery, anaesthetic technique and postoperative management. Important in this assessment is an accurate history of exercise tolerance and life style. Dyspnoea at rest or on minimal exertion or the presence of central cyanosis indicate severe respiratory disease. Vitalography is useful in defining the problem and assessing the response of airways resistance to treatment. An arterial carbon dioxide tension of 6·7 kPa (50 mmHg) or greater is an indication for admission to intensive care after thoracic or abdominal surgery and usually intermittent positive-pressure ventilation (IPPV) is required. Local anaesthetic techniques should be considered for surgery and postoperative pain relief in patients with severe respiratory disease. High spinal or epidural block, however, can adversely affect the circulation and also significantly embarrass intercostal muscle activity. General anaesthesia is, therefore, often the method of choice for major abdominal or thoracic surgery, certainly for those who are going to be electively ventilated afterwards.

Upper Respiratory Tract Infection

Upper respiratory tract infection increases the perioperative risks considerably. There is irritability of the airway and respiratory defence mechanisms against infection are impaired. This situation may persist for several weeks after a common cold has disappeared. Except for emergency surgery it is therefore normally unacceptable to administer general anaesthesia to patients with a current or recent upper respiratory tract infection. In order to avoid wastage of resources patients booked for elective surgery should be instructed to report immediately if they have a cold or sore throat so that their admission can be postponed in time for the bed to be reallocated.

Asthma

Asthmatics can occasionally develop severe bronchospasm during anaesthesia. It is important that elective surgery is performed only during a period of remission. If the asthma is not well controlled, the treatment must be reviewed. The therapeutic regimen which has been found to be optimum for the patient should be continued until he is transferred to the operating theatre. More important than which agents are used for premedication is that the patient is adequately sedated and that there is good cholinergic blockade.

Smoking

Smokers should be advised to abstain before and after surgery. There are several relevant adverse effects of smoking. The most important is that postoperative respiratory morbidity is increased by up to six-fold. Stopping smoking for 12–24 h improves oxygen transport, cardiovascular function and wound healing due to elimination of carbon monoxide and nicotine. Stopping for 1 week considerably decreases bronchial irritability but at least 6 weeks are required to bring about any improvement in small airways disease, hypersecretion of mucus, tracheobronchial clearance or immune response.

Tuberculosis

It is important to identify patients with active tuberculosis so that cross-infection by contamination of anaesthetic equipment can be avoided.

Cardiovascular Disease

There are many factors in relation to surgery which may adversely affect cardiovascular function. Some of these factors are: anxiety, pain, premedication, induction and general anaesthetic agents, airway stimulation, muscle relaxant and reversal agents, IPPV, local analgesia, surgical stimulation or manipulation, blood loss and replacement, decreased body temperature, fluid and electrolyte abnormalities, acid–base and blood gas changes, bacteraemia and endotoxaemia. Whether by direct or reflex action, these may alter myocardial contractility, cardiac rate or rhythm, vascular tone or venous return. The important end results are the adverse effects on cardiac output and myocardial oxygenation.

Maintaining cardiac output and myocardial oxygenation is obviously always of high priority, especially in the presence of pre-existing cardiovascular disease. Due consideration to diagnosis, treatment and stabilization preoperatively can often make a greater difference to the outcome than any subsequent efforts.

Myocardial Infarction

Patients who have suffered a recent myocardial infarction, whether complicated or not, have a very high risk of perioperative reinfarction. As shown in *Table* 13.2 this risk decreases as the interval between infarct and surgery increases until at 6 months the risk has almost returned to normal. Reinfarction in relation to surgery carries a mortality of 50%. This risk does not seem to be influenced by the use of local analgesic techniques. It is important to realize that up to 30% of myocardial infarctions are not recognized, either because they are clinically silent or as a result of an atypical presentation. For this reason preoperative electrocardiography is justified in all in-patients over 40 years of age and non-urgent surgery is not justified within 6 months of a patient having had a myocardial infarction.

Table 13.2 Reinfarction rate in relation to surgery

Time from previous infarct	*Reinfarction rate*
Within 3 months	30%
3–6 months	15%
Over 6 months	5%

Cardiac Failure

Surgery in patients with uncontrolled congestive cardiac failure carries a very poor prognosis. Treatment with diuretics is usually indicated and sometimes digoxin is required. Particular attention must be given to the cause and any exacerbating factors, e.g. hypertension, tachyarrhythmias and any other influences which have an adverse effect on cardiac output and myocardial oxygenation. Severe refractory cardiac failure requires intensive therapy and only very urgent life-saving surgery can be contemplated. Such a state may be precipitated by an acute surgical condition in a patient with cardiovascular disease, particularly if there has been a period of shock. In this situation it is necessary to monitor and optimize the ventricular filling pressure and this requires a central venous catheter. If there is a predominantly left ventricular problem, a pulmonary artery balloon catheter is required to measure the pulmonary artery wedge pressure which normally reflects the left ventricular filling pressure. Inotropic and/or vasodilator therapy may then be required. If there is severe pulmonary oedema, oxygenation can often only be maintained with artificial ventilation, high inspiratory oxygen concentrations and sometimes positive end-expiratory pressure (PEEP).

Arrhythmias

Cardiac arrhythmias may be the presenting sign of several significant underlying disorders. Coronary artery disease is the most common cause, but other causes include valvular heart disease, cardiomyopathy, myocarditis, ventricular hypertrophy, thyrotoxicosis and phaeochromocytoma. Many factors in relation to surgical conditions, surgery and anaesthesia can precipitate or exacerbate cardiac arrhythmias in a susceptible individual. Cardiac output and myocardial oxygenation can be compromised because of the adverse effects on heart rate, atrioventricular transport or pattern of ventricular contraction. When time allows patients with significant dysrhythmias should be treated preoperatively and often a period of stabilization is beneficial. Treatment involves drug therapy, cardioversion or insertion of a pacemaker depending on the particular problem. Occasionally insertion of a temporary pacemaker to cover the immediate perioperative period is indicated for those with particular conduction defects.

Cardiac Pacemaker

The use of diathermy should be avoided where possible in patients with pacemakers because of potential problems. Misinterpretation of a diathermy current can lead to false inhibition of pacemakers in the 'on demand' mode. This can be avoided by switching the pacemaker to the 'fixed rate' mode. With permanent pacemakers this is usually done by use of a magnet placed on the skin over the implanted generator. Secondly, because the pacemaker lead may act as an aerial, currents may be induced in the system when diathermy is used. It is possible that these currents could induce ventricular fibrillation or cause damage to the pacemaker. The chances of this happening, however, are small if bipolar diathermy is used or if the active electrode is kept at least 15 cm away from the pacemaker and the indifferent electrode plate is placed as far as possible from the pacemaker and in a direction which ensures that the diathermy dipole will be at right angles to that of the pacemaker system.

Valvular Heart Disease

The operative risk in those with valvular heart disease is increased depending on the severity of the disease. The degree to which the lesion is interfering with cardiac function must be assessed and any sequelae noted. Cardiac failure and arrhythmias must be controlled. A full understanding of the haemodynamic effects of the particular lesion is necessary so that correct supportive measures can be defined and those influences which have an adverse effect can be avoided. Again the ultimate priority must be to maintain myocardial oxygenation and good cardiac output. Valvular heart disease or the presence of artificial valves causes a predisposition to subacute bacterial endocarditis and prophylactic antibiotic therapy should be prescribed when any procedure associated with a risk of bacteraemia is being done. Patients with prosthetic heart valves and those with mitral stenosis complicated by atrial fibrillation are usually on long-term oral anticoagulant therapy. This must be reviewed preoperatively.

Hypertension

Patients suffering from hypertension are particularly at risk of cardiovascular instability and myocardial or cerebral damage during anaesthesia. No patient should go for surgery without a record of blood pressure. All those noted to be hypertensive ought to be started on 4-hourly recordings because anxiety can have a dramatic effect on an isolated measurement. If hypertension is sustained, the patient is best stabilized on therapy preoperatively. Elective surgery ought to be postponed if the diastolic pressure is 110 mmHg or greater and the advice of a cardiologist sought. Although essential hypertension is usually the cause, the possibility of renal disease, coarctation of the aorta, phaeochromocytoma or Cushing's syndrome ought to be borne in mind. If the patient has malignant hypertension, surgery can only be contemplated if his life is immediately at risk from the surgical condition. In any patient with hypertension, sequelae such as cardiac failure, myocardial ischaemia or renal impairment can occur and may require treatment preoperatively. All antihypertensive therapy should be continued until the patient goes to the operating theatre. The fluctuations which occur during surgery are much less in the well controlled hypertensive. It is important to note that the risks associated with hypertension are not limited to general anaesthesia and the above applies equally to local anaesthesia. The sympathetic outflow block which occurs with subarachnoid or extradural block can lead to profound hypotension. Vasoconstrictor drugs used with local anaesthetics can also precipitate marked hypertension.

Phaeochromocytoma

Rapid fluctuations in blood pressure can occur during and immediately after resection of a phaeochromocytoma. Attention to certain details can reduce this problem. There must be good blood pressure control with effective alpha-adrenergic blockade preoperatively. As the constrictor effect on capacitance vessels is relieved blood volume expansion may be required. The intraoperative management requires continuous monitoring of arterial and central venous pressure, with the careful use of a short-acting hypotensive agent such as sodium nitroprusside to deal with acute rises in blood pressure. Adequate consideration must be given to the ventricular filling pressure as the catecholamine effect is removed.

Anaemia

In treating acute blood loss, blood volume replenishment is of a higher priority than making good the red blood cell deficit. Where time and blood availability permits, a haematocrit value of 0·30 is optimal. In patients with chronic anaemia presenting for elective surgery, the cause must be found if possible and treatment instituted with iron, folic acid or hydroxycobalamin as appropriate. Time must be allowed for such therapy to produce an adequate response. When surgery is more urgent, a haemoglobin of 10 g/dl need not delay the operation. If the haemoglobin is less than 10 g/dl the following points must be considered. Although anaemia reduces the oxygen-carrying capacity of blood and causes a compensatory increase in cardiac output, this is not normally significant at haemoglobin levels of greater than 8 g/dl. Those with renal failure usually tolerate lower haemoglobin levels. Patients with cardiorespiratory disease may need higher haemoglobin levels. Because of the problem of circulatory overload and because transfused blood does not reach its full oxygen-carrying capacity for several days, blood should only be transfused for chronic anaemia if it can be given slowly and if it can be given 48 h before surgery. Otherwise it may be better to leave blood transfusion until the operation when blood can be given to replace losses. It is important to be aware of the significance of the oxygen dissociation curve in this situation. For a given haemoglobin level, a shift of the curve to the left which causes a fall in the P50 (oxygen tension when haemoglobin saturation is 50%) of the blood by only 0·5 kPa (4 mmHg) requires the cardiac output to be doubled in order to maintain the same level of tissue oxygenation. Factors which affect the position of the dissociation curve, such as acid–base status, carbon dioxide level and body temperature may be as important as the haemoglobin level.

Polycythaemia

The care of polycythaemic patients requiring surgery needs careful consideration. It is not always appreciated that the effect of increasing haematocrit on blood viscosity is semi-logarithmic and viscosities of 5 or 6 times normal have been recorded in patients with polycythaemia. Increased blood viscosity and hypertension cause increased cardiac work and there is a predisposition to thromboembolic disorders. It is important to find the cause and to reduce the haematocrit before surgery. Ideally the haematocrit ought to be reduced, by repeated venesection if necessary, over several weeks but when surgery cannot wait a more modest venesection with colloid replacement at the time of surgery ought to be considered in severe cases.

Haemoglobinopathy

All patients of negro origin and those originating from Eastern Mediterranean countries, the Middle East or India ought to be screened for sickle-cell disease. Blood transfusion preoperatively may be indicated and all efforts made to avoid hypoxia, acidosis or circulatory stasis.

Haemostatic Defects

In any patient with a history or signs suggestive of a bleeding tendency, the following tests may help exclude a haemostatic defect: tourniquet (Hess) test, bleeding time, clotting time, platelet count, prothrombin time and kaolin cephalin clotting time. If a problem is confirmed and there is no obvious cause, the advice of a haematologist is normally required.

Gastrointestinal Disease

Several points in relation to gastrointestinal disorders are relevant to anaesthesia. Many conditions are associated with a risk of regurgitation and the possibility of pulmonary aspiration, especially at the time of anaesthetic induction or during recovery. In those particularly at risk, a nasogastric tube should be used to reduce the volume of the gastric or oesophageal contents and an H_2-receptor antagonist given to reduce the acidity. Fluid and electrolyte disturbances, acid–base imbalance and poor nutritional states may all cause cardiovascular instability and problems in relation to the use of anaesthetic agents and muscle relaxants. As far as possible fluid and electrolyte losses should be replenished preoperatively. Serum potassium is particularly important. Occasionally, abdominal distension caused by intestinal obstruction can be so great that it causes severe respiratory embarrassment.

Obesity

Obese patients are more susceptible to perioperative complications and surgical mortality is doubled. A full respiratory and cardiovascular assessment is necessary. Oxygenation can become a problem as a result of merely adopting the supine position, without the additional reduction in functional residual capacity that occurs under general anaesthesia. Obesity is associated with an increased cardiac output, hypertension and cardiomegaly. Obese patients are often diabetic.

Liver Disease

In patients with liver disease, tests of hepatocellular function and information on the response to previously administered sedatives or analgesics can be helpful in gauging the likely impairment of drug metabolism. Encephalopathy must be graded and may dictate special postoperative support, as deterioration often occurs, at least initially. Blood glucose control is often impaired and ought to be monitored. When there is gastrointestinal haemorrhage, attention must be given to blood volume replacement and efforts to avoid absorption of breakdown products. Vitamin K ought to be administered parenterally but haemostatic function may still be defective because of inadequate synthesis of coagulation factors due to hepatic cellular damage. In addition, there may be thrombocytopenia due to hypersplenism and bone marrow depression. Renal function must be assessed and, because of the danger of deterioration in relation to surgery in those with liver disease, attention must be given to prophylaxis. The best prophylaxis is to monitor urine output hourly throughout the perioperative period and to treat oliguria when it occurs, without delay. The infectivity of patients in whom hepatic disease is secondary to viral infection must be determined whenever possible.

Renal Disease

The current serum potassium level must be known in patients with renal failure having surgery. The danger is of a high serum potassium precipitating cardiac arrest. This is most likely to occur after the use of suxamethonium which causes a further rise in the serum level. Hyperkalaemia must be corrected by exchange resin, glucose and insulin therapy or dialysis, if necessary. Water and sodium excretion is often abnormal and uraemia can cause vomiting and diarrhoea so that dehydration or fluid overload with pulmonary oedema and cardiac failure can occur. Anaemia is a common finding and is due to bone marrow depression, gastrointestinal bleeding or haemolysis. Low haemoglobin levels are well tolerated and blood transfusion with its obvious problems must only be considered in extreme cases and where time and the facility to deal with the fluid load exists. Likewise a degree of metabolic acidosis may be acceptable. Hypertension is common and if it is not well controlled, the drug therapy must be reviewed. Other problems may include pericarditis, a bleeding tendency due to platelet and capillary defects and there is an increased incidence of hepatitis B virus carrier state.

Diabetes Mellitus

Patients with diabetes mellitus may present several problems perioperatively. Blood glucose control requires special attention and the cardiovascular and renal complications need to be evaluated. *Table* 13.3 outlines the perioperative requirements with regard to blood glucose control. Those normally on oral therapy, having major surgery, may require insulin if there is sepsis or if control is normally poor. Diabetics on insulin, having minor surgery, ought to be first on the operating list. The morning insulin should be withheld preoperatively and when the patient has fully recovered from the anaesthetic he is given a reduced dose of insulin along with a snack. The principles of management for insulin-dependent diabetics having major surgery is summarized in *Table* 13.4.

Table 13.3 Diabetes mellitus

	Minor surgery	*Major surgery*
Diet alone	Check blood glucose	Check blood glucose
Oral therapy	Omit on day of surgery	Omit on day of surgery
	Monitor blood glucose	Monitor blood glucose
	Recommence therapy when able to eat	May require insulin regimen
Insulin therapy	Withhold preop. insulin	Normally require i.v. regimen

Table 13.4 Insulin-dependent diabetes—major surgery

Stabilize preoperatively
No s.c. insulin on day of surgery
I.v. infusion—dextrose
Insulin by i.v. infusion
Monitor blood glucose and serum K
Adjust insulin and K administration

Thyroid Disease

A retrosternal goitre can compress or displace the trachea. This may cause intubation difficulties and occasionally respiratory obstruction, which may not present until after induction of anaesthesia. Tracheal involvement may be seen on a plain chest radiograph but sometimes views of the neck and thoracic inlet are required to define the problem. Indirect laryngoscopy is required to exclude vocal cord palsy. Surgery in an uncontrolled hyperthyroid patient carries the risk of precipitating a thyroid crisis. Elective surgery ought to be postponed until the patient is stabilized on therapy. Urgent surgery can be carried out using beta-blockade and potassium iodide, intravenously if necessary. It is important that these patients receive adequate preoperative sedation. Larger doses than normal may be required because of the usually very anxious state and because of the increased rate of drug elimination. Similarly, patients who are hypothyroid ought to receive treatment before surgery if possible. This, however, takes time. Myxoedematous patients have a limited cardiac reserve and require reduced doses of drugs because of a slower rate of distribution and metabolism.

Myasthenia Gravis

The main problems in patients with myasthenia gravis are impaired respiratory activity, reduced ability to cough and clear secretions, dysphagia, regurgitation and pulmonary aspiration. Perioperative control may require anticholinesterase therapy to be given parenterally. Several points ought to be remembered. The ratio of parenteral dose to equivalent oral dose is 1:30. Excessive secretions and bradycardia are more often a problem with parenteral therapy and a vagolytic agent such as atropine is likely to be required. Atropine must always be given simultaneously if the intravenous route is used. Anticholinesterase requirements are usually less during bed rest but are increased in the presence of infection. It is unwise to operate in the presence of a chest infection except in an emergency. Patients with myasthenia gravis are very sensitive to the action of muscle relaxants and the anaesthetic must be planned with this in mind. Postoperative airway protection or ventilatory support may be required after major surgery. This is more likely in those with a long history of myasthenia gravis, those with chronic respiratory disease, those on high-dose therapy, and those with a vital capacity which is reduced or demonstrates fatigue.

Carcinoid Syndrome

If a patient with carcinoid syndrome has severe diarrhoea, fluid and electrolyte replenishment must be adequate. The danger with carcinoid tumours is the sudden appearance of extreme fluctuations in blood pressure, cardiac arrhythmias or bronchospasm. Precipitating factors are anxiety, hypotension and handling of the tumour, especially hepatic secondaries or a pulmonary primary. Bronchospasm can be resistant to treatment. Occasionally these patients have pulmonary or tricuspid valve stenosis due to endocardial fibrosis. The biggest problem arises when the condition is not diagnosed preoperatively and therefore a high index of suspicion is required.

Drug Therapy

All preoperative drug therapy should be reviewed with respect to dosage, toxicity, pertinence, efficacy and whether or not to continue perioperatively. Drugs can be listed in three categories as shown in *Table* 13.5.

Table 13.5 Preoperative drug therapy

Preoperative decision	*Drug therapy*
1. Continue up to and including morning of operation	Treatment of: cardiovascular disease respiratory disease epilepsy Parkinsonism thyroid disorders Corticosteroids—*see* text
2. Discontinue	Monoamine oxidase inhibitors Oral anticoagulants—*see* text
3. Continue with caution	Tricyclic antidepressants Lithium Levodopa Ecothiopate iodide Sedatives and tranquillizers

Steroids

Patients on steroid therapy for longer than 2 weeks preoperatively and those who have been on steroid therapy for more than 1 month within the past year may have induced adrenal insufficiency and require cover for surgery. Hydrocortisone 100 mg 1 h preoperatively is all that is required for minor surgery. For major surgery this is repeated 6-hourly for 24–72 h postoperatively.

Oral Anticoagulants

Oral anticoagulants should be stopped before any surgery which has a potential for causing significant bleeding, particularly if not amenable to external pressure. Even using vitamin K, reversal can take up to a week and in urgent cases fresh frozen plasma is required. When anticoagulant prophylaxis is required perioperatively heparin should be used.

Contraceptive Pill

Oestrogen-free contraceptive pills should not be discontinued. Oestrogen-containing pills should be discontinued for 4 weeks before major elective surgery or any operation on the legs. When this is not possible prophylaxis with heparin is required. Contraceptive pills need not be discontinued before minor surgery not involving the legs, if the procedure is short and there is early mobilization.

Diabetic Therapy

The perioperative management of diabetes mellitus is outlined above.

Alcohol

Heavy alcohol drinkers are tolerant to the effects of anaesthetic agents. The possibility of liver or cardiac damage must be excluded. The symptoms of acute withdrawal are sometimes severe and it is important to note that only a very small amount of ethanol is required to alleviate the condition.

Drugs Addiction

Drug addicts can become seriously ill during withdrawal and narcotic support should obviously be provided perioperatively. Hepatitis B and AIDS virus carrier state should always be determined.

Specific Anaesthetic Problems

Hypersensitivity Reactions

Hypersensitivity reactions can be anaphylactic which requires previous exposure to the agent or anaphylactoid which can occur on first exposure to the agent. Since anaesthetic drugs are often given as an intravenous bolus, reactions can be sudden and severe with cardiovascular collapse and/or intense bronchospasm both of which can be very resistant to treatment. Although more common in those with a history of allergy or asthma, the occurrence is unpredictable. Often several drugs have been given prior to a reaction and it may be impossible to determine which is responsible. All drugs which are suspect for the individual must be avoided subsequently if possible.

Atypical Plasma Cholinesterase

The neuromuscular blocking effect of suxamethonium is prolonged in patients with atypical plasma cholinesterase. Homozygous inheritance of the atypical enzyme occurs in 0·05% of the population and apnoea lasting several hours results if suxamethonium is given. In most cases the condition can be confirmed by measuring the plasma cholinesterase level and its dibucaine number. When a case is identified family investigation is necessary.

Malignant Hyperpyrexia

Malignant hyperpyrexia is a very rare condition which is often fatal and occurs in susceptible individuals in response to many of the drugs used in relation to anaesthesia. Suxamethonium and halothane are the most potent of the trigger agents which include all the volatile agents. The susceptibility is due to an inherited muscle cell defect which causes intense and sustained activity within the cells when exposed to a trigger agent. Body temperature rises rapidly and there is hypoxia, hypercapnia, metabolic acidosis and hyperkalaemia. Treatment involves active cooling and supportive measures aimed at maintaining oxygenation and restoring biochemical normality. The only specific treatment is intravenous dantrolene. Susceptibility can often be detected from the family history of problems or death associated with anaesthesia. Confirmation requires muscle biopsy challenge tests.

Porphyria

Porphyria is an inherited disorder of prophyrin metabolism and a severe attack can cause respiratory paralysis, convulsions or coma. Several drugs may precipitate an acute episode in patients who suffer from the condition. Thiopentone and methohexitone are the most relevant to anaesthesia.

Dystrophia Myotonica

Dystrophia myotonica is an inherited disorder which causes muscle weakness and an inability to relax the muscle after contraction. Anaesthetic agents such as thiopentone which cause respiratory depression can very easily cause respiratory failure. Suxamethonium and neostigmine can exacerbate myotonia. These patients are also susceptible to cardiac irregularities under anaesthesia.

Airway Problems

Airway problems arising under anaesthesia are much less difficult to manage if they are anticipated. The difficulties which can arise are: refractory upper airway obstruction after induction of anaesthesia, complications of airway irritability, difficult tracheal intubation and tracheal obstruction. Careful preoperative evaluation, measures to ameliorate the particular problem and proper preparation for the anaesthetic can reduce the risk involved.

Refractory upper airway obstruction after induction is not always predictable but is more likely to occur in patients with anatomically bulky tissues in the tongue, neck or jaw, or those with a pathological space-occupying lesion involving the upper airway such as enlarged tonsils, haematoma, oedema, infection or tumour. Even greater trouble can be anticipated if there is also immobility of the neck or temporomandibular joints as can be caused by arthritis, contractures, fractures or muscle spasm. Nasal obstruction, bleeding into the airway or risk of regurgitation also make handling this situation more difficult as do features which make it hard to fit a mask to the face and form a seal.

Airway irritability is associated with respiratory tract infection, smoking, asthma and the presence of secretions, blood or regurgitated material. The possible consequences have already been mentioned.

Anatomical features which make tracheal intubation difficult include: increased posterior or anterior mandibular depth, decreased mandibular length, obtuse mandibular angles, short muscular neck, protruding upper teeth, long, high, arched palate and narrow, deep mouth. Any pathology which causes distortion or decreased mobility of the mandible or cervical spine or any pathology which occupies, distorts or compresses the mouth, pharynx, larynx or trachea is likely to impede intubation. In cases of suspected difficulty, previous anaesthetic records can be invaluable and a thorough examination of the upper airway including radiography, indirect laryngoscopy and, possibly, attempted direct laryngoscopy may be necessary.

Lesions involving the trachea or main bronchi capable of causing serious obstruction under anaesthesia need not necessarily cause clinically significant obstruction preoperatively. Posture, venous congestion, and altered pulmonary dynamics may increase the degree of obstruction dramatically. Tracheal intubation occasionally makes the problem worse, particularly if the lower end of the tube impinges on the lesion. It is important to define the anatomical extent of the lesion preoperatively and to identify any factors which increase the obstruction.

Emergency Surgery

When the surgical pathology demands an emergency operation, the preoperative preparation is dictated by the urgency of the surgery. Judgement is required in deciding the correct priorities and the optimum time for intervention. The highest priorities must include establishing a clear airway, adequate ventilation and oxygenation, restoration of blood volume and circulatory support. In the bleeding patient, restoration of blood volume may not be possible before surgery to arrest the bleeding. Poor myocardial function resulting from a period of shock is common and continuing hypotension and low cardiac output does not necessarily indicate continuing hypovolaemia. Uncontrolled concomitant medical conditions may contribute to cardiovascular and metabolic derangements. Assessment must, however, be rapid, selective and guided by pointers as they arise and priorities may change as factors come to light.

Because of the risk of regurgitation and pulmonary aspiration during anaesthesia, patients having surgery should, whenever possible, be fasted for 6 h before induction. Because of the problem of hypoglycaemia, children should only be fasted for 4 h. When surgical intervention is urgent, the risk of regurgitation obviously has to be balanced against the risk of delay. It is also relevant that, in patients suffering from acute gastrointestinal pathology, trauma, severe pain, shock or heavy sedation, the stomach may still be full after 6 h. Although it is often impossible to empty the stomach completely, the insertion of a stomach tube to reduce the contents is beneficial, as are efforts to reduce the acidity.

Day-case Surgery

For patients to have minor surgery under general anaesthesia, regional nerve block or sedation on a day-case basis, there must be adequate accommodation, facilities, equipment and staffing. Careful patient selection and efficient preoperative assessment are necessary. Only patients who are normally healthy or who have minor systemic disease not interfering with normal activities are suitable. This includes those with medical conditions which have been adequately investigated, accurately defined and well controlled on therapy. Social circumstances must also be adequate and there must be a responsible adult available to care for them at home. Initial assessment must be carried out at the time of the outpatient consultation before booking for day-case surgery. This requires a full history and examination, including blood pressure measurement. Arrangements must be made to have any necessary investigations done before admission. Instructions to the patient must be given verbally and in writing with regard to preoperative fasting, transport and escort arrangements for going home and postoperative instructions. The latter includes avoiding driving, operating machinery and ingestion of alcohol for 24 h after the procedure. Final assessment is carried out on the day of admission and there must be sufficient time for this to be done properly. Use of a check-list type record increases the efficiency of this process. The anaesthetist must be informed as early as possible of any potential problems. Premedication is only occasionally required.

Postoperatively, pain relief normally takes the form of simple oral analgesics which can be continued by the patient at home. Sometimes the need for parenteral analgesics or antiemetics may delay discharge or involve the services of the general practitioner or community nurse in the patient's home. All patients must be assessed by a member of the medical staff before being discharged and must be alert, communicating well and walking comfortably unaided. If doubt exists as to fitness for discharge, overnight admission must be arranged and this is required in 2–3% of cases.

Informed Consent

The patient has a right to decide whether he will accept or reject the treatment proposed. Explanation of the diagnosis and treatment, including perioperative procedures and their consequences, as well as a disclosure of risks involved is necessary for the patient to make an informed choice. The degree of disclosure of risks is a matter of clinical judgement and may in some instances be limited by the danger of psychological detriment to the patient. However, if the patient is of sound mind and asks specifically about the risks involved, he must be answered truthfully and as fully as he requires and in a language which he can understand. The explanation given to children must be as detailed as they are capable of dealing with. It is a common mistake to underestimate a child's ability to cope with a truthful account. Full explanation having been given, written or witnessed consent by the patient is required for both surgery and anaesthesia. To administer anaesthesia without consent constitutes an assault. If the patient is not capable of giving consent, it must be obtained from the next of kin. If the patient is under 16 years of age, consent must be obtained from a parent or guardian. In an emergency situation when the patient is unable to give consent because, for example, he is unconscious and the next of kin cannot be contacted, the patient should be given any treatment that is immediately necessary in his best interest.

Premedication

Preoperative anxiety is the main reason for premedication but often explanation and reassurance are what is really required. When relief of anxiety is the only requirement, an oral benzodiazepine such as temazepam is most effective with few side-effects. Due to the limited amount of water which can be allowed preoperatively to help swallow tablets and the fact that they are often taken in the supine position, a high percentage of tablets and capsules given as premedication do not reach the stomach. An elixir is therefore more effective.

Papaveretum plus hyoscine is the most commonly prescribed intramuscular premedicant. This has several effects which may be beneficial for some patients. The combination has a powerful sedative and amnesic effect. Papaveretum provides preoperative pain relief and allows some assessment of the effect of a narcotic in the individual patient. The analgesic effect is beneficial during the anaesthetic and immediate postoperative period. Hyoscine has an antiemetic action and its anticholinergic effect reduces parasympathetic reflex activity such as excessive production of secretions or bradycardia which can occur in response to intubation, suxamethonium or certain surgical stimuli. The disadvantages are: a very dry mouth, postoperative drowsiness, occasionally nausea and vomiting and the fact that an injection is required.

Children up to 1 year of age need only be given atropine intramuscularly. Older children are often given trimeprazine which is a phenothiazine and atropine for its anticholinergic effect orally.

Excessively anxious patients may be difficult to sedate safely. A benzodiazepine such as midazolam titrated intravenously in small increments is usually very effective but should be reserved for the immediate preoperative period.

Preparation for Theatre

As a safeguard against disastrous accidents certain points need to be checked before the patient is finally anaesthetized. The most efficient way of doing this is by a check list which is part of the nursing process in preparing a patient for theatre. The following must be confirmed: identification, consent, site of operation, appropriate fasting and removal of false teeth, contact lenses, hearing aids, jewellery, hair clips, make up and nail varnish. Vulnerable sites, for example injuries or arthritic joints, must be noted and those handling the patient warned. A final check on the patient's condition is necessary in case of sudden deterioration and when blood is likely to be required it is necessary to check that it is available.

With regard to appropriate fasting, children fasted for longer than 4 h preoperatively are in danger of developing hypoglycaemia. If the period of fasting is likely to be longer than 4 h, a glucose drink should be given 4 h preoperatively or an intravenous infusion of dextrose set up.

ANAESTHESIA

The objective of anaesthesia is to eliminate the ordeal for the patient during surgery, to provide adequate operating conditions and to maintain physiological homeostasis. General anaesthesia implies that the patient loses consciousness and hence there is complete absence of suffering during the procedure. The perception of pain may be separately abolished by local anaesthetic block, while sedation and systemic analgesia are used to alleviate anxiety and discomfort. In addition, there are two major prerequisites for surgery. There must be good access to the operation site and there must be no movement, either voluntary or reflex. To achieve these conditions, especially for abdominal or thoracic surgery, muscle relaxation is usually required and this can be provided by deep general anaesthesia, neuromuscular block or local anaesthesia. The patient may be affected by many deleterious influences arising from the anaesthetic, surgery or pre-existing pathology. The airway must be protected and pulmonary ventilation maintained. Adequate blood volume, circulation and oxygenation must be ensured. This requires comprehensive preoperative preparation, an awareness of the possible complications of the anaesthetic and procedures involved, constant monitoring and the institution of appropriate corrective measures. Another important consideration is the reversal of the anaesthetic process. Recovery should ideally be smooth and rapidly complete with minimum distress and discomfort.

General Anaesthesia

A patient who is unconscious but not deeply anaesthetized exhibits several responses to painful stimuli which can be harmful and which can make surgery very difficult. Most of these reflexes are abolished under deep anaesthesia. The use of muscle relaxants allows surgery to be performed at a much lighter plane of anaesthesia. Neuromuscular blockade prevents reflex skeletal muscle activity which causes movement, increased abdominal muscle tone, vomiting and laryngeal spasm. If the patient is only lightly anaesthetized profound autonomically mediated cardiorespiratory responses still occur and adequate analgesia is required if these are to be avoided. Anaesthesia, analgesia and muscle relaxation are therefore the three components of balanced anaesthesia and this normally involves the use of several agents. All of these have unwanted effects which have to be considered along with the requirements of the surgery and any relevant problems the patient may have, before selecting the technique to be employed.

Induction of Anaesthesia

Intravenous induction of anaesthesia is normally preferred because it is smooth, fast and least disturbing. The most commonly used drugs are thiopentone sodium, methohexitone sodium, etomidate and propofol. The duration of unconsciousness is normally between 2 and 10 min and the initial recovery is mainly due to redistribution within the body causing a fall in the concentration of the drug in the brain. Metabolism and elimination are, however, relevant in relation to hang-over effect, drug interactions and accumulation with repeated doses. Breakdown of etomidate and propofol is rapid, whereas complete metabolism of thiopentone and methohexitone takes many hours. These drugs are very poor analgesics and are not normally used for maintaining surgical anaesthesia. Each agent has its own profile of adverse effects. Hypotension and respiratory depression are common and usually dose related. Methohexitone, etomidate and propofol can cause pain on injection and hypersensitivity reactions can occur with any of the intravenous anaesthetic agents.

Induction using an inhalational agent may be preferable for some children or for those with potential airway problems, but most patients find it unpleasant. Any of the inhalational anaesthetic agents can be used. Cyclopropane is the most rapid and has very little smell but it is highly explosive and great care is required in its use.

If there is doubt as to whether the upper gastrointestinal tract is empty, the airway and lungs must be protected by an endotracheal tube during anaesthesia. The danger of pulmonary aspiration of stomach or oesophageal contents then only exists during the critical period before the endotracheal tube is inserted and the cuff inflated. When muscle paralysis is induced prior to intubation, the cough reflex is lost and the glottis lies open. Vomiting is not possible at this stage because of neuromuscular blockade but passive regurgitation can occur. To protect the lungs during this period the induction technique must include preoxygenation, cricoid pressure and the use of a muscle relaxant of rapid onset and short duration. There must be adequate assistance for the anaesthetist and proper equipment, including good suction apparatus and the facility to tip the patient head down quickly.

The Airway

As the level of anaesthesia deepens, muscle relaxation increases and the supraglottic airway often becomes occluded due to the tongue falling back, especially when the patient is supine. Pulling the chin up and extending the head is sometimes all that is required to clear the airway but often this is not enough and the jaw has to be thrust forward with considerable force to alleviate the obstruction. In order to do this the mouth must be opened to disengage the teeth and increase the mobility at the temporomandibular joints. The insertion of an artificial oropharyngeal airway usually solves the problem but at light levels of anaesthesia it may not be tolerated. A nasopharyngeal airway is sometimes more successful and usually causes less irritation. Occasionally, however, it can create nasal bleeding and exacerbate the airway problem. Bacteraemia can also result from trauma to the nasal mucosa.

The following points are important when trouble in maintaining the airway is expected. The higher the alveolar oxygen concentration which exists when ventilation becomes difficult, the greater is the period available in which to solve the problem. A slow induction gives more time to deal with the complication as it develops and if severe intractable airway occlusion does occur suddenly, retreat to a phase of anaesthesia at which reversal of the obstruction occurs ought to be possible before severe hypoxaemia supervenes.

Laryngeal spasm can occur without warning, particularly under light anaesthesia and in patients with a predisposition such as smokers and those with a current or recent upper respiratory infection. Precipitating factors include any painful surgical stimulation and glottic irritation due to instrumentation, premature insertion of an artificial airway and the presence of secretions, blood or vomit. To alleviate spasm the cause must be removed and anaesthesia increased. When it is severe, 100% oxygen under slight pressure must be administered with the jaw held firmly forward. Only rarely is it necessary to give a muscle relaxant and pass an endotracheal tube.

Bronchospasm is likewise more likely to occur under light anaesthesia and is more common in patients with asthma, chronic obstructive airways disease or acute respiratory infection. Constriction of the small airways can be triggered by the intravenous administration of certain drugs, the introduction of a tracheal tube or any of the factors which can cause laryngeal spasm. The management of bronchospasm includes removing stimulation and deepening the level of anaesthesia when possible. If it persists, a beta-2 stimulant such as salbutamol should be given slowly intravenously. Aminophylline and hydrocortisone may be added if necessary. In severe cases IPPV with 100% oxygen is required. Sometimes bronchospasm is very resistant to treatment and occasionally so intense that oxygenation is impossible and death results.

The presence of secretions, gastrointestinal contents or blood in the upper airway can cause respiratory embarrassment due to irritation, obstruction or pulmonary aspiration. The results of aspiration depend on the nature of the material entering the lower respiratory tract. Immediate problems arise if it causes blockage of the airways or if it is acidic. Acid aspiration syndrome includes the rapid onset of intense bronchospasm, cardiovascular collapse and the development of the clinical picture of adult respiratory distress syndrome (ARDS). The mortality is very high. It is therefore important to deal with foreign material in the upper airway immediately. The patient must be tipped head down and turned to the lateral position. The rapid use of suction is essential and reflex laryngeal spasm or bronchoconstriction must be treated accordingly. If aspiration of the material does occur, tracheal intubation and endotracheal suction is indicated. Early administration of steroids (methylprednisolone 30 mg/kg i.v.) may prevent massive pulmonary capillary damage. Physiotherapy, bronchoscopy and treatment of infection may be required later. In addition, if acid has entered the bronchial tree, cardiovascular resuscitation with intravenous colloid and careful attention to central venous pressure is required and IPPV with positive end-expiratory pressure (PEEP) may be necessary.

Tracheal Intubation

Intubation of the trachea is necessary in order to administer IPPV, to protect the lungs from contamination or to provide access for operations on the head and neck. A tracheal tube also secures the airway and provides a route for endotracheal suction. Disposable, cuffed, oral tubes are the most commonly used. The size refers to the internal diameter; 8·0 or 8·5 mm is used for female adults and 9·0 or 9·5 mm for males. For children below the age of 5 or 6 years uncuffed tubes are used and the ideal fit is that which is snug so that aspiration is prevented but not so tight that a leak cannot be produced by a slightly exaggerated inflation pressure. The Macintosh laryngoscope, which has a curved blade, is the most commonly used, but for babies a straight-bladed laryngoscope is usually preferred. A muscle relaxant is normally given to provide good conditions for intubation. With the patient's head on a pillow and shoulders on the mattress, the head is extended and the neck flexed to give the optimum position for subjects with normal anatomy. The laryngoscope blade is used to displace the tongue to the left and the tip advanced anterior to the epiglottis until it reaches the vallecula. The handle of the instrument is then pulled in an antero-inferior direction in relation to the patient, while resisting the rotational pressure on the blade as shown in *Fig.* 13.1. The endotracheal tube is passed from

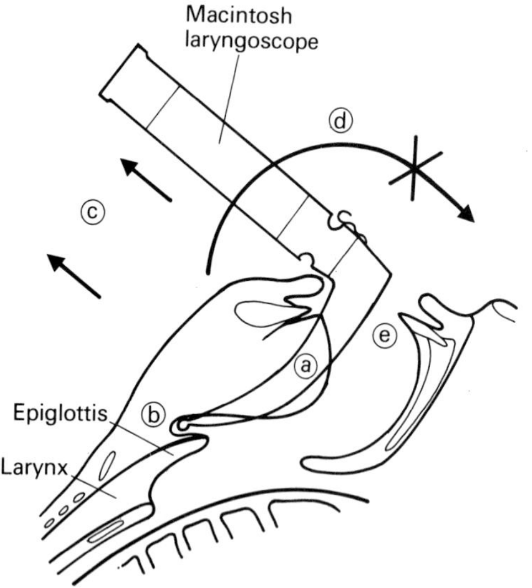

Fig. 13.1 Use of laryngoscope for tracheal intubation. This diagram illustrates the correct placement of a curved laryngoscope blade and the direction of the force which must be applied to the handle for optimum visualization of the larynx without risk of trauma. The following points are indicated: *(a)* Tongue displaced to left by blade. *(b)* Tip of blade in vallecula. *(c)* Direction of pull on handle. *(d)* Tendency to rotation which must be resisted. *(e)* Gap between upper incisors and blade.

the side, maintaining vision of the tip and the larynx throughout. It is a common mistake to overestimate the length of the trachea and pass the tip of the tube beyond the carina. This dramatically interferes with oxygenation as it causes venous admixture of about 50% of the cardiac output. To avoid this it is important to advance the tube through the larynx until the entire cuff is below the vocal cords and no further. The best confirmation that the tube is in the trachea is to see a vocal cord lying against the tube before withdrawing the laryngoscope. The cuff is expanded with enough air to form an adequate seal and no more. The seal required is that which prevents leakage around the tube when the lungs are inflated to about twice the normal tidal volume.

When difficulty in passing an endotracheal tube is anticipated it is unwise to administer a muscle relaxant until either the larynx has been visualized or it has been demonstrated that manual ventilation using a face mask is possible. The airway may become compromised when paralysis occurs, however, and when major problems are expected the safest technique it to intubate under local anaesthesia with the patient awake, using either the conventional laryngoscope as described above or a fibreoptic instrument. This requires the patient's cooperation and an alternative is to use a mainly gaseous induction until the patient is deeply anaesthetized when an attempt to visualize the larynx can be made, while spontaneous respiration is maintained. Backward pressure on the larynx and the use of a malleable introducer is helpful. When this is unsuccessful a gum elastic bougie can sometimes be introduced first and then used as a railroad for the endotracheal tube. Sometimes difficulty with intubation is not expected and only becomes obvious after the muscle relaxant has been given. This is a more formidable problem if there is also obstruction to pulmonary ventilation through a face mask or if there is a coexisting regurgitation risk.

General Anaesthetic Agents

General anaesthesia is usually sustained by the use of inhalational agents. It is common practice to use a combination of nitrous oxide with one of the volatile anaesthetic agents. Nitrous oxide, which is a gas at room temperature and pressure, has a very powerful analgesic effect but a very weak hypnotic action. It has relatively few adverse effects and any action on cardiovascular or respiratory function is usually negligible. In order to ensure that the gas mixture contains adequate oxygen the inspired concentration of nitrous oxide is usually limited to 67%. This does not give adequate anaesthesia on its own and it is necessary to add the very strong hypnotic effect of halothane, enflurane or isoflurane. These are the three volatile agents in common use and all of them produce a degree of muscle relaxation, but have relatively weak analgesic action. They are liquids at room temperature and require special vaporizers. To provide the necessary fine control of administration, the vaporizers are accurately calibrated and compensate for changes in temperature and gas flow. All three have unwanted actions, most of which are dose related and *Table* 13.6 illustrates the profile of each agent in relation to cardiorespiratory effects.

Isoflurane has little direct effect on the heart. It causes least susceptibility to arrhythmias and its hypotensive effect is almost entirely due to vasodilatation. This is in contrast to halothane and enflurane which drop the blood pressure mainly by decreasing myocardial contractility and therefore reducing cardiac output. The main disadvantages of isoflurane are its respiratory irritant effect and its current high cost. Arrhythmias are less of a problem with enflurane than with halothane but enflurane causes greater myocardial depression. Because of its tendency to produce abnormal electro-encephalograph activity, enflurane is avoided in epileptic patients. Massive liver-cell necrosis is a very rare complication of halothane anaesthesia. Because of the lack of specificity of the clinical presentation and the pathological changes, the exact incidence is not known but it is certainly less than 1 in 10 000. The risk is greater and the onset more rapid if halothane anaesthesia is repeated within a 3-month period. It is also more common in females, in the obese and in patients with organ-specific autoimmunity. None of the above inhalational agents is inflammable.

Intravenous supplements are often given in order to reduce the concentration of volatile agent required and consequently decrease dose-related side-effects. Opioids are commonly used for this purpose because they also alleviate the stress response to surgery and produce a smoother and more comfortable recovery. Fentanyl and alfentanil are particularly suitable because neither has significant cardiovascular effects and both have a short duration of action. Alfentanil is eliminated more quickly than any other opioid agonist. It is therefore suitable for short procedures or when postoperative respiratory depression is a particular concern. If, in addition, a benzodiazepine such as midazolam or a butyrophenone such as droperidol is used, the volatile agent can often be eliminated and this is desirable in certain situations. Anaesthesia in a patient with cerebral oedema is

Table 13.6 Cardiorespiratory effects of the volatile anaesthetic agents

	Halothane	*Enflurane*	*Isoflurane*
Irritant effect	+	+	+++
Respiratory depression	+	++	++
Myocardial depression	++	+++	+
Hypotension	+	++	++
Heart rate	Decreased	Increased	Increased
Susceptibility to arrhythmias	+++	++	–

Key: – no risk;
+ minimal;
++ moderate;
+++ significant.

an example of such a situation because all the volatile agents cause a rise in intracranial pressure.

Ketamine is a unique anaesthetic agent which can be given intravenously or intramuscularly. It produces complete analgesia and a condition known as dissociation anaesthesia. The airway and respiration are well maintained. Its main disadvantages are that it can cause vivid dreaming, hallucinations, emergence delirium and hypertension. It is used mainly for repeated minor procedures in children and it is very useful when dealing with trapped casualties.

Anaesthetic Apparatus

For reasons of safety, convenience and cost, most operating theatres have a piped delivery system for oxygen and nitrous oxide. A large liquid oxygen reservoir normally supplies an entire hospital and banks of cylinders provide the nitrous oxide and reserve oxygen. Gauges on the anaesthetic machine (*Fig.* 13.2) measure the pipeline pressure for each gas and the normal supply pressure is 4 bar (60 lbf/in^2). Each anaesthetic machine carries at least one reserve cylinder of oxygen and one of nitrous oxide. Pressure gauges indicate when the cylinders need replacement and regulators reduce the pressure of the gas coming out of the cylinders to 4 bar. When the pipeline gas is being used the cylinders must be closed. If the oxygen supply fails, the fall in pressure is detected by a device which produces an audible alarm. A needle valve for each gas controls its flow which is measured by a rotameter. Gases emerging from the rotameters join a common pathway which leads to the vaporizers. The proportion of gas which passes through the vaporizing chamber containing the volatile agent is controlled by the switch which is used to set the concentration. The final anaesthetic mixture then emerges from the fresh gas outlet of the machine to be conducted to the patient by one of several possible breathing systems.

The Magill, Bain, Lack, T-piece and circle systems are commonly used in current practice for delivering the gases to the patient and these are illustrated in *Fig.* 13.3. All may

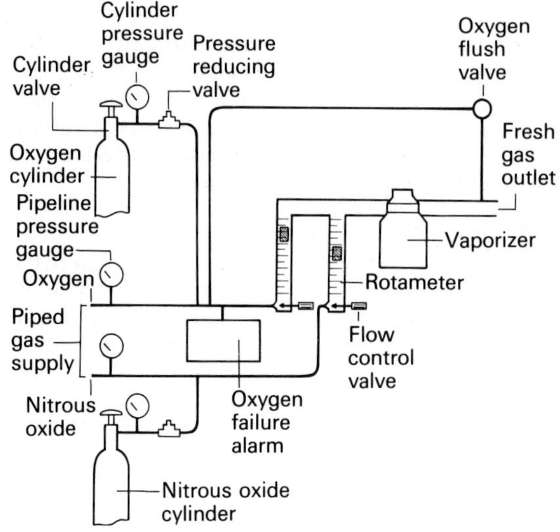

Fig. 13.2 Diagrammatic representation of the components of a basic anaesthetic machine.

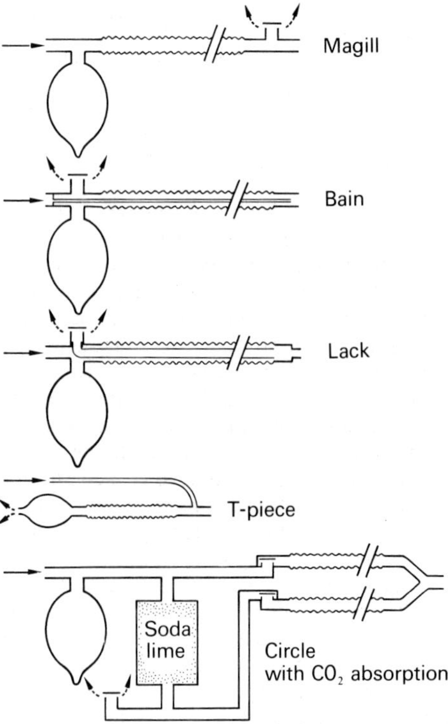

Fig. 13.3 Common anaesthetic breathing systems. Anaesthetic gases enter as indicated by the solid arrows on the left when the system is connected to the fresh gas outlet of the anaesthetic machine. A mask or endotracheal tube, attached to the outlet on the right of the diagram, delivers the gas mixture to the patient and the expired gas escapes as shown by the broken arrows.

be used with spontaneous respiration or to provide manual ventilatory support. The Magill and Lack systems, however, are more efficient for spontaneous respiration, while the Bain is more efficient for manual ventilation and it can also be adapted for use with an automatic ventilator. The T-piece arrangement is used for small children and babies. It causes very little resistance to breathing, the dead space is low and continuous positive airway pressure (CPAP) or positive end-expiratory pressure (PEEP) can be applied. Circle systems with carbon dioxide absorption can be operated with very low flows of fresh gas but they are clumsy and complex. Their use, however, is increasing because of the high cost of newer anaesthetic agents, an increasing awareness of the dangers of pollution and better gas monitoring facilities. In addition, the inspired gas is warm and has a high water vapour content. Other systems deliver gas which is cold and completely dry and this increases body heat loss and causes drying of the respiratory mucosa and inspissation of secretions.

Muscle Relaxants

Relaxation of skeletal muscle may be required to permit endotracheal intubation, to facilitate IPPV or to abolish the reflex muscle contraction which occurs in response to surgical stimulation. Muscle relaxant drugs act by blocking the postsynaptic acetylcholine receptors in the neuromuscular junction. The agents in general use are suxamethonium, tubocurarine, alcuronium, pancuronium, atracurium and vecuronium. Suxamethonium produces profound relaxation of rapid onset and short duration. It is commonly used for tracheal intubation, especially when speed and ideal conditions are necessary or when continuing neuromuscular block is not required. Bradycardia and postoperative muscle pains are common side-effects of suxamethonium and its use is precluded in some conditions because of the rise in serum potassium, intraocular pressure and intracranial pressure which occur. It is also contraindicated in patients with atypical plasma cholinesterase, myotonia dystrophica or a susceptibility to malignant hyperpyrexia. The other agents are different from suxamethonium in that they do not cause an initial depolarization of the postsynaptic membrane and they are therefore referred to as 'non-depolarizing'. All act for longer than 20 min and normally require reversal. Each differs in its cardiovascular effects and method of elimination. Blood pressure is most influenced by tubocurarine which causes hypotension and pancuronium which causes an increase in blood pressure and heart rate. These attributes may be useful or undesirable depending on the requirements of a particular case. Vecuronium and atracurium are least likely to have a prolonged action in renal failure and atracurium is the drug of choice when hepatic function is severely impaired. In both situations, monitoring the degree of neuromuscular blockade with a nerve stimulator helps avoid overdosage.

Intermittent Positive-pressure Ventilation

Automatic ventilation is necessary for long operations or if muscle relaxation is required. Arterial carbon dioxide tends to rise during prolonged anaesthesia if the patient is breathing spontaneously. Neuromuscular block causes paralysis of the respiratory muscles. When IPPV is first instituted, hypotension is common especially in less fit and hypovolaemic patients. The sudden rise in intrathoracic pressure and fall in arterial carbon dioxide impedes venous return and reduces myocardial contractility. Cardiovascular adaptation takes time and to avoid the fall in blood pressure, ventilation should be introduced at a low tidal volume and gradually increased to the desired level, with careful monitoring. Attention must be given to other factors acting simultaneously such as the induction and anaesthetic agents which also cause hypotension. There is a large variety of automatic ventilators currently available, employing several different mechanisms to inflate the lungs. The compression of a bellows, using electrical power or high-pressure gas, is a common method and this is illustrated in *Fig.* 13.4. The expiratory valve is closed during the inspiratory phase and

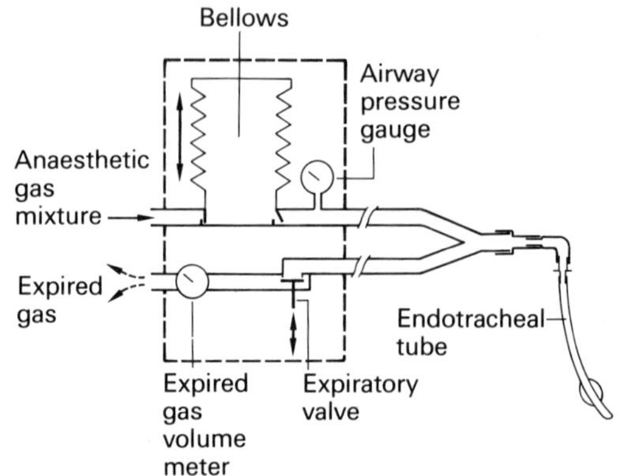

Fig. 13.4 Diagrammatic representation of a simple ventilator.

then opens to allow the patient to exhale passively. The operator can normally manipulate the composition of the inspired gas, the tidal volume and the frequency of ventilation. In many models the ratio of inspiratory to expiratory time can be adjusted either directly or indirectly. All ventilators have a gauge which measures airway pressure, but the other parameters displayed depend on the particular machine. The ventilating frequency is usually set at 10–12 inflations per minute in adults and progressively greater in children up to 25–40 in neonates. The tidal volume is adjusted until observation and auscultation of the chest indicates that expansion is adequate. This normally gives a tidal volume greater than the 7–8 ml/kg necessary to produce normocapnia in a patient with normal lungs. This excess inflation prevents atelectasis during long periods of ventilation and ensures that most patients will be hypocapnic which increases the safety margin and reduces the amount of anaesthetic and muscle relaxant required. Monitoring the airway pressure can detect changes in the lung resistance or compliance, obstruction or leakage in the ventilator system or the need for further muscle relaxant.

Reversal and Extubation

The non-depolarizing muscle relaxants competitively block neuromuscular transmission and their action can be overcome by increasing the acetylcholine available at the junction. Reversal is achieved by the use of neostigmine which inhibits the breakdown of acetylcholine by acetylcholinesterase. Intravenous neostigmine causes increased acetylcholine, not only at the neuromuscular junction, but at all cholinergic nerve endings. This results in the unwanted muscarinic effects of acetylcholine which include bradycardia, salivation and intense intestinal contraction. These effects must be blocked by giving atropine or glycopyrrolate along with the neostigmine. Reversal of the neuromuscular block is not possible when the concentration of muscle relaxant is high. There must therefore be some return of neuromuscular function before the neostigmine is given, if reversal is to be successful.

If good respiratory effort does not return after termination of the anaesthetic and reversal of the muscle relaxant, the endotracheal tube must be left in situ and IPPV continued until improvement occurs. There are three common reasons. Hypocapnia in a patient who is still unconscious usually results in continuing apnoea. Inadequate reversal of the muscle relaxant causes shallow respiration which is gasping and diaphragmatic in nature and often accompanied by marked tracheal tug on inspiration. Depression due to opioid drugs normally causes a low respiratory rate, but it may take the form of continuing apnoea or intermittent respiration which occurs only when the patient is aroused. In addition to breathing adequately, patients who are in danger of vomiting or who have any upper airway problem must also be awake enough to maintain their own airway and protect the lungs with a good cough reflex before it is safe to remove the endotracheal tube. These patients are best extubated in the lateral position. Oxygen 100% is administered to all patients and the pharynx is cleared by suction under direct vision before removal of the tube. As the endotracheal tube is removed there must be suction at the ready and assistance standing by to tip the patient head down instantly should the need arise. The mandible is held forward and a face mask firmly applied so that 100% oxygen can be administered under slight pressure until regular breathing and a secure airway is established. Irritability with coughing, breath holding, straining, vomiting and laryngeal spasm is common at this stage and it is important to keep the pharynx clear of secretions or any foreign material. Severe laryngeal spasm is a particularly serious problem and more likely to occur in small children. The safest way to ensure a clear and protected airway is to allow the patient to wake up properly before removing the endotracheal tube.

Local Anaesthesia

Local anaesthesia can be used as an alternative or in addition to general anaesthesia for surgery. Total inhibition of afferent transmission of surgical stimuli by blocking nerve conduction can prevent the neuro-endocrine responses to surgery which may be possible under general anaesthesia. Analgesia usually persists into the early postoperative period and with some techniques this may be extended. In addition to the desired effect at the site of injection, however, local anaesthetics can exert widespread actions on the body and these may be particularly hazardous for some patients. General anaesthesia has the advantage of speed and 100% efficiency. Controlled ventilation is easily instituted where necessary, assuring oxygenation and carbon dioxide elimination. The circulatory insult in patients with cardiovascular disease is often more easily controlled under general anaesthesia than when major central neural block with local anaesthetic is used. Whether local or general anaesthesia is safer in a particular case depends on the type of surgery, the block required and the specific problems related to that patient.

Local anaesthetic agents inhibit membrane depolarization in all excitable tissues and hence block neuronal transmission of impulses. All types of nerve fibres are affected. Preganglionic fibres are the most sensitive and then, in order of decreasing sensitivity, pain, temperature, touch, proprioception and motor fibres. Only a small number of agents are used in current practice and these are listed in *Table* 13.7. All these can produce toxic effects if injected into a blood vessel or if an absolute overdose is administered. The maximum safe doses quoted relate to healthy individuals of average build. The dose which results in systemic toxicity varies according to the rate of absorption from the injection site and this depends very much on the blood flow. The volume of distribution and rate of metabolism are also important. All these factors are affected by the physical state of the patient. The first sign of toxicity is often numbness or tingling of the tongue or around the mouth, followed by light-headedness. The patient may feel very anxious and experience tinnitus before becoming drowsy. At higher blood levels there is loss of consciousness, convulsions and apnoea. Cardiovascular collapse eventually occurs due to myocardial depression, vasodilatation and hypoxia. Treatment is aimed at maintaining a clear airway and oxygenation, with artificial ventilation if necessary. Intravenous midazolam, diazepam or thiopentone is used to control convulsive activity. Hypotension is treated with intravenous fluid and, if severe, ephedrine may be required.

Table 13.7 Local anaesthetic agents

Agent	*Use*	*Maximum safe dose* (for peripheral use)
Lignocaine	Surface infiltration Peripheral nerve block Caudal	3 mg/kg (or 7 mg/kg with vasoconstrictor)
Bupivacaine	Epidural Spinal Peripheral nerve block	2 mg/kg
Prilocaine	Surface infiltration Peripheral nerve block Intravenous regional anaesthesia	5 mg/kg (or 8 mg/kg with vasoconstrictor)

Adrenaline is often added to local anaesthetic agents to produce vasoconstriction and slow down the rate of absorption. This reduces toxicity and prolongs the duration of action. The concentration of adrenaline should not be more than 1:200 000 and the maximum safe dose is 0·5 mg. Much smaller doses injected into a blood vessel cause tachycardia and cardiac arrhythmias. Felypressin is an equally effective alternative vasoconstrictor which is less cardiotoxic. Because of the risk of tissue ischaemia, neither should be injected near end-arteries and they should not be used for ring blocks or intravenous regional anaesthesia.

Sedation

Sedation is commonly used to allay anxiety and discomfort and hence increase the patient's ability to cooperate during minor procedures or operations under local anaesthesia. Sedation can be given orally, intramuscularly or intravenously as described under premedication. Intravenous titration of a short-acting agent is a safe method of giving adequate sedation without risk of overdosage, provided that the increments are small and enough time is allowed to assess the effect before each administration. Elderly patients can be very sensitive to the effects of sedative drugs and incremental doses as low as 0·5 mg midazolam, for example, may be necessary whereas in fit young individuals 2·5 mg is appropriate. Sedation given without due care exposes the patient to many of the risks of general anaesthesia, especially airway obstruction and aspiration of vomit. Not all patients behave as expected unfortunately. Sometimes confusion and removal of inhibitions as a result of sedation can lead to a total loss of cooperation. If analgesia is required, an opioid in dilute solution can be administered in small boluses, again with frequent assessment of the effect. It is important to realize that respiratory depression may not present until after the procedure when stimulation is no longer present. Although rousable, the patient may lapse into sleep and apnoea when left alone. Short-acting opioids should therefore be used if large doses are likely to be required.

Spinal and Epidural Anaesthesia

Subarachnoid and epidural anaesthesia are suitable for abdominal surgery but more so for operations involving the lower abdomen, pelvis, perineum and lower limbs. Cardiovascular disease or hypovolaemia is a contraindication to their use for anaesthesia above the 3rd lumbar segment because block of the autonomic sympathetic outflow results in vasodilatation causing relative hypovolaemia, loss of peripheral vascular resistance and hypotension. Other contraindications are problems with haemostasis, local sepsis or contamination at the site of insertion and to a lesser extent pre-existing spinal or neurological pathology. Equipment and expertise for cardiopulmonary resuscitation must always be readily available. An intravenous infusion is established and at least 500 ml crystalloid or colloid given before the procedure. The blood pressure is measured throughout and more plasma expansion may be required if hypotension occurs. A vasoconstrictor drug such as ephedrine must also be at hand. Pulmonary blood flow is often affected causing changes in the matching of ventilation and perfusion. Oxygen should therefore be administered routinely. The importance of impeccable sterility during the insertion and top-up procedures must be emphasized. Postoperative headache is more common if a large needle is used for spinal or if dural puncture occurs with an epidural needle. The incidence is reduced if the patient is kept well hydrated and remains supine for 24 h.

Spinal Anaesthesia

The patient is placed in the lateral or sitting position, and the back arched to give maximum flexion of the lumbar vertebral column. Except in difficult cases, a 25-gauge spinal needle is used and the point of insertion is in the midline halfway between the tips of the spinous processes of the 3rd and 4th lumbar vertebrae. One space above or below may be used when trying to achieve a higher or lower block. The needle is advanced in the sagittal plane in a slightly cephalad direction through the supraspinous and interspinous ligaments and the ligamentum flavum which stretches across the interlaminar foramen. Less resistance is then felt as it crosses the epidural space and a definite snap is usually felt as the dura and arachnoid membranes are punctured to enter the subarachnoid space. In difficult cases, particularly when due to calcification of the ligaments, a paramedian approach is often more successful. When the needle has entered the subarachnoid space, the stilette is removed and cerebrospinal fluid should emerge. The spinal anaesthetic agent is then injected and the needle removed before repositioning the patient to give the desired distribution of the agent. The level of spread depends on the characteristics of the anaesthetic solution, the volume injected, the way in which it is injected and the posture of the patient. After 15 min the patient can be repositioned for surgery without affecting the distribution. Bupivacaine is the most commonly used agent. It is supplied in a special preparation containing 5 mg/ml, with no preservative, and mixed with glucose to give a solution with a specific gravity which is greater than that of cerebrospinal fluid. The dosage range is 2–4 ml and the duration of analgesia varies from 45 min to 3 h depending on the degree of block required.

Epidural Anaesthesia

Epidural block is more difficult to perform and less predictable than spinal. A catheter can be inserted, however, to give top-up doses so that the duration of the block is not a limiting factor, as it is with spinal anaesthesia, and furthermore it can be extended for postoperative analgesia. There are two additional dangers with epidural anaesthesia and these are inadvertent intravascular or subarachnoid injection. Comparatively large volumes of local anaesthetic agent are used which result in immediate toxic manifestations if injected into a vessel. Intrathecal injection results in a total spinal block with cardiovascular collapse, loss of consciousness and respiratory arrest. Catheters which appear to be correctly placed initially and produce a normal block can very occasionally deliver a subsequent top-up into the subarachnoid space.

An 18- or 16-gauge Tuohy needle is used to direct the epidural catheter upwards or downwards in the epidural space, as shown in *Fig.* 13.5. In the lumbar region insertion of the needle is as described for spinal injection, using either a midline or paramedian approach, but it is important to stop in the epidural space and great care is required to avoid puncturing the dura mater. Several methods are used to ascertain precisely when the tip of the needle emerges from the dense ligamentum flavum and enters the lax tissues of the epidural space. Pressure, applied to the plunger of a syringe filled with air or saline and attached to the needle, is commonly used to identify the loss of resistance which occurs at that point. Devices such as the Macintosh balloon are also used. Once the needle is in place with the end aperture facing in the desired direction, the catheter is fed in. After careful inspection for blood or cerebrospinal fluid, a bacterial filter is attached and a small test dose of local anaesthetic agent is injected as a final check. The agent used is now almost exclusively bupivacaine, usually without adrenaline. This produces a block which is maximal by about 30 min and lasts for 2–4 h. The solution tends to fall in

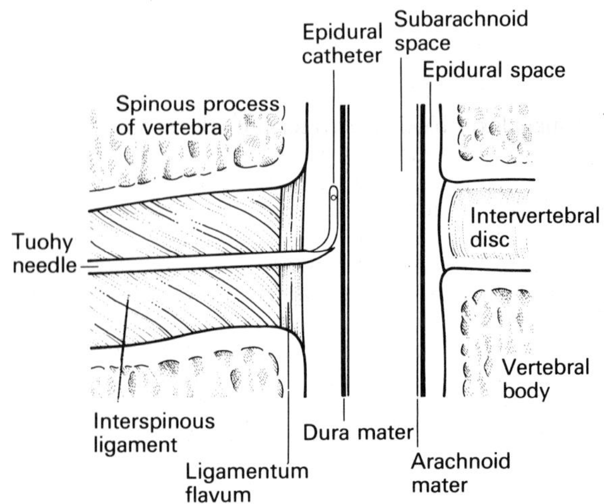

Fig. 13.5 Use of a Tuohy needle to introduce an epidural catheter.

the epidural space and the extent of the block is therefore dependent on the patient's posture, as well as the concentration of the drug and the volume used.

Thoracic epidural anaesthesia is difficult to perform and it is potentially dangerous. It must only be attempted by those who have acquired considerable experience and skill using the lumbar approach. For postoperative use, close supervision by adequately trained nursing staff in an intensive care or high dependency unit is essential. The problems with insertion are that the thoracic spinous processes are very oblique, the epidural space is narrow and overshoot can easily cause spinal cord injury. Dosage is smaller and more critical than is the case with lower blocks and a fall in cardiac output is liable to occur due to blocking of the cardiac as well as vascular sympathetic supply. Nevertheless, perfect analgesia can be produced, with the patient fully alert and cooperative. Given the appropriate staff and conditions, thoracic epidural analgesia is justified in selected patients having major upper abdominal or thoracic surgery or after chest trauma, particularly when sputum retention is likely.

When anaesthesia of the sacral nerve roots is sufficient, as is the case when operating on the anus, vulva, vagina or penis for example, a caudal epidural block can be used. Access to the epidural space is gained by passing a needle through the sacral hiatus and up the sacral canal. 20–30 ml of local anaesthetic solution is required. Catheterization by this route is not advisable but a block of sufficient duration to give good analgesia in the immediate postoperative period can be obtained using a single dose of bupivacaine. Problems with this technique are the difficulty with sterility, the unpredictable height of the block and the fact that large doses are required and intravascular injection can occur.

Local Anaesthesia for Hernia Repair

A field block using 0·5% lignocaine or prilocaine with adrenaline is a useful technique for inguinal or femoral herniorrhaphy in patients who are in poor condition. The 12th thoracic, iliohypogastric and ilio-inguinal nerves are blocked by injection of 30 ml deep to the external oblique aponeurosis, 1·5 cm medial to the anterior superior iliac spine. 20 ml is injected 1·5 cm above the midpoint of the inguinal ligament again deep to the external oblique and this anaesthetizes the genital branch of the genitofemoral nerve. The neck of the sac may be infiltrated at this time or later when it is exposed. The subcutaneous tissues are infiltrated with a further 20 ml from the spine of the pubis along the line of the incision and upwards towards the midline to block contralateral nerves.

Brachial Plexus Block

Brachial plexus block is used for procedures on the arm and there are two commonly used approaches. The axillary route is by far the safest in inexperienced hands. 20–40 ml of local anaesthetic is injected into the axillary sheath as high as possible. Half is injected to one side of the axillary artery and half to the other. To prevent distal spread, the perivascular sheath is compressed just below the site of injection. If anaesthesia in the distribution of the musculocutaneous nerve is required this must be blocked separately. Supraclavicular brachial plexus block is produced by injecting 20–30 ml of local anaesthetic on to the brachial plexus as it crosses the first rib behind the subclavian artery. The needle is inserted 1 cm above the midpoint of the clavicle lateral to the pulsation of the subclavian artery and advanced backwards, inwards and downwards at 80° to the skin, until either paraesthesiae is felt by the patient or the needle impinges on the first rib. The risk of pneumothorax is a major disadvantage of this technique.

Intravenous Regional Anaesthesia

Intravenous regional anaesthesia is a simple and reliable method which can be used for surgery on an upper or lower limb. The procedure requires minimal skill but a knowledge of the signs of local anaesthetic toxicity and its treatment is required. Resuscitation equipment and the ability to use it must be at hand. An intravenous cannula is inserted distally in the limb to be anaesthetized. Secure venous access must also be established elsewhere. A cuff is applied proximally, the limb is then exsanguinated and the cuff inflated to 50 mmHg above systolic pressure. Prilocaine 0·5% plain is the safest solution but lignocaine 0·5% plain is also used; 0·6 ml/kg is injected slowly into the intravenous cannula in the isolated limb. Care must be taken to ensure that the cuff remains inflated for at least 20 min after the injection. If the cuff causes discomfort a second cuff should be used below it in the analgesic part of the limb and the original cuff removed.

Cardiovascular Homeostasis

Oxygenation of the vital organs must always be the first priority. This requires perfusion of the tissues with oxygenated blood. The primary consideration when dealing with cardiovascular problems is therefore the cardiac output. Its main determinants are shown in *Fig.* 13.6 which also lists some of the many physiological, pathological and pharmacological influences which may exist in relation to surgery and anaesthesia.

A tendency to hypotension is common under anaesthesia and this may be due either to vasodilatation or a reduced cardiac output. Vasodilatation can be caused by the induction agent, volatile anaesthetic, muscle relaxant or autonomic reflex activity. If hypotension is accompanied by poor peripheral perfusion, giving cold, pale extremities with poor capillary refill, it usually indicates that cardiac output is inadequate. Poor cardiac output can be caused by impaired myocardial contractility or inadequate ventricular filling. Myocardial depression is frequently a problem with high concentrations of halothane or enflurane and poor venous return often results from hypovolaemia, vascular dilatation or IPPV. Hypotension is normally treated by attending to the underlying problem and by infusion of fluid, except when there is evidence of cardiac failure or fluid overload. The effect of transfusion must be continually assessed and due consideration given to the estimated fluid loss, the volume already given and the central venous pressure.

The most common causes of a rise in blood pressure are intubation of the trachea and light anaesthesia. The possibility of hypercapnia must always be remembered. Acute rises in blood pressure are often seen in patients with pre-existing hypertension, especially if it is not well controlled preoperatively. Drugs which increase blood pressure such as pancuronium, adrenaline and ketamine should be avoided in these patients. Myocardial work and hence oxygen demand is increased when the blood pressure rises and therefore myocardial ischaemia or failure may occur. Hypertension increases surgical bleeding and there is also a risk of cerebrovascular catastrophe. Blood pressure may be controlled with adrenergic blocking drugs. Labetalol which blocks both alpha and beta receptors is often used. Other agents include sodium nitroprusside, trimetaphan and nitrates, all of which are short-acting vasodilators also used to produce deliberate hypotension for certain procedures when an avascular field

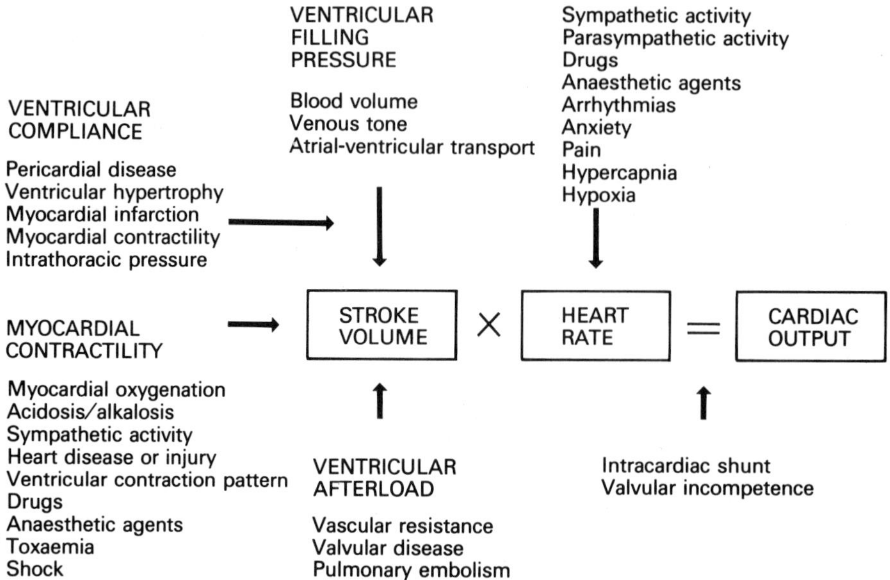

Fig. 13.6 The main determinants of cardiac output.

is required. Hydralazine is a vasodilator which can rapidly control hypertension and it has a long duration of action.

Changes in heart rate and rhythm are important because of the effect on cardiac output and myocardial oxygenation. Alterations in autonomic balance caused by a drug or reflex activity is often responsible, but the most serious causes are hypoxia and hypercapnia which must be excluded first. Specific treatment may be required but elimination of the cause is often more important.

Bradycardia is a common complication of halothane and suxamethonium but can also result from stimuli, such as pulling on the bowel mesentery, which increase vagal activity. Cardiac output drops as the stroke volume approaches its maximum and at very low heart rates there is a danger of progression to asystole. Atropine or glycopyrrolate are normally given when the heart rate falls to 40 beats/min. As the rate of the sinoatrial node falls another focus can take over and atrioventricular nodal rhythm is very common under anaesthesia. The ventricular rate may be normal in nodal rhythm, but occasionally the effect on the atrial transport mechanism results in a significant fall in cardiac output. Treatment is as for bradycardia.

Many patients have a modest tachycardia at induction due to preoperative anxiety or premedication with atropine or hyoscine. Arising during anaesthesia, an increased heart rate may result from a sympathetic response to surgical stimulation especially under light anaesthesia. Other causes include hypovolaemia, hypercapnia, pyrexia and drugs such as pancuronium or adrenaline. As the heart rate increases above 140 beats/min the cardiac output may begin to fall but the rate at which this occurs varies greatly, particularly in heart disease. The decreased diastolic time leads to reduced ventricular filling and therefore stroke volume. There is increased myocardial work but decreased coronary blood flow, which occurs mainly during diastole. Treatment is directed at the cause but specific therapy is necessary if there is concern about the cardiac output or myocardial ischaemia. Supraventricular tachycardia sometimes responds to vagal stimulation produced by pressure applied over the carotid sinus. Alternative treatment depends on the nature of any other cardiac problems, previous treatment and the urgency of the situation and includes practolol or another beta-adrenergic antagonist, digoxin, verapamil or synchronized direct current shock. Ventricular tachycardia is more serious and should be treated immediately with lignocaine or direct current shock.

Ventricular ectopic beats are common under halothane anaesthesia and usually disappear if halothane is replaced by another agent. Treatment with lignocaine is indicated if frequent ectopic complexes are occurring, particularly if they are multifocal or tending to encroach on the preceding T-wave.

Blood Loss

Haemorrhage does not normally produce any clinical effects until more than 10% of the patient's blood volume has been lost. The heart rate then increases, but the blood pressure is initially maintained by compensatory vasoconstriction. With decreasing venous return, the cardiac output begins to fall. After 20% blood loss, hypotension may emerge and eventually tissue perfusion is compromised. When 30% of the blood volume is lost, the circulation is usually so poor that tissue oxygenation is grossly inadequate. The resulting cellular hypoxia causes the pathological changes of shock, with organ failure and damage. Renal failure, disseminated intravascular coagulopathy and adult respiratory distress syndrome are common sequelae of severe shock. These are the consequences of acute blood loss in otherwise healthy individuals. Both local and general anaesthesia dramatically affect the compensatory response to blood loss. The same sequence of events occurs under anaesthesia, but hypotension occurs after much smaller losses, especially in less fit patients.

The effects described are mainly due to loss of volume rather than red blood cells. If blood volume can be maintained with intravenous infusion of fluid the above sequence is prevented. Which particular fluid is used is not important in the short term, but colloid solutions, such as those containing gelatin, hetastarch, human albumin or dextran 70, remain in the circulation for longer than crystalloid solutions. Red blood cells only become important as the haematocrit falls significantly below 0·30. Until then oxygen transport can be sustained, provided the blood volume is adequate and the heart is capable of increasing its output. Transfusion of red cells is therefore only necessary after at least 20% of the blood volume has been lost and they are normally given as stored whole blood or plasma reduced blood. All red cell preparations, except fresh whole blood, are deficient in coagulation factors and platelets. These may be provided in the form of fresh frozen plasma and platelet concentrate and are necessary if blood loss is massive, if there are pre-existing deficiencies or if there is a consumption coagulopathy. The amount given is guided by clinical assessment of the bleeding, coagulation studies and platelet counts.

The volume of blood lost during surgery can be estimated by weighing swabs and measuring the amount in the reservoir of the suction apparatus and 25% is usually added for other losses, such as that on the drapes. In neonates, the total blood volume may be less than 200 ml and therefore very small losses are significant. Swabs are weighed meticulously before any drying occurs and a small fluid trap is placed in the suction line near to the nozzle. When accurate measurement of the loss is not possible, replacement is based on clinical assessment of the patient's circulating blood volume. Normovolaemia is indicated by satisfactory blood pressure, heart rate and peripheral perfusion. Often, however, vasoconstriction persists after replenishment and fluid overload can occur while the peripheral perfusion remains poor. Careful attention must be given to the central venous pressure and the judicious use of a vasodilator may be indicated after the blood pressure has recovered. If the patient has suffered a period of shock, myocardial contractility may be depressed due to ischaemic damage, circulating depressant substances and metabolic factors. Therefore, adequate cardiac output may not return immediately when the blood volume is restored. In this situation a rising central venous pressure usually indicates that sufficient fluid has been given. Inotropic support may be required if the central venous pressure is high and sustained. Causes such as hypoxia, acidosis, hyperkalaemia, hypocalcaemia, or high intrathoracic pressure due to IPPV or pneumothorax should be eliminated first.

Rapid transfusion of large volumes of stored blood may give rise to complications because of its low temperature and the high content of potassium, citrate and microaggregates. A blood warmer should be used if more than 2 units are to be given quickly. This prevents hypothermia and the adverse effects on the heart of the low temperature and the high extracellular potassium. Intravenous boluses of calcium can be given to offset the transient lowering of ionized calcium caused by high plasma levels of citrate. If more than 3 units of stored blood are being transfused, it should be administered through a 20-micron filter. This removes the aggregates which can interfere with pulmonary function by microvascular obstruction. These filters also remove useful reversible platelet aggregates and must not therefore be used when giving fresh blood or platelet concentrate.

Body Temperature

Unless efforts are made to conserve heat, body temperature tends to fall during surgery. This is particularly so in small children and during long procedures, especially if a body cavity is open or if large volumes of cold fluid are infused. Anaesthesia depresses the thermoregulatory centre in the hypothalamus. Alteration of skin flow, manipulation of metabolic rate, sweating and shivering are the mechanisms by which body temperature is normally controlled. These may be directly affected by general anaesthetic and neuromuscular blocking agents. There are also many factors which encourage heat loss. Patients tend to be lightly covered, the drapes often become wet and evaporation from the operation site and respiratory mucosa adds considerably to the heat loss.

The environmental temperature must never be less than 24 °C. The ideal temperature for high risk adults is 28° C and 30° C for neonates, but this is uncomfortable and stressful for staff and there is invariably a compromise. The following measures can be used to reduce heat loss in those at risk: placing a warming blanket below the patient, covering all exposed parts with insulating material, warming all fluids administered, including surgical fluids, and warm humidification of the inspired gases. Neonates, especially the premature, become hypothermic very readily. Their surface area to volume ratio is high, they have little subcutaneous insulating fat, they do not shiver and to increase heat production they rely on metabolism in brown fat which is depressed under anaesthesia. Body temperature must be monitored and care taken to ensure conservation of body heat on the table and also during transportation and recovery.

Monitoring

All patients must be monitored under anaesthesia to ensure adequate oxygen delivery, respiration and circulation as well as an appropriate plane of anaesthesia. To check that adequate oxygen continues to be delivered to the patient, the supply pressure gauges, flowmeters and anaesthetic system connections must be constantly reviewed. Basic respiratory monitoring includes observation of the reservoir bag excursion, chest movement and respiratory pattern. When a ventilator is in use, the airway pressure displayed on the gauge and air entry assessed by auscultation are important. The cardiovascular state is continually checked by observation of skin colour and peripheral perfusion, palpation of a peripheral pulse, measurement of the blood pressure and monitoring the electrocardiograph. A precordial stethoscope is routinely used in small children and babies. The level of anaesthesia is gauged from the respiratory pattern, the position and size of the pupils and a knowledge of the anaesthetic dosage. In addition, lacrimation, sweating, tachycardia, increased blood pressure or reflex movement must be noted as possible indications of inadequate depth. The above is the basic monitoring which is essential for safe anaesthesia. How much more than this is employed depends on the patient's pathology and general fitness, the operation being performed, the anaesthetic technique and the availability of equipment.

An in-line oxygen analyser with an alarm may give added protection against hypoxic gas mixtures. Measurement of the expired minute volume gives more information about the patient's ventilation on IPPV and capnography may be used to assess carbon dioxide elimination. The end tidal partial pressure of carbon dioxide normally reflects the arterial level. Blood gas analysis provides a more accurate picture of alveolar gas exchange. Pulse oximetry is a non-invasive technique which provides a display of arterial oxygen saturation. For a given level of circulation and oxygen-carrying capacity, the saturation reflects the oxygen delivery to the tissues. It therefore provides a continuous, final check on all systems 'up-stream'. When cardiac output may be compromised, measurement of urine output gives an indication of not only renal function but also renal blood flow which normally reflects the entire circulation. Monitoring central venous pressure enables transfusion to an optimum ventricular filling pressure and this is important when there is large blood loss or when the myocardial performance is suspect. Occasionally a balloon flotation catheter is required to measure pulmonary artery wedge pressure to assess more reliably the filling pressure of the left ventricle. Arterial cannulation is justified in high-risk patients and enables continuous instantaneous display of the systemic arterial pressure and its wave form. Access for multiple blood gas analysis is also secured. Cerebral function monitoring may be useful when the circulation of the brain is at risk. To avoid heat injury to the patient the temperature of any water blanket, blood warmer and humidification system must be frequently checked.

POSTOPERATIVE CARE

The potential for problems postoperatively is great and a high standard of care is required. This is as important to the health of the individual as good surgery and safe anaesthesia. An awareness of the risks is essential, including those peculiar to the individual or the particular operation, as well as those common to all patients. Care must be directed primarily at prevention, early diagnosis and treatment of complications. The basic priority is again to ensure optimum respiratory function, oxygenation and circulation. Postoperative pain can cause intense suffering and also plays a significant role in the aetiology of pulmonary sequelae. Potent analgesia invariably has its own risks, but a conscientious and well informed approach by the staff involved can provide adequate and safe pain relief using simple methods in the vast majority of cases.

Immediate Recovery Phase

During the immediate recovery phase, the patient regains consciousness. More important, at this stage, is the return of normal respiratory drive and muscle activity to give adequate pulmonary ventilation through a patent airway which is guarded by vital protective reflexes. This can be a period of cardiorespiratory flux, as the decreasing influence of anaesthetic agents is replaced by the increasing effects of pain, discomfort, rewarming and analgesic drugs. A high standard of care during recovery is essential. The period of unconsciousness should be as short as possible and the patient must be closely observed by well trained staff in an adequately equipped recovery area. High risk patients should be transferred straight to intensive care.

In the early stages, attention must be focused primarily on the airway. The patient is normally nursed in the lateral position, with the jaw held forward, and must not be left unattended until capable of protecting the airway and responding to simple commands. Oxygen is administered routinely and suction apparatus must be at hand. Respiration is continuously monitored by the nurse attending the patient. Gas movement with respiration is assessed by watching the condensation on a transparent oxygen mask, by feeling or listening in front of the mouth or by auscultation over the larynx. Obstruction is detected by listening for added sounds and observing the pattern of chest movement. Cardiovascular monitoring includes observation of skin colour and perfusion, palpation of a peripheral pulse and serial measurement of arterial blood pressure. An anaesthetist should be readily available during this period and there must be immediate access to full resuscitation equipment.

Problems in relation to the airway, such as obstruction, irritability and vomiting are common and management is similar to that under anaesthesia. Unless measures are taken to prevent it, obstruction of the airway in the pharynx often occurs, due to the tongue being flaccid in the unconscious patient. As the level of consciousness lightens, irritability can complicate the problem by causing coughing, straining, breath holding, vomiting or laryngeal spasm. This may be exacerbated by stimuli such as an artificial airway, foreign material or excessive suction. For this reason an oropharyngeal airway often has to be removed earlier than it would otherwise have been and maintaining the upper airway may require considerable skill and effort.

As described in relation to reversal and extubation, hypoventilation in the absence of upper airway obstruction is commonly due to hypocapnia in an unconscious patient, residual neuromuscular block or respiratory depression caused by an opioid drug or volatile anaesthetic agent. Even if previously normal, respiration can deteriorate during this period when stimulation is no longer being applied. Respiratory drive can also be obtunded due to severe hypercapnia or excessive oxygen administration to susceptible individuals with chronic lung disease. Other causes of inadequate ventilation are pulmonary oedema, retained secretions, pneumothorax, severe bronchospasm and abdominal distension. Management initially includes ensuring a clear airway, administering a high inspired oxygen concentration and stimulating the patient. If respiration is grossly inadequate, IPPV should be instituted. An assessment of the following factors may be useful in making a diagnosis: pre-existing pathology, agents used for anaesthesia, respiratory effort, pattern of respiration, physical examination of the chest and, if necessary, nerve stimulator testing, blood gas analysis and chest radiography. Small doses of naloxone will reverse the respiratory depressant effects of opioids and may be diagnostic. Doxapram, a respiratory stimulant, may be used to treat other causes of central respiratory depression, provided hypocapnia can be excluded. Incomplete reversal of a non-depolarizing muscle relaxant may respond to a small supplement of neostigmine, with atropine, and if this is not effective ventilation must be supported until recovery occurs. Too much neostigmine may exacerbate the problem. If difficulties persist when the patient is awake, the cause is less likely to be central respiratory depression and, if muscle power is good, residual paralysis can be excluded.

Hypoxaemia and Oxygen Therapy

Modest hypoxaemia in the first 2 h postoperatively is common in patients breathing air. The major cause is a continuation of the factors which alter the distribution of ventilation and blood flow in the lungs during anaesthesia. There is an increased proportion of the pulmonary blood flow either perfusing poorly ventilated alveoli or not taking part in gaseous exchange at all. The effect of this on arterial oxygenation is greater if the mixed venous oxygen content is low due to an inadequate cardiac output or increased oxygen utilization, as may occur during shivering. Mismatching of ventilation and perfusion of this nature is usually worse after abdominal or thoracic surgery and often lasts for several days. The main reason is a reduction in the functional residual capacity of the lungs resulting from the wound pain increasing muscle tone and abdominal distension restricting the diaphragm. Minor degrees of collapse are common and add to the problem. Other causes of hypoxaemia are hypoventilation as described above and diffusion hypoxia. The latter occurs in the first 5 min after nitrous oxide is discontinued, and is due to the gas entering the alveoli from the blood much faster than nitrogen diffuses in the opposite direction. The result is that alveolar oxygen is diluted and the concentration falls. This is not normally significant in fit patients and is easily prevented by administration of 100% oxygen for a few minutes.

Oxygen should be administered routinely until the patient is awake. This should be extended to at least 2 h after major surgery or if the patient suffers from respiratory or cardiac pathology, which is likely to exacerbate the hypoxaemia or increase vulnerability to low oxygen tensions. After major abdominal or thoracic surgery oxygen therapy may have to be continued for 24 h or more. It may be discontinued on the day after surgery, if the patient is relatively free of pain and able to sit up, take deep breaths and cough effectively. There must be no evidence of sputum retention or atelectasis. If cardiac output is suboptimal, if there is pulmonary oedema or a pulmonary ventilation problem, oxygen must be given. When doubt exists as to the requirement of oxygen therapy, blood gas analysis is useful. This investigation is of more value if the inspired concentration is accurately known (*vide infra*). The arterial oxygen tension can then be compared with the predicted value.

Oxygen is usually given by a mask, such as the Hudson or the Mary Catterall (MC), which does not administer a constant known percentage of oxygen, because of variable dilution of the oxygen by air drawn in during inspiration. This is not usually important because the requirement for routine postoperative use is a concentration of somewhere between 35 and 60%. Unless there is additional lung pathology 35% is sufficient to ensure an adequate arterial level of oxygen and toxicity is unlikely to occur if less than 60% is given. For more accurate administration of oxygen at a constant known percentage, a high air flow oxygen enrichment (HAFOE) mask, such as the Ventimask, can be used. A specific mask or entrainment jet delivers only one concentration and several models are available for different values from 24% up to 60%. Accurate masks delivering low inspired oxygen concentrations are essential for patients with chronic lung disease who have lost normal ventilatory control and depend on moderate hypoxaemia to stimulate respiration. Such patients require enough oxygen to avoid serious hypoxaemia but not so much that the arterial oxygen tension approaches normal and removes respiratory drive.

When longer term oxygen therapy is required, humidification is necessary, especially for patients with sputum retention or who are mouth breathing. Attempts to humidify oxygen delivered to the jet of a mask are counterproductive. The entrained air is not humidified and condensed water interferes with the function of the jet. Efficient humidification usually requires a blower humidifier of the heated water or ultrasonic type. The best of the nebulizing humidifiers, such as the Inspiron 2305, are a reasonable compromise. Although they do not produce as good humidification, they are cheap, small, light, safe and easy to use.

Restlessness and Confusion

Hypoxia causes restlessness and confusion and vice versa. Breaking this vicious cycle by successfully administering oxygen to the patient is one of the major challenges which can present in the recovery area or later in the surgical ward. Constant supervision and the use of the minimum constraint commensurate with the application of a mask or nasal cannulas is required in the first instance. If the patient remains confused while breathing 60% oxygen, blood gas analysis is required. A low cardiac output is another common cause which must be excluded. Pain or a full bladder in the presence of residual anaesthetic effects is often a significant factor. Other possible causes include hypercapnia, hypo- or hyperglycaemia, endotoxaemia, septicaemia and alcohol or drug withdrawal.

Postoperative IPPV

When high-risk patients have major thoracic or abdominal surgery, IPPV is often continued electively in the postoperative period. Normal blood gas exchange can usually be achieved more easily and the work of breathing is eliminated. This often results in reduced oxygen consumption and better arterial levels and there is, therefore, less demand on cardiac output. Myocardial oxygenation may be improved, as the work load is reduced and the oxygen supply increased. Positive intra-alveolar pressure reduces any tendency to pulmonary oedema, while good pulmonary expansion and easy access to secretions helps prevent collapse. Adequate analgesia and sedation can be given to allow the patient to rest.

For postoperative IPPV, the patient must be admitted to an intensive care unit and constantly supervised. There are also additional risks and disadvantages which have to be considered. The complications of artificial ventilation include machine failure, inadvertent extubation, pneumothorax and pulmonary sepsis. Cardiac output can be compromised, as a result of the high mean intrathoracic pressure impeding venous return. This is only significant when there are other adverse influences on the circulation or when there is a problem with gaseous exchange requiring high inflation pressures or PEEP. Weaning from ventilation is less often a problem than is feared. Ideally, before IPPV is discontinued there should be cardiovascular stability without inotropic support, good blood gas tensions with 40% inspired oxygen, no evidence of pulmonary collapse and good analgesia with the subject alert. If the patient can maintain adequate spontaneous respiration unaided, take deep breaths and cough effectively, the endotracheal tube can usually be removed. The duration of IPPV can be from a few hours up to two days or more, if there are postoperative complications. The vast majority of patients, however, are ventilated only until the day after surgery. A major factor is how easily adequate analgesia can be achieved without depressing respiratory drive and ability to cough.

The use of elective ventilation varies between units and depends on the facilities available and the experience of the staff involved. The following are some of the factors which are regarded as relative indications for postoperative IPPV:

1. A major surgical procedure of long duration, particularly if there is massive blood loss, metabolic upset or hypothermia.
2. Severe respiratory disease especially if obstructive in nature or if there is no ventilatory reserve, as indicated by a raised arterial carbon dioxide tension or severely limited exercise tolerance.
3. A poor cardiovascular state, due to heart disease or the surgical condition.
4. Severe sepsis.
5. Gross obesity.
6. Compromised cerebral state especially if caused by cerebral oedema.
7. Difficult analgesia.

Cardiovascular Complications

There is a high incidence of cardiovascular problems in the early recovery period and hypotension is the most common.

The implications of a low blood pressure in terms of cardiac output, the management of hypotension and the importance of ventricular filling pressures are described in relation to cardiovascular homeostasis and blood loss under anaesthesia. The most frequent adverse influence during recovery is the residual effect of anaesthetic drugs, particularly the volatile inhalational agents which cause myocardial depression and vascular dilatation. Hypotension resulting from this often occurs as sympathetic activity subsides due to the withdrawal of surgical stimulation or the administration of analgesics. Other causes are the relaxation of vasoconstriction with rewarming, venous pooling caused by changes in posture, true hypovolaemia due to fluid or blood loss, autonomic responses to pain or sympathetic blockade produced by top-up doses of epidural local anaesthetic. A low blood pressure accompanied by a central venous pressure which is high and sustained indicates that cardiac function is compromised. This can be caused by an arrhythmia or myocardial depression due to drug action, hypoxia, metabolic effect or heart disease. Two important causes of this picture which require immediate attention are pneumothorax and cardiac tamponade. Bacteraemia, endotoxaemia and septicaemia produce hypotension by effects on vascular tone and myocardial contractility. A fall in blood pressure may also be the presenting sign of hypoglycaemia, adrenal cortical insufficiency and hypersensitivity reactions.

Treatment of hypotension must take into consideration the underlying cause, previous fluid management and the filling pressure of both ventricles. Provided there is not a specific left ventricular problem or a risk of pulmonary oedema, the filling pressure in both sides is usually assumed to be represented by the central venous pressure (CVP) which is assessed by examination of the external jugular veins or measured by means of a central venous catheter. Transfusion of fluid is the treatment for hypovolaemia whether relative or real. Modest expansion of blood volume also improves the cardiac output if it is reduced as a result of impaired myocardial contractility, provided the filling pressure is not already high. Great care is required because overtransfusion of a small amount can exacerbate the problem. When doubt exists as to the suitability of giving fluid, a 200 ml aliquot is infused. The cardiovascular state must then be assessed and this includes measurement of the CVP. This is repeated until there is either an improvement in cardiac output or an increasing CVP indicates that overload is imminent.

When hypotension is a persistent or recurring problem, it is important to measure urine volume hourly, as in all high-risk patients. Urinary output is a very valuable index of the circulation as well as renal function and should be monitored in patients with hepatobiliary or renal disease, major injuries or severe sepsis. Urine volume measurement is also indicated after major vascular or cardiac surgery or any severe hypoxic or hypovolaemic episode. Sodium and water retention postoperatively is a normal stress response, but in these high-risk patients oliguria of less than 30 ml/h has to be treated because of concern for the cardiovascular or renal state. A low urine output in a patient with a patent urinary catheter can be due to dehydration, renal hypoperfusion or incipient renal failure. In most cases renal hypoperfusion is a reflection of the cardiac output. If there is corroborative evidence of dehydration or low cardiac output, appropriate treatment should be given. When oliguria persists in a well-hydrated patient with a normal blood pressure and good peripheral perfusion, a small dose of a loop diuretic, such as frusemide 10 mg, should be given. An increased dose (40 mg) is given if there is no response within 30 min. When oliguria persists a central venous catheter should be inserted for pressure measurement. If it is low or normal, aliquots of fluid may be given provided there is no sustained rise in the central venous pressure. Large quantities of fluid should not normally be given unless there is evidence of a deficit. A dopamine infusion through the central line at a rate of up to 5 μg/kg/min should be instituted if urine output does not improve.

Hypertension, abnormalities of heart rate and rhythm and cardiac failure are all possible complications during postoperative recovery. The causes, significance and treatment have been described in relation to preoperative care and anaesthesia and apply equally to the postoperative period. It is important to stress that any cardiovascular abnormality which arises may have a sinister underlying cause, such as hypoxia or hypercapnia.

A potentially fatal dysrhythmia causing cardiac arrest can arise in a diseased heart, especially in relation to an episode of severe ischaemia or infarction without any other cause. This, however, cannot be assumed to be the case when such cardiovascular collapse occurs postoperatively. As well as instituting basic maintenance resuscitation, diagnosing the electrical state and using direct current shock or drug therapy to re-establish sinus rhythm, it is vitally important to identify any precipitating factor. The following are examples of conditions which must be treated before resuscitation can be successful: catastrophic blood loss, metabolic acidosis, hyperkalaemia, acute airway obstruction, tension pneumothorax and cardiac tamponade.

Postoperative Analgesia

Complete analgesia without risk of complication is a guarantee which cannot be claimed by any of the techniques used for postoperative pain relief. Pain resulting from thoracic or abdominal incisions is particularly difficult to treat safely and the importance of this in relation to pulmonary sequelae must be emphasized. Pulmonary collapse, caused by poor expansion and sputum retention, is the usual precursor of postoperative bronchopneumonia. Pain inhibits both deep breathing and effective coughing and also, by increasing abdominal tone, reduces the pulmonary functional residual capacity and this encourages alveolar collapse. Patients in severe pain are reluctant to move and this encourages venous stasis and therefore venous thromboembolism. Early mobilization is also important in reducing the severity and duration of the pain itself. For a given operation, the intensity and duration of postoperative pain varies greatly between individuals, as does their response to it. Anxiety has a major influence on the pain threshold and other discomforts such as nausea, vomiting, dry mouth, and the presence of a nasogastric tube can add to its misery.

The vast majority of patients are treated postoperatively with systemic opioid analgesia. Which particular drug is given and its route, and whether it is administered intermittently or by continuous infusion are relatively unimportant compared with the dosage. Individual requirements and sensitivity to respiratory depression can vary up to 30-fold. The initial prescription must take into account the patient's age, weight, sex and general physical state. Any habits likely to stimulate tolerance and factors which may increase sensitivity or interfere with drug elimination should also be considered. Subsequent dosage must be titrated to the effect. This means frequent assessment of the patient and review of the requirement. Medical and nursing staff must be familiar with the pharmacology of the drug which is used, particularly its side-effects and pharmacokinetics in relation to the method of administration. The opioid drugs effectively increase the pain threshold and reduce the psychological response to pain. All cause respiratory depression, nausea and vomiting which are dose related. Vasodilatation may result from a slight inhibitory effect on the vasomotor centre and stimulation of histamine release. This does not normally cause significant hypotension unless, for example, the patient is hypovolaemic. Suppression of the cough reflex is an effect which is confined to the morphine derivatives. Other opioid side-effects include dysphoria, sweating, itching, dry mouth, dizziness, miosis, urinary retention and constipation. There is reduced bowel peristalsis, increased sphincteric action and delayed gastric emptying. Increased pressure in the biliary ducts from contraction of the sphincter of Oddi can aggravate biliary colic and this is a particular problem with the morphine group. Opioids should be avoided if possible in patients with a head injury or increased intracranial pressure. The hypercapnia which may result further raises the intracranial pressure and miosis makes assessment more difficult. A reduced dosage may be required when there is hepatic failure and extreme caution is necessary if opioids are administered to patients with limited respiratory reserve.

By far the most common method of administration of systemic opioid analgesics is conventional intermittent intramuscular injection. This is not ideal, but with appropriate care adequate analgesia can usually be achieved. Modest doses should be administered frequently by injections which are given before intolerable pain returns. This avoids the peaks during which there is a risk of respiratory depression and troughs during which there is inadequate analgesia due to the time lag between injection and effect. The standard dose of morphine (*vide supra*) is 0·1–0·2 mg/kg and it normally acts within 15–30 min with a peak effect at 45–90 min. If circulation is poor the onset and peak are both delayed. Its average duration of action is 4 h. Injections may be required much more often than 4-hourly initially. Small intravenous injections, producing a peak effect after about 20 min, should be used to gain control of pain in the early stages. The patient should be regularly visited by nursing staff looking for signs of respiratory depression or excessive drowsiness and assessing the need for further analgesia. The aim should not necessarily be to abolish pain but to reduce it to a tolerable level. Patients normally wait too long before requesting analgesia. Injections should be given when the pain is beginning to increase and this is established by observation and examination, as well as asking the patient. The increased pain associated with physiotherapy and dressing changes etc. should be anticipated and adequate analgesia ensured. In difficult cases the use of other means of analgesia such as entonox by inhalation or intercostal nerve block should be considered for these procedures. Medical staff must provide clear instructions, with enough flexibility for the nurses to give adequate analgesia under normal circumstances. Prescriptions must be regularly reviewed and intravenous boluses given when necessary.

Other parenteral methods of administering systemic opioid analgesics include continuous infusion or patient-controlled systems by the intravenous, intramuscular or subcutaneous route. Each has advantages but none of these techniques is universally established in use for routine postoperative analgesia in the general ward. Provided an adequate loading dose of drug is given, a continuous intravenous infusion delivered by syringe pump quickly achieves a constant blood level. Titration is easier and troughs of inadequate analgesia are avoided. This method is commonly used in intensive care and high dependency units. Patient-controlled therapy requires a delivery device such as the Cardiff Palliator which delivers a preset dose in each bolus and limits the number of doses in a given period as well as the minimum time between each. Other systems provide a basal continuous infusion with added patient-controlled boluses, up to a maximum.

The various opioid drugs differ in their potency, onset of action and duration. None, however, is significantly superior to the others in analgesic effect or in relation to side-effects. Buprenorphine may be given sublingually and can produce effective analgesia of long duration. It has some antagonist activity and is best avoided if another opioid has previously been given. Although respiratory depression is less likely to occur with buprenorphine than morphine, it is not reversed by naloxone and is therefore more difficult to treat. Parenteral opioid therapy is usually not required for more than 48 h except after upper abdominal or thoracic surgery. Oral analgesics are usually substituted as the level of pain subsides. Slow-release morphine can be given orally when severe pain persists but normally codeine, dihydrocodeine or dextropropoxyphene-paracetamol compound are adequate. Non-opioid analgesics such as paracetamol are sufficient for mild pain. These oral preparations may be used from the start after less painful minor procedures. Pethidine 1 mg/kg intramuscularly is commonly used for postoperative analgesia in children. Papaveretum 0·2–0·3 mg/kg intramuscularly is often used for older children and for severe pain. Paracetamol elixir orally is sufficient for milder pain. Babies under 5 kg weight or under 3 months of age should not be given opioid drugs. Analgesia is not normally required but paracetamol may be used if necessary.

Local analgesic techniques have the potential to provide total pain relief, but each has risks or limitations which prohibit more widespread use. Catheters are used in the epidural space or directly in the wound, for example, to provide continuing analgesia. Single dose nerve conduction blocks are used to cover periods of intense pain as may occur immediately postoperatively or during physiotherapy. Some local anaesthetic techniques, spinal or caudal block for example, performed primarily for the operative procedure can give useful early postoperative analgesia, if bupivacaine is used.

Total analgesia, produced by boluses or an infusion of bupivacaine through a thoracic epidural catheter, is of considerable benefit after major thoracic or abdominal surgery for patients with severe respiratory disease. It enables them to cough effectively, take deep breaths and cooperate fully at physiotherapy, even if there is some intercostal muscle paralysis. Mobility is improved and, with the release of reflex muscle tone, the functional residual capacity improves. Respiratory complications are less likely to occur and IPPV can often be avoided by using this method of analgesia. There are, however, prerequisites and complications which limit its use and these are described earlier in this chapter.

Small doses of opioid drugs injected intrathecally or epidurally can give prolonged good analgesia without affecting other sensory, motor or autonomic nerve conduction. This avoids many of the problems which occur with bupivacaine and epidural opioid administration is now widely used. Acute respiratory depression which may be delayed for up to 18 h after injection can occur, however, and close monitoring is necessary. Morphine has the longest duration of action by this route and a dose of 2 mg can be effective for more than 12 h. It is, unfortunately, the most likely to cause central depression of respiration and diamorphine is safer. Preservative-free preparations must be used.

Intercostal and paravertebral nerve blocks are used to provide temporary analgesia, for example for physiotherapy, after thoracic or upper abdominal surgery, if the incision does not cross the midline. The pain resulting from rib fractures or a troublesome chest drain is also treated by these methods. Intercostal block is easily achieved with 3 ml of 0·25% bupivacaine injected adjacent to each nerve. The needle is inserted 7 cm from the midline of the back to make contact with the lower border of the rib. It is then carefully moved down on the rib, with a slight upward angulation, until it slips under the lower edge. The local anaesthetic is injected between 1 and 3 mm deep to the rib margin. Pneumothorax is a particular danger. Intercostal nerve block can be performed under direct vision at the end of a thoracotomy. If a cryoprobe is used analgesia lasting several weeks can be produced.

Minor Complications

Patients frequently suffer significant discomfort and inconvenience as a result of minor postoperative complications. These are particularly resented, if occurring in relation to minor surgery, when a return to normality soon after the procedure is expected. Many patients experience postoperative nausea and vomiting. Occasionally this gives rise to serious problems due to pulmonary aspiration or fluid and electrolyte losses. The possibility of an underlying cause must always be borne in mind. Some patients are very susceptible and may vomit after the most minor of procedures. Identifiable factors associated with postoperative vomiting include opioid analgesics, fear, pain, gastrointestinal surgery and premature ingestion of fluids during recovery. Commonly used antiemetics are prochlorperazine, perphenazine, cyclizine and metoclopramide. None is significantly superior and all have side-effects such as drowsiness, hypotension and dystonia which preclude routine prophylactic use. Fixed combinations of opioid and antiemetic should not be prescribed on a regular basis, as overdosage with the antiemetic frequently occurs. Patients very often complain of headache, backache, drowsiness or dizziness after surgery under general anaesthesia. Headache also occurs surprisingly frequently after procedures under local anaesthesia. Persistent hiccuping is a much less common complaint but one which can be very distressing and often resistant to therapy. Sore throat and hoarseness are common after tracheal intubation and trauma to the lips, teeth or larynx can also occasionally occur. Complications of intravenous injection or cannulation include bruising, haematoma, phlebitis, superficial venous thrombosis and thrombophlebitis. Up to 50% of patients who have suxamethonium may experience muscle pains on the day after and in some this can be severe and incapacitating. More serious and fortunately less common postoperative sequelae include peripheral nerve palsies due to pressure injury, corneal ulceration caused by drying or abrasion and laryngeal oedema or granulomas following intubation. Persistent psychological upset can occur after a difficult induction, awareness during the procedure or emergence delirium.

Further Reading

Campbell D. and Spence A. A. (1985) *Norris and Campbell's Anaesthetics, Resuscitation and Intensive Care*. Edinburgh, Churchill Livingstone.

Commission on the Provision of Surgical Services: Guidelines for Day Case Surgery (1985). London, Royal College of Surgeons of England.

Dodson M. E. (1985) *The Management of Postoperative Pain*. London, Arnold.

Eriksson E. (1979) *Illustrated Handbook in Local Anaesthesia*. London, Lloyd-Luke.

Grant I. S. (1985) Intercurrent disease and anaesthesia. In: Smith G. and Aitkenhead A. R. (ed.) *Textbook of Anaesthesia*. Edinburgh, Churchill Livingstone, pp. 464–491.

Lee J. A., Atkinson R. S. and Watt M. J. (1985) *Sir Robert Macintosh's Lumbar Puncture and Spinal Analgesia—Intradural and Extradural*. Edinburgh, Churchill Livingstone.

The Medical Protection Society Annual Report 1985. Section on informed consent. No. 93, pp. 17–19.

Schneider A. J. L. (1983) Assessment of risk factors and surgical outcome. *Surg. Clin. North Am.* **63**, 1113–1126.

14 Cutaneous Disorders and Malignancy

W. Frain-Bell and A. Cuschieri

A surgeon need not aspire to be a specialist in diseases of the skin but should be able to recognize the more common dermatoses and skin tumours and also to know which of the various abnormal changes in the skin are associated with systemic disease. This chapter has been compiled with this principle in mind, reference being made by name only to those less common conditions which are the province of the dermatologist and are dealt with in dermatological textbooks.

It is necessary, however, to be able to diagnose dermatitis (eczema), to appreciate the various constitutional patterns of response such as in atopic dermatitis, to know how contact dermatitis is investigated, to determine the relevance of irritant and allergic factors and to be familiar with the basic principles of treatment. Knowledge of the common dermatoses is essential.

Common Benign Dermatoses

Dermatitis (Eczema)
1. Atopic
2. Seborrhoeic
3. Discoid
4. Varicose/stasic
5. Contact
6. Universal/exfoliative

Psoriasis
Acne Vulgaris
Infection
1. Bacterial
2. Viral
3. Fungal
4. Infestations

Erythemas
Urticaria

Of the tumours of the skin by far the most common are the various forms of viral wart, seborrhoeic keratosis, and the accompanying acanthomas and cutaneous papillomas, melanocytic naevi, cysts and lastly, the tumours associated with age and exposure to carcinogens, such as solar ultraviolet as in basal-cell carcinoma, solar keratosis and squamous-cell carcinoma.

The erythemas are those reactions of the skin in which erythema is a major component associated with variable amounts of oedema, blister formation or haemorrhage (e.g. purpura) as the result of the response of the cutaneous blood vessels (vasculitis) to certain factors such as drugs, infection and various forms of systemic disease.

Lastly, there are specific and non-specific changes in the skin which are known to be associated with abnormality of other body systems. Most of these are relatively uncommon but no less important since their recognition can sometimes be of significant help in the diagnosis of an acute or chronic surgical problem.

COMMON BENIGN DERMATOSES

Dermatitis (Eczema)

Here the diagnosis is made on the presence of certain changes in the skin and the type of dermatitis on additional factors such as those of history and distribution. The range of morphological changes include erythema, oedema, vesicle/bulla, exudation in the acute phase of the response; and thickening/lichenification with variable scaling and pigmentation in the chronic phase (*Fig.* 14.1). Certain of these changes are more commonly found in one pattern of dermatitis than in another, and this information, when combined with history and distribution, allows for the definition of the following constitutional types.

In *atopic dermatitis* there is usually a history of other forms of atopy such as hay fever and/or asthma in the subject or near relative. Although the onset of the dermatitis may be delayed into childhood and occasionally adult life, approximately 60% are affected during the first year of life and 90% by the time they reach the age of 5 years. It is important, however, to remember that all dermatitis in the infant is not of the atopic type. The persistence of the reaction and subsequent affection of the skin of the cubital and popliteal fossae helps to confirm the diagnosis. In its most severe form it may continue late on into adult life but in most affected subjects it fluctuates in severity and at different sites over variable periods during childhood, adolescence, and adult life. The atopic dermatitis sufferer usually has a dry skin (xeroderma) and is therefore particularly liable to develop hand dermatitis (*Fig.* 14.1*b*) following exposure to skin irritants, especially of degreasing type; this is of importance in the career guidance of the atopic subject. Colonization of the skin, affected with atopic dermatitis, by *Staphylococcus*

Histological illustrations in this chapter are by courtesy of Dr J. Rogers, Ninewells Hospital, Dundee.

aureus is common and there is the additional predisposition to certain virus infections, such as warts, molluscum contagiosum and rarely the severe form of widespread superinfection with the virus of herpes simplex or vaccinia in Kaposi's varicelliform eruption. This is related to certain defects of cell-mediated immunity. The relevance of food allergy to the state of atopic dermatitis is still not clear, although it is probably of importance in some children. Also, there is little evidence as yet that the environmental allergens such as grass pollen, house dust, moulds, etc. relevant to an associated hay fever and asthma, play a part in the chronic dermatitis. Similarly the elevated serum IgE levels found in over 80% of subjects with atopic dermatitis have yet to be shown to have pathogenic significance.

Treatment of this form of constitutional dermatitis will entail the regular use of various concentrations of cortisone-containing topically applied preparations. Unless these preparations are used with care and the amounts controlled by regular consultation and reduced in parallel with clinical improvement, percutaneous absorption of the steroid will lead to suppression of pituitary/adrenal function likely to be of particular relevance in operative surgical procedures. Atrophy of the skin will also occur from the injudicious use of this topical therapy and may raise problems in healing of surgical incisions and the ease with which the skin is traumatized, particularly over relatively avascular areas such as the skin over the shin. Similar cutaneous changes are encountered after long-term systemic steroid therapy.

Seborrhoeic Dermatitis

Many individuals have minimal evidence of seborrhoeic dermatitis in the form of an irritating scaly erythema of the scalp, often localized to one or two persistent areas with occasional involvement of the eyebrows, presternal and interscapular skin. In some subjects the reaction will become more widespread and persistent going on to involve the facial creases, behind the ears, around the forehead, at the line of division with the hair-bearing scalp and in the pubic area. There is also a liability to develop intertrigo which is an inflammation of approximating skin surfaces as in the axillae, groins, submammary and intergluteal skin. Superimposed yeast infection is common—made that more

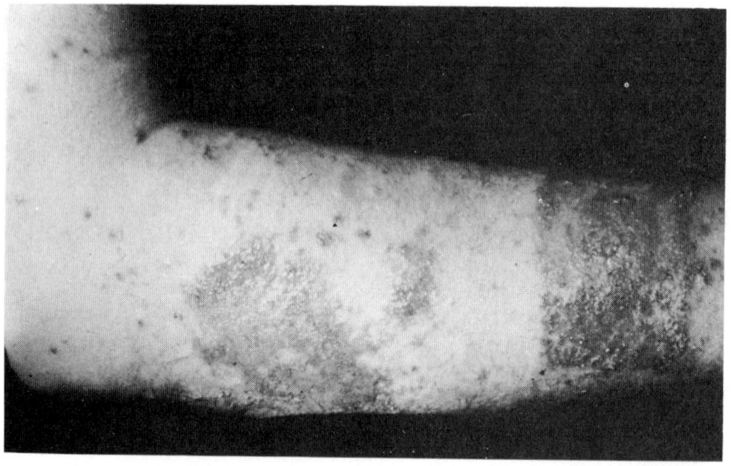

a

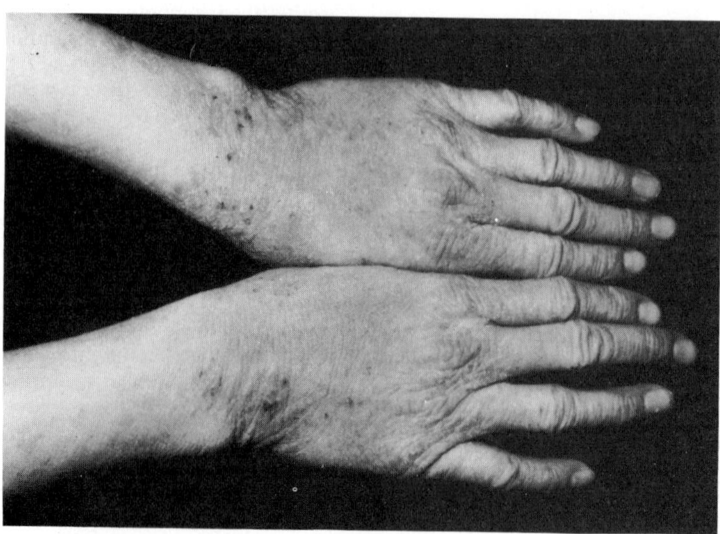

b

Fig. 14.1 *a, b,* Eczema (dermatitis). In acute/subacute eczema (*a*) the skin changes are in the form of erythema, oedema, papules and vesicles, with thickening of the skin and accentuation of the skin lines in the chronic stage (*b*). [*continued over*]

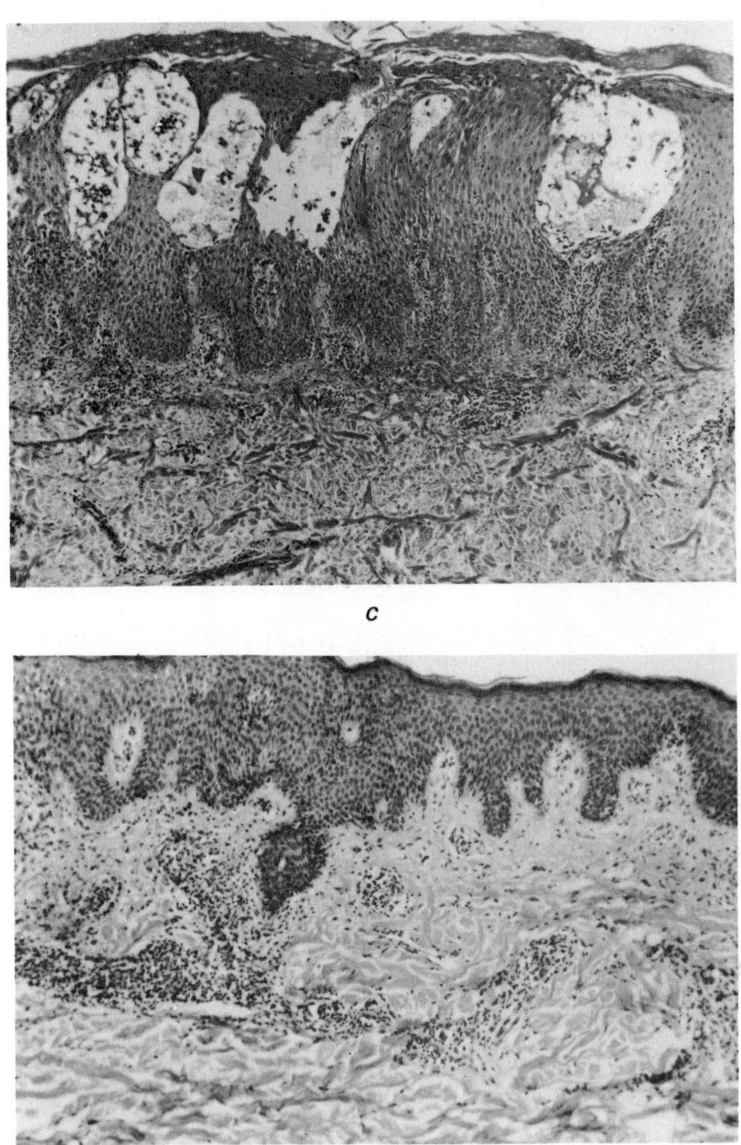

[*Fig. 14.1 continued*] *c, d,* Acute and chronic eczema (dermatitis). In the acute stage (*c*) the epidermis is disorganized by the presence of spongiotic vesicles and normal maturation of cells from basal layer to stratum corneum is impossible. A mild inflammatory infiltrate is present in the upper part of the dermis. In the chronic stage (*d*) the epidermis regains its normal distribution but some spongiosis and acanthosis remain. A dense perivascular lymphocytic infiltrate is present in the upper dermis.

likely if topical steroid preparations are used for any length of time in the flexures without the concomitant inclusion of anti-yeast substances such as nystatin.

The seborrhoeic subject is particularly liable to pyogenic infection of the hair follicle/sebaceous gland unit—in its mildest form as staphylococcal folliculitis with the tendency to progress to boil (furuncle) and even carbuncle formation in some subjects. Such a state of follicular infection, if chronic, raises obvious problems for surgery in both patients and staff.

Discoid Dermatitis

This is sometimes called nummular dermatitis because of the coin-shaped appearance of the discrete patches of dermatitis. This form of dermatitis appears in a number of different ways and the purist might choose to argue against the use of the qualifying term 'discoid' for all these, but in practical terms there are advantages in using the term for all dermatitis reactions which present with this morphological pattern. The distribution is that of bilateral symmetrically placed lesions over the limbs in particular, with or without affection of the back of the hands. The trunk may also be affected. It is likely that the appearance of discoid eczema on the skin of the back of the hands and fingers is frequently a reaction to physicochemical irritants. Middle-aged and elderly males are prone to develop a form of discoid dermatitis which appears first on the distal half of the leg; there may or may not be an associated varicosity of the veins. Subsequent spread is to the arms, particularly the extensor aspects, and later also to the trunk.

Varicose and Stasis Dermatitis

Reference has already been made to the discoid pattern of dermatitis not uncommonly developing in male subjects with uncomplicated varicose veins of the legs, preceded often by a stage of skin irritation with the later development of dermatitis. There is much to be said for restricting varicose dermatitis as a label to this form of presentation and using stasis dermatitis for that with a history of previous deep thrombosis leading subsequently to stasis oedema, pruritus and dermatitis. Stasis dermatitis is thus a response of the skin of the distal third of the leg spreading soon up the legs, associated in many subjects with episodes of superficial phlebitis and cellulitis, leading to chronic induration and ultimately stasis ulceration (*Fig.* 14.2). Varicose ulceration is discussed in Chapter 57.

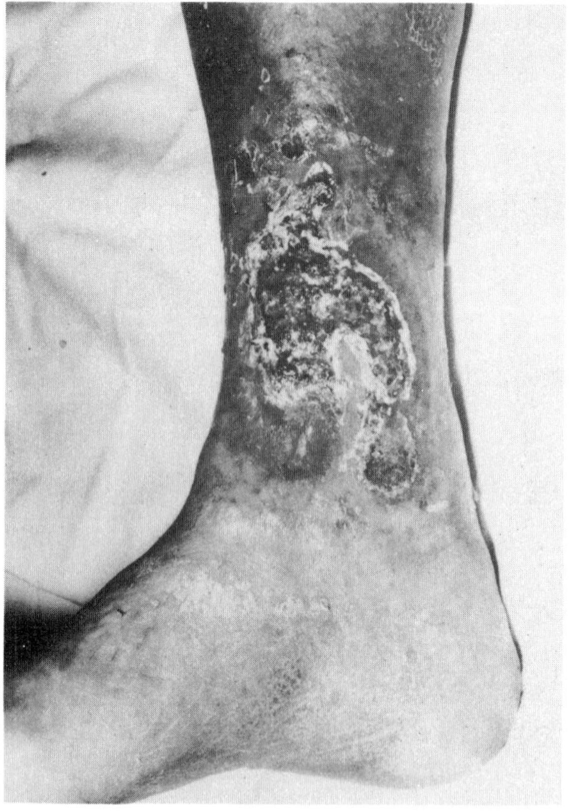

Fig. 14.2 Chronic stasis ulceration of the leg.

Contact Dermatitis

Having defined the constitutional patterns of reaction, we come to what is a dermatitis occurring at a site in contact with a substance capable of acting either as a physicochemical irritant or as an allergic sensitizer, or both. The eruption will occur, initially anyway, at sites of maximum contact, such as the hands. Confusion sometimes arises when, e.g. a contact dermatitis of the hands triggers off a relapse of one of the constitutional patterns of dermatitis, e.g. atopic or seborrhoeic, leading to a spread of the reaction along the distribution of the constitutional response additional to the primary contact site. The importance here lies in recognizing the presence of the contact factor so that investigation and guidance can be directed towards this aspect.

Contact dermatitis occurs most commonly as a result of irritant factors and much less commonly due to specific contact allergens. However, the irritant dermatitis can lead to easier absorption of environmental allergens so that contact allergy develops later, superimposed on the original irritant dermatitis. The skin patch test technique is therefore used to determine the presence or not of a contact allergen and is based on the application of the substance to the skin under an occlusive patch in a concentration which is known not to produce an irritant response in normal subjects. The production of a localized patch of dermatitis (*Fig.* 14.3*d*) some 24–48 h later indicates contact cell-mediated allergic sensitivity. It has to be appreciated, however, that the substance may not be a contact allergen for an individual as demonstrated by a negative skin patch test but yet be responsible for the contact dermatitis since the concentration to which the subject is environmentally exposed is such that it produces a contact irritant dermatitis.

The technique of skin testing is illustrated in *Fig.* 14.3. The appropriate dilution of the substance is applied to the skin, usually of the back, by means of an occlusive patch test which aids percutaneous absorption and the skin is examined usually 48 h later. A positive response indicating delayed type of cell-mediated contact allergic sensitivity is in the form of morphological dermatitis (*Fig.* 14.3*d*) with histological features of eczematous changes in the epidermis and lymphocytic infiltration around the dermal blood vessels (*Fig.* 14.1*c*). Certain substances produce contact dermatitis only after exposure of the skin to ultraviolet radiation or to light; the technique used in this instance is called the photopatch test and is similar to the skin patch test except in so far as a third patch is required which is removed after 24 h, while the other two patches are kept closed, and irradiated with appropriate amounts of radiation of wavelengths related to the absorption spectrum of the test substance. A positive reaction (indicating either photoallergy or phototoxicity) occurs only at the irradiated site.

The range of substances in appropriate dilutions which will cover the majority of common contact allergens is available for skin testing when the subject's history does not point to a specific contact factor (*Table* 14.1).

Table 14.1 European standard series of contact allergens

CC	Control WSP
C1	Potassium dichromate 0·5%
C2	Cobalt chloride 1%
C3	Nickel sulphate 5%
C4	Formaldehyde 1% in H_2O
C5	PPD 0·5%
C6	Balsam of Peru 25%
C7	Turpentine 10% in olive oil
C8	Neomycin sulphate 20%
C9	Parabens 15%
C10	Colophony 60%
C11	Wool alcohol 30%
C12	Epoxy resin 1%
C13	Mercapto mix 2%
C14	Thiuram mix 1%
C15	Black rubber mix 0·6%
C16	Carba mix 3%
C17	Ethylene diamine 1%
C18	Fragrance mix 8%
C19	Benzocaine 5%
C20	Quinoline mix 6%
C21	Paratertiary butyl phenol formaldehyde resin 1%
C22	Primin 0·01%

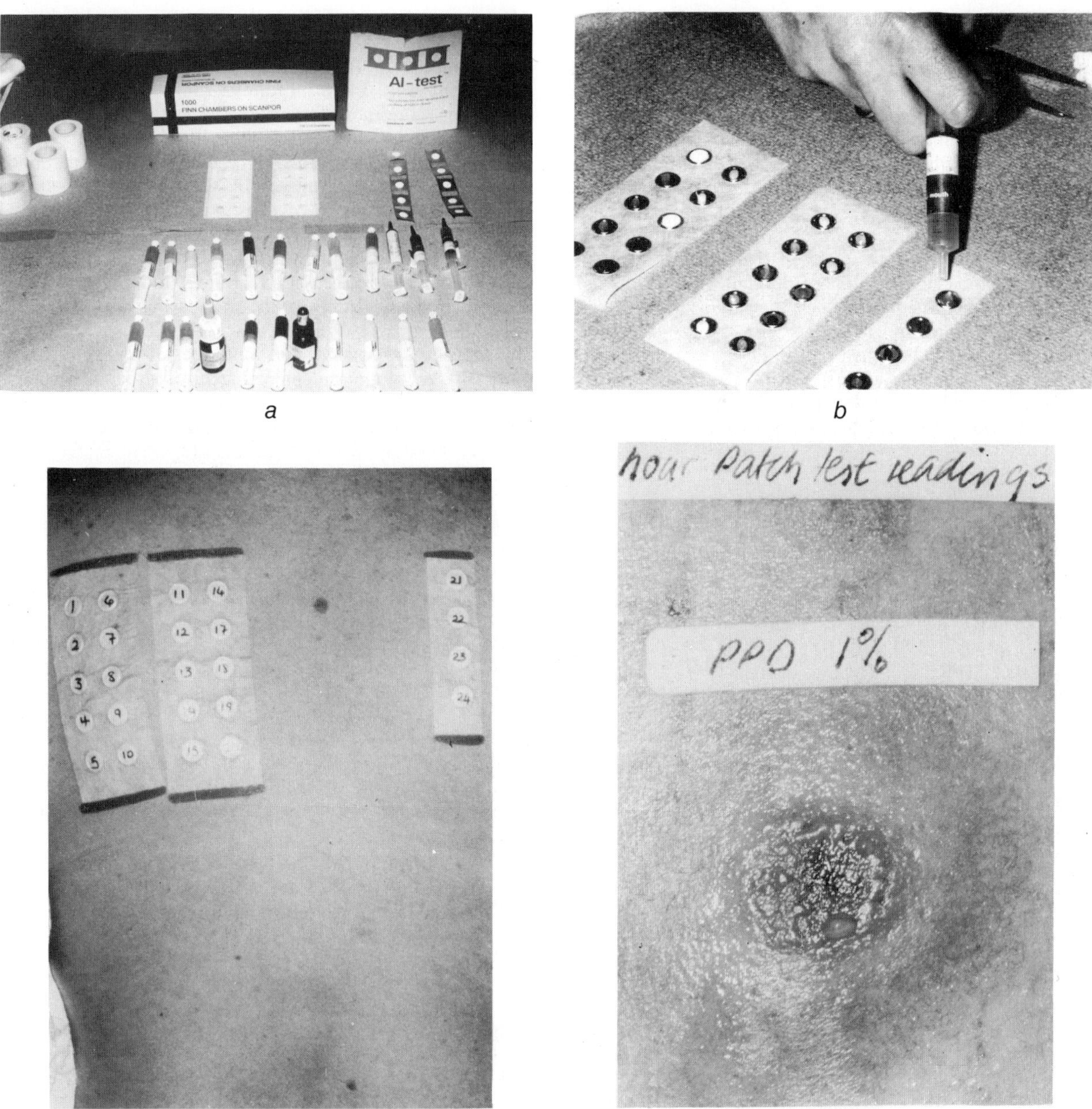

Fig. 14.3 Finnchamber. The technique of skin patch testing. The test materials are refrigeration-stored syringes (*a*), applied in measured amounts to the centre of each Finnchamber (*b*), and applied to the skin of the back for 48 h (*c*). A positive response is indicated by localized eczema (*d*).

Universal dermatitis in which the whole skin is affected may occur as an extreme form of the patterns of reaction already described or as an indication of disturbance of another body system, e.g. as part of systemic reticulosis, and here the term 'exfoliative dermatitis' is often applied. In the assessment of such a condition investigations need to be directed towards contact, systemic and constitutional factors.

Treatment

The treatment of these various forms of dermatitis involves the use of topical steroid suppression along the lines indicated in the treatment of atopic dermatitis, with the addition of appropriate antibiotic or antibacterial substances in the presence of secondary infection, the use of anti-yeast preparations in flexural intertrigo, and the avoidance of potent steroid substances on the skin of the face.

Psoriasis

Psoriasis affects 1–2% of the population and occurs at all ages and in both sexes. A family history of psoriasis is common and the mode of inheritance is thought to be most probably by means of an autosomal dominant trait with incomplete penetrance. There is an increase in the frequency of certain HLA antigens and it is likely that the gene which determines susceptibility to develop psoriasis is inherited along with the genes of histocompatibility. This genetic predisposition results in the development of the cutaneous condition only in those individuals who are, in addition, exposed to other unknown factors which may include certain infections. While some authorities believe dermal changes precede the characteristic epidermal dysplasia of psoriasis, others feel the primary event is the movement of polymorphonuclear leucocytes from the dermal papillae into the epidermis in response to abnormally high concentrations of chemoattractants present in the upper epidermal layers. As a result of increased epidermal cell proliferation the cutaneous lesions develop which consist of variable sized well-demarcated erythematous papules and plaques with surface silvery scaling (*Fig.* 14.4*a*). The individual lesions may be small as in guttate psoriasis, but commonly form large plaques classically distributed on the elbows, knees and scalp, although any part of the body skin can be affected. Pruritus is uncommon except in the elderly. Affection of the body flexures may occur in the elderly and in those who as a result of obesity are liable to develop flexural intertrigo. A dystrophy of both finger and toe nails is common (*Fig.* 14.4*b*). Psoriasis can be a disabling and distressing condition, both for the patient and for the family, but is usually not serious or life-threatening, except in the acute pustular or universal erythrodermic forms, both of which may be precipitated by the use and subsequent withdrawal of systemic corticosteroid drugs. The patient with the erythrodermic form of reaction may demonstrate systemic changes such as cardiovascular insufficiency, impaired temperature regulation, protein and water loss and malabsorption as a result of the shunting of blood from the gut to the erupting skin.

Psoriasis is associated with a number of types of arthropathy. It may mimic rheumatoid arthritis although serologically these patients are rheumatoid factor negative. Other forms of arthropathy include mono and multiple large joint

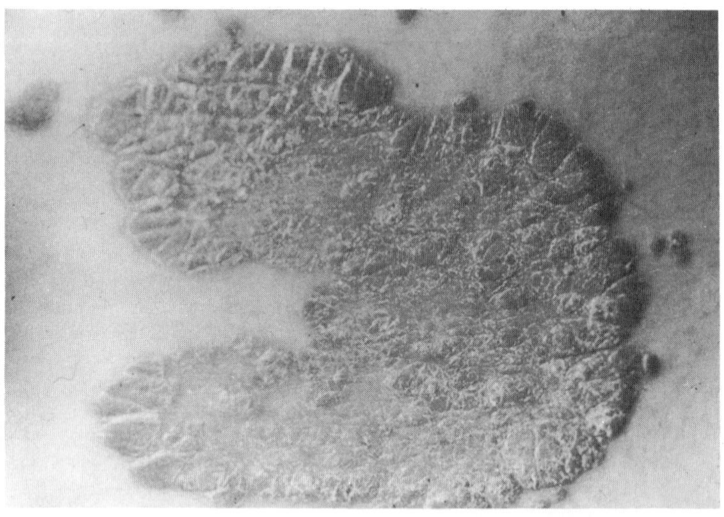

a

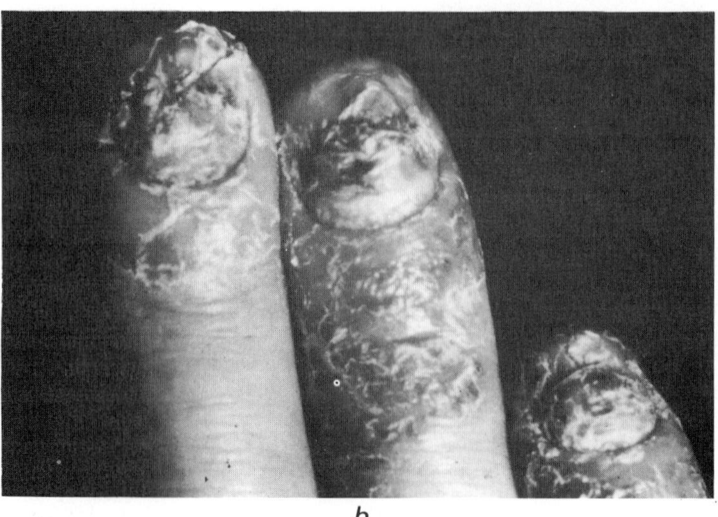

b

Fig. 14.4 Psoriasis. The lesion in psoriasis is well-demarcated from the surrounding normal skin, is reddish in colour, with a variable amount of surface silvery scaling (*a*). The commonly associated dystrophy of nails consists of pitting with subungual thickening and a variable colour change in the nail plate (*b*). [*continued over*]

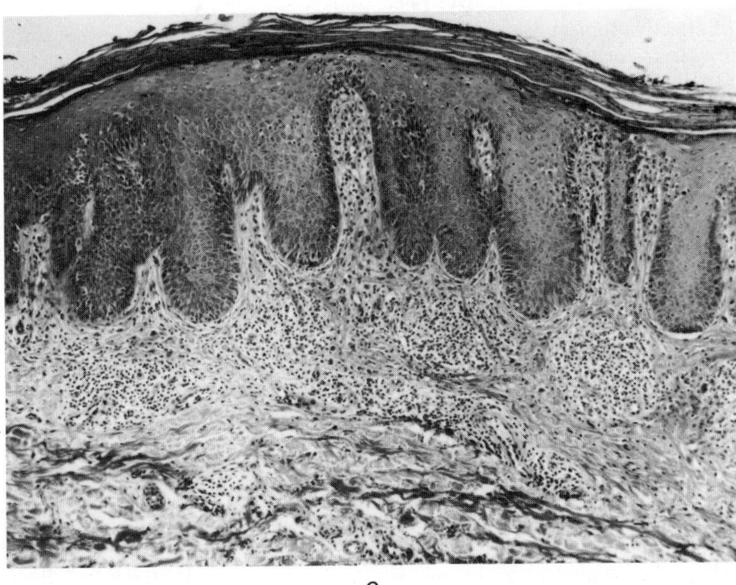

c

[*Fig. 14.4 continued*] *c*, This section shows elongation and clubbing of the rete pegs and elongation of dermal papillae. On the right the thin supra-papillary plate allows inflammatory cells to infiltrate the parakeratotic stratum corneum and form small linear micro-abscesses.

types, sacro-iliitis and ankylosing spondylitis as well as the distinctive progressive distal joint arthropathy. In all forms of psoriatic arthropathy the rheumatoid factor is serum negative.

Treatment involves the topical application of substances which affect epidermal cell proliferation probably through action on cellular DNA, such as tar and dithranol, along with phototherapy using the shorter wavelength ultraviolet (UV-B 290–320 nm), sunburn wavelengths and photochemotherapy where the irradiation is by means of the longer ultraviolet (UV-A 320–400 nm) in combination with the oral or topical application of photoactive substances such as the psoralens. Opinions vary as to the justification for the regular topical application of the corticosteroids but they are probably best restricted to short-term treatment of localized lesions—the systemic administration of these drugs should be avoided. The administration of the retinoid group of drugs such as etretinate is effective in the treatment of psoriasis and in particular of the more severe forms. Also, in the future the combination with psoralen photochemotherapy (PUVA) should allow for the relative reduction of dosage of both the etretinate and the UV irradiation, thus minimizing unwanted side-effects. Antimetabolites, such as methotrexate, are effective in the treatment of the severe forms of psoriasis and are usually confined to those cases which have proved unresponsive to other forms of therapy.

Acne Vulgaris

This affects to a variable degree the majority of adolescents at some time during their developing years and does continue on into adult life in approximately 5% of those affected and may still trouble a few on into middle age. Persistence of the condition for many years is particularly seen with the severe form of cystic acne conglobata.

First seen with the onset of puberty, when in both sexes androgen production is increased as a result of which the sebaceous glands are stimulated to secrete sebum which then allows for growth within the follicles of bacteria such as *Propionibacterium acnes*. The aetiology of acne would appear in the main to be due to an increased sebum excretion which is androgen mediated, along with hyperkeratinization of the pilosebaceous duct, the stimulus to which may be hormonal or may also be due to the direct action of sebaceous lipid modified by the bacteria which colonize the duct. These organisms, which are present both on the skin surface and in the pilosebaceous duct, are *Propionibacterium acnes* (*P. acnes*), *Staphylococcus epidermidis*, and *Pityrosporum ovale*, with the *P. acnes* being the most important one, and thus the use in treatment of topical benzyl peroxide along with oral antibiotics, both of which have the action of reducing the number of bacteria and affecting their physiological activity. The presence of these bacteria and the enzymes which they produce affect the structure of the wall of the pilosebaceous unit and are also responsible for the subsequent inflammatory reaction which leads to the classic acne papule and pustule. In the minority of subjects the acne may be of the severe acne conglobata type leading to scarring which may be hypertrophic and is characterized by the presence of nodulocytic lesions and sinuses and double comedones. This is sometimes associated with hidradenitis suppurativa and pilonidal cysts.

Certain external environmental factors will affect the acne process, such as exposure to oils and halogenated hydrocarbons, occlusive cosmetics and localized friction. Acne may also be a feature of certain endocrine disorders as in Cushing's syndrome and adrenal virilism and of liver disease and may be caused or aggravated by drugs such as the corticosteroids, epanutin, rifampicin, lithium, chlorpromazine and, in the past, iodides and bromides.

Treatment is directed towards control of the bacteria and the over-production of sebum which leads to blockage of the sebaceous gland duct. The efficacy of treatment is likely to increase with the development of measures directed against the production of sebaceous secretion and which can be used without unwanted side-effects in both sexes. Benzyl peroxide is probably the most effective topical preparation and will reduce colonization with *P. acnes*. In addition, the long-term administration orally of antibiotics such as tetracycline and erythromycin is widely used. Of more recent times the advent of the retinoids, and in particular isotretrinate has resulted in the availability of effective treatment for the most troublesome and severe forms of acne. In some subjects ultraviolet irradiation is useful but any improvement is usually not maintained for any length of time after the irradiation is stopped.

INFECTIONS OF THE SKIN

Bacterial Infections

Impetigo is commonest in the younger age groups and in the child may be bullous but in most instances the thin-walled subcorneal blister soon breaks to form the classic yellow crusted lesion (*Fig.* 14.5); central clearing with the joining together of neighbouring lesions may result in a circinate eruption mimicking a fungal infection. In temperate climates the organisms tend to be staphylococci or mixed infection with streptococci with the latter predominating in hotter countries. With a streptococcal infection the possibility of acute nephritis developing must be remembered.

Staphylococcal infection of the hair follicles leads to folliculitis, boils and carbuncles, depending on the site and subsequent spread of the infection (*Fig.* 14.6).

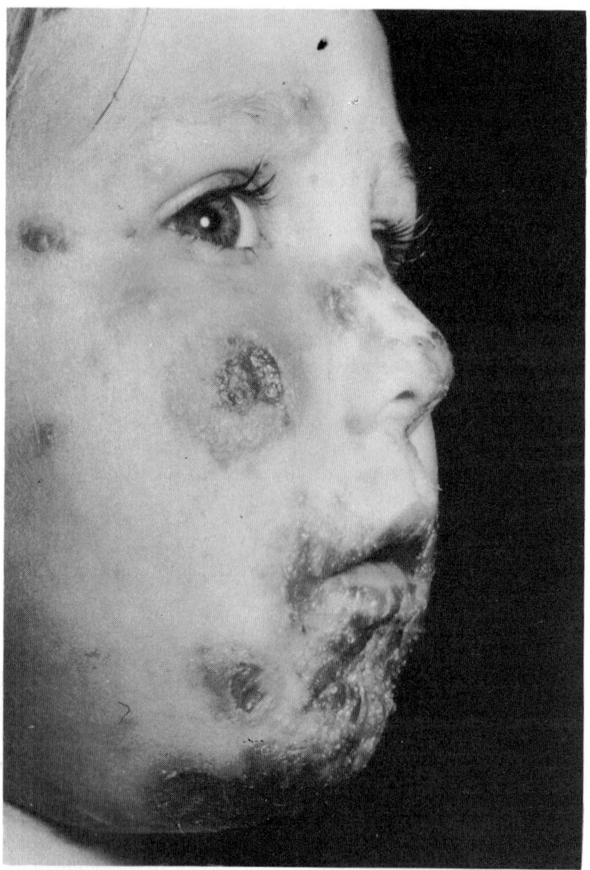

Fig. 14.5 Impetigo. Most commonly seen in children; presenting with or without initial flaccid blisters which soon rupture to form discoloured crusted areas.

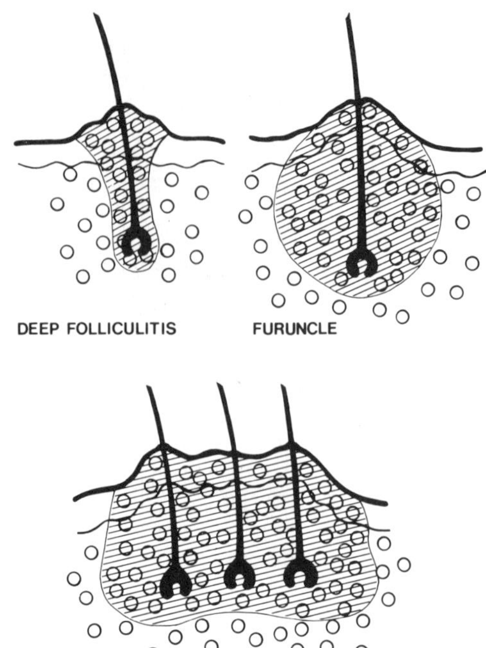

Fig. 14.6 This illustrates diagrammatically the localization of the reaction of inflammation in folliculitis, furuncle (boil) amd carbuncle.

Toxic epidermal necrolysis resembles scalding of the skin with the development of widespread areas of erythema and raw, tender patches occurring as a result of infection of the skin with staphylococci which produce a toxin causing the epidermal splitting (*Fig.* 14.7).

Treatment. Treatment for the simple case of impetigo, folliculitis and boils consists of the isolation of the responsible organisms, the use of appropriate topical antibiotic or antibacterial substance, and the assessment of the carrier state for the organism, where indicated. Systemic antibiotic therapy is used where nephritogenic streptococci are isolated and where the infection is widespread or deeply invading one or more follicle.

Persistent or recurring infection usually occurs if there are factors which alter the skin soil, such as infestations, itchy dermatoses as in atopic dermatitis or, more rarely, systemic diseases, such as diabetes or immune deficiency.

Viral Infections

Of these the most common is the human wart virus producing a range of usually multiple, benign tumours which vary in appearance, being often filiform or digitate on the face and neck, raised and 'verrucous' on the fingers and hands, depressed into the skin of the sole (plantar verruca) and sometimes small and flat with a brownish colour (plane warts) or as a plaque consisting of tightly packed, small warts (mosaic warts). Diagnostic difficulties usually only arise in the adult with a single warty tumour or with the plantar callosity which in the adult is more commonly seen than plantar verruca. In the verruca paring of the lesion will demonstrate the interruption of the epidermal ridge pattern and the presence of capillary bleeding points. Warts will eventually clear spontaneously in many cases and this justifies the use in the first instance of wart paints, and if this fails freezing with carbon dioxide snow or liquid nitrogen.

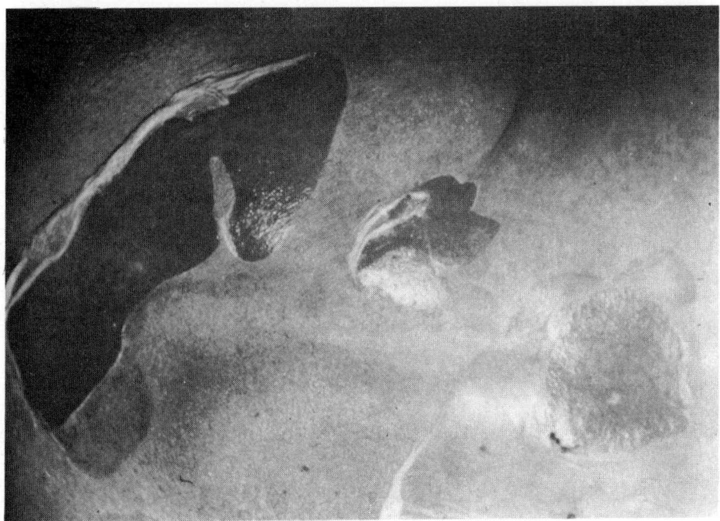

Fig. 14.7 Toxic epidermal necrolysis. Presents as flaccid scald-like blisters, soon rupturing to leave extensive raw red areas.

Curettage and electrocautery are effective in digitate and filiform lesions and may be required in the occasionally persistent plantar verruca in the adult. Surgical excision or radiotherapy should be avoided.

The herpes simplex virus (Type I in non-genital and Type II in genital herpes) infection most commonly presents as recurrent, relatively mild reactions, particularly on the face, in the form of grouped vesicles on a swollen erythematous base with subsequent crusting; occasionally with adenitis or erythema multiforme. This recurrent form is due to the persistence, following the primary infection of the virus, in the sensory nerve ganglion and its subsequent reactivation from time to time. Occasionally the affection presents with linear lesions, particularly in the lower thoracic or lumbar regions (zosteriform herpes simplex) then requiring differentiation from herpes zoster. The primary infection may present in early childhood as a severe herpetic gingivostomatitis with pyrexia and systemic upset. A severe widespread disseminated vesicular eruption is occasionally seen in the atopic form to which the term 'eczema herpeticum' is given. Treatment, which is only partially effective, consists of acyclovir. This agent has been reported to reduce the severity and frequency of recurrent herpes simplex infections, as well as being of great value in primary herpes infections including eczema herpeticum. Topical antibiotics may be of value in controlling secondary infection.

In herpes zoster ('shingles') the virus from a primary or subclinical attack of chicken pox remains dormant being reactivated by a subsequent unknown stimulus leading to the development of the herpes zoster eruption which is preceded by 3 or 4 days of localized discomfort with aesthesia or pain over the involved neural segment and is usually in the form of a unilateral and segmental collection of vesicles on an erythematous base which become pustular, associated with systemic upset and lymphadenitis. Affection of the ophthalmic branch of the trigeminal nerve requires attention to be paid to the ocular involvement. Widespread lesions may develop (disseminated zoster) and indicate a possible lymphoreticular disorder, such as a malignant reticulosis. Persistent pain (post-herpetic neuralgia) after the eruption has healed may occur particularly in the elderly subject. The possibility of pressure by a tumour on the posterior root ganglia needs also to be considered.

Fungal Infections

Infection of the skin by a fungus (tinea; ringworm) leads to eruptions which vary depending on the site affected, the type of fungus (seed), and the affected individuals's response (soil). The source of the infection is usually directly or indirectly from an infected human or animal (domestic or farm). The hair, nails and skin may all be involved. Factors which predispose to fungus infection are sweating and friction. The types of fungus (dermatophyte) belong to three main genera: microsporum, epidermophyton and trichophyton. The commonest clinical presentation is that of an infection of the skin of the feet (tinea pedis, athlete's foot) and varies in severity from a mild irritation and scaling of the skin of the toe webs (particularly the 3rd and 4th webs) to a more acute response which may in parts be vesicular with involvement of the skin of all toe webs, spreading down on the neighbouring skin of the sole and eventually to involve all or part of both feet. An associated reaction of the skin of the hands may follow and even some form of erythema of the skin of the trunk and limbs, both of which may be the result of an immunological response to the presence of the fungus. In this type of presentation involvement of the nails is less commonly seen than in chronic affection of the skin of the feet and/or hands. Affection of the skin of the groin (tinea cruris; Dhobi's itch) may occur in association with either of the forms of affection of the feet and will also vary in severity and degree of chronicity. Affection of the skin of the trunk and limbs, head and neck, other than the hands and feet and skin flexures, tends to be due to infection from an animal source and presents in the form of one or more irritating scaly chronic plaques which in time clear the centre but maintain an active spreading periphery (tinea circinata; tinea corporis) (*Fig.* 14.8*a*). A variable pustular element is common and ranges from a mild to the most acute response where pustulation is marked and associated with a boggy swelling of the skin particularly well seen on the hairy parts of the beard and scalp (kerion) (*Fig.* 14.8*b*). Confirmation of the clinical diagnosis depends on the

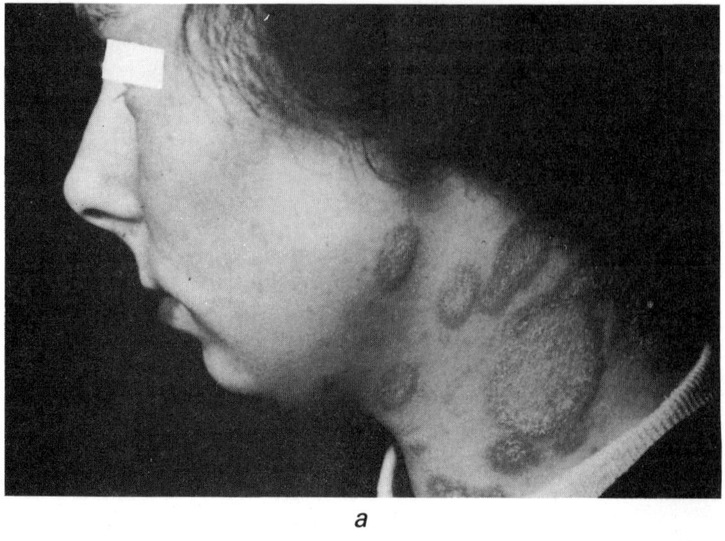

Fig. 14.8 *a*, Tinea circinata. Erythematous scaly patches with central clearing and active spreading edge. *b*, Kerion. Boggy swelling of the chin with multiple pustules.

demonstration of mycelium in samples of skin, nails or hair by direct microscopical examination and definition of the responsible fungus by subsequent cultural studies. Treatment involves control of the circumstances leading to the skin maceration and the topical or systemic administration of fungistatic preparations.

Yeast infection of the skin, particularly with *Candida albicans*, is common and as with fungus infection (dermatomycoses) is an interaction between seed and soil in that yeast infection occurs most often when the skin is exposed to increased moisture, maceration and repeated minor trauma. Most commonly this leads to chronic paronychia or to monilial intertrigo in the form of red, raw-looking moist reactions with peripheral scaling and outlying pustules, particularly if the latter has been treated with topical steroid preparations without the addition of appropriate anti-yeast ingredients such as nystatin. An associated diabetic condition should be excluded. Systemic mucocutaneous candidiasis is rare but when suspected indicates a search for a possible immune deficiency (Chapters, 5, 78).

The treatment of cutaneous monilial infection is that of the inflammatory intertrigo as well as the specific treatment of the candida infection by the topical application of preparations containing nystatin or amphotericin B.

Acquired Immune Deficiency Syndrome (AIDS)

In addition to Kaposi's sarcoma, patients suffering from the acquired immune deficiency syndrome appear at high risk of developing a number of dermatological conditions. These include xeroderma, chronic acneiform folliculitis, seborrhoeic dermatitis, vasculitis, and troublesome fungal, bacterial and viral infections. These last two conditions may be early indications of the development of AIDS.

Cutaneous Tuberculosis

Lupus vulgaris caused by *Mycobacterium tuberculosis* is rare nowadays. The typical soft apple-jelly nodules consist of tuberculous granulation tissue covered by atrophic epidermis. In addition, fibrosis is a prominent feature and the lesion extends mainly by direct centrifugal spread but satellite lesions are not infrequent and result from lymphatic spread. Two other mycobacteria are associated with chronic ulcerating lesions of the skin. *Mycobacterium ulcerans* causes a chronic necrotic ulcer with overhanging edges which develops from the breakdown of an initial subcutaneous nodule. The lesion which occurs typically in the lower limbs bears little histological resemblance to tuberculosis. Infection of skin abrasions by *Mycobacterium marinum (balnei)* is usually acquired in swimming pools. The ulcers or granulomatous nodules are often solitary, occur commonly on the elbow or knee and tend to heal spontaneously.

THE ERYTHEMAS

The erythemas result from a reaction of the small cutaneous blood vessels leading to a range of morphological changes, such as macules, papules with a background of oedematous

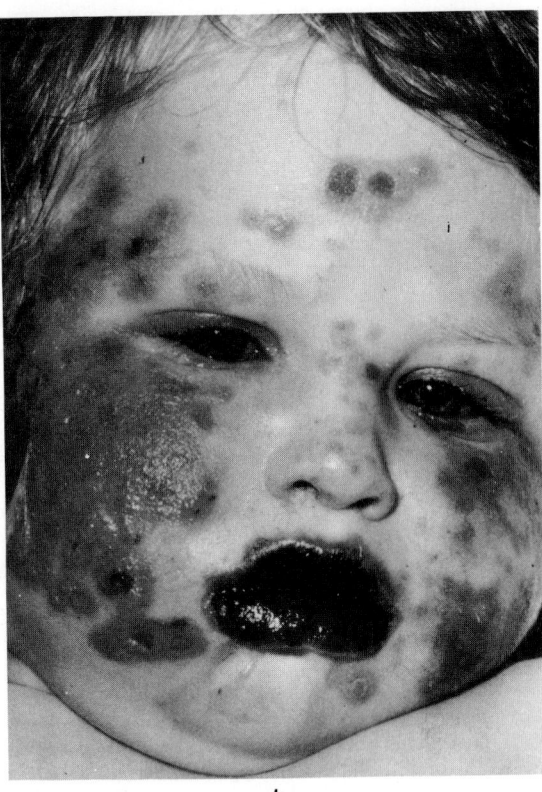

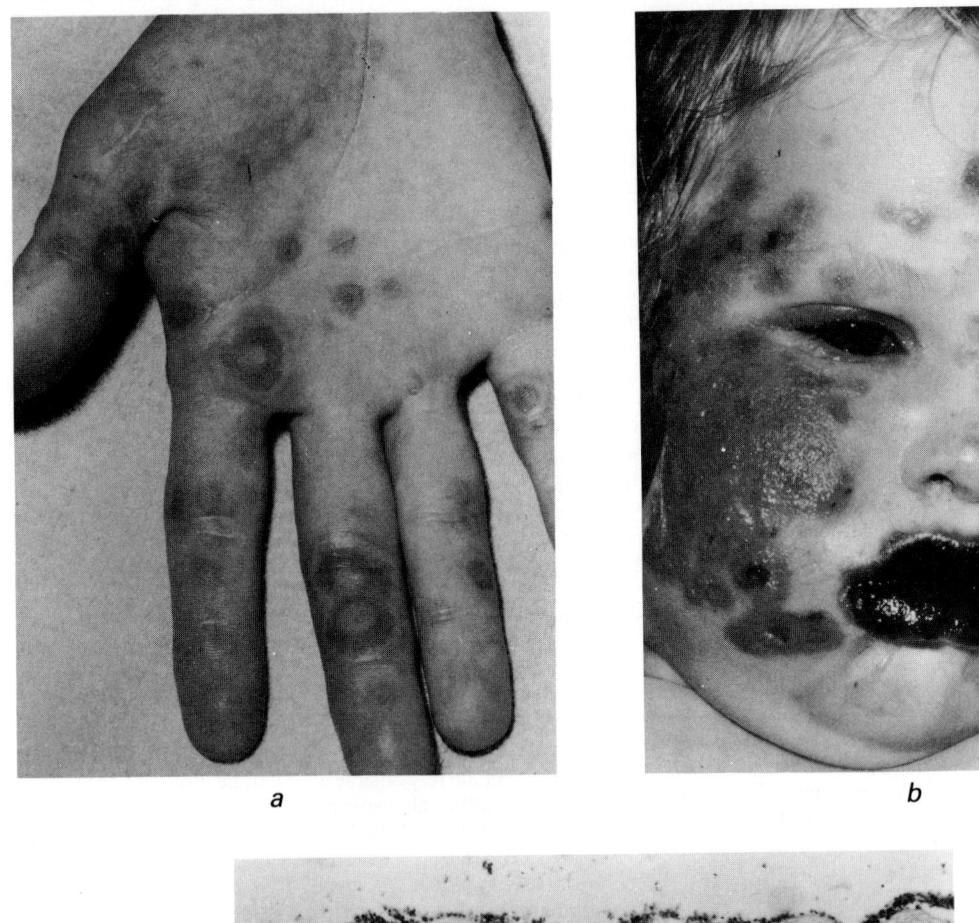

a b

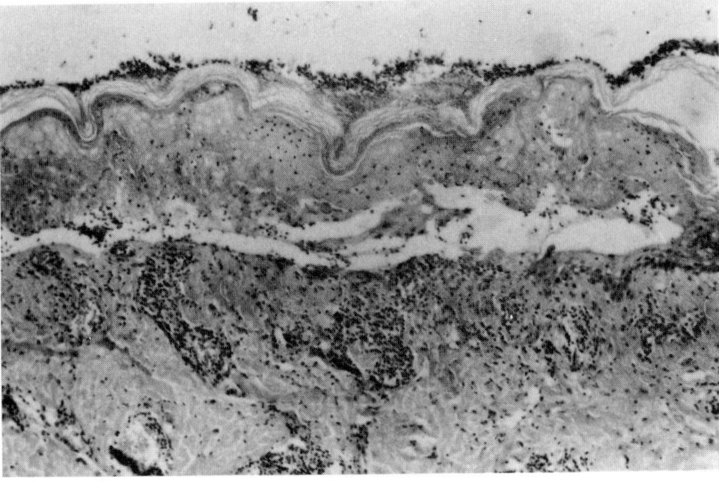

c

Fig. 14.9 a and b, Erythema multiforme. In the common mild form, the lesions are those of macules and papules and iris target lesions with extensive blistering and affection of the mucous membranes in the most severe form. c, In this severe example the entire epidermis is necrotic and has separated from the dermis where anti-inflammatory changes are present.

erythema. When the reaction is more acute, vesicles or larger bullae may also appear in association with a variable amount of destruction of the epidermis, best seen in the more acute forms of erythema multiforme and in toxic epidermal necrolysis (Lyell's disease). Purpura and other evidence of blood vessel wall damage, such as haemorrhagic bullae, may also be seen. In the erythemas, therefore, the morphological changes, and thus the descriptive labels applied, will depend on the severity of the reaction and the effect on different layers of the skin. With the exception of erythema marginatum, said to be specifically associated with acute rheumatism, many of the other forms are associated with infection, drug administration, or systemic disease, or not infrequently found to be idiopathic.

Erythema Multiforme

In its mildest and most commonly seen form (*Fig.* 14.9*a*) presents as a bilateral symmetrically distributed eruption, consisting of macules, papules, iris (target) lesions, with a background of erythema and oedema, over the limbs especially the extensor aspects, the face and to a variable extent on to the trunk. In the more acute form the reaction of the skin is more widespread, with bullae which are often haemorrhagic, being seen and with subsequent loss of epidermis, affection of the mucous membranes, particularly the buccal mucosae and lips, and symptoms and signs of a general systemic upset, classically seen in the Stevens–Johnson syndrome (*Fig.* 14.9*b*). Some examples of erythema multiforme are not infrequently idiopathic although the eruption can be attributed to infection, drug administration, or systemic disease. A not uncommon association is that of recurrent erythema multiforme with recurrent attacks of herpes simplex infection.

Erythema Nodosum

This presents in the form of erythematous nodules of 2·5–5·0 cm in diameter, which are painful as well as being tender to touch and most commonly seen on the anterior aspects of the shins but can appear also, but less frequently, on the skin of the thighs and upper limbs. An associated systemic upset is variable and may be absent. The erythematous nodules are variable in number and may continue to appear over a period of a number of days, the whole reaction, however, often being present for no longer than 3–4 weeks and usually less if the patient is confined to bed during the first week or two. The individual lesions as they clear present colour changes similar to those seen in a resolving bruise. Erythema nodosum may be associated with infection such as streptococcal or tuberculous or as a manifestation of sarcoidosis or in association with drug administration.

Erythema Induratum

Now less commonly seen with the reduction in incidence of tuberculous infection, it presents with indurated nodules and plaques on the back of the calves of the legs leading to a varying amount of tissue destruction and scarring and usually, although not invariably, accompanied by an abnormal reaction to cold as demonstrated by livedo reticularis or cutis marmorata. Differential diagnosis is from other forms of nodose erythema and is based on histological evidence of a tuberculous granuloma.

Of the remaining relatively rare erythemas, investigations are directed towards the exclusion or otherwise of systemic disease.

Toxic Epidermal Necrolysis (Lyell's Disease)

Also termed 'scalded skin syndrome' and already referred to in discussion of impetigo where the necrotic change in the epidermis is due to staphylococcal infection. It may also occur with the characteristic widespread loss of surface skin as a result of a reaction to the therapeutic administration of certain drugs such as allopurinol, sulphonamides, penicillin, phenylbutazone and phenolphthalein.

Treatment. Relatively easily treated with appropriate systemic antibiotics, it becomes, however, of much more serious clinical significance when drug induced and a fatal outcome may occur in 25% in this instance.

URTICARIA

The lesion seen in urticaria is a localized swelling of the skin as a result of oedema of the dermis presenting in the form of an itching, erythematous papule which rapidly enlarges to form the characteristic urticarial wheal with central pallor and surrounded by erythema; separate lesions may coalesce to form rings with central clearing. There may be an associated, usually asymmetrical, localized swelling of, e.g. part of the face (angio-oedema) and less often large subcutaneous swellings (giant urticaria) which may occur on any part of the body. It is likely that histamine is responsible for the wheal in most cases of chronic urticaria, although other substances, such as serotonin, kinins, prostaglandins, anaphylatoxin and acetylcholine, will produce a similar form of cutaneous response. Acute urticaria, as seen, e.g. in penicillin allergy and in serum sickness, is of sudden onset with widespread urticarial wheals and lasting for a number of days; on occasions this may lead on to chronic urticaria. The majority of cases of chronic urticaria are idiopathic and may last with fluctuating severity for months and even years. The remainder are examples of physical urticaria (i.e. due to pressure, heat, cold or light) and, cholinergic urticaria in which exercise, heat and emotion are precipitating factors.

Chronic idiopathic urticaria is more commonly seen in the atopic and in the female, although by no means exclusively so. A specific responsible allergen, be it dietary or otherwise, is rare, although aspirin will aggravate the condition in about one-third of the cases acting by degranulation of mast cells. A relatively uncommon association with bowel candidiasis has been reported. It is therefore not yet known whether this form of urticaria is mediated by pharmacological or immunological mechanisms.

In the physical urticarias a relatively small group occur as a result of exposure to heat or to cold, the latter presenting in a number of different forms. In hereditary cold urticaria the inheritance is as an autosomal dominant, starting soon after birth and lasting throughout life and precipitated by a cold environment. Symptomatic cold urticaria occurs in paroxysmal cold haemoglobinuria or in association with cold agglutinins or with cryoglobulinaemia, e.g. in myeloma or systemic lupus erythematosus. In idiopathic cold urticaria the onset is usually delayed until early adult life, the urticaria developing as a result of direct contact with cold substances such as a piece of ice.

Urticaria following exposure of the skin to sunshine (solar urticaria) is rare although an urticarial wheal is not an uncommon feature of the response of the skin to light in polymorphic light eruption which is the commonest of the photodermatoses to affect females. It can indicate the presence of a photoactive substance in the skin as a result of accumulation of a metabolic product, such as porphyrin as in erythropoietic protoporphyria or of a therapeutically administered photoactive substance.

Investigation of chronic urticaria is usually unrewarding and although an urticarial skin response may be part of the cutaneous manifestations of certain systemic diseases, the finding of such is rare.

Hereditary Angio-oedema

A dominantly inherited reduction in functioning C_1 esterase inhibitor which results in the formation of kinins and other vasoactive peptides leading to gross oedema induced by trauma or drugs. The resultant subcutaneous pruritus-free swellings are first seen in childhood. They may last for a number of days. Involvement of the gastrointestinal or upper respiratory tracts may result in colic or asphyxia respectively. The latter may prove fatal in the absence of treatment. Prophylactic therapy involves the use of epsilon aminocaproic acid (EACA), danazol or stanozolol. In the acute attack fresh frozen plasma replacement of C_1 esterase inhibitor may be of value.

DRUG ERUPTIONS

The possibility that a reaction of the skin may be due to a substance administered as part of treatment or investigation of a disease requires consideration. It is unfortunate, therefore, that there are still no reliable laboratory tests which will allow for confirmation or otherwise of the diagnosis of drug eruption suspected on clinical grounds.

The question of a drug eruption arises where there is the development, usually fairly rapidly, of an eruption, perhaps preceded by pruritus for a day or two. The rash which is bilateral and symmetrical consists of an admixture of erythema, oedema and morbilliform lesions, and if more severe, blisters and purpura with other evidence of skin vessel damage, usually spreading rapidly and often associated with the development or increase in symptoms of systemic disturbance. The human skin is limited in its patterns of reaction and therefore an eruption may well be common to a number of drugs although certain drugs have a tendency to produce specific skin lesions. The continued administration of a drug which is unsuspected as being responsible for a reaction of the skin may result in universal affection of the skin (exfoliative dermatitis, erythroderma) which would then constitute an emergency situation with the subject becoming progressively more unwell with pyrexia, rigors, and the metabolic and physiological effects associated with widespread skin change. It is also important to remember that systems other than the skin may be affected and thus disturbance of any of these systems requires evaluation at the same time.

Reference in passing has already been made to the part played by exposure to light in the production of contact dermatitis. It is also important in certain reactions of the skin following parenteral administration of drugs. Certain drugs are also able to photosensitize, leading to eruptions which are confined to the exposed skin. Those most commonly involved are the phenothiazines, the thiazide diuretics, the non-steroidal anti-inflammatory groups of drugs, the tetracyclines, amiodarone, and of more recent times probably also the retinoids. In most instances a phototoxic mechanism is involved although on occasions an immunologically-based photoallergic response may be implicated. However, the mechanisms involved in the light-induced drug eruption tends most often to be that of the phototoxic type where, following absorption by the substance of appropriate wavelengths of ultraviolet radiation, the resultant skin changes will depend on the structures involved and the depth in the skin at which the reaction takes place. In most instances, however, it tends to be in the form of a dusky erythema reaction which mimics sunburn, usually associated with burning discomfort, and with certain drugs the subsequent development of pigmentation which may persist. Some subjects, however, will develop only pigmentation of the skin without any preceding erythema reaction and thus drug-induced photosensitivity always requires to be considered as a possible cause of skin pigmentation. One of the characteristics of the phototoxic response is that it is liable to occur in any individual who takes adequate quantities of the drug and at the same time is exposed to light containing adequate amounts of UVR, whereas the photoallergic response will be triggered off by relatively small amounts of the responsible allergen and appropriate wavelengths of UVR.

The technique of phototesting is used to determine the wavelengths of UVR or light responsible for the reaction of the skin. This information can be of help in the assessment of the aetiological factors whereas in the porphyria the excess amounts of photoactive porphyrin which accumulate in the skin react to parts of visible light (400–600 nm).

The commonest skin carcinogen is ultraviolet light and the incidence of basal-cell and squamous-cell carcinomas is directly related to the amount of exposure to UVR, as is skin ageing and premalignant changes such as dryness, solar keratosis and senile purpura. It is likely also the UVR plays a part in the development of malignant melanoma.

CUTANEOUS CHANGES IN GASTROINTESTINAL DISEASE

Reference is made later to changes in the skin which raise the possibility of malignancy within the gastrointestinal tract. There remain, however, a number of other skin conditions which are known to be associated with gastrointestinal disease:

Aphthous ulcers	Hereditary haemorrhagic telangiectasia
Benign mucosal pemphigoid	Blue rubber-bleb naevi
Vitiligo	Malignant papulosis
Pyoderma gangrenosum	Henoch–Schönlein purpura
Dermatitis herpetiformis	Kaposi's sarcoma
Acrodermatitis enteropathica	Pseudoxanthoma elasticum
Behçet's syndrome	Ehlers–Danlos syndrome

Recurrent oral ulceration is seen in ulcerative colitis, Crohn's disease, malabsorption syndromes, and Behçet's syndrome.

Benign Mucosal Pemphigoid (Cicatricial Pemphigoid)

The vesiculobullous element is a common feature of many cutaneous reactions but in two specific conditions the blister element predominates, those of pemphigus and pemphigoid. The level of blister formation differs in that in the former it is intra-epidermally situated and in the latter subepidermal. A variant which is called 'benign mucosal pemphigoid' develops in addition to the bullous lesions on the skin, affection of the eyes and the mucous membrane of the mouth and perineal area leading to subsequent scarring. The reaction may spread down to involve the lining of the oesophagus.

Vitiligo

In vitiligo areas of depigmentation occur at various sites in the skin, as a result of destruction of the pigment-forming melanocytes. It is a common condition affecting 1–2% of the general population with an association with other autoimmune conditions, such as pernicious anaemia, and atrophic gastritis, hyperthyroidism, thyroiditis, adrenal insufficiency, some forms of uveitis and sympathetic ophthalmia.

Pyoderma Gangrenosum

This can occur on any skin site in approximately 10% of patients with ulcerative colitis and, more rarely, with Crohn's disease and presents in the form of erythematous swellings with pustulation which lead to the development of indurated plaques with undermined edges and areas of ulceration (*Fig.* 14.10).

Dermatitis Herpetiformis

This is a pruritic eruption consisting of attacks of erythematous wheals usually with blisters, affecting the skin of the elbows and extensor forearms, knees, shoulders, sacrum and scalp. More commonly seen in adult males, it tends to last for a number of years, and is usually adequately controlled by dapsone (diamino-diphenyl-sulphone) and occurs as a result of disturbance of immune mechanisms, deposits of IgA being present at the dermo-epidermal junction. It is frequently associated with coeliac disease and malabsorption.

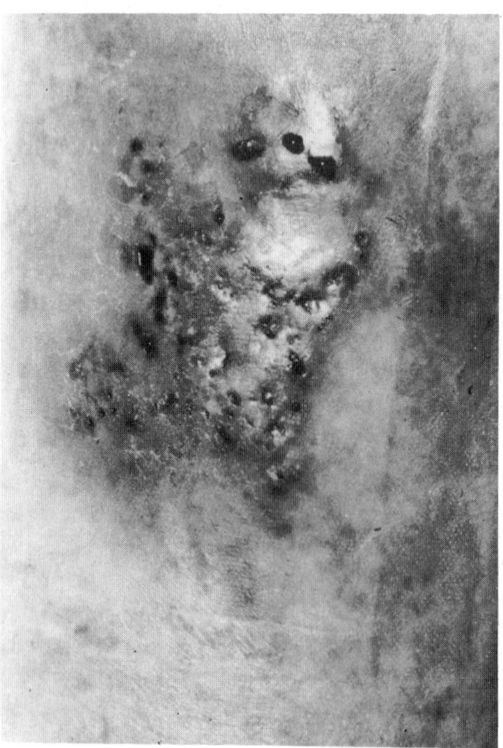

Fig. 14.10 Pyoderma gangrenosum. Epithelial proliferation with multiple necrotic ulceration and both the involvement in the skin and the gut have been shown to benefit from a gluten-free diet.

Acrodermatitis Enteropathica

This is a recessively inherited disorder which presents in infancy with an erythematous eruption with vesicles, pustules and crusting, with secondary candida infection affecting particularly the skin around the mouth and anogenital region, fingers and scalp; there is an associated diarrhoea and alopecia. It is due to zinc deficiency probably as a result of a defect of gastrointestinal zinc absorption, although an abnormality yet to be defined may be common to both the bowel and the skin.

Behçet's Syndrome

In this condition recurrent ulcers appear both on the buccal mucosa and genitalia and may be associated with cutaneous lesions resembling erythema nodosum and with superficial migratory thrombophlebitis. Along with affection of the cardiac, respiratory and central nervous systems, gastrointestinal ulceration may occur.

Hereditary Haemorrhagic Telangiectasis (Weber–Osler Disease)

This is discussed in Chapters 29 and 73.

Blue Rubber-bleb Naevus Syndrome

Consists of rubbery, compressible, blue subcutaneous nodules appearing especially in the skin of the limbs and trunk as a special form of cavernous haemangioma. They are associated with similar lesions in the gastrointestinal tract which may be responsible for melaena.

Malignant Atrophic Papulosis (Degos's Syndrome)

This condition is rare and consists of the development of crops of pink dome-shaped papules which subsequently develop an atrophic porcelain white centre as a cutaneous manifestation of an endovasculitis which also affects the gastrointestinal tract leading to abdominal cramps, vomiting and enteritis, and ultimately haemorrhage, perforation and peritonitis.

Henoch–Schönlein Syndrome (Anaphylactoid Purpura)

This is a manifestation of leucocytoblastic vasculitis; it affects children and young adults with a purpuric eruption which may be initially an urticarial erythema and occurs particularly on the skin of the lower extremities and buttocks but may also affect the trunk, arms and face. There is frequently joint pain and renal and abdominal complications, the latter being associated with colic, haemorrhage and intussusception (*see* Chapter 73).

Kaposi's Sarcoma (Multiple Idiopathic Haemorrhagic Sarcoma)

This is characterized by the presence in the skin (particularly of the distal parts of the lower limbs) of bluish red nodules and pigmentation, leading to lymphoedema and perhaps ulceration. Other parts of the skin may be affected as may other organs including the gastrointestinal tract, leading to haemorrhage and melaena. Ultimately, a reticulosis may develop. Kaposi's sarcoma presents as a manifestation of AIDS. The morphological features are quite unlike the classic form. They tend to be widespread and multiple affecting any skin or mucosal site. Early lesions are small, reddish brown to purple, simulating a bruise. Early lesions therefore provide diagnostic problems.

Pseudoxanthoma Elasticum

This condition is both a recessive and dominantly inherited

abnormality of elastic fibres which results in cutaneous lesions, retinal changes in the form of angioid streaks and changes in the blood vessels which may lead to cardiovascular problems and because of involvement of the arteries of the gastric mucosa, to gastrointestinal haemorrhage. The lesions of the skin which are most commonly found on the sides of the neck, axillae and groin consist of soft, yellowish papules in confluent plaques in a skin which appears soft, lax and wrinkled.

Ehlers–Danlos Syndrome

This condition is both dominantly and recessively inherited and consists of a connective-tissue defect which leads to fragility of the skin and blood vessels as a result of which the skin is hyperelastic and some joints hyperextensible. As with pseudoxanthoma elasticum, gastrointestinal haemorrhage may occur.

ENDOCRINE DISEASE AND THE SKIN

Pituitary

In acromegaly the skin is coarse, greasy, pigmented and thickened, along with hypertrichosis, whereas in hypopituitarism there is hypopigmentation and thinning of the skin and loss of sexual hair. In addition, there are the characteristic and diagnostic cutaneous features of Cushing's syndrome with striae, hirsuties, pigmentation, acne and purpura, with a tendency to develop chronic fungal infection due to *Trichophyton rubrum* or *Tinea versicolor.*

Thyroid

In hyperthyroidism the skin is warm and sweating and there may be a complaint of irritation with an increased incidence of alopecia areata and vitiligo, and a tendency to scalp hair fall of the telogen effluvium type. Pigmentary changes are variable. Pretibial myxoedema (*Fig.* 14.11) occurs in association with thyrotoxicosis, usually following treatment, in the form of thickened waxy plaques with prominent hair follicles situated over the anterior aspect of the lower legs resulting from the accumulation of acid mucopolysaccharide in the dermis. In hypothyroidism (myxoedema) on the other hand, the skin is dry, pale, coarse and swollen, with loss of scalp and eyebrow hair.

Adrenals

In addition to the pigmentation of Addison's disease, which is widespread but often accentuated on exposed skin and at sites of friction, there are the changes of adrenal virilism to be considered such as hirsuties, acne and male pattern baldness.

Diabetes Mellitus

Certain skin conditions are associated with the development of diabetes such as infection, particularly with candida, and later ischaemic changes; also, vitiligo, xanthomatosis, necrobiosis lipoidica and diabetic dermopathy.

In necrobiosis lipoidica there develops a thickened plaque which is yellowish in colour in the centre and violaceous at the periphery, gradually becoming atrophic with telangiectases and a tendency to ulcerate. Most commonly seen on the shins it can appear on other parts of the legs and in the skin elsewhere. In diabetic dermopathy red papules or small nodules develop on the skin of the lower legs which may ulcerate to leave small depressed scars and pigmentation.

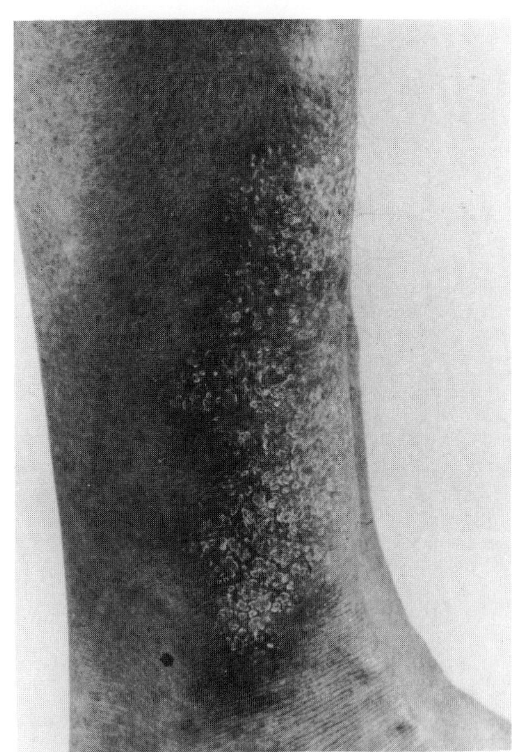

Fig. 14.11 Pretibial myxoedema. A thickened waxy plaque with prominent hair follicles, most commonly seen over the anterior aspects of the lower legs.

METABOLIC ABNORMALITIES AND THE SKIN

Porphyria

In hepatic porphyria, porphyria variegata, congenital erythropoietic porphyria and erythropoietic protoporphyria, abnormal amounts of porphyrins accumulate in the skin which then combine with light to produce certain characteristic cutaneous changes. In hepatic porphyria there is increased skin fragility (*Fig.* 14.12*a*) with blisters, milia (*Fig.* 14.12*b*), scarring and hyperpigmentation, increased growth of hair, and in more severe cases, sclerodermatous changes. In the rare congenital erythropoietic porphyria the destruction of tissue is that much greater. In erythropoietic protoporphyria on the other hand, particularly as it presents in the UK, the symptoms are often greater than the signs in that there is complaint of severe discomfort and often pain in the exposed skin associated with swelling which may be minimal, leading to thickening of the skin particularly over the knuckles, with accentuated skin lines and fine linear scarring on the face.

Hyperlipidaemia

In disturbances of lipid metabolism various forms of xanthomas may be seen in the skin. Plane xanthomas, as xanthelasma, occur on the eyelids or in the palmar creases or sides of neck or trunk and are to be found in association with Types II, III and IV hyperlipidaemia. The tuberous xanthomas (*Fig.* 14.13), on the other hand, appear as raised nodules over the extensor aspects of joints and on the buttocks and are associated with Types II and III hyperlipidaemia. They may show a particular predilection for extensor tendons (tendinous xanthomas) such as those

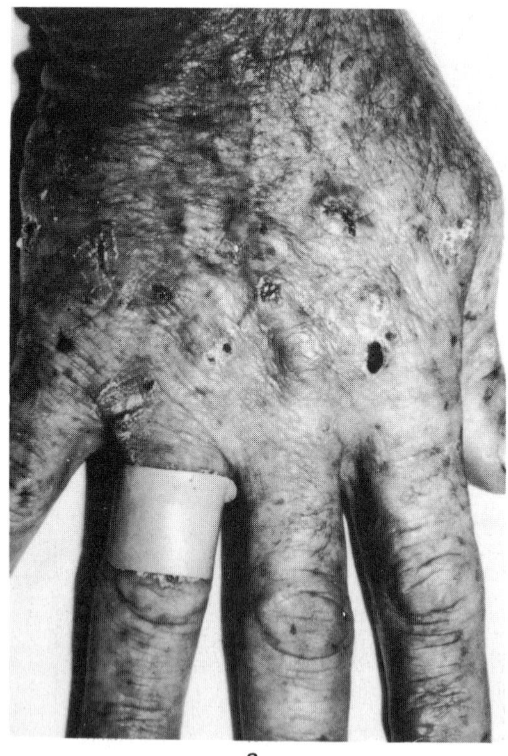

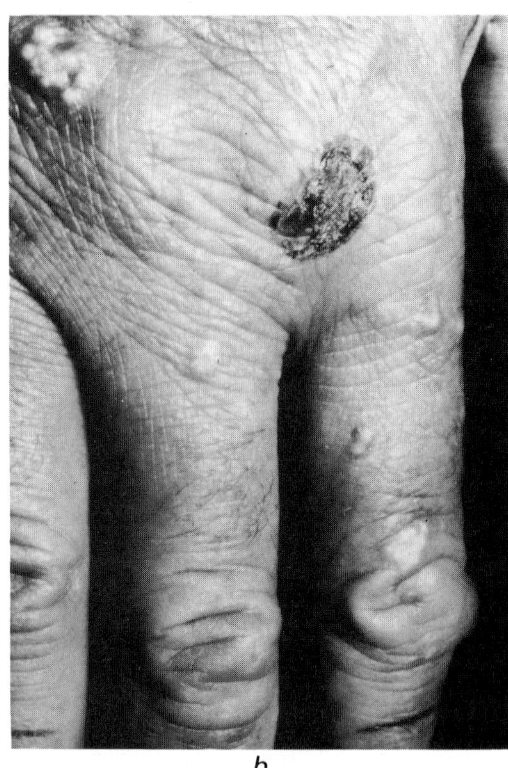

Fig. 14.12 Hepatic porphyria. Changes resulting from increased fragility of the skin (*a*); blister formation and multiple milia (*b*).

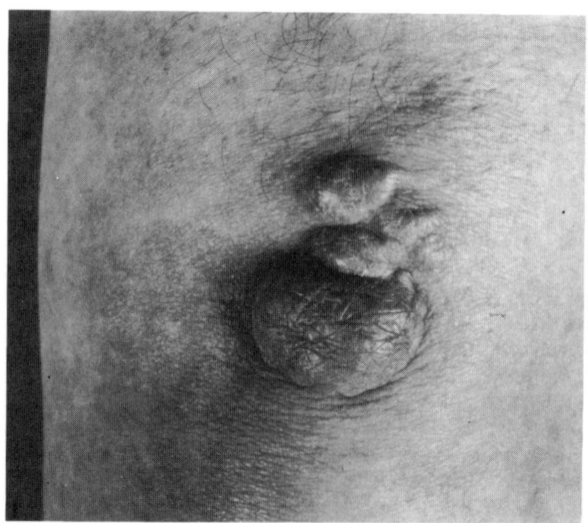

Fig. 14.13 Cutaneous xanthoma. Yellow or orange coloured nodules in the skin of the elbow.

over the knuckles and around the elbows and in this instance are associated with Types II and III hyperlipidaemia. In the eruptive xanthomas there is sudden rapid development in the skin of smaller yellow papules associated with diabetes and Types I, II, III and IV hyperlipidaemia.

Other Metabolic Disorders

The conditions resulting from disorders of amino acid metabolism are rare, such as alkaptonuria, Hartnup's disease, etc., but most have cutaneous changes which, although not always diagnostic, draw attention to the possibility of such metabolic errors.

CUTANEOUS VASCULITIS

A number of conditions with both cutaneous and systemic affections are due to inflammatory reactions of the blood vessels and reference has already been made to examples of these, such as Henoch–Schönlein purpura, erythema multiforma, erythema nodosum and erythema induratum. Also, there are polyarteritis nodosa and granulomatosis vasculitis in the form of Wegener's granulomatosis and temporal arteritis, all of which may have extensive involvement of other systems additional to the changes seen in the skin. The inability to determine specific causal factors makes classification of the 'vasculitis' difficult.

Lupus erythematosus, dermatomyositis and scleroderma can be grouped together as collagen-vascular disorders. In lupus erythematosus the reaction may be confined to the skin (*Fig.* 14.14) or as the acute systemic form which involves many of the body systems. In scleroderma there is once again a cutaneous form called morphoea as well as systemic scleroderma. The latter often presents as Raynaud's phenomenon which may be the only manifestation for some years to be followed by the sclerodermatous tightening and atrophy of the skin of the fingers and hands, also noticeable on the face, particularly around the mouth, perhaps with the development of numerous spider angiomas. Involvement of the oesophagus leads soon to dysphagia. Additional symptoms arise depending on the severity of the affection of other systems.

CUTANEOUS MANIFESTATIONS OF MALIGNANCY

Certain cutaneous signs and symptoms suggest the possibility of underlying malignant disease. Direct invasion by malignant cells, as in Paget's disease or secondary cutaneous metastases from a distant primary cancer, are referred to later. Skin haemorrhage in the form of purpura, petechiae and ecchymosis may occur in leukaemia and the dysproteinaemias. In generalized pruritus or a chronic widespread idiopathic pruritic eruption (although in the majority of instances it will be found to be benign and unconnected with systemic disease), systemic malignancy must always be excluded. Persistent severe infection of the skin, to which the leukaemia patient is particularly prone, may be manifested by viral infection (herpes simplex and herpes zoster), chronic candidiasis, systemic fungal infection or chronic boils. Increased viscosity may present as Raynaud's phenomenon or erythromelalgia. In addition, there are a number of more specific skin conditions (skin markers) which when present raise the possibility of systemic malignancy.

These are:

Acanthosis nigricans
Dermatomyositis
Acquired ichthyosis
Acquired hypertrichosis lanuginosa ('malignant down')
Pachydermoperiostosis
Exfoliative dermatitis/erythroderma
Bowen's disease
Erythemas: erythema gyratum repens/glucagonoma syndrome
Arsenical keratosis/pigmentation/basal-cell epithelioma
Reticulohistiocytoma
Carcinoid
Palmoplantar keratoderma (Howell–Evans syndrome)
Gardner's syndrome
Peutz–Jeghers' syndrome
Thrombophlebitis migrans
Multiple seborrhoeic keratosis (Leser Trélat)
Others

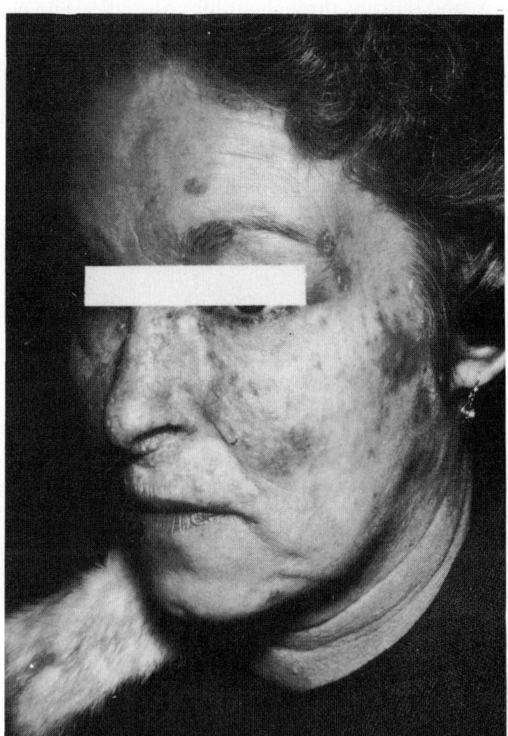

Fig. 14.14 Chronic cutaneous lupus erythematosus. Chronic patches of persistent erythema, telangiectasia, follicular plugging and scarring.

Acanthosis Nigricans

In this condition, which is greyish-brown or black in colour, a roughness of the skin develops with thickening and accentuation of the skin lines. It affects particularly the axillae but may also appear on the back, groins (*Fig.* 14.15), umbilicus and nipples. A less marked benign form presents in early childhood and similar changes again less marked can be seen in the flexures of certain dark complexioned obese individuals (pseudo-acanthosis nigricans). Its appearance therefore in a non-obese adult, particularly if also affecting the palms and mouth, strongly suggests associated malignancy, particularly of the gastrointestinal tract.

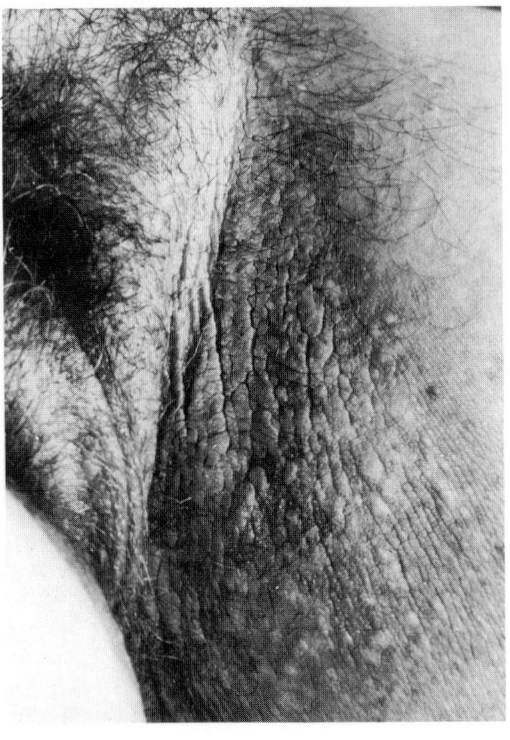

Fig. 14.15 Acanthosis nigricans. Thickening of the skin which is brown or black in colour, with accentuation of the skin lines.

Dermatomyositis

This is an inflammatory condition of the skin and the muscles associated with malignancy in 30% or more of affected subjects. The myositis element may be minimal or undetectable but when present consists of aching and weakness of the muscles leading to difficulty in sitting up in bed or climbing stairs. There is often erythema and oedema of the face, particularly around the eyes, with a purplish-red heliotrope colour. Elsewhere there is an affection particularly of light-exposed areas with erythema, telangiectasis and atrophy. On the hands there is often periungal telangiectasis with scaly lesions over the knuckles.

Acquired Ichthyosis

Dryness of the skin (mild ichthyosis; xeroderma) is common and not infrequently associated with atopy and as such is benign, and remains throughout life. Also in certain elderly subjects the skin becomes dry and itchy with advancing years. Very rarely, however, an adult will suddenly develop widespread dry scaling of the skin, often with an element of increased pigmentation which may be associated with a reticulosis and particularly Hodgkin's disease.

Acquired Hypertrichosis Lanuginosa ('Malignant Down')

This is very rare and manifests as a sudden appearance of fluffy lanugo hair, particularly on the face, ears and upper trunk.

Pachydermoperiostosis

May be primary and as such a rare inherited developmental defect. In secondary pachydermoperiostosis the affection of the skin and the bones can be due to an underlying malignant tumour, most often a bronchogenic carcinoma. The skin of the ears, lips and tongue may become enlarged and thickened with increased folding of the scalp (cutis verticis gyrata) in association with clubbing of the fingers and toes and painful subperiosteal new bone formation of the tibia, radius and phalanges. There may also be palmar and plantar hyperkeratosis and hyperhidrosis.

Exfoliative Dermatitis/Erythroderma

Universal skin changes either in the form of dermatitis or persistent scaly erythema and oedema (erythroderma) may be due to a reticulosis which should be suspected once the more common causes, such as contact allergic sensitivity or drug-induced reaction, have been excluded.

Bowen's Disease

When this form of intraepidermal epithelioma appears on exposed skin it is probably due to long-term UVR exposure. When, however, it is noted on covered areas, and particularly if multiple, then previous ingestion of inorganic arsenic is a possibility. There may also be an associated tendency to develop malignancy of one or more systems and particularly the respiratory, gastrointestinal or genito-urinary systems.

Erythemas

The relationship between the erythemas and systemic disease has already been referred to. In one of these, erythema gyratum repens, the erythema reaction moves slowly over the body surface producing a pattern resembling the grain of wood. It is particularly associated with malignant disease of the breast and lung.

Necrolytic Migratory Erythema (Glucagonoma Syndrome) (Fig. 14.16)

The eruption is in the form of a figurate erythema with superficial blisters spreading out from the skin of the perineum over the lower abdomen and buttocks. It is due to a glucagon-secreting tumour of the alpha cells of the pancreas.

Arsenical Keratosis/Pigmentation and Basal-cell Carcinomas

Previous ingestion of inorganic arsenic may lead to the development of small hard keratoses on the palms and soles in association with 'raindrop' pigmentation and the appearance of multiple basal-cell carcinoma on both exposed and covered skin. These cutaneous changes draw attention to the necessity for the investigation of other systems for the presence of malignant change.

Reticulohistiocytoma

In this rare condition firm, brown-yellowish nodules develop in the skin of the face, ears and fingers, in association with arthritis which may be severe and mutilating.

Carcinoid Syndromes

These are discussed in Chapter 73.

Palmoplantar Keratoderma (Howell–Evans Syndrome)

This is usually a benign thickening of the skin of the palms and soles (tylosis) arising as a result of a dominantly inherited trait or due to external physical factors in predisposed individuals. However, it has also been reported in association with oesophageal carcinoma in the members of two families.

Gardner's Syndrome

In this syndrome there is an association between multiple

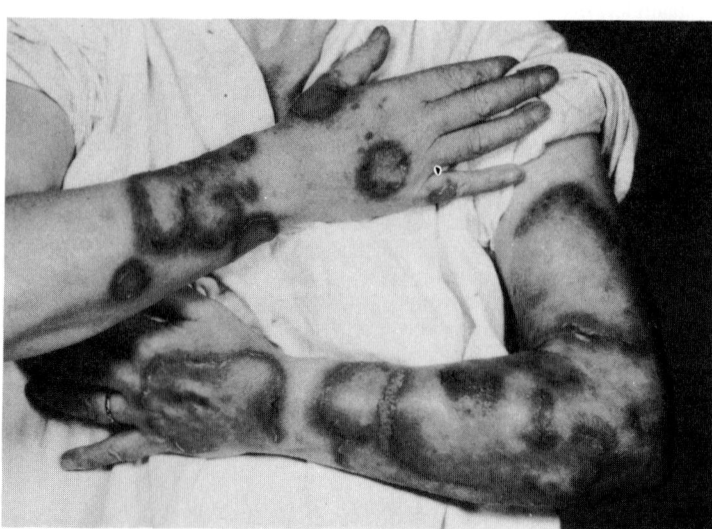

Fig. 14.16 Necrolytic migratory erythema (glucagonoma syndrome). Figurate erythema with superficial blistering.

Table 14.2 Benign and malignant tumours of the skin

Based on Sanderson K. V. and Mackie Rona (1980) Tumours of the skin. In: Rook A., Wilkinson D. S. and Ebling F. J. E. (ed.) *Textbook of Dermatology*, 3rd ed. Ch. 66. Oxford, Blackwell.

The term tumour is used in the broad context of a swelling.

Superficial benign epithelial tumours
- Verrucous naevus
- Naevus comedonicus
- Naevus sebaceus
- Seborrhoeic keratosis
- Stucco keratosis
- Skin tag
- Acquired digital fibrokeratoma
- Intra-epidermal epithelioma (Borst–Jadassohn)
- Harber's syndrome
- Clear-cell acanthoma
- Kerato-acanthoma
- Pseudo-epitheliomatous hyperplasia—seen in margin of chronic ulcers and chronic cutaneous TB

Hair follicle tumours
- Trichofolliculoma
- Inverted follicular keratosis
- Tricholemmoma
- Tricho-epithelioma
- Multiple eruptive milia
- Pilomatrixoma
- Trichogenic adnexal tumour
- Trichodiscoma

Sebaceous gland tumour
- Naevus sebaceus
- Senile sebaceous hyperplasia
- 'Sebaceous' cyst
- Steatocystoma multiplex
- Sebaceous adenoma
- Sebaceous carcinoma

Cysts of the skin
- Keratinous cyst
  - Epidermoid
  - Tricholemmal
- Dermoid
- Milium
- Steatocystoma multiplex
- Eccrine hidrocystoma
- Apocrine hidrocystoma
- Bartholin's cyst
- Myxoid cyst of the skin
- Branchial cyst

Sweat gland tumours
- Syringoma
- Eccrine hidrocystoma
- Eccrine acrospiroma
- Eccrine hidradenoma
- Syringo cystadenoma papilliferum
- Hidradenoma papilliferum
- Erosive adenomatosis of the nipple
- Apocrine hidrocystoma
- Nodular apocrine hidradenoma
- Dermal cylindroma
- Spiradenoma
- Adenoid cystic carcinoma of skin
- Hidradenocarcinoma

Premalignant conditions
- Solar keratosis
- Disseminated superficial actinic porokeratosis
- Cutaneous horn
- Bowen's disease
- Multicentric pigmented Bowen's disease
- Intra-epidermal carcinoma of the eyelid margin
- Arsenical keratosis
- Erythroplasia of Queyrat
- Leucoplakia
- Leucokeratosis of the lips
- Post-irradiation keratoses
- Tar keratoses

Basal-cell tumours
- Basal-cell naevus
- Premalignant fibro-epithelial tumour (Pinkus)
- Basal-cell carcinoma

Squamous-cell carcinoma

Paget's disease of the nipple

Extramammary Paget's disease

Metastatic malignant tumours

Melanocyte tumours
- Lentigo
- Melanocytic naevi
  - Common forms
    - Junctional
    - Compound
    - Intradermal
  - Special forms
    - Oculocutaneous
    - Sutton's naevus
    - Pigmented hypertrichotic
    - Congenital
- Neurocutaneous melanosis
- Juvenile melanoma
- Dermal melanocytosis
  - Mongolian spot
  - Blue naevus
  - Ota's naevus
- Melanotic freckle
- Precancerous melanosis
- Malignant melanoma

Fibrous tissue tumours
- Dermatofibroma (histiocytoma)
- Disseminated dermatofibroma
- Keloids and hypertrophic scars
- Nodular fasciitis
- Elastofibroma
- Juvenile fibromatosis
- Fibrous hamartoma of infancy
- Desmoid tumour
- Dermatofibrosarcoma protuberans
- Fibrosarcoma
- Epithelibid sarcoma
- Pseudosarcoma

Blood vessel tumours
- Granuloma telangiectaticum
- Glomus tumour
- Multiple progressive angioma
- Haemangiopericytoma
- Kaposi's sarcoma—AIDS related
- Lymphangiosarcoma of Stewart and Treves
- Malignant angio-endothelioma
- Diffuse malignant proliferation of vascular endothelium

Nerve and nerve sheath tumours
- Neuroma cutis
- Neurofibromatosis
- Neurofibroma
- Neurolemmoma
- Neurofibrosarcoma
- Cutaneous meningioma

Leiomyoma

Leiomyosarcoma

Osteoma cutis

Crostis lymphoma

Merkel cell tumours

sebaceous cysts, polyposis of the colon, dental abnormalities, osteomas of facial bones and skin fibromas, with a tendency for malignant changes to develop in the intestinal polypi.

Peutz–Jeghers' Syndrome

This is discussed in Chapter 73.

The appearance of radiodermatitis, e.g. following X-ray irradiation of cavernous haemangiomas of the skin of the neck may indicate subsequent malignant change in an underlying structure, such as the thyroid gland.

BENIGN AND MALIGNANT TUMOURS OF THE SKIN

It is important to recognize with confidence the relatively small number of benign or malignant tumours which are most commonly seen.

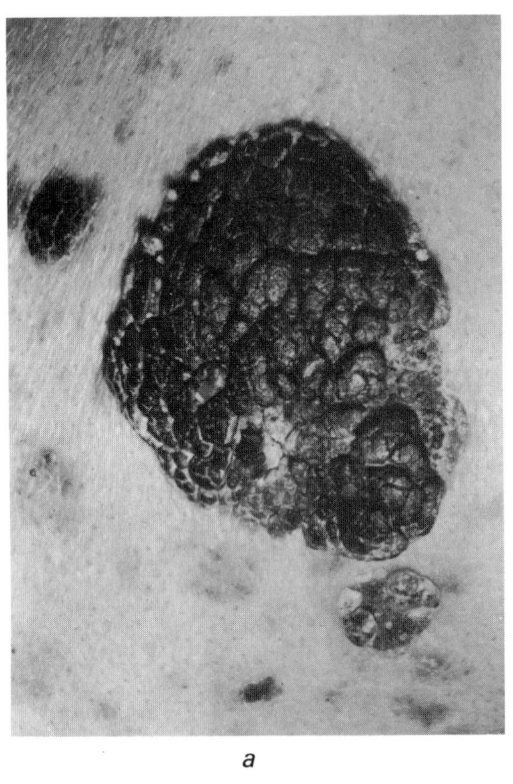

a

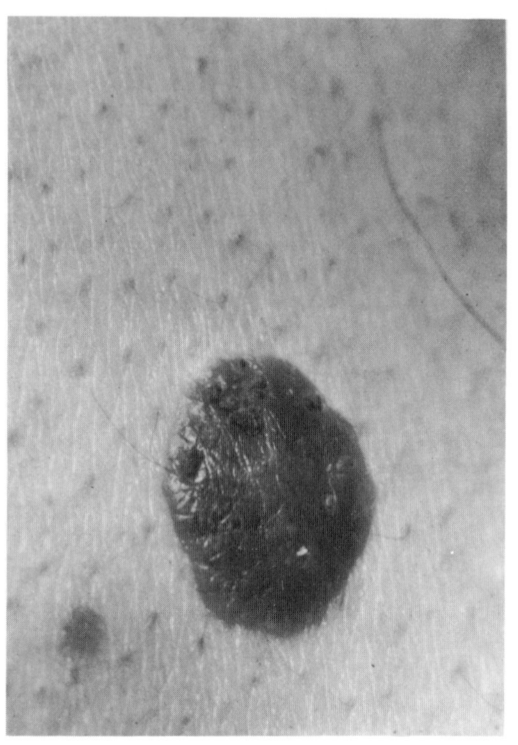

b

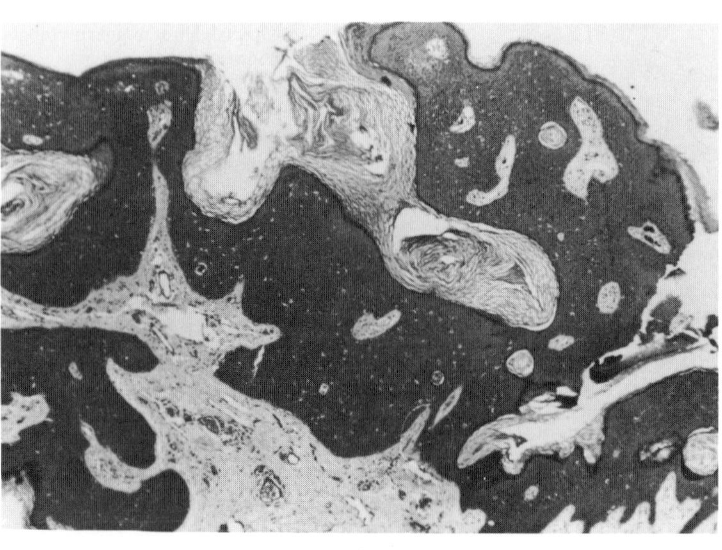

c

Fig. 14.17 Seborrhoeic keratoses. Variable-sized stuck-on warty plaques (*a*); sometimes the lesion is more smooth surfaced and less warty with keratin plugs to be seen in the follicular orifices (*b*). *c*, The closely packed, dark staining, basiloid cells of this superficial tumour are associated with tortuous, keratin-filled cysts which extend from the surface into the tumour mass and mimic keratin cysts when cross-sectioned.

The ability to diagnose these on clinical grounds alone helps to avoid unnecessary treatment of benign lesions and also allows for decisions to be made with regard to treatment and prognosis without the prior necessity for biopsy. It is also possible to make a clinical diagnosis with many of the other tumours listed in *Table* 14.2 but this may not always be possible on morphological grounds alone and histological studies are necessary before a definitive label can be attached.

Seborrhoeic Keratoses, Skin Tags

Considered to be dominantly inherited, seborrhoeic keratoses are often numerous, affecting both sexes equally, increasing in number from middle age onwards. They range in size from a few mm to 2–3 cm, and from small, flat, yellowish spots to large, warty plaques which appear stuck on to the skin (*Fig.* 14.17*a*). Some examples are, however, smooth-surfaced and domed but with follicular orifices which contain keratin plugs (*Fig.* 14.17*b*). They are commonly seen on sebaceous gland containing sites. They tend to be pedunculated and not keratotic when seen around the eyes or in the body flexures. Skin tags are related to, if not a form of, seborrhoeic keratosis and are commonly seen on the skin of the neck and trunk particularly in middle-aged women. A profuse eruption of seborrhoeic keratosis may follow a dermatosis, such as dermatitis, and may rarely be a cutaneous manifestation of systemic malignancy.

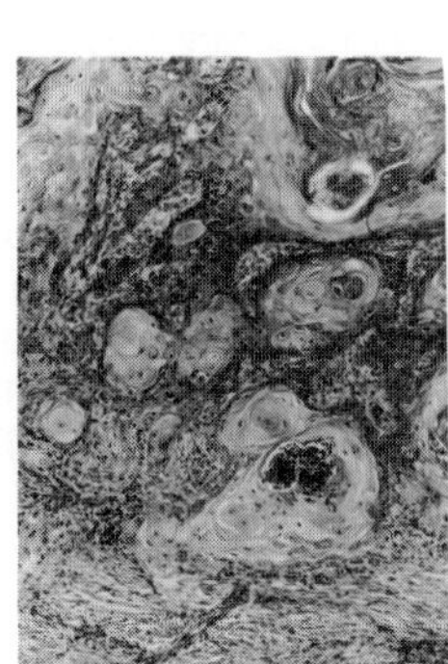

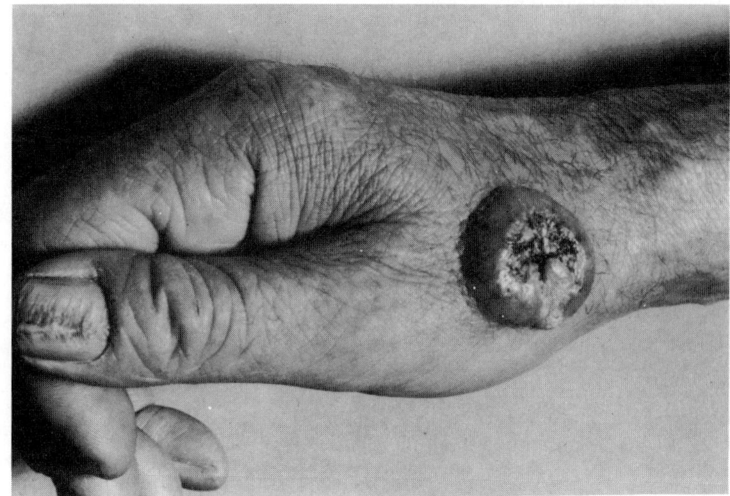

a

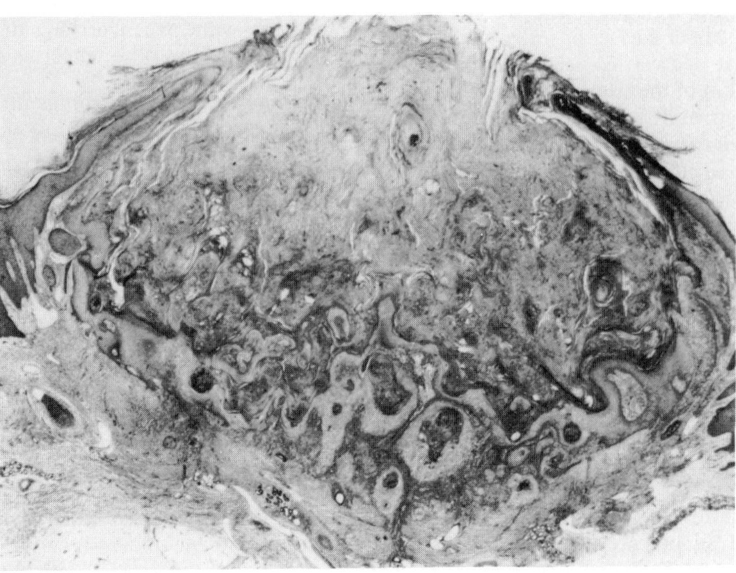

b

Fig. 14.18 *a*, Kerato-acanthoma. Enlarging flesh-coloured nodule with central keratin plug. *b*, The cytological details of this lesion are essentially the same as in a keratinizing squamous carcinoma but sagittal section of the whole lesion plus the short clinical history may permit a firm diagnosis. The magnified insert (*a*) shows detail of the lower edge of the lesion where large keratinal cells are invaded by polymorphs.

Kerato-acanthoma

A relatively common benign tumour usually of the exposed skin of males in particular and of the middle-aged and elderly. It seems likely that cutaneous carcinogens such as UVR and tar can be aetiological factors as may also infection in association with minor skin injuries.

It originates from pilosebaceous follicles, starting as a skin-coloured or reddish papule which soon rapidly enlarges reaching its maximum in about 4 weeks when it presents as a variable-sized (usually 1–2 cm diameter) fleshy smooth nodule usually with some telangiectasis and a central keratin-filled crater. Having reached its maximum size spontaneous resolution then takes place usually over the next 3 months by means of a gradual increase in the central keratin plug in parallel with flattening of the surrounding fleshy circumference to leave a puckered crenated scar. This natural history may vary, with the total duration being that of many months or with recurrence after curettage or excision or apparent resolution (*Fig.* 14.18).

Epidermal or Epithelial Naevi

These are localized developmental defects of the epidermis and its adnexal structures, such as the sebaceous and apocrine sweat glands and the hair follicles. They tend to be defects of predominantly one or other structure and thus the major component usually determines the distinctive clinical appearances. In the verrucous naevi (naevus unius lateralis) there is excessive development of the epidermis. In the *sebaceous naevus*, as the name implies, the sebaceous gland dysplasia predominates resulting in the development of a slightly raised yellow or yellowish-brown plaque, usually present at birth and commonly found in the scalp and neighbouring skin of the forehead, temple and around the ears. Basal-cell carcinoma develops in 20% and therefore prophylactic excision is indicated. In *naevus syringocystadenoma papilliferum* the defect involves the apocrine gland, most commonly presenting as a plaque with a papillomatous and warty surface on the skin of the face or scalp, where part of the lesion may be that of cicatricial alopecia. It is less commonly seen on the skin of the trunk and limbs. Malignant change may develop in 10%, usually basal-cell carcinoma but squamous-cell carcinoma has been reported.

In some middle-aged and elderly subjects, so-called senile sebaceous hyperplasia occurs in the form of yellowish, rounded papules, symmetrically distributed over the skin of the forehead and temples. Although the term 'sebaceous adenoma' is also used for these papules, it can refer to a single lesion, once again most commonly found on the face or scalp, and consisting of a collection of incompletely differentiated sebaceous cells.

Cysts

The term 'sebaceous cyst' is often misused for all common cysts of the skin and particularly those seen on the scalp. Preferably, however, it should be confined to those cysts seen in steatocystoma multiplex (an hereditary autosomal dominant disorder) and all other cysts arising from the pilosebaceous follicle should be referred to as keratinous cysts of either epidermoid or pilar type in which the former only has a lining identical with the stratification of the epidermis. The differences in histological features are illustrated in *Fig.* 14.19. The epidermoid cyst is a dome-shaped swelling usually skin-coloured but yellowish if the cyst is near the surface and freely movable over the underlying structures. It can be single but is more often multiple, and is found especially in the skin of the face, neck, shoulders, chest, scrotum or scalp. They are usually fixed to the epidermis; there may be a central keratin-filled punctum. The majority of epidermal cysts arise from retained secretions but some follow trauma and are due to implantation of epidermis into the deeper tissues (implantation dermoid). Congenital dermoid cysts are not uncommon in the skin and subcutaneous tissues and occur in embryonic cleavage lines. They are lined by squamous epithelium and may contain tissues arising from the embryonic germ layers.

With the pilar cyst there is frequently a family history with an autosomal dominant pattern of inheritance and a tendency to be restricted to one area, such as the scalp. All cutaneous cysts can and often become secondarily infected and patients often present with this complication when the treatment is surgical evaluation. Elective excision of the cyst is often required to prevent recurrence of the infection. The indication for removal of cutaneous cysts is commonly for cosmetic reasons but some have a high nuisance value especially those on the scalp. Unless the cyst wall is removed completely recurrence is inevitable.

Milia

Milia are small subepidermal cysts which are composed of lamellated keratin, and are usually white but may be yellowish in colour, lying immediately beneath the epidermis and particularly seen on the skin of the face. Sometimes they can be diagnostically useful in that they can be a sequelae of a bullous eruption and as such may be seen in the exposed skin of the face and backs of the hands in hepatic porphyria.

Histiocytoma (Dermatofibroma)

This is a common benign tumour usually affecting the skin of the limbs, particularly in the female. It consists of a single but occasionally multiple, small, firm nodule which is attached to the epidermis, freely movable over the underlying tissues, with a colour range from pink or red to brown and ivory-white when of long duration. It is thought to follow insect bites or other forms of minor trauma.

Dermatofibrosarcoma Protuberans

This is a tumour arising from fibroblasts which is locally malignant, affecting the sexes equally and thought sometimes to follow trauma. Most commonly found on the trunk and the flexures, it presents usually in early adult life as a dermal nodule or nodules which are skin-coloured or red, which coalesce as the lesion grows to form a plaque with irregular protuberant swellings. Spread to regional lymph glands is rare and metastases are very uncommon.

Keloid

This condition is best considered as a complication of healing in a skin wound. It is commonly encountered in dark-skinned races and can cause extreme unsightliness which is particularly distressing to female patients. The keloid consists of a mass of fibrous tissue covered by an attenuated and densely adherent epidermis and is prone to recur particularly after total excision. Treatment is by subtotal excision through the outermost limit of the lesion with meticulous suture of the skin edges and topical steroid injection, although the efficacy of the latter in preventing recurrence has not been proven. However, the local injection of triamcinolone at the early immature stage is often followed by reduction in size or complete flattening (*see* Chapter 1). Keloids are said to respond to topical or intralesional steroid providing this is administered within 6 months of the onset of the keloid.

Desmoid Tumour

This is a slow growing fibrous tumour which arises usually in the muscle walls of the anterior abdominal wall but may affect the pelvic or axillary regions. The natural history of the tumour has not been established although there are reported instances when the desmoid tumour was observed to be locally invasive. Treatment is by adequate local excision. Recurrence is common and may necessitate extensive surgery, such as hemipelvectomy for pelvic lesions causing severe pain from involvement of nerves by the tumour.

Ganglion

This is strictly speaking a subcutaneous swelling. There is still controversy with regard to the aetiology of these cystic lesions. Although they are often considered as degenerative lesions, others maintain that ganglia are benign tumours of tendon sheath or joint capsule. The cyst which may be uni- or multilocular contains a glairy clear viscous fluid and the cyst wall is composed of fibrous tissue without a true endothelial lining. Often the ganglion is attached at some point to a joint capsule but there is no communication between the interior of the cyst and the joint cavity or the tendon sheath.

Ganglia occur most commonly on the dorsum of the wrist of adults but may be found in the palm, fingers, ankles and foot. Usually they are painless but occasionally the patient complains of discomfort and slight pain. A deeply situated ganglion in the wrist or palm may cause median or ulnar nerve compression with the development of motor and

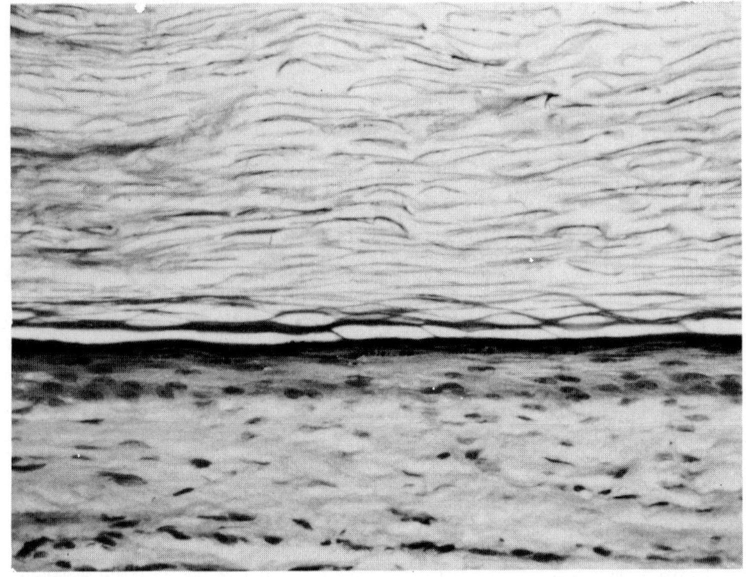

a

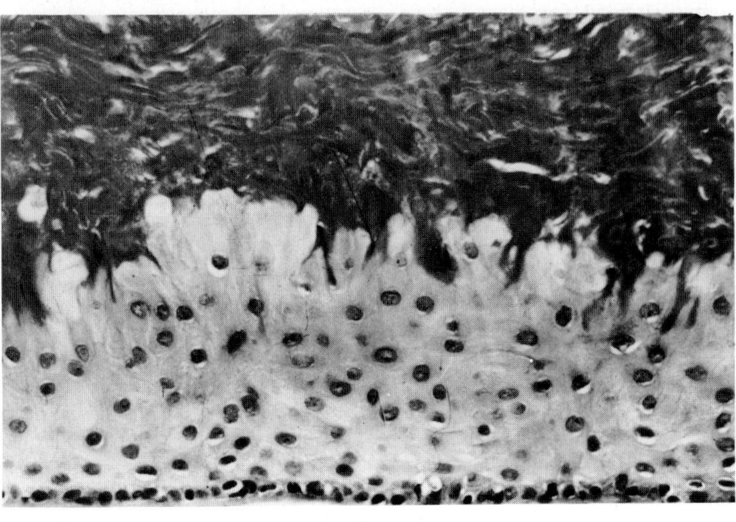

b

Fig. 14.19 *a*, The compressed wall of an epidermal cyst produces compact layered keratin through a granular layer as in normal epidermis. *b*, The wall of a pilar cyst produces a more amorphous type of keratin from swollen hair follicle cells. No granular layer is present.

sensory impairment. Treatment of ganglia is by excision which can be difficult and requires to be complete if recurrence is to be avoided.

Lipoma

This ubiquitous tumour is composed of fat cells, indistinguishable from those of normal adipose tissue, and is commonly encountered in the subcutaneous plane most commonly of the back, shoulders and upper arm. Lipomas are usually localized, lobulated and encapsulated by a thin fibrous capsule and are often observed to dimple when displaced laterally through the overlying skin. Most constitute soft fluctuant subcutaneous swelling although in some the fibrous stroma is more pronounced, resulting in a firmer consistency (fibrolipoma). Other sites of occurrence include the submucosal layer of the intestinal tract (when they may become pedunculated and initiate an intussusception), inter- and intramuscular compartments, subperiosteal region and extradural space.

Diffuse lipomas are less frequently encountered. These are not encapsulated and are typically found in the neck. Dercum's disease is a rare condition of diffuse overgrowth of adipose tissue occurring in menopausal women, usually affecting one of the limbs. The diffuse adipose thickening is tender and for this reason the condition is also known as 'adiposis dolorosa'.

The treatment of lipomas is by local excision.

Calcifying Epithelioma of Malherbe (Pilomatrixoma)

This peculiar benign tumour, usually of the face or upper limbs, consists of a hard well-defined spherical fibrous lesion located in the dermis or subcutaneous layer surrounding a calcified core which often causes a crackling sensation on compression of the tumour. Treatment is by local excision.

Neurofibroma

A neurofibroma may be solitary but when multiple (neurofibromatosis, Von Recklinghausen's disease) it is dominantly inherited and commonly associated with multiple café-au-lait spots. The single lesion is usually first seen in adult life and multiple neurofibromatosis in later childhood or early adolescence; they arise from peripheral nerves and their supporting structures, and may be associated with renal, endocrine and skeletal abnormalities.

Leiomyoma

Leiomyomas arise from smooth muscle in the form of variable-sized dermal nodules, red or brown in colour, most often seen in the trunk, and are subject to pain which may be precipitated by touch, temperature change, or emotional disturbances.

Cutaneous Haemangioma

These hamartomatous lesions include the capillary angioma ('port-wine-stain') which is the commonest birth mark and the *cavernous angioma* ('strawberry mark'). The latter may be present at birth but does not usually appear until a few weeks later, first as a small red macule which slowly increases in size to reach the final strawberry shape and appearance at about 6 months of age (*Fig.* 14.20). Most commonly affecting females, it remains usually unchanged, perhaps increasing in size with the growth of the child, and then starts to resolve spontaneously with the appearance of pale areas, and increasing flaccidity, 60% having disappeared by the third year and most of the remainder by 6–7 years of age. Treatment is usually not required. Superficial ulceration or bleeding may rarely occur and the former may lead to a less satisfactory cosmetic result. Extensive angiomas of this type can be associated with thrombocytopenia and surgical excision is then indicated, if feasible.

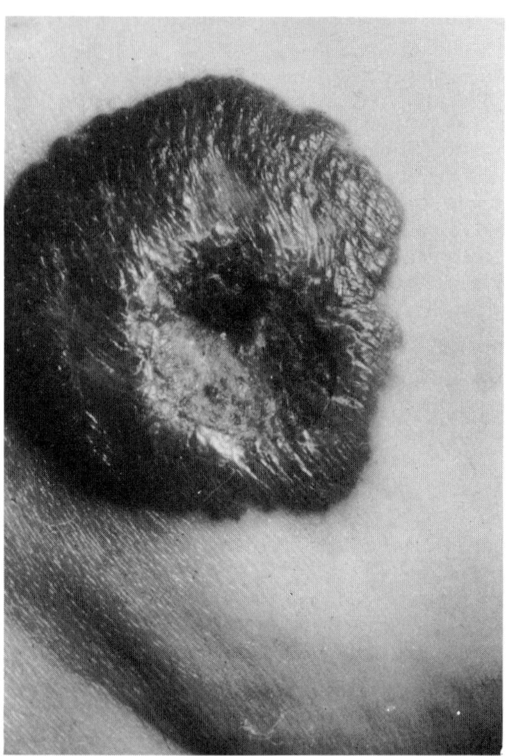

Fig. 14.20 Cutaneous haemangioma (strawberry mark). Reddish, well-demarcated lesion showing evidence of early spontaneous resolution.

There is a rare variant of cavernous haemangioma affecting usually the lower limbs and consisting of a diffuse arteriovenous malformation which involves the various muscular compartments and leads to an overgrowth of the limb. Extensive varicose veins and varicose ulcers develop in time. The massive blood flow through the affected limbs results in a hyperkinetic circulation and cardiac enlargement. Surgical treatment is difficult and local excision of the malformation is often impossible. Amputation is often resorted to.

Glomus Tumour

The glomus tumour consisting of vascular channels surrounded by glomus cells and nerve fibres, is a relatively uncommon, usually single, painful pink or purple nodule, most commonly seen on the extremities. In a subungual situation the pain can be severe leading usually to earlier diagnosis and treatment. Sometimes multiple, when the tumours are then found to be deeper in the dermis, bluish and usually not painful.

Cutaneous Lymphangioma

The most commonly seen form of lymphangioma is lymphangioma circumscriptum which appears as a group of small deeply situated vesicles in which there may be a vascular component (haemolymphangioma). It can be associated with disorders of the main lymphatic vessels. Surgical excision is often followed by recurrence.

Lymphangiosarcoma of Stewart and Treves is a malignant tumour of vascular endothelium occurring in association with postmastectomy lymphoedema and presenting as dusky blue nodules.

Granuloma Telangiectaticum (Pyogenic Granuloma)

This is a commonly seen nodule made up of proliferating capillaries, often following trauma, and usually rapidly growing. It occurs in both sexes and at any age, and is usually reddish in colour and ulcerates and bleeds easily; it may be pedunculated. Situated most often on the skin of the hands and feet, and particularly on fingers or toes, but may appear elsewhere on the face, trunk and limbs. It does not usually disappear spontaneously and therefore requires preferably to be excised, although curettage and diathermy may be successful.

Mastocytosis

Mastocytosis, which is characterized by an erythematous or pigmented papular eruption, may be purely cutaneous with localized and generalized forms or systemic with infiltration of internal organs. Involvement of the gastrointestinal tract may result in nausea, vomiting, abdominal pain and diarrhoea. Patients with systemic involvement may rarely develop mast-cell leukaemia or other malignancies.

Premalignant Changes

In the production of such changes it is no longer sufficient to consider environmental sunshine exposure in view of the current widespread use of artificial sources of irradiation in solaria and with sunbeds and also of phototherapy and in particular photochemotherapy in the treatment of psoriasis.

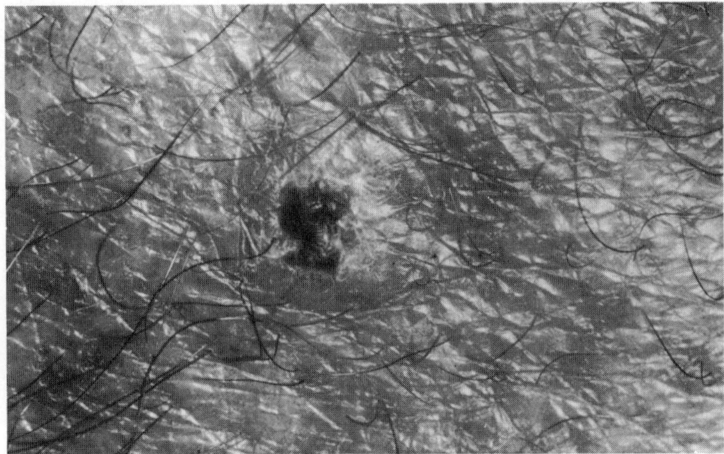

a

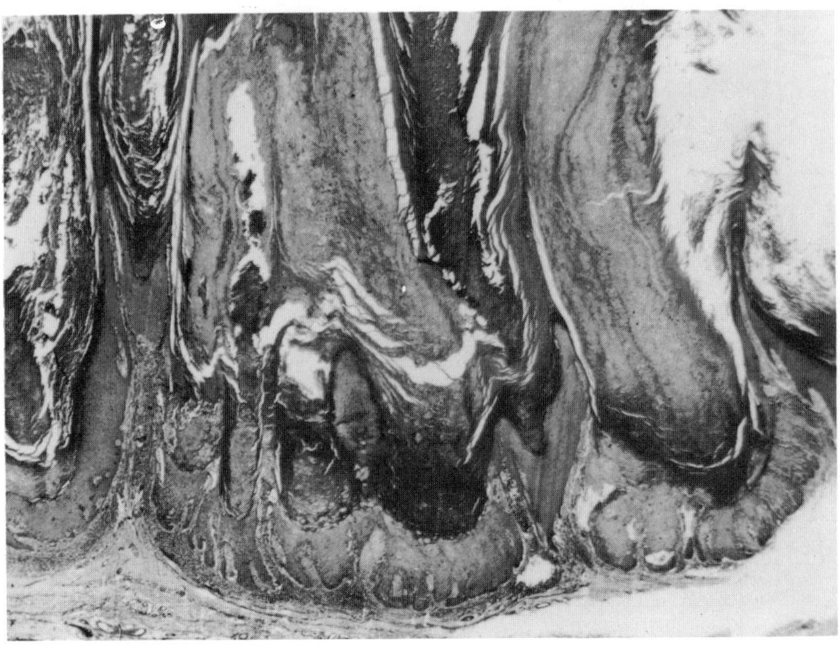

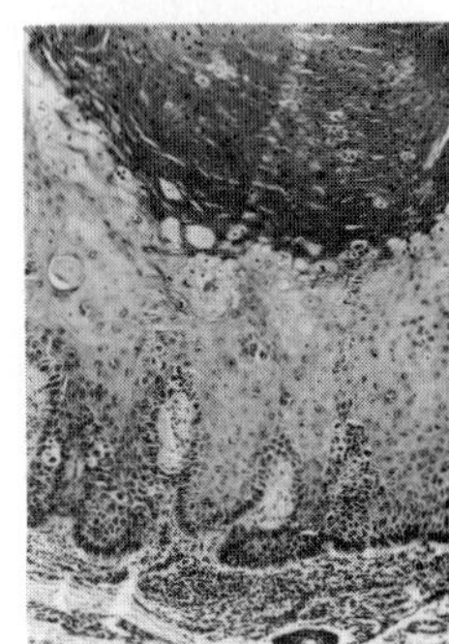

b

Fig. 14.21 *a*, Solar keratosis. *b*, This example shows a horny mass of alternating orthokeratotic and parakeratotic cells above an acanthotic epidermis which in the magnified insert on the right can be seen to consist of dark staining active cells in the basal zone and bizarre keratinized cells replacing the spinous and granular layers.

Skin ages mainly as a result of the accumulated effect of UVR exposure leading eventually to premalignant changes in the form of dryness, loss of elasticity, and patchy hypopigmentation and hyperpigmentation, haemorrhages (senile purpura), and ultimately localized areas of abnormal keratin formation (early solar keratosis). The solar keratosis is thus most commonly seen on exposed skin sites, such as the backs of hands, rim of ears, and the face, and in the older age groups, but is seen earlier in those with fair complexion and of Celtic origin, and in particular if resident for any length of time in a part of the world with greater amounts of sunshine than their country of birth. It is an irregular, crusted lesion which may be flat or raised, with variable horn formation, and on the face often appears as rough,

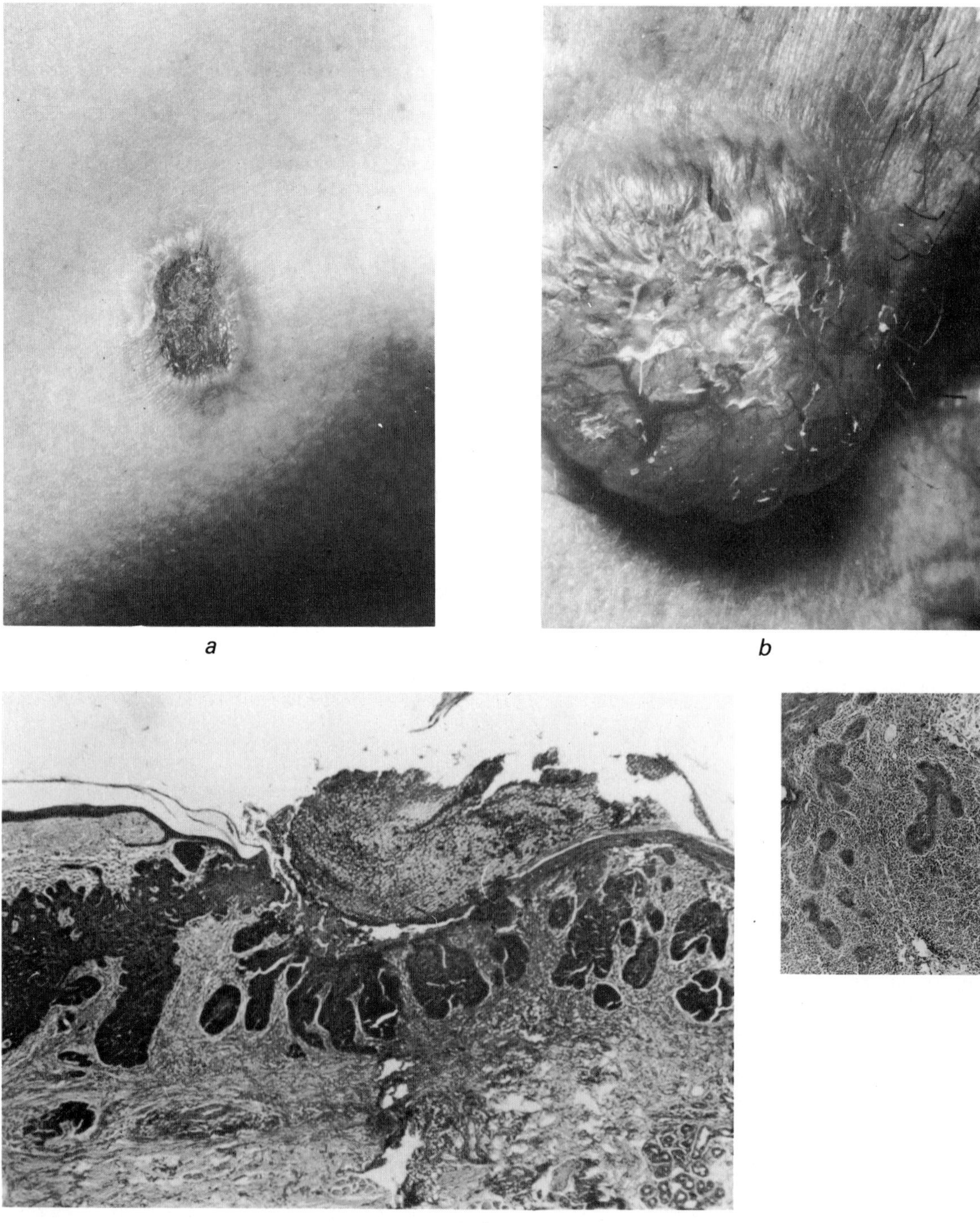

Fig. 14.22 *a*, Basal-cell epithelioma (rodent ulcer). Central ulceration with pearly border with surface telangiectasis. *b*, Cystic basal-cell epithelioma. Cystic-looking nodule with surface telangiectasia and pearly border. *c*, Columns of dark staining basal cells penetrate into the dermis and spread out below the epidermis at the edge of elevated centre which is covered by a thick crust. In higher magnification palisading of cells at the edge of the tumour masses is present.

yellow or dirty brown scaly plaques (*Fig.* 14.21). It is potentially malignant but frequently fails to progress towards squamous-cell carcinoma in the life time of the affected subject. Similar UV ageing of the lips, especially the lower lip, is much more likely to lead to squamous-cell carcinoma as is the leucoplakia of the buccal mucosa. Carcinogens additional to UVR, such as tar, inorganic arsenic, ionizing radiation, radiant heat and chronic skin ulceration, may all lead eventually to malignant change. The development of squamous-cell carcinoma should be suspected when the lesion becomes indurated and feels firm on palpation with the induration appearing to extend beyond the visual margin of the lesion; in time the central keratotic crust is shed to produce either central ulceration or an otherwise eroded induration margin with perhaps a purulent exudate in the base.

Intra-epidermal Epithelioma (Carcinoma)

As seen in Bowen's disease this forms scaly, sometimes erythematous plaques, most commonly appearing on the skin of the trunk. The lesions are often multiple, slow growing and their slightly raised margin is sharply demarcated from the neighbouring normal skin. Another example of intra-epidermal carcinoma is Paget's disease of the nipple, although in this instance it is in fact a cutaneous extension of an intraduct carcinoma (*see* Chapter 60).

Basal-cell Carcinoma

Developing from the basal cells, this is the commonest malignant tumour of the skin. It is locally destructive but rarely metastasizing. Basal-cell carcinoma is more common in males after the age of 40 years and occurs predominantly on the upper and central parts of the face. Exposure to UV light and/or some modifications of the cells of an adnexal structure are considered to play a part in the development of this type of tumour. Starting usually as a small translucent papule, it goes on to develop a number of different forms. Basal-cell carcinoma may be solitary or multiple. The nodulo-ulcerative form is that most commonly seen (*Fig.* 14.22*a*), but the lesion may be pigmented, cystic (*Fig.* 14.22*b*), superficial and morphoeic. It is usually slow growing. The possibility of local invasion becomes important when the tumour is located in the skin around the eyes, nose or ears.

Treatment of basal carcinoma is either by surgical excision (with primary closure or skin grafting) or radiotherapy and equally good results are obtained by either. Surgery is preferable when the lesion is adjacent to cartilaginous structures and radiotherapy is the treatment of choice when the extent and site of the lesion would necessitate extensive plastic surgical reconstruction and in the frail and elderly patient. Several other treatment modalities have been used: cryodestruction, topical chemotherapy (5-fluorouracil), chemical cautery (zinc chloride paste) etc. Recurrence after treatment is rare and most such instances represent new lesions.

There is also Moh's Chemosurgery which is a technique developed in North America which has become established there for the control at light microscopic level of the excision of tumours where the edge of the lesion is clinically indistinct. In the main, this applies to a small number of carefully selected basal-cell carcinomas. The technique involves serial horizontal excisions of the lesions with histological examination by frozen section of the undersurface of each layer. This process is continued until the area is confirmed to be cancer-free when mercurochrome is applied and the wound left to heal by secondary intention.

Squamous-cell Carcinoma (*Fig.* 14.23)

This is a more aggressive tumour than basal-cell carcinoma and may spread especially to regional lymph nodes and sometimes further afield. Squamous-cell carcinoma occurs in sites exposed to UV radiation and some 75% of cases are confined to the head (ears, temples and lips). The other common sites are the dorsum of the hand and the perianal margin. The lesion may assume several macroscopic forms from a fleshy fungating lesion to a hard punched-out ulcer with an indurated base. Squamous-cell carcinoma is the usual type of neoplasm that develops in irradiated skin, around old chronic sinuses, scars and ulcers (Marjolin ulcer).

The treatment of squamous-cell carcinoma is along the lines described for basal-cell lesions. There is still controversy, however, regarding the management of cases (usually in the head and neck) presenting with associated enlargement of the regional lymph nodes. Individual biopsy of these nodes is inadvisable as it obviates the benefits of block dissection. Some advocate primary block dissection at the time of excision of the primary. Others favour a period of observation (3–4 weeks) after excision of the primary lesion and proceed to block dissections if the lymphadenopathy does not regress.

Melanocytic Naevi

The lentigo is a common brown or dark brown macule, usually, but not necessarily, first seen in childhood, permanent, but sometimes fading with the passage of the years. The majority do not show transition towards a junctional melanocytic naevus although this can occur in childhood.

The melanocytic naevus is common, often first seen in childhood, and increasing in number throughout life with a reduction in old age. It appears in a variety of forms (*Fig.* 14.24), the term 'junctional' being used when the proliferation of naevus cells is confined to the epidermal/dermal junction (*Fig.* 14.25*b*) in comparison with the 'dermal' form where collections of cells are seen only in the dermis and 'compound' when both sites are involved (*Fig.* 14.25*c*). These are benign lesions although malignant melanoma may rarely develop and especially in the junctional form. The congenital pigmented naevus, which is present at birth (*Fig.* 14.26) may affect extensive areas of the skin and has a greater potential for malignant change.

Malignant Melanoma

Incidence

There has been a remarkable rise in incidence of and mortality from melanoma in all white populations surveyed since 1955. This increase has averaged 5% each year during this period. In a number of countries, e.g. North America, Australia, UK, Scandinavian countries, etc., melanoma has been shown to occur more frequently in communities living close to the equator. Thus, the highest incidence is found in Queensland, Australia (40 new cases/100 000 per annum). In England and Wales the incidence now averages 10 new cases/100 000 as opposed to 5/100 000 new cases annually in Scotland. In the UK, melanoma is now commoner than Hodgkin's disease and although it is still far less frequent than other skin cancers, e.g. squamous-cell carcinoma, it accounts for the majority of deaths due to cutaneous malignancy.

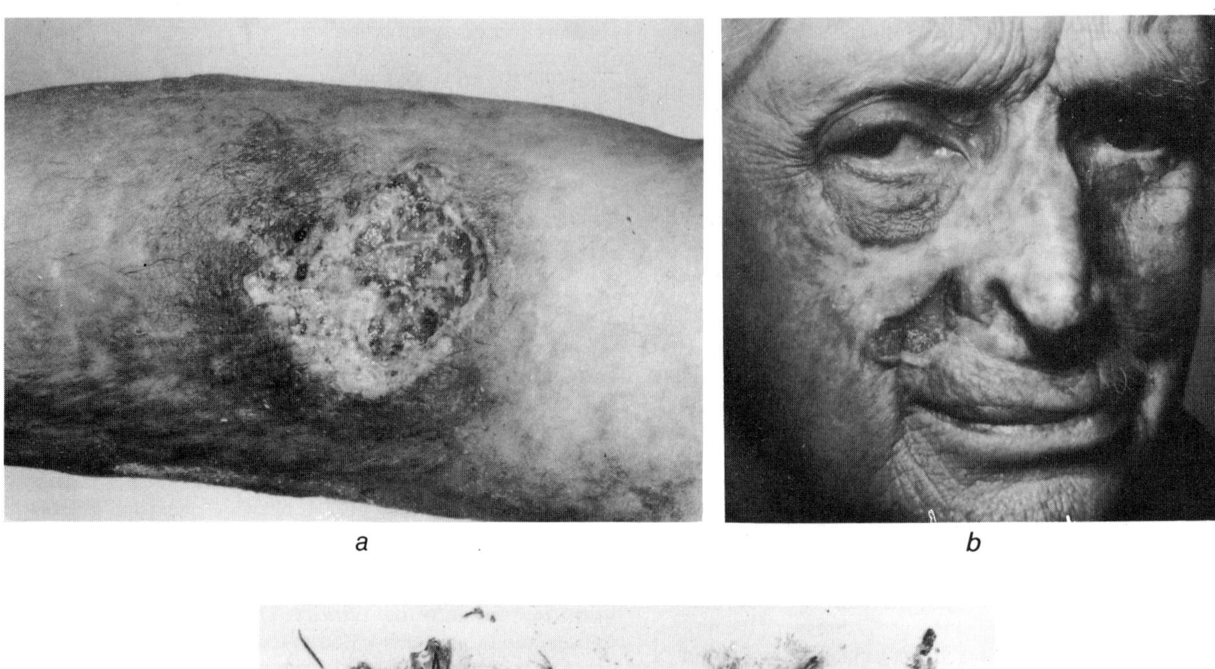

a b

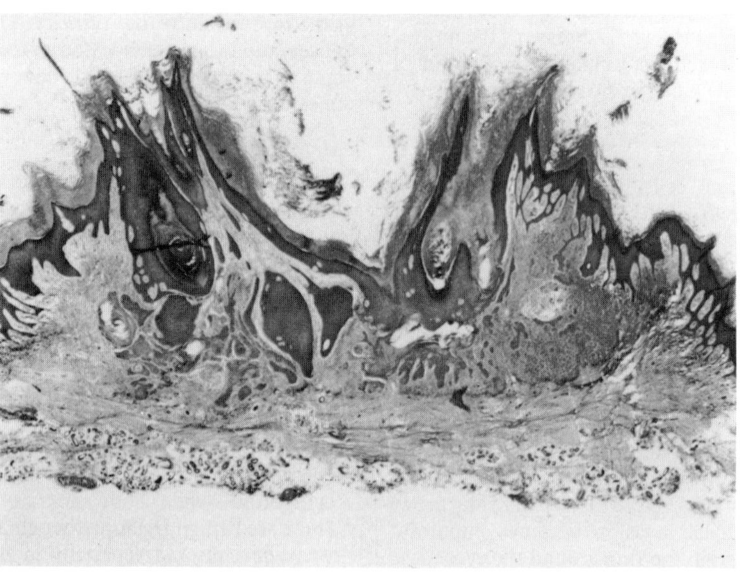

c

Fig. 14.23 Squamous-cell carcinoma. *a*, Chronic indurated ulcer with thickened rolled edge. *b*, Squamous-cell carcinoma in a patient with lupus vulgaris. *c*, The epidermis shows papillomatosis and columns of dysplastic squamous cells penetrate deep into the dermis.

Aetiology

The aetiology of melanoma remains speculative. The association with chronic exposure to sunlight (ultraviolet light) is not as direct and clear cut as with squamous-cell carcinoma. Melanoma tends to develop in fair-skinned individuals who tan poorly and get easily sunburnt. The current thinking suggests that short bursts of heavy exposure to sunlight may act as the promoting agent and are more important than chronic gradual exposure which may, indeed be protective by inducing a sun tan. A recent report demonstrated a high incidence of melanoma in office workers exposed to fluorescent light. This requires confirmation as the amount of radiation in the *total* ultraviolet range from these lamps is small. Whereas the increasing use of sunbeds to achieve a skin tan is likely to be followed by a rise in the incidence of squamous-cell carcinoma, it is not known whether it predisposes to melanoma. Some argue that the tan acquired in this way may be protective by preventing acute sunburn in these individuals.

Genetic factors are important. The disease is common amongst individuals of the Celtic race and there is a family history in 3–6% of patients. In some cases there is a familial history of abnormal naevi and, more rarely, the dysplastic naevus syndrome.

In Western countries, melanoma is more common in social class I. Hormonal factors may be operative as indicated by the presence of oestrogen and progesterone receptors in some melanomas and the higher incidence of the disease during the reproductive period in women.

Pathology

Five clinicopathological types of melanoma are recognized,

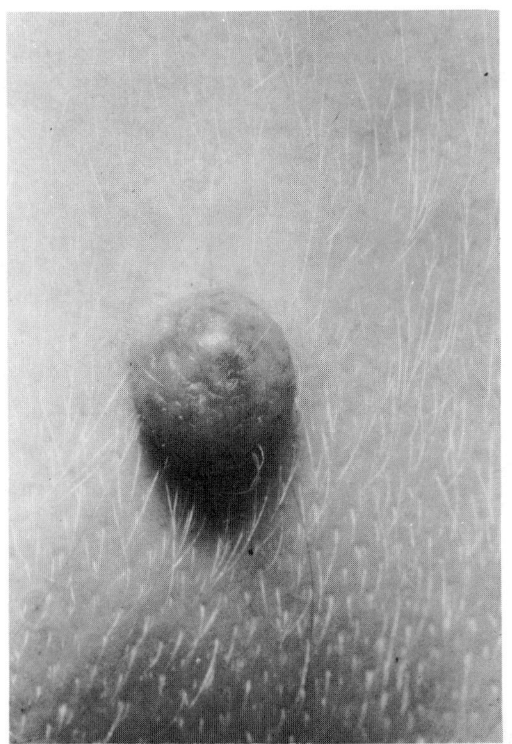

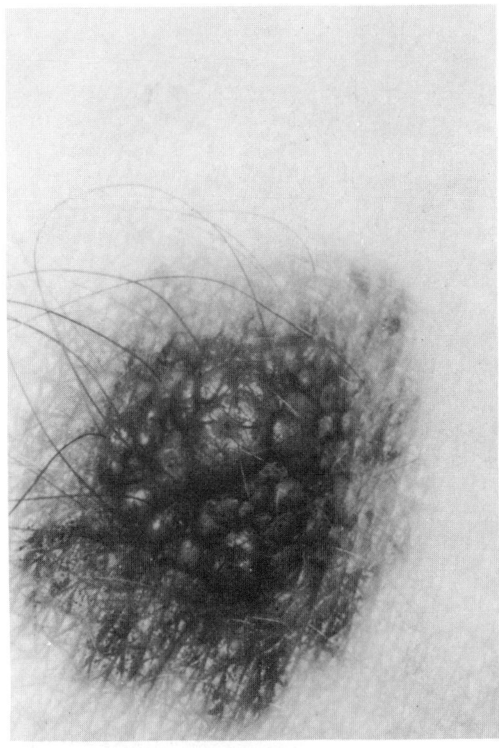

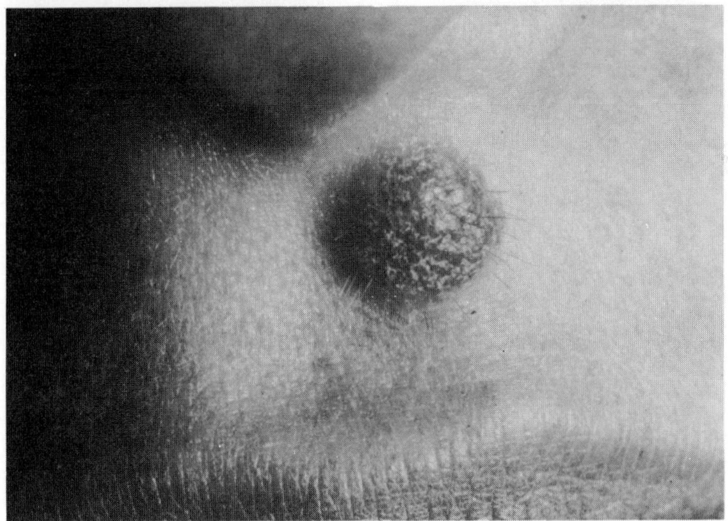

Fig. 14.24 Melanocytic naevi. Some common forms of this benign tumour.

four of which are cutaneous:

- Malignant lentigo (lentigo maligna, Hutchinson's melanotic freckle)
- Acral lentiginous melanoma
- Superficial spreading melanoma
- Nodular melanoma
- Mucosal melanoma

The superficial spreading melanoma commonly arises in pre-existing moles (cirça 30%).

MALIGNANT LENTIGO. (*Fig.* 14.27 *a-b*) This is considered by some to be a distinct disease from the other cutaneous melanomas since its epidemiological features are similar to those of squamous-cell carcinoma in that there is an association with chronic exposure to sunlight. Pathologically, the tumour is confined to the epidermis. It most commonly affects the skin of the face or back of the hand of middle-aged and elderly subjects presenting in the form of a flat brown to dark brown patch, which may be slightly raised with some colour variation in different parts and an irregular margin. Slowly growing, it carries an excellent prognosis after local excision. Untreated, it may change to a more aggressive and invasive tumour, such a development being manifested by pigmentary changes and eventually localized nodule formation (*Fig.* 14.27*c*). It accounts for 6–11% of all melanomas in white races.

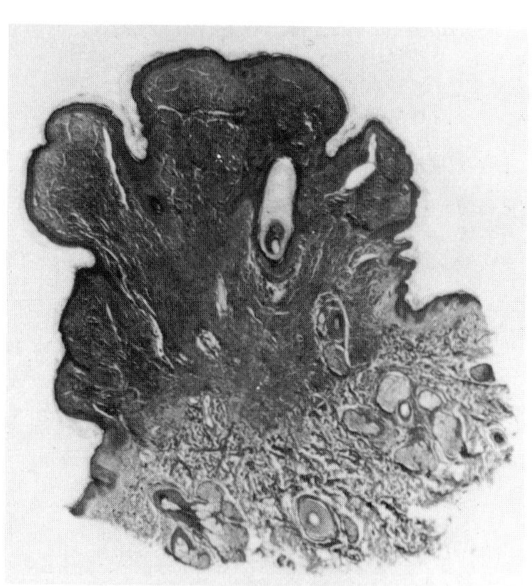

a

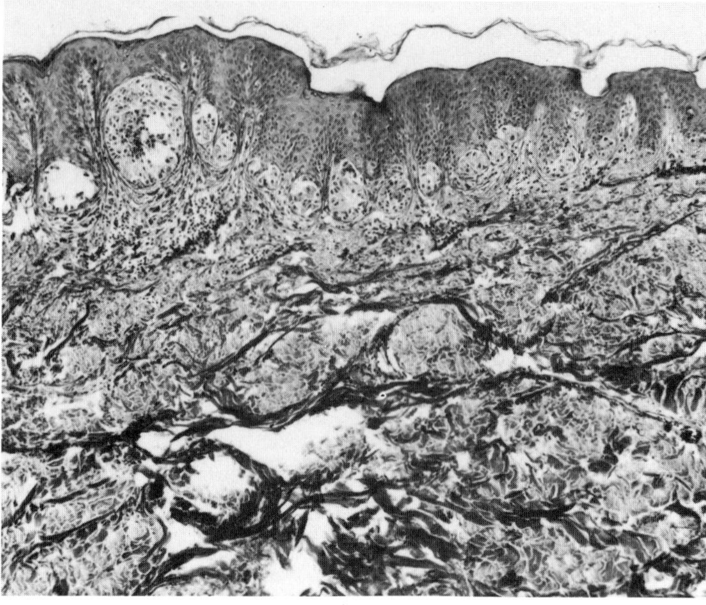

b

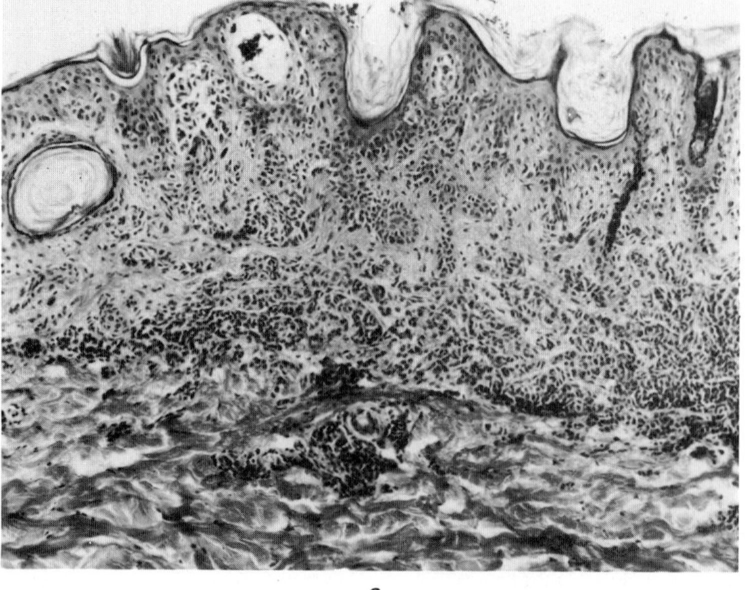

c

Fig. 14.25 *a*, Intradermal melano-naevus. In this papillomatous lesion no naevus cells remain within the epidermis but the dermis is packed with columns of naevus cells which tend to become spindle shaped in the deeper areas then disappear completely in the lower dermis. *b*, Junctional naevus. The naevus cells are arranged in orderly pockets along the lower margin of the epidermis. *c*, Compound naevus. In addition to the pockets of naevus cells within the epidermis, columns of polygonal naevus cells are present in the upper dermis.

ACRAL LENTIGINOUS MELANOMA. This develops in the nail bed and on the palmar surface of the hands and plantar aspect of the feet. It forms a flat/brown black macular lesion and when it occurs beneath the nail, it can be mistaken for a subungual haematoma. It is the clinicopathological type which affects black people when they develop melanoma. When diagnosed, they are usually thick lesions and carry a poor prognosis. It is the rarest form of melanoma in white individuals, accounting for 0·6–1% of cases.

SUPERFICIAL SPREADING MELANOMA. This is the commonest reported clinicopathological type (65%). This melanoma spreads horizontally for a varying period before growth occurs in a vertical direction with the formation of nodules and ulceration. It affects any part of the body and is usually seen in the 4th to 5th decade as a pigmented lesion which has been growing slowly over a number of months or years, which then becomes mildly itching or sore and exhibits deepening pigmentation and an inflammatory reaction related to the advancing irregular edge (*Fig.* 14.27*d,e*). The lesion may have depigmented areas, usually near the centre. The lesion is usually greater than 0·5 cm at the time of diagnosis and is then palpable with distinct nodules within it. Superficial spreading melanoma has a better prognosis than the nodular variety (*vide infra*). However, this is not the result of any intrinsic difference in the biological aggressiveness between the two types, but is simply a reflection of the thickness of the lesion, the nodular type being generally thicker and therefore more advanced. There are no survival differences between superficial spreading and nodular melanomas of the same measured thickness.

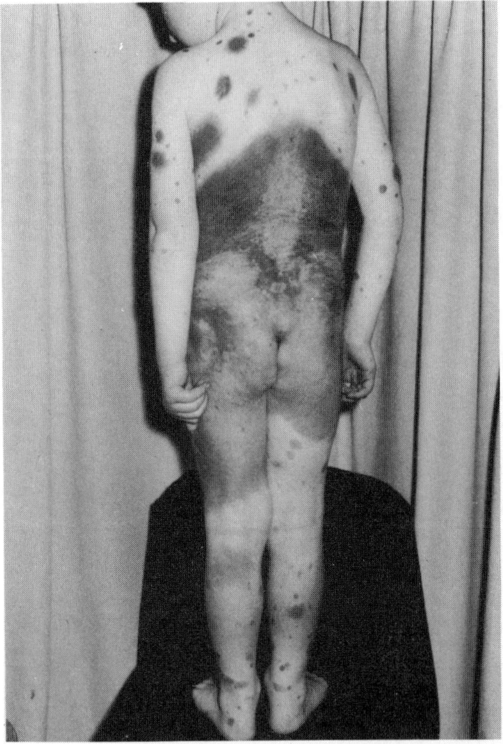

Fig. 14.26 Congenital pigmented naevus.

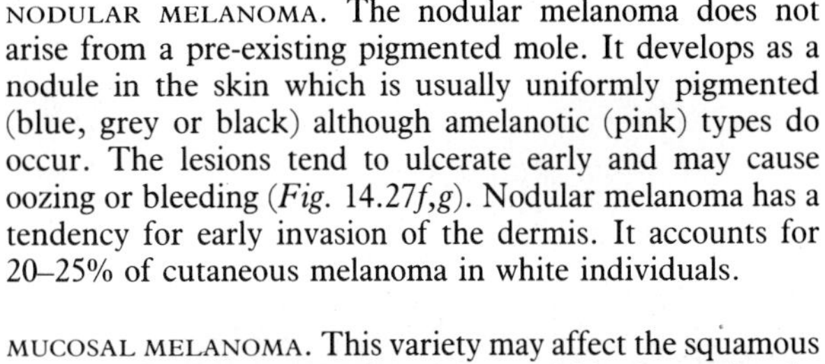

NODULAR MELANOMA. The nodular melanoma does not arise from a pre-existing pigmented mole. It develops as a nodule in the skin which is usually uniformly pigmented (blue, grey or black) although amelanotic (pink) types do occur. The lesions tend to ulcerate early and may cause oozing or bleeding (*Fig.* 14.27*f,g*). Nodular melanoma has a tendency for early invasion of the dermis. It accounts for 20–25% of cutaneous melanoma in white individuals.

MUCOSAL MELANOMA. This variety may affect the squamous mucosa of the anorectum, vagina and labia. It carries the worst prognosis and disseminates early.

Microstaging of Melanoma

This was introduced by Breslow and forms a reliable indicator of prognosis and affects the local management of the disease. The thickness of the lesion is measured in millimetres. The initial microstaging which is still used in some centres is shown in *Table* 14.3.

Table 14.3 Effect of Breslow's microstaging on regional node metastases and survival

Thickness of lesion	*Incidence of nodal involvement*	*5-year survival*
<0·75 mm	0	100%
0·76–1·5 mm	10%	80–90%
1·6–3·0 mm	20%	60%
>3·0 mm	40% or more	<50%

More recently, the cut-off for the good prognosis tumours has been extended to 1·0 mm as the tumours which fall within this category still carry a 95–100% 5-year survival.

Clark introduced the histological levels of microstaging (*Fig.* 14.28). The levels are outlined in *Table* 14.4. Level I is melanoma in situ which is also referred to as atypical melanocytic hyperplasia or premalignant melanosis. The two microstaging systems are complementary and the information from both gives the best estimate of prognosis. It is important to realize that a given tumour thickness does not

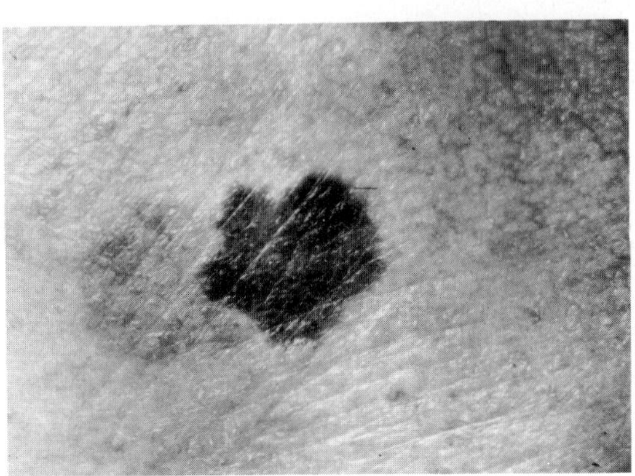

a

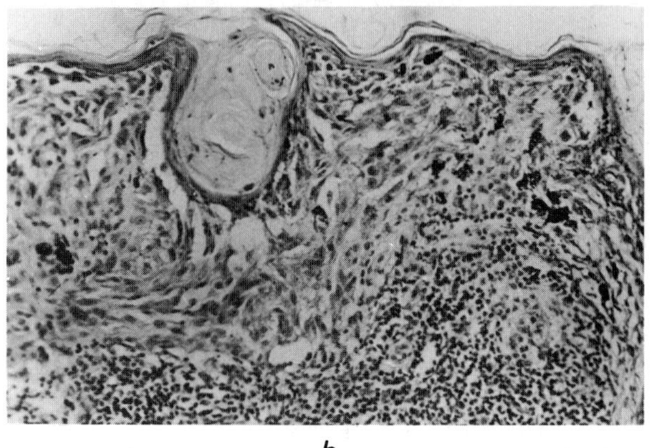

b

Fig. 14.27 *a*, Lentigo maligna. Clinical lesion, this is most commonly seen on the face. *b*, Lentigo maligna. The epidermis is almost completely replaced by abnormal spindle-shaped melanocytes. Dark staining masses of melanin are seen in macrophages immediately below the epidermis and there is a dense inflammatory infiltrate. Any such atypical melanocytes within the dermis would indicate [*continued over*]

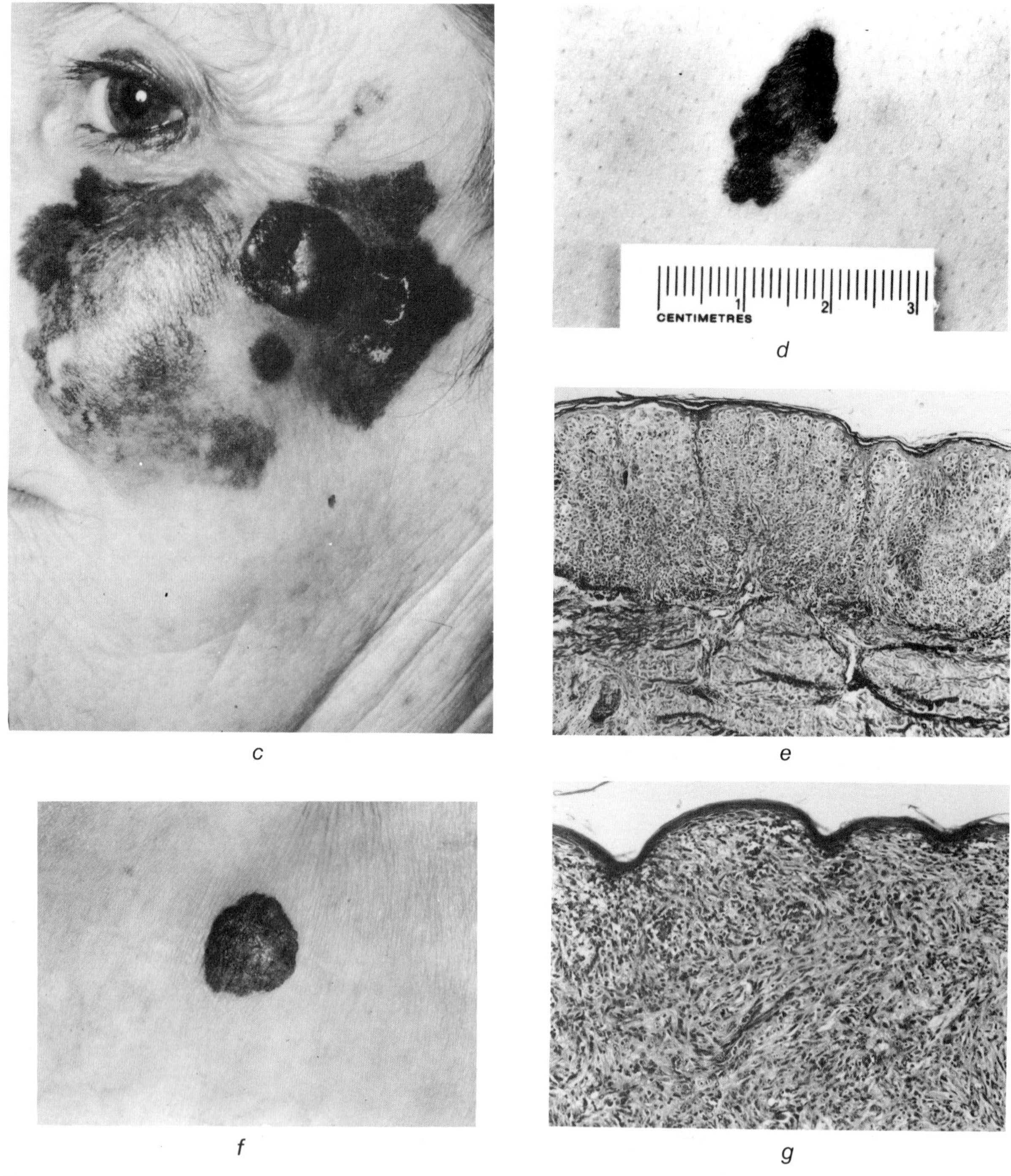

[*Fig. 14.27 continued*] *c*, Lentigo malignant melanoma. *d*, Superficial spreading melanoma—clinical appearance. *e*, Superficial spreading melanoma. The epidermis is almost completely replaced by atypical melanocytes which obliterate the rete pegs and dermal papillae but do not penetrate below the papillary dermis. *f*, Nodular melanoma—clinical lesion. *g*, Nodular melanoma. The surface of this nodular lesion shows an epidermis eroded from below by a mass of atypical epithelioid and spindle-shaped cells which show a fine dusting of melanin pigment.

always correspond to the same level of histopathological grading. Thus a 1·7 mm lesion with a level IV will carry a worse prognosis than a lesion of identical thickness but with a lesser Clark grade, such as level III.

Other Prognostic Risk Factors

In addition to tumour thickness and level of invasion, prognosis is adversely affected by the following:

SITE. Melanomas of the upper back, posterior arm, posterior neck, and posterior scalp (BANS) carry a worse prognosis than lesions situated elsewhere in the body.

ULCERATION. Ulceration width $>3\,mm^2$.

HISTOLOGICAL FEATURES. Mitoses $>6/mm^2$, minimal or absent lymphocytic response and the presence of microsco-

Table 14.4 Clark's histological staging and prognosis

Level of involvement		*Histological node involvement*	*5-year survival*
I	Melanoma does not penetrate the basement membrane (in situ)	0	100%
II	Melanoma extends into the papillary dermis	5%	90–100%
III	Melanoma reaches the junction between the papillary and reticular dermis	10–30%	80–90%
IV	Melanoma extends into the reticular dermis	30–40%	60–70%
V	Melanoma extends into the subcutaneous fat	60–70%	15–30%

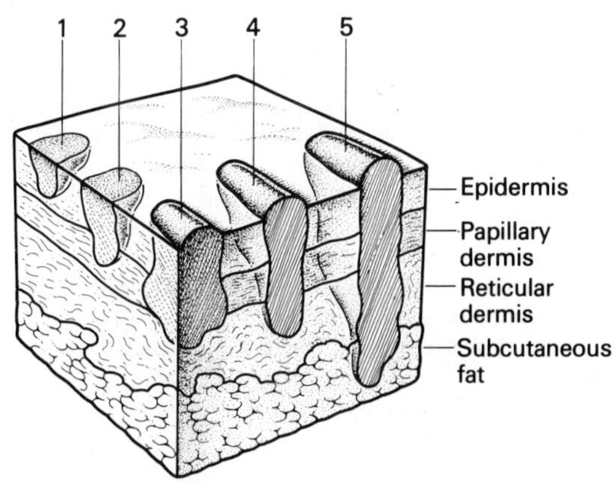

Fig. 14.28 Diagrammatic representation of Clark's levels of invasion of the skin by melanoma.

pic satellites. The latter are uncommon in thin lesions and frequent in thick lesions (37%).

HISTOLOGICAL NODE INVOLVEMENT. Involvement of the regional nodes is accompanied by a significant reduction in the 5-year survival. The prognosis is particularly bad if four or more of the regional nodes are involved.

PREGNANCY. Pregnancy worsens the prognosis but subsequent pregnancy in women who had melanoma treated previously has no effect on survival.

Clinical Features

Melanoma is extremely rarely encountered before puberty although the median age has fallen dramatically during the last two decades. It is now one of the commoner tumours in young adults. The disease is more frequent in females. This sex difference is especially marked in England and Wales. There are differences in the site distribution between the sexes, melanomas being more common in the legs in females and more frequent in the trunk, head and face in males (*Fig.* 14.29).

The signs and symptoms which are suggestive of the development of a melanoma in a pre-existing mole are shown in *Table* 14.5. It is important to stress, however, that every pigmented lesion is suspect especially if irregular in surface, pigmentation and outline. If there is a clinical doubt, excision biopsy of the lesion with immediate frozen section or urgent paraffin histology (within 24–48 h) is mandatory.

METASTATIC MELANOMA WITH UNKNOWN PRIMARY. Some patients present with nodal metastases, visceral involvement or both in the absence of a detectable primary lesion. It is presumed that spontaneous regression of primary lesion after it has metastasized has occurred in these patients. The

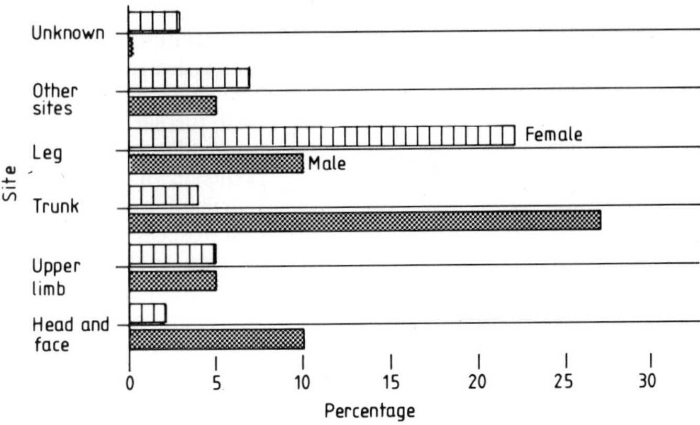

Fig. 14.29 Site distribution of melanoma.

Table 14.5 Clinical features indicative of the development of a melanoma in a pre-existing mole

Change in size	
Change in outline	Irregular
Change in elevation	Thicker, more palpable, nodules
Change in colour	Increasing pigmentation, depigmentation, irregular pigmentation
Change in surrounding tissues	Pigmented halo, satellite lesions
Development of symptoms	Itching, awareness of lesion, serous discharge and bleeding

prognosis is similar to that of stage II and III patients with a known primary.

INTRANSIT METASTASES. These are usually encountered in patients with recurrent locoregional disease. They consist of pigmented nodules more than 5 cm from the original scar but not beyond the regional nodes. Systemic deposits develop in 90% of patients with nodal deposits and in 70% with intransit deposits.

CLINICAL STAGING. In terms of the degree of advancement of the disease at the time of presentation, three clinical stages are recognized as follows:

- Stage I — The melanoma is confined to the primary site—primary lesion with or without satellites within a radius of 5 cm of the primary.
- Stage II — Metastatic involvement of a regional lymph node (single group) or intransit cutaneous metastases.
- Stage III — Involvement of two or more groups of lymph nodes, disseminated cutaneous disease or visceral involvement.

Treatment

This consists of biopsy of suspicious lesions with microstaging, surgical treatment of the primary, management of the regional lymph nodes, regional perfusion and systemic chemotherapy.

BIOPSY AND MICROSTAGING. Whenever possible, an excisional biopsy with a surrounding margin of normal skin and including subcutaneous fat should be performed. This is submitted either for frozen section or urgent paraffin histology to confirm the diagnosis and to establish the thickness of the lesion in millimetres and its Clark's level. The ellipse should be in the direction of the lymphatic drainage.

TREATMENT OF THE PRIMARY. The extent of the local excision and its depth remain controversial although there is general agreement that wide excisions in all cases are inappropriate.

Low-risk Lesions: A 1·0 cm margin is advocated for lesions which are thinner than 0·76 mm and have not extended beyond level II. The deep fascia is not included in the excision.

Intermediate Lesions: These range in thickness from 0·76 to 1·5 mm and may extend to level IV. The excision margins vary between 2 and 5 cm depending on the prognostic factors. Thus lesions in the BANS area, lesions extending to Clark's level IV and ulcerating primaries will require a wide margin. The deep fascia is not included in the excision.

Advanced Lesions: A 5·0 cm excision is indicated for lesions greater than 3·0 cm in depth. Some would advocate removal of the deep fascia to ensure clearance at the base of the tumour. Others believe that excision of the deep fascia is inadvisable and may enhance spread.

MANAGEMENT OF THE REGIONAL LYMPH NODES. The results of two prospective studies have shown no benefit from elective node dissection in stage I disease. There is therefore no indication for routine block dissection of lymph nodes. However, regional block lymphadenectomy is generally advised in the following:

- Certain Stage I patients: Head and neck lesions >0·75 mm thick. Recurrent lesions. Lesions of intermediate thickness in both sexes (0·8–3·0 mm).
- All Stage II patients: Including those in whom a primary tumour cannot be found (occult melanoma).

It is debatable whether block dissections should be done in patients with lesions > 4 mm thick or stage III disease as the long-term survival is not altered by this treatment. It is important to stress, however, that the results of clinical trials of block dissections in patients with histologically involved nodes are awaited and surgical practice may have to be altered in light of the findings of these studies some of which are nearing completion.

REGIONAL PERFUSION. This is applicable to tumours of the limbs and is designed to achieve a high local concentration of cytotoxic drugs with minimal systemic toxicity. Efficacy is improved further by incorporating an oxygenator in the circuit in addition to a heat exchanger to enable hyperthermic perfusion of the isolated limb with well oxygenated blood delivering a high concentration of antineoplastic drugs. Retrospective reports indicate the benefit of this form of treatment especially in locally recurrent neoplasms with multiple skin deposits (intransit metastases). It has also been used as an adjunct to surgical treatment in thick lesions, stage II and stage III disease. There is, however, at present no evidence to show that combined treatment with surgery and regional perfusion in these patients is superior to surgery alone.

The complications of isolated hyperthermic limb perfusion include myelosuppression (since it is virtually impossible to completely isolate a limb), oedema of the extremities, infection, vascular injuries and hepatitis.

SYSTEMIC CHEMOTHERAPY. This involves exhibition of cytotoxic agents, immunotherapy and endocrine treatment. At the moment there is no evidence that adjuvant chemotherapy and immunotherapy carries any survival advantages over surgery alone in patients with stage I and II disease. These treatment modalities are therefore applicable only to patients with advanced disseminated disease.

Cytotoxic Therapy: The drugs which have some activity are dimethyltriazeno-imidazole-carboxamide (DTIC; dacarbazine), the nitrosoureas (BCNU, CCNU and methyl CCNU), cyclophosphamide, adriamycin, vindesine and bleomycin. DTIC appears to be the most effective single agent and is especially useful for pulmonary secondaries and lymph node involvement. It is administered intravenously (250 mg/m^2/day) for 5 days. Its main disadvantage is the severe gastrointestinal toxicity which results in diminished tolerance because of severe nausea and vomiting. These can, however, be largely prevented by the administration of lorazepam. Vindesine gives similar response rates and is far less toxic than dacarbazine. More recently, combination cytotoxic therapy (DTIC + vindesine, bleomycin + vincristine + CCNU + DTIC) has been shown to enhance the duration of the response and it is likely that this approach will be used in preference to single agent treatment in the future.

Immunotherapy: Intralesional injection of BCG, purified tuberculin, vaccinia, dinitrobenzene and *C. parvum* results in regression of the injected cutaneous nodules in 75%. However, the combination of immunotherapy (BCG and other immune stimulant drugs such as levamisole) with cytotoxic therapy or surgical excision does not improve the results of these treatment modalities when administered alone.

Hormone Treatment: Following the demonstration of oestrogen and progesterone receptors in some melanomas, treatment with anti-oestrogens (e.g. tamoxifen) and stilboestrol has been advocated in patients with systemic disease and response rates of 16–22% have been reported.

Malignant Subcutaneous Tumours

These include fibrosarcoma and liposarcoma. It is still debatable whether a liposarcoma ever arises as a malignant degeneration in a benign lipoma. Both liposarcoma and fibrosarcoma often extend deeply into the muscular compartments of the extremity and tend to recur even after wide excision. Although growth is much less vigorous than in the case of osteogenic sarcoma, metastases do occur. If the tumour recurs after wide and deep local excision, amputation is advisable. Both fibrosarcoma and liposarcoma do not respond to radiotherapy.

Metastatic Carcinoma

Some malignant tumours tend to produce skin metastases more frequently than do others; the incidence of cutaneous metastases is between 3 and 4%. Such metastases occur most commonly with primary malignancy in breast, stomach, lung, large intestine, kidney, prostate gland, ovary, liver and bone. The deposits appear to be inflammatory in nature and somewhat more vascular than the surrounding skin. Also with certain tumours and especially with carcinoma of the lung there may be a widespread dissemination with emboli of malignant cells resulting in the sudden appearance in the skin of numerous nodules, particularly in the scalp and on the trunk. Cutaneous metastases invariably indicate a bad prognosis.

Further Reading

Balch C. M., Soong S. J., Milton G. W. et al. (1982) A comparison of prognostic factors and surgical results in 1786 patients with localized (stage I) melanomas treated in Alabama, USA and New South Wales, Australia. *Ann. Surg.* **196,** 677–684.

Breslow A. (1981) Prognosis in cutaneous melanoma: tumour thickness as a guide to treatment. *Pathol. Annu.* **15,** 1–14.

Fitzpatrick T. B., Eisen A. Z. et al. (1986) *Dermatology in General Medicine,* 3rd ed. New York, McGraw-Hill.

Rook A., Wilkinson D. S., Edling F. J. C. (ed.) (1986) *Textbook of Dermatology,* 4th ed. Oxford, Blackwell.

Rosin R. D. and Westbury G. (1979) Isolated limb perfusion for malignant melanoma. *Practitioner* **224,** 1031–1036.

Shuster S. (1978) *Dermatology in Internal Medicine.* London, Oxford Medical Publications.

Section 2

Trauma

15 *Trauma—General Considerations*

S. R. Shackford and D. B. Hoyt

INTRODUCTION

Trauma, accidental or intentional injury, is the principal public health problem in most countries. Each year, more than 140 000 Americans die and approximately 80 000 are permanently disabled as a result of injury. The number of deaths occurring annually in the USA due to trauma is over three times the number of combat fatalities which occurred during the whole of the nine-year Vietnam conflict. Trauma is the leading cause of death between the ages of 1 and 44. It is responsible for 79% of the deaths occurring between the ages of 15 and 24. Because it commonly affects children, adolescents and young adults, trauma results in the loss of more productive work years than cancer and heart disease combined. The cost to society, both directly, in terms of health care costs, and indirectly, in terms of the loss of goods and services, amounts to billions of dollars annually. The cost to the individual in terms of pain, suffering, incapacitation, disfigurement and loss of self-esteem is inestimable.

If the number of fatalities due to trauma is plotted as a function of time after injury, three peaks appear. The first peak, which consists of approximately 50% of all trauma-related deaths, contains those patients who die instantaneously or very soon after injury. These fatalities are generally due to an injury or a combination of injuries considered to be lethal, such as a brainstem laceration or a ruptured heart. Since survival from such injuries is considered to be unprecedented, improvement in the instantaneous or immediate mortality rate can only be attained by accident prevention or measures aimed at decreasing the severity of the insult, such as motor vehicle safety restraints. The second peak, which contains approximately 30% of trauma fatalities, occurs within hours of injury and is usually due to severe haemorrhage. Considerable reduction in the number of people dying during this period can occur if there is rapid transport from the scene of the accident to a hospital fully staffed and equipped to care for victims suffering severe injuries. The development of a 'systems' approach to trauma care has resulted in a significant reduction in the mortality of patients dying within hours of injury. A trauma system operates within a geographical region (i.e., city, county, state) and provides for rapid transport of victims of major trauma to specified hospitals within that region. These specific hospitals are called trauma centres because they have concentrated resources and expertise to treat severely injured patients immediately and effectively. The integration of prehospital care, rapid transport and immediate surgical treatment within a trauma system has been demonstrated to reduce preventable deaths due to trauma from 20–30% to 2–9%. The third peak in trauma deaths occurs days to weeks after injury and is usually due to infection and multiple organ failure. Reduction in late mortality can be anticipated with a better understanding of the immune depression which occurs after acute injury.

BIOMECHANICS OF INJURY

Injury occurs by deformation of tissues beyond their failure limits producing structural damage and alteration of function. Injury can be produced by penetrating or non-penetrating trauma. The amount of energy delivered and the area of application of that energy are major determinants of the amount of tissue damage.

Penetrating trauma involves the application of energy focused over a small area. The most common penetrating injuries are produced by knives (stab wounds) and firearms (gunshot wounds). Other less common forms of penetrating injury include impalement, which occasionally accompanies a motor vehicle accident or a fall, or a fragment injury produced by shards of glass or pieces of metal or wood. The severity of any penetrating injury is directly related to the amount of kinetic energy applied by a projectile at the time of impact or entry. The formula for kinetic energy is $KE=wv^2/2g$, where w is the mass or weight of the projectile, v is the velocity of the projectile, and g is gravity. As can be seen by the formula, velocity of the projectile is paramount in determining the degree of tissue damage. Low-velocity projectiles are considered to be those whose initial, or muzzle, velocity is less than 1200 feet per second (fps); medium-velocity projectiles are those with a muzzle velocity of 1200–1500 fps; and high-velocity projectiles are those with a muzzle velocity of over 2500 fps. *Table* 15.1 displays the amount of kinetic energy produced by commonly used firearms. It is important to remember that each fragment of a bullet which has shattered on impact should be considered as a projectile dissipating kinetic energy to tissues.

Non-penetrating or blunt trauma distributes energy over a much larger area than penetrating trauma. Blunt trauma may be associated with rapid acceleration, as occurs when a pedestrian is struck by a car, or rapid deceleration, which occurs in high-speed motor vehicle accidents or falls. Due to

Table 15.1 Weight of projectile, muzzle velocity, and approximate maximum kinetic energy of frequently used firearms

Description (calibre)	*Projectile weight (grams)*	*Muzzle velocity (feet per second)*	*KE ($ft/lb \times 10^2$)*
Pistols			
0·22 short	29	1000	0·5
0·38 special	158	870	1·8
9 mm Luger	125	1150	2·6
0·45	250	860	2·8
0·357 magnum	158	1430	5·0
0·44 magnum	240	1470	8·1
Rifles			
0·22 long	40	1150	0·8
5·56 mm M–16	55	3250	9·1
0·30–30 Winchester	170	2200	12·8

differential inertia, such deceleration or acceleration can produce extreme degrees of strain at points of anatomical fixation. In addition, severe direct deformation of tissue occurs at the points of impact. Strain can be produced along the longitudinal axis of a structure (tensile strain) producing a stretch or compression deformity. Opposing forces applied across the longitudinal axis of a structure (shear strain) cause fracture or tearing. As with the projectile velocity in penetrating trauma, the rate of loading or strain rate is an important determinant of tissue damage. The tolerance of biological tissues to injury is lessened at higher rates of loading. For example, bone will fail at a lower strain applied at higher rates. For these reasons, it is easy to understand how high-speed motor vehicle accidents can produce such severe injury.

Knowledge of the biomechanics or the mechanism of injury is extremely important in directing the initial management of and diagnostic approach to trauma victims. Knowing the forces involved in an accident helps to establish a threshold of awareness and increase the 'index of suspicion' of certain specific injuries.

MANAGEMENT OVERVIEW

Trauma care can be considered to consist of five phases: prehospital phase; early hospital or resuscitation phase; operative phase; intensive care phase; and convalescent or rehabilitative phase.

Prehospital Phase

Trauma patients can be categorized into three groups according to severity of injury: those which are rapidly fatal, those which are potentially fatal, and those which are not fatal. The first group includes patients who have rapid exsanguination, massive head injury, cervical cord transection or major airway disruption and produce death inevitably in less than 10 minutes. Most prehospital care will be unable to effect a change in the mortality associated with this kind of injury. Approximately 5% of traumatic injuries and 50% of *deaths* fall within this category. The third group which accounts for approximately 80% of trauma patients includes those injury categories which are minor or confined to the soft tissue and isolated extremity fractures. This group rarely has a major abdominal or thoracic injury. Urgent treatment is not essential, and these patients will survive without significant disability even with prolonged delays before definitive therapy.

The real impact of prehospital care is on the *second* group who are salvageable if medical care is provided quickly. Prehospital care can be divided into basic and advanced life support skills.

Basic Life Support

Basic life suport skills in which all prehospital personnel are trained include extrication, spinal protection, splinting, control of external haemorrhage and basic cardiopulmonary resuscitation.

Extrication is concerned with removing the victim from the immediate vicinity of the accident while providing immobilization of the spine and extremities to prevent further injury.

Spinal protection includes strapping the patient to a back board and immobilizing the head with sandbags and tape.

Immobilization of extremities with splints prevents further damage to vessels, nerves and soft tissues and may reduce the extent of haemorrhage around the fracture. Control of external bleeding can be achieved with firm pressure applied over the wound. Tourniquets should be avoided if at all possible.

Basic cardiopulmonary resuscitation is an important basic life support skill, but is often ineffective in severely injured patients. Airway control and effective ventilation is a more important priority and without it, cardiac massage is of little value. Cardiopulmonary resuscitation should always be tried in multiply injured patients, but should not delay transfer.

In summary, basic life support skills are aimed at stabilization but are limited in dealing with problems which most significantly impact on mortality.

Advanced Life Support

Because haemorrhage and injuries to the head and chest are responsible for early mortality after trauma, management of the airway, hypovolaemic shock and severe head injuries emerge as essentials skills for advanced life support.

Airway

The patient who answers when questioned has an adequate airway and can be assumed to be able to protect that airway from aspiration. However, a patient who is unconscious secondary to hypovolaemia or a significant head injury should be assumed to be at risk for aspiration, hypoxia and hypercarbia, and requires control of the airway.

Intubation of the airway assures protection from aspiration, control of gas exchange, and the ability to hyperventilate in order to control intracranial pressure in patients who are comatose (Glasgow Coma Score ≤8, *Table* 15.2).

Circulation

Following establishment of an airway and adequate ventilatory exchange, the next priority then becomes maintenance of circulation. This is assessed by determining the blood pressure by palpation and the peripheral perfusion by evaluating the time required for capillary refilling. Inability to palpate a radial pulse corresponds to a central arterial blood pressure of less than 80 mmHg. Delayed capillary refilling (determined by compression of the digital capillary bed and watching for refilling in less than two seconds) is also a sound clinical indicator of shock. If a patient has peripheral evidence of hypoperfusion and a blood pressure less than 90 mmHg, between 20–40% of the circulating blood volume is lost. For an adult male, this translates to 1–2 L.

Peripheral intravenous catheters should be inserted and resuscitation begun with isotonic crystalloid solution, i.e., Ringer-lactate. In addition, a MAST (Military Antishock Trousers) suit can be applied and, although of questionable significance when transport times are less than 15 min, it should be used when transport times are likely to be longer than 15 min or intravenous access is impossible. Transport should *never* be delayed to start intravenous lines.

External haemorrhage should be tamponaded by direct pressure and fractures splinted prior to or during transport.

Brain Resuscitation

The final aspect of prehospital care concerns the management of severe head injury. Establishing an airway and initiation of hyperventilation are the first line of therapy for severe head injury and remain the mainstay of treatment. In addition, restitution of circulating blood volume to maintain cerebral perfusion pressure is of obvious importance.

Resuscitation Phase

The transfer of patient care from prehospital to inhospital teams should occur in an organized fashion with a report which rapidly details the mechanism of injury, the obvious injuries, the patient's vital signs, and significant treatment started by the prehospital personnel. Assessment and treatment then follow a logical sequence based upon protocol and clinical judgement.

Primary Survey: Assessment

During the primary survey, life-threatening conditions are identified and management is begun simultaneously. The airway is reassessed and cleared of blood, vomitus and foreign body. Evaluation of the airway requires constant attention to the possibility of a cervical spine fracture which means that hyperextension and hyperflexion of the neck must be avoided. Adequacy of ventilatory exchange is assessed by auscultation. If there is inadequate ventilatory exchange (i.e., obvious distress or respiratory rate greater than 35), the patient should be ventilated with a bag valve device connected to a mask until definitive airway control can be obtained with an endotracheal tube or cricothyroidotomy.

Immediately life-threatening injuries which can compromise ventilation and perfusion include: open pneumothroax, tension pneumothorax, massive haemothorax and a massively crushed chest. If any of these entities are present, definitive airway management is an essential part of therapy.

Estimation of blood volume deficit and cardiac status are next in the initial assessment. Blood pressure, pulse, skin perfusion, urine output, mental status and central venous pressure are useful indicators of a haemodynamic status. The initial survey is limited to assessment of the first three. A 15–20% blood volume loss will cause a drop in the blood pressure. With a 30% volume loss, the blood pressure will be in the range of 60–80 mmHg. With a 40% volume loss it will be less than 50 mmHg. The pulse rate will be elevated and the skin pale and cool in advanced stages of hypovolaemia.

Once the gravity of hypovolaemia is appreciated, resuscitation should begin immediately. This should include infusion of Ringer-lactate through large-bore intravenous catheters (at least two lines should be started) and application of the MAST. Rapid infusion of 1–2 L of Ringer-lactate promptly re-establishes and maintains normal blood pressure in patients who have lost less than 15% of their blood volume and who do not have persistent bleeding.

If the initial infusion of 2 L of Ringer-lactate fails to restore blood pressure or perfusion, the patient has a deficit of greater than 15% of the circulating blood volume and one must give blood promptly in addition to Ringer-lactate. This may require transfusion with uncrossmatched blood (type O, Rh negative) in severely hypotensive patients. Uncrossmatched type specific blood can be used if the patient's blood type is known and the circumstances demand it.

Sources of external exsanguinating haemorrhage should be controlled with direct pressure on wounds. Splinting of fractures will reduce blood loss at the fracture site. Significant intrathoracic or intra-abdominal bleeding should be suspected in patients without fractures or evidence of external haemorrhage.

A brief neurological examination utilizing the components of the Glasgow Coma Score (*Table* 15.2) and determination of pupillary size completes the primary survey. Based on

Table 15.2 Glasgow coma score

Eye opening	
Spontaneous	4
To voice	3
To pain	2
None	1
Verbal response	
Orientated	5
Confused	4
Inappropriate words	3
Incomprehensible	2
None	1
Motor response	
Obeys command	6
Localizes pain	5
Withdraws (pain)	4
Flexion (pain)	3
Extension (pain)	2
None	1
Total	3–15

this assessment, a patient with a Glasgow Coma Score of 8 or less should receive aggressive brain resuscitation in concert with other aspects of initial resuscitation.

Secondary Survey

The secondary survey is directed at identification of suspected and unsuspected injuries and involves performing a thorough physical examination. A history should be obtained, if possible. This begins with the report given by the prehospital personnel and should include the mechanism of injury, the patient's vital signs and those treatments given by the prehospital personnel. Knowing the mechanism of injury, the physician can judge those areas of the body which may have sustained the greatest energy transfer and modify the investigations appropriately. In addition, any information regarding the patient's pertinent past medical history, including allergies, medications, known past illness and the time of the last meal should be determined.

A blood specimen should be sent for type and crossmatch and haematocrit determination. An arterial blood gas analysis should also be performed to assess the acid–base status and adequacy of ventilation. Blood should be held in the event that a toxicology screen or other biochemical investigations are deemed necessary.

The skull and head are palpated for haematomas, lacerations and fractures. The eyes are evaluated for pupillary reactivity, and the ears are checked for haemorrhage. The mouth is examined for retropharyngeal haematomas and aspirated foreign bodies. The neck is evaluated for venous distension or tracheal deviation (indicating increased intrathoracic pressure) and palpated for obvious cervical fractures. Penetrating injuries in the neck should not be probed. Cranial nerve function should be determined and recorded.

Inspection of the anterior and posterior aspects of the chest will identify penetrating or sucking chest wounds and the paradoxical movement of a flail chest. Palpation will reveal crepitus and rib or sternal pain, indicating *probable* fractures. The chest is auscultated at the apex for pneumothorax and at the base for haemothorax. Distant heart sounds in conjunction with distended neck veins may indicate cardiac tamponade.

The abdominal examination determines whether there is injury significant enough to warrant surgical intervention. The initial examination may be misleading and may give no indication of the patient's condition several hours later. Hence, close observation and frequent re-evaluation of the abdomen is important, particularly if definitive diagnostic procedures such as diagnostic peritoneal lavage are not immediately available. Inspection of the abdomen for bruising or abrasions may suggest underlying organ injury. Penetrating wounds should be marked with radiopaque markers. Auscultation is generally not helpful unless bowel sounds are absent, thereby raising the suspicion of significant visceral injury. The presence of pubic or iliac crest pain, pelvic instability, or perineal haematomas should raise suspicion of a major pelvic fracture.

The extremities should be assessed for tenderness, ecchymosis, crepitus, skin integrity and the presence of peripheral pulses and neurological deficit. Evaluation for vascular injury should include inspection and palpation of the neck, supraclavicular spaces, groins and all extremities for large expanding haematomas, particularly in conjunction with nearby penetrating injury or broken bones—indicating possible disruption of major artery.

Neurological examination should include motor and sensory evaluation, as well as continued re-evaluation of the patient's level of conciousness, pupillary size and Glasgow Coma Scale.

In summary, the secondary survey allows a more complete evaluation of all potential injuries and provides the basis for development of a care plan for definitive management.

Monitoring

During the initial resuscitation an awareness of the adequacy of treating hypovolaemic shock, respiratory distress and intracranial hypertension has to be appreciated and monitored. Minimal monitoring in patients with significant head injuries should include an intracranial monitoring device, a Foley catheter, a central venous catheter, and an arterial line. These monitors allow one to check the administration of asanguineous fluid and blood to physiological end points such as blood pressure, central venous pressure, urinary output and arterial pH and base deficit.

The arterial line is also useful to monitor gas exchange in patients with significant chest and abdominal injuries who are in respiratory distress. A central venous pressure monitor is invaluable in early detection of increased intrathoracic pressure such as that which occurs with pericardial tamponade and tension pneumothorax. Constant electrocardiographic monitoring is indicated in all patients with significant injury.

Where to Resuscitate

Although the majority of patients with multiple trauma, either blunt or penetrating, will be best served by resuscitation in an emergency room or trauma resuscitation space, a small group of patients is best served by direct transfer to the operating room where resuscitation can be accomplished and surgical management effected within 15 min of arrival. The indications for operating room resuscitation in our institution include: (1) all patients in full cardiac arrest; (2) all patients who are haemodynamically unstable, unresponsive to prehospital volume administration; (3) all patients with major external haemorrhage uncontrollable by direct pressure or other means; (4) all patients with massive soft-tissue injury that will require surgical intervention or at least maintenance of a sterile environment (i.e. evisceration, traumatic amputation, massive degloving injuries); (5) all patients transferred from another facility with a definitive diagnosis which requires immediate operation. In our experience, such an operating room resuscitation is required in 6% of patients admitted to a major trauma centre.

Rapid volume resuscitation and open chest cardiac massage can be rewarding in patients with cardiac arrest who have at least one vital sign present (a palpable pulse, evidence of cardiac activity or respiratory excursion). If one vital sign can be reliably established, this aggressive form of therapy is warranted.

A more important group of patients are those sustaining penetrating trauma, particularly to the chest who, despite prehospital resuscitative efforts, remain hypotensive. Immediate surgical management is often needed and unnecessary delay by transfer to another resuscitation area only adds to the potential mortality. Treatment is best accomplished in the operating room with a full team including the anaesthetist, surgeon, operating room technician and nursing staff.

In summary, the early hospital care, or the resuscitation phase, should follow an orderly set of priorities which include a primary survey, with assessment of airway, breathing, circulation, neurological disability and a complete exposure of the patient to assess all injuries. Simultaneous with this resuscitative effort, life-threatening problems identified during the primary survey are treated, shock management is initiated, the cervical spine stabilized and external haemorrhage controlled. The secondary survey should then proceed with a complete evaluation of the head, face, neck, chest, abdomen, perineum, rectum, extremities and nervous system. Laboratory and radiological investigations should be decided upon and performed in priority order. Whether the patient should be resuscitated in the operating room or in the emergency room should be determined by the patient's overall condition and the severity of injury.

Operative Phase

Surgical procedures are directed at arresting haemorrhage, removing destroyed or devitalized tissue, repairing injured soft tissues and stabilizing fractures. The distinction between the resuscitation and operative phases can be artificial, especially in the severely injured or moribund patient. Control of the airway and support of the circulation may occur simultaneously with resuscitative thoracotomy and laparotomy in patients who suffer cardiopulmonary arrest after trauma. Similarly, simultaneous operations by two or three separate teams are often a necessity in patients who suffer major multiple system injury. Simultaneous operations are life saving and serve to decrease operative time and the risk of subsequent anaesthesia. The importance of early and expeditious operation in trauma patients requiring surgery cannot be overstated. Lack of recognition of the need for operation and/or a delay in surgical management are the leading causes of morbidity and preventable deaths due to trauma. In addition, early operation, such as for stabilization of fractures, has been shown to decrease morbidity, duration of hospitalization and cost.

Intensive Care Phase

Patients who have suffered severe injury with or without operation will require a period of intense observation and care. This may entail something as complex as mechanical support of ventilation and circulation or something as simple as experienced observation of vital signs in a high-risk patient. During this phase, particular attention is paid to cardiopulmonary function, fluid and electrolyte balance, and coagulation parameters. Invasive monitoring of left and right ventricular function, intracranial pressure and arterial and venous pressures is common. Such intense observation and monitoring allows for early recognition of problems and early institution of therapy. As in the early hospital phase, delays in recognition or management often lead to disastrous complications or death.

Rehabilitation Phase

Rehabilitation is the process by which biological and psychosocial functions are restored sufficiently to allow an injured person to enjoy the maximum of autonomy. The object is to return patients to the level of function which existed prior to the injury. Rehabilitation requires a team approach which often draws on the skills of the neurosurgeon, orthopaedic surgeon, plastic surgeon, occupational therapist, physiotherapist and social worker.

16 Complications in Trauma Management

R. C. MacKersie, D. B. Hoyt and M. M. Sedwitz

Complications associated with the management of acutely-injured patients can be classified into: (1) complications related to the specific organ or injury involved; (2) complications that are common to the management of any surgical patient; and (3) complications that are unique or more closely related to trauma care. This chapter will deal primarily with the latter category. Complications common to general surgery patients and those related to specific traumatic injuries are discussed in other sections of this textbook.

The most serious avoidable complications that occur in multiply-injured patients are the results of delay in diagnosis, delay in treatment, or missed injuries. The components of successful management of multiply-injured patients include: (1) rapid transport to definitive care facilities; (2) immediate management of any ventilatory or circulatory embarrassment; (3) a well ordered thorough diagnostic evaluation; and (4) early operative intervention when indicated for both diagnostic and therapeutic reasons. Avoidable deaths and complications after trauma can be minimized by rapid transport, rapid referral, rapid diagnosis, and rapid definitive treatment.

COMPLICATIONS DURING INITIAL RESUSCITATION

Missed injuries and delay in diagnosis that occur during the initial resuscitation of the trauma patient may be related to inexperience, incomplete initial assessment, or poor serial observation. The diagnosis of an injury is usually preceded by the suspicion of its existence, and inexperience in the resuscitation and evaluation of trauma patients often manifests itself as an inappropriately low index of suspicion. Mechanisms of injury, associated occupant death in the case of vehicle accidents, location of wounds, age of the patient, clinical status as observed in field, and associated complaints all have bearing on the clinician's first estimate as to the likelihood of a particular injury. Failure to consider these factors in the initial evaluation may result in serious injuries being overlooked.

All trauma patients, regardless of outward appearance, require a complete, head to toe physical examination. The tendency to limit examination to the face, neck and anterior torso should be avoided. Perineal lacerations, penetrating wounds to the back, posterior knee dislocations, and precordial icepick wounds are all examples of injuries that can be overlooked as a result of an incomplete initial examination.

During the initial evaluation patients require close serial observation to assess the physiological effects of resuscitation. This includes continuous evaluation of ventilation, circulation, and level of consciousness. Patients intubated for respiratory distress with an undiagnosed tension pneumothorax, for example, may actually be worsened by such a manoeuvre. Failure to improve under these circumstances should prompt immediate re-evaluation. Similarly, a decreasing level of consciousness during the early phase of resuscitation may suggest a severe closed head injury that was not previously suspected.

Early complications related to respiratory failure may be anticipated and avoided in many situations. Patients with closed head injury and Glasgow Coma Scores of 8 or less require intubation for both airway protection, and hyperventilation to help reduce intracranial pressure. Patients with Glasgow Coma Scores of 9 to 12 and a diminishing level of consciousness can also be expected to require early intubation. Airway complications associated with severe maxillofacial or neck injuries, and inhalation injuries when associated with airway oedema may also be avoided by early endotracheal intubation.

Failure to appreciate the degree and aetiology of shock in the early phase of trauma resuscitation is a common pitfall. Sources of non-hypovolaemic shock such as tension pneumothorax, cardiac tamponade, and myocardial contusion, must be quickly distinguished from hypovolaemic shock. Vital signs are reliable indicators of shock, but hypovolaemia may occur initially in the absence of hypotension, widened pulse pressure, or increased pulse rate. One sensitive indicator of perfusion in the trauma patient is base excess obtained from arterial blood gases. Worsening or failure to improve a base excess during the resuscitation phase is indicative of either continuing haemorrhage or inadequate resuscitation. Although crystalloids are the mainstay of initial fluid resuscitation, patients with profound or recurrent hypotension should receive blood products early in their course. Failure to maintain oxygen-carrying capacity by red cell transfusion can lead to severe haemodilution and may precipitate cardiac arrest, particularly in elderly patients.

Many injuries fail to manifest any clinical signs or symptoms and may lead to disastrous consequences if overlooked. These occult injuries usually occur in association with other more easily detectable injuries, and may be suspected and diagnosed by this association. For example: penetrating injuries in close proximity to a vessel, or associated with an anatomically related neurological deficit, may not present with any significant haematoma, bleeding, or diminution of downstream pulses. Serious vascular injuries not otherwise suspected, including arterial transection, may be diagnosed by arteriography. Similarly, posterior knee dislocations have a high associated incidence of popliteal artery trauma, often without any clinical manifestation. Routine arteriography should be performed in all posterior knee dislocations because of this common association. Abdominal injuries may be associated with skeletal injuries. Left-sided 9th–10th rib fractures and lumbar spinous process fractures are associated with a 20–30% incidence of intra-abdominal injury. The appropriate diagnostic measures should be undertaken despite the absence of clinical signs when patients present with these associated skeletal injuries. Occult genito-urinary injuries can be easily diagnosed with contrast studies and may occur in the complete absence of any clinical manifestation such as haematuria. In the case of major axial or anterior/posterior deceleration injuries, complete arterial intimal disruption with renal artery occlusion may occur. In penetrating trauma, injuries to the kidney or ureter may occur in the absence of haematuria and should be suspected on the basis of wound proximity.

Resuscitation and evaluation of the patient with multiple injuries require a variety of minor surgical procedures and the frequent prehospital use of devices that act to ensure airway patency and improve blood pressure. A list of these various diagnostic and therapeutic interventions and their related complications as shown in *Table* 16.1.

Endotracheal intubation has been shown to be the most effective way of maintaining an airway in the prehospital setting. Accidental oesophageal intubation, while uncommon, must be considered in any patient who has been intubated in the field. A rapid check for tube position including auscultation, palpation of the balloon at the suprasternal notch and inspection by direct laryngoscopy if needed, should be performed in every patient intubated prior to arrival in the resuscitation area. The use of the oesophageal obturator airway has been shown to be substantially less effective than endotracheal intubation in providing for adequate ventilation. Its use has been abandoned in many trauma centres.

The major complication associated with peripheral venous access, including upper and lower extremity cutdowns, is septic phlebitis. Resuscitation of critically-injured patients usually occurs in the emergency department and under less than perfectly aseptic conditions. In one review of septic phlebitis, 70% of the involved intravenous catheters were inserted in the emergency department. A policy of routine removal and replacement of all resuscitation lines including percutaneous central venous catheters, will reduce the incidence of septic catheter complications.

The use of percutaneous subclavian vein catheterization in trauma patients has the potential to cause serious complications, particularly so since the ease of venous cannulation in hypovolaemic patients may be impaired. Prospective studies of subclavian catheterization in patients with clinical

Table 16.1 Technical complications associated with trauma resuscitation

Intervention	*Complication(s)*
Oesophageal obturator airway	Hypercapnia, tracheal intubation, hypoxia, acidosis
Endotracheal intubation	Oesophageal intubation traumatic intubation
Positive-pressure breathing	Precipitation of tension pneumothorax air embolism (when associated with lung laceration)
Cutdown intravenous lines	Injury to greater saphenous nerve injury to median nerve injury to brachial artery infection
Percutaneous subclavian central line	Pneumothorax haemothorax/haemorrhage infection
Intercostal intubation	Intra-abdominal or diaphragmatic injury improper placement retained haemothorax infection lung laceration
Diagnostic peritoneal lavage	False positive/false negative lavage bladder, gastric perforation bowel or vascular perforation infection
Arterial lines	Digital ischaemia infection local bleeding
MAST suits	Respiratory embarrassment ? exacerbation of intracranial hypertension compartment syndrome limited patient access

shock has suggested that the complication rate is in fact, relatively low (approximately 5%) and is directly related to the experience of the physician placing the line.

Complications related to radial and femoral arterial lines occur in about 7% of patients. These complications include digital ischaemia, site inflammation, catheter sepsis, and site bleeding. In one large series there was no difference between the complication rate with the femoral and radial artery sites. The most common complication was digital ischaemia and this responded promptly to removal of the associated catheter, without necessitating surgical thromboendarterectomy or producing actual tissue necrosis.

Complications associated with the insertion of chest tubes for the evacuation of blood or air, may be minimized by careful attention to detail in regard to the site of insertion, and meticulous aseptic technique. The majority of thoracic injuries associated with haemo- or pneumothorax may be treated by the insertion of large bore (36–40 F) straight chest tubes. The temptation to place low lying chest tubes should be avoided since: (1) they offer little additional advantage to the evacuation of blood from the pleural space; and (2) are more commonly associated with diaphragmatic penetration and injury to the spleen or liver. Failure to evacuate a haemothorax completely may be the result of either improper tube placement or inadequate tube size. The treatment of clotted haemothorax after the correct positioning of intercostal tubes is somewhat controversial. While it is true that spontaneous resolution of the clotted haemothorax will occur in most cases, these patients are often febrile and have prolonged hospital courses. Many centres now favour the early operative evacuation of the large clotted haemothorax.

Complications related to diagnostic peritoneal lavage have been drastically reduced by the adaptation of the open method for catheter placement. The so-called closed method, in which the catheter with a trocar stylet is forced through the infraumbilical midline fascia resulted in a high incidence of complications (6–8%), including bowel perforation and large vessel injury, and has been abandoned in most centres. The open method utilizes a small fascial incision and the passage of the peritoneal dialysis catheter under direct vision. The complication rate using this method has been reported at between 0 and 2%. Prior to the placement of peritoneal dialysis catheters, all patients require decompression of the bladder, usually by Foley catheterization, and many will similarly require decompression of the stomach by nasogastric intubation. Failure to do so can lead to gastric or bladder perforation.

Improper technique in peritoneal lavage may result in both false negatives and false positive interpretations. The former may occur when the catheter is passed into the preperitoneal space (space of Retzius), not making contact with the peritoneal cavity. The latter may occur in the presence of a major pelvic fracture with anteriorly dissecting retroperitoneal haematoma, and may be avoided by a supra-umbilical approach. False positives may also occur as a result of poor haemostasis during catheter placement, particularly when used for penetrating trauma, when the interpretation relies on a relatively low red blood cell count in the lavage fluid.

Military antishock trousers (MAST) are used frequently to increase systolic blood pressure in hypotensive patients. They have the potential for increasing intra-abdominal pressure as well, and the associated decrease in diaphragmatic excursion may lead to respiratory embarrassment, particularly in patients with thoracic injuries. The prolonged use of MAST (more than 4 h) in patients with lower extremity orthopaedic injuries, has also been associated with the development of compartment syndromes.

MASSIVE TRANSFUSION

The salvage of patients with major injuries often requires the transfusion of one or more circulating blood volumes to sustain circulation during resuscitation and treatment. As the amount of transfused blood increases, complications may develop that are not as commonly associated with more moderate blood replacement that occurs during elective surgery. Complications related to massive transfusions are listed in *Table* 16.2.

Table 16.2 Complications associated with massive blood transfusions

Acidosis
Decreased oxygen delivery
Hypothermia
Hypocalcaemia
Microembolization, ? pulmonary injury
Dilutional thrombocytopenia
Coagulopathy
Disseminated intravascular coagulation (DIC)
Transfusion reactions

The metabolic changes that accompany massive transfusions are related to the chemical changes that occur in banked blood. Acidosis as a result of shock and hypoperfusion may be exacerbated in massive transfusion by the increased amount of lactic acid present in stored blood. This acid load is rapidly metabolized in patients who can be adequately resuscitated, however, and the routine administration of alkalinizing solutions to treat acid–base imbalances is not indicated.

The reduction in 2,3-diphosphoglycerate (2,3-DPG) that occurs in banked red cells acts to increase haemoglobin affinity for oxygen and thereby decreases oxygen transport. The effect in massive transfusion appears to be limited, as 2,3-DPG levels quickly return to normal following resuscitation. The effects of pH on the oxyhaemoglobin dissociation curve appear to be quantitatively more important than 2,3-DPG shifts.

Hypothermia caused by the rapid infusion of large quantities of cold, banked blood may act to exacerbate acidosis, increase myocardial irritability, and worsen coagulopathy. While the use of conventional blood warmers will prevent transfusion-associated hypothermia, the slow infusion rate associated with these devices make their use impractical in patients with massive haemorrhage. Very recently, high flow rate heat exchangers have become available, designed to warm large volumes of crystalloid and blood products to 37 °C.

Hypocalcaemia related to the rapid infusion of citrate in banked blood, has been a concern in massive transfusions, but rarely is identified as a clinical problem. This is explained by the fact that elevation of citrate levels requires a high transfusion rate (approximately one unit every five minutes), and even when elevated, citrate levels fall rapidly following transfusion. In addition, calcium is rapidly mobilized from bone, maintaining plasma levels under most circumstances. The routine administration of calcium during blood transfusion is therefore not usually indicated.

The pulmonary embolization of microaggregates has been cited as a potential problem of blood transfusion. Fibrin, and degenerating platelets and white cells have been thought to contribute to the pulmonary injury seen in association with shock and trauma. No correlation has been established between the degree of pulmonary injury and the volume of blood transfusion, and the need for micropore filters (Bently, Pall, Swank) in major trauma has not been well established.

The major defect in blood coagulation following massive transfusion occurs as a result of dilutional thrombocytopenia. Stored blood is a poor source of platelets, there are limited platelet stores in the body, and the capacity of the bone marrow to respond to increased demand is limited. In one study of patients receiving an average of 33 units of blood, there was a strong correlation between the volume of transfused blood and the platelet count. Although bleeding times in normal patients are prolonged with platelet counts below 100 000/mm^3, adequate surgical haemostasis can usually be achieved with platelet counts greater than 50 000. Each unit of administered platelets will elevate platelet count by 10 000–15 000/mm^3.

Dilution of coagulation factors in massive transfusion may also result in coagulopathy. Factors V and VIII are the most labile in banked blood. Patients with significant elevations in prothrombin or partial thromboplastin times require the additional administration of fresh frozen plasma and/or cryoprecipitate to correct this dilutional coagulopathy. In patients receiving packed red cells, the administration of one unit of fresh frozen plasma for every five units of red blood cells may reduce the incidence of coagulopathy during massive transfusions.

A rare but devastating haematological complication of massive transfusion is disseminated intravascular coagulation (DIC). This syndrome can be initiated by many disease states including massive soft-tissue trauma, brain injuries, prolonged shock, and reactions to mismatched blood. The diagnosis of DIC is supported by persistent thrombocytopenia, increased fibrinolytic activity and diminution of clotting factors. Replacement of clotting factors and platelets and the treatment of identified causes are the mainstay of therapy.

The use of whole blood versus blood component products for massive transfusion is controversial. Studies of moderate blood replacement in major elective surgery have failed to demonstrate any difference in coagulopathy between whole blood and packed cells, but similar studies of blood components in massive transfusion are lacking. The use of fresh, whole blood avoids many of the metabolic problems associated with the use of banked blood. Acidosis is reduced, clotting factors and platelets are replenished, oxygen-carrying capacity is unimpaired, and microaggregate formation is minimized. However, practical limitations of obtaining same-day type specific whole blood in large quantities limits the use of fresh whole blood in many communities.

Because of the delay associated with obtaining cross-matched blood in patients who require massive transfusions, two alternatives are commonly used: low-titre O negative blood, and type-specific uncrossmatched blood. The increasing use of component therapy has limited the titration of Group O blood, in many areas, and the potential exists for transfusion reactions in blood with high anti-A or anti-B antibody titres. In addition, the transfusion of large amounts of 'universal donors' blood may lead to later incompatibilities when blood typed and crossmatched from the patient's original sample is later administered. The use of type-specific, unmatched blood appears to be a better alternative for use in patients requiring massive transfusion. Its use in trauma patients has been examined and found to be virtually without major complications. In patients profoundly hypotensive who require blood transfusion within the first five to ten minutes of resuscitation, type O blood may be preferable.

Autotransfusion of shed blood in trauma patients has been shown to be effective in reducing transfusion requirements. In general, however, the use of anticoagulants (citrate-phosphate-dextrose) limits autotransfusion to about 3000 ml. Beyond that point, clinically significant DIC or coagulopathy may occur. Autotransfusion is most useful for intrathoracic haemorrhage, where blood can be collected from intercostal tubes. Its use in abdominal trauma has been restrained due to the potential for blood contamination by associated gastrointestinal injuries.

IMMUNOSUPPRESSION AND INFECTION

Late mortality accounts for as much as 30% of traumatic deaths. The greatest threat to severely injured patients surviving their initial injuries is infection. Post-traumatic sepsis, in several studies, accounts for as much as 80% of all non-neurological deaths following trauma. Although the metabolic and endocrine response to injury has been closely studied, we have a poor understanding of why some patients are susceptible to and succumb to sepsis following injury while others seem to tolerate a similar degree of injury without significant complications. The current hypothesis is that a defect in the immunological defence occurs following injury, which allows opportunistic micro-organisms to gain a foothold and convert what would normally be a mild subclinical infection into a lethal one.

Immunosuppression in the Burn Injury

Evidence accumulated in recent years supports the above hypothesis for one form of trauma — major thermal injuries. Patients with greater than 40% total body surface area burns are universally immunocompromised. The immune defects include: (1) transient depression of immunoglobulin production, both primary and secondary; (2) activation of the complement system, both alternative and classic pathways (production of complement split products with immunoregulatory capabilities such as C3A and C5A); (3) depression of neutrophil function (phagocytosis, chemotaxis, intracellular killing); (4) depletion of fibronectin and serum opsonic activity; (5) long-term depression of T-cell lymphocyte response with increased T suppressor cells; (6) reduced monocyte/macrophage function with increased suppressor macrophage function; (7) increased immunosuppressive prostaglandin E production and depressed phagocytosis; (8) release of endotoxin tissue-degradation products, cytokines and lymphokines with immunosuppressive properties; and (9) decreased skin test reactivity to standard recall antigens.

The degree of immunological compromise in burn patients appears to correlate directly with the degree of injury and the subsequent incidence of sepsis. Experiments designed to boost the immune responsiveness in burned animals show a reduction in sepsis with the return of immunocompetence as measured by return of the helper/suppressor

T-cell ratio towards normal. The best indicators of susceptibility to sepsis in burn patients appear to be the occurrence of circulating suppressor proteins, decreased monocyte/macrophage activity, and reduced lymphocyte response with subpopulation shifts characterized as an increase in suppressor cells and decrease in helper cells. Skin testing, although indicative of immune suppression, is far too sensitive to predict subsequent sepsis.

Immune Defects in Trauma in General

As with burns, it is clear that major operative, blunt or penetrating trauma are all accompanied by some degree of immunological compromise. Specific defects which can be noted in this population include: (1) increased circulating suppressor proteins; (2) early decrease in skin reactivity; (3) decreased neutrophil chemotaxis and intracellular killing; (4) complement activation with generation of complement products and complement-mediated increased vascular permeability leading to multiple organ failure; (5) increased suppressor cell and inhibitory macrophage activity; (6) decreased opsonic protein, particularly fibronectin, and depressed reticuloendothelial system function; and (7) decreased T-cell response to mitogens following trauma. In addition, multiple other non-immunological variables are at least empirically associated with sepsis in trauma patients. These include the number of organs injured, the number of units of blood administered, the length of the operative procedure, the severity of injury and physiological state as indicated by traditional trauma scoring systems. Immune function is also decreased in the very young and in the very old and in patients with poor nutritional status. Steroids suppress the inflammatory response. Antibiotics, such as tetracycline, chloramphenicol, clindamycin, streptomycin, gentamicin, kanamycin and neomycin inhibit cell-mediated immunity. Anaesthetic agents such as halothane, cyclopropane, ether and nitrous oxide can inhibit both B- and T-cell function and increase the spread of tumours, depress allergic responses and inhibit phagocytosis. There is also very good evidence from experiences with organ transplantation that the simple administration of blood products is also immunosuppressive (*see* Chapters 10 and 78). The isolation and quantification of the immune defect produced by injury has been hampered by the multiplicity of factors and the dissimilarity in patterns of injury.

Injury Severity and Immune Depression in the Development of Sepsis

Despite the complexity of quantitating multiple injuries, it has been shown that the tendency to develop the immunosuppressed state can be correlated with the severity of injury, as calculated by an anatomical injury severity score (ISS). Although patients at risk for sepsis can be identified on the basis of injury severity scores, the value of these scores in predicting sepsis on an individual basis has yet to be demonstrated. The severity and duration of shock may also be associated with an immunosuppressed state. Patients at risk for sepsis require close monitoring for clinical signs of infection, thorough diagnostic evaluation and aggressive management of identified infections in order to prevent what would normally be a subclinical infection from developing into an uncontrolled septic state.

The best indicators to date of the immunosuppressed state which leads to an increased risk for sepsis following injury include decreased T-cells with decreased helper cells and increased suppressor cells, a pattern which is sustained until the time that the patient's septic risk goes away. Of equal significance is the emergence of immunosuppressive peptides which are generated by injury and emerge as quickly as thirty minutes following injury. Their presence and ability to inhibit immune function can be similarly correlated with infection risk.

Clinical Infections

As with any perioperative patient, pulmonary infection and complications relative to atelectasis and impairment of ventilation are a persistent problem, particularly with thoracic and upper abdominal injuries. Patients with pulmonary contusions and multiple rib fractures are at high risk for subsequent superinfection of these injured areas. Daily chest radiographs and sputum Gram stains should be performed on all seriously injured patients. The development of an infiltrate on chest radiography or the development of purulent secretions is indicative of a significant infection. Antibiotics should be started early in accordance with Gram stains or based on institutional bacterial sensitivities and adjusted later on the basis of culture reports. The use of prophylactic antibiotics should be avoided.

As portals of bacterial entry, monitoring devices, including ventriculostomies for intracranial pressure, central lines and Swan–Ganz catheters for haemodynamic monitoring, central and peripheral intravenous lines for volume resuscitation and nutritional support and Foley catheters for monitoring urinary output all have the potential for producing severe infections. This is particularly true for instrumentation and monitoring devices placed during the resuscitation phase since these devices are often placed under less than sterile conditions. The risk of catheter-related sepsis in trauma patients may be reduced by the early removal or replacement of all resuscitation lines.

The post-traumatic infections which are the most difficult to evaluate are those in patients who develop fever and leucocytosis several days following injury and operation. Careful evaluation of all potential sources of infection must be performed early, and repetitively if necessary. Wounds, catheter and chest tube sites, urine, sputum and blood are all evaluated as potential sources. Less common infections such as sinusitis, meningitis, septic phlebitis involving central veins, and fungal infection should also be considered.

Determining the presence of an intra-abdominal infection may be difficult, particularly in patients following abdominal surgery. Patients may continue to have peristalsis and minimal physical findings, yet have significant intra-abdominal infection. Computerized tomography is useful in localizing intra-abdominal abscesses or fluid collections. Its applicability as a means of definitive diagnosis in the septic patient, however, appears to be more limited. Acalculous cholecystitis is a potentially life-threatening complication that occurs following major trauma, often in patients receiving parenteral nutrition. Ultrasonography or radionucleotide scans may be useful in the diagnosis.

The development of multiple organ failure (MOF), characterized by pulmonary, renal, CNS, cardiovascular and gastrointestinal system failure, is usually an indirect manifestation of uncontrolled sepsis from a site that is either unappreciated or inadequately controlled. Patients who develop multiple organ failure require aggressive localization of any potential source of infection. Exploratory laparotomy may be necessary to identify an intra-abdominal source. Using MOF as the only indication for operation, laparotomy will be successful in finding the septic focus in approximately 50% of patients. Failure to treat adequately an infectious source in patients developing multiple organ failure following trauma is almost universally fatal.

In general, the traumatized patient is characterized by an immunosuppressive defect, and the infectious complications can be classified relative to either time of onset or final outcome. The outcome will be determined by the patient's degree of immunosuppression and this is probably related to the amount of injury sustained. The best approach to patients following massive injury who subsequently become septic is a thorough, aggressive search for the underlying source of infection and treatment according to the principles of débridement, drainage and utilization of antibiotics.

POST-TRAUMATIC RESPIRATORY FAILURE

Acute respiratory failure occurring after trauma is a frequent complication, and may be produced by a variety of causes. The three major categories: obstruction, ventilatory failure, and impairment of gas exchange are outlined in *Table* 16.3 with their more common aetiologies. Airway obstruction is often associated with craniofacial injuries either secondary to severe airway oedema or the inability to protect and maintain a patent airway in an unconscious patient. Aspiration of gastric contents or foreign bodies, another cause of obstruction, is also frequently associated with craniofacial injuries. Penetrating neck injuries may produce substantial expanding haematomas and produce obstruction secondary to airway compression. The majority of these injuries are apparent at initial evaluation and most require early endotracheal intubation or cricothyroidotomy.

Table 16.3 Causes of post-traumatic respiratory failure

Obstructive causes
Craniofacial injuries
Closed head injury—inability to protect airway
Aspiration/foreign body
Expanding neck haematoma
Burns
Causes of ventilatory failure
CNS injury
Cord trauma
Diaphragmatic rupture
Severe flail chest
Malnutrition
Causes of gas exchange derangements (ARDS)
Neurogenic
Sepsis
Fat embolus
Microemboli/shock/massive transfusion
Pulmonary contusion
Aspiration
Inhalation injury
Oxygen toxicity

Ventilatory failure can likewise be produced by CNS lesions producing flaccid paralysis. High cervical cord trauma at the C2 or C3 level may produce phrenic nerve paralysis and result in a total absence of ventilatory capacity. Spinal cord injuries between C5 and T10 are also capable of producing varying degrees of limitation in ventilatory capacity secondary to impairment of intercostal and abdominal musculature. Patients with these lower cord injuries may not initially present with ventilatory failure but are at high risk for subsequent respiratory complications.

Acute respiratory failure secondary to flail chest is usually associated with an underlying pulmonary contusion, but massive disruptions of the chest wall alone may impair ventilatory capacity. Patients with extended disruptions of the skeletal chest wall, particularly in the older age group, may benefit from operative rib stabilization using external struts or K wires.

Gas exchange abnormalities frequently occur following shock and trauma and are the most common cause of respiratory failure. The so-called adult respiratory distress syndrome (ARDS) was originally described by Ashbaugh in 1967, having reported acute respiratory distress in twelve patients without underlying lung disease. Since that time, it has become clear that ARDS may develop in a wide variety of clinical situations (*Table* 16.3). The clinical features of ARDS are characterized by hypoxia, increased arteriovenous pulmonary shunting, an increased physiological dead space, and decreased lung compliance. Pulmonary artery pressures and central venous pressures are usually within normal limits. Chest radiographs initially show a diffuse interstitial pulmonary oedema pattern which may progress to more severe consolidation as intra-alveolar oedema occurs. At the microscopic level, fluid first accumulates in cuffs around the small bronchioles, with microvascular congestion and intravascular aggregates of fibrin, platelets and leucocytes. In the later stages of ARDS, fibroblast proliferation and the deposition of collagen produces intra-alveolar and interstitial fibrosis.

The common pathway in the production of pulmonary oedema in ARDS is an increase in pulmonary microvascular permeability. This results in increased fluid and protein flux across the pulmonary capillary endothelium. The precise mechanisms by which this permeability leak is produced has been the subject of intensive investigation for the past several years. Various mechanisms have been proposed. Neurogenic pulmonary oedema and pulmonary oedema that occurs secondary to contusion are most likely the result of stretched capillary pores. This leak may occur as a result of either direct injury, in the case of pulmonary contusion, or because of extremely high pulmonary microvascular pressures produced by a diffuse alpha-adrenergic discharge, in the case of neurogenic pulmonary oedema.

Sepsis is probably the most common clinical event that leads to the development of ARDS, and is the major cause of late mortality in trauma patients. Numerous mediators of septic lung injury have been studied. These include cellular elements such as lymphoctyes, polymorphonuclear leucocytes, platelets and macrophages. Humoral mediators include complement, histamine, lysosomal enzymes, superoxide radicals, coagulation products and arachidonic acid metabolites, among others. It has become clear that there is an intricate relationship between these mediators. No one mediator alone is responsible for producing the pulmonary injury, nor is any single mediator indispensable to the process.

The overall mortality of ARDS remains quite high, and has been essentially unchanged in the last two decades. The reported mortality for ARDS in trauma patients varies between 30 and 40%, but mortality may be as high as 90% in patients with more severe derangements in gas exchange. Many patients go on to develop multiple organ failure with renal, hepatic and cardiac involvement.

There is, as yet, no specific therapy for ARDS. Pharmacological studies using vasodilators, steroids, and non-steroidal anti-inflammatory agents are under investigation, but the clinical effectiveness of these agents has yet to be demonstrated. One recent clinical investigation using prostaglandin E infusion in patients with ARDS showed improvement in early mortality associated with its use. Further trials are in progress.

The primary ventilatory derangements in ARDS are hypoxia and acidosis. Management should be directed at maintaining adequate oxygenation, and reducing or limiting the degree of pulmonary oedema. Mechanical ventilation utilizing positive end-expiratory pressure (PEEP) acts to improve oxygenation by increasing functional residual lung capacity. To date there is no conclusive evidence of any direct effect of PEEP on capillary permeability, or on the level of pulmonary oedema *per se*. PEEP has the additional advantage of maintaining arterial oxygenation in the face of decreasing inspired oxygen concentration, thereby limiting the potential for pulmonary oxygen toxicity.

Fluid therapy in ARDS should be directed at maintaining cardiac output and renal perfusion. It is desirable in the face of a pulmonary microvascular leak, to maintain pulmonary capillary wedge pressures as low as possible consistent with adequate perfusion, since elevation of these pressures may act to increase the level of oedema and worsen gas exchange. The choice of fluid for volume resuscitation in the face of ARDS remains controversial. There is no conclusive experimental or clinical data to favour the use of crystalloid versus colloid solutions in the treatment of ARDS. A sound approach is to use blood products to maintain oxygen-carrying capacity and crystalloid solutions to maintain intravascular volume.

The recognition, localization and treatment of a septic source remains the most important factor in limiting the pulmonary injury in post-traumatic patients who develop ARDS in association with clinical sepsis. Commonly, occult intra-abdominal infections in patients with injuries to the gastrointestinal tract often represent the precipitating cause. In many instances patients develop bronchopneumonia on top of their ARDS, often with resistant hospital organisms. Careful monitoring of sputum Gram stains, cultures, daily chest radiographs are important for the early detection of secondary respiratory infections. Patients with central nervous system injuries seem particularly prone to develop respiratory infections.

WOUND PROBLEMS

The majority of traumatic wounds can be managed using conventional methods of irrigation, removal of foreign material, débridement of divitalized tissue, and either meticulous primary closure, delayed primary closure, or closure by secondary intention. The degree of contamination and the amount of devitalized tissue may be greater for certain types of traumatic wounds, however, and the risks for subsequent infection and further tissue loss correspondingly higher.

Close-range Shotgun Wounds

The ballistic design of shotgun shells favours the dispersion of energy into tissues at close range. The relatively wide area of injury associated with these wounds, particularly at close range, frequently leads to large areas of tissue necrosis. In addition, shell materials and interposed portions of clothing may be driven into the depths of the wound by the force of the typical shotgun blast. Because of these factors, all close-range shotgun injuries require mandatory exploration and careful removing of shell casings, wadding, or clothing material. Pellets not encountered in the exploration and débridement of the central wound do not require removal.

With the exception of head and neck injuries, the early closure of shotgun wounds has been associated with a 50% incidence of the development of serious infections. These wounds, therefore, are generally best treated by delayed primary closure. In many instances repeated débridement will be required because of additional tissue necrosis. Occasionally split-thickness skin grafting will be required for areas of larger skin loss. The principles regarding the operative exploration and diagnostic workup of shotgun wounds involving the thorax or abdomen are in general similar to those for other forms of penetrating trauma to these areas.

Degloving Injuries

Degloving injuries involve the separation of skin and subcutaneous tissue from the underlying muscle and fascia by the application of pressure and shearing force to the surface of the skin. The severity of these wounds varies from the elevation of a relatively minor skin flap to the complete circumferential detachment of skin and subcutaneous tissue from the underlying fascia. These injuries most commonly involve the lower extremity and are often associated with vehicle accidents. Management of associated injuries including fracture stabilization and repair of neurovascular injuries takes precedence over repair of the associated degloving injury.

Appropriate choices of management of degloving injuries will depend on the area of separated tissue, degree of contamination, degree of crush injury involved, associated injuries, and the location of the flap base (proximal vs. distal). Injuries associated with a relatively small flap, proximally based, with minimal crush and contamination, may occasionally be treated by vigorous irrigation, débridement and careful closure over closed suction drains. The majority of these injuries, however, involve larger flaps with significant crush and contamination. These more extensive injuries, and those that involve distal-based flaps are prone to subsequent infection and tissue necrosis. In a review of degloving injuries of the extremities and trunk, Kudsk et al. (1981) had the best results in treating degloving injuries by harvesting of either full or split-thickness skin grafts from the degloved section, thorough débridement of the underlying tissue and immediate grafting. They had a better than 90% take of grafts when performed in this manner. All patients who had simple reduction and closure of the avulsed flap showed progressive necrosis of this flap within the first few days. Over half of these wounds became infected. The majority of large avulsion flaps, particularly those involving crush injury or distally based flaps, are best treated by early thorough irrigation and débridement, and grafting using skin harvested from the involved flap segment.

Delayed Primary Closure for Traumatic Injuries

Delayed primary closure was developed over two hundred years ago as a means of reducing the incidence of wound infection in military injuries. Despite the development of antibiotics, the incidence of wound complications associated with primary closure in wounds that involve severe contamination, foreign bodies, or devitalized tissue, remain unacceptably high, and there continues to be an important place for delayed primary closure in the management of these wounds.

The term 'delayed primary closure' (DPC) refers to the structured closure of skin and subcutaneous tissue several days following traumatic or incisional wounds. The goal of DPC is to allow anatomically acceptable wound closure early in the post-injury course, without the inconvenience and delay associated with secondary healing. The well-documented superior resistance to infection in DPC wounds appears to be related to higher partial oxygen tensions and higher blood flows measured in these wounds as opposed to wounds closed primarily.

The initial treatment of contaminated wounds and wounds that involve devitalized tissue involves removal of retained foreign material, vigorous débridement, and irrigation with high-velocity stream, usually with antibiotic solution. Following initial irrigation and débridement, wounds to be treated by DPC are generally packed loosely with either sterile gauze or gauze containing antiseptics such as iodoform, acriflavine or xeroform. Operative dressings are generally left undisturbed unless repeated débridements are anticipated, or there are clinical indications of underlying infection. The timing of delayed primary closure is important and not completely agreed upon in the literature. Empirical clinical and experimental data suggest that the optimum time for delayed primary closure is between four and six days following initial incision or injury. Additional information may be gathered in the case of unfavourable wounds by quantitative bacterial cultures. pH monitoring has been used also in an attempt to define better high-risk wounds. In general, these techniques are not practical for performance on a daily basis and the decision regarding which wounds may be safely closed by delayed primary techniques rests with the experience of the surgeon.

If wounds are without obvious signs of infection by the fourth to sixth day, they may be closed by a variety of techniques. Large wounds may require limited undermining of the flaps, and suture approximation. Wounds that can easily be closed without tension may be loosely approximated using microporous skin tape. The advantages of this method are patient comfort and convenience, in addition to providing for a relatively loose closure allowing the egress of any entrapped serous fluid. The vast majority of traumatic and incisional wounds that show no sign of active infection after 4–6 days can be successfully managed in this manner. Wounds that fail on delayed primary closure are treated in an open manner and allowed to heal by secondary intention.

Necrotizing Infections

The term 'necrotizing fasciitis' often refers to a family of diseases with names such as bacterial synergistic gangrene, streptococcal or gas gangrene, necrotizing myonecrosis, and necrotizing cutaneous mucormycosis. While these may be associated with surgical incisions or leg ulcers, they are most commonly associated with traumatic injuries, often very minor ones. The clinical presentation may be subtle in its earlier stages and usually consists of erythema, oedema, and pain out of proportion to the physical findings. As the disease progresses, fascial necrosis occurs with devascularization of the skin and subcutaneous tissue as a result of microthrombosis of the penetrating vessels. In these later stages there are often associated haemorrhagic bullae and local anaesthesia of the skin. Crepitus is present on occasion and the patients are usually quite toxic with leucocytosis, tachycardia and hyperpyrexia. This is an immediately life-threatening condition. The diagnosis is best made by operative exploration of the involved wound, and may be confirmed by Gram stain smears, bacteria cultures, or frozen section biopsy. The majority of these infections are caused by mixed aerobic and anaerobic organisms with streptococci being present in most cases.

The most important prognostic factor in the treatment of necrotizing infections is early recognition and wide surgical débridement. Findings at exploration may vary from severe fascial and/or muscle devitalization to more limited subcutaneous oedema and ischaemia. Wide surgical débridement of all devitalized skin and fascia is necessary to control infection. The majority of these infections do not involve significant amounts of muscle tissue and so amputation can usually be avoided. Antibiotics including high-dose penicillin, aminoglycosides, and coverage for anaerobes are given empirically and adjusted as indicated by antibiotic sensitivity reports. Hyperbaric oxygen may be a valuable adjunct in the treatment of many of these infections but should not be considered a substitute to surgical débridement.

Wounds that are at high risk for saprophytic contamination such as injuries created by gardening or farm implements should be examined for the presence of a mycotic infection, particularly when there is a lack of response to initial antibiotic and surgical treatment. Mucor and rhizopus may produce invasive infections and require the addition of amphotericin B to the therapeutic regimen.

Mortality from necrotizing infections is extremely variable and ranges between 10 and 40%. Age, arteriosclerosis, diabetes mellitus and delay in diagnosis are factors associated with increased mortality. Infections originating in the extremities have a better prognosis than those originating in the head, neck or trunk.

Further Reading

Baker C. C., Peterson S. R. and Sheldon G. F. (1979) Septic phlebitis: a neglected disease. *Am. J. Surg.* **138**, 97–103.

Collins J. A. (1974) Problems associated with the massive transfusion of stored blood. *Surgery* **75**, 274–295.

Flint L. M., Cryer H. M., Howard D. A. et al. (1984) Approaches to the management of shotgun injuries. *J. Trauma* **24**, 415, 419.

Gervin A. S. and Fisher R. P. (1984) Resuscitation of trauma patients with type-specific uncrossmatched blood. *J. Trauma* **24**, 327–331.

Gottrup F., Fogdestam I., and Hunt T. K. (1982) Delayed primary closure: an experimental and clinical review. *J. Clin. Surg.* **1**, 113–124.

Jacobs L. M. and Hsieh J. W. (1984) A clinical review of autotransfusion and its role in trauma. *JAMA* **251**, 3283–3287.

Kudsk K. A., Sheldon G. F. and Walton R. L. (1981) Degloving injuries of the extremities and torso. *J. Trauma* **21**, 835–839.

Rinaldo J. E. and Rogers R. M. (1982) Adult respiratory-distress syndrome. *N. Engl. J. Med.* **306**, 900–909.

Tranbaugh R. F. and Lewis F. R. (1982) Respiratory insufficiency. *Surg. Clin. North Am.* **62**, 121–132.

17 *Soft-tissue Injuries of the Neck*

R. C. Mackersie

The neck is an anatomically complex region that acts as a conduit for multiple structures, including vital components of the vascular, neurological, respiratory and digestive systems. The density and relative vulnerability of these structures dictates that injuries to this region be given a high priority in the management of multiply-injured patients. The frequency of serious injury and the diagnostic challenge that neck trauma presents has generated considerable controversy regarding the 'best' diagnostic approach. The policy of mandatory operative exploration of all penetrating neck injuries was developed as a result of wartime experience that demonstrated reduced mortality with this approach. More recent civilian experience has shown similar results utilizing a policy of selective operative management. Developments in prehospital care, rapid transport to designated facilities, and improvements in non-invasive diagnostic methods have further acted in synergistic fashion to reduce the morbidity and mortality in patients with neck injuries.

INITIAL RESUSCITATION

The propensity for respiratory compromise in patients with vascular or tracheal injuries makes the early establishment of a secure airway essential. Approximately 10% of patients with neck injuries will have some degree of airway compromise. Upper airway obstruction may be caused by haematoma, laryngeal fractures, soft-tissue swelling, or bleeding. Many patients with blunt injuries will have associated craniofacial trauma. Endotracheal intubation is mandatory in patients with significant obstructive signs and should be considered as a prophylactic measure with injuries capable of producing obstruction. The establishment of a surgical airway via cricothyroidotomy is often necessary in patients who cannot be easily intubated by the oral or nasal route.

Hypovolaemic shock is treated by the establishment of large-bore i.v. cannulas and the infusion of Ringer-lactate or type-specific blood. Obvious external haemorrhage from cervical wounds can often be controlled by direct pressure. Massive external haemorrhage from major vascular wounds requires more direct digital control by the insertion of a gloved finger through the wound. Blind clamping in an effort to control haemorrhage is dangerous and should not be attempted.

Overlooked occult haemorrhage from seemingly innocuous penetrating neck wounds is a dangerous pitfall. Wounds at the base of the neck may produce massive internal bleeding into the mediastinum and/or pleural space. Exsanguinating haemorrhage from these injuries can occasionally be controlled by direct pressure, but may require an immediate anterolateral thoracotomy for proximal vascular control.

Following initial resuscitation, patients who are haemodynamically stable must be assessed for the need for operative intervention. The details of this assessment will be discussed, but during this period, any manoeuvre that may act to exacerbate or produce recurrent haemorrhage should be avoided. Probing of the injury beneath the platysma muscle may disrupt haemostasis. Similarly, gagging or coughing also increases the risk of recurrent haemorrhage and nasogastric tube placement should therefore be deferred. Patients with suspected or known vascular injuries undergoing operative exploration should undergo skin cleansing and be draped prior to anaesthetic induction in the event that straining during induction disrupts local haemostasis. The risk of venous air embolism during this phase of treatment can be minimized by maintaining patients with suspected venous injuries in the supine position with gentle pressure on the cervical wound.

METHODS OF EVALUATION

The need for operative intervention is the central question that must be addressed by any method undertaken to evaluate neck injuries. This need can be determined on the basis of clinical findings (*Table* 17.1). While this list is not universally agreed upon, the presence of any of these findings is associated with a high incidence of reparable injuries. A small percentage of patients will present with active bleeding, shock, or an expanding haematoma and require immediate operative intervention. Other patients with superficial (to the platysma) wounds or absence of swelling or other clinical signs (in the case of blunt trauma) will require no further evaluation.

For clinically stable patients, non-invasive studies (radiographs, arteriography, contrast radiographs, computerized tomography, endoscopy) may serve several purposes. They

Table 17.1 Indications for operative intervention in the management of neck injuries

Vascular injuries
Hypotension/shock
Active external bleeding
Large or expanding haematoma
Distal pulse deficit
Bruit
Hemispherical deficit or hypoperfusion
Significant haemothorax or haemomediastinum
Peripheral nerve lesion adjacent to major vascular structures
Aerodigestive injuries
Subcutaneous air/crepitus
Air emanating from wound
Unexplained blood in aerodigestive tract
Respiratory stridor
Dysphagia/hoarseness
Neurological injuries
Cranial nerves: VII, IX, X, XI, XII
Impaired diaphragmatic motion — phrenic n.
Brachial plexus deficits

may be used for localization of a known or suspected lesion and aid in planning the operative approach. They may also be used, with varying degrees of reliability, to exclude potential injuries. In the case of arteriographic embolization or occlusion, the procedure may also be therapeutic.

Chest and simple anteroposterior and lateral neck films are routinely obtained in all patients with penetrating injuries. Occult haemorrhage into the chest, associated pneumothorax, or cervical soft-tissue air all are relatively reliable indicators of serious injury.

Arteriography is perhaps the most widely used invasive method. In high cervical injuries, arteriography has been found to be very accurate. The reliability of arteriography in excluding mediastinal vascular injuries has been questioned, however, due to the size and orientation of the aorta and great vessels. Arteriographic definition of venous injuries has not been found to be particularly accurate.

The use of contrast oesophagography in the evaluation of cervical oesophageal injuries is controversial. Because of the fascial investments of the cervical oesophagus, the sensitivity of contrast extravasation in defining injury is not necessarily as high as it is for the intrathoracic oesophagus where effluent from a laceration or perforation tends to be less contained. While oesophagography is used in some centres, several investigators have found the incidence of missed injuries associated with this method as high as 50% in patients who were eventually explored. Most of these patients, however, had clinical evidence of an aerodigestive injury. Similarly, oesophagoscopy has not proven to be a reliable means of excluding injury with a reported sensitivity in several small studies of only 40–50%. Although the sensitivity of combined endoscopy and oesophagography may be somewhat higher, the clinical utility of negative oesophageal studies remains to be defined.

PENETRATING NECK INJURIES

For purposes of diagnostic strategy and operative approach, the neck has been divided into three zones (*Fig.* 17.1).

Injuries that occur above the angle of the mandible

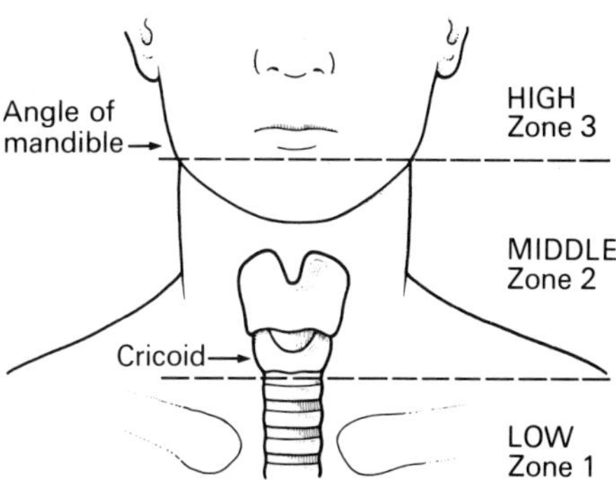

Fig. 17.1 Classification of neck injuries.

(Zone 3) may involve the petrous or cavernous portions of the internal carotid artery, the vertebral artery or deep branches of the external carotid artery. Wide exposure of this area and distal vascular control may be difficult to obtain. Routine exploration as a diagnostic manoeuvre may be both hazardous and inaccurate. Gunshot wounds account for the majority of these injuries, and patients may present with haematoma or haemorrhage from the mouth, nose, throat or the wound. There are often associated neurological injuries.

Arteriography is the diagnostic method of choice for Zone 3 injuries. It has proven to be both highly sensitive and specific, and a negative study obviates the need for vascular exploration. The intracranial circulation can be assessed in the event that carotid ligation becomes necessary. Embolization may be indicated for inaccessible branches of the external carotid artery, the vertebral artery or a thrombosed internal carotid in a comatose patient. Patients with very high carotid lesions, in whom ligation is anticipated, may be candidates for extracranial–intracranial bypass.

Zone 1 injuries occur at the base of the neck and, like Zone 3 injuries, do not allow easy accessibility from an operative standpoint. Injuries in Zone 1 may involve proximal carotid, subclavian or innominate vessels, and patients are at risk for exsanguinating haemorrhage which may be occult if the blood tracks into the chest or mediastinum. Thirty-nine per cent of patients with Zone 1 vascular injuries presented with unexplained shock in a series by Flint et al. (1973). It is of note also that 32% of patients in this series had no clinical signs suggesting a major vascular injury.

Management strategy for Zone 1 injuries consists of early operative exploration for patients with obvious clinical signs of major vascular injury (shock, major external or intrathoracic or mediastinal bleeding, pulse deficit or anatomically related neurological deficit). The role of ancillary studies, particularly arteriography, in the management of asymptomatic Zone 1 injuries remains controversial. While the principles of exclusion arteriography may apply to injuries of the subclavian or distal carotid vessels, the reliability of angiography in excluding innominate or proximal carotid injuries remains to be determined. Earlier series advocating diagnostic exploration on the basis of proximity did not rely on preoperative arteriography. More recent studies suggest that asymptomatic Zone 1 patients with negative arteriograms may be safely managed without operative exploration.

A variety of incisions have been used to gain exposure and vascular control for thoracic inlet injuries (*Fig.* 17.2). The operative approach will be determined by the specificity of

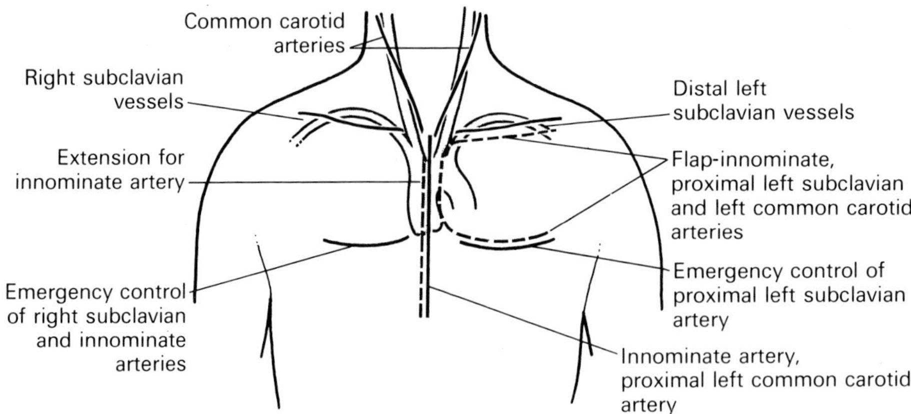

Fig. 17.2 Operative approaches for Zone 1 injuries to the neck.

localizing signs, preoperative arteriography, or associated intrathoracic injuries. Transverse clavicular incisions are used for access to distal subclavian injuries. Proximal access to right subclavian or innominate vessels is best obtained through a median sternotomy with supraclavicular lateral extension for additional exposure. Left proximal subclavian injuries will generally require an anterolateral thoracotomy for control. 'Trapdoor' or 'book' incisions simply combine an anterior thoracotomy with a median sternotomy and supraclavicular extension for wide exposure to left-sided and aortic arch injuries. More distal carotid injuries can be best approached via an anterior sternocleidomastoid incision.

It is injuries to Zone 2 that have generated the greatest controversy regarding their management. The experience gained during the Korean and Viet Nam conflicts with these injuries demonstrated the value of routine exploration in reducing morbidity and mortality, and was subsequently applied to civilian trauma. As experience was gained, the policy of mandatory exploration in patients with no clinical signs or symptoms of underlying injury was re-examined because of the high incidence of negative explorations. Many centres now follow a policy of selective exploration of Zone 2 injuries.

Table 17.2 Mandatory versus selective neck exploration

Mandatory exploration
For
Risk of injury is high
Diagnosis can be made with certainty
No delay in diagnosis or treatment
Minimizes hospital time and cost
No significant morbidity with negative exploration
Against
Many negative explorations
Significant morbidity with negative exploration
More costly than selective management
Injuries may still be missed
Selective exploration
For
Avoids unnecessary explorations
No significant mortality with delayed treatment
Cost and hospital time less than or equal to mandatory exploration
Non-invasive studies are very accurate in defining significant injuries
Against
Incurs potentially dangerous delay
Serious injuries may be missed with non-invasive studies
Requires more hospital resources

The controversy regarding mandatory versus selective neck exploration remains unresolved. The principal arguments for each approach are summarized in *Table* 17.2. The debate is one of diagnostic methods, not therapy. There is no role for the non-operative management of patients with clinically suspected vascular or aerodigestive injuries.

A summary of results for selective and mandatory exploration policies in several recent series is presented in *Table* 17.3. Although there are minor variations in clinical indications for operative exploration, and the utilization of ancillary studies, the bulk of this experience suggests that there is little difference in clinical outcome between these policies. More extensive literature reviews of earlier studies also support the contention that policies using selective and mandatory neck exploration produce similar clinical results. The author prefers mandatory exploration for all Zone 2 injuries that penetrate the platysma. Patients with isolated neck wounds not found to have significant injuries can be managed on the ward postoperatively and discharged within 24–48 h, minimizing hospital time and expense, and maximizing diagnostic efficiency.

SPECIFIC INJURIES

The repair of most arterial injuries can be accomplished by lateral arteriorrhaphy, primary re-anastomosis, or autologous graft interposition. Ligation is rarely indicated for major vessels except in cases of certain carotid lesions, or when a patient's condition demands a short operative time. Vertebral artery ligation can also be performed in most cases without sequelae. Major venous injuries should be repaired when possible, but ligation generally does not lead to significant morbidity, and can be performed safely. Smaller veins should be ligated without attempts at repair. Vascular injuries are further discussed in Chapter 20.

Lacerations of the larynx and trachea are repaired primarily. Mucosal approximation should be performed carefully with fine absorbable sutures to avoid intraluminal granulation tissue. Tracheal rings and cartilage can be reapproximated using non-absorbable extramucosal sutures.

Table 17.3 Cumulative results: Mandatory versus selective management

	Total patients	*Patients explored*	*Negative exploration*	*Total deaths*	*Deaths, explored*	*Deaths, observed*
Mandatory	477	408 (85%)	231 (56%)	16 (3·3%)	16 (3·3%)	0 (0%)
Selective	316	148 (47%)	29 (19·6%)	12 (3·8%)	10 (3·2%)	2 (0·6%)

Oesophageal and Pharyngeal Injuries

Cervical injuries to the oesophagus and pharynx are repaired in one or two layers and drained using soft Penrose or closed suction drains. More distal oesophageal injuries may be primarily repaired if diagnosed early. Late repair of intrathoracic oesophageal injuries should not be attempted. These injuries are best treated by wide drainage and oesophageal diversion and exclusion as outlined by Urschel et al. (1974).

Neurological Injuries

Injuries to the cord, cranial nerves, brachial plexus, or intracranial structures may occur with neck injuries, particularly with gunshot wounds. A brief neurological examination should be performed whenever possible to both identify specific nerve injuries and heighten the index of suspicion for involvement of adjacent vascular structures. Lacerations of major nerves are débrided and repaired primarily whenever possible. Interposition nerve grafts may be required in cases that involve more extensive tissue loss.

BLUNT NECK INJURIES

Blunt neck injuries are caused most commonly by a direct blow to the thyroid or cricoid cartilage either as the result of motor vehicle or 'clothes-line' accidents. Injuries to the larynx, trachea, pharynx, or oesophagus may result. Patients may present with airway obstruction, hoarseness, dysphagia, subcutaneous air, laryngeal deformities, blood in aerodigestive tracts, haematoma, or simply soft-tissue swelling. Signs of vascular injury are similar to those for penetrating injuries. Airway obstruction often requires placement of a surgical airway. In the presence of severe laryngotracheal trauma a cricothyroidotomy often is not feasible, and tracheostomy will be required.

Non-invasive diagnostic methods are used initially in clinically stable patients, and include contrast radiography and computerized tomography. The cervical spine must also be carefully evaluated in the initial assessment. Arteriography, bronchoscopy and oesophagoscopy may be indicated.

Vascular injuries are given highest priority and neck exploration is performed on the basis of arteriographic findings. Oesophageal and pharyngeal lacerations are repaired and drained. Laryngeal fractures are generally repaired with the use of a stent.

COMPLICATIONS OF CERVICAL TRAUMA

Massive haemorrhage leading to hypovolaemic cardiac arrest and complications arising from spinal cord injuries are the leading causes of mortality in patients with cervical trauma. Missed injuries, involving the oesophagus, may lead to fistula formation, abscess, and occasionally to mediastinitis. Undiagnosed vascular injuries have produced late sequelae including arteriovenous fistula and false aneurysms. Glottic or subglottic stenosis may result from laryngeal and tracheal injuries.

Further Reading

Ayuyao A. M., Kaledzi Y. L., Parsa M. H. et al. (1985) Penetrating neck wounds mandatory versus selective exploration. *Ann. Surg.* **302,** 563–567.

Belinkie S. A., Russell J. C., DaSilva J. et al. (1983) Management of penetrating neck injuries. *J. Trauma* **23,** 235–237.

Bivins B. A., Procter C. D., and Bell R. M. (1985) Arguments against mandatory exploration. In: Dailey R. H. and Callhan M. (ed.) *Controversies in Trauma Management.* Edinburgh, Churchill Livingstone.

Elerding S. C., Manart F. D. and Moore E.E. (1980) A reappraisal of penetrating neck injury management. *J. Trauma* **20,** 695–697.

Flint L. M., Snyder W. H., Perry M. O. et al. (1973) Management of major vascular injuries in the base of the neck. *Arch. Surg.* **106,** 407–413.

Golueke P. J., Goldstein A. S., Sclafani S. J. et al. (1984) Routine versus selective exploration of penetrating neck injuries: a randomized prospective study. *J. Trauma* **24,** 1010–1014.

Merion R. M., Harness J. K., Ramsburgh S. R. et al. (1981) Selective management of penetrating neck trauma. *Arch. Surg.* **116,** 691–696.

Narrod J. A. and Moore E. E. (1984) Selective management of penetrating neck injuries. *Arch. Surg.* **119,** 574–578.

Obeid F. N., Haddad G. S., Horst H. M. et al. (1985) A critical reappraisal of a mandatory exploration policy for penetrating wounds of the neck. *Surg. Gynecol. Obstet.* **160,** 517–521.

Urschel H. C. et al. (1974) Improved management of esophageal perforation; exclusion and diversion in continuity. *Ann. Surg.* **179,** 587.

18 *Chest Injuries*

S. R. Shackford

INTRODUCTION

Blunt trauma, such as that sustained in motor vehicle accidents, falls or explosions, characteristically produces multiple injuries, with significant trauma to the chest occurring in 35–40% of patients. Chest injury after traffic accidents has been implicated as the sole cause of death in 10–15% of fatalities and was found to be a significant contributing factor in 50–60% of deaths. The mortality rate of an isolated chest injury is less than 10%, but increases to 35% with major injuries to two or more additional organ systems.

Generally, penetrating injuries of the chest are seen less frequently than blunt injuries, comprising 10–30% of the chest trauma seen at many trauma hospitals, although this incidence is significantly higher in some urban centres. Approximately 75% of these injuries are produced by stab wounds. However, the frequency of gunshot wounds of the chest is increasing, paralleling the increasing use of firearms in assaults, robberies and suicides. The mortality rate of a stab wound of the chest is 2–3% while that of a gunshot wound is 15–20%.

INITIAL MANAGEMENT

The initial management of patients with suspected chest injury differs in no significant way from the initial management of any injured patient. That is, an adequate airway is established, breathing is assured, haemorrhage is controlled, and intravenous access is established. In the patient with suspected chest injury, particular attention should be paid to the respiratory rate, respiratory effort, auscultatory findings, appearance of the neck veins, position of the trachea and the results of palpation of the chest wall. Abnormalities should lead one to suspect injuries which could be immediately life threatening such as airway obstruction, massive haemothorax, open pneumothorax, tension pneumothorax and pericardial tamponade. Such injuries must be treated immediately, without delay for confirmatory laboratory tests of radiography. For example, tachypnoea and dyspnoea associated with diminished breath sounds, distended neck veins and a tracheal shift away from the site of suspected injury suggest the presence of a tension pneumothorax which will require immediate decompression. Similarly, hypotension associated with distended neck veins, a parasternal knife wound and no tracheal shift suggest pericardial tamponade requiring immediate decompression.

A chest radiograph should always be a part of the initial evaluation and management of a patient with suspected chest injury. Careful examination of the chest film should always include inspection of the lung parenchyma, mediastinal structures and thoracic cage. After insertion of an endotracheal tube, a central venous catheter, a nasogastric tube or a tube thoracostomy, the radiograph should be repeated to check the tube position and to confirm that the desired result (i.e., gastric decompression or lung re-expansion) has taken place.

During the initial evaluation of blunt chest trauma, an electrocardiogram should also be obtained to screen for possible myocardial contusion.

Finally, all patients with a suspected chest injury should have an arterial blood gas analysis performed. The arterial P_{O_2} and P_{CO_2} are invaluable in alerting one to the early signs of ventilatory failure (hypoxia and/or hypercarbia) which may not be clinically apparent. In addition, the blood gases are also extremely useful in guiding mechanical ventilatory support allowing one to modulate the fraction of inspired oxygen and the mechanically delivered rate and tidal volume. The pH and base deficit assist in determining the magnitude of the lactic acidosis which invariably accompanies hypovolaemioc shock and in determining the effectiveness of fluid and blood resuscitation in restoring perfusion and relieving the acidosis.

One general principle which deserves emphasis is that the ultimate outcome of any severely injured patient is dependent not only on the specific injury or constellation of injuries sustained and how these injuries are managed, but also upon the physiological reserve of the patient. This reserve depends, in large part, on the patient's age and state of health prior to injury. The older the patient and the more serious the pre-existing disease, the less reserve and the more likely the possibility of rapid deterioration. Expeditious resuscitation and evaluation are, therefore, extremely important so that the patient's condition is not further compromised by delay in management.

MECHANISM OF INJURY

The forces involved in producing significant blunt chest trauma are many and varied. The concussive effects of a direct blow to the thoracic cage, such as that produced by a steering wheel or dashboard, may injure the chest wall as well as the underlying viscera. There is speculation that chest wall concussion may produce shock or stress waves similar to those produced by blast injury. These waves may be reflected by the posterolateral chest wall and focused at areas other than those directly under the area of impact. With greater energy transfer, concussive forces may produce crush injuries of the thoracic cage and may be associated with rupture of the alveoli or tracheobronchial tree, especially if the glottis is closed at the time of impact. Rapid horizontal deceleration, as occurs frequently in motor vehicle accidents, or rapid vertical deceleration, as occurs in falls from great heights, can produce significant shearing forces at points of anatomical fixation. Shearing, stretching and torsion are particularly damaging to the great vessels of the thorax. These forces will frequently fracture or tear the relatively non-compliant intimal layer of the artery leading to pseudoaneurysm or rupture.

INJURIES OF THE THORACIC CAGE

Rib Fractures

Rib fractures are the most common injury sustained after blunt chest trauma. A rib can be broken after relatively insignificant trauma, such as a fall against a table or a curb. This is particularly true in older patients. With ageing, the chest wall loses compliance and relatively insignificant compressive forces tend to fracture the more 'brittle' ribs.

Rib fractures may be a subtle indication of a more serious associated injury. For example, a fracture of the first rib is a hallmark of severe trauma and it has been associated with major chest, abdominal and vascular injuries. It stands to reason that fracture of the first rib would be associated with significant energy transfer since it is anatomically well protected by the clavicle anteriorly and the scapula and associated musculature posteriorly. Therefore, the presence of a first rib fracture should alert one to the possibility of associated life-threatening injuries such as traumatic thoracic aortic pseudoaneurysm or a ruptured abdominal viscus. When one sees a first rib fracture, consideration should be given to obtaining arch aortography and performing diagnostic peritoneal lavage. Similarly, fractures of the lower ribs should arouse suspicion of hepatic or splenic injury. A 20% incidence of splenic rupture has been described with a fracture of any one or a combination of the tenth through the twelfth ribs on the left.

Rib fractures can lead to significant complications if inappropriately or inadequately treated. Since the pain of rib fractures can be intense, the discomfort frequently leads to splinting, poor inspiratory effort and ineffective cough which eventually result in atelectasis and pneumonia. Elderly patients or those with emphysema are particularly vulnerable to these complications. One can get a reasonable idea of how severely the pain is compromising the patient's ability to ventilate by measuring the tidal volume and the forced vital capacity. A tidal volume of less than 5 ml/kg or a forced vital capacity of less than 10 ml/kg is evidence of significant compromise. Three or fewer broken ribs can be treated with intercostal nerve blocks while four or more are best treated with epidural anaesthesia using either morphine or 0·5% bupivacaine. With adequate pain relief there should be an increase in the tidal volume and vital capacity and an improvement in the cough effort. Attempts to stabilize the fractured ribs with tape or binders may result in more splinting and further compromise gas exchange. Complications of rib fracture include haemothorax, pneumothorax, atelectasis and pneumonia.

Sternal Fractures

Sternal fractures are associated with a sharp blow to the anterior chest, such as that caused by the automobile steering wheel during abrupt deceleration. The incidence of sternal fractures is low, occurring in approximately 5% of patients with severe chest injury. The mortality rate has been reported to be as high as 30%. This relatively high mortality rate is due to the presence of associated chest injuries which include traumatic pseudoaneurysm of the thoracic aorta, ruptured oesophagus, myocardial contusion, ruptured bronchus and flail chest. Therefore, all patients with a sternal fracture should be carefully examined for the presence of associated intrathoracic injuries. The diagnosis of a sternal fracture can be suspected by the mechanism of injury and the presence of localized, usually severe, tenderness on palpation. Treatment is directed initially at pain relief to ensure an effective inspiratory effort. Approximately 25% of patients will eventually require operative reduction and fixation because of persistent pain, chest wall deformity, or chest wall instability.

Subcutaneous Emphysema

The presence of subcutaneous emphysema in a trauma patient is usually an indication of visceral injury. Air can enter the subcutaneous tissue through a laceration in the parietal pleura associated with a simple pneumothorax, through an external wound, or it can dissect up out of the mediastinum subsequent to a ruptured oesophagus or bronchus. The air itself is benign and will be reabsorbed with time after treatment of the primary problem. Intercostal intubation may be indicated in a patient with subcutaneous emphysema and rib fractures, especially if a general anaesthetic is contemplated. The chest tube is essential to reduce the potential for a tension pneumothorax when positive airway pressure is applied to the lung.

Flail Chest

Flail chest injuries are common, occurring in approximately 20% of patients with severe blunt chest injury. A flail chest results from multiple contiguous, comminuted or segmental rib fractures. It can also occur without rib fractures when there is separation of ribs from the sternum associated with disruption of the ligamentous attachments of the ribs to the transverse process of the vertebral bodies. Similarly, a sternal 'flail' results when there is bilateral disruption of the rib attachments to the sternum. These types of injuries produce a segment of chest wall which is responsive to changes in the pleural pressure rather than to the muscular action of the chest cage. This 'flail' segment moves paradoxically during inspiration and expiration. That is, it moves inward with inspiration (when pleural pressure is negative) and outward with expiration (when pleural pressure is positive). In the past, a generally accepted tenet was that this paradoxical respiration was a key factor in the pathophysiology of flail chest. Paradoxical respiration led to 'pendulluft', a to-and-fro movement of air between the lungs which necessarily impaired tidal flow and interfered with ventilation. Historically, all attempts at treating flail chest were aimed at stabilizing the chest wall in an effort to arrest the paradoxical movement of the flail segment. Initially, this took the form of taping or strapping the fractured ribs. Later, various forms of internal stabilization utilizing orthopaedic devices were tried, but without much success in decreasing the mortality rate of 30–40%. Tracheal intubation and positive-pressure ventilation were eventually utilized to managed flail chest. These modalities provided for internal pneumatic stabilization of the chest wall by inducing an alkalotic apnoea while ensuring that there was optimal gas exchange. Tracheostomy and mechanical ventilation for 3–5 weeks was required to allow for proper healing of the rib fractures. This innovation in technology did not significantly change the overall mortality rate which remained at about 30%. In addition, an added morbidity arose because of the complications associated with tracheostomy, prolonged intubation and mechanical ventilation.

Subsequent improvements in respiratory therapy coupled with a better understanding of the underlying pathophysiology improved the treatment of flail chest. The use of intermittent mandatory ventilation (IMV) and constant positive airway pressure (CPAP) lessened the time of mechanical ventilation and helped to decrease the morbidity associated with prolonged mechanical ventilation. These advances in understanding of the pathophysiology led to treatment of flail chest without intubation and mechanical ventilation. Rather than placing the emphasis on trying to re-establish the stability of the chest wall, efforts were made to treat the frequently associated pulmonary contusion, and to be very aggressive with pain relief and chest physiotherapy. This regimen resulted in significant improvements in mortality and morbidity by decreasing the number of patients receiving tracheostomy and mechanical ventilation and by lessening the duration of mechanical ventilation and the duration of hospitalization.

Non-ventilatory management of flail chest injuries requires constant physician input and a skilful intensive care unit nursing staff. Constant attention is paid to the patient's respiratory status beginning at the time of admission to the hospital. Mechanical problems such as airway obstruction or haemopneumothorax are quickly alleviated. An arterial blood gas measurement is done while the patient is breathing room air. On the basis of the clinical findings and the arterial blood gas results, an initial decision regarding therapy is made. If the patient manifests respiratory distress and hypoxaemia, he is intubated and CPAP, with or without IMV, is initiated. If the patient is not in respiratory distress and has an arterial oxygen tension of greater than 8·6 kPa (65 mmHg), a more conservative approach is used. Tidal volume, vital capacity and respiratory rate are measured prior to administration of pain relief. After pain relief with either epidural anaesthesia or intercostal nerve blocks, measurements of tidal volume and vital capacity are repeated. With effective analgesia, patients should demonstrate an increase in tidal volume and vital capacity and a decrease in respiratory rate.

Chest physiotherapy, incentive spirometry, and postural drainage are coordinated with periods of maximum pain relief. Within 72 h, the need for regional anaesthesia decreases, and pain can be relieved adequately with systemic analgesia such as intramuscular morphine sulphate or oral codeine.

Patients with flail chest should not be transferred from the intensive care area until their pain is well controlled, their cough is effective, and their tidal volume is adequate. This usually requires 2–5 days depending on the nature of their chest injury and the magnitude of their associated injuries. If at any time during the initial evaluation or subsequent therapy the patient's pulmonary status deteriorates, ventilator support should be initiated. This support is individualized according to the patient's needs. If the patient is hypoxaemic but ventilating adequately (as evidenced by normocarbia, respiratory rate of less than 30), CPAP delivered by mask or endotrachael tube is instituted. If ventilation is a problem (as evidenced by carbon dioxide retention, tachypnoea, or respiratory distress), IMV is added.

Ventilatory support is essential for some patients with flail chest injuries. These patients manifest clinical respiratory distress early in their hospital course. They have a moderate degree of ventilation-perfusion inequality and intrapulmonary shunting and their hypoxaemia improves only slightly when supplementary oxygen is administered. Intubation and CPAP are lifesaving in these patients. If intubation and respiratory support are not provided, the arterial $P\text{O}_2$ continues to fall and, later, the arterial $P\text{CO}_2$ rises. The latter is an indication of advanced respiratory failure and mandates immediate ventilatory support. Patients with flail chest injuries who are not in clinical respiratory distress on admission to the hospital may have mild hypoxia due to mild ventilation–perfusion inequality which improves with supplementary oxygen. Such patients will benefit from conservative management.

INJURIES INVOLVING THE PLEURAL SPACE

Simple Pneumothorax

Pneumothorax occurs when air, usually originating from the pulmonary alveoli or small airways, accumulates in the pleural space. It is common after penetrating or blunt injury. Approximately 90% of patients with a pneumothorax due to blunt injury have an associated rib fracture. Physical findings include diminished breath sounds, hyper-resonance on percussion, decreased respiratory expansion on the side of injury and, occasionally, soft-tissue crepitus. A chest radiograph is confirmatory and should always be performed in a stable patient prior to treatment. Traumatic pneumothorax should be treated by intercostal intubation. Since a coexisting haemothorax is common, a large tube should be placed to ensure complete evacuation of air and blood. The use of prophylactic antibiotics has been advocated by some to prevent empyema.

Tension Pneumothorax

A tension pneumothorax is created if air continues to accumulate in the pleural space to the point that the pressure in the pleural space exceeds ambient (atmospheric) pressure (i.e., there is positive intrapleural pressure). Positive intrapleural pressure will create a significant impediment to ventilation and circulation since normal tidal flow to the affected lung and venous return to the heart are dependent upon a pressure gradient created by negative intrapleural pressure. Therefore, a tension pneumothorax will produce symptoms of both respiratory and haemodynamic compromise. A tension pneumothorax can be caused by an oblique laceration of the lung or bronchus which acts as a one-way valve allowing air to accumulate but not to escape from the pleural space. Currently, the most common cause of a tension pneumothorax is positive-pressure ventilation of a patient with a simple pneumothorax. The application of several positive-pressure breaths to a lung with even a small air leak will rapidly convert a simple to a tension pneumothorax. The diagnosis should be readily apparent from the physical examination. Dyspnoea with or without tachypnoea is usually present. The involved hemithorax is hyper-resonant and breath sounds are decreased. In advanced stages there is hypotension associated with cervical venous distension and tracheal shift toward the contralateral hemithorax. If the patient is receiving positive-pressure ventilation there may be massive subcutaneous emphysema. A chest radiograph is seldom needed to make the diagnosis, but if obtained it will show moderate depression of the hemidiaphragm, mediastinal shift toward the contralateral hemithorax and widening of the intercostal space (*Fig.* 18.1). Treatment consists of immediate decompression with a large-bore needle placed in the second intercostal space in the midclavicular line. The needle should be left in place until intercostal intubation has been placed in the fourth space in the midaxillary line.

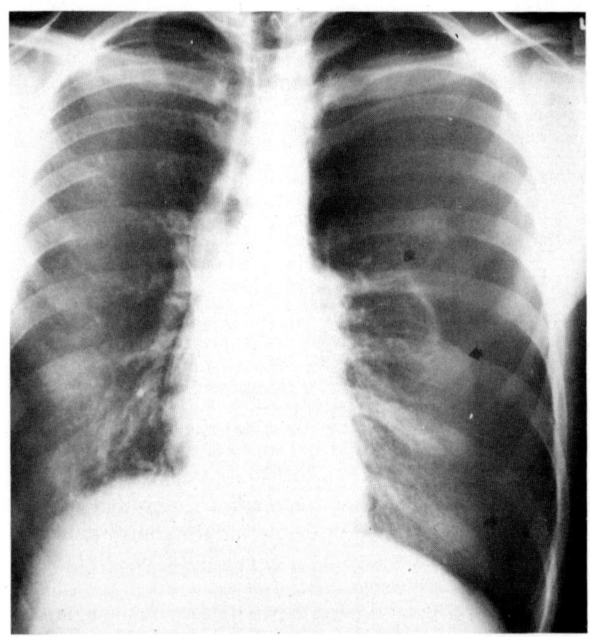

Fig. 18.1 Left tension pneumothorax. Note the tracheal and mediastinal shift to the right of midline, the collapsed lung (arrows), the widened intercostal spaces, and the depressed left hemidiaphragm. (By courtesy of Dr Linda Olson.)

Open Pneumothorax

Open pneumothorax is rarely encountered in civilian practice. When it does occur, it is usually due to close range shotgun blasts or impalement in which a chest wall defect is created. The chest wall defect allows for equilibration between the atmospheric pressure and the pleural pressure. Loss of the pressure gradient impairs ventilation and decreases venous return. If the chest wall defect is large there will be no effective alveolar ventilation since air will preferentially enter the pleural space through the chest wall defect with each inspiration instead of entering the airway. This produces a 'sucking chest wound'. Diagnosis is obvious by inspection. Treatment consists of immediate coverage of the defect with petrolatum-impregnated gauze. This creates a closed pneumothorax, which should be treated by intercostal intubation. In most cases, definitive exploration and chest wall débridement in the operating room will be required.

Haemothorax

Haemothorax, blood accumulating within the pleural space, occurs in approximately 50–75% of patients with severe blunt or penetrating chest trauma. Bleeding may be minimal or massive dependent upon the organ injured. Small lung lacerations or puncture wounds infrequently bleed massively because of the low pressure in the pulmonary circulation and because the lung has a high concentration of tissue thromboplastin. Bleeding from an intercostal artery can be extensive, especially if it is incompletely transected or tangentially lacerated such that vasospasm is ineffective in slowing or stopping bleeding. Patients may present in shock or be relatively asymptomatic depending upon the magnitude of haemorrhage. Breath sounds are decreased on the involved side, especially if there is an associated pneumothorax. The supine chest radiograph (*Fig.* 18.2) will show a diffuse haziness compatible with fluid density which will layer out on a decubitus or upright film. Adequate treatment requires intercostal intubation which must be large enough to ensure evacuation of all blood. Residual haemothorax will clot and eventually organize into a fibrothorax which can severely restrict the expansion of the involved lung. Simple intubation will be satisfactory treatment of most patients with haemothorax. However, massive initial return (greater than 1000–1200 ml) or significant continued haemorrhage (greater than 100–200 ml/h for several hours) are an indication for emergency thoracotomy to control bleeding.

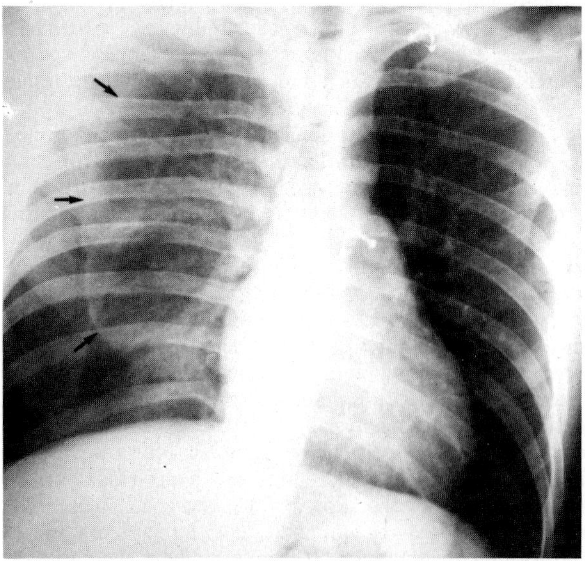

Fig. 18.2 Right haemopneumothorax. Note the diffuse haziness in the right hemithorax which contains blood compared to the clear hemithorax on the left. Note the collapsed right lung (arrows). (By courtesy of Dr Linda Olson.)

Intercostal Intubation

The most effective way of evacuating the thorax of blood and air in trauma patients suffering a haemopneumothorax is with a tube thoracostomy. Thoracentesis may be ineffective in completely removing a haemothorax leading to an increased risk of fibrothorax.

The patient should be placed in the supine position with the involved thorax slightly elevated on a folded sheet or blanket. The fifth or sixth interspace is generally selected since it will provide for adequate drainage of blood. The proposed site should be thoroughly scrubbed, prepared with iodine or alcohol, draped and infiltrated with local anaesthetic. A large tube (No. 36 F) is used to ensure complete evacuation of blood. A small incision is made in the skin of the interspace one level below the site of proposed pleural entry and a tract developed through the subcutaneous space to just over the top of the rib. The interspace below is selected to provide a 'shutter' closure effect to prevent recurrent pneumothorax when the tube is discontinued. The pleural space is entered over the superior aspect of the rib to avoid the neurovascular bundle which runs along the inferior aspect. A clamp, rather than a trocar, is used to enter the pleural space. A trocar is not used because it may injure the underlying lung or diaphragm. Prior to insertion of the tube it is prudent to insert a gloved finger into the chest to confirm entry into the pleural space. The tube is then directed along the tract while ensuring that all drainage holes are within the chest. It is then connected to a drainage system, sutured in place and covered with a sterile dressing. Tube position is confirmed by radiography.

INJURIES OF THE LARGE AIRWAYS

Major injuries of the tracheobronchial tree are believed to be rare. The true incidence is unknown because many patients die prior to reaching the hospital. This is particularly true of patients with penetrating injuries who rapidly exsanguinate because of injuries to the adjacent pulmonary vessels. In addition, a group of patients with blunt injury do not present acutely but develop symptoms referable to the lesion later in life.

Tracheobronchial disruption due to blunt trauma occurs within one inch of the carina in greater than 80% of cases and carries a mortality rate of approximately 30%. The typical tear is circumferential; vertical tears along the cartilaginous junction are less frequent. The mechanism of injury is thoracic compression which produces bursting and shearing forces.

Patients generally present in one of two ways. In the first, the bronchus ruptures into the pleural cavity causing a pneumothorax, which can be massive. These patients will be in mild to moderate respiratory distress. Presenting symptoms include haemoptysis, subcutaneous or mediastinal emphysema and, occasionally, cyanosis. Physical findings include decreased breath sounds and hyper-resonance. A second form of presentation is much less acute. The bronchial rupture does not communicate with the pleural space, but with the mediastinum. If there is a rent in the pleura, it is small or seals quickly. Respiratory distress in this group is uncommon. Some patients may complain of mild haemoptysis. There may be subcutaneous emphysema in the neck and auscultation of the chest may reveal a crunching sound with each heart beat (Hamman's sign) indicative of mediastinal emphysema. Healing of the rupture frequently results in stricture with airway obstruction and atelectasis. Bronchiectasis and suppuration may follow.

A chest radiograph will frequently reveal findings suggestive of a torn bronchus. Among these are: pneumothorax with or without subcutaneous and mediastinal emphysema (*Fig.* 18.3); air surrounding the course of a bronchus, and obstruction in the course of an air-filled bronchus. Bronchoscopy will confirm the diagnosis of tracheobronchial injury and should be considered in any patient with blunt chest trauma who has suggestive clinical or radiographic findings. In those patients who present acutely and who are in moderate respiratory distress, the procedure should be done by a thoracic surgeon in an operating room prepared for urgent thoracotomy.

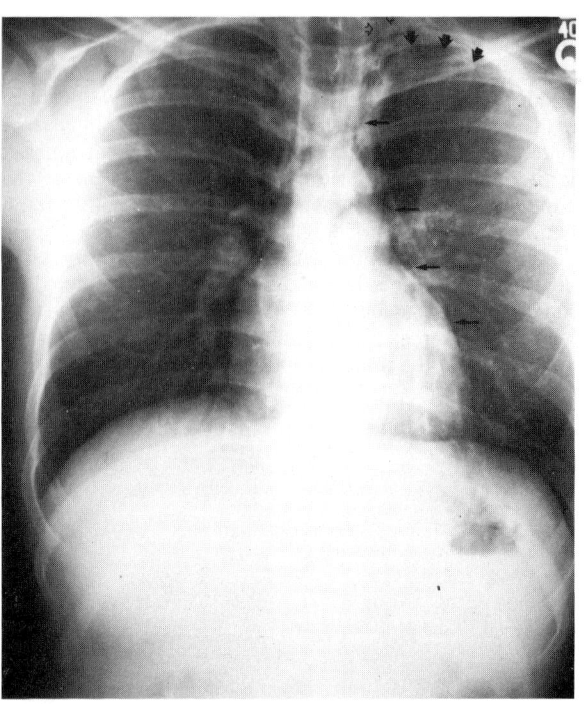

Fig. 18.3 Mediastinal and subcutaneous emphysema and a left apical pneumothorax associated with a small bronchial tear. The pneumomediastinum is outlined by the arrows along the cardiac silhouette, the pneumothorax by the arrows at the apex of the left lung and the subcutaneous air by the open arrows in the neck. (By courtesy of Dr Linda Olson.)

Treatment depends on the extensiveness of the disruption and the patient's clinical course. Complete disruption requires emergency thoracotomy and repair. If bronchoscopy reveals a tear of less than one-third of the circumference of the bronchus and the lung is re-expanded with simple intercostal intubation, surgery may not be required.

INJURIES OF THE PULMONARY PARENCHYMA

Pulmonary Contusion

Pulmonary contusion is one of a spectrum of parenchymal injuries produced by compressive forces acting on the lung. Contusion results in haemorrhage and oedema formation in the alveoli and interstitium without accompanying major parenchymal disruption as occurs in pulmonary laceration, pulmonary haematoma or traumatic lung cavitation. Contusion occurs in up to 70% of patients with severe blunt chest trauma. The mortality rate is variable and depends upon associated injuries, underlying lung disease and patient age. The mortality rate of an isolated pulmonary contusion ranges from 14 to 40%.

There is now substantial evidence to suggest that the changes associated with pulmonary contusion are similar to those produced by blast injury. High-pressure waves and thoracic compression disrupt the pulmonary capillary membrane resulting in a capillary 'leak' phenomenon in the area of the injury. The extravasation of blood and plasma into the alveoli and interstitium results in decreased compliance of both the injured and the adjacent uninjured lung. The decrease in compliance leads to hypoventilation and ventilation–perfusion inequalities. Alveolar flooding causes an increase in intrapulmonary shunting which is partially compensated by hypoxic vasoconstriction. These microvascular changes result in hypoxaemia, the degree of which is dependent upon the amount of lung which is injured. The decrease in compliance increases the work of breathing. In addition, the pain associated with the chest injury decreases the patient's inspiratory and cough effort resulting in atelectasis, retention of secretions and further reduction in compliance. If the patient is unable to meet the demands of increased ventilatory work because of age or associated injuries, respiratory failure ensues.

Diagnosis is usually based upon the mechanism of injury, arterial blood gas analysis and chest radiography. The radiographic changes occur within 1 h of injury in 70% of patients while in the remainder there is a time lag of between 4 and 6 h. The classic finding is a poorly defined infiltrate suggesting both alveolar and interstitial oedema (*Fig.* 18.4). The most marked changes may occur in and around the hilar structures. This may be due to a concentration of forces produced by the refraction and reflection of stress waves by the mediastinal structures and the rigid thoracic cage. Depending on the severity of injury and the treatment, resolution can begin within 48–72 h, but may require 2–3 weeks to be complete.

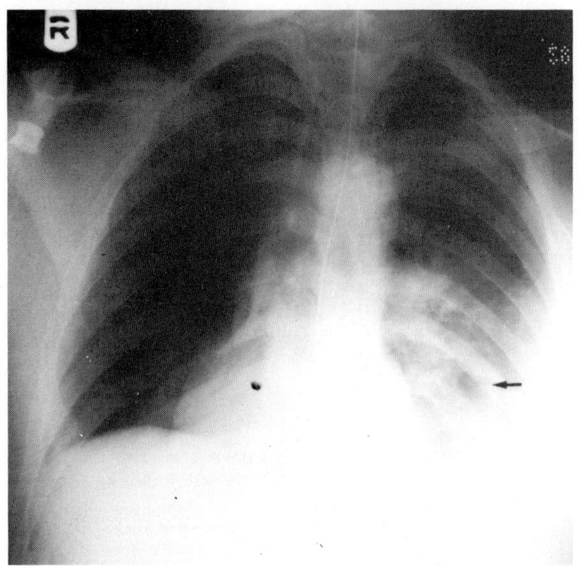

Fig. 18.4 Pulmonary contusion. Note the diffuse haziness in the left lower lobe. There is also a traumatic pulmonary pneumatocele within the contusion (arrow).

The treatment and the prognosis of pulmonary contusion is dependent upon the severity of the lung injury, and the nature and severity of associated injuries. Initially, attention is turned to treating the life-threatening injuries. This may require the infusion of large quantities of fluid and blood. Resuscitation of patients in shock, especially those with an insult to the pulmonary microvasculature, should be done judiciously, titrating the amount of resuscitative fluid to physiological end-points such as cardiac filling pressures, mean arterial pressure and urinary output. It is important to keep these patients in a 'dry state' to attempt to decrease pulmonary interstitial oedema. For these reasons, patients with pulmonary contusion should be monitored closely. An arterial line allows access to blood gases as well as close observation of the blood pressure. A pulmonary artery catheter is indicated in those patients with severe associated injuries who require significant amounts of fluid. Measurement of the pulmonary capillary wedge pressure, the cardiac output and the mixed venous blood gases is invaluable in discerning trends and initiating therapy in these critically ill patients. Fluid and blood should be administered to maintain oxygen delivery at a sufficient level to meet the metabolic demand as evidenced by the base deficit and the mixed venous oxygen tension. The type of asanguineous solution used is not critical since both crystalloid and colloid will leak during the stage of microvascular injury and increased capillary permeability. Over-zealous resuscitation results in an increase in the pulmonary capillary hydrostatic pressure and the accumulation of oedema fluid in the injured lung which will serve to exaggerate the problem and worsen the clinical picture. Patients who manifest any signs of respiratory failure should be intubated and mechanically ventilated until compliance and gas exchange return to normal. The period of ventilatory support may be as short as 48 h in patients with small contusions and no associated injuries or as long as several weeks in those patients with septic complications who develop protracted capillary leak phenomenon. Neither prophylactic antibiotics nor steroids are indicated for a contusion secondary to blunt trauma. Corticosteroids have been shown to decrease bacterial clearance from the lung.

Pulmonary Laceration

Pulmonary laceration is common after penetrating injury but rare after blunt chest trauma. In non-penetrating trauma the mechanism is similar to that which produces contusion but is much more severe. Occasionally, a spicule of bone from a fractured rib may cause the laceration. Patients usually present in respiratory distress with haemoptysis of varying degree. This should alert one to the presence of a more severe injury than pulmonary contusion in which haemoptysis is uncommon. A chest radiograph will show a haemopneumothorax in addition to a pulmonary contusion.

Treatment consists of insertion of a chest tube to drain the haemothorax and expand the lung. With a large laceration there may be a significant air leak which occasionally will require a second chest tube. Bronchoscopy should be performed in those patients with haemoptysis to rule out a ruptured bronchus.

Patients who require mechanical ventilation and who have significant air leak due to a lung laceration present a major problem. Changes in pulmonary compliance associated with the injury 'stiffen' the lung parenchyma causing the tidal ventilation delivered under positive pressure to follow the path of 'least resistance' and, thus, to be directed out through the laceration and to be effectively lost from the patient. The leak decreases alveolar ventilation and can result in elevated arterial carbon dioxide tension. In addition, the high flows through the parenchymal laceration prohibit healing and prolong the need for ventilator support. This problem can be addressed by using high-frequency positive-pressure ventilation to allow for adequate oxygenation and ventilation at lower mean airway pressures. This form of mechanical support is usually associated with a decrease in the size of the air leak and more rapid healing of the inury, If, however, a significant leak persists, or the lung fails to re-expand, or if haemorrhage from the chest tube persists at a significant rate (usually greater than 100–200 ml/h), thoracotomy is indicated. As with pulmonary contusion, prophylactic antibiotics and corticosteroids are not indicated.

Pulmonary Haematoma

A pulmonary haematoma is produced by bleeding into a pulmonary laceration which is contained by the parenchyma or the pleura. The mechanism of injury and the presenting symptoms are similar to pulmonary contusion, although haemoptysis is more frequent in patients with a pulmonary haematoma. The chest radiograph helps to distinguish the two lesions as a haematoma has a better defined margin than contusion and tends to assume a more spherical shape due to the elasticity of the surrounding uninjured lung (*Fig.* 18.5). Occasionally, the haematoma will have a central lucency if there has been an associated tear in an airway. Resolution will generally occur within 2–3 weeks during which time the patient may have intermittent low grade fever. Treatment is conservative with antibiotics reserved for those patients with a documented infection.

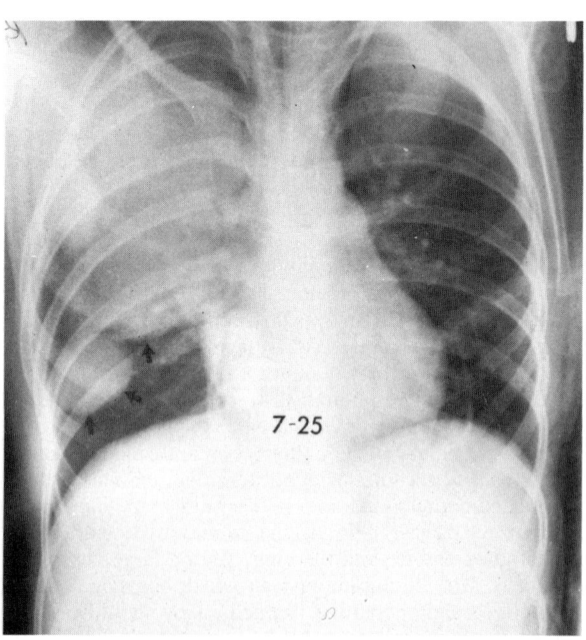

Fig. 18.5 Pulmonary haematoma. Note the well-defined margins of this lesion (arrows) as compared to a pulmonary contusion (*Fig.* 18.4). (By courtesy of Dr Linda Olson.)

Traumatic Pulmonary Pneumatocele

More rare than a pulmonary haematoma, a pulmonary pneumatocele is formed when the disruptive force ruptures a small bronchus without producing significant haemorrhage. This results in the formation of a pulmonary cavity. A pneumatocele as an isolated injury is tolerated well. Patients may have mild chest pain, dyspnoea and haemoptysis. A chest radiograph will show an air-filled cavity which may have an air fluid level on upright film (*Figs.* 18.4, 18.6). It is important to rule out a pre-existing lesion such as a pulmonary abscess or tuberculosis. If the chest film is only suggestive and questions remain, computerized tomography is helpful in establishing the diagnosis. The course is benign in the vast majority of patients with only 4 infections occurring in the 40 cases reported in the world's literature up to 1981. Prophylactic antibiotics are not recommended. Conservative management with pulmonary toilet and observation are indicated. Resolution is slow, requiring up to 16 weeks.

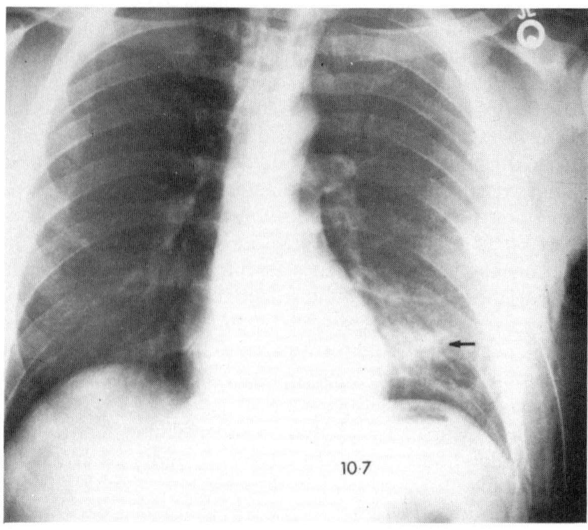

a

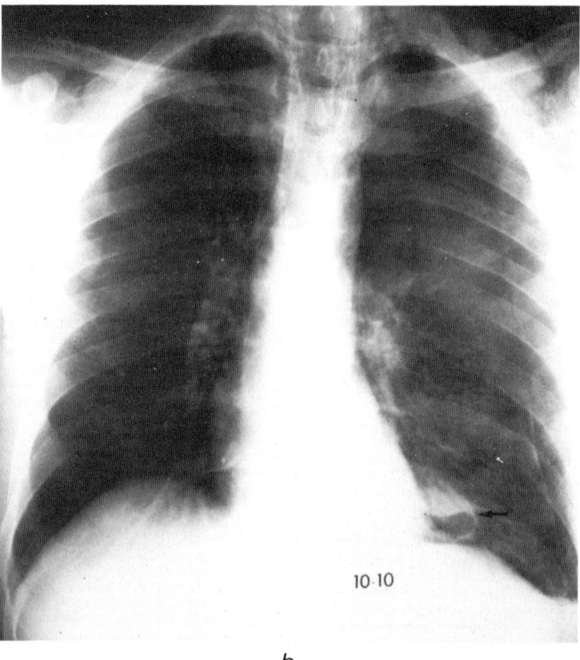

b

Fig. 18.6 Traumatic pulmonary pneumatocele. This lesion began as a small pulmonary contusion (*a*). Over 36 h it developed a cystic appearance (*b*). (By courtesy of Dr Linda Olson.)

Injury of the Thoracic Aorta

Traumatic rupture of the thoracic aorta occurs in 10–15% of automobile accident fatalities. Approximately 80% of victims with this injury will die at the scene of the accident or in transit to the hosptial. Of the patients reaching hospital 30%

will die in 6 h, 50% within 24 h, and 90% within 10 weeks if no surgical treatment is rendered. Major teaching centres report treating 1–4 patients per year with this injury.

Although the term 'rupture' implies that bursting forces due to aortic compression and elevation of the intraluminal pressure are primarily responsible for the injury, other forces associated with rapid deceleration are operant. These include horizontal and transverse shear and torsion stress. Shear forces effect damage at points of fixation due to unequal rates of deceleration. All of these forces combine to disrupt the intima and media to form a pseudoaneurysm contained only by the adventitia.

The most common sites of aortic injury after blunt trauma are the descending aorta just distal to the origin of the left subclavian artery and the ascending aorta just proximal to the innominate artery. Because injuries of the ascending thoracic aorta are frequently associated with severe cardiac injuries and death, the majority of patients surviving long enough to receive surgical treatment have injuries located between the origin of the left subclavian and the ligamentum arteriosum.

The clinical presentation is extremely variable. Patients may have no sign of significant trauma or be in extreme distress as a result of multiple injuries to the chest, abdomen and extremities. Thoracic injuries frequently associated with aortic rupture include flail chest, first rib fracture, sternal fracture and severely displaced clavicle fracture or sterno-clavicular dislocation. Patients most frequently complain of chest or back pain. On physical examination, dyspnoea, dysphagia or hoarseness may occasionally be found due to compression of associated structures. It is important to note blood pressure and pulse character in each of the upper and lower extremities. This is because a 'pseudocoarctation' of the aorta may be produced when the distal portion of fractured intima prolapses into the aortic lumen, in which case there will be upper extremity hypertension with attenuation of the pulse in the lower extremities. A thorough neurological examination is extremely important, as patients may present with paraplegia or paraparesis as a consequence of compression of the intercostal arteries supplying the spinal cord. In addition, neurological dysfunction of the lower extremities is a recognized complication of the surgical management of the lesion. Hence, it is important to document neurological function in all patients suspected of having this injury prior to the institution of any treatment.

Diagnosis of a ruptured thoracic aorta requires a high index of suspicion based on the mechanism of injury (i.e., rapid deceleration) and the presence of associated injuries (i.e., sternal fracture or flail chest). The chest radiograph is very useful as a screening procedure, but definitive diagnosis requires arch aortography. Radiographic findings on a plain film suggestive of aortic injury are those which indicate the presence of a mediastinal haematoma and include: superior mediastinal widening equal to or greater than 8 cm on a standard 100-cm anteroposterior projection; shift of the trachea to the right of midline; loss of the sharp contour of the aortic knob; obliteration of the medial aspect of the left upper lobe; opacification of the clear space between the aorta and the pulmonary artery; and depression of the left mainstem bronchus (*Fig.* 18.7). Widening or loss of the paravertebral stripe and displacement of the nasogastric tube to the right of midline also suggest mediastinal haemorrhage. Less reliable associated findings, which are not necessarily indicative of mediastinal haemorrhage, include: left haemothorax, fracture of the first or second ribs; and clavicle fracture. Of all the plain film findings, widening of the superior mediastinum is generally considered to be the most sensitive. It is important to remember that these findings may be extremely subtle and, on occasion, may be totally absent, especially if the film is taken very soon after the accident. Therefore, consideration of the mechanism of injury and sound clinical judgement must play an important role in the selection of patients for aortography. Aortography can be performed rapidly and skilfully in most trauma centres and is mandatory, in stable patients, before proceeding to the operating room. The aortogram will establish the diagnosis and provide valuable information regarding the location and extent of the injury (*Fig.* 18.8). Percutaneous transfemoral aortography is a very low risk procedure with an incidence of serious contrast reactions of less than 0·1% and an incidence of local complications (i.e., vessel injury, thrombosis, haematoma, embolization) of less than 0·5%.

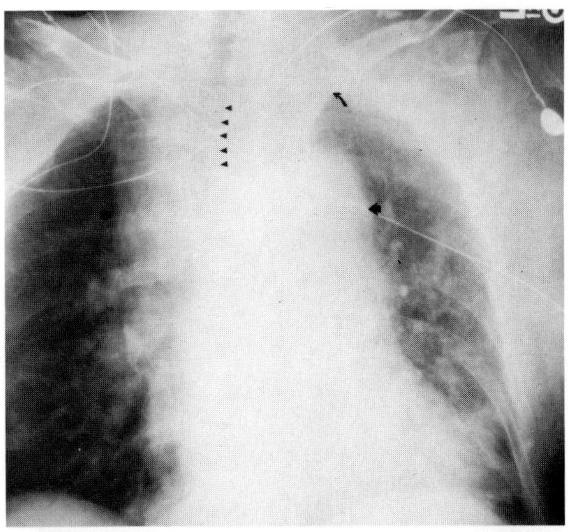

Fig. 18.7 Traumatic aortic rupture. Note the widening of the superior mediastinum (thick arrow), shift of the trachea to the right of midline (small arrow heads) and the obliteration of the medial boarder of the apex of the left lung producing an 'apical cap' (curved arrow).

Recently, computerized tomography has been advocated as being useful in the diagnosis of thoracic aortic rupture. However, the sensitivity and specificity of this modality in the diagnosis of aortic trauma is unknown. Moreover, injuries of the major aortic branches occasionally occur in association with aortic rupture and these would be missed with computerized tomography. For these reasons, arch aortography remains the only definitive diagnostic procedure for thoracic aortic rupture.

Treatment of thoracic aortic injury is surgical. Surgical repair requires left thoracotomy with or without partial left heart bypass.

Perioperatively, it is important to avoid hypertension. For this reason, insertion of an arterial cannula and a central venous monitor is mandatory. Either a peripheral long line placed through the femoral vein or antecubital fossa or an internal jugular line should be inserted. The subclavian route is to be avoided as the mediastinal haematoma may be entered and decompressed. Excessive administration of crystalloid and blood should be avoided. If the patient is

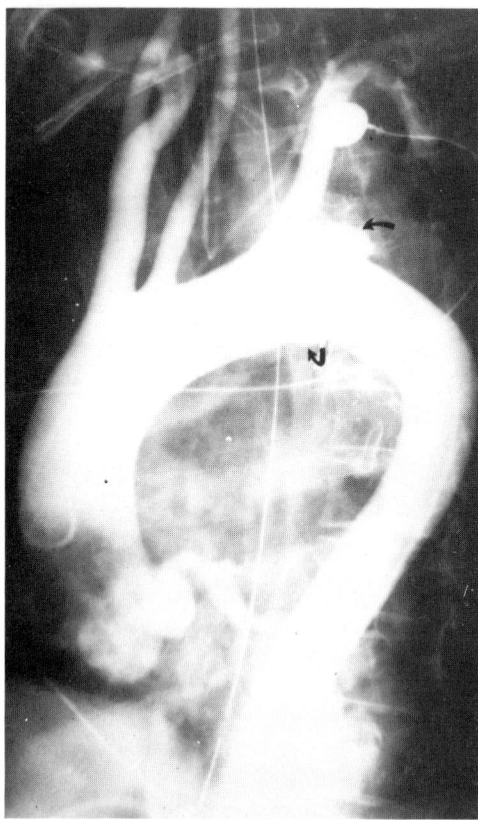

Fig. 18.8 Traumatic aortic rupture. Percutaneous transfemoral aortography (oblique view) demonstrating extravasation of dye just distal to the take-off of the left subclavian artery (arrows).

stable, procedures and manipulations which cause pain and anxiety and which can raise the systolic pressure should be postponed until after the patient is anaesthetized. If the patient is hypertensive, pharmacological manipulation of the blood pressure is indicated.

CARDIAC INJURIES

Myocardial Contusion

There is little agreement among clinicians regarding any aspect of myocardial contusion. The true incidence is largely unknown, probably because there is no unanimity concerning diagnostic criteria. Controversy also surrounds the significance of a contusion once discovered and its ultimate prognosis.

Myocardial contusion has been thought to occur in up to 75% of patients sustaining major blunt chest injury, although it has only been reported in 15% of patients with fatal chest injuries. Based upon several large series, 'clinically significant' myocardial contusion occurs in approximately 5–15% of patients with severe chest trauma. By 'clinically significant' is meant that the patient suffers a potentially life-threatening cardiac complication or death with contusion proven at autopsy. Post-mortem findings vary from petechial haemorrhages of the epicardium to myocardial rupture. Classically the contusion is haemorrhagic and well circumscribed. It may be full thickness or partial thickness and may involve more than one chamber. Contusion may even progress to liquefaction necrosis resulting in late rupture with tamponade or, if the septum is involved, late septal defect.

The injured myocardium is dysfunctional and prone to arrhythmias or conduction delay as well as abnormalities in wall motion. These factors can induce cardiac failure which may only become manifest during surgery for an associated injury. Other complications include pericarditis and pericardial effusion, with or without tamponade.

The mechanism of injury is usually a sternal blow, such as that produced by a steering wheel during rapid deceleration. Other frequently cited mechanisms include kicks, punches and falls. Rarely, the trauma is seemingly insignificant.

There are no classic signs or symptoms. Patients frequently complain of chest pain which is not relieved by vasodilators. Physical examination may reveal tenderness over the anterior chest associated with bruises or abrasions. However, signs of external thoracic trauma are frequently lacking. Auscultatory findings of murmur or rub are infrequent.

The chest radiograph is not helpful other than revealing associated injuries. Because there are no universally accepted diagnostic criteria of a myocardial contusion, the sensitivity and specificity of the various diagnostic modalities used to determine the presence of a contusion are highly variable. Controversy exists as to which modalities to utilize in a patient with blunt chest trauma in whom a contusion is suspected. An electrocardiogram (ECG) is generally accepted as the first step. The most frequent abnormalities noted are ST–T wave alterations (usually elevation of the ST segment) and sinus tachycardia. Supraventricular and ventricular arrhythmias, sinus and AV nodal dysfunction, and right and left bundle-branch blocks have been reported. The false negative rate of ECG ranges from 7 to 17% while false positives occur in up to 60%. Sinus tachycardia and ST–T wave changes may be due to hypovolaemia, hypoxia, pain and anxiety, all of which are frequent after severe trauma and probably account for the high false positive rate of ECG.

Measurement of the concentration of the myocardial band in the total creatinine phosphokinase (CPK–MB) level has been suggested as being helpful in the diagnosis of myocardial contusion. Since skeletal muscle injury frequently accompanies injury to the chest and since skeletal muscle contains approximately 1·1% CPK–MB, a level of greater than 2–5% CPK–MB has been suggested as being diagnostic. However, it is now well documented that CPK–MB elevations can occur without any clinical or post-mortem evidence of cardiac injury.

Radionuclide imaging utilizing technetium pyrophosphate has been useful to diagnose experimentally induced left ventricular myocardial contusion. The failure of scans to successfully diagnose contusion in man can be attributed to a number of factors. First, there are no diagnostic criteria as to what constitutes a positive scan. Secondly, pyrophosphate is a bone-scanning agent. Contusions, especially of the thin-walled right ventricle, may be obscured by the ribs or sternum. Thirdly, experimentally induced contusions are probably more severe and, thus, more easily seen than those occurring in the majority of trauma patients.

The most promising of the new techniques is two-dimensional (2-D) echocardiography. The right ventricle, which is the chamber most commonly injured, can be easily visualized. Wall motion abnormalities, intramural haematoma, intracavitary thrombus, pericardial effusion, and valvular dysfunction have all been seen. This procedure is inexpensive and can be done quickly and non-invasively at the bedside.

Once the diagnosis is suspected, patients should be monitored. Patients who have an isolated chest injury without major thoracic trauma can be monitored with a central venous catheter, daily 12-lead ECGs, and continuous ECG monitoring for 48–72 h. Supplemental oxygen may be administered. Arrhythmias should be treated aggressively. However, there are no data to support the use of prophylactic lignocaine. Patients with more severe injuries, especially those who require surgery, should be more invasively monitored with a pulmonary artery catheter and an arterial line placed prior to surgery. Emergency surgery to control haemorrhage or sepsis will eliminate factors which aggravate hypotension and hypoxia and would otherwise adversely affect myocardial function. Clinical judgement should dictate when patients no longer require monitoring and are fit for discharge. Follow-up visits should include a physical examination and ECG. If an abnormality had been noted on 2-D echocardiogram while the patient was hospitalized, a 2-D echocardiogram should be obtained in follow-up. Patients with a myocardial contusion who have a benign hospital course have a much better prognosis than patients suffering a myocardial infarction.

Cardiac Rupture

Cardiac rupture after blunt trauma is usually fatal. Patients generally succumb to exsanguination if the pericardium is ruptured or to tamponade if the pericardium is intact. The extent and severity of damage to the heart are probably related to the phase of the cardiac cycle at the time of injury. Late diastole or early systole are periods of increased vulnerability because the chambers are full and the valves are closed. Rapid compression of the heart during these periods can result in rupture of one or more chambers, laceration or perforation of the ventricular septum or injury to the mitral or aortic valve.

Ventricular rupture is usually fatal, probably because the pressure within the ventricle is higher than that in the atrium resulting in more rapid exsanguination or development of cardiac tamponade. Therefore, those patients surviving long enough to reach the hospital usually will have atrial injury. Atrial rupture usually occurs in the appendage since it is the weakest and thinnest part.

Cardiac rupture should be suspected in any patient with blunt chest trauma who manifests the signs and symptoms of pericardial tamponade, i.e. rising central venous pressure, hypotension, narrowed pulse pressure, muffled heart sounds, or a moderate decrease in blood pressure during inspiration.

No single laboratory test or radiograph is diagnostic of cardiac rupture. Rather, the diagnosis is based upon a high index of suspicion combined with the clinical presentation. Performing unnecessary diagnostic tests can be harmful, particularly if it requires transport of the patient to a part of the hospital poorly equipped to care for critically ill patients. In a stable patient suspected of having a cardiac injury, central venous pressure monitoring is extremely important. Portable chest radiography, ECG and portable 2-D echocardiography can be helpful in determining the nature of associated chest injuries and the extent of the cardiac insult in the stable patient. These studies, if desired, should be obtained as soon as possible after the patient's arrival.

Should the stable patient develop tamponade, volume infusion should be initiated, while plans for definitive therapy are being made. Volume expansion will temporarily increase filling pressure and cardiac output, even with moderate degrees of tamponade. This may allow enough time for transport to the operating room. If no surgeon is immediately available, pericardiocentesis should be undertaken to relieve tamponade. It should be remembered that pericardiocentesis is not definitive therapy and that cardiorrhaphy is still required.

Cardiac Valvular and Septal Defects

Valvular and septal defects do occur after blunt trauma but are infrequently encountered in clinical practice because they are often associated with ventricular or atrial rupture and death. Their presentation may be acute or chronic. Cardiac murmurs in patients who sustain blunt chest trauma and who have evidence of cardiac injury require investigation. A 2-D echocardiogram, measurement of intracardiac pressures or a formal cardiac catheterization may be required to make the diagnosis.

Penetrating Cardiac Injuries

Injuries of the heart are encountered in 2–4% of penetrating chest and abdominal injuries. Once thought to be universally fatal, penetrating cardiac trauma currently has a survival rate of 30–81%. This is largely due to improvements in prehospital care and advances in cardiac surgery. Most cardiac injuries which survive long enough to be treated are secondary to stab wounds. Survival is generally better after stab wounds because there is usually only a single chamber injury, there is little loss of cardiac tissue, the pericardial defect is small allowing tamponade rather than rapid exsanguination to develop, and the associated injuries are minor. Approximately 30–50% of patients with gunshot wounds of the heart who survive transport will eventually die secondary to severe cardiac and associated injuries.

As with cardiac rupture, penetrating cardiac injuries present with signs of either exsanguination and hypovolaemic shock or tamponade. Heart sounds may be muffled, although this is not a constant finding. Management principles are identical to those outlined for cardiac rupture.

INJURIES OF THE OESOPHAGUS

Traumatic perforation of the oesophagus from externally applied forces is rare. This is due, in part, to its protected location and, in part, to its elasticity and mobility within the thorax. While penetrating trauma can occur at any point, oesophageal rupture after blunt trauma most often occurs in the distal third just above the gastro-oesophageal junction. This area of the oesophagus has been demonstrated to be relatively weak. Rupture is probably produced by a sudden increase in intraoesophageal pressure due to blunt upper abdominal or lower chest trauma. Since the cricopharyngeus and the lower oesophageal sphincter are usually closed, this rapid rise in pressure causes the oesophagus to rupture at its weakest point.

The condition of the patient at the time of presentation is dependent upon the site of rupture and the degree of contamination. The amount of contamination is generally related to the delay in presentation. Injuries to the cephalad thoracic or cervical oesophagus, especially those produced by instrumentation, may have little contamination and be benign compared to those occurring in the distal oesophagus which are usually associated with contamination from gastric juices. Therefore, patients may be relatively asymptomatic with only mild dysphagia or chest pain. On the other hand, there may be moderate abdominal and chest pain, dyspnoea, and signs of hypovolaemia progressing to shock as mediastinitis develops. There may be decreased breath sounds over the involved hemithorax secondary to an associated haemopneumothorax or pleural effusion. Hamman's sign often is present due to the associated pneumomediastinum. A chest radiograph may show pneumothorax, haemothorax, or pneumomediastinum. A barium or Gastrografin swallow is a necessity to confirm the diagnosis and to localize the lesion.

Treatment should be vigorous and expeditious. Large-bore venous access is required since much intravascular volume can be lost in the inflammatory process within the mediastinum. Because of the potential for continued contamination, a nasogastric tube should be placed. Broad-spectrum antibiotics, with coverage for salivary anaerobes, should be started as soon as possible. If a pneumothorax or haemothorax is present, it should be drained preoperatively. The upper two-thirds of the thoracic oesophagus are approached with a right thoracotomy, while the lower third is approached through a left thoracotomy. Débridement, repair and coverage of the repair with pleura or an intercostal muscle flap, wide drainage and oesophageal exclusion with a cervical oesophagostomy and a gastrostomy are considered by many to be the best therapy. Early diagnosis and treatment are the most important factors in obtaining survival rates of 50–70%. (*See also* Chapter 66.)

19 *Abdominal Injuries*

D. B. Hoyt and R. C. Mackersie

INTRODUCTION

In civilian life, the majority of abdominal injuries are due to blunt trauma, secondary to high-speed automobile accidents. Penetrating injuries, although often associated with wartime combat, are seen with increasing frequency in hospital emergency departments, particularly in urban areas. The failure to manage abdominal injuries successfully accounts for the majority of *preventable* deaths following multiple injuries. Failure to recognize occult abdominal haemorrhage and to control bleeding successfully from intra-abdominal organs leads to significant morbidity, and such injuries account for approximately 10% of traumatic deaths that occur annually in the USA.

There are many mechanisms which account for abdominal injuries. The recognition of two major groups—penetrating and non-penetrating— is of greatest importance for treatment and has direct implications for the diagnostic work-up and therapy.

The abdomen encompasses a large area of the body, from the diaphragm superiorly to the infragluteal fold inferiorly, including the entire circumference of this region. Penetrating or blunt injury to the back may result in significant intra-abdominal injury as well. Multiple system injuries, particularly those involving the central nervous system, chest and musculoskeletal system are often associated and may obscure injury to the abdominal contents and symptoms from this area. In patients with multiple system trauma in whom specialty consultation is needed, the overall responsibility for treatment must reside with one physician, preferably the general surgeon. The importance of *repeated* assessment of a patient suspected of having intra-abdominal injury cannot be over-emphasized.

Experience shows that accurate categorization of injuries allows the development of treatment protocols which minimize wasted time and improve efforts in preoperative and intraoperative management of abdominal injuries.

ANATOMICAL CONSIDERATIONS

A practical knowledge of the contents of the abdomen is important. Assessment of the abdomen is influenced by its differing anatomical features. For evaluation purposes, the abdomen should be divided into four areas: intrathoracic abdomen, true abdomen, pelvic abdomen and the retroperitoneal abdomen (*Fig.* 19.1). With the exception of the true abdomen, all the other areas are difficult to assess on physical examination.

The intrathoracic abdomen is that portion of the upper abdomen which lies beneath the rib cage. Bony and cartilagenous structures make this portion essentially inaccessible to palpation. Its contents include the diaphragm, liver, spleen and stomach. Each may be injured when blunt or

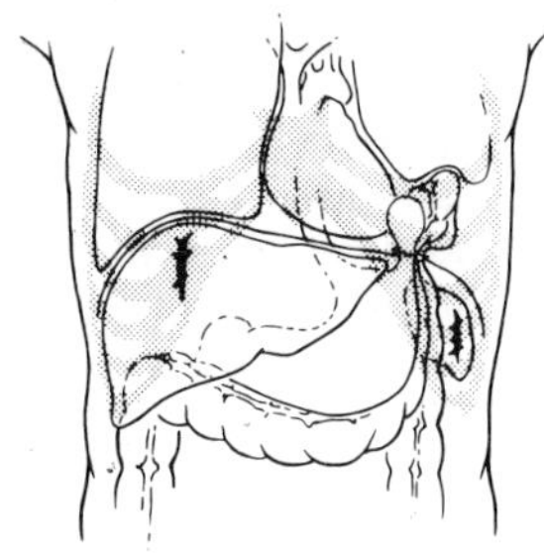

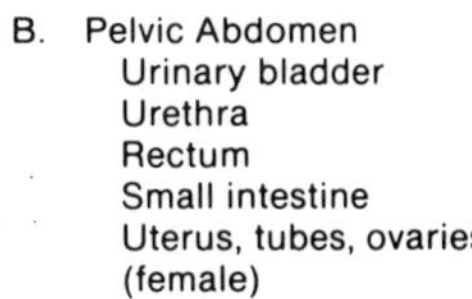

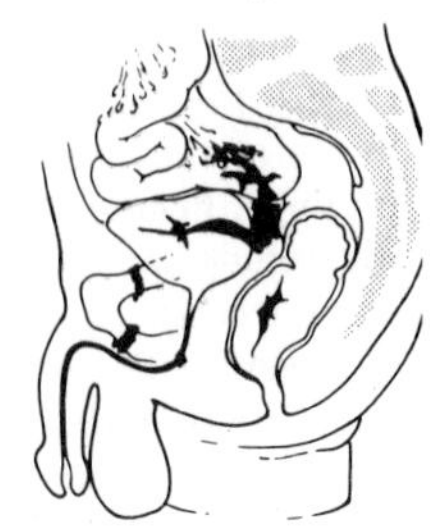

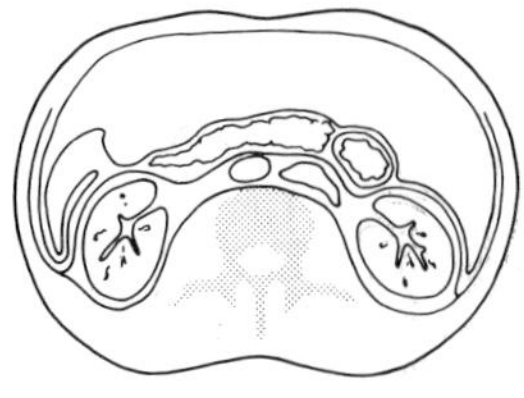

Fig. 19.1 Contents of the abdomen. (After Hardy J. D., ed. 1977. *Rhoads' Textbook of Surgery*, 5th ed. Philadelphia, Lippincott.)

Table 19.1 Aetiology of abdominal injuries

Penetrating	*Blunt*	*Iatrogenic*
Stab wounds	Crush injury	Endoscopic
Gunshot wounds	Blast injury	External cardiac massage
Shotgun wounds	Seatbelt syndrome	Peritoneal dialysis
		Paracentesis
		Percutaneous transhepatic cannulation
		Liver biopsy
		Barium enema

penetrating injury is delivered to the rib cage. Peritoneal lavage becomes useful in evaluating this area of anatomy.

The pelvic abdomen lies in the hollow of the pelvis and is surrounded on all sides by the bony pelvis. Its contents include the rectum, bladder, urethra, small bowel, and in females the uterus, tubes and ovaries. Trauma to the pelvis, particularly pelvic fractures, may damage the organs within, and penetrating injuries of the buttocks may injure any or all of the pelvic organs. Injury to these structures may be difficult to diagnose because of the lack of physical findings. As such, suspected injuries to this area of the abdomen must be investigated using adjunctive procedures such as bladder catheterization, urethocystography and sigmoidoscopy.

The retroperitoneal abdomen contains the kidneys, ureter, pancreas, second and third portion of the duodenum, and the great vessels, the aorta and vena cava. Injury to these structures may occur secondary to penetrating or blunt trauma as well. The kidneys may be damaged by injury to the lower ribs posteriorly, and any of these structures may be damaged by crushing injuries to the front or sides of the trunk. Again, injury to these structures may result in few physical findings, and physical examination and peritoneal lavage are of little or no help. Evaluation of the retroperitoneal abdomen requires utilization of radiographic procedures including intravenous pyelography, angiography and computerized tomography. In addition, serum amylase determinations may be helpful.

Finally, the true abdomen contains the small and large intestines, the bladder when distended, and uterus when gravid. Injuries to any of these organs is usually manifested by pain from peritonitis and is associated with abdominal findings. Peritoneal lavage is a useful adjunct when suspecting injury, and a plain abdominal film might be helpful when free air is present.

In summary, the abdomen consists of four distinct anatomical areas, each one which is suspected of sustaining injury must be investigated systematically with the knowledge of limitations of physical examination, and the appropriate X-ray or diagnostic procedures which may reveal the diagnosis.

CLASSIFICATION OF INJURIES

The classification of abdominal injuries based upon aetiology is extensive (*Table* 19.1). Classifications involving the amount of injury or the number of organs injured or the association of extra-abdominal injuries are not practical from the standpoint of diagnosis or treatment of abdominal injuries. It is more useful to categorize injuries into penetrating and non-penetrating, as this correlates best with the likelihood of significant intra-abdominal injury, the speed with which diagnosis and treatment must be accomplished and the associated mortality and morbidity.

Penetrating Wounds

With the availability of hand guns, this has replaced the knife as the most common cause of significant penetrating injury to the abdomen. Significant intra-abdominal injury occurs about 80% of the time following a gunshot wound, whereas significant injury occurs approximately 20–30% of the time following stab wounds. The frequency of injury following penetrating abdominal trauma is shown in *Table* 19.2.

Injuries to both thoracic and abdominal cavities occur in 25% of patients with penetrating wounds of the abdomen, and conversely, patients with penetrating wounds of the thorax can often have significant intra-abdominal injury since the wound may traverse the diaphragm and result in abdominal injury. Whether selective management or mandatory laparotomy is the best method for treating stab wounds is debated and discussed further below. Most agree that gunshot wounds to the abdomen should be explored as the probability of significant intra-abdominal injury is so high. The difference in injury potential is a function of the increased kinetic energy associated with a gunshot wound.

Blunt Trauma

Incidence of blunt abdominal trauma is increasing because of the increased automobile and motorcycle accident rate. The car remains the cause of non-penetrating trauma in at least 60% of patients with this injury. The incidence of specific organ injuries is listed in *Table* 19.3.

Table 19.2 Frequency of injury in penetrating abdominal trauma

Organ	*Per cent*
Liver	37
Small bo	26
Stomach	19
Colon	17
Major vascular	13
Retroperitoneal	10
Mesentery and omentum	10
Spleen	7
Diaphragm	5
Kidney	5
Pancreas	4
Duodenum	2
Biliary system	1
Other	1

Table 19.3 Frequency of injury in blunt abdominal trauma

Viscera	*Per cent*
Spleen	25
Kidney	12
Intestine	15
Liver	15
Retroperitoneal haematoma	13
Mesentery	5
Pancreas	3
Diaphragm	2
Urinary bladder	6
Urethra	2
Vascular	2

The sudden application of pressure to the abdomen is more likely to rupture a solid organ than a hollow viscera, and this accounts for the greater incidence of solid organ injury. More elastic tissues of the young tolerate trauma better than the less resilient or fixed tissue of older people and accounts for the difference in significant intra-abdominal injury following blunt trauma in children and adults.

Iatrogenic Injuries

Significant intra-abdominal injury can follow iatrogenic causes already listed in *Table* 19.1, and these represent a variety of commonly performed diagnostic and therapeutic procedures that can lead to significant intra-abdominal injury. The principles of diagnosis and treatment are no different from other traumatic injuries.

PREHOSPITAL CARE

Little can be done for patients with abdominal injuries in the field. For penetrating wounds, sterile dressings should be applied and the patient carefully monitored. Any foreign bodies imbedded in the trunk should not be removed as major bleeding might follow removal. Evisceration is best left undisturbed, except to apply a sterile dressing and protect the patient from further injury. General features of stabilization and evaluation include ensuring an adequately functioning airway, inserting intravenous lines, preferably in the upper extremity, and the beginning of fluid resuscitation.

HOSPITAL CARE AND DIAGNOSIS

Diagnosis and treatment should proceed concurrently following established protocols, many of which already have been reviewed. In the patient with suspected abdominal injury, the history of injury as well as the physical examination remain important factors in the surgeon's decision-making process.

DIAGNOSIS: HISTORY

Penetrating injuries present less diagnostic challenges other than whether or not to explore the abdomen. An attempt should be made to establish details of the weapon involved. Blunt trauma assessment can be greatly aided by accurate history. Obtaining a history from the paramedical team that the patient was involved in an automobile accident in which the steering wheel was impacted strongly suggests the possibility of duodenal or pancreatic trauma. If the patient has sustained rib fractures on the lower left chest there is a 20% chance of associated splenic injury and with rib fractures on the right there is 10% chance of liver injury. Back pain associated with a compression fracture of the upper limb or spinal region carries an associated 20% chance of significant renal injury. This, in combination with the aspects of physical diagnosis and adjuncts to physical diagnosis as discussed below, assists in the initial assessment of abdominal injury.

RESUSCITATION

The ABC of emergency resuscitation, airway, breathing and circulation should be initiated. A patent functioning airway must be established, particularly in the comatose patient prior to evaluation of the abdomen. If necessary, an endotracheal tube is placed and assisted ventilation begun. Upper extremity, large-bore i.v. cannulas are started and resuscitation begun with Ringer-lactate. Blood samples are drawn for basic studies including Hb, PCV, urea and electrolytes, amylase and blood for type and cross-match. Arterial blood gas is determined and repeated to assess ventilatory status and acidosis. An early rapid assessment of the abdomen is performed.

The key objective of the physical diagnosis of abdominal injury is to identify the need for operation. The precise determination of organ injury is unnecessary. Physical examination becomes the determination of intra-abdominal bleeding or peritoneal irritation. Unfortunately, because of anatomical constraints, evaluation of bleeding or peritoneal irritation may not be determined by examining the abdominal wall. Associated injuries often cause tenderness and spasm in the abdominal wall and make this diagnosis complex. Lower rib fractures, pelvic fractures, or abdominal wall contusion may mimic the signs of peritoneal irritation and it may be impossible to determine if there is significant intra-abdominal bleeding or peritoneal irritation from a ruptured viscus.

Since the primary manifestation of solid organ injury is haemorrhage, particularly following blunt trauma, the patient should be monitored closely during the initial assessment and resuscitation for evidence of continuing or refractory haemorrhagic shock. If this is a real suspicion, a MAST suit should be applied and further evaluation of the patient should occur in the operating room. A patient who remains haemodynamically stable allows for complete evaluation including physical examination, peritoneal lavage and adjunctive radiographic and laboratory evaluation.

PHYSICAL EXAMINATION

Physical assessment should proceed in an orderly fashion. The patient should be evaluated for signs of blunt trauma and for penetrating wounds. Small abrasions or areas of ecchymosis may represent warnings of significant intra-abdominal injury. All the penetrating wounds should be marked with radio-opaque clips and a subsequent radiograph taken to delineate the trajectory of the bullet or path of the knife and allow for an intelligent assessment of the likelihood of associated injury. The abdominal wall and back should be carefully inspected and posterior ecchymosis should raise the possibility of retroperitoneal injury. Absence of bowel sounds may be helpful to assess significant peritoneal irritation from blood or intestinal contents. This is more often likely to be a late finding following injury.

The patient's respiratory pattern should be evaluated. Halted, laboured breathing may be from diaphragmatic irritation or accompany upper abdominal injury. It may be a clue to significant abdominal trauma. Pain in the shoulder with inspiration (Kehr's sign) on the left side corresponds with irritation of the diaphragm from bleeding. Palpation may reveal localized tenderness, spasm or rigidity of the abdominal wall. This finding or direct rebound tenderness should make the clinician very suspicious of significant intra-abdominal injury. In the conscious patient, suprapubic tenderness and pelvic lateral wall tenderness are assessed for, indicating a pelvic fracture. Inspection of the perineum and urethral meatus for blood raises the possibility of pelvic fracture as well. The passage of a Foley catheter should be delayed until radiographic evaluation of the pelvis and urethra can be made.

As assessment continues, an indwelling urinary catheter and a sample of urine are sent to the laboratory to evaluate for microscopic haematuria. If one is suspicious of injury to the lower urinary tract, bladder or urethra because of an associated pelvic fracture, catheterization should be delayed until urethrography is performed to rule out injury to the urethra. Rectal examination is performed. Sphincter tone is evaluated. The integrity of the rectal wall, the position and mobility of the prostate are evaluated, and the examining finger should be tested for the presence of gross or occult blood. A nasogastric tube is passed, aspirated and tested for blood.

Interpretation of Physical Findings

Injuries of the organs in the intraperitoneal portion of the abdomen can occur in vascular organs, solid organs and hollow organs. Interpretation of the physical findings associated with these different structures is often a function of the amount of time that each of these types of organs require to create peritoneal irritation.

The spectrum of injury can go from a patient with rapid intra-abdominal bleeding, secondary to a mesenteric artery laceration, with no physical findings except hypovolaemic shock to a patient with immediate peritoneal irritation from inflammation following injury to the stomach or colon. Small intestinal injury may not produce significant intra-abdominal findings for 24 h. Because of the spectrum with which the interpretation of physical findings may present, frequent re-evaluation becomes an essential component of any management protocol which rests short of definitive diagnosis.

ADJUNCTIVE STUDIES FOR ASSESSMENT OF ABDOMINAL TRAUMA

Several laboratory, radiological studies and ancillary diagnostic procedures are useful in evaluating a patient suspected of abdominal injury.

Laboratory Studies

Laboratory tests of value in the evaluation of a patient with abdominal trauma include haematocrit, urine analysis and serum amylase. White count, serum creatinine, glucose and electrolyte determinations are often obtained for baseline values but have little contribution to early management. The diagnosis of massive haemorrhage is usually obvious and haematocrit merely confirms this. Urine analysis will indicate the presence of microscopic haematuria. In blunt trauma, greater than 30–50 RBC/mm^3 should lead to radiographic evaluation of the kidneys and urinary bladder. Serum amylase can be normal in the face of major pancreatic injury or enteric injury, but elevated values should raise suspicion of significant intra-abdominal injury. Serum amylase can be elevated in patients without significant visceral injury. Any suspicion of pancreatic or duodenal injury should ultimately be ruled out in the patient with a history of epigastric trauma with a contrast study.

Radiological studies of potential value in the evaluation of abdominal trauma include abdominal plain films, urethrography and cystography, IVU, CT scan, radionuclide scans, ultrasound and angiography.

All injuries from penetrating trauma should be evaluated with a plain radiograph with radio-opaque markers to allow evaluation of the injuring trajectory. In blunt trauma, plain radiographs may delineate fractures with associated visceral injury potential, show free intraperitoneal air, retroperitoneal 'stippling', associated duodenal injury or loss of the psoas shadow indicating retroperitoneal bleeding.

The ancillary procedures of computerized tomography (CT), ultrasound, angiography and radionuclide scanning continue to be evaluated. At present, CT has real value in the accurate evaluation of solid organ injuries (liver, spleen) and contrast-enhanced CT has great accuracy in the delineation of intra-abdominal bleeding. The accuracy of CT in evaluating viscus injury is unclear, and this is still under evaluation. Ultrasound, angiography, and radionuclide scanning have limited value in the *early* management of a trauma patient and are best left for serial observation during non-operative management of solid organ injuries such as subcapsular haematoma of the liver or splenic haematomas. Injuries to the retroperitoneal organs such as the kidneys and bladder are best evaluated by IVU and cystography. Angiography is indicated when significant arterial injury is suspected based on IVU.

Abdominal Paracentesis and Peritoneal Lavage

Peritoneal lavage is the standard technique used to detect significant intra-abdominal haemorrhage following blunt trauma and can be used to evaluate significant intra-abdominal injury following stab wounds. Its applicability following low-velocity gunshot wounds is unclear, and it has no place in the management of high-velocity gunshot wounds. Abdominal paracentesis can be used instead of peritoneal lavage when intra-abdominal haemorrhage is suspected. It should be emphasized that a negative abdominal paracentesis is of no diagnostic significance, and it is best to practice peritoneal lavage.

Peritoneal lavage, like paracentesis, is of greatest value in those patients whose physical findings may be difficult to evaluate. The specific indications for peritoneal lavage include unconscious trauma patients with signs of abdominal injury, patients with high-energy transfer-suspected intra-abdominal injury and equivocal physical findings, patients with multiple injuries and unexplained shock, patients with non-contiguous or thoraco-abdominal injuries, patients with spinal cord injury, and intoxicated patients in whom abdominal injury is suspected. Contraindications include patients with previous abdominal operations, pregnancy, morbid obesity and patients with an obvious surgical abdomen. An additional indication includes patients who are candidates for intra-abdominal injury who have equivocal diagnostic findings, and will be undergoing prolonged general anaesthesia for other injuries and unavailable for continued re-evaluation.

A pelvic radiograph should be taken before performing peritoneal lavage when pelvic fractures are suspected, so that, if necessary, the incision can be made in the supra-umbilical position. This avoids a false positive test from passing the catheter through the pelvic haematoma, which has dissected onto the anterior abdominal wall below the umbilicus.

Lavage is rarely used with gunshot wounds. Essentially all gunshot wounds are explored by laparotomy. When local exploration of the stab wounds is positive for peritoneal penetration, peritoneal lavage can be performed. In blunt trauma, peritoneal lavage is considered positive when 5–10 ml of grossly bloody aspirate is obtained or when the lavage fluid has greater than 100 000 RBC/mm^3. Evaluation of lavage fluid in stab wounds should be based upon a protocol. In general, greater than 5 000–10 000 RBC/mm^3 is considered a positive lavage and laparotomy should follow.

Technique of Peritoneal Lavage

Prior to initiation of peritoneal lavage, the bladder should be emptied by drainage with a catheter. The abdomen is prepared with povidone-iodine and draped with sterile towels. The midline of the lower abdomen is infiltrated with lignocaine and epinephrine, and a small incision is made and carried down to the linea alba. This is incised and a peritoneal dialysis catheter is placed and seated against the peritoneum and the peritoneum is penetrated. Once the peritoneum is entered, the stylet is withdrawn and the catheter directed at a 45° angle into the pelvis. The catheter is aspirated, and if the aspirate returns 5–10 ml of non-clotting blood, the study is positive. If little or no blood is aspirated, a 1000 ml bag of normal saline or Ringer-lactate is slowly infused into the peritoneal cavity. Once infused, the empty i.v. bottle is placed on the floor allowing the intraperitoneal fluid to siphon back into the bottle. Grossly bloody fluid indicates a positive lavage and pink fluid is sent for a cell count with greater than 100 000 red cells being considered positive.

Generally accepted criteria for a positive peritoneal lavage in blunt trauma include grossly bloody fluid, red blood cell count greater than 100 000/mm^3, white cell count greater than 500/mm^3, amylase greater than 200 units, and the presence of bile, faeces or bacteria. A rough index of cloudiness in the lavage fluid is the ability to read news print through the fluid in the i.v. tubing. If the words can be read, the lavage is considered to have less than 100 000 RBC/mm^3 and a formal count should be obtained.

ESTABLISHING PRIORITIES AND INDICATIONS FOR SURGERY

It is the unique job of the general surgeon caring for the trauma patient to integrate various specialties that may be called upon to participate in the care of the multiply-injured patient. This may often require a two-team approach, for instance, with the simultaneous management of a major intracranial injury and intra-abdominal injury.

Indications for laparotomy include signs of peritoneal injury, unexplained shock, evisceration of a viscus, a positive diagnostic peritoneal lavage, and deterioration of findings during routine follow-up.

In preparation for laparotomy certain aspects to protect the patient from severe hypotension during the early stages of surgical exploration must be kept in mind. Vascular access must be secure. If the patient has suffered major blood loss, central venous catheterization should be performed. Arterial cannula should be placed to allow perioperative recording of the blood pressure. Broad-spectrum antibiotics should be given as soon as the decision to perform laparotomy is made, and these should be continued into the postoperative period, determined by the operative findings and the presence of associated injuries. Hypothermia is often a problem in patients who have prolonged intra-abdominal operations for multiple injuries and have large volumes of transfusion. Anticipating the need for warming is important.

OPERATIVE APPROACH

The operative approach for abdominal trauma is straightforward. A midline incision is preferred. There are few reasons to deviate from this. This allows extension into a median sternotomy in the event that more proximal control of the vena cava or aorta is needed. In addition, the patient should be routinely cleaned from the sternal notch to the midthigh to allow harvesting of the saphenous vein for any encountered vascular injury.

Once the abdomen is opened, obvious blood and clot is removed by packing all four quadrants of the abdomen and sequentially removing these from the lower abdomen first and next from the upper abdomen. Any area that is found to be the source of haemorrhage can be repacked. Additional inflow occlusion can be accomplished by clamping the aorta at the diaphragmatic hiatus. Obvious leaking hollow viscus wounds are rapidly sutured and contamination is thereby minimized during the course of the operation. Retroperitoneal haematomas may be the source of exsanguinating haemorrhage if rupture into the free peritoneal cavity has occurred. If not, these can be left for investigation at a later time, depending on the location. Haematomas of the pelvis associated with pelvic fractures should not be disturbed. Stable haematomas in the perinephric space lateral to the midline that are not expanding are best left undisturbed. Central haematomas that may involve injury to the major vascular structures, pancreas or duodenum are noted and exploration of these is carried out after control of injuries within the peritoneal cavity.

Once haemorrhage has been controlled by packing and ongoing contamination has been controlled, time must be taken to allow re-establishment of the patient's circulating blood volume and cardiac output. Prolonged sustained periods of hypotension should be avoided at all costs and this can generally be done with packing. Once the intra-abdominal injuries have been repaired, a complete thorough exploratory laparotomy methodically investigating the entire abdominal contents is performed.

SPECIFIC INJURIES—DIAPHRAGMATIC INJURIES

Following blunt trauma, the diaphragm is involved in about 4% of injuries and most commonly involves the left hemidiaphragm. The right hemidiaphragm can be involved and massive visceral herniation is possible. All should be repaired to avoid the long-term consequence of herniation that may be fatal to the patient. The diagnosis is suspected when respiratory distress and radiological evidence of pleural effusion are not relieved by intercostal catheter decompression or when an upright radiograph demonstrates visceral herniation.

Penetrating injuries between the nipples and below the costal margins should be assumed to have penetrated the diaphragm. At the time of exploratory laparotomy in blunt or penetrating trauma, the entire diaphragmatic surface should be explored to rule out injury. Simple holes may be repaired with interrupted horizontal mattress sutures and larger lacerations or actual defects may have to be repaired with prosthetic material.

Repair of acute traumatic diaphragmatic rupture is accomplished through the abdomen because of the potential for associated intraperitoneal injuries. Defects discovered at a later time are satisfactorily dealt with by a transthoracic approach. The complications of diaphragmatic rupture result primarily from missing the injury and presentation later with incarceration and possible strangulation of intestinal viscera.

Spleen

The spleen is the intra-abdominal organ most frequently injured in blunt trauma. It is often accompanied by rib fractures on the left side. The spleen lies in the left upper quadrant of the abdomen and in the intrathoracic abdomen. It lies to the left and slightly behind the stomach. During increased intra-abdominal pressure accompanying blunt trauma compression of the spleen may occur between the anterior wall and the posterior rib cage. The history is helpful if the patient can describe a blow, fall or sports injury to the left chest, flank or left upper abdomen. Likewise, in penetrating trauma, a wound of entry or exit in this area should raise suspicion. Clinical signs may often be surprisingly few and one must often maintain a high index of suspicion based on injury mechanism. The clinical picture of splenic injury includes signs of blood loss, left upper quadrant abdominal pain, and pain in the left shoulder (Kehr's sign).

Adjunctive laboratory studies are in general not helpful. Leucocytosis and decreased haematocrit will occur, but these are not specific for splenic injury. Plain abdominal films may show enlargement of the splenic shadow and medial displacement of the stomach. Radionuclide scanning and CT scanning can reveal significant splenic injury but should only be pursued with an understanding of what therapeutic plan will follow if these tests are positive. Peritoneal lavage should be performed when there is the possibility of splenic injury. This becomes the indication for laparotomy.

The management of splenic trauma has been the subject of major re-examination over the past decade, and emerging is an increased appreciation of the danger of intra-abdominal abscess and postsplenectomy sepsis following routine splenectomy. The recognition of fatal pneumococcal septicaemia in patients undergoing splenectomy has led to an interest in splenic salvage. The spectrum of injury may vary from a simple laceration or contusion without capsular disruption to total fragmentation of the spleen.

During the course of laparotomy, the spleen is evaluated for haemorrhage. If haemorrhage from the spleen is appreciated, one must make a decision regarding splenic salvage. Essential to the success of splenic salvage is adequate mobilization of the spleen from its attachments. Care must be taken during the course of mobilization to prevent further injury. Once mobilized, the tail of the pancreas is freed from the posterior retroperitoneum and the spleen is delivered into the abdominal incision. Ongoing bleeding can be controlled from the spleen during mobilization by digital compression. Capsular tears of the spleen can be controlled by topical haemostatic agents. Lacerations into the splenic substance can be controlled with interlocking absorbable sutures. Major lacerations of the splenic substance involving less than 50% of the splenic tissue can be treated with segmental splenic resection. Splenic salvage should not be pursued if the patient has protracted hypotension or if undue delay is anticipated in attempting to repair the spleen and the patient has other severe injuries. With penetrating injury damage to adjacent structures such as stomach, pancreas, colon and diaphragm must be considered and investigated.

Non-operative management of splenic trauma in adults is a possible option if the patient presents more than 12 h after injury and is haemodynamically stable with no other signs of abdominal injury. A non-invasive radiographic test, such as radionuclide scan or CT scan should be performed and the patient followed sequentially. Complications following splenectomy include early transient thrombocytosis which resolves spontaneously over 1–3 months. Anticoagulation should not be utilized. Delayed haemorrhage, pancreatitis and subphrenic abscess also occur. The incidence of subphrenic abscess is probably increased by postoperative drainage and most would advise against it.

Postsplenectomy Sepsis

The other complication following splenectomy is postsplenectomy sepsis. It is clear that fatal pneumococcal septicaemia in children under the age of 4 is a real risk. The incidence of life-threatening sepsis in adult patients also seems to be increased. The significance of the clinical incidence is less easy to define. When splenectomy is indicated or required, postoperative follow-up and management are essential. Immunization with the polyvalent pneumococcal vaccine and booster immunization every three years should be done. In addition, prophylactic antibiotics should be used at any time the patient is to undergo instrumentation such as during dental repair or surgery.

These patients should be advised of their increased potential risk for postsplenectomy sepsis and should carry an identification card to alert health care workers of this possibility whenever they have an infection. All infections should be considered as emergencies and treated with antibiotics.

Liver Injuries

The liver is the largest organ in the abdominal cavity and is commonly damaged in blunt and penetrating abdominal trauma and in thoraco-abdominal injuries. Because of its size, injuries sufficient to lacerate liver are associated with injuries to other organs in about 80% of cases. Spontaneous haemostatic mechanisms which characterize liver tissue may contribute to the constant observation that 85% of liver injuries are not bleeding at the time of laparotomy and patients tolerate these injuries very well. Most liver injuries will in fact require only documentation and in most cases no drainage. The minority of liver injuries therefore require definitive surgical care. These, however, present as complex a problem to the surgeon as any other injury.

The history is helpful in that there is usually an indication of blunt energy transfer, particularly to the right rib cage or upper abdomen. Physical findings may be minimal in that early bleeding may not cause peritoneal irritation. The abdomen may or may not be distended. Any patient who is hypotensive after blunt abdominal trauma must be suspected of having a severe liver injury. Likewise, a patient who has a history of being in shock at the scene following blunt trauma should be suspected of having a major liver injury.

Peritoneal lavage will be most helpful in establishing the diagnosis and if lavage is positive, laparotomy is indicated. In haemodynamically stable patients or those with contraindication to peritoneal lavage, CT scanning is most precise in evaluating subcapsular haematomas and lacerations. Documentation of this and the high association of other organs injured should lead one to laparotomy in the event of a positive CT scan.

Injuries vary from capsular tears and non-bleeding lacerations, to large fractures and lobar destruction, with extensive parenchymal disruption and hepatic artery and venous injuries. The type of injury dictates the amount of surgical therapy required. The principles of management of liver injury are the same, regardless of the severity of injury. They involve control of bleeding, removal of devitalized tissue and establishment of adequate drainage.

Simple lacerations which have stopped bleeding at the time of surgery do not require drainage unless they are deep into the parenchyma with the high possibility of postoperative biliary leakage. Subcapsular haematomas can be simply evacuated if there is no associated parenchymal injury (*Fig.* 19.2). Lacerations which continue to bleed despite attempts at local control will require opening the liver wound—a tractotomy. The depths of the liver wound are explored and specific vessels and biliary radicals individually ligated.

In the event that bleeding continues despite segmental ligation of parenchymal vessels, the porta hepatis should be compressed (Pringle manoeuvre). If the bleeding stops it can be assumed to be from the portal veins or hepatic artery. If the bleeding continues, it is assumed to be coming from the hepatic veins. The portal triad can also be intermittently clamped to allow visualization during placement of sutures as parenchymal vessels are ligated.

When selective ligation fails, ligation of the hepatic artery is an alternative. It may produce dramatic haemostasis without subsequent liver failure. This should be done as close to the liver as possible and only as a last resort.

An alternative for deep lacerations with persistent bleeding is resectional débridement of the segment of the liver. This is accomplished with finger fracture, removing devitalized liver or a portion of the segment, whole segment or lobe to allow access and control of bleeding. This will be required in approximately 5–8% of all liver injuries. Subsegmental resection may be adequate; if segmentectomy or lobectomy is required, a knowledge of the anatomy is imperative in order not to compromise inflow or outflow to the remaining segments.

A decision should be made early, the blood bank notified and adequate help and exposure obtained. Exposure is best accomplished by complete division of the capsular attachments. Finger fracture through the parenchyma with individual ligation of vessels and biliary radicals as they are encountered after adequate control of the porta hepatis is the best technique.

Inability to control bleeding by clamping the porta hepatis implies significant retrohepatic vena caval bleeding or bleeding from the hepatic veins. If this is unilobular, then débridement and resection should be sufficient. With bilobar involvement or uncontrollable haemorrhage from a single lobe, early consideration should be given to the placement of the intracaval shunt (*Fig.* 19.3). To accomplish this, the sternum is split and a chest tube is placed through the right atrium. Proximal and distal control are obtained above and below the liver, above the renal veins. This will allow better visualization of hepatic vein and vena caval lacerations which can be directly suture ligated.

In the event that parenchymal or hepatic vein bleeding cannot be controlled and the patient remains difficult to resuscitate, packing of the injury and resuscitation is most

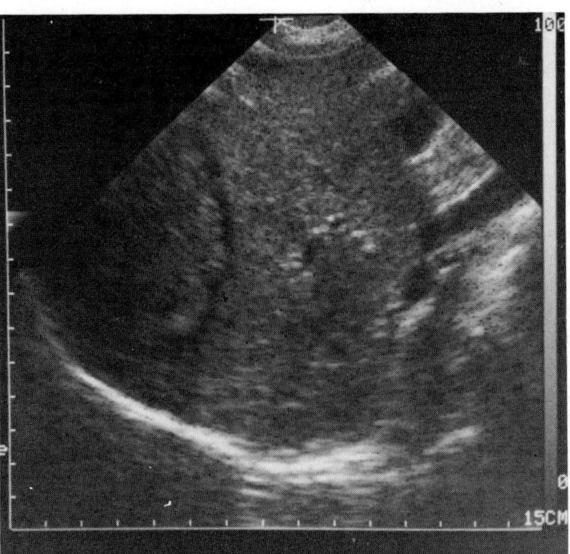

a

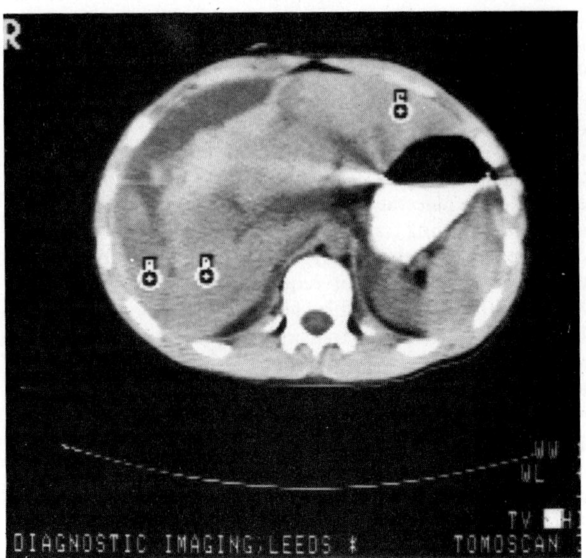

b

Fig. 19.2 *a*, Ultrasound of liver, showing large haematoma. *b*, CT scan of liver in same patient showing encapsulated haematoma and underlying liver damage.

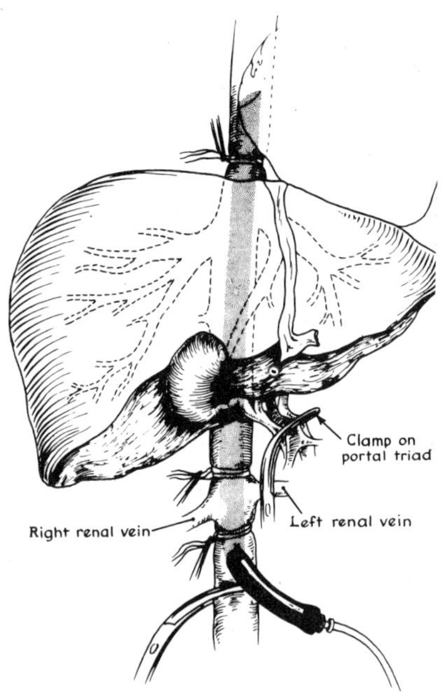

Fig. 19.3 The placement of a caval catheter may be achieved by introducing the catheter into the abdominal vena cava as shown or by a route through the atrial appendage if the chest has been opened.

appropriate. Subsequent removal of the packs 24–72 h postoperatively can be followed with resection and suture ligation in a resuscitated patient.

When haemostasis is achieved, non-viable tissue should be débrided and the area drained. When extensive parenchymal damage or central penetrating injuries are encountered, active drainage with sump tubes is indicated. T tubes in the common duct have no place unless the extra hepatic biliary tree is injured.

Significant complications following liver injury include pulmonary complications, coagulopathy, hypoglycaemia, jaundice, biliary fistulas, haemobilia and subdiaphragmatic and intraparenchymal abscess formation.

Although disseminated intravascular coagulation and impaired liver synthesis can be implicated in the aetiology of the coagulopathy following liver resection the most important factor is usually hypothermia and inadequate blood component replacement. Patients undergoing major hepatic resection following trauma need continuous glucose infusion during the early postoperative period. Hypoalbuminaemia, though present, does not require albumin administration but should be treated with aggressive nutritional support. Hyperbilirubinaemia is transient and will peak in two to three weeks and usually does not go above 10 mg/dl. Intrahepatic and subphrenic abscesses can develop, particularly when large amounts of débridement have been necessary and are diagnosed with clinical signs of sepsis and imaging with ultrasound or CT. Biliary fistulas usually close spontaneously. Haemobilia is a rare complication which presents with intrahepatic bleeding into the bile ducts and can be diagnosed with endoscopy and treated with arteriography.

Stomach Injuries

Injuries of the stomach are very rare in blunt trauma and common in penetrating trauma. The stomach is intrathoracic, partially protected by the rib cage and relatively difficult to diagnose. Any penetrating wound in this area should be suspected of causing injury to the stomach and requires investigation of the anterior and posterior surface at the time of laparotomy.

During initial evaluation, insertion of a nasogastric tube and aspirate positive for blood may point to a gastric injury and should raise suspicion.

The intraoperative evaluation of stomach injury includes good visualization of the oesophageal hiatus, evaluation of the anterior portion of the stomach, division of the gastrocolic ligament, and complete visualization of the posterior aspect of the stomach. Penetrating wounds are débrided and primary closure performed. Maceration of the stomach from significant penetrating or blunt injury may require gastric resection.

Postoperative complications include intra-abdominal abscess, particularly in the lesser sac, but are rare. The other complication of gastric injury is gastric fistula. The treatment is immediate reoperation and repair using healthy tissue.

Duodenal Injury

Isolated injury to the duodenum usually does not cause significant hypotension and signs of peritonitis may be delayed if the retroperitoneal duodenum is injured. Failure to recognize this injury is associated with high morbidity and mortality caused by abscess formation in the lesser sac. Entry wounds between the xiphoid and umbilicus suggest possible injury to the duodenum and non-penetrating duodenal injury may be caused by crushing injuries where intraperitoneal and extraperitoneal duodenum is macerated or contused against the spine. A closed loop compression of an airfilled loop following a seatbelt injury can account for maceration injury often seen in the duodenum. History of trunk injury or localized blow to the epigastrium with handle bars, steering wheel or fist should suggest these types of injury.

Adjunctive diagnostic tests might include hyperamylasaemia. This occurs in about half of the patients with blunt injury to the duodenum as a result of extravasation of intra-abdominal pancreatic amylase. Elevated serum amylase following blunt trauma is not diagnostic of an injury but raises suspicion and necessitates further diagnostic study. Abdominal radiographs may suggest duodenal injury showing obliteration of the psoas shadow, absence of air in the duodenal bulb, or air in the retroperitoneum outlining the kidney. Psoas muscle and lumbar spine abnormalities such as spastic lordosis in association with transverse process fractures, indicate major injury in this area.

Definitive diagnosis requires contrast duodenography or CT scanning with contrast. Extravasation of contrast material is an absolute indication for laparotomy. Distortion of the duodenum indicates significant injury and is a relative indication for laparotomy. The radiographic picture of an intramural duodenal haematoma is not an indication to operate immediately.

Intraoperative evaluation of the duodenum requires complete mobilization of the duodenum (Kocher manoeuvre). The hepatic flexure of the colon is taken down to expose the anterior aspect of the second portion of the duodenum and inspection of the third and fourth portions of the duodenum at the base of the transverse colon should be done. Retroperitoneal haematomas in the area of the duodenum must be explored and the lesser sac should be entered to exclude associated pancreatic injuries.

Limited perforations or simple lacerations of the duodenum within six hours of injury are treated with primary closure. After six hours the risk of duodenal leak increases. Suction decompression of the duodenum with a transpyloric nasogastric tube, tube jejunostomy or tube duodenostomy is advisable if repair is in any way compromised.

If the laceration of the first and second portion of the duodenum is extensive and primary closure would be associated with obstruction, Roux-en-Y jejunoduodenostomy is indicated. Multiple or extensive lacerations that narrow the lumen and jeopardize the vascularity of the duodenum are best managed by pyloric exclusion. The proximal duodenum is defunctionalized by closing the pylorus and establishing gastric drainage with a gastrojejunostomy. Wounds of the first and second portion of the duodenum are closed primarily and the duodenum drained with a tube duodenostomy. The area around the duodenum is also drained.

Pancreaticoduodenectomy is occasionally indicated for massive injury in the right upper quadrant in which the proximal duodenum cannot be repaired. This is usually accompanied by maceration of the head of the pancreas and thereby becomes the indication for pancreaticoduodenectomy.

The distal duodenum (third and fourth portions) can be primarily closed as with the proximal duodenum if the injury is dealt with within six hours of injury. For injuries longer than six hours or with maceration of the distal duodenum, resection of the third and fourth portions of the duodenum and duodenal jejunostomy should be performed.

Duodenal haematomas confirmed by radiocontrast study can be expected to resolve and management consists of nasogastric suction until peristalsis returns and slow introduction of solid food. Persistent duodenal obstruction will require operative treatment.

Other than postoperative bleeding, the most significant complication following duodenal injury is the development of a duodenal fistula which occurs in 5–10% of the patients following anastomosis. Unlike a gastric fistula, it is generally managed non-operatively with nasogastric suction, nutritional support and aggressive stoma care. In addition, antibiotics are indicated if infection occurs. Uncomplicated fistulas will close in six weeks and should be treated operatively if they persist beyond six weeks.

Pancreatic Injuries

Blunt trauma to the abdomen from direct kick or blow or seatbelt injury may crush the pancreas over the vertebral column. Epigastric and posterior penetrating wounds can likewise penetrate the pancreas and are often associated with significant injuries involving the kidney, vena cava and colon. This is of particular concern in that enzymatically active pancreatic juice increases the possibility of anastomotic leak following these injuries if they are not recognized and treated appropriately. The shared blood supply between the pancreas and duodenum makes the likelihood of these two injuries occurring in combination very high.

Diagnosis is by history and associated clinical findings, although these may be non-existent. Suspicion must be raised and serial re-evaluation undertaken if there is any doubt. Elevation of serum and urinary amylase following blunt injury is not diagnostic, but a persistent elevation suggests pancreatic injury and this must be ruled out. Contrast duodenography may reveal widening of the C-loop. A loss of the psoas shadow, anterior displacement of the stomach and duodenum from a pancreatic phlegmon, and left pleural effusion are all suggestive of a pancreatic injury but not specifically diagnostic. CT scanning is of potential value but its role is still unclear.

Patients seldom undergo laparotomy because of pancreatic injury alone. Instead, they are generally operated on because of intraperitoneal blood loss or peritonitis. At the time of laparotomy, the pancreas should be examined and any evidence of adjacent injury seen (i.e., duodenal haematoma, haematoma in the transverse mesocolon or any evidence of trauma to the anterior wall of the stomach or spleen). Any retroperitoneal haematoma around the pancreas should be explored, and retroperitoneal bile staining indicating a concurrent duodenal or biliary tract injury must be investigated. If there is any evidence that the pancreas has been contused, it should be drained. Injury to the body and tail, which is refractory to simple débridement, should be treated with splenectomy and distal pancreatectomy. Injuries to the midportion of the pancreas can theoretically be treated with pancreaticojejunostomy, but little is to be gained over splenectomy and distal pancreatectomy in this circumstance.

Penetrating wounds to the right of the superior mesenteric vein should be treated with débridement and direct suture ligation of areas of bleeding. Débridement must be conservative in that bile ducts may be injured and blood supply compromised.

Significant injury to the head of the pancreas or to the right of the superior mesenteric vessels will be associated with a 30–60% probability of temporary pancreatic fistula and this should be accepted. Severe trauma to the head of the pancreas in association with duodenal injuries should be treated with débridement of the pancreas, closure of the duodenal wound, and pyloric exclusion as described above. Extensive damage to the head of the pancreas and duodenum may require total pancreatoduodenectomy. Wide drainage is the rule and should be anticipated even when the pancreas is only locally débrided. This should be accomplished with sump drains brought out to the flank and left in place until drainage has stopped.

The most common complication of pancreatic injury is a persistent pancreatic fistula, and if well controlled should close spontaneously unless there is obstruction to the pancreatic duct.

Small Intestine Injuries

Injuries to the small intestine occur in approximately 15–20% of the patients who require laparotomy after blunt trauma. The postulated mechanisms are: (1) crushing injury of the bowel between the spine and the blunt object, such as a steering wheel or handle bars; (2) deceleration shearing of the small bowel at fixed points such as the ileocaecal valve and around the mesenteric artery; and (3) closed loop rupture caused by increased intra-abdominal pressure. Injuries to the small intestine are present in approximately 25–30% of the patients who require laparotomy after penetrating trauma. Diagnosis is often either directly apparent secondary to peritoneal injury, or indirectly due to bleeding from the raw surface of the enterotomy. Antibiotics should be started preoperatively.

At operation, significant bleeding will be the first priority. After application of packs and vascular control of exsanguinating haemorrhage, non-crushing clamps should be applied to prevent further leakage. The small bowel should be carefully examined from the ligament of Treitz all the way to the ileocaecal valve.

Contusion of the antimesenteric wall of the bowel may

result in delayed perforation and seromuscular sutures can be used to imbricate the contusion into the lumen.

Mesenteric haematomas which extend up to the bowel should be incised and evacuated such that the underlying bowel can be adequately examined.

Single holes from stab wounds or shotgun pellets can be closed without débridement. Since penetrating injuries in general occur in pairs, careful examination of the bowel wall on the opposite side must be done to avoid missing any small perforations. If two adjacent holes are found, they can be connected across the bridge of bowel and a transverse closure effected so as not to narrow the lumen. Large lacerations are débrided and closed. Transection of the small bowel is débrided and closed in routine fashion and the mesenteric defect should be closed to prevent herniation. Any large segments of bowel that are devascularized or have multiple defects should be resected and reanastomosed.

Patients are maintained on postoperative decompression with a nasogastric tube until peristalsis returns and feeding is then begun.

Major complications include intra-abdominal abscess, anastomotic leakage, enterocutaneous fistula, as well as intestinal obstruction. Intra-abdominal abscess must be drained. If obstruction occurs early it can generally be treated conservatively with a nasogastric tube, but may require reoperation. Enterocutaneous fistulas can be treated conservatively if the output is low and should be expected to close spontaneously with parenteral nutrition.

Injuries to the Colon and Rectum

The greatest number of injuries to the colon and rectum are the result of penetrating or perforating trauma. Blunt trauma accounts for only about 5% of colonic injuries. The amount of force required to damage the colon is considerable and as such, the colon is relatively refractory to blunt injury. Rectal injuries can occur in association with pelvic fracture and any patient with a significant pelvic fracture has to have the possibility of rectal injury considered in addition to evaluation of other pelvic viscera, such as the bladder, distal ureters, and vagina.

Signs and symptoms are not specific for injury to the colon and rectum but will create peritoneal irritation, tenderness and occur relatively early following injury. Laboratory studies are not helpful, radiological studies may show free air in the peritoneal cavity. Peritoneal lavage is of value if intraperitoneal colonic injury is present and may return fluid with blood or bacteria. If the injury is confined to the extraperitoneal colon and rectum, lavage is of no value. Extraperitoneal colonic or rectal injury is extremely difficult to diagnose. A high degree of suspicion has to be maintained. The possibility of rectal injury has to be considered in any patient with penetrating trauma to the lower abdomen or buttocks. Digital examination is essential. The presence of blood on examination is strong evidence for colon or rectal injury, and proctoscopic and sigmoidoscopic examinations should be performed. About 95% of colon injuries are caused by gunshot, shotgun or stab wounds, and whenever the possibility of colonic injury is entertained, prophylactic antibiotics should be started intravenously immediately. The number of doses continued postoperatively is determined by the degree of colon injury.

The central debate in the operative management of colonic injury is between primary repair of low-risk colonic injuries versus repair and proximal colostomy or resection and colostomy.

Primary repair can be selected when known associated complicating factors have been excluded. Complications increase in primary repair when there is preoperative hypotension, intraperitoneal haemorrhage exceeding a litre, more than two associated organs injured (hepatic, pancreatic, splenic are the most dangerous), significant faecal spillage, or more than six hours have lapsed since injury. Many patients with low-risk penetrating colon injuries can be treated with primary closure or resection and primary anastomosis following these guidelines. All high-risk colon injuries or those associated with severe injuries as indicated above should be treated with resection and colostomy. An alternative or compromise between colostomy and primary repair has been advocated with exteriorization of the repaired segment. The success of this technique varies and it is probably of no great benefit over exteriorization alone. Postoperative complications include abscess formation, anastomotic leak, peristomal hernia, and the morbidity and mortality associated with colostomy closure.

The morbidity and mortality from rectal injuries is primarily due to inadequate initial therapy and the complications associated with delayed sepsis. Rectal injury must be suspected when there is any penetrating injury or a sacral fracture that produces a pelvic ring disruption. Sigmoidoscopic examination is essential.

The principles of operative management include: (1) placement of the patient in the lithotomy position which allows simultaneous exposure of both the perineum and abdomen; (2) wide débridement of all dead and devitalized tissue; (3) a totally defunctioning colostomy (simple loop colostomy is inadequate); (4) rectal wall closure if possible; (5) retrorectal drainage with coccygectomy when necessary to attain adequate rectal drainage; and (6) distal rectal stump wash-out. Antibiotics, nutritional support and repeat débridement are also indicated.

Complete rectal destruction is an indication for a primary abdominal perineal resection, with packing which should be removed in approximately 48 h. Complications following rectal injuries include pelvic abscesses, urinary or rectal fistulas, rectal incontinence and stricture, and loss of sexual function and urinary incontinence.

Retroperitoneal Haematomas

Management of the retroperitoneal haematoma in patients with multisystem trauma has for years been a source of confusion and controversy. The optimum management of retroperitoneal haematoma depends on a number of factors including aetiology, location and other associated injuries.

The retroperitoneum can be divided into anatomical zones for purposes of decision making (*Fig.* 19.4). Central retroperitoneal haematomas (Zone 1) are associated with pancreaticoduodenal injuries or major abdominal vascular injury. Flank or perinephric haematomas (Zone 2) may be associated with injuries to the genito-urinary tract, or in the case of penetrating trauma, with injuries to the colon. Zone 3 injuries, which are confined to or originate from the pelvis, are most often associated with pelvic fractures. Retroperitoneal haematomas in Zone 1 regardless of aetiology or size, are explored because of the high incidence of associated major vascular, pancreatic or duodenal injuries, and the high morbidity and mortality if these are overlooked.

Zone 2 haematomas caused by penetrating injuries should be explored if: (1) they are expanding, (2) they are adjacent to the colon and may be concealing an occult colonic injury, (3) preoperative evaluation with either nephrotomography or computerized tomography has demonstrated a major renal injury. Proximal control of the renal pedicle should be

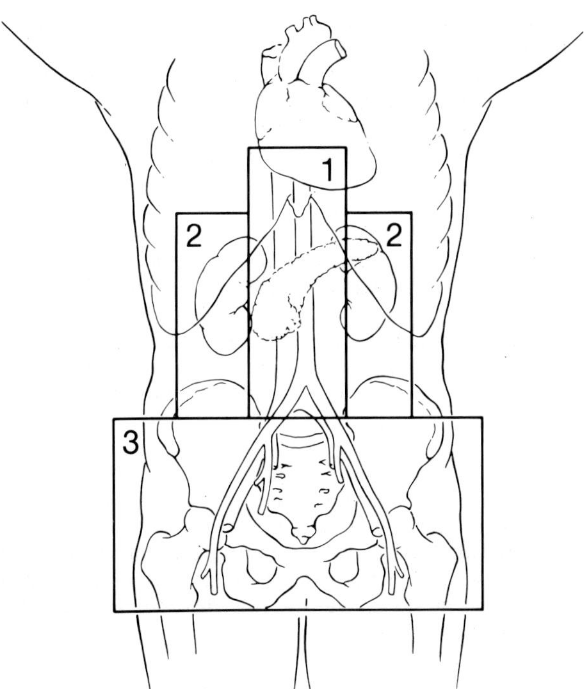

Fig. 19.4 Zones of the retroperitoneum (*see text*).

gained in any exploration of a perinephric haematoma. Zone 2 haematomas caused by blunt trauma can be left alone if they are not expanding and the IVU is normal.

Zone 3 retroperitoneal haematomas are generally explored in patients with penetrating injuries in order to exclude major vascular injuries. Local bleeding encountered at exploration under these circumstances is generally easy to control and the associated injuries can be identified. Patients with Zone 3 haematomas secondary to blunt trauma usually have associated pelvic fractures, and exploration of the haematoma can be hazardous. There is often extensive injury to the rich presacral venous and arterial circulation. Incision of the peritoneum destroys the tamponade effect, and dissection in the haematoma may produce catastrophic bleeding. Discrete bleeding points can rarely be identified. Exploration of these haematomas is associated with an increased transfusion requirement and a high mortality.

Management of Pelvic Fractures

Pelvic fractures continue to be a major cause of morbidity and mortality in patients with blunt abdominal injury. Pedestrian and motor vehicle accidents account for the majority of these injuries, with an associated mortality between 10 and 25%. Massive haemorrhage and coagulopathy continue to account for 40–60% of the mortality in this group of patients.

Pelvic fractures have been classified by a number of different schemes. The most useful classification is that by Trunkey (*Fig.* 19.5). Type I injuries represent comminuted or crush fracture of the pelvis and involve three or more elements of the pelvic rings. These fractures have the highest morbidity and mortality and are accompanied by massive haemorrhage and severe soft-tissue injury. Type II fractures are unstable injuries and involve at least two breaks in the pelvic ring. These include diametric fractures with cephalad displacement of the hemipelvis (Malgaigne), and 'open book' fractures. Type III pelvic fractures are stable fractures generally involving a single element in the pelvic ring or fractures of the pubic rami.

The initial management of the patient with pelvic fractures will depend on associated injuries. In patients with severe pelvic fractures who are haemodynamically unstable, intracavitary haemorrhage must be excluded using conventional means, including radiological studies and diagnostic peritoneal lavage. The incidence of false positive peritoneal lavage is high in this group of patients due to free dissection of blood out from the pelvis into the abdominal cavity and passage of the lavage catheter into an expanded preperitoneal space filled with haematoma. The latter can be minimized by performing diagnostic peritoneal lavage through a supraumbilical midline incision. Laparotomy is performed immediately for patients with positive lavage. Intra-abdominal visceral injuries are treated, and the pelvic haematoma is not explored.

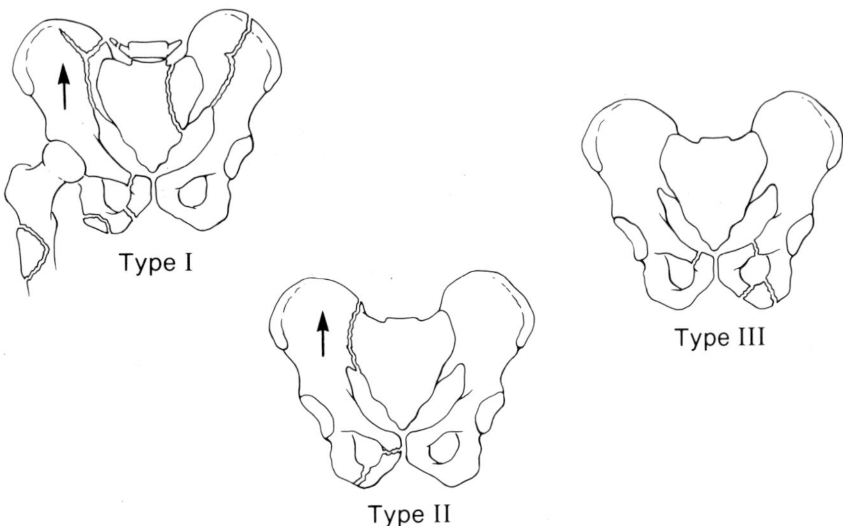

Fig. 19.5 Pelvic fracture classification (*see text*).

Control of ongoing pelvic retroperitoneal bleeding represents the greatest challenge in these patients and is the main cause of mortality. Both arterial and venous bleeding may be present and patients may lose in excess of 20 units of blood into a major pelvic injury. Methods of haemorrhage control that have been developed in recent years include: (1) application of the military anti-shock trousers (MAST), (2) pelvic arteriography and arterial embolization, and (3) early reduction of the pelvic fracture using external pelvic fixation.

The use of MAST for early control of haemorrhage has resulted in increased survival and appears to decrease transfusion requirements. MAST suits have been most often used for 'field resuscitation', but have more recently been advocated for extended use in hospital for non-operative control of venous retroperitoneal pelvic bleeding.

Pelvic arteriography and embolization plays an important role in the early management of massive or persistent pelvic retroperitoneal haemorrhage. Embolization is a safe and effective means of non-operative control and has resulted in reduced morbidity and mortality. The selection of patients for arteriography depends on the magnitude of pelvic haemorrhage, and should be performed when transfusion requirements become high.

In patients with unstable pelvic fractures and wide displacement, early reduction by external pelvic fixators can serve to reduce discomfort and subsequent transfusion requirements. The role and timing of early pelvic fixation have not been clearly defined in relationship to the other modalities outlined.

The best algorithm for management of haemorrhage from pelvic fractures utilizes early arteriography. Indications are recurrent hypotension following initial resuscitation (attributed to the pelvic fracture) or if the transfusion requirements exceeds 6 units within the first two hours following injury. Patients should be maintained in the MAST suit until arteriography can be performed. Following arteriography patients remain in the MAST suit while any hypothermia and coagulopathy are corrected. Pelvic external fixation is performed in selected cases where there is wide fracture displacement.

Ligation of the hypogastric artery for control of pelvic haemorrhage has been advocated in the past. Because of the rich arterial supply this is an ineffective manoeuvre for control of arterial haemorrhage and arteriography is preferable. There is no effect on venous bleeding by hypogastric ligation.

Pelvic fractures associated with deep perineal lacerations, or rectal or vaginal lacerations are classified as compound pelvic fractures. These injuries are associated with a high incidence of septic complications and carry a mortality of approximately 50%. The primary source of contamination is the faecal stream, and complete diversion is necessary to reduce septic complications. A double-barrelled colostomy should be performed after adequate control of the retroperitoneal haemorrhage has been obtained. A loop colostomy does not provide complete diversion and should not be used under these circumstances.

Urinary Tract Injuries—General

Because of its location, injuries to the genito-urinary tract are often clinically silent and are frequently overlooked in the face of more obvious abdominal or thoracic injuries. An awareness of the subtle manifestations of genito-urinary injuries is necessary to avoid missed injuries. The physical examination is unreliable in diagnosing urinary tract injuries, but these injuries are amenable to radiological diagnosis. Systematic orderly evaluation of the urinary tract reduces the chance of missing injury and limits the number of unnecessary retroperitoneal explorations for minor trauma.

Different criteria should exist for initial evaluation of the urinary tract in blunt vs. penetrating trauma. In blunt trauma, fractures of the lower portion of the rib cage or spinous processes fractures have been associated with increased incidence of renal injuries. Findings of a flank haematoma or ecchymosis on physical examination or associated solid viscus injuries found at laparotomy are also associated with increased incidence of significant renal trauma.

Penetrating trunk trauma, particularly that to the back or the flank, has the potential of significant renal injury without any obvious clinical manifestations. A high index of suspicion should exist with any penetrating trauma in the vicinity of the renal tract despite outwardly negative clinical signs.

Bladder catheterization allows evaluation of the presence and degree of haematuria. The presence of haematuria, either microscopic or gross, is indicative of urinary tract injury, but the absence of haematuria does not exclude the presence of a urinary tract injury. Of patients with penetrating injuries to the renal tract 15–20% will not present initially with haematuria, and renal artery occlusion may occur in blunt trauma without associated haematuria. Urinalysis remains, however, the most sensitive screening test.

Intravenous pyelography (IVP) is usually the next step in the radiological evaluation of renal injuries. The degree of haematuria necessary to prompt further evaluation by IVP has not been clearly defined. Penetrating injuries in the vicinity of the urinary tract should be evaluated with intravenous pyelogram regardless of the presence of haematuria. Patients who have sustained major axial or anteroposterior deceleration injuries should undergo evaluation using IVP regardless of the findings on urinalysis.

The majority of patients with blunt trauma and haematuria are found to have a normal IVP. Current data suggests that 50 RBCs per high-powered field distinguishes between patients with minor and potentially major urinary tract trauma. This results in a decreased number of intravenous pyelograms performed without apparent increased missed urinary tract injuries.

Retrograde cystography is used to diagnose rupture of the bladder. Rupture of the bladder should be suspected in a patient with haematuria and lower pelvic or abdominal trauma. Patients with pelvic fractures involving the anterior arch are particularly prone to have an associated bladder injury. Cystography is performed by the infusion of 250 ml of contrast under gravity flow. If no injury is apparent initially, additional contrast may be necessary to delineate the injury. Intra- and extraperitoneal bladder rupture can usually be differentiated using these methods.

Retrograde urethrography (RUG) is used to define suspected urethral tears, which occur predominantly in males. Absolute indications for performing retrograde urethrogram include blood at the urethral meatus and free floating prostate. A high index of suspicion for urethral injuries should also exist in male patients who present with large perineal haematomas or other perineal injuries. Patients who are suspected of having urethral rupture should not be catheterized. Retrograde urethrogram is performed by slow infusion of undiluted contrast material through a small Foley catheter with a balloon inflated in the meatal fossa. Extravasation is seen with injury.

Computerized tomography is being used increasingly to evaluate patients with a variety of abdominal and retroperitoneal injuries, and has been found useful in the preoperative staging of renal injuries. Patients in whom the results of IVP are either indefinite or abnormal should be followed up with a CT scan.

Renal Injuries

The kidney is the most commonly injured part of the urinary tract. Classification of renal injury is divided into minor and major injuries, minor injuries comprising approximately 85% of the cases. Renal contusions comprise the vast majority of minor renal trauma and can almost invariably be treated without operation. Major renal trauma includes deep cortical medullary lacerations with extravasation and large perinephric haematomas, and vascular injuries of the renal pedicle. Microscopic or gross haematuria is usually present but it is of note that the degree of haematuria in most seriously injured patients is a poor predictor of the degree of renal injury.

With penetrating injuries, approximately 80% will require laparotomy for associated intra-abdominal injuries. The problem at laparotomy is the decision to whether to explore a perinephric haematoma. If the patient's condition has not allowed adequate preoperative evaluation with IVP, it is best to explore all perinephric haematomas produced by penetrating injuries. Perinephric haematomas associated with blunt injuries are not explored unless they are pulsatile or expanding. The incidence of nephrectomy under these circumstances has been shown to be greatly reduced with a transabdominal approach and vascular control of the renal pedicle prior to mobilization of the kidney.

In patients suspected of having renal injury because of an abnormal or indefinite IVP, evaluation using computerized tomography provides a more precise definition of the degree of renal injury. The use of computerized tomography under these circumstances allows some patients with isolated renal injuries to be managed non-operatively. Patients with suspected major renal vascular trauma are further evaluated using arteriography.

Indications for operative exploration in patients with penetrating trauma include a suspected renal injury found at laparotomy with incomplete preoperative staging and patients with IVP or CT scans demonstrating renal pedicle injury, urinary extravasation, or parenchymal laceration with significant perinephric haematoma. Indication for operative intervention in patients with blunt trauma is more controversial, but in general includes patients with large renal lacerations and extravasation, renal pedicle injuries, or patients with large or expanding perinephric haematoma.

The increasing use of CT scanning may allow more patients with both blunt and penetrating renal injuries to be managed non-operatively. However, the precise definition of non-operative injury has not as yet, been determined.

Operative options at the time of exploration for renal trauma include a nephrectomy, partial nephrectomy, and repair of transcapsular lacerations using omental and/or peritoneal patch grafts.

Ureteral Injuries

Injury to the ureter is uncommon and occurs mostly with penetrating trauma. The presence of haematuria in ureteral injury is not a consistent finding. Ureteral injury is generally suspected preoperatively by the location of the penetrating injury, or in the case of blunt injury with the presence of concomitant intra-abdominal or other genito-urinary tract injuries. In 80–85% of cases of ureteral injury, IVP will confirm the diagnosis; 15–20% of ureteral injuries are not demonstrated on IVP and require demonstration by retrograde ureterography. Many ureteral injuries are missed at initial evaluation and present late as urinomas with associated fever, flank mass and pain, or as a urinary fistula, often presenting as urine extravasation through the cutaneous site of the penetrating injury.

In patients whose clinical condition does not allow for preoperative IVP, the diagnosis of ureteral injury may be made at the time of laparotomy by chromo-ureterography. This is accomplished by the intravenous injection of 5 ml of methylene blue or indigo carmine dye. Extravasation of the blue-tinged urine into the operative field usually serves to confirm the presence of ureteral injury and to locate its site.

Surgical options for repair of injured ureters include uretero-ureterostomy, or ureteral reimplantation into the bladder. In cases of extensive ureteral loss, autotransplantation of the kidney into the iliac fossa may be necessary for injuries to the upper third of the ureter. Middle third injuries may require reimplantation of the damaged ureter into the normal ureter across the midline, or renal and bladder mobilization to allow for a tension-free anastomosis. Long segment ureteral losses in the lower third may be managed by the creation of an anterior bladder flap tube into which a shortened ureter may be reimplanted.

Bladder Injuries

The majority of bladder injuries occur as a result of blunt external trauma, and should be strongly suspected in patients with haematuria and pelvic fractures. Bladder rupture may be extraperitoneal or intraperitoneal. The former is usually a result of perforations by adjacent bony fragments from the site of the pelvic fracture, and the latter the result of rupture of the dome that occurs when a full bladder sustains a direct blow. Diagnosis is made by cystography. Intravenous pyelography is often necessary to evaluate the upper urinary tract. The possibility of ureteral injury should be considered also in any patient with a bladder injury.

Repair of intraperitoneal rupture of the bladder is accomplished via a transabdominal approach, and includes a suprapubic cystostomy with drainage.

The management of extraperitoneal rupture of the bladder is more controversial. Some investigators have advocated the non-operative management of extraperitoneal rupture by the use of prolonged Foley catheter drainage. Non-operative management usually requires that the patient have no intra-abdominal injuries, no significant local haemorrhage and no urinary tract infection. A 20–25% complication rate has been reported with non-operative management of extraperitoneal bladder rupture. Patients with severe pelvic fractures and massive retroperitoneal bleeding are best managed non-operatively. A delayed repair of their extraperitoneal rupture may be required once the retroperitoneal bleeding is controlled and their condition stabilized. These patients are at very high risk for haemorrhagic complications associated with dissection into the retroperitoneal pelvic haematoma.

Injuries to the Urethra

Disruption of the urethra is an injury found mostly in men, and associated with either pelvic fractures or so-called straddle injury. Posterior urethral tears are present in approximately 10% of pelvic fractures. Ruptures of the anterior urethra are generally associated with straddle injuries and are often isolated lesions. Urethral injuries are suspected on the basis of mechanism, associated pelvic fracture, perineal haematoma or perineal injury, blood at the urethral meatus, and displacement of the prostate gland. Diagnosis is made by a retrograde urethrogram. Intravenous pyelography is generally performed in patients with associated injuries. The majority of patients with rupture of the posterior urethra will have a complete tear. About half the patients with anterior urethral injuries will have complete tears.

The initial management of the urethral injuries has undergone significant change in the past several years. Conventional early urethral realignment has given way to initial bladder decompression by suprapubic cystostomy and a delayed urethroplasty. Delayed repair has served to markedly diminish the incidence of stricture, impotence and incontinence associated with urethral repair at the time of injury.

Complications of Genito-urinary Trauma

Stepwise systematic evaluation of suspected genito-urinary injuries will result in a low incidence of delayed diagnosis, and the associated haemorrhagic and infectious complications.

Early complications of genito-urinary injury include haemorrhage, urinary extravasation, and infection. Haemorrhage may be massive with severe renal injuries and can result in exsanguination. Urinary extravasation from renal fracture, ureteral lacerations and bladder rupture, may result in retroperitoneal urinomas. These collections are prone to infection and may lead to abscess formation. Patients with large retroperitoneal haematomas, associated urinary extravasation, and urinary tract infection can result in seeding of the haematoma and eventually abscess formation and sepsis.

Late complications of genito-urinary trauma include hypertension, arteriovenous fistula and pyelonephritis with renal injuries; stricture formation and hydronephrosis with ureteral transections, and stricture, incontinence and impotence, with disruptions of the urethra.

20 *Vascular Trauma*

Marc M. Sedwitz and S. R. Shackford

HISTORICAL PERSPECTIVE

Vascular injuries are a major cause of morbidity and mortality in the trauma patient. The approach to the management of serious arterial and venous injuries and their complications has been developed in large part through the cumulative military experience since World War II. Nevertheless, few arterial injuries were reconstructed prior to the Korean conflict and DeBakey reported a 49% amputation rate following arterial ligation, during World War II. The amputation rate was reduced to 13% during the Korean War experience with vascular trauma as a result of frequent use of arterial repair. The lessons of the Vietnam War experience expanded our ability to treat vascular trauma aggressively with good success. The shortened evacuation time which minimized ischaemia, the repair of accompanying venous injuries, and the availability of experienced surgeons all contributed to the high success rate. Since that time, the technological advancements in angiography, non-invasive imaging, Doppler examination, and improved prosthetic grafts and suture materials have added to the successful management of these difficult problems.

AETIOLOGY

The majority of vascular injuries in the civilian experience are the result of direct penetrating or blunt trauma. However, another increasingly frequent cause of vascular injury is iatrogenic in nature, as the need for interventional diagnostic and therapeutic procedures increases. Penetrating injuries (primarily stab and gunshot wounds) comprise the majority of the vascular injuries seen in the urban setting. However, as the frequency of motor vehicle accidents increases the resultant vascular injuries secondary to blunt trauma will increase also.

The trauma produced by a bullet is proportional to its energy which in turn is related to the velocity of the projectile (energy = 1/2 mass × velocity^2). A high-velocity missile will not only produce significant direct injury but will also produce a cavitational and suction effect (blast injury) that can disrupt the intima of the vessel more extensively than may be initially apparent and produce major complications. Severe blunt trauma frequently produces fractures, dislocations, and tremendous crushing forces that may disrupt the adjacent neurovascular bundle. Rapid deceleration injuries from motor vehicle accidents or falls may result in powerful forces of torsion, compression and stretching that lead to significant vascular injury. The descending thoracic aorta, hepatic veins and renal arteries are particularly vulnerable to these kinds of deceleration forces.

PATHOPHYSIOLOGY

A vessel may be lacerated, transected, contused, or may go into spasm. Arterial laceration is the most common type of vascular injury from penetrating trauma. Any arterial injury can produce a haematoma, form a pseudoaneurysm, decompress into a venous channel to form an arteriovenous fistula, or thrombose. Transection of an artery often induces retraction of the intima and media which act to control the exsanguinating haemorrhage. Since the intima is the weakest layer of the artery, its disruption can lead to thrombosis in the absence of external signs of blood loss or significant haematoma suggestive of vascular injury. Traumatic arterial spasm is a rare entity that cannot be diagnosed with certainty, but represents a myogenic reaction independent of the autonomic nervous system in medium-sized muscular arteries. If not recognized early, these injuries can lead to significant morbidity from ischaemia.

INITIAL PREOPERATIVE EVALUATION

Successful management of traumatic vascular injuries depends upon the expedient evaluation and effective treatment of the patient. This includes management of the airway, vigorous resuscitation with crystalloid infusion, and appropriate attention to any other accompanying life-threatening injuries. Although most vascular injuries are diagnosed promptly, others may be more insidious and require a high index of suspicion. It is clear that the burden of investigation rests upon the surgeon to be sure that an occult injury is not missed. A diminished or absent distal pulse, a history of persistent arterial bleeding, a large or expanding haematoma, major haemorrhage with hypotension, an injury to anatomically related nerves, or a bruit at or distal to a suspected injury, alone or in combination are useful in the diagnostic evaluation. Signs of severe distal extremity ischaemia such as: pain, pallor, pulselessness, paralysis, and paraesthesias are helpful in determining the urgency of repair.

In the setting of prolonged extremity ischaemia, time is of critical importance. Whereas brain tissue dies within minutes in the face of acute ischaemia, muscle and peripheral nerve tissue may tolerate anoxia for 4–6 h. Delay in diagnosis and failure to act promptly will lead to a low flow state with intravascular stasis, activation of intravascular coagulation and thrombosis. This eventually causes irreversible damage to skeletal muscle, peripheral nerves and visceral organ function.

The presence of pulses does not exclude major vascular injury. Distal pulses may be present in over 25% of cases of proximal arterial injury. The arterial pulse wave may be propagated through soft clot, an intimal flap or by way of collateral blood flow around a thrombosed vessel. In this setting there may even be absent clinical signs of ischaemia.

Doppler flow studies can be a valuable adjunct for the evaluation of suspected vascular injury. A monophasic arterial flow signal, a stepdown in Doppler pressure measurements, or a decrease in flow velocity support a clinical suspicion of injury.

Biplanar angiography can confirm, localize and aid in identifying surgical options in vascular trauma. Secondly, angiography has provided an increased rate of positive surgical explorations by excluding the presence of injury. The accuracy of angiography is between 92% and 98% with the majority of errors occurring when there are false positive interpretations. A review of neck and extremity angiography for vascular trauma correctly evaluated the absence of significant vascular injury even though an injury was clinically suspected. More importantly, angiography disclosed a 20% incidence of clinically unsuspected vascular injuries. Thus, exclusion arteriography is helpful in the management of vascular trauma to avoid unnecessary exploration in a stable patient with equivocal signs of arterial injury. Digital subtraction angiography (DSA) has also been useful in the evaluation of the trauma patient. The advantages of intra-arterial DSA as compared to conventional angiography include the use of less contrast material, a shorter time for the procedure, and cost effectiveness. The accuracy of intra-arterial DSA has been described and may be a valuable tool for extremity injuries.

The effective initial management of vascular injuries may be simplified by Brink's classification. Category I represents patients in shock from ongoing haemorrhage, category II are vascular injuries occurring in haemodynamically stable patients who have potential for significant morbidity, and category III represents a clinically suspected injury in a stable patient. According to Brink, category I patients require immediate operative intervention. Sources of haemorrhage will usually be obvious following penetrating trauma. However, major blunt trauma can be particularly perplexing. The classic dilemma of managing combined thoracic and abdominal trauma in the unstable hypotensive patient supports laparotomy prior to angiography when no obvious source of bleeding is discovered by chest radiography or intercostal intubation. Category II and III patients merit thorough and rapid evaluation often including angiography as part of the initial evaluation.

After the initial management of the trauma patient obvious sources of external bleeding can be controlled in most cases with manual compression or packing. Blind clamping and the use of a tourniquet are to be condemned. Blind probing of a stable wound should not be attempted unless a suspected vascular injury can be immediately controlled. Since shock and associated injuries often contribute to overall morbidity and mortality, these problems often demand priority in saving the patient's life. The patient in the operating room usually will undergo general anaesthesia. Intubation should be careful and can be hazardous particularly when the patient has vascular injuries of the neck and great vessels. The patient should undergo skin preparation and draped broadly with consideration given to the sources of autogenous vein and artery for subsequent repair. In extremity injuries the use of a shunt has permitted long delays in repair of the vascular injuries until other life-threatening injuries or stabilizing orthopaedic procedures are completed.

OPERATIVE MANAGEMENT

Incisions should be vertical with transverse extensions at the joint creases. They should be placed parallel to the vessel and should incorporate resection of previous scars which can be a principal source of wound complication. Division of arterial and venous collaterals should be avoided. It is preferable to remove the contralateral saphenous vein in dealing with major lower extremity arterial and venous injuries. Obtaining proximal and distal control prior to evacuating the haematoma is paramount in dealing with vascular injuries. The use of balloon catheters has been invaluable when proximal or distal control has been difficult. Systemic heparin at a dose of 50–75 units/kg is generally administered prior to clamping unless other injuries contraindicate its use. Regional heparinization may be utilized in cases that prohibit systemic anticoagulation. It cannot be overstated that balloon catheter thrombectomy is essential prior to vascular repair in order to prevent postoperative problems. Administration of antibiotics is standard therapy prior to and following surgery. Repair usually can be performed by simple lateral arteriorrhaphy or resection of a short segment (<2 cm) of artery with primary anastomosis. The remainder of injuries require replacement with either autogenous saphenous vein or prosthetic material (PTFE or Dacron). Accompanying venous injuries, particularly to the deep femoral and popliteal veins, should be repaired to maximize the chances of success when the artery is repaired.

MANAGEMENT OF SPECIFIC INJURIES

Vascular Injuries of the Intrathoracic Aorta and Great Vessels

Injuries to the arch and great vessels are usually caused by penetrating rather than blunt trauma. The morbidity and mortality of these injuries are among the highest in vascular trauma. Most of these patients expire prior to arrival at the hospital from profound shock secondary to massive haemorrhage.

Successful management of these injuries depends upon aggressive resuscitation, often utilizing lower extremity intravenous lines, early intubation, prompt diagnosis and rapid surgical control of haemorrhage. Diagnostic signs suggestive of great vessel trauma are: (*a*) cardiac arrest; (*b*) persistent shock; (*c*) cardiac tamponade; (*d*) a mediastinum widened to >8 cm; (*e*) recurring haemothorax; (*f*) blunting of the aortic knob; (*g*) pleural capping; (*h*) deviation of the mainstem bronchus; (*i*) displacement of the nasogastric tube; (*j*) neurological deficits; (*k*) pulse deficits, or (*l*) bruits. However, about one-third of these injuries have no obvious clinical sign of vascular trauma, except for a penetrating cutaneous wound. High-grade arteriography is useful, but should not delay surgery in a haemodynamically unstable patient.

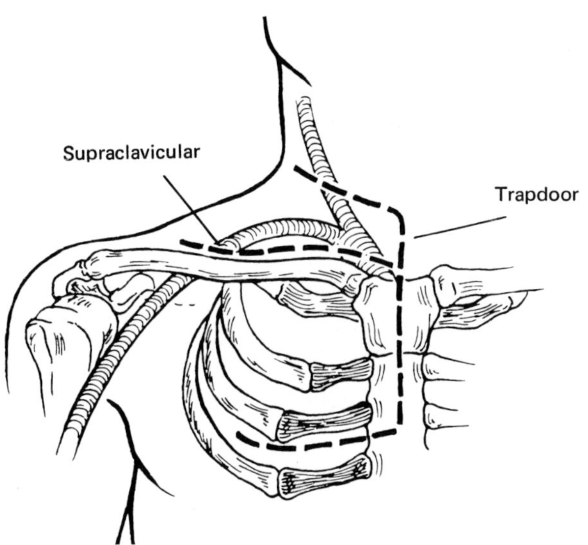

Fig. 20.1 The 'trapdoor' approach to the great vessels.

Wide preparation of the neck and chest is essential. Injuries to deep mediastinal vessels require a median sternotomy. Often this incision can be extended into the supraclavicular fossa or obliquely anterior to the sternocleidomastoid muscle in the neck. The proximal left subclavian artery can be difficult to repair and a 'trapdoor' or 'book' thoracotomy extension may be made into the left third or fourth intercostal space or a left lateral thoracotomy performed (*Fig.* 20.1).

During repair of the innominate artery the need for maintaining cerebrovascular flow by placing a shunt has been considered. Scant distal back bleeding, stump pressures in the carotid artery <60 mmHg, or EEG changes during intraoperative monitoring suggest the need for placing a shunt to maintain cerebral blood flow prior to repair of the innominate or carotid artery.

The majority of thoracic pseudoaneurysms produced by blunt trauma occur at the aortic isthmus. If untreated and unrecognized the pseudoaneurysm has an unpredictable course, and may rupture from hours to months later. Aortography is the only definitive test to identify this problem although CT scans have been helpful. The use of a Gott shunt, femoral–femoral bypass or left ventricular assist device can maintain flow to the kidney and prevent spinal cord ischaemic complications. Cardiopulmonary bypass has not often been required.

Innominate Vascular Injury

Innominate vascular injuries are most frequently caused by penetrating trauma. Three-quarter of these patients present with shock. Bypass is the preferred method of repair when a large mediastinal haematoma is discovered. With major trauma many surgeons utilize prosthetic material for repair of the great vessels. However, the saphenous vein is still commonly used. If there is significant contamination, the use of ligation and extrathoracic bypass (carotid–carotid, subclavian–subclavian, axillary–axillary, subclavian–carotid) through uncontaminated tissue planes has been used successfully to avoid prosthetic graft material. Accompanying injuries to the superior vena cava (SVC) and innominate vein are common. A shunting procedure during repair of the SVC may be required.

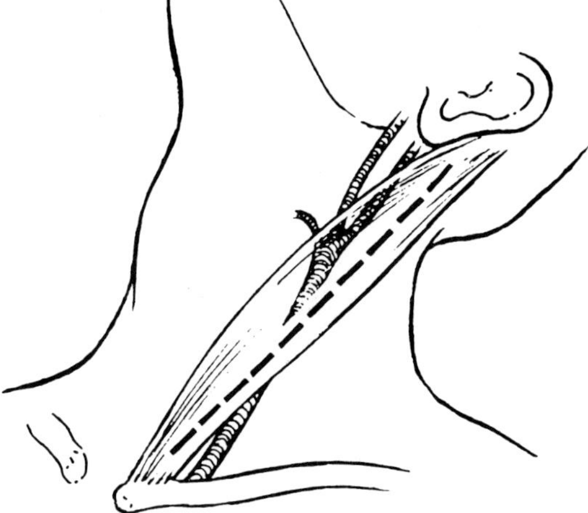

Fig. 20.2 Incision to approach carotid vessels.

Both SVC and innominate vein injuries may be a source for air embolization. In the event of this complication, immediate direct aspiration of air from the pulmonary artery right ventricle and atrium, and SVC is required. Innominate vein injuries should be repaired, whenever possible, since serious sequelae can result from ligation.

Subclavian Vascular Injuries

Penetrating trauma continues to be responsible for the majority of subclavian vascular injuries. Mortality from these injuries has declined to 4·7%. The majority may be repaired by primary anastomosis or an interposition graft. The 'book' thoracotomy, into the third or fourth intercostal space is the most useful incision.

Blunt trauma that produces fractures of the clavicle and the underlying first rib can produce significant injury to the subclavian vessels situated between these bony elements. The incidence of subclavian injuries with first rib and clavicular fractures is reported to be 14%. Subclavian vascular injuries often have accompanying spinal cord or brachial plexus injuries which are responsible for significant and sometimes devastating disability.

Carotid Artery Injuries (*Fig.* 20.2)

Management of carotid artery injuries represents a most important aspect in the treatment of neck trauma. Significant carotid trauma is often complicated by injury to other arterial or venous structures as well as to the larynx, pharynx, trachea, oesophagus, salivary glands, thoracic duct and adjacent cranial and cervical nerves. Carotid artery injuries due to penetrating trauma often present with haemorrhage, haematoma and shock. The common carotid artery is most frequently injured. The neurological status of the patient is a critical factor that determines therapeutic options for management. Controversy exists as to whether restoration of cerebral blood flow in the presence of a neurological deficit can convert an area of ischaemic infarct into a haemorrhagic one. A 40% operative mortality has been noted in patients with preoperative coma. However, recent studies suggest an aggressive approach to revascularization of the carotid artery injury even in the setting of a moderate to severe neurological deficit. For instance, a significant clinical improvement has been observed in two-thirds of patients presenting with coma who underwent revascularization. Reversal of neurological deficits has also

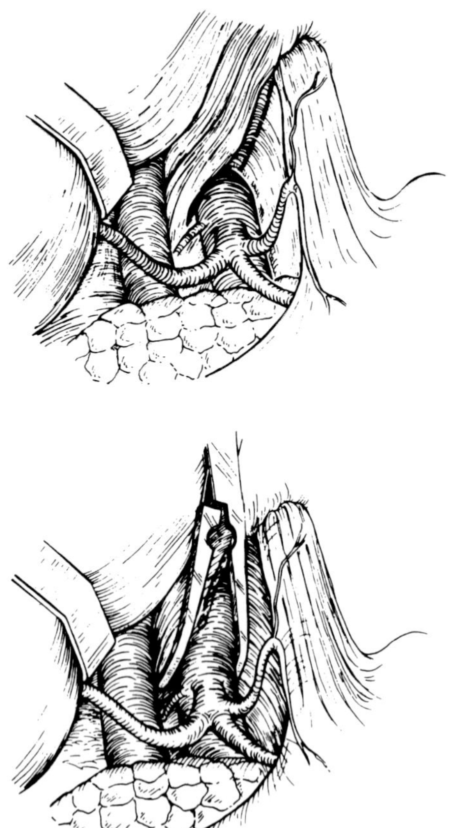

Fig. 20.3 To gain access to the supracoeliac aorta, the liver is retracted upward, the stomach downward and the posterior peritoneum incised. The muscular crus of the diaphragm is incised (broken line).

been reported in patients who have undergone extracranial-to-intracranial (EC–IC), bypasses for high cervical or intracranial internal carotid injuries. However, major carotid artery injuries should be ligated in the setting of profound neurological deficit or coma.

Blunt trauma to the carotid artery can be difficult to diagnose since patients often have accompanying closed head injuries or other complications of blunt trauma. The neurological sequelae of blunt carotid trauma may be slower to develop than with penetrating injuries since it is usually an intimal disruption or mural contusion that leads to slow thrombosis or subsequent embolization. Limb paralysis in an alert patient, a lucid interval, transient ischaemic attacks, Horner's syndrome, or a history of forceful trauma to the neck producing a haematoma are symptoms highly suspicious of blunt carotid trauma. These deficits may occur hours to days after a reported injury. Resection of the damaged artery and an interposition graft with autogenous tissue or primary anastomosis is recommended. The patient with a dense stroke and occlusion is unlikely to benefit from operation.

Vertebral Artery Injuries

Traumatic injury of the vertebral artery is rare because of the protection offered by its anatomical course through the cervical vertebrae. Although more commonly injured by penetrating trauma, blunt trauma with fracture of the cervical spine can produce vertebral artery injury. Suspicion of a vertebral artery injury demands immediate angiography. Trauma to the vertebral artery may produce significant haemorrhage, thrombosis or development of a pseudoaneurysm or arteriovenous fistula. The latter two complications cannot be effectively treated by ligation alone. However, angiographic embolization using detachable balloon catheters has effectively treated these difficult problems.

Intra-abdominal Vascular Injuries

Infrarenal and supracoeliac aortic injuries can be approached directly and efficiently following proximal control of the aorta in the chest or at the subdiaphragmatic hiatus (*Fig.* 20.3). The highest mortality and greatest challenge occurs with injuries of the suprarenal aorta when significant accompanying visceral injuries are encountered. Access for control and repair of suprarenal aortic injuries is through a midline or thoracoabdominal incision with reflection of the left colon, spleen and pancreas to the right (*Fig.* 20.4). It is essential that repairs be performed expeditiously since prolonged ischaemia to the kidneys and liver can cause postoperative complications. In general these organs tolerate up to 60 min of warm ischaemia. Cooling of the abdomen with 4 °C Ringer-lactate lavage is essential to prolonging the ischaemic tolerance of the liver and kidneys.

Primary repair of the aorta is often possible. The use of prosthetic material should be avoided when gross contamination of the abdomen is present. Extra-anatomical reconstruction is an important alternative if direct repair will be compromised by risk of infection.

It cannot be overstated that these patients benefit greatly from aggressive resuscitation and blood replacement. Use of the cell saver may be of critical importance. Protecting the patient from tissue hypoxia, hypothermia and acidosis can prevent coagulation problems which lead to further haemorrhage and perpetuate coagulopathy.

Injuries to the visceral vessels are rare. They represent 1–5% of all vascular injuries from penetrating trauma. All visceral blood vessels should be repaired whenever possible. In general, these injuries are repaired primarily and occasionally require a vein patch or an interposition graft. Ligation of an important visceral artery demands angiographic knowledge that collaterals exist which will continue to perfuse the gastrointestinal tract. However, injuries to the coeliac axis may be treated with ligation at its origin. Ligation of the superior mesenteric artery is poorly tolerated and every attempt at repair must be pursued. The inferior mesenteric artery has sufficient collateral flow to permit ligation without complications. However, in elderly patients, the inferior mesenteric artery may be an important source of blood supply to the colon, especially if the superior mesenteric artery is compromised.

Hepatic artery injuries can usually be repaired by primary anastomosis. Hepatic artery ligation proximal to the origin of the gastroduodenal artery is usually well tolerated without adverse sequelae. Results of ligation distal to this point are unpredictable. The status of any injury to the portal vein must also be determined prior to arterial ligation. The splenic artery may be ligated without accompanying injury to the spleen, but attempts at repair of the vessel are advised.

Renal Artery Injuries

Prompt repair of renal artery injuries is essential to maximize and preserve renal function. Although penetrating trauma is more common, renal artery thrombosis is seen more often from blunt trauma. The stable patient with haematuria should undergo an intravenous pyelogram. If there is no visualization of a kidney on IVP the patient

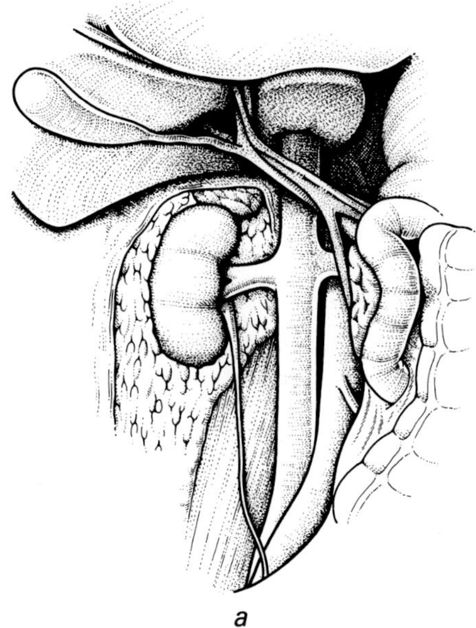

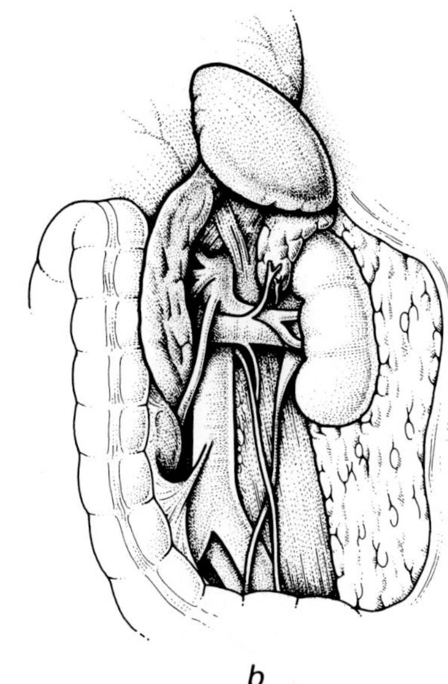

Fig. 20.4 *a*, Exposure of upper abdominal aorta and visceral vasculature by reflection of the right colon and head of pancreas and duodenum. *b*, Exposure of the infra and supra renal cava as well as portal vein by reflecting the left colon, spleen and pancreas. (After Blaisdell F. W. and Trunkey D. D. (ed.) *Abdominal Trauma*, Vol. 1, New York, Thieme-Stratton Inc.)

requires renal arteriography and surgery. Suspected renal artery injuries are best approached by exposing the abdominal aorta and obtaining control of the renal artery and vein. If delay in diagnosis or repair has been substantial, nephrectomy may be necessary. Many renal artery injuries are insidious since they present with few external signs of injury and without haematuria. In virtually all cases renal artery repair should be attempted. Autotransplantation or *ex vivo* renal artery repair may be contemplated in an attempt to salvage the kidney with complicated injuries.

Injuries to the Extremities

Femoral artery injuries are the most common of the lower extremity. They frequently are caused by penetrating trauma, but can also be caused by fractures, dislocations, and by iatrogenic injury from cardiac catheterization or placement of intra-aortic balloon pumps. Femoral artery injuries often have accompanying venous and nerve injuries. The importance of deep vein reconstruction in addition to arterial repair cannot be overemphasized. Failure to perform venous repair appears to be a significant determinant of late morbidity. When the profunda femoris artery is injured repair should be attempted since the superficial femoral artery may become occluded from subsequent atherosclerotic vascular disease. The popliteal vessels are particularly prone to blunt trauma injury from fractures and dislocations. The amputation rate for injuries in this area ranges up to 61%. Concomitant popliteal vein injury plays an important role in the success of vascular reconstruction. Expeditious repair of both the vein and artery is therefore essential.

Although the ideal sequence of repair in patients with combined orthopaedic and popliteal vascular injuries is sometimes unclear, vascular repair should precede external fixation when there is threatened limb loss. Early heparinization and the use of mannitol to minimize muscle compartment swelling are valuable adjuncts. The use of a Javid shunt has been utilized to maintain distal blood flow to the extremities, while other life-threatening injuries are being repaired. Heparin should be continued in the postoperative period to enhance vein patency. Injury to the small vessels below the trifurcation represents an occasional management dilemma. When both tibial arteries are injured the amputation rate may reach 65%, whereas with injury to only one vessel the rate is much lower. Angiography in this area is important in defining the sites and extents of all the injuries. This is particularly true with multiple pellet wounds from a shotgun blast. If arteriography demonstrates only a single isolated arterial injury below the knee without active bleeding, pseudoaneurysm or arteriovenous fistulas, and the patient has no other signs of distal ischaemia then observation without surgical intervention is justified. On the other hand, any patient who demonstrates ischaemia, bleeding, or a vascular complication of the injury must undergo immediate exploration and repair of the artery. If a vein graft is required for repair, it should be harvested from the contralateral extremity.

Vascular injuries in the upper extremity are extremely common. Not only are these injuries caused by penetrating trauma but are also caused by the increasing use of the brachial artery approach for angiography and cardiac catheterization, and by the techniques of arterial blood gas monitoring. Long bone fractures with and without joint dislocations are another source of potential vascular trauma (*Fig.* 20.5). In children the brachial artery is particularly vulnerable to injury from supracondylar fractures of the humerus.

Most upper extremity vascular injuries do not produce limb-threatening ischaemia and the diagnosis can be established by physical examination or angiography. Injuries to the axillary and brachial arteries require immediate exploration and can usually be treated by thrombectomy and primary repair with or without a vein patch (*Fig.* 20.6). Injuries to the radial and ulnar arteries are usually easy to repair but can be ligated if an intact palmar arch is present. Fasciotomy of the forearm may be needed to maximize successful repairs in cases of advanced ischaemia.

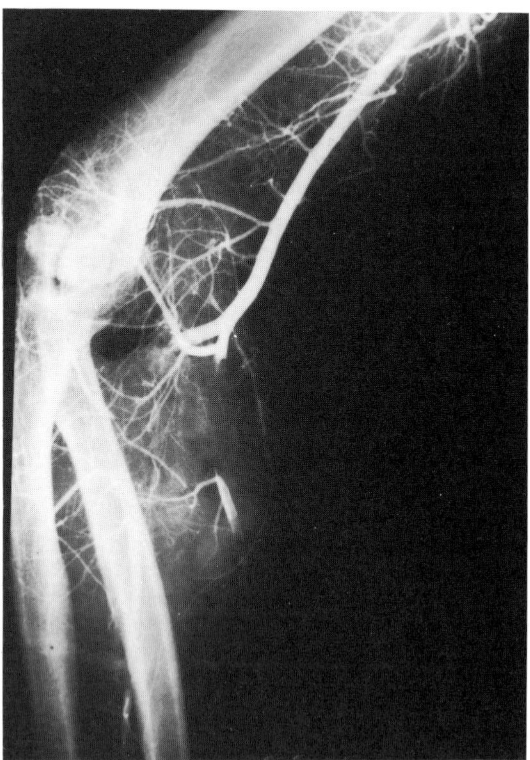

Fig. 20.5 This patient sustained a severe crush injury to an elbow resulting in a massive haematoma, complete transection of the proximal ulnar artery and contusion/thrombosis of the proximal radial artery. Circulation was restored using a reversed autogenous saphenous vein graft between the brachial and radial arteries.

Intra-abdominal Venous Injuries

Historically, intra-abdominal venous injuries have been a complicated and frustrating problem for the trauma surgeon. The high mortality (35–53%) and morbidity of these injuries is correlated with the location of the injury. The presence of associated vascular and visceral injuries, the aetiology of the injury, and the presence of shock upon arrival to the hospital are critical variables which determine survival. Venous injuries can be more difficult to manage than arterial injuries. The exposure of the injury is often poor. Veins require delicate handling when being sutured and will not tolerate tension. Blind occlusion of large veins with clamps often results in increased haemorrhage since the intraluminal pressure is increased and exacerbates the arterial bleeding. Venous repairs are often thrombogenic and can lead to venous insufficiency and pulmonary embolism. Prosthetic material has worked poorly in the venous circuit. However, with the use of a ringed PTFE graft and creation of an accompanying arteriovenous fistula to maintain flow through the graft, patency of many repairs can be improved.

Suprarenal vena caval wounds often involve the hepatic veins. Ligation of a simple hepatic vein appears to be well tolerated. Most hepatic vein injuries have been managed by primary repair after mobilization and division of the hepatic ligaments. Severe injury has often required occlusion of the suprahepatic and infrahepatic caval and portal veins. This manoeuvre, which abruptly terminates cardiac blood return, is not well tolerated by the patient for long periods and can cause death in the hypovolaemic patient. Vascular isolation

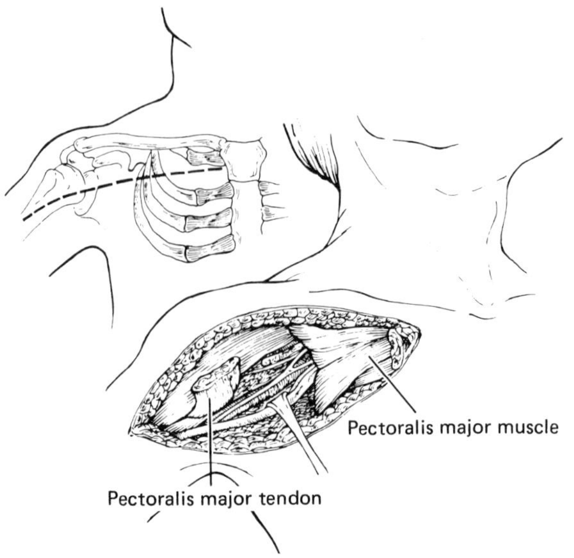

Fig. 20.6 Approach to axillary artery.

of the retrohepatic cava has been described with extension of the midline laparotomy incision into a median sternotomy and placement of an atriocaval shunt. Control of bleeding by packing or occlusion of inflow into the injury site is essential prior to insertion of the shunt. However, few patients survive this injury even with an atriocaval shunt.

In contrast, infrarenal caval injuries have only one-half the mortality of their suprarenal counterparts. These injuries can be more easily approached by mobilizing the right colon and reflecting the duodenum. Ligation of the infrarenal vena cava is an alternative that is well tolerated despite increased venous insufficiency in the lower extremities.

In all cases, portal vein and superior mesenteric vein injuries require attempts at repair. Both injuries are similarly lethal (mortality 54–71%). While portal vein ligation has been reported to be well tolerated in 90% of cases, some patients without sufficient collaterals develop intestinal infarction and portal hypertension after ligation. A series from San Francisco General Hospital stresses 'second look' operations at 24–48 h after ligation to evaluate small bowel viability. The same report advocates measurement of portal pressures to help determine the need for a portal-systemic venous shunt.

MAJOR VASCULAR INJURIES AND PELVIC TRAUMA

The high mortality (30–60%) of pelvic fractures is secondary to unrelenting haemorrhage. Multiple lacerations of both small and medium-sized arteries and veins are the source of exsanguinating haemorrhage in the pelvis. Success in managing these patients requires rapid assessment, vigorous resuscitation, and reversal of the systemic effects of prolonged shock.

Haemorrhage can at least be minimized by compression of the pelvic area with a use of MAST suit. In the same way, early external fixation of the pelvis provides immobilization and amelioration of the bleeding caused by movement of unstable large bony fragments. Patients who continue to require massive transfusions despite control of intra-abdominal and intrathoracic bleeding sources are candidates for early therapeutic embolization of pelvic arterial bleeding in the angiography suite. Hypogastric artery ligation has few advocates, as it has been shown to be almost totally ineffective. However, it represents the last manoeuvre prior to packing the pelvis and re-exploring the patient later.

ACUTE AND CHRONIC SEQUELAE OF VASCULAR INJURY

Haemorrhage

Bleeding subsequent to arterial repair is uncommon, occurring in less than 5% of cases. It may present as frank haemorrhage from the operative incision or as a rapidly expanding haematoma. In virtually all cases the cause is a technical error, resulting from inadequate haemostasis in the wound or from too widely spaced sutures in the vascular repair. Rarely, bleeding may be due to a missed arterial or major venous injury. Patients who develop this complication should be returned to the operating room immediately for evacuation of surrounding haematoma, identification and correction of the problem.

Thrombosis

Occlusion of a vascular repair is the most frequently encountered acute complication of vascular surgery. Depending on the vessel involved and the type of repair (i.e., lateral arteriorrhaphy, interposition grafting, etc.), thrombosis occurs after arterial repair for trauma in approximately 10% of cases. If late thromboses are included, the incidence rises to about 20%. Early thrombosis is due to a technical problem, most commonly stenosis of the repair. Other causes include intimal dissection with prolapse and missed injury. Because these technical problems are easily corrected if discovered early, it is prudent always to perform completion arteriography at the initial operation. Thrombosis presents with a loss of distal pulses associated with signs of ischaemia (i.e., pallor, poikilothermia, pain, paralysis, paraesthesia). If pulses that were initially present disappear, the diagnosis is thrombosis and there is no need for confirmatory arteriography. These patients should be returned as soon as possible to the operating room for thrombectomy and completion arteriography. On the other hand, if pulses were never palpable after the repair and the patient is hypothermic, vasospasm may be present. In such cases, every effort should be made to rewarm the patient and improve perfusion to the extremity. If pulses do not return, either arteriography or exploration should be considered.

Arteriovenous Fistula

Arteriovenous fistula after arterial trauma occurs in 2–7% of cases. The most common causes are fragment, shrapnel or shotgun wounds. A myriad of systemic physiological changes occur as flow increases through the fistula—going from the high pressure arterial system to the low pressure venous system. Among these changes are increases in the cardiac output, heart rate, central venous pressure and blood volume. Local changes in the area of the fistula include dilatation of the proximal artery and the distal vein, distal varicosities and extremity oedema. Most of these changes are reversible with correction of the fistula. Patients may present with signs of venous stasis disease, arterial insufficiency or frank congestive heart failure. Often the physical findings are very suggestive of the diagnosis. These findings include a palpable thrill and an audible bruit or machinery type murmur. Occlusion of the fistula may cause a decrease in the elevated pulse rate (Nicoladani–Branham's sign). Arteriography should always be performed preoperatively to confirm the diagnosis, localize the lesion anatomically and determine the presence of any associated pathology. The treatment is surgical as less than 2% will close spontaneously.

Pseudoaneurysm

The incidence of pseudoaneurysm following trauma is difficult to ascertain since they are often reported in association with arteriovenous fistulas. A pseudoaneurysm may cause symptoms by encroachment on local structures as it expands or it may present acutely with rupture, distal embolization or thrombosis. Arteriography should be obtained preoperatively to define the anatomy and associated pathology. Surgical resection with end-to-end anastomosis or interposition grafting is the treatment of choice.

Infection

Infection of an arterial suture line is a disastrous complication which often leads to haemorrhage and eventual amputation. Factors leading to infection include closure of a contaminated wound, inadequate soft-tissue coverage of an arterial repair and inadequate débridement of a traumatized, contaminated vessel. This complication is best avoided by vigorous cleansing of contaminated wounds, aggressive débridement of devitalized tissues, coverage of arterial repairs with soft tissue, which is not under tension, and administration of broad-spectrum antibiotics, preferably begun preoperatively.

Compartment Syndrome

A compartment syndrome is the result of trauma or severe prolonged ischaemia which leads to swelling within a closed space. This contained swelling produces a rise in tissue hydrostatic pressure to the point that blood flow is compromised. If untreated, a compartment syndrome will result in myonecrosis and limb dysfunction. The most common areas involved are the anterior compartment in the lower leg and the volar compartment in the forearm. Since nerve tissue is more susceptible to ischaemia than is muscle tissue, initial symptoms include paraesthesias and pain in the involved extremity. Pain may be severe, especially when the limb is passively moved. Pulses may be palpable even in advanced stages and generally are not reliable indicators of the severity of the syndrome. If one suspects a developing compartment syndrome, compartmental pressure should be determined. This can be done by insertion of a plastic cannula or a wick catheter directly into the involved muscle or muscle group. Surgical decompression or fasciotomy is indicated in those patients with a compartmental pressure of greater than 40 mmHg initially or a pressure of 30 mmHg which is sustained for greater than four hours. If compartmental pressures cannot be obtained, one must proceed based upon the clinical situation. For example, if a patient with a popliteal artery injury undergoes revascularization of the lower extremity approximately 10–12 h after injury and develops a tense anterior compartment associated with a peroneal nerve palsy and loss of sensation in the distribution of the peroneal nerve (first web space), fasciotomy is indicated. The treatment of a compartment syndrome should not be postponed since irreversible myonecrosis with resultant contracture will occur within 12 h.

21 Treatment of the Burns Victim

Martin C. Robson

The burn injury can be one of the most serious and devastating forms of trauma that man can sustain. Millions of people around the world are hospitalized for the treatment of burns each year and thousands die. The daily cost of care for a burns victim is tremendous. The economic loss to any nation is staggering and must be measured not only in currency but in the permanent loss of millions of productive years. This loss is magnified by the fact that 50% of major burns occur during the formative and productive years.

Destruction of the skin by heat results in severe local and systemic physiological alterations. The management of the burns victim requires understanding of the pathophysiology, diagnosis and treatment not only of the local skin injury, but also of the derangements that occur in the haemodynamic, metabolic, nutritional, immunological and psychological homeostatic mechanisms. Proper patient care demands that the burn wound, the accompanying systemic changes and alterations produced by treatment be conceptually viewed as dynamic interrelated processes, not as isolated phenomena.

The burns victim requires a recovery period extending over months or years, even with successful treatment. The evaluation and treatment of diverse physiological changes over a prolonged time requires a team of health professionals and paraprofessionals. Indeed, the recognition of the need to develop highly specialized teams and burn care facilities has been the major advance in the management of burns in the past quarter-century. The UK has been one of the world leaders in this development.

Final success or failure of treatment of the burns victim is difficult to measure. Survival or death is not necessarily an adequate yardstick. Death of the victim with a nearly total body surface injury, hands and face burned beyond recognition, and so deep as to preclude fully functional reconstruction and rehabilitation, may not be considered failure. Similarly, survival without consideration of the functional and social rehabilitation of the victim should not be our only measure of success. The burns team must treat the patient as a whole person and measure success or failure, not on how they understand and treat the burn, but on how they understand, treat and rehabilitate the burned person.

EVALUATION OF THE BURNS VICTIM

The first essential in treating a burns victim is to determine the severity of the injury in that individual and then to decide the level of expertise necessary to care for him. A carefully performed history and physical examination specifically modified for the burns victim must be rapidly performed.

The ultimate determinants of the severity of the burn injury are the volume of tissue destroyed and whether the victim in his particular state of health can withstand it. The guidelines which help us to evaluate this are the victim's age, the extent of the burn, the depth of the injury, the area of the body involved, whether an associated inhalation of noxious gases occurred at the time of burning, and whether or not co-morbid factors are present in addition to the burn

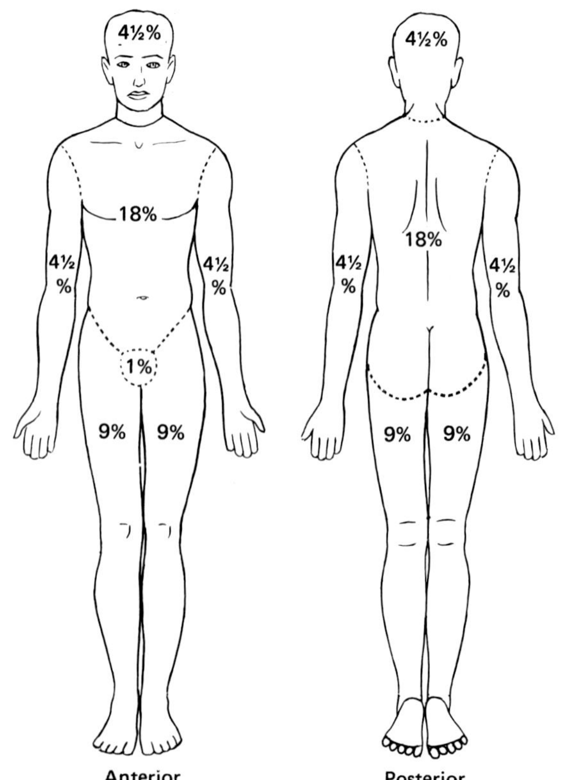

Fig. 21.1 Rule of Nines for the adult patient.

BURN SHEET

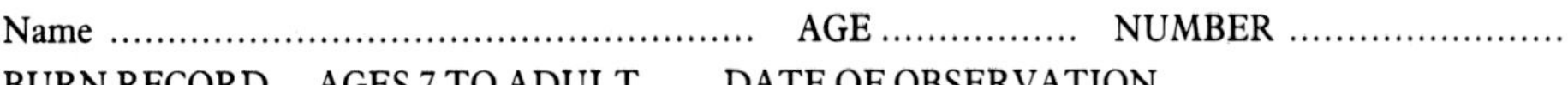
Name .... AGE .... NUMBER ....
BURN RECORD. AGES 7 TO ADULT. DATE OF OBSERVATION ....

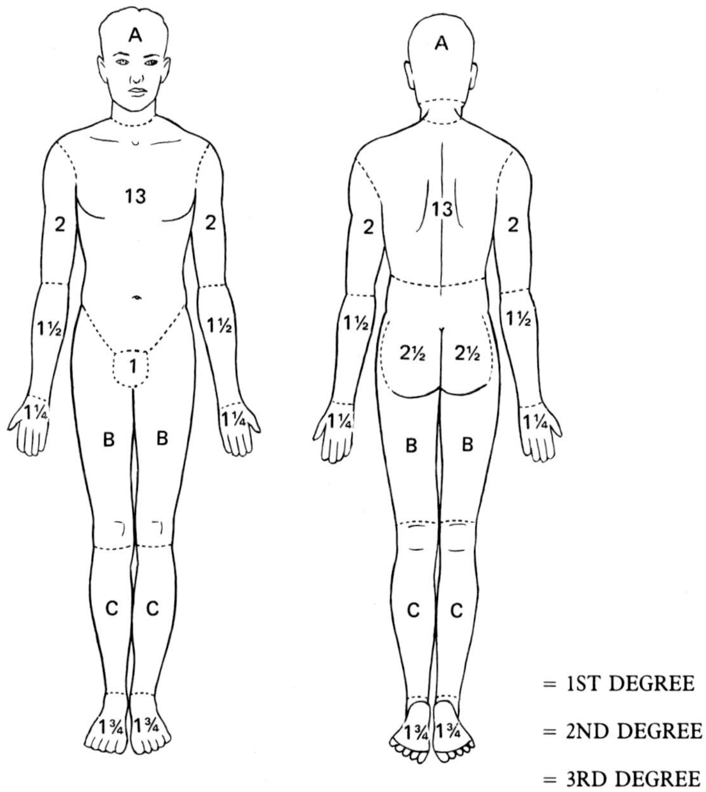

= 1ST DEGREE

= 2ND DEGREE

= 3RD DEGREE

RELATIVE PERCENTAGES OF AREAS AFFECTED BY GROWTH

AREA	AGE 10	15	ADULT
A ½ OF HEAD	5½	4½	3½
B ½ OF ONE THIGH	4¼	4½	4¾
C ½ OF ONE LEG	3	3¼	3½

% BURN BY AREAS

PROBABLE 3RD° BURN	HEAD ... NECK ... BODY ... UP. ARM ... FOREARM ... HANDS .... GENITALS ..... BUTTOCKS ..... THIGHS ..... LEGS ...... FEET ......
TOTAL BURN	HEAD ... NECK ... BODY ... UP. ARM .... FOREARM ... HANDS .... GENITALS ..... BUTTOCKS ..... THIGHS ..... LEGS ...... FEET ......

Fig. 21.2 Burn size chart modified from Lund and Browder.

injury which will affect the treatment or eventual outcome of the victim.

Age

All large series report that burns at the extremes of age carry a greater morbidity and mortality. The age of the patient determines the natural thickness of the skin and also dictates the amount of stress a person can withstand. A good guideline is that burns in people under the age of 3 or over the age of 60 years tend to be more severe.

Extent

The extent of the burn surface involved can be determined by careful observation and should be graphically recorded. This is important not only for diagnosis and treatment but also for prognosis and statistics. It is customary to record the extent of injury in terms of percentage of body surface area involved. A rough estimate of the extent can be made by using the Rule of Nines (*Fig.* 21.1) but more detailed assessment requires careful mapping on a specialized form (*Fig.* 21.2). Children require modification of either of these

BURN SHEET

NAME .... AGE .... NUMBER ....

BURN RECORD. AGES—BIRTH—7½ DATE OF OBSERVATION ....

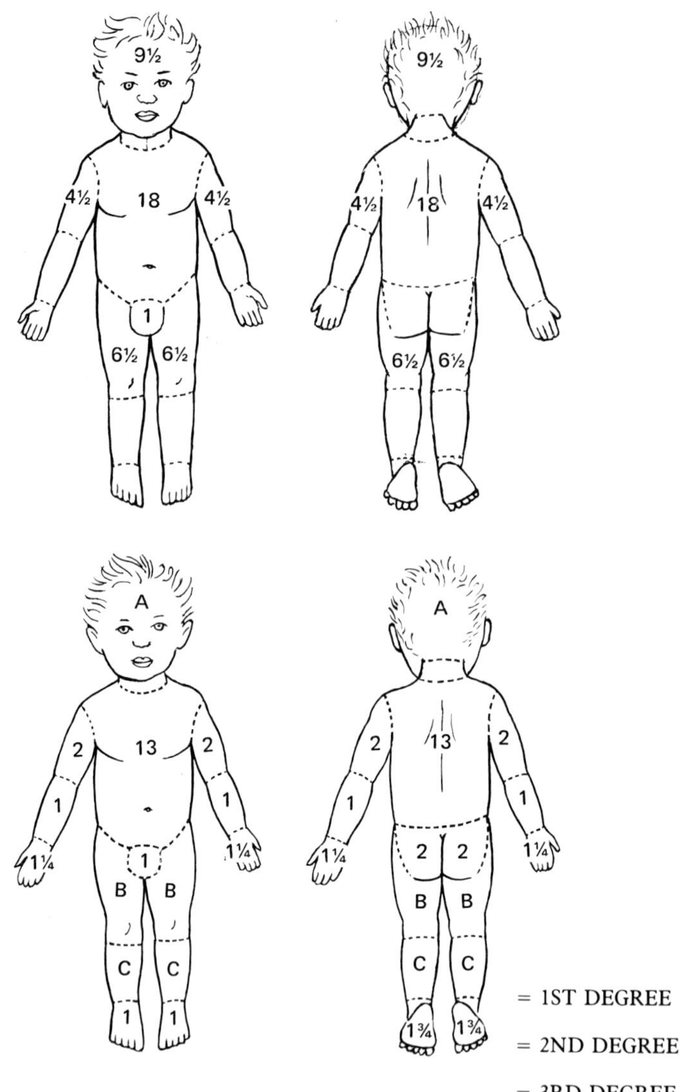

RELATIVE PERCENTAGES OF AREAS AFFECTED BY GROWTH

AREA	AGE 0	1	5
A ½ OF HEAD	9½	8½	6½
B ½ OF ONE THIGH	2¾	3¼	4
C ½ OF ONE LEG	2½	2½	2¾

% BURN BY AREAS

PROBABLE 3RD° BURN	HEAD ... NECK ... BODY ... UP. ARM ... FOREARM ... HANDS .... GENITALS ..... BUTTOCKS ..... THIGHS ..... LEGS ...... FEET ......
TOTAL BURN	HEAD ... NECK ... BODY ... UP. ARM ... FOREARM ... HANDS .... GENITALS ..... BUTTOCKS ..... THIGHS ..... LEGS ...... FEET ......

SUM OF ALL AREAS .... PROBABLY 3RD° .... TOTAL BURN ....

Fig. 21.3 Modifications in estimation of burn size required for children.

methods because of their head–chest size discrepancies and limb differentials compared with the adult (*Fig.* 21.3).

Depth

Since the volume of tissue destroyed is ultimately important, the depth as well as the extent of injury is evaluated. Unfortunately, this is impossible to estimate correctly. Although many elaborate tests have been proposed to evaluate depth of burning, none have proved totally reliable. Depth of the injury is non-uniform throughout the burn's extent and the depth may be progressive with time. Knowledge of the aetiological agent and time of exposure is helpful in determining the depth of injury. Scald burns, other than those due to immersion, tend to be more superficial than contact or flame burns. Chemical and electrical burns tend to be deep even though they may initially appear superficial. Erythema and thin watery blisters are associated with superficial burns, while thick-walled steam blisters and dry, leathery eschar are associated with deeper burns. However, appearance may be deceptive as will be discussed later under pathophysiology.

Sensation is not as helpful as once thought for differentiating burn depth. Even full-thickness burns have pressure sensation because the pressure receptors, Paccinian corpuscles, are located beneath the dermis. Pin prick is absent in deep burns; it can also be absent in burns of moderate depth. Therefore, it is not a good predictor of full-thickness injury as was often reported.

For the initial treatment of the burns victim it is only necessary to separate those injuries which are truly superficial and will heal rapidly from those which are deeper and will require hospitalization and specialized care. The full extent of the injury will reveal itself between the fourth and fourteenth day after the thermal insult.

Location

The location of the burn injury is important. Burns of the face and neck, hands, feet and perineum carry specific problems in their treatment, reconstruction and eventual rehabilitation. These areas are considered primary areas. Significant burns of the primary areas become major by location, regardless of the total body extent or depth of the injury.

Inhalation Injury

The associated inhalation of noxious gases which caused pulmonary damage increased the mortality in the McIndoe Regional Burns Unit from 13·9% to 58%. Thus, suspicion of inhalation should be determined on initial evaluation. Victims injured in a closed space are likely to develop pulmonary symptoms. Similarly, patients who present with singed nasal vibrissae, conjunctivitis, pharyngeal oedema, carbonaceous sputum, bronchorrhoea, or hoarseness are considered suspect.

Co-morbid Factors

Associated trauma at the time of burning increases the severity of the burn. Also, existing disease states prior to the thermal event can help determine the treatment and outcome. Cardiovascular, respiratory, renal, or metabolic diseases can complicate care and increase mortality. Seizure disorders and alcohol or drug abuse tend to predispose patients to burn and complicate their treatment.

Categorization

Using the above criteria, burns can be categorized conveniently for determination of severity. The classification adopted by the American Burn Association is presented in *Table* 21.1. Additional useful information prior to the initiation of treatment includes the history of the victim's immunizations, especially against tetanus, any history of known allergies, and the social circumstances surrounding the burn. Suicide or homicide attempts, child abuse, and the inability of the victim to care for himself may all influence the initial evaluation of the burns victim and assist in determining the level of expertise necessary for proper treatment.

PATHOPHYSIOLOGY OF THE LOCAL BURN INJURY

Within the limits of biological variability, human skin will tolerate temperatures up to 40 °C for brief periods of time. Temperatures above this level result in a logarithmic increase in tissue destruction, irrespective of the time of exposure. The depth of burning is determined by the combination of the burning agent, temperature and the time of exposure. Three concentric zones of significant thermal injury have been described by Jackson (*Fig.* 21.4). In the centre of the injury at the point of contact with the heat, cells are immediately destroyed by coagulation. Next, there is a zone of injured cells which might under ideal circumstances survive, but usually progress to tissue death over

Table 21.1 Classification of thermal burns

	Major Burn	*Moderate Burn*	*Minor Burn*
Size partial-thickness	>25% adults >20% children	15–25% adults 10–20% children	<15% adults <10% children
Size full-thickness	>10%	2–10%	<2%
Primary areas	Major harm if involved	Not involved	Not involved
Inhalation injury	Major burn if present or suspected	Not suspected	Not suspected
Associated injury	Major burn if present	Not present	Not present
Co-morbid factors	Poor risk patients	Patient relatively good risk	Not present
Miscellaneous	Electrical injuries		
Treatment environment	Usually specialized burn care facility	General hospital with designated team	Often managed as outpatient

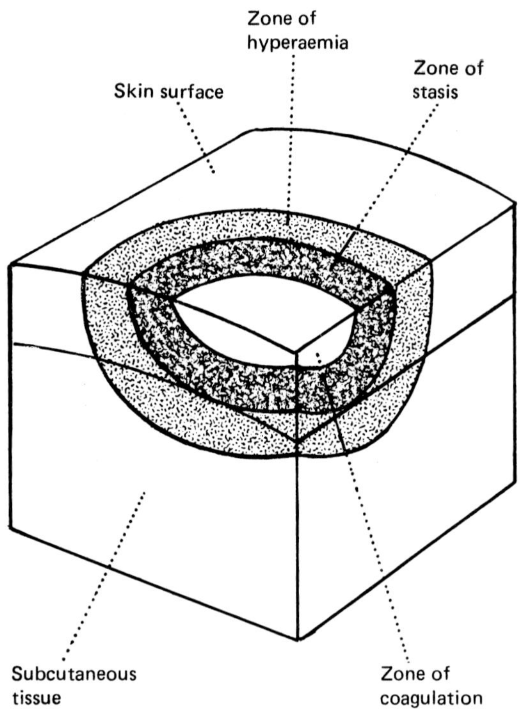

Fig. 21.4 Three zones within a major burn (after Jackson).

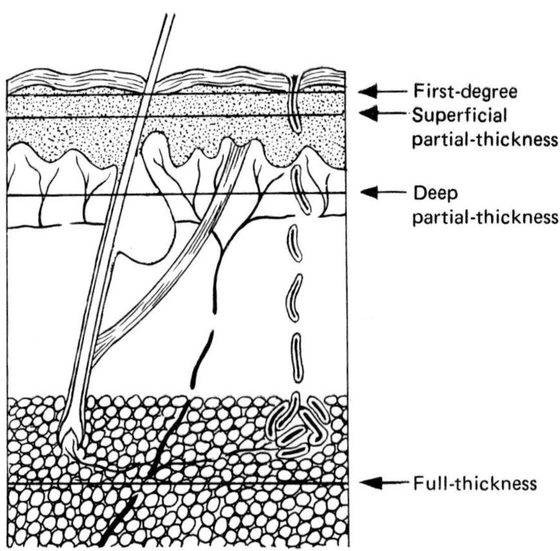

Fig. 21.5 Schematic diagram of skin demonstrating depth of burn.

24–48 h. This zone has been labelled the zone of stasis. Finally, there is a zone of tissue known as the zone of hyperaemia which has been minimally injured but will recover over a period of 7 days.

Clinically, the amount of cells in the skin that are destroyed or injured is reflected in the functional capacity of the skin. Therefore, the depth of burning is important. Although in any given area the depth will vary depending on the blood supply, thermal conductivity and evaporative water loss from this skin, it is easier to view burns as a uniform injury. The superficial or first-degree burn is characterized by erythema and discomfort only. Within a few days the outer injured cells peel off the totally healed skin with no scarring. The second-degree burn is best divided into two subsections: superficial partial-thickness and deep partial-thickness (*Fig.* 21.5). The superficial partial-thickness injury is characterized by blisters. Removal or breaking of the blisters results in weeping from the burn surface. Since the basal layers of the skin are not destroyed in this injury, regeneration is prompt and these burns usually heal in 14–17 days in the absence of infection. The deep partial-thickness burn is more severe with many areas of marginally viable tissue. This skin will only survive and heal under the most optimal conditions. The third-degree or full-thickness burn contains totally destroyed skin. Whereas the more superficial injuries are characterized by increased vascularity, this is an avascular injury. Coagulation necrosis of the cells, thrombosis of vessels, and accumulation of fluids and cellular infiltrate in the margins of the wound characterize the injury. This burn cannot heal itself. Total-thickness skin loss can only be restored by ingrowth from the margins of the wound or by application of skin grafts from non-burned portions of the body. Finally, fourth-degree injuries involve death or injury to subcutaneous tissues such as fat, fascia, muscle or bone.

Cytological damage occurs as protein is denatured by rising temperatures. Many of the changes are reversible. Only at temperatures in excess of 45 °C does denaturation exceed the ability of the cell to repair the damage. At this temperature thermolabile enzyme systems are blocked and when the enzyme activity decreases to 50% of normal, cell death occurs. The response of the cells involved in burns is neither uniform nor static. The blood supply and local environment of the wound will help to determine the cells' response. Additional trauma, oedema, decreased vascular supply or bacterial invasion will further injure or destroy cells that initially survive the thermal insult.

In addition to cell damage, there are both immediate and delayed vascular and cellular inflammatory responses at the burned site. Accumulation of fluid in the burn wound is a prominent feature of thermal injury. The fluid and electrolyte shift within the wound is related to the type and severity of the injury. This appears to be secondary to a series of mediators released following the thermal insult. These mediators include vasoactive amines, prostaglandins, thromboxanes and leukotrienes. Immediately, a spasm of venules, vasoconstriction of arterioles, and dilatation of capillaries occur. Capillaries and venules become permeable in the burned area allowing leakage of fluid, electrolytes, and proteins. The immediate response is followed within 6 h by a delayed response with venular dilatation and further capillary permeability. The most rapid fluid loss occurs during the first 12 h post-burn and is accompanied by cell margination and emigration as seen in inflammation from other causes. Another cause of loss of fluid into the burn wound (besides capillary permeability) is the breakdown of the cell membrane by the thermal injury which injures the sodium pump. This results in an increase in intracellular sodium and water and an efflux of potassium.

There is a local cellular response accompanying the fluid response. Neutrophils emigrate from vessels into the tissues and are attracted by chemotaxis to the site of the injury. Monocytes migrate into the area and tissue macrophages differentiate in the area as needed for repair. The wound macrophages are the cells which control healing by release of a number of substances such as angiogenesis factor and growth factor.

SYSTEMIC RESPONSE TO LOCAL INJURY

As the above events are occurring at the local site of burning, systemic changes also take place. The functions of all organ systems will eventually be altered due to the effects of a major burn. Some of the changes are related to burning itself, and some are in response to the stress of injury.

Cardiovascular Response

Among the most immediate and most severe changes are those in the heart and blood vessels. A precipitate drop in cardiac output of up to 50% occurs. Although this was originally thought to be due to an unknown myocardial depressant factor, it now appears to be secondary to changes in the interstitium in the wound and adjacent unburned tissue. There is an increase in interstitial oncotic pressure due to release of osmotically active cellular elements. When this osmotic gradient occurs across an injured basement membrane, massive oedema can occur. As blood volume and plasma volume fall, further decreases in the cardiac output occur until levels of as little as 20% of normal are reached. A direct toxic effect of the burn or burn byproducts can cause myocardial failure of either the left heart, right heart, or both. This initial cardiac effect appears to be self-limited, and the cardiac output returns toward normal within 36 h in patients surviving their burns.

The fluid shifts in the local burn area are accompanied by total body fluid shifts in the larger injuries. Almost total body capillary permeability occurs in patients with greater than 30% body surface area burns. The lung vasculature may be the only tissue spared. The fluid-electrolyte-protein loss renders Starling's hypothesis ineffective and the fluid enters a functional third space. This represents an overall haemodynamic defect. Fully 60% of the extracellular fluid volume may be lost in a major burn through capillary permeability, the intracellular fluid shifting into the heat-injured cells, and evaporation following destruction of the skin barrier. Most of the loss occurs within the first 8–12 h but massive fluid losses continue for at least 48 h after injury. Added to these losses specific for the burn injury is the obligatory fluid loss by respiration and urine. The fluid loss to the outside and to the inside functional third space results in haemodynamic instability or burn shock. The understanding of burn shock was necessary before adequate resuscitation techniques could be devised.

Besides the fluid portion of the vascular system, the systemic cellular elements also have a predictable response. Progressive anaemia occurs beyond that predicted in response to direct red-cell destruction by heat. Red-cell survival is decreased and the normal hypoxic stimulus for haemopoiesis appears to malfunction. Red-cell trapping by the reticuloendothelial system and losses through capillary permeability and thrombus formation further diminish the red-cell mass. Platelet changes postburn are biphasic. An initial thrombocytopenia is followed by a prolonged thrombocytosis. The thrombocytopenia is accompanied by hypofibrinogenaemia and a brief state of diffuse intravascular coagulopathy. As will be discussed later, neutrophils are affected by burn injury and this affects the systemic host defences.

Renal Response

Renal function is altered in the burn victim as in any trauma victim. The posterior pituitary releases ADH, causing maximal reabsorption of water in the renal tubules. Maximum sodium reabsorption occurs simultaneously because of aldosterone release from the adrenals. This combination results in excretion of a small amount of concentrated urine containing a decreased sodium concentration.

The injured cells in the burn wound release increased amounts of myoglobin, haemoglobin and toxic products which are presented to the kidney. If an adequate glomerular filtration rate is not maintained, or if renal ischaemia occurs, these products cannot be effectively removed and acute tubular necrosis ensues. This is the basis of renal failure which was previously a common accompaniment of burn shock.

If volume losses are replaced by a similar fluid and volume to that being lost, renal blood flow is maintained. This results in an adequate glomerular filtration rate and urine volume. Since urine volume reflects solute load and glomerular filtration rate, decreased renal function is almost inevitably a result of inadequate fluid and electrolyte replacement. It has been shown that a urine rate of 30–50 ml/h in an adult and 1·2 ml/kg/h in a child are adequate for the kidney to remove the toxic breakdown products and maintain function during the period of haemodynamic instability.

Pulmonary Response

The pulmonary system is exposed to a lack of oxygen secondary to combustion and this may be aggravated by inhalation of noxious stimuli at the time of injury. The hypoxia is a stimulus for release of injurious free oxygen radicals as well as arachidonic acid metabolites. Although the heat is dissipated before it can cause a pulmonary burn, it does cause damage to the upper airway leading to oedema and obstruction. As the burns victim becomes oedematous and his cardiac output falls, the vascular space contracts leading to a ventilation : perfusion imbalance. This leads to inadequate peripheral perfusion and lactic acidosis. The prolonged poor perfusion results in cell damage and thrombosis in the capillaries. As resuscitation re-establishes adequate flow, these products are pushed back into the venous circulation to be cleared by the already injured lungs. To effect the resuscitation, large volumes of salt-containing fluid are given resulting in a weight gain of 15–20% making the chest wall heavy and hard to move. This excursion may be further limited if an unyielding, leathery eschar is present on the anterior thorax. Unless severe smoke inhalation occurs, there does not appear to be altered permeability in the lungs so lung water is usually not increased. This allows large volumes of resuscitation fluid to be used without risking pulmonary oedema. The level of the diaphragm may be elevated by a reflex ileus, further decreasing the intrathoracic volume.

All burn victims show a degree of hyperventilation. Ventilation is about twice normal with minute volumes up to 14 L at a ventilatory rate of 20/min. This is due to increased oxygen needs and a ventilation:perfusion imbalance. In addition, burns of over 40% total body surface area develop restrictive disease with a mild to moderate decrease in lung volume, a decreased vital capacity and an increase in pulmonary resistance.

Gastrointestinal Response

The initial response of the gastrointestinal tract to a major burn is a reflex ileus due to splanchnic vasoconstriction. If decompression is not instituted, acute gastric dilatation, vomiting and possible aspiration occurs. Gastroduodenal mucosal ulceration is a frequent occurrence in the burns victim. This may not always be clinically evident. The ulceration appears not to be due to true hyperacidity. Gastrin does not appear to be increased in the burn patients. However, the ulcerations seem to be due to a relative hyperacidity, and during the first 72 h postburn patients seem to have a higher basal acid output than later in their burn course.

Liver function is altered following thermal injury. These changes are probably due to altered circulation and hypoxia and the effects of toxic waste products. Liver biopsies have shown cloudy swelling and evidence of glycogenolysis as early as 3 h after burning.

Musculoskeletal Response

Direct injury to the fascia, tendon, muscle and outer cortex of bone can occur at the time of burning. Localized or generalized osteoporosis and demineralization may result from the burn *per se* or secondary to prolonged immobilization. New periosteal bone growth, myositis ossificans, and heterotopic bone formation have all been reported in the burns victim.

Neuroendocrine Response

Adrenaline and noradrenaline are released in great amounts following thermal trauma. This appears to be a protective mechanism, since the mortality is higher in burn victims who cannot sustain this increased response. The adrenal cortex also responds with increased secretion of 17-hydroxycorticosteroids. These corticosteroids remain elevated as in a standard stress reaction until the patient is healed. Mineralocorticoids, specifically aldosterone, increase to conserve the decreasing sodium ion lost to the third space at the time of injury. This helps to prevent hypovolaemia by conserving sodium ions.

Metabolic-nutritional Response

The metabolic rate of the burns victim is greatly accelerated. Oxygen consumption is increased and nitrogen losses magnified. Associated with this hypermetabolic response are protein catabolism, ureagenesis, lipolysis, and increased gluconeogenesis. As the water-holding lipid in the skin is destroyed, evaporative water losses increase at a tremendous energy expense. The resultant cooling of the body results in shivering, thus adding to the energy demand. However, these mechanisms do not totally explain the hypermetabolism, and prevention of the evaporative water loss by external heat or impermeable dressings does not eliminate the hypermetabolism.

The hypermetabolic state following burning results in profound catabolism with decreased glucagon : insulin ratios and extreme intracellular cation alterations. Intracellular sodium concentration rises and will remain high unless at least 5000 calories/day are administered. A negative nitrogen balance accompanies the hypermetabolism and the nitrogen requirements may be as high as 20 g of nitrogen/m^2 body surface burn/day during the first month postburn.

A diet containing a calorie:nitrogen ratio of 100 : 1 appears to be effective in countering the hypermetabolic response. Also, the metabolic rate can be lessened by administration of high-dose morphine, anaesthesia, and early wound closure.

Immune Response

The systemic immune responses are altered by burning. Defects have been identified in both the cellular and humoral immunological defence mechanisms. Impaired cellular immunity is suggested by an overall lymphocytopenia with a relative increase of T-suppressor cells, a decrease in interleukin-2, and an observed delayed rejection of allograft skin. Humoral defects such as depression of the immunoglobulins and complement titre have been documented. Recent isolation of an immunosuppressive peptide isolated from burn victims' serum has shed some light on immune system abnormalities. How this is related to the concept of a burn 'toxin' which is released by burn tissue is not presently understood.

There are other changes in the normal host defence mechanism seen following thermal injury. The inflammatory reaction is depressed, neutrophil chemotaxis inhibited, and phagocytosis is less than optimal. In addition, once phagocytosis occurs, the intracellular enzymatic killing of the bacteria is decreased.

Psychiatric Response

Victims respond to the psychological stresses attendant with major trauma in individualized patterns. These patterns may be more dependent on the patient's pre-burn personality than on a response specific for burning. Situational depression is a uniform response, but true psychosis is unusual. Temporary toxic psychotic symptoms accompany the other physiological alterations such as shock, hypoxia, water imbalance, electrolyte disturbance and sepsis. Iatrogenic factors such as inadequate relief of pain and anxiety, injudicious use of drugs and sleep deprivation can all trigger various responses of the psyche.

The above responses can be expected from any major burn. Other local and systemic alterations are seen as complications occur. These will be discussed in the complications section of this chapter.

EMERGENCY (CASUALTY) DEPARTMENT TREATMENT

The initial treatment of the burns victim is contingent upon proper evaluation and the understanding of the local and systemic pathophysiological alterations. The same attention to cardiorespiratory function, haemorrhage and associated injuries given to any trauma patient must be directed to the burns victim.

The emergency department treatment will depend upon the category of burn. Minor burns can be totally treated in an ambulatory setting. For these patients, the treatment consists of tetanus prophylaxis, burn wound infection prophylaxis and analgesia. In patients who have had effective tetanus immunization within the past five years, a tetanus toxoid booster should be administered. In patients not previously immunized against tetanus, human antitetanus immune globulin should be given for passive protection and standard active immunization begun. In the minor burn wound, true burn wound sepsis is rare except that due to the β-haemolytic streptococcus; thus only systemic penicillin during the 72 h of wound oedema is necessary. This boosts the host's defence against the streptococcus during the period of time that the normal skin antistreptococcal fatty acids are inactivated by oedema. Topical antibacterials are unnecessary. The wound needs only to be cleansed with a bland soap and carefully dressed. In the smaller wounds, the decision as to whether or not to débride blisters is a matter of individual preference. The wound can be easily dressed by applying a non-adhering gauze next to the wound followed by a bulky absorptive dressing. The parts should be immobilized in a safe functional position. The wound must then be inspected at 24 h and periodically until healing occurs. The minor burn will usually be a superficial partial-thickness injury and thus quite painful. Therefore, a consideration of analgesia completes the initial treatment.

Moderate and major burns require hospitalization. Therefore, the emergency department treatment is not definitive. It is important that the initial emergency care does not complicate later definitive treatment. Immediate treatment of the impending vascular collapse is begun by introducing a large bore needle or plastic catheter into a peripheral or central vein, preferably through unburned skin. If a cut-down is necessary, the area should be carefully prepared and the integumentary wound left unclosed to prevent infection. Blood is drawn for cross-match, blood count, electrolytes, glucose and urea nitrogen. Arterial blood gases and pH are obtained if there is any suspicion of inhalation injury or respiratory dysfunction. An infusion of buffered electrolyte solution is begun at a rapid rate. Initial monitoring of the resuscitation is performed by inserting an indwelling urinary catheter attached to a closed draining system.

Following this initiation of resuscitation, the adequacy of respiration is evaluated. If respiratory distress is present, the most likely early cause will be a deep burn with an unyielding eschar about the anterior and lateral chest. When present, it is relieved by a chest escharotomy to release the restriction of rib motion and increase the thoracic excursion, thus improving ventilatory function. Inhalation of steam or noxious gases can cause epiglottal and/or pharyngeal oedema resulting in upper airway obstruction requiring intubation; the nasal tracheal route is most convenient since the tube may be required for extended periods of time. Tracheostomy is best avoided in the emergency treatment unless mandated by associated injuries such as severe facial fractures or a flail chest.

An encircling eschar can cause vascular embarrassment to the extremities due to the development of obligatory oedema in the deeper tissues. Elevation of the extremities may alleviate this if it is minimal but a surgical escharotomy or enzymatic decompression is usually necessary. The need for release to prevent avascular necrosis and the adequacy of escharotomy can be monitored by repeated checking of capillary refill or by use of a Doppler flow meter.

Relieving pain and anxiety may be considered once the state of shock and the respiratory status have been evaluated. Analgesics are given intravenously since intramuscular absorption is unpredictable during the period of decreased cardiac output and massive fluid translocation. Small, frequently repeated dosages of narcotics and tranquillizers are quite effective. The medication may decrease gastrointestinal motility but this is rarely significant since a reflex ileus exists as a result of the splanchnic vasoconstriction. A nasogastric tube is used for gastric decompression until the ileus resolves.

Tetanus prophylaxis and antistreptococcal measures are instituted in the moderate and major burns as outlined for the minor burns. However, further infection prophylaxis is necessary for the larger and deeper burn wound. Reverse isolation measures are used to begin aseptically the burn wound management. Cold saline or water for 15–20 min is helpful in decreasing oedema and pain in the wound. Blisters are best débrided since they are hard to maintain intact in the larger burn wounds. If the blister is broken, serum and desquamated cells form a crust that is susceptible to bacterial invasion. Following débridement the wound is dressed with a topical antibacterial agent. In choosing the initial burn wound management it is helpful to know the desires of the physicians who will provide definitive treatment since the various wound dressings have different advantages and disadvantages.

Once these initial steps are complete, consideration of transfer to a definitive care facility is undertaken. The sample categorization listed in *Table* 21.1 can help determine where the patient will receive his definitive care. Transfer procedures and 'en route' treatments are best agreed upon prior to the individual event so that this aspect of the victim's care can proceed smoothly.

DEFINITIVE TREATMENT

Resuscitative Fluid Management

Initial guidelines to the amount and rate of fluid replacement are provided by the weight of the patient and percentage of the total body surface area injured. However, these are only guidelines and it is more important to understand the pathophysiology of decreased cardiac output and extracellular fluid volume loss. Rigid application of the various formulae which have been proposed is not useful and ignores the individual variability of patients.

To determine the resuscitative fluid replacement, one must recall that the greatest loss of fluid occurs during the first 8–12 h postburn and then continues more slowly over the next 12–16 h. Simultaneous measurements of the cardiac output, plasma volume and extracellular fluid have demonstrated that plasma volume replacement and the return of a normal cardiac output depend only on the rate of fluid replacement. Because of the capillary permeability, colloid replacement seems to be of no benefit in the immediate postburn period. Osmotic pressure cannot be built up over a freely permeable membrane. Therefore, since sodium seems to be the ion that is lost to the circulation in disproportionate amounts, sodium ions and not colloid appear to be the key to resuscitation.

Many formulae have been advanced to predict how and when the sodium ion-containing solution is administered. Critical analysis of the formulae reveal that the total volume replacement varies only 2% over 48 h and the total millimoles (milliequivalents) of sodium vary only 6% during the same period. All formulae give approximately 0·52 mmol of sodium/kg body weight/% body burn. In order to compensate the obligatory loss from the vascular compartment this must be given at a rate exceeding 4·4 ml/kg/h. When the sodium ion is replaced in this amount and at this rate, cardiac output returns to normal by 24 h postburn. This occurs whether the sodium ion is in a hypotonic, isotonic, or hypertonic solution.

Following return of the cardiac output at 24 h, there remains a plasma gap. This amounts to approximately 0·35–0·5 ml/kg/% body burn. By 24 h capillary integrity returns and Starling's hypothesis appears to be restored. Therefore, colloid can be used to replete the plasma volume. By 30 h, both cardiac output and plasma volume should be returned to normal and effective resuscitation completed. Further administration of sodium appears only to aggravate the oedema. So from 30 h until gastrointestinal peristalsis returns, free water can be given to maintain a normal serum sodium level and cover the obligatory insensible losses.

Adequacy of fluid and electrolyte resuscitation is determined by clinical observation and not by the ability to fulfil an arbitrary formula. A urine output of 30–50 ml/h in the adult or 1·2 ml/kg/h in the child is the best monitoring parameter. If the urine output does not reach these levels the fluid input must be increased. Urine flow in excess of these parameters prior to mobilization of the oedema reflects fluid overload. In addition to the urine output, the burns victim who is being adequately resuscitated should have a clear, lucid sensorium, a pulse rate less than 120, and a haematocrit less than 60%.

The use of the central venous pressure monitoring catheter or Swan–Ganz monitoring of the pulmonary wedge pressure has not proved useful in the acute resuscitation period. Because of the total body capillary leak and the tendency for the left ventricle to go in and out of failure for brief periods of time, these pressure indices do not necessarily reflect the true volume situation.

Based on the above considerations, acute resuscitation can be effective by beginning a buffered balance salt solution at a rate exceeding 4·4 ml/kg/h. At the end of the first hour the amount is adjusted based on the urine output. This is continued for 24 h and at that time dextrose and water replaces the salt solution. Colloid is added to replace the remaining plasma volume deficiency. This approach covers all fluid, protein and electrolyte losses in the adult and leads to an adequately resuscitated patient.

In the child of 10 kg body weight or less, the maintenance fluid requirements are often greater than that required for burn loss replacement. Therefore, in these children the maintenance fluid requirements are calculated using 100 ml/kg body weight of a fluid containing 3 mmol sodium ion/100 ml and 2 mmol potassium ion/100 ml. In addition, 2 ml/kg/% body surface burn are required to replace the loss due to thermal injury. Plasma may be useful in infants to provide passive immunization, so 1/4 of their burn fluid loss is replaced with plasma.

Respiratory Management

Emergency escharotomy should have been performed in the emergency department. The adequacy of this must be evaluated. To be effective an escharotomy requires multiple incisions in both the vertical and transverse directions and the incisions need to extend into the neighbouring unburned tissue.

All major burns victims require high-flow humidified oxygen (10 litre/min) with an FIO_2 approaching 100%. This allows the dissipation of carboxyhaemoglobin within a short period of time. All patients deserve monitoring with periodic arterial blood gas determinations during the first 18–24 h postburn.

Upper airway oedema of the pharynx, epiglottis and vocal cords is evaluated. This is easily done by mirror indirect largyngoscopy or, when available, by fibreoptic bronchoscopy. If mild oedema is noted, intermittent positive-pressure breathing with a bronchodilator may be a useful adjunct to the humidified oxygen. Meticulous atraumatic pulmonary toilet must also be carried out. If significant laryngeal oedema is seen intubation is recommended via the nasotracheal route with a low-pressure cuffed endotracheal tube.

These measures should suffice for the uncomplicated burns victim. Those developing inhalation injury, progressive pulmonary insufficiency, or other respiratory problems will be discussed under pulmonary complications.

Metabolic and Nutritional Needs

To overcome the negative nitrogen balance attendant with the major burn at least 20 g/m^2 body surface area burn/day during the first month post injury and approximately 15 g of nitrogen/m^2/day during the second month must be given to the patient. Rapid wound closure decreases this loss since once this is achieved, the protein loss falls to 4 g/m^2/day. Since maintenance of the burns victim in a cool dry environment adds to the metabolic needs and nitrogen catabolism, it is best to avoid this. Environmental temperatures between 32 and 34 °C have been demonstrated to increase the urinary excretion of nitrogen.

In addition to the protein needs, non-protein calories must be provided. These can be determined by giving 25 kcal/kg body weight plus 40 kcal/% body surface area burn to the adult. The child needs more calories/kg body weight and the infant needs as much as 90–100/kg. In the victim with a major burn, this amount of calories can be rarely given consistently without resorting to supplemental tube feedings. If more than 5000 cal/day are required, a tube is placed in the stomach and, as soon as the ileus is resolved, tube feeding is instituted on a 24-h continuous basis. Solutions containing up to 1·5 cal/ml with an osmolar concentration of not more than 600 are well tolerated. This regimen decreases the need for parenteral hyperalimentation.

Vitamin supplementation and fat must be provided. One gram of ascorbic acid, 50 mg of thiamine, 50 mg riboflavine and 500 mg of nicotinamide plus twice the daily requirements of vitamins A and D appear to be sufficient. The standard tube feedings contain adequate amounts of fat but elemental diets and parenteral regimens may be deficient. Trace metals must also be provided if less than full tube feedings are used for alimentation.

Protecting the Gastrointestinal Tract

The reflex ileus usually subsides by 48–72 h. Once the gastric contents are not being removed, protection of the gastric mucosa is a consideration. Even though the complications of the gastrointestinal tract are not due to true hyperacidity, controlled studies have shown that neutralization of the gastric contents and maintenance of the gastric pH above 7·0 protects against clinically significant complications of stress ulceration (antacids or H_2-blockers).

Immune Considerations

The concept of using immunotherapy to prevent or correct the defects in host response has been popular. The early use of whole blood or plasma may passively affect the immune response but this has not been of documented value except possibly in infants. Gammaglobulin injections have also been tried in children at a dose of 1 ml/kg body weight on alternate days during the first week postburn.

The use of hyperimmune or convalescent serum to provide passive immunization has been documented experimentally. However, this carries the risk of allergic reaction or anaphylaxis, as does the use of any antiserum. Active immunization by vaccination has had several recent trials. If this is used for specific bacterial species such as *Pseudomonas aeruginosa,* it must be a polyvalent vaccine because of the tendency of new strains emerging for which the vaccine is not effective. Even large clinical series reporting the use of polyvalent vaccines have concluded that active immunization is not a very effective means of preventing the infectious complications in the burns victim.

One of the most useful and practical means of boosting the immune system is by adequate nutritional support. Failure of the body's response to common skin antigens and prolonged acceptance of skin allografts have been used as proof of impaired cellular immunity in the burns victim. Anergy can be reversed by preventing or correcting the negative nitrogen balance and providing greater than 5000 cal/day. Similarly, the well-nourished patient appears to reject skin allografts at a normal rate. Therefore, close attention to the metabolic and nutritional needs will serve a double purpose.

A host defence defect, which occurs following thermal trauma and is unrelated to immunity, is the loss of the normal antibacterial properties of skin. Normal skin secretes sebum which contains high levels of fatty acids, particularly oleic acid which destroys streptococci. Any break in the skin or inflammation which results in serum accumulation or the presence of local oedema inactivates sebum and allows rapid multiplication of streptococci. Therefore, a necessary treatment to reverse this host defect is the administration of systemic prophylactic penicillin during the oedematous phase of the burn injury. This period usually lasts for approximately 72 h and the use of systemic antibiotics beyond this period in the uncomplicated burn appears unwarranted. Also since these antibiotics are only given for the specific defence defect, they should be specific for the streptococcus and not be broad spectrum. Further use of antibiotics is reserved for the treatment of infectious complications as will be discussed later.

The Burn Wound

Attention to the burn wound must not take precedence over the life-saving support of other systems in the burn wound victim. Therefore, discussion of the treatment of the burn wound has been reserved to this point. However, the *sine qua non* of treatment of the burns victim is treatment of the wound itself and the eventual success or failure of how the other systems respond will depend on how well one treats the burn wound. Proper treatment of the wound begins with doing no harm to the injured cells so that any tissue still viable after the initial thermal event can survive. As these protected surviving injured cells are recovering, the necrotic cells not capable of recovery must be removed and replaced. Closure of the burn wound with viable cells to provide a functional and aesthetically satisfactory coverage as rapidly as possible seems like a reasonable goal for the burn wound treatment.

Initial cooling, cleansing, and débridement of the burn wound were discussed under emergency department treatment (p. 318). The definitive care team must determine which part of the wound is non-viable and when the wound should be closed. Determination of the wound viability is one of the most difficult problems facing the burn surgeon today. No method to determine the depth of burn is absolute. Therefore, since one wishes to do no harm to the remaining viable cells, an absolute approach to burn wound management is difficult. This is not a serious problem in the small circumscribed burn wound or even one up to 15–20% total body surface area. For these wounds, if one feels they include dead cells deep into the reticular dermis, even though they may not be full-thickness, one is justified in early excision of the necrotic tissue and closure of the wound.

Full-thickness excision and coverage of burn wounds above 15–20% have been reported. However, these are associated with increased blood loss, frequent episodes of sepsis and, except in rare reports, a high morbidity and mortality. As the burn wound exceeds 35–40% of the body surface area, full-thickness excision and autografting become an arithmetic problem. Available donor sites for coverage decrease as the size of excision increases.

An alternative to full-thickness burn wound excision exists. Based on the concentric zones of injury elucidated by Jackson, an intradermal or tangential excision can be performed. Janzekovic has championed this approach and reported on 4370 patients treated by tangential excision and grafting 3–5 days postburn. She lists as advantages for this method: (1) removal of only necrotic tissue, (2) salvage of injured tissue that would otherwise have progressed to necrosis, and (3) preservation of the biological properties of the dermis and prevention of contractures by immediate skin grafting. In addition, she states that when the amount of donor site tissue is limited, this technique can remove necrotic tissue to the level of viable cells and temporary coverage can be provided by allograft skin while the surviving deep dermal elements recover to provide skin continuity.

The theoretical advantages of full-thickness excision of truly necrotic skin and partial-thickness excision of deep dermal burns are ideal for the treatment of the burn wound. Tangential excision offers nothing if the burn wound is large and full-thickness. For the large partial-thickness injury, tangential débridement should be beneficial. In some centres it has appeared to reduce the morbidity and mortality. However, all the theoretical advantages are difficult to attain in the practical clinical situation. Removal of *only* dead tissue is not easy. In fact, several pathological studies have been reported showing that up to 50% of the tangential shavings contain viable skin. Bleeding can be of staggering amounts and portals of infection are opened if the tangential débridement is performed after the wound has been colonized. Graft take in controlled studies has been documented to be less than optimal on the tangentially excised wound. Finally, the decreased hospital stay and the increased cost effectiveness suggested by proponents of this treatment have yet to be corroborated by controlled studies except for burns less than 40%.

Since determination of definitely non-viable tissue is difficult and the various types of excision and closure have not proved to be a panacea in the larger burn wounds, an alternative approach is available. This approach allows the patient to be supported while the burn wound evolves and reversibly injured cells heal. It demands protection of the wound from bacterial invasion, the major deterrent to healing. Infection prophylaxis of the burn wound is part of the local treatment of every wound. The skin is never sterile and cannot be readily sterilized. It is colonized by both a resident and transient flora (*Table* 21.2). These bacteria are in the depths of the skin, in tubules of sebaceous glands and around hair follicles. Therefore, cultures of the skin surface rarely reflect the skin's bacterial population. Infection prophylaxis is aimed at preventing an increase in colonization from exogenous transient flora or proliferation of resident flora to levels sufficient to cause burn wound sepsis. Two prophylactic measures have been mentioned. Tetanus immunization and systemic penicillin therapy during the oedema phase are both given to prevent infection.

The next decision must be how to dress the burn wound. The choices include excision with skin dressing as previously discussed, occlusive dressings, exposure, and semi-open techniques with topical chemotherapy. True occlusive dressing methods are infrequently used today. To be effective, the dressing must be carefully constructed and applied using meticulous aseptic technique. Following careful cleansing and débridement of the wound, an inner layer of fine mesh or impregnated gauze is placed next to the burn to allow drainage. Next a bulky absorptive material is applied and carefully immobilized by a non-distensible inelastic wrap. The dressing remains intact to protect the wound and is only changed if wound exudate soaks through it, or odour,

Table 21.2 Bacteriology of normal skin

- I. Resident flora
  - A. Aerobic Gram-positive cocci
    1. *Micrococcus luteus*
    2. *Staphylococcus epidermidis*
  - B. Coryneform group
    1. *Corynebacterium xerosis*
    2. Lipophilic diphtheroids
  - C. Fungi
    1. *Pityrosporum ovale*
    2. *Pityrosporum orbiculare*
  - D. Anaerobic bacteria
    1. *Propionibacterium acnes*
- II. Transient flora
  - A. Aerobic Gram-positive cocci
    1. *Staphylococcus aureus*
    2. *Streptococcus pyogenes*
    3. *Streptococcus faecalis*
  - B. Aerobic Gram-positive rods
    1. *Corynebacterium pyogenes*
    2. Mycobacterium spp.
    3. Bacillus spp.
  - C. Fungi
    1. *Candida albicans*
    2. Other candidas
    3. Dermatophytes
    4. Phycomycetes
  - D. Enteric bacteria
    1. *Pseudomonas aeruginosa*
    2. *Escherichia coli*
    3. *Enterobacter aerogenes — Klebsiella pneumoniae*
    4. *Proteus mirabilis*
  - E. Anaerobic bacteria
    1. *Peptostreptococcus constellatus*

pain or fever demand wound inspection. This method was based on the concept of protecting the wound from exogenous bacteria. However, since all skin contains a bacterial level of 10^3 organisms/g of tissue, the occlusive dressing does not prevent multiplication of these organisms in a warm moist environment and wound sepsis from endogenous sources.

To reverse the problem seen with occlusive dressing, exposure therapy was introduced in the UK by Wallace in 1949. With this method, a dry eschar forms over the burn wound and acts as a physiological dressing. This prevents access of bacteria to the underlying wound and the dryness of the eschar will not support bacterial growth on its surface. To use this method, a reverse isolation technique is necessary to attempt to decrease the exposure to exogenous contamination, especially during the time required for eschar formation. In Sweden circulating warm air beds hasten the eschar formation.

Several major disadvantages prevent universal acceptance of this method. As with the occlusive dressing method, the only bacteria from which the victim is protected are those from exogenous sources and these are not the major offenders. The eschar does not remain an intact barrier but often develops cracks which break the theoretical barrier. In addition to not being a totally effective means of infection prophylaxis, there is evidence that desiccation of the injured cells in the zone of stasis is deleterious to their survival and that burn wounds treated by exposure become deeper over the first 24–48 h. Chiefly because neither the occlusive dressing nor the exposure methods were effective in preventing the complications of burn wound sepsis, the semi-open technique with topical chemotherapy has evolved. Once it was realized that the prevention of infection in the burn wound involved the maintenance of an equilibrium between endogenous as well as exogenous bacteria and factors of host resistance, it became obvious that the goal was to prevent the numerical proliferation of bacteria. As the balance of bacteria is upset by the burn injury, organisms proliferate to levels greater than 10^5 organisms/g of tissue and migrate through the tissue. These proliferating organisms surround and occlude blood vessels leading to thrombosis and an avascular burn wound sepsis. Topical chemotherapy seems to be the only rational approach to prevent the numerical proliferation of bacteria and therefore is the mainstay of infection prophylaxis in most centres today.

Any suitable topical chemotherapeutic agent for treatment of the burn wound should prevent desiccation, not produce pain, be non-allergenic and non-toxic, and, most importantly, be bactericidal but not injure viable cells in the burn wound. Unfortunately, none of the topical agents now available fulfil all these criteria. All have advantages and disadvantages. None has totally prevented bacterial proliferation. The present three most commonly used topical chemotherapeutic agents worldwide are: silver sulphadiazine, silver nitrate solution, and mafenide acetate.

Regardless of the topical agent chosen to be used in the semi-open method for infection prophylaxis, its efficacy should be monitored by constant surveillance of the bacterial flora of the burn wound. This is most effectively achieved by quantitative and qualitative analysis performed or burn wound biopsies. The bacteria isolated from the biopsies can be tested against the various topical agents available. The test bacteria are spread over an agar plate and the topical chemotherapeutic agents are placed into wells in the agar. Zones of inhibition predict an agent's effectiveness. Using objective results of bacterial control, one can decide which agent is best for a given victim at a given time. There is no chemotherapeutic agent of choice and there never can be one. The bacterial flora of a given wound in a given burns unit are continuously changing and must be monitored for effective infection prophylaxis.

If early excision of the necrotic tissue is not elected and topical chemotherapy is the method of burn wound treatment, the non-viable tissue must still be removed. Historically, eschar separation occurred spontaneously between the 10th and 14th postburn days. This spontaneous separation was due to bacterial autolysis. Successful control of wound sepsis by topical chemotherapy has resulted in prolonged adherence of the eschar. Therefore, a definite plan to remove the necrotic tissue as soon as definite non-viability has been established becomes necessary. Physical removal of the non-viable tissue may take the form of full-thickness excision, intradermal débridement, daily surgical cleansing of the loosening eschar, or enzymatic dissolution of the eschar.

Daily débridement following removal of the topical agent can be done in hydrotherapy. This allows softening of the eschar so that the non-viable tissue can be gently cut away. An advantage of this technique is that it is relatively pain-free and does not require repeated anaesthesia, even in children. Enzymatic agents periodically gain popularity as a means to débride necrotic tissue. These enzymes are said to digest dead collagen while sparing viable collagen. A major deterrent to their use is the reported high incidence of bacterial proliferation when enzymes are used to dissolve the eschar. This tendency toward sepsis can be controlled if the enzymatic agent is used concomitantly with topical antibacterial agents.

Once the necrotic tissue has been removed from the burn wound, closure can proceed. If the injury is partial-thickness, closure will occur spontaneously by regeneration from epidermal elements in the dermis. The full-thickness defect will require closure by autografts. When donor sites are not sufficient for autograft coverage, temporary closure of the burn wound is achieved with biological dressings. These temporary biological dressings applied to the burn wound render it less painful, reduce fluid and protein loss from the wound surface, and preserve bacteriological control while donor sites re-epithelize prior to re-use.

Allograft skin, xenograft skin, and amniotic membranes have been demonstrated to be effective as temporary biological dressings. These are applied to the burn wound following removal of the eschar and remain in place from 48 to 96 h. Each can be useful in buying time for the burns victim. Allografts and amniotic membranes seem to be more effective than xenografts at maintaining bacterial control of the burn wound because they more readily allow vascular ingrowth. In addition to temporary biological dressings, synthetic and biosynthetic dressings are now available to serve as temporary skin substitutes. The most effective of these is a bilaminate composite dressing comprised of nylon mesh and silicone bonded to a collagen peptide coating. It must be remembered that these biological or biosynthetic dressings are only temporary, and permanent closure with autograft skin should remain the goal of burn wound treatment.

Sheets of autograft skin should be used for permanent wound closure whenever possible. Priority areas for grafting should be the face, especially the eyelids, the neck, the hands and the various flexion creases of the body, e.g. the popliteal fossa. When donor sites are limited, the sheet graft can be 'meshed' so it can be expanded 1·5–9 times its original size. Meshed grafts are a compromise to the best wound closure and should not be used on the face, hands, feet, or flexor aspects of the body. Successful skin grafting requires that the grafts be applied to a satisfactory bed. This means a bed that contains 10^5 or fewer bacteria/g of tissue and no streptococci. This can be determined preoperatively by quantitative and qualitative bacterial cultures of tissue biopsies from the wound bed. It can also be predicted by the successful application of a skin allograft applied as a 'test' or a prognosticator of autograft acceptibility. Following application of the autograft to a properly receptive bed, several days of immobilization are necessary. This combination of therapeutic manoeuvres should result in greater than 95% success in permanent closure of the burn wound.

Preservation of Function

Successful treatment of the burns victim means not only survival but also the return to society as a functional human being. Contraction is a normal component of wound healing. Myofibroblasts with contractile properties are found in the granulating wound following thermal injury. If the contracture is severe enough, a pathological contracture results. Prevention of contracture, therefore, becomes an important part of the definitive care of the burns victim. Prevention is more desirable and effective than later correction of deformity. The principles of prevention of contracture and preservation of function are practiced immediately upon admission. These include splinting at all times in the optimal position to avoid contracture. Larson has shown that the position of comfort is the position of contracture and that the burn wound will shrink until it meets an opposing force. Positioning, splinting and range of motion exercises are begun immediately and continued until wound closure.

At the time of wound closure, adequate amounts of skin are applied maintaining the proper positioning and splinting. Following adherence of the grafts, prolonged pressure is applied by specially constructed elastic garments. The pressure appears to reduce hypertrophic scarring, increase pliability and preserve contouring. Splints are maintained especially at night-time and range of motion exercises continued until the newly healed collagen is matured. By maintaining a closely regulated schedule for 9 months to 1 year following wound closure, a much more functional result is obtained and the need for reconstructive procedures markedly reduced.

COMMON COMPLICATIONS DUE TO BURN INJURIES

The previous section discussed treatment of the major burn victim when only the normal physiological responses to thermal trauma were present. Complications can occur in every physiological system secondary to burn injury. Many of these complications are unique and thus their management must be understood to care successfully for the burns victim.

Renal Failure

Acute renal failure can occur only after prolonged and profound shock from unrecognized or untreated hypovolaemia following the thermal burn. It should rarely occur if the principles of resuscitation are understood. Following an acute burn, oliguria or anuria should not be diagnosed as renal failure but only as insufficient volume replacement. Increasing the sodium-containing electrolyte solution to an adequate amount to achieve 30–50 ml/h urine flow will flush the renal tubules. The fluid input should be pushed until urine output results. If fear of overloading is present, a pulmonary wedge pressure can be obtained. Only if this is elevated should the increased rate of resuscitation be slowed. Diuretics are of little help in this situation and should be reserved until hypovolaemia is absolutely corrected.

Inhalation Injury

Inhalation of heat, noxious gases and incomplete products of combustion may be the most lethal component of thermal injury. Several syndromes are associated with such inhalation and cause complications to the pulmonary response. The first group of victims develop pulmonary complications within moments of injury and often die at the site of the fire. This complication is due to asphyxia because the combustion consumes the oxygen available to the victim. Davies reported that the UK Fire Research Station has shown the concentration of O_2 close to the seat of a fire can be as low as 2%. At this concentration, death ensues in 45 sec. The problem is worsened because the oxygen-deficient inspired air contains carbon monoxide which combines with the haemoglobin molecule thus further decreasing the availability of oxygen to the tissue. CO levels can reach 30 000 ppm which causes death within minutes. Adding to the hypoxia is the inhalation of HCN contained in smoke. This causes rapid tissue hypoxia plus hyperventilation.

Another immediate complication arising from inhalation is the oedematous response discussed in the previous section. This can become worsened if, in addition to the heat, noxious gases such as sulphur dioxide and hydrochloric acid are present to cause bronchial spasm. This combination of oedema, largyngeal spasm and bronchospasm often cause immediate death.

The next group of patients with pulmonary complications develop respiratory symptoms several hours after admission. These are the patients suspected on initial evaluation to have suffered significant inhalation injury. This group develops progressive hypoxia and hypercarbia, and may have high levels of carboxyhaemoglobin. Initial high-flow humidified oxygen may not suffice as treatment. Further hypoxaemia, restlessness, tachypnoea and wheezing occur. This degree of significant inhalation injury may be diagnosed by fibreoptic bronchoscopy or by a radioactive xenon lung scan. However, these are not necessary and a clinical diagnosis is suggested by a $P\text{O}_2$ of less than 10 kPa (75 mmHg) within 72 h postburn in a well-resuscitated patient or a rapidly falling $P\text{O}_2$ in the presence of a slowly increasing $P\text{CO}_2$. In these patients, vital capacity, minute ventilation, maximum expiratory flow volume curves and effective compliance must be maintained. When high flow oxygen, CPAP (continuous positive airway pressure) mask and bronchodilators fail to show improvement, intubation may be required. An increasing pulmonary resistance and right-to-left pulmonary shunt along with increased work of breathing may require mechanical ventilation. The goal of ventilation is to use the lowest FIO_2 level possible to maintain a $P\text{aO}_2$ greater than 7·3 kPa (55 mmHg). The FIO_2 should be maintained less than 40–50%. If this cannot be done, one must add positive end-expiratory pressure. Steroids have not been shown to be helpful in treating smoke inhalation and in several studies have indeed been shown to be harmful. Secondary bacterial invasion of these injured lungs must be watched for and treated when it occurs.

There are other pulmonary complications not necessarily related to inhalation. These are atelectasis, pneumonia, pulmonary emboli, emphysema, bronchiectasis, pneumothorax and pulmonary oedema. Therefore, meticulous toilet must be maintained throughout the course of treatment of the burns victim and bronchoscopy should be utilized when appropriate. Finally, respiratory failure can occur with systemic sepsis as part of the multiple organ failure syndrome. These patients require intubation and mechanical ventilation. However, despite high oxygen concentrations, pressures and increased positive end-expiratory pressures the patient sometimes cannot adequately be ventilated and succumbs.

Burn Stress Pseudodiabetes

The complication occasionally seen as a result of the metabolic and nutritional responses is a syndrome of hyperglycaemia, glycosuria without ketonuria, acute dehydration, shock, coma and renal failure. Hyperglycaemia is common following trauma because of the increased catecholamine response and a decreased sensitivity to insulin. Combine this with the hyperglycaemia resulting from the necessary caloric replacement of a major burn and one can understand how the syndrome can occur. Careful monitoring of the blood sugar and liberal use of insulin can usually prevent the solute diuresis and subsequent dehydration with a rising blood urea nitrogen and serum sodium, and central nervous system symptoms.

Gastrointestinal Complications

Despite the initial intubation and subsequent treatment with antacids, gastroduodenal ulceration occurs in upwards of 80% of patients with major burns. However, clinically significant bleeding is becoming less common as burn wound sepsis is controlled. Once bleeding occurs it is usually brisk and difficult to control. Neutralization of gastric contents to above pH 7·0 may help. However, if bleeding cannot be rapidly controlled, operative intervention is necessary. Gastric resection is reported to be the most effective management of significant bleeding except in children where vagotomy and drainage have been successful.

Lower intestinal bleeding can also complicate the burn injury. Ulcers of the mucosa and muscularis mucosa of the colon have been reported. Colonoscopy has proved an aid in identifying the source of bleeding. Intra-arterial pitressin may control colonic bleeding. The question of candida in the aetiology of these ulcerations has been raised since they have not been seen in a centre where antifungal oral medication is a routine part of the management of all burn victims.

Compression of the distal portion of the duodenum by the superior mesentery artery may result in partial or complete duodenal obstruction in the debilitated catabolic patient. This results in post-feeding fullness, bile-stained vomitus and failure to gain weight. The syndrome is best prevented by beginning promptly on the fourth postburn day to replace the patient's nutritional needs. Once the symptoms begin, the diagnosis is confirmed by cinefluoroscopy of the duodenum following ingestion of a barium meal. Treatment can often be effective by passing an intestinal tube by fluoroscopy beyond the obstruction and instituting enteral hyperalimentation. Failure to pass the tube requires parenteral hyperalimentation. If operation becomes necessary, a duodenojejunostomy relieves the problem.

Biliary stasis leading to an acalculus cholecystitis may occur in the immobile burns victim who is being hyperalimented. This should be suspected in patients with right upper quadrant pain, unexplained vomiting, or fever of an unknown origin. It appears more commonly in patients with sepsis who may develop metastatic emboli to their gallbladder. This complication can be serious because perforation often occurs without warning and emergency cholecystectomy or cholecystostomy becomes necessary.

Hepatitis is a leading cause of death in the burns victim who survives the initial hospitalization. Multiple blood transfusions add to the risk of infection with hepatitis B and non-A non-B viruses. Also, several anaesthesias may be required during the course of management, exposing the patient to the dangers of drug-induced hepatitis. This complication must be watched for during the convalescent period and for a year postburn.

Infectious Complications

The most frequent complications of the major burn are due to bacterial, viral or fungal infection. As infection in the burn wound is beginning to be understood and controlled, pulmonary infection is becoming the leading cause of death. The pulmonary infection supervenes on the lung already compromised by the complications of inhalation of noxious gases. These will not be reiterated here. However, worldwide, the leading infectious complication remains burn wound sepsis.

Burn wound sepsis is an imbalance in the normal equilibrium between bacteria and host resistance, resulting in a numerical increase in bacteria. As bacteria increase from the normal level of 10^3 organisms/g of tissue to levels of greater than 10^5/g, they break out of the hair follicles and glands and migrate through the tissue colonizing along the dermal–subcutaneous interface. Levels of growth in excess of 10^5

bacteria/g of tissue constitute 'burn wound sepsis', and levels of 10^8 to 10^9 bacteria/g may be associated with lethal burns. Surface swabs are deceptive since the process of proliferation occurs in the subeschar plane. Blood cultures also may be deceptive since lethal burn wound sepsis can occur without spread of viable organisms into the bloodstream and without secondary visceral lodgement. This is especially likely to be the case for Gram-negative organism burn wound sepsis. If the burn wound sepsis is due to Gram-positive organisms, bloodstream invasion is more likely, although negative blood cultures do not provide security.

Burn wound sepsis can occur from bacteria arising in the wound from both exogenous and endogenous sources. Regardless of the source of bacteria, quantitative bacterial cultures of wound biopsies have been a useful guide to management. These biopsies must contain the eschar-viable tissue interphase. In addition, histological biopsies processed to allow the depth of invasion are important. The presence of bacteria in normal adjacent unburned tissue determines invasive burn wound sepsis. There are clinical aids to the diagnosis; some of these, such as verdoglobin in the urine or fluorescence of wound bacteria with ultraviolet light, are of historical interest only since they require such overwhelming bacterial invasion. The diagnosis can and should be made much earlier by newer techniques, such as the rapid slide estimate of bacterial quantification or histological evaluation.

Several clinical signs suggestive of the systemic response to burn wound sepsis exist. Hyper- or hypothermia must be considered a possible sign of sepsis especially if the temperature is greater than 39 °C or less than 36·5 °C. Congestive heart failure occurring in someone who is not considered to be fluid overloaded should be considered to be secondary to wound sepsis until proven otherwise. Similarly, the unexpected onset of respiratory distress or pulmonary oedema must be assumed to be secondary to sepsis. The onset of unexplained ileus after 48 h postburn is suggestive of sepsis. An onset of mental confusion or a mental status change requires that sepsis be eliminated in the aetiology. Finally, a deepening or worsening of the burn wound is probably due to microbial proliferation and invasion.

Laboratory aids which are helpful in diagnosing systemic sepsis include the presence of greater than 10^5 bacteria/g of tissue on biopsy of the wound or invasion of bacteria into normal tissue histologically. Blood cultures obviously are helpful when positive. Blood glucose levels have been helpful since levels of over 7·28 mmol/l (130 mg %) are statistically associated with septicaemias from Gram-positive organisms, whereas the presence of a blood glucose of less than 6·16 mmol/l (110 mg %) suggests Gram-negative septicaemia. A depressed white blood cell count of less than 4000 or a markedly elevated count of greater than 30 000 suggests sepsis. Azotaemia without dehydration or obstructive uropathy and with no history of nephrotoxic drugs is often associated with burn wound sepsis. In the immediate postburn period, thrombocytopenia and transient disseminated intravascular coagulopathy are common. This usually corrects itself by 24 h. The presence of thrombocytopenia, hyperfibrinogenaemia, or fibrin split-products in the blood after 24 h is an indication of sepsis.

The infections discussed to this point have been bacterial in origin. Fungi and viruses also cause infection in the burn patient. Prominent among these is candida. Candida burn wound invasion is common. However, bloodstream invasion is rare except when the patient's ecology has been upset by prolonged use of multiple antibiotics or a parenteral hyperalimentation line that has been abused. The presence of candida in the burn wound may not have clinical significance but the finding of it in the bloodstream or in the urine of a non-catheterized patient should be considered an indication for antifungal therapy. Similarly, the presence of a fluffy yellow exudate seen on the patient's retina is diagnostic of candidaemia. Viral burn wound sepsis also occurs. The cases reported carry an extremely high mortality. The presence of vesicular lesions at the periphery of the wound should raise suspicion of viral invasion.

The treatment of burn wound sepsis begins with prevention. The standard treatment of débridement, tetanus prophylaxis, systemic penicillin for the oedematous phase, topical chemotherapy, removal of necrotic tissue, and adequate nutrition to maintain the immune response, are all means of preventing burn wound sepsis. Since these measures have become routine in most burn centres, the incidence of burn wound sepsis has markedly decreased. The trend toward earlier excision and wound closure, especially when this can be effected with autograft skin, has helped to eliminate the severity of burn wound sepsis seen when eschar was allowed to remain in place for a period of weeks. However, if the bacteria proliferate to larger numbers in the burn wound, invasive sepsis into the systemic circulation must be treated. The early sign of invasion is at the subeschar uninjured tissue interface. Once systemic sepsis is present, the entire burns victim must be supported. Haemodynamic support is necessary to prevent vascular collapse. The cardiac decompensation, pulmonary oedema and respiratory distress may require intubation and ventilatory support. Nutrition must be maintained and this becomes difficult since ileus accompanies the sepsis. Parenteral alimentation may be necessary.

Systemic antibiotics are of little value in trying to control the bacterial level in the burn wound following the oedematous phase. The vascular changes of the full-thickness burn with local occlusion of small vessels prevent the adequate delivery of potent systemic antibiotics to the foci of bacterial growth. Even though they are not helpful in controlling infection confined to the burn wound, systemic antibiotics are necessary when systemic sepsis develops. Close monitoring of antibiotic blood levels is necessary because proper blood levels are difficult to maintain in the hypermetabolic burns victim.

The burn wound may require excision to control the septic focus. Other foci must be sought. Most common of these is suppurative thrombophlebitis. When systemic sepsis occurs in the burn patient and the burn wound is not the source, all veins which have been previously cannulated should be examined and, if suspicious, should be opened and/or excised. Other foci of infection often overlooked in the burns victim are the heart valves and the meninges. Reports of acute bacterial endocarditis and meningitis are becoming more frequent as understanding of the burn wound infection control is improving.

DIFFERENCES SEEN IN CHEMICAL BURNS AND ELECTRICAL INJURY

Chemical Burns

Tissue damage secondary to a chemical depends on: (1) the concentration of the agent, (2) the quantity of the agent, (3) the length of time the agent is in contact with the tissue, (4) the degree of tissue penetration, and (5) the specific mechanism of action. The principal difference between thermal burns and chemical burns is that in the chemical burns tissue destruction continues as long as contact is maintained unless the agent is inactivated by its reaction with the tissue. This means that chemical burns are usually deeper than they initially appear and progress with time. Fluid resuscitation is often underestimated.

The initial treatment of a chemical burn is dilution of the chemical with water. This is best delivered by continuous running water or by prolonged hydrotherapy in large volume tanks for 12 h. Neutralizing agents should not be used since they cause exothermic reactions and increased tissue damage. Following the 12 h of initial dilution, local care of the wound with débridement, topical chemotherapeutic agents and eventual wound closure is the same as for the thermal burn. The exception is the chemical burn involving the eyes. These injuries require initial copious irrigation with saline and consultation with the ophthalmologist.

Electrical Injury

Electrical injury is due to the flow of electrons through a conductor. Electrons seek the path of least resistance through the conductor. Collisions of electrons with conductor particles change electrical energy into thermal energy or heat. If the conductor is tissue in the human body, this produces an electrical injury.

The effects of passage of an electric current through the body depend on the type of current, the voltage of the current, the resistance offered by the tissue, the amperage of current flowing through the tissue, the pathway of the current through the body and the duration of contact. The relationship between the current flow in amperage, voltage and resistance measured in ohms is expressed by Ohm's Law (Current = Voltage/Resistance). More importantly, the actual heat generated by passage of current through a conductor is determined by Joule's Law (Heat = Voltage × Current). Combining the two laws one can predict the damage occurring with electrical injury. Tissue resistance to electrical current increases from nerve to vessel to muscle to skin to tendon to fat to bone.

There are several types of injury seen after contact with an electrical source. The arc injury is a localized injury caused by intense heat or flash at the termination of current flow. This often occurs on flexor surfaces of joints where current exits and re-enters skin, attempting to find the shortest pathway. The major type of injury is that due to heat generated as current flows through tissue. This type of injury is worse in tissue with high resistance. The vessels thrombose as current passes rapidly along them. The full extent of this type of current injury is insidious and not immediately appreciated. The third type of injury is the flame burn which occurs if the heat generated from the electricity is high enough to cause ignition of the victim's clothing.

There are some special effects of electrical injury which differentiate them from other thermal trauma. Anoxia and ventricular fibrillation can cause immediate death. Also both early and delayed rhythm abnormalities may occur. There is a high risk of renal failure compared with thermal burns because of haemoglobin and myoglobin deposits in the renal tubules. This requires a higher urine flow (75 ml/h in adults). The urine must be alkalinized to keep the haemoglobin and myoglobin in a more soluble state. Tetanic muscle contractions accompany the passage of electricity and may be strong enough to fracture bones, especially the spine. Spinal cord damage can occur secondary to such a fracture and can also occur late due to a demyelinating effect of the current. Intraperitoneal damage can occur to the gastrointestinal tract secondary to the current. This frequently leads to bowel perforation and peritonitis. Because of the progressive vessel thrombosis, delayed rupture of major vessels has been reported. There are finally late effects which accompany these injuries. Chief among these is cataract formation which is delayed days to months postinjury.

Treatment for the victim of an electrical injury usually begins with cardiopulmonary resuscitation, since cardiac standstill or ventricular fibrillation is common. Fluid replacement is begun with a buffered alkaline salt solution at a volume and rate to achieve a urine output of 75 ml/h. No type of replacement formula can serve even as a rough guideline because the injury is more extensive than can be predicted by the skin damage. Monitoring is easier in the electrical injury since total capillary permeability does not occur. Therefore, the use of central venous pressure monitoring and measurements of pulmonary wedge pressure is more helpful than in a major thermal injury in which capillary leaking is predominant. An osmotic diuretic such as mannitol is useful if significant haemoglobinuria or myoglobinuria is present. Associated injuries, such as bony fractures, must be treated. For wound management, the non-viable tissue is débrided early. This will have to be repeated as the progressive destruction continues. Intravenous fluoroscein and illumination of the wound with ultraviolet light has proved helpful in delineating viable and non-viable tissue at the time of débridement. The best topical chemotherapeutic agent for the electrical injury is the one with the best penetrating ability and the one most effective against clostridia. These characteristics describe mafenide acetate cream (Sulfamylon) better than other agents. Fasciotomies should be performed liberally. However, despite release of this compression, vascular thrombosis frequently leads to major amputations.

FUTURE TRENDS FOR IMPROVING TREATMENT OF THE BURNS VICTIM

The greatest chance to improve statistics for burn victims in the future is prevention. Recent advances in the USA such as the routine use of nonflammable materials for children's nightclothes have significantly reduced the severity of injury. Laws to make all clothes nonflammable seems like an attainable goal. Similarly, legislation to govern the amount of heat delivered from household hot water systems would decrease the number of scald burns occurring in the home. Finally, fabrication standards to prevent public meeting areas from being constructed with materials known to produce toxic substances upon incineration will prevent severe smoke inhalation.

Several major blocks in solving the plight of the burns victim are obvious. All treatment and prognoses are based on the amount of injured tissue present. Although charts are available to determine the extent of the burn wound, these are not extremely accurate. New techniques of planimetry and computer analysis and storage will soon allow accurate reproducible mapping of the surface extent of the burn. However, there are still no effective means available to determine the depth of the wounds. Dyes such as Patent blue or fluoroscein have not been reliable at differentiating depth. Work with a fibreoptic perfusion fluorometer may improve this usage in the future. Reflected light imaging, laser Doppler fluorometry, high-frequency ultrasonic imaging, and portable xenon-133 washout scans are being evaluated as means to predict accurately which cells are non-viable postburn.

Once the amount of truly non-viable tissue can be determined, the zones of injury in the burn wound can be accurately delineated. The cells in Jackson's zone of stasis can then be pharmacologically manipulated to increase their survival. Pilot studies in this field have shown that the progressive sludging and thrombosis in the zone of stasis is not affected by antisludging or anticoagulant drugs such as heparin or low molecular weight dextran. However, inhibitors of certain arachidonic acid metabolites seem to prevent sludging and decrease the progressive dermal ischaemia. Agents which inhibit prostaglandin and thromboxane synthesis can experimentally increase dermal perfusion and salvage the zone of stasis. Other mediators of the inflammatory response such as leukotrienes, vasoactive amines, and free oxygen radicals have been demonstrated to be present in the burn wound early after injury. Understanding the role of these mediators and modulating their effects pharmacologically may significantly lessen the volume of tissue destroyed by thermal trauma.

Manipulation of the immune defence mechanisms will alter the course of the burns victim. In the past year, many of the immune defects seen following a major burn and thought to be inherent in the burns injury, have been totally reversed by providing adequate nutrition to the patient. If the current suspense surrounding the 'burn toxin' can be solved, many of the systemic effects of the injury may be lessened or may disappear. Recent elucidation of an immune suppressive factor found in the serum of burn victims may be a step in explaining this problem. If a polypeptide substance which appears to cause the myocardial depressant effect and drop the cardiac output can be identified in human beings as it has been in mice, then an antidote to that peptide can be developed. Immunomodulators which can specifically reverse various lymphocyte and phagocyte abnormalities seen postburn are being evaluated in clinical trials. These may allow one to isolate the exact immune defect in a given victim, and prevent or reverse it.

Finally, if a burn wound of any size could be covered without further stressing the burns victim, then the morbidity and mortality would rapidly diminish. The present need to use autograft skin is often the difference between survival and death. Several exciting experimental developments are underway. Epidermal and dermal cells are being grown in tissue culture. Some evidence exists that as these are grown, they lose their antigenicity. Theoretically, these cultured epidermal and dermal cells could be sprayed onto the burn wound to effect resurfacing. If the antigenicity could be overcome, a tissue culture bank could be developed to resurface any victim upon demand. The use of allograft skin has been shown to be useful for long periods of time with the aid of immunosuppression. A single case has been reported in which tolerance was achieved with this technique and when the cyclosporin was withdrawn the allografts remained permanently in place. Artificial skin is being investigated in many laboratories worldwide. The one which appears most successful is undergoing a multicentre clinical trial in the US. This compound is made of a collagen-glycosaminoglycan complex temporarily covered with a silicone sheet. It forms a 'neodermis' by becoming vascularized on an excised wound. Once this occurs, the silicone sheet is replaced by an epidermal autograft or tissue cultured coherent epithelial sheets. These new substitutes for the victims' own skin may ease the plight of the burn surgeon.

Further Reading

Brown J. M. (1977) Inhalation injury and progressive pulmonary insufficiency in a British burns unit. *Burns* **4**, 32.

Davies J. W. L. (1975) The fluid therapy given to 1027 patients during the first 48 hours after burning. I & II. *Burns* **1**, 319.

Davies J. W. L. (1986) Toxic chemicals versus lung tissue—an aspect of inhalation injury revisited. *J. Burn Care Rehab.* **7**, 213.

Demling R. H. (1985) Medical Progress—Burns. *N. Engl. J. Med.* **313**, 1389.

Jackson D. McG. (1953) The diagnosis of the depth of burning. *Br. J. Surg.* **40**, 588.

Janzekovic Z. (1975) The burn wound from the surgical point of view. *J. Trauma* **15**, 42.

Larson D. L., Abston S., Evans E. B. et al. (1971) Techniques for decreasing scar formation in the burned patient. *J. Trauma* **11**, 801.

Robson M. C., Krizek T. J. and Wray R. C. (1979) Care of the thermally injured patient. In: Zuidema G. D., Ballinger W. F. and Rutherford R. B. (ed.) *The Management of Trauma*, 3rd ed. Philadelphia, Saunders.

22 Reconstructive and Plastic Surgery

Martin C. Robson and Robert W. Parsons

The branch of medicine dealing with reconstructive and plastic surgery is broad and difficult to define. In the active sense, plastic means formative or capable of moulding. Surgeons working in reconstructive and plastic surgery are moulding the integument and musculoskeletal framework with the aim of correcting deformity. Deformity can be real or imagined and may result from congenital, acquired or psychological sources. Often, deformities include defects which must be covered or filled. Procedures in this field of surgery are often divided between reconstructive and aesthetic. Sir Harold Gillies defined these as follows: reconstructive surgery attempts to restore the individual to the normal, while aesthetic surgery attempts to surpass the normal.

Although the origins of plastic surgery are difficult to trace in a direct line, it is customary to note that Susruta described operations for reconstruction of the amputated nose in the 6th and 7th century BC, that the Ebers Papyrus contained records of the reconstructive procedures in ancient Egypt, and that Celsus used advancement flaps at the beginning of the Christian era. In the sixteenth century Gaspare Tagliacozzi wrote a milestone treatise on reconstruction of the nose using an arm flap. Modern plastic surgery as a coherent discipline can trace its roots directly to the 19th century work of Carpue, von Graefe and Dieffenbach. Skin grafting was developed by Reverdin in France and by Lawson and Pollock in England.

War has always been a major stimulus to reconstructive surgery and many of these earlier developments were in response to war injuries. The modern specialty involving reconstructive and plastic surgical procedures really began in the wake of the First World War as a result of the leadership of Sir Harold Gillies in the UK, along with Kazanjian, Blair and Ivy in the USA. The Second World War saw the emergence of numerous surgeons who devoted themselves entirely to the practice of reconstructive and plastic surgery and firmly established its place in modern medicine.

WOUND HEALING

The goal in the correction of deformity is not only closure of the defect but also the attaining of the finest, least noticeable scar possible. The healing of wounds, described in Chapter 1, must be totally understood by the surgeon dealing with deformity. Controlling inflammation and deciding upon the proper choice of healing by first intention, second intention, or third intention is the first step. Removing the deterrents of ideal wound healing may require more than the rudiments of wound healing. Of importance are the use of proper débridement, atraumatic technique, and placement of the scar in the same direction as the skin lines when possible. The age of the patient, the region of the body, the type of the skin, and avoidance of haematoma, dead space and infection are likewise significant.

Simplicity is often a virtue. Whenever possible, closure of wounds by direct approximation and primary healing is desirable, whether dealing with a primary injury or a reconstructive procedure. Often, however, defects exist which cannot be directly sutured. In such situations grafts or flaps are required. Traditionally, closure by grafts is considered first; then the possibilities of local flaps and distant flaps are evaluated, choosing the simplest method which will produce the desired result. More recently, with the better understanding of the safe use of axial and musculocutaneous flaps, these have assumed a more prominent place in the hierarchy of techniques. In addition, closure or reconstruction by the free transfer of composite tissue using microvascular anastomosis has become increasingly common as its complication rate has become comparable to that of myocutaneous flaps. Direct closure, grafts, flaps, free tissue transfer and occasionally planned healing by secondary intention comprise the armamentarium of the reconstructive and plastic surgeon.

SKIN GRAFTS

Grafting of skin from distant parts of the body for wound closure was one of the greatest advances in reconstructive surgery. In a few short years from 1869 to 1876, most of what a surgeon needs to know about skin grafting was presented. In 1869 Reverdin reported hastening the healing of the granulating wound by application of small 'epidermic' grafts. The following year, George Lawson and George David Pollock presented papers to the Clinical Society of London in which Lawson described the full-thickness skin graft and enumerated the conditions essential for grafting large portions of skin; while Pollock described the first grafts on burn patients, the first allografts, and the first allograft rejection. Lawson's conditions for graft survival are as applicable today as when they were written:

1st 'That the skin should be applied to a healthy granulating surface'.

2nd 'That skin *only* should be transplanted, and that special care be taken that there is no fat adherent to it'.

3rd 'That the portion of skin should be accurately and firmly applied to the granulating surface'.

4th 'That the new skin should be kept in its new position without interruption, and that it should be lightly covered with a layer of lint, and over this is a small compress of cotton wool . . . '.

Definition and Classification

A skin graft by definition is a segment of skin (epidermis and dermis) which has been totally separated from its blood supply and transplanted from its normal bed (donor site) to a new area (recipient site). A split-thickness or partial-thickness skin graft includes epidermis and part, but not all, of the dermis (*Fig.* 22.1). A full-thickness skin graft includes epidermis and full thickness of the dermis. A composite graft, although not strictly a skin graft, includes the full thickness of the skin and a portion of the underlying tissue such as subcutaneous tissue, muscle, cartilage or bone. Another classification is by the source of the graft. An autograft is a graft transplanted from one area to another in the same individual, while an allograft (homograft) is transplanted from one individual to another in the same species. A xenograft (heterograft) is transplanted from one individual to another individual of a different species.

Split-thickness Grafts

These grafts can vary in thickness depending on the amount of dermis included (*Fig.* 22.1). Thin split-thickness grafts contain little dermis and are cut only to the level of the subpapillary vascular plexus. Medium-split thickness grafts are the most commonly used, and are cut to the layer of the dermal plexus. Thick split-thickness grafts contain most of the dermis, approximately three-quarters thickness. The thickness of the graft is relative, depending on the age and sex of the patient and the region of the body of the donor site. Clinically, the translucency of the graft and the pattern of bleeding from the donor site help determine the thickness. The thicker the graft, the more opaque it becomes. The thinner translucent graft will come from a bed with many closely-spaced, fine, bleeding points of the subpapillary plexus. Thicker grafts cut at a deeper layer leave a bed with fewer, larger vessels from the dermal plexus.

Split-thickness skin grafts are best used to cover large denuded surfaces or on granulating wounds. They are also used when wound contraction is of no consequence. A great advantage of these grafts is that their donor sites heal themselves from the remaining skin appendages, such as hair follicles and sweat glands. This allows harvesting of grafts of almost any size needed to close a defect. The thickness of the graft is one of preference of the surgeon but several guidelines are helpful. The thinner the graft, the higher is the chance of survival on the recipient site. Thinner grafts have fewer cells to be nourished prior to establishment of the blood supply. Also, since the undersurface of the graft has a higher density of vessels, vascular ingrowth can proceed more rapidly. Also the donor site of a thin split-thickness graft will epithelize more rapidly.

Thin grafts have some disadvantages. The thinner the graft the more the interface of the fibrous tissue between the graft and the recipient site will contract during the maturation phase. Therefore, the wound beneath a thicker split-thickness graft will contract much less and the recipient site under a full-thickness graft minimally, if at all. Thicker grafts will more closely resemble their donor site in colour, texture and hair distribution.

Full-thickness Grafts

Skin grafts which include the full thickness of the dermis tend to resemble normal skin better than split-thickness grafts. They provide more padding, a better colour match, a more nearly normal hair pattern, and inhibit wound contraction in the recipient site. Because they require ideal conditions for survival they must be placed in a vascular recipient site. Their thickness requires more nourishment prior to the establishment of vascular integrity.

The major disadvantage of full-thickness grafts is that their donor sites cannot heal spontaneously since no skin appendages are left behind. Therefore, the size of the graft is limited to dimensions which will allow primary closure of the donor site. If this practice is not followed, the donor site from a large full-thickness graft must be closed by a split-thickness graft. Only rarely is this approach used.

Composite Grafts

Occasionally a skin defect requires underlying supportive tissue as well as skin. Most frequently this is reconstructed with a flap as will be discussed later. However, if the area of loss is small enough a skin graft containing underlying tissue

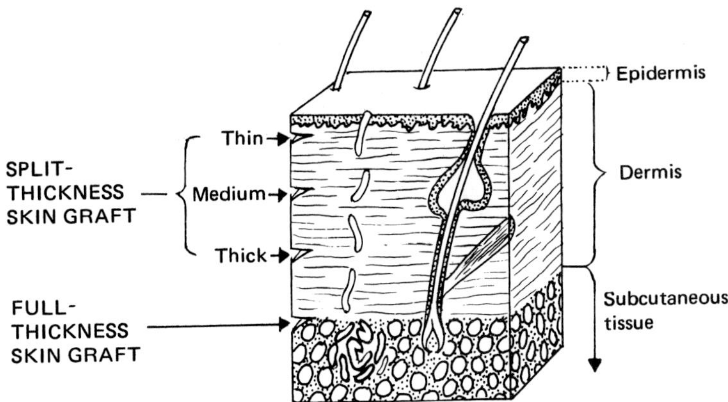

Fig. 22.1 Skin grafts are described as split-thickness or full-thickness depending on the amount of dermis included in the graft. Split-thickness grafts are further divided dependent upon their thickness.

(a composite graft) can be used. The risk of non-vascularization of this type graft severely limits its usefulness. However, if no portion of the graft is more than 0·5 cm from the wound edge, the survival rate is good. The blood supply to a composite graft is through its margin instead of its base, which accounts for the strict size limitation.

Survival of a Skin Graft

A skin graft, like any graft, must obtain a blood supply from its recipient site to survive. Therefore, the recipient site must be capable of providing the necessary vascularity. Bare cortical bone, bare tendon and bare cartilage cannot do this, and are unacceptable recipient sites for skin grafts. Heavily irradiated tissue, fibrotic longstanding granulation tissue and ischaemic tissue with arteriosclerotic changes are relatively poor recipient beds.

Once a skin graft is transplanted to a recipient bed it has a finite period of time to become revascularized. This process begins as the skin graft absorbs fluid like a sponge. The saturated graft is like an *in vivo* tissue culture. During this plasmatic phase, a fibrin network is formed between the graft and the recipient bed which holds the graft in place.

Within the first 48 h, connections are established between the bed and the empty 'ghost' vessels on the underside of the graft. Whether this is due to neovascular budding into the empty vessels as a pathway of least resistance or due to chance attachment by inosculation is not fully resolved at this time. However, between 12 and 48 h blood flow is returned to this graft and it becomes pink and attains the ability to blanch on pressure.

Total vascularization is achieved by new vessels growing into the graft. These new vessels initially follow the vascular channels already existing in the graft. As the vascular attachments are re-established, continuity of the lymphatic system is restored. Maturation of the skin graft occurs over a period of time as in any wound. This depends on the collagen maturation described in Chapter 1 and not on the vascularization. The new skin graft needs to be supported during the maturation phase for optimal results.

Causes of Failure

Good contact between the skin graft and its recipient bed is necessary for vascularization of the skin graft. The leading cause of failure of the skin grafting procedure is prevention of good contact by haematoma or seroma. Because of this, meticulous haemostasis of the bed is necessary before applying a graft. Topical haemostatic agents such as thrombin or epinephrine may be useful adjuncts. If adequate haemostasis cannot be attained, a delay of 24–48 h prior to application of the graft is better than application of the graft to an oozing bed. Inspection of the graft by the second or third day allows one to remove any collection of fluid preventing contact of the graft with the bed.

Improper immobilization between the graft and the recipient site is another frequent cause of failure. Movement between the graft and the bed injures the budding capillaries and prevents vascularization. Tie-over bolster dressings help immobilize the graft especially on concave recipient surfaces. Convex surfaces can usually be dressed with the proper immobilizing dressings without tie-overs. If a recipient site such as the chest cage is in constant movement, complete exposure of the graft is the most satisfactory treatment. This prevents shearing as the dressing and the recipient bed move in an asynchronous manner.

Grafting on to an unacceptable or poor bed may result in graft failure. As stated previously, cortical bone, bare cartilage and bare tendon cannot accept the graft. Bacteria can also make a bed unacceptable. Numerous experimental and clinical studies have shown that if a potential graft bed contains greater than 10^5 organisms/g of tissue the chance of skin graft survival markedly decreases. This is true for all organisms except the β-haemolytic streptococcus; any level of streptococci in a wound will jeopardize a successful application of the skin graft.

Infection occurring following a skin grafting used to be a common cause of graft failure. Today it remains a distant fourth as an aetiology. If the recipient bed contains 10^5 or fewer bacteria/g of tissue and no β-haemolytic streptococci at the time of graft application, it is rare to lose a graft because of

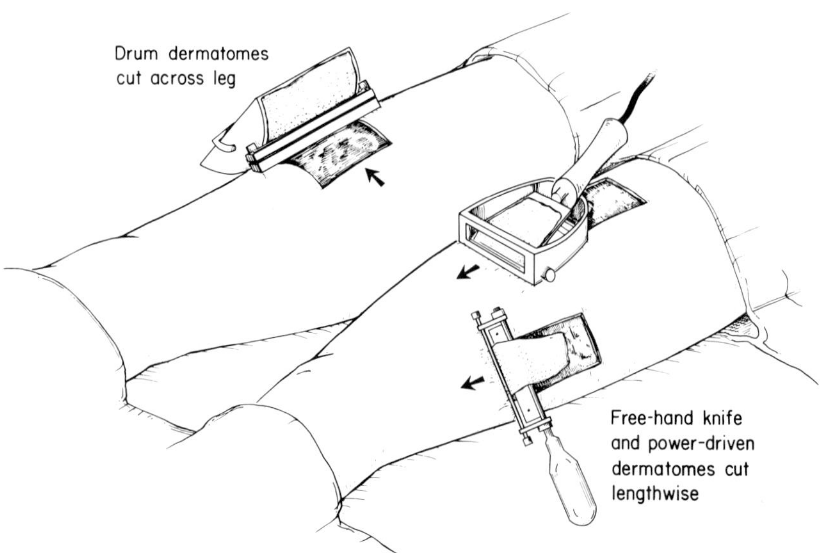

Fig. 22.2 Examples of available instruments to cut split-thickness skin grafts.

infection. However, infection continues to be considered the cause of skin graft loss by the neophyte. The reason for this is that, regardless of the true cause of loss, a non-vascularized graft becomes a perfect pabulum for bacteria and secondary infection intervenes. If a graft is not inspected until late, the loss will be interpreted as having been caused by infection.

Techniques of Skin Grafting

Split-thickness skin grafts can be procured by various modifications of three basic methods: free hand excision, the use of a dermatome, or a power driven 'hair clipper' dermatome (*Fig.* 22.2). The graft is transferred to a properly prepared recipient site and tailored to the wound. It may be secured in place by sutures, adhesive strips, a dressing, or simply by rapidly forming fibrin. A proper dressing for immobilization is applied unless the decision has been made to treat the graft by exposure.

Full-thickness and composite grafts are obtained with a scalpel. Exact patterns of the defect to be grafted are transferred to the donor site, outlined and incised. Any adherent fat must be meticulously removed from the undersurface of a full-thickness graft to assure optimal survival.

Postoperative care of the skin graft is as important as the operative technique. The graft should be inspected by 48 h using an aseptic technique. Any fluid found beneath the graft should be aspirated or evacuated by making a small nick in the graft to express it. If fluid is not removed by 96 h, evidence has been presented that the graft epithelizes on the undersurfaces preventing satisfactory vascularization. The graft must be immobilized and protected for at least 5–7 days. Oedema should be prevented in the recipient bed for 4 to 6 months. This becomes of great practical importance to grafts to the lower extremity.

The Donor Site

Choosing the donor site for a skin graft requires some thought. The colour, texture, vascularity, thickness and hair-bearing nature of the skin varies from one area of the body to another. In general, the nearer the donor site is to the recipient site, the more closely the skin will match. Skin grafts to the face taken from above the clavicle tend to retain their natural blush state, whereas those from below the clavicle tend to take on a yellowish or brownish hue. The donor site of a split-thickness skin graft is like a partial-thickness burn or deep abrasion. It must be protected from trauma and bacteria in order to epithelize satisfactorily. Many dressings are satisfactory for the donor sites, including impregnated fine mesh gauze, biological membranes such as xenograft skin, or modified parachute silk. The important thing is that bedclothes do not stick to it, the patient does not lie on it, and that it does not become macerated.

SKIN FLAPS

As stated earlier, deformities and defects are best corrected or closed by primary approximation whenever possible. Skin grafting is usually thought of as a second choice. However, cases exist where skin grafting is either not possible or not desirable. The area in need of reconstruction may lack the vascularity necessary to support a skin graft. Bare bone, tendon, cartilage, irradiated tissue and ischaemic wounds are all examples of such areas. Tissue to reconstruct these defects must carry its own blood supply. When two surfaces must be reconstructed, an inherent blood supply is necessary. An example of this is the full-thickness loss of an eyelid or cheek or the full-thickness loss of the chest wall. There are also situations where a skin graft could theoretically close a defect but would not serve the final purpose as well as vascularized composite tissue. Such is the case when deeper tissue is desired for contouring but the defect is too large for a composite graft or when padding is required over a bony prominence. Occasionally a skin graft will correct a deformity or close a defect but is not the most desirable type of reconstruction. This is true if future surgery will be necessary beneath the reconstructed area, if near-normal sensation is required of the reconstructed tissue, or if the hoped-for aesthetic result cannot be achieved by a skin graft. In all of these circumstances reconstruction can be effected by a skin flap.

Definition and Classification

A skin flap by definition is a segment of skin and subcutaneous tissue which is transferred from its original position on the body to another site while maintaining its own inherent vasculature for nourishment. In some cases deeper tissue such as muscle or bone is carried with the skin flap. All flaps have a 'pedicle' which is their vascular base of attachment.

In order to understand skin flaps, a thorough knowledge of their blood supply is necessary. There are two main anatomical patterns of blood supply to the skin. The first of these depends upon vessels from the aorta or its major branches which lie deep to the muscles. Perforating branches through the muscles or along fascial planes become the *musculocutaneous* and *fasciocutaneous arteries*, and terminate by supplying the dermal-subdermal plexus of the skin (*Fig.* 22.3). This vascular pattern forms the predominant blood supply to the skin in humans. In the other anatomical

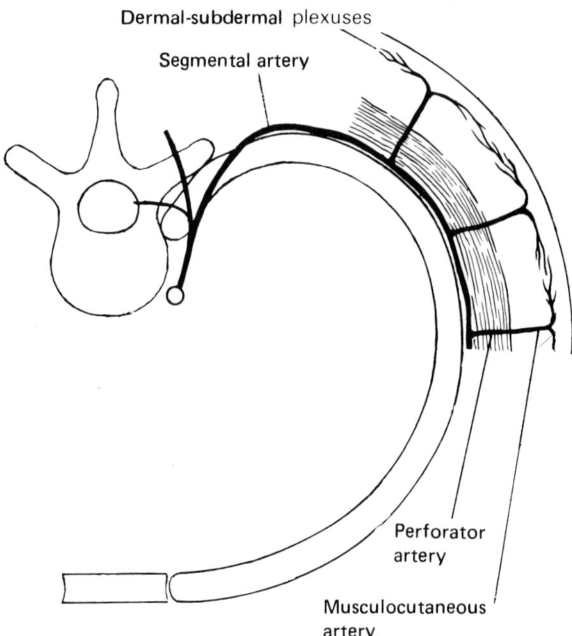

Fig. 22.3 Schematic representation of musculocutaneous artery perforating the muscle to supply the dermal-subdermal vascular plexus.

pattern, vessels from the aorta or its major branches form *direct cutaneous arteries* which lie superficial to the muscles and parallel to the skin for long distances, and supply the dermal-subdermal plexus directly (*Fig.* 22.4).

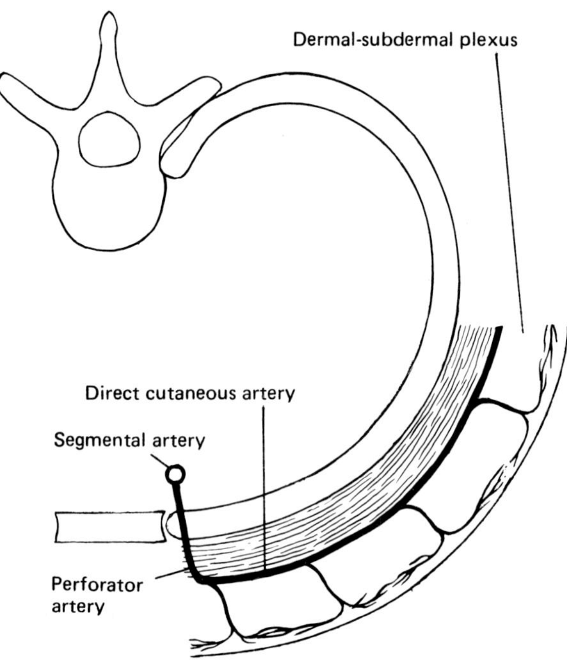

Fig. 22.4 Schematic representation of direct cutaneous artery paralleling the skin superficial to the muscle layer.

A *cutaneous* or *random pattern flap* is a flap based on a blood supply from musculocutaneous arteries penetrating perpendicularly into its base, supplying the length of the flap through the longitudinal dermal-subdermal plexus (*Fig.* 22.5). The surviving length of this flap is limited by the perfusion pressure in the vessels.

An *axial* or *arterial pattern flap* receives its blood supply from a direct cutaneous artery which enters its base and runs longitudinally within the flap (*Fig.* 22.6). The length of the flap is determined by the length of the direct cutaneous artery supplying it, plus an additional random portion at the termination of the artery supplied by the dermal-subdermal plexus.

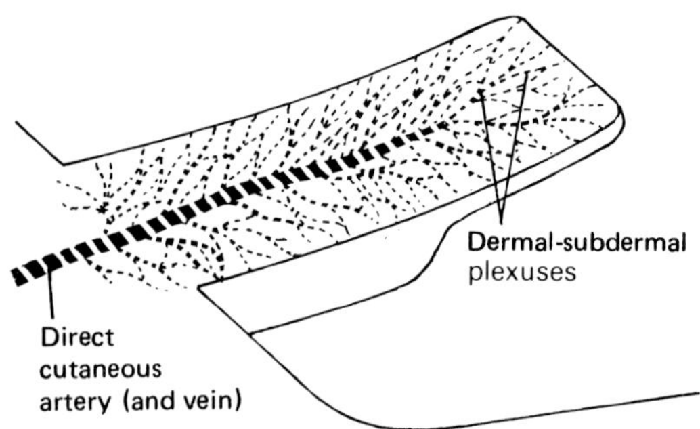

Fig. 22.6 Axial or arterial pattern flap being supplied by a longitudinal direct cutaneous artery.

A third type of flap, the *musculocutaneous* or *myocutaneous flap* has been described more recently. If a muscle is adequately supplied with blood flow through a single dominant vascular pedicle, the muscle with its overlying skin and subcutaneous tissue can be raised as a flap and transferred as a unit on the segmental vascular pedicle. In this case a large area of skin can be transferred on multiple muscle perforators fed by the pedicle without the limitations imposed on cutaneous or random flaps. Likewise a fasciocutaneous flap may be raised by including the vascularized fascia in the same way.

Any of these types of flaps can be transferred by dividing its vascular pedicle and re-anastomosing it in a recipient site. When this technique is used, the flap is classified as a *free-flap*. A free-flap is not considered a graft since vascularization and nourishment is immediately re-established through the pedicle.

Cutaneous (Random) Pattern Flaps

In the past, most skin flaps were of the cutaneous or random pattern type. These flaps lack an anatomically recognized arteriovenous system. Therefore, they have strict length limitations. The length cannot survive beyond the blood

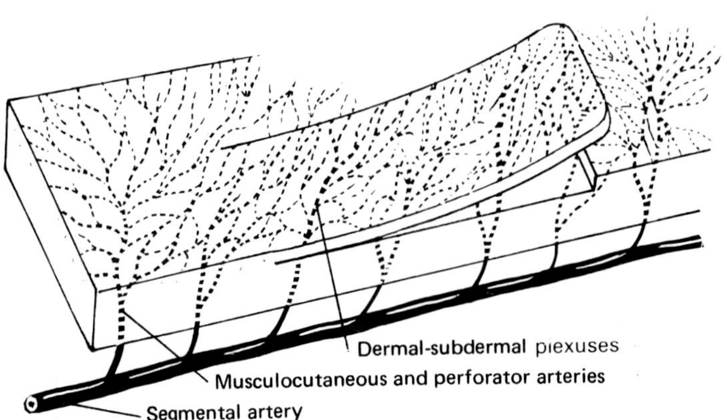

Fig. 22.5 Cutaneous or random pattern flap being supplied by a perpendicular musculocutaneous artery in its base.

supply of the dermal-subdermal anastomotic plexus perfused by the perforating musculocutaneous arteries without special conditioning of the flap. Unfortunately, there are no simple rules or formulae to predict the exact safe length: base width ratio for survival. The flap can be conditioned to survive to greater lengths by performing a preliminary procedure on the flap to enhance the blood supply to a specific area of tissue. The preliminary procedure is known as a *delay* because transfer of the flap to its final recipient site is delayed. It consists of partially dividing the blood supply to the flap 2–4 weeks before its actual transfer. The purpose of the delay is to condition the extra length of the flap to survive in a state of relative hypoxia at the time of transfer. The exact physiological mechanisms of how a delay procedure works have been widely studied but are not well understood.

Cutaneous pattern flaps can be subclassified as local flaps or flaps from a distance. The local flaps can be of the simple advancement variety (*Fig.* 22.7), or can rotate around a pivot point. Flaps of the latter variety are either rotation flaps, transposition flaps, or interpolation flaps (*Fig.* 22.8). The advancement flap is elevated and stretched forward into a new position. It depends upon the elasticity of the skin and is of limited value. Rotation, transposition and interpolation flaps all have in common a pivot point and an arc through which the flap can be rotated. The radius of the flap is the line of greatest tension of the flap. The understanding of the pivot point and the flap's arc are paramount in planning any of these flaps.

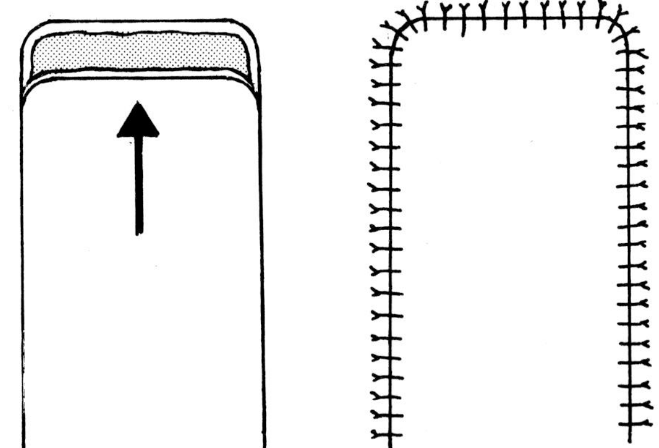

Fig. 22.7 Advancement type cutaneous pattern flap.

Flaps from a distance used for reconstruction may be applied to the defect directly as when an arm flap is brought to the nose, or can be brought to the defect indirectly in multiple stages using a carrier. An abdominal flap initially attached to the arm as a carrier and later transferred via the arm to the nose would be an example of a distant flap being transferred indirectly. Distant flaps transferred by an indirect means are rapidly becoming of historical interest only as other techniques such as axial flaps, musculocutaneous flaps, and free-flaps are becoming more commonly utilized.

Axial (Arterial) Pattern Flaps

Since axial or arterial pattern flaps are supplied by a specific longitudinal arteriovenous network, traditional length:base width ratios play no role in the designing of the flap. In fact, no skin is necessary at the base of these flaps, and the artery

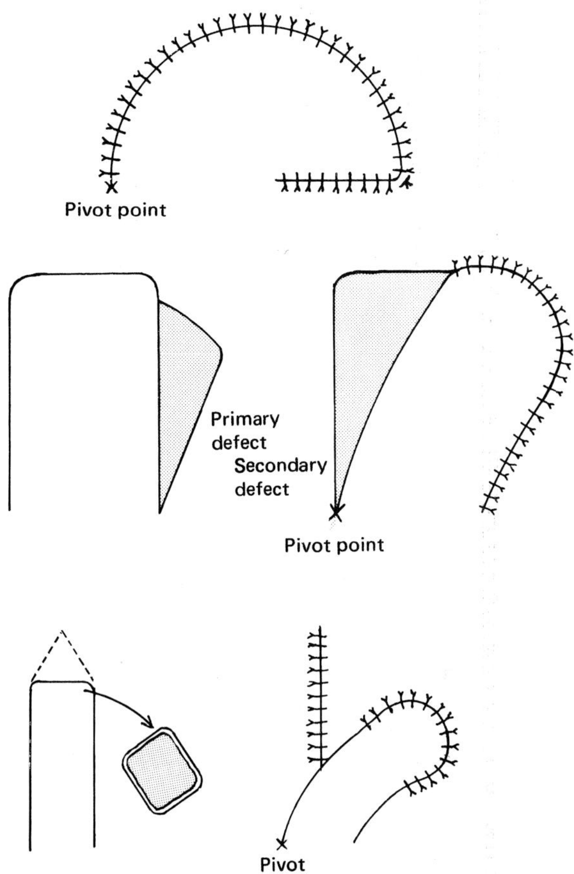

Fig. 22.8 Examples of rotation, transposition and interpolation cutaneous pattern flaps.

and vein alone can serve as the base of pedicle. This type of axial flap is called an island flap. Often, the nerve is preserved with the vessels in the pedicle making it a neurovascular island flap.

Axial flaps have become very popular in reconstructive surgery. The key to their use is an exact knowledge of the anatomy of the direct cutaneous arteries. Since the skin is unimportant in the flap's base, the pivot point becomes the artery itself and the arc of the flap can be 360° within the reach of the artery. This type of flap is not universally useful because there are a limited number of direct axial arteries with known cutaneous vascular territories.

Musculocutaneous (Myocutaneous) Pattern Flaps

Since axial pattern flaps are limited by the small number of known cutaneous vascular territories and since the remainder of the body's skin is supplied by perforating musculocutaneous arteries, Owens suggested elevating the muscle with its longitudinal segmental artery to supply an overlying skin flap. McCraw et al. have described musculocutaneous vascular territories over all regions of the body. Using these known musculocutaneous vascular territories, an axial compound flap of skin, subcutaneous tissue and muscle can be designed for almost any defect. The bulk of the muscle in the flap can often be a disadvantage and the loss of the normal function of the muscle transferred in the flap may be so disabling as to contraindicate the use of a specific flap.

Free-flaps

With the advent of microvascular surgical techniques in the late 1950s, it became feasible to anastomose arteries and veins of less than 1 mm diameter. Therefore, experimental transfers of skin flaps were performed in the 1960s and by 1973 the first successful free-flap transfer was reported in the human. Since that time, reports of reconstructive procedures using free-flaps have become increasingly frequent. Success rates of greater than 90% for this type of flap transfer are reported by some surgeons. It appears not to be justified when other means of reconstruction such as skin grafts, cutaneous, axial or musculocutaneous flaps are equally satisfactory. It requires specialized teams of personnel, specialized equipment and increased operating time. However, the free-flap frequently does provide the best solution for a reconstructive problem and occasionally may be the only salvage for a particular patient.

Characteristics of Skin Flaps

All types of skin flaps have certain characteristics which help differentiate their reconstructive results from skin grafts. The skin of a flap tends to maintain its original colour and texture. This can be an obvious cosmetic advantage, especially on the face. Hair growth, sebaceous secretion, sweating and sensation are fairly well preserved in skin flaps. Sweating and sensation may be temporarily absent but usually recover to an extent. In most instances, flaps tend to be more durable than skin grafts. This is especially true over a bony prominence or other pressure points. Finally, flaps tend to grow in proportion to total body growth. Although bulk is one of the advantages of flaps, excessive bulk can be a disadvantage. An axial pattern flap requires all the subcutaneous tissue of the donor site to be transferred since the direct cutaneous artery is just superficial to the muscle. A fasciocutaneous flap requires a similar amount of tissue. A musculocutaneous pattern flap obviously requires the muscle and subcutaneous tissue to be transferred. It should be remembered, however, that the denervated muscle will atrophy following transfer. If too much bulk will still be a problem in the reconstruction, three possible solutions exist. A cutaneous pattern flap can be used, which will be thinner since it need only carry enough subcutaneous tissue to protect the dermal-subdermal vascular plexus. Alternatively, secondary procedures can be used to 'debulk' the subcutaneous tissue at a future time after the flap has successfully survived its transfer. Another solution is to transfer only the muscle as a flap and cover it with a split-thickness skin graft.

Requirements for Flap Survival

The single most important requirement for flap survival is adequate nutrient blood flow. The flap is planned and the transfer procedure executed so that sufficient inflow of arterial blood and outflow of venous blood for all of the tissue comprising the flap is maintained. There are several principles for the surgeon to keep in mind to maximize the chance of fulfilling this requirement. Flaps should be designed, whenever possible, so that a large vessel enters the base of the flap. Milton has shown that a flap will survive to a 50% greater length when this can be done. The density of the vascular supply to the skin and subcutaneous tissue decreases as one proceeds caudally from the head. Therefore, flaps can more safely be relied upon in the head and neck area than in the foot. When possible cutaneous pattern flaps should be aligned so that their bases are more cephalad than their tips. Collateral cutaneous anastomoses of vessels across the ventral and dorsal midlines of the body are scarce. Therefore, cutaneous flaps should not be designed so that their blood supply is required to cross the midline. However, it is possible to design certain fasciocutaneous and musculocutaneous flaps which do cross the ventral midline. Finally, age must be a consideration. Advancing age is associated with a higher incidence of arteriosclerosis and therefore skin may have a relative degree of ischaemia in the elderly.

If the arterial inflow to a flap can be predicted to be insufficient, it can be augmented by a delay procedure as discussed previously. Insufficient venous outflow is usually due to one of the conditions listed under 'complications' in the next section. However, occasionally inflammatory oedema or oedema due to stasis will impede the venous outflow. Changing the position of the patient to take advantage of gravity may facilitate the egress of blood and oedema as will intermittent compression of the flap.

Since adequate arterial inflow to the flap is vital to its survival, it is helpful to know if this requirement has been met at the time of flap elevation and transfer. The best test for this at present is the use of fluorescein dye. Fluorescein absorbs light in the ultraviolet range and emits light in the visible range with a yellow hue. Intravenous injection of fluorescein dye (15 mg/kg body weight) will travel into all areas of the body being perfused. After 10–15 min the flap in question is inspected under ultraviolet light. All areas of the flap being adequately perfused will give the yellow hue. Those areas failing to appear yellow under the ultraviolet light are not receiving adequate arterial inflow.

Causes of Skin Flap Failure

Once a flap has been properly designed and elevated and the arterial inflow substantiated by the fluorescein dye test, the flap should survive transfer. However, failure can still occur if there are complications. Suturing a flap into place under excessive tension can cause necrosis of the flap. The tension can interfere either with venous outflow or, if excessive, arterial inflow. Kinking of the flap at the time of transfer or postoperatively similarly can cause vascular compromise. Most frequently kinking results in venous embarrassment and can be corrected if recognized before irreparable damage has occurred. Pressure on a flap can obviously lead to necrosis. A mild to moderate degree of inflammatory oedema occurs in all flaps. If this is inhibited by a tight constricting dressing, vascular compromise will occur. However, often an even amount of compression is of aid to a flap to help prevent excessive kinking or to overcome the oedema of gravity. A great deal of surgical judgement is necessary to differentiate between adequate compression and excessive pressure. Until this judgement is attained, it is probably best to leave most flaps free of dressings. Just as a haematoma will spell disaster for a skin graft, it may totally destroy a flap. Often the haematoma is difficult to diagnose in the flap because of the normal degree of postoperative oedema. However, since the consequences are so dire, any patient in whom a significant haematoma is suspected should be returned to the operating theatre for formal exploration and evacuation of the blood and clots. Infection is not a common cause of flap failure. The speed and ease with which bacteria multiply to critical levels of $>10^5$ organisms/g of tissue are diminished by the excellent blood supply with its accompanying cellular and humoral host defence factors. However, when infection does occur it can destroy a flap. In the well-vascularized flap, infection is most frequently due to the β-haemolytic streptococcus. If erythema and warmth herald a streptococcal cellulitis, intravenous penicillin can often abort the infection. Infection more commonly occurs in the marginally vascularized flap or the flap which is jeopardized by tension or kinking. In this situation, anaerobic infections can occur. These infections are insidious and may be responsible for a slowly increasing necrosis of what initially appeared to be a satisfactory flap.

The Skin Flap Donor Site

Just as in skin grafting, donor site considerations are important in using skin flaps. When possible, an adjacent donor site is preferred to allow a local flap instead of a distant flap. As a general rule, axial pattern flaps are preferred to cutaneous or random flaps. The location on the body in relation to the total body vasculature has previously been discussed. Another important consideration is that the donor site must be able to spare the tissue to be transferred without serious loss of function.

If a thick, durable cover is required in a potential donor site, it would be ill-advised to sacrifice needed functional coverage using that specific donor site. Similarly, as previously mentioned, it is contraindicated to use a muscle with a critical function as a donor muscle for musculocutaneous pattern flap.

Closure of the flap donor site is another consideration. In the advancement flap and often in the rotation type flap, no defect occurs in the donor site. Some other donor defects can be closed by direct approximation. Still others will require a skin graft for closure. It is the mistake of a neophyte to try to avoid skin grafts in flap donor sites. Often the use of a graft will be the difference between success and failure of the flap, since direct closure of the donor site may require just enough tension to jeopardize the flap's vascularity. Occasionally, tertiary closure of a donor site is indicated. Allowing granulation tissue to form often decreases the deformity of the donor site defect, after which tertiary closure by a delayed skin graft may give the most satisfactory result.

SCAR REVISION

Scar formation is the fundamental phenomenon of wound healing in most human tissues including the dermis. An understanding of normal wound healing, described in Chapter 1, and insight into the factors which make a scar less than optimal are both essential to planning scar revisions. All scars must proceed through the inflammatory, proliferative and maturation phases of wound healing, and will therefore require time to reach their final appearance. A normal scar which appears hypertrophic at 6 weeks may be quite satisfactory after 6–12 months. If the mature scar is not satisfactory, application of the basic principles of reconstruction can then be expected to result in an improved scar.

The most common reasons for unacceptable scars are an unfavourable direction of the original wound or incision in regard to the normal lines of skin tension, failure of proper dermal approximation and a pathological extension of normal wound contraction which results in a contracture.

The simplest scar revision consists of excising the scar and reapproximating the wound edges. If the excessive scarring was due to an improper direction of the original wound, the wound direction should be realigned so that the new scar will fall in the lines of minimum resting tension. As a general rule, these lines will run perpendicular to the fibres of the underlying muscle. Often, realigning a scar to the minimum resting skin tension lines will allow it to become almost invisible. When the wound is reapproximated, the dermis is carefully approximated with an inverted suture (*Fig.* 22.9). This supports the tissues until the tensile strength of the new collagen is sufficient to prevent spreading of the scar. Although a degree of wound contraction is a normal part of wound healing, contracture is preventable. Placing the direction in the lines of minimum resting tension will greatly help. The line of contracture can be lengthened either by excising the old scar as an ellipse, thus elongating each side of the wound slightly, or by adding tissue by introducing a skin graft or a flap.

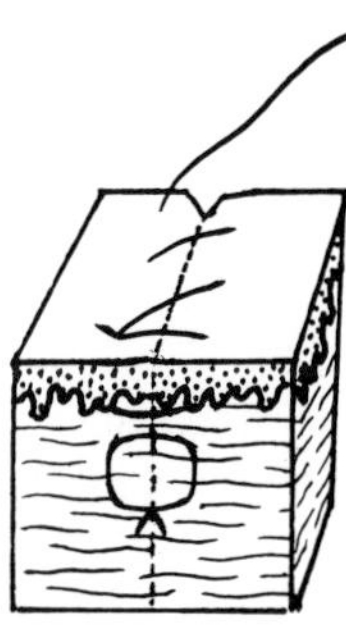

Fig. 22.9 Technique of wound closure with inverted suture in dermis to provide keystone to the repair.

An unacceptable scar may be due to a deficiency in tissue. If the original wound was closed under excessive tension, a widened hypertrophic or depressed scar, or a contracture would be expected. When the scar is incised or excised, the edges retract widely and the tissue deficiency becomes apparent. A split-thickness or full-thickness skin graft will replace the deficiency and improve the scar. Skin grafts are useful for scar revision in areas where previous scars or skin grafts are of poor quality or have a poor colour match. Following excision, a carefully tailored full-thickness skin graft will improve the quality and colour match. If a previous skin graft appears as a patch on the face, the skin graft and surrounding skin are removed and a new graft covering a full aesthetic unit such as the forehead or cheek, is used for resurfacing.

Skin flaps are sometimes indicated for scar revision. A depressed scar may require a flap for bulk. A scar may be atrophic due to ischaemia and a flap with its inherent blood supply may be required to increase the vascularity of the revision. Finally, just as with a skin graft, a flap may improve a scar by adding tissue to relieve tension.

Z-PLASTY

The Z-plasty is a technique by which two triangular skin flaps are interchanged in position to gain length along a scar or skin fold at the expense of the adjacent tissues. Understanding of the geometry and principles of the Z-plasty allows the reconstructive surgeon to lengthen a contracted scar, obliterate a web contracture, add to an area of deficient tissue and change the direction of a scar, thus giving him an important technique of scar revision. The incisions are designed with three lines of equal length: a central member, and two limbs extending from its ends to resemble the letter

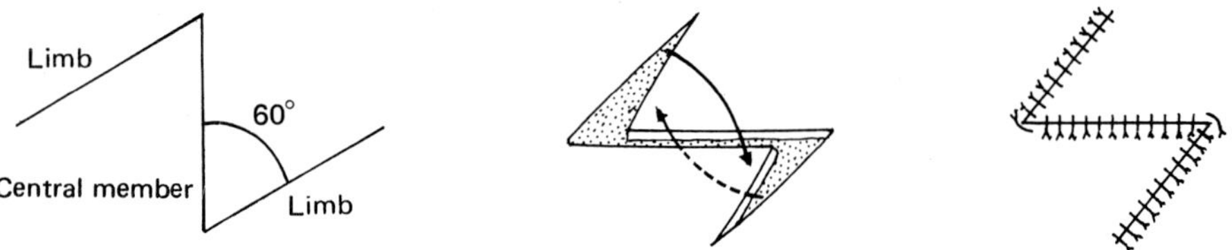

Fig. 22.10 Design of 60°–60° angle Z-plasty showing interpolation of flaps and final configuration.

Z or its mirror image. The angles formed by the limbs with the central member can vary depending on the desired final result; angles of 60° can be shown mathematically to give the maximum practical increase in length. When the flaps are mobilized and transposed the flap bases lie along the line formerly occupied by the central member, resulting in a gain in length (*Fig.* 22.10). This gain in length is approximately 25% for 30° angles, 50% for 45° angles and 75% for 60° angles. Further details of the design and use of the Z-plasty may be found in McGregor's text.

CHRONIC ULCERATING WOUNDS

Large ulcerating wounds often are difficult to close. Two types of ulcerating wounds which reconstructive surgeons are frequently called upon to treat are pressure ulcerations overlying bony prominences and vascular ulcers of the lower extremities. These wounds, and all ulcerating wounds, have in common, granulation tissue. Since granulation tissue does not exist in the absence of bacteria, these wounds are chronically contaminated. Their management requires understanding of the role of bacteria in their pathogenesis and its successful control.

Pressure Ulcerations

These lesions are sometimes called 'decubitus ulcers'. However, the term is too limiting since a pressure ulceration can occur over any bony prominence whether or not the body is in the decubitus position. In fact, a pressure ulcer can be caused iatrogenically by application of too tight a bandage. Pressure ulcerations begin with erythema and oedema in the skin overlying a pressure point such as a bony prominence. The sequence of events from redness of the skin to complete dissolution is so rapid as to suggest that localized infection with its attendant bacterial enzymes may be part of the aetiology. Compression of the tissue has been shown to render the area susceptible to localization of small amounts of bacteria circulating in the blood or lymphatic systems. Ischaemia and denervation also play a role in the pathogenesis. Each of these predisposes the tissue to bacterial invasion.

Because evidence shows that bacteria play a significant role in pressure ulcerations, patients who are bedridden or have ischaemia or denervated areas of their bodies need infection surveillance not only of their skin but of their urinary tract and bloodstream as well. Prevention of pressure is of paramount importance. Patients should have their positions changed at least every 2 h. If turning is not possible, a water or gel-filled mattress has been documented to be of value in decreasing susceptibility to pressure ulcerations. In addition to elimination of pressure, hygiene and infection surveillance, general nutrition is important. Prevention or correction of anaemia and any negative nitrogen balance is of proven usefulness.

Once the area becomes an ulcerated lesion with granulation tissue the goal is to débride the necrotic tissue and restore the wound to bacterial equilibrium with a bacterial level of 10^5 or fewer organisms/g of tissue and no streptococci present. Topical antibacterials and biological dressings are used as with any chronic granulating wound. These principles have been enumerated for the burn wound in Chapter 20. The wound can then undergo definitive closure either by direct approximation, flap coverage, or a skin graft. Flaps have most frequently been utilized because of the necessity to provide bulk. Local flaps of the rotation or transposition type are most common. Recently, the musculocutaneous flaps have been demonstrated to be very effective. Regardless of the flap chosen, the general principles for operative management of a pressure sore are: (1) removal of the ulcer with a surrounding rim of normal tissue; (2) removal of the underlying bony prominence; and (3) closure with a well-vascularized skin flap.

Leg Ulcers

The generic term, leg ulcer, has helped make these lesions difficult to manage. Many aetiological factors can be responsible for these ulcers and differentiation is important to understanding their treatment. A brief differential diagnosis of leg ulcers by aetiology is listed in *Table* 22.1. Successful management of leg ulcers includes conservative measures carried out in the preoperative period, operative measures and postoperative measures. Without special regard to each of these, treatment of any leg ulcer is unlikely to be satisfactory. Topical treatment to decrease the tissue bacterial level is begun during the conservative period. Certain additional measures are necessary depending on the aetiology of the ulcer. Oedema must be removed from feet with venous stasis ulcers and this is best done by elevation. However, elevation of the foot is harmful in ischaemic ulcerations such as those seen with arteriosclerosis, vasculitis, or diabetes. Underlying vascular disorders must be diagnosed and corrected, if possible. Non-invasive arterial and venous evaluation techniques have greatly aided this diagnosis. In addition to the non-invasive studies, arteriography may be required.

Table 22.1 Differential diagnosis of leg ulcer

I. Venous hypertension
II. Arterial—ischaemia
   a. Hypertensive—Martorell
   b. Arteriosclerotic
III. Trauma
IV. Vasculitis
V. Blood dyscrasias
   a. Sickle-cell anaemia
   b. Leukaemia
VI. Diabetes mellitus

The operative management of leg ulcers has become much easier since the recognition of the role of tissue bacteria in the success of skin grafts. Once the underlying structures such as tendon and bone are adequately covered by granulation tissue containing 10^5 or fewer bacteria/g of tissue and no streptococci, almost all leg ulcers can be successfully closed by a split-thickness skin graft. If ischaemia prevents adequate granulation tissue and bare tendon or bone exists in the depth of the wound, a vascularized skin flap may be necessary. In the past, distant cutaneous flaps often were required in the form of a cross-leg flap to cover an ischaemic ulcer on a lower extremity. However, today most of these lesions can be effectively closed by a musculocutaneous flap or a free-flap.

Postoperative measures are important after closing the leg ulcers. Skin grafts on the lower extremities must be protected from hydrostatic pressure and oedema for a minimum of 4–6 months. Therefore, the patients should wear customized pressure gradient elastic stockings delivering 30–40 mmHg pressure evenly to the leg. In addition, local hypoxia must be prevented in a patient whose ulcer is due to sickle-cell anaemia. This can be done by repeated blood transfusions, keeping the patient's haematocrit greater than 35% and his reticulocyte count less than 2% during the time of complete graft maturation. An educational programme for the patient, helping him to understand the aetiology of his ulcer and the preventive measures he may use in the future, completes the reconstruction of this common problem.

LYMPHOEDEMA

Swelling of the extremities due to lymphoedema may be primarily, due to lymphatic dysplasia, or secondary (acquired), due to proximal obstruction. The cause of primary lymphoedema is not known. It appears to be about twice as common in females as compared with males. Primary lymphoedema can be classified as congenital, lymphoedema praecox, or lymphoedema tarda. Congenital lymphoedema is present at birth. If it is both congenital and hereditary, it is known as Milroy's disease. Lymphoedema praecox, the most common form of lymphoedema, appears in childhood or early adult life. Lymphoedema tarda, on the other hand, does not appear until middle or later life. All three types of primary lymphoedema are probably due to a congenital defect since lymphangiography reveals lymphatic dysplasia. The most common abnormality seen is hypoplasia of the lymphatics. This abnormality accounts for approximately 87% of the cases. Hyperplasia exists in about 8% of the cases and true lymphatic aplasia is seen in about 5%.

The treatment of primary lymphoedema consists of both conservative non-operative measures and surgical procedures. The key to conservative management is the reduction of swelling and the prevention of its recurrence. Elevation of the extremity is basic and may be combined with distal-to-proximal massage or intermittent mechanical compression. Elastic support at about 30–40 mmHg is essential whenever the extremity is dependent and may be best achieved with custom knitted elastic hose. Minor infections in the lymphoedematous extremity must be prevented. Because the oedema fluid inactivates the body's natural defence mechanisms against the β-haemolytic streptococcus, long-term prophylactic penicillin therapy may be indicated. Minor trauma and fungal infestations, must be avoided.

Surgery for the treatment of primary lymphoedema can be divided into two different approaches. Attempts to re-establish lymphatic drainage include burying a dermal flap or transferring an omental flap into the area deficient of lymphatics. Recently, microsurgical techniques have been used to construct lymphaticolymphatic or lymphaticovenous anastomoses. None of these attempts have been routinely successful. The other surgical approach involves excision of the lymphoedematous tissue and wound closure with skin grafts or flaps. At present this gives the most predictable result in the treatment of primary lymphoedema. (*See also* Chapter 57.)

Secondary lymphoedema results from an acquired obstruction of lymphatic channels in the proximal portion of the extremity. It can be due to a post-traumatic or postsurgical obstruction, metastatic malignancy to the inguinal or axillary lymph nodes, or to infectious or parasitic disease in the nodes (*see* Chapter 4). The history is usually suggestive of the cause and lymphangiography is diagnostic. Whereas hypoplasia or aplasia is usually present in primary lymphoedema, large lymphatic trunks with tortuosity and dermal backflow are seen in the secondary case.

Conservative non-operative measures are unlikely to be successful in secondary lymphoedema. Operations to bypass the blocked lymphatics should be performed early. These procedures include skin flaps, musculocutaneous flaps and omental flaps designed to bridge the obstruction. It must be admitted that the cosmetic results of these procedures are not always satisfactory although the complication of repeated infection can be reduced.

FACIAL TRAUMA AND FRACTURES OF THE FACIAL SKELETON

These topics are fully discussed in Chapters 25 and 26. Some of the basic principles of plastic and reconstructive surgery are emphasized here. Trauma to the soft tissues and skeleton of the face often occurs in association with other injuries. The immediate priorities are an adequate *airway*, control of *bleeding* and evaluation of the state of *consciousness*. The possibility of intracranial and cervical spine injury must be evaluated, as well as life-threatening trauma to other parts of the body. The treatment of the facial trauma itself, even if extensive, is relatively less urgent. The preliminary examination must include evaluation of facial nerve function and the possibility of injury to the parotid duct, the eye and the lacrimal apparatus. Contact lenses should be looked for, and removed if found. When necessary, definitive treatment may be delayed until more urgent injuries are treated.

The basic management of all facial soft-tissue wounds begins with thorough irrigation and haemostasis. Fracture lines may be noted in the depths of the lacerations and these wounds may provide access for open reduction and fixation. Foreign material must be searched for and removed. Devitalized tissue is minimially débrided, keeping in mind that the vascularity of the facial tissues often permits survival of fragments of tissue with little attachment. Bony fragments with any attachment whatsoever should be allowed to remain in place. The skin margins usually require little excision, but bevelled edges should be squared off to prevent irregularities in the scars. Dirt and other foreign particles embedded in the skin in abrasions and blast injuries require thorough removal. It may be necessary to use a scrub brush or even primary dermabrasion to avoid disfiguring traumatic tattooing.

If the facial nerve branches are injured, the severed ends

may be identified and sutured using magnification and fine suture materials. When parotid duct injury is suspected the duct may be cannulated from its oral opening and a fine tube left in place over which the severed ends of the duct are approximated. The lacrimal canaliculi may also be repaired over fine polyethylene tubing.

The wounds should be accurately closed in layers, approximating the mucosa, the muscles and the skin. Closure should begin by accurately joining known points, using as landmarks the irregularities of the laceration itself and features such as the hairline, eyebrow, vermilion border of the lip and nasolabial fold. The final result can be seriously marred by minor inaccuracies in the closure of these anatomical features. The eyelids may be repaired by the technique of Mustarde, using a pull-out suture of nylon for the conjunctiva and accurately suturing the 'grey line' of the tarsal border. (*See also* Chapter 31.)

Flaps of skin resulting from a slicing injury may tend to become elevated during healing, producing the 'trap door' deformity as the circumferential scar contracts. If quite small, such flaps should be primarily excised and the resulting defect closed in the same manner as a fusiform excision of a skin lesion; otherwise, secondary revision is usually preferred to primary Z-plasties or other local manoeuvres.

Wounds, which at first appear to involve major tissue losses, will often close quite completely when the 'jigsaw puzzle' is put together by this type of meticulous closure. When there is an avulsive loss of skin, it is frequently desirable to obtain wound closure with a split-thickness skin graft and plan for secondary reconstruction. A great deal of experience and judgement is required to decide on primary reconstruction of traumatic defects. Full-thickness losses of the cheek and jaw region may call for the use of distant flaps such as the deltopectoral axial flap or the trapezius myocutaneous flap. Because of the resulting aesthetic defect the forehead is usually avoided as a flap donor site except for reconstructon of major nasal losses.

The facial skeleton is largely accessible to observation and palpation. Early examination of injuries, before swelling is extensive, will usually permit quite accurate diagnosis of the skeletal injury. Dysaesthesia in the distribution of the infraorbital or mental nerve suggests a fracture through the region of its foramen; the subjective complaint of a change in the occlusal bite points to a maxillary or mandibular fracture. Trismus is most commonly the result of a depressed zygomatic arch fracture.

The nasal bones, orbital rims, zygomatic arch and the border of the mandible are subcutaneous and readily palpated, and the nasal septum is visible by speculum examination. The anterior and lateral walls of the maxilla and the surface of the mandible are palpable intraorally. The motion of the temporal mandibular joint can be appreciated by palpation on the anterior wall of the external auditory canal. Displacement of the maxilla or mandible results in malocclusion which is readily appreciated subjectively by the patient and visible intraorally. Significant asymmetry should be looked for; depression in the malar area and a shift of the nose from the midline both suggest underlying fractures. Malar depression is often best appreciated by looking over the brow from above. Fractures of the orbital floor may present with enophthalmos, diplopia, or restriction of upward gaze as a result of entrapment of the inferior rectus muscle.

Radiological examination is confirmatory of the clinical findings and may reveal additional unsuspected injury. The most useful views are the Waters projection for the evaluation of maxillary and zygomatic fractures, the submentovertical view for the zygomatic arches, and the Townes technique for the subcondylar region of the mandible. The Panorex examination and oblique views of the mandible are useful for fractures of the body and ramus. An occlusal dental film will help in assessing palate fractures. Tomograms may be needed in some orbital floor and condylar fractures (*see* Chapter 26). Computed tomography is increasingly used for neurosurgical diagnosis and can provide the most exact diagnosis of facial fractures. Unsuspected fractures are often revealed and clinical judgement is extremely important to determine which fractures require surgical treatment.

FACIAL PARALYSIS

Partial or complete paralysis of the facial nerve may be congenital or may occur as a result of injury, tumour excision or disease. When the conditions of a traumatic or surgical wound permit, primary suture of the nerve trunk or its branches, using appropriate magnification, is the most satisfactory treatment. When a segment of the nerve is missing, a graft of branches of the cervical plexus or the sural nerve may be used to bridge the gap. If the wound is not satisfactory for these techniques as a primary procedure, the severed ends may be identified and tagged with sutures or haemostatic clips for secondary repair after primary healing of the wound. Nerve crosses using the ipsilateral hypoglossal or spinal accessory nerve have been advocated and may succeed in giving static tone to the face. They are less satisfactory than grafting because they result in mass facial movement of the paralysed side. In addition, they require sacrifice of the normal function of the donor nerve.

When paralysis has been present for more than a year, the degeneration of motor end-plates makes both spontaneous recovery and surgical repair of the nerve unlikely. Reconstructive procedures to substitute for facial muscle function are indicated to protect the eye, improve oral continence and support the sagging tissues of the face. Techniques for reconstruction include static suspension, dynamic substitution, mechanical or prosthetic devices, and creation of wrinkle lines and skin folds to improve appearance.

Palpebral function and protection of the cornea are the most important considerations in the upper face. The widened palpebral fissure may be narrowed by a permanent lateral tarsorrhaphy to suspend the lower lid or by a fascial strip to suspend the border of the lid from the medial tarsal ligament to the lateral orbital wall. The temporalis muscle and fascia can be transferred to provide dynamic suspension of the lower lid and may be used in both the upper and lower lids to allow voluntary closure of the eye (*Fig.* 22.11). This dynamic method is the most generally satisfactory procedure available. Other methods include insertion of a wire spring to allow upper lid closure and implantation of a gold weight in the upper lids for closure by gravity.

Suspension of the corner of the mouth and nasolabial fold area by autogenous fascia lata, either as a sheet or as strips, is one of the more common approaches to provide static support for paralysis of the lower face (*Fig.* 22.11). This is often combined with face-lifting techniques to eliminate excess skin and elevate the sagging side of the face or with dynamic techniques such as temporalis and masseter muscle transfers. Thompson has advocated previously denervated palmaris longus or short toe extensors, neurotized from the normal side, and nerve grafts from the normal side have

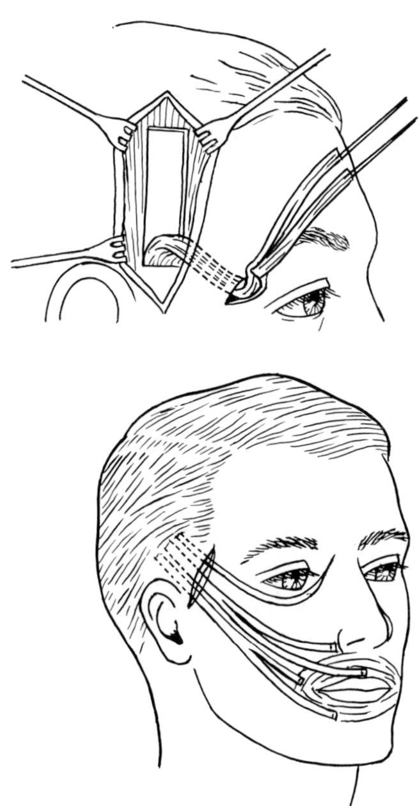

Fig. 22.11 Showing how temporalis muscle-fascial unit can be used to provide dynamic function to paralysed orbicularis oculi, and fascia lata grafts can give static support to paralysed muscles of lower face.

been attempted. These latter techniques have given inconsistently reproducible results and have not become widely used.

Other techniques used for facial paralysis include neurectomy and myomectomy of the hyperactive normal side, selectively excising segments of nerve, muscle or both. The most satisfactory results have been with neurectomy of the frontal branch for forehead asymmetry. Return of the hyperactivity has been common in the cheek. There is no procedure or combination of procedures which can restore the paralysed face to normality, and often the achievement of symmetry in repose is a major challenge. By selecting procedures to meet the individual requirements of patients, however, marked improvement is possible.

HEAD AND NECK TUMOURS

Reconstructive and plastic surgery has a major role to play in the management of head and neck tumours. Large and potentially mutilating resections are often necessary, yet it is important to re-establish a continent, functioning mouth and a presentable appearance.

Skin carcinomas of both the basal-cell and squamous-cell types may require only local excision with an appropriate margin, with primary closure. The fusiform excision should be planned along the normal lines of minimum skin tension. Often, however, closure will require a skin graft or a local flap which must be carefully planned to avoid disfigurement. As always, adequate resection is paramount and the reconstructive techniques must then be adapted to the defect. Excision should be combined with neck dissection when a carcinoma has metastasized to the cervical lymph nodes.

In malignant melanoma, the work of Clarke and Breslow in relating the depth of invasion and thickness of the tumour to metastases has made decisions on management more straightforward. If the tumour has not invaded the reticular dermis and is less than 0·75 mm in depth, local excision is adequate treatment when no cervical lymph nodes are palpable. With invasion into the reticular dermis and when the depth of invasion is greater than 1·5 mm, an elective node dissection improves the prognosis. If invasion has reached the level of the subcutaneous fat, elective node dissection is again not indicated because of the frequency of blood-borne metastases. However, involved lymph nodes should be excised (*see* Chapter 14).

In the resection of an intraoral carcinoma there is often a large defect which may involve a portion of the jaw as well as the lips, cheek, floor of mouth, tongue or palate. To obtain closure and function the surgeon needs to have available a number of flaps which can be raised and moved primarily. The forehead flap, based upon the superficial temporal and postauricular arteries on the ipsilateral side, has been a versatile tool for intraoral reconstruction in the past. The deltopectoral flap has been commonly used for reconstruction of the neck, floor of the mouth, chin and lips. Both the forehead and deltopectoral flaps are axial flaps based upon direct cutaneous arteries. The trapezius myocutaneous flap can serve in many situations as an alternative to the deltopectoral flap, and the latissimus dorsi and pectoralis major myocutaneous flaps have been used with increasing frequency. Some intraoral defects, especially in areas of radiation damage, are best closed with a free-flap which can be anastomosed to vessels outside the area of radiation damage. Free composite osteocutaneous and osteomyocutaneous flaps have permitted some of the most satisfactory and elegant reconstructive results following resection of the tongue, floor of mouth and jaw.

CONGENITAL ANOMALIES

Congenital anomalies of the head and neck and external parts of the body are a natural part of the scope of plastic surgery because the prime surgical requirement for correction is frequently a repositioning or remodelling of abnormal structures, or the construction of absent features. A knowledge of normal structure and function is the essential basis for the correction of these abnormalities. The most common congenital problems treated by plastic surgeons include cleft lip and palate, embryological abnormalities of the branchial arches and clefts, thyroglossal duct anomalies, hypospadias and congenital hand anomalies (*see* Chapters 23 and 25).

Microtia

The external and middle ear are formed from elements of the first and second branchial arches. While microtia may be seen clinically as an isolated finding, it is usual to discover an associated abnormality of the temporomandibular joint or other stigmata of a more involved branchial arch syndrome. These include underdevelopment of the maxilla, mandible, temporal bone, zygoma, and muscles of mastication, expression and palatal movement, as well as macrostomia. These syndromes are usually grouped under the title of hemifacial or craniofacial microsomia. A hereditary syndrome involving these structures bilaterally is called mandibulofacial dysostosis (Treacher Collins syndrome).

Reconstruction of the external ear is begun at age 4–6 years. The usable portions of the microtic ear are repositioned and a framework of carved costal cartilage or alloplastic material is placed beneath the hairless skin in the proper location. After some months the ear is brought out from the side of the head using the skin graft posteriorly. The external auditory canal and middle ear are not reconstructed in unilateral microtia because present techniques cannot bring hearing to within the necessary 20 dB of normal for binaural hearing. In bilateral middle ear anomalies with significant conduction deafness, early use of bone-conducting hearing aids is essential for normal development of the auditory cortex

Hypospadias

Hypospadias is approximately as common as cleft lip and palate, occurring in some degree in about 1 in 300 live male births. The urethra may end anywhere along its penile course. It is fortunate that the most severe degrees of hypospadias are the least common. Hypospadias is usually associated with chordee, a downward deflection of the shaft of the penis caused by fibrous scar-like tissue which may be embryologically related to the missing distal corpus spongiosum. Newborns with hypospadias should never be circumcised because the preputial skin is invaluable for the corrective surgery. In the past, correction was usually performed in stages. The first procedure was correction of the chordee, after which urethral construction was done in one or two steps with urinary diversion through the perineal urethrostomy. Single stage corrections such as those described by Mustarde and by Horton and Devine have become increasingly popular in recent years. The incidence of complications such as fistulas and strictures remains significant in all present techniques of surgery (*see* Chapter 84).

AESTHETIC SURGERY

Aesthetic surgery may be defined as surgery intended to improve the appearance of the patient. As such, it would encompass both the correction of disfigurement, as in scar revisions, and the enhancement of normal appearance through cosmetic surgery. The dividing line between these areas is sometimes indistinct. All of plastic surgery may be considered aesthetic in so far as it strives to achieve the most pleasing possible result.

The concept of body image is important in aesthetic surgery. A person's body image may be considered as simply the way the individual views his physical appearance in the mind's eye. Our body images change as we grow and age, influenced by the perceptions of what is considered normal, attractive and desirable in our culture, and our reactions to expressions of admiration or disapproval in those around us. The body image may be seriously disrupted by disfigurement; it may or may not be 'realistic' in relation to the perception of others. The basic goal of aesthetic surgery is to change the appearance of the patient in order to correct disequilibrium in the body image.

The selection of patients for aesthetic surgery is crucial, since a pathological body image may be more appropriately treated by psychiatry than surgery. Gillies is reported to have said that vanity is the best reason for aesthetic surgery. Patients who simply want to feel better about their appearance are much more likely to achieve their goals than those looking for secondary gain in the form of business or personal success. Cosmetic surgery has not yet saved a foundering marriage or transfused professional talent. If the patient's goals are unrealistic the surgeon cannot be successful.

Prominent Ears

Prominent or protuding ears are a common problem resulting from congenital absence of the antehelical fold or an excessively high concha or both. Surgery to correct this problem is highly successful. It may be done before the child starts school, or with local anaesthesia at 7 or 8 years of age.

Rhinoplasty

The nose reaches its adult shape during adolescence, with the development of mature facial bone form, and indeed may be considered in this sense a secondary sexual characteristic. As the most prominent and central feature of the face, it is not surprising that requests for surgical improvement in its appearance are common. The appearance of the nose is largely determined by the underlying bony and cartilaginous skeleton. Injury, disease and developmental events which alter the nasal skeleton result in the variation seen clinically in patients requesting surgery.

Except in conditions such as rhinophyma, surgery is concerned with alteration of the nasal skeleton, allowing the skin to shrink and drape itself over the new nasal contour. The operation is done through intranasal incisions, often with regional and topical anaesthesia. Operative steps tailored to the individual patient may include removal of bony cartilaginous hump, narrowing of the nasal bones, repositioning of the nasal bones and septum, and careful trimming of the lateral and alar cartilages. The final result must appear symmetrical, properly proportioned and in the midline of the face. A great deal of skill may be required to achieve this result. In other cases a lack of support may call for bone and cartilage grafts, judicious narrowing of the nostril floors and excisions at the alar base.

Surgery for the Ageing Face

In an era when Western society seems to place ever-increasing emphasis on youthfulness, requests for aesthetic surgery are becoming more and more common from both men and women. The progressive loss of turgor and elasticity in the facial skin, and relaxation in the subcutaneous musculo-aponeurotic system result in sagging of the eyelids, increased palpebral fat accumulations, facial wrinkling and jowl formation and relaxation of the skin and platysma muscle in the neck. Patients may have very specific requests for improvement or may need correction in all areas. Virtually all of these operations may be done with either local infiltration anaesthesia using epinephrine, or with general anaesthesia which may include hypotensive techniques.

In many cases the patient's objective may be realized by excision of the redundant skin of the eyelids with removal of the fat protrusions beneath the orbicularis oculi muscle. Care must be taken to avoid producing ectropion by excision of too much skin from the lower lids. If the brows are significantly ptotic, elevation by skin excision just above the eyebrow or a forehead lift through a coronal incision may be required.

The face lift procedure involves elevating the skin of the cheek and neck through an incision hidden in the hair, and following the contours of the preauricular area. The thin fascia of the subcutaneous musculo-aponeurotic system may be plicated with sutures or dissected and advanced, and the platysma muscle may also be tightened or partially excised to eliminate the folds in the anterior neck. Localized fat accumulations in the submental and submandibular region may be excised. All of this dissection must be done with great care to avoid injury to the branches of the facial nerve and haemostasis must be meticulous to avoid postoperative haematoma. The skin is advanced and the excess excised before closing the wounds.

Fine wrinkling is effaced temporarily following face lifting by the postoperative oedema, but is not eliminated. Radial wrinkles about the mouth have been treated by dermabrasion, but the most successful elimination of fine wrinkles follows chemical peeling of the skin produced by the application of a phenol-containing solution.

Reduction Mammoplasty

Operations to correct excessively large breasts have been a part of the surgical repertoire for many years. Women with gigantomastia are subject to upper back pain, an involuntary round-shouldered posture, painful cutting-in of the brassière straps on the shoulders and submammary intertrigo, as well as self-consciousness and interference with physical activity. When the deformity is moderate the nipple and areola may be transposed on a pedicle with excision of the hyperplastic tissue inferiorly or laterally. More severe degrees of ptosis and enlargement may require removing the nipple-areolar complex and replacing it at the end of the operation as a free graft on the reconstituted breast mound, following amputation of the excess breast fat. The operation is uniformly successful in correcting the patient's complaints and the aesthetic result with modern techniques is generally quite good.

Augmentation Mammoplasty

Breast augmentation for mammary hypoplasia, or to increase the size of small normal breasts, has become increasingly popular since the availability of relatively inert soft implants made from dimethylpolysiloxane. These may consist of a thin silicone rubber shell filled with a silicone gel or with saline. The implant is placed between the breast and pectoral fascia through either a short submammary incision or an areolar incision. The implants rapidly are incorporated into the body image, but of course remain a foreign material encased in scar capsule from a physiological point of view. If the capsule remains thin the appearance and feel of the augmented breasts is quite natural; however, in as many as one-third of the patients, one or both capsules become thickened and contracted. In some cases it is necessary to rupture the scar capsule by manual compression (closed capsulotomy) or to do a second surgical procedure (open capsulotomy).

Breast Asymmetry

Asymmetry of the breasts is quite common, but of usually minor degree. When it is significant enough to prompt the request for surgery the operation should be tailored to the individual patient. Some women may require reduction mammoplasty on the larger side, some augmentation of the hypoplastic side, and some a combination of both. Unilateral hypoplasia may be associated with a small or absent pectoralis major muscle which contributes to the deformity.

Gynaecomastia

Enlargement of the male breast commonly occurs at puberty without evidence of endocrine abnormality. Small degrees of subareolar enlargement may spontaneously subside in a year or two. However, feminine breast development in an adolescent male is often a source of great concern and requires surgical correction. This is generally done through an incision at the margin of the areola, the breast tissue being removed in segments if necessary. The skin of the breast shrinks appropriately after removal of the excess tissue except in the most severe hypertrophies.

Body Sculpturing

A variety of operations have been devised to remove the redundant and ptotic skin folds which may remain after massive weight loss, or to improve the body contours distorted by localized accumulations of fat. Reduction mammoplasty and mastopexy, sometimes done for these indications, have already been discussed. The loose abdominal skin present after multiple pregnancies or weight loss may be dealt with by abdominoplasty. Using a low transverse incision, the skin is mobilized to above the rib margins and advanced, with excision of the excess. The umbilicus is left *in situ* on the abdominal wall and brought through a new opening in the skin. Other body sculpturing procedures are less satisfactory because of scarring and difficulty in attaining a truly aesthetic result. These include excision of flabby ptotic skin of the buttocks in the gluteal crease, 'thigh lifts' using an anteromedial incision below the groin, and excision of skin folds from the arms.

RECENT ADVANCES AND THE WAY AHEAD

Reconstructive and plastic surgery has been a discrete specialty for only a brief time. During the past fifty years the principles outlined in this chapter have been applied to numerous deformities. In addition to the specific problems discussed, the field includes skin malignancies, burns, and congenital and acquired hand deformities. These have been covered in other sections of the text and, therefore, not repeated here.

Because the specialty is young, it is constantly changing as old principles are applied to new problems and new discoveries are made. Several recent advances will help to guide the reconstructive and plastic surgeons in the years ahead.

Wound Healing

The basic aspects of wound healing described in Chapter 1 are fundamental to the entire scope of reconstructive surgery, providing understanding of observed phenomena and allowing the planning of new clinical approaches to wound problems. The same is true for new advances in wound healing research. The recent discovery that there are at least four different types of collagen, found in different ratios in different tissues, will probably lead to the ability to modify and control chemically some aspects of healing and scar formation. Agents such as colchicine, steroids, and β-aminopropionitrile, which interfere with collagen synthesis and cross-linking, are research tools which will guide the development of clinically useful drugs to modify the healing response. The observation that some fibroblasts have structural and physiological characteristics of smooth muscle cells (myofibroblasts) is already suggesting clinical applications in the management of patients. In addition, a number of factors such as vitamin A and scarlet red may enhance epithelization. With further development these new research findings may permit the clinical control of undesirable scar effects, not only in skin but in conditions such as oesophageal stricture and cirrhosis.

Craniofacial Malformations

During the past decade new horizons have opened in the treatment of congenital malformations involving the skull and facial bones. The cranium enlarges and is moulded by the growth of the brain, laying down new bone along the cranial sutures. The pattern of cranial and facial growth seems to be determined by the cranial base. When the cranial and craniofacial suture lines close and fuse prematurely, this normal growth and expansion is distorted. The resulting deformities of Crouzon's disease, Apert's syndrome, unilateral plagiocephaly, and other syndromes have until recently been refractory to surgical management.

The pioneering work of Tessier in devising a combined intracranial and extracranial approach to these problems has led to a new and highly specialized field of surgical endeavour. At first these osteoplastic procedures were done only in adults, but early correction is now seen as an advantage to try to foster normal growth. The strip craniectomies of the cranial sutures, done for many years by neurosurgeons to prevent deformity, have been extended to the frontosphenoid and fronto-ethmoid sutures, and only the cranial base itself remains inaccessible. The enlarged cranium of the controlled hydrocephalic can also be reduced. This type of surgery requires a team of highly specialized surgeons and supporting professionals, and is therefore concentrated in major centres. There is real hope that in the future many of the severe craniofacial abnormalities will be prevented by early intervention.

In the wake of this technical advance has come new research in bone grafting and bone healing. Differences in the vascularization, survival and absorption of membranous and endochondral bone grafts are being investigated. The mechanisms of the induction of new bone formation by implantation of demineralized bone powder, coralline hydroxyapatite, and other substances are under study, as well as the role of periosteum in bone regeneration. The possibility of inducing regeneration in bony defects is a tantalizing goal, as yet unachieved with regularity.

Genitalia Reconstruction

The development of musculocutaneous flaps has allowed genital reconstruction to be advanced. Gracilis musculocutaneous flaps from the medial thighs can provide tissue for construction of a vagina or penis following radical tumour ablation. The inherent blood supply of these flaps make the reconstruction safe even in the face of heavy irradiation.

In addition to these advances in genitalia reconstruction following tumour ablation, surgeons have been able to apply microsurgical techniques for trauma cases. Amputation of the penis as a result of a deviant act or self-mutilation is no longer an unreconstructible disaster. Successful replantation can be accomplished with microanastomoses of both vessels and nerves.

A final application of advances in flap surgery for genital reconstruction has been in cases of gender dysphoria. Gender reassignment surgery to provide female or male external genitalia is now quite successful.

Reconstruction of the Breast

Reconstruction after a mastectomy for cancer is becoming a frequent procedure with the development of new surgical techniques. There should be no reason for the cancer surgeon to compromise his treatment of the patient to permit reconstruction. If there is sufficient skin remaining the plastic surgeon may simply create a breast mound with an implant, and reconstruct the nipple-areolar complex with tissue from the remaining side or grafts from the ear, groin or genital regions. Additional skin to replace scar and radiation damage may be obtained with the latissimus dorsi musculocutaneous flap, the medially based thoraco-epigastric flap, or by covering the area with omentum and using a split-thickness skin graft. When a radical mastectomy has been done the latissimus dorsi muscle can provide tissue to fill out the infraclavicular hollow. All of these techniques simply provide more adequate skin cover for a breast mound created by an implant. The transverse rectus abdominus myocutaneous flap can provide both skin cover and an adequate breast mound for most patients. It is much more difficult technically, however, and associated with more potential complications. Fear of hiding a recurrence is probably not justified since the skin remains accessible to examination and the deep chest wall is not a frequent site for residual tumour.

There also has been a trend in recent years to advocate subcutaneous mastectomy, simple mastectomy, or 'total mastectomy' for patients with premalignant disease in situ carcinoma of the breast. In such cases, the nipple itself should have a core of tissue removed to excise the ducts. There is usually no shortage of skin for reconstruction, and indeed there is sometimes an excess which must be tailored. Reconstruction is done using either subcutaneous or submuscular implants, with nipple-areolar reconstruction as needed.

Bone Replacement

Great strides have been made in the replacement of bony defects. Induction of bone formation has been mentioned. Long bones and mandibular reconstruction is being undertaken with microvascular anastomoses. The pectoralis major myocutaneous flap carrying a vascularized rib, and direct arterial osteocutaneous flaps from the rib, scapula and iliac crest, have provided reliable ways to reconstruct the mandible after radiation and in other difficult situations. Segments of fibula are transferred to large bone defects created by radical tumour ablation or trauma. The anastomoses of the interosseous vessels supplying the fibula to appropriate recipient vessels provides for an immediately viable bone graft capable of growth. This capability will revolutionize tumour surgery of the head and neck and sarcomas.

Further Reading

McDowell F. (1977) *The Source Book of Plastic Surgery.* Baltimore, Williams & Wilkins.
McGregor I. A. (1980) *Fundamental Techniques of Plastic Surgery and their Surgical Applications*, 7th ed. Edinburgh, Churchill Livingstone.

Section 3

Head and Neck Surgery

23 *Swellings of the Neck*

A. G. D. Maran and P. M. Stell

INTRODUCTION

The head and neck is an intricate anatomical region, and many of its structures have highly complex and important physiological functions. Of the many deformities and diseases of this area, those of most interest to the general surgeon are the congenital lesions, trauma and tumours.

Because of the highly complex anatomy and physiology of this area, different specialties have developed to deal with different problems since no clinician alone can deal effectively with all disease in this area. Indeed the management of many disorders of the head and neck entails the co-operative effort of specialists from several disciplines. Examples of interdisciplinary co-operation include the treatment of carcinoma of the pharynx by an otolaryngologist and a plastic surgeon, the combined efforts of an oral surgeon and an otolaryngologist in the treatment of tumours of the upper jaw, and of a plastic surgeon and an orthodontist in the management of cleft palate.

Although diseases of the head and neck may be discussed from several different angles, there are certain common threads running through most of these diseases. These include disordered respiration and deglutition, disordered sensation, and the necessity of providing a satisfactory cosmetic outcome, since most of the operations on the head and neck are carried out on a visible and highly emotive part of the anatomy.

Because many of the operations on the head and neck interfere with the patient's respiration, swallowing, or external appearance, reconstructive surgery plays a large part in surgery of the head and neck. Reconstruction may also be needed to restore normal or near-normal appearance. The restoration of normal function is usually aimed at achieving a normally functioning oral cavity or pharynx. The functions of the oral cavity may be interfered with by congenital lesions (e.g. cleft palate), by trauma, or by the resection of tumours. Restoration of a normally functioning oral cavity, with respect to both speech and deglutition, entails the restoration of a competent oral seal, stable upper and lower jaws, normal dentition and a tongue of normal bulk and mobility. These essential components of a normally functioning oral cavity are restored by appropriate corrective procedures on both the bony skeleton and soft tissues. Ablative operations which cause deformity of the external appearance must also be minimized. Often this requires the restoration of both bony contours and soft-tissue outline.

Investigations

The investigations of a patient with a disease of the head and neck include the investigation of disordered physiology, radiology and endoscopy.

The investigation of disordered physiology in the head and neck seldom includes the use of biochemistry, as it does for so much of abdominal surgery, and indeed the common biochemical parameters are seldom abnormal in disease of the head and neck, apart from patients with a prolonged period of severe dysphagia for food, when the patient may become dehydrated, hypoproteinaemic and hypokalaemic.

On the other hand, disorders of the head and neck often interfere markedly with many physiological functions which can be tested. Objective and accurate methods for the testing of hearing, balance and sight have been in established clinical use for a long time. These tests are often very important in the preoperative investigation of a patient with disease of the head and neck, e.g. a careful examination of the visual acuity, visual fields and ocular muscles may establish the presence of involvement of the orbit by a tumour of the maxillary antrum. Tumours may also interfere with one or both phases of speech: phonation produced by the larynx, and articulation by the mouth. Tests of disordered function in these areas are much less often used and are much less refined, but this area would almost certainly be a fruitful one for research.

Radiology, as in other parts of the body, may be required to give information about certain static structures, and may also help in the elucidation of disordered physiology. The important static structures are the bones and cartilage of the head and neck, though it is often possible to outline the soft tissues, such as the soft palate, and the cervical oesophagus. The important radiological abnormalities of the bones and cartilage of the head and neck include fractures and invasion of the bones of the facial skeleton by tumours arising in neighbouring soft tissue. Thus, for instance, destruction of the bony outlines of the maxilla is virtually always seen in tumours of the maxillary antrum, and invasion of the mandible (an important event both for treatment and prognosis) occurs in about 15% of malignant tumours within the mouth. Radiology also contributes significantly to the elucidation of disordered physiology, notably of swallowing, but also of the larynx, where appropriate techniques may demonstrate loss of mobility of the internal structures of the larynx, an important consideration which affects both the treatment of tumours and the long-term prognosis.

CT scanning and magnetic resonance are of most use where endoscopy is impossible or operative exploration not recommended. In head and neck disease they have a very large part to play in the investigation of nasopharyngeal tumours and other tumours around the base of the skull. They are useful techniques in investigating the spread of maxillary cancer but they have little part to play in the investigation of the oropharynx, larynx, hypopharynx or oral cavity. Endoscopy and the simple clinical examination skills accompanied by fine-needle aspiration biopsy, can achieve more than the radiological high technology offered by these modalities.

Endoscopy also forms an important part of the investigation of many patients with disease of the head and neck. Examination of the inside of the laryngeal and pharyngeal cavities was developed towards the end of the 19th century and was established by the 1930s. Bronchoscopy and oesophagoscopy were introduced into clinical practice at the same time. These methods still remain very valuable, particularly for the investigation of patients with tumours of this area, both to assess the extent of the tumour and to allow an adequate piece of tissue to be obtained for biopsy. The more recently developed flexible endoscopes may have a part to play in assessment of disease of the larynx and pharynx, though their place has not as yet been defined. It seems unlikely that they will replace rigid endoscopy of this area. Flexible endoscopes also allow other structures within the head and neck, notably the nasopharynx, nasal cavity and the interior of the maxillary antrum, to be examined. Nasoendoscopy is also used for the assessment of velopharyngeal patency in patients with cleft palates.

The accuracy and definition of laryngoscopy may also be improved by the addition of the operating microscope in the technique of microlaryngoscopy which allows more accurate definition and photography of a tumour.

Perhaps the most useful advance in the investigation of head and neck disease has been the increasing reliability of fine-needle aspiration biopsy. This is because of the increasing number of pathologists who are specializing in cytology. It is such a specialized technique that these specimens cannot be sent to a general pathology laboratory and there have to be only a few people interested in the technique in any centre. Accuracy rates of over 95% are essential if a service is to be established. False negatives are always interpreted in the light of clinical findings and this is where the 'errors' come. In tumour investigation false positives would be very serious and would bring the service into question.

Very little work seems to have been carried out in the use of tumour markers in the investigation of head and neck cancer. The relationship between nasopharyngeal cancer and the Epstein–Barr virus (EBV) is becoming increasingly sophisticated. In Hong Kong it is now being used as screening for cancer amongst high-risk persons such as first-degree relatives. An elevated serum titre of IgA to the viral capsid antigen (VCA) of 1:10 or greater may be the first indication of subclinical nasopharyngeal carcinoma. It is the practice now to admit such patients for multiple nasopharyngeal biopsies even in the absence of symptoms or signs, especially when titres of other EBV-specific antibodies are also elevated. This has also been the only tumour where imprint smears are of use. Nodes are removed from patients with nasopharyngeal carcinoma and imprint smears made for staining for the nuclear anti-Epstein–Barr virus (EBNA) in the tumour cells before submitting the specimen for histopathology.

CONGENITAL NECK LUMPS

Lymphangiomas

The cystic hygroma (*Fig.* 23.1) is one of the lymphangiomatous tumours which include simple lymphangiomas and cavernous lymphangiomas. These may be combined with haemangiomatous elements.

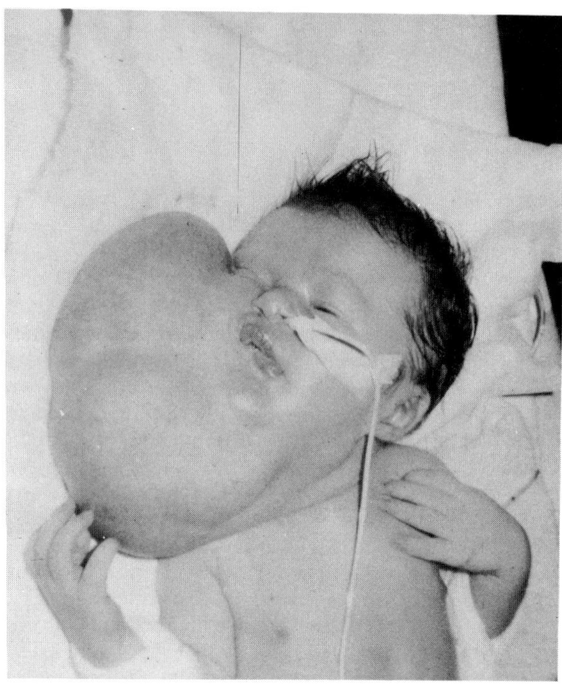

Fig. 23.1 Cystic hygroma.

Embryology

The lymph system arises from five primitive sacs (two jugular sacs, two posterior sciatic sacs and a single retroperitoneal sac) developed from the venous system. Endothelial buds from these extend centrifugally to form the peripheral lymphatic system.

There are two theories of origin of lymphangiomas: either they may be sequestrations of lymphatic tissue derived from portions of the primitive sacs, which retain their rapid proliferative growth potential and have no connection to the normal lymph system or they may arise from endothelial fibrillar membranes which sprout from the walls of the cyst, penetrate surrounding tissue, canalize and produce more cysts.

Pathology

Lymphangiomas have been classified into three groups:

1. Lymphangioma simplex, composed of thin-walled capillary-sized lymphatic channels.
2. Cystic hygroma, composed of cysts varying in size from a few millimetres to several centimetres in diameter.
3. Cavernous lymphangioma, composed of dilated lymphatic spaces often with fibrous adventitia.

The smaller lymphangiomas occur in the lips, tongue and cheek where the tissue planes are tighter, whereas the cystic hygroma has more space to expand into the tissue planes of the neck. Simple lymphangiomas can occur anywhere in the mouth as pale, soft, fluctuant lesions; they form one-third of all lymphangiomatous tumours. More common are cavernous lymphangiomas which form 40% of these lesions, mainly occurring in the tongue. At the base of the tongue they must be differentiated from a lingual thyroid, a lingual carcinoma or an internal laryngocele. They also occur on the lateral border. Some cheek lesions reach an enormous size and are very difficult to eradicate since total excision produces an unacceptable cosmetic defect.

A cavernous lymphangioma of the floor of the mouth can be part of a cystic hygroma or may be a ranula. Macrocheilia usually affects only the upper lip.

Cystic hygroma forms 30% of the whole. It consists of large, multinodular cystic masses which may communicate or be isolated. The walls are thin and the contained fluid can be clearly seen. A hygroma occurs in the cervicofacial region spreading into the cheek, mouth, tongue, parotid and even the ear canal.

Histologically the cyst is lined by a single layer of flattened endothelium, with fetal fat and cholesterol crystals. They are rare tumours forming 0·5% of large series of neck lumps. There is no sex or side predominance. Two out of 3 are noted at birth, and 9 out of 10 before the end of the second year.

Thirty-five per cent of lymphangiomas of all types occur in the cheek, tongue and floor of mouth, 25% in the neck and 15% in the axilla.

Clinical Features

Most of these tumours manifest themselves at birth or shortly afterwards. Lymphangiomas in the mouth can first appear in adult life as can recurrences of cystic hygromas after surgery in infancy. Recurrences usually occur on the periphery of the facial area where the main mass originally presented, such as the ear, parotid or posterior triangle.

While size alone is the prominent first symptom and sign, if the cyst is big enough it can cause stridor. In very large cysts a lateral displacement of the trachea and even mediastinal widening may be seen on the radiograph.

Sudden increase in size due to spontaneous haemorrhage may be fatal. Brachial plexus compression with pain and hyperaesthesia may also occur.

Treatment

Cystic hygroma should be excised. Other treatments described include aspiration, incision and drainage, injection of sclerosants and radiotherapy.

Incision and drainage should only be done for infection which is rare. Injection with sclerosants should be avoided because of the proximity to major vessels and nerves; it also thickens the walls and tissue planes and makes surgery much more difficult.

Young patients should not be irradiated because of the dangers of retarded bone and tissue growth and thyroid malignancy. Surgery should only be delayed in the premature infant; delay in otherwise healthy infants only leads to continuing morbidity and increased mortality. It has been suggested that complete regression occurs in 15% but other authors claim never to have seen this.

No operation should be done without a preoperative chest radiograph to rule out mediastinal involvement. Damage to the facial, hypoglossal and accessory nerves may be difficult to avoid. It is difficult to get a good cosmetic result in huge cysts because of the tissue displacement and the large amount of skin that must be removed.

Intraoral lymphangiomas should be removed from an external approach since they are almost certainly much more extensive than expected. Lymphangiomas of the base of the tongue can often be dealt with by coagulation diathermy, repeated if necessary. Cryosurgery may also be helpful. Lymphangioma of the upper lip should be dealt with by a lip shave and vermilion advancement and excision of muscle and cyst to produce a lip of acceptable size.

Recurrences usually appear within the first 9 months in about 10–15% of patients. The recurrence rate is higher with cavernous lymphangioma than with cystic hygroma. The problem with the latter is residual cysts growing with the patient.

Midline Dermoid Tumours

Pathology

There are three varieties of dermoid cyst in the head and neck:

1. The epidermoid cyst which has no adnexal structures is lined by squamous epithelium and may contain cheesy keratinous material. This is the commonest variety.

2. The true dermoid cyst (*Fig.* 23.2) which is lined by squamous epithelium and contains skin appendages such as hair, hair follicles, sebaceous glands and sweat glands. These are either congenital or acquired. The congenital type is derived from ectodermal differentiations of multipotential cells pinched off at the time of closure of the anterior neuropore. It therefore occurs along lines of fusion. The

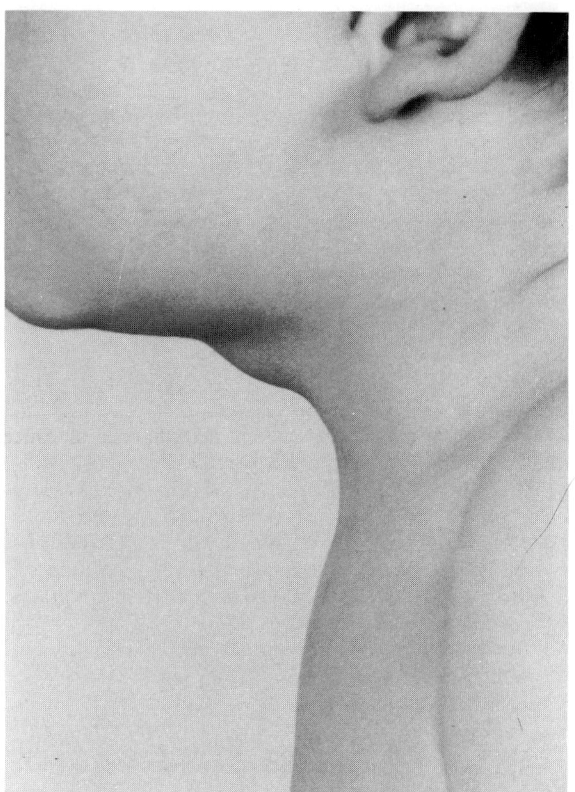

Fig. 23.2 True dermoid cyst in the sublingual region.

acquired type is due to implantation of epidermis at the time of a puncture type of injury. It is often solid with cystic spaces containing sebaceous material.

3. The teratoid cyst can be lined by squamous or respiratory epithelium and it contains elements formed from ectoderm, endoderm and mesoderm—nails, teeth, brain, glands, etc. This is the rarest variety in the neck and is nearly always diagnosed in the first year of life.

Twenty per cent of all dermoid cysts are found in the neck, and 30% in the head and face. Dermoids form 30% of all midline cysts and there is no sex predominance.

Clinical Features

These cysts present as solid or cystic masses in the midline of the neck between the suprasternal notch and the submental region. They can also occur lateral to the submandibular gland. Painless swelling is the only symptom, but if the cyst is large, minor obstructive symptoms can occur.

About 20% of dermoids occur in the mouth, either deep to the mylohyoid (sublingual) or superficial to it (submental). They present in the second and third decades, but are probably present since birth.

Treatment

Complete excision is usually easy and should be done in all cases.

Thyroglossal Duct Cysts (*Fig.* 23.3)

The commonest midline neck cyst is a remnant of the thyroglossal duct. This cyst can occur anywhere in the area bounded by the foramen caecum above, the manubrial notch inferiorly and the anterior borders of the sternomastoid laterally.

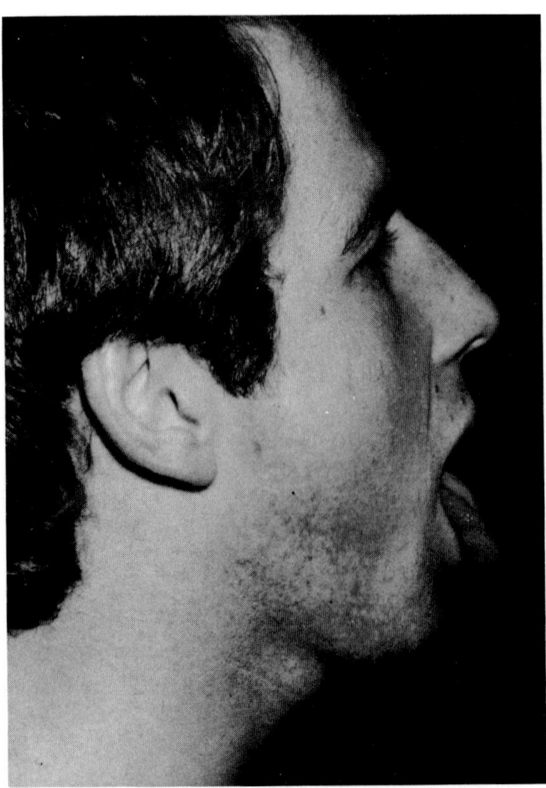

Fig. 23.3 Thyroglossal cyst with upward displacement on protrusion of the tongue.

Embryology

The thyroid anlage arises from the floor of the primitive pharynx midway between the first and second pharyngeal pouches. It becomes a hollow tube that soon loses its lumen to become solid as it migrates to the lower neck. The distal end divides into two portions which become the lobes of the thyroid gland; the stalk, if it persists, becomes the thyroglossal duct and pyramidal lobe. The duct atrophies at the sixth week, but persists at the top end as the foramen caecum. If it does not atrophy it remains as a persistent thyroglossal duct. Since the tongue develops later than the thyroid anlage, the thyroglossal duct is buried deep in the foramen caecum, and since the hyoid bone develops even later, the duct can run in front, behind and usually through the bone.

Pathology

Men and women are equally affected. The age range is from 4 months to 70 years with a mean of 5½ years. Ninety per cent are in the midline and 10% are to one side of the midline; of these 95% are on the left and 5% are on the right. Their site is as follows:

Prehyoid	75%
Thyroid cartilage level	15%
Suprahyoid	5%
Cricoid level	4%
Base of tongue	1%

The duct is always subcutaneous and spontaneous fistula formation is rare. A fistula is usually the result of infection, attempted drainage of a misdiagnosed abscess, or inadequate removal of the hyoid. The cyst and the duct are lined by squamous epithelium, but thyroid tissue is rarely found in the wall.

Clinical Features

Ninety-five per cent present with a painless cystic lump which moves on swallowing or protruding the tongue. The cyst is mobile in all directions and usually is transilluminable. If it is low in the neck the subcutaneous tract can often be seen. Five per cent present with tenderness and rapid enlargement due to infection.

Fistula is present in 15% of cases and is usually the result of a previous operation or an infection.

Suprahyoid cysts may be mistaken for a submental adenitis or a dermoid. Prehyoid cysts are nearly always dumb-bell or bar shaped and can push the base of the tongue upwards causing dysarthria. If the cyst is near the surface of the tongue base it must be distinguished from a lingual thyroid or a carcinoma. Cysts low in the neck must be differentiated from a thyroid adenoma by a thyroid scan. Other diagnoses to be considered are sebaceous cyst and lipoma.

Treatment

Thyroglossal duct cyst should be removed, including the central portion of the hyoid bone (Sistrunk's operation). Small openings into the vallecula consequent on removing the bone can easily be closed.

Thyroglossal Duct Carcinoma

Over 100 cases of thyroid carcinoma arising in a thyroglossal duct cyst have now been described. The tumour is always a papillary thyroid carcinoma. Most presented as benign cysts, and the diagnosis was only made by histology.

There is a slight female preponderance (4:3) and the peak age incidence for women is 30–40 and for men 50–60 years. Only 10% have metastases compared to 40–50% for carcinoma arising in an ectopic thyroid.

The treatment is local excision followed by suppressive doses of thyroxine.

Branchial Cysts (*Fig.* 23.4)

Origin

There are four theories of the origin of branchial cyst but because of the complicated development of the neck none has been proven by embryological investigation. Most of the theories have attempted to correlate clinical findings with known embryological facts but none can stand close scrutiny.

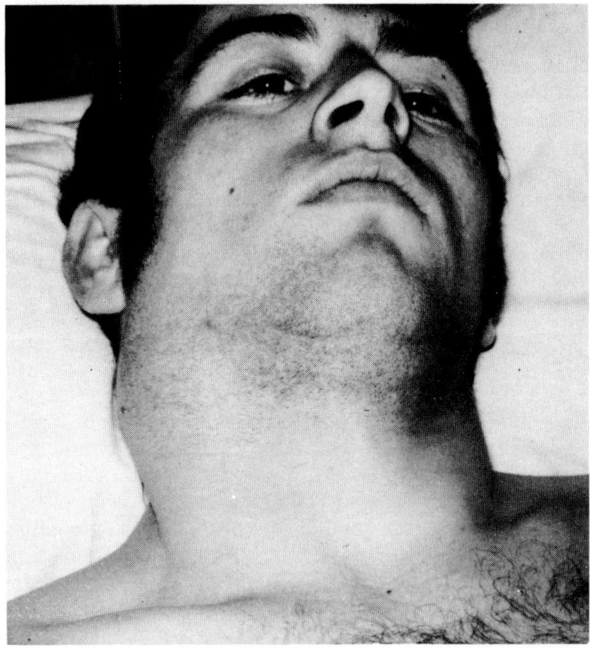

Fig. 23.4 Right-sided branchial cyst. The swelling was noted by the patient after an upper respiratory tract infection.

1. Branchial Apparatus Theory

These cysts may represent remains of the pharyngeal pouches or branchial clefts or a fusion of these two elements.

A 2-week-old embryo has on each side 6 branchial arches, 5 branchial clefts and 5 pharyngeal pouches. These arrangements are not parallel, but tend to come together at the sixth arch. The first and second arches are important, the third and fourth less so, and the fifth and sixth vestigial.

The second pharyngeal pouch forms the palatine tonsils; the second arch grows downwards on its lateral side to meet the fifth arch, thus enclosing the second, third and fourth clefts forming the cervical sinus of His. By the sixth week the branchial apparatus has disappeared, having formed the ear, tongue, hyoid, larynx, tonsils and parathyroids.

Origin from the third or fourth pouches is unlikely, as they would have to pass over the hypoglossal nerve to reach the skin and would be severed by the upward movement of that nerve during development.

A fourth arch pouch tract would also have to pass below the subclavian artery on the right and the aortic arch on the left.

A third arch pouch should have its internal opening in the pyriform fossa and a fourth arch pouch below this. These have never been described, so that origin from these pouches can be discounted.

Origin from the first pouch is possible because high branchial cysts have been described lying under the parotid gland with an internal opening between the bony and cartilaginous meatus. If the branchial apparatus theory were to be upheld one would expect many more cysts to have internal openings; it is a popular misconception that many branchial cysts have an internal opening. One would also expect more cysts to be present at birth. Not only has this only once been described but the peak age incidence is in the third and fourth decades which is late for a congenital lesion (cf. thyroglossal duct cysts).

2. Cervical Sinus Theory

This is an extension of the previous theory and considers that branchial cysts represent remains of the cervical sinus of His which is formed by the second arch growing down to meet the fifth. It is unlikely that this is true for those with an internal tract since this is closed by a fusion of its ectodermal lining from within towards the surface. This makes an internal opening difficult to achieve.

3. Thymopharyngeal Duct Theory

Cysts may be a remnant of the original connection between the thymus and the third branchial pouch from which it takes origin. The originator of this theory presumed that the hyoid bone constituted the lower level of branchial derivatives. Not only is this false but a persistent thymic duct has never been described. Furthermore, no branchial cyst has ever been described deep to the thyroid gland nor have there been any examples of tracts between the pharynx and the thymus.

4. Inclusion Theories

Finally it has been suggested that the cyst epithelium arises from lymph-node epithelium or that the cysts are the result of epithelial inclusion in lymph nodes. The following facts support this theory:

a. Most branchial cysts have lymphoid tissue in the wall and are found in the parotid and also the pharynx.

b. The peak age incidence is later than expected for a congenital condition.

c. A branchial cyst in a neonate is rare.

d. This theory also explains why a branchial cyst rarely has an internal opening or at best a tract with an ill-defined termination. However, a skin pit, usually found in the lower neck, does have a big tract, with no cysts in the tract and no internal opening. These pits are probably unconnected with branchial cysts and are probably due to malfusion in the development of neck skin.

In summary, therefore, cysts with a proven internal opening are probably derived from the second or first branchial pouch, but the majority, without an internal opening, are probably due to epithelial remnants in lymph nodes. The lesion is therefore probably neither 'branchial' nor 'congenital'.

Clinical Features

Sixty per cent occur in men and 40% in women; the peak age incidence is the third decade, the range being from 1 to 70 years. Two out of three are on the left side. Two per cent are bilateral. Two-thirds are anterior to sternomastoid in the upper third of the neck and the remainder are in the middle and lower thirds, the parotid, the pharynx and the posterior triangle.

The presenting features are:

Continuous swelling	80%
Intermittent swelling	20%
Pain	30%
Infection	15%
Pressure symptoms	5%

Seventy per cent are cystic on palpation and 30% are solid.

Pathology

Cysts are usually lined by stratified squamous epithelium but may be lined by non-ciliated columnar epithelium. More than 80% have lymphoid tissue in the wall; this may be due to chronic infection or may indicate origin from a lymph node. The cyst contains straw-coloured fluid in which cholesterol crystals can be found.

Treatment

Branchial cysts should be removed.

A carotid angiogram may be considered to exclude a chemodectoma if there is direct or transmitted pulsation and the cyst feels solid.

Branchial fistulas and tracts should be dealt with by an elliptical excision of the pit and an initial dissection of the tract to as high a level as possible. A second skin incision should then be made at the highest level of dissection to complete the removal—the so-called 'step-ladder' method.

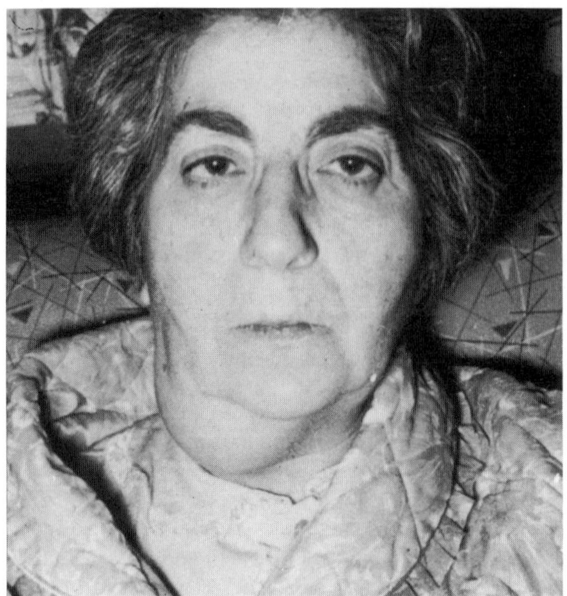

Fig. 23.5 Laryngocele.

Laryngocele (*Fig.* 23.5)

A laryngocele is a large air-containing sac arising from the laryngeal saccule.

Pathology

In the UK the incidence is approximately 1 per 2½ million population per year. The sex incidence is 5:1 in favour of men and the peak age incidence is 50–60 years. Eighty-two per cent occur in Caucasians. Eighty-five per cent are unilateral and 15% bilateral. They can be external (30%) where the sac arises from the laryngeal ventricle and expands into the neck through the thyrohyoid membrane, internal (20%) where it arises from the laryngeal ventricle and stays within the larynx, presenting in the vallecula, or combined (50%). Laryngoceles are lined by columnar ciliated epithelium whereas simple laryngeal cysts are lined by squamous epithelium.

It has long been held that laryngoceles are due to 'blowing' hobbies or jobs such as trumpet playing or glass blowing. A careful review of the published cases reveals at most 4 patients were subject to these habits so that this theory appears to be untrue. Of more importance is the coexistence of a carcinoma of the larynx which acts as a valve allowing air under pressure into the ventricle.

Lower animals have air sacs, e.g. the cheek pouch of monkeys, the fish pouch of pelicans, the tracheal sacs of emus, the syrinx of male quacking birds, etc. Lateral laryngeal sacs are well developed in certain anthropoid apes and are a means of enabling the animal to rebreathe while holding its breath for long periods.

Laryngoceles in man, therefore, are almost certainly atavistic remnants corresponding to these lateral air sacs. On occasion they become manifest due to an increase in intralaryngeal air pressure due to blowing or coughing.

Clinical Features

The commonest presenting features are hoarseness and a swelling in the neck. The third commonest symptom is stridor which can come on very suddenly over a period of a few days or even hours in a patient who had previously only mild symptoms for months or years. Other presenting symptoms are dysphagia, sore throat, snoring, pain or cough. Ten per cent present with infected sacs—pyoceles—and because of the mixture of infection and air on the radiograph a diagnosis of gas gangrene is sometimes made. On palpation, the swelling, which is usually large and over the thyrohyoid membrane, can be emptied easily.

A plain radiograph of the neck is diagnostic showing an air-filled sac. To diagnose smaller laryngoceles one must keep the condition in mind and radiograph every patient with hoarseness since this is the commonest presenting symptom. This radiograph should be done with the glottis open since the detection rate falls markedly when the larynx is under tension. All patients with a laryngocele should have a careful laryngoscopy to exclude carcinoma.

Treatment

All laryngoceles should be removed because of the danger of laryngeal obstruction. The most thorough method is to remove the superior half of the thyroid ala, after raising a perichondrial flap, to get at the neck of the sac. The ventricle is closed and the closure is reinforced by the perichondrial flap.

If the patient presents with a pyocele this should be treated with antibiotics before surgery.

INFECTIVE NECK LUMPS

Tuberculous Cervical Adenitis (*Fig.* 23.6)

Pathology

The condition is not common in the USA or Europe, but it is still common in Asia and Africa. There are 32 000 new cases of tuberculosis (TB) in the USA each year and 5% of these (1600) get cervical lymphadenitis.

Where the incidence of TB is low, primary infections are acquired later, so that tuberculous nodes occur in young adults. In the UK, the maximum age incidence is 5–9 years, but 1 in 3 occur over the age of 25 years.

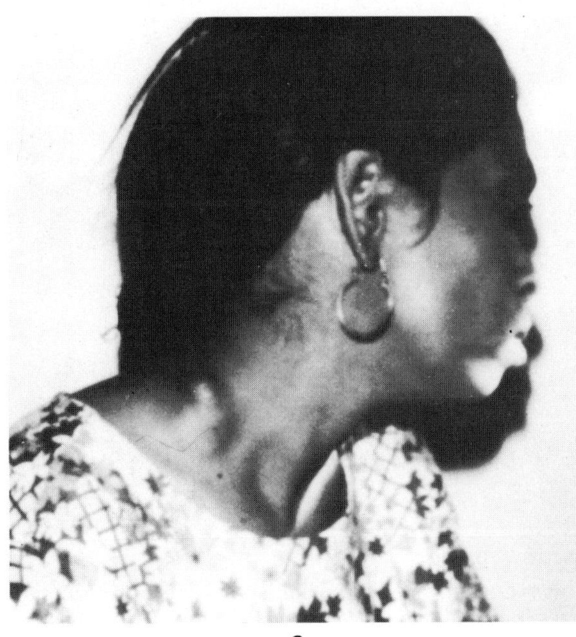

a

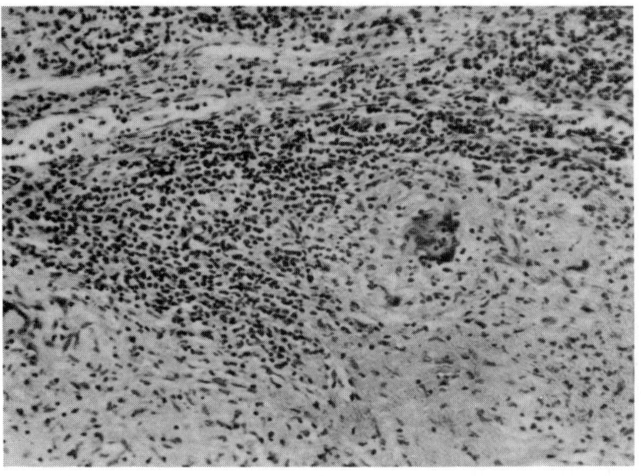

b

Fig. 23.6 *a*, Tuberculous lymph nodes affecting the posterior cervical group. *b*, Histology of the excised nodes from the same patient showing a tubercular follicle.

The bacillus is usually of the human variety, compared to the situation 40 years ago when the bovine type was commonest; atypical mycobacteria (*see* Chapter 5) may also cause lymphadenopathy. The bacillus reaches the lymph nodes by direct drainage or by haematogenous spread. The incidence of coexisting pulmonary TB is less than 5%. In one series almost half of the excised tonsils showed evidence of TB, and it thus appeared that the tonsil was the source and that the cervical adenitis was precipitated by an attack of acute tonsillitis. Once the bacillus has entered the host further exposure is not necessary to trigger off the adenopathy.

Clinical Features

Most patients give a fairly long history and usually seek medical advice because the lumps have become painful. In Asia the presentation is different: 20% have discharging sinuses, 10% a cold abscess and 10% are adherent to the skin; these patients usually have a negative chest radiograph.

Ninety per cent are unilateral and 90% involve only one node group, the commonest being the deep jugular chain followed by the nodes in the submandibular region and then those of the posterior triangle.

Diagnosis is by a positive tuberculin skin test, demonstration of acid-fast bacilli in the biopsy and growth of *Mycobacterium tuberculosis* from the biopsy. In the USA patients should also have histoplasmin and coccidioidin skin tests (*see* Chapter 39). The differential diagnosis is between lymphoma and metastatic cancer. The absence of a primary tumour in a young adult and the length of history usually makes the latter diagnosis improbable.

Treatment

The treatment is an excisional biopsy followed by 9–12 months of antituberculous chemotherapy. If the nodes are very large and matted local removal is dangerous since the nodes are often attached to the internal jugular vein. A functional neck dissection should then be done preserving the sternomastoid, accessory nerve, and jugular vein if possible. In a child it is usually wise to remove and examine histologically the tonsils before removing the lymph nodes.

If removal is not followed immediately by chemotherapy a sinus forms with persistent drainage and later ugly scars.

Sarcoidosis

Sarcoidosis presenting as cervical adenitis with no other manifestation of the disease is extremely rare. The neck nodes are not often involved in this condition even when it is generalized. It is almost impossible, therefore, to make a preoperative diagnosis and a biopsy is always needed. The histological characteristic is the absence of caseation. Other clinical and radiological findings will confirm the diagnosis. The Kveim test is now seldom used.

Neck Space Infections

Neck space infections are very rare and there is confusion about how many neck spaces there are—estimates vary from 13 to 20. A fascial space is an area of loose connective tissue bounded by dense connective tissue called fascia. It is a matter of opinion how thick connective tissue must be before it is called fascia and this is where the disagreement as to the number of spaces arises. Knowledge of the anatomy of the areas in which infection tended to collect was important in the pre-antibiotic days from the point of view of routes of spread, complications, and surgical drainage, but nowadays knowledge of three spaces will allow management of 90% of patients.

Retropharyngeal space: This space lies between the

pharynx and the posterior layer of the deep fascia which bounds the prevertebral space. It separates the pharynx from the vertebral column and extends from the base of the skull to the posterior mediastinum as far as the bifurcation of the trachea. Anteriorly it connects with the pretracheal space so that infections can spread via this latter space to the anterior mediastinum. However mediastinitis due to a retropharyngeal abscess is rare. In the infant this space contains one or two lymph nodes.

The lateral pharyngeal space is more commonly known as the parapharyngeal space; it lies lateral to the pharynx connecting with the retropharyngeal space posteriorly. Laterally it is bounded by the lateral pterygoid muscles and the sheath of the parotid gland. It extends from the base of the skull to the level of the hyoid bone where it is limited by the sheath of the submandibular gland. This sheath is also connected to the sheaths of the stylohyoid muscle and the posterior belly of the digastric muscle.

The parapharyngeal space is bounded anterosuperiorly by the pterygomandibular raphe and the spaces around the floor of the mouth anteroinferiorly. This space is prone to infection because of its close connection to the tongue, teeth, parotid, submandibular gland and tonsils.

The submandibular space is bounded above by the mucous membrane of the floor of the mouth and tongue and below by the deep fascia that extends from the hyoid to the mandible. It is divided into two by the mylohyoid muscle so that the submandibular gland, which is wrapped around the mylohyoid muscle, extends into both parts of the space. The space superior to the mylohyoid muscle is called the sublingual space and contains the sublingual gland. The space inferior to the muscle is the submaxillary space which contains the gland. Anteriorly lies the submental space between the two anterior bellies of digastric.

Infections of this space are known as Ludwig's angina.

Clinical Features and Management

Retropharyngeal Abscess

This occurs in children and adults. In infants it is due to a lymphadenitis secondary to an upper respiratory tract infection. The child has a sore throat; examination shows a swelling behind an otherwise normal tonsil. The temperature is elevated to 38–39 °C and the child is ill. The swelling may obstruct the posterior nares and push the soft palate down. Respiratory obstruction is an ever-present danger because a child's spine is short and his larynx is high. (In a 9-month-old infant, the epiglottis is at the level of the atlas.)

Radiographs of the neck show a large retropharyngeal swelling. Treatment is by incision and drainage in the tonsil position.

In an adult, a retropharyngeal abscess usually signifies a tuberculous infection of the cervical spine. It is of insidious onset with a low-grade fever. Pus must be obtained to confirm the diagnosis which is also suggested on a radiograph of the cervical spine. Treatment is by antituberculous chemotherapy.

Parapharyngeal Abscess

This is more common in adults than children. It is a complication of tonsillectomy or tonsillitis in about 60% of patients and a complication of infection or extraction of the lower third molar in a further 30%. Infection of the petrous apex can rarely rupture directly into the space. Infection of the mastoid tip can also enter the space via the digastric sheath but is exceedingly rare now.

There is fever and marked trismus because of involvement of the medial pterygoid muscle. The tonsil is pushed medially but looks normal. The most marked swelling is in the neck at the posterior part of the middle third of the sternomastoid muscle. Each patient should be given at least 48 h treatment with an antibiotic, but as by the time most patients have a swollen neck, incision and drainage will be required (*Fig.* 23.7).

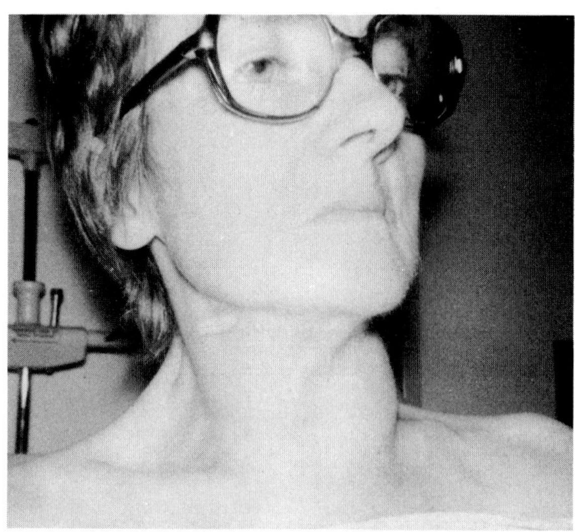

Fig. 23.7 Parapharyngeal abscess.

Ludwig's Angina

This is a rapidly swelling cellulitis of the floor of the mouth and submandibular space secondary to soft-tissue infection, tonsillar infection and infection of the lower premolar and molar teeth. Over 80% of patients have dental disease and in these patients the lower molars are set eccentrically with the roots closer to the inner than to the outer side of the jaw, or the roots of the second and third molars may lie inferior to the mylohyoid line. Root abscesses of these teeth therefore drain into the submaxillary rather than sublingual space. This space may be affected with minimal discomfort from the tooth, pain comes from tension within the bone but if this gives way and drains there is no dental pain. In cases of dental origin the most usual organisms are *Streptococcus viridans* and *Escherichia coli.*

When the infection spreads to the sublingual space the floor of the mouth becomes very swollen and appears as a roll of oedematous tissue rising to the level of the biting edge of the teeth. The tongue is elevated posterosuperiorly and respiratory obstruction is a danger. The patient is very ill with a temperature of over 38·2 °C (101°F) with pain, trismus and salivation.

Treatment is by antibiotics; incision and drainage should be postponed as long as possible because pus is seldom found.

Infectious Mononucleosis

Pathology

This condition is probably caused by the Epstein–Barr virus although a similar disease can be caused by cytomegalovirus infection. It is infectious, common in young people and spread by personal contact, such as kissing.

The disease is self-limiting, but it has been postulated that it is an atypical benign form of leukaemia. Atypical mononuclear cells derived from lymphocytes form 10–20% of white cells in the peripheral blood and infiltrate the spleen and lymph nodes (and occasionally the liver, brain, kidneys and bone marrow).

Clinical Features

The presenting symptom is often a sore throat with high fever, anorexia and general malaise. The tonsils enlarge and are covered by exudate. The cervical lymph nodes are enlarged and rubbery. Skin rashes, mild jaundice, aseptic meningitis and peripheral neuropathies may occur. Prolonged debility and depression often complicate recovery. More than 10% of mononuclear cells are found on the blood film and a monospot test is positive. Even in the absence of jaundice the serum bilirubin and aminotransferases may be raised.

Treatment

Antibiotics are contraindicated, especially ampicillin which often causes a skin rash in this condition. To prevent relapse, patients should not be allowed back to work if there is persistent adenopathy. Tracheostomy is sometimes required for upper airway obstruction.

Toxoplasmosis

In a patient with all the clinical manifestations of infectious mononucleosis and a negative monospot test, this diagnosis must be considered. It is due to infection with the small protozoon *Toxoplasma gondii.* Children can acquire it from their pets since infection is widespread among many domestic and wild animals in Europe and South America. Pregnant women can pass it on to the fetus causing death in utero, premature birth or congenital malformations, including macular degeneration and ocular nystagmus. Diagnosis is made serologically or by lymph-node biopsy.

The illness can last a few days or less commonly weeks or months.

Treatment is by pyrimethamine and a sulphonamide.

Brucellosis

Pathology

The host for the brucella is the cow for *Brucella abortus,* the pig for *B. suis* and the goat for *B. melitensis.* Man contracts brucellosis by contact or by consuming products from these animals. It is commonest in farmers, vets and abattoir workers.

Clinical Features

The varied symptoms make diagnosis difficult. Common symptoms are: an unexplained undulating fever of the Pel–Ebstein type which continues for some weeks and subsides only to return a few weeks later, sweating, debility, fatigue, anorexia, sore throat and headache. Examination reveals neck node enlargement, hepatosplenomegaly and arthralgia. Diagnosis rests largely on suspicion and is confirmed by agglutination tests.

Treatment

The acute form responds to tetracycline and chloramphenicol, but the chronic form is resistant.

TUMOURS OF NEUROGENOUS ORIGIN

Peripheral Nerve Tumours

The neural crest differentiates into the Schwann cell and the sympathicoblast; this latter cell gives rise to paraganglionic cells from which arise chemodectomas and glomus jugulare tumours, and ganglionic cells from which arise benign and malignant ganglioma. The Schwann cell gives rise to the Schwannoma (neurilemoma) and the neurofibroma (*Table* 23.1). Nerve tumours are rare, forming only about 1% of all head and neck tumours.

Table 23.1 Neurogenic tumours arising from neural crest cells

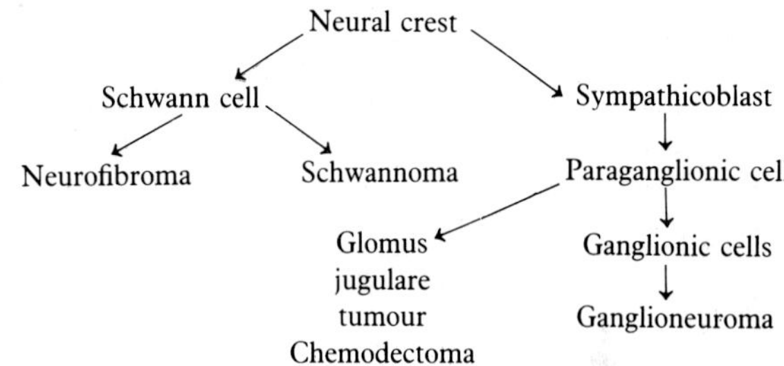

Pathology

The thin outer sheet of nerve is called the neurilemma and the inner sheath of Schwann is the neurolemma. Tumours arising from the inner nerve sheath are often called neurilemomas which is wrong, as is neuronoma. The correct name is Schwannoma and these are clinically different from neurofibroma.

Peripheral nerve tumours are commoner in the head and neck than the rest of the body and are commonest in the lateral part of the neck. They arise from the cervical and brachial plexus and ninth to twelfth cranial nerves, but most commonly from the vagus within the carotid sheath. They are all commoner in women than men. The differentiating features between Schwannoma and neurofibroma are shown in *Table* 23.2.

Histologically, Schwannomas show well-developed cylindrical bands of Schwann cells and delicate connective tissue fibres with a tendency toward pallisading of the nuclei about a central mass of cytoplasm (Verocay bodies). This is known as Antoni type A tissue whereas Antoni type B tissue is a loosely arranged stroma in which the fibres and cells form no

Table 23.2 The differences between Schwannoma and neurofibroma

Schwannoma	*Neurofibroma*
Solitary	Usually occur as part of the syndrome of multiple neurofibromatosis
Never associated with von Recklinghausen's syndrome	Often associated with von Recklinghausen's syndrome
Painful and tender	Asymptomatic
Encapsulated	Non-encapsulated
Seldom malignant	8% malignant

distinctive pattern. These two types may be mixed with one predominating. No neurites traverse the lesion.

Neurofibromas show a compact arrangement of spindle type cells arranged in streams and twists. They can present as cutaneous or subcutaneous masses or as a deep-seated plexiform neuroma involving major nerve trunks.

Other neurogenous tumours—ganglioneuroma, Schwannoma, glioma, meningioma, paraganglioma, neuronaevi—occur more often in patients with neurofibromatosis than in the general population. This suggests that neurofibromas are derived from a disseminated neuroblastoma or aberrantly migrating neural crest cells.

Gangliomas are also called ganglioneuromas; they are very rare. They usually arise from a cervical sympathetic ganglion; are firm, smooth, well encapsulated and microscopically contain ganglion cells and neurites. Twenty-five per cent are estimated to be malignant and these neuroblastomas grow relentlessly.

Postoperative neuromas are the result of amputation or trauma to the nerve. They are not true tumours but represent attempts by the damaged nerve to repair itself; the axis cylinders become enmeshed in Schwann cells and scar tissue. If this process becomes hyperactive the neuroma becomes clinically obvious and the patient experiences localized pain and tenderness.

Malignant change in nerve sheath tumours in the head and neck is very rare: only 1 sarcomatous change in a series of 303 of solitary nerve tumours. But such change occurs in from 10 to 15% of patients with multiple neurofibromatosis. The only thing that differentiates a neurogenous sarcoma from a fibrosarcoma is its origin from a nerve trunk.

Surgery in neurofibromatosis does not predispose to sarcomatous change. Rapid growth suggests malignant change; pain and paraesthesiae occur when a large nerve is involved. These tumours do not metastasize to regional lymph nodes, but to the lungs. Two in three recur locally and may metastasize later. Low-grade tumours grow slowly and anaplastic ones quickly.

Clinical Features

These tumours enlarge slowly over a period of years with no symptoms and a painless neck mass as the only sign. While the tumour remains benign there is no interference with nerve function apart from pressure on the sympathetic chain which soon shows as a Horner's syndrome. Even when the tumour becomes malignant, the nerve may still function even when the tumour reaches a large size. Diagnosis is from other lateral neck masses; an angiogram is usually required. If the tumour presents as a pharyngeal mass diagnosis is from other parapharyngeal space tumours such as deep lobe parotid tumours, minor salivary gland tumours, chemodectoma, lymphoma and hibernoma.

Treatment

The diagnosis of a solitary nerve tumour is made by excising it which is also the treatment.

The nerve with which the tumour is associated only becomes evident at operation in 1 patient out of 4. The nerve may be stretched over the capsule of the tumour or less commonly the tumour can lie in the central core of the nerve with the fibres spread around it. Every effort should be made to preserve the nerve.

Postoperative neuromas must be excised to distinguish them from recurrent cancer.

The best treatment for malignant nerve tumours is en bloc excision of the area. The cure rate varies from 80% for well-differentiated malignant Schwannoma to only 20% for the undifferentiated type.

Chemodectomas

Nests of non-chromaffin paraganglionic cells derived from the neural crest occur on the carotid bulb, the jugular bulb, in the cavity of the middle ear, in the ganglion nodosum of the vagus nerve, the adventitia of the ascending aorta, the aorta, the innominate and pulmonary arteries and in the ciliary ganglion of the orbit. Carotid body cells act as chemoreceptors so that it is suggested that tumours of these cells be called chemodectomas.

The only condition that affects chemoreceptor tissue is neoplasia.

Pathology

There is a high incidence of chemodectoma in Peru where most of the population live at altitudes of 2000–5000 m. This is probably due to the fact that chronic hypoxia at high altitudes leads to carotid body hyperplasia. A raised incidence has also been noted in other series from high altitude sites such as Colorado and Mexico City.

In other areas this tumour is rare: there have been just over 500 cases described in the literature.

The average age of presentation ranges from 35 to 50 years, the youngest reported case being 12 years. The sex incidence is roughly equal.

There is a striking family history in 10% of cases. There is a tendency to bilateral tumours, tumours of other similar cells and concurrent phaeochromocytoma. Twenty-five per cent are bilateral in those with no family history.

The globular or ovoid tumour is firmly adherent to the bifurcation of the common carotid artery, but seldom grows to more than 4–5 cm. The cut surface is homogeneous, solid and grey-brown in colour.

Histology shows a marked similarity to the architecture of the normal carotid body: large uniform epithelioid cells surrounded by a vascular stroma. There are capillaries (shown by silver staining) in the fibrous septa between the cell nests. These tumours are non-secreting.

Proven metastases are very rare, there being only 30 cases reported and not all of these stand scrutiny. There have been no reports of autopsies in which the death of the patient was attributed to a chemodectoma of the carotid body. Many of the cases claimed as malignant have in fact turned out to be due to metastases from a papillary carcinoma of the thyroid.

Clinical Features

All patients present with a painless lump in the neck which is palpable in the region of the carotid bulb. The lump is said to move from side to side but not up and down—this is not helpful because nearly all neck lumps in this area exhibit this mobility be they cystic or neoplastic.

There is always a long history varying from 4–5 to 7 years. This is helpful in differentiating a lump in this site from a lymphoma or a metastatic node, but is compatible with a tuberculous node or a branchial cyst. About 30% of patients have a pharyngeal mass pushing the tonsil medially and anteriorly; this mass should not be biopsied.

The normal site of growth of the tumour is from the inner aspect of the notch of the bifurcation of the carotid artery causing displacement and separation of the internal and external carotid arteries (*Fig.* 23.8). If growth occurs mainly on the medial side (which is the usual side of origin) a pharyngeal swelling occurs with no lateral neck swelling. The tumour may grow up the vessels to the base of the skull.

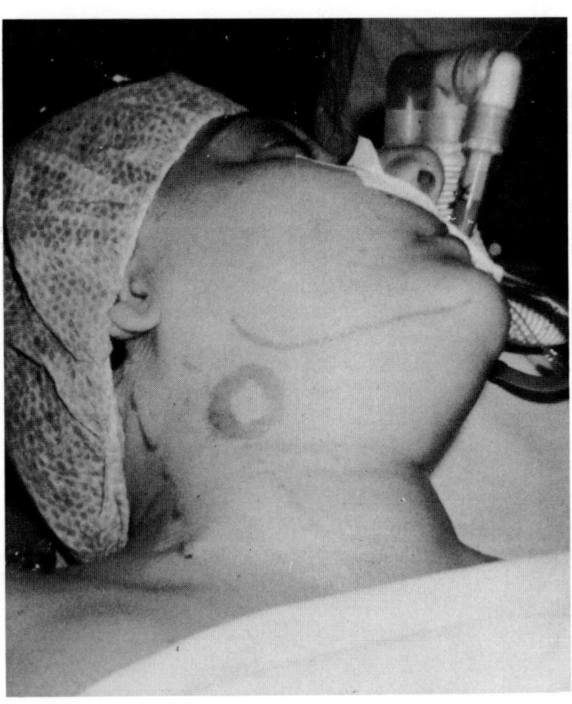

Fig. 23.8 Carotid body tumour. The surface markings outline the sternomastoid and the mandibular margin.

The mass is firm and rubbery and usually demonstrates transmitted rather than expansile pulsation. A bruit may be present and the mass may decrease in size with carotid compression to refill in stages with each pulsation. Rarely, patients complain of mild dysphagia or discomfort. Large tumours may involve the ninth, tenth, eleventh and twelfth cranial nerves and occasionally the sympathetic chain, causing a Horner's syndrome.

Diagnosis

The diagnosis is usually erroneously made at an operation for biopsy of a neck mass. The diagnosis can be made provisionally on the history of a longstanding neck mass in a young patient and on physical examination. Whenever it is suspected a carotid angiogram (*Fig.* 23.9) should be done for the following reasons:

1. To see if there is separation of the internal and external carotid arteries with a tumour circulation in the mass. The feeding vessel arises from the external carotid or vertebral artery.
2. To determine the extent of the tumour.
3. To see if there is cross circulation. If the tumour is to be resected and the artery grafted it is essential to know about cross circulation so that the patient and the surgeon can balance the risk of the procedure against the possible benefits.

An angiogram nowadays in young fit people carries very little risk. The radiologist should use fast injection rates and rapid serial filming.

In the capillary phase there is an internal blush and the draining veins are usually dilated. The differentiation between chemodectoma and glomus vagale tumour is based only on the position of the tumour. The technique can be enhanced by the use of subtraction techniques.

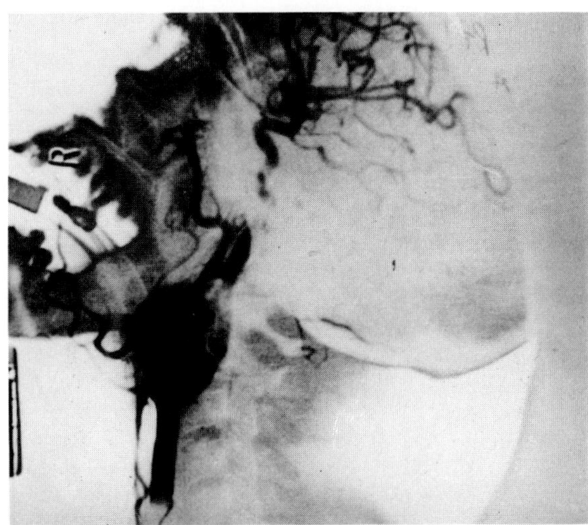

Fig. 23.9 Angiogram of a carotid body tumour.

Treatment

From 1930 to 1950 various reported series put the operative mortality rate at around 35% and the morbidity rate at 45% including frequent hemiplegia. It was concluded 'that it would seem doubtful whether anything more than a diagnostic biopsy should be done where tumours are without symptoms and growing slowly'. With advances in arterial surgery, carotid bypass, hypothermia and a better understanding of the physiology of cerebral blood flow allowing better selection, the mortality from the operation has fallen dramatically. Most would now agree that the mere presence of a carotid body tumour does not justify an attempt at removal, but removal is indicated for:

1. Tumours which are histologically and clinically malignant and which are resectable.
2. Tumours growing aggressively.
3. Patients in good health under 50 years of age with a small or medium-sized tumour.
4. Those tumours which have extended into the pharynx and palate and are interfering with swallowing, speaking and breathing.

Since no patient has died from the tumour the indications for surgery should be as conservative as possible.

It was originally thought that chemodectomas and all related tumours were radio-resistant, but some have now been shown to respond to radiotherapy. Radiotherapy should therefore be used in patients who should have surgery but who refuse, for poor-risk patients, or in metastatic disease.

Glomus Vagale Tumours

This tumour is extremely rare. It presents as a mass at the angle of the jaw, rather too high for a diagnosis of branchial cyst and too low for a diagnosis of a parotid neoplasm. Some cause pain and discomfort and a few a pharyngeal mass. Angiography shows an abnormal tumour circulation from the external carotid, at a higher location than that of a carotid body tumour. Removal of this tumour is much more difficult and potentially dangerous than removal of a carotid body tumour and if diagnosed is probably best referred to a surgeon who has experience in their removal.

After removal the patient will have a vocal cord paralysis

and should be offered a Teflon injection soon after the operation to improve glottic closure.

MALIGNANT NECK MASSES (*Fig.* 23.10)

The main malignant problem to be considered is secondary carcinoma metastatic to the lymph nodes in the neck.

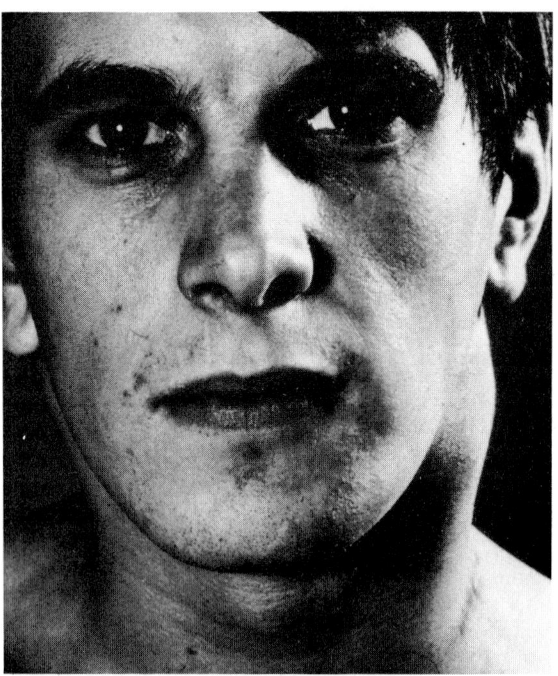

a

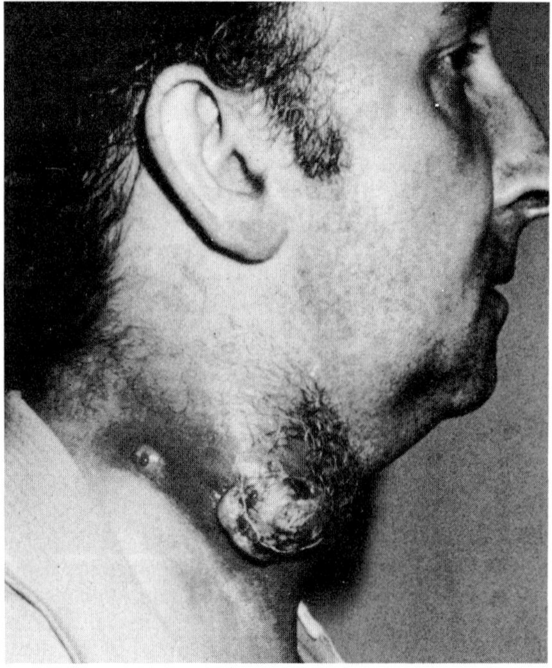

b

Fig. 23.10 *a*, Malignant neck nodes N1b. *b*, Malignant neck nodes N3.

Many carcinomas of the head and neck sooner or later metastasize to the lymph nodes of the neck which form a barrier that prevents further spread of the disease for many months. A carcinoma of the head and neck is assigned a stage which depends not only on the extent of the primary tumour (and the presence of distant metastases) but also on enlargement of the cervical lymph nodes. The current classification suggested by the UICC is shown in *Table* 23.3. This is a useful classification but is subject to some criticism. There is a great deal of observer error so that different observers only agree on the presence of palpable lymph nodes in about 70% of patients. Furthermore the value of the a and b categories is doubtful since these categories depend on a clinical opinion as to whether tumour is present in a palpable node or not and must therefore be entirely subjective; previous reports show that only 60% of palpable nodes contain tumour. The N3 grade is very contentious. There is little agreement of what is 'fixed'. Also the structure to which the node is fixed is important. For example a node fixed to skin has a very different prognosis than one fixed to the skullbase. Finally, the progression from N0–N3 suggests that the prognosis diminishes in that order whereas the prognosis for bilateral nodes (N2) is usually much worse than that for fixed nodes (N3).

Table 23.3 Clinical staging of cancer of head and neck

N—Regional lymph nodes
N0—Regional lymph nodes not palpable
N1—Movable homolateral nodes
  N1a—Nodes not considered to contain growth
  N1b—Nodes considered to contain growth
N2—Movable contralateral or bilateral nodes
  N2a—Nodes not considered to contain growth
  N2b—Nodes considered to contain growth
N3—Fixed nodes

For these reasons the AJC cervical lymph node classification is preferable. This is shown in *Table* 23.4. This classification puts emphasis on size which is more directly related

Table 23.4 AJC recommendations for lymph node staging

NX—Minimum requirements to assess the regional nodes cannot be met
N0—No clinically positive node
N1—Single clinically positive homolateral node 3 cm or less in diameter
N2—Single clinically positive homolateral node more than 3 cm but not more than 6 cm in diameter, or multiple clinically positive homolateral nodes, none more than 6 cm in diameter
N2a—Single clinically positive homolateral node more than 3 cm but not more than 6 cm in diameter
N2b—Multiple clinically positive homolateral nodes, none more than 6 cm in diameter
N3—Massive homolateral node(s), bilateral nodes, or contralateral nodes(s)
N3a—Clinically positive homolateral node(s), none more 6 cm in diameter
N3b—Bilateral clinically positive nodes (in this situation, each side of the neck should be staged separately; i.e. N3b: right, N2a; left, N1)
N3c—Contralateral clinically positive node(s) only

to prognosis. A node under 3 cm is N1 and a node 3–6 cm is N2. It is considered that any node more than 6 cm is automatically fixed to adjacent structures or consists of matted series of nodes and so the word fixation never appears. The N3 grade not only has nodes larger than 6 cm but includes the almost inevitably fatal bilaterally positive nodes and contralateral positive node.

The approximate distribution of patients between the four categories NO–N3 is shown in *Table* 23.5. The four categories of the UICC classification will be used as convenient headings to discuss various aspects of the management of metastatic nodes in the neck.

Table 23.5 Approximate incidence of lymph node metastases

NO	70%
N1	20%
N2	5%
N3	5%

Patients with No Palpable Metastases (NO)

Over 40 years ago it was suggested that when an operation was carried out for a carcinoma of the mouth, the nodes in the neck should be cleared at the time without waiting for involvement to become evident, i.e. a so-called elective neck dissection.

The pathological argument supporting this concept is that some lymph nodes may be involved by tumour (occult nodes) and still be impalpable. The incidence of such occult nodes at various sites is given in *Table* 23.6.

Table 23.6 Incidence of occult nodes

Supraglottic larynx	15%
Pyriform sinus	40%
Base of tongue	20%
Transglottic	10%
Glottic with a fixed cord	5%

It may be that elective neck dissection has some place in the patient who is unlikely to return for follow-up and has a tumour with a known high incidence of occult nodes such as the pyriform fossa, whereas there can be little or no reason to operate on a patient who can readily attend for follow-up and who has a tumour such as a laryngeal carcinoma where the incidence of occult nodes is small. In laryngeal carcinoma the incidence of occult nodes is in the region of 10–15% so that if all these patients are submitted to radical neck dissection 85–90% will suffer the increased morbidity and mortality associated with this operation to no purpose. Furthermore, there is some evidence that a patient with a laryngeal carcinoma with no palpable nodes in the neck is better treated by radiotherapy so that the issue of prophylactic neck dissection for laryngeal carcinoma scarcely arises in any case.

All these arguments may in any case now be becoming superfluous because it appears that elective irradiation of the entire neck can sterilize the vast majority of occult nodes. Elective neck irradiation drastically reduces the recurrence in the same side of the neck in patients with carcinoma of the mouth, oropharynx, pyriform fossa and supraglottic larynx.

Unilateral Neck Nodes (N1)

It is generally accepted, at least by surgeons, that surgery is required to control lymph-node metastases in the neck. The standard operation for dealing with metastatic nodes in the neck is that of radical neck dissection described by Crile in 1906; a further classic paper describing the indication, the technique and the complications was that of Hayes Martin.

Although the technique of radical neck dissection has been standard for many years several changes have taken place within the last 10 or 15 years, notably in the use of combined radiotherapy and surgery, in various technical modifications to reduce the incidence of complications, and in the so-called functional neck dissection.

Prevention of Complications

The incidence of major complications after radical neck dissection is low. The major potentially lethal complications of radical neck dissection are wound breakdown and infection, necrosis of the skin flaps and rupture of the carotid arteries. It is also well known that these complications are increased by previous radiotherapy. Two major modifications of technique have been introduced over the last 10 years to combat the major lethal complications—modifications of the incision and protection of the carotid sheath.

In the patient who has been irradiated, particularly one in whom a fistula is likely to form because a carcinoma in the larynx, pharynx or mouth has been resected, the carotid sheath should be protected. Two methods have been described: muscle flaps and free grafts of dermis. The former method is safer than the latter. The favourite muscle to use is the levator scapulae which derives its blood supply from superiorly and anteriorly. At the end of the radical neck dissection it can therefore be divided at its inferior and posterior limits and be turned forward to be stitched over the carotid sheath, protection being completed by stitching the muscle graft to the posterior belly of the digastric superiorly and the remnant of the sternomastoid muscle inferiorly.

Functional Neck Dissection

Attempts have been made to reduce the morbidity after a radical neck dissection by the so-called functional, conservative techniques. The long-term morbidity after radical neck dissection is due to the removal of the accessory nerve. Removal of both internal jugular veins can cause a very unsightly swelling of the face, in addition to dangerous increase in intracranial pressure on rare occasions. In a functional neck dissection the entire aponeurotic system of the neck, with its lymph nodes included, is removed preserving the sternomastoid muscle, the accessory nerve and the internal jugular vein. Although superficially attractive, this operation has not stood the test of time. In the N0 neck it carries the same recurrence rate as the full radical neck dissection and does not leave the patient with a stiff shoulder. On the other hand surgery on the N0 neck has virtually been abandoned in favour of elective radiation.

In the N1 neck, the recurrence rate after radical neck dissection is 25% and, although various claims were made by several authors that the recurrence rate after functional neck dissection was anything from 0 to 10%, it was difficult to understand how by removing less one got less in the way of recurrence. It has now been established that the true recurrence rate is very much higher after functional neck dissection if it is performed in a node positive neck and it has largely been abandoned.

It is of course well known that a restricted neck dissection of this type is indicated in papillary carcinoma of the thyroid gland, a tumour which does not rupture the capsule of the gland and therefore can be dealt with by a modified neck dissection, using a single transverse incision and preserving the sternomastoid muscle, the accessory nerve and the submaxillary space with sacrifice of the internal jugular vein.

The Occult Primary

One further problem to be discussed is the pathology, diagnosis and treatment where a lymph node in the neck is found to contain carcinoma but the primary site is apparently unknown.

Cancer presenting with a node in the neck is mainly a disease of men (men:women 4:1) with a maximum age incidence of 65 in men and 55 in women. Between one-third and one-half of all such nodes are replaced by squamous carcinoma, one-quarter by undifferentiated or anaplastic carcinoma and a similar number by adenocarcinoma if the supraclavicular nodes are involved, followed by a small number of miscellaneous tumours, including melanomas, thyroid gland tumours, etc.

In about one-third of patients a primary tumour can be found by investigation at the time of presentation. The primary sites in order of frequency are as follows: nasopharynx, tonsil, base of the tongue, thyroid gland, supraglottic larynx, floor of the mouth, palate and pyriform fossa (head and neck sites); bronchus, oesophagus, breast and stomach.

Careful follow-up will later reveal a primary site in up to one-third of patients. These primary sites are rather more commonly found in the head and neck than anywhere else and the sites are again those in the above list. The relative frequency of the various sites is as shown in *Table 23.7*.

Obviously the frequency of involvement of these sites will depend to some extent on the interest of the individual surgeon.

Table 23.7 Relative frequency of primary sites

Site	%
Oropharynx	15%
Nasopharynx	15%
Thyroid	20%
Hypopharynx	10%
Lung	20%
Gastrointestinal tract	10%
Miscellaneous distant sites	10%

In earlier times a malignant node in the neck has been called a branchiogenic carcinoma, that is a carcinoma arising in a branchial remnant. Twenty-eight cases were recorded by Crile as being branchial carcinomas but no real search was made for a primary tumour. The nose and throat were examined in some patients; in one the branchial carcinoma was said to have extended into the pyriform fossa and one had a nasopharyngeal carcinoma which was thought to be irrelevant. Chest radiographs were taken in only 11 (and in 3 of these definite metastases were present which may well have been lung primaries); radiographs of the skull and jaws were taken in 'several cases' only. As a result of Crile's paper many patients with a malignant node in the neck were thought to have a branchial carcinoma; since Crile had shown that treatment of this was difficult and the survival poor, it became standard practice to confine investigation to excision of the node; if squamous carcinoma was found a diagnosis of branchial carcinoma was made, no primary tumour was looked for and little further was done.

Hayes Martin was the chief opponent of this policy and urged strongly that a biopsy should be the last investigation to be done and that a search for a primary tumour must be made. He showed that these tumours were virtually always secondary to a primary tumour of the head and neck which could be treated, although he stated that a branchial carcinoma might be a real entity.

A diagnosis of branchial carcinoma might be legitimate in the following circumstances:

1. Survival without recurrence for 5 years after surgical eradication.
2. Autopsy proof that mouth, pharynx, larynx, trachea, oesophagus, lungs, nasopharynx, tonsils, salivary glands and thyroid gland (the last three by serial section) are free from primary cancer. At autopsy the nasopharynx is difficult to inspect satisfactorily—even more difficult than it is in life—and the nasal sinuses, even those most accessible to the pathologist, are seldom opened. A tiny epithelioma of the tonsils, a microscopic cancer of the thyroid gland or a miniature scar carcinoma of the lung apex, may require serial section for their detection. No recorded case of branchiogenic carcinoma has satisfied this criterion.
3. Demonstration of a carcinoma in a branchial cyst known to be of long standing, the patient surviving for 5 years symptom-free.
4. Histological proof of origin from tissues in branchial vestiges.
5. The tumour must be situated anterior to the border of the sternomastoid muscle.

Tumours satisfying all the above criteria are extremely rare, but a few cases have been recorded which seem likely to be true branchial carcinomas.

Investigations

The steps to be followed are those used in the investigations of any patient with an undiagnosed lump in the neck (*Fig. 23.11*). In patients with suspected secondary malignancy in the cervical lymph nodes, the areas to be covered include:

1. Primary sites: head and neck
   Inspection, palpation, radiology, endoscopy, biopsy, cytology, and supravital staining.
2. Cervical lymph nodes
   Inspection, palpation, pattern, level, aspiration, excision, morphology, histology.
3. Other primary sites
   General physical examination, radiology, laboratory tests, endoscopy, biopsy, cytology.

The lists of radiological investigations were formidable at one time but experience has shown that apart from the chest, imaging any area from which there are no symptoms or signs shows a very low yield and often results in unnecessary delay and expense in treatment.

Endoscopy is to be meticulous and should be illuminated by fibreoptics, particularly when examining the nasopharynx, the bronchi and the oesophagus. If no primary tumour is found a blind biopsy should be taken of the posterior wall of the fossa of Rosenmüller and of the pyriform fossa on the same side. It is also preferable to remove the tonsil on the same side and have it examined by multiple sections.

Supravital staining with toluidine blue may be useful in

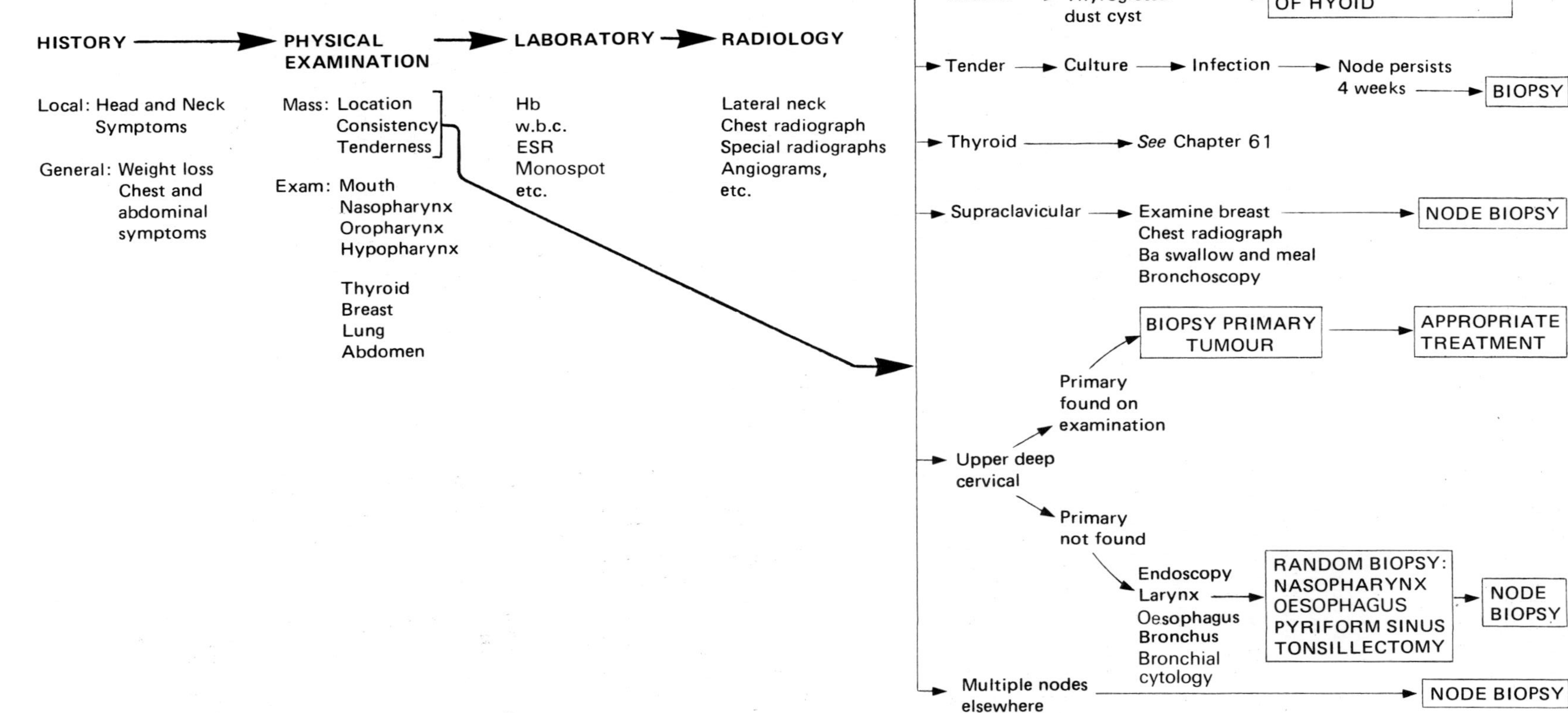

Fig. 23.11 Flow chart for the investigation of a patient with a lump in the neck.

showing up areas of abnormal epithelium in sites normally lined by squamous epithelium such as the tongue, but is of little value in sites such as the larynx which are normally lined in part by respiratory epithelium.

If the above regimen of clinical examination and endoscopy does not provide an answer to the site of the primary tumour, fine needle aspiration biopsy of the gland should be carried out.

If aspiration biopsy does not give a satisfactory answer excisional biopsy must be contemplated; such a biopsy must always excise the lymph node entirely, and an incisional biopsy must never be carried out. Even then there may be serious consequences of excision including:

1. Local and possibly general spread of the disease.
2. Compromise of a subsequent neck dissection or irradiation.
3. Additional scar tissue causing difficulty in accurate palpation.
4. A false sense of security for the patient who feels that the lump has been removed.

It cannot be too strongly emphasized that excisional biopsy of a node in the neck should seldom be necessary and Hayes Martin's statement still holds true—'an enlarged lymph node should never be excised as the first or even an early step in diagnosis'; 'if, as a last resort, a cervical node must eventually be removed for diagnosis the operation must be performed by a surgeon who is able and willing to treat the primary cancer if it is later found somewhere in the head and neck'.

Management

In nearly all series, the treatment of the node with a truly occult primary has almost always been accompanied by postoperative radiotherapy. If the tumour is large and the biopsy shows a squamous carcinoma with extracapsular spread, radiotherapy should be carried out. If one discrete node in the upper part of the neck is involved a radical neck dissection should be carried out, whereas if there is more than one node involved, or nodes in the lower part of the neck, radiotherapy is given; supraclavicular nodes are not treated further because it is presumed that they are secondary to a visceral carcinoma. This policy provides a survival rate of about 35%.

In those patients where the primary tumour is not found it is essential to repeat the search for a primary tumour at frequent intervals after the neck nodes have been treated. Large series have shown that the primary lesion was later found in about 30%, whereas a further 40% died with metastatic disease and no evidence of a primary lesion. Of the survivors, 20% show no further evidence of any malignant disease at any time after treatment of the neck nodes. This again, however, raises the possibility of the existence of branchogenic carcinoma. It would be unlikely that a primary head and neck tumour would disappear on removal of the metastasis. This is dormancy reversed! Total removal of a cancer arising in heterotopic squamous epithelium in a lymph node could well result in a long-term cure. The follow-up needs to be continued for a very long time, since the primary tumour, particularly if it is in the tonsil, may not appear for many years and also patients with one head and neck tumour have up to a 1:3 chance of getting another one.

Bilateral Neck Nodes (N2)

Bilateral neck nodes are not common, occurring in about 5% of head and neck cancers overall, more commonly from tumours of the base of the tongue, the supraglottic larynx and the hypopharynx. It is generally agreed that the presence of bilateral neck nodes is a very bad prognostic sign and survival rates fall to about 5% in the presence of such an event. Despite this low survival rate many surgeons have advised staged or simultaneous bilateral neck dissection.

For the last 10 years or more it has been appreciated that it may not be necessary to stage operation on the two sides so that it is possible to carry out a neck dissection on both sides at the same sitting with reasonable safety, although the complication rate may be high. Formation of fistulas, sepsis, skin slough and facial oedema which tend to persist, are the most important complications. The postoperative death rate is about 10% and half the patients die of uncontrolled local disease. Patients with supraglottic carcinoma and bilateral neck nodes have a reasonable prognosis, whereas nearly all other tumours, particularly of the mouth, the oropharynx and the hypopharynx, when associated with bilateral neck nodes, have an extremely bad prognosis, and surgery probably does not influence the natural history of the disease.

The most feared complication after bilateral neck dissection is increased intracranial pressure. It has been shown that tying one internal jugular vein produces a three-fold increase of the intracranial pressure, whereas tying the second side produces a five-fold increase; the intracranial pressure then tends to fall over about 8 days but not to normal. Furthermore, the pressure falls quite rapidly within the first 12 h so that if the patient can be got over this period he is probably out of immediate danger. The methods to be used to avoid this complication include:

1. Removal of CSF (which is dangerous).
2. Keeping the patient in the sitting position.
3. Avoiding dressings which compress the neck.
4. Infusion of mannitol.

It should be noted that the treatment and prognosis for a patient in whom a node appears on the second side of the neck some time later is quite different from the patient who suffers from bilateral neck nodes at the time of presentation, and a 5-year survival rate of 30% can be achieved in this case.

Fixed Nodes (N3)

The presence of fixed nodes is an uncommon event occurring in about 5% of all patients with head and neck cancer. The word 'fixed' itself is one which is subject to individual interpretation and indeed very few nodes are truly fixed. A node is unlikely to be fixed until it becomes very large, i.e. 6 cm or more in diameter, and is rarely fixed when it is smaller than this. It has generally been thought that the presence of fixed nodes contraindicates surgery, but this is probably not absolutely true. If the tumour is fixed to or invades the jugular vein, the patient is almost certainly incurable, since nearly all patients will die of distant metastases and it must therefore appear that such invasion is indeed a contraindication to useful treatment: it is, however, difficult to predict.

Fixation to the base of the skull in the region of the mastoid process and to the branchial plexus is also almost certainly a contraindication to treatment. Fixation to the skin is not necessarily a contraindication and it is possible to resect the tumour with the overlying skin which is replaced with a myocutaneous flap. On occasion, this has produced long-term survival and certainly may give very helpful palliation.

A review of a small number of patients with fixed nodes being treated by preoperative radiotherapy and surgery showed that a few patients survived, but the only ones to do so were those in whom examination of the specimen after radical neck dissection showed that the tumour had been sterilized by radiotherapy; the remaining patients all died.

When a tumour invades the arterial tree, resection of this vascular system has been described. If the common carotid artery is replaced by a vein graft the operative mortality is high. Despite the occasional survivor reported by the highly skilled, this technique does not appear to have become generally accepted.

THE WAY AHEAD

Benign Neck Masses

Whilst it may produce little clinical dividend there is still a place for investigation into the anatomy and embryology of some of the benign diseases of the neck, notably branchial cyst. The most frequent opinion is that this lesion is congenital in origin is almost certainly wrong.

Malignant Neck Nodes

No significant advance in the management of malignancy in the neck nodes can be expected from conventional surgery or radiotherapy or a combination of the two. The improvements in prognosis which were originally hoped for from prophylactic neck dissection have not occurred, although the real answer could only be provided by a controlled prospective trial, which remains to be done. Similarly prophylactic neck irradiation for the patient without palpable metastases offers promise, but again a controlled trial is lacking.

In the treatment of the patient with established lymph-node metastases in one side of the neck the supremacy of surgery was recently challenged by radiotherapists. It may be that radiotherapy can sterilize small nodes, but carefully controlled investigations are needed to determine the place of radiotherapy: some radiotherapists would also have to report their results in terms of 5-year survival rather than the nebulous concept of 'control' after an unspecified interval.

Another question to be answered by a trial is the place of pre- and postoperative radiotherapy. Despite initial enthusiasm for preoperative radiotherapy for the majority of head and neck tumours, recent careful trials have shown that in fact the survival rate for tumours of all head and neck sites is not increased by preoperative radiotherapy.

The results of trials using postoperative radiotherapy in various sites are awaited.

In summary, there are several forms of treatment which have been advocated very strongly, but which have not been subjected to a clinical trial before they were introduced. Because the number of patients with head and neck cancer is small, it is very difficult for one man to run a trial in one centre, so that multicentre trials are needed, with all their problems. Despite these difficulties such trials can be organized and it is a great pity that repeated attempts are made to introduce new forms of treatment without a proper trial.

Perhaps the greatest advance which could be achieved in the next few years would be general acceptance of the fact that if a man over the age of 50 presents with a single node in the upper part of the neck, the head and neck, the naso-, oro, and hypopharynx *must* be examined particularly carefully *before* a biopsy is taken of the node. To do otherwise almost always leads to death of a patient who otherwise had a reasonable chance of cure.

Further Reading

Batsakis J. G. (1979) *Tumours of the Head and Neck. Clinical and Pathological Considerations.* 2nd ed. Baltimore, Williams & Wilkins.

Djalilian M., Weiland L. H., Devine K. D. et al. (1973) Significance of jugular vein invasion by metastatic carcinoma in radical neck dissection. *Am. J. Surg.* **126,** 566.

Emery P. J. et al. (1984) Cystic hygroma of the head and neck. A review of 37 cases. *J. Laryngol. Otol.* **98,** 613.

Ferlito A. et al. (1984) Assessment and treatment of neurogenic and non-neurogenic tumours of the parapharyngeal space. *Head Neck Surg.* **7,** 32.

Howie A. J. et al. (1982) The definition of branchial cysts, sinuses and fistulae. *Clin. Otolaryngol.* **7,** 51.

McGuirt W. F., McCabe B. F. and Krause C. J. (1979) Complications of radical neck dissection. A survey of 788 patients. *Head Neck Surg.* **1,** 481.

Ranadive N. U. et al. (1984) Thyroglossal cyst. *Postgrad. Med.* **30,** 175.

Shreedhar R. et al. (1984) Carcinoma arising in a branchial cyst. *Br. J. Surg.* **71,** 115.

Spiro R. H., Derose G. and Strong E. W. (1983) Cervical node metastases of occult origin. *Am. J. Surg.* **146,** 441.

Stell P. M., Dalby J. E., Singh S. D. et al. (1984) The fixed cervical lymph node. *Cancer,* **53,** 336.

24 *The Salivary Glands*

A. G. D. Maran

SURGICAL ANATOMY

There are four main salivary glands—two submandibular and two parotids—and multiple minor salivary glands. These minor glands occur throughout the entire upper respiratory tract, notably in the palate and base of tongue.

The parotid gland has been likened to a lump of bread dough poured over an egg whisk—the dough representing the glandular tissue and the egg whisk the facial nerve. Most of the parotid gland lies above the nerve (the superficial lobe), the nerve lies totally surrounded by parotid tissue and the parotid tissue below the nerve is the deep lobe or retromandibular portion (*Fig.* 24.1). The parotid is invested in periparotid fascia which supports it from the zygoma and becomes continuous with the masseter fascia anteriorly and the sternomastoid fascia posteriorly. Within this fascia lie 15–20 lymph nodes, swelling of which may mimic parotid tumours.

The facial nerve emerges from the mastoid at the stylomastoid foramen lateral to the styloid process and immediately enters the parotid. There are several ways to identify it during parotidectomy but the two most reliable are as follows:

1. The tragal cartilage of the external ear has a pointed end and the facial nerve lies 1 cm inferior and 1 cm medial to this landmark under the temporomasseteric fascia.
2. If the posterior belly of the digastric muscle is followed up to the mastoid process the facial nerve bisects the angle formed by the bony tympanic plate and the muscle. As soon as the nerve passes the styloid process it proceeds anterolaterally in the gland before dividing into its upper and lower divisions two-thirds of the way to the mandible. The two divisions are the temporozygomatic and the cervicofacial branches, which divide into peripheral branches. The nerves to the forehead muscles and the upper and lower lids

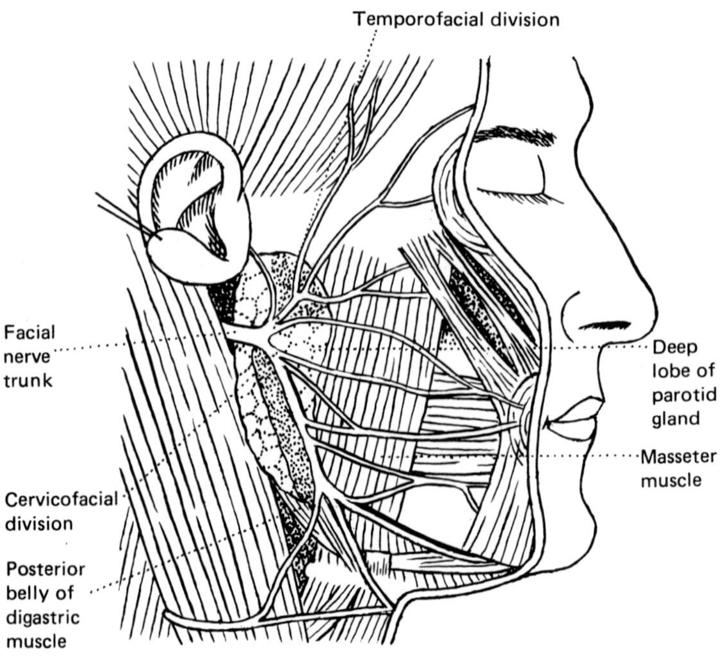

Fig. 24.1 Surgical anatomy of the parotid salivary gland.

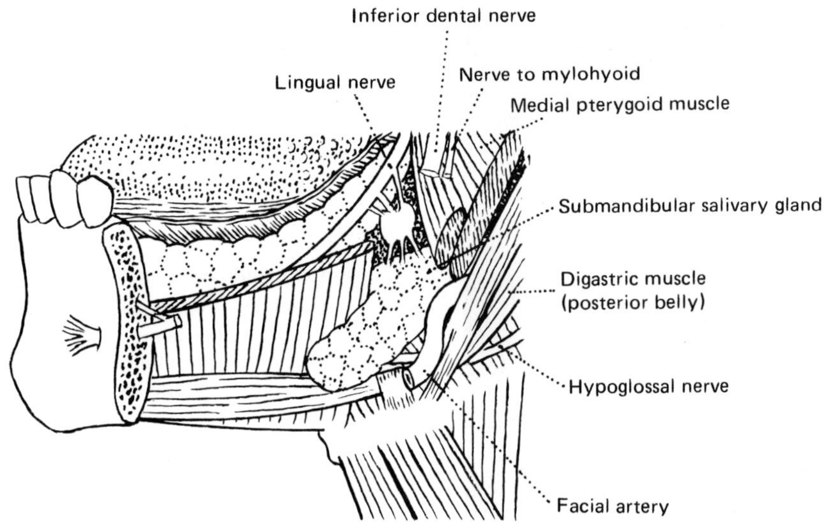

Fig. 24.2 Surgical anatomy of the submandibular salivary gland.

arise from the temporozygomatic branch and the buccal branch, and nerves to the upper and lower lips arise from the cervicofacial branch. Variations are common but the above configuration is the most usual.

The retromandibular portion of the gland lies in the parapharyngeal space along with the carotid sheath, the vagus nerve, the sympathetic trunk and fat. Masses in this space, which lies lateral to the tonsil, may arise from any of these structures and may present in the pharynx or externally.

The submandibular gland lies under the mandible on the mylohyoid muscle (*Fig.* 24.2). The posterior part bends around the posterior border of the muscle and from this part arises the duct which runs on the floor of the mouth to open at the frenulum of the tongue. In the deeper part lie the lingual nerve, the submaxillary ganglion and the hypoglossal nerve all of which should be preserved during removal. On the surface of the gland lies the lower branch of the facial nerve and damage to this causes weakness of the lower lip on this side. The facial artery is enmeshed in the substance of the gland posteriorly and can be found one finger's breadth anterior to the angle of the mandible.

Minor salivary glands occur throughout the upper respiratory and alimentary tracts, the commonest sites being in the buccal mucosa, the floor of the mouth and the tongue. They also occur in the nasopharynx, tonsil and supraglottic larynx.

SURGICAL PATHOLOGY

There are two features of salivary gland tumours which make them unique. First, some tumours occur only in the salivary glands and nowhere else in the body, and secondly as well as benign and malignant tumours there are some which have very variable biological behaviour. These two facts and also the difficulty of histopathological interpretation have led to a profusion of classifications none of which have been universally accepted.

The common benign tumours are the pleomorphic and monomorphic adenomas and the common malignant ones, the adenoid cystic carcinoma and malignant pleomorphic adenomas. Adenocarcinomas are rare and there is considerable doubt as to whether squamous-cell carcimona exists at all. Areas that look like squamous-cell carcinoma occur both in malignant mixed-cell tumours and mucoepidermoid tumours. Tumours of variable malignancy are the mucoepidermoid tumour and the acinic-cell tumour. Rarer tumours are haemangioma, lymphangioma, sarcoma, lipoma, lymphoma, and metastatic tumours.

The commonest non-tumorous condition is sialectasis which is the background in which calculi form. Some medical disorders and certain allergies can cause sialomegaly and a number of conditions can mimic sialomegaly with no actual abnormality of the glands.

Of increasing interest is Sjögren's disease which as well as being the second most autoimmune disease has close links with lymphoma.

BENIGN TUMOURS

1. Pleomorphic Adenoma

This is also known as a mixed-cell tumour and comprises 60% of all salivary gland tumours. In the parotid it forms 90% of all benign tumours and in the submandibular and minor salivary glands it constitutes less than 50% of all tumours but is the commonest benign tumour. The sex distribution is equal and the peak age incidence is in the fifth decade. In the parotid it is usually unilateral but bilateral tumours can occur. In the minor salivary glands the only site in which it presents with any frequency is the palate.

The tumour grows slowly with long quiescent periods and short periods of rapid growth. Some patients may have ill-defined local discomfort but it is usually symptomless, apart from the lump. Pain and facial paralysis should arouse the suspicion of malignancy.

The capsule of compressed normal parotid tissue varies in thickness and the tumour extends into the capsule in a lobulated fashion (*Fig.* 24.3). This is why shelling out the tumour leads to the risk of local recurrence which may be in several sites since some of the lobules in the capsule can be left behind. The cut surface of the tumour is greyish-white or blue with possible cyst formation and haemorrhage. Ten

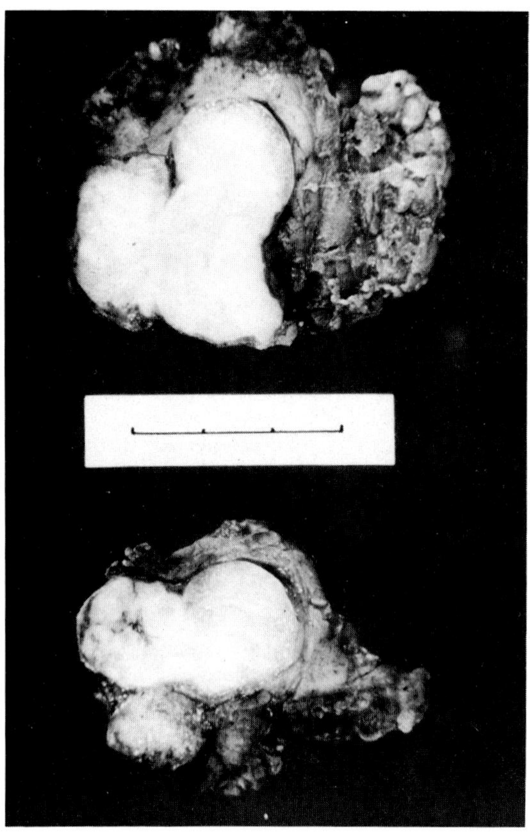

Fig. 24.3 Pleomorphic adenoma. The tumour is seen to extend into the capsule which consists of compressed normal parotid tissue varying in thickness.

per cent of tumours are highly cellular and although showing no malignant propensity such a tumour is more liable to recur.

The tumours contain epithelial and mesodermal elements (*Fig.* 24.4). The mesodermal parts arise from the myoepithelial cell which is a contractile cell surrounding the tubules draining individual acini.

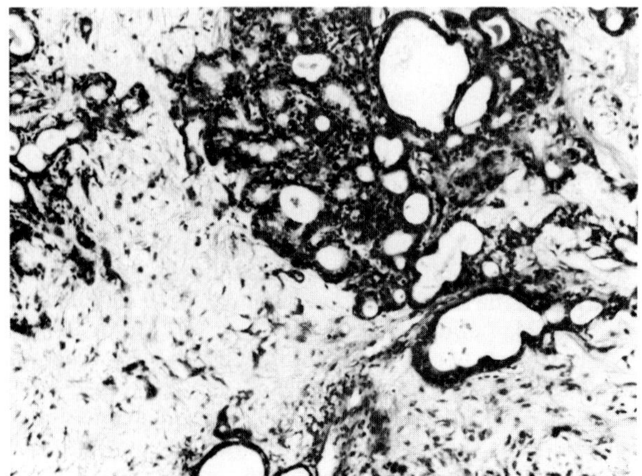

Fig. 24.4 Photomicrograph of a pleomorphic adenoma showing epithelial and myoepithelial (mesodermal) components.

Pleomorphic adenoma is a tumour of high implantability. If the capsule is ruptured during removal, then tumour will implant on the residual parotid. This will cause recurrences which are apparently multifocal but this is a geographic rather than a pathological notion. In the management of the recurrent tumour, the nerve will be involved and the sheath may need to be stripped. Although these tumours are not very radiosensitive, surgery for recurrence should always be followed by irradiation.

2. Monomorphic Adenoma

a. Papillary cystadenoma lymphomatosum (*Warthin's tumour*) is invariably benign and is only seen in the parotid gland. It is much commoner in males, the male:female ratio being 7:1. The peak age incidence is in the seventh decade and 10% are bilateral but rarely synchronously. They are soft and cystic and are often fluctuant. The tumour probably arises from parotid tissue included in the lymph nodes which are usually present within the parotid sheath.

b. Oncocytoma arises from oncocytes which are derived from intralobular ducts or acini. They may undergo a diffuse multinodular hyperplasia known as oncocytosis. It is seen most frequently in the sites of minor salivary glands and the diagnosis must be borne in mind in the presence of lumps in the nasopharynx and larynx, especially in elderly males. It is also known as oxyphil-cell adenoma. It rarely undergoes malignant change.

MALIGNANT TUMOURS

1. Adenoid Cystic Carcinoma

This is the commonest and may arise from any salivary tissue; it is, however, more common in minor than in major glands. It comprises 31% of minor salivary gland tumours, 2% of parotid gland tumours and 15% of submandibular gland tumours. Twenty-five per cent of parotid tumours are malignant with 14% proving to be adenoid cystic carcinomas. The submandibular gland has 47% incidence of malignancy and 31% of these are adenoid cystic carcinoma. Sixty-five per cent of minor salivary gland tumours are malignant and 38% of these are adenoid cystic carcinoma.

The maximum age incidence is in the sixth decade and there is an equal sex incidence. The commonest presenting feature is pain and the tumour may be present for some years before diagnosis. It is some time before a mass becomes palpable or evident in many cases and the patient may spend a few years visiting different specialists with regard to facial pain.

The incidence of lymph-node involvement from direct or contiguous invasion rather than from emboli is low (15%). It tends to spread along nerve sheaths and this accounts for the large numbers of preoperative facial paralyses (18%). Distant metastases, especially to the lungs, is another feature of this tumour indicating that vascular dissemination is more important than lymphatic spread. Forty-three per cent of patients with adenoid cystic carcinoma have distant metastases and two-thirds of these are in the lungs.

The 5-year survival rate varies from 60 to 80% but few series record more than a 30% 10-year survival.

2. Adenocarcinoma

Adenocarcinoma forms 3% of parotid tumours, and 10% of submandibular and minor salivary gland tumours. The sex incidence is equal and it is one of the commoner salivary gland tumours in children.

There are three basic histological patterns—tubular, papillary and undifferentiated. The last type is usually very biologically aggressive and metastasizes distantly. There is also a 23% incidence of preoperative facial paralysis.

3. Squamous-cell Carcinoma

This is a rare tumour in the salivary glands and almost never occurs in the minor glands. Two-thirds of the patients are men and the maximum age incidence is in the seventh decade. It is an aggressive tumour and shows no tendency to encapsulation. It grows rapidly causing pain, facial paralysis, skin fixation and ulceration. About one-half of the patients have metastatic lymph glands when first seen It arises from the duct system and some pathologists deny its existence considering them all to be high-grade mucoepidermoid carcinomas. The other possible error is that the tumour started in a parotid lymph node as metastasis from another head and neck site.

4. Malignant Pleomorphic Adenoma

This has been used synonymously with carcinoma ex-pleomorphic adenoma (carcinoma arising from a mixed tumour). These designations signify two separate entities.

The true malignant pleomorphic adenoma is very rare and presents in two forms: the first is the benign pleomorphic adenoma which inexplicably metastasizes and the second is the carcinosarcoma of salivary glands that metastasizes with two types of elements. Both are rarities.

The carcinoma arising in a mixed-cell tumour is commoner and represents 1–6% of lesions of the mixed-cell category. It is commonest in the parotid, then the submandibular followed by the minor salivary glands of the palate, lip, paranasal sinuses, nasopharynx and tonsil. The original mass will usually have been present for 10–15 years and even when malignancy supervenes the tumour may remain grossly encapsulated.

It has the worst prognosis of any salivary gland malignancy. There is an accelerated recurrence rate and a high incidence of metastases (30–70%).

Not many series report a 5-year survival rate of more than 40%.

TUMOURS OF VARIABLE MALIGNANCY

1. Mucoepidermoid Tumour

Since this was first described in 1945 debate has continued about its biological classification. This can be summarized as follows:

a. One view is that it is always a carcinoma whose behaviour is related to its histology. Low-grade or well-differentiated tumours act like benign mixed-cell tumours—intermediate ones are more aggressive and high grade or undifferentiated tumours metastasize early and carry a poor prognosis.

b. The more recent view is that behaviour is not related to histological appearance and apparently benign ones can eventually metastasize while initially aggressive ones can disappear with the appropriate treatment. For this reason the word 'tumour' is applied rather than 'carcinoma'.

Mucoepidermoid tumours can arise in any salivary tissue and constitute 4–9% of salivary gland tumours. Nine out of 10 involve the parotid gland. In minor salivary glands, the palate is the commonest site, followed by the buccal mucosa, the tongue, the floor of mouth, the lip and the tonsil.

The age range at presentation is very wide and it is the commonest salivary gland tumour in childhood. The sex incidence is equal and the peak age incidence is in the fourth decade.

If low-grade tumours are excluded there is almost a 50% incidence of lymph-node metastases. Five-year survivals of around 40% for intermediate and high-grade tumours are reported.

2. Acinic-cell Tumour

This accounts for between 2 and 4% of all parotid gland tumours and like Warthin's tumours it may be bilateral (3%). It is rarely found outside the parotid gland. It is not uncommon in childhood but the peak age incidence is the fifth decade.

They are derived from two cell sources: (*a*) the reserve cells of the terminal tubules, or (*b*) the intercalated ducts. It may also occur in intra-parotid lymph nodes and this feature is also similar to Warthin's tumour.

It exhibits a variable biological behaviour but survival rates of around 90% at 5 years make it a much more benign tumour than mucoepidermoid. Attempts to predict biological behaviour from histomorphological findings have not been fruitful but about 10% do metastasize.

RARE TUMOURS

1. Haemangioma

Less than 20 cases of haemangioma of the parotid gland have been reported. The parotid may, however, be involved in haemangiomas occurring primarily elsewhere, e.g. the skin overlying the gland and the infratemporal fossa.

Spontaneous regression definitely occurs in some tumours so that no treatment should be offered until the age of 7 or 8 and then only if the tumour is enlarging.

2. Lymphangioma

There are three types of lymphangioma—simple lymphangioma, cavernous lymphangioma and cystic hygroma. The thin-walled lymph spaces invade the parotid and adjacent tissue and do not replace the glandular parenchyma. The tumours are soft and fluctuant and usually transilluminate.

Ranulas in the floor of the mouth may be either blocked minor salivary glands or cavernous lymphangiomas. The latter are more prone to recurrence after excision because of the virtual impossibility of total excision. Cystic hygromas almost always involve the parotid gland and the submandibular space and may require several excisions for total removal.

3. Sarcoma

Sarcomas may be part of the rare malignant mixed-cell tumour spectrum but salivary glands can also be involved in osteogenic and chondrosarcomas of the mandible.

4. Lipoma

This must be differentiated from fatty infiltration which is usually bilateral while lipomas are usually unilateral. It lies lateral to the parotid but the rare tumour of brown fat, the hibernoma, can occur in the parapharyngeal space. Removal is uncomplicated unless it extends into the anterior compartment of the face in which case the terminal branches of the nerve can be at risk.

5. Metastatic Tumours

The parotid lymph nodes may be involved by spread from carcinomas of the scalp and facial skin, especially melanomas. Adenocarcinoma from the digestive tract or urogenital system may present as parotid gland metastases.

6. Salivary Gland Heterotopia

Heterotopic islands of salivary gland tissue have been described in a number of sites in the head and neck—pituitary gland, middle and external ear, mastoid bone, thyroglossal duct cyst, capsules of the thyroid and parathyroid glands, mandible, lymph nodes and the sternoclavicular joints. If these develop to any size then they become manifest as a lump or as an interference with function (e.g. conductive deafness).

7. Basal-cell Adenoma

This is the isocellular counterpart of the mixed-cell tumour. It may be misdiagnosed as an adenoid cystic carcinoma. It can occur in any salivary tissue but is usually in the parotid.

8. Myoepithelioma

This is possibly a one-sided dominance of myoepithelial cells in a mixed tumour. Malignant variants have never been described and it tends to occur in young adults.

9. Sjögren's Disease

In 1888 Dr Mikulicz descibed a syndrome consisting of enlargement of the parotid, submandibular and lacrimal glands. Over the next few years the following were added and Mikulicz disease became Mikulicz sydrome—tuberculosis, syphilis, sarcoidosis, recurrent parotitis of unknown aetiology and actinomycosis. Some years later, mucous gland atrophy in the nose, larynx and vulva were added to the syndrome.

In 1933, Sjögren, a Stockholm ophthalmologist, described the triad of xerostomia, keratoconjunctivitis sicca and arthritis. In 1952, Godwin described benign lymphoepithelial lesion. Whether this exists or not is still a subject for debate and most immunologists now hold the view that it is merely part of Sjögren's disease. It is also held that it is a localized form of Sjögren's disease within the parotid gland. Lymphocytes aggregate around the ducts and lumens become obliterated.

Sjögren's syndrome can be divided into two types:

a. Primary Sjögren's syndrome or the sicca syndrome which consists of xerostomia and xerophthalmia which has a much higher risk of developing into lymphoma.

b. Secondary Sjögren's syndrome which is the complete triad in 48% of cases, rheumatoid arthritis being the accompanying autoimmune disorder but SLE, scleroderma and polymyositis are also seen.

Sjögren's syndrome is a multisystem disease, not only involving the mouth, the eyes and the parotid gland but causing atrophic gastritis, chronic pancreatitis, autoimmune liver disease and renal tubular acidosis.

The laboratory tests that are positive in their diagnosis are usually a high ESR, a raised IgG on protein profile, a positive antinuclear factor and a positive rheumatoid factor. There are several specific antigens for the condition which, however, cannot readily be tested.

Definitive diagnosis is by means of sublabial biopsy where minor salivary glands are sampled from the back of the lower lip and periductal lymphocytic infiltration is seen.

The immunological abnormality is a defect of the suppressor helper T-cell ratio with a depression of T suppressor cell activity. This allows the escape of autoantibody-secreting clones of B-cells. The antigen is probably the duct which in turn has been altered by a cytomegalovirus infection.

There is a 1:6 chance of lymphoma developing and if it does develop in the parotid gland, the 2-year survival rate is 0%.

Primary lymphoma arising in the parotid glands is much more benign than lymphoma arising in the sicca syndrome and over 80% will be alive at 4 years.

SIALECTASIS

This is the salivary gland analogue of bronchiectasis. Both diseases are of unknown aetiology and involve a progressive destruction of the alveoli and parenchyma of the gland accompanied by duct stenosis and cyst formation as the alveoli coalesce.

Most cases are thought to be congenital and in childhood it may mimic mumps—but mumps seldom recurs. Fifty per cent have no symptoms after childhood and only a small proportion require treatment.

The typical presentation is painful enlargement of one salivary gland shortly after eating. It takes a few hours to regress and is made worse by eating again. Attacks come in runs lasting for days or weeks with long free periods of remission. These attacks are due to the main ducts being blocked by stones or epithelial debris. The parotid is a serous gland low in calcium and so the epithelial debris seldom calcifies but in the mixed submandibular glands the epithelial debris from the necrotic ducts and alveoli calcifies and stone formation is common. In bronchiectasis the epithelial debris is coughed up and in sialectasis it forms 'mud' that blocks ducts and may become calcified.

Diagnosis is confirmed radiologically by sialography which shows two varieties—fusiform or globular (saccular). Fusiform patterns are similar to bronchographic patterns in bronchiectasis namely cyst formation and duct stricture. An example of globular sialectasis is seen in *Fig.* 24.5. This has been shown to be due to lipiodol escaping from the alveoli and ducts and being deposited in the stroma of the gland.

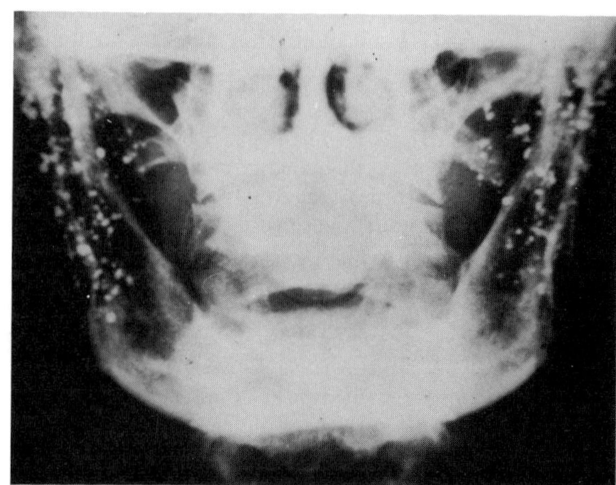

Fig. 24.5 Bilateral parotid sialogram showing diffuse saccular sialectasis.

This is the pattern seen in Sjögren's disease and it is now held as further evidence of primary duct damage possibly by CMV.

INFECTIONS

The commonest infection of the parotid glands is due to the mumps virus. While other infections with bacteria are classically described in debilitated patients in the postoperative phase, parotitis is occurring with increasing frequency in otherwise fit patients. It is never primarily bacterial however in this group; it is due to echo and Coxsackie virus infection. If the infection is not aborted in its early stages with antibiotics then parotid abscess will result. Since the infection is confined within the parotid capsule it becomes tense and is very painful.

INVESTIGATIONS

History

The age of the patient is obviously important because mumps is much commoner in children than in adults. Although mumps can be predominantly unilateral, such a presentation should make one suspect a diagnosis of congenital sialectasis rather than mumps—especially if it happens twice.

It is important to establish if the condition affects one gland or more than one. Tumours are unilateral (*Fig.* 24.6) apart from Warthin's on very rare occasions. Sialectasis also usually affects only one parotid gland although bilateral submandibular involvement is sometimes seen. Diffuse enlargement (sialomegaly) is caused not only by sialectasis but also benign lymphoepithelial lesion, drug allergies a number of systemic conditions (*see below*) while tumours are always localized masses.

If the swelling is related to eating then it is likely to be due to calculous disease secondary to sialectasis (*Fig.* 24.7). No other sialomegalies are related to eating. The duration of swelling due to calculi is variable and may last from under an hour to several days. Benign tumours grow slowly although if bleeding occurs inside a cystic tumour, such as a pleomorphic adenoma, then the patient may become alarmed at a growth spurt. Malignant tumours increase in size fairly rapidly and are often associated with facial weakness.

Pain is a characteristic feature of duct obstruction by a calculus or infection (e.g. mumps). Benign lymphoepithelial lesion is often uncomfortable rather than painful as are allergic reactions. Adenoid cystic carcinoma typically presents with pain which may result in the patient seeing specialists in various disciplines associated with facial pain.

Systemic conditions such as myxoedema, diabetes, Cushing's disease, hepatic cirrhosis, gout and alcoholism, may be associated with painless sialomegaly. More recently parotomegaly as a feature of bulaemia and also of AIDS has been reported. Drugs such as thiouracil, phenylbutazone, isoprenaline, Distalgesic and high oestrogen contraceptive pills can also cause sialomegaly.

Finally, enquiry should be made into other symptoms

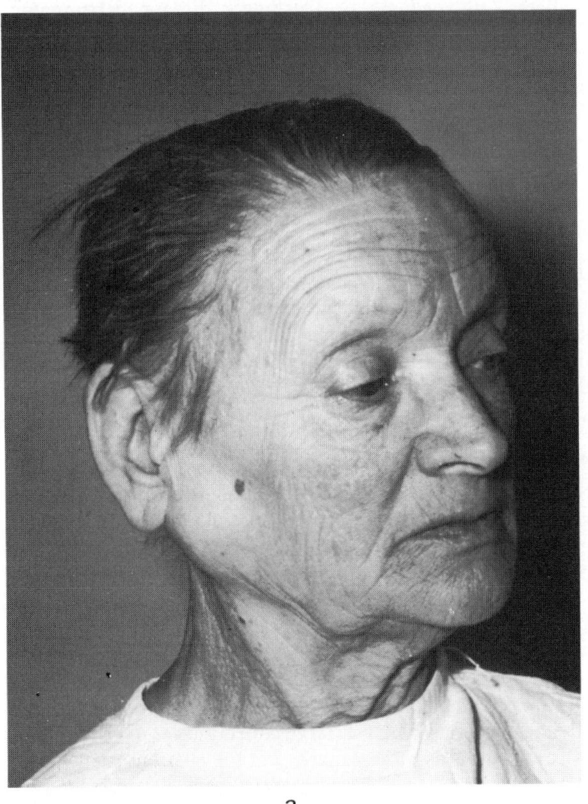

a

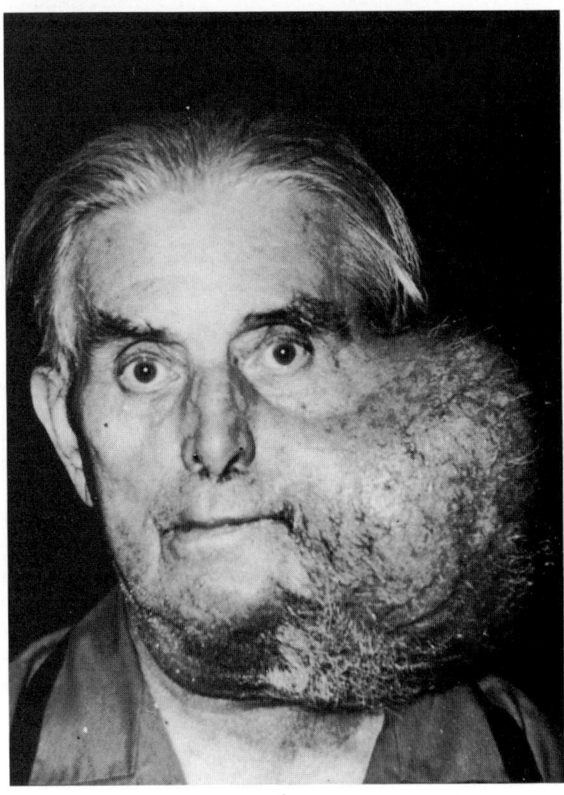

b

Fig. 24.6 *a*, Pleomorphic adenoma of the right parotid gland. *b*, Large pleomorphic adenoma of the left parotid gland. Despite the size, there is no paralysis of the facial nerve.

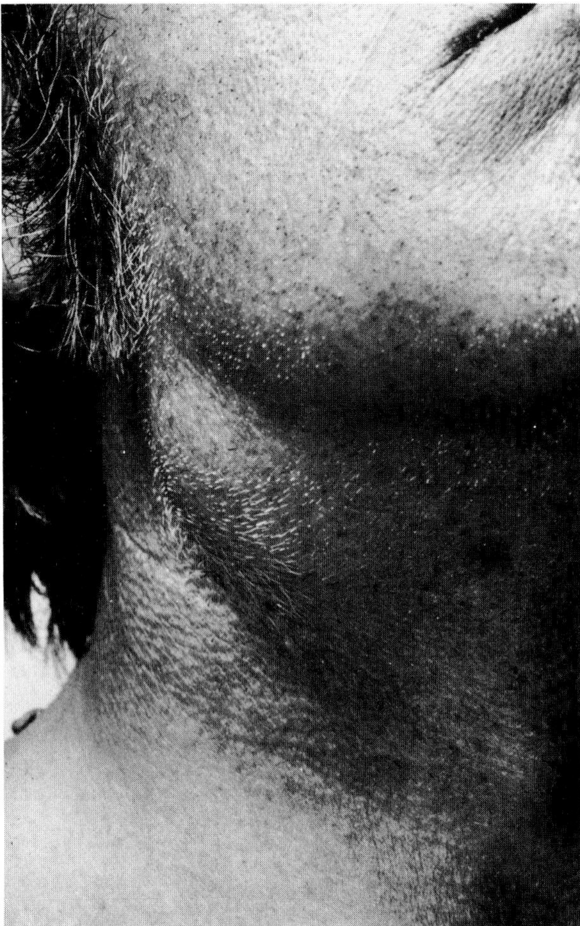

Fig. 24.7 Enlargement of the right submandibular salivary gland due to calculous disease. Attacks of pain and swelling were precipitated by meals.

the patient may have because sarcoidosis and tuberculosis can enlarge a gland, as can hydatid disease in appropriate countries.

Examination

Inspection should reveal which area is involved and whether it is one gland or more than one. Establish whether it is a local mass or a diffuse swelling. Skin involvement should make one suspect a malignant tumour as should any facial weakness.

On palpation decide whether it is solid or cystic—cystic masses may be Warthin's tumours, cystic pleomorphic adenomas, branchial cysts or parasitic cysts. Solid tumours can be smooth or irregular but this gives little help as to diagnosis because pleomorphic adenomas are often irregular and knobbly. Benign tumours are always mobile and any fixation should raise the strong suspicion of malignancy. In assessing any parotid mass one should ask the patient to clench his teeth so that the masseter is contracted; this allows one to assess if the swelling is in fact a hypertrophied masseter and it also allows one to see whether or not the mass is inside the muscle (haemangioma or myxoma) or outside it. Complete examination of all the salivary glands is essential to decide whether the mass is single or multiple and whether or not other glands are affected (as in Sjögren's disease).

No examination of this area is complete without examining the pharynx. Parapharyngeal tumours are either dumb-bell, in which case they present in the pharynx and also in the superficial lobe of the parotid, or deep lobe only, in which case they present primarily in the pharynx pushing the tonsil and/or palate medially.

All salivary glands should be palpated bimanually. In the submandibular area stones may be felt or moved and in the parotid area pressure on a sialectatic gland may express pus from the duct.

Clinical diagnosis of a salivary gland mass is usually not difficult but the following rarities should be kept in mind since they may mimic sialomegaly.

1. Hypertrophic masseter.
2. Winged mandible (in the first arch syndrome).
3. Dental cysts.
4. Branchial cysts.
5. Myxoma of the masseter.
6. Neuroma of the facial nerve.
7. Facial vein thrombosis.
8. Temporal artery aneurysm.
9. Lipoma.
10. Lymphangioma.
11. Mandibular tumours.
12. Mastoiditis.
13. Lymphadenitis of the pre-auricular node.
14. Sebaceous cyst.

Laboratory Tests

The appropriate endocrine tests should be done to exclude diabetes, myxoedema or Cushing's disease. Rheumatoid factor and hypergammaglobulinaemia are often found in Sjögren's disease. Uric acid levels will be raised in gout. If sarcoid is suspected, a Kveim test is required. In all cases a full blood count and ESR should be done. Salivary flow rates will be less than 0·5 ml/min in Sjögren's disease. The Schirmer's test also shows a decrease in tearing (<5 mm in 5 min).

Radiology

a. Plain Films

Parotid stones are almost always radiotranslucent, while submandibular stones are nearly always radio-opaque. Intra-oral films should be done in both cases. Plain films are also useful in differentiating many of the extra-salivary causes of sialomegaly.

b. Sialography

Sialography is the most useful radiological investigation of salivary gland disease but it must be performed by an experienced radiologist since artefacts can be created both by traumatic cannulation and by overfilling the gland.

Its main use is in the assessment of a suspected sialectasis. In congenital saccular sialectasis the characteristic snow-storm appearance is seen. There is extravasation of radio-opaque material at the intralobular duct level and strictures and clubbing of the duct system may be demonstrated. In advanced cystic sialectasis large collections of dye are seen in the cysts and this is most marked in the post-emptying films. Both of these types of sialectasis can be mimicked by overfilling.

Pure duct stenosis is nearly always an iatrogenic artefact caused by traumatic cannulation. Some patients may stenose their parotid ducts by biting their cheeks but submandibular duct stenosis can only be caused by operative interference in the floor of the mouth or by traumatic cannulation.

Sialography in tumour assessment is valueless; it can, however, give some idea of deep lobe involvement and also whether or not the mass is indeed within the parotid, if combined with CT scanning.

c. Angiography

This is sometimes required in the investigation of tumours of the parapharyngeal space in order to differentiate salivary gland tumours from chemodectoma of the carotid or a nerve sheath tumour both of which have a characteristic tumour circulation. Its use here has largely been superseded by CT scanning.

d. Scanning Techniques

The early hopes that salivary gland scanning with technetium 99m pertechnetate have not been fulfilled. The finding that all tumours were 'cold' apart from Warthin's has not been substantiated in the longer term and the technique is accompanied by an unacceptably large number of false positive and false negative results.

CT scanning with sialography shows up deep lobe displacement well.

e. Biopsy

On no account should a discrete salivary gland mass be subjected to incisional biopsy. Since there is a 9 out of 10 chance that a single parotid mass is a pleomorphic adenoma incising it is not only unnecessary but will almost certainly lead to a later recurrence. The only acceptable biopsy in such cases is by parotidectomy. If, however, there is skin involvement and undoubted malignancy then incisional biopsy is acceptable. Some cytologists are becoming expert in evaluating fine-needle aspiration biopsy but it is too early to give the technique general recommendation.

Neither should a parapharyngeal mass be biopsied through the pharynx. If the mass is a chemodectoma the bleeding will be uncontrollable and if it is a salivary gland tumour, the recurrence will be unacceptable.

On the other hand diffuse enlargement of a salivary gland is probably not due to a tumour and if a diagnosis has not been made after clinical, radiological and laboratory studies an incisional biopsy may be done. If Sjögren's disease is suspected then a sublabial minor salivary gland biopsy is diagnostic.

Minor salivary gland tumours presenting in the oral cavity and upper respiratory tract have a high chance of being malignant. They are surface tumours and therefore incisional biopsy is to be preferred to excisional biopsy. This policy carries no risk of implantation but it does mean that patients with benign tumours will be subjected to a later local excision. On the other hand this practice ensures that a correct treatment plan can be formulated and discussed with the patient if the tumour is malignant with no danger of false security in that the tumour has been 'removed'.

TREATMENT POLICY

Benign Tumours

a. Parotid

The treatment of benign tumours of the parotid has passed through several phases during the last 30 years. Enucleation carried a high recurrence rate and so it was followed by enucleation and postoperative radiation. This policy was often unacceptable in the young who were not only given a long time for potential and undoubted recurrences but the risk of radiation-induced cancer was added. Recurrence rates were much lower in those series in which 'enucleation' meant not merely the extracapsular removal of the tumour but removal of the mass together with a good cuff of normal parotid tissue.

Since a proportion of facial weaknesses was due to these techniques, especially extracapsular enucleation, as well as the other risks, total superficial parotidectomy was next advocated. This was very successful in terms of prevention of recurrence and the nerve was safe in the hands of skilled operators because the first step in the operation is identification of the facial nerve and its two main branches. It became evident, however, that the procedure was often too extensive, e.g. removal of the upper portion of the parotid gland for a small tumour at the ear lobe seems unnecessary. Now, therefore, a hemisuperficial parotidectomy is often done (i.e. all the parotid tissue lateral to one main branch, either upper or lower, of the nerve).

b. Submandibular

Benign tumours in this gland are rare and are often misdiagnosed; the cause of the mass is often an enlargement of one of the overlying lymph nodes. This does not alter the fact that the operation of choice is simple removal of the submandibular gland taking care to preserve the mandibular branch of the facial nerve, the lingual nerve and the hypoglossal nerve.

c. Parapharyngeal Salivary Tumours

The approach which is vetoed on grounds of recurrence risk and also damage to surrounding structures is the intraoral one. If the tumour is of the dumb-bell variety then an ordinary superficial parotidectomy is commenced. The superficial lobe is left pedicled to the deep lobe at one of two places, depending on where the deep lobe tumour is—either between the upper and lower divisions of the nerve or below the lower division. Thereafter the nerve and its branches, to the extreme periphery, are dissected from their medial surface so that either the upper and lower branches can be separated, giving access to the parapharyngeal space, or the lower branch is lifted up and access gained by this route. The deep lobe is removed by finger dissection quite easily because there is an area of very loose areolar tissue lateral to the pharyngeal mucosa. What is occasionally difficult is the removal of a bulky tumour from behind the vertical ramus of the mandible. In this case simple forward dislocation of the mandible doubles the retromandibular space; if, however, even more room is required then a mandibular osteotomy at the angle can be performed with later wiring. But it is almost never necessary.

d. Minor Salivary Gland Tumours

Once the diagnosis has been established by incisional biopsy removal depends on the site. In all sites, apart from the hard palate, local removal with primary closure is usually straightforward. On the hard palate there is always the possibility of extension into bone from the deep surface of the tumour. It would, however, be unnecessary to make a hole in the palate with the consequent necessity to wear an obturator for every patient. This operation is reserved for highly cellular pleomorphic adenomas whose proven recurrence rate is more than 50%. Other tumours are removed locally—the bare area on the palate can be closed with a split-thickness skin graft or left to re-epithelize.

Malignant Tumours

a. Parotid

Radiation has little place to play in the primary treatment of malignant salivary gland tumours. It does, however, have an increasingly important part to play as an adjuvant to surgery especially in adenoid cystic carcinoma which until recently has been considered radioresistant.

Whatever else is done in the management of malignant parotid tumours there is little doubt that the whole parotid must be removed. What else is removed with it depends on the size and position of the tumour. It will be clear whether or not to remove the temporomandibular joint, the vertical ramus of the mandible, the mastoid, the external auditory meatus, or skin. What is not so well established is what to do about the facial nerve. If the nerve is free of tumour then it should be dissected out and left intact. This situation is rarely possible, however, because what one often finds is a nerve totally enmeshed in tumour with no apparent functional loss in the way of facial weakness. When the nerve is removed immediate attempts should be made to bridge the gap with a nerve graft using the great auricular nerve which has the same diameter as the main trunk of the facial nerve. If this fails then later attempts to rehabilitate the facial paralysis can be done (provided the patient is clear of tumour) using a cross-face anastomosis technique. It is very rarely possible in parotid surgery to carry out faciohypoglossal anastomosis because the necessary piece of facial nerve is almost always removed.

In adenoid cystic carcinoma, the nerve excision should be wide because the tumour infiltrates nerve sheaths and eventually travels intracranially. The facial nerve should be removed well into the mastoid, drilling it out of its bony canal. The great auricular and the auriculotemporal nerve should also be removed.

In the rare case of nodes being palpable in the neck a radical neck dissection is performed but if no nodes are palpable elective neck dissection is contraindicated.

The role of postoperative radiotherapy is not defined but consideration should be given to its use if margins of clearance are in doubt. A facial nerve graft, however, will not be affected by postoperative radiotherapy but in animal experiments preoperative radiotherapy adversely affects the success of nerve grafts.

b. Submandibular

The operation here is wide removal of the submandibular gland, including the submental fat, the digastric and the tail of the parotid. Depending on the extent of the tumour the mandible or skin may have to be removed also. Consideration may also have to be given to a full radical neck dissection.

As in the parotid, if the tumour is adenoid cystic carcinoma then the lingual and hypoglossal nerves should be excised as far proximally as possible.

Postoperative radiotherapy may also be considered.

c. Parapharyngeal Tumours

These tumours will almost certainly affect the superficial lobe of the parotid and so the same considerations apply as laid down in the parotid section (*see above*).

d. Minor Salivary Glands

The treatment of malignant tumours of minor salivary glands, which are almost invariably adenoid cystic carcinoma, depends on the site. If it is in the oral cavity then it will require a very extensive excision and reconstruction. This tumour is traditionally thought to give good 5-year survival and poor 10-year survival. It is now considered that this is because most of the large series are written up from specialists who get tertiary referrals. This means that the tumour had been inadequately treated for some years before they come to the expert. It is now being shown in various publications that if these tumours are treated by wide excision when first seen, then the outlook is very good because this group of patients do not seem to have the risk of development of further tumours in the head and neck that patients with squamous carcinoma of the head and neck have.

Tumours of Variable Malignancy

Mucoepidermoid tumour and acinic-cell tumour present as apparently simple benign tumours and diagnosis is made after the excision is performed as outlined in the section on treatment of benign tumours. Further surgery is not indicated unless the margins are in doubt and primary postoperative radiotherapy is not advised. The patient should be followed at monthly intervals for the first year and 2-monthly intervals for a further 4 years in an attempt to detect recurrence. If it does recur then malignant potential is presumed and wide field excision is undertaken followed by postoperative radiotherapy.

Rare Tumours

a. Haemangioma

Less than 20 of these have been described in the parotid and excision by means of a parotidectomy is usually possible. If, however, it turns out to be a haemangioma of the infratemporal fossa rather than the parotid the operation should be abandoned because of risk to the facial nerve and the second procedure should be via a Weber Fergusson approach, lifting back the cheek and also the zygoma in order to obtain a better approach to the infratemporal fossa. Since this scars the face, however, it should not be done unless the tumour is giving rise to troublesome symptoms due to size.

b. Lymphangioma

This usually forms part of a previously treated cystic hygroma. The lymphangioma is usually superficial to the parotid and is easily removed without the usual exposure of the facial nerve. Where difficulty arises this is anterior to the parotid as it extends into the cheek; here the terminal branches of the nerve may be damaged but three landmarks may be useful.

i. The zygomaticotemporal division crosses the zygoma midway between the ear and the lateral canthus of the eye.

ii. The buccal branch runs parallel to the parotid duct and 1 cm superior to it.

iii. The mandibular branch of the facial nerve crosses the facial artery (which is 2·5 cm anterior to the angle of the mandible), 1 cm below the lower border of the mandible.

In the submandibular region a lymphangioma is usually a cavernous lymphangioma of the submaxillary space and is best approached intraorally.

c. Lipoma

This lies superficial to each gland and is easily removed without nerve damage although in the face it may go far anterior to the parotid putting the terminal branches at risk (*see above*).

d. Sarcoma

This usually arises from the mandible and pushes one of the salivary glands outwards. Osteogenic sarcoma should be excised, irradiated and treated with long-term cytotoxic therapy. Chondrosarcoma behaves with variable malignancy and if it recurs after mandibulectomy then little can be done.

e. Lymphoma

If a lymph node removed from a salivary gland region proves to be lymphomatous then the usual steps of staging the disease by lymphangiography and laparotomy should be commenced. It is rare for an actual salivary gland to be infiltrated by lymphoma.

f. Benign Lymphoepithelial Lesion

Bouts of pain and swelling should be treated at first with anti-inflammatory drugs and if severe, consideration should be given to the use of steroids in short courses. If one gland enlarges and stays enlarged then it should be removed but it is seldom necessary to use surgery for this condition apart from the situation of enlargement leads to the suspicion of malignancy. The malignant transformation in this condition is to an anaplastic carcinoma. Fewer than 30 such cases have been described and half have been in eskimos (the 'eskimoma').

Sialectasis

The treatment of this falls into three stages depending on the severity of the attacks.

1. If the attacks of pain are mild and infrequent and if the swelling subsides in a few hours then the patient should be advised to finish each meal with a citrus drink in order to try to expel debris from the ducts. This is also helped by massage in the direction of the duct.

Many patients have no further trouble after the diagnostic sialogram which flushes the ducts. Over 50% will resolve with this treatment.

2. If stones are present it depends in which gland they are and where in each gland they are.

a. In the submandibular gland, stones in the duct can be removed from the intraoral route by cutting down on the stone in the duct and marsupializing the duct open. If they are in the body of the gland then the whole submandibular gland should be removed.

b. In the parotid gland a stone in the duct is very rare and can be removed intraorally. If the attacks persist after conservative therapy then a total parotidectomy should be carried out. A superficial lobectomy is insufficient and often results in a postoperative salivary fistula. This is because unlike parotidectomy for tumour, diseased cystic deep lobe is left behind. The residual deep lobe in a non-sialectatic gland is denervated and stops secreting.

COMPLICATIONS OF PAROTIDECTOMY

1. Frey's Syndrome

Frey's syndrome consists of discomfort, sweating and redness of the skin overlying the parotid area occurring during and after eating. It is due to the severed ends of parasympathetic secretomotor fibres growing into the skin; when the patient eats, these fibres are stimulated (as they formerly were for the production of saliva) and they cause vasodilatation and sweating.

If asked about the symptoms 60% of post-parotidectomy patients will admit to some degree of this but only 20% of patients actually complain of it. Spontaneous resolution within 6 months is usual but a small number of patients require active treatment. This takes the form of a tympanic neurectomy which divides the parasympathetic pathway.

2. Nerve Damage

This is best avoided by using the landmarks to identify and preserve the facial nerve referred to previously in this chapter (p. 362). In addition to these anatomical landmarks, identification of the nerve is aided by a facial nerve stimulator.

If the nerve is deliberately sacrificed at the time of excision then the gap should be bridged with a graft of the great auricular nerve. If only the main trunk is divided and only one or at the most two distal branches require joining proximally then a facial–hypoglossal anastomosis is advised.

Other rehabilitative procedures are tarsorrhaphy, fascial sling procedures and unilateral face lift.

3. Salivary Fistula

This is a theoretical possibility in all superficial parotidectomies where a normal deep lobe is left in situ with a cut surface. Its occurrence, however, is extremely rare and it only seems to occur if a sialectatic deep lobe is left behind. It also occasionally occurs after open biopsy.

Most cases settle in a few weeks and anticholinergic drugs to cut down secretion seem to be of little value. Before removing the deep lobe it is worth trying to persuade a radiotherapist to administer the few hundred rads necessary to dry it up.

4. Cosmetic Deformity

After a total parotidectomy a considerable retromandibular depression occurs. This can be filled by turning up a muscle flap from sternomastoid to fill the area.

Further Reading

Batsakis J. G. and Regezi J. A. (1978) The pathology of head and neck tumours: salivary glands Part I. *Head Neck Surg.* **1**, p. 59 Parts II, III and IV in succeeding volumes).

Mason D. K. and Chisholm D. M. (1975) *Salivary Glands in Health and Disease.* Philadelphia, Saunders.

Thackray A. C. (1955) Sialectasis. *Arch. Middlesex Hosp.* 5, p. 151.

25 *Surgery of the Face*

J. C. McGregor

PRINCIPLES

Introduction

The face represents the most important aesthetic area of the body. Physical excellence or imperfection can have profound effects on an individual's life and the reaction of others. It is not just skin that is important, for facial appearance depends on the underlying bone, cartilage framework and facial muscle activity. Because of its very rich blood supply surgical incisions usually heal rapidly and flaps of varying types and sometimes outrageous dimensions are usually successful. Surgery should be none the less performed carefully since the result of bad surgical techniques can be, at best unattractive, and at worst a disaster.

Technique

Gentle handling of the tissues with skin hooks and fine forceps reduces tissue damage and improves the chance of prompt healing. Incisions should be at right angles to the skin surface except in hair-bearing skin where bevelling in the line of the hair shafts preserves the hair follicles and prevents bald patches. Skin sutures should be 5 or 6–0 gauge and should not be tied so tight as to cause strangulation. Removal at 4–5 days ensures that suture marks will not remain permanently. The use of subcuticular sutures or steri-strips may be employed when desired and in certain situations, such as the eyelid, may give excellent cosmetic results. There is no conclusive evidence on a long-term appraisal regarding the superiority of any suture material over silk in the production of scars. Particular care should be taken in the alignment of skin edges at key positions such as the eyebrow and lip and in the horizontal approximation of wound edges to prevent stepping.

Where elective incisions have to be made it is wise to place them in natural crease lines or in a direction where the lines of selective skin tensions run. Some examples are shown in *Figs.* 25.1–25.11. Scars may also be concealed by placing them within a hairline, below lash margins, or behind the ear. On other occasions they may be avoided by making incisions in other sites. Thus the floor of the orbit is approached through incisions in the inferior conjunctival fornix, the nose through the intranasal incisions and the jaws through incisions in the buccal sulcus.

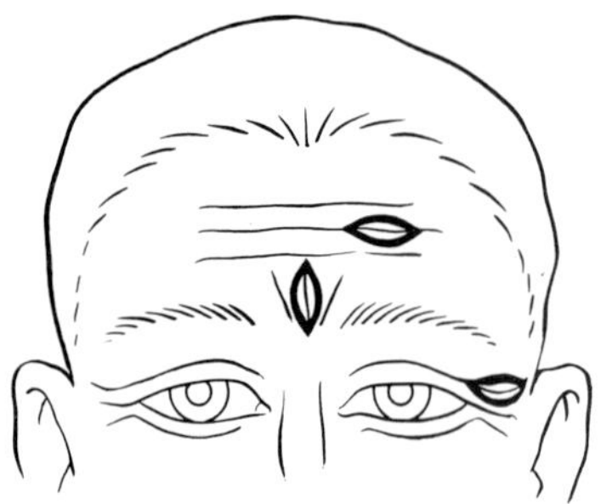

Fig. 25.1 Elliptical excisions on the forehead and temple. (*Figs.* 25.1–25.11 from *British Journal of Surgery*, 1974, **61**, 566.)

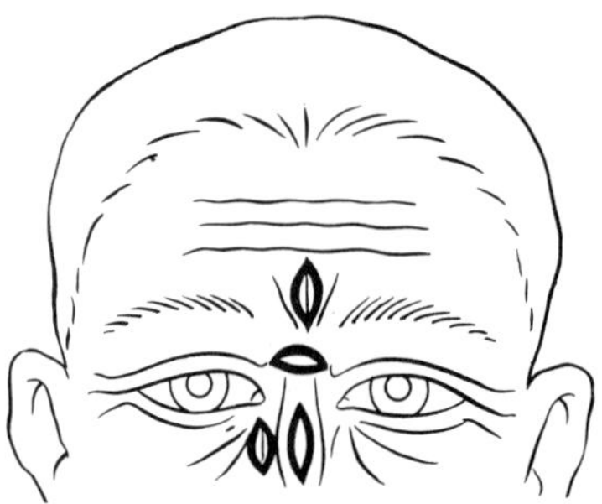

Fig. 25.2 Elliptical excisions on the nose.

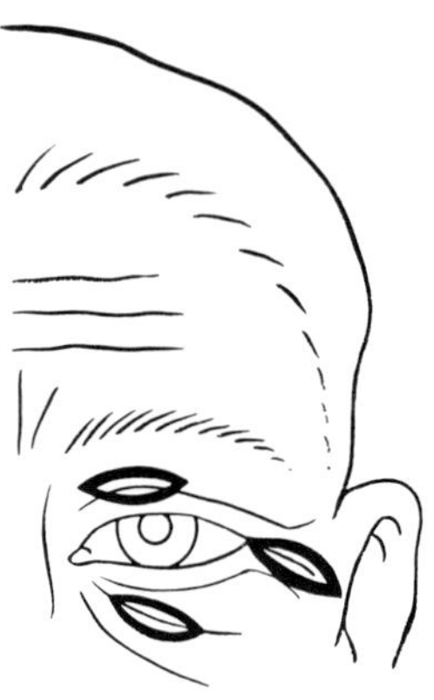

Fig. 25.3 Elliptical excisions on the eyelid.

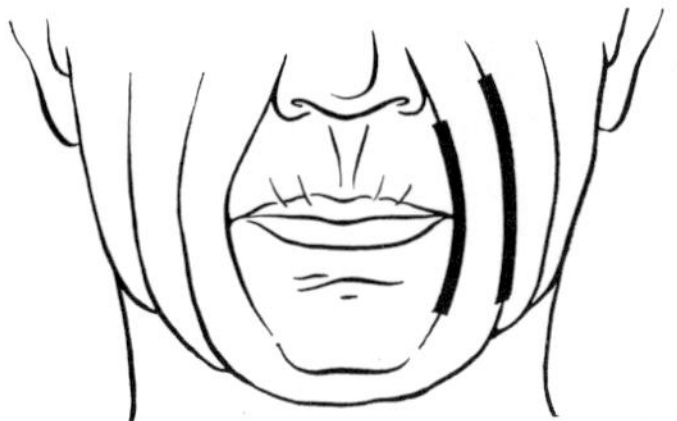

Fig. 25.4 Lines of relaxed skin tension on the cheeks.

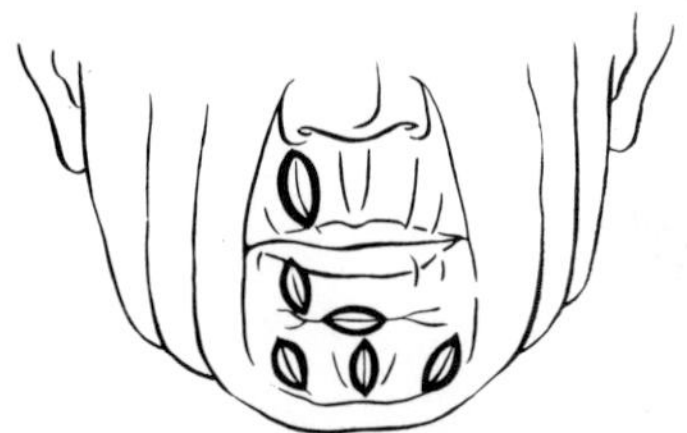

Fig. 25.5 Elliptical excisions on the chin.

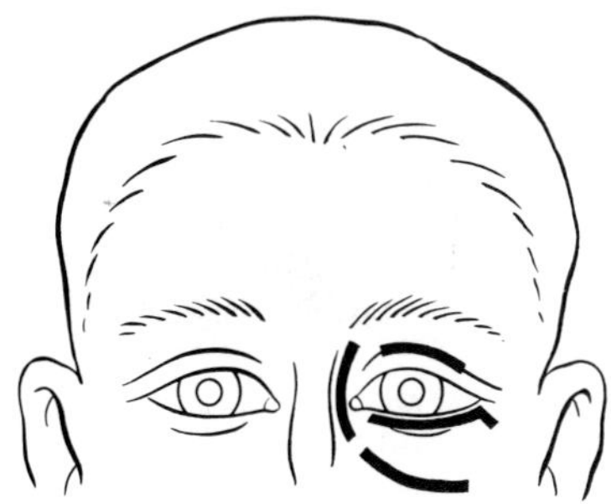

Fig. 25.6 Incisions for exposure of the medial and inferior walls of the orbit and for surgery in the levator muscles.

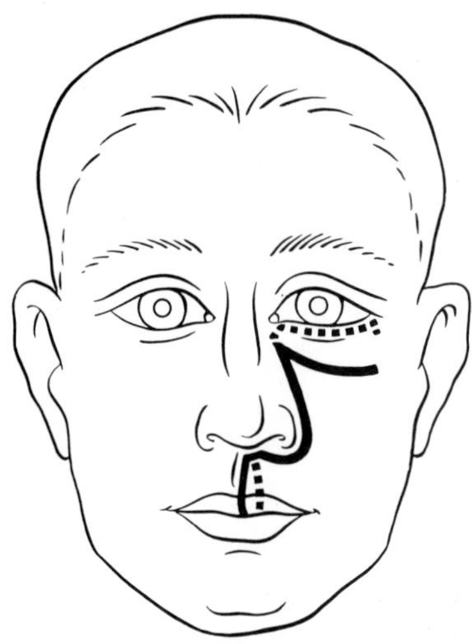

Fig. 25.7 The classic Ferguson incision.

In situations where closure of defects directly cannot be achieved, either because of the size or because of unacceptable tissue distortion, grafting or flaps must be considered.

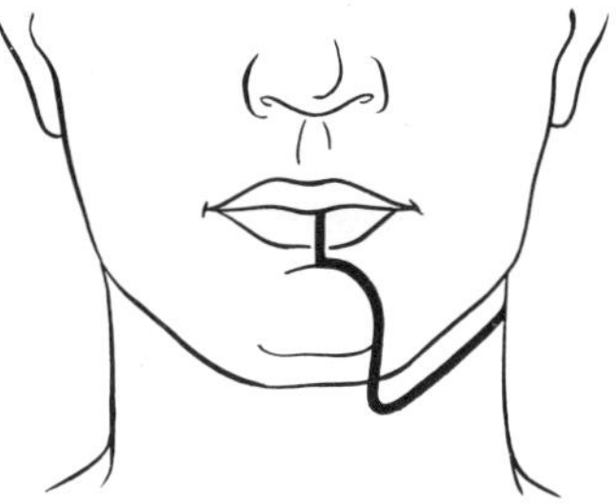

Fig. 25.8 The lip-splitting incision used for wide access to the mandible, tongue and floor of the mouth.

Fig. 25.9 The 'flying bird' incision for correction of deformities of the alar cartilage.

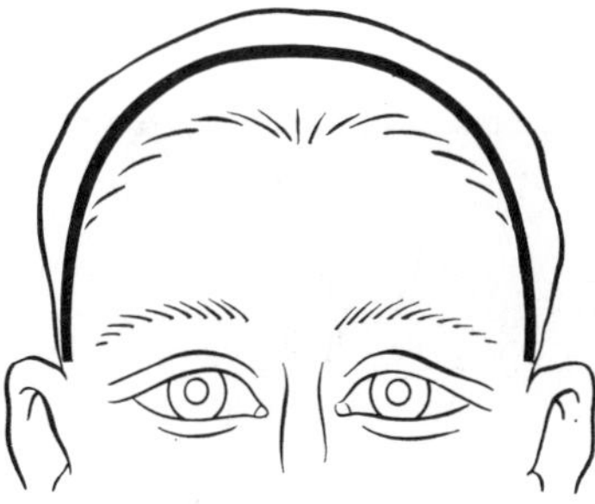

Fig. 25.10 The coronal incision for exposure of frontal bones and sinuses.

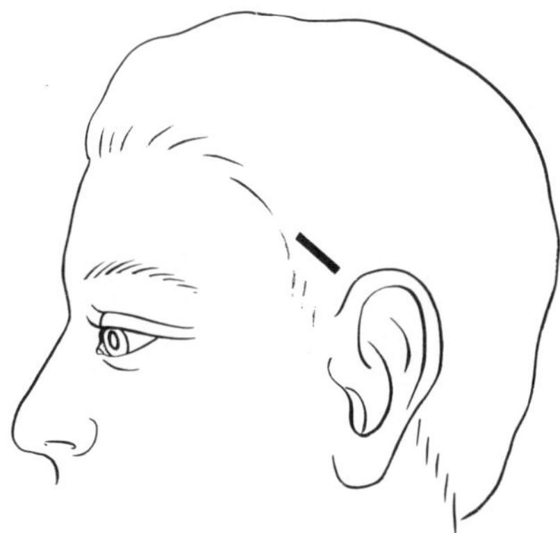

Fig. 25.11 The Gillies temporal approach for elevation of fractured molars.

GRAFTS

Split-skin grafts, though easy to obtain (*Figs.* 25.12–25.14), are not in general satisfactory from a cosmetic point of view. The colour can vary from being very pale to very pigmented. The reasons for pigmentation in split-skin grafts are unknown. The large donor site caused by use of the forehead temporal artery flap, requires to be split-skin grafted and represents a significant cosmetic blemish which may be unacceptable (*Fig.* 25.15). In the emergency situation, where tissue loss exists and in the management of the burned face, split-skin grafting may be useful (*Fig.* 25.16).

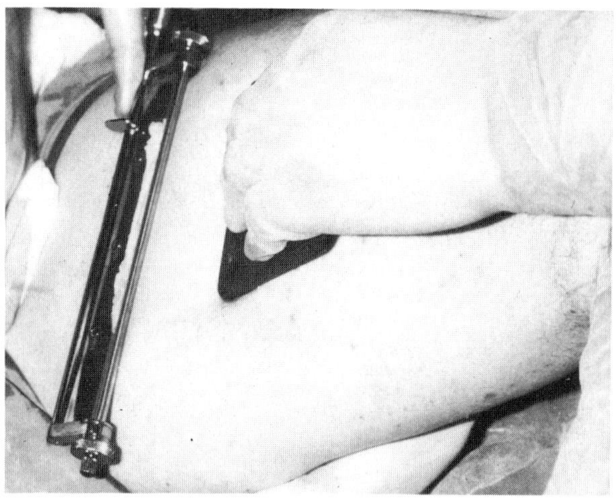

Fig. 25.12 Split-skin graft being cut from thigh with hand-held knife.

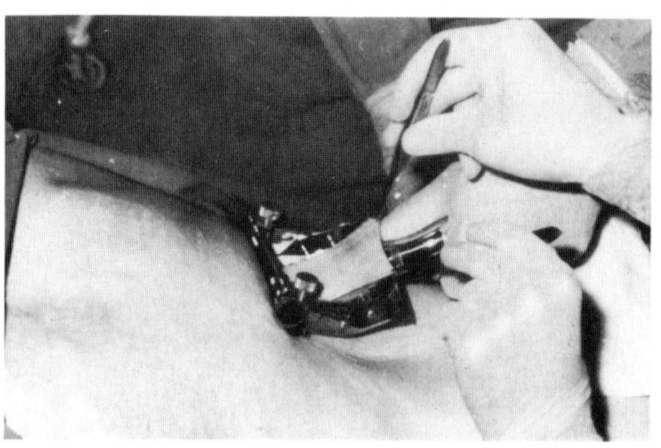

Fig. 25.13 Split-skin graft being cut using an electrical dermatome.

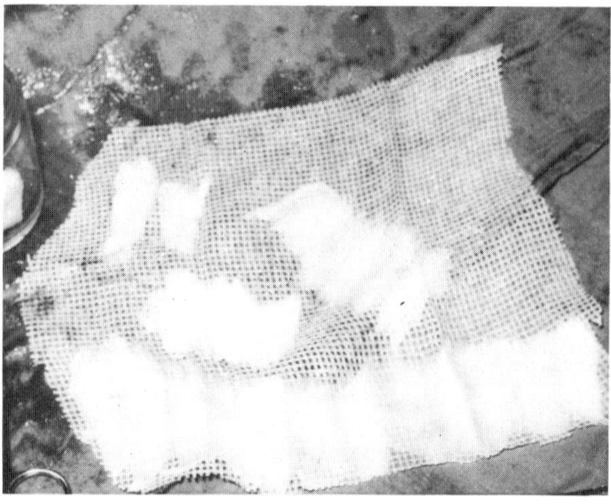

Fig. 25.14 Skin graft laid out on tulle. It may be stored in a sterile container at 4 °C for 2–3 weeks.

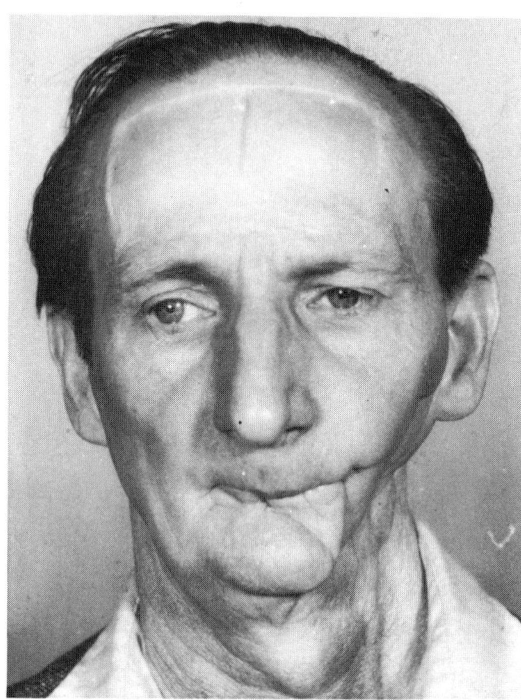

Fig. 25.15 Skin-grafted forehead following use of a flap for intra-oral reconstruction and partial mandibulectomy.

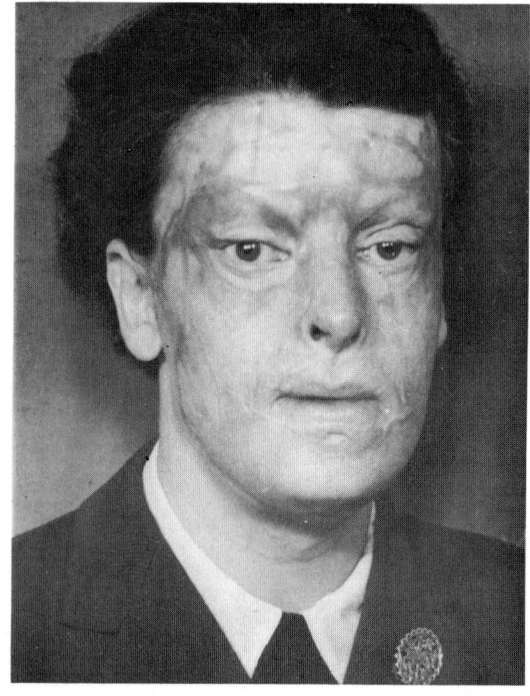

Fig. 25.16 A severe burn of the face showing repair by skin grafting.

Full-thickness grafts have certain advantages with regard to repair of facial defects. Not only does the colour tend to remain consistent with the donor site but they do not contract like split-skin grafts. These grafts may be obtained from retro-auricular, pre-auricular, nasolabial or supraclavicular skin. The colour obtained from these sites can usually be satisfactorily matched with the facial skin (*Fig.* 25.17). In the planning of facial repair, it is useful to consider the face as a series of aesthetic units. Not only should scars be placed if possible at junction lines between units, but grafts (or flaps) should be planned to lie appropriately.

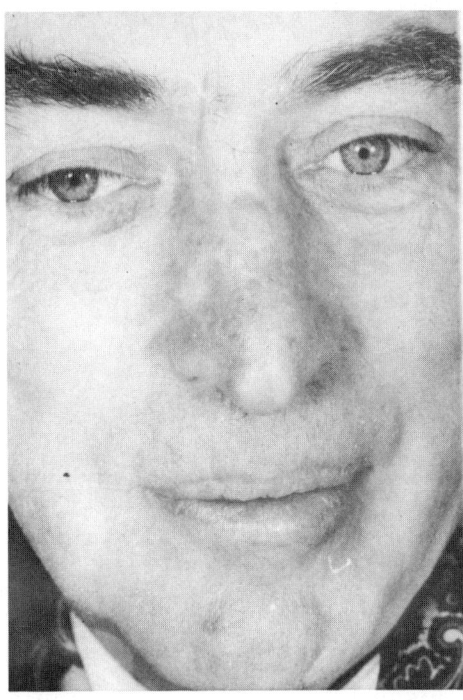

Fig. 25.17 Retro-auricular full-thickness grafts have been used to resurface defects on the right side of the nose following excision of a rodent ulcer.

FLAPS

Flaps have many uses and many designs in facial reconstruction. Flaps can be divided into:

1. Local random pattern flaps
2. Axial pattern flaps
3. Musculocutaneous flaps
4. Microvascular or free flaps.

Local Flaps

This is the simplest form of reconstruction and many designs are possible due to the excellent blood supply in the face. Some examples are shown (*Figs.* 25.18–25.19). In general, provided care is taken to avoid creating tissue distortion and recognition of aesthetic units, the cosmetic results are usually good. Flaps which have their bases superiorly may remain oedematous for a long time. It is worth waiting up to 1 year to allow for improvement.

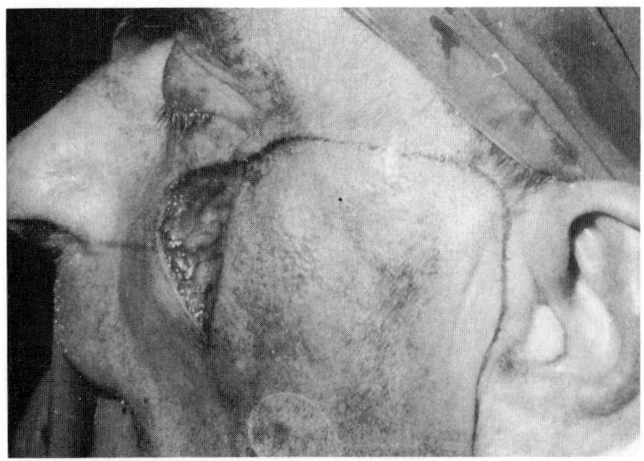

a

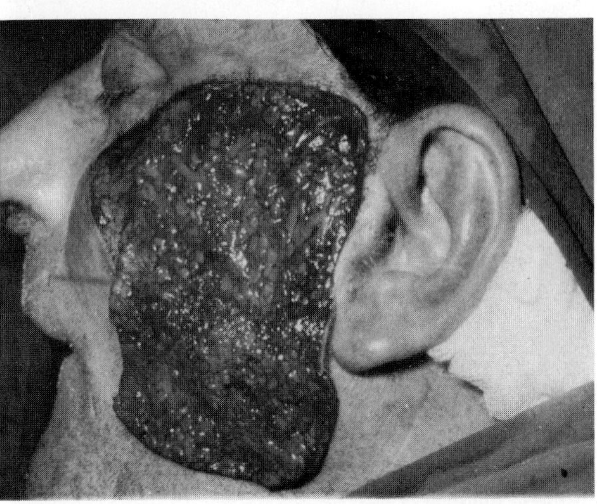

b

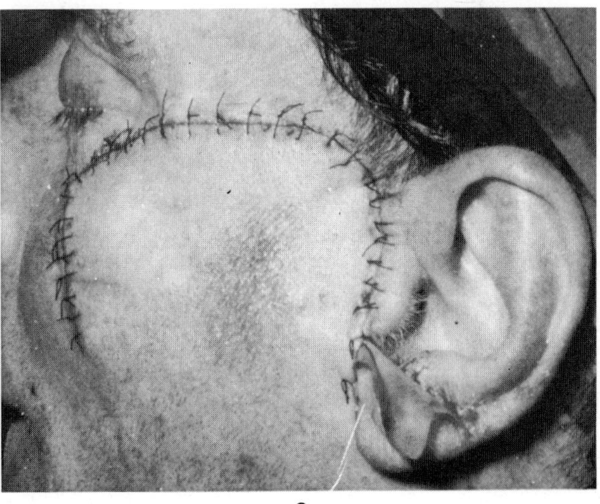

c

Fig. 25.18 Resurface of a defect of the cheek by means of a transposition cheek flap.

Axial Flaps

The temporal artery or forehead flap has for a long time provided a safe and useful means of repair of both extra- or intraoral defects. In the external face it can provide a source

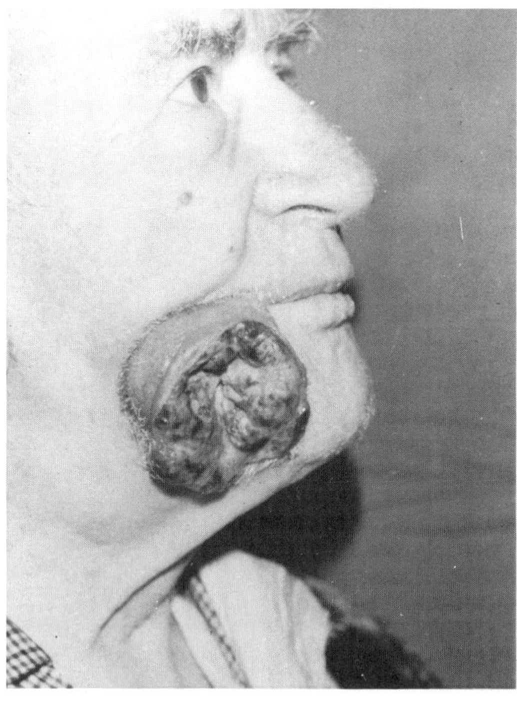
a

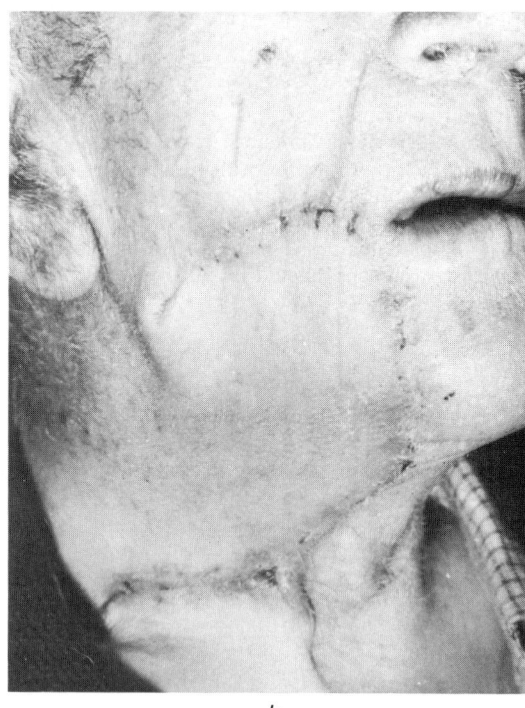
b

Fig. 25.19 *a,b*, Squamous carcinoma and repair by transposition neck flap (elderly man with lax skin).

of tissue for repair of orbital, cheek, nose and even lip (*Fig.* 25.20). It is extremely safe. The need to graft the donor site in the forehead is a disadvantage and represents a significant cosmetic blemish.

The deltopectoral flap, based on the intercostal perforators, remains a still useful though more unpredictable axial flap. The secondary defect requires to be grafted and the flap on most occasions can reach the zygomatic regions. It may be useful to combine with a forehead flap to produce a full-thickness repair (*Fig.* 25.21).

Musculocutaneous Flaps

These flaps have the great merit of using muscle-perforating vessels to augment the overlying skin.

There are a number of musculocutaneous flaps which can be used in facial surgery. They have the advantage of excellent blood supply. Examples of this include the sternomastoid, trapezius, latissimus dorsi and pectoralis major musculocutaneous flaps (*Figs.* 25.22–25.23). These can be used for both intra- and extraoral repairs. They are a good source of well vascularized tissues and the secondary defects can often be relatively insignificant. The majority of reconstructions carried out using musculocutaneous flaps are rapid, simple and safe. In situations where previous radiotherapy or infections exist, musculocutaneous flaps can be very effective because they introduce well-vascularized tissue. Muscles can also be used without skin.

Microvascular Flaps

The advent of microsurgery in plastic and reconstructive surgery has further increased the possibilities in facial surgery. The cosmetic results, however, are not necessarily better than by using other methods. When, however, particular problems of soft tissue or bone framework exist, there are good indications. For example, in severe hemifacial atrophy soft tissue may be augmented by using omentum or free latissimus dorsi muscle flap (*Fig.* 25.24). Vascularized bone, if required for mandible reconstruction, can be obtained using a free iliac crest bone graft. In facial palsy some improvements may be possible using free vascularized and innervated muscle flaps though the results may be both unpredictable and difficult to measure.

THE BONY SKELETON

The aesthetic appearance of the face is dependent on the underlying bone structures as, for example in acromegaly where the lower jaw may be unduly prominent. Abnormalities may be congenital, as in Crouzon's disease, or acquired, as a result of trauma or excisional surgery. Orbitocraniofacial surgery is probably the newest major surgical field. Much of the credit for this specialty belongs to Paul Tessier (Paris) but Sir Harold Gillies performed the first craniofacial procedure in England in 1949. This kind of surgery carries significant risks of morbidity and mortality and should be carried out in specialist units by highly trained teams. The results can be impressive (*Fig.* 25.25).

TRAUMA

The compulsory wearing of front seat belts in the UK has reduced the incidence of facial injuries resulting from road traffic accidents. Careful preoperative assessments are essential and other coexisting major system injuries identified if present. A full radiographical examination should be done to assess fractures or foreign bodies. Care should be taken with

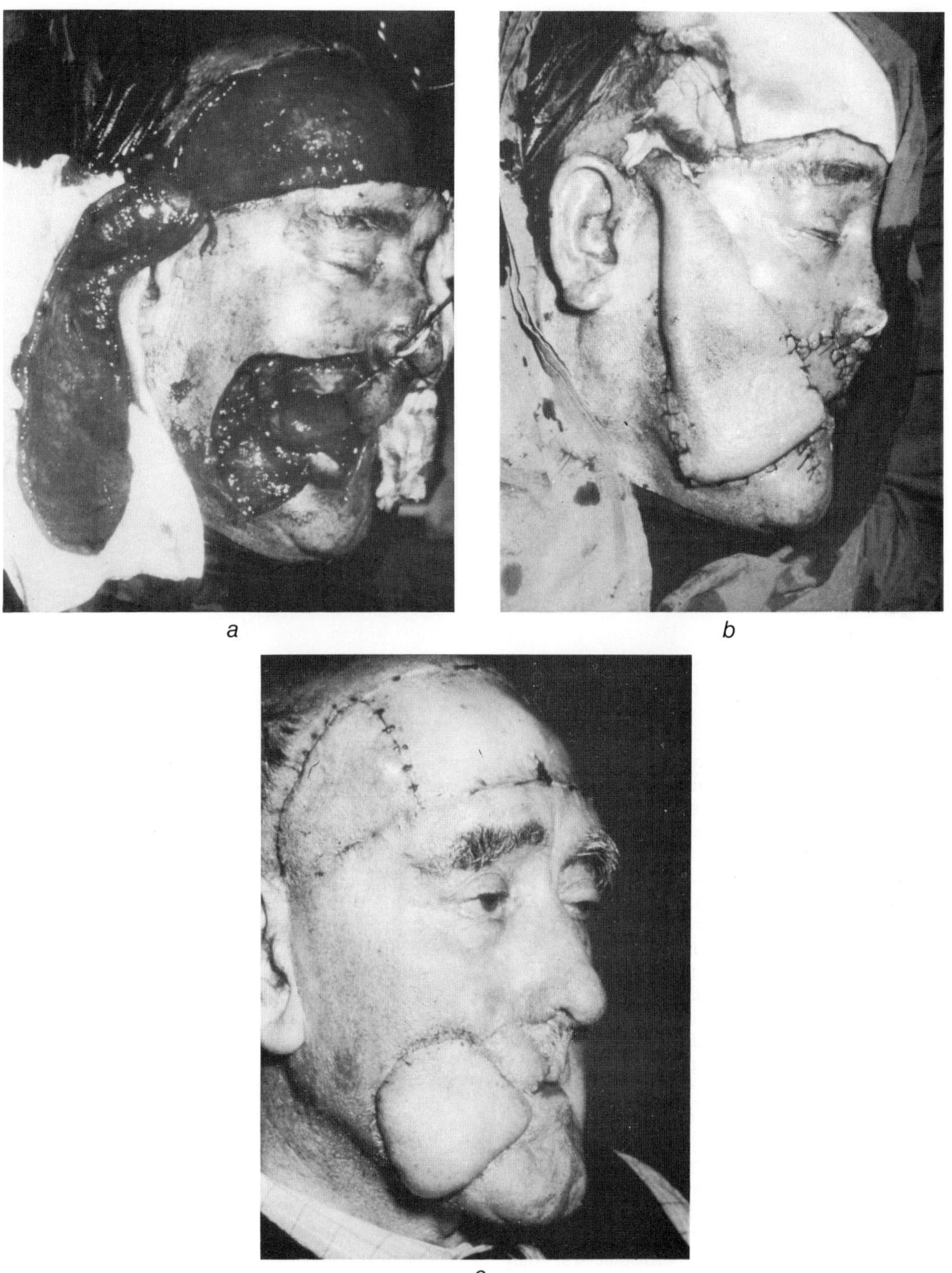

Fig. 25.20 *a,b,c,* Forehead flap in use for resurfacing a defect of the lip. Division of the pedicle occurs at 3 weeks. Further trimming of the flap could improve appearance.

any injuries near the eye. If there are lacerations of the eyelids and the lids are too swollen to inspect the globe, this should be deferred until the patient is anaesthetized. Attempts to prise open the lids in the conscious patient can raise the intraocular pressure to dangerous levels.

Treatment

Facial lacerations can leave very obvious and disfiguring scars which can have enormous impact on the patients' quality of life. The best results are obtained in conditions where there is good anaesthesia, good light, delicate instru-

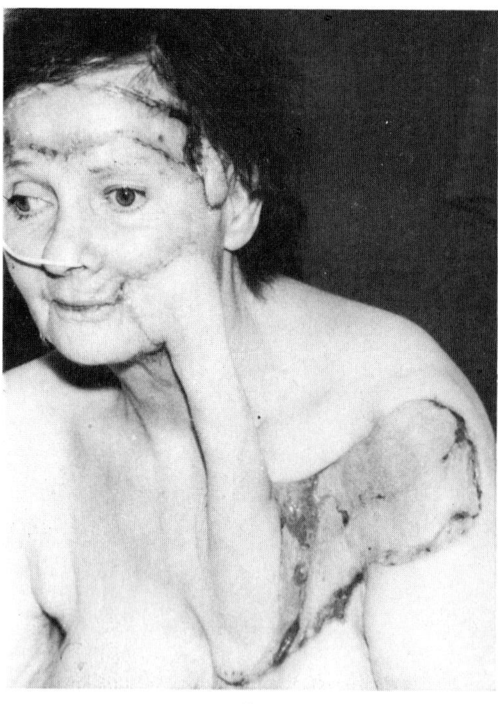

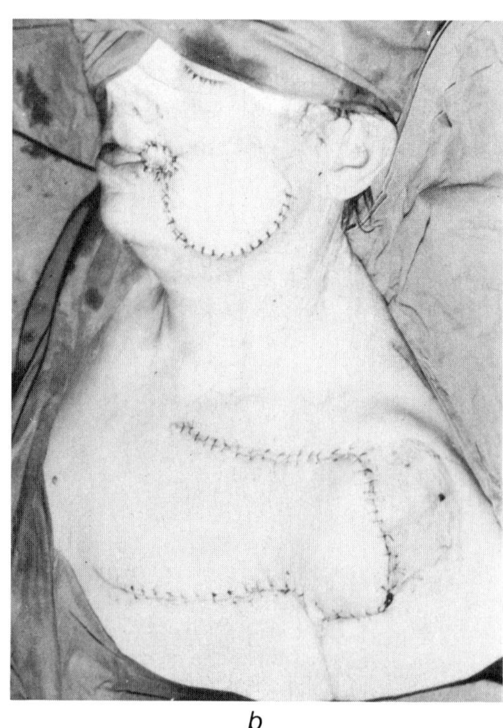

Fig. 25.21 *a*, A deltopectoral flap used in conjunction with a forehead flap which is providing internal lining. *b*, Division of pedicle and inset of flap into cheek and return of unused pedicle to chest.

ments and fine sutures. Primary treatment includes adequate wound toilet. Failure to remove all the dirt and grit can lead to permanent tattooing (*Fig.* 25.26). Every effort must, therefore, be made to scrub dirt from wounds. On occasions, when dirt has been deeply ingrained (as after explosions) it may be necessary to use a scalpel to pick out the particles. These techniques must not, of course, be applied in the case of corneal or scleral pigmentation. Having done all necessary wound toilet, careful repair is carried out. If large soft-tissue defects occur, split-skin grafts or flaps can be used provided the surgeon's experience is such that the necessary decisions can be made. Divided branches of the facial nerve or major salivary ducts are best repaired at the time of injury. The use of an operating microscope may be invaluable in repairing these structures.

Scar Revision

It is important to wait several months and even as long as one year to allow for spontaneous improvements. Red, thick scars may pale and soften, rendering revisions less likely. This process may be aided by regular massage with a bland ointment. Injection of steroids into hypertrophic scars may hasten their resolution. Secondary surgery may involve the correction of errors in primary management such as malalignment or ingrained pigment. Contracture bands, or scars lying in an unfavourable position, may be released or changed using Z or W plasties.

Burns

Burns to the face are relatively common though in most instances are superficial. There is often considerable oedema within the first 48 h. These burns are kept exposed. Primary excision of facial burns is not done except when there is obvious full-thickness destruction of the eyelid and potential risk of exposure of the eye. In these cases some form of protective flap cover is necessary. Hypertrophic scarring may be treated initially by wearing some form of pressure garment for several months as this may cause considerable flattening of raised scars. The late reconstruction of the burned face, by means of grafts and flaps, may take years of work. Microvascular free-flap transfer may considerably speed up the repair. It is important to remember that any burn may be associated with inhalation of smoke or toxic gases and the recognition and treatment of this is of paramount importance. Tracheostomy is rarely required.

NEOPLASIA

The face is subject to the whole range of skin tumours, both benign and malignant. Benign lesions include the various papillomas, moles and epidermoid or sebaceous cysts. All of these are usually easy to excise with good cosmetic results.

The exposed situation of the face probably renders it a favourable site for the various malignancies. Solar keratosis may be a premalignant situation for squamous carcinoma as can radiation damage from other causes.

Squamous carcinoma is fairly common on the lateral parts of the facial skin and ear. Excision must include at least 1 cm of healthy tissue. Repair of defects can be difficult. Full-thickness defects of the nose or cheek require repair of internal lining as well as external cover. This may involve grafting the undersurface of a flap or using two flaps. The lower eyelids may be repaired by a variety of flaps including cheek rotation flaps and flaps from the upper lids. Support and lining may be obtained using nasal and septal chondromucosal free grafts. Functional reconstruction of the upper

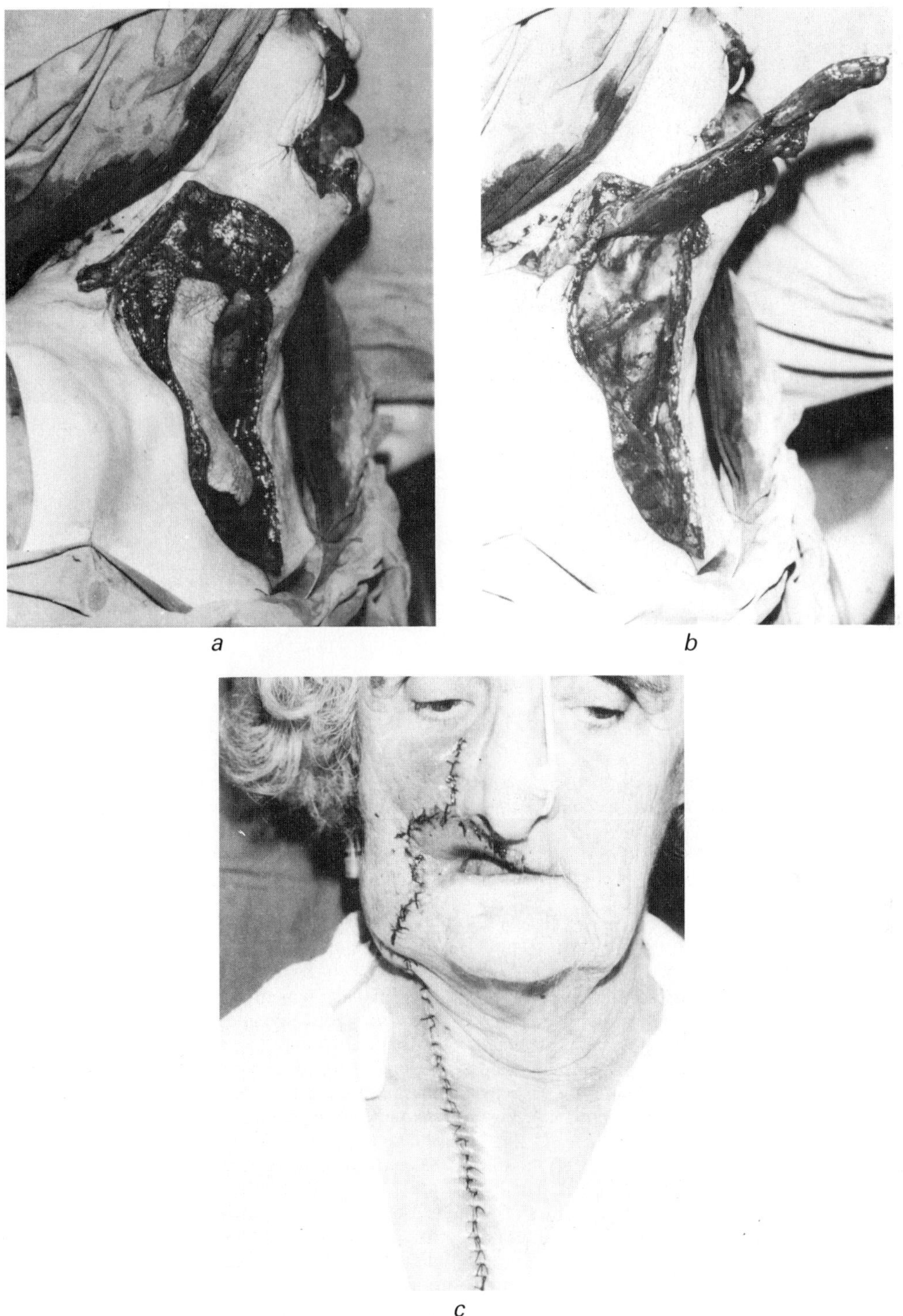

Fig. 25.22 *a,b,c,* Rodent ulcer of the right oral commissure. Repair by sternomastoid muscle flap with island of skin which is brought into defect under bridge of intact skin.

lid can be obtained by using part of the lower lid as a switch flap rotated through 180°. Defects of the lip after excision of squamous-cell carcinomas are repaired by direct approximation if the defects are small. Larger defects require local advancement flaps or switch flaps. Cancer is more common in the lower lip and is related to outdoor occupations and excessive sun exposure. Premalignant leucoplakia changes may be treated by mucosal excision and repair by advancement of buccal mucosa anteriorly. This procedure, sometimes known as a 'lip shave', usually produces a good cosmetic appearance.

Basal-cell carcinomas can be found in all parts of the body

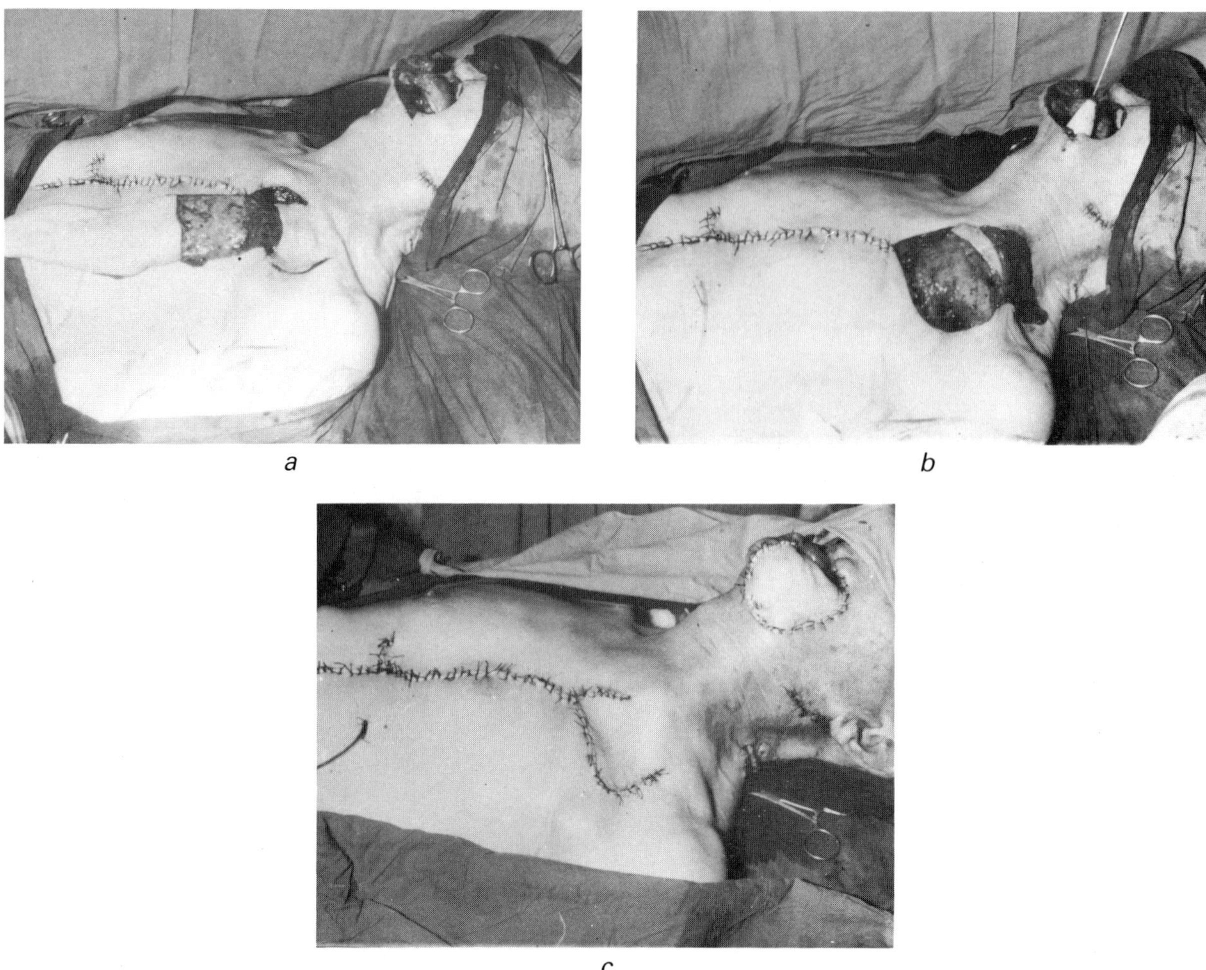

Fig. 25.23 *a,b,c,* Rodent ulcer of left corner of mouth with repair of defect with an island pectoralis major myocutaneous flap.

skin but are most common in the middle third of the face (nose, eyelids and cheeks). This slowly growing tumour rarely metastasizes but is capable of progressive local tissue erosion (*Fig.* 25.27). Lesions in the inner canthus, alar creases and in the region of the auditory meatus are particularly prone to being neglected or treated inadequately. Pigmented rodent ulcers may mimic melanomas (*Fig.* 25.28).

Excision with a margin of 3–4 mm of healthy tissue around the visible lesion margins, is advisable. Repair by grafts or local flaps may be done according to the size, site or depth of the defect. When uncertainty about surgical clearance is possible, the use of frozen sections and skin grafts (rather than flaps) is a wise approach. On the other hand, where there is no possibility of surgical cure, the use of a flap may allow postoperative radiotherapy or delay the occurrence of external ulceration of the tumour.

Malignant melanoma of the facial skin is probably slightly less common than in other sites. Contrary to belief, pathology rarely indicates malignant change in a pre-existing mole. Moles occur very commonly in the face. Any sudden increase in size, change in pigmentation, bleeding or itch should be looked on as suspicious. The prognosis is, to a great extent, unpredictable but pathological assessment of tumour depth is probably of value as would be the presence of regional nodal spread. In the elderly, the gradual appearance of flat pigmented patches may be considered to be a possible premalignant melanoma (lentigo maligna) (*Fig.* 25.29). Consideration should be given to excising such lesions, particularly if any raised nodules develop. The margin of excision for facial melanomas tends to be less than it might be in other sites because of a desire not to deform the face unduly. A margin similar to that for squamous-cell cancers is probably advisable with reconstruction by flap or graft.

Both squamous-cell carcinoma and malignant melanoma may metastasize to the regional lymph nodes. A radical neck dissection should form part of the primary operation if nodes are involved. It is usually considered that prophylactic neck dissection does not confer any advantages in patient survival.

CONGENITAL ANOMALIES

A large number of congenital abnormalities of the face can occur. These may involve skin, subcutaneous tissues or bone and may affect special regions such as the nose, lips, ears and mouth. Severe psychological problems can occur as a result of deformity so there may be real pressure to deal with them at an early age. Careful counselling of parents and

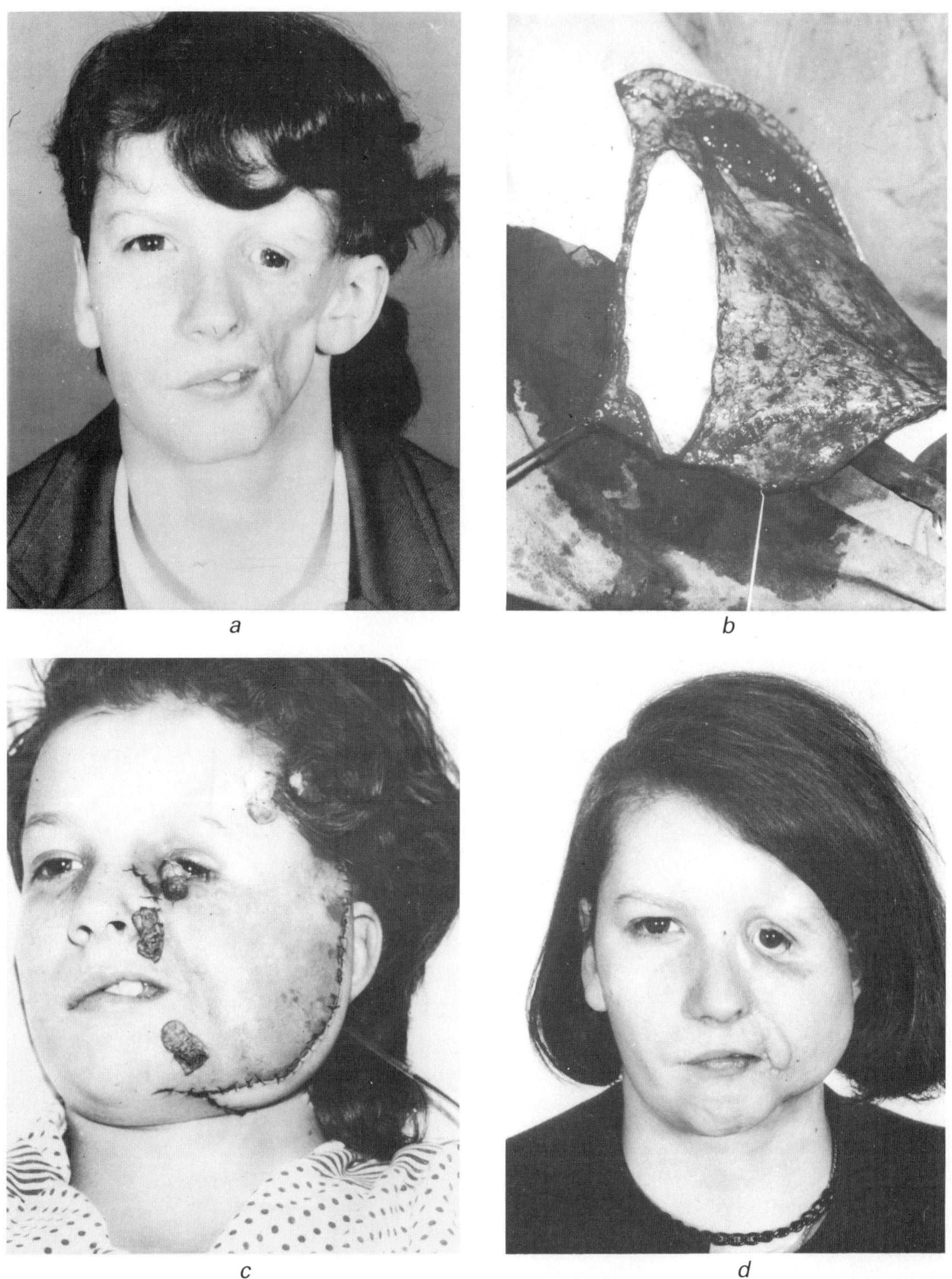

Fig. 25.24 a, A young girl with severe hemifacial atrophy; b, A latissimus dorsi myocutaneous flap is raised with a skin island; c, A microsurgical transfer to the cheek is performed using the muscle as a subcutaneous implant; d, The clinical appearance after several years. Several minor adjustments have been made. (By courtesy of *Journal of Royal College of Surgeons of Edinburgh*.)

patients is usually advisable. Surgery is best done by surgeons trained in paediatric plastic surgical techniques.

1. Pigmented Vascular Naevi

Three types commonly occur:

a. Port Wine Stain

This well-recognized lesion is a capillary haemangioma lying in or just beneath the dermis (*Fig.* 25.30). It is usually flat and skin texture is normal but irregularities do occur rendering cosmetic cover by creams less satisfactory. Some

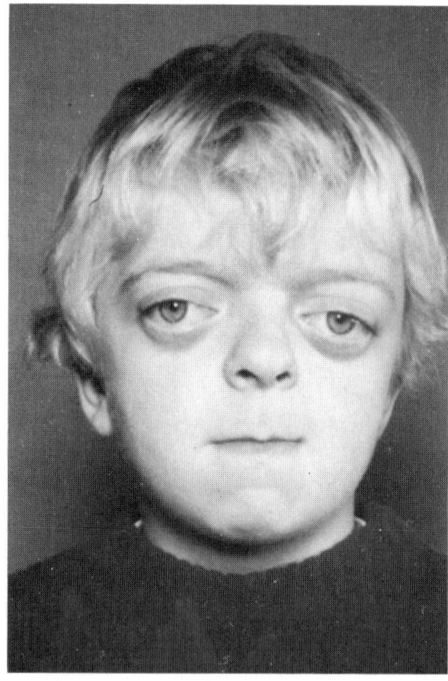

a

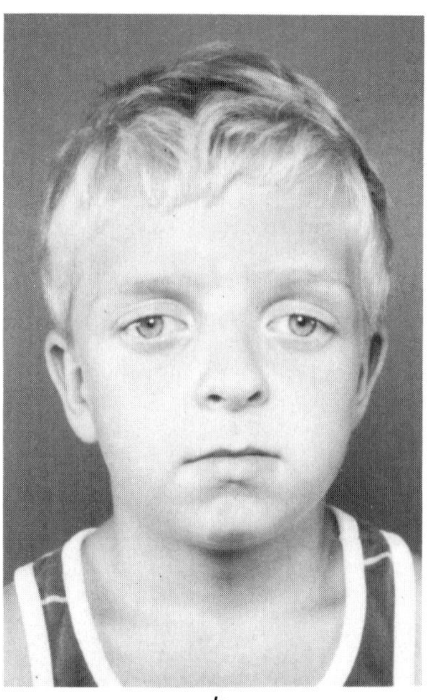

b

Fig. 25.25 *a*, Crouzon's preoperative; *b*, Crouzon's after Le Fort III advancement. (By courtesy of Dr I. T. Jackson.)

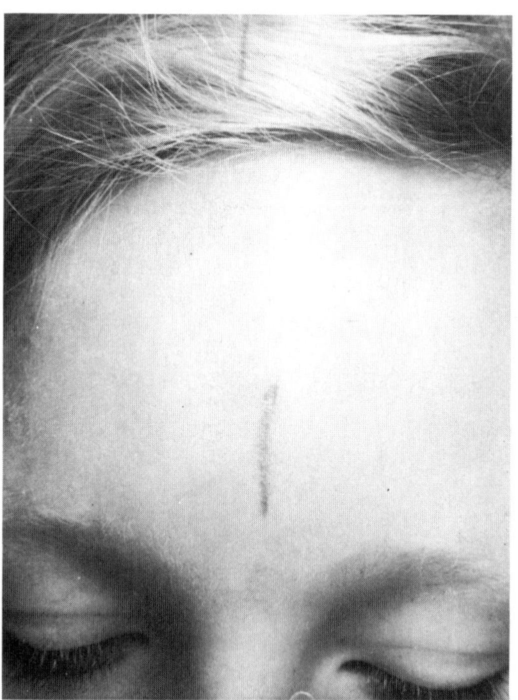

Fig. 25.26 Pigmented scar after failure of initial wound cleaning.

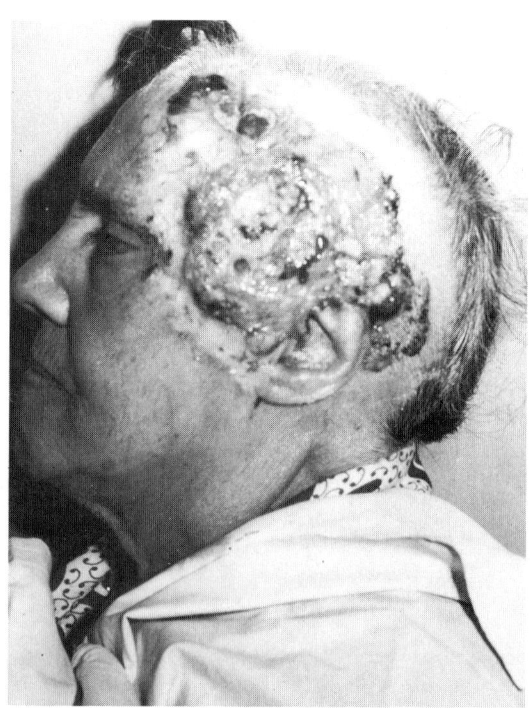

Fig. 25.27 Longstanding rodent ulcer showing extensive local tissue erosion.

excellent results may be obtained by careful excision and full-thickness grafting, provided attention is given to meticulous techniques and anatomical zones. The use of tattooing with flesh-coloured pigments can give reasonable but unpredictable results while lasers, at present, are not widely available but may offer an important future solution.

b. The Strawberry Naevus

This usually occurs shortly after birth and can enlarge at an alarming rate for several months. If left it generally resolves spontaneously after several years (*Fig.* 25.31). Reassurance rather than early surgery is advised unless the lesion is in the eyelids and threatens to or occludes the vision in an eye.

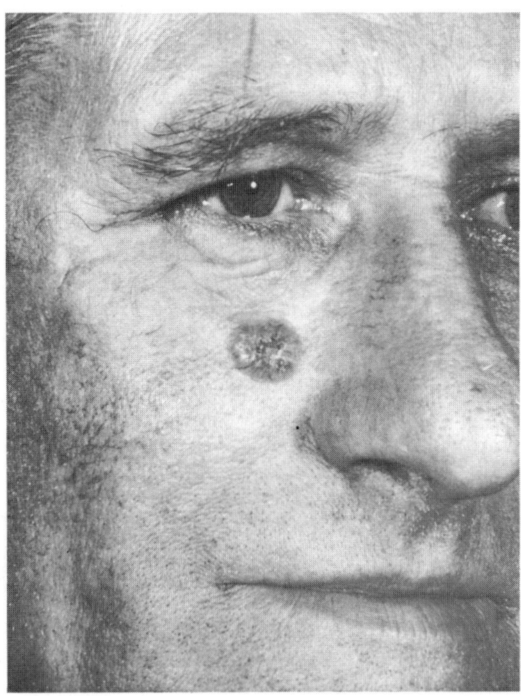

Fig. 25.28 Pigmented basal-cell carcinoma.

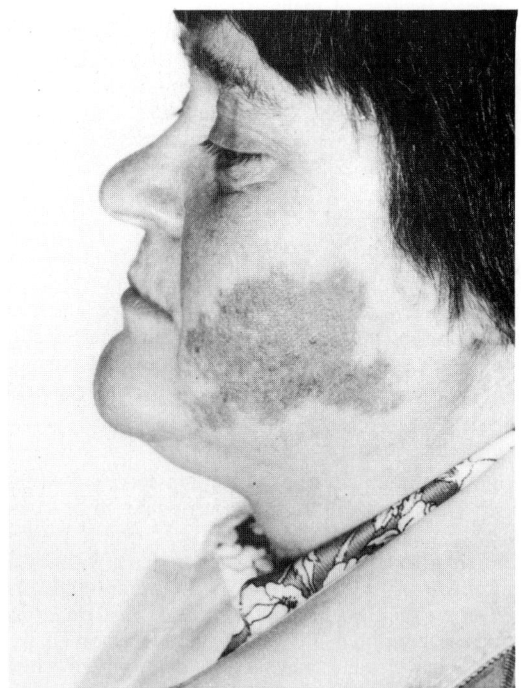

Fig. 25.30 Port wine stain.

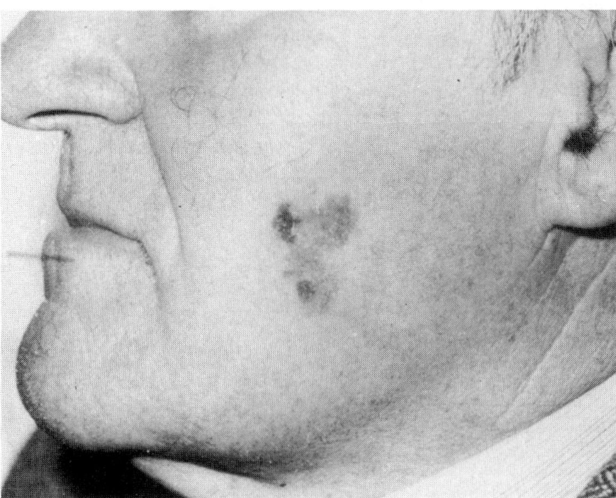

Fig. 25.29 Lentigo maligna of the cheek.

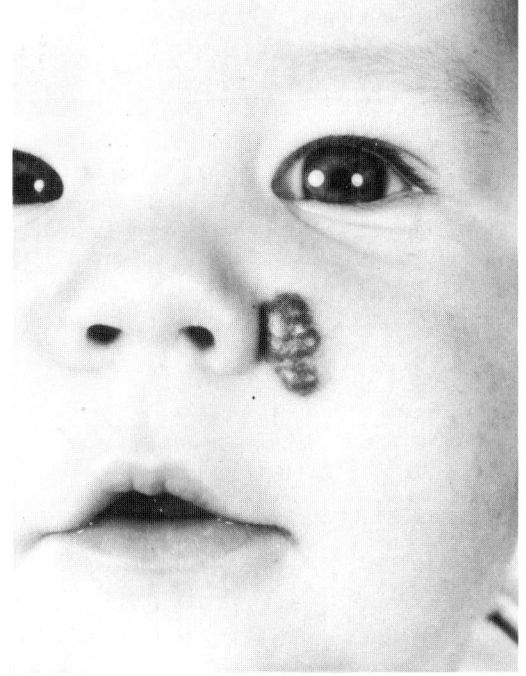

Fig. 25.31 Strawberry naevus.

Haemorrhage is extremely rare and ulceration which can occur is readily treated by conservative methods. Surgery may be used to tidy up any redundant papery skin which remains after resolution. Histologically it presents a varied picture of large vascular spaces in and deep into the dermis with capillary elements.

c. *Cavernous Haemangioma*

This consists of large vascular spaces at the subdermis level usually of a venous nature. Sometimes there is an element of lymphangioma and overlying strawberry components and it is worth while allowing time for any resolution. When the lesions persist there is a limited place for cryosurgery but the results can be disappointing. Surgery can be difficult and it is advisable to consider carefully the risks as opposed to the cosmetic problems. Angiography is itself not without risk but may be necessary to delineate the vascular channels and components, be they arterial or venous.

Proximal ligation of main arteries may be dangerous as well as inadequate since the result may be an opening up of alternative anastomotic pathways. Embolization, using small emboli of plastic balls or autogenous muscle may, in carefully selected cases, be the answer. This technique should only be done by specialists working in properly equipped hospitals. Bone changes may occur in association with large haemangiomas either through direct involvement or because of increased local vascularity.

2. Pigmented Non-vascular Naevi

Pigmented naevi have already been discussed and usually present no problems. Large congenital naevi may occur and can represent significant cosmetic blemishes. Excision and repair by direct closure, grafts or flaps may be required.

3. Congenital Anomalies of the Nose

The most common deformities are in association with cleft lips (*see later*). Surgical procedures may have to be staged in order to take account of the growing child. Minor congenital notches of the nostril margin can be dealt with by local advancement flaps. One other fairly common deformity which is frequently misdiagnosed and mistreated is the midline nasal dermoid. Persistence of a developmental midline epithelial element may be found anywhere from the base of the columella to the glabella. A fistulous tract passes downwards and may extend as far as the anterior cranial fossa. An extradural abscess may occur. These lesions often present as a midline cyst or pit with protruding hair. The correct treatment is a careful and tedious dissection to trace the tract to its outer limits. Exceptionally a craniotomy may be required.

4. Congenital Lesions affecting the Ears

a. Preauricular Sinuses and Accessory Auricles

As a result of the complex development of the auricle from the first and second branchial arches, maldevelopment may give rise to sinuses and accessory parts of cartilage. The latter are usually early excised (unless they are required to reconstruct a malformed ear). Recurrent abscesses may be the presentation of sinuses. Careful surgical excisions are usually effective.

b. Prominent or Bat Ear

This is the commonest congenital anomaly and one which causes considerable distress in the Western but not the Eastern world. The deformity occurs in varying degrees and may be associated with a failure of cartilage folding to create an antihelical fold or with a relative excess of conchal cartilage. The former abnormality is treated fairly readily by various operations designed to create a new fold. The surgical approach to them is usually through the posterior skin. Folding of the cartilage can be achieved by insertion of non-absorbable horizontal mattress sutures or by scoring the anterior surface of the cartilage. This releases tension and enables the cartilage to bend in the opposite direction. Where the deformity is due to conchal excess, excision of an appropriate amount of cartilage may give satisfactory correction.

c. Cryptotia and Microtia

These deformities occur less commonly. In the former the cartilage framework, though present, is partly buried under the scalp skin. Reconstruction involves release and resurfacing with local skin flaps. Microtia is where the ear is congenitally absent apart from rudimentary soft tissue. Reconstruction is very difficult and the results can be disappointing. The provision of a prosthetic ear may be a better solution.

5. Cleft Lip and Palate

Bearing in mind the complex functions which are concentrated in the face it is hardly surprising that the development of this region is subject to a bewildering assortment of anomalies. It is beyond the scope of this section to describe the detailed development of the face and related structures, though a few general points should serve as a basis for understanding the treatment of some of the major deformities.

Pathology

While there is a good deal of disagreement on the detailed formation of the face, His's original concept of the fusion of several processes is helpful as regards the position of the various clefts which may affect it. These are indicated in *Fig.* 25.32. While clefts of the upper lip are relatively

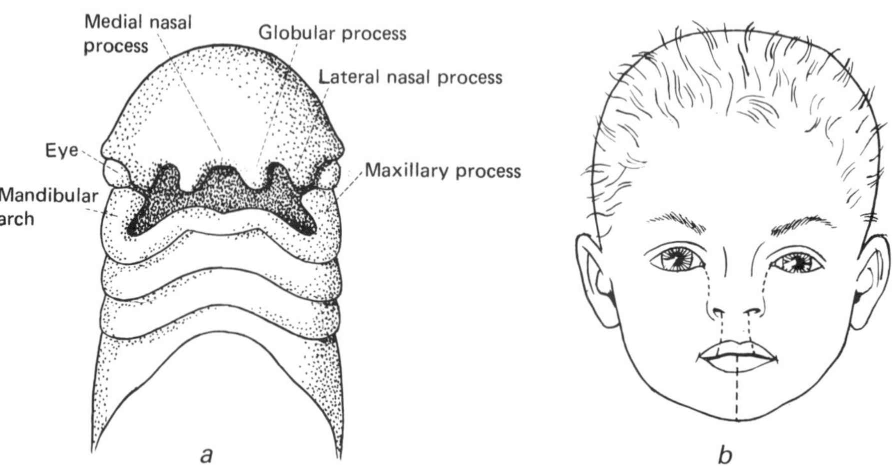

Fig. 25.32 *a*, His's concept of facial development; *b*, Lines of cleft formation resulting from faulty fusion.

common, midline clefts of the lower lip and jaw and oblique facial clefts are extremely rare and are not considered further. Clefts of the lip may be uni- or bilateral and from a simple vermilion notch to a complete cleft involving the floor of the nostril. They also vary in the extent to which they involve the underlying hard tissues.

The palate may be divided into primary and secondary palates on embryological grounds. The primary palate consists of two parts: (*a*) the central lip; and (*b*) the premaxillae as far as the incisive foramen, so that a complete cleft of the primary palate involves the soft tissues of the lip and nostril floor as well as the alveolus and anterior portion of the hard palate, i.e. the structures formed from fusion of the medial and lateral nasal processes and the maxillary processes. The secondary palate is the rest of the hard palate and all of the soft palate and develops quite differently, 10–12 days later, by the fusion of two processes from the maxillae which swing upwards when the tongue descends and fuse from backwards. Clefts of the secondary palate vary in degree from behind forwards.

Clefts of the Primary Palate

Since the primary palate is formed by about the 35th day and the secondary palate by the 47th day, it is obvious that clefts in this region will have an influence on subsequent development. This results in a complex deformity which comprises more than a simple cleft in the structures. Thus the lip on the medial side of the cleft is short in vertical height as is the columella. The alveolus on the medial side slopes upwards and tends to be rotated anteriorly and towards the normal side, while the alveolus on the lateral side is short and retroposed. This causes a flaring or lateral displacement of the alar base while the nasal tip and septum are displaced towards the normal side (*Fig.* 25.33). In bilateral clefts the philtrum or central lip is short in vertical height, as is the whole columella which pulls down the tip of the nose. Unrestrained growth of the central stem leads to protrusion of the whole premaxillary complex (*Fig.* 25.34). A further complicating factor in the treatment is the fact that these are not simple clefts in otherwise normal tissues.

There is also a tissue deficiency, and a lack of growth potential persists throughout the growth period causing further deformity, such as maxillary retrognathism. In recent years attention has been focused on the absence of muscle in the central lip in complete bilateral clefts, and abnormal disposition and attachment of the fibres of the orbicularis oris in both unilateral and bilateral clefts (*Fig.* 25.35).

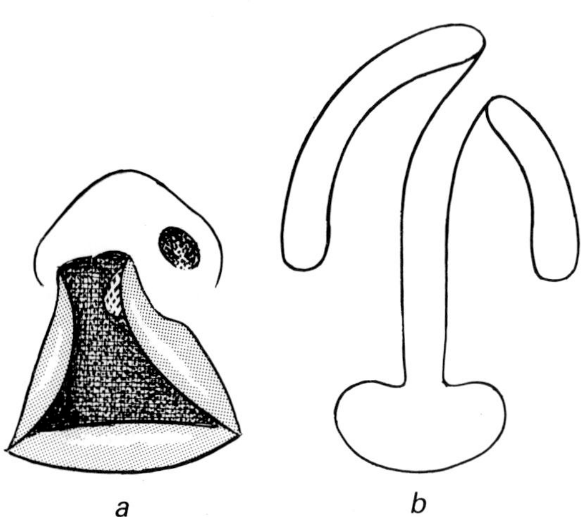

Fig. 25.33 *a*, External deformity in unilateral cleft; *b*, Distortion of alveolar arches.

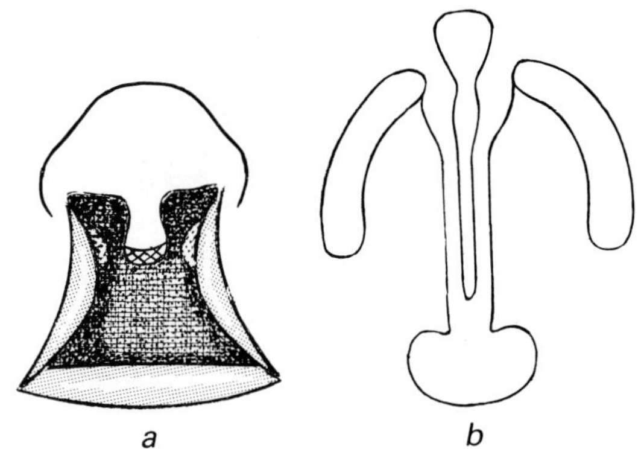

Fig. 25.34 *a*, External deformity in unilateral cleft; *b*, Distortion of alveolar processes and protruding premaxilla.

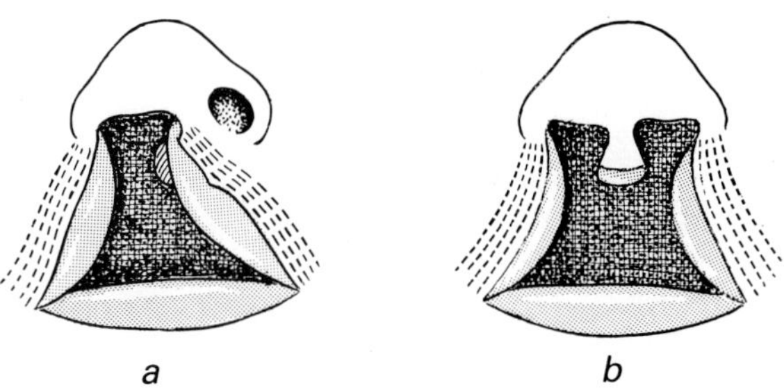

Fig. 25.35 Disposition of fibres of orbicularis in: *a*, Uni- and *b*, Bilateral cleft lips.

Orthodontic Treatment

The alveolar deformities can be considerably reduced by presurgical orthodontic treatment which makes the surgery of cleft lip considerably easier and subsequently more accurate. The infant is fitted with a dental plate which facilitates feeding in cases of cleft palate as well as reducing the dental deformities. Success demands the skilled and dedicated attention of an orthodontist experienced in this work.

Where presurgical orthodontic treatment is available the timing of cleft lip repair is dictated by the response to the orthodontic treatment, being carried out when the orthodontist feels he has achieved the optimal correction. The operation is usually carried out between 3 and 6 months and is usually combined with repair of the anterior palate, i.e. as much of the hard palate as is reasonably possible. In the absence of presurgical orthodontics most surgeons operate at about 3 months, though some prefer to do so considerably earlier. Clefts of the secondary palate should be repaired later between 12 and 18 months. This provides the child with an intact mechanism by the time he starts to speak and produces better speech results.

Repair of Cleft Lip

There are many surgical techniques for cleft lip repair. For the unilateral cleft Millard's rotation/advancement operation gives excellent results (*Fig.* 25.36). This technique preserves

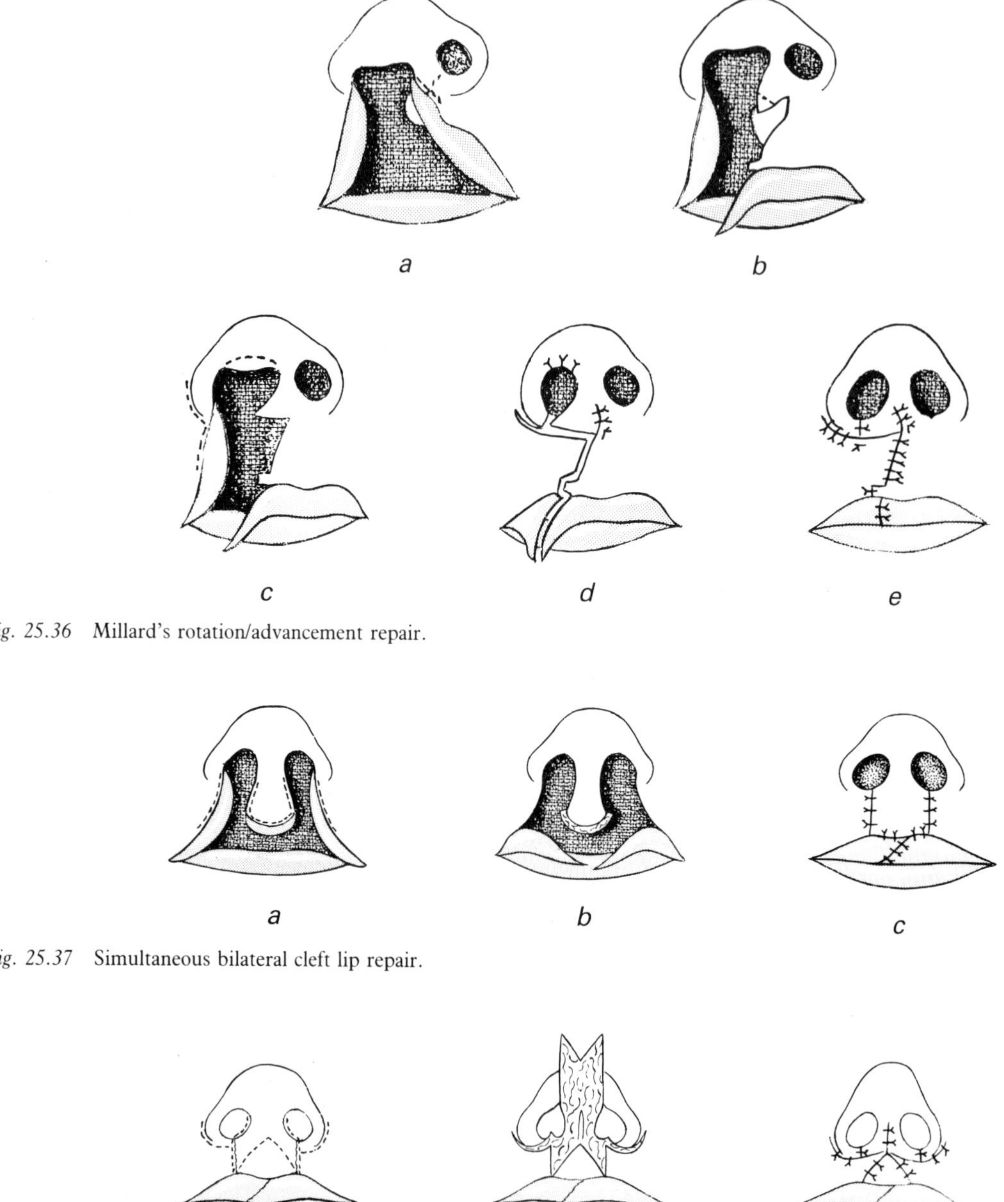

Fig. 25.36 Millard's rotation/advancement repair.

Fig. 25.37 Simultaneous bilateral cleft lip repair.

Fig. 25.38 The fork flap procedure to lengthen the columella, correct the alar flare, reconstruct the muscle sphincter and improve the shape of the philtrum.

the natural landmarks which are always present and places them in their normal position. It lengthens the medial side of the cleft as well as the columella on the cleft side, corrects the alar flare and provides a balanced lip and a greatly improved nose. The bilateral cleft is a different problem: attempts to increase the vertical height of the central lip causes horizontal tightness, for, while there is sufficient tissue available for this type of rearrangement in a unilateral cleft, there is not enough to do it on both sides. A lip which is symmetrical if slightly short, but slack enough horizontally must be accepted. *Fig.* 25.37 indicates how this can be achieved while not discarding any tissue at all. This procedure does not lengthen the columella, and leaves an unnaturally square and wide philtrum with flaring alar bases. All of this is corrected at a second operation at 4–5 years when the orbicularis muscle fibres can also be freed from the alar bases and sutured together to reconstruct the oral sphincter (*Fig.* 25.38).

Repair of the Secondary Palate

Clefts of the secondary palate are repaired in 2 layers. The nasal layer consists of mucous membrane which is mobilized

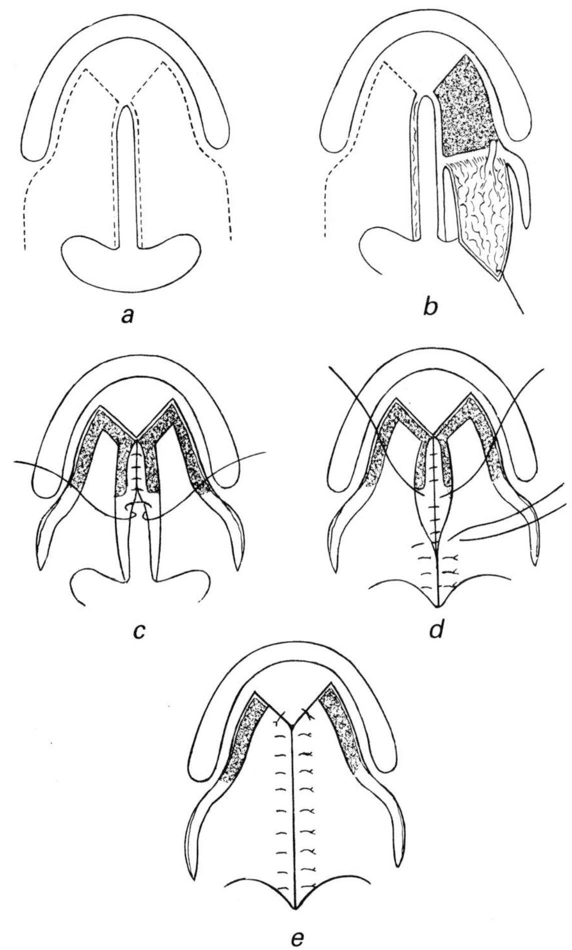

Fig. 25.39 V to Y repair of cleft palate.

from the upper surface of the hard palate by special dissectors and posteriorly from the soft palate. Additional mucosa, when required, is available on the vomer. The oral layer consists of mucoperiosteum anteriorly and of palatal mucosa on the soft palate. By raising flaps, as indicated in *Fig.* 25.39, it is possible to achieve a V to Y lengthening of the palate to facilitate velopharyngeal closure which is vital if the typical speech deformity characterized by nasal escape is to be avoided. It is also vital to release the levatores palati from their abnormal attachments to the posterior nasal spines and to unite them to each other, thereby reconstructing the normal levator sling mechanism.

The exposed bone on the hard palate lateral to the flaps granulates and epithelizes very rapidly. The area which presents most difficulty in closure is usually the junction between the hard and soft palates, and there are a number of more or less complicated flaps described to deal with this problem.

Secondary Corrective Surgery

While it is usually possible to obtain an acceptable result on the lip at the primary operation for unilateral clefts, a secondary procedure is almost routine for bilateral clefts. Many minor 'trims' can be required for the perfect result, including correction of excess vermilion, marginal notches and irregularities of the mucocutaneous junction. Secondary procedures on the nose are also often required, including adjustment of the alar base, correction of tip asymmetry and straightening of the nasal septum and bony framework. To an increasing degree, secondary work is also being advocated for correction of the underlying maxillary deformities, and this is considered in Chapter 21.

In some cases of cleft palate there are residual speech defects following the primary repair. The most usual and typical stigma is nasal escape due to inadequate closure of the velopharyngeal opening. This can be shown in some cases by lateral radiographs which show a failure of contact between the soft palate and the posterior pharyngeal wall, but obviously this will not be demonstrated where the gap is to each side of the midline. Direct observation and assessment of the function of this region is readily made during speech by using a child's cystoscope passed through the nose under local anaesthesia (nasendoscopy). Where there is nasal escape a number of operations are available for lengthening the soft palate and of building the posterior pharyngeal wall forward by implants or flaps. Other varieties of pharyngoplasties using flaps seek to narrow the gap or to improve the function in this area. Assessment of the merits of different operations is not easy.

Acknowledgement

Mr David Maisels kindly gave permission for diagrams and material used in the previous edition to be included or modified.

Further Reading

General Techniques of Wound Care, Skin Grafts and Flaps

Bell R. C. (1973) *The Use of Skin Grafts.* Oxford, Oxford University Press.
Converse J. M. (1977) *Reconstructive Plastic Surgery I.* 2nd ed. Philadelphia, Saunders.
Daniel R. K. and Terzis J. K. (1977) *Reconstructive Microsurgery.* Boston, Little Brown.
Grabb W. C. and Myers M. B. (1975) *Skin Flaps.* Boston, Little Brown.
Mathes S. J. and Nahai F. (1982) *Clinical Applications for Muscle and Musculocutaneous Flaps.* St. Louis, Mosby.
O'Brien B. Mc. (1977) *Microvascular Reconstructive Surgery.* Edinburgh, Churchill Livingstone.
Zoltan J. (1984) *Atlas of Skin Repair.* London, Karger.

Craniofacial, Cleft Deformities and Trauma

Converse J. M. (1977) *Reconstructive Plastic Surgery 2 and 4.* 2nd ed. Philadelphia, Saunders.
Edwards M. and Watson A. C. H. (1980) *Advances in the Management of Cleft Palate.* Edinburgh, Churchill Livingstone.
Jackson I. T. (1981) *Recent Advances in Plastic Surgery 2.* Edinburgh, Churchill Livingstone.
Jackson I. T. et al. (1982) *Atlas of Craniomaxillofacial Surgery.* St. Louis, Mosby.

Skin Tumours

Grabb W. C. and Smith J. W. (1973) *Plastic Surgery*. 2nd ed. Boston, Little Brown.
Milton G. W. (1977) *Malignant Melanoma of the Skin and Mucous Membranes*. Edinburgh, Churchill Livingstone.

Congenital

Mustarde J. C. (1971) *Plastic Surgery in Infancy and Childhood.* Philadelphia, Saunders.
Pruzansky S. (1961) *Congenital Anomalies of the Face and Associated Structures*. Springfield, Ill., Thomas.
Serafin D. and Georgiade N. G. (1984) *Paediatric Plastic Surgery*. Vol. 1. St. Louis, Mosby.

Burns

Heimbach D. M. and Engrav L. H. (1984) *Surgical Management of the Burn Wound*. New York, Raven Press.
Hummel R. P. (1982) *Clinical Burn Therapy. A Management and Prevention Guide*. Bristol, Wright.

26 *Injuries of the Maxillofacial Skeleton*

Paul F. Bradley

INTRODUCTION

The face is a key part of the anatomy in a social animal such as homo sapiens, and injuries to it are significant for a variety of reasons both physical and emotional. The visage is extensively utilized for expressive purposes. It also harbours the entry to the respiratory and gastrointestinal tracts, together with the portals of vision, hearing and smell. Injuries may materially interfere with the functions of communication, breathing, eating, speaking, sight and hearing. Interference with the airway may be life threatening in occasional instances.

Deformity of the face, whether it is temporary or permanent, can be most distressing because it threatens to disrupt social contact so that the psychological management of the patient must be remembered, with reassurance playing a significant part. Maxillofacial injuries tend to incite more fear in the subject than trauma elsewhere as it is harder to divorce oneself from a condition which is so close to the centre of consciousness.

As the face is commonly unprotected by clothing, it is especially exposed to trauma. In addition, facial bones are vulnerable as they are quite thin because lightness is important in an animal which holds its head erect, such as man.

Fortunately, the area has an excellent blood supply, so that injuries heal well with a lack of secondary infection, and fractures unite far more quickly than in the long bones. However, at the time of the acute injury the abundant blood supply may create problems, particularly in the scalp, tongue and lips where haemorrhage can be profuse. Control is usually prompt, however, with conventional measures of pressure combined with clamping of any major arterial bleeding points. The speed of healing of facial bone fractures provides a minimum of inconvenience for the patient but does mean that definitive reduction should be carried out within 10 days, otherwise malunion may well occur.

All of the above features stress the importance of maxillofacial injury. It behoves any doctor to be beware of the signs and symptoms of such injury and their initial treatment. This is especially true of the casualty officer.

HISTORY

As always a good history can be most helpful in piecing together a picture of the accident, and with it an appreciation of the sort of injuries to be expected. It may not be possible to obtain this from the subject due to impairment of speech or defect of consciousness. A relative's testimony or that of an ambulance man may be very useful in filling in some of the missing data.

It is particularly important to establish the following:

A. Mechanism of Injury

Information on this aspect can aid in determining the possible sites of injury and their severity and nature. It is meaningful to divide the various mechanisms into three main groups related to the causative kinetic energy (Lindahl's classification).

1. Kinetic Energy of the Individual exerted on to the Facial Structures

This is seen most typically in falls, and is commonest in the young and elderly. A typical example in the adult is shown in *Fig.* 26.1*a* which illustrates the so-called 'parade ground fracture'. This occurs when someone faints, as for example a soldier on parade, and falls directly on to the point of chin. Here there may typically be a laceration below the chin, fractures of the thin condylar necks of the lower jaw, and often a midline fracture. In the elderly, one should be mindful of possible medical causes for such falls. Myocardial infarction or cerebrovascular accident particularly should be excluded as these may be of major importance, especially if an anaesthetic is planned. In the child the elasticity of the facial bones is remarkable but fractures can occur. The maxilla is relatively protected by the cranium as the face has as yet failed to grow downwards and forwards to its full degree. Fracture of the upper jaw in the young child, if it does occur, is often accompanied by a skull fracture for this reason (usually a group 3 causative mechanism).

2. Kinetic Energy expended on to the Individual

The causative incident here is a blow which most typically may be caused by a fist, kick or sporting equipment such as a tennis racquet. Such incidents are commonest in young adolescents and adults. It is helpful to know whether a single blow was administered or whether multiple traumas occurred. Two typical examples are shown in *Fig.* 26.1*b*. The first one comprises a localized blow, as by a racket in this case, over the zygomatic arch causing a fracture of its most prominent part.

The second example shows a more powerful and diffuse

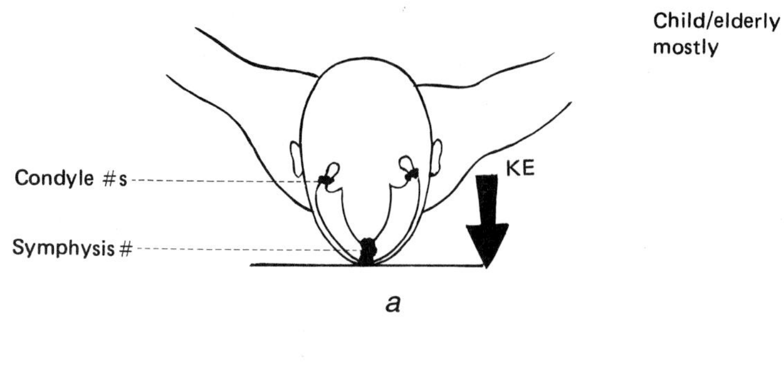

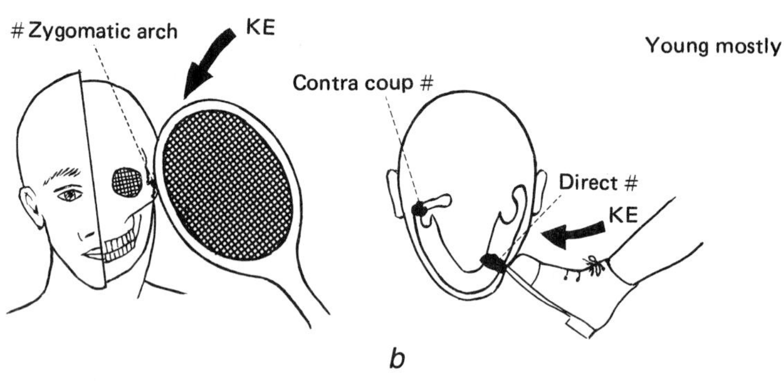

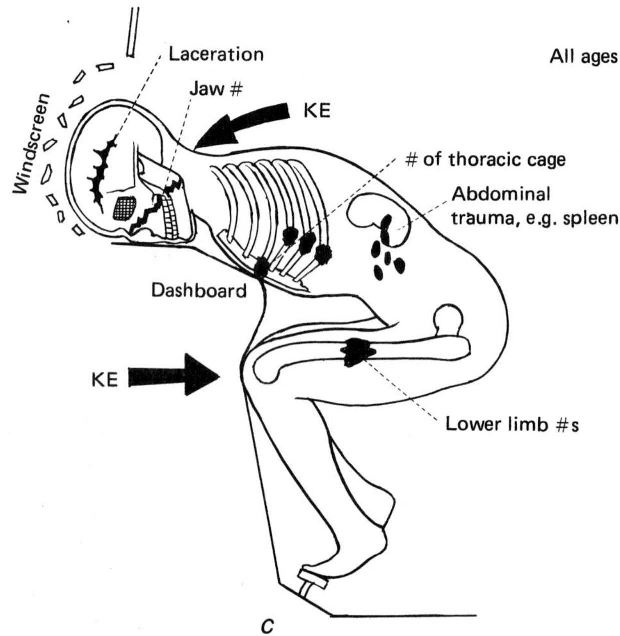

Fig. 26.1 Mechanism of facial injuries: kinetic energy onto facial structures (Lindahl's classification). *a*, Of individual, e.g. fall. *b*, Onto individual, e.g. sports and assault. *c*, Combination, e.g. RTA.

force in the form of a kick administered over the horizontal ramus of the jaw producing a direct injury at the site of impact and a *contre-coup* injury on the opposite side in the thin condylar region.

3. Combination of Kinetic Individual Energy of the Individual and Kinetic Energy exerted on to the Individual

In this instance the body may be thrown against an object which has its own individual momentum. Such a combination produces a major degree of disruptive energy and can be responsible for severe and multiple injuries. The most common example is the road traffic accident which may of course occur in all age groups. Fortunately road traffic trauma is tending to decrease due to lowering of speed limits and the compulsory use of front seat belts. It is in this group that the most severe injuries are likely to occur, and also that combination with injury in other regions is most likely. *Fig.*

26.1*c* shows how a maxillofacial injury may be combined with other conditions in the context of a front-seat passenger without seat belt. The face is commonly impacted against the upper part of the dashboard resulting in skeletal injuries to any of the facial bones. Soft-tissue laceration occurs due to the shattering of the windscreen. Impact of the thoracic region against the main dashboard can result in a variety of injuries, particularly rib fractures and sternal fractures.

The abdomen may also share in such trauma with the possibility of rupture of intra-abdominal organs, particularly the spleen.

Lastly, the lower limb may be thrust forcibly against the lower part of the dashboard structures, again with the possibility of a variety of lesions but perhaps most typically fractures of the patella or long bones.

B. Functional Deficit Noted

One should record whether the patient has noted any particular problems since the incident or whether these have been observed by onlookers. One should know whether the patient was rendered unconscious at any time. Retrograde or post-traumatic amnesia should be inquired into as indication of possible cerebral damage. Enquiries should be made as to whether any pain is noted in the facial region and for nasal discharge, failure of teeth to occlude, visual problems, particularly double vision and numbness of the facial dermatomes. One should also enquire for pain in other regions, and particularly for any difficulty in moving the neck. It is vitally important to pick up a cervical fracture early, as neurological damage can occur in an unstable case during further examination, or, more particularly, as a result of administration of a general anaesthetic with relaxant during treatment of a facial fracture.

C. Previous Treatment

If the patient has been seen at a previous hospital then normally a casualty card will accompany him. One should note whether any tetanus prophylaxis has been given and fluid replacements. The administration of antibiotics is also of significance.

D. General Medical History

It has previously been mentioned that medical conditions may be significant as a cause of a fall so that enquiries should be made of any previous cardiac, neurological or endocrinological problems.

Other conditions which are particularly important in trauma patients include: steroid medication or adrenal pathology as there is a danger of Addisonian crisis after trauma unless steroid supplements are adequate, and also diabetes because jaw injuries may preclude the taking of a full diet.

EXAMINATION

A number of schemes for examining a possible maxillofacial injury have been advocated. The simplest and the one most unlikely to miss signs, is to start at the top of the scalp and work down steadily level by level until the chin is reached. *Prior to detailed examination of the facial region, the neck should be checked as moving the head could produce neurological damage in undetected cervical fracture.* The hand should be gently run down the back of the neck palpating each neural spine and also searching for any areas of tenderness in the associated longitudinal muscles.

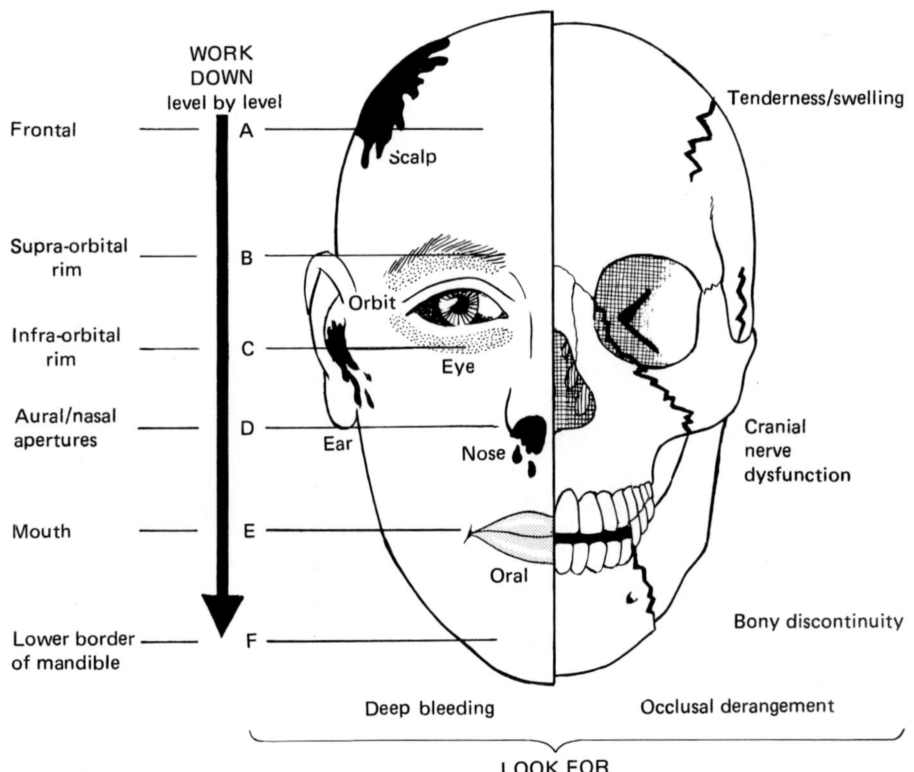

Fig. 26.2 Examination of facial injury.

The following features should be specially looked for (*Fig.* 26.2):

A. Tenderness and Swelling

The tissues are likely to be tender to palpation and often swollen in an area of injury although this sign does not, of course, indicate definite skeletal damage. It does, however, alert one to the need for further checking at the particular site.

B. Deep Bleeding

Facial lacerations will, of course, leave superficial traces of blood but there are certain sites where deep bleeding may be detected and are particularly significant:

1. Haematoma of the Scalp

This may indicate an underlying skull fracture, e.g. of the frontal bone.

2. Aural (*Fig.* 26.3)

Bleeding from the ear may occur in a fracture of the middle cranial fossa or more locally a rupture of the tympanic membrane or disruption of the walls of the bony meatus. The latter can occur when the condylar head is driven forcibly back after a blow on the lower jaw.

3. Circumorbital (*Fig.* 26.4)

Bleeding can arise within the orbit as a result of fracture of any of the bones contributing to this structure, particularly the frontal bone, ethmoids, nose, maxilla and zygoma. Deep bleeding tends to be confined to the limits of the orbit by the orbital septum which is a condensation of connective tissue in continuity with the tarsal plates. This characteristic distribution is known sometimes as 'panda eyes' or in the USA as 'racoon eyes'.

4. Subconjunctival Haemorrhage (*Fig.* 26.5)

Local trauma to the sclera can produce a small localized haemorrhage, but a haemorrhage where it is impossible to discern the posterior limit even when the eye is moved to the contralateral side indicates bleeding coming from within the orbit and spreading underneath the conjunctiva. This again indicates a fracture somewhere within the orbit, i.e. frontal bone, nasal bones, maxilla or zygoma. It may be either lateral or, less commonly, medial and this gives some indication of which bone is involved. Bilateral subconjunctival haematomas may also occur in strangulation.

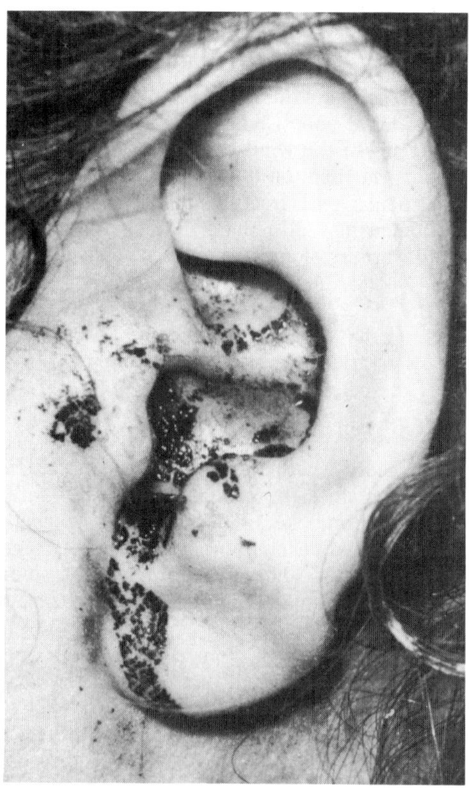

Fig. 26.3 Aural bleeding indicates a fracture of the bony meatus or rupture of the drum. Middle cranial fossa fracture should be excluded.

5. Nasal Bleeding (Epistaxis) (*Fig.* 26.6)

The nose may bleed after relatively minor trauma in some individuals. However, it should alert one to the possibility of skeletal fracture of the nose or of one of the bones which contribute to the maxillary sinus which is in continuity with the nose, particularly the maxilla and zygoma. Unilateral nose bleeding or epistaxis is particularly significant.

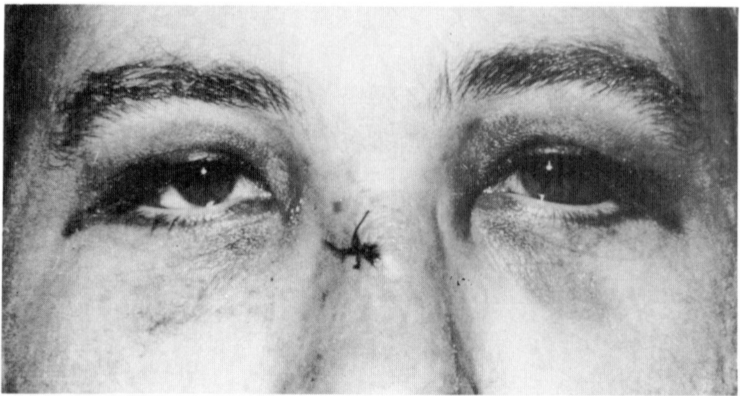

Fig. 26.4 Circumorbital ecchymosis ('panda eyes') is due to bleeding within the orbit being confined by the orbital septum and is seen in fractures of the maxilla, zygoma, ethmoids or frontal bone.

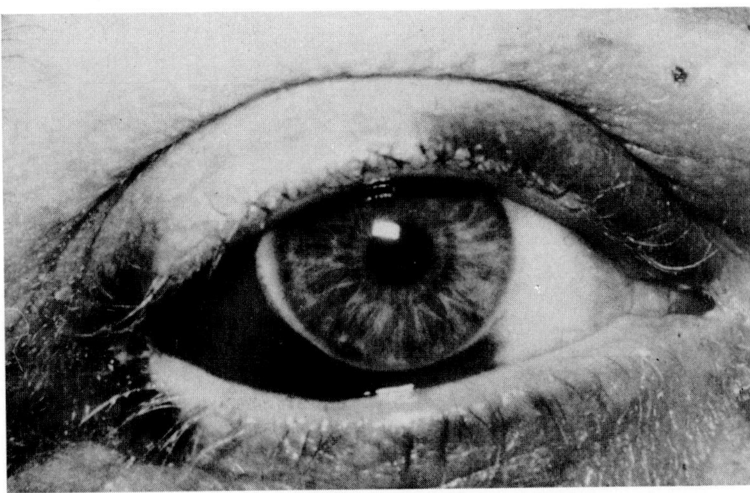

Fig. 26.5 Subconjunctival haemorrhage without posterior limit is due to blood tracking forward under the conjunctiva from injury to the orbit, almost always a fracture.

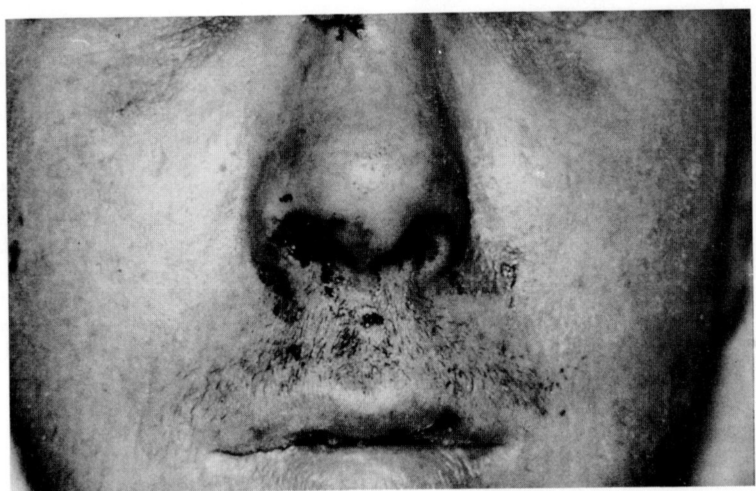

Fig. 26.6 Epistaxis may be a result of trauma to the nose or bleeding from the aural cavities in fractures of the maxilla or zygoma.

It is very important to differentiate epistaxis from leakage of CSF which may occur in high level maxillary and nasal fractures involving the region of the cribriform plate. Such leakage indicates the risk of meningitis. In the early stages CSF may be mixed with blood and nasal catarrh. Later it is present alone and has a characteristic pale amber appearance leaving a faint stain on the skin. Biochemical estimation of glucose and protein levels can be undertaken as confirmation.

6. *Intraoral* (*Fig.* 26.7)

A haematoma in the lingual sulcus related to the mandible is said to be pathognomonic of fracture of the mandible as this area is protected from direct trauma and is only likely to be affected if the bone is fractured. Haemorrhage in the region of the greater palatine foramen is Guérin's sign and indicates a fracture through the region of the greater palatine canal, i.e. a maxillary fracture.

C. Bony Discontinuity (*Fig.* 26.8)

It may be possible to detect a step of a displaced fracture of the facial bones. However, oedema occurs very rapidly in the facial region so that after an hour or so post-injury, it may not be possible to detect lesser degrees of bony discontinuity. Sites of particular importance are:

1. *Frontal Bone*

It may be possible to detect depressed fractures of this bone.

2. *Supraorbital Rim*

Fracture of the frontal bone may give rise to a step at this site. Steps in the region of the frontozygomatic suture occur often in zygomatic fracture but can be very difficult to palpate.

3. *Infraorbital Rim*

Steps at this stage may occur in pyramidal fractures of the maxilla or zygomatic fracture.

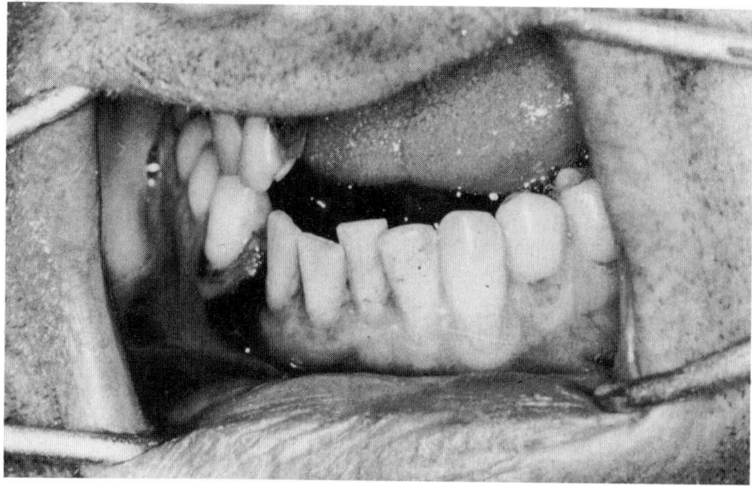

Fig. 26.7 Lingual haematoma in mandibular fracture (between the lower right lateral incisor and canine).

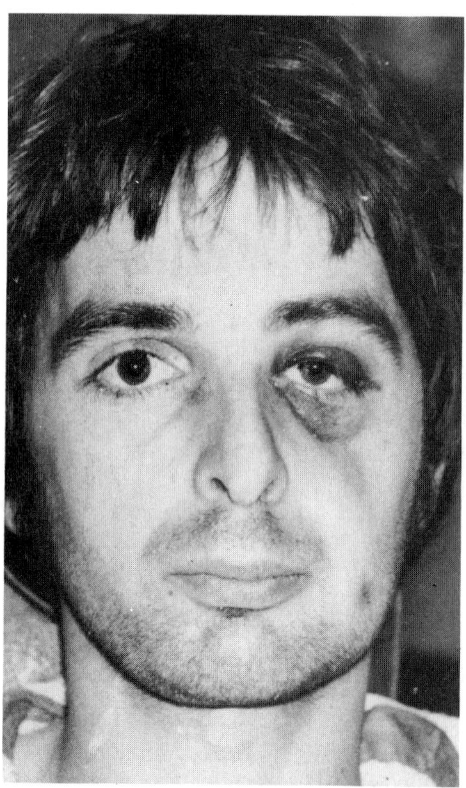

Fig. 26.8 Obvious step over a depressed fracture of the left zygoma.

4. Mandibular Lower Border

It is important to palpate the whole of the lower border of the mandible for any discontinuity. A useful adjunctive test is to place a finger in the external auditory meatus and ask the patient to open and close the jaw. Normally the condyle should be felt to move in and out of the fossa but in the case of a fracture-dislocation this will not be palpated.

D. Cranial Nerve Dysfunction

A simple rapid testing of cranial nerves should always be carried out in facial injury although the finer points of such an examination may not be practicable in an injured patient. Of particular importance are:

1. Disturbance of Extraocular Movements

These can occur in orbital fractures where the most inferior muscles may be entrapped, notably the inferior rectus (*Figs.* 26.9 and 26.14). More widespread disturbance can occur where the nerves of supply (cranial nerves III, IV and VI) together with the frontal branch of V are disturbed in fractures through the superior orbital fissure (superior orbital fissure syndrome).

Fortunately the optic nerve is usually well protected by a dense ring of bone but occasionally this may be disrupted in this so-called orbital apex syndrome. The significance of pupillary changes in cranial injury is well recognized. Local injury to the eye in the form of a traumatic iritis can also produce a sluggish or even dilated pupil. Testing both direct and consensual reflexes may help to determine in pupillary changes whether the basic defect is in the afferent limb, i.e. optic nerve, or in the efferent limb, i.e. oculomotor nerve.

2. Disturbance of Fifth Nerve Function

Sensory loss should be sought over the main distribution of the trigeminal nerve. Disturbance in the infraorbital area may indicate involvement in either the nasal, labial or palpebral branches and may occur where any fracture extends through the region of the infraorbital foramen or canal, as in fractures of the maxilla or zygoma. Disturbance of mental sensation may well occur in fractures of the mandible as the inferior alveolar nerve traverses a large length of the lower jaw between the mandibular and the mental foramen.

3. Loss of Facial Nerve or Auditory Function

Disturbance in function of these may occur in fractures of the middle cranial fossa. It is important in cases of facial lacerations to check that there has been no loss of VII nerve function or related branches. If this has occurred then peripheral nerve repair is likely to be required.

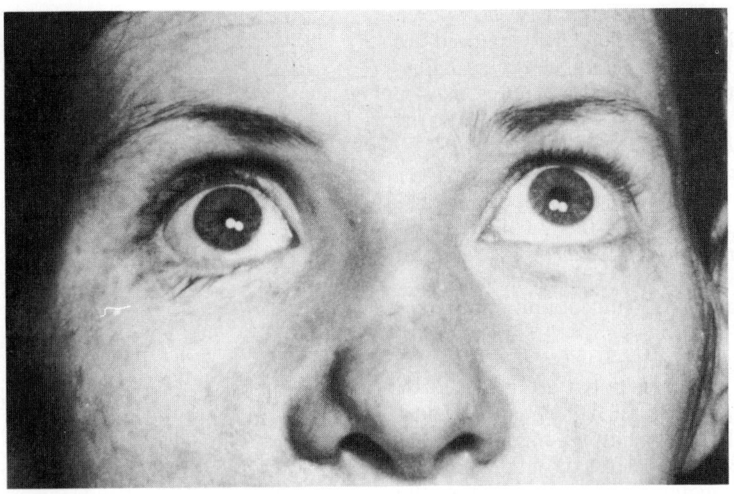

Fig. 26.9 Failure of elevation of right eye on looking upwards due to entrapment of inferior oblique muscle in a fracture of the orbital floor.

E. Disturbance of Dental Occlusion

A displaced fracture of the jaws involving the dental alveolar segment is likely to cause a derangement of the occlusion of the teeth (*Fig.* 26.10). There may well be a step in the occlusal plane. Some slight experience may be necessary in certain cases as one may not know in a particular case whether the patient has a pre-existing malocclusion, such as an open bite. In these cases examination of the teeth for wear facets is very helpful in determining where pre-existing contacts occurred. Where front teeth have never met, the small tubercles which are present at eruption may persist on the incisal edges. Particular occlusal disturbances seen in individual fractures are described in relevant sections.

RADIOGRAPHIC EXAMINATION OF MAXILLOFACIAL INJURY

It is probably true to say that if a facial fracture is not detectable by clinical examination then there will be little indication for treatment. Radiographic examination is, however, an important investigation for any patient with a suspected facial fracture. It can be particularly helpful when facial swelling is at its height, obscuring bony deformity; it may take as much as 4 or 5 days for such swelling to regress after a major injury. Radiographs enable one to assess the full extent of injury and this is most valuable in treatment planning. It is important to detect stable undisplaced fractures which do not require treatment for medicolegal reasons. The fact that a blow occasioned in an assault was sufficiently powerful to cause bony injury has legal significance.

A word of caution is necessary in ordering detailed radiographic examination early in the management of patients with multiple injuries. A number of facial views, particularly those utilized in examination of the upper jaw (occipitomental views) require the patient to be turned on his face. This may be unsafe and impracticable in a severely injured patient, particularly one who is unconscious or who may have spinal injuries. Alternative views not requiring the

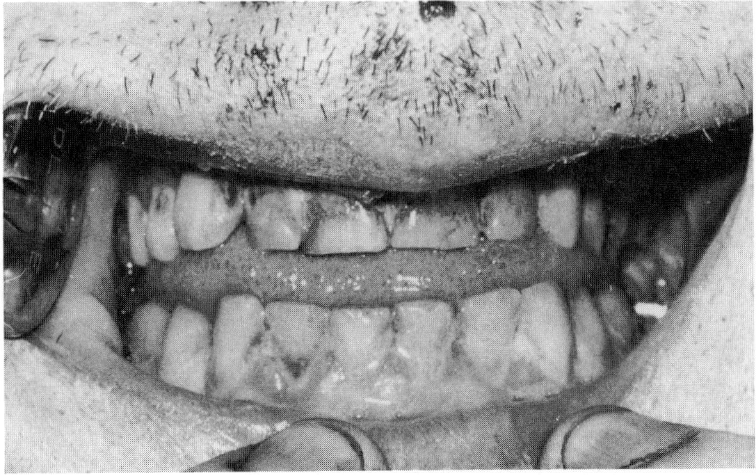

Fig. 26.10 Disturbance of dental occlusion. Anterior open bite, as here, can occur in fractures of the maxilla or in bilateral fracture of the mandibular condyles.

prone position may have to be obtained in these cases, even though they prove somewhat inferior. Also in such instances, the emphasis is thrown on careful clinical examination to establish the fracture pattern. Tomography may be useful in complex cases as this can be carried out without the need for turning the patient.

A general principle of fracture radiography is that for certain diagnosis two views at right angles to each other are required. This should be observed in the maxillofacial region as far as possible, particularly in the mandible where an undisplaced fracture may be very hard to detect save in an angulation near to the plane of the discontinuity itself.

Mandible

Classically, lateral views of the lower jaw are provided by *right* and *left lateral obliques* (*Fig.* 26.11) which are taken with the relevant side of the face against the film but rotated so as to throw the image of the opposite side of the mandible clear. A tomographic view requiring a special apparatus, the *orthopantomogram* (OPG) has tended to supplant lateral oblique views, where it is available, as it shows the whole of the lower jaw from condyle to condyle in one continuum (*Fig.* 26.12).

In either case a further radiograph at right angles is needed to observe the principle previously stated. A *posteroanterior view* of the mandible is best as the vertical ramus areas show clearly being nearest to the film (*Fig.* 26.13). This requires the subject to be face downwards, and if this is inadvisable an *anteroposterior* may be substituted.

The midline region of the mandible is poorly seen on lateral obliques, while in the OPG of posteroanterior projections the image of the cervical vertebrae is superimposed. To overcome this certain intraoral views, which involve placing a film in the mouth, are available, such as the *true occlusal* film showing the outline well and the *oblique occlusal* taken at an angle revealing bony detail well. Dental *periapical* films are useful in examining the relationship of a fracture to individual teeth and detecting root damage, but may be difficult to obtain in a severely injured patient due to the precision of placement necessary.

The condylar areas tend to be superimposed on the image of the base of a skull and a specialized anteroposterior view is helpful, namely the *Towne's view* or even better the *reverse Towne's*. In cases of difficulty *transcranial condylar* radiographs may be needed.

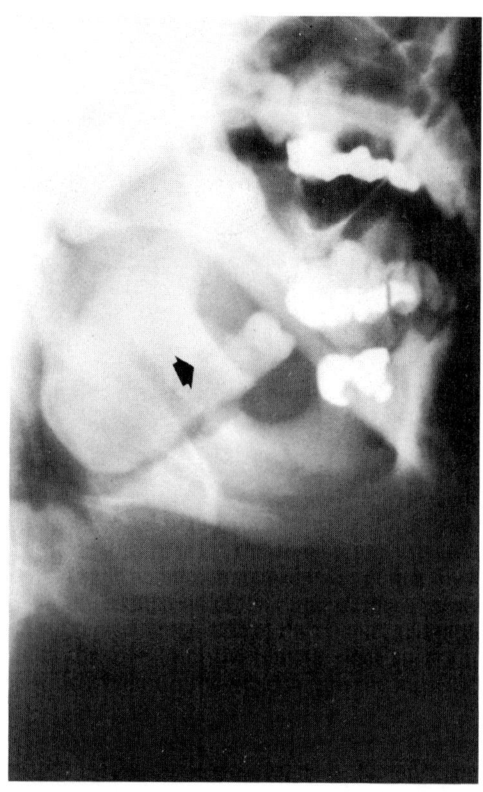

Fig. 26.11 Lateral oblique radiograph of mandible showing fracture. This is 'horizontally unfavourable' in its obliquity allowing upward displacement of the proximal fragment under the influence of the elevator muscles (pterygomasseteric sling) as shown by the arrow.

Maxilla

Standard anteroposterior views of the skull, such as the occipitofrontal view, cause superimposition of the dense petrous part of the temporal bones over the lower parts of the orbit and maxilla, so that their usefulness is limited, although the supraorbital margin can be well seen and the area of the frontomalar sutures. For proper delineation of the maxilla and zygoma it is necessary to displace the image

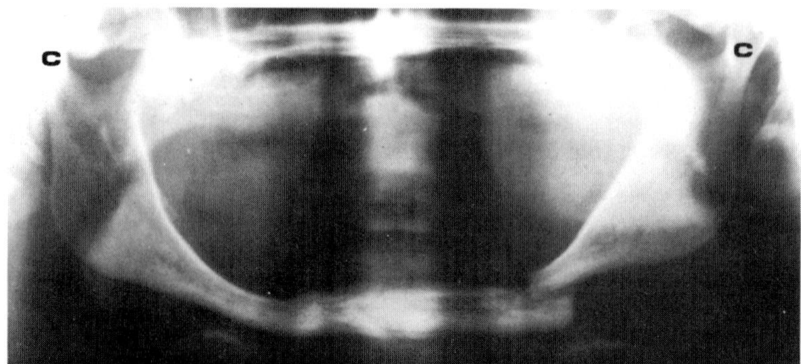

Fig. 26.12 Orthopantomograph (OPG) showing fracture of the left body in an elderly subject with an atrophic mandible. The OPG, if available, is preferable to the lateral oblique views as it shows the whole mandible from condyle to condyle indicated (c).

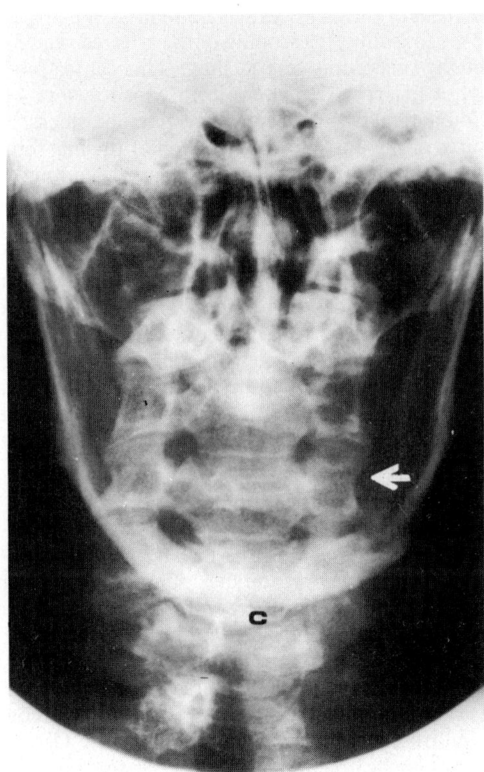

Fig. 26.13 Postero-anterior view of the mandible of the same fracture as in *Fig.* 26.12. This shows that the obliquity of the fracture is 'vertically unfavourable' allowing inward displacement of the proximal fragment under the influence of the pterygomasseteric sling (arrow). Cervical spine outlines (c) tend to be superimposed over the anterior mandible and here a dental occlusal film can be very helpful.

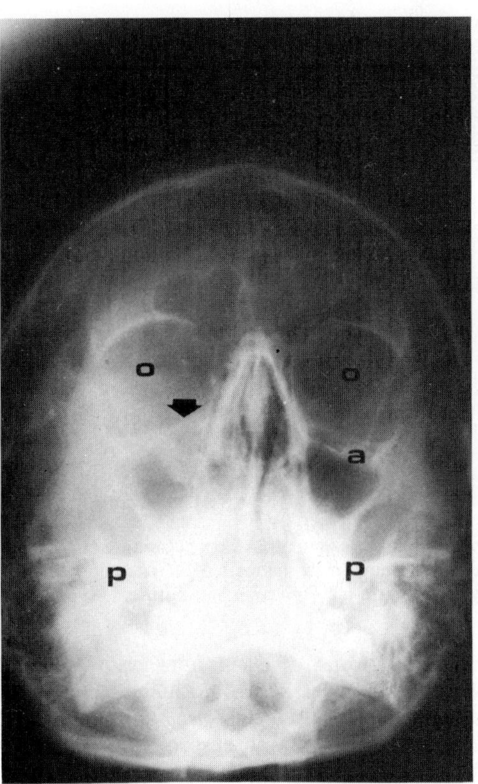

Fig. 26.14 Occipitomental radiograph showing right-sided orbital blow-out fracture (arrow). Note the clear antrum on the contralateral side A. The orbits are indicated O. In this view the dense petrous part of the temporal bone (P) is projected away from the mid-face whereas in a conventional postero-anterior view of the skull (occipitofrontal) there is superimposition.

of the petrous temporal bone away from the area of interest. The following radiographs are helpful.

1. Occipitomental (*Figs.* 26.14, 26.15)

This shows vertical displacement at the orbital margin.

2. Thirty Degree Occipitomental (*Fig.* 26.16)

This view has greater 'tip' and one is viewing the inferior orbital margin almost from below so that horizontal displacement can be judged.

If the patient cannot be turned on his face for the occipitomental view, which involves placing the chin (menton) and nose on the film while shooting the rays through the occiput (hence the term occipitomental) then a view may be taken with the patient lying face upward, but in the reverse direction, i.e. *mento-occipital*. Definition on this view is very much inferior to the true occipitomental as the facial structures are furthest away from the film and hence show magnification and lack of clarity. It is, however, well worthwhile undertaking in the circumstances indicated.

3. Lateral Facial Bones

This shows fracture lines running through the region of the frontomaxillary suture lines or nasal septum, and also any steps in the line of the pterygoid plates.

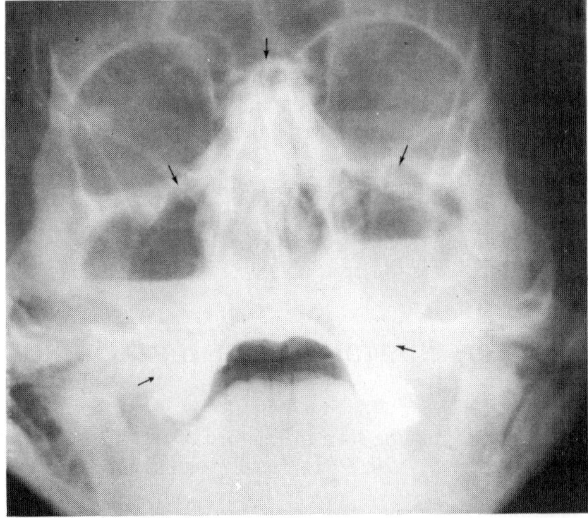

Fig. 26.15 Occipitomental radiograph showing blood in both antra as a result of a Le Fort II fracture of the maxilla. Arrows indicate the fracture sites.

Zygoma

The same views as for the maxilla are indicated, namely the *occipitomental* and *30° occipitomental* with the addition of the

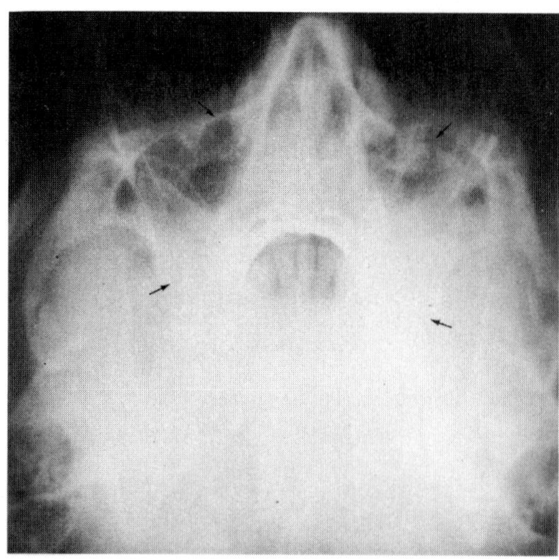

Fig. 26.16 The same case of Le Fort II fracture as *Fig.* 26.15 but occipitomental shows more angulation (30° occipitomental). Radio-opacity of the antra now appears more diffuse.

submentovertical which is taken from below showing the zygomatic arch outlines. Occasionally in a case where fracture is uncertain a *rotated occipitomental* taken from one side of the midline may help. In suspected 'orbital blow-out' tomography is usually needed.

Nose

1. Occipitofrontal

Shows mediolateral displacement of the nasal bones and the position of the nasal septum. An AP view of the skull is an alternative if the patient cannot be turned on his face.

2. Lateral of Nasal Bones

This is useful in establishing the presence of a fracture, although care should be taken not to interpret the normal suture between the frontal and nasal bones as a discontinuity. Clinical examination is of more importance than radiographs in nasal fractures and the signs are detailed in the following section.

The various radiographs detailed above are summarized in *Table* 26.1. Those views requiring the patients to be in the prone position are marked with a P and alternatives are suggested if this is not advisable.

SIGNS OF INDIVIDUAL FACIAL FRACTURES

Mandible

The signs that may be seen in fracture of the mandible are summarized in *Fig.* 26.17. Especially significant are:

1. Deranged Occlusion

If the patient has teeth or wears dentures then in a displaced fracture it is likely that the dental occlusion will be altered. In the normal state the mandible is in a state of balance between the elevator muscles (pterygomasseteric sling) and the depressor muscles (digastrics and mylohyoids). When fracture occurs the mandible may be separated into different segments, each of which may be displaced by the actions of one group of muscles alone so that the normal balance is disrupted. A typical example of this is shown in *Fig.* 26.17.

Fractures of the condyles, vertical ramus and angle region are prone to exhibit telescoping of the affected region by the pull of the pterygomasseteric sling. This causes premature contact of the posterior molar teeth which may be on both sides in bilateral fractures or unilateral in one-sided fracture. Fractures in the posterior body region of the mandible tend to have the minor fragment pulled upwards and inwards by the sling. Bilateral fractures of the anterior part of the mandible may allow the symphyseal region to be pulled downwards and backwards by the digastric muscles with a risk of airway obstruction. Midline fractures of the mandible may allow both sides to collapse in somewhat under the influence of the mylohyoid muscles. The degree of displacement that occurs depends on the mobility within the fracture site and also the obliquity of the fracture. A fracture may be described as horizontally favourable or unfavourable depending on whether displacement is discouraged or encouraged in the particular plane.

2. Deranged Mental Sensation

The inferior dental nerve runs through a large part of the lower jaw from the mandibular foramen to the mental foramen. It may be traumatized in this course by fractures and sensory impairment may occur. This may be total (anaesthesia) or partial where the patient has a sense of touch but cannot perceive pinprick (paraesthesia) or where light touch and pinprick can be felt but the sensation feels different from the other side (dysaesthesia). Occasionally sensation may be accentuated by comparison with the other side (hyperaesthesia) but this is more usually seen during a phase of nerve recovery.

3. Haematoma Formation

It is usual to see some degree of haematoma formation in the region of a fracture. Lingual haematoma is almost certainly pathognomonic of fractured mandible, as this area is protected from external trauma.

Fractures of the condyle of the mandible usually exhibit tenderness over the pre-auricular region, and there may be unilateral premature contact of molar teeth on the affected side if telescoping of fragments has occurred. In fracture-dislocation a finger in the external auditory meatus while the patient opens and closes the mandible will detect that no movement is felt in the glenoid fossa on the affected side.

Maxilla

There are three classic fracture sites of the maxilla as described by Le Fort. They are shown in *Fig.* 26.18, together with their associated signs. The classic Le Fort fracture lines are:

1. Le Fort (Low Level or Guérin) Fracture

This fracture line starts at the lateral aspect of the pyriform fossa and extends above the roots of the teeth under the zygomatic buttress and across the pterygoid plates low down. It also traverses the lower part of the nasal septum. It separates the dentoalveolar part of the maxilla from the rest of the cranial skeleton. The fragment may be surprisingly mobile (floating maxilla). There is usually evidence of haematoma formation in the buccal sulcus throughout its extent. Epistaxis is common as the fracture lines run through the antral cavities which communicate with the nose. Dental occlusion may be deranged and the classic malocclusion is that of an anterior open bite, as with all maxillary fractures.

Table 26.1 Facial fractures

Site	*Signs* (not always present)	*X-rays*	*Treatment*	*Immobilization or union*
Mandible	Deranged dental occlusion. Disturbed mental sensation. Sublingual haematoma	1. Right and left lateral obliques of mandible or OPG. 2. PA Mandible (P). 3. Occlusal (true and oblique). 4. Towne's view for condyles (ideally Reverse (P))	Intermaxillary fixation (IMF) Skeletal fixation in unstable cases	Unilateral 4 weeks Bilateral 6 weeks. Unilateral condyle 10 days
Maxilla Le Fort I Maxilla Le Fort II Maxilla Le Fort III	Anterior open bite I, II, III. Circumorbital ecchymosis II, III. Subconjunctival haemorrhage II, III. Epistaxis I, II, III. Disturbed infraorbital sensation II. Guérin's sign I	1. Occipitomental (P) 2. 30° Occipitomental (P) 3. Lateral of facial bones	Craniomaxillary Fixation, plus IMF	4 weeks
Zygoma	Circumorbital ecchymosis. Subconjunctival haemorrhage. Unilateral epistaxis. Lack of cheek prominence. Disturbed infraorbital sensation. Trapped coronoid. Diplopia	1. Occipitomental (P) 2. 30° Occipitomental (P) 3. Submentovertical	Elevation by temporal approach Skeletal wiring in unstable cases	4 weeks
Orbital blow-out	Disturbed infraorbital sensation. Diplopia. Muscle entrapment. Enophthalmos	1. Occipitomental (P) 2. 30° Occipitomental (P) 3. Tomography orbits	Pack antrum and/or orbital floor implant or graft	3 weeks
Nasal bones	Epistaxis. Asymmetry of nose. Circumorbital ecchymosis. Subconjunctival haemorrhage	Lateral nasal bones Occipitofrontal (P)	Reduction by: Walsham's forceps, Ashe's forceps. POP splint or lead plates	3 weeks

N.B. (P) indicates that this view requires the patients to be turned face downwards which may be contraindicated in a major trauma case. Alternative, if inferior, views in these cases are:

PA mandible : AP mandible.
Reverse Towne's view : Towne's view.
Occipitomental : Mento-occipital.
Occipitofrontal : AP skull.

2. Le Fort II Fracture (Pyramidal)

A higher level fracture such as the Le Fort II is often characterized by major facial oedema. This fracture courses across the nasal bones into the medial part of the orbit and then across the anterior aspect of the maxilla in the region of the infraorbital foramen to cut across the pterygoid plates near their mid point. There is an associated fracture across the nasal septum. As the fracture runs through the orbit there is commonly circumorbital ecchymosis ('panda eyes') and subconjunctival haemorrhage. Epistaxis is likely to occur and CSF leak may be present. An anterior open bite is the classic occlusal deformity.

3. Le Fort III Fracture (high level or craniofacial dysjunction)

This is a very major injury where the whole of the maxilla and the zygoma is sheared off the rest of the cranium. There is commonly major facial oedema. Circumorbital ecchymosis and subconjunctival haemorrhage are likely to occur. A hooded appearance of the upper eyelids may occur as the maxilla can be driven downwards and backwards along the plane of the sphenoids taking with it the suspensory ligaments of Lockwood which support the eyes. There is a great risk of CSF rhinorrhoea due to the high level fracture running through the region of the cribriform plate and posterior walls of the frontal sinuses.

It should be emphasized that the classic Le Fort fracture sites are not always found and it is not uncommon to see fractures at different levels on two sides or for fractures to be present at two or more sites.

Zygoma

In the USA this fracture is often known as a 'trimalar' fracture as there are usually three main fracture sites, i.e. at the frontomalar suture, at the zygomatic arch and in the region of the zygomaticomaxillary suture close to the infraorbital foramen. The important signs are summarized in *Fig.* 26.19. They are:

1. Circumorbital ecchymosis and subconjunctival haemorrhage.
2. Sensory changes in the regions of the infraorbital

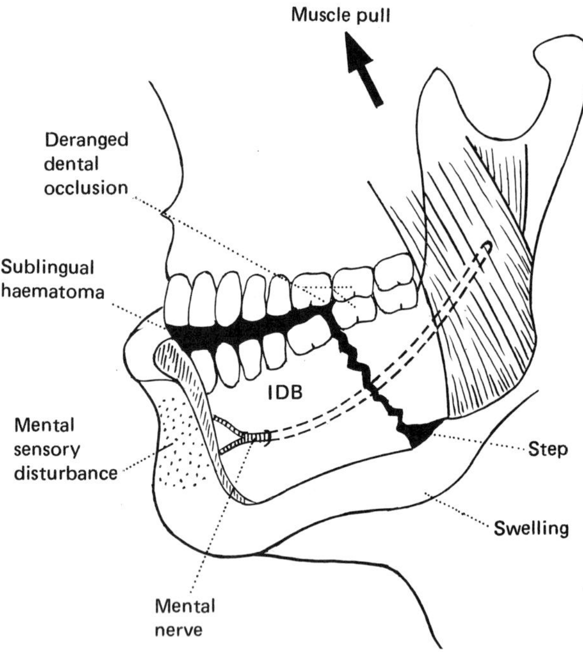

Fig. 26.17 Signs of fracture of mandible. IDB, Inferior dental bundle comprising inferior dental nerve and vessels.

nerve. These are also commonly seen in Le Fort's II fractures of the maxilla.

3. Unilateral epistaxis.
4. Lack of normal cheek prominence due to depression.
5. Interference with lateral movements of the mandible due to impingement on the coronoid process (may occur in arch fractures particularly).
6. Ocular disturbance.

As part of the fracture site involves the orbital floor it is common for bruising to occur in the most inferior extra-ocular muscles, i.e. the inferior oblique and inferior rectus. This may produce some defect of function of these muscles with resulting double vision or diplopia. In simple bruising this will settle with time but if the muscles are actually entrapped in the fracture site such improvement does not occur and defective elevation of the eye is usually obvious.

One must be aware of the orbital 'blow-out' fracture where the floor of the orbit caves into the antral cavity (*Fig.* 26.20). This may occur alone (pure 'blow-out') or in combination with other neighbouring fractures (impure orbital 'blow-out'). Entrapment of the inferior oblique may occur. In major 'blow-out' fractures where a major degree of orbital fat prolapses into the antrum, fat atrophy and scarring may produce a progressive diplopia and loss of prominence and lowering of the eye (enophthalmos). This may occur some weeks or even months after the actual fracture.

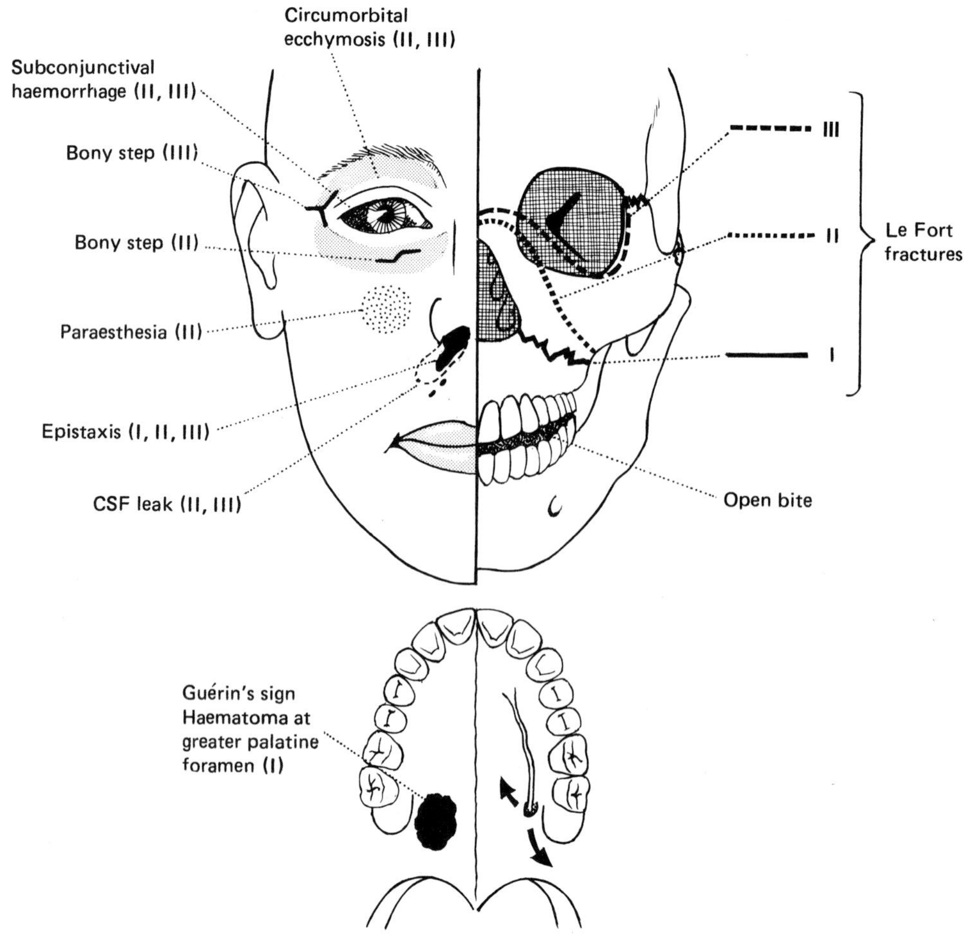

Fig. 26.18 Signs of fracture of maxilla.

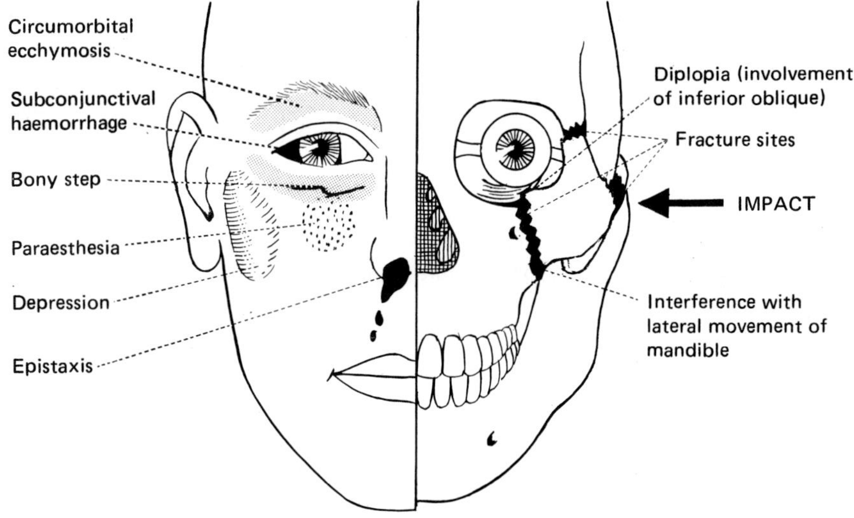

Fig. 26.19 Signs of fracture of zygoma.

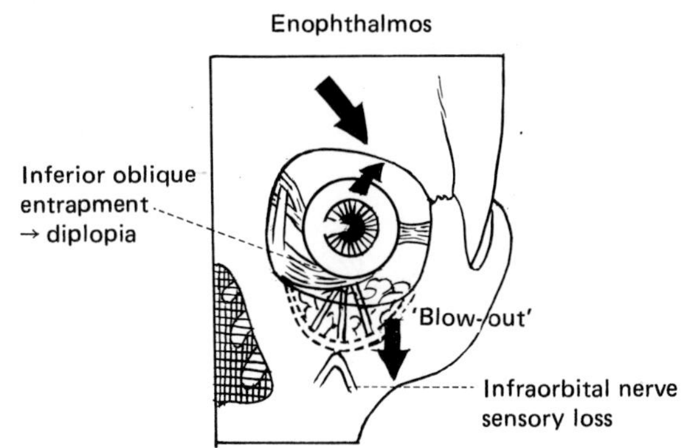

Fig. 26.20 Orbital 'blow-out' fracture.

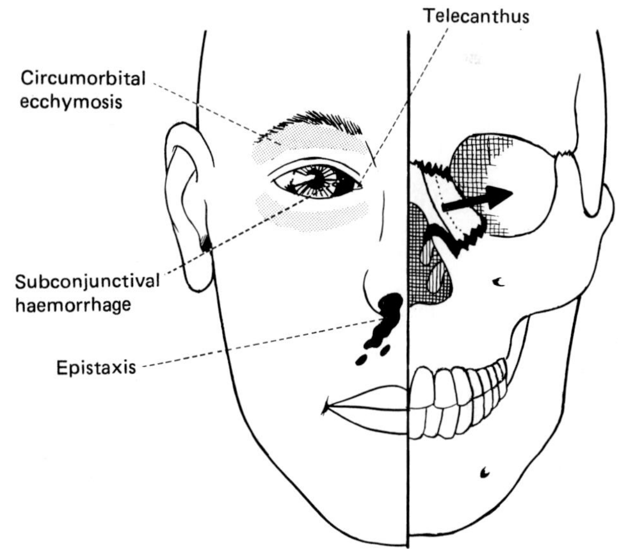

Fig. 26.21 Nasal bone fracture.

Nose

Lateral blows tend to displace the nose to the contralateral side. Anterior trauma tends to result in a depression of the nasal bridge and widening of the intercanthal distance. Circumorbital ecchymosis and medial subconjunctival haemorrhage is likely. Epistaxis is obviously very common and will be bilateral (*Fig.* 26.21). Septal deflection may occur so that the interior of the nose should always be inspected to detect this fracture and also a septal haematoma which requires urgent drainage to prevent cartilage necrosis.

TREATMENT OF MAXILLOFACIAL INJURIES

Primary Treatment

It should be emphasized that a maxillofacial injury must be seen in the context of the patient's general status and other injuries. In multiple trauma cases it is often good policy to delay definitive treatment of the maxillofacial injury until the full extent of the patient's other injuries is established and stabilization is obtained of the major systems. There is a real danger in subjecting a patient to general anaesthesia shortly after major trauma unless this is necessary for life-threatening injury such as a ruptured spleen or a middle meningeal haemorrhage. One normally has about 10 days before a provisional union occurs in which definitive reduction and fixation may be carried out. Simple maxillofacial injuries on their own can, of course, be treated without delay. There are, however, certain emergencies which may present initially in a maxillofacial injury and which require primary treatment. They are:

1. Obstruction of the Airway (*Fig.* 26.22)

An unstable bilateral fracture of the anterior part of the mandible may allow the attachment of the tongue to be posteriorly displaced under the influence of the digastric muscles as shown in *Fig. 26.22a*. A fracture of the maxilla with gross posterior displacement may occlude the nasal airway and force the soft palate down on to the dorsum of the tongue, again with obstruction (*Fig.* 26.22*b*). Such events require emergency measures. The mouth should be

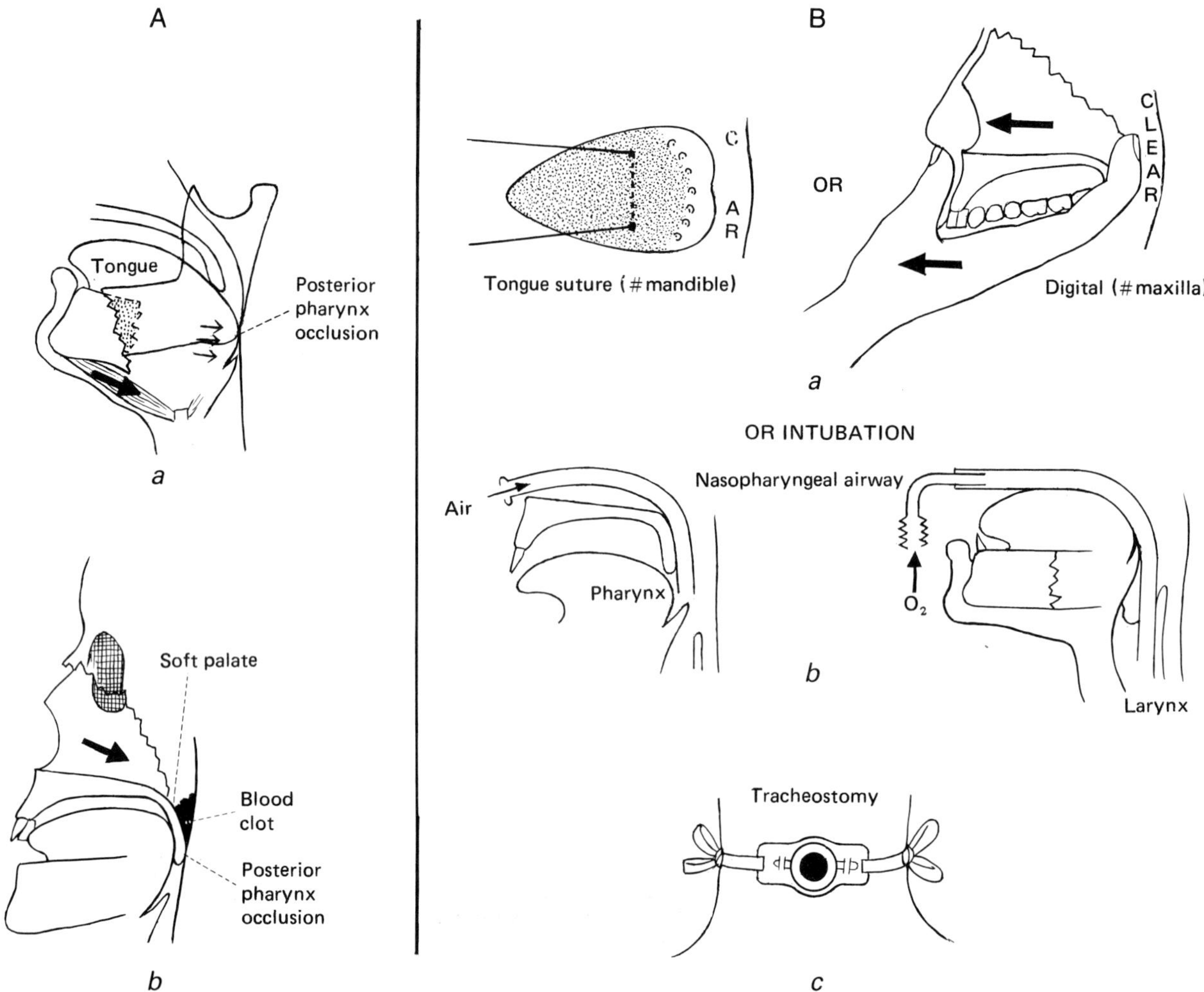

Fig. 26.22 Airways obstruction. A, Problem. *a*, Displaced bilateral fracture of mandible. *b*, Fractured maxilla displaced backwards and downwards. B, Remedy. *a*, Immediate. *b*, Intermediate. *c*, Long-term.

cleared of blood and debris manually and suction applied. If the tongue has fallen back it may be brought forward by pushing a finger behind it and inserting a large tongue suture through the dorsum of the tongue or grasping it with a towel clip. A posteriorly displaced maxilla may be brought forwards and upwards by two fingers passed behind the soft palate to quickly bring the jaw forward. After these initial measures attention must be given to obtaining a more permanent airway. In the case of maxillary injury nasopharyngeal airways may be passed through both nostrils and may suffice. An alternative measure, which is likely to be necessary with an unstable mandible or combination injuries is to intubate the patient. After this, consideration can be given to the need for tracheostomy although it should seldom be necessary to perform an emergency tracheostomy without the presence of an endotracheal tube.

2. Bleeding (*Fig.* 26.23)

Major life-threatening haemorrhage is seldom a feature of maxillofacial injury. Indeed in a patient who shows signs of hypovolaemia, such as a lowered blood pressure, one should exclude other injuries more likely to give this picture, such as a ruptured spleen.

Arterial bleeders or a venous ooze may be encountered. Pressure packs held firmly in place for approximately 10 minutes will usually deal with the problem, but a persistent arterial bleeder requires clamping.

Occasionally in maxillary or nasal fractures, nose bleeding may be very profuse. Anterior nasal packing may be tried but often it is necessary to pass bilateral postnasal packs. The technique for this is illustrated in *Fig.* 26.23*c*. It involves passing a soft rubber catheter down the nasal cavity so that it can be grasped behind the soft palate and pulled forward through the mouth. This enables a tape to be attached to it which connects with a postnasal pack. Traction on the rubber catheter brings the pack round the back of the soft palate to lodge in the posterior nares. The traction tape is tied to the face as is also a small tape acting as a tail which is left tied to the corner of the mouth to enable eventual removal of the pack. A Foley type catheter can be used as an alternative or there are now purpose designed inflatable nasal catheters on the market. Postnasal packs should not normally be left for longer than 48 h because of the risk of infection, although this is minimized by prescription of antibiotics. Following the insertion of the postnasal pack conventional anterior nasal packs should be inserted to reinforce their effect.

In a very occasional case even the above measures may fail

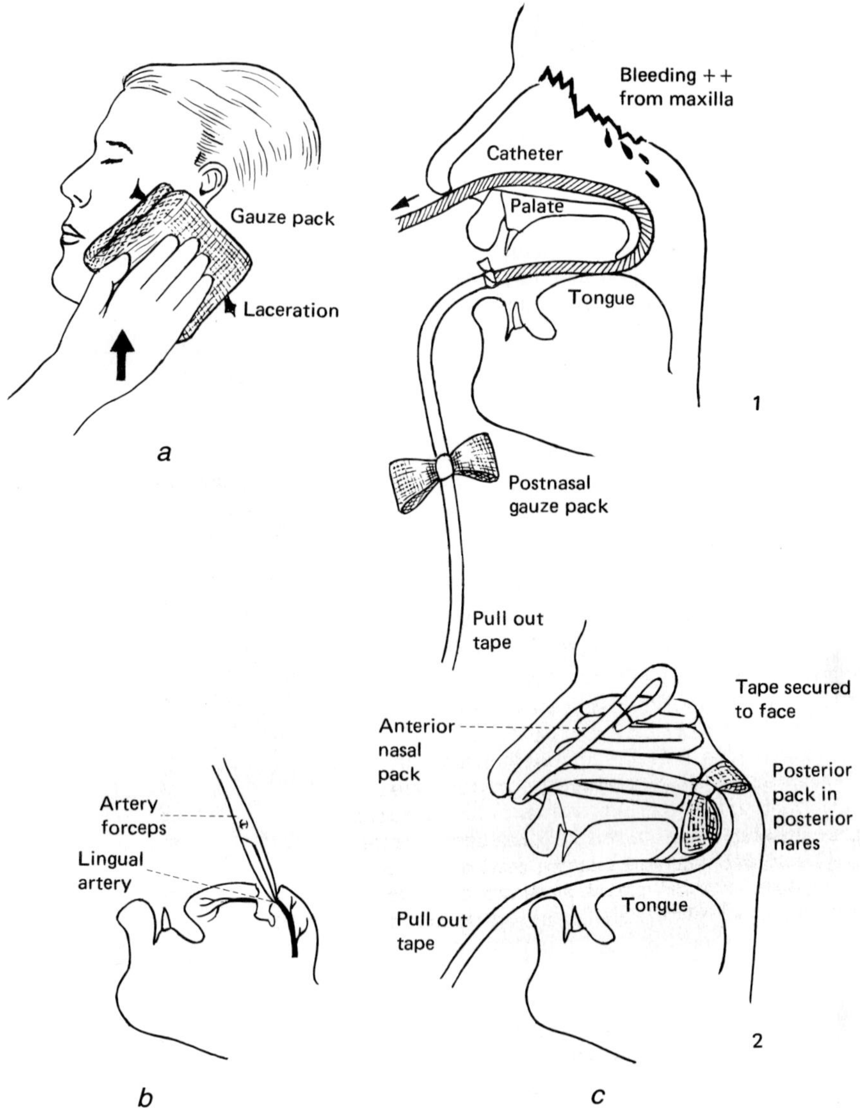

Fig. 26.23 Control of bleeding. *a*, Pressure. *b*, Clamping arterial bleeders. *c*, Nasal packing for persistent epistaxis, e.g. fracture of maxilla 1. Introduction. 2. Secured (leave $\simeq$48 hours + antibiotic).

to arrest bleeding, and consideration may need to be given to ligation of the external carotid artery on the affected side. This is often not as effective as might be hoped because of the crossover circulation from the opposite side, but may help in the overall control of a difficult situation.

3. *Pain Relief*

Surprisingly many maxillofacial injuries are not very painful in the early stages. Presumably this is due to trauma of the peripheral nerve branches at the fracture site. Narcotics may be indicated, but great care should be given in administrating opiates in cases of head injury, lest changes of consciousness are obscured and pupillary changes masked. Conservative doses of pentazocine can be administered with caution.

The use of supportive bandages to help discomfort is a traditional first aid method. The Barton bandage has a time-established place in the history of primary treatment. Such supports, however, can provoke more pain and disturbance unless they are very carefully applied. A crêpe bandage gently taken from under the chin to over the crown of the head and then around transversely, with turns going under the external occipital protuberance, can provide a gentle support in some cases. It can be reinforced with stretch Elastoplast. The majority of cases, however, do not need these measures.

4. *Prevention of Infection*

In high level fractures of the maxilla and naso-ethmoidal fractures, it is as well to give protection against possible meningitis associated with CSF leak. This is given in the first few days even though definitive diagnosis of CSF leak has not been established. Medication with a sulphonamide such as sulphadimidine in a dose of 1 g qds is usual as this agent is released into the CSF. It is usually combined with 6-hourly doses of penicillin.

In compound fractures either externally or into the mouth antibiotic medication is indicated, usually with penicillin.

Where facial laceration may have been contaminated with dirt there is a need to provide protection against tetanus (*see* Chapter 5).

Fracture of Mandible

If the patient has teeth then intermaxillary fixation (IMF) is employed to fix the teeth of the mandible to those in the maxilla. Dental occlusion provides a good guide to accurate reduction. Eyelet wiring or the use of arch bars or the employment of cap splints (*Fig.* 26.24) may be indicated. Eyelet wires are used where there is a good dentition, but arch bars will help where gaps are present. Cap splints are particularly helpful in more complex fractures. Where the patient has no teeth, Gunning splints can be constructed which are secured to the jaws themselves usually by peralveolar wires in the upper and circumferential wires in the lower. It is of great help in the construction of Gunning splints to have the patient's dentures, and the casualty officer should obtain these for the oral surgeon when he first sees the patient. Even if the dentures have been broken they can still prove of considerable use.

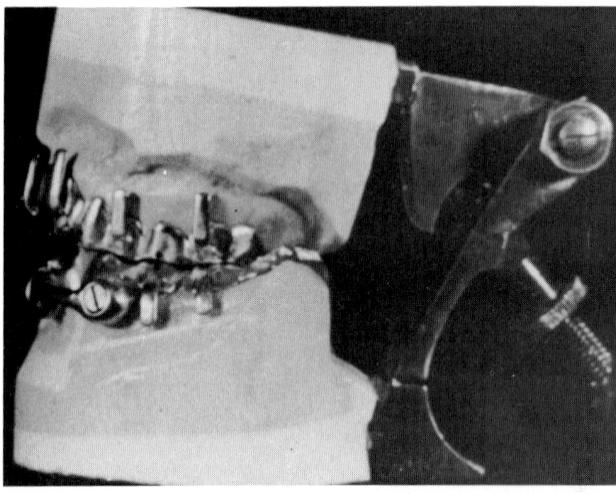

Fig. 26.24 Cap splints. The jaws are immobilized together (intermaxillary fixation) by passing wires around the hooks on the upper and lower splints.

In unstable fractures, IMF alone may be insufficient for control, so that open reduction is indicated with skeletal fixation by lower border or upper border wiring, bone plating or, alternatively pinning. Fixation after mandible fracture is approximately 4 weeks in unilateral cases but may require 6 weeks in bilateral cases or even longer in grossly comminuted fractures, atrophic mandibles or very elderly patients. Unilateral fractures of the condyle may only require 10 days' fixation. Fractures of the condyle normally only require treatment if the patient is unable to attain centric occlusion.

Fracture of Maxilla

It is not sufficient in fractures of the maxilla to carry out intermaxillary fixation as mandibular movements will be transmitted to the maxilla and there is a real danger of pumping organisms through the region of the cribriform plate with a risk of meningitis. After reduction with Rowe forceps, cranial fixation should be undertaken and ideally this is to the maxilla (craniomaxillary fixation). A 'halo' or Levant type frame (*Fig.* 26.25) or plastic headcap is used and this is linked to the splint in the upper jaw via projection bars and universal joints. Alternatively, in minimally displaced fractures, internal suspension wires may be used and either attached to the pyriform aperture or over the zygomatic arches or from the frontal bone above the frontomalar suture. The site of the origin of the suspension wire must obviously be above the known fracture site. Four weeks is normally sufficient for union of a fractured maxilla.

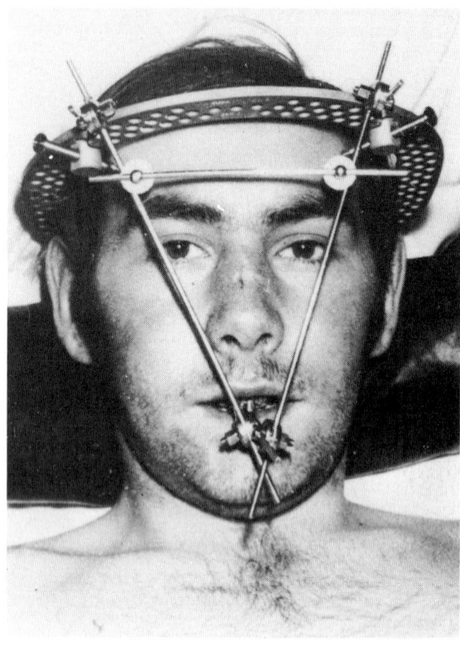

Fig. 26.25 A 'halo' frame providing craniomaxillary fixation for a fracture of the maxilla.

Fracture of Zygoma

The majority of simple zygomatic fractures can be reduced via an incision in the temporal region which passes through the temporalis fascia allowing an instrument to be slipped down beneath the zygomatic arch. The instrument (an elevator) can then lift up the displaced part (*Fig.* 26.26). Union is normally complete in about 4 weeks. More complex fractures may require exposure of the fracture sites at the frontomalar suture and/or infraorbital margins with direct skeletal wiring.

An orbital blow-out fracture in isolation can often be remedied by opening the antrum and placing a pack in it which is removed after 2–3 weeks via an oral route. An alternative method which may be necessary in more complex orbital blow-out fractures is direct surgical exposure of the orbital floor through an infraorbital or eyelid incision with insertion of a graft to the defect or more usually a Silastic implant.

Nasal Fracture

Reduction is carried out with Walsham's forceps for the nasal bones and frontal processes of the maxilla (*Fig.* 26.27). Ashe's septal forceps are used to attempt to reposition the displaced septum in the vomerine groove although this can be difficult. Immobilization of the fracture is obtained with a plaster-of-Paris nasal splint which is left on for 5–7 days.

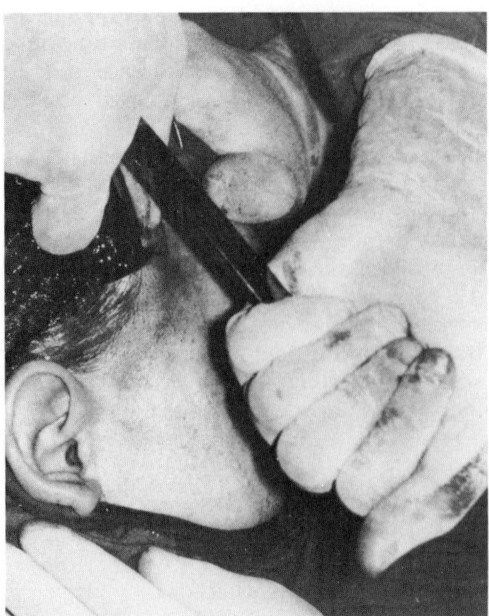

Fig. 26.26 Elevating a fracture of the zygoma by the Gillies temporal approach.

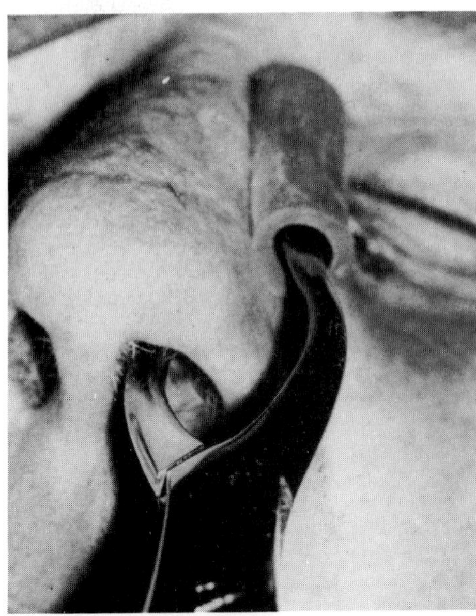

Fig. 26.27 Reduction of a nasal bone fracture with a Walsham's forceps.

In unstable cases, lead plates and a vertical mattress suture of wire can be used. It can be difficult to obtain adequate control of a displaced nasal septum, and if the healed position is inadequate then a subsequent operative procedure several weeks after fracture union can be carried out in the form of a submucous resection or septal repositioning.

Occasionally the insertion of the medial canthal ligaments may be disrupted together with a small related fragment of bone. In these cases surgical exposure may be necessary together with wiring which needs to be carried out with a special technique in view of the thin nature of the bone. Nasal fractures are considered further in Chapter 29.

CONCLUSION AND WAY AHEAD

In general, fractures of the facial skeleton heal well due to the excellent blood supply of the area. Indeed, prompt recognition is necessary as definitive reduction needs to be undertaken within 10 days of injury because a degree of early union will be encountered after this time. This behoves a knowledge of the signs and symptoms of such injuries in those responsible for the management of trauma victims. It is, however, vital to take into account other coexisting conditions, particularly in the central nervous system, thorax and abdomen, which should take precedence because of their life-threatening nature. Facial injuries do not constitute an emergency unless they threaten the airway or are a source of haemorrhage. Should malunion occur due to inevitable delay, as for example in a severe head injury, a range of procedures are now available for eventual osteotomy and definitive reduction.

Prevention is obviously the ideal form of management. Legislation to ensure the wearing of front seat belts has brought about a significant reduction in maxillofacial trauma and this may be enhanced further by the general use of rear seat belts.

Management will be helped by extension of knowledge of the mechanisms of traumatic damage. For example, a better understanding of compartmentalization within the orbital fat is leading to improved insight into orbital blow-out fractures.

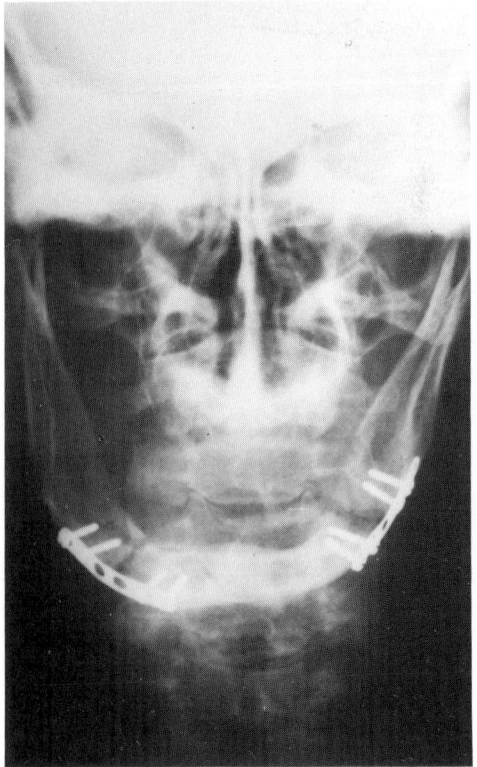

Fig. 26.28 Fracture of an atrophic mandible on postero–anterior X-ray showing treatment by compressive bone plating. Bone plates are particularly useful where one wishes to avoid inter-maxillary fixation either because it would not give a precise reduction or because of poor patient compliance as in a mentally disturbed subject.

Accurate radiographic diagnosis is obviously a preliminary to good reduction. Tomography helps greatly in more difficult cases. CT scanning is finding an increasing role, as in orbital injuries where it may localize unusual sites of blow-out and of course, very importantly, in the evaluation of concomitant head injuries.

Bone plating techniques are becoming more widely used in maxillofacial practice. Compressive plates are now available (*Fig.* 26.28) although their use requires very careful technique to avoid the creation of occlusal discrepancies. It may be possible to dispense with intermaxillary fixation in many cases. This may be very valuable in mentally compromised patients or where there is a risk of ankylosis due to prolonged immobilization as in intracapsular condylar fractures, or in the presence of other injuries as in the thorax requiring a free airway. Additionally, many subjects wish to return to activity as soon as possible in a time of economic recession where prolonged convalescence can lead to a deterioration in clientele in self-employed occupations or even job loss.

There is a growing awareness that a combined craniofacial approach may be necessary in certain instances. This particularly applies to severe nasoethmoidal injuries associated with damage to the anterior cranial fossa in the region of the posterior walls of the frontal sinuses and the cribriform plate. Co-operation between neurosurgeons and maxillofacial surgeons has led to improved management in this field. Indeed, growing mutual understanding between all those specialties dealing with the victims of trauma is a continuing aim to provide optimal therapy for our patients.

Further Reading

Killey H. C. Revised by P. Banks (1987) *Fractures of the Middle Third of the Facial Skeleton.* Bristol, Wright.
Killey H. C. Revised by P. Banks (1983) *Fractures of the Mandible.* Bristol, Wright.
Rowe N. L. and Williams J. L. (1985) *Maxillofacial Injuries*, Vols. 1 and 2. Edinburgh, Livingstone.

27 The Oral Cavity

P. M. Stell and A. G. D. Maran

PATHOLOGY

Lesion presenting within the oral cavity may arise from three groups of tissue:

1. The teeth.
2. The bone of the mandible and maxilla.
3. The epithelial lining of the mouth, with the underlying connective tissue.

1. The Teeth

Tumours of the teeth are of course the concern of the dentist. All that is given here, therefore, is a brief list of the lesions (*Table* 27.1).

Table 27.1 Tumours of the teeth (adapted from Lucas)

1. *Lesions consisting of odontogenic epithelium*
   Ameloblastoma
   Adenomatoid odontogenic tumour
   Calcifying epithelial tumour
   Calcifying odontogenic cyst
2. *Lesions consisting of odontogenic epithelium and mesenchyme*
   Ameloblastic fibroma
   Ameloblastic sarcoma
3. *Lesions consisting of odontogenic epithelium and calcified dental tissues*
   Odonto-ameloblastoma
4. *Lesions consisting of calcified dental tissues, but without odontogenic epithelium*
   Complex odontome
   A tumour-like mass of enamel, dentine and cementum
   Compound odontome
   Dens invaginatus (dilated odontome)
   A developmental malformation in which an invagination of enamel is formed in a tooth
   Enameloma
   A developmental malformation consisting of small ectopic deposits of enamel on a tooth
   Dentinoma
   A tumour-like lesion in which the only calcified tissue is dentine
   Cementoma
   A basically fibrous lesion in which cementum or cementum-like tissue is also present
5. *Lesions consisting of odontogenic mesenchyme*
   Fibroma
   Myxoma

2. The Bone of the Mandible and Maxilla

The tumours which may arise from bone are shown in *Table* 27.2.

Osteoma

An osteoma is a growth consisting of cancellous or compact bone, which, in the jaws, may occur as a circumscribed mass growing outwards from the bone or as a dense mass growing within the bone. The mandible is involved more often than the maxilla, and the tumour occurs more often in adults over the age of 40. The osteoma is benign and does not recur after complete removal.

Torus Palatinus and Mandibularis

These are non-neoplastic bony outgrowths occurring from the palate and the mandible respectively. They are both quite common, the palatal torus being commoner than that of the mandible. They are said to be more common in certain races, such as Eskimos and Mongoloid races, than in Caucasians. A torus palatinus usually arises in adolescence and always involves the midline. It presents as a flat ridge of bone, which is usually removed. The lesion is entirely benign.

Osteosarcoma

Osteogenic sarcoma is the commonest primary malignant tumour of bone, but it is a comparatively rare tumour in the jaws. Sarcomas of the mandible are commoner than those of the maxilla and usually occur between the ages of 10 and 30. It presents as a swelling which enlarges fairly rapidly and

Table 27.2 Tumours arising from bone of mandible and maxilla

BONE
- Osteoma, osteomatosis
- Osteoid osteoma and osteoblastoma
- Torus palatinus and torus mandibularis
- Osteosarcoma

GIANT-CELL LESIONS
- Giant-cell tumour of bone
- Giant-cell lesions in hyperparathyroidism

SECONDARY TUMOURS

which may be accompanied by pain and numbness of the lip due to involvement of the inferior alveolar nerve. If the tumour occurs in the maxilla it usually invades the nose and orbit rapidly. The sarcoma is highly malignant and metastasizes early to lungs, brain and other bones. The survival rate after treatment, usually by radical surgery, is in the region of 20%.

Secondary Tumours

Metastases may occur to the mandible from a wide variety of primary tumours.

3. Lesions of the Epithelial Lining

a. Benign Lesions of the Oral Mucosa

Traumatic Ulcer

This ulcer is usually caused by biting the cheeks or by the sharp edge of a broken tooth or poorly fitting dentures. The cause should be eliminated, and thereafter a traumatic ulcer should heal in a week, but if it does not, a biopsy should be taken to rule out malignancy.

b. Recurrent Oral Ulceration

Leaving aside those ulcers associated with generalized disease, and those with obvious local causes, such as biting, and ill-fitting dentures, there are many recurrent aphthae with no obvious cause. Recurrent oral ulceration (ROU) is a common disease, and it is said that almost 1 in 5 of the population will suffer the disease at some time in their life; the disease is commonest in the third, fourth and fifth decades and is twice as common in women as in men.

ROU has been divided into major and minor types. In the minor form a single ulcer or a small crop of ulcers appears on the mucosa several times a year, runs a short painful course and heals in a week without scarring. The major form, which is uncommon, is usually one of persistent, multiple ulceration which may persist for years, and is incapacitating (*Fig.* 27.1).

A third form of ROU has recently been recognized, termed herpetiform ulceration. The ulceration begins as a pinhead point, gradually enlarges and coalesces; the ulcers may invade any part of the mouth or pharynx, are commonest in women and persist for a year or two (*Fig.* 27.2).

If extra-oral sites are involved the disease is described as Behçet's syndrome. The original syndrome was oral and genital ulceration with iridocyclitis, but vascular, joint, neurological and gastrointestinal manifestations have been added since.

The relative incidence of the various idiopathic forms of ROU is 65% minor ROU, 10% major ROU, 10% herpetiform, and 15% Behçet's disease. Recurrent oral ulceration may also be due to some underlying disease such as deficiency of vitamin B_{12} or folic acid, iron deficiency, ulcerative colitis or coeliac disease. Jejunal biopsy showed the 'flat' pattern typical of coeliac disease in 20% of patients with recurrent aphthae. Aphthous stomatitis is extremely common in tropical sprue; indeed the word 'sprue' is derived from the Dutch word 'spruw' meaning an aphthous ulcer.

The cause of ROU has not yet been established. Infection by the virus herpes simplex has often been suggested, but this has been disproved. Recently, adenovirus type 1 has been implicated by culturing the virus, and *Streptococcus sargens* has also been implicated but the latter organism is often found in normal people.

Allergy to food has not been associated with ROU, except for allergy to milk protein (casein, alpha and beta lactalbumin) and gluten in the major form. High levels of circulating antibodies to oral mucosa were found in 75% of patients with disease using the tanned red cell haemagglutination technique.

There is considerable support for the theory that cell-mediated immunity to oral mucosal antigens (or more likely to some antigenically cross-reacting microbial antigen) are concerned in the pathogenesis of recurrent ulceration and Behçet's syndrome. A significantly increased frequency of HL-A5 antigen has been found in patients with Behçet's disease.

To the list of causes must now be added the administration of beta-blocking agents, particularly propranolol (Inderal), which can cause multiple or single ulcerated areas in the mouth, surrounded by marked hyperaemic reaction but which resembles aphthous ulcers.

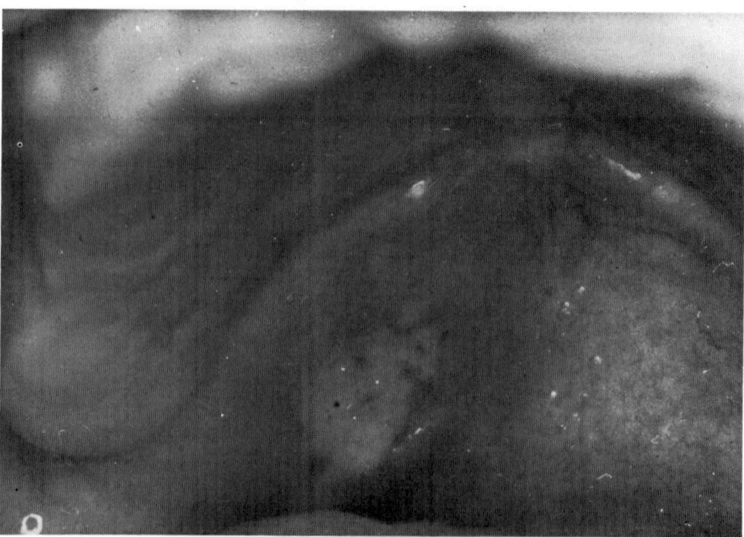

Fig. 27.1 Recurrent aphthous ulceration (major type) affecting soft palate.

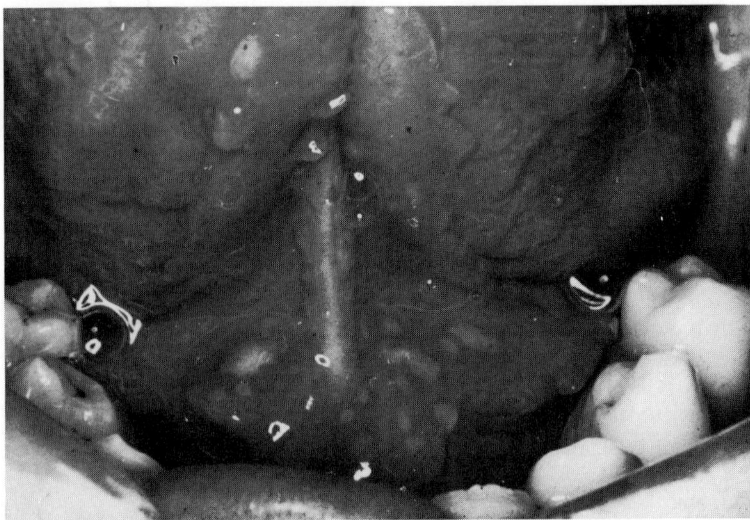

Fig. 27.2 Recurrent aphthous ulceration (herpetiform type) affecting anterior floor of mouth and ventral surface of tongue.

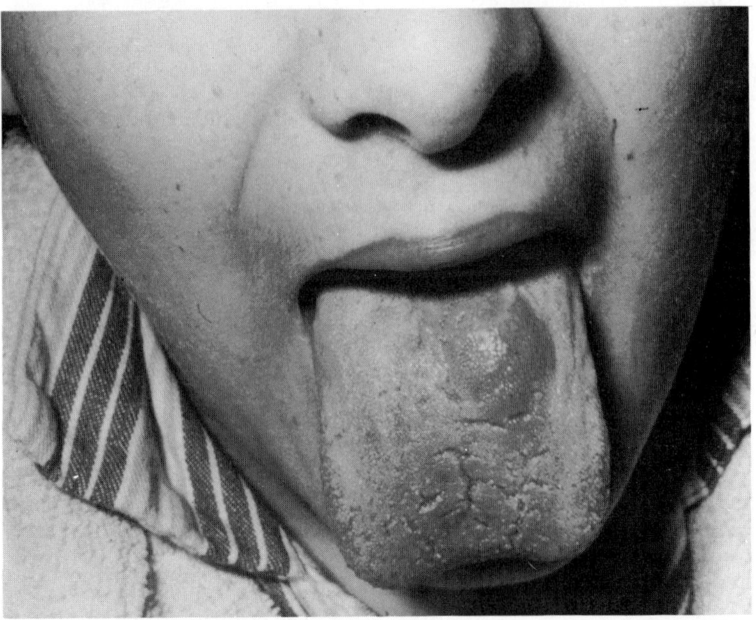

Fig. 27.3 Median rhomboid glossitis.

The treatment of ROU has been unsatisfactory. Topical steroids are the most widely used. Topical hydrocortisone hemisuccinate sodium (Corlan) reduces the number of ulcer days and the number of new ulcers by half compared with an inert placebo. Topical tetracycline is the treatment of choice for herpetiform ulcers. Recurrent aphthae can occur in women in the premenstrual week and are then usually controlled by oestrogens, for example ethinyloestradiol 0·2 mg daily. A new approach has been the administration of the immunopotentiating drug levamisole.

c. *Specific Tongue Lesions*

Median Rhomboid Glossitis (*Fig.* 27.3)

This is a lesion of the tongue consisting of a smooth, red, rhomboid area lying immediately anterior to the foramen caecum. It has been said that this represents a remnant of the tuberculum impar, but more recently it has been suggested that the disease is due to infection by the *Candida albicans*. The condition should be treated by firm reassurance that it is not malignant, and by a fungicidal drug.

Geographic Tongue

Large or small areas of the dorsal surface of the tongue show atrophy of the filiform papillae, resulting in a smooth, red mucosal surface in which the fungiform papillae become visible as little red elevations. The borders of the smooth area are usually accentuated by a 'marginal' hypertrophy of the filiform papillae. In a matter of weeks or months the area becomes normal again, but the lesion may then become apparent somewhere else on the tongue. The cause is unknown.

Geographic tongue is a harmless lesion not requiring treatment other than reassurance.

Hairy Tongue

Hairy tongue is a common, but still not completely understood, condition of the tongue, characterized by a hairy, black-brown or yellow aspect of the dorsal surface of the tongue. Micro-organisms (the streptothrix) may play a role as well as changes in the physiological movements of the tongue. Smoking seems to be a promoting factor. Treatment consists of mechanical cleaning of the tongue with a toothbrush twice or more a day, starting at the posterior end of the tongue and moving gently towards the tip. This is often combined with a fungicidal lozenge.

d. Benign Tumours of the Oral Mucosa

The lining of the mouth is entirely squamous epithelium, with many minor serous and mucinous glands, overlying the underlying muscle. Tumours may occur from any of these elements.

Squamous-cell Papilloma

Squamous-cell papillomas are fairly common between the ages of 20 and 50, occurring almost exclusively in the region of the soft palate and uvula. They are usually single, but multiple papillomas may occur. Malignant change does not occur.

Salivary Tumours

Most tumours of salivary origin occurring within the mouth are malignant, and with the exception of the hard palate, salivary tumours are very uncommon; virtually the only benign tumour to arise here is the pleomorphic adenoma.

Granular-cell Tumour (myoblastoma)

This tumour arises from skeletal muscle, but there is some controversy as to its true nature. It may be a true benign tumour, but many consider it to be either a degenerative or regenerative lesion. The tumour was originally thought to be derived from skeletal muscle, but electron microscopy suggests that the myoblasts more probably arise from Schwann cells. Two types are known: the first occurs on the gum pads in the newborn, and is a separate entity (congenital epulis). It has an 8:1 predominance in girls, and is three times more commonly seen in the upper jaw than the lower. The second occurs in the adult beneath the mucous membrane of the upper aerodigestive tract (*Fig.* 27.4). The maximum age incidence is between 30 and 40, and the tumour is slightly more common in women than in men.

This latter lesion can affect many sites including the skin and the larynx and the gastrointestinal tract, but one-third of all reported cases occur within the mouth, the tongue being much the most common site.

The mucosa overlying a granular-cell myoblastoma, on about 2 occasions out of 3, shows the appearance of pseudo-epitheliomatous hyperplasia. It is very important to differentiate this from true malignancy which does not occur in this lesion. Local excision is the treatment of choice.

Epulides

An epulis is a granuloma occurring on the gums. The following types have been described.

1. Congenital.
2. Fibrous.
3. Pregnancy.
4. Giant cell.

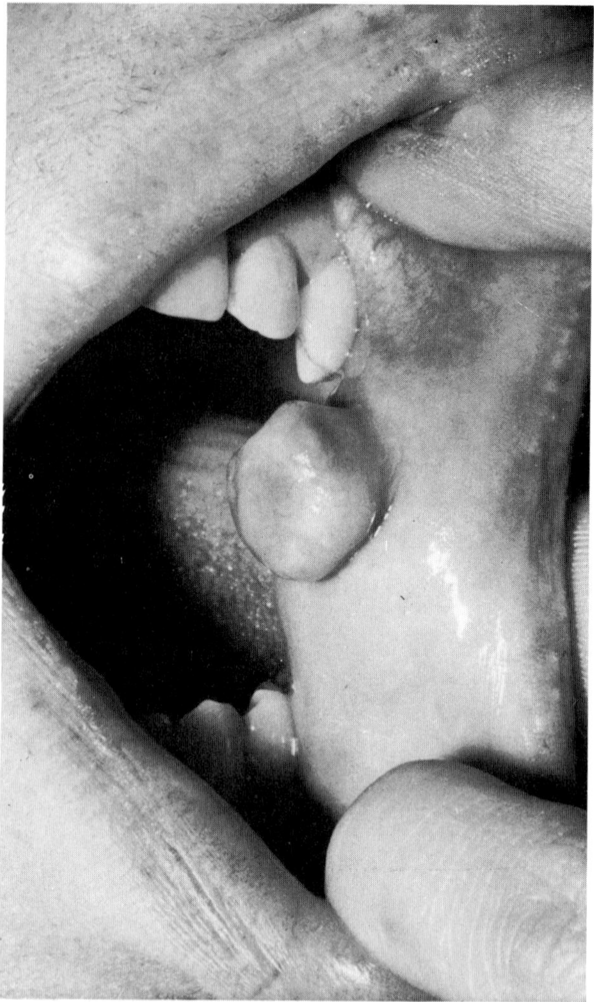

Fig. 27.4 Granular-cell myoblastoma arising beneath the buccal mucosa.

1. The congenital epulis. This has been referred to above under granular-cell tumour. It is a benign lesion which is removed locally and does not recur.
2. The fibrous epulis affects any age, and both sexes equally. The lesion is predunculated and arises from an interdental papilla in response to caries of an adjacent tooth. The lesion is treated by excision and treatment of its cause.
3. The pregnancy granuloma resembles a pyogenic granuloma. It appears about the third month of pregnancy on the gums of pregnant women suffering from gingivitis. It resolves once the pregnancy is over.
4. The giant-cell epulis or osteoclastoma occurs usually between 30 and 40, and affects women more than men. It arises more often from the anterior part of the alveolus than the posterior, and on the lower jaw more often than the upper. The cause of the lesion is unknown: histology shows a large number of giant cells. Treatment may require the removal of an adjoining tooth. The differential diagnosis includes the 'brown' tumour of hyperparathyroidism.

Haemangioma

Cavernous haemangiomas can occur at any point in the oral cavity, but are probably more common on the tongue than elsewhere. They have no predilection for any particular age or sex, and many are seen in patients over the age of 40.

Ranula (*Fig.* 27.5)

Ranulas are of two varieties, simple or plunging. The simple ranula is a true retention cyst of one of the minor salivary glands lining the oral cavity. The plunging ranula extends beyond the mucous membrane into the floor of the mouth and into the fascial planes of the neck. Its tendency to extend is thought to be due to the extravasation of mucus.

Dermoid Cysts

Only about 2% of all dermoids occur in the mouth; they may be either sublingual or submental in position and manifest themselves in the second or third decades of life.

Leucoplakia

The term 'leucoplakia' is an entirely clinical one and means nothing more than a white patch. Histologically,

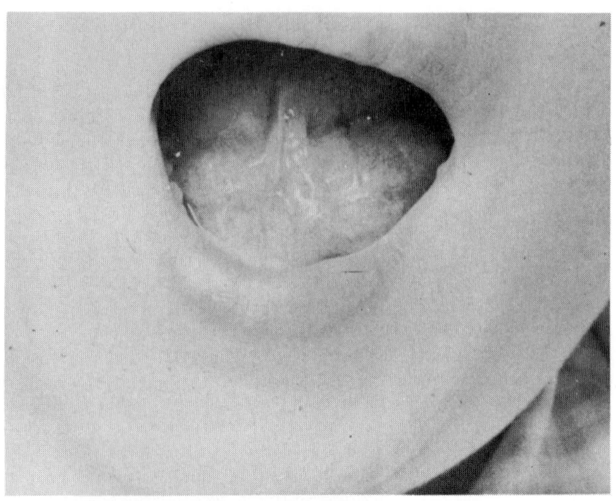

Fig. 27.5 Simple ranula.

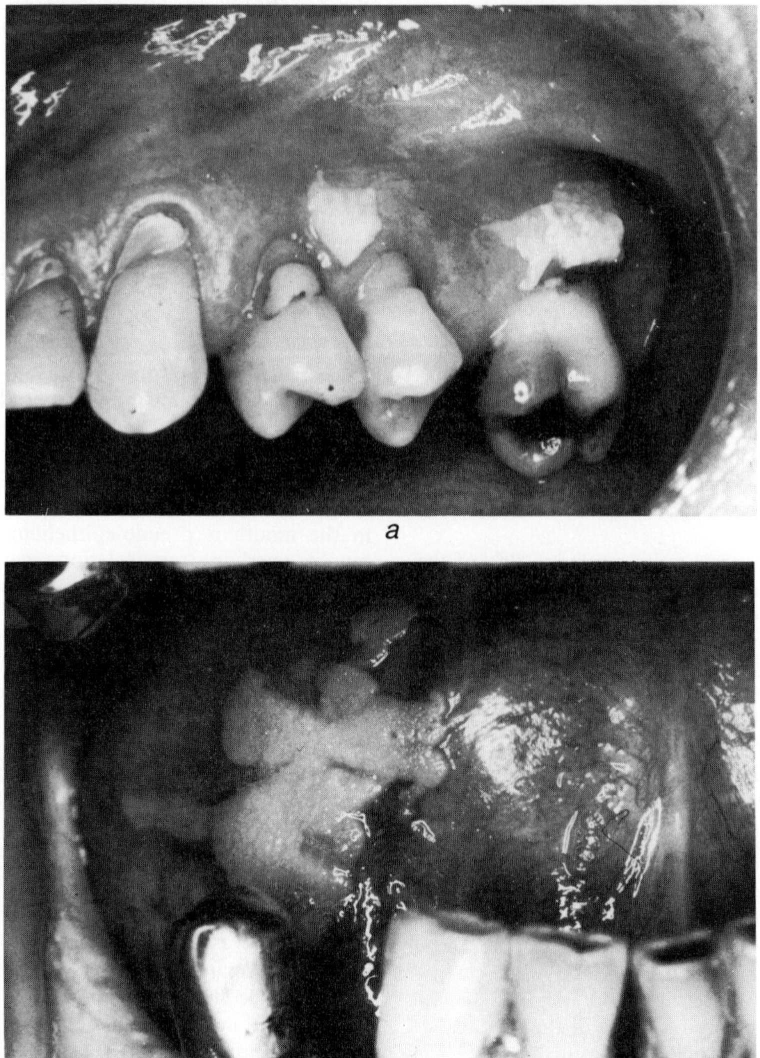

Fig. 27.6 Simple keratosis (benign white patches) due to mild irritation. *a*, Frictional keratosis of gingiva due to excessive toothbrushing. Note erosion at cervical margins of the teeth. *b*, Frictional keratosis of the lateral border of the tongue due to ill-fitting gold crown [*continued over*]

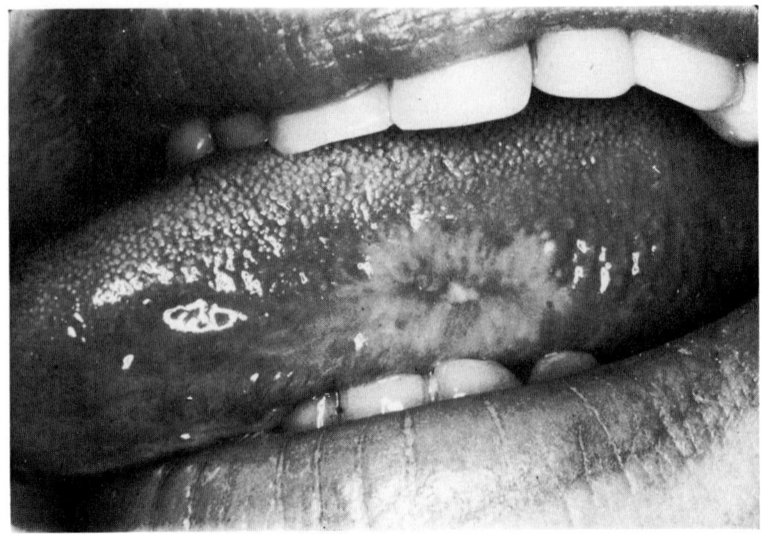

c

[*Fig. 27.6 continued*] *c*, Frictional keratosis of the lateral border of the tongue. (*Figs.* 27.6–27.11, 27.15 supplied by Professor D. M. Chisholm, Department of Dental Surgery, Dental School, Dundee.)

such a white patch may be divided into one of three basic categories:

1. A simple keratosis arising as a response to mild irritation (*Fig.* 27.6).
2. Various combinations of hyperkeratosis, parakeratosis and acanthosis.
3. A hyperkeratotic lesion with, in addition, dyskeratosis and possible progression to a carcinoma-in-situ (*Fig.* 27.7).

There is little correlation between the clinical appearance of the white patch and its histological features, so that histology is essential in deciding whether a white patch is entirely benign, or whether it is likely to proceed to frank squamous carcinoma. The proportion of patients with leucoplakia which progresses to carcinoma varies in different series reported, but a figure of approximately 10% would be generally acceptable.

Leucoplakia in the mouth is quite common: 80% of the lesions are found in men, most commonly between 50 and 60. The buccal mucosa, including the commissures, is the most common site (60%) followed by the alveolar mucosa, the tongue, the lip, the palate, the floor of the mouth and the gingiva in that order. Its cause is basically unknown, though it is widely believed to be due to irritation, such as ill-fitting dentures, or abuse of tobacco or alcohol.

The following factors are associated with a higher risk of progression to malignancy:

1. Length of history.
2. Female sex.
3. A combination of irritant factors, due to:
   a. Electrical potential differences due to dissimilar dental restorations.
   b. Excessive alcohol consumption, and
   c. Excessive use of tobacco.
4. Site: Lesions of the margin or base of the tongue.
5. The erosive type of leucoplakia.

The differential diagnosis includes the following:

1. Benign squamous-cell hyperplasia which is usually restricted to the hard palate and is a reactive response in patients with ill-fitting dentures.
2. White sponge naevus (*Fig.* 27.8), or Heck's focal epithelial hyperplasia. Both of these diseases are extremely uncommon.
3. Lichen planus, a chronic mucocutaneous disease affecting not only the skin but also the oral mucosa in a higher proportion of patients. The lesion may be reticular, erosive, or plaque in appearance. This disease is only rarely premalignant.

Erythroplakia

Some patches in the mouth are red rather than white in appearance. Although the term 'erythroplakia', like leucoplakia, has no histological significance, the incidence of epithelial dysplasia and progression to invasive carcinoma is much commoner in red lesions than in white (*Fig.* 27.9).

An important histological feature of some benign lesions in the mouth is pseudo-epitheliomatous hyperplasia: the mucosa overlying certain lesions may show an exaggerated epithelial response which superficially resembles squamous-cell carcinoma. This lesion is entirely benign, however, and it is important that it be recognized by both pathologist and clinician. It occurs in the mucosa overlying the following lesions: benign squamous-cell hyperplasia, granular-cell myoblastoma and keratoacanthoma.

TREATMENT. After a firm histological diagnosis has been established, these mucosal lesions are treated by removing the diseased mucosa. This can be done by simple stripping or by cryosurgery. If the defect after stripping is large, it should be grafted by the quilting technique.

e. Malignant Tumours

The approximate distribution of tumours within the oral cavity can be seen from *Table* 27.3. The vast majority of tumours within the mouth are malignant, and about 95% of malignant tumours are squamous-cell carcinomas; the remaining 5% consist of salivary tumours (which constitute about 80% of this group) and malignant melanoma.

Although tumours of the lip are theoretically to be included with tumours of the mouth, they really constitute an entirely different problem, discussed separately in Chapter 14.

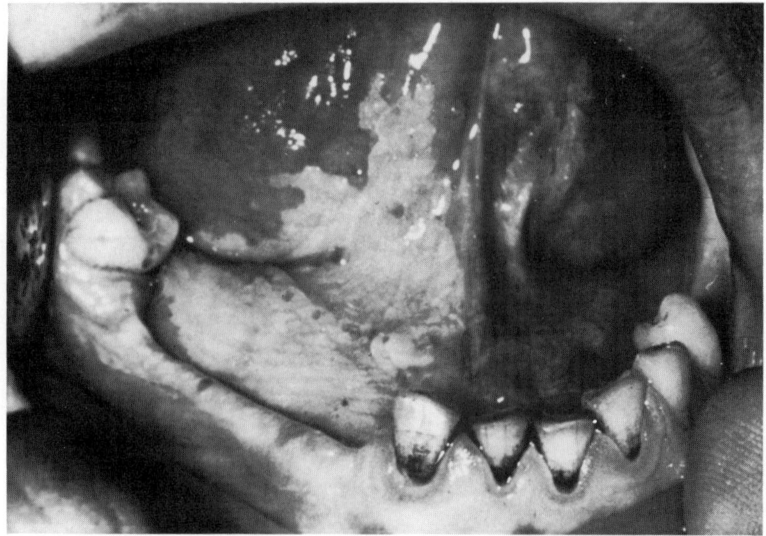

a

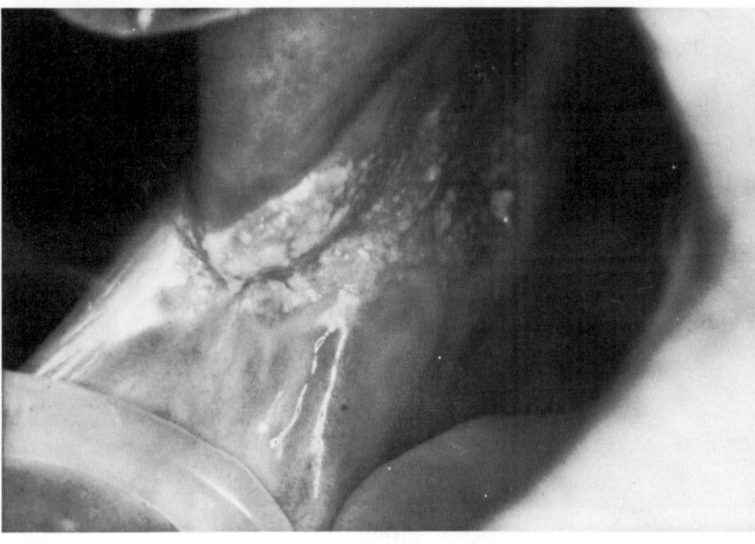

b

Fig. 27.7 Premalignant white patches. *a*, Sublingual keratosis affecting right surface and floor of the mouth. Aetiology was unknown. *b*, Chronic hyperplastic candidosis (speckled leucoplakia) affecting right angle of the mouth.

Oral cancer accounts for 1% of cancer deaths in England and Wales, and for 5% of such deaths in the USA. The annual incidence of oral cancer is approximately 2500 in England and Wales and 23 000 in the USA. The incidence has fallen quite dramatically in England and Wales, at about 3% per annum for the last 20 years. Until about 30 years ago the disease was one almost exclusively of men with a male to female ratio of 10:1 or more, but the disease has remained constant in women whilst it has fallen dramatically in men, so that the sex incidence in England and Wales is now approaching equality.

It is strange that a site which is so readily accessible to examination should show such a high frequency of advanced tumours: the vast majority of tumours are over 2 cm in size when first seen, but a recent series shows that 70% of all oral cancers are not recognized as such by general dental or medical practitioners. Screening techniques have been shown to be more or less valueless in the detection of early oral cancer.

The cause of oral cancer remains unknown, though it is commonly said that heavy smoking and drinking are associated with this tumour. This is rather difficult to correlate with the fact that the use of tobacco and alcohol has increased markedly in the Western world in the last 30 years at a time when the incidence of the tumour has been falling by about 3% per annum. It is also well known that chewers of betel nuts and tobacco, and those who smoke cigars with the lighted end inside the mouth are all highly susceptible to oral cancer. Even here, however, there may be other factors which are important such as poor nutrition and poor dental hygiene.

Several different TNM Classifications have been devised

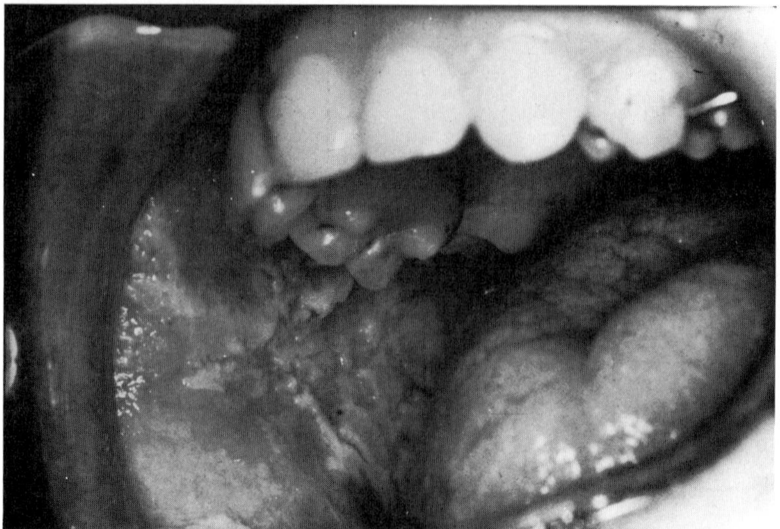

Fig. 27.8 White sponge naevi (familial white-folded dysplasia). This is a developmental lesion affecting the buccal mucosa and is entirely benign.

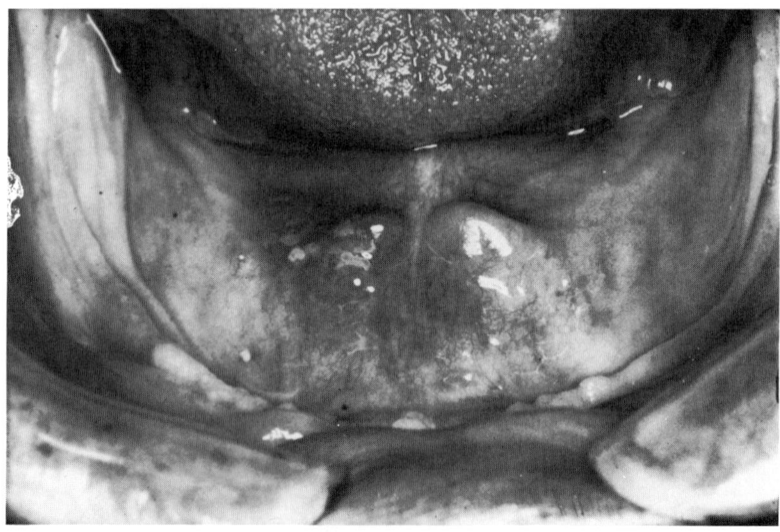

Fig. 27.9 Speckled lesion (i.e. alternate areas of leucoplakia and erythroplakia) affecting right floor of mouth close to the submandibular duct orifice. Biopsy revealed early invasive squamous-cell carcinoma.

Table 27.3 Relative incidence of squamous-cell carcinoma in the mouth

Tongue	30%
Floor of mouth	15%
Alveoli (upper and lower)	15%
Buccal mucosa	15%

Table 27.4 TNM classification of oral cavity cancer

T1	≤2 cm
T2	>2–4 cm
T3	>4 cm
T4	Extension to bone/muscle, etc.
N1	Homolateral movable node(s)
N2	Contra- or bilateral movable node(s)
N3	Fixed node(s)

for reporting oral cancer. None of these is entirely satisfactory but the current UICC method is shown in *Table* 27.4.

The sites of origin of squamous-cell carcinoma within the mouth are the following: the buccal mucosa, the gum (gingiva and alveolar mucosa), the tongue and the floor of the mouth.

Forty per cent of patients have lymph-node metastases on admission, the submandibular and jugulo-omohyoid nodes being those most often involved. Distant metastases (to the lung and occasionally to the liver) are very uncommon at first presentation, occurring in only about 1%, but ultimately distant metastases are a reasonably common cause of death.

The presence of palpable lymph nodes in the neck, if they are invaded by tumour, significantly affects the prognosis. About 60% of patients with oral tumours may be cured if there are no palpable nodes in the neck, but this survival rate falls to 30% in the presence of unilateral involved nodes and to 1% for bilateral nodes.

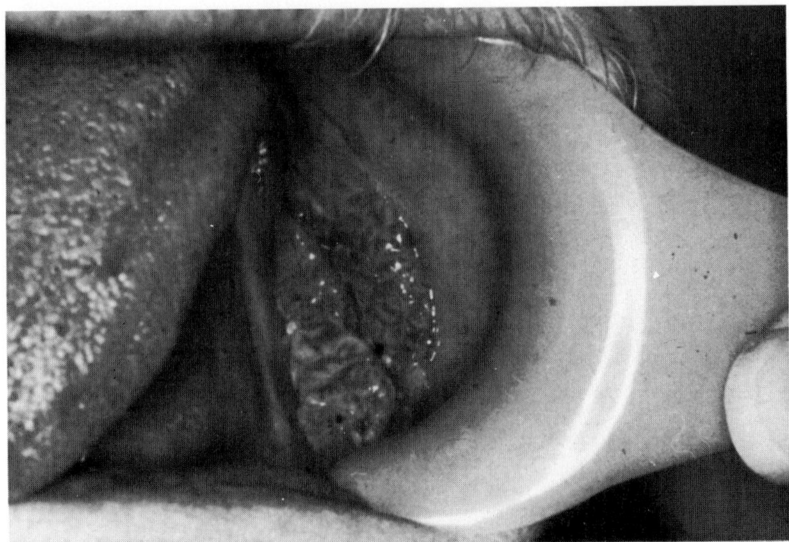

Fig. 27.10 Squamous-cell carcinoma of the right buccal mucosa—the exophytic type.

Carcinoma of the Buccal Mucosa

Carcinoma of the buccal mucosa is an aggressive tumour affecting older patients. The sex and geographical variation in incidence is wide and is related to differing standards of oral hygiene and the chronic use of local irritants such as tobacco and betel nuts.

There are three distinct clinicopathological types of buccal carcinoma:

1. Exophytic (*Fig.* 27.10).
2. Ulcero-infiltrative.
3. Verrucous.

The exophytic is the most common and the verrucous type the least. All varieties are well to moderately differentiated and are frequently associated with surrounding areas of hyperkeratosis. Most of these tumours arise from the mucosa lying against the lower third molar tooth.

Exophytic carcinomas occur most commonly at the level of the buccal commissure, whereas ulcero-infiltrative carcinomas occur further posteriorly in the mouth, presenting as a deep excavating ulcer which involves the buccinator muscle early. Both types ultimately invade deeply, ulcerate through the skin, invade the adjacent bones and extend to the pterygomaxillary fossa. The latter event is associated with trismus and is virtually always incurable.

A verrucous carcinoma is a low grade squamous-cell carcinoma which more often occurs on the buccal mucosa than in any other area of the body (75%). It represents less than 5% of all oral cancers, and may also affect the lower alveolus. It usually presents as an indolent slowly growing area of leucoplakia. It is important that it be recognized for the following reasons:

1. It is often underdiagnosed as being benign.
2. It carries the most favourable prognosis of all forms of oral cancer.
3. It is important that it must not be treated by radiotherapy. This tumour, if it is treated by radiotherapy, always recurs, and, on about 25% of occasions, anaplastic degeneration is induced by the radiotherapy leading to rapid progress, metastases and death. The microscopic picture of the tumour is quite distinctive.

The three lesions which must be distinguished from carcinoma are:

1. Kerato-acanthoma, which is very rare in the oral cavity.
2. Squamous papilloma.
3. Pseudo-epitheliomatous hyperplasia, which was described above and which may be associated with granular-cell tumours, benign epithelial hyperplasia and kerato-acanthoma.

In addition to local spread, buccal tumours metastasize by lymphatics, most commonly to the submandibular nodes on the same side; invasion of the deep cervical nodes is uncommon. Such metastases occur in 50% of cases, but this only applies to the exophytic and ulcero-infiltrative types, since metastasis from a verrucous carcinoma has only rarely been recorded. Death from carcinoma of the buccal mucosa is almost always due to local recurrence rather than distant metastases.

Carcinoma of the Gums (gingiva and alveolar mucosa) (*Figs.* 27.11 and 27.12)

Carcinomas at this site form approximately 10% of all oral malignant tumours. They generally occur in the premolar and molar regions of the lower jaw. Carcinomas of the maxillary antrum may also infiltrate the upper gingiva and in some of these cases it may be impossible to decide whether the tumour arose in the antrum or in the mouth.

Most of these tumours are well differentiated, but tend to spread widely within the mucosa, and are thus usually ulcerated, although exophytic varieties are also common. Almost half of carcinomas of the gum involve the underlying bone and this occurs early in the ulcerating type.

These tumours also metastasize to the submandibular nodes, on approximately 30% of occasions.

Five per cent of tumours at this site are non-squamous in type: about 6% of all minor salivary gland tumours arise on

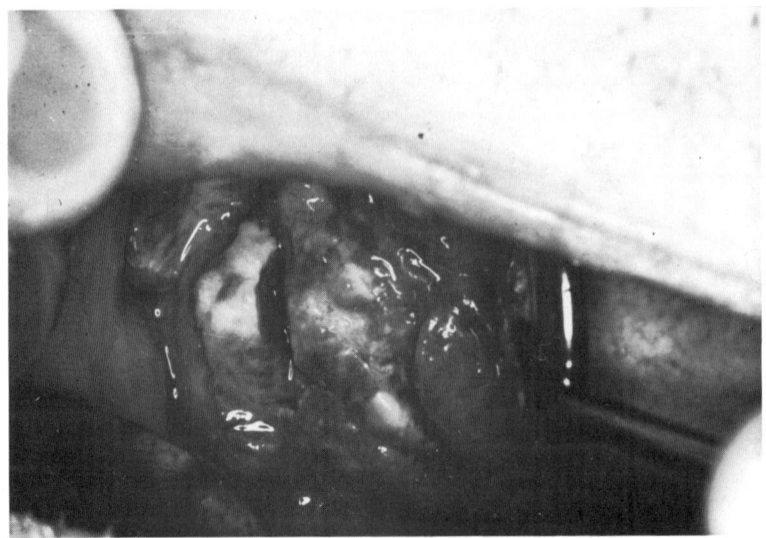

a

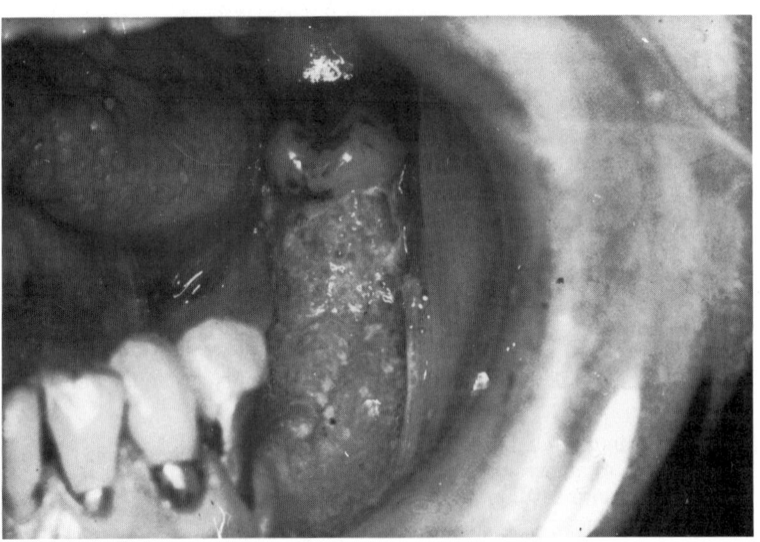

b

Fig. 27.11 *a*, Squamous-cell carcinoma of the right alveolar ridge of the mandible. *b*, Squamous-cell carcinoma of the left alveolar ridge of the mandible.

the gum, muco-epidermoid carcinoma and adenoid cystic carcinoma being much the most common.

Carcinoma of the Tongue

Carcinoma of the tongue constitutes about half of all oral cancers. Of tumours of the tongue 97% are squamous cell in type, the remainder being salivary tumours and connective-tissue tumours. Squamous-cell carcinoma is predominantly a disease of men in the middle years of life. Poor oral hygiene, the use of tobacco and alcohol and coincident syphilis have all been said in the past to be important but syphilis now is very rarely seen coexisting with carcinoma of the tongue. The symptoms and findings and biological behaviour of carcinoma of the tongue vary considerably with the site, particularly between the anterior two-thirds and the posterior one-third; carcinomas of the posterior third of the tongue are considered in tumours of the oropharynx (p. 427).

The common sites of involvement of the tongue are as follows:

1. The anterior free third (30%) (*Fig.* 27.13).
2. The middle third including the lateral border and ventral surface of the tongue (65%) (*Fig.* 27.13).
3. Dorsum of the tongue (5%).

These tumours are infiltrative, ulcerative and exophytic, and virtually all are greater than 2 cm in diameter when the patient first presents (*Fig.* 27.14).

Tumours arising from the ventral surface extend directly to, and involve, the floor of the mouth, and are then difficult to differentiate from tumours arising primarily at this site.

The presenting symptoms of carcinoma of the tongue are shown in *Fig.* 27.13.

Tumours of the tongue may be infiltrative or exophytic but whichever the type, there is usually deep infiltration,

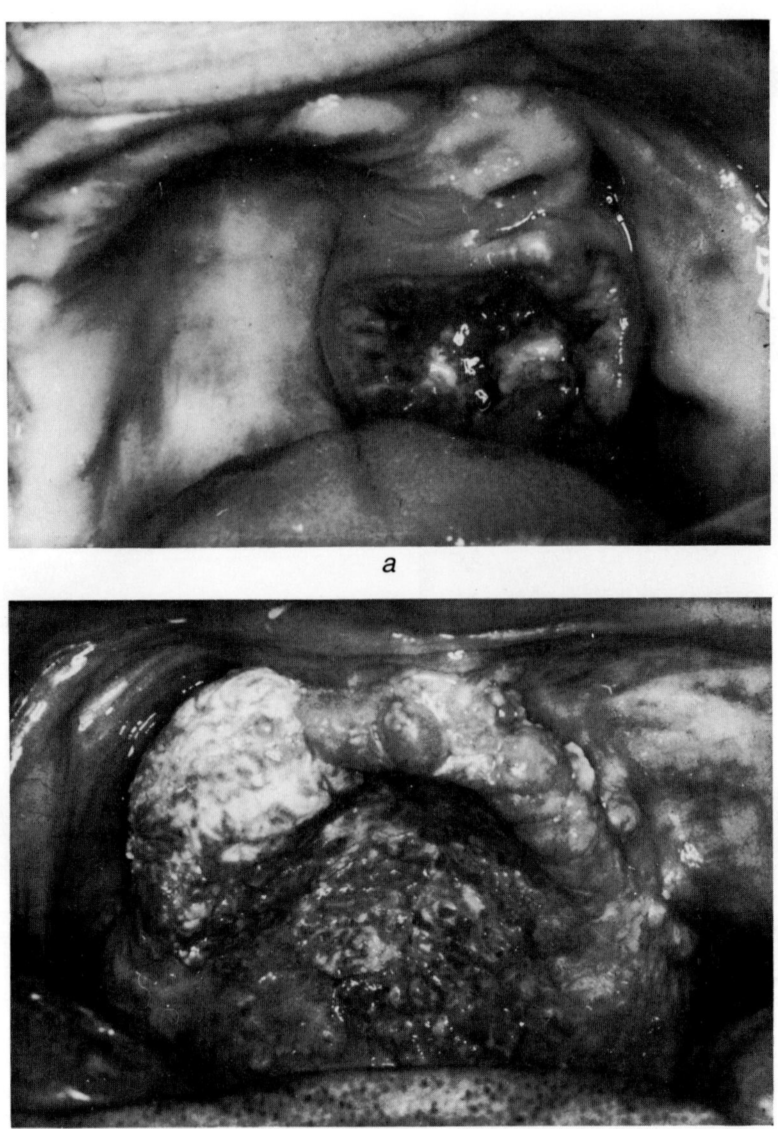

Fig. 27.12 *a*, Squamous-cell carcinoma of the left alveolar ridge of the maxilla. *b*, Squamous-cell carcinoma of the right alveolar ridge of the maxilla with wide field change in palate and left side.

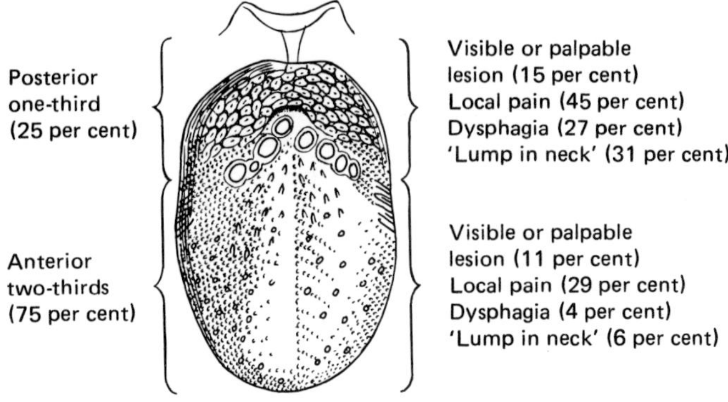

Fig. 27.13 Presenting symptoms in carcinoma of the tongue.

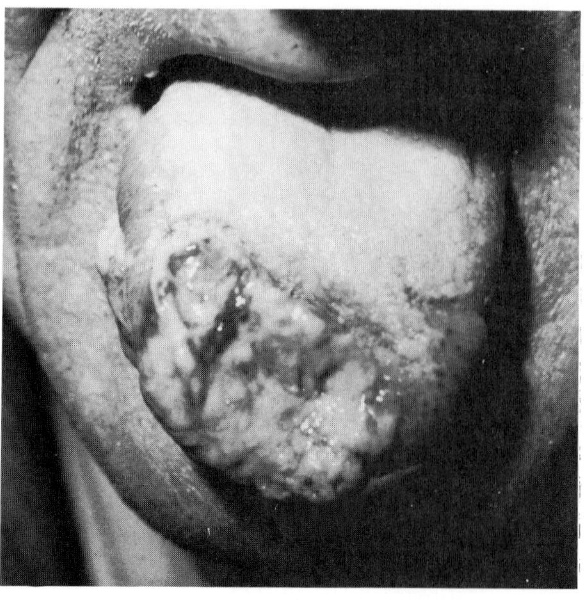

a

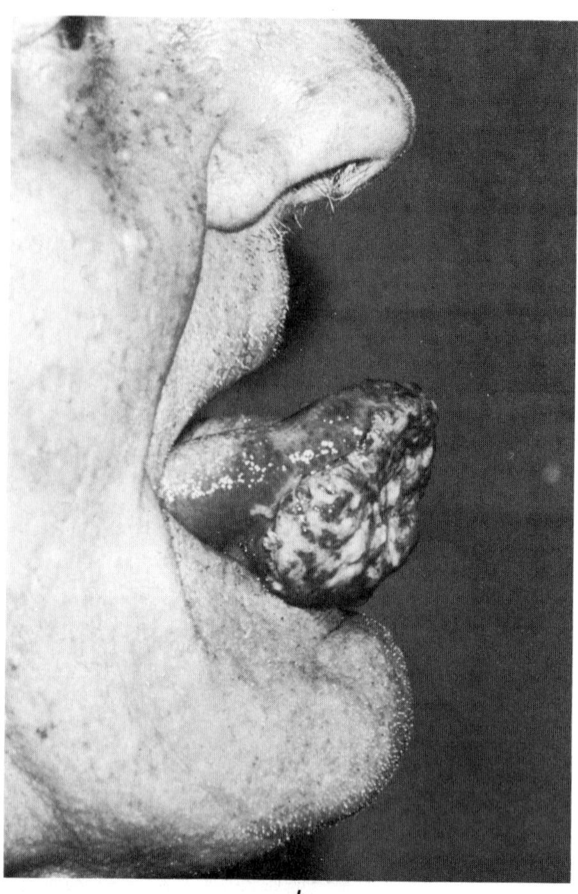

b

Fig. 27.14 *a*, Carcinoma of the anterior third of the tongue. *b*, Carcinoma of the ventral surface of the tongue.

which is better felt than seen. These tumours are usually moderately to well differentiated.

Recurrence after resection of carcinoma of the tongue is relatively high, and probably almost half the patients undergoing resection of a carcinoma of the tongue will suffer local recurrence due to invasion by fingers of the tumour between the interlacing muscle bundles of the tongue.

Squamous-cell Carcinoma of the Floor of the Mouth (Fig. 27.15)

Between 10 and 15% of oral carcinomas occur at this site, which is the second most common site for squamous-cell carcinoma in the oral cavity. The most common site is the anterior part of the floor of the mouth, midline tumours of the anterior part of the floor of the mouth being relatively uncommon, at least in England and Wales.

These tumours tend to infiltrate widely to involve the gums, the tongue and the muscles of the diaphragm of the floor of the mouth. Once the tumour reaches the mandible it can spread along the periosteum. In the anterior part of the floor of the mouth spread inferiorly is limited by the mylohyoid diaphragm, but in the posterior one-third of the gutter this diaphragm is absent and the tumour can then spread readily into the tissues of the submandibular triangle.

These tumours metastasize to the digastric nodes, and the jugulo-omohyoid node, but only rarely to the submental node. Distant metastases are also rare. These carcinomas are usually well differentiated, and the prognosis is affected more by the size and extent of the primary lesion than by its histological appearance. Multifocal carcinoma is common, and 20% of these patients have a second primary carcinoma at some other site, more than half of these being the head and neck. The incidence of lymph-node enlargement in this disease varies between 35 and 70% in various reported series, but examination of radical neck dissection specimens shows that in 30% of these the node is enlarged due to infection and not to the presence of the tumour.

Squamous-cell Carcinoma of the Hard Palate

Tumours of the soft palate are discussed elsewhere (*see* Chapter 28). True squamous-cell carcinomas of the hard palate, as distinct from those of the upper alveolus, are exceedingly uncommon in the UK, but are common in India due to the smoking of the chutta (a type of cigar) with the burning end inside the mouth. The vast majority of tumours of the hard palate in the UK are of salivary origin. Approximately 75% of malignant minor salivary gland tumours occur at this site: 40% of these are adenoid cystic carcinomas, 25% adenocarcinomas, 20% muco-epidermoid carcinomas, the remainder being miscellaneous types, including malignant mixed tumours and acinic-cell tumours.

INVESTIGATIONS

1. History

A painful ulcer or a painless lump is usually the presenting complaint of a patient with an oral tumour. If there is pain then the patient will also complain of difficulty in eating and difficulty in speaking. If there is any fixation of the tongue, difficulty will also be found in propelling food backwards out of the mouth into the pharynx. Any lesion near the alveolus will result in difficulty in wearing dentures and perhaps toothache and non-healing sockets after extractions. An ulcer may also cause halitosis. Generally speaking the more anterior the lesion, the quicker the patient will seek

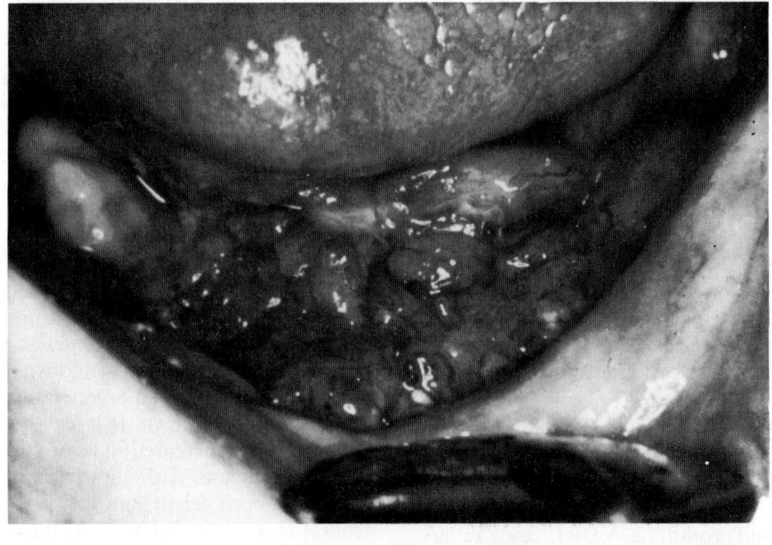

a

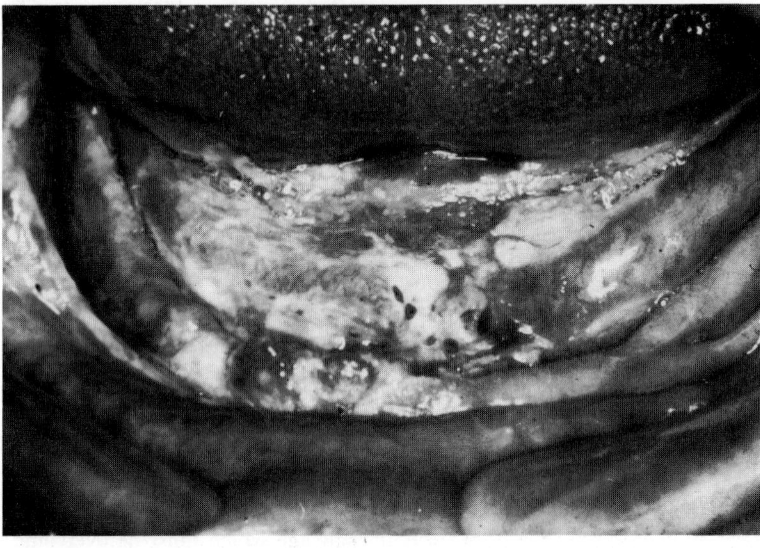

b

Fig. 27.15 *a*, Squamous-cell carcinoma of the floor of the mouth. *b*, Extensive squamous-cell carcinoma of the anterior alveolar ridge of mandible and floor of the mouth.

advice. An enlarged neck gland may be noticed especially in the submandibular area.

2. Examination

Observation will give information regarding the nature (exophytic or ulcerative) and site of the lesion. Asking the patient to move the tongue from side to side and behind the upper teeth will allow the degree of fixation to be assessed.

Palpation is an integral and necessary part of examination of the oral cavity. Tongue ulcers are like icebergs, in that while a small proportion of the tumour is visible there may be three or four times the volume in the deeper tissues of the tongue. This is only assessed by palpation. Similarly, lesions of the buccal mucosa must be assessed for invasion and again this is only possible by bimanual palpation.

Staging is based on size and so this should be recorded. The extent of induration is included in this estimate of size.

Nerve involvement is important to assess. Tongue anaesthesia means involvement of the lingual nerve and since this lies deep then its involvement means extensive spread of tumour. In the hard palate, anaesthesia suggests tumour invasion of the greater palatine nerve and such patients are incurable. Nerve involvement is usually seen in adenoid cystic carcinoma which has a predilection for nerve sheath extension.

Mandibular involvement is best assessed radiologically, but an accurate note must be made of the relation of the tumour to bone, and any fixation must be noted.

Finally the neck should be palpated for metastatic nodes. These usually lie in the submandibular area or the upper deep jugular chain, but the tongue has direct drainage also to the jugulo-omohyoid node in the lower part of the neck. Lesions in the posterior part of the oral cavity can spread to retropharyngeal nodes. Often the only sign of this is pressure of the enlarged node on the sympathetic chain resulting in a Horner's syndrome.

While the diagnosis of an oral cancer is rarely in doubt and can readily be confirmed by biopsy, it is sometimes of interest to use the metachromatic staining properties of 2% toluidine blue. If this dye is left in contact with a suspected tumour for 30 sec and the mouth is then rinsed out, carcinoma remains stained blue while normal tissues are not.

The state of the teeth is an important consideration if radiotherapy is to be used since caries in an irradiated jaw generally increases the risk of osteoradionecrosis.

3. Laboratory Investigations

These do not play a major part in the investigation of oral tumours: a full blood count, ESR, urea, electrolytes and proteins usually suffice. Since there is a tenuous relation between oral tumours and syphilis a VDRL and TPHA (*see* Chapter 5) should not be forgotten. If tuberculosis is diagnosed from the biopsy then a Mantoux test should be performed.

4. Radiology

Plain films should be taken of each half of the mandible and also an orthopantogram. As well as tumour involvement of the mandible note should be made of the state of the teeth (if any), root abscesses, periapical infections and retained roots. All of these facts are important considerations in the use of radiotherapy.

If the tumour is on the palate, then tomograms of the maxillary sinuses should be performed to assess any invasion of the hard palate.

If spread to the retropharyngeal area is suspected, CT scan is useful.

About 10% of all patients with an intra-oral squamous-cell carcinoma have invasion of the mandible, but this proportion rises to 30% or more if the tumour arises from or involves the alveolus. The radiological changes include:

a. An irregular defect with a permeative margin (due to invasion).
b. A smooth defect with a well-defined margin (due to erosion).
c. Floating teeth.
d. Pathological fracture.
e. Displaced bone fragments.
f. An expanded inferior dental canal.

5. Biopsy

Biopsy should either be performed without anaesthetic or with a general anaesthetic. Local infiltration anaesthesia is not recommended as the increase in tissue pressure may spread the tumour. Large exophytic tumours can be biopsied without anaesthesia but patients with ulcerative lesions need a general anaesthetic which also allows accurate assessment of spread.

Care should be taken to biopsy a representative piece of the tumour—not the necrotic centre or a dysplastic edge.

In the case of a lump on the cheek or palate an incisional biopsy should be performed so that an accurate wide field excision can be planned if the tumour is malignant. Incisional biopsy of surface tumours carries no risk of implantation provided that it is not extended too deeply.

TREATMENT POLICY

Untreatable Patients

In some series as many as 20% of patients are untreatable. The reasons include: distant metastases, refusal by the patient, very advanced local disease (invasion of the whole tongue, widespread invasion of the mandible, etc.), bilateral neck glands and poor general condition.

Factors Governing Treatment

There are no definite indications for the use of either surgery or radiotherapy as primary treatment. In general, surgical treatment is required for larger tumours, particularly those invading the mandible, tumours recurrent after radiotherapy and tumours associated with palpable neck glands. Combination of planned preoperative radiotherapy followed by surgery has shown that as the preoperative dose of radiotherapy is increased so is the cure rate, but so also is the complication rate. Although trials of this method of treatment have been carried out for some years it has not gained general acceptance because no information is available regarding the effect of planned postoperative radiotherapy on survival rates.

Radiotherapy seldom rescues a patient with recurrences after surgery but surgery for failed radiotherapy succeeds in about 1 in 3 cases, usually at the price of a crippled oral cavity. If excision or grafting of the jaw is required it is preferable that the jaw should not have been irradiated. If neck glands are palpable a radical neck dissection should be performed, provided they are unilateral, but if they are bilateral the 5-year survival rate is almost nil, so that it is doubtful if any treatment should be undertaken. Fixed glands are not generally a contraindication to radical neck dissection as the structure to which they are fixed can often be removed.

Problems of Surgery

The primary problem is the correct assessment of spread so that adequate excision can be done. Since all tissues in the mouth apart from the hard palate and alveoli are soft then quite deep extension of an apparently small superficial lesion can occur.

Rehabilitation of the oral cavity after surgery presents a challenge which must be overcome. If the excision of soft tissue and bone can be arranged so that the patient can wear teeth, good rehabilitation will be achieved. If the patient has teeth, he can articulate and eat even with a scarred tongue and floor of mouth, but without teeth, mobility of the tongue becomes increasingly important. Replacement of soft tissue by a flap is needed when more than half the tongue is excised or when less than 1 cm of the floor of the mouth remains. Various flaps are available and great experience is needed to know which is suitable. The anterior part of the floor of the mouth can be replaced by nasolabial flaps and the lateral part over the alveolus by lingual flaps. Extensive defects require repair by distant flaps. Axial flaps such as the deltopectoral or temporal flap were very popular until recently but have now almost completely passed into history and have been replaced by musculocutaneous flaps. The work horse is undoubtedly the pectoralis major musculocutaneous flap (*Fig.* 27.16). The flap consists of a pedicle of muscle bearing the pectoral branch of the acromiothoracic artery on its deep surface and with an island of skin at its distal end. The flap is elevated up to the clavicle, passed under the skin of the upper part of the chest and lower part of the neck and finally through the surgical defect beneath

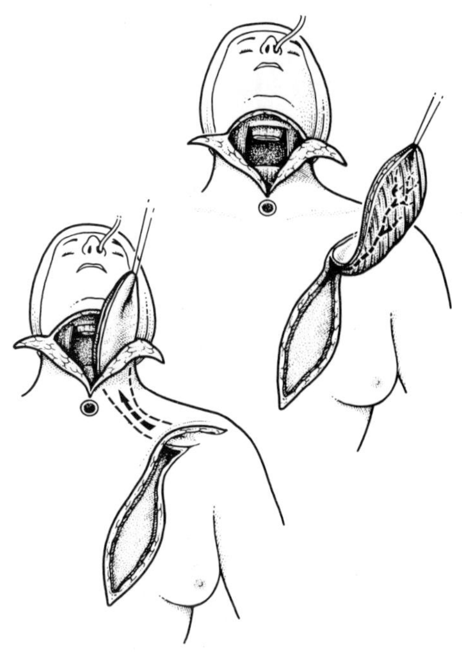

Fig. 27.16 Pectoralis major myocutaneous flap used to reconstruct defects of the cheek, floor of the mouth and pharynx, although the reconstruction after pharyngolaryngectomy is nowadays better achieved by a vascularized graft of jejunum.

the mandible so that the skin island lies in the mouth and the muscle pedicle lies over the carotid sheath.

Removal of any part of the upper jaw is easily rehabilitated with a prosthesis and a denture, but if any of the lower jaw is lost a satisfactory denture cannot be worn. A denture also needs a good sulcus on both sides of the alveolus.

It might be thought that loss of bone in the lower jaw could be made good with a graft. This is certainly the case in benign conditions but in malignant disease where the dental state is nearly always appalling and the tissues unhealthy and infected, the same conditions do not apply. On occasion primary bone grafts must be used but the problems are generally so great that the trend now is to leave a strut of the patient's own mandible rather than to excise completely and graft.

Marginal mandibulectomy (*Fig.* 27.17) is only applicable to tumours invading the mandible posterior to the mental foramen. If the tumour invades the anterior part of the mandibular arch between the two mental foramina and it is not possible to preserve the lower strut of cortical bone this part of the mandible must be replaced because if it is not the patient is unable to swallow even his own saliva in addition to having a very unsightly cosmetic deformity. This is probably one of the two most difficult areas of reconstruction in head and neck surgery. Several techniques are available, the most popular at the present time being some form of inert metal prosthesis, a musculocutaneous flap containing a piece of bone (such as the trapezius flap with the spine of the scapula) or a free graft of skin and bone whose artery and vein are reanastomosed by microvascular surgery in the neck, the most popular at present being the forearm flap containing a segment of radius based on the radial artery.

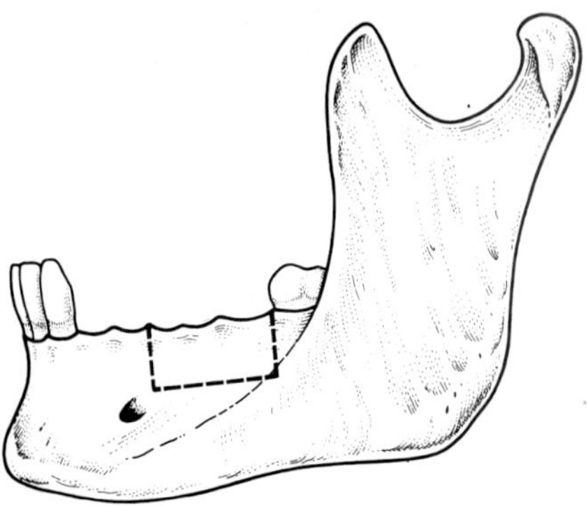

Fig. 27.17 Diagrammatic representation of marginal mandibulectomy performed for tumours invading the mandible posterior to the mental foramen.

Problems of Radiotherapy

In many parts of the world radiotherapy is not always available. A full course of radiotherapy to the oral cavity causes mucositis and a painful mouth for some weeks after treatment, but this is of little consequence if a cure is achieved.

The relationship between radiotherapy and the teeth is important to understand. Radiotherapy has no direct cariogenic effect on the teeth but it tends to cause periodontal disease. It is this which causes marginal caries. Thus if a patient with intact teeth is irradiated he should have at least a 6-monthly dental check for the rest of his life. If he fails to do this and if caries starts then pulpitis and apical abscess formation quickly follow. This is much more serious in the irradiated than in the unirradiated mandible because of the risk of osteoradionecrosis. This condition is always liable to occur if even an edentulous mandible is irradiated but if infection from a tooth occurs then an irradiated mandible may well be completely lost through necrotic dissolution.

It is therefore wiser to extract all teeth and retained roots before irradiating an oral cavity. This seldom meets with any resistance from the British patient because patients with an oral cancer either have no teeth or badly diseased teeth. Perhaps the greatest problem of radiotherapy in the oral cavity, however, is the diagnosis of recurrence. If radiotherapy fails it does so in the deepest part of the tumour where oxygen tension is lowest. If the surface mucosa heals it is difficult to know whether deep induration is viable or non-viable tumour.

28 *The Larynx and Pharynx*

P. M. Stell and A. G. D. Maran

THE LARYNX

The larynx is an important organ whose functions include phonation, protection of the lower respiratory tract during swallowing and initiation of the cough reflex. The diseases of the larynx of interest to the general surgeon include trauma, vocal cord paralysis and tumours.

Trauma and Stenosis

Acute Laryngeal Trauma

The causes of laryngeal injury include road traffic accidents, stab wounds, falling on to a sharp edge, and blows to the neck from sports such as karate and basketball. The larynx is normally protected by the projecting mandible, so that a prerequisite of such injuries is that the neck is extended. A direct blow then forces the cartilaginous framework of the larynx posteriorly against the cervical spine. In the young the cartilages are elastic and may therefore recoil so that the resulting injury is a dislocation or a laceration of the vocal cord. With increasing age, however, the cartilages calcify and ossify so that they fracture.

Laryngeal fractures may be classified into four types:

1. Supraglottic fractures (*Fig.* 28.1).
2. Glottic fractures.
3. Cricotracheal separation (*Fig.* 28.2).
4. Combined comminuted fractures.

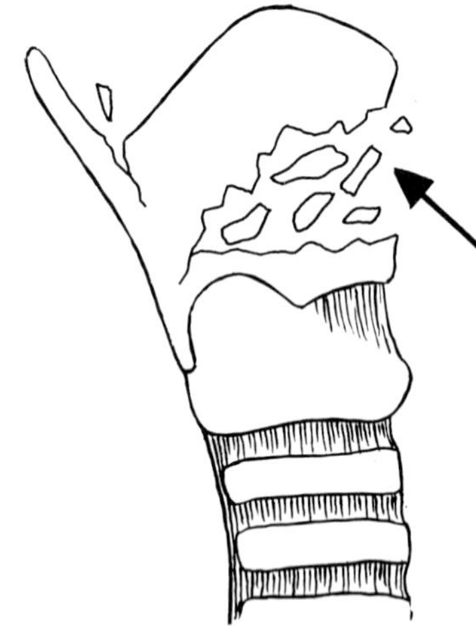

Fig. 28.1 Supraglottic fracture and displacement. The direction of the force is outlined by the arrow. Displacement of the supraglottic structures is backwards and upwards.

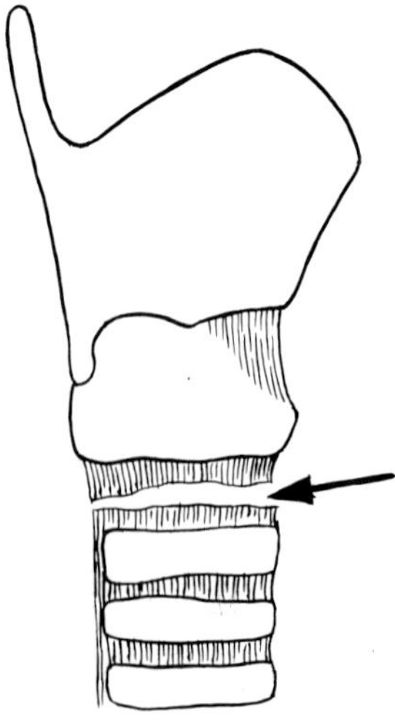

Fig. 28.2 Cricotracheal separation which is the only common injury to the trachea and results in an inferior displacement of the trachea.

Diagnosis of Laryngeal Injury

A laryngeal injury must be diagnosed in the acute phase. A patient with a laryngeal injury is usually seen in the emergency room and often has multiple injuries. The management of life-threatening injuries must obviously take precedence, but those dealing with patients who sustain multiple injuries must have a healthy suspicion of laryngeal injury. Injury to the larynx should be suspected if the patient has difficulty in breathing, surgical emphysema of the neck, or loss of the laryngeal prominence. All of these are easy clinical features to elicit and must be looked for in every seriously injured patient. The reason for this is that acute injuries to the larynx can almost always be managed successfully with restoration of the normally functioning larynx, whereas if the larynx is allowed to heal, fibrosis and scarring occur which is always difficult and sometimes impossible to treat with restoration of a normally functioning larynx.

Further investigations include laryngoscopy and radiographs, notably plain films and laryngography.

Treatment

The principles of treatment of laryngeal trauma in the acute phase are as follows:

1. Exploration. The wound should be explored, non-viable cartilage should be excised and mucosal lacerations are sutured. A tracheostomy should be established well below the fracture site to secure an airway as any exploration of the larynx results in oedema and respiratory obstruction.
2. Fractures are reduced where possible.
3. After reduction of fractures the fragments are stabilized by internal fixation by a solid laryngeal stent, which must be left in place for at least 6 weeks.
4. Mucosal lacerations of the vocal cord are kept apart during the healing phase by a sheet of tantalum plate (a McNaught keel), left within the larynx and removed 3 weeks later.

Discontinuity of the larynx and trachea due to crico-tracheal separation is dealt with by re-anastomosis.

Chronic Laryngotracheal Stenosis

Stenosis of the larynx and trachea is an uncommon lesion but an important one, which interferes with speech and breathing, and the ability to clear secretions from the lower respiratory tract. Its causes include acute injury to the larynx which has gone unrecognized, tracheostomy, infections, such as tuberculosis, and tumours.

The most frequent stenoses are those affecting the glottic area, and those affecting the cricoid area and the upper part of the cervical trachea together.

Investigations

These include direct and indirect laryngoscopy, but the most helpful investigation is radiology, particularly laryngography. This is a double contrast dye technique. The larynx is anaesthetized with local anaesthetic, and radio-opaque dye is instilled into the larynx. This demonstrates the various parts of the larynx and allows mobility to be detected by screening. Xerography is also helpful in these patients.

Stenoses at the glottic level are dealt with by opening the larynx by an external approach (laryngofissure) and division of the adhesions. A tantalum plate is left within the larynx to hold the raw areas apart while they heal (*Fig.* 28.3), and is removed 3 weeks later.

Stenoses of the cricoid and upper trachea are dealt with by resection of the stenosed area and re-anastomosis of the trachea to the lower border of the cricoid or thyroid cartilages.

Vocal Cord Paralysis

The muscles which move the vocal cords are, with one exception, supplied by the recurrent laryngeal nerve, a branch of the vagus. Since the left recurrent laryngeal nerve arises in the chest, intrathoracic disease may cause a vocal cord paralysis, as may disease in the neck.

Because of its longer path the left recurrent laryngeal nerve accounts for 80% of all paralyses. About 5% of paralyses are bilateral. Men are affected 8–10 times more commonly than women, possibly because malignant disease is the commonest cause.

The causes are shown in *Table* 28.1.

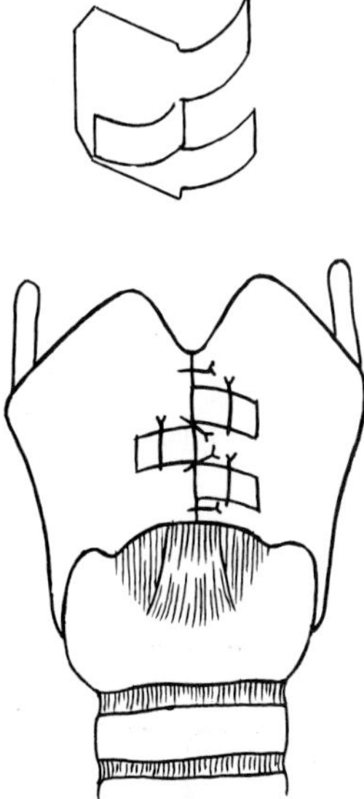

Fig. 28.3 Tantalum plate (McNaught keel) used to prevent laryngeal stenosis after frontal laryngectomy. The plate is left in situ for 3 weeks and then removed after reopening of the neck wound. The patient's tracheostomy is allowed to close soon after removal of the plate.

Table 28.1 Causes of paralysis of the recurrent laryngeal nerve

Malignant disease	25%
Surgical trauma	20%
Non-surgical trauma	10%
Inflammatory	15%
Idiopathic	15%
Neurological	5%
Miscellaneous	10%

Malignant Disease

One in four paralyses of the recurrent laryngeal nerve is due to cancer, and of these 50% are lung cancer, 20% oesophageal cancer and 10% thyroid cancer. The remainder include various uncommon tumours of the head and neck and metastases.

Surgical Trauma

Permanent vocal cord paralysis after thyroidectomy should now be a rare event. The incidence of permanent paralysis rises, however, with repeat operations. Other surgical causes include resections of the oesophagus and lung for carcinoma, surgery of the carotid artery, surgery for congenital heart disease, radical neck dissection and operations for pharyngeal pouch.

Idiopathic Causes

The cause of recurrent laryngeal paralysis is not found in about 15% of cases and many of these are assumed to be due to a viral neuropathy. Epidemics of this paralysis occur coincident with outbreaks of influenza and of other viral diseases. It may also occur as a complication of infectious mononucleosis.

Types of Vocal Cord Paralysis

For reasons which are not entirely understood either the muscles which abduct the vocal cord from the midline may be involved alone in a lesion of the recurrent laryngeal nerve, or all the muscles may be involved. If the abductors only are involved, the vocal cord is fixed in the midline (*Fig.* 28.4), whereas if all muscles are involved the vocal cord is fixed in a position half-way between the midline and that which it adopts in the full maximal inspiration, this being known as the 'cadaveric position' (*Fig.* 28.5). There are thus four possible types: unilateral abductor paralysis, unilateral total paralysis, bilateral abductor paralysis and bilateral total paralysis.

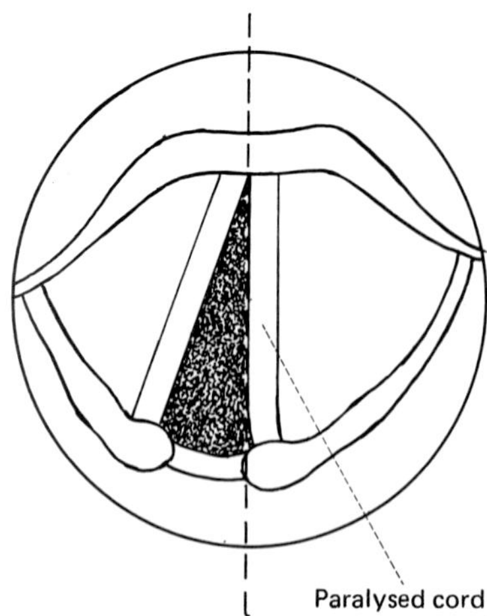

Fig. 28.4 Unilateral abductor paralysis. The paralysed cord lies in or close to the midline.

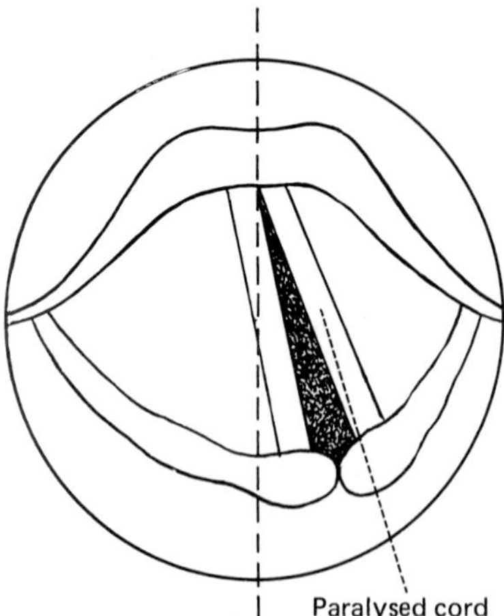

Fig. 28.5 Unilateral complete paralysis. The unaffected cord often crosses over the midline to the paralysed side.

Investigations

HISTORY. The type of voice depends on the position of the vocal cords. A whisper suggests a total paralysis, whereas a fairly normal voice suggests an abductor paralysis.

Stridor, especially on exertion, occurs in bilateral abductor paralysis, and aspiration in bilateral total paralysis.

EXAMINATION. Consideration of the causes indicates what to look for in general examination of the patient. A full head and neck examination must always be done: indirect laryngoscopy is very important to determine the position of the cords.

RADIOLOGY. A chest radiograph including tomograms should always be done. A barium swallow is also advisable and a thyroid scan should be done if a thyroid mass is palpable.

Radiographs of the base of the skull, the petrous bones and nasopharynx may also be needed.

LABORATORY STUDIES. These have a very limited value. Every patient should have full blood indices measured: the differential white count, film and ESR may be of help in the lymphomas or tuberculosis. If mononucleosis is suspected, Paul–Bunnell and monospot tests are done: other viral studies can be started but since a change in titre is the finding of diagnostic significance, these take time. Neuropathy only occurs in well-established previously diagnosed diabetes so that a glucose tolerance test is not needed. With the rise in incidence of venereal disease, a VDRL and TPHA should be done (*see* Chapter 5).

ENDOSCOPY. Most patients require nasopharyngoscopy and biopsy of the fossa of Rosenmüller, oesophagoscopy, direct laryngoscopy to assess if immobility of the cord is due to a muscle paralysis or a joint fixation, and bronchoscopy. If a mediastinal cause is suspected mediastinoscopy may be done.

Treatment

UNILATERAL ABDUCTOR PARALYSIS. In this case, one vocal cord is paralysed in the midline. The voice is almost normal, and stridor and aspiration do not occur. Apart from speech therapy no treatment is usually needed.

UNILATERAL TOTAL PARALYSIS. In this case, one vocal cord is paralysed in the cadaveric position. The patient is hoarse, but, what is more important, he cannot cough efficiently.

Unless the cause is a carcinoma, nothing should be done for 6 months, except speech therapy. If the paralysis is due to a carcinoma, especially of the lung, then the distress of a weak voice and inefficient cough should be alleviated immediately with injection of Teflon lateral to the vocal cord to make the larynx competent so that the patient can cough.

BILATERAL ABDUCTOR PARALYSIS. Since this usually occurs after a thyroidectomy, immediate re-exploration of the neck should be considered to see if the recurrent nerves have been caught in a ligature applied to the inferior thyroid artery.

The voice is good but there is stridor on exertion so that a tracheostomy is required. If a speaking valve is applied to the tracheostomy tube the patient can speak normally. Some patients cannot tolerate a permanent tracheostomy and for them a cordopexy is available.

The principle of this operation is to resect one arytenoid cartilage (to widen the airway) and to anchor the vocal cord laterally. The operation may be carried out endoscopically or by a variety of external approaches.

BILATERAL TOTAL PARALYSIS. The cause is usually a serious CNS disease such as bulbar paralysis. These patients are not only aphonic but, because they cannot produce a positive subglottic pressure, the swallowing is incoordinated. As the patient cannot cough either, he aspirates food and is in constant danger of pneumonitis. A tracheostomy is usually needed for bronchial toilet and a nasogastric tube for feeding. Injection of Teflon into one vocal cord may help a little as may cricopharyngeal myotomy. A total laryngectomy may be needed to protect the lungs.

Tumours of the Larynx

Pathology

Tumours of the larynx may be malignant or benign, but benign tumours constitute 5% or less of all laryngeal tumours. Benign tumours are predominantly papillomas, but chondromas, granular-cell myoblastomas and other rare tumours can occur.

Squamous-cell carcinoma forms the vast majority of malignant laryngeal tumours: rare tumours include verrucous carcinoma, undifferentiated carcinoma, adenocarcinoma (including adenoid cystic carcinoma) and the sarcomas, notably fibrosarcoma.

Approximately 90% of laryngeal carcinomas occur in men with a peak age incidence between 55 and 65. The incidence in men has fallen progressively for the last 30 years, so that the disease is now becoming relatively more common in women. It is widely stated that laryngeal carcinoma is caused by heavy smoking, but this statement is difficult to reconcile with the falling incidence of this tumour.

The larynx may be divided into three regions: the supraglottis (mainly the epiglottis and the vestibular folds), the glottis (mainly the vocal cords) and the subglottis (the region below the vocal cords ending at the lower border of the cricoid cartilage) (*Fig.* 28.6). Approximately 40% of laryngeal carcinomas affect the supraglottic space, 60% the glottic area and 5–10% the subglottic area.

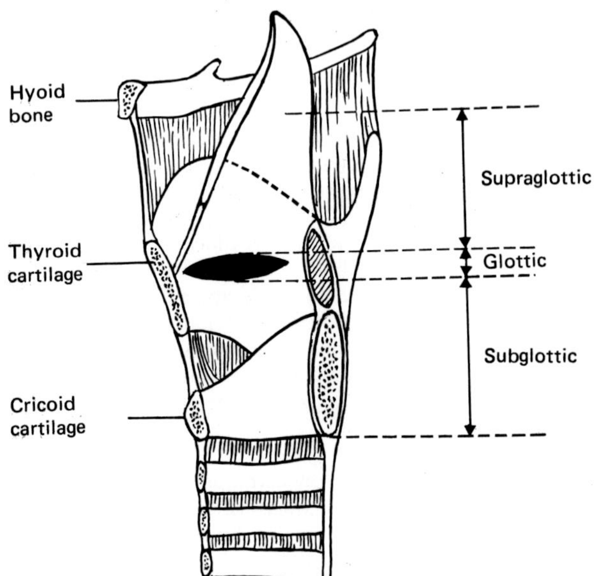

Fig. 28.6 Subdivision of the larynx used for the classification of laryngeal tumours.

Supraglottic carcinomas tend to remain localized to the epiglottis and seldom spread inferiorly on to the vocal cords. They spread anteriorly through the epiglottic cartilage into the space in front of this cartilage, the pre-epiglottic space. About 35% of patients with a supraglottic carcinoma have a palpable lymph gland in the neck when first seen, but distant metastases, as in all laryngeal carcinomas, are extremely uncommon (less than 1%).

Glottic carcinomas remain localized to the vocal cord for many months. A vocal cord carcinoma may spread along the vocal cord and down the opposite side, but spread above and below the vocal cord only occurs later in the disease. Because the vocal cords are poor in lymphatics these tumours rarely metastasize to the gland in the neck, and almost never distantly. For this reason they have a very good prognosis.

Subglottic carcinoma is uncommon; it usually presents with stridor due to obstruction of the upper airway by the bulk of the tumour. These tumours produce fixation of the vocal cord in about 30% of cases, but 20% metastasize to a lymph node in the neck; furthermore, they have a fairly high incidence of distant metastases, either to lungs or bones, so that these tumours tend to behave more like bronchial tumours than laryngeal tumours.

A further laryngeal tumour is that sometimes described as being 'transglottic' and sometimes as 'multiregional'. This is an extensive tumour affecting all the divisions of the larynx, and probably arising as a field change all over the larynx. This tumour invades the cartilaginous framework of the larynx widely, extends posteriorly into the pharyngeal mucosa, and metastasizes to the lymph nodes in the neck on about 1 occasion in 3.

Laryngeal tumours may be staged by the TNM system, the basis of which is as follows:

T1—tumour limited to the site of origin with normal mobility.

T2—tumour spreading from the site of origin to a neighbouring site (e.g. a tumour of the vocal cord spreading to the subglottic space).

T3—tumour limited to the larynx but with fixation of the vocal cord.

T4—extension of the tumour beyond the larynx to neighbouring structures, mainly the pharynx.

Nodes in the neck are also staged into N0, N1, N2 and N3 (*see* Chapter 23).

Investigations

HISTORY. The main symptom is hoarseness; dysphagia with pain in the ear usually indicates involvement of the pharynx, and difficulty in breathing indicates a large tumour involving the subglottic space.

EXAMINATION. This includes general examination, and examination of the larynx itself, looking for the extent of the tumour and paralysis of the vocal cords. It is also very important to palpate the neck for enlarged lymph nodes.

Radiology

The methods in use include the following: plain films, to demonstrate erosion of the cartilaginous framework; tomograms, mainly to assess the size of the lesion; CT scans to show the soft-tissue extent of the tumour and also any invasion of cartilage. Laryngography, that is a double-contrast technique, and xerograms have now been almost totally abandoned in carcinoma.

Endoscopy

A laryngoscopy is carried out to assess the limits of the tumour, and to obtain a biopsy. Microlaryngoscopy may be used to allow the larynx to be examined under magnification which, it is claimed, improves the diagnostic accuracy.

Most (95%) patients with laryngeal carcinoma are suitable for treatment. The contraindications include distant metastases (1%), possibly very advanced age and poor general condition, refusal by the patient and finally very advanced disease.

Both radiotherapy and surgery are available for the treatment of the vast majority of tumours. Practice differs between the USA and the UK: in the USA surgery is used for primary treatment very much more often than in the UK, where virtually all patients are treated in the first place by radiotherapy.

Supraglottic tumours in the UK are generally treated primarily by radiotherapy and those tumours which recur after this are treated by total laryngectomy. Very advanced tumours, particularly if associated with lymph nodes in the neck, should be treated primarily by total laryngectomy and radical neck dissection. Small tumours confined to the epiglottis may be treated by a supraglottic laryngectomy preserving the vocal cords so that the patient can speak normally after the operation.

Glottic tumours should virtually all be treated by radiotherapy which has outstanding results: approximately 95% of patients should be cured of their tumour. In the unlikely event of recurrence after radiotherapy a partial hemilaryngectomy can usually still be carried out, again with preservation of the voice.

Subglottic tumours are uncommon so that it is not easy to know what is the correct thing to do. Certainly some of these tumours can be controlled by radiotherapy and this is probably the treatment of choice for small or moderate-sized lesions, with total laryngectomy being reserved for recurrence.

Finally, the large transglottic, or multiregional tumour, often must be treated primarily by total laryngectomy, particularly if associated with enlarged lymph nodes in the neck. Indeed, the laryngectomy may be carried out as an emergency since such patients often present with stridor. If a tracheostomy is done in these circumstances there is a high risk of implantation of tumour into the stoma, an event which is almost always untreatable.

Aftercare and Follow-up

Patients who have been treated for a laryngeal carcinoma either by radiotherapy or by surgery should be followed up:

1. To detect a recurrence of the tumour within the larynx or in the lymph nodes in the neck.
2. To detect any complication of treatment such as perichondritis after radiotherapy, inhalation after partial laryngectomy or stricture of the pharynx.

Recurrence after radiotherapy, either at the primary site or in the nodes is treated by surgery as appropriate, i.e. total laryngectomy or radical neck dissection. Recurrences after surgery can seldom be treated by radiotherapy, however, and in this event there is usually little which can be done to help the patient.

An important part of the rehabilitation of the patient after total laryngectomy is the restoration of his voice. This may be done by teaching the patient oesophageal speech, by various artificial electronic devices, or by creating deliberately a tracheopharyngeal fistula which allows air to pass through the trachea into the pharynx to produce vibration.

THE PHARYNX

The pharynx consists of three parts: the nasopharynx, the oropharynx and the hypopharynx. These areas are shown diagrammatically in *Fig.* 28.7.

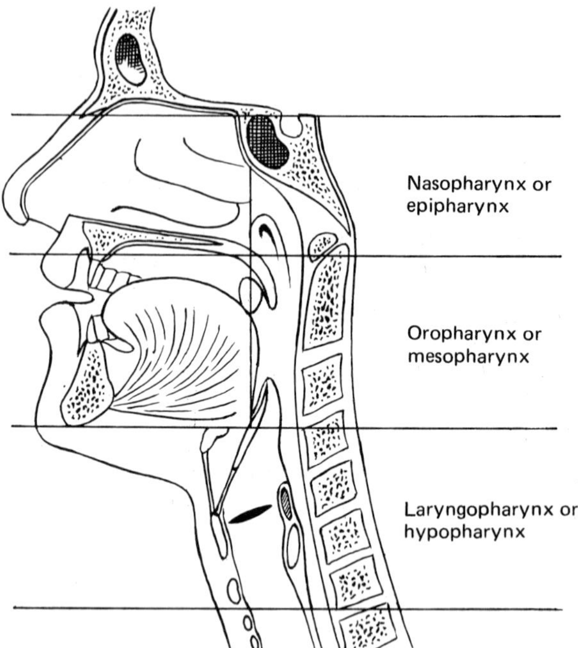

Fig. 28.7 Divisions of the pharynx.

The Nasopharynx

The diseases of surgical interest are 'adenoids' and tumours.

Adenoidectomy

Adenoidectomy is the commonest operation in the UK. Many children suffer from obstructive symptoms in the upper respiratory tract, associated with recurrent infections, nasal obstruction and deafness. It is felt that the adenoids may contribute to this syndrome by blocking drainage from the nose and the Eustachian tubes. However, there is no certain evidence that the adenoids are either enlarged or infected. Furthermore, the sole criterion of the benefit of this operation is the mother's opinion, and this is of very doubtful validity. There is almost certainly a place for this operation, but that place remains to be defined.

Surgical Pathology

Nasopharyngeal cancer is very common in China, accounting for 30% of malignant neoplasms. Elsewhere it is rare. American-born second generation Chinese have a lower risk of nasopharyngeal cancer than those born in China.

Familial clustering occurs suggesting the influence of a shared environment. It is suggested that the configuration of the Chinese nasopharyngeal vault may allow carcinogens to be deposited in the fossa of Rosenmüller. The Epstein–Barr virus may also have a role in the generation of a nasopharyngeal cancer. Although significant titres to Epstein–Barr virus are only present in 45% of patients with early nasopharyngeal carcinoma, the titres are elevated in 100% of patients with advanced disease.

The male:female ratio is about 2:1 and the maximum age incidence is 30–60 years.

Squamous-cell carcinoma, well or poorly differentiated, accounts for two-thirds of all tumours: non-Hodgkin's lymphomas form most of the rest.

The incidence of lymph-node metastases in squamous-cell carcinoma is shown in *Table* 28.2.

Table 28.2 Incidence of lymph-node metastases in nasopharyngeal carcinoma

N0	*N1*	*N2*
55%	30%	15%

Benign Tumours

The only benign tumour of any importance in the nasopharynx is the nasopharyngeal angiofibroma. This is a tough, rubbery tumour usually arising from the lateral wall of the nasopharynx. It virtually always occurs in boys and its maximum age incidence is at puberty. Histologically, the tumour consists of vascular spaces with no contractile elements in their walls, surrounded by fibrous tissue. Although these tumours are histologically benign they grow and expand anteriorly into the nose and the orbit.

Investigations

History

One in three patients present with nasal symptoms such as epistaxis or rhinorrhoea, 1 in 5 with deafness, 1 in 5 with lymph-node metastases, 1 in 10 with pain and the remainder with cranial nerve palsies, speech and swallowing problems, hoarseness and eye symptoms.

Examination

The nasopharynx is examined with a postnasal mirror. The tympanic membrane is examined for indrawing and the presence of fluid in the middle ear. The cranial nerves and the cervical sympathetic nerves are also assessed. Finally the neck is palpated.

Radiology

Plain films of the base of the skull should be examined for bone destruction which can be seen in about 30%. The foramen lacerum, carotid canal, greater wing of the sphenoid and the petrous apex are the likely sites of bone destruction. Patients with cranial nerve paralysis show bony destruction five times more commonly than patients with no cranial nerve paralysis. Carcinoma also invades bone more commonly than lymphoma or sarcoma. Tomograms will be required to delineate the extent of destruction including CT scans.

The circulation of a nasopharyngeal angiofibroma should be demonstrated by an angiogram. Greater detail can be shown by a subtraction angiogram.

Biopsy

A biopsy of a carcinoma is taken under general anaesthesia. An angiofibroma must not be biopsied.

Treatment Policy

Radiation is the treatment of choice for squamous-cell carcinoma and the lymphomas. The neck should be included in the field whether or not the neck glands are palpable.

A radical neck dissection is reserved for cases where lymph glands are not controlled by radiotherapy and where enlarged nodes appear after the primary has been controlled.

If the primary tumour recurs then a further course of radiotherapy can often be given. Chemotherapy and cryosurgery have a place in pain relief in such cases.

Nasopharyngeal angiofibromas should be treated by surgery because if they are left alone they expand into neighbouring cavities, notably the orbit, causing blindness. Such tumours should therefore be removed. Much the best approach is a Le Fort I osteotomy carried through the maxilla and the lower part of the nasal cavity on both sides just above the alveolus. The alveolus and hard palate are left pedicled on the palatine artery and are then displaced downwards giving extremely good access to the nasopharynx and to the cavities into which the tumour can extend, such as the sphenoid sinus, the pterygopalatine fossa, etc. The tumour can thus be grasped with an obstetric volsellum and be removed by finger dissection. Once bleeding has been controlled the alveolus is fixed to the upper part of the maxilla with wires.

The Oropharynx

Tonsillectomy and tumours are the points of surgical interest at this site.

Tonsils

The tonsils form part of a circle of lymphoid tissue, Waldeyer's ring, surrounding the respiratory tract. They form a functional part of the gut-associated lymphoid tissue system.

Tonsillitis is a common disease of childhood. The organisms isolated from the pharynx include the Gram-positive cocci (usually the haemolytic streptococci) and viruses, including adenoviruses, the Epstein–Barr virus and herpes simplex. The tonsils when they are removed show evidence of viral infection only within the tonsil itself.

Tonsillitis is a short-lived infection characterized by pyrexia, dysphagia, sore throat and otalgia. Its important complications include peritonsillar abscess, rheumatic fever and acute glomerulonephritis. The pathogenesis of the latter two is unproven, but they may be immunological phenomena.

Recurrent tonsillitis causing repeated loss of schooling is often treated by tonsillectomy, but there is virtually no objective evidence on which to assess the place of this operation. Tonsillectomy is also indicated for quinsy, and for the rare infant with cor pulmonale due to massive hypertrophy of the tonsils and adenoids.

Tumours of the Oropharynx

Surgical Pathology

The oropharynx is lined by squamous epithelium which contains minor salivary glands: it also contains the tonsil in its lateral wall. Epithelial, salivary tumours and lymphomas can occur at this site.

The relative incidence of the three different types of oropharyngeal tumour are shown in *Table* 28.3.

SQUAMOUS-CELL CARCINOMA. The annual incidence of carcinoma of the oropharynx in the UK is 8 per million. For

Table 28.3 Histological types of oropharyngeal tumours

Epithelial tumours	
Squamous-cell carcinoma	75%
Lympho-epithelioma	5%
Reticuloses:	
Non-Hodgkin's lymphomas	15%
Miscellaneous, including salivary tumours	5%

reasons which are not known, the rate in the USA is much higher than this, being 60 per million. The maximum age incidence is 70 and there is a male:female ratio of 10:1. The relative site incidence of this tumour is shown in *Table* 28.4 and the incidence of lymph-node metastases in *Table* 28.5.

Table 28.4 Site incidence of oropharyngeal tumours

Tonsil	70%
Base of tongue	20%
Posterior oropharyngeal wall	5%
Remainder	5%

Table 28.5 Incidence of nodes in the neck in oropharyngeal carcinoma

N0	*N1*	*N2*	*N3*
35%	30%	5%	30%

LYMPHOMAS. Non-Hodgkin's lymphomas form 15% of all oropharyngeal tumours: their maximum age incidence is 70, and these tumours are twice as common in men as in women. The incidence of the various different forms of non-Hodgkin's lymphoma in the oropharynx using the Kiel classification is shown in *Table* 28.6.

Table 28.6 Lymphomas of the oropharynx
Incidence of separate types (n = 79 cases)

Centroblastic	56%
Centroblastic/Centrocytic	18% (14% nodular; 4% diffuse)
Immunocytoma	14%
T-cell	78%
Lymphoblastic	3%
Unclassified	2%

Non-Hodgkin's lymphomas of the tonsil form half of all lymphomas of the upper respiratory tract: lymphography reveals disease below the diaphragm in as many as 35% of patients in some series. Half of all patients suffer a relapse after the primary treatment but virtually never at the primary site. Recurrent disease is much more common at non-lymphoid sites, such as the gastrointestinal tract, bone, skin, liver and lungs, than at distant lymphoid sites, such as the mediastinum and retroperitoneal nodes.

SALIVARY GLAND TUMOURS. Salivary gland tumours can occur at any site in the oropharynx, but the soft palate immediately superior to the tonsil is much the commonest site. At least half of these tumours are malignant, adenoid cystic carcinoma forming the vast majority.

Investigations

Investigations include history and clinical examination, radiology (of the local area and of the chest) and biopsy.

Although laparotomy is often carried out for staging of Hodgkin's disease, it appears to be unnecessary in the non-Hodgkin's lymphomas and the requisite information can be obtained by lymphography and percutaneous liver biopsy.

Treatment Policy

SQUAMOUS-CELL CARCINOMA. Approximately 20% of patients with oropharyngeal carcinoma are incurable for the following reasons:

Highly anaplastic tumours	Distant metastases
Bilateral neck glands	Patient's refusal
Trismus	Advanced age (say over 75 years)
Horner's syndrome	Poor general condition

Treatment of a tonsillar carcinoma depends on the presence or absence of palpable lymph nodes. The patient with no palpable glands in the neck should be treated primarily by radiotherapy, but if the patient has enlarged glands he must be treated by surgery.

The standard procedure for oropharyngeal carcinoma is the so-called commando operation (jaw-neck dissection, hemimandibulectomy, etc.). After resection of the involved area, with the adjacent portion of the mandible, and in continuity with the products of a radical neck dissection, the resected area is usually replaced.

Tumours of the base of the tongue are usually poorly differentiated and should be treated by radiotherapy in view of the poor differentiation of the tumour, the reconstructive problems of replacing the base of the tongue, and difficulties in defining the margin of the tumour since such a tumour invades widely beneath the mucosa into the muscles of the tongue.

NON-HODGKIN'S LYMPHOMAS. These tumours must be treated by radiotherapy provided that there is no disease below the clavicle. If there is disseminated disease the local disease is usually still treated by radiotherapy but chemotherapy is given for the metastases.

SALIVARY TUMOURS. Although some tumours, particularly the small ones, may occasionally regress with radiotherapy, the vast majority of these tumours require surgery, which must be at least as extensive as that for a squamous-cell carcinoma at the same site.

Diseases of the Hypopharynx

Globus Hystericus

PATHOLOGY. It is said that the symptoms of this disease, i.e. a 'lump in the throat' are caused by spasm of the cricopharyngeal sphincter and an electromyogram of this muscle does indeed show increased activity. Radiology will show a variery of lesions of the foregut, extending as far as the stomach, the commonest being hiatus hernia in 1 patient in 3. One patient in five shows an osteophyte of the cervical spine indenting the pharynx.

CLINICAL FEATURES. The patient is usually a middle-aged woman who complains of discomfort when swallowing saliva, and which is often relieved by swallowing food: it is always felt in the midline just above the suprasternal notch.

Clinical examination is entirely normal.

RADIOLOGY. If the pharyngeal soft-tissue shadow posterior to the trachea on a lateral radiograph of the soft tissues of the neck is narrower than the body of the vertebra behind it, the patient can reasonably be reassured that there is no organic disease present and be reviewed 2–3 weeks later. If the symptoms persist for more than 3 weeks a barium swallow and meal and an oesophagoscopy much be done.

TREATMENT. The best and often the only treatment necessary for this disease is strong reassurance that the patient does not have any serious disease particularly cancer. Antacids are useful if the symptom is clearly associated with reflux oesophagitis.

Sideropenic Dysphagia and Pharyngeal Pouch

These are dealt with in Chapter 67.

Tumours of the Hypopharynx

Surgical Anatomy

The hypopharynx consists of three parts: the postcricoid area, the pyriform fossa and the posterior wall.

Surgical Pathology of Squamous-cell Carcinoma

LOCAL SPREAD. Tumours of the pyriform fossa extend through the thyrohyoid membrane to invade the carotid sheath, or through the cricothyroid membrane to invade the thyroid gland. A palpable neck mass in this disease may be direct extension of the tumour and not an enlarged lymph node: this should be confirmed by asking the patient to swallow. These tumours also rapidly invade the aryepiglottic fold and false cord, structures rich in lymphatics, and pass through these to invade and fix the vocal cord, causing hoarseness.

These tumours behave like oesophageal tumours and show significant mucosal spread of 10 mm on average.

A postcricoid carcinoma may, in the late stages, invade the prevertebral fascia. Vocal cord paralysis is also fairly common (approx. 10%) and is usually due to extension of the tumour outside the oesophagus to invade the tracheo-oesophageal groove. Because of the close proximity of the thyroid gland to the cervical oesophagus invasion of the latter gland occurs commonly.

LYMPH-NODE METASTASES. Cancer of the hypopharynx has a notorious propensity to metastasize to the lymph nodes of the neck, and indeed an involved node may be the presenting symptom, particularly of tumours of the pyriform fossa. The incidence of lymph-node metastases in hypopharyngeal carcinoma is shown in *Table* 28.7.

Table 28.7 Incidence of lymph-node metastases from hypopharyngeal carcinoma

	N0	*N1*	*N2*	*N3*
Pyriform fossa	20%	70%	5%	5%
Postcricoid	70%	20%	5%	5%

Aetiology

Known contributory factors include: sex (postcricoid carcinoma is commoner in women), geography (postcricoid carcinoma occurs rarely in continental Europe and North America), sideropenic dysphagia and previous radiation.

Investigations

HISTORY. The symptoms include dysphagia for food, sore throat, hoarseness, otalgia and loss of weight. There may also be a history of previous radiotherapy for thyrotoxicosis.

EXAMINATION. The pharynx and larynx are examined with a laryngeal mirror. The extent of a tumour of the pyriform fossa can be seen, and a paralysis of the vocal cord, an important physical sign, is also detected.

The neck is then examined carefully for enlarged lymph nodes. It is also very important to move the larynx from side to side over the vertebral column for two reasons: to assess fixation to the prevertebral fascia; laryngeal crepitus is lost in patients with postcricoid carcinoma.

RADIOLOGY. Plain lateral soft-tissue films of the neck and a barium swallow are performed in every case to define the extent of the tumour. CT scans are also very useful in showing the invaded nodes in the mediastinum.

ENDOSCOPY. The purpose of an endoscopy in a patient with a hypopharyngeal carcinoma is to assess the extent of the disease and to obtain a biopsy.

In the patient with carcinoma of the pyriform fossa the following points are noted:

Spread of the tumour into the upper end of the post-cricoid space, to or beyond the midline of the posterior pharyngeal wall and to the base of the tongue.

In a postcricoid carcinoma the following points require attention:

1. The lower extent of the tumour, measured with reference to the incisor teeth. This is needed to decide whether the tumour is operable, and to decide what method of pharyngeal replacement is to be used.
2. The mobility of the pharynx over the prevertebral fascia, which is assessed by palpation.

Treatment

One patient in four with a hypopharyngeal carcinoma is untreatable due to the following factors:

1. Poor general condition and advanced age.
2. Fixation of the tumour to the prevertebral fascia.
3. Fixation of the vocal cord in postcricoid carcinoma.
4. Bilateral neck glands: treatment does not affect the natural history of the disease in the presence of involved glands on both sides of the neck, and surgery only makes the patient more miserable.
5. Distant metastases.
6. Refusal of the patient.

In practice the patient, who is not treated, usually shows more than one of these unfavourable factors.

COMBINED SURGERY AND RADIOTHERAPY. One of the most recent fashions in the treatment of head and neck cancer has been to administer preoperative irradiation in order to reduce local recurrence by implantation and dissemination by veins and lymphatics. Although the concept is attractive, a recent controlled trial has shown that this procedure does not increase survival rates. This form of treatment is now very much less popular than it used to be.

RADIOTHERAPY. Patients without enlarged lymph nodes have a 20% chance of surviving for 5 years when treated with radiotherapy, but in the presence of enlarged nodes the cure rate is negligible—less than 5%. Radiotherapy, therefore, should be reserved for the patient without enlarged nodes, and with a small tumour. Conversely, surgery will be needed as the primary form of treatment for large tumours with enlarged cervical nodes and for tumours which recur after radiotherapy.

CHEMOTHERAPY. The remarks made about chemotherapy in the treatment of cancer of the oral cavity (Chapter 27) apply with even more force to the treatment of pharyngeal and laryngeal tumours.

SURGERY. Management of Lymph Nodes. For the patient with secondarily involved lymph nodes, the operation of radical neck dissection has stood the test of time.

Resection of the Primary Tumour: The operation advised depends on the site of the primary tumour.

Tumours of the pyriform fossa may require laryngectomy and partial pharyngectomy or total pharyngolaryngectomy. It is not necessary always to do a total pharyngectomy, and it is possible to preserve enough pharyngeal mucosa in 2 patients out of 3 for closure of the defect in the same manner as after total laryngectomy for laryngeal carcinoma. The patient is thus spared the problem of pharyngeal reconstruction. When this is not possible (usually because the tumour has invaded the postcricoid space) a total pharyngolaryngectomy with pharyngeal reconstruction is necessary.

Tumours of the postcricoid region should be treated surgically. A total pharyngolaryngectomy is required with resection of part or all of the oesophagus if the tumour extends into the cervical oesophagus, which it usually does.

Pharyngeal Repair: A resected pharynx must be reconstructed. Two techniques are available depending on whether it is necessary to resect the entire oesophagus in addition. If a total pharyngolaryngo-oesophagectomy has been carried out the most satisfactory solution is to mobilize the stomach and the first two parts of the duodenum. The graft is transferred to the neck either through the posterior mediastinum or through the right side of the chest, and the fundus of the stomach is anastomosed to the base of the tongue. The operation has a high operative mortality of about 15%, but fistulas are very uncommon thereafter, and the swallowing is very good—normal swallowing is restored within days of the operation and, furthermore, the patient continues to be able to swallow if he gets a local recurrence in the neck. For smaller tumours it is usually not necessary to resect the entire oesophagus, and only the cervical part of the oesophagus needs to be replaced. Since the last edition of this book the rather unsatisfactory multi-stage method of repair using deltopectoral flaps which had a high incidence of stenosis has been abandoned. This flap was replaced by the use of the pectoralis major musculocutaneous flap which had the advantage of a slighly lower incidence of stenosis and only required one stage. This, in turn, has been largely abandoned in favour of an ileal loop. Towards the end of mobilization of the pharynx and larynx (along with a neck dissection if necessary) a second general surgical team opens the abdomen and prepares a loop of ileum on a vascular pedicle. Once the specimen is removed the ileal loop is transferred to the neck, its artery and vein are reanastomosed by microvascular techniques to whichever vessels are suitable (the facial artery and vein being the most usual) and finally the bowel ends are anastomosed with the oropharynx above (often by end-to-side anastomosis) and to the oesophagus below by end-to-end anastomosis. In competent hands the success rate should be at least 95% and the mortality of this particular procedure is virtually nil. For tumours confined to the neck, this is now the treatment of choice.

THE WAY AHEAD

Laryngeal trauma is uncommon but it is a potent source of disability. The vast majority of patients are young, and only 2 out of 3 recover normal speech, swallowing and respiration. The incidence of chronic stenosis could be reduced by greater protection of the neck in motor vehicles, and by greater awareness by casualty officers of the possibility and seriousness of laryngeal trauma. Very few of these injuries are diagnosed in the acute phase. Every casualty officer should examine the multiple injured patient for loss of the laryngeal prominence and surgical emphysema of the neck.

Rehabilitation of the voice after total laryngectomy remains an area for development. About 60% of patients develop a satisfactory oesophageal voice: the remaining 40% must rely on an electronic device or a tracheo-oesophageal shunt. What is needed is an implantable device capable of producing a noise, similar to the output of the normal larynx, which could then be articulated by the normal mechanism.

Since the last edition of this book the surgical challenge of replacement of the gullet after resection of tumours of the pharynx has largely been solved by methods discussed above.

Further Reading

Alberti P. W. and Bryce D. P. (1976) *Centennial Conference of Laryngeal Cancer*. New York, Appleton-Century-Crofts.
Stell P. M. (1973) Cancer of the hypopharynx. *J. R. Coll. Surg. Edin.* **89**, 20–30.
Stell P. M. (1976) Tumours of the oropharynx. *Clin. Otol.* **1**, 71–91.

29 The Nose and Paranasal Sinuses

P. M. Stell and A. G. D. Maran

CONGENITAL ANOMALIES

Posterior Choanal Atresia

The obstruction is at the posterior end of the nose, a few millimetres anterior to the bony edge of the hard palate. There is a higher incidence of unilateral atresia with preponderance of the right side and the disease is commoner in girls than boys. There is persistence of the bucconasal membrane formed at the posterior end of each nasal sac. Multiple abnormalities may be present affecting the head, heart and alimentary system.

Unilateral atresia may cause few symptoms at birth and may not be diagnosed for years. It usually causes a continuous mucoid, at times purulent, rhinorrhoea. It is treated by a transpalatal resection after the age of 6 months. Bilateral atresia causes respiratory difficulty at birth with cyanosis, temporarily relieved by crying and aggravated by feeding. Usually an oral airway must be inserted. Intranasal choanotomy is then performed as soon as possible. The diagnosis is confirmed by the lack of aeration or bubbling through the nose, the inability to pass a fine catheter or probe, or by radiographs with a contrast medium.

Congenital Neoplasms of Neurogenic Origin

Gliomas and Encephaloceles

These have a similar origin (*Fig.* 29.1). Both contain glial tissue but the encephalocele is lined with meninges and communicates directly with the brain. The glioma is firmer and usually arises from the lateral wall of the nose, while the encephalocele extends from the roof and may show pulsation and changes in size on straining. A glioma may cause nasal obstruction, obstruction to the nasolacrimal duct, broadening of the bridge of the nose, or a frank external tumour depending on the site of the defect. Imaging will demonstrate bony or intracranial involvement with every lump on or in the nose in infancy. The glioma can be removed completely with no complications, but the encephalocele requires closure of the dural defect which, if small, can be closed extradurally.

EPISTAXIS

The blood supply to the nasal cavity is derived from branches of both the internal and external carotid arteries.

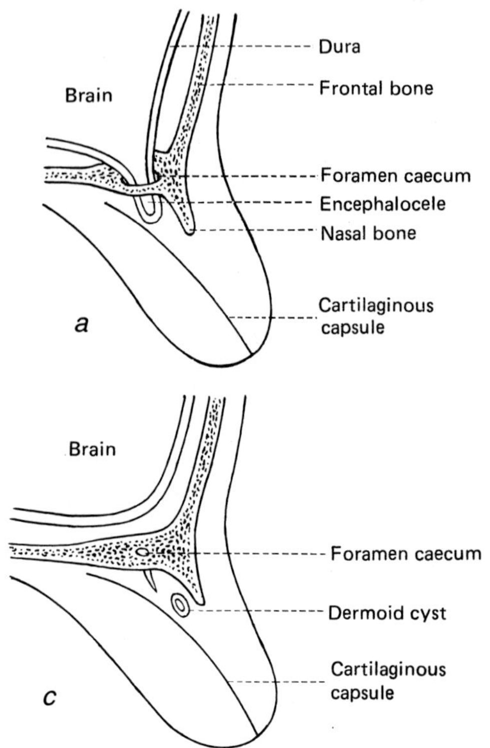

Fig. 29.1 Relationship between *a*, Encephalocele, *b*, Glioma and *c*, Dermoid cyst.

The upper parts of the nose are supplied by branches from the internal carotid artery, and the rest from the external carotid artery.

Surgical Pathology

The cause of an epistaxis is not determined in about 85% of patients. The known causes will now be discussed in greater detail.

Hereditary Haemorrhagic Telangiectasia

The gene of this hereditary disease is completely dominant and the defect may be passed from either parent to a child of either sex. The presenting symptom in virtually all the patients is epistaxis. Telangiectases may occur on any mucous membrane or anywhere on the external surface of the body. The nasal mucosa is most commonly affected but lesions are frequently found in the tongue, palate, lips, buccal mucosa, pharynx and conjunctiva. There are two basic vascular abnormalities: first, localized areas in the capillaries, where the walls have been reduced to the endothelial layers only, perhaps due to an inherited lack of elastic tissue, and secondly visible dilatations of arterioles and capillaries leading to arteriovenous fistulas, such as may be found in the lungs. Bleeding always occurs from the summit of the telangiectases and never extravasates into the surrounding tissue. Thus, the factors which determine whether the lesions bleed or not are to be found in the state of the overlying epithelium and not in the vessels themselves. It is this fact which has led to the forms of treatment which attempt to modify the overlying epithelium.

Infections

Epistaxis may occur in any infection due to the accompanying hyperaemia but certain infectious diseases are classically responsible for epistaxis. These include rheumatic fever, nasal diphtheria, smallpox, whooping cough, scarlet fever and typhoid fever. Epistaxis in children may also be due to the presence of an intranasal foreign body.

Tumours

The only important benign tumour causing epistaxis is the juvenile angiofibroma.

Malignant tumours are well known to cause a bloodstained nasal discharge, though not all do.

Coagulation Defects

These may be due to liver disease or anticoagulants and appear to be responsible for about 5% of epistaxis. The most important diseases are leukaemia, haemophilia, von Willebrand's disease, polycythaemia, macroglobulinaemia, myeloma and thrombocytopenia. The bleeding may also be due to administration of anticoagulants.

Idiopathic

The so-called idiopathic group includes about 85% of patients. These patients can be divided into those who bleed from the antero-inferior part of the septum (Little's area) in children, and those from the superior part of the nose in the elderly. The exact pathology of bleeding from Little's area in children appears to be related to two factors: hyperaemia of the upper respiratory tract in children, and nose picking and repeated rubbing of an area where the mucosa is stretched over cartilage and bone.

In the elderly it is commonly thought that the cause of the epistaxis is hypertension, but careful studies have shown that the blood pressure in these patients is no higher than in an age- and sex-matched controlled population. Whilst the hypertension may initiate the bleeding, its persistence and severity are explained not by the elevated blood pressure but by the inability of the large vessels to contract.

Management

The management of epistaxis is divided into two phases: arrest of the haemorrhage and treatment of the underlying cause.

Arrest of Haemorrhage

The bleeding may be stopped by one of three methods:

1. Local cautery (chemical or electrocoagulation).
2. Packing of nose with gauze or by an inflatable balloon.
3. Arterial ligation.

Ligation of the anterior and posterior ethmoidal artery and/or the maxillary artery in the infratemporal fossa is preferable to the insertion of a postnasal pack.

An uncommon specific disease causing epistaxis also requires specific treatment as appropriate.

NASAL POLYPS

Pathology

The aetiology of nasal polyps is not completely clear.

It used to be thought that nasal polyps were a consequence of allergy but it has been shown recently that this is true in only 30%, and that most probably chronic infection is the causative factor in the rest. Ninety per cent arise from the ethmoid air sinuses.

The present pathogenetic theory holds that polyps develop as a consequence of rupture of the epithelium as a result of tissue pressure from an oedematous and infiltrated nasal mucosa. The infiltrated and oedematous lamina propria prolapses caudally in the form of granulation tissue; the vascular stalk is established and at the same time epithelization of the prolapsed tissue takes place from the edges of the ruptured epithelium. At this stage a small polyp has formed. Mucous glands then grow from the epithelium into the depths of it. At the same time the volume of the polyp increases, probably due to gravity and the haemodynamic conditions of congestion of the venous discharge through the thin stalk. Through passive growth of the polyp the characteristic, very long, tubular ducts arise and this explains the much lower density of glands than observed in the normal nasal mucosa. With increasing age of the polyp, fibrosis and round-cell infiltration of the stroma increase, the glands degenerate and become cystic.

Malignant degeneration of nasal polyps does not occur, but nasal polyps can arise secondary to malignant disease in the nose. A unilateral polypus, especially if accompanied by a bloodstained purulent discharge, should be treated with suspicion. The tissue removed at polypectomy should always be submitted to histological examination.

Polyps usually form in the middle meatus (*Fig.* 29.2), particularly near the ostia of the sinuses, and sometimes in the roof of the nose; it is not clear why they are never seen on the septum, in the lower meatus nor in the lower respiratory tract. Nasal polyps are frequently accompanied by bronchial asthma, and, as such, are an expression of a disorder of the entire respiratory tract which must be treated as one unit. Often nasal polyps are harbingers of asthma, which develops later.

In a number of patients with nasal polyposis, particularly if combined with non-atopic bronchial asthma, intolerance

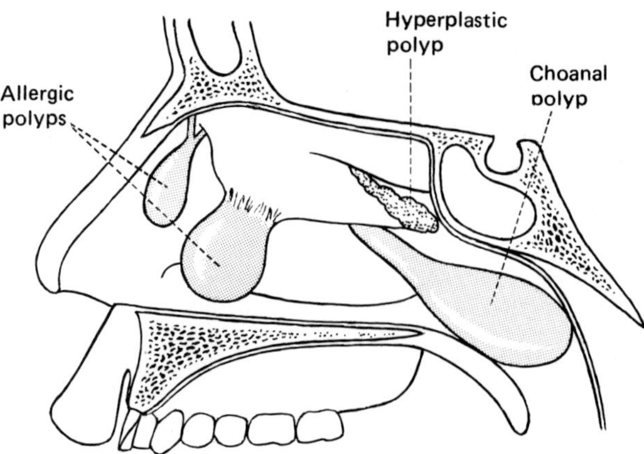

Fig. 29.2 Types of nasal polyps.

for aspirin, with often a crossed intolerance to indomethacin, pyrazones and coal tar dyes, is encountered. Ingestion of these substances can lead to severe and even fatal dyspnoea and respiratory arrest; they should, therefore, be used with great care in these patients. The pathogenesis of this syndrome is not quite clear, but there is evidence that it is related to the inhibitory action these compounds exert on the biosynthesis of prostaglandins.

Nasal polyps occur rarely during childhood. If nasal polyps are found in a child, they must be suspected to be the first symptom of mucoviscidosis (*see* Chapter 71).

One out of every 10–20 children with mucoviscidosis suffers from nasal polyposis. The polyps can be present at a very young age, even in the second year of life. In about 15% of the patients with mucoviscidosis an allergy is demonstrable. If this combination is present then nasal polyps are found in 1 out of every 3 patients.

Nasal polyps also occur in the rare Kartagener's syndrome (bronchiectasis, situs inversus and nasal polyps). They have also been described in children with Peutz–Jegher's syndrome of pigmented spots on the skin, especially around the mouth, and polyposis of the gastrointestinal tract.

A specific type of polypus is the antrochoanal polyp which occurs especially in the second and third decades of life, but can also occur in children. The polyp is solitary, arising from the maxillary antrum (most frequently from the lateral wall) and passes via the ostium and the nasal cavity into the nasopharynx. Histologically, the polyp does not differ from other nasal polyps. The choanal polyp can reach an enormous size and has a marked tendency to recur; a Caldwell–Luc operation is usually necessary in order to eradicate it.

Treatment

Polypectomy can be carried out either under local or general anaesthesia. If the nasal polyps are the result of a chronic maxillary sinusitis a Caldwell–Luc operation (removal of maxillary sinus mucosa and intranasal antrostomy) is often carried out at the same time. If there have been multiple recurrences, an external ethmoidectomy may be indicated.

If the nasal polyps are due to atopy this should be treated in the usual manner. Purulent infections of the nasal mucosa should be treated with antibiotics. This is even more important than usual since every patient with polyps is a potential sufferer from asthma. Corticosteroids have an extremely powerful effect, but it is not usually justifiable to prescribe oral corticosteroids over a period of years for this chronic disorder.

NASAL INJURIES

Septal Haematoma and Abscess

Pathology

A septal haematoma is a collection of blood between the septal cartilage and the mucoperichondrium, usually on both sides of the nose. Since cartilage in contact with blood under any form of pressure necroses drainage must be instituted immediately to avoid nasal collapse. Furthermore, a septal haematoma almost always precedes a septal abscess.

Treatment

A septal haematoma or abscess should be widely incised and evacuated immediately, after which the incision must be held open with a small rubber drain and the nose must be packed to hold the mucosa against the cartilage. The patient should be treated for at least a week with appropriate antibiotics.

Nasal Fractures

Pathology

There are 3 types of nasal injury depending on the force and direction of the blow.

1. Class I Fracture

From the minimal force either the septal cartilage fractures between its fixed points (the nasal bone and maxillary spine) or the thin distal end of the nasal bone is depressed giving an impression of deviation.

2. Class 2 Fracture (*Fig.* 29.3)

From a greater force the thick proximal part of the nasal bone fractures. This is associated with a C-shaped fracture

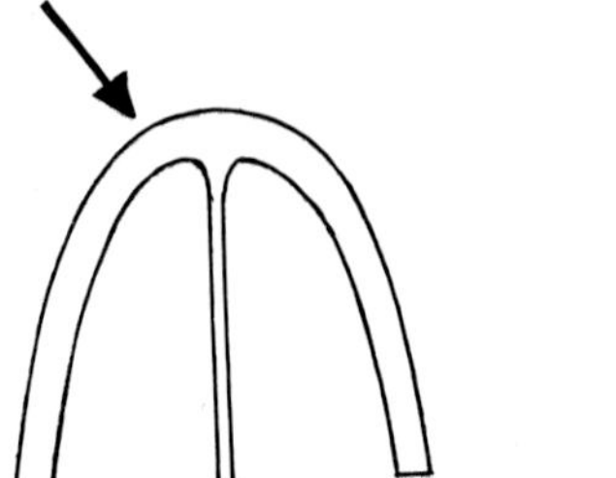
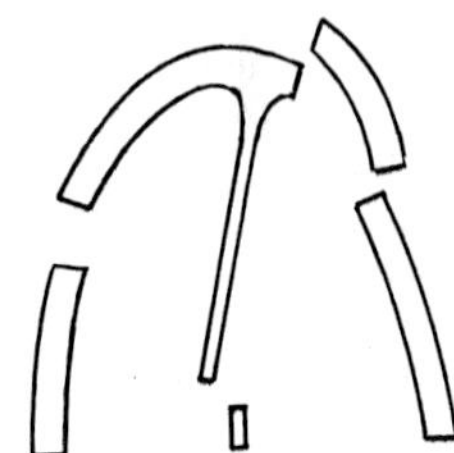

Fig. 29.3 Lateral displacement injury with fracture of the septum and both nasal bones.

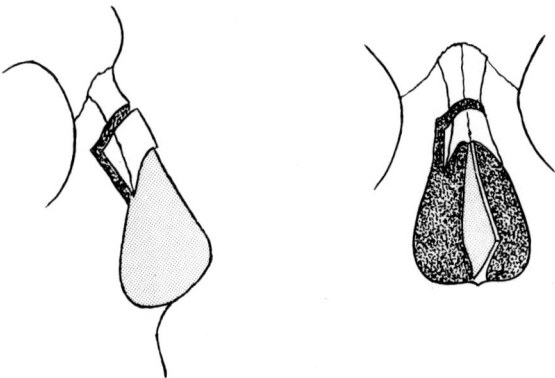

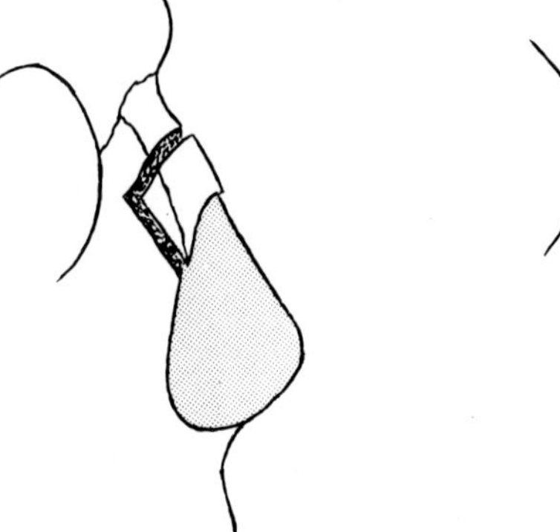

Fig. 29.4 Diagram of a moderate frontal injury which is commonly associated with a septal fracture.

of the perpendicular plate of the ethmoid and septum. They tend to overlap and so simple manipulation is not sufficient. A satisfactory long-term result can only be achieved by surgery to the septum in addition to manipulation of the nasal bones.

3. *Class 3 Fracture* (*Fig.* 29.4)

The severest force, usually from the front pushes the nasal bones into the ethmoid sinus and under the frontal bone. The medial wall of the orbit is thus disrupted as may be the cribriform plate. There will be apparent telecanthus, a shortening and gross deformity of the nose and an altered nasofrontal angle. There may be CSF leak, tearing, diplopia and blindness.

The deformity requires immediate open reduction.

Clinical Features

A history of trauma to the midface accompanied by epistaxis, a noticeable deformity and nasal airway obstruction are the usual complaints. Nasal obstruction suggests skeletal displacement or a septal haematoma. Nasofrontoethmoidal complex fractures may produce diplopia and epiphora.

The amount of swelling, ecchymosis and deformity seen on examination is usually directly proportional to the magnitude of the trauma. The fractured nose is commonly exquisitely tender. The absence of bony crepitus on palpation does not rule out a fracture, since the fragments are usually impacted due to swelling. The nasal swelling is commonly accompanied by peri-orbital swelling and ecchymosis, as well as occasional subscleral haemorrhage.

The nasofrontoethmoidal complex fracture is characterized by marked deepening of the nasion, severe swelling and telecanthus. There may be apparent telecanthus, an illusion created by the absence of the normal ridge lent by the dorsum of the nose between the eyes. Normally the eyes should be separated from one another by approximately the length of one eye (30–35 mm). In traumatic telecanthus the medial canthal ligaments are displaced laterally, giving the appearance that the eyes are likewise displaced. If the fracture continues through the cribriform plate or fovea ethmoidalis, a CSF rhinorrhoea may complicate the fracture.

Nasal fracture accompanied by avulsion of tissue is fortunately rare.

Detailed pretraumatic photographs of the patient may be helpful in making an accurate assessment of the injury. Radiographs are of limited diagnostic value as vascular markings and previous fractures may confuse the physician. Radiographs, however, may be important medicolegally.

Treatment

Reduction and fixation should be done as soon after the injury as possible, because of the tendency of these fragments to become stabilized rapidly. Closed reduction may be readily performed under local anaesthesia.

The procedure has two goals: the septum must be straightened, thereby opening the airway, and the bony pyramid must be restored to its pretraumatic configuration. Both goals may be thwarted because of pre-existing deformity.

Maintenance of position is accomplished by intranasal packing and an external splint.

Most lacerations of the mucosa require no suturing. Synechiae or webs may be avoided by the insertion of a Silastic sheet on each side of the septum. In compound injuries involving the skin, a layered closure resulting in everted wound edges should be done.

Complications

Airway obstruction may result from septal deflection, a combination of septal and bony deformity, or scar tissue. It is virtually impossible to manipulate a distorted or fractured septum back into position and so open reduction is necessary. This may be performed at the time of injury but usually it is better to allow the soft-tissue swelling to subside over a period of about 2 weeks and then to operate. The operation of septoplasty involves detaching the nasal septum from its dislocated position and replacing it in the midline. Formerly only the obstructing portion of septum was removed (the SMR or submucous resection operation) but this is done less frequently now because of loss of support and subsequent collapse of the nose. The septoplasty operation also corrects any external nasal deformity in the cartilaginous part of the nose.

External nasal deformity due to malposition of the nasal bones is the result of undiagnosed nasal bone fracture probably hidden by oedematous, overlying soft tissues or failure of nasal manipulation. Although a seemingly simple manoeuvre, nasal manipulation only succeeds in completely straightening about 50% of fractured nasal bones. Bony deformity is corrected by osteotomies performed through small intranasal incisions.

The operations of septoplasty and nasal osteotomy form the basis of the rhinoplasty operation. Also involved in rhinoplasty may be modification of the nasal tip cartilages which is performed for either purely cosmetic reasons or to repair the growth deformities secondary to cleft lip and palate. Profile deformities are corrected by inserting grafts of cartilage (usually homografts cartilage from SMR operations) or bone (either rib or iliac crest).

Synechiae should be divided when diagnosed and the raw surfaces kept apart by a sheet of Silastic.

Persistent epiphora may occur after fractures of the nasofrontoethmoid complex and usually requires a dacrocystorhinotomy for its correction.

TUMOURS

Surgical Pathology

Incidence

Cancer of the maxilla constitutes 1/500 of all cancers and so is relatively rare both in the UK and in the USA; it is much commoner, however, in Africa. Two men are affected to every woman and the average age at first diagnosis is 55. Cancer of the ethmoids and nasal fossa are as common as each other and together are as common as maxillary cancer. Cancer of the sphenoid and frontal sinuses is very rare and will not be discussed further. The site incidence and histological types are shown in *Fig.* 29.5.

Aetiology

There are no true precancerous conditions of the nose and sinuses, but there are certain occupations which are prone to nasal cancer, the best known being the furniture industry. Until 1924, when arsenicals were removed from the processing, workers in the chrome and nickel industries were prone to nasal cancers. It has recently been shown that workers in the furniture and shoe industries in the UK are also prone to adenocarcinoma of the ethmoids.

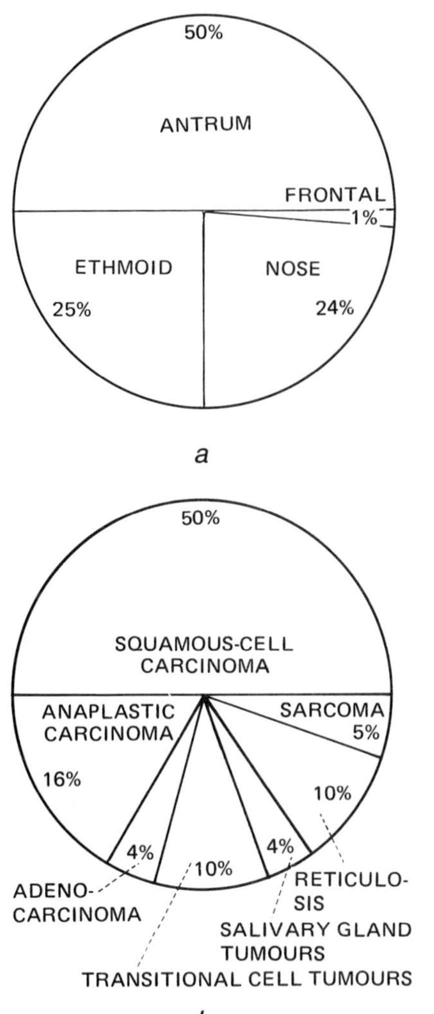

Fig. 29.5 *a*, Site incidence of cancer of the nose and sinuses. *b*, Histological types of tumours of the nose and sinuses.

SQUAMOUS-CELL CARCINOMA. Squamous-cell carcinoma of the maxillary antrum presents in two forms—antro-alveolar tumours, some of which are ectopic salivary gland tumours, and antro-ethmoidal tumours.

Tumours of the lower half of the antrum (antro-alveolar tumours) usually present with dental symptoms because of invasion of the alveolus. These tumours do not usually invade the base of the skull or orbit; 5% have an enlarged node in the neck, most commonly in the submandibular region. Antro-ethmoidal tumours often involve the orbit—probably in at least half the cases (*Fig.* 29.6), and involvement of the infraorbital nerve is also common. About 5% have an enlarged lymph node, most commonly an upper deep cervical node.

Cancers of the nasal fossa affect the septum and lateral wall with roughly equal frequency: cancers of the floor of the nose are less common. Involvement of the orbit is rare and occurs only in tumours of the lateral wall, and involvement of the cranial nerves is very rare. Enlarged lymph nodes occur in 5% of patients. The submandibular nodes being most commonly involved.

One patient in three ultimately dies of metastases, the commonest sites being, in descending order: the abdominal viscera, the lungs and bones. One patient in five develops a second primary tumour, the commonest site being the bronchus.

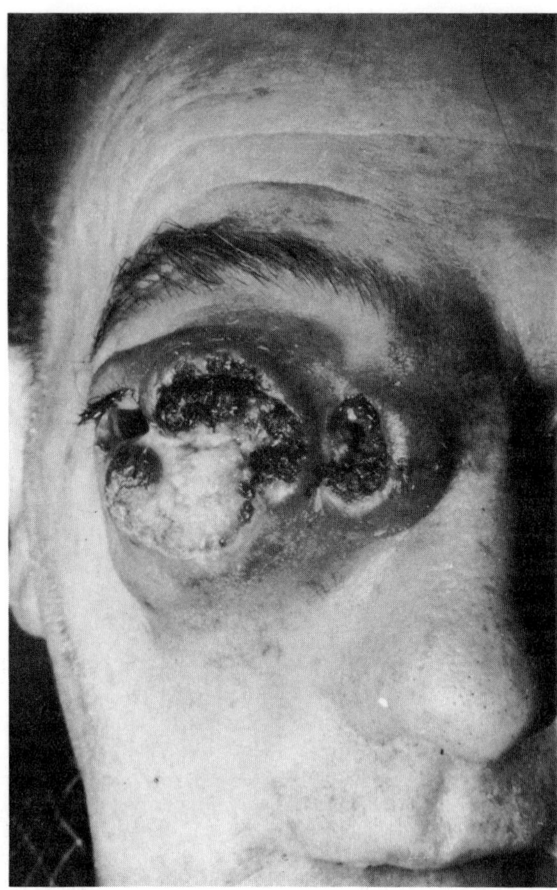

Fig. 29.6 Carcinoma of the ethmoids invading the orbit.

TRANSITIONAL-CELL CARCINOMA. Transitional-cell tumours behave in one of three ways. First, the benign tumour which presents as a polypoidal mass in one nostril and has a marked propensity to recur after removal, but which never becomes malignant. Secondly, the tumour which after repeated removal becomes frankly malignant and invasive. Finally, there is the tumour which is a transitional-cell carcinoma from the beginning.

ADENOCARCINOMA. Adenocarcinomas of the nose and sinuses are uncommon except in certain workers in the furniture industry; they tend to be of low-grade malignancy, and although they invade locally into the orbit and base of skull they seldom metastasize to lymph nodes or to a distance. Any adenocarcinoma of the respiratory tract should be suspected of being secondary to a primary elsewhere, most often a renal adenocarcinoma—before radical treatment of such a tumour is undertaken. Therefore, a primary in the kidney and bowel should be excluded.

SALIVARY TUMOURS. The commonest salivary tumours to occur in the nose and sinuses are the adenoid cystic carcinoma, muco-epidermoid tumours and pleomorphic adenomas. Any salivary gland tumour in the nose and sinuses behaves in a much more aggressive fashion than a similar tumour in a major salivary gland, and from the point of view of treatment all salivary gland tumours occurring within the nasal cavity and sinuses should be regarded as being malignant.

Rare Tumours

1. *Plasmacytoma* may occur in its solitary form at any point in the upper respiratory tract, the commonest site being the nose. Only very rarely does a solitary soft-tissue plasmacytoma progress to multiple myeloma. It is usually treated by radiotherapy, although there is no real evidence that radical treatment is necessary.
2. *Reticuloses.* These occur in the nose, almost always in the form of reticulum-cell sarcoma, but are rare. Radiotherapy is the treatment of choice.
3. *Fibrosarcoma.* In the nose and sinuses this tumour tends to be only moderately aggressive and locally malignant, and metastases are uncommon. The treatment is to give a full dose of radiation followed by operation as for carcinoma.
4. *Sarcoma.* Osteogenic sarcoma of the maxilla is treated by radiotherapy and surgery but a chondrosarcoma is completely radioresistant and should be treated by maxillectomy.
5. *Melanoma.* This is derived from the neural crest. The usual site of origin is the middle or inferior turbinate, and these tumours usually present with epistaxis, although a polypoidal mass may form which is usually not pigmented. About 4 out of 10 of these patients will have a node in the neck at some stage of the disease.
6. *Olfactory neuroblastoma.* This tumour also arises from the neural crest and presents as a polypoidal mass which arises from the upper part of the nose, and which bleeds readily. As it arises from the olfactory nerve, invasion into the anterior cranial fossa readily occurs through the cribriform plate, but systemic metastases are very unusual. Radiographs often show calcification of the tumour. Unlike other neural tumours this tumour responds well to radiotherapy.
7. *Pseudotumours.* Three granulomatous lesions occur in the nose and may be confused with tumours. They all usually affect the lower end of the nasal septum.

a. Bleeding haemangioma of the nasal septum—this is a cavernous haemangioma which has a propensity to recur if resection is not adequate.
b. Granuloma pyogenicum—a foreign body granuloma.
c. Granuloma gravidarum—a granuloma occurring in pregnant women, usually affecting the gingiva, but occasionally occurring in the nose. It resolves spontaneously after delivery.

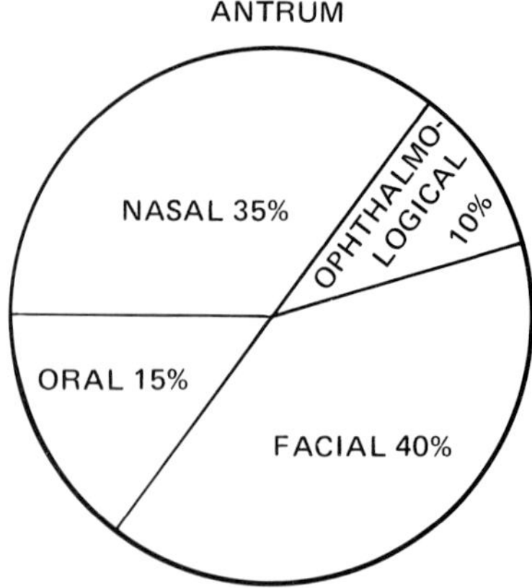

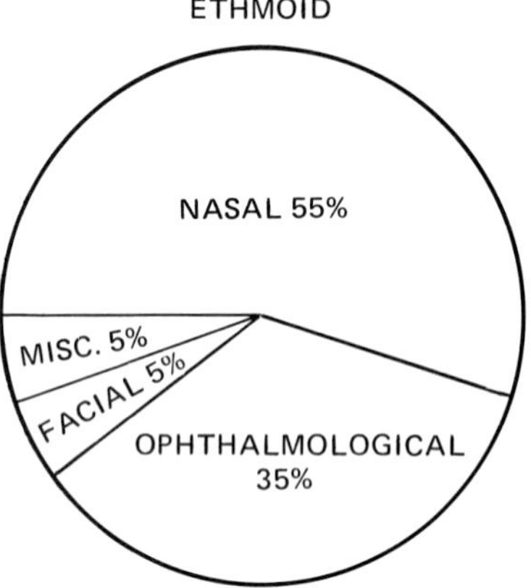

Fig. 29.7 Presenting symptoms of tumours of the nose and sinuses.

Investigations

History

The presenting symptoms and their relative frequency in cancer at different sites are shown in *Fig. 29.7*.

Examination

The face is examined for fullness of one cheek, numbness of the cheek and ptosis due to a Horner's syndrome caused by pressure on the cervical sympathetic chain by a lateral retropharyngeal node. The nose, nasopharynx and mouth are inspected for evidence of tumour and for numbness of the hard palate indicating involvement of the greater palatine nerve. The pharynx and larynx are examined for evidence of ninth and tenth cranial nerve palsies. Finally, the hard palate, the buccal sulcus and the anterior surface of the antrum are palpated.

The eyes are examined for proptosis and for ophthalmoplegia, preferably by an ophthalmologist.

The neck is palpated for enlarged nodes, and the abdomen is also palpated, first to see if there is a primary elsewhere and secondly to exclude a metastasis—the abdominal viscera being the commonest site.

Radiology

Virtually all patients have evidence of bone destruction because all these tumours are diagnosed late. If bone destruction is seen on plain films, tomography should be done. All patients should have CT scanning to assess spread into the sphenoid sinus and anterior cranial fossa. Magnetic scanning is not so useful as bone erosion is the important information. Chest radiographs should be taken to exclude secondaries and to assess the general health.

Other Investigations

If a myeloma is suspected the plasma proteins should be estimated, and the urine examined for Bence Jones protein. If there is a watery nasal discharge, it is examined for the presence of cerebrospinal fluid—this can be done simply with a Clinistix, or by injecting fluorescein into the CSF and seeing if it appears in the nose. The most sophisticated method is to put a tampon in the nose, inject radioactive albumin into the CSF, and estimate the radioactive content of the tampon.

Biopsy

This is best done by the intranasal route, although it is also possible via a Caldwell–Luc approach.

Treatment Policy

About 20% of patients are incurable due to various general and local factors. The patient may be a very poor surgical risk, or distant metastases may be present or he may refuse to have a disfiguring operation.

It is difficult to be dogmatic about methods of treatment, which certainly differ between the USA and the UK. Recent developments in craniofacial surgery have extended the scope for surgery in these tumours.

The only thing which can be said with certainty is that combined radiotherapy and surgery must be used—either alone gives poor results.

The radiotherapy is usually given first—6000 rad in 6 weeks is the ideal. There is only one exception to this—the patient with clinical or radiological invasion of the malar bone. If such a patient is irradiated, osteitis occurs with deterioration in the patient's general condition, and the end result is widespread sequestration of the malar bone causing a very bad deformity.

Four to six weeks after radiotherapy the patient has an operation tailored to his need, taking into account the extent of the disease and the patient's age and general condition.

A tumour of the lower half of the antrum involving the palate but not the orbit is best managed by a partial maxillectomy removing all the hard palate, the alveolus and the medial wall of the antrum up to and including the middle turbinate.

Tumours of the upper half of the jaw (antro-ethmoidal) can be managed by total maxillectomy and orbital removal but craniofacial techniques are now used. The combined approach allows removal of both ethmoid labyrinths and since the optic nerve can be isolated and seen, orbits may be preserved that otherwise would be removed. Intracranial extension no longer dictates inoperability but involvement of brain is usually fatal.

Tumours in the nasal fossa are usually high on the lateral wall and are best treated as antro-ethmoidal tumours. Uncommon tumours low on the lateral wall, floor and septum are best exposed by a sublabial rhinotomy followed by excision of the involved area with a wide margin.

The above combined therapy applies only to squamous-cell carcinoma. The lymphoid tumours are obviously managed by radiotherapy alone, whilst salivary gland tumours are usually radioresistant and should have an operation—the technique being tailored to the extent and site of the tumour as outlined for carcinoma.

Involved neck nodes should be included in the treatment fields. If they do not respond to the radiotherapy a radical neck dissection should be carried out if the primary is controlled; these patients have a poor prognosis, however—few patients with a maxillary carcinoma and nodes in the neck survive for 5 years, and there have been no reports of 5-year survival for an ethmoidal carcinoma with enlarged nodes at the time of presentation.

Osteoma (*Fig.* 29.8)

The osteoma is the commonest benign tumour of the paranasal sinuses, being present on radiographs of 1% of all frontal sinuses (*Fig.* 29.9). It is also occasionally found in the ethmoid sinuses.

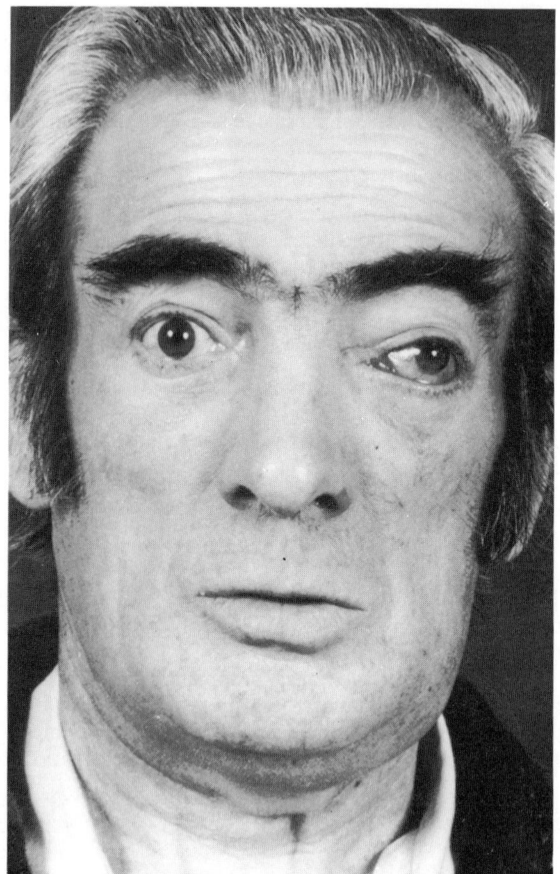

Fig. 29.8 Osteoma of the frontal/ethmoid sinuses displacing the eyeball.

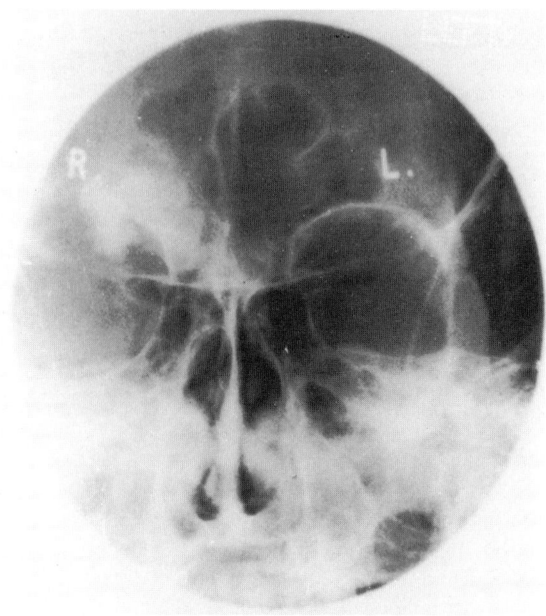

Fig. 29.9 Radiograph of frontal osteoma.

The tumour is thought to arise from persistent embryonal periosteum at the junction of endochondral and membranous bones. Histology shows these tumours to be either 'ivory', composed of hard, dense, compact bone, or 'spongy' with a periphery of compact bone surrounding a cancellous lamellar centre.

An osteoma may present with:

1. External deformity
2. Displacement of the eyeball
3. Headache
4. Chronic infection
5. Recurrent meningitis if the posterior wall of the sinuses is eroded.

Radiology shows the typical well-defined calcified mass.

If the osteoma is causing symptoms it should be removed. The frontal sinus is opened by elevating an osteoplastic flap, and the osteoma is broken off at its pedicle.

THE WAY AHEAD

Two obvious fields for development in this area are the treatment of simple, common nasal polyps, and the measurement of nasal function.

Several theories have been proposed as to the cause of nasal polyps, but none has been proved. It is very unlikely that the long-held view that nasal polyps are due to infection and/or allergy is the full story. If it were, treatment of this common disorder would be easy. Unfortunately, a fairly large number of patients with nasal polyps suffer repeated recurrences, which are very difficult to manage. Radical surgery on the sinuses is certainly not the answer, and although recurrent nasal polyps can be controlled by corticosteroids these obviously have disadvantages in the long run.

Until the fundamental mucosal defect causing nasal polyps is understood logical and successful treatment for nasal polyps will not be available.

There is at the moment no universally accepted commonly used method of assessing the nasal flow rate (rhinometry). Numerous methods have been proposed over the last century, a sure sign that no single one is satisfactory. The air flow through the nose is very complex, being linear on inspiration and turbulent on expiration. There is a diurnal variation in the patency of the nasal airways and there is a cycle whereby one nostril opens up as the other closes.

On top of this there are enormous variations in nasal resistance due to psychological, hormonal and environmental factors. Whether these difficulties can ever be overcome in an effort to provide a simple, reproducible and generally acceptable method of measuring nasal resistance is doubtful. Such a method is badly needed, however, in the assessment of nasal obstruction, a symptom which may vary from a mild occasional nuisance to permanent misery. Logical decisions about the treatment of many nasal conditions and assessment of the efficacy of such treatments can really only be made on the basis of such measurements.

30 The Ear

M. S. McCormick

Most ear conditions are seen and dealt with by an otolaryngologist but there are occasions when a general surgeon will either have to manage the patient or decide on the priorities of management if there are multiple problems. He may also be asked to assess problems when specialist advice is not available. There are four groups of conditions which the general surgeon may be asked to assess in this regard. He should be able to differentiate the urgent from the non-urgent and identify serious signs and symptoms when present. We shall now consider in turn affections of the ear caused by trauma, infection, tumours and, finally, facial nerve paralysis.

SURGICAL ANATOMY

The pinna is composed of a convoluted piece of elastic cartilage to which the skin is tightly applied. This not only gives it its characteristic appearance but also explains why inflammatory lesions of the pinna are extremely painful. The cartilage of the pinna and the external auditory meatus are contiguous and abut with the bony meatus of the temporal bone itself. The external ear is on average 27 mm long and ends at, and is separated from, the middle ear by the tympanic membrane. Sound entering the ear canal is absorbed by the tympanic membrane and energy is then transferred to the inner ear via three ossicles, the malleus, incus and stapes. This mechanism provides a mechanical advantage of 23:1 from the cantilever system of ossicles and also the comparative areas of the tympanic membrane and the opening into the inner ear at the oval window. Perforations of the tympanic membrane or ossicular discontinuity will therefore result in deafness due to failure of conduction of sound through to the inner ear.

The inner ear houses in dense ivory bone, the sensory end-organs of the cochlea and the vestibular apparatus subserving hearing and balance respectively, and each supplied by its own division of the eighth cranial nerve. The structure of these differing end-organs is similar in that each is encased in a bony hard capsule and the sensory epithelium is contained in a membranous tube filled with endolymph, which is itself bathed in perilymph. It is common, therefore, that conditions affecting the inner ear should produce not only deafness but also dizziness.

The facial nerve accompanies the divisions of the eighth nerve in the internal meatus. As the cochlea and vestibular nerves supply the end-organs, the facial nerve enters the middle ear and curves through at almost a right angle to run horizontally through the middle ear in close proximity to the oval window. It then turns inferiorly, courses through the mastoid bone and the floor of the external meatus, to exit from the base of the skull at the stylomastoid foramen and then anteriorly to enter the parotid gland which it divides into a superficial and deep lobe.

Perhaps of more importance are the contiguous structures to the middle ear and mastoid which may be involved in disease processes which spread from the site of origin. The limits of the mastoid air-cell system are defined by a thin plate of bone which separates the middle ear cleft from the meninges of the middle and posterior cranial fossa. The anterior bony meatal wall is related to the temporomandibular joint and parotid gland. In the floor of the middle ear lies the jugular bulb and anterior to this, the canal for the carotid artery as it enters the skull.

TRAUMATIC LESIONS

External Ear

1. Lacerations

Often a through and through laceration of the pinna follows injury. This should be repaired in layers, i.e. cartilage and skin, trimming back the cartilage when necessary to get good apposition and closure of both layers. Dexon or vicryl should be used for cartilage. If the skin looks non-viable it is wise to be conservative and await events as often 'non-viable skin' will survive because of the excellent blood supply to the ear. Indeed often large portions or even the whole pinna may be sewn back in place following traumatic avulsion or excision. The success of such a 'composite graft' is not unusual.

2. Haematoma

This is a common sporting injury which results in a collection of blood between the perichondrium and cartilage of the pinna. It is cosmetically obvious, very painful and if not dealt with, will result in avascular necrosis of the cartilage with subsequent deformity of the pinna. Infection and subsequent healing by fibrosis produces a pinna not dissimilar to a florette of a cauliflower ('cauliflower ear').

If small these may be aspirated but often the haematoma

requires evacuation by incision and drainage. The perichondrium is then closely reapplied to the cartilage by either packing and pressure dressing or by through and through mattress sutures which maintain contact between the perichondrium and the cartilage (*Fig.* 30.1).

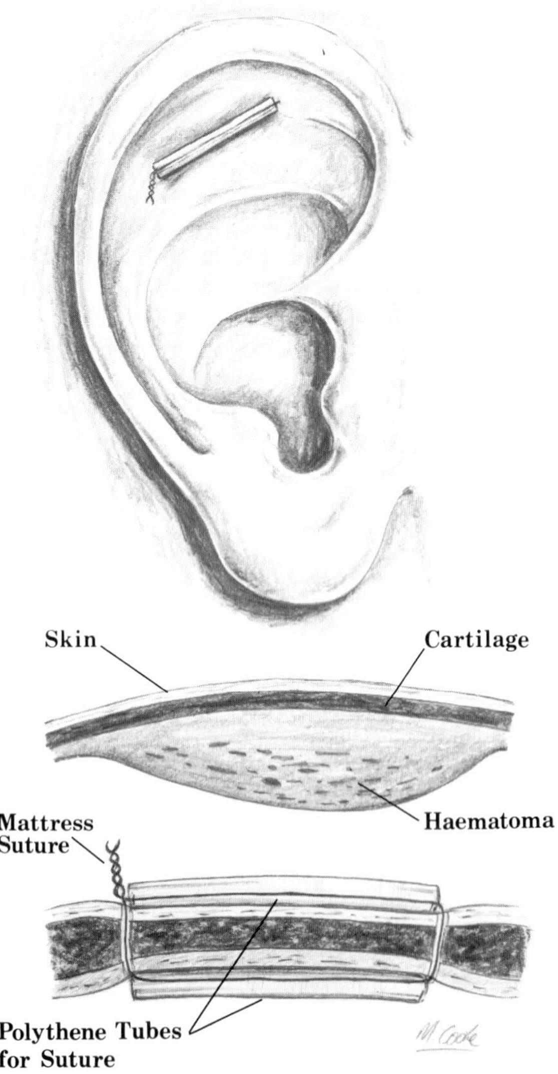

Fig. 30.1 Treatment of auricular haematoma.

3. *Self-induced or Iatrogenic Injury*

Patients often complain that the ears have bled after they have used cotton buds for cleaning. Also following otoscopy or syringeing the external ear canal may be injured. Often the injury is only to the ear canal itself and the patient can be reassured accordingly. However, care is needed when severe deafness or dizziness is reported. An otologist's opinion should then be sought.

4. *Foreign Bodies*

Most foreign bodies can be syringed from the external ear by using water at body temperature and a syringe with a nozzle that can direct the jet of water along the posterior ear canal wall. This avoids any risk of injury to the tympanic membrane. Perhaps the only exception to syringeing is a vegetable foreign body which may swell with water. Direct instrumentation and removal is necessary in these cases.

5. *Fractures*

The anterior bony meatal wall may be fractured by a frontal blow to the mandible, forcing the head of the mandible through the glenoid fossa into the meatus. Treatment is only necessary if the canal is stenosed; however, this is not urgent.

Middle Ear

1. *Blast Injury*

The increase in terrorist use of explosives has resulted in a concomitant increase in blast injuries. The sudden and extreme changes in pressure caused by a bomb blast may rupture the tympanic membrane. A perforation may similarly follow a slap on the ear or other sporting injuries. There are no characteristic features apart from fresh blood around the ragged edges of the perforation. Although the defect may be sizeable it is common for these perforations to heal spontaneously; therefore a conservative approach is usually adopted. The patient is advised to keep the ear dry so that otitis media does not impair subsequent healing. If spontaneous repair does not take place then surgical repair, a tympanoplasty, will be necessary. If the ossicular chain has been disrupted or damaged this may also be repaired.

2. *Penetrating Injuries*

The external ear has a double curve between the cartilaginous and bony portions, thus most injuries of this area cause an otitis externa only. Occasionally instrumentation, syringeing or other sharp objects used by patients to clean their ears may perforate the tympanic membrane. These are usually small and heal spontaneously.

Welders occasionally report that a spark of hot metal has entered their ear and examination will confirm perforation of the tympanic membrane. These rarely heal and indeed in these cases surgical repair often fails. However, the acute management is as for other perforations of the tympanic membrane, i.e. keep the ear dry and await spontaneous healing.

Inner Ear

1. *Blast Injury*

A bomb blast may not only rupture the tympanic membrane but there may also be a compressional effect in the cochlea. This may be the result of the extreme noise which may damage the cochlea or the direct pressure effect on the sensory end-organ. The damage in the ear may be minor or severe and occasionally results in total destruction inside the ear. Total deafness, a roaring tinnitus and disabling vertigo should arouse the examiner's suspicions in this regard. Inner ear resuscitation with the use of steroids, vasodilatation with praxilene and carbon dioxide inhalations are advised by some but their scientific value is unproven.

2. *Fractured Base of Skull*

The temporal bone may be fractured by a severe head injury, usually after a road traffic accident. Bleeding from the ear is almost pathognomonic of a fractured temporal bone. Cerebrospinal fluid (CSF) otorrhoea is often also seen. This implies that there is an abnormal communication between the middle ear and the subarachnoid space. Prophylactic antibiotics should be commenced and continued for

7–10 days. Examination of the ear may reveal a fracture line and fresh blood in the external meatus or, more commonly, blood in the middle ear will be seen, a haemotympanum. The direction of the fracture line determines the severity of the injury. Longitudinal fractures represent 80% of fractures and extend through the middle ear and disrupt the tympanic membrane. Often the ossicular chain is involved but damage to the inner ear and facial nerve is rare. It is often possible to repair the damage in the middle ear at a later date.

In contrast, however, transverse fractures (20%), traverse the middle ear, the cochlea and internal meatus. This results in a profound permanent sensorineural hearing loss and a facial paralysis.

Management

The diagnosis is essentially clinical as radiology often fails to demonstrate the fracture line. Prophylactic penicillin and sulphadimidine are prescribed to prevent meningitis. If a CSF fistula persists then it may be necessary for a neurosurgeon to seal the dura at the site of injury if spontaneous closure does not occur. The assessment of any deafness present may be difficult due to the patient's general condition associated with the closed head injury. However, a guide to any hearing loss can be obtained by simple clinical testing with the spoken voice in the test ear, and also with Weber's tuning fork test. An activated tuning fork is placed on the forehead. If the inner ear is totally destroyed by the fracture then hearing will only be possible in the good ear and therefore sound will be heard in the opposite side to the fracture. If, however, the injury has produced only a conductive as opposed to an inner ear deafness, the Weber's test will lateralize to the ear with the conductive hearing loss, i.e. the fractured middle ear.

The management of facial nerve paralysis is dealt with later in the chapter.

OTITIS MEDIA

There are various types of otitis media but in fact only one of these types produces life-threatening complications. A *cholesteatoma* is an abnormal collection of squamous epithelium in the middle ear cleft. It is usually preceded by childhood otitis media. The accumulation of debris within the middle ear cleft may become infected and this is in effect a localized abscess within the confines of the middle ear. Osteolytic enzymes are produced which not only erode the ossicles within the middle ear producing conductive deafness, but may also erode the bony confines of the temporal bone, exposing dura and causing meningitis and extra- or intradural brain abscess. Furthermore the cholesteatoma can erode into the inner ear and cause labyrinthitis, total deafness and vertigo if the semi-circular canals are involved, or a facial paralysis if the facial nerve canal is eroded. Most patients with ear symptoms will have sought the advice of a specialist in this regard unless they have ignored the symptoms and present as a matter of urgency with a severe complication as indicated above.

Management

History

There is usually a long history of chronic ear problems regarding discharge and deafness. The advent of a facial weakness or dizziness requires the urgent attention of an otologist. Headache is not a common feature of uncomplicated otitis media and its presence may indicate an intracranial complication.

Examination

Otological examination usually reveals a foul-smelling otorrhoea and debris obscures the tympanic membrane. It is important to assess adequately facial nerve function and also to look for focal neurological signs such as homonymous hemianopia or ataxia as seen in temporal lobe or posterior fossa abscess.

Radiology

Most radiography is unhelpful in assessing a cholesteatoma. Indeed the radiologist will often report a poorly pneumatized sclerotic mastoid bone as indicating infection, when in fact the ear may only be scarred by past infection and be completely quiescent. However, a CT scan is the investigation to perform when an intracranial complication is suspected.

Audiometry

Audiological tests will confirm or refute your clinical impressions regarding deafness, but if this is available then usually a specialist will also be available.

Treatment

Uncomplicated cholesteatoma is a localized problem within the middle ear and mastoid. Treatment requires a mastoidectomy where the honeycomb of cells in the mastoid is drilled away using the operating microscope and a high-speed drill with cutting burrs. A cavity is created which expands the external meatus into the mastoid cellular system so that the disease is exteriorized and intracranial complications are therefore prevented. It is the aim in modern otology to reconstruct the middle ear sound conduction mechanism at surgery so that the ear should not only be rendered safe but be useful audiologically. If the facial nerve is involved removal of the disease matrix from around the nerve is performed and the swelling of the nerve sheath is also reduced by decompression of the nerve in its bony canal.

A subperiosteal abscess over the mastoid process is the commonest complication of otitis media. It may be the result of acute fulminant otitis media in younger children or caused by a cholesteatoma. Incision and drainage of the abscess is a matter of urgency and should be combined with mastoid surgery. If specialist help is not available the abscess should be drained, treatment with antibiotics commenced and the patient referred to an otologist.

A common problem exists in the differential diagnosis of post auricular swelling due to a mastoid abscess and lymphadenitis secondary to scalp infection or otitis externa. If a primary cause of infection is not obvious then specialist advice is needed.

Intracranial complications are treated on their merits and surgery on the ear is performed as soon as the patient's general condition permits, but often burr hole aspiration of an abscess is performed under the same anaesthetic as mastoidectomy. The urgency and seriousness of these complications must be emphasized, and specialist advice should be sought immediately.

TUMOURS

Surgical Pathology

Tumours of the external ear and meatus present early because of pain or visible ulceration; therefore diagnosis, management and results of treatment are good. However, tumours of the middle ear and mastoid present late, are difficult to treat, have a very poor prognosis, but fortunately are rare.

Ulcerating tumours of the external ear are either basal-cell or squamous carcinomas. Most occur in adult males who have an outdoor occupation. Basal-cell tumours (rodent ulcers) are locally invasive, may be aggressive but do not metastasize. In contrast, the squamous carcinoma metastasizes to the pre- and postauricular lymph nodes.

Within the meatus occasional benign tumours of the ceruminous glands occur and these require complete excision. The commonest 'tumours' seen in the external ear are ivory osteomas. These are often multiple, are present in both ear canals and are often seen in those who swim in relatively cold water, for example surfers, etc. They are completely benign and cause symptoms only if they narrow the external meatus sufficiently to cause stenosis and retention of debris.

Cancer of the mucosa in the middle ear is usually preceded by a prolonged history of otorrhoea. Most are squamous carcinomas (70%) whilst the remainder are composed of adenocarcinomas, melanomas or sarcomas. They are usually painless and present with a complication, such as facial paralysis.

Occasional vascular tumours from the internal carotid or, more commonly, the jugular vein involve the middle ear. Often the patient complains of a pulsatile tinnitus due to transmitted vascular sounds to the cochlea.

Management

History

Ulcerating tumours on the pinna usually present no problems regarding diagnosis. The onset of pain or bleeding in an ear which has discharged intermittently for many years should be viewed with some suspicion as middle ear cancer is notoriously difficult to diagnose. A high index of suspicion and biopsy of any 'granulation tissue' is indicated.

Vascular tumours cause conductive deafness and pulsatile tinnitus. If very large, e.g. glomus tumour arising from chemoreceptor cells in the jugular bulb, then a jugular foramen syndrome may be present, i.e. paralysis of the ninth, tenth and eleventh cranial nerves causing hoarseness, weak shoulder movement and asymmetry of movement of the soft palate.

Examination

Lesions of the pinna are obvious but growths in the external meatus and middle ear are very difficult to assess as often a bleeding polyp fills the canal. Examine fully the facial nerve and compare its function with the other side, remembering to immobilize the contralateral side. Examine also the parotid and mastoid areas as well as the upper deep cervical lymph nodes for lymphatic metastases. The rest of the cranial nerves should also be examined if a glomus tumour is suspected.

Radiology

A plain radiograph of the base of the skull may show destruction or expansion of the jugular bulb or other foramen by tumour. Likewise, mastoid radiographs may show erosion in tumours of the external and middle ear. Tomography is helpful in defining how far the tumour has spread anteriorly and CT scanning will show intracranial spread. One specific contraindication to surgery is extension of growth medial to the carotid canal in the anterior petrous temple bone.

Contrast radiology, i.e. angiography, or CT scan with contrast is helpful in vascular tumours, not only identifying the size of the lesion but also feeding vessels may be identified and even embolized (angiography) at the time of investigation. Nuclear magnetic resonance imaging is a non-invasive highly accurate method of illustrating soft-tissue growths and will undoubtedly add much to the investigations of this kind in the future. However, if such a facility does exist then undoubtedly a specialist otologist will be available for advice.

Biopsy

If a carcinoma is suspected then biopsy of granulation tissue should be performed. If, however, there is no preceding otorrhoea and a bleeding polyp is protruding from the ear canal, it might be more appropriate to perform contrast radiology before biopsying a vascular lesion.

Treatment

Lesions of the pinna can be treated with radiotherapy or surgery but as a biopsy is necessary surgical excision and biopsy is usually simpler and quicker to perform, e.g. wedge excision (*Fig.* 30.2).

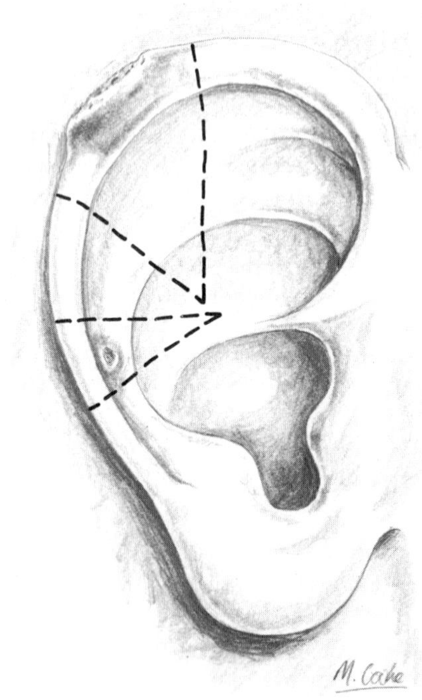

Fig. 30.2 Wedge excision of ulcer.

Cancers of the middle ear and mastoid can be removed by petrosectomy if the tumour is still confined to the temporal bone. This is a major operation with considerable mortality and morbidity. It is necessary usually to excise the pinna as well as the temporal bone lateral to the internal carotid artery. It is also necessary to graft any dural defects produced and also provide skin flap cover for the resected area. This is best done by a rotation scalp flap. Postoperatively the patient is not only deaf and dizzy, but also has a complete facial palsy. Radiotherapy is often used postoperatively. Despite such heroic surgery the prognosis is poor in this condition.

FACIAL NERVE PARALYSIS

Surgical Pathology

Facial nerve paralysis has a profound effect on patients as the ability to express his emotions is lost as a result of the paralysed face. As some lesions must be treated urgently it is important to be able to differentiate those that require immediate treatment from those where no treatment is indicated.

Facial nerve paralysis can result from damage to the facial nerve at any point along its course. Included in this is the supranuclear path of the fibres in the brainstem. A cerebrovascular accident at this level produces not only hemiparesis but also a facial nerve paralysis which is characteristic in that the forehead, which has bilateral cortical representation is spared from paralysis. However, the diagnosis in this regard is usually obvious. A lower motor neurone facial palsy may be the result of a lesion from any point from the brainstem to its peripheral destination. The common causes are listed in *Table* 30.1.

Table 30.1 Causes of facial nerve paralysis

Traumatic	Temporal bone fracture following surgery to the ear or parotid facial lacerations
Infective	Viral—herpes zoster 'Ramsay Hunt syndrome'. Bacterial—otitis media, cholesteatoma
Tumours	Benign—cerebellopontine angle tumours, acoustic neuroma, meningioma Malignant—carcinoma of the middle ear, malignant parotid tumours
Idiopathic	Bell's palsy

Management

In managing a patient with a facial palsy it is of the utmost importance to exclude treatable causes before making a diagnosis of 'Bell's palsy'.

History

Obvious diagnosis such as temple bone fracture, past history of ear infections or the presence of a lump in the parotid gland, will help establish the diagnosis. Note should also be taken of symptoms relating to the various divisions of the facial nerve (*Table* 30.2).

Examination

Clinical examination of the ear for cholesteatoma or carcinoma will show an obvious abnormality and a specialist's urgent attention should be sought. A lump in the parotid gland should not pose any diagnostic problems regarding the aetiology of the facial paralysis as it is almost certainly a malignant tumour. If the ear drum looks intact, look for vesicles as seen with a herpes zoster infection, the 'Ramsay Hunt syndrome'.

Table 30.2 Facial nerve branches

Branch	*Destination*	*Symptoms*	*Test*
1. Greater superficial petrosal nerve	Lacrimal glands	Dry eye	Schrimer's tearing test
2. Nerve to stapedius	Stapedius muscle	—	Tympanometry (audiometry)
3. Chorda tympani	Taste fibres anterior 2/3 of tongue	Loss of taste. Metallic taste on tongue	Taste testing
4. Terminal branches to muscles of facial expression	Face	Paresis or palsy	Movements of face

It is important to examine the facial movements fully to assess whether there is a complete paralysis or merely a paresis and whether this has affected all the divisions of the nerve. In doing so remember always to immobilize the contralateral side of the face when testing each branch of the facial nerve, i.e. the forehead, the eye, the cheek, the lips and the chin. Difficulty may arise in the patient with a severe injury to the soft tissues of the face, e.g. Le Fort fractures of mid-face. Bruising and oedema may obscure any facial movements. Remember also to examine the parotid for a small malignant lump, the neck for metastases, intraorally for signs of disease affecting the parotid duct and also any extension of a tumour in the deep lobe of the parotid. This may be visible as a mass bulging into the pharynx usually above and behind the tonsil pushing the soft palate forward. It is of vital importance to know the onset of paralysis in relation to trauma and also whether some movement albeit slight, is present. If movement is present then undoubtedly the facial nerve is intact and it must be assumed that recovery will proceed. If after injury paralysis was delayed then likewise it can be assumed that the facial nerve is intact and recovery will occur. If paralysis is complete and was immediate following trauma or surgery it must be assumed until proven otherwise that the nerve has been divided and appropriate surgical action must be taken immediately.

Radiology

If the ear drum is intact and normal but there is a history of deafness, tinnitus and vertigo, radiographs of the internal auditory meatuses may show signs of an acoustic neuroma or a cerebellopontine angle tumour. CT scanning is diagnostic if intracranial disease is suspected.

Audiology

If an acoustic neuroma is suspected there are various sophisticated tests of hearing which can be performed which help to distinguish between hearing loss produced by diseases of the cochlea as opposed to diseases of the nerve.

Facial Nerve Function Tests

If the face is totally paralysed it may be possible to stimulate the peripheral branches of the facial nerve as they pass close to the skin as long as the nerve has not 'degenerated'. It is possible to do this scientifically using electromyography or electroneuronography. All these tests will indicate whether the injury to the nerve is a neuropraxia and recovery will be prompt and usually complete or whether the nerve has degenerated and recovery will therefore be by regeneration, take many months rather than weeks and also be incomplete. Tests of the various branches of the facial nerve may also help to indicate the site of the lesion if in the temporal bone. Further recovery of facial nerve function is first noted by the recovery of the stapedius muscle.

Treatment

Treatment if any, depends on the diagnosis. The management of cholesteatoma and tumours has already been dealt with. If herpetic infection of the geniculate ganglion and the facial nerve is suspected then treatment with acyclovir is appropriate as this improves the long-term outlook in this debilitating condition. Malignant tumours of the parotid are dealt with on their own merits according to general surgical principles in relation to the patient's age, general condition, and the presence of other metastases etc.

In traumatic facial paralysis much depends on the possible site of the lesion and the results of electrical testing.

1. Surgical laceration of the parotid

In this case it is highly likely that the nerves have been transected by the injury and immediate exploration of the parotid is required. The facial nerve trunk is found in the usual manner and the peripheral branches are also found if possible and sutured end to end. If, however, only a few divisions of the nerve have been cut it is acceptable not to explore as the muscles will reinnervate from the remaining cross-branching intact fibres of the nerve.

2. Temporal bone fracture

The onset of a facial nerve paralysis immediately following a fractured temple bone usually indicates a transverse fracture of the bone through the internal auditory meatus. Recovery is poor in these conditions so once the patient's general condition permits and with the confirmatory electrodiagnostic evidence of degeneration, an exploration of the ear is performed. Principles of surgical management in this respect are to establish the continuity of the nerve, elevate any fragments of bone which may be penetrating the nerve sheath, decompress any contused segments of the nerve and finally to graft the facial nerve if totally disrupted.

3. Bell's palsy

If no obvious cause for the facial paralysis has been found and radiology has excluded intracranial problems, then it must be assumed that the paralysis is idiopathic. There is debate as to the management of patients with this condition but 95% have a good recovery no matter what treatment. If the paralysis is complete and electrical testing suggests degeneration then a short course of steroids is exhibited. Care must always be used in the elderly, hypertensive or diabetic patient. Some prefer to decompress the facial nerve in its horizontal and vertical portions in the middle ear but there is no convincing evidence that this gives better results than steroids or indeed no treatment at all.

Facial nerve grafting

Many surgeons are now familiar with the techniques of microvascular and microneural repair using the operating microscope. In repair of the facial nerve in the temporal bone or the parotid the great auricular nerve is often used as it is in the line of incision and easily harvested. Care is taken to get sharp ends to the peripheral nerve stump and the graft before apposition with either sutures or biocompatible glue. Recovery of function takes 12–24 months. There are alternative reanimation procedures which can be used for the long-term paralysed face or in those where a facial nerve graft is not suitable. Included in this respect are fascial sling procedures, face lift procedures or anastomosis of other cranial nerves to the distal facial nerve, e.g. hypoglossal or accessory to facial anastomosis.

Summary

Most causes of facial nerve palsy are obvious and few require urgent treatment. Foul-smelling otorrhoea usually indicates cholesteatoma and vesicles on the tympanic membrane are diagnostic of the Ramsay Hunt syndrome. In the remainder electrical testing of the facial nerve will identify those whose nerves are degenerate and in whom consideration to decompression of the nerve should be given. The investigation and management of other cases are probably best dealt with by a specialist.

31 *Ocular Trauma*

Jeffrey S. Hillman

INTRODUCTION

The position of the eye on the surface of the body renders it especially vulnerable to injury both in isolation and in association with more extensive facial injury. It is important for the general surgeon to be acquainted with the range of ophthalmic injuries and to examine patients with them in mind, for delayed diagnosis and treatment will often reduce the chance of a favourable outcome with a retained and functioning eye. Failure to diagnose eye injury and refer appropriate cases for specialist management is more commonly due to failure to elicit a history, perform a simple clinical examination or measure visual acuity than to lack of specialized skills or equipment.

The eye is afforded good protection by the bony orbit, fractures of which have been considered in Chapter 26. The lids by their reflex action also offer protection but they are easily lacerated. Specialist surgical repair may be required for lacerations through the lid margin which need accurate alignment to avoid notching and for medial lid lacerations involving the lacrimal canaliculus.

Classification of eye injuries:

1. Contusion
2. Perforation
3. Foreign body
4. Chemical.

CONTUSION

The force of a large object such as a football is usually taken by the margins of the bony orbit but that of a smaller object, such as a squash ball, and the concussion wave of an explosion may be taken directly upon the globe.

Corneal Abrasion

Abrasion of the cornea is demonstrated by the instillation of a small amount of fluorescein dye from a sterile paper-impregnated strip when the area denuded of epithelium takes up the yellow stain. After extensive abrasions the single instillation of a short-acting local anaesthetic drop, e.g. benoximate, may be necessary to relieve pain and lid spasm and allow examination. Healing occurs spontaneously over 24 h and is helped by the lubricant effect of antibiotic ointment.

Hyphaema

When haemorrhage occurs into the anterior chamber between the iris and the cornea the blood is at first diffuse but later settles with a fluid level. The source of the bleeding is commonly damage to the iris root which may be torn from its attachment to the ciliary body (iridodialysis). Hyphaema indicates intraocular damage and the need for specialist examination of the intraocular contents to assess the extent of the damage and to watch for traumatic glaucoma (which may follow damage to the drainage angle of the anterior chamber). Repeated and persistent hyphaema may lead to corneal bloodstaining—a brown opacification from the absorption of haemosiderin into the corneal stroma.

Lens Displacement

Lens subluxation or dislocation is demonstrated on rapid side-to-side eye movements when the inertia of the vitreous body is transmitted by the unsupported lens to the iris causing it to wobble (iridodonesis). With subluxation it may be possible to see the curved edge of the lens crossing the pupil when the eye is examined with an ophthalmoscope set with a high + lens, e.g. +8 dioptres. After severe contusion injury, rupture of the lens capsule may cause the lens to become cataractous, the opacity appearing black against the blurred red fundal reflex when viewed with the ophthalmoscope set for lens examination.

Vitreous Haemorrhage

In mild form vitreous haemorrhage may appear as a large number of vitreous 'floaters' but when extensive it may considerably reduce visual acuity. On ophthalmoscopic examination there will be a dimness or possibly complete loss of fundal reflex and detail.

Retinal Damage

Retinal oedema (commotio retinae) appears as an area of fundal blanching usually in the lower retina when it is asymptomatic or in the macular region when there is disturbance of central vision and fall in acuity. It is usually self-limiting but occasionally the affected retina may develop degenerative changes. Haemorrhage may be found in the retina or in the preretinal space. Contusion injury may produce peripheral retinal tears which may later progress to detachment of the retina. Such tears are only seen after full dilatation of the pupil with mydriatic drops.

Choroidal Rupture

With severe contusion the choroid at the posterior pole may split along a crescentic path concentric with the disc. This is associated with degeneration of the overlying retina and will destroy central vision if the macula is involved. The exposure of the underlying sclera causes the area of rupture to appear as a white crescent.

Avulsion of the Optic Nerve

The optic nerve may be torn from its attachment at the posterior pole by a sudden violent rotatory movement of the eye or a sudden increase in intraocular pressure may expel the nerve like a cork from a bottle. The disc is replaced by a deep white hole and visual loss is profound. Fundal view is usually obscured by extensive vitreous haemorrhage.

Globe Rupture

The globe may be ruptured by a severe contusion injury with a small hard object such as a golf ball. The rupture may be seen across the cornea or may be confined to the posterior segment of the globe when it will not be visible on external examination. Visual acuity will be markedly reduced and the eye will appear collapsed often with vitreous haemorrhage. Intraocular pressure will be low when compared with the fellow eye but this should be assessed with extreme caution if damage is not to be increased.

PERFORATION

Perforation of the eye may be purely corneal or scleral or may cross the limbus to be corneoscleral. It may occur with or without lid injury and it is important to be aware that a small and apparently insignificant lid wound may overlie a serious perforation of the underlying globe which will be missed unless specifically looked for. This is a special risk in the case of injury with a dart or glass spicule from a shattered windscreen. Most perforating injuries have a wound which is easily visible but the small wound of a dart may require examination with a slit lamp microscope for confirmation. Visual acuity is usually impaired and intraocular pressure reduced but the latter should be assessed only with the same strict caution as in suspected globe rupture. All eyes with perforating injuries should be radiographed to exclude an intraocular foreign body.

Corneal Perforation

The cornea adjacent to a laceration often appears opalescent from corneal oedema especially if some hours old. Prolapse of the iris via the wound is common and this distorts the pupil giving a peak which 'points' to the wound. Hyphaema will be present to a varying degree depending upon the amount of damage to iris and ciliary body. Shallowness of the anterior chamber from loss of aqueous may be identified by comparison with the fellow eye. Mild damage to the lens may cause localized opacification visible with the ophthalmoscope set with a high + lens. This may be stationary or may progress slowly to full opacification of the lens (cataract). Disruption of the anterior lens capsule will release flocculent white lens matter into the anterior chamber with immediate cataract formation.

Conjunctival Laceration

In all conjunctival lacerations it is important to exclude an underlying scleral perforation and this may need wound exploration under local anaesthetic drops or general anaesthetic.

Scleral Perforation

The overlying conjunctiva will be lacerated and haemorrhagic. Within the lips of the wound appears darkly pigmented choroid and through the wound may be found prolapsing vitreous gel. External haemorrhage from the choroid or ciliary body is common and may be profuse and internal haemorrhage into the vitreous will interfere with the ophthalmoscopic view of the fundus and reduce visual acuity. The retina may be detached by direct trauma or by subretinal haemorrhage.

Sympathetic Ophthalmitis

This is a rare but serious complication of perforating eye injury in which uveal tissue (iris, ciliary body or choroid) has been damaged or entrapped in the wound. An autoimmune hypersensitivity develops to the patient's own uveal pigment giving a severe chronic granulomatous uveitis in both the injured and the fellow eye appearing some weeks or months after injury. Sight may be lost in both eyes. The fellow eye is almost completely protected by enucleation of the injured eye within 14 days of injury and so a decision has to be made at about the tenth day whether to retain or enucleate the injured eye. The serious risks of sympathetic ophthalmitis have to be balanced against the apparent visual potential of the injured eye and for this reason blind perforated eyes are usually ultimately removed. If there is delay in the diagnosis and repair of a perforating injury then the poor appearance of the eye at this time of assessment carries a correspondingly greater chance that prophylactic enucleation will be considered necessary. The incidence of this complication has been reduced by prompt and meticulous wound toilet and closure and the outcome improved by control with long-term systemic steroids should signs of uveitis appear in the fellow eye. Enucleation of the excitor eye at the stage of sympathetic ophthalmitis often fails to halt the process.

FOREIGN BODY

The history of the nature of injury is particularly important in the diagnosis of intraocular foreign body as the entry wound is often small and the immediate effect upon visual acuity not marked. Delayed diagnosis is commonly the subject of litigation. Radiography is essential in all cases where there is the least reason to suspect foreign body and especially when there is a history of something striking the eye whilst hammering.

The site of entry may be scleral or corneal and may require slit-lamp microscope examination for its detection. The foreign body may come to rest anywhere along its track depending upon its size and velocity and a small, high-velocity particle may give a double perforation to arrest in the orbital tissues. When the foreign body lies within the cornea or anterior chamber or in the iris it may be easily visible on direct inspection. Arrest within or passage through the lens may immediately produce a localized opacity which may spread throughout the lens over following weeks to produce a mature cataract. On entering the posterior compartment the foreign body may lie in the vitreous or impale the posterior wall of the eye when vitreous haemorrhage may result from retinal or choroidal vascular damage. Full pupil dilatation is essential for examination of the lens, including that part which is normally hidden by the iris, and for examination of the fundus. Gross intraocular infection is uncommon with an intraocular foreign body because of the sterilizing effect of frictional heat developed on passage through the air, but antibiotic cover and antitetanus prophylaxis are routine.

The presence of a missed intraocular foreign body may become evident by the development of later complications. The most common reason for the patient to return for reassessment is a gradual fall in visual acuity with the development of cataract. With retained metal intraocular foreign bodies, particular syndromes may develop depending upon the composition of the metal.

Siderosis

This is a delayed response to the retention of an iron-containing foreign body. Chemical dispersion occurs within the eye and a small foreign body may have dissolved by the time that siderosis is established. Brown iron staining occurs within the cornea, the iris and in the capsule of the lens which subsequently opacifies. Iron deposition within the peripheral retina leads to degeneration with depression of the electroretinogram and gradual failure of vision. Late removal of the foreign body may fail to halt the siderosis.

Chalcosis

A retained foreign body containing a high percentage of copper induces an acute suppurative inflammatory reaction which is highly destructive to the eye. If the copper content is lower then gradual dispersal of copper throughout the eye produces chalcosis. The cornea develops a blue-green deep peripheral ring and the lens develops a sunflower-shaped opacity, both similar to the appearances found in hepatolenticular degeneration. The iris assumes a greenish hue and brown particles may be seen on slit-lamp microscope examination of the vitreous. In the retina lustrous deposits have occasionally been described along the retinal vessels. The fall in vision associated with chalcosis is largely due to the lens changes.

CHEMICAL INJURY

The effects of harmful chemicals upon the eye depend upon the nature of the chemical as well as the duration and degree of contact and with the ease of penetration. Some agents have a predominantly surface action whilst others exert their main effects after penetrating the eye. The corneal epithelium offers a barrier to water-soluble molecules and the stroma offers a barrier to fat-soluble molecules but those molecules with both hydrophilic and lipophilic components cross the cornea with relative ease.

The range of potentially harmful chemicals used in the home, in industry and in agriculture, together with those used deliberately to cause injury in the pursuit of crime or warfare, is vast. Some specific agents merit particular attention.

Strong Acids

These have a strong surface action producing an immediate chemical burn with coagulation of the epithelium in the affected area—usually the lower cornea and conjunctiva because of the protective upward rolling of the eye. Penetration is often not marked.

Strong Alkalis

These produce more severe injuries than acids because of penetration associated with the destruction of cell membranes and their action continues for some time after the injury. Clinically they produce conjunctival epithelial loss and oedema and corneal ulceration and opacification. Burns with powdered lime or lime-containing plaster have a prolonged corrosive action if all contaminating particulate matter is not meticulously removed from the conjunctival sac

Ammonia

This is one of the most damaging chemical agents and is widely used as a refrigerating agent in freezers, as a cleansing agent and increasingly as an immobilizing weapon for criminal purposes. It produces marked conjunctival and corneal oedema which progresses to scarring and has a high penetration rate causing gross intraocular damage which often destroys the eye.

The general principles involved in the emergency management of chemical injury are the rapid dilution and removal and in some cases neutralization of the chemical. Prolonged irrigation (for 5–10 min timed by a clock) should be instituted as soon as possible, preferably at the place of injury rather than delay whilst awaiting transfer to an accident or ophthalmic unit. On arrival at such a unit the irrigation should be repeated without delay. Water is a suitable irrigating fluid and special buffered irrigating fluid is preferable only if it can be obtained in adequate quantity and without delay. The further management after irrigation requires specialist ophthalmic care and depends upon the nature of the chemical.

Section 4

Neurosurgery

32 Principles of Pathophysiology, Diagnosis and Management

H. Alan Crockard

INTRODUCTION

For many general surgeons and physicians, neurological signs, epilepsy, coma and neural trauma, produce concern and irrational fear which is only a fraction below that of the population at large, yet these same persons diagnose and treat cardiogenic shock, oesophageal varices and hepatorenal failure. Part of the problem has been a preservation of neurological mysticism but a greater fault has been ignorance of basic pathophysiological mechanisms which produce the neurological signs and which can be ameliorated in many instances by the attention to first aid details. Of course there are many fine points of neurology which require the very keenest diagnostic acumen but it is vitally important for patient management that those involved in their care recognize symptoms and signs which are caused by lesions requiring urgent medical or surgical intervention. Sometimes neurological signs and symptoms appear rapidly and the patient obviously deteriorates; on other occasions the complaint may have been present for many years. Thus, another basic requirement apart from the appreciation of various combinations of symptoms and signs, is the ability to recognize those which require urgent attention and those where minutes or hours are not so important. A patient may have epileptic seizures about once a month for 10 years but a totally different complexion on the disease process is provided by the additional history of morning headaches associated with vomiting and increasingly blurred vision. It will not be the purpose of this section to act as a small neurological and neurosurgical textbook; rather the authors have attempted to emphasize common neurological and neurosurgical problems encountered in normal surgical practice and to outline the primary care of these conditions as well as explaining the basis of the modern neurosurgical approach to the disease.

Neurological science is rapidly expanding and the authors have attempted to indicate possible lines of progress in the understanding and treatment of the disease processes. If symptoms and signs are learned by heart their retention may be tenuous; for that reason the basic pathophysiology responsible for the symptoms and signs will be explained. The aims of therapy, methods of investigation, the various types of surgical procedure, postoperative care and complications will also be covered in this first chapter, while the succeeding chapters will concentrate on specific neurosurgical problems. These occur in every branch of medical practice and another purpose of this section is to emphasize that the further improvement and widening scope of patient care can only come about by cross-fertilization between various specialties.

PATHOPHYSIOLOGY

Intracranial Contents

The non-compressible intracranial contents are housed within a semiclosed box, the cranium. There are 700–900 ml of glia, 500–600 ml of neuronal tissue and these constitute the bulk of the intracranial contents. Blood (100–150 ml) two-thirds of which is on the venous side, cerebrospinal fluid (100 ml) and extracellular fluid (75 ml) are important, apart from their nutritive functions to the neuroglial mass, by the fact that their volume can be altered to accommodate increasing 'brain' mass due to tumour or brain swelling. This ability to alter their volumes to accommodate changes in other compartments is referred to as *compliance*. Without this ability, an increase of 1 ml in intracranial volume would effectively raise intracranial pressure by 200 mmHg. Compliance is not infinite, however, and eventually a change in volume of any of the intracranial constituents results in a rise in pressure (*Fig.* 32.1).

Intracranial Pressure

Intracranial pressure (ICP) is not a static measurement as suggested by the recording of an individual lumbar puncture pressure, but varies with respiratory cycle and the systolic/diastolic changes in blood pressure. Any rise in intrathoracic or intra-abdominal pressure is transmitted directly to the cranial contents via the neck veins and the dural venous sinuses, which are devoid of valves. The position of the head relative to the rest of the body will also have a profound effect on ICP. For all these variations and fluctuations, however, the normal ICP is about 10 mmHg (130–150 mm H_2O) when the subject is lying down but when standing may be negative. In health and when the patient is lying horizontally on his side the pressure in the lumbar theca will approximate to that in the cisterna magna and the lateral ventricles. Careful measurement, however, with accurate instruments will show a slight gradient of pressure from the ventricles to the lumbar theca but the variation is extremely small. If there is a spinal cord tumour, a mass in the posterior fossa, or an obstruction along the CSF pathways

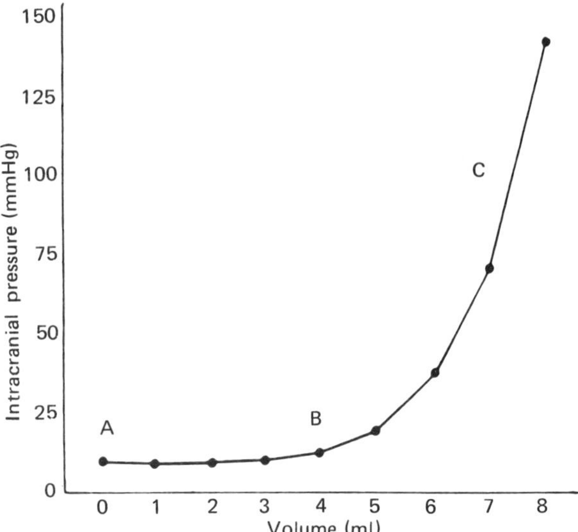

Fig. 32.1 The pressure/volume curve illustrates the changes of volume which may occur with no increase in pressure (A–B). Beyond the point of inflexion (B) a slight volume change is associated with marked pressure variation. Patients with tumours, head injuries, or strokes must be treated as if they have no compliance (B–C).

then pressure differentials develop within the CSF pathways and lumbar puncture pressure is not only dangerous to perform but erroneous in result. The most accurate and informative method of assessing ICP is by attaching a ventricular catheter inserted through a burr hole to a pressure transducer, and using this technique, it is possible to detect raised pressure associated with tumours or head injuries or the effects of anaesthetic inhalational agents. The addition of carbon dioxide to the inhaled gas mixtures will dilate intracranial blood vessels, raise the intracranial volume and possibly increase ICP. The expansion of an intracranial haematoma or the acute obstruction of the CSF pathways will also increase one of the volumes with a shift to the right along the pressure volume curve (*Fig.* 32.1), eventually exhausting the compensating mechanisms and causing a rise in ICP. Normally there is a great difference between mean arterial blood pressure and intracranial pressure so that the cerebral perfusion pressure is always more than adequate to allow for adequate perfusion of the cerebral capillaries. However, on the decompensated part of the pressure volume curve a slight change in intracranial volume may produce a large change in ICP and produces either focally or generally a reduction in cerebral perfusion. This, in turn, will produce oedema, increasing brain bulk, further raising the ICP and establishing a vicious circle.

The pressure may not be raised continuously or may appear to be normal until the arterial carbon dioxide level changes or the patient raises his intracranial blood volume by coughing (*Fig.* 32.2). In such a situation the patient may have a normal ICP for most of the time, but 'moves' along the pressure volume curve to the decompensation point and beyond during coughing or increased carbon dioxide tension due to a pneumonia. Thus the pressure volume curve of compliance is fundamental to the understanding of the rapidly changing levels of consciousness in the patient with intracranial pathology.

Brain Shift and Herniation

Elevated ICP, if severe, will compromise the circulation in the supra- and infratentorial compartments and if the latter is affected, the resultant medullary ischaemia will produce a rise in systemic blood pressure, a bradycardia and a slowing of the respiratory rate (the Cushing response). It is also associated with increased drowsiness. If there is a rise in the pressure in the supratentorial compartment relative to the posterior fossa or if the pressure in the posterior fossa exceeds that in the cervical spine, then portions of brain may herniate downwards and impact the tentorial opening or foramen magnum. Tentorial herniation, in which the uncus of the temporal lobe is forced into the tentorial opening, occludes the posterior cerebral arteries and compresses the third nerve as well as producing midbrain ischaemia. At the foramen magnum, the cerebellar tonsils may be impacted in the craniocervical junction producing signs of medullary failure. Injudicious lumbar puncturing in the presence of papilloedema for a tumour, or chronic subdural abscess may convert a moderate diffusely elevated pressure problem into one of a pressure gradient across the tentorium or at the foramen magnum and causing a dramatic and often irreparable deterioration in the patient's condition. In the supra-

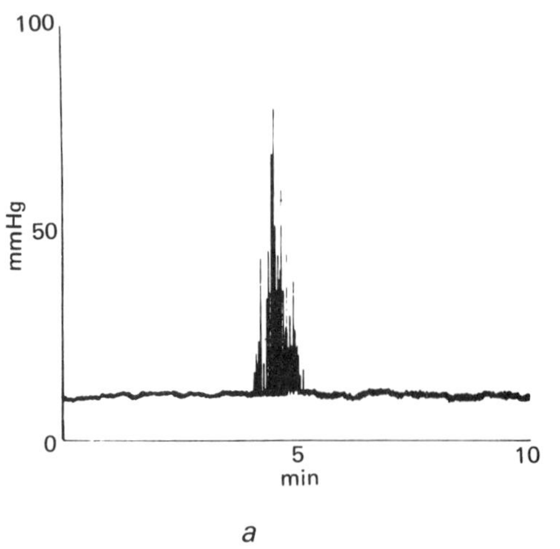

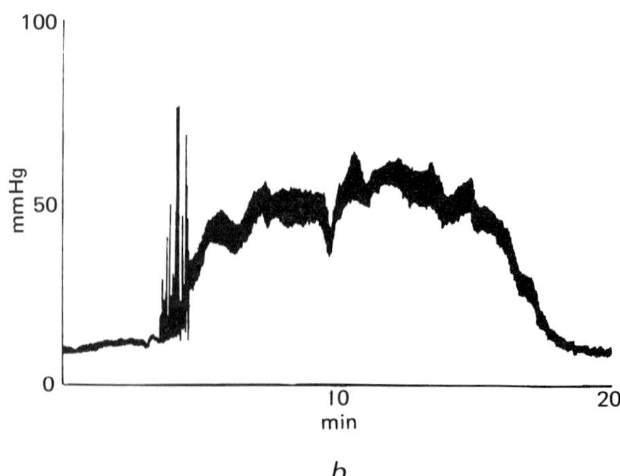

Fig. 32.2 *a*, The effect of coughing on normal intracranial pressure is transient. *b*, A patient at or beyond the point B on the pressure/volume curve (*Fig. 32.1*) may seriously impair cerebral perfusion by coughing.

tentorial compartment, if a tumour or haematoma expands in one cerebral hemisphere it will cause brain distortion. With the associated raised pressure, there may be unilateral uncal herniation and compression of the midbrain against the tentorial opening on the opposite side which is clinically manifest by clouding of the level of consciousness, dilatation of the pupil on the side of the lesion due to the third nerve compression and a hemiparesis on the opposite side (most usually) or the same side (occasionally). This latter phenomenon of ipsilateral hemiparesis is a 'false localizing sign' due to the tentorial compression of the cerebral peduncle on the side opposite to the compressing mass.

Cerebrospinal Fluid Pathways and Circulation

Most of the CSF is manufactured by the choroid plexus, the rest is the bulk flow of extracellular fluid produced in the microcirculation and draining into the ventricular system. The choroid plexus is situated in the lateral, third and fourth ventricles with the most in the bodies of the lateral ventricles. CSF formation and its flow are dependent on a pressure gradient; the fluid passes from both lateral ventricles through the third and the aqueduct of Sylvius into the fourth ventricle and then into the subarachnoid space. Most of the fluid is absorbed by the arachnoid granulations which abut into the sagittal sinus, but about 20% is absorbed along the nerve root sheaths in the spine. The absorption of CSF, like its production, is pressure-dependent and both these factors make the estimation of the total manufacture of CSF in any time period difficult but it is thought to be about 500 ml/day. If the balance between production and absorption is altered or there is a block in the CSF pathways at any level a problem will develop. *Hydrocephalus* is the term used to describe the excessive accumulation of CSF within the head. It may be due to an overproduction of CSF such as by the rare choroid plexus papilloma; usually it is due to obstruction in the CSF pathways in the aqueduct of Sylvius, at the outlet of the fourth ventricle or externally between the midbrain and the tentorium as a result of infection, trauma, congenital defects, or distortion produced by tumours or cysts. Impairment of the absorptive properties of the arachnoid granulations due to infection or blockage with blood breakdown products will also produce the condition. In the author's understanding it is always associated with a persistent or intermittently raised pressure no matter how small; 'hydrocephalus ex vacuo', is a misnomer for cerebral atrophy and use of the term to cover non-pressure situations has produced confusion. This is not to say that the obstructed CSF may not find alternative routes for absorption; some children for instance, with aqueduct stenosis may not need treatment or may require only intermittent drainage.

The effects of the condition will depend on how complete the obstruction is and how rapid its onset. The sudden obstruction of the aqueduct by a clot may produce coma in less than 12 h, whereas the patient with normal pressure hydrocephalus may present months or years after the onset. In childhood, an expanding head may be the first clue, but in the adult increasing drowsiness, ataxia and incontinence may be the first indications of the development of the condition. As the ventricles continue to expand, the supratentorial compartment enlarges, compressing the midbrain against the tentorial notch, affecting the quadrigeminal plate, resulting in loss of upward gaze, and, in the advanced condition, the 'sunset eyes' of the late hydrocephalic child. An intraventricular tumour may produce local ventricular dilatation behind it, resulting in unilateral expansion, distortion and brain shift. Obstruction in the fourth ventricle may produce cerebellar tonsillar herniation in the same way as supratentorial expansion may result in uncal herniation at the tentorium. The prolonged effects of hydrocephalus are white matter damage, neuronal loss, cranial nerve palsies, pituitary and hypothalamic damage, idiocy, paraplegia and tetraplegia. A rarer complication of CSF pathway obstruction is *syringomyelia* due to the expansion of the spinal central canal. It is often associated with the Arnold–Chiari malformation which predisposes to obstruction at the foramen magnum but may also occur distal to an intramedullary cord tumour or as a late effect of spinal cord trauma.

Cerebral Blood Flow and Metabolism

One-fifth of the cardiac output is directed to supply the brain's metabolic needs which are almost exclusively aerobic and therefore require high glucose and oxygen inputs. The removal of waste products and the lactic acid produced by the anaerobic glycolysis is an equally important function of cerebral blood flow. In the normal state, flow is directly related to metabolic requirements; thus the grey matter has a flow four times that of white matter and at the level of the microcirculation, fluctuations in flow are produced by extracellular pH changes; the accumulation of lactic acid will lower pH and dilate the arterioles. Blood carbon dioxide levels act through the same mechanism and its accumulation results in a cerebral vasodilatation. Less than 2% of the energy requirement for normal neuronal function can be derived from sources other than aerobic glycolysis and thus the maintenance of an adequate flow to the brain is a priority. The normal cerebral blood flow of about 50 ml/100 g/min is remarkably constant over a wide range of blood pressure, intracranial pressure and blood oxygen levels in the normal situation and this ability to control its blood supply is referred to as *autoregulation*. One of the first effects of trauma, infection, tumour or stroke is to abolish this control either focally in the area of the lesion or generally to the whole brain; thus the supply of blood becomes dependent on systemic blood pressure and cardiac output. Even so, there are wide tolerances built into the system and normal cellular function, as judged by electrical activity, may still exist at reduced cerebral blood flow until a critical point at around 20 ml/100 g/min, when electrical activity ceases. The cells may still survive, however, but if the blood flow drops below 8 or 10 ml/100 g/min, cell membranes are disrupted and recovery is not possible. These blood flow values apply to grey matter; those for white matter are very much lower, but as death of the neuronal body will result in the demise of the axon, these higher flow values must be considered to be the critical levels below which flow may not drop without serious consequences. Obviously the same effects may be produced by lack of oxygen or glucose.

Another factor which is important in the understanding of cerebral pathophysiology is the normal function of the capillary bed. According to Starling's Law a pressure drop of about 20 mmHg between the arterial and venous ends is required for the normal function of the microcirculation. As with the blood flow, there is a very adequate safety margin in the normal situation with a 90 mmHg differential between arteries and veins, the terminal arterioles reducing this to about 30 mmHg. A reduction in the blood pressure, as with a cardiac arrest or a rise in venous pressure due to venous thrombosis, airway obstruction or a general rise in intracranial pressure due to diffuse oedema or a cerebral tumour, will upset this homoeostasis and prevent normal microvascular function. The blood–brain barrier will break down, extracellular fluid will accumulate producing a further rise in local pressure and a vicious circle ensues. This phenomenon may occur focally, as around a tumour, producing focal oedema, or develop generally as after a cardiac arrest or an anoxic episode. After such a mishap it is vitally important to realize that the normal homoeostatic mechanisms such as autoregulation and normal microcirculatory functions are no longer present and that cell survival is dependent on an adequate blood pressure, a reduction in intracranial pressure, the maintenance of normal or higher than normal blood oxygen levels with a reduction in carbon dioxide. Hypercapnia which can easily be tolerated in the normal situation may result in 'steal' phenomenon around an infarct or tumour, further worsening the situation, and is the explanation of the frequently observed clinical picture of neurological deterioration in the presence of chest infection in the unconscious patient.

Brain Swelling and Oedema

After trauma, cardiac arrest or an anoxic episode, the loss of autoregulation allows a greater than normal volume of blood to circulate through the head owing to vasoparalysis. As mentioned earlier, this will result in a raised intracranial pressure, and if one could examine the brain in the living individual with this condition it would appear to be very swollen, although measurements of the brain tissue itself would suggest that at this stage there is little or no oedema. This is the stage of brain swelling which may subside with little sign of oedema. The situation is rarely so simple and there may be areas of contusion, laceration or ischaemia which develop brain oedema and the water content of the brain itself increases. Following head injury, with the breakdown in blood–brain barrier, intravascular fluid is extravasated into the extracellular compartment resulting in vasogenic oedema. Damaged astrocytes may accumulate water intracellularly and this is known as cytotoxic oedema. Ischaemic oedema may contain vasogenic and cytotoxic elements. Anti-oedema agents will be of little value in brain swelling as the increase in brain volume is due to an expansion of the vascular compartment. Steroid therapy has been shown to be useful in peri-tumour or peri-infarct oedema but not in trauma.

Neuroendocrine Problems

Because of the association of the hypothalamus and pituitary, abnormalities in the area may not only produce endocrine problems, but also signs of raised intracranial pressure, epilepsy, chiasmal compression or hydrocephalus and endocrine diseases. With increasing awareness and more sophisticated tests, the detection of microadenomas producing prolactin and other hormones causing a secondary amenorrhoea and galactorrhoea must be considered by every clinician.

Lesions around the hypothalamus will affect the appetite, temperature and mood as well as interfering with the drainage of CSF. The hormonal imbalances themselves may result in abnormal mental states and the expansion of the tumour if such there be, may also produce mental changes.

Apart from the specific hormone releases from the hypothalamus and pituitary, current research is emphasizing more and more the endocrine status of the whole brain. The discovery of endorphins and their role in the modification and appreciation of pain in the last few years has been a classic example, and further research has shown that these same substances also modulate hypothalamic and pituitary functions. The presence and function of acetylcholine, noradrenaline and gamma-aminobutyric acid are well known but other substances such as prostaglandins, vasoactive substances and the biogenic amines are found in varying quantities throughout the brain and increasingly the concept is being accepted that these chemical transmitters modulate neural function. The neurosurgeon has little defence against the friendly gibe of the endocrinologist that the brain is one of the body's major endocrine organs.

SURGICAL NEUROLOGY

It is not within the scope of this book to go into every neurological sign, rather the purpose is to draw attention to various symptoms and signs which may point to a condition requiring acute therapeutic intervention. As with the abdomen or the thorax, one symptom or sign taken in isolation is rarely as important as a combination, thus headache by itself or vomiting in isolation or the occasional complaint of blurred vision may not amount to anything of significance but, taken as a combination, they require investigation to exclude raised ICP. The rate of change of symptoms and signs, that is, the speed of onset or the rate of development, again is more important than the intensity of any one symptom. The rapid expansion of a small intracranial haematoma may soon render the patient senseless while the slowly growing meningioma, which has been present for 10 years, may assume massive proportions before clinical suspicions are raised.

The production of clinical signs and symptoms is a complex matter and depends on the organization of the nervous system with more sophisticated and complex controls being superimposed on a simple reflex arc. The most obvious example of this is the difference between an upper and lower motor neurone lesion, for instance damage to anterior horn cells or motor root results in a flaccid weakness in the affected muscle. However, if the upper motor neurone above the anterior horn cell is involved, the muscle may not function with voluntary control but there is increased tone in the affected muscle due to the unchecked activity of extrapyramidal reticular fibres which also influence the anterior horn cell. A cerebellar lesion may produce an apparent weakness of the muscle but more obviously an uncoordinated movement because of its ability to convert the desired movement into an accurate and smoothly performed function. Interruption of the sensory input at any level will also affect the 'biofeedback loops' and prevent an accurate movement of the limb, say, without visual supervision. Finally, lesions in the frontal cortex may abolish any desire to move the arm and result in apparent paralysis to all except noxious stimuli. In higher mental functions this also pertains, so that the most recently acquired and complex skills may be the first to disappear after diffuse injury or infection and the last to return. Epilepsy may be regarded as the surfacing of normally inhibited, inappropriate electrical activity which may develop as a result of an irritative focus and whose manifestations will depend on the site of the focus as well as its spread throughout the brain. Unconsciousness and alertness, sleep and wakefulness are highly complex neurophysiological phenomena influenced by a vast number of factors affecting the reticular system in the midbrain and brain stem. The essence of diagnosis, therefore, must be the pinpointing of the site or sites of the lesion before appropriate diagnostic and therapeutic action can be undertaken.

Alteration in Consciousness

One of the most frequent problems encountered by the clinician is to decide whether a patient is normally responding and fully aware of his surroundings and the problem is equalled by the difficulty in conveying to his colleagues exactly what he means by the descriptive terms used in his account of the patient's condition. Terms like 'semi-conscious', 'semi-comatose' and 'stuporose' have vastly differing meanings to different persons and so it is important to tabulate exactly what the clinician finds. *Fully conscious implies being fully aware of and interacting in an appropriate fashion to one's environment.* The patient may, however, have an organic mental state which though allowing him to be conscious, impairs his intellect, his personality or his memory. If he is not fully conscious, the clinician must ask himself how unconscious. The Glasgow Coma scale (*Table* 32.1) and the classic textbook by Plum and Posner are useful guides. They have chosen five levels of 'coma' ranging from drowsiness, response to verbal commands, flexion to painful stimuli, extension to painful stimuli and no response to painful stimuli. The description of the clinical state must be followed by a search for the cause. Has the patient got a neurological disease or a metabolic disease? Is there any suggestion of drug or alcohol ingestion? Is there any chest disease or cardiovascular illness which would result in diminished cerebral perfusion? Most important, too, is the determination of whether the level of consciousness is improving or deteriorating.

Table 32.1 Assessment of level of consciousness using the Glasgow Coma Scale

Eye opening		
Spontaneous	4	E
To speech	3	
To pain	2	
Nil	1	
Best motor response		
Obeys	6	M
Localizes	5	
Withdraws (flexion)	4	
Abnormal flexion	3	
Extensor response	2	
Nil	1	
Verbal response		
Orientated	5	V
Confused conversation	4	
Inappropriate words	3	
Incomprehensible sounds	2	
Nil	1	
Coma score (responsiveness sum = 3–15 (E + M + V))		

Epilepsy

The generalized convulsion of grand mal seizure may be provoked by a wide variety of intracranial pathology, metabolic disease or cardiorespiratory difficulties and may not help in the localization of the condition. Focal epilepsy or Jacksonian fits, where consciousness is not lost and the seizure affects the face or arm, etc., may provide the clinician with a clue as to the site of the lesion responsible for the phenomenon. Unusual epigastric sensations, peculiar sense of taste in the mouth or smell, the feeling of being in a familiar place or situation (*déjà vu*) may indicate the temporal lobe as the site of the lesion. There are obviously many manifestations of epileptic phenomena which are beyond the scope of this section; it is important for the clinician when confronted with an unusual phenomenon to ask himself, 'Is it epileptic?' 'Is it ischaemic?' 'Is it hysterical?'

Raised Intracranial Pressure

There are many causes of raised intracranial pressure and while mention has already been made of the cardinal signs, the diagnosis and treatment are so important that its features are reiterated. Altered consciousness may be one of the later signs associated with raised intracranial pressure but the patient may have a preceding history of headaches, worse in the morning (as the condition progresses waking the patient) and associated with vomiting. Later, blurring of vision, difficulty in focusing, or a visual field defect may be noted. The patient may have difficulty with memory, or a change in personality. In the child, the parents may have noticed a truncal ataxia or unsteadiness on its feet, there may occasionally be some neck rigidity and increased tone in all the limbs. Examination must always include fundoscopy to detect papilloedema and retinal haemorrhages. Acutely raised intracranial pressure may present with the signs of tentorial or foramen magnum herniation. Plain radiographs of the skull may show signs of prolonged or chronically raised ICP such as copper beating, erosion of the dorsum sellae, widening of the sutures, pineal shift or extraneous calcification.

Spinal Cord Compression

The three cardinal signs of cord compression as a result of extradural compression by a disc or a tumour or by the expansion of intradural cyst or tumour compressing the cord or a spinal tumour itself are the history and signs of sensory changes, limb weakness and sphincter disturbances. In the acute situation all three may occur together but in the slowly progressive condition there is usually a clue in the history as to whether the lesion is extradural or intradural. The former often presents with pain or paraesthesia of some duration followed by loss of muscle power and finally bladder disturbance. This latter function is controlled by fibres which lie in the most central part of the cord and thus intramedullary lesions, i.e. lesions within the spinal cord itself, may present with bladder dysfunction at an early stage. *It is important to realize that once the stage of loss of sphincters has been passed, the chances of cord recovery following surgical decompression are limited.* It is important, therefore, to suspect and diagnose it at as early a stage as possible. Plain radiographs of the spine may show erosions of the pedicle, collapsed vertebrae, a kyphos, or a soft-tissue mass associated with the vertebral body destruction.

Localization

a. Cranial Nerves

The cranial nerves may be involved in an intracranial mass or in a fracture along the base of the skull and thus a knowledge of their distribution is helpful in localization. Loss of sense of smell, for instance, may be associated with fractures of the anterior fossa, with a CSF fistula following trauma, or meningiomas of the olfactory groove, but these are relatively rare compared to the frequency of involvement of the optic nerve, the optic chiasma and the optic radiation in intracranial pathology. The nerves associated with eye movements are also closely involved both anatomically and in response to damage of the second cranial nerve. Deteriorating visual acuity may indicate increasing papilloedema, progressive optic atrophy, or macular degeneration; examination of the visual fields is of the utmost importance. A bitemporal visual field loss suggests a pituitary lesion while a homonymous hemianopia indicates damage in the optic radiation or occipital cortex. Quadrantanopia, i.e. loss of a quadrant of vision, may be easily missed and so all four quadrants must be carefully tested. Scotomas may also indicate intracranial pathology but are more usually due to intraocular conditions. Reactions of the pupils, conjugate eye movements and the ability to accommodate are complete neurological functions which require the function of several cranial nerves as well as midbrain structures. Unequal pupils or a dilating pupil on one side may indicate compression of the ipsilateral third nerve by uncal herniation into the tentorium. In traumatic cases, however, it is well to remember that direct injury to the eye can lead to a traumatic mydriasis which may be incorrectly thought to be due to third nerve compression from uncal herniation. The sixth cranial nerve is particularly vulnerable to raised intracranial pressure as it has the longest intracranial course and a lateral gaze palsy will result. Conjugate upward and downward eye movements are controlled from the midbrain and loss of upward eye gaze may indicate tentorial compression in hydrocephalus or a midbrain lesion. Within the cavernous sinus run the third, fourth, sixth and branch of the fifth cranial nerves and with the cavernous sinus syndrome all are, to some extent, affected. The cerebellopontine angle is another area where a group of cranial nerves may be affected by the same lesion and so the fifth, seventh and eighth may be, to some extent, involved with the progression of an acoustic neuroma. Brainstem lesions often present with one or more of the lower cranial nerves involved unilaterally or bilaterally with loss of palatal and gag reflexes.

b. Supratentorial Lesions

Half of the patients who present with supratentorial lesions may have a history of epilepsy or present with a seizure but there are other signs which may indicate which particular area is involved, such as occipital, parietal, temporal or frontal, depending on which function is affected. Dysphasia obviously occurs in lesions around the Sylvian fissure on the dominant hemisphere. Mental confusion may point to a frontal defect. A parietal lobe defect, apart from weakness, may demonstrate signs of disturbed body image where the patient may not be able to identify correctly the position of a contralateral limb with closed eyes and may not be able to process the information coming from two simultaneously touched areas of the body on opposite sides (sensory extinction). Asked to draw a clock, the patient may be quite unable to do so.

c. Infratentorial Lesions

Infratentorial lesions often present with signs of raised intracranial pressure as the aqueduct, the fourth ventricle or the tentorium is quickly obstructed by an expanding mass. Cranial nerves are often involved at an early stage. Lesions in the cerebellum, particularly in the midline, will result in ataxia, and nystagmus is very often present.

PRINCIPLES OF THERAPY

The Unconscious Patient

Careful repeated observations and nursing of the highest quality must be the minimum requirement in the management of neurosurgical patients. Attention to the airway in the unconscious patient is absolutely essential; with careful monitoring of the vital signs it is common experience to observe marked changes in level of consciousness, limb responses to painful stimuli, etc. in response to small changes in arterial oxygen and carbon dioxide and fluctuations in blood pressure. Thus the most important part of the therapeutic management of neurosurgical patients must be the maintenance of an adequate cerebral perfusion pressure, adequate oxygenation or hyperoxia and arterial carbon dioxide levels at or below normal levels. Unless an endotracheal tube is in position, patients should be nursed in the three-quarter prone position so that oropharyngeal secretions can drip out of the mouth; if possible an oropharyngeal airway should be strapped in position. Frequent chest physiotherapy, humidification of the inspired gases and tracheal toilet are absolutely essential. Restlessness in the unconscious patient may be due to the distended bladder, the undetected or untreated fracture and attention to these factors may greatly reduce the restlessness. A bed with padded cot sides should be used in preference to limb restraint which adds to the patient's confusion and restlessness. A nasogastric tube may be passed to decompress the gastrointestinal system in the presence of paralytic ileus; once gastric function has returned, the same tube may be used to supply the patient's fluid and calorie requirements. In the early stages careful fluid replacement may be supplied by the intravenous route using 5% dextrose or Hartmann's solution but not isotonic saline; it is absolutely essential to avoid overhydration and excess Na^+ intake as this will increase cerebral oedema. The patient should be turned at least 4-hourly with attention to pressure areas. Care should be taken to prevent corneal abrasions and a wise precaution is to apply antibiotic impregnated ointment regularly. Mouth care is absolutely essential and the fact that parotitis is such a rare problem in neurosurgical units nowadays is a tribute to the high nursing care.

The Paralysed Patient

Care of the quadriplegic or paraplegic patient is another situation demanding the highest nursing care and attention to small detail, if the patient is not to succumb to intercurrent infections and bed sores. All the anaesthetic skin must be treated with the utmost care, pressure areas must be carefully treated and the patient moved frequently to prevent pressure sores. In traumatic paraplegia or quadraplegia great care must be taken in moving the patient so that the head, shoulders and pelvis are moved as one piece or else further movement at the fracture site may damage further the injured cord. Hypotension may occur due to damage to the sympathetic outflow, and, as with the intracranial contents, so also the spinal cord requires a minimum perfusion pressure to maintain its blood flow. Bladder catheterization will be necessary in the first few days.

Reduction of Intracranial Pressure

As mentioned earlier, a very small reduction in intracranial volume may be sufficient to reduce the ICP (*see Fig.* 32.1) and hence minor, almost insignificant manipulations may go a long way to alleviating the condition. In the acute situation, the airway is vital. Endotracheal intubation, sedation and, in extreme cases, muscle relaxation and controlled ventilation, are the most effective ways of rapidly reducing ICP. The head injury or restless patient with a tumour may not lie sufficiently still during the CT scan and intravenous sedation to diminish the restlessness may also increase the ICP. As such it is much more prudent to embark on the investigation following skilled induction of anaesthesia and controlled ventilation with a mild degree of hypocapnia. Osmotic dehydration is another method of rapid reduction in ICP and mannitol 20%, 1–1·5 g/kg body weight, given as an intravenous bolus, will produce a reduction in ICP within 10 min. Prolonged administration has certain problems, particularly electrolyte imbalance, for which the patient may require up to 130 mmol potassium per day replacement as the proximal renal tubular function is inhibited by this hyperosmolar agent. Nevertheless, it is a most useful agent and in conjunction with ventilation provides one of the most rapid 'medical' decompressions, but its place in prolonged therapy is doubtful.

In the less acute situation, particularly for the oedema surrounding a tumour, steroids have been successful in reducing ICP. Intravenous dexamethasone 16–20 mg (0·25 mg/kg body weight) followed by 4–8 mg 4–6-hourly, can produce a change in the patient's clinical state within an hour. Though frequently used in trauma, there is no clinical or experimental evidence to support the claims that steroids have any effect on traumatic cerebral oedema; however, there is some evidence, particularly from the laboratory, to suggest their value in ischaemic oedema. The danger of gastrointestinal haemorrhage may be reduced with the use of alkali; more recently, H_2 antagonists such as cimetidine have been shown to be effective. Raised ICP due to ventricular obstruction is best treated by CSF drainage and a burr hole with insertion of a ventricular catheter attached to a closed external drainage system may relieve the pressure safely. A situation which will persist for longer than a few days should be treated definitively by the insertion of a shunt system.

The prolonged treatment of raised ICP presents some problems. Examples of this are patients with benign intracranial hypertension or inoperable tumours. Prolonged use of steroids leads to the complications associated with high dose steroid therapy.

Control of Epileptic Seizures

In the acute situation it is vital to control the airway and prevent the patient damaging himself. The next priority is to attenuate the fit or at least prevent a second one. For this, intravenous diazepam 10 mg initially is most useful. It is important to control the fits even if this should require endotracheal intubation and respiratory assistance due to the high dose of anticonvulsants given. A patient may die during status epilepticus and so, if intravenous diazepam is unsuccessful, induction of anaesthesia with high dose barbiturates and muscle relaxation may be required. If the patient has had one fit, then therapy must be directed to prevent a second fit and for more prolonged control of the situation phenytoin and phenobarbitone are most widely used. It is important to remember that phenytoin is only very slowly absorbed, that intramuscular injection does not raise the blood level any better than oral administration and therapeutic levels may not be attained for 2 days. Intravenous phenytoin 1 g stat, followed by 0·5 g 6-hourly may achieve therapeutic levels quicker but diazepam or phenobarbitone cover must be used until the blood levels are sufficiently high. Chlormethiazole, 40–100 ml of an 0·8% infusion over 5–10 min, is recommended.

Infection

Bacterial infection of the CNS produces such devastation that it is important to diagnose and treat the condition appropriately from the earliest possible stage. Following trauma, infection is introduced by fractures through the air sinuses; the paranasal sinuses often contain Gram-positive cocci, particularly pneumococci and staphylococci, and it is appropriate to prescribe ampicillin or flucloxacillin, while fractures involving the ear may cause a Gram-negative infection and thus chloramphenicol or gentamicin should be considered. Postoperatively the infection is often due to a *Staphylococcus albus* from the patient himself, often sensitive to ampicillin or flucloxacillin. Neonates and young children with septicaemia may develop meningitis caused by *E. coli* and gentamicin should be considered. Prior to antibiotic therapy, swabs for culture of a discharging wound, nasal sinuses, etc. should be taken, and if there are no signs of raised intracranial pressure, a lumbar puncture for a sample of CSF must be examined and cultured. Antibiotic therapy must be vigorous and should be administered by the intravenous route in the initial stages to maintain constant high blood levels. More than one antibiotic may be used if the infecting agent has not been determined and while this is frowned on by bacteriologists the consequences of inadequately treated meningitis leave the clinician little choice; besides, the weight of clinical experience would be in favour of a degree of controlled polypharmacy. Abscesses will be dealt with in a subsequent chapter.

INVESTIGATIONS

So often the temptation is to perform a battery of tests without adequate consideration. As many of these are complex, prolonged and have associated morbidity, it is important before embarking on the more complex investigations to ask 'What do I want to know? What are the hazards? Is it worth the risk?' Some of the more common neurological investigations are considered under separate headings, but it will be obvious that any ill or unconscious patient must have baseline measurements of haematology, blood chemistry, blood gases and urinalysis. An adequately penetrated chest radiograph is also necessary in coma.

Lumbar Puncture

Lumbar puncture is a most useful test providing information on the CSF, its pressure and whether or not a block exists along the CSF pathways. *It is contraindicated if there is any suggestion of raised intracranial pressure* or a clinical suspicion of a spinal block—this latter possibility should only be investigated in a neurosurgical centre where an emergency or decompressive operation can be performed. Removing fluid from the CSF pathways may cause a deterioration in the patient by uncal or foramen magnum herniation and should this occur, the patient may lose consciousness during the investigation. Rapid instillation of an equivalent amount of saline may sometimes reverse the deterioration. In the neonate, ventricular tap may be performed to obtain CSF and in expert hands a cisternal or lateral cervical puncture between C1 and C2 may be used.

Examination of the CSF obtained will provide much information in cases of sudden unconsciousness. In the absence of trauma to the head, blood in the CSF, especially if there is associated xanthochromia, is diagnostic of a subarachnoid haemorrhage or intracranial bleed. Cloudy fluid containing numerous white cells will favour a bacterial meningitis. The diagnosis may be more subtle and the CSF findings in a variety of conditions are shown in *Table* 32.2.

Table 32.2 Diagnosis of meningitis by examination of CSF obtained by lumbar puncture

Disease	*Colour*	*Cells*	*Protein* (g/l)	Sugar	Culture
Bacterial					
Acute	Turbid	Polymorphs 1–10 × 10^3	↑ 2–5	N or ↓	+VE
Resolving	Clear	Polymorphs ↓ Lymphocytes 10–100	Reducing	N	—
Tuberculosis bacterial meningitis (TBM)	Clear	Lymphocytes 200–400	↑ 0·8–20	↓	+VE
Viral	Clear	Lymphocytes 100–200	N	N	−VE
Fungal	Clear	Lymphocytes 50	N or ↑	↓	+VE
Subarachnoid haemorrhage	Xanthochromia	Red cells White cells	↑	N or ↑	−VE

Electrical Studies

The electroencephalogram (EEG) is available in most large hospitals and is very useful in the diagnosis of encephalitis, poisonings and metabolic causes of coma. An epileptic focus may be identified and there is typically a low voltage record over a subdural haematoma; slow waves may be detected over an infarct or tumour. For many neurosurgical problems, however, it is an investigation of limited value. Computer analysis of the EEG has value as a research tool. Evoked cortical potentials are 'average enhanced signals' detected from the brain after repeated electrical stimulation of a peripheral nerve (somatosensory evoked response—SER) or by visual or auditory stimuli to the eye or ear. SER is useful in assessing cord function after injury; it may be related to cerebral flow and metabolism in head trauma and subarachnoid haemorrhage. Auditory evoked response may define brainstem function in addition to the inner ear, and visual evoked responses can accurately test the visual pathways and are diagnostic in multiple sclerosis. More recently averaging techniques have been employed to motor responses after magnetic stimulation of the motor cortex. This allows anterior spinal cord monitoring.

Nerve conduction studies may be useful in differentiating between an entrapment neuropathy and a toxic or metabolic cause.

Radiology

Adequate plain radiographs of the skull and cervical spine should be obtained in all patients in whom trauma is suspected. Penetration and positioning are very important and unless the views are true anteroposterior and lateral, skull fractures and pineal shift will be missed (60–80% of unconscious adults with traumatic intracranial haematoma have a skull fracture and inadequate radiography may miss the fracture). In spinal conditions also, plain radiographs must be of the highest quality.

Brain scans using technetium 99 are relatively inexpensive and a useful screening device for detecting infarcts and tumours, but the test lacks the sensitivity and localization of a CT scan.

Perhaps one of the most exciting new tools available to clinicians for the examination of head and spine is computer axial tomography (CT scan), examples of which are seen in succeeding chapters. It has revolutionized the understanding and management of so many conditions that the time is approaching when lack of this investigation may be considered less than optimal for the unconscious patient.

Angiography is still an important neurological investigation and is absolutely indicated in vascular diseases, subarachnoid haemorrhage and meningiomas. Nowadays a retrograde femoral catheter technique with selective catheterization is preferred and in subarachnoid haemorrhage it is advisable to study all four major vessels to identify multiple aneurysms. For vascular lesions of the spinal cord spinal angiography should be performed by an expert in the field. Smaller quantities of dye may be injected, reducing the risks, using digital subtraction angiography. The technique may also be employed to intravenous injections of the dye. The picture quality is now as good as conventional angiography.

The ventricular system, cisterns and subarachnoid spaces have been investigated by introducing air either by lumbar puncture or through a burr hole. Both procedures require anaesthesia and even in expert hands have a significant morbidity. With the advent of the CT scan, the indications for the investigation are becoming fewer.

Myelography with iodized oil or more recently a water-soluble contrast Metrizamide is useful for investigating the contents of the spinal-dural sac or of extradural lesions compressing the cord. The patient should be screened prone and supine, and the test should not be performed if there is a possibility of a posterior fossa tumour or foramen magnum herniation.

Magnetic resonance imaging (nuclear magnetic resonance scans) have provided unrivalled views of the intracranial contents, particularly the posterior fossa and the spinal cord. It is now the investigation of choice for spinal tumours and syringomyelia. The expense of the system, however, will curtail its widespread usage for some time. Within this neurosurgical section, examples of this investigation have been used so that the reader may compare the quality with CT scans or radioisotopes.

NEUROSURGICAL PROCEDURES

Anaesthesia

As already mentioned earlier in the chapter, respiratory inadequacies, hypotension, hypercapnia, coughing and struggling will all without exception cause a deterioration of the neurosurgical patient. It is absolutely essential therefore that any procedure requiring anaesthesia in a patient suspected of intracranial disease must minimize these potential hazards. If the patient is having a non-neurosurgical procedure, e.g. facial surgery, or internal or external limb fracture fixation, then the clinician must decide whether the procedure is sufficiently urgent or necessary in the patient with the head injury and suspected raised ICP. The patient who has an intracranial problem requiring neurosurgery must also have neuroanaesthesia of the highest order. The general principles are given below. It is preferable that a cuffed, non-kinkable endotracheal tube is passed and in most cases muscle relaxants and controlled ventilation with moderate hypocapnia (P_{CO_2} 30–35 mmHg) will provide an excellent operative field and optimal cerebrovascular conditions. Inhalational agents, such as halothane, act extremely quickly and can be reversed rapidly but all produce some degree of intracranial vasodilatation and, in the situation of raised ICP, present a potential and actual hazard. Intravenous anaesthetic agents are preferable but require skill in their use. In the surgery of vascular tumours, arteriovenous malformations and dissection of an intracranial aneurysm, elective hypotension may be employed; this, however, must be the domain of the expert as is postoperative therapeutic hypertension to improve the flow in ischaemic cerebral tissue.

Surgical Procedures

No attempt is made in this section to describe the techniques involved in neurosurgical operations; however, some procedures are so common that indications for their use are given. Techniques are developing rapidly and alternative approaches to classic problems have become popular.

It is obvious that the expansion in neurosurgery requires both its practitioners and other clinicians to explore constantly the possibilities of combined approaches and the neurosurgeon finds himself frequently working with vascular, ophthalmic, otological, maxillofacial, thoracic, orthopaedic and plastic surgeons.

Perhaps the simplest and oldest neurosurgical procedure is the *burr hole* and it is lifesaving in extradural haematoma where removal of the clot will rapidly reduce ICP. Burr holes for post-traumatic haematomas have been taught classically as frontal, parietal and temporal or both sides but with the advent of the CT scan it is possible to site the burr hole exactly over the clot with much more accuracy, eliminating the 'woodpecker' element in the procedure. The burr hole is also required for ventricular puncture, ventriculography or burr hole biopsy, but has disadvantages, in that during a biopsy haemorrhage cannot be controlled and if the hole is incorrectly sited, a false negative diagnosis may be made.

Using a *craniotomy*, the flap can be sited to provide good exposure of a tumour or allow brain retraction to expose the circle of Willis for aneurysm surgery. Lesions in or around the ventricular system will require a transcortical approach through a 'silent' area.

Posterior fossa surgery is performed by midline or paramedian incision and an occipital craniectomy.

Before the improvements in anaesthesia, posterior fossa explorations were inevitably performed in the sitting position with high risk of air embolism but with improved anaesthesia and controlled ventilation, more and more posterior fossa explorations are performed in the prone position with neck flexion.

Hydrocephalus is treated by shunting procedures, ventriculo-peritoneal, ventriculo-atrial and only in exceptional cases ventriculo-pleural. The ventricular catheter must be sited in the anterior horn of the lateral ventricle in front of the foramen of Monro, which marks the anterior limit of the choroid plexus, to avoid growth of the latter into the ventricular shunt with occlusion of the drainage hole. the ventricular catheter is connected to a pump or flushing device which may contain a pressure-operated slit valve. The drainage tube may also have a slit valve.

The classic approach for hypophysectomy is by a transcranial operation but with the advent of the operating microscope, more and more *pituitary* surgery, both for microadenomas and for large suprasellar tumours, is being performed by a trans-sphenoidal approach (either midline or initially through the ethmoids).

Acoustic tumours, if large, must be removed by a posterior fossa approach but smaller ones may be removed very satisfactorily by an otological approach through the petrous bone. With careful teamwork the facial nerve can be preserved in many instances.

Cerebrospinal fluid fistulas present a variety of differing technical problems and tax the ingenuity of the clinician. The exact site of leak must be determined to decide whether a transcranial approach or one through the affected air sinus is best.

There are several different surgical approaches for diseases of the *spine and vertebral column*.

For decompression or removal of intradural tumours a posterior approach with multilevel laminectomy is required. A very wide laminectomy carries the risk of subsequent scoliosis or kyphosis and the amount of bone removed must be very limited, particularly in children. Surgery for the prolapsed disc can be quite limited and need not affect the stability or strength of a spine. If a vertebral body or a disc is the problem then an anterior approach, transorally for the odontoid region, lateral to the oesophagus for the cervical spine, an anterolateral or transthoracic approach for the thoracic spine, are examples of the differing skills required.

Arteriovenous malformations or fistulas may be successfully excised using microscopic techniques but many are so widespread and involve deep structures that removal is too hazardous; some of these are successfully embolized following selective catheterization.

Generalized or focal *ischaemia* may be improved using an extracranial–intracranial anastomosis.

Congenital facial deformities or head and neck malignancy may need a combined approach.

POSTOPERATIVE CARE AND COMPLICATIONS

Following a neurosurgical procedure, postoperative observations are absolutely vital: the level of consciousness, pupillary response and limb movements and any change which may herald the accumulation of an intracranial clot.

Respiratory function and chest physiotherapy play a major role in the success or failure of intracranial procedures, thus great emphasis may be placed on their meticulous care in the immediate postoperative period. Pyrexia postoperatively in the neurosurgical patient may be due to blood in the subarachnoid space, a chest infection or a urinary infection. Fortunately meningitis, wound infections, etc. are relatively rare. Postoperatively, epilepsy is a major complication and some surgeons administer anticonvulsants prophylactically before an intracranial surgical operation.

It is obvious that the postoperative care of neurosurgical patients is similar in all ways to the preoperative management and requires dedication from medical and nursing staff.

DIAGNOSIS OF BRAIN DEATH

With increasing use of organ transplant techniques as well as scarcity of high technology resources it has become imperative that clinicians have medicolegal guidelines to aid in the diagnosis of brain death. Often the diagnosis is obvious but difficulties arise with patients requiring cardiopulmonary assistance, those who have taken barbiturates overdose, other poisons, asphyxiation or following cold water drowning. In such cases it is desirable to have at least two experienced clinicians not involved in the original resuscitation or the planned organ transplantation to give their opinion.

Electrocerebral silence in EEG records may be useful but it is not diagnostic of brain death, especially in barbiturate coma; it has, therefore, been omitted from the guidelines suggested by the World Federation of Neurologists. These are:

1. Total absence of response to nociceptive stimulation of the dermatomes supplied by the cranial nerves.
2. Absence of spontaneous breathing with complete reliance upon artificial respiration.
3. Absence of corneal reflex.
4. No response to vestibular stimulation using 20 ml of ice water for each test.
5. Fixed and dilated pupils.
6. Absence of oculocardiac reflex.
7. The above findings must be present for minimum period of 6 h from their first demonstration.

Further Reading

Crockard H. A., Hayward R. and Hoff J. T. (1985) *Neurosurgery: The Scientific Basis for Clinical Practice.* London, Blackwell Scientific Publications.

Hayward R. (1980) *Essentials of Neurosurgery.* Oxford, Blackwell.

Jennett W. B. and Teasdale G. (1980) The Management of Head Injuries. In: *Contemporary Neurology*, 3rd ed., Vol. 15. Philadelphia, Davis.

Plum F. and Posner J. B. (1972) Diagnosis of Stupor and Coma. In: *Contemporary Neurology*, 2nd ed. Philadelphia, Davis.

Symon L. (1979) Neurosurgery. In: Rob C. and Smith R. (ed.) *Operative Surgery*, 3rd ed. London, Butterworths.

Trubovich R. (1979) Management of acute intracranial disasters. *Int. Anesthesiol. Clin.* **17**, Nos. 2 and 3.

33 Congenital Malformations of the Central Nervous System and its Coverings

Kenneth Till

INTRODUCTION

Congenital malformations occur more commonly in the central nervous system of liveborn babies than elsewhere in the body. The lesion may be at once obvious, notably with scalp or skull swellings and myelomeningocele. Others may be hidden and without overt disturbance of function, as with many spinal cord malformations. Although a malformation may be apparent or suspected at birth, a period of observation is often justified before investigations are started. This is so, for example, when a dermal sinus is found or craniosynostosis is suspected. It is indeed a feature of many malformations that, whether recognized at birth or not, their ill effects may not develop until much later, even occurring in adult life. Examples of this are: aqueduct stenosis causing insidious development of hydrocephalus with long delayed overt signs; a dermoid cyst growing very slowly and only revealing its presence as an expanding lesion years later; a lipoma attached to the lower spinal cord causing neural damage in later life.

Most CNS malformations are associated with an agenesis or underdevelopment of neural tissue (of which agenesis of the corpus callosum is an example (*Fig.* 33.1*a*) and hence are not amenable to surgical treatment. It is important, however, to be aware of another feature of such malformations, which is that the lesions are often multiple; each of these may influence prognosis and management and some may require surgical intervention. Thus an apparently innocuous and unimportant birthmark in the skin of the lower back may be the only clue to the presence of gross spinal cord malformation; conversely, extensive surgery may be contemplated for a child with hypertelorism, yet be of doubtful value if the child has, in addition, agenesis of the corpus callosum and mental retardation.

Congenital malformations of the CNS and its coverings may therefore often be the concern of the neurosurgeon (as well of course as the paediatrician) not merely in infancy but throughout childhood.

ABNORMALITIES OF THE SKULL AND SCALP IN INFANTS

The visible or palpable lesions which may be found in newborn infants include scalp angioma, dermoid cyst, dermal sinus, haematoma (subperiosteal or subgaleal), meningocele (usually occipital, occasionally frontal or nasal), encephalocele (occipital or nasal), scalp defect, skull defect, and rare scalp tumours (sarcoma, haemangiopericytoma, neurofibroma). The familiar 'strawberry' naevus has no deeper significance, whereas the naevus flammeus of face and scalp may be accompanied by significant abnormalities of meninges and cerebrum (the Sturge–Weber syndrome). Except in the neoplastic group, diagnosis is usually possible by simple inspection. Developmental abnormalities are nearly always in the midline, although meningoceles and encephaloceles may extend asymmetrically. These latter lesions characteristically are inconstant in size and in underlying tension, and a bone defect beneath them can usually be palpated in the skull.

Dermoid cysts, visible and palpable through the skin, usually lie in the region of the anterior fontanelle and in later childhood rest in a shallow hollow external to the periosteum. An intracranial extension of a cyst in this region is very rare. A *skin* or *dermal sinus*, on the other hand, is usually found in the occipital region and may appear to be a simple dimple, possibly with a tuft of hair emerging from it. By sliding the scalp over the bone the tethering of the sinus to the underlying tissue can be revealed by the puckering of the skin. It must then be assumed that the sinus extends into the posterior fossa (where it may end blindly or expand into a dermoid cyst) until surgical exploration proves otherwise (*Fig.* 33.1*b*, *c*).

Subperiosteal haematoma is a rare sequel to birth trauma and can be diagnosed when the extent of the fluctuant swelling is limited by the vault sutures. The haematoma cannot extend further because the periosteum is firmly adherent to the sutures. It may be confused with the even rarer cerebrospinal fluid leakage (which, being necessarily associated with a dural tear and skull fracture, has greater significance for treatment and prognosis). The correct diagnosis may of course be obtained by aspirating the fluid, but it is far wiser to await events, when resolution of a haematoma within a few weeks, or the failure to do so of a CSF collection will provide the answer.

A *congenital scalp defect* is usually in the region of the vertex, and at birth may appear either as a healing scar or as an open granulating area, and may be superficial or involve all layers of tissue down to the dura. A *congenital skull defect* without overlying scalp lesion probably never occurs.

Neoplasms of the scalp or skull are nearly always solid, may grow with alarming speed, involving all tissue layers

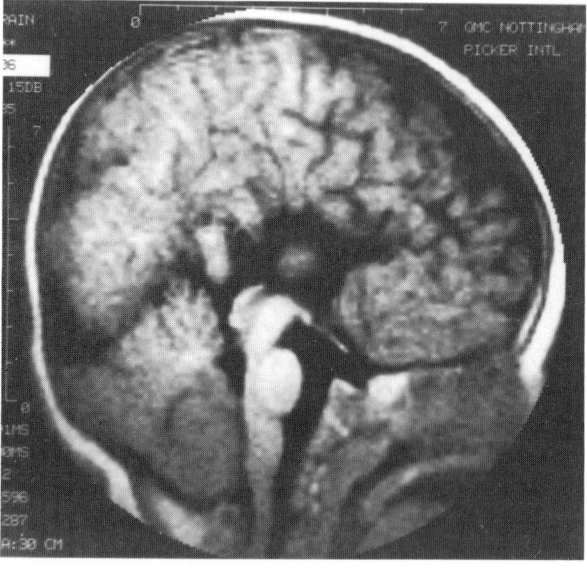

a

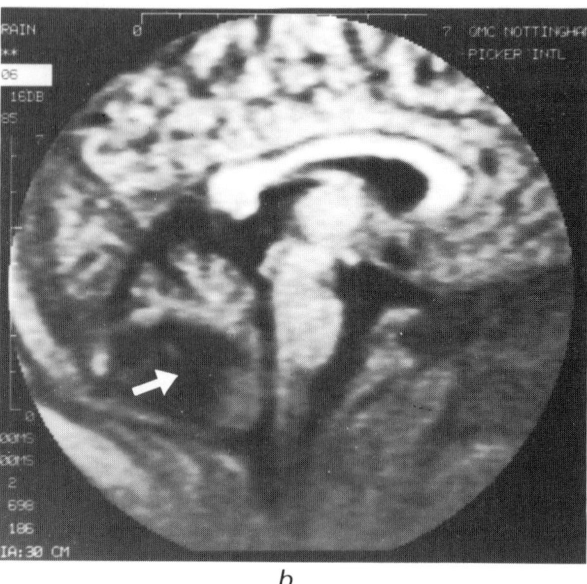

b

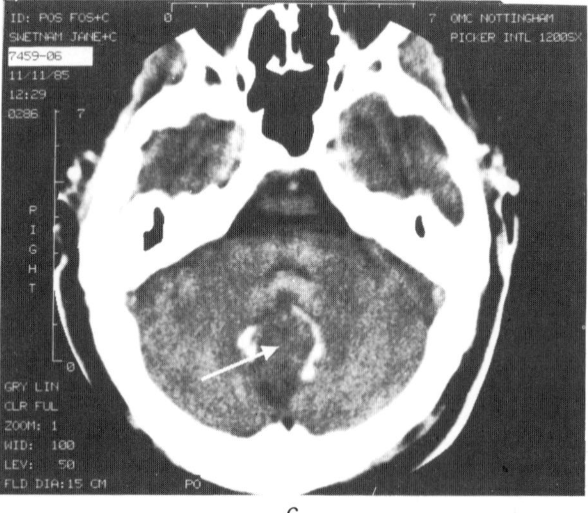

c

Fig. 33.1 *a*, Agenesis of the corpus callosum. MRI, lateral view. (C.f. *b* which shows a normal corpus callosum) *b*, Dermoid cyst in posterior fossa (*arrowed*), MRI, lateral view, showing large midline defect in the cerebellum. *c*, CT scan: spherical lesion with partially calcified wall.

except the underlying skull in the early stages but may occasionally regress and disappear as do the scalp angiomas.

Diagnosis

Plain skull radiographs may reveal an underlying bone defect. With a meningocele or encephalocele this defect has a smooth border with unthickened rim, but the rim is thickened with an adjacent 'tramline groove' when the lesion is a dermal sinus passing intracranially. There is so little calcification in the neonate's skull, however, that abnormalities such as these as well as fractures may not be apparent. Repeated radiography will then be necessary after a few weeks if the clinical situation permits such a delay. Repeated radiography is of particular importance when the circumstances suggest that a fracture may be present. Because a fracture may be the only evidence of injury, it may have medicolegal relevance but, in addition, alerts the clinician to the possibility of a 'growing fracture' in later infancy.

Treatment

The *superficial angioma*, or '*strawberry naevus*', regresses and has usually disappeared by the age of one year, and thus no treatment but reassurance is required. *Dermoid cysts* over the anterior fontanelle, having no intracranial extension, grow very slowly. Their removal is simple but operation becomes even safer if delayed for six or more months. *Dermal sinuses*, in contrast, present a potentially very serious hazard, because of the risk of intracranial infection, either meningitis or, if the cyst lies more deeply, an abscess within the cyst. Indeed it is not rare for the sinus to be overlooked until meningitis develops in later childhood, or a localized scalp swelling with inflammation and perhaps discharge of pus draws attention to the lesion. Investigation by CT or MRI (*Fig.* 33.1*b*, *c*) together with angiography (to discover in particular the relation of the venous sinuses to the dermal sinus or cyst) should be carried out before operating.

The sinus is then exposed down to the bone and thence into the posterior fossa. Complete removal is sometimes not possible, when complex venous sinuses render the attempt too dangerous. A solid mass which is suspected of being a scalp or skull *neoplasm* should at first be observed for a few weeks before deciding upon biopsy or attempted removal. If the rate of growth is rapid the baby's life is unlikely to be saved, whereas spontaneous regression, even after initial increase in size, may occur and the hazards of operation avoided. If the lesion remains unchanged or simply grows with the child then further investigation and operation when the child is larger can be undertaken.

An *encephalocele* or *cranial meningocele* may cause difficulty in nursing or feeding the baby, either because of the size of the swelling or (commonly) because there is considerable tenderness. Hence excision may be necessary soon after birth, and of course is a matter of urgency when there is actual or potential breakdown of the cyst coverings and the risk of CSF leakage. The glial tissue within an encephalocele has little or no function. Its removal may be essential if adequate skin covering is to be achieved, but often some or all the tissue can be replaced within the skull through the bone defect. Tight dural closure, which is important for a successful outcome, may be facilitated by this replacement. If the lesion is small and covered by healthy skin and not apparently tender, delay in treatment is wise because this allows the study of any associated malformations and may reveal the presence of progressive hydrocephalus. In all cases, however, operative treatment should only be undertaken with expert anaesthetic and nursing services available.

CRANIOSYNOSTOSIS

Definition

Craniosynostosis is a condition of premature fusion of one or more sutures in the vault or base of the skull. This occurs after a period of retarded growth of dura and bone in the region of the affected sutures. Deformity of the skull results from the localized impairment of growth, and is usually of a characteristic and easily recognized shape. Often there are associated malformations, particularly of the maxilla and the digits; over fifty distinct syndromes have been described. Normal skull growth and shape are mainly determined by the growth of the brain, particularly during the first six months of life. The localized impairment of bone growth in craniosynostosis is accompanied by compensatory increase of skull volume elsewhere because in most forms of the disorder the brain's potential for growth is normal. For example, synostosis affectingly only the sagittal suture prevents the skull from widening normally; increased growth at the coronal and lambdoid sutures allows the skull to enlarge in the anteroposterior diameter, thus attaining a normal volume.

Aetiology

Some types of craniosynostosis are inherited through autosomal dominant genes, but most cases arise sporadically, probably as mutations. The child then has a 1 in 20 chance of his or her offspring suffering from similar or related disorders.

Diagnosis

An apparent abnormality of skull shape, or marked right/left asymmetry or a circumference below the 3rd centile, all indicate the need for plain radiographs. Although a correct diagnosis can often be made by simple inspection, radiological confirmation is essential because there are wide normal familial and racial variations. The suspicion of craniosynostosis may arise at or soon after birth. If radiographs do not show abnormality, they should be repeated after one or two months. An abnormally small head with normal sutures suggests a diagnosis of primary microcephaly. The radiological changes in craniosynostosis occur in sequence as follows. There is first a reduction in the number and size of the digitations, the suture gradually becoming a linear narrow 'gap' between the adjacent bones; at the same time the edges of the bones thicken. There follows a bridging of the gap by bone, the fusion of the bones often remaining incomplete even in the late stages of the condition, a reminder that bony union is not the primary abnormality but is the end of a process which began with impaired growth much earlier. Bone in the neighbourhood of the premature fusion or even elsewhere may show 'digital' or convolutional markings; these are not an indication of raised intracranial pressure but appear to be part of the growth disorder.

Longstanding low intracranial pressure, such as may follow shunt treatment for hydrocephalus, may lead to diminished skull growth, with inactive sutures and, occasionally, fusion across sutures.

Types of Craniosynostosis

The *sagittal suture* is the vault suture most commonly affected; impaired growth along it leads to a reduced transverse or coronal diameter, with a compensatory increase in the anteroposterior diameter, resulting in the shape known as scaphocephaly (*Fig.* 33.2*a*).

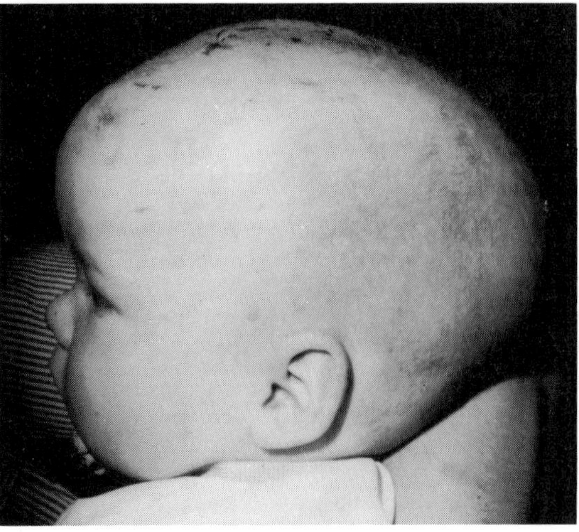

a

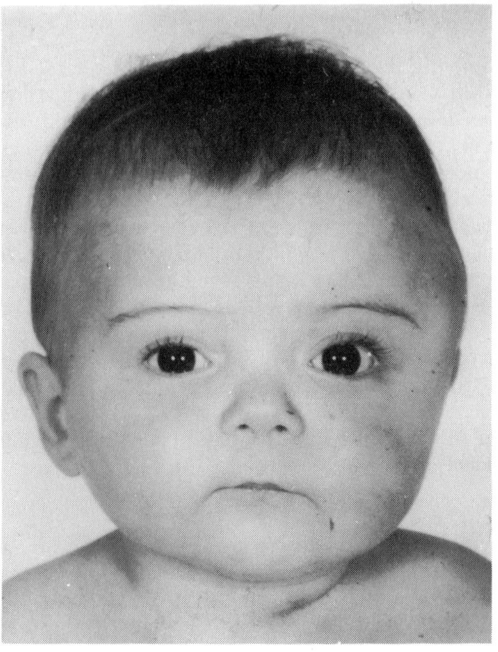

b

Fig. 33.2 Craniosynostosis. *a*, Scaphocephaly due to premature fusion of the sagittal suture. *b*, Brachycephaly due to premature fusion of coronal sutures.

Bilateral *coronal synostosis* is the next most frequently occurring type. The anterior fossae are small because not only are the frontal bones poorly developed but growth at the frontonasal and frontosphenoid sutures is retarded. The anteroposterior diameter of the head is thus diminished, while the brain's increase in bulk leads to an increase in transverse diameter (*Fig.* 33.2*b*).

Bilateral coronal synostosis may occur alone, but more commonly is part of complex craniofacial malformations. These include Apert's syndrome (when there is also syndactyly in all four extremities) and Crouzon's syndrome (with underdevelopment of the maxilla). When both coronal and sagittal sutures are affected the head is not only broad but has a prominent or even pointed forehead. If the impairment of growth begins *in utero* while the anterior fontanelle is large, the deformity becomes gross (*turricephaly*).

Craniosynostosis of only one coronal suture (usually combined with impaired growth at the frontonasal and frontosphenoid sutures of the same side) causes frontal asymmetry, with a flattened frontal bone and shallow orbit (*frontal plagiocephaly*).

Metopic suture synostosis occurs normally around the time of birth. If the fusion of the frontal bones occurs prematurely *in utero* the skull becomes pointed and narrow anteriorly, with flattened frontal bones and, sometimes, hypotelorism. The posterior part of the head is normal; the overall shape is thus triangular (*trigonocephaly*).

'*Total*' craniosynostosis affects synchronously all the vault sutures and most of the sutures of the skull base, and results in the head being round and small, not obviously abnormal in shape. Plain radiographs show widespread convolutional marking, probable evidence of longstanding raised intracranial pressure. The brain, having at first normal growth potential, is reduced in size through the failure of the skull to grow adequately; this is therefore a form of secondary microcephaly.

Lambdoid suture synostosis is extremely rare except as part of total craniosynostosis.

Signs and Symptoms

In addition to the abnormal head shape, the retarded skull growth may so restrain brain bulk that intracranial hypertension develops in later infancy or childhood. Thus headache, papilloedema, secondary optic atrophy and eventually mental retardation may occur. Primary optic atrophy can arise from orbital deformity. These sequelae are, however, usually seen only in bicoronal and total synostosis and in a small proportion of children with Apert's or Crouzon's syndromes. The shallow orbits which result from impaired growth at the coronal and orbital roof sutures cause proptosis, often with incomplete lid closure. Stenosis of the nasolacrimal ducts is present in such patients and may require treatment. The high arched palate of many children with bicoronal synostosis is accompanied by choanal atresia, with mouth breathing and frequent upper respiratory tract infections.

Treatment

When the type of craniosynostosis is one likely to restrict cerebral growth, the principal aim of treatment is to ensure adequate increase of skull volume. An increase of orbital volume in affected cases is an associated aim. Improvement of skull shape and facial appearance is, in these cases, of secondary importance. The brain's rapid increase in bulk during the first few months of life is used to increase skull volume and improve craniofacial disproportion after appropriate freeing of bone structures has been achieved by operation. Surgery must therefore be undertaken before the age of three months if maximum benefit is to be obtained, because the intracranial forces diminish rapidly after that. After the age of about six years major reconstructive surgery is necessary when the deformity is sufficiently disturbing to the child's mental and physical health and the risks of the procedure are fully accepted by the parents.

Sagittal craniosynostosis is best treated, before the age of 6 months, by a linear craniectomy, removing a strip of bone 1–1·5 cm in width over the sagittal sinus. The bone edges are waxed and then covered with a thin layer of film, made from nylon or silastic rubber. This covering, inserted to prevent bony union across the gap, is secured with tantalum clips or silk sutures through the bone. The craniectomy must extend beyond the coronal suture anteriorly and the lambda posteriorly; the gap then rapidly widens and continues to do so for at least six months, while it is gradually filled by bone growing from the underlying dura.

Bilateral coronal synostosis requires craniectomy along the site of the fused suture, carrying the bone release to the zygomatic process of the frontal bone and then medially in the roof of the orbit towards the midline. The superior orbital margins and the frontal plate of bone are thus released to allow forward growth of the anterior part of the skull vault. The lateral canthus may be advanced at the same time and secured in its new position by a strut of bone. If the operation is carried out early enough in infancy, brain growth will ensure an improvement in skull shape and in the depth of the orbits.

Combined sagittal and *coronal craniosynostosis* requires both operations described above. Through a bicoronal scalp incision the scalp is reflected anteriorly and posteriorly to allow adequate exposure of the areas of bone to be excised.

Total craniosynostosis, if diagnosed in infancy, or if discovered in later life with evidence or suspicion or impaired cerebral growth compression, should be treated by extensive bilateral craniotomy, the main purpose of which is to allow decompression by creating large free flaps of bone on each side by means of linear craniectomies.

Major advances in craniofacial reconstructive surgery, pioneered mainly by Tessier, are increasingly used, especially in the treatment of Apert's and Crouzon's syndromes in later childhood. It has at the same time become increasingly apparent that complex cranioplasties are possible in the infant, both permitting normal cerebral growth and using that growth to achieve improved craniofacial proportions.

HYDROCEPHALUS

Impairment of CSF circulation leads to ventricular enlargement, which is the type of hydrocephalus amenable to surgical treatment (*Fig.* 33.3*a*). Obstruction of CSF flow, and thus an increase of intracranial pressure, may arise from:

1. *Occlusion of the basal arachnoid spaces* secondary to arachnoiditis caused by prenatal or perinatal subarachnoid haemorrhage. A similar hydrocephalus develops occasionally in later life following intracranial haemorrhage from an aneurysm, and after a posterior fossa operation, when leakage of blood into the CSF pathways may provoke arachnoiditis.
2. *Stenosis of the aqueduct of Sylvius*, usually a congenital malformation (*Fig.* 33.3*b*).

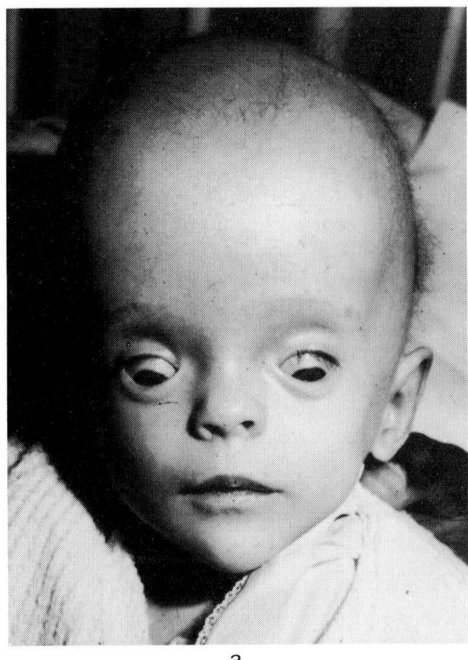

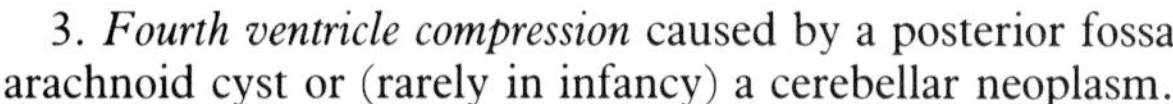

3. *Fourth ventricle compression* caused by a posterior fossa arachnoid cyst or (rarely in infancy) a cerebellar neoplasm.

4. *Congenital occlusion of the exit foramina of the fourth ventricle (Dandy–Walker syndrome).*

5. *Arnold–Chiari malformation*, in which the brain stem is elongated and extends, together with part of the cerebellar hemispheres, into the upper cervical canal (*Fig.* 33.3*c*). The exit foramina of the fourth ventricle are then in the cervical canal; the return of CSF to the intracranial subarachnoid space through the 'crowded' foramen magnum may then become obstructed.

The diagnosis of congenital hydrocephalus may not be apparent until the baby is several months old. The clinical condition then resembles that of *acquired* hydrocephalus such as may follow meningitis, head injury, or the development of an intracranial neoplasm. Hydrocephalus arising from overproduction or malabsorption of CSF is extremely rare.

Symptoms and Signs

Obstruction to the CSF pathways leads to an increase of intraventricular pressure, which enlarges the ventricles while compressing the cerebral mantle and, in the infant, causes abnormally rapid skull growth. After the first year of life undue head enlargement from raised intracranial pressure remains possible throughout childhood but the rate of growth is much reduced. A baby with even advanced hydrocephalus usually shows little disturbance of brain function; the diagnosis therefore depends mainly upon recognizing the increased head size, the abnormal rate of growth, the increased tension over the fontanelle (which is often larger than normal), and the abnormal percussion note. Impaired venous drainage within the skull causes distension of the scalp veins. A limitation of upward gaze and a tendency for the eyes to maintain a downward direction (the 'setting sun' sign) are present in advanced cases and are almost pathognomic of hydrocephalus (*Fig.* 33.3*a*).

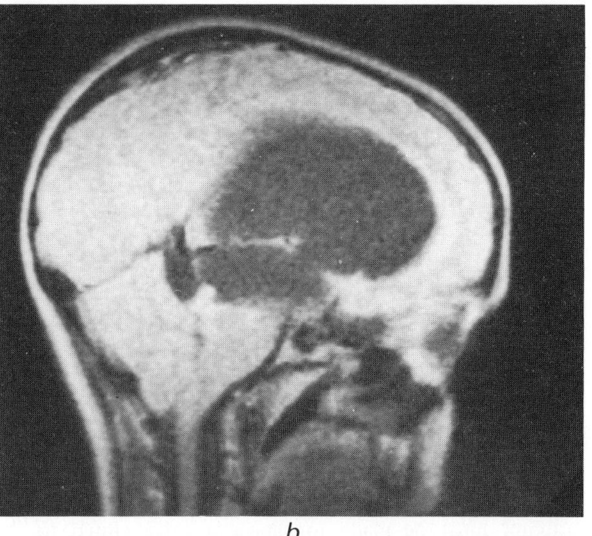

b

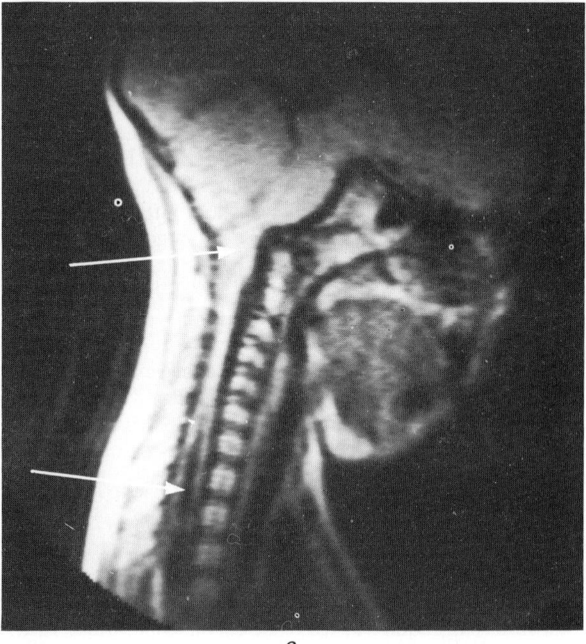

c

Fig. 33.3 *a*, Hydrocephalus. An example of advanced hydrocephalus showing shiny scalp, distended veins and down-turning 'sunset' eyes. *b*, Hydrocephalus due to aqueduct stenosis. MRI, lateral view, showing dilated lateral and third ventricles, with normal small fourth ventricle. *c*, Arnold–Chiari malformation. MRI, lateral view, showing elongated medulla, extending into upper cervical spinal canal (*arrowed*). The patient also had a syrinx in the upper thoracic cord.

The hydrocephalic baby is usually fully alert (the presence of the anterior fontanelle and the ease with which the skull can enlarge ensure that the intracranial pressure does not rise far above normal); this condition contrasts with that of the baby with recent head injury, subdural effusion or cerebral neoplasm. Vomiting may occur, but like the other classic signs of raised intracranial pressure (papilloedema and impaired cerebration) is rare in the infant with hydrocephalus.

Treatment

Hydrocephalus is treated by diversion of the ventricular CSF either to the abdominal cavity where it is absorbed through the peritoneal membrane or to the bloodstream in the right cardiac atrium. The maintenance of ventricular pressure between appropriate limits and of the rate of flow of CSF are achieved by a one-way valve with a built-in resistance, of which many types now exist. The most commonly used are the Hakim–Cordis, Heyer–Schulte, Holter and Pudenze devices. The valve, placed between a silicone catheter in the lateral ventricle and another in the atrium or peritoneal cavity, should be inserted as soon as possible after the diagnosis of progressive hydrocephalus has been made. When the diagnosis is made in later childhood after the anterior fontanelle has closed, the choice of a valve with the right characteristics is particularly critical because excessive reduction of ventricular pressure is likely to cause symptoms of intracranial hypotension and, more importantly, collapse of the cerebral mantle with rupture of veins. In all cases an attempt must be made to choose a valve suited to the pressure and flow requirements of the patient.

The satisfactory maintenance of a shunt over a period of years with correct pressure and flow rate, free from infection and blockage, requires regular review of the child's condition and development. Even when there are no signs or symptoms of undue intracranial pressure and no abnormal rate of skull growth, the maintenance of as near normal a ventricular size as possible (checked by MRI or CT) is important for a satisfactory outcome. It is probable that maximum cerebral maturation in the young child is only achieved if the ventricular size is not much greater than normal. This ideal is seldom realized, but a change of valve to one of lower resistance may be advisable if ventriculomegaly persists, even when the child appears to be progressing satisfactorily.

When the hydrocephalus is more complex (for example when it is associated with an arachnoid cyst or the Dandy–Walker syndrome) it may be necessary to drain the CSF from more than one region; thus hydrocephalus with a posterior fossa arachnoid cyst is best treated by a cyst–peritoneal or cyst–atrial shunt.

Complications of Shunt Treatment

These are not rare; about 50% of the children treated for the first time will require at least one further operation. In the immediate postoperative period excessive reduction of intracranial pressure may cause bleeding into the ventricles or the subarachnoid space. This occurs through collapse of the cerebral mantle and rupture of cortical or subependymal veins. This complication is less likely if CSF has not been allowed to escape during the operation. Occlusion of the shunt, at any time, even years after the procedure, may happen rapidly or slowly. The blockage usually is at the ventricular end where choroid plexus may grow into the end of the catheter, or where reduction of ventricular size has caused cerebral tissue to occlude the openings in the catheter. Blockage may also develop at the lower end of the shunt through peritoneal reaction or, in the case of a ventriculo–atrial shunt, where the child's growth has brought the cardiac catheter out of the heart into the superior vena cava. Only rarely is the valve itself blocked, but those with a slit mechanism may slowly increase resistance to flow and hence cause further ventricular enlargement.

Infection associated with a shunt may occur early if operative technique has been faulty but also may develop months or years later from blood-borne organisms which grow in the lumen of the shunt and thence pass into the bloodstream or the peritoneal cavity. The only indications of such infection are occasional pyrexia, vague malaise, and, most commonly, a slowly progressive anaemia. Repeated cultures of blood (obtained if possible after pumping the valve), or of CSF, are sometimes necessary to confirm the diagnosis.

Disconnection of the valve from the ventricular or lower catheter may follow trauma or be the result of the child's growth and at first causes only intermittent dysfunction. There is relative shortening of the lower catheter as the child grows; the lower end of the catheter is drawn into the superior vena cava where both occlusion and infection are more likely to develop. A peritoneal catheter is inserted with a length sufficient for considerable body growth.

Ulceration of the scalp over a valve is rare but is particularly likely in a small baby. Careful placement of the valve away from the skin incision, the choice of a small valve, and the use of a bone defect in which to place the valve all help to avoid this complication.

Future Trends

Progress in the treatment of hydrocephalus will come from a better understanding of CSF dynamics and of methods of continuous control and adjustment of intracranial tension and ventricular size.

CONGENITAL MALFORMATIONS OF THE BACK

The formation of the spinal cord, nerve roots, and their coverings is a simultaneous development of derivatives from entoderm, mesoderm and skin ectoderm. It is for this reason that malformations of neural structures are nearly always accompanied by abnormalities of skin and bone. These visible or radiologically demonstrable lesions thus often provide the clue to the existence of hidden neural maldevelopment. The conditions which may be encountered include diastematomyelia (split cord), elongated cord with short filum terminale (a form of tethered cord), intraspinal lipoma, dermal sinus and dermoid cyst, neurenteric cyst, and tethering bands between cord and surrounding structures.

Diagnosis

The abnormalities listed above may all be associated with lower limb or sphincter disorders by the time the baby is born. They may also cause progressive lower limb sensory and motor changes, sphincter weakness and abnormal spinal curvatures in later childhood. It is because these later developments can be prevented by early diagnosis and treatment, that attention to the superficial signs in an otherwise normal child is so important. The skin over the lower back nearly always shows a 'birth mark'; this may be an area bearing an abnormal growth of hair (the so-called 'fawn's tail'), a pigmented area, a capillary naevus, a dermal sinus, or a subcutaneous lipoma (*Fig.* 33.4).

The baby may be born with inequality of the dimensions of the lower limbs, usually most obvious in the feet, one of which is likely to show talipes. Many children are, however, not brought for advice until they begin to walk, when limp or clumsiness of gait is noticed. There is sometimes a slowly progressive weakness of one lower limb. In later life backache or urinary incontinence may direct attention to the correct diagnosis.

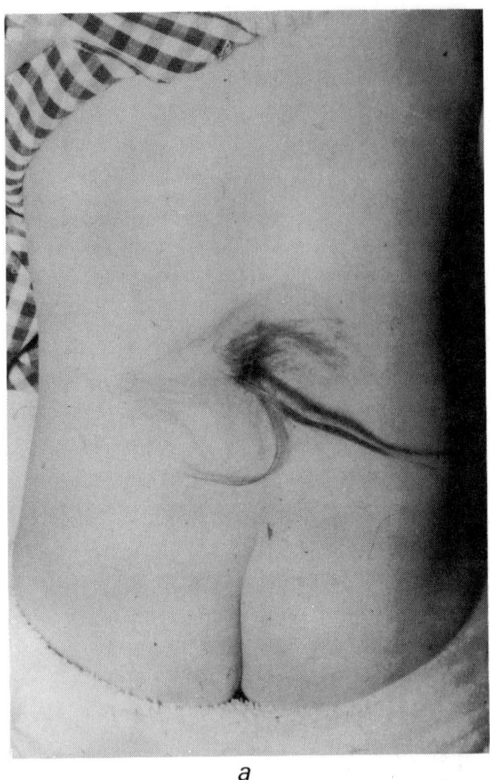

a

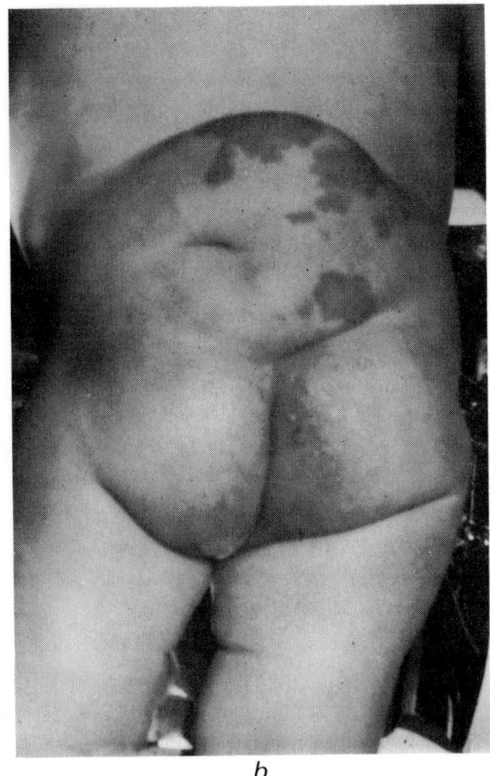

b

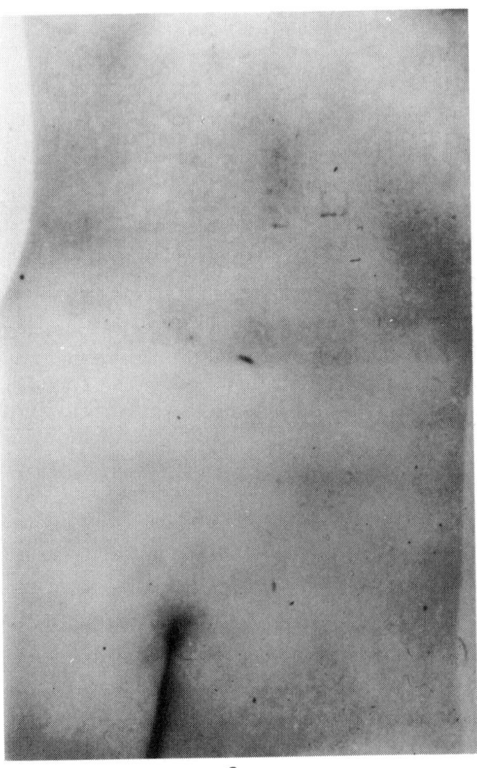

c

Fig. 33.4 Spinal dysraphism. *a*, Hairy back, 'fawn's tail'. *b*, Subcutaneous lipoma and capillary naevus. *c*, Dermal sinus.

Management

The early diagnosis of these forms of 'occult', spinal dysraphism is, as mentioned above, important if irreversible deterioration is to be avoided as the child grows.

Once the presence of skin abnormality, lower limb asymmetry or sphincter disturbance has been detected, plain radiographs of the *whole* spinal column should be obtained. It is not rare to find bony malformation at more than one level. In a neonate a delay of one or two months before radiography is wise, in order to obtain better detail of any abnormality. If the radiographs are of good quality and normal, there is very little likelihood of a cord or nerve root lesion being present. If the radiographs show developmental abnormalities such as a widened spinal canal, midline bony spur within the canal (*Fig.* 33.5), deficient intervertebral discs or abnormal spinal curvatures, then further investigation is indicated. Myelography following the injection of air or metrizamide into the cisterna magna has been the usual way of demonstrating such abnormalities as elongated cord, thickened filum terminale, immobilization of the cord by fibrous bands, cysts or dermal sinus. *Fig.* 33.5*b* shows an example of a metrizamide myelogram demonstrating a thick short filum with a conus divided into two and lying in the sacral region. CT and MRI can provide even better detail of these structures (*Fig.* 33.6).

The surgical procedure which should follow the discovery of these abnormalities has as its aim the removal of potentially harmful lesions (dermoid cyst, neurenteric cyst, dermal sinus, midline bony spur) and the freeing of the cord from restraining structures such as fibrous bands, short filum, and, whenever possible, intradural lipoma. Even when the child displays no sign of cord or root disorder, spinal

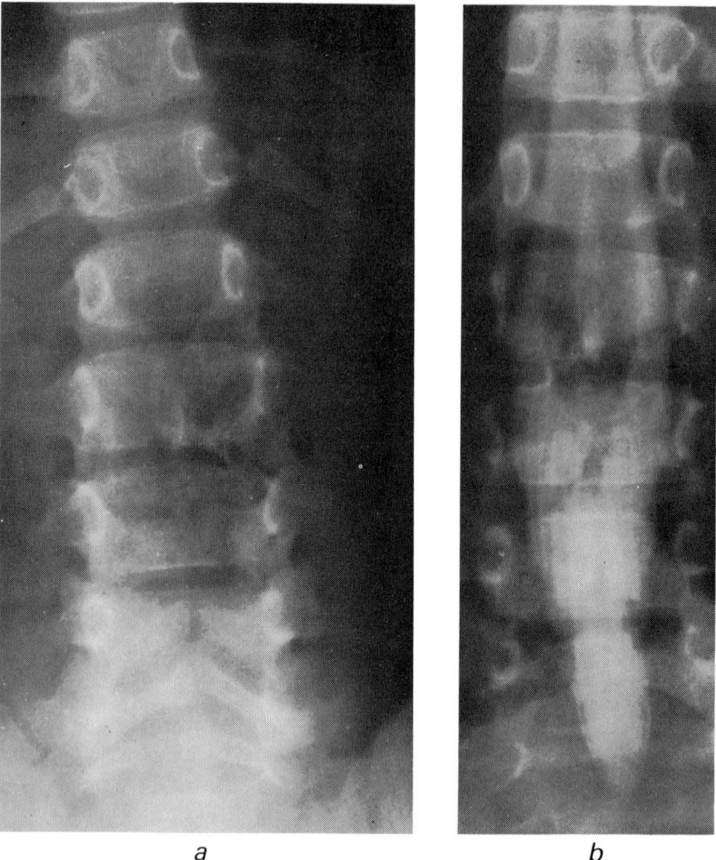

Fig. 33.5 Spinal dysraphism. *a*, Radiograph showing wide spinal canal, midline bone spur. *b*, Metrizamide myelogram showing divided cord and low-lying conus with thickened filum.

exploration should be carried out as a prophylactic measure, since the probability of later neuronal damage is quite high. More debatable are the indications for intervention when root and cord involvement with a lipoma has been demonstrated. To free the neural structures from fatty tissue is difficult and the risks of damage are high. When deterioration is known to have occurred, the attempt must be made. How the lipoma causes neural damage is poorly understood, but the arrest of deterioration after freeing the nerves and cord cannot be doubted. If therefore limbs and sphincters are intact, the author's opinion is that operation should not be undertaken, but the child's condition should be checked every few months during the growing period.

Genetic Factors

The genetic significance of parents having a child with occult spinal dysraphism is the same as with spina bifida cystica. Thus there is a 1 in 20 to 1 in 25 chance of any further children being born with anencephaly or spina bifida cystica.

Counselling is therefore very important, together with the possibility of diagnosis in early pregnancy.

SPINA BIFIDA CYSTICA

This, the commonest spinal malformation, refers to meningocele (in which there is a dural sac containing arachnoid and CSF but no neural elements) and the much commoner myelomeningocele, in which there are nerve roots and usually spinal cord, often with much loss of function in these structures.

These malformations and more severe forms such as myeloschisis result from a failure, during the 20th to the 28th days after conception, in the sequence of neural groove formation, invagination, neurulation and neural crest differentiation. The variety of possible outcomes is great, but only the two commonly encountered in surviving babies will be considered here. Myelomeningocele (*Fig.* 33.6*b*) is nearly always associated with the Arnold–Chiari malformation of the hind brain (*see Fig.* 33.3*c*) and hence with hydrocephalus. The functions of the grossly distorted (and often deficient) nerve roots and lower cord are always impaired. This may be revealed by talipes developing in utero, dislocation of the hips, lower limb weakness, or incompetence of anal and bladder sphincters. However, many of the other nerves reach their appropriate destinations and function normally. It is the probability of damage to these nerves in postnatal life that led to the policy of early operation, in order to protect them from trauma and infection.

Diagnosis

When operative treatment is regarded as necessary within 24 hours of birth (*see below*) then complete assessment of the sac contents is not possible. The overt lesion is a swelling on the back, covered by skin or thin membrane and containing

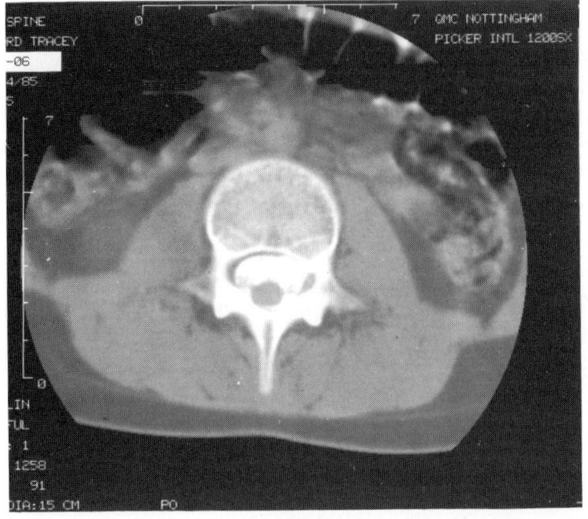

a

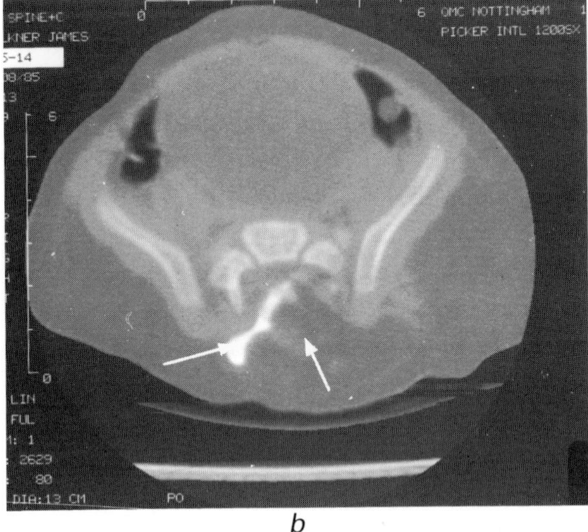

b

Fig. 33.6 *a*, Spinal dysraphism. CT scan, sacral canal. The filum is grossly thickened. Nerve roots of the cauda equina are shown. *b*, Spinal dysraphism. CT scan, sacral canal, after contrast medium injection. The wide canal is largely occupied by a low attenuation lipoma on the left, attached to the cord anteriorly and extending outside the canal posteriorly. A meningocele sac lies on the left.

fluid. The mass may extend over one to five vertebral segments and is most commonly centred at the lumbar or thoracolumbar levels and less often in the lumbosacral region. The bone defects (spina bifida) always involve more vertebral segments than are overlain by the cyst. Neural elements including the malformed cord may be visible within or in the wall of the sac, and the widely separated bifid spinous processes can be seen and palpated; talipes, weak lower limbs, and patulous anus are evident by direct inspection and indicate the impaired nerve supply to the affected muscles. Important associated abnormalities (which are likely to effect the policy of management) include hydrocephalus and kyphosis, the latter resulting from vertebral anomalies and weakness of erector spinae muscles. In 30% of babies with myelomeningocele there is malformation of the urinary tract, such as ureteral duplication, solitary kidney, neuropathic bladder. Plain spine radiographs are required to define the bone abnormalities and the degree of kyphosis.

Management

The diagnosis of myelomeningocele or anencephaly in early pregnancy is possible by ultrasonography or by estimation of alpha-fetoprotein levels in blood or amniotic fluid. This early diagnosis is particularly important if a previous pregnancy has produced such a malformed foetus or baby, in order that the parents may be offered the opportunity to consider a termination of the pregnancy.

The early operative treatment of *meningocele* is only necessary if the covering of the sac is so thin that leakage of CSF has occurred or is threatened, or if the sac is so large that handling and feeding the baby is difficult. On the other hand the early repair of a myelomeningocele and the provision of skin and fascial covering to protect the cord and roots undoubtedly reduces the chance of damage from trauma or infection. Therefore an early decision about treatment has to be made. Certain features have been found to reduce substantially the chance of survival into later childhood, even when every modern resource is available for the care of the child. These features of such prognostic importance are: (1) Marked hydrocephalus at birth (a head circumference 2 cm greater than the 97th centile); (2) Kyphosis; (3) A spinal lesion extending over more than 5 segments; (4) A lesion extending into thoracic levels; (5) The presence of ventriculitis; (6) Additional gross anomalies such as cardiac malformation.

Babies with one or more of these features have been excluded from operative treatment by many paediatric and neurological surgeons, in the belief that false hopes should not be raised, that misplaced effort and fruitless allocation of resources should be avoided, and that it is wrong to assist the survival of individuals with gross handicaps and very limited capacity to enjoy life. The questions posed by these matters are complex and must be answered by individual doctors practising in this field, assisted by the attitudes of parents and of society in general. The doctor's attitude and his recommended management should be determined only after he has acquired experience of the length and quality of survival which follow different methods of management and different criteria for selection, unless he eschews selection and treats all babies with myelomeningocele. Although the family circumstances are among the many factors to be taken into account, it is self-deception to suppose that either parent is in a position soon after the birth to consider the matter calmly and knowledgeably. My own view is that although it is agreed that some babies with the adverse features will survive, the overall distress and suffering in such cases is a small fraction of that which would be caused by avoiding selection. Once the decision to operate upon the spinal lesion has been made, it is important that total care is provided; this means treatment of hydrocephalus when indicated, of hip dislocation, talipes, paraparesis and urinary tract involvement. At the same time the parents' need for considerable support must be recognized and attended to.

Operative Treatment

The objectives of operation are to replace the neural structures of the myelomeningocele within the spinal canal, where they should be surrounded by subarachnoid space (CSF) and covered externally by dura, fascia and skin. These objectives cannot always be realized. The canal has no bony or cartilaginous roof but is usually sufficiently capacious. The dural lining of the sac is often plentiful and can be swung as a flap to cover the neural elements. The lateral lumber fascia may similarly be dissected and reflected to cover the dura. The skin defect which remains after the thin membrane of the sac has been removed is often very large. It may be necessary to rotate large skin flaps based on buttock and trunk in order to obtain closure of the defect.

Associated progressive hydrocephalus, which is present in 70% of babies with myelomeningocele, may prevent successful healing of the back lesion unless treated by a shunt, preferably at the same time as the back operation.

Investigation of the urinary tract should be carried out after a few weeks, when satisfactory progress is being made following the initial treatment.

Orthopaedic surveillance is important from an early stage. The particular nature of any muscle imbalance and the probable hypoaesthesia of the skin, together with the need to protect the healing back lesion will all modify the more orthodox orthopaedic measures.

Acknowledgements

I am grateful to Professor B. S. Worthington and Dr Ian Holland, from whose department at the University and Medical School of Nottingham *Figs.* 33.1*a*, *b*, *c*, 33.3*b*, *c* and 33.6*a*, *b* were supplied.

34 *Intracranial Emergencies, Trauma, Vascular Accidents, Infections*

H. Alan Crockard

INTRODUCTION

The presentation of a patient with altered or deteriorating level of consciousness or the development of a hemiparesis or an epileptic fit will be encountered by most medical practitioners during the course of their practice. For some patients, no therapy will help, in others, however, attention to simple details such as the care of the airway, correction of blood gases and blood pressure will improve the patient's condition. The problem with many neurosurgical emergencies is that they only come to attention after the neuronal damage has been done. The aim of management must therefore be threefold; prevention of secondary pathophysiological effects, such as brain swelling and vascular spasm, the diagnosis of the cause of the catastrophe, and the prevention of further deterioration due to rebleeding, further fits, etc. The general measures in the care of the unconscious patient have already been mentioned in Chapter 32 as have been the principles regarding the treatment of raised ICP. This chapter will concentrate on three of the more common intracranial emergencies, head injuries, vascular accidents and intracranial infections. In many cases, the cause of the patient's deterioration is not immediately obvious and the diagnosis may be clouded by drugs, or alcohol, hysteria or incorrectly observed signs and so a high level of awareness of the causes and the characteristics of various common neurological conditions is essential.

Unconsciousness may be caused by a wide variety of systemic illnesses and thus the clinician must examine for and exclude diabetes, cardiac problems, hepatic or renal failure as well as systemic or pulmonary infections or latent blood loss.

The purpose of this chapter is to outline the pathophysiology, diagnosis, management and indications for surgery in these three major neurosurgical emergencies.

HEAD INJURIES

Epidemiology and Definitions

Injuries to the head are extremely common, either as single injuries or part of generalized trauma to the body following road traffic accidents, etc. Ten per cent of the case load in an Accident and Emergency Unit will be head injuries, but the vast number of these are relatively minor requiring reassurance and first aid. One-fifth of head injuries attending emergency units are admitted and of these admissions, 2–3% will die. One-third to one-half of the deaths occur before the patients reach hospital and another one-third die within 24 h of admission. Over one-half of the patients are less than 30 years of age and it is a disease of male preponderance. Road traffic accidents, either to vehicular users or pedestrians, are the more common cause, but in the very young and very old, falls and accidents in the home produce a significant number. Industrial accidents, leaving aside the transport injury, produce relatively few head injuries as compared to limb, hand and back injuries.

Vehicular failure accounts for less than 10% and pre-existing medical conditions (myocardial infarction, subarachnoid haemorrhage, epilepsy) only account for 1 in 2000 head injuries. Alcohol or drugs is an increasing problem and in one study, one-half of the patients admitted unconscious with head injuries had significant blood alcohol levels. Apart from alcohol, human error, misjudgement or carelessness are the most common predisposing causes for head injury.

Head injuries may be classified as *closed head injuries*, where the scalp is intact and there is no communication of the intradural contents with the atmosphere so that there is no CSF leak from nose or ear. The closed head injury may be due to the moving head striking a surface such as the road or if the head itself is struck by a moving object such as a stone or a bottle. Brain damage is most severe if the head is free to move and the acceleration/deceleration injury or whiplash mechanisms may produce severe or fatal injuries with no head impact. Occasionally the head may be crushed between two surfaces producing a compression type of injury but this is relatively rare. *Open head injuries* imply a communication between the intradural contents and the atmosphere, and are often caused by impact with a small sharp object.

A skull fracture is an index of the severity of the impact and should alert the medical practitioner to the likely associations or complications such as haematoma, CSF leak, meningitis, etc. Treatment of the fracture itself is rarely indicated; treatment of the brain is always indicated.

Fractures may be linear (single or multiple) or complicated with or without depression. In a penetrating injury there may be multiple small bony fragments and foreign bodies carried into the depths of the wound (*Figs.* 34.1, 34.2). Occasionally in the young child, suture diastasis occurs instead of skull fracture.

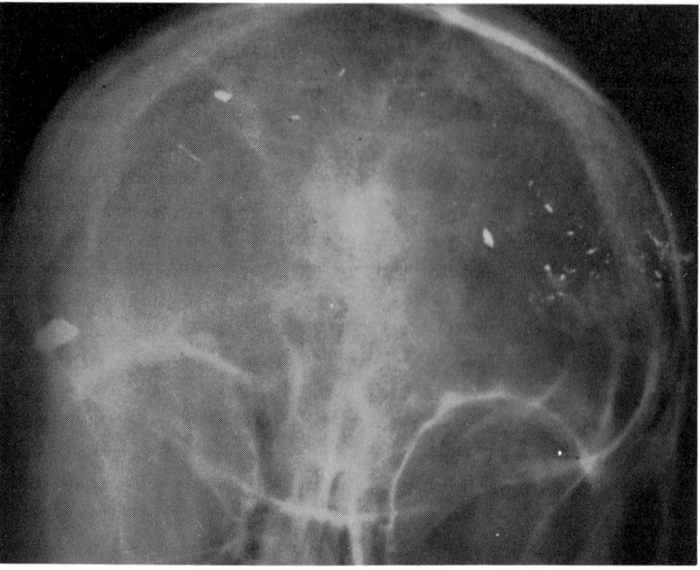

Fig. 34.1 Side-to-side cranial gunshot wound with entrance in the left frontotemporal area. Metallic fragments spread intracranially.

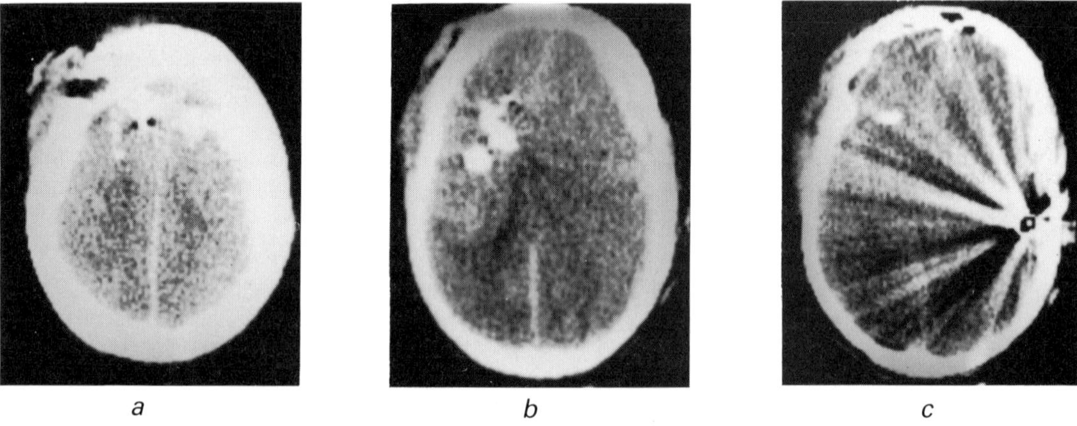

Fig. 34.2 *a, b, c,* CT scan of same patient showing the extent of the injury from right frontotemporal to left parietal. The metallic fragments cause the sun-ray appearances.

Patterns and Pathology

There are *patterns of injury* of the brain, skull, face and the whole body which are well-recognized results of specific injuring mechanisms, and it is important to bear this in mind in the management of severe head injury so that other serious injuries are not to be missed. It must always be remembered that the head is attached to the body and its injury must be viewed in the context of trauma to the whole organism. In the acceleration/deceleration type of injury produced by a vehicular accident, there is a large amount of rotation at the craniospinal axis resulting in a whiplash injury; the face and the cervical spine will also be injured and chest injuries, or injuries to the lower limb at the acetabulum, patella, or lower leg may be present in 25% of cases. Often the motion is not entirely unidirectional and there is a rotational element as well as anteroposterior acceleration/deceleration. The brain injury may include subfrontal, temporal and surface contusions, white matter damage due to tearing of the fibres and also focal areas of damage around blood vessels, dural edges and bony prominences. Intradural damage may extend from the frontal poles to the upper cervical spine and include cranial nerve and cervical root damage.

Brainstem injuries though classically described by clinicians because of the 'brainstem signs', are always associated with diffuse white matter damage extending well beyond the area of the brainstem. The classic feature of diffuse white matter damage is widespread axonal injury and is demonstrated histologically by retraction balls and degeneration of long fibre tracks in the cerebral hemispheres, the brainstem and spinal cord, together with focal lesions in the corpus callosum and rostral brainstem. Impact to the face will result in fractures and as the 'wedge' of facial bones is driven inwards, it will tend to 'slide' backwards and downwards damaging the base of the skull, creating dural tears and CSF leaks. More severe displacement will result in brain damage to the subfrontal areas, optic chiasma and hypophyseal hypothalamic areas.

Extradural haematomas (*Fig.* 34.3), that is between the bone and the dura, are usually due to damage to a major artery, such as the middle meningeal. Except in the very young, rupture of the middle meningeal artery is almost invariably associated with a bone fracture across the line of the middle meningeal artery. Occasionally, bilateral extradural haematomas may result from a torn sagittal sinus, but usually this type of injury is associated with massive intradural damage and the extradural component is relatively minor in comparison. Extradural haematomas cause increased intracranial pressure, distortion and herniation of the brain, with compression of the brainstem. In theory they may continue to expand until intracranial pressure is similar to blood pressure, thereby abolishing cerebral perfusion.

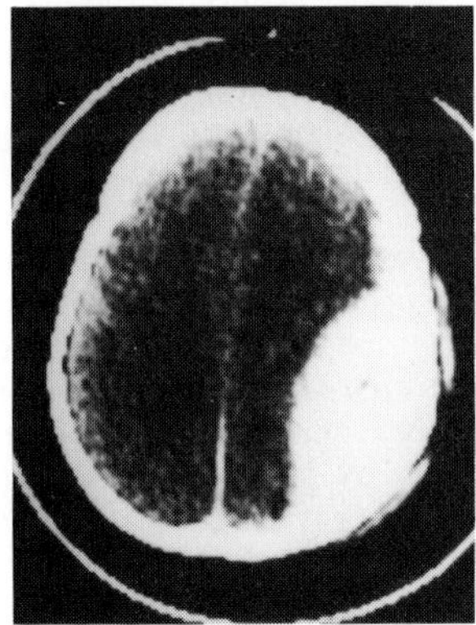

Fig. 34.3 CT scan—extradural haematoma.

Classically traumatic *intradural haematomas* have been divided into acute and subacute, subdural and intracerebral haematomas, but with the advent of the CT scan and systematic pathological studies, the distinctions between these has been blurred. The acceleration/deceleration forces and rotational components will produce maximal damage on the surface of the brain causing contusions and bleeding from veins and arteries but the damage may extend deep into the substance of the brain and often the acute subdural haematoma is merely the surface manifestation of damage which may extend down to the ventricular system, hence the term 'burst lobe' (*Fig.* 34.4). The difference, therefore, between an acute and subacute subdural haematoma is essentially a clinical one of manifestation by clinical signs at a different time scale following the impact. Both are associated with brain damage, contusion and laceration and arterial and venous injuries. They are clinically, pathophysiologically and biochemically different from *chronic subdural haematoma* (*Figs.* 34.5, 34.6), which is a low-pressure collection of tea-coloured fluid, surrounded by thick secreting membranes. Initially a clot forms on the surface of the brain owing to a torn bridging vein, then lysis leads to the accumulation of degradation products which are hyperosmolar and therefore attract water, causing the 'clot' to increase in volume. A capsule or membrane forms around it preventing the dissipation of the degradation products. Unlike the acute or subacute haematomas, the process takes weeks or months and the original head injury may have been forgotten or ignored.

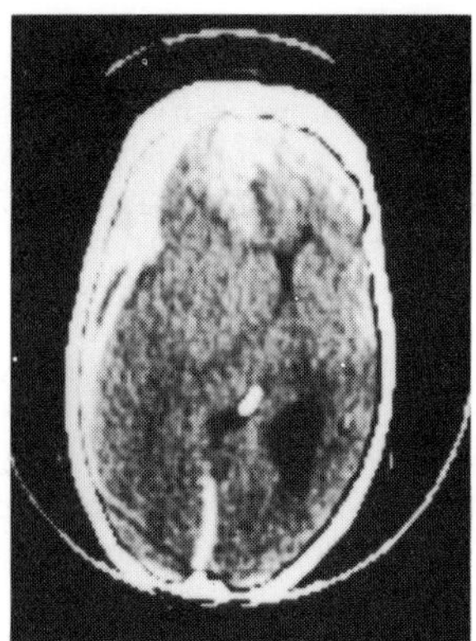

Fig. 34.4 Subdural haematoma associated with intracerebral damage.

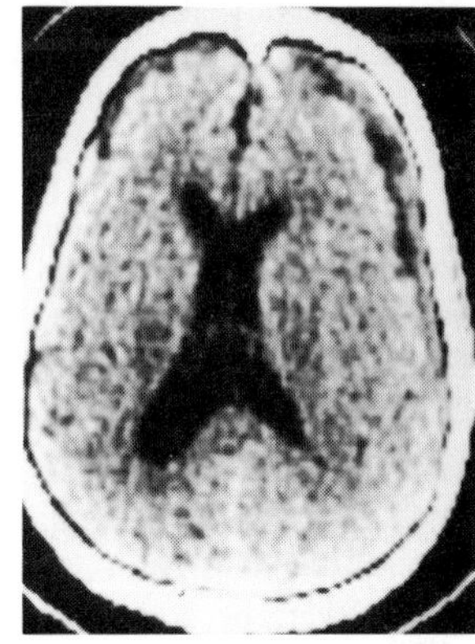

Fig. 34.5 Chronic subdural haematomas; right side larger than left.

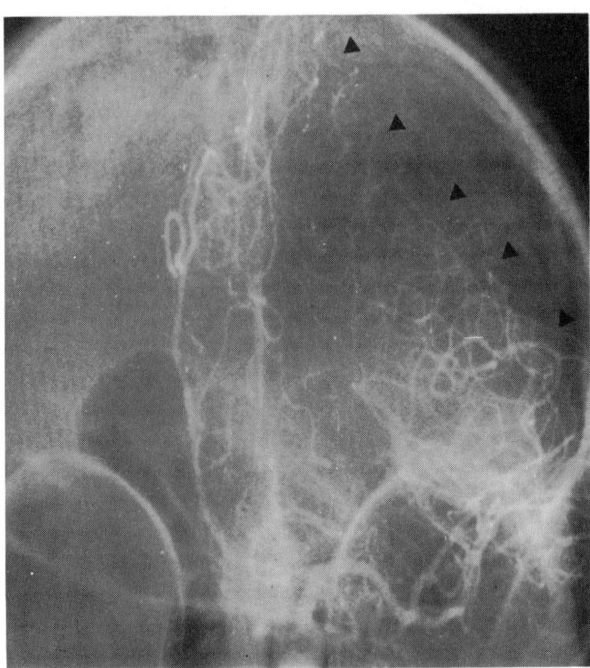

Fig. 34.6 Angiogram showing subdural haematoma.

Both the diffuse white matter damage and intracranial haematoma with associated contusions and lacerations are primary effects of the injury but they in turn produce *secondary complications* so that if the patient survives the first insult he may succumb to the epiphenomena. As a result of the injury, there will be *brain swelling* due to an increase in blood volume. As this occurs within a confined unyielding space, the intracranial pressure will rise. Experimental studies have shown that at the time of impact or shortly after there is a temporary fall in cardiac output, the duration and degree of which depend on the initial injuring energy. These two phenomena (decreased cardiac output and raised intracranial pressure) have the combined effect of reducing cerebral perfusion, producing ischaemic damage on the surface, the so-called border zone infarcts and also damage in the hippocampus, basal ganglia and hypothalamic and brainstem nuclei. Obstruction of the airway, chest damage and hypoventilation will all compound the situation by producing anoxia which will further add to the cerebral insult.

Anoxia and focal or generalized reduction in cerebral perfusion will interfere with cellular metabolism and cell membrane function, and water will accumulate; capillary damage will increase permeability and all these factors will result in *brain oedema*.

In theory, the secondary phenomena of anoxia, decreased perfusion and oedema could be avoided and to emphasize this Jennett has referred to this group as those who 'talk and die'; others emphasize these avoidable factors by referring to them as the 'second accident'.

Assessment of Severity

A review of a small series of case notes in any hospital will reveal a wide variation in the descriptions of its severity and the expected outcome. Severe head injury or coma mean different things to different specialists. The same is true of all injuries and in an effort to standardize descriptions and assessments of severity, an international scale has been adopted. The *abbreviated injury score (AIS)* can therefore be applied to each injury of the limb, the abdomen, the head, etc. and the total score can be shown to relate closely to the expected outcome given the patient's age. From a neurological and neurosurgical point of view, however, this classification is too generalized and it is difficult to assess between 'serious but likely to survive' and 'serious unlikely to survive', AIS 3 and 4 (*Table* 34.1). Various coma scales have been devised in an attempt to quantify the neurological sequelae of injury and the most successful to date has been the *Glasgow Coma Scale* which enables degrees and types of impaired consciousness to be described by clearly defined terms which do not depend on arbitrary levels of consciousness. It is based on three features—eye opening, verbal response and motor response (*see Table* 32.1). Coma is defined as 'no eye opening, no comprehensible verbal response and not obeying commands'. Those with a score of 7 or less are in coma whereas patients with 9 and above are not in coma. Obviously a detailed description of the patient requires examination of the pupils, blood pressure, respiratory pattern and detailed description of limb movements but the adoption of this coma scale throughout the world has allowed, for the first time, comparisons to be made internationally, as well as emphasizing to the individual clinician the importance of objective measurements in seriously ill patients.

Table 34.1 Abbreviated injury scale (AIS)

AIS 0	No injury
AIS 1	Minor injury
AIS 2	Moderate injury
AIS 3	Severe injury (not life-threatening)
AIS 4	Serious injury (life-threatening, survival probable)
AIS 5	Critical injury (survival uncertain)
AIS 6	Maximum injury (currently untreatable)

The Severe Head Injury

Assessment

Upon admission of the patient with severe head injury, immediate resuscitation must be set in motion and this will be described subsequently. In parallel and equally important is the assessment of the individual patient and this must include obtaining a good history of the events that caused the accident. (How far did the patient fall? How fast was the car moving? What was the patient's clinical state soon after the incident? Is he improving or deteriorating? Is there any history of pre-existing disease or ingestion of drugs?) All this must be obtained if possible from the ambulance men, policemen or relatives who accompany the patient. It is so easy to brush these people aside in the urgency of resuscitation, thereby losing vital information. The patient who has tripped, fallen and hit his head may have limb injuries as well as a head injury; someone who has fallen 6 metres or been knocked down by a car must be assumed to have multiple injuries until proven otherwise.

On admission the patient should be placed on a trolley, stripped of all his clothing and *examined back and front* for obvious bruises, swellings and deformities. He must be moved as a whole with head, shoulders and pelvis being moved together to minimize the risks of spinal cord damage.

He should be kept on the trolley throughout the initial resuscitation, repeated examinations and radiographs, as excessive movement during the early phase produces needless pain, increases shock and the likelihood of further bleeding into bruised muscles, thoracic cavity or retroperitoneally. To examine the back the patient is rolled onto one side and bruises, swellings and abrasions noted. Rapid palpation of the spinal column will detect any gross step kyphos.

The patient's *level of consciousness*, verbal response and spontaneous limb movements call for special attention and annotation. (Is he orientated for place and time? Will he respond to questions, or simple commands? If not, do any or all of his limbs move to painful stimuli by flexion or extension?) Pupil size and response, respiratory rate and rhythm, pulse and blood pressure are also noted. From this rapid initial examination an indication of the severity of injury is obtained and noted down, for it is the change of these clinical signs which may indicate an improvement following therapy or deterioration due to the expansion of an intracranial haematoma. Examination may be complicated by alcohol, a cervical spinal injury or facial fractures. Thus, in assessing the patient it must be emphasized that a combination of physical signs more closely reflects the condition than a physical sign taken out of context. Alcohol or other drugs will depress the level of consciousness and one of the major problems in the initial period is to decide if the patient's coma is due to the head injury or due to the blood alcohol level. If the latter can be rapidly determined it will greatly assist the clinician. *Unreactive pupils* may indicate brain death but if the limbs move spontaneously or flex to pain another cause must be found for this unexpected sign, such as facial fractures producing chiasma damage and hence the lack of light reaction. Direct damage to an eye will produce a traumatic mydriasis and lead to unequal pupils. Unequal pupils may also be due to damage to cervical sympathetic as part of a whiplash injury causing a Horner's syndrome with a small pupil on the affected side making the normal pupil appear larger. *Limb movements* must be carefully noted and assessed in conjunction with the other physical signs. Do all limbs move spontaneously? Purposefully? Only in response to pain? Does the patient flex or extend the limb(s)? A common error is to blame an intracranial haematoma for a monoparesis, while the cause may be plexus injury. A spinal injury as well as affecting limb movements may also produce a profound hypotension which may be attributed incorrectly to concealed haemorrhage, but the presence of warm peripheral extremities despite the low blood pressure may be a clue in this condition.

Injuries of the head, face and neck should be carefully examined and obvious lacerations on the face and within the hair line carefully noted. Lacerations of the scalp must be carefully examined and probed prior to suturing to exclude foreign bodies and unsuspected fractures or depressed fractures. A soft swelling in the temporal region should alert one to the possibility of an underlying temporal fracture. A generalized, soft swelling of the scalp may indicate an extensive subgaleal haematoma usually associated with a fracture line across the sagittal sinus. A 'doughnut' type swelling, often interpreted as a depressed fracture, is more usually due to a haematoma in the tissues outside the skull. Examination of the face, jaw and inside of the mouth is very important.

Fractured teeth, or dental plate, signs of intraoral bleeding may indicate possible aspiration of intraoral contents into the lungs.

Airway obstruction will be caused by a fractured mandible or by a retropharyngeal haematoma. The Le Fort III type of fracture must be suspected with frontal impacts to the face and a mobile middle third of the face detected by gripping the upper incisors and attempting to move the maxilla in and out. Examination of the neck for any swellings indicating great vessel damage should be performed. Expansion of a haematoma may compress the trachea and obstruct the airway. Increasing swelling at the root of the neck may be due to mediastinal bleeding which is tracking upwards. Crepitus in the region indicates surgical emphysema from a bronchial or tracheal fracture or undetected penetrating injury.

Respirations must be carefully observed and having established an unimpeded airway, the respiratory pattern, rate and rhythm should be assessed; shallow grunting respirations with unequal movements of the sides of the rib cage will indicate a flail chest; diaphragmatic breathing alone may be due to a cervical cord lesion; marked hypoventilation is seen in drug addicts, barbiturate overdosage and alcohol intoxication. Occasionally, hypoventilation may be due to the inappropriate administration of analgesia in the early post-injury period. Classically, the unconscious head injury exhibits tachypnoea and hyperventilation, while those with extensive 'brainstem' damage may display periodic respiration. Thus in the immediate post-injury period with the unconscious head injury, quiet normal respiration is uncommon and should be carefully studied to exclude any unsuspected airway obstruction, cord damage or drug ingestion.

Arterial blood gases are most useful both in diagnosing and managing the condition. The closed head injury characteristically has a low arterial carbon dioxide and low to normal oxygen levels. A raised carbon dioxide level usually indicates airway obstruction; a low oxygen may indicate a pulmonary shunt.

The *abdomen and pelvis* must be examined carefully for signs of a ruptured viscus or intra-abdominal bleeding. The unconscious patient will require a urinary catheter and if inserted at an early stage this will demonstrate the presence or absence of haematuria. Examination of the *limbs* to ascertain the peripheral pulses and colour of distal parts, particularly if there is a deformity, is important in the initial phase so that ischaemic damage to the limb may be avoided, and, if the limb is broken, it should be immobilized as quickly as possible. Care should be taken not to insert an intravenous line into a fractured limb.

Resuscitation and Treatment

While the general principles for resuscitation will be similar for all severely injured patients it must be emphasized that treatment must be provided according to each patient's needs. There is an increasing tendency in some 'shock, trauma units' for a conveyor belt attitude to be adopted. While this approach will ensure the inclusion of most of the steps required in resuscitation there is a danger of inappropriate and dangerous therapy when it is used as a fixed code. Fluid overload producing 'Da-Nang lung' is such an example and there are numerous examples of patients intubated, paralysed and ventilated before a full assessment of their condition. Meticulous care must be taken to ensure the appropriate therapy for each individual patient.

The first task in resuscitation is to secure an *adequate airway*. If the patient is drowsy with no facial or pharyngeal damage, no airway may be needed but the patient should be nursed in the three-quarter prone position to prevent subsequent tracheal soiling. If he is unconscious or has oropharyngeal damage then some form of airway will be required. The very least that should be inserted is an oropharyngeal airway, having cleaned out the mouth and pharynx and ascertained if there are any loose teeth. If there are a lot of secretions or oropharyngeal bleeding, an endotracheal tube should be passed with care. Emergency tracheostomy is rarely required when the services of a skilled anaesthetist are available. A fractured larynx or trachea obstructed by a solid object which will not be dislodged by suction tubing are two obvious examples where a tracheostomy is absolutely indicated but such instances are few and far between. Having inserted the airway, its position is carefully checked to exclude any further airway obstruction ensuring that it is in the trachea and not in a bronchus and that both lungs are aerating equally. *The care of the airway is the chief preventive factor in reducing mortality and morbidity following trauma.* Having established an airway then most traumatized patients benefit from oxygen with humidification supplied by a mask (*Fig.* 34.7).

Some patients will require *controlled ventilation* or ventilatory assistance and the indications for its use are outlined in Chapters 6 and 13.

Some authorities consider that ventilation should never be used; others advocate its use on practically all head-injury patients for prolonged periods. In the author's opinion controlled ventilation, to be effective, must be instituted early and its maximum effect is produced over the first 48 or 72 h at the stage of brain swelling due to increased blood volume. Thereafter there is little evidence that it improves

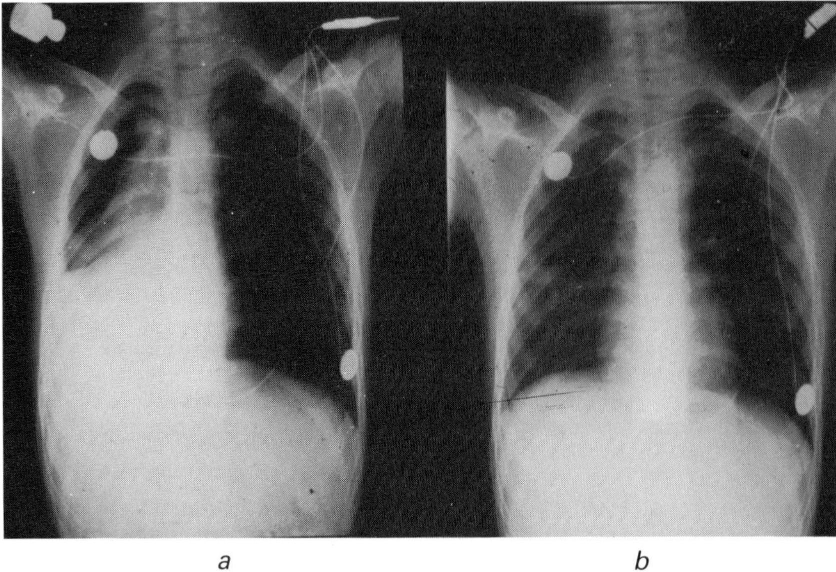

Fig. 34.7 Chest problems compound intracranial damage. *a*, A major bronchus obstructed with mucus resulted in a right lower lobe collapse. *b*, Vigorous physiotherapy relieved the situation.

intracranial conditions, unless there is a separate pulmonary problem. The aim of controlled ventilation in the acute head injury patient is to reduce intracranial pressure by abolishing coughing and struggling which impede venous return, to improve pulmonary toilet, to increase blood oxygen levels and, with muscle relaxation, to abolish shivering, decerebrate spasms and hyperthermia which may utilize up to 30% of the inspired oxygen. The price for these benefits is the loss of neurological signs at an evolutionary period in the disease with the possibility of masking the signs of an increasing intracranial haematoma, though the increasing availability of CT scanning is reducing this risk. Thus, a decision to use controlled ventilation must be carefully weighed and decided for each individual and each location. A form of therapy used in a highly equipped major accident centre may be impracticable in another setting. There are certain situations in which controlled ventilation is beneficial, and these are tabulated in *Table* 34.2. If after a period of resuscitation the pupils remain or become fixed and dilated the situation is hopeless and controlled ventilation should cease.

With multiple injuries, a central venous line is preferable to prevent fluid overload and at the same time effectively and rapidly replace circulating blood volume.

A severe closed head injury may require little *fluid replacement* but it is extremely useful in the initial period to have a fluid line available. Careful fluid balance must be maintained

Table 34.2 Indications for controlled ventilation

Cranial gunshot wound
Associated chest injury
Aspiration pneumonitis
Emergency reduction ICP
Control of epilepsy
Diffuse brain swelling, especially in children

and a urinary catheter should be inserted to ensure accurate fluid balance. The cranial missile injury or multiple injuries may require blood in the resuscitation period, but the severe closed head injury will not. A bolus of *mannitol* has been shown experimentally to improve the cardiovascular haemodynamics and survival if given early after injury, but there is little evidence that long-term administration reduces intracranial pressure. The problem of rebound and of increasing the size of the haematoma are theoretical objections to its use but again in the experimental situation in the presence of a brain laceration the blood/CSF ratio is maintained, suggesting that the osmotic effect is still present. Over the last decade *dexamethasone* has been used throughout the world in the treatment of the closed head injury, without any substantial, experimental or clinical evidence that it has any beneficial effect on traumatic cerebral oedema at normal or high doses. Steroids are considered useful if there has been any pulmonary inhalation. Antacid therapy has been used traditionally to prevent stress-induced erosive gastritis and haematemesis. This practice is being changed to the use of cimetidine both as a prophylactic measure and in the treatment of established erosive gastritis. Routine prophylactic antibiotics should not be given but if there is a CSF leak or evidence of an aspiration pneumonitis then appropriate antibiotics should be given. *Anticonvulsants* are not prescribed routinely. However, if there is an extensive open wound the risks of epilepsy are sufficient to merit early institution therapy. Early epilepsy, i.e. within the first 24 h, should be treated; intravenous diazepam 10–15 mg may stop the fit but will not prevent further fits and other anticonvulsant therapy must be used. Status epilepticus must be adequately controlled and in the head injury patient will probably require controlled ventilation as well as adequate anticonvulsant therapy. Epilepsy in the early post-traumatic period may indicate an intracranial lesion such as a laceration or haematoma and a space-occupying lesion must be excluded.

Analgesia and sedation present persistent problems in the patient with multiple injuries. Reduction of the fracture and splintage will go a long way to reduce pain. Infiltration of local anaesthetic around fractured ribs will also improve respiration as well as reducing pain and unless there is a very definite indication for analgesics these should be withheld in the unconscious patient as should sedation for restlessness. Again, the unconscious patient's restlessness may be made worse by restraint or by the undetected distended bladder. Meticulous attention should be given to the skin over the pressure areas, all inspired gases should be humidified, the eyes should be protected to prevent drying of the cornea or corneal abrasions, mouth care is also essential, a urinary catheter or a sheath arrangement in the male is desirable.

Close observation at quarter-hourly intervals of the severe head injury is mandatory in the early post-injury period, together with careful notes of the patient's condition. A chart based on the Glasgow Coma Scale is most useful for recording the patient's progress. Inevitably head injuries will be admitted to hospitals not completely equipped to deal with every aspect of their treatment and for the severe injury or the unconscious patient with multiple injuries a major intensive care unit in a trauma centre is the ideal place for management.

The temptation is to *transport* the patient as rapidly as possible from the receiving hospital, but no patient should be transferred until fully examined and resuscitated and after having discussed the patient's condition with the specialist in the receiving hospital, transportation should then be organized. The airway must be scrupulously guarded during transport and if possible an endotracheal tube should be inserted. In the patient with severe pulmonary injury as well as head injury, transportation with controlled ventilation accompanied by an anaesthetist is desirable. The same holds true for the gunshot wound of the head. Only with this level of care can the incidence of patients who 'talk and die' be reduced during the transportation period. If the patient is not transferred until a pupil is fixed and irresponsive to light, the damage may be irreversible.

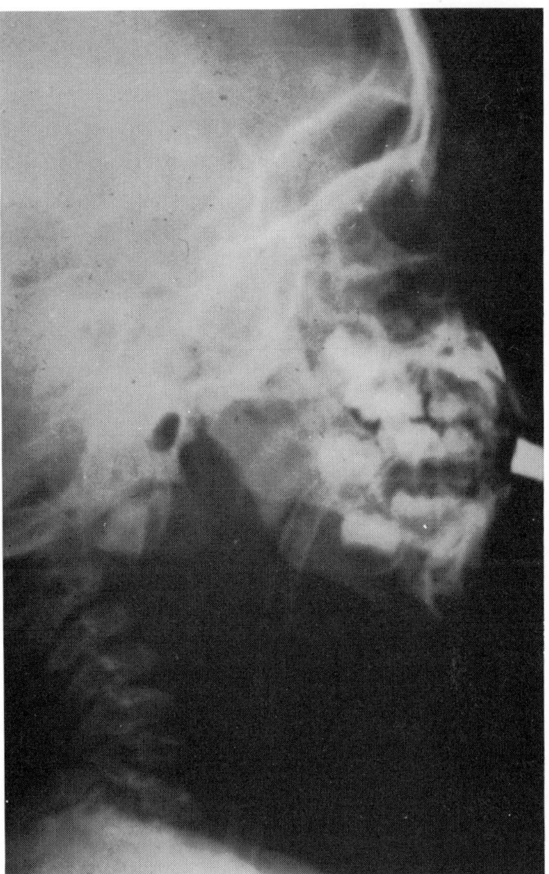

Fig. 34.8 Neck injury associated with a closed head injury. Note the fracture-dislocation of the odontoid peg; the endotracheal tube is pushed forwards by a large haematoma.

Investigations

For the patients with multiple injuries, there is an understandable desire to proceed as rapidly as possible to the radiology department where every conceivable radiograph is taken. This approach is to be resisted and the patient should not be moved from the resuscitation area until that process is complete. Occasionally with penetrating chest injuries or deterioration of ventilation, despite an endotracheal tube and underwater chest drainage, urgent radiology is required and in many trauma units this facility is available in the resuscitation area. As far as head injuries are concerned, clinical signs are more important to the clinicians than the presence or absence of skull fractures. For the unconscious head injury patient the minimum radiological requirements in the initial period are a *skull radiograph* (anteroposterior and lateral), *cervical spine* (*Fig.* 34.8) as far down as T1 and a *chest radiograph*. Unless these films are of good quality, they may be potentially hazardous. Thus, extradural haematomas in the adult are almost invariably associated with skull fracture (95%) but a poor quality radiograph may mask the fracture and lull suspicions. Good anteroposterior and lateral skull radiographs will reveal most vault fractures, some basal fractures, depressed fractures, foreign bodies, pineal shift, intracranial air (*Fig.* 34.9) and fluid levels in the sphenoid sinus (indicating dural tear and CSF leak). Cervical spine radiographs without clear views of C6, C7 and T1 will miss the areas most likely to be damaged in the acceleration/deceleration type of injury. For facial fractures suitable

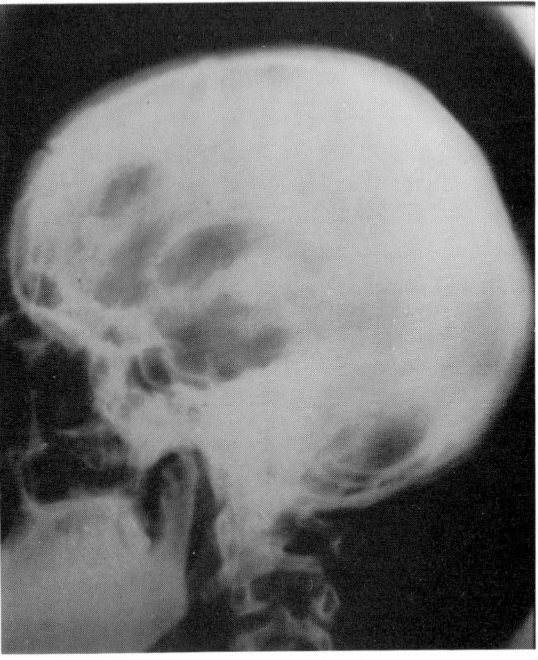

Fig. 34.9 Traumatic intracranial air in the subarachnoid space and ventricles. There is a frontal fracture but the air entered through bilateral petrous bone fractures.

views must be taken but it should be remembered that many of these views require good patient co-operation and unless there is a good indication, these radiographs may be delayed until later. The advent of computerized tomography has added a new dimension to diagnosis and management of the severe head injury (*Table* 34.3). Some would claim that it has made obsolete the need for skull radiographs, but there will be many places in the world where immediate availability of CT scan for all head injuries is out of the question and therefore some guidelines may be given as to which patients would most benefit from such an investigation. The availability of the CT scan makes angiography in the early post-injury period unnecessary in most severe injuries but as with plain radiographs, unless the CT scan is of good quality, the study is of little value. Therefore, if the patient is very restless a decision will have to be made as to the advisability of anaesthetizing the patient. Thus the clinician must ask himself if the information to be obtained is worth the risks involved in the investigation.

Table 34.3 CT scans in head injuries

In First 6 Hours
Unconscious with focal signs
Conscious with focal signs
Fluctuating level of consciousness
Deteriorating level of consciousness
Coma. Differential diagnosis
Epilepsy focal or general
Depressed fracture
Penetrating injury. Missile, shrapnel, etc.
Combined head and facial injury
In First Week
Repeat scan at 3 days in all above
Postoperative
Investigation CSF leaks
Intracranial infection
In First Month
? Intracranial infection
? Hydrocephalus
? Chronic subdural collections

Emergency Surgery

1. Suture of Scalp Laceration

Hair around the laceration should be clipped, the area thoroughly cleaned and the laceration probed for fractures, linear or depressed, which may have been missed on the plain skull radiograph. If there is a depressed fracture it must be explored and débrided under full operating conditions. In the absence of fractures the wound may be cleaned and sutured to appose the galea, subcutaneous tissue and skin.

2. Indications for Surgery during the First Day

If there is a deteriorating level of consciousness with a linear fracture through the temporal bone and focal signs, a patient may require an emergency burr hole to save his life. The decision to perform the operation in the general surgical unit, or whether to transfer him to a neurosurgical service will depend on the availability and the expertise of staff. *Patients with deteriorating levels of consciousness should not be placed in ambulances for long journeys*. On the other hand, it is quite common in the acute situation for a simple burr hole to be inadequate to cope with an intracerebral haematoma or 'burst lobe' and so the services of a neurosurgeon will be required. If possible the situation should be discussed with a neurosurgeon. Missile injuries will require expert neurosurgical care as will open and closed depressed fractures, and for any of these conditions early consultation and neurosurgical advice should be sought.

3. Anaesthesia

In a few deeply unconscious patients or in an extreme situation, burr holes may be required under local anaesthetic and there are many instances where this has been life-saving, but is not an ideal form of treatment, however, and with the general availability of highly trained anaesthetists even the simple burr hole is better managed under general anaesthesia. Induction of anaesthesia in the unconscious patient, with the probability of raised intracranial pressure is a delicate procedure, which, if inexpertly handled may cause irrevocable damage, such as coning. It is vitally important to prevent hypoxia or coughing and thus endotracheal intubation with controlled ventilation and the avoidance of inhalational agents such as halothane are the general principles of good neuroanaesthesia in the trauma situation.

4. Surgical Technique

Details of craniotomy, elevation of depressed fracture, craniocerebral missile injury, etc. are beyond the scope of this book but brief details are given as to the positioning of burr holes required for the evacuation of intracranial haematoma in an emergency situation. Temporal burr holes should be placed low in front of the ear and just above the zygomatic process. If an extradural haematoma is detected, another burr hole may be required in the posterior parietal region to help in the removal of the clot.

Active bleeding from the middle meningeal artery will necessitate a craniectomy which in its simplest terms is an enlargement of the temporal burr hole using bone rongeurs, but it may be necessary to convert the burr holes into a craniotomy for a satisfactory evacuation of the clot and haemostasis. Frontal and parietal burr holes should be placed 3–4 cm from the midline and in the acute situation it is wise to perform bilateral burr holes unless clinical signs or the CT scan indicate precisely the position of the clot. It must be emphasized, however, that with the current availability of CT scans close to major Accident and Emergency Departments, the indications for performing 'blind' burr hole is receding. It is preferable to intubate and ventilate the patient, administer a bolus of mannitol, perform appropriate CT scans and then plan a craniotomy.

Complications of Head Injury

Intracranial Haematoma

About 1 or 2% of all the patients admitted with head injuries have intracranial haematomas. As mentioned earlier, in the acute phase the distinction is merely between the extradural and intradural, as many of the intradural haematomas have components of the acute subdural haematoma, intracerebral clots and 'burst lobes'. Occasionally extradural and intradural are found in the same patient. Frequent neurological observations, good skull radiology to demonstrate fractures and a high degree of awareness will aid early detection and the unconscious patient with lateralizing signs, will usually be found to have an intracranial haematoma. There are some features which may help to distinguish between the extradural haematoma alone and the intradural clot. Classically the patient with an *extradural haematoma* may present after a relatively minor injury to the side of the head, is dazed, has a lucid interval then lapses into unconsciousness (*see Fig.* 34.3).

On the other hand the patient with an *intradural haematoma* may be unconscious from the time of injury, is less likely to have a lucid interval and is more prone to epilepsy (2% incidence of epilepsy in extradural haematoma, compared with 18% in intradural haematomas) (*Fig.* 34.10). Extradural haematomas are more common in younger patients while intradural clots are more common in patients over 40 years of age. Skull fractures are common in both groups. The siting of the clot is more closely related to the clinical signs than the position of the skull fracture. *Intracranial haematoma should be suspected in all those patients in coma with focal signs with a skull fracture and those who have not fully recovered consciousness 6 h after the injury*. If the injury has been severe, the haematoma or laceration may extend into the ventricular system. The outlook in such instances is very poor as it indicates brain damage to midline structures usually involving the hypothalamus or midbrain structures. The traumatic subarachnoid haemorrhage has little in common with the spontaneous subarachnoid bleed in terms of clinical course and prognosis. In the traumatic situation while the blood may be an irritant, the prognosis is that of the head injury.

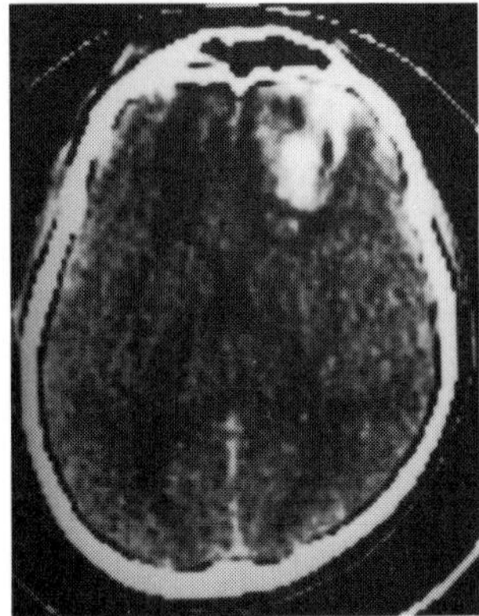

Fig. 34.10 Traumatic intracerebral haematoma in the right frontal area.

Depressed Fractures and Cranial Defects (*Fig.* 34.11)

Depressed fractures may be simple or compound, the former indicating that the skin is intact, the latter associated with a laceration and together they account for 10% of all the head injuries referred to neurosurgical units in the UK.

The indications for surgery in the closed depressed fracture are few; the risk of epilepsy is not reduced by operation, but when there are focal signs there is usually a contusion or small haematoma associated with the fracture and the elevation of the depressed fragments with removal of the clot may improve the neurological signs. Depressed fractures in the forehead may be elevated for cosmetic reasons. With *compound depressed fractures* however, there is a very significant risk of secondary brain infection and all of these *require surgery as soon as possible*. Infection after depressed fracture is usually associated with delayed operation because the severity of the injury was not appreciated initially. Treatment of depressed fractures should be performed by neurosurgeons, as the results from the Korean War show, where the incidence of infection was reduced from 41 to 1% by immediate evacuation of casualties to a neurosurgical unit. The same experience has been described in Belfast in the treatment of missile injuries while delayed diagnosis in civilian injuries in Scotland resulted in an infection rate of 10% in compound depressed fractures. The principles of surgery include adequate exposure, removal of all foreign material, evacuation of haematoma, small bone fragments, dural closure with the help of temporalis fascia or fascia lata, and adequate skin closure. Some authorities recommend the

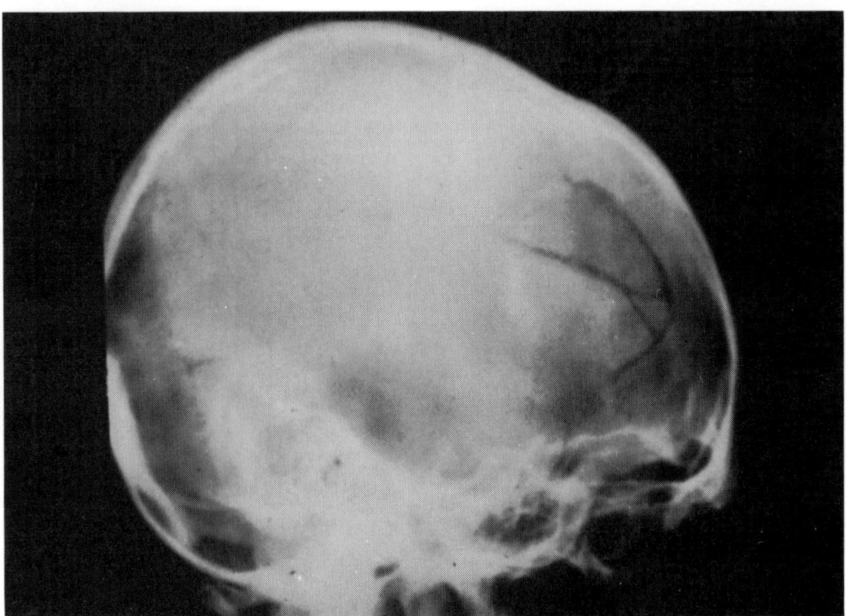

Fig. 34.11 Frontoparietal depressed fracture.

repositioning of the sterilized loose bone fragments to reduce the need for a subsequent cranioplasty and while this may be used occasionally, it is this author's opinion that a subsequent cranioplasty is a safer procedure.

There are many different methods of repairing skull defects, each having its proponent with split rib graft being one of the more popular methods involving living tissue. It does, however, require a thoracotomy and it seems to this author to be a major procedure for a minor defect. Acrylic plates either preformed or poured as cold setting material have been widely used and are generally satisfactory. Metallic cranioplasty with tantalum plates has been advocated for over 20 years but recently the introduction of *titanium* and accurate preforming techniques have provided a lightweight but strong cranioplasty which can be screwed into position using an on-lay technique and allows follow-up scanning without metallic artefact. Defects around the forehead with associated cranial facial injury can be repaired with strips of titanium which can also be used as a form of internal fixation for the unstable facial fracture (*Fig.* 34.12). An additional advantage of the titanium cranioplasty is that the metal is non-magnetic and will not interfere with subsequent magnetic resonance imaging.

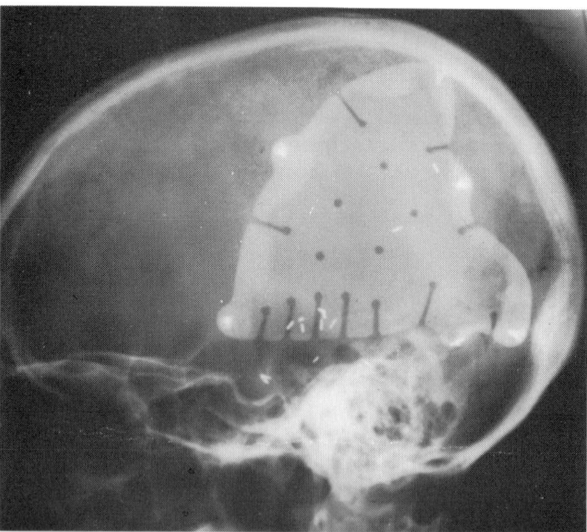

Fig. 34.12 Titanium plate cranioplasty.

Craniofacial Injuries (*Fig.* 34.13)

While head injuries may be life-threatening, craniofacial injuries rarely are so serious, but delay in the diagnosis and treatment of craniofacial injury is often due to inadequate examination and will lead to gross facial, orbital and dental deformities which may not be easily corrected in the recovery period. Craniofacial injuries may be divided into those involving only soft tissues, such as eyelids, eyes, tongue and pharynx, and those in which the facial skeleton is damaged, with maxillary and malar fractures which may affect the orbital contents trapping muscles in the fractures and, for instance, producing diplopia. Frontal impacts as well as leaving unstable facial fractures will result in injuries to the naso-ethmoidal complex, the orbital roof and fractures through the frontal bone and frontal sinus. These are almost invariably associated with dural lacerations and subfrontal

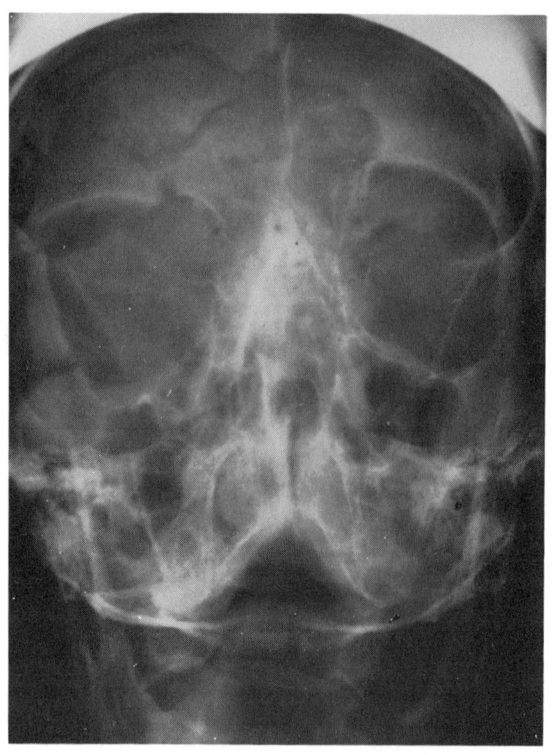

a

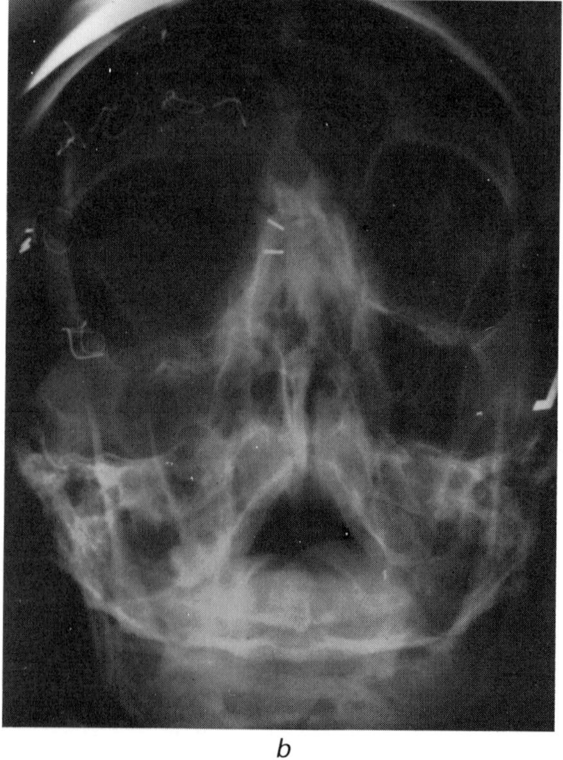

b

Fig 34.13 *a*, Extensive facial injuries with compound frontal fractures. *b*, Definitive surgery for intracranial débridement and correction of facial fractures performed at first operation.

brain damage and in severe cases may be associated with chiasmatic, pituitary stalk and hypothalamic damage. Occasionally urgent maxillofacial help is required to secure the airway and the arrest of haemorrhage with intranasal packs. Surgery within the first 24 h should be considered for the reduction of a severely displaced maxilla to improve the airway, stabilization of an anterior bilateral fracture of the mandible and intraoral haemorrhage, often a manual reduction. The eyelids and eyes should be attended to after resuscitation, if possible, and the adequate débridement, cleansing of wounds and accurate apposition of wound edges will go a long way to reduce postoperative scarring. If anaesthesia is required for a neurosurgical procedure such as a compound depressed fracture then maxillofacial correction can be considered at the same time. As with other branches of trauma management, teamwork is essential with co-operation at the highest level between the various specialties. Faciomaxillary injuries are considered in Chapter 26.

Cerebrospinal Fluid Fistula

With fractures involving the base of the skull there is a high incidence of CSF leak. This pertains particularly to those with significant facial injuries. In the acute post-injury period the loss of CSF may escape attention as there will be considerable bleeding from the nose and mouth. Occasionally, fluid may not leak externally but is swallowed by the patient as it leaks into the posterior pharynx.

Rhinorrhoea is the commonest presentation and is due to fractures involving the cribriform plate, the naso-ethmoid complex and occasionally fractures into the sphenoid sinus. Fractures involving the petrous bone either in the middle or posterior fossa components may result in otorrhoea. Very occasionally CSF may leak out through the orbit and present as tears. In the severe head injury with craniofacial involvement the rhinorrhoea may be profuse and a lateral skull radiograph performed during the resuscitation period may show air intradurally or intraventricularly and fluid levels in the sphenoidal sinus. *Reduction of the maxillary fracture may significantly reduce the rhinorrhoea.* In many patients with CSF fistula the escape of fluid has reduced significantly or stopped within 48 h. The possibility of a CSF fistula must always be borne in mind and the diagnosis made by a close examination of the skull films to detect fracture and testing with Dextrostix any clear fluid from the ear, nose or eye. (If there is blood mixed with the fluid a false positive result will be obtained.) All patients in whom a CSF fistula is suspected or diagnosed should be treated with a broad-spectrum antibiotic after culture of the normal flora of the nose, mouth and ears. If after 48 h the fistula persists, or if there is a severe leak of fluid earlier, the neurosurgeon should be involved. The indications for a dural repair will vary from patient to patient and neurosurgeon to neurosurgeon but in most cases a repair is indicated if the leak persists for 7–10 days. Prior to surgery it is important to obtain good radiographic evidence of the exact site of the fracture thought to be the site of the fistula.

Tomograms of the appropriate area of the base of the skull may be indicated. Metrizamide cisternography with CT scanning has proved effective in some cases and more accurate in localization in skilled hands than radio-isotope tags inserted into the CSF pathways. If highly skilled otorhinolaryngology is available the actual site of the leak in the anterior nasal passages may be confirmed by direct inspection and use of minute Dextrostix pledglets inserted into the nasal passages. If the fracture involves the cribriform plate there will be a loss of smell. Otorrhoea is often associated with deafness or vestibular nerve signs. An intracranial approach for dural repair is indicated in the anterior cribriform plate area for extensive fracturing involving the frontal sinuses, but transethmoidal or transphenoidal approaches should be considered in fistulas involving the sphenoid or posterior ethmoidal air sinus. The exact site of the fracture on the petrous bone must be determined to decide whether a middle or posterior fossa approach is required. Occasionally if the fracture involves the mastoid air sinuses a transmastoid approach can be used.

Infections

Intracranial infections will be considered subsequently.

Hydrocephalus

The advent of the CT scanner and intracranial pressure monitoring techniques have added a new dimension to the understanding of ventricular dilatation following head injury. In many cases the ventricles are reduced to slits during the first 48 or 72 h owing to generalized brain swelling. Very occasionally in the acute situation, a deteriorating level of consciousness may be due to aqueductal or fourth ventricular obstruction by blood. In such circumstances a burr hole and ventricular drainage may result in a dramatic improvement in the patient's condition. More usually, however, ventricular dilatation is not noted until weeks or months after the injury and the question then arises as to whether the patient has hydrocephalus (either high or normal pressure) or whether the ventricular dilatation is secondary to atrophy. An indication that hydrocephalus may be present can be obtained from the history of a patient whose rate of recovery has slowed down, i.e. a previously continent patient becoming incontinent, the development of staggering and walking with a broad-based gait. In such patients monitoring the intracranial pressure has shown the 'B' wave pattern of raised pressure and they may benefit from the insertion of a CSF shunt. It is probable that the incidence of hydrocephalus after intracranial emergencies such as trauma, haemorrhage or infection has been underdiagnosed, and a significant number of patients might benefit from the insertion of a shunt (*Fig.* 34.14).

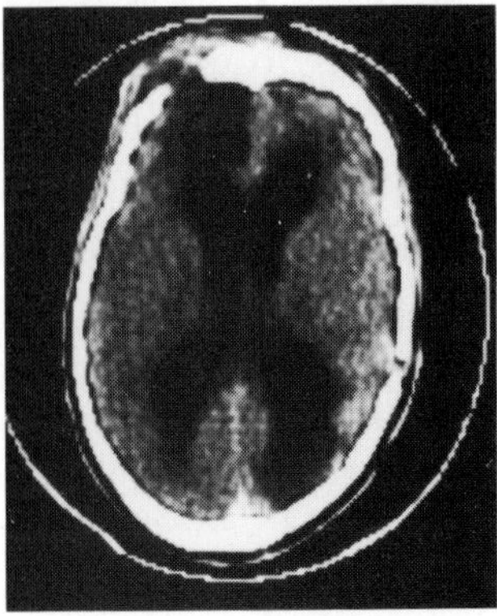

Fig. 34.14 Late effects of head injury. Cortical atrophy, ventricular dilatation and porencephalic cyst.

Epilepsy

As previously mentioned epilepsy may indicate the presence of a haematoma, but even in its absence epilepsy is a common post-traumatic complication the exact incidence of which varies with the severity of the injury. Thus in the severe missile injury 40% of the patients will eventually develop epileptic seizures, while only 5% of closed head injuries will develop this complication. Jennett's classic studies demonstrated the risk of epilepsy associated with the type of injury and the time following injury.

Early epilepsy, i.e. a fit occurring during the first week, is usually focal and a quarter of such cases will go on to develop *post-traumatic epilepsy*. In the early post-injury period there is a danger that *status epilepticus* may develop. Epilepsy after the first week is considered late epilepsy. In the closed head injury it is very much less common than early epilepsy but once established further fits may occur. The risks of epilepsy are higher in those who have had a post-traumatic amnesia of more than 24 h, dural penetration, intracranial haematoma, missile injury or early epilepsy. It can be a considerable disability in those who have otherwise made a good recovery.

Cranial Nerve Palsy

Any cranial nerve or any combination of cranial nerves may be damaged in head injury but the most common to suffer are the first, second, sixth, seventh and eighth. In cases of diplopia and deafness as well as facial palsy, it is important to ascertain if the defect is due to nerve transection, nerve compression or to entrapped muscles as in the diplopia due to fractures involving the orbital floor. Decompression of the facial nerve, surgical attention to the middle ear ossicles or freeing of a trapped inferior rectus muscle are valuable surgical manoeuvres.

Endocrine Disturbances

While diabetes insipidus is relatively rare following closed head injury, it is probable that a number of head injury patients suffer subclinical damage to the pituitary and hypothalamus. The supraoptic nucleus is particularly vulnerable as shown in recent experimental and clinical studies, and the pituitary stalk may be sectioned or a subsequent pituitary infarction may occur due to hypoperfusion, hypoxia and oedema. A significant number of children who have had severe head injuries become obese and display hypogonadism. Amenorrhoea following trauma for 2 or 3 months is often noted. In the acute situation diabetes insipidus may develop but a more common electrolyte disturbance is hyponatraemia thought to be due to the inappropriate secretion of antidiuretic hormone.

Coexisting or Predisposing Diseases

As mentioned earlier a predisposing disease such as a myocardial infarction or stroke as the cause of a head injury is relatively rare. Nevertheless, in the elderly patient it is important to exclude these possibilities. A history of diabetes or epilepsy should be sought. By far the most common predisposing condition is intoxication with alcohol or drugs.

The Minor Head Injury

For every one severe head injury treated, there may be 100 patients with less severe head injuries who have attended the hospital. Many of these patients require little more than reassurance but some will require admission and observation, and it is unfortunate that this difficult decision is often left to those with least experience. The *indications for admission* will vary from patient to patient and from area to area but there are certain conditions for which admission is indicated (*Table* 34.4).

Patients who have been stunned for a few seconds or are unconscious very briefly, have recovered fully and are accompanied by intelligent caring relatives may be discharged into the care of their relatives, who have been warned about signs of intracranial haematoma. Head injuries in infants and toddlers are a difficult problem. Many children curl up and go to sleep following an injury. Is this a normal response or is the drowsiness due to raised intracranial pressure? Fortunately it is rarely the latter. Children also have a tendency to vomit after head injury and there is a higher incidence of epilepsy in the same way that they are prone to febrile convulsions. If there are no abnormal neurological signs such a child may be discharged into the care of an intelligent mother who should be warned of the signs of increasing intracranial pressure and told to return if she is worried.

Table 34.4 Minor head injury: indications for admission

Altered level of consciousness
History of a fit following injury
Neurological signs
CSF fistula
Skull fracture on radiography
If the clinician is in doubt

Post-traumatic Syndromes

Post-concussional Syndrome

This was first described in the 1930s and applied to patients with a variety of persisting symptoms following head injury, the most common of which were headache, dizziness, impairment of memory, lack of concentration, depression and anxiety. It is more common in road traffic accidents than in sporting injuries. Medical opinion has been divided into those who have regarded them as malingerers and those who are convinced that there is an organic basis for the syndrome. Litigation obviously enhances the number and degree of symptoms but there is little doubt that there is an organic basis for some of their complaints.

A whiplash injury may be associated with the post-concussional syndrome in the patients who have suffered an acceleration/deceleration injury. There is intense neck pain, occasionally nystagmus, as well as the symptoms already described.

Psychiatric Syndromes

If the patient survives a major brain injury with extensive focal and generalized damage he is unlikely to be the same person. Intelligence levels drop, actions are often less inhibited and social graces may decline and attention span is very limited. Some children become hyperactive and virtually unmanageable, at least temporarily. In a few children and more commonly in adults a hypoactive state develops with loss of drive, initiative and depression.

Hydrocephalus

The incidence of the complication following injury has already been covered in Chapter 3.

Epilepsy

Already mentioned earlier in this chapter (*see* p. 476).

Prognosis

As mentioned earlier, using the Glasgow Coma Scale after

resuscitation period, those with a scale of 7 or less are severely disabled permanently and many will be a burden on their family or society if they survive the initial trauma. There are other factors which help in the assessment of outcome.

Age is by far the most important: the 50-year-old patient, unconscious for 24 h may never work again, whereas the 10-year-old, unconscious for 3 weeks, may have a successful career. It is not a sliding scale with age, thus adolescents have a considerably better outlook than those over 40 years of age. The association of other injuries must also be taken into consideration when assessing outcome, and again the young and previously healthy can withstand the injury much better than those in middle life. 'Recovery' has many components, the main three being physical, mental and social. Most physical recoveries will have taken place in the first 6 months after injury but improvements in the mental state and social behaviour may be slower. Jennett and Bond have described an 'Outcome Scale' and shown that 80% recovery is achieved in the first 6 months.

VASCULAR ACCIDENTS

Introduction

Cerebrovascular disease is the third commonest cause of death in Western Society and accounts for 1600 deaths per million of the population; one-half are due to cerebral thrombosis and embolism, one-third die from cerebral haemorrhages and 5% are caused by subarachnoid haemorrhage. Cerebrovascular disease is closely related to raised blood pressure and the incidence is falling in the USA, has been stationary in the UK and is increasing in Japan. The maximum reduction in mortality has been in females and is directly related to the control of blood pressure. In India there is a high incidence of cerebrovascular disease in the young in the absence of hypertension or diabetes. The *risk factors* associated with cerebrovascular disease are *hypertension* and *diabetes*, while elevated blood lipoproteins, so closely related with extracranial arterial disease, does not seem to be as closely associated with intracranial vascular disease. *Bood viscosity* is a major risk factor and population studies have shown that the group with the lowest risk from stroke are people who are normotensive with a low normal haematocrit. *Platelet microemboli* propagated on atheromatous plaques or due to changes in platelet adhesiveness are another risk factor. *Associated cardiac disease* causing hypotension, emboli in fibrillation, or low output states following myocardial infarction, must all be considered in the evaluation of cerebrovascular disease. Over one-half of the patients with heart disease will eventually have a cerebral infarction.

Strokes

A stroke may be defined as 'a focal neurological deficit due to a vascular lesion'. The causes are legion and some of the more common ones are listed in *Table* 34.5. In the over 60s, cerebral thrombosis and infarction are the most common causes (*Fig.* 34.15), while in children, trauma, epilepsy, tumours or a rare vasculitis may be implicated. The physiological requirements of neural tissue in terms of blood flow and energy supply have already been mentioned in the introductory chapter and form the basis of the diagnosis and management of the condition. Strokes may become a 'surgical problem' for two reasons. First, patients subjected to surgery may develop strokes in the postoperative period and

Table 34.5 Some causes of strokes

Thrombosis
Embolus
Cerebral haemorrhage
Subarachnoid haemorrhage
Hypoperfusion—cardiovascular
Hypoxia, hypercapnia—cardiorespiratory
Hypertension
Tumour
Trauma
Systemic diseases—diabetes
Intoxications—alcohol, barbiturate
Arteritis—giant cell, moya moya, etc.
Inflammatory diseases—granuloma
Infections
Venous thrombosis

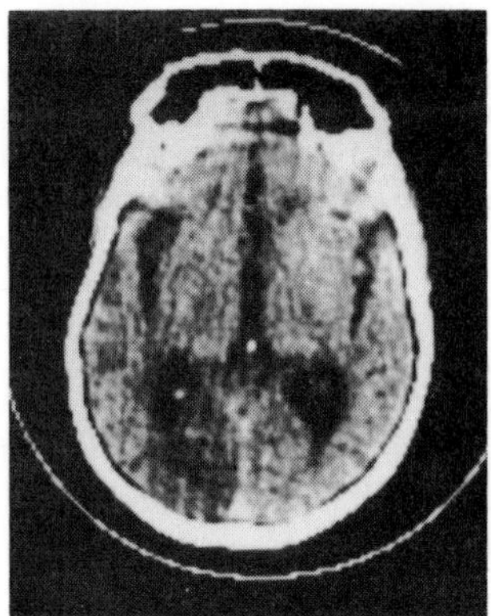

Fig. 34.15 CT appearance of a stroke showing low attenuation area supplied by a major vessel (left posterior cerebral).

so it is imperative that all surgeons have a working knowledge of the disease, its prevention and management. The second reason is that some strokes can be prevented or ameliorated by surgery and the indications for surgical intervention and pre- and postoperative management of these conditions will also be mentioned. A stroke which occurs in the carotid territory is characterized by a hemiplegia with a third nerve palsy and if the patient is conscious there may be a homonymous visual field defect. Lesions in the vertebrobasilar circulation are manifest by bulbar signs, such as difficulty or abnormal respiratory patterns and pinpoint pupils.

Strokes in Surgical Wards

Causes

In the context of the assessment of the surgical patient examination of the cerebrovascular system is of vital importance. Preoperatively its presence must be taken into consideration to decide if the patient is really fit for the proposed surgery.

Postoperatively the patient may have a stroke due to a *cardiac problem* causing pump failure and in this context it is worth remembering that a patient in atrial fibrillation has half of the expected cardiac output. Emboli may emanate from the heart following a myocardial infarct or after cardiac surgery. Half of the patients with heart disease will eventually have cerebral infarctions. Another common postoperative problem which may lead to a stroke is *fluid imbalance*; a patient who is dehydrated preoperatively and then inadequately transfused in the postoperative period will have marked *increased viscosity*. Less commonly over-correction of blood loss resulting in an over-generous red cell mass may occur and all these factors predispose to intravascular clotting. Inadequate pulmonary function and abnormal arterial blood gases are perhaps the commonest postoperative complication and the *hypoxia or hypercarbia* produced may be all that is required to tip the balance in favour of a stroke in an elderly patient. *Metabolic problems* are another common postoperative surgical problem which may predispose to a stroke; the diabetic patient may be less than adequately controlled after surgery and major hepatic or renal surgery may predispose to a stroke. Occasionally the stroke may be iatrogenic in that a *drug overdose* may be inadvertently administered, e.g. narcotics to those with poor pulmonary function or hepatorenal failure. Inadequate control of heparin or dicoumarol in the postoperative period may lead to intracerebral clots. Hypotension or hypertension are other common iatrogenic problems predisposing to a stroke. *Air embolism* must be considered, particularly in procedures such as air insufflation of uterus and Fallopian tubes.

During intracranial operation on venous sinuses or in patients in the sitting position, air may be sucked into the venous system.

Surgery for Stroke

Unless the stroke is due to a large intracerebral haematoma causing pressure and distortion *there is little that surgery can offer the patient with the completed stroke*. For many people there may be no premonitory signs but in 20% of patients this final neurological catastrophe is preceded by a transient ischaemic attack. A *transient ischaemic attack* (TIA) is a focal disturbance of cerebral circulation, often repetitive, which results in a period of impaired function lasting a short time and recovering without residual disability (Ross Russell). The differential diagnosis of a TIA must include focal epilepsy, migraine, diabetes, acute hypertension and generalized cerebral ischaemia but the main problems are in the extracranial portions of the vertebral and carotid arteries. Those in the carotid distribution often affect the middle cerebral artery territory producing weakness and clumsiness or numbness of the contralateral arm and leg. Occasionally there may be transient blindness (amaurosis fugax). Those in the vertebrobasilar territory cause vertigo often associated with extension or rotation of the neck, and there may be diplopia, ataxia or dysarthria.

There are a variety of pathophysiological mechanisms by which a transient ischaemic attack may be provoked. Systemic hypotension is an obvious example but a very rare cause of the condition. Compression of the extracranial artery by fibrous band or cervical spondylosis is also implicated but the two most commonly accepted factors are *platelet emboli* forming on and breaking away from atheroma and *vascular stenosis and occlusion* leading to hypoperfusion of the circle of Willis and producing either carotid or vertebrobasilar insufficiency depending on the configuration of the vessels, the degree of stenosis and changes in systemic blood pressure. It may be that a combination of the embolic and haemodynamic mechanisms occur in transient ischaemic attacks.

Angiography of patients reveals that two-thirds have multiple lesions, one-third have a stenotic lesion in the internal carotid and one-fifth show vertebral artery stenosis. In a further one-fifth of patients, no occlusion may be found and about 5% have an intracranial vascular lesion.

Since its first successful description in the early 1950s by Eastcott and his colleagues endarterectomy of affected vessels in the neck has been a widely employed technique throughout the world. The indications for its use, its success and its complications, however, have required a great deal of careful analysis to separate fact from fiction. An asymptomatic bruit over one carotid in a healthy, young, normotensive patient may not be sufficient cause to recommend a vascular procedure, no more than in the patient with the completed stroke in the acute situation in whom a carotid bruit is found. It is well to remember that patients presenting with cerebral atherosclerosis or transient ischaemic attacks have usually other signs of generalized atherosclerosis and their *mean survival as a population is 4 years from the date of the first ischaemic attack*. The cause of death in over half the patients is a *myocardial infarction*. Significant and lasting relief can be provided for many patients by medical treatment alone such as the control of blood pressure and stopping smoking. Hypertensive patients with normal pulses and no bruits are best treated by an antihypertensive and antiplatelet therapy. In young patients (less than 60 years of age) who have a bruit, angiography should be performed to outline the origins, cervical and intracranial portions of the four major vessels. Having established the diagnosis, the decision for surgery must be made for each individual patient and each individual medical centre.

There is no doubt that teams dealing with the problem on a regular basis have much better results. With an overall operative mortality of 1·5% there is no significant difference between medical and surgical management of patients with unilateral stenosis. Surgery is recommended for patients with bilateral stenosis or in unilateral stenosis and contralateral occlusion (*Table* 34.6).

Table 34.6 Therapy for strokes and cerebrovascular insufficiency

Medical	*Surgical*
Unfit for surgery	Fit for surgery
Completed stroke	Normotension
Acute stroke	Localized vascular lesion
Transient ischaemic attacks	Transient ischaemic attacks
Hypertension	Extracranial carotid disease
Vascular disease	Intracranial vascular insufficiency
Blood disorders	
Widespread intracranial disease	
Widespread extracranial vascular disease	
Dementia: vascular insufficiency	

Extracranial/Intracranial Anastomosis

Since the pioneering work of Donaghy, many surgeons throughout the world have become skilled in the successful suturing of vessels 1 mm in internal diameter. This skill has been greatly used in free skin flaps and repair of amputations and has been advocated as an operation to improve or counter cerebral ischaemia. The evaluation of the technique is still far from complete and there is no doubt that there are many operations performed throughout the world with dubious indications at present. Some would advocate its use in dementia due to cerebral atherosclerosis but there would

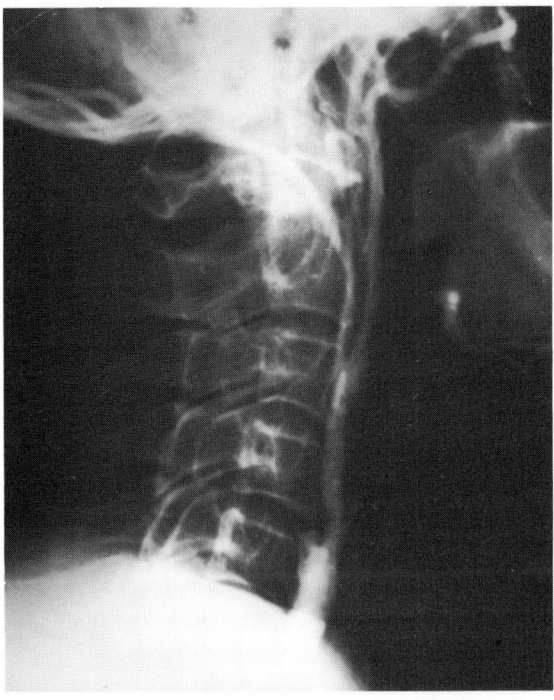

a

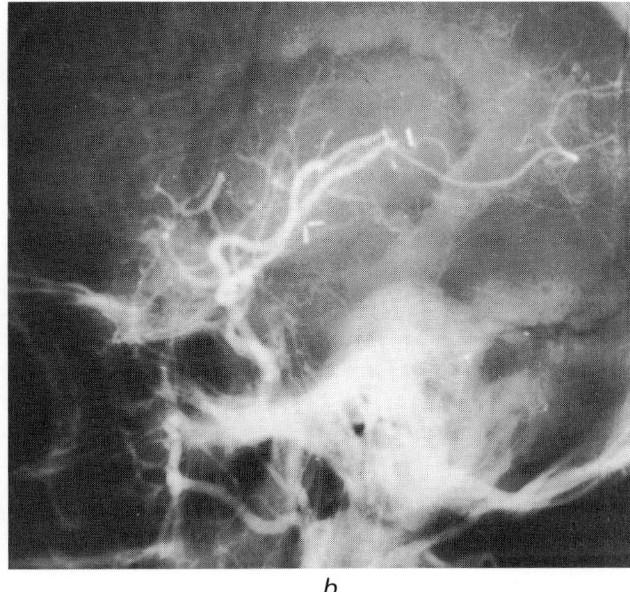

b

Fig. 34.16 Intracranial and extracranial vascular disease in a patient. *a*, Note occlusion of internal carotid with dependence on vertebral arteries. *b*, An extracranial/intracranial vascular anastomosis to improve blood supply and stop the patient's transient ischaemic attacks.

seem to be few physiological or objective clinical data to support this claim. There are undoubtedly some cases of transient ischaemia with multiple extracranial vessel disease in whom an extracranial/intracranial anastomosis abolishes symptoms (*Fig.* 34.16), but it must be emphasized that the procedure should only be considered after sufficient study and thought has been given to the major vessels in the neck. The excision of an intracranial vessel in which there is a giant aneurysm may be another rare indication for this procedure.

A recent international prospective study of patients undergoing extracranial/intracranial anastomosis following transient ischaemic attacks has failed to produce any evidence that surgery has any benefit over medical therapy over a five-year period. This has called into question the widespread use of the operation. It is a rare example of an international prospective study to evaluate a surgical procedure in the same rigorous way that a new drug should be assessed.

Intracranial Haemorrhage

Non-traumatic intracranial haemorrhage may occur within the brain substance, usually the subcortical white matter, or on the surface of the brain underneath the covering membranes of the brain, the so-called subarachnoid haemorrhage. Having bled it may extend from within outwards or vice versa, may rupture into the ventricular system, spread through the subarachnoid system or rupture into the subdural space. As with any other cerebrovascular accident, an intracranial haemorrhage is a sudden event with the abrupt onset of clinical signs and associated with a high mortality. Many of the affected patients have generalized arteriopathies, are hypertensive and their peak presentation is between 40 and 60 years of age. It has been traditionally the domain of the physician but over the last 20 years with improvements in diagnosis and operative techniques, surgery has been shown to play a significant part in the management of selected cases. Treatment, diagnosis and surgery must be available early. The purpose of this section is to outline the general principles in the pathology and natural course of events following intracranial haemorrhage so that the risks for each individual patient developing complications can be assessed, to allow an objective assessment of their treatment.

Subarachnoid Haemorrhage

Subarachnoid haemorrhage is a clinicopathological syndrome produced by blood in the subarachnoid space. It is due to the *rupture of an aneurysm* in over half the cases, while in a quarter no cause is found. Hypertension rupturing a small vessel accounts for 15%, arteriovenous malformations are present in 5% and less frequent causes are as diverse as blood dyscrasias, infections, tumours, angiopathy, intoxications and vitamin deficiencies.

Typically, the onset is abrupt with severe headache, neck stiffness, vomiting, photophobia in the mild cases and altered consciousness ranging from drowsiness to coma with focal neurological signs in the more severely affected. In the classic syndrome, the diagnosis should be relatively straightforward and it may be confirmed, having excluded papilloedema, by a lumbar puncture which will reveal evenly bloodstained CSF with a xanthochromic supernatant if the lumbar puncture is delayed for 12–24 h after the ictus. Such a diagnosis is only made in a quarter of patients on admission. The other major differential diagnoses include meningitis, brain tumour, cerebral haemorrhage or thrombosis. Systemic disease or a metabolic cause for coma may often be sought, particularly because of the glycosuria that often

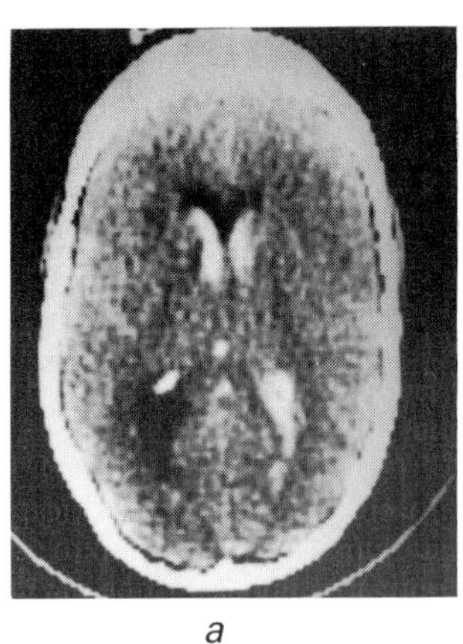

a

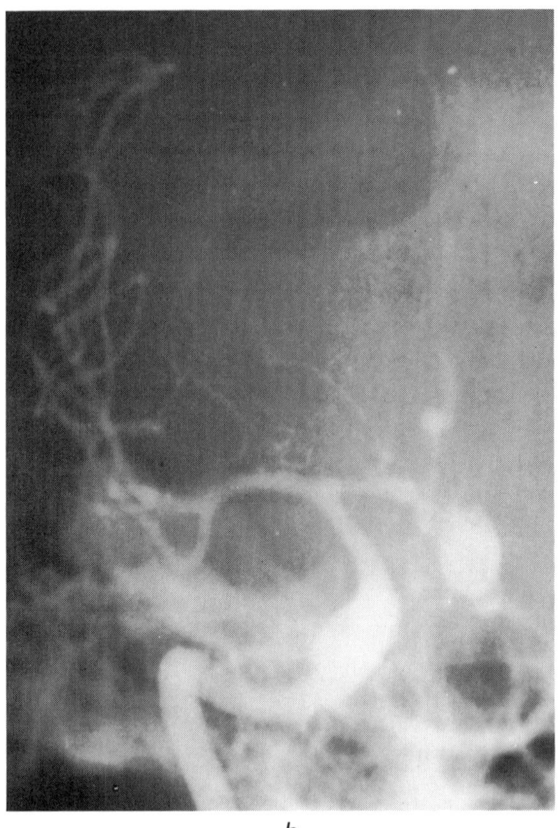

b

Fig. 34.17 *a*, CT scan of interventricular blood in a patient with a subarachnoid haemorrhage. *b*, Angiography revealed an anterior communicating artery aneurysm with marked spasm of the anterior cerebral artery.

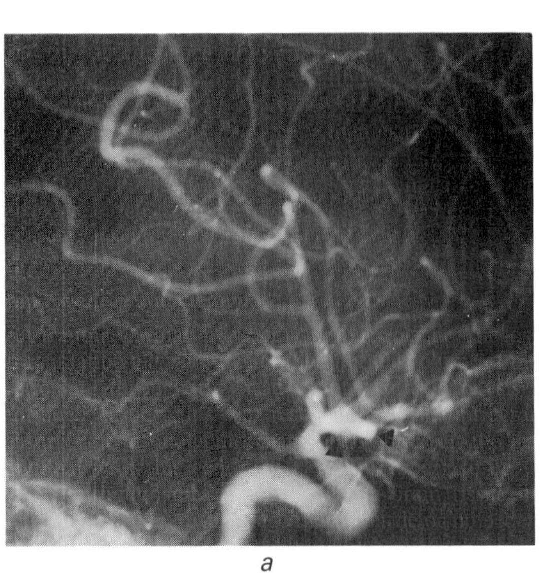

a

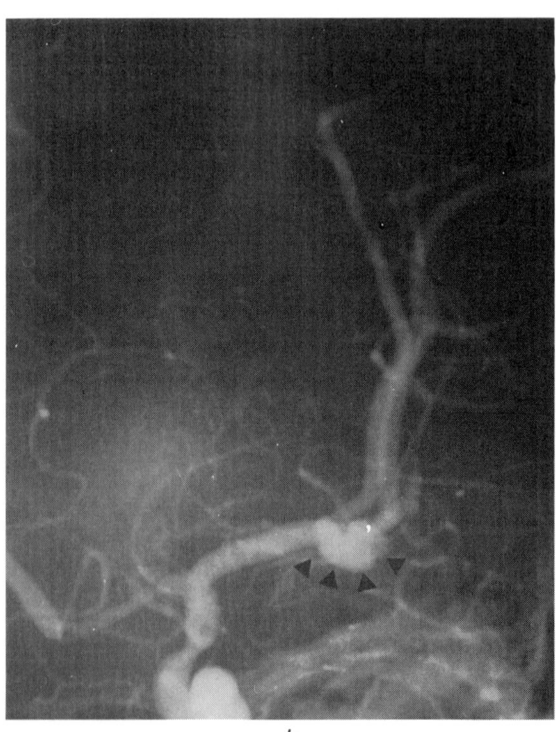

b

Fig. 34.18 *a*, *b*, More than one view will be required to successfully delineate an aneurysm, and unless the arteriography is of the highest quality optimal treatment is not possible.

accompanies subarachnoid haemorrhage. The elucidation of the subarachnoid haemorrhage requires radiological investigations such as CT scan and angiography (*Fig.* 34.17). In patients less than 30 years of age the cause is more likely to be an angioma or arteriovenous malformation, while patients aged between 40 and 60 years are more likely to have a ruptured aneurysm; in patients over 65 years hypertension is a significant cause. Males and females are equally affected, apart from the over 60s when females predominate.

Cerebral Aneurysms

Aneurysms of the major intracranial blood vessels are relatively rare but their rupture accounts for 28% of the cerebrovascular deaths in people less than 60 years of age. Their exact incidence is difficult to determine. In Western society there are 1–2 per 10 000 of the population per year diagnosed as having a subarachnoid haemorrhage due to an aneurysm. But with increasing awareness of the syndrome of subarachnoid haemorrhage and the ready availability of non-invasive tests such as CT scanning, it is confidently predicted that many more will be diagnosed each year, and the true incidence may be 10–12 per 10 000 per year. Haemorrhage from aneurysms is rare before the age of 20 with a sharp increase in incidence between 40–60, falling off rapidly thereafter. The aneurysms are usually saccular, often multilobular (*Fig.* 34.18) and are found at major branches of the circle of Willis. Over 90% of the aneurysms are concentrated on the anterior part of the circle of Willis, the most common site being the internal carotid artery (*Fig.* 34.19). Aneurysms of the posterior circulation account for 5–7% (*Fig.* 34.20). Most are classified as berry aneurysms, are associated with hypertension and atheroma, but a few may be due to embryological variants, or even rarer causes such as mycotic aneurysm due to bacterial endocarditis or trauma to a major cerebral vessel. Berry aneurysms gradually develop and rarely cause trouble until they are 5 mm in diameter. Thereafter there is a real possibility of their rupture. About 2% of all aneurysms continue to grow and present much later as space-occupying lesions, producing cranial nerve palsies, cavernous sinus syndromes or epilepsy. They are larger than 30 mm and defined as giant aneurysms. The actual rate of expansion of the aneurysm is obviously variable but in those cases in which angiography is being performed before a haemorrhage, it would seem that the rate of growth is over a period of years rather than months.

Aneurysms are often single but 1 person in 5 will have multiple aneurysms. Mirror image aneurysms are particularly common in the middle cerebral artery territory where 1 in 3 will be so affected. For this reason alone, *four vessel angiography must be performed in all cases* of subarachnoid haemorrhage.

Small aneurysms are often unsuspected until the presenting subarachnoid haemorrhage. Occasionally an internal carotid artery aneurysm may compress the oculomotor nerve producing localized supraorbital pain and a third nerve palsy, and in such patients, emergency angiography should be performed to define the aneurysm prior to its rupture. The rupture of the aneurysm may vary from a slight leakage of blood to a more major event with an associated haematoma and it is obvious that survival will depend on the severity of this event. Overall 10–12% of patients who have a subarachnoid haemorrhage due to a ruptured berry aneurysm will be dead before their admission to hospital. A significant proportion of the survivors will be moribund and the *overall mortality due to this first bleed from the aneurysm is 40%*. Of those who survive the first haemorrhage 35% will be dead within a year from a recurrent haemorrhage. Considered another way, *only half of those who survive a first haemorrhage will be alive 5 years later if not surgically treated.* The overall mortality rises to 64% with the second haemorrhage, and to 84% with the third bleed. Recurrence of haemorrhage from the aneurysm is most common during the first 6 weeks after the presenting haemorrhage with a peak 7–14 days later. Treated by bed rest alone only 40% will survive a year and the aim of therapy, therefore, must be to prevent the aneurysm bleeding again either by encouraging thrombosis and fibrosis in the aneurysm or by excluding it from the circulation by a surgical procedure. This then is the dilemma presented in the management of the subarachnoid haemorrhage: the more delayed, the fitter the patient will be to survive the operation, the more likelihood of the aneurysm producing the final fatal bleed before the surgery is performed. Thus, for each patient the risks of delay versus urgent surgery must be carefully weighed up by specialists in the field.

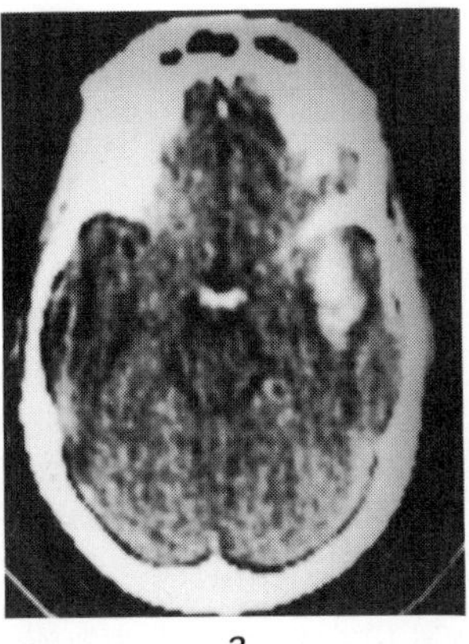

a

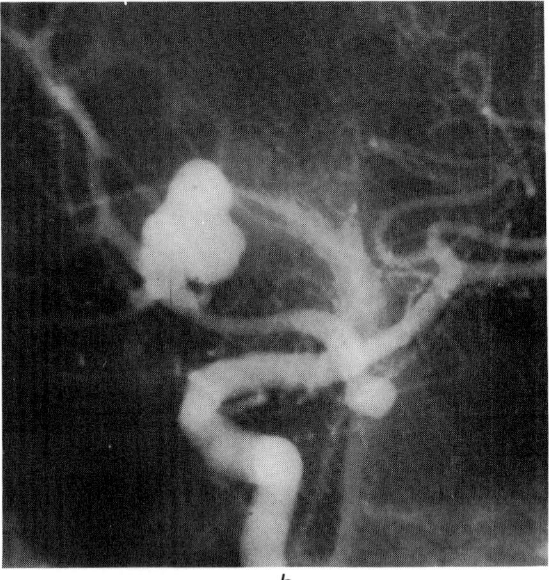

b

Fig. 34.19 *a*, Spontaneous intracranial haemorrhage. *b*, Due to a ruptured middle cerebral artery aneurysm. Note the associated internal carotid aneurysm (20% of patients have multiple aneurysms).

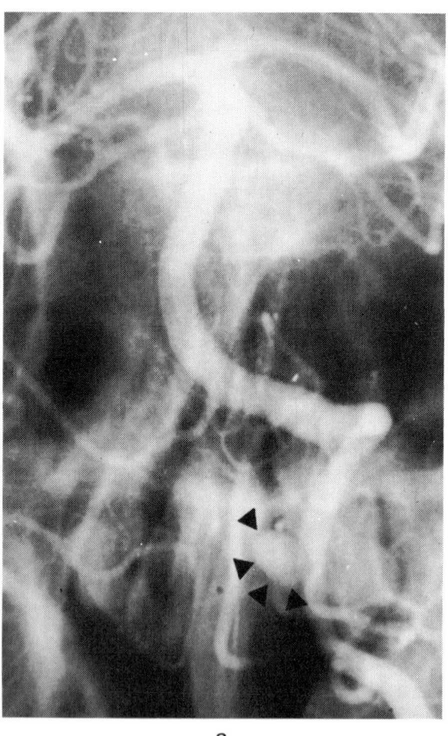
a

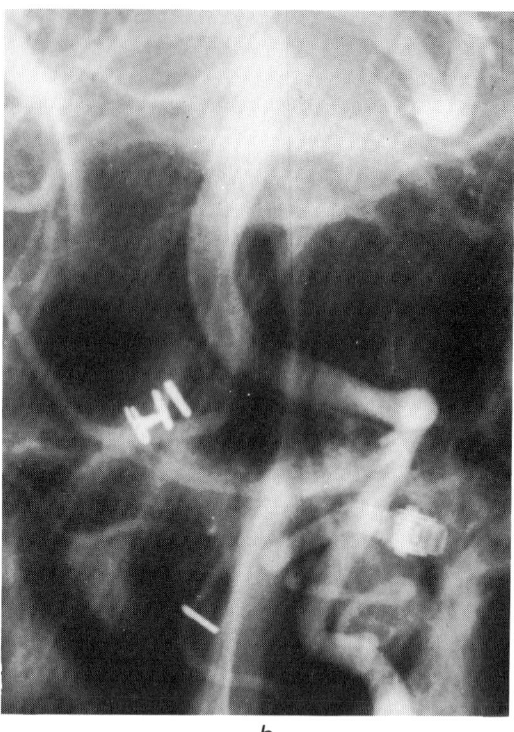
b

Fig. 34.20 *a*, Vertebral arteriography revealed an aneurysm at the origin of the posterior inferior cerebellar artery. *b*, At operation an angled Heifetz clip successfully occluded the aneurysm and preserved the posterior inferior cerebellar artery and this was confirmed by postoperative angiography.

Following the subarachnoid haemorrhage there are a series of pathophysiological changes and complications which may develop on which depends the outcome in terms of survival or its quality. As blood escapes from the ruptured vessel it will produce an acute rise in intracranial pressure which reduces the cerebral perfusion pressure producing focal and generalized ischaemia. As the pressure rises the midbrain and brainstem will be compressed causing bradycardia, a reduction in cardiac output, changes in pulmonary function and in severe cases neurogenic pulmonary oedema. There will be a massive increase in circulating catecholamines, a reduction in renal function and a glycosuria. The blood vessels surrounding the ruptured aneurysms may go into spasm producing intense focal ischaemia. Blood escaping from the aneurysm may produce a clot, causing brain shift and coning. Epilepsy may occur. Gastric haemorrhages from acute gastric erosions are common and there are cardiac changes ranging from conduction abnormalities to electrocardiographic changes indistinguishable from a myocardial infarction. Following these immediate complications there may be focal or generalized brain swelling as a result of the initial ischaemia or as a result of persisting vasospasm (*see below*).

There may be areas of infarction usually related to intense spasm in the parent vessel to which the aneurysm is attached and it is estimated that between 45–70% of patients who have subarachnoid haemorrhage will have *ischaemia* or actual *infarctions*. *Arterial spasm* following subarachnoid haemorrhage has been a condition which has challenged and puzzled researchers for many years and there would appear to be two distinct components, an initial spastic response developing immediately after the haemorrhage and lasting a few hours, and the spasm that occurs after the initial event and is maximal between the fifth and tenth days. Clinically it is manifested by gradual deterioration in the patient's conscious level and the development of focal neurological signs, the appearance on CT scan of large areas of low attenuation and an angiographic appearance of poorly filling intracranial vessels. If sufficiently severe, large areas of infarction will be produced and a significant proportion of the mortality and morbidity following subarachnoid haemorrhage is due to this complication. The exact mechanism is not yet understood but requires three components: a damaged blood vessel, blood in the subarachnoid space, especially a clot around the aneurysm, and some brain damage.

Late complications following subarachnoid haemorrhage may be the direct result of the complications already mentioned. In addition, there is the important and often under-diagnosed complication of *post-haemorrhagic hydrocephalus*. The blood in the subarachnoid space produces adhesions around the tentorium or obstructs the arachnoid granulations to produce hydrocephalus. In the first week or so after haemorrhage many patients have dilated ventricles which resolve spontaneously, but in a few patients the process continues and they may survive the haemorrhage to present subsequently with normal pressure hydrocephalus. It is important therefore that all patients who have had a subarachnoid haemorrhage have a CT scan 6 months after the ictus.

With so many complications, the potential rebleeding, the general health of the patient and the presence of other systemic diseases make the analysis of various forms of treatment difficult. The adoption of an internationally accepted classification has allowed sufficient data to accumulate to provide valid information on the natural history of the disease and thus allow comparison of the efficacy of the various forms of therapy. The classification of Hunt and Hess (*Table* 34.7) is the most generally accepted variant of Botterell's original classification. The aim of therapy therefore must be directed at maintaining or improving the patient's original presenting grade in the Hunt and Hess classification and if surgery is employed then the operative mortality or morbidity expected from the surgeon should be less than that accruing from the untreated disease. Obviously aneurysms must be treated in specialized units by neurosurgical teams practised in their management; this is not the field for the occasional operator. *Treatment of subarachnoid haemorrhage* consists initially of the care of the unconscious patient and attention to the pathophysiological changes described in Chapter 32.

Table 34.7 The Hunt and Hess grading system for subarachnoid haemorrhage (After Hunt and Hess (1968) Surgical risks as related to time of intervention in the repair of intracranial aneurysms. *J. Neurosurg.* **28**, 14–21).

Grade 1	Asymptomatic. Slight headache and neck stiffness
Grade 2	Severe headache and neck stiffness. No neurological signs or neurology
Grade 3	Drowsy, confused, or mild focal deficit
Grade 4	Stupor. Hemiparesis. Vegetative disturbances
Grade 5	Coma. Decerebrate rigidity

Bed rest, analgesia for headaches, anti-emetics for vomiting and the avoidance of direct light to help the photophobia are all general measures aimed at alleviating the symptoms. Often the patient's blood pressure is raised when first admitted and the problem is that of deciding whether the hypertension is a pre-existing condition or secondary to the raised intracranial pressure and impaired cerebral perfusion. Vigorous control of blood pressure should be avoided; if there are cardiac abnormalities on ECG then a beta-blocking drug may improve the cardiac status as well as reducing the blood pressure. Small doses of chlorpromazine (25 mg) may allay the patient's anxiety as well as reducing the blood pressure. Dexamethasone 4 mg 4-hourly may reduce the complications of ischaemia. The risk of further haemorrhage may be reduced by the careful administration of antifibrinolytic agents such as tranexamic acid or EACA. Patients in Grades 1 and 2 (Hunt and Hess classification) should proceed rapidly for further investigation, identification of the aneurysm and surgery. Grade 5 patients are too ill and should be treated conservatively until their condition improves. The problem has always been Grades 3 and 4. If a patient is deteriorating, having presented in Grade 1 there is a likelihood that he has an intracranial haematoma or there is progressive arterial spasm. Investigation should be carried out quickly and if a haematoma is present, surgery for the removal of the haematoma should be carried out. If, however, the patient presents in Grades 3 and 4 and shows signs of improving, angiography should be delayed as long as possible.

These are difficult decisions and ones that must be carefully weighed up by a team experienced in the management of the problems.

Surgery has been revolutionized by the use of the operating microscope and the availability of a wide variety of spring clips. It is possible with the magnification and good lighting provided by the microscope to identify perforating vessels, distinguish them from adhesions, identify accurately the neck of the aneurysms and place exactly a clip to occlude it. Operative mortality will vary with the site of the aneurysm but averages 5–10% for internal carotid artery aneurysms, 10–20% for anterior communicating artery aneurysms and 20–30% for basilar aneuryms. The choice of materials for manufacture of the clip has now become an important issue with the advent of magnetic resonance imaging. Deaths have already been described following the investigation in the postoperative period of patients with ferromagnetic aneurysm clips. Indirect surgical procedures such as carotid ligation and proximal arterial clipping are being used less and less as surgeons become experienced with the operating microscope. Occasionally the aneurysm has no neck and in these circumstances the defect is wrapped in gauze, soaked in a biological cement.

INFECTIONS OF THE NERVOUS SYSTEM

Introduction

Infections of the CNS are fairly common and are caused by bacterial, fungal, parasitic, rickettsial and viral organisms which produce inflammatory changes in the brain and its surrounding membranes which may result in diffuse changes such as meningo-encephalitis or more localized pathology as in a brain abscess or tuberculoma. *Many of the central nervous system infections can be cured by early, aggressive and appropriate treatment.* Delay in diagnosis often results in therapeutic failure and while they often present a difficult diagnostic problem occurring in patients already suffering from other systemic diseases, it is important to suspect and exclude a CNS infection when there is any history of increasing headaches, clouding of consciousness, pyrexia or meningeal irritation. It is impossible in this chapter to cover adequately the protean aspects of CNS infections; guidelines of the more common diseases, their presentation and management are given.

The diseases produced may be a meningitis, an encephalitis, meningo-encephalitis, cerebritis, ventriculitis or abscess formation. Meningitis or ventriculitis will cause obstruction to the fluid pathways and interfere with the absorption of CSF and hydrocephalus is a frequent complication. The cranial nerves at the base of the brain may be involved in the inflammatory process resulting in nerve palsies. Surface veins or the dural sinuses may be involved and thrombosis or thrombophlebitis may occur, particularly in the young. Encephalitis or cerebritis will always produce brain oedema, brain swelling, brain shift and the possibility of tentorial or foramen magnum herniation; viral illnesses may produce areas of necrosis.

Bacterial Infection

The usual infecting organisms are the staphylococcus, streptococcus, pneumococcus, *E. coli* and proteus. Infections with pseudomonas and klebsiella species are less common and are often secondary to inadequately treated infections or general debilitation. The organisms gain entrance by bloodborne infection from an antecedent infection, such as a pneumonia, or a septicaemia in an infant. Fractures, especially around the paranasal air sinuses, and penetrating wounds will predispose to the infection. Infections around the paranasal sinuses may also cause a meningitis. Postoperative infections after a craniotomy or more commonly the infection of CSF shunt system or reservoir are more usually due to the commensal *Staphylococcus epidermidis*.

With the exception of shunt infections, bacterial meningitis is usually an acute *fulminating illness characterized by fever, headache, nausea and vomiting and nuchal rigidity*. Ten per cent of patients lapse into coma at an early stage and focal or generalized epileptic seizures are noted early in 20% of the patients. Lumbar puncture may show a raised pressure, cloudy CSF with numerous polymorphs, raised protein and a low sugar (*Table* 32.2), and in over 90% of the cases culture will reveal the organism.

A CT scan at this stage may be unremarkable but is a useful baseline to compare subsequent events such as abscess formation or hydrocephalus (*Fig.* 34.21). Adequate antibiotic therapy must be given after a CSF sample is obtained and before the results of the culture are known. It is important that the therapy chosen should penetrate the blood–brain barrier, although this will be impaired in an inflammatory reaction and some idea of the infecting organism can be made from the presumed cause of the meningitis. The paranasal air sinuses often contain streptococci or pneumococci, while the mastoid air cells or middle ear may produce *E. coli* or proteus and appropriate antibiotics should be used. Intravenous infusions are usually sufficient to obtain high blood levels with good penetration into the CSF spaces for flucloxacillin and related antibiotics. If, however, Gram-negative bacteria are suspected, such as in neonatal meningitis, then aminoglycosides should be used and because of their low penetration to the CSF spaces, intrathecal administration is recommended for them. The classic regimen of sulphonamides, crystalline penicillin and chloramphenicol is a well-tried combination when in doubt and a favourite of a former generation, but there are, however, many organisms which are resistant to penicillin and with the availability of more powerful broad-spectrum antibiotics the emphasis on triple therapy is receding. If a blood-borne route is suspected, especially in the presence of abdominal sepsis or mastoid infection, bacteroides can often be cultured with selective techniques and it is for this reason that metronidazole should be added to the antibiotics in severe meningitis or brain abscess (*see below*). If aminoglycosides are used, blood levels should be in the therapeutic range and this can be performed quite rapidly in most large laboratories to allow adjustment to a therapeutic range. Too often failure with the aminoglycosides is due to inadequate therapy based on dosage calculated from the body weight and not on blood levels. Frequent lumbar punctures (every 24–48 h) during the first week will confirm the efficiency of therapy and a falling white cell count, a change from polymorphonuclears to mononuclear cells with a fall in CSF protein will indicate success. Rising white cell counts or failure to fall may indicate inappropriate antibiotic therapy, loculation, hydrocephalus or a brain abscess. Other therapy that may be used during the acute bacterial stage are steroids to reduce brain oedema and improve CSF transport and absorption through the arachnoid villi. If there is much brain swelling, intravenous mannitol may also be employed. In the presence of a shunt system or any foreign material left at operation this must be removed and other means of removing the CSF, such as daily ventricular aspiration of fluid, must be considered. Antibiotic therapy must be continued until the cell count has fallen and until the temperature has returned to normal for several days. Careful monitoring of renal and liver function is required especially with the use of streptomycin or the aminoglycosides. Cephalosporins should not be used. Anticonvulsants must be employed if there have been any fits. Careful monitoring of the patient's progress is absolutely essential to detect the development of hydrocephalus.

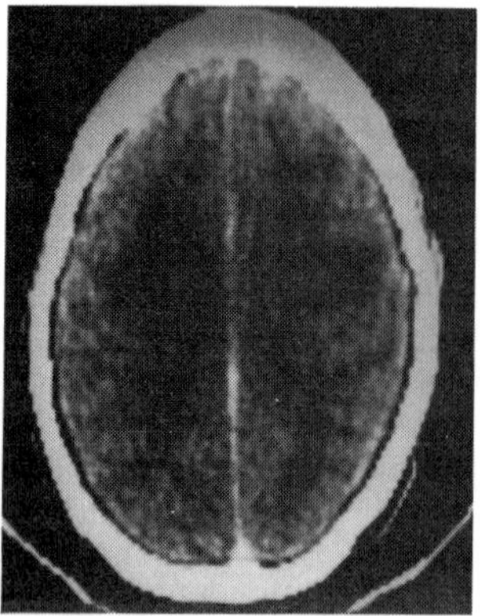

Fig. 34.21 Meningitis and cerebritis producing diffuse oedema.

The Immunosuppressed Patient

Patients being treated for Hodgkin's disease or leukaemias by radiotherapy or those with sarcoid or diabetes are particularly susceptible to meningitides of unusual varieties such as those caused by nocardia and pseudomonas as well as those caused by fungi such as cryptococci and candida.

Careful examination of the CSF, cultures in aerobic and anaerobic conditions and cytospin techniques for concentrating the organism all must be employed in such patients.

Since the writing of the first edition, the increase in patients suffering from AIDS (acquired immune deficiency syndrome) has produced many patients requiring neurosurgical evaluation and treatment and in certain hospitals in New York and Miami, admissions have been as common as those due to trauma. Any patient with multiple intracranial abscesses or recurrent intracranial infection must be carefully evaluated for this complication.

Tuberculous Meningitis

Unlike bacterial meningitis the course of tuberculous meningitis may be insidious, develop over 2 weeks but again is characterized by headache, fever, drowsiness and neck stiffness. Well over half the patients will have signs of pulmonary tuberculosis on a chest radiograph and a third may have evidence of miliary spread. Cerebrospinal fluid reveals numerous lymphocytes, a low sugar content and, after cytospin, organisms positive to Ziehl–Neelsen stain may be identified. The best results will obviously come from laboratories well versed in the technique, while the average laboratory may identify the organisms on smear in less than 10% of cases. CSF culture will be positive in well over half but unfortunately the result is not to hand for weeks. Treatment therefore of tuberculous meningitis must be with triple therapy from the time that it is suspected and must be continued for 6 months. The classic triple therapy of PAS, isoniazid and streptomycin has been replaced by isoniazid 300 mg daily with rifampicin 600 mg daily and ethambutol 25 mg/kg daily. Hydrocephalus, cranial nerve palsies and epilepsy are common complications and any indication of ventricular enlargement on the CT scan may indicate that a shunt is required.

Fungal Meningitis

A cryptococcus or candida infection may produce signs and symptoms mimicking tuberculous meningitis. Examination of the CSF will reveal essential differences (*Table* 32.2). Careful culture and a high index of suspicion are required if these causes of meningitis are to be successfully treated.

Amphotericin B 0·5 mg/kg intravenously, daily, is required for a period of 8–10 weeks. The drug itself is toxic and may produce confusing signs such as fever and drowsiness with the development of renal failure and electrolyte abnormalities.

Brain Abscesses

Though a relatively uncommon form of infection of the CNS, brain abscesses are a diagnostic and therapeutic challenge. If detected early and treated vigorously the patient will survive. However, it is a sad reflection on the level of detection when a community review of the disease revealed the overall mortality, including those undetected until postmortem, is still over 60%. Brain abscesses are usually secondary to sepsis elsewhere in the body and in the USA blood-borne infections from chest or abdominal disease are the most common. Infection of the paranasal air spaces or chronic suppurative otitis media (CSOM), however, is the most common cause in the UK although this is rapidly changing towards the American pattern with improved attention to 'glue ears'. Trauma, either direct penetration of the brain substances or dural tears associated with fractures of the air sinuses, are relatively less common causes of abscesses. Postoperative abscesses are mercifully rarer still. The common sites for abscesses are the temporal and frontal lobes where over half of the abscesses are found. Posterior parietal, occipital and cerebellar abscesses are very rare as are those around the thalamus. Multiple abscesses are found in immunosuppressed patients and those with cardiac abnormalities, such as Fallot's tetralogy. The population most at risk are those in the fourth to sixth decades.

There is an inverse relationship between the length of history and mortality. Those with signs and symptoms of less than 2 weeks usually have a cerebritis, intense oedema formation with brain shift (*Fig.* 34.22), and a mortality of 70%, while those with a history extending over several months present as a 'tumour' and have a well-localized abscess with little oedema surrounding it (*Fig.* 34.23). Survival is also related to the level of consciousness at the time of presentation; those with a rapidly deteriorating level of consciousness have a poor prognosis regardless of treatment, whereas those with focal signs, such as epilepsy or hemiparesis, can expect a good outcome. There is no typical history and a high index of suspicion of a change in level of consciousness, epilepsy, hemiparesis in a patient known to have sepsis or a head injury in the recent past must alert the clinician to the possibility of intracranial sepsis and the presence of an abscess. Lumbar puncture should be deferred until a *CT scan* excludes the presence of a mass lesion. Occasionally an angiogram will be required to differentiate between an abscess and a vascular tumour but indications for this latter examination are becoming fewer and there is certainly *no place for ventriculography* in the identification of an abscess nowadays.

Treatment of the abscess has been revolutionized by the presence of the CT scan which allows careful monitoring. During the state of cerebritis with no pus, recent work has shown that successful treatment may be achieved by CT scan-monitored antibiotic therapy. However the surgical principle of drainage of pus must be followed intracranially, as in other parts of the body, and this should be accompanied by appropriate antibiotic and anticonvulsant therapy.

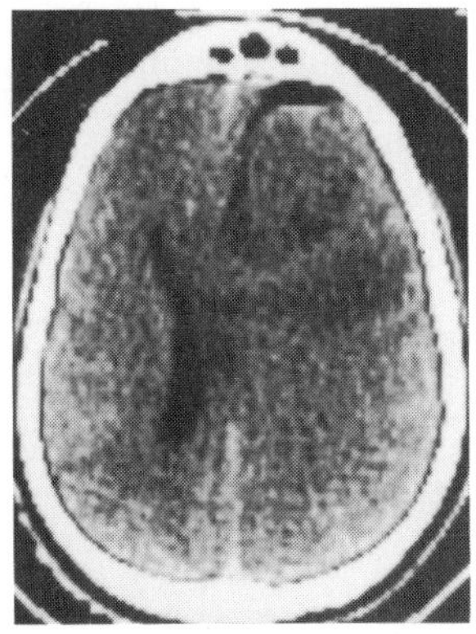

Fig. 34.22 An acute abscess showing air and fluid as it extended from the frontal sinus. The infection is not well demarcated from the surrounding brain.

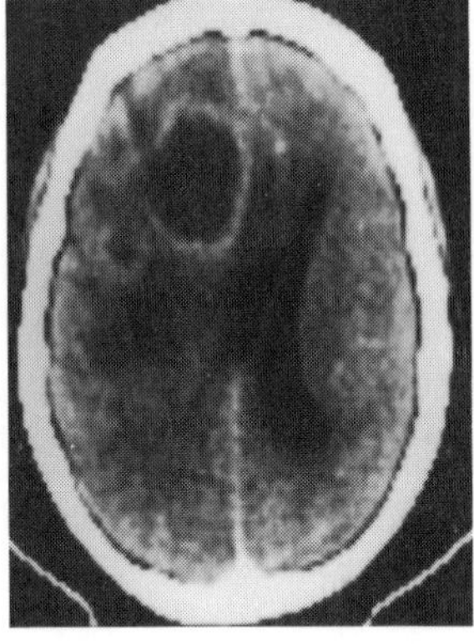

Fig. 34.23 A chronic abscess cavity with several daughter cavities; the capsule enhances and the lesion is well demarcated.

Excision of the wall of the abscess, classically taught, may be less important than previously considered. It does not reduce the risk of epilepsy and the associated morbidity with the attempted removal of the abscess wall means that it should be considered only routinely in infratentorial abscesses in the cerebellum related to middle ear infections.

Spinal Abscesses

Spinal abscesses are usually epidural, caused by the extension of a vertebral osteomyelitis or haematogenous spread from a distant source. The patient is acutely ill with local spinal tenderness, rapid progression from girdle pain to impaired cord function over a few days. Lumbar puncture reveals raised protein and myelography outlines the site of the abscess. An emergency laminectomy is required with drainage of the abscess and specific antibiotic therapy instituted and continued over 6–8 weeks. Spinal subdural abscesses are relatively less common and treated by drainage of subdural pus by lumbar puncture if possible and antibiotic therapy.

Viral Infections

Viral encephalitis has usually an abrupt onset, characterized by a fever, rapid loss of consciousness and in many cases epileptic fits. One-third to one-half of the affected patients will have a history of an upper respiratory tract infection in themselves or members of their family, and there is a seasonal incidence in late spring and autumn. One of the most devastating is that caused by herpes simplex virus which produces an acute necrotizing encephalitis, affecting the temporal and frontal lobes and from which up to one-half of the patients die and many of the survivors have severe deficits (*Fig.* 34.24).

Diagnosis is on CT scan appearances of bitemporal oedema, bilateral temporal slow waves on EEG and a positive biopsy. Antiviral titres are not diagnostic without acute and convalescent serum with a 3-week interval. Treatment with antiviral agents has been advocated using adenine arabinoside A (Ara-a) 15 mg/kg for 10 days, and while initial results were encouraging the outcome in larger series is more dubious.

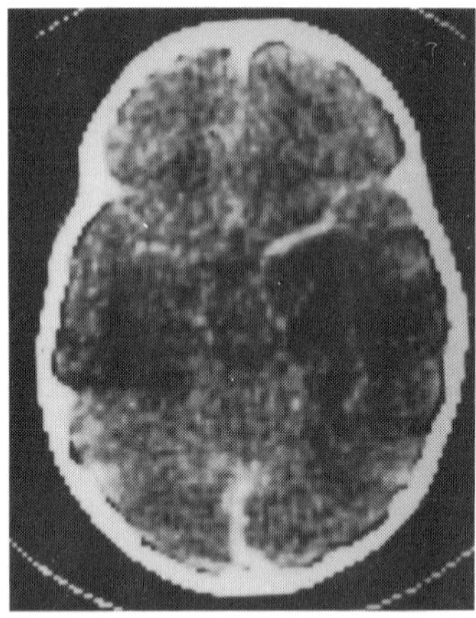

Fig. 34.24 *Herpes simplex* encephalitis showing bilateral temporal lobe oedema and necrosis.

Tuberculoma

Tuberculomas are extremely uncommon in Europeans but may represent 20% of all the 'brain tumours' presenting in Indian neurosurgical practice. It is characterized by its insidious onset and development of focal signs of epilepsy. CT scan (*Fig.* 34.25) and angiography help to make the

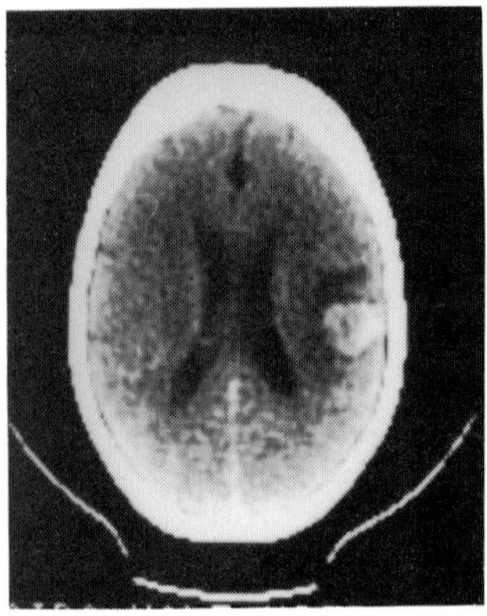

Fig. 34.25 A tuberculoma presents a solid mass which may be mistaken for a tumour.

Parasitic Infections

Protozoan infections are perhaps one of the commonest causes of headaches, drowsiness and pyrexia. There are still 300 000 000 people living in areas where malaria has not been eradicated and 10% of all deaths in infants in Africa are due to this infection. Trypanosomiasis causes sleeping sickness and is prevalent in central and eastern Africa. Toxoplasmosis is another common protozoal infection affecting the CNS. It may be in a congenital form when the fetus is infected in the last 6 months (infection before this results in a stillbirth). It affects the brain and the eyes, causing periventricular necrosis, hydrocephalus and multiple areas of cerebral calcification.

An acquired form of toxoplasmosis results in a meningo-encephalitis and hepatitis.

Metazoan infections such as hydatid (*Echinococcus granulosus*) may infest the brain and while it is common in sheep in certain areas, it is a relatively uncommon intracranial infection in man. Tapeworm infections such as *Taenia solium* may produce fits and multiple areas of calcifications in the brain. In some parts of the world it may account for 10% of the patients investigated for brain tumour. Trichinosis also acquired from ingestion of pork may present with signs and symptoms suggestive of bacterial meningitis.

Further Reading

Crockard H. A., Hayward R. and Hoff J. T. (1985) *Neurosurgery: The Scientific Basis of Clinical Practice*. London, Blackwell Scientific Publications.

Symon L. (1978) Neurosurgery, In: Rob C. and Smith R. (ed.) *Operative Surgery*, 3rd ed. London, Butterworths.

Trubovich R. (ed.) (1979) Management of acute intracranial disasters. *Int. Anesthesiol. Clin.* **17**, Nos. 2 and 3.

Head injuries

Jennett W. B. and Teasdale G. (1980) *Management of Head Injuries*. Vol. 15. In: *Contemporary Neurology*. Philadelphia, Davis.

Odling-Smee W. and Crockard H. A. (1980) *Trauma Care*. London, Academic.

Vascular

Ross Russell R. W. (1984) *Cerebral Arterial Disease*, 2nd ed. London, Churchill Livingstone.

Vinken P. J. and Bruyn G. W. (ed.) (1972) Vascular diseases of the nervous system. *Handbook of Clinical Neurology*, Vols. 11 and 12. Amsterdam, North Holland.

Infections

De Louvois J., Gortvai P. and Hurley R. (1977) Bacteriology of abscesses of the central nervous system. *Br. Med. J.* **2**, 981–984.

McClelland C. J., Craig B. F. and Crockard H. A. (1978) Brain abscesses in Northern Ireland: A 30-year community review. *J. Neurol. Neurosurg. Psychiatry* **41**, 1043–1047.

Pons V. G. and Hoff J. T. (1980) In: Wilson C. B. and Hoff J. T. (ed.) *Infections of the Central Nervous System in Current Surgical Management of Neurological Disease.* Boston, Little Brown.

35 *Tumours of the Nervous System*

David G. T. Thomas

Tumours of the nervous system occur within the skull, the spinal canal and on peripheral nerves. Any cell in the brain, spinal cord or peripheral nerve may give rise to a tumour, as may any of the soft-tissue or bony surrounding structures. Metastatic tumours occur both as a result of local invasion of the nervous system and by blood-borne seeding from distant primary tumours. These tumours collectively form a very heterogeneous pathological collection, each with its own distinctive morphological appearance and characteristic natural history. There is a limited reserve of function in the normal nervous system, and once this is exhausted failure of function results. Therefore, whatever their cell of origin and their particular anatomical site, these neoplasms tend to present clinically with symptoms due either to general raised intracranial pressure or spinal compression, or with recognizable clinical syndromes due to specific loss of neurological function.

In most cases of nervous system tumours, specialized investigations, especially neuroradiological studies, are required to confirm the clinical diagnosis and to direct the surgeon in operative management. Certain tumours whose biological behaviour is benign can be cured by neurosurgery. Others have a poor prognosis due either to their histological malignancy or to the disabling and fatal brain damage they can cause owing to their specific site in the nervous system. In the latter case histologically benign neoplasms can behave biologically in a malignant fashion with a poor clinical prognosis in spite of treatment.

INCIDENCE, EPIDEMIOLOGY, AETIOLOGY

Neurological tumours are not uncommon. The incidence of tumours of the nervous system is approximately 10–15/100 000, with about 80% being intracranial tumours of varying kinds, and of these about half are primary brain tumours. In patients coming to autopsy in developed countries, about one-third of all such tumours have been undiagnosed in life. In this undiagnosed group about two-thirds are asymptomatic and death has been due to other causes, while in the remaining one-third the terminal neurological syndrome has been misinterpreted. About 2% of deaths in Europe and the USA are due to brain tumours.

Nervous system tumours occur more commonly with increasing age, with a peak incidence in childhood at 5–9 years and a second peak at 50–55 years. The type of tumour occurring varies with age. In infancy and childhood the most common tumour of the nervous system is the medulloblastoma. This is a malignant, primitive cell tumour of the cerebellar vermis. Certain other posterior fossa tumours, i.e. ependymoma and choroid plexus papilloma in the fourth ventricle and astrocytoma in the cerebellar hemisphere, are also characteristic tumours of childhood, as are the less common astrocytomas of optic nerve, hypothalamus and brainstem. Neuroblastomas of the adrenal medulla are other rare nervous system tumours occurring in children, and are highly malignant. However, meningioma, neurilemoma and pituitary adenomas, all relatively frequent in adults, are virtually unknown in childhood. Tumours of the cerebral hemisphere are also rare in children.

In adolescence and early adult life the pattern changes and tumours of the supratentorial, intracranial compartment are most common. Germinoma and teratoma of the pineal region, as well as craniopharyngioma, commonly present at this stage in life. Congenital spinal tumours, dermoid or lipoma, often present at this time. In the next two decades (20–40 years) astrocytoma and oligodendroglioma of the cerebral hemispheres are the most common brain tumours, while haemangioblastoma is the most common cerebellar tumour encountered. Primary tumours of the spinal cord, ependymoma and astrocytoma, as well as neurilemoma of the spinal roots, may also present in this age group.

In the older age groups (50–70 years), the more malignant cerebral gliomas (anaplastic astrocytoma, glioblastoma) become more common, as do cerebral metastases. Intracranial meningiomas and neurilemomas of the acoustic nerve, as well as pituitary adenomas, are relatively frequent in these older patients. Spinal meningiomas and spinal extradural metastases also become more common in this age group.

Peripheral nerve tumours, apart from neuroblastoma in childhood (itself a rare tumour), are much rarer than intracranial or spinal nervous system tumours at any age.

Certain nervous system tumours are found more commonly in men than women. There is an overwhelming male predominance in germinoma and teratoma of the pineal region. There is a slight preponderance in men of medulloblastoma, most kinds of glioma, craniopharyngioma, epidermoids and dermoids, as well as vascular malformations. Metastatic carcinoma in the brain and spine, due principally to the frequency of primary bronchogenic carcinoma, is also more common in men. In women there is a preponderance of meningiomas, which is slight in the intracranial compartment but is very marked in the spinal canal.

The aetiology of nervous system tumours remains unknown, although chemicals used in the rubber industry, head injury, radiation therapy to the head and previous toxoplasma infection have all been put forward as possible causal factors in particular types of nervous system neoplasms.

TUMOUR TYPES AND PATHOLOGY

Classification of nervous system tumours is based on histological identification of cell type and of tissue architecture in the neoplasm. When these tumours are grouped by cell of origin, it is possible to reduce the very wide variety of types found, some common, some very rare, to a relatively small number of categories (*Table* 35.1).

Neuroepithelium

The most common nervous system tumours are those arising from neuroepithelial cells of brain, spinal cord and peripheral nerve. The normal glial cells, that is astrocytes, oligodendrocytes and ependymal cells, in any region of the brain or spinal cord can give rise to tumours known collectively as '*gliomas*', all of which are malignant to a greater or lesser degree. These tumours account for 40–50% of brain tumours and 15% of spinal tumours (*Table* 35.2). Cells of the choroid plexus and of the pineal can also give rise to tumours, which are intrinsic within the brain. Neuronal cells can also, much more rarely, give rise to tumours, e.g. the malignant neuroblastoma of the adrenal medulla. Primitive, embryonal, neuroepithelial cell types are recognized in two relatively common and highly malignant nervous system tumours, the glioblastoma and the medulloblastoma.

Table 35.1 Types of nervous system tumours: Classified by cell of origin

1. NEUROEPITHELIUM: 'GLIOMAS', astrocytomas, oligodendroglioma, ependymoma, medulloblastoma; neuronal tumours
2. NERVE SHEATH: neurilemoma (Schwannoma), neurofibroma
3. MENINGES: meningioma
4. LYMPHOMA
5. BLOOD VESSEL: Haemangioblastoma
6. GERM CELL: Germinoma, teratoma
7. OTHER MALFORMATIONS: Craniopharyngioma, epidermoid, dermoid, colloid cyst
8. VASCULAR MALFORMATION: Arteriovenous malformation, cavernous angioma
9. ANTERIOR PITUITARY: Pituitary adenoma
10. EXTENSION FROM REGIONAL TUMOUR: chordoma, glomus jugulare
11. METASTASIS

Table 35.2 Comparative frequency of different types of nervous system tumours

Tumour Type	*Cranial*	*Spinal*
Glioma	50%	15%
Neurilemoma/neurofibroma	6%	12%
Meningioma	16%	15%
Haemangioblastoma	2%	1%
Craniopharyngioma or dermoid	3%	5%
Arteriovenous malformation	1%	5%
Pituitary adenoma	8%	
Metastases	12%	45%
Other	2%	2%

Histological Grading of the Gliomas

The most widely used system for grading gliomas is that of Kernohan and Sayre which distinguishes four categories, I, II, III and IV, indicating increasing degrees of malignancy. This is determined on histological examination by the degree of pleomorphism of cells, the presence and increased number of mitotic figures and of atypical mitosis, as well as by an assessment of disordered features in tissue architecture including necrosis, vascular hyperplasia and cellularity.

These tumours spread by diffuse local infiltration and, occasionally, by seeding within the CSF pathways. They virtually never spread to cause metastases in other parts of the body. Therefore staging, as applied in the TNM classification of many other solid tumours, is not applicable to gliomas.

Nerve Sheath

Tumours can arise from the Schwann cells (neurilemoma), or fibroblasts (neurofibroma), in cranial nerves, spinal roots or peripheral nerves, and together constitute about 6% of intracranial tumours and about 12% of spinal tumours (*Table* 35.2). These neoplasms affect particularly the eighth cranial nerve (acoustic neurilemoma), the dorsal spinal roots and peripheral nerves. They may occur sporadically or in association with other neuroectodermal abnormalities in von Recklinghausen's disease. They are usually well encapsulated, sometimes cystic tumours which appear benign histologically. However, they may, depending on their site, cause clinically serious disability or death.

Meninges

Tumours of the meninges, after the gliomas, are the most common nervous system neoplasms, accounting for about 16% of intracranial and 15% of spinal tumours (*Table* 35.2). They arise from the meningeal covering of the brain and spinal cord, and their cell of origin can be arachnoidal, pial, dural or, in some cases, endothelial. Most meningiomas are attached to the dura near the venous sinuses, either in the vault or the base of the skull, or in the spinal canal. Others can arise within the ventricles of the brain from the tela choroidea of the choroid plexus. Usually they are well-encapsulated tumours, although sometimes they grow *en plaque* as a sheet spreading over the cerebral surface. Typically they have a benign histological appearance, which varies according to their cell of origin. Sometimes sarcomatous change can occur, with local invasion of brain or bone.

Lymphoma

Primary cerebral lymphoma is a rare tumour and the cell of origin of these tumours remains controversial. These are malignant neoplasms and the group includes microglioma and reticulum-cell sarcoma. They occur with increased frequency in patients on long-term immunosuppression, especially in those who have received organ transplants.

Blood Vessels

Haemangioblastoma, which occurs most commonly in the cerebellum but which can occur in the cerebral hemisphere or in the spinal cord, comprises about 2% of intracranial and 1% of spinal tumours (*Table* 35.2). These neoplasms are often associated with the congenital anomalies of von Hippel–Lindau disease. It is formed of blood vessels and intervening, fat-filled stromal cells, and often contains a fluid-filled cyst cavity. It is usually well encapsulated and histologically benign.

Germ Cell

Embryonic tumours, arising from germ cells, are found mainly in the pineal region. These are rare, malignant tumours, occurring predominantly in men, and about 60% of them are *germinomas*, with a histological appearance identical to that of seminoma of the testis, graded II–III on the Kernohan scale. The *teratoma*, which is the next most common pineal region tumour, contains tissue derived from more than one embryonic cell layer and is generally Grade I.

Other Malformations

Several other congenital embryonic malformations can result in tumours in the nervous sytem. The craniopharyngioma accounts for about 3% of intracranial tumours. It arises from the vestigial remnants of the craniopharyngeal duct (Rathke's pouch) either within the pituitary sella or in the suprasellar region. Commonly it is cystic and contains fluid, with the appearance of engine oil, containing cholesterol crystals, while the solid tumour is often calcified. Epidermoids and dermoid cysts are rare tumours which occur intracranially at the base of the skull and in the spinal canal, often in the region of the conus at the lower end of the spinal cord. Epidermoid cysts contain pearly white fluid, while dermoids contain soft, cheesy material, as well as in some cases dermal elements like hair or teeth. The colloid cyst occurs within the third ventricle of the brain, close to the foramen of Monro, and can cause acute, sometimes fatal, hydrocephalus. Lipomas can occur in the corpus callosum and in the conus of the spinal cord or in the spinal extradural space. The spinal lipomas are often associated with spinal dysraphism. Epidermoids, dermoids and lipomas constitute about 5% of spinal tumours (*Table* 35.2).

All these embryonic malformations increase in size very slowly and histologically appear benign. However, when they do eventually present clinically, they may cause functional disability which may be serious, or even disastrous, to the patient. Their operative surgical treatment, because of their particular locations, may also be technically difficult and hazardous.

Vascular Malformation

Congenital malformation of the vascular tree can produce arteriovenous malformation and cavernous angioma. Because these lesions may behave as expanding neoplasms in the brain or spinal canal, as well as causing vascular syndromes due to haemorrhage or ischaemia, they are generally grouped with other tumours of the nervous system.

Anterior Pituitary

Pituitary adenomas constitute about 8% of intracranial tumours (*Table* 35.2), and arise from the cells of the anterior pituitary gland. They may be subdivided, by the staining of their cytoplasm with its contained secretory granules, as acidophilic or basophilic or as chromophobe adenomas. More recently, immunohistochemical methods have become available to stain specifically for pituitary hormones, like growth hormone or prolactin, in such adenomas. Generally they appear benign histologically, but carcinomatous change can occasionally occur.

Extension from Regional Tumour

Tumours which occur at the base of the skull, outwith the nervous system, may invade locally and so present as nervous system tumours. Relatively benign tumours, e.g. chordoma or glomus jugulare tumours, can behave in this way. Because of their site and potential for recurrence, surgical treatment of these neoplasms can be very difficult. In the spinal canal relatively benign lesions, e.g. eosinophilic granuloma or solitary myeloma, can behave in this way.

Metastases

Metastatic tumours of the nervous system are diagnosed with increasing frequency. They account for 12–20% of cerebral tumours and about 45% of spinal tumours. Secondary intracranial deposits may be caused by spread from distant visceral tumours or sometimes by direct spread from carcinomas of the nasopharynx, lacrimal gland or skull sinuses. Carcinomatous meningitis can also occur due to seeding of cells deposited in the CSF pathways. Spinal extradural metastases occur, due either to spread from distant tumours or to direct invasion of bone and extradural tissue.

PATHOPHYSIOLOGY OF NERVOUS SYSTEM TUMOURS

Cranial Tumours

The internal volume of the adult human skull is approximately 1500 ml, and about 90% of this space is occupied by brain. The brain, which itself is 80% water, is incompressible. Only about 10% of the intracranial volume is occupied by CSF or blood, which may be displaced. Any space-occupying lesion within the skull, including all forms of intracranial tumour, rapidly take up the reserve of volume available by displacement of CSF and cause increase in intracranial pressure as well as shift of brain within the skull. Raised intracranial pressure gives rise to a classic triad of clinical symptoms which includes headache, due to stimulation of sensitive nerves in the dura, vomiting, due to stimulation of centres in the medulla and outflow through the vagus nerves to the gut, and visual failure, due to papilloedema of the optic disc caused by increased pressure transmitted along the optic nerve sheath. Brain shifts also occur due to local mass effect of tumour or to generalized increase in pressure. Within the skull there are dural septa, namely the falx in the midline and the tentorium between the middle and posterior cranial fossae, which are firm and unyielding. Brain may herniate past the margins of these septa. Tentorial herniation, with its premonitory signs of unilateral dilatation of the pupil due to direct pressure on the third nerve from the uncus of the temporal lobe as it is forced by raised pressure down through the tentorial hiatus, can lead to rapidly fatal midbrain dysfunction coupled with occlusion of the posterior cerebral artery. This phenomenon of 'coning' can also occur when the cerebellar tonsil is forced by pressure gradients to herniate through the foramen magnum of the skull and to compress fatally the medulla with its vital centres. Either form of pressure cone may be precipitated by injudicious lumbar puncture in the presence of raised intracranial pressure (ICP). If the effects of brain herniation do not lead to fatal midbrain or medullary failure, eventually a terminal state is reached where ICP is equal to systemic arterial blood pressure and cerebral circulation ceases, due to 'pseudo-occlusion' of the carotid and vertebral vessels as they enter the skull. Blockage of the normal CSF pathways by small tumours, particularly at their narrowest points, i.e. the foramen of Monro, the aqueduct of Sylvius and the outlet foramina of the fourth ventricle, may give rise to hydrocephalus and a consequent rise in ICP out of all proportion to the size of the obstructing tumour. Acute hydrocephalus can produce very severe headache, with screaming attacks, neck stiffness, opisthotonos and, in some cases, apnoea. Chronic hydrocephalus produces the triad of headache, vomiting and papilloedema, which commonly may be associated with ataxia of gait and dementia.

In addition to the effects of raised ICP, intracranial tumours may cause local brain dysfunction, with specific effects characteristic of particular locations. Any supratentorial tumour, either in the cerebral hemispheres or in the surrounding structures may cause epilepsy. The epilepsy may be focal or generalized, motor or sensory. In many cases where a slowly growing, infiltrative glioma develops, epilepsy as a symptom may precede by several years the development of other features. Failure of brain function, particularly dysphasia, hemiparesis and visual loss, are also common presenting features. Tumours in the infratentorial compartment exert their local effects on cerebellum, medulla and lower cranial nerves, and cause, for example, ataxia, severe vomiting, deafness and difficulty in swallowing.

Spinal Tumours

The spinal cord is contained within the bony spinal canal. The reserve of volume available within the spinal cord, particularly in the dorsal spine, is relatively even more restricted than in the skull. The reserve of function available within the spinal cord, and its capacity to recover after insult, is also more limited than that of most parts of the brain. Spinal cord compression due to spinal tumour is therefore often an even more acute process than the development of raised ICP and focal brain dysfunction due to brain tumour. Both motor and sensory function are affected, with a distinct segmental component *at the level of the lesion* and additional loss of function *below the lesion*.

Peripheral Nerve Tumours

Tumours on peripheral nerves occur outside the spinal canal in the trunk or limbs, and do not grow within a constricted bony compartment. However, they do generally cause local pain, and, eventually, motor or sensory dysfunction in the nerve distribution.

CLINICAL DIAGNOSIS OF NERVOUS SYSTEM TUMOURS

Cranial Tumours

The presenting symptoms of patients with brain tumours tend to be those due to raised ICP or to local brain dysfunction, or to a combination of both.

Symptoms due to Raised Intracranial Pressure

Headache

Headache associated with brain tumour is frequently most noticeable in the early morning and lessens as the day wears on. It is usually not constant. The headache is often exacerbated by movement or by coughing and as time progresses it becomes more severe. Often it is bifrontal or occipital, but sometimes it appears to be localized to the site in the skull where an underlying tumour is later found. In some patients, where the pain is due to acute hydrocephalus, the pain is so severe that the patient cries out.

Vomiting

Vomiting associated with brain tumours is frequently worse in the early morning. It is sometimes associated with nausea, but not with abdominal discomfort. Tumours which impinge directly on the fourth ventricle may cause almost constant vomiting, and infants and children with posterior fossa tumours are not infrequently dehydrated and emaciated for this reason.

Failure of Vision

Visual failure with loss of visual acuity due to papilloedema, particularly when it comes on gradually, may be tolerated by the patient who may present only when virtually blind. Examination shows papilloedema, often with exudates and haemorrhages, with sometimes optic atrophy. Field defects, particularly bitemporal hemianopia due to pituitary tumours, may present following traffic accidents or failure at ball games due to defective vision.

Mental Change

Changes in conscious level, ranging from apathy or drowsiness to coma, may be due to raised ICP. Changes in alertness or in mood may be reported by the patient's relatives or friends.

Diplopia

Partial IIIrd or VIth nerve palsies may occur with incipient brain herniation at the tentorial notch. The patient may complain only of diplopia on lateral gaze, but examination will confirm partial oculomotor or abducens palsies. Such symptoms indicate a precariously poised brain and require urgent investigation.

Acute Brain Herniation

In some cases the first noticeable effect of a brain tumour will be sudden brain herniation, with 'coning' at the tentorium or foramen magnum, resulting in an apnoeic attack. Frequently such attacks are fatal, but in some cases they remit spontaneously. When this happens and the patient is brought to hospital, urgent further investigation and treatment are indicated.

Specific Brain Tumour Syndromes

Neuroepithelial Tumours—'Gliomas'

CEREBRAL HEMISPHERE TUMOURS.

Frontal Lobe (*Fig.* 35.1*c*, *d*): Mental changes, with emotional lability and facetiousness, are often early symptoms. In the left, dominant hemisphere dysphasia accompanies the spastic hemiparesis which develops as the tumour involves the posterior frontal lobe. Epilepsy, either as focal motor manifestations in the contralateral face and limbs or as a generalized convulsion, frequently occurs. Early signs are the presence of abnormal grasp reflexes, and slight facial weakness or hemiparesis, with papilloedema.

Corpus Callosum (*Fig.* 35.1*b*): Dementia, with incontinence and bilateral pyramidal tract signs are features of this glioma which spreads through the corpus callosum to affect both frontal lobes.

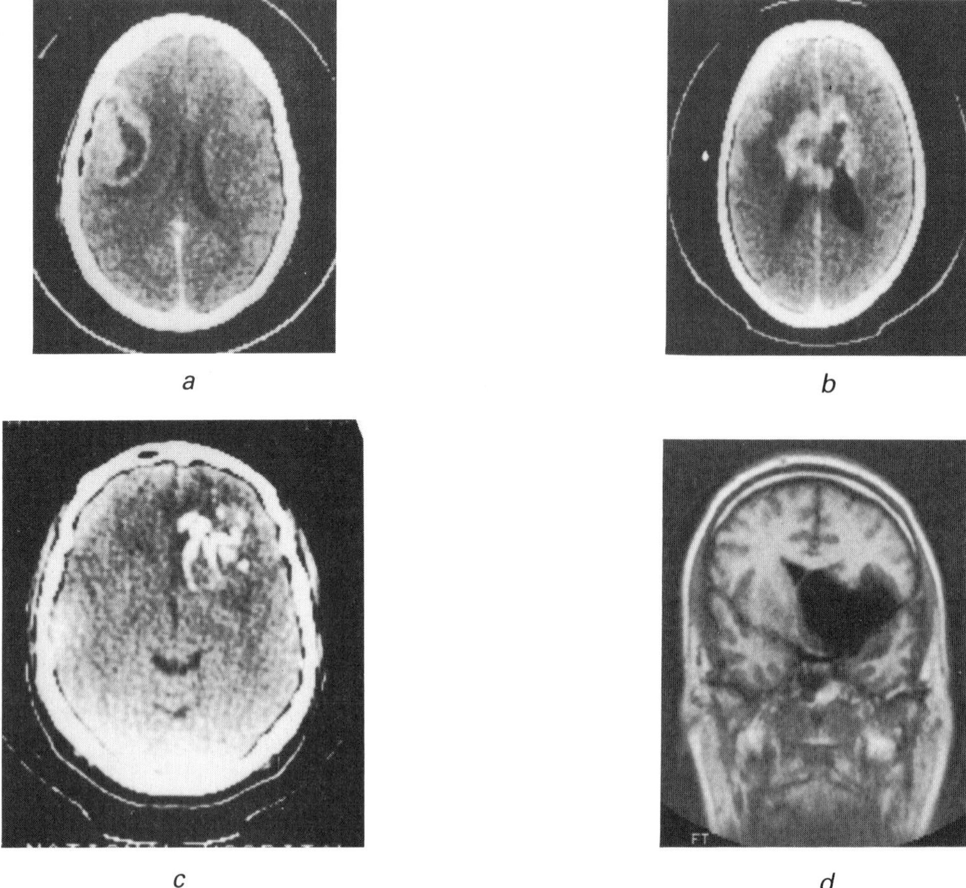

Fig. 35.1 CT scans of glioma. *a*, Left temporal. *b*, Corpus callosum. *c*, Right frontal, partly calcified tumour. *d*, MRI scan, T_1 weighted image coronal plane low-grade frontal tumour.

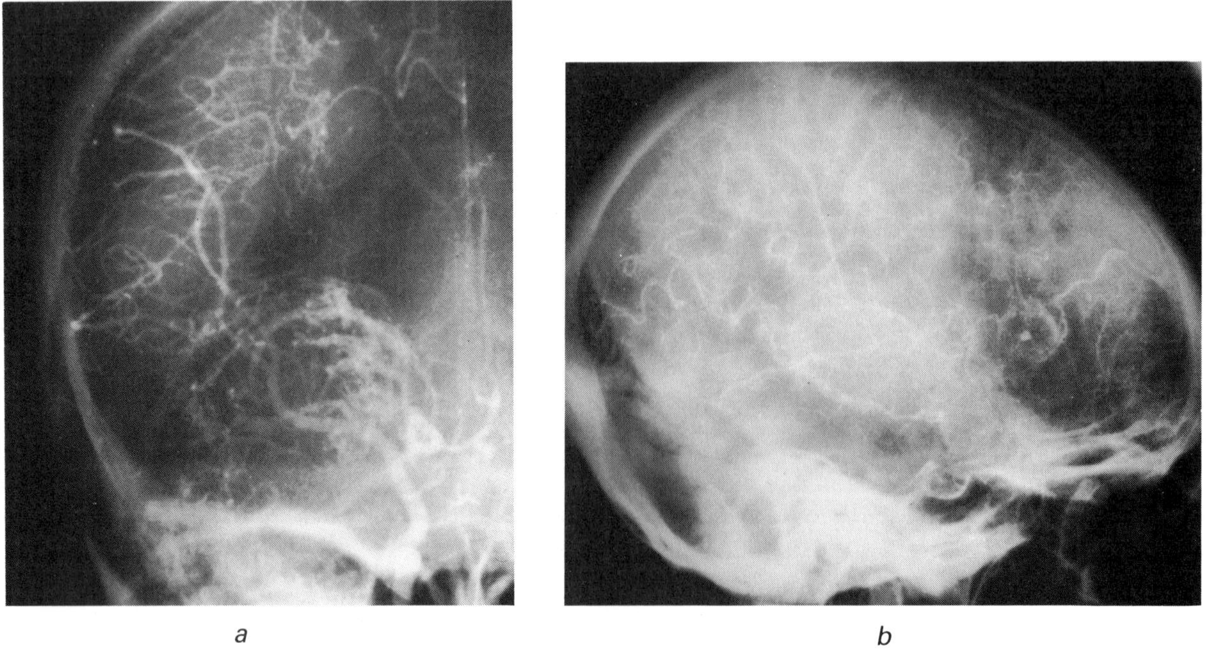

Fig. 35.2 Carotid angiogram. *a*, Right carotid injection, AP projection. Pathological circulation in glioma of temporal region. *b*, Right carotid injection, lateral projection. Pathological circulation in metastasis in posterior frontal region.

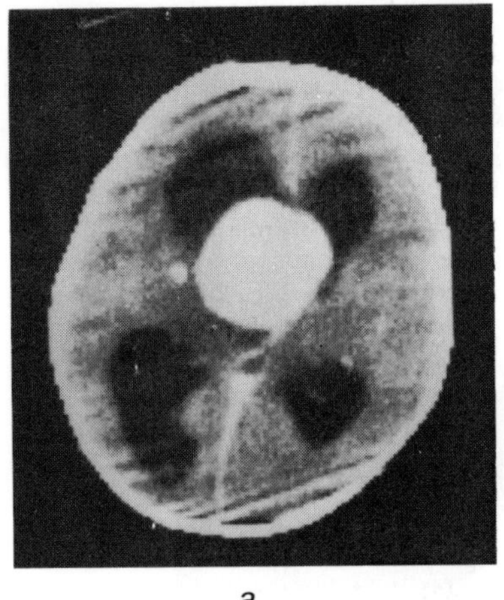
a

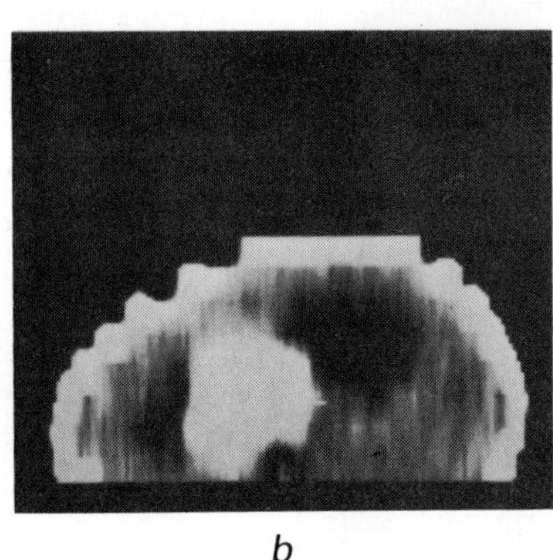
b

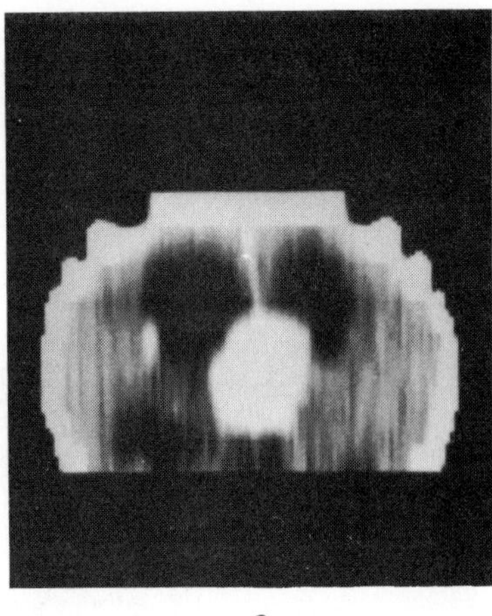
c

Fig. 35.3 CT scan. Glioma of third ventricle region, with associated massive hydrocephalus. *a*, Conventional CT scan cut, horizontal brain section. *b*, Sagittal reconstruction. *c*, Coronal reconstruction.

Parietal Lobe: Involvement of the sensory cortex leads to neglect of the contralateral side of the body with often visual inattention as well. In the dominant, that is usually the left, hemisphere, parietal tumours cause receptive dysphasia, while in the right hemisphere general capacity for orientation of the body image and left-right discrimination is disordered.

Occipital Lobe: Tumours in the occipital lobe cause a homonymous hemianopia, which often presents late, only when the patient has developed other features due to raised ICP.

Temporal Lobe (*Figs.* 35.1*a*, 35.2*a*): Hemiparesis, homonymous hemianopia, dysphasia in the dominant hemisphere, and epilepsy are features of gliomas in the temporal lobes. Often the epilepsy is of a specific 'temporal lobe' type. It may take the form of feelings of fear or pleasure, olfactory or gustatory hallucinations, or repetitive psychomotor movements.

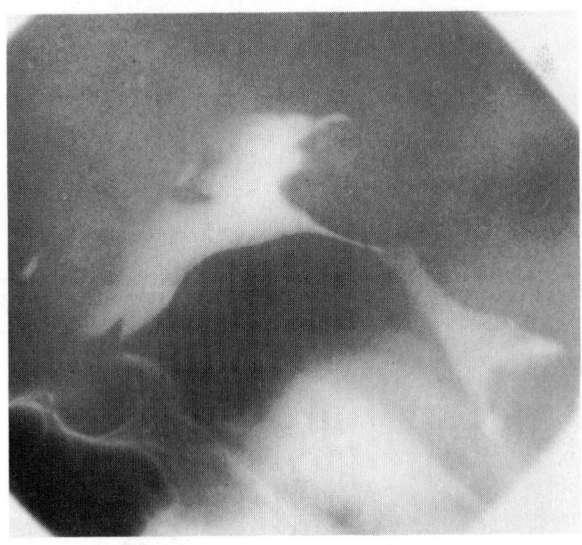

Fig. 35.4 Ventriculogram. Lateral projection, showing third ventricle, aqueduct and fourth ventricle. Pineal region tumour outlined in posterior third ventricle.

THIRD VENTRICLE REGION TUMOURS.
Optic Chiasma, Hypothalamus, Pineal, Thalamus (*Figs.* 35.3, 35.4): Gliomas can occur in the hypothalamus or optic chiasma, particularly in children. These may present with failure of growth, loss of appetite or failure of temperature control or by causing diabetes insipidus often with visual failure or with symptoms of raised ICP, particularly when there is associated hydrocephalus (*Fig.* 35.3).

Germinomas and teratomas of the pineal region grow at the posterior end of the third ventricle. Gliomas can also occur in the posterior third ventricle and mimic pineal tumours by causing pressure on the quadrigeminal plate. These tumours all usually cause palsy of upward gaze, ptosis and dilatation of the pupils.

Gliomas which grow in the thalamus and basal ganglia generally cause contralateral sensory and motor deficits, before producing symptoms due to raised ICP.

BRAINSTEM (*Fig.* 35.5). Glioma affecting the brainstem causes progressive, but in some cases fluctuating, lower cranial nerve palsies associated with symptoms due to disturbance in the long tracts passing through the stem to the body. Change in facial sensation (trigeminal (V) nerve), diplopia (abducens (VI) nerve), facial weakness (facial (VII) nerve), deafness (acoustic (VIII) nerve), or difficulty in swallowing and speaking (glossopharyngeal (IX) nerve, vagus (X) nerve, hypoglossal (XII) nerve), alone or in combination may be the presenting symptoms. Spastic weakness of the limbs, sensory loss or ataxia may also be features. Hydrocephalus or increased ICP are unusual. Children and adolescents are those generally affected and the history is usually short.

CEREBELLUM AND FOURTH VENTRICLE. Cerebellar Astrocytoma, Medulloblastoma and Ependymoma (*Fig.* 35.6*b*, *c*, *d*, *e*, *f*). Cerebellar dysfunction is an early sign of most cerebellar astrocytomas which involve the lateral lobes of the cerebellum. Ataxia of the limbs, most marked on the side of the tumour, and nystagmus are found. Usually there are

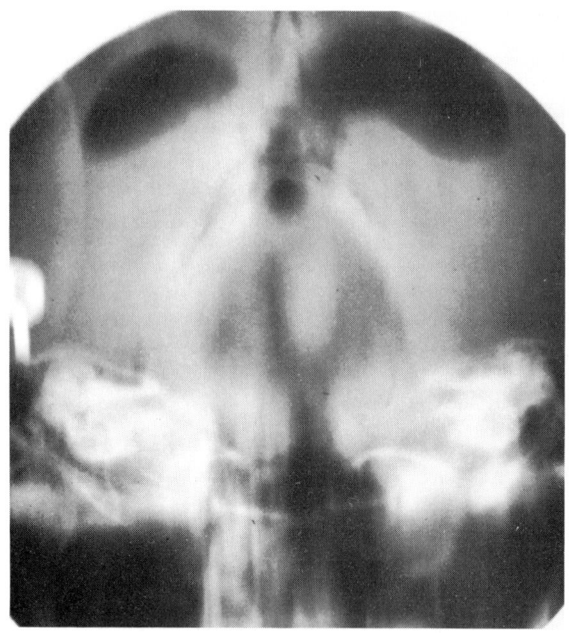

Fig. 35.5 Air encephalogram. Tomogram in AP projection shows asymmetrical enlargement of brainstem by intrinsic glioma, more marked on the left.

associated signs of hydrocephalus and raised ICP with papilloedema and sometimes optic atrophy in those children who, as is found not infrequently, have a long history measured in months or one to two years. In adults, haemangioblastoma and metastasis in the cerebellar hemisphere present with very similar symptoms, but generally a shorter history.

Tumours of the cerebellar vermis and fourth ventricle—medulloblastoma and ependymoma principally—tend to have a much shorter history and to present with different

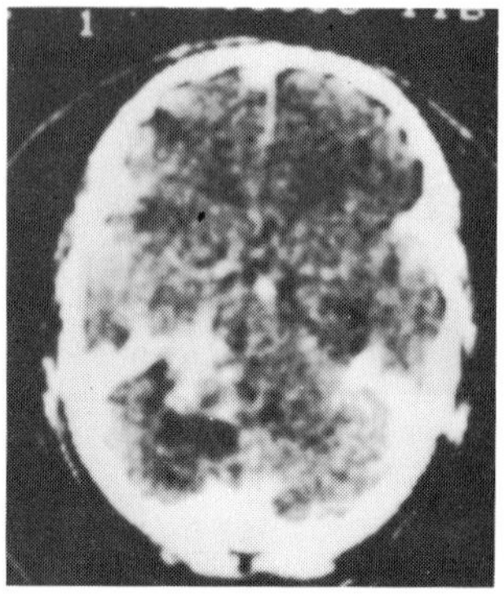

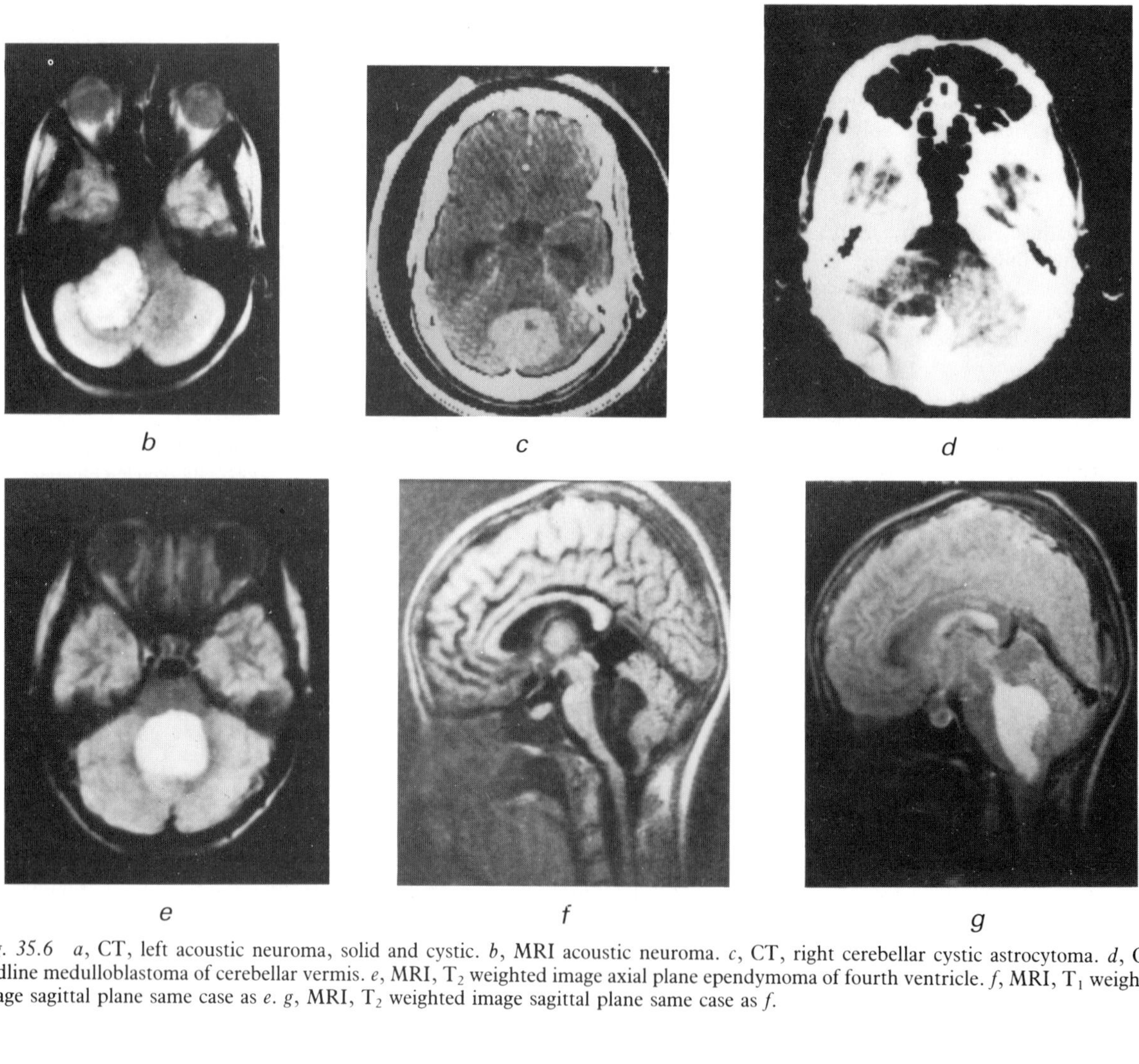

Fig. 35.6 *a*, CT, left acoustic neuroma, solid and cystic. *b*, MRI acoustic neuroma. *c*, CT, right cerebellar cystic astrocytoma. *d*, CT, midline medulloblastoma of cerebellar vermis. *e*, MRI, T_2 weighted image axial plane ependymoma of fourth ventricle. *f*, MRI, T_1 weighted image sagittal plane same case as *e*. *g*, MRI, T_2 weighted image sagittal plane same case as *f*.

symptoms. The midline cerebellar functions are disordered and often there is severe truncal ataxia, such that the infant or child cannot stand or sit. Vomiting, headache and neck stiffness are other features due partly to hydrocephalus and raised ICP and partly to local pressure within the posterior fossa.

Neurilemoma

Acoustic Neurilemoma (*Fig.* 35.6*a, b*). Unilateral, progressive deafness is the first symptom of neurilemoma growing in the acoustic (VIII) nerve. Gradually the tumour grows larger, expanding the internal acoustic meatus and filling the cerebellopontine angle and causing cerebellar ataxia and sometimes hydrocephalus as well as depression of the corneal reflex (VII nerve) and sensory loss in the face (V nerve).

Meningiomas

CRANIAL VAULT. Parasagittal, Convexity (*Fig.* 35.7*a*): Meningiomas which arise from the anterior part of the sagittal sinus or the anterior part of the dural falx tend to cause only mental symptoms, due to bifrontal brain dysfunction and sometimes only present very late when symptoms of raised ICP supervene. Tumours which arise from the dura over the middle third of the sagittal sinus frequently present early with focal epilepsy, often with associated weakness in the contralateral foot. Meningiomas in the more posterior part of the sinus tend to be silent clinically, until raised ICP with hemianopia leads to their detection. Tumours arising in the anterior frontal convexity of the cranial vault may produce only mental changes, or focal epilepsy and hemiparesis if sited more posteriorly.

BASAL. Sphenoid Wing, Olfactory Groove, Suprasellar (*Fig.* 35.7*b*): Meningiomas which arise at the inner portion of the sphenoid wing involve the optic nerve, the carotid artery and cranial nerves of the cavernous sinus (III, IV, V, VI), and result in ophthalmoplegia, visual failure and proptosis. Tumours at the outer end of the ridge expand into the

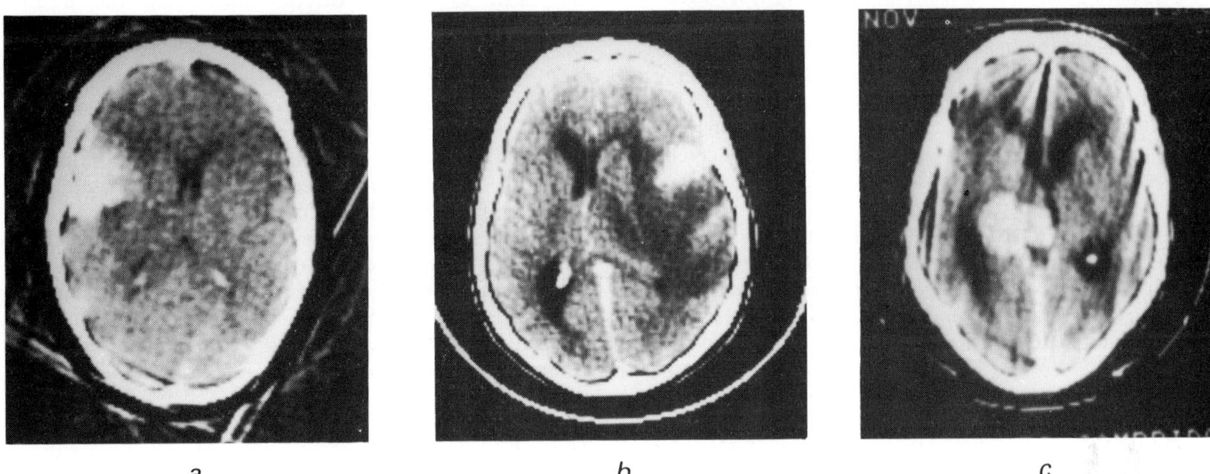

a b c

Fig. 35.7 CT scans of meningioma. *a*, Left, vault. *b*, Right, outer sphenoid wing. *c*, Left, tentorium.

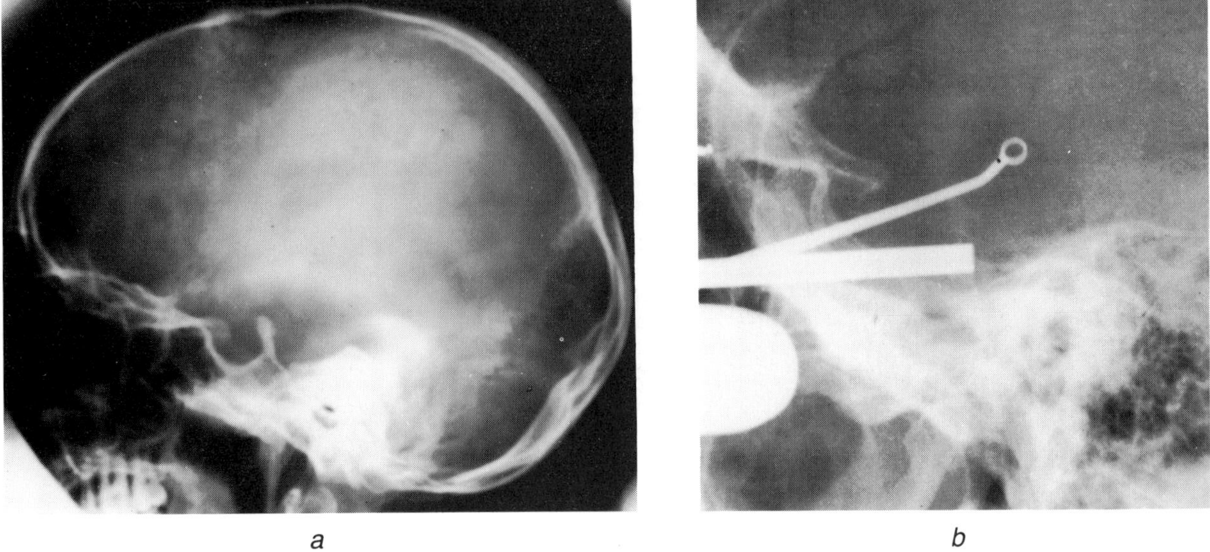

a b

Fig. 35.8 Plain skull radiograph. Lateral (*a*) Slight enlargement of pituitary fossa, due to pituitary microadenoma. *b*, Massive erosion of pituitary fossa, due to chromophobe adenoma. Peroperative radiograph at trans-sphenoidal tumuor removal.

Sylvian fissure and impinge on the posterior frontal and temporal lobes. Symptoms of facial or limb weakness, or, on the left side, dysphasia may be caused, sometimes associated with temporal lobe epilepsy.

Meningiomas of the olfactory groove region cause anosmia, which is rarely complained of by the patient, until symptoms of raised ICP arise. In this situation a tumour can cause optic atrophy on the ipsilateral side due to direct optic nerve pressure, with contralateral papilloedema (Foster–Kennedy syndrome).

Suprasellar meningiomas arise from the dura of the tuberculum sellae and cause symptoms early due to compression of the optic chiasma, with bitemporal field loss similar to that found with other tumours of this region (pituitary adenomas, craniopharyngioma).

Posterior Fossa Meningiomas, Clivus, Foramen Magnum, Cerebellopontine Angle, Tentorium (*Fig.* 35.7*c*): Meningiomas which arise from the dura of the skull base at the clivus or foramen magnum present with multiple lower cranial nerve palsies, in association with long tract signs in the limbs, while laterally placed tumours in the cerebellopontine angle cause deafness (VIII nerve), facial weakness (VII nerve), or sensory changes in the face (V nerve). Tumours arising from the tentorium may give rise to symptoms due to pressure on the cerebellum, i.e. ataxia and cranial nerve palsies, or to pressure upwards on the cerebral hemisphere, i.e. epilepsy and hemianopia.

Meningiomas at other Sites, Intraventricular, Sylvian Fissure: Meningiomas can arise within the lateral ventricles or deep in the Sylvian fissure, not attached to dura. The symptoms they give rise to are usually hemiparesis with features of raised ICP.

Pituitary Adenomas

CHROMOPHOBE ADENOMA (*Figs.* 35.8*b*, 35.9*a*, *b*, *c*). Non-functioning pituitary adenomas generally present as tumours with symptoms due to their space-occupying effect, although they can in some cases present with the endocrine features of hypopituitarism. Suprasellar extensions of such adenomas compress the optic chiasma and cause bitemporal hemianopia, frequently associated with headache and optic atrophy. Occasionally there is haemorrhage into chromophobe pituitary adenomas, 'pituitary apoplexy', which causes sudden increase in visual loss with severe headache and systemic upset.

FUNCTIONING MICROADENOMA (*Fig.* 35.8*a*). Functioning pituitary tumours tend to present differently, often at an earlier stage while still microadenomas (less than 10 mm in diameter). The adenomas which produce growth hormone present with acromegaly, and those producing ACTH with Cushing's disease. Microadenomas producing prolactin cause amenorrhoea, galactorrhoea and infertility in women. These functioning tumours can also cause headache, and may increase in size to cause chiasmal compression.

Craniopharyngioma

These congenital cystic tumours may present in adolescence or early adult life, or sometimes much later in adult life. In younger patients bitemporal hemianopia and papilloedema associated with failure of growth and diabetes insipidus are the common presenting syndromes. In the older age group, hydrocephalus, due to obstruction of the foramen of Monro, may lead to mental deterioration being the leading symptom.

Intracranial Metastases (*see Fig. 35.2b*)

Single or multiple intracerebral or intracerebellar metastases can present in ways similar to primary gliomas in the same sites. Metastatic carcinoma can also cause a diffuse infiltration of the subarachnoid space, 'carcinomatous meningitis', which presents with headache, vomiting, meningism and varying cranial nerve palsies associated with long tract signs. Bony metastases at the base of the skull can produce similarly varied constellations of cranial nerve palsies, associated with headache. The cerebellopontine angle is a not uncommon site for such deposits, with deafness (VIII nerve), facial numbness (V nerve), and facial weakness (VII nerve).

Special Investigations of Cranial Tumours

The investigation of a patient with symptoms suggestive of an intracranial tumour is performed in two stages. Initially, screening tests are applied to establish the presence or absence of a tumour. These tests, plain skull radiograph, EEG, isotope scan and computerized axial tomogram (CT) or magnetic resonance imaging (MRI), can be performed as an outpatient or inpatient procedure. If a tumour is disclosed, a second phase of investigation is required. This

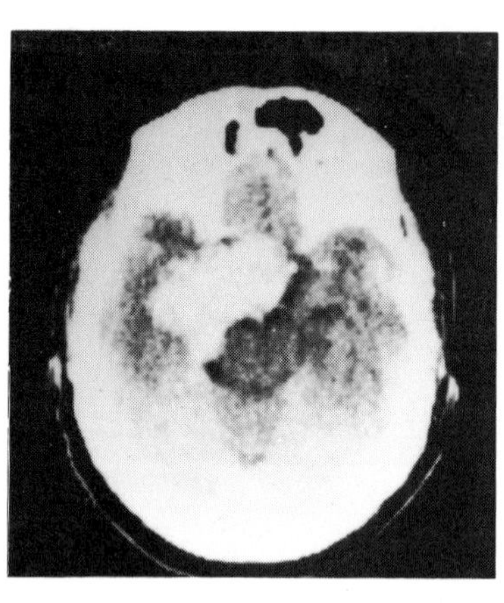

a

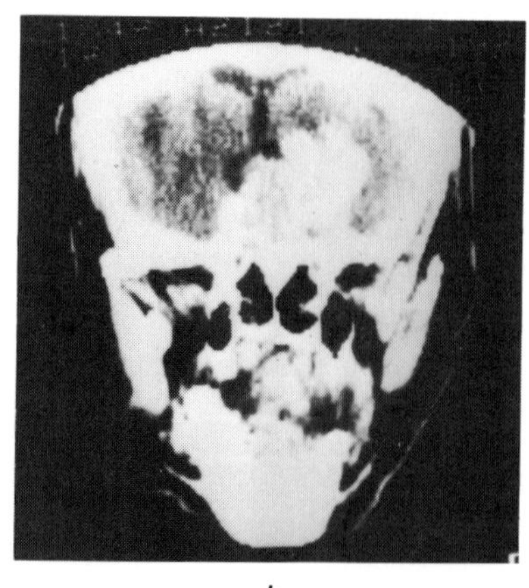

b

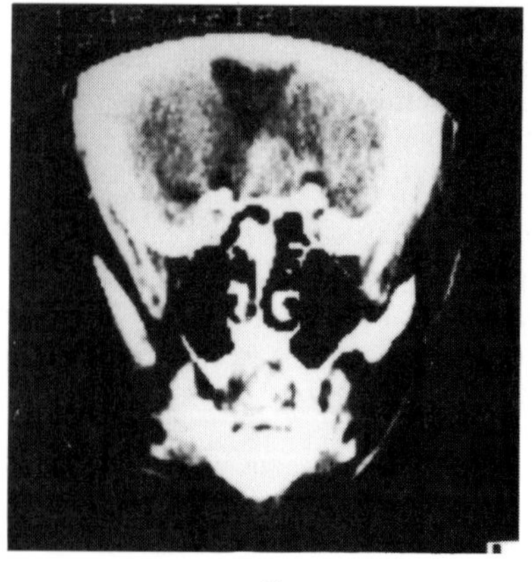

c

Fig. 35.9 CT scans of pituitary tumours. *a*, Conventional scan, large suprasellar and left temporal extension. *b*, Coronal scan, same case as *a*, large suprasellar extension into third ventricle. *c*, Coronal scan, moderate suprasellar extension.

involves use of invasive neuroradiological procedures such as angiography, pneumoencephalography and ventriculography.

Plain Skull Radiograph

Plain skull radiography is the initial, very important, step in neuroradiological investigation. Erosion of the dorsum sellae shown in a lateral film may confirm the presence of chronically raised ICP, while shift of a calcified pineal gland in the anteroposterior film may lateralize a supratentorial tumour. Enlargement of the pituitary fossa may indicate the presence of a pituitary adenoma (*Fig.* 35.8) or a craniopharyngioma. Other pathognomonic changes which appear on plain films are erosion of the internal auditory meatus by acoustic neurilemoma, enlargement of the optic canal by optic nerve glioma or sclerosis of the skull vault or sphenoid ridge associated with meningioma. Cerebral metastases may be diagnosed on the basis of multiple lytic or sclerotic lesions in the skull vault or base, associated with primary or metastatic tumours visible on chest radiography.

Electroencephalogram (EEG)

An EEG is useful in identifying focal brain abnormalities, particularly in patients presenting with epilepsy. Serial studies may indicate an increasing organic abnormality in the brain.

Isotope Scan: Computerized Axial Tomogram (CT)

Isotope encephalography depends on the entry of radioactive material into diseased areas of brain where tissue permeability is selectively altered. Intracranial tumours may be demonstrated and localized (*Fig.* 35.10).

CT scan has improved on isotope scan. It is non-invasive in the co-operative patient, although the restless patient may require general anaesthesia. The CT scan shows the site of an intracranial tumour relative to the ventricular system and skull, as well as the degree of 'enhancement' following intravenous injection of radiological contrast material (*see Figs.* 35.1, 35.3, 35.6, 35.7, 35.9, 35.11). Information is thus obtained about cystic elements of a tumour, about peritumoral oedema in surrounding brain, as well as an impression of its relative vascularity.

Angiography

Injection of iodine-containing contrast material into the carotid or vertebral arteries, usually through a femoral catheter, demonstrates the intracranial arteries. The method involves a small morbidity and mortality. Sometimes angiography reveals diagnostic tumour circulation (*see Fig.* 35.2). But even if it does not achieve this it usually reveals details of the feeding vessels of the tumour which are important technically for planning operative surgery.

Pneumo-encephalography/Ventriculography

These methods involve injection of air or of positive radiological contrast material into the subarachnoid space by lumbar puncture or into the lateral ventricles through a burr hole. The CSF pathways are outlined and these methods are particularly important in the demonstration of tumours of the third ventricle and pineal regions, as well as those in the suprasellar and cerebellopontine angle regions (*see Figs.* 35.4, 35.5).

Other Investigations

Blood tests, for example hormone assay in cases of pituitary tumour or erythrocyte sedimentation rate in metastatic

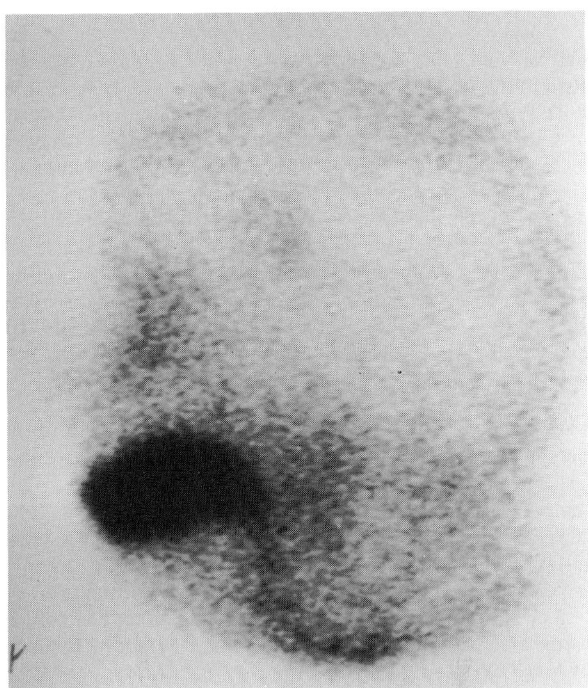

Fig. 35.10 Isotope brain scan. Left lateral. Tumour (solitary cerebral metastasis) in posterior frontal region.

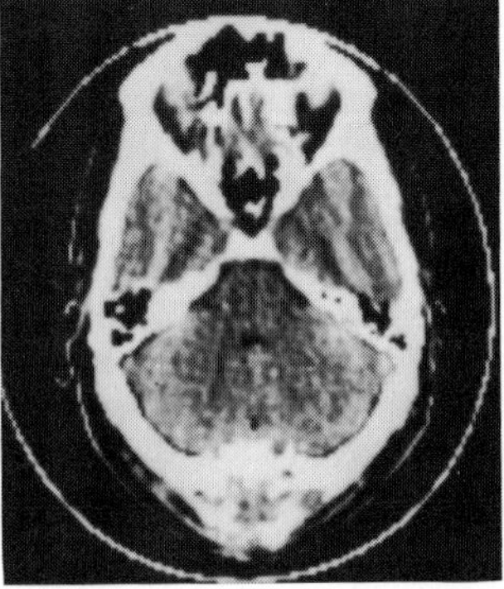

Fig. 35.11 CT scan. Solitary myeloma of occipital bone.

tumour, may play an important part in diagnosis of specific tumours. CSF examination may lead to positive cytological diagnosis, e.g. in some cases of pineal germinoma and medulloblastoma or in carcinomatous meningitis, or it may reveal a very high protein level, as in acoustic neurilemoma. However, lumbar puncture is unsafe in the presence of any intracranial tumour with raised ICP, and ventricular puncture through a burr hole may be necessary.

SPINAL TUMOURS

The cardinal symptoms of spinal tumours are local pain at the site of the lesion with loss of neurological function at and below this level. Spinal tumours may arise within the dura (intradural), be in the substance of the cord (intramedullary), in the subarachnoid space (extramedullary), or be outside the dura (extradural).

Symptoms due to Spinal Compression

Pain

Pain in the neck or back due to spinal tumour, whether due to bony involvement (primary or metastatic bone tumour) or to spinal root involvement (neurilemoma or meningioma), is localized at the level of the lesion. Pain due to intramedullary tumours (astrocytoma, ependymoma, angioma) is more diffuse within the neck or back. Often the pain is worse at night, possibly due to redistribution of associated oedema fluid with recumbency. Frequently the pain is severely exacerbated by coughing or straining. Exercise may provoke pain or loss of function in patients with spinal angioma. In many cases the pain predates symptoms due to loss of neurological function by months or even years.

Loss of Neurological Function

Spinal compression causes, at the segmental level of the lesion, bilateral loss of motor power, loss of sense of pain, temperature, vibration and position and loss of tendon reflexes. Below the lesion, due to dysfunction in the long tracts of the cord, there is loss in motor function, sensation, hyper-reflexia and dysfunction in bladder and bowel sphincters causing urinary retention and constipation. Where the compression is caused by a laterally placed tumour a Brown-Séquard syndrome may result. This consists of unilateral segmental features and crossed long tract signs with loss of motor function and sense of vibration and joint position on the side of and up to the level of the lesion, with contralateral loss of pain and temperature below the lesion.

In the adult, because the skeleton has outgrown the spinal cord, the segmental spinal cord level differs from that of the bony vertebral level. Below the axis (C2), in the neck and thorax, the approximate segmental level of the cord can be obtained by adding two to the vertebral level. The spinal cord ends in the conus, which is at the level of the lumbar vertebrae L1–2, so that the lumbar spinal segments lie at T11–12 vertebral levels, with the sacral cord level at L1–2 vertebrae. Below this level the lumbar and sacral nerve roots form the cauda equina. It is often possible to deduce accurately the level of spinal compression from clinical examination, but neuroradiological investigations are essential in confirming the diagnosis and in planning surgical treatment.

Acute and Chronic Spinal Compression

When loss of neurological function due to spinal compression develops quickly, over days or hours, it can only be reversed by urgent investigation and treatment. If motor power, sensation and sphincter function are lost acutely, so that the patient cannot stand or walk and is in urinary retention, a surgical emergency exists. Unless the compression is relieved in a matter of hours function cannot be restored.

Chronic spinal compression may give rise to progressive symptoms over weeks, months or even years. When the final stage of complete loss of function is reached diagnosis and relief of compression also demand emergency treatment. However, usually the patient presents at an earlier stage. Even if all function has been lost there is a better prospect for reversing the effects of chronic rather than acute spinal compression.

Specific Spinal Tumour Syndromes

Intradural Extramedullary Tumours

NEUROFIBROMA. Any spinal level may be affected by this tumour of the spinal roots, which is usually intradural and presents with pain and loss of function due to spinal compression. In the cervical region combined intradural and extradural components are often found, while thoracic tumours are sometimes wholly extradural. The extraspinal part of the tumour may present as a mass in the neck or mediastinum, discovered by palpation or on routine chest radiography. In some cases the stigmata of von Recklinghausen's syndrome, i.e. café-au-lait patches in the skin or subcutaneous nodules, are apparent and indicate the possibility of multiple tumours.

MENINGIOMAS. Spinal meningiomas arise from the inner surface of the dura and occur chiefly in the dorsal spine and in middle-aged or elderly women. Usually there is a history over many months of pain and gradual loss of function.

Intradural Intramedullary Tumours

ASTROCYTOMA, EPENDYMOMA ('GLIOMAS'); HAEMANGIOBLASTOMA. Spinal astrocytoma causes swelling of the cord over several segments, often in the cervical or upper dorsal region, resulting in loss of function over several spinal segments, as well as pain and loss of neurological function in the sphincters and in the legs. Ependymoma may also occur in the cord in the cervical or dorsal region but commonly arises in the lumbosacral region in the conus or in the filum terminale. They cause local pain as well as flaccid paralysis and sensory loss in the legs and loss of sphincter function. These tumours may seed through the subarachnoid space in the spinal canal or to the subfrontal region. Haemangioblastoma is a comparatively rare intramedullary spinal tumour, generally slow growing and only spreading locally.

EPIDERMOID, DERMOID, LIPOMA. These tumours occur mainly in the lumbosacral region. Some epidermoids probably result, years later, from skin implanted at previous lumbar puncture by needles not correctly fitted with a stilette. Dermoids and lipomas are congenital tumours, often associated with degrees of spinal dysraphism ranging from spina bifida occulta to meningomyelocele, in which embryonic rests later cause symptomatic tumours. Their clinical symptoms often resemble those of conus or cauda equina ependymomas, and they present in children and young adults.

ANGIOMA. Angiomas of the spinal dura or spinal cord may present with ictal onset of pain and loss of function due to spinal subarachnoid haemorrhage. Often, however, they present with symptoms of progressive spinal compression with pain and fluctuating loss of function. They may occur at any spinal level and in patients of any age.

Extradural Extramedullary Tumours

PRIMARY AND METASTATIC MALIGNANT TUMOURS. Secondary deposits of carcinoma are the most frequent cause of extradural spinal tumours. They occur either in the bone of the body or lamina of the vertebra, causing pathological fracture or collapse, or in the extradural tissue as a cuff which encircles and constricts the spinal theca. Bronchus, breast and prostate are particularly common sources, and the primary may be known or be latent when the spinal secondary presents with pain and loss of function. They occur particularly in middle-aged and elderly patients. Myeloma, other reticuloses and sarcoma may also cause spinal compression, with or without bony involvement, as may direct spread of tumour from lung or retroperitoneal tissue. Chordoma is another rare, primary tumour of spinal column which causes extradural spinal compression.

Special Investigations of Spinal Tumours

Plain Radiograph

Plain radiograph of the spine, including oblique and tomographic views when necessary, may reveal diagnostic appearances in patients with spinal tumours. Neurofibroma often causes erosion of the pedicle of a vertebra, or widening of an intervertebral foramen. Large cervical or intrathoracic dumb-bell extensions of neurofibroma may appear as soft-tissue shadows. Spinal meningioma only occasionally causes bony erosion, but may show pathological areas of calcification. Intramedullary tumours often cause widening of the bony spinal canal over several segments, sometimes with thinning of the laminae. Spina bifida may be identified in association with many cases of dermoid or lipoma. Often extradural metastases cause fracture and collapse of the vertebral body (*Figs.* 35.12, 35.13) or erosion of the pedicle or lamina at the affected level. This may be associated with other bony metastases on skeletal survey or with evidence of primary or secondary lung tumour.

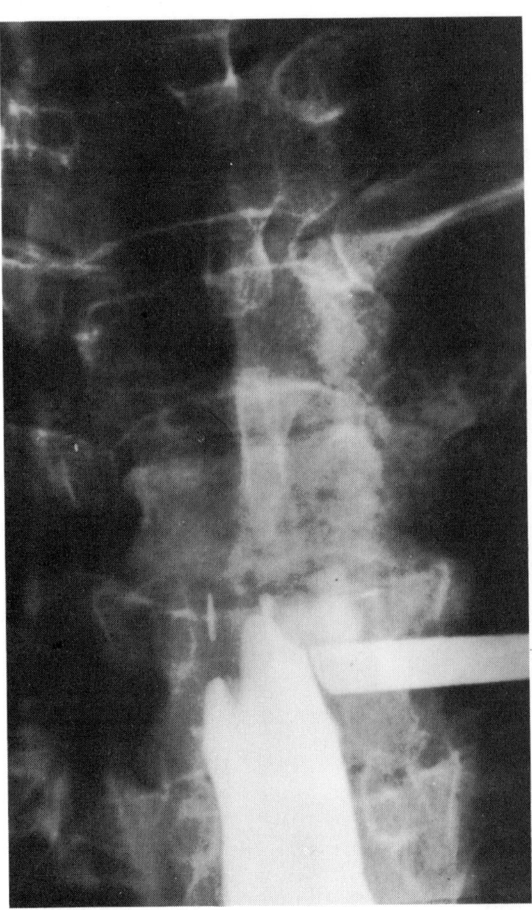

Fig. 35.12 Myelogram, thoracocervical junction AP projection. Spinal metastasis. Complete extradural block to Myodil contrast material at level of marker. Bony erosion in pedicles of vertebra above this level.

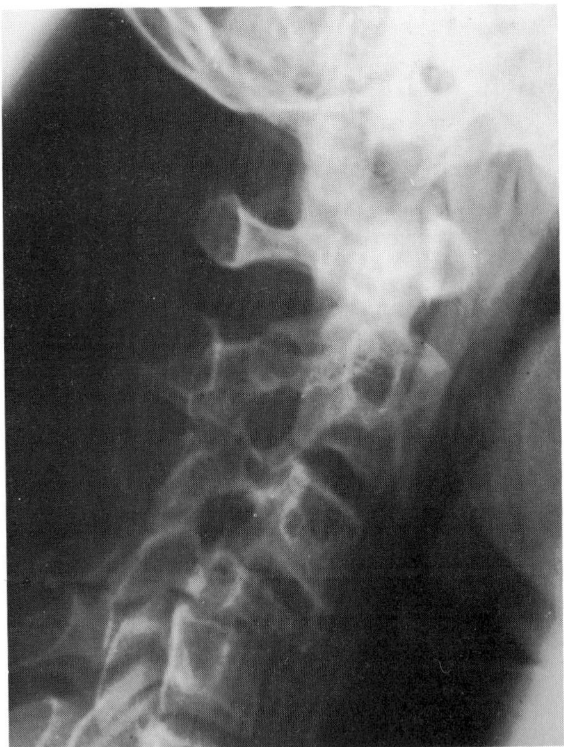

a

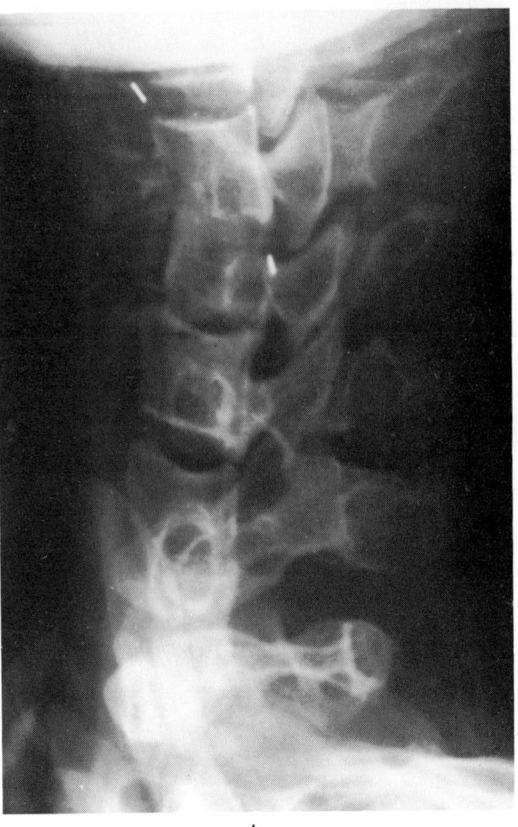

b

Fig. 35.13 Cervical spine, plain radiograph, lateral projection. *a*, Pathological fracture with subluxation of 4th cervical vertebra, due to solitary metastasis. *b*, Postoperative appearance following tumour removal and fusion with iliac bone graft.

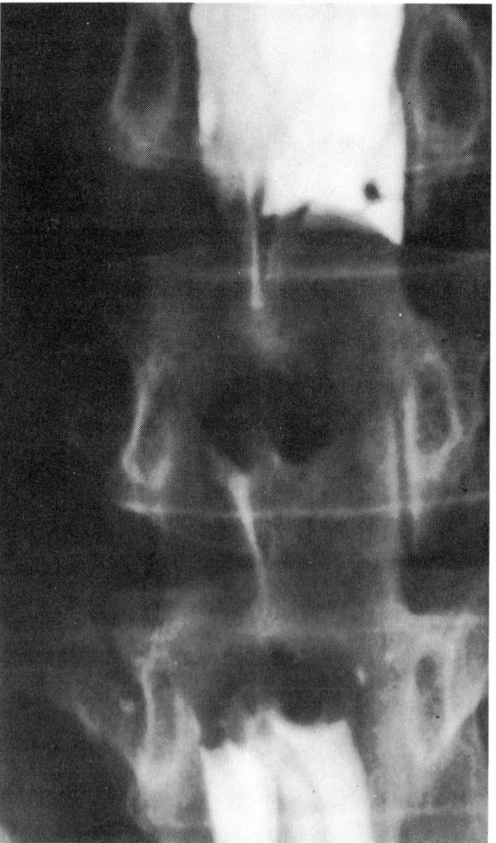

Fig. 35.14 Myelogram, lumbar spine AP projection. Intradural neurofibroma of cauda equina.

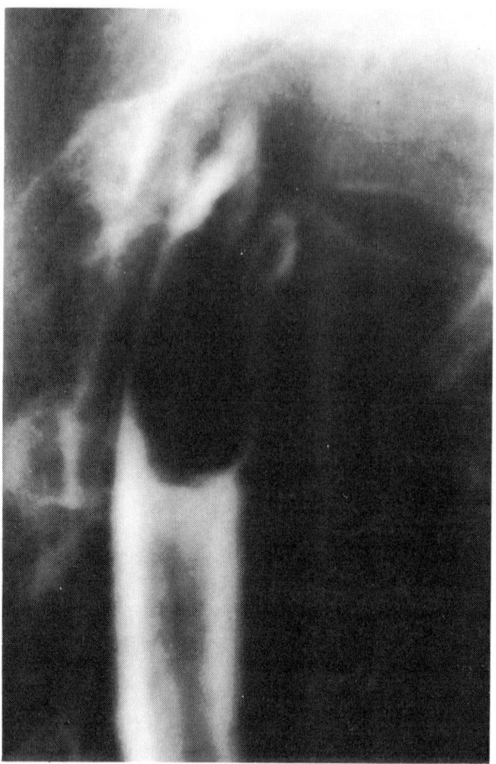

Fig. 35.15 Myelogram, thoracic spine lateral projection, Intradural meningioma.

Myelography

Positive contrast materials, either Myodil or newer water-soluble media (e.g. metrizamide) are used to outline the spinal subarachnoid space and to demonstrate blocks due to spinal compression. Intradural and extradural tumours tend to produce characteristic types of blocks visible on myelography (*Figs.* 35.12, 35.14, 35.15, 35.16). Other deformities in the spinal cord, e.g. abnormal vessels of an angioma, may be demonstrated (*Fig.* 35.17*a*). The contrast is generally injected by lumbar puncture, although it may be necessary to use cisternal or lateral cervical puncture if the lumbar theca is obstructed by tumour or if it is desired to get contrast above the level of a complete spinal block. Specimens of CSF are obtained for biochemical and cytological diagnosis at the time of myelography. Myelography can precipitate deterioration in patients with spinal tumour with rapid increase in loss of function. It is therefore desirable that the investigation is performed when both patient and surgeon are prepared to proceed to surgery immediately, if this proves necessary.

Spinal Angiography

Angiography of the spinal arteries can reveal spinal tumours, and is particularly helpful in cases of vascular neoplasms, e.g. haemangioblastoma, and in spinal angioma (*Fig.* 35.17*b*). The procedure carries an appreciable neurological morbidity and is done only with a view to subsequent surgery.

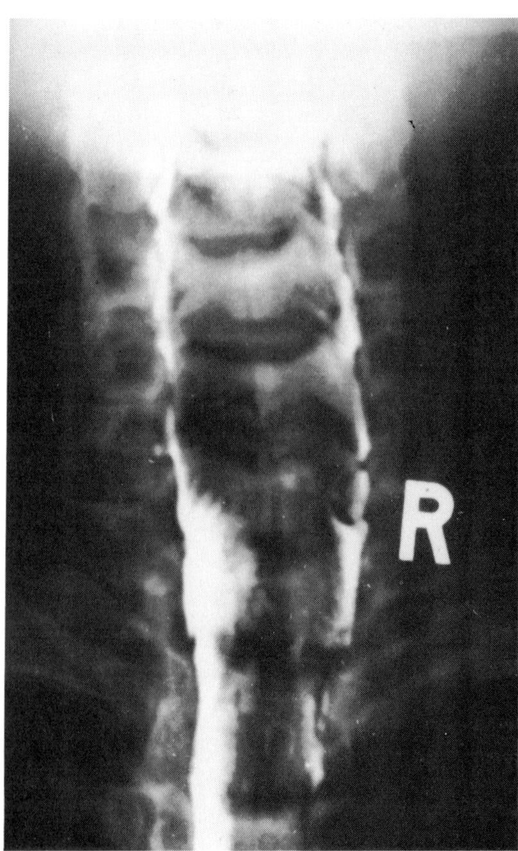

Fig. 35.16 Myelogram, cervical spine AP projection. Intramedullary astrocytoma of spinal cord, with massive widening of cord shadow.

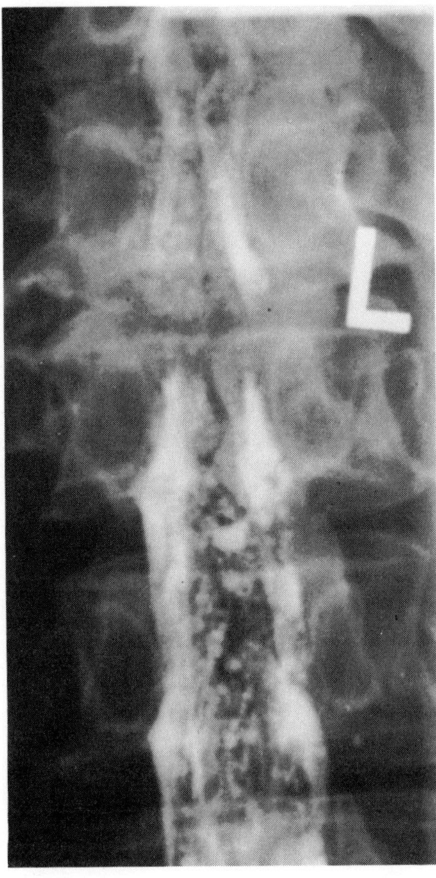

a

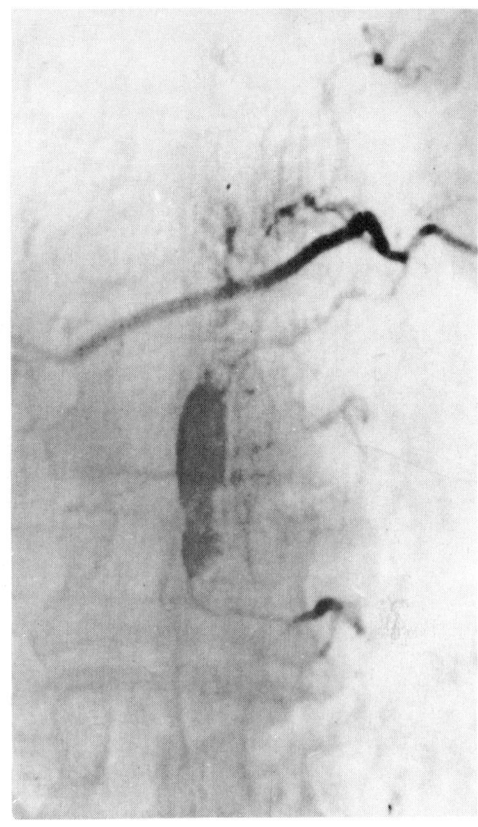

b

Fig. 35.17 a, Myelogram, thoracolumbar spine AP projection. Arteriovenous malformation, irregular serpiginous markings on cord. b, Spinal angiogram, AP projection. Arteriovenous malformation, feeding artery and draining veins.

Other Investigations

Examination of the CSF from below the level of a complete spinal block shows it to be yellow, and with a very high protein level, often in excess of 1 g/100 ml (normal <40 mg/100 ml). If the pressure is measured it may be raised and characteristically shows no fluctuation with compression of the jugular veins in the neck (Queckenstedt's test). Cytological examination may reveal tumour cells, particularly in cases of ependymoma.

CT scan of the spinal cord is possible, and in some cases can reveal tumour, e.g. cystic intramedullary astrocytoma. However, resolution of the cord within the bony spinal canal is difficult and this method is not used routinely. Endomyelogram, by percutaneous puncture of the cord and injection of contrast material into cystic intramedullary tumours, is possible and useful in selected cases.

Peripheral Nerve Tumours

The presenting symptoms of patients with peripheral nerve tumours are those of local mass effect or of loss of function, alone or in combination.

Symptoms due to Local Mass Effect

The patients may notice a lump in the subcutaneous tissues of the limbs or trunk, which very gradually increases in size. Often the lump is painless but sometimes it is tender and on percussion by the finger it may be possible for the surgeon to elicit local pain and paraesthesiae which shoot down the peripheral nerve distribution (Tinel's sign). Sometimes large, otherwise silent, peripheral nerve tumours may present by obstruction of the trachea, oesophagus or vessels in the neck or by mediastinal obstruction in the chest.

Symptoms due to Loss of Function

Sensory loss or paraesthesiae in the cutaneous distribution of a peripheral nerve may be early symptoms of tumour. Later, motor function may be impaired causing paralysis and tendon reflexes become depressed.

Specific Peripheral Nerve Tumour Syndromes

Neurilemoma, Neurofibroma

Tumours may arise from the Schwann cells or from the fibroblasts of any peripheral nerve. They may be single or multiple, particularly in association with von Recklinghausen's disease (*Fig.* 35.18). Often they present as painless subcutaneous nodules without neurological symptoms.

Neuroblastoma

This tumour arises from sympathetic nervous tissue in the adrenal medulla or, occasionally, elsewhere in the retroperitoneal or retropleural spaces. It is a not uncommon tumour of infancy and childhood, and metastasizes early and widely to liver, bone and orbit. The presenting symptoms are

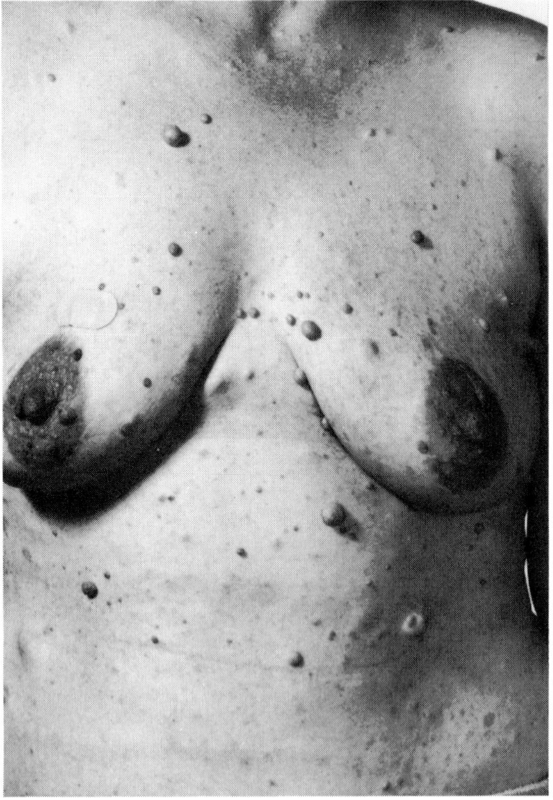

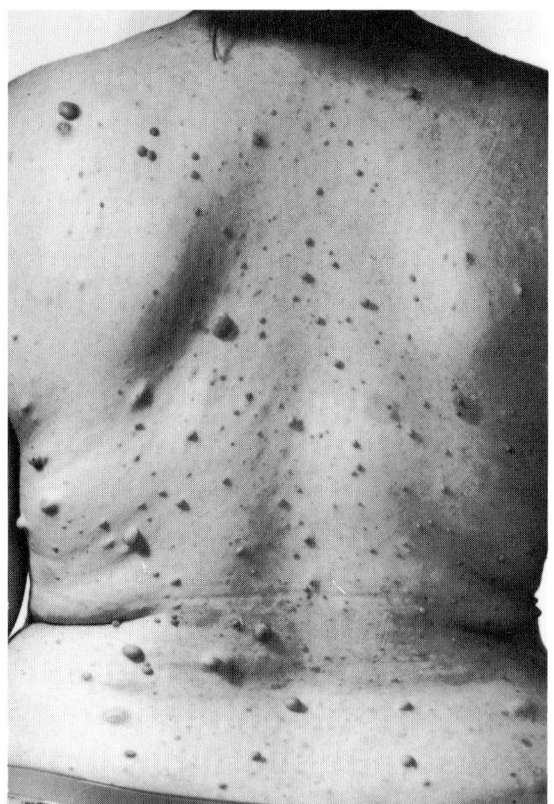

Fig. 35.18 Von Recklinghausen's disease of nerves.

protean and range from abdominal enlargement, with pain and vomiting, to generalized weakness, fever and weight loss. Metastases may present while the primary remains latent, with masses in the lymph nodes, skull or orbits.

Traumatic Neuroma

A relatively common, non-neoplastic, cause of palpable peripheral nerve tumours is trauma. Healed scars in the overlying skin or history of closed trauma indicate that this is the probable cause of the mass. Tinel's sign (*see above*) is often positive and there is loss of function, sometimes total, in the nerve distal to the lesion.

Special Investigations of Peripheral Nerve Tumours

Plain Radiograph

Spinal radiography may demonstrate dumb-bell extensions or associated multiple tumours in cases of neurofibroma. A radiograph of the neck or chest may reveal soft-tissue masses which, on biopsy, prove to be peripheral nerve tumours.

Electromyography (EMG)

Electrophysiological tests of nerve conduction may be used to confirm dysfunction in a peripheral nerve, and may indicate the site of the lesion within the nerve or relative to its central connection with the anterior and posterior roots of the spinal cord.

Other Investigations

The histamine flare reaction, in some cases, is useful in determining the site of the lesion in relation to the dorsal root ganglion. Urinary catecholamines are elevated in many cases of neuroblastoma. Nerve growth factor may be elevated in familial cases of multiple neurofibromatosis associated with von Recklinghausen's disease.

TREATMENT OF NERVOUS SYSTEM TUMOURS

Cranial Tumours

Surgery

Surgery of intracranial tumours depends on accurate preoperative localization by neuroradiological investigation, because it is difficult to change the operative approach once the skull has been opened. Particularly careful technique is required in neurosurgery to lessen the chance of brain damage by retraction or by postoperative haematoma or infection. Burr hole exploration is employed for needle biopsy or drainage of a cyst, while craniotomy through the cranial vault or occipital craniectomy in the posterior fossa are used to expose larger areas for more extensive tumour removal. Trans-sphenoidal, translabyrinthine and transclival surgery can be employed to approach certain basal skull tumours directly. Shunt operations, in which the CSF is artificially drained through a tube passed from the lateral ventricles to the vena cava or peritoneum, are also employed in the surgical management of certain tumours. In the majority of cases synthetic glucocorticoids, dexamethasone or betamethasone, are used as adjuvants to control cerebral oedema before, during and after surgery.

Cerebral Hemisphere Gliomas

These diffusely invasive tumours cannot be removed completely and the extent of tumour resection is a matter of surgical judgement based on the site of the lesion in relation to vital structures and on the age and general neurological condition of the patient. Even where preoperative diagnosis of highly malignant glioma with poor prognosis seems certain, most neurosurgeons seek histological confirmation by biopsy in order to avoid leaving occasional patients with undiagnosed benign tumours untreated. Tumours arising in critical areas, for example beneath the speech areas in the parietal region of the dominant left hemisphere, are generally biopsied only. However, in the frontal, temporal or occipital regions it is possible to perform decompressive lobectomy and in other areas it is often possible to debulk the glioma by drainage of cyst fluid or local removal of necrotic tumour. Such surgical internal decompression relieves the symptoms of raised ICP and allows further palliative treatment of malignant tumours with adjuvant radiotherapy and chemotherapy.

Third Ventricle Region Tumours: Brainstem Gliomas

Gliomas in the third ventricle or thalamus and pineal region germinomas and teratomas, as well as gliomas of the brainstem, are usually demonstrated unequivocally by neuroradiological investigation. Commonly these inaccessible tumours are not biopsied. A shunt is performed to relieve hydrocephalus, where this exists, before further treatment with radiotherapy. In cases where the diagnosis is in doubt or where there is a special indication, e.g. presence of a large cystic element or failure to respond to radiation, these lesions may be directly approached at surgery.

Cerebellum and Fourth Ventricle Region Tumour

Astrocytomas of the cerebellar hemisphere, which are often simply small nodules lying in the wall of a fluid-filled cyst, can in some cases be totally removed by surgery. Tumours in the midline of the cerebellum, that is medulloblastoma, ependymoma and choroid plexus papilloma, can only be removed partially and often a shunt is required to relieve hydrocephalus prior to adjuvant radiotherapy.

Acoustic Neurilemoma

Small acoustic nerve tumours may be removed through the labyrinth with deafness as the only side-effect. More usually these tumours are too large to be removed safely in this way and an intracranial approach is required. Radical curative removal is the aim of surgery for this benign tumour. However, there is a morbidity due to damage to the adjacent normal facial nerve (facial paralysis in some cases) and other lower cranial nerves as well as risk of mortality due to damage to vital structures in the brainstem or to its blood supply.

Meningiomas

These benign tumours, when they occur in the cranial vault, are excised radically with a wide cuff of surrounding normal dura in order to prevent recurrence. This treatment is usually curative, although it is associated with a small morbidity and mortality. Recurrence can occur, particularly with parasagittal tumours. However, basal tumours present more technical operative problems and total removal with acceptable morbidity may, in some cases, be impracticable. There is a small place for radiotherapy in irremovable or recurrent meningiomas.

Pituitary Adenomas

Large pituitary adenomas, particularly those with irregular suprasellar extensions, are generally approached by transfrontal craniotomy and partially or subtotally removed. Rapid decompression of the optic chiasma is thereby achieved and postoperative radiotherapy is given to reduce the risk of recurrence from remaining tumour. Smaller tumours, with more limited suprasellar extensions, as well as functioning microadenomas may be approached from below through the trans-sphenoidal route. In many cases of microadenoma it is possible to restore normal pituitary function by selective total removal of the encapsulated tumour sparing compressed normal pituitary.

Craniopharyngioma

Partial removal at craniotomy, with subsequent radiotherapy is generally the optimum surgical management of craniopharyngioma. In some cases more radical surgery may be justified and in others lesser procedures, e.g. simply drainage of cyst fluid, may be warranted.

Intracranial Metastases

Single intracranial metastases in the cerebral hemispheres or in the cerebellum may be removed at craniotomy, for palliation of symptoms and for diagnosis. Local recurrence, in spite of postoperative radiotherapy, is common, unless the primary tumour or other metastases cause the patient's death first. Multiple metastases, in those cases where the differential diagnosis from multiple cerebral abscess can be made on radiological grounds, are not usually subjected to surgery.

Radiotherapy

Postoperative radiation is of benefit in the treatment both of primary and secondary malignant brain tumours, and in the treatment of pituitary adenomas and craniopharyngiomas which have been partially removed.

Malignant Brain Tumours, Gliomas, Medulloblastoma, Metastases

The total amount of radiation which may be given to the brain without serious complications is limited to about 5500 rad, given in 5 daily fractions in 6 consecutive weeks. Beyond this dose radiation necrosis, at any time from 3 months to 5 years later, causes unacceptable brain damage and morbidity. Gliomas of the brain are usually treated postoperatively with whole brain irradiation, with a higher dose in the tumour area. In spite of such treatment these tumours recur. The reported results for surgery and adjuvant radiotherapy for cerebral gliomas are in the following ranges: Grade I–II tumours 58–86% survival at 1 year, 31–64% at 3 years and 20–50% at 5 years; Grade III–IV tumours 20–40% at 1 year, 0–16% at 3 years and 0–9% at 5 years. The median survival for Grade III–IV gliomas with surgery alone is approximately 6 months.

Radiotherapy for medulloblastoma and other malignant posterior fossa tumours, as well as for pineal region and brainstem tumours, is performed in a similar way. However, in medulloblastoma, ependymoma and germinoma of the pineal region whole neuraxis radiation, i.e. brain and spinal cord, is given to reduce the risk of spread of tumour within the CSF pathways. The optimum results in medulloblastoma for surgery with radiotherapy are 25–40% 5-year survival, and 10–25% 10-year survival.

Cerebral metastases, whether solitary or multiple, may be treated with palliative whole brain irradiation.

One recent promising development in radiotherapy for cranial tumours is the use of radiation sensitizers, e.g.

misonidazole, to increase the radiation damage to tumour cells which are otherwise relatively protected by hypoxia, while not increasing undesirable radiation necrosis in normal surrounding brain.

Benign Tumours, Pituitary Adenomas, Craniopharyngioma

Radiotherapy, at total doses in the order of 4500 rad, is commonly given to the pituitary region following partial removal of pituitary adenoma. In non-functioning tumours this decreases both the bulk of residual tumour and the risk of late recurrence. It may be beneficial in reducing excessive hormone production in some cases of functioning pituitary adenomas where surgery has not been fully effective. Craniopharyngiomas are less radiosensitive than pituitary neoplasms but postoperative radiotherapy does decrease the recurrence rate also in these tumours.

Chemotherapy

Malignant Brain Tumours

Chemotherapy of cerebral glioma increases survival to a modest but significant extent. The nitrosourea group of drugs (BCNU, 1,3-bis-(2-chloroethyl-1-nitrosourea) and CCNU (1(2-chloroethyl)-3-cyclohexyl-1-nitrosourea) and procarbazine are effective agents when given either as adjuvant therapy following radiation treatment or later at the time of recurrence of malignant glioma. These agents prolong median survival by a few months, with 15% survival at 2 years. These drugs are also modestly effective against recurrent medulloblastoma. Methotrexate, when given by intrathecal injection, is a chemotherapy agent which is useful in carcinomatous or leukaemic meningeal infiltration.

Spinal Tumours

Surgery

Surgical approach to spinal tumours is generally by posterior laminectomy, directly at the level of the lesion, as determined by clinical and radiological findings. In occasional cases a lateral or anterior approach to the spine, through the abdomen, chest, neck or mouth may be indicated to provide a direct route to the tumour, with minimum spinal cord retraction.

Neurofibroma, Meningioma

These benign intradural tumours are totally excised, after laminectomy and dural opening have been performed. Technically the emphasis is on minimal retraction of spinal cord during piecemeal 'gutting' of the tumour followed by complete removal of tumour capsule and its attachments in order to reduce the risks of recurrence.

Astrocytoma, Ependymoma (Gliomas)

These malignant tumours, which lie in the substance of the spinal cord, are approached by laminectomy and opening of the dura. Often they are cystic and fluid may be aspirated. This, together with partial removal or biopsy, achieves a degree of internal decompression. Postoperative radiotherapy is generally given.

Epidermoids, Dermoid, Lipoma

Total or subtotal removal of these slow-growing intradural intramedullary tumours is facilitated in some cases by the use of the operating microscope. Internal decompression, coupled with the decompression provided by laminectomy, usually relieves the symptoms of pain and loss of function.

Angioma

Preoperative spinal angiography can in cases of dural angiomas reveal the feeding arteries and draining veins so that these can be identified directly at laminectomy and ligated prior to excision of the dural lesion. Other types of spinal angiomas affect the substance of the cord, and thus their removal at laminectomy is technically more difficult and carries more neurological morbidity.

Malignant Extradural Tumours

Acute spinal compression due to a cuff of metastatic tumour may be relieved by laminectomy and removal of the extradural tumour. This achieves rapid decompression of the spinal cord. Cases where the malignant tumour has invaded the body of the vertebra and caused collapse with bony compression anteriorly are more difficult to relieve by posterior laminectomy. In selected cases, where the prognosis for life of the underlying malignancy is a year or more, it is appropriate to consider the more major operations of lateral or anterior decompression with removal of the diseased vertebral body and spinal fusion with a bone graft.

Postoperative radiotherapy to the site of spinal metastasis, as well as the primary site, may be indicated.

Radiotherapy

Malignant Tumours, Astrocytomas, Ependymoma (Gliomas)

Gliomas of the spinal cord are sensitive to radiation, but unfortunately the normal cord is, like the brain, susceptible to radiation necrosis. Local radiation to the site of biopsy or partial removal of spinal astrocytoma is helpful in delaying recurrence of symptoms, and may produce additional improvement over and above that seen after surgical decompression. Radiotherapy to spinal ependymoma is also beneficial in delaying local recurrence and, by use of neuraxis

Table 35.3 Results of treatment of different types of tumour

Cranial			
Glioma	Operative mortality approximately 2–10%		
	Median Surival		
	1-yr survival	3-yr survival	5-yr survival
Grades I–II	58–86%	31–64%	20–50%
Grades III–IV	20–40%	0–16%	0–9%
Neurilemoma	Operative mortality approximately 2–5% Recurrence rate approximately 10% at 10 yr		
Meningioma	Operative mortality approximately 5% Recurrence rate approximately 2–25% (according to site) at 10 yr		
Craniopharyngioma	Operative mortality approximately 2–20% Recurrence rate approximately 30% at 10 yr		
Pituitary adenoma	Operative mortality approximately 1–2% Recurrence rate approximately 10% at 10 yr		
Metastases	Operative mortality approximately 10% Median survival 3–6 months. 1-yr survival 10–25%		
Spinal			
Glioma	Operative mortality less than 1% Recurrence rate 5–20% at 5 yr		
Neurilemoma	Operative mortality less than 1% Recurrence rate less than 1%		
Meningioma	Operative mortality less than 1% Recurrence rate less than 1%		
Metastases	Operative mortality approximately 5–10% Median survival 6–12 months. 1-yr survival 25–40%		

radiation, in reducing distant CSF seeding in other parts of the spinal canal or in the subfrontal region.

Extradural Metastasis

Following urgent surgery for acute spinal cord compression due to extradural metastasis local radiotherapy is of use in delaying recurrence. Where the symptoms of spinal compression are less acute, and where the diagnosis is known with reasonable certainty, it can sometimes be best to treat the patient with radiotherapy at the outset and to defer surgery. With spinal metastases from certain radiosensitive tumours, for example myeloma or teratoma of the testis, this form of management can often relieve symptoms without surgery. However, in some cases, deterioration occurs during radiotherapy and this is an indication for urgent decompressive laminectomy.

Chemotherapy

Systemic chemotherapy has a part to play in the treatment of some metastatic tumours, e.g. myeloma. Intrathecal chemotherapy, e.g. with methotrexate, is also beneficial in certain cases of meningeal infiltration by carcinoma or in recurrent spinal ependymomas.

Peripheral Nerve Tumours

Surgical exploration and excision of peripheral nerve tumours is carried out by the most direct route in the limb or trunk, having regard to surrounding structures.

Neurofibroma

The peripheral nerve is exposed, and where possible a plane of cleavage is developed between the tumour and the peripheral nerve and the neoplasm is removed. If it is not possible to separate the two structures it may be reasonable to totally excise the tumour and parent nerve if the sacrifice in function is only cutaneous sensation or motor function in an unimportant part. However, in nerves supplying the limbs it is often not reasonable to sacrifice the nerve and the best that can be achieved is partial removal. In many cases this will improve symptoms and recurrence will be long delayed. Rarely neurofibromas become malignant and may metastasize, requiring local radiotherapy.

Neuroblastoma

Early and radical surgery is desirable for these adrenal, retroperitoneal tumours and in many cases this may be curative. When skeletal or other metastases are present the prognosis is very poor. Early postoperative radiotherapy and adjuvant chemotherapy are indicated.

Traumatic Neuroma

Following nerve division by injury there is a loss of function and formation of a traumatic neuroma at the site of nerve injury. Exploration, with excision of the neuroma and resuture of the nerve, is usually indicated.

THE WAY AHEAD

The treatment of malignant intracranial and spinal tumours is likely to improve in the future with developments of new methods in surgery and adjuvant modes of therapy. More accurate removal of brain tumours with the aid of peroperative CT scan control and by use of laser or ultrasonic techniques, coupled with improved magnification and illumination obtained under the operating microscope, are already available on a research basis. New forms of radiation employing proton and neutron particles have been used in place of megavoltage X-rays. These methods have properties which may confer particular advantages in particular forms of tumour. Radiation-sensitizing drugs which counteract the protective effect of hypoxia on tumours have been developed and other classes of drugs which may sensitize tumours, e.g. by impeding repair in damaged neoplastic cells, may be discovered in the future. Chemotherapy drugs available now have only modest effects in most tumours, but information has become available about the desirable pharmacological properties of better agents and such drugs may possibly be arrived at by synthesis or extraction from biological products. Newer non-invasive methods of investigation, either by scan or by biochemical assay, may allow both earlier diagnosis of brain tumour and also earlier detection of recurrence, so that further treatment may be given. Such developments in treatment offer hope for improved results in both benign and in malignant nervous system tumours.

Further Reading

Northfield D. W. C. (1973) *Surgery of the Central Nervous System*. Oxford, Blackwell.
Russell D. S. and Rubinstein L. J. (1977) *Pathology of Tumours of the Nervous System*. London, Arnold.
Symon L. (1979) In: Rob C. and Smith R. (ed.) *Operative Surgery: Neurosurgery*. London, Butterworths.
Thomas D. G. T. and Graham D. I. (ed.) (1980) *Brain Tumours: Scientific Basis, Clinical Investigation and Current Therapy*. London, Butterworths.

36 Spinal Injury and Disc Problems

Julian T. Hoff

ANATOMICAL AND PHYSIOLOGICAL CONSIDERATIONS

Of the 33 vertebrae normally found in man, only 24 have functional movement. Most of the movement of the spine occurs in the cervical and lumbar regions, while the thoracic spine is relatively immobile. Movement during flexion and extension is greatest in the lower cervical and lumbar segments, and is maximal during rotation in the upper cervical and lumbar segments. Each vertebra consists of a body, which bears weight, and the posterior elements (laminae, spinous process, pedicles, transverse processes), which provide flexibility and stability of the vertebral column. The spinal canal is ovoid in shape with its greater dimension in a longitudinal plane. The canal assumes a more triangular shape in the lumbar region.

The intervertebral disc consists of two parts. The circumferential annulus is dense fibrous tissue of great strength; the central nucleus is fibrocartilage with little tensile strength, but with substantial elasticity. Fibrocartilage may be fragmented acutely or degenerate gradually with time, and it heals slowly because of poor blood supply. The nucleus is about 80% water at birth; it gradually dehydrates and loses its elasticity with age. The annulus, on the other hand, heals well and is buttressed by heavy anterior and posterior longitudinal ligaments for added strength. Intervertebral disc disease may occur at any level from C1 to S1. The cervical and lumbar areas are affected most often, while thoracic disc disease is uncommon.

The spinal cord occupies about one-half of the spinal canal, is centrally placed, and moves rostrally and caudally a few mm during flexion and extension of the neck. Side-to-side motion is restricted by the tethering effect of the intradural dentate ligaments. It is supplied with blood by radicular arteries which arise from the vertebral artery and thyrocervical trunk in the neck, from intercostal arteries in the thorax, and from lumbar arteries in the low back. An arterial confluens, the artery of Adamkiewicz, is typically found in the T10–L2 region, often on the left side. It supplies the lower thoracic cord and conus medullaris.

The spinal cord terminates as the conus at L1–2. Dorsal and ventral nerve roots emerge from the conus separately, pass within the lumbar sac to their respective intervertebral foramina and exit from the spinal canal. The roots join to form a true nerve within the neural foramen. Sacral nerve roots are medial and central within the lumbar sac, adjacent to the filum terminale, which is the pial-arachnoid structure that anchors the conus to the caudal end of the spinal canal.

Three fibre tracts of the spinal cord are important clinically (*Fig.* 36.1). The corticospinal tract carries motor fibres from the cortex to lower motor neurones, crossing the midline at the decussation of the pyramids in the medulla. The dorsal columns carry sensory fibres conveying position, vibratory and light touch sensation from the dorsal roots to the opposite cerebral cortex through a decussation in the brainstem. The spinothalamic tract transmits pain and temperature sensation from the contralateral side across the midline of the cord, within two or three segments of each dorsal root entry zone, to the ipsilateral thalamus. Lower motor neurones are located in the ventral horns of the spinal cord grey matter.

The C1 nerve root emerges from the spine above C1; the

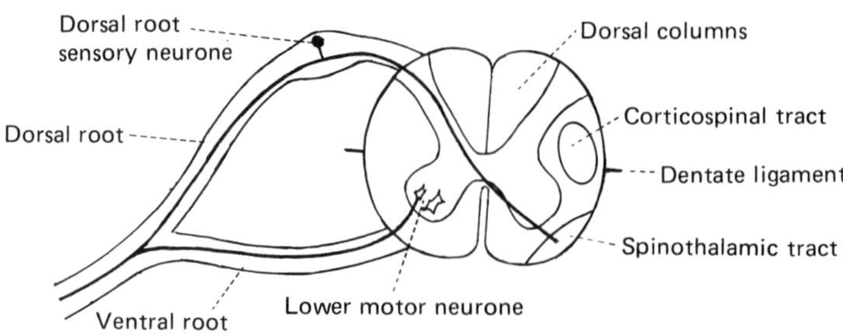

Fig. 36.1 Diagram of transverse section of spinal cord showing important clinical anatomy.

C2 root emerges below the C1 vertebra. Hence the root that emerges from the spine between C5 and C6 vertebrae is the C6 root. C8 emerges between C7 and T1 and the T1 root emerges below the T1 vertebra. Lumbosacral nerve roots carry on the same relationships to the vertebrae determined by emergence of the T1 nerve root below the T1 vertebra. That is, the L4 nerve root emerges below L4, and the S1 root emerges below S1.

Because a root (e.g. L4) passes laterally toward the neural foramen as it descends within the spinal canal, it passes the adjacent intervertebral disc (e.g. L4–5) at its extreme lateral edge, hugging the pedicle of the vertebra laterally (*Fig.* 36.2). The nerve root (e.g. L5), which descends to the next lowest foramen, passes across the disc space (e.g. L4–5) more medially, in a vulnerable location to diseases involving the disc.

Sensation about the deltoid area is basically related to the C5 root, while sensation in the thumb is a C6 root function. A normal biceps jerk requires an intact C6 root; the triceps jerk is dependent upon the C7 root, and intrinsic muscles of the hand allowing abduction and adduction of the fingers are

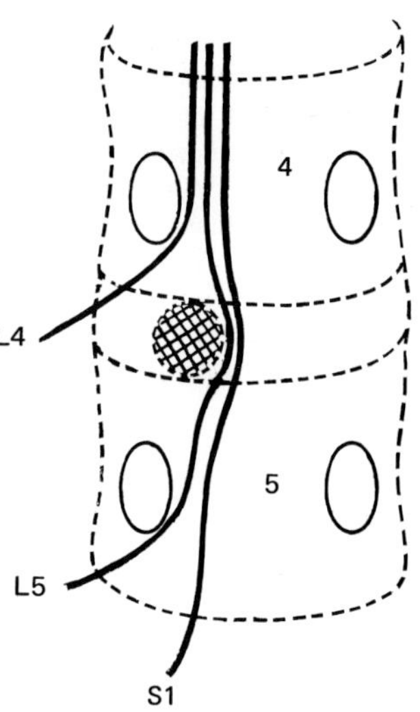

Fig. 36.2 Diagram of the lumbar spine and nerve roots. Note the relationship of the L5 nerve root to the L4–5 disc space.

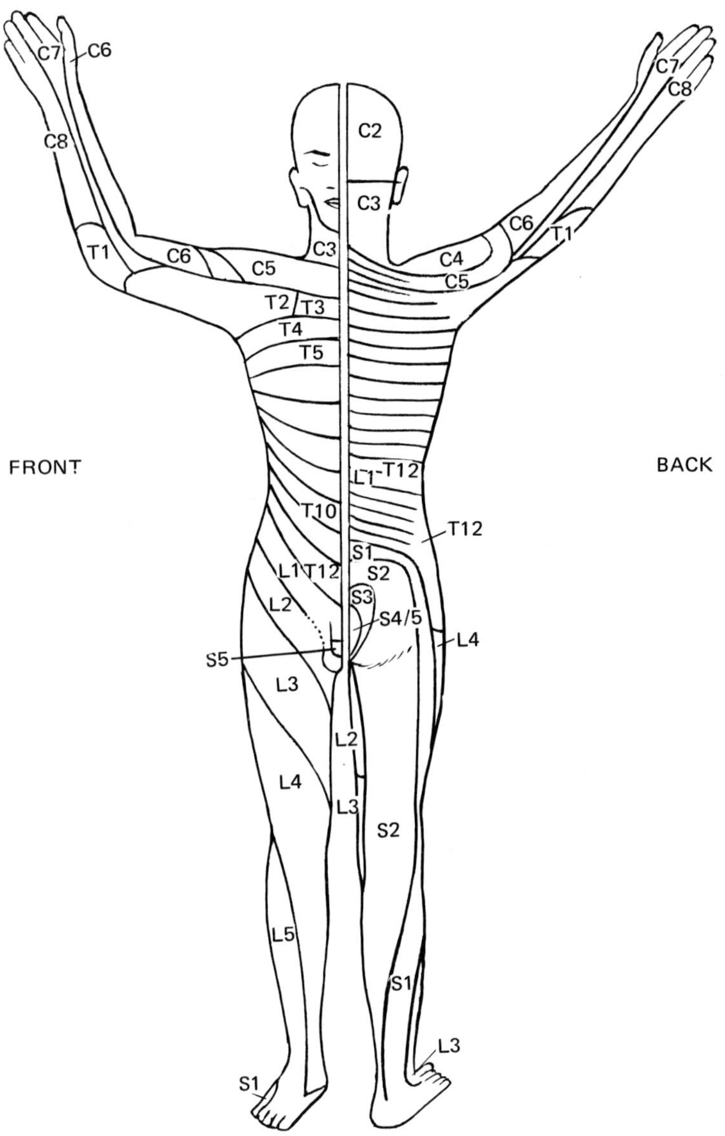

Fig. 36.3 Diagram of the dermatomal pattern in man.

innervated by C8. The T10 dermatome is at the level of the umbilicus anteriorly. The sensory distribution of L5 is on the medial aspect of the foot and the great toe. S1 sensation is experienced over the lateral aspect of the foot, the 5th toe, and the sole of the heel (*Fig.* 36.3). Pain or sensory deficit in those dermatomal areas implies involvement of either L5 or S1 fibres. Plantar flexion is primarily an S1 motor function; dorsiflexion of the foot is an L5 function. The ankle jerk is primarily dependent upon S1, while the knee jerk depends upon L3 and L4. The L5 fibres may contribute to both or neither reflex.

SPINE AND SPINAL CORD INJURY

Traumatic injury of the spinal cord may result from vertebral fracture/dislocation, hyperextension of the cervical spine in the presence of a narrow spinal canal, and herniation of intervertebral disc material into the canal. Neurological involvement ranges from mild and transient to severe and permanent. A spine injury should be suspected in all patients with multiple injuries, particularly of the head. Spinal tenderness and/or deformity, weakness of any or all extremities, respiratory distress, and arterial hypotension are particularly good indicators of a spinal cord injury.

Clinical Findings

1. Neurological

Clinical findings may include root, cord or combined signs and symptoms. Radiculopathy is characterized by motor and sensory impairment in the corresponding myotome and dermatome. Pain in the dermatome of a compressed root may be intense and easily aggravated by movement.

Traumatic myelopathy demonstrates more clinical variability. It usually is manifested as one of four syndromes (*Fig.* 36.4): (*a*) Transection of the cord is accompanied by arreflexia, flaccidity, anaesthesia and autonomic paralysis below the level of the lesion. Arterial hypotension is characteristic when the transection is above T5 and it may be exaggerated by postural changes. Transection is often termed a 'complete' lesion. (*b*) Partial or 'incomplete' injury may result in the Brown-Séquard syndrome which implies a sagittal hemisection of the cord. Ipsilateral loss of motor function, position and light touch sensation, and contralateral loss of pain and temperature sensation below the level of injury are typical. (*c*) When the cord is squeezed but incompletely transected, as in a hyperextension injury, the central cord syndrome may appear. Characteristically motor function and pain-temperature sensation are lost in the upper extremities, while these functions are relatively preserved in the lower extremities. (*d*) The anterior spinal artery syndrome includes loss of all cord function below the lesion except for position, vibratory and light touch sensations transmitted by the dorsal columns. This clinical picture of an incomplete lesion usually arises when the anterior spinal artery is occluded, perhaps from an acutely ruptured cervical disc in the midline.

Signs and symptoms of cauda equina compression are those of radiculopathy except that many roots are usually involved. Bladder distension from detrusor muscle paralysis, flaccidity of the anal sphincter and loss of perineal sensation are common.

2. Other System Responses

Acute spinal cord injury is normally accompanied by a variety of systemic responses in addition to those occurring in the nervous system. Ventilation may be profoundly affected. If the cord lesion is above C3 apnoea ensues, accounting for the high mortality of this injury at the scene of the accident. Involvement of the cord from C4 and below, on the other hand, produces variable respiratory disturbances, but survival is likely because spontaneous ventilatory effort can be initiated. Often, however, tidal volume is insufficient in injuries involving C4–C6, causing progressive hypoxia and carbon dioxide retention. Airway obstruction, atelectasis and pneumonia are common complications soon after injury. Assisted ventilation is almost always necessary for days to weeks in patients with cervical spinal cord injury.

Ileus is usual after spinal cord and cauda equina injury. Gastric distension follows, especially when coupled with air swallowing by the anxious patient. Distension may be severe, requiring nasogastric suction to relieve it. Similarly, bladder distension is common because bladder and pelvic floor muscles are flaccid. Distension may be severe enough to cause compression of the vena cava and pelvic veins, impairing venous return to the heart and contributing to systemic hypotension.

Blood pressure is usually low if the cord injury is high enough (T5 and up) to eliminate much of the sympathetic nervous system and the vasomotor tone it provides. Tachycardia is a common compensatory response to hypotension. Postural hypotension is an early hazard in patients with

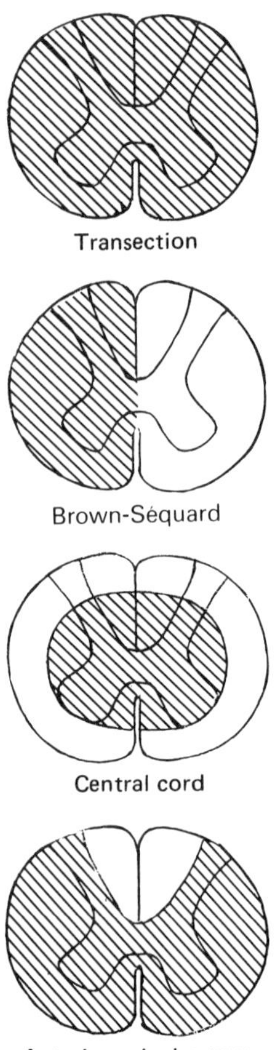

Fig. 36.4 Diagram of the common lesions found in spinal cord injury. The hatched areas represent the site of injury.

spinal cord injury because some routine procedures (e.g. myelogram, nursing care) necessitate position changes. Hypotension is controlled by the administration of intravenous fluids. Colloid is preferred to reduce the definite threat of vascular overload and pulmonary oedema.

Temperature control may be severely compromised, particularly in children, because of absent sweating and cutaneous vasomotor activity below the level of cord injury. Patients become vulnerable to environmental temperature change if the body surface area for heat exchange is significantly changed.

Diagnosis

While radiographic examinations of the spine are essential, further insult to the already-injured cord may result during these procedures. Thus, any patient with a suspected spinal injury should be moved by two or more persons standing on the same side, their arms beneath the patient's body. The two lift the patient simultaneously while two additional persons exert gentle traction on the head and feet to maintain neutral alignment of the patient's spine. The patient should not be turned to the lateral position; rather, lateral views are taken across the table (*Fig.* 36.5). When an injury to the cervical spine is suspected, the head and neck should be immobilized before the films are taken. This is best done by placing the patient on a spine board with the head fixed to it or with cervical traction in neutral position. Flexion should be avoided specifically. The C7–T1 level must be visualized which may require pulling the patient's shoulders downward, or a transaxillary 'swimmer's'-view, or tomography. The patient with a thoracolumbar injury can also be immobilized effectively on a spine board and should be maintained immobile until the stability of the fracture has been determined.

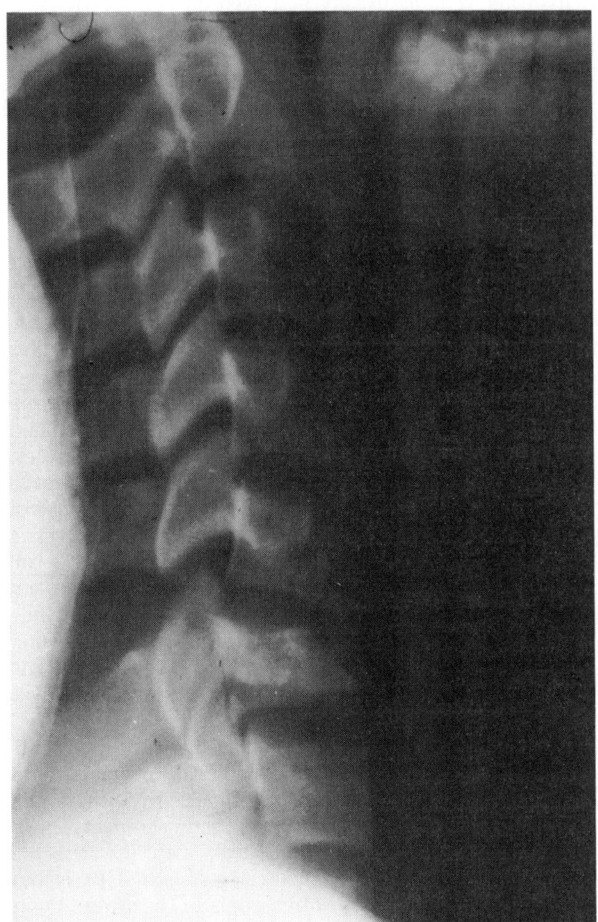

Fig. 36.5 Cervical radiograph, lateral view. The fracture at C6 is obvious on plain film.

Tomography provides a more detailed study of the spinal injury and may reveal fractures and/or dislocations not apparent on plain films. Most patients with spinal cord injury should undergo this examination, particularly when routine films are either normal or inadequate. Computerized tomography of the spine, with and without contrast, offers a non-invasive method for studying the spine and spinal cord, and will be used more in the future.

Treatment

The objectives of treatment are to protect undamaged structures, to restore function to reversibly damaged neural tissue, to correct spinal alignment, and to achieve permanent spinal stability. Hence reduction and immobilization of the fracture/dislocation must receive top priority.

Cervical spine malalignment can almost always be reduced by skeletal traction alone. If the spinal canal is not realigned, cord and root function will rarely improve. Furthermore, bony healing will be unsatisfactory unless the fragments are realigned.

In cervical fracture/dislocations skull tongs are an effective means of applying traction. They should be seated percutaneously through the outer table of the skull in line with the mastoid tips. Weight can be added gradually then, maintaining pull on the spine in neutral position. Frequent lateral view radiographs are essential during this procedure to assure good reduction. If ligamentous injury is severe small amounts of weight may distract the fracture and injure the cord more. It is thus good policy to begin with 2·3 kg (5 lb) and confirm its effect before proceeding further. Usually soft tissues are relatively intact, though, and weight may be added as necessary to reduce the fracture. Once the spinal injury is reduced, traction should be maintained to immobilize the spine. Frequent follow-up films are taken to confirm correct position. In order to heal, the usual cervical spine injury requires 6 weeks to 4 months of immobilization, either by skeletal traction in bed or by external fixation. To mobilize patients with neck injury as soon as possible (particularly the elderly) a 'halo' skull fixation device incorporated into a lightweight plastic jacket is effective.

Occasionally a cervical fracture cannot be reduced by traction alone without jeopardizing remaining cord function. Open reduction, usually by the posterior approach combined with a fusion procedure, may be necessary in certain instances. Fractures of the thoracic and lumbar spine should also be reduced as soon as possible. Bed rest often suffices, but open reduction and internal fixation of the fracture may be required.

Transection of the spinal cord causes complete loss of voluntary sensory and motor function below the lesion. The same clinical picture may result, rarely, when the cord is physiologically transected but not anatomically divided. That state of 'physiological transection' may last up to 24 h, but hardly ever beyond that. Thus, cord function which is lost completely for more than 24 h cannot be expected to return, no matter what therapy is rendered. If any cord function is preserved after injury, then some degree of function can return, provided the cord and spine are protected from secondary injury. In fact, up to 85% of patients who have some clinical evidence of cord function 24 h after injury can eventually walk. These simple facts underscore the absolute need for careful physical examination of the patient with a spinal cord injury not only immediately after injury, but also repetitively thereafter.

Indications for early operation on patients with spinal cord injury are therefore straightforward: (1) Inability to reduce the fracture/dislocation satisfactorily by closed methods (this is an unusual circumstance); (2) neurological deterioration in a patient with an incomplete cord lesion initially; and (3) severe compression of the spinal cord by an intraspinal mass shown by myelogram which persists despite reduction of the fracture/dislocation (e.g. disc material) and causes complete loss of cord function within 24 h of injury. Open wounds, such as those inflicted by stabbings and gunshots, should also be débrided and closed whether the lesion is complete or incomplete. Early operation to fuse the spine is warranted, particularly in elderly patients, when early mobilization and rehabilitation are mandatory.

Prognosis

The patient with an incomplete cord injury can be expected to walk again provided early care is protective and rehabilitation is well planned. Patients with complete lesions, however, rarely recover function below the lesion. Rehabilitation in them is directed toward self-care and vocational readjustment. Most persons with these handicaps can eventually achieve independence. Life expectancy is shortened slightly in paraplegics, and significantly in quadriplegics, because of the long-term problems associated with care of insensitive skin leading to pressure sores and recurrent urinary infections due to bladder neck obstruction eventually producing upper urinary tract infections and impaired renal function. The types of bladder disturbances and their management are discussed in Chapter 83.

DISC PROBLEMS

Cervical Disc Disease

If the nucleus of a cervical intervertebral disc extrudes through the annulus and posterior longitudinal ligament, adjacent neural structures may be compressed. Compression of the spinal cord may result in paraplegia or quadriplegia, depending on the segment involved, and compression of a spinal root may cause paralysis and sensory loss in structures of the upper extremity innervated by it. The severity of the clinical syndrome depends upon the site and severity of compression by the displaced disc fragment. Often the annulus and adjacent ligaments hold, preventing complete extrusion of the fragmented disc, but tear sufficiently to allow the disc to bulge into the spinal canal or foramina.

The annulus may rupture and the nucleus herniate into the spinal canal or neural foramen acutely. Often, however, the nucleus does not extrude, but simply fragments and progressively degenerates. The disc space gradually narrows, the joint becomes looser, and the cartilaginous end-plates of the adjacent vertebrae abut and wear more quickly. Bony spurs develop at the joint in reaction to the increased mobility and decreased elasticity. If a bony spur (osteophyte) forms in the neural foramen, the nerve root passing through may be chronically irritated and compressed. If the osteophyte forms within the spinal canal, then the cord itself may be compromised. Formation of osteophytes around the joints of vertebrae is termed 'spondylosis'. Cervical spondylosis is common and may even be 'normal' in ageing persons. Radiographic evidence of cervical spondylosis exists in 85% of people over 65 years of age.

The onset of symptoms and signs of an extruded disc fragment may be acute or insidious. Acute symptoms may follow trauma or may be unrelated to trauma. Neck and radicular discomfort occur simultaneously, but spinal cord symptoms are rare. There is usually limitation of neck motion, with tenderness over the brachial plexus and straightening of the normal cervical lordosis. Decrease in a deep tendon reflex is common with or without weakness in the muscles supplied by the compressed root. There is also hypoaesthesia or hyperaesthesia in the dermatomal pattern of the affected root. With foraminal osteophytes, episodes of cervical discomfort recur over many months or years before radicular symptoms occur. Interscapular aching and sub-occipital headaches are common complaints. The signs and symptoms of cervical spondylotic myelopathy are those of progressive spastic paraparesis with some limitation of neck motion, mild to moderate sensory changes in the lower extremities, weak and wasted upper extremities, and cervical dermatomal sensory loss.

Plain radiographs may be within normal limits (except for straightening of the cervical lordosis) or may demonstrate narrowing of a disc space. Radiographs may show osteophytic formation at the appropriate neural foramen with disc narrowing. This is usually best seen on oblique views. In cervical spondylosis, there is usually radiological evidence of osteophytes and disc narrowing at multiple levels, and in most cases the sagittal diameter of the cervical spinal canal is narrowed. The height of the canal as measured on a lateral view plain radiograph of an adult should normally be 16 mm or more (*Fig.* 36.6).

Myelography may show a small ventral extradural defect obliterating a nerve root cuff. In cervical spondylosis, the myelogram shows bar-like ventral defects at the disc space, usually occurring at multiple levels and sometimes associated with apparent widening of the cord shadow on the anteroposterior projection. Electromyography may confirm the diagnosis and localize the lesion more specifically, particularly when myelographic defects are multiple.

Cervical disc disease must be differentiated from inflammatory diseases affecting the soft tissues and joints of the pectoral girdle, such as subdeltoid and subacromial bursitis, Tietze's syndrome and cervical sprains; cervical rib and scalenus anterior syndrome, nerve entrapment syndromes in the upper extremities, such as carpal tunnel syndrome and tardy ulnar palsy; coronary insufficiency and angina pectoris; neoplasms of the pulmonary apex, e.g. Pancoast tumours; neoplasms of the brachial plexus; neoplasms of the cervical cord and medullocervical junction; fractures, dislocations, or subluxations of the cervical spine; and inflammatory disease of the cervical theca, such as arachnoiditis, sarcoidosis and Pott's disease.

Initially, cervical disc disease should be treated medically unless there is evidence of spinal cord compression or motor loss in an extremity secondary to root compression. Adequate medical therapy for patients suffering from radiculitis includes immobilization of the neck with mild traction exerted on the neck in a neutral position. This is best achieved with continuous or interrupted (2 h in and 1 h out) halter cervical traction. Analgesics, tranquillizers and local heat are frequently used in combination with traction. Cervical traction is applied in the neutral position. The weight

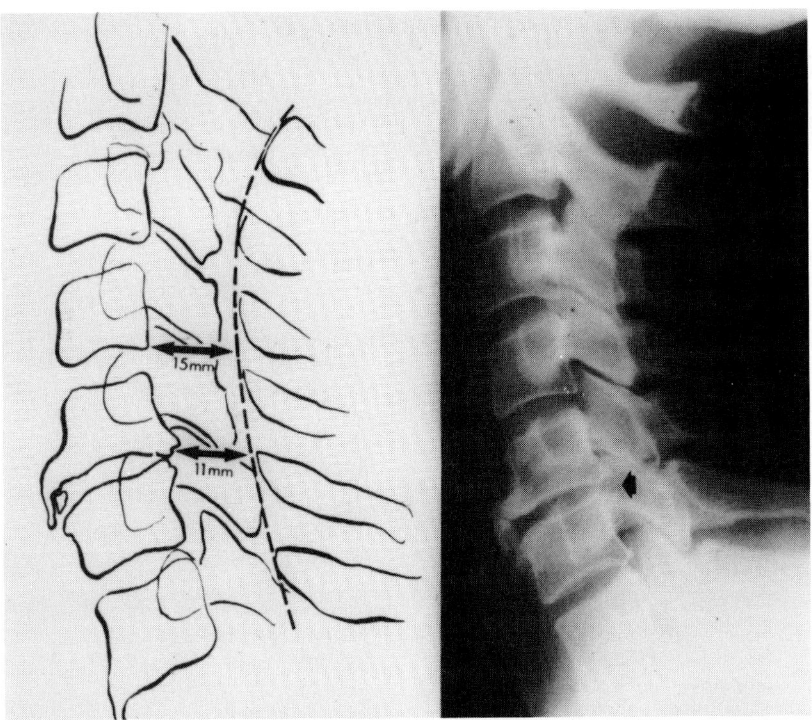

Fig. 36.6 Cervical radiograph and diagram to show a narrowed spinal canal (11 mm in this case) and the method used to measure it.

used generally ranges from 2·3 to 4·5 kg (5–10 lb), depending on the size of the patient.

There are two methods of treating cervical disc disease surgically: (1) posterior decompression of the nerve roots, spinal cord, or both; and (2) anterior decompression of nerve roots, spinal cord (or both), with or without fusion. The choice is based on consideration of a particular patient's anatomical lesion. It may occasionally be necessary to use both an anterior and posterior approach.

Seventy-five per cent of patients will recover following an adequate trial (10–14 days) of medical therapy, even though some will continue to have cervical or interscapular discomfort or mild paraesthesias. Some will have recurrence of their radicular symptoms on return to full activity. In many cases, these patients can be managed for years with intervals of cervical traction and a cervical collar, but some will require surgical therapy. For the 25% who do not respond to conservative therapy, operation is required.

Improvement follows operative treatment of a cervical disc in approximately 80% of patients who fail to respond to medical treatment. Surgical treatment of cervical spondylosis with myelopathy results in improvement in 50% of cases and arrest of the disease in many of the remainder.

Thoracic Disc Disease

The nucleus of a thoracic disc may extrude into the spinal canal as a result of forceful trauma. Because the canal is small in relation to the spinal cord within it, cord compression results from disc rupture. Paraplegia is often abrupt and may be permanent. More often, though, osteophyte formation secondary to a degenerated thoracic disc accounts for spinal canal narrowing. Then evidence of cord compression is more gradual and progressive. Treatment for a thoracic disc is primarily surgical. The offending disc or spur is best removed by an anterior or lateral approach.

Lumbar Disc Disease

If the nucleus of a lumbar intervertebral disc extrudes through the annulus and posterior longitudinal ligament, nerve roots may be compressed. Sensory loss, dermatomal pain, motor loss in the myotome(s) innervated by those root(s), and loss of tendon jerk(s) may result. The severity of the syndrome produced depends upon the site and severity of root compression. Occasionally the entire cauda equina may be compressed, resulting in complete loss of motor and sensory function including bowel and bladder sphincter control. Sometimes disc rupture may occur in the midline, compressing centrally placed sacral nerve roots preferentially, without involvement of laterally placed lumbar roots.

Fragmentation of a lumbar disc may occur without extrusion of the nucleus. In that event, elasticity of the joint is reduced and mobility is increased. The annulus may then simply bulge without tearing. As time passes, osteophytes form around the degenerated disc and may encroach upon the spinal canal and root foramina. Lumbar stenosis is the end result, a spondylotic condition common in the elderly.

Over 90% of clinical problems arise from the L4–5 and L5–S1 intervertebral areas, with most of the remainder from L3–4. Lumbar disc disease rarely involves higher levels. Pain is usually chronic, but the onset may be acute when associated with frank herniation. There may be back pain, leg pain, or both. The radiation of low back pain into the buttock, posterior thigh and calf is usually the same with disease at the L4–5 or L5–S1 interspaces. This radiating pain may be aggravated by coughing, sneezing, or the Valsalva manoeuvre. Bending or sitting accentuates the discomfort, whereas lying down characteristically relieves it. Most commonly the pain is described as aching, but frequently has a sharp or shooting element. Numbness of the leg(s) is present in fewer than one-third of patients. Rarely, bowel and bladder sphincteric disturbances are noted.

Palpation usually reveals tenderness over the sciatic notch, popliteal fossa, or both. Paravertebral muscles may be in spasm. Straight leg raising produces back or leg pain that is accentuated by dorsiflexion of the foot. Ipsilateral leg pain produced by contralateral straight leg raising is highly suggestive of a lumbar disc herniation. Weakness of dorsiflexion of the great toe is a common finding, especially with L4–5 disease. Weakness of plantar flexion, on the hand, suggests L5–S1 disease. Weakness of the quadriceps may occur with L3–4 herniation. Atrophy may be present if nerve roots have been chronically compressed. Hypoaesthesia on the dorsum of the foot is common; it occurs on the outside of the foot more often with L5–S1 disease, and on the medial aspect of the foot with L4–5 disease. The ankle jerk is commonly depressed with S1 root compression, but may also be reduced when the L5 root is compromised. A depressed knee jerk suggests an L3–4 lesion.

Plain films of the lumbosacral spine will identify congenital or acquired bony changes. Disc space narrowing is an unreliable sign of symptomatic disease since narrowing of the disc space may occur without clinical symptoms. Myelography is diagnostic in 80–90% of cases of lumbar disc disease (*Fig.* 36.7). It is useful to localize the disease and exclude the presence of an intraspinal tumour. False-positive and false-negative findings may occur. Electromyography may confirm the diagnosis when myelography is equivocal. Occasionally, epidural injections of anaesthetics, steroids, or both may localize the symptomatic level precisely and reduce symptoms at the same time. Lumbar discography and epidural venography are other tests which may be diagnostic in selected cases. The recent advent of computerized tomography of the spine, coupled with injection of radio-opaque contrast material into the spinal fluid,

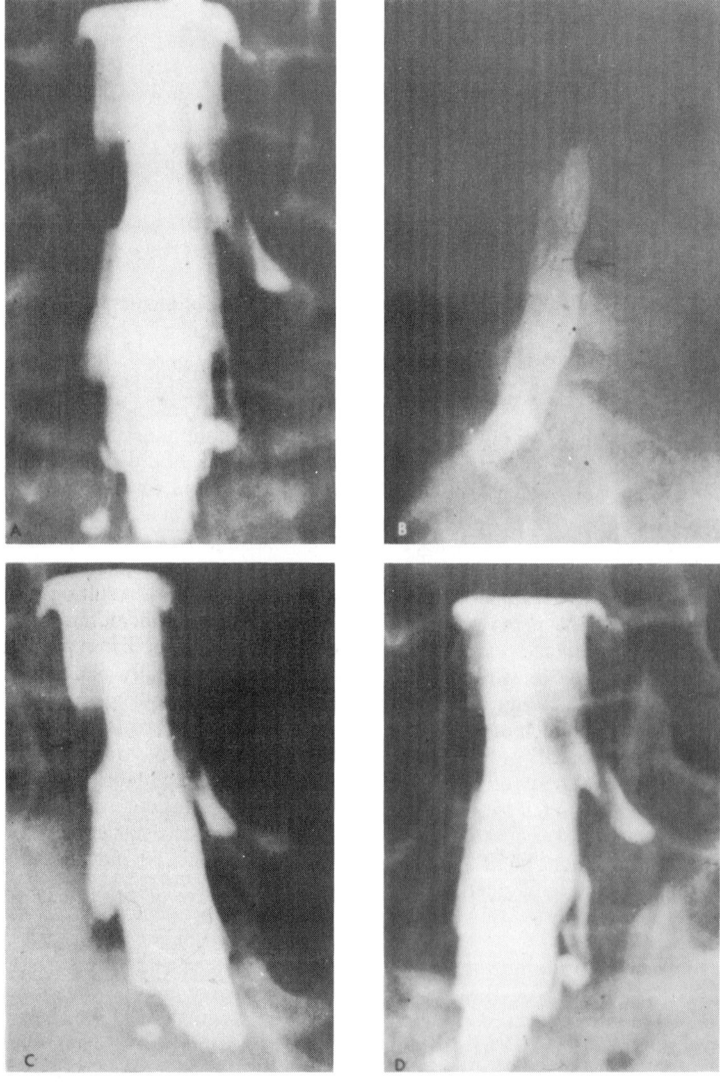

Fig. 36.7 Lumbar myelogram. AP, lateral and oblique views. Note the defect in the radio-opaque column overlying the L4–5 disc space. The L5 nerve root is compressed by a ruptured disc fragment.

will likely provide high specific diagnosis with little risk to the patient in the near future.

The advent of magnetic resonance imaging (MRI) has had an impact on diagnostic procedures for spine diseases. The test is non-invasive and has the potential to replace myelography and CT scanning completely. The resolution of MR images is of sufficient quality even at this early stage to indicate that the procedure will be highly advantageous in the future. *Fig.* 36.8 demonstrates the usefulness of lumbar spine MRI in a 30-year-old female with a history of a previous disc operation at L5–S1. She developed recurrent pain related to a herniated lumbar disc seen clearly at L4–5, one level above the previous disc herniation.

Back pain with radiation to the leg has many causes besides lumbar disc disease: (1) bony abnormalities such as spondylolisthesis, spondylolysis and lumbar spondylosis; (2) primary and metastatic tumours of the cauda equina, spine and pelvis; (3) inflammatory disorders, including abscess, arachnoiditis and spondylitis; (4) degenerative lesions of the spinal cord and peripheral neuropathies; (5) peripheral vascular occlusive disease, and (6) gynaecological problems, such as endometriosis.

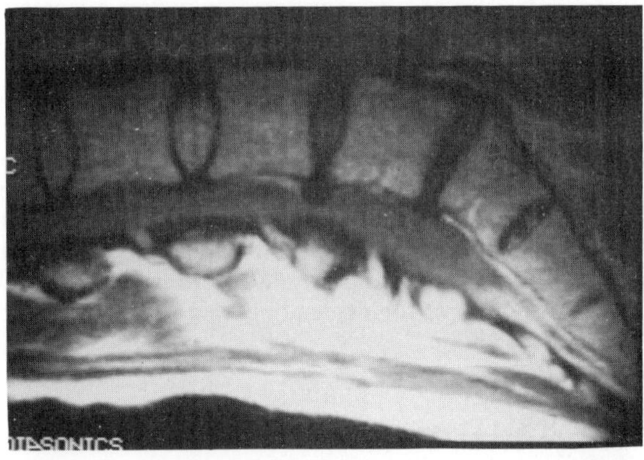

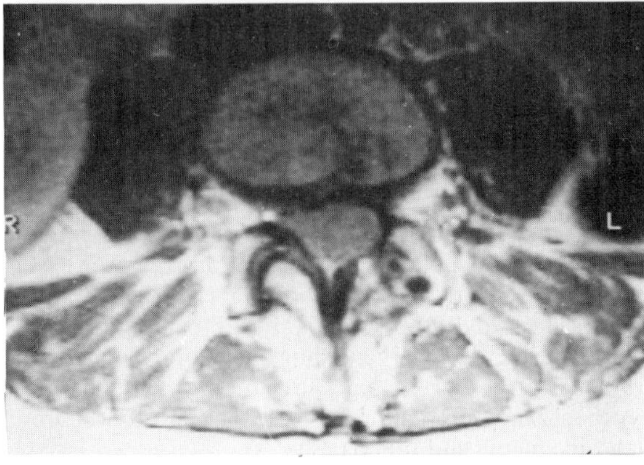

Fig. 36.8 Magnetic resonance imaging. An extruded lumbar disc is clearly seen in the sagittal and transverse slices. (Images by courtesy of UCSF/RIL and Diasonics MRI, South San Francisco, California.)

Medical treatment is indicated in all patients who do not have progressive weakness or sphincter disturbances. Bed rest, local heat, analgesics and skeletal muscle relaxants are usually effective in a few days. Pelvic traction during bed rest may relieve muscle spasm. Physical therapy and limited exercise often help when the acute episode passes. A corset or back brace partially immobilizes the patient and can prevent recurrent muscle spasm. Most patients improve with medical treatment sufficiently to return to full activity. The lumbar disc syndrome may recur intermittently with stress or exertion. Recurrences may be treated identically, often successfully.

Surgical treatment is indicated in patients with a progressive neurological deficit, chronic disabling pain or both. The acute onset of weakness or sphincter disturbance constitutes an emergency, demanding prompt diagnosis and early operation. About 10% of patients with lumbar disc disease will require operation sometime during the course of the disorder. If myelography demonstrates an extruded disc fragment which accounts for the clinical signs and symptoms, then 85% of patients will recover completely after surgical treatment. If the syndrome is not typical, the myelogram equivocal and the patient poorly motivated to improve, operation is less effective. Emotional factors, including litigation and industrial injury, play an important role in the eventual outcome, whether the treatment is medical or surgical.

VASCULAR INJURIES OF THE SPINAL CORD

Occasionally after aortic surgery or cardiac surgery involving the bypass procedures, the patient recovers consciousness but is found to have a weak or insensitive leg or occasionally is paraplegic. More rarely a patient may quite inexplicably develop an anterior spinal artery syndrome following a minor anaesthetic procedure and in retrospect it has been associated with a drop in blood pressure during induction or during uncontrolled haemorrhage. All these rare but well-recognized complications are the result of impairment of the blood supply of the spinal cord and great care must be taken in the elderly to ensure that the blood pressure remains adequate. The blood supply of the spinal cord being rather tenuous is impaired further by marked osteophytes or a narrowing of root canals as is found in achondroplasia and interruption of the arteries of Adamkiewicz may produce disastrous results. Surgery around the lumbar region therefore should preserve what appear to be minor lumbar arteries if possible.

Vascular injuries of the spinal cord may occur spontaneously in dissecting aneurysm or in patients with embolic disease. Acute decompression sickness is associated with spinal cord damage which has now been shown to be due to the accumulation of the gas bubbles in the extradural venous complex obstructing the venous return from the cord.

Further Reading

Guttmann L. (1976) *Spinal Cord Injuries. Comprehensive Management and Research,* 2nd ed. Oxford, Blackwell, p. 694.
Holdsworth F. (1970) Fractures, dislocations and fracture-dislocations of the spine. *J. Bone Joint Surg.* **53B**, 1534.
Rothman R. H. and Simeone F. A. (1975) *The Spine*. Philadelphia, Saunders, p. 900.
Yashon D. (1978) *Spinal Injury*. New York, Appleton-Century-Crofts, p. 395.

37 *The Surgery of Pain*

Michael P. Powell

INTRODUCTION

Neurosurgeons have been involved closely in the management and control of pain since the birth of the specialty. Based on the theory of transmission of nociceptive impulses in the spinal nerve roots and cord, the first pain procedure, dorsal rhizotomy, was performed in 1888 by Bennett. Spiller and Martin performed the first anterolateral cordotomy in 1911, although Gowers had made the observation that the spinothalamic tract would constitute the pathway for the transmission of pain 25 years earlier. Despite extensive research the physiology of pain remains incompletely understood. Nevertheless our understanding has improved considerably with important contributions such as the 'Gate Theory' of Melzac and Wall and the more recent identification of endorphins and enkephalins.

Over the last decade there has been considerable improvement in the pharmacological control of pain. Clinicians involved in pain control, in particular oncologists and radiotherapists, now have a very wide armamentarium of drugs on which they may call. Their demands on surgical methods of pain control have been reduced considerably as a result.

Surgery for pain is also changing. Improved understanding of pain pathways has suggested new approaches, and new technology has allowed the use of more sophisticated methods to alter pain pathways. Pain surgery often uses currently fashionable techniques. Stereotactic lesioning of pain control was an offshoot of the stereotactic lesioning for movement disorders which were developed and perfected in the 50s, 60s and early 70s. The popularity of the transcutaneous nerve stimulation may reflect the improvement in miniaturized electronics which has become available over the past two decades.

This chapter outlines the anatomical and physiological pathways in the transmission of the nociceptive impulse. The methods currently available for altering and suppressing the transmission of nociception will be outlined and their relative merits discussed. Emphasis will be given to those techniques in most common usage, but brief mention will be made of some of the lesser used and of newly introduced procedures which have not yet reached common practice.

Because pain control is frequently difficult to achieve, 'pain' patients benefit from a multidisciplinary approach with anaesthetists, neurologists and oncologists providing a balanced clinical opinion. The ideal of complete and lasting pain relief without loss of normal sensation is and probably will remain unattainable; each therapeutic approach must be a compromise. Surgery is considered only after a long and exhaustive search for an alternative. The percentage of pain relief must be compared against the risks of the procedure which may be considerable. The expected duration of analgesia must be compared to the prognosis of the patient.

Interruption of pain pathways may not only reduce or abolish the connections of the pain receptors to the brain, but will also alter neuronal responses by reducing input, altering the pattern of discharge from relay nuclei such as within the dorsal horn laminae, and disturb feedback as well as the relationship of the descending modulating pattern of impulses.

ANATOMY AND PHYSIOLOGY

A brief description of the current understanding of pain perception forms a useful basis to the understanding of its control.

Peripheral Reception

Skin Receptors

There is no specific receptor type of nerve ending that subserves pain alone; instead nociception is served by high threshold mechano- and thermoreceptors which respond to pressure, heat and other toxic stimuli by alteration in their firing patterns. The nerve endings are unmyelinated nerve terminals in the dermis and surrounding hair follicles. In deeper organs, mechanoreceptors such as those around joints, ligaments and other tissues are used.

Peripheral Nerves

Nociceptive impulses are transmitted to the spinal column via unmyelinated C fibres (less than 1 μm in diameter) and small myelinated fibres known as Aδ. These larger fibres are between 1 and 14 μm in diameter. Their cell bodies lie in the dorsal root ganglia.

Dorsal Root Ganglia

The majority of nociceptive fibres enter the spinal cord via the dorsal root to synapse in the laminae of the dorsal horn on specific cells. The cells that serve pain fibres in the ganglia are the B-cells.

Dorsal Root Entry Zone

The sensory fibres enter the spinal cord via the dorsal root entry zone (DREZ) which is a site of major interest in pain control. It is at this level that the integration and modification of the nociceptive impulse seems most likely to occur as suggested by Melzac and Wall, in their gate control theory.

The dorsal horn of the central grey matter of the cord is split up into a number of morphologically different areas (*Fig.* 37.1). Electrophysiological studies show that nociceptive fibres synapse at various of these levels, in particular level I and, to a lesser extent, level II. Fibres also project from level V before being transferred to the contralateral side in Area X across the median raphe.

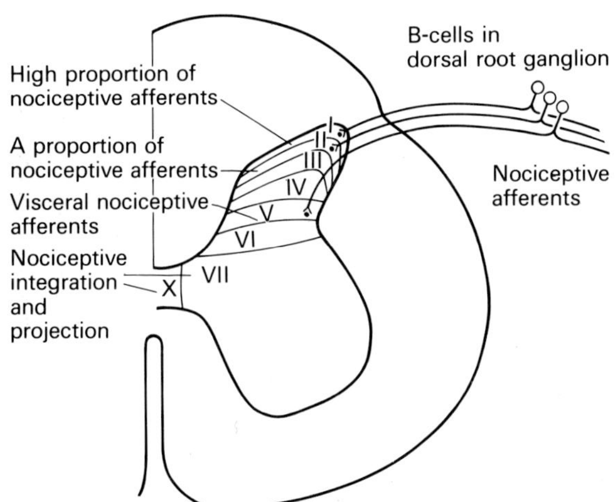

Fig. 37.1 Nociceptive inputs to cat lumbar cord grey matter laminae (modified from Rexed).

Spinothalamic Tract

The now integrated modified pain impulse is transmitted by the spinothalamic tract in the ventrolateral funiculi of the spinal cord (*Fig.* 37.2). The most important nociceptive pathway is the lateral spinothalamic tract which lies just anterior to the dentate ligament on the anterolateral border of the spinal cord. From this tract, which includes temperature, a major component, fibres project to various nuclei within the brain substance.

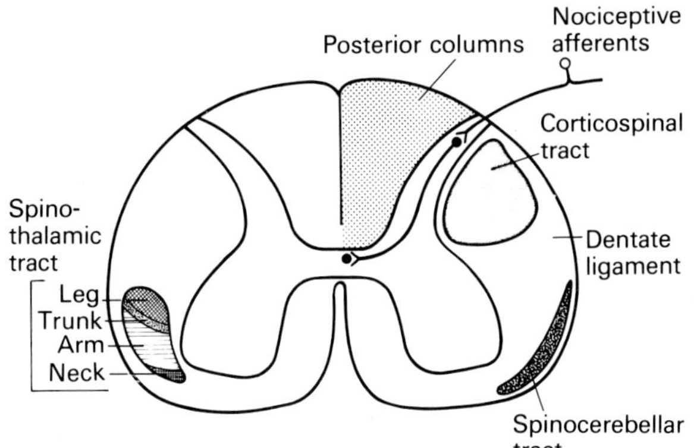

Fig. 37.2 Tracts within the spinal cord at C1–2.

Midbrain

The mesencephalon centre, though small in volume, contains not only major pathways such as the spinothalamic tract, but also other tracts involved in pain modulation such as the spinoreticulothalamic tract. The spinothalamic tract itself lies at the dorsolateral angle of the tegmentum and is only 0·65 mm^2 in cross-section. Fibres are organized in strictly somatotopic fashion with distal areas such as the foot represented most laterally. It is of interest to note that a tract contains only 10% of the fibres carried in the upper cervical region. The remaining 90% leave the tract in the lower midbrain. The spinothalamic pathway is closely related to the central grey matter surrounding the aqueduct (the peri-aqueductal grey, PAG) with which it also makes synaptic contact. The PAG is known to be an effector of the emotional response to noxious stimuli.

Spinothalamic Projections

The spinothalamic tract projects to a number of different nuclei, in particular the parafascicular and the intralaminar nuclei of the brainstem, and others of the reticular formation. Projections to the peri-aqueductal grey nuclei (PAG) in the region of the midbrain, and the wall of the third ventricle are of current interest in pain control. Fibres from the thalamus must project to the cortex, but it is well known that stimulation of the sensory area of the cortex only occasionally produces pain. Furthermore, removal of the entire primary somatosensory area seldom has any effect on pain or temperature sensibility. It is only a small cortical area, the secondary somatosensory area, that seems to have any pain perception.

There appears to be two different pathways subserving pain within the brain, an 'old' pain pathway with slow response projecting to brainstem nuclei and 'new' that projects directly to the thalamus. The 'old' pathway is present in all vertebrates and considered to provide basic physiological responses to pain without true pain perception.

Descending Pathways in Pain Control

There is considerable recent interest in the function of modulating descending pathways within the central nervous system which effect a reduction in nociceptive input projecting to the brain. High levels of enkephalins are found in these areas.

Modulating pathways start directly at the spinal level from small collaterals from the proprioceptive fibres which pass via the dorsal root to the dorsal column and to the gracile and cuneate nuclei. These collaterals pass back from the dorsal column to cause inhibition at the dorsal horn.

Within the dorsal column nuclei there are further areas associated with inhibition as well as two areas within the brainstem reticular formation and within the thalamus itself. The spinal pathways for these systems are unknown, but are thought to descend with the dorsal lateral funiculus on a bilateral basis. Some evidence also exists to suggest that cortical inhibition of pain can occur at various levels in the nociceptive response, and effected at the dorsal horn.

These pathways and tracts described in the preceding paragraphs are summarized in *Fig.* 37.3.

Future Developments

The recent discovery of opiate transmitters within the CNS gives the neurophysiologist and clinician the challenge to control pain by entirely physiological means. The exact role

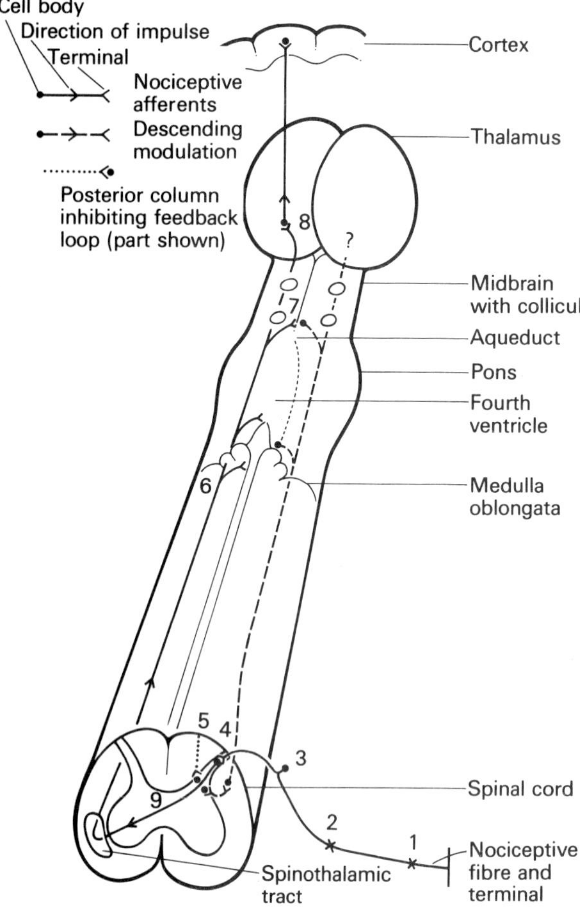

Fig. 37.3 Summary diagram of pain pathways.

of enkephalins and their site of action remains to be quantified. There is, however, a strong connection between sites of nociceptive impulse modification and areas of high concentration of enkephalins. Experimentally applied enkephalins in very small doses at specific sites have a profound analgesic effect, although they have many side-effects.

Also of considerable interest are the connections of these pain-modulating centres with sites involved in hormonal control, an important example of which being the pituitary gland. In clinical practice it has been known for many years that hypophysectomy can control the pain of metastatic deposits, even in hormone-independent tumours.

Currently, there is great interest in the frontal projections in pain pathways, and it remains to be seen whether these connections will have any significant part to play. Certainly there is historic precedent in the use of frontal leucotomy and tractotomy in pain control, although these methods have been abandoned.

PAIN CONTROL

Principles

Pain is caused by many different diseases, is generated in different ways and perceived in different forms. To achieve pain control all aspects must be considered before the clinician embarks on an attempt at control.

Pain associated with malignant disease may make the life of the patient intolerable. It may be due to an irremovable primary, metastases, direct invasion of sacral and brachial plexuses, or the effect of chemotherapy or radiotherapy on peripheral nerves. Because the pain may be intolerable and life span limited its control must be radical.

'Benign' pain may be caused by nerve damage and neuromas, or by causalgia or by deafferentation rather than from a pain-producing lesion. 'Benign' pain is a complex problem to deal with and it may be extremely difficult to control. Any solution ought to attempt long-term control without altering function significantly.

Set out in *Table* 37.1 are some of the myriad of procedures used to control pain, the indications for the procedures (*Table* 37.2) and the factors that must be considered before a procedure is embarked upon (*Table* 37.3). In practice, the simpler peripheral nerve blocks are the most frequently used

Table 37.1 Pain control procedures

1. Peripheral Procedures
   a. Nerve blockade
      i. Surgical
      ii. Thermal (radiofrequency or cryoprobe)
      iii. Chemical (alcohol or phenol)
   b. Sympathectomy
      i. Surgical ganglionectomy
      ii. Chemical ganglionectomy
      iii. Peripheral sympathetic blockade (guanethidine)
2. Central Lesions
   a. Ascending lesions
      i. Surgical
      ii. Thermal (e.g. dorsal root ganglionectomy and tractotomies
   b. Descending control modification
      i. Dorsal column stimulation
   c. Central stimulation of pain centres (e.g. peri-aqueductal grey)
3. Depot release of pain control substances (e.g. spinal catheters)
4. Hormone manipulation (e.g. hypophysectomy)
5. Counter-irritation (? transcutaneous nerve stimulation)

Table 37.2 Causes of pain

1. Uncontrolled origin (e.g. irremovable primary)
2. Axonal loss or neuroma formation
3. Causalgia
4. Deafferentation

Table 37.3 Considerations in choice of pain control procedure

1. Ease of performing the procedure
2. Direct morbidity of the procedure
3. Percentage success in pain control
4. Duration of that success
5. The side-effects of the procedure itself

procedures. Pain usually recurs, but the nerve blocks are as easy to repeat.

Counter-irritation is a useful non-invasive or minimally invasive pain control method, transcutaneous nerve stimulation (TNS) being particularly successful in the management of benign pains. This may work by peripheral stimulation of pain-modulating central pathways, via the large sensory A fibres. Acupuncture may stimulate a central pain modulating pathway in the same way.

'Central' lesions are performed much less frequently. Rhizotomy for the control of paroxysmal neuralgias are undertaken by most neurosurgical centres while others are performed by surgeons with a special interest in pain. It is possible that depot release systems will become routine procedures in malignant pain control. Electrode implantation for long-term stimulation or for 'lesioning' of brain nuclei, are procedures that are performed by only a handful of specialist neurosurgical centres throughout the world.

Specific Pain Control Procedures

A general outline of specific procedures to control pain are given.

Peripheral Nerve Blocks

Peripheral nerve blockade by surgery, heat or chemicals forms a major part in the control of benign and malignant pains and paroxysmal neuralgia. Trial procedures with local anaesthetic are often made before long-term blockade is attempted. Chemical blocks with alcohol and phenol are commonly used. Radiofrequency heat lesions can be used for deeply situated nerves. The operator can stimulate the nerve prior to forming the heat lesion. It is particularly indicated for use in trigeminal neuralgia, in posterior rami blocks for intravertebral joints of the lumbar spine and for dorsal root ganglion blockade.

Sympathetic Blockade

Causalgias, axonal loss and neuroma pains may respond to pain control procedures that alter the sympathetic input to these areas. Chemical ganglionectomy, e.g. the stellate ganglion block, is frequently performed for dysaesthetic limb pain. Surgical sympathectomy is much less frequently performed. Certain limb dysaesthesias may be managed by instillation of guanethidine into the exsanguinated arm under tourniquet control.

Counter Irritation

Transcutaneous nerve stimulation (TNS) is of current interest because of its ability to control nociceptive pain or deafferentation pain of many types. It is particularly useful in the treatment of chronic pain such as sciatica.

Dorsal Rhizotomy

The severance of dorsal roots, dorsal rhizotomy, for pain control has already been mentioned in the introduction as one of the earliest methods of pain control but because of disappointing results it is now performed chiefly for the control of post-thoracotomy pain. It has been argued by its supporters that the failure to control pain for a long period of time may be because of insufficient severance of enough relevant nerve root, although the recent identification of high threshold afferent, non-myelinated nociceptive fibres in the ventral roots (making up 25–35%) may be responsible for the recurrence of pain. A modification, rhizidiotomy, where the dorsal rootlets are cut on their ventral surface and also over the pia of the dorsal root entry zone, is recommended by Sindou in France.

Chemical rhizotomy, using intrathecal phenol, is an elegant non-surgical way of effecting pain relief in the short term. The method described by a number of authors, in particular Nathan, involves lumbar puncture and careful positioning prior to the introduction of phenol. The major complication of the technique is the loss of bladder control, but in patients with short prognosis from unremitting malignant pain, this may be an acceptable risk.

Dorsal Root Entry Zone (DREZ) Lesions

With the identification of the DREZ as a major site of nociceptive integration, there has been an expanding interest in the control of deafferentation pain by lesions in the area (Nashold). The procedure is thought to block the input and integration of the pain impulse at the dorsal root level. In deafferentation, where the dorsal horn cells discharge without input, the lesion destroys their autonomous discharge. The particular indication is in deafferentation pain resulting from brachial plexus avulsions and herpes zoster. The technique involves a number of radiofrequency lesions made in the DREZ of the spinal cord which has been exposed at laminectomy.

Excellent results are claimed with 80% pain relief. Complications arise from the risk of an extensive cervical laminectomy and cord manipulation. There is also the danger of ipsilateral leg weakness and/or loss of joint position sense if the lesion extends into the corticospinal tract and/or dorsal columns which lie close to the DREZ. Further experience has shown that 15% of patients have recurrence of their pain.

Commissural Myelotomy

This procedure aims to interrupt the median raphe and thus stop spinothalamic transmission as the impulse crosses from the dorsal laminae to the contralateral spinothalamic tract. Only small series have been reported, in total approximately 200 cases, mostly for malignant pain of visceral origin, particularly central, rectal and bladder pain. Pain relief for up to a year is claimed.

Anterolateral Cordotomy

Spiller first performed open anterolateral cordotomy in 1911 with the aim of interrupting the spinothalamic nociceptive transmission. The procedure rapidly gained neurosurgical acceptance as the treatment of choice for malignant pain, particularly involving the limbs. Visceral pain, in particular pelvic pain, is less well controlled. The technique can be performed either under general or local anaesthesia. At laminectomy an incision is made in the spinothalamic tract to the depth of 5 mm, usually employing a special knife. Pain relief is reported at 80%, but there are a number of complications, including respiratory failure, hypotensive crises, sphincter disturbance and contralateral paresis. Mirror image pain developing later is also reported, as well as recurrent altered or abnormal patterns of pain which can be extremely difficult to control. Because of recurrence the place of open cordotomy in the treatment of benign pain must be considered with care, and even in the treatment of malignant pain percutaneous techniques are employed more frequently.

Percutaneous Cordotomy

High cervical percutaneous cordotomy has largely replaced the open procedure. It was first introduced by Mullen in

1963 who initially used a strontium-90 needle to make the lesion, although it is now performed using radiofrequency generated heat lesions. The indications are the same as for the open procedure. A lateral high cervical puncture is performed under fluoroscopic control. The needle is guided through the dura into the contralateral C1–2 space anterior to the dentate ligament. The cord is entered and stimulated to identify the physiological position within the cord tracts. Once the needle is within the correct area lesions are made to produce hemi-anaesthesia in the contralateral side (*Fig.* 37.4). Results are good, between 75–80% success. Lesions last for approximately two years. Complications of the procedure include loss of ipsilateral limb power, usually in the leg, and unsteadiness of the gait is also reported. If bilateral lesions are made the patient must be carefully observed for the loss of respiratory drive in the hours following the procedure.

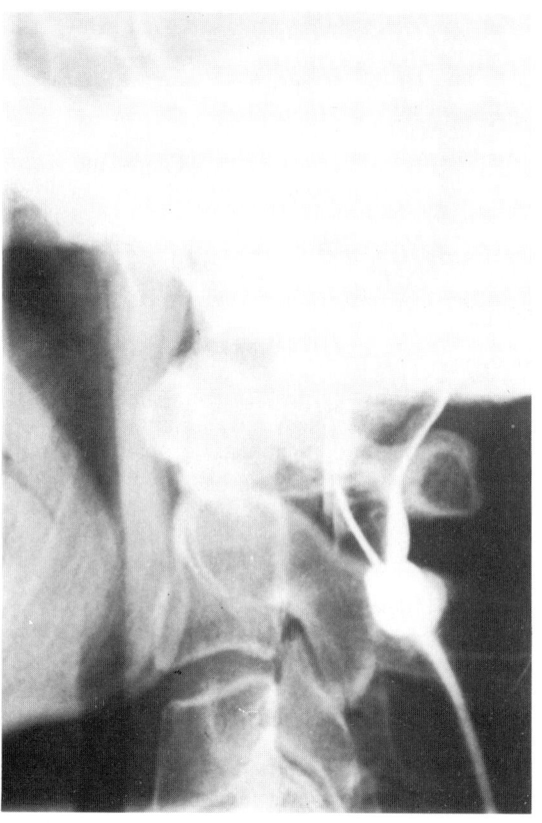

Fig. 37.4 Lateral cervical radiograph during percutaneous cordotomy. Spinal needle in C1–2 interspace. Contrast outlines back of cord, dentate ligament and anterior surface of cord.

Medullary Tractotomy

Before the popularity of stereotactic thalamic lesioning and, more recently, percutaneous cordotomy, a number of different medullary sites were discovered where at open operation the spinothalamic tract could be divided. The sites are of historic interest, for lesions made in these areas had a high incidence of complications including death. Medullary tractotomy for the control of anaesthesia dolorosa is an exception.

Mesencephalic Tractotomy

Open techniques for mesencephalic tractotomy have now been abandoned in favour of stereotactic techniques. Very occasionally a variety of lesions involving the midbrain are used in pain control for extensive cancer pain (unilateral or bilateral) involving head, neck and arms. Approximately 50% of cases respond well to mesencephalic tractotomy. Mortality is low, approximately 3·5%, but morbidity is high at 37%. Pain relief may be greater than the measure of anaesthesia achieved. In malignant conditions the effect is usually sufficient to last the life of the patient, but in benign pain the effects tend to wear off after 3–5 years. Side-effects include dysaesthetic pain in at least 15%. Other complications include gaze palsies, from the relationship of the site of the lesion to the superior colliculus.

Stimulation of the Peri-aqueductal Grey

Stimulation of the PAG has been recommended as an alternative to midbrain lesioning. The use of stereotactically implanted long-term electrodes has now been tried by a number of groups. The stimulation causes a reduction in sensation of chronic pain, rather than inhibiting sensation of any new acute pain. Seventy-five per cent success is claimed by one author, Ray, but other authorities are more cautious. Deafferentation pain does not respond. Its major use may be in the treatment of chronic back pain and sciatica which is refractory to all other forms of treatment. The procedure is still very much in the experimental stage.

Posterior Thalamic Lesions

Brain lesions for pain control are performed rarely. Various stereotactic lesions sites within the thalamus have been used. The main terminations to the spinothalamic and quintothalamic tract (from the spinal nucleus of the Vth cranial nerve) are found at the intralaminar group of nuclei, in particular the parafasicular nucleus and the nucleus limitans. These sites, with the adjacent ventro-posterior (lateral and medial) nuclei have been the subject of much research. Lesions made within the VMP and the VPL produce non-specific effects with variable and at best partial relief of pain, although loss of vibration joint position sense and cutaneous light touch from non-noxious stimuli are common. Lesions in either the intralaminar group of nuclei are more reliable in pain control producing consistent analgesic results. Careful stimulation before the lesion is made allows adjustment of target site and improves results. One Japanese authority, Sano, claims considerable success from his lesions made bilaterally in intramedullary laminae; others are more cautious.

Thalamic Stimulation

This technique, attractive on theoretical grounds, is still under investigation and not an accepted form of pain control.

Dorsal Column Stimulation

Dorsal column stimulation with implanted extradural wires is a recent development in pain control, and acts by stimulation of the descending pain-modulating pathways in the dorsolateral funiculus, or by direct retrograde stimulation of dorsal columns which modify nociception at the dorsal horn. Neuropathic pain of 'chronic' back patients responds to DCS. It may also be used for phantom limb pain. The chronic 'back' patient is often refractory to all other methods of pain control and therefore any response in this difficult group is welcomed.

Depot Release Systems

A catheter is inserted in the lumbar subarachnoid and epidural spaces and allows the drug to diffuse directly onto the roots through the dura. Intraventricular use is a future possibility and has been tried in certain pain centres, in particular in Paris where a good success rate is reported. It is particularly useful for short-term pain relief from widespread malignant disease. Subcutaneous slow-release pumps may be attached to the catheter.

Alternative Methods of Pain Control

Metastatic deposits from carcinoma of breast and prostate have long been known to respond to hormone manipulation. As a result of recent improvement in anti-oestrogens such as tamoxifen therapy, and equal success with simple procedures such as subcapsular orchidectomy, the use of pituitary ablation is less common than a few years ago. Nevertheless it remains a useful adjunct in pain control. It is of particular interest that pituitary ablation performed for other tumours also has a percentage success in controlling cancer pain, possibly by interrupting hypothalamic–pituitary axis for enkephalins.

Hypophysectomy can be performed by a number of different routes, but in patients with disseminated malignancy the least complex procedure is undoubtably indicated. Fluoroscopic or stereotactic placement of needles, electrodes or cryoprobes trans-nasally into the pituitary fossa have been described. The response to pain is good in 40% of patients; reasonable result is expected in a further 30%. Relief can be immediate or develop slowly over a number of days. The patients need hormone replacement following this form of surgery. Complications include CSF rhinorrhoea and diabetes insipidus.

PAROXYSMAL NEURALGIAS

The cutaneous sensory cranial nerves V, VII (nervus intermedius), IX and X can be the origin of paroxysmal neuralgias. Of these by far the most common is trigeminal neuralgia (or tic douloureux) which comprises over 95%. Glossopharyngeal neuralgia contributes about 1·4% and VII and X neuralgias even less. Trigeminal neuralgia is characterized by a severe and lancinating pain in a division of the trigeminal nerve. It occasionally affects more than one division, but most commonly affected is the mandibular division. There are no clinical signs and sensation is entirely normal. Pain is triggered by a number of minor stimuli such as cold winds, cold water, talking or eating. These devastating pains can cause major changes in the life of the sufferer.

Aetiology

In the majority of cases the abnormality lies between the dorsal root entry zone of the Vth nerve on the pons and the trigeminal ganglion. A vascular abnormality is frequently found, such as loops of the anterior inferior cerebellar artery or ectatic loops of the basilar artery which compress the nerve tract. This observation was first reported by Dandy in 1934 but since then Janetta has noted these abnormalities in as many as 88% of his operative series. Post-mortem studies have attempted to analyse the frequency of abnormal vascular loops, but in the absence of dynamic pulsation the results are difficult to interpret. Demyelination is found frequently, often in relation to a compressing loop. Sometimes this may be merely a small plaque at the dorsal root entry zone or within the ganglion itself. In most series there are a small proportion of posterior fossa cerebropontine angled tumours noted, usually acoustic neuromas and small meningiomas at the entrance of Meckel's cave. Paget's disease of the skull either with foramen ovale overgrowth or basilar invagination make up a smaller proportion. Finally in most series there are a small number of patients with multiple sclerosis and others suffering from the severe burning discomfort of post-herpetic neuralgia.

Pain is generated in relatively short crescendos as a response to minor stimuli which stop of their own accord. This observation, in combination with the response to anticonvulsants, suggest that neuronal epileptiform discharge may be the cause of pain. The evidence that the myelin sheath is lost at a number of sites, further suggests the possibility that the innocuous stimulus is strengthened and its pulse train widened by the effect of reverberating impulses passing between demyelination sites. The success of a number of different procedures in the control of trigeminal neuralgia may be ascribed to their causing further demyelination.

Management

The treatment of trigeminal neuralgia reflects the overall management of pain.

1. Drug Treatment: The majority of patients respond satisfactorily to anticonvulsants, in particular carbamazepine. This drug can be built up until either the pain responds or the side-effects become too great or too sustained. Occasionally it is found that the patient breaks through carbamazepine control. Other anticonvulsants such as phenytoin can be tried.

2. Peripheral Procedures: Nerve blockade or section is frequently used as a first-line management. In the mandibular division, pain can be managed by dental blocks, in the maxillary division by infraorbital avulsion, in the ophthalmic division by section of the supraorbital nerve. Nerve blockade may be simple to perform but its effectiveness seldom lasts for more than one year. It leaves the face anaesthetic in a division which may become intolerable to patients from the sensation of 'dead woodiness'.

Percutaneous Rhizotomy at the Gasserian Ganglion

Most neurosurgeons favour percutaneous procedures in which the foramen ovale is entered, using radiofrequency heat lesions to coagulate the ganglion, but chemical rhizotomy is also performed either with absolute alcohol or phenol (both these drugs are difficult to control) and glycerol (*Fig.* 37.5).

Good results are reported in over 80% of most large series. The pain relief lasts over a number of years and recurrence, in the region of 10%, can be treated by repeated coagulation. Deep anaesthesia seldom remains, thus sparing the patient the 'woody' feeling mentioned with the denervation procedure. If deep anaesthesia does occur in the ophthalmic division the cornea may be at risk and require protection.

Following his work on glycerol markers in Meckel's cave prior to stereotactic radiosurgery, Hakanson at the Karolynska Institute in Stockholm, noted that a substantial number of his patients achieved pain relief before the definitive treatment. This led him to use absolute glycerol for ganglionlysis. This chemical has had a surprising success and is being strongly promoted at present. It acts slowly but has an excellent response in over 85% of cases. There is a very low incidence of side-effects and anaesthesia of the skin is not achieved. The recurrence rate is small.

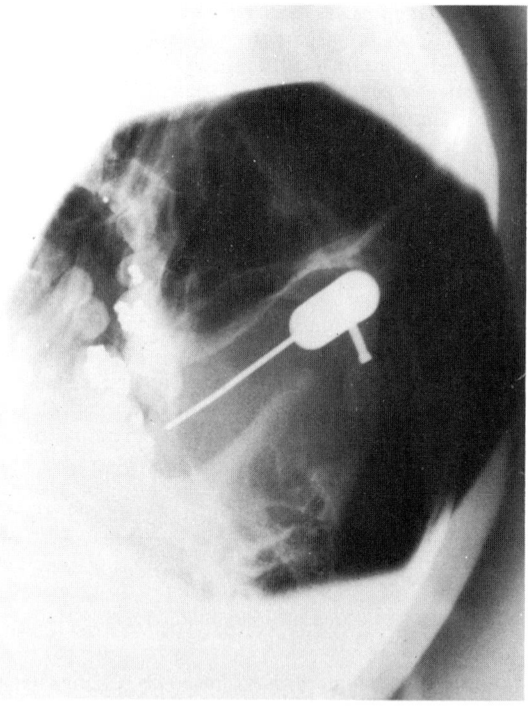

a

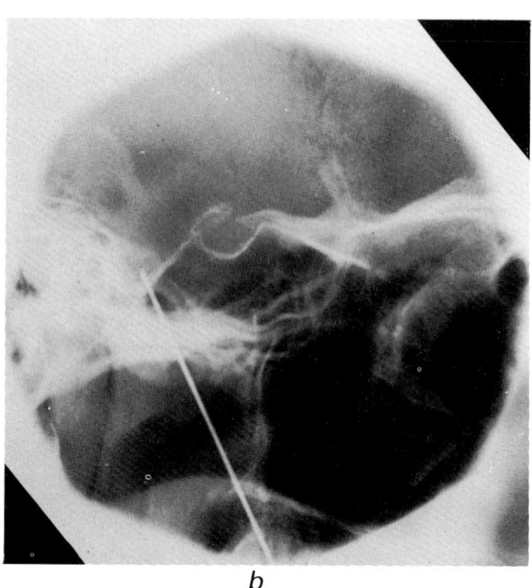

b

Fig. 37.5 Percutaneous trigeminal coagulation. *a*, Base of skull radiograph showing needle in foramen ovale. *b*, Lateral skull radiograph showing needle through foramen ovale to back of clivus.

Other Methods

Recent reports of stimulation of the trigeminal nerve outside the foramen ovale have been made. A percutaneous implant of a stimulator wire is brought out in much the same way as transcutaneous nerve stimulation or dorsal column stimulation. It is too early to assess the results.

A number of different approaches to the ganglion have been used in the past. Of these, the extradural subtemporal route of Frazier is deservedly the best known and was used by most neurosurgeons until development of percutaneous techniques and the reduction in mortality and morbidity of posterior fossa procedures. A small temporal craniectomy is used and the ganglion identified medial to the foramen spinosum. The relevant division of the trigeminal ganglion can then be sectioned under direct vision.

Janetta recommends the removal of the compressing loops of any artery found in the region, at the same time packing off the nerve. It is probable that this relieves both the stimulus to the nerve from the vascular compression and also causes a small amount of demyelination sufficient to block the impulse reverberating. Good initial results are reported.

Anaesthesia Dolorosa

Occasionally pain develops in the anaesthetic face after an ablative procedure on the trigeminal nerve. This deafferentation pain is extremely difficult to treat satisfactorily. In the event of surgical solution becoming necessary, medullary tractotomy may be performed.

The results of this procedure, as might be expected, are not particularly good and both percentage pain relief and recurrence of pain are both relatively high. There is also a high incidence of complications, in particular for contralateral sensation and ipsilateral motor power. Medullary tractotomy is infrequently performed.

CONCLUSION

A number of pain-controlling procedures have been described and have been related to the way in which they affect pain pathways by interruption, stimulation or modification. It should be remembered that some procedures are commonly performed every day in every district general hospital, some are occasionally performed in a few centres, and some rarely performed by a mere handful of dedicated 'pain' surgeons.

For the clinician, pain patients are often difficult subjects to treat, and have an undeserved reputation for posing problems of interpretation and management. However, a balanced view of their specific problems, associated with a carefully planned treatment tailored to their specific needs can be rewarded by complete change in the patient's life for the better, and their undying gratitude.

Further Reading

Melzac R. and Wall P. D. (1965) Pain mechanisms: a new theory. *Science* **150**, 971–79.

Wall P. D. and Melzac R. (ed.) (1984) *Textbook of Pain*. London, Churchill Livingstone.

White J. C. and Sweet W. H. (1969) *Pain and the Neurosurgeon*. Springfield Ill., Thomas.

Section 5

Thoracic Surgery

38 Introduction to Thoracic Diseases

R. A. Clark

EMBRYOLOGY AND CONGENITAL ABNORMALITIES

During the fourth week of intrauterine development a midline groove appears on the ventral surface of the foregut immediately caudal to the hypobronchial eminence (future epiglottis) from which the respiratory tract will develop. Starting caudally a diverticulum becomes progressively separated from the foregut leaving only a small patent connection (the laryngeal aditus) just below the hypobronchial eminence. Maldevelopments during this phase may result in oesophageal atresia, tracheal stenosis or a tracheo-oesophageal fistula. The distal end of the diverticulum soon divides equally into the right and left lung buds. The respiratory epithelium and mucus glands arise from the diverticulum while the cartilage, muscle, elastic tissue, blood vessels and lymphatics develop from the splanchnic mesoderm on the ventral surface of the foregut into which the diverticulum grows. The developing trachea and bronchi derive their blood supply from the dorsal aorta and upper posterior intercostal arteries and their autonomic innervation from the vagus nerve and sympathetic chains, an arrangement which persists into adult life.

Initially the two lungs buds are symmetrical but by the 5-mm stage the adult asymmetry is evident with the left bud lying more transversely. Soon both tubes give off an anterior diverticulum (the right middle and the left upper/lingular divisions) and by the 15-mm stage the right bud has divided further giving a craniodorsal branch (right upper division) and the adult pattern of three right and two left lobes is laid down. Additional primary branching of the stem bronchi may give rise to an accessory lobe, e.g. a cardiac lobe, or a segmental bronchus may be derived directly from the trachea or stem bronchi, i.e. the apical division of the right upper lobe arising from the trachea. By birth, 18 bronchial generations have been formed by successive divisions, often unequal, of the daughter bronchi.

Among the types of accessory lobes described are:

1. The tracheal lobe arising from and communicating with the trachea.
2. Dissociated lung masses situated in the abdomen or neck, and
3. Interlobar sequestration (lower accessory lobe).

The third has the greatest clinical significance.

The sequestrated lobe may consist of a single large cyst or a mass of ill-defined tissue firmly adherent to the posterior segment of a normal lower lobe (90% left) and having its own blood supply from the aorta passing through the pulmonary ligament. The abnormality may present as a tension cyst soon after birth or as a variable radiological shadow. Opinions vary as to whether these are true accessory lobes with an independent origin or whether they represent a portion of lung which has become detached from a normal lobe. Rarely an extralobar sequestration of lung occurs which shares the pulmonary artery supply of its associated lung.

Early in fetal life deepening furrows (fissures) divide the lung mesenchyme into lobules around each primary bronchial division (future lobes). If separation is incomplete vascular bridges between adjacent lobes may persist into the adult and present problems at lobectomy. Failure of segregation results in a single-lobed lung.

Normally the azygos vein lies medial to the lung bud curling anteriorly above the right hilum. Occasionally the developing lung bud pushes the vein laterally when it becomes embedded within the right upper lobe and a deep fissure separates a segment of lung, 'the azygos lobe', which may be visible radiologically.

Agenesis of one lung is compatible with normal life until the third or fourth decades when emphysema usually develops in the remaining lung. In true agenesis the ipsilateral pulmonary artery is absent but there is often a small bronchial stump surrounded by hypoplastic or cystic lung tissue. The remaining lung may lack lobulation and grows to twice its normal size displacing the heart and mediastinum to the contralateral side. Occasionally one lung may be hypoplastic. Agenesis of both lungs has been described in an 8-month-old fetus.

The early lung buds contain a loose vascular network which drains into the sinus venosus and cardinal veins, i.e. the future systemic venous system. Later, after the septum primum has divided the primitive atrium, a single vessel develops and connects the primitive pulmonary circulation with the left atrium. Many of the pulmonary venous anomalies encountered in the adult may be traced to maldevelopment at this stage with persistence of some drainage into the systemic veins and right atrium.

The common terminal and origins of the primitive left and right pulmonary veins are progressively absorbed into the developing atrium until two veins from each side open separately into the fully developed left atrium. Abnormal pulmonary veins may arise from arrested or excessive absorption at this stage.

The pulmonary arteries arise from the sixth branchial arch arteries and by the sixth week receive their blood supply wholly from the right ventricle. Soon the right artery only supplies the right lung but on the left the connection with the aorta persists until birth as the ductus arteriosus.

The primitive pleural spaces (the pericardioperitoneal canals), into which the lung buds grow, are in continuity with the primitive pericardium and the peritoneal cavity. With the rapid growth of the lungs the pericardium becomes separated from the pleural cavity, a process which may be incomplete (usually on the left) or which may produce developmental abnormalities, i.e. pleuropericardial cysts. The development of the diaphragm gradually closes the pleuroperitoneal openings although they may persist (usually on the left) as true diaphragmatic hernias.

DIAPHRAGM

The closure of the pleuroperitoneal canals completes the diaphragm which is a composite structure derived from several elements, some of them paired, as shown below.

Source	*Structures derived*
Septum transversum	The central tendon and parts of the sternal, costal and lumbar muscle
Pleuroperitoneal membranes (2)	Small dorsolateral muscle segments
Costal and sternal chest wall (2)	Varying amounts of sternal and costal muscle

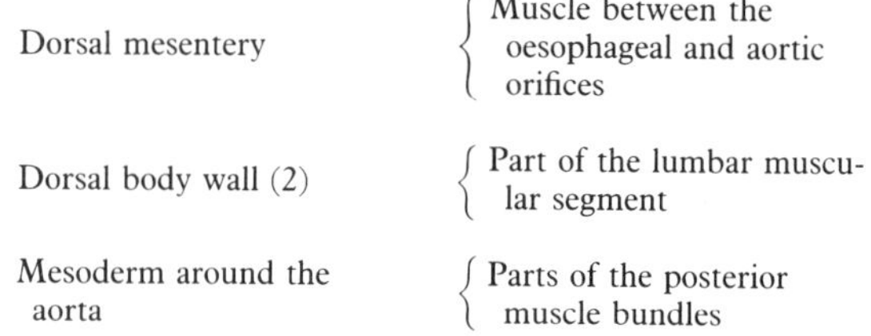

Source	*Structures derived*
Dorsal mesentery	Muscle between the oesophageal and aortic orifices
Dorsal body wall (2)	Part of the lumbar muscular segment
Mesoderm around the aorta	Parts of the posterior muscle bundles

The septum transversum forms the bulk of the adult diaphragm. The motor supply is entirely through the phrenic nerve (C3, C4, and C5, the segmental origin of the septum transversum) but the intercostal nerves carry some sensory fibres from the lateral aspects of the diaphragm. Any infection, injury or compression which involves the phrenic nerve during its extended course may cause diaphragmatic paralysis. Within the diaphragm, the phrenic nerves form a series of arcades (*Fig.* 38.1) and these should be avoided during operations involving the diaphragm. The muscle fibres are situated peripherally around an unyielding central tendon which is pulled down when the muscle contracts.

The developing diaphragm contains five major openings: three permanent—the oesophageal, the aortic and the inferior vena caval—and two transient—the pleuroperitoneal canals—which may persist as true developmental hernias (usually left) with abdominal and thoracic organs in direct contact (*Fig.* 38.1). Such hernias are not, as was originally thought, synonymous with herniation through the foramen of Bochdalek (*Fig.* 38.1). The latter arise as a result of inadequate development of the diaphragmatic muscle in the region of the lumbocostal trigone; the abdominal and thoracic contents being separated by the peritoneal and pleural membranes. Similar defects may occur in the region of the sternocostal triangles, i.e. herniation through the foramen of Morgagni, while muscular maldevelopment may be re-

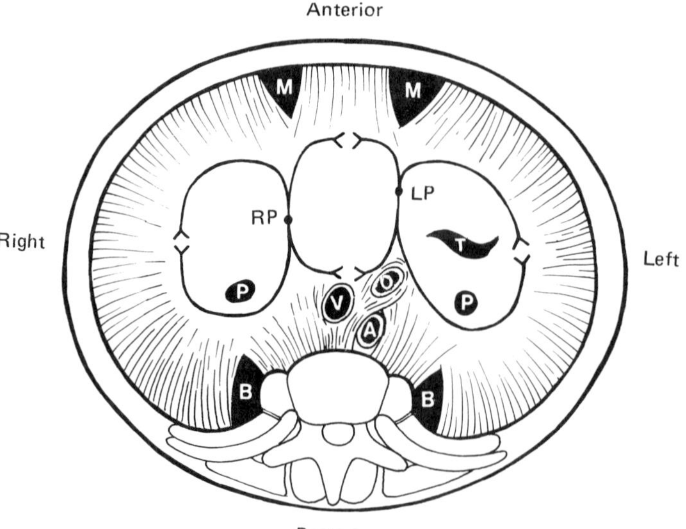

Fig. 38.1 Schematic representation of the under surface of the diaphragm to illustrate the phrenic nerve arcades and the various normal orifices and pathological defects. A = aortic orifice, O = oesophageal hiatus, V = inferior vena caval orifice, LP = left phrenic nerve, RP = right phrenic nerve. The potential defects are B = lumbosacral trigone (Bochdalek's hernia), M = sternocostal trigone (Morgagni's hernia), P = pleuroperitoneal canals (true diaphragmatic hernia) and T = traumatic tears leading to diaphragmatic hernia.

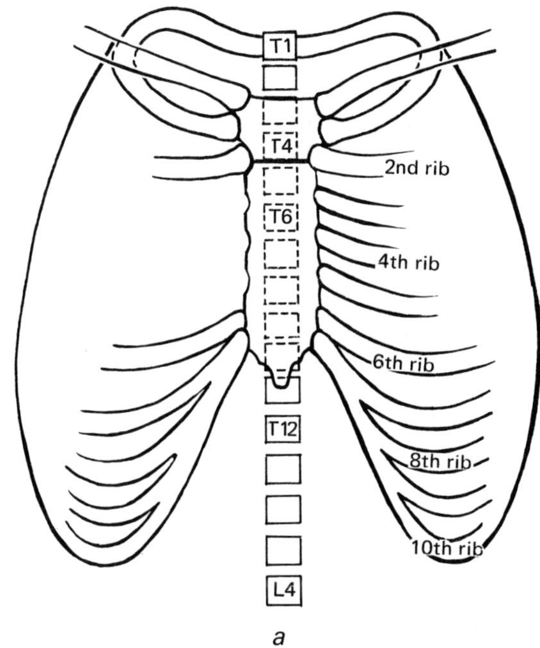

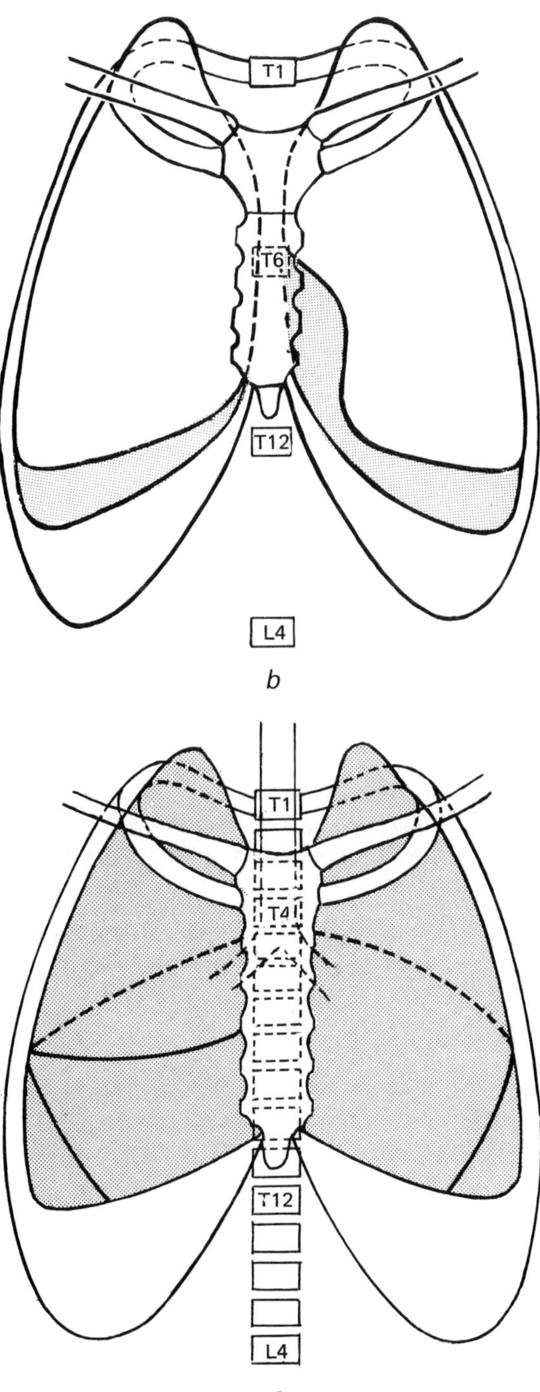

Fig. 38.2 Surface anatomy of: *a*, Ribs and costal margin (on expiration); *b*, Pleural reflections and costodiaphragmatic recesses; *c*, Lung fissures and tracheal bifurcation (on expiration).

sponsible for some oesophageal hernias. In an eventration of the diaphragm part (usually right) or the whole (usually left) of a hemidiaphragm is devoid of muscle fibres and moves paradoxically with respiration. Following trauma, diaphragmatic rupture is most likely to involve the central tendon with herniation of the abdominal contents through the tear.

SURFACE ANATOMY

While there is considerable variation in the position of the costal margin depending on the stature, obesity or posture of the patient, *Fig.* 38.2 outlines some of the important relationships within the thorax. As a result of the obliquity of the ribs and the curvature of the thoracic spine the suprasternal notch lies at the level of the 3rd thoracic vertebra, the lowest part of the costal margin (in the anterior axillary line) is level with the 3rd lumbar vertebra, and the anterior end of the 7th rib approximates to the disc space between the 10th and 11th thoracic vertebrae (*Fig.* 38.2*a*).

With inspiration not only do the ribs rotate upwards and outwards but the thoracic vertebral column increases in length and the manubrium is lifted outward and upward to a maximum of 5 cm. When ankylosing spondylitis involves the joints of the thorax, expansion of the cage is considerably restricted and respiration becomes dependent on diaphragmatic movements, making upper abdominal surgery hazardous. Kyphosis and scoliosis considerably alter the shape of the rib cage, distorting the pulmonary architecture, restricting movement and impairing function.

The position of the diaphragm varies greatly, being higher in obesity and pregnancy, causing rotation of the heart which may suggest cardiomegaly on a chest radiograph. At the end of expiration the right hemidiaphragm is usually one intercostal space above the left, the apex of the dome usually lying at the level of the disc between the 10th and 11th thoracic vertebrae. During quiet breathing the diaphragm moves about 1·5 cm but with deep inspiration the excursion may increase to up to 10 cm.

The pleura are separated by a few millilitres of watery fluid which is continually being formed and reabsorbed by the pleura. The fibroelastic parietal pleura is readily separated over the apex and mediastinum but separation is less easy from the lateral and anterior walls and is most difficult over the diaphragm. The pleura heals readily after surgery often without adhesion and can successfully combat simple infections. Gross thickening and fibrosis of the pleura may compress the lung, restricting movement, but the thickened rind can usually be easily stripped allowing re-expansion of the lungs. While the visceral pleura is devoid of pain fibres the parietal pleura has a rich nerve supply and irritation causes pleuritic pain.

The blunt apices of the lung with their covering layers of pleura protrude for 2·5–3·5 cm above the junction of the medial third with the lateral two-thirds of the clavicle. Here they are partially protected by the suprapleural membrane which spreads out from the transverse process of the 7th cervical vertebrae to the inner borders of the 1st ribs separating the pleura from the subclavian vessels. The cervical pleura and apices of the lung may be damaged during surgery to the lower neck or by clumsy attempts at introducing central venous lines or pacemakers with a subsequent pneumo- or haemothorax.

The costomediastinal pleural reflections start behind each sternoclavicular joint, move medially to the midmanubrial level then continue downward close to the midline as shown in *Fig.* 38.2*b*. On the left, at the level of the 4th cartilage, it curves laterally behind the ends of the 4th–6th costal cartilages. The position of the costomediastinal reflection is important when planning a mediastinotomy.

The mediastinal pleura is interrupted by the hilum where the parietal and visceral layers are continuous on the superior, anterior and posterior aspects but inferiorly the two layers are carried downwards for a short distance as the pulmonary ligament. Large arteries arising directly from the aorta may traverse the pulmonary ligaments to supply sequestrated segments of the lower lobes. Behind the hilum, on the right, there may be an elongated recess of the parietal pleura between the oesophagus and the anterior surface of the vertebral column.

The costodiaphragmatic recess runs inferolaterally from behind the xiphoid process to the level of the 10th rib in the midaxillary line then ascending posteriorly to the body of the 12th thoracic vertebrae. During quiet breathing the lungs do not completely fill the costodiaphragmatic recesses, the two layers of parietal pleura being in apposition for up to 7·5 cm in the midaxillary line. A liver biopsy through the right 9th and 10th intercostal spaces should be performed at the end of a full expiration to prevent lung damage.

In a pneumothorax the intercostal draining tube is best sited in the 2nd intercostal space anteriorly or through the 3rd intercostal space in the midaxillary line so as to catch the air rising to the top of the lungs. In contrast, post-thoracotomy, empyema and malignant pleural effusion drains should be sited at the base of the lungs as this is where the fluid tends to collect.

The internal mammary arteries arise from the subclavian arteries and pass anteriorly over the cervical pleura and behind the first costal cartilage 1·5 cm from the sternal edge descending vertically to the 6th costal cartilage where it divides into musculophrenic and superior epigastric arteries. At mediastinotomy the artery is identified, ligated and divided.

The intercostal vessels and nerves lie in the costal groove on the inferior surface of the ribs giving posterior, lateral and anterior cutaneous branches. Division or injury to the cutaneous nerves may result in distressing postoperative symptoms and in any surgical approach this should be borne in mind.

At operation the posterior end of the oblique fissure is found at a lower level than described in many anatomical texts, lying opposite the head of the 5th or 6th rib. From here it spirals inferolaterally until it reaches the anterior diaphragmatic surface at the junction between its medial third and lateral two-thirds. On the right the transverse

Table 38.1 Bronchial tree

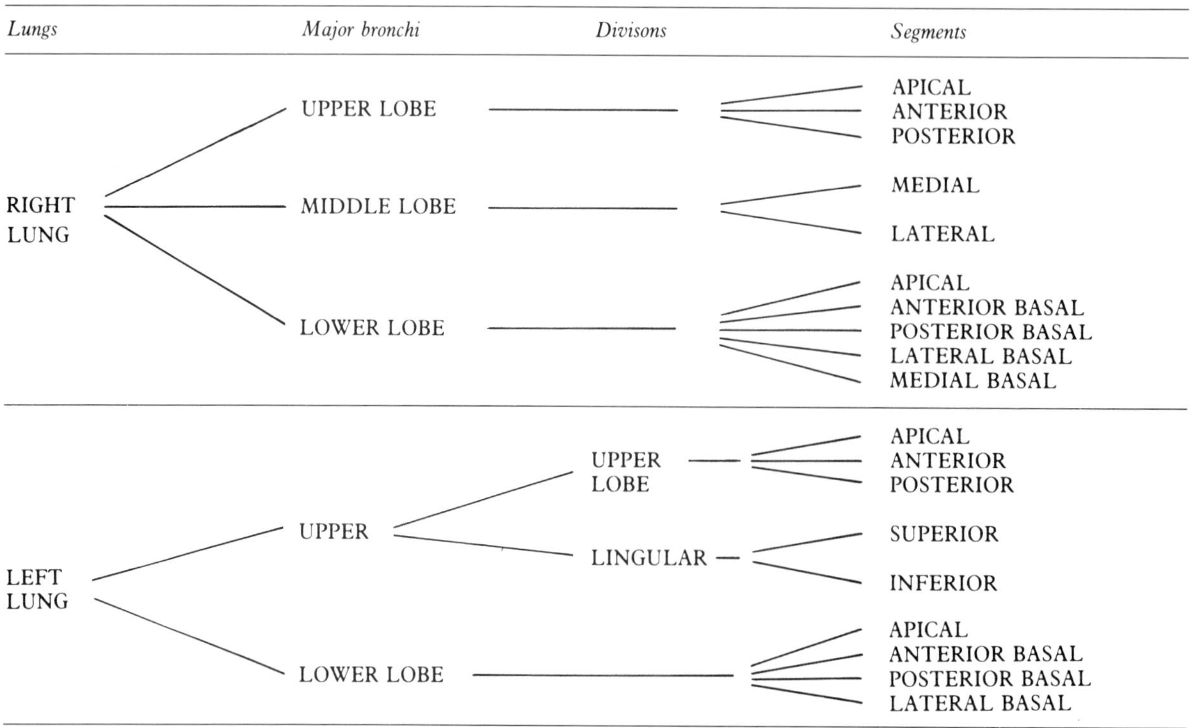

Lungs	*Major bronchi*	*Divisons*	*Segments*
RIGHT LUNG	UPPER LOBE		APICAL ANTERIOR POSTERIOR
	MIDDLE LOBE		MEDIAL LATERAL
	LOWER LOBE		APICAL ANTERIOR BASAL POSTERIOR BASAL LATERAL BASAL MEDIAL BASAL
LEFT LUNG	UPPER	UPPER LOBE	APICAL ANTERIOR POSTERIOR
		LINGULAR	SUPERIOR INFERIOR
	LOWER LOBE		APICAL ANTERIOR BASAL POSTERIOR BASAL LATERAL BASAL

fissure runs horizontally on the anterior surface at the level of the 4th costal cartilage (*Fig.* 38.2*c*). Clinically the upper lobes are found anteriorly above the 4th rib with the right middle lobe and lingula filling the lower anterior chest. The lower lobes occupy the posterior surface below the 5th rib but above this level are the posterior segments of the upper lobes. The major lobar and segmental bronchi are shown in *Table* 38.1 and reference should be made to standard anatomical texts for details of their surface anatomy.

Half the trachea lies in the thorax and being tethered only at the larynx and carina there is considerable mobility during both respiration and movement. Above the suprasternal notch it lies in the midline but deviates slightly to the right in the thorax before dividing at the level of the 5th thoracic vertebra (*Fig.* 38.2*c*).

HILAR RELATIONSHIPS

While there are similarities in the anatomy of the two hila, differences exist which have surgical significance (*Fig.* 38.3). The phrenic nerves pass just anterior to both hila lying between the mediastinal pleura and the pericardium while the vagus nerves run behind the hila where they give off their pulmonary branches. The oesophagus and azygos vein lie behind the right hilum before the latter arches forward above the hilum in close proximity to the right main bronchus and pulmonary artery to join the superior vena cava. The descending aorta lies behind the left hilum and with the ascending and arch of the aorta forms a loop through which emerges the left main bronchus. This arrangement may make pneumonectomy leaving a short left bronchial stump difficult if the aorta is dilated or atheromatous. The left main bronchus rarely divides before the hilum but the right upper lobe bronchus may arise under the vena cava less than 2 cm from the carina.

The left vagus nerve crosses anterior to the arch of the aorta just lateral to the ligamentum arteriosum. Here it gives off the left recurrent laryngeal nerve which curves backwards and upwards around the arch of the aorta. The main vagal trunk then passes posteriorly above the left pulmonary artery. While the left pulmonary artery is shorter it is easier to ligate since the right passes behind the ascending aorta and superior vena cava making exposure more difficult. The left bronchial arteries usually arise from the descending aorta and give branches to the oesophagus and trachea. The main right bronchial artery often arises from the medial aspect of the descending aorta, hooking up over the origin of the left main bronchus before crossing the carina to reach the anterior surface of the right main bronchus. The superior vena cava lies anterior and the right atrium below the right hilum. The pulmonary trunk lies anterior and the left atrium below the left hilum.

The superior pulmonary veins lie in front of the pulmonary arteries and bronchi in both hila. The short left pulmonary artery passes transversely, anterior to the left main bronchus as the latter passes obliquely downwards and laterally (*Fig.* 38.3*a*). In the left hilum the artery arches

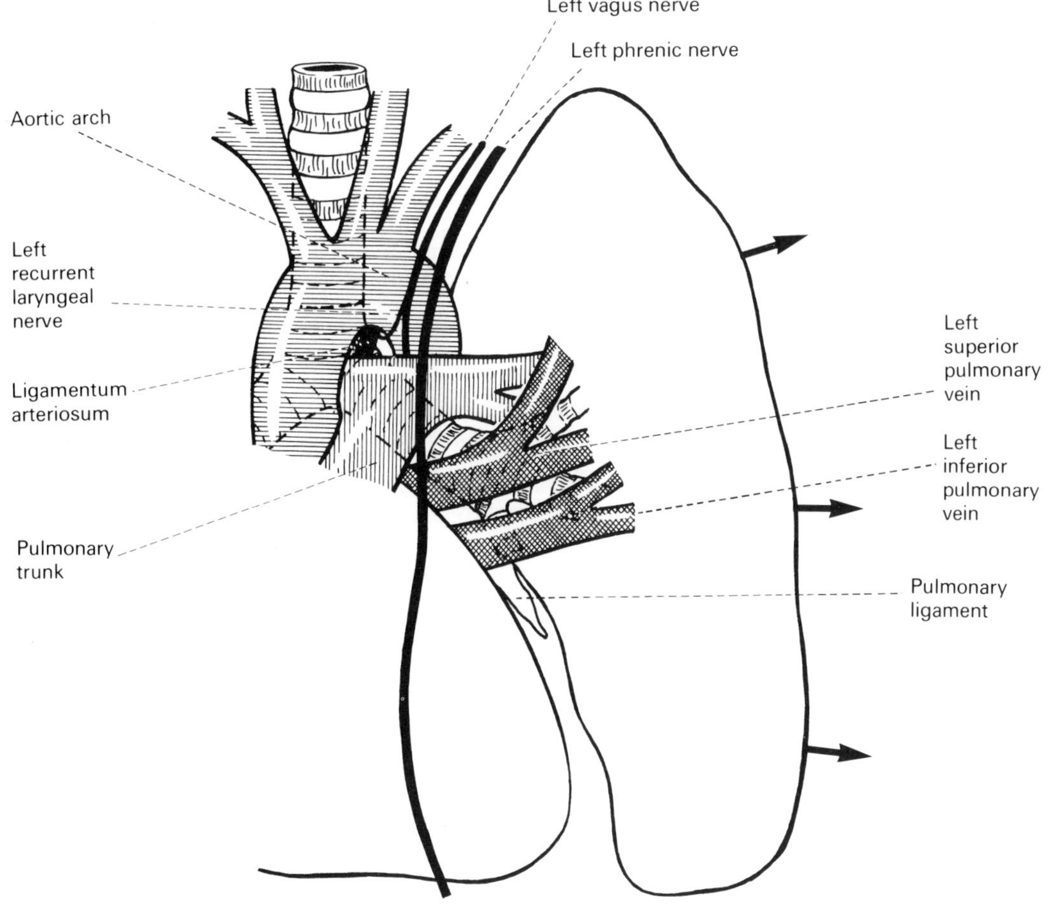

[*See over*]

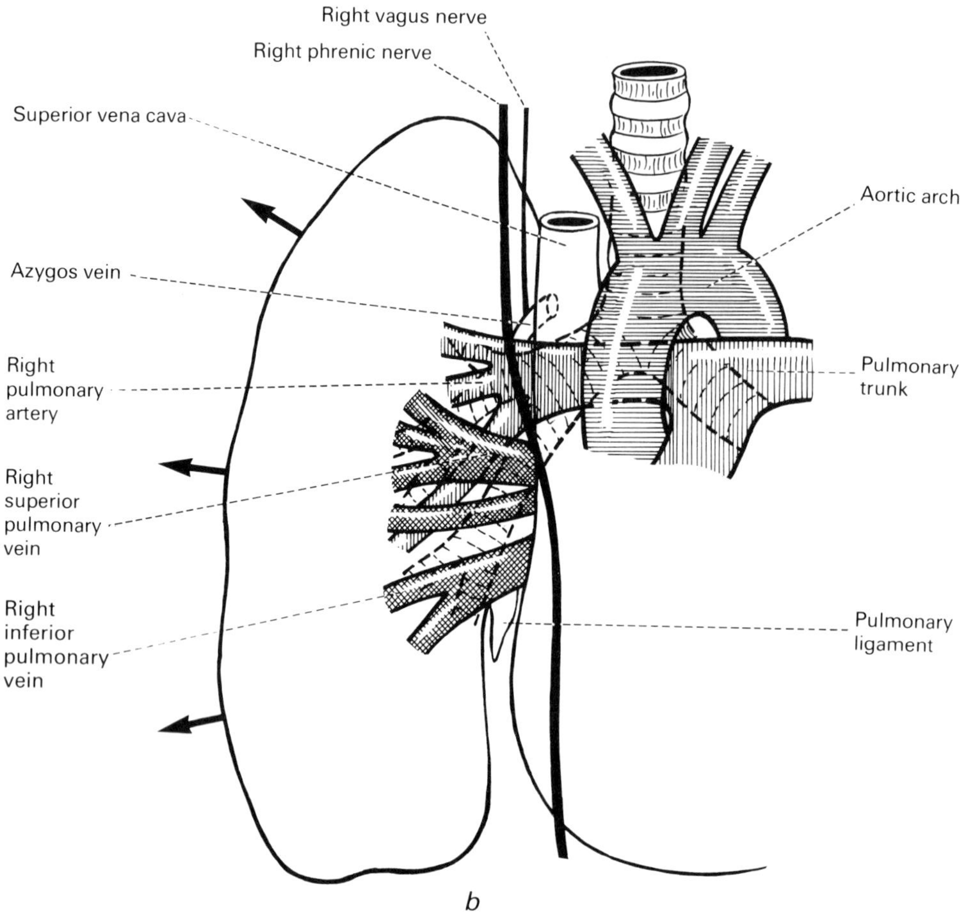

Fig. 38.3 Hilar anatomical relationships: *a*, Left; *b*, Right.

above the bronchus coming to lie posteriorly to it in the fissure. In the right hilum (*Fig.* 38.3*b*) the artery lies anterior to the main bronchus where it gives off a branch to accompany the right upper lobe bronchus before passing posterolateral to the intermediate bronchus in the intralobar fissure. The superior pulmonary veins, pulmonary arteries and bronchi are easily accessible by an anterosuperior approach. The inferior pulmonary veins on each side lie inferior and posterior to the other hilar structures and can be located in the attachment of the pulmonary ligaments to the hila. Occasionally the three tributaries of the left inferior vein do not join until near the pericardium when separate ligation may be necessary. The middle lobe vein may appear as a separate entity in the right hilum. Segmental resections require a knowledge of the anatomy of the bronchopulmonary segments which have been described in detail by Kent and Blades.

LYMPHATICS

The lungs are richly supplied with lymphatic channels which surround the bronchi and blood vessels, form a plexus beneath the visceral pleura and permeate the bronchial walls. When distended, in lymphangitis carcinomatosa or pulmonary oedema, the full extent of the network becomes apparent and the vessels may become visible radiologically. The constant expansion and relaxation of the lungs help to pump the lymph towards the hilum, flow being directed by simple valves. The vessels communicate freely and some lymph flows outwards to the subpleural plexus before returning through the lung to the hilar region, a fact which may have importance in the pleural spread of bronchial carcinoma. Lymphoidal tissue is found at each bronchial bifurcation from the respiratory bronchioles inward, although true lymph nodes only appear at the level of the segmental bronchi.

The lymph having drained into the lobar (hilar) nodes, then passes to the tracheobronchial chain which surrounds the bifurcation of the trachea, its exact destination depending on the lobe or segment of origin, the distribution having been described in detail by von Hayek. The inferior tracheobronchial nodes lie within the angle of the carina where they receive lymph from both sides, a factor which may contribute to the contralateral spread of tumour described at mediastinoscopy. Nodes above and lateral to the bifurcation are usually larger on the right. The aorta and left pulmonary artery isolate several of the left upper tracheobronchial nodes forming the para-aortic subgroup. These nodes lie in close relationship to the origin of the left recurrent laryngeal nerve and receive drainage from the apical segment of the left upper lobe. The two paratracheal chains receive drainage from their respective tracheobronchial nodes, the trachea, the oesophagus and the upper mediastinal structures and send efferent vessels to the deep lower cervical nodes. On the left the paratracheal nodes are closely related to the ascending recurrent laryngeal nerve. Enlargement of the deep cervical nodes may be indicative of an underlying pulmonary pathology and biopsy may be diagnostic. The lymph finally enters the venous system at the junctions of the subclavian and internal jugular veins either independently or having joined the right lymphatic or thoracic ducts. In addition to the principal drainage some lymph from the lower lobes passes via the pulmonary ligaments to nodes in the posterior mediastinum or through the diaphragm into the retroperitoneal chain. Enlarged intrathoracic nodes rarely suppurate although caseous tuberculous nodes may erode through a bronchial wall, while if the nodes are adherent to bronchi, pulmonary vessels or a persistent ductus arteriosus they may present problems during surgery.

Fluid and protein from the pleural space is drained principally through lymphatics in the mediastinal pleura into the parasternal and para-aortic chains. There are channels through the diaphragm which facilitate the spread of fluid and infection from the abdomen to the pleural space but not in the reverse direction. Lymph from the parietal pleura and chest wall drains into nodes around the internal mammary vessels (parasternal), at the heads of the ribs or into the anterior or posterior mediastinal chains.

The thoracic duct enters the thorax through the aortic orifice and runs up the posterior mediastinum between the aorta and azygos vein to the level of the seventh thoracic vertebrae where it crosses obliquely behind the oesophagus before proceeding along the left oesophageal border into the neck where it joins the venous system. Chylothorax may result from either surgical or traumatic damage to or tumour invasion of the duct.

DEFENCE MECHANISMS

The cellular lining and submucosa of the respiratory tract form a very delicate structure, which requires an efficient defence system if it is to be protected from the numerous irritants and contaminants contained in the air to which it is continually exposed. Large particles, greater than 5–7 μm, are trapped in the hairs and tortuous passages of the nasal cavity or settle out in the oropharynx. Certain irritants (noxious gases) and some types of a particulate matter entering the nose, pharynx, larynx, trachea or larger bronchi may activate the sneeze, gag or cough reflexes, thereby preventing material from gaining access to, or remaining within, the respiratory tract or cause the subject to withdraw from the contaminated area. These reflexes may be suppressed by drugs (analgesics, hypnotics), alcohol overdose, general or local anaesthesia or head injury which may predispose to damage from inhalation or aspiration of foreign material including gastric contents. Following chemical or viral tracheitis the mucosa may exhibit increased sensitivity to minimal stimuli for several months.

The elastic tissue within the bronchial walls permits the bronchial tree to distend in every plane during inspiration, returning to resting levels on expiration, an action which milks material within the bronchial lumen towards the trachea. This action may be aided by the peristaltic movements of the bronchial muscles. In bronchiectasis these mechanisms are lost and material collects within the damaged bronchi favouring subsequent infection.

The respiratory tract is lined by ciliated epithelium. A mucus blanket, 5 μm thick, rests on the tips of the cilia. This blanket is constantly being moved up the bronchial tree, at a rate of between 5 and 20 mm/min, by the rhythmic beating of the cilia carrying with it any particulate or foreign material deposited on its surface, to be swallowed on reaching the pharynx (mucociliary escalator). The cilia move in a watery fluid which facilitates their action. Anything which (*a*) impairs cilial action, e.g. smoking, (*b*) alters the composition of the bronchial mucus, e.g. chronic bronchitis, (*c*) damages the ciliated epithelium, e.g. bronchiectasis, squamous metaplasia, or (*d*) dries the blanket, e.g. breathing non-humidified air through a tracheostomy, will interfere with this delicate mechanism. Atmospheric air is both warmed and humidified within the nasal passages preventing such damage.

As yet our knowledge of the functions of the bronchial secretions is incomplete. By coating the mucosal surface they undoubtedly prevent excessive water loss, protect the cells from inhaled irritants and form the mucus blanket. They also contain compounds with antimicrobial activity including: (*a*) lysozyme which lyses bacteria; (*b*) lactoferrin which has a bacteriostatic action; and (*c*) interferon with antiviral activity. Submucosal plasma cells secrete respiratory IgA which is active against viruses and possibly some bacterial agents. Deficiency of IgA or one of the above compounds may be responsible for some cases of recurrent chest infections.

Non-pathogenic bacteria, spores or small particles entering the distal respiratory tract are engulfed and removed by the specialized alveolar macrophages. These cells may be damaged or inactivated by cigarette smoke, inhaled irritants or alcohol. The effect of smoking on the macrophages has been implicated in the pathogenesis of some forms of emphysema (*see* Chapter 39).

Invasion of the respiratory tract by pathogenic bacteria is followed by the rapid outpouring of polymorphonuclear leucocytes, lymphocytes and fluid rich in antibodies from the pulmonary circulation. Any disorders which interfere with the formation or activity of these agents will predispose to respiratory infection.

THE FUNCTIONS OF THE LUNG

While ventilation has attracted most attention the lungs may have other functions although our understanding of them is incomplete. The lungs contain a high concentration of trypsin and as more than 90% of the blood passes through them on each circuit this has suggested a possible role in the removal and destruction of foreign and degenerate proteins from the circulation. In the absence of α_1-antitrypsin, required to deactivate trypsin, the lungs may undergo autodigestion with the formation of basal bullae. Various roles within the endocrine system have been attributed to the lungs, namely: (*a*) the storage of histamine and noradrenaline; (*b*) the synthesis, release and metabolism of hormones, such as the prostaglandins; (*c*) the conversion of angiotensin I into angiotensin II; and (*d*) the destruction of bradykinin. Some drugs may be metabolized in the lungs, e.g. lignocaine, and the association of simple pulmonary eosinophilia with certain drugs has been attributed to an allergic response following their concentration in lung tissue prior to deactivation. The larynx and bellows action of the lungs are essential for speech and communication and voice changes resulting from involvement of the recurrent laryngeal nerves may be the first indication of pulmonary pathology.

Respiration

The processes involved in the exchange of oxygen and

carbon dioxide within the lungs cannot be considered in isolation from the transport of these gases by the blood or their utilization or production at cellular level. Normally the composition of venous and arterial bloods are kept within narrow limits, in spite of considerable variations in the utilization and production of the respiratory gases, by means of a sensitive feedback mechanism and the complex integration of the pulmonary, circulatory and nervous responses.

Respiration will be considered under four headings: (1) the transport of oxygen and carbon dioxide within the blood; (2) factors influencing gas exchange within the lungs; (3) the mechanics of breathing; and (4) the nervous and chemical control of respiration.

1. Oxygen and Carbon Dioxide Transport by the Blood

At both alveolar and tissue level the exchange of oxygen and carbon dioxide with the blood occurs by simple diffusion and requires the maintenance of adequate concentration gradients to be effective. However, only a small proportion of either gas is carried in simple solution, where it is in direct equilibrium with the external gases. The majority form reversible combinations with the blood constituents which act as a reservoir to maintain the levels in solution. Blood gas estimations record the total content of each gas, whether as a solute or in combination.

As 98% of the oxygen is carried as oxyhaemoglobin it is the amount of haemoglobin which determines the capacity of the blood to carry oxygen and this may be reduced by more than half in severe anaemia. In contrast, the degree of saturation is independent of the haemoglobin concentration and depends on the oxygen tension gradients in the lungs and the tissues. Thus 15 g of haemoglobin with a saturation of 97% will carry 20 vol % while 7·5 g of haemoglobin with the same saturation (97%) will only carry 10 vol %.

The relationship between the oxygen tension and haemoglobin saturation is defined in the oxygen dissociation curve (*Fig.* 38.4) which is sigmoidal rather than linear, a significant factor in the smooth exchange of oxygen in the lungs and tissues. At rest the arterial (97%) to venous (75%) saturation difference is around 25% but this hides a 60% change in oxygen tensions, i.e. 98 mmHg arterial to 40 mmHg venous. Thus as the oxygen tension in the tissues is about 40 mmHg compared to 98 mmHg in arterial blood and in the alveolar gas about 100 mmHg compared to 40 mmHg in venous blood, a pressure gradient of 60 mmHg exists at both sites to facilitate adequate gas exchange.

On exercise there is an increase in the concentration of both hydrogen ions and carbon dioxide and a rise in temperature within the tissues, each of which will shift the dissociation curve to the right and lead to the release of more oxygen in the tissues for a given oxygen tension. As more oxygen is utilized the tissue oxygen tension falls, increasing the blood to tissue oxygen gradient and facilitating oxygen transfer. The resultant lower oxygen saturation and tension in venous blood increases the oxygen gradient at alveolar level, increasing its uptake.

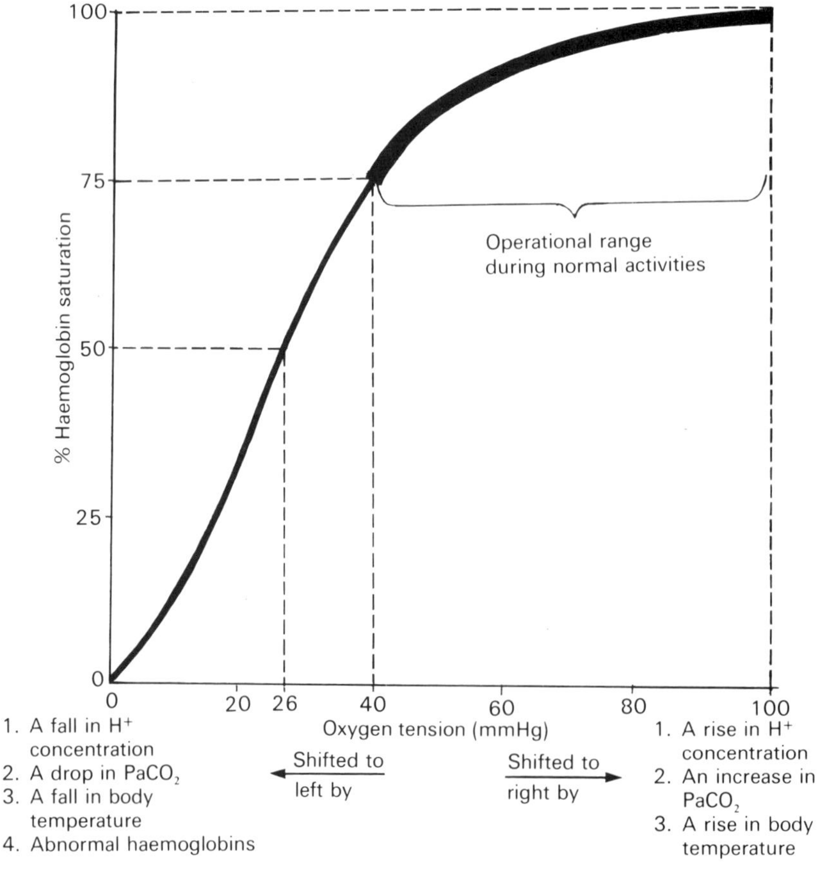

Fig. 38.4 Standard oxygen dissociation curve at pH 7·4 and 37 °C.

The oxygen dissociation curve is shifted to the left if there is a fall in hydrogen ion concentration, a drop in the carbon dioxide tension or in the body temperature, following exposure to carbon monoxide or in presence of abnormal haemoglobins making it more difficult to release oxygen from the blood.

The greater solubility of carbon dioxide means that a 6 mm pressure difference between arterial (40 mmHg) and venous (46 mmHg) blood is sufficient to permit adequate uptake from the tissues and elimination in the lungs. In the tissues carbon dioxide rapidly enters red blood cells where it either combines with haemoglobin to form carbamino-haemoglobin (which, while it accounts for only 6–7% of the total carbon dioxide content of venous blood, carries 20–30% of that delivered to the alveolar gas) or forms carbonic acid under the influence of carbonic anhydrase. The carbonic acid dissociates into hydrogen ion, which is taken up by reduced haemoglobin, and bicarbonate, which diffuses into the plasma. The lower alveolar gas tension favours release of carbon dioxide and a reversal of the chemical processes described above.

2. Gas Exchange

The features of alveolar gas exchange under resting conditions are shown in *Fig.* 38.5. During quiet breathing a red cell takes approximately 0·75 sec to pass through the pulmonary capillaries (transient time) during which time gas exchange has been completed.

Ideally each alveolus would receive its appropriate share of the inspired air and pulmonary circulation, the respiratory rate being adjusted to keep the alveolar tensions of oxygen at 100 mmHg and carbon dioxide at 40 mmHg.

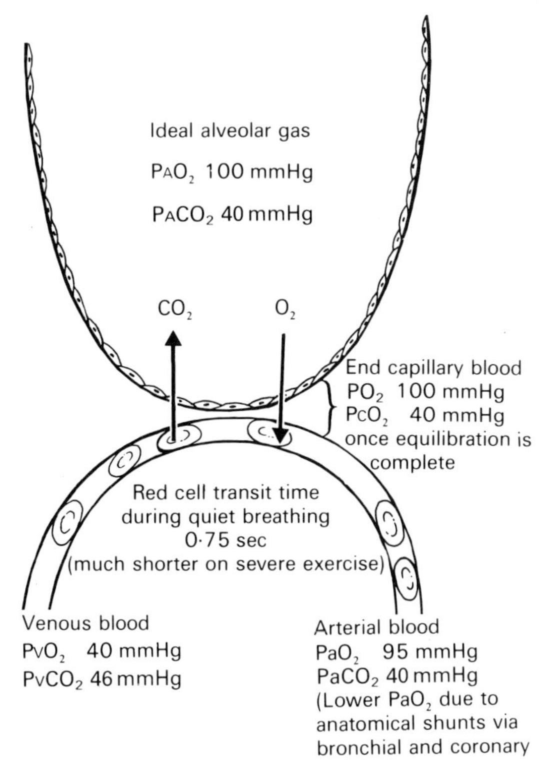

Fig. 38.5 Schematic representation of the alveolar–capillary gas exchange.

Factors which depress the activity of the respiratory centre (anaesthetic agents, hypnotics, analgesics) or impair the degree of respiratory movement (myasthenia gravis, poliomyelitis or severe kyphoscoliosis) may reduce overall alveolar ventilation to such a degree that the alveolar tension of carbon dioxide rises and that of oxygen falls leading to hypercapnia and hypoxia.

Even in healthy subjects there is a degree of mismatching of ventilation and perfusion, some alveoli being well ventilated but poorly perfused while the reverse situation occurs in others. When standing erect the ratio of ventilation to perfusion varies as you move down the lung. A change of posture, i.e. lying supine, alters the pattern of ventilation and perfusion seen in the lungs due in part to the redistribution of blood flow to the dependent areas. The mismatching of ventilation and perfusion becomes more evident in disease and is a major factor underlying the functional abnormalities found in chronic bronchitis.

The movement of air from the mouth to the alveolus is made up of two components: (1) *Transport*, involving the flow of air through the bronchial tree as far as the alveolar ducts; and (2) *Gas mixing*, by which gas diffuses into the alveoli from the alveolar ducts. Maldistribution of inspired air may result from disorders in either component. Bronchial obstruction by mucosal oedema, muscle spasm, secretion or fibrosis as occurs in chronic bronchitis may impede air flow to some areas, while marked dilatation of the air spaces as seen in emphysema, will interfere with gas mixing. Perfusion of poorly ventilated areas in chronic bronchitis and emphysema effectively increases the degree of venous shunting leading to a fall in the oxygen tension. However, the slight rise in carbon dioxide tension which occurs results in sufficient hyperventilation to reduce the arterial carbon dioxide to normal levels. In the presence of severe ventilation perfusion imbalance as may be seen during an acute exacerbation of chronic bronchitis carbon dioxide retention may also occur.

Embolization or thrombosis of pulmonary vessels is associated with well-ventilated but poorly perfused alveoli but unless the area involved is large this has little effect on the blood gases.

The arterial oxygen tension is a little lower than that at the end of the pulmonary capillaries due to the drainage of blood from the coronary and bronchial systems directly into the left atrium usually accounting for about 6% of cardiac output. This percentage is increased: (*a*) in the presence of a right-to-left anatomical shunt due to congenital heart disease; or (*b*) by the passage of blood through non-ventilated lung, i.e. in lobar pneumonia or atelectasis (physiological shunt). Both mechanisms cause hypoxia, but have little effect on the carbon dioxide level.

Given the normal oxygen tension gradient between alveolar air and capillary blood equilibrium occurs across the membrane even if the transit time is considerably reduced as in severe exercise. Thickening of the membrane by alveolar fluids, oedema or proliferation of alveolar cells, as may occur in left ventricular failure, fibrosing alveolitis, sarcoidosis or paraquat poisoning, may impair the transport of oxygen resulting in hypoxia initially present on exercise, but later occurring at rest. Hyperventilation and the more rapid diffusion of carbon dioxide ensure normal or reduced arterial levels of this gas.

3. The Mechanics of Breathing

During quiet breathing only inspiration is associated with active muscular contraction, expiration occurring as a result of the elastic recoil of the lungs and chest wall. The main respiratory muscles are the diaphragm and intercostal muscles which are augmented during forced inspiration or forced expiration by the accessory muscles of respiration, including neck, shoulder girdle and abdominal muscles. The descent of the diaphragm normally increases the longitudinal thoracic diameter and accounts for most of quiet inspiration. This action is impaired in severe emphysema where the diaphragm is low and flat permitting little, if any, downward movement, and indeed, traction by the diaphragm may result in indrawing of the lower costal margin during inspiration which may further embarrass ventilation. Patients who have paralysed intercostal muscles, e.g. following poliomyelitis depend on diaphragmatic respiration in which case an acute abdomen or abdominal surgery may be associated with severe respiratory difficulties.

During inspiration the intercostal muscles rotate the ribs upwards and outwards along an axis through their sternal and vertebral connections, increasing the anteroposterior and transverse diameters of the chest. During forced inspiration the upper ribs are stabilized by the action of the accessory muscles of the neck while in forced expiration the lower ribs are fixed through contraction of the rectus muscles, making the movements of the other ribs more efficient.

The energy expended in moving air within the respiratory tract depends on the combined resistances of the abdominal contents and the elastic and viscous forces of the chest wall and lungs. Elastic recoil causes the lungs to collapse and the chest wall to expand on opening the chest, the two opposing forces being balanced only at the end of quiet expiration.

The distensibility or compliance of the chest wall or lungs refers to the force required to produce a given change in their volume, the relationship for both being linear over the range of ventilation (normally 0·2 L/cm of water for each). The lower the compliance the greater the force required. Therefore factors which reduce the compliance of either the chest wall (obesity, thoracoplasty or kyphoscoliosis) or of the lung (pneumonia, atelectasis, oedema, fibrosis, pulmonary resection and some anaesthetic agents), will increase the work of breathing.

Air flow within the bronchial tree is independent of the compliance, being proportional to the pressure gradient between the alveoli and the atmosphere and the total cross-sectional area of the bronchial tree at any given level. Any narrowing of the respiratory tract, i.e. from laryngeal spasm, secretions, bronchospasm, fibrosis, mucosal oedema or tumour will impede air flow and increase the work of breathing. During quiet breathing 90% of air flow is laminar, however, the flow becomes progressively more turbulent the faster the rate of respiration thereby greatly enhancing the effort required.

The alveoli are prevented from collapsing during respiration by a lipoprotein (surfactant) which, by decreasing

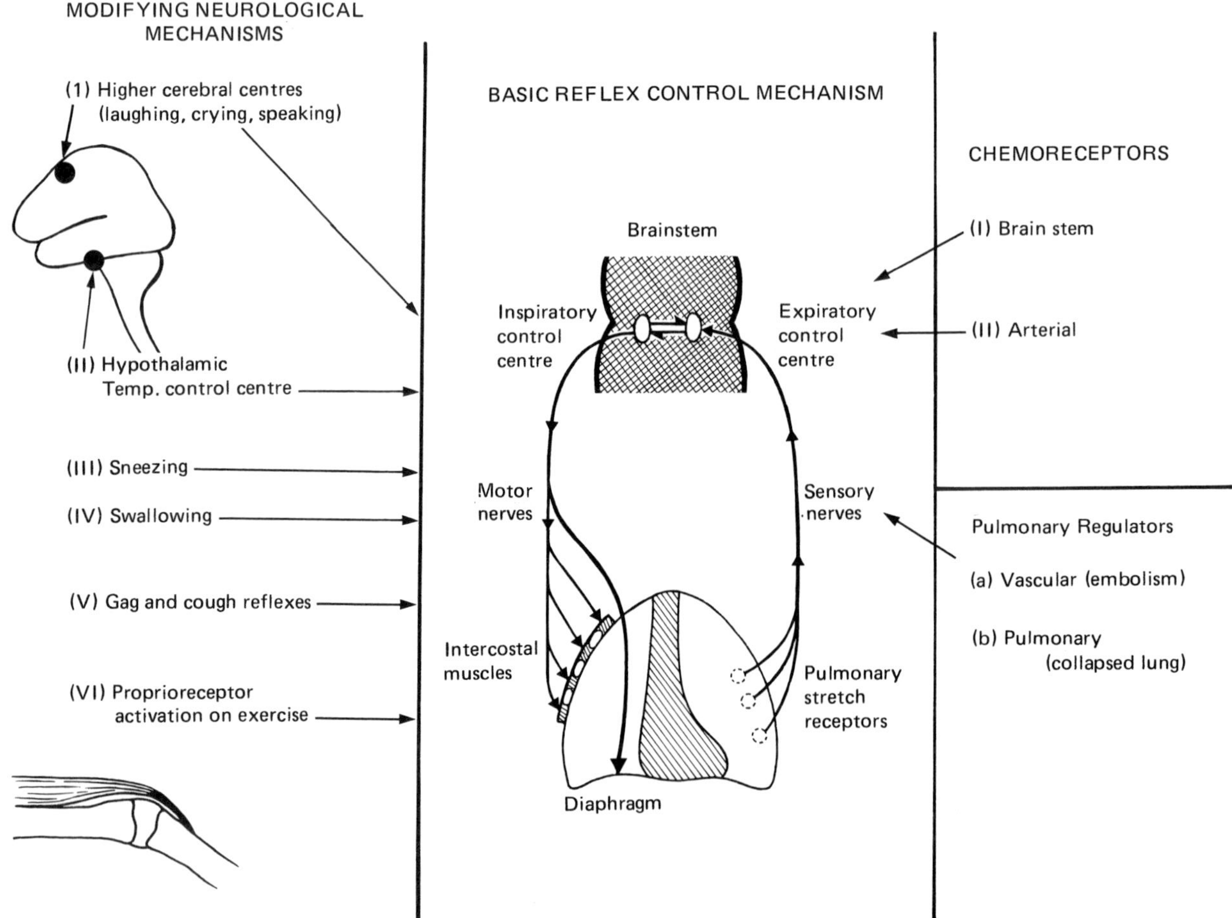

Fig. 38.6 Control of respiration.

surface tension on expiration and increasing it on inspiration, stabilizes the pressure within the alveolar spaces. In the absence of surfactant, as in the respiratory distress syndrome of the newborn, the alveoli collapse on expiration requiring enormous pressures for re-expansion.

4. The Nervous and Chemical Control of Respiration (*Fig.* 38.6)

Breathing is controlled by the respiratory centre, a loosely knit collection of neurones within the reticular formation of the medulla oblongata, which is influenced by several reflex and chemical mechanisms. The depression of brainstem activity by hypnotics, anaesthetics, sleep or vascular disorders will reduce ventilation. During quiet breathing, in animals, the inspiratory component of the respiratory centre initiates inspiration, but vagal afferent impulses (the Hering–Breuer reflex) from the distending lung reach the expiratory component which then inhibits further inspiration.

Activation of lung receptors following a pneumothorax reflexly stimulates the inspiratory centre leading to tachypnoea. Distension of the pulmonary vascular bed, e.g. due to left ventricular failure, or the obliteration of the pulmonary arteries, e.g. by multiple small emboli, both lead to rapid shallow respiration through vagally-mediated reflexes. Impulses arising (*a*) from the higher cerebral centres, during speaking, crying or laughing, (*b*) from the hypothalamic temperature control centre during pyrexia, or (*c*) from local sensory endings in swallowing, coughing or sneezing, all act on the respiratory centre to modify ventilation. Increased ventilation on exercise is initiated by afferent impulses arising in the muscles and joints involved.

In the normal subject the carbon dioxide and oxygen tensions and the hydrogen ion concentration of arterial blood are kept within narrow limits through constant monitoring by central and peripheral chemosensitive areas which reflexly act on the respiratory centre modifying ventilation. The major sites for chemical regulation are the chemosensitive areas on the anterolateral surfaces of the medulla oblongata which respond to changes in the hydrogen ion concentration within the CSF. Changes in carbon dioxide tension may act directly on the chemoreceptors as well as by altering the hydrogen ion concentration within the CSF. An increase in the hydrogen ion concentration or a rise in the arterial carbon dioxide tension above 40 mmHg both stimulate the respiratory centre increasing the respiratory rate, provided the inspired oxygen tension remains normal. At altitude, hypoxia stimulates respiration and with acclimatization the respiratory centre becomes adjusted to a lower trigger threshold for carbon dioxide tension.

The peripheral chemoreceptors of the carotid and aortic bodies account for about 20% of the resting respiratory drive. These areas respond to changes in arterial oxygen tension although in normal subjects a fall in the inspired oxygen concentration to below 16% (atmospheric 20·89%) is required before there is any significant increase in ventilation. While responding to variations in the hydrogen ion concentration and carbon dioxide tension within the arterial blood the peripheral receptors are less sensitive than the brainstem chemoreceptors to these changes.

The reduced oxygen and elevated carbon dioxide tensions associated with either alveolar hypoventilation, e.g. drug overdose, or significant ventilation-perfusion imbalance, e.g. chronic bronchitis, may both stimulate respiration by activating the chemoreceptors. In severe hypoxia, if the carbon dioxide tension rises above 70 mmHg the chemoreceptors become less sensitive to this stimulus allowing the hypoxic drive to predominate. Under these circumstances the injudicious use of high inspired oxygen concentrations may abolish this drive and lead to fatal respiratory depression.

LUNG FUNCTION TESTS

Lung function tests can be of considerable value in assessing overall lung function but their accuracy depends upon the co-operation of and active participation by the patient. The simplest tests, while being clinically the most valuable, are relatively insensitive, requiring significant functional impairment before changes are detected. Sophisticated tests may detect impairment earlier but are not readily available. Both types of information may be useful: (*a*) in confirming the diagnosis; (*b*) in assessing the severity of the disease; or (*c*) in predicting and following the response to treatment. Discussion will centre around the measurements of ventilatory function, static lung volumes, transfer factor and exercise performance with reference to the value of blood gas analysis, all of which are simple and easy to perform.

Measurements of *ventilatory function* are made using a spirometer (or vitalograph) or a peak flow meter (or gauge). Spirometry measures (*a*) the total volume, and (*b*) the rate of flow of air during a forced expiration performed after a maximum inspiration. Two measurements are made: (*a*) the forced vital capacity (FVC) which is the total amount of air expired, in litres, and (*b*) the forced expiratory volume (FEV_1) which is the volume (in litres) expired in a given time, usually one second. The FEV_1 may be expressed as a percentage of the FVC (the FEV_1/FVC ratio) to give a useful indicator of functional impairment. The results are compared with predicted values which take into account the height, age and sex of the patient. Two patterns of abnormality may be found, the obstructive and the restrictive.

In obstructive airways disease (chronic bronchitis, emphysema or asthma) both the FVC and the FEV_1 are reduced but the effect on the latter is more marked, causing a fall in the FEV_1/FVC ratio. If spirometry is repeated after the administration of a bronchodilator or following a period on high doses of corticosteroids it may show an improvement in the FVC, FEV_1 or both indicating a degree of reversibility which may be of significance in diagnosis (distinguishing asthma from chronic bronchitis) or when planning treatment. In restrictive lung disease (fibrosing alveolitis, sarcoidosis or pulmonary oedema) there is an equal reduction in both the FVC and FEV_1 so that the FEV_1/FVC ratio remains normal and there is no improvement with bronchodilators.

The peak flow meter or gauge records the maximum rate, in litres/minute, at which air can be expired following a full inspiration, the peak expiratory flow rate (PEFR). The PEFR is reduced in airways obstruction but may be normal in restrictive lung disease. The peak flow gauge is portable and permits serial measurements of the PEFR at set times during the day whether at home or work. This is particularly useful in asthma when it will (*a*) give a guide to the natural history of the disease, (*b*) help in identifying trigger factors and (*c*) aid in assessing the most effective treatment regime.

The *static lung volumes* are measured by rebreathing air containing a known concentration of an inert gas (usually helium), until equilibrium is reached between the gas in the spirometer and that in the lungs. The most important measurements are: (*a*) the amount of air in the lungs at the end of a full inspiration (in litres), the total lung capacity

(TLC); and (*b*) the volume of air remaining after a maximal expiration (in litres), the residual volume (RV). The RV may be expressed as a percentage of the TLC, the RV/TLC ratio, giving a measure of the amount of air trapped in the lungs at the end of expiration. Predicted values for each of these parameters are available taking into account the patient's height, age and sex. While the TLC and RV are both increased in emphysema, the RV is raised to a greater extent, producing elevation in the RV/TLC ratio, which may exceed 70% in severe cases (predicted usually below 35%) indicating the degree of air trapping which may be present. Similar but less marked changes, in TLC, RV and RV/TLC ratio, may be found in asthma and chronic bronchitis. In restrictive lung disease (fibrosing alveolitis, sarcoidosis) the TLC is reduced while the RV remains normal or is reduced.

The *transfer factor* (T_{CO}) is a measure of the rate, in ml/min/mmHg, at which carbon monoxide passes from the atmosphere into the red blood cell. Several factors may influence this process of which the following are the most important: (*a*) airflow obstruction (chronic bronchitis and asthma) which affects gas movement from the mouth to the terminal bronchi; (*b*) emphysema which increases the distance for diffusion between the terminal bronchi and the alveolar membrane; (*c*) increased thickness of the alveolar capillary membrane (fibrosing alveolitis, sarcoidosis, paraquat lung) which delays the passage into the capillaries; (*d*) the total area of alveolar-capillary membrane available for gas exchange which is reduced in emphysema and following pneumonectomy; (*e*) the amount and composition of the haemoglobin, anaemia reducing while polycythaemia increases the rate; and (*f*) the cardiac output, the quicker the flow, the faster the uptake. The transfer factor is a crude measurement which is affected by a variety of diverse conditions and is not solely a measure of diffusion across the alveolar-capillary membrane as was originally taught. The results should be interpreted in the light of the clinical findings and the pattern from the other respiratory function tests.

Lung size is important, the T_{CO} increasing throughout childhood and falling following pneumonectomy. To overcome this Krogh introduced the transfer coefficient (K_{CO}) which divides the transfer factor (T_{CO}) by the alveolar volume.

In spite of these difficulties measurements of the transfer factor and K_{CO} are valuable in interstitial lung disease, i.e. fibrosing alveolitis and sarcoidosis, both as an indicator of severity and in assessing response to treatment.

Two techniques are available for measuring the transfer factor: (*a*) the single breath method in which the patient takes a single breath of a mixture containing 0·2–0·3% carbon monoxide and holds his breath for a set time; and (*b*) the steady-state method where the patient breathes from a bag containing a very low concentration of carbon monoxide until equilibrium is reached. The steady-state method gives lower readings but has the advantage that it can be performed during exercise when defects in diffusion may first be detected, i.e. early sarcoidosis.

The pattern of ventilatory function, static lung volumes and transfer factor expected in the main types of respiratory disorder are summarized in *Table* 38.2.

The ability to *perform exercise* can give useful information about the overall respiratory function bearing in mind the results may be affected by the patients' cardiovascular and locomotor state and their general fitness. Standard tests record the number of stairs climbed or the distance walked within a set time usually 6 or 12 min. Repeat testing may indicate the response to medical treatment or training regimes, i.e. in chronic obstructive airways disease. In many asthmatic patients with inadequate symptomatic control vigorous sustained exercise over a short period usually five minutes may induce bronchospasm, which can be recorded as a drop in the FEV_1 or in the peak expiratory flow rate. This test may be diagnostic in children with asthma and may be repeated at subsequent clinic visits to assess the response to treatment. More sophisticated tests using a treadmill or bicycle ergometer will distinguish between cardiovascular and respiratory problems.

Blood gas analysis in which the oxygen and carbon dioxide tensions and the hydrogen ion concentrations in arterial blood are measured using special electrodes can give valuable information, provided the instruments are properly serviced and calibrated. Some patients with established chronic bronchitis have reduced oxygen and raised carbon dioxide tensions even when clinically at their best. The management of severe infective exacerbations or postoperative respiratory complications in patients with established chronic bronchitis often requires repeated blood gas analysis, as the inspired oxygen concentration given will depend on the arterial hydrogen ion concentration and the carbon dioxide tension. In contrast, patients with primary emphysema ('pink puffers') usually have a normal oxygen, but reduced carbon dioxide tension. In early interstitial lung disease, e.g. fibrosing alveolitis, the blood gases may be normal when resting with both the oxygen and carbon dioxide tensions falling on exercise, a pattern which later

Table 38.2 Changes in pulmonary function tests in obstructive and restrictive lung disorders

	FVC	*FEV*	*FEV_1/FVC*	*TLC*	*RV*	*RV/TLC*	*T_{CO}*
1. *Obstructive airways disease*							
Chronic bronchitis	↓	↓↓	↓	N or ↑	N or ↑	↑	↓
Emphysema	↓↓	↓↓↓	↓↓	↑↑	↑↑↑	↑↑	↓↓
Asthma	↓	↓↓	↓	N or ↑	N or ↑	↑	N or ↑
2. *Restrictive lung disease*							
Fibrosing alveolitis	↓↓	↓↓	N	↓	N or ↓	N or ↑	↓↓
Sarcoidosis	N or ↓	N or ↓	N	N	N	N	↓

↓ reduced, ↑ increased, N normal.

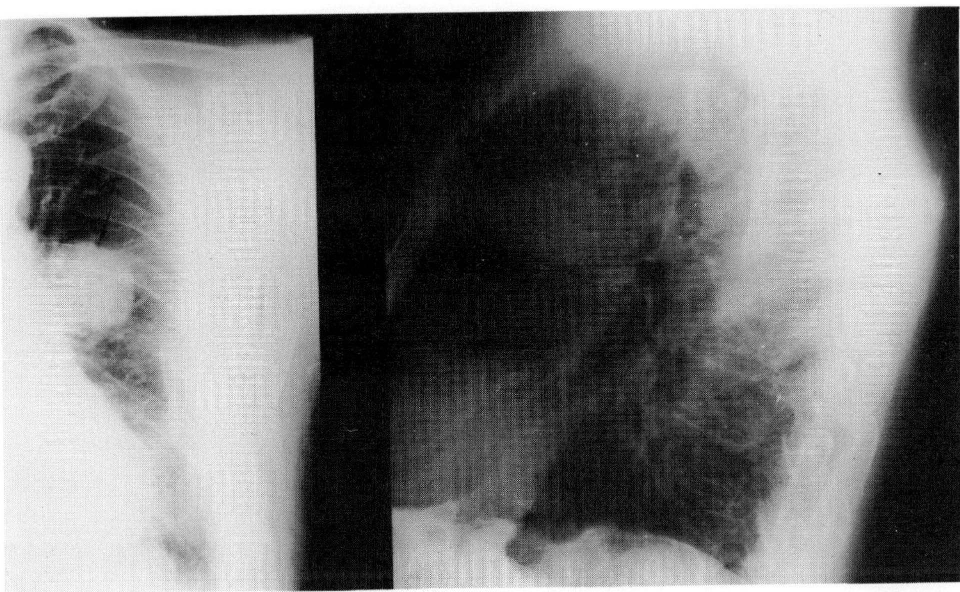

Fig. 38.7 Postero-anterior and lateral films demonstrating a pulmonary lesion, the exact location of which can only be determined by examination of both views.

becomes established at rest. Even when breathing 100% oxygen in the presence of a significant right-to-left anatomical shunt the resting arterial oxygen tension remains low (usually below 120 mmHg).

RADIOLOGY

The radiological examination forms the cornerstone of investigations in thoracic medicine. Considerable information as to the nature, extent and segmental distribution of a disease can be obtained from postero-anterior and lateral films (*Fig.* 38.7). While a peripheral lesion may be well defined, the definition of centrally placed lesions may be blurred by secondary collapse or consolidation. Careful inspection of the soft-tissue shadows, bony structures, mediastinal and hilar regions and the area behind the heart may yield additional information. Comparison with previous films or repeating the radiograph at a later date will reveal the development, rate of change or resolution of pulmonary lesions (*Figs.* 38.8, 38.9, 38.10).

Prompt referral for a chest radiograph of patients who develop new and persistent or have a change in their respiratory symptoms can assist in early diagnosis and treatment of thoracic diseases. Miniature radiography for mass population screening is no longer feasible. However, surveillance of selected groups of patients, who are at risk of developing respiratory diseases, e.g. immigrants, alcoholics, or who if they develop diseases such as tuberculosis may disseminate them widely, i.e. nurses, teachers, should be considered.

In acutely ill or immobile patients it may be necessary to take a portable anteroposterior film which has the disadvantage of greater scatter of radiation producing an enlarged distorted cardiac outline. Penetrated postero-anterior films may give better resolution of lesions (*a*) in the region of the vertebral column and mediastinum, or (*b*) if they are obscured by the heart, pleural effusions, breast shadows or diaphragms. An apical lordotic view improves visualization of apical lesions while rib lesions and early diffuse lung disease may be better seen on oblique films. A lateral decubitus film, with the patient lying on his side, will allow the displacement of a non-encysted effusion permitting better visualization of the diaphragm and underlying lung. The introduction of a small pneumoperitoneum may occasionally help in defining diaphragmatic or subdiaphragmatic lesions (*Fig.* 38.11).

Lateral, anteroposterior or oblique tomography, by providing a series of films set at different depths, may help to define a lesion in the lung or mediastinum or may indicate any narrowing or distortion of the trachea or main bronchi. Cavitation (*Fig.* 38.12), calcification (*Fig.* 38.13) and satellite lesions may help distinguish a tuberculoma from carcinoma; the presence of an air crescent may indicate an aspergilloma and feeding vessels may be discernible in arteriovenous abnormalities.

The dynamic movements of the heart, lung and diaphragm can be observed during fluoroscopy (screening). Phrenic nerve paralysis or eventration of the diaphragm appears as elevation of the involved hemidiaphragm which moves paradoxically on sniffing or deep breathing. Mediastinal shift with ventilation may be seen in a tension pneumothorax or obstructive emphysema when it may be the first indication of an inhaled foreign body in children. A barium swallow, under screening, in patients with chest disease, may reveal displacement or indentation of the oesophagus by nodes or tumour, a mega-oesophagus or oesophageal diverticulum with pulmonary overspill, a tracheo-oesophageal fistula, the presence and nature of diaphragmatic herniation or the position of the left hemidiaphragm in cases of effusion or collapse (*Fig.* 38.14).

Angiography, through a catheter in the pulmonary artery, may be helpful: (*a*) in defining a pulmonary arteriovenous anomaly; (*b*) in the diagnosis and assessment of selected cases of suspected pulmonary embolus; and (*c*) in establishing arterial dilatation as the cause of hilar enlargement. Occasionally aortic or selected bronchial angiography is useful in outlining aortic aneurysms, studying the bronchial

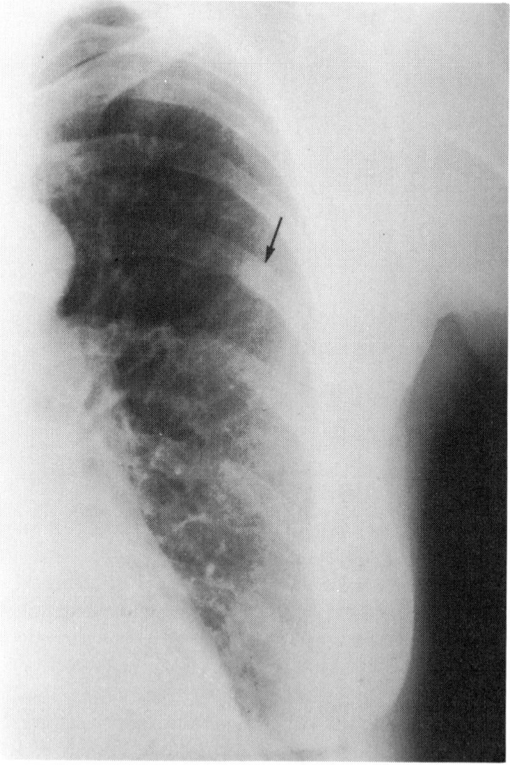

a

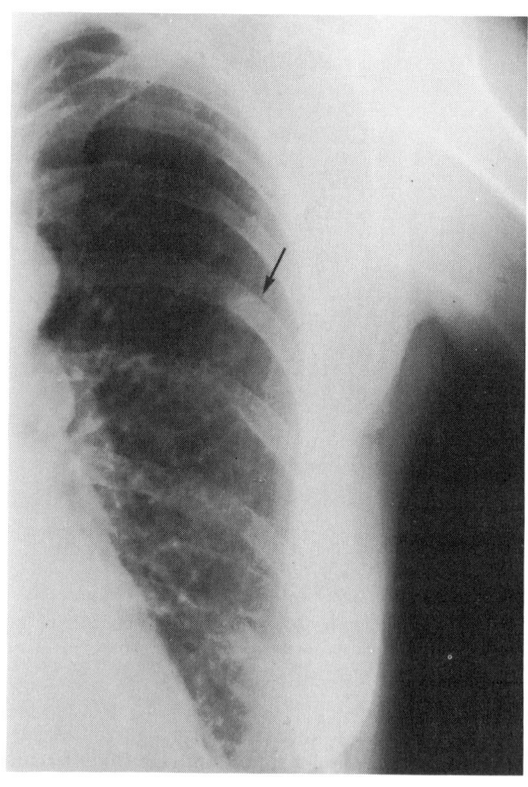

b

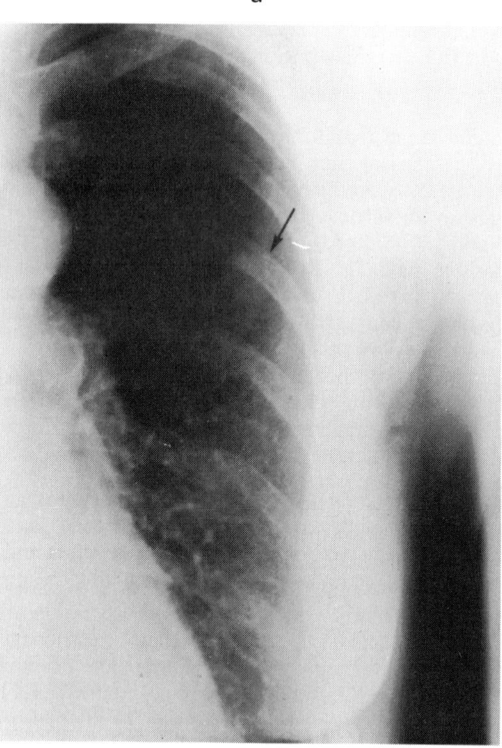

c

Fig. 38.8 *a, b, c*, Radiographic series over a period of 2½ years in a patient treated for carcinoma of the larynx by radiotherapy. Progressive increase in size of the well-circumscribed lesion led to a decision for surgical intervention. Left upper lobectomy was performed and histological examination showed the lesion to be an adenocarcinoma.

blood flow or defining the blood supply to a sequestrated lobe.

Bronchography is a valuable investigation, the technique used depending on the experience of the operator. In children it is best performed under general anaesthesia. The right side should be outlined first taking postero-anterior and right lateral films, followed by the outlining of the left bronchial tree with further postero-anterior and oblique films. Interpretation requires a detailed knowledge of bronchial anatomy. Bronchography is most useful in (*a*) confirming the diagnosis in a case of suspected bronchiectasis (*Fig.* 38.15); (*b*) defining the extent of bronchiectatic involvement during preoperative assessment; or (*c*) showing the distribution and severity in established bronchiectasis to aid in the planning of medical treatment, i.e. postural drainage. A bronchogram may help distinguish between middle lobe collapse or consolidation and a loculated effusion in the oblique or horizontal fissures. The bronchial glands may appear as diverticular in chronic bronchitis but bronchography is rarely indicated in this condition. Bronchograms are of little help in bronchial carcinoma.

BRONCHOSCOPY

Direct visualization of the bronchial tree at bronchoscopy can yield invaluable information although considerable experience is required in order to interpret the appearances. The main indications for bronchoscopy are outlined below.

1. In Diagnosis

a. *Radiological abnormalities* including:
Prominent hilar shadows, lobar or segmental collapse, persistent consolidation, discrete pulmonary lesions,

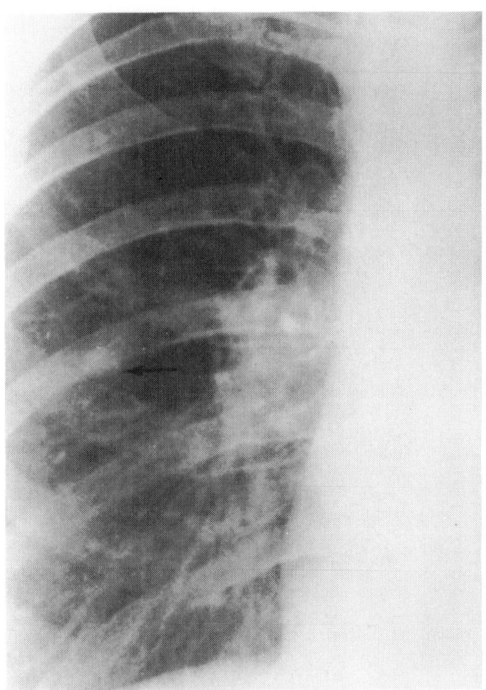

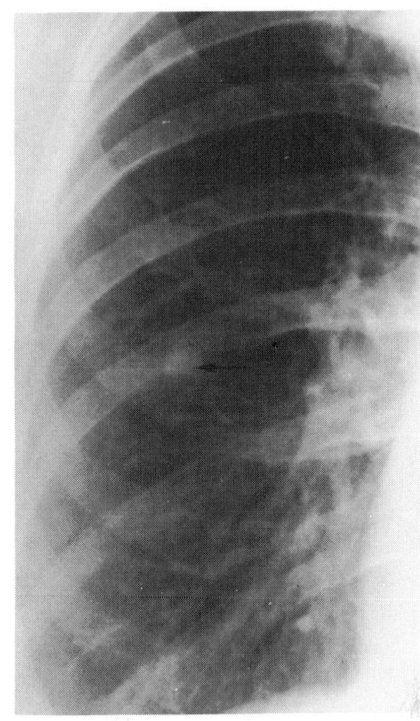

Fig. 38.9 Lesion in the right midzone showing no change in size over a 2-year period. The lesion is presumed benign and no active measures were taken except for regular radiological review.

diffuse lung shadowing (transbronchial lung biopsy), some cases of pleural effusions.

b. Abnormal symptoms and signs
Hoarseness with a bovine cough, recurrent haemoptysis, recurrent infections at the same site, persistent cough without cause, possible foreign body inhalation, stridor, a persistent rhonchus over a major bronchus, suspicion of a ruptured bronchus.

c. Follow-up to other investigations
Positive sputum cytology with a normal chest radiological appearance.

2. In Investigation

a. Limited broncho-alveolar lavage to obtain bronchial secretions for bacteriological, histological and cytological examination may have diagnostic significance.
b. The assessment of regional function by measuring air flow and gas concentrations from different bronchi.

3. In Preoperative Assessment

a. To determine the operability of a carcinoma by examining the state of the cords, any tracheal indentation or carinal broadening, its position in relation to the carina, and in assessing whether a lobectomy or pneumonectomy may be indicated.

b. To determine the site of persistent bleeding, i.e. which segmental or lobar brochus is involved.

4. In Treatment for the Removal of:

a. Retained secretions following drug overdose, during assisted ventilation, in acute or chronic respiratory failure and lung abscess.

b. Gastric juices after aspiration.

c. Inhaled foreign bodies.

d. Bronchial casts following bronchial lavage in severe asthma.

5. In Research

a. To obtain bronchial secretions and alveolar cells by bronchial lavage to determine their composition and function in health and disease.

b. To study bronchial mobility and its modification by various drugs.

While complications are infrequent bronchoscopy is best avoided in status asthmaticus, severe superior vena caval obstruction, if tuberculosis is suspected or is still active, or in the presence of an uncorrected bleeding diathesis.

Attention should be paid to the movement of the cords, the patency and mobility of the tracheobronchial tree, the state of the mucosa, the presence of any obstruction and the nature of the bronchial secretions, each finding being recorded. Bronchial or lung biopsies, pus or secretions from the bronchial tree, or washings from bronchial lavage should be obtained and sent for the appropriate examinations. The appearances in bronchial carcinoma, tuberculosis, bronchiectasis, foreign bodies and chronic inflammation may be diagnostic and are well illustrated in Stradling's monograph on bronchoscopy. The site of a tumour may affect its operability as may the occurrence of hilar, paratracheal and subcarinal gland involvement. The orifice containing a blood clot or from which blood is emerging may indicate the lobe or segment involved although the cause of the bleeding may not be visualized. Inflammation and oedema around an organic foreign body may make immediate removal difficult

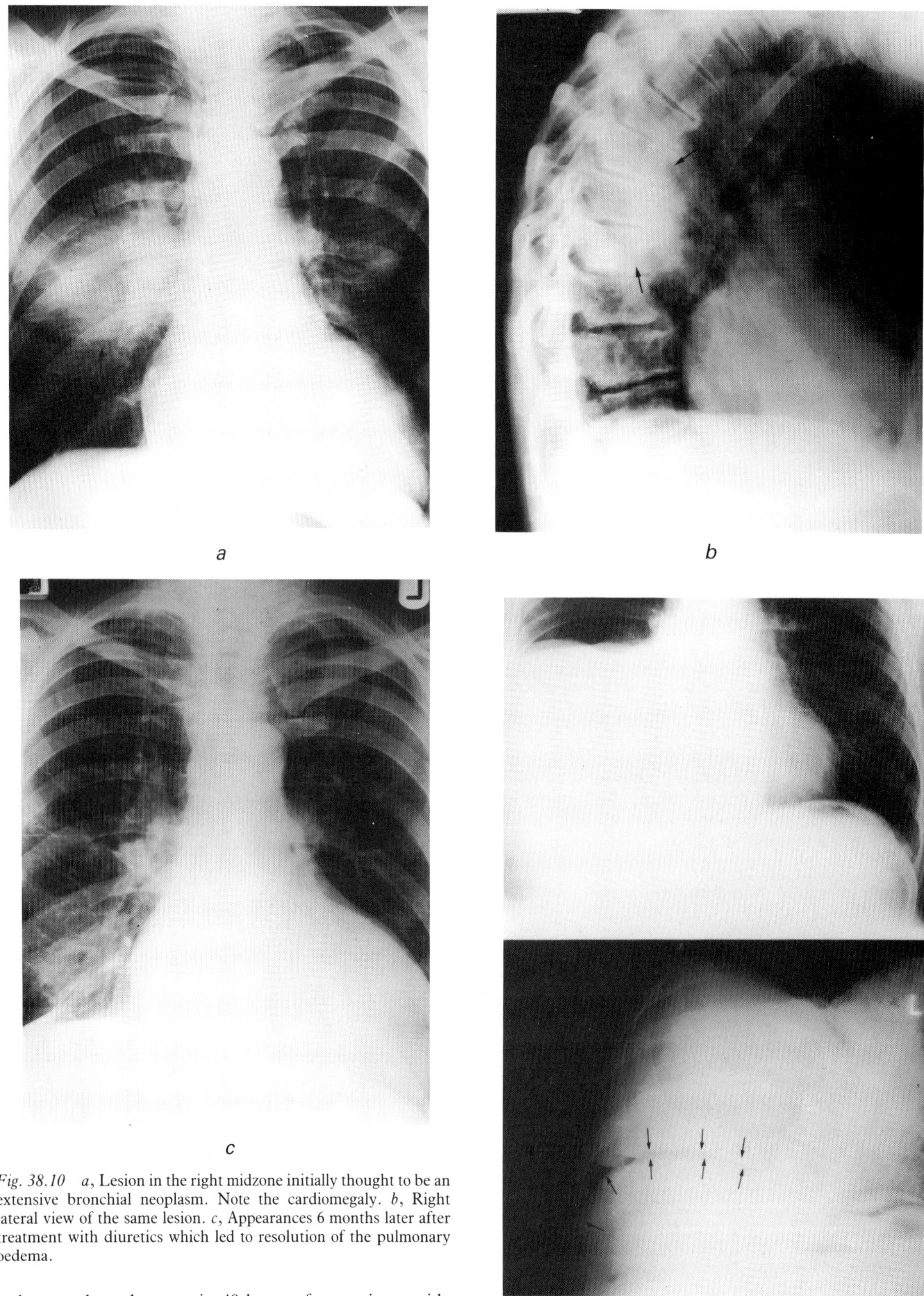

Fig. 38.10 *a*, Lesion in the right midzone initially thought to be an extensive bronchial neoplasm. Note the cardiomegaly. *b*, Right lateral view of the same lesion. *c*, Appearances 6 months later after treatment with diuretics which led to resolution of the pulmonary oedema.

Fig. 38.11 Value of pneumoperitoneum in defining supradiaphragmatic from infradiaphragmatic lesions. This patient had an infrapulmonary effusion.

and repeat bronchoscopy in 48 hours after corticosteroids and antibiotics may be necessary.

Two types of bronchoscope are available: (*a*) the rigid; and (*b*) the flexible fibroscope, and expertise in the use of

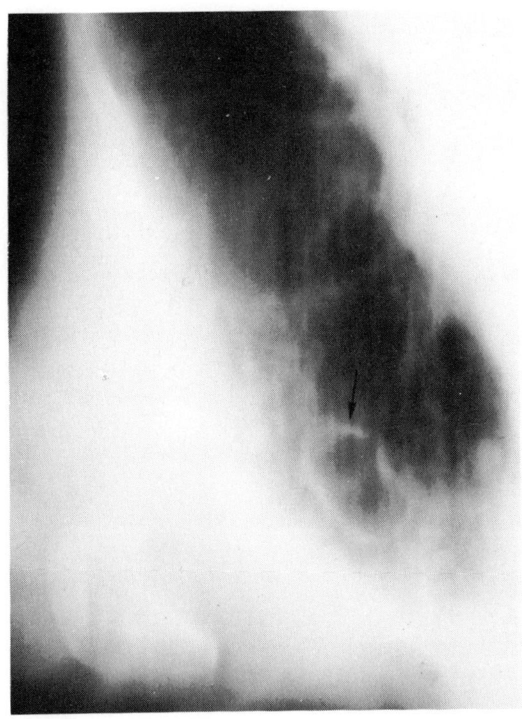

Fig. 38.12 Tomogram showing a cavitating lesion.

both is desirable (*Fig.* 38.16). The rigid instrument permits the taking of larger biopsies from accessible lesions, the better removal of secretions and the easier control of bleeding. Used in conjunction with the newer fibreoptic telescopes, which can be withdrawn for cleaning, it enables good visualization. The rigid instrument is essential for the removal of foreign bodies. The fibreoptic instrument has several advantages: (*a*) it can be passed transnasally at the bedside of severely ill patients with little distress; (*b*) it gives better visualization, particularly of the upper lobe and lingular bronchi; (*c*) it can be passed through an endotracheal tube in patients on ventilators for aspiration of secretions or diagnosis; and (*d*) its fine forceps may be safely passed transbronchially in order to biopsy solid peripheral or diffuse lung lesions. However, smearing of the lenses by blood or secretions may present problems. Although the fibroscope has increased the number of segmental bronchi seen, visualization is still limited to a circumscribed arc of 5–6 cm around each hilum and many peripheral lesions remain outwith the field of view (*Fig.* 38.17). Both instruments may be passed using either general or local anaesthesia depending on the facilities available and the skill of the operator.

Complications which are rarely serious include: (*a*) damage to teeth from the rigid instrument; (*b*) haemorrhage which is usually slight but biopsy of a vascular adenoma may present problems; (*c*) anoxia during and after the procedure as a result of: (i) obstruction by the bronchoscope; (ii) the effects of the sedation; and (iii) suppression of the cough reflex by the local anaesthesia; and (*d*) laryngeal oedema due to trauma or the use of too large an instrument (in children).

BIOPSY TECHNIQUES

Lung Biopsy

In diffuse lung disease a histological diagnosis may be important to the management of the case and several biopsy techniques are available. Transbronchial lung biopsy during fibreoptic bronchoscopy has the advantages of simplicity, permitting biopsies from different areas with few complications, but the biopsies are small which may make interpretation difficult. The trephine biopsy, using a high-speed drill, was introduced by Steel and can give good results in experienced hands but pneumothorax may be a problem. Several methods using percutaneous cutting needles (Tru-cut, Vim–Silverman) have been advocated although the incidence of complications (haemorrhage and pneumothorax) is higher. The diagnostic yield for each of these methods are roughly

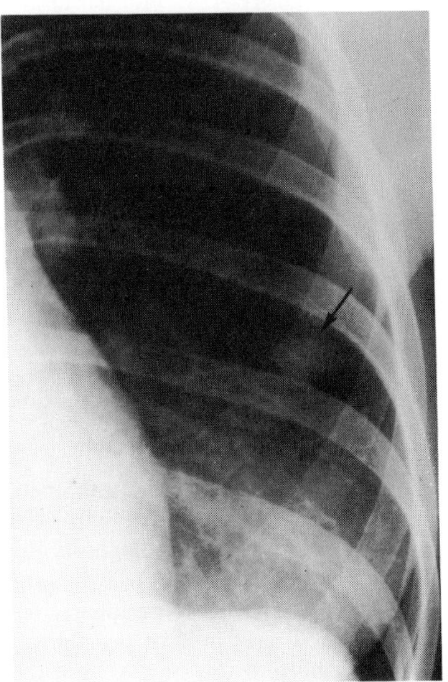

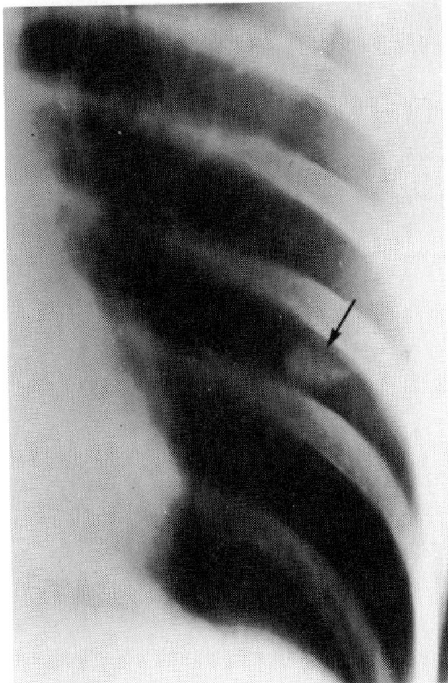

Fig. 38.13 Calcification in a tuberculoma, present in the PA film and obvious in the tomogram.

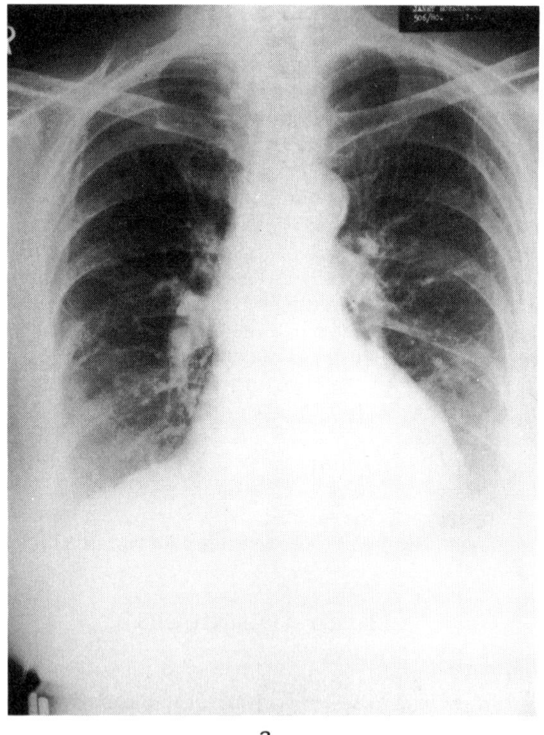

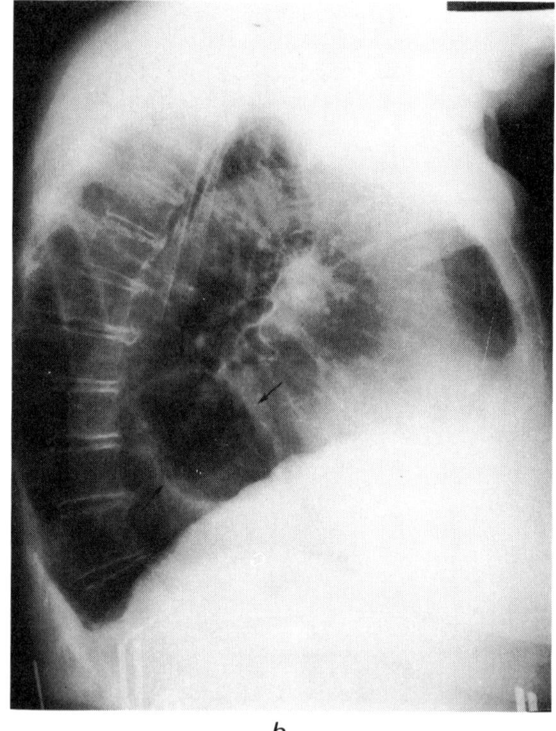

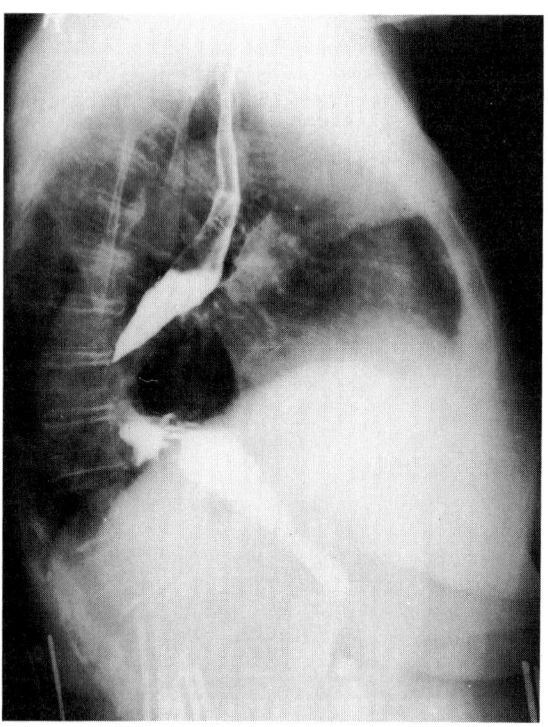

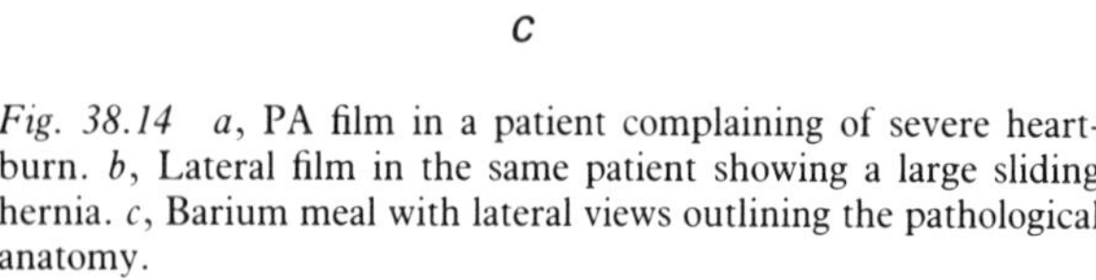
Fig. 38.14 *a*, PA film in a patient complaining of severe heartburn. *b*, Lateral film in the same patient showing a large sliding hernia. *c*, Barium meal with lateral views outlining the pathological anatomy.

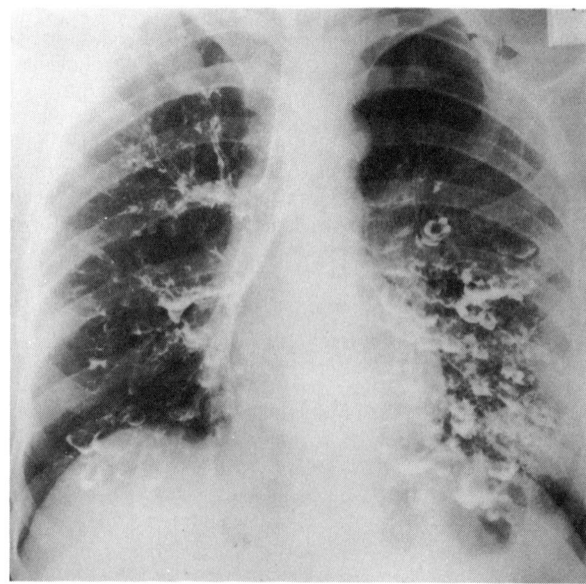
Fig. 38.15 Bilateral bronchogram showing extensive saccular bronchiectasis. (By courtesy of Dr Paul Grech.)

comparable. In difficult cases a thoractomy and open lung biopsy, taken from an area with obvious disease, will provide adequate tissue for diagnosis although accompanied by a recognizable morbidity.

The diagnosis of solid peripheral lesions beyond bronchoscopic view may present problems. At fibreoptic bronchoscopy a blind brush biopsy from the feeding segmental bronchus may give a cytological diagnosis or the flexible biopsy forceps may be screened into the lesion but this is

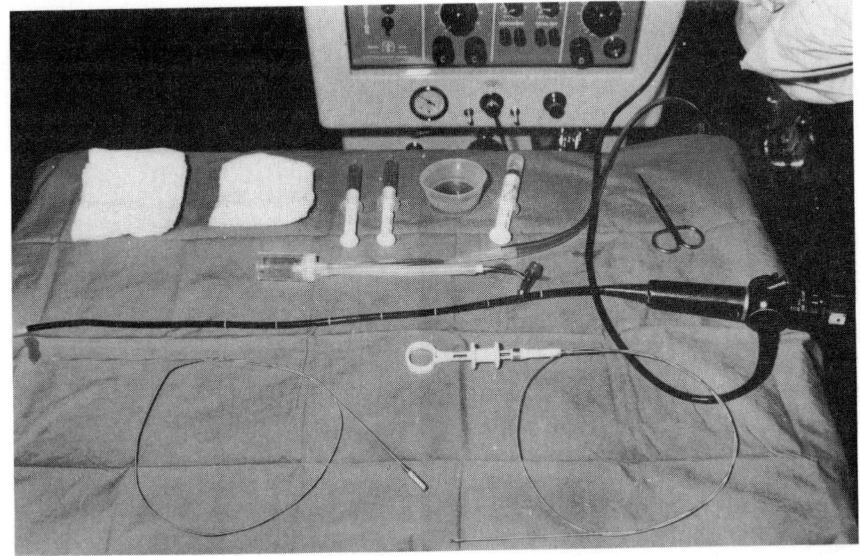

a

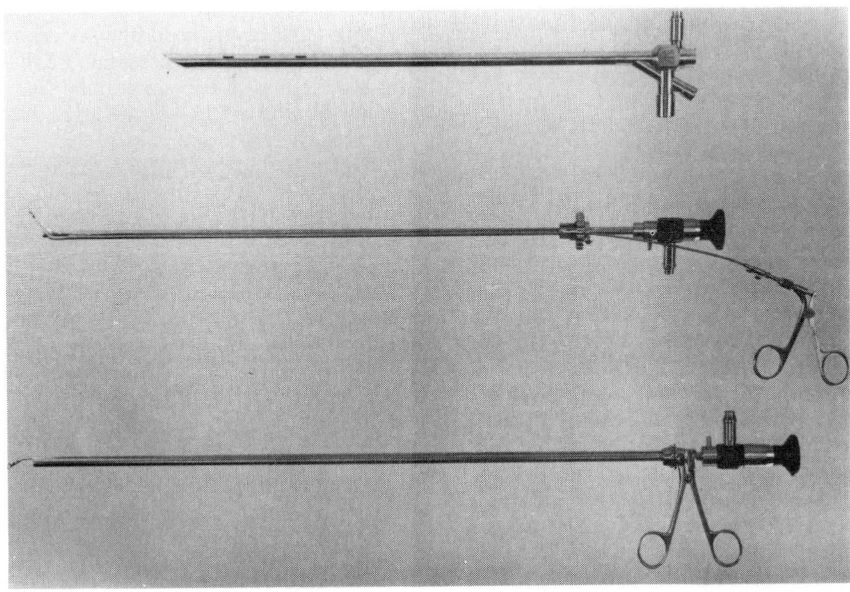

b

Fig. 38.16 *a*, *b*, Bronchoscopes and biopsy forceps.

often time consuming. An alternative approach is the aspiration needle biopsy which involves the percutaneous passage of a needle into the lesion under fluoroscopic control and the aspiration of material for cytological and histological examination. Complications include pneumothorax and slight haemoptysis but there is no evidence to suggest tumour spread along the needle tract. Thoracotomy and resection may be necessary if the diagnosis remains in doubt.

Pleural Biopsy

If a pleural effusion has a malignant or tuberculous aetiology then a pleural punch biopsy using an Abrams' needle (*Fig.* 38.18) may be diagnostic but the lack of specific histological features in other causes of a pleural effusion limits its value. The biopsy should only be performed in the presence of pleural fluid. Aspiration of fluid for cytology, biochemical analysis and bacteriological culture should be done concurrently. In the absence of fluid, solid pleural lesions may be biopsied using a Vim–Silverman or Menghini needle. If other methods fail thoracotomy and open pleural biopsy may be necessary.

Node Biopsy

The supraclavicular and axillary lymph nodes may be enlarged in some diseases which either arise in the lungs or have associated pulmonary abnormalities, e.g. bronchial

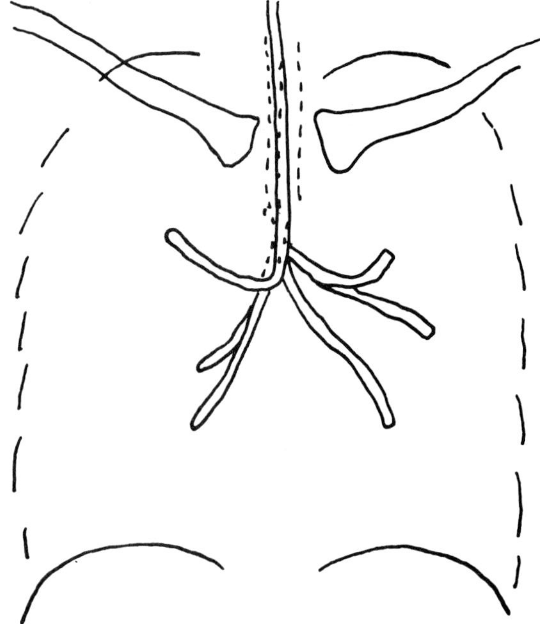

Fig. 38.17 A composite line drawing constructed from several radiographs taken during fibreoptic bronchoscopy with the tip of the bronchoscope in the most accessible bronchus to each lobe. (By courtesy of British Journal of Radiology.)

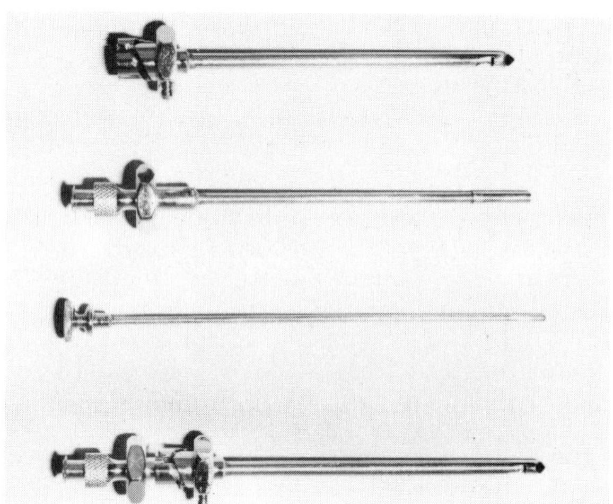

Fig. 38.18 The Abrams' needle.

neoplasm, tuberculosis, sarcoidosis, lymphoma when a node biopsy may be diagnostic. Recently, the percutaneous aspiration of material from these nodes for cytological examination has been introduced although it has not been fully evaluated. Routine scalene node biopsy in the preoperative assessment in malignancy is unhelpful.

Mediastinoscopy

Under general anaesthesia the superior mediastinum in the vicinity of the trachea is explored through a midline incision in the supraclavicular notch. Nodes from the subcarinal chain, both hilar groups and the paratracheal region or malignancy close to the trachea may be biopsied but lesions anterior to the great vessels, i.e. the thymus, are beyond reach. Encouraging results have been reported in tuberculosis, sarcoidosis, lymphoma and hilar or mediastinal malignancy. Mediastinoscopy has been used in the routine preoperative assessment in patients with malignancy when up to a third of cases were considered inoperable due to mediastinal node involvement at times on the contralateral side. Complications include haemorrhage, which may be severe, left recurrent laryngeal nerve palsy, surgical emphysema, pneumothorax and tumour seedling in the incision scar.

Mediastinotomy

Through a short vertical parasternal incision the anterior ends of the 2nd and 3rd ribs are resected, the internal mammary artery ligated and divided at either end of the wound and the mediastinal pleura displaced laterally, allowing inspection and biopsy of lesions in the paratracheal and hilar regions without the morbidity associated with thoracotomy. Lesions in the anterior and posterior mediastinum, hilar and paratracheal regions may be palpated and biopsied under direct vision without the possibility of excessive haemorrhage which can occur with mediastinoscopy. This may be invaluable in diagnosing mediastinal lesions and in the preoperative assessment of potentially resectable bronchial tumours when the finding of malignancy in frozen sections of hilar or mediastinal nodes may prevent further surgical intervention. Inspection of the pleural cavity and lung surface is also possible following introduction of an endoscope and collapse of the lung (double lumen tube) by the anaesthetist.

Thoracoscopy

The introduction of a thoracoscope into an artificially induced pneumothorax has been used to inspect and biopsy pleural lesions but it has never gained universal acceptance, thoracotomy being preferred. However, it may be of some value in the investigation of a pleural effusion when other methods have failed.

Cytology

While a histological diagnosis is preferable useful information may be obtained from the cytological examination of sputum, bronchial secretions or pleural fluid, provided the necessary expertise in the interpretation is available.

SPUTUM

Valuable information may be obtained by studying the quantity and macroscopic appearance of sputum. The degree of purulence, the presence, persistence, nature and amount of haemoptysis (pure blood, mixed with sputum, rusty sputum) or the appearance of casts, needs to be recorded. A stained smear of sputum is easy to prepare and may show the causal agent, irrespective of previous antibotic therapy, considerably in advance of the culture results, i.e. in tuberculosis. The film may also show eosinophils, asbestos bodies, *Pneumocystis carinii* or *Entamoeba histolytica*.

Sputum culture, as well as demonstrating the causal agents, will indicate their sensitivity to standard antibiotic therapy. The suspected diagnosis should be given to the bacteriologist as special procedures may be necessary, i.e. specific culture media for tuberculous and fungal infections and anaerobic culture for lung abscesses or actinomycosis. Laryngeal swabs and gastric or bronchial aspiration may be used to obtain suitable specimens.

SKIN TESTING

The tuberculin skin tests have proved valuable in assisting diagnosis, tracing contacts and in epidemiological studies of tuberculosis. The three methods used, the Mantoux, Heaf and Tine tests, all involve the intradermal implantation of tubercular protein which induces a delayed hypersensitivity reaction in patients who have had either a BCG vaccination or a past or present infection with the tubercle bacillus. The resultant induration is measured and must be above a preset level to indicate an infection, i.e. a Mantoux greater than 10 mm by 10 mm, as mild non-specific reactions are frequent. There is a delay of 3–8 weeks between infection and the test becoming positive. Patients with impairment of Type IV immunity, i.e. infants, the elderly, those with lymphoma, sufferers from the acquired immune deficiency syndrome (AIDS) or patients on steroids may have a negative test in the presence of rampant tuberculosis.

The formation of a sarcoid granuloma 6 weeks after the intradermal injection of sarcoid material (Kveim Test) can confirm the diagnosis of sarcoidosis although the test is negative in 25% of cases. As steroids suppress the reaction the Kveim test is best performed before starting treatment. Delayed hypersensitivity skin tests may also be of value in suspected cases of histoplasmosis, blastomycosis, hydatid disease, berylliosis or coccidioidomycosis.

An immediate Type I reaction (wheal and flare) on skin testing to commonly encountered or specific antigens may indicate an allergic basis for asthma, particularly in children. An immediate (Type I) or delayed (Type III) reaction to *Aspergillus fumigatus* may be helpful in distinguishing between the different clinical responses to this fungus.

COMPUTERIZED TOMOGRAPHY

Since 1975 computerized tomography of the thorax has been used increasingly for the investigation of chest wall, pleural, pulmonary and mediastinal abnormalities. Its clinical impact has been less impressive in the thorax than in the brain, abdomen and pelvis, largely due to the relative accuracy of routine chest radiography. Several clinical situations have now been identified in which computerized tomography provides useful diagnostic information.

The various mediastinal structures are particularly well separated, the aorta, the great arteries and veins, the pulmonary arteries and the trachea and bronchi, usually being identified without difficulty (*Fig.* 38.19*a*, *b*, *c*). If there is any suggestion of abnormality of the aorta, intravenous infusion of contrast medium will opacify the vessel. The ability of computerized tomography to evaluate the density of a mediastinal mass will be of value in distinguishing between cystic and solid lesions and between tissues of different density, such as fat and tumour. It has considerable value in the identification of mediastinal lymphadenopathy and may thus enable the clinician to assess quantitatively the effect of treatment in conditions like lymphoma. It is not capable of distinguishing between lymphadenopathy due to secondary spread and reactive hyperplasia which limits its usefulness in the preoperative assessment of bronchial carcinoma.

The place of computerized tomography in the investigation of parenchymal lung disease has not yet been fully evaluated although it is possible to identify pulmonary parenchyma, intrapulmonary vessels and normal bronchi. It certainly provides a more sensitive method for detecting pulmonary metastasis than conventional radiography. This, however, will only affect patient management when a lung tumour is discovered for the first time or where further apparently malignant nodules are discovered in a patient who was thought previously to have only one. It is, therefore, particularly suitable for the investigation of a patient for whom excisional surgery is planned for an apparent solitary lung metastasis. It can also be used in the situation where a patient has positive sputum cytology but no radiological or endoscopic evidence of where in the lung the primary is situated.

Other clinical situations where it may provide helpful information are: (*a*) in the investigation of a solitary pulmonary nodule, where previously unsuspected calcification has been demonstrated, even when conventional tomography has failed to do so; (*b*) in the diagnosis of pleural shadows when effusions and plaque are particularly well visualized (*Fig.* 38.19*d*); and (*c*) in showing the extent and degree of invasion of a malignant mesothelioma.

SCANNING TECHNIQUES

Lung Scans

Radio-isotope scanning has been used to study and quantify regional ventilation and perfusion in normal and diseased lungs. While a useful adjuvant in selected cases, such scans are rarely diagnostic by themselves.

Two methods are in common usage for studying perfusion:

1. Microspheres of human albumin usually labelled with technectium-99^{m} (half-life of 6 h) and large enough to lodge in the pulmonary capillaries, are injected intravenously, the resultant scan reflecting the pattern of perfusion. Within 8 h the particles have been broken down and removed from the pulmonary circulation. Radiation is minimal.
2. When the insoluble, inert gas xenon-133 (half-life of 5 days) is injected intravenously in saline, it completely diffuses into the alveolar gas during its first passage through the lungs and an immediate gamma scan will show the pattern of perfusion. The xenon is rapidly excreted.

Ventilation may be studied by the inhalation of krypton-81^{m} (half-life of 13 sec) or an isotope of xenon (133, 125 or 127), both gases being inert and insoluble. Krypton gives better definition but the short half-life limits its usefulness. A scan taken after a single deep inspiration will show the initial distribution of inspired air. Serial scans while breathing the gas until it is evenly distributed (wash-in) and again throughout its elimination will give valuable information about the pattern of ventilation and the rate of filling and emptying of poorly ventilated areas.

The rapid excretion of xenon allows sequential ventilation and perfusion scans to be taken which may then be compared and quantified to give regional ventilation-perfusion ratios. When standing erect there is a greater blood flow to the bases with proportionally more air going to the upper zones giving a higher ventilation-perfusion ratio at the apex than at the base. The pattern alters when lying down as more blood goes to the dependent areas.

The volume of the lungs, together with the low energy of the radiation emitted, necessitates scanning in several planes if maximum information is to be obtained. The size of the heart and mediastinal structures affects the appearances in the anterior scans while the largest volume of lung is seen on the posterior views.

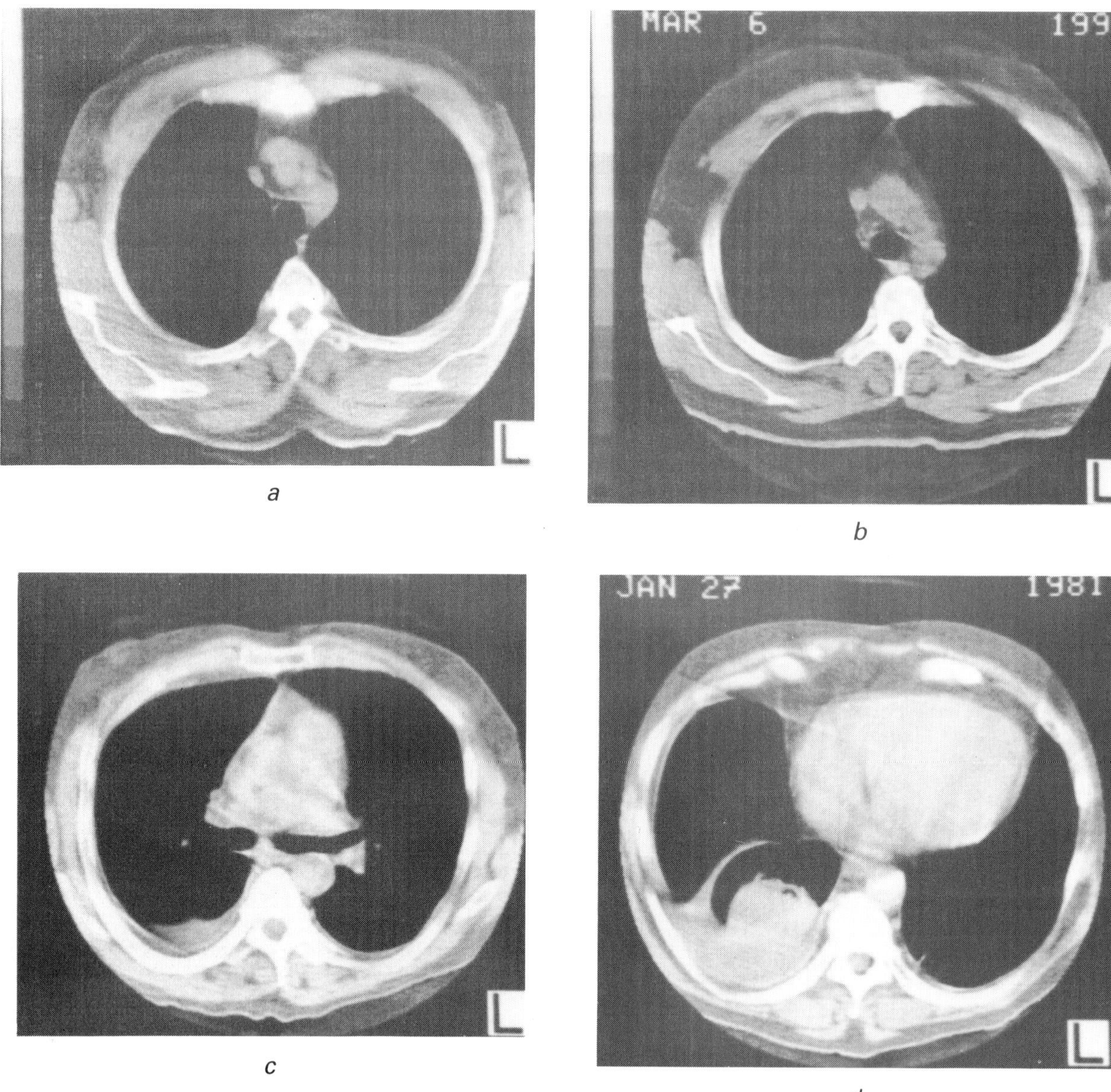

Fig. 38.19 CT thoracic scan at various levels. *a*, CT scan through the upper mediastinum showing clear lung fields, a normal trachea and normal great vessels. *b*, CT scan showing normal aortic arch, normal trachea and clear lung fields. *c*, CT scan at the level of the tracheal bifurcation showing the main carina (normal), the descending thoracic aorta behind the left main bronchus and a right-sided pleural effusion lying in the paravertebral gutter. *d*, CT scan just above the diaphragm showing the heart and descending aorta; there is a large right-sided pleural effusion in the paravertebral gutter with fluid extending into the oblique fissure and considerable shrinkage of the right lower lobe.

A recent chest radiograph, preferably on the day of the scan, and a full clinical history are essential for the accurate interpretation of ventilation and perfusion scans. The appearances in various clinical states are summarized in *Table* 38.3.

If a pulmonary embolus is suspected several points are important if the scans are to be correctly interpreted.

1. A normal perfusion scan virtually excludes the diagnosis.
2. In a patient with a normal chest radiograph a filling defect on the perfusion scan is usually diagnostic.
3. When there is radiological evidence of collapse or consolidation it is essential to have both ventilation and perfusion scans.
4. It is difficult and often impossible to make the diagnosis in the presence of significant emphysema.
5. Serial scans may be helpful in demonstrating fresh emboli or the resolution of existing ones.

When considering surgery for bullous emphysema or bronchial carcinoma the function of the remaining lung is important and lung scans may give valuable information. If a child is suspected of having inhaled a foreign body, but the radiograph is normal, xenon ventilation and perfusion scans may be diagnostic. In the presence of a right-to-left anatomical shunt some microspheres bypass the lungs lodging (transiently and without causing damage) in the brain, liver, spleen and kidney and the radiation from these organs has been used as a measure of the size of the shunt. Chest

Table 38.3 Isotope scanning in pulmonary disease

Disease	*Perfusion scan*	*Ventilation scan*
1. *Pulmonary thrombo-embolism*	Segmental defect often larger than any radiological lesion	80%—normal 10%—smaller and 10%—larger ventilatory changes compared with perfusion defect
2. *Pneumonia*		
a. Bronchial	Defects less than radiological change	Ventilation defects equal to perfusion defects
b. Lobar	Defects the same as radiological changes	
3. *Emphysema*		
a. Generalized	Diffuse patchy filling defects	Poor ventilation over same areas
b. Bullae	Large defect over affected area	Poor ventilation with delayed filling of affected area
4. *Foreign bodies*	The initial xenon scan is normal but thereafter the xenon is retained in the affected area	Poor or absent filling of affected area
5. *Right-to-left anatomical shunts*	Microspheres give normal pattern but less intense	Normal

deformity sufficient to impair respiratory movement will affect the findings. Lung scans are of no value in the interstitial lung diseases, e.g. fibrosing alveolitis, sarcoidosis.

Aerosol Lung Scans

The inhalation of radioactive particles from an aerosol (usually containing technetium-99^{m}) will give some information about ventilation but is likely to be most useful in studying mucociliary clearance in health and disease although the evaluation of the method is incomplete.

Scanning of Other Organs

Bronchial carcinomas, particularly the small cell anaplastic (oat-cell) tumour, often metastasize early, and staging of the tumour is becoming increasingly important when planning treatment. When asymptomatic, recourse to bone, brain and liver scanning may demonstrate hidden deposits and prevent unnecessary thoracotomy.

Any cause of rapid bone metabolism will show up as an area of increased activity on a *bone scan*. If coned X-rays of the area show no evidence of benign disease, a 'hot spot' is usually indicative of a bony metastasis, the scan often picking up the deposit many weeks before the appearance of any radiological abnormality. Bone scans are positive in 10% of bronchial neoplasms where there is no evidence of spread clinically, radiologically or on any other scans. A negative bone scan does not exclude bony secondaries.

Bone scanning will establish a metastatic cause for bone pain permitting palliative radiotherapy or show the extent of bony involvement when there is radiological evidence of bone metastases. Previous radiotherapy causes decreased uptake while serial scans have shown regression of deposits with chemotherapy in breast and prostatic tumours but not as yet with bronchial neoplasms. Occasionally pulmonary metastases from an osteogenic sarcoma take up the isotope and appear on the scan.

The radio-isotope (DTPA) *brain scan* may give corroborative evidence of a metastatic deposit in the presence of a neurological deficit, i.e. personality change or monoplegia, but the appearances may be confused with a cerebral vascular accident. The scans are most helpful when there are multiple discrete peripheral deposits. The CT scan and magnetic resonance imaging give better resolution, being capable of defining small asymptomatic secondary deposits and distinguishing between metastases and other cerebral space-occupying lesions. Occasionally a cerebral abscess complicates chronic pulmonary sepsis, i.e. bronchiectasis, when a CT scan may be helpful.

A radio-isotope liver scan rarely shows evidence of hepatic secondaries unless the liver function tests, and in particular the alkaline phosphatase are deranged. Deposits bigger than 1·5 cm may be visualized, but by this stage hepatic metastases are often detectable clinically. Ultrasound liver scanning is more sensitive and a patient with an abnormal isotope liver scan should have the findings confirmed by an ultrasound scan which will distinguish between cystic and solid lesions. An upper abdominal CT scan may give useful information regarding the presence of hepatic and adrenal secondaries in cases of potentially operable bronchial carcinoma. A single solid lesion visible on a liver scan may be biopsied in order to obtain a histological diagnosis. In a difficult case with abnormal scans laparoscopy with inspection and biopsy of the liver may be contemplated prior to thoracotomy being undertaken.

Respiratory problems may complicate amoebic or bacterial liver abscesses while pulmonary hydatid disease is often associated with hepatic involvement and isotope and ultrasound liver and upper abdominal CT scans may be helpful in such cases. A liver biopsy may be diagnostic in sarcoidosis, lymphoma and in disseminated miliary tuberculosis of the elderly but it should always be preceded by a liver scan.

Thyroid Scanning

This may be helpful in diagnosing retrosternal or ectopic thyroid tissue within the chest.

MISCELLANEOUS INVESTIGATIONS

Biochemical tests are of limited value in respiratory disease. As yet there is no simple marker to help in the diagnosis and follow-up of bronchial carcinomas. Although some bronchial tumours, particularly the small cell anaplastic type exhibit endocrine function with the secretion of hormones such as ACTH and vasopressin, assays of these hormones are not generally available to enable their use in the management of these cases. Urinary 5-hydroxyindole acetic acid may be elevated in a carcinoid bronchial adenoma. Hypercalcaemia and hypercalciuria can occur in sarcoidosis, a high ESR in myelomatosis and hypogamma-globulinaemia in recurrent respiratory infections. The protein content of a pleural effusion distinguishes between exudates and transudates.

Raised serum antibodies to respiratory viruses, mycoplasma or rickettsia may be helpful in diagnosing an atypical or viral pneumonia. A positive antinuclear factor, LE cells or rheumatoid factor are found in some cases of fibrosing alveolitis. Precipitating antibodies to specific organic antigens can determine the causal agents and confirm the diagnosis in extrinsic allergic alveolitis, e.g. farmer's lung. Precipitins to *Aspergillus fumigatus* are found in an aspergilloma.

The ECG is rarely diagnostic in respiratory disease although right ventricular hypertrophy and strain may occur in cor pulmonale or in massive pulmonary embolus.

Further Reading

Collins J. V., Dhillon D. P. and Goldstraw B. (1987) *Practical Bronchoscopy*. Oxford, Blackwell Scientific Publications.

Felson, B. (1973) *Chest Roentgenology*. Philadelphia, Saunders.

Von Hayek H. (1960) *The Human Lung*, trans. V. E. Krahl. New York, Hafner.

Kent E. M. and Blades B. (1942) The surgical anatomy of the pulmonary lobes. *J. Thorac. Surg.* **12**, 18.

Stradling P. (1986) *Diagnostic Bronchoscopy*, 5th ed. Edinburgh, Churchill Livingstone.

West J. B. (1985) *Respiratory Physiology—The Essentials*, 3rd ed. Baltimore, Williams & Wilkins.

39 *Pulmonary Infections*

R. A. Clark

BRONCHIECTASIS

Bronchiectasis is defined as chronic irreversible dilatation of the large or medium-sized bronchi (4th to 9th generations) which can be shown on bronchography and may be confirmed by examination of resected or post-mortem lung specimens. It is not a single entity, there being several causal mechanisms with differing clinical and radiological presentations. While the details of each pathological process are not fully understood two factors are common to them all;

1. An outward tension applied to the exterior of the bronchial walls, and
2. A weakening of the bronchial walls.

1. The outward tension may develop in several ways.

a. During acute respiratory infections in infancy the smaller bronchi may become blocked by mucopus with collapse of the lung parenchyma distal to the obstruction. The resultant loss of lung volume increases the tension in the unaffected areas, with the application of stretch to the outside of the bronchial walls which, if damaged, will dilate. In the adult the bronchi are larger and less easily blocked while gas exchange develops between alveoli, through the alveolar pores, permitting the ventilation of affected areas from healthy neighbouring tissue and preventing lung collapse.

b. Chronic suppurative pneumonias, including some adenoviral and influenzal infections in childhood, grumble on with progressive destruction of the smaller bronchi and lung parenchyma producing a loss of lung volume with increased tension and stretch applied to the bronchial walls in the absence of any significant bronchial obstruction.

c. The obstruction of a major bronchus initially causes segmental or lobar collapse which is soon followed by the accumulation of fluid in the affected bronchi and alveoli which tends to restore the lung volume. If the obstruction is not relieved quickly suppuration invariably supervenes with considerable tissue destruction and healing by fibrosis, both of which increase the tension applied to the bronchial walls in the affected area.

2. Weakening of the wall results from damage to bronchial muscle or elastic tissue. The usual cause is infection which invades the wall with destruction of both elements, often occurring as part of the same process which produced the damage to the peripheral lung tissue. In some bronchiectatic cysts there may be little evidence of any normal bronchial architecture although the damage is usually less severe.

In Chagas' disease, when the causal organism, *Trypanosoma cruzi*, dies toxins are released which destroy the bronchial parasympathetic ganglia causing a loss of bronchomotor tone, a factor which has been implicated in the bronchiectasis complicating this disorder.

Classification

Traditionally, bronchiectasis has been classified according to the type of bronchial dilatation seen on bronchography, e.g. cylindrical, saccular or cystic, but this has proved unsatisfactory. Although attempts at a classification based on clinical and pathological findings are incomplete the following scheme forms a framework for discussion.

1. Postinfective bronchiectasis
   a. Follicular
   b. Saccular
2. Postcollapse bronchiectasis
   a. Proximal obstruction
   b. Distal obstruction
3. Post-tuberculous bronchiectasis
4. Allergic bronchiectasis
5. Congenital bronchiectasis
   a. Arrested development
   b. Cilial dysfunction
6. Immune deficiency syndromes
7. Pseudobronchiectasis

1a. Postinfective Follicular Bronchiectasis

This invariably develops in children under the age of 7 with symptoms occurring before puberty. Two-thirds of cases follow measles or whooping cough while grumbling adenoviral or influenzal infections account for many others. Pathologically the bronchi show cylindrical dilatations with thickened walls, peribronchial fibrosis, peripheral destruction and collapse, a generalized lymphocytic infiltration, epithelial ulceration and fibrous thickening of the pleural and interlobar septa.

1b. Postinfective Saccular Bronchiectasis

In this there is often a history of a severe bronchopneumonia in childhood although the symptoms develop much later. Bronchiectatic and normal bronchi are interspersed within the same lobe and although the smaller bronchi of the involved segments are destroyed collateral ventilation between normal and diseased areas leads to compensatory emphysema in the affected alveoli so that there is little loss of lung volume. There are numerous, pus-filled, saccular dilatations in continuity with medium-sized bronchi. The bronchial architecture of these cysts is completely disrupted, their walls consisting of fibrous granulation tissue with an ulcerated squamous epithelium.

2. *Postcollapse Bronchiectasis*

a. The obstruction of a segmental or lobar bronchus by a bronchial neoplasm, foreign body, adenoma or hilar gland enlargement (usually tuberculous), if not relieved quickly, is followed by suppuration, abscess formation, fibrosis and collapse within the affected area. The larger bronchi lying distal to the obstruction become bronchiectatic presenting as dilated, pus-filled, 'finger-like' swellings.

Even if the obstruction is relieved and the lobe or segment re-expands, e.g. following the removal of a foreign body, or the resolution of tuberculous glands, bronchiectasis may still develop as a result of parenchymal and bronchial damage which occurred during the obstruction (middle lobe syndrome).

b. Rarely, bronchiectasis develops after a viral or atypical pneumonia in adults if there has been peripheral collapse due to diffuse obstruction of the smaller bronchi by thick mucopus with coincidental damage to the walls of the proximal bronchi.

3. *Post-tuberculous Bronchiectasis*

Lung destruction and fibrosis are characteristic features of pulmonary tuberculosis resulting in contraction of a lobe or segment with distortion of the proximal bronchi. When the tuberculous process involves the bronchial walls (tuberculous endobronchitis) the resultant suppuration, caseation and fibrosis weaken the bronchi, predisposing them to bronchiectasis. These changes are most frequently seen in the upper lobes where they are often asymptomatic.

4. *Allergic Bronchiectasis*

In allergic bronchopulmonary aspergillosis damage occurs at the sites of impaction of mucus plugs. These plugs may contain small quantities of the fungus, *Aspergillus fumigatus*, which provokes a destructive allergic reaction within the bronchial walls. There is an associated collapse of the distal lung. After treatment with corticosteroids the obstruction and collapse resolve but areas of bronchiectasis remain. Future episodes occurring in different segments result in bronchiectasis scattered throughout the medium-sized bronchi of both lungs.

5. *Congenital Bronchiectasis*

a. Congenital bronchiectasis resulting from the *arrested development* of the smaller bronchi and alveoli undoubtedly occurs but its frequency is disputed. Symptoms begin in early childhood. The affected lobe or lung is small, adherent to the chest wall and supplied by hypoplastic pulmonary arteries. The proximal bronchi while containing their normal complement of elastic tissue, muscle and cartilage present as dilated tubular structures. There is little recognizable parenchymal tissue.

In a sequestrated lung segment the bronchi are bronchiectatic.

Arrested parenchymal development between birth and 8 years may produce unilateral emphysema (MacLeod's syndrome) in which bronchiectasis features prominently.

b. Cilial Dysfunction

A hereditary defect of cilial ultrastructure has been found in patients with Kartagener's syndrome (bronchiectasis, sinusitis, male infertility and transposition of the viscera). Dysfunction of cilia interferes with the activity of the respiratory ciliated epithelium and mucus blanket (mucociliary clearance) predisposing to recurrent infections and diffuse bronchiectasis.

6. *Immune Deficiency Syndromes*

Any condition which leads to a reduction in immunity, including the acquired immune deficiency syndrome (AIDS) leaves the patient open to recurrent respiratory infection of varying severity. The overall result of which is to cause a loss of peripheral lung tissue and a weakening of the bronchial walls. Treatment is mainly supportive.

7. *Pseudo-bronchiectasis*

Some respiratory infections produce viscous pus which obstructs the smaller bronchi causing alveolar collapse. A bronchogram in the acute phase may reveal dilatation of the proximal bronchi which return to normal size with resolution of the infection leaving no evidence of permanent damage (pseudo-bronchiectasis).

General

Several years may elapse between the causal illness and the onset of symptoms and although the affected bronchi are all damaged in the same episode, the presentation of overt disease may vary between segments, clinical symptoms developing in some areas only after resection or collapse in others. There is no evidence to suggest that the 'spill-over' of pus from bronchiectatic segments produces bronchiectasis in other areas even though it may predispose to progressive bronchitis.

Bronchiectasis is multilobar in 70% of cases and often involves both lungs. The posterior basal segment of the left lower lobe is most frequently affected while the anterior and apical segments of that lobe are often spared. When the lingula is involved there is usually concomitant disease in the left lower lobe.

Defence Mechanisms

Bronchiectasis disrupts the bronchial defence mechanisms in a variety of ways:

1. The rhythmic expansion and relaxation of the bronchi so important in the movement of secretions up the bronchial tree and which is dependent on the elasticity of the bronchial walls is impaired in bronchiectatic segments due to the destruction of elastic tissue.
2. The ciliated epithelium is often ulcerated or replaced by squamous metaplasia interfering with the action of the mucus blanket (mucociliary clearance) essential for the removal of inhaled particles.
3. Bronchomotor tone is lost or impaired due to inhibition or destruction of the bronchial muscle. Where the normal bronchial architecture is destroyed the resultant thin-walled cysts lack support and may dilate during expiration.
4. During normal coughing the bronchi narrow and the intrabronchial pressure rises helping to propel material into and up the trachea. Cinefluorographic studies have shown a normal cough response in cylindrical bronchiectasis but in cystic or saccular disease the proximal portions of the affected segments may collapse with dilatation and sputum retention distally.

5. Whether the patient is standing, sitting or lying the effect of gravity is to retain secretions in the lower lobes. In the presence of basal bronchiectasis this action is an additional factor in the retention of secretions. Gravity may be put to useful effect during postural drainage.

Unless the secretions produced and retained in bronchiectatic segments are effectively drained they form an ideal culture medium for bacterial growth.

Functional Effects

Emphysema

Compensatory emphysema may develop as a result of the causal illness by one of two mechanisms:

1. If there is significant parenchymal destruction and most of the bronchi in an area are affected, segmental or lobar collapse may ensue in which case the alveoli in the surrounding lung will dilate to fill the void.
2. When bronchiectatic and normal bronchi are interspersed within a lobe, then even if there is destruction of the smaller bronchi lung collapse may be prevented by collateral ventilation between alveoli in normal and diseased areas. Gas exchange occurs freely during inspiration but is impeded on expiration so that the alveoli in affected areas become progressively distended.

In addition, the grumbling infective bronchitis which results from spillage of infective material from bronchiectatic segments into otherwise normal lungs may lead to progressive parenchymal destruction with loss of lung volume in the affected area and secondary compensatory emphysema in the adjacent lung tissue.

Bronchopulmonary Blood Flow

In the presence of grumbling inflammation the bronchial arteries hypertrophy and the blood flow through them is greatly increased. As the arteries arise directly from the aorta the blood within them is at systemic pressure. As a result of these factors haemoptysis of varying degrees is a common feature. At the same time the anastomoses between the bronchial and pulmonary arteries enlarge, allowing extensive shunting of systemic blood into the pulmonary circulation and increasing the pulmonary arterial pressure which reduces the pulmonary blood flow and diverts desaturated blood away from the diseased area. Large shunts may considerably increase left ventricular output occasionally leading to left ventricular hypertrophy and cardiac decompensation.

Ventilation-perfusion Ratios

Studies of regional lung function suggest that both ventilation and perfusion are reduced in the affected areas. When a whole lung is involved, with the other side functioning normally, the diseased area may receive a third of the ventilation while contributing less than 10% to oxygen uptake. The overall lung function depends on the amount of lung involved, the degree of accompanying bronchitis, emphysema or asthma, and the age and smoking habits of the patient. Lung function may be significantly improved following curative resection.

Clinical Features

Some cases remain asymptomatic, only being picked-up on routine chest radiography or during post-mortem examination. Many patients complain of cough with sputum production going back to childhood. This may occur for 2–3 weeks after a 'cold' or be present every day with increased severity during exacerbations. The cough is worse in the mornings and is aggravated by running, laughing, stooping or eating. Patients often sleep on their affected side so as to reduce nocturnal symptoms. The daily sputum volume varies, at times exceeding 200 ml and may be doubled with inpatient physiotherapy and postural drainage. The sputum volume and colour are important in assessing the severity and activity of the disease. In severe cases the production of large quantities of foul-smelling sputum may interfere with the patient's social life.

Bronchiectasis may present as a recurrent pneumonia and pleurisy involving the same area with associated malaise, fever and flu-like symptoms. Chronic parenchymal suppuration often produces a gnawing ache over the affected area with failure to thrive in children, and cachexia, weight loss and malaise in adults.

Blood-streaked sputum is common in adults but rare in childhood. Pure haemoptysis, often intermittent and at times severe, without an obvious cause, may be the presenting feature in 'dry bronchiectasis' which is often associated with limited disease, i.e. middle lobe. The haemoptysis may result from the erosion of a calcified hilar gland (broncholith) through the bronchial wall.

The physical findings vary from 'normal' to extreme emaciation with a multiplicity of signs although the latter is rare nowadays. Coarse crepitations in the same area over several months or during recurrent chest infections, at times associated with a pleural rub, are characteristic of the infective form. The features of collapse, consolidation or fibrosis may be superimposed. Finger clubbing occurs but is not a constant finding even in advanced disease (*Fig.* 39.1). Wheeze, reversible to bronchodilators, may predominate and needs to be distinguished from asthma. The degree of dyspnoea and wheeze usually reflects the extent of the associated bronchitis and emphysema. In severe cases there may be cyanosis, laboured respirations with use of the accessory muscles and right heart failure.

Chronic sinusitis often complicates bronchiectasis being particularly troublesome in advanced cases. Brain abscesses, although a classic complication, are now uncommon. In severe cases amyloidosis may develop and periodic checks for proteinuria and hepatosplenomegaly backed up by rectal biopsy are advisable.

In the majority of cases (93%) postero-anterior and lateral chest radiographs, supplemented by tomography where indicated, show abnormalities which, taken in conjunction with the history and clinical findings, suggest bronchiectasis. The more obvious changes are:

1. *Crowding of the lung markings* (often behind the heart), with associated 'tramlining' (tubular shadows). If patent, the thickened walls of the dilated bronchi are separated by air-filled spaces but in the presence of excessive secretions a banding effect with rounded lower margins is observed.
2. *Hairline cystic shadows* (1–2 cm) occur in 13% of cases and in the presence of excessive secretions fluid levels may be seen (*Fig.* 39.2).
3. *Persistent collapse or fibrosis of a lobe or lung.* If the affected area lies behind the heart it may not be clearly visible unless a penetrated PA film is taken although an increased radiotranslucency from compensatory emphysema in the left upper zone may be seen.
4. *Recurrent pneumonic shadowing* at the same site, clearing between infections.

Less obvious changes include: (*a*) partial collapse of a lung or lobe with an elevated hemidiaphragm, mediastinal

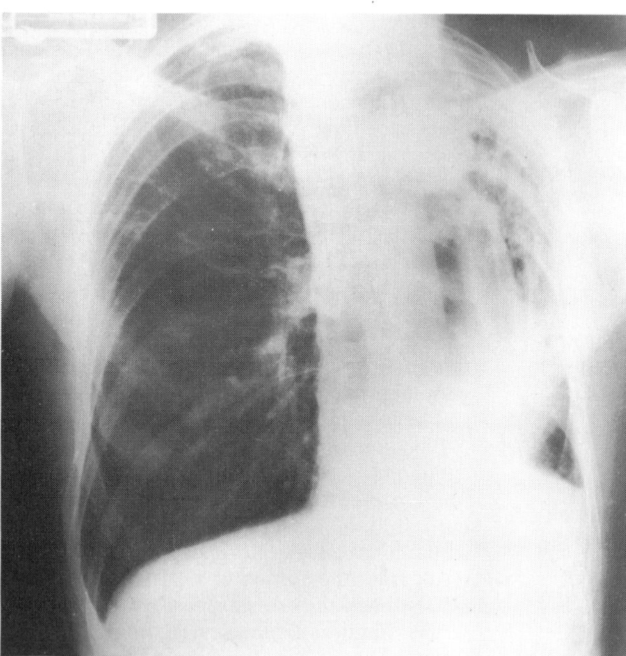

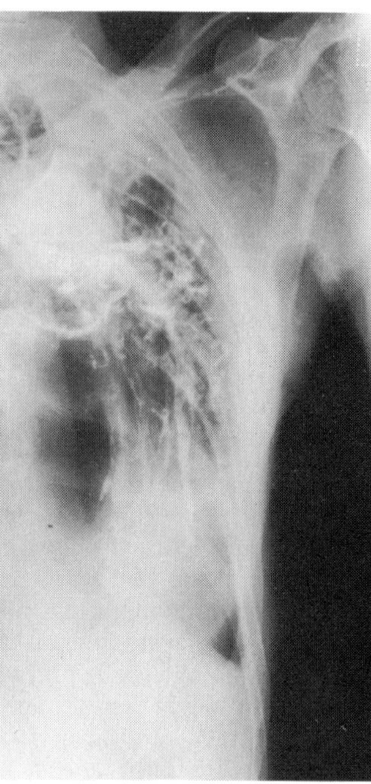

Fig. 39.1 Contracted fibrotic left lung with bronchiectatic change from previous tuberculosis.

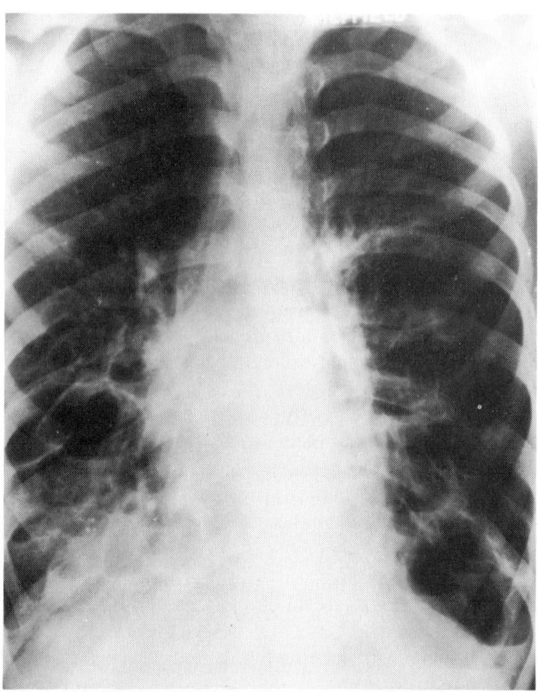

Fig. 39.2 PA chest film showing extensive ring shadows throughout both lower lobes; several of the ring shadows show fluid levels representing saccular bronchiectasis. (By courtesy of Dr Paul Grech.)

shift or altered position of the interlobar fissures, (*b*) small pulmonary arteries feeding the bronchiectatic segment, (*c*) localized emphysema, and (*d*) pleural thickening overlying a diseased area.

Bronchography may be necessary to confirm the diagnosis, the technique used depending on the experience of the investigator. For good bronchograms adequate preparation is essential which may mean a short spell in hospital for intensive physiotherapy, postural drainage and chemotherapy, followed by full explanation of the procedure and adequate premedication. In the presence of excessive secretions bronchoscopy to remove sputum and spray the bronchial tree with local anaesthetic, often ensures better results. The smaller the airways the greater the risks and bronchography is rarely justified under the age of 3. In children, general anaesthesia and endotracheal intubation are essential, with careful observations after the procedure in case acute airways obstruction should develop.

The right lung should be examined first with careful positioning to ensure complete filling of all segmental bronchi and postero-anterior and right lateral films taken. After filling the left bronchial tree further postero-anterior and left oblique films are taken. Normal bronchi appear as parallel line shadows which become progressively smaller with each division. There is no alveolar filling leaving a 3–5 mm clear rim around the chest wall (*Fig.* 39.3). In bronchiectasis there may be loss of side branches, premature blunting and various forms of bronchial dilatation. In saccular bronchiectasis the bronchi appear as dilated (up to 4 times normal), finger-like projections rarely extending below the hemidiaphragm with no peripheral filling (*Fig.* 39.4). Sac-like dilatations opening off the main bronchi are a feature of cystic bronchiectasis (*Fig.* 39.5). With cylindrical disease the smaller bronchi are involved, being tortuous and ending with bead-like terminations (*Fig.* 39.6). The bronchi may appear tortuous without obvious dilatation but may become frankly bronchiectatic following resection or collapse in other areas.

Bronchography is useful in: (*a*) confirming the diagnosis in the presence of normal or minimal radiological change; (*b*) investigating haemoptysis where bronchiectasis is a possibility; and (*c*) localizing and determining the extent of the disease when considering surgery or postural drainage.

The diagnosis of bronchiectasis is straightforward in a

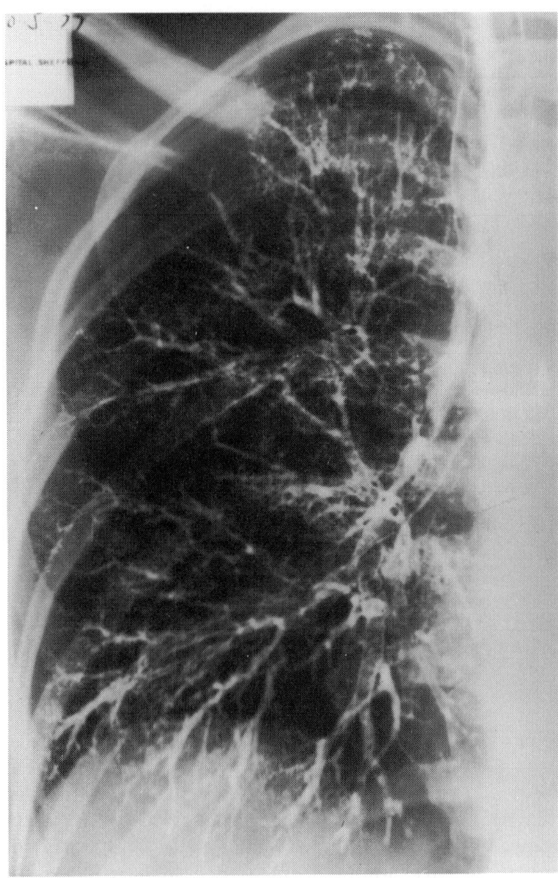

Fig. 39.3 PA view of a normal right bronchogram performed via an intratracheal catheter positioned in the right main bronchus. (By courtesy of Dr Paul Grech.)

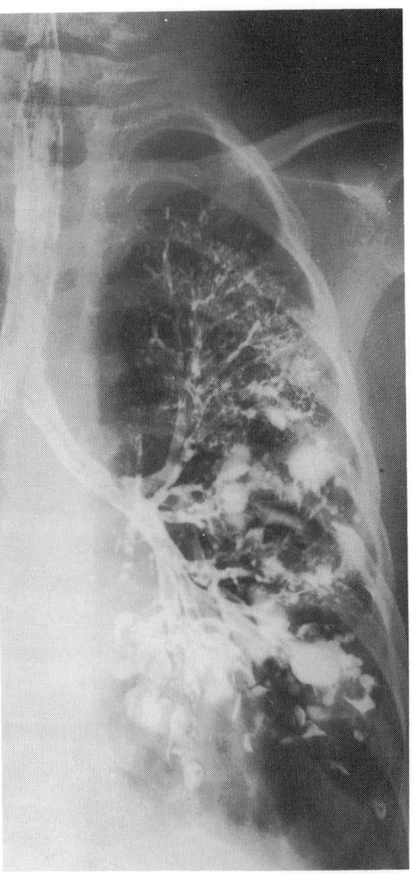

Fig. 39.4 Left bronchogram showing extensive saccular bronchiectasis of the lingular and left lower lobe bronchi. (By courtesy of Dr Paul Grech.)

patient with cough and sputum since childhood, persistent crepitations in the same area, finger clubbing, and tram-lining on radiography. When presenting in older patients it may be confused with chronic bronchitis or asthma but delineation is essential to allow appropriate treatment. Tuberculosis can cause or complicate bronchiectasis.

Management

Although the incidence of bronchiectasis appears to be falling preventive measures continue to be essential. Vaccines against whooping cough and measles, improved management of neonatal and infantile bronchiolitis and the early treatment of childhood infections have all contributed. Effective treatment of tuberculosis, prophylactic chemotherapy in tuberculin-positive and BCG vaccination in tuberculin-negative children remain important. An awareness of the possibility of foreign body inhalation, particularly in children, with prompt investigation and intensive physiotherapy to promote early re-expansion of any segmental or lobar collapse are important factors.

In severe bronchiectasis major problems may result from: (*a*) the constant discomfiture, excessive sputum production and bad breath necessitating jobs which avoid personal contact; (*b*) repeated time off school or work interfering with education and employment opportunities; (*c*) the limitations on sporting and social activities; and (*d*) an adverse effect on marital prospects. The older patients adapt better but depression remains a frequent complication.

Surgical resection is curative, provided all the diseased areas can be excised, leaving reasonable pulmonary function. Medical measures may control but not eradicate the disease and secondary bronchitis, emphysema or asthma often devlelop. Unfortunately, the cases which respond least well to conservative measures usually have extensive involvement which prevents surgical intervention.

Successful medical management depends on effective postural drainage backed up by appropriate antibiotic therapy. Good drainage clears the secretions, controlling infection and reducing the chance of secondary damage. As co-operation is essential, it is important to educate the patient as to the nature of his disease and the rationale behind drainage which is often best achieved by a spell in hospital during which correct positioning can be demonstrated, breathing exercises taught and a close relative instructed in basic physiotherapy. Bronchography will show the diseased areas and indicate the appropriate posture. Privacy is essential, permitting free expectoration without embarrassment. A bronchodilator aerosol taken 10–15 min before drainage may relieve bronchospasm and improve the results. The frequency depends on the severity, profuse sputum production may require drainage several times a day but when symptoms are restricted to 'colds' once daily during the infection may be sufficient. The procedure is tedious and the patient requires frequent encouragement from his doctor.

There is considerable variation in the antibiotic require-

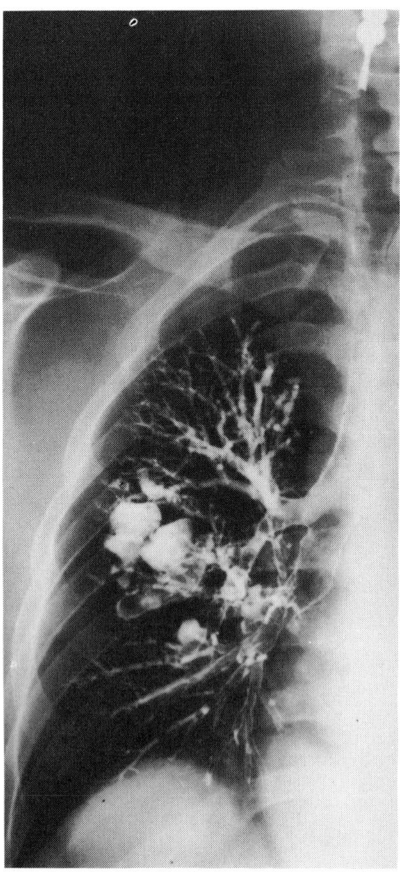

Fig. 39.5 PA view of a right bronchogram performed through the cricothyroid route (note needle at the cricothyroid membrane). The anterior branch of the upper lobe bronchus is affected with cystic bronchiectasis. (By courtesy of Dr Paul Grech.)

ments. Some patients need treatment only for acute infections while others benefit from broad-spectrum antibiotics, either daily or throughout the winter months, with appropriate changes during exacerbation. Where possible treatment should be guided by the results of sputum cultures but these may be unhelpful because of: (*a*) previous antibiotic therapy; (*b*) the presence of anaerobes not easily cultured; or (*c*) overgrowth by mixed commensal organisms. In severe cases it may not be possible to keep the sputum clear of pus. Early discharge after an exacerbation often helps prevent secondary infection. The repeated culture of species of klebsiella, pseudomonas or proteus presents major problems with the danger of permanent superinfection by these organisms necessitating barrier nursing during hospital admissions.

Surgical resection should be considered at an early stage in cases of severe or recurrent haemoptysis, recurrent disabling pneumonia, persistent cough with significant sputum production or lobar collapse due to bronchial obstruction, provided that the patient is young, otherwise fit, with a reasonable respiratory reserve and the disease is restricted to one lobe or lung.

In cases where the disease is multilobar but not extensive careful assessment is required before considering surgical intervention. The response to medical treatment, the age and general condition of the patient, the degree of respiratory reserve and the extent of upper respiratory tract involvement are important factors. Distorted but not obviously bronchiectatic segments on bronchography may become frankly diseased after resection of other areas. Bilateral disease is not an absolute contraindication to surgery provided selective segmental resection leaves adequate functioning lung. Occasionally it may be justified to remove a badly damaged lobe even in the presence of minor disease elsewhere. Saccular bronchiectasis with lobar collapse responds better than cylindrical disease with compensatory emphysema.

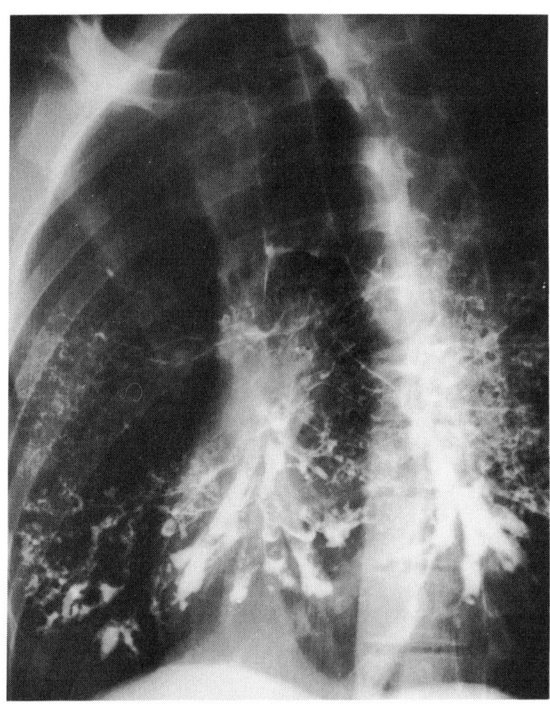

Fig. 39.6 Inhalation bronchogram showing cylindrical bronchiectases of all the bronchi of both lower lobes (By courtesy of Dr Paul Grech.)

Careful preoperative preparation is essential, including sputum checks for tuberculosis, a full otolaryngological assessment and intensive physiotherapy, postural drainage and antibiotic therapy leading up to surgery. Operative mortality is low (1%) although the postoperative period is often stormy with collapse, atelectasis and sputum retention necessitating intensive physiotherapy. Cough and sputum production persist in up to 40% of cases but is usually less severe and several factors may be responsible including: (*a*) failure to remove all the diseased areas; (*b*) postoperative collapse with fresh damage; (*c*) associated bronchitis and emphysema; and (*d*) re-infection from chronic sinusitis.

The place of surgery requires careful evaulation. Results in children suggest 50–75% are cured or improved but 10–40% later develop bronchitis. A comparison of medical and surgical treatment over 16–25 years showed that one-third of each group were symptom-free with a few deaths from severe disease in the medical group. Surgery undoubtedly benefits selected cases but the criteria for referral have become increasingly stringent with improvements in medical control.

Each case must be considered according to the individual circumstances but *Table* 39.1 indicates the principles of management.

Table 39.1 Management of bronchiectasis

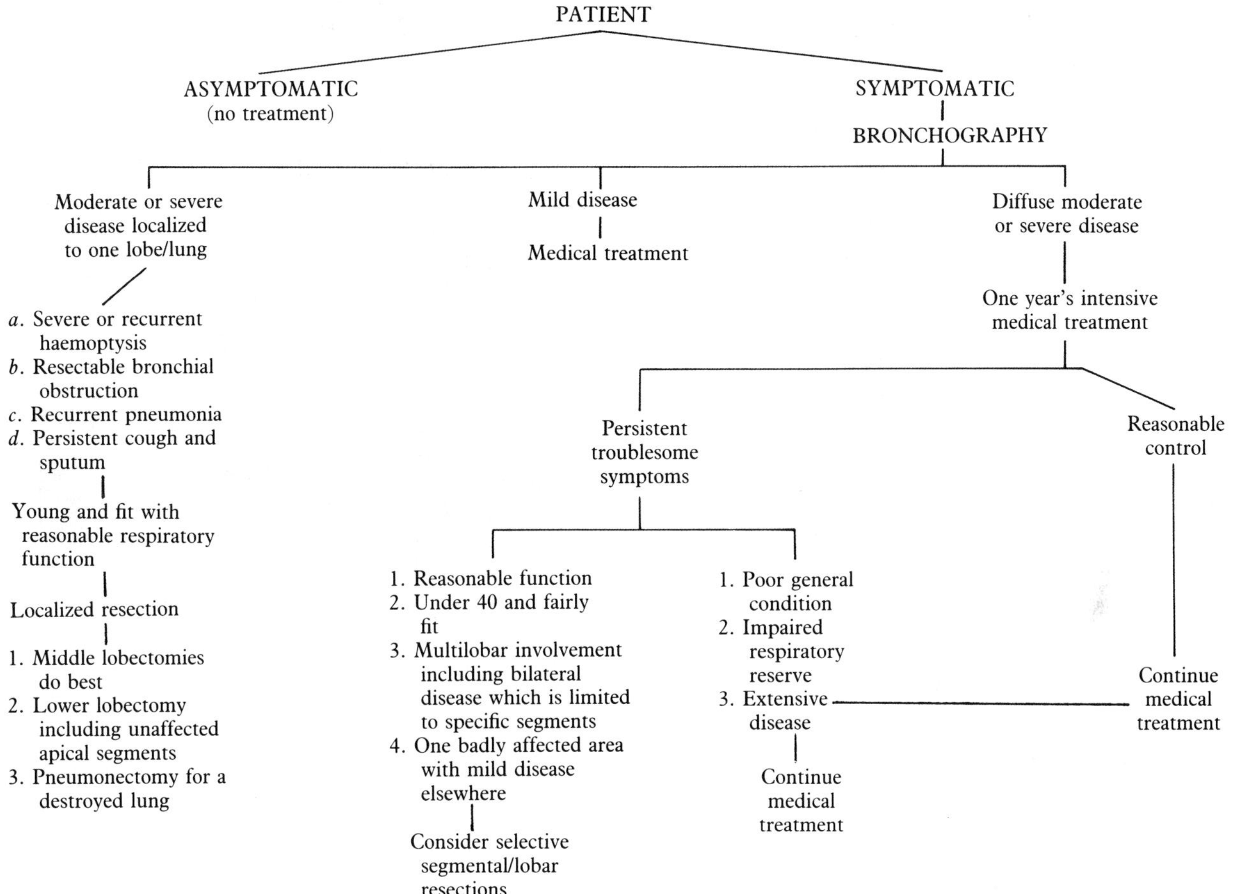

LUNG ABSCESS

Any process which causes lung suppuration may produce an abscess although the definition is usually restricted to necrotic cavitating lesions caused by pyogenic organisms, excluding tuberculosis, fungal infections and cavitating tumours. Following the introduction of antibiotics the incidence has fallen but a chronic abscess causing emaciation, cerebral sepsis or amyloidosis may still be encountered in the third world. The mode of infection varies considerably, the chief causes being:

1. *Aspiration* of infected material from the oropharynx or nasal cavity.
2. *Bronchial Obstruction* to a major bronchus by tumour; foreign body or glands predisposing to distal suppuration.
3. *Suppurative Pneumonias*, particularly staphylococcal and klebsiella infections.
4. *Infected Infarcts* either resulting from septic emboli or due to secondary infection of a pulmonary infarct.
5. *Chest Trauma* by the implantation of infected material or by secondary infection of a haematoma.
6. *Transdiaphragmatic Spread* from hepatic or subphrenic sepsis.
7. *Lung Cysts or Bullae* which become secondarily infected.

Aspiration

Previously, aspiration was the commonest cause but now bronchial obstruction due to carcinoma predominates. For aspiration to produce an abscess three conditions must be fulfilled:

1. *A source of infected material* which is usually the mouth, 80 per cent have dental sepsis causing pyorrhoea or tartar masses. Tonsillectomy and dental extraction were formerly responsible for 25% of cases but improved techniques have reduced their importance.
2. *Impairment of the defence mechanisms* due to: (1) depression of the cough or gag reflexes by drugs, anaesthesia, alcohol, epileptic fits or electroconvulsive therapy; (2) disruption of the action of the ciliated epithelium and mucus blanket by smoking or anaesthetics; or (3) ineffective coughing following thoracic or abdominal surgery or due to general debility.
3. *Bronchial obstruction*: the inhaled material must be large enough to obstruct a bronchus causing distal collapse. The mass will lodge in the most dependent segment, which is usually one of the axillary segments of the right upper lobe or the apical segment of the right lower lobe (*Fig.* 39.7).

Suppuration and necrosis develop distal to the obstruction and spread circumferentially destroying most tissue, including blood vessels, which lie in the path. An abscess may

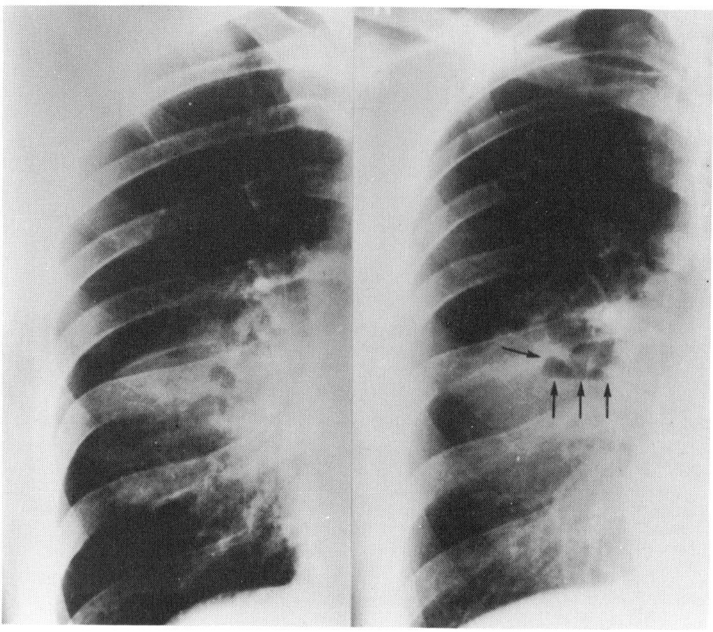

Fig. 39.7 Aspiration lung abscess in the apical segment of the right lower lobe.

rupture into a bronchus with the expectoration of pus, or into the pleura causing an empyema which may be associated with a persistent bronchopleural fistula. With treatment most abscesses heal leaving a fibrotic scar but large cavities may persist, becoming secondarily infected. An untreated abscess may be multilocular spreading across interlobar fissures, its interior traversed by ridges of undestroyed tissue and containing numerous pouting bronchial openings.

The initial symptoms, fever, rigor and malaise, are nonspecific and may be modified by antibiotic therapy. Later, cough, haemoptysis, deep-seated pain and pleurisy may develop. Intrabronchial rupture is followed by the expectoration of large quantities of foul-smelling pus. When a lung abscess follows oral, otolaryngeal or abdominal surgery there has usually been a stormy postoperative period with respiratory symptoms beginning within a few days of the operation.

Examination of the chest may be normal. Chest expansion may be diminished, the percussion note impaired or bronchial breathing, crepitations or a transient pleural friction rub heard on auscultation. Localized tenderness in the intercostal segments overlying an abscess is a useful but transient sign. Finger clubbing may occur usually in chronic cases.

The initial radiograph often suggests a segmental or lobar pneumonia but after the intrabronchial rupture and the expectoration of pus a fluid level develops within a round or oval opacity. A chronic cavity may have an irregular outline with variable surrounding infiltration and no fluid levels. The radiological picture may resemble: (*a*) a cavitating bronchial carcinoma, but the walls of the latter tend to be thicker and more ragged; (*b*) a hiatus hernia when the position and appearance on barium swallow are important; or (*c*) cavitation of a rheumatoid nodule or an area of progressive massive fibrosis when the history and biochemical tests may be helpful.

The complications of lung abscesses—severe haemoptysis, cerebral abscess, cachexia, weight loss and amyloid—are now rare in western countries.

A neutrophil leucocytosis of 20 000–30 000 is common.

Aspiration lung abscesses are rarely caused by a single organism and various combinations of anaerobic (bacteroides, fusobacterium and streptococci), microaerophilic (streptococci) and aerobic (klebsiella, haemophilus, pseudomonas and intestinal bacteria) organisms may be identified if special culture techniques are used. Organisms with proteolytic activity (*Borrelia vincentii* or clostridia species) may produce putrefaction.

Bronchoscopy may be helpful to exclude bronchial obstruction due to tumour, foreign bodies or glands, and to clear secretions from the bronchial tree.

The majority of aspiration lung abscesses respond to postural drainage, physiotherapy and large doses of intramuscular benzylpenicillin but antibiotic treatment may have to be modified in the light of the organisms isolated and their sensitivities. Healing usually occurs leaving a fibrous scar although treatment may need to be continued for 2–3 months. Very occasionally surgical drainage may be required in severely ill patients failing to respond to medical treatment. A chronic cavity or a fibrotic lobe may need to be resected and if there is any doubt about a possible underlying neoplasm exploratory thoracotomy should be undertaken.

Improved dental hygiene, preoperative treatment of respiratory infections, advances in oral and otolaryngeal surgery, better anaesthesia and improved postoperative care, have all contributed to the falling incidence.

Bronchial Obstruction

Obstruction of a major bronchus by tumour, foreign body or glandular enlargement, unless relieved quickly, invariably leads to segmental or lobar suppuration. The symptoms, signs and radiographic appearances suggest an unresolving pneumonia. Bronchoscopy will indicate the nature of the obstruction and will permit removal of a foreign body. It may be difficult to distinguish between a cavitating tumour and a proximal neoplasm with a distal abscess but, if feasible, both should be resected.

Suppurative Pneumonias

Lung abscesses most frequently complicate staphylococcal or klebsiella infections although any pneumonia may cause suppuration given suitable conditions.

The incidence of staphylococcal lung abscesses is highest at the extremes of life. In the elderly they usually occur as part of a staphylococcal bronchopneumonia, a precursor of which is often influenza. The mortality is high. There are multiple small peribronchial abscesses from which the inflammation rapidly spreads causing considerable lung destruction. If the process is arrested there may be extensive residual fibrosis.

Children tend to develop a staphylococcal lobar pneumonia which is less severe than the bronchopneumonias of the elderly. Abscesses form and during coughing and crying they may become inflated through a check-value mechanism producing tension pneumotoceles (*Fig.* 39.8). These may (*a*) compress the lung causing respiratory embarrassment, or (*b*) rupture into the pleural space forming a pyopneumothorax. The former usually respond to conservative measures but occasionally require surgical deflation while the latter needs drainage and systemic antibiotics.

Suppurative klebsiella pneumonias usually start in the right upper lobe and unless treated effectively with antibiotics to which the organism is sensitive, rapidly spread to the remaining lung producing extensive destruction, abscess formation and fibrosis. Elderly males are principally affected although the incidence is falling. If the destroyed lobes are the site of persistent or recurrent infection resection may be necessary.

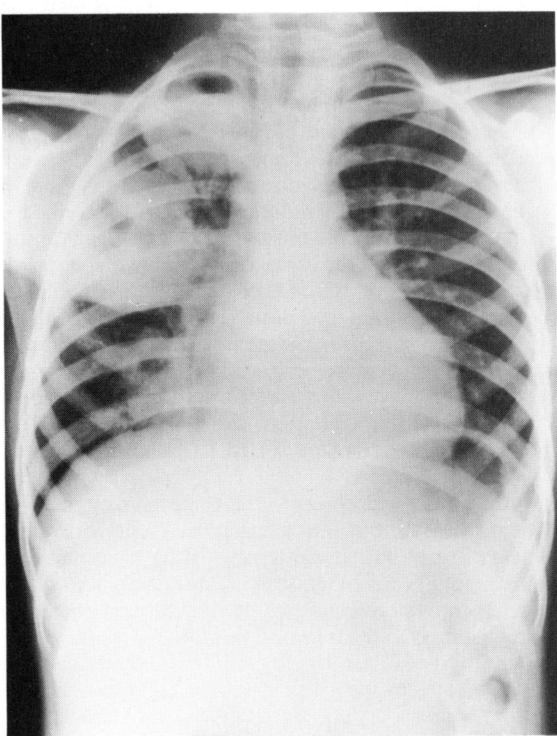

Fig. 39.8 Multiple staphylococcal abscesses of the right lung in a child.

Infected Infarcts

Septic emboli most frequently arise from an infected venous cannula and less commonly from thrombophlebitis of the pelvic or lower limb veins or infective endocarditis involving the right side of the heart or a ductus arteriosus. The result is usually numerous small peripheral abscesses but occasionally a larger artery is involved with segmental suppuration.

Although the majority of pulmonary infarcts are aseptic a few become secondarily infected with airborne bacteria. Diagnosis may present a problem and exploratory thoracotomy and resection may be necessary (*Fig.* 39.9).

At thoracotomy when a lobectomy is being undertaken the remaining lung is usually mobilized and care must be taken to prevent the residual lung rotating on its pedicle when its blood supply may become impaired leading to pulmonary infarction and suppuration necessitating emergency thoracotomy and resection.

Chest Trauma

Lung abscesses may follow open chest wounds with or without foreign body implantation or closed chest trauma due to infection of a haematoma or contused lung tissue. Management is usually conservative.

Transdiaphragmatic Spread

A subphrenic abscess invariably produces paralysis and elevation of the hemidiaphragm with basal atelectasis and a 'sympathetic' pleural effusion. Infection may spread to the effusion (empyema) or the lung (suppurative pneumonia) or the abscess may rupture through the diaphragm into the lower lobe with expectoration of pus. Initial treatment is directed towards the subphrenic infection, but an empyema will need draining and the lung abscess may require excision.

When amoebiasis affects the right lobe of the liver inflammation may spread through the diaphragm often pro-

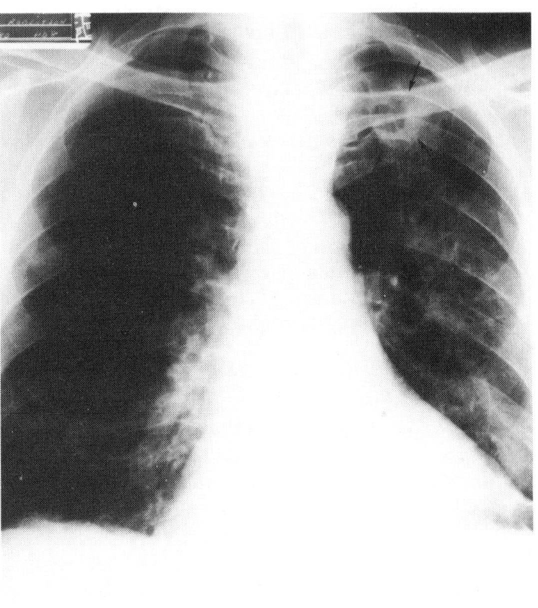

Fig. 39.9 Abscess in the left upper lobe resulting from an infected cavitating pulmonary infarct.

ducing pleural adhesions which may prevent the formation of an effusion or empyema. The right lower lobe may become infected by direct spread or by the transdiaphragmatic rupture of an hepatic abscess. The resultant lung abscess eventually ruptures into a bronchus with the expectoration of a thick reddish-brown liquid ('anchovy' or 'chocolate' sauce). A fistula may connect the biliary and pulmonary systems with the expectoration of bile. The amoebiasis should be treated medically (*see* Chapter 4) before any hepatic or pulmonary surgery is undertaken.

Lung Cysts or Bullae

If a hydatid cyst becomes secondarily infected either in situ or after intrabronchial rupture an abscess forms which is usually surrounded by considerable parenchymal inflammation and segmental or lobar resection is often necessary.

Infected bullae or cysts may resemble a lung abscess radiologically and present diagnostic difficulties. The patient is usually less severely ill although the radiological appearances are slower to resolve due to poorer drainage. Surgery is rarely indicated.

PULMONARY HYDATID DISEASE

Of the hydatid onchospheres (embryos) which gain entry to the portal circulation (*see* Chapter 4) only 10–20% pass through the liver to lodge in the pulmonary circulation. These develop into classic hydatid cysts with an outer laminated ectocyst and inner germinal layer from which the primitive adult worms are formed. Apart from a thin rim of fibrous tissue (pericyst or adventitia) they provoke little host response.

The lower lobes are most frequently involved (55%) and in 20% the pulmonary lesions are bilateral. Some reports have suggested concomitant liver involvement in up to 70% of cases. The pulmonary hydatid cysts are usually round or oval but may be indented by any rigid structure they encounter during their slow growth. Occasionally the cyst fills a hemithorax. The cysts appear as white, pearly-grey patches just beneath the pleural surface.

Spontaneous bronchial or pleural rupture or spillage at operation may be followed by the formation of daughter cysts in the lungs, pleura or mediastinum. Infection of an intact or ruptured cyst (lung abscess) with its surrounding pulmonary inflammation usually results in the death of the parasite. Rarely the parasite dies in situ when the cyst walls may calcify. Spontaneous healing occasionally follows rupture with expectoration of the cyst. Hepatic cysts may: (1) suppurate, the infection spreading through the diaphragm with the formation of an empyema or lung abscess; or (2) rupture into the pleura with dissemination to form daughter cysts.

Clinical Features

Pulmonary hydatid cysts are often symptomless presenting on routine chest radiography. Pleural pain and cough are the commonest symptoms although compression may produce dyspnoea or dysphagia. Occasionally severe dyspnoea occurs with a small cyst, the mechanism being uncertain. Haemoptysis usually precedes intrabronchial rupture when clear salty fluid, containing portions of membrane or pearly cysts, is expectorated. Occasionally a large fragment of the cyst wall can block a main bronchus causing acute respiratory distress. Intrapleural rupture is accompanied by severe pleuritic pain. Allergic reactions (itch, urticaria and wheeze) often precede while anaphylactic shock may follow either bronchial or pleural rupture. A lung abscess invariably follows intrabronchial rupture with continuing cough and sputum production. Hepatic or diaphragmatic pain with associated hepatic tenderness and fever may precede transdiaphragmatic rupture or spread of infection from a liver cyst.

A dense, round or oval, clearly demarcated shadow, which if small may resemble a neoplasm or if large fill the hemithorax, is the commonest radiological finding (*Fig.* 39.10). A small leak prior to rupture may produce an 'air halo' between the cyst wall and pericyst (adventitia). Following intrabronchial rupture with partial expectoration, the redundant laminated layer may curl up and float on the surface of the fluid (the 'water-lily' sign). Rarely a cyst calcifies (*Fig.* 39.11). An abscess with surrounding lung collapse or consolidation usually follows rupture although occasionally resolution occurs. Diaphragmatic paralysis or a pleural effusion may precede or follow intrapleural rupture or transdiaphragmatic spread.

In endemic areas a dense cyst on chest radiography is highly suggestive while the 'air halo' and 'water lily' signs are diagnostic. If clear, salty fluid is expectorated it should be examined for parts of the laminated layer, brood capsules and small worms. Details of the Casoni, complement-fixation and the newer immunological tests are given in Chapter 4. Both the Casoni (90%) and the hydatid complement-fixation tests (85%) are more likely to be positive in the presence of complications, and both the tests may remain positive for several years after successful resection. Blood eosinophilia is found in 20% of cases. Liver scans may be helpful in confirming concomitant liver involvement (70%). When the diagnosis is suspected aspiration needle biopsy should be avoided as anaphylactic shock or pleural dissemination may result.

Treatment

Initially treatment is medical (*see* Chapter 4). Surgery is advisable if there is no response to medical therapy as rupture may cause anaphylaxis, dissemination or chronic pulmonary sepsis. Where possible the cyst should be removed intact. Three procedures are available: (*a*) resection of the cyst after careful aspiration of a little fluid and instillation of ether, 20% sodium chloride, 10% formalin or 0·5% silver nitrate to kill the parasite; (*b*) following exposure of the superficial wall the proximal intrabronchial pressure is raised sufficiently to extrude the cyst in toto; or (*c*) lobectomy for a ruptured cyst with secondary infection. An empyema or a transdiaphragmatic fistula may require excision.

PULMONARY TUBERCULOSIS

Pulmonary tuberculosis must be considered in its world context where it remains a major problem with a high mortality. Effective chemotherapy, BCG vaccination and environmental improvements have drastically reduced the incidence in western countries. However, inadequate treatment has produced strains of *Mycobacterium tuberculosis* resistant to some of the first-line drugs in several third world countries. The incidence in children and adolescents has reached low levels in the western world in contrast to the third world where these age groups remain a problem. A major source of new cases in Britain and Europe is the breakdown of quiescent primary foci or healed lesions

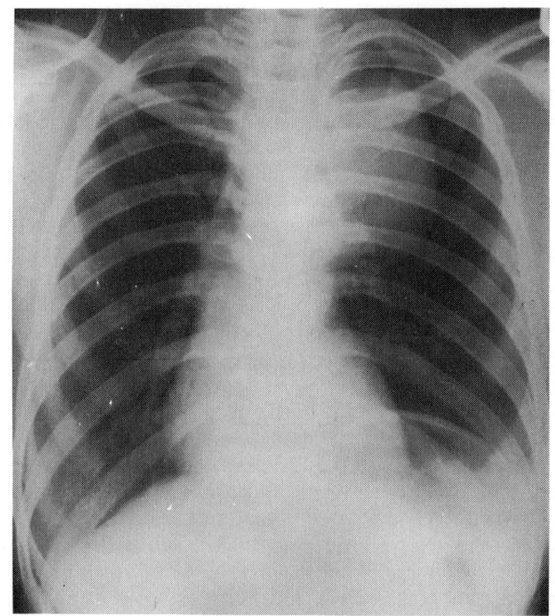

Fig. 39.10 Hydatid cyst in the left upper lobe. The shadow is homogeneous and presents a clear-cut outline. (By courtesy of Dr Paul Grech.)

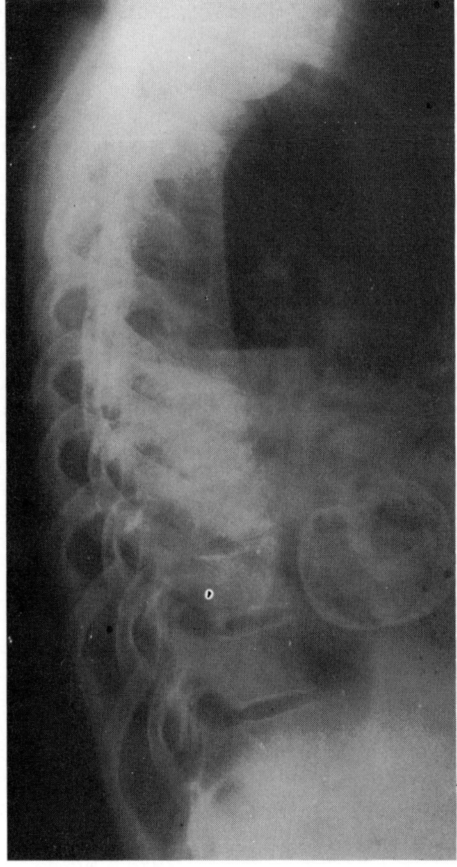

Fig. 39.11 Left lateral chest film showing two calcified hydatid cysts in the left lung. There is also a fluid level posteriorly indicating secondary infection in one of the cysts. (By courtesy of Dr Paul Grech.)

inadequately treated in the past in patients whose immune response has decreased either as a result of the ageing process or because they have developed a debilitating disease, e.g. diabetes, chronic alcoholism. The speed of modern travel, the increased mobility of the population and long incubation period mean that immigrants (or tourists) contracting the disease in endemic areas may present many months later in their new environment, the second major source of new cases in Britain.

Pulmonary tuberculosis usually results from airborne spread of the human *M. tuberculosis* from open cases of the disease. The initial reaction, the primary complex, may (1) heal with calcification; (2) lead on to the various forms of postprimary pulmonary disease; or (3) involve other organs by haematogenous spread.

The primary complex consisting of peripheral pneumonitis and regional gland involvement may follow inhalation of a single organism in susceptible cases. Any part of the lung may be involved although the upper lobes are preferred in adults. After the initial acute reaction the bacilli are engulfed by alveolar macrophages. There is early spread to the lymph nodes where most bacilli are arrested, only a few gaining entry to the general circulation. After 3–8 weeks the patient develops hypersensitivity to the tubercular protein, the tuberculin test becomes positive and the macrophages release their contained bacilli. A classic granulomatous lesion develops containing epithelial cells, Langhans giant cells, lymphocytes and fibroblasts with caseation (cheesy necrosis which results from hypersensitivity to the tubercular protein). The reaction usually subsides over several months with fibrosis and calcification but the scar may contain viable organisms capable of reactivation under suitable conditions. Most primary infections are asymptomatic or associated with a mild respiratory illness. Occasionally malaise, weight loss, fever, erythema nodosum or phlyctenular conjunctivitis may occur. The radiological appearances are variable; the pneumonitis may predominate with little glandular involvement but in children and Afro-Asians the glandular component often overshadows any lung lesion (*Fig.* 39.12).

Lobar collapse or occasionally obstructive emphysema may result from pressure by the enlarged hilar nodes while localized tuberculous endobronchitis, in the vicinity of a node, may lead to bronchial stenosis. The intrabronchial rupture of a gland with aspiration of tuberculous material may result in an acute exudative lesion (epituberculosis) which is the result of either a hypersensitivity reaction to the tubercular protein or less commonly a caseous pneumonia. These complications may be symptomless although cough and wheeze are commonly found. Chemotherapy, corticosteroids and postural drainage usually produce slow resolution and bronchoscopy is rarely indicated. Thoracotomy may be necessary to relieve obstructive emphysema or stridor and if the damage has caused bronchiectasis surgical resection may be required at a later date (*Fig.* 39.13).

A change in the tuberculin status from negative to positive while under observation is diagnostic of primary tuberculosis. With an extensive primary lesion, tubercle bacilli may be identified on smears or cultures of sputum or gastric washing but this is unusual.

When hilar or paratracheal glandular enlargement predominates, whether unilateral or bilateral, gland biopsy may be necessary to exclude a lymphoma. Reports from South Africa suggest mediastinoscopy may be helpful, otherwise mediastinotomy or thoracotomy should be considered.

Infants and young children developing a primary lesion or who react strongly to a tuberculin test should be prescribed

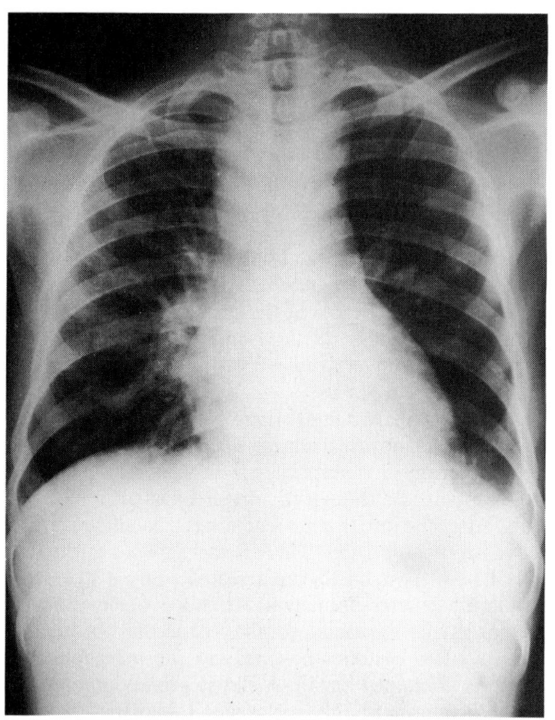

Fig. 39.12 Mediastinal glandular involvement and a small left-sided basal effusion due to primary TB in a 20-year-old African. Note that there is little radiological evidence of parenchymal involvement.

prophylactic antituberculous chemotherapy to prevent progression to the potentially lethal miliary or meningeal forms of the disease.

Occasionally the primary lesion merges into postprimary pulmonary tuberculosis. More commonly, haematogenous spread leads to: (*a*) miliary tuberculosis with widespread organ involvement; (*b*) pleural involvement producing an effusion; (*c*) the apical lesions of classic postprimary tuberculosis; or (*d*) focal infection of other organs, e.g. bones, kidney which may present as active disease only after the lapse of several years.

Postprimary pulmonary tuberculosis is the most important source of continuing infection in any community. It may arise from: (*a*) direct extension of a primary lesion; (*b*) reactivation of a healed primary lesion; or (*c*) haematogenous spread to the apices from a primary lesion (commonest cause). In an active case the following pathological stages are occurring side by side: *pre-exudative* with vasodilatation, interstitial oedema and swollen macrophages; *exudative* with varying degrees of oedema, fibrinous exudation, histiocytic, lymphocytic and leucocytic infiltration; *caseation* where necrosis occurs with the formation of a cheesy debris; *productive* when epithelioid, histiocytic and Langhans giant cells encircle a caseous area and early fibrotic containment begins; *fibrotic* during which fibrosis, often commencing peripherally, invades the tubercles; *cavitation* when liquefaction and expectoration of caseous material leads to cavity formation, the walls of the cavities being lined by soft, caseous material.

There are no specific clinical features, the presentation depending on the nature and extent of the disease. Mild debility may pass unnoticed, the patient being picked-up on routine radiography. The insidious progression of malaise, anorexia and weight loss over several months suggests tuberculosis. The development or worsening of a cough, which does not respond quickly to antibiotics, requires further investigation. The sputum may be mucoid, purulent or bloodstained and occasionally severe haemoptysis follows involvement of a major vessel. Nagging chest pain is common. In advanced disease dyspnoea and wheeze may occur. Recurrent colds with intervening malaise or pneumonia which fails to respond to treatment are frequent presentations. The classic night sweats are encountered less often than previously. Many patients complain of dyspepsia and a routine chest radiograph is always advisable in such cases.

The patient's general condition may be good in minimal disease but in the advanced stages they are pale, cachectic, flushed and pyrexial. The most characteristic signs are post-tussive crepitations at the apices, but these may be absent or replaced by the features of pneumonic consolidation. In chronic fibrocaseous disease the trachea and mediastinum may be drawn to the affected side.

The earliest radiological signs are usually unilateral or bilateral soft apical shadows which gradually extend and become confluent. Small cavities develop which are best seen on tomography. The soft infiltrates may be superimposed on a background of calcified, fibrotic scarring. In fibrocaseous disease there are large thick-walled cavities with extensive fibrosis. Residual fibrosis may shrink the upper lobes with shift of the upper mediastinum and elevation of the hilar shadows. The radiological appearances may be classified as minimal, moderate or advanced depending on the extent of the soft shadowing and degree of cavitation (*Figs.* 39.14, 39.15, 39.16).

The history, physical findings and radiological appearance often suggests the diagnosis which may be confirmed from direct smears or culture of sputum or gastric washings. The tuberculin test is usually strongly positive but may be negative in advanced disease. A therapeutic trial on antituberculous chemotherapy may be justified on the clinical findings and tuberculin reaction in the absence of sputum confirmation.

The majority of cases respond well to antituberculous chemotherapy although considerable pulmonary fibrosis may still follow treatment. In western countries sputum-positive cases are usually hospitalized until negative but once treatment is commenced most patients soon cease to be infectious and isolation is not universally feasible, particularly in developing countries. Severe cases may require bed rest but early mobilization is desirable.

The scope for surgical intervention varies considerably. In western countries surgery is restricted to cases with: (*a*) resistant organisms; (*b*) persistent infection in a badly damaged lung; or (*c*) failure of cavity closure after 2 years' chemotherapy, attention being paid to the state of the contralateral lung and segmental or lobar resections being preferred. Resections (including pneumonectomies) and thoracoplasties still have a place in the third world in the treatment of progressive or persistent infections due to inadequate chemotherapy or resistant organisms. Usually 3 months' chemotherapy should be given before any surgical intervention and continued for the appropriate time postoperatively to lessen the risks of dissemination or empyema.

A *tuberculoma* is a dense, slowly growing, peripheral tuberculous granuloma usually 1–3 cm in diameter which is often asymptomatic, being picked up on routine radiography. It must be differentiated from benign or malignant neoplasms and hydatid disease. Radiologically its outline is poorly defined and its density variable. Tomography may reveal calcification or small adjacent satellite lesions. The lesion may have been present in a radiograph taken months or years earlier. The tuberculin test is usually strongly positive but may be negative. Tubercle bacilli are rarely obtained from sputum smear or culture. In a fit patient where the diagnosis is in doubt thoracotomy is indicated followed by wedge or segmental resection of the tuberculoma. If suspected preoperatively some authorities suggest chemotherapy before the operation but in any event chemotherapy should be given for the appropriate time postoperatively. If surgery is contraindicated the diagnosis may be established by percutaneous aspiration needle biopsy or antituberculous chemotherapy may be given and the response assessed.

Chest Wall Tuberculosis

A cold abscess or tuberculous sinus of the chest wall usually arises as a result of pus tracking from caseous lymph nodes in the anterior or posterior intercostal or mediastinal chains or from tuberculous osteitis of a vertebra. It may also follow

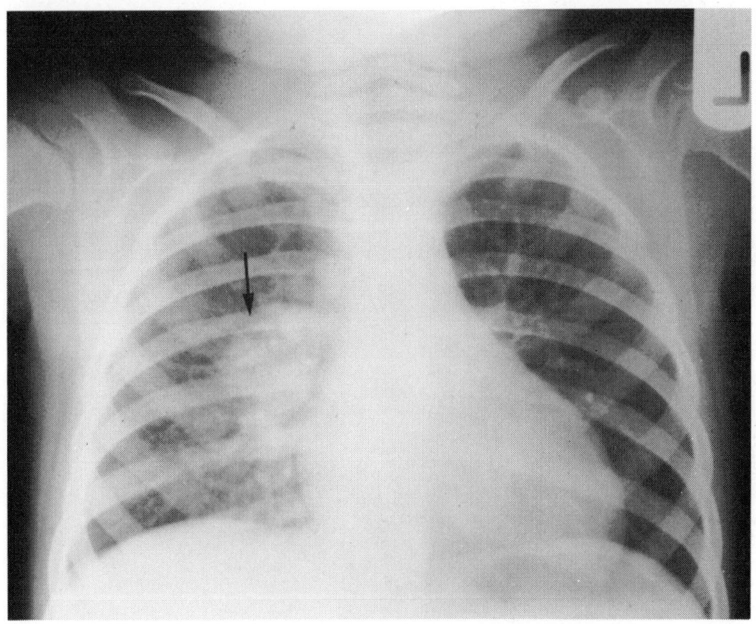

a

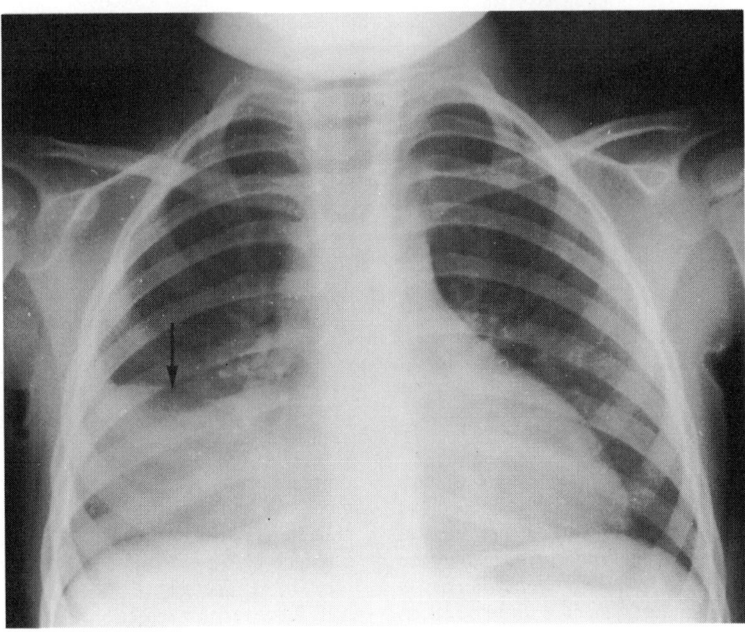

b

Fig. 39.13 *a*, Primary pulmonary TB with glandular involvement in a child aged 3 years. *b*, Three months later; poor response to treatment resulting in progression of the disease with middle lobe collapse/consolidation. [*continued over*]

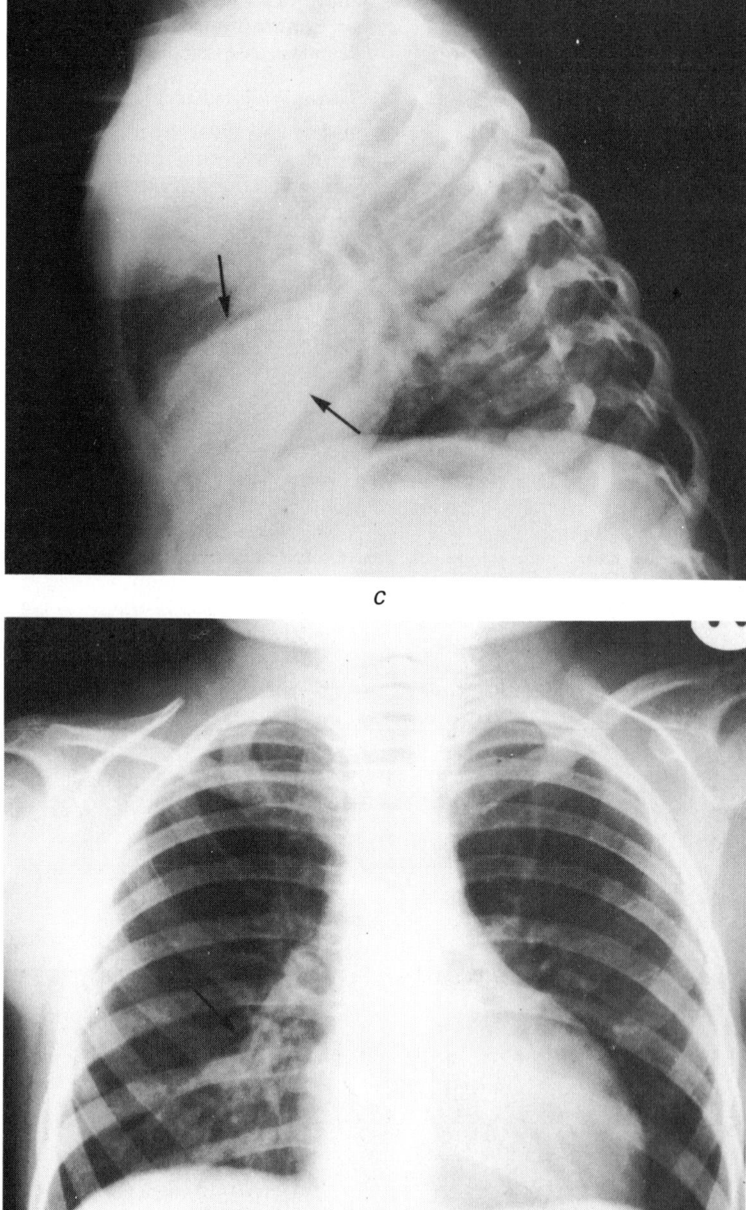

c

d

[*Fig. 39.13 continued*] *c*, Lateral view of the collapse/consolidation. *d*, One year after (*b*) and (*c*) following successful chemotherapy: there is considerable improvement but increased striation is visible in the right lower zone suggesting early bronchiectatic change.

reactivation of pulmonary disease previously treated with recurrent artificial pneumothoraces in the days before adequate chemotherapy was available and where pleural involvement had occurred. The ribs and cartilage may be infected as part of the spread. Response to chemotherapy is usually good but if surgery is undertaken care must be taken to explore the tracks fully and remove any caseous nodes. A preoperative sinogram may be helpful.

The Late Effects of Pulmonary Tuberculosis

Tuberculosis often leads to considerable fibrosis, destruction and bronchiectasis in a segment, lobe or lung and if this gives rise to persistent symptoms, resection should be considered provided the function of the remaining lung is satisfactory. Severe or recurrent haemoptysis from an area of 'dry' bronchiectasis or following the erosion of a broncholith, may warrant resection. An aspergilloma resulting from fungal superinfection of a persistent cavity is best resected although residual lung function often prevents this. Pleural fibrosis or calcification may require decortication to allow full re-expansion (*Fig.* 39.17). Patients are still encountered with a fixed, fibrotic, calcified hemithorax following pre-

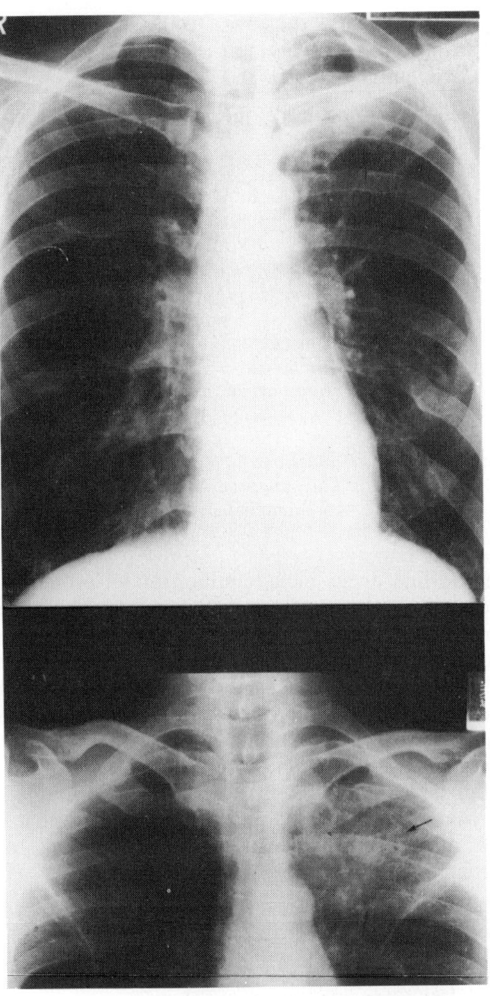

Fig. 39.14 Minimal TB in the left upper lobe, better visualized in the apical view (*below*).

vious artificial pneumothoraces although there is usually little that can be done to improve this situation. Thoracoplasty is compatible with normal life, particularly in non-smokers, although underlying bronchiectasis may aggravate any associated bronchitis. Rarely infection around a thoracoplasty or plumbage material may require further surgical intervention.

Antituberculous Chemotherapy

The introduction of effective drug regimens has revolutionized the management of tuberculosis. It is important that any regimen: (*a*) uses a combination of drugs which takes into account the resistance patterns of the local organisms, and (*b*) that it is modified in the light of the sensitivity tests when these become available. As there may be a delay of 3–6 months before the sensitivity results are known the initial regimens should include at least three drugs to which the organism is likely to be sensitive. Failure to adhere to these two principles will lead to the emergence of resistant strains.

To be effective a regimen must be: (*a*) taken regularly; (*b*) continued for sufficient time. Regular treatment may include intermittent regimens taken 2 or 3 times weekly under supervision. With the falling incidence of tuberculosis it is becoming increasingly difficult to persuade patients to continue treatment for sufficient time once the initial improvement has been achieved. Failure to take regular treatment for sufficient time may lead to relapse.

The first effective regimens combine streptomycin, para-aminosalicylic acid (PAS) and isoniazid:

Streptomycin 0·5–1 g daily for 3 months
Isoniazid 300 mg daily } For 18–24 months
PAS 10–15 g daily }

In spite of their tremendous impact such regimens had three major disadvantages:

a. Daily injections of streptomycin for 3 months are uncomfortable and lead to hypersensitivity reactions in patients and nursing staff.

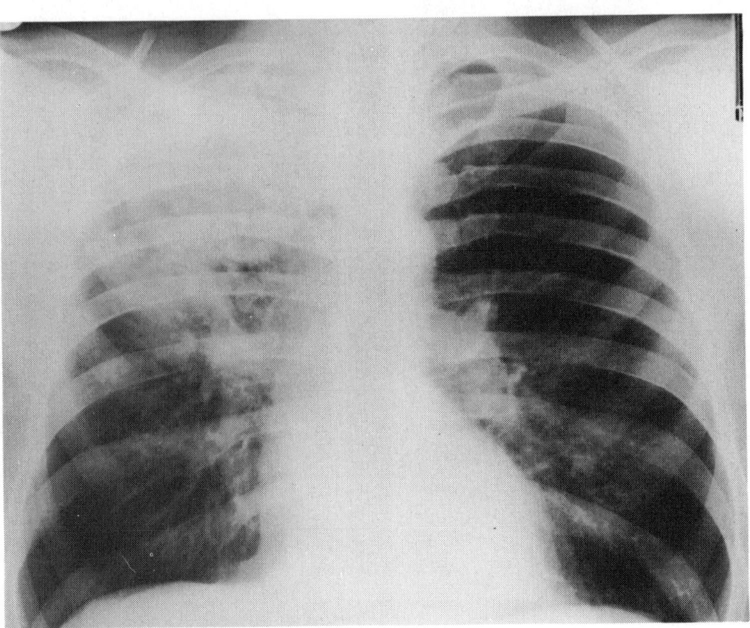

Fig. 39.15 Moderate right upper zone TB in an alcoholic.

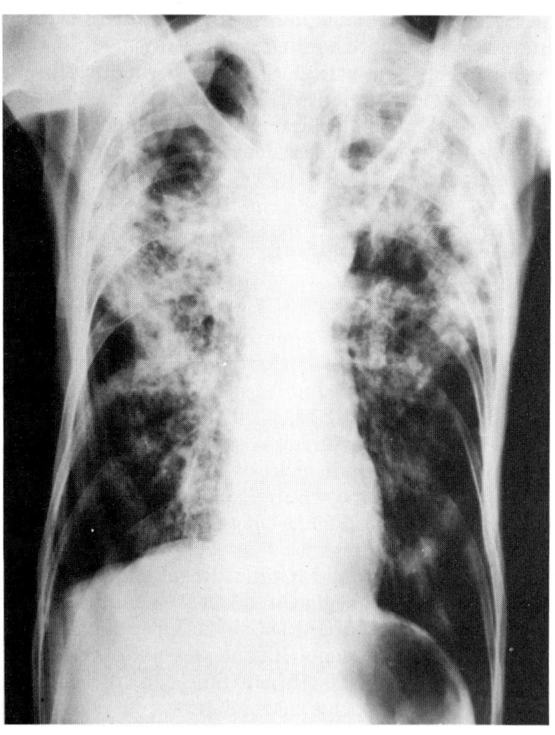

Fig. 39.16 Advanced bilateral cavitating TB. The patient was an alcoholic and weighed 5 stones at the time of death.

b. PAS frequently causes gastrointestinal upsets which were at times unacceptable to the patient, and

c. The length of the course.

In spite of this, such regimens are cheap and effective treatments.

Several drugs have been developed possessing varying antituberculous activity as shown below:

	First-line drugs
Bactericidal	Isoniazid Rifampicin Streptomycin (in an alkaline pH) Pyrazinamide (in an acid pH)
Bacteriostatic	Ethambutol Thioacetazone Para-aminosalicylic acid (PAS)

Second-line drugs include ethionamide, prothionamide, capreomycin, vibramycin and cycloserine. Their mode of action is incompletely understood.

First-line drugs are those in common usage while second-line drugs are reserved for resistant cases. In principle bactericidal drugs (those which destroy the organism in situ) are preferred to bacteriostatic (those which interfere with the organism's reproduction allowing the body's defence mechanisms to deal with the infection).

In consequence various regimens (similar to that shown below) have been built around the combination of isoniazid and rifampicin.

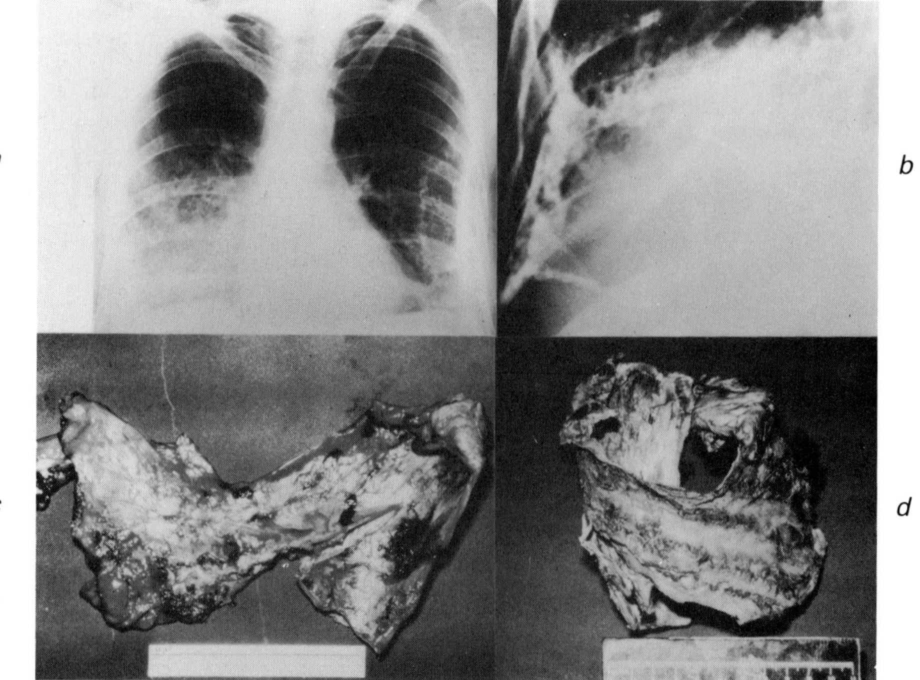

Fig. 39.17 This 32-year-old male presented 10 years after a full course of antituberculous therapy for pulmonary TB. *a*, PA chest film showing bilateral calcified pleural reactions. *b*, Tomogram of the right lower zone showing extensive calcification. *c*, Resected calcified pleura immediately after decortication. *d*, Fixed specimen 24 h later showing rib indentations.

Rifampicin 450 mg (under 50 kg) 600 mg (over 50 kg) Isoniazid 300 mg	Daily for 9 months
plus	
Streptomycin 1 g (3 days weekly) or Ethambutol 15 mg/kg daily	For the first 3 months only

In general, these regimens have few side-effects, are well tolerated giving 100% cure within 9 months and have become standard therapy in many western countries. A major disadvantage is their cost.

Ethambutol can cause retrobulbar neuritis if used in high doses or for longer than 3 months. This usually recovers once the drug is stopped. As the drug is excreted by the kidney ethambutol should be used only as a second-line drug and then with extreme caution in patients with renal failure. However, there have been reports recently of irreversible ocular damage occurring within days of starting on the standard dose of ethambutol (15 mg/kg/day). Because of these potential problems guidelines for the use of ethambutol have been drawn up by the British Thoracic Society (Citron and Thomas) which everyone using the drug is advised to follow.

Recent reports have suggested that pyrazinamide 20–30 mg/kg may be at least as effective as ethambutol when used during the first 2–3 months of treatment. If this is confirmed then pyrazinamide is likely to replace ethambutol in standard chemotherapy regimens.

Trials in which streptomycin plus pyrazinamide have been added to rifampicin and isoniazid suggest that cure can be achieved within 6 months.

In many third world countries intermittent regimens using various combinations of isoniazid, streptomycin, PAS, rifampicin, ethambutol and thioacetazone have been introduced in an attempt to treat widespread disease within a limited budget. Such regimens have the advantage of administration 2 or 3 times weekly under supervision. Similar regimens (as illustrated below) may be used in western countries to treat patients who have defaulted from previous follow-up or who are considered unreliable.

Streptomycin 1 g twice weekly Isoniazid 600 mg twice weekly Pyridoxine 10 mg twice weekly	For 18–24 months

(Pyridoxine is added to counteract the effect of large doses of isoniazid on pyridoxine metabolism.)

PULMONARY ACTINOMYCOSIS

The two bacteria *Actinomyces israelii* and *Nocardia asteroides* which cause actinomycosis both produce similar chronic respiratory infections. The characteristics of each organism are described in Chapter 5. *N. asteroides* accounts for only 10% of cases of pulmonary actinomycosis.

A. israelii lung infections usually result from the inhalation of infected material from the oropharynx but are occasionally due to the spread of actinomycosis from the abdomen or cervicofacial region. Nocardia gains entry by the inhalation of spores from the soil.

Pulmonary actinomycosis starts insidiously as a peripheral focus in a lower lobe. The advancing lesion crosses fascial planes to involve other lobes or extends to the pleura where it forms either an empyema or pleural adhesions with the subsequent invasion of the chest wall and the formation of chronic sinuses. The involved lung is densely fibrotic and honeycombed with small abscesses. Fever, toxaemia, malaise, weight loss, cough with bloodstained sputum, and pleuritic pain develop and become progressively worse. Not only is tuberculosis mimicked but it may coexist. Radiologically there are varying-sized cavitating pneumonic shadows which may be associated with a pleural effusion or rib periostitis (*Fig.* 39.18).

A. israelii infections may be diagnosed by the presence of sulphur granules in either the sputum or pus from a sinus, or the organism may be cultured using anaerobic or microaerophilic techniques. *N. asteroides* has to be grown using aerobic cultures.

High doses of penicillin for several months cure *A. israelii* infections. *N. asteroides* usually responds to sulphonamides but sensitivity tests are important. It may be necessary to drain an empyema or resect damaged lung after the completion of medical treatment.

PULMONARY FUNGAL DISEASE

Recent therapeutic changes have increased the importance of the respiratory fungal diseases while improved investigative techniques have advanced our understanding of them. The introduction of new drugs has had two effects:

1. Prolonged usage of broad-spectrum antibiotics affects the bacterial flora of the respiratory tract allowing colonization by fungi which may later invade the lung parenchyma with subsequent widespread dissemination.
2. Corticosteroids and cancer chemotherapy impair both cellular and humoral immunity permitting growth of organisms normally rejected.

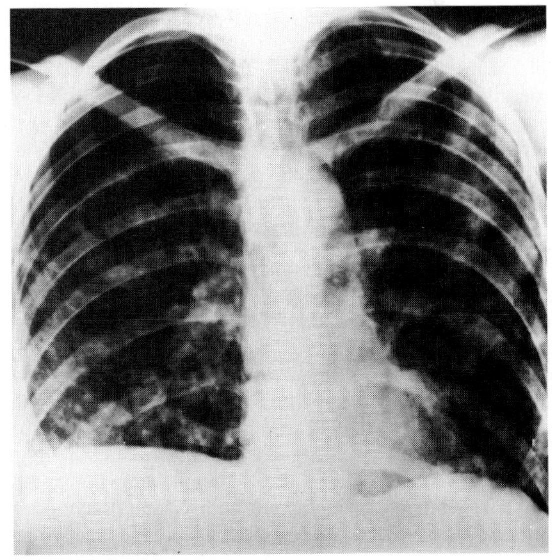

Fig. 39.18 This 16-year-old male developed ileocaecal actinomycosis a few weeks after an appendicectomy. A month later he developed a cough and a chest film showed diffuse patchy consolidation throughout both lung fields. There is also a right pneumothorax. (The more common radiological appearance of pulmonary actinomycosis is massive consolidation.) (By courtesy of Dr Paul Grech.)

Table 39.2 Fungal infections of the respiratory tract

Group	*Organism*	*Distribution*	*Infection*
Yeast-like fungi	*Candida albicans*	Worldwide	Opportunistic
	Cryptococcus neoformans	Worldwide	Opportunistic
Filamentous fungi	*Aspergillus fumigatus* (and other species)	Worldwide	Opportunistic
	Mucor (several species)	Worldwide	Opportunistic
Diamorphic fungi	*Coccidioides immitis*	South-Western USA	Parasitic
	Histoplasma capsulatum	Worldwide (Rare in Britain)	Parasitic
	Blastomyces dermatitis	Eastern USA, Africa	Parasitic
	Paracoccidioides brasiliensis	South America (Central America)	Parasitic
	Sporotrichum schenckii	South Africa, France, USA	Parasitic

Suppression of the immune response either induced intentionally in order to prevent tissue rejection following organ transplantation or occurring as part of the acquired immune deficiency syndrome (AIDS) has been a further factor in the increasing incidence of fungal infections of the lung.

Only a few fungi cause respiratory disease in man. The majority are inhaled as spores from their natural habitat, the soil. Some being ubiquitous are found worldwide, e.g. aspergillus, others require specialized soil conditions, e.g. coccidioides, while others prefer soil rich in bird or bat excreta, e.g. histoplasmosis. Candida lives symbiotically with man requiring altered immunity before producing disease. Person-to-person spread is rare.

The resultant infection may be:

1. *Opportunistic*, where impaired defence mechanisms or lung fibrosis permits the growth of otherwise harmless organisms. Such infections occur worldwide, e.g. moniliasis, or
2. *Parasitic*, where the fungus invades normal lung tissue usually producing a subclinical primary infection which rarely progresses to chronic disease, e.g. coccidioidomycosis. Most of these fungi are endemic in specific regions but the speed of modern travel means they may present anywhere. These organisms are highly infectious and present problems to laboratory workers handling specimens.

The nature of the lesions produced by fungi varies from necrosis and fibrosis resembling fibrocaseous tuberculosis, e.g. coccidioidomycosis, through bronchitis and pneumonia, e.g. moniliasis, to the allergic manifestations of aspergillosis.

The diagnosis may be difficult, particularly in opportunistic infections where, with the exception of an aspergilloma, there are no distinctive clinical or radiological features, and is usually based on exclusion in the presence of repeated heavy cultures of the fungus. Post-mortem diagnoses require special histological staining. Most of the parasitic fungi have a specific delayed skin test although in acute cases it may be necessary to make the diagnosis from smears, cultures or animal inoculations.

In opportunistic infections antibiotic, steroid or cytotoxic therapy should be modified to allow recovery of the host's defence mechanisms. Amphotericin B is a good broad-spectrum antifungal agent for inhalation or intravenous use but side-effects (nephrotoxicity) limit its usefulness (*see* Chapter 5). Less toxic drugs, 5-fluorocytosine, and the imidazoles (econazole and miconazole), have been developed, although their exact role still has to be determined. With limited disease or for residual lung fibrosis surgical resection may be indicated.

The incidence of each disease varies considerably. In endemic areas, the parasitic fungi may infect 80–90% of the population, e.g. coccidioides, of which 20–25% have mild symptoms but only 0·1–0·2% progress to serious disease.

At present it is not possible to produce a complete classification of the respiratory fungal infections but *Table* 39.2 serves as a framework for discussion.

Moniliasis (Candidiasis)

Although oropharyngeal and laryngeal candidiasis are fairly common, bronchopulmonary involvement is unusual even in chronically debilitated patients or those receiving long-term antibiotics, high-dose steroids or cytotoxic therapy. *Candida albicans* is usually responsible although other species may be involved. Three types of pulmonary moniliasis have been described.

1. *Monilial bronchitis* occurs in infancy, fibrocystic lung disease or debilitated elderly patients. The bronchial walls are studded with greyish-yellow plaques containing fibrin, hyphae and spores. Clinically there is an irritating cough productive of scanty 'milky' sputum with basal striations or normal appearances on radiography. Diagnosis depends on repeated culture of the fungus from the sputum.

2. *Monilial Pneumonia.* Rarely a necrotic pneumonia develops in severely debilitated patients giving patchy ill-defined shadows radiologically. The patient has a fever with tachycardia, dyspnoea and a cough productive of blood-stained sputum. The fungus is repeatedly obtained on sputum cultures.

3. *Generalized Moniliasis.* Occasionally following aggressive antibiotic, steroid or cytotoxic therapy, particularly in the presence of an indwelling venous cannula, a severe generalized candidal infection develops. Monilial pyaemia occurs with septic infarcts and abscesses developing in many organs including the lungs. The prognosis is poor, the diagnosis often being made at post-mortem.

When considering pulmonary moniliasis the patient's general condition is important, i.e. in terminal carcinoma treatment should be supportive. Where possible, antibiotic, steroid or cytotoxic therapy should be modified. If the organism is sensitive 5-fluorocytosine is the drug of choice. Otherwise intravenous and inhaled amphotericin B together with nystatin inhalations, may be tried.

Cryptococcosis (Torulosis)

Cryptococcus neoformans is found worldwide. While most infections occur in patients suffering from chronic diseases, i.e. diabetes, alcoholism, occasionally healthy subjects are infected. The inhaled fungus sets up a symptomless subpleural focus with hilar gland enlargment (resembling primary tuberculosis) which is often self-limiting with complete resolution. The lesion may:

1. Form a localized granuloma with a well-defined fibrous capsule and central caseation. This is usually symptomless, being mistaken for a neoplasm on routine radiography, or

2. Spread by progressive infiltration to produce cavitating consolidation. If the pleura is involved an empyema may develop. The clinical picture resembles tuberculosis with malaise, cough, sputum, chest pain and soft cavitating opacities on radiography.

Haematogenous spread can occur at any stage with the development of a chronic grumbling meningitis (resembling tuberculous meningitis) or lesions in other organs. The meningitis is often the presenting feature and in any case of pulmonary cryptococcosis lumbar puncture is essential before commencing treatment.

Special stains are required to identify the organism in smears of sputum or CSF. Culture is confirmatory but skin and complement fixation tests are unhelpful.

5-Fluorocytosine penetrates the blood–brain barrier and has improved the prognosis in cryptococcal meningitis. It can be tried in progressive lung lesions as an alternative to intravenous amphotericin B. Solitary lesions are best resected to establish the diagnosis and prevent spread to the meninges. Destroyed lung from progressive pulmonary disease may require resection after a period of medical treatment.

Aspergillosis

The inhalation of spores of *Aspergillus fumigatus*, which reach their peak in the damp winter months, is the usual cause of aspergillosis but other species may be involved. *A. fumigatus* is a common laboratory contaminant and several sputum cultures may be necessary to confirm the diagnosis. Immediate and delayed skin tests and serum precipitins can be useful in distinguishing between the different disease entities. The clinical, radiological, immunological and mycological findings are all important when diagnosing aspergillosis.

Several disease entities are encountered:

a. Hypersensitivity Reactions

1. Asthma

This may take the form of acute type I allergic asthma following exposure to large concentrations of spores when the immediate skin test is usually strongly positive.

Alternatively, allergic bronchopulmonary aspergillosis may develop, the principal features of which are recurrent asthmatic attacks associated with malaise, cough productive of bronchial casts, sputum and blood eosinophilia, and transient shadows on radiography (*Fig.* 39.19). Permanent proximal bronchial damage (bronchiectasis) occurs at the site of the impaction of the casts. The immediate and delayed skin tests are positive in 40% and precipitins in 10%. Long-term corticosteroids may be required to control the symptoms. Antifungal agents have little place in therapy.

2. An Extrinsic Allergic Alveolitis

This may follow exposure to *A. clavatus* (malt worker's lung which resembles farmer's lung) where the reaction occurs mainly at alveolar level. Several hours after exposure the patient becomes dyspnoeic with malaise, fever, cough, weight loss and generalized aches. Radiologically there are diffuse patchy shadows and the respiratory function tests show a restrictive pattern of ventilation with a reduction in the transfer factor. Serum precipitins to *A. clavatus* are invariably present. Recovery usually follows removal from exposure although if the symptoms are severe steroids may be required. Relapse occurs following re-exposure to the fungus.

b. Aspergilloma

Any chronic cavity, e.g. tuberculous, may become secondarily infected with *A. fumigatus* which grows on necrotic debris to form a mycelial mass. There is little surrounding reaction, the mass gradually filling and distending the cavity. There is usually a small crescentic halo of air above the mass, best seen on tomography (*Fig.* 39.20). Cough, intermittent haemoptysis and expectoration of brown sputum containing the fungus is the usual presentation. The haemoptysis is occasionally severe. Systemic upset, fever, malaise and weight loss may occur. The fungus can be grown from the sputum and precipitin tests are invariably strongly positive. While resection is desirable the disease which produced the cavity has often compromised lung function making surgery impracticable. Steroids and co-trimoxazole have been tried with varying success. Amphotericin B by inhalation or intravenously or 5-fluorocytosine may control the disease if they can penetrate the fungus ball. Miconazole has been used over several months to prevent reinfection, but relapse invariably occurs once the drug is stopped due to the ubiquitous nature of the organism.

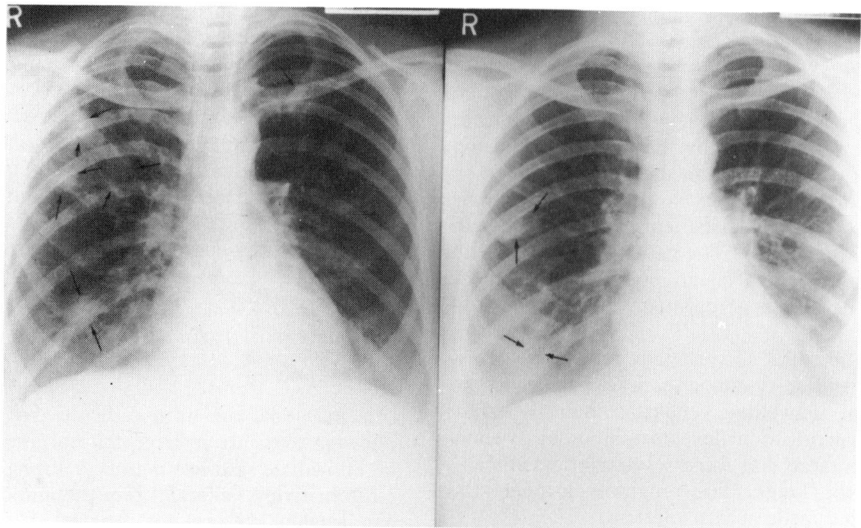

Fig. 39.19 PA chest films of the same patient demonstrating the changing pattern of pulmonary infiltrates in bronchopulmonary aspergillosis.

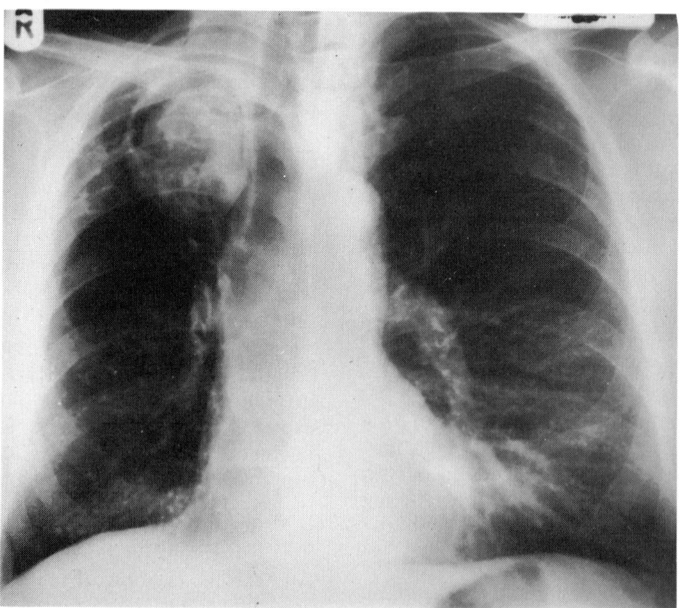

Fig. 39.20 PA chest film showing a large mass lying loose inside an old cavity in the right apex. The mass is outlined by air inside the cavity and it can be shown to move when the patient changes position. Diagnosis: aspergilloma.

c. *Pneumonic Aspergillosis*

Diffuse pneumonic shadowing or lobar consolidation may develop in debilitated subjects with immune deficiency. The infection may be fulminating with rapid haematogenous spread to many organs and generalized toxaemia. Alternatively, there may be a good tissue response with the formation of multiple small abscesses when cough, sputum, malaise and fever predominate. The fungus may be cultured from sputum, bronchial washings obtained at bronchoscopy or material obtained from an aspiration lung biopsy. Precipitating antibodies are often present and a rising titre is diagnostic. Intravenous amphotericin B is the treatment of choice, but if the organism is sensitive 5-fluorocytosine may be tried. The newer imidazoles (particularly econazole) are producing encouraging results. The resection of an infected lobe may be considered although the risk of developing a bronchopleural fistula is high.

Mucormycosis

Mucormycosis usually causes destructive skin lesions with involvement of the upper respiratory tract and meninges. Occasionally the lungs are involved, usually in drug addicts or following splenectomy for malignancy. Pneumonia or localized bronchial invasion followed by erosion into the pulmonary vessels may occur. Clinically there is cough, haemoptysis and pleurisy with ill-defined diffuse shadowing on radiography. The organism can be obtained from smears or culture of sputum. Prognosis is poor but intravenous and inhaled amphotericin B or surgical resection should be considered.

Coccidioidomycosis

Inhalation of the chlamydospores of *Coccidioides immitis* produces a primary infection in up to 84% of the population in endemic areas. Occasionally the primary lesions spread directly or breaks down later to give progressive lung disease.

Primary Infection

Within 3 weeks the chlamydospores release spherules which produce localized subpleural inflammation. This is usually asymptomatic resolving within 2 months to leave a small scar which may later calcify. Occasionally mild respiratory symptoms (pyrexia, cough with bloodstained sputum, pleurisy, malaise and headache) may develop and rarely erythema nodosum or erythema multiforme occurs. Scattered soft shadows with hilar adenopathy are seen radiologically. A single dense lesion resembling a tumour or tuberculoma may persist requiring resection for diagnosis.

Progressive Pulmonary Coccidioidomycosis

This may be acute or chronic with an overall mortality of 60% within two years.

The *acute* form is associated with rapid intrapulmonary dissemination causing acute bronchopneumonia, necrosis and oedema. The systemic effects predominate with anorexia, weight loss, fever, malaise and the signs of a bronchopneumonia. There are diffuse patchy or confluent shadows radiologically. Should healing occur it produces extensive fibrosis, bronchiectasis and cavity formation. Haematogenous spread, particularly in infants or the elderly, produces miliary foci (resembling tuberculosis) in many organs and is usually rapidly fatal.

More frequently a *chronic* infection occurs with the formation of granulomas, which are surrounded by fibrous walls and contain a mass of caseating material. Satellite lesions are common. Rupture into a bronchus may produce a chronic cavity. Similar granuloma are found in skin, bone, lymph nodes and brain. There is progressive malaise, cough and sputum with radiological evidence of solid or cavitating lesions.

Coccidioidomycosis has to be distinguished from tuberculosis and tumour. Histologically, spherules are present but may be difficult to identify in chronic lesions. Sputum culture or guinea-pig inoculation can be helpful. The coccidioidin skin test produces a reaction within 72 h but may be negative in severe disseminated disease. In endemic areas a calcified primary complex on radiography with negative tuberculin but positive coccidioidin test is diagnostic. Precipitin, complement-fixation or immunofluorescence antibody tests may be helpful in acute cases.

Most patients need no treatment. In progressive disease intravenous and inhaled amphotericin B may be helpful. Surgical resection of local pulmonary or bone lesions or drainage of an empyema may be necessary.

Histoplasmosis

The incidence of histoplasmosis shows considerable variation, being 85% in some areas of central USA, 10–15% in river valleys in India and Malaysia with only sporadic cases occurring in the UK and then usually as a result of previous travel or exposure to imported material, e.g. cotton. *Histoplasma capsulatum* prefers soil rich in bird or bat excreta and has been responsible for several minor epidemics of respiratory illness in cavers and poultry workers, e.g. cave sickness. While most infections follow the inhalation of spores, young children may be infected through the alimentary tract leading to severe disseminated disease with miliary mottling on chest radiography and recovery of the organism from bone marrow or liver biopsy.

A primary lesion consisting of parenchymal and glandular components (resembling a primary tuberculous focus) follows inhalation of the fungus. The organism is taken up by and then destroys the macrophages causing a local reaction and caseation. The enlargement and necrosis of the regional glands is milder than in tuberculosis but may still lead to right middle lobe collapse or subsequent erosion of a phlebolith through the bronchial wall with haemoptysis. Most primary lesions heal rapidly with fibrosis and calcification but in older patients resolution may take up to 2 years with the production of a solid primary lesion consisting of layers of fibrosis and necrosis which may be mistaken for a tumour. Blood-borne dissemination may occur at any stage and is believed to account for the characteristic disseminated calcified opacities seen on chest radiography (*Fig.* 39.21). The majority of primary foci are asymptomatic although there may be mild influenzal symptoms which settle rapidly. Rarely, fever, malaise, weight loss, chest pain, cough and haemoptysis may develop and last for several months. Radiologically, localized or diffuse pneumonic shadowing with hilar adenopathy which heal with fibrosis and later calcification may be seen.

Rarely (0·2%) either acute or chronic *progressive pulmonary histoplasmosis* follows the primary lesion. The *acute* form consisting of a progressive caseating pneumonia with exten-

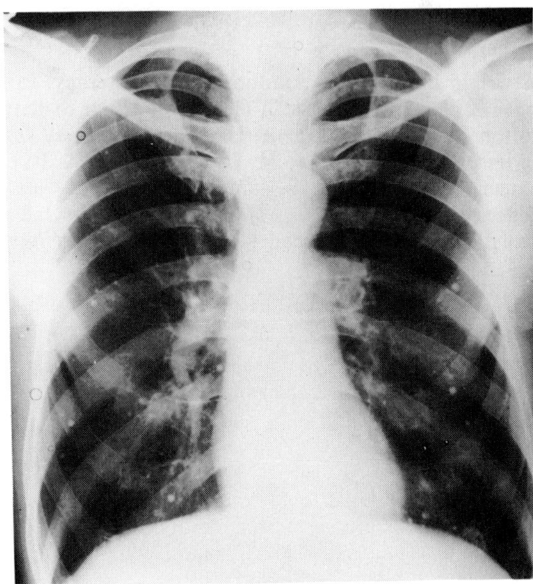

Fig. 39.21 Chest film showing small round opacities in the lower parts of both lungs. The calcification is dense and appears homogeneous although with magnification some of the nodules consist of a central core surrounded by a halo of decreased density which is characteristic of histoplasmosis. (By courtesy of Dr Paul Grech.)

sive lung destruction and severe systemic upset has a high mortality and must be distinguished from tuberculosis.

The commoner *chronic* form affects the upper lobes with progressive caseation, fibrosis and cavity formation resembling tuberculosis. Blood-borne dissemination leads to chronic granuloma in other organs. The clinical features include increasing debility, weight loss, dyspnoea, a chronic productive cough, intermittent haemoptysis, the signs of pneumonia or cavitation over the upper lobes and a radiological picture suggesting fibrocaseous tuberculosis.

The organism may be identified from smears, culture or guinea-pig inoculation of sputum or gastric washing. The histoplasmin test becomes positive within 8 weeks but may be negative in severe cases. Complement-fixation, agglutination or precipitin antibody tests may be helpful. Treatment with intravenous amphotericin B is required for progressive symptomatic disease. Isolated granuloma may need surgical resection.

North American Blastomycosis

This disease, which principally affects forestry and agricultural workers, was first isolated along the eastern seaboard of the USA but subsequently found in Africa and is thought to have reached America at the time of the slave trade. The spores of *Blastomyces dermatitis* produce a granulomatous caseating lesion in the lower lobes with regional gland enlargement. Haematogenous spread may involve other organs. The initial infection may be asymptomatic or produce acute respiratory symptoms of varying severity. The primary lesion may heal with calcification or extend producing either an acute fulminating pneumonia or chronic fibrocaseous disease with progressive disability clinically resembling tuberculosis. An empyema or a chronic chest wall sinus may develop. The radiological findings include pneumonic shadowing, fibrocaseous destruction with cavitation, miliary mottling and hilar gland enlargement. Tuberculosis frequently coexists. Accessible lesions, e.g. skin, should be biopsied and sputum sent for culture and guinea-pig inoculation. The intradermal blastomycin test produces a delayed reaction but may be negative in severe cases. Serological tests are unreliable. Intravenous amphotericin B is the drug of choice but stilbamidine is a useful alternative.

Paracoccidioidomycosis

Infection with *Paracoccidioides brasiliensis* is largely restricted to Southern and Central America. Primary infections principally involve the mucocutaneous junctions with considerable disfiguration. Inhalation may lead to lung involvement with small granulomas, extensive pneumonia or chronic suppuration, cavitation and fibrosis. Rarely blood-borne spread produces miliary lung lesions.

The diagnosis may be obtained by biopsying an accessible lesion, sputum culture or immunofluorescent studies. An intradermal skin test is available and the complement-fixation test may be positive in acute cases. Intravenous amphotericin B may effectively control the infection although reactivation may occur several years later. Reports using miconazole are encouraging.

Sporotrichosis

In South Africa, France and Southern USA sporotrichosis is endemic. *Sporotrichum schenckii* lives in soil and usually enters the body through skin abrasions causing a subcutaneous granulomatous nodule with local lymphatic spread and blood-borne dissemination. Only rarely are the lungs involved either by haematogenous spread or direct inhalation, with the production of chronic thin-walled cavities and satellite granuloma. Skin biopsy, sputum culture, mice inoculation or the sporotrichin skin test may be helpful in diagnosis. The skin lesion responds to high doses of potassium iodide while pulmonary sporotrichosis may be arrested by intravenous amphotericin B permitting later surgical resection of the damaged lung.

Further Reading

Cartwright R. Y. (1980) Antifungal Chemotherapy. In: *Opportunistic Mycoses of Various Body Sites*. New York, Wiley.

Citron K. M. and Thomas G. O. (1986) Ocular toxicity from ethambutol. *Thorax* **41**, 737–739.

Crofton J. W. and Douglas A. C. (1981) *Respiratory Diseases*, 3rd ed. Oxford, Blackwell.

Sanderson J. M., Kennedy M. C. S., Johnson M. F. et al. (1974) Bronchiectasis—the results of surgical and conservative management. *Thorax* **29**, 407.

Spencer H. (1984) *Pathology of the Lung*, 4th ed. Oxford, Pergamon.

Toman K. (1979) *Tuberculosis—Case Finding and Chemotherapy. Questions and Answers.* Geneva, WHO.

40 Disease of the Pleura, Spontaneous Pneumothorax and Emphysema

R. A. Clark

PLEURAL EFFUSION

A pleural effusion exists when there is an abnormal amount of fluid within the pleural space detectable on clinical or radiological examination. The pleura are normally kept moist by a thin layer of fluid (up to 15 ml), which is constantly being formed and reabsorbed (with an hourly turnover of up to 500 ml). A collection of 100–300 ml is necessary for radiological and at least 500 ml for clinical detection.

An effusion will develop when the equilibrium between formation and absorption is disturbed. The factors governing the exchange of fluid are the same as at any capillary/tissue interface, namely:

1. *The capillary hydrostatic pressure* which is dependent on the venous pressure. An increase in systemic venous pressure, e.g. congestive cardiac failure or constrictive pericarditis, may be an important factor in the formation of an effusion. If there is a concomitant rise in the pulmonary venous pressure, e.g. left ventricular failure, then the effects are additive but cor pulmonale alone has little effect.

2. *The colloidal osmotic pressure* is proportional to the molar concentrations of the proteins such that the lower molecular weight proteins, i.e. albumin, have the greatest effect. Any cause of hypoproteinaemia, e.g. the nephrotic syndrome or liver disease, will reduce the pressure and encourage the formation of an effusion. Proteins from the pleural space drain solely into the lymphatic system principally through the mediastinal pleura, a process encouraged by exercise. Although the turnover of protein is slower than water and electrolytes, 1 g of albumin may be exchanged in 24 h. In normal subjects the pleural fluid contains 10–20 g/l or protein and this rises in the presence of increased capillary permeability, i.e. pleural inflammation. Decreased reabsorption may be as important as increased output in the formation of some effusions.

3. *The capillary permeability* is increased in pleural inflammation, i.e. pneumonia or pulmonary infarction, allowing more fluid and protein to enter the pleural space.

4. *Lymphatic drainage*. Cells and protein leave the pleural space via the lymphatic system and any impairment of lymphatic drainage, i.e. lymph node infiltration (tumour), a maldeveloped lymphatic system (yellow nail syndrome) or increased venous pressure (congestive cardiac failure), will encourage the formation of an effusion.

A pleural effusion is always a manifestation of local or systemic disease. Its size may vary from just sufficient to blunt the costophrenic angle to large enough to fill a hemithorax with displacement of the heart and mediastinum to the contralateral side. The effusion may (*a*) lie free within the pleural space when it will gravitate to the most dependent part; (*b*) become loculated within an interlobar fissure; or (*c*) become encapsulated by adhesions anywhere in the pleural space. Not all effusions arise directly from a pathological process, 'sympathetic effusions' being a collection of clear fluid in response to a lesion within the thorax, e.g. an empyema, or abdomen, e.g. a subphrenic abscess. The composition of an effusion often varies from area to area.

An asymptomatic effusion may be picked up on routine radiography. The usual presentation is of progressive dyspnoea which may be associated with pleuritic pain or a dull ache. There may be fever and toxaemia which settles after aspiration. Cough and haemoptysis usually indicate an underlying pulmonary cause.

The physical findings in a moderate or large effusion lying free in the pleural space, are diminished expansion, stony dullness, diminished or absent breath sounds and reduced vocal fremitus and resonance over the affected side. A pleural friction rub may be audible at the top of an effusion with an area of bronchial breathing a little lower. If large there may be shift of the heart and mediastinum to the contralateral side. A subpulmonary effusion presents with the features of an elevated hemidiaphragm. If the effusion lies within an interlobar fissure there may be no abnormal findings.

Radiologically, blunting of the costophrenic angle may be the only finding. A small effusion may be distinguished from pleural thickening and its size determined by a lateral decubitus film when the fluid will run down and collect as a puddle in the most dependent part. Large effusions show the characteristic axillary tail with a concave upper border (the upper margin is at the same level right round the effusion but in the PA chest film the fluid in the axilla is seen end on and appears as a dense concave shadow). In a large effusion the hemithorax may appear opaque with the mediastinum shifted to the opposite side (*Fig.* 40.1).

It may be difficult to distinguish an infrapulmonary effusion from an elevated hemidiaphragm. Such effusions are seldom completely loculated and fluid will be displaced in a decubitus film. If loculation has occurred a small artificial pneumoperitoneum (*see Fig.* 38.11, p. 544) or the gastric air bubble will help delineate the lower margin of the diaphragm.

Interlobar effusions may present bizarre appearances on the PA radiograph but a lateral film usually shows the characteristic round or oval shadow in line with a fissure (*Fig.* 40.2). Occasionally a bronchogram may be necessary to distinguish an effusion from collapse or consolidation of the right middle lobe.

While the causes of a pleural effusion are numerous, the patient's age and environmental circumstances will influence the likely aetiology. Thus tuberculosis would be more likely in an adolescent from the third world than in an elderly western male. Similarly the size of the effusion and whether it is unilateral or bilateral will be of diagnostic significance. The major causes for each group are set out below.

Unilateral Effusions

	Small to moderate effusions	*Large effusions occupying most of a hemithorax*
Frequent causes	Secondary malignancy (50%) Bacterial pneumonia Cardiac failure Pulmonary infarction Tuberculosis Connective-tissue disorders	Secondary malignancy (66%) Tuberculosis Cardiac failure Empyema Haemothorax
Less frequent	Pneumothorax Lymphoma Subphrenic abscess Pancreatitis Primary pleural tumours Fungal infection Viral infection Post-myocardial infarction	
Rare	Drug induced (methysergide, practolol nitrofurantoin) Lung abscesses Bronchiectasis Amoebiasis Yellow nail syndrome	

Bilateral Effusions

These usually suggest a systemic cause:

1. *Most commonly a transudate:* Congestive cardiac failure; Hypoproteinaemia (nephrotic syndrome, liver disease); Constrictive pericarditis; Meigs's syndrome; Myxoedema.
2. *Some may be exudates:* Multiple pulmonary infarcts; Connective-tissue disorders; Secondary malignancy; Rarely, tuberculosis.
3. Alternatively, there may be separate causes on each side, i.e. pulmonary infarct on one side and congestive cardiac failure on the other.

An indication as to the aetiology may be obtained from the history. Pleuritic pain suggests inflammation prior to the effusion, i.e. pneumonia or pulmonary infarction, while a dull ache may accompany malignant infiltration. Dyspnoea out of keeping with the size of the effusion may indicate underlying cardiac or pulmonary disease and haemoptysis suggests carcinoma, pulmonary infarction or pneumonia. Peripheral oedema might indicate cardiac failure or hypoproteinaemia. In difficult cases, some help may be obtained from the mode of onset and duration (the more rapid the more acute), any abdominal symptoms (pancreatitis or perforated bowel), recent abdominal surgery (subphrenic abscess, pneumonia or infarction), previous mastectomy (secondary malignancy), occupation (including exposure to asbestos many years previously), travel (amoebiasis), contact with tuberculosis or drug history (remembering an effusion may develop after drug withdrawal).

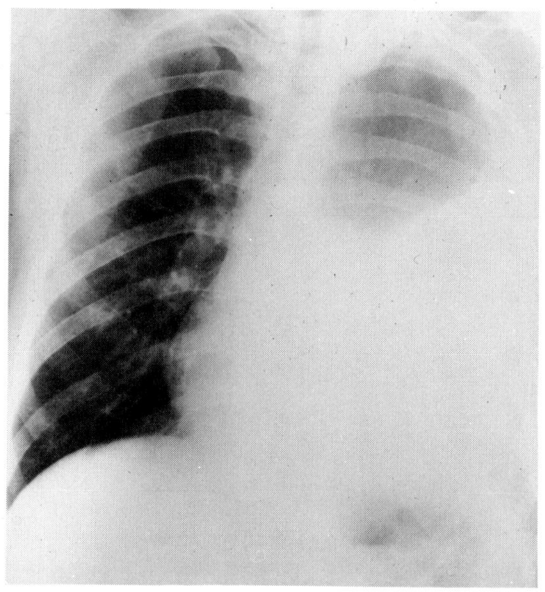

Fig. 40.1 Large left pleural effusion with mediastinal shift to the right.

A comprehensive physical examination is essential with special attention being paid to lymphadenopathy or clubbing, the signs of cardiac failure, constrictive pericarditis or hypothyroidism, any breast or abdominal masses, abdominal tenderness or scars and the occurrence of ascites or a deep venous thrombosis.

A chest radiograph taken after aspiration or in the lateral decubitus position may indicate an underlying pulmonary lesion while a previous film may give a valuable lead (*Fig.* 40.3).

Smear, culture and animal inoculation of sputum, tuberculin or fungal skin tests, bronchoscopy, electro- and echocardiography, ventilation and perfusion lung scans, and immunological tests (rheumatoid factor, antinuclear factor and LE cells) may give valuable diagnostic leads.

Aspiration of a little fluid (20–30 ml) from an area of maximum dullness confirms the diagnosis and its appearance may give an indication as to the aetiology:

1. *Transudates.* Usually clear, light straw-coloured fluid which fails to clot. Protein less than 30 g/l. Systemic cause, e.g. congestive cardiac failure or hypoproteinaemia.
2. *Exudates.* Clear but darker yellow clotting on standing. Protein greater than 30 g/l. Local cause, e.g. tumour, infection.
3. *Bloodstained.* Traumatic pleural taps will cause fresh bleeding. Continuous aspiration of old, dark red blood is characteristic of malignancy but may also occur in tuberculosis, infarction and pancreatitis.
4. *Frank blood* (haemothorax). Pure blood usually follows chest trauma, including ruptured aorta.

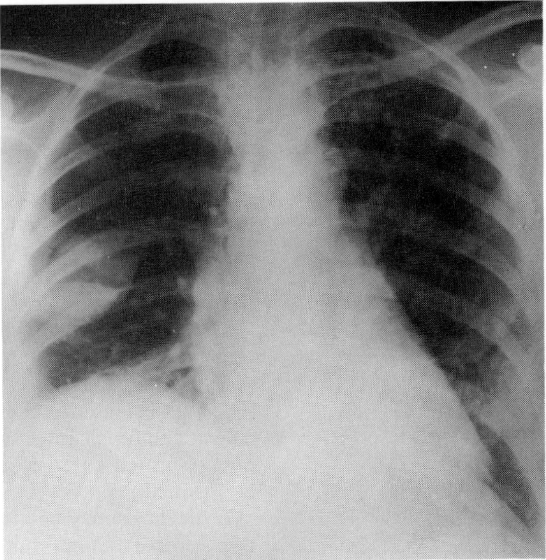

a

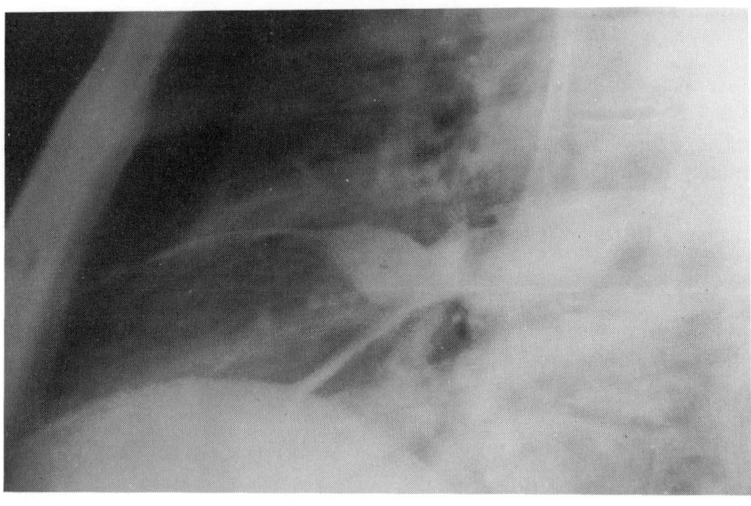

b

Fig. 40.2 Interlobar pleural effusion. (*a*) An opacity is seen in the right midzone, better visualized in the lateral projection; (*b*) where it proved to be due to two lamellar shadows along the transverse and oblique fissures. (By courtesy of Dr Paul Grech.)

5. *Turbid*. Indicative of a high cell count as found in pneumonic effusions.

6. *Frank pus* (empyema). Frankly purulent fluid of varying viscosity. There is no clear demarcation between turbid effusions and an empyema.

7. *Opalescent effusions*. Shimmering whitish semitranslucent due to a high cholesterol level. A rare feature of longstanding effusions of whatever cause, i.e. malignancy, tuberculosis or nephrotic syndrome.

8. *Chyle* (chylothorax). White and oily due to the collection of lymph secondary to involvement of the main lymphatic canals (e.g. damage or involvement of thoracic duct).

A large volume of fluid may be aspirated either for diagnostic purposes or to relieve symptoms (dyspnoea, fever). The needle is usually inserted in the posterior axillary line just below the upper level of dullness with the patient leaning forward. For loculated effusions the site may be determined from postero-anterior and lateral films or the procedure may be done under fluoroscopic control. The needle size will depend on the nature of the fluid. Failure to obtain sufficient fluid usually results from: (*a*) aspiration at too low a level resulting in hitting the diaphragm which may be elevated from pulmonary collapse; or (*b*) loculation with adhesions. The initial aspiration should be limited to 1 litre in adults (less in children) as too rapid or too large an aspiration may precipitate: (*a*) unilateral pulmonary oedema (the exact mechanism being uncertain); (*b*) respiratory distress and pain; (*c*) tachycardia; or (*d*) hypotension. Other less acute complications include pneumothorax, haemorrhage or infection. Occasionally a 'sympathetic effusion' may be tapped instead of the main collection.

Aliquots of the aspirate should be sent for cytological, biochemical and bacteriological examination.

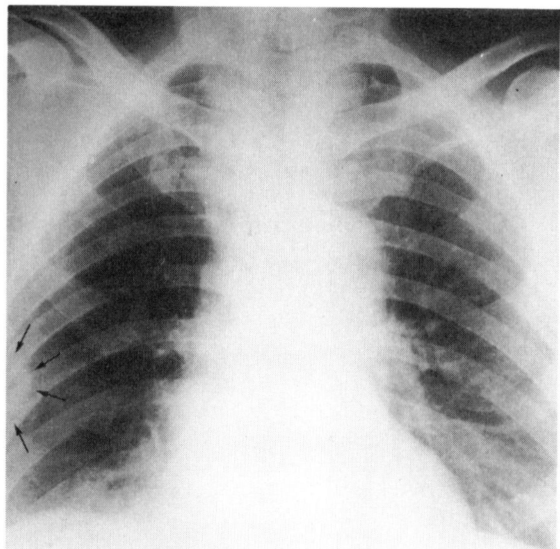

Fig. 40.3 Peripheral right lower lobe shadow discovered after tapping of right pleural effusion. The lesion was a carcinoma.

Cytology

While the total cell count is of little value, differential cell counts may provide useful information. Malignant cells may be identified. However, inexperienced cytologists may misinterpret the appearance of the mesothelial cells giving a false positive reading. While a high lymphocyte count is common to both tuberculosis and secondary malignancy, mesothelial cells are frequently found in the latter but not in the former. Neutrophilia is found in pneumonic effusions. Some effusions have a high eosinophil count which has little diagnostic significance.

Biochemical Analysis

Biochemical analysis of pleural fluid for diagnostic purposes is of limited value. A protein level below 30 g/l suggests a transudate and above this level an exudate but around the cross-over point the picture is blurred. A low glucose level (below 1·7 mmol/l, 30 mg/100 ml) is often found in rheumatoid arthritis but also occurs in malignancy and empyema. A high amylase is associated with pancreatitis but is also found in a ruptured oesophagus. The fat content is high in chylothorax and the cholesterol may be elevated in a chronic effusion. The rheumatoid factor is present in most cases of rheumatoid arthritis but is also found in some cases of malignancy and tuberculosis.

Bacteriological Examination

This may be by smear of sulphur granules or pus (fungi or actinomycosis), culture for anaerobes, aerobes, fungi or tuberculosis (positive in only 25% of tuberculous effusions) or animal inoculation (tuberculosis). Close co-operation with the bacteriologist is essential.

Pleural Biopsy

The introduction of a closed pleural biopsy technique using the Abrams' needle (*see Fig.* 38.18) has proved a simple, safe and effective means of diagnosing pleural effusions of tuberculous (80%) or malignant (60–70%) origin particularly if 3 or 4 biopsies are taken each time and the procedure repeated if necessary. The lack of distinctive histological features in other causes has limited its usefulness. The biopsy should only be attempted in the presence of fluid. If a bleeding diathesis is suspected this should be corrected first. Complications (pneumothorax, slight bleeding) are rare.

Pleural effusions are always the manifestation of disease and should never be considered idiopathic. If, in spite of extensive investigation, the diagnosis remains in doubt, thoracoscopy with direct visualization and biopsy of the pleura or open biopsy at thoracotomy should be considered. The latter is most valuable in suspected tuberculosis, secondary malignancy, empyema and fungal infections. Alternatively, the patient may be followed up with the investigations repeated at a later date. A two-year follow-up of 27 cases of undiagnosed effusion led to the diagnosis in 16 (60%), the major causes being secondary malignancy, tuberculosis and fungal infections. If tuberculosis is suspected but not confirmed a trial of antituberculous chemotherapy may be justified.

A diagnosis may be made on clinical ground, e.g. congestive cardiac failure, but the effusion fails to respond to appropriate treatment, i.e. diuretics, when further investigation may indicate a different aetiology.

Factors which may be important in the diagnosis or management of specific types of pleural effusion are considered below.

Congestive cardiac failure is the commonest cause of a transudate (*Fig.* 40.4). It may develop within 24 h of elevation of the venous pressure and is more likely to occur if both the systemic and pulmonary venous pressures are raised. Initially unilateral, usually on the right, it may become bilateral if the failure remains uncontrolled. Provided the dyspnoea is not severe, a trial of diuretics without aspiration is often justified.

Most *pulmonary infarcts* involve the pleural surface with subsequent inflammation and the formation of a small to moderate effusion which is usually clear, yellow fluid but

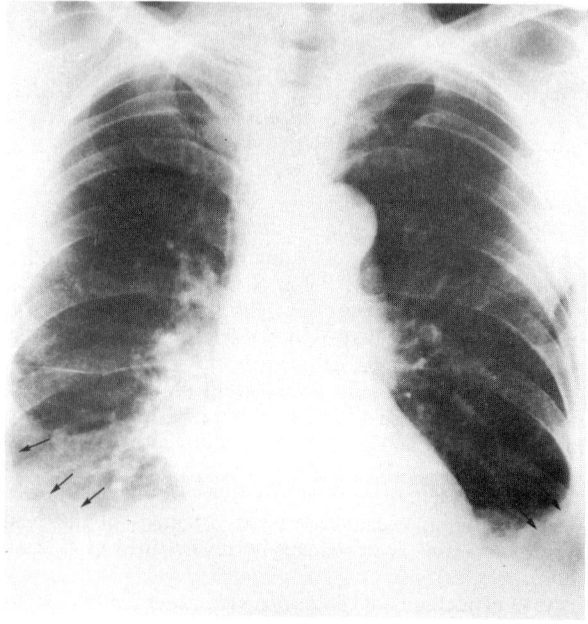

Fig. 40.4 Bilateral basal pleural effusions and a prominent horizontal fissure due to cardiac failure.

may be bloodstained. Most effusions are self-limiting and rarely require aspiration. The diagnosis depends on identifying the underlying infarction by lung scans or pulmonary angiography.

Eighty per cent of *subphrenic abscesses* develop a 'sympathetic effusion' which contains polymorphs but no organisms. The effusion should be aspirated, the abscess drained, and antibiotics given to lessen the risk of an empyema.

Hepatic amoebiasis may cause a 'sympathetic effusion' but more often pleural adhesions develop which allow the infection to spread directly to the right lower lobe.

A pleural effusion, usually on the left, may complicate up to 10% of cases of *severe acute pancreatitis* the fluid often being bloodstained and having a high amylase content. The mechanism remains in dispute.

Ascites secondary to cirrhosis is often associated with bilateral effusion which arise from a combination of: (*a*) hypoproteinaemia; and (*b*) the direct passage of fluid through the diaphragm via the lymphatics or diaphragmatic defects. Rarely an ovarian tumour is associated with ascites and bilateral pleural effusions which resolve after resection of the tumour (*Meigs's syndrome*).

Peritoneal dialysis may be complicated by bilateral effusions.

Ten per cent of patients with *acute rheumatic fever* develop a small or moderate, transient pleural effusion, at times bilateral, which usually requires no treatment.

A protracted unilateral effusion requiring repeated aspiration may be the first manifestation of *rheumatoid arthritis*. The fluid, which may be opalescent, has a low glucose content and is usually positive for the rheumatoid factor. Pleural rheumatoid nodules may be visible on thoracoscopy. At post-mortem pleural adhesions are common in rheumatoid arthritis and are believed to result from recurrent pleurisy or effusions. Bilateral effusions occasionally complicate *systemic lupus erythematosus* and may be the presenting feature.

Pleural involvement in a *bacterial pneumonia* may progress to the formation of a serous effusion which should be suspected if fever persists in spite of appropriate antibiotic therapy. The frequency with which an effusion develops depends on the causal organism, i.e. 10% with pneumococcal, 35% with anaerobic and 50% with staphylococcal pneumonias. The turbid fluid is rich in neutrophils but an organism is rarely cultured from it. The effusion may: (1) remain serous, resolving without complications; (2) cause pleural fibrosis with restriction in lung function; or (3) develop into an empyema. In view of the latter possibility such effusions should be aspirated to dryness, when the fever invariably settles.

Pleural effusions are infrequent in *viral infections* and when they occur they are usually small and only detected radiologically. The diagnosis depends on showing a rising viral antibody titre.

Pleurisy and pleural effusions occur early in actinomycosis as a prelude to an empyema and chest wall involvement. Sulphur granules in pus or sputum are diagnostic of *Actinomyces israelii* infections.

Pleural effusion may complicate primary coccidioidomycosis, blastomycosis, histoplasmosis or cryptococcosis and if suspected special culture media will be required.

Tuberculous pleural effusions may arise: (*a*) during the course of the primary complex in children (7%) when the effusion is often small and self-limiting, resolving over 3–4 months without residual fibrosis or calcification; (*b*) as the main postprimary tuberculous manifestation in adolescents; or (*c*) as a complication of postprimary pulmonary tuberculosis. The pleura are usually studded with small tubercles, the effusion resulting from the combination of an inflammatory exudate and a hypersensitive reaction to the tubercular protein.

Classic adolescent tuberculous effusions which develop within a year of the primary complex are still frequently encountered in the third world but have become uncommon in western countries. Several weeks of vague ill-health, pleural pain and fever are usual but progressive dyspnoea may be the presenting feature. A pleural rub may be heard, particularly if the effusion is small. The effusion is the principal radiological abnormality, the lung fields and hilar shadows often appearing normal. The tuberculin test is strongly positive. The pleural fluid is rich in lymphocytes, but smears of centrifuged debris are rarely positive and culture of the organism is difficult. Closed pleural biopsy using the Abrams' needle is positive in 70–80% of cases. Treatment with chemotherapy, pleural aspiration (repeated as necessary), and breathing exercises usually ensures rapid and complete recovery but inadequate treatment or delayed diagnosis can lead to pleural thickening or calcification which requires decortication.

If a postprimary tuberculous cavity ruptures into the pleural space a pneumothorax and effusion results but this has become rare with good chemotherapy. The chest radiograph shows a hydropneumothorax with the underlying pulmonary lesion. If inadequately treated there is the danger of developing a tuberculous empyema with progressive contraction and fibrosis of the hemithorax. A similar situation resulting from previous artificial pneumothorax treatment may still be encountered. When treating a tuberculous empyema, resection of the affected lobe or a pleuropneumonectomy may be necessary.

Most *malignant pleural effusions* result from the secondary involvement of the pleura from primary tumours arising in other organs, primary pleural tumours accounting for but a few. The effusion is an exudate which is formed as a result of increased capillary permeability and obstruction to the lymphatic and venous drainage. The pleura are usually studded with metastatic deposits, direct invasion being uncommon. Bronchial and breast primaries are the commonest followed by pancreatic, stomach and uterine. The effusion may be the first indication of malignancy with little evidence of the primary site, or result from the extension of a previously diagnosed lesion. It may herald the end of many symptom-free years in a breast carcinoma which had been previously resected. At autopsy a third of patients dying of Hodgkin's disease have a pleural effusion but the cause may be other than metastatic spread, i.e. infection. Effusions may also complicate some lymphomas. With lymphomas and some extrathoracic primaries, i.e. breast, the effusions may be bilateral. When complicating lymphangitis carcinomatosa the effusions are often bilateral and add to the patient's distress.

There may be few symptoms if the effusion is small or slowly developing. However, most malignant effusions collect over a few days with increasing dyspnoea, nagging chest pain and cough. A careful history and examination may reveal the site of the primary lesion. A post-aspiration chest radiograph may show metastatic pleural deposits or enlarged mediastinal nodes (lymphomas). Occasionally the fluid is a clear, yellow exudate but more often it is uniformly bloodstained. Cytology may show malignant cells or lymphocytes but a normal cytological report does not exclude tumour. Closed pleural biopsy (Abrams' needle) may confirm the diagnosis and give some indication of histological type. In difficult cases the diagnosis may be made by thoracoscopy or at exploratory thoracotomy.

Most malignant pleural effusions cause considerable distress, i.e. dyspnoea and chest pain, but are difficult to control as they often reaccumulate rapidly following aspiration in spite of the variety of therapies on offer. As yet there is no consensus as to the best means of treatment and controlled trials are urgently needed. A few cases respond to hormone therapy (some breast tumours), systemic cytotoxic chemotherapy (some breast, ovarian and small-cell bronchial carcinomas or lymphoma), radiotherapy (some lymphomas) or pleural resection (the occasional mesothelioma) but the majority require palliative measures. Repeated aspiration only depletes the patient's proteins. Intubation and drainage have been reported to induce adhesions and prevent recurrence in 50% of cases. Aspiration followed by instillation of sclerosing agents, e.g. tetracycline, mepacrine and talc or the organism *Corynebacterium parvum* to induce an inflammatory reaction have their advocates. Cytotoxic agents, e.g. mustine, 5-fluorouracil, thiotepa or bleomycin may be instilled, the best results occurring if the fluid contains a high cell count and if the aspiration and drainage are carried out over several days using an indwelling drainage tube. Some authorities consider that systemic corticosteroids reduce the rate of reaccumulation as well as improving the patient's mental state. If the above methods fail and the patient's condition remains good with a favourable prognosis pleurodectomy may be considered but this is accompanied by a significant morbidity. If the diagnosis is made at thoracotomy, pleurodectomy or pleural abrasion should be considered to facilitate the formation of adhesions.

CHYLOTHORAX

The collection of chyle (lymphatic fluid) within the pleural space following rupture or trauma to the thoracic duct or the right bronchomediastinal trunk, although comparatively rare, is increasing in frequency. The fluid is rich in protein, fat, fat-soluble vitamins, water and electrolytes and its repeated aspiration often causes emaciation, hypoproteinaemia and lymphopenia.

The major causes are:

1. *Surgical trauma*. The technical advances in thoracic and oesophageal surgery have increased the chance of trauma to the lymph ducts although a chylothorax complicates less than 0·005% of such operations. The risks are greatest with surgery in the vicinity of the left subclavian artery. Block dissection of neck glands or scalene node biopsy have also been implicated. If the injury is recognized at the time of surgery and the duct ligated chylothorax does not develop.
2. *Trauma*. Sudden hyperextension of the spine may lead to rupture of the thoracic duct just above the diaphragm. Chlylothorax may also complicate falls, compression injuries or blows to the trunk, stab or gunshot wounds and severe episodes of coughing or vomiting.
3. *Obstruction* to the thoracic duct from enlarged lymph nodes usually secondary to malignancy (gastric carcinoma, follicular lymphoma), but occasionally from tuberculosis or filariasis may cause a chylothorax. Rarely, thrombosis of the left subclavian vein, aortic aneurysm or benign lymphangioma have been implicated.
4. *Miscellaneous*. Congenital fistulas, birth injury or chylous ascites are rare causes.

Two to ten days may elapse between rupture and the formation of a chylothorax during which time chyle is believed to collect in the posterior mediastinum. While longer latent periods have been described (6½ years) these cases probably represent re-rupture at the site of a previous scar. Up to 2·5 litres of chyle may be produced daily.

The sudden onset of dyspnoea and pyrexia without toxaemia is the usual presentation. The clinical and radiological features are those of an effusion. The aspirate is characteristically white and oily with a high fat content, and can usually be easily distinguished from an opalescent effusion. Occasionally the ingestion of a lipophilic dye, which when absorbed rapidly passes into the chyle, may be used to establish the diagnosis. The effusion rapidly reaccumulates and repeated aspirations may lead to cachexia and death. In chronic cases a fibrous rind may limit chest expansion.

There is a 50% chance of spontaneous closure. Conservative management may necessitate frequent aspirations but a time limit should be set to prevent excessive emaciation from nutrient loss. Ligation of the thoracic duct is safe and effective due to its extensive communications with the right bronchomediastinal trunk and the azygos, intercostal and vertebral veins. Some workers advocate drainage of the pleural space by intubation and suction followed by the instillation of talc or other sclerosing agents to induce pleurodesis and improve the results of conservative treatment.

EMPYEMA

The incidence of empyema has fallen since the introduction of antibiotics for the treatment of pulmonary infections. Early diagnosis and effective therapy are essential if the fixed, fibrotic hemithorax characteristic of a chronic empyema is to be avoided. Of the sources of infection shown below pulmonary infections remain the most important.

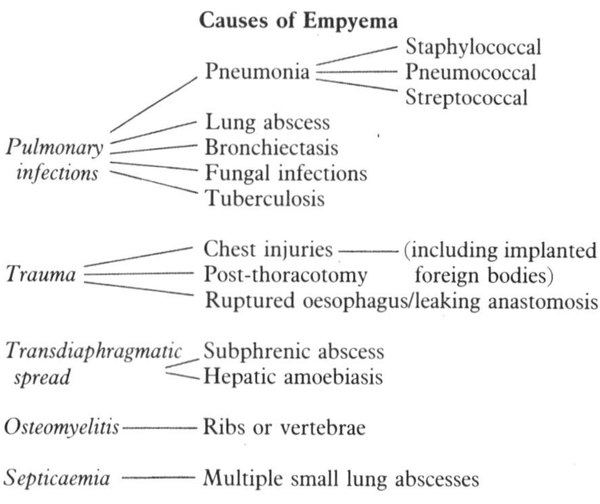

'Dry pleurisy' may be the first indication of pleural inflammation although this is quickly followed by the outpouring of fluid rich in protein and polymorphs but frank purulence must develop before an effusion is referred to as an empyema. The empyema may lie free in the pleura space or be encapsulated by fibrinous pleural adhesions which arise as a local defence mechanism often encouraged by antibiotic therapy. Continued accumulation of pus compresses the lung with shift of the mediastinum to the opposite side. Fluid may be absorbed making the pus more viscous. Fibrin is continually deposited on the pleural surfaces producing a thickening rind, the deeper layers of which become fibrotic and avascular permitting easy stripping during surgical decortication. Adequate treatment at this stage will produce full re-expansion of the lung with gradual resolution of the pleural inflammation and no functional impairment.

The transition from an acute to chronic empyema is arbitrary, periods of between 6 and 12 weeks having been suggested. The continual formation and fibrosis of the pleural rind progressively restricts chest wall and diaphragmatic movement, eventually producing a shrunken, flattened, immobile hemithorax with overlapping ribs and scoliosis to the affected side. Adhesions may loculate the viscous pus. At this stage it may be difficult to aspirate pus even for diagnostic purposes. There may be considerable subpleural alveolar destruction and fibrosis leading to permanent functional impairment, even if lung re-expansion is achieved. Brain abscesses, bone marrow suppression or amyloidosis may result from the chronic inflammation.

The term 'pyopneumothorax' refers to the situation where there is air and pus within the pleural space. This may occur: (*a*) if the empyema discharges into a bronchus forming a bronchopleural fistula; (*b*) if the empyema results from the rupture of a lung abscess or cyst (hydatid) again with the formation of a bronchopleural fistula; (*c*) following pleural aspiration if the lung is bound down by fibrotic rind and unable to re-expand; or (*d*) if the empyema contains gas-forming organisms usually associated with implanted foreign bodies, i.e. clostridial species.

Occasionally an empyema erodes through the chest wall forming a collar-stud abscess which may break down giving a discharging fistula in continuity with the empyema cavity (empyema necessitatis).

The pathological process is modified according to the infecting organism. Streptococcal infections produce thin pus with few adhesions and considerable toxaemia while a pneumococcal empyema becomes rapidly encapsulated with less systemic upset. Empyemas secondary to lung abscesses often contain mixed anaerobic, microaerophilic and aerobic organisms capable of producing putrefaction with foul-smelling pus. An empyema associated with spreading infection distal to a bronchial carcinoma may go unnoticed in the patient's general deterioration.

Clinical Presentation

The clinical features of acute and chronic empyemas are considered separately.

Acute

The patient may present with a pyrexia or a respiratory infection which has failed to respond or has relapsed during or after treatment. There may be a history of recent thoracic or abdominal surgery, trauma or liver disease. A sudden deterioration in a child with staphylococcal pneumonia or severe pleurisy in hydatid disease may herald the development of an empyema.

Fever, rigors, a swinging temperature, malaise, anorexia, weight loss and pleurisy, followed by a gnawing chest pain, are common but may be modified by antibiotic therapy, i.e. into a low-grade grumbling pyrexia. Cough is unusual except with a bronchopleural fistula when large quantities of pus may be expectorated. Dyspnoea may arise if there is lung compression.

The signs of an empyema lying free within the pleural space are those of a pleural effusion, but encapsulated lesions in the interlobar fissures, mediastinum or subpulmonary area may produce no abnormal signs. Finger clubbing can develop within 2–3 weeks. Occasionally a collar-stud abscess (empyema necessitatis) develops usually in relation to the anterior end of the 5th costal cartilage.

A leucocytosis of 15 000–30 000 is common. Pus, aspirated through a wide-bore needle, should be cultured for anaerobic, microaerophilic and aerobic organisms, including fungi and tuberculosis, but previous antibiotic therapy may affect the results.

Radiologically, a free-lying empyema resembles a pleural effusion and, if large, the entire hemithorax may be opaque. PA and lateral films are necessary to localize an encapsulated lesion which has different features depending on its site: (*a*) lying posteriorly and at the base of the pleural cavity it may appear triangular (*Fig.* 40.5) whereas in other parts of the cavity its outline is oval with the base along the chest wall; (*b*) interlobar lesions are usually dense, round or elliptical shadows in the plane of the fissures which may be confused with lobar collapse or consolidation but can be distinguished on bronchography; (*c*) dense oval or round shadows around the heart, mediastinum or diaphragm may be difficult to diagnose; (*d*) a multilobar empyema may have several segments separated by a considerable distance; (*e*) occasionally an encapsulated empyema may induce a 'sympathetic' serous effusion which obscures the underlying lesion. The fluid level of a pyopneumothorax (*Fig.* 40.6) may simulate a lung abscess but an empyema has a sharper outline and lacks a segmental or lobar distribution. Iodized oil injected into the cavity will define its dimensions prior to treatment.

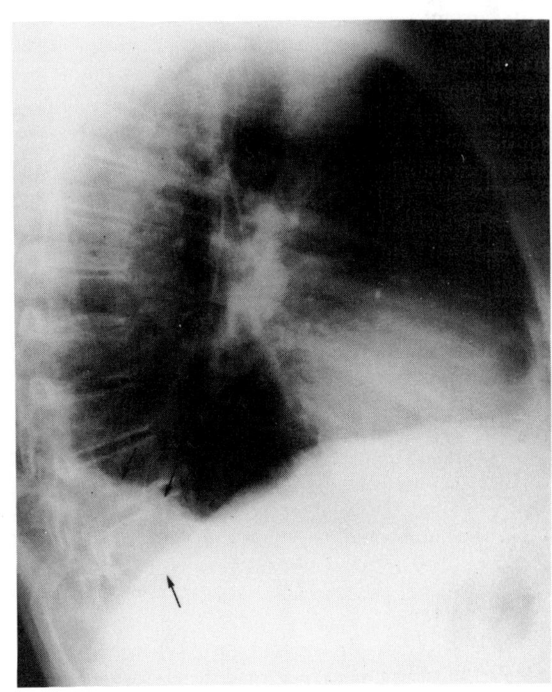

Fig. 40.5 Empyema right base posteriorly. Triangular outline.

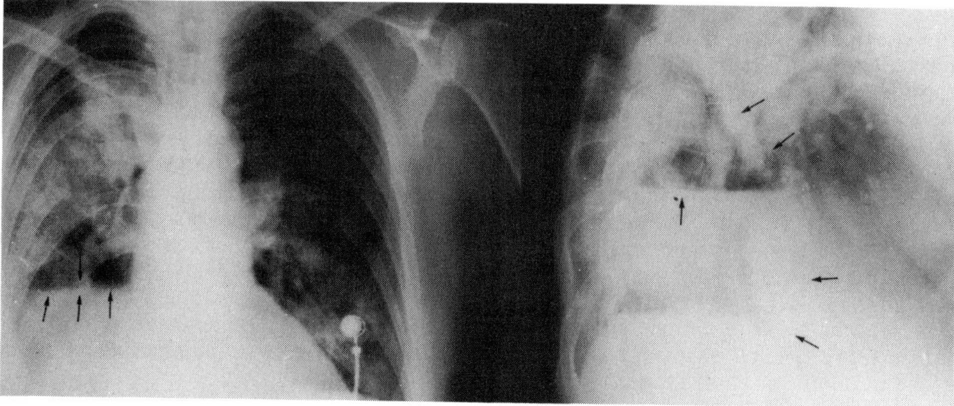

Fig. 40.6 Right-sided pneumonia with pyopneumothorax. The limits of the empyema are outlined by the arrows in the lateral film.

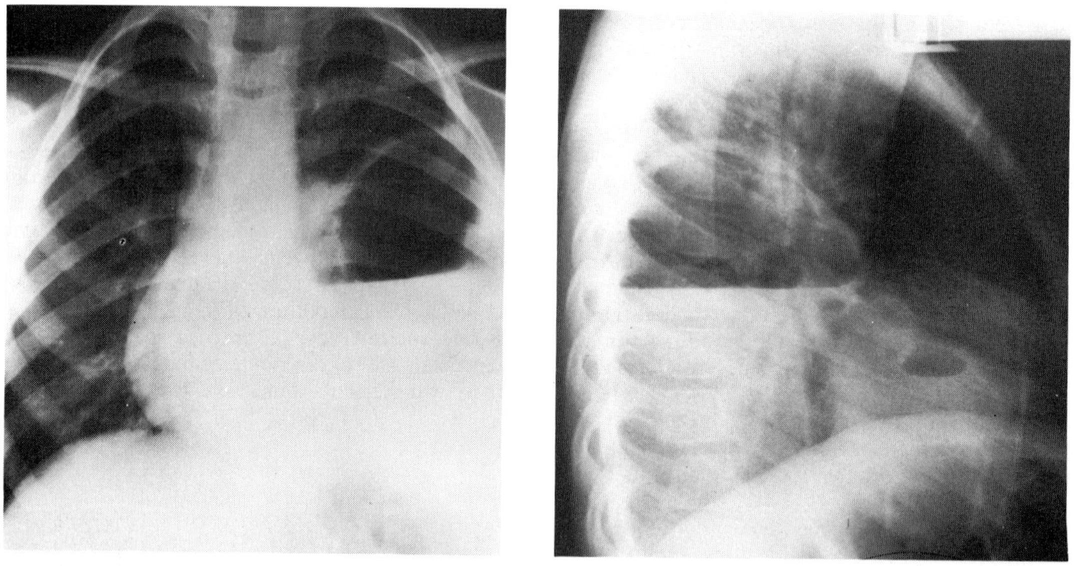

a

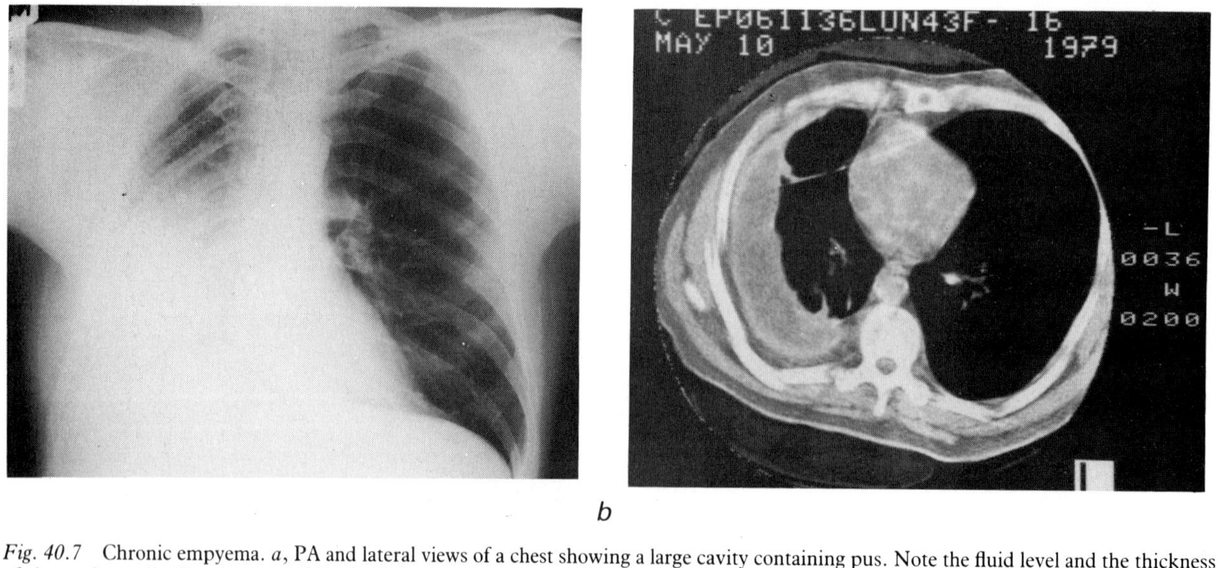

b

Fig. 40.7 Chronic empyema. *a*, PA and lateral views of a chest showing a large cavity containing pus. Note the fluid level and the thickness of the cavity wall. (By courtesy of Dr Paul Grech.) *b*, PA radiograph and CT scan of a patient with chronic empyema and a contracted hemithorax.

Chronic

A chronic empyema most frequently follows inadequate treatment of the acute phase. Less commonly it results from: (*a*) a persistent bronchopleural fistula; (*b*) a retained foreign body; or (*c*) an insidious infection due to tuberculosis, fungi or actinomycosis.

Generalized toxaemia, malaise, anorexia, weight loss, grumbling pyrexia, gnawing chest pain and cutaneous fistulas are common. A persistent cough productive of sputum, particularly when lying on the contralateral side, or an aspiration pneumonia in the 'good lung', are features of a persistent bronchopleural fistula.

Progressive pleural fibrosis produces a shrunken, immobile hemithorax with scoliosis to the affected side. Finger clubbing is common. When bronchopleural and cutaneous fistulas coexist air is expelled through the skin sinus on coughing. A normochromic, normocytic anaemia and leucopenia are common. The features of amyloidosis may be superimposed.

Radiologically, there is dense pleural opacification, elevation of the hemidiaphragm, crowding of the ribs (some of which may show periostitis) and a shift of the mediastinum to the affected side. Fluid levels, which may be multiple with a loculated empyema, occur with bronchopleural or cutaneous fistulas or after aspiration. Pleural calcification may complicate a tuberculous or post-traumatic empyema (*Figs.* 40.7, 40.8).

Pleural aspiration is often difficult but any pus or sputum should be sent for bacteriological examination, including cultures for tuberculosis and fungi, as a prelude to treatment.

When planning treatment the state of the underlying lung, which may be visible radiologically, is important and bronchoscopy to exclude bronchial obstruction (tumour or foreign body) and bronchography to indicate any bronchiectasis should be considered.

Treatment

Acute

When the pus is thin the pleural space should be aspirated to dryness through a wide-bore needle and a broad-spectrum antibiotic given both intrapleurally and systemically, the antibiotic chosen depending on the sensitivities of the organism. Daily aspirations should be continued until the pus ceases to recollect. Vigorous physiotherapy, including breathing exercises, will aid lung re-expansion and encourage good chest movement. If repeated aspirations are difficult a wide-bore intercostal tube with drainage to an underwater seal system may be considered.

If the lung fails to re-expand with aspiration there are two alternatives:

1. *Rib resection*. A generous segment of a rib which lies just above the bottom of the cavity is resected and the cavity fully explored with the removal of all the pus and fibrin deposits. Biopsies from the cavity wall should be sent for pathological and bacteriological examination. The resulting cavity may be drained either by means of: (*a*) a closed system in which a wide-bore tube is left in the space and connected to an underwater seal drainage bottle to which gentle suction may be applied if necessary; or (*b*) an open system where a short length of wide-bore tubing discharges into dressings or a stoma bag. As the volume of pus draining decreases the closed system may be converted into an open one and the tube gradually shortened as the cavity diminishes in size. Aggressive physiotherapy is essential while antibiotic therapy should be guided by the results of the bacteriological investigations, and given for sufficient time if reinfection is to be prevented.

2. *Thoracotomy and decortication*. When the empyema is loculated or if there is an extensive fibrinous rind thoracotomy with excision of the empyema (decortication and removal of all the pus and fibrin clots) is required. Apical and

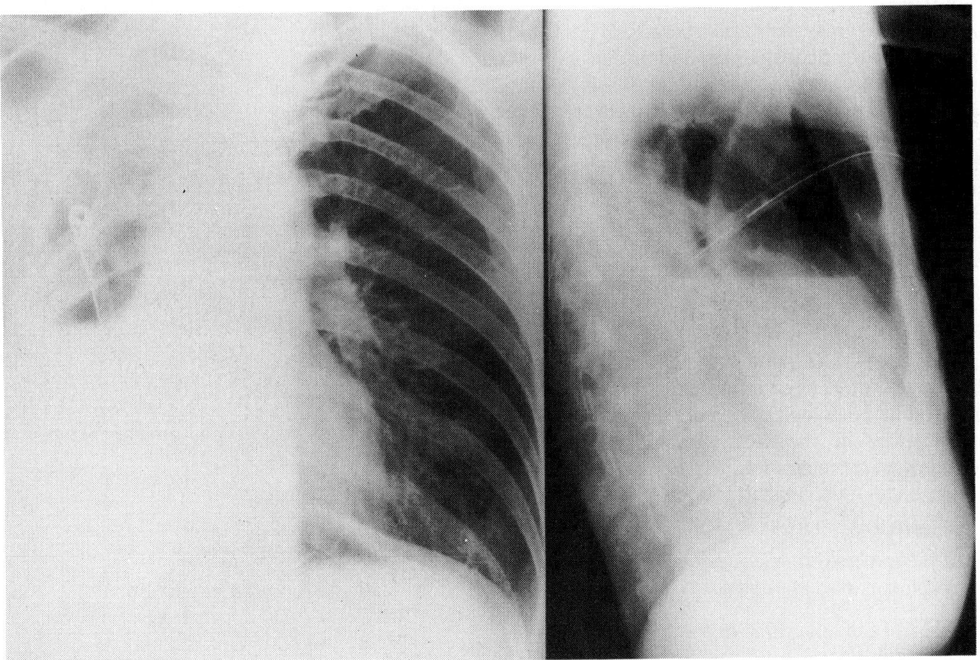

Fig. 40.8 Right postpneumonectomy chronic empyema.

basal drains connected to underwater seal systems ensures adequate drainage and lung re-expansion. Appropriate antibiotic therapy and vigorous physiotherapy are essential.

Most bronchopleural fistulas close spontaneously with adequate treatment. A wide-bore drainage tube connected to an underwater seal drainage system may be fitted with a one-way valve to facilitate physiotherapy and patient mobility during the day. Adequate closure of the cavity checked if necessary by sinograms is essential before removal of the tube if reinfection and chronicity are to be avoided. Fibrinolytic agents have no place in the treatment of empyemas.

Chronic

Aspiration is of little value in treating a chronic empyema. Rib resection and drainage can be effective, particularly in improving the condition of severely ill patients prior to thoracotomy.

When considering thoracotomy the patient's physical state and the condition of the underlying lung are important. If these are good then decortication and excision of the empyema and any cutaneous sinuses followed by free drainage usually ensures full re-expansion although there may be permanent functional impairment due to alveolar destruction and fibrosis.

If there is underlying bronchiectasis, pulmonary fibrosis, a lung abscess or bronchial obstruction due to a resectable tumour or foreign body, then lobectomy plus decortication or pleuropneumonectomy should be considered provided the overall lung function permits. Occasionally a limited thoracoplasty or a muscle flap may be used to obliterate the residual cavity.

When the lesion is extensive, the lung function impaired or the patient's general condition poor, it may be impossible to eradicate an empyema and rib section followed by open drainage via a wide-bore tube may be beneficial.

Post-pneumonectomy Empyema

The development of a leak in the bronchial stump left after pneumonectomy invariably leads to infection of the fluid filling the hemithorax. If this occurs at an early postoperative stage then the leak may be closed surgically at times using a muscle flap. With adequate toilet and drainage of the hemithorax and appropriate antibiotic therapy this may prevent a chronic empyema developing. However, once infection is established in the hemithorax chronicity ensues and the only treatment available is open drainage by a wide-bore tube.

TUMOURS OF THE PLEURA

The pleural cavities are lined by mesothelial tissue, the exact embryological origin of which remains in doubt. It contains both mesothelial and connective-tissue elements and tumour may arise from both. Histologically, epithelial and fibrous elements may coexist in the same tumour, suggesting perhaps a common mesothelial origin.

Pleural tumours may be classified in various ways, but a useful clinical division is between:

1. Localized pleural lesions (plaques).
2. Diffuse malignant mesothelioma.

1. Localized Pleural Lesions (*Fig.* 40.9)

Microscopically, these are usually firm well encapsulated lesions of either the parietal or visceral pleura, but they may occasionally be nodular or pedunculated. Commonly they have the histological appearance of a fibroma, but they can resemble a lipoma, haemangioma or a pericytoma. In some instances there is marked cellularity and pleomorphism suggesting a fibrosarcoma or a liposarcoma while in most

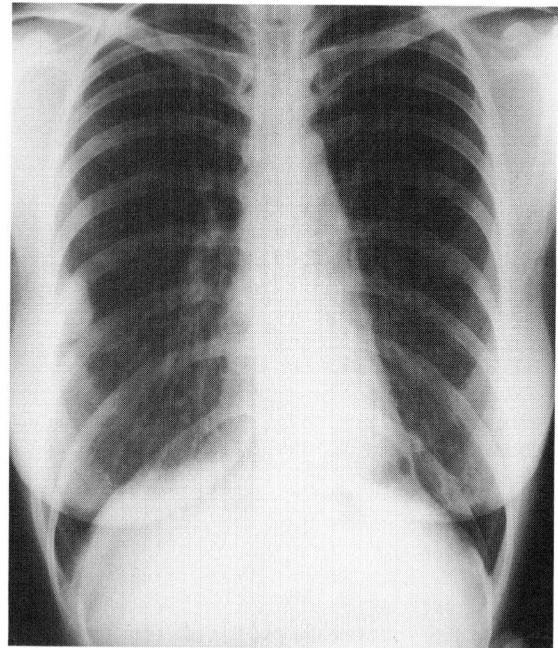

a

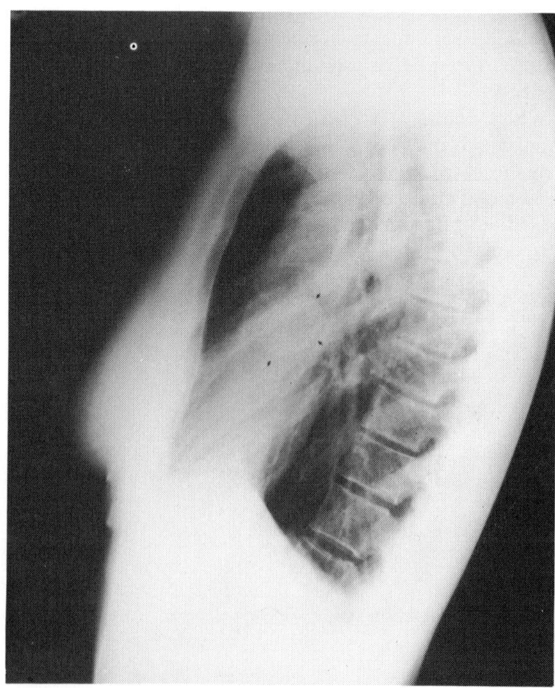

b

Fig. 40.9 *a*, PA, *b*, lateral radiographs of a benign pleural tumour.

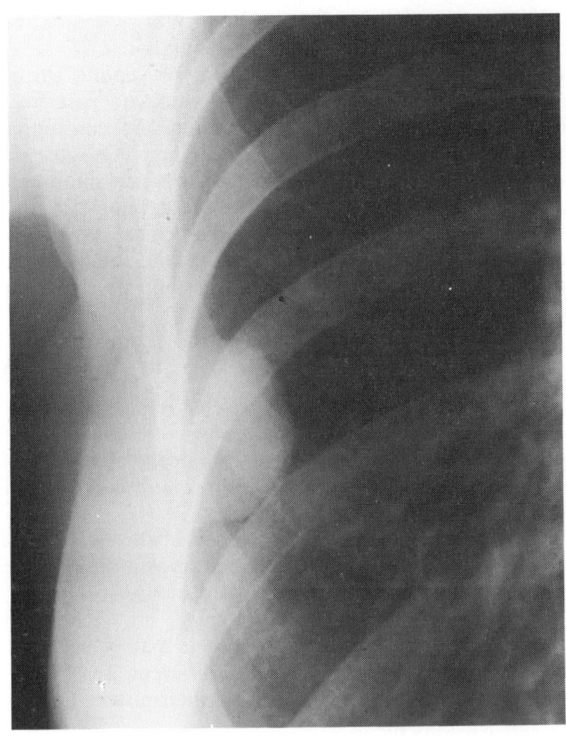

c

Fig. 40.9 *c*, close-up radiograph of a benign pleural tumour.

instances they are benign. In time or in a lesion recurring after previous local resection they may become locally invasive. They vary in size from a centimetre to a large mass filling most of the hemithorax.

2. Diffuse Malignant Mesothelioma

The incidence of these tumours has increased over recent years in line with the increasing industrial use of asbestos which is now known to be the major causal factor although 20–30 years may elapse between exposure and the appearance of the tumour. Asbestos exposure has also been associated with the development of localized fibrous pleural plaques, but there is no evidence that malignant mesotheliomas develop from these lesions. Very rarely, non-industrial malignant mesotheliomas occur.

The tumour gradually spreads out as a thick yellow-grey fibrotic sheet to encase the lung. The underlying lung or chest wall may be infiltrated and there is a tendency for the tumour to grow along the tracks of the needle biopsies or through thoracotomy scars on to the skin surface. The pericardium may become involved by direct extension leading clinically to constrictive pericarditis. The contralateral pleura and peritoneum may also be involved by direct spread. In the early stages large bloodstained pleural effusions are common, but as the tumour advances the fluid tends to be replaced by tumour tissue. Mediastinal and hilar gland involvement occurs in up to 80% of cases, and blood-borne spread to the liver, contralateral lung, bone, adrenal, and meninges, originally thought to be rare, is not infrequently found at autopsy. Various histological features, i.e. adenocarcinoma, sarcomatous, undifferentiated, polygonal, have been described, and although the tumours are often mixed, one particular cell type usually predominates.

Clinical Features

Localized pleural lesions rarely produce symptoms and are often diagnosed by chance on a routine chest radiograph. The commonest symptoms are dyspnoea, chest pain and cough, although occasionally they may be associated with joint pains, chills, pyrexia and finger clubbing. Pleural effusions rarely occur with this type of tumour.

There are no characteristic features associated with a diffuse malignant mesothelioma although a history of exposure to asbestos should always be sought. Breathlessness and chest discomforture are the commonest symptoms often associated with a large pleural effusion. Cough, weight loss and haemoptysis are less common presenting features. Pain may be a very severe persistent symptom. The affected lung becomes constricted with shift of the mediastinum to that side. Abdominal distension with palpable hard masses may occur if the peritoneum is involved. The disease progresses relentlessly with a prognosis of 12–24 months.

Investigations

The diagnosis may be suspected from the chest radiological appearance. Localized pleural lesions are often peripherally situated, rounded, homogeneous opacities, which usually have a clear-cut outline (*Fig.* 40.9*a*). Oblique views and computerized tomography may give further helpful information. A diffuse malignant mesothelioma presents a different radiological appearance with a hazy pleural opacity varying in size and distribution, which is often accompanied by a pleural effusion. The tumour may eventually spread to involve the lung parenchyma, mediastinum and diaphragm. Computerized tomography gives a good picture of the extent of pleural involvement and will also indicate the presence of an effusion even in an extensive mesothelioma (*Fig.* 40.10). Any effusion should be aspirated and its cellular content examined. The diagnosis of mesothelioma can be difficult unless histological proof is obtained either by needle biopsy or biopsy at thoracotomy, but the risk of tumour implantation along the needle track or in the thoracotomy scar has to be borne in mind.

Management

Diffuse malignant mesothelioma is a prescribed industrial disease, and patients suspected of suffering from it should be referred to the Medical Boarding Centre (Respiratory Diseases).

Treatment

The appropriate treatment for localized pleural lesions is surgical excision, which usually presents no difficulty although recurrence can occasionally occur. Diffuse malignant mesothelioma is more difficult to manage. Radical pleuropneumonectomy may offer a chance of cure in a few less aggressive cases diagnosed at an early stage. Large pleural effusions should be drained with instillation of cytotoxic agents to reduce the risk of recurrence. Once direct infiltration of the lung, diaphragm or mediastinum has occurred surgery is inappropriate. Unfortunately these tumours are usually resistant to both radiotherapy and chemotherapy. Adequate analgesia for relief of chest pain is essential together with appropriate supportive measures for terminal care.

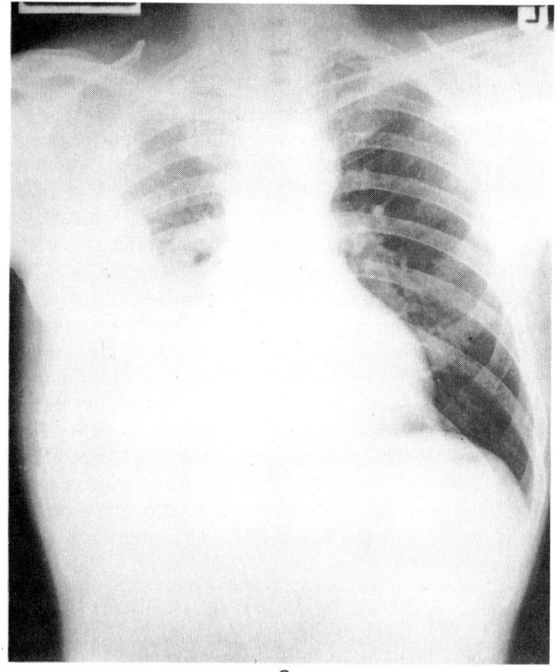

a

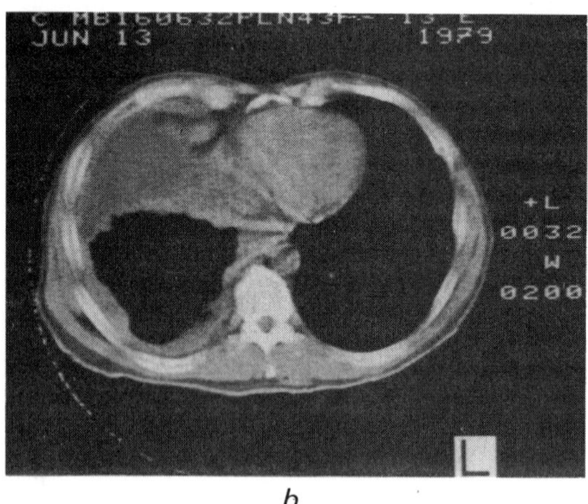

b

Fig. 40.10 *a*, PA chest radiograph and *b*, CT scan of a patient with a diffuse malignant mesothelioma.

SPONTANEOUS PNEUMOTHORAX

Pneumothorax (air in the pleural space) was recognized in the nineteenth century usually as a complication of pulmonary tuberculosis. With the advent of chest radiography the frequent occurrence of spontaneous pneumothorax not associated with active tuberculosis was recognized. A pneumothorax may be: (1) *localized*, when the volume of air and amount of lung collapse is limited by pleural adhesions; or (2) *generalized*, when the whole lung recoils towards the hilum with the air lying free in the pleural space. Various terms may be used to describe a pneumothorax: (1) *closed*, indicating closure of the pleural tear preventing further escape of air; (2) *open*, when air continues to pass freely between the lung and pleural space throughout respiration; and (3) *valvular*, where air freely enters the pleural space on inspiration but becomes trapped on expiration due to closure of the leak. A *tension pneumothorax* develops from the valvular type when its progressive enlargement, which may occur rapidly, causes displacement of the mediastinum, kinking of the great vessels and increasing respiratory and cardiovascular distress.

Several factors may predispose to the development of a spontaneous pneumothorax of which the following are the most important:

1. The formation of *subpleural blebs* containing air which has leaked through congenital defects in the alveolar walls and tracked up to collect at the apices, often bilaterally (common in young adults).
2. The development of a *bulla* as part of chronic bronchitis, generalized emphysema, in α_1-antitrypsin deficiency or in paraseptal or postfibrotic emphysema (*Fig.* 40.11).
3. Following diffuse *air trapping* in generalized emphysema or severe asthma when there may be leakage of air through the rupture of alveoli in different areas.
4. *Hyperinflation* of alveoli during intermittent positive-pressure ventilation.
5. *Progressive dilatation and rupture* of congenital cysts (*Fig.* 40.12), the pneumatoceles of childhood staphylococcal pneumonias or occasionally of the cysts which may accompany tuberculosis, carcinoma, honeycomb lung or pneumoconiosis.

An unusual variety is associated with menstruation although the causal mechanism remains uncertain.

Clinical Features

Spontaneous pneumothoraces are most common in two age groups: (1) apparently healthy, but usually thin adolescents,

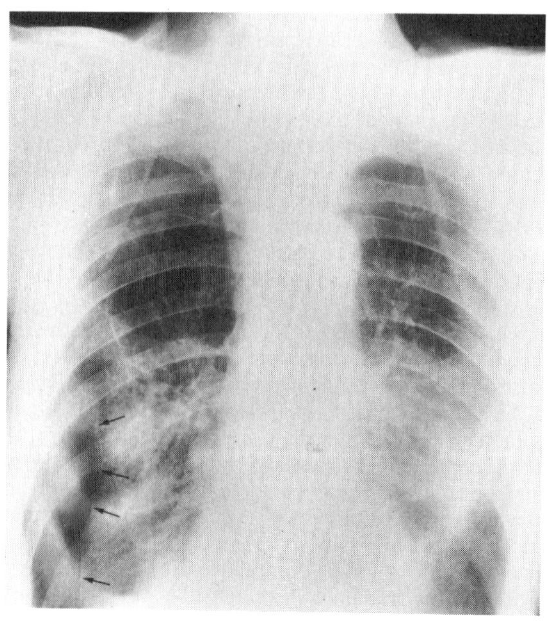

Fig. 40.11 Right localized pneumothorax in a chronic bronchitic.

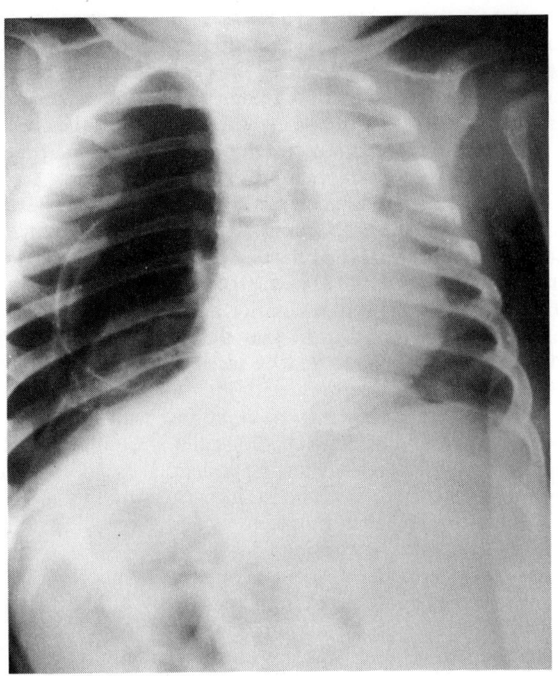

Fig. 40.12 Tension cyst in a child with an associated tension pneumothorax causing mediastinal shift to the left side.

and (2) the older patients with chronic bronchitis and emphysema. The sudden onset of unilateral pleuritic chest pain and dyspnoea is the commonest presentation. These symptoms are only rarely associated with exercise. In an otherwise healthy adult the dyspnoea may soon abate although there may be no radiological improvement. Alternatively, worsening dyspnoea is indicative of progressive lung collapse and may be the first sign of a tension pneumothorax, other features of which are increasing anxiety, restlessness, cyanosis, hypotension, tachycardia, clammy extremities and shock. In severe asthma or during assisted ventilation a deterioration in the patient's condition should alert the clinician to the possibility of a pneumothorax, the signs of which may be masked and a radiograph is often required to establish the diagnosis. Between 3 and 5% of patients sustaining a pneumothorax also suffer significant intrapleural haemorrhage which is associated with greater systemic effects, i.e. malaise, hypotension and pronounced tachycardia.

The physical signs of air in the pleural space are a hyperresonant percussion note, diminished movement and faint or absent breath sounds on the affected side. Occasionally, in a small pneumothorax, there may be a clicking sound in time with the heart beat. In a tension pneumothorax the chest wall may be distended on the affected side, with shift of the trachea and apex beat to the opposite side made worse by expiration (*Fig.* 40.12).

Occasionally a subpleural bleb ruptures but the visceral pleura remains intact. After tracking to the hilum, air enters the mediastinum from where it may spread to the neck producing the distinctive crepitus of subcutaneous (surgical) emphysema.

Investigations

A standard chest radiograph is the only relevant investigation. If the patient is not severely distressed erect posteroanterior films taken on inspiration and expiration will demonstrate the extent of the pneumothorax (*Fig.* 40.13).

Treatment

There are several methods of treatment, the choice being dictated by the clinical and radiological findings, but even with a small pneumothorax admission for observation should be considered because of the possibility of rapid progression from a small to a tension pneumothorax.

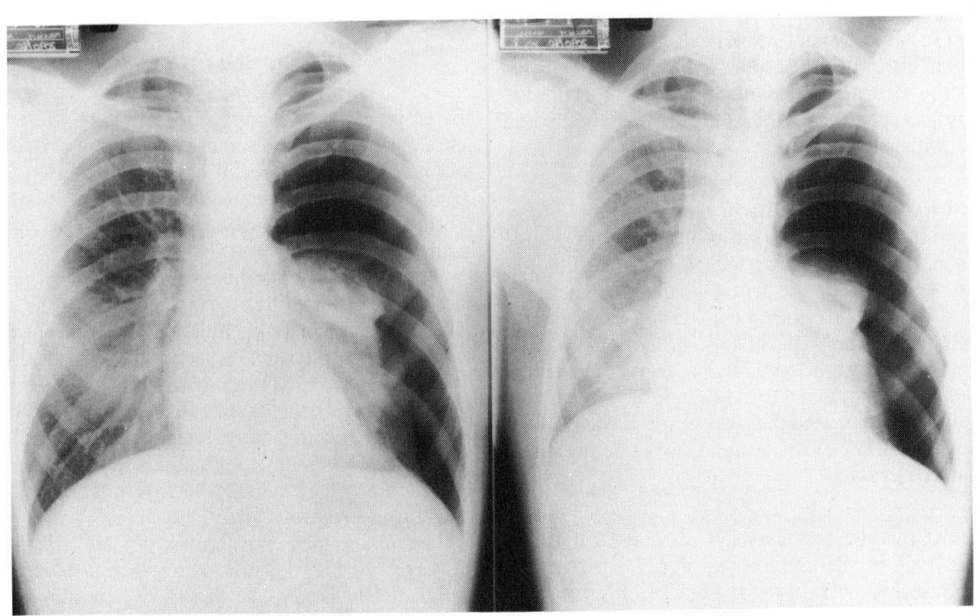

a b

Fig. 40.13 Large left pneumothorax with mediastinal shift during expiration (*b*).

1. Conservative Management

A fit patient with a small pneumothorax may safely be observed without intubation. Some clinicians advocate oxygen therapy in the belief that it aids resolution. Once it has been established that the pneumothorax is static or resolving the patient may safely be discharged without further treatment. At least one-quarter of patients treated in this way will present later with a recurrence of their spontaneous pneumothorx.

2. Needling

In patients distressed from, or in whom there is a rapidly developing tension pneumothorax the insertion of a large-bore needle, cannula or tube into the affected hemithorax may be lifesaving, relieving the situation until more permanent treatment can be instigated.

3. Aspiration

Simple aspiration of the air using a wide-bore needle in the 2nd intercostal space in the midclavicular line, a suction apparatus and a one-way valve has its advocates although it has not found general acceptance.

4. Intercostal Drainage

This is the treatment of choice for the majority of cases. It is a simple, safe technique when carried out properly and usually produces a rapid re-expansion of the lung. There are several points of importance regarding the technique which should be stressed.

a. SITE OF INSERTION. The second intercostal space in the midclavicular line is one of the safest and most popular sites of insertion, and is particularly suitable for the patient with a pneumothorax, as it provides better drainage of the apex. For cosmetic reasons the midaxillary line in the 4th or 5th space may be preferred in young females. A basal drain in the 8th or 9th intercostal space is required if there is a localized basal pneumothorax.

b. ANAESTHESIA. A local anaesthetic is all that is required but the chest wall should be anaesthetized in layers down to and including the pleura and the infiltrating needle should be inserted into the pleural cavity to check that the space contains air at the chosen site.

c. CHOICE OF DRAIN. The majority of clinicians now use a sterile polythene tube which has a radio-opaque marker and several side holes. This may be inserted: (*a*) with the aid of a metal trocar passed through the centre of the drain; or (*b*) through a metal cannula introduced using a separate trocar. Some clinicians favour the Malecot type of catheter which has to be inserted through a trocar using an introducer in order to flatten out the flanges. Although it is easy to introduce small-bore tubes into the pleural space such tubes tend to kink and obstruct as the patient moves or breathes and they should be avoided.

d. INSERTION. If the site for insertion has been carefully chosen on the basis of the radiological appearance, most drains can be inserted with perfect safety. Care must be taken when inserting a basal drain to avoid pushing the introducer through the diaphragm into the abdominal cavity.

e. MANAGEMENT. When the drain is connected to the underwater seal system there should be an immediate stream of bubbles as the lung inflates. This will continue until full inflation is obtained at which point the patient will experience some pleuritic chest discomfort. Thereafter the air leak usually diminishes although some patients continue to leak large quantities of air even with the lung inflated. A confirmatory chest radiograph should be taken shortly after the drain is inserted. If the lung is fully inflated no further action is required. If the lung is partially aerated consideration should be given to applying gentle suction to the chest drain. If there has been no aeration and the drain is correctly placed it must be assumed that the major bronchi to the affected lung are obstructed by secretions, and therapeutic aspiration bronchoscopy carried out. If general anaesthesia is used, bronchoscopy may be combined with forced inflation of the lung. The drain should be left in situ until there is no further air leak even when the patient takes a deep breath or coughs. If there is a persistent and continuing air leak beyond 7–10 days then thoracotomy and surgical closure of the fistula should be considered.

A second episode of spontaneous pneumothorax on the same side may be managed in the same way. If three or more pneumothoraces have occurred then some form of pleurodesis is required. This is most commonly achieved by a small lateral thoracotomy at which any localized bullae can be ligated or oversewn. Occasionally a limited resection of a bullous area may be necessary. If the surface of the parietal pleura is then abraded with a dry gauze swab, diathermy or painted with Bethidine, this will produce adhesion between the lung and the parietal pleura. Excision of the parietal pleura is a more extensive procedure with a higher morbidity.

The insufflation of sterile powdered talc, kaolin, or irritating chemicals, e.g. mepacrine, tetracycline, into the pleural space through the intercostal tube when the pneumothorax is still present, is also an effective way of producing pleurodesis. Views differ as to the advisability of this procedure which can be extremely painful.

EMPHYSEMA

In emphysema the air spaces distal to the terminal bronchioles are irreversibly increased in size above the normally accepted limits as a result of either dilatation or destruction of their walls. This definition embraces a number of distinct entities, the pathogenesis of the majority being incompletely understood.

The terms 'centrilobular' and 'panacinar' may be used to describe specific types of emphysema. The centre of the lobules are principally involved in the centrilobular form while the emphysema is diffusely spread throughout the affected segment in the panacinar type. Air spaces of more than 1 cm in diameter are referred to as bullae or cysts, the terms often being interchangeable. Emphysema may be unilateral or bilateral, segmental, lobar or generalized.

There is impairment of both ventilation and perfusion in any emphysematous area.

Ventilation. The transference of gas through the distal air spaces occurs by diffusion; a process which becomes less efficient the larger the space. When the bronchus to an emphysematous area is obstructed ventilation occurs by diffusion from neighbouring alveoli via the alveolar pores, further increasing the inefficiency of the gas exchange.

Perfusion. Three mechanisms: (1) attenuation and destruction of the capillary bed; (2) increased tension within the emphysematous cyst impeding capillary blood flow; (3) hypoxia in the emphysematous space causing reflex vasoconstriction of the feeding arterioles—acting individually or in concert have been suggested as causes for the reduction in blood flow seen in emphysematous areas.

It is not possible to give a complete classification of emphysema, but the major types are listed below.

Types of Emphysema

Causal mechanism	*Type of emphysema*
a. Overinflation	Senile Fibrotic scarring Compensatory
b. Atrophy or hypoplasia	Paraseptal MacLeod's syndrome Lung agenesis
c. Destruction	α_1-antitrypsin deficiency 'Primary emphysema' Associated with chronic bronchitis
d. Check valve	Obstructive emphysema Tension cysts Bullae

Senile Emphysema

With age the elasticity of the lungs declines, predisposing to a generalized dilatation of the air sacs which has little functional significance.

Fibrotic Scarring

The alveoli around small areas of fibrosis, e.g. tuberculous scars, become distended and cysts can form, which, if lying subpleurally, may rupture causing a spontaneous pneumothorax.

Compensatory Emphysema

This refers to the hyperinflation of a segment, lobe or lung which follows collapse, fibrotic contraction or resection in another area. If the cause of the collapse, e.g. a foreign body, can be removed and the lung re-expands then the emphysema resolves.

Compensatory emphysema has importance in two contexts:

a. DIAGNOSIS. As a collapsed left lower lobe lies behind the heart it may be missed on routine radiography but an increased hypertransradiancy in the left upper zone from compensatory emphysema may be instrumental in making the diagnosis.

b. POSTOPERATIVE FUNCTION. The success of any lung resection is dependent upon the state of the remaining lung. In a healthy child requiring lobectomy for obstructive emphysema the residual lung will expand to fill the void without significant alteration in function. In contrast, many patients undergoing resection for bronchial carcinoma have impaired function due to chronic bronchitis and emphysema. Any postoperative compensatory emphysema will aggravate the situation and a detailed preoperative assessment of respiratory function is essential in order to ensure a reasonable quality of life after surgery.

Paraseptal Emphysema

This occurs along connective-tissue septa, particularly down the anterior lung margin, and is thought to result from atrophy in the surrounding lung tissue lessening support and allowing the alveoli to distend. Clinically it has significance as a cause of spontaneous pneumothorax or giant bullae.

MacLeod's Syndrome

MacLeod's syndrome is a condition in which there is unilateral panacinar emphysema resulting from damage to the lung parenchyma occurring between birth and 8 years of age, the other lung being unaffected. Few patients recall any childhood illnesses although the syndrome has been shown to follow measles and tuberculosis. Most patients are asymptomatic, being diagnosed on routine chest radiography. Occasionally the affected lung may be the site of persistent or recurrent infection when pneumonectomy may be considered. Alternatively, pneumonia in the unaffected lung may cause sufficient additional functional impairment to bring the disorder to light. Clinically the percussion note is hyperresonant and the air entry diminished over the affected lung.

Radiologically there is unilateral hypertransradiancy with a decrease in hilar and peripheral vascular markings and a shift of the mediastinum to the unaffected side on expiratory films. Pulmonary angiography confirms a small pulmonary artery while bronchography shows a bronchiectatic bronchial tree. There is reduced ventilation, the affected lung accounting for only 10% of the oxygen uptake. Other causes of unilateral hypertransradiancy, e.g. congenitally absent pectoral muscles, mastectomy, must be excluded. If the remaining lung is healthy there are usually few problems but any respiratory infection should be promptly treated.

Lung Agenesis

Agenesis of one lung leads to considerable enlargement of the other, the disorder presenting as progressive emphysema in the third or fourth decades.

α_1-Antitrypsin Deficiency

The lung contains high concentrations of the proteolytic enzyme trypsin, which is thought to play an important role in the removal of foreign and damaged proteins from the circulation. In congenital α_1-antitrypsin deficiency the levels of this enzyme may be insufficient to deactivate the available trypsin. Following an insult to the lung, e.g. by smoking, a process of autodigestion begins with the progressive destruction of alveolar tissue and the formation of large bullae initially in the lower lobes (*Fig*. 40.14). Patients usually present between the ages of 30 and 50 with progressive dyspnoea and a radiograph showing basal bullous emphysema. Resection of the affected lobes may produce temporary improvement but the process inevitably recurs in the remaining lung. As α_1-antitrypsin levels and phenotype measurements are readily available family studies are recommended with genetic counselling and advice to affected youngsters regarding smoking.

Primary Emphysema (vanishing lung, 'pink puffers')

In this condition generalized panacinar involvement arises from widespread destruction of the alveolar walls producing varying sized air sacs. There may be pathological evidence of

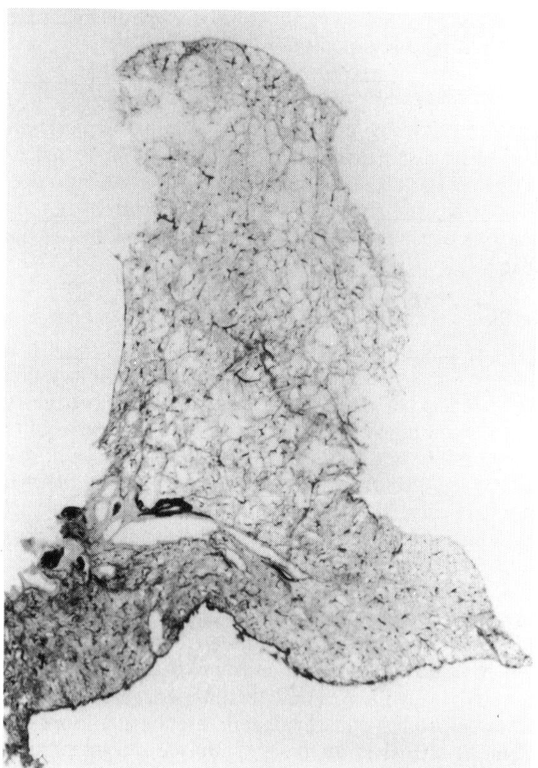

Fig. 40.14 Slice through the right lower lobe in a patient with α_1-antitrypsin deficiency showing diffuse emphysematous change.

associated chronic bronchitis. The disease progresses remorselessly to early death from respiratory failure with few signs of cardiac decompensation.

Primary emphysema is believed to develop as a result of autodigestion although the mechanism is not fully understood. The constituents of cigarette smoke or inhaled irritants are believed to induce an inflammatory reaction at the level of the terminal bronchioles and alveolar sacs, which leads to an accumulation of alveolar macrophages and white blood cells in the affected area. Both types of cell are rich in proteolytic enzymes normally used to destroy ingested foreign proteins and bacteria. Other constituents of cigarette smoke damage both the alveolar macrophages and the white blood cells leading to the local release of high concentrations of these proteolytic enzymes. Under normal circumstances the blood contains antiproteolytic enzymes which deactivate any proteolytic enzymes that are released in the lungs.

Unfortunately, cigarette smoke contains agents which inactivate the antiproteolytic enzymes undermining this defence mechanism. Thus the released proteolytic enzymes embark on a process of progressive autodigestion of terminal bronchi and alveolar spaces replacing them by emphysematous cysts.

The patient expends considerable energy in hyperventilating to maintain his arterial oxygen tension. The chest remains hyperinflated throughout respiration and during inspiration there may be paradoxical indrawing of the lower ribs resulting from the action of the flattened diaphragm. Air entry is poor but there may be few added sounds. The liver may be palpable due to the downward displacement of the diaphragm.

Treatment is mainly supportive using bronchodilators and oxygen. Whole lung radiotherapy, carbimazole, and sedation have advocates, but have not found general acceptance. A few of the younger patients with primary emphysema and some cases of α_1-antitrypsin deficiency have undergone heart/lung transplantation, and the initial results are encouraging.

As well as primary emphysema (pink puffers) the spectrum of chronic obstructive airways disease includes the syndrome of the 'blue bloater' which presents as another distinct clinical entity. In such cases the principal pathological findings are those of chronic bronchitis namely:

1. Considerable hypertrophy of the bronchial submucosal mucus-secreting glands leading to irregular irreversible narrowing of the bronchi, thereby impeding airflow.
2. An increase in the number of epithelial mucus-secreting goblet cells with their extension down to the smaller bronchi.
3. A change in the composition and quantity of the mucus produced. The thick tenacious mucus interferes with the normal mucociliary clearance and causes blockage of the distal bronchi with collapse and infection.

Emphysema may or may not be present but when it occurs it develops by the same mechanism as in primary emphysema.

In spite of their cyanosis, hypoxia and polycythaemia, blue bloaters are lethargic, obese and hypoventilated. Rhonchi are usually present. Cardiac failure, which occurs early, is thought to result from the effects of profound hypoxic episodes occurring during sleep. The disease progresses rapidly with a 75% mortality within 5 years. Treatment is supportive with advice regarding smoking and occupation, bronchodilators, antibiotics (when necessary) and domiciliary oxygen for 12–15 h per day.

The clinical features of primary emphysema (pink puffers) and blue bloaters are compared below:

	Pink puffers	*Blue bloaters*
Dyspnoea	Marked (at rest)	On exercise
Cough	Mild	Marked
Sputum	Scanty	Daily ++
Recurrent infections	Uncommon	Frequent
Respiration	Hyperventilation	Hypoventilation
Appearance	Thin	Obese
Colour	Pink	Cyanosed
Use of accessory muscles	+++	+
Percussion note	Increased +++	Normal or increased +
Cardiac failure	Develops late	Occurs early

Radiologically, there is a considerable difference between the findings in the two groups. Pink puffers show hyperinflated lungs, with low, flat, poorly moving diaphragms, a long, narrow heart, prominent hilar vessels with a loss of peripheral lung markings and bullae (*Fig.* 40.15). The blue bloater may have a normal chest radiograph or show evidence of irregular patchy fibrosis with few of the features associated with emphysema (*Fig.* 40.16) and studies have shown a poor correlation between the radiological appearances and the pathological findings of emphysema in these cases.

The results of the respiratory function tests differ between the two groups as shown below:

	Pink puffers	*Blue bloaters*
FEV_1 (forced expiratory volume in one second)	Reduced+++	Reduced++
FEV_1 Response to bronchodilators	Poor	Less than 10%
FVC (Forced vital capacity)	Reduced++	Reduced+
FEV_1/FVC ratio	Reduced++	Reduced++
TLC (Total lung capacity)	Increased+++	Normal or increased+
RV (Residual volume)	Increased+++	Increased+
RV/TLC ratio	Increased+++ (often over 70%)	Increased+
Carbon monoxide transfer factor	Reduced+++ (often below 50% of predicted)	Reduced+
Arterial Blood Gases		
P_aO_2	Normal	Reduced++
P_aCO_2	Reduced+	Increased++

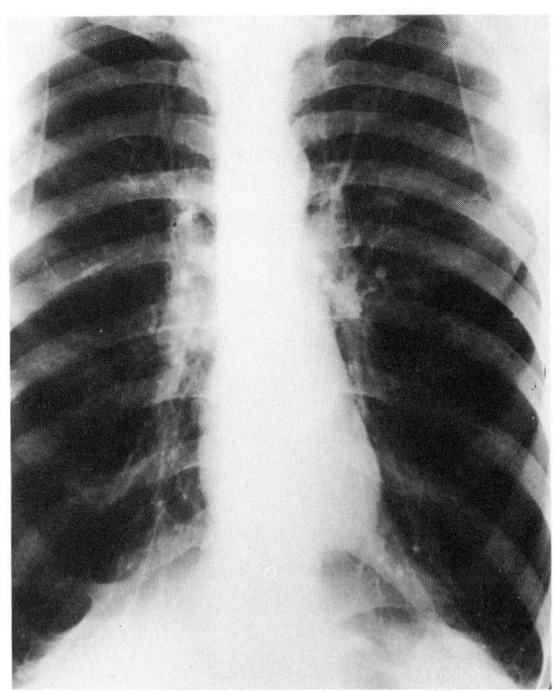

Fig. 40.15 PA film of a pink puffer with a long narrow heart, low diaphragm, general loss of lung architecture and widening of the rib spaces.

While pink puffers and blue bloaters form distinct clinical entities within the spectrum of chronic obstructive airways disease most patients present a mixed picture showing varying combinations of chronic bronchitis and emphysema. Many show some improvement in respiratory function following the inhalation of a bronchodilator which is often more evident with regards forced vital capacity (FVC) than the forced expiratory volume (FEV_1), in contrast to the picture seen in asthma. Nevertheless it indicates a reduction in the work of breathing and points to a potential for clinical improvement.

Before thoracotomy every patient should undergo the respiratory function tests shown in the above table together with an exercise test, i.e. a 6-minute walking test or an

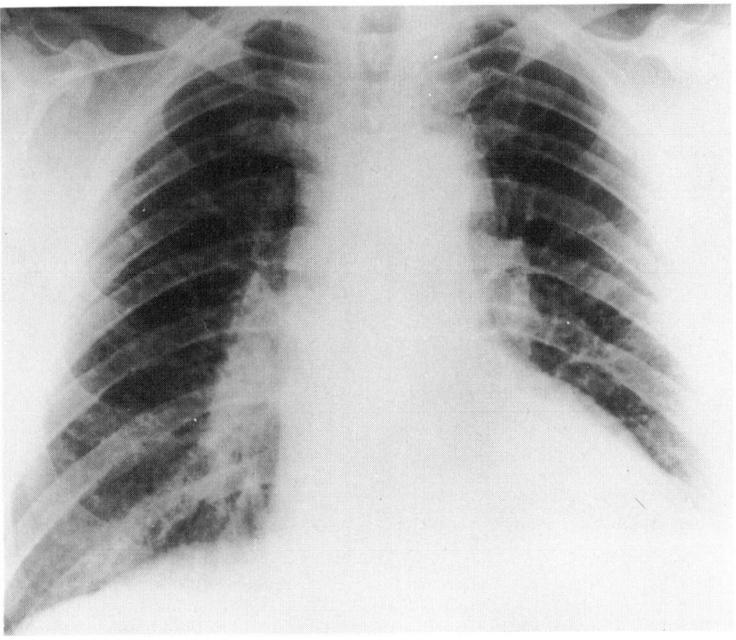

Fig. 40.16 PA film of a blue bloater showing a big heart and prominent pulmonary arteries but the diaphragm is not depressed and there is good lung architecture.

assessment of their ability to climb stairs, to gauge their overall functional status. An FEV_1 of below 1 litre which cannot be improved by bronchodilators or an RV/TLC ratio over 70% are contraindications to surgery. Blood gases indicate the preoperative status and give a baseline in case of postoperative problems. Maximum respiratory function should be achieved preoperatively using bronchodilators, physiotherapy, oxygen, antibiotics and occasionally short courses of high-dose steroids.

Obstructive Emphysema

Partial obstruction of a bronchus may lead to segmental or lobar emphysema through a check valve mechanism, i.e. the air entering during inspiration cannot fully escape on expira-

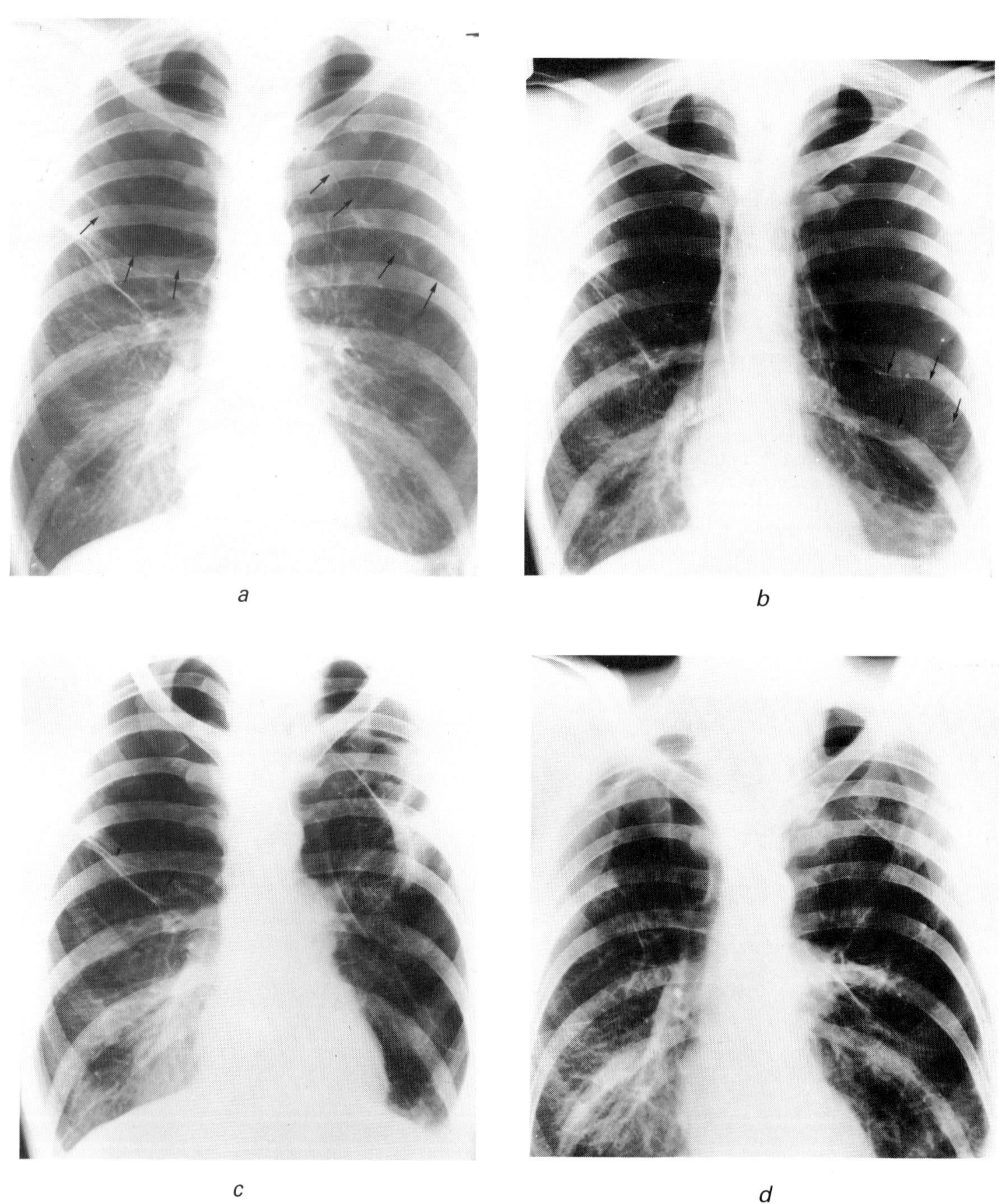

Fig. 40.17 *a*, Large emphysematous bullae in both apices. Chest film taken in 1971. *b*, Follow-up film in 1974 demonstrating compression of the left lower lobe by the expanding bullae. *c*, 1975, marked radiological improvement after a Monaldi procedure on the left side. The procedure improved the patient's breathlessness considerably. *d*, Follow-up film in 1979 after a Monaldi procedure on the right side. The patient is now active and fairly mobile.

tion causing 'air trapping'. It may be the earliest sign of an inhaled foreign body (particularly in children) and rarely of bronchial carcinoma. Radiologically there is an area of hypertransradiancy which fails to deflate on expiration, causing a shift of the mediastinum to the contralateral side. Xenon slowly enters the zone during a ventilation scan but becomes trapped following the perfusion study. Usually the emphysematous phase is followed by deflation and infection in the affected area, but occasionally the obstructive emphysema progresses with compression of normal lung tissue and dyspnoea which may require surgical relief. Rarely, unilateral or bilateral obstructive emphysema arises from obstruction in the mediastinum, e.g. enlarged bronchogenic cyst or tuberculous glands, when exploration may be necessary.

Tension Cyst

In infancy the partial obstruction of a bronchus feeding a congenital cyst may lead to its progressive enlargement with compression of the surrounding lung causing acute dyspnoea when resection of the cyst may be life saving.

Emphysematous Bullae

Many apical bullae result from paraseptal or postfibrotic emphysema. Basal bullae may complicate α_1-antitrypsin deficiency. Of greater clinical importance are the giant bullae, which occur most frequently in association with primary emphysema or chronic bronchitis.

A bulla may protrude from the lung being attached by a narrow pedicle, when resection and obliteration of the stem can be readily achieved or, alternatively, it may be broadly based lying either superficially where it is covered by pleura or deep within the lung when much of a lobe or segment may be involved.

A bulla may arise as a result of the destructive process which caused the background emphysema or through two distinct check-valve mechanisms:

1. Partial obstruction of the feeding bronchus causes trapping of air during expiration, or
2. Blockage of the feeding bronchus when ventilation occurs by collateral drift from surrounding air spaces, the air readily entering during inspiration but becoming trapped on expiration.

As a bulla enlarges the tension within it may increase with progressive compression of the surrounding lung.

Most apical bullae are asymptomatic, being picked up on routine radiography (*Fig.* 40.17) and need only periodic review. They may cause spontaneous pneumothorax and if this is recurrent, obliteration of the bullae and pleural abrasion or pleurodectomy may be indicated. Rarely a large bulla causes chest discomfort when surgery may be helpful.

The majority of giant bullae occur in patients with long-standing chronic obstructive airways disease. Their appearance may lead to a worsening in the patient's condition although it is often difficult to assess their contribution to the overall functional impairment. If the respiratory function is reasonable a period of observation and full medical treatment for the underlying obstructive airways disease, i.e. bronchodilators, physiotherapy, antibiotics, oxygen and occasionally corticosteroids should be encouraged. This often produces significant clinical improvement but should the patient's condition continue to deteriorate or if the initial impairment is severe surgical treatment for the bullae should be considered. There is no reliable preoperative way of assessing the response to surgery but as much information as possible should be obtained before making the final decision. Thus:

1. Detailed respiratory function tests.
2. Radiology, including whole lung tomography to define the extent of a bulla and determine the state of the remaining lung.
3. Bronchoscopy and, if possible, bronchospirometry to indicate the state of the bronchial tree and the contribution made by the bullous areas to ventilation, and
4. Ventilation and perfusion scanning to define the bulla and give information about the remaining lung.
5. Thoracic CT scanning at full inspiration and expiration may give valuable information about the bulla and its effect on the surrounding lung tissue.

All have a place depending on what is locally available. Surgery is indicated:

1. If the bulla is ventilated but not perfused when it only adds to the dead space, or
2. When the bullae are compressing lung which would otherwise contribute meaningfully to respiratory function.

Various surgical procedures are available depending on the patient's condition and the extent of the disease.

1. If the patient is severely disabled with a large superficial bulla, a one-stage Monaldi procedure with the introduction of a catheter into the space to allow gradual deflation over several weeks should be considered. Operative mortality is low and significant functional improvement may be obtained even though symptoms are likely to recur at a later date (*Fig.* 40.17).
2. Thoracotomy with excision or deroofing of the bulla and oversewing of the feeding bronchi should be considered if the patient's condition permits this. Some surgeons advise pleurodectomy or pleural abrasion to prevent the possibility of a subsequent spontaneous pneumothorax (*see Fig.* 40.12).
3. Apart from a few cases of α_1-antitrypsin deficiency lobectomy is rarely justified as it removes lung which is potentially functional.

Following thoracotomy the postoperative course may be stormy depending on the underlying obstructive airways disease. Adequate analgesia and aggressive physiotherapy are essential. If respiratory failure ensues controlled oxygen therapy will be required. The operative and immediate post-thoracotomy mortality for severe cases is between 10 and 15%.

With careful selection considerable subjective improvement can be obtained which may be reflected in improved respiratory function tests. The concurrent diseases are usually progressive and respiratory failure or recurrence of bullae develop in time, but if the quality of life has been improved in the intervening period intervention will have been justified.

Further Reading

Brody J. S. and Snider G. L. (1985) *Current Topics in the Management of Respiratory Diseases*, Vol. 2. Edinburgh, Churchill Livingstone.

Clee M. D. and Clark R. A. (1982) *Medical Problems associated with Tobacco Smoking*, Ch. 11, Sect. 114. International Encyclopaedia of Pharmacology & Therapeutics. Pergamon.

Collis J. Leigh, Clarke D. B. and Abbey Smith R. (1976) *D'Abreu's Practice of Cardiothoracic Surgery*, 4th ed. London, Arnold.
Flenley D. C. (1979) Chronic bronchitis and emphysema. *Medicine*, 3rd Series.
Lowell J. R. (1977) *Pleural Effusions—A Comprehensive Review*. Baltimore, University Park Press.
Manfredi F., Rosenbaum D. and Childress R. H. (1965) Diffuse malignant mesothelioma of the pleura. *Am. Rev. Resp. Dis.* **92**, 269.

41 *Tumours of the Lung*

A. J. Mearns

BRONCHIAL CARCINOMA

Carcinoma of the bronchus presents a major challenge to medical management in the latter half of the 20th century. Although in countries like Great Britain the number of cases seems to have reached a plateau in the last 10 years, the overall mortality is still 80% within one year of diagnosis. Operative treatment gives the best results in terms of survival for carcinoma of the bronchus, but the resectability rate for non-small cell carcinoma of the lung is of the order of 10% and for small cell carcinoma of the lung is 1% or less.

The assessment of patients with carcinoma of the bronchus demands a high index of suspicion for symptoms so that any early presentation may result in selection for surgical excision, as this offers the best hope of 5-year survival: 60% Stage 1 and 30% overall for all surgical resections. The incidence in Great Britain is of the order of 40 000 cases per annum, and with only 10% suitable for operative resection there is a demand for alternative forms of treatment. Approximately 40% of patients receive treatment with either radiotherapy or chemotherapy or a combination of the two. Thus more than 50% of patients receive no curative treatment whatsoever (*Fig.* 41.1). As the majority of patients will receive no active therapeutic intervention demands fall upon services for the palliative control of symptoms, particularly of pain, and for terminal care.

The diagnosis, staging and treatment of carcinoma of the bronchus involves most of the disciplines of medicine: physicians, surgeons, radiologists, radiotherapists, pathologists, cytologists and the newer specialty of medical oncologist. The emerging services of counselling, mutual support groups and hospice care all have an important role in the care of patients with carcinoma of the bronchus.

Incidence

Accurate descriptions of primary lung cancer were made at the beginning of the 19th century but little further progress was made for 100 years. More extensive clinical reports and reviews appeared in the early 20th century at which time the importance of bronchoscopy in the diagnosis of bronchial carcinoma was realized. Surgery of the thorax was developing and culminated in the first successful pneumonectomy being performed in 1933.

There has been an increasing recognition of the importance of carcinoma of the bronchus as the 20th century progressed. Unfortunately the initial dominance of pulmonary tuberculosis as the major cause of haemoptysis probably obscured the real incidence of bronchial carcinoma earlier. As the social and epidemiological control of tuberculosis began to have an effect and then finally with streptomycin and further antituberculous drugs, cure was effected, the true prevalence of carcinoma of the bronchus was understood and appreciated. As the incidence of tuberculosis fell and the specialization of chest physicians and chest surgeons developed particularly with the spread of the skill of rigid endoscopy, diagnostic rates increased.

The major series reported on between the wars were based on autopsy findings. Although the accuracy of death certification has been disputed, the autopsy recordings are regarded as reliable but inevitably highly selected. Such data confirmed an increasing incidence of bronchial carcinoma. As the technological advances occurred after the Second World War they were applied to the diagnosis and management of carcinoma of the bronchus. Cytology developed in the 1960s and imaging techniques, ultrasound, computerized

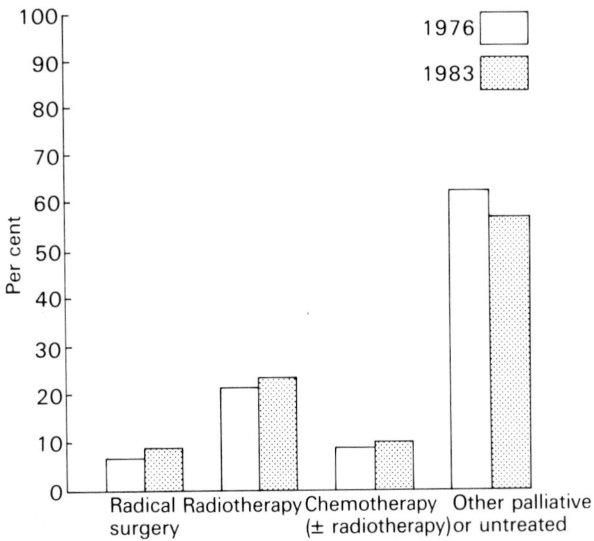

Fig. 41.1 Distribution of initial treatment decisions in the management of carcinoma of the bronchus. 1976: 2360 cases; 1983: 2511 cases. Less than 50% of patients received active intervention. (By permission of the Yorkshire Regional Cancer Registry.)

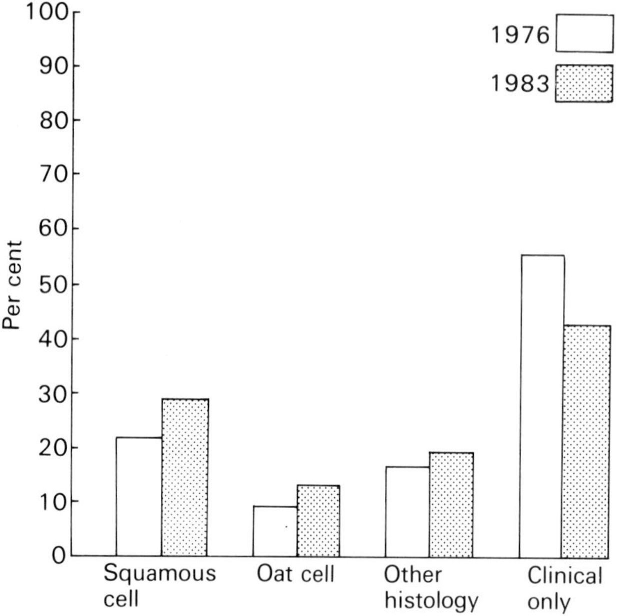

Fig. 41.2 Distribution of histological grouping of carcinoma of the bronchus. 1976: 2360 cases; 1983: 2511 cases. There is an increase from 45% to 58·4% in the proportion of histologically confirmed diagnoses over 7 years. (By permission of the Yorkshire Regional Cancer Registry.)

tomography and radionuclide scanning were applied in the 1970s. Fibreoptic bronchoscopy developed in the 1970s and is now a widespread skill. These techniques have all added to our understanding of carcinoma of the bronchus, e.g. the histological diagnosis of bronchial carcinoma is now made more often (*Fig.* 41.2).

The extraordinary rise in the mortality from carcinoma of the bronchus identified in the 20th century has been particularly noted in the economically developed countries. The incidence is higher in males than females; although presently the rates in men are stable; the rates in women continue to increase. A major proportion of cancer deaths in men and women is attributable to carcinoma of bronchus. In 1930 the mortality for men with carcinoma of the bronchus was estimated to be 10 in 100 000 of the population, in the UK today it remains over 10 times this number. Estimates have been made from mass radiography compaigns of between 1 and 3 men in a thousand of the population over 45 suffer from bronchial carcinoma.

One change in the epidemiology that has taken place is a shift in the mean age at presentation in adult males. The mean age of presentation has now shifted from the 6th decade to the 7th decade. An increasing number of patients are presenting in the 8th and 9th decades (*Fig.* 41.3).

Aetiology

Although extensive laboratory experimentation has been carried out in animals, so far the models have been poor and correlation with human disease has not helped our understanding. This has been felt to be because there is poor data about risk to human beings, although it is probably much more to do with the difference in the biology in men and the animal models rather than true discrepancies in the data collection. However, several specific aspects of the aetiology in man are well recognized.

Atmospheric Pollution

Mortality rates from lung cancer in urban communities are much higher than for people from non-urban areas and epidemiology suggests that this is not due simply to differences in smoking habits. The increasing incidence of the disease was first noticed in industrial Eastern Germany after the First World War. Since then the observation has been repeatedly made that the occurrence rates correlate closely with atmospheric pollution and population density. The disease is more common in social class 5 and decreases in incidence with higher social class.

Occupational Factors

There is a higher mortality from bronchial carcinoma in particular industries. Workers with uranium and pitchblende miners had a higher mortality than predicted, but with improved ventilation and the removal of radon gas these levels have fallen. Workers exposed to chromium, nickel, arsenic and haematite also have raised standardized mortality rates for bronchial carcinoma. That exposure to asbestos is the most important factor responsible for the development of mesothelioma of the pleura is now established. The incidence of bronchial carcinoma in workers exposed to asbestos is raised above normal; however, in combination with smoking there seems to be an additive effect and the incidence is ten times higher when exposed to the combined risk of smoking and asbestos.

Smoking

The individual patient's contribution to his lung cancer is principally through the smoking of cigarettes. When smoking habits have been compared, it has been demonstrated repeatedly that those who have lung cancer are much heavier smokers than a control group matched for age, sex and economic status. There are many other aetiological factors and the relationship between smoking habits and the risk of lung cancer is not a simple one. Factors such as the extent of inhalation of the cigarette smoke and type of tobacco smoked are also important. The risk to pipe smokers is much less than that for cigarette smokers, but it is still higher than for non-smokers. Overall it seems that pipe smoking increases the mortality from lung cancer by a factor of about 5 and cigarette smoking by a factor of about 10, though this enhanced mortality is more marked in heavy smokers. There is now clear evidence from countries in which the cigarette consumption is rising that the mortality from bronchial carcinoma is following closely the smoking habits of the nation.

Interesting health educational experiments are carried out occasionally on the medical profession and an informed drive was made in the 50s and 60s to estimate the incidence of carcinoma of the bronchus in doctors and to educate them out of the smoking habit. A subsequent fall in the incidence of carcinoma of the bronchus in doctors was recorded. This is powerful epidemiological evidence that health education works and that smoking does have a causal relationship with lung cancer. Even now this is in dispute from some quarters but the health education has continued and there is a steady reduction in smoking throughout the population.

The histological changes in the bronchial mucosa which are found in cigarette smokers have been extensively investigated. The more important changes appear to be the abnormality of ciliary action extending to loss of cilia, basal-cell hyperplasia and the appearance of atypical cells with irregular hyperchromatic nuclei. These histological appearances, particularly the basal-cell hyperplasia and the squamous

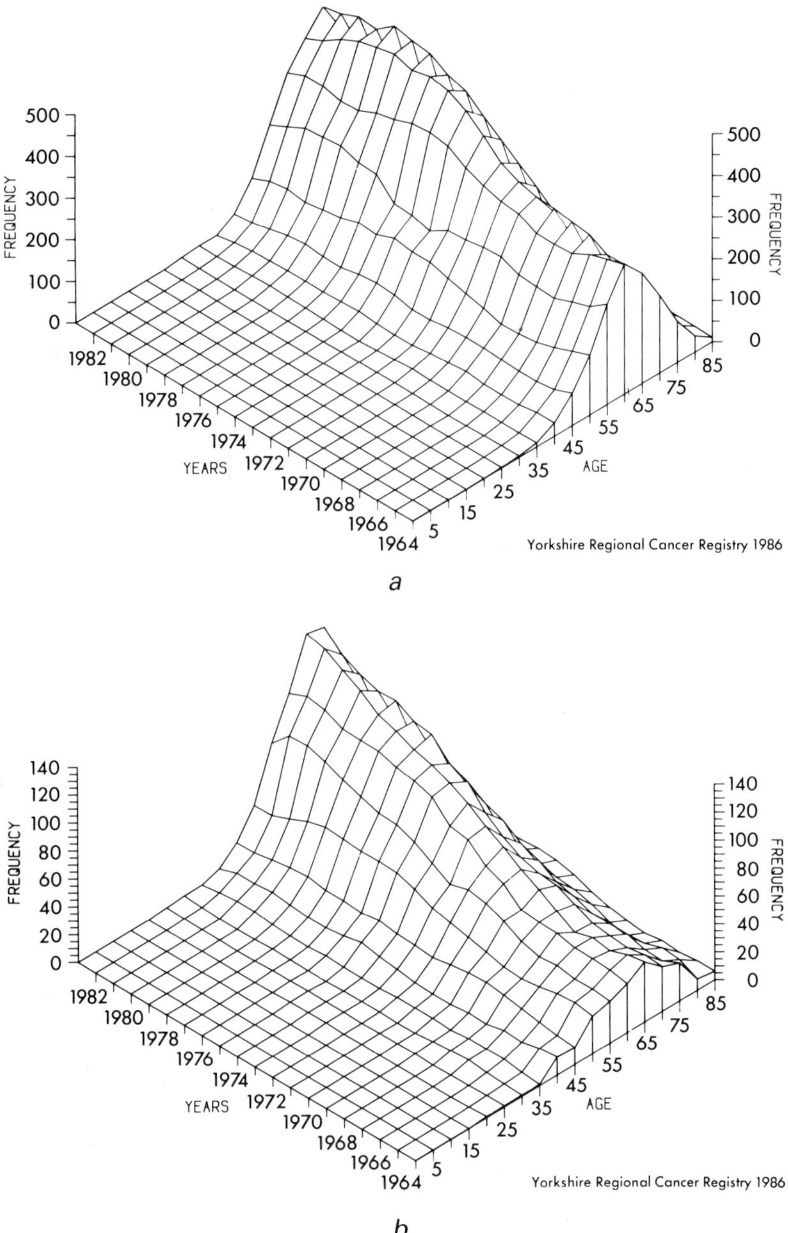

Fig. 41.3 Carcinoma of the bronchus. *a*, Male age distribution, 1964–83. *b*, Female age distribution, 1964–83. Frequency is expressed as cases per hundred thousand. The peak incidence for men has moved from 60 years of age to 70 years of age over 18 years. The total incidence rate for men in 1976 was 118/100 000 and for women 30·8/100 000. For 1983, the total incidence rate for men was 114/100 000 and for women 38·9/100 000. (By permission of the Yorkshire Regional Cancer Registry.)

metaplasia, indicate instability of the mucosa and may be considered as premalignant. The tumours which develop in this situation are squamous or small cell or the anaplastic bronchial carcinomas—the link with adenocarcinoma is more tenuous. The relationship of bronchial carcinoma to disease, such as pulmonary tuberculosis and chronic bronchitis, is difficult to ascertain. There is no doubt that bronchial carcinoma may arise at the site of previous scarring, particularly in patients who have had tuberculous infection. There is little to suggest that the incidence of bronchial carcinoma is higher in patients who have had previous tuberculous infection. The situation is complicated by the fact that more smokers than non-smokers suffer from both pulmonary tuberculosis and chronic bronchitis and any increase in the incidence of bronchial carcinoma may be related more to their smoking habits than to other diseases.

Pathology

The bronchial carcinomas arise from the bronchial and bronchiolar epithelium. The basal or bronchial germinal cells are the progenitors of intermediate cells and amine precursor uptake decarboxylation (APUD) cells. The intermediate cells develop into the ciliated bronchial mucus-secreting cells and under abnormal conditions into squamous epithelial cells. Normal bronchial mucus-secreting cells under abnormal conditions undergo metaplasia to squamous cells. Ciliated cells also undergo metaplasia to become mucus secreting in response to irritation. Occasionally APUD cells may secrete mucus and in a malignant tumour derived from these cells malignant squamous cells may occasionally be found. Bronchiolar epithelium consists of Clara cells, ciliated columnar and cuboidal shaped cells together with scattered APUD cells. All three types can give rise to tumours. Bronchiolar–alveolar-cell cancers arise both from bronchiolar epithelium and from type 2 pneumocytes; therefore, occasionally bronchiolar–alveolar tumours are composed of mucus-secreting cells, some columnar but non-mucus-secreting cells, and a few bear close resemblance to the peg-shaped Clara cells.

The World Health Organization Classification (*Table* 41.1) is a general classification designed to be a guide to all people working with light microscopy. As more sophisticated techniques are not available throughout the world it was felt that a general agreement should be based upon the information that can be gleaned from light microscopy with standard histological staining techniques. As an increasing understanding of the pathology and natural history of lung carcinoma has been obtained, the histological classification has an important value for prognosis and in making management decisions about patterns of treatment.

Premalignant Changes

Atypical epithelial proliferation has been shown to be associated with several different types of lung tumour. The most common is the squamous metaplasia and dysplasia proceeding to carcinoma-in-situ. Atypical epithelial proliferation may also occur in the vicinity of scars and in association with interstitial fibrosis; this is particularly the case in the peripheral malignancy associated with asbestos exposure. In this group of carcinomas which are mostly peripherally situated, adeno-, adenosquamous and occasionally undifferentiated alveolar-cell carcinomas occur. On occasion such tumours may be multifocal.

Table 41.1 Histological classification of lung cancer, WHO 1981

Malignant epithelial tumours

Squamous-cell carcinoma (epidermoid carcinoma)
Variant:
a. Spindle-cell (squamous) carcinoma

Small-cell carcinoma
a. Oat-cell carcinoma
b. Intermediate-cell type
c. Combined oat-cell carcinoma

Adenocarcinoma
a. Acinar adenocarcinoma
b. Papillary adenocarcinoma
c. Bronchiolo-alveolar carcinoma
d. Solid carcinoma with mucus formation.

Large-cell carcinoma
Variants:
a. Giant-cell carcinoma
b. Clear-cell carcinoma

Adenosquamous carcinoma

Carcinoid tumour

Bronchial gland carcinoma
a. Adenoid cystic carcinoma
b. Muco-epidermoid carcinoma
c. Others

Others

Squamous Carcinoma

The incidence of squamous-cell carcinoma in some series is as high as 60%. Unfortunately most series are highly selected and real epidemiological evidence of a gross population reported with carcinoma of the bronchus is lacking; but a population study with a histological maximum of identification of 60% showed that squamous carcinoma of the bronchus occurred in approximately 40% of the histologically identified tumours (*Fig*. 41.2). Recent international opinion has concluded that spindle-cell carcinoma previously included in the anaplastic group of carcinomas is a variant of squamous carcinoma. This intelligence has come from electron microscopy and immunohistochemical studies. Squamous carcinomas occur mainly in the large bronchi and form a large proportion of central growths. They lend themselves to biopsy at bronchoscopy more easily perhaps than more peripherally situated tumours. Such tumours grow slowly and spread mainly in the extra-cartilaginous parts of the bronchial wall and invade adjacent lymph glands in continuity. Squamous-cell growths undergo central necrosis and may cause a crescentic cavitation within a tumour mass seen on radiography. This sign is diagnostic of squamous carcinoma of the bronchus. Squamous-cell carcinomas grow in the walls of bronchiectatic and abscess cavities and they have been described in relation to scarring in the periphery; however, recent observation suggests that adenocarcinoma is much more commonly related to scar tissue. Squamous carcinomas tend to bulk up and obstruct the lumen causing progressively obstructive emphysema and then total obstruction of the bronchus with absorption collapse and quite commonly secondary distal inflammatory disease. Squamous-cell carcinoma is usually only associated with hypercalcaemia as a manifestation of non-metastatic endocrine syndromes associated with malignant disease of the bronchus.

Small-cell Carcinoma

Considerable debate has taken place over the years to identify small-cell carcinoma as a distinct entity. It is now described as embracing three cell types: oat-cell carcinoma which has a lymphoid type of picture and carries a slightly better prognosis than the intermediate-cell carcinoma which seems to be much more aggressive, and the combined oat-cell carcinoma describes those histological patterns where the oat-cell appearance is mixed with adeno- or squamous features elsewhere in the tumour. The degree of aggression of the malignant process seems to be that of the oat-cell component.

It has been particularly important in the last ten years to identify histologically the group of small-cell carcinomas because although the prognosis remains poor we have been able to shift the disease-free interval by approximately nine months with aggressive chemotherapy. The quality of life of these patients has been improved. The previously expected survival proportion of histologically diagnosed oat-cell carcinoma was 50% at 3 months and 20% at one year. With modern chemotherapeutic regimes we now have a survival proportion of 20% at 2 years.

Oat-cell carcinoma tends to occur centrally and it is derived from the APUD cells present in the bronchial tree. Histologically they are related to the bronchial carcinoid tumours. Indeed there is a form of oat-cell carcinoma which may pursue a more indolent course but does eventually metastasize. Such tumours form an intermediate group both in structure and behaviour between bronchial carcinoids and the malignant oat-cell group. Occasionally there may even be amyloid in the stroma of a small-cell carcinoma which is more typical of the bronchial carcinoid tumour.

Adenocarcinoma

Adenocarcinoma is a well-recognized category for carcinoma of the lung but the categorization is very much dependent upon a primary definition of what is a gland? The difficulty is that histologically a gland may be described as a collection of cells which are of a secretory nature which discharge their product into the lumen, i.e. an acinus or tube. On the other hand, a gland can consist of a single secretory cell. These problems are addressed by the adenocarcinoma group for all four types of tumour. Although these tumours can occur centrally there is an increasing frequency of presentation as more peripheral tumours and ultimately the bronchiolar carcinoma presents only as a peripheral lesion. Adenocarcinomas in the periphery of the lung are related to and often arise in relation to lung damage and when so, are commonly described as scar carcinomas. They are an important group to diagnose, often detected on an incidental chest radiograph as they are one of the more favourable groups of tumours responding to resection. Bronchiolar–alveolar-cell carcinoma is a rare type of tumour and accounts for 1–2% of malignant tumours of lung in some series. It seems to occur with equal frequency in both sexes and was initially described as arising from the Clara cell in the bronchial mucosa. This type of tumour may occur as multiple or single greyish-white nodules and often as mucus-secreting tumours; they tend to infiltrate locally. An entire lobe of a lung may be replaced by tumour tissue. Unfortunately the diagnosis is commonly only suspected when a patient has had a long period of antibiotic thereapy and there has been failure of resolution of a suspected inflammatory process; indeed if an inflammatory process fails to resolve radiologically within the expected period of time, i.e. 3–4 weeks, bronchiolar–alveolar carcinoma should be suspected. As these tumours present late because of this peculiar characteristic they are often unresectable. However, in the small group of patients that do present with incidentally identified peripheral lesions and resection is undertaken, the prognosis is good.

Large-cell Carcinoma

Large-cell carcinoma is now given a specific category. Giant-cell and clear-cell carcinoma are histological descriptions and diagnosed only after biopsy or resection. The prognosis is not good as they are thought to be relatively anaplastic, present late and represent an aggressive form of malignant disease.

Adenosquamous Carcinoma

This is a histological identification again and is designed to embrace the truth of the microscope that various patterns of tumour can be found in bronchial carcinoma which fit both definitions. Their behaviour pattern is intermediate between the squamous and adenocarcinomas.

Carcinoid Tumour

Carcinoid tumour is a tumour of the APUD cells which occur in the bronchi. This may occur centrally or peripherally. It is a slow growing tumour which spreads by direct invasion over a long period of time. Very occasionally metastases are reported but this is unusual. These tumours respond to surgical resection and indeed most local resections and reconstructions are done for this type of tumour. It represents one end of the spectrum for the APUD-type cell tumour and is relatively benign. The prognosis in the resected condition is excellent, as high as 70% survival at 5 years. Rarely the bronchial carcinoid tumours may give rise to a similar syndrome to that associated with intestinal carcinoid tumours. There is occasionally a more unusual form of short-chain polypeptide output.

Bronchial Gland Carcinoma

This group of slow growing tumours occurs predominantly in the major bronchi. There are essentially two types: the adenoid cystic carcinoma and the muco-epidermoid carcinoma. The adenoid cystic carcinoma has been called the cylindroma which is a description of the microscopical findings and it is related to tumours that grow in the salivary glands. Such tumours were described in the bronchus as early as 1877. These tumours should be considered as low-grade bronchial carcinomas. They grow beneath the bronchial epithelium and extend directly into the subjacent bronchial wall and continue to spread in the peribronchial tissue. They very rarely present within the lumen of the bronchus but essentially they cause occlusion of the bronchus and trachea by extrinsic infiltration and compression. They spread in the perineural lymphatics and metastasize late to the lung. The majority of these patients present late, but there are reports of aggressive tracheal and major bronchial resection and reconstruction with some long-term survivors. Approximately 60% are operable at presentation. The mortality is of the order of 20% because proximal tracheobronchial surgery is technically difficult and demanding and the long-term survival is almost always complicated by late recurrence although survivors as long as 16 years are reported.

Muco-epidermoid tumour of the bronchus is a locally malignant condition and should be identified with the bronchial carcinomas. Microscopically they vary in appearance. They may contain clumps of squamous-cell type with identifiable intercellular bridges. In other parts of the tumour groups of mucus-secreting cells may form acini or be intermixed with epidermoid cells. In young adults muco-epidermoid tumours behave as the salivary gland muco-epidermoid tumours and are locally invasive. Occasionally in adults muco-epidermoid tumours progress to become the adenosquamous cell lung carcinoma. This tumour is a very rare occurrence. The local behaviour is that of bronchial obstruction by polypoid extrusion into the bronchus.

Clinical Features

The majority of patients with bronchial carcinoma are males over the age of 50 but the range is wide and occasional cases have been recorded even in the first and second decades of life. The average duration of symptoms before diagnosis is about six months, but a small percentage of patients have no symptoms at all, the diagnosis being made as a chance radiographic finding. Unfortunately the initial symptoms tend to be non-specific—cough, tiredness, anorexia and weight loss—making early diagnosis difficult.

Symptoms

Most patients who develop lung cancer are smokers and it is quite likely that they will have had a morning cough for many years. If there has been a change in their coughing habit then this should be investigated further. The amount and type of sputum produced in bronchial carcinoma varies widely and may be frankly purulent owing to secondary infection. Haemoptysis requires full investigation even if there is merely a trace of blood in the sputum. Massive haemoptysis is not a frequent occurrence with primary bronchial carcinoma but persisting minor haemoptysis is one of the more common presentations. Many patients present with chest pain, sometimes quite unrelated to the pulmonary opacity. Pleuritic pain may be associated with secondary pneumonia due to bronchial obstruction, while more continuous pain occurs with chest wall invasion or metastatic rib deposits. Mediastinal invasion has been reported to produce central discomfort deep within the chest. Breathlessness may be due to a variety of factors—bronchial obstruction, pulmonary collapse, pleural effusion, lymphangitis, diaphragmatic paralysis—or merely to concomitant chronic bronchitis. Some patients with alveolar-cell carcinoma present with copious, thin, mucoid sputum, but such specificity is rare. Often patients present with symptoms due to complications of their disease, *vide infra*.

Physical Signs

Many lung tumours produce no abnormal physical signs at all. The commonest signs in the chest are consequent on bronchial obstruction and are, therefore, those of pulmonary collapse and consolidation. There may be evidence of pleural effusion and chest wall invasion may cause local tenderness. A common form of spread for carcinoma of the lung is via the lymphatics. The lymph drainage deposits of malignant cells may accumulate in the right paratracheal nodes and extend up into the neck and can present in the scalene node. The right paratracheal nodes are closely applied to superior vena cava and SVC obstruction from thoracic inlet obstruction with extension to the supraclavicular nodes is quite common. Careful examination of the neck and abdomen is necessary in all patients with a suspicion of malignant disease of the lung.

Manifestations of Bronchial Carcinoma

i. DIRECT INVASION. Primary bronchial carcinoma is commonly a locally invasive disease and the structures adjacent to the site of origins are commonly invaded. Thus the diaphragm, mediastinum and chest wall are immediately available. Also structures in the chest wall (*Fig.* 41.4), particularly ribs, intercostal nerves, brachial plexus, sympathetic chain and pericardium are commonly involved especially in the late stage of the disease. Invasion of the sympathetic chain at the level of the first rib can produce Horner's syndrome (*Fig.* 41.5). Invasion of the hilum particularly on the left side will commonly cause hoarseness from damage to the left recurrent laryngeal nerve. Damage to the right recurrent laryngeal nerve is uncommon as this does not truly enter the thoracic cavity but it can occur as a product of a right-sided apical tumour invading the floor of the posterior triangle. Invasion of the phrenic nerve produces diaphragmatic paralysis (*Fig.* 41.6) and it is not uncommon for patients to notice a change in their effort tolerance.

Direct invasion of the pericardium predisposes to effusion and cardiac dysrhythmia and often atrial fibrillation. Pleural involvement produces pleural effusion and direct spread will involve the chest wall producing pain and occasionally a

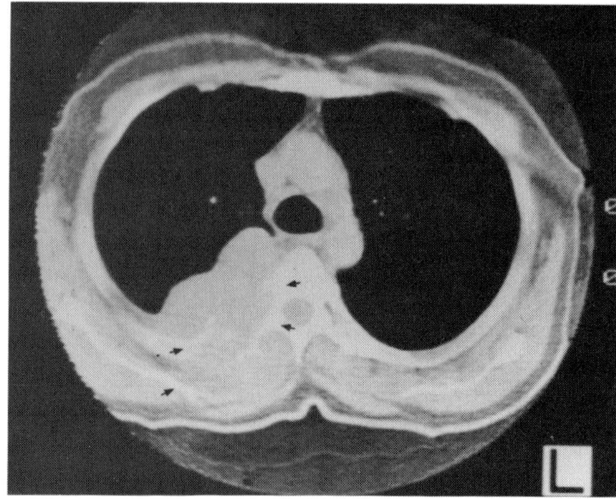

Fig. 41.4 CT scan showing extensive chest wall invasion.

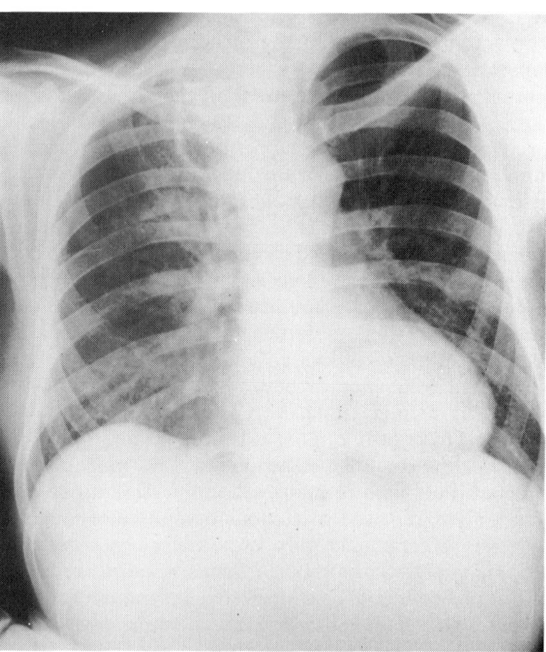

a

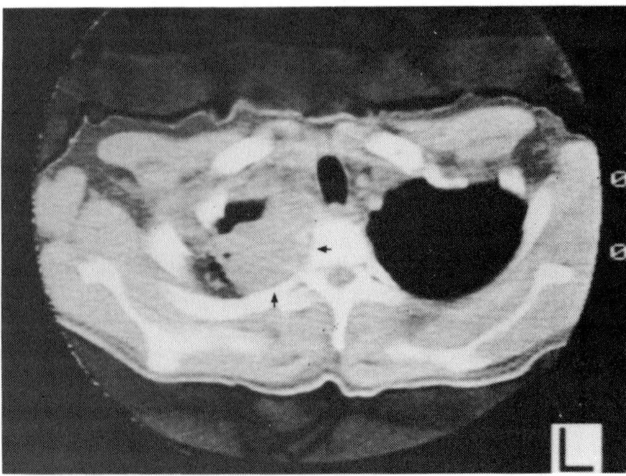

b

Fig. 41.5 *a*, PA chest radiograph and *b*, CT scan showing an apical bronchial carcinoma producing Pancoast's syndrome.

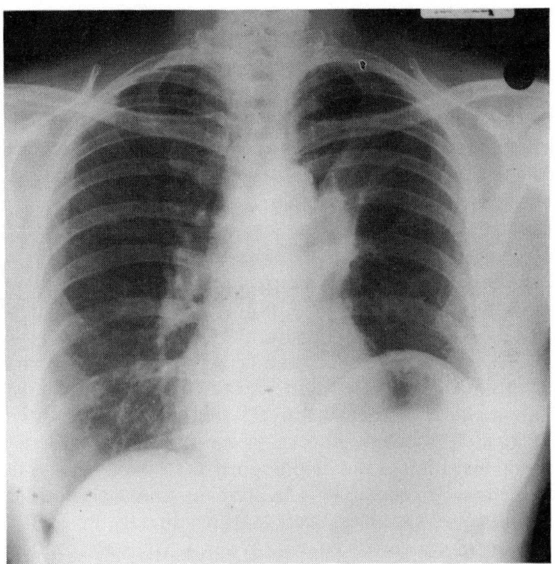

Fig. 41.6 PA chest radiography showing a left hilar tumour with phrenic nerve paralysis.

Table 41.2 Non-metastatic syndromes in bronchial carcinoma

Endocrine
Gynaecomastia
Hormone secretion—ADH, ACTH, parathormone, insulin, TSH
Neurological
Cerebellar degeneration
Myasthenic syndrome
Neuropathy
Musculoskeletal
Myopathy
Finger-clubbing
Hypertrophic osteoarthropathy
Cutaneous
Dermatomyositis
Scleroderma
Acanthosis nigricans
Circulatory
Non-bacterial endocarditis
Gammaglobulin abnormality
Purpura
Thrombophlebitis migrans

mass in the chest wall. Invasion of the apex of the lung to involve the brachial plexus and produce Horner's syndrome, pain and paralysis of the function of the arm, particularly involving the 7th/8th roots, produces a condition known as Pancoast's syndrome (*Fig.* 41.5). More commonly, simple invasion of the chest wall at the level of the second intercostal nerve will produce pain down the medial aspect of the arm in the distribution of the intercostobrachial nerve. This sign is often missed and patients have treatment to non-existent disease of the shoulder. Superior vena caval obstruction is rarely a product of right upper lobe tumour with direct invasion; more commonly it results from lymph-node involvement at the inlet. Initial SVC obstruction produces a feeling of fullness in the face on rising in the morning, occasionally puffy eyes, and goes on to produce a plethoric face with venous distension. The hands have a bluish tinge whilst the feet remain pink and venous collaterals are generated over the front of the chest wall.

ii. METASTATIC SPREAD. The more common carcinomas of lung all produce metastases. Small-cell carcinoma commonly presents with metastases apparent—the metastatic spread is often the cause of the symptoms. Non-small-cell carcinoma occasionally presents with metastatic spread. The common sites of deposition of metastases in carcinoma of the bronchus are brain, bone, liver and the contralateral lung. Involvement of brain, liver and bone are bad prognostic signs. Unfortunately on simple clinical assessment patients may be deemed operable, however CT scanning of brain and ultrasound of liver commonly rejects a further 10% of patients as having occult metastases. These patients are believed to contribute to the early postoperative mortality. With better case selection from the use of these imaging techniques the early mortality associated with the resected group will be lessened. Thus the long-term prognosis for the operative group should improve although of course less patients will be found suitable for operative treatment.

iii. NON-METASTATIC SYNDROMES. By definition this is a group of syndromes associated with the carcinoma of the bronchus where metastatic spread is not apparent. The incidence of these syndromes is thought to be as high as 10% and full understanding of the pathological mechanisms is not yet apparent. *Table* 41.2 lists the described conditions that can occur. The majority are based on occasional papers usually collected personally over time or even single case reports. A number of the non-metastatic syndromes are relatively common—inappropriate ADH and ACTH secretion, cerebellar degeneration and other neuropathies, finger clubbing, hypertrophic osteoarthropathy, thrombophlebitis migrans and hypercalcaemia. The other manifestations are much less common.

Endocrine: These usually arise late in the course of bronchial carcinoma and are seen more often with oat-cell carcinomas than with any other variety. Bilateral adrenal cortical hyperplasia is the commonest endocrine manifestation of bronchial carcinoma and is due to the production of ACTH by the tumour itself. This leads to very high concentrations of cortisol in the plasma and eventually to the clinical features of Cushing's syndrome. Oat-cell and occasionally squamous-cell carcinomas have been demonstrated to produce a parathormone-like substance which induces hypercalcaemia. The clinical picture is of polyuria, thirst, constipation and mental confusion. Antidiuretic hormone may be secreted again by oat-cell tumours producing water retention and hyponatraemia. Other hormones which have been identified on rare occasions as being produced by bronchial carcinomas are 5-hydroxytryptamine, thyroid stimulating hormone and an insulin-like hormone. Gynaecomastia is seen rarely in bronchial carcinoma and is usually accompanied by hypertrophic osteoarthropathy.

Neuromuscular: Various forms of neuropathy and myopathy may occur in bronchial carcinoma and include cerebellar degeneration with ataxia, dysarthria and extrapyramidal symptoms. Sensory and motor neuropathies occur, the latter often taking the form of weakness of the limb girdle muscles.

Cutaneous: Dermatomyositis has been recorded in various forms of tumour and certainly occurs in patients with bronchial carcinoma. Scleroderma (systemic sclerosis) may produce specific lung abnormalities but is also found in association with bronchial carcinoma, as is the skin condition called acanthosis nigricans.

Skeletal: Hypertrophic osteoarthropathy is a syndrome characterized by pain in the wrists and ankles which are tender and hot to the touch; there may occasionally be profuse sweating, Raynaud's phenomenon and gynaecomastia and, in the great majority of cases, gross finger clubbing is present. The syndrome is most often associated with carcinoma of the bronchus but may also occur with pleural fibroma and pulmonary sepsis, but the pathogenesis is unclear. The lesion is characterized radiologically by the presence of periosteal elevation and new bone formation, particularly at the wrist and ankle. The manifestations disappear immediately if the primary tumour is resected. Vagotomy may also relieve the symptoms should the lesion prove unresectable.

Circulatory: Thrombophlebitis migrans is probably the commonest of the circulatory complications of bronchial carcinoma, though also seen with many other tumours. Other conditions which have been reported are purpura, non-bacterial endocarditis and abnormalities in the gamma-globulins.

Diagnosis

Chest Radiography

This is the crucial investigation in patients suspected of having bronchial carcinoma. One of the most common appearances is unilateral enlargement of the hilar shadow but the opacities produced by bronchial carcinoma vary considerably and include: a small round nodule, an obvious large mass, an irregular density or an infiltrative lesion (*Fig.* 41.7). Usually the margin is poorly defined and there may be streaky densities running from the main mass into the surrounding lung, or towards the hilum. Cavitation occurs, particularly in squamous-cell carcinoma and may be identified with greater certainty by tomography. The inner wall of such a cavity is often irregular and may be quite thin (*Fig.* 41.8). In squamous carcinoma the cavitation is not always a function of liquefaction and consequently an air fluid level may not occur; the cavitation is sometimes eccentric and is characteristic of such tumours.

A common radiological appearance is that of collapse or consolidation distal to what may be quite a small endobronchial tumour (*Fig.* 41.9). A pulmonary tumour may also be totally obscured by a concomitant pleural effusion. The mediastinum must be looked at with great care because of the frequency of metastatic spread to the lymph glands. Enlargement of the pericardial silhouette is suggestive of pericardial effusion. Phrenic nerve invasion produces unilateral elevation of the diaphragm and its paralysis should be confirmed by screening. The bony cage must also be closely examined as the chest wall may be directly invaded with erosion of the involved rib. When a tumour invades the mediastinal glands and then spreads along or obstructs the lymphatics into both lungs, this may be seen as bilateral hilar enlargement with streaky shadows extending into both lung fields. This is called lymphangitis carcinomatosa (*Fig.* 41.10).

Sputum Cytology

Population screening by sputum cytology has been undertaken, particularly in high-risk groups. It is a particularly valuable investigation but requires the samples to be collected and handled appropriately and the skill and experience of the cytologist is crucial. Only 30–40% of bronchial carcinomas are visible at bronchoscopy but positive sputum cytology may be found in 50–60% of patients with bronchial carcinoma. False negatives are common, and the more specimens that are examined the higher is the positivity rate. In good hands false positives should be quite rare. This technique is particularly suitable for patients in whom

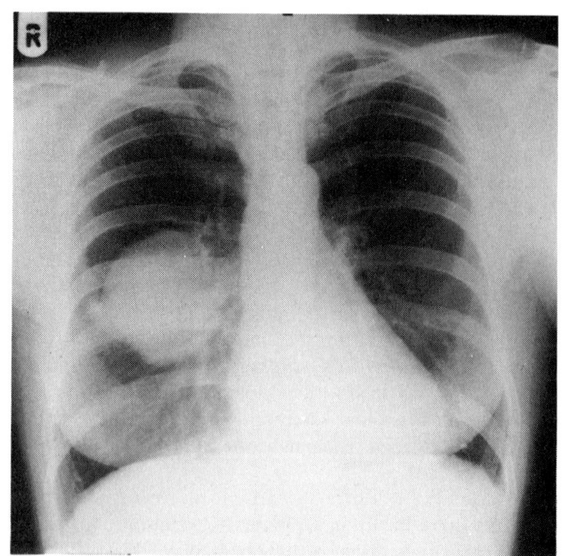

a

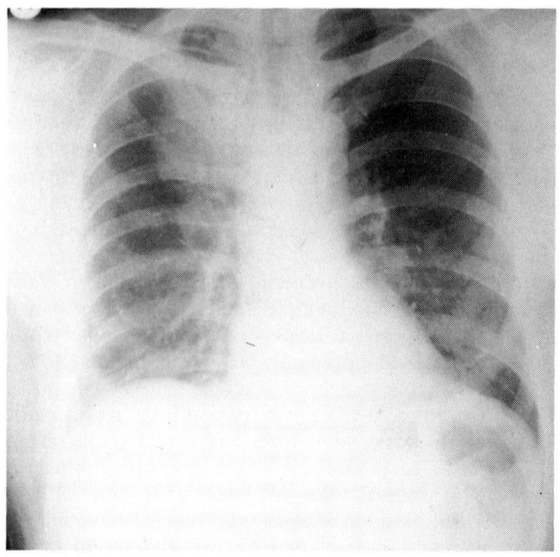

b

Fig. 41.7 *a*, *b*, PA chest radiographs showing typical bronchial carcinoma.

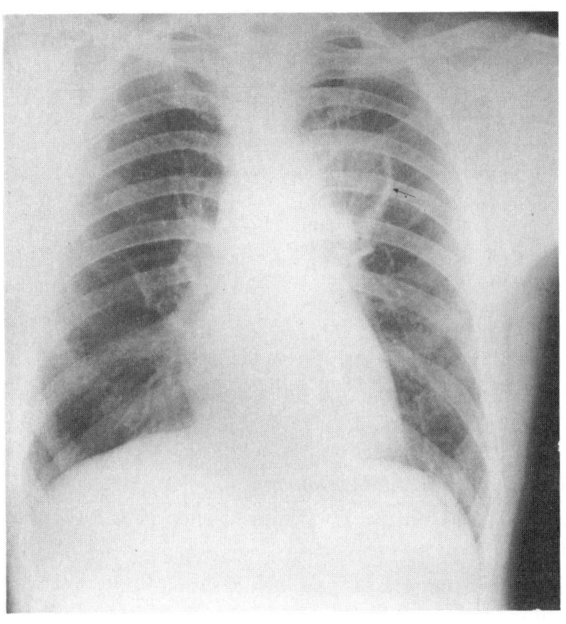

a

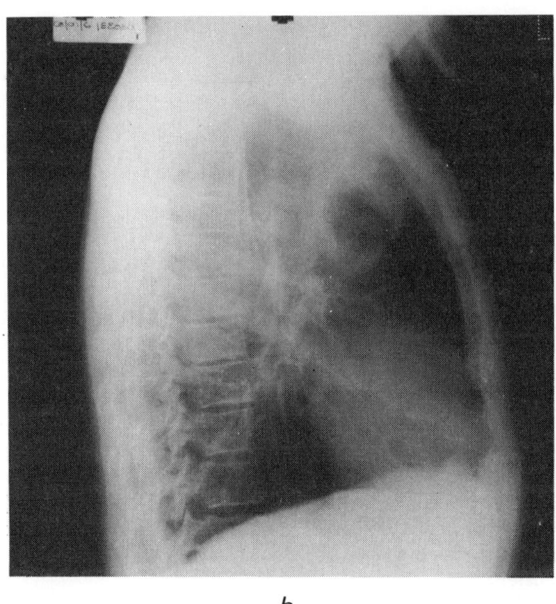

b

Fig. 41.8 *a*, PA and *b*, lateral chest radiographs showing a large cavitated squamous carcinoma.

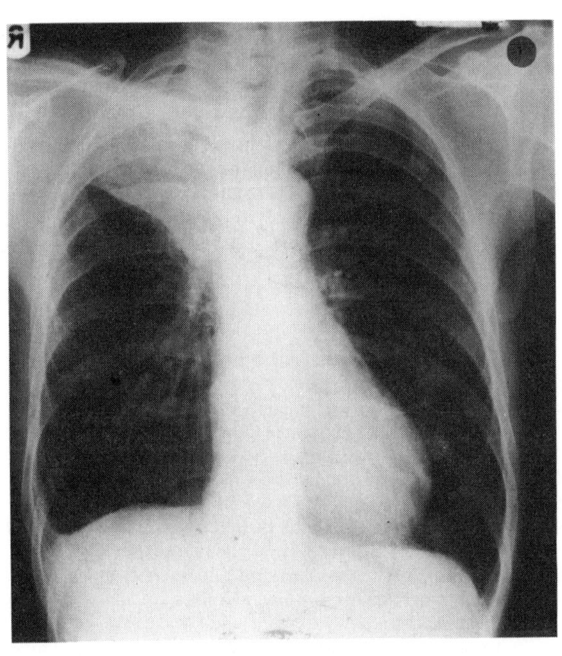

a

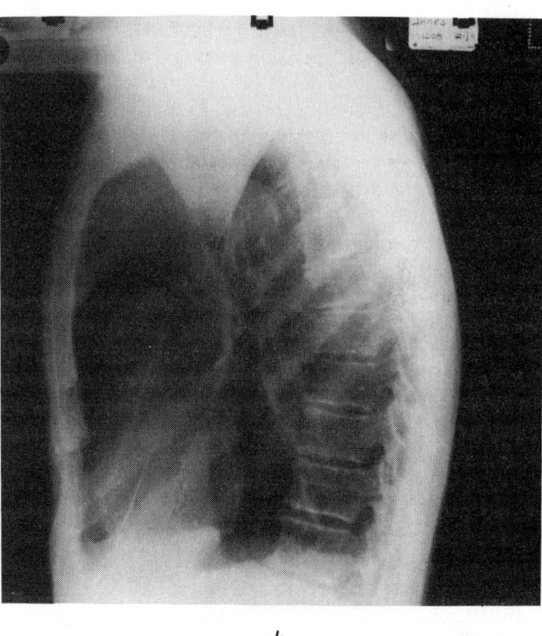

b

Fig. 41.9 *a*, PA and *b*, lateral radiographs showing right upper lobe collapse due to a small obstructive bronchial carcinoma.

bronchial carcinoma is strongly suspected but bronchoscopy has not confirmed the diagnosis.

Bronchoscopy

Bronchoscopy permits direct examination of the vocal cords, trachea, main lobar and segmental bronchi and often, sub-segmental bronchi. It allows direct biopsy of visible tumours (about 40% of all bronchial carcinomas) and sampling of secretions and cells from more peripheral lesions. There may also be indirect evidence of the presence of a tumour, such as external compression, distortion of a bronchus or widening of the carina.

The advent of the fibreoptic bronchoscope has enabled a great many physicians with varying experience to practice bronchoscopy without general anaesthesia and with a minimum of disturbance to the patient. There has been considerable discussion as to the relative merits of rigid and fibreoptic bronchoscopy—the facility to use both is clearly

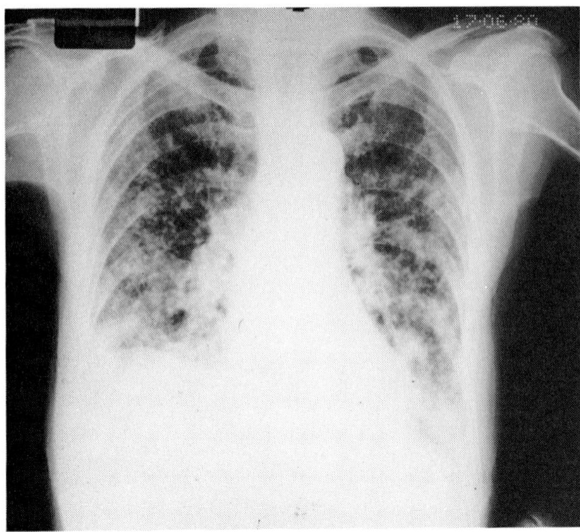

Fig. 41.10 Chest radiograph showing widespread lymphatic carcinomatosis.

best. The modern rigid bronchoscope has excellent optics and can take biopsies from within the upper lobe segmental bronchi under direct vision with ease. It is easier to use for manipulative procedures within the bronchial tree, such as the removal of foreign bodies. It is, however, usually passed under general anaesthesia. The obvious advantages of the flexible fibreoptic bronchoscopes are their ease of insertion—usually transnasally under local anaesthesia—and their ability to inspect the segmental and subsegmental bronchi in the upper lobes. It is possible to carry out many procedures through the flexible bronchoscope which previously required rigid bronchoscopy—biopsy, cytology, bronchography, and, in particular, transbronchial biopsy of peripheral pulmonary lesions under radiographic control is possible. The combination of endoscopic biopsy of visible bronchial tumours with aspiration of secretions from the involved bronchus, brush biopsy, transbronchial biopsy and sputum cytology, may take the positivity rate in patients with lung cancer over 80% when clinical staging for active treatment is undertaken. Extensive investigatory procedures when active interventional treatment is not proposed is not cost effective.

Other Investigations

Percutaneous needle biopsy under radiographic control, is a further technique utilized by some clinicians in the investigation of peripheral lesions. It carries with it the danger of pneumothorax and haemothorax. This technique is now improving in yield when executed under CT scanning control.

Most other investigations available for carcinoma of the lung are more appropriate to evaluation for resection and staging for radiotherapy or chemotherapy and for follow-up. CT scanning is becoming increasingly popular as a primary diagnostic tool, but this is probably inappropriate because unless management decisions are being undertaken it is an expensive procedure that adds little to the presumptive diagnosis. Histological confirmation of lung cancer now approaches 60% of all cases (*see Fig.* 41.2).

Many patients referred for diagnosis because of the possibility of lung cancer will, in fact, have a non-neoplastic disease. Bronchiectasis, tuberculosis, pneumonia and lung abscess may at times show features suggestive of a lung tumour. The correct diagnosis will usually be reached as long as the appropriate investigations are performed. Greater diagnostic difficulty is presented by the solitary pulmonary nodule. A rounded, peripheral shadow may be due to a primary bronchial carcinoma, a hamartoma, tuberculosis, metastatic tumour and a variety of other conditions, such as rheumatoid disease, fungal infection and even pulmonary embolism. Previous chest radiographs should always be sought and may be of great value in determining the age of the lesion. If all the usual diagnostic measures fail to give a positive answer, then exploratory thoracotomy may become necessary. Where it is felt that the lesion has a high probability of not being a bronchial carcinoma, observation may be appropriate or percutaneous biopsy under radiographic control attempted.

Staging of Bronchial Carcinoma

This is based on the TNM classification (*Table* 41.3) and involves:

Clinical—diagnostic staging (before thoracotomy and initiation of treatment)

Surgical—evaluation staging (includes the above data together with information obtained at exploratory thoracotomy)

Table 41.3 Definitions for staging bronchogenic carcinoma

TO	No evidence of primary tumour.
TX	Tumour proven by the presence of malignant cells in bronchopulmonary secretions but not visualized roentgenographically or bronchoscopically, or any tumour that cannot be assessed.
TIS	Carcinoma-in-situ.
T1	A tumour that is 3·0 cm or less in greatest diameter, surrounded by lung or visceral pleura, and without evidence of invasion proximal to a lobar bronchus at bronchoscopy.
T2	A tumour more than 3·0 cm in greatest diameter, or a tumour of any size that either invades the visceral pleura or which has associated atelectasis or obstructive pneumonitis extending to the hilar region. At bronchoscopy, the proximal extent of demonstrable tumour must be within a lobar bronchus at least 2·0 cm distal to the carina. Any associated atelectasis or obstructive pneumonitis must involve less than an entire lung, and there must be no pleural effusion.
T3	A tumour of any size with direct extension into an adjacent structure such as the parietal pleura, the chest wall, the diaphragm or the mediastinum and its contents; or a tumour demonstrable bronchoscopically to involve a main bronchus less than 2·0 cm distal to the carina; or any tumour associated with atelectasis or obstructive pneumonitis of an entire lung or pleural effusion.
N0	No demonstrable metastases to regional lymph nodes.
N1	Metastases to lymph nodes in the peribronchial or the ipsilateral hilar region, or both, including direct extension.
N2	Metastases to lymph nodes in the mediastinum.
M0	No distant metastases
M1	Distant metastases such as in scalene, cervical, or contralateral hilar lymph nodes, brain, bones, liver or contralateral lung.

Occult carcinoma	*Stage 1*	*Stage 2*	*Stage 3*
TX N0 M0	T1S N0 M0	T2 N1 M0	T3 any N or M
	T1 N0 M0		N2 any T or M
	T1 N1 M0		M1 any T or N
	T2 N0 M0		

Post-surgical treatment—pathological staging (used to assign a pathological classification to those patients who have a resection). This is carried out on all resected specimens and indeed is the basis of effective TNM staging.

Re-treatment staging (assessment before further treatment for recurrent or progressive disease) and autopsy staging.

Management

Surgery

The best prospect of cure for any individual patient with bronchial carcinoma is operative resection although only 10% of patients are suitable for such treatment. There is unfortunately an exploratory thoracotomy rate which approaches 25%. Investigation of a patient when the possibility of surgical resection is raised, must be designed to limit this unnecessary exploratory thoracotomy rate.

CONTRAINDICATIONS. Extrathoracic metastases, whether they are in brain, liver, bone, skin or cervical lymph nodes contraindicate surgery. Spread of a primary lung tumour to the other lung is a further contraindication.

Resectability is a function of safe dissection within the mediastinum and the effective excision of the tumour with its lymph drainage. Simple guides to resection manifest themselves on a chest radiograph with the closeness of the tumour mass to the mediastinum, particularly whether it is confluent with the aorta in the left chest. Involvement of the chest wall may cause Horner's and Pancoast's syndromes. Recurrent laryngeal or phrenic nerve palsy are relative contraindications. There is an aggressive approach which suggests that patients with a Pancoast's tumour can have a local resection which includes the brachial plexus as a palliative procedure for a directly invasive process. This is suggested as the best way of handling the pain. There is some reservation about such a procedure. The advantages of CT scanning of the brain have shown that in surgical series some 10% of patients have occult cerebral metastases at the time of resection. It is an expensive procedure to screen 100 patients with CT scans of the head in order to save 10 patients from surgery.

Ultrasound of the liver is a much more reasonable and cheap facility and now tends to be available in most hospitals for screening for liver secondaries. The cost of screening the cohort to find some 10% of patients when secondaries are not obvious is feasible. Similarly, bone scanning may detect the presence of occult bone secondaries, but again it is an expensive procedure with a small return of the order of 5–8%. The intrathoracic lymphatic spread is a most important manifestation of malignant disease. Routine mediastinoscopy and left anterior mediastinotomy, where appropriate, is used in most units as a routine assessment for resectability. Mediastinoscopy particularly gives access to the paratracheal node group which is essentially the main drainage from the chest; some 70% of tumours drain to this node group. Left anterior mediastinotomy allows access to the left hilum at the level of the aortic arch and the pulmonary artery can be explored for resectability and biopsies taken. Extracapsular metastases of the lymph nodes are a bad prognostic sign, indicating a 50% mortality at 6 months in non-small-cell carcinoma. Such involved nodes, if found, contraindicate resection.

Recent work with CT scanning has shown that a resolution of around 5 mm for mediastinal nodes is not a good discriminant for the presence or absence of malignant invasion of the nodes. CT scanning is not recommended for evaluation of mediastinal nodes but it is of value to image mediastinal confluence. Thoracic tomography is probably of equal value.

Invasion of Pleura and Chest Wall: Invasion of the visceral pleura is classified as T2 tumour and involvement of the parietal pleural as T3. The prognosis is poorer in this group of patients. Occasionally the tumour spreads directly across the pleura, attacks the chest wall and causes pain. It is not unreasonable ethically to resect a lobe or even a lung with a piece of chest wall *en bloc*; but the long-term prognosis is usually poor. The presence of pleural effusion indicates a T2/T3 tumour and the prognosis is poor. Individual surgeons have tried aggressive combined therapy, particularly using radiotherapy locally, before and after resection to treat these patients. The number of cases treated is small, the trials are few and the outcomes uncertain. Mostly such operations are done on an individual basis, the decision taken is guided very much by professional integrity, the relationship between the patient and the surgeon and their mutual expectations, and the advice of other medical attendants.

Carcinoma of the Main Bronchi: The common bronchial carcinoma involving the main bronchi to within 1·5 cm of the main carina is resectable. As the tumour margin approaches the carina prospects for resectability lessen. The decision to resect is then about the technical competence of the surgeon, the unit and the estimated biological activity of the tumour. For the muco-epidermoid and the adenoid cystic carcinoma resection of the main bronchus and side wall of the trachea with reimplantation of the bronchi, even excision of the carina, if feasible, may be undertaken. However, this is an uncommon situation as the majority of patients have relatively aggressive squamous carcinomas and do not present as suitable cases for resection. However, the commonest tumour associated with resection at the carina and tracheal wall is the well-differentiated squamous carcinoma which is the most frequent lesion of the proximal tracheo-bronchial tree.

Poor Respiratory Function: Recently the development of differential lung perfusion scanning has been demonstrated to be an accurate predictor of the proportionate loss of lung function after pneumonectomy. It is now becoming more and more routine to use this measurement and produce an estimate of the patient's potential respiratory function postoperatively. This has been an important step forward because patients are often seen to have poor respiratory function on first impression. However, should the lesion be shown to have grossly reduced the function of the affected lung, it is likely that the patient will not suffer greatly the loss of such a lung as he has already had a physiological trial of life on one lung. Consequently, of itself, poor respiratory function is not a contraindication to surgery. The sputum load associated with chronic bronchitis is much better coped with by modern technology. A patient with a predictable postoperative sputum load can be electively given a minitracheostomy for care of a postoperative sputum retention. A period of physiotherapy preoperatively and a minitracheostomy postoperatively makes it quite feasible to take patients successfully through pulmonary resection who would not have been thought suitable in the past.

All patients with the prospect of pneumonectomy should have FEV_1 and FVC measurement and attention paid to their initial discrepancy against the prediction nomogram. Differential perfusion scan should be used to predict the postoperative figures. A majority of patients can manage on approximately 35% of their predicted figures. As the normal figures are very much a function of height, age and sex there is no simple rule of thumb for safe resection.

Recent statistical observations have suggested that the problem of a recent myocardial infarction is a major predictor of postoperative myocardial dysfunction and death. It is recommended that no patient should have a thoracotomy for malignant disease within three months of the insult and that no patient should have a thoracotomy for benign condition within six months of a myocardial infarction. After six months the incidence of perioperative myocardial reinfarction falls to levels appropriate to the age and sex of the patient.

There is an increasing number of patients in the 8th decade presenting with carcinoma of the bronchus and increasingly these patients are being found suitable for resection.

OPERATIVE TECHNIQUE. Good thoracic surgery requires close co-operation between the surgeon and the anaesthetist. Modern anaesthetic techniques must include the ability to monitor closely the patient's condition throughout the procedure. This is facilitated by continuous monitoring of the ECG and the intra-arterial and central venous pressures in appropriate patients. The anaesthetist must be able to control ventilation throughout the procedure and the ability to ventilate either lung individually may be of great assistance in certain procedures.

Access to the lung is best achieved by lateral or posterior thoracotomy. The latter approach is seldom used today as its primary value for secretion control has been pre-empted by the use of the double-lumen endotracheal tube. Thoracotomy is performed at the level of the 5th or 6th rib. The ribs are separated with a self-retaining retractor. Because of the lymphatic drainage of the lung it is generally felt that lobectomy is the minimum safe resection, although it is well known that lesser procedures, such as segmental resection and even wedge resection, may produce an apparent cure of bronchial carcinoma. Even lobectomy is suitable only for relatively small or peripheral tumours. Removal of the entire lung by pneumonectomy is required for hilar tumours and peripheral tumours which have spread across the oblique fissure. Using all available diagnostic methods the surgeon should have a tissue diagnosis preoperatively in 70–80% of cases. Of the remainder, the diagnosis will be clear in a considerable proportion at the time of surgery. If there is any doubt then it may still be reasonable to perform lobectomy, but pneumonectomy should not be performed without first making a histological diagnosis wherever possible by frozen section, the tissue being obtained ideally by wedge excision rather than incision biopsy. Thorough preoperative screening, including the use of mediastinoscopy, should eliminate the majority of those patients who will be unsuitable for surgical resection. Thus of all patients in whom operation is undertaken, 10% proven unresectable is a desirable limit. Direct invasion of pericardium, diaphragm, pleura and even chest wall, does not preclude *en bloc* resection and it is occasionally compatible with long-term survival.

COMPLICATIONS OF PULMONARY RESECTION. All patients who undergo this sort of surgery are liable to the usual complications of a major operative procedure. Such problems as superficial wound infection, venous thrombosis and pulmonary embolism may be prevented by suitable prophylaxis; others such as myocardial infarction are not preventable but a recent history of infarction, severe angina and uncontrolled hypertension are important predictors of such postoperative problems. The complication rate tends to rise with the age of the patient, much of this rise being associated with the deterioration of the cardiovascular system. Certain specific complications occur following thoracic procedures and they are worthy of further mention.

In the normal course of events following lobectomy two tubes are used to drain the pleural space on the resected side. Initially there will be some blood loss and commonly there will be an air leak for 24 h. Within 48 h the basal drain can be removed and after 24 h of no air leak the second drain can be removed. At this point the residual lobe should fill the space on the operated side. There will be some shift in the mediastinum and elevation of the diaphragm appropriate to the loss of volume on that side. When a patient has had pneumonectomy there are two choices of initial management. One is to use a tube to drain the hemithorax on the resected side. The tube is kept clamped over the next 24 h with a one-minute release in each hour, and possibly some blood will spill out through the underwater seal. In normal circumstances the bleeding will be minimal and the mediastinum will shift during the subsequent 24 h and the intercostal tube is removed the next day. At this point there will be a shift in the mediastinum and elevation of the diaphragm on the resected side. There will be a fluid level in the space usually at mid-hilar level. Over the subsequent weeks this air will absorb, the mediastinum will come across and at 3 months there may well not be an air fluid level in this space. The alternative early management is that the chest is closed at operation and in the immediate postoperative period with the patient breathing spontaneously a needle is introduced into the space and air is aspirated under aseptic technique and manometric control until the pressure in the space on the resected side is negative in both phases of respiration. The patient will be watched for 24 h for any evidence of occult bleeding and a further chest radiograph taken the following morning. After this time the course of events should be as described for the tube drainage group.

There are two specific problems associated with a pneumonectomy: (1) infection in a closed space which may come from an infected wound or have been acquired at operation; (2) bronchopleural fistula when the bronchial stump leaks into the space, space fluid enters the bronchial tree; air will accumulate and infection be transferred to the pneumonectomy space.

Empyema of the Pleural Space: This may follow a wound infection, and one becomes suspicious if the patient becomes ill with a pyrexia and a raised white cell count but there is no evidence of a bronchopleural fistula. The space is aspirated and if infection is confirmed, the space should be drained and two-tube irrigation set up for a week. With modern antibiotics and good bacteriology it should be possible to sterilize the space by continuous flushing. The space should be explored and decorticated and the two-tube flushing with antibiotic solution for a week should sterilize the space. Should the space remain infected at three weeks the patient should have an open stoma produced. At six months a thoracoplasty involving six or seven ribs should be quite adequate to obliterate this space. This procedure may seem drastic but it can be carried out with relatively few problems and a low mortality and it is surprising how acceptable cosmetically a thoracoplasty under such circumstances can be.

Bronchopleural Fistula: These commonly occur at about the 10th day and presently have an incidence of 5–10%. There is a classic change in the chest radiograph when the fluid level which was previously seen on a chest radiograph is seen to be lower and there is an increase in the darkness on the film of the air in the space. A further amount of air has come via the fistula into the space and produced an increased translucency to X-rays. The mediastinum may well have moved back to the midline and the fluid level dropped because the volume is now larger and some space fluid may have been coughed up.

If the patient coughs up space fluid, it will be coloured appropriate to the time since operation as the blood left in the space passes from being frank-red blood though the process of blood breakdown to the brown haemosiderin-loaded fluid after two weeks. The presence of space fluid in the sputum pot is the most important clinical sign.

The patient is ill with a temperature, often has a tachycardia and has a persistent cough usually productive of space fluid and demonstrates the appropriate radiological changes.

A high index of suspicion is necessary for successful treatment is dependent on early intervention. The patient's chest should be re-explored, the stump of the bronchus be identified, dissected back and re-sutured and a muscular flap with a viable neuromuscular bundle should be brought down and sutured over the stump. The patient should then have seven days of irrigation of appropriate antibiotic fluid, through two tubes to sterilize the space. This is usually adequate to deal with this problem. Small fistulas, especially on the left side, can be managed with two-tube irrigation and cicatrization of the bronchial stump. Such cicatrization is done with 20% sodium hydroxide for 2 min and then neutralized by 50% acetic acid.

If there is a persistent infection in the space the patient will require a stoma and ultimately a thoracoplasty. These complications should add only minimally to the 10% mortality which results from pneumonectomy.

Surgical Emphysema: This is to be expected when the scapula is lifted as the chest wall is explored but it is usually only local and is simply absorbed over 4 or 5 days. Occasionally air is extravasated, particularly following lobectomy, and is of no particular consequence as long as the cavity is adequately drained and the air leak ultimately stops. Very occasionally there is a peripheral air leak that persists; it is usually associated with a small communicating bronchiole that passed across the fissure, and was cut across at lobectomy. A limited apical thoracoplasty to obliterate the space and close the fistula may be necessary.

Haemorrhage: Postoperative bleeding occurring after pneumonectomy almost always is from the bronchial arteries. Rarely, a disastrous haemorrhage may occur from a pulmonary artery and it is usually too late for re-operation. The problem of pulmonary artery bleeding is usually an interoperative problem which is rarely disastrous but it is the only cause of intraoperative death. The bleeding into the pneumonectomy space requires re-exploration and evacuation. Occult haemorrhage from the bronchial vessels can cause a clotted haemothorax; this should be suspected if the appropriate mediastinal shift has not occurred and the patient required volume support for occult blood loss. It may be wise to evacuate the space.

Herniation of the Heart: The pericardium is often opened during pneumonectomy and portions of the pericardium may require excision if involved by tumour. If the resulting defect is large the heart may herniate right out of the pericardium producing sudden circulatory collapse due to the distortion of the great vessels. Urgent re-operation is required.

Retention of Secretions: This is not the problem it formerly was. Modern elective use of minitracheostomy in patients who are likely to have a secretion problem postoperatively makes for simple access on the ward for aspiration of secretions. Should any patient unexpectedly manifest a secretions load a minitracheostomy can be inserted under local anaesthesia in the ward without difficulty. All thoracic surgical units should have physiotherapists and junior staff who are wholly familiar with the management of sputum load and minitracheostomy should be available in the ward for immediate insertion. With this particular facility now becoming widely available less patients will require postoperative ventilation for respiratory failure.

The major contribution to good postoperative patient cooperation has been the recent advances in pain relief. These have been the use of cryoanalgesia of the intercostal nerves and the increasing use of infusion pumps for morphine delivery.

In the past it has been very unusual for patients with pneumonectomy ever to get off ventilators if they had respiratory failure. With modern jet ventilation and minitracheostomy and a combination of the two which is now developing this problem should have a much better outcome in the future.

RESULTS. Factors which Influence the Outcome.

Delay in Diagnosis: There is evidence from several reported series that patients in whom the diagnosis is made at routine radiography when they are asymptomatic, have a better prognosis than those patients who have presented because of symptoms related to their tumour.

Histological Type: The prognosis in squamous and adenocarcinoma is equivalent except that women with resected adenocarcinoma seem to have the best prognosis. The prognosis in anaplastic carcinoma is much worse. Few patients with small-cell carcinoma are offered operation, but the small group of patients who do have resections seem to show a survival proportion equal to the overall resected group outcome.

Tumour Size: There is a distinct relationship between tumour size and survival rate. If a tumour under 2 cm is surgically resected then this patient should have a 5-year survival rate of about 40%. If on the other hand the tumour is greater than 5 cm in diameter the 5-year survival is about 10%. (This is acknowledged in the TNM classification: T1<3 cm; T2>3 cm.)

Lymph Node Involvement: There is a steady decrease in survival rate as each successive group of lymph nodes is involved. Thus direct invasion of local lymph nodes in the pulmonary parenchyma does little to diminish 5-year survival. As soon as hilar or mediastinal glands are involved the 5-year survival declines sharply, particularly if there is perinodal invasion (N1 prognosis is better than N2).

Direct Invasion of Mediastinum and Chest Wall: It has already been indicated that such invasion reduces the chance of a cure. It applies particularly to involvement of mediastinal structures, such as pericardium, aortic wall, superior vena cava and recurrent laryngeal nerve. Chest wall invasion is often surgically treatable and occasionally compatible with long-term survival (T3+/−M1 poor prognosis).

Vascular Invasion: It has been demonstrated that 5-year survival in patients with vascular invasion is likely to be under 10%. When there is no evidence of either vascular or lymph node involvement the 5-year survival rate may rise to over 60%. Such invasion is common in anaplastic tumours.

Type of Resection: If it is possible to remove the tumour by lobectomy then this carries with it an operative mortality of 4% and a 5-year survival of around 40%, though the range is quite wide. Pneumonectomy is a more major undertaking but is required for the more extensive tumour. It carries with it an operative mortality of 8–12% and the 5-year survival is about half that for lobectomy. There are marked differences in the surgical approach to the management of the patient who is found at operation to have an extensive bronchial carcinoma. In some patients there is involvement of a structure which renders the tumour entirely unresectable. These patients do badly and their management is considered further in the next part of this chapter. If there is extensive mediastinal glandular involvement, it is still possible to carry out resection of the primary tumour with enucleation of the gland masses (N2 disease). A true *en bloc* dissection is difficult because of the unpredictability of the lymphatic drainage. It is believed by some that palliative resection is entirely appropriate in this situation and may assist further therapeutic measures by reducing tumour bulk. The alternative view is that incomplete surgical resection is inappropriate and that palliation by radiotherapy without resection is more appropriate. It is obvious that the morbidity and mortality of this type of surgery will vary according to how aggressive a policy is adopted.

The tumour with the best prognosis will be the small well-differentiated squamous or adenocarcinoma which can be apparently completely removed by lobectomy—the 5-year survival may reach 60% in such patients (T1,N0). The overall survival at 5 years in surgically resected patients is usually 25–30%.

Radiotherapy, Chemotherapy and Immunotherapy

Research continues using various combinations of radiotherapy, chemotherapy and immunotherapy to try and modify the course of non-resectable malignant disease of the lung. The pattern of behaviour of the different cell types is so established that a simple management classification has grown up: small-cell and non-small-cell carcinoma. Small-cell carcinoma is very sensitive to both local radiotherapy and chemotherapy. Considerable short-term responses and a limited shift in the survival time have been gained in small-cell carcinoma. There has been no benefit from chemotherapy applied to non-small-cell carcinoma. Radiotherapy remains a legitimate approach to non-small-cell carcinoma that is confined to the thorax.

The doubling time of the tumour, i.e. the time required to double its size, is related to the histological type, being longest in adenocarcinoma (mean about 170 days) and shortest in small-cell carcinoma (mean about 33 days). Small well-differentiated squamous-cell carcinomas have the best prognosis following resection as they tend to grow slowly and metastasize late. In contrast, small-cell tumours grow rapidly and disseminate early, often before the diagnosis is made. Thus, when comparing outcomes of the different modalities of treatment it is important to realize that the separate tumour groups have differing and distinctive characteristics.

Difficulties in staging bronchial tumours add to the problems. Every effort should be made to obtain evidence of intrathoracic and distant spread when assessing patients for a given treatment regime. Unfortunately, post-mortem studies have shown that 20% of patients dying in the immediate postoperative period, after an apparently successful resection, had soft-tissue metastases not recognizable by current screening techniques.

IMMUNOTHERAPY. Considerable effort has been applied during the last 20 years to pursue chance observations that patients who had infected spaces tended to live longer and perhaps this was evidence of some form of immuno-enhancement. Levamisole and *Corynebacterium parvum* have been used specifically in carcinoma of the bronchus and have not made any difference to long-term survival. Likewise intrapleural BCG has also failed to give any benefit.

Immunotherapy as an approach to the management of carcinoma of the lung, both small-cell and non-small-cell, has not demonstrated an improvement in survival proportion.

RADIOTHERAPY. Radiotherapy is now generally administered by megavoltage equipment (supervoltage) enabling the administration of a higher dose of radiation which can be more accurately directed, thereby reducing the danger of both skin reaction and damage to other tissues, e.g. bone. Small-cell carcinomas are the most radiosensitive, followed by large-cell anaplastic and squamous cell, with the adenocarcinomas responding poorly. The total dose of radiation depends partly on the histological type but mainly on whether curative treatment is being attempted or merely palliation undertaken. The treatment usually consists of daily fractions (around 200 rad) given 5 days a week for 2–6 weeks depending on the dose required, e.g. 3000–4000 rad in radical treatment. The field irradiated usually includes a section of the adjacent mediastinum as well as the tumour mass. When treating centrally placed or mediastinal lesions care has to be taken not to over-irradiate the radiosensitive spinal cord thereby causing radiation myelitis.

The complications of radiotherapy to bronchial neoplasms include:

1. Oesophagitis which occurs within 6 weeks of starting irradiation. It is often helped by antacid mixtures which contain a topical anaesthetic (Mucaine). Rarely, its severity is such as to cause cessation of radiotherapy.
2. Pneumonitis which is seen as transient soft shadows on chest radiography occurring within a few weeks of the treatment. It may be either symptomless or associated with cough and dyspnoea when the symptoms may be helped by oral steroids.
3. Pulmonary fibrosis, commencing 4–8 months after treatment. It may be asymptomatic, appearing on routine radiography or present as cough and dyspnoea. Respiratory function tests show a restrictive pattern, i.e. reduced FEV_1, FVC, lung volumes and transfer factor. Steroids may reduce the symptoms but will not affect the fibrosis.
4. Rarely, transient nausea and anorexia may occur but

these are easily controlled with anti-emetics and rapidly settle after treatment.

5. Carditis and pericarditis are rare complications occurring between 6 and 12 months after treatment.

Radiotherapy is usually contraindicated in the presence of a large pleural effusion. Any respiratory infection should be treated and surgical wounds allowed to heal before commencing treatment.

Treatment may be classified as curative, palliative or adjuvant.

Curative Radiotherapy: Curative radiotherapy is only possible in operable equivalent cases. Those cases who have either an operable tumour but have refused surgery or who have an inoperable but localized intrathoracic tumour, e.g. too close to the carina to be resectable. Radical treatment is contraindicated if the tumour is large, when there is extensive mediastinal involvement, in the presence of distant metastasis and in patients whose general condition is poor. In operable equivalent cases some reports have claimed a success rate following radical radiotherapy which is comparable to that of resection but the results from most centres are less favourable. Many clinicians reserve aggressive radical radiotherapy for the fit younger patients preferring to defer treatment in the elderly until symptoms develop.

Palliative Radiotherapy: In palliative radiotherapy the object is to relieve symptoms and improve the quality of life. Good results are obtained in controlling haemoptysis, relieving superior vena caval obstruction (effective in 70% of cases with late recurrence in 20%) and in some cases of distressing cough and dyspnoea. Treatment may relieve occlusion of a major bronchus. Bone pain is often helped at least temporarily by palliative irradiation.

With spinal deposits paraplegia is a possiblity. Non-small-cell carcinoma of the bronchus is not sufficiently radiosensitive to allow for rapid decompression so laminectomy is still the more effective procedure. Radiotherapy is reserved for slowly evolving or stable compression syndromes. Some radiotherapists would use dexamethasone cover and treat on a daily assessment basis and only proceed to decompression if the evidence showed further deterioration of spinal cord function.

Non-small-cell carcinoma is notoriously resistant to chemotherapy and no enhancement of radiotherapy has been demonstrated in combination trials.

It has been suggested that palliative radiotherapy might be offered to elderly patients with resectable tumours as an alternative to the risks of surgery but many clinicians prefer to keep such patients under review, treating their symptoms as they arise.

Cerebral secondaries may be treated palliatively with good short-term results. In small-cell tumours, cerebral secondaries are common and some radiotherapists advocate prophylactic brain irradiation as part of the initial management of such cases.

Adjuvant Radiotherapy: Radiotherapy may be given as an adjuvant to surgery or chemotherapy. Preoperative radiotherapy can make surgery more difficult and may increase the postoperative complications without any measurable benefit. An exception is the Pancoast's tumour. Studies involving routine postoperative radiotherapy have failed to show any definite advantage. However, individual cases may benefit and a young patient with minimal residual mediastinal disease following resection may be considered for radical radiotherapy.

Hyperbaric oxygen in combination with radiotherapy has not shown any benefit. Likewise the use of electron affinic diffusible compounds, e.g. misonidazole, do not increase the survival proportion or improve apparent local control.

There is a little evidence that neutron therapy will help in treating bronchial carcinomas.

Radiotherapy to the primary lesion followed by small-dose total-body irradiation has been advocated for small-cell carcinomas but the results of controlled trials are awaited.

Unfortunately the results of radiotherapy in bronchial carcinoma have not been significantly improved by the technical advances of the past twenty years. Only a few highly selected patients benefit from radical (curative) treatment but where palliation is required radiotherapy can be of value.

Recently major studies have begun to try and estimate the place for postoperative radiotherapy in node-positive disease. It is to be hoped that in the next ten years the place of radiotherapy in combination with resection will be evaluated by randomized controlled trials.

CHEMOTHERAPY. The observation that small-cell anaplastic carcinomas respond to a number of cytotoxic drugs (cyclophosphamide, methotrexate, lomustine, vincristine, doxorubicin, procarbazine, V.P.16-epipodophyllotoxin and ifosfamide) has stimulated interest in this field. Survival may be prolonged from 6 months to upward of 2 years. However, all the available drugs can produce toxic side-effects and patient compliance with treatment regimens of 12 months or more may present problems. The clinician is faced with encouraging continuance with a therapy for which there is no evidence of lasting benefit. Any regimen should be safe but effective and acceptable to the patient without seriously impairing the quality of life. A transient poor quality of life needs a good trade-off to be recommended.

The response of squamous-cell, large-cell anaplastic and adenocarcinomas of the bronchus to cytotoxic drugs has so far been disappointing.

The side-effects of chemotherapy may be divided into: (i) early, which may follow each treatment and last for a variable time (stomatitis, nausea, vomiting, malaise); or (ii) delayed, starting some time after commencing treatment (marrow depression, alopecia, infection, neurotoxicity, depression, weight loss).

Cytoxic drugs may be administered as single agents, in combined regimens or as part of adjuvant therapy.

Single-agent Chemotherapy: Single-agent chemotherapy is used to assess tumour response to that drug. Several drugs, e.g. vindesine, ifosfamide, are currently under investigation in squamous-cell, large-cell anaplastic and adenocarcinomas of the lung. A reduction of more than 50% in tumour size indicates a significant response. No present single-dose regime has proved effective in any large group of patients.

Combination Chemotherapy: Research has shown that the most effective regimens in small-cell carcinoma involve non-cross-resistant combinations of active drugs given simultaneously, e.g. vincristine, methotrexate and cyclophosphamide or doxorubicin, methotrexate and 5-fluorouracil. The optimal time between courses depends on the drugs used and the response obtained. Whichever drug combinations have been used with or without adjuvant radiotherapy, the mean survival time has not yet exceeded 16–18 months and relapses frequently follow cessation of treatment. Further work is needed to establish the most effective regimens, the frequency of administration and the duration of treatment.

Recently, the concept of alternating chemotherapy regimens using two drug combinations, e.g. (i) cyclophosphamide, methotrexate, vincristine, and (ii) doxorubicin plus procarbazine, has been applied to treating small-cell tumours. The groups may be used alternately or one may be given for a set period, e.g. three months, and then the other for a similar time. Such regimens are beneficial in the lymphomas but controlled studies in bronchial carcinoma are awaited.

Pulsed therapy using four agents taken over three days at three weekly interval for six pulses has recently been developed. Patient compliance is good and the side-effects tolerable when a period of recovery with no treatment is part of the planning.

Adjuvant Chemotherapy: Many regimens used to treat small-cell tumours include radiotherapy to the primary lesion given either before starting chemotherapy or after two or three pulses of the drugs. Initial reports suggest a beneficial effect although the results of further controlled trials are awaited.

The place of surgery in the treatment of small-cell carcinoma has been debated ever since two studies comparing radiotherapy with surgery showed a 4% 10-year survival in the radiotherapy group and nil in the surgical. Other workers have suggested up to 30% 5-year survival following resection of localized small-cell tumours. Trials are currently under way looking at the value of surgery plus combination chemotherapy in the management of resectable small-cell carcinomas. It takes national organizations to get such data and there is a large potential for bureaucratic difficulties of co-ordination. This suggests that much co-operation is necessary between interested physicians and surgeons in order that these evaluations may be carried out. Cynics suggest that this may not be possible.

Laser Therapy

Lasers are becoming increasingly popular and are being applied to the management of bronchial carcinoma. They are designed to deliver heat energy at a point in a controlled manner. The local heat injury has its effect by evaporation of tissues. Instruments designed to deliver laser energy via fibreoptic instruments and modifications of the original rigid bronchoscope are available. They are designed to burn away tissue and thus may be useful for clearing blocked bronchi. In a small group of patients where their luminal obstruction is a function of true ingrowth of tissue rather than extrinsic compression, laser therapy may well increase the internal diameter and thus the delivery of extra air flow to the lung should it still be functioning. Lasers are very limited in their value as it is end-stage palliation where they are indicated. Presently laser therapy is under evaluation. In the next few years clear indications will manifest themselves and lasers may find a limited place to maintain patency of the bronchi in end-stage malignant disease of the bronchus. Already small trials are going ahead evaluating a combination of laser therapy to increase bronchus patency and local radiotherapy to try to control peribronchial disease. It is very difficult to produce randomized control trials with this group of patients but it is the only way for us to evaluate the varied treatment.

Terminal Care

In many patients dying of lung cancer there is a slow deterioration over several months with considerable physical and mental distress. Palliative radiotherapy should be used where applicable to relieve symptoms. The control of pain is important and it is essential to administer analgesics regularly, preferably at a frequency which prevents the pain from breaking through. Various combinations of analgesics including acetylsalicylic acid, paracetamol, codeine phosphate, dextromoramide, dextropropoxyphene, phenazocine, dipipanone, papaveretum, morphine, diamorphine and prochlorperazine may be used. Treatment of respiratory infections will depend on the patient's general condition. Mental distress and anxiety may be helped by corticosteroids (prednisolone) chlorpromazine (Largactil) or cocaine (in various mixtures). Finally, the patient's family should be considered as they may require considerable medical nursing or social support.

Patients with recurrent laryngeal nerve palsy may be helped by an injection of Teflon paste into the affected cord. This may be carried out under local anaesthetic. Patients are helped by the return of the effective cough and improved phonation.

Increasingly there is a hospice movement growing up in the western world and the terminal care of carcinoma of the bronchus is commonly making use of such services.

QUALITY OF LIFE ESTIMATES. As the patients with carcinoma of the bronchus have such a poor prognosis and many treatments are debilitating, measurement of the quality of life is important. A number of scales have been developed to estimate pain and subjective symptoms; such scales are usually linear and completed by the patient. Much criticism has been made of these scales and they are not generally accepted. The Karnovsky Scale is a ten-point evaluation of dependence and is much more widely accepted because of the apparent objective aspect. More recently in Great Britain a matrix has been proposed. This matrix combines an eight-point physical viability scale and a four-point psychological index in an eight by four matrix. The squares of the matrix are weighted and the patient is evaluated with quality of life proportion at any point in the evolution of his disease. This matrix may then be given a third dimension in time. The quality of life index is incorporated into the actuarial curves by averaging the index for individuals in the survival proportion. This new index is then plotted as quality adjusted life years (QALY). This method of evaluation of effective therapy is developing rapidly and has value for the management of carcinoma of the bronchus. There is a further input to this equation and that is cost; the gross cost can be estimated of a treatment group and then the outcome in QALY terms expressed.

RARE LUNG TUMOURS

Hamartoma occurs as a rare lung tumour and even more rarely it can occur endobronchially. Hamartoma is a disorganized group of locally appropriate cells that do not form a co-ordinate structure and it takes the form of a tumour. The most common type is chondromatous. It is diagnosed on radiography (*Fig.* 41.11), where it is seen as a discrete lesion; often flecks of calcium are seen at tomography. Hamartomas grow slowly and if there is any doubt about the diagnosis they are simply enucleated without lung resection.

Very occasionally hamartomatous malformations occur in the bronchus and can be a predisposing cause of bronchiectasis. They are found at excision of the bronchiectatic lobe.

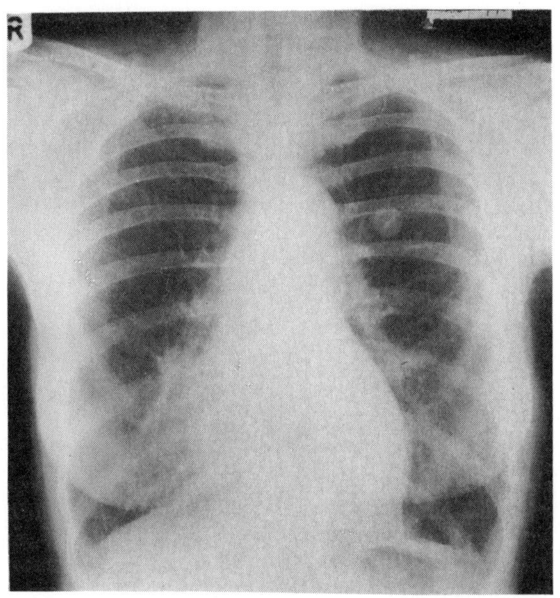

Fig. 41.11 PA chest radiograph showing a chondroma.

Occasionally they may be removed endobronchially when there is confidence in the histological diagnosis at biopsy. They are of little importance and are easily dealt with. Their diagnosis is usually suspected before excision.

Lymphoma

Primary Hodgkin's Disease of the Lung

This may arise in peribronchial lymph nodes and may eventually invade the bronchi. The patients tend to be young and may be asymptomatic at the time of diagnosis. Cough, haemoptysis, chest discomfort, pyrexia and itch may occur as presenting symptoms. The radiological appearance is of a unilateral and fairly well-circumscribed shadow which rarely cavitates. The diagnosis is occasionally made at bronchoscopy but more often by mediastinoscopy, mediastinotomy or thoracotomy. Where there is doubt about the diagnosis, surgical resection may be indicated but such tumours are sensitive to combination chemotherapy and radiotherapy.

In patients with generalized Hodgkin's disease the lung is involved in almost half. There are several radiological patterns: (i) enlargement of the hilar glands with streaky opacities spreading out into the lung; (ii) a lobar pattern of infiltration; (iii) irregularly disseminated nodules which may occasionally cavitate; (iv) disseminated rounded lesions which can be similar to tuberculosis. The diagnosis can usually be made by biopsy of an accessible gland. Surgical treatment has little to offer.

Non-Hodgkin's Lymphoma

Secondary involvement of the lung in generalized non-Hodgkin's lymphoma is common. Pleural deposits are commoner than are those in the lung; but the clinical and radiological manifestations are similar to those of Hodgkin's lymphoma. Primary pulmonary lymphosarcoma is extremely rare. It is a relatively benign form of the disease with most patients being over 40 years old at presentation. It appears radiologically as a discrete rounded opacity and the clinical features are also non-specific: cough, haemoptysis and chest discomfort. The diagnosis is not suspected in the majority of patients and most are operated on because it is thought that the lesion is a bronchial carcinoma. Surgical resection, radiotherapy and chemotherapy may all be used, and the prognosis is usually quite good.

Sarcoma

Primary pulmonary sarcomas are very rare and the diagnosis may be difficult to establish. The pathologist may have problems in differentiating them from anaplastic carcinomas and another source of error is the possibility of an occult extrathoracic primary sarcoma with pulmonary metastases. Various malignant mesodermal tumours have been described in the lung, including fibrosarcoma, neurofibrosarcoma, leiomyosarcoma and rhabdomyosarcoma. They occur in a younger age group than does bronchial carcinoma and are often asymptomatic for a considerable period. With increasing size they will produce cough, haemoptysis and chest discomfort. Metastases are relatively uncommon but local invasion and pressure effects will eventually be seen. Surgical excision is the treatment of choice wherever possible, although some of the tumours may also be radiosensitive.

There is a particular variety of lung tumour called a carcinosarcoma in which there is a mixture of malignant epithelial and sarcoma-like tissue. The histological pattern is variable and there may even be elements of striated muscle. Isolated examples of pulmonary melanoma, lipoma, plasmacytoma and haemangiopericytoma have been recorded but are pathological curiosities. They usually have no specific radiological or diagnostic features and should be dealt with where possible by surgical excision.

Pulmonary Arteriovenous Fistula

This abnormality is also occasionally called a vascular hamartoma since it is a malformation rather than a tumour. It is due to the persistence of fetal anastomoses between the arterial and venous sides of the pulmonary circulation. About 20% of cases have multiple fistulas and the supplying vessel is occasionally systemic. The haemodynamic effect of the fistula is a shunt of unoxygenated blood with a fall in Pa_{O_2} while the Pa_{CO_2} remains normal.

This condition is not uncommonly a problem of hereditary telangiectasia which is inherited as an autosomal dominant.

Small pulmonary arteriovenous fistulas are asymptomatic but if there is a major shunt then there will be cyanosis and breathlessness. On examination there may be finger clubbing, polycythaemia, and in about half of the cases, there is a murmur immediately over the lesion. Radiologically the lesion will appear as a rounded or lobulated opacity which may be multiple (*Fig.* 41.12*a*). Tomography is helpful but the diagnosis is made by pulmonary angiography (*Fig.* 41.12*b*). Treatment of a symptomatic solitary arteriovenous fistula in the past has been surgical. Recent developments have demonstrated that it can be quite simply obliterated using transvenous embolization techniques. This is now the method of choice as very effective reductions of shunt are obtained by the radiologist.

Previously at thoracotomy the aim was to ligate and divide the abnormal vessels and to peel them out of the lung without lung resection. The prognosis was very good but the operation was often tedious and occasionally incomplete. Embolization techniques are effective and if anything more complete because of the continuous radiological visualization of the vasculature which is most difficult at open

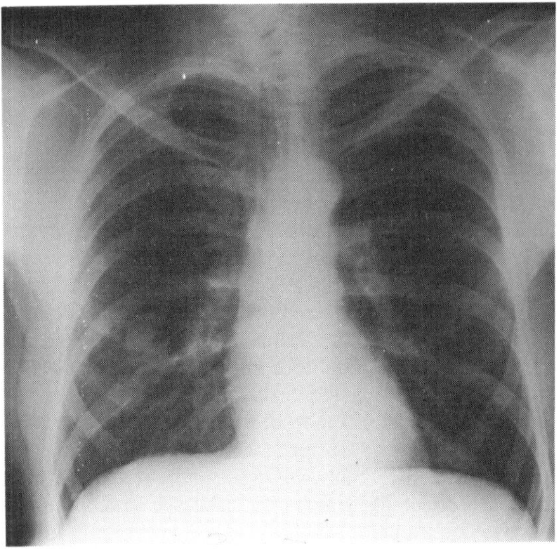

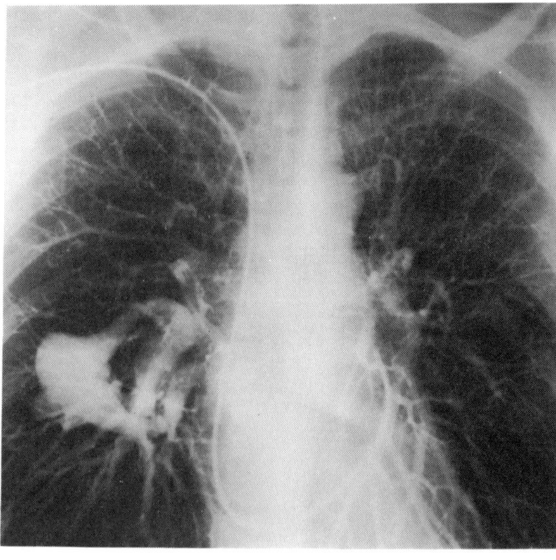

a b

Fig. 41.12 *a*, PA radiograph and *b*, angiogram of a solitary pulmonary arteriovenous fistula.

operation. The radiologist is also able to deal with multiple fistulas much more easily. It is likely that thoracotomy for arteriovenous fistulas will become unnecessary.

Tumours of the Trachea

Involvement of the lower trachea by carcinoma originating in the bronchial tree is not uncommon, but primary tumours of the trachea are rare. Benign tracheal tumours have a similar spectrum to the endobronchial lesions—fibroma, chondroma, leiomyoma and also papilloma and haemangioma. The most common malignant tracheal tumour is the squamous-cell carcinoma. The cylindroma or adenoid cystic carcinoma occasionally occurs and less common malignant tumours are small-cell and muco-epidermoid carcinomas.

Clinically these tumours present with cough, sputum, haemoptysis and dyspnoea. Stridor is often present, and may be aggravated in the supine position. Many patients are treated as bronchitics or asthmatics at the time of initial presentation and their chest radiography may well be normal. Diagnosis is made by tracheal tomography (*Fig.* 41.13) and bronchoscopy. The latter may be hazardous, particularly if general anaesthesia is used. Steps must be taken to ensure that there is an adequate airway if biopsy is undertaken as bleeding and oedema may compromise the airway very rapidly. A pedunculated benign tumour may be safely resected through the bronchoscope but malignant tumours require surgical resection. Excision greater than 5 cm of trachea may be accomplished with end-to-end anastomosis using suprahyoid release. Tracheal prostheses are still at the experimental stage.

Metastatic Pulmonary Tumours

The pulmonary capillary bed constitutes a very effective filter interposed between the pulmonary and systemic circulations. The reasons that determine the survival and multiplication of tumour cells within the pulmonary capillaries are poorly understood. Some tumours have a predilection to metastasize to the lungs. These include melanoma, osteogenic sarcoma, neuroblastoma, hypernephroma and carcinomas of various organs, such as breast, colon, ovary and prostate. Malignant cells may lie dormant in the lung for years after their primary tumour has been dealt with and growth may apparently commence after a long interval. It is more likely that the late appearance reflects the growth rate of the original tumour.

The metastatic nodule usually causes no symptoms. It may rarely present in the bronchus when cough or haemoptysis occur. The pulmonary deposits, when multiple, will interfere with parenchymal function. Although pulmonary

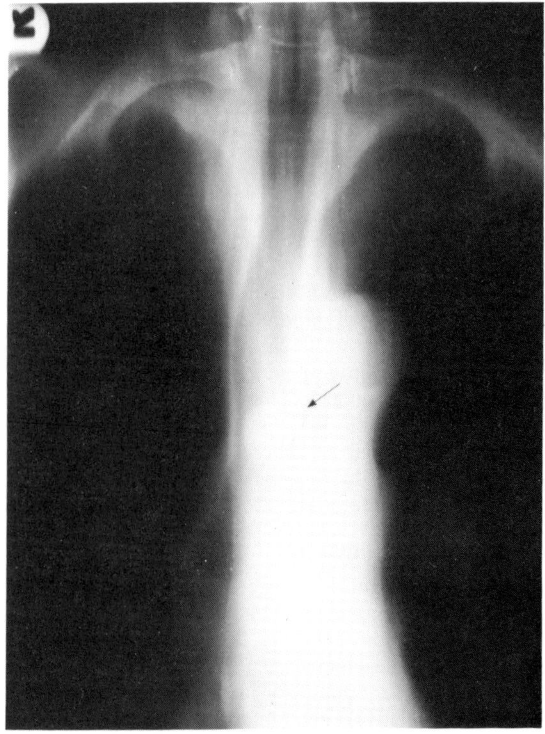

Fig. 41.13 Tracheal tomogram showing a rounded tumour 3 cm above the bifurcation.

metastases are usually multiple and bilateral, haemoptysis is uncommon. If they involve the pleural surface of the lung then the patients may complain of pleuritic pain or an effusion may develop. Few pulmonary metastases are visible at bronchoscopy but sputum cytology or bronchial brushings may occasionally be helpful.

The vast majority of pulmonary metastases are quite unsuitable for surgical treatment as they are multiple and occur in the terminal stages of the patient's disease. There are three main situations where surgical treatment may be undertaken:

1. The Solitary Nodule

Excision of a metastatic pulmonary tumour is not infrequently undertaken on the assumption that it is a primary lung tumour. The situation is further complicated by the inability of the pathologist to be certain whether a lesion, such as an isolated adenocarcinoma within the lung, is a primary lung tumour or metastasis from an adenocarcinoma in some other site.

2. Excision of a Solitary Metastasis

It is well recognized that isolated pulmonary metastases from tumours elsewhere in the body occur. Attempted resection of such a lesion, however, would only be undertaken in certain circumstances: (i) If the primary tumour has been completely dealt with and there is no evidence of local recurrence or other metastases; (ii) The pulmonary metastasis should be solitary. Multiple metastases within one lobe may be worth considering with regard to surgical treatment. Whole lung tomography or computerized axial tomography must be done in order to avoid operating on patients who have multiple or bilateral metastases; (iii) There should be a time interval between the treatment of the primary tumour and the management of the metastasis. It is common practice to wait several months following treatment of the primary in order to avoid putting the patient through an unnecessary operation should there be local recurrence at the site of the primary or the development of multiple metastases. Patients with the longest intervals between treatment of their primary and resection of their metastases have the best prognosis.

The tumours which most often fulfil these criteria are sarcomas, particularly osteogenic sarcoma, hypernephroma, and carcinoma of the colon. Surgical resection should be as limited as possible and in this situation wedge or segmental resection is acceptable.

3. Reduction of Metastatic Tumour Mass

In certain patients it may be justifiable to resect large multiple metastases even though surgical cure is impossible. This is particularly the case when it is thought that the tumour and the metastases are likely to be sensitive to chemotherapy. Recently the use of median sternotomy has been advocated to approach both lungs at one operation.

Further Reading

Crofton J. W. and Douglas A. C. (1981) Tumours of the lung. In: *Respiratory Diseases*, 3rd ed. Oxford, Blackwell.

Overholt R. H., Neptune W. B. and Ashraf M. M. (1975) Primary cancer of the lung: a 42-year experience. *Ann. Thorac. Surg.* **20**, 511.

Pearson F. G., Todd T. R. J. and Cooper J. D. (1984) Experience with primary neoplasms of the trachea and carina. *J. Thorac. Cardiovasc. Surg.* **88**, 511–518.

Shields T. W. (1983) *General Thoracic Surgery*, 2nd ed. Philadelphia, Lea & Febiger.

Shore D. B. and Paneth M. (1980) Survival after resection of small cell carcinoma of the bronchus. *Thorax* **35**, 819–822.

Smyth J. F. (ed.) (1984) *The Management of Lung Cancer*. London, Arnold.

Spencer H. (1985) *Pathology of the Lung*, Vol. II, 4th ed. Oxford, Pergamon.

42 Diseases of the Mediastinum

A. J. Mearns

ANATOMY

The mediastinum is defined as that part of the thorax contained between the two pleural sacs and divided somewhat arbitrarily into four areas as indicated in *Fig.* 42.1.

Superior Mediastinum

This is the area bounded anteriorly by the manubrium and posteriorly by the first four thoracic vertebrae. The superior boundary is the thoracic outlet formed by the first thoracic vertebra, the first ribs and the superior margin of the manubrium. The inferior boundary is an artificial plane drawn from the manubriosternal angle to the lower border of the fourth thoracic vertebra. Through the superior mediastinum pass the arch of the aorta and its three branches, the brachiocephalic veins, the superior vena cava and vena azygos, the trachea and oesophagus, the thoracic duct, vagus, phrenic, recurrent laryngeal and sympathetic nerves. It also contains part of the thymus gland and several lymph nodes.

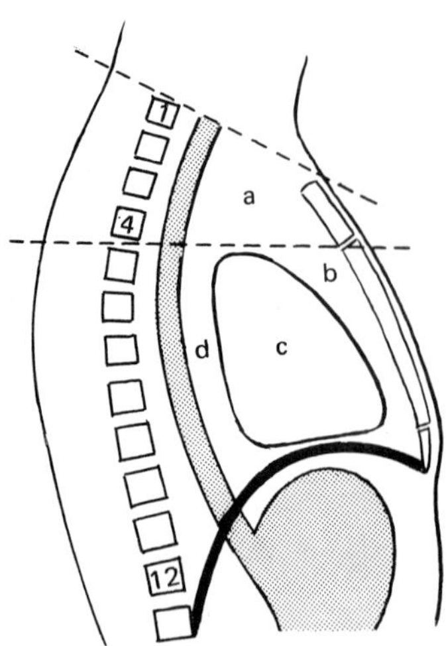

Fig. 42.1 Anatomy of the mediastinum. *a*, Superior. *b*, Anterior. *c*, Middle. *d*, Postérior.

Anterior Mediastinum

This lies between the body of the sternum and the pericardium. Its main contents are the lower part of the thymus gland, lymph nodes and fat.

Middle Mediastinum

This area of the thorax is occupied by the heart, the intrapericardial portion of the great vessels, the pericardium itself, the phrenic nerves and their accompanying pericardiacophrenic vessels.

Posterior Mediastinum

This is the remaining mediastinum bounded anteriorly by the pericardium, above by the line from the manubriosternal

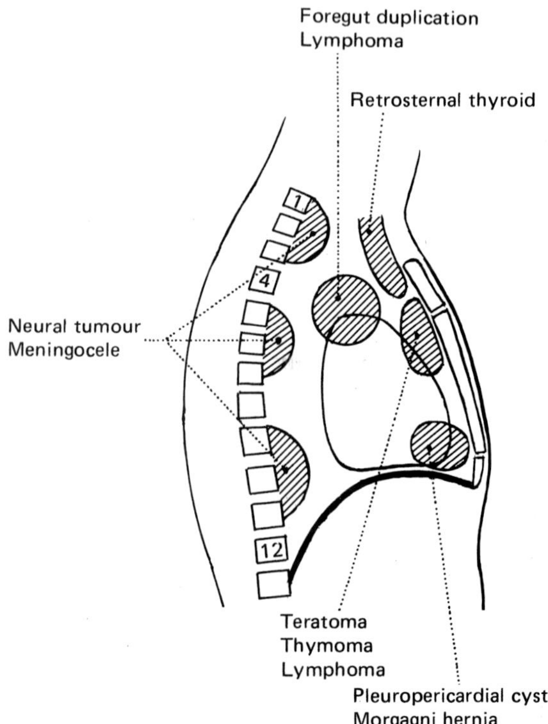

Fig. 42.2 Pathological anatomy of the mediastinum.

angle to the fourth vertebra, and the diaphragm below. It contains the descending thoracic aorta and its branches, the azygos and hemiazygos veins, the thoracic duct, various lymph nodes, the oesophagus, the vagus and sympathetic nerve trunks.

The anatomical divisions of the mediastinum being arbitrary, are not of major clinical import; but the exact situation of any mediastinal opacity on the chest radiograph is important in establishing the likely diagnosis. The situation of the more common mediastinal lesions is indicated in *Fig.* 42.2.

LESIONS OF THE MEDIASTINUM

In the superior mediastinum the commonest tumour is a retrosternal extension of an enlarged thyroid gland; occasionally ectopic thyroid tissue is found in the mediastinum. The latter is entirely detached from the cervical thyroid gland and has a separate mediastinal blood supply. Arterial aneurysms and oesophageal tumours occur in the superior mediastinum but are considered in detail in the appropriate chapters. The most common mass lying posteriorly in the superior mediastinum is a neurogenic tumour. Radiological opacities around the trachea are most often due to lymph node enlargement from a wide variety of pathological processes: tuberculosis, sarcoidosis, lymphoma and bronchial carcinoma, etc. Such lymph node involvement, particularly lymphoma, may also extend into the anterior compartment. The common anterior mediastinal lesions, i.e. thymic tumours and teratomas, may also extend into the superior mediastinum behind the manubrium.

The range of differential diagnoses in anterior mediastinal lesions is small, there being few structures in this area. Thymic cysts and tumours are the commonest abnormalities encountered. The germ-cell tumours are the other major group of solid tumours occurring in this area. When the mass lies anteriorly at the level of the diaphragm two other possibilities must be considered, namely pleuropericardial cyst and a hernia through the foramen of Morgagni. Lymphoid tumours, lymph-node enlargement, cystic hygroma and ectoptic thyroid may occur in this space.

Most abnormalities arising in the middle mediastinum originate in the heart and great vessels and have to be distinguished from enlargement of one or other of the cardiac chambers. Primary tumours of the pericardium are rare. Foregut duplications and thymic tumours may overlie the middle mediastinum in the straight radiograph.

Oesophageal pathology and aneurysms of the descending thoracic aorta are amongst the most common abnormalities in the posterior mediastinum but are not described further in this chapter. Of those lesions normally considered to be of posterior mediastinal origin, neural tumours are the most common and are typically situated in the paravertebral area. Cystic lesions related to the trachea or oesophagus may represent one or other variety of duplication of the foregut. Although a great variety of disorders occurs in the mediastinum, the majority are relatively benign cysts and tumours. There are many abnormalities of developmental origin as a product of the complexity of the embryology of this area, witness the complexities of cardiovascular development and the migration of the thyroid and thymus glands during development.

Pulmonary, spinal, chest wall, and metastatic tumours occasionally invade the mediastinum directly.

CLINICAL FEATURES

The clinical effect produced by a mediastinal mass depends on a variety of factors, particularly site, size and rate of growth. Cysts and benign tumours usually enlarge slowly and may be completely asymptomatic even when large. Eventually this type of growth will compress adjacent structures, but interference with function is a late phenomenon. In contrast, malignant tumours, aneurysms and infections tend to produce more dramatic symptoms and signs. The mediastinum contains structures vital to several different systems of the body, all of which may be affected by an enlarging mediastinal mass.

Respiratory

It is common for a retrosternal goitre to cause both tracheal compression and displacement at the level of the thoracic outlet (*Fig.* 42.3); but symptoms of tracheal air flow obstruction as stridor and breathlessness occur late. The narrowing needs to reach the critical diameter of the trachea to generate the Reynolds number* for the system. At this time the air flow is turbulent, thus stridor is present and the work of breathing is increased. Direct invasion of the tracheal lumen in malignant thyroid disease causes such physical signs much earlier in the disease process. Lymphoid tumours may surround, compress and invade the trachea and main bronchi producing stridor and dyspnoea. The trachea may occasionally be compressed by a neurogenic or other solid tumour enlarging within the thoracic outlet.

Cough is a symptom which may be produced when there is tracheal or bronchial invasion or compression. Haemoptysis is not commonly associated with mediastinal tumours

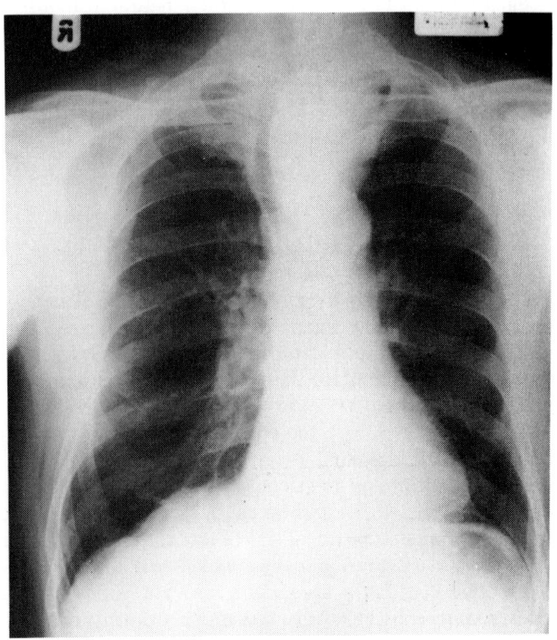

Fig. 42.3 PA chest radiograph demonstrating a large retrosternal goitre with displacement of the trachea.

*Reynolds Number (Re) is a dimensionless quantity: Re=V*Dp/u where V is the averaged velocity across the tube, i.e. trachea, D is the diameter of the tube, p is the density of the fluid, i.e. air, and u is its viscosity.

unless there is malignant invasion of the tracheobronchial tree. Aortic and brachiocephalic aneurysms may distort and compress the trachea and may produce a more dramatic form of haemoptysis on rare occasions. Large mediastinal tumours may also cause stridor and dyspnoea.

Cardiovascular

Compression, displacement or invasion of the heart or great vessels may cause various cardiac symptoms and signs including tachycardia and arrhythmias. Obstruction of the superior vena cava with typical venous congestion in head, neck and upper limbs is most often due to metastatic bronchial carcinoma but may also occur with other solid superior mediastinal tumours such as lymphoma and thymoma. Anterior mediastinal masses press upon the right ventricular outflow and pulmonary artery to produce a systolic murmur in inspiration.

Alimentary

Hernia through the foramen of Morgagni is usually asymptomatic but if stomach, small bowel or colon enters the hernia obstructive symptoms may be produced. Dysphagia is the most common alimentary symptom of mediastinal tumours, but is more often due to primary oesophageal disease or extrinsic compression of the oesophagus by metastatic mediastinal glands. Large benign posterior mediastinal tumours often displace the oesophagus but dysphagia is a late symptom.

Neurological

The phrenic, vagus and recurrent laryngeal nerves may be invaded directly by malignant mediastinal tumours or by metastatic tumour from bronchial carcinoma. Horner's syndrome is seen occasionally with neural tumours at the thoracic outlet. Posterior mediastinal neural tumours are usually benign and although they may involve one or more intercostal nerves, they do not often produce pain in the distribution of that particular nerve. About 10% of neural tumours have a dumb-bell like extension through the intervertebral foramina and this may cause spinal cord compression.

RADIOLOGICAL FEATURES

The standard postero-anterior chest radiograph is not ideal for assessment of the mediastinum. A normal mediastinal outline radiographically can conceal an opacity of considerable size. It is, therefore, common for mediastinal abnormalities not to be observed radiologically until they are of sufficient size to change the outline of the mediastinum on the postero-anterior film. A good lateral film is essential in the assessment of any suspected mediastinal opacity. While tomography may be of assistance in the accurate identification of pulmonary opacities, it is of less value in the mediastinum. When a suspected mediastinal abnormality cannot be clearly identified in the lateral film both anteroposterior and lateral tomography may be of assistance. Contrast media will delineate radiologically various other mediastinal structures and this will at times assist in accurate identification of the site and nature of a mediastinal opacity.

1. Barium Swallow

Barium swallow is indicated in any patient presenting with dysphagia but may also be useful in patients with a superior or posterior mediastinal mass to demonstrate exactly where the oesophagus is in relation to the lesion and whether there is any oesophageal displacement or compression.

2. Computerized Tomography (CT scanning)

This technique is particularly suitable for the localization and identification of mediastinal abnormalities. It can indicate the exact site, size, shape and density of a mediastinal cyst or tumour and can often detect invasion of surrounding structures. CT scanning may also be used to identify vertebral abnormalities and the presence of relatively small gland masses in the mediastinum. In a patient with a suspected thyroid mass it will demonstrate whether or not there is continuity with the cervical thyroid.

3. Aortography

Suspicion of an aneurysm of the great vessels is the indication for aortography. This investigation may also be indicated occasionally to demonstrate the relationship of the arch of the aorta or the great vessels to a particular mediastinal abnormality. However, contrast enhancement of CT scanning and digital subtraction arteriography (DSA) are replacing formal catheterization in many centres.

4. Venography

Venography of the superior cava is not usually necessary to confirm the presence of caval obstruction as the clinical picture is typical. Where the clinical features are less obvious, or where a good collateral circulation has developed, it is relatively easy to inject dye into the great veins to confirm the diagnosis. Occasionally, individual veins may be selectively cannulated and dye injected to demonstrate a tumour circulation—this can be done in patients with myasthenia gravis who are suspected of having thymic tumours.

5. Other Radiological Investigations

Screening of the patient may assist in the diagnosis of some cardiovascular abnormalities and should also be done to confirm the presence of paradoxical movement of the diaphragm when phrenic nerve paralysis is suspected. Pulmonary arteriography will confirm extrinsic compression of the pulmonary artery as a cause of a systolic murmur. Doppler ultrasound scanning now allows turbulent flow to be detected non-invasively. The indications for invasive angiography continue to fall as the non-invasive techniques become more widely available.

Artificial pneumomediastinum at one time gained some popularity as a method of delineating mediastinal lymphadenopathy but is rarely used today. Lymphangiography may occasionally be helpful and is still used to identify tumour invasion of nodes as the resolution of CT scanning is not adequate for this task.

OTHER INVESTIGATIONS

1. Bronchoscopy

This is of value in mediastinal disease to confirm suspected tracheal or bronchial compression, and to exclude primary tracheobronchial pathology.

2. Mediastinoscopy

This is an invasive investigation which carries with it a low morbidity and is extremely useful in making a histological diagnosis without resort to thoracotomy. The mediastinoscope is inserted in the pretracheal plane and a limited area of the mediastinum is accessible in this way. Anterior mediastinoscopy, to inspect the retrosternal space, has been replaced by anterior mediastinotomy (*vide infra*).

Mediastinoscopy has great value when there is a suspicion of the following problems:

a. Lymphadenopathy due to sarcoidosis, tuberculosis and bronchial carcinoma. Mediastinoscopy gives access for biopsy to paratracheal, tracheobronchial and even carinal lymph nodes.

b. Mediastinal lymphoma—this investigation is particularly appropriate in this condition where a combination of chemotherapy and radiotherapy is now usually employed in preference to radical surgery.

c. Idiopathic mediastinal fibrosis.

d. Occasionally a bronchogenic cyst may accidentally be drained; they do not recur afterwards.

3. Anterior Mediastinotomy

This involves a small incision to either side of the sternum directly over the costal cartilage which is removed to create a window for extra or intrapleural inspection and palpation. Commonly, the left second costal cartilage is excised for access to the anterior mediastinum and left hilar area in staging of carcinoma of the bronchus. It is also of great value for the histological identification of all accessible lesions of the anterior mediastinum to confirm the diagnosis before planned resection. Access is via either right or left second to sixth costal cartilage excision.

DISEASES OF THE MEDIASTINUM

Tracheal and oesophageal disease, aneurysms of the heart and great vessels are discussed elsewhere. Lymphadenopathy associated with such diseases as tuberculosis and sarcoidosis commonly occur and are diagnosed at mediastinoscopy or mediastinotomy. Tuberculosis is treated effectively by modern chemotherapy. Sarcoidosis is a self-limiting disease which may require steroids to contain the more severe symptoms and to minimize the end-stage fibrotic problems.

Thyroid

Mediastinal thyroid tissue is most commonly found as the retrosternal extension of a multinodular goitre. Ectopic thyroid tissue is rare, but presents usually as an anterior mediastinal opacity which has no continuity with the cervical thyroid tissue and often derives its blood supply from the mediastinum. The siting of this ectopic thyroid tissue is related to the complicated developmental migration of the thyroid, islands of which may be found anywhere from the base of the tongue to the pericardium. Clinically, ectopic thyroid is usually asymptomatic and is a chance radiological finding. A retrosternal extension of a multinodular goitre will displace the structures in the superior mediastinum, particularly the trachea and oesophagus, which may eventually be compressed. Thus dyspnoea can occur, but dysphagia is a late symptom and is associated more often with malignant thyroid tumours. Ectopic thyroid tissue must always be suspected of being nodal deposits from well-differentiated malignant disease of the thyroid.

a. Investigations

In the postero-anterior chest film a rounded mediastinal opacity will be seen (*Fig.* 42.3) which is situated anteriorly in the lateral film. There may occasionally be calcification within thyroid cysts and tumours. Barium swallow should be carried out if there is dysphagia. A radioisotope thyroid scan may indicate functioning thyroid tissue within the thorax. A negative scan excludes neither retrosternal extension of a cervical goitre nor ectopic thyroid tissue. Computerized tomography of the neck and mediastinum may be helpful in accurate localization of the thyroid and any retrosternal extension.

b. Management

Retrosternal extensions of multinodular goitres derive their blood supply from the neck and can almost always be safely enucleated through a standard low cervical incision. Occasionally the retrosternal element may be so large that it cannot be delivered through the thoracic outlet without splitting part or all of the sternum. The diagnosis of a retrosternal thyroid should certainly be made preoperatively and it is very helpful to the surgeon to know whether or not a retrosternal extension is in continuity with the main thyroid mass. When an anterior mediastinal mass is not in continuity with the cervical thyroid tissue it should be approached either by median sternotomy or lateral thoracotomy.

Parathyroid

Parathyroid adenomas occurring within the mediastinum are rare, being found in less than 5% of patients with hyperparathyroidism. The explanation of this ectopic parathyroid tissue is related to the fairly complicated developmental migration of the parathyroid tissue. As with parathyroid adenomas in the neck, the diagnosis is suspected on clinical and biochemical grounds and these tumours are very rarely visible on routine radiography. It is occasionally possible to demonstrate a tumour circulation by selective angiography, but multiple sampling from the veins of the neck and mediastinum for estimation of parathormone levels may give a more accurate indication of the site of the parathyroid adenoma. Recently DSA has been shown to have value as an imaging technique for parathyroid tissue. Surgical exploration involves complete examination of the neck before the sternum is split and the mediastinum explored.

Preoperative injection of methylene blue may aid the identification of the parathyroid gland at open operation.

Thymus

The thymus gland has right and left lobes closely bound together which may overlap each other to some extent. It lies anteriorly in the superior mediastinum and extends both superiorly into the neck in front of the left brachiocephalic vein and also inferiorly into the anterior mediastinum where its lower poles are closely related to the pericardium. Its relative size is greatest in the full-term infant when it is as large as the heart itself, but after puberty the thymus undergoes fatty degeneration to a varying extent. It derives a blood supply from the internal thoracic arteries and the venous drainage is into the left brachiocephalic vein. In the young child the size and shape of the thymus varies considerably and the gland is subdivided into lobules by fibrous septa. In the elderly, it may be represented by just two strands of rather unimpressive fatty tissue. In the child, the thymus can be recognized to have a cortex and a medulla, the former contains predominantly lymphocytes, whereas the latter has epithelial cells and Hassall's corpuscles. The function of the thymus gland has been the subject of an enormous amount of research over the last 20 years and has still not been completely clarified. Some aspects of its function are of considerable relevance to surgeons. The thymus plays a vital role, particularly in childhood, in determining the immunological competence of the individual. It is at the height of its activity as the modifier of thymic lymphocytes, the T-cells, during neonatal period. These T-cells influence other lymphocytes, the B-cells to produce immunoglobulins in response to antigenic stimulation. The lymphocytes are from the bone marrow initially and develop into the two distinct populations, T-cells and B-cells. T-cells develop their identity in the neonatal period after passing through a thymic phase. The T-cells then migrate to colonize the T-cell area of the lymph nodes, the paracortical area. Recently, subpopulations of T-cells have been identified: helper and suppressor, which influence the B-cell accordingly. The normal ratio of helper to suppressor T-cells is 2:1, this ratio is reversed in the immunocompromised patient. Thymic agenesis is characterized by an absence of T-cells and a failure of cell-mediated antibody response. Further subsets of lymphocytes are being identified as the monoclonal antibody marker techniques develop. Rapid changes in our understanding in this area are likely to continue for some time.

The part played by the thymus in myasthenia gravis is still not fully understood but thymectomy appears to reduce the production of the motor end-plate antibodies which block the response to acetylcholine. Thymectomy has also been demonstrated on occasions to influence the course of other diseases, such as polymyositis and subacute sclerosing panencephalitis. Pathological abnormalities in the thymus gland have been recorded in many diseases—in particular thyrotoxicosis, systemic lupus erythematosus, acquired haemolytic anaemia and hypogammaglobulinaemia. Thymic involution is in general associated with immunological deficiency states and thymic hyperactivity, both hyperplasia and neoplasia, with disease processes such as myasthenia, myocarditis and polymyositis.

Thymic Cysts

These are usually relatively small, asymptomatic, benign lesions which occur anteriorly in the mediastinum. In adults thymic cysts are often small but may be multiple and have an attachment to the thymus gland. Small cysts are lined by ciliated epithelium or by columnar cells, larger ones by flattened epithelial or cuboidal cells. It remains unclear whether these cysts are derived from branchial pouch remnants or whether they differentiate from the thymic tissue. The majority of patients are asymptomatic but children with large thymic cysts may develop respiratory distress. Chest radiography shows a well-defined rounded opacity lying within the anterior mediastinum or anterior portion of the superior mediastinum (*Fig.* 42.4). On occasions the mass may be closely related to the pericardium and angiocardiography may be needed to define the extrapericardial position, CT scanning should demonstrate a well-defined fluid-containing opacity and may assist considerably with the diagnosis (*Fig.* 42.5). Even though most of these thymic cysts are asymptomatic, surgical excision is recommended. The reasons for this are several—doubt about the diagnosis, the possibility of malignancy and the likelihood of enlargement. The latter may occur with considerable rapidity if there is haemorrhage into the cyst. Median sternotomy gives excellent access to these thymic lesions and is now the preferred incision. They can also be excised with little difficulty through a lateral thoracotomy. Surgical excision establishes the diagnosis and thymic cysts do not recur.

Thymic Tumours

These are the most common anteriorly situated tumours in the mediastinum but have also been reported around the hila and even within the lung. One of the problems with a thymic tumour is that there is considerable difference of opinion regarding the correct pathological classification. Some can confidently be called benign and others malignant but a considerable number are on the borderline between the two. Similarly, some tumours are clearly of epithelial

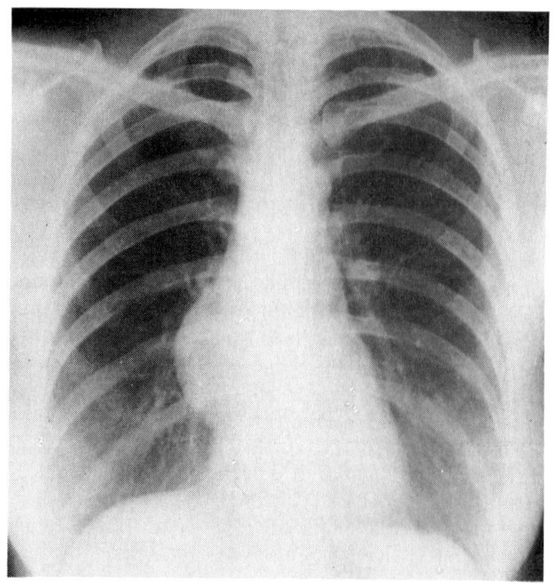

a

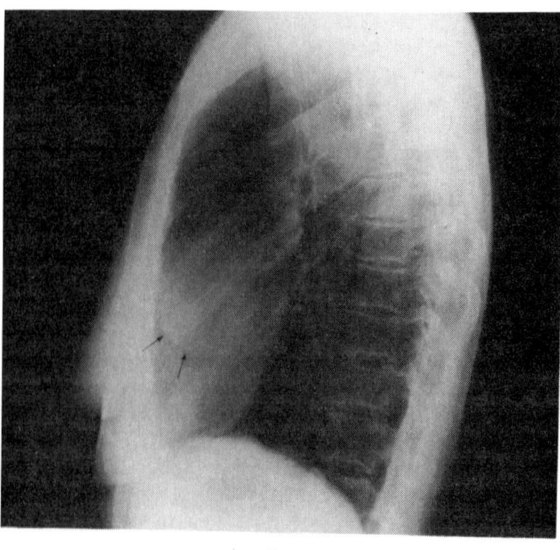

b

Fig. 42.4 *a*, PA and *b*, lateral chest radiographs showing an anterior mediastinal thymic cyst.

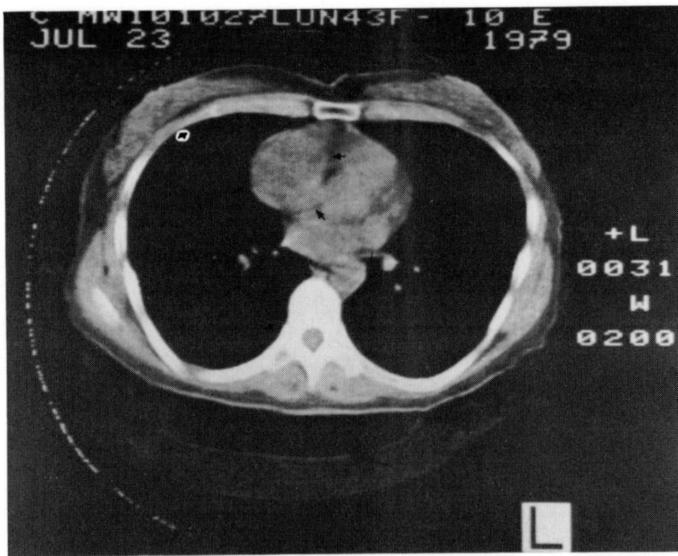

Fig. 42.5 CT scan of the same patient as in *Fig.* 42.4.

origin whereas others consist almost entirely of lymphoid tissue. The most common appearance is a mixture of the two varieties with one or other element predominating. A clinical subdivision is also possible on the basis of whether or not myasthenia gravis is present. Another peculiar aspect of thymic tumours is that their clinical behaviour may bear little relationship to the pathological appearance. A small encapsulated and apparently benign tumour may recur locally or even on a more widespread basis. In contrast, apparently infiltrative malignant tumours, even when incompletely resected, may be compatible with prolonged survival. In general, local invasion at the time of surgery is a poor prognostic factor associated with local recurrence, though distant metastases are quite unusual. Classification as malignant or benign for thymoma is therefore best used descriptively about the behaviour of the individual lesion.

Thymoma (without Myasthenia)

The majority of such patients are asymptomatic. Even when symptoms occur, they are often non-specific—chest pain, cough and occasionally breathlessness. Superior vena caval obstruction and hiccup have been reported. Radiologically, a thymoma does not have a characteristic appearance and the presence of any anterior mediastinal mass should suggest this diagnostic possibility. Tomography is of limited value but may demonstrate the presence of calcification in about 10% of such tumours.

TREATMENT. Any opacity suspected of being a thymoma should be surgically excised. The contraindication is clear-cut evidence of invasion of the great vessels demonstrated either by the presence of caval obstruction with a cavogram supporting invasion rather than compression, or by an arteriogram indicating invasion of the aorta or its branches. CT scanning may be helpful in this situation. The most suitable incision is a median sternotomy, though such tumours can also be removed without difficulty through a thoracotomy. Even benign thymic tumours may be adherent to surrounding structures and because of the possibility of local recurrence, excision *en bloc* with adjacent pericardium and pleura may be needed. Radiotherapy is an important adjunct to the management of patients who have thymic tumours which are towards the lymphomatous end of the spectrum. It is certainly indicated in irresectable tumours or those which have been incompletely resected. Combination chemotherapy has also been tried, but the response is unpredictable; presently no clear-cut recommendations are apparent.

The Thymus and Myasthenia Gravis

The pathogenesis of myasthenia is still not fully understood but it is probable that part of the disease process is related to the production of an antibody which blocks the effect of acetylcholine at the motor end-plate. These antibodies are not produced within the thymus but it has been recognized for over 80 years that patients with myasthenia gravis have abnormalities of the thymus gland.

The diagnosis, clinical features and medical management of myasthenia are outwith the scope of this book. Some 75–80% of patients with myasthenia may derive some benefit from thymectomy, about half getting a satisfactory remission. The pathological appearance of the thymic gland in the majority of myasthenics shows some degree of hyperplasia particularly of the lymphoid elements but between 10 and 20% of myasthenics are reported to have thymomas. These are usually small—under 2 cm—and may not be visible on routine chest radiography. Computerized tomography may pick up quite small thymic tumours and they may also be identified by selective cannulation and angiography through the thymic vein. An important recent development has been the demonstration that patients with acquired myasthenia gravis benefit temporarily by plasmapheresis. This is due to the washing out by plasma exchange of the motor end-plate antibodies, levels of which in the blood can now be measured by assay. After plasmapheresis the benefit lasts for several weeks and includes significant improvement in respiratory function.

Access for operative excision of the thymus is the subject of some debate. For simple excision of the thymus the cervical approach is recommended by some authorities, as the more major procedure of sternotomy is thought to be unnecessarily injurious. Median sternotomy gives excellent access and is the incision of choice in a patient with suspected thymic tumour. It is, however, an incision which does have a certain morbidity, including the unpleasant, though not very frequent, complication of mediastinal infection with sternal dehiscence. Division of the upper half of the sternum, extending to the second or third intercostal space, has never gained much popularity although access is adequate. A wide excision of the thymus is the best approach and if there is a tumour present, a block of mediastinal tissue including both pleura and pericardium should be removed. These measures are justified because the principal problem with thymic tumours is their propensity to local recurrence.

The mortality from elective thymectomy should now be nil as long as the postoperative care is appropriate. The benefit from thymectomy is not immediate and patients will usually still require their anticholinesterase drugs in the early postoperative period. Steroid therapy and even immunosuppression may be of assistance to the patient, combined with thymectomy and plasmapheresis, in inducing remission. The best results are obtained in young females in whom the disease has been diagnosed relatively recently and who do not have a thymic tumour. It should also be noted that the development of myasthenia following excision of a thymoma has been recorded but is by no means a common occurrence.

Teratoma and Extragonadal Germ-cell Tumours

By definition teratoma contains tissue from all three germinal layers though the degree of representation of each layer may vary considerably. The most common mediastinal teratoma is the dermoid, which derives principally from the ectodermal layer and is usually cystic. Its development in this situation is thought to be related to the complexity of the embryology of the mediastinum. These lesions are rarely found anywhere other than anteriorly in the mediastinum and probably arise from cells originating in the area of the third branchial pouch and cleft. The solid tumours may contain an odd mixture of adult and embryonic tissue, with varying degrees of maturity.

Presentation

Most mediastinal teratomas are symptomless and are found on routine chest radiography. Infection occasionally occurs in the cystic variety of tumour but malignant change is much the most important complication. About one-third of dermoid cysts and two-thirds of solid teratomas may eventually become malignant. Occasionally, pathognomonic symptoms occur, such as the coughing up of hair or sebaceous material but in general when symptoms arise they are due to compression of surrounding mediastinal structures.

Investigations

Most of these tumours are symptomless and are chance radiographic findings. They are rounded homogeneous shadows which have a well-defined margin and lie anteriorly in the mediastinum (*Fig.* 42.6). They may extend very considerably laterally to displace the lung, particularly in infants. Calcification is present in about one-third of these tumours and recognizable teeth may occasionally be seen. The presence of a fluid level is an indication of a fistulous communication with the lung or tracheobronchial tree. It is not usually necessary to undertake further sophisticated investigation but tomography and computerized tomography will delineate the opacity accurately and may give more information about the nature of its contents.

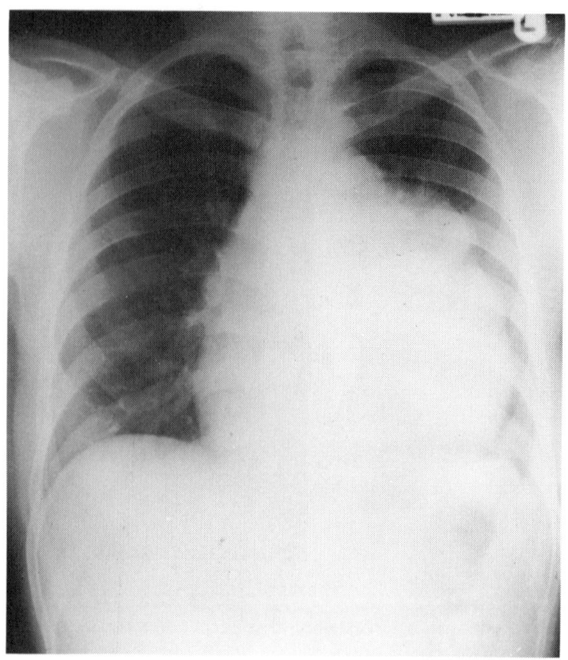

Fig. 42.6 AP chest radiograph of an adult with a large benign teratoma.

Management

Surgical exploration and removal of the lesion is always the treatment of choice. There are several reasons for this—up to 30% of the relatively benign dermoid cysts become malignant whereas the proportion is very much higher for the solid teratomas, particularly in men. Although teratomas tend to enlarge gradually, they occasionally enlarge quite rapidly and produce pressure effects. The other problem is simply doubt about the diagnosis and it is very important in patients with mediastinal tumours that an accurate pathological diagnosis is made in order that all appropriate therapy may be given.

Surgical access to the anterior mediastinum is best obtained by median sternotomy, particularly when it is suspected that an anterior mediastinal tumour is malignant. Benign teratomas usually project to one or other side of the mediastinum and can easily be removed by an appropriate lateral thoracotomy. Patients in whom the teratoma has apparently involved the pericardium, have also been recorded and it is not unusual for portions of the pericardium and pleura to need to be resected in order to be sure of mediastinal clearance. The surgical removal of a teratoma is a simple procedure which involves little dissection unless either infection or malignant change has occurred. If a benign teratoma is excised completely then local recurrence is unusual, but there is a much higher incidence of this complication and even of more distant metastases if the lesion is malignant.

Previously teratoma classification embraced a rarer group of primary mediastinal tumours now identified as of germ-cell origin. Earlier opinion that these tumours might be metastatic from primary tumours of the gonads no longer obtains; their primary mediastinal origin is now widely accepted. They are consequently categorized as germ-cell tumours of the mediastinum.

The category includes seminoma, embryonal-cell tumour

and choriocarcinoma; less commonly, teratocarcinoma, endodermal sinus-yolk sac-tumours and germ-cell tumours of mixed histology occur.

Although they may present in much the same way as any anterior mediastinal tumour, their behaviour tends to be more aggressive with invasion of surrounding structures and early distant metastases, particularly to the lungs. As with chorionepitheliomas elsewhere, chorionic gonadotrophin may be secreted and occasionally gives rise to gynaecomastia and testicular atrophy.

Complete surgical excision offers the best chance of survival, and may be followed by radiotherapy and chemotherapy. In patients with mediastinal seminoma good results have been obtained by irradiation and chemotherapy without surgical resection. However, the patient requires an initial histological diagnosis. Therefore the usual approach is that of effective excision as the investigative and therapeutic singular event. Initial anterior mediastinotomy may often have produced the histological information if the diagnosis of germ-cell tumour was not suspected.

Modern solid tumour chemotherapy often involves an operative debulking procedure, so that modern management of malignant teratoma and germ-cell tumours of the mediastinum usually involves a major operative excision.

Neurogenic Tumours (*Table* 42.1)

Approximately 75% of tumours of the posterior mediastinum are of neurogenic origin. Benign tumours arising from the nerve sheath take two forms, the neurofibroma and neurilemmoma. Neurofibroma is non-encapsulated and shows a tangle of neurofibrils of schwannian origin. Neurilemmoma is encapsulated and consists of Antoni type A and B tissue with collections of foamy macrophages. It is not unusual to see elements of neurofibroma and neurilemmoma within the same specimen. Malignant change may occur in the neurofibroma to fibrosarcoma of neural origin. Sarcomatous change in neurilemmomas is very rare, although occasional local recurrence may occur after resection.

Table 42.1 Neurogenic tumours of the mediastinum

Benign	*Malignant*
Nerve Sheath Origin	
Neurilemmoma	Malignant Schwannoma–neurogenic sarcoma
Neurofibroma	
Autonomic Ganglia	
Ganglioneuroma	Neuroblastoma–sympathetico-blastoma Ganglioneuroblastoma–partially differentiated neuroblastoma
Paraganglion System	
Sympathetic	
Phaeochromocytoma true paraganglionoma	Malignant phaeochromocytoma
Parasympathetic	
Non-chromaffinoma–chemodectoma	Malignant paraganglionoma

Tumours of the sympathetic nervous system demonstrate variable differentiation between individual tumours and often within the same tumour. Neuroblastoma is more common in children, it tends to occur in the upper posterior mediastinum, is unencapsulated, and often infiltrative at presentation. There is a more differentiated form of tumour of the sympathetic nervous system called a ganglioneuroblastoma or a differentiated neuroblastoma; this is to identify the less aggressive aspect of the tumour which is encapsulated, appears lobular and is usually not infiltrative at presentation. The benign form occurs in adults as a ganglioneuroma. This is the most common form of tumour of the sympathetic nervous system. Grossly the presentation is of a smooth well-encapsulated mass in the posterior mediastinum which on cross-section usually has a fibrous yellow/grey appearance.

Survival is directly poportional to the differentiation at microscopy. Effective resection will cure ganglioneuroma. Solid tumour chemotherapy is developing apace for the neuroblastomas of childhood and cure rates are rising.

Presentation

Most patients with neural tumours are entirely asymptomatic and the diagnosis is made as a chance radiographic finding. Very large neural tumours may produce pressure symptoms, such as dyspnoea, cough, or dysphagia. Root pain in the distribution of the involved nerve is uncommon but Horner's syndrome may be produced by involvement of the cervical sympathetic chain at the thoracic outlet. Extension of neural tumours through the intervertebral foramina may press upon the spinal cord. Patients with multiple neurofibromatosis, Von Recklinghausen's disease, may have intrathoracic and mediastinal manifestations of their disease. A recent major population survey in multiple neurofibromatosis has suggested that previous estimates of rates of malignant change have been exaggerated.

Investigations

Mediastinal neural tumours are posteriorly situated, have a 'D'-shaped hairline outline, and are of uniform density (*Fig.* 42.7). Up to 20% of patients have associated rib and vertebral abnormalities, apart from the local effect of a large tumour pressing on the posterior end of the ribs. Barium swallow examination may demonstrate oesophageal displacement in those patients with large tumours but bronchoscopy is unhelpful. A neural tumour in the upper and middle posterior mediastinum is accessible at mediastinoscopy. Trucut type biopsy is particularly useful via this route to the level of the seventh thoracic vertebra. Routine tomography is not very helpful but computerized tomography may assist in the identification of vertebral abnormalities and tumour extending into the vertebral foramina.

Neuroblastomas of the mediastinum are somewhat less aggressive than those in the retroperitoneum, but they do secrete catecholamines which can be estimated in a urine sample. Recently, a new biochemical test has been evaluated. Neurone-specific enolase is an enzyme present in the serum in patients with neural tumours. It is most valuable to have a high probability of diagnosis before thoracotomy so that the operation is properly executed. Both these tests should be done in children with posterior mediastinal masses. It is also wise to use these estimates if the adult disease is thought to be progressive.

Management

In general the policy with patients suspected of having

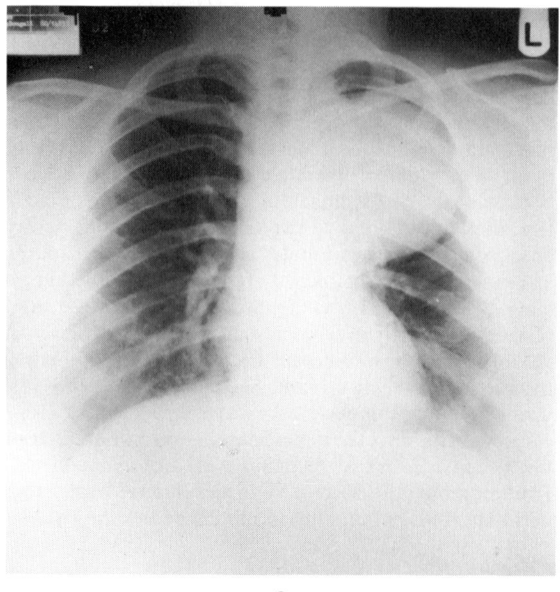

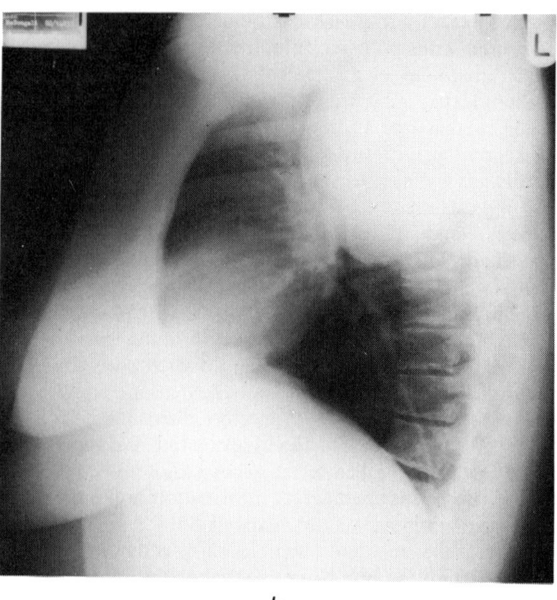

Fig. 42.7 *a*, PA and *b*, lateral chest radiographs in a patient with a benign ganglioneuroma.

mediastinal neurogenic tumours has been to advise thoracotomy and resection of the tumour because of doubt about the diagnosis and the possibility of malignancy. Certainly if a tumour is enlarging, it should be excised as it will produce pressure effects on surrounding structures. Of patients who have neurogenic tumours, particularly ganglioneuromas, 10–15% have direct extension of their tumour into intervertebral foramina. Such patients should have the initial thoracotomy with excision of the intrathoracic mass and a careful attempt to remove the intraforaminal aspect. Should this not remove all the tumour a second stage planned procedure, a laminectomy or fenestration with extradural exploration, should follow immediately. Excellent results follow such a combined procedure. In patients who have generalized neurofibromatosis the presence of a typical posterior mediastinal opacity is not sufficient indication for exploratory surgery but resection is required if the lesion is enlarging.

Operation is carried out through a posterolateral thoracotomy at a level appropriate to the site of the tumour. Immediate complications of surgery are few and consist principally of incomplete resection and the consequences of division of the sympathetic nerves near the thoracic outlet. Recurrence after apparently complete resection of a benign lesion is quite unusual. Other than rapid growth, there are no features which distinguish a malignant from a benign tumour. If the latter type of tumour is excised completely, no further treatment is required.

Neuroblastoma is often large at presentation; although the use of radiotherapy is declining it is still used to reduce tumour mass before operation. Postoperatively pulsed chemotherapy is used. Cis-platinum-based regimes are given at monthly intervals for six pulses in neuroblastoma. Presently the 5-year survival proportion in neuroblastoma is 60–70% with operative removal and chemotherapy.

Spontaneous regression and maturation phenomena have been described in neuroblastoma. The mechanisms are ill understood but when the phenomena occur the prognosis is markedly improved.

TUMOURS OF THE PARAGANGLION SYSTEM. Chemically active and inactive tumours occur. The phaeochromocytoma is rare in the mediastinum, and if symptoms are present various manifestations of hypertension, hypermetabolism and diabetes may occur. Such symptoms associated with a mediastinal mass suggest an active phaeochromocytoma. Either or both adrenaline and noradrenaline may be produced, vanilylmandelic acid is the main urinary excretion product. This should be estimated in the 24-hour urine output. Urinary and serum catecholamine estimation is now the preferred confirmatory test as this test has a positive test probability of disease present of >90%. One per cent of phaeochromocytomas present in the thorax, usually in the paravertebral gutter. The approach at removal is the routine for paravertebral tumours associated with the precautions for removal of phaeochromocytomas below the diaphragm, i.e. the use of alpha- and beta-blockade. The tumour is usually highly vascular and this response affects the surrounding tissues. The tumour is a reddish-brown, soft, glandular structure. Effective removal of the benign lesion is curative, but the malignant lesion carries a very poor prognosis.

Chemodectomas are rare; they may be found in the posterior mediastinum or associated with the viscera. This soft tumour is richly vascular, uncommonly malignant, and should be removed *en bloc* if possible. Occasionally, excision of the tumour is not feasible, a biopsy must be done. Radiotherapy is given when malignancy is confirmed.

Thoracic Meningocele

The thoracic meningocele is a cystic lesion arising from the spinal meninges protruding through an intervertebral defect. It extends beneath the pleura and presents a radiological appearance very similar to a neurogenic tumour though rather more translucent (*see Fig.* 42.7). Two-thirds of patients with intrathoracic meningoceles also have multiple neurofibromatosis and almost all have vertebral or rib abnormalities adjacent to the opacity. These are usually in the form of kyphosis, scoliosis, or bone defects. If the diagnosis is suspected then it may easily be confirmed by myleography. Treatment of choice is surgical excision, though if the lesion is large, it may be complicated by a spinal fluid fistula.

Pleuropericardial Cysts

Thin-walled cysts containing clear fluid are occasionally found in the anterior cardiophrenic angle. They are closely related to the pericardium and are probably due to developmental abnormality when a lacunar cavity fails to fuse to the main pericardial sac. They have been given various names including pericardial coelomic cysts and springwater cysts. They are seen more often on the right side of the chest than on the left and are usually asymptomatic.

Presentation

The great majority are detected as a chance radiographic finding. Amongst those with symptoms chest discomfort is commonest, followed by dyspnoea and cough. Clinical signs are rare, but when the cyst is very large dullness to percussion over the anterior chest wall and diminished air entry at the base anteriorly may be noted.

Investigations

Radiographically they present as smooth, round opacities usually at the right cardiophrenic angle. The lateral film demonstrates that they occupy the anterior angle between the sternum and the diaphragm. The principal differential diagnosis is from a hernia through the foramen of Morgagni. Barium enema and computerized tomography may be helpful in resolving the diagnosis.

Management

It may be difficult to make a firm diagnosis without surgical intervention. If an irrefutable diagnosis could be made without thoracotomy, there would be no justification for removal of the cysts. Resection presents no technical difficulty and no patient should come to harm from this procedure. Occasionally a communication exists between the cyst and the pericardium but no problems arise because of this. If previous films are available which show that the opacity has been present, unchanged in size, for several years, then operation is probably not justifiable. In this situation the diagnosis may be confirmed by aspiration of the cyst, with the removal of the typical clear fluid. Malignant change does not occur.

Cystic Duplications of the Foregut

There are two principal varieties of foregut duplications, which between them account for 10% of all mediastinal cysts and tumours. The first arises from a relatively localized abnormality at the stage of development when the tracheobronchial tree is growing from the primitive foregut wall. The resulting duplication may be either in the wall of the oesophagus—a gastroenteric or enterogenous cyst—or in the wall of the tracheobronchial tree—a bronchogenic cyst. These cysts develop within the muscle of the foregut canal and are almost always lined by ciliated columnar epithelium. The second variety develops much earlier in fetal life as part of a more diffuse congenital lesion called the split notochord syndrome, and is commonly associated with vertebral and sometimes with spinal cord abnormalities. It is thought that these defects are the result of varying degrees of adhesion between endoderm and ectoderm so that the ectodermal cells from which the notochord develops are split into two separate centres. In this way cystic lesions develop in association with congenital scoliosis or hemivertebrae. The duplication may occasionally lie low in the posterior mediastinum and be associated with thoracoabdominal abnormalities, such as mesenteric duplications. Such a lesion is called a neuroenteric cyst.

a. Bronchogenic Cysts

These may also be called bronchial cysts and arise as a result of abnormal budding of the bronchial pathways during development. They are thin-walled and often merely have some connective tissue and a little smooth muscle in the wall. They may also contain cartilage and glandular elements. Cysts which have not been infected are filled with clear, yellow, or milky fluid and they may be classified according to their location: (1) Paratracheal—attached to the tracheal wall just above the bifurcation. (2) Carinal—the attachment is at the level of the carina and the cyst is often adherent to the anterior oesophageal wall. (3) Hilar—the cyst is attached to one or other main bronchus. Occasionally bronchogenic cysts are also found attached to lobar bronchi.

Presentation

The majority of these cysts are asymptomatic and the abnormality is diagnosed on routine radiography or an incidental film. As the cysts enlarge they may cause pressure symptoms, in particular respiratory distress, cough and dysphagia. Occasionally infection occurs and there may be a fistula between the cyst and the tracheobronchial tree. This complication may produce systemic disturbance with haemoptysis and purulent sputum.

Investigations

Standard postero-anterior and lateral chest radiographs demonstrate a smooth rounded, homogeneous mediastinal opacity, usually situated just anterior to the vertebral column. The presence of a fluid level indicates a fistula into the tracheobronchial tree. A barium swallow may be helpful in demonstrating that the cyst is anterior to the oesophagus and may in fact displace it. Bronchoscopy is usually carried out but demonstrates little more than tracheobronchial compression on occasions.

Management

Preoperatively the diagnosis can rarely be made with complete certainty. When doubt exists thoracotomy and surgical excision are indicated. Any cyst that is producing pressure symptoms should obviously be removed forthwith.

b. Enterogenous Cysts

Developmentally these are segments of the alimentary tract which have separated completely or partially from it. They tend to be lined by mucosa similar to that of the foregut—usually columnar but occasionally squamous. Two types are recognized: (1) Oesophageal cysts: these lie either within or very close to the wall of the oesophagus and are lined by ciliated columnar epithelium. They probably represent true duplication and share a common blood supply with the oesophagus. Their usual site is at the middle third of the oesophagus more frequently on the right than on the left. (2) Neuroenteric cysts: these are cystic structures lying in the posterior mediastinum separate from the oesophagus. They have a variable epithelium and a muscular wall resembling that of the intestine. They have a fibrous posterior attachment to the spine and are commonly associated with vertebral abnormalities. These are the cystic derivatives which are part of the split notochord syndrome. Because the vertebral column and the foregut elongate at different rates, the final position of the cyst is often caudal to that of the vertebral defect. Accordingly radiographs of the cervical and upper thoracic spine may be required to demonstrate the vertebral abnormalities. These cysts also tend to present as a chance radiological finding and are usually asymptomatic. The complications of infection and tracheobronchial obstruction are seen occasionally as with bronchogenic cysts. One additional complication is that mediastinal cysts lined by gastric-type mucosa are prone to all the complications of peptic ulceration. Because of these potentially serious complications and the difficulty of making an unequivocal diagnosis, surgical excision at thoracotomy remains the treatment of choice.

Lymphoma

Mediastinal involvement occurs in up to 50% of patients with Hodgkin's disease and in 10–20% of patients with non-Hodgkin's lymphoma. The mediastinal abnormality is part of the generalized lymphomatous disease and involves particularly the superior and anterior mediastinum.

Presentation

A proportion of these patients present with lymphoma elsewhere and the mediastinal abnormality is noted on routine chest radiography. Where the mediastinal masses reach a considerable size pressure effects may be noted, particularly cough, dyspnoea and stridor. Sometimes the mediastinal mass is large enough to produce superior vena caval obstruction.

Investigations

Chest radiography will demonstrate whether the mass is paratracheal, hilar or anterior mediastinal. Further investigation is directed principally towards making a histological diagnosis and determining the extent of the disease elsewhere in the body. Bronchoscopy is relatively unhelpful in most cases other than demonstrating tracheobronchial compression. Mediastinoscopy will usually provide a histological diagnosis, and will also serve to distinguish lymphoma from other causes of multiple lymph gland enlargement in the mediastinum, particularly sarcoidosis, metastatic carcinoma and primary pulmonary tuberculosis. Giant-cell hyperplasia of the lymph glands may occur and is an important differential diagnosis as it is a self-limiting condition requiring no treatment.

Management

The details of management of lymphoma are discussed in Chapter 71. The majority of patients will respond to a greater or lesser extent to intermittent combination chemotherapy with or without radiotherapy. Surgical treatment has little to offer in that the disease is generalized though it is thought by some that reduction in tumour bulk may improved the efficacy of the chemotherapy. Dramatic pressure symptoms such as caval obstruction or stridor are usually taken as an indication for urgent chemotherapy and radiotherapy.

Rare Mediastinal Tumours

Mediastinal cysts and tumours present a particularly interesting diagnostic challenge, partly because of their relative rarity and partly because of the difficulty of being certain of the preoperative diagnosis even when apparently typical clinical and radiological appearances are present. Many of the conditions already discussed in this chapter are uncommon but the differential diagnosis is further lengthened by the occurrence of several more groups of even rarer mediastinal tumours (*Fig.* 42.8). As one would expect, any area of the body that contains fat and fibrous tissue may occasionally produce lipomas, fibromas, and their malignant counterparts, the liposarcoma and fibrosarcoma. Similarly, there is a wide variety of vascular and lymphatic tissue in the thorax which can produce many unusual tumours, usually classified according to their cellular composition. Thus a vascular tumour consisting of capillaries alone is called a capillary haemangioma except where the vessels are widely dilated when it becomes a cavernous haemangioma. If one or other cell group within the vessel wall predominates then the tumour may be called a haemangio-endothelioma. These are relatively benign tumours. However, the malignant angiosarcoma and haemangiopericytoma have been reported. They can occur in any age group and in any part of the mediastinum. If they involve the posterior mediastinum then extension on to the vertebral bodies and into the spinal canal can cause insuperable problems.

Angiography may be necessary for the diagnosis, but CT scanning and digital subtraction angiography (DSA) are increasingly used as alternative imaging techniques. Surgical excision is the treatment of choice but is a high risk procedure in the more extensive tumour.

A slightly more common and rather different tumour is the lymphangioma or cystic hygroma which is seen particularly in children. As the name suggests they are benign cystic tumours which occur in the anterior mediastinum and have a good prognosis. The aetiology is not fully understood—they may arise from lymphoid tissue normally present in the area or may grow from mesodermal rests which produce abnormal lymphoid channels. The cystic hygroma is a particular variety of lymphangioma developing in relation to the lymph vessels of the jugular or iliac region; such a mediastinal lesion is usually associated with a cervical hygroma. They consist of a number of cysts of varying size, lined with epithelium and the walls may contain smooth muscle and lymphocytes. The contents are clear or straw-coloured fluid. Standard chest radiographs may show a mass extending from the hilar area well up into the neck, and cystic spaces may be visible in it. Occasionally there is involvement of the pericardium with the production of chylopericardium. Early surgical removal is the treatment of choice.

The thoracic duct itself has occasionally been the site of cystic change but the diagnosis has never been made preoperatively. There are two varieties: (i) degenerative: these are usually found incidentally in the elderly at the time of autopsy. They may be multiple and the presence of atherosclerosis and calcification has been recorded; (ii) lymphangiomatous: this may also produce single or multiple cyst-like spaces filled with chyle. They occasionally rupture into the pleura and may cause spontaneous chylothorax. Enhanced CT scanning or DSA may assist in the diagnosis if other dilated lymphatic channels can be identified. Lymphangiography would obviously be diagnostic but is rarely considered in the investigation of an undiagnosed mediastinal mass.

Mediastinitis

Mediastinitis is not a diagnosis in itself and is a complication of another primary condition. The commonest cause is perforation of the oesophagus which may be either spontaneous or traumatic and this is dealt with in Chapter 65.

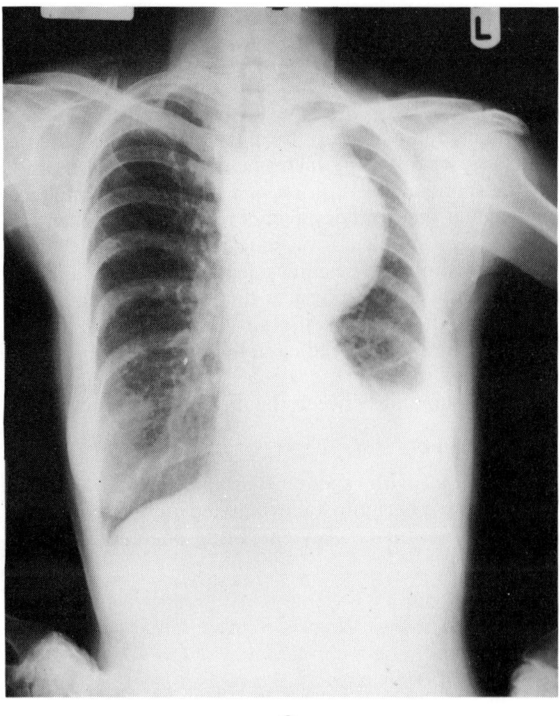

a

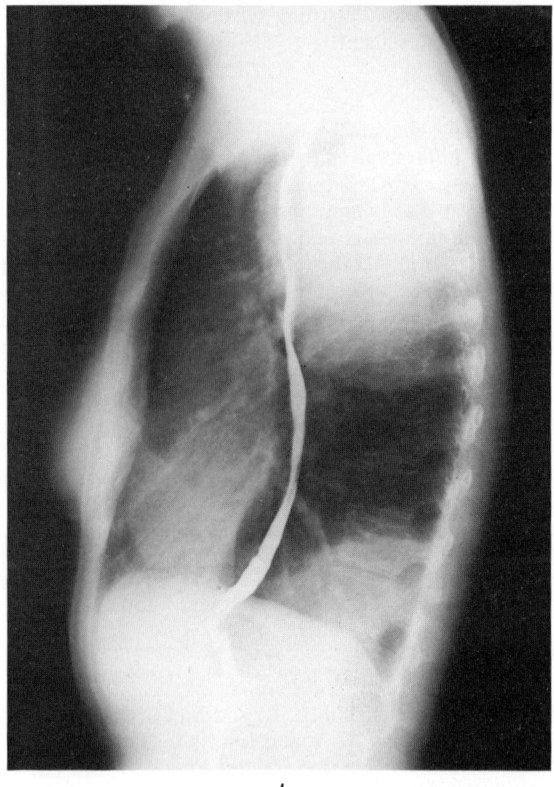

b

Fig. 42.8 *a*, PA and *b*, lateral barium radiographs of a patient with a malignant mediastinal sarcoma and left pleural effusion.

The formation of pus within mediastinal lymph nodes secondary to infection of the lungs or oesophagus, may lead to acute mediastinitis as can vertebral tuberculosis or osteomyelitis. The clinical features are those of severe systemic upset with chest pain, rigors, pyrexia, dyspnoea and sometimes cyanosis and dysphagia. The mediastinal pleura is involved and a pleural effusion develops. This may proceed to a pyopneumothorax and mediastinal emphysema may also be seen. The management consists of treatment of the primary condition, antibiotics and surgical drainage of any abscess or pyopneumothorax.

Idiopathic Mediastinal Fibrosis

This condition is sometimes called chronic fibrous mediastinitis and its aetiology is still not understood. It may be related to retroperitoneal fibrosis and perhaps even to other fibrosing diseases, such as Riedel's thyroiditis, Dupuytren's contracture and possibly sclerosing cholangitis. The term midline fibroses has been suggested as a group description. The coexistence of two or more of these conditions has now been recorded more than once and the term multifocal fibrosclerosis has been suggested. An immunological mechanism for this process has been postulated but has not yet conclusively been demonstrated nor has there been any consistent evidence of an infective basis although histoplasma has been isolated in a few cases. The drug methysergide which has been used in the treatment of migraine is associated with the production of both retroperitoneal and mediastinal fibrosis. The condition is characterized by the appearance of masses of hard white tissue infiltrating diffusely throughout the mediastinum but not invading the heart or lungs. It is seen most frequently in the superior mediastinum in men and obstruction and compression of the tracheobronchial tree, great veins, oesophagus and pulmonary vessels may occur.

Presentation

The clinical features are insidious and are mainly due to compression of the superior vena cava and innominate veins. The veins of the head, neck and upper limbs become distended and the face and neck swell, particularly when the patient is lying flat. There may be swelling of the eyelids, subconjunctival oedema, headache, breathlessness and epistaxis. With the passage of time venous collateral channels develop, some of which are clearly visible on the abdominal wall and some of the clinical features resolve.

Complications

Extensive fibrosis around the trachea or bronchi may produce increasing dyspnoea, stridor and eventually death. If the pulmonary vessels are involved recurrent infection and haemoptysis may be produced. The pulmonary arteries and veins may be involved in the disease process.

Investigations

Chest radiography may be relatively unimpressive, showing merely some broadening of the superior mediastinum. Bronchoscopy may find evidence of compression of the tracheobronchial tree and pulmonary angiography may occasionally be helpful. Venography of the superior vena cava will confirm the extent of the obstruction and the collateral circulation. Barium swallow may demonstrate oesophageal involvement.

Management

The principal problem is the differentiation from malignant mediastinal infiltration and this can usually only be made either at mediastinoscopy, mediastinotomy or thoracotomy. Steroid therapy and immunosuppression have been exhibited without impressive clinical results. Surgical treatment has little to offer in that the fibrosis is widely infiltrating and cannot usually be resected. Caval obstruction has been treated by a venous bypass from the left brachiocephalic vein to the right atrial appendage. Patency rates are low in this condition because the disease progresses. An adequate collateral circulation will normally develop in time. Occasionally there is a localized area of mediastinal fibrosis which can be removed surgically. The disease is not necessarily progressive and some patients undergo slow improvement as collateral venous channels develop. If stricture of the tracheobronchial tree, oesophagus or pulmonary vessels occurs, then the outlook is not good.

Mediastinal Emphysema

This is a condition produced by rupture of an air-containing viscus either within the mediastinum or in a position where the air may track into the mediastinum. It is seen most commonly following rupture of the oesophagus, either spontaneously or following instrumentation. It is also produced by the spontaneous ruptures of a subpleural pulmonary cyst or bulla. If the overlying pleura remains intact then air may track in the subpleural plane to the hilum and thence into the mediastinum. The clinical features depend on the aetiology but the classic physical finding is of crepitus in the tissues of the neck as the air tracks upward out of the mediastinum. Chest radiography demonstrates a translucency produced by the air between the pleura and the mediastinum and between the mediastinal structures.

Management

All patients with spontaneous mediastinal emphysema should have a barium swallow carried out to see whether the oesophagus is intact. Any coexisting pneumothorax should be drained.

Further Reading

Bush S.E., Martinez A. and Bagshaw M. A. (1981) Primary mediastinal seminoma. *Cancer* **48**, 1877.

Davidson K. G., Walbaum P. R. and McCormack R. J. M. (1978) Intrathoracic neural tumours. *Thorax* **33**, 359–367.

Glenn W. L., Liebow A. A. and Lindskog G. E. (ed.) (1976) The mediastinum and mediastinal tumours. In: *Thoracic and Cardiovascular Surgery with Related Pathology*, 3rd ed. Englewood Cliffs, Prentice-Hall, pp. 405–453.

Holmes Sellors T., Thackray A. C. and Thomson A. D. (1976) Tumours of the thymus. *Thorax* **22**, 193–220.

Le Roux B. T. (1960) Mediastinal teratoma. *Thorax* **15**, 333–338.

Sabiston D. C. and Oldham H. N. (1976) The mediastinum. In: Sabiston D. C. and Spencer F. C. (ed.) *Gibbon's Surgery of the Chest*, 2nd ed. Philadelphia, Saunders.

43 *Disorders of the Chest Wall, Tracheostomy and Minitracheostomy*

A. J. Mearns

CONGENITAL ANOMALIES OF THE THORACIC CAGE

Congenital abnormalities of the bony thorax are often incidental findings on routine chest radiography, e.g. a midthoracic rib with a bifurcated anterior end which may be fused with the rib above or below (*Fig.* 43.1*a*). There may be complete absence of one or more ribs but an accessory or cervical rib is more common (*Fig.* 43.1*b*). When such costal anomalies occur they are sometimes associated with defects of the vertebral bodies, such as hemivertebrae and with thoracic and neurological defects. The majority of these abnormalities are of little clinical significance and only if extensive do they present a clinical problem.

1. Pectus Excavatum

This is a deformity of the anterior chest wall characterized by depression of the sternum (*Fig.* 43.2). It may be localized to the lower sternum but most often begins at the manubriosternal junction. The ribs are abnormal in that the posterior ends are unusually horizontal and the anterior ends rather vertical. The costal cartilages are thought to grow in a disordered manner such that they are too long and accommodations occur in other structures within the chest wall.

Symptoms directly due to this physical abnormality are rare. Patients may be very conscious of the unusual shape of their chest wall and be unwilling to participate in activities such as swimming and sunbathing. Cardiorespiratory problems can occur in severe pectus excavatum but most patients with moderate to severe degrees of depression, even with displacement of their heart to the left, have no clinical disability whatsoever. There is an increased incidence of chronic bronchitis and pulmonary infection in the older age group and an ejection systolic murmur may be audible at the left sternal edge. Routine pulmonary function tests usually show that lung volumes and dynamic function are within

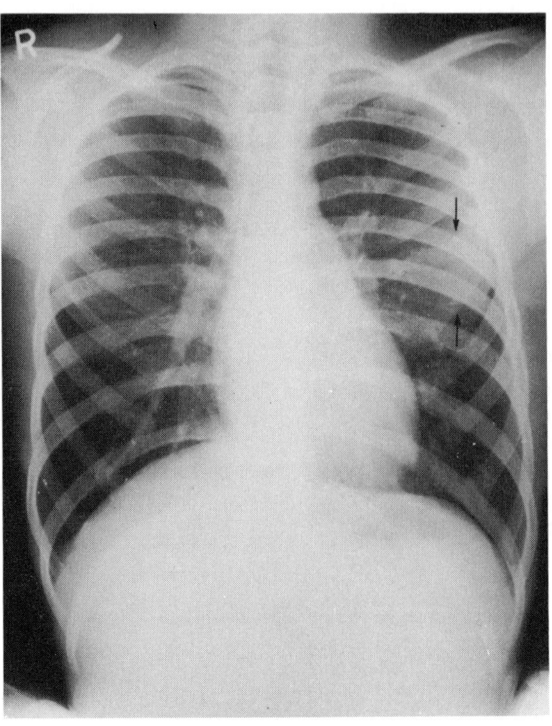

a

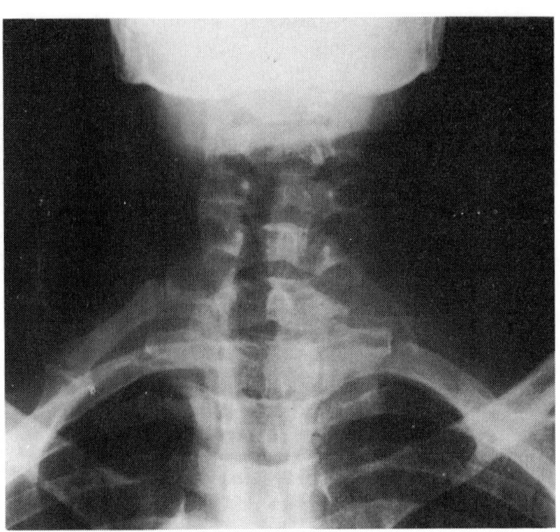

b

Fig. 43.1 *a*, Bifid fourth left rib anteriorly—congenital anomaly noted on a routine PA chest radiograph. *b*, AP radiograph of thoracic outlet showing a cervical rib articulating with the first rib on the right side.

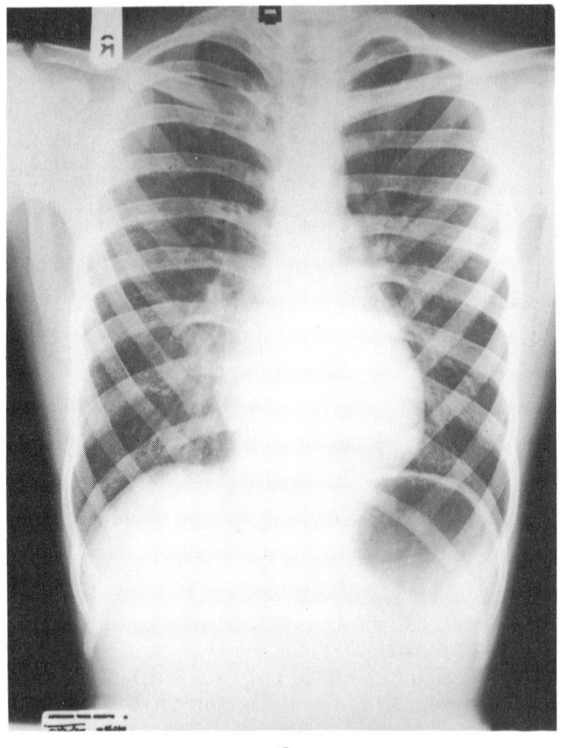

a

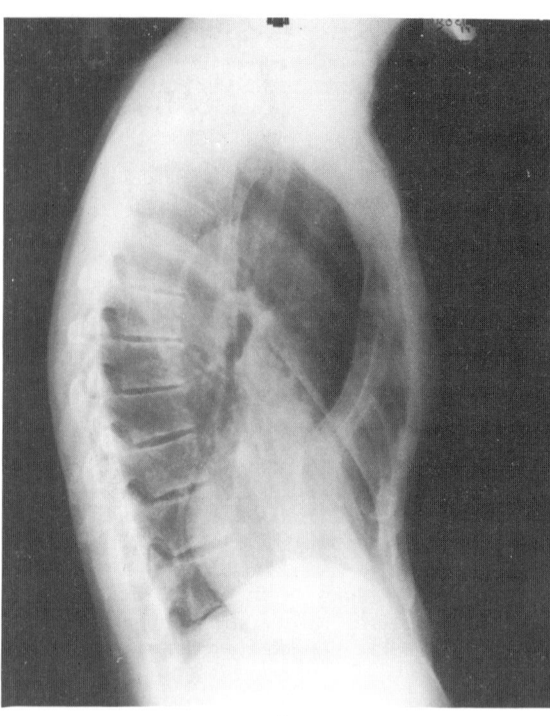

b

Fig. 43.2 *a*, PA and *b*, lateral chest radiographs showing the typical bony deformity associated with pectus excavatum.

normal limits. The degree of abnormality may be assessed clinically and radiologically—the latter by measuring the distance between the body of the sternum and the vertebral column in the lateral chest radiograph.

Treatment

The condition so rarely causes symptoms that the indications for treatment are usually cosmetic. There is no general agreement with regard to the optimum timing for surgical correction; some surgeons operate in early childhood, but there is always the possibility of asymmetrical growth of costal cartilage continuing. There will not be further growth after the mid teens. As the decision to operate is almost always cosmetic it should be decided by the individual and not the parents. The case for masterful inactivity is strong in the growing years. Breast development in the pubescent girl often modifies her attitude to minor deformity which may no longer be so obvious.

The potential hazards of major reconstructive surgery—anaesthesia, infection, pulmonary embolism, etc.—must always be borne in mind when considering such cosmetic surgery. The operation under general anaesthesia consists of two parts: (*a*) *Mobilization*—a bilateral submammary incision gives excellent access from sternal notch to ninth costal cartilages. The involved costal cartilages, usually the third to the seventh or eighth, are resected subperichondrially. A sternal osteotomy is done at about the manubriosternal junction and the body of the sternum elevated as far as is required; (*b*) *Fixation*—the sternum needs to be stabilized in its new anterior position. Wiring at the site of the osteotomy may be sufficient in the infant or young child but the older patient requires more secure internal fixation. External fixation is no longer practised as with modern implant materials so few complications occur. Most methods of internal fixation rely on retrosternal struts, plates or steel wires resting on the rib ends at either side. These internal fixation devices are removed after the anterior chest wall has united. Patients are usually discharged on the fourth day. The strut is removed electively at day surgery after 18 months.

2. Pectus Carinatum

This is also known as 'pigeon' or 'keel' chest deformity and is much less common than pectus excavatum. It may be associated with vertebral abnormalities. Two main varieties are seen: (*a*) at manubrial level, in which case the manubrium and the body of the sternum are almost at right angles to one another; (*b*) at a much lower level near the xiphisternum (*Fig.* 43.3). The deformity may be either symmetrical or asymmetrical—in the latter the sternum lies obliquely with depression of the costal cartilages on one side and elevation on the other. Again it seems likely that asymmetrical growth of the costal cartilages is responsible. Genuine cardiorespiratory abnormalities are rarely associated with this condition and the reason for surgical correction is cosmetic.

Treatment

The operative technique is similar to that for pectus excavatum, using general anaesthesia and bilateral submammary incisions. The involved costal cartilages may be dealt with either by multiple chondrotomies or resection. The sternum will require an osteotomy in order to allow it to fall back towards the vertebral column. It is not usually necessary to employ struts, pins or plates to maintain the reduction, as long as adequate mobilization has been obtained.

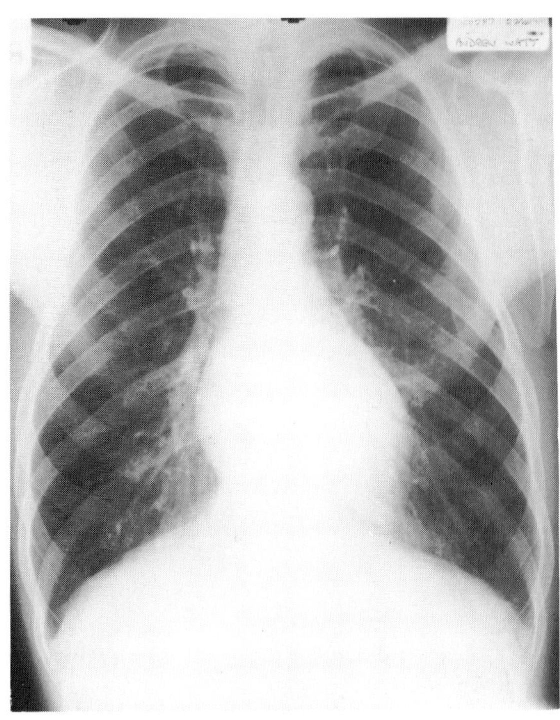

a

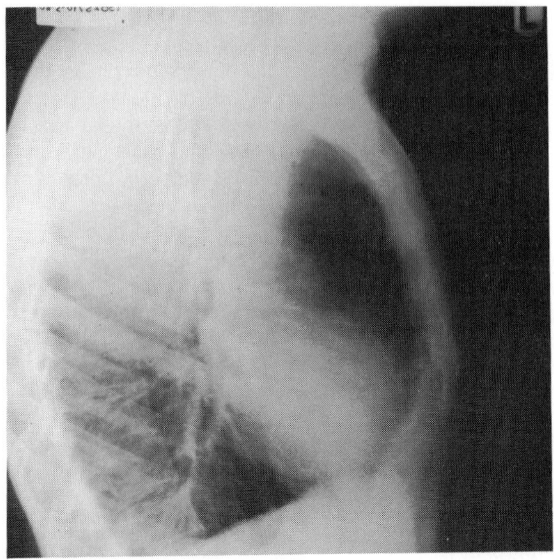

b

Fig. 43.3 *a*, PA and *b*, lateral chest radiographs showing the thoracic deformity of pectus carinatum.

3. Cleft Sternum

Embryologically the sternum is a paired mesenchymal structure which becomes cartilaginous and migrates towards the midline. There are three major components, the manubrium, the body and the xiphoid, each having separate centres of ossification. Failure of fusion of the sternum may lead to a cleft in the midline and there may be associated defects of the diaphragm, pericardium and abdominal wall. If the heart is exposed then the condition is termed 'ectopia cordis'. Such patients usually have other congenital heart disease in the form of septal defects, valvular abnormalities, or even the tetralogy of Fallot. If the operation is carried out in infancy, satisfactory closure of the cleft sternum can be obtained, but in later life much more complex surgical procedures may be required.

Thoracic Outlet Syndrome

The thoracic outlet is the space bounded anteriorly by the manubrium sterni, the first ribs laterally and the first thoracic vertebra. This is a narrow channel through which pass various important structures. These structures may be adversely affected by congenital abnormality as well as degenerative processes, tumours and trauma. The various conditions which can produce symptoms and signs of compression in this area may be grouped together under the term 'thoracic outlet syndrome'. This includes accessory cervical ribs, the scalenus anterior syndrome and may also include symptoms due to hyperabduction and thrombosis of the subclavian vein (*see* Chapter 52).

INFECTIONS OF THE CHEST WALL

Osteomyelitis

Primary osteomyelitis of the ribs or sternum occurring through haematogenous spread from a soft-tissue infection elsewhere in the body is now unusual. A destructive osteomyelitis of the sternum can occur as a complication of median sternotomy, the most common organisms responsible being staphylococci. Tuberculosis and fungal infections can occasionally involve the chest wall by direct extension from underlying infection of the lungs, pleura or lymph nodes. Treatment consists principally of the institution of appropriate antibiotic therapy and, on occasion, surgical resection of the involved segment of rib or cartilage. Occasionally chronic infections of the sternum fail to respond to simple measures and radical chest wall resection may then be required in order to eliminate the infection.

Infections of the Soft Tissues

The skin and subcutaneous tissues of the chest wall are subject to all the common infections which occur anywhere in the body. More serious are the deeper chest wall infections which are now uncommon. Subpectoral and subscapular abscesses, usually due to streptococci or staphylococci, originate in the ribs or the scapula. They require appropriate antibiotic therapy and surgical drainage. If an empyema within the pleural space is not treated appropriately then it may occasionally rupture into the subcutaneous tissues and present as an empyema necessitatis. Cold abscess of the chest wall may present similarly as a collar stud abscess.

TUMOURS OF THE CHEST WALL

Bone and Cartilage

The most common chest wall tumours are the chondromas and chondrosarcomas which originate in the costal cartilages. They often occur close to the costochondral junction and present as a visible and palpable swelling in this area. Radiologically a chondroma usually shows expansion of the rib but the cortex remains intact. Chondrosarcomas, by contrast, tend to have a more destructive effect on the surrounding bone. Surgical treatment consists of resection of a block of chest wall—this may be a relatively limited resection if the appearances are typically benign, but chondrosarcomas are very prone to local recurrence even after what appears to be a radical resection. Other tumours do occur in the bony thorax but are less frequent—osteogenic sarcoma probably accounts for about 10% of malignant chest wall tumours, being mainly a tumour of the long bones in adolescence. The radiographic appearance is fairly typical with a dense cortex and the radiating subperiosteal calcification so often seen with this type of tumour in other sites. Myeloma is occasionally seen as an apparently solitary lesion in a vertebra or a rib but is more commonly encountered as multiple lytic lesions. The radiographic appearance is of expansion of the rib with central translucency. These tumours are best dealt with by a combination of radiotherapy and chemotherapy, although it may be appropriate to resect a solitary rib lesion if the diagnosis is in doubt. Other lesions occasionally encountered in ribs are Ewing's tumour, eosinophilic granuloma and monostotic fibrous dysplasia. Primary pulmonary and pleural tumours may invade the chest wall and produce bone destruction. The majority of tumours in ribs and thoracic vertebrae are not primary but metastatic, arising from primary tumours in other viscera—particularly breast, lung, thyroid and prostate. The majority of these metastases, with the exception of the prostatic type, produce bone destruction and a pathological fracture is quite often the presentation. Radiotherapy or chemotherapy may offer effective palliation.

Tumours of Soft Tissues

These tumours may arise in any of the soft tissues of the chest wall—skin, subcutaneous fat, breast, connective tissue or muscle. Lipomas of the chest wall do not usually present a major diagnostic problem as they have a typical clinical appearance, particularly on palpation. They occasionally arise in the deeper planes of the chest wall and a diagnosis may not be clear until they are explored surgically. The malignant tumour of fat, the liposarcoma, is also seen in the chest wall—it is slow-growing and should be excised widely as local recurrence is the main problem. Fibromas occur in the chest wall as well as in the pleura and multiple thoracic neurofibromas may be found as part of the syndrome of von Recklinghausen's disease. Other tumours which have been reported are haemangiomas, haemangiopericytomas, desmoid tumours, rhabdomyomas and rhabdomyosarcomas. These are all rare and the diagnosis is often unclear until biopsy or surgical excision. With all such tumours a relatively wide margin of normal rib and intercostal muscles, including the underlying pleura, is best resected. If radiologically or at operation the appearances are suggestive of a malignant tumour, then the excision should be extended to include an apparently normal rib above and below whenever possible. Large areas of the chest wall may require excision in such surgical procedures and the resulting defects of ribs or sternum may be reconstructed with rib grafts, Marlex mesh, or an acrylic plate.

MISCELLANEOUS CHEST WALL DISORDERS

Lung Hernia

A lung hernia or pneumatocele is the protrusion of pulmonary tissue outwith the normal pleural boundaries (*Fig.* 43.4). This may occur through the chest wall via an intercostal space, at the apex through the thoracic outlet or through the diaphragm. These hernias are seen following trauma and surgery, and may also occur spontaneously. The most common variety other than following surgery is the intercostal lung hernia which is usually either alongside the sternum or the vertebral column where the intercostal muscles are relatively incomplete. A congenital deficiency of Sibson's fascia, the aponeurosis overlying the apex of the lung, may allow herniation of the lung into the neck. This usually develops in adults, particularly those with bronchitis and emphysema, and is occasionally seen in people whose occupation involves maintaining high expiratory pressures, such as trumpeters and glassblowers. These hernias are usually asymptomatic but may require surgical repair.

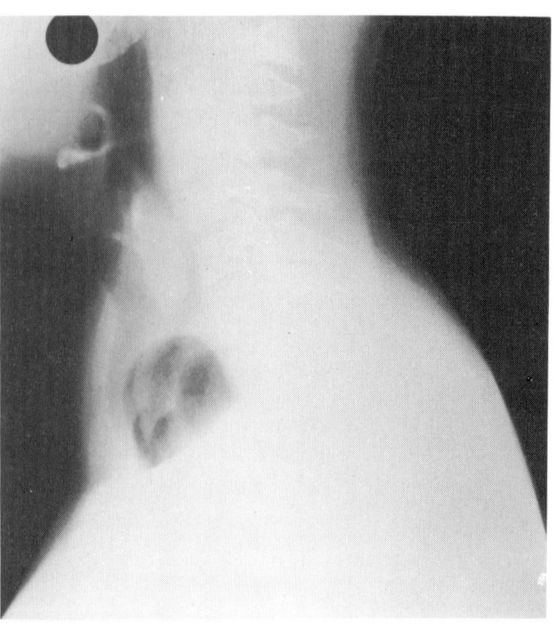

Fig. 43.4 Lateral radiograph of the neck showing a cervical lung hernia displacing the trachea.

Costochondritis

In 1921 Tietze described a syndrome of painful swelling in the area of the second or third costochondral junction. There is tenderness and some swelling over the costal cartilages but no inflammatory change in the skin. Radiography of the area is unhelpful and no treatment is required. It has been reported that surgical resection provides complete relief but it is very unusual for the symptoms to be sufficiently severe to warrant such interference.

TRACHEOSTOMY

The operation of tracheostomy has been known and practised for hundreds of years but had an unenviable reputation in its earlier days, being performed almost entirely for high respiratory obstruction due to foreign bodies, 'croup' or one of the 'quinsies'. The operation made a major contribution to the management of laryngeal diphtheria in the 19th century but as diphtheria antitoxin became available it was used less and less. With the epidemic of poliomyelitis in the 1950s the value of intermittent positive-pressure ventilation on a long-term basis was appreciated and the interest in tracheostomy changed from use in relieving upper airway obstruction to providing access for mechanical ventilation. Experience confirmed the use of routine tracheostomy for the control of bronchial secretions. In patients who were deeply unconscious or unco-operative following some intracranial incident or particularly following recoverable head injuries control of respiratory secretions is vital for recovery.

Tracheostomy through the second and third ring of the trachea was increasingly preferred over the cricothyroid membrane incision. The standard tracheostomy tube was too large and caused disturbance of the function of the glottis and quite obvious speech abnormalities were commonly present, after use of cricothyroidotomy for intubation. Consequently cricothyroid membrane intubation for access to the trachea was abandoned. However, more recently the use of a simple catheter at the level of the cricothyroid membrane for the aspiration of secretions and the delivery of oxygen has been further developed as minitracheostomy. Minitracheostomy at the level of the cricothyroid membrane should now be the treatment of choice for simple control of bronchial secretions.

1. Indications

The majority of patients may be ventilated quite easily in the short term by the passage of an endotracheal tube through the mouth. If ventilation is proposed to take any length of time i.e. 12 h or more, the formal passage of a nasotracheal tube is indicated. The modern nasotracheal tubes made of the inert plastics allow ventilation for 2–3 weeks without difficulty. The previous indications for tracheostomy to sustain the ventilation of the patient are becoming less necessary as confidence with these inert plastic endotracheal tubes develops. However, tracheostomies are still required for long-term ventilation and if there is any supraglottic stenosis or as a final pathway as a tracheostome for laryngectomy or pharyngolaryngectomy. Occasionally it is necessary to perform a tracheostomy and use a cuffed tube to prevent the soiling of the bronchi from pharyngeal overspill to the trachea.

2. Surgical Technique

a. *Standard Tracheostomy*

The formal tracheostomy operation should be carried out electively and be performed in an operating theatre under local or general anaesthesia with all facilities available. Unless the patient has supratracheal obstruction, an endotracheal tube will usually be in situ at the time of tracheostomy. Occasionally elective tracheostomy my be necessary before proceeding to an operative procedure and this may be carried out under local anaesthetic with no prior general anaesthesia. This is the formal approach for the unintubatable patient who requires a general anaesthetic with endotracheal ventilation.

The patient should be supine with a support under the shoulders, allowing maximum extension of the head and neck. The standard approach is a 2–3 cm transverse incision 2 cm above the sternal notch. The deep fascia is divided in the midline and the infrahyoid muscles separated. The thyroid isthmus is exposed and the pretracheal fascia divided to display the trachea down to about the fourth ring. The thyroid isthmus normally covers the second and third tracheal rings and may have to be mobilized and retracted upwards. If the isthmus is bulky or the access poor, it should be clamped and divided in the midline and the two halves secured by suture. Access may be considerably improved by traction with a sharp hook in an upwards direction on the first tracheal ring. Before any incision is made in the trachea, the surgeon must check that the correct sizes of tracheostomy tube are available, that the cuff inflates properly and that the correct catheter mounts and connections are available. Complete haemostasis is advisable before making the tracheal incision.

Although various tracheal incisions have been described over time and there was an enthusiasm for a 'U'-shaped flap in the tracheal wall previously, long-term experience has demonstrated that such flap types of tracheostomy unfortunately have been associated with a higher incidence of late tracheal stenosis. The theoretical short-term advantage of the ease of access when the need for reinsertion arises during the first 48 h after tracheostomy is outweighed by the problems of late tracheal stricture. Therefore the present recommendation is for a short vertical incision adequate for the insertion of the tracheostomy tube having gauged the size necessary. Adult males usually take a 39 or a 42 F, whilst the female trachea accepts 33 or 36 F.

Structures at risk during standard tracheostomy are few but the thyroid isthmus can be tied without difficulty. However, in small children before the angle of descent of the ribs is fully established the innominate vein lies high on the trachea and is at risk; similarly, the apical pleura may be breached.

b. *Minitracheostomy* (*Fig.* 43.5)

Minitracheostomy is performed (*Fig.* 43.6) with the patient supine with the head extended on a flexed neck. It is unusual for the patient to require general anaesthesia, but elective minitracheostomy for postoperative bronchial toilet in patients with a secretion load is increasingly being used. The minitracheostomy is inserted at the end of the elective procedure prior to extubation. (*See also* p. 165).

With the head extended on a flexed neck the cricothyroid membrane is palpated and a small amount of local anaesthetic introduced. The surgeon stands immediately behind the patient's head or to the side and the guarded knife, held with the cutting edge pointing caudally, is used to make a vertical incision straight through the cricothyroid membrane. The introducer is then passed into the trachea and the minitracheostomy tube, usually a 4 mm paediatric tube with a flange, is passed over the introducer into the trachea. The introducer is removed and the flange fixed, either by direct suturing or tapes (*Fig.* 43.5*b*). Once the minitracheostomy tube is in situ a 12 F gauge catheter can be passed and secretions aspirated. A 14 F gauge catheter can be wedged in the tracheostomy tube and humidified oxygen delivered more accurately than has previously been possible.

3. Management

The management of the minitracheostomy is simple and demands minimal care. There was a theoretical risk with the original Mark I design as there was no fixed flange. The possibility existed of losing the minitracheostomy tube into the adult bronchus, but it very rarely happened. It was usually associated with a failure to suture the split ends carefully to the skin.

The standard tracheostomy is indicated for the patient who requires long-term ventilation. This is executed with the cuffed standard tracheostomy tube. Earlier designs induced the local complication of pressure necrosis, but over the years improved quality of tracheostomy cuffs and finally development of the low-pressure high-volume cuff have virtually eliminated the late endotracheal stenosis and tracheomalacia from necrosis of tracheal cartilage. Occasionally the end of the tube may be driven into the wall causing local necrosis and even fistulous involvement of the innominate artery. Careful attention paid to the ventilatory attachment to the tracheostomy tube and the swinging arm control to take the weight of the ventilator attachments to hold the tracheostomy tube in the unstressed midline position should eliminate that sort of problem.

Bronchial toilet is executed via both tracheostomy and minitracheostomy tubes without difficulty using sterile soft catheters of the appropriate size. Catheter design has recently developed to stop the use of the endhole catheter which tends to engage against the bronchial wall as suction is applied. Venturi flow catheters and side-aspirating catheters are available for use with suction down endotracheal, tracheal and tracheostomy tubes. Aspiration suction must only be applied as the catheter is withdrawn. Catheters should be introduced disconnected from the suction or with the suction side vented and the catheter occluded until withdrawal starts.

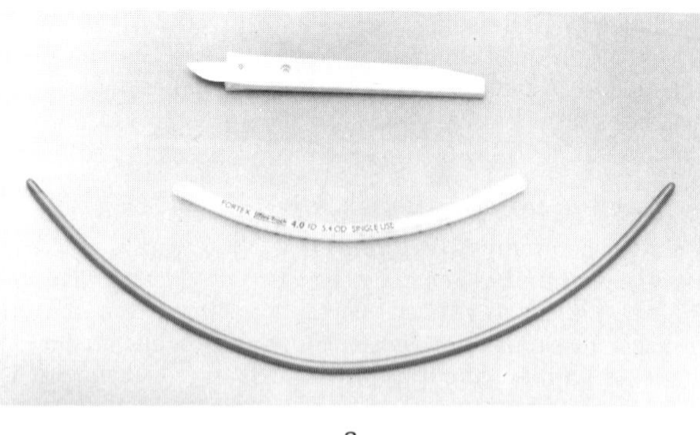

a

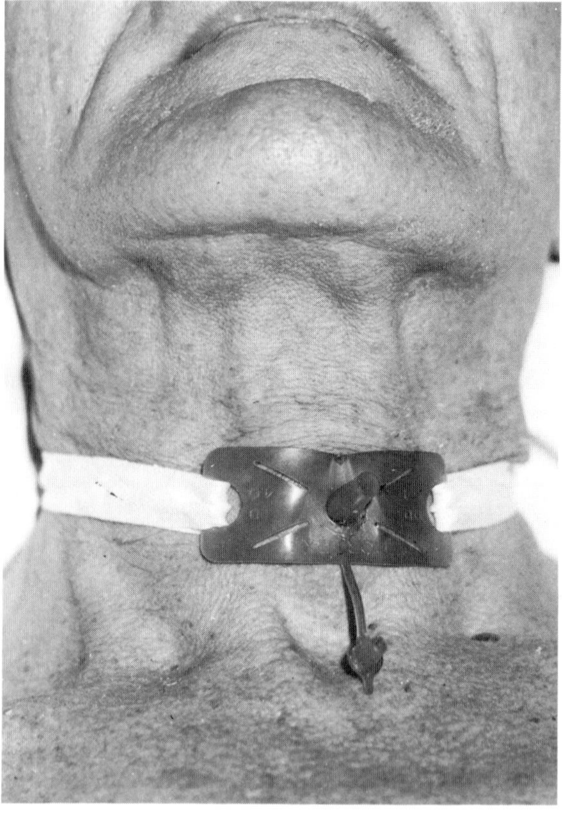

b

Fig. 43.5 *a*, The minitracheostomy set consists of a guarded knife, an introducer and a cannula. Mark I design. *b*, Minitracheostomy in position. Mark II design.

Any standard tracheostomy tube must be presented with well humidified air or oxygen when either breathing spontaneously or being ventilated. When the minitracheostomy is being used to introduce oxygen into the trachea this oxygen must be adequately humidified. The use of the open minitracheostomy tube purely for access for secretions does not require humidification because the flow characteristics dictate that the major air flow will be through the larynx rather than through the long narrow minitracheostomy tube. Removal of the tube is simple and a dry dressing is all that is needed. The wound heals in 72 h. Occasionally a weaning period is necessary and a whole range of devices is available for maintaining access to the trachea and to allow the patient to speak.

4. Complications

The complications of tracheostomy are very occasionally fatal and nearly always are caused by avoidable technical error. There is a small mortality associated with the operation itself because of the trying circumstances under which occasionally it is executed. The problems of anoxia associated with difficulties in establishing an airway in very difficult circumstances may be very trying. Occasionally bleeding may present problems, particularly in small infants when the higher position of the innominate vein is not appreciated.

a. Displacement of the Tube

For 48 h after standard tracheostomy the track between the skin and the tracheostome is not fully established and should the tracheostomy tube be displaced in this early period reinsertion of the tube can be difficult. It should be a strict rule that no tracheostomy tube is formally changed within 72 h. The tracheostomy tube should be checked for its position and function on immediate insertion and sutured or tied firmly in position at this time. Incorrect reinsertion of the tube will be quite inadequate if the initial indications for the tracheostomy still obtain. Any attempt to ventilate in a misplaced tube will meet high resistance and the ventilator pressures will rise. Under these circumstances ventilated air can be forced into the tissues and surgical emphysema develop. Tracheostomies in the first 48 h must be in the care of skilled and aware attendants. It is inevitable that patients on ventilators will be in intensive care wards and that nurses will be in constant attendance. Good training and understanding from the bedside staff is vital. In the acute situation during this early period re-intubation by the endotracheal method to re-establish the airway is best. Then the tracheostomy tube can be reintroduced at leisure. It was this complication that led to the Björk flap type of procedure which makes the early period much safer should the tube be displaced. However, with the increased bedside skills in the management of tracheostomy the late complications of Björk flap of tracheal stenosis is presently a more significant risk than the problem of early dislodgement of the tracheostomy tube.

b. Pneumothorax

Pneumothorax is a complication of any ventilated patient. It can complicate the tracheostomy in small children when the

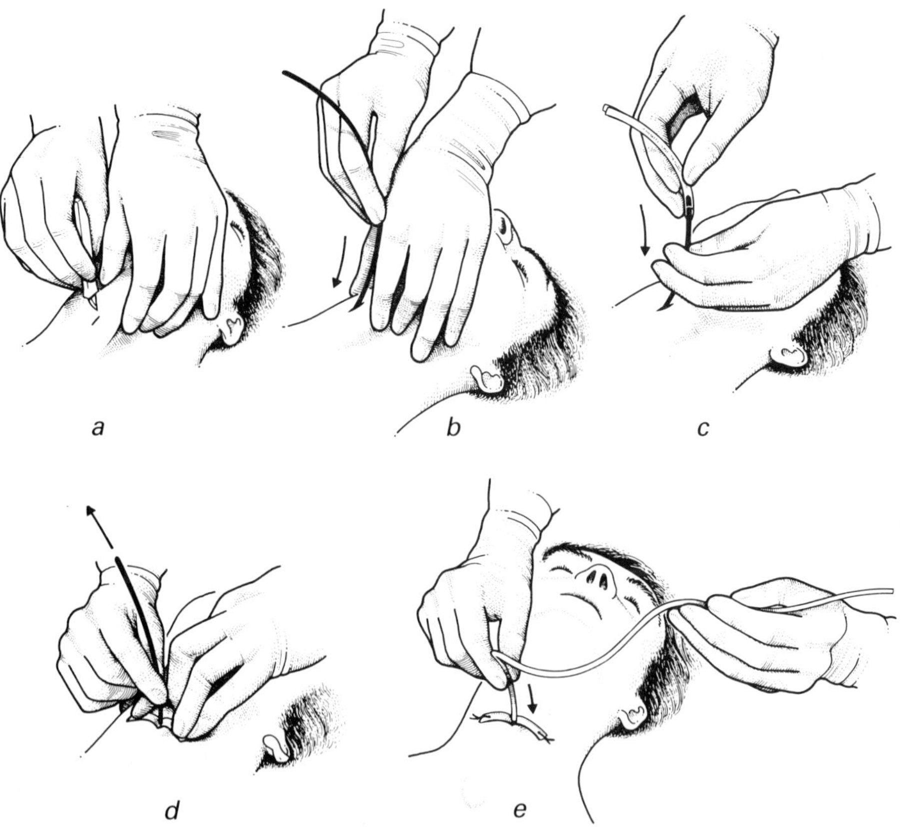

Fig. 43.6 *a*, Minitracheostomy is performed with a guarded knife and a vertical incision is made in the cricothyroid membrane. *b*, The introducer is inserted into the trachea and *c*, the minitracheostomy cannula is passed over the introducer into the trachea. *d*, With the flanges firmly sutured to the skin access is simple for aspiration of secretions or the introduction of humidified oxygen (*e*). The illustrations are of the Mark I design (*see Fig.* 43.5*a*).

apical pleura is closer to the tracheotomy site, and thus may be opened at operation because of the late descent of the ribs. The ribs are horizontal in the infant and the angle of descent, i.e. the angle between the upper border of the first thoracic vertebra and the first rib in full expiration, although the descent begins at 6 months of age, is not complete, i.e. 60°, until the child is 7 years old.

c. *Haemorrhage*

Haemorrhage occurring during the operative procedure should be completely controlled before the tracheal incision is made. Late haemorrhage causes more tracheostomy-related deaths than any other complication. Classically the haemorrhage is from the brachiocephalic artery or the origin of the right common carotid artery. It occurs because of pressure necrosis by the tracheostomy tube through the anterior tracheal wall into the major artery which is its immediate relation. This is due to angulation of the tracheostomy tube and is wholly avoidable. This complication is usually fatal within a few minutes, death more often being due to drowning rather than to exsanguination. Sometimes there is a significant but brief spontaneous arterial haemorrhage which may be taken as a warning of impending disaster. There are occasional reports of this complication being temporarily controlled by insertion of a finger into the stoma and digital compression of the relevant artery against the sternum, but survival is rare.

d. *Tracheal Stricture*

Stricture of the trachea related to tracheostomy occurs at three sites—the level of the stoma, the level of the cuff and at the tube tip. It is hoped that with intelligent use of low-pressure cuffs at least one of these sites will now be relatively rare. The reported incidence of tracheal stenosis varies considerably but is probably at least 10%, though few of these constrictions have clinical significance. Severe strictures require excision.

e. *Tracheo-oesophageal Fistula*

The incidence of this complication is fortunately low, previous estimates about 1 in 200, and is usually related to prolonged assisted ventilation, overinflation of the cuff and the presence of a nasogastric tube in the oesophagus. It is a complication which in itself carries a high mortality but nevertheless can be surgically repaired. The incidence of this complication is falling with the use of low-pressure high-volume cuffs and fine-bore enteral feeding tubes.

THE WAY FORWARD

Minitracheostomy is likely to become a routine procedure to be performed by junior doctors under local anaesthesia in the wards. Bronchoscopy for bronchial secretion control will become a thing of the past. Developments of jet oscillation for oxygen delivery via the standard tracheostomy and minitracheostomy will become an elective form of respiratory support, although the humidification of jetted gases remains a problem.

Further Reading

Matthews H. R. and Hopkinson R. B. (1984) Treatment of sputum retention by minitracheotomy. *Br. J. Surg.* **71**, 147–150.
Shields T. W. (1983) *General Thoracic Surgery*. Philadelphia, Lea & Febiger.

Section 6

Cardiac Surgery

44 Introduction

P. O. Daily and M. M. Mitchell

PREOPERATIVE CARE

A wide variety of patients present for cardiac surgery. This generally includes children with congenital defects and adults with acquired valvular disease, combined valvular and coronary artery disease, pure coronary artery disease or its sequelae, and great vessel disease such as aortic aneurysms. The cardiac status of the 'elective' patient may vary from one of full compensation to controlled decompensation. The preoperative assessment must be carefully tailored to accommodate individual needs. A careful medical history and complete physical examination should be obtained in every case and most patients must undergo specialized haemodynamic and angiographic investigations. Preoperative echocardiograms are generally also performed on most patients. It is essential for the surgeon and cardiologist to co-operate in making as accurate an assessment of the cardiac anatomy as possible. This has obvious implications in the field of congenital heart surgery but also extends to the evaluation of adults with acquired heart disease, e.g. an elderly patient scheduled to undergo valvular heart surgery may have many non-specific symptoms. In such circumstances, it is important to study the coronary artery anatomy as well as to evaluate the diseased valve. Failure to recognize coronary artery disease preoperatively may have catastrophic consequences in the operating theatre. Similarly, it is essential to recognize associated diseases such as peripheral vascular disease (especially carotid disease), pulmonary compromise, renal disease, haematological disorders, and other diseases which may require special management in conjunction with cardiac surgery.

Blood samples should be obtained routinely for sequential multiple analysis (SMA), haematological evaluation and for cross-matching. Thus, the following serum levels should be available preoperatively.

Biochemical Survey

Sodium, potassium, chloride, CO_2, blood urea nitrogen (BUN), creatinine, total calcium, phosphate, uric acid, alkaline phosphatase, total bilirubin, conjugated bilirubin, cholesterol, total triglycerides, total lipids, total protein, albumin, glutamic oxaloacetic transaminase (SGOT), lactate dehydrogenase (LDH) and creatine phosphokinase (CPK) with myocardial iso-CPK.

Hematological Survey

Haemoglobin, red cell count, white cell count with differential, haematocrit, mean corpuscular volume, mean corpuscular haemoglobin concentration, platelet count, bleeding time, prothrombin time, partial thromboplastin time, blood group, sickle-cell preparation.

When indicated, renal function should be assessed by creatinine clearance and fractional sodium excretion tests. Adult patients should undergo pulmonary function tests (*see* Chapter 38) and, if indicated, baseline arterial blood gas determinations. In some practice settings, it may be useful to have a standardized preoperative check list form available for completion on the evening before operation. This will ensure that all tests have been performed and that the blood bank has the necessary blood available. Errors of omission can largely be minimized by having preprinted orders for preoperative care, immediate postoperative care, transfer out of the intensive care unit, and transfer from the post-coronary care unit to the regular floor, and, finally, discharge orders. Blanks can be provided for variations in medications and laboratory tests can be selectively ordered as needed.

Anticoagulants, aspirin and related drugs such as dipyridamole (Persantine) and sulfinpyrazone (Anturan) should be discontinued 7–10 days prior to operation. Similarly, potassium-losing drugs and other cardiac medications should be withdrawn, if possible, over one or two days preoperatively. The dosage of anti-arrhythmic drugs can usually be reduced prior to operation, but if this is clinically unacceptable, the serum levels should be obtained for postoperative comparison. This may be particularly useful in the management of patients on procainamide (Pronestyl) or quinidine. Preoperative withdrawal of digoxin is recommended by many authorities, to ensure that any postoperative arrhythmias are not due to digitalis toxicity. In most patients the withholding of digoxin on the day of surgery is sufficient, if serum digoxin levels are non-toxic. Patients with angina usually present on a variety of nitrates. These drugs may be withheld preoperatively, provided the patients are closely monitored and the drugs are available if needed. In the past, propranolol was considered a myocardial depressant with the potential to decrease cardiac output in the immediate postcardiopulmonary bypass period. However, recent evidence suggests that this is not the case and, indeed, may be advantageous. In the preoperative phase it reduces the effect of increased emotional stress on the myocardium and permits a smoother and easier anaesthetic induction. In the postoperative period the drug also suppresses a variety of tachyarrhythmias. In similar fashion, calcium channel blockers should not be precipitously withdrawn. Minor tranquillizing drugs may be used especially in patients with coronary artery insufficiency whose myocardial oxygen requirements may exceed the available supply.

An honest and open discussion of the risks and benefits of surgery with the patient and his family constitutes informed consent. A class for patients and their families regarding the disease process, surgical procedure and intensive care unit practices and procedures can be enormously helpful in alleviating the many apprehensions which normally accompany heart surgery. Such classes are best conducted by the appropriate nursing staff.

PERIOPERATIVE MANAGEMENT

A. Anaesthesia for Cardiac Surgery

The goals of the anaesthetist in the perioperative period are, in order of priority, to minimize the risks of patient mortality and morbidity, provide optimal conditions for the surgical procedure, minimize discomfort to the patient, and generally expedite the accomplishment of the intended surgical intervention. The fundamental effects for which the anaesthetist aims during the anaesthetic are amnesia, analgesia, muscle relaxation, and maintenance of autonomic nervous system balance. In order to achieve these goals and effects, the anaesthetist needs to make an accurate preoperative assessment of the patient, and understand the requirements of the surgical procedure. He needs to be expert at establishing vascular access and using modern monitoring techniques. The anaesthetist also needs to be expert in the use of not only anaesthetic drugs and adjuncts but also vasodilators, cardiotonic drugs and pressors, drugs and techniques for the treatment of cardiac arrhythmias, management of bleeding disorders, pulmonary physiology and respiratory care, and the management of various concurrent medical problems, e.g. diabetes mellitus or renal failure.

During the preoperative visit, the anaesthetist seeks to gather the information that he needs, and to inform and educate the patient. He reviews and confirms the surgeon's assessments and findings by examining the patient and reviewing the medical records. Direct communication with the surgical team in the preoperative period and discussion of the special features of the planned procedure is generally very useful, and for unusual procedures and/or especially ill patients is essential. Surgical, nursing and anaesthesia personnel must work together as a team to assure a good outcome of the procedure.

Establishment of a close interpersonal relationship between the anaesthetist and patient during the preoperative visit can go a long way towards alleviating the patient's anxiety and securing his co-operation. Generally the prescription of some sedative preoperative medication is also useful in promoting a smooth transportation of the patient into the operating room, establishment of monitoring modalities, and induction of anaesthesia. In fact, appropriate preoperative medication may be essential to prevention of a catastrophic exacerbation of the patient's condition due to anxiety and stress. On the other hand, care needs to be exercised in order to avoid dangerous over-sedation and risk of myocardial and respiratory depression.

For infants less than 3 months old, preoperative sedation is most often not required. Gentle, reassuring body contact with the anaesthetist or a nurse and a pacifier to suck on is often enough to allow establishment of essential monitoring and induction of anaesthesia by inhalation agent with a mask. Older infants up to 20 kg in weight can be induced with rectally administered sodium pentothal 40–50 mg/kg or methohexitol 20–25 mg/kg, or with ketamine 8–12 mg/kg intramuscularly with atropine 0·05 mg/kg mixed in the same syringe. These techniques require strict attendance of the anaesthetist to monitor for respiratory depression and are not suitable for application outside the operation room suite in the absence of an anaesthetist. Older paediatric patients may benefit from the administration of oral premedication such as diazepam 0·05–0·15 mg/kg 60–90 min prior to the expected time of induction of anaesthesia. They are then persuaded to accept establishment of an intravenous catheter and induction with intravenous agents, or induction with an inhalation agent by mask.

Premedication of adult patients for cardiac surgery is usually heavy, with the exception of patients with significant pericardial disease, stenotic valvular disease, or advanced mitral valve disease with pulmonary involvement. Morphine 0·08–0·12 mg/kg with scopolamine 0·002–0·005 mg/kg can be used, or some other sedative in an appropriate dose can be substituted for the scopolamine.

Careful attention needs to be shown to the management of the patient's chronic medications. Beta-blocking agents, calcium channel blockers, nitrates, and most antihypertensive drugs should be continued right up to the time of surgery, including doses due the morning of surgery. Anticoagulants and diuretics need to be discontinued several days prior to surgery. Appropriate blood levels tests need to be done to guide dosage management and assure therapeutic non-toxic levels of other drugs, such as digoxin.

Essential monitoring needs to be established before the induction of anaesthesia. This includes a precordial stethoscope to monitor breath and heart sounds, the electrocardiogram (ECG) to monitor for arrhythmias and ischaemia, both direct invasive arterial pressure and a back-up blood pressure by cuff, and at least central venous pressure, if not pulmonary artery pressure and thermal dilution cardiac output. Frequently, several ECG leads are monitored simultaneously to improve detection of ischaemia. Arterial blood gas (ABG) monitoring is also essential. Baseline and frequent intraoperative ABG, serum electrolyte, and haematological values should be obtained. The activated clotting time (ACT) and/or other measurement of clotting function should also be monitored. A pulmonary artery catheter (PAC) should be placed in patients with congestive heart failure, high-grade coronary artery disease, significant carotid artery or aortic disease, pulmonary hypertension, unstable circulation, or in whom unusual surgical bleeding or clotting problems are expected such as with repeat procedures. A PAC is relatively contraindicated in patients with abnormal cardiac anatomy, severe pulmonary hypertension (due to increased risk of pulmonary artery perforation), tricuspid or pulmonary valve disease (especially if a surgical procedure is planned for the tricuspid or pulmonary valves), or if the patient is a cardiac transplant recipient or donor.

There are several basic anaesthetic techniques commonly used for cardiac surgery. For paediatric patients, inhalation anaesthetics are often used, typically but not exclusively, halothane. Usually considerably less than one MAC (minimum alveolar concentration) is required of the potent inhalation agent and nitrous oxide is either not used or limited to 50% inspired concentration or less. Liberal doses of non-depolarizing muscle relaxants (e.g. 0·15 mg/kg of pancuronium) and supplemental narcotics (e.g. 20–50 μg/kg of fentanyl) are used. The patient is expected to require continued intubation and mechanical ventilation for about 24 h. For the simpler, shorter procedures, the dose of narcotics can be limited to 10 μg/kg and the muscle relaxants reversed at the end of the procedure to allow earlier extubation.

For adults with coronary artery disease undergoing surgical revascularization who have good ventricular function, a fairly standard anaesthetic technique using some narcotics (e.g. 25 μg/kg or less of fentanyl, 2·5 μg/kg or less of sufentanil, 0·25 mg/kg or less of morphine, or an equivalent dose of some other narcotic) in conjunction with a potent inhalation agent and muscle relaxant is often used. Induction of anaesthesia can be accomplished expeditiously with sodium pentothal or some other rapid acting intravenous agent. Nitrous oxide is generally limited to 50% or less. If they are haemodynamically stable, the patient can be extubated a couple of hours after surgery is finished.

Less healthy patients with compromised ventricular function and/or valvular disease are most often anaesthetized with a high dose narcotic and 100% oxygen technique in order to maximize haemodynamic stability. Up to 120 μg/kg of fentanyl, equivalent doses of sufentanil, or as much as 2 mg/kg of morphine may be used with this technique. If morphine is used, the rate of administration should be limited to no more than 5 mg/min to avoid marked vasodilatation due to release of histamine. Fentanyl and sufentanil should be administered slowly at first to avoid milder vasodilatation and bradycardia, and then can be given quite rapidly. Typically about half of the total narcotic dose will be given before intubation of the trachea, another quarter of the total dose before sternotomy, another increment just after initiation of cardiopulmonary bypass, and the remaining narcotic after the patient has been weaned from cardiopulmonary bypass and is relatively stable. The timing of the administration of muscle relaxants can be critical with high-dose narcotic techniques. If not given soon enough during the induction of anaesthesia, the patient may become so rigid as to prevent adequate ventilation (even with vigorous positive-pressure ventilation), and if given too soon the patient may remember being paralysed. A second smaller dose of muscle relaxant is typically given just after initiation of cardiopulmonary bypass. High dose narcotic/oxygen techniques commit the patient to a period of postoperative mechanical ventilation (typically about 24 h).

Irrespective of the particular technique employed, the hallmark of a good anaesthetic is a smooth induction and stable maintenance of surgical anaesthesia without significant pre-incision cardiovascular depression, or reflex hypertension and tachycardia due to sympathetic stimulation with the skin incision and/or sternotomy. This is best achieved with a deliberate pace during the induction of anaesthesia, and close attention to and monitoring of the patient with particular attention to pre-load, after-load, and heart rate, and maintenance of optimal ABGs and laboratory parameters.

Thoughtful and judicious use of vasodilators, pressors, and cardiotonic, depressant, and anti-arrhythmic drugs as adjuncts to careful adjustment of anaesthetic drug administration is frequently necessary. Maintenance of body temperature is important, especially for procedures where cardiopulmonary bypass is not used, and in the period after weaning from cardiopulmonary bypass. This is particularly critical in smaller paediatric patients.

The anaesthetist's responsibilities do not end when the patient leaves the operating room. A smooth safe transition to care in the postoperative intensive care unit requires a complete communication of the important information about the patient's condition that the anaesthetist has acquired during the preoperative and intraoperative period to the personnel that will be attending the patient postoperatively. Frequently the anaesthetist remains intimately involved in the patient's care, especially respiratory care, for several days.

B. Principles of Cardiopulmonary Bypass and Deep Hypothermia with Circulatory Arrest

The establishment of cardiopulmonary bypass (CPB) represents a highly unphysiological situation. Notably, in most situations the flow is non-pulsatile. Additionally, the average perfusion pressure across the systemic vascular bed is probably somewhat less than in the normal situation. A number of incompletely understood and highly complex responses of the body to this highly abnormal situation occur. These, in part, represent the so-called humoral amplification systems which includes the activation of complement, and the formation of anaphylatoxins C3A and C5A with their attendant adverse effects. Additionally, heparinization does not totally prevent microcoagulation. This, in turn, may also result in activation of the clotting cascade. Some of the principal responses include activation of fibrinolysis and activation of the kallikrein–bradykinin system. Furthermore, after the conclusion of cardiopulmonary bypass, the heparin and protamine interaction may also exacerbate some of the above aspects of the humoral amplification systems. Consequently, because of the unphysiological nature of CPB, it appears that the length of time of CPB is directly related, at least partially, to an individual's ability to recover from the effects of CPB. Also, decreasing age of the patient (less than 4 years) is associated with worsening of the above effects.

Current methods of CPB involve improved bubble oxygenators. More recently, effective membrane oxygenators which prevent a direct blood–gas interface are available, although, in some membranes it is probable that there is still a blood–gas interface within the membrane. Most of the pumping mechanisms consist of roller pumps which may result in some damage to the blood components. As the blood passes through the pump heads and oxygenator, whether bubble or membrane, and through various filters to remove microaggregates, additional damage occurs to the blood and blood components. This is further exacerbated by passing through cardiotomy suckers which adds to the significant shear forces which have incompletely understood effects on blood and blood components and may, in part, elicit activation of the humoral amplification systems.

Standard connections to the heart–lung machine may involve venous cannulation by a single cannula which has a 'double stage' component inasmuch as part of the cannula is in the inferior vena cava and a second part of the cannula lies in the right atrium to allow return of blood from that area as well as from the superior vena cava. While the advantage of a single cannula is obvious, it is possible that if, for any reason, the venous return line is partially obstructed, systemic venous blood will enter the right atrium and ventricle and rewarm these areas as well as the interventricular septum to the same temperature as the systemic venous blood. This is particularly apt to occur when the heart is displaced, e.g. to expose the mitral valve through an incision in the area of the right superior pulmonary vein or when the apex of the heart is elevated and deviated toward the patient's right for exposure of the circumflex coronary artery or its obtuse marginal branches. A preferred alternative is separate cannulation of the superior and inferior vena cava with introduction of the cannulas through the right atrial wall or directly into the cavae themselves. With bicaval cannulation return of systemic blood flow into the right heart can be precluded by umbilical tapes passed around the outside of the venae cavae to occlude them by compression against the caval cannulas. Typically, arterial cannulation is instituted by direct cannulation of the ascending aorta by a variety of commercially available cannulas. In some situations, such as atherosclerotic or dissecting aneurysms of the ascending aorta, femoral artery cannulation is mandatory. For left heart bypass, venous cannulation of the left atrium and arterial cannulation of the femoral artery or distal thoracic aorta is occasionally performed. It is usually necessary to prevent distension of the left heart during CPB when the left ventricle is not ejecting. This can be accomplished by pulmonary artery, left atrial, or left ventricular venting. The goal is to prevent pulmonary venous pressure from exceeding 10 mmHg. If this level is exceeded for a significant period of time, pulmonary oedema may occur. Furthermore, decreased perfusion of subendocardial tissues with variable degrees of myocardial infarction may occur.

Priming of the heart–lung machine to establish the perfusate typically is accomplished in adults with a variety of crystalloid solutions which may include the addition of osmotic agents such as plasminate and mannitol. It is frequently possible in adult patients to perform the entire operation without the addition of any foreign blood products, whatever, and to avoid their use in the postoperative period by using cell-saving devices. However, in smaller children and infants and, in particular, neonates, some use of blood components is required. An additional advantage of haemodilution is that of increased tissue perfusion. Formulae are available for computing the required addition of red blood cells in order to arrive at a predetermined haematocrit for the perfusate in the case of children and neonates.

Prior to cannulation, heparinization is carried out by intravenous administration of 300 units of heparin/kg of body weight. Activated coagulation times are then monitored on a regular basis to determine the adequacy of heparinization and whether or not additional heparin may be required during the period of cardiopulmonary bypass. Sufficient flow rates during perfusion are essential in order to ensure the adequacy of tissue oxygenation. Obviously, the flow rates are dependent upon body temperatures. It is highly desirable, in most instances, to lower body temperature to 25–30 °C in order to decrease the oxygen requirements. For example, the oxygen requirement at 28–30 °C is reduced to approximately 50% of that at 37 °C. The advantages are that lesser flow rates can be utilized which result in decreased pressures to which the blood is exposed (theoretically decreasing damage to the blood), decreased bleeding while on CPB, and reduced likelihood of disruption of the tubing system. Furthermore, should an unanticipated brief period of circulatory arrest be required, enhanced central nervous system protection is provided by the hypothermia. While various flow rates have been used successfully, general guidelines are as follows:

37 °C, approximinately 2 L/min/m^2
30 °C, 1·8 L/min/m^2
25 °C, 1·7 L/min/m^2
20 °C, 1·6 L/min/m^2

This corresponds, roughly, with 80–90 ml/kg/min at normothermia to 40–50 ml/kg/min at 20 °C. In infants, however, increased flow rates are required to equal approximately 2·5–2·8 L/min/m^2 at normothermia with corresponding changes at the lower temperatures. During the period of cardiopulmonary bypass, it is essential to monitor the adequacy of oxygenation. This can be assessed by continuous monitoring of the oxygen saturation of the venous return blood ($SV{O_2}$). However, it should be recognized that significant arteriovenous shunting can result in superficially elevated oxygen saturations in the systemic venous blood. Adequate urine output along with electroencephalographic monitoring further ensure adequate tissue perfusion. It is also important to maintain a mean arterial pressure of 60–90 mmHg.

At the conclusion of cardiopulmonary bypass and after removal of the arterial cannula, protamine is administered to reverse the effects of heparin. Usually 3 mg/kg of body weight of protamine is administered. However, continued monitoring of the activated clotting time may indicate the need for additional protamine.

As mentioned above, occasionally significant reactions are observed with the heparin/protamine reaction which in part may be related to the activation of complement. These reactions usually result in substantial hypotension associated with elevated pulmonary vascular resistance and, at times, can be lethal unless specifically dealt with by the administration of pressors and an increase in preload. It is noteworthy that it appears not to matter whether the protamine is administered intravenously or intra-arterially since the protamine heparin reaction *per se* appears to result in complement activation. Diabetic patients who have been using NPH insulin are particularly likely to have a protamine reaction based on an acquired allergy to protamine which appears to be different from the above described reaction.

C. Myocardial Protection

Protection of the myocardium is critical if the heart is to withstand the combined effects of the underlying pathology and the trauma of operative intervention. No time is allowed for the severely injured myocardium to recover as it must resume full function in the immediate postoperative period if the patient is to survive.

There are three major areas which require attention in order to achieve maximum myocardial preservation.

Preoperative Phase

This is the area which is most frequently neglected.

1. Myocardial reserve and performance must be at optimum levels preoperatively. Factors affecting myocardial reserve include:

a. Oxygen transport, which can be improved by correcting anaemia, an abnormal pH, respiratory depression, low cardiac output or hypovolaemia.

b. Cardiac rate is important in optimizing cardiac output in that either sinus bradycardia or tachycardia may result in decreased cardiac output. Furthermore, arrhythmias may also compromise cardiac output and should be corrected if possible preoperatively.

c. Preload abnormalities (preload is defined as the ventricular end diastolic volume). Preload is influenced by the inotropic and chronotropic state of the heart and by intravascular volume and can be improved by attention to these parameters.

d. Afterload abnormalities (afterload is defined as the resistance to shortening of the myocardium fibres). Systemic hypertension may increase afterload and should be controlled preoperatively.

e. Myocardial contractility (which is independent of preload and afterload) is affected by abnormal sympathetic tone or electrolyte imbalance. Both medications and/or acidosis can cause a decrease in myocardial contractility and must be corrected.

2. The precise haemodynamic dysfunction of the heart must be accurately defined preoperatively by angiography of the coronary arteries and heart chambers. The surgeon must be fully aware of any abnormalities which may affect the myocardium.

3. Coexisting diseases should be evaluated and dealt with as far as possible before cardiac surgery.

Anaesthesia Phase

The critical period is the induction of anaesthesia, during which a fixed amount of oxygen is available to the myocardium. The prime aim, therefore, is to avoid an excessive oxygen demand and to provide adequate ventilation. Stress increases myocardial oxygen consumption by producing sympathetic overactivity and catecholamine release and hence increased afterload and myocardial contractility. Stress must therefore be minimized by selecting specific drugs for each patient.

Intraoperative Phase

The precise method of myocardial protection may be selected based upon the anticipated period of myocardial ischaemia. For short procedures such as aortic valvotomy, which should require no more than 15 min of myocardial ischaemia, can be performed by reduction of the perfusate temperature to 28–30 °C prior to cross-clamping of the aorta. Following aortic cross-clamping, the heart may be allowed to beat or electrically fibrillated, if desired. For pulmonary valvotomy, the aorta may be left unclamped with the heart allowed to continue to beat. For longer periods of myocardial ischaemia, two principles are important. The first is the desirability to obtain more rapid cardiac arrest to avoid depletion of the myocardial energy stores. This can be accomplished with a variety of cardioplegic solutions which, invariably, are hypothermic (less than 10 °C). Recently it has been advocated to induce cardioplegia in patients who have significant depletion of myocardial energy stores with normothermic cardioplegic solution and also to use normothermic cardioplegic solution, again just prior to removal of the aortic cross-clamp. At the present time, however, the use of warm cardioplegic solution pre- and post-procedure is not widely employed.

The second principle of myocardial protection is the *maintenance* of cardiac hypothermia after cardiac arrest and hypothermia has been induced by a cold cardioplegic solution. This may be facilitated by systemic hypothermia to 20 °C. Selective cardiac hypothermia can be accomplished with topical saline at 4 °C or with a cooling jacket that surrounds the ventricles which contains an enclosed circuit through which cold saline (4 °C) is continuously circulated to maintain myocardial hypothermia. Saline slush placed around the ventricles has also been used but has been associated with an unacceptable incidence of phrenic nerve paresis and if used for more than one hour may result in significant myocardial damage secondary to frostbite.

The exact composition of the cardioplegic solution has received extensive attention both in the laboratory and clinically. While changes are continually being made in the cardioplegic solution, the characteristics that are desired include the rapid induction of cardiac arrest without depletion of myocardial energy stores, the avoidance of myocardial oedema, the avoidance of destabilization of the cell membrane, and the delivery of an appropriate substrate to the myocardium for continued metabolism. Additional controversy exists as to whether or not the cardioplegic solutions should be crystalloid or contain red blood cells for the delivery of oxygen to the myocardium. However, since in most cases the temperature of the cardioplegic solution is less than 10 °C, there is evidence that oxygenation of a crystalloid solution may be as effective as blood cardioplegia in the delivery of oxygen to the myocardium given the reduced metabolic rate. From a clinical standpoint, it appears that crystalloid cardioplegia solution with or without blood is acceptable. For neonates and infants undergoing cardiac surgery with cross-clamp times of more than 20 min, it is not clear whether or not cardioplegia adds additional significant protection compared to profound cardiac hypothermia by itself. It is probable that the inappropriate administration of cardioplegic solution may result in substantial myocardial damage. Specifically, delivery of the cardioplegic solution at excessive pressure may result in significant myocardial oedema.

An optimal temperature range for myocardial hypothermia has not been precisely defined but extensive investigation suggests that myocardial preservation is enhanced at lower temperatures provided that freezing is avoided. In the clinical setting, however, it has proved extremely difficult, if not impossible, to obtain and maintain myocardial temperatures at 10 °C or less. The maintenance of myocardial hypothermia depends upon preventing rewarming which can occur from both the interior of the heart as well as the exterior. Interior rewarming of the right heart occurs because of return systemic venous blood entering the right atrium and right ventricle. This results in a rewarming of the right heart, including the interventricular septum, to temperatures approximately the same as the perfusate. As discussed previously, this can be prevented by placing separate cannulas into the superior and inferior venae cavae either through the right atrium or by direct caval cannulation followed by occlusion of the venae cavae against the caval cannulas with tapes passed around them.

Since true, non-coronary collateral blood flow is extremely low, most left-sided cardiac rewarming, if caval tapes are used, occurs from blood entering the pulmonary venous system through bronchial collaterals or, in the case of patients with cyanotic heart disease, major aortopulmonary collaterals. The effect of left-sided return blood flow is identical to that on the right in that rewarming to the temperature of the perfusate occurs. Left-sided rewarming may be prevented by pulmonary artery venting or, if not adequate, by direct left atrial or left ventricular venting. In certain patients with particularly large aortopulmonary collaterals, control prior to initiating cardiopulmonary bypass may be necessary. For excessive bronchial arterial flow, silastic tapes placed around each of the pulmonary veins to occlude them can be utilized after the initiation of pulmonary artery venting. The prevention of exterior cardiac rewarming may be obtained by the use of continuous pericardial lavage with cold saline (4 °C). This, however, results in the problem of the saline obscuring the operative field and of mixing of the saline with the perfusate resulting in unwanted additional haemodilution. Also, blood may be lost with removal of the saline. When cold saline is instilled in only the posterior pericardium, the anterior aspect of the heart, which includes the majority of the right ventricle, will be subjected to rapid rewarming.

Maintenance of more complete myocardial hypothermia may be obtained by keeping the anterior aspect of the heart covered with cold sponges. The use of a cooling jacket, however, will ensure adequate coverage of the ventricular myocardial muscle mass and, at the same time, prevent mixing of the myocardial coolant and the perfusate. Exterior rewarming primarily occurs because of conduction of heat from the aorta which affects the posterior aspect of the heart, from the lungs which affects the lateral aspects, and from the liver through the diaphragm which affects the inferior wall. The anterior myocardium is rewarmed by convection from contact with room air and by radiation of heat from the operating room lights.

The methods in the foregoing discussion will preclude these potential causes of rewarming.

In the majority of centres performing cardiac surgery at present, cardioplegia combined with some form of selective myocardial hypothermia is utilized as the primary method of myocardial protection in most procedures. However, it should be mentioned that with mild to moderate systemic hypothermia of 25–30 °C, intermittent aortic cross-clamping may be utilized for the performance of distal coronary anastomoses. Typically, proximal anastomoses are performed with the aorta unclamped and the heart beating. This method has resulted in operative mortality and perioperative myocardial infarction rates comparable to those obtained with cardioplegia and myocardial hypothermia.

At the conclusion of the intracardiac portion of the procedure, it is essential to remove all retained left-sided air. A variety of methods and manipulations are successful in doing so. The general principles involve placement of the patient in the Trendelenburg position to prevent cerebral embolization of any ejected air. It is necessary to have a vent in the ascending aorta at a location which represents the highest point with respect to gravity. Prior to release of the aortic cross-clamp, caval tapes are removed and the left side of the heart is filled from blood passing through the right heart and pulmonary artery. As this occurs, air is aspirated from the left atrium, left ventricle and the ascending aorta. After several aspirations the aortic cross-clamp is removed. Also, it is useful to have the anaesthetist hyperinflate the lungs and roll the operating table from side to side to facilitate removal of air which may have been aspirated into the pulmonary veins.

After defibrillation, the patient is maintained in the Trendelenburg position until all of the left-sided air has been aspirated or removed from the air vent in the ascending aorta. During the period of air removal and with the heart beating, intermittent compression of the left atrium forces any retained air into the left ventricle from which it is ejected into the aorta and out through the aortic air vent. The operating table should be levelled only after it is certain that all of the air has been removed from the left heart. This is probable when, during three separate, consecutive periods of compression of the left atrium, no air bubbles are observed exiting the aortic vent site.

POSTOPERATIVE CARE

General Management

The patient returning from the operating room is accompanied by the anaesthetist and surgeon to the intensive care unit and is greeted by two nurses, one of whom will subsequently be responsible for the patient and the other will assist in the initial few minutes. A member of the respiratory care team is also present to provide the necessary ventilator adjustments. Transport is accomplished with both ECG and arterial pressure monitoring in progress.

Most patients returning to the unit are physiologically in the phase of rewarming and are generally on constant infusions of medications (such as nitroprusside) which cause peripheral vasodilatation. Thus, large volumes of fluid will be required to maintain an adequate cardiac output. Moving the patient usually drops the central venous pressure by pooling a large amount of the blood volume, and this event, coupled with recovery of the myocardium itself, usually results in an observed drop in the central venous pressure by the time the patient has returned to the intensive care unit. Care must therefore be taken to ensure adequate volume status.

Ventilatory function is another priority. Usually patients are ventilated in the uncomplicated case overnight, especially if the anaesthetic technique employed is that of high dose narcotics. A tidal volume of 10–15 ml/kg of body weight allows for the initial ventilator setting to be modified according to the arterial blood gases.

Pre-load requirements vary greatly between individuals and depend largely on the pre-existing state of cardiac function. Patients with diminished cardiac reserve usually require higher filling pressures to maintain cardiac output. Basic water requirements can be met with the amounts depicted in *Table* 44.1. The amounts given are on an hourly basis so that adjustments can be made more easily when indicated. After the basic water need has been met, additional fluid replacement will be discussed below. Where indicated, placement of a flow-directed pulmonary artery catheter intraoperatively can be especially helpful in estimating the volumes needed to maintain an adequate cardiac output. Left-side filling pressures can also be estimated by the pulmonary artery catheter or measured directly by a left atrial line placed at surgery. Decreased left ventricular compliance which may accompany mitral stenosis, for example, results in increased atrial dimensions which in turn require larger filling volumes. If the cardiac output is marginal and the inotropic state of the myocardium precariously low so that renal function may consequently be impaired, it is helpful if a cardiac output thermodilution catheter is used. In the routine case, however, the chest tube output of blood

Table 44.1 Fluid replacement for adults after cardiac surgery

	Total fluids ml/m²/h	*Type fluid*	*Potassium replacement* mEq/m²/24 h
Day of operation	20	5% D/W	10
Postop. day 1	30	5% D/W	20
Postop. day 2	30	5% D/W	20
Postop. day 3	40	5% D/0·25 NaCl	10

1. All fluid for flushing of i.v. lines and delivery of medications must be subtracted from above amounts.
2. Balanced salt solutions should be used for flushing of intra-arterial lines (to prevent spasm and pain) and should be kept to a minimum (3 ml/h).
3. Oral feedings should be started as soon as tolerated with corresponding decreases in i.v. fluids.

is replaced volume for volume (with plasmanate if the haematocrit is greater than 32 and with blood if it is less than 32) in sufficient quantities to maintain the central venous pressure at near preoperative levels and the urine output at approximately 20 ml/h/m^2 or 0·5–1·0 ml/kg/h. Potassium is replaced as indicated in *Table* 44.1 and is maintained at a serum level of 4·0–4·5 mmol/L. A standardized postoperative note is completed immediately, taking care to note the positions of chest tubes and pacing wires.

Routine antibiotic prophylaxis is instituted preoperatively on the morning of operation and continues until the evening of the second postoperative day and consists of an intravenous cephalosporin 1 g every 6 h in adult patients. The antibiotic is discontinued 48 h postoperatively. Cimetidine, 300 mg i.v. every 6 h, is given to patients with prior history of gastrointestinal bleeding or those considered at risk of 'stress ulceration' due to the severity of the disease or prolonged illness.

Ventilatory support is recommended until the morning following operation, when weaning from the ventilator utilizing intermittent mandatory ventilation (IMV) is commenced. If adequate blood gases are obtained, the patient is extubated and a treatment protocol is started which consists of chest percussion, ultrasonic nebulization and incentive spirometry. The chest tube is removed on the first day if the output is serous and less than 20 ml/h. The peripheral intravenous lines and urinary catheter are removed at this time as well. The central venous line is kept in place until the patient is transferred from the intensive care unit and until the serum potassium is within normal limits, since oral potassium supplementation can be particularly uncomfortable in the early postoperative phase.

Routinely, on the afternoon of the first postoperative day or on the morning of the second postoperative day the patient is transferred to a monitored ward (telemetry) and incentive spirometry is continued. Ambulation is imperative and helps to decrease the degree of lung atelectasis. Chest radiography is performed twice weekly. Diuresis with frusemide (Lasix) my be required to restore the patient's preoperative weight. The usual fluid overload results in a 2–3 kg (5–7 lb) increase in weight. Small pleural effusions are generally not tapped unless there is a significant degree of respiratory embarrassment.

All patients with prosthetic valves are commenced on oral anticoagulants immediately following removal of the chest tubes. Patients with aortic porcine or bovine xenografts are maintained on anticoagulants for a period of 6 weeks and those with mitral xenografts for a period of 3 months. New evidence suggests lifelong anticoagulation may be necessary with all heterografts, however. In cases of mechanical valve replacement anticoagulant therapy is necessary indefinitely. Antiplatelet therapy with persantine and aspirin is given for a period of one year to all patients after coronary bypass grafting. A randomized prospective study has indicated that this regimen results in enhanced graft patency. In the uncomplicated first-time procedure, the patient is discharged from the hospital on the fifth to seventh postoperative day, and even sooner in some children (ASD, VSD).

SPECIFIC MANAGEMENT OF POSTOPERATIVE PROBLEMS

For the majority of patients undergoing cardiac surgical procedures, with a routine approach to postoperative management, uncomplicated convalescence is the rule rather than the exception. However, patients who are older, present with compromised left ventricular function, and have significant associated diseases affecting the lungs, liver and kidneys, and who also may have generalized vascular disease often represent substantial problems in postoperative management. For these patients it is best to approach each system separately so as to provide an organized, complete approach to the patient which will enhance the probability of postoperative recovery. As an example of this approach, management of the cardiovascular system will be discussed.

Cardiovascular System

Because of its utmost importance with respect to survival, management of the cardiovascular system assumes first priority. The most important consideration with respect to the cardiovascular system is the maintenance of cardiac output adequate to meet the metabolic demands of the patient as a whole. It has been demonstrated that cardiac indices less than 2 L/min/m^2 in paediatric patients and less than 1·5 L/min/m^2 in adult patients are associated with a significantly increased operative mortality rate. The primary determinants of cardiac output are:

1. Cardiac rate and rhythm
2. Preload
3. Inotropic state of the heart
4. Afterload

These terms have already been defined. For proper management of patients with a compromised cardiovascular system, adequate monitoring is essential. This includes continual measurement of the central venous pressure or right heart filling pressure as well as continuous monitoring of the systemic arterial pressure. The ability to assess cardiac index is also mandatory and can be performed most readily by the transvenous insertion of a Swan–Ganz catheter for thermodilution cardiac output determination as well as intermittent measurement of pulmonary artery wedge pressure to estimate left heart preload. In patients in whom compromised cardiac output is present preoperatively or intraoperatively, it is prudent also to leave in a left atrial line for direct measurement of left heart preload which may be removed postoperatively. Additional monitoring includes regular assessment of the patient's neurological status and measurement and recording of urinary output. Indirect evidence of an adequate cardiac output is afforded by regular determination of peripheral perfusion based on the quality of the peripheral pulses, skin temperature, and colour of the extremities. An additional valuable adjunct is the use of a pulmonary artery fibreoptic catheter which allows continuous monitoring of mixed venous oxygen saturation. Assuming oxygenation is constant, changes in cardiac output will be immediately reflected by changes in saturation of the mixed venous blood. This information can be displayed digitally and recorded continuously. Additional essential information includes regular sampling of arterial blood gases.

Manipulation of the determinants of cardiac output is by two basic approaches. The first is to optimize the volume of the intravascular space for controlled preload. The second is by pharmacological manipulation of cardiac rate and rhythms, contractility and afterload. Based on the Starling relationship, left and right heart filling pressures must be optimized in order to improve cardiac output. For the restoration of the intravascular volume it is necessary to distinguish crystalloid from colloid requirements for appropriate replacement of fluids. As mentioned, the requirements for water and, especially, sodium in the postoperative period are markedly reduced. Therefore, unless there is an additional loss of body water and electrolytes, the total water replacement should be restricted to that described in *Table* 44.1. Although somewhat arbitrary, if the haematocrit is greater than 32, additional volume expansion should be performed by colloid solutions such as plasmanate or salt-poor albumin. Also, a synthetic colloid solution such as Hespan may be administered. With reduced levels of the haematocrit, red blood cells may be given. Current practice entails the use of blood components rather than whole blood. Unless there is significant postoperative bleeding, whole blood is rarely administered. Once right- and left-side filling pressures have been optimized based upon cardiac index determinations, additional increases of cardiac output are obtained by pharmacological or mechanical means.

Pharmacological agents used for manipulation of the determinants of cardiac output can be grouped into three major classes: (1) antiarrhythmic agents; (2) inotropic agents; (3) afterload reduction agents. Since many of these agents directly or indirectly affect the autonomic nervous system, it is important to understand their specific effects on the autonomic system (*Table* 44.2).

Cardiac arrhythmias may significantly compromise cardiac output by affecting cardiac rate and function. However, before pharmacological manipulation, a determination should be made regarding whether or not the arrhythmia is compromising cardiac output. If so, underlying causes such as hypoxaemia, acidaemia, and mechanical cardiac causes such as tamponade or residual cardiac defects should first be eliminated. The appropriate antiarrhythmic agent may then be selected based upon the underlying arrhythmia and associated cardiac rate as outlined in *Table* 44.3.

After optimizing preload and control of cardiac rate and rhythm, inotropic agents and afterload reduction may further improve cardiac output. The correct use of these agents is dependent upon frequent assessment of cardiac output and calculation of systemic vascular resistance based upon the following formula:

$$\text{SVR} = \frac{(\text{Aortic mean pressure} - \text{central venous pressure})}{\text{cardiac output (L/min)}} \times 80$$

$$(\text{normal range} = 800\text{–}1200 \text{ dynes/sec/cm}^{-5})$$

After the initiation of intravenous inotropic agents (*Table* 44.4) reduction of excessively high SVR is necessary for further increases of cardiac output (*Table* 44.5).

Table 44.2 Adrenergic receptors

α_1. Vasoconstriction
α_2. Inhibit norepinephrine release

β_1. Tachycardia, increased contractility
β_2. Relaxation of smooth muscle

'Dopaminergic'—increase renal and mesenteric blood flow

Table 44.4 Inotropic agents

Drug	*Action* α_1	β_2	*Cardiac* β_1 *inotropic/chromotropic*		*Dose*
Dopamine†	+*	+	++	+	2–10 μg/kg/min
Dobutamine	0	?	++	+	5–20 μg/kg/min
Adrenaline	+	0	++	++	0·01–0·1 μg/kg/min
Noradrenaline	+++	0	++	0	0·01–0·10 μg/kg/min
Isoproterenol	0	0	++	+++	0·01–0·20 μg/kg/min
Calcium chloride	0	0	++	0	10–30 mg/kg over several minutes

* 10 μg/kg/min or greater.
† Stimulates 'dopaminergic' receptor sites to dilate renal and mesenteric vessels at doses of 1–2 μg/kg/min.

Table 44.3 Antiarrhythmic agents*

	Drug	*Indications*	*p.o. dose*	*i.v. dose*	*Half-life*
CLASS I					
Effect on depolarization	Quinidine	PACs, PVCs, maintain sinus rhythm	300–600 mg 6-hourly	5–10 mg/kg	5–7 h
	Procaine	PVC, recurrent VT	250–750 mg 4-hourly	10–15 mg/kg	2·5–4·7 h
	Xylocaine	Frequent PVCs, multiple PVCs, coupled PVCs, VT, VF		20–50 μg/kg/min	1·2–2 h
CLASS II					
β-adrenergic blockage	Propranolol	SVT, AF with rapid VR	10–100 mg 6-hourly	0·1 mg/kg	4–6 h
CLASS III					
Prolonged duration of action potential	Bretylium	Refractory VT and fibrillation	—	5 mg/kg	4–17 h
CLASS IV					
Slow channel calcium blockage	Verapamil	SVT, atrial fibrillation/flutter	30–180 mg 6-hourly	75–150 μg/kg	3–7 h
	Nifedipine	Same	10–40 mg 4–6-hourly	5–15 mg/kg	3 h
Digoxin		SVT, atrial flutter or fibrillation with rapid VR	0·25 mg/d	0·50–0·75 mg/kg	1·7 d

*Specific directions detailing the use, dose, administration and side-effects should be consulted before administering these medications.
PAC, Premature atrial contractions; PVC, Premature ventricular contractions; VT, Ventricular tachycardia; VF, Ventricular fibrillation; SVT, Supraventricular tachycardia; AT, Atrial fibrillation.

Table 44.5 Vasodilators (after load reduction)

Drug	*Site of action*	*Dose (i.v.)*	*Duration*
Nitroglycerine	Venous	10–20 μg/min	Transient
Nitroprusside	Arterial and venous	25–400 μg/min	Transient
Diazoxide	Arterial	100–300 mg 6-hourly	4–12 h
Hydralazine	Arterial	5–40 mg 6-hourly	4–8 h

1. Doses per kg body weight are not used because of wide variations in doses.
2. Doses for adult patients only.

MECHANICAL REDUCTION OF AFTERLOAD

In addition to pharmacological manipulation of afterload, an ingenious mechanical device, the intra-aortic balloon, was developed in 1961 by Moulopoulos and Kolff. The intra-aortic balloon consists of a catheter inserted via the femoral artery into the descending thoracic aorta with a balloon attached at its end. The balloon is triggered by the electro-cardiographic signal to inflate during diastole (*Fig.* 44.1). As an alternative to suturing of a graft on the femoral arteries depicted in *Fig.* 44.1, the femoral artery can be exposed directly but insertion of the balloon may be carried out by the use of percutaneous techniques. These avoid the time

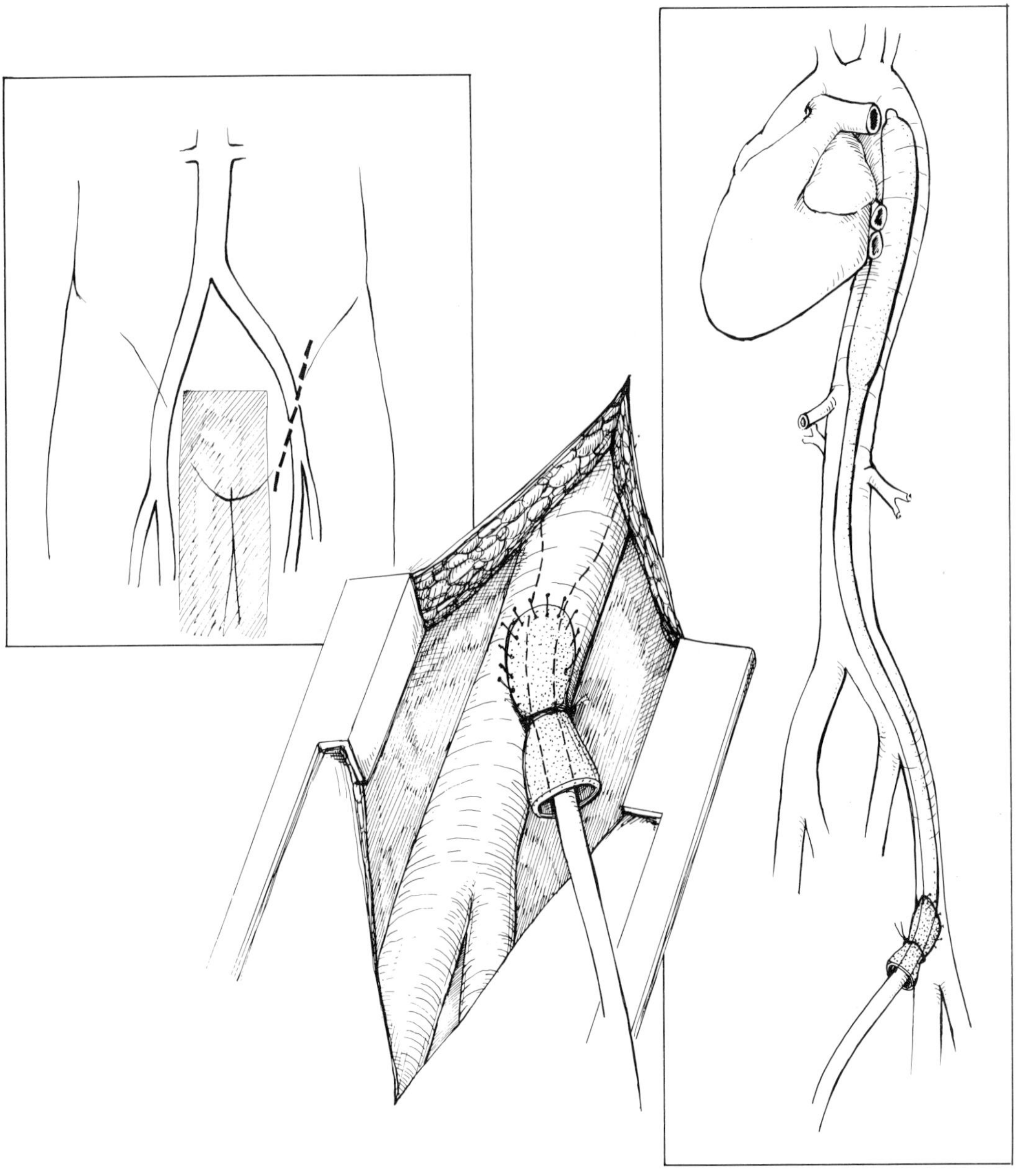

Fig. 44.1 Diagrammatic representation of details pertaining to the incision, insertion and placement of intra-aortic balloon.

required to suture a graft in place and also eliminate the possibility of infection of a foreign substance. However, it should be emphasized that if the artery is exposed directly and percutaneous techniques are used to insert the balloon, removal should be accomplished by direct visualization of the artery and suture closure of the insertion site of the artery at the time of removal.

The intra-aortic balloon provides diastolic augmentation usually for 1–3 days postoperatively, but has been used for more than 30 days. Low molecular weight dextran 50 ml every six hours is routinely used while the balloon is in place. At the time of balloon removal Fogarty embolectomy catheters are passed proximally and distally to ensure adequate inflow and runoff. Heparin is used whenever compromise in the distal flow is suspected.

Several complications may arise from intra-aortic balloon pump insertion and use. The most common of these is compromise of blood flow to the extremity in which the balloon is inserted. Therefore, frequent observation for adequate blood supply to that extremity must be carried out. When severe peripheral vascular disease precludes the insertion of the intra-aortic balloon pump through either femoral artery, cannulation of the ascending aorta with direction of the balloon pump into the descending thoracic aorta may be performed. The net increase in cardiac output by intra-aortic balloon pump varies from 15 to 20%.

Occasionally, however, this degree of augmentation is inadequate and, therefore, for the severely failed left ventricle, an extracorporeal left ventricular assist device may be necessary which is connected between the left atrium and aorta. In some instances of right ventricular failure, a right ventricular assist device may be indicated, as well. Rarely, both right and left assist devices may be necessitated.

Although used infrequently to date, the use of a total heart replacement device such as the Jarvik 7 can provide support for the patient until a donor heart becomes available, assuming the patient meets the criteria for cardiac transplantation.

Further Reading

Balderman S. C., Bates R. J. and Anagnostopoulos C. E (1977) Cardiac valve replacement: Improved survival related to air exclusion and myocardial protection. *Ill. Med. J.* **151**, 2, 113–116.

Ballance C. A. (1920) *The Bradshaw Lecture on the Surgery of the Heart*. London, Macmillan.

Brothwell D. and Sandison A. T. (1967) *Disease in Antiquity*. Springfield, Ill., Thomas. pp. 474–488.

Carrel A. and Guthrie C. (1906) Résultats du patching des artères. *C. R. Soc. Biol. (Paris)* 1009.

Lamberti J. J., Anagnostopoulos C. E., Al-Sadir J. et al. (1976) Mechanical circulatory assistance for the treatment of complications of coronary artery disease. *Surg. Clin. North Am.* **56**, 83-94.

Lin C. Y. and Benson D. W. (1976) Cardiac anaesthesia for lethal disease of the ascending aorta. In: Anagnostopoulos C. E. (ed.) *Lethal Diseases of the Ascending Aorta*. Baltimore, University Park Press, pp. 129–143.

Lin C. Y., Little A. and Anagnostopoulos C. E. (1980) Potassium propranolol and cardiac surgery. Paper presented at International Anaesthesia Society Conference, Hamburg.

Rehn L. (1897) Veber, Penetrierende Herzwondeu und Herznaht. *Arch. Klin. Chir.* **55**, 315.

Williams D. H. (1897) Stab wound of the heart and pericardium—suture of the pericardium—patient alive three years afterwards. *Med. Rec.* **51**, 437.

45 *Acyanotic Congenital Heart Disease*

P. O. Daily

INTRODUCTION

Cyanosis is a clinical manifestation of the presence in the circulation of more than 5 g/100 ml of reduced haemoglobin; and in patients with congenital heart disease it is usually due to shunting of blood from the venous (right) to systemic (left) circulation. All other congenital heart defects are acyanotic. These lesions can be categorized by the presence or absence of a left-to-right shunt, non-shunting lesions causing pressure or volume overload primarily of the right heart, left heart or great vessels, and primary myocardial disease (*Table* 45.1). Shunting defects include patent ductus arteriosus, atrial septal defect, ventricular septal defect, and atrioventricular canal anomalies. Pure pulmonary stenosis and Ebstein's anomaly represent lesions occurring in the right side of the heart without a shunt. Congenital mitral and aortic valve anomalies represent lesions occurring on the left side of the heart without a shunt. Coarctation of the aorta, aortic arch anomalies and coronary artery anomalies represent lesions of the great vessels occurring without a shunt. Obstructive and non-obstructive cardiomyopathy represents primary myocardial disease. This chapter deals with the anatomy, physiology, diagnosis and surgical treatment of the acyanotic congenital heart defects.

PATENT (PERSISTENT) DUCTUS ARTERIOSUS

The term 'ductus arteriosus' was first recorded in the 16th century. Although surgical interruption of the ductus is a standard cardiac surgical procedure today, medical manipulation with prostaglandins and indomethacin is evolving, particularly in the sick premature newborn.

Anatomy and Physiology

The ductus arteriosus is a normal fetal communication between the aorta just distal to the left subclavian artery and the pulmonary artery just to the left of the bifurcation of the pulmonary trunk. In utero, the ductus diverts blood from the high resistance pulmonary circulation to the aorta and low resistance placental vascular bed where gas exchange

Table 45.1 The diagnosis of acyanotic congenital heart defects

Acyanotic

Shunt Absent			Shunt Present
Right Heart	**Left Heart**	**Great Vessels**	
•Pulmonary Stenosis •Ebstein's Anomaly	•Mitral and •Aortic Valve Anomalies •Obstructive Cardiomyopathy	•Coarctation •Aortic Arch Anomalies •Coronary Artery Anomalies	•ASD •VSD •A-V Canal •PDA

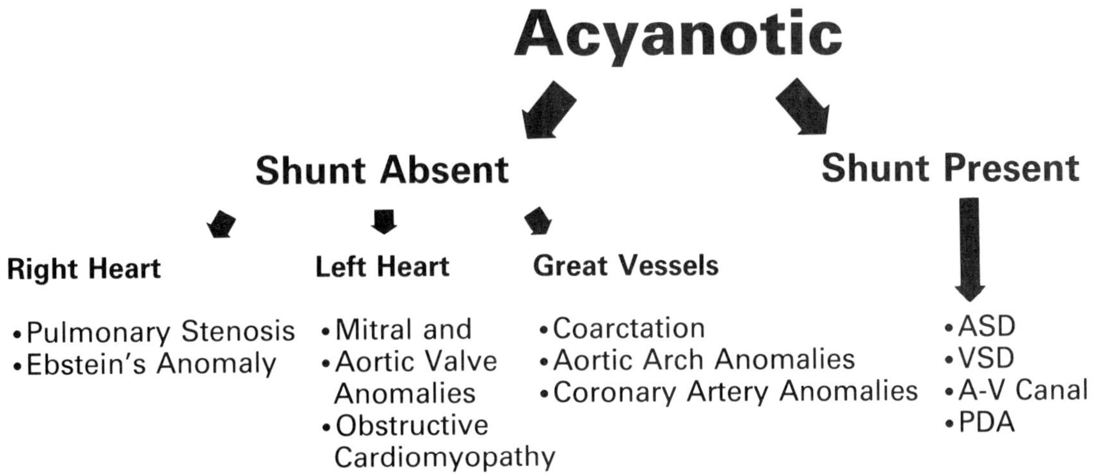

takes place. At birth, the sudden drop in pulmonary vascular resistance and increase in oxygen tension resulting from the onset of respiration is accomplished by contraction of the medial smooth muscle and functional closure of the ductus. Additionally, vasoactive substances such as bradykinin and endogenous catecholamines facilitate closure whereas prosta-glandins relax ductal smooth muscle, contributing to patency. The increased incidence of ductal patency in prema-ture infants may relate to the increased sensitivity of ductal tissue to prostaglandins. In full-term infants ductal tissue is more responsive to oxygen tension, promoting ductal closure. By eight weeks anatomical closure occurs in 88% of infants by subintimal fibrosis and thrombosis, eventually leading to the formation of a connective-tissue band, the ligamentum arteriosum.

The physiological disturbance produced by a persistent ductus arteriosus is dependent on the size of the ductus and the pulmonary vascular resistance. If the ductus is small, ductal flow is minimal and chiefly from left to right (*Fig.* 45.1*a*), and there is no accompanying increase of pulmonary artery pressure or vascular resistance. If the communication is large but pulmonary vascular resistance remains normal, a large left-to-right shunt occurs, causing volume overload of the left heart. If the ductus is large and pulmonary vascular resistance is increased, severe pulmonary hypertension is present accompanied by right to left ductal shunting (*Fig.* 45.1*b*). This results in pressure overload of the right heart with no increased load on the left heart. Ductal closure after six months of age is rare. Natural history is related to the size of the ductus with congestive heart failure as the primary cause of death with larger ducti and endocarditis with smaller ones. The death rate has been estimated at 30% in the first year with a decrease to 1%/year through the third decade increasing to 4%/year in subsequent decades.

Diagnosis

Although infants may present with congestive heart failure and older patients with dyspnoea on exertion, most patients are asymptomatic. Symptoms and physical signs vary, depending upon the magnitude of the shunt, the status of the pulmonary vasculature and the direction of the shunt. The characteristic continuous 'machinery' murmur of patent ductus arteriosus is produced by a large left-to-right shunt with normal pulmonary artery pressure. In the presence of pulmonary hypertension, the left-to-right shunt may no longer be large and may occur chiefly during systole. If pulmonary hypertension is severe, resulting in right-to-left flow, cyanosis (more severe in the lower half of the body) may occur.

Chest radiograph shows cardiomegaly, left atrial enlargement and increased pulmonary vascular marking. Left atrial enlargement and left ventricular hypertrophy are present on ECG. Right ventricular hypertrophy may be seen in the presence of pulmonary hypertension. Increased left atrium : aorta ratio on echocardiography in premature infants indicates an enlarged persistent ductus.

Cardiac catheterization is necessary when the diagnosis is in question, when there is a possibility of associated intracardiac defect, or when evidence of pulmonary hypertension is present. The diagnosis may be made by catheter position if it passes from the pulmonary artery through the ductus to the aorta. Oxygen saturation will be higher in the pulmonary artery than in the right ventricle. Pulmonary artery pressure is usually normal but may be elevated. An aortogram will demonstrate a left-to-right shunt, and a right ventriculogram or pulmonary angiogram a right-to-left shunt if present. If contrast radiography is deemed necessary, it can be easily performed at the bedside by injecting contrast material in the infant's aorta at the same time that a portable chest roentgenogram is obtained. Cardiac catheterization is generally not indicated in newborns where the increased left atrial to aortic ratio can be determined by echocardiography.

Treatment

The standard treatment is surgical division if an adequate-sized structure is present. This is done electively between the ages of 2 and 5 years or subsequently when discovered. If untreated, complications from infective endocarditis or heart failure may occur. As a rule, the presence of a ductus arteriosus is sufficient indication for operation. Pulmonary vascular disease may result from persistent ductus arteriosus and, if severe enough to cause reverse ductal shunting,

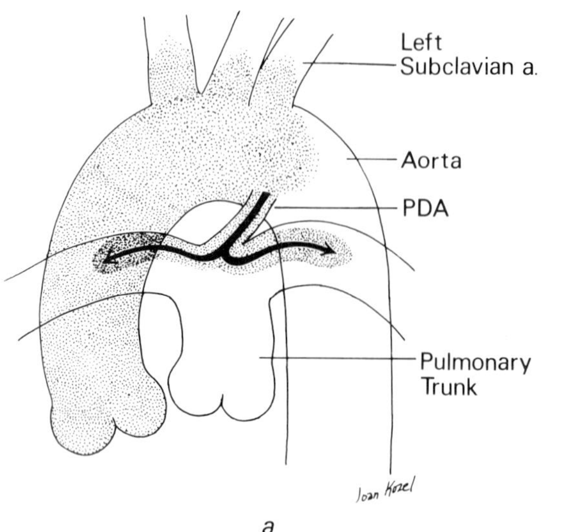

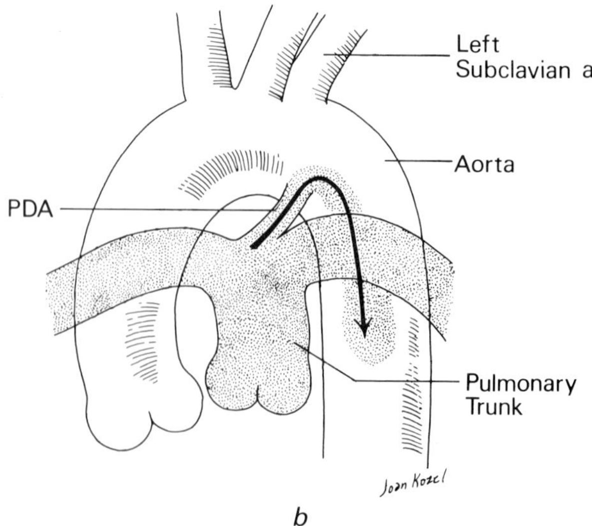

Fig. 45.1 The physiology of patent ductus arteriosus. *a*, Usual physiology with left-to-right shunting through the ductus. *b*, Right-to-left shunt through a ductus arteriosus.

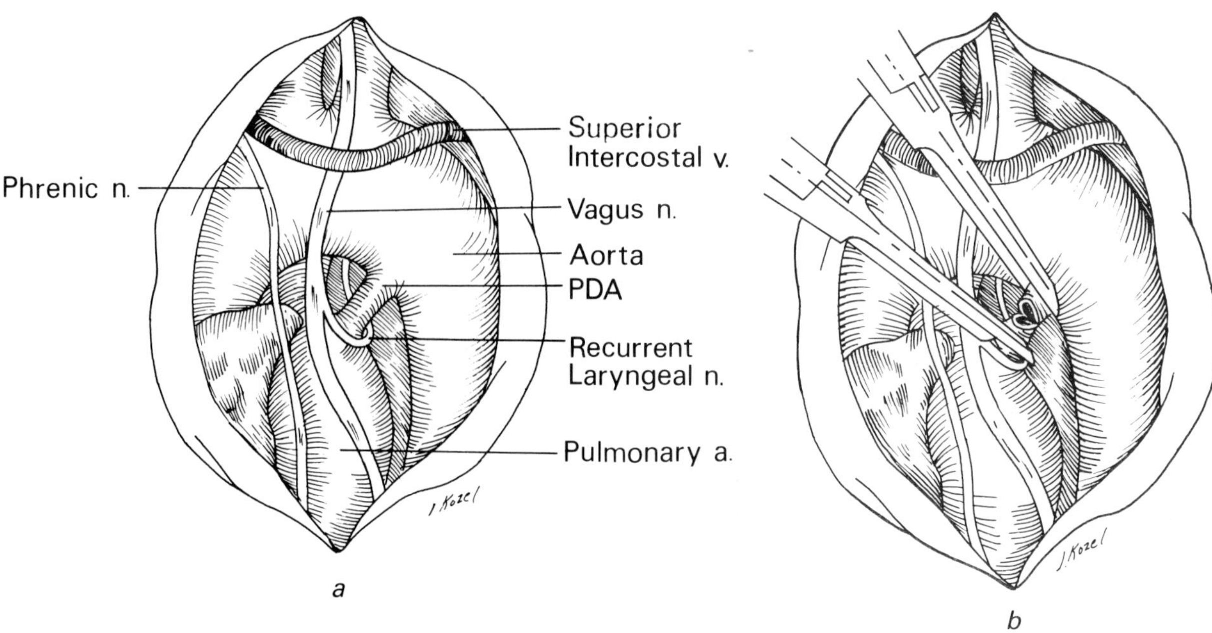

represents a contraindication to closure. In the premature infant the primary surgical indication is ventilator dependency. Left atrial enlargement by echocardiography is confirmatory of the diagnosis.

The chest is entered through a left 4th intercostal space posterolateral incision (*Fig.* 45.2). The ductus is exposed by incising the mediastinal pleura posterior to the phrenic nerve and the vagus nerve. The ductus is isolated by sharp dissection with careful attention to the recurrent laryngeal nerve coming from the vagus around the ductus. A pair of Pott's ductus clamps is placed allowing ample room between them for suturing. The ductus is divided with scissors and closed in two rows. In an adult with a large or calcified ductus, mobilization of the aorta proximally and distally may be prudent. In premature infants or patients with a small ductus, ligation or silver clip closure probably has no higher a recurrence rate than division.

Elective division of a patent ductus arteriosus in a child has a mortality of less than 1%. In children with other cardiac anomalies or in the adult, the mortality is higher and may approach 5% depending on the nature of the associated lesions or haemodynamic abnormalities. In the premature infant surgical ductal closure is associated with a low operative mortality (1%) but the hospital mortality may approach 20% because of other problems associated with prematurity such as the respiratory distress syndrome. In small babies, it is essential that the left pulmonary artery is not mistaken for the large ductus at the time of ligation. It is equally important to distinguish the aortic arch from the patent ductus. Complications are unusual but include phrenic nerve injury, recurrent laryngeal nerve injury and chylothorax.

The premature infant with respiratory distress syndrome and patent ductus arteriosus appears to benefit from closure of the ductus and reduction of pulmonary blood flow. Medical closure with indomethacin is often successful during the first week of life; if not, surgical ligation should be performed within 10 days of intubation. If the effects of patent ductus can be controlled medically it is desirable to do so since 80–100% in premature infants will close spontaneously. Prostaglandin E_1 and E_2 produce relaxation of the ductus and are useful in temporarily palliating cyanotic infants with pulmonary outflow obstruction dependent on this communication for survival. Medical manipulation of the ductus arteriosus reduces the urgency of operative intervention in congenital heart disease.

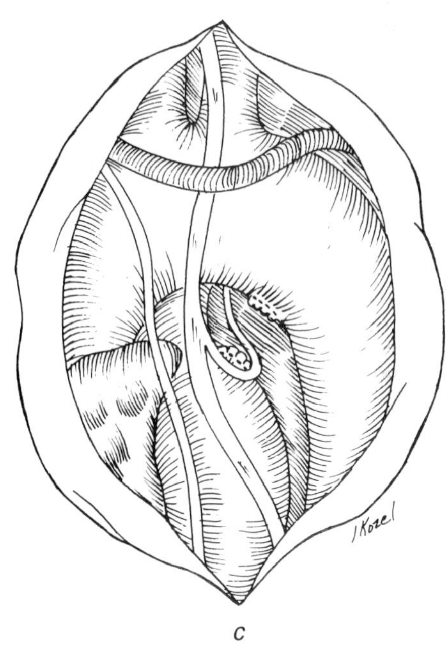

Fig. 45.2 Patent ductus arteriosus. *a*, Anatomy as viewed through a left thoracotomy. *b*, Clamping and division of the ductus after the recurrent laryngeal nerve has been isolated and protected. *c*, Completed operation with the ductus arteriosus oversewn.

COARCTATION OF THE AORTA

Coarctation of the aorta, a congenital constriction of the aorta, usually occurs just distal to the left subclavian artery. Although first described anatomically over 200 years ago and clinically in 1875 by Wernicke, the first successful corrections were performed by Craaford and Gross working independently in 1945. The incidence of isolated coarctation is 5–8% of congenital heart disease.

Anatomy and Physiology

The narrowing in coarctation may occur anywhere in the aorta but is most commonly just distal to the left subclavian artery. Depending on its relationship to the ductus, it has been classified as preductal, postductal and juxtaductal. It is generally juxtaductal in newborn infants. More complicated variations, including interrupted aortic arch, will not be discussed.

Significant obstruction results in hypertension in the upper extremities and hypotension in the lower extremities. Most of the flow to the lower body occurs through dilated collateral arteries, including the internal mammary, intercostal, lateral thoracic and subscapular arteries. In rare instances, preductal coarctation with a large patent ductus arteriosus results in differential cyanosis of the lower extremities. Common coexisting congenital heart defects include bicuspid aortic valve, patent ductus arteriosus, ventricular septal defect and mitral valve abnormalities. In addition, aneurysms of the circle of Willis may sometimes occur.

Diagnosis and Natural History

The child or adult with coarctation of the aorta is often asymptomatic. If symptoms are present, they are usually related to the hypertension. The infant with severe coarctation usually presents in the early weeks of life in critical condition with congestive heart failure. Physical examination reveals absent or reduced pulsations in the femoral

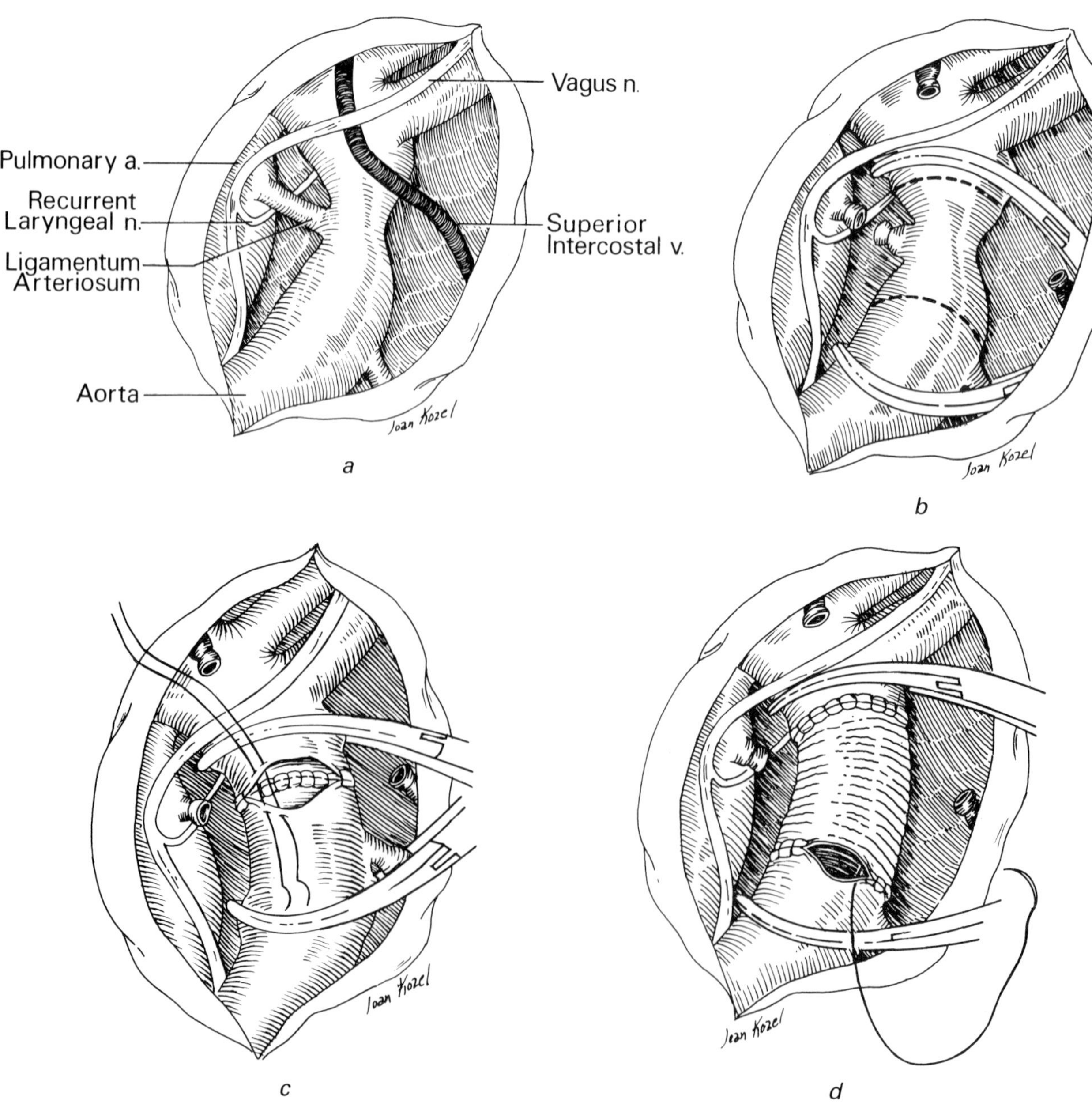

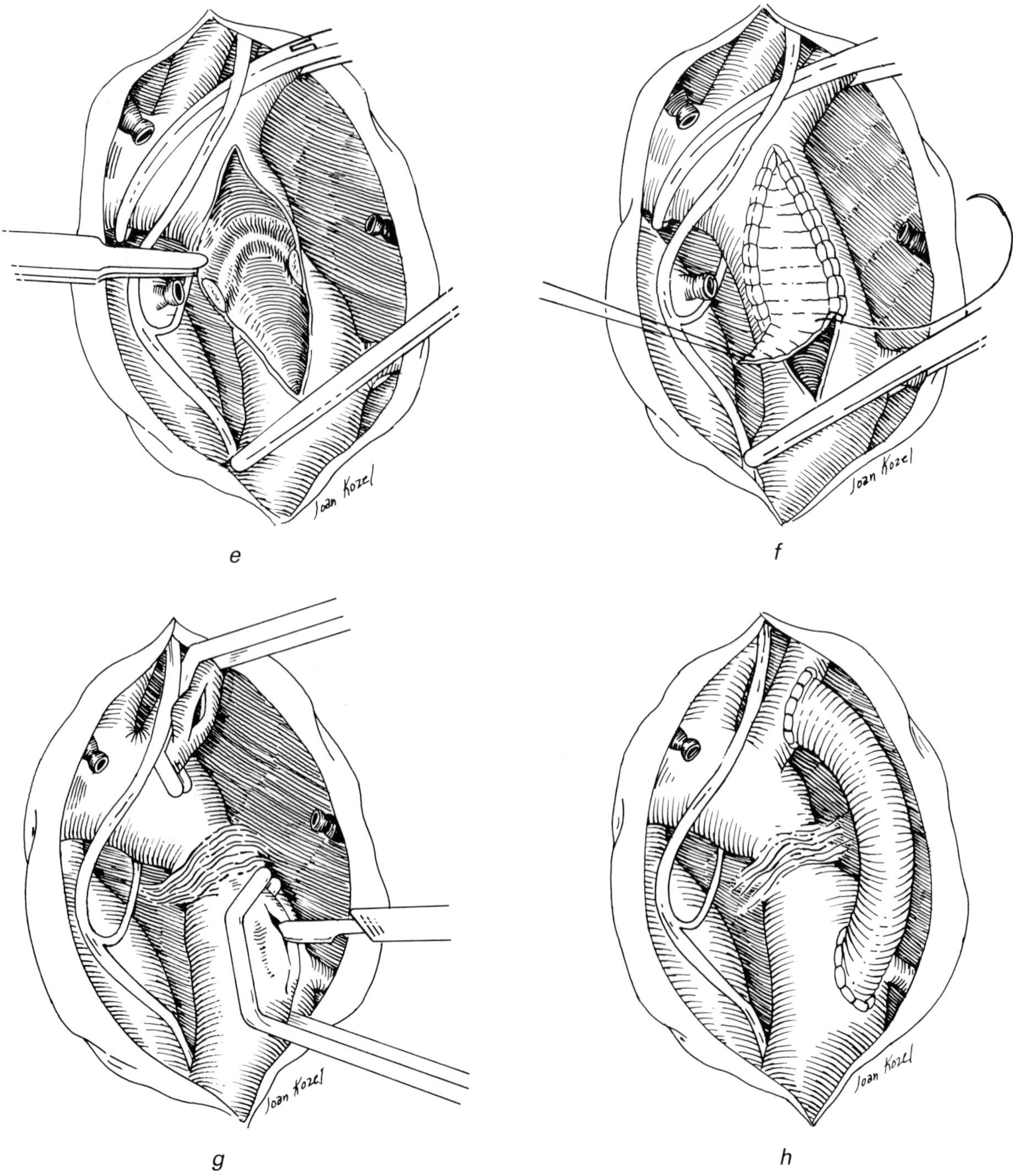

Fig. 45.3 Coarctation of the thoracic aorta. *a*, Anatomy as viewed through a left thoracotomy. *b*, Clamps applied, patent ductus arteriosus or ligamentum arteriosum divided. *c*, End-to-end anastomosis performed. *d*, Alternative repair by replacing long coarctation segment with Dacron graft. *e*, Coarctation in infant with aorta open. *f*, Patch aortoplasty performed over coarctation segment. g, Clamps placed and incisions made for subclavian to descending aorta jump graft in reoperation for coarctation. *h*, Bypass graft in place.

arteries, decreased blood pressure in the lower extremities and non-specific systolic murmur at the upper left sternal border and back. Sometimes, in older children or adults, pulsations or flow murmurs over dilated collateral vessels may be noted. Using the Doppler ultrasonic device, a pressure gradient in the infant or child of more than 20 mmHg between upper and lower extremities is virtually pathognomonic.

Chest radiography shows varying degrees of cardiac enlargement. Dilatation proximal to the coarctation combined with poststenotic dilatation may produce the 'reverse 3' sign of the upper left mediastinal shadow. Notching of the undersurface of ribs indicates enlarged intercostal arteries providing collateral flow.

The ECG may be normal or may show left ventricular hypertrophy. Echocardiography and cardiac catheterization are not necessary for the diagnosis of coarctation but are useful to exclude associated intracardiac defects. If the diagnosis is not obvious, an aortogram should be performed. Aortography also defines the length and degree of narrowing which is beneficial for intraoperative management with respect to the need for a tube graft.

Of all infants born with isolated coarctation of the aorta, approximately 15% require surgery in the first 12 months of life because of the development of severe congestive heart failure. Of those who survive the first year, approximately 20% die between the first and second decade of life and by the age of 50, 80% have expired. The optimal age for correction is in childhood between 2 and 4 years of age. Under the age of 2, there is a significantly increased incidence of re-coarctation and after the age of 6, there is increased probability of the persistence of hypertension with increasing age at the time of correction. When congestive heart failure is refractory to medical management in infancy, repair of the coarctation is indicated. There is controversy as to whether or not a subclavian flap procedure or primary end-to-end anastomosis allows for optimal growth. It is conceivable that with the performance of end-to-end anastomoses with polydioxinone suture, the incidence of re-coarctation may be significantly decreased. In larger children, over the age of 2, primary end-to-end correction is preferred, when appropriate. However, if a long segment coarctation is present, prosthetic graft insertion may be necessary. When coarctation is associated with other defects, in particular ventricular septal defect, the coarctation should be repaired first. If severe congestive heart failure persists, that defect could be repaired within three to four days as opposed to banding of the pulmonary artery. In a great majority of cases, repair of the coarctation will allow adequate medical management of the patients until they have reached a larger size. Since the longevity of patients with untreated significant coarctation is half that of the normal population, operation is recommended for older patients unless there are important contraindications.

The more common causes of death in isolated coarctation are congestive heart failure, bacterial endocarditis, aortic rupture, and rupture of intracranial aneurysms.

Treatment

In the critically ill infant, operation is urgent. The presence of severe failure dictates prompt surgical intervention unless it is relieved by a brief trial of medical therapy. Even so, there is no real advantage in postponing the surgery for several weeks or months.

Operative mortality is less than 2% in the older child or adult, but may approach 20% in the infant with severe congestive heart failure and associated defects. Postoperative complications include haemorrhage, infection, chylothorax, visceral arteritis with abdominal pain, and re-coarctation (most commonly in infants). Blood pressure usually returns to normal in a few weeks, but 5–10% of patients will remain hypertensive despite an adequate operation. The cause is not clear but may involve renal mechanisms through the renin–angiotensin system. Paraplegia is rare (0·4%) in first-time operations but is seen more frequently at reoperation.

Operation is performed through a left 3rd or 4th intercostal space posterolateral incision (*Fig.* 45.3*a*). The superior intercostal vein is divided, the aorta dissected proximal and distal to the narrowed segment to allow clamp placement, and the ductus or ligamentum arteriosum divided (*Fig.* 45.3*b*). If possible, the intercostal arteries are not divided. The recurrent laryngeal nerve is carefully preserved.

The exact technique depends on the age and anatomy of the patient. For a standard postductal short segment coarctation in the older child or adult, resection and end-to-end anastomosis by continuous suture is performed (*Fig.* 45.3*c*). In the younger patient the anterior wall of the suture line should be interrupted to allow growth and reduce the chance of recurrent coarctation. If the coarcted segment is long, a Dacron graft may be necessary (*Fig.* 45.3*d*). Aortoplasty with patch graft is useful in the long segment coarctation and in infants (*Fig.* 45.3*e,f*). Bypass graft from the left subclavian artery to the descending thoracic aorta may be useful for a recurrent coarctation with difficult adhesions (*Fig.* 45.3*g,h*). Others prefer the use of the subclavian artery as a patch.

AORTIC ARCH ANOMALIES

Abnormalities in this group include anomalies of position, course and composition of the aorta and its branches, abnormalities of length, size or continuity of the aorta, and anomalies of the pulmonary artery system. Although the number of distinct abnormalities is large, those requiring surgical intervention are few. Most lesions are asymptomatic and are merely anatomical curiosities. The three vascular rings requiring surgical intervention due to oesophageal or tracheal compression are: double aortic arch, right aortic arch with left ligamentum arteriosum, and left aortic arch with retro-oesophageal subclavian artery. Aortic arch anomalies are rare and represent only 1–2% of congenital heart disease.

Anatomy and Physiology

The commonest aortic arch anomaly to cause symptoms is double aortic arch (*Fig.* 45.4*a*). It occurs when neither of the embryological aortic arches regresses. The ascending aorta, therefore, bifurcates with usually a smaller arch to the left and anteriorly and a larger arch to the right and posterior to the trachea and oesophagus. These limbs then rejoin to form the descending aorta producing a ring around the oesophagus and trachea. With right aortic arch and left ligamentum arteriosum, the aorta passes to the right of the trachea and oesophagus while the ligamentum passes to the left behind the trachea and oesophagus to join the pulmonary artery anteriorly thus completing the vascular ring (*Fig.* 45.4*b*). A retro-oesophageal right subclavian artery does not truly constitute a vascular ring (*Fig.* 45.4*c*). In this lesion the right subclavian artery arises as a separate last branch off the arch of the aorta. It passes behind the oesophagus and proceeds to the right and superiorly. Although many authors feel this lesion may cause symptoms due to posterior impingement on the oesophagus, others feel that this anomaly is almost never a cause for symptoms.

Diagnosis

These patients present with recurring symptoms of tracheal or oesophageal obstruction or both. A history of repeated aspiration pneumonia, respiratory distress following eating or drinking, persistent or recurring stridor, or relief from symptoms by hyperextension of the head is characteristic. Symptoms usually start in infancy or early childhood. The indication for operation is the presence of symptoms.

The diagnosis can usually be made by the combination of

history, chest radiography and barium swallow. By outlining the direction and level of compression of the oesophagus most anomalies can be diagnosed. Although frequently performed, there is no absolute necessity for aortography or bronchography. Only those patients with significant symptomatology should undergo surgery. This is particularly true in the first six months of life. After that time, symptoms are usually less severe and may disappear with time.

Treatment

There is agreement that the infant with severe symptoms of respiratory or oesophageal compression and a double aortic arch benefits from interruption of the arch. This is accomplished usually through a left 4th interspace posterolateral incision since the left anterior arch is usually diminutive in size. The recurrent laryngeal nerve should be identified, the ligamentum arteriosum divided, and the descending thoracic aorta, left and right aortic arches and arch branches identified. Vascular clamps may be applied to the left arch which is then divided and the ends oversewn. The oesophagus and trachea should be dissected free from surrounding tissue and the ends of the arch attached to surrounding tissues so as to provide maximum decompression of the trachea and oesophagus. Even so, symptoms may persist for weeks to months following operation owing to the compression changes in the underlying trachea and oesophagus.

With a right arch, left ligamentum arteriosum, and retro-oesophageal left subclavian artery, the ligamentum is divided as well as the retro-oesophageal left subclavian artery. The artery is divided at the level of the aortic arch. Again the trachea and oesophagus should be dissected free from surrounding structures.

If it is clear that a retro-oesophageal right subclavian artery is causing symptoms of compression, division of this vessel is probably indicated. The approach is similar to those described above. Operative mortality is low (less than 10%). However, after surgery, symptoms may persist with slow improvement over several months. Ultimately, relief of symptoms is usually complete.

PULMONARY STENOSIS

Obstruction to outflow from the right side of the heart may occur at the ventricular level, the infundibular level, the valvular level or the pulmonary artery level. The more complicated lesions such as pulmonary atresia, primary infundibular stenosis, the 'two-chambered' right ventricle and supravalvular pulmonary arterial stenosis will not be dealt with in this chapter. The commonest lesion is pulmonary valvular stenosis with intact ventricular septum. It comprises 8–10% of all congenital cardiac defects. Today, with safe cardiopulmonary bypass, valvular pulmonary stenosis is repaired under direct vision or by percutaneous transvenous balloon dilatation.

Anatomy and Physiology

Pulmonary valvular stenosis represents a continuum of malformations of the pulmonary valve. This varies from mild fusion of the valve leaflets to a conical funnel-shaped valve with only primitive commissures. The valve opening, therefore, may be as small as 1 or 2 mm or nearly normal. In addition, there may be secondary hypertrophy of the right ventricular outflow tract in the infundibular region as well as dilatation of the proximal main pulmonary artery. The valve ring itself is adequate in size. Poststenotic dilatation of the pulmonary artery is almost always present but is not necessarily related to the degree of valvular stenosis.

Physiologically, pulmonary stenosis results in high pressures in the right ventricle and secondary hypertrophy of the right ventricular muscle mass. Since there is no communication through the ventricular septum, the pressure in the right ventricle may equal or exceed that of the left ventricle. Because of the increased pressure load on the right ventricle, right-sided heart failure may eventually occur.

Diagnosis

If the pressure in the right ventricle is less than 13·3 kPa (100 mmHg), patients are usually asymptomatic. The lesion is picked up by the presence of a heart murmur. With severe stenosis symptoms may vary from mild exertional dyspnoea to frank heart failure. Physical examination may reveal evidence of right ventricular enlargement. A prominent right ventricular impulse on palpation accompanied by a thrill may be found. Auscultation reveals a systolic ejection murmur loudest in the 2nd left intercostal space near the sternal border. This may be accompanied by an ejection systolic click. Prominent venous pulsations in the neck may be observed. Cyanosis is absent except in severe stenosis with an atrial communication.

Radiological examination reveals evidence of right ventricular enlargement. The most striking finding is enlargement of the main pulmonary artery due to poststenotic dilatation. In addition, right atrial enlargement may be seen in half the cases. Pulmonary vascularity is usually normal. It may be diminished if significant right-to-left atrial shunting is present.

The ECG reveals right atrial enlargement characterized by peaked P waves, right ventricular hypertrophy, sometimes accompanied by a 'strain' pattern, and right axis deviation.

M-mode echocardiography is of limited value both in establishing the diagnosis and in determining the severity of obstruction.

Cardiac catheterization is necessary to establish a definitive diagnosis, determine the severity of obstruction, and rule out associated anomalies. A resting peak systolic pressure of over 4 kPa (30 mmHg) in the right ventricle and a systolic gradient greater than 2 kPa (15 mmHg) between the pulmonary artery and right ventricle is abnormal. By a combination of right ventricular angiography and pressure recording while withdrawing the catheter from the pulmonary artery peripherally to the right ventricle proximally, the exact site of obstruction can be identified. During angiography, the infundibulum can be observed to see if it relaxes during diastole. If it does not, some element of infundibular obstruction is present and may have to be dealt with at operation. If relaxation occurs, the infundibular hypertrophy is considered to be compensatory to the pulmonary valvular obstruction and will resolve after relief of the valvular obstruction. The severity of obstruction is often reflected by the right ventricular systolic pressure: right ventricular pressure less than 6·65 kPa (50 mmHg) is mild, right ventricular pressure between 6·65 kPa (50 mmHg) and the left ventricular pressure is moderate, and right ventricular pressure greater than that of the left ventricle is severe.

Neonates who become symptomatic with severe pulmonary stenosis have a 14% death rate within one month without surgery. Infants who have moderate pulmonary stenosis are likely to have progression of the pulmonary stenosis to severe after the age of 2. Mild pulmonary stenosis after the age of 2 is much less likely to progress. However, when

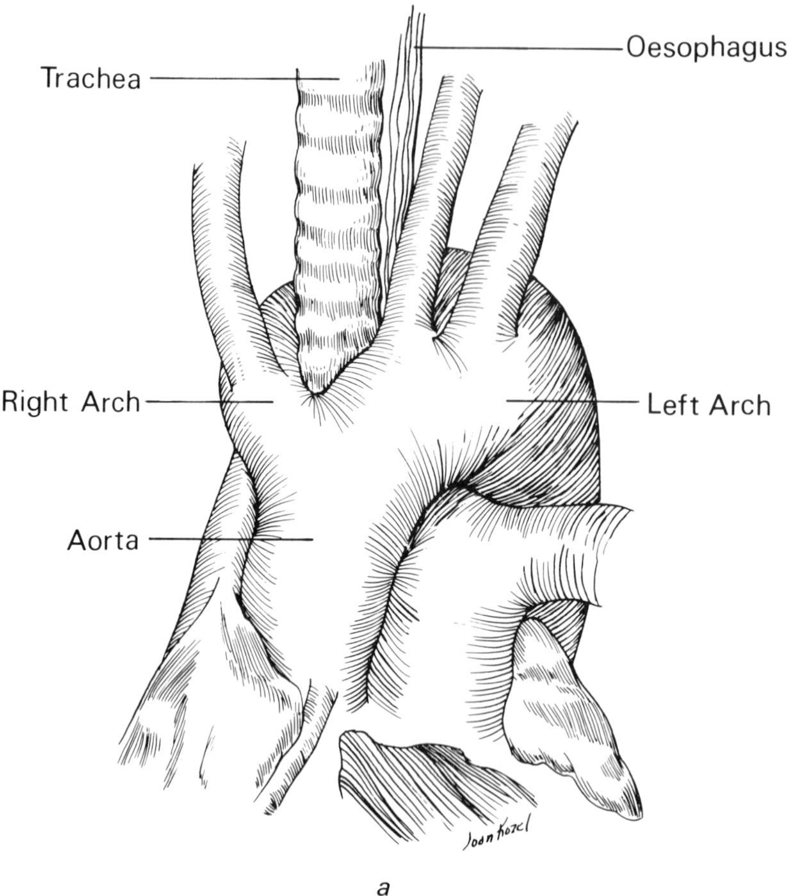

Trachea
Oesophagus
Right Arch
Left Arch
Aorta
Joan Kozel

a

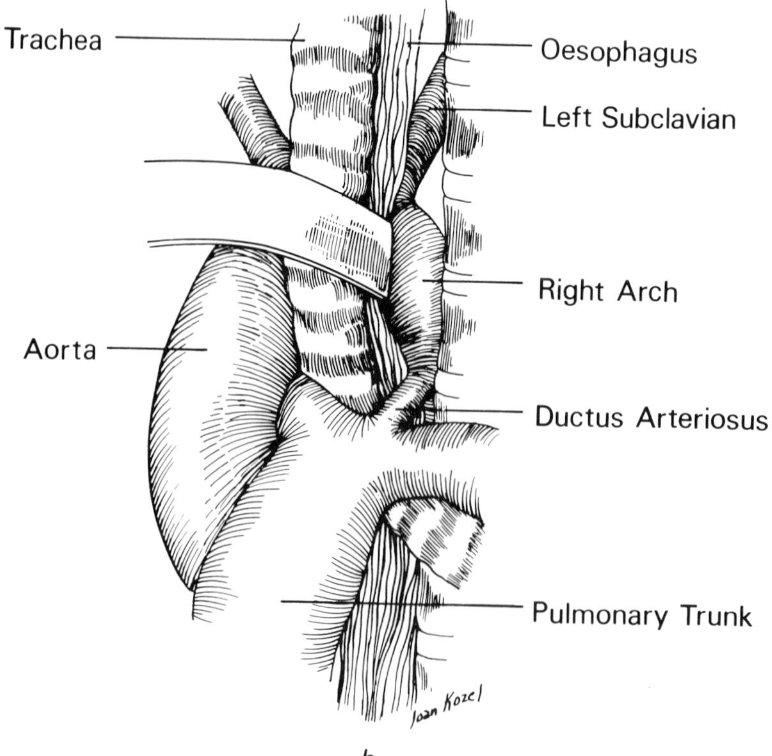

Trachea
Oesophagus
Left Subclavian
Right Arch
Aorta
Ductus Arteriosus
Pulmonary Trunk
Joan Kozel

b

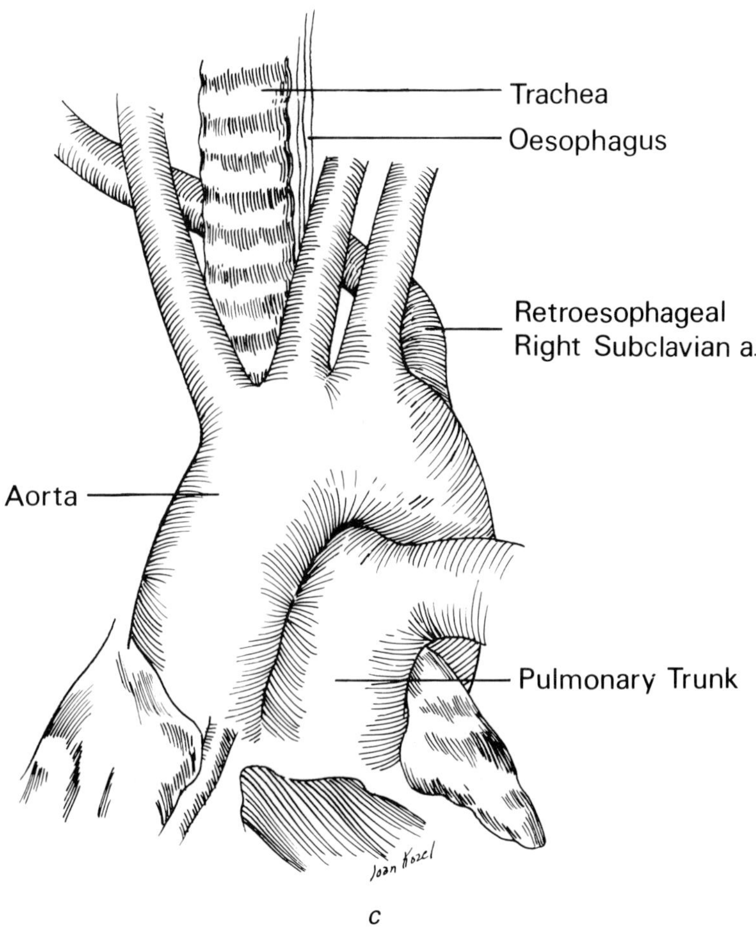

Fig. 45.4 Aortic arch anomalies. *a*, Double aortic arch. *b*, Right aortic arch with left ductus arteriosus. *c*, Retro-oesophageal right subclavian artery.

symptoms are present or in the case of severe stenosis, as based on the above criteria, surgery is indicated.

Treatment

Infants with heart failure or with suprasystemic pressures in the right ventricle require immediate valvotomy. Patients with mild stenosis usually do not require an operation. Moderate stenosis in an asymptomatic individual with no signs of right ventricular enlargement or failure can be followed by means of serial ECGs and chest radiographs. With the development of right ventricular hypertrophy or heart failure, operation should be performed.

Pulmonary valvotomy is performed through a midline sternotomy incision using cardiopulmonary bypass. The pulmonary artery is opened and the valve incised along the lines of its commissures to the annulus (*Fig.* 45.5). The infundibular area should be evaluated to ensure that there is no significant infundibular obstruction. Occasionally, when significant annular stenosis occurs, an outflow patch will be necessary. Pulmonary insufficiency is well tolerated as long as pulmonary artery pressure is normal. The surgeon, therefore, should ensure that there is an adequate opening regardless of the production of pulmonary insufficiency.

When surgery is necessitated in the first six months of life, the mortality has been reported to range between 10 and 50%. After the age of 1 year, mortality is much lower and is approximately equal to the risk of cardiopulmonary bypass.

ATRIAL SEPTAL DEFECT

The first heart defect to be repaired using cardiopulmonary bypass was an atrial septal defect performed by Gibbon in 1952 on Cecilia Bavolik. Cardiopulmonary bypass allows adequate visualization and good repair of the defect, including the more complex forms. Atrial septal defects account for about 7% of congenital heart disease.

Anatomy and Physiology

The three most common anatomical variants of atrial septal defect are: ostium secundum, ostium primum and sinus venosus. Ostium primum defects are a form of endocardial cushion defect and will be discussed later. The ostium secundum septal defect is an elliptical hole between the right and left atrium, occurring usually at the site of the foramen ovale in the midportion of the atrial septum. Sinus venosus defects occur high in the atrial septum near the orifice of the superior vena cava and are frequently accompanied by anomalous drainage of the right upper lobe pulmonary veins into the superior vena cava close to the right atrium. Ostium

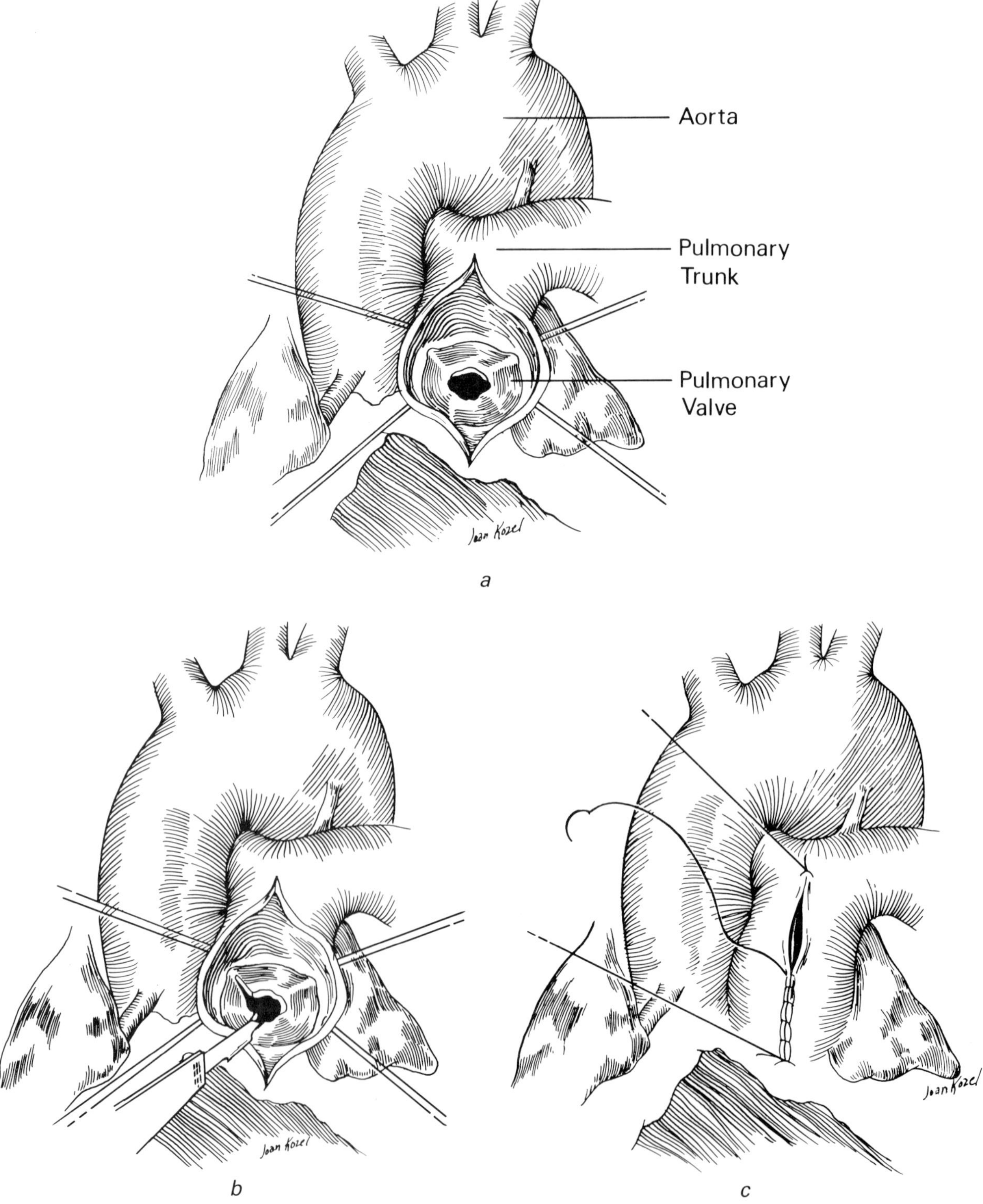

Fig. 45.5 Pulmonary stenosis. *a*, Anatomy. *b*, Pulmonary artery opened and pulmonary valve incised. *c*, Pulmonary artery closed with a running suture.

secundum defects represent failure of the septum secundum to close the ostium secundum in the region of the foramen ovale. This defect can be quite large and encompasses nearly the entire postero-inferior margin of the atrial septum. Sinus venosus defects represent a failure of fusion of the left valve of the sinus venosus with the posterosuperior portion of the atrial septum.

The physiological outcome of atrial septal defects is a left-to-right shunt. The direction and magnitude of the shunt are dependent on the relative pressures in the right and left atria which, in turn, are dependent on the compliances of their respective ventricles. The normally greater compliance of the right ventricle as compared to that of the left, favours left-to-right shunting across the defect. In addition, a small amount of right-to-left shunting may also occur. Despite a large pulmonary blood flow, e.g., three or four times systemic blood flow, pulmonary resistance usually remains low or normal in children. Occasionally, in adults, increased pulmonary resistance may occur, resulting in severe pulmonary hypertension and a net right-to-left shunt, frequently indicating irreversible arteriolar changes.

Diagnosis

Although patients occasionally present with symptoms of dyspnoea, the majority are asymptomatic at the time that the defect is detected. Characteristically, there is fixed splitting of the second heart sound due to delayed emptying of the right ventricle. Increased flow across the pulmonary valve produces a systolic murmur along the left sternal border.

The electrocardiogram shows evidence of right atrial enlargement and right ventricular hypertrophy. The chest radiograph also shows evidence of enlarged right atrium and right ventricle. In addition, the pulmonary artery is enlarged and there are increased pulmonary vascular markings. The left atrium is usually not enlarged, in contrast to other left-to-right shunts (PDA, VSD). The echocardiogram shows evidence of right ventricular volume overload characterized by an enlarged right ventricular end-diastolic dimension and paradoxical septal motion.

Cardiac catheterization is necessary for a definitive diagnosis of atrial septal defect, to define its anatomy, to quantify the shunt and to rule out associated lesions. The position of the catheter as it passes from the right atrium to the left atrium may suggest the type of defect. If the catheter passes in the midatrium it is most likely a secundum defect; if it passes low in the atrium, it raises the possibility of a primum atrial septal defect. The pressures in the right and left heart are usually normal. With a large atrial septal defect the left atrial and right atrial pressures are equal. Dye dilution and oxygen saturations show evidence of a predominantly left-to-right shunt and can be used to quantify the shunt. A pulmonary or left atrial angiocardiogram will demonstrate shunting of contrast into the right atrium and any coexistent anomalous pulmonary veins. In the case of sinus venosus defects, the lower portion of the superior vena cava also becomes opacified following contrast injection into the pulmonary artery because of the partial anomalous pulmonary venous return. A left ventricular injection should be performed to rule out an associated ventricular septal defect or an endocardial cushion defect with its characteristic 'gooseneck' deformity of the left ventricular outflow tract.

Untreated, the early prognosis is good with less than 1% dying in the first year. However, in the ensuing decades, mortality is increased so that by the age of 40, less than 50% are alive. The usual cause of death is progressive congestive heart failure with or without irreversible pulmonary vascular disease. Spontaneous closure may occur with atrial septal defect and is most likely to occur in the first year of life. Subsequent to the first year, spontaneous closure is quite rare. When closure does occur, it appears to be more common in smaller defects rather than the larger ones.

Treatment

If a patient is asymptomatic the definitive repair can usually be deferred until the age of 3–6 years. Occasionally, in a younger child with failure to grow and progressive heart failure, earlier intervention is necessary. In the older child or adult, the atrial septal defect should be repaired when diagnosed. Untreated, this lesion may eventually result in pulmonary hypertension, supraventricular arrhythmias, heart failure and a higher operative risk. If the pulmonary hypertension is severe, to the extent that a large right-to-left shunt exists, repair is contraindicated.

The mortality rate for repair of an atrial septal defect of the secundum or sinus venosus type is less than 1%. In the older patient with some degree of pulmonary hypertension this risk is increased.

During total cardiopulmonary bypass an incision is made in the right atrium posteriorly. The defect is visualized and the anatomy defined (*Fig.* 45.6*a*). If small, and especially in children, the defect can usually be repaired by primary suture (*Fig.* 45.6*b*). If the defect is large, especially in adults, a patch may be necessary. In sinus venosus defects with anomalous pulmonary venous drainage, a patch is used to close the defect and reroute the pulmonary venous return into the left atrium (*Fig.* 45.6*c*,*d*). Occasionally, due to narrowing of the superior vena cava, an additional patch will be necessary on the right atrial caval junction in order to reduce this narrowing. Care should be taken in placing any sutures in the region between the coronary sinus and tricuspid valve (the area of the AV node) and at the superior anterior rim of the defect where the aortic valve may be found. It is safe to repair a simple secundum atrial septal defect under normothermia with the heart fibrillated, although standard anoxic techniques are frequently used.

Definitive repair of atrial septal defect in the first few years of life should produce a life expectancy comparable to that of the matched general population. However, in older patients, repair of atrial septal defect usually does not result in a life expectancy equal to the general population. This is particularly true in repair of atrial septal defects in patients aged 60 years or older.

VENTRICULAR SEPTAL DEFECTS

Currently these defects are repaired using cardiopulmonary bypass. Ventricular septal defect as an isolated lesion comprises about 15% of congenital heart disease.

Anatomy and Physiology

Ventricular septal defects may be categorized into four variants depending on their anatomical location (*Fig.* 45.7*a*). The supracristal ventricular septal defect occurs between the crista supraventricularis and the pulmonary valve. The infracristal ventricular septal defect located just caudal to the crista supraventricularis comprises 80% of ventricular septal defects seen at operation. The atrioventricular canal type of ventricular septal defect occurs somewhat more posteriorly and inferiorly than the infracristal variety. The fourth type of ventricular septal defect is the muscular variety. This may consist of multiple defects anywhere in the muscular portion of the ventricular septum.

The major physiological derangement in isolated ventricular septal defect is shunting of blood from the left to the right ventricle. The degree of this shunt is directly related to the size of the defect. When the defect is large the degree of flow through the ventricular septal defect is determined by the relative resistances of the pulmonary and systemic circulation. If a large defect is allowed to continue, pulmonary hypertension may eventually occur with pulmonary vascular changes. This may result in reversal of the direction of the shunt. Once a right-to-left shunt occurs in uncomplicated ventricular septal defect (Eisenmenger's complex) closure of the ventricular septal defect is contraindicated. A persistent ventricular septal defect may be complicated by the development of infective endocarditis. Supracristal or infracristal ventricular septal defects may also be complicated by prolapse of the aortic valve leading to progressive aortic regurgitation.

Diagnosis

The symptoms with which a patient presents are determined by the size of the shunt, the state of the pulmonary vascular bed and the changes that occur in these two parameters with time. Patients with small defects are usually asymptomatic. In the first year of life, symptoms from left ventricular failure such as tachypnoea, poor feeding and easy fatigability and recurrent pulmonary infections are usually secondary to large left-to-right shunts. These usually appear after the early months of life as pulmonary vascular resistance falls and the shunt increases. With appropriate medical management, the failure can usually be controlled and elective repair then performed at a later date. It is particularly desirable to manage infants with ventricular septal defects medically because of the relatively high spontaneous closure rate. For example, ventricular septal defects in children 1 month of age or less have an 80% probability of closing. This decreases to 50% by 6 months of age and 25% by 1 year of age. After 6 years of age, there is a very low probability of spontaneous closure. However, when medical management does not suffice, primary repair should be undertaken at any age except in the case of multiple ventricular septal defects for which pulmonary artery banding is indicated in the age group of 6 months or less. Of those infants with large ventricular septal defects that are not managed surgically, approximately 9% die in the first year. The death rate then stabilizes until the second and third decades when it increases again. At that point, Eisenmenger's syndrome develops and 50% have usually succumbed by the age of 35. The usual cause of death is congestive heart failure or recurrent pulmonary infections. Occasionally the cardiac failure is refractory and surgical intervention is necessary in infancy. Children in the pre-school age may remain asymptomatic or present with mild to moderate exertional dyspnoea and tiredness. The typical physical findings are: a palpable thrill and a loud pansystolic murmur along the left sternal border with maximal intensity in the 3rd or 4th interspace, a split second heart sound with accentuated pulmonary component if the pulmonary artery pressure is elevated, and a diastolic flow murmur at the apex if the shunt flow is larger, resulting in a pulmonary-to-systemic flow ratio greater than 1:7–2:1.

The ECG shows evidence of left or combined ventricular hypertrophy in the presence of a large left-to-right shunt with normal pulmonary artery pressures. If pulmonary hypertension is present, the right ventricular hypertrophy predominates. The chest radiograph shows enlargement of the left atrium and left ventricle, prominence of the main pulmonary artery, and increased pulmonary vascularity. Two-dimensional echocardiography may identify moderate or large ventricular septal defects; however, its reliability for quantitating the defect size is still open to question.

Cardiac catheterization is useful in detecting associated anomalies and in defining the location and size of the ventricular septal defect, and the degree of shunt. Oxygen saturations and dye dilution curves detect and quantitate the shunt. Pulmonary artery pressures are documented, and the ratio of pulmonary to systemic vascular resistance is calculated. A pulmonary to systemic vascular resistance ratio greater than 0·70 indicates increased operative mortality and likelihood that the pulmonary hypertension may persist.

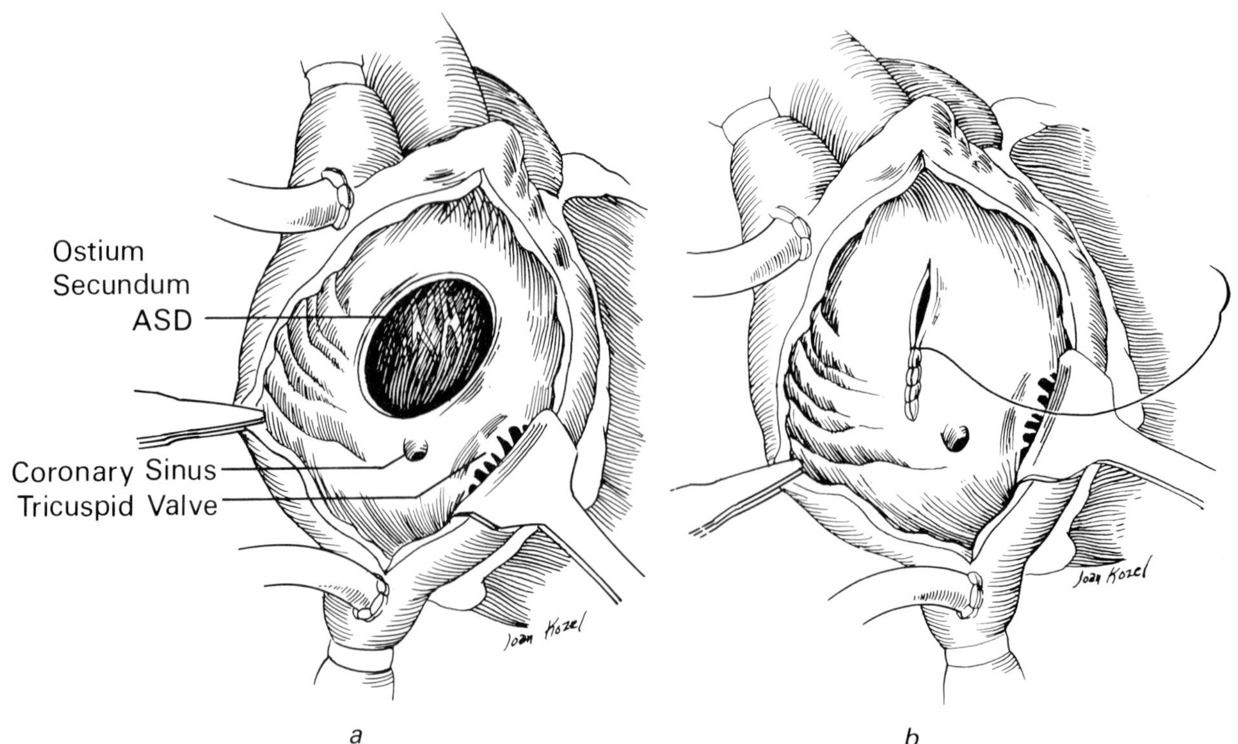

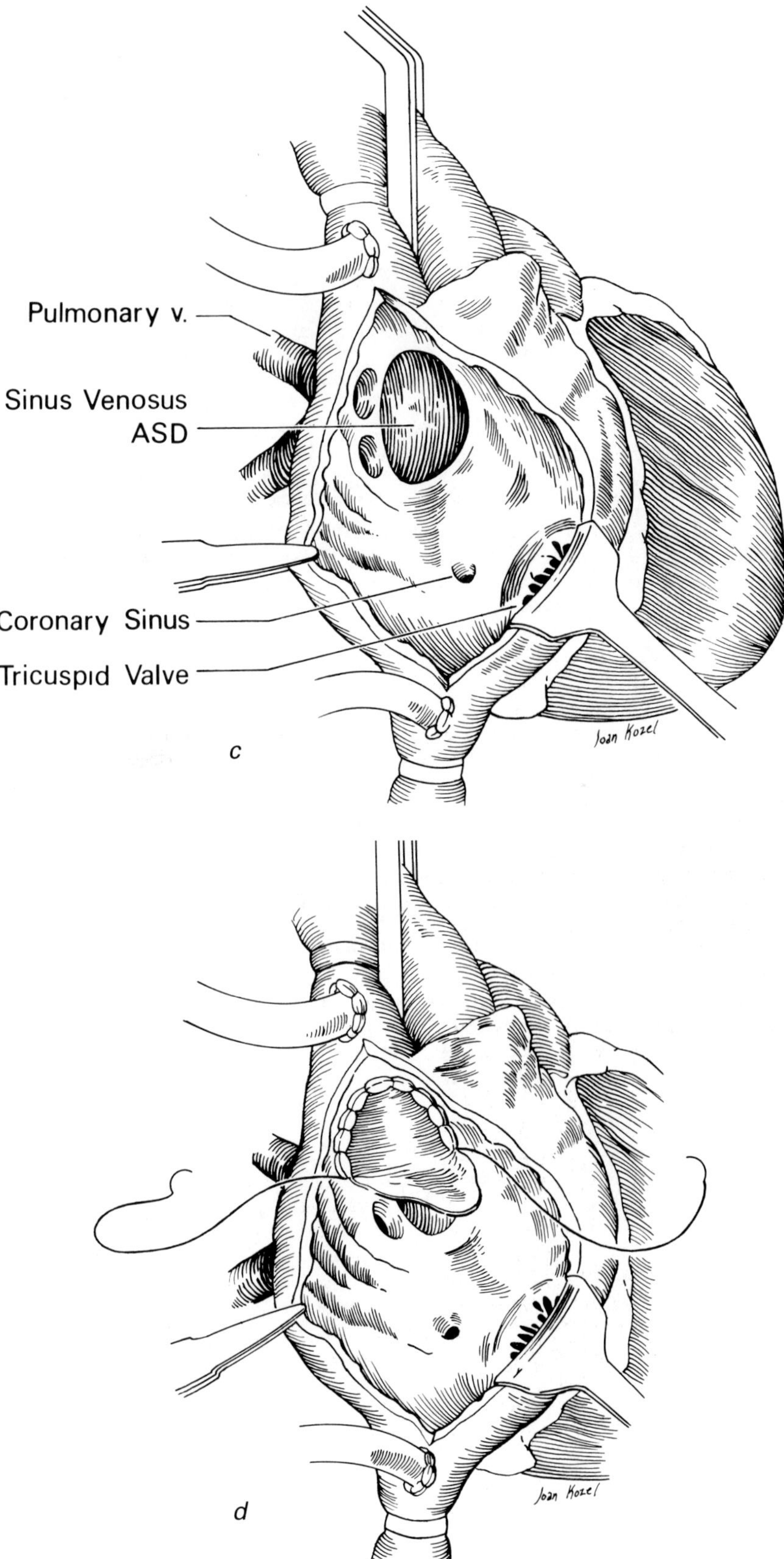

Fig. 45.6 Atrial septal defects. *a*, Anatomy of secundum atrial septal defect. *b*, Secundum atrial septal defect being repaired with a running suture. *c*, Anatomy of sinus venosus atrial septal defect. *d*, Patch closure of sinus venosus atrial septal defect redirecting pulmonary venous flow to the left atrium.

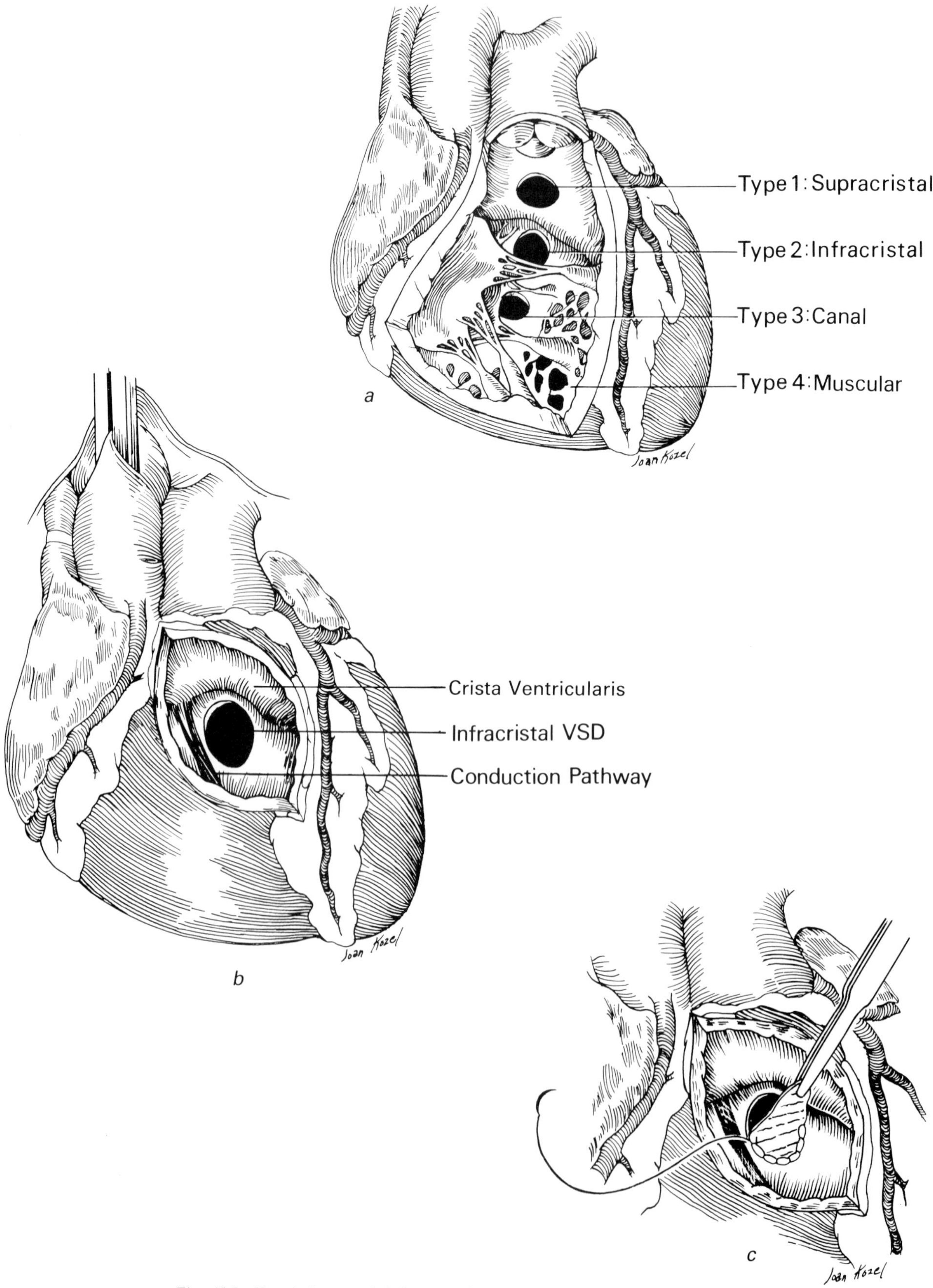

Fig. 45.7 Ventricular septal defects. *a*, Anatomical classification of ventricular septal defects. *b*, Infracristal ventricular septal defect anatomy demonstrating the conduction pathway. *c*, Patch closure of infracristal ventricular septal defect.

Treatment

Small defects with a pulmonary-to-systemic flow ratio of 1·5:1 or less in a small child may not require surgery. There is a good chance that these defects will become smaller or may even close spontaneously. The risk of pulmonary hypertension is nil. A moderate defect with a large left-to-right shunt in a stable infant should also be followed medically until 2–3 years of age at which time it may be corrected electively after a repeat catheterization. A large defect in an infant with refractory cardiac failure needs urgent total corrective surgery. Pulmonary banding is performed only when the defects are multiple and of the muscular type. Such defects are difficult to close in small babies. If the septal defect is accompanied by markedly elevated pulmonary vascular resistance, surgical correction is contraindicated.

A mortality of less than 2% is expected with correction of a ventricular septal defect. In the infant with severe failure this mortality may approach 10%. Permanent heart block can occur following closure of a ventricular septal defect but usually has an incidence of less than 1·0%. Nevertheless, it is a potential complication especially in atrioventricular canal types of defects. Persistent heart block for 2 weeks or more following surgery may necessitate placement of a permanent pacemaker.

The operation is performed with the patient on total cardiopulmonary bypass (*Fig.* 45.7*b*). The defect may be approached through a ventriculotomy with interrupted or continuous sutures to effect patch closure of the defect (*Fig.* 45.7*c*). Alternatively, an incision is made through the right atrium and repair carried out through the tricuspid valve, usually with continuous polypropylene sutures securing a prosthetic patch. It is particularly important to avoid placing sutures deeply in the posterior and inferior rim of the defect in order to avoid the atrioventricular conduction system.

ATRIOVENTRICULAR CANAL

Anatomy and Physiology

Atrioventricular canal anomalies represent a continuum of defects. In its simplest form, this is composed of an atrial septal defect lying low in the atrial septum with or without a cleft in the anterior leaflet of the mitral valve (*Fig.* 45.8). This complex is known as ostium primum atrial septal defect or partial atrioventricular canal. Its repair is relatively straightforward. In its most complicated form, this anomaly is comprised of a low lying atrial septal defect that is confluent with a ventricular septal defect, and clefts and deformity of the atrioventricular valves. In complete atrioventricular canal defects the left-sided atrioventricular valve consists of three leaflets: left superior, left lateral and left inferior leaflets. The medial aspects of the left superior and left inferior leaflets are adjacent to the interventricular

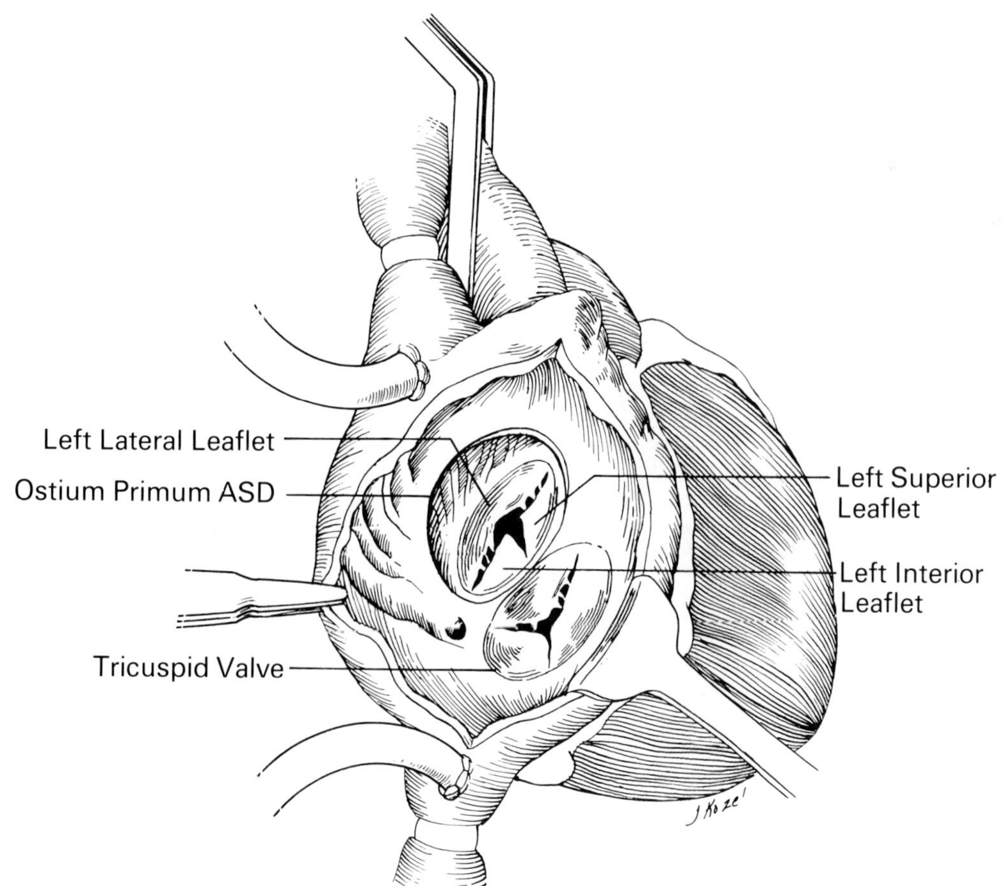

Fig. 45.8 Incomplete atrioventricular canal or ostium primum atrial septal defect composed of a low-lying atrial septal defect and cleft of the anterior leaflet of the mitral valve.

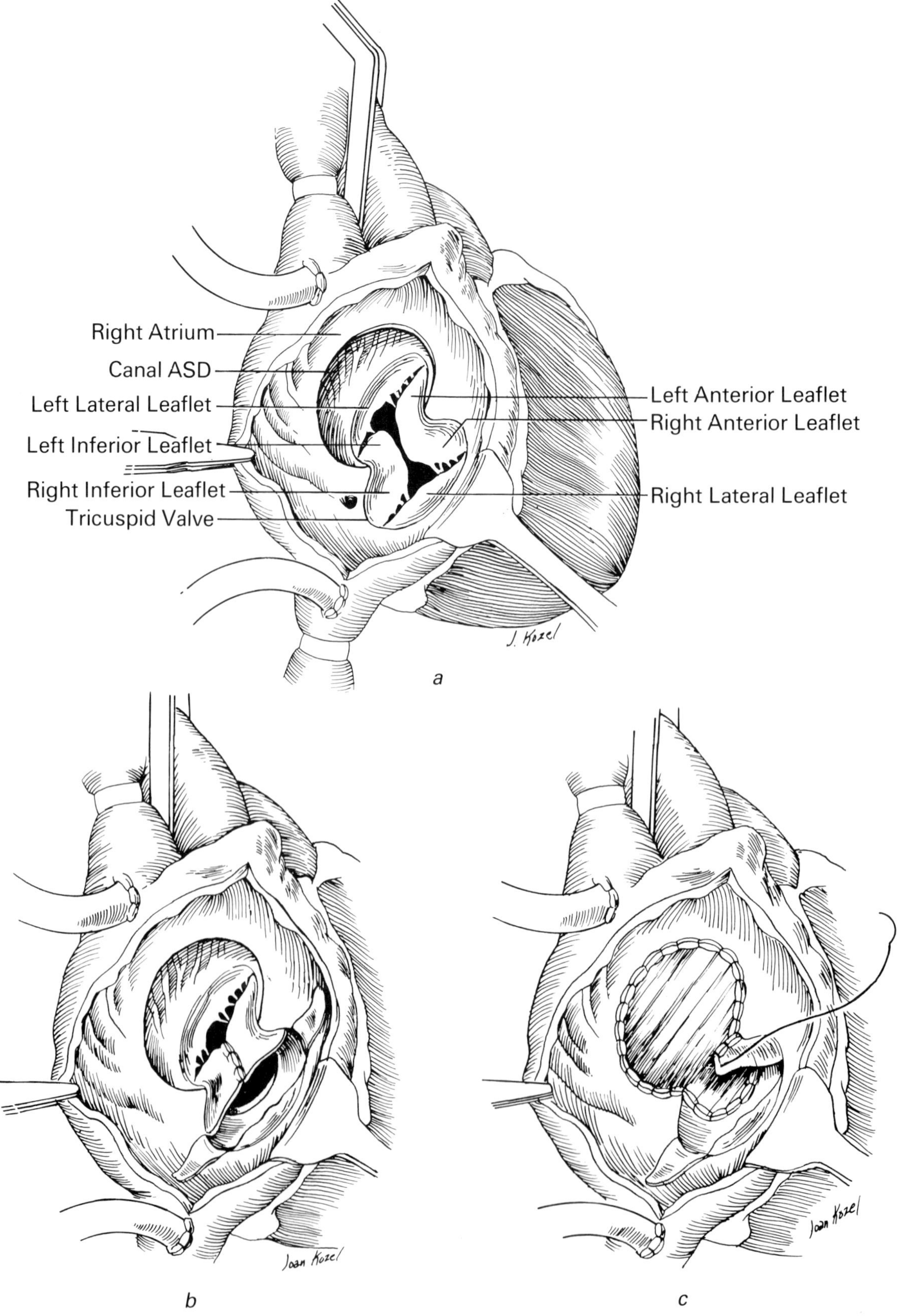

Fig. 45.9 Complete atrioventricular canal. *a*, Anatomy of the complete atrioventricular canal type three. Repair of complete atrioventricular canal: *b*, The common leaflet is divided and the mitral portion reconstructed. *c*, A patch closing the ventricular and atrial septal defects is in place and the anterior portion of the tricuspid valve leaflet is being sutured to the patch at the appropriate level.

septum. The right atrioventricular valve, likewise, has three corresponding leaflets: right superior, right lateral and right inferior leaflets (*Fig.* 45.9*a*). The variations in complete atrioventricular canal are dependent upon the degree of overriding of the left superior leaflet over the interventricular crest. When there is no overriding the defect has been characterized as Rastelli Type A. With an intermediate degree of overriding, the chordae tendineae from the left superior leaflet attach to papillary muscles on the right side of the heart, which corresponds with Rastelli Type B. With more severe overriding, of the left superior leaflet, there are no chordae tendineae attached to the crest of the septum corresponding to Rastelli Type C (*Figs.* 45.8 and 45.9*a*,*b*,*c*). Patients with a partial atrioventricular canal without significant mitral regurgitation have a natural history similar to that for secundum atrial septal defects. However, with increasing degrees of mitral regurgitation, the mortality in infancy may be elevated to 20% without surgical correction. With complete atrioventricular canal and, in particular, with significant degrees of mitral regurgitation, there is an 80% mortality by age 2 years. The mode of death is usually congestive heart failure, with or without superimposed pulmonary infections. Pulmonary vascular disease occurs in 90% of patients by one year with complete atrioventricular canal.

The physiology of these defects is that of a combination of left-to-right shunting, mitral insufficiency and varying degrees of pulmonary hypertension. There is left-to-right shunting of blood through the atrial septal defect, and, in complete atrioventricular canal, through the ventricular septal defect as well. Severe pulmonary hypertension with elevated pulmonary vascular resistance is usually present in complete common atrioventricular canal. Pulmonary vascular obstructions tends to occur fairly rapidly after the first or second year. Occasionally, the right ventricle or left ventricle may be hypoplastic.

Diagnosis

The ECG is diagnostic. Left axis deviation with a right bundle-branch block pattern, and a vectorcardiogram revealing a counterclockwise loop in the frontal plane strongly suggest atrioventricular canal anomalies. In addition, first-degree heart block is common. The chest radiograph shows right atrial and biventricular enlargement with a prominent pulmonary artery and increased pulmonary vascularity. The echocardiogram reveals apparent extension of the anterior leaflet of the mitral valve through the plane of the ventricular septum and disappearance of large portions of the ventricular septum accompanied by what appears to be a single large atrioventricular valve. Cardiac catheterization with complete atrioventricular canal usually shows systemic pressures in the pulmonary artery with evidence for left-to-right and right-to-left shunting at the atrial and/or ventricular levels. A left ventriculogram reveals mitral regurgitation and the characteristic deformity of the left ventricular outflow tract giving the appearance of a 'gooseneck'.

Treatment

The operative mortality and results of surgical correction of ostium primum atrial septal defect are generally similar to those of secundum atrial septal defects. Complete atrioventricular canal has a different surgical prognosis. Early attempts at repairing complete atrioventricular canal carried a mortality of 50% or higher. However, recent series in children over 2 years of age show a mortality of less than 10%. In the absence of irreversible pulmonary vascular changes complete repair should be accomplished as soon as possible. Pulmonary artery banding has been attempted to reduce the pulmonary artery pressure and blood flow in this lesion; however, the results have been variable owing to its variable effects on the mitral regurgitation.

Operation is performed utilizing total cardiopulmonary bypass with exposure of the defect through a right atriotomy (*Fig.* 45.9*a*). A patch is sutured to the ventricular septum attempting to avoid the area of the atrioventricular node. The left superior leaflet is divided forming a mitral and a tricuspid portion. Extra valve substance is left on the mitral side of the leaflet (*Fig.* 45.9*b*). The cleft is repaired commonly with Teflon or pericardial-supported sutures, and the leaflet is reattached to the ventricular septal patch at the appropriate level. It should not be attached low near the rim of remaining ventricular septum since the normal level of attachment is higher. Some have advocated using a small strip of pericardium to buttress the closure of the cleft in the valve as well as its attachment to the septal patch. In a similar manner, the tricuspid leaflet is attached to the septal patch and the atrial portion of the patch sutured (*Fig.* 45.9*c*). An alternative approach is to use a prosthetic patch to close the ventricular septal defect with attachment of the patch to the bridging left superior leaflet. A separate patch, preferably of pericardium, is then utilized to close the atrial septal defect. In the infant, valve replacement with a prosthetic valve is undesirable. In the older child with a deficiency of mitral valve leaflet tissue, a prosthetic valve should be used only when absolutely necessary. The results of concomitant prosthetic valve replacement of the mitral valve with this lesion have thus far been discouraging. In addition to the usual complications of cardiopulmonary bypass in an infant, this lesion carries an increased risk of heart block and peristent mitral regurgitation.

CONGENITAL ANOMALIES OF THE CORONARY ARTERIES

The two anomalies to be discussed in this section are anomalous origin of the left coronary artery from the pulmonary artery and congenital coronary artery aneurysms and fistulas. Anomalous origin of the left coronary artery from the pulmonary artery was first reported by Abbott in 1908. The clinical syndrome was described by Bland in 1933 and has subsequently been referred to as the Bland–White–Garland syndrome. Surgical therapy for this lesion included pericardial poudrage and ligation of the coronary artery at its origin from the pulmonary trunk. Since 1964, however, some methods for arterial revascularization of the coronary artery have been advocated. Either saphenous vein bypass grafting or subclavian artery anastomosis has been performed. We advocate the latter for its growth potential.

Since the widespread use of cardiopulmonary bypass, the most frequent technique for repair includes ligation of the fistula with repair of the aneurysm or saphenous vein bypass grafting of the distal vessel.

Anatomy and Physiology

Anomalous origin of the left coronary artery from the pulmonary artery results in myocardial ischaemia or infarction after birth. Also, mitral regurgitation is frequent because of papillary muscle ischaemia and left ventricular dilatation. If pulmonary hypertension is present for a while, the high pulmonary artery pressure is transmitted to the left coronary artery. This promotes perfusion of the left ventricular myocardium and at the same time allows for the development of collateral circulation from the right coronary artery. If this situation does not occur, death in early infancy from myocardial infarction and/or heart failure is the rule. In those that survive and continue to have low pressures in the pulmonary artery, blood will flow from the right coronary artery through collaterals to the left coronary artery and into the pulmonary artery. This results in a left-to-right shunt through the coronary artery bed with a total myocardial flow less than that provided by a two-coronary system. The child with this physiology may continue for some time with signs and symptoms related to myocardial ischaemia but without suffering a fatal myocardial infarction. In less than 10% of the cases, the right coronary artery may also arise from the pulmonary trunk. This is usually an incidental post-mortem finding.

Coronary artery fistulas usually occur (65%) between the right coronary artery and the right ventricle or right atrium. They may also involve the left anterior descending or circumflex branch opening into the right heart chambers. This condition results in a left-to-right shunt due to flow of blood from the coronary artery to the right side of the heart. This results in a left-to-right shunt, usually without symptoms, unless pulmonary-to-systemic blood flow is greater than 1·5:1.

In addition to these lesions, a single coronary artery may supply the distribution of both normal coronary vessels.

Diagnosis

The infant with anomalous origin of the left coronary artery usually presents with cardiomegaly and heart failure. Death may occur within the early months of life from massive myocardial infarction. Those who develop adequate intercoronary collateral circulation may do well for several years. Between these two groups are patients who present during early childhood with mild heart failure. Physical findings in this lesion are dependent on the degree of damage to the left ventricle. If little or no damage has occurred as in the rare cases with abundant intercoronary collaterals, the physical examination may be normal. Patients who have suffered a myocardial infarction have gross cardiomegaly and may present with evidence of a left ventricular aneurysm. In addition, a murmur of postinfarction mitral regurgitation may be present. The ECG resembles that of the adult with arteriosclerotic heart disease. It often shows evidence for acute or recent anterolateral myocardial infarction. The chest radiographs show left ventricular enlargement and pulmonary venous congestion in the infant or child who has had severe myocardial damage. In patients with adequate collateral circulation and a large left-to-right shunt increased pulmonary vascularity may be observed. Two-dimensional echocardiography may suggest the diagnosis by failure to demonstrate the left main coronary artery as it normally arises from the aortic root. Cardiac catheterization will show absence of a left coronary artery originating from the aortic root, and delayed filling of the left coronary system via the intercoronary collaterals in a retrograde fashion emptying into the pulmonary artery. The shunt from the coronary system to the pulmonary artery is usually small; even in those with adequate collateral flow the pulmonary to systemic flow ratio is often less than 2:1.

Coronary artery aneurysms and fistulas may be found incidentally at post-mortem examination. If large, the fistula results in significant shunting of blood from the abnormal coronary artery to the receiving right heart chamber. Signs and symptoms of failure may be present but symptoms related to myocardial ischaemia are unusual. The electrocardiogram may be normal or may reveal left ventricular and

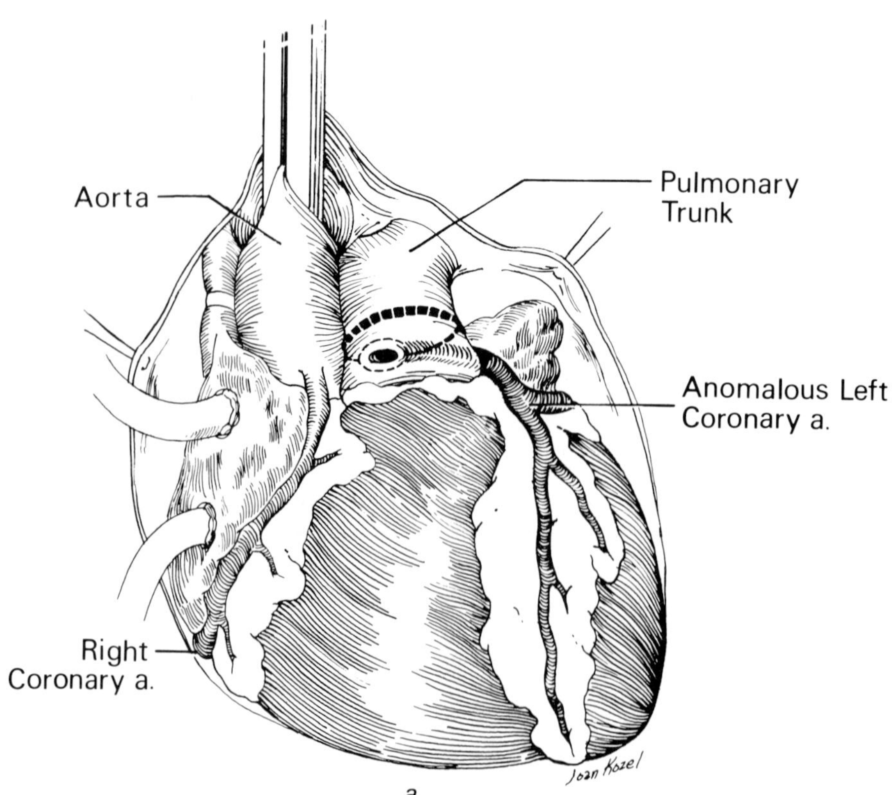

a

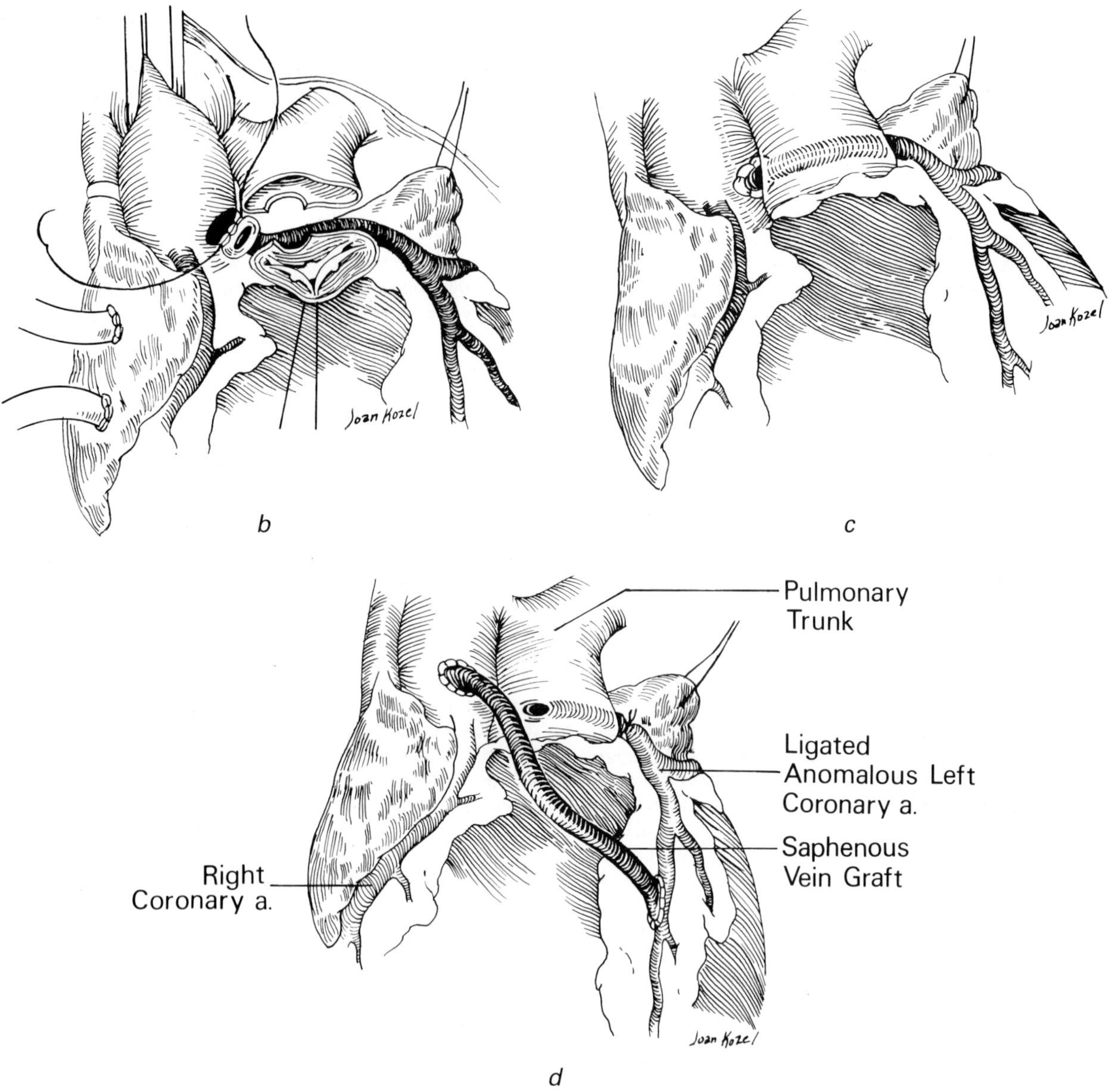

Fig. 45.10 Anomalous origin of the left coronary artery from the pulmonary artery. *a*, Anatomy and incision for removal of the left coronary artery ostium from the pulmonary artery and re-anastomosis to the aorta. *b*, Pulmonary artery divided and left coronary artery ostium anastomosed to the aorta. *c*, Anastomosis to the aorta completed. *d*, Saphenous vein bypass graft from the aorta to the anomalous left coronary artery with ligation proximally.

left atrial enlargement due to volume overload. Right ventricular enlargement may also be present. The chest radiograph may reveal cardiac enlargement and increased pulmonary vascularity. The aneurysm, even if large, is often not recognizable. The diagnosis is made by cardiac catheterization and arteriography. In most cases the right heart pressures are normal and the shunt is small. Occasionally the shunt may be large with elevation of right-sided and pulmonary arterial pressures. Coronary angiography will delineate the aneurysm, site of fistula formation and feeding vessels.

Treatment

Infants with the classic symptom complex of the Bland–White–Garland syndrome and anomalous left main coronary artery, run the risk of sudden death from myocardial infarction and ventricular arrhythmia. These patients should be treated as an adult with severe coronary heart disease and possible myocardial infarction. Congestive heart failure should be treated medically. If at all possible, operation should be deferred until the patient is 2–3 years old, at which time definitive repair can be accomplished by one of several methods of revascularization. Cooley described an operation which can be used even in the infant. This involved transecting the pulmonary artery, excising a cuff of the pulmonary artery around the anomalous origin of the coronary, anastomosing the cuff of pulmonary artery to the aorta primarily, and then re-approximating the pulmonary artery (*Fig.* 45.10*a*,*b*,*c*). Long-term follow-up is not available. Other procedures which are commonly done in the older child or adolescent include anastomosis of the left subclavian artery to the left coronary artery, use of the left subclavian artery as a free graft between the aorta and the left coronary artery when it will not reach directly, and use of saphenous vein bypass grafting (*Fig.* 45.10*d*). The procedure of choice in the older patient is left subclavian artery to coronary grafting. If correction is performed under the age of 2 years because of severe symptomatology, operative mortality is quite high, ranging from 10 to 50%. It is recommended in infants who are particularly ill to simply perform ligation of the anomalous left coronary artery at its origin from the pulmonary artery. Revascularization by one of the above methods can be performed as a secondary procedure. After the age of 2, revascularization can be undertaken with a very low operative mortality and it appears that with procedures other than saphenous vein grafting, long-term survival is possible.

Operations for coronary artery aneurysm and fistula should be performed ideally during the pre-school age; in an older individual, it should be done at the time of diagnosis. The risk of non-operative treatment of this lesion includes progressive enlargement with rupture (rarely), the development of endocarditis, and, in the patient with a large shunt, the development of failure from a large left-to-right shunt.

In most instances treatment can be accomplished by placing several horizontal mattress sutures with pledgets underneath the coronary artery ligating the fistula (*Fig.* 45.11*a*,*b*). If the aneurysm is large, it should be plicated. If the fistula cannot be closed easily by the mattress suture technique, the aneurysm may be opened. The fistula opening, which may be multiple, is identified and closed primarily from within the aneurysm (*Fig.* 45.11*c*,*d*,*e*).

In a review of the literature, hospital mortality for repair of coronary arterioventricular fistula was 4%. Hospital mortality for repair of anomalous origin of the left coronary artery ranges from 17 to 59%, primarily relating to the preoperative myocardial damage.

CONGENITAL AORTIC STENOSIS

Aortic stenosis may occur at the subvalvular, valvular and supravalvular level.

Anatomy and Physiology

Obstruction of left ventricular outflow may occur at the subvalvular level due to either muscular obstruction or a membrane. In addition, obstruction may occur due to deformities of the valve itself or narrowing of the supravalvular obstruction, present in more than half of patients, in valvular aortic stenosis. The lesion consists of thickening of the valve leaflets with varying degrees of fusion at the commissures (*Fig.* 45.12). The majority of these patients have fusion of the commissure between the right and left coronary cusps, producing a bicuspid valve with an eccentric narrowed opening. Infants who become symptomatic after 1 year of age are subject to sudden death with the incidence varying from 2 to 20%. However, it seems to occur predominantly in those with severe, as opposed to lesser degrees of aortic stenosis. When mild, this abnormality may go undetected for years until the patient develops calcification and further stenosis at age 30–40 years. The second most common type of obstruction is discrete subaortic stenosis and usually consists of a ring of fibrous tissue located several mm below the aortic valve (*Fig.* 45.13). Only rarely is subvalvular aortic stenosis a problem with respect to symptomatology in infancy. Supravalvular aortic stenosis is the result of an obstructing ridge of fibrous tissue growing into the ascending aorta immediately distal to the aortic sinuses (*Fig.* 45.14). From the external surface, the aorta may appear only mildly indented. Such children may have associated peripheral pulmonary artery stenoses as well as craniofacial deformities and hypocalcaemia. Muscular obstruction beneath the aortic valve, commonly known as idiopathic hypertrophic subaortic stenosis, will be discussed in Chapter 50.

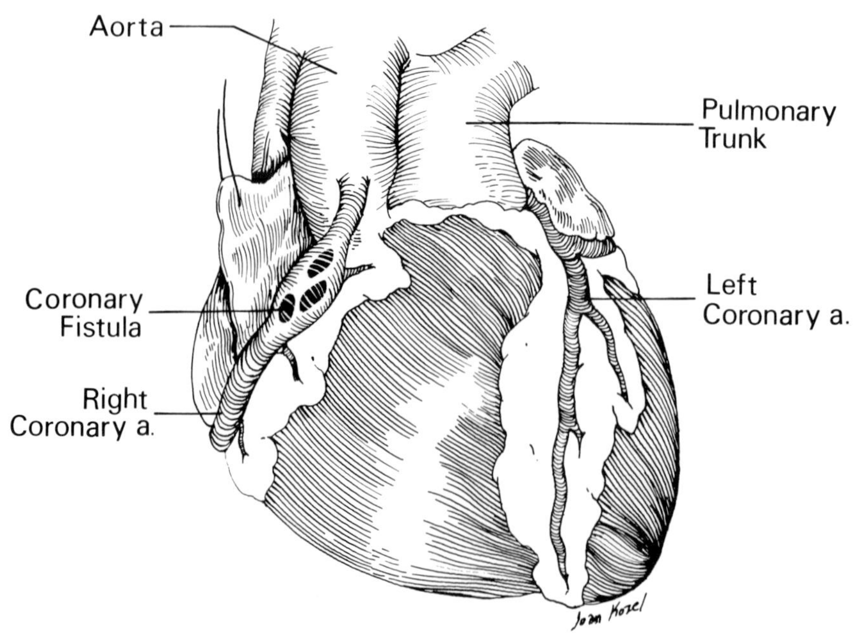

a

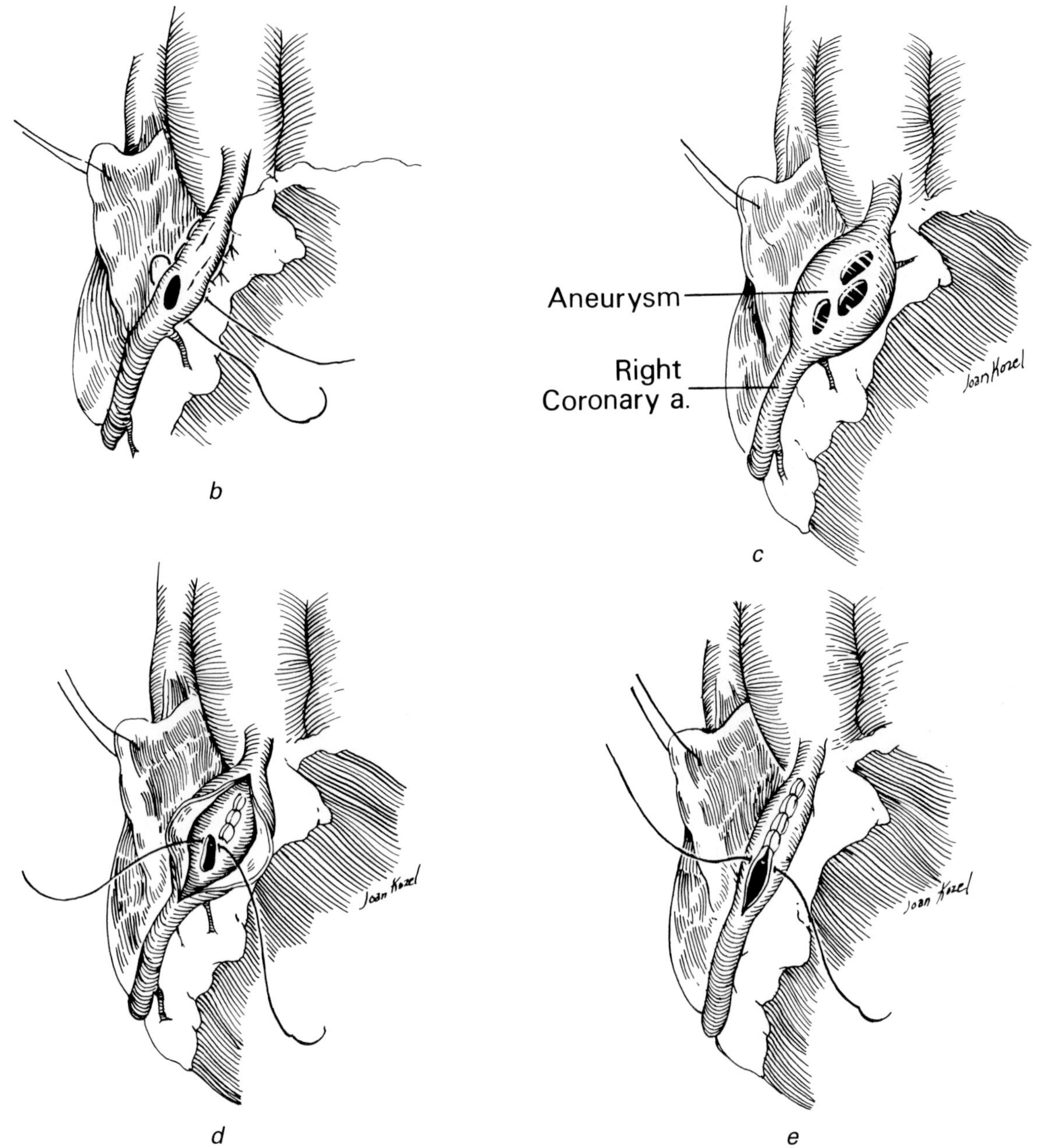

Fig. 45.11 Coronary artery fistula and aneurysm. *a*, Coronary fistula from the right coronary artery to the right heart. *b*, Fistula ligated with mattress sutures placed underneath the coronary artery. *c*, Anatomy of coronary artery aneurysm and fistula from the right coronary artery to the right heart. *d*, Aneurysm opened and fistula oversewn from within the artery. *e*, Coronary artery aneurysm plicated and closed.

The basic physiology of all of these fixed lesions is obstruction to left ventricular outflow. This results in elevation of pressure within the left ventricle. In response to the increased work of the left ventricle, its myocardium hypertrophies. In order to maintain adequate cardiac output in the face of the fixed aortic obstruction, the systolic pressure of the left ventricle increases. With exercise, these pressures may be more than twice that of the aorta. In addition, since the systolic phase of the cardiac cycle increases with increasing obstruction, there is less diastolic filling time for the coronary arteries. The combination of decreased coronary flow in the face of increased ventricular work and hypertrophy may result in myocardial ischaemia.

Diagnosis

Severe congenital aortic stenosis may result in heart failure, dizziness or fainting episodes with exertion, chest pain due to coronary insufficiency and even death. Physical examination reveals a systolic thrill and ejection murmur loudest over the 2nd right intercostal space or suprasternal notch, transmission of the murmur into the carotid vessels and decreased atrial pulses with delayed upstroke. An ejection systolic click may be present if the stenosis is valvular and mild. Not infrequently, there may be a faint early diastolic murmur of aortic regurgitation along the left sternal border.

The ECG reveals evidence of left ventricular hypertrophy, and, when the stenosis is severe, a strain pattern may be present. The chest radiograph may reveal normal heart size with or without aortic poststenotic dilatation. With progression of time, it shows evidence of left ventricular enlargement and pulmonary congestion in the presence of cardiac failure. The M-mode echocardiogram differentiates valvular from subaortic stenosis, and the two-dimensional echocardiogram can identify all four types of aortic stenosis. An estimate of the systolic pressure gradient can be derived from the left ventricular end-systolic diameter-wall thickness ratio or from the ratio of the aortic valve orifice to the aortic diameter.

Cardiac catheterization is necessary to determine the severity and location of the aortic stenosis. By withdrawing the catheter from the left ventricle to the aorta, the exact location of the obstruction as well as its severity can be identified. A left ventriculogram will also localize the obstruction and show mitral insufficiency, if present. An aortogram will demonstrate the presence of aortic insufficiency and associated coronary anomalies.

Treatment

Infants with cardiac failure who do not respond to medical management should undergo operation on an urgent basis. A gradient across the left ventricular outflow tract of 60 mmHg or greater is also an indication for operation even in the relatively asymptomatic patient. Progressing left ventricular hypertrophy shown by serial electrocardiography and by echocardiography necessitates early operation. The relief of discrete *subvalvular membranes* or supravalvular aortic stenosis is usually permanent. Relief of valvular aortic stenosis, however, appears to be temporary. A significant number of these patients will develop calcification, and further stenosis of their aortic valve in later life will make them candidates for eventual valve replacement. A significant complication that can occur following valvulotomy is the production of aortic insufficiency. It is, therefore, better to accept a mild to moderate residual gradient across a deformed aortic valve rather than to attempt complete ablation of a pressure gradient at the risk of producing aortic

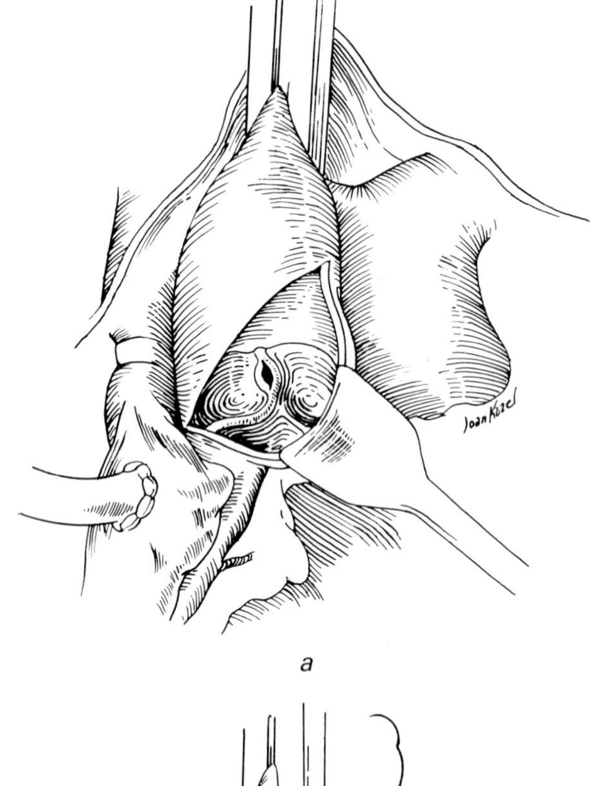

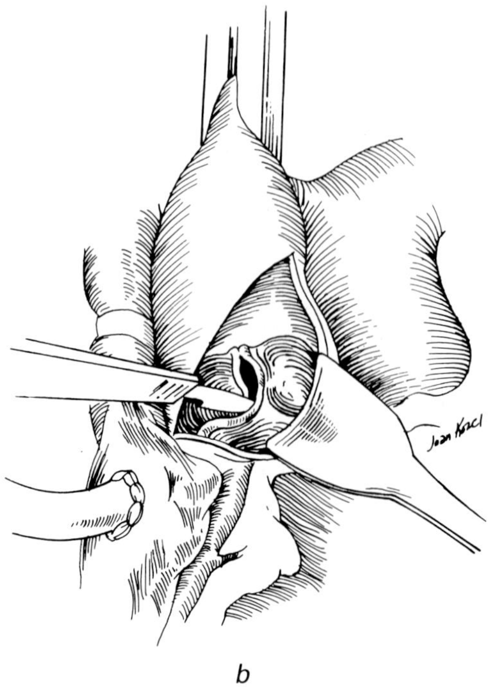

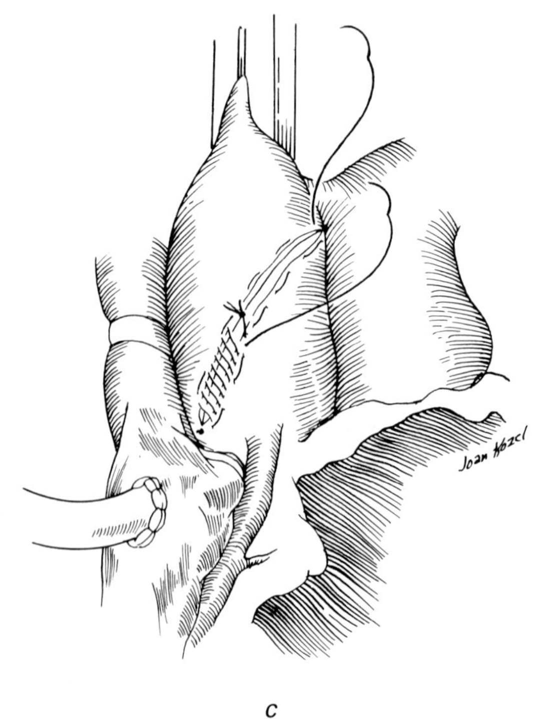

Fig. 45.12 Valvular aortic stenosis. *a*, Anatomy as viewed through a reverse hockey stick aortotomy. *b*, Valve incised by scalpel. *c*, Aortotomy closed.

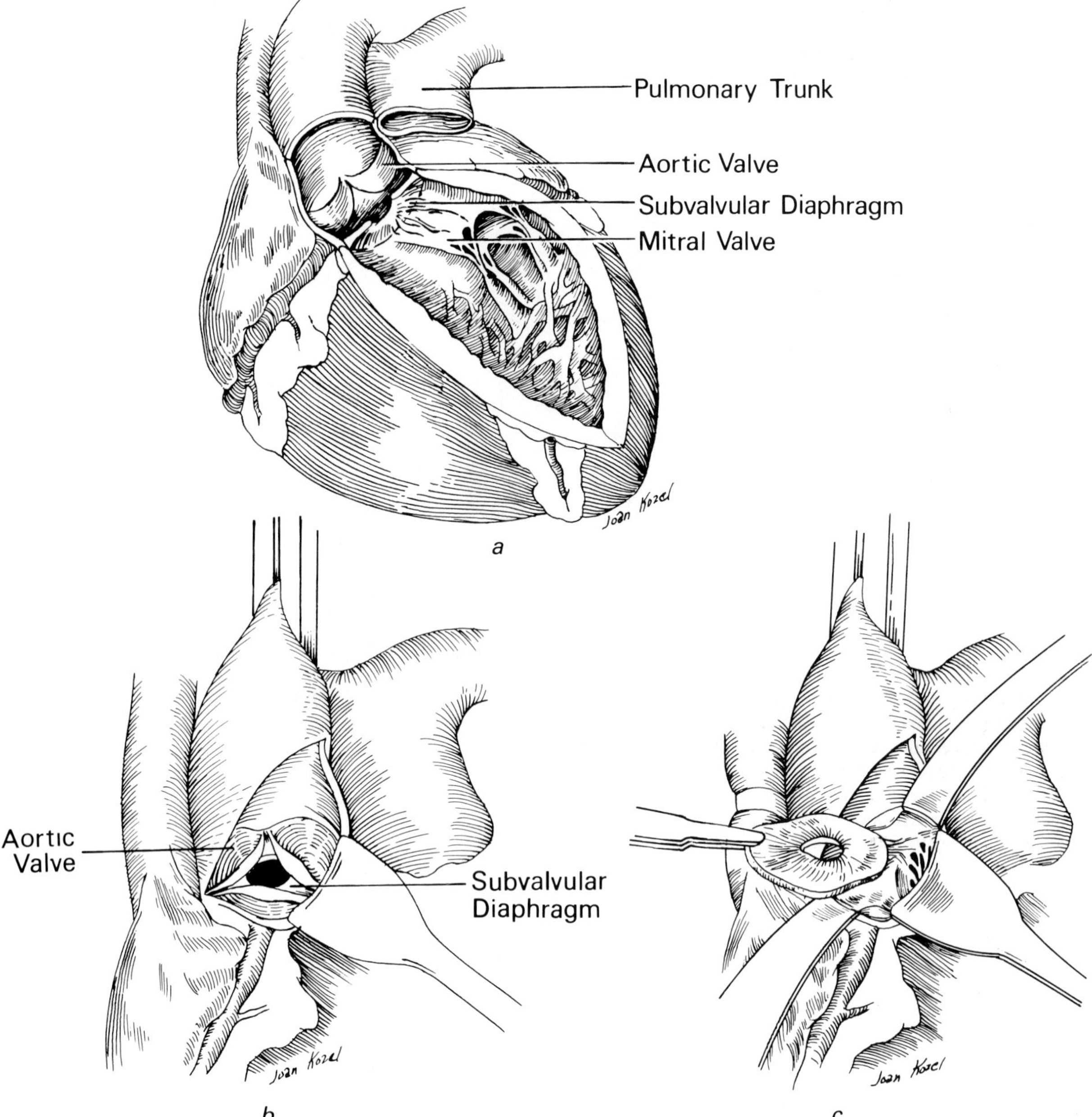

Fig. 45.13 Subvalvular aortic stenosis. *a*, Anatomy of the subvalvular diaphragm. *b*, View of the subvalvular diaphragm through an aortotomy. *c*, Subvalvular diaphragm excised severing fibrous bands connecting the diaphragm to the mitral valve.

insufficiency. Although an extremely rare complication, heart block may occur following resection of a subaortic membrane.

The operations for all these lesions are performed with cardiopulmonary bypass. Valvular stenosis is corrected by a transaortic approach. The valve is inspected and incisions are made along the lines of fused commissures to within 1 or 2 mm of the aortic annulus (*Fig.* 45.12*b*,*c*). Care should be taken to avoid the production of aortic insufficiency. In the case of a bicuspid valve the incomplete commissure between the right and left coronary cusps should not be incised. Such an incision will result in aortic insufficiency due to destruction of the suspension of these valve leaflets. In the case of discrete subvalvular aortic stenosis access is obtained through an aortotomy by retracting the leaflets of the aortic valve carefully. An artist's conception of the membrane is visualized and excised in *Fig.* 45.13*b*,*c*. Care must be taken not to damage the mitral or aortic valve to which the membrane is frequently attached and to avoid injury to the area of the atrioventricular node. Rather than sharply excising the subvalvular membrane, it can be removed in a fashion similar to endarterectomy. This is particularly important in the area of its attachment to the mitral valve leaflet so as to avoid damage to the anterior mitral valve leaflet. Following removal of the subvalvular membrane in this fashion, it is desirable to perform a myotomy with or without myectomy in the area of the commissure between the right and left coronary leaflets as performed after

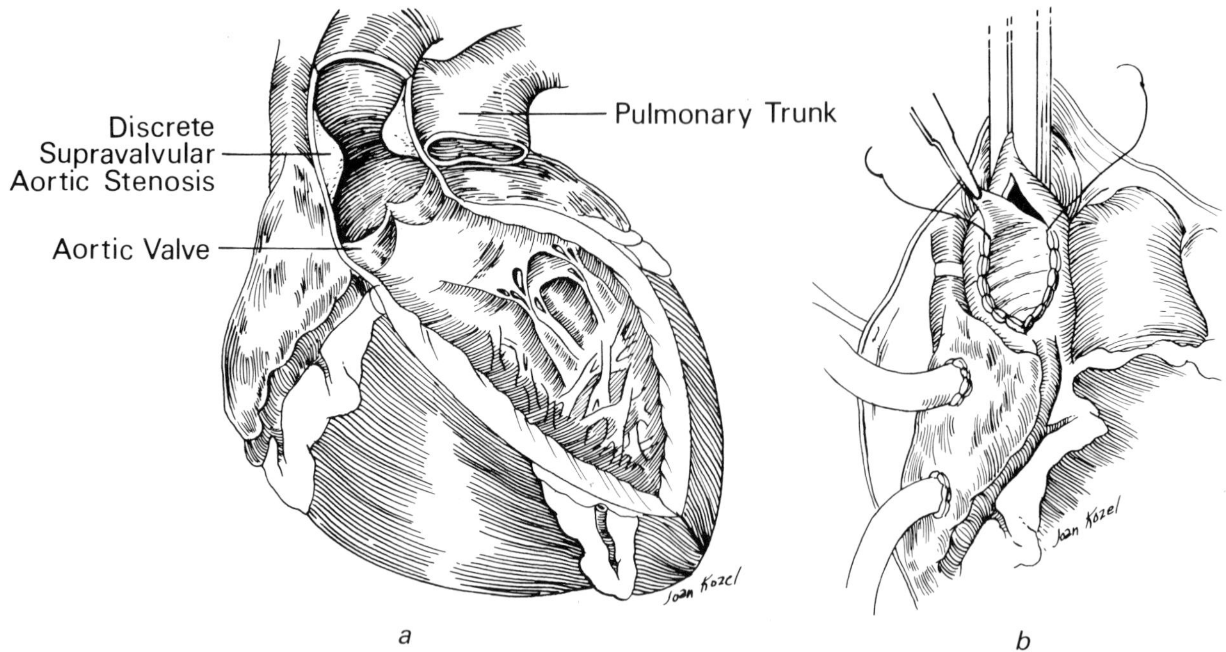

Fig. 45.14 Discrete supravalvular aortic stenosis. *a*, Anatomy of supravalvular aortic stenosis. *b*, Patch repair for supravalvular aortic stenosis.

idiopathic hypertrophic subaortic stenosis. In the case of supravalvular aortic stenosis of the localized type the ridge of tissue is excised and a suitable patch placed to reconstruct an adequate outflow (*Fig.* 45.14*b*). In the case of diffuse narrowing of the ascending aorta a long patch must be used to open this area adequately. In this particular lesion, there is no discrete area of obstruction to be excised. In some instances, however, there is a ridge of thickened aortic tissue which can be removed. Furthermore, if the stenosis is severe, it is desirable to use a bilobed patch with extensions into the non-coronary and right coronary sinuses. In the case of the right coronary sinus, it is important to protect the right coronary artery. The surgical results with valvotomy in infancy range from an operative mortality of 10–50% with the majority of the survivors requiring reoperation over a period of three or four to ten years. When performed in older age groups, longer periods of palliation are obtained before valve replacement is necessitated. Also, in groups over 1 year of age, the risk is very low with an operative mortality of only 1–2%. The operative risk with discrete subvalvular aortic stenosis is approximately 2–4%. Eighty per cent of patients undergoing this procedure are alive at follow-up at 15 years. The operation is effective also in relieving the aortic outflow gradient. It is very rare to have to perform surgery for supravalvular aortic stenosis in infancy. In older children, this can be done with a mortality of 3–5% and, again, it is definitive with respect to relief of the lesion.

CONGENITAL ABNORMALITIES OF THE MITRAL VALVE

Several unusual lesions may affect the mitral valve in an isolated manner. They account for less than 0·5% of congenital heart disease. Congenital mitral stenosis may be due to a variety of lesions varying from mitral atresia to a small but normally constructed mitral valve. The small mitral valve and annulus associated with the hypoplastic left heart syndrome is usually fatal. Other lesions producing stenosis usually result in decreased exercise tolerance, dyspnoea on exertion, heart failure, and recurrent pneumonias by the age of 2–3. The physical examination reveals typical findings of mitral stenosis, namely, right ventricular impulse and an apical diastolic rumble with presystolic accentuation. Chest radiography shows left atrial enlargement with pulmonary congestion. Also, the pulmonary veins may enter the left atrium via a common pulmonary venous trunk with small orifice (cor triatriatum) resulting in similar high-pressure and low-pressure chambers. The ECG will show a 'P mitrale' as demonstrated by a broad notched P wave. The echocardiogram shows abnormal anatomy and restricted movement of the valve. The exact severity of the lesion, however, is difficult to quantify by this technique. Cardiac catheterization is still necessary to quantitate the degree of obstruction, identify the anatomy of the valve, and rule out associated defects. The surgical treatment depends upon the anatomy of the valve apparatus. In young children, mitral valvuloplasty would be ideal if at all possible. This may temporize the defect until the child reaches an age at which a prosthetic valve may be implanted.

A supravalvular ring of connective tissue may divide the left atrium into a proximal high-pressure and a distal low-pressure atrial chamber. Both lesions present with the same signs and symptoms as valvular mitral stenosis and may be strongly suspected echocardiographically. The diagnosis is made by left atrial angiography demonstrating two distinct left atrial chambers with unequal pressures. In supravalvular ring, the left atrial appendage is situated in the proximal high-pressure chamber; in cor triatriatum, it is located in the distal low-pressure chamber. Excision of the ring or membrane separating the atrial chambers can be accomplished with excellent long-term results.

The parachute mitral valve is another cause for congenital

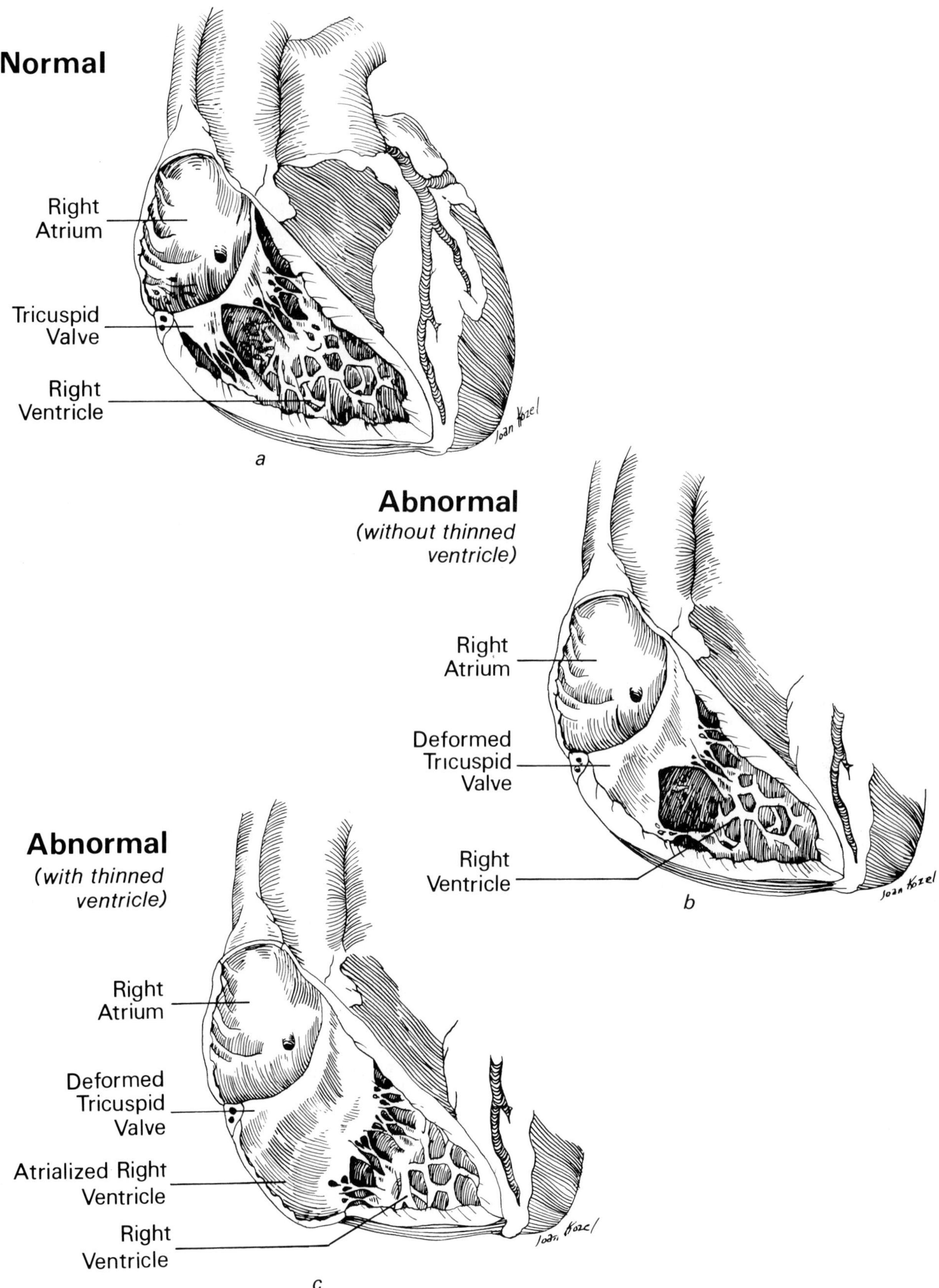

Fig. 45.15 Ebstein's anomaly of the tricuspid valve. *a*, Anatomy of a normal tricuspid valve. *b*, Ebstein's anomaly with no thinning of the ventricle but tricuspid valve deformity. *c*, Ebstein's anomaly consisting of valve deformity and atrialization of the right ventricle.

mitral stenosis. The hallmark is a single papillary muscle into which the chordae tendineae from both mitral valve leaflets attach. Again, the clinical signs and symptoms are those of valvular mitral stenosis. Echocardiography may demonstrate this lesion. Surgical treatment is difficult. It may be possible to divide the papillary muscle so that the chordae tendineae from each valve leaflet insert to their own portion of the papillary muscle but the effectiveness of this approach is not known. In older children or adults, valve replacement may be necessary.

The double orifice mitral valve is a lesion commonly seen associated with other congenital anomalies. It has been reported in endocardial cushion defect. Although it may present as mitral insufficiency usually the accompanying mitral valve abnormalities produce a net effect of obstruction. This lesion rarely presents in an isolated manner for surgical consideration. Isolated congenital mitral regurgitation is rare and on occasion improves with medical therapy.

CONGENITAL ABNORMALITIES OF THE TRICUSPID VALVE (without necessary cyanosis)

The most interesting abnormality of the tricuspid valve is Ebstein's anomaly. Over 500 cases of this anomaly have been reported. Ebstein's anomaly represents less than 1% of congenital heart disease.

Tricuspid insufficiency as an isolated anomaly is rare. It is usually associated with other more severe anomalies of the right heart. A transient form of this lesion may occur in the newborn. Its aetiology and pathogenesis remains unknown. With proper medical therapy this physiological disturbance disappears. The clinical manifestations of tricuspid insufficiency include extreme cardiomegaly, congestive heart failure, hepatomegaly and tachypnoea. A pansystolic murmur is heard most prominently at the right lower sternal border. Chest radiography and ECG show right axis deviation, right bundle-branch block and right atrial enlargement. Cardiac catheterization will reveal tremendous enlargement of the right atrium and right ventricle with significant tricuspid regurgitation. Surgical therapy in these infants is usually not successful.

Tricuspid stenosis is also rare as an isolated lesion and more commonly occurs with associated right heart abnormalities. The presenting symptoms are similar to those of tricuspid atresia with cyanosis usually present. Corrective surgery has occasionally been reported with this lesion.

Anatomy and Physiology

Although the exact anatomy of Ebstein's anomaly of the tricuspid valve is variable, there are two characteristic features. The valve tissue itself, especially the anterior leaflet, is redundant. The medial and posterior leaflets are adherent to the ventricular wall and are displaced for a variable distance into the right ventricular cavity. Thus, the origin of the free portion of the valve leaflet occurs some distance away from the atrioventricular junction. The portion of right ventricle to which the leaflets are attached is known as the atrialized portion of the right ventricle. Although the remainder of the right ventricle is usually of normal formation and thickness, the atrialized portion may be paper thin (*Fig.* 45.15). Associated anomalies of the right heart are common. The physiology of this lesion is quite variable. Cyanosis, if present, is due to an associated right-to-left shunt at the atrial level due to some obstruction at the tricuspid orifice. Patients appearing with cyanosis in infancy have an extremely poor outlook with a 50% mortality. Those who survive the initial period do relatively well until succumbing to congestive heart failure, sudden death secondary to an arrhythmia, and cerebral abscess or paroxysmal embolus with or without stroke. Physiologically, there may be obstruction and/or insufficiency of the tricuspid valve itself. Cyanosis may disappear in early life but usually recurs. If there is no atrial communication, cyanosis is not a feature of this lesion.

Diagnosis

Since the anatomy and physiology of Ebstein's anomaly are quite variable, so are the presenting features. Symptoms may be minimal; however, the patient usually presents with cyanosis, a heart murmur, and severe congestive heart failure. With time, the cyanosis disappears. However, between the ages of 5 and 10 it usually recurs. One hallmark of Ebstein's anomaly is the frequent occurrence of paroxysmal supraventricular tachycardia. This occurs in about 25% of these patients. On auscultation, a triple or quadruple rhythm is common. The most frequent murmur is that of tricuspid insufficiency presenting as a pansystolic murmur at the lower right sternal border.

The ECG usually presents with either a right bundle-branch block pattern or evidence of the Wolff–Parkinson–White syndrome. Arrhythmias include supraventricular tachycardia, nodal rhythm, atrial flutter and fibrillation and occasionally, premature ventricular contractions. The P waves are usually peaked, indicating right atrial enlargement. Echocardiography is useful for the diagnosis in that it shows a prominent tricuspid valve whose closure occurs later than that of the mitral valve. The chest radiograph is quite variable; right atrial enlargement is characteristic, and may be massive. Left atrial enlargement is absent. The aorta and pulmonary artery are usually normal or small, and the pulmonary vascular markings may be reduced.

Cardiac catheterization entails a high risk due to the danger of provoking arrhythmias. The diagnosis is facilitated by recording an intracavitary ECG with a catheter electrode. Simultaneous recording of the ECG and pressure by catheter into the right ventricle may reveal an area with a right atrial pressure but a right ventricular muscle potential. Selective angiocardiography, with injection of contrast into the right ventricle, usually demonstrates the displacement of the tricuspid valve and the site of the atrialized right ventricular chamber. Cardiac catheterization also helps determine the degree of tricuspid stenosis and insufficiency, the severity of shunting across an associated atrial septal defect, if present, and may uncover any previously unrecognized associated anomalies of the right heart.

Treatment

Treatment of Ebstein's anomaly is determined by the degree of valvular abnormality. Many patients may not need surgical intervention for as long as they are relatively asymptomatic. In some symptomatic patients, some type of valvuloplasty can be performed by plicating the thinned portion of the right ventricle and reconstructing the tricuspid valve. In most others, plication of the right atrium and the thin portion of the right ventricle must be accompanied by tricuspid valve replacement.

Further Reading

Patent Ductus Arteriosus

Clyman R. I. and Heymann M. A. (1981) Pharmacology of the ductus arteriosus. *Pediatr. Clin. North Am.* **28**, 77.
Kirklin J. W. and Barratt-Boyes B. G. (1986) Patent ductus arteriosus. In: *Cardiac Surgery*. New York, Wiley, pp. 679–697.

Coarctation of the Aorta

Clarkson P. M., Nicholson M. R., Barratt-Boyes B. G. et al. (1983) Results after repair of coarctation of the aorta beyond infancy: A 10 to 28 year follow-up with particular reference to late systemic hypertension. *Am. J. Cardiol.* **51**, 1481.
Metzdorff M. T., Cobanoglu, A., Grunkemeier G. L. et al. (1985) Influence of age at operation on late results with subclavian flap aortoplasty. *J. Thorac. Cardiovasc. Surg.* **89**, 235.

Aortic Arch Anomalies

Kirklin J. W. and Barratt-Boyes B. G. (1986) Interrupted aortic arch. In: *Cardiac Surgery*. New York, Wiley, pp. 1070–1080.
Roesler M., de Leval M., Chrispin A. et al. (1983) Surgical management of vascular ring. *Ann. Surg.* **197**, 139.

Pulmonary Stenosis

Griffith B. P., Hardesty R. L., Siewers R. D. et al. (1982) Pulmonary valvulotomy alone for pulmonary stenosis: Results in children with and without muscular infundibular hypertrophy. *J. Thorac. Cardiovasc. Surg.* **83**, 577.
Lababidi Z. and Wu J. (1983) Percutaneous balloon pulmonary valvuloplasty. *Am. J. Cardiol.* **52**, 560.
Polansky D. B., Clark E. B. and Doty D. B. (1985) Pulmonary stenosis in infants and young children. *Ann. Thorac. Surg.* **39**, 159.

Atrial Septal Defect

Cockerham J. T., Martin T. C., Gutierrez F. R. et al. (1983) Spontaneous closure of secundum atrial septal defect in infants and young children. *Am. J. Cardiol.* **52**, 1267.
Hairston P., Parker E. F., Arrants J. E. et al. (1974) The adult atrial septal defect: Results of surgical repair. *Ann. Surg.* **179**, 799.
Meyer R. A., Korfhagen J. C., Covitz W. et al. (1982) Long-term follow-up study after closure of secundum atrial septal defect in children: An echocardiographic study. *Am. J. Cardiol.* **50**, 143.

Ventricular Septal Defect

Albus R. A., Trusler G. A., Izukawa T. et al. (1984) Pulmonary artery banding. *J. Thorac. Cardiovasc. Surg.* **88**, 645.
Corone P., Doyan F., Gaudeau S. et al. (1977) Natural history of ventricular septal defect: A study involving 790 cases. *Circulation* **55**, 908.
Doty D. B. (1983) Closure of perimembranous ventricular septal defect. *J. Thorac. Cardiovasc. Surg.* **85**, 781.
Soto B., Becker A. E., Moulaert A. H. et al. (1980) Classification of ventricular septal defects. *Br. Heart J.* **43**, 332.

Atrioventricular Canal

Piccoli G. P., Gerlis L. M., Wilkinson J. L. et al. (1979) Morphology and classification of atrioventricular defects. *Br. Heart J.* **42**, 621.
Studer M., Blackstone E. H., Kirklin J. W. et al. (1982) Determinants of early and late results of repair of atrioventricular septal (canal) defects. *J. Thorac. Cardiovasc. Surg.* **84**, 523.

Congenital Anomalies of the Coronary Arteries

Donaldson R. M., Raphael M. J., Yacoub M. H. et al (1982) Hemodynamically significant anomalies of the coronary arteries: Surgical aspects. *Thorac. Cardiovasc. Surg.* **30**, 7.
Moodie D. S., Fyfe D. and Gill C. G. et al. (1983) Anomalous origin of the left coronary artery from the pulmonary artery (Bland–White–Garland syndrome) in adult patients: Long-term follow-up after surgery. *Am. Heart J.* **106**, 381.
Urrutia-S C. O., Falaschi G. and Ott D. A. (1983) Surgical management of 56 patients with congenital coronary artery fistulas. *Ann. Thorac. Surg.* **35**, 300.

Congenital Aortic Stenosis

Binet J. P., Losay J., Demontoux S. et al. (1983) Subvalvular aortic stenosis. Long-term surgical results. *Thorac. Cardiovasc. Surg.* **31**, 96.
McKay R. and Ross D. N. (1982) Technique for the relief of discrete subaortic stenosis. *J. Thorac. Cardiovasc. Surg.* **84**, 917.
Sink J. D., Smallhorn J. F., Macartney F. J. et al. (1984) Management of critical aortic stenosis in infancy. *J. Thorac. Cardiovasc. Surg.* **87**, 82.

Congenital Abnormalities of the Mitral Valve

Gardner T. J., Roland J. M., Meill C. A. et al. (1982) Valve replacement in children. A fifteen-year perspective. *J. Thorac. Cardiovasc. Surg.* **83**, 178.
Pass H. I., Sade R. M., Crawford F. A. et al. (1984) Cardiac valve prostheses in children without anticoagulation. *J. Thorac. Cardiovasc. Surg.* **87**, 832.

Congenital Abnormalities of the Tricuspid Valve

Danielson G. K. and Fuster V. (1982) Surgical repair of Ebstein's anomaly. *Ann. Surg.* **196**, 499.
Kirklin J. W. and Barratt-Boyes B. G. (1986) Ebstein's malformation. In: *Cardiac Surgery.* New York, Wiley, pp. 889–910.
de Leval M. (1983) Tricuspid valve. In: Stark J. de Leval M. (ed.) *Surgery for Congenital Heart Disease.* New York, Grune & Stratton, pp. 453–466.

46 Cyanotic Congenital Heart Disease

P. O. Daily

Central cyanosis in congenital heart disease is due to the shunting of systemic venous blood into the systemic arterial circulation. This may be obligatory, i.e. determined by intracardiac connections which permit no other pathway for the venous blood, or be dependent on intracardiac mixing of blood, through defects, determined by pressure relationships which in turn are determined by morphological features. Examples of these lesions are:

Obligatory Connections
- Transportation of the great arteries and corrected transposition
- Total anomalous pulmonary venous connection

Common Mixing
- Univentricular heart
- Common atrium
- Atresia of either atrioventricular valve
- Pulmonary atresia with intact ventricular septum
- Truncus arteriosus

Dependent Intracardiac Mixing
- Fallot's tetralogy
- Pulmonary atresia with ventricular septal defect
- Pulmonary stenosis with atrial septal defect
- Double outlet right or left ventricle with pulmonary stenosis
- Ebstein's anomaly

Cyanotic congenital heart disease may be encountered at any age, but is frequently noted in infancy and early childhood. Although the history, physical examination, ECG and chest radiograph provide important clues to the diagnosis, the latter is only possible by cardiac catheterization and selective angiocardiography, supported by techniques such as nuclear angiography and echocardiography.

A complete morphological and physiological diagnosis is essential to the planning of treatment. Since so many conditions exist, it is necessary to use a comprehensive analytical approach. Although some conditions are immediately recognizable, e.g. with selective angiocardiography, it is important to employ a routine approach to analysis—the steps employed in assessing morphology are shown in *Table* 46.1.

Table 46.1 Diagnosis of congenital heart disease

A. Define atrial status
B. Describe atrioventricular junction
  i. Connections
  ii. Mode of connection
  iii. Ventricular morphology
  iv. Relation of chambers in ventricular mass
C. Describe ventriculo-arterial junction
  i. Connections
  ii. Relation of arterial valves and great arteries
  iii. Morphology of outflow tracts
D. Define additional anomalies

TRANSPOSITION OF THE GREAT ARTERIES

This is defined as the condition of atrioventricular concordance together with ventriculo-arterial discordance, i.e. the morphological right atrium connects with the morphological right ventricle via a tricuspid atrioventricular valve but the right ventricle then connects with the aorta. Similarly, the left-sided connections are: left atrium to left ventricle to pulmonary artery. There are thus parallel pulmonary and systemic circulations, and survival depends on cross mixing between the circulations, e.g. bronchial collaterals, an atrial or ventricular septal defect, a patent ductus arteriosus, or combinations thereof. Such additional anomalies are not uncommon and greatly affect the natural history and clinical features. Anomalous origin, course and single or multiple coronary arteries are frequent.

So-called 'simple transposition' is the most common situation. There is no ventricular septal defect and the ductus usually closes very early in infancy. Mixing of blood then only occurs across the atrial septum, usually a patent foramen ovale and bronchial collaterals. Since the mixing is poor, the infant presents with deep cyanosis within hours or days after birth. The natural history is that 80% of infants survive the first week but by two months only 17% are alive. At the end of one year, the survival is approximately 4%.

If a ventricular septal defect is present, better mixing is possible but at the expense of possible excessive shunting of blood into the pulmonary circulation with resulting lung congestion, heart failure and pulmonary hypertension. The combination of increased pulmonary flow and/or pressure and cyanosis is associated with early development of pulmonary vascular disease which may become irreversible by the age of 1 year. When pulmonary stenosis coexists with a ventricular septal defect and transposition, the lung vasculature is 'protected'. Intracardiac mixing is good and, providing the stenosis is not so severe as to cause underperfusion of the lungs, then survival beyond infancy is usual. For all forms of transposition of the great arteries, the survival is 55% at 1 month, 15% at 6 months, and 10% at 1 year reflecting improved survival when there is enhanced mixing by an atrial septal defect, ventricular septal defect, or patent ductus arteriosus.

Diagnosis and Treatment

Diagnosis requires cardiac catheterization and angiocardiography—often on an emergency basis. Once the diagnosis is established, a balloon-tipped catheter is inserted via a peripheral vein, guided into the right atrium and across the patent foramen ovale into the left atrium. The balloon is then inflated and pulled rapidly back across the atrial septum, which is torn at the inferior margin of the foramen ovale. This Rashkind technique of balloon atrial septostomy is effective in increasing intracardiac mixing in young infants, but after the first months of life the atrial septum thickens and the operative creation of an atrial septal defect by the Blalock–Hanlon closed technique is needed if increased mixing is required (*Table* 46.2).

Since the vast majority of patients with transposition present in early infancy, balloon atrial septostomy is the usual standard technique. After balloon septostomy, survival is 85% at 3 months.

Further Surgical Treatment

Further treatment is aimed at the conversion of the parallel circulation into a series circulation, where systemic venous blood proceeds to the lungs and pulmonary venous blood to the rest of the body. This can be achieved by rearrangement of flow at the atrial, ventricular or great artery level.

Atrial Redirection of Flow

Venous inflow is redirected within the atrium by the insertion of a specially shaped baffle (the Albert–Mustard operation (*Fig.* 46.1)) or by a technique which utilizes the tissue of the atrial septum and free wall (Senning). The techniques are applicable at all ages, can be performed with a low early risk and can be combined with simultaneous correction of associated anomalies. The best results are achieved in 'simple' transposition. Atrial switching using the Senning or Mustard technique is associated with an operative mortality as low as 1·5% in recently reported series.

Ventricular Redirection of Flow

When transposition coexists with a very large ventricular septal defect, an intraventricular patch can be inserted to redirect flow. This is rarely done.

The more usual ventricular redirection is used when transposition coexists with a high ventricular septal defect and left ventricular outflow tract obstruction (LVOTO). A tunnel patch reconnects the left ventricle via the septal defect to the aorta and continuity between the right ventricle and pulmonary artery is achieved by placing a valved external conduit (*Fig.* 46.2). This approach is not generally applicable in infants, is confined to the VSD/LVOTO combination and there are early and late complications related to the external RV-PA conduit. However, in selected patients satisfactory early results have been obtained. Operative mortalities have been reported ranging from 20 to 50%.

The surgical creation of pulmonary arterial stenosis, i.e. pulmonary artery banding to relieve heart failure due to a large ventricular septal defect with transposition can also

Table 46.2 Plan of treatment with simple and complicated transposition of the great arteries

Simple transposition

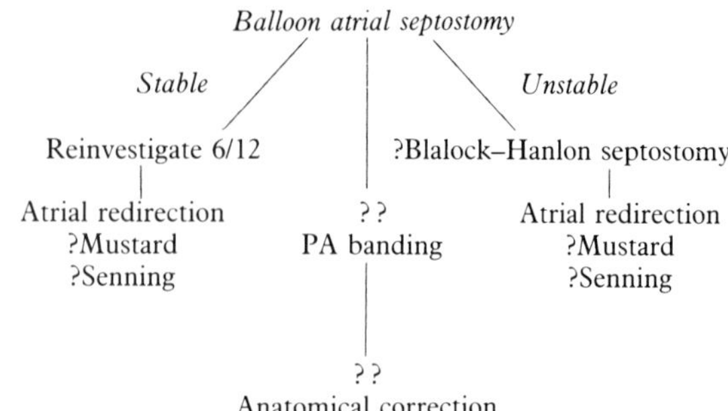

Transposition of the great arteries/ventricular septal defect

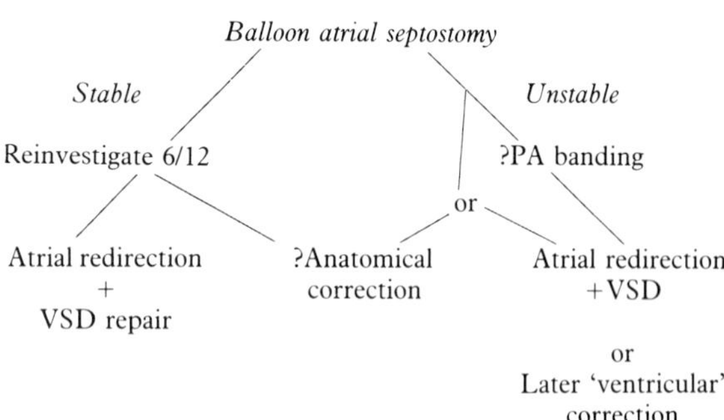

Transposition of the great arteries/ventricular septal defect/ pulmonary stenosis

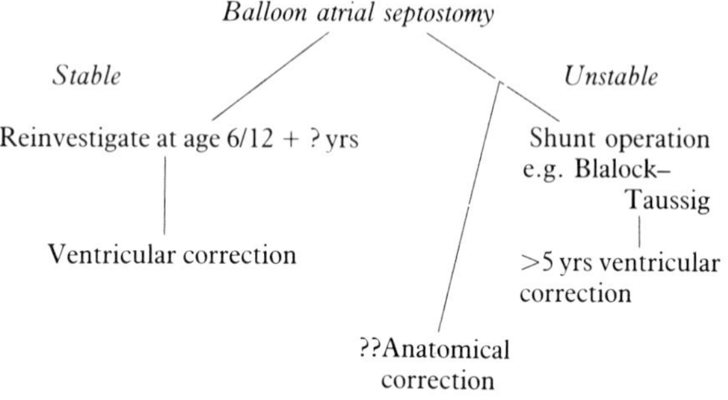

have this ventricular redirection technique applied at subsequent 'correction'.

Great Arterial Redirection of Flow

Reconnection of the aorta and pulmonary artery to their appropriate ventricle combined with repositioning of the coronary arteries is probably the ideal solution to transposition. With simple transposition, left ventricular pressure falls rapidly after birth as pulmonary vascular resistance decreases. The muscle mass of the left ventricle reduces commensurately and the ventricle rapidly loses the ability to support systemic pressure, the immediate consequence of anatomical arterial 'correction'. Recent reports of arterial switching for simple transposition of the great vessels have been associated with operative mortalities as low as 15%. Operation in the neonatal period allows arterial switching before the left ventricle becomes unable to support the

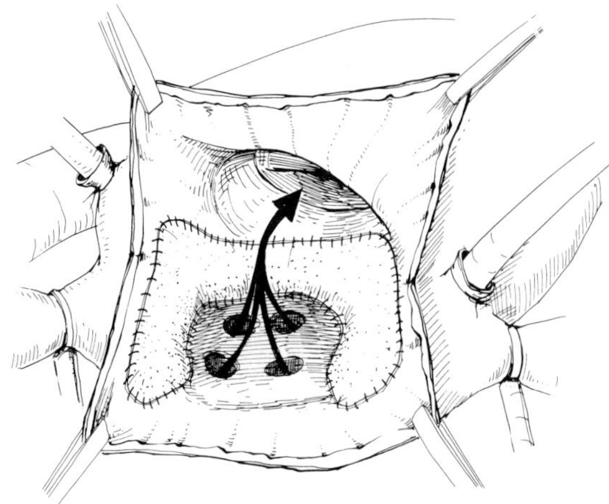

Fig. 46.1 The Albert–Mustard operation.

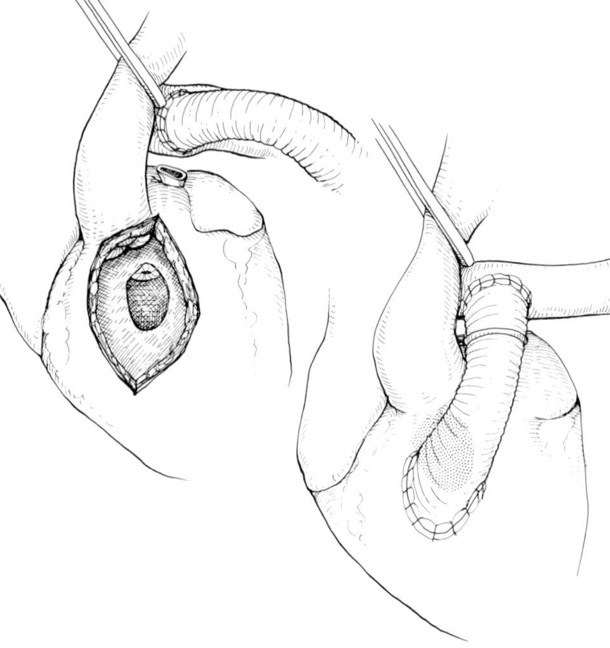

Fig. 46.2 The Rastelli procedure.

systemic circulation. This is associated with the persistence of elevated pulmonary vascular resistance in the neonatal period. With ventricular septal defect without left ventricular outflow obstruction, arterial switching has been associated with an operative mortality of zero in a small series of 6 patients to as high as 40%. However, the combined operative mortalities for pulmonary artery banding followed by arterial switching have been consistently at 15% or above. This does not compare favourably with the 1–2% mortality associated with atrial switching by either the Senning or Mustard approach.

Thus this form of correction to date has mostly been applicable when there is a high left ventricular pressure, e.g. with LVOTO (±VSD) but without pulmonary vascular disease. LVOTO can be induced with pulmonary artery banding in simple transposition prior to anatomical correction.

Early results with anatomical correction have been moderately encouraging and it may be that this will prove the direction for future development.

CORRECTED TRANSPOSITION

Corrected transposition is defined as that condition in which there is a discordant atrioventricular and discordant ventriculo-arterial connection, i.e. right atrium to anatomical left ventricle to pulmonary artery, and left atrium to anatomical right ventricle and aorta. The circulations are thus in series and functionally 'corrected'. In 1–5% of patients there are no associated defects so there are no underlying physiological sequelae. However, ventricular septal defect is present in approximately 80% and clinically significant pulmonary stenosis in 25% and the two occur together relatively frequently. Thus, the clinical presentation of the patients is related to cyanosis in those with ventricular septal defect and pulmonary stenosis and excessive pulmonary blood flow without pulmonary stenosis. Additional associated defects are atrial septal defect with a single ventricle and regurgitation of the systemic AV valve. Ten to thirty per cent develop heart block over a period of time.

Surgical treatment in this situation requires repair of the associated defects which usually are ventricular septal defect and relief of pulmonary stenosis. The site of the coronary arteries and conduction system complicates the repair and the long-term results are not wholly satisfactory. The right ventricle remains the systemic ventricle; the tricuspid valve, which is anatomically abnormal, is often incompetent and there are late problems of arrhythmias. There is also doubt about the long-term functional adequacy of valved external conduits which may sometimes have to be inserted. Operative mortalities have ranged from 10 to 40% in various series and are associated with the severity of the underlying defects. More recently there has been an overall improvement in operative mortality rates to less than 10%.

PULMONARY STENOSIS/ATRESIA WITH INTACT VENTRICULAR SEPTUM

Pulmonary stenosis is among the common congenital cardiac anomalies. However, pulmonary atresia represent only 1–2%. In pulmonary stenosis, there is usually no cyanosis unless right ventricular outflow tract obstruction is severe enough so that right-to-left shunting occurs at the atrial level across a patent foramen ovale or atrial septal defect. This most obviously is the case also with atresia of the pulmonary valve.

This condition presents very early in infancy and generally carries a bad prognosis especially if the right ventricle is tiny. In pulmonary atresia, the right ventricle is small but thick-walled and harbours supra-systemic pressures. Its muscle is dysplastic and there are usually myocardial sinusoids connecting the ventricular cavity with the coronary vessels. Less commonly, the right ventricle is of nearly normal size or even large, and has a normal inlet tricuspid valve.

At birth the pulmonary circulation is dependent on patency of the ductus arteriosus and remains so unless a systemic artery to pulmonary artery shunt is created or the right ventricular outflow obstruction is relieved to the extent that it is then able to perfuse the lungs.

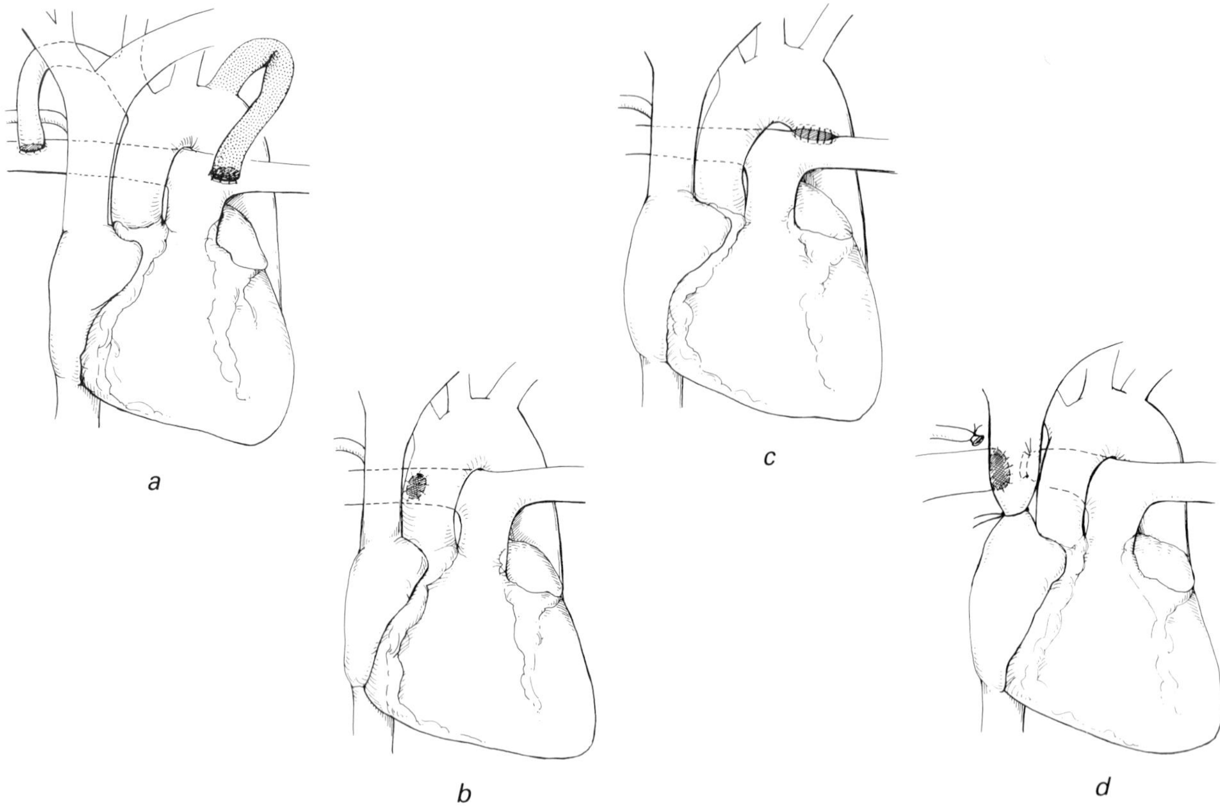

Fig. 46.3 Extracardiac shunts for cyanotic congenital heart disease. *a*, Proper right subclavian to pulmonary artery (Blalock–Taussig) and improperly left kinked subclavian to pulmonary artery anastomosis. *b*, Waterston shunt between the ascending aorta and right pulmonary artery. *c*, The Potts shunt between the descending aorta and left pulmonary artery and modified Blalock–Taussig shunt with Gore-Tex graft. *d*, The Glenn shunt between the superior vena cava and right pulmonary artery.

Treatment

This remains a major problem. Infusion of prostaglandin E during the first week of life maintains or increases duct patency and pulmonary blood flow and reduces metabolic acidosis as well as arrhythmias. For these reasons, it is usually started prior to and continued through surgery. The type of surgery is controversial but the best results have been when pulmonary valvotomy has been combined with arterial shunt (*Fig.* 46.3). The atrial shunt is not closed at this stage.

The aim of this surgical approach is to maintain pulmonary blood flow and hence systemic arterial oxygenation while decompressing and providing an outflow for the obstructed right ventricle. This not only improves right ventricular function but also allows it to grow. Survivors of operation in infancy require a second stage outflow reconstruction combined with atrial septal repair.

Survivors of operation in infancy require a second stage outflow reconstruction combined with atrial septal repair. The mortality associated with the palliation of pulmonary atresia in infancy is 10–15%. Operative mortality for the second stage which includes closure of the atrial septal defect, pulmonary outflow tract opening, and closure of any previous aortopulmonary shunts varies from 10–25%.

The results of surgical correction of cyanotic pulmonary stenosis and atrial septal defect when the stenosis is less severe are more predictable and satisfactory. The timing of operation depends on clinical progress, size of right ventricle, degree of cyanosis and severity of right ventricular hypertension.

TOTAL ANOMALOUS PULMONARY VENOUS CONNECTION

This is characterized by lack of connection of the pulmonary veins with the left atrium. It represents approximately 2% of congenital anomalies. Pulmonary venous blood enters the heart directly through venous tributaries of the right atrium, e.g. superior vena cava (45%), coronary sinus (25%) or portal/hepatic veins (25%) or mixed (5%). There is thus mixing of systemic and pulmonary venous blood in the right atrium. Blood then enters the right and left ventricles, the latter from the left atrium via an atrial septal defect. The degree of cyanosis, therefore, depends on the resistance to flow through the lungs. Obstruction to pulmonary venous drainage, most typically when the veins drain below the diaphragm and through the liver, results in severe pulmonary hypertension and marked arterial desaturation. Such infants become critically ill and cyanosed within hours or days after birth. Survival after birth is related to the degree of pulmonary venous obstruction. With more severe examples of pulmonary venous obstruction, only 50% survive 3 months and 20% survive the first year of life.

Treatment

Gross cyanosis in infants with total anomalous pulmonary

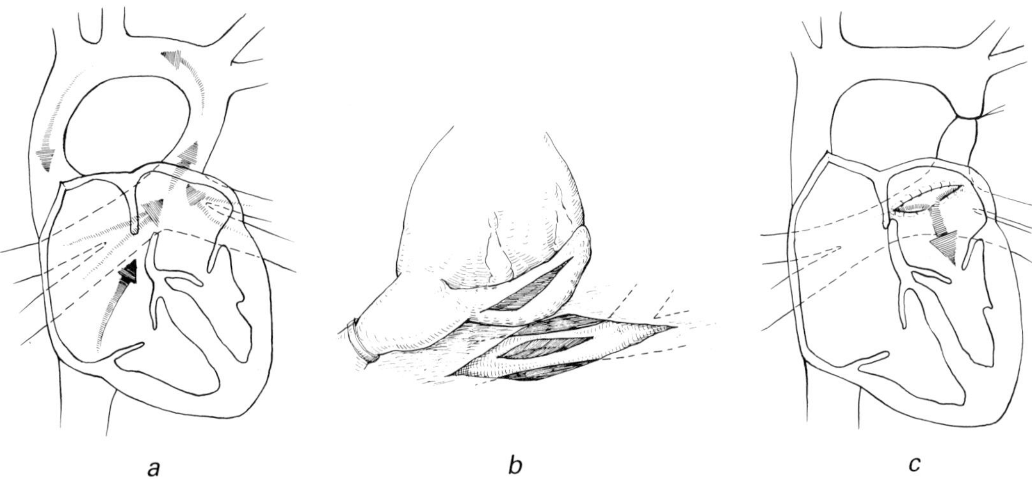

Fig. 46.4 Total anomalous venous return to superior vena cava. *a*, Preoperative circulation. *b*, Operative exposure. *c*, Postoperative circulation. The Malm approach through the right, with enlargement of the left atrium is often necessary.

venous connection may be a sign of unfavourable haemodynamics and morphology, and early operative correction is necessary. In recent years, the results of corrective surgery have improved most notably in the infants with supradiaphragmatic type of drainage. The operative procedure involves direct connection of the pulmonary veins to the left atrium, a feasible proposition since the veins usually join together to form a confluent retrocardiac sinus (*Fig.* 46.4). In addition, enlargement of the left atrium is carried out through the Malm right atrial approach. The same approach is carried out when venous return is below the diaphragm into the portal/hepatic veins. After establishing connection of the pulmonary veins to the left atrium, it is necessary to ligate the common venous channel to eliminate anomalous drainage and also to close the always present atrial septal defect.

That operative results are still only moderately good is probably due to the small size of the left heart in some patients, or to pulmonary vascular obstruction in some older subjects. Operative mortality in the first year of life varies from 9% to as high as 40% and averages 15%. When the anomalous pulmonary venous return is mixed, i.e. into separate sites to the extent that a confluent retrocardiac sinus is not present, surgical repair is difficult.

ATRIOVENTRICULAR VALVE ATRESIA

Mitral atresia, usually associated with gross underdevelopment of other left heart structures or single ventricle, has a bad prognosis. Since attempts at treatment are, at present, not generally indicated the condition is not discussed further.

Right atrioventricular valve orificial atresia (*tricuspid atresia*) does not have such a gloomy prognosis and various means of treatment have been developed.

In most instances, this forms part of the univentricular heart syndrome, a condition in which both AV valves actually or *potentially* communicate with a single ventricular chamber which communicates, in turn, with an outlet chamber. The aorta and pulmonary artery arise from the ventricle or outlet chamber in a variety of ways.

Systemic venous blood crosses an interatrial septal defect, mixes with pulmonary venous blood and enters the ventricle via the mitral orifice.

The clinical picture is determined by the site of origin of the great arteries and by the presence of any obstruction to flow. Often, and more frequently with normally related great arteries, there is obstruction to blood flow to the lungs which are oligaemic; consequently, the patient presents with cyanosis. Less commonly, but more often with transposed great arteries, pulmonary blood flow is excessive and the presenting clinical picture is that of early left heart failure with only minimal cyanosis.

Treatment of Tricuspid Atresia

Palliative surgery in infants depends upon the extent of pulmonary blood flow. If deficient, it can be augmented by a shunt operation; if excessive, it can be decreased by banding of the main pulmonary artery. Shunts are either arterial or venous, examples of arterial shunts are the Blalock subclavian artery-to-pulmonary artery shunt, the Waterston ascending aorta-to-right pulmonary artery shunt or the Potts descending aorta-to-left pulmonary shunt. An example of a venous shunt is the Glenn superior vena cava-to-right pulmonary artery anastomosis (*see Fig.* 46.3). Although venous shunting has theoretical advantages, it is also difficult to perform in small infants.

In recent years, the principle of right atrial to pulmonary artery continuity has been developed. The essence of the operation (Fontan procedure) is to utilize the right atrium as the venous pumping chamber, closing the atrial defect and establishing continuity with the lungs by a conduit which either contains a valve mechanism or which is placed to an outlet chamber (closed off from the ventricle) and making use of a naturally present pulmonary valve. That the right atrium can support pulmonary flow is not in doubt, but only if resistance to pulmonary flow is normal or low.

After the first clinical successes, it is now apparent that several contraindications to the Fontan procedure exist. These include small pulmonary arteries, increased pulmonary vascular resistance, increased left atrial pressure secondary to mitral valve regurgitation or left ventricular dysfunction and, probably, age less than two years. No valves are required in the atrial to pulmonary artery circuit. While the loss of atrial contraction may decrease flow, success has been obtained in cases of persistent atrial fibrillation. In more recent clinical series, operative mortalities of less than 10% for the Fontan procedure, or a variation thereof, have been obtained. In many instances, significant levels of physical activity are possible. Long-term survival is enhanced by the elimination of late mortality associated with persistent severe cyanosis.

COMMON MIXING AT VENTRICULAR LEVEL

Univentricular Heart

Previously there has been no general agreement as to the precise definition of univentricular heart or single ventricle. Primarily, this is because of the fact that considerable variability of ventricular anatomy occurs in a spectrum of hearts that have been characterized as single ventricle ranging from essential absence of ventricular septum to hearts in which both ventricles are clearly present but one is markedly larger than the other. The confusion is compounded by the addition of hearts with only a single AV valve such as in mitral or tricuspid atresia. In order to clarify the definition of univentricular hearts, R. H. Anderson has suggested that the connection of both AV valves to a single ventricular cavity be the primary criterion establishing the diagnosis of univentricular heart. If, for example, both AV valves connect to an anatomical left ventricle, this would be characterized as double inlet left ventricle or, more rarely, double inlet right ventricle. In both anatomical types, the great vessels may be normally related, dextro-transposed, or laevo-transposed. By convention, it has been agreed that when one valve and at least 50% of the other AV valve is overriding a single ventricular cavity, then the diagnosis is established. While tricuspid atresia can also be classified as univentricular heart with this classification, those hearts with a single AV valve are best considered in the appropriate category such as tricuspid or mitral atresia.

The clinical presentation is determined by the relative magnitudes of systemic and pulmonary blood flow, the presence of pulmonary hypertension and/or obliterative pulmonary vascular disease, intracardiac flow streaming (preferential or otherwise), AV valve function, presence of associated anomalies, e.g. subaortic and subpulmonary stenosis or anomalies of venous connection, and heart rhythm disturbances.

The natural history of univentricular heart is, at least in the early years of life, less severe than tricuspid atresia, for example, with 50% of patients surviving to four years. However, only infrequently do individuals reach their twenties.

In planning therapy, a precise assessment of anatomy and haemodynamics is required. Surgery, if indicated, may then be purely 'extracardiac' and palliative, or aimed at a more radical intracardiac approach. This remains a developing area with, as yet, encouraging results only.

Surgical Principles

1. Purely palliative techniques relate to the status of the pulmonary blood flow; systemic–pulmonary shunts to increase it, or pulmonary artery banding to reduce excessive flow.

2. The application of the modified Fontan technique has been mentioned under Tricuspid Atresia.

3. Septation of the ventricle is theoretically the most corrective approach. Its applicability technically depends on the anatomy of the AV valves; the position of the great arteries and coronary arteries; the ability to locate the conduction system—either visually, electrophysiologically or by anatomical knowledge and, probably most importantly, the function of the newly created ventricles whose septal component consists of a non-contracting synthetic material.

To date there has been relatively little total experience accumulated with septation for univentricular heart. In two larger series, the operative mortality has ranged from 10 to 47%. However, when the results for septation are examined for all types of univentricular heart, the operative mortality at the University of Alabama has been 36% and at the Mayo Clinic 47%. Furthermore, there were 18% late deaths for an accumulated mortality of 65% in the Mayo Clinic experience. In a larger series of the Fontan procedure for varieties of univentricular heart, the operative mortality has been near 10%. Furthermore, late survival after the Fontan procedure for univentricular heart seems to be better than that following septation. It is, therefore, difficult to argue that septation should continue to be performed except in highly selected circumstances based on precise anatomy and physiology.

COMMON MIXING AT GREAT ARTERIAL LEVEL

A single outlet heart is that situation when the ventricle (univentricular heart) or both ventricles eject blood, either directly, via a ventricular septal defect or via an outlet chamber into a single great artery.

Pulmonary atresia with ventricular septal defect is discussed in conjunction with tetralogy of Fallot (*see below*).

Truncus arteriosus (*Fig.* 46.5) is defined as the condition whereby a single artery arises from the heart and this artery gives rise, in its proximal part, to the systemic, pulmonary and coronary arteries. There is a single, often tricuspid or quadricuspid, thick and sometimes functionally abnormal semilunar valve. A large high ventricular septal defect is also present. The anatomy of the pulmonary arteries varies. The right and left arteries may arise from a short main vessel originating from the truncus or they may arise separately from the truncus. Sometimes there is stenosis of the orifices of the pulmonary arteries. Occasionally, the truncal valve is stenotic or incompetent.

Patients with truncus arteriosus have very poor survival in infancy with no more than 10–15% surviving beyond one year. However, for those who do survive beyond one year, survival into the third decade of life is not uncommon and is usually associated with the development of Eisenmenger's sydrome. Ebert has reported a mortality of 16% in infants 6 months of age or less undergoing correction of truncus arteriosus. Most others, however, have experienced a significantly higher operative mortality approaching 50% in infancy, particularly within the first six months of life. In the largest reported series the operative mortality was 29% of 167 cases. Since patients having correction of truncus arteriosus in infancy require a conduit, generally a valved conduit, a second operation is invariably necessary to enlarge the conduit, with or without a valve.

TETRALOGY OF FALLOT

In 1888 Fallot described a specific congenital anomaly of the heart. He described a tetrad of ventricular septal defect, right ventricular infundibular stenosis, right ventricular

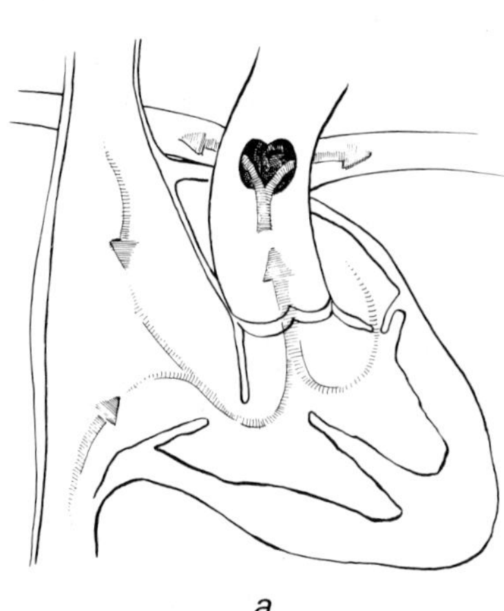

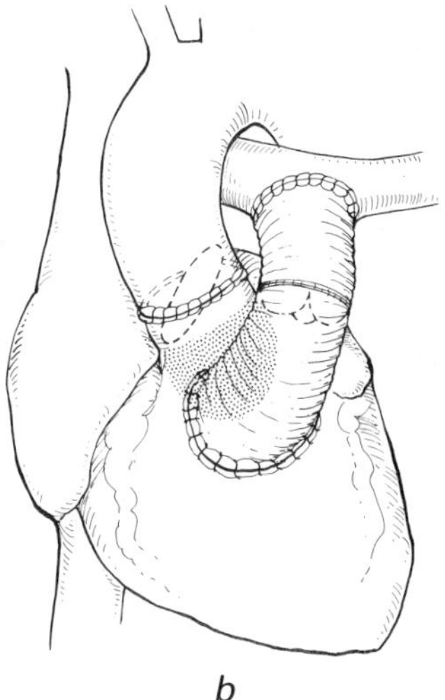

Fig. 46.5 Truncus arteriosus. *a*, Preoperative circulation. *b*, Postoperative appearance.

hypertrophy and dextroposition of the aorta. In recent years various investigators have suggested separate classification from the classic description, but it is probably easier to accept anatomical differences into the classification of tetralogy of Fallot as 'variations'.

Analysis for the entire group of tetralogy of Fallot reveal that in the absence of operative intervention only 50% reach the age of 7 years, 20% reach 14 years and not many more than 10% survive to 21 years.

It appears that the primary defect in tetralogy of Fallot relates to abnormalities in the development of the interventricular septum. Together, these abnormalities result in infundibular stenosis and ventricular septal defect. Secondarily, right ventricular hypertrophy occurs because of the pulmonary outflow tract stenosis. Various degrees of aortic overriding are related to variations in the abnormalities of the interventricular septum. Without operative intervention, 25% of patients with tetralogy of Fallot die in their first year. This is increased to 40% by the third year and 70% by the tenth year. Relatively few, however, die in the first month. In the subsets of tetralogy of Fallot with absent pulmonary valve and pulmonary atresia, 50% die in the first year.

Anatomy of the Four Components of Tetralogy of Fallot

1. Ventricular Septal Defect

The defect is between the infundibular and ventricular septal components and its diameter is usually similar to the diameter of the aortic root. The defect may be delineated by a complete muscular rim or may have its postero-inferior margin consisting of tricuspid annulus and membranous tissue. Inferiorly the defect is related to the septal cusp of the tricuspid valve and superiorly to the non-coronary cusp of the aortic valve. Conducting tissue enters the ventricle from the atrioventricular node through the fibrous trigone and proceeds closely related to the inferior margin of the septal defect.

2. Right Ventricular Outflow Obstruction

The anterior displacement and rotation of the infundibular septum, hypertrophy of the septal and parietal extensions of this septum, and variable development of the free wall of the infundibulum, narrow the outflow tract in varying degrees. (In most cases the infundibulum is of normal length, although narrowed; less commonly, it is shortened.) Right ventricular outflow obstruction usually also involves stenosis and/or hypoplasia of the pulmonary annulus, valve and arteries. In practical terms, this results in three main types of infundibular stenoses: (i) localized stenosis at the infundibular inflow. Usually, this localized ostium is lined with thick fibrous endocardium. Beyond this, the infundibulum is of normal length with the negligible hypertrophy of the free wall and an infundibular 'chamber' is seen on the angiograms; (ii) diffusely narrowed infundibulum of approximately normal length; (iii) the hypoplastic infundibulum which is short and narrow, resulting in the ventricular septal defect coming into close proximity to the pulmonary valve.

Some degree of pulmonary valve stenosis is always present in tetralogy of Fallot. This stenosis varies from minimal to severe, rarely atresia. The latter may be acquired after birth. The cusp anatomy is usually abnormal, being bicuspid in nearly 50% of cases.

The degree of valve stenosis does not necessarily correlate with the size of the pulmonary valve annulus although if this is of small diameter the valve must be severely stenotic.

Obstruction within the pulmonary arteries may be present and can occur as a localized narrowing of either or both the right and left pulmonary artery orifices or rarely as peripheral branch stenoses. Sometimes there is absence of one pulmonary artery, usually the left.

3. Right Ventricular Hypertrophy

Hypertrophy of the body of the right ventricle is a secondary phenomenon as is that of the wall of the right atrium. Hypertrophied ventricular muscle bundles within the ventricular body may rarely produce further obstruction, and then right ventricular pressure becomes higher at the apex than near the septal defect.

4. Dextroposition of the Aorta

This consists of clockwise rotation and rightward displacement of the aortic valve and dextro-anterior deviation of the distal infundibular septum. In normal hearts, the aortic valve overrides the right ventricle by its right one-third, the proximal part of the infundibular septum deviates from the line of the muscular septum by approximately 30° to accommodate this normal overriding. In tetralogy of Fallot, due to the dextroposition of the aorta, more of the aortic valve overrides the right ventricle. In approximately 10% of cases the aortic valve arises almost exclusively from the right ventricle. The authors define the great artery connection as to be that of double outlet ventricle when one of the great arteries and 90% of the other vessel arise from the same ventricle.

Associated Conditions

The tricuspid valve is usually normal. Occasionally accessory tissue is attached to the underside of the infundibular septum and may partially occlude the ventricular septal defect.

Atrial septal defect or patent foramen ovale is present in approximately 30% of patients and a persistent left superior vena cava in about 5%. Approximately 25–30% of patients have a right aortic arch.

Anomalies of the coronary arteries may occur, the most important being the origin of the anterior descending artery from the right coronary artery. When present, this artery runs across the right outflow tract to reach the anterior interventricular groove. It is thus vulnerable to accidental injury during right ventriculotomy at the time of open-heart surgery.

Persistent ductus arteriosus occurs in less than 5% of patients.

In older patients, aortic regurgitation may be present, probably being secondary to dilatation of the relatively unsupported aortic annulus or to prolapse of one of the aortic cusps.

There is a variable degree of development of aortopulmonary collateral vessels related in general to the reduction in pulmonary flow. In severely cyanotic patients there is an extensive network of fine systemic vessels entering the lungs from bronchial, intercostal, internal mammary, pericardial, mediastinal and, rarely, the coronary arteries. These collateral vessels communicate with the pulmonary arteries and therefore participate in gas exchange. Shunt volumes of up to 20% of the left heart output may reach the lungs in this way. Rarely, there are large aberrant arteries, termed aortopulmonary collaterals, arising directly from the aorta.

Haemodynamics

The right ventricular outflow obstruction results in a variably reduced pulmonary blood flow and right-to-left shunting across the ventricular septal defect of varying severity. The degree of shunting is determined by the relative resistances in the systemic circulation and right outflow. This relationship is variable in the individual patient, e.g. systemic resistance falls during exercise or anaesthesia, infundibular obstruction can increase on exercise or excitement. In some infants and children, the right-to-left shunt may suddenly increase in a paroxysmal manner unrelated to exercise.

Right and left ventricular pressures are equal since the ventricular septal defect is large and non-restrictive. If the ventricular septal defect is restrictive because of partial closure by an accessory tricuspid valve tissue, right ventricular pressure exceeds left ventricular pressure.

Clinical Considerations in Tetralogy of Fallot

Cyanosis and Clubbing

The systemic arterial oxygen in content or saturation is determined by the relative volumes of oxygenated left ventricular blood and desaturated shunted blood from the right ventricle which mix together. Cyanosis depends on the level of desaturated haemoglobin in arterial blood. Therefore, anaemic patients may not be cyanosed despite a significant right-to-left shunt. Alternatively, polycythaemic patients are cyanosed with only a moderate shunt.

The degree of cyanosis is, therefore, explicably variable over time in any one patient, and in general from patient to patient. Cyanotic attacks which are associated with severe tissue hypoxia, may cause unconsciousness or even death. Intravenous or subcutaneous morphine can relieve an attack, or propranolol can be given either acutely or on a continuous basis. However, the ideal treatment is to increase pulmonary blood flow surgically.

Classically a right outflow ejection murmur heard maximally in the left second or third intercostal spaces is present. The more severe the obstruction, the less prominent is the murmur. During a cyanotic attack the murmur diminishes and may even become inaudible.

Diagnosis

Definitive diagnosis is by cardiac catheterization and angiocardiography. Biventricular angiograms are essential to define AV valve, ventricular septal ventriculo-arterial anatomy and connections. We prefer oblique views to profile intracardiac septa and combine these with craniocaudal views to define the anatomy of the pulmonary arteries. Information about morphology so obtained is essential in the decision-making process regarding the technique of surgical intervention.

Indications for Operation

The indication for surgical intervention in tetralogy of Fallot is the establishment of the diagnosis in view of the relatively poor natural history without surgical intervention.

The usual clinical picture in patients with tetralogy is of cyanosis and restricted exercise tolerance. Occasionally, in infants, a ventricular left-to-right shunt is present though this progressively reduces as right outflow obstruction increases with age. A right-to-left shunt and cyanosis then develop, accompanied frequently by compensatory polycythaemia. A coexisting atrial left-to-right shunt indicates rare coexisting total or partial anomalous pulmonary venous return.

Chronic tissue hypoxia reduces resistance to infection, and polycythaemia may cause spontaneous venous or arterial thrombosis. Cerebral abscess is a significant risk.

In general, tetralogy represents such an abnormal haemodynamic state with such a poor prognosis that operative correction should always be considered. The most important consideration is selection and timing of the method of correction. There are wide anatomical and clinical manifestations and surgical management must be individualized.

Operative management may be by palliative operation with total correction at a later date or by primary total correction. Palliative operations are directed towards increasing pulmonary blood flow. This is gained either by a systemic–pulmonary artery shunt or by decreasing the degree of right outflow obstruction.

Systemic–pulmonary Artery Shunts

More recently, there has been an increased tendency to perform aortopulmonary shunting by the establishment of a Gore-Tex graft from the subclavian artery arising directly from the aorta to the ipsilateral pulmonary artery. The

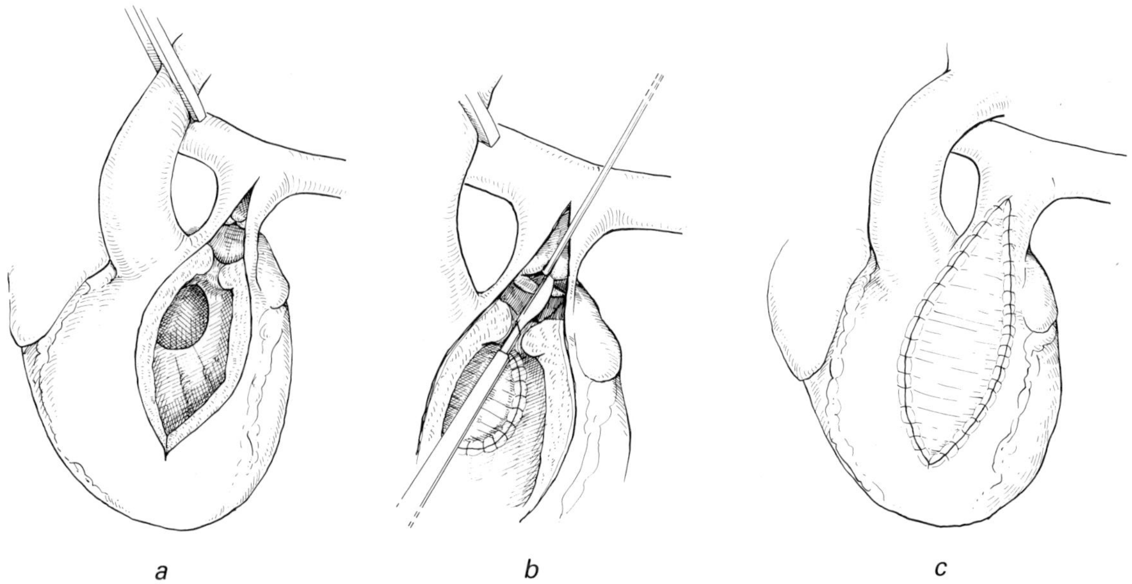

Fig. 46.6 Tetralogy of Fallot. *a*, Operative appearance of ventricular septal defect, outflow and pulmonary valve obstruction. *b*, Repair of ventricular septal defect and valvotomy. *c*, Outflow patch.

advantages of this approach are that the subclavian artery is preserved, minimal dissection is required to perform the procedure, rates of patency have been acceptable, and closure of the shunt at definitive correction is relatively easy. Alternatively, the classic Blalock–Taussig procedure can be performed. The Waterston, Potts and Brock procedures are performed much less frequently. Overall, the mortality for aortopulmonary shunting is typically less than 2% (*Fig.* 46.3).

Decreasing Right Outflow Obstruction (Brock Operation)

The right ventricle is exposed and, by means of a valvulotome inserted into the ventricle, the outflow stenosis is reduced by pulmonary valvotomy and/or removal of portions of the muscular infundibular stenosis.

Total Correction of Tetralogy of Fallot

This is an 'open' operation, where the ventricular septal defect is closed and the right outflow obstruction completely relieved (*Fig.* 46.6).

Operative policy varies from centre to centre but must take into account the relative risk of the operative approach which in turn relates to the age and size of the patient and to the individual intracardiac anatomy.

A reasonable policy is to perform palliative operation in the first six months of life unless the intracardiac anatomy appears quite ideal for complete correction, i.e. a localized infundibular stenosis with well-developed infundibular chamber beyond the stenosis, and with fair-sized pulmonary valve annulus and pulmonary arteries.

After infancy, one-stage correction is preferred, although occasionally detrimental intracardiac morphology favours staged approach. Second-stage correction is ideally completed before the age of 4 years. Operative incremental risk factors relate to whether or not there are significant problems with the pulmonary arteries such as branch stenosis or agenesis of the left pulmonary artery, major associated anomalies, and more than one previous operation. Earlier reported operative mortalities associated with total correction of tetralogy of Fallot have been as high as 15–20%. More recently, levels under 5% are commonplace. In a large experience reported from the University of Alabama, the overall mortality for all procedures with all subsets of patients was 10·5%. However, for total correction in a more recent group the mortality was under 5%.

PULMONARY ATRESIA WITH VENTRICULAR SEPTAL DEFECT

In this condition there is no direct communication between the right ventricle and the pulmonary artery. There is right-to-left shunting. Pulmonary blood flow is from the aorta, through large and/or small collaterals and, frequently, a patent ductus arteriosus.

This condition is related to tetralogy of Fallot. The morphology of tetralogy is present with variable infundibular development and dextroposition of the aorta as previously described. The haemodynamics and clinical presentation are essentially similar but more extreme than with tetralogy. The clinical presentation depends on the anatomical source and volume of pulmonary blood flow, and the major factor determining feasibility of operative improvement is also the morphology of the pulmonary arteries.

The anatomy of the pulmonary arterial tree depends on whether or not derivatives of the embryonic 6th aortic arches are present. A patient with pulmonary atresia in whom a persistent ductus arteriosus is the source of pulmonary blood flow and which communicates with normally developed intrapericardial pulmonary arteries, represents a much less complex problem than a patient *who has no 6th arch derivatives*, i.e. no main right pulmonary artery; no pulmonary trunk and no intrapericardial left pulmonary artery. In these patients the pulmonary blood supply is derived from numerous systemic–pulmonary collateral arteries which arise either from the aorta directly or from its major branches. Such collaterals join with pulmonary arteries within the lung. A combination of this and 6th arch development may occur and there may be no intrapulmonary connection between vessels to the different sources.

In patients with 6th arch derivatives central pulmonary artery development is variable. The source of pulmonary blood may be single, e.g. a persistent ductus arteriosus, or may be via multiple systemic arteries which communicate with the central pulmonary arteries. Larger aortopulmonary collaterals often have stenoses at the point of anastomosis with pulmonary arteries. However, they may cause pulmonary vascular disease.

The various complexities of the pulmonary blood supply in patients with pulmonary atresia and ventricular septal defect demand detailed selective angiocardiographic studies. The presence and size of any intrapericardial pulmonary arteries must be known. The major aortopulmonary collaterals must be located. The haemodynamic status of the pulmonary vasculature must be assessed. When the 6th arch derivatives are present and there are well-developed intrapericardial pulmonary arteries, pulmonary vascular resistance is usually low. Where there are large aortopulmonary collaterals and absent or hypoplastic intrapericardial pulmonary arteries, the pulmonary vascular resistance may be high and has to be calculated. In surgical terms, the important resistance is that at the site to which the right ventricle will be connected in the corrective operation.

As with tetralogy, associated defects of the atrial septum, systemic venous connections, coronary arteries and a right aortic arch occur.

Indications for Operation

Newborn infants with pulmonary atresia and ventricular septal defect often present with cyanosis due to decreasing pulmonary flow as the ductus arteriosus becomes smaller. Occasionally, infants with this condition may have heart failure due to excessive pulmonary blood flow through the collaterals.

More commonly, the right-to-left shunt and relatively low total pulmonary flow causes hypoxia, cyanosis and reduced exercise tolerance, and the risk of complications as previously described.

Emergency surgery consisting of aortopulmonary shunting, e.g. using a central Gore-Tex graft from ascending aorta to pulmonary trunk, is necessary for the newborn infant whose ductus arteriosus may be closing. Prostaglandin E infusion before and during the operation helps maintain ductal patency during this critical period.

Complete correction involves repair of the ventricular septal defect and establishing continuity between the right ventricle and pulmonary arteries. The latter usually involves the insertion of a homograft valve. Because of this it is desirable to delay total correction until the age of 5 or so when a homograft valve sufficient for adulthood, namely 20–25 mm, may be inserted.

Operative correction or palliation is contraindicated if the pulmonary resistance exceeds 10 units/m^2 body surface area or if there is lack of suitably sized pulmonary arteries to permit distal anastomosis.

Further Reading

Transposition of the Great Arteries

Castaneda A. R., Norwood W. I., Lang P. et al. (1984) Transposition of the great arteries and intact ventricular septum: Anatomical repair in the neonate. *Ann. Thorac. Surg.* **38**, 438.

Kanter K. R., Anderson R. H., Lincoln C. et al. (1985) Anatomic correction for complete transposition and double-outlet right ventricle. *J. Thorac. Cardiovasc. Surg.* **90**, 690.

Moulton A. L., de Leval M. R., Macartney F. J. et al. (1981) Rastelli procedure for transposition of the great arteries, ventricular septal defect, and left ventricular outflow tract obstruction. *Br. Heart J.* **45**, 20.

Penkoske P. A., Westerman G. R., Marx G. R. et al. (1983) Transposition of the great arteries and ventricular septal defect: results with the Senning operation and closure of the ventricular septal defect in infants. *Ann. Thorac. Surg.* **36**, 281.

Corrected Transposition of the Great Arteries

Danielson G. K. (1983) Atrioventricular discordance. In: Stark J. and de Leval M. (ed.) *Surgery for Congenital Heart Defect.* New York, Grune & Stratton, pp. 387–396.

Hwang B., Bowman F., Malm J. et al. (1982) Surgical repair of congenitally corrected transposition of the great arteries: Results and follow-up. *Am. J. Cardiol.* **50**, 781.

Westerman G. R., Lang P., Castaneda A. R. et al. (1982) Corrected transposition and repair of associated intracardiac defects. *Circulation* **66**, 1–197.

Pulmonary Atresia with Intact Ventricular Septum

Bull C., de Leval M. R., Mercanti C. et al. (1982) Pulmonary atresia and intact ventricular septum: A revised classification. *Circulation* **66**, 266.

Cobanoglu A., Metzdorff M. T., Pinson C. W. et al. (1985) Valvotomy for pulmonary atresia with intact ventricular septum. A disciplined approach to achieve a functioning right ventricle. *J. Thorac. Cardiovasc. Surg.* **89**, 482.

Coles J. G., Freedom Rm., Olley P. M. et al. (1984) Surgical management of critical pulmonary stenosis in the neonate. *Ann. Thorac. Surg.* **38**, 458.

Lewis A. B., Wells W. and Lindesmith G. G. (1983) Evaluation and surgical treatment of pulmonary atresia and intact ventricular septum in infancy. *Circulation* **67**, 1318.

Total Anomalous Pulmonary Venous Connection

Hammon J. W. jun., Bender H. W. jun., Graham T. P. jun. et al. (1980) Total anomalous pulmonary venous connection in infancy: Ten years' experience including studies of postoperative ventricular function. *J. Thorac. Cardiovasc. Surg.* **80**, 544.

Hawkins J. A., Clark E. B. and Coty D. B. (1983) Total anomalous pulmonary venous connection. *Ann. Thorac. Surg.* **36**, 548.

Tricuspid Atresia

Brux J. L., Zannini L., Binet J. P. et al. (1983) Tricuspid atresia. Results of treatment in 115 children. *J. Thorac. Cardiovasc. Surg.* **85**, 440.

Fontan F., Deville C., Quaegebeur J. et al. (1983) Repair of tricuspid atresia in 100 patients. *J. Thorac. Cardiovasc. Surg.* **85**, 647.

Tandon R. and Edwards J. E. (1974) Tricuspid atresia. A re-evaluation and classification. *J. Thorac. Cardiovasc. Surg.* **67**, 530.

Single Ventricle

Ebert P. A. (1984) Staged partitioning of single ventricle. *J. Thorac. Cardiovasc. Surg.* **88**, 908.

Moodie D. S., Ritter D. G., Tajik A. H. et al. (1984) Long-term follow-up after palliative operation for univentricular heart. *Am. J. Cardiol.* **53**, 1648.

Stefanelli G., Kirklin J. W., Naftel D. C. et al. (1984) Early and intermediate-term (10-year) results of surgery for univentricular atrioventricular connection ('single ventricle'). *Am. J. Cardiol.* **54**, 811.

Truncus Arteriosus

DiDonato R. M., Fyfe D. A., Puga F. J. et al. (1985) Fifteen-year experience with surgical repair of truncus arteriosus. *J. Thorac. Cardiovasc. Surg.* **89**, 414.

Ebert P. A., Turley K., Stanger P. et al. (1984) Surgical treatment of truncus arteriosus in the first six months of life. *Ann. Surg.* **200**, 451.

Tetralogy of Fallot

Arciniegas E., Farooki Z. Q., Hakimi M. et al. (1980) Results of two-stage surgical treatment of tetralogy of Fallot. *J. Thorac. Cardiovasc. Surg.* **79**, 876.

Ilbawi M. N., Grieco J., DeLeon S. Y. et al. (1984) Modified Blalock–Taussig shunt in newborn infants. *J. Thorac. Cardiovasc. Surg.* **88**, 770.

Rosenthal A., Behrendt D., Sloan H. et al. (1984) Long-term prognosis (15 to 26 years) after repair of tetralogy of Fallot: I. Survival and symptomatic status. *Ann. Thorac. Surg.* **38**, 151.

Zhao H. X., Miller D. C., Reitz B. A. et al. (1985) Surgical repair of tetralogy of Fallot. *J. Thorac. Cardiovasc. Surg.* **89**, 204.

Ventricular Septal Defect with Pulmonary Atresia

Haworth S. G. and Macartney F. J. (1980) Growth and development of pulmonary circulation in pulmonary atresia with ventricular septal defect and major aortopulmonary collateral arteries. *Br. Heart J.* **44**, 14.

Kirklin J. W., Blackstone E. H., Kirklin J. K. et al. (1983) Surgical results and protocols in the spectrum of tetralogy of Fallot. *Ann. Surg.* **198**, 251.

Piehler J. M., Danielson G. K., McGoon D. C. et al. (1980) Management of pulmonary atresia with ventricular septal defect and hypoplastic pulmonary arteries by right ventricular outflow construction. *J. Thorac. Cardiovasc. Surg.* **80**, 552.

47 *Acquired Valvular Heart Disease*

C. E. Anagnostopoulos and W. Y. Moores

The development of cardiac surgery for acquired diseases of the aortic and mitral valve began prior to the era of cardiopulmonary bypass. A 'closed' operation to dilate the fused valve leaflets in mitral stenosis was attempted successfully in 1923 by Cutler at the Peter Bent Brigham. The first successful true mitral 'valvotomy' was in 1925 by Sir Henry Souttar of the London Hospital. For a number of reasons this early success with closed technique lay dormant for over 20 years until Bailey, Harken and Glenn devised instruments for transventricular or transatrial dilatation of both the aortic and mitral valves in the late 1940s. The precise development of valvular surgery awaited the development of cardiopulmonary bypass in 1952. Following this, many different procedures for repair and replacement of heart valves were devised.

Currently valvular heart disease has taken two directions. Valve replacement today is a safe procedure when patients are correctly selected. Its long-term success depends on the continuing development of newer, more durable prosthetic valves with a lower incidence of thromboembolism. Another direction of the field is the development of newer techniques for repair of the diseased valves. The results of valve surgery are therefore constantly improving and evolving.

ACQUIRED AORTIC VALVE DISEASE

Anatomy and Physiology

The aortic valve cusps are semilunar in shape and attached to a fibrous sleeve, the aortic fibrous ring (*Fig.* 47.1). There are no chordae as in the mitral valve for support; it maintains stability by its form and long attachment to the margin of the aorta. The aortic valve has three cusps, an arrangement which offers the maximum unobstructed cross-

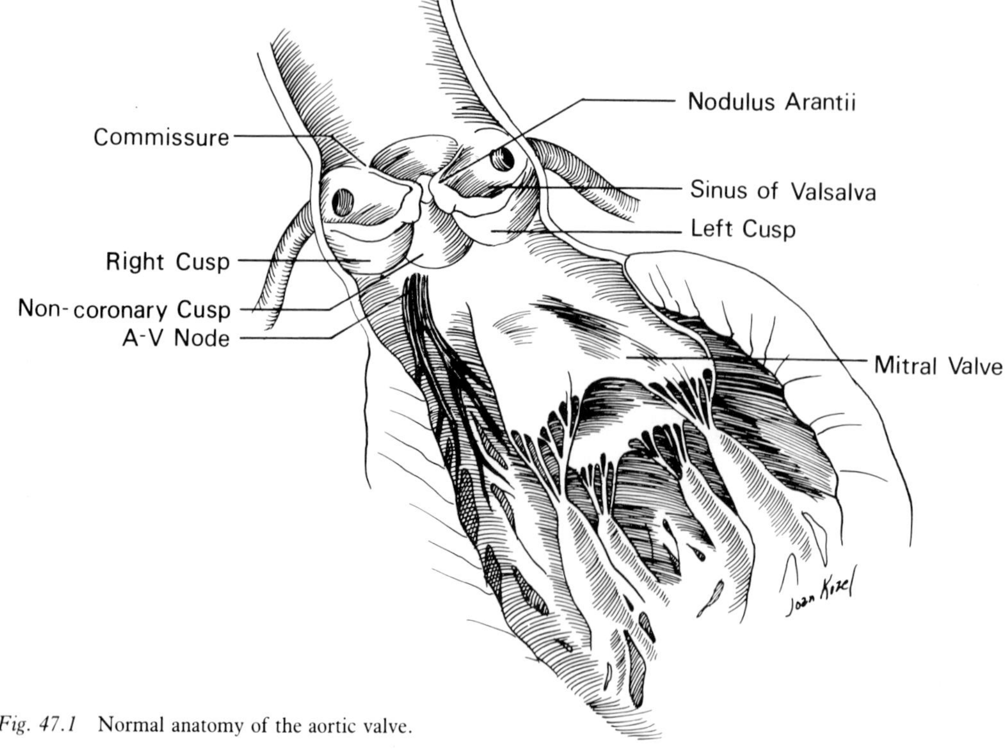

Fig. 47.1 Normal anatomy of the aortic valve.

sectional area when the valve is open (compared to bicuspid or quadricuspid valves), with minimal distortion of the cusps when closed. The right aortic sinus of Valsalva above the cusp gives rise to the right coronary artery anteriorly, the left sinus to the left coronary artery posteriorly, and the lateral cusp and sinus are the non-coronary ones. The free margins of the valve cusps meet in areas called commissures. The free margin itself is composed of a centrally located fibrous nodule, the nodulus Arantii, surrounded on each side by a very thin half-moon shaped area termed the lunula. The anterior leaflet of the mitral valve is adjacent to the left and the non-coronary cusp. The conduction pathway (atrioventricular node, bundle of His and posterior radiation), is in the ventricular septum at the junction of the non-coronary and right coronary cusps.

The function of the semilunar valve is much like that of a parachute. At the end of the ejection phase of ventricular systole an infinitesimally short period of reverse blood flow towards the ventricle snaps the aortic valve cusps together preventing regurgitation of blood past the aortic valve into the ventricle. During systole eddy currents are formed in the sinuses of Valsalva that tend to keep the valve cusps away from the vessel wall. They float freely in the bloodstream approximately half way between the vessel wall and their closed position. Therefore, the valve is not only designed to prevent regurgitation, but also is so structured as to prevent the cusps from blocking the coronary ostia.

When the primary defect is aortic stenosis, there is a decrease of the cross-sectional area at the level of the aortic valve due to fusion, fixation, and stiffening of the valve leaflets. Whereas in an adult this area is normally about $3{\cdot}0\,cm^2$, in aortic stenosis it is usually reduced to less than $1\,cm^2$. Narrowing of the aortic valve orifice produces a pressure gradient across the aortic valve. The left ventricle is forced to contract more vigorously in order to force enough blood through the stenotic valve. As a result there is hypertrophy of the left ventricular muscle. When a severe obstruction has been present for some time, left ventricular failure may occur. There is elevation of the end-diastolic pressure in the left ventricle and, often, elevation of the left atrial and pulmonary artery pressures. The failing left ventricle can no longer maintain a normal cardiac output through the stenotic valve. The pressure gradient between the left ventricle and aorta may be decreased at this point in time as left ventricular failure occurs; the typical murmur may also be diminished or absent then.

In aortic regurgitation the primary defect is regurgitation of blood into the left ventricle early in diastole. Left ventricular volume is increased. Forward blood flow is decreased as part of the effective cardiac output returns to the left ventricle. In severe aortic insufficiency, as the left ventricle fails, there is elevation of the end-diastolic pressure, as well as elevation of mean left atrial and pulmonary arterial pressures. There is also widening of the pulse pressure as diastolic pressure in the aorta decreases.

Aetiology of Disease States

Rheumatic fever is probably the most common acquired aortic valve disease. Acutely there is inflammation extending through the valve cusps. The oedema and cellular infiltration of the acute process progress to fibrosis and thickening with deformation of the valve. The valve leaflets become fused at the commissures. Eventually more and more of the free edges of the cusps become fused resulting in a small opening at the centre of the valve. Subsequent calcification is common.

Calcific aortic valve disease may be a result of trauma to a congenitally deformed valve from turbulent blood flow. In some series up to 50% of patients dying of aortic stenosis in adult life exhibited calcification of a congenitally deformed valve. The most common deformity is the congenitally bicuspid aortic valve. These patients may demonstrate some calcification by the age of 20. Some patients, however, present with a murmur of aortic stenosis in midlife with no prior history of either heart murmur or rheumatic fever. This group probably represents calcification in a valve that has degenerated owing to accelerated ageing.

Syphilis, subacute bacterial endocarditis, trauma and Marfan's syndrome are less common causes of aortic regurgitation. Syphilis causes dilatation of the ascending aorta secondary to infiltration by inflammatory cells around the vasa vasorum of the aorta. The muscular and elastic layers of the aortic media are destroyed. Aortic regurgitation occurs when the aortic root is involved by dilatation. This is a relatively uncommon cause of aortic regurgitation nowadays. Subacute bacterial endocarditis is more common. Aortic regurgitation is produced by perforation of a valve leaflet or disruption of normal leaflet suspension. Vegetations may also appear on the valve cusps preventing apposition and occasionally resulting in septic emboli. Penetrating trauma can produce aortic regurgitation by directly injuring the valve leaflets. Blunt trauma can also produce aortic regurgitation when a sharp blow to the chest occurs with the valve closed. A sudden increase in pressure against the closed aortic valve may detach a cusp from its commissural attachment.

Marfan's syndrome is an inherited disease, one of the features of which is cystic degeneration of the medial layer of the aorta. This eventually leads to dilatation of the ascending aorta with annular dilatation and secondary valvular regurgitation. The classic presentation of these patients is a tall physique with elongated arms and legs, long fingers, hyperextensible joints, subluxation of the lens of the eye, high arched palate, prolapse of the mitral valve and a tendency toward dissection of the ascending aorta. Treatment of the aortic lesion in this disease usually requires replacement of the valve and ascending aorta with reimplantation of the coronary arteries into the prosthetic ascending aorta.

Diagnosis

Even moderate to severe aortic valve disease may progress for some time without symptoms. When aortic stenosis does give rise to symptoms, they consist of effort syncope or dizziness, angina pectoris and dyspnoea occurring in that order. Syncope may in fact be a very early serious symptom even in children. Symptoms of angina or syncope may occur as a reduced and relatively fixed amount of cardiac output cannot keep up with the demand placed on the heart with exercise. In its terminal stages, frank congestive heart failure may be the supervening symptom. One disquieting aspect of aortic stenosis is a 10–20% incidence of sudden death. This may be related to arrhythmias. In addition to their underlying disease, a significant number of these patients develop coronary artery disease in the 'normal' course of events, or infective endocarditis becomes superimposed on the deformed valve. The latter may follow dental procedures performed without antibiotic prophylaxis.

In regurgitation, symptoms include sweating, palpitations, fatigue, angina and dyspnoea on exertion. As the left ventricle fails symptoms of pulmonary congestion and right heart failure become prominent.

Physical examination in aortic stenosis reveals evidence of left ventricular hypertrophy, a harsh ejection-systolic murmur often preceded by an ejection click in the right 2nd intercostal space with radiation to the carotid arteries. A prominent thrill may be palpable in the same location. With advanced aortic stenosis and calcification of the valve the aortic component of the second heart sound is decreased or absent and no ejection click is audible. The blood pressure may be low–normal with a decreased pulse pressure and sluggish upstroke. In aortic regurgitation the typical murmur is an immediate diastolic murmur which is often loudest in the left 4th intercostal space. Many of these patients with severe leakage across the valve have a loud left ventricular third heart sound followed by a short diastolic murmur (Austin–Flint). This presumably is caused by the regurgitant jet of blood from the aortic valve pushing the anterior leaflet of the mitral valve into the stream of blood going from the left atrium to the left ventricle in diastole. The pulse pressure is wide as a result of an increased systolic pressure and a decreased diastolic pressure in the aorta. The pulse has a 'water-hammer' or 'pistol-shot' quality as a result of the rapid high upstroke with a rapid fall off in diastole.

The ECG may show evidence of left ventricular hypertrophy and strain in both aortic stenosis and regurgitation. The chest radiograph will show evidence of left ventricular enlargement in aortic stenosis with poststenotic dilatation of the ascending aorta. Note, however, that the heart may remain normal in overall size until cardiac failure supervenes. In aortic regurgitation, however, considerable overall enlargement of the heart is obvious, depending on the regurgitant volume and degree of associated cardiac failure. Both lesions may show calcification in the region of the aortic valve although it is more common in aortic stenosis. This is best appreciated by image intensification fluoroscopy although when heavy calcification is present it is visible in the lateral view on the plain radiograph.

Echocardiography is very useful in screening patients with aortic valve disease. Findings of calcification and decreased excursion of the valve in aortic stenosis, as well as changes in contractility and thickness of the ventricle, may be used to estimate the severity of the disease. Two-dimensional echocardiography can give a rough estimate of the aortic valve area. In the presence of significant aortic regurgitation there may, in addition, be fluttering of the anterior leaflet of the mitral valve in diastole. The standard and two-dimensional echocardiograms are useful in detecting a bicuspid aortic valve.

The quantification of aortic stenosis or regurgitation requires cardiac catheterization, although a reasonable estimate of regurgitation can be made using the newer Echo and Doppler flow techniques. Simultaneous measurement of pressure in the left ventricle and aorta will quantitate the gradient across a stenotic aortic valve. A gradient of more than 50 mmHg is indicative of severe aortic stenosis in the presence of a reasonable cardiac output. Since cardiac outputs vary it is important to calculate actual valve areas using both gradients and cardiac outputs prior to assigning a severity classification to the aortic stenosis. A calculated aortic valve area of less than $1{\cdot}5\,cm^2$ is considered mild aortic stenosis, less than $1\,cm^2$ is moderate aortic stenosis, and less than $0{\cdot}5\,cm^2$ severe aortic stenosis. Left ventricular end-diastolic pressure may be elevated in aortic stenosis but is more commonly increased in aortic regurgitation. Elevation of left atrial, pulmonary artery, and right heart pressures may result. An aortic root angiogram is used to detect and roughly quantitate the degree of aortic regurgitation. Rapid complete filling of the left ventricle within one diastole indicates severe leakage across the aortic valve. A left ventriculogram is obtained to determine the contractility of the left ventricle and the ejection fraction may be calculated. Simultaneous coronary angiography should be performed especially in patients over 40 years of age whether they have symptoms of angina or not. An atrial septal defect or patent foramen ovale should be looked for to avoid problems with venous line air at surgery.

Indications for Operation

To understand the indications for operation in aortic valve disease it is necessary to be familiar with the natural course of the disease itself. Acute aortic regurgitation results in a sudden volume load on the left ventricle. Since there is no compensatory hypertrophy, there is early dilatation and failure of the left ventricle, as well as possible coronary ischaemia and sudden death. Medical management is unsuccessful in these patients and emergency aortic valve replacement is necessary. Chronic aortic regurgitation, however, is an insidious process that gradually results in ventricular failure. These patients can be watched carefully for a period of time until there is evidence of hypertrophy. Once a patient has hypertrophy or severe failure in the presence of aortic regurgitation, the ventricle will frequently not recover to a normal state even after the volume load on the ventricle is relieved. Fifty per cent of patients with more than 100 mmHg pulse pressure or less than 40 mmHg aortic diastolic pressure are dead within 2 years. Seventy-five per cent of patients are alive 5 years after a diagnosis of moderate aortic regurgitation is made. Fifty per cent are still alive at 10 years. With mild aortic regurgitation 95% of patients are alive at 10 years.

Once a patient shows evidence of decompensation, the course is usually rapidly downhill. If valve replacement must be performed in the patient with uncompensated left ventricular failure, the morbidity and mortality are greatly increased. Therefore, patients with aortic regurgitation should undergo replacement of the aortic valve before they develop symptoms of significant failure.

Patients with aortic stenosis may remain asymptomatic despite marked reduction in valve area. Relatively large gradients across the aortic valve may be well tolerated for years if left ventricular function remains relatively unimpaired. Nevertheless, the 5- and 10-year survival following the diagnosis of aortic stenosis is only 40% and 20% respectively. Two problems demand cautious observation in these patients. First, there is an increased incidence of sudden death in patients with moderate to severe aortic stenosis. Second, when symptoms of syncope, angina or severe breathlessness occur, the average survival is only 2 years. Therefore, patients with haemodynamically severe aortic stenosis or who have developed symptoms of angina, syncope, or congestive heart failure or signs of cardiac enlargement should undergo early valve replacement.

Risks and Complications

The operative mortality for elective aortic valve replacement is less than 5%. The incidence of postoperative embolism, thrombosis, or prosthetic valve infection is small. In patients with severely decompensated left ventricles, especially with aortic regurgitation, the operative mortality is significantly higher, approaching 20%. Even though a patient may have an acutely decompensated left ventricle in the presence of aortic stenosis, removal of the pressure gradient by replacement with a prosthetic valve will fequently produce dramatic improvement.

Potential complications following valve replacement are paravalvular leak and infection. Paravalvular leakage may occur due to insecure seating of the valve at the time of operation, disruption of sutures, or disruption of a friable annulus. The incidence of this complication is less than 5% in most large series. Infection of a prosthetic valve is a serious complication. The incidence of this complication in several large series is between 0·5 and 4%. The specific type of therapy and prognosis depend on the infecting organism. Staphylococcus is the most common organism causing prosthetic endocarditis within 60 days of valve replacement, whereas streptococcus is more common beyond that 60-day period. An attempt at prolonged intravenous antibiotic treatment of these organisms is warranted since a significant

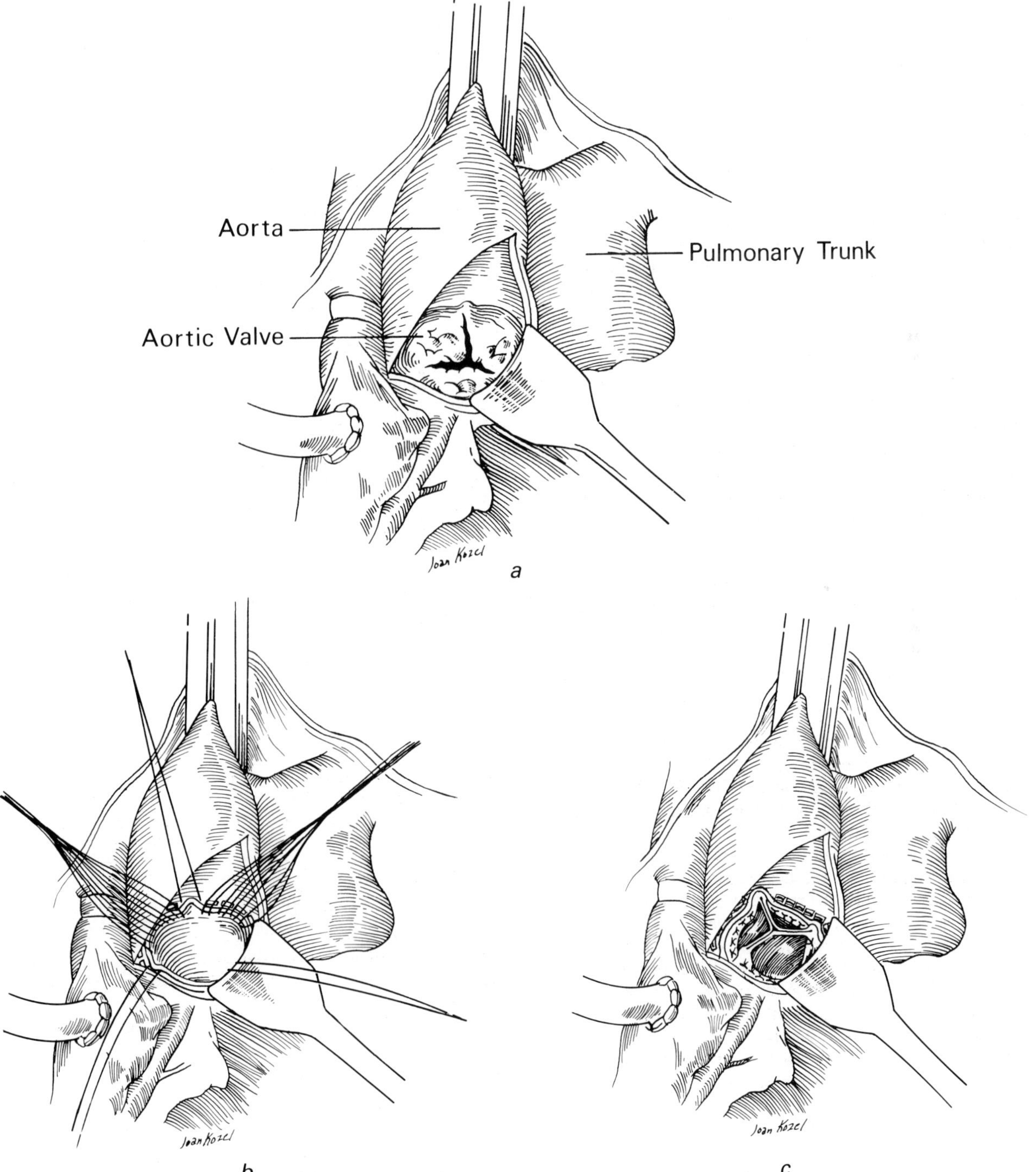

Fig. 47.2 Aortic valve replacement: *a*, A calcified stenotic aortic valve as viewed through a reverse hockey stick aortotomy. *b*, The aortic valve has been excised and some of the valve sutures have been placed in the aortic annulus. Three stay sutures have been placed at the commissures for retraction and a vein retractor is exposing the area. *c*, A porcine heterograft valve has been lowered into position and the sutures tied and cut.

number of these patients will respond to antibiotic therapy. Fungus infection and certain Gram-negative organisms have shown relatively few signs of responding to antibiotic therapy alone. When these organisms are involved, especially in the presence of a new paravalvular leak, early valve replacement is currently being recommended. If the patient does not respond dramatically to a trial of antibiotic therapy or if failure is present, valve replacement with wide débridement of the infected annulus should be carried out. All patients with prosthetic valves should be covered by antibiotics for dental or genito-urinary procedures, or other surgical procedures which may result in bacteraemia.

Other complications are related to the specific type of valve used. The varying rates of thrombosis and embolism with mechanical bioprosthetic valves will be discussed later. Likewise, degeneration in bioprosthetic valves will also be discussed at the end of this chapter.

Operative Technique for Aortic Valve Replacement

Aortic valve replacement is performed through a midline sternotomy incision using cardiopulmonary bypass. In the presence of severe aortic regurgitation, the surgeon must be prepared to cross-clamp the aorta if the heart fibrillates once bypass has begun, to prevent massive dilatation of the left ventricle. In addition, a sump catheter (or vent) is placed into the left ventricle or through the left atrial appendage, the right superior pulmonary vein, or the pulmonary artery to decompress the left ventricular chamber. The patient is cooled to 24–28 °C and the aorta cross-clamped. The aortic valve is exposed through a reverse hockey stick incision extending down into the non-coronary sinus of Valsalva (*Fig.* 47.2*a*). Although myocardial preservation may be obtained with continuous coronary artery perfusion, this technique is almost never used and has been replaced by the more effective technique of intermittent perfusion with one of the many cardioplegia agents available. The latter have the advantage of placing the heart in diastolic arrest. In addition, the heart itself may be cooled topically with 4 °C saline, ice slush, or a local cooling device. The aortic valve is excised leaving a small rim of valve tissue for suturing. In some cases with extensive calcification this is not possible. If the valve annulus is of adequate size horizontal mattress sutures with pledgets are placed circumferentially beginning in the region of the left coronary orifice (*Fig.* 47.2*b*). Care is taken to avoid injury to the conduction system in the area of the junction of the right and non-coronary cusp and the mitral valve in the area of the left and non-coronary cusp. If the annulus is small, simple sutures may be necessary to avoid narrowing it. Techniques are also available for enlarging the annulus when necessary by incision of the normal mitral or ventricular septum. The choice of valve is up to the individual centre. The valve is then lowered into place and the sutures tied and cut (*Fig.* 47.2*c*). If the ascending aorta is narrow, especially when a porcine heterograft valve is used, a patch may be necessary to enlarge the ascending aorta. As the patient is rewarmed to normothermia, the aortotomy is closed and air is carefully evacuated from the left heart and continuously from the ascending aorta. Once the heart has resumed its own rhythm and is ejecting blood into the aorta, the vent evacuating air from the aorta is removed. The patient is then gradually weaned from cardiopulmonary bypass.

Results of Operation

Five-year survival following aortic valve replacement is influenced by many factors. A 5-year survival of 75–85% has been reported with the Ross homograft, the Bjork–Shiley disc valve, the Starr–Edwards ball valve, and the porcine heterograft valve. The survival rate of patients with primary aortic regurgitation is worse than those with aortic stenosis. Some of the factors related to a decreased survival following valve replacement include: patient's age, the presence of congestive heart failure preoperatively, the patient's functional class, cardiac enlargement, elevated left atrial or pulmonary artery pressure, the presence of concomitant coronary artery disease, and the presence of depressed left ventricular function as measured by cardiac index and left ventriculogram. The type of aortic valve prosthesis used probably does not have a significant effect on long-term survival.

The quality of life following aortic valve replacement may be influenced by the type of prosthesis used. Long-term anticoagulation is necessary to prevent thromboembolism with most types of prosthesis. There is a small but definite incidence of anticoagulant-related morbidity and mortality from bleeding. The patient taking anticoagulants must have frequent blood tests and refrain from activities which might result in serious injury with potential bleeding. The porcine heterograft valve is associated with a lower incidence of thromboembolism and originally was thought to eliminate the necessity for anticoagulation. However, many patients even with this valve in the aortic position are now being anticoagulated long term to prevent degeneration related to microscopic clotting on the leaflets. Furthermore, it is now known that porcine heterograft valve degeneration requiring replacement occurs. No fewer than 9 of our last 100 patients to receive such valves required replacement within 2½ years of the initial procedure, leading to the use of the Bjork–Shiley valve more frequently.

ACQUIRED DISEASE OF THE MITRAL VALVE

Anatomy and Physiology

The normal mitral valve consists of an anterior and a posterior leaflet (*Fig.* 47.3) as well as two commissural leaflets. The edges of the leaflets are extremely thin and delicate. A small distance from the edge are fine nodules called the noduli Albini. These nodules mark the area of coaptation of the valve leaflets. There are three sets of chordae tendineae attaching the mitral valve to the ventricle and preventing the valve from inverting into the left atrium during systole. The first set of chordae arise from the apices of the papillary muscles and insert into the edges of the valve leaflets. The second set of chordae attach to the ventricular surface of the valve leaflets in the area of the noduli Albini. These chordae are thicker and stronger than the first-order chordae and are the mainstays of the valve mechanism. The third-order chordae originate from the ventricular wall and attach closer to the valve annulus. Each leaflet receives chordae from more than one papillary muscle and each papillary muscle sends chordae to more than one leaflet.

Normally there is no gradient across the mitral valve, nor is there any regurgitation. The normal adult mitral valve area is 4–6 cm^2.

In the normal heart the opened valve leaflets are close to each other during ventricular filling or during operative induced fibrillation or arrest. This is most likely due to the presence of eddy currents behind the valve leaflets. With normal P–R intervals the increase in ventricular pressure at the beginning of ventricular contraction causes the mitral valve to close. When the P–R interval is long the mitral

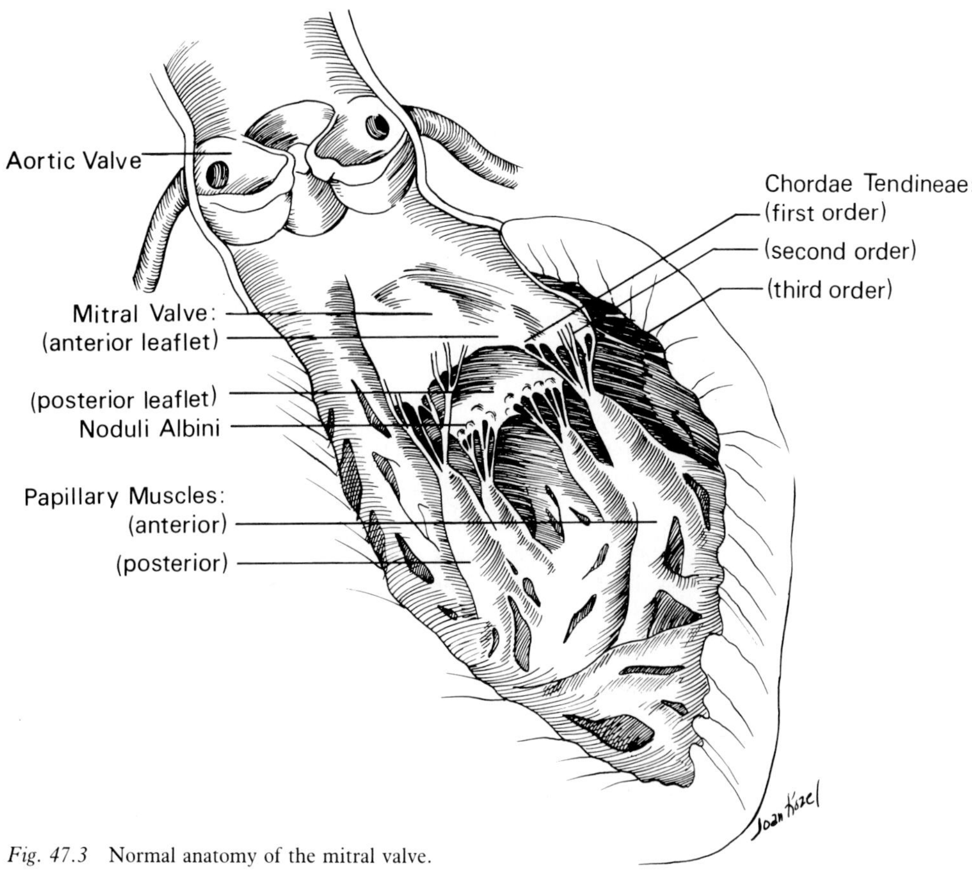

Fig. 47.3 Normal anatomy of the mitral valve.

valve closes as a result of atrial relaxation with a lowering of left atrial pressure in relation to ventricular pressure.

When the mitral valve becomes stenotic with a valve area of less than 2·5 cm^2 there is obstruction to the free flow of blood from the left atrium to the left ventricle in diastole. This causes a rise in pressure in the left atrium and a significant pressure gradient between the left atrium and left ventricle at the end of diastole. With more significant mitral stenosis (a valve area of less than 1 cm^2) there is a reduction in cardiac output, a further elevation in left atrial pressure, and an elevation in pulmonary vascular resistance. Eventually this leads to elevated right heart pressures which can produce tricuspid regurgitation. With a valve area of 0·5–1 cm^2 cardiac output becomes relatively fixed and can no longer be increased with exercise or exertion. These patients may demonstrate symptoms at rest. With tachycardia, there is decreased time for filling of the left ventricle owing to the stenotic orifice. This leads to a further reduction in cardiac output. With longstanding mitral valve disease the development of atrial fibrillation is common, and, in addition, there is a very significant risk of mural thrombus formation with systemic embolization. A left atrial pressure greater than 30 mmHg will exceed the oncotic pressure of plasma in the pulmonary capillaries. Transudation of fluid into the interstitium of the lung produces pulmonary oedema and Kerley's B lines on radiography.

Mitral regurgitation results in a portion of the left ventricular volume leaking into the left atrium during systole. With the following diastole part of the regurgitant volume, in addition to normal forward flow, fills the left ventricle. This results in dilatation of both the left atrium and left ventricle with left ventricular hypertrophy as the inevitable consequence. Although there is a very raised left atrial pressure during ventricular ejection (it may be as high as 90 mmHg), the mean left atrial pressure is usually not as elevated as with mitral stenosis because of left atrial and pulmonary venous capacitance and elasticity. With severe longstanding mitral regurgitation, elevation of pulmonary vascular resistance and right heart pressures may follow. These patients may develop a 'giant left atrium' if the process continues for a significant period of time. The extent of left atrial enlargement, however, is not related to the degree of mitral regurgitation but to the variable compliance of the chamber. These patients may develop atrial fibrillation and are at risk of systemic embolism, although the incidence is less than in those with predominant mitral stenosis.

Aetiology of Disease States

The most common valvular cardiac lesion is mitral stenosis. Although no history of rheumatic fever is obtained in 50% of patients with this lesion, this is considered the most common aetiology. Women are affected more frequently than men. Due to current effective antibiotic prophylaxis in patients with streptococcal pharyngitis, the incidence of rheumatic valvular disease has declined significantly, particularly in Western countries. Although rheumatic fever affects all areas of the myocardium, pericardium and valve tissue, the significant lesion in most patients is an active valvulitis. The pathological changes of the mitral valve include fusion of commissures, fibrosis and retraction of the valve leaflets with eventual calcification, and fusion and shortening of the chordae tendineae. Congenital mitral stenosis is rare.

The symptoms of rheumatic valve involvement do not usually occur for 10–12 years following an attack of rheumatic fever. The most likely cause for this delay is that the initial inflammatory reaction in and around the valve leads to turbulent flow. Valve destruction progresses due to the altered haemodynamics in the area of the valve. A second possibility, recurrent episodes of rheumatic fever, is unlikely. Concomitant myocardiopathy and pericarditis occasionally occur.

Unlike mitral stenosis, mitral regurgitation has several possible aetiologies. Rheumatic fever is probably the most common. Mild degrees of valve involvement may be accompanied by massive dilatation of the mitral valve annulus.

Mitral valve prolapse is an increasingly recognized syndrome. This defect rarely results in significant mitral insufficiency. It is frequently associated with anginal symptoms, or dysrhythmias, and rarely with embolism.

Less common causes of mitral regurgitation are infective endocarditis, ruptured chordae tendineae, and papillary muscle necrosis secondary to myocardial infarction with resulting rupture of chordal attachments. Mitral regurgitation is also associated with myxomatous degeneration of the valve, Marfan's sydrome, Libman–Sachs endocarditis, and various connective tissue and metabolic diseases affecting the mitral valve. Hurler's syndrome, Ehlers–Danlos syndrome, amyloidosis and sarcoidosis have all been associated with mitral regurgitation.

Diagnosis

Patients with mitral stenosis present with a history of increasing frequency and severity of dyspnoea on exertion, orthopnoea, and paroxysmal nocturnal dyspnoea. Frequent episodes of left heart failure with pulmonary oedema and even haemoptysis are not unusual. Haemoptysis may be an early symptom due to rupture of bronchial pulmonary venous anastomoses with bleeding into the tracheobronchial tree.

Acute exacerbation of symptoms commonly accompanies exercise, pregnancy, a serious infection, or the onset of atrial fibrillation. Frequently, the diagnosis is first made in women during pregnancy when there is increased demand on the heart for cardiac output to the fetus. Intermittent episodes of atrial fibrillation may be brought to the physician's attention by the occurrence of a systemic embolus.

Symptoms of mitral regurgitation are similar to those of mitral stenosis but are usually less severe. When mitral regurgitation occurs as a result of an acute episode, such as papillary muscle necrosis from myocardial infarction, emergency surgical intervention is often necessary.

The physical findings of mitral stenosis in patients in sinus rhythm include: an apical delayed diastolic murmur preceded by the opening snap of the mitral valve, an accentuated first heart sound and an accentuated pulmonary component to the second heart sound. In addition, when the valve leaflets are extremely immobile or calcified, the first heart sound may be reduced and the opening snap may be absent or minimal. A diastolic thrill may be palpable at the apex. In isolated mitral stenosis the normal left ventricle may be difficult to palpate at the apex whereas obvious enlargement of the right ventricle can be appreciated.

In mitral regurgitation cardiac palpation reveals the dynamic precordial movement of an enlarged left ventricle. There is a pansystolic murmur at the apex radiating to the left axilla. Due to the large volume of blood crossing the mitral valve there may be a loud third heart sound followed by a short diastolic murmur.

The ECG of mitral valve disease may show various supraventricular rhythm disturbances. Atrial fibrillation and flutter are common. The 'P mitrale' consists of a P wave longer than 0·12 sec with two separate peaks. Left ventricular hypertrophy may be recorded in mitral regurgitation, and right ventricular hypertrophy commonly in mitral stenosis with associated pulmonary hypertension.

The chest radiograph in mitral stenosis shows enlargement of the left atrium (demonstrated in both posterior-anterior and lateral projections) enlargement of the left pulmonary artery and left atrial appendage, the latter giving a smooth projection to the left heart border, increased pulmonary venous vascular markings in the upper lung fields and interstitial pulmonary oedema as demonstrated by Kerley's B lines. In contrast, in mitral regurgitation there is usually enlargement of the left ventricle. Massive enlargement of the left atrium may also be seen and as with mitral stenosis prominence of the upper lobe veins and Kerley's B lines may be noted. Calcification in the region of the mitral valve may be identified on image intensification fluoroscopy or, when heavy, may be noted in both posterior-anterior and lateral chest radiographs.

Echocardiography is an excellent technique for studying the mitral valve. Evidence of delayed emptying of the left atrium, abnormal motion of the mitral valve leaflets due to commissural fusion, increased thickness or calcification of the valve leaflets, and enlargement of the left atrium may all be seen in mitral stenosis. Two-dimensional echocardiography may provide an estimate of the mitral valve area. With mitral regurgitation, volume overload of the left ventricle may be recorded, but the echocardiogram is less useful in this condition than in mitral stenosis. Mitral valve prolapse and mitral valve vegetations may often be identified by echocardiography, as well as other forms of mitral pathology involving abnormalities of the chordae tendineae and calcification of the annulus.

Cardiac catheterization in mitral stenosis may reveal elevation of right heart pressures. Left atrial pressure measured directly or indirectly by pulmonary artery wedge pressure is usually elevated, particularly on exercise. Pulmonary vascular resistance may be elevated. Left heart catheterization reveals a pressure gradient between the left atrium and left ventricle in end-diastole with a decrease in the calculated mitral valve area. The left atrial pressure tracing in mitral stenosis will show 'a' giant a wave (the pressure wave produced by atrial contraction in sinus rhythm) and in mitral regurgitation a giant V wave (the pressure wave produced by ventricular systole). Left ventriculogram will demonstrate the severity of mitral regurgitation. Concomitant coronary angiography should be performed for its own indications or in otherwise asymptomatic patients over the age of 40. An atrial septal defect or patent foramen should be looked for to avoid surprises at surgery with possible air in the venous lines.

Indications for Operation

Once more it is important to recognize the natural history of the valve lesion to determine when an operation should be recommended. In mitral stenosis the asymptomatic patient may remain so for 10–20 years. However, patients in the New York Heart Association functional class III and IV treated medically have a 5-year survival rate of approximately 60 and 15% respectively. It is clear therefore that patients who are asymptomatic should be treated medically and that patients in functional class III and IV are candidates for surgical treatment. Patients in functional class II may be treated either medically or surgically depending on their degree of disability and their surgical prognosis. Patients with pulmonary artery aneurysm may be inoperable.

Pure mitral regurgitation carries a similar prognosis to mitral stenosis (overall 5-year survivals of 75–80%). However, the combination of mitral regurgitation and mitral stenosis reduces the 5-year survival to approximately 60%. A mild decrease in mitral valve area (for example, 2 cm^2) becomes extremely significant in the presence of increased mitral valve flow due to the presence of significant mitral regurgitation. Because of the poorer prognosis for medical therapy of the combined lesion, earlier surgical intervention is indicated.

Risks and Complications of Mitral Valve Operations

The operative mortality for mitral valve replacement in the otherwise uncomplicated patient is currently less than 5%. With newer techniques for myocardial preservation during cardiopulmonary bypass this mortality will probably approach the mortality of cardiopulmonary bypass alone (approximately 1%). One complication unique to mitral valve replacement is that of ventricular rupture. It has been reported to occur at the thin attachment of the atrium to the ventricle in the posterior atrioventricular sulcus or in the midportion of the left ventricle overlying the papillary muscle. It is caused by overzealous resection of the mitral annulus or papillary muscle in most instances. It may also be caused by the strut of a porcine heterograft valve especially after an episode of cardiac massage postoperatively or transventricular sump drains, or posteriorly placed stiff pericardial tubes. This complication may occur acutely in the operating room or hours to days postoperatively. Survival is rare in the delayed type of rupture; however, in the operating room with immediate reinstitution of cardiopulmonary bypass and careful repair from within, after temporary removal of the prosthesis and avoidance of the circumflex coronary artery survival is possible. Intra-aortic balloon should be used postoperatively to allow for less ventricular tension.

Delayed complications following mitral valve replacement are: prosthetic valve infection, prosthetic valve thrombosis, embolism, and degeneration of a bioprosthetic valve. Aside from prosthetic valve infection which occurs in up to 3% of valve replacements, the incidence of the other complications appears to be related to the specific valve prosthesis being used. The bioprosthetic valves were thought to have a lower incidence of valve thrombosis and embolism, but recent figures challenge this view. In addition, the longevity of these valves is currently in question.

Operative Techniques

'Open' mitral commissurotomy with the use of cardiopulmonary bypass has gained in popularity in the last 10 years. In combination with plastic repairs of the subvalvular mechanism, open commissurotomy can provide significant palliation. The patient is placed on cardiopulmonary bypass and the left atrium exposed through an incision just posterior to the interatrial groove. The mitral valve leaflets are retracted until the areas of the fused commissures are identified. Cautious incision in the two commissures is carried out until the valve leaflets have been divided up to a few millimetres from the valve annulus to avoid division of the unsupported commissural leaflets. At this time the subvalvular mechanism is inspected. Frequently there is fusion of the chordae and shortening. When simple fusion is present the chordae can be separated by incision with a scalpel. When there is concomitant shortening, the papillary muscle can also be divided with scalpel incision. A few centres have reported repair of elongated chordae tendineae by incising the papillary muscle and suturing the redundant chordae into the muscle itself. In cases of annular dilatation a Carpentier ring, a flexible Duran ring, or a Wooler annuloplasty can be used to circumferentially tighten the mitral valve annulus. The left ventricle is then filled with fluid or blood through a transaortic perforated sump tube, and the valve checked for competency. If regurgitation is mild or absent and an adequate valve area has been obtained, the atrium is closed and the air is carefully evacuated from the left side of the heart. If, however, severe mitral insufficiency has been produced, prosthetic replacement of the mitral valve is necessary.

Exposure for mitral valve replacement is usually achieved through the same approach (*Fig.* 47.4*a*). A midline sternotomy incision is preferred for both types of procedures. The valve is excised leaving a rim of valve tissue on the mitral annulus, especially in the region of the posterior leaflet. In areas of severe calcification, a rongeur may be necessary to completely débride annular calcification. Horizontal mattress sutures with or without pledgets are then placed circumferentially in the mitral annulus and subsequently through the sewing ring of a prosthetic valve (*Fig.* 47.4*b*). Valve sizers are available for each type of prosthetic valve in order to determine the correct size of prosthetic valve to insert. Usually, a valve one size smaller than the largest size that can be placed through the valve annulus is selected. If a heterograft valve is used a dental mirror is inserted through the orifice of the prosthesis to assure that no sutures have been inadvertently wrapped around a strut. The prosthetic valve is then lowered into position and the sutures tied and cut (*Fig.* 47.4*c*). The left atrium is then closed while air is vented from the left ventricle and ascending aorta. Air is repeatedly evacuated from the left ventricle, the left atrium and right superior pulmonary vein, and ascending aorta while the heart resumes normal cardiac action. Bjork–Shiley valve discs are oriented appropriately posteriorly by rotation to avoid impingement on the septum upon opening. In uncomplicated mitral regurgitation with no deficiency of valve leaflet tissue, an annuloplasty may be all that is necessary to provide valve competency.

Results of Operation

Results with Bjork–Shiley and Starr–Edwards valves are similar. The 5-year survival following mitral valve replacement is in the 70–85% range. There are few series with long-term follow-up of open mitral commissurotomy. The limited data available indicate that the 5-year survival is approximately 95% with 90% of patients in functional class I and II. An additional 5% of patients require valve replacement less than 5 years following commissurotomy. With the more extensive valvuloplastic procedures being used currently these results will improve.

ACQUIRED DISEASE OF THE TRICUSPID VALVE

Isolated disease of the tricuspid valve is rare. Rheumatic involvement of the tricuspid valve along with the mitral or aortic valve, or functional tricuspid regurgitation as a result of right heart dilatation from longstanding mitral and aortic valve disease is more common. These lesions may be divided into three categories: *organic disease* of the tricuspid valve,

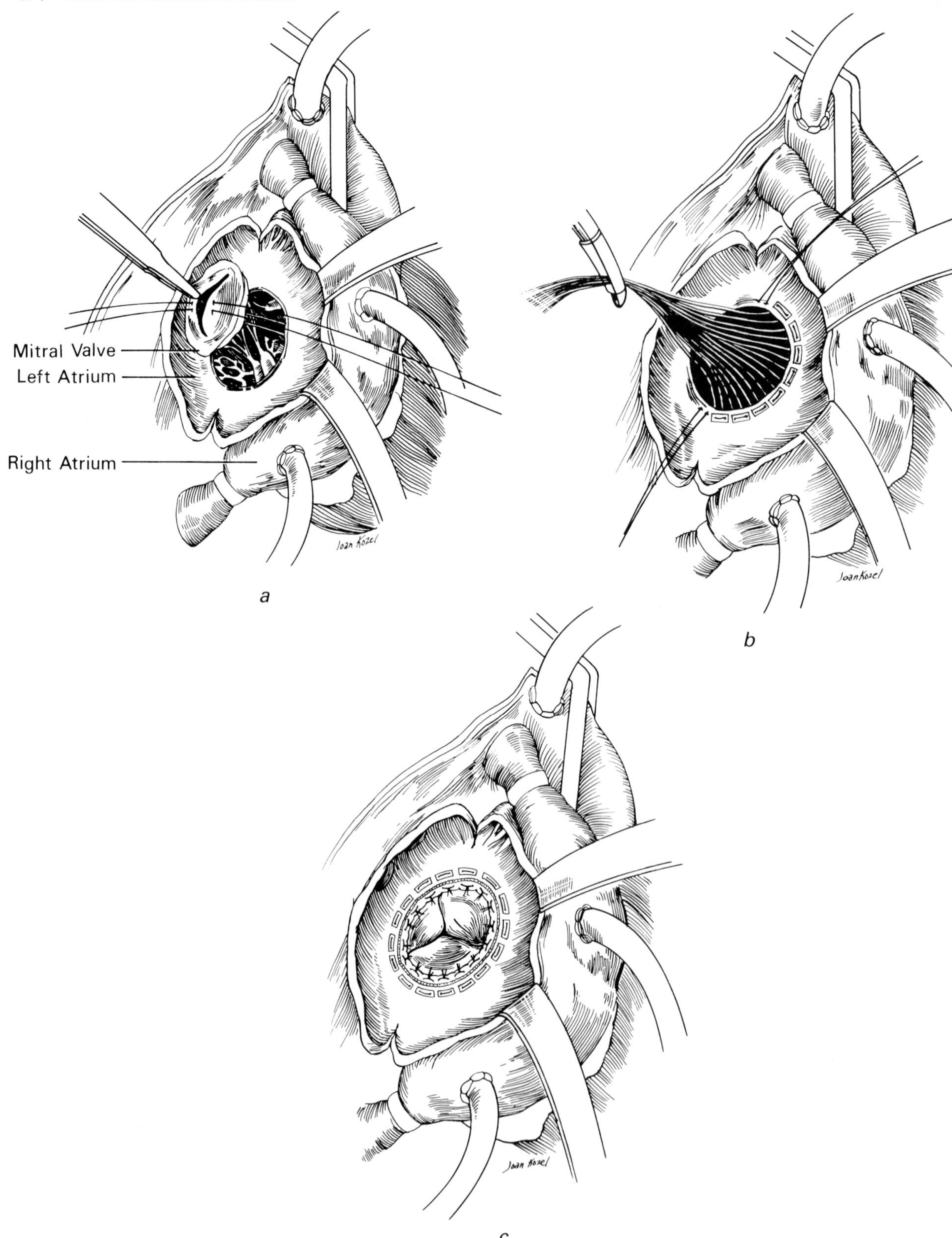

Fig. 47.4 Mitral valve replacement: *a*, Exposure for excision of the diseased mitral valve is obtained through a left atriotomy by retracting the atrial wall with two bladder retractors. The valve has been partially excised and the chordae tendineae will be divided at the level of the tips of the papillary muscles. *b*, The valve has been excised and two stay sutures have been placed in the annulus, one adjacent to the aortic valve and one 180° opposite. Part of the pledgeted valve sutures have been placed through the annulus. *c*, The porcine heterograft mitral valve has been lowered into position and the sutures tied and cut.

functional reversible disease of the tricuspid valve, and *irreversible functional disease* of the tricuspid valve. Patients with significant tricuspid regurgitation or stenosis present with findings of severe peripheral oedema, hepatosplenomegaly, ascites, and abnormal jugular venous pulsations. A murmur of tricuspid valve disease may be mistaken for one of mitral origin if the patient is not examined carefully.

Chest radiography reveals multichamber enlargement from the related multivalvular disease as well as right atrial enlargement. The ECG may show a peaked P wave secondary to delayed right atrial activation. Cardiac catheterization will show an elevated right atrial pressure with an end-diastolic gradient between the right ventricle and right atrium. An elevated right atrial 'a' wave (the pressure wave secondary to atrial contraction) is found. Although tricuspid valvulotomy is occasionally successful, replacement is usually necessary.

Tricuspid regurgitation is the result of rheumatic valvulitis or dilatation of the right ventricle and tricuspid annulus. It may also be caused by blunt chest trauma or infective endocarditis. The physical findings of distended neck veins and a pulsating liver along with ascites and peripheral oedema may be found with severe tricuspid regurgitation. A pansystolic murmur maximal along the lower right sternal border and significantly louder during inspiration may be heard. Chest radiography and ECG are similar to tricuspid stenosis. But specific enlargement of the right atrium is more common in tricuspid stenosis. Both the right atrium and ventricle are enlarged in regurgitation. Cardiac catheterization is notoriously ineffective for determining the degree of tricuspid insufficiency owing to induced insufficiency by the catheter.

Patients with organic stenosis of the tricuspid valve usually require valve replacement or commissurotomy. Tricuspid regurgitation, however, may be organic or functional. *Organic tricuspid regurgitation* may be treated by either valve replacement or valvuloplasty (Carpentier full ring, Duran Flexible ring, Cooley partial ring, or De Vega suture). If caused by infection then tricuspid valvectomy is compatible with long-term survival in the absence of left heart valve disease. Functional tricuspid regurgitation should be assessed before and after repair of other valves. If there is marked improvement when the patient is weaned from cardiopulmonary bypass following repair of the aortic or mitral valve, nothing further need be done. If there is still significant tricuspid regurgitation or if the patient has been jaundiced preoperatively, tricuspid annuloplasty should be performed. If significant tricuspid regurgitation is left untreated, then postoperative morbidity and mortality are increased.

The porcine heterograft valve has markedly improved the results of tricuspid valve replacement recently. This is the valve of choice in the tricuspid position because of the significantly lower incidence of thrombosis, obstruction and embolism. The techniques are similar to those of mitral annuloplasty and replacement. Heart block will be avoided if the septal leaflet of the tricuspid valve is preserved for suture placement.

The operative mortalities for aortic and mitral valve replacement, mitral and tricuspid valve replacement and triple valve replacement are similar. The 5-year survival for patients with organic tricuspid valve disease is significantly better than with functional tricuspid valve disease (70% versus 40%). This probably reflects the extensive deterioration of the ventricle which accompanies functional dilatation of the tricuspid annulus. Earlier operation will be necessary to salvage additional patients from this group.

THE WAY AHEAD

Future improvements in the surgical treatment of valvular heart disease depend on better myocardial preservation during cardiopulmonary bypass and improvements in the bioengineering of the newer prosthetic cardiac valves. With the use of cardioplegia solutions, myocardial function can be preserved for the 1–2 h necessary for any valve repair or replacement procedure. These techniques have allowed the surgeon two or more hours of safe operating time in a bloodless field with a relaxed myocardium. With safe aortic cross-clamping for this period of time, the surgeon can do a meticulous job of either reconstruction or replacement of one or more valves, and of simultaneous coronary revascularization or ventricular reconstruction or repair of coexisting congenital defects.

The development of better and safer prosthetic heart valves is the most important aspect of current therapy for acquired valvular heart disease.

The original ball valve prosthesis consisted of a stellite cage with a Silastic ball. Subsequently, to promote endothelization of the base and sewing ring and to reduce trauma to blood elements, the sewing ring and struts of the cage were covered with cloth. With time, contact of the ball with the cloth on the inner surface of the struts led to degeneration and increased trauma to blood elements. The final stage in the development of the ball valve, therefore, was to place an inner track of stellite inside the cloth-covered strut which formed the major structural support of the valve (*Fig.* 47.5). This inner track of stellite eliminated cloth wear. The original ball was composed of uncured Silastic. A significant number of these early balls degenerated due to absorption of plasma lipids. Distortion of the shape of the ball or ball-valve variance led to malfunction of the valve and disintegration of the ball led to catastrophic embolization. The second stage of the development of the ball was to cure the Silastic and impregnate the ball with barium. This eliminated distortion of the shape of the ball and allowed fluoroscopic determination of the movement of the ball within the cage. The final stage in ball design was to change the construction to a hollow stellite device. The hollow stellite ball in the track valve cage represents the final stage, thus far, in the development of the Starr–Edwards ball valve prosthesis.

The most commonly used disc valve is the Bjork–Shiley tilting disc valve prosthesis (*Fig.* 47.6). The original valve introduced in 1969 was composed of a Delrin disc in a stellite cage encircled by a Teflon sewing ring. In 1971 the composition of the disc was changed to pyrolytic carbon. Other improvements in valve construction included: changing the shape of the disc to a convex–concave structure to reduce turbulence and increased angle of opening, moving the pivot point 2·5 mm to allow clearance between the disc and the ring, enlarging the smaller of the two openings by 40% to reduce stagnation, and including the inlet strut as an integral part of the valve structure to increase the mechanical strength of the valve. The valve also now has a radio-opaque marker in the disc to allow fluoroscopic determination of disc movement and a rotating cage to allow positioning of the disc for maximum clearance of the ventricular or aortic wall once the valve has been sutured in place.

A newer mechanical valve which has recently been introduced has adopted a unique design. The St Jude Medical bi-leaflet valve (*Fig.* 47.7) is constructed entirely of pyrolytic carbon with two centrally hinged biconvex leaflets. This design results in a central opening with the smallest gradients and largest effective orifice areas of any mechanical

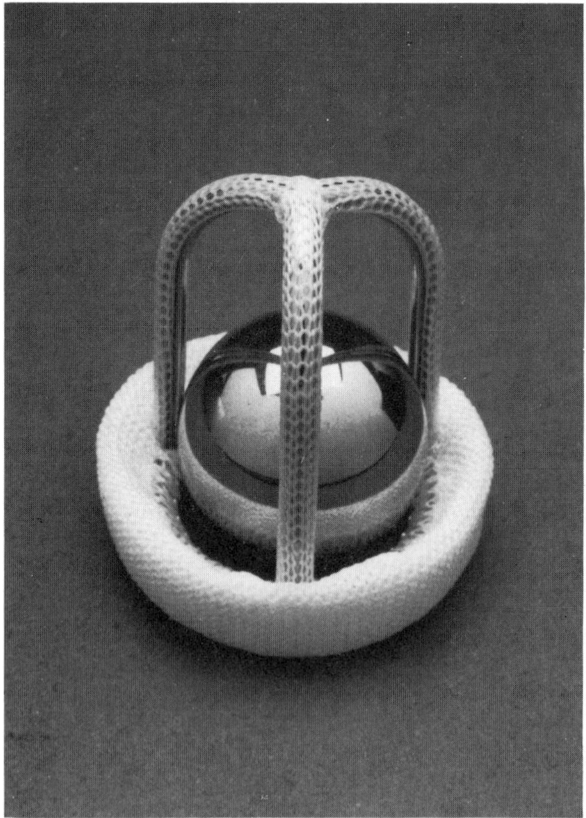

Fig. 47.5 Starr–Edwards 2400 aortic valve prosthesis.

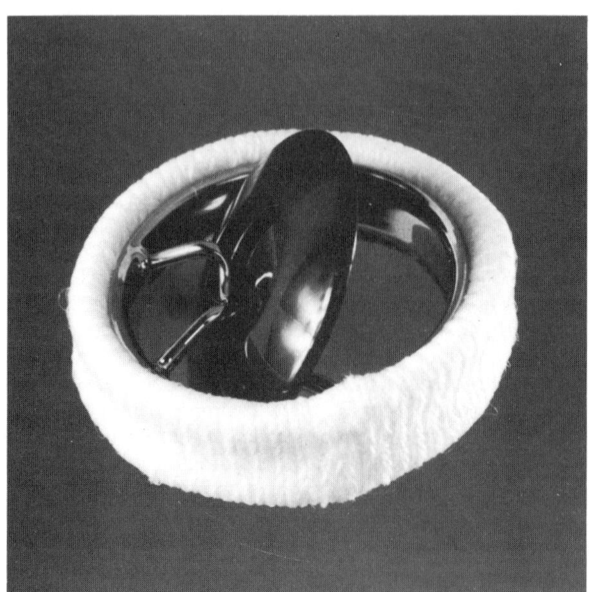

Fig. 47.6 Bjork–Shiley tilting disc valve prosthesis.

prosthetic valve. Long-term studies should be available in the near future. Initial laboratory testing, however, indicates that the valve is structurally sound and haemodynamically

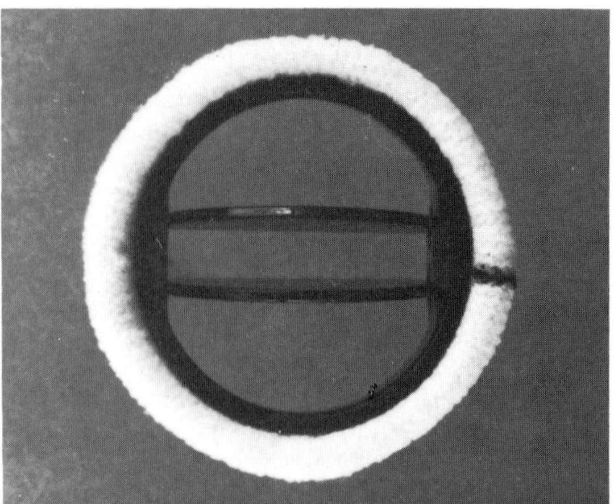

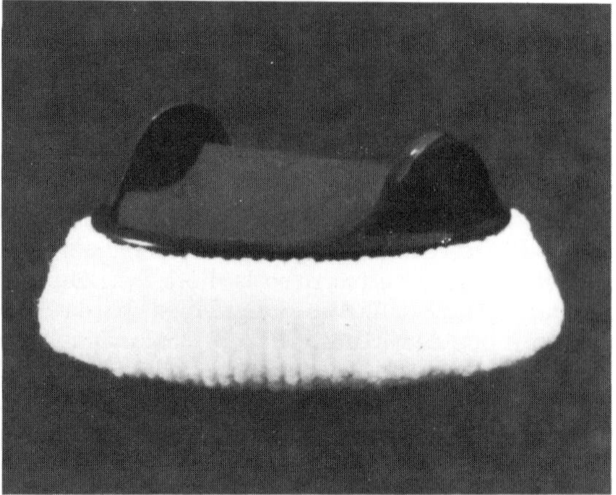

Fig. 47.7 St Jude Medical bi-leaflet valve.

effective. Tissue valves, or bioprostheses, have also undergone continued development and testing. Fresh aortic homograft valves were the first stage in the development of tissue valves. These valves were implanted as free grafts in the subcoronary position. A high incidence of valve failure and valve infection led to preoperative preparation of these valves by sterilization in various antibiotic solutions. Procurement in most centres other than some in Great Britain and New Zealand continued to be a problem and this led to the development of the formaldehyde preserved porcine heterograft valve. Although sterility was assured and rejection eliminated by the use of formaldehyde, tissue deterioration was found to occur in over 60% of the valves at 2 years. In 1970, glutaraldehyde was used as a tanning agent. This preservation technique, in combination with a flexible stent, provides the basis of porcine heterograft valves implanted today. Glutaraldehyde provides stabilization of collagen cross-linkage and the flexible stent allows for opening and closing of the leaflets and ventricular contraction with symmetrical distribution of stress.

The two most common porcine heterograft valves used today are the Hancock and the Carpentier–Edwards. The Hancock valve has been used for a longer period of time and has undergone modification. The original valve consisted of an aortic valve removed from a single pig. One leaflet of the pig aortic valve, however, contains a muscle bar which

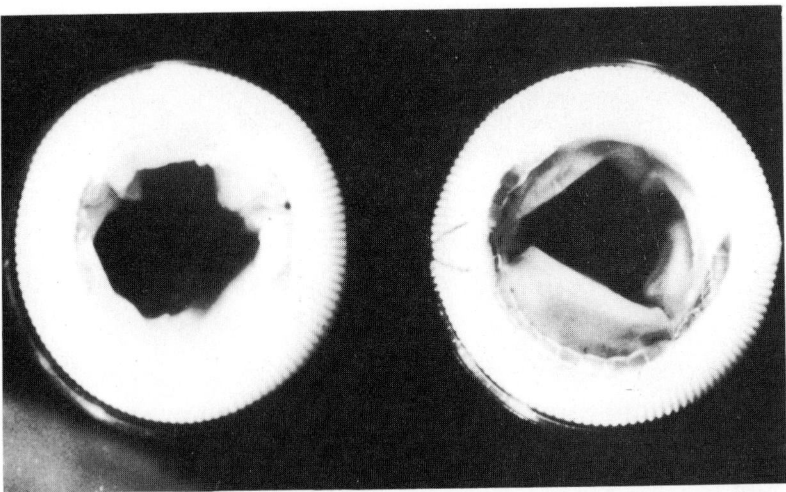

Fig. 47.8 Hancock porcine heterograft valve. A comparison of the modified orifice valve (left) with the older model with a muscle bar obstructing the outflow.

results in incomplete opening of that leaflet. The newer model, modified orifice Hancock valve, circumvents this problem by substituting a leaflet from a second pig for the muscle bar leaflet (*Fig.* 47.8). This improvement has resulted in enlargement of the effective orifice area. The valves are mounted on a Dacron-covered semiflexible stent and are fixed with glutaraldehyde. The Carpentier–Edwards valve is preserved in a similar manner with glutaraldehyde (*Fig.* 47.9). The stent upon which the valve is sewn is designed to be flexible at the sewing ring as well as at the commissures. This more flexible stent allows for reduced stress on both the base and the commissures of the valve leaflets.

A third porcine heterograft valve developed was the Angell–Shiley. This valve incorporates one of 70 different anatomical configurations of stent to approximate more closely the actual porcine aortic root from which the valve was removed. The resulting sewing ring is not circular in shape. In the Ionescu–Shiley bovine pericardial heterograft valve, pericardium is used to construct the leaflets rather than porcine aortic valve tissue (*Fig.* 47.10). The construction of the leaflets allows more complete opening than the other heterograft valves and better haemodynamic performance. The authors have used this valve successfully in small patients in the mitral position.

The choice of which type of prosthetic valve to implant in a patient depends on multiple factors. The surgeon must consider the haemodynamic performance of the valve, the durability of the valve, the necessity for the use of anticoagulation and the incidence of thrombosis, structural failure and embolism (*Table* 47.1). All of these factors will determine the best valve for each particular patient. For aortic valve replacement, the homograft, Bjork–Shiley and Starr–Edwards ball valves have all proved durable in clinical use. Thrombosis and structural failure are rarely a problem with these valves in the hands of experts. Although the Starr–Edwards valve has good haemodynamic function, its major disadvantages are a higher incidence of embolism than other valves and a requirement for lifelong anticoagulation. The Hancock and Edwards porcine heterograft valves have not proved their long-term durability. Indeed, recent studies of histology by light and electron microscopy show that the majority of these valves have evidence of collagen degeneration from 2 months to 6 years after implantation.

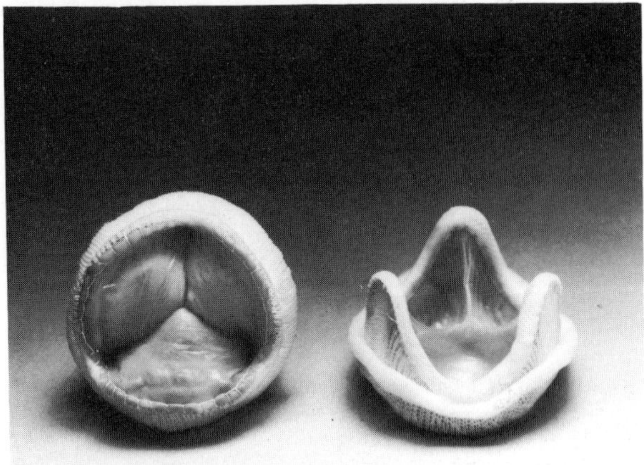

Fig. 47.9 Carpentier–Edwards porcine heterograft valve.

Although valve failure is relatively uncommon so far, a few recent reports indicate that valve degeneration and calcification may increase dramatically with time. The advantage of the heterograft valves is a low incidence of embolism. In small sizes in the aortic position these valves tend to have a higher gradient than an equivalent sized mechanical prosthesis. The Bjork–Shiley valve is a durable valve with excellent haemodynamic performance even in small sizes. It does require lifelong anticoagulation and carries a risk of sudden catastrophic thombosis if anticoagulants are discontinued. The rate of embolism with this disc valve is comparable to the heterograft valve. The St Jude valve is too new for adequate evaluation. In the aortic position it has excellent haemodynamics even in very small sizes. Early reports indicate no problem with thrombosis, but structural failure and embolism have been reported. Durability *in vivo* is unproven; however, pulse duplicator testing *in vitro* has shown excellent durability. The Ionescu–Shiley pericardial heterograft valve has demonstrated excellent haemodynamic function even in small sizes and a low rate of embolism. However, structural failures have occurred with a frequency comparable to the heterograft valves. In the mitral position

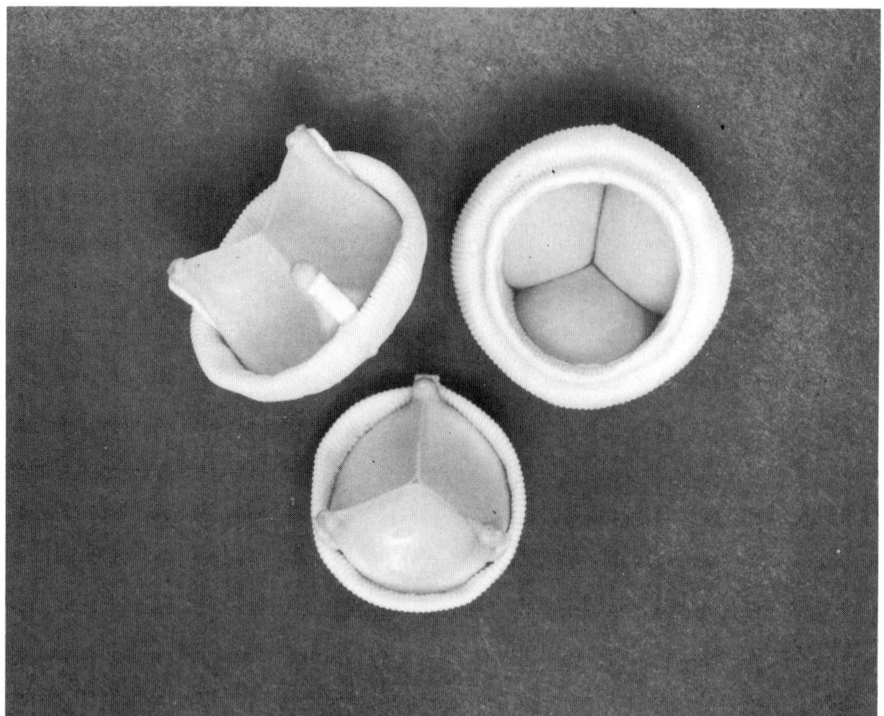

Fig. 47.10 Ionescu–Shiley pericardial heterograft valve.

the Starr–Edwards ball valves have again demonstrated durability over 10 years. Although haemodynamics are good, there is a significant incidence of embolism despite the use of lifelong anticoagulation. The heterograft valves have similar properties in the mitral position as in the aortic position. Although it was initially thought that anticoagulation would be unnecessary, recent data indicates that patients in atrial fibrillation run the risk of systemic emboliza-

Table 47.1 Comparison of commonly used prosthetic heart valves

Valve	*Thrombosis* (%/yr)	*Structural failure* (%/yr)	*Embolism* (%/yr)	*Haemodynamics*	*Advantages*	*Disadvantages*
Aortic						
Starr–Edwards 1200/60	0	0	5	Low gradients	Durable	Anticoagulation
Starr–Edwards 2400	0	0	3	Moderate gradients	Durable	Anticoagulation
Bjork–Shiley	0·3	0	0·7	Low gradients in small sizes	Durable Good haemodynamics	Anticoagulation
St Jude	0	0	0	Low gradients in small sizes	Excellent haemodynamics	?Durability
Hancock	0–0·1	0·2–2	0·5–2	High gradients in small sizes	Low embolism No anticoagulation	?Durability
Carpentier–Edwards	0	0·2–1	0–1	High gradients in small sizes	Low embolism No anticoagulation	?Durability
Ionescu–Shiley	0	0·6	0·2	Low gradients in small sizes	Excellent haemodynamics Low embolism No anticoagulation	?Durability
Mitral						
Starr–Edwards 6120	0·1	0	6	Low gradients	Durable	Anticoagulation
Starr–Edwards 6400	0	0	5	Low gradients	Durable	Anticoagulation
Bjork–Shiley	1·3	0	1·2–4·2	Low gradients	Durable	Anticoagulation Thrombosis
St Jude	0	0	0·9	Low gradients in small sizes	Excellent haemodynamics	?Durability
Hancock	0–0·2	0·5–2	1–3	Low gradients	?Anticoagulation	?Durability
Carpentier–Edwards	0·1	0·1	0·1–2	Low gradients	?Anticoagulation	?Durability
Ionescu–Shiley	0	0·6	0·9	Low gradients in small sizes	Excellent haemodynamics No anticoagulation	?Durability

tion. In addition, the long-term durability of this valve is currently being questioned. The Bjork–Shiley disc valve has been shown to be durable with excellent haemodynamic function. There is a significant risk (probably less than the ball valves) of systemic embolization. The newer model Bjork–Shiley valve may reduce this even further. The greatest risk to patients with this valve is sudden catastrophic thrombosis upon cessation of anti-coagulation for whatever reason. Thus heparin is indicated during such episodes as other surgery. The St Jude valve in the mitral position has the same characteristics as in the aortic position with a very low incidence of systemic embolization so far. The Ionescu–Shiley valve also has the same properties as in the aortic position.

Recent reports of very high rates of valve degeneration and calcification in children when a porcine heterograft valve has been implanted raise serious doubts as to this valve's future in that population. As high as 20% of aortic and mitral valves implanted in children have calcified. In addition, 10% of heterograft valves inserted in a conduit have shown degeneration, although a major advantage of the heterograft valve was once thought to be its usefulness in children since it did not require anticoagulation.

When deciding which valve to insert in a patient, the surgeon must also be concerned about the risks of lifelong anticoagulation. Haemorrhagic complications occur in up to 3% of patients per year, half of which are fatal. The decision to implant a mechanical prosthesis in a patient, therefore, involves more than merely a consideration of frequent blood tests to monitor anticoagulation therapy or restriction from vigorous athletics in children with the risk of injury and excessive bleeding. The risk of haemorrhage, frequently fatal, in patients on long-term anticoagulation must be considered prior to making the final determination of which valve to insert.

In time, a valve free from the risks of thrombosis, structural failure, and embolism, with excellent haemodynamic function in even the smallest sizes, composed of substances that will provide excellent durability, and not requiring anticoagulation will be developed. Until then, the surgeon must choose the most appropriate valve for each patient based on their advantages and disadvantages.

Further Reading

Balderman S. C., Bates R. J. and Anagnostopoulos C. E. (1977) Cardiac valve replacement: Improved survival related to air exclusion and myocardial protection. *Ill. Med. J.* **151**, 113.

Bjork V. O. and Henze A. (1979) Ten years experience with the Bjork–Shiley tilting disc valve. *J. Thorac. Cardiovasc. Surg.* **78**, 331.

Carpentier A., Chauvaud S., Fabiani J. N. et al. (1980) Reconstructive surgery of mitral valve incompetence: Ten-year appraisal. *J. Thorac. Cardiovasc. Surg.* **79**, 338.

Copeland J. G., Griepp R. B., Stinson E. B. et al. (1977) Long-term follow-up after isolated aortic valve replacement. *J. Thorac. Cardiovasc. Surg.* **74**, 875.

Ferrans V. J., Spray T. L., Billingham M. E. et al. (1978) Structural changes in glutaraldehyde-treated porcine heterografts used as substitute cardiac valves. Transmission and scanning electron microscopic observations in twelve patients. *Am. J. Cardiol.* **41**, 1159.

Karp R. B., Cyrus R. J., Blackstone E. H. et al. (1981) The Bjork–Shiley valve. *J. Thorac. Cardiovasc. Surg.* **81**, 602.

Kloster F. E. (1975) Diagnosis and management of complications of prosthetic heart valves. *Am. J. Cardiol.* **35**, 872.

MacManus Q., Grunkemeier G. L., Lambert L. E. et al. (1978) Non-cloth-covered caged-ball prostheses. *J. Thorac. Cardiovasc. Surg.* **76**, 788.

Myerowitz P. D., Lamberti J. J., Replogle R. L. et al. (1979) Delayed complications following heterograft valve replacement. *Bioprosthetic cardiac valves.* Deutsches Herzzentrum Munchen, pp. 335–340.

Nicoloff D. M., Emery R. W., Arom K. V. et al. (1981) Clinical and hemodynamic results with the St Jude medical cardiac valve prosthesis. *J. Thorac. Cardiovasc. Surg.* **82**, 674.

Oyer P. E., Stinson E. B., Reitz B. A. et al. (1979) Long-term evaluation of the porcine xenograft bioprosthesis. *J. Thorac. Cardiovasc. Surg.* **78**, 343.

Rapaport E. (1975) Natural history of aortic and mitral valve disease. *Am. J. Cardiol.* **35**, 221.

Salomon M. W., Stinson E. B., Griepp R. B. et al. (1977) Mitral valve replacement: Long-term evaluation of prosthesis-related mortality and morbidity. *Circulation* **56**, Suppl. 2, Pt 2, 94–101.

Teply J. F., Grunkemeir G. L., Sutherland H. D. et al. (1981) The ultimate prognosis after valve replacement: An assessment at twenty years. *Ann. Thorac. Surg.* **32**, 111.

Zusman D. R., Levine F. H., Carter J. E. et al. (1981) Hemodynamic and clinical evaluation of the Hancock modified-orifice aortic bioprosthesis. *Circulation* **64**, Suppl. 2, Pt 2, 189–91.

48 *Surgery for Coronary Atherosclerosis*

W. Y. Moores and C. E. Anagnostopoulos

Atherosclerosis of the coronary arteries and the myocardial complications which result from this arterial disease produce a rate of death and disability which has reached epidemic proportions in western society. Furthermore, cardiac sudden death, which is usually the result of coronary atherosclerosis, is often not reported as a fatal infarction. Thus, the total number of deaths due to coronary atherosclerosis is higher than these figures would indicate.

Though risk factors which predispose to the development of coronary artery disease have been statistically documented, a unitary concept for the aetiology of coronary atherosclerosis has not emerged. Identifiable risk factors include hereditary characteristics such as male sex, a positive family history of coronary artery disease, hypertension, hyperlipidaemia and diabetes. Environmental, and possibly modifiable, risk factors include cigarette smoking, a diet high in cholesterol, saturated fatty acids and calories, and obesity. Hereditary risk factors are poorly controllable and, unfortunately, the concept of retarding coronary artherogenesis by modification of environmental risk factors has not been a practical success, partially because of deeply ingrained patterns of life style and diet. Therefore, the search has continued for pharmacological and surgical means of alleviating the public health problem that the symptomatic and life-threatening manifestations of coronary atherosclerosis represent.

Anatomy (*Fig.* 48.1)

The left main coronary artery (LMCA) arises from the left coronary sinus of the aortic root, courses posterior to the pulmonary artery, and after a length which is usually 6–15 mm, divides into its major branches, the left anterior descending (LAD) and circumflex (Cx) arteries. The LAD is the continuation of the LMCA and runs anteriorly in the interventricular sulcus, giving off branches to the anterolateral left ventricular wall called diagonals and branches to the septum called septal perforators. The LAD then continues toward, and usually around, the apex of the heart to communicate with the terminal branches of the posterior descending artery. The LAD often is epicardial in location but its initial 2 cm are covered in epicardial fat. The middle third of the LAD may be intramyocardial or even run within the septum, making surgical exposure difficult.

The Cx coronary artery arises at right angles to the LMCA–LAD axis and runs anterior to the left atrial appendage in the left atrioventricular groove. It lies beneath the great cardiac vein and gives off branches at acute angles which run onto the lateral and posterolateral aspect of the left ventricle. In 10% of cases the posterior descending artery is the distal continuation of the circumflex. Though the lateral circumflex branches may run intramyocardially it is uncommon for posterolateral branches to do so.

The bifurcation of the LMCA is quite commonly a trifurcation with the third division arising between the LAD and Cx and supplying the anterolateral left ventricle. This vessel has been termed a lateral division, high lateral, first marginal or intermediate artery (INT) and quite commonly runs intramyocardially.

The right coronary artery (RCA) arises from the right coronary, or anterior sinus. Approximately 50% of the time there is a separate orifice for a conus vessel which runs over the pulmonary outflow tract to communicate with the LAD. The main RCA runs in the right atrioventricular groove giving off branches to the right ventricle, and terminally dividing into the posterior descending coronary artery (PDA) and a posterior lateral branch to the left ventricle, the posterior ventricular branch. The PDA runs in the posterior intraventricular groove and provides septal perforators. The main RCA may be intra-atrial but an intramyocardial location is unusual for the PDA and almost never occurs with posterior ventricular branches of the RCA.

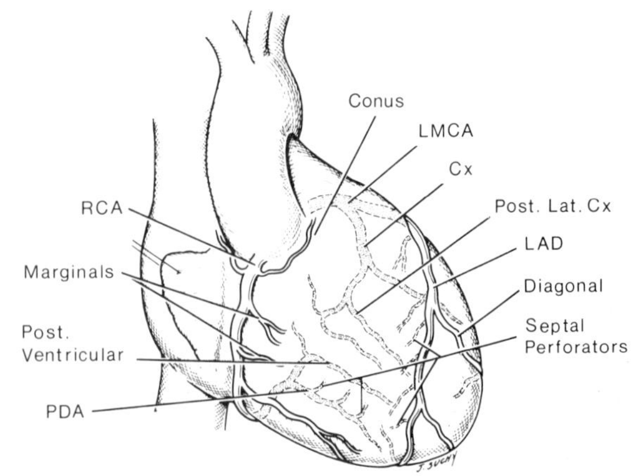

Fig. 48.1 Coronary artery anatomy.

The distribution of the major coronary arteries tends to be reciprocal and many patterns of dominance have been identified. However, in general, the anterior descending supplies the anterior and anterolateral aspect of the left ventricle and the anterior two-thirds of the septum, roughly 50% of the left ventricular myocardium. The RCA and Cx supply the posterior aspect of the left ventricle and demonstrate an inverse relationship in the size of the two vessels.

In the surgical setting, when the RCA provides both the PDA and the major posterolateral branch to the left ventricle, it is a 'right dominant system'; when the RCA gives off the PDA but no other left ventricular branch it is called 'co-dominant'; and when the PDA originates from the circumflex it is considered a 'left dominant' system.

Pathology

The pathological entity producing the vast majority of obstructive coronary artery disease is atherosclerosis. The early arterial lesion tends to be focal, is usually non-circumferential, and histologically appears as lipid-filled macrophages. The more mature lesion contains fibrous elements and subendothelial lipids, mostly cholesterol and other sterols, either free or contained within macrophages. Calcification may occur. The most common pattern for atheroma is a lipid accumulation associated with a fibrous layer on its luminal side. In an older atheroma predominantly fibrous layers may alternate with lipid layers, a characteristic which has led to the speculation that atheroma formation occurs episodically. The details of atherogenesis, however, are incompletely understood, though abnormalities of lipid metabolism and platelet complexes have been implicated by circumstantial evidence.

Atherosclerosis in the arterial wall does not necessarily produce stenosis or obstruction of the vessel. However, as the lesion increases in thickness it tends to do so at the expense of the vessel lumen and only extends slightly into the media of the artery. This characteristic sparing of most of the media makes possible the surgical technique of endarterectomy for removing some atherosclerotic obstructions. Though stenotic atherosclerotic lesions are common, it appears that total obstruction is often due to associated thrombosis. The pathophysiology of progression to total thrombosis is not entirely clear but usually the underlying atherosclerosis has reduced the vessel lumen by more than 25%. In some cases, the fibrous endothelium overlying the lipid accumulation may be seen to have ruptured and it is possible that lipid exposure may trigger thrombosis. However, thrombotic lesions are also seen in the presence of an intact endothelium. Haemorrhage into atheromatous plaques has also been thought to cause progression to occlusion. In some patients aneurysmal dilatation of coronary arteries may be seen along with obstructive lesions. The clinical significance of these areas is not clear though it is suspected that embolization from these aneurysmal segments may occur.

The distribution of atherosclerosis within the coronary arteries is not uniform and tends to occur proximally, particularly in the LAD and circumflex systems. In the RCA the most common areas of severe disease are the proximal one-third of the vessel and distally between the marginal and posterior descending branches. However, any area of any vessel may be involved. Advanced coronary atherosclerosis, particularly in the diabetic or hyperlipidaemic patient, may be manifest as disease both proximally and distally, but severe distal disease without any proximal involvement is quite uncommon. Intramyocardial segments of coronary arteries tend to be less involved with atherosclerosis than epicardial segments.

Pathophysiology

The aetiology of coronary atherosclerosis is probably metabolic and its basic pathology is arterial. However, clinical manifestations do not occur until the arterial disease produces anatomical limitations of blood flow through the coronary vessels to such an extent that ischaemia or infarction of the myocardium results.

Cardiac muscle has a high metabolic oxygen requirement and a high rate of arterial blood flow, three times that of the rest of the body. Myocardial anaerobic metabolism is very inefficient and under basal conditions the myocardium extracts 65–75% of the oxygen from coronary arterial blood. Therefore, significant increases in oxygen consumption must be accompanied by an increase in coronary flow.

Because of systolic intramyocardial wall tension and the epicardial to endocardial direction of coronary arterial flow, a high proportion of the myocardial blood flow occurs during diastole. After experimental coronary artery occlusion, subendocardial flow decreases faster than epicardial flow and is slower to recover with reperfusion. Experimentally and clinically, the subendocardium is the region most susceptible to ischaemia.

The level of myocardial oxygen consumption determines the need for oxygen supply. Myocardial oxygen consumption is positively related to:

1. Intramyocardial wall tension. Wall tension is positively related to the impedance to ventricular ejection or 'afterload'. Also, to produce a given intraventricular pressure the intramyocardial wall tension developed must increase as the end-diastolic volume of the ventricle increases, a relationship described by the law of LaPlace. Then, intramyocardial wall tension is positively related to end-diastolic volume or 'preload'.
2. Heart rate.
3. Contractile state of the myocardium (rate of fibre shortening).

The state of oxygen balance, i.e. the presence or absence of ischaemia in any segment of myocardium is determined by oxygen demand as well as by oxygen supply. Patients with aortic stenosis, idiopathic hypertrophic subaortic stenosis, or systemic hypertension with severe left ventricular hypertrophy and high myocardial oxygen needs, may exhibit myocardial ischaemia without obstructive coronary disease. Because the pathological anatomy of the coronary arteries is only one of many factors influencing myocardial oxygenation, the determination of what is a 'significant' degree of arterial stenosis is not always simple. A given coronary artery may be sufficient to supply myocardial oxygen needs to the 80-year-old sedentary retiree but not to the 42-year-old jogger. In general, we consider lesions angiographically occluding greater than 70% of the vessel lumen to be 'significant'. However, it is possible with the use of stress testing to demonstrate ischaemia distal to some 50% lesions in large vessels, particularly if the lesion is characterized by a long segment of obstruction.

Clinical Presentation

The clinical presentations of patients with coronary artery disease tend to fall into the major groups of angina pectoris, myocardial infarction, sudden death and the asymptomatic or mildly symptomatic patient.

Angina Pectoris

Originally used to refer to chest pain associated with heart disease, the term 'angina' is most useful if we use it to refer to any subjective sensation caused by myocardial ischaemia but unassociated with myocardial infarction. Cardiac pain is thought to be caused by afferent sympathetic nerve stimulation, though the details of the neuro-anatomy are unknown. Many different kinds of chest, arm, neck, jaw, or back pain may be caused by myocardial ischaemia, or profound ischaemia may produce no pain at all. One of the major problems in dealing with coronary disease is that the relationship between myocardial ischaemia and symptoms is very imprecise.

Natural history data from the Framingham study show that if patients with angina are taken as a group, 30% will die within 8 years and 44% of those deaths will be sudden. And, of patients with angina suffering myocardial infarction, only 15% lose their symptoms of angina.

The clinical syndromes representing angina can be divided into two useful subgroups: stable angina, indicating a chronic clinical syndrome where symptoms are brought about with a known activity or amount of exertion, and unstable angina, a term which has been used to describe a variety of clinical syndromes characterized by symptoms progressively worsening in severity.

Myocardial Infarction

Ischaemic events progressing to myocardial necrosis may be classified into the subgroups of non-transmural and transmural infarction. Non-transmural infarction often occurs without an acute change in coronary anatomy when, under conditions of increased myocardial oxygen utilization, a 'watershed' area of myocardium becomes severely ischaemic and infarction results. Transmural infarction is more often associated with progression to total occlusion of the supplying coronary artery. However, it is important to note that total occlusion of a vessel does not necessarily lead to transmural or even subendocardial infarction. Also, transmural infarction may occur without total coronary occlusion or acute change in coronary anatomy. Rarely, coronary spasm may result in myocardial infarction without the presence of a fixed obstruction.

The natural history of patients suffering a myocardial infarction is a grim one. For 80% of patients who have their first infarction, it will represent their first symptom of coronary artery disease, and between 30 and 40% of patients suffering an infarction will die within one month of that event. For those surviving, the mortality over the next 5 years is approximately 5% per year according to the Framingham and Health Insurance Plan of Greater New York studies of large populations.

Sudden Death

In most studies of the phenomenon of sudden death, three-quarters of male deaths and one-half to two-thirds of female deaths are due to coronary artery disease. In 30–50% of these patients, death is the first manifestation of heart disease. The pathophysiology of this event is not always clear. Acute thrombi in major vessels without histological infarction, thrombi with infarction and platelet aggregates, have all been documented at post-mortem examination following sudden death. However, in the majority of cases post-mortem examination demonstrates no acute histological change. Arrhythmias and acute ventricular failure may both play a role in causing sudden cardiac death.

The Asymptomatic or Minimally Symptomatic Patient

An aggressive approach to the diagnosis of coronary artery disease will identify patients with severe disease but without incapacitating symptoms. This creates some difficult therapeutic decisions as it is not easy to make the asymptomatic patient feel better! However, long-term follow-up studies of patients with angiographically proven coronary disease have now shown that the survival of patients with coronary artery disease is closely related to coronary artery anatomy and left ventricular function and only slightly related to symptoms. Data from Proudfit's classic study (*Table* 48.1) shows that the chances of a severely symptomatic patient with single vessel disease surviving 10 years are almost twice as great as the patient with three critically obstructed vessels and minimal symptoms. Unfortunately, the incidence of sudden death and sudden myocardial infarction make management solely based on clinical symptoms a gamble.

Table 48.1 Angiographic coronary anatomy, symptoms and survival (from Proudfit et al., 1978)

	% Survival at 10 years by symptoms	
Coronary arteries with >70% stenosis	*Angina classes 1 and 2**	*Angina classes 3 and 4**
1	62·3%	62·5%
2	47·4%	36·8%
3	32·4%	19·7%
LCA	26·7%	23·8%

*NYHA Classification.

Evaluation of the Patient with Coronary Disease

The imprecision in the relationship between clinical symptomatology and coronary anatomy and the strong correlation between coronary anatomy, left ventricular function and patient prognosis make cardiac catheterization including coronary arteriography and left ventriculography the cornerstone of the evaluation of the patient with coronary artery disease. Chest pain, or 'angina' is a ubiquitous symptom, and some patients thought to have 'anginal' symptoms or even myocardial infarction may have normal coronary arteries. Definitive diagnosis and prediction of the likely natural history of the patient's disease must be based on arteriography.

Angiographically, patients with coronary artery disease are evaluated to determine:

1. The number of vessels significantly (greater than 70%) obstructed. Long-term follow-up has shown large differences in survival of patients divided into groups with single, double, or triple vessel disease and though any large grouping will include patients with varying prognoses, these distinctions are the most useful thus far.
2. Left ventricular function: Indices of ventricular function include: left ventricular end-diastolic pressure (LVEDP), ejection fraction, and subjective evaluation of segmental wall motion abnormalities.
3. Viability of the myocardium distal to critical stenoses.
4. The presence or absence of coronary spasm.

The patient who may also be a surgical candidate is, in addition, evaluated for the quality and size of the vessels distal to critical obstructions.

In patients where arteriographic demonstration of anatomy leaves unanswered questions, non-invasive, dynamic studies of myocardial physiology may be useful. For example: (1) thallium and pyrophosphate radionuclide scans may help define whether a non-functioning myocardial segment is ischaemic or infarcted; (2) exercise thallium scanning or stress testing with ECG monitoring can be useful to document or confirm ischaemia in a patient with non-occlusive coronary lesions of uncertain physiological significance; (3) if positive, preoperative thallium and ECG exercise testing provides a non-invasive means of monitoring revascularization postoperatively; (4) ventricular function may be non-invasively monitored with blood pool scanning and echocardiography.

In patients who are surgical candidates, the renal, hepatic and pulmonary systems are carefully evaluated. A complete neurological examination is carried out and the carotid arteries are evaluated for bruits. There are no absolute contraindications to coronary artery revascularization, although relative contraindications include situations where a patient has severe diffuse left ventricular impairment, symptoms of congestive heart failure, no angina, and technically unfavourable coronary anatomy.

MEDICAL MANAGEMENT OF CORONARY ARTERY DISEASE

Current medical management of coronary artery disease is based on the principles of risk factor control, prevention of possible intra-arterial thrombotic complications, treatment of spasm, and relief of acute or chronic ischaemia by maintaining a favourable myocardial oxygen balance.

Risk Factors

Dietary and Serum Lipid Management

Demonstration that the prevalence of coronary artery disease in a population has a positive correlation with total caloric intake, dietary cholesterol and saturated fats and serum levels of cholesterol and triglycerides has led to the speculation that alteration in diet and in serum lipid levels might retard the development of atherosclerosis and its complications. Definitive proof of such a hypothesis is difficult and the studies required are quite time consuming, but the Finnish Mental Hospital study does provide evidence that the mortality rate from coronary heart disease in males may be reduced by replacing dietary dairy fats with vegetable oils, thus reducing cholesterol intake and replacing saturated fatty acids with polyunsaturated fatty acids. The evidence of the efficacy of dietary therapy is not iron clad and in no study does dietary management eliminate the complications of atherosclerosis. However, there has been no demonstration of adverse effects from cholesterol-lowering diets and nutritional management continues to be part of the treatment of any patient with coronary artery disease.

Pharmacological management can be used to lower serum lipid levels in patients with hyperlipoproteinaemias unresponsive to dietary therapy. Clofibrate, nicotinic acid and anionic bile acid-binding resins such as cholestyramine and colestipol are medications currently available that have been shown to lower serum lipid levels in selected groups of patients. The effect of these agents, however, has not been clearly demonstrated to decrease atherogenesis and they are associated with side-effects, possibly with an increased incidence of gallbladder disease and cancer.

Further, it must be kept in mind that dietary management and pharmacological alteration of serum lipid levels have not been shown to induce regression of angiographically demonstrated coronary arterial lesions or to alter the natural history of coronary artery disease once angiographically demonstrated critical obstructions have developed.

Hypertension Control

Systemic hypertension is statistically associated with the development of coronary atherosclerosis. Though antihypertensive therapy has not been clearly shown to reduce the incidence of coronary arterial lesions or clinical disease it can reduce the symptoms from coronary artery disease by reducing myocardial oxygen consumption and may have a beneficial effect on atherogenesis.

Cigarette Smoking

Though the pathophysiological mechanism is unclear, cigarette smoking appears to hasten the development of atherosclerosis. Further, the incidence of vein graft occlusion following operation for peripheral vascular disease is increased in the persistent smoker. Though the same demonstration has not been made following aortocoronary vein grafting, cessation of smoking is part of the management of any patient with coronary artery disease whether or not they are a candidate for surgery.

Alteration of Life Style

Though the development of coronary atherosclerosis has been correlated with certain personality characteristics (the so-called 'Type A' personality), changes in life style have not been shown to decrease the mortality or morbidity from coronary artery disease or to reduce progression of atherogenesis.

Exercise Training

Individuals with sedentary jobs appear to have a higher statistical incidence of coronary atherosclerosis than those with occupations requiring more physical activity. Also, physically fit individuals appear to be able to engage in a higher level of activity at a lower heart rate and blood pressure, thus increasing the capacity for activity of the patient with ischaemic heart disease. However, physical training does not eliminate atherosclerosis and there is little current evidence that it materially affects the natural history of angiographically documented coronary disease.

Control of Thombotic Mechanisms and Spasm

Antiplatelet Agents

Circumstantial evidence derived from pathological, epidemiological and physiological studies has led to theoretical considerations of a possible role played by blood platelets in atherogenesis and in the pathophysiology of myocardial infarction and sudden cardiac death. The logical speculation that antiplatelet agents might prove useful in the treatment of patients with coronary artery disease has led to a number of clinical trials. Previous prospective studies of aspirin therapy for patients following myocardial infarction, both in the UK and in the USA, have demonstrated no statistically significant advantage of aspirin though there was a trend toward a lower mortality in the treatment groups. However, recent reports from the Mayo Clinic have demonstrated the beneficial effects of aspirin and dipyridamole on vein graft patency. A multi-centre trial of sulfinpyrazone therapy following myocardial infarction seemed to show a statistically significant decrease in mortality in the treatment group for the first 8 months after infarction though statistically significant differences in the composition of the treatment and control groups indicate that more data are needed. Clofibrate studies indicate a possible lowering of cardiac morbidity and mortality with treatment though whether results are due to the lipid-lowering or antiplatelet effects of the drug are unclear and an increase in cancer deaths in the treatment group is worrisome. Antiplatelet agents do not eliminate coronary artery disease but may help reduce the incidence of sudden death. There is as yet no evidence that the natural history of the patient with angiographically demonstrated coronary artery disease is at all altered by antiplatelet therapy.

Control of Spasm

It is becoming increasingly apparent that coronary spasm plays a role in production of angina in some patients. Spasm may occur in angiographically normal arteries but usually is superimposed on an atherosclerotic lesion which may range from mild disease to severe obstruction. Patients with ischaemia on the basis of spasm, a situation often associated with rest pain, usually experience amelioration of symptoms when treated with calcium flux antagonists, such as nifedipine. Nifedipine also has been effective for some patients with exercise-induced angina, though the response is less predictable than for individuals with rest pain. The range of clinical syndromes appropriate to be treated with these agents has not yet been defined, and calcium flux antagonists represent a possible avenue of further advance in anti-anginal therapy.

Reduction of Myocardial Oxygen Consumption

Since ischaemia is an imbalance between myocardial oxygen supply and demand it is a logical conclusion that reduction in myocardial oxygen consumption might prevent or reverse ischaemia in the patient with coronary artery disease.

Beta Blockade

The use of beta-adrenergic-blocking agents such as propranolol and practolol has been shown to decrease heart rate, blood pressure, myocardial contractility and myocardial oxygen consumption. Beta-blocking agents represent a major advance both in the control of the chronic symptoms of coronary artery disease and in the treatment of acute ischaemic episodes. Further, there is some evidence to indicate that beta blockers may reduce the incidence of sudden death in the first 2 years after myocardial infarction, probably through an anti-arrhythmic effect. Symptomatic patients with coronary artery disease should have a trial of propranolol therapy whether or not operation is contemplated. However, pharmacological beta blockade has not been demonstrated to alter favourably the natural history of angiographically documented coronary artery disease.

Nitrites

Though experimentally nitrites produce coronary vasodilatation and an increase in coronary flow, their effect in the patient with coronary artery disease appears to be mediated through venodilatation, a decreased venous return, a decreased left ventricular end-diastolic volume or 'preload', and a resulting decrease in myocardial oxygen consumption. Sublingual nitroglycerin is the most commonly used agent but in recent years long-acting nitrites, nitropaste and intravenous nitroglycerin have been more commonly used for the prevention and management of acute ischaemia.

Pharmacological or Mechanical Afterload Reduction

Decreasing the impedance to aortic ejection decreases the myocardial wall tension which must be developed and, therefore, myocardial oxygen consumption. Clinically, this can be accomplished on a chronic basis with a large number of antihypertensive agents. In situations of acute ischaemia afterload reduction is usually managed with intravenous nitroprusside or nitroglycerin infusion. Pharmacological reduction of afterload is limited by the requirement that the systemic blood pressure be adequate to perfuse the heart and other organs. This quandary can sometimes be resolved with the use of the intra-aortic balloon pump (IABP). A balloon catheter is placed in the descending aorta. The balloon inflates during diastole, increasing the diastolic arterial pressure, increasing coronary flow and possibly redistributing flow to poorly perfused areas of myocardium. The balloon then deflates just prior to ejection, thus reducing the impedance to left ventricular ejection. Use of the IABP has been a major advance in treatment of coronary artery disease both in the patient suffering from acute ischaemia and in postsurgical management of the failing left ventricle (*see* p. 645).

The recent addition of pharmacological agents generally classified as calcium channel blockers has added to the medical management available for treatment of coronary artery disease. These agents have been quite effective in relieving the symptoms of occlusive coronary artery disease and are not currently used merely for the relief of suspected coronary spasm. These agents can be problematic in the perioperative period since they work as vasodilators and negative inotropic agents; reports exist showing adverse peripheral vascular collapse in patients treated with these agents as part of their chronic medical treatment. Adequate follow-up studies attesting to the efficacy of these agents in prolonging survival in coronary artery disease are not currently available.

SURGICAL TREATMENT OF CORONARY ATHEROSCLEROSIS

History

The demonstration of selective coronary arteriography by F. Mason Sones made direct methods of revascularization possible. Although right coronary endarterectomy had been performed by Bailey without arteriography as early as 1957, accurate attempts at direct revascularization must be based on the knowledge of the precise location of significant obstructions. Early attempts at removing stenotic lesions by endarterectomy or endarterotomy and patch grafting were sometimes effective and in fact Dr Sabiston's first patient was still alive 15 years later. Favaloro at the Cleveland Clinic Foundation and Johnson and others in Milwaukee, Wisconsin, ushered in the era of direct revascularization by their demonstration of the feasibility of bypassing obstructions with segments of saphenous vein, while leaving the host coronary arterial system largely intact. Green followed the same principle and utilized the internal mammary artery as the conduit. Advances in the theory and the practice of direct revascularization have been rapid since its inception, and today direct revascularization is the most commonly performed cardiac surgical procedure in the world.

Operative Technique

The goal of the surgical treatment of coronary artery disease is to prevent myocardial ischaemia or infarction by establishing functioning bypass grafts distal to critical coronary artery stenoses without effecting a decrement in left ventricular function or a complication of another organ system. An understanding of some of the technical issues involved in performing coronary artery bypass surgery is essential not only for the prospective cardiac surgeon, but also for any physician who might exert input into a patient's decision to undergo myocardial revascularization. The explosion of the clinical application of coronary artery bypass grafting throughout the world has led to the development of many variations in operative technique.

Preoperative Period

The patient with coronary artery obstruction is in a potentially unstable situation from the time he enters the hospital until functioning grafts are in place. Preoperative anxiety increases the risk of the patient developing an ischaemic episode. Therefore, the pharmacological prophylaxis against myocardial ischaemia, propranolol and long-acting nitrates, are not decreased prior to surgery. Nitropaste is applied routinely prior to operation and the patient is sedated with morphine and barbiturates. On the day prior to surgery an extensive review of the procedures to be followed on the day of operation is made with the patient so that unfamiliar situations do not arise to increase anxiety. In the operating room, arterial and central venous pressure catheters are placed under local anaesthesia. Only for patients with severe pre-existing left ventricular dysfunction are Swan–Ganz type catheters placed in the preoperative period.

Preliminary Techniques and Cardiopulmonary Bypass

The operation is performed through a median sternotomy. When the internal mammary artery is to be used as a graft, it is dissected from the chest wall with the use of haemoclips and electrocautery but the pedicle is left intact proximally and distally. A standardized cannulation technique is then carried out. Alternative cannulation techniques include single right atrial cannulation and venting of the left atrium, pulmonary artery or aorta (*Fig.* 48.2). During cardiopulmonary bypass heparinization is maintained with doses of 1 mg/kg every hour. Oxygenation during cardiopulmonary bypass is accomplished with a membrane type oxygenator, the system primed with a balanced electrolyte solution. During normothermic perfusion a minimum flow of 2·4 L/min/m^2 is maintained. When hypothermia is established and peripheral resistance increases flows are decreased to maintain a systemic arterial pressure of 60–80 mmHg.

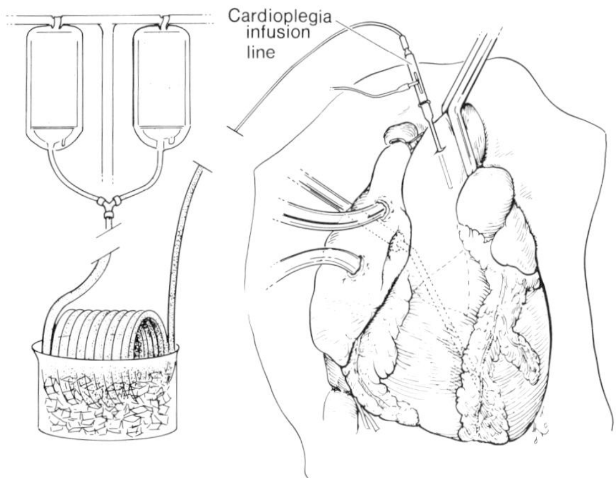

Fig. 48.2 Cannulation for coronary artery disease.

Myocardial Protection

Since the major goals of direct coronary revascularization are to protect myocardium and maintain left ventricular function it is critical that the operation itself does little or nothing to injure the myocardium. However, performance of anastomoses involving the small coronary vessels requires a still, unobscured field for optimal results. The distal (graft to coronary) anastomoses are performed during aortic occlusion. To protect the myocardium during the period of ischaemia, cold potassium cardioplegic solution (potassium chloride 1·193 g, magnesium chloride 3·253 g, and procaine hydrochloride 0·273 mg/l of Ringer's solution at less than 10 °C) is instilled under pressure into the aortic root immediately following aortic cross-clamping until the heart is completely flaccid (*Fig.* 48.2). This technique is designed to abruptly arrest electrical and mechanical activity within a few seconds of aortic cross-clamping and to keep the myocardium cold. Metabolic activity is then minimized and depletion of high-energy phosphate compounds during ischaemia inhibited. Infusion of cardioplegia is briefly repeated after completion of each anastomosis in order to maintain the low myocardial temperature and prevent wash-out of the cardioplegic solution by collateral flow. Although the classic cardioplegia solution has been a hyperkalaemic one, similar to the solution specified above, additional refinements in the application of these solutions has resulted in some improved results using hyperkalaemic solution with oxygenated blood (blood cardioplegia). Oxygenation of crystalloid non-blood containing cardioplegia has also proved efficacious.

The tourniquets around the caval cannulas and the action of the left atrioventricular vent minimize the problem of myocardial rewarming by the systemic or pulmonary return of warm blood. In cases with aortic clamping of longer than 30 min adjunctive measures are used to decrease the rate of myocardial rewarming by non-coronary collaterals and include: (1) systemic hypothermia (25–28 °C) which also allows temporary decreases in the perfusion pressure which decreases collateral flow; (2) topical hypothermia with cold (4 °C) saline, ice slush, and/or a cooling pad. Use of these techniques has provided consistent myocardial protection and clinical recovery of left ventricular function has been excellent following periods of aortic occlusion of up to 80 min in cases of pure revascularization.

Grafting Techniques

During cannulation the saphenous vein is dissected from the leg by the surgeon's assistants. When an internal mammary artery is to be used, the distal attachments are divided following cannulation, and the flow assessed at normotension.

Cardiopulmonary bypass is then established and the heart and vessels examined. Sites of ventricular scar are noted and the coronary vessels identified. The surgeon must depend on the arteriogram to define accurately the location of the coronary obstructions. The epicardium or myocardium overlying the vessels to be grafted is then divided with a scalpel to expose the vessel wall. In general, an attempt is made to place the graft distal to any atherosclerotic lesions, even if they are not occlusive. However, that is not always possible and distally diseased vessels are commonly grafted, particularly where the arteriogram shows an adequate lumen to be present.

The decision having been made as to which arteries are to be grafted, the saphenous vein segments are then prepared. The distal ends are cut at a 45° angle. If the long axis of the distal venotomy does not measure at least 10 mm in length, a small longitudinal slit is made in the heel of the vein to lengthen it.

The distal anastomoses are usually constructed during a single period of aortic cross-clamping with cardioplegic protection. However, some surgeons prefer to perform the proximal anastomoses first to decrease cardiopulmonary bypass time and still others have obtained excellent results utilizing the older, intermittent aortic occlusion technique. This latter technique relies on mild systemic hypothermia (30–32 °C), and relatively short periods of occlusion (6–10 min) with myocardial reperfusion between ischaemic episodes. A 7-mm longitudinal coronary arteriotomy is made and the anastomoses constructed in an interrupted fashion with siliconized braided silk suture material, 12 sutures per anastomosis. Sutures are placed in the vessel wall and arranged around the anastomosis in an orderly fashion. The sutures from one side are placed through the graft wall and tied down in order. All the sutures on the opposite side are then placed through the graft (*Fig.* 48.3) before any are tied. The vessel is then probed and the remaining sutures tied down. This technique ensures that the surgeon will have an accurate view for placement of all sutures and that tension is not placed on the wall of the coronary vessel by traction on a suture. However, many other surgeons use continuous monofilament suturing techniques successfully for distal vein to coronary anastomoses. The most posterior grafts, posterolateral circumflex and posterior right coronary branches, are grafted first. The procedure is then continued from posterior to anterior through the lateral circumflex and diagonal branches to the anterior descending. When an internal mammary artery graft is scheduled that anastomosis is performed last. When all the distal anastomoses have been completed the cross-clamp is removed from the aorta. Occasionally in situations where severe atherosclerosis involves the ascending aorta, the proximal anastomoses are constructed under the single cross-clamping to minimize trauma to the aorta.

When the aortic clamp is removed the arterial pressure is increased in order to perfuse the native, still obstructed, coronary circulation at a higher pressure while the vein graft lengths are measured and the proximal anastomoses are being completed. The grafts are as short as possible consistent with the size of the heart. Grafts to branches of the left coronary system are brought off the left side of the ascending aorta at an angle which enables them to curve around the pulmonary artery. Grafts to the right coronary artery follow a course similar to that of the native right coronary artery in the right atrioventricular groove (*Fig.* 48.4). A 4 to 5 mm punch is used to create an aortic opening and a continuous 5/0 synthetic monofilament suture used to complete the anastomosis.

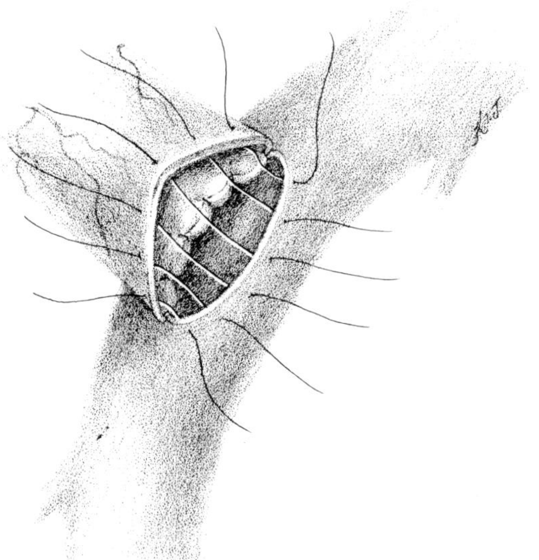

Fig. 48.3 Vein graft anastomosis.

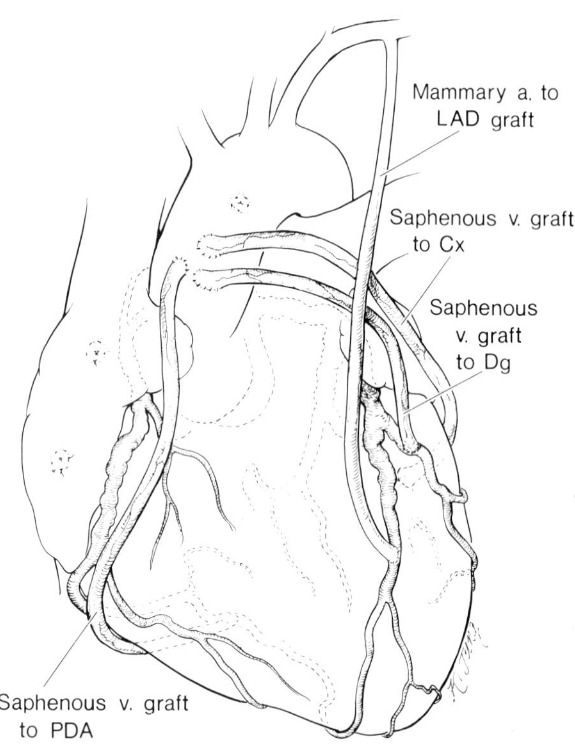

Fig. 48.4 Completed internal mammary artery and saphenous vein grafts.

Conduit Selection and Grafting Patterns

With rare exceptions, bypass grafts are constructed with either the left or right internal mammary artery (IMA) or segments of the long saphenous vein. Postoperative studies of direct IMA to coronary anastomoses performed at the Cleveland Clinic Foundation have demonstrated a 95% patency rate of grafts studies at least 4 years after surgery, confirming this favourable attribute. More recent studies from the Cleveland Clinic Foundation evaluating ten-year follow-up in patients with internal mammary artery grafts have demonstrated a beneficial effect on patient survival as well as graft patency. Disadvantages of the IMA include the more extensive procedure required to obtain the graft, making it less suitable in unstable patients, the associated left pleurotomy and slight decrement in postoperative pulmonary function which results, and the relatively small size of the IMA, which limits the potential maximum flow through the graft. However, the IMA flow is sufficient as long as the IMA is larger than the recipient vessel, and the IMA has been demonstrated to increase in size with time. Therefore, the IMA is the authors' primary choice for grafting the left anterior descending coronary artery. That decision is modified by the relative contraindications of: (1) a recipient vessel twice as large as the IMA; (2) marked left ventricular hypertrophy, (3) haemodynamic instability prior to bypass; (4) an IMA flow of less than 60 ml/min measured at normal tension; (5) severe chronic obstructive lung disease; and (6) an age greater than 70 years old. The IMA is particularly useful in grafting vessels with diffuse disease or limited outflow and when the LAD is larger than the IMA, the IMA can be used to graft diagonal or proximal circumflex branches.

The right internal mammary artery, proximal end in situ, can sometimes be used to graft the LAD or proximal RCA, with the left internal mammary artery then available for diagonal or circumflex branches.

Despite the favourable characteristics of the internal mammary graft and its recent increased usage, segments of long saphenous vein remain the standard conduits for coronary revascularization. Most patients have an adequate length of vein in one extremity; it is readily obtained and technically easy to work with. One disadvantage is the size discrepancy between the saphenous vein and the recipient vessel which leads to a lower velocity of flow through the conduit and may contribute to early graft occlusion. Therefore veins of greater than 10 mm in diameter are not used as simple grafts except in desperation. Veins of less than 4 mm in size have been demonstrated to have a high rate of early thrombosis and consequently are avoided where possible. Simple aorta to coronary artery vein grafts with one proximal and one distal anastomosis are the standard approach. However, sequential grafts with one proximal and multiple sequential distal anastomoses are used with the following indications: (1) paucity of available vein; (2) severe atherosclerosis of the aorta making a small number of proximal anastomoses desirable; (3) necessity for multiple grafts to small vessels, each having limited run-off. In this situation the most distal anastomosis is constructed to the largest vessel in the hopes that flow will be maintained to the intermediate vessels which individually might have too small a run-off to support a single graft. Spatial relations of vessels are appropriate for the construction of bridge grafts involving the diagonal and left anterior descending, multiple circumflex branches, and the posterior descending and posterior ventricular branches of the right coronary artery. The third, least desirable, pattern is that of multiple distal anastomoses with one proximal anastomosis to the aorta and multiple proximal vein to vein anastomoses. These are referred to as 'Y-grafts' and are used when multiple distals are needed, proximal anastomoses to the aorta are contraindicated and the spatial arrangement of the distal vessels as not suitable for segmental grafting (*Fig.* 48.5).

In cases of reoperation or where patients have undergone saphenous vein stripping, the usual conduits may not be available. Alternatives include: (1) free IMA grafts: dividing the IMA from the subclavian may enable the conduit to reach distal vessels which the in situ graft will not; (2) short saphenous vein; (3) cephalic vein: the arm vein is quite a thin vessel; especially in women and must be dissected carefully; (4) homologous umbilical vein; (5) Gore-Tex grafts. (4) and (5) are used infrequently and only when no alternative can be found. Reports of their success are mixed with a patency rate of only about 50%, and are of preliminary interest only.

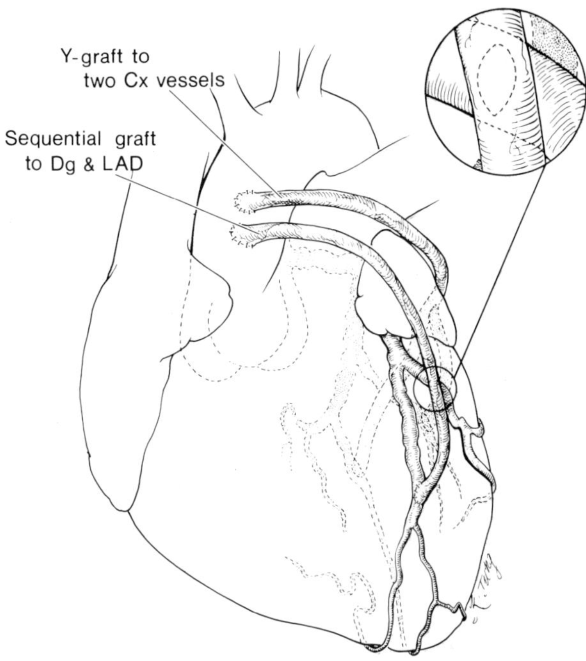

Fig. 48.5 Sequential and Y-grafts.

There is no simple answer to the question of which coronary arteries can be, or should be grafted. In general, the authors graft all coronary vessels 1 mm or greater with a greater than 50% proximal obstruction and viable myocardium distally.

As bypass grafting techniques have improved, the use of endarterectomy has declined and now the authors occasionally use endarterectomy accompanied by vein bypass grafting for completely obstructed right coronary arteries. The multiple left ventricular branches of the anterior descending, and circumflex coronary arteries provide a hazard to endarterectomy of the left coronary system.

Post-bypass Management

Post-bypass haemodynamic management is carried out according to the principle of minimizing myocardial oxygen consumption and is individualized according to the patient's preoperative left ventricular function, coronary anatomy and the extent of revascularization possible. Left atrial pressure is kept as low as is consistent with a good mean arterial pressure and cardiac output, usually less than 12 mmHg. Obviously, patients with preoperative left ventricular dysfunction will not always have a normal left atrial pressure postoperatively, but post-bypass left atrial pressure should be lower than preoperative left ventricular end-diastolic pressure. The cardiac rate and rhythm are regulated as necessary with atrial or occasionally, atrial-ventricular sequential pacing. Hypertension is treated with small boluses of nitroglycerin and, if needed, continuous nitroprusside infusion to decrease the impedance to left ventricular ejection. The post-bypass intraoperative period should be used to examine ventricular function visually and haemodynamically. The heart should not become distended, segments viable preoperatively should contract well and left atrial pressure should be lower than preoperative left ventricular end-diastolic pressure at an equivalent systemic pressure. If grafts are functioning distal to the critical stenoses and myocardial protection has been adequate, ventricular function should be improved post-bypass. If that is not the case an accurate diagnosis of the problem should be made while still in the operating room. The ECG and visual inspection of the heart may be used to localize an area of ischaemic myocardium. Inadequate protection during ischaemia, intracoronary air, graft dysfunction, technical error, coronary embolization, coronary dissection and the presence of a stenotic lesion not appreciated at angiography are all potential causes of myocardial dysfunction post-bypass. If the area of myocardium not functioning satisfactorily is well perfused with blood and is still dysfunctional an injury to the myocardium must be assumed to have occurred. Rather than treat this unusual situation with inotropic support alone our approach is to institute IABP support to attempt to limit the area of injury. Inotropic agents are sometimes used for patients with severe preoperative ventricular dysfunction who have not suffered intraoperative injury but in whom we wish to maintain a low ventricular end-diastolic pressure. Also, patients with severe intraoperative injury may not respond entirely to IABP support and may need inotropic support as well. The use of IABP support is not without complications and other surgeons may favour the use of inotropic agents prior to inserting an inter-aortic balloon pump.

Once post-bypass haemodynamics have stabilized, heparinization is reversed with protamine, the cannulae removed, haemostasis obtained, and two mediastinal drainage tubes are placed. The pericardial fat pad is brought over the grafts and sutured to the diaphragm to cover and protect the grafts, the sternum approximated with wire and the subcutaneous tissues and skin closed with continuous suture material.

With careful post-bypass intraoperative assessment unpleasant haemodynamic surprises in the early postoperative period are rare. Serum enzymes and a 12-lead ECG are checked upon arrival in the intensive care unit and continuous monitoring of mean arterial pressure and left atrial pressure is routine. Patients with severe haemodynamic difficulties are monitored with intermittent cardiac output determinations as well. Cardiac dysfunction which has its onset in the intensive care unit is usually due to cardiac tamponade from retaining clot and re-exploration is indicated after early graft occlusion is ruled out by repeat ECG criteria.

SURGICAL RESULTS

Perioperative Morbidity

The major categories of postoperative complications and their frequency of occurrence are listed in *Table* 48.2. The decrease in the incidence of reoperations for haemorrhage and in postoperative respiratory insufficiency is probably in part due to modern membrane type oxygenators, their decreased trauma to blood elements and to fewer intraoperative blood transfusions. The incidence of stroke, defined as either a transient or permanent neurological deficit, has been relatively constant since 1970 and even though the deficit was temporary in approximately half the cases, potential

Table 48.2 Complications following myocardial revascularization. Cleveland Clinic Foundation (from Loop et al., 1979)

Complication	*1967–1970*	*1972*	*1978*
Perioperative infarction	7·1%	4·3%	1·2%
Stroke	2·0%	1·3%	1·7%
Wound complication	2·0%	2·4%	0·8%
Respiratory insufficiency	5·0%	1·8%	0·7%

neurological complications remain a major risk and continuing challenge. Wound complications represent a problem but the incidence has declined to approximately 1%.

The incidence of perioperative infarction can be quite variable, depending upon the criterion used to make the diagnosis. Defining perioperative infarction as the presence of new Q waves correlated with postoperative serum enzyme elevations yielded figures listed in *Table* 48.2. Defining perioperative infarction in this manner will obviously exclude some patients who suffered small infarcts or non-transmural infarcts, or had scattered, non-focal areas of damage at the time of surgery. However, the clinical significance of the 'missed' perioperative infarcts is unclear. For 102 Cleveland Clinic Foundation patients who survived perioperative infarcts with new Q waves the 5-year survival was 94%.

Operative Mortality

Operative mortality is related to the extent of disease and preoperative ventricular function. *Table* 48.3 lists the operative mortality rate for 3000 cases of elective myocardial revascularization performed at the Cleveland Clinic Foundation in the years 1976–1978 grouped by extent of disease and severity of left ventricular impairment. Other surgical groups have confirmed the reproducibility of such results.

Table 48.3 Operative mortality. First 1000 elective revascularization patients per year 1976–1978. Cleveland Clinic Foundation

Extent of disease (Vessels > 70% stenosis	*Operative mortality*
Single vessel	0·5%
Double vessel	1·0%
Triple vessel	1·1%
LMCA	1·1%
Left Ventricular Contraction	
Normal LV	0·8%
Mild impairment	0·9%
Moderate impairment	1·6%
Severe impairment	1·9%

Graft Patency

IMA and saphenous vein graft patency rates for patients undergoing surgery at the Cleveland Clinic Foundation in the years 1971–1973 and undergoing postoperative catheterization are shown in *Table* 48.4. These are probably

Table 48.4 Graft patency in patients undergoing surgery, 1971–1973. Cleveland Clinic Foundation (from Loop et al., 1979)

Surgery to catheterization intervals	*Patients studied*	*Grafts studied*	*Per cent patent*
Vein Graft			
< 7	122	191	72·25
7–12	426	733	81·45
13–24	557	977	83·42
25–36	101	168	85·71
37–48	74	127	72·87
>48	200	341	70·38
IMA Grafts			
< 7	59	59	89·83
7–12	131	133	97·74
13–24	148	150	93·33
25–36	25	26	100·00
37–48	23	23	91·30
>48	38	38	94·74

minimum patency rates as many asymptomatic patients did not undergo re-study.

Ninety-eight patients in this group underwent more than one postoperative catheterization and of 123 vein grafts patent at the first study, 109 (88·6%) remained patent at the second study, with a mean interval between the catheterizations of 42 months. Of 58 IMA grafts patent at first recatheterization, 54 (93·1%) remained patent after a mean interval of 33 months. In general, vein grafts to the LAD have a slightly higher patency rate than grafts to the circumflex and right coronary vessels.

The probable causes of early and late graft failure are multiple. Technical events, inadequate host vessel run-off and saphenous vein damage appear to be related to early failure. Late histological changes in vein grafts which include intimal hyperplasia and vein graft atherosclerosis may produce vein stenosis or occlusion. Progression of atherosclerotic disease in the host coronary vessels, secondarily limiting outflow probably also contributes to the progressive fall-off in late patency. To summarize, a high percentage of vein graft occlusion appears to take place in the first year after surgery. However, there is a continuing slow drop in the patency rate with time, as indicated by serial studies of vein grafts. IMA grafts appear to have a very high early patency and a low rate of late occlusion. Late atherosclerosis of IMA grafts has not yet been documented angiographically.

Relief of Angina

Symptom improvement has a strong correlation with graft patency. Of patients found to be completely revascularized at recatheterization (functioning grafts distal to all stenoses greater than 70% in major vessels), approximately 90% are asymptomatic. Even incomplete revascularization is helpful as approximately 60% of patients with at least one functioning graft are asymptomatic at late follow-up and 30% have mild angina. Further, ventriculographic studies of patients asymptomatic at late follow-up and with functioning grafts indicate that most patients have not suffered interval myocardial infarction, which also could account for a lack of angina. In general, 60–70% of patients undergoing coronary revascularization can be expected to be asymptomatic at 5 years following surgery.

Long-term Survival

Follow-up of the first 1000 patients undergoing isolated coronary revascularization procedures at the Cleveland Clinic Foundation each year from 1971 to 1973 has demonstrated a 5-year survival of 92·2% of these 1000 patients. As shown in *Table* 48.5, 5-year postoperative survival was adversely affected by poor preoperative ventricular function and the extent of preoperative coronary atherosclerosis. Survival was also adversely affected by incomplete revascularization.

Table 48.5 1971–1972 Surgical patients. Cleveland Clinic Foundation (from Loop et al., 1979)

Five-year actuarial survival	*Survival* (%)
All patients	92·2%
LV contraction	
Normal or mild impairment	93·0%
Moderate or severe impairment	84·2%
Completeness of Revascularization	
Complete	93·8%
Incomplete	88·0%
Extent of Disease	
Single vessel	96·5%
Double vessel	93·6%
Triple vessel	89·8%

INDICATIONS FOR MYOCARDIAL REVASCULARIZATION

Indications for any operation, myocardial revascularization included, fall into the broad categories of symptom relief and prolongation of patient survival. The most generally accepted indication for coronary bypass surgery is coronary atherosclerosis producing angina which is severe enough to limit the patient's life-style despite medical therapy. As mentioned above, myocardial revascularization has been shown to be statistically very successful in alleviating angina. Indications based on the hope of prolonging patient survival are more complicated and controversial.

Proudfit's classic study of 601 patients with angiographically documented coronary artery disease treated non-operatively and followed for a minimum of 10 years contains the largest patient population and the longest and most complete follow-up of any study of the natural history of coronary atherosclerosis. Further, patients who were surgical candidates were selected as a subgroup. The 5-year survival of these surgical candidates separated by preoperative extent of disease is shown in the third column of *Table* 48.6. Since pharmacological beta blockade was not used extensively in the USA until the early 1970s the management of these patients did not always include these pharmacological agents, a theoretical disadvantage in trying to compare their outcome with that of surgically treated patients. More recent medical series, compiled in the era of beta blockers, contain fewer patients who have been followed for much shorter periods. However, 5-year actuarial survival concerning the Veterans Administration Hospital Cooperative Study non-surgical group and 4 year survival concerning the non-surgical group from a matched series reported from Seattle, Washington are also contained in *Table* 48.6.

Table 48.6 Five-year actuarial survival of three series of medically treated patients and Cleveland Clinic Foundation surgically treated patients

Extent of disease	*VA medical group*	*Seattle medical group*	*CCF medical group (surgical candidates)*	*CCF surgical group 1971–1973*
Single vessel	83	93	88	96·5
Double vessel	87	76	69	93·6
Triple vessel	70	75	57	89·8

Survival expressed in per cent.

The European Coronary Surgery Study Group randomized males less than 65 years of age with mild or moderate chronic angina and good ventricular function into medical and surgical treatment groups. *Table* 48.7 contains recently reported 5-year survival data concerning some of these patients.

Table 48.7 Survival of patients followed for 5 years. European Coronary Surgery Study Group

Extent of disease	*Medical group*	*Surgical group*
Double vessel	87·5	91·6
Triple vessel	84·8	94·9
Left main	61·7	92·9

Survival expressed in per cent.

Definition of patient subgroups for the purpose of analysing survival data has usually been on the basis of the number of vessels with angiographically significant (>70%) obstruction, as this characteristic appears to be the single most accurate predictor of survival in patients with coronary artery disease treated non-surgically. However, these subgroups are extremely heterogeneous in nature since such a simple classification system does not take into account angiographic characteristics such as the length of the obstructions, non-significant disease, the size and distribution of the vessels diseased, or ventricular function. Also, some non-invasive characteristics can contribute to survival prediction.

SINGLE VESSEL DISEASE

The three non-surgical groups in *Table* 48.6 indicate a 5-year survival of 83–93% for patients with single vessel disease. Proudfit further documented a 75% 10-year survival for this angiographic subgroup and a worse prognosis for isolated LAD stenosis, recording an 80·8% 5-year and 53·7% 10-year survival.

Five-year survival following surgery for patients with single vessel disease in the 1971–1973 cohorts was 96·5%. For those patients revascularized for isolated LAD obstruction survival was 98·3% compared to 93·0% for RCA and 88·7% for circumflex disease. The lower survival of patients with RCA and Cx grafts may be due to progression of atherosclerosis in the non-grafted LAD. Revascularization for single vessel disease is widely accepted in the face of incapacitating symptoms but controversial in other settings since statistical survival prolongation has not been clearly demonstrated. Our own view, based on our 5-year surgical results, is that we recommend operation for patients with single vessel disease if the vessel and area of myocardium at risk are large even if the patient is not totally disabled by symptoms. Recently, coronary catheter angioplasty has been reported by Grundzig for such patients with good results.

DOUBLE VESSEL DISEASE

Double vessel disease carried a 5-year survival ranging from 69 to 87% in the medical studies in *Table* 48.6 and a 50% survival in Proudfit's 10-year data. The authors' surgical patients had a 93·6% 5-year survival. These data encourage a tendency to recommend revascularization for double vessel disease for reasons of statistical survival prolongation, though this is a concept not universally agreed upon. Data from the Seattle Heart Watch study appear to support this view.

The European Cooperative Study Group did not demonstrate significant prolongation of survival at 5 years for surgically treated patients with double vessel disease. However, this was in part because of a relatively favourable survival of the medical group, brought about by the high survival of medically treated patients with double vessel disease but without significant LAD obstruction. Medically treated patients with double vessel disease, including significant LAD obstruction, had a survival comparable to that of medically treated patients with triple vessel disease.

TRIPLE VESSEL DISEASE

The situation is more clear cut for patients with three vessel disease, as data from a number of centres indicate statistical prolongation of survival for surgically treated patients. The 5-year survival of the authors' surgically treated patients is 89·8% compared to the 57–75% survivals in the *Table* 48.6 medical groups. The European Coronary Surgery Study Group reported significant prolongation of survival at 5 years for their surgically treated patients. The authors recommend surgery for patients with triple vessel disease even in the absence of severe symptoms.

LEFT MAIN CORONARY ARTERY STENOSIS

Significant stenosis of the LMCA is a lethal anatomical situation with the most favourable series showing a 61·7% 5-year survival without surgery. Review of the first 300 LMCA patients undergoing surgery at the Cleveland Clinic showed an 88·6% 5-year survival. The authors recommend surgery for all patients with a 70% stenosis of the LMCA even if they are asymptomatic.

UNSTABLE ANGINA

Unstable angina is a term which has been used to describe a variety of symptom complexes. However, since unstable symptoms may be representative of a number of pathophysiological situations ranging from no myocardial ischaemia at all to complete myocardial infarction, relatively precise clinical criteria for 'unstable angina' are necessary for comparisons of therapy. The clinical criteria for unstable angina as defined by the National Cooperative Study of Unstable Angina are: a new or changing angina pattern, admission to a coronary care unit, transient ECG changes associated with angina, no new Q waves or enzyme elevations, no myocardial infarction within 3 months and an age less than 71 years. The anatomical causes of unstable angina include atherosclerotic obstruction, atherosclerotic obstruction with superimposed spasm and pure coronary spasm. There is no simple solution to the problem of unstable angina, but the authors' general principles of management of unstable symptom complexes are:

1. Relieve Ischaemia

Aggressive pharmacological management with nitrates, beta blockade and sedation will almost always control acute ischaemia. If these techniques are unsuccessful and if ECG changes demonstrate that the symptoms are clearly due to myocardial ischaemia intra-aortic balloon pump (IABP) support is the next step. In clinical situations where unstable angina seems likely to be due to coronary spasm, nifedipine is instituted and beta blockade is stopped.

2. Establish an Anatomical and Physiological Diagnosis

Once the acute symptoms are controlled, ECG and radionuclide scanning criteria are used to rule out acute myocardial infarction. If infarction has not occurred or if infarction has occurred but evidence of ischaemia persists, coronary arteriography is undertaken. If a completed infarction is documented and no evidence of ongoing ischaemia exists, catheterization is carried out at an interval ranging from 1 to 6 weeks. Once the coronary anatomy has been defined, the usual indications for surgery are applied.

3. Operation

With rare exceptions, the authors try to avoid undertaking revascularization in the face of either acute infarction or persistent ischaemia. If pharmacological and IABP support is unsuccessful in relieving acute ischaemia, the authors will occasionally undertake emergency revascularization in this difficult situation. They have found that the mortality for emergency operations for acute ischaemia is higher than for elective cases and particularly in women the incidence of perioperative myocardial infarction is increased when operation is undertaken in the face of ischaemia. Availability of modern non-operative management techniques has made emergency revascularization for acute ischaemia rarely necessary.

Progression of Disease and Reoperation following Direct Revascularization

Bypass grafts are intended to maintain or increase blood flow distal to obstructive coronary lesions which exist at the time of operation, but do not prevent the development of further obstructions. Indeed, progression of atherosclerotic lesions in both saphenous vein grafts and the host coronary circulation appears to be the major factor limiting the effectiveness of revascularization. It is critical that physician and surgeon impress upon the patient that atherosclerosis is a systemic and potentially progressive disease and that risk factor control may have an effect upon graft patency, future symptoms, and longevity following surgery. Indications for recatheterization following surgery are essentially the same as those prior to operation with the exception that the authors recommend routine coronary arteriography at 1 and 5 years postoperatively.

Reoperations for coronary atherosclerosis are technically more difficult than initial procedures due to the scarring which complicates cannulation and vessel identification. A review of over 500 reoperations for revascularization at the Cleveland Clinic Foundation demonstrated an increased operative mortality but a graft patency rate and symptom response which approaches that of primary operations. Therefore, the indications for reoperation are not vastly different from those for primary procedures.

SURGICAL COMPLICATIONS FOLLOWING MYOCARDIAL INFARCTION

Ventricular Aneurysm

Myocardial infarction which produces transmural necrosis of an area of ventricular wall may lead to the formation of a left ventricular aneurysm. Acute aneurysm formation may occur early after infarction and angiographically appears as a large area of paradoxical expansion during systole. If the patient survives the acute event the area of infarction may progress to a chronic fibrous aneurysm, which is a large thinned-out scar, clearly delineated from surrounding muscle by obliteration of endocardial trabeculations and often containing mural thrombus. Few patients with acute aneurysms undergo catheterization, though the development of an acute aneurysm does place the patient at risk of cardiac rupture. A small group of patients with acute aneurysms has undergone surgery at the University of Chicago with excellent survival. However, chronic aneurysms constitute the vast majority of those approached surgically.

Most aneurysms are anterolateral or anteroseptal in location, and result from left anterior descending stenosis or occlusion. Posterior true aneurysms occur between the posterior papillary muscle and the interventricular septum but only constitute 2–3%, probably because the patient with a large posterior infarction is likely to suffer papillary muscle damage as well and not survive the peri-infarction period. Rarely a posterolateral aneurysm will occur in the circumflex distribution. False aneurysms have been documented in a few patients who survived postinfarction ventricular rupture.

Ventricular aneurysms produce a severe haemodynamic disadvantage. The amount of functioning left ventricular muscle is decreased, a large akinetic scar is present and inefficient left ventricular contraction is associated with a high end-systolic ventricular volume, an increase in intramyocardial wall tension and therefore, high myocardial oxygen consumption. The natural history of left ventricular aneurysms is a grim one with 60–73% of patients dead within 3 years of diagnosis. Presenting symptoms and operative indications include: (1) angina pectoris; (2) congestive heart failure; (3) ventricular arrhythmias; (4) systemic embolization. Sixty to seventy-five per cent of aneurysm patients will describe angina, which may occur even with single vessel disease. Congestive heart failure is the next most common surgical indication with ventricular arrhythmias or systemic embolization being the major surgical indication in less than 5% of cases.

Aneurysmectomy is performed through a median sternotomy with cardiopulmonary bypass. Aortic cross-clamping or ventricular fibrillation is used to avoid systemic embolization. Following removal of mural thrombus and clearly delineated scar tissue the ventricle is repaired with two or three layers of suture and any indicated grafting procedures are then carried out. From 1972 to 1976, 400 patients underwent aneurysmectomy at the Cleveland Clinic Foundation with an operative mortality of 3% for isolated aneurysmectomy and 3·4% for aneurysmectomy and revascularization.

Bypass grafting of critically stenotic coronary arteries supplying non-aneurysmal regions of myocardium is an important aspect of the surgical treatment of the patient with an aneurysm, and has a positive effect on long-term survival. For 349 consecutive surgical patients undergoing aneurysmectomy between 1962 and 1972 at the Cleveland Clinic Foundation the 7-year survival was 69% for patients with single vessel disease, 65% for patients with multiple vessel disease and 50% for those with multiple vessel disease and incomplete revascularization.

Cardiac Rupture

Cardiac rupture, a complication in approximately 8% of fatal myocardial infarctions has occasionally been diagnosed and treated with success. It occurs more frequently in older, hypertensive patients, 2–5 days following a first myocardial infarction and may be preceded by recurrent pain and enzyme elevation as well as increasing pericardial effusion and infarct expansion on echocardiography.

Ventricular Septal Rupture

Ventricular septal rupture is an uncommon but dramatic complication of myocardial infarction which usually occurs within the first week following infarction and presents as a sudden haemodynamic deterioration accompanied by a new systolic murmur. The rupture usually occurs in the distal septum, anteriorly or apically following anterior infarction and posteriorly following inferior wall infarction. It is usually the patient's first infarction, a history of hypertension is common, as is single vessel coronary disease.

Diagnosis at the bedside may be established with the use of a Swan–Ganz pulmonary artery catheter to demonstrate a left-to-right shunt. Cardiac catheterization is then performed to document the coronary anatomy and to establish whether or not the mitral valve apparatus is intact.

Management of this condition is surgical closure of the rupture. However, some judgement must be exercised as to the timing of the operation. In the critically ill patient initiation of IABP support may stabilize the haemodynamic situation sufficiently to allow catheterization and to aid intra-operative and postoperative haemodynamic management. However, IABP support is not a substitute for surgery. Because of tissue friability following an infarction there are technical advantages to delaying surgery to 3 or 4 weeks postinfarction and a few patients with small shunts and good residual myocardial function may maintain stable haemodynamics on medical management and allow the surgeon to temporize. However, once the need for inotropic agents or IABP support arises, continued deterioration is inexorable unless the defect is urgently repaired.

Operative approach is based on the following technical principles:

1. Approach to the defect is through the infarct, allowing maximum preservation of viable myocardium.
2. Anterior rupture can often be closed by direct suture using the right ventricular wall to close the defect or by sewing a prosthetic patch into the septum.
3. Posterior septal rupture following inferior infarction presents a more complicated problem as the geometry of the diaphragmatic wall leaves less muscular tissue available for use in closing the defect. Prosthetic material can be used both as a septal patch and also as replacement for the infarcted inferior wall, which relieves tension from suture lines and contributes to a stable closure.
4. Stenotic arteries supplying viable myocardium are grafted.

Operative mortality for patients who require operation acutely following infarction ranges from 25 to 50% and is increased for patients with posterior septal rupture when compared to those with anterior defects. More recently operative mortality has improved, mainly due to technical facility in repairing posterior defects. Patients able to survive to a month postoperatively may be corrected with a risk of approximately 10%. Long-term follow-up data do not include large patient numbers but most operative survivors are either asymptomatic or minimally symptomatic. Long-term survival (5–8 years) ranges from 63 to 89% in some reported series.

Mitral Insufficiency

There is a wide spectrum of mitral valve dysfunction associated with coronary artery disease. As the long axis of the ventricle shortens during systole papillary muscle contraction prevents prolapse of the mitral valve leaflets and subsequent mitral regurgitation. Ischaemia of the papillary muscle may prevent normal stabilization of the valve leaflets and regurgitation may ensue. Further, infarction and rupture of the papillary muscle may allow prolapse of the leaflet and florid regurgitation.

Papillary muscle rupture following myocardial infarction usually occurs in the first week following the infarct and is characterized by a new systolic murmur and haemodynamic deterioration. The posterior papillary muscle is usually involved, following an infarct in the area of a dominant right coronary artery. Diagnostically it is necessary to distinguish this condition from ventricular septal rupture. Rarely, the two mechanical defects occur together. Catheterization with left ventriculography and coronary arteriography will establish the diagnosis and demonstrate the coronary anatomy.

Haemodynamic deterioration following papillary muscle rupture is an indication for immediate operation. IABP support can be helpful in reducing the risk of catheterization and operation but is not a substitute for mitral valve replacement or repair. As with ventricular septal rupture an occasional patient with a favourable anatomical situation and a small infarction may remain stable and operation may be deferred 4–6 weeks.

The technical aspects of mitral valve repair or replacement following papillary muscle rupture are based on the lack of chamber enlargement and annular scarring which is seen in patients with a more chronic form of mitral valve dysfunction. Although replacement has been preferred over repair in the past, recent improved results using mitral valve repair in these situations have been reported. If replacement is used, then a low profile disc type valve is used because of the favourable haemodynamics of small valve sizes of this design, and Teflon-backed horizontal mattress sutures are used to sew the valve to the thin annulus. Revascularization of critically obstructed coronary arteries is combined with valve replacement.

Mitral valve dysfunction may also occur in patients with coronary artery disease but without infarction and frank papillary muscle rupture. Ischaemia of the papillary muscles may occur intermittently, producing severe mitral regurgitation which may be acutely improved by relief of ischaemia and afterload reduction. Such mitral dysfunction can often be improved by revascularization, which may relieve papillary muscle ischaemia, and may improve left ventricular function, thus reducing ventricular size. It is unusual to be forced to undertake mitral valve replacement for ischaemic mitral valve disease without the presence of frank papillary muscle rupture.

Post-infarction Shock

Patients with cardiogenic shock following myocardial infarction present with arterial hypotension, a decreased urinary output, decreased peripheral perfusion and a cardiac index of less than 2 L/min. When caused by myocardial insufficiency without the presence of a mechanical lesion, such as septal rupture or papillary muscle infarction, this condition predicts a mortality of greater than 90%. Intra-aortic balloon counterpulsation alone has been shown to improve haemodynamics for a few days, but not the long-term outlook. Consequently, Buckley and colleagues at the Massachusetts General Hospital initiated a programme of initial IABP support followed by myocardial revascularization for this very critically ill group of patients. It is their concept that in a patient with a large myocardial infarction, there may be a marginal zone of ischaemic myocardium around the infarct which, if successfully revascularized, could improve left ventricular function enough to sustain life. Their initial results have indicated a survival rate of between 40 and 50%, a remarkable accomplishment with these critically ill patients.

Emergency Revascularization for Myocardial Infarction

Myocardial infarction may often be a progressive event with haemodynamic instability caused by the initial ventricular dysfunction contributing to further loss of myocardium. Based on this concept a number of groups have treated selected patients in the throes of myocardial infarction with emergency revascularization, i.e. surgery with 4–6 h after the onset of symptoms, without the indications of a mechanical defect or cardiogenic shock. It has been the hope that this treatment would reduce infarct size and possibly reduce arrhythmia formation. Some initial encouraging results have been reported, but it must be realized that there are many factors at work selecting the patient populations. Therefore, results are difficult to interpret regarding application of the general concept of revascularizing an acute myocardial infarction. It is clear that under some circumstances revascularization of an infarct can be detrimental to the patient and in the past mortality from this approach has been high. This must still be considered a controversial indication for revascularization. Recently acute streptokinase infusion has been proposed, with surgery for symptom recurrence.

On occasion, urgent percutaneous transcoronary angioplasty (PTCA) has been used effectively in some centres.

Further Reading

Anturane Reinfarction Trial Research Group (1978) *N. Engl. J. Med.* **298**, 289.

Barratt-Boyes B. G., White H. D., Agnew T. M. et al. (1984) The results of surgical treatment of left ventricular aneurysms: An assessment of the risk factors affecting early and late mortality. *J. Thorac. Cardiovasc. Surg.* **87**, 87.

Bates R. J., Beutler S., Resnekov L. et al. (1977) Cardiac rupture—challenge in diagnosis and management. *Am. J. Cardiol.* **40**, 429.

CASS Principal Investigators and their Associates (1983) Coronary artery surgery study (CASS): A randomized trial of coronary artery bypass surgery: Survival data. *Circulation* **68**, 939.

CASS Principal Investigators and their Associates (1984) Myocardial infarction and mortality in the coronary artery surgery (CASS) randomized trial. *N. Engl. J. Med.* **310**, 750.

Chesebro J. H., Fuster V., Elveback C. R. et al. (1984) Effect of dipyridamole and aspirin on late vein-graft patency after coronary bypass operations. *N. Engl. J. Med.* **310**, 209.

European Coronary Surgery Study Group (1980) Prospective randomized study of coronary artery bypass surgery in stable angina pectoris. Second interim report of the European Coronary Surgery Study Group. *Lancet* **2**, 492.

Hammermeister K. F., DeRouen T. A., Murray J. A. et al. (1977) Effect of aortocoronary saphenous vein bypass grafting on death and sudden death. *Am. J. Cardiol.* **39**, 925.

Kannel W. B. and Feinlab M. (1972) Natural history of angina pectoris in the Framingham study. *Am. J. Cardiol.* **29**, 154.

Kay J. H., Zubiate P., Mendez M. A. et al. (1980) Surgical treatment of mitral insufficiency secondary to coronary artery disease. *J. Thorac. Cardiovasc. Surg.* **79**, 12.

Loop F. D., Cosgrove D. M., Lytle B. W. et al. (1979) An 11-year evolution of coronary arterial surgery (1967–1978). *Ann. Surg.* **190**, 444.

Loop F. D., Lytle B. W., Cosgrove D. M. et al. (1986) Influence of the internal mammary graft on postoperative cardiac events and 10 year survival. *N. Engl. J. Med.* **314**, 1.

Mock M. B., Ringqvist I., Fisher L. D. et al. (1982) Survival of medically treated patients in the coronary artery surgery study (CASS) Registry. *Circulation* **66**, 562.

National Cooperative Study Group (1977) Unstable angina pectoris—National Cooperative Study Group to compare medical and surgical therapy. I. Report of protocol and patient population. *Am. J. Cardiol.* **37**, 896.

Turpeinen O. (1979) Effect of cholesterol-lowering diet on mortality from coronary heart disease and other causes. *Circulation* **59**, 1.

Vlodaver Z. and Edwards J. E. (1971) *Prog. Cardiovasc. Dis.* **14**, No. 3.

49 *Cardiac Transplantation*

D. R. Zusman, E. B. Stinson and P. O. Daily

HISTORY

Clinical experience with cardiac transplantation began in January 1964, when Hardy performed the first human orthotopic cardiac transplant, a xenograft, from a chimpanzee to a man in a patient who was in terminal cardiogenic shock. Satisfactory cardiac output could not be achieved and the patient eventually died. Barnard, in December 1967, performed the first cardiac transplant using a human donor. The patient survived 17 days.

This initial experience heralded a worldwide enthusiasm for the procedure with more than one hundred transplants being performed during the next 12 months by 64 teams in 22 countries. However, a majority of these cases were performed at Stanford. The results were initially poor, for no one was capable of appreciating the degree of difficulty in postoperative care and the problems associated with infection and rejection following transplantation.

A new interest in cardiac transplantation occurred in 1978 which has been sustained. Over 350 cases were performed in 1985, the majority using orthotopic rather than heterotopic techniques. The number of transplant procedures per year, both worldwide and at Stanford University Medical Center are reflected in *Fig.* 49.1.

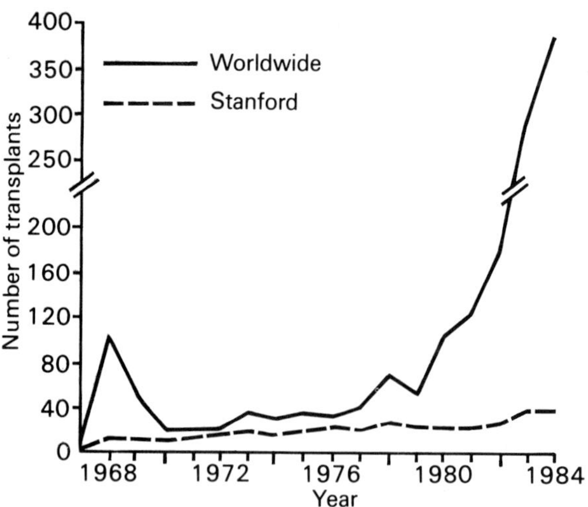

Fig. 49.1 Comparison of number of cardiac transplant procedures worldwide and at Stanford University Medical Center.

There have been four principal areas of development leading to sustained improvement in clinical results over the past 15 years. These include the effectiveness of topical cardiac cooling for myocardial protection which has helped in distant donor procurement; improvement in the diagnosis of cardiac rejection by applying the relationship of histopathological changes in endomyocardial biopsies; the introduction of antithymocyte globulin both rabbit and horse; and, finally, further improvements in immunosuppression with the introduction of cyclosporine and the appreciation of its associated toxicities.

The experience that the authors have had at Stanford and, presently, at Sharp Memorial Hospital/UCSD provides the data for this chapter. Included in this discussion will be recipient and donor selection, operative techniques for both the donor and recipient, the principles of both early and late postoperative management, xenograft transplantation and the association of malignancy in transplanted patients, and the survival and rehabilitation rates.

RECIPIENT SELECTION

Selection criteria have become more stringent with accumulated experience and have been refined to identify potential recipients most likely to benefit from the operation. The goal of preoperative evaluation is the identification of individuals most likely to benefit in terms of survival and rehabilitation following transplantation. Such individuals are those with end-stage cardiac disease for which no efficacious or clinically proven form of treatment other than biological heart transplantation exists. These patients also have a prognosis of survival limited to several months. The most common aetiological diagnoses of recipients who have undergone transplantation include coronary artery disease or idiopathic cardiomyopathies (*Table* 49.1).

Personnel capable of accurate assessment of such patients include a cardiologist, a pulmonary specialist, social worker, and a transplantation coordinator. Complete cardiovascular evaluation includes angiography, cardiac catheterization and, in some cases, endomyocardial biopsy to exclude treatable causes of disease.

The general criteria for the selection of potential heart transplantation candidates include: (1) objective evidence of advanced physical incapacitation due to documented, isolated heart disease; (2) a limited life expectancy estimated to

Table 49.1 Stanford cardiac transplantation recipient diagnosis

Coronary artery disease	156
Cardiomyopathy	178
Valve disease with CM	19
Congenital heart disease	6
Coronary artery emboli	2
Cardiac tumour	1
Post-traumatic aneurysm	1
Myocarditis	1
Sarcoid	2
	366

a duration of weeks to months; (3) unanimous agreement that medical therapy has been optimal and that no surgical procedure, other than transplantation, could offer realistic expectation of functional improvement and extension of life; and (4) strong family support to aid the recipient emotionally during the pre- and postoperative period and for the rest of his or her life.

Multiple patient-related factors have come to be recognized as adversely affecting the outcome of heart transplantation. These features constitute relative or absolute contraindications to transplantation: (1) age over 60 years; (2) severe pulmonary hypertension as defined by elevated pulmonary vascular resistance of greater than 8–10 Wood units unresponsive to prostaglandin E_1 administration or nitroprusside; (3) severe irreversible hepatic or renal dysfunction; (4) active systemic infection; (5) separate systemic illness; (6) recent (less than 6 weeks) and unresolved pulmonary infarction; (7) diabetes requiring insulin for control; (8) severe peripheral or cerebral vascular disease; (9) active peptic ulcer disease; and (10) history of behaviour abnormality.

The restraints reflect the 'state of the art' in heart transplantation and the necessity for indefinite immunosuppression and will be subject to modification with further developments in control of the immune process.

THE CARDIAC DONOR

The requirement for a viable heart, undamaged by prolonged periods of ischaemia necessitates the use of a neurologically dead patient. The concept of brain death was recognized in California by legislative action in 1974. Presently, confirmation by two physicians, not necessarily neurologists or neurosurgeons, is necessary to declare a patient as brain dead.

The majority of cardiac donors have sustained irreversible cerebral damage as a result of closed head injuries. The remainder have suffered either gunshot wounds to the head or spontaneous intracranial haemorrhage. Donors over 35 years of age are considered unsuitable due to evidence suggesting asymptomatic atherosclerosis involving the donor coronary arteries.

Recipient matching is based on: (1) ABO compatibility; (2) absence of positive lymphocyte crossmatch; and (3) less than a 20% discrepancy between donor and recipient body mass for heart transplantation. If the recipient candidate has not had previous surgery or blood transfusions, or if the preoperative cytotoxic lymphocyte screen is negative, then it is acceptable to perform the cytotoxic lymphocyte crossmatch post transplant. This should be the exception rather than the rule.

PREOPERATIVE MANAGEMENT OF DONORS FOR HEART TRANSPLANTATION

Brain death is often accompanied by loss of motor tone with resultant hypotension. This may be due to hypovolaemia or myocardial injury/dysfunction. High urine output from diabetes insipidus may contribute to hypovolaemia, hypernatraemia, and hypercalaemia. Haemostatic temperature control is often lost and the patient becomes hypothermic. Neurogenic pulmonary oedema may also occur. When first evaluating a potential donor, the adequacy of cardiac function is initially determined by the mean arterial pressure, the central venous pressure, and the state of tissue perfusion, i.e., urine output. One reviews the chest radiograph, electrocardiogram, and performs a physical examination to rule out any pathological murmurs or chest trauma. Although ST–T segment abnormalities are often present in severely brain-injured patients, if the myocardial MB–CPK fraction is not elevated, then it is felt that the heart is not likely to be injured. However, we have proceeded with coronary arteriography and left ventriculograms in order to determine myocardial injury, when warranted.

Every effort is made to maintain a stable and adequate blood pressure with the judicious use of volume replacement and minimal vasopressors. The goal of 'pressor therapy' is to maintain the mean arterial pressure at or greater than 70 torr. It is extremely important to have a central venous line or Swan–Ganz catheter in the early management of patients so one can determine the systemic vascular resistance as well as maintain adequate filling pressures. Commonly, when first contacted about a potential donor, the patient is often hypovalaemic due to diabetes insipidus. If the patient is well perfused with a normal or increased CVP and one cannot wean dopamine to less than 2·5 mg/kg/min, alpha-agents should be instituted. Inability to wean the dopamine at this point indicates a contractility problem and the heart should not be used for transplantation.

OPERATIVE TECHNIQUE FOR DONOR CARDIECTOMY AND ORTHOTOPIC HEART TRANSPLANTATION

The operative technique for the donor cardiectomy is as follows: The patient is brought to the operating room and a standard median sternotomy incision is performed. The pericardium is opened vertically and suspended laterally. The heart is examined for evidence of contusion, coronary artery disease, valvular disease, or congenital anomalies. The recipient team is informed of the findings and, at appropriate times, the cardiectomy is then undertaken.

The donor heart is removed without cardiopulmonary bypass. The patient is systemically heparinized with 30 000 units of heparin. The azygos vein and superior vena cava are tied and cut. The aorta is cross-clamped and 1 L of cold cardioplegia is infused into the ascending aorta and topical cold saline applied. The inferior vena cava is cut within the pericardium. The heart is then excised by cutting the pulmonary veins and the pulmonary artery and aorta. The donor heart is then cooled by immersion in cold saline at 3–4 °C. Functional integrity of the donor sino-atrial node, though anatomically denervated, is preserved by appropriate tailoring of the donor atrial anastomotic lines.

Ischaemic times of 3 h have been tolerated without apparent ill effect. In the laboratory, hearts preserved in this manner for 24 h and stored at 3–4 °C have produced a satisfactory cardiac output after transplantation. Prior to implantation, the donor heart is trimmed of fat and vessels are tailored to size. The superior vena cava is tied and an incision is made from the inferior vena cava upwards towards the right atrial appendage so as to leave intact the sino-atrial node. Implantation of the heart is begun in the left atrium. When this anastomosis has been completed, the right atrial anastomosis is performed; part of the inter-atrial septum is, thus, doubly sewn. A catheter is now placed into the left atrial appendage. The left ventricle is continuously flushed with cold saline as the aortic anastomosis is performed. This has the effect of both cooling the heart and removing air from the left atrium and ventricle. When the aortic anastomosis is completed, the cross-clamp is removed. The caval snares are released and the pulmonary artery anastomosis is then completed. The heart generally resumes spontaneous sinus rhythm, otherwise an electrical shock is required for defibrillation (*Fig.* 49.2).

The early postoperative care for cardiac recipients differs very little from that of routine cardiac surgical patients except for the institution of myocardial inotropic support, because of temporary depression of donor cardiac output and the administration of immunosuppressive drugs.

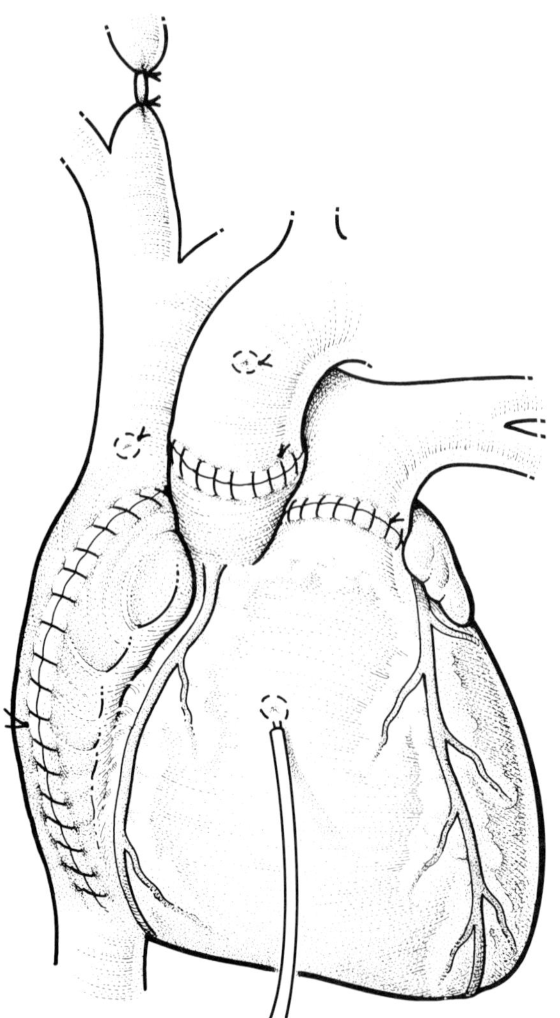

Fig. 49.2 Implantation of the donor heart.

Suppression of the immune response after cardiac transplantation is required on an indefinite basis. The heart is subjected to host immune responses that result in acute but reversible rejection episodes in most cases during the early postoperative period. During the late postoperative interval, the threat of acute rejection, although attenuated, nevertheless persists and, therefore, necessitates chronic maintenance of immunosuppression.

Immediately after transplantation, we use a four-drug protocol (*Table* 49.2). Patients are placed on cyclosporin A, the metabolite of a fungal product. Patients are given 12–16 mg/kg as a preoperative dose and then maintained on a divided dosage of 10 mg/kg orally q.i.d. A cyclosporin level is obtained three times weekly in order to maintain therapeutic levels. A level of 200–300 ng/ml trough is maintained for the first 30 days and then 50–150 ng/ml, thereafter. Horse ATG 10 mg/kg/day is given for the first week and circulating T-lymphocytes are maintained at less than 5% during this time. Patients are given a loading dose of imuran (4 mg/kg preoperatively), a cytotoxic agent, and then maintained on 2 mg/kg orally daily. The dosage is adjusted according to the circulating white cells. Finally, prednisone 0·8–1·0 mg/kg/day in divided dosages are given. The dosage is subsequently decreased by 0·1 mg/kg/week until a maintenance level of 0·2 mg/kg/day is obtained for the ensuing months.

An attempt was made to maintain patients on either low-dose prednisone during the initial post-transplant period or possibly withdrawing prednisone on a long-term basis. However, the incidence of rejection episodes increased dramatically, necessitating the reinstitution of steroids.

The toxicity of such generalized immunosuppression accounts for the greatest proportion of morbidity and mortality after cardiac transplantation. The most important complications consist of infection but others, such as osteoporosis and aseptic necrosis may also be influential factors in determining rehabilitation status. Infectious complications have constituted the most common cause of death in most series. The magnitude of this problem is indicated in *Table* 49.3 as experienced at Stanford University. It was noted that a total of 249 infections in the 173 cyclosporin patients have been diagnosed. Opportunistic pathogens and mixed infections are common. Given the high incidence of infection, especially in the early postoperative period when high-dose immunosuppression is required, demands aggressive diagnosis and treatment for successful management. Surveillance for infection, therefore, is maintained at all times. Frequent chest radiographs are obtained because the majority of infections are pulmonary in location.

Patients who develop low-grade fevers obtain urgent transvenous endomyocardial biopsy to rule out possible rejection. If this is unrewarding or if a pulmonary infiltrate is noted, transtracheal aspirates (TTA) are performed. Specimens are sent for Gram stain, KOH, AFB, silver stain for *Pneumocystis carinii*, direct fluorescent antibody for Legionella, aerobic and anaerobic bacterial cultures, viral cultures, Legionella and fungal cultures. Antibiotics for pulmonary infection are never begun until a TTA, bronchoscopy or transthoracic needle aspirate are done. Serology for cytomegalovirus, herpes virus, toxoplasmosis, and cryptococcus in addition to urine, sputum, and throat swabs for

Table 49.2 Heart transplantation—Adult protocol

Immunosuppression	*Loading dose*	*Maintenance dose*	*Lab. work*	*Biopsy*	*Acute rejection* (1st and 2nd episodes)	*Ongoing rejection*
Solu-Medrol	500 mg i.v. after CPB 125 mg i.v. q 12° × 3 doses	See prednisone	ECG once a week		1 g i.v. × 3 days with biopsy on day 5–7 post-rejection episode	1 g i.v. × 3 days (+ RATG) and re-biopsy (if rejection does not resolve, retransplant)
Prednisone		0·8 mg/kg taper by 0·1 mg/week until 0·1 mg/kg reached *after* discharge			Prednisone held at current patient dosage during 3 days of Solu-Medrol i.v.	Increase prednisone dosage after Solu-Medrol
Cyclosporin-A	16 mg/kg preop. 12 mg/kg/day preop. for renal insufficiency	9 mg/kg/day (until result of first Cyclosporin level)	Cyclosporin level q MWF 200–300 ng/ml (trough) —1–30 days 50–150 ng/ml (trough) — > days	Weekly and p.r.n. for increased temperature	No change	No change
ATG (either rabbit or horse, not both together)	Horse i.v. 10 mg/kg/day × 7 days		E-rosette count q day Circulating T lymphocytes < 5%, d/c after T-cell recovery		Not given for 1st or 2nd rejection episodes	Rabbit 2·5 mg/kg/day i.m. × 3 days (individualized)
Imuran	4 mg/kg preop.	2 mg/kg	WBC and platelets q day until stable, then MWF (WBC diff. only if indicated)		No change in dosage	No change in dosage

Table 49.3 Stanford cardiac transplantation infections 15 December 1980–1 January 1986

1.	Bacterial	98
2.	Viral	88
	Titre rise only	27
3.	Fungal	26
4.	Protozoan	6
5.	Nocardia	4

shed CMV are carried out weekly and may be helpful in identifying the pathogen. In patients with non-diagnosed elevated temperatures or leucocytosis, a white blood cell scan, a lung CT scan or a lumbar puncture may be indicated.

Due to this aggressive approach, a relatively high degree of success has been achieved in the treatment of infections in the cardiac recipients, including those caused by unusual organisms. The success rate for infections with nocardia, aspergillosis, and pneumocystis has been achieved as a result of this approach.

The frequency of infection correlates directly with doses of immunosuppressive drugs required for continued suppression of the host immune response. After the first postoperative year, the overall rate of serious infections is 0·03 episodes per 100 patient days in contrast to a rate of 1·24 per 100 patient days for the first 3 months. These data underscore the importance of prompt diagnosis and appropriate treatment of infection in the achievement of long-term survival after cardiac transplantation.

ACUTE CARDIAC REJECTION

The frequency of acute cardiac graft rejection episodes is highest in the early postoperative period and averages 1·73 episodes per 100 patient days during the first 3 months. It diminishes, markedly, thereafter, to a level of 0·10 episodes per 100 patient days after the first year. Because only approximately 7% patients fail to exhibit acute rejection after transplantation, early diagnosis and reversal of rejection by appropriate augmentation of immunosuppression are essential for survival.

Early histological changes seen in rejection include mild cellular infiltration, infiltration with intracellular myocardial oedema, infiltration with myocyte necrosis, and the irreversible, severe form of infiltration, myocyte necrosis and marked haemorrhage. The goal of effective management of acute graft rejection is early diagnosis and reversal of this process before morphological injury of myocytes has occurred.

Prior to the era of cyclosporin which has been found to preserve left ventricular function, the diagnosis of acute rejection was made clinically on the basis of ECG changes, a diastolic gallop, and generalized decrease in QRS voltage. However, the gold standard presently used for the diagnosis of cardiac allograft rejection is the right ventricular endomyocardial biopsy. This is performed in the operating room during the early postoperative period at weekly intervals or at any time when suspicion of rejection is entertained. It is performed by percutaneous transvenous Seldinger technique under image intensification. More than 5000 such biopsy procedures have been performed without serious complications. Appropriate augmentation of immunosuppression for acute rejection is then associated with rapid resolution of histological changes over a period of six days.

There is currently no simple, non-invasive reliable technique to diagnose rejection. As systolic and diastolic function are currently being evaluated by echocardiography and findings are being correlated with rejection, it is necessary to obtain an echocardiogram with each cardiac biopsy. In order to assess the diastolic function at times of acute rejection, the isovolumic relaxation period (IVR) is calculated from an M mode echophonocardiogram and compared with the results of the ECG and endomyocardial biopsy. When the endomyocardial biopsy is normal, the IVR period is 78 ± 12 msec. Changes in systolic function do not reliably reflect the appearance of endomyocardial biopsy when a 10% reduction in IVR is used as a criterion for acute rejection. For this reason we still use the endomyocardial biopsy as confirmation for acute rejection.

Acute rejection episodes associated with histopathological evidence for rejection and biopsy specimens are signs of impaired graft performance and require augmentation of immunosuppression consisting of pulses of Solu-Medrol (1 g) intravenously daily for 3 days. Prior use of actinomycin D or systemic heparinization is no longer required. With such regimens, over 90% of acute rejection episodes can be successfully reversed. However, should patients have continuing, ongoing rejection, an additional 3 g of Solu-Medrol are given. Should this prove to be unsuccessful, rabbit ATG is sometimes required (2·5 mg/kg i.m. for 3 days). Response to therapy is determined by repeat cardiac biopsy 72 h following the third dose of Solu-Medrol or rabbit antithymocyte globulin. If performed earlier, a therapeutic response may not be observed. Late postoperatively, acute episodes of rejection are less frequent and usually less severe than those observed early after transplantation. Effective management can usually be achieved by simple augmentation and then gradual tapering of the dosages of oral prednisone. Only occasionally is high dose pulse therapy required.

LATE POSTOPERATIVE MANAGEMENT

Many transplant recipients have preoperative renal dysfunction that may be aggravated by cardiopulmonary bypass and cyclosporin. The following measures greatly reduce the incidence of renal failure post-transplant: (1) administration of less than 18 mg/kg of cyclosporin preoperatively if the creatinine clearance is abnormal; (2) monitoring of daily serum cyclosporin levels for the first week postoperatively aiming for 150–250 ng/ml for the first month and then 50–100 ng/ml thereafter; (3) use of mannitol during cardiopulmonary bypass and then postoperatively with each dose of cyclosporin; (4) maintenance of optimal CVP, i.e. high inflow and outflow; (5) use of renal effective doses of dopamine; and (6) use of diuretics as required to maintain a urine output of at least 1 ml/kg/h.

One particular late postoperative complication is noteworthy. This is the problem of accelerated graft atherosclerosis (AGAS), a major limiting factor in long-term survival in the early experience. This accelerated form of coronary atherosclerosis appears to be due to donor coronary myointimal proliferation with associated fibrosis and subsequent atherosclerotic degeneration. The pathogenesis is thought to be related to immunologically mediated injury of the donor coronary arterial endothelium. The resultant reparative process, if uncontrolled, can then progress to complete arterial occlusion of major coronary arteries. The consequences of this form of graft atherosclerosis include ischaemic dysfunction with congestive heart failure, myocardial infarction, and sudden death.

Patients are later placed on platelet antagonists (dipyridamole) which appear to reduce the time-related incidence of graft atherosclerosis. The detection of advanced occlusive disease is considered an indication for elective retransplantation of the heart in recipients without other complicating factors. This has been attempted several times with minimal increase in morbidity and mortality. The disease process is diffuse and, therefore, precludes aortocoronary bypass grafting.

To identify significant predictors of accelerated graft atherosclerosis, a stepwise Cox univariant and multivariant regression analyses were performed. The results indicated that the number of rejection episodes and total prednisone dose were significant determinants of AGAS in cyclosporin-treated groups; age and HLA A2 mismatch were significant predictors in the azathioprine treated group. Thus, subgroups at high risk for late development of AGAS can be identified.

Patients are discharged on an average of 3–4 weeks after transplantation and then evaluated in the outpatient clinic at twice-weekly intervals for 1–2 months, then once weekly. In the absence of complications, they are seen at monthly intervals. Those with uncomplicated late postoperative courses return to their geographical origins or referrals and remain under the care of their private cardiologist.

All patients, however, are readmitted at annual intervals for invasive evaluation which includes coronary arteriography, left ventriculography, cardiac catheterization, and endomyocardial biospy.

LYMPHOMA

The risk of lymphoma in immunosuppressed transplant recipients is many times higher than that of the general population. Lymphoma of the diffuse histiocytic type is over 350 times more common among transplant recipients than in the general population. A striking feature of post-transplant lymphomas is their relatively short induction period and high frequency of central nervous system involvement. Renal and cardiac transplant patients have a similarly increased incidence of neoplasia, but cardiac transplant recipients have a higher risk for developing lymphoma.

Several risk factors for post-cardiac transplantation lymphomas have been suggested, including age less than 40 years, idiopathic cardiomyopathy as primary disease process, repeat transplantation, cyclosporin immunosuppression, use of rabbit ATG in combination with cyclosporin, and EBV infection.

Cyclosporin in particular may be linked to the role of EBV in the aetiology of post-transplant lymphoma. Cyclosporin produces greater variation in titres of antibody to EBV than does conventional immunosuppression. Furthermore, it has been shown *in vitro* that cyclosporin inhibits cytotoxic response of the cytotoxic/suppressor T cell population to autologous EBV-infected B lymphocytes. Clinically, this may render patients more vulnerable to primary EBV infection or EBV reactivation.

XENOGRAFTING

To secure a donor population is one of the most difficult problems in organ transplantation. All transplant centres are suffering from a lack of donors.

Among heterogeneous animals, those most closely related to man are orangutans, gorillas, chimpanzees, followed by gibbons, baboons, and Japanese macaques. New evidence based on biochemical comparisons of blood and the proteins manufactured by both man and ape indicate an even closer kinship. Two members of the monkey family, in fact, chimpanzees and baboons, offer man a complete range of blood types. Baboons have groups A, B, and AB but not O; chimpanzees have A and O but not B or AB. This close blood tie may prove to be the answer to the greatest problem of supply that threatens to limit the range of transplantation surgery even after the immune barrier has been overcome. It is to the non-human species that many scientists are now looking. To bridge the gap that does exist between man and monkey, one of the world's greatest geneticists, Dr Joshua Lederburg, at Stanford University, offered this solution, 'A vigorous and eugenic programme, not of man, but of some non-human species, to produce genetically homogeneous material as a source for spare parts. The technical problems of overcoming the immune barrier would be immensely simplified if the heterografts came from a genetically constant source. The more so if the animal supplying the grafts could be purposefully bred for this utility.'

It was naturally presumed that the anthropoids, such as the orangutan, gorilla, and chimpanzee, would be the best donors. However, orangutans and gorillas had to be excluded from the study as they are internationally protected animals. Many researchers challenge the idea of non-human transplantation but there exists an impression that the challenge has become neglected along with the development of non-human transplantation because no promising result has been obtained due to the difficulty in controlling the rejection which occurs in non-human to human transplantation.

Techniques of removing and transferring organs from monkey to man have already been developed in several laboratories. In October 1963, Dr Keith Reemstma, of Tulane University, transplanted the first technically successful kidney transplant between chimpanzee and a human being. The first non-human to human heart transplantation was performed by Dr Hardy on 23rd January 1964, at University Hospital in Jackson, Mississippi. Both transplanted organs survived only a short period of time.

The first and foremost difficulty in heterotransplantation is the hyperacute rejection phenomenon caused by preformed antihuman–human donor antibodies present in the blood of humans. Dr Chibo from the Heart Institute of Japan tried to discover the relationship between serological data which showed compatibility and survival time using dogs and their family species. Her work established a clear relationship between the data and survival length. Dr Bailey of Loma Linda tried to apply these serological conditions to primates and man for these tests were quite essential for detecting antibodies in the recipient population.

There may be the possibility of clinical application if a man and a primate pair with good concordance are selected. Even from the immunological aspects of primates, the primary candidate for non-human donor seem to be, again, the chimpanzee. However, even if using a chimpanzee as a xenodonor, the probability of finding a concordant individual is 5%, as low as 1·1% with the baboon and 2% with a Japanese macaque. It is necessary to discover the next stage

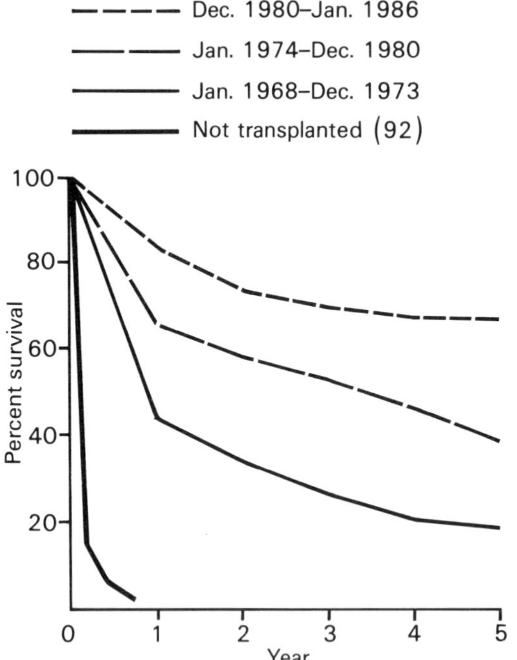

Fig. 49.3 Survival rates after cardiac transplantation. Note improvement over the years.

of screening test which would improve donor selection. However, before transplantation is actually performed between man and primate, it seems necessary to carry out transplantation experiments and serological testing as simulation between primates and different species.

SURVIVAL AND REHABILITATION

Patient survival rates calculated for the entire series of 400 patients is illustrated in *Fig.* 49.3. Survival at one, two, three, four and five years postoperatively is 83, 74, 69, 65, and 53% respectively. Sixty-six patients are currently living more than 5 years after transplantation, 14 are living more than 10 years after transplantation, and the longest more than 16 years after operation.

The survival of patients officially selected as potential recipients who died before suitable donor became available is also illustrated in *Fig.* 49.3. The average survival in this group was 47 days.

Two indications for cardiac retransplantation have been identified; one is accelerated graft atherosclerosis and the other, recurrent acute rejection episodes. The primary causes of death among Stanford patients are summarized in *Table* 49.4.

The rehabilitation status of long-term surviving patients in this series has been assessed, defining rehabilitation as the restoration of physical and psychosocial capacity sufficient to provide the recipient with the option of returning to active employment or other activity. Eighty-seven per cent of patients living one year or more after transplantation, thus analysed, have been rehabilitated and most have returned to active employment.

Table 49.4 Stanford cardiac transplantation cyclosporin patients. Cause of death (n=166)

Infection	16
Rejection	8
Malignancy	4
Coronary artery disease	5
Acute graft failure	4
Pulmonary hypertension	1
CVA	2
Cerebral oedema	1
Hepatic failure	1
	42

Further Reading

Barnard C. N. (1967) A human cardiac transplant. *S. Afr. Med. J.* **41**, 1271.

Brumbaugh J., Baldwin J. C. et al. (1985) Quantitative analysis of immunosuppression in cyclosporine-treated cardiac transplant patient with lymphoma. *Heart Transplantation* **4**, 307.

Caves P. K., Stinson E. B. et al. (1973) Diagnosis of human cardiac allograft rejectors by serial cardiac biopsy. *J. Thorac. Cardiovasc. Surg.* **66**, 461.

Dawkins K. D., Oldershaus P. J. et al. (1985) Noninvasive assessment of cardiac allograft rejection. *Transplantation Proc.* **XVII**.

Hunt S. A. (1983) Complications of heart transplantation. *Heart Transplantation* **III**.

Kosek J. C., Bieber C. P. and Lower R. R. (1971) Heart graft arteriosclerosis. *Transplantation Proc.* **3**, 512.

Lower R. R. and Shumway N. E. (1960) Studies on orthotopic transplantation of canine heart. *Surg. Forum* **11**, 18.

Myers B. D., Ross J. et al. (1984) Cyclosporin–A associated chronic nephropathy; a potentially irreversible renal injury. *N. Engl. J. Med.* **311**, 699.

Oyer P. E., Stinson E. B. et al. (1983) Cyclosporin in cardiac transplantation. A two and one-half year follow-up. *Transplantation Proc.* **XV**, Suppl. 1.

Shumway N. E. (1983) Recent advances in cardiac transplantation. *Transplantation Proc.* **XV**.

Stinson E. B. et al. (1969) Cardiac transplantation in man. III. Surgical aspects. *Am. J. Surg.* **118**, 182.

50 *Miscellaneous Conditions of the Heart and the Great Vessels*

J. Levett and W. Y. Moores

OCCLUSIVE DISEASE OF THE AORTA AND ITS MAJOR BRANCHES

Occlusive disease of the aorta and its major branches is rarely encountered in routine adult cardiac surgical practice. Congenital deformity of the aorta, such as coarctation, is an exception and is usually treated by simple excision or bypass of the narrowed segment. Most often this is accomplished without the aid of cardiopulmonary bypass. However, in the absence of preoperative evidence of good collateral flow, such as rib notching or large intermuscular collaterals, femoral cannulation and partial cardiopulmonary bypass may be needed, especially in the adult, if spinal cord ischaemia is to be avoided. Another helpful criterion in the planning of the operative procedure with respect to the need for bypass is intraoperative distal thoracic aortic pressure following clamping; if the mean pressure is below 50 mmHg, bypass appears to offer a greater margin of safety. If the aorta and subclavian arteries lend themselves to partial occlusion a graft may be adequate between them (*see* Chapter 45).

Localized obstruction to various major branches of the aorta has been recognized for many years. Atherosclerosis is the most common cause but others include syphilis, collagen vascular disease, thromboangiitis obliterans and trauma. Takayasu, in 1908, described a syndrome in young Oriental women who presented with multiple occlusions of the arch vessels. Typically the symptoms are of arterial insufficiency related to the distribution of the affected artery and the diagnosis is confirmed by aortography. Treatment may involve thromboendarterectomy for vertebral and carotid lesions and graft replacement or bypass for lesions in other vessels, such as the innominate and subclavian arteries.

Occlusive atherosclerotic disease of the carotid arteries is encountered in cardiac surgical practice and requires special concern. The typical patient presents with a history suggestive of transient ischaemic attacks together with angina or evidence of coronary artery disease. In such instances, an arch aortogram and coronary arteriography are required before a decision can be made as to the sequence of operative intervention. The choice depends largely on the symptomatology. If preinfarction angina is the greatest threat, and no recent 'carotid' symptoms exist, then coronary revascularization may be performed utilizing slightly higher flow and pressure on cardiopulmonary bypass than normally. If the cardiac symptoms can be controlled by intensive medical therapy, as occurs most commonly, and the carotid disease is symptomatic, then carotid endarterectomy can be safely performed first. Cardiopulmonary bypass equipment should be available during this procedure in case life-threatening coronary ischaemia occurs during anaesthesia. Controversy still surrounds the combined approach of carotid endarterectomy immediately followed by coronary bypass. The available literature is scarce, but suggests that there is no greater morbidity or mortality in the combined approach. However, there are theoretical objections such as the reactivity of the cerebral vessels to altered flow (non-pulsatile flow is present during cardiopulmonary bypass). Furthermore, when a cerebrovascular accident does occur, it is usually haemorrhagic, suggesting a greater friability of the cerebral vessels which may be related to cardiopulmonary bypass. The optimum, mean carotid pressure required during a typical three-vessel coronary revascularization procedure (which usually takes about 90 min on bypass) is unknown. The authors prefer simultaneous procedures when symptoms involving both cardiac and cerebral ischaemia are present.

ANEURYSMS OF THE THORACIC AORTA

Aneurysms of the aorta are generally atherosclerotic in origin although syphilitic aneurysms may rarely be encountered. Dilatation of the ascending aorta due to Marfan's syndrome or other collagen diseases may also occur and this may occasionally involve the aortic valve.

Treatment of these aneurysms is determined by size and symptoms. A 7-cm ascending aortic aneurysm has at least a 50% 2-year rupture rate. Evidence of increasing size radiographically is a clear indication for replacement. Often aneurysms produce symptoms such as cough or dysphagia secondary to compression of posterior structures. In the presence of massive dilatation of the ascending aorta, aortic valvular dysfunction may ensue and this demands a more extensive operative procedure. The extent of the saccular component must be carefully assessed. Occasionally atherosclerotic aneurysms are shown to involve the entire aortic arch, often with concomitant aortic valvular disease or coronary artery disease.

Replacement of the aortic arch has been among the most challenging and difficult feats in cardiovascular surgery.

Much controversy still exists as to the safest and most reliable technique. Two general methods have been employed. The first involves constant cardiopulmonary bypass with selective cannulation of the arch vessels. The second method consists of total hypothermic circulatory arrest with cerebral anoxia. Both techniques have inherent advantages and disadvantages, and it appears that the results are not strikingly different. The early experience utilizing selective cannulation and moderate hypothermia was dismal, presumably owing to the effects of high non-pulsatile flow in the cerebral circulation. A common result postoperatively was intracerebral haemorrhage. Low flow in the range of 600–700 ml/min in each cerebral vessel yielding a mean arterial pressure of 50–60 mmHg dramatically improved survival in this procedure. The development of deep hypothermia and circulatory arrest during the early era of aortic arch replacement was designed to solve this troublesome problem of cerebral circulation but in many centres was complicated most commonly by severe coagulopathy since the core body temperature is reduced to under 15 °C. However, it is not clear whether the unfavourable early experience with this technique is entirely explained on this basis since impressive results continue to appear in the literature. Techniques not involving extracorporeal circulation, but employing a variety of temporary shunts, have been described for years, but are not easily standardized for routine practice. The major indication for total replacement of the aortic arch is expanding aortic aneurysm. These patients should obviously be referred if possible to centres highly experienced in the operative management of this unique entity.

AORTIC DISSECTION

Acute aortic dissection, the most common lethal catastrophe involving the aorta, is a condition characterized by haemorrhagic intramural separation of the aortic media. Its incidence is probably much greater than generally appreciated, since it often presents as sudden chest pain followed by death. Awareness that the diagnosis of acute aortic dissection must be considered in the differential diagnosis of all cases of sudden chest pain is the first step in controlling the catastrophic sequelae of this condition. It is twice as common in men as in women. The majority of patients are in the 4th–7th decades.

Dissection of the aorta most commonly occurs in hypertensive patients but at least 20% of patients give no history suggestive of hypertension. Pregnancy is known to be an independent risk factor, but the reasons are poorly understood. Generalized stigmas of atherosclerosis are usually not present, and long-standing dilated atherosclerotic aneurysms tend to rupture rather than dissect. Cystic medial necrosis of the aorta has been noted in many patients with dissection.

Though the aetiology of dissection of the aorta remains a mystery, it is a devastating disease that can literally affect all organ systems. Rapidly lethal within hours of its onset, it represents a true indication for emergency therapy. The early era of cardiac surgery was fraught with dismal results in the treatment of the disease, and this eventually led to the adoption of temporary or long-term medical therapy for both acute and chronic aortic dissection involving both the ascending and descending aorta. This therapy, aimed at decreasing the blood pressure by the use of constant infusion of drugs, such as trimetaphan or sodium nitroprusside, combined with a negative inotropic agent, such as propranolol, was advocated by Wheat and forms the mainstay of therapy which is also utilized in the management of patients eventually treated surgically.

The identification of the site of aortic dissection is of great importance in the management of the disease. If the history and physical signs warrant arteriography, care should be taken if possible to define the site of the intimal tear and plan appropriate management. The surgical classification of dissection is best limited to two types, those which involve the ascending aorta (Type A) and those which do not (Type B). This conceptual scheme has practical implications as well since it indicates the type of operation and the choice of incision. Dissections involving the ascending aorta require median sternotomy with total cardiopulmonary bypass and those of the descending aorta demand a left thoracotomy with partial bypass techniques. The purpose of the operative procedure is not often curative but is aimed always at preventing the lethal sequelae. In the case of dissections involving the *ascending aorta*, therefore, therapy is aimed, first, at replacing the aortic segment since risk of impending rupture into the pericardium is extremely high (*Fig.* 50.1*a*) and, secondly, at safely repairing or replacing the aortic valve since dilatation results in severe aortic regurgitation. An *arch intimal tear* which dissects in a retrograde fashion

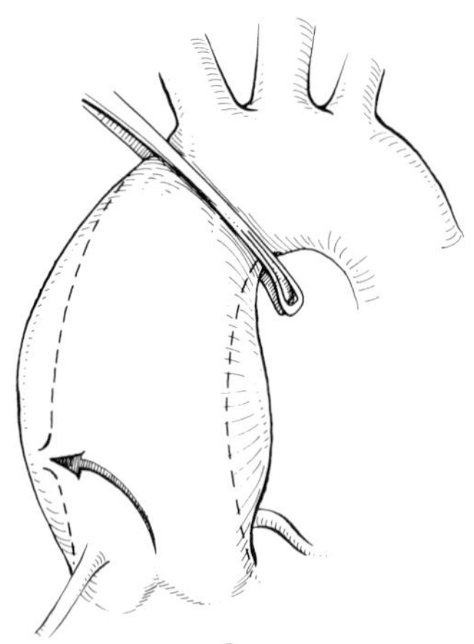

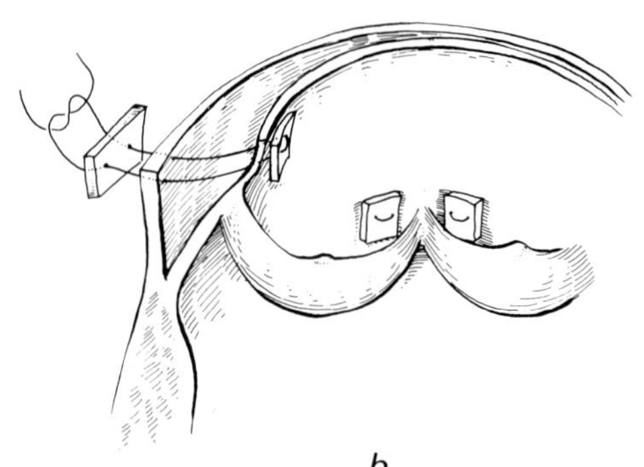

Fig. 50.1 Acute aortic dissection, intimal tear (*a*) and detail of commissural supporting sutures (*b*).

into the ascending aorta does not always require replacement of the site of the tear itself (unless recent enlargement or bleeding is seen in the arch) but rather of the ascending aorta with correction of the aortic valvular apparatus. Often arch dissections will result in proximal and distal progression of the dissection process, but therapy is aimed always at assuring that the immediate life-threatening abnormality is corrected. Prolonged medical therapy is indicated in stable arch dissections. It is unclear why rupture of the ascending aorta is more common than rupture of the arch itself. It may be related to the structural support offered by the surrounding branches and structures.

Dissection of the *ascending aorta* complicated by aortic regurgitation is, therefore, best treated by femoral cannulation, replacement of the ascending aorta and either replacement of the valve or resuspension of the leaflets (*Fig.* 50.1*b*). Occasional composite valve and graft placement with coronary reimplantation is indicated (*Fig.* 50.3). In cases of friable acute aortic dissections the 'Teflon-sandwich' technique is indicated (*Fig.* 50.2). Arch dissections are treated in the same manner if involvement of the ascending aorta is present and continuing symptoms persist despite medical therapy. The treatment of dissections involving the *descending aorta* and/or arch alone remains, however, quite controversial. The risk of rupture of the descending thoracic aorta is lower than that of the ascending aorta. Furthermore, in the absence of sequelae, such as arterial insufficiency to peripheral organs due to intimal flaps, patients can be managed quite well on medical therapy alone. Replacement of the descending thoracic aorta is fraught with a variety of complications which actually result in a higher mortality than replacement of the ascending aorta and valve. The partial bypass techniques employed during the repair may cause increased afterload on the heart when the aortic clamp is placed. This may result in cardiac strain and therefore requires special care. Femoral vein cannulation with placement of a long venous cannula into the right atrium is employed, but this may limit the volume return to the pump necessitating, in some cases, decompression of the heart directly through the pulmonary artery. The pulmonary complications resulting from a collapsed heparinized lung are also substantial. Furthermore, there is no convincing data to suggest that the routine surgical treatment of an uncomplicated Type B acute aortic dissection is better than

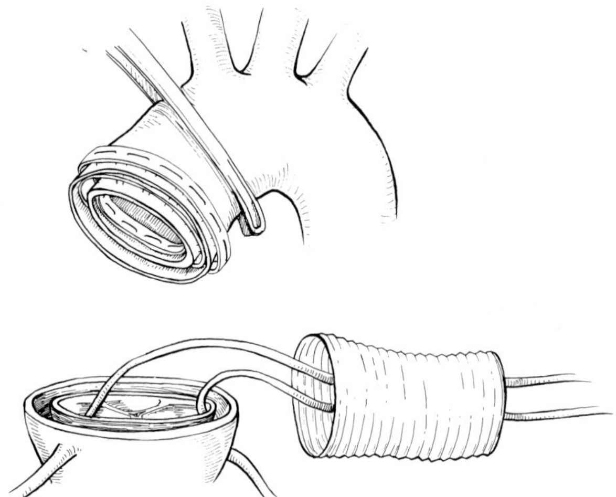

Fig. 50.2 Detail of 'Teflon-sandwich technique' in preparation of distal anastomosis in cases of friable acute aortic dissections.

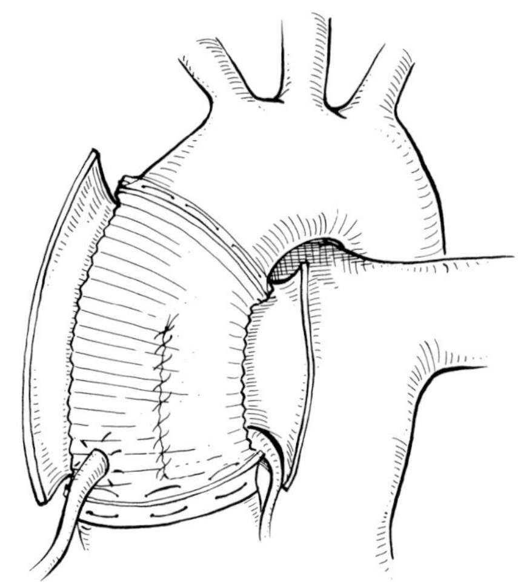

Fig. 50.3 Composite valve and graft placement with coronary reimplantation.

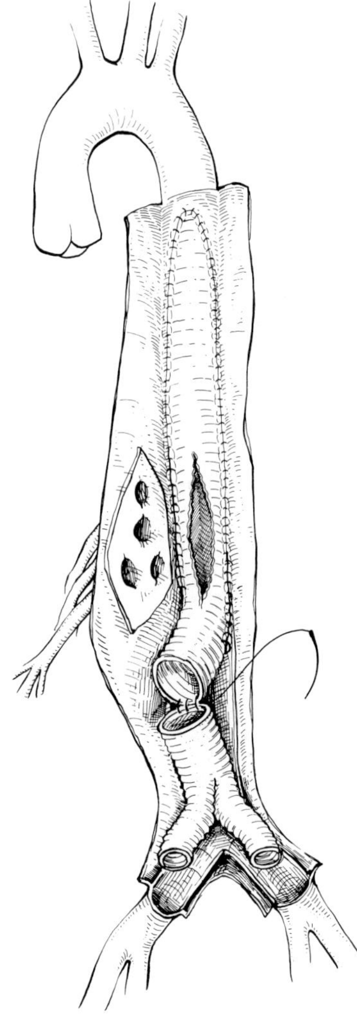

Fig. 50.4 Extensive thoraco-abdominal replacement with preservation of intercostal, spinal and visceral arterial supply, modified from Crawford.

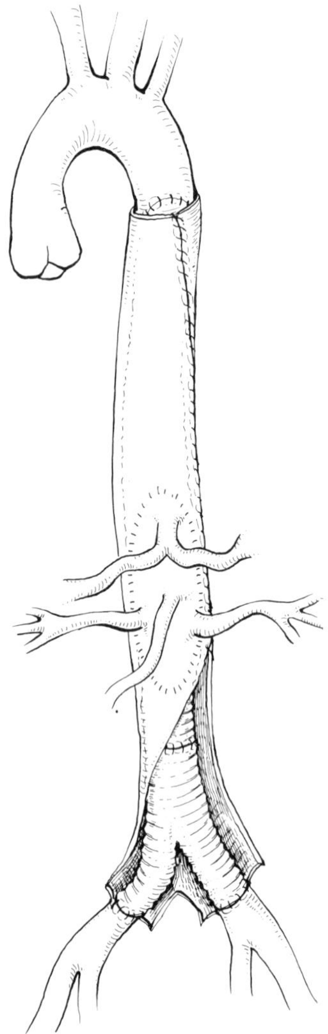

Fig. 50.5 Aortic wrapping following extensive thoraco-abdominal resection.

medical therapy. Newer extensive surgical techniques involving entire thoraco-abdominal aortic replacement with visceral and renal artery attachment (*Figs.* 50.4, 50.5) as well as limited techniques such as the insertion of stiff grafts rapidly ligated onto the aorta, both without extracorporeal bypass or heparinization, may improve surgical results. The acute surgical mortality of Type A dissections is 10–15% and for Type B this rises to 15–30%. The incidence of redissection among Type B dissections treated medically is slightly higher. Type B acute aortic dissections treated medically may result in expanding aneurysms, true 'dissecting aneurysms'. Progression of symptoms is an indication for surgery which can often be quite difficult technically at this point.

In summary, dissections should be rapidly diagnosed on clinical grounds, confirmed by arteriography and treated pharmacologically, whether or not surgery is to follow. The exception is the patient in shock. The indications for surgical intervention include most acute Type A dissections, arch dissections with continuing neurological symptoms or expansion and Type B dissections which are associated with specific organ involvement or continuing pain (failure of

Table 50.1 Indications for surgical or medical therapy for dissecting aortic aneurysms

Surgical

1. Resistant shock	10. Impending rupture on radiographical examination
2. Overwhelming aortic valve insufficiency	11. Carotid obstruction
3. Saccular aneurysm	12. Normotension
4. Tamponade	13. Marfan's syndrome
5. Myocardial ischaemia	14. Pregnancy
6. Reversible central nervous system syndromes	15. Coarctation
7. Pulmonary artery obstruction	16. Failure of medical therapy (pain, anuria)
8. Right bundle-branch block	
9. Resistance to antihypertensive agents	

Medical

1. No clear-cut origin of dissection visible on angiography in the absence of overwhelming aortic insuficiency or tamponade
2. A stable B dissection with previously untreated hypertension and especially serious concomitant pulmonary disease
3. A stable redissection in a patient improperly treated since first dissection
4. Multiple simultaneous dissections
5. Clotted false lumen
6. Unavailable cardiac surgical facilities.

medical therapy). Chronic Type B and arch dissections are repaired if they are expanding or symptomatic. The results at the University of Chicago indicate a 66% 30-day operative survival and 90% 30-day medical survival in a series of 60 prospectively treated patients whose 5–10 year follow-up indicates 50% survival among surgical patients and 30–40% among those treated medically according to the authors' recommendations (*Table* 50.1). This represents an encouraging trend in the treatment of a disease whose outlook untreated was 50% 48-hour survival and survival either with medical or surgical therapy until 1975 was 50% at 2½ years.

CARDIAC NEOPLASMS

Primary cardiac neoplasms may be classified as benign or malignant. Approximately 75% are benign and myxomas account for 50% of the benign group. Myxomas are more common on the left side of the heart. Rhabdomyoma is the most frequent cardiac neoplasm of children and the second most common benign tumour. Malignant tumours account for 25% of primary cardiac neoplasms and generally include various types of sarcoma. Metastatic tumours of the heart are more common than primary cardiac neoplasms and are found 20–30 times more frequently.

Signs and symptoms of cardiac tumours are related to local invasion, systemic manifestations and peripheral embolization. Pericarditis, chest pain, congestive heart failure, pulmonary hypertension, arrhythmias, fever, weight loss, anaemia and thrombocytopenia have been reported. The classic findings of mitral stenosis on clinical examination in a patient with left atrial myxoma have been described many times. Diagnosis in the modern setting is based on M-mode and two-dimensional echocardiography which has been found to be quite accurate and has therefore supplanted routine cardiac catheterization in some centres such as the authors' because of the risk of embolization with the latter procedure.

Treatment of these tumours is safely accomplished using cardiopulmonary bypass with resection of a margin of endocardium around the fibrovascular stalk. The complication rate is low if attention is paid to avoidance of perioperative tumour embolization.

IDIOPATHIC HYPERTROPHIC SUBAORTIC STENOSIS

This is a condition characterized by marked left ventricular hypertrophy, which is most striking in the ventricular septum. The upper posterior part of the septum bulges into the left ventricular outflow tract. Obstruction to outflow results when the anterior mitral leaflet impinges on this posterior part of the septum in systole. Histologically, marked disarray of myocardial architecture and bizarre hypertrophy of the individual myocytes is almost always seen. It has a strong familial tendency.

Left ventricular outflow obstruction is not always present in idiopathic hypertrophic subaortic stenosis at rest. When present, however, it is variable and may change, depending on the contractile state of the left ventricle, its end-diastolic volume and the arterial blood pressure. An increase in contractile state, reduction of end-diastolic volume and a fall of arterial blood pressure all tend to increase the gradient.

The diagnosis is easily established by M-mode echocardiography, which demonstrates asymmetric septal hypertrophy and abnormal systolic movement of the anterior mitral leaflet. Cardiac catheterization is required to assess the severity of the outflow obstruction and allow pharmacological and physiological provocation.

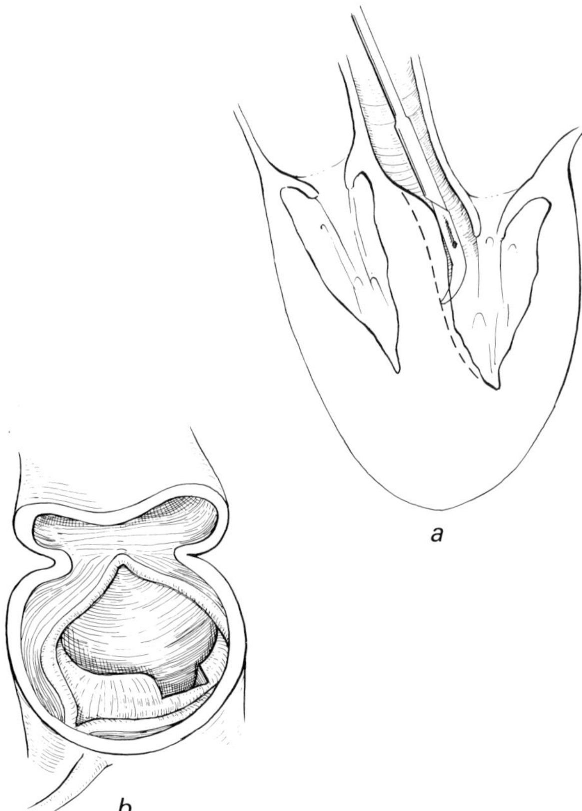

Fig. 50.6 The Morrow operation for idiopathic subaortic stenosis (*a*). *b*, The result of myotomy after operation near the junction of right and left aortic cusps.

Most patients can be managed medically with long-term therapy with propranolol. However, symptomatic patients with resting outflow gradients greater than 60 mmHg require surgery. The surgical approach is the one described by Morrow, which involves excision of a tunnel of muscle from the ventricular septum along the line between the right and left coronary cusps, through a transaortic approach (*Fig.* 50.6).

PULMONARY EMBOLECTOMY FOR MASSIVE EMBOLISM

Although pulmonary embolectomy without cardiopulmonary bypass was attempted for many years following Trendelenburg's report in 1908, successful pulmonary embolectomy became possible only after the development of cardiopulmonary bypass in the 1950s. Presently, the increasing use of heparin anticoagulation in hospitalized medical and surgical patients has made the need for pulmonary embolectomy very rare although we are confronted with occasional patients who present with refractory hypotension and documented massive pulmonary embolism. Attempts to remove these emboli with suction catheters with or without cardiopulmonary bypass have been partially successful and if the patient is relatively healthy and not responsive to medical therapy, a central pulmonary embolus may be removed using cardiopulmonary bypass. These patients are often found to have emboli in both pulmonary arteries and both sides should therefore be carefully explored. An inferior vena cava filter should be inserted or vena caval interruption should be performed at the same time to protect the patient from further emboli. Occasional patients with recurrent emboli can go on to develop increased pulmonary resistance. Recent reports from the University of California, San Diego, have substantiated that pulmonary artery thromboendarterectomy using circulatory arrest can benefit these patients significantly.

CARDIAC TRAUMA

In patients who arrive alive in an emergency room following stab or gunshot wounds to the heart, the outlook is good for eventual survival, following control of bleeding with or without cardiopulmonary bypass. The patient typically presents with an entry point in the thorax or upper abdomen, in severe shock and cardiac tamponade manifested by distended neck veins, distant heart sounds, paradoxical pulse and elevated central venous pressure. Immediate needle aspiration through the subxiphoid route of as little as 10 or 20 ml of blood or clots will often result in increased blood pressure and permit rapid transport to the operating room. Four large-bore intravenous cannulas should be inserted and the patient intubated if necessary. The patient should then be transported to the operating room for appropriate treatment; emergency room thoracotomy is to be discouraged and is reserved for the moribund patient who fails to develop a blood pressure after appropriate volume replacement. A median sternotomy in the operating room is preferred so that all cardiac chambers are immediately accessible and if a wound is present that demands cardiopulmonary bypass easy cannulation is possible. The principle of early therapy is accessibility to the wound and most of such repairs can be accomplished without cardiopulmonary bypass. The right ventricle and right atrium are most commonly injured. Ninety per cent survival in patients who arrive alive in the operating room with cardiac trauma has been achieved.

Cardiac contusion secondary to blunt trauma is being recognized with increasing frequency today, especially in patients with multiple trauma from automobile accidents. It must be suspected with chest injuries involving multiple rib fracture, sternal fracture or aortic injury. The ECG may show non-specific ST and T wave changes, MB-CPK enzymes may be elevated, and technetium pyrophosphate myocardial imaging is helpful in diagnosis and follow-up. The patient suspected of having cardiac contusion should be observed in hospital.

PERICARDIAL DISEASE

The pericardium may be congenitally absent either completely or segmentally, with small portions of the left side most often missing. Pericardial cysts and diverticula may occur as well as rare primary neoplasms of both the benign (teratoma) and the malignant (mesothelioma, sarcoma) variety. The pericardium is more commonly involved with metastatic tumour.

Pericarditis may result from a variety of causes including viruses (Coxsackie viruses A and B, influenza viruses A and B), tuberculosis, pyogenic infection, irradiation, uraemia, rheumatoid disease and postcardiac trauma. The most common group, however, is idiopathic, although many such cases may in fact be viral.

Surgery is indicated for pericarditis when cardiac motion and filling is impeded by pericardial constriction.

Constrictive pericarditis is diagnosed at cardiac catheterization which reveals equalization of cardiac chamber pressures in diastole, elevated right atrial pressure, with an M-pattern in the right atrial pressure pulse and an early diastolic dip in otherwise elevated ventricular diastolic pressure, producing a 'square-root' sign. The most common presenting symptom of constriction is severe fatigue or dyspnoea on exertion. Calcification may or may not be present. Surgery is aimed at removal of the pericardium anteriorly to the level of the phrenic nerves laterally, with stripping of the epicardium from the surface of the heart and great arteries, veins and atria. Posteriorly, the pericardium should be removed if it appears to be thickened and constrictive. Reconstriction under such circumstances does not occur. The operation is best performed on cardiopulmonary bypass since manipulation of the unsupported heart often depresses myocardial function. An advantage of this technique is the relative ease of identifying the proper plane for dissection when the ventricle is not distended. After removal of the pericardium down to the epicardial layer during the initial dissection, it is often advisable to strip the remaining epicardium from the heart surface if this can be done without excessive bleeding or difficulty. Care should be taken at all times to avoid injuring the coronary arteries.

If hospital deaths are excluded (5–15%), long-term survival can be quite satisfactory with an excess of 80% of patients living beyond five years in some series.

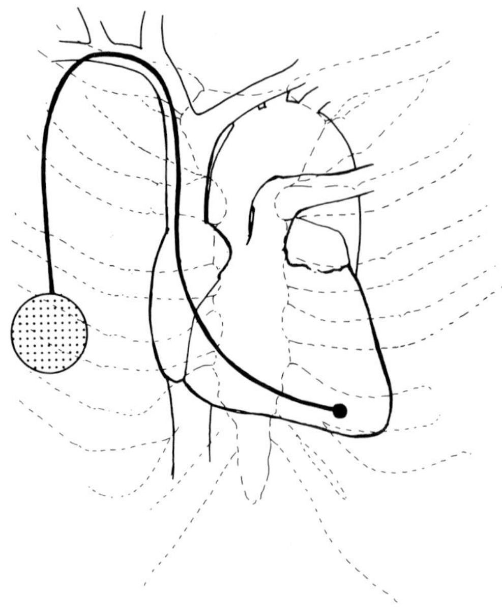

Fig. 50.7 Right ventricular apical placement of permanent intravenous pacemaker.

PACEMAKERS FOR HEART BLOCK AND RELATED ARRHYTHMIAS

Since the introduction of implantable pacing systems in the late 1950s, pacemakers have been used with increasing frequency in a variety of conditions. Indications for permanent pacing include complete heart block from a variety of causes and symptomatic sick sinus syndrome as well as several other symptomatic or life-threatening arrhythmias. Modern pacemakers are easily implanted using epicardial or transvenous electrodes and the present displacement rate of transvenous leads is quite low.

The decision to implant a pacemaker is followed by consideration of the type of unit to be implanted, the type of lead, and the site of implantation. Cosmetically, small thin units are preferred and generally ventricular inhibited demand units are used. Transvenous leads are usually placed via the cephalic vein in the deltopectoral groove (*Fig.* 50.7). Newer units are completely programmable and allow modification of not only the heart rate, but sensing and output thresholds. The newest addition to the hardware of pacing devices provides permanent sequential pacing of the atria and ventricles in a manner that simulates sinus rhythm. This technique can be especially helpful in patients with poor left ventricular function with increased ventricular compliance, as may be seen in aortic stenosis, for example. The atrial 'J'-shaped wire is inserted transvenously and hooks into the right atrial appendage In growing children the leads are most commonly inserted directly into the myocardial mass utilizing epicardial pacer leads. Complications such as infection, perforation or embolism are very rare and indications have expanded constantly since the first days of permanent intrathoracic pacing by Glenn of Yale University.

SURGERY FOR RESISTANT VENTRICULAR TACHYCARDIA

Because the prognosis for chronic ventricular tachycardia can be devastating in drug-resistant cases of Wolff–Parkinson–White syndrome, or pure ventricular tachycardia (with or without ischaemic heart disease) and since the development of electrophysiological techniques for invasive preoperative or epicardial and endocardial perioperative 'mapping' of the focus of such arrhythmias, surgical techniques for control of such problems have been developed. They involve (1) identification and transections of accessory conduction pathways for control of resistant WPW syndrome (approximately 50% long-term success rate in a series of 37 patients with 100% survival), (2) ventricular endocardial 'stripping' after aneurysmectomy (approximately 83% long-term success and 93% survival in two series of 50 patients), and (3) ventricular *arrhythmia focus 'incision'* patients without aneurysms (68% long-term success and 74% survival in a series of 19 patients).

Further Reading

Bickerstaff L. K., Pairolero P. C., Hollier L. H. et al. (1982) Thoracic aortic aneurysms: A population-based study. *Surgery* **92**, 1103.

Crawford E. S. and Crawford J. L. (1984) *Diseases of the Aorta Including an Atlas of Angiographic Pathology and Surgical Technique.* Baltimore, Williams & Wilkins.

Daily P. O., Dembitsky W. P., Peterson K. L. et al. (1987) Modifications of techniques and early results of pulmonary thromboendarterectomy for chronic pulmonary embolism. *J. Thorac. Cardiovasc. Surg.* **93**, 221–33.

DeBakey M. E., McCollum G. H., Crawford E. S. et al. (1982) Dissection and dissecting aneurysms of the aorta: Twenty-year follow-up of 527 patients treated surgically. *Surgery* **92**, 1118.

Guiraudon G. M., Klein G. J., Gulamhusein S. et al. (1984) Surgical repair of Wolff–Parkinson–White syndrome: A new closed-heart technique. *Ann. Thorac. Surg.* **37**, 67.

Harken A. H. and Josephson M. E. (1984) Surgical management of ventricular tachycardia. In: *Tachycardias, Mechanisms, Diagnosis, Treatment.* Josephson M. E. and Wellens H. J. J. (ed.) Philadelphia, Lea & Febiger.

Larrieu A. J., Jamieson W. R., Tyers G. F. O. et al. (1982) Primary cardiac tumours: Experience with 25 cases. *J. Thorac. Cardiovasc. Surg.* **83**, 339.

McCaughan B. L., Schaff H. V., Piehler J. M. et al. (1985) Early and late results of pericardiectomy for constrictive pericarditis. *J. Thorac. Cardiovasc. Surg.* **89**, 340.

McKenna W., Deanfield J., Farugui A. et al. (1981) Prognosis in hypertrophic cardiomyopathy: Role of age and clinical electrocardiographic and hemodynamic features. *Am. J. Cardiol.* **47**, 532.

Morrow R. G. (1978) Hypertrophic subaortic stenosis. Operative methods utilized to relieve left ventricular outflow obstruction. *J. Thorac. Cardiovasc. Surg.* **76**, 423.

Phibbs B., Friedman H. S., Graboys T. B. et al. (1984) Indications for pacing in the treatment of bradycardias. Report of an independent study group. *JAMA* **252**, 1307.

Section 7

Vascular Surgery

51 *Introduction*

D. Charlesworth

ARTERIOSCLEROSIS

Arteriosclerosis, hardening of the arteries, is a process which occurs with advancing years and in which the normal constituents of the arterial wall—smooth muscle, collagen and elastic fibres—are replaced by fibrous tissue. The lining of the arteries, the intima, is disrupted, thickened and in places overlies accumulations of lipid-containing cells. These, at first discrete areas of fatty infiltration, are called plaques and the material within them atheroma. As time passes the plaques may increase in size and partially or completely block the lumen of the artery, or they may disintegrate leaving a crater, 'an ulcerated plaque' in which small friable clots of blood may form. At any time during the process of arteriosclerosis the artery may:

1. Become completely or partially blocked;
2. Develop small clots which form on the damaged intima and in ulcerated plaques may break free and be washed downstream until arrested at a point where their dimensions exceed those of the artery; such clots are referred to as emboli.
3. Undergo destruction of the architecture of its wall reducing its stength to a point at which the elastic limits are exceeded and the artery becomes dilated. At certain points in the arterial tree, presumably where the stresses are greatest, dilatation can be so gross that an 'aneurysm' is formed.

The symptoms and signs associated with arteriosclerosis are a consequence of these three occurrences:

A. Gradual obstruction of the lumen will reduce the supply of blood to all those points supplied by the artery in question. If it is an iliac or femoral artery the patient may complain of pain on exercise—'intermittent claudication'. A complete obstruction of either or both these arteries may reduce the supply of blood to such an extent that the patient complains of pain at rest and eventually the foot may be so deprived of blood that it dies—gangrene.

Obstruction of specific arteries will produce characteristic symptoms and signs:

1. The coronary arteries —angina and myocardial infarction.
2. The mesenteric arteries—abdominal pain after food and malabsorption.
3. The renal arteries—hypertension.
4. The branches of the aortic arch and extracranial carotid arteries—transient ischaemic attacks, stroke, or claudication in the muscles of the hand and forearm.

B. Emboli arising from ulcerated plaques in the internal carotid arteries may cause transient ischaemic attacks and strokes. Emboli arising in aneurysms may cause acute ischaemia in the leg (aortic and popliteal aneurysms). (Probably the commonest site at which emboli originate is the left atrium where they form as a result of dyshrythmias rather than atherosclerosis.)

C. The natural history of aneurysms depends on the specific type:

1. Aortic aneurysms occur in that portion of the abdominal aorta between the renal arteries and the bifurcation. Such aneurysms may extend into one or both iliac arteries and rarely may extend upwards beyond the renal arteries to the level of the diaphragm or into the thoracic aorta—'thoraco-abdominal aneurysms'. By far the commonest complication is spontaneous rupture.
2. Popliteal aneurysms are rare, often bilateral (two-thirds) and sometimes they are associated with an abdominal aortic aneurysm (one-third). They may: (*a*) rupture; (*b*) thrombose, leading to gangrene; (*c*) press on the popliteal nerves occasioning paraesthesia in the lower leg and foot.

The clinician must learn to recognize the symptoms and to detect the presence of arteriosclerosis and its complications by clinical examination. It must be borne in mind that arteriosclerosis in the peripheral arteries is almost always associated with arteriosclerosis in the coronary arteries and that symptoms may arise when an artery is only partially occluded (a stenosis) and the pulses are present distally.

Clues to the presence of a stenosis are decreased pulse pressure and a bruit over the artery in question. The bruit is caused by vibrations in the arterial wall which are at a frequency within the audible range and which in turn are created by perturbations in the blood downstream from a stenosis.

Much of the difficulty and problems that a clinician has are in estimating the hydraulic effects of stenoses. When a stenosis becomes so tight that over 50% of the area of cross-section of the lumen is obliterated it will have an adverse effect on flow which gives rise to both symptoms and signs.

The effect which a stenosis has on flow also depends upon the rate of flow. A patient who has no symptoms when he walks slowly may have severe symptoms if he hurries. The picture is further complicated because there is a natural tendency for small arteries to dilate when the main artery is blocked and they supply a variable, and often surprisingly good, collateral circulation which may mask the effects of the obstruction in the main artery.

Aetiology

Who gets arteriosclerosis? The answer is probably that we all do, and rather surprisingly it is unique to human beings. However, the process is not a uniform one, the age at which it starts varies considerably and it may be twenty or thirty years before symptoms manifest themselves. In some people the process is accelerated both in the age of onset and rate of decline. Such patients are likely to be cigarette smokers and there is a direct correlation between the number of cigarettes smoked each day and the severity of the problem. There is a less obvious connection between arteriosclerosis in the peripheral arteries and hypertension, hyperlipidaemia, diet and exercise. This is in contrast to coronary arteries where there does seem to be a correlation with hypertension and hyperlipidaemia. Diabetics whose symptoms start when young and who are dependent upon insulin get a characteristic thickening and obliteration of small arteries in the extremities and, if they live long enough, atherosclerosis in their main arteries. Late-onset diabetes is associated with arteriosclerosis and in some cases may be a consequence of it. The pattern of arteriosclerosis is similar to that which occurs in normal people of the same age. The incidence of diabetes in patients who have symptoms of peripheral vascular disease is about 10–12% in Great Britain but rises to 30–40% in some series reported from Europe and North America.

Arteriosclerosis affects all large arteries but has a predilection for certain sites (*Fig.* 51.1).

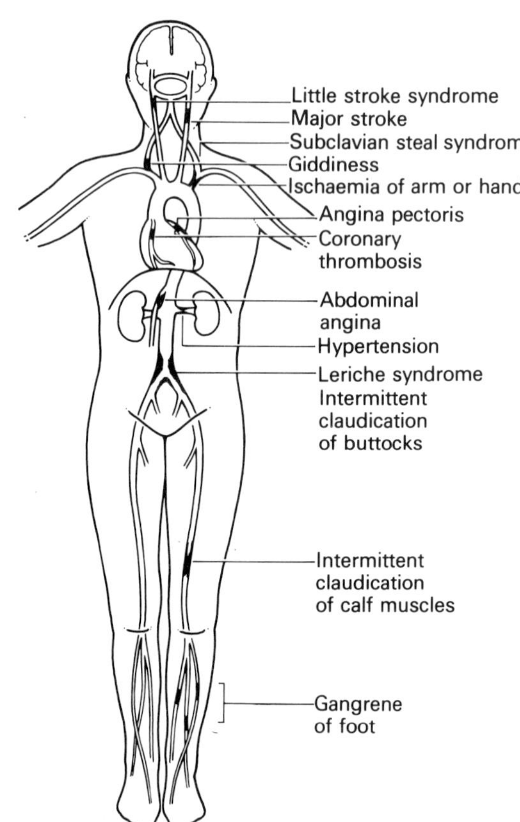

Fig. 51.1 Predominant sites and clinical syndromes of arteriosclerosis obliterans.

Management

The treatment of patients who have 'peripheral vascular disease' is essentially surgical but that doesn't mean one would commend operation to all patients; whether or not one does so depends on the severity of the symptoms and the prognosis. (If we take extreme examples: (*a*) one would hesitate to recommend an operation to an elderly patient who had claudication, but could walk over 200 metres and whose general health was poor; (*b*) if the same patient had a large tender and painful abdominal aneurysm then one would advise operation on the basis that the prognosis would be very poor without surgery.)

In a small number of patients the symptoms may suggest peripheral vascular disease but the signs may be absent or at variance with the diagnosis, whilst in other patients there may be more than one cause for the symptoms. If on the basis of the symptoms an operation is indicated, which operation will give the best result will depend on which arteries are affected and the extent of disease both proximal to and distal to the principal site of obstruction. In order to make a proper decision the surgeon will need more information, information which can in turn be obtained from specialized investigations.

Investigations

These may fall into two broad categories:

A. Test of general health and fitness for operation.

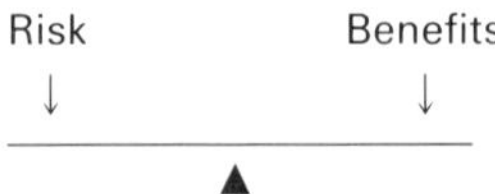

If one thinks of the problem as a balance, factors which increase the risk v. the benefits of operation (e.g. in the example given earlier the risks include advanced age, myocardial ischaemia, respiratory disease, whilst the benefits might at best be a doubling of the distance which the patient can walk without a rest), it helps one to arrive at a reasonable course of action.

B. Tests designed to reveal the topography of the arteries and the consequences of any discontinuation within them.

Visualization of the arteries (to be more precise the visualization of the lumen of the arteries) can be achieved in several ways:

1. Angiograms—injection of radio-opaque dye directly into an artery. Usually a narrow catheter is introduced into the aorta (translumbar aortogram) or the common femoral artery (Seldinger technique) and dye is delivered into the lumen of the aorta.

Good resolution can be obtained but the method can be painful and is not without complication. Computer-enhanced images of arteries can be produced after intravenous injection of dye. The resolution is, at present, less good than that which is obtained by conventional intra-arterial injection.

Radio-isotopes can also be given and images of arteries produced using a gamma camera. The magnetic nuclear resonance is characteristic to each type of atom and images of tissues within the body can be built up with a nuclear magnetic resonance scanner (NMR). Refinement of the current machines may well displace conventional arteriography. Pictures of arteries can be obtained using pulsed ultrasound and some sort of device which records the coordinates at which signals are recorded. Images can be obtained in two dimensions and are particularly useful when assessing aneuryms of the abdominal aorta and lesions within the extracranial carotid arteries.

Tests of function are useful in that they provide objective evidence to support a patient's own testimony about his limitations and can be used to reassess function after treatment.

To measure the effects of a stenosis two pieces of information are necessary: its size in relation to the artery, often expressed as a percentage: Area of stenosis/Area of artery × 100%, and the velocity of flow through the stenosis, because this affects the hydraulic consequences. Test of function tells us something about a stenosis at different rates of flow (velocity).

The common techniques are:

1. Response to exercise—step tests, walking, and measurement of flow before and after exercise, plethysmography.
2. Direct measurement of velocity from ultrasound signals.
3. Ratio of systolic pressure in ankle to that in arm.
4. Waveform analysis of Doppler shifted ultrasound signals. Most surgeons use a combination of clinical examination, functional assessment and arteriograms to derive information, on the basis of which, they can choose the most appropriate treatment and form a reliable prognosis.

Principles of Management

Arteriosclerosis cannot be reversed by medicines nor can aneurysms be reduced in size or their walls made stronger by drugs. (It is interesting to speculate that there is an association between copper deficiency and failure to cross-link collagen fibres. Certain inherited metabolic defects, Ehlers–Danlos syndrome, are characterized by lack of collagen or elastic fibres and the presence of multiple aneurysms. The mechanism by which cross-linking of collagen is achieved is a complex one including several enzymes as well as copper and in the majority of aneurysms there is no known biochemical defect.) It is sensible to make sure that patients who have peripheral vascular disease and ischaemic heart disease are given the best possible treatment for their hearts, bearing in mind that β-blockers can make claudication worse; also to eliminate anaemia and polycythaemia, both of which can highlight peripheral vascular disease. Almost all patients with arteriosclerosis smoke and can be expected to improve if they stop smoking. Long-term treatment of chronic occlusive vascular disease by anticoagulants is valueless as are vasodilators. Antiplatelet drugs are thought to reduce the incidence of transient ischaemic attacks in patients with carotid stenoses and to inhibit the adherence of platelets to prostheses. Prostacyclin has proved to be disappointing in management of vasospastic disorders. Various drugs purport to alter the deformability of red cells (and hence improve flow through capillaries), reduce the viscosity of blood, or to improve gaseous exchange within the tissues. Opinions about their efficacy vary. In practice the management of patients who have symptoms and signs of peripheral vascular disease is predominantly surgical, with the provisos already mentioned with regard to claudication. For aneurysms, acute and chronic ischaemia with and without gangrene, the management is by operation.

In principle the intention is always the same, to restore the flow of blood, but in practice there are various ways of achieving this.

1. Disobliteration of an artery, endarterectomy, angioplasty by balloon dilatation or by laser. It is too soon to judge what the place of lasers will be in future, and the long-term results of angioplasty are not known. Angioplasty by balloon dilatation is useful for short stenoses particularly in the iliac arteries; it gives less reliable results when used in the superficial femoral artery. It has been used in both carotid and coronary arteries but at the moment most surgeons prefer endarterectomy.
2. The commonest, most successful and apparently most durable operation is bypass. In the aorta and iliac arteries one can expect over 95% of bypasses to be patent after five years and over 70% at ten years, whilst in the superficial femoral artery bypasses made with saphenous vein remain patent in the majority of cases (70+% after five years when 'run-off' is good). If an artificial artery is used (prosthesis), the results of femoropopliteal bypass are less good but when 'run-off' is normal 50–60% remain patent after four years. A large variety of prostheses are available to be used as substitutes for arteries; in general the large diameter vessels, 8 mm, can be replaced successfully but prostheses of less than 5 mm diameter give poor results. For vessels of this size saphenous vein is used where possible. Modifications of human and animal arteries have proved to be disappointing when used as substitutes in human beings (the majority either occlude early or become aneurysmal).

Skill and experience are required to choose the most appropriate treatment for individual patients and meticulous technique is mandatory if good results are to be obtained from operation.

52 Vascular Disorders of the Neck and Upper Limb

P. H. Dickinson and John Chamberlain

It is appropriate to consider vascular disorders of the neck and upper limb in a single chapter because these two territories share a common blood supply through the innominate, left common carotid and left subclavian arteries. A reduction of blood flow in any of these vessels can cause ischaemia of the arm and the brain either alone or in combination. However, in spite of this close relationship, the vascular disorders of neck and upper limb are, for the sake of clarity, described in separate sections of this chapter.

THE NECK

Cerebral Ischaemia in Extracranial Cerebral Artery Disease

Pathophysiology

Cerebral ischaemia, secondary to disease of the extracranial cerebral arteries, may be precipitated by secondary thrombosis or embolism of the intracranial arteries or by a significant reduction in total cerebral blood flow. The result of ischaemia is infarction of the brain tissue which, once established, is irreversible. Temporary ischaemia is demonstrated by the full recovery which follows transient ischaemic attacks (TIAs), the commonest clinical manifestation of extracranial cerebral artery disease. A TIA is defined as a short-lived focal disturbance of neurological function lasting typically 2–15 min, but occasionally up to 24 h, in patients with vascular disease leaving them without deficit and tending to recur.

Atherosclerosis is the commonest disease of these arteries, less commonly they are affected by tortuosity, coils, kinks, fibromuscular dysplasia or arteritis. Atherosclerosis characteristically causes a localized plaque in the wall of the artery which may narrow the artery or ulcerate. Narrowing may progress until finally the artery is occluded by thrombosis which extends from the primary site of disease proximally and distally to the next important branches where the collateral flow will, in most instances, limit its extension. Portions of this consecutive thrombus may break off to form emboli which pass distally to occlude the smaller arterial branches, or possibly, direct extension of the thrombus itself may block them.

On an ulcerated plaque, platelets adhere where they combine with fibrin to form a thrombus. Thrombi and atheromatous debris may be dislodged at intervals forming emboli which may lodge in retinal or cerebral arterial branches. Emboli from the heart are generally larger and may occlude an extracerebral artery itself, such as the common carotid artery at its bifurcation. The outcome of embolism will depend, among other factors, upon its frequency, the size and number of emboli and the site of impaction. There may be a cumulative effect from repeated embolization which can also influence events.

A reduction in total cerebral blood flow may be the precipitating mechanism which causes ischaemia, but the arterial lumen must be reduced appreciably before it interferes with normal blood flow; for example, about 75% reduction in cross-sectional area in one internal carotid artery. The resulting reduced cerebral blood flow cannot respond adequately to stresses such as arterial hypotension and hypoxia; consequently in these circumstances, variations in blood pressure and blood gas tensions may precipitate an attack of cerebral ischaemia.

The pathological and clinical effects resulting from these mechanisms will be influenced by a number of factors, other than those already specifically mentioned, including the age of the patient, the state of the other cerebral arteries and, most importantly, the collateral circulation.

The circle of Willis acts as a distribution network for blood entering the brain and variations in its anatomy can have a significant influence on the outcome of disease in its feeding arteries. A 'normal' circle is present in only 52% of brains; anomalies, such as absence or hypoplasia of the posterior communicating artery, are frequent. They are more common in the anterior to posterior links than right-to-left anastomoses. Deviations from the normal anatomy remain relatively unimportant until the blood flow is decreased; inadequate anastomoses can then present a serious hazard by restricting collateral flow. It may be one of the reasons why some patients with a single occluded cerebral artery develop a complete stroke whilst others with several occluded arteries remain symptom-free.

Clinical Features

The clinical picture of cerebral ischaemia varies from patient to patient and in the same patient on different occasions. The cooperation of an experienced neurologist is essential, particularly to assist in the elucidation of the diverse symptoms and signs of cerebral ischaemia, and to help distinguish them from those due to other neurological disorders. None the less, the surgeon must be aware of the numerous clinical manifestations of cerebral ischaemia and be able to assess the role of surgical treatment both in general terms and in the individual patient. It is emphasized, however, that the decision whether or not a particular patient requires surgical treatment not only involves a careful consideration of the symptoms and signs, but also of other factors including age, occupation, smoking habits, mental state, general health, diabetes, family history of strokes and the presence of vascular disease elsewhere in the body. Several of these constitute significant risk factors which will be mentioned again later.

Cerebral ischaemia may be sudden and catastrophic in its onset followed by death, or by a crippling hemiplegia. Those patients who partially recover, but have a serious neurological deficit, rarely, if ever, require surgery. In fact, the evidence is that operation makes this group worse. Fortunately TIAs, by definition, are followed by full recovery. It is in the management of patients with TIAs where the surgeon has a vital part to play. The prime object of surgical treatment is to prevent a permanent stroke, but to stop the attacks themselves is of immediate and equal importance to the patient.

Cerebral ischaemic attacks may be conveniently divided into those which occur in the territory of the brain supplied by the carotid arteries (the cerebral hemispheres and retinae), and those which occur in the area supplied by the vertebrobasilar arteries (the brainstem, the cerebellar hemispheres and occipital lobes of the cerebral hemispheres). Both can be involved in the same patient either simultaneously or in separate attacks.

Carotid Artery Territory

Ischaemia is invariably unilateral because one side usually predominates though both carotid arteries may be diseased. Visual disturbances (due to retinal artery occlusion) occur on the same side as the arterial lesion, the clinical effects of hemisphere ischaemia occur on the opposite side of the body.

Transient neurological disturbances are the common early clinical manifestations of ischaemia and may consist of ipsilateral blindness (amaurosis fugax) and contralateral motor and sensory disturbances such as numbness and tingling and loss of power in the face, arm and leg. If the dominant hemisphere is affected, dysphasia is common. The duration of a TIA may vary from a few minutes to several hours. It is generally accepted that an attack of longer than 24 h will be accompanied by permanent tissue changes and should be classified as a stroke. The frequency and number of attacks are variable. Some patients may have attacks occurring at intervals over several years and suffer no residual neurological defect, whereas others may develop a permanent deficit after only one or two attacks. The attacks may stop spontaneously, probably due, in some instances, to complete occlusion of the involved artery and consequent cessation of microembolization. However, in most patients, especially in those with internal carotid artery stenosis, the condition is steadily progressive. Published work shows a variable incidence of stroke. A rate of 7% of completed stroke incidence in patients with TIAs per year of follow-up is the currently accepted figure. It has been suggested that TIAs resulting from vertebrobasilar artery disease tend to follow a more benign course, but several authors dispute this.

Vertebrobasilar Territory

Because the single basilar artery supplies both sides of the hindbrain, symptoms and signs are bilateral and extremely variable. There may be relatively mild symptoms of light-headedness and dizziness or more severe symptoms of vertigo, diplopia, paraesthesiae, ataxia, dysarthria and bilateral alternating limb weakness. Drop attacks, in which the patient falls to the ground without losing consciousness and can pick himself up immediately, are a characteristic feature. When the affected artery supplies both the arm and the brain, features of ischaemia in both areas may be combined. The cerebral symptoms usually predominate, the arm ischaemia merely causing some tiredness or aching of the limb after exercise. Occasionally cerebral symptoms follow excessive use of the arm ('subclavian steal').

Examination of the patient with symptoms of ischaemia in either territory may reveal reduced or absent pulses and a thrill or bruit in the region of arterial narrowing in the neck or arm. The fingers may show colour or nutritional changes and the systolic blood pressure in the affected arm may be lower than on the opposite side. On ophthalmoscopic examination an embolus in a branch of the retinal artery may be seen if the examination is performed during an attack of amaurosis fugax.

Investigations

All patients should have routine blood examination, chest, skull and cervical spine radiographs, electrocardiogram, and electroencephalogram. The exclusion of a diabetic state and hypercholesterolaemia are also necessary. Brain scanning using $^{99}\mathrm{Tc}^{m}$ may be performed and will detect already established brain infarcts.

When the diagnosis of a significant lesion in an extracerebral artery is made on clinical grounds, or following the use of screening techniques to be described below, and surgical treatment is being considered, arteriography is essential. It is the only special investigation necessary in the symptomatic patient. Arch arteriography by retrograde catheterization through the femoral or brachial arteries to give four-vessel visualization is preferred to direct puncture of the common carotid or vertebral arteries because these latter procedures carry a greater risk and provide only limited information. Arterial lesions are often multiple so it is important that the four arteries which supply the brain are clearly visualized and that the intracranial circulation, particularly the anastomotic circulation in the circle of Willis, is fully assessed. The site of the lesion, its extent and morphology are shown with a high degree of accuracy. More recently with the advent of digital subtraction angiography (DSA), biplanar views of the extra- and intracerebral circulation can be produced using an intravenous bolus injection of contrast medium. This procedure is virtually free from risk of the serious complications of death or permanent stroke which occur not infrequently with conventional angiography, and is now beginning to replace other 'non-invasive' methods of investigating the extracerebral vessels. DSA or other less risky methods of investigation should be used first for routine screening of extracerebral arterial disease in patients with disease at other sites (e.g. coronary artery disease, abdominal aortic aneurysm, etc.), and in other doubtful cases.

Numerous non-invasive methods have been devised, some still being in the experimental stage. Most of them have been designed to study blood flow in the internal carotid artery, either directly in the neck by a variety of ultrasound techniques including phonangiography (the visual analysis of a carotid bruit) and ultrasonic imaging or, indirectly, by measuring blood flow in its first intracranial branch, the ophthalmic artery. Flow and pressure in this vessel can be assessed by: bilateral oculoplethysmography which measures the pulse pressure in the retinal arteries and compares the affected side with the opposite side; supra-orbital Doppler examination; or facial thermography. These indirect methods are of limited value because they can only detect, but not distinguish between, an occlusion or a high-grade stenosis (i.e. one that has a greater than 50% diameter reduction or a 75% or more reduction in cross-sectional area) sufficient to reduce intracranial internal carotid artery flow. The inability to distinguish between an occlusion, which in most cases is not amenable to surgical correction, and a high-grade stenosis which can be corrected by operation is an obvious drawback. Further drawbacks of these methods are, that they cannot identify patients with bilateral severe stenoses or occlusions and they cannot identify a non-flow-reducing stenosis or an ulcerating lesion. Direct methods on the other hand, especially when used in combination, such as ultrasonic imaging and pulsed Doppler spectrum analysis (Duplex Scanning) offer a more accurate assessment, being able to distinguish between normal, stenotic and occluded arteries and also to localize the site of a lesion. Using these methods a diagnostic accuracy of about 90% compared with contrast arteriography has been claimed. Such sophisticated techniques are not yet available for routine use except in some major centres but the simpler more limited methods still have an important screening function. If they detect a significant stenosis then contrast arteriography should follow.

Computerized tomography is used to detect areas of cerebral infarction but its precise role in the investigation of cerebral ischaemia has yet to be determined.

Non-invasive techniques offer a safe method of investigation and are especially suitable for the screening of patients with an asymptomatic bruit or of patients with other arterial lesions requiring major surgery in whom an internal carotid artery stenosis is suspected. Some surgeons now believe that an internal carotid artery stenosis should always be excluded before embarking on coronary artery grafting or other forms of major vascular surgery because of the increased risk of postoperative stroke in those who have an internal carotid artery stenosis (*see* Chapter 48).

OCCLUSIVE DISEASE OF THE EXTRACRANIAL CEREBRAL ARTERIES

The Innominate and Proximal Subclavian Arteries

Pathophysiology

Arteritis is a rare cause of occlusion of the aortic arch branches in Western countries but is commoner in Russia and the Far East. It characteristically affects young women and usually involves more than one aortic branch.

Atherosclerosis is the commonest cause of aortic arch disease in Western countries. It generally begins as a localized plaque at the origin of an aortic branch or at the origins of the right subclavian or right common carotid arteries. Sometimes the disease originates in the arch itself and extends to involve the orifices of one or more branches. Stenosis of these arteries can gradually progress to complete occlusion, the effect of which will depend upon the pattern of collateral blood flow. Innominate artery occlusion extends only to its bifurcation where patency is maintained by retrograde flow from the right common carotid artery into the subclavian artery. The extent of proximal subclavian artery occlusion is limited by reversed blood flow in the vertebral artery.

An ulcerating lesion of the innominate and proximal subclavian arteries may cause embolization of the brain or upper limb. Stenosis or complete occlusion reduces cerebral blood flow either directly or, indirectly, by causing reversed flow in the right common carotid or vertebral arteries ('subclavian steal'). Clinical effects are not common because of the excellence of the collateral circulation unless there is an associated internal carotid artery stenosis. The reduction of blood flow to the arm is generally insufficient to produce significant symptoms and signs unless the arm is strenuously exercised.

Clinical Features

The pattern of symptoms and signs will depend upon which artery is affected and the type of lesion present—ulcerative, stenotic or occlusive, for example, an ulcerating lesion of the innominate artery may cause episodes of hand ischaemia and carotid territory TIAs. Stenotic or occlusive lesions of the innominate or proximal subclavian arteries may result in symptoms and signs of subclavian steal, namely episodes of vertebrobasilar territory ischaemic symptoms in association with tiredness and aching of the arm, a bruit in the supraclavicular fossa, unequal radial pulses and a difference in the systolic blood pressure between the arms.

Investigations

Arch arteriography is essential. Views in different planes and subtraction films will help to pick out small areas of roughening and ulceration. Delayed films may demonstrate retrograde flow in the vertebral and common carotid arteries (*Fig.* 52.1). Retrograde flow in the absence of clinical features, a not unusual radiological finding, is not an indication for surgery.

Treatment

Surgical treatment is rarely necessary unless there is repeated microembolism. Of those with haemodynamically significant lesions, demonstrated by clinical examination or on arteriography, probably less than 8% require surgery. However, 85% of patients with symptoms and who had an associated internal carotid artery stenosis, were relieved of their symptoms by carotid thromboendarterectomy.

For those relatively few patients selected for operation on the innominate or proximal subclavian arteries there is a choice of surgical procedure, using either an extra- or intrathoracic approach. In the early days of vascular surgery local thromboendarterectomy through a transthoracic incision was the preferred method. If there were multiple occlusions various bypass procedures from the aortic arch were employed. Intrathoracic operations, however, have a higher risk and in an attempt to reduce the mortality and morbidity extrathoracic methods were introduced. The most popular current procedure for proximal subclavian artery occlusion is a common carotid artery to subclavian artery bypass (saphenous vein or Dacron tube graft) through a neck incision. Other surgeons prefer transposition procedures, e.g. the left subclavian artery beyond the block is divided and the distal cut end anastomosed to the left common carotid artery. A return to thromboendarterectomy of the innominate artery or the proximal left subclavian artery through a median sternotomy or a lateral thoracotomy has been advocated by Wylie and his colleagues in San Francisco.

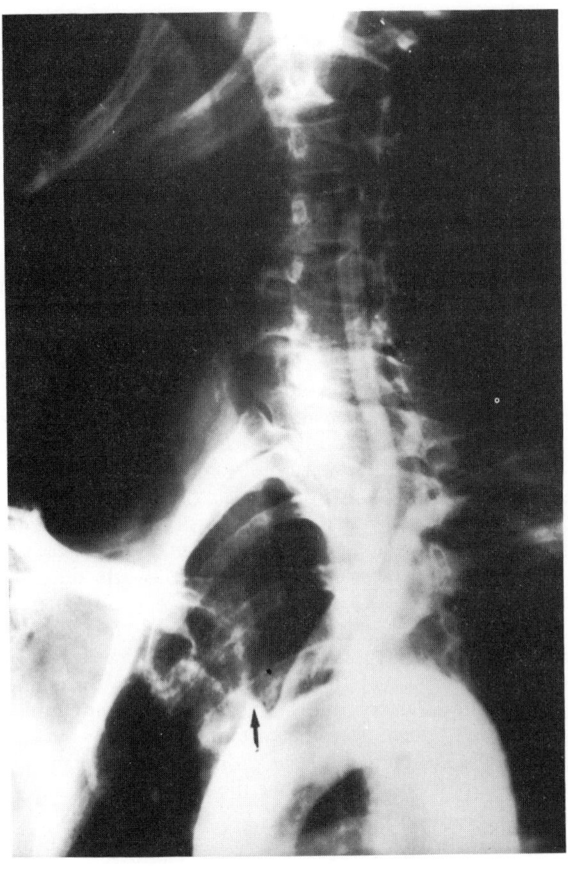
a

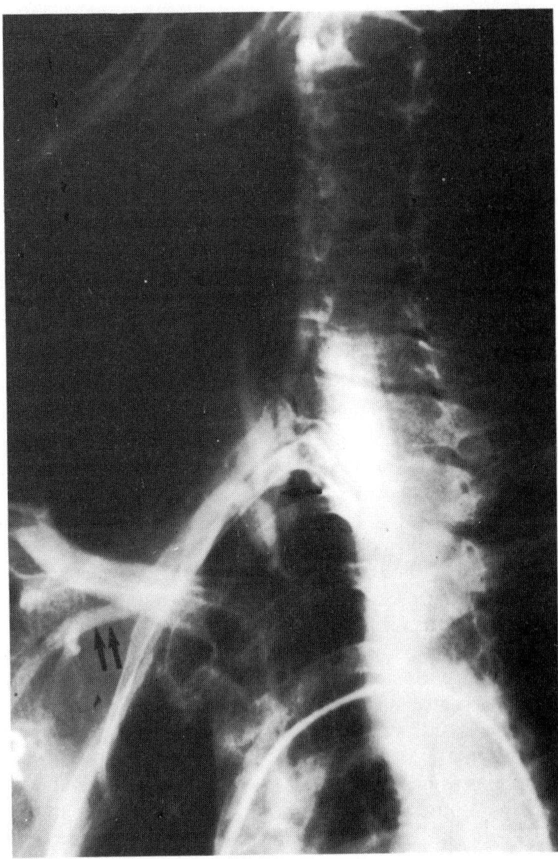
b

Fig. 52.1 Arch arteriogram. *a*, Early filling phase shows stump of occluded innominate artery. *b*, Late phase shows retrograde filling of the right subclavian artery from the right vertebral and common carotid arteries.

The Vertebral Artery

Pathophysiology

The vertebral arteries may be occluded by atherosclerosis, kinks, bands, fibromuscular dysplasia or osteophytes secondary to degenerative disease of the cervical spine. Movements of the head and neck may aggravate the effects of occlusive disease.

An atherosclerotic plaque is generally confined to the first few millimetres of the artery. If a stenosis proceeds to complete occlusion the resultant thrombosis spreads to the level of the second cervical vertebra where muscular branches maintain its patency. Obstruction of a single vertebral artery is symptomless because adequate cerebral blood flow is maintained through the other vertebral artery and the carotid system.

Clinical Features

Symptoms of vertebral artery insufficiency alone are rare; most symptomatic patients have an accompanying internal carotid artery stenosis which dominates the clinical picture. Ischaemic symptoms in vertebrobasilar artery territory, such as vertigo, occur when both arteries are diseased. There is sometimes a relationship between the onset of symptoms and simply turning the head, the patient falling to the ground in a typical drop attack. On examination a bruit may be heard near the vertebral artery origin at the root of the neck.

Investigations

The usual site of disease at the origin of the artery can only be clearly demonstrated by arch arteriography. Care is necessary to avoid direct injection of the contrast medium into the mouth of the artery otherwise hind brain infarction may result; the catheter tip must be kept well within the subclavian artery. Direct needle puncture arteriography has now largely been abandoned for the following reasons: there is danger of brainstem ischaemia if too concentrated a dose of contrast medium is given; a number of arteriovenous fistulas have been reported following the use of this technique; and the origin of the artery cannot be adequately visualized by this method.

Treatment

Only rarely is reconstruction indicated and, when it is, the right vertebral artery is chosen because of the easier access. A cervical approach to the origin of the artery is made and a thromboendarterectomy performed with or without a patch graft of vein or Dacron to repair the arteriotomy.

The Common Carotid Artery

Pathophysiology

The common carotid artery may be narrowed at its origin or at its bifurcation and often there are associated lesions of the internal and external carotid arteries. In the right common carotid artery the primary lesion is invariably at the bifurcation. Atherosclerosis is responsible for all right common carotid and most left common carotid artery stenosing lesions. Arteritis is a rare cause of proximal stenosis in the left common carotid artery. Should stenosis at any of the sites proceed to a complete block, the pattern of occlusion will vary according to the site of the primary disease and the collateral blood flow. Proximal occlusion will cause thrombosis which will extend up to, but not involve, the bifurcation because flow will be maintained in the internal carotid artery from the external carotid artery. Should thrombosis begin at the bifurcation, as is most likely, and there is associated disease of its two branches, all three vessels will be occluded.

Clinical Features

These will vary according to the site of the original disease and the pattern of occlusion. Proximal stenosis or even complete occlusion may be asymptomatic, provided that collateral blood flow is maintained through the external carotid artery. Stenosis of all three arteries is likely to cause symptoms of hemisphere and retinal ischaemia. Sudden occlusion in association with inadequate collateral blood flow can result in a hemiplegia, or at best, severe symptoms of hypoperfusion. Reduced or absent pulsation will be noted on palpation of the artery in the neck and a bruit may be heard over it. Ulcerating lesions rarely, if ever, occur in the proximal common carotid artery. Distal ulcerating lesions behave in the same manner as similar lesions in the internal carotid artery with which they will probably be associated.

Investigations

Arch arteriography is necessary to demonstrate the extent of the occlusion and the condition of the other cerebral arteries, in particular the internal and external carotid vessels.

Treatment

Operation is indicated if the patient has symptoms of cerebral ischaemia. The type of arterial reconstruction will be determined by the arteriographic and operative findings. Thromboendarterectomy is generally possible on the right side and may be extended if necessary into the internal and external carotid arteries. In the presence of complete occlusion of the right internal carotid artery, restoration of flow through the external carotid artery will help to improve the overall cerebral blood flow. On the left side a bypass graft or transposition procedure, combined with a limited thromboendarterectomy, may be preferred, thus avoiding the need to open the chest to reach the origin of the artery.

The Internal Carotid Artery

The internal carotid artery is the most common of the extracranial cerebral arteries to be affected by disease with resulting ischaemia of the brain. It is not surprising, therefore, that it has received most attention from physicians and surgeons throughout the world. Since the first report of a case of internal carotid stenosis treated by operation in 1954 (Eastcott, Pickering and Rob) many large series have been reported and much has been written about this relatively tiny lesion.

Pathophysiology

An atherosclerotic plaque in the first centimetre or two of its course is the most common lesion of the internal carotid artery (*Fig.* 52.2); more rarely it is affected by tortuosity, coils, kinks, fibromuscular dysplasia or aneurysm. Reduced perfusion of the hemisphere and retina, microembolism, or complete occlusion with extension of thrombus to the intracranial branches are possible sequelae. The atherosclerotic lesion may be confined to the internal carotid artery or it may also involve the distal common carotid artery and the origin of the external carotid artery.

Whether or not a stenotic lesion produces a sufficient reduction in cerebral blood flow to cause ischaemic symptoms depends upon a number of factors which have already been discussed. The lumen must be reduced to a diameter of less than 1 mm before the blood flow is sufficiently impaired to produce cerebral ischaemia. Lesser stenoses will be more significant if there is occlusion of the contralateral internal carotid or other cerebral arteries.

The risk of a stenotic lesion causing sudden thrombus in the whole length of the carotid artery is an ever present one. The thrombus will extend from the origin of the artery to at least its first intracerebral branch, the ophthalmic. The consequences of such an episode will depend upon the factors which have already been discussed, including the extent of the intracranial internal carotid artery thrombosis and the efficiency of the collateral blood flow. Complete internal carotid artery occlusion may be quite symptomless; it is a well-known fact that arteriography may reveal a complete occlusion in a patient with no evidence of cerebral ischaemia past or present. None the less, in the presence of internal carotid artery stenosis, the risk of a sudden complete stroke is high whether due to thrombosis, embolism or hypoperfusion. More than 75% of patients who suffer permanent strokes have had TIAs and, as already has been stressed, there is a 7% incidence of completed stroke per

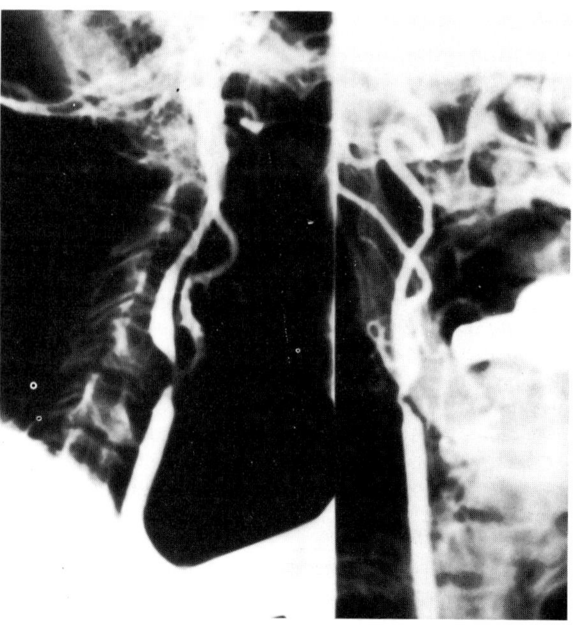

Fig. 52.2 Carotid arteriogram in two planes showing a tight atherosclerotic stenosis at the bifurcation of the common carotid artery involving the origins of both the internal and external carotid arteries.

year of follow-up in patients with TIAs. The greatest risk of a stroke developing is in the year following the first TIA, especially in the first 2 months.

Clinical Features

The classic presentation is of recurrent TIAs though, unfortunately, a sudden complete stroke may be the first manifestation. The significance of TIAs and their relationship to future stroke production cannot be over-emphasized and their early recognition and investigation are vital.

Transient ischaemic attacks due to internal carotid artery disease have already been described. Their recognition is usually not difficult though they do have to be differentiated from the clinical features of other neurological disorders, such as migraine and focal epilepsy. Transient ischaemic attacks resulting from vertebrobasilar artery disease must also be differentiated.

A bruit in the neck may be a useful confirmatory sign, but there is not always one present even in the presence of a severe stenosis. If there is a bruit present it does not necessarily indicate a significant lesion; there may be a louder bruit on the symptomless side. Amaurosis fugax accompanied by the ophthalmoscopic sighting of a retinal embolus is diagnostic.

Investigations

When the clinical features point firmly to the diagnosis of a significant stenosis and particularly when surgical intervention is urgent, investigation should proceed immediately to arch arteriography. If the diagnosis is in doubt, or in asymptomatic cases, or where there may be a contraindication to surgery, non-invasive methods of investigation should be used in the first instance. If they suggest a significant stenosis then digital subtraction angiography or arch arteriography should be recommended.

Treatment

When the surgical correction of internal carotid artery stenosis by thromboendarterectomy (the procedure now adopted by the vast majority of surgeons) was first introduced, questions were raised about its safety and, indeed, the necessity for such a procedure, for comparatively little was known then about the natural history of the disease. Over the past 25 years since carotid reconstruction was introduced, a vast amount of information has accumulated. There is now little doubt among most clinicians that internal carotid artery thromboendarterectomy can be a safe and effective method of treatment. Mortality in experienced hands is less than 2% and the incidence of postoperative stroke is also less than 2%. The effectiveness of the procedure is clear: most patients lose their TIAs and the risk of stroke can be reduced from 40% to 1–3%. The case for operation seems unassailable but it must be emphasized that mortality and morbidity figures may be higher, especially in less experienced hands. However, internal carotid thromboendarterectomy is now firmly established as the routine treatment for most cases of symptomatic internal carotid artery stenosis. How may the procedure be kept safe?

The main problem at operation is the maintenance of adequate cerebral blood flow while the vessels are clamped. In the early stages of development, the operation was done as quickly as possible under hypothermia. Now, a careful, meticulous operation is done with cerebral vascularization maintained by a variety of methods which include the maintenance of a slightly raised blood pressure, systemic heparinization and the routine or selective use of a shunt. The method selected depends upon the individual choice of the surgeon. Continuous EEG monitoring during operation is employed by some surgeons who do not routinely use a shunt or other method of support. Extreme care is necessary at operation to avoid dislodging a thrombus or atheromatous debris from the site of the lesion during manipulation of the artery and before the clamps have been applied.

For all patients, measures should be taken to deal with associated hypertension. The control of hypertension should be a gradual process otherwise a full stroke may be precipitated from hypoperfusion of the brain. There may be some patients in whom surgery is contraindicated and in these patients there may be some help gained by anticoagulation for 3–6 months during which time an ulcerated plaque may re-epithelize. More recently attention has focused on the use of antiplatelet agents, either aspirin in low dose, 75 mg daily, with or without the addition of dipyridamole (Persantin) 100 mg q.d.s., or sulphinpyrazone (Anturan) 100 mg q.d.s. There is some evidence that these agents may be effective in reducing the incidence of stroke, particularly in male patients.

The Asymptomatic Internal Carotid Artery Bruit

Quite understandably the success of internal carotid thromboendarterectomy in stopping TIAs and, more importantly, preventing strokes has encouraged some surgeons to consider prophylactic surgery in asymptomatic cases. The asymptomatic internal carotid artery stenosis is generally discovered while the patient is being investigated for other manifestations of peripheral vascular disease or when radiological examination reveals an asymptomatic lesion on the opposite side to a symptomatic one.

Results have been presented, mainly from the USA and Continental countries which suggest that patients with an asymptomatic internal carotid artery stenosis are at high risk of developing TIAs or a completed stroke which may be fatal. The figures suggest that the risk is appreciably higher than that which follows operation for asymptomatic disease. Several surgeons are now following an aggressive policy in these cases. However, other figures, particularly from the UK, suggest that patients with an asymptomatic bruit are not so much at risk and a more cautious approach is recommended.

Should a patient with an asymptomatic bruit over the internal carotid artery be investigated? The answer is 'yes' and this can be done by non-invasive methods. The use of Duplex scanning or digital subtraction angiography has allowed safer screening of these patients. DSA itself may demonstrate a significant lesion but if the picture quality is not adequate for surgery then arteriography may follow, following the demonstration of a lesion by these other techniques (*Fig.* 52.3). Evidence is now accumulating to suggest that patients with stenoses >75% should be offered prophylactic surgery as they are at greater risk of developing a stroke.

The External Carotid Artery

The external carotid artery provides an important collateral blood flow through the ophthalmic artery in cases of complete or near-complete occlusion of the internal carotid artery. Its importance is underlined by the number of reconstructive procedures which have been designed to maintain its patency particularly in the presence of complete occlusion of the internal carotid artery. Mention has already been made of the value of restoring blood flow through the

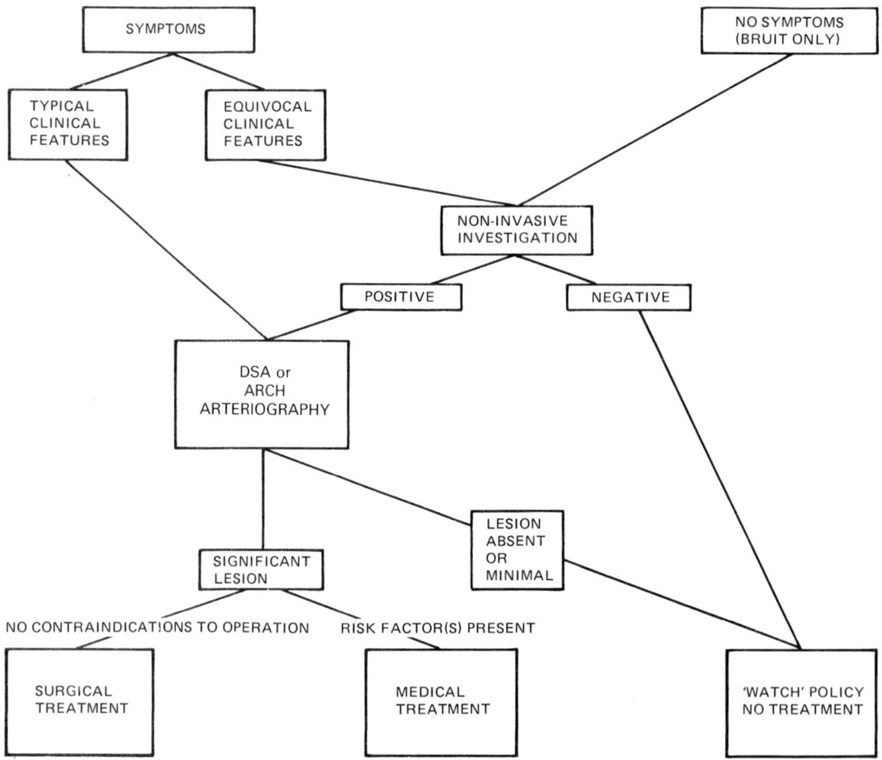

Fig. 52.3 Internal carotid artery stenosis. Scheme of management.

external carotid artery by thromboendarterectomy or bypass of the completely occluded common carotid artery.

In 1969 Yasagil introduced the operation to anastomose the superficial temporal artery to the cerebral branch of the middle cerebral artery, with the hope that the revascularization of the cerebral circulation might relieve symptoms due to complete internal carotid occlusion. However, the results of a recent International Multicentre trial of the procedure of external carotid to internal carotid bypass (EC–IC shunt) has concluded that the procedure does not reduce the risk of stroke, either fatal or non-fatal and for the majority of patients this procedure has no significant benefit. The risks of this surgery are simply not worth taking although there might be a small subgroup, whose TIAs are related to reduced flow, which might benefit from this procedure but these are difficult to define; certainly this operation can no longer be advised for the majority of patients with carotid occlusion or disease not accessible from the neck by conventional endarterectomy.

The Results of Surgery for Cerebral Ischaemia

Carefully planned and controlled surgery of the extracerebral cranial arteries, especially in the patient with TIAs, will achieve rewarding results. Patency rates of over 90%, low mortality, and low postoperative stroke incidence have been reported from several centres, although less satisfactory figures from other centres underline the continuing need for careful selection of patients and for skilled surgery.

Among several factors which increase the risks of surgery are hypertension, bilateral internal carotid artery disease, symptomatic peripheral vascular disease at other sites, heart disease and diabetes. The presence of one or more of these risk factors results in a significant rise in postoperative morbidity.

There is no doubt, however, that surgery will remove distressing symptoms in the majority of cases and reduce the threat of a crippling stroke. There is also an improvement in the mental state of the patient which can be readily observed by the clinician and the patient. This clinical impression has now been supported by investigation using neuropsychological testing.

Operation is contraindicated for those patients with an acute total occlusion of the internal carotid artery, particularly in the siphon section, and a serious neurological deficit because of the high operative mortality (over 60%). In those patients with evolving strokes, there is the danger of worsening the neurological deficit. The dangers of operation in the acute state result from intracranial haemorrhage and cerebral oedema following revascularization of an infarcted area of the brain.

Disobliteration of the chronically occluded internal carotid artery has resulted in patency rates of less than 40% and in fact may be dangerous (because of the danger of cerebral haemorrhage or embolism from the dislodgement of clot during mobilization of the artery) where there is little or no neurological deficit. The operation is pointless if the patient is already hemiplegic.

Other Disorders of the Extracranial Cerebral Arteries

Tortuosity, Coils and Kinks

Elongation of the extracranial cerebral arteries with consequent coiling or kinking is quite common. Tortuosity of the innominate artery or common carotid artery is a not-infrequent clinical observation in a thin, elderly, hypertensive female who complains of a pulsatile swelling low in the neck, usually on the right side. She has probably been referred with the diagnosis of a carotid or innominate artery aneurysm, but more careful clinical examination, which can be confirmed by an ultrasound scan, reveals a prominent tortuous artery only. Reassurance can normally be given without resorting to arteriography; only the hypertension may need treatment.

Tortuosity of the vertebral artery is uncommon but the internal carotid artery is quite often tortuous, coiled or kinked. Tortuosity and coiling may occur at any age and are unrelated to hypertension; they are probably congenital in origin and become exaggerated with ageing. Kinking, on the other hand, is thought to be an acquired condition and occurs in older patients with atherosclerosis and hypertension. Tortuosity and coiling are asymptomatic and do not require treatment. If a patient with cerebral ischaemic attacks is found on investigation to have a kinked internal carotid artery and no other lesion, then surgical correction of the kink will be necessary.

Surgical correction of kinking is aimed at removing the kink and straightening out the artery by shortening it. This is done by removing a segment containing the kink (which may have an atherosclerotic plaque on it) and joining the two ends by direct anastomosis or, preferably, the proximal end is ligated and the distal end sutured to the side of the common carotid artery which ensures wider anastomosis.

Fibromuscular Dysplasia

This is a rare disease of the internal carotid artery, being found in only 0·25–0·68% of patients undergoing carotid arteriography. It is usually bilateral and affects middle-aged women almost exclusively, causing transient attacks of cerebral ischaemia or, even less frequently, a sudden stroke. A high-pitched bruit over the internal carotid artery is a characteristic feature. The diagnosis is made on arteriography which shows either classic beading of the internal carotid artery, a localized stenosis, or a tubular stenosis.

Treatment is necessary in the presence of ischaemic attacks. Gradual dilatation of the affected artery through a small incision in the carotid bulb is the preferred method of treatment and good results are reported.

Injury

Injury to the arteries in the neck occurs in civilian practice and on the battlefield with equal frequency. The majority result from penetrating injuries due to stabbing, gunshot and shrapnel wounds. Closed injuries following blows to the head or neck are less common. Penetration of the internal carotid artery by an ingested foreign body sticking in the throat is a rare cause.

Open wounds generally result in laceration or complete division of the artery, the most commonly affected being the common carotid artery. Closed injuries cause intimal tears, likely to be followed by thrombosis. The immediate effects of injury vary considerably. Death of the patient may result from uncontrolled bleeding, from asphyxia due to pressure of a haematoma, or from severe cerebral ischaemia. The surviving patient may be hemiplegic. Neurological sequelae may be delayed for hours or days, or they may be absent altogether. Arteriovenous fistula and false aneurysm are possible delayed effects.

Immediate surgical exploration and repair of the damaged artery is necessary in the majority of cases. Simple side suture or end-to-end anastomosis may be possible for incised wounds. Lacerated wounds tend to cause more arterial damage and if a long segment has to be excised, a graft replacement will be necessary. A vein graft is preferred to a prosthetic graft because of the dangers of infection. Closed injuries associated with intimal tearing and thrombosis are treated by thrombectomy and repair of the intima or excision of the injured segment if the damage is extensive.

Generally there will be no time nor need for arteriography but where the situation does not seem urgent, as in a closed injury with minor or no cerebral ischaemic symptoms, arteriography may be helpful in determining the site, type and extent of the injury.

There is controversy concerning the role of surgery in patients with an established neurological defect. Some surgeons maintain that restoration of cerebral blood flow may be harmful by causing haemorrhage into an infarcted area of the brain. On the other hand, instances have been reported where reversal of a hemiplegia has resulted following restoration of blood flow. The timing of surgical intervention is critical, the earlier the intervention the more likely recovery will be complete.

Aneurysm

Aneurysm is rare in the extracranial cerebral arteries. Often a suspected aneurysm proves to be no more than a tortuous carotid artery on careful examination. Most aneurysms are either atherosclerotic or post-traumatic in origin. However, there is a rising incidence of false aneurysm following carotid endarterectomy.

The clinical features are of a pulsatile swelling in the neck associated in some cases with cerebral ischaemic attacks due to microembolism. Fixed neurological deficits and rupture are other reported complications.

Treatment is usually necessary and should consist of excision of the aneurysm with restoration of arterial continuity by direct end-to-end anastomosis, graft replacement, or patch angioplasty.

Arteriovenous Fistula

Pathophysiology

An arteriovenous fistula in the neck is almost always traumatic in origin, only rarely is it congenital. A penetrating injury such as a stabbing or gunshot wound is the usual mechanism but occasionally a closed injury of the neck may be responsible. In recent years a number of cases of fistula have followed needle puncture arteriography of the common carotid and vertebral vessels.

An arteriovenous fistula of the carotid is generally found between it and the internal jugular vein. Vertebral arteriovenous fistulas occur between the second part of the artery and its accompanying plexus of veins or between its first or third parts and the adjacent segment of internal jugular vein.

Clinical Features

The patient complains of a loud buzzing or pulsating noise in the head on the side of the injury. Dizziness may be a feature but neurological symptoms are usually absent. A thrill can be felt and a bruit heard at the site of the fistula and for a variable distance away from it. Occasionally a pulsatile swelling may be present. Compression of the common carotid artery proximal to a carotid–jugular fistula will result in the disappearance of the bruit and thrill. Vertebral artery compression is more difficult so that confirmation of the diagnosis may require arteriography. Arteriography is necessary in all cases of arteriovenous fistula both to confirm the diagnosis and to localize accurately the site of the lesion.

Treatment

Carotid–jugular fistula is treated by excision of the fistula and repair of both artery and vein; surgical access is usually straightforward. A vertebral arteriovenous fistula is more difficult to reach, particularly if the second or third parts of the artery are affected. Repair of artery and vein is not necessary as one vertebral artery can be sacrificed with no danger of neurological sequelae. The second part of the vertebral artery is exposed by removing parts of two, three or more cervical transverse processes. The artery and veins are ligated on either side of the fistula which is then excised. Excellent results have been reported using this technique with no serious postoperative complications.

Vertebral arteriovenous fistula following needle puncture arteriography should no longer occur because most radiologists now prefer retrograde catheterization of the subclavian artery.

Carotid Body Tumour (*see also* Chapter 23)

This is a rare but important tumour; errors in diagnosis or treatment may cause death or permanent disablement.

Pathophysiology

A carotid body tumour is one of the group of tumours which were given the name 'chemodectoma' by Milligan in 1950. Chemodectomas arise in chemoreceptor organs which are situated in various parts of the body and are sensitive to changes in the chemical compositions of arterial blood. In the neck they may arise from the carotid body situated at the bifurcation of the common carotid artery or in the glomus vagale or glomus jugulare at the base of the skull.

A carotid body tumour usually grows slowly, surrounding the internal and external carotid arteries, separating them at their origins but occasionally displacing them anteriorly or medially. It may gradually extend upwards along the internal carotid artery to the base of the skull. These tumours are generally extremely vascular, deriving their blood supply mainly from numerous tiny branches of the external carotid artery. Some tumours are sufficiently vascular to pulsate, others are fibrotic, less vascular and non-pulsating. The degree of penetration of the artery wall varies, some merely displacing the adventitia, others penetrating into the media occasionally narrowing the arteries themselves. This variation in structure is one of the main reasons why these tumours offer such a challenge to the operator. The microscopic picture is also variable. The classic picture is of groups of polyhedral cells arranged in alveolar fashion separated by vascular connective tissue trabeculae. Other tumours contain much more connective tissue which scatters the tumour cell groups. Mitotic figures are not present. The question of malignancy is a controversial one. There may be local infiltration or spread to neighbouring lymph nodes and distant metastases have been reported. Generally, however, the tumours are slow growing, well circumscribed and encapsulated.

Clinical Features

A small, symptomless swelling in the carotid triangle is the most common form of presentation. The possibility of a carotid body tumour must always be considered when examining a lump in the carotid triangle. Occasionally a patient fails to report to a doctor until the tumour has reached a large size when pressure symptoms may be present. The patient sometimes complains of a pulsating noise in the ear on the affected side, particularly when lying in bed. There may be a history of blackouts or attacks of dizziness.

A carotid body tumour may be found on both sides. One is usually larger than the other, the second generally being found on routine examination, the patient having been unaware of its presence.

Chemodectomas may be multiple. It is not unusual for a patient who has had treatment for a glomus tympanicum, a glomus jugulare, or a glomus vagale to be found to have, at follow-up, a tumour in the carotid triangle. Patients are thus occasionally referred by otolaryngologists or radiotherapists following treatment for other chemodectomas.

On examination a tumour is felt in the carotid triangle at the level of the angle of the jaw. It is usually firm and transmits pulsation from the carotid arteries. Occasionally it is large, soft and exhibits expansile pulsation. It may be movable from side to side, but not up and down as do many other cervical swellings. A thrill may be felt on palpation and a bruit heard on auscultation. If the tumour is of the locally infiltrative variety there may be evidence of cranial nerve palsies, such as hemiatrophy of the tongue or vocal cord paralysis.

A carotid body tumour must be distinguished from other swellings in the carotid triangle, such as an enlarged lymph node, a lowly situated tumour of the parotid salivary gland, or a prominent or tortuous carotid artery. When the diagnosis of a carotid body tumour cannot be excluded on clinical grounds, arteriography is necessary. Diagnostic exploration of a doubtful lump in the carotid triangle must be avoided.

Investigations

A tortuous common carotid artery in the anterior triangle of the neck in a thin, elderly, hypertensive female may be thought to be a carotid body tumour on simple examination. An ultrasound scan will identify such cases and avoid the need for a carotid arteriogram which has increased risks in these patients.

A carotid arteriogram is essential in all cases of suspected carotid body tumour and will establish the diagnosis beyond doubt. The classic arteriographic picture is of a vascular tumour separating the origins of the internal and external carotid arteries in the 'goblet' fashion (*Fig.* 52.4). If the main part of the tumour lies posteriorly, as it occasionally does, then there may be no separation of the vessels. The vascular tumour is then seen to be displacing the vessels anteriorly or medially.

If the surgeon explores a lump in the carotid triangle because he has considered the diagnosis of a carotid body tumour to be unlikely, he must, nevertheless, keep the possibility of such a tumour in mind at operation. If he unexpectedly finds a vascular tumour closely related to the carotid vessels, he should withdraw and not attempt biopsy or excision. Serious complications have resulted from such incautious explorations. It is safer and wiser to discontinue the operation and have a carotid arteriogram done later.

Treatment

In the younger patient a carotid body tumour should be excised, preferably by a surgeon trained in vascular surgery techniques. In the elderly, poor-risk patient, with a small, slow-growing, symptomless tumour, no treatment except simple observation is necessary. Between these two extremes is a group of patients who require careful consideration before a decision is made; for example, they may be old, have other disabling diseases, or they may have chemodectomas at other sites.

If a tumour is large and causing symptoms but the risks of surgery seem high, radiotherapy may be tried. Unfortunate-

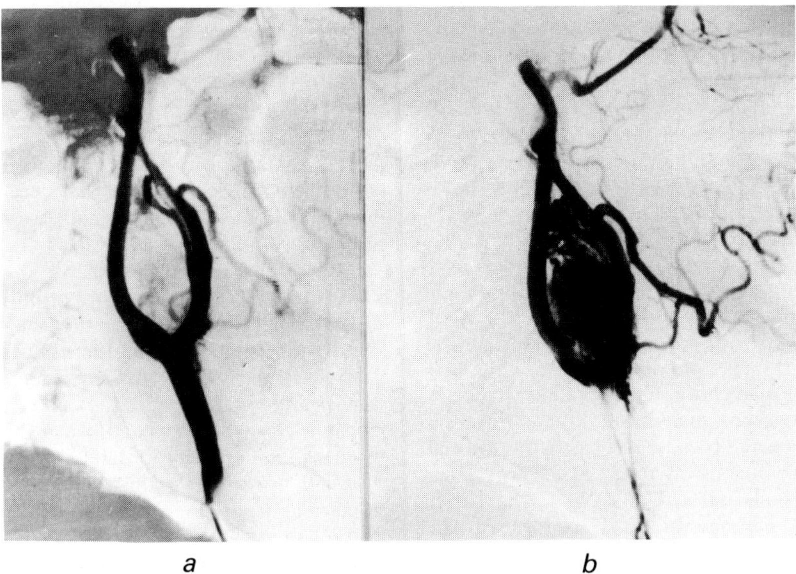

Fig. 52.4 Subtraction films of a carotid arteriogram showing a carotid body tumour. *a*, Early filling phase shows the typical separation of the internal and external carotid arteries by the tumour ('goblet' deformity). *b*, Late filling phase showing the pathological circulation within the tumour.

ly, the results are not encouraging, and are not without risk of cranial nerve damage or even damage to, and subsequent occlusion of, the carotid arteries themselves. If a patient already has an inoperable chemodectoma at another site there is generally little purpose in excising a carotid body tumour unless it is causing intolerable symptoms. In such patients radiotherapy may be given.

When surgery is judged to be the best form of treatment in a given case, the patient must be clearly told of the risks of surgery on the one hand and the risks of leaving the tumour or of radiotherapy, on the other. Unfortunately the surgeon will have little indication of how easy or difficult the operation might be before he has exposed the tumour. Operation can prove easy and straightforward, with simple excision of the tumour through the classic subadventitial plane, or it may be difficult and demanding. If the tumour is of the infiltrative type with deep penetration of the arterial wall, resection of the bifurcation and replacement by a vein graft may be necessary. In such cases, there is obviously an increased risk of complications, the most serious of which is a hemiplegia. With careful use of vascular surgery techniques it should be possible to avoid serious trouble in the majority of cases. Should the internal carotid artery be injured during the course of operation, it is essential to administer systemic heparin immediately and put a temporary intraluminal shunt into the internal carotid artery. In this way, clotting in the carotid system will be avoided and adequate blood flow will be maintained to the hemisphere whilst excision of the tumour is completed and the artery repaired by a vein graft. The results of excision of a carotid body tumour are usually excellent.

Glomus Jugulare and Glomus Vagale Tumours

These tumours arise in relation to the jugular bulb (glomus jugulare) or the vagus nerve (glomus vagale). They may extend upwards into the temporal bone, the middle or inner ear, or intracranially, or downwards in the neck.

Clinical Features

If the main extension is upwards, aural symptoms, such as loss of hearing, tinnitus, aural bleeding and vertigo will cause the patient to visit his doctor, who is likely to refer him to an otorhinolaryngologist.

When extension is downwards into the neck the patient will present with a tumour in the upper part of the carotid triangle which may be difficult to distinguish from a carotid body tumour. A buzzing or pulsating noise in the head is often a feature of these tumours. Cranial nerve palsies may accompany either upward or downward extending tumours; the most commonly affected are the IXth, Xth and XIth cranial nerves so the patient may have an absent pharyngeal reflex, vocal cord paralysis and shoulder drop (the jugular foramen syndrome). Diagnosis should be confirmed in all cases by arteriography. Tomographic pictures of the base of the skull will help to determine whether or not bone involvement has occurred.

Treatment

Tumours extending into the temporal bone, middle and inner ear are dealt with by an otorhinolaryngologist but tumours in the neck may well be referred to a general or vascular surgeon.

Neck tumours can be excised with remarkably little residual cranial nerve damage. If extension into the skull has occurred more extensive surgery will be necessary requiring the help of a neurosurgeon or an otorhinolaryngologist. Inoperable tumours should be treated by radiotherapy, though the response is generally disappointing.

Carotid Sinus Syndrome

In those rare individuals who have hypersensitive carotid sinuses, bradycardia, asystole or hypotension (causing fainting) may result from slight pressure (such as the wearing of a tight collar or merely turning the head) on the carotid bifurcation. These attacks must be differentiated from the more common cause of fainting, such as vasovagal attacks, postural hypotension, heart disease and cerebrovascular disease. Patients with fainting attacks due to pressure on the carotid sinus in whom asystole lasts more than 2 sec, the heart rate slows more than 30%, or the systolic blood pressure falls by more than 30 mmHg, will require treatment. The most effective method is surgical denervation of the carotid sinus. In over half of the cases bilateral operation will be necessary.

THE UPPER LIMB

Upper Limb Ischaemia

Upper limb ischaemia, as an entity, understandably receives less attention from surgeons than lower limb ischaemia, because it is less common and because reconstructive arterial surgery is performed comparatively rarely in the arm, even for symptomatic cases of occlusive disease of the larger arteries. Nevertheless, a more systematic approach to the problems of upper limb ischaemia is needed than has generally been accorded in the past, particularly when it is remembered how important this part of the body is to the individual. Severe ischaemia in the upper limb can cause a degree of disability which far exceeds that which results from a comparable circulatory deficit in the leg, and the total loss of an arm is a tragedy from which the patient can never fully recover.

Pathophysiology

Although similar disease processes may affect the arteries of the arm and leg there are fundamental differences in pathophysiology and clinical presentation. In the leg, atherosclerosis of the larger arteries is common, and early symptoms invariably take the form of muscle effort pain (intermittent claudication) followed, often much later if at all, by colour and nutritional changes in the toes. In the arm, by contrast, atherosclerosis and other forms of chronic arterial occlusion (with the possible exception of the late effects of trauma) are less common, although atherosclerosis of the innominate and proximal subclavian arteries can be the cause of arm ischaemia (as well as of cerebral ischaemia) as has already been discussed in the first section of this chapter. It is the digital, less commonly the palmar, arteries which are frequently the first and, in many disorders, the only arteries to be affected in the upper limb; they may be narrowed or blocked by spasm, microemboli, local thrombosis, or various forms of arteritis, all of which may cause cyclical colour changes and discomfort in the fingers. The greater efficiency of the collateral circulation in the upper limb is also a significant factor in determining the difference between the effects, both pathophysiological and clinical, of ischaemia in the leg and in the arm.

Trauma is the most common single cause of severe upper limb ischaemia which it can precipitate by a variety of mechanisms: direct injury to the artery from blows, penetrating wounds or avulsion, resulting in interruption of continuity or thrombosis; spasm and arteritis of the digital and palmar arteries from vibrating tools and hypothenar hammer injury; and embolism from intrinsic trauma of the subclavian artery by a cervical rib, first rib or clavicle.

Acute ischaemia due to major embolism from the heart, or less frequently from lesions in the more proximal arteries, follows the same pattern in the arm as in the leg but is less common. Microembolism, secondary to injury or atherosclerosis, occurs more frequently in the upper limb and is often the cause of acute ischaemic attacks, mainly affecting the fingers.

Clinical Features

The commonest signs of ischaemia in the upper limb are colour changes in the fingers, which may be followed later by infection, ulceration or gangrene. These digital manifestations of arterial insufficiency are generally referred to as Raynaud's syndrome, regardless of the cause. They may herald serious underlying disease or merely be manifestations of a mild cold sensitivity of little clinical significance.

There is potential danger in using the term Raynaud's syndrome when the symptoms and signs are strictly unilateral. In most cases of Raynaud's syndrome the changes are clearly bilateral and the underlying cause benign or chronic. The diagnosis of Raynaud's syndrome may give a false sense of security to the clinician and further investigation and treatment is delayed. However, when the symptoms and signs are confined to one side the underlying cause, often a digital artery embolism, is of serious significance. The emboli may have originated in a subclavian artery damaged by compression, or from an atherosclerotic plaque in a proximal artery. With no further warning the next embolus may be larger and occlude a major artery with resulting extensive ischaemia. Many cases are delayed because the general practitioner diagnoses Raynaud's disease and prescribes vasodilator pills; this delay may lead to limb loss. Appreciation of the possible serious significance of unilateral digital ischaemia will prevent such a catastrophe by promoting urgent investigation and treatment in cases of so-called 'unilateral Raynaud's'. It is best to avoid the term 'Raynaud's syndrome' altogether when referring to unilateral digital ischaemia (UDI).

Acute ischaemia, which is invariably unilateral, can be caused by injury, major embolism, microembolism, acute thrombosis or, rarely, acute aortic dissection.

Injury and major embolism in particular can result in extensive ischaemia affecting the whole arm. The patient is suddenly aware that the limb, or part of the limb, has become lifeless and numb. The first reaction is to shake it and rub it in an attempt to bring it back to life. The fingers are white or blue and will not move. Pain is a variable feature but can be intense. Subsequent events depend, in particular, on the efficiency of the collateral circulation and the state of the distal arterial tree. Considerable improvement may occur quite spontaneously or in response to modest conservative measures if the circumstances are favourable. In others, where there is an inadequate collateral circulation or where the distal tree has already been blocked by multiple small emboli or becomes blocked by propagated thrombus, the ischaemic area rapidly turns cold, and the pallor or cyanosis changes to a characteristic mottling, followed soon afterwards by blistering of the skin and gangrene. A line of demarcation develops between dead and living skin. Muscle groups, such as the flexors of the forearm, become swollen, tender and hard and at a later point contract with resulting flexion of the appropriate joints. Peripheral pulses are reduced or absent beyond the site of arterial occlusion.

Microembolism does not initiate this sequence of events in its earlier stages. A finger or fingers may become suddenly pale, numb and cold but usually recover quite quickly though some may remain discoloured for several days. Recurrent microembolism causes a series of ischaemic attacks which may be cumulative in their effect, resulting eventually in more extensive and permanent ischaemia. The significance of recurring microembolism will be discussed later when considering the vascular complications of thoracic outlet compression.

The source of an embolus may be obvious if there is evidence of heart disease and if the embolus is a large one. The subclavian artery may be suspected if a bruit is heard over it or there is a pulsatile swelling in the supraclavicular fossa. The distribution of palpable and absent pulses is a guide to the site of impaction of a larger embolus. The introduction of Doppler ultrasound has facilitated more precise localization of blocked and patent arteries, both large and small.

Sudden thrombosis in a large or medium-sized artery affected by atherosclerosis may be suggested by a slower, possibly less dramatic onset, a previous history of vascular insufficiency in the limb, and evidence of other manifestations of atherosclerosis.

Acute aortic dissection will be suspected if the patient has chest pain and the arterial pulses in other limbs are absent or fluctuating, but differentiation from major embolism from the heart can be difficult.

Episodic symptoms and signs of ischaemia may be unilateral or bilateral. The importance of recognizing unilateral episodic ischaemia has already been stressed and will be discussed in more detail later.

Episodic digital ischaemia is the most common clinical manifestation of bilateral upper limb arterial insufficiency. It was first described by Raynaud in 1862 and has since been generally referred to as Raynaud's phenomenon. It is characterized by sequential colour changes and discomfort in the fingers of both hands on exposure to cold. Though bilateral, one side may predominate in the early stages. The sequence of colour changes, which usually begin at the ends of the fingers and spread proximally, is of pallor followed by cyanosis and then, as the circulation returns, redness. The third stage of rubor is often accompanied by tingling, burning or pain. This precise pattern is by no means always present but, whatever the sequence of symptoms and signs, the clinical picture of Raynaud's phenomenon is unmistakable. The term 'Raynaud's phenomenon' should be reserved for this episodic digital ischaemia, or 'asphyxia', as Raynaud himself described it; whereas the term 'Raynaud's syndrome' should imply the presence of bilateral digital ischaemia in any of its forms.

As time passes there may be loss of tissue with characteristic pulp atrophy and other clinical manifestations of chronic ischaemia, presently to be described.

The peripheral pulses will be present in most instances and there will be no anatomical abnormality in the supraclavicular region. There may be further clinical evidence of a connective tissue disorder or other systemic disease.

Chronic ischaemic changes occur, in advanced stages of the Raynaud's syndrome, as a delayed effect of trauma, and in severe chronic obliterative disease of the large and medium arteries. There may be the usual colour response to cold but many of the changes remain permanent or 'fixed'. Joint stiffness, cyanosis or rubor, thinning or thickening of the skin, infection, ulceration and gangrene of the fingers are usual. Aching, heaviness, muscle fatigue and loss of power of the limb (often referred to collectively as 'claudication') are a feature of advanced cases of larger artery occlusion, ischaemic signs in the fingers being less common in this group. Joint contractures due to muscle fibrosis may complicate unsuccessfully treated or neglected cases of major embolism and arterial injury. Arterial pulses will be reduced or absent in varying degree depending upon the underlying cause of the chronic ischaemia.

Causalgia, Sudeck's atrophy and other forms of sympathetic dystrophy exhibit some of the clinical features of chronic ischaemia and should be included in the differential diagnosis of painful, discoloured fingers.

Investigations

A careful history and examination will determine the cause in a number of cases. If an injury or an embolus from the heart is clearly the cause of acute ischaemia, no special investigation is necessary and operation should not be delayed. If thoracic outlet compression or proximal artery disease is suspected a radiograph of the thoracic outlet will confirm whether or not there is a bony abnormality and an arch arteriogram will help to identify the source of a non-cardiac embolus and the site, nature and extent of the arterial occlusion.

In bilateral episodic and in chronic ischaemia more time will be available for detailed investigation which should include: full blood examination, estimation of the ESR, blood viscosity and plasma fibrinogen level, serological tests for auto-antibodies, Rose–Waaler and cold agglutinins, a radiograph of the chest and, in some cases, barium examination of the gastrointestinal tract, intravenous pyelography and skin and muscle biopsy. Arch arteriography is necessary in all unilateral cases and selected bilateral cases when the source of trouble is thought to be in the proximal arteries. Distal arteriography will demonstrate the pattern of palmar and digital artery occlusion but is not diagnostic and is not necessary as a routine. Doppler ultrasound will help to identify occluded and patent segments of artery and has the virtue of being simple and non-invasive.

Causes of Upper Limb Ischaemia

Raynaud's Syndrome

The causes of Raynaud's syndrome comprise a heterogeneous group of disorders, few of which require operative treatment. The surgeon may have patients referred with ischaemia of the fingers for diagnosis by the general practitioner, or be asked for his opinion on definitive surgical treatment in highly selected cases by physician colleagues. Reconstructive arterial surgery has no place in the treatment of these disorders (except in unilateral cases when the term 'Raynaud's' should not be used) and upper thoracic sympathectomy has a limited role. The surgeon is often required merely to deal with local sepsis or to remove tissue for biopsy.

PATHOPHYSIOLOGY. A list of groups of disorders which may be responsible for Raynaud's syndrome is shown in *Table* 52.1. The causes are: primary (where there is no associated digital artery disease), and secondary (where there is an underlying disease of the digital arteries). It is clear that the pathological changes which can occur from such a diversity of causes will be extremely variable.

The response of the digital arteries to cooling varies in different individuals, most people experience colour changes in their fingers on exposure to cold at some time in their lives. The colour changes are due to spasm of the digital arteries resulting from vasomotor sympathetic activity which is fully reversible. Although vasomotor activity plays an important part in all cases of Raynaud's syndrome it is not the basic underlying cause, even in primary Raynaud's

Table 52.1 Causes of Raynaud's syndrome

Primary
Constitutional disturbance of the finger circulation (e.g. hereditary cold fingers, acrocyanosis)
Raynaud's diseases (Lewis' 'local fault' in the digital arteries)
Secondary
Connective tissue disorders (e.g. systemic sclerosis, systemic lupus erythematosus, polyarteritis nodosa, rheumatoid arthritis, dermatomyositis, polymyositis)
Atherosclerosis
Thromboangiitis obliterans
Cold injury (e.g. frostbite)
Occupation disorder (hypothenar hammer syndrome, vibration white finger syndrome)
Haematological disease (e.g. polycythaemia vera)
Drugs (e.g. ergot, beta-blockers, contraceptive pill)
Malignant disease
Others (e.g. serum hepatitis, chronic renal failure)

syndrome. Sympathetic vasomotor overactivity is not now considered to be a major cause.

In some individuals the normal sympathetic vasomotor response to cooling is exaggerated (constitutional Raynaud's syndrome) and in others there is a 'local fault' in the digital arteries which is independent of sympathetic vasomotor control (Raynaud's disease). Both of these disorders follow a benign course, but in Raynaud's disease some endothelial proliferation occasionally occurs in the digital arteries though this does not lead to nutritional changes in the fingers. If ulceration or gangrene does occur in patients with Raynaud's disease then the diagnosis should be questioned. With the availability of improved diagnostic techniques more patients, thought originally to have Raynaud's disease, have subsequently been found to have an associated connective-tissue disease. It is now suggested that all patients with Raynaud's syndrome should be regarded as running a high risk of having an underlying autoimmune disease.

Secondary Raynaud's syndrome follows a less benign course than primary Raynaud's syndrome and permanent ischaemic changes in the fingers are common. The different diseases which can cause secondary Raynaud's syndrome precipitate digital ischaemia by a variety of pathological processes in the digital arteries or circulating blood, but the end result is always the same, digital artery occlusion leading eventually to ischaemia and the possibility of infection, ulceration and gangrene. Vasculitis is common to all autoimmune disorders, the histological features of which vary considerably in the individual diseases. Atherosclerosis in the digital arteries, rare before the age of 50 years, causes thrombosis which is characteristically segmental in distribution, but this is not specific to the disease; segmental thrombosis is also seen in thromboangiitis obliterans, vibrating tool disease and in frostbite years after the original injury. The role of microembolism in digital ischaemia has already been discussed. Increased blood viscosity may be an important factor in some of the diseases which cause Raynaud's syndrome but probably not in Raynaud's disease.

To summarize: although the basic pathophysiology of Raynaud's syndrome remains unsolved it is considered that there are two fundamental mechanisms at play. In some cases there is an exaggerated vasoconstrictor response to cold by otherwise essentially normal digital arteries (primary Raynaud's syndrome) and in others there is a normal cold-induced vasoconstrictor response acting upon a diseased artery in which there is reduced blood flow due to luminal narrowing or obstruction (secondary Raynaud's syndrome). Most authorities are now in favour of this latter mechanism in the majority of cases.

CLINICAL FEATURES. The clinical recognition of Raynaud's syndrome offers little difficulty. The story of colour changes in the fingers on exposure to cold or occasionally by emotion are instantly recognizable although the exact pattern may vary. The distribution of colour changes may differ amongst the fingers, and the thumbs are not affected.

The age, sex and occupation of the patient are noted and a careful history taken with particular regard to duration of symptoms, response to cold and exposure, previous injury, acute ischaemic episodes, drug taking, and the presence of signs or symptoms, such as joint swellings and dysphagia, which might indicate the presence of an autoimmune disease. If the patient has used vibrating tools during the course of his occupation, vibration white finger (a prescribed industrial disease since April 1985), will be suspected.

Examination of the patient may reveal very little, particularly in early cases and in the warm environment of the examination room. It may be necessary to see the patient on several occasions before any signs in the hands are observed. Artificial exposure to cold is not always successful in reproducing colour changes. In more advanced cases there may be tapering of the finger ends, ulceration or gangrene. Coarsening of the skin of the fingers, joint stiffness, subcutaneous calcification, telangiectasis of fingers, neck and face, puckering of the periorbital skin, and pinching of the nose will suggest scleroderma. Raynaud's syndrome in association with rheumatoid arthritis is often an early feature so that joint changes may not necessarily be found in patients with this disease. The peripheral pulses will be normal unless there is a unilateral cause for the ischaemia (if the symptoms and signs appear to be unilateral the cardiac state must be assessed and the neck examined for a cervical rib, subclavian artery occlusion or aneurysm).

When a patient manifesting Raynaud's phenomenon is a young woman with a long history of poor circulation and in whom there are no nutritional changes in the fingers, Raynaud's disease is the probable cause. However, if the symptoms and signs first appear in middle age a connective-tissue disorder is likely. The underlying cause of Raynaud's syndrome may be impossible to determine on clinical grounds alone; fortunately there are now available a wide range of investigations which will help to unravel this diverse syndrome.

INVESTIGATIONS. Blood is taken for routine examination and other tests including estimation of the ESR, which is characteristically raised in autoimmune disease; estimation of the plasma fibrinogen level and blood viscosity; a search is made for cryoproteins, paraproteins and cold agglutinins and a full immunological survey for auto-antibodies is carried out. Radiological examination of the chest and an electrocardiogram are also done routinely. In suspected cases of systemic sclerosis radiographs of the hands, feet and elbows to detect calcification, and barium studies of the gastrointestinal tract and an intravenous pyelogram to demonstrate interference with smooth muscle activity, are done. Microscopy of the nail folds may reveal characteristic changes in the capillary loops in connective-tissue disorders. Skin, muscle or renal biopsy may be diagnostic in systemic sclerosis, dermatomyositis, polymyositis and polyarteritis nodosa. Brachial and arch arteriography have a limited role in the investigation of Raynaud's syndrome but are important if the symptoms and signs appear to be unilateral.

TREATMENT. Clearly it is important to determine the underlying cause of the syndrome if at all possible before treatment is given.

If a diagnosis of primary Raynaud's disease is made then little active treatment is necessary and the patient can be reassured and given a favourable prognosis. General advice on the care of the hands, the avoidance of unnecessary exposure to cold and damp, and the importance of not smoking is emphasized. In some circumstances a change of occupation may be wise. Vasodilator drugs are often prescribed but they are not generally effective. The benefits of upper thoracic sympathectomy are of short duration; operation now plays little part in the treatment of primary Raynaud's syndrome.

The larger group of patients with secondary Raynaud's syndrome due to autoimmune disease poses a greater problem in management. In the majority of cases response to treatment is disappointing or shortlived, and the progress of the disease is depressingly downhill. Vasodilators are of little value, though the calcium channel-blocking agent, nifedipine (Adalat), a potent vasodilator, in a dose of 10 mg t.d.s., has proved helpful and side-effects are few. Unfortunately, the manufacturers (Bayer) warn against its use in women of child-bearing age; this is disappointing when it is realized that 60–90% of Raynaud's sufferers are women. Temporary relief may be obtained from oral guanethidine and phenoxybenzamine or from intra-arterial reserpine or guanethidine. Injection of 15–20 mg of guanethidine into a dorsal hand vein with the arterial circulation interrupted by a tourniquet for about 20 min is a more acceptable procedure than intra-arterial therapy when treatment can be repeated. Prostaglandins have been used with beneficial effects in severe vasospastic disease and corticosteroids may be helpful in early cases of systemic sclerosis. Reduction of plasma fibrinogen and the lowering of blood viscosity, either by defibrination with snake venom enzymes or by plasma exchange, may be useful; plasma exchange has been reported to give encouraging early results, with healing of digital ulcers, reduction in pain and reduced frequency of attacks. Upper thoracic sympathectomy can be helpful in patients with painful ischaemia due to thrombosis of the digital arteries secondary to atherosclerosis and thromboangiitis obliterans, but rarely for those with an autoimmune disease.

In an acute exacerbation of Raynaud's syndrome, which often punctuates the slow downhill course, treatment in hospital with intravenous heparin and low molecular weight dextran has proved helpful in some cases, though the improvement is generally of short duration. Frostbite, a relatively uncommon cause of Raynaud's syndrome, should be treated with heparin, low molecular weight dextran and corticosteroids. Other causes of secondary Raynaud's syndrome, such as polycythaemia vera and malignant disease, will require specific treatment. Patients with vibration tool disease should be encouraged to modify their occupation.

Occlusion of the Distal Subclavian, Axillary and Brachial Arteries

The commonest causes of occlusion in these arteries, in order of frequency, are: injury, embolism and atherosclerosis. Unsuccessfully treated or untreated cases of injury and embolism can result in severe symptomatic occlusion in spite of the usual efficiency of the upper limb collateral circulation. This underlines the importance of urgent and effective treatment in the acute stage.

INJURY. Reference has already been made to the fact that trauma is the commonest cause of upper limb ischaemia. The principles of management of arterial injuries in the upper limb are the same as those for similar injuries in the leg and elsewhere. Arterial injuries are considered in detail in Chapter 55 but there are some features particular to the arm which merit special consideration here.

Diagnostic arterial catheterization of the brachial artery has emerged in recent years as the most frequent type of injury to result in symptomatic arterial occlusion of the arm. An awareness of the problem should lead to a reduction in the incidence of injury and of subsequent chronic ischaemia by the adoption of better techniques and by ensuring early surgical intervention in the acute stage.

Injuries in the shoulder region, a feature of motor cycle accidents, can be accompanied by severe stretching or avulsion of the brachial plexus. The resultant neurological complications may overshadow an associated injury of the subclavian or axillary arteries. An avulsion injury of one of these arteries may be remarkably silent at first, with little or no bleeding and with the distal blood flow maintained through an effective collateral circulation. The ends of the artery retract and the adventitia closes over thus sealing the vessel. Significant bleeding may be absent or delayed but if it does occur large amounts of blood may accumulate in the axilla or thorax before becoming clinically obvious. If in cases of brachial plexus injury the distal pulses are reduced or missing, a damaged subclavian or axillary artery must be suspected and surgical exploration carried out as soon as possible. In doubtful cases arteriography is helpful.

Supracondylar fractures of the humerus, particularly in children, may be accompanied by loss of or diminution of the wrist pulses. Spasm must never be presumed to be the cause of the arterial occlusion. If there is not an immediate return of normal pulsation after reduction of the fracture urgent exploration of the brachial artery should be undertaken. Delay will be discouraged if the tragic consequences of a Volkmann's ischaemic contracture are remembered.

Intra-arterial injection of anaesthetic drugs remains a constant threat in spite of the great care exercised by anaesthetists. Heparin (10 000–15 000 units) should be administered immediately, preferably through the same needle as the anaesthetic was given. This should be followed by a continuous intravenous infusion of low molecular weight dextran and heparin for several days.

The long-continued use of crutches may lead to thrombosis and chronic occlusion of the axillary artery. It should rarely be encountered nowadays if correct preventive measures are adopted.

MAJOR EMBOLISM. No longer should major embolism of the upper limb be treated conservatively. Emergency embolectomy should be undertaken even in the very ill patient, using local anaesthesia, if necessary. The earlier the operation is done the more likely will the circulation be restored to normal; failure to act quickly may result in loss of the arm.

CHRONIC OCCLUSIVE DISEASE of the larger arm arteries from whatever cause will require surgical treatment if ischaemic symptoms are disabling. This may be upper thoracic sympathectomy or arterial reconstruction. The most favoured reconstructive procedure is a saphenous or basilic vein bypass. Excellent long-term results have been achieved. It has been found that after reconstructive operations for atherosclerotic occlusion in the arm, progress or acceleration of the disease does not occur as it tends to do in the leg.

The effects of intrinsic injury due to compression of the subclavian artery will now be considered separately.

Thoracic Outlet Compression

PATHOPHYSIOLOGY. We are concerned principally with the vascular effects of thoracic outlet compression; the much more common neurological effects will be referred to only briefly.

Compression of the second or third parts of the subclavian artery may be caused by a cervical rib, the clavicle, an abnormal first rib (congenital abnormality, fracture with callus formation or tumour), or the scalenus anterior muscle. The commonest of these causes is a complete bony cervical rib, the artery being nipped between the rib and the scalenus anterior muscle. Only rarely does the scalenus anterior muscle itself cause narrowing. The artery may also be compressed between an abnormal first rib and the clavicle or between a normal first rib and a clavicle deformed by a tumour or previous injury. Although compression of tissues between a normal clavicle and a normal first rib may cause pain, paraesthesiae and muscular weakness (costoclavicular syndrome) or venous obstruction, the subclavian artery is not affected. The axillary artery may be compressed by the pectoralis minor muscle but this must be exceedingly rare.

Compression causes gradual narrowing of the subclavian artery which in its early stages is symptomless. The arterial wall thickens due either to fibrosis or to the development of atherosclerosis, adding to the mechanical narrowing. The artery may suddenly occlude completely due to thrombosis (*Fig.* 52.5) or, alternatively, slowly dilate beyond the stenosis. Dilatation is due to turbulence of the blood flow which causes lateral stresses on the wall of the artery just beyond the stenotic area, eventually leading to the formation of an aneurysm. On the inner wall of the post-stenotic aneurysm small thrombi may collect which can subsequently dislodge forming emboli (*Fig.* 52.6). Showers of small emboli settling in the digital arteries will cause ischaemic episodes which superficially resemble Raynaud's phenomenon, but the symptoms and signs are unilateral, often only one or two fingers are affected, and the period of ischaemia is longer than in a typical Raynaud attack. If a detached piece of thrombus from an occluded subclavian artery or from a post-stenotic aneurysm is large, the radial, ulnar, brachial or even axillary arteries may be blocked (*Fig.* 52.7). Repeated or multiple small emboli may occlude the medium-sized arteries, such as the radial and ulnar, by aggregation. The aneurysm itself may become completely occluded by thrombus.

Sudden thrombosis of the subclavian artery results in propagated clot extending proximally and distally as far as the next major collateral. Proximally this may be to the vertebral artery orifice and if pieces of thrombus break off they may pass up the vertebral artery and cause infarction in the hind brain or, less frequently, pass up the common carotid artery to cause retinal and hemisphere ischaemia. Distal propagation of thrombus may be extensive and can be difficult to remove at operation, particularly if there has been delay of more than 24 h between the onset of occlusion and exploration.

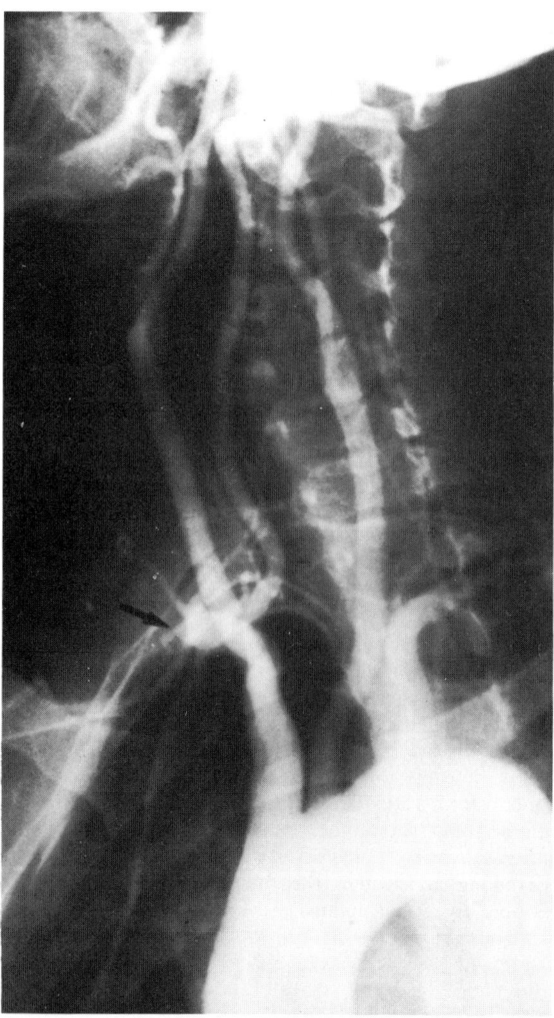

Fig. 52.5 Arch arteriogram showing complete occlusion of the first part of the right subclavian artery due to compression by a cervical rib.

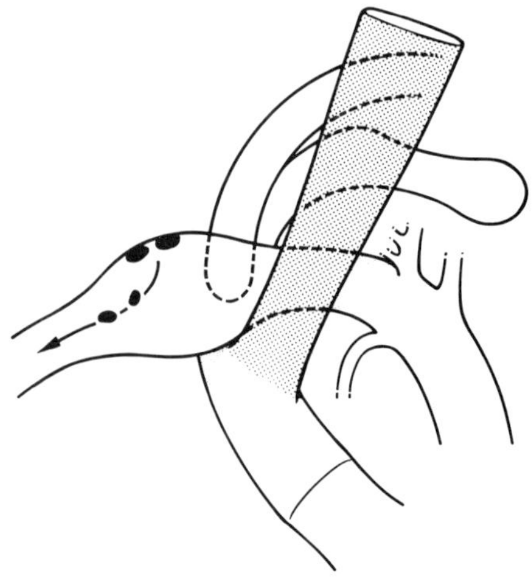

Fig. 52.6 Diagram showing post-stenotic dilatation of the subclavian artery secondary to compression by a cervical rib. Mural thrombus is present in the aneurysm, portions of which may break off to form emboli.

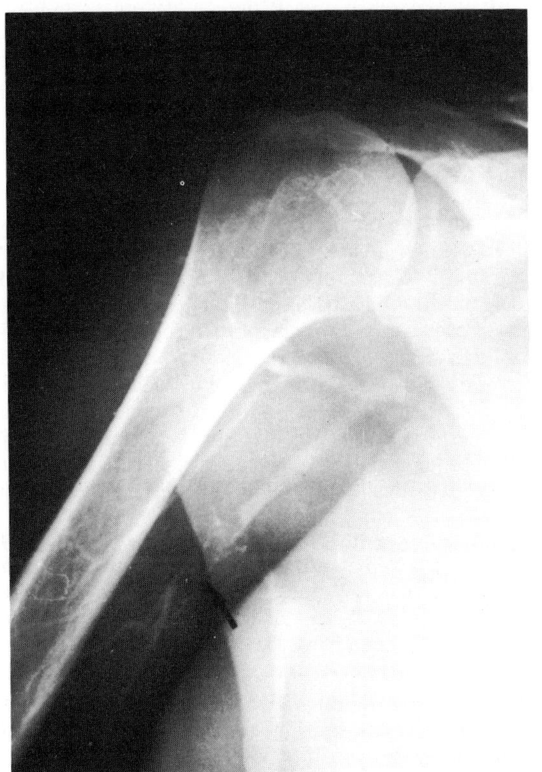

Fig. 52.7 Same patient as in *Fig.* 52.5. The brachial artery has filled through collaterals and emboli are shown within its lumen. These are detached portions of the thrombus which occluded the first part of the subclavian artery.

Thrombosis of the subclavian and axillary veins may result from thoracic outlet compression and is a more frequent occurrence than arterial thrombosis from the same cause.

CLINICAL FEATURES. These are neurological or vascular; only rarely do they occur together in the same individual. Neurological symptoms and signs result from stretching or compression of components of the brachial plexus—most commonly the lower roots—by a cervical rib or abnormal first rib. Pain and paraesthesiae in the fingers, hand or arm, and muscular weakness and wasting are common neurological features. They must be differentiated from similar symptoms and signs resulting from cervical spondylosis, cervical disc protrusion or carpal tunnel compression.

Vascular symptoms and signs are due to pressure on the subclavian artery and are strictly unilateral. They may vary from recurrent episodes of minor digital ischaemia to sudden massive ischaemia of the whole limb. Episodes of ischaemia are likely to increase in frequency and severity, each one adding to the residual ischaemic effects of previous attacks.

A cervical rib or other bony abnormality may be visible or palpable just above the clavicle. There may be a palpable thrill or bruit over the subclavian artery. A symptomless pulsatile swelling may be the only clinical feature. The subclavian and more distal pulses may be reduced or absent and the blood pressure in the affected arm will be lower than the opposite normal side, or may be unrecordable. Movements of the arm, shoulder, head and neck may cause temporary disappearance of the radial pulse. This is a not uncommon finding in normal individuals so it must be regarded with some caution; it is only likely to be significant if quite minor alterations in posture result in disappearance of the radial pulse.

INVESTIGATIONS. Radiographs of the neck, shoulder and thoracic outlet followed by arch arteriography should be routine in all cases of thoracic outlet compression associated with definite or possible vascular involvement. Patients presenting with venous obstruction require phlebography. Nerve conduction studies and electromyography are often done in neurological cases but some authorities discount their value and emphasize that clinical assessment remains the most important factor in diagnosis and the choice of treatment.

TREATMENT. Patients with neurological symptoms only should be treated by correction of faulty posture and with shoulder girdle strengthening exercises. There is often an accompanying psychological element and, as the neurological symptoms and signs themselves may be difficult to differentiate, the surgeon should seek the advice of a neurologist before embarking on surgical treatment. When surgical treatment is necessary, resection of an abnormal bony structure such as a cervical rib plus resection of the first rib is the recommended procedure. When there is no bony abnormality resection of the first rib alone is advocated.

The presence of vascular complications demands immediate attention; the need for surgical treatment is urgent. The aims of operation are: to remove the compressing structure or structures, to repair the subclavian artery and to restore the distal circulation by removing emboli and propagated thrombus. All of these can generally be done through a single transverse incision one finger's breadth above the clavicle though, on occasions, it may be necessary to extend the wound downwards and to divide the clavicle. The longer the delay between onset of symptoms and operation the more difficult will it be to clear the distal arterial tree. A balloon catheter passed distally through a subclavian arteriotomy in the neck may be all that is necessary in early cases; others may require additional arteriotomies lower down. Multiple emboli and adherent thrombus, particularly in the radial and ulnar arteries, may be impossible to remove and an upper thoracic sympathectomy will be necessary in addition to the local repair of the subclavian artery.

The type of subclavian artery reconstruction selected will depend upon the operative findings. A post-stenotic aneurysm should be excised and continuity restored by end-to-end anastomosis or by the interposition of a vein graft. Lesser degrees of dilatation can be corrected by simple arteriotomy and excision of part of the wall, removing at the same time any mural thrombus present. Stenosis, if not severe, may not require repair but nevertheless the artery should be opened. There have been a number of case reports of the unexpected finding of unsuspected, impalpable thrombus in the lumen of the artery in cases of quite minor narrowing and where the thrombus was not visible on preoperative arteriograms. Severe narrowing will require arteriotomy and vein patch, thromboendarterectomy or excision and vein graft replacement.

The Symptomless Cervical Rib

A cervical rib which is not causing symptoms should generally be left alone. A cervical rib occurs in 0·4% of the population (70% are bilateral) but is only symptomatic in

10% of instances; most individuals with a cervical rib go through life without complications from the rib. However, there are circumstances where serious consideration must be given to removing a symptomless rib. If a patient with bilateral ribs has had vascular complications from one rib it is generally advisable to remove the opposite symptomless rib. A somewhat similar situation arises when a close relative, often a brother or sister, of a patient who has suffered vascular complications is found on routine screening to have a cervical rib. The following case illustrates this problem:

A girl, aged 14 years, was admitted to hospital with ischaemia of the hind brain due to vertebral artery embolism from a subclavian artery thrombosis secondary to a cervical rib. After a difficult and anxious time the patient made a complete neurological recovery without the need for surgical intervention. The offending rib was removed soon afterwards and the damaged portion of subclavian artery replaced by a saphenous vein graft. The parents were understandably concerned when a younger sister was found on radiography to have bilateral complete cervical ribs and they requested that the ribs be removed. This was done and she made an uneventful recovery. When seen recently, several years after operation, she was symptom-free and expressed relief that the ribs had been removed when she was young.

Aneurysm

Aneurysms below the level of the clavicle are rare, most of those described have been traumatic, mycotic or congenital in origin. The reason for the low incidence of atherosclerotic aneurysm in the arm is obscure but is probably related to the fact that atherosclerosis in the upper limb arteries is comparatively uncommon and possibly due to the absence of any particular points of fixation of the arteries below the level of the clavicle.

Most aneurysms of whatever type should be excised because of the danger of rupture, thrombosis or embolism; continuity is restored by direct anastomosis or by means of a vein graft.

Arteriovenous Fistula

Arteriovenous fistulas may be congenital, acquired (mostly post-traumatic) or therapeutic. Arteriovenous fistula of the limbs is fully covered in Chapter 78; therefore the subject will not be discussed any further in this section.

Axillary/Subclavian Vein Thrombosis

Massive venous thrombosis (phlegmasia caerulea dolens) is a rare cause of ischaemia of the arm. The most commonly encountered venous problem is thrombosis of the axillary or subclavian veins which may occur apparently spontaneously, or in association with thoracic outlet compression, or following excessive or unusual use of the arm ('effort' thrombosis). This latter cause is illustrated by the following case history:

A bank manager, aged 35 years, was admitted to hospital with swelling and cyanosis of the right arm which he noticed immediately after completing a strenuous game of squash. The patient stated that the arm felt heavy and numb but there was no pain and he could move it normally. Examination revealed a blue, swollen right arm in which the subcutaneous veins of the elbow, upper arm and shoulder were distended. There was no abnormality in the neck and the arterial pulses were normal. The axillary vein (which in some cases can be felt as a tender cord) was not palpable. Radiographs of the neck and shoulder were normal. The patient was given heparin and low molecular weight dextran by intravenous drip for 5 days followed by oral warfarin for 3 months. Full recovery followed.

No special investigation is necessary in the majority of cases. In refractory and chronic cases, infra-red photography may demonstrate more clearly the pattern of distended veins which are acting as collaterals. Phlebography may be helpful in determining the site, extent and nature of the venous block. Only occasionally is operation necessary, either to excise a compressing structure, such as a cervical rib or first rib, or to remove thrombus from within the vein.

Cyanosis and oedema of the hand ('oedème bleu') may occur as a result of a reluctance to use the limb after quite trivial injury. It is seen most commonly in young hysterical women but may be found in men, particularly if litigation is pending. Occasionally it is self-inflicted, the patient causing swelling of the arm by tying string or a band around it. Treatment must be directed to the underlying psychological problem and operation studiously avoided.

THE WAY AHEAD

In extracranial cerebral artery disease the wider use of non-invasive methods of investigation will enable more information to be gained about the natural history of the atherosclerotic lesion. The current prophylactic element in the surgical treatment of transient ischaemic attacks may be extended to include some cases of asymptomatic internal carotid artery stenosis, particularly those with tight lesions, if it can be confirmed that operation significantly lowers the incidence of stroke in such patients. On the other hand, controlled trials presently being conducted comparing surgical and non-surgical treatment of carotid artery stenosis are awaited with interest; the results might indicate that non-operative treatment should play a more prominent role in the future. Improved ultrasonic imaging will enable the more dangerous tightly stenotic and ulcerating lesions to be detected with increased frequency and clarity than at present, thereby reducing the need for routine arteriography with its greater risks. Wider availability of digital subtraction arteriography will lead to a more detailed knowledge of the morphology of atherosclerosis and should allow an improved assessment of the cerebral collateral circulation; it may replace conventional angiography in the selection of patients for surgical treatment.

In the field of upper limb ischaemia the most likely advance will be in the further elucidation of the numerous causes of secondary Raynaud's syndrome by means of improved immunological testing. It is to be hoped that the causes of the many underlying autoimmune diseases will become known and that prevention of some and more effective treatment of others will become possible. Microvascular techniques will extend the range of arterial reconstruction in the arm to include the palmar and digital arteries. As a direct result of the developments mentioned the prognosis in vascular disorders of the neck and upper limb is likely to be improved significantly over the next few years.

53 *Aorto-iliac Disease*

D. Charlesworth

Arteriosclerosis affects all parts of the aorta but the more gross manifestations of the process are seen predominantly at the bifurcation of the abdominal aorta and in the common iliac arteries. This portion of the aorta is less elastic than the thoracic aorta, its wall contains more collagen and the geometry of the bifurcation may create, in certain circumstances, secondary flow phenomena which in turn produce rapid oscillations in the stresses on the wall. The response of the wall to these stresses may be an alteration in the ratio of smooth muscle to collagen, increased fibrosis, and consequently changes in the transport of lipoproteins across the wall. Whatever the mechanism the result is the same, the diameter of cross-section of the lumens of the aorta and iliac arteries are reduced and flow, initially at high velocities and later even when the patient is at rest, is reduced. In some patients, and for reasons which are obscure, the aorta dilates between the renal arteries proximally and the bifurcation and an aneurysm is formed.

The vast majority of patients who have generalized arteriosclerosis and in whom the abdominal aorta and its bifurcation are involved fall into one of three broad categories:

Group 1 Those patients in whom the bifurcation is affected and the distal vessels are virtually normal.
Group 2 Those who have generalized arteriosclerosis with occlusions and/or stenoses in both the aorto-iliac segment and the superficial femoral arteries.
Group 3 Those who have abdominal aortic aneurysms.

Group 1. The first group of patients tend to present with symptoms in their fourth and fifth decades, 10 years or more before the second group develop symptoms. The presenting symptom is intermittent claudication, which commonly affects both legs, with pain in the calf, thigh and buttocks. In men this symptom may be accompanied by impotence (Leriche syndrome). The prognosis is poor, about 40% of such patients can be expected to lose a leg due to gangrene within 5–10 years and the majority also have coronary artery disease. The incidence of hyperlipidaemia is much higher in this group of claudicants than in those who present in their sixth decade.

The characteristic clinical findings are absent or diminished femoral pulses. A thrill or bruit also suggests a stenosis proximal to the point at which the artery is examined. The diagnosis can be made from the history and clinical findings and in cases of doubt from investigations. The differential diagnosis includes sciatica from a prolapsed intervertebral disc, or spinal stenosis, arthrosis and metastases in the spine.

Simple non-invasive tests may help, ankle/arm pressure ratios of less than one would be considered abnormal; and analyses of the Doppler shifted ultrasound waveforms recorded after insonnation of the common femoral arteries may reveal a reduction in pulsatility (energy).

Management

This depends entirely on the severity of the symptoms and the prognosis. A young man with symptoms can be expected to get worse slowly but unless the symptoms interfere with the quality of life there is no immediate indication for operation. One may expect some improvement if the patient stops smoking, loses weight and where appropriate, e.g. in hyperlipidaemia, alters his diet. If the symptoms are severe, affect the patient's lifestyle or there is no evidence of improvement after a period of 6–12 months' observation it is reasonable to recommend operation.

Investigations will include a careful check on general health including an electrocardiogram. Many centres particularly in the USA now recommend more sophisticated tests of cardiac function because of the high incidence of coronary artery disease and because deaths associated with the operation are, in the vast majority of instances, due to myocardial infarction.

Before embarking on an operation it is essential to know whether or not the patient has angina and/or has had a myocardial infarct. If the patient is known to have ischaemic heart disease it is appropriate to assess the severity. A cardiologist should consider whether the patient is suitable for a coronary artery bypass, and whether, if immediate operation is necessary, the anaesthetist is confident he can manage the problems. A further degree of difficulty arises from the fact that many patients have coronary artery disease but have no symptoms, and the question arises, if a screening test for coronary artery disease shows it to be present, what should be done?

Opinions vary considerably as to the best way of managing patients who have atherosclerosis in both peripheral and coronary arteries. Policy varies from an aggressive one of recommending coronary artery bypass for even those patients who have covert cardiac disease to one in which only patients with severe symptoms are investigated. It is sound practice to work closely with cardiologists, cardiac surgeons and anaesthetists, then to discuss each patient individually before deciding on a particular course of action.

The essential investigation in the case of patients with diffuse disease is an aortogram, done by the translumbar route, or by retrograde catheterization, or by intravenous angiography with computer enhancement of the image DVA. The radiologist's choice is a matter of personal preference and the practical difficulties of using the Seldinger technique in a person who has an obstruction in the iliac arteries.

From the angiograms the surgeon needs to know:

1. The precise site and extent of the block.
2. The state of the arteries proximal to the block, in particular the condition of the renal and mesenteric arteries.
3. The state of the arteries downstream.

(In the case of an isolated lesion in the aorta the arteries downstream are, by definition, normal; the implications of multisegmental disease will be discussed later.)

Operation

The choice of operation is modified by the patient's general condition, his age, extent of disease and the prognosis. Essentially the choice lies between endarterectomy and bypass, with, in some circumstances, balloon angioplasty or laser angioplasty as alternatives. A bypass procedure gives excellent results both in terms of function and in the duration of 'cure'. Usually all three arteries, aorta and both common iliacs are affected, even if there is a complete block in only one, and hence replacing all three simultaneously with a bifurcated graft is reasonable. One can anticipate that 90–95% of bifurcation grafts will remain patent for over five years and over 70% over ten years. When only one iliac artery is bypassed it is necessary to replace the contralateral one in a large percentage of patients within a few years.

The surgical approach to the aortic bifurcation is usually transperitoneal and a prosthesis made from Teflon or Dacron is used. Such prostheses are made from a woven or knitted material and in the latter case a velour knit produces a material which is both strong and porous. The dimensions of the prosthesis are chosen to match the patient's own arteries, commonly 16 mm trunk with two 8 mm diameter limbs. The straight part of the prosthesis is joined to the aorta below the renal arteries either end to end, or end to side, and the limbs to either the common iliacs or to the common femorals according to the extent of the atheroma. The site, at which the distal anastomosis is made, makes no difference to the results provided that the external iliac artery is free from atheroma when an aorto-iliac graft is inserted. The mortality from this operation is between 1 and 2%, death, in most cases, follows a postoperative myocardial infarction.

Endarterectomy is appropriate when there is a short, limited block in one iliac artery. This may be done through an arteriotomy—so-called open endarterectomy, or 'closed' where a wire loop is used to strip out a core of atheroma (*Figs*. 53.1, 53.2). In either case the artery may be closed directly or a patch inserted (an angioplasty). The results are good but in general are less durable than bypass and the modern tendency is to do a bypass by choice. It is possible to dilate an artery using a balloon (balloon angioplasty), a technique which has gained popularity since the introduction of carefully engineered balloons of finite diameter. The technique is particularly useful when there is a short stenosis

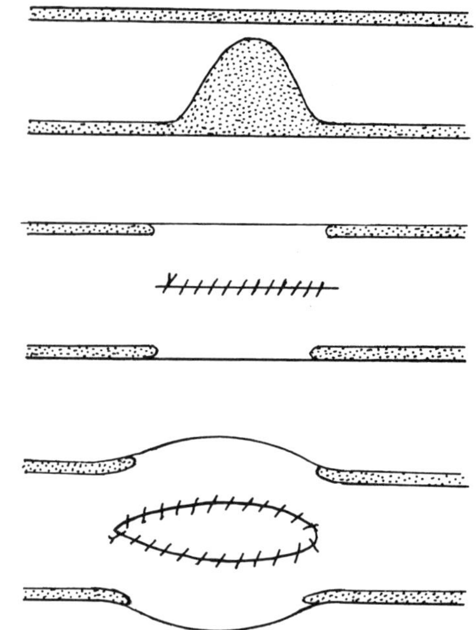

Fig. 53.1 Demonstrates the principles of an endarterectomy in which the atheromatous plaque is removed. The arteriotomy may be simply closed by a suture or deliberately widened by an angioplasty, using vein or synthetic materials.

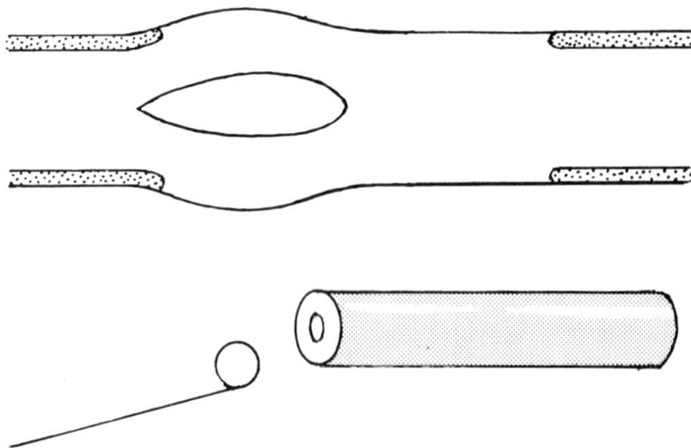

Fig. 53.2 Demonstrates the principle of the ring stripper which produces a core of atheromatous material from an occluded vessel. The instrument is introduced via a longitudinal arteriotomy.

in a large artery and the patient is thought to be unfit for operation.

It is difficult to give precise figures for the results of percutaneous transluminal angioplasty in the circumstances we are considering. A substantial number of patients have been followed up but in the majority of cases the patients had 'multisegmental' problems and insufficient data is produced to allow separate analyses of those with an isolated iliac or aortic occlusion. One can expect 90% patency after an angioplasty with negligible mortality and a low 2·5–5% incidence of complications. Cumulative patency rates of 90% at one year and 80% at three years are reported.

A recent development is the use of lasers in angioplasty. Precisely controlled pulses of laser energy are directed at atheromatous plaques the process being controlled by X-rays or done under direct vision (fibreoptic arterioscopy).

Management of Patients in Group 2

The essential feature of these patients is that arteriosclerosis is widespread—so-called 'multisegmental disease'. These patients are usually in their sixth or seventh decade (average age of onset of symptoms of claudication in men is 64 years).

The demands they make of their legs and their expectations vary considerably and the surgeon's approach is usually to 'wait and see'. Approximately 40% of patients in this age group have intermittent claudication which improves with time, i.e. as the collateral circulation improves. Operation is indicated for those who have symptoms of pregangrene—pain in the feet when lying horizontal, 'rest pain'—or who deteriorate progressively and find their symptoms intolerable.

The essential investigations are similar to those for Group 1 patients. However, the presence of ischaemic heart disease or respiratory disease is not regarded as an absolute contraindication to operation. Patients who have ischaemic feet, with pain at rest and patches of frank gangrene face an amputation and the morbidity associated with mid-thigh amputation outweighs by far that of even the most extensive reconstruction.

Whilst claudication occurs in patients who have an occlusion in the iliac or superficial femoral arteries, rest pain is more usually associated with an occlusion at two points in the arterial tree, e.g. both the aorto-iliac segment and superficial femoral arteries.

The surgeon has several options open to him, and his choice is influenced by his wish to achieve the best possible results without mortality or morbidity. Usually he achieves this by repairing the proximal block and then waits to see the effect before considering repair of the distal block (*Fig.* 53.3):

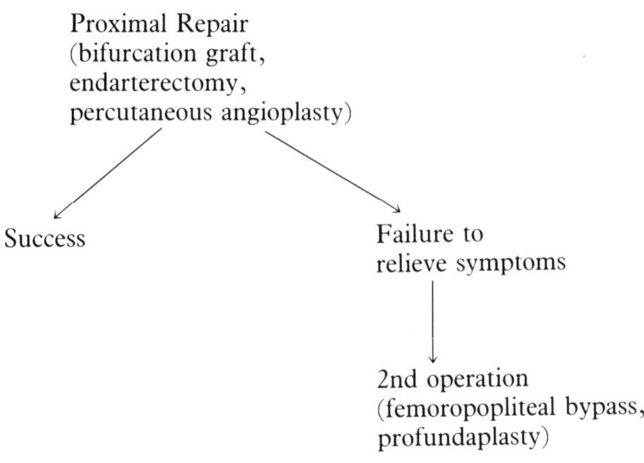

Obviously it is both possible and desirable to combine some of these procedures and the usual combinations are:

A. Transluminal angioplasty plus femoropopliteal bypass.
B. Transluminal angioplasty plus profundaplasty.
C. Aortofemoral bypass plus profundaplasty.
   The majority of reconstructions of this type remain patent but in as many as 50% the symptoms remain unchanged.
D. Aortofemoral bypass plus femoropopliteal bypass.
   This operation, which gives excellent results, is a formidable one and suited only to very experienced vascular surgeons.

When the aorta and iliac arteries are stenosed and this is combined with an occlusion in the arteries downstream it is helpful to have some objective evidence of the dynamic effect of the upstream stenosis. Patients who have 'multisegmental disease' and who complain of intermittent claudication present a difficult problem, because it is often difficult to know which of two or more stenoses is the principal constraint on the circulation. Tests which illustrate the topography of the arteries, angiograms etc., may reveal a stenosis, the dynamic effects of which can only be guessed at. What is needed in these circumstances are tests of function.

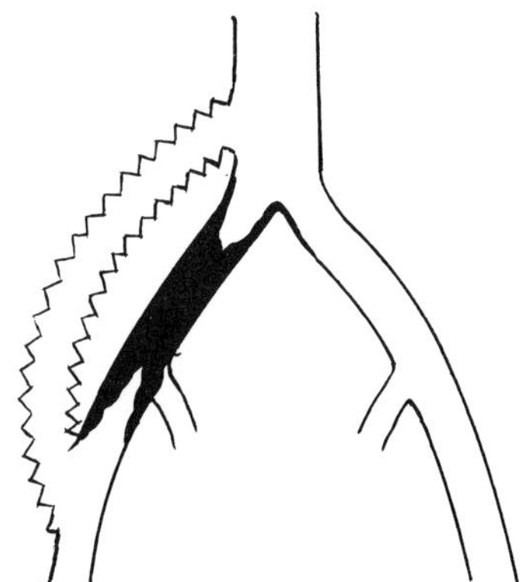

Fig. 53.3 Shows a unilateral aorto-iliac bypass graft for an occluded common iliac segment.

1. Measurements of arterial pressure. The difference in pressure between two points in an artery is influenced by the velocity of flow and the dimensions of any stenosis in the artery. Advantage is taken of this in the papaverine test. Pressures in the aorta and common femoral arteries are recorded simultaneously both before and after the rate of flow has been increased by an injection of papaverine. A difference of over 10 mmHg at rest and 25 mmHg after papaverine is taken to indicate the presence of a 'significant' stenosis.

Systolic pressure at the knee or ankle can be compared with that at a point of reference in the arm and the difference expressed as a ratio, the ankle/arm pressure index. It is a useful means of identifying an occlusion but is of little help in identifying which of two lesions has the greater dynamic effect, and one cannot distinguish at what level an occlusion lies on the basis of this test alone. A ratio of less than 1 is taken to be abnormal, patients who have pain at rest usually have lower values than claudicants but there is considerable overlap.

2. When an artery is insonnated by a beam of ultrasound the sound waves are scattered, those which are scattered from a moving object (i.e. red cell) are reflected at a different wavelength, the Doppler shift. The Doppler shift frequency is a measure of the velocity of the blood and a velocity v. time trace can be obtained. This pulse waveform can be analysed by various mathematical techniques to measure the damping effect on the pulse wave produced by a stenosis. The precise mathematical method, Fourier analysis, Laplace transformation or principal component analysis, is probably not so important. All these methods are comparable, no one having a considerable advantage in terms of accuracy over another. What is important is that all these methods, and for that matter direct measurements of pressure, are influenced by an obstruction in the arteries downstream from the point of insonnation. Each method is reliable when stenoses of over 70% are involved. Stenoses of less than 50% (area) probably have little or no effect on the circulation, so

difficulties arise in the case of stenoses between 50% and 70%.

ABDOMINAL AORTIC ANEURYSM

Aetiology

The aetiology of abdominal aortic aneurysm is degenerative atheromatous disease. Atheroma leads to weakening of the vessel wall, with fibrosis, destruction of the internal elastic lamina and loss of collagen, all of which may progress to localized dilatation. Abdominal aortic aneurysms are remarkably constant in their extent, usually from 2–3 cm below the renal arteries to the aortic bifurcation and on occasions extending into the common iliac arteries. Under 5% of abdominal aortic aneurysms involve the renal arteries or extend more proximally into the thoracic aorta.

It is probable that in some cases, aneurysmal formation may not be due to atheroma but involves a process of unknown aetiology and in which case the appearances are characteristic—so-called inflammatory aneurysms. These make up about 12% of abdominal aneurysms. The appearance of an inflammatory aneurysm is typical, with dense fibrous tissue extending beyond the limits of the aneurysm itself into the retroperitoneal tissues. There is dense plasma-cell and round-cell infiltrate in the adventitia of the aorta and beyond. It has been suggested that the inflammatory aneurysm is a result of an autoimmune process, and that all aortic aneurysms may result from a similar pathological onset. However, it is unusual to note progression of any autoimmune process after operation although the diseased segment of aorta has been left in situ. True infective aortic aneurysms are rare but salmonella organisms are occasionally cultured from the intra-aortic thrombus.

Clinical Features

In most cases of abdominal aortic aneurysm, peripheral arterial disease is not severe and it is normal to feel all the pulses distal to the aneurysm. Peripheral arterial occlusions are noted in less than 20% of patients with aortic aneurysms, which is a lower figure than might be expected in patients with generalized arterial disease. There is also evidence that patients with aortic aneurysm have a lower mortality from coronary and cerebral arterial disease than is to be expected.

Patients with an abdominal aneurysm are usually over 60 years of age, and the incidence of aneurysms increases with age. Once an aneurysm has developed it will continue to dilate and eventually rupture (Chapter 55). Such evidence as there is suggests that the increase in diameter is not regular (neither linear nor exponential) but is sporadic. Periods of apparent quiescence are succeeded by times of rapid expansion. In over 50% of patients who have an abdominal aortic aneurysm measuring more than 6 cm in diameter one can anticipate that the aneurysm will rupture within two years. In the UK about 1·5% of patients who come to post-mortem have an intact aortic aneurysm and about 0·5% of all deaths are due to rupture of an abdominal aortic aneurysm.

Approximately one-third of aneurysms are asymptomatic and are found coincidentally on clinical examination, at operation or are seen on plain radiographs of the abdomen. About one-half of the patients with abdominal aneurysms complain of pain which may be sited in the abdomen or in the back, less usually in the legs (sciatica) and rarely in the testes.

On examination a pulsatile swelling may be felt in the epigastrium or left lumbar region. If the aneurysm is large, it may well be visible and can extend into the pelvis.

Management

In patients in whom the diagnosis is in doubt ultrasound scans, plain films of the abdomen and CT scans are helpful. CT scans are particularly useful if there is a question of the aneurysm extending above the renal arteries. Angiograms are not absolutely necessary, and opinions vary as to whether the additional information which may be obtained outweighs the risks involved.

Natural History of Aneurysm

Patients in whom an aneurysm is discovered should be advised to have it resected; if the aneurysm is symptomatic then operation should be carried out without delay.

Abdominal aortic aneurysm may rupture into the retroperitoneal space or intraperitoneally; more rarely they rupture into the duodenum or the vena cava (*see* Chapter 55).

Arteriovenous fistulas between the aorta and inferior vena cava or between iliac arteries and veins usually results from the erosion of an aneurysm. Erosion of a degenerative atheromatous aneurysm into the gut is rare and more commonly it arises from a false aneurysm, which forms at the site of anastomosis after insertion of a prosthesis. Traumatic fistula may be caused by penetrating injury or accidental damage during lumbar intervertebral disc surgery.

The clinical features associated with an aortocaval fistula include rapidly progressive cardiac failure, bruit, and palpable thrill present over the fistula, venous congestion with oedema in the legs and occasionally pulsating veins in the legs. Arteriography will confirm the diagnosis and may outline the sac of the false aneurysm.

Operation

Abdominal aortic aneurysms should be managed surgically where possible. Using the transperitoneal approach the aorta is cross-clamped above the aneurysm. Then the common iliac arteries are clamped and the aneurysmal sac opened and a prosthesis inserted. Prostheses are usually made from Dacron or Teflon and may be a simple tube or a bifurcation graft (trouser-graft) (*Fig.* 53.4). The bifurcation graft is inserted from the aorta above to the common iliac arteries

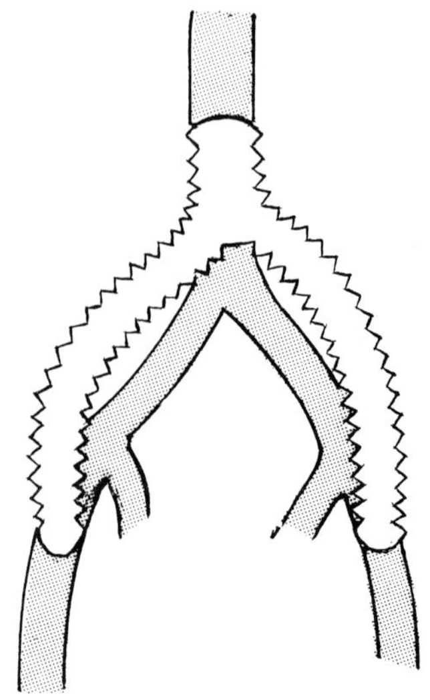

Fig. 53.4 Where the iliac vessels are bilaterally occluded a Y-graft or trouser graft of Dacron will bypass the affected segments and is normally taken to the common femoral vessels.

below, or to the common femoral arteries. The operative mortality for elective surgery of abdominal aortic aneurysms is less than 2% in the hands of competent vascular surgeons.

Complications of Surgery

These include myocardial infarction, renal failure, coagulopathies, and acute ischaemia of the bowel and lower limbs. Renal failure can occur in patients even if the aneurysm and the operative resection do not involve the renal arteries directly. The mortality from renal failure is greatly increased if the renal arteries are involved and resection necessitates re-implantation of the renal arteries into the graft. (In such patients re-implantation of the superior mesenteric artery may also be required.) It is inevitable that the inferior mesenteric artery is ligated in the course of the operation and this may lead to ischaemia of the descending colon, particularly if the superior mesenteric and coeliac arteries are also narrowed by atheroma. In this case there will be an inadequate collateral blood supply via the marginal arteries to the colon. Ischaemic colitis presents with diarrhoea, often bloody and may progress to gangrene and perforation of the colon. Some surgeons prepare the colon by irrigation prior to aortic surgery with this complication in mind. In those patients with arterial disease distal to an aneurysm, repair may be followed by acute ischaemia of the lower limbs. This has been attributed to emboli (thrombus and atheromatous debris thrown off in the course of operation 'trash foot'), and attempts to reverse the changes by catheter embolectomy should be made if suspicions are raised by the appearance of the feet immediately after operation.

Results

Late results are good with excellent long-term patency and a life expectancy equal to that of the general population of similar age. Occasionally one sees infection in a prosthesis, about 1–2% which may present as a sinus in the groin, secondary haemorrhage, or as an abscess surrounding the graft. Low grade infection at the site of an anastomosis can lead to the formation of a false aneurysm. When such an aneurysm occurs at the proximal anastomosis an aorto-duodenal fistula may form. The management of these septic complications is difficult and involves removal of the prosthesis and construction of some form of extra anatomic bypass.

RUPTURED ABDOMINAL AORTIC ANEURYSM

This diagnosis must be borne in mind in any patient presenting with severe pain in the abdomen or back and in whom there are signs of hypovolaemic shock. In obese patients who are shocked the aneurysm may be impalpable. Some patients may present with a history of pain present for over a day or two, whilst others will present with sudden onset of symptoms and signs of blood loss. Approximately half the patients with a ruptured aortic aneurysm survive to reach hospital and about half of these survive operation.

The site of rupture is usually through the posterior wall of the aneurysm with leakage into the retroperitoneal space. Intraperitoneal rupture of an aneurysm is associated with massive blood loss and is usually immediately fatal.

The differential diagnosis is from mesenteric vascular accidents, perforation of a hollow viscus, dissecting aneurysm or a myocardial infarct. Less commonly, but particularly in obese patients the condition may be mistaken for peritonitis, ureteric colic and a prolapsed intervertebral disc.

Management

If a patient is suspected of having a ruptured abdominal aneurysm 6 units of blood should be cross-matched and the patient transferred to the operating theatre. There is some advantage to administering fresh frozen plasma (2 units) as soon as possible. The incidence of coagulopathy is fairly high and most vascular surgeons give fresh frozen plasma and platelets in addition to whole blood. It is essential to limit the volume of intravenous clear fluids because haemodilution contributes to the coagulopathy.

It has been suggested that a pressurized suit which encompasses the abdomen and legs is an advantage and will allow a patient with a ruptured aortic aneurysm to be transported more safely, but convincing evidence of this is lacking.

At operation rapid control of the aorta proximal to the aneurysm (and if possible between aneurysm and renal arteries) must be obtained. After this the blood pressure can be stabilized by infusion of whole blood and plasma. Most surgeons use a prosthesis made from woven Dacron or Teflon; this is impervious to fluids and helps restrict further losses which might occur if a porous prosthesis (velours and knitted types) were used.

Deaths which occur in the course of operation usually follow cross-clamping of the aorta and are probably due to the additional stress a high after-load places on an ischaemic myocardium. Others die from uncontrollable bleeding which may be associated with a coagulopathy. After operation deaths result from myocardial infarction, pneumonia and renal failure.

The results of operation will depend on the policy of selection employed at each centre. In some hospitals all patients are resuscitated for 12–24 h and only the survivors of this policy are operated on and included in mortality statistics. If all patients are operated upon who reach hospital alive and one includes deaths in transit in the statistics, then only a half of all patients with a ruptured aneurysm reach hospital alive and about one-half survive operation. These figures can be improved considerably by excluding patients over 75 years of age and ones who present with a systolic pressure of less than 90 mmHg. However there are patients whose ages exceed this figure and who have profound hypotension who survive. It is difficult to exclude any patient on the grounds that their inclusion would have an adverse effect on mortality statistics.

The incidence of deaths from renal failure has been reduced dramatically, by ensuring that the period of hypotension is kept to a minimum, and renal failure is treated promptly. After operation the blood pressure, central venous pressure, urine output, serum electrolytes and packed cell volume are measured at regular intervals. Anuria or oliguria associated with a rise in blood urea, creatinine and potassium should be countered promptly. A close liaison with expert nephrologists has virtually eliminated renal failure as a cause of death in our practice. Measures to counter renal failure include fluid and salt restriction, use of ion exchange resins, peritoneal dialysis and renal dialysis. The vast majority of cases of renal failure are caused by prolonged hypotension (prerenal) and can be expected to recover in time. Late complications include infection of the prosthesis and aortoduodenal fistulas. The incidence of thrombosis in bifurcation grafts is low and, thankfully, so is the incidence of infection. However, one can expect to see both problems in a busy practice and reoperation may be necessary.

Infected Vascular Grafts

This problem may present at any time up to ten years after the original operation. Symptoms may be dramatic—haematemesis from an aorto-enteric fistula, false bleeding from an aneurysm in the groin or in rare instances the prosthesis may become cannibalized by the intestine. Usually the patient presents with an insidious onset of vague symptoms, he feels unwell, has backache and often loses weight. In the case of a perigraft infection, without haemorrhage a CT scan is probably the most helpful investigation. When a bifurcation graft is infected it is essential that it is removed and circulation restored by an extra anatomical bypass. The overall mortality from this complication is 25% but, in the presence of an aorto-enteric fistula the mortality is over 40%.

Occluded Vascular Grafts

Inevitably some reconstructions of the aorta and iliac arteries will occlude in time. The incidence of occlusion is low but is known to be associated with:

A. Unilateral reconstructions—bypass or endarterectomy.
B. Patients in whom there were further occlusions distal to the common femoral at the time of the original bleeding.

Occlusion in one or both limbs of a bifurcation graft occurs in approximately 10% of the total number of limbs (i.e. bifurcation grafts × 2) within 5 years. There is no evidence to suggest that the type of prosthesis influences this.

Patients in whom a prosthesis has occluded may:

1. Have no symptoms.
2. Have recurrence of claudication.
3. Claudicate at such a short distance that the symptom is intolerable.
4. Develop pain at rest.

Patients in the latter two groups require investigation and treatment. Treatment consists of either replacing the original prosthesis or doing a thrombectomy. Either operation may be combined with some form of distal reconstruction to improve 'run-off'.

SUMMARY

The surgery of the infrarenal aorta and iliac arteries can be technically difficult, particularly when the arteries are heavily calcified. This is also true when iliac aneurysms are present and in the case of inflammatory aneurysms. Careful selection of the appropriate operation for each patient allied with good surgical technique can produce excellent long-lasting results.

Further Reading

Bell P. R. F. and Tilney N. L. (eds.) (1984) *Vascular Surgery*. London, Butterworths.
Berguer J. J. and Yao J. S. T. (eds.) (1985) *Reoperative Arterial Surgery*. New York, Grune & Stratton.
Greenhalgh, R. (ed.) (1983) *Diagnostic Techniques and Assessment Procedures in Vascular Surgery*. London, Grune & Stratton.

54 Vascular Disease of the Lower Limbs

P. R. F. Bell

Vascular problems affecting the lower limbs are extremely common. The most serious is occlusive arterial disease caused by atherosclerosis leading to chronic ischaemia which particularly affects heavy smokers, diabetics and the elderly. Rarer causes of vascular insufficiency include Buerger's disease, aneurysm of the femoral or popliteal arteries, entrapment of the popliteal artery and cystic adventitial degeneration of that vessel. Acute ischaemia caused by embolism from a central source is also very common and eminently treatable if recognized in time. Vasospastic and inflammatory problems can also affect the blood supply to the lower limb.

ATHEROSCLEROSIS

The pathology of this condition has already been described in Chapter 51. The consequence is ulceration of the intima followed by thickening of the arterial wall and progressive stenosis leading to occlusion of segments of the artery. In the lower limb the commonest sites for occlusion are: the femoral artery in the adductor canal immediately above the knee, the origin of the profunda femoris artery, the popliteal trifurcation and in the individual tibial or peroneal vessels (*Fig.* 54.1). The reason why these sites are particularly prone to stenosis is not understood. Various risk factors have already been mentioned but from the practical point of view the commonest are smoking, diabetes and a family history of vascular problems.

The disease is an essentially benign one and the majority of those afflicted will not lose their limbs provided that the patient is prepared to stop smoking. This is an important point to remember when considering treatment, which will be discussed later. As the stenosis in any particular segment of the artery progresses, collateral circulation through small branches above and below the stenosed area provides an alternative pathway for blood (*Fig.* 54.2) which allows the limb to be retained and claudication to remain mild. If the disease progresses then gangrene will eventually supervene and limb loss occur.

Clinical Presentation

This problem can present in one of two ways—a chronic picture of progressive reduction in the circulation culminating in limb loss or an acute presentation with the possibility of imminent gangrene.

Chronic Presentation—Intermittent Claudication, Rest Pain and Gangrene

The patient gives a classic history of pain which starts after walking a defined distance. When he stops and rests the pain is relieved but returns when he starts to walk again. The time taken for the pain to disappear and the distance the patient can walk is a guide to the severity of the disease. The longer it takes for the pain to disappear and the shorter the distance walked, the worse is the problem. Gradually, if the condition progresses the distance the patient can walk will become less and less until eventually pain will be present even at rest, at this point the circulation has reached the point where there is insufficient blood to nourish the skin.

Claudication is diagnosed by taking a proper history, but it is possible to confuse it with other causes of pain in the leg which include hip and knee disorders, diseases of the spine, particularly slipped disc, various neuropathies, venous problems and the interesting condition of spinal claudication. All of these have a particular history which will help to distinguish them from true claudication, which never causes pain at rest in the thigh or calf. Pain at rest only occurs with severe disease and then usually in the foot or toes. In

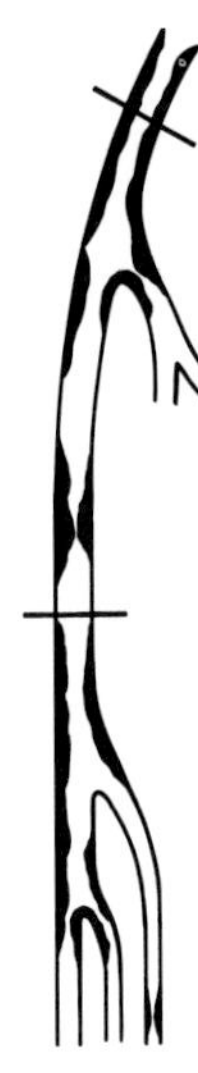

Fig. 54.1 Sites of atheromatous stenosis in the lower limb.

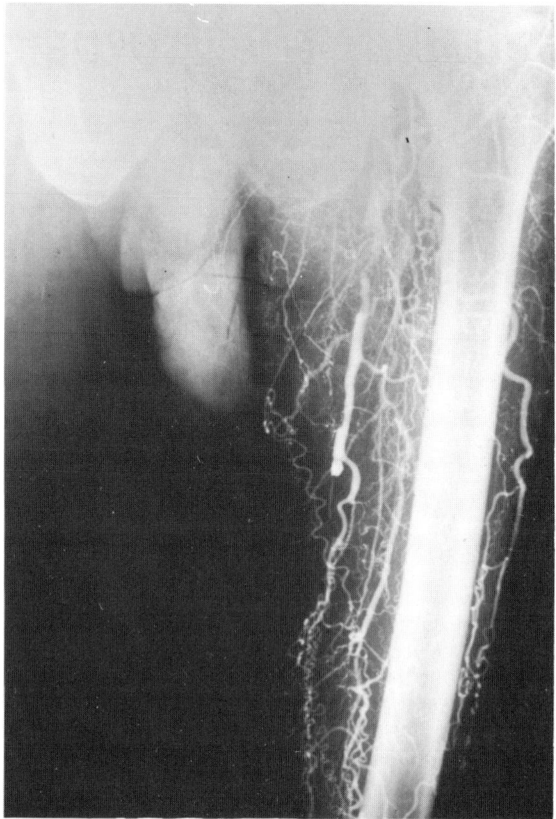

Fig. 54.2 An arteriogram showing extensive collateral channels.

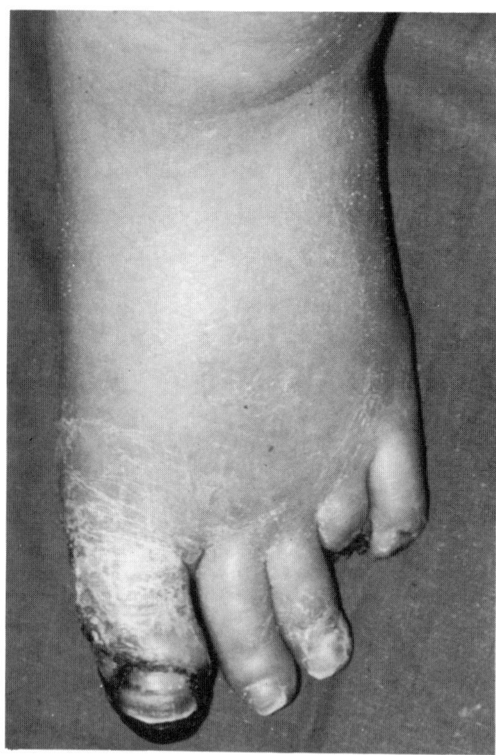

Fig. 54.3 A foot with chronic ischaemia; note the dry skin, minor gangrene and loss of the fourth toe.

addition, the pain is never made worse by movements of the spine, hip or knee. For these reasons a full examination of the joints and spine as part of a routine examination of the lower limb is mandatory. Peripheral neuritis usually produces a classic history. The patient says that he feels as though he is walking on glass. Venous disease usually causes an aching pain on standing or a bursting pain on walking if venous obstruction is present. Swelling of the ankles is also a common subsidiary symptom. Spinal claudication can usually be distinguished from true claudication by taking a careful history. The patient will complain that after walking a certain distance pain occurs down the back of the leg in the distribution of the sciatic nerve, ischaemia of which causes the symptoms.

PHYSICAL SIGNS. The patient may have evidence of chronic ischaemia, such as ulceration of the toes, dry gangrene, pressure sores, areas of inflammation due to infection entering the foot through a cut, loss of hair, reduction of temperature, and possible pallor (*Fig.* 54.3). Although the femoral pulse may be palpable distal pulses will normally be found. Depending upon the degree of ischaemia, elevation of the foot will lead to blanching and emptying of the veins which become guttered. When blanching has occurred, if the leg is then allowed to dangle over the side of the bed, it will slowly get pinker, the veins will fill and it will become a dusky red. The time taken for blanching to occur is an indication of the severity of the disease, the more rapid the blanching the worse the disease (Buerger's test).

Acute Presentation

The patient will usually give a history of claudication over the previous years but will present with a sudden onset of severe pain in the leg and foot with pallor, coldness, possible loss of sensation or numbness and difficulty in movement of the foot with stiffness. These are all signs of acute ischaemia but can also be caused by arterial embolization which is discussed later. The physical signs are fairly dramatic, the foot looks mottled with a very poor capillary circulation (*Fig.* 54.4). If the mottling does not disappear on compression this is a bad sign indicating a poor prognosis. The foot is usually very cold, sensation may be poor and movements of the foot may be difficult indicating that dangerous ischaemia is occurring.

Management of a Patient with Intermittent Claudication

Patients with intermittent claudication do not usually need active surgical treatment unless their disability is causing severe symptoms. The relatively benign course of the disease must be emphasized and the possibility of making a patient worse by operative intervention always remembered. With these points in mind and for the purpose of treatment, patients should be divided into clinical groupings which will decide whether subsequent investigations take place. For convenience a division into mild, moderate and severe claudication ought to be made. This is entirely a clinical decision and is based upon the taking of a proper history and examining the patient. Investigations are not usually required to place the patient in one of these groups. The definition of mild claudication varies but a patient can walk usually several hundred yards and the problem does not significantly interfere with his job or life style. Moderate claudication means the patient can usually walk more than 100 yards and the symptoms are interfering with his life style or work but he can manage if pushed to do so. Severe

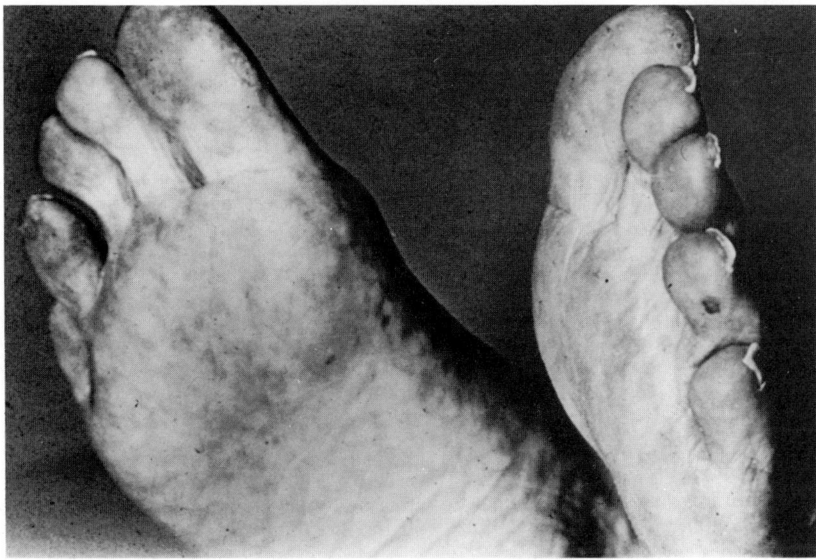

Fig. 54.4 Acutely ischaemic feet, mottled and pale.

claudication usually occurs when a patient can walk less than 100 yards and when this occurs serious interference with work or leisure is obvious. A fourth category—rest pain or gangrene will occur when the circulation has reached a point where it is not sufficient to maintain nutrition even at rest. At this point the patient is in danger of limb loss and some form of interventional therapy is usually required. In general, patients who have mild or moderate claudication do not require surgical treatment whereas those with severe claudication or rest pain normally do.

Treatment of Mild or Moderate Claudication

Conservative treatment is usually indicated for patients in these groups. Most importantly the doctor should explain to the patient the exact nature of the disease, he should also point out that the symptoms he has, do not mean imminent limb loss. This reassurance alone is often sufficient to alleviate the patient's symptoms, as some 'friend' has often told him that he knew of an acquaintance who after these symptoms lost a leg! Having explained the disease to the patient it then needs to be said that drugs in general do not help this condition. There is no concrete evidence to show that improvement will occur following a course of any particular drug. There is, however, some evidence that the patient should take regular exercise and stop smoking. The doctor should be specific about the exercise that needs to be taken and explain to the patient exactly what he has to do. The calf muscles in particular, need to be exercised and walking or heel-raising exercises are generally the ones to be preferred. Some forms of activity such as cycling do not usually exercise the correct muscles and will not help the patient. More important, stopping smoking must be emphasized very strongly, pointing out that if the patient persists he may move into the rest pain group with a possible amputation as the end point. When advice to stop smoking is given this should not be done in a dictatorial or sanctimonious fashion. Smoking is an addiction and those who suffer from it must be given help to stop. It is no use saying sternly 'Go away and stop smoking' as those who are addicted cannot do so. Help from such wide sources as Stop Smoking Support Groups, Acupuncture, Hypnosis, etc. should be available and should be actively used if success is to be obtained. There is ample evidence to show that those patients with vascular disease of the lower limbs, who stop smoking and exercise regularly, will double or treble the distance they can walk within a relatively short time. It is important to emphasize that the process of collateral build-up can take as long as six months and the treatment should not be written off as unsuccessful until an appropriate length of time has passed. Apart from this advice no other investigations, invasive or otherwise, are necessary except perhaps to measure the patient's haemoglobin, take a chest radiograph and possibly an exercise ECG. These tests are done because of the high risk of cardiovascular and respiratory disease in these patients.

Treatment of Severe Claudication and Rest Pain

Conservative measures will by now have been tried without success. In general drugs do not work in this condition but these will be referred to again later. Because the patient is likely to require an operation a thorough cardiovascular assessment has to be made because of the likelihood that anaesthesia will be needed. This will involve an assessment of the heart, lungs and the carotid circulation. This is done not to avoid an operation but to allow the anaesthetist to make any provisions that may be necessary to make the operation as safe as possible. Generally speaking, and particularly where rest pain is present, an operation cannot be avoided as the consequence of failed reconstruction or failure to reconstruct, is amputation which of course requires anaesthesia anyway.

Special Investigations

Although an impression of the severity of the ischaemia and the level of occlusion has already been made on clinical grounds more precise information is now necessary before surgical or other intervention is possible. The aim must be to try and confirm the clinical findings and to assess the adequacy of inflow and outflow into the lower limb.

Confirmation of the Site of Occlusion and Assessment of Outflow

Measurement of the ankle pressure can be useful as an approximate indication of outflow. This is often compared with the brachial pressure to give a ratio of the ankle/brachial pressure index which is normally near to 1. Patients with mild claudication usually have an index of about 0·6 while with rest pain and gangrene it usually falls below 0·4. Measurement of these pressures can be very helpful as they provide information which might be useful if conservative treatment is decided upon. For example, if the pressure is less than 50 mmHg at the ankle or if the index is less than 0·4, healing of an ulcer is highly unlikely without some form of surgical intervention. By the same token if the index is of the order of 0·6 or the ankle systolic pressure is over 75 mmHg then healing may well occur. Although pressures are useful, the only accurate way to assess the level of the occlusion and the quality of the run-off is by outlining the arteries in some way. There are two ways of doing this, intravenous arteriography (digital subtraction angiography (DSA)) and conventional arteriography. DSA necessitates the injection of large quantities of contrast into a central vein. Computer controlled X-rays are then taken to visualize the arterial system. Although this technique gives good pictures of the carotid and large central vessels the results with distal vessels do not usually offer sufficient detail to allow proper assessment of the site of the occlusion or the outflow. As a result, the investigation for assessing the site of obstruction and the outflow in the lower limb remains conventional arteriography, by direct injection of contrast medium into the aorta. Two techniques are used, the translumbar injection of contrast medium which requires general anaesthesia, or retrograde insertion of a catheter via a femoral artery into any part of the aorta or its branches (Seldinger technique) which can be performed under local anaesthesia. Generally speaking the Seldinger technique is to be preferred, but sometimes the catheter cannot negotiate a stenosis of the iliac artery and a translumbar procedure has to be used. Arteriograms should not be ordered lightly as they are potentially dangerous. They can lead to haemorrhage, damage to vessels, thrombosis and distal embolization and should only be used as a prelude to interventional therapy by surgery or other means. When properly performed the arteriogram will provide information about the adequacy of proximal vessels, the site of the occlusion and the state of the run-off vessels in the leg, all of which will influence the decision to operate.

Inflow

As previously mentioned many of these patients have combined diseases of the aorto-iliac segment and distal vessels. Before operating on the lower limb, inflow of blood into the distal vessels has to be confirmed as adequate. This cannot be done by simply palpating the femoral pulses or by looking at the arteriogram although these two parameters are the ones which are often relied upon. If there is any doubt at all about the adequacy of the inflow vessels on arteriography then some form of inflow test should be performed. A number of tests have been described using the Doppler probe with frequency analysis of the waveform. Measurement of various components of the waveform has been suggested as useful, including transfer function, pulsatility index, and principal component analysis but none of these can discriminate the difficult case. The advantage of these methods is that they are non-invasive. The best test, however, is the direct measurement of pressure through a needle placed into the femoral artery. This has to be compared with pressure measured in the radial artery, using a needle inserted at the wrist. A pressure drop between the two of 10 mmHg or more at rest is significant. In order to sharpen the test further the patient is usually given 20 mg of papaverine directly into the femoral needle. This causes vasodilatation of the distal arterial bed which accentuates any fall in pressure across a potential stenosis. A fall of more than 20% is significant and means proximal disease (*Fig.* 54.5). In these circumstances the patient should not have a distal operation until the proximal stenosis has first of all been dealt with in one way or another.

Adequacy of the Graft

The best graft for lower limb arterial bypass is the patient's own saphenous vein. Before making the decision to operate one has to ensure that it is present and not varicose.

The decision to proceed further will therefore depend upon a number of risk factors, including the severity of the disease, the site of the obstruction, the adequacy of inflow, the adequacy of the outflow, the presence of the long saphenous vein, the fitness of the patient for surgery, the presence or absence of diabetes and the smoking history (*Table* 54.1). In most cases some of these factors will be less than optimal. A decision to proceed to reconstructive surgery may still be made if the alternative is amputation. If, however, a patient has moderate to severe claudication then an operation should not be performed unless as many of these factors as possible are acceptable. Assuming adequate

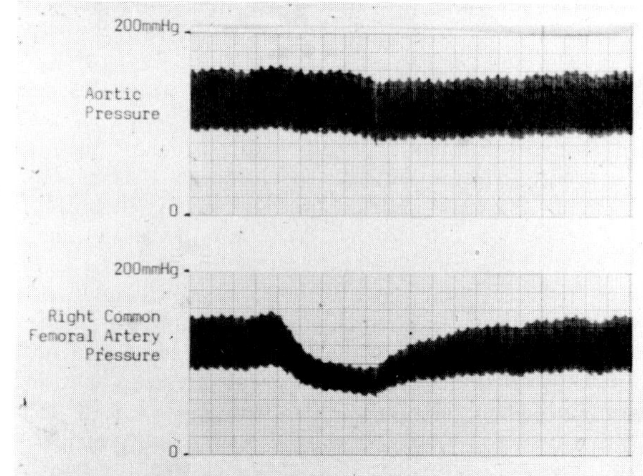

Fig. 54.5 Significant fall in pressure in the femoral artery following the injection of papaverine, indicating a serious proximal stenosis.

Table 54.1 Risk factors and successful surgery

Severity of the disease
Adequate inflow
Adequate outflow
Availability of long saphenous vein
Site of obstruction
Patient's general condition
Diabetes
Continued smoking

inflow the treatment decided upon will depend on the site of the obstruction.

Femoropopliteal Occlusion

This type of obstruction is bypassed using a graft extending from the femoral artery above to the popliteal artery below (*Fig.* 54.6). The best results are obtained by using the patient's own long saphenous vein which is reversed for the procedure. If the saphenous vein is not available or is varicose, other grafts are available made from either synthetic materials such as Dacron or Polytetrafluoroethylene (PTFE) (*Fig.* 54.7) or, alternatively, human umbilical vein appropriately treated and covered in a net of Dacron (*Fig.* 54.8). The obstruction in the artery can be bypassed either above or at the knee providing there is a distal patent segment to which the graft can be stitched. The popliteal artery is exposed through a medial incision either above or below the knee. The results of this type of operation are good with five-year graft patency rates of about 70% for long saphenous vein and 50% for synthetic grafts.

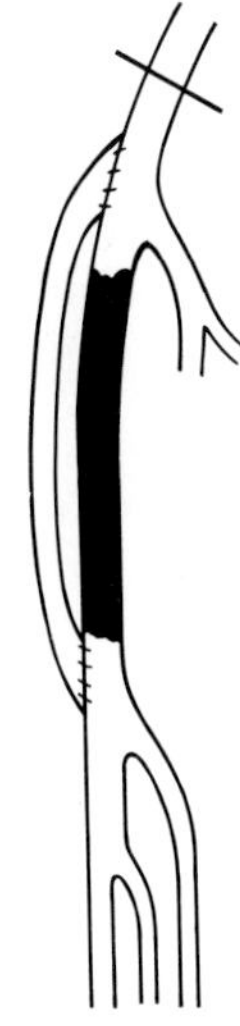

Fig. 54.6 Femoropopliteal bypass for obstruction of the femoral artery.

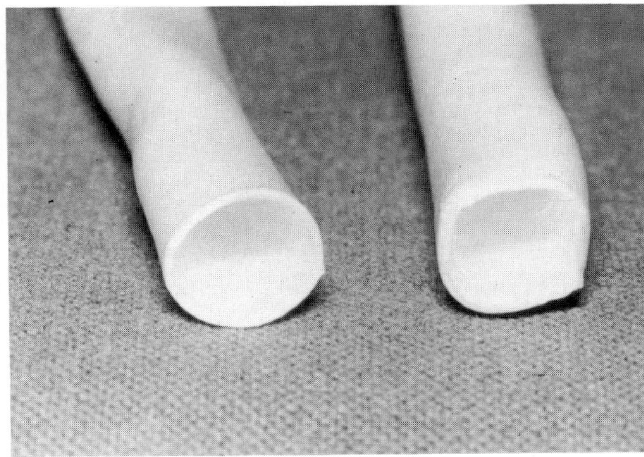

Fig. 54.7 Grafts made from PTFE; the right is the older thick-walled type and the left the newer thin-walled graft.

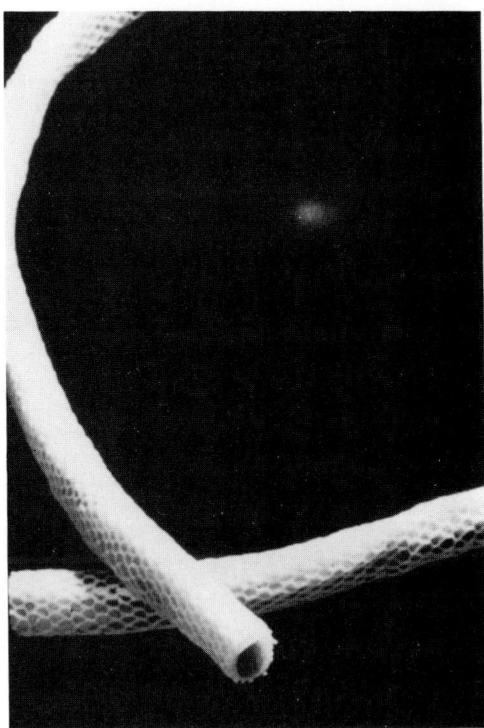

Fig. 54.8 Human umbilical vein graft.

Femorodistal Grafts

If the obstruction lies more distally at the popliteal trifurcation or beyond, then the chances of success are proportionally less, being worst when only single vessel run-off is available (*Fig.* 54.9). For this reason the operation should not usually be performed for claudication unless it is severe. If, however, rest pain or gangrene is present then this procedure can produce adequate limb salvage in appropriate cases but only if the long saphenous vein is available. Various authors have used human umbilical vein and PTFE but the success rate of approximately 25% at 2 years is not appealing. For the operation to be reasonably successful long saphenous vein from groin to midcalf or ankle can be used providing the in situ method is used. In this technique the long saphenous vein is exposed in its entirety or through a series of sequential incisions, all its branches are ligated and the valves destroyed with a special stripper (*Fig.* 54.10). This needs careful attention to detail otherwise the vein can be seriously damaged. By doing this, blood can be made to flow in a retrograde fashion down the vein, the upper end of which is sutured to the front of the femoral artery. Distally the narrower part of the vessel can then be sutured end-to-side to the available patent artery at midcalf or ankle. This is a difficult technique and magnification with a loupe is usually required for the distal anastomosis. Unless the vein is available or there is good run-off to an intact plantar arch in the foot, primary amputation should be considered. Techniques are currently being evolved to try and assess the likelihood of success by measuring the resistance to flow prior to reconstruction.

Profundaplasty

In situations where the inflow is adequate the profunda artery is stenosed at its origin and there are no distal vessels

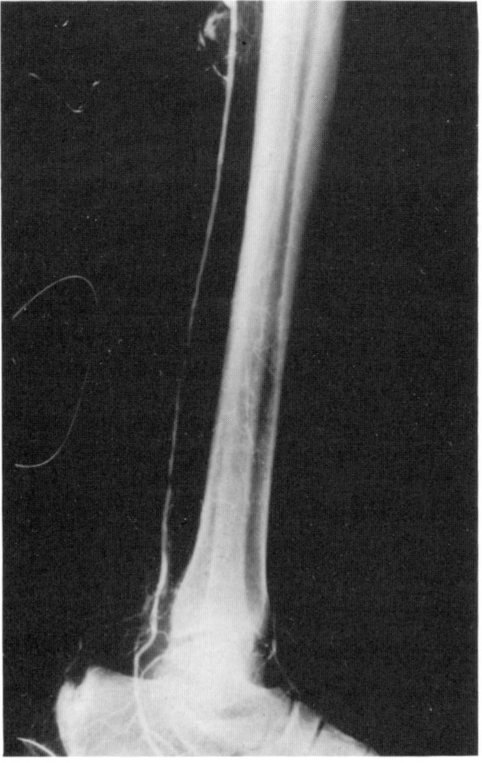

Fig. 54.9 Arteriogram showing single vessel run-off into the foot.

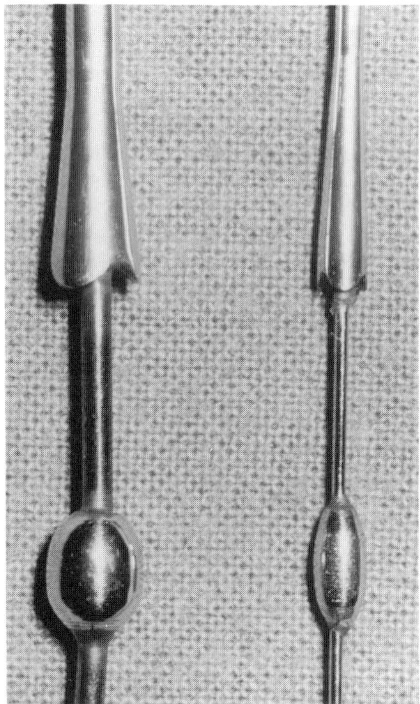

Fig. 54.10 Strippers used to destroy the veins prior to in situ bypass grafting.

available for reconstruction, the possibility of profundaplasty should be borne in mind. Significant stenosis of the origin of the profunda femoris artery is best defined by oblique arteriograms of this region (*Fig.* 54.11). Profundaplasty using a patch of Dacron or vein to widen the origin of that vessel can be successful if reasonable collaterals are available lower down the leg (*Fig.* 54.12).

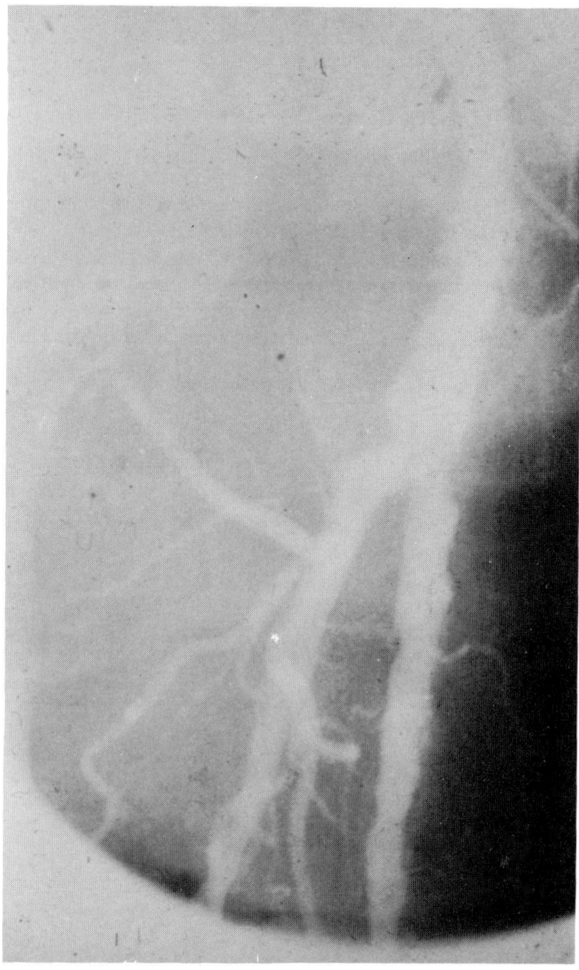

Fig. 54.11 Oblique arteriogram showing stenosis of the profunda femoris artery at its origin.

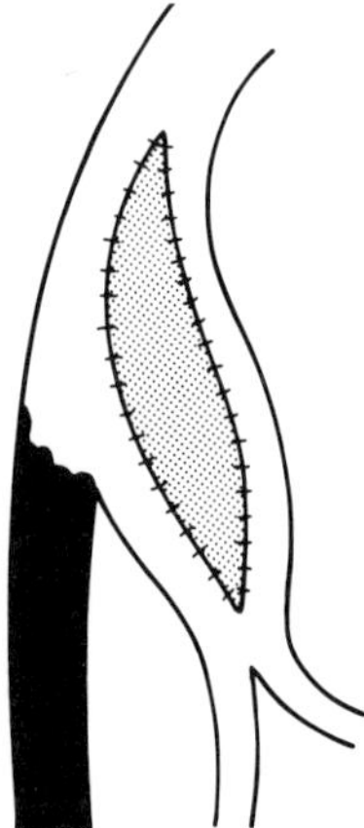

Fig. 54.12 Profundaplasty using a Dacron patch.

Revascularization of the Isolated Popliteal Segment

Occasionally, the popliteal artery behind the knee appears on arteriography as a patent segment. Above it the vessel is

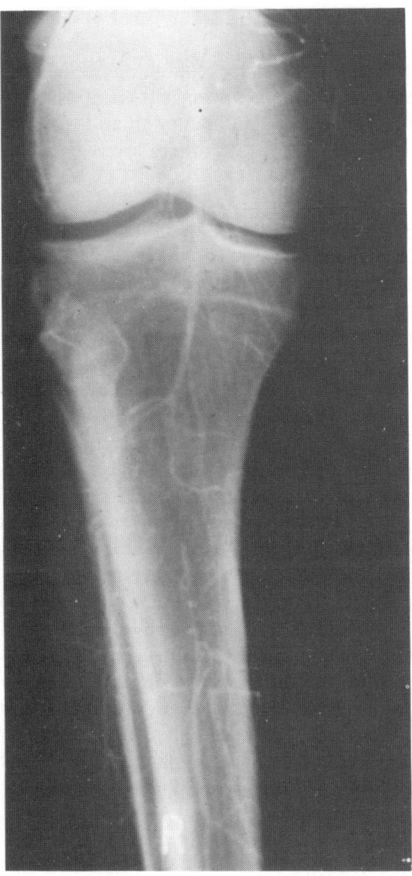

Fig. 54.13 Arteriogram showing isolated popliteal segment.

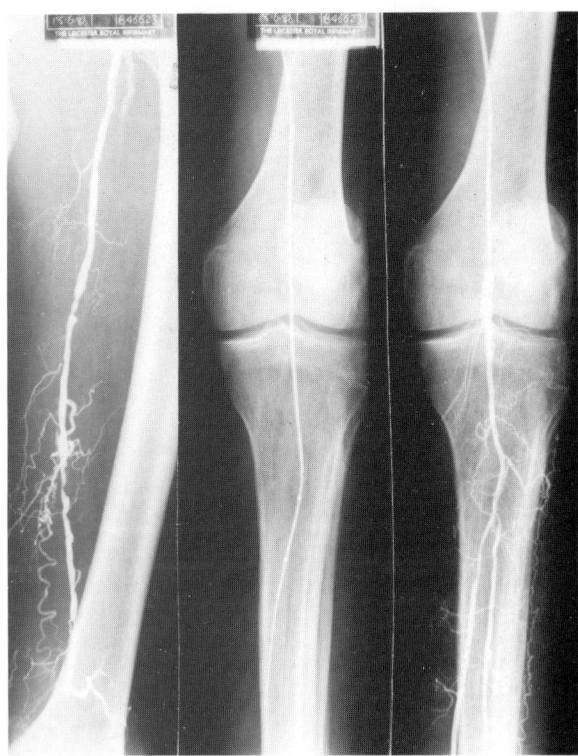

Fig. 54.14 Transluminal angioplasty for femoropopliteal occlusion. On the left the arteriogram shows occlusion of the femoral artery above the knee with multiple stenoses. The middle picture shows the passage of the angioplasty catheter below the occlusion. The right-hand picture shows the result after angioplasty with good revascularization.

blocked and distally there are no good run-off vessels (*Fig.* 54.13). If this is the case then reintroducing blood to this closed segment using either vein, PTFE or human umbilical vein graft can be useful. In patients who have gangrene or ulcers on their toes, it may usefully revascularize a limb for a sufficient length of time to allow localized amputations to heal and thereby provide limb salvage.

Other Treatments

Transluminal Angioplasty

This technique, popularized by Gruntzig has revolutionized the treatment of some types of arterial disease in the lower leg. By introducing a Silastic catheter with an inflatable balloon of a predetermined size at its tip, directly into the artery it is possible to stretch the narrow area and recanalize the vessel. The technique is particularly suitable when applied to proximal strictures in the iliac artery but can also be used to dilate short strictures or obstructions of the superficial femoral or popliteal vessels. The method requires local anaesthesia and very significant improvements to the circulation can be obtained (*Fig.* 54.14). It is not generally suitable for distal stenoses below the knee level. The technique is, however, not without complications. It is possible to make the patient worse by internal dissection, distal embolization or even rupture of the vessel concerned; however, the problems are few and these can be dealt with if necessary by arterial surgery at the time. More recently, areas of total occlusion have been removed by laser treatment prior to angioplasty thereby possibly expanding the indications for this technique.

Drug Treatment of Chronic Arterial Disease

In general drugs are of little use for the treatment of rest pain, gangrene or claudication. Various drugs have been tried including prostacyclin, and a variety of vasodilators without any evidence of prolonged success.

Sympathectomy

This operation was used extensively some years ago to treat patients with vascular disease. Unfortunately the operation has not been successful probably because the patient's circulation is already maximally dilated at the time of the procedure. It never improves claudication but may occasionally help some patients with rest pain. For this reason surgical sympathectomy has largely been abandoned except for vasospastic disease, hyperhidrosis and occasionally Buerger's disease; phenol sympathectomy, on the other hand, is used extensively to treat patients with rest pain. Such patients are often elderly, the circulation is stable, they may have some skin loss but the problem is not progressive. Phenol in water is administered to the patient through a lateral injection using a long lumbar puncture needle. The needle skirts the vertebral column and enters the plane immediately in front of the lumbar fascia which contains the sympathetic trunk (*Fig.* 54.15). When phenol is injected into this plane it produces an effective sympathectomy which although not increasing the blood flow to the foot

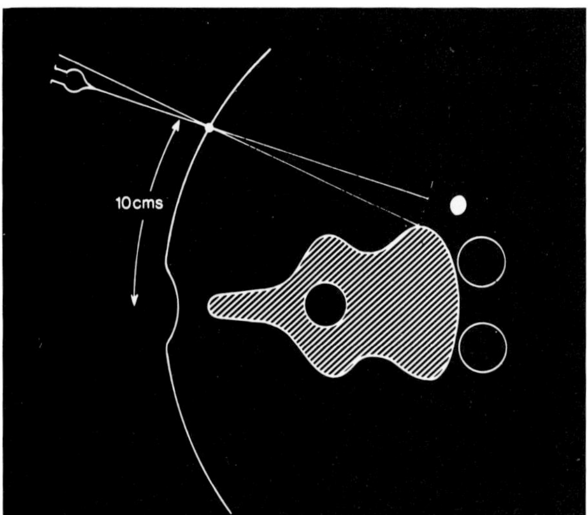

Fig. 54.15 Phenol sympathectomy. Phenol is injected around the sympathetic chain after passing a needle through the lumbar fascia.

does relieve rest pain in many cases, probably by interfering with afferent sensory circuits.

BUERGER'S DISEASE

Dispute has raged for many years as to whether this is merely a collection of symptoms representing a more severe form of atherosclerosis or whether it is a distinct entity. The critical features are that medium to large arteries are involved in young men who are heavy smokers. Progression to amputation is inevitable and any form of treatment is merely palliative. In addition, the pathology of the affected arteries usually shows an inflammatory reaction involving both vein and artery with giant-cell infiltration. Whether this is a primary pathological lesion or secondary to the gangrene and infection accompanying the disease remains a matter for discussion. Generally speaking direct arterial surgery does not help these patients and may even result in an acceleration of the problem. At best a surgical sympathectomy is usually all that is available to these patients who continue to smoke in spite of efforts to try and make them stop.

RARE CAUSES OF CLAUDICATION OR REST PAIN

Two other conditions usually presenting in young males are worth bearing in mind when considering claudication with absent distal pulses. The first is popliteal entrapment syndrome where the popliteal artery passes medial to and beneath the medial head of gastrocnemius muscle leading to constriction of the vessel. In the second condition, cystic medial degeneration, a mucinous cyst develops in the wall of the popliteal artery, again at the level of the knee, causing constriction of the lumen and eventual occlusion of the vessel itself. The treatment of the first condition is simple and merely involves releasing the artery, the second requires incision and aspiration of the cystic material or bypass grafting.

ACUTE ISCHAEMIA OF THE LOWER LIMB

There are four main causes of acute ischaemia, arterial embolization, acute thrombosis superimposed on atheromatous stenosis, a popliteal aneurysm and trauma. Trauma is covered elsewhere and the others are discussed below.

Clinical Presentation

The patient will present with a sudden onset of severe pain in the foot and calf. The pain will be excruciating, require strong analgesia and progress quite quickly to numbness and stiffness of the foot. Where the lesion has been caused by atheroma there will often be a previous history of claudication which will not usually be the case with embolus. The pulse must be felt to exclude atrial fibrillation which is a common cause of embolus and a recent history of myocardial infarction sought. On inspection the foot will be mottled, blue and cold (*see Fig.* 54.4). If the mottling becomes a confluent staining which cannot be dissipated by pressure this is a very bad sign suggesting tissue death. As the condition deteriorates the patient will lose sensation in the foot and leg and movements will eventually cease. At this stage death of the limb has occurred and infection with wet gangrene is not far away. Pulses may be completely absent or palpable only at the femoral level in the groin.

A popliteal aneurysm may be easily felt either pulsating or as a thrombosed sac. In this event the other limb should always be examined as there will usually be an aneurysm there as well giving a clue to the diagnosis. If the foot or toes are covered with small red circular areas which look like a rash the possibility of minute emboli from a proximal aneurysm should be considered.

Management

In such a patient a differential diagnosis between embolus, thrombosis and popliteal aneurysm, has to be made. If there is any doubt about the cause (and there usually is) an angiogram done without delay can be helpful. It may show popliteal aneurysm or at least its sac with thrombus in it or demonstrate an embolus with its characteristic rounded edge (*Fig.* 54.16). In the case of atheromatous thrombosis some collateral vessels may be seen.

Arterial Embolus

If the patient is fibrillating or if there has been a recent myocardial infarct without a previous history of claudication then a presumptive diagnosis of embolus is made. The patient should be fully heparinized using 10 000 units of heparin 6-hourly given by a continuous infusion pump. The services of an anaesthetist should be available and an embolectomy performed under local infiltration anaesthesia with light sedation. General anaesthesia is rarely necessary. The femoral artery should be exposed through a transverse incision after controlling the vessels, and a Fogarty catheter (No. 3) passed distally into the profunda femoris and superficial femoral arteries in turn until all clot has been removed *and there is good back bleeding* (*Fig.* 54.17). It is very important not to inflate the balloon too much as this merely damages the intima. Just sufficient to withdraw clot is all that is required. Passing a larger catheter (No. 4) proximally may be necessary if bleeding from the common femoral artery is inadequate or if the vessel is blocked. If the catheter does not pass easily to the ankle this means the cause is usually atheroma and attempts to bulldoze through with the Fogarty catheter are to be resisted. Under these circumstances, back bleeding will be poor and the cause is usually

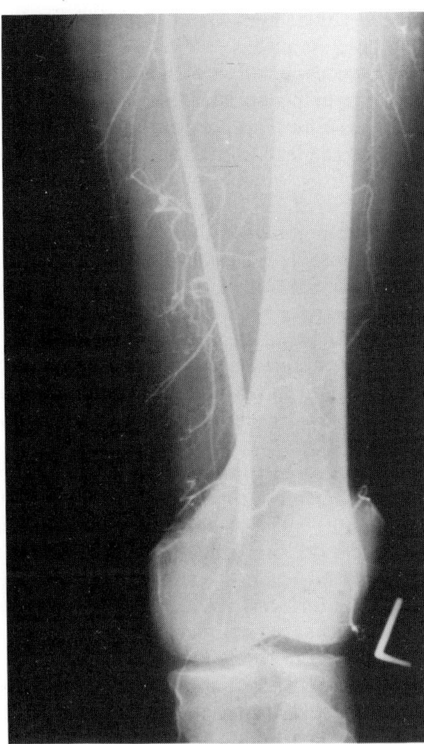

Fig. 54.16 Arteriogram showing thrombus in the popliteal artery from an embolus.

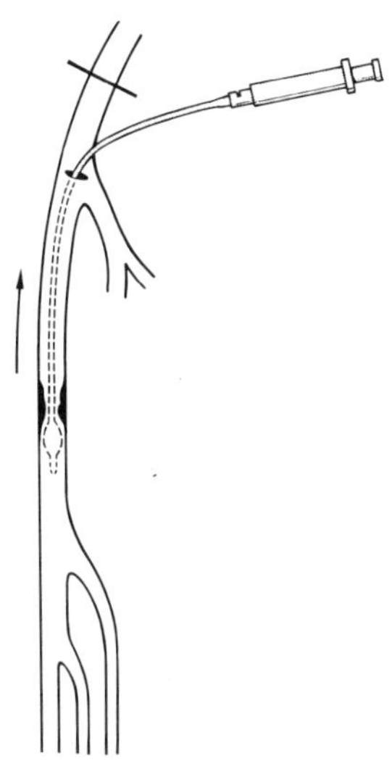

Fig. 54.17 The femoral artery has been opened with a transverse incision and a Fogarty embolectomy catheter inserted. The catheter is withdrawn removing the clot with it.

due to atheroma. In this event some form of reconstructive procedure will be needed and the patient will then have to be anaesthetized. If an embolus can be removed less than 12 h after occlusion then the results are excellent. If as is often the case the diagnosis has not been made early enough, then the results are relatively poor. In cases where the leg is revascularized after periods of prolonged ischaemia, lower limb fasciotomy is usually necessary to prevent muscle infarction when inevitable swelling occurs. All four compartments should be widely opened. Heparinization should continue for 7 days followed by long-term warfarin therapy.

Acute Thrombosis Superimposed upon Atheromatous Disease

This is a difficult condition to treat and initial heparinization should be the rule. The arteriogram will show the level of the lesion and the patient should then be carefully observed from hour to hour. He should not be left overnight without observation as in the morning the leg may be dead. Signs of an improving situation due to collateral build-up include the return of a capillary circulation and the maintenance of sensation and movement. If this occurs for 24 h then the patient's leg will usually recover and secondary treatment can then be undertaken later. If, however, there is any deterioration or failure to improve then active treatment must be the rule. Recent studies using a low dose of streptokinase injected directly into the thrombus (6000 u/h for 6 h) through a catheter passed down the affected artery have been quite successful and is to be recommended in these situations (*Fig.* 54.18). If this fails or if there appears to be a reasonable run-off below the obstruction then angioplasty for short segments of occlusion will also result in a marked improvement. For more severe disease some form of bypass grafting as previously mentioned, will usually help the limb. This is a high-risk group, however, and the chances of limb loss can be 40–50% if management is not accurate and prompt.

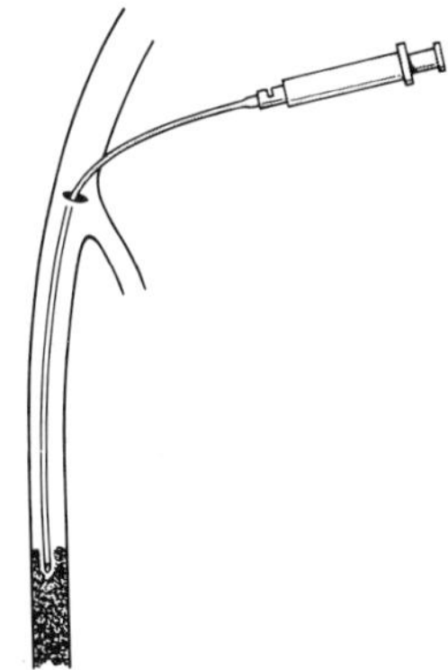

Fig. 54.18 Low dose streptokinase infused directly into the thrombus.

Aneurysm of the Aortofemoral or Popliteal Arteries

These lesions often present with a warning shower of emboli which appear as small very painful haemorrhagic lesions in the foot or toes which often resolve slowly. This must not be taken as a good sign but rather as a warning that an operation is necessary before further embolization and limb loss occurs. An alternative presentation, particularly with a popliteal aneurysm, is acute ischaemia due to thrombosis of the sac or thrombus passing distally into the foot. In these circumstances the patient has to be watched carefully. If the circulation improves and the sac has thrombosed no further treatment is required. If, however, deterioration occurs or the sac remains patent with a risk of further embolization, the aneurysm should be exposed through a medial or posterior approach, opened and replaced with a graft of Dacron or saphenous vein. If this is done the results are very good as

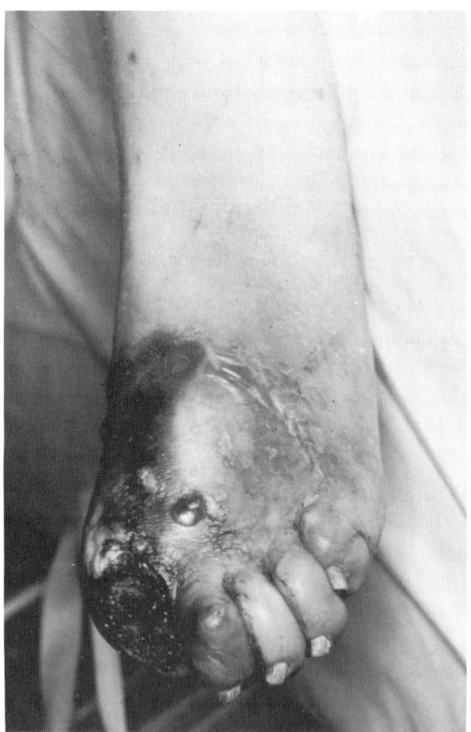

Fig. 54.19 Diabetic gangrene; severe infection with lymphangitis.

the vessels are usually large and it is relatively easy to find an outflow channel onto which to sew the graft.

DIABETIC FOOT

Diabetics, especially those with juvenile onset disease, are particularly prone to vascular problems. They are of course prone to any type of vascular disorder and can present in any of the ways already described. They are, however, also prone to a peculiar kind of local ischaemia due to their inability to combat infection following minor trauma often in the presence of diabetic neuropathy. Two clinical presentations occur, in one case the patient will present with a severely inflamed swollen foot with lymphangitis, early gangrene, and suffer inappropriately little pain (*Fig.* 54.19). On examination all pulses are present. This is a dangerous condition which can lead to anaerobic infection and progress to extensive gangrene which requires immediate amputation if life is to be saved. Wide-spectrum antibiotics must be given immediately in large doses taking account of the likelihood of anaerobic infection. A suitable combination is gentamicin and metronidazole with penicillin. The foot should be watched carefully and any localized area of pus drained and dead tissue excised widely. Infection spreads rapidly and not infrequently whole rays of the foot need to be removed with the area left open to drain. With this aggressive approach excellent results can be obtained (*Fig.* 54.20).

In the second type of presentation the patient has large vessel disease with absent pulses. This situation is more serious and results again from trauma and superimposed infection, but blood supply is so poor that the ultimate prognosis for the limb is bad. Once again antibiotics should be given and an arteriogram performed. Some form of limb salvage procedure has to be undertaken followed by excision of the affected areas of the foot and toe leaving the wounds to drain and heal. Secondary amputations with skin grafting might be necessary. Unfortunately, the limb salvage in this type of diabetic foot tends to be poor.

AMPUTATIONS

The end point of failed vascular surgery or indeed if vascular surgery is inappropriate is an amputation. The aim must always be to do an amputation early rather than late and give the patient a chance to rehabilitate himself before he becomes so ill that this is not possible. Generally speaking, distal amputations are contraindicated because they tend not to heal unless some form of simultaneous vascular reconstruction is also possible. The best amputation, which affords good rehabilitation is a below-knee procedure. Alternatives such as through-knee or above-knee amputations do not give such good results. Amputations through

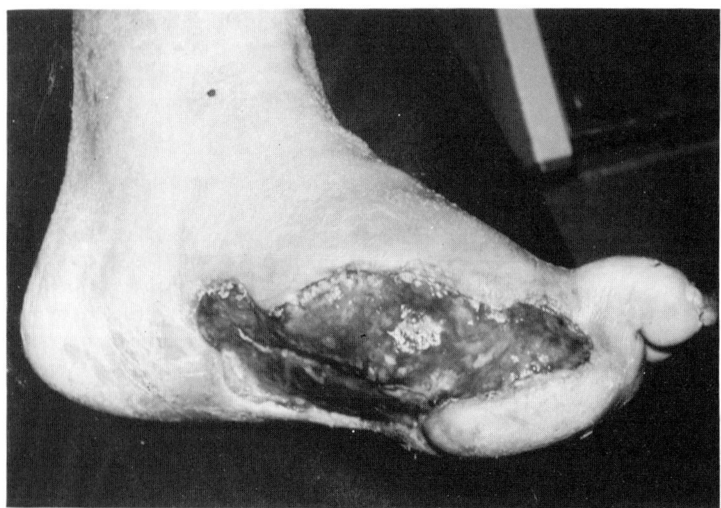

Fig. 54.20 Diabetic foot recovering after extensive removal of infected and gangrenous tissue.

the foot and ankle should be avoided in these patients unless an associated revascularization procedure is being performed.

Above-knee Amputation

This procedure is usually undertaken in patients where tissue loss is such that a below-knee or distal amputation will not heal. These amputations usually heal when done through equal anterior and posterior flaps at approximately 11 inches from the trochanter. Prostheses are improving but in older people this type of procedure tends to make rehabilitation difficult.

Through-knee and Gritti–Stokes Amputations

These procedures are popular with some surgeons and do provide good rehabilitation, especially with the new evolving prostheses. They are not, however, universally performed and tend to be relatively unpopular.

Below-knee Amputations

This procedure is a difficult operation and satisfactory healing rates can only be obtained if the surgeon concerned is experienced. About 75–80% should heal if case selection is appropriate (*Fig.* 54.21). Various methods of trying to assess whether the flow of blood in the skin and muscles is adequate to allow healing to take place have been investigated. These include measurements of blood flow, tissue oxygen tension, thermography and pressure measurement. Unfortunately although useful guidance can be obtained, absolute cut off points are not available and in spite of these sophisticated tests there are still a percentage of amputations which fail to heal and have to be converted later to above-knee procedures. A classic below-knee amputation involves the fashioning of a long posterior flap which contains most of the vessels and muscles. The flap is then folded over the bones to form an even stump (*Fig.* 54.22). Recently, attempts to produce better healing have led to the introduction of the skew flap amputation making use of the areas where the blood supply is thought to be best.

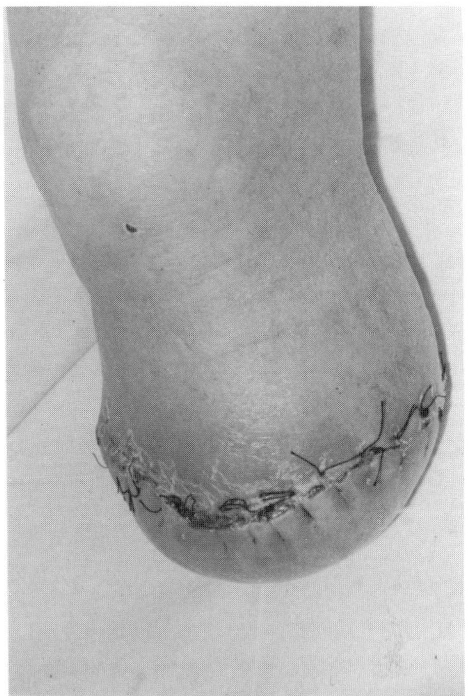

Fig. 54.21 Healing below-knee amputation stump.

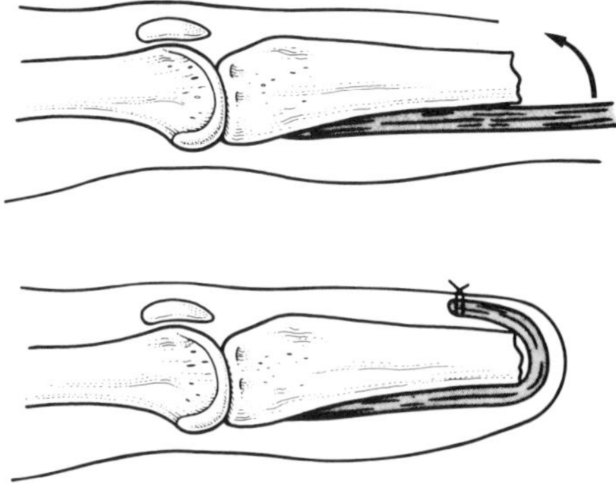

Fig. 54.22 Below-knee amputation. Posterior flap incorporating the muscles is used to cover the tibial stump.

Distal Amputations

Amputations through the ankle or mid-tarsal area or toes should only be performed if the blood supply can be improved. Generally speaking the Syme's amputation should not be done for patients with peripheral vascular disease. Transmetatarsal procedures are undertaken using a sole flap very similar to that used for below-knee amputations. Toes are removed using equal anterior and posterior flaps and in general sutures should not be used to close the skin, this being best done with pieces of steristrip or other skin adhesives.

Rehabilitation of the amputee is extremely important and the surgeon performing the procedure is responsible for making sure that satisfactory facilities for limb fitting and rehabilitation are available.

REST PAIN WITH PULSES IN NON-DIABETICS

This curious condition sometimes causes pain in the leg of a patient who is non-diabetic, is found to have severe pain with tiny areas of skin loss but all peripheral pulses are present. This presentation is probably due to platelet embolization from areas of aorta or larger vessels where plaques have formed. Treatment is by giving antiplatelet drugs or in some cases removing the area of platelet embolization if this can be found. Conventional arteriography is not useful for this but labelling of platelets with indium may show up a hot spot which could be excised.

VASOSPASTIC DISORDERS AND ARTERITIS

Raynaud's phenomenon and various other types of immune arteritis do affect the foot. If Raynaud's disease is present it usually affects both hands and feet, rarely the feet alone are involved. In severe cases where blistering is present with tissue loss, surgical sympathectomy is the answer although it should not be performed bilaterally in males because ejaculation is thereby prevented. For acrocyanosis which presents with extensive cold blue feet sometimes extending up to the leg and knee area, sympathectomy may again be useful in selected cases. Patients with various types of arteritis such as those caused by lupus erythematosus, polyarteritis or scleroderma are hard to treat. Even though the underlying condition is treated, the foot lesions do not usually respond and direct surgery or sympathectomy rarely help.

Further Reading

Borozan P. G., Schuler J. J., Spigos D. G. et al. (1985) Percutaneous angioplasty of the lower extremities. In: Jamieson C. (ed.) *Current Operative Surgery—Vascular Surgery*. London, Baillière Tindall, pp. 63–74.

Buonocore E., Meaney T. F., Borkowski G. P. et al. (1981) Digital subtraction angiography of the abdominal aorta and renal arteries. *Radiology* **139**, 281–216.

Couch N. (1984) Amputation and rehabilitation: the geriatric and diabetic leg amputee. In: Bell P. R. F. and Tilney N. L. (ed.) *Vascular Surgery*. London, Butterworth, pp. 230–247.

Darling R. C., Buckley C. J., Abbott W. M. et al. (1974) Intermittent claudication in young athletes: popliteal artery entrapment syndrome. *J. Trauma* **14**, 543.

Evans L. E., Webster M. W., Brooks D. H. et al. (1981) Expanded polytetrafluoroethylene femoropopliteal grafts: 48 months follow-up. *Surgery* **89**, 16.

Jamil Z., Hobson R. W. II, Lynch T. G. et al. (1984) Revascularization of the profunda femoris artery for limb salvage. *Am. J. Surg.* **50**(2), 109–111.

Leader (1985) Neurospinous claudication. *Lancet* **2**, 704.

Levine A. W., Bandyk D. F., Boner P. H. et al. (1985) Lessons learned in adopting the in-situ saphenous vein bypass. *J. Vasc. Surg.* **2**(1), 145–153.

Macpherson D. S., Evans D. H., Bell P. R. F. (1984) Common femoral artery doppler wave forms: A comparison of three methods of objective analysis with direct pressure measurement. *Br. J. Surg.* **71**, 46–50.

Ratliff D. A., Clyne C. A. C., Chant A. D. B. et al. (1984) Prediction of amputation wound healing: the role of transcutaneous P_{O_2} assessment. *Br. J. Surg.* **71**, 219–223.

Towne J. B. (1984) Management of foot lesions in the diabetic patient. In: Rutherford R. B. (ed.) *Vascular Surgery*. London, Saunders, pp. 661–669.

55 *Emergency Non-traumatic Vascular Conditions*

M. G. Walker

ARTERIAL EMBOLISM

Arterial embolism is the most frequent cause of acute ischaemia which may be completely reversible if diagnosed and treated promptly. It occurs most often against a background of cardiac decompensation. Organized thrombus, often from a heart chamber, is dislodged, commonly impacting and obstructing a vessel at a bifurcation. The majority of emboli travel to the lower extremities, about half lodging in the common femoral artery. The patients are often elderly and frail, almost 80% of them having some form of cardiac decompensation. About half will have atrial fibrillation, most frequently in association with ischaemic heart disease. One-third will have had a proven myocardial infarction, one-quarter a previous embolism. Other causes of atrial fibrillation such as rheumatic fever, thyrotoxicosis and hypertension are less frequently implicated. Subacute bacterial endocarditis produces multiple emboli, and prosthetic heart valves are also a source of emboli. Mural thrombi from atherosclerotic lesions may break away. Cardioversion may also result in embolization.

The diagnosis is usually straightforward, thrombosis and embolism being easily distinguished from one another. Difficulty may arise, however, as to the cause of ischaemia where there is no obvious source of embolus, especially if there is a background of known peripheral vascular disease. In such cases of acute-on-chronic ischaemia, arteriography is of great help in establishing the diagnosis and determining the correct treatment.

Obstruction of the circulation produces sudden ischaemia of the affected part which, if not relieved, may result in gangrene. The degree of ischaemia depends on the site and duration of the obstruction and the nature of the collateral circulation. Pain, followed by coldness, pallor and numbness and a varying degree of paralysis is the rule. It should be remembered that not infrequently the embolic event occurs during sleep, resulting in presenting symptoms of a motor or sensory nature. Occasionally 'silent' embolism occurs; the patient being unaware of the condition.

Clinical examination reveals usually a waxy pallor, empty veins, coldness and absence of pulses distal to the site of obstruction. Motor and sensory loss to a varying degree are also evident. Differential diagnosis should not prove too much of a problem. The chief conditions to be borne in mind are: acute arterial thrombosis, dissecting aneurysm, deep vein thrombosis, venous gangrene, drug abuse.

A careful history and physical examination are usually enough to establish the diagnosis in most patients. Because of the frequency of underlying cardiac problems, electrocardiography and chest radiography should be arranged. Full blood count, blood sugar, urea and electrolytes should be estimated and Doppler ultrasound assessment of the affected limb recorded. Arteriography is only necessary when there is doubt as to whether the problem is thrombotic or embolic.

The prime consideration should be of life rather than limb salvage. Having made the diagnosis, it is important to institute supportive measures to correct any existing cardiac decompensation as far as is possible. Digitalis, diuretics, anti-arrhythmic drugs are all used as necessary. Maintenance of blood pressure is also vital. Unless contraindicated, systemic heparinization should be implemented immediately. This helps to prevent further propagation of thrombus and also, hopefully, lessens the chance of an associated deep vein thrombosis. Since the advent of the Fogarty catheter, limb salvage has improved dramatically but the overall mortality remains approximately 25%. In view of the usual poor general condition of the patient, the procedure of arterial embolectomy is most frequently carried out under local anaesthesia. Only when embolism is associated with a near terminal event, or when massive gangrene is present, is embolectomy contraindicated.

As a general rule, the longer the duration of occlusion the greater the degree of ischaemia, but there are frequent and significant exceptions to this concept (*Fig*. 55.1). The condition of the patient's limb, when initially seen, is the real determinant of limb salvage. Lack of motor activity associated with a 'wooden' feel to the muscle bulk is a contraindication to surgery. When there is advanced ischaemia as evidenced by early rigor, the amputation rate is high but limb salvage not impossible. Complications with restoration of flow in such a case relate to the return of acidotic blood to the heart, hypotension and fatal arrhythmias occurring. Renal failure may also ensue. Maintenance of blood pressure by volume replacement and cardiac support is necessary.

The common femoral, superficial and profunda femoris arteries are displayed via a vertical groin incision. An arteriotomy is made over the common femoral artery sufficient to allow visualization of the profunda orifice. Local thrombus is removed and then with care and never using force, the Fogarty catheter is passed distally down the profunda and superficial femoral arteries. It is vital to ensure

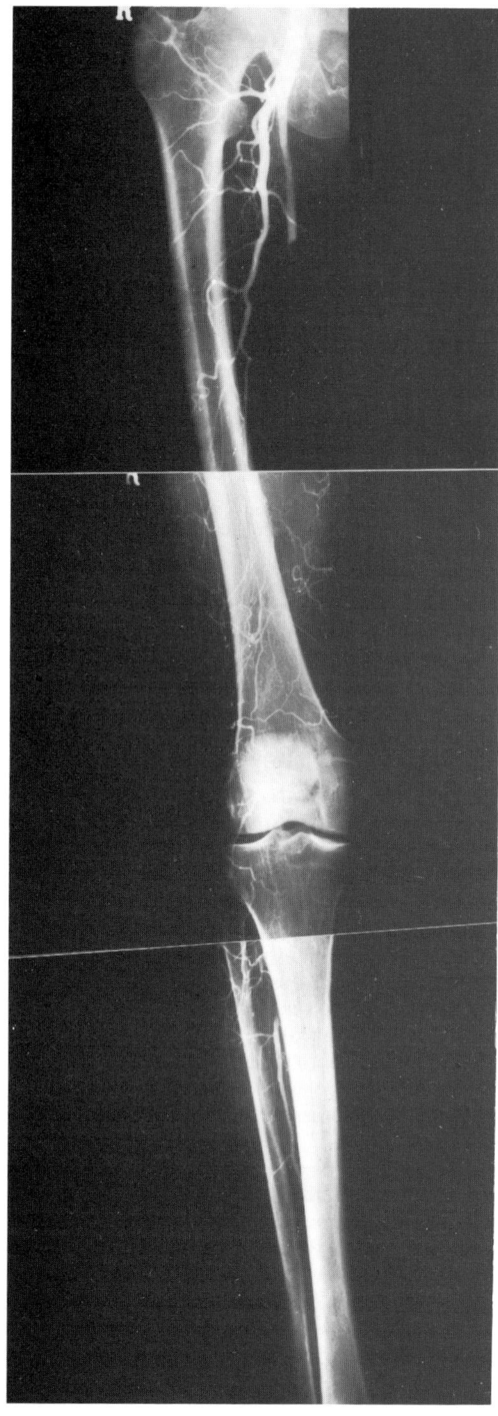

a

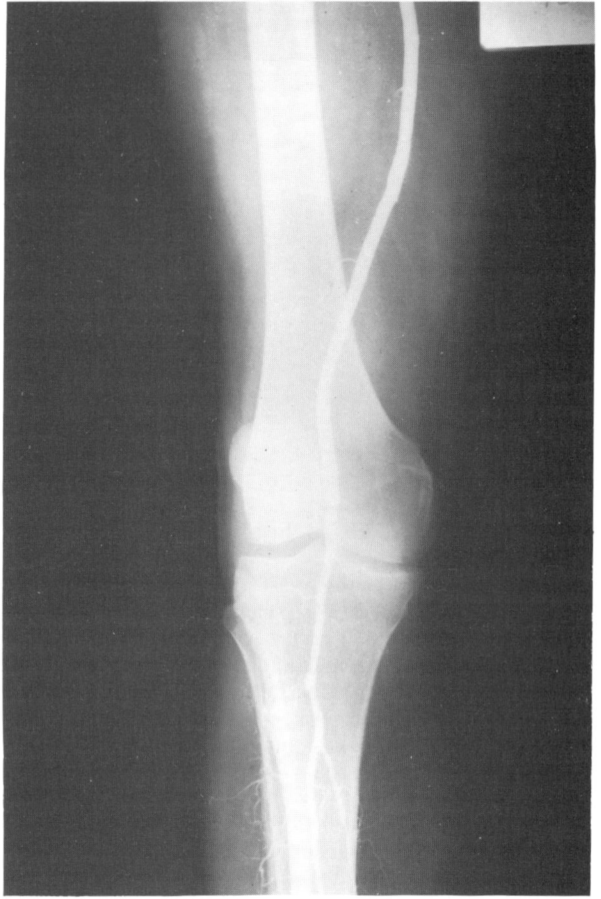

b

Fig. 55.1 Thrombectomy 3 weeks after the initial embolic/thrombotic event resulted in patency of the superficial femoral, popliteal and peroneal arteries and relief of rest pain. *a*, Preoperative and *b*, postoperative arteriograms.

patency of the profunda femoris as it may represent the sole source of blood supply to the lower limb. The catheter should be passed on two or three occasions and patency of the distal arterial tree confirmed, especially the popliteal trifurcation, by operative arteriography as back-bleeding is an unreliable sign. Care should be taken when inflating the balloon in the calf as over-distension may result in serious vessel damage. As the catheter is withdrawn, the balloon size has to be adjusted and this 'feel' is only gained through experience. The arteriotomy is closed with a continuous suture, though on occasion an autogenous vein patch graft may be necessary where stenosis seems apparent. Occasionally it may be necessary to expose the popliteal artery at the same time in order to guide the catheter beyond its trifurcation, either by direct manipulation or arteriotomy. Where there has been delay in revascularization or swelling is present, then fasciotomy is indicated. Heparin therapy is recommenced postoperatively for 2–3 days and the patient then given oral anticoagulants for 6 months or so. By such measures, limb salvage rates of 95% are achieved.

Saddle embolism of the abdominal aortic bifurcation is dealt with by the same approach, exposing both common femoral arteries. The diagnosis is usually suggested by the sudden onset of pain and coldness in the lower limbs, with loss of the common femoral pulses. Arteriography is not indicated. Local anaesthesia is used. Before passing the catheter proximally, the contralateral common femoral artery is occluded to prevent possible embolization to that limb from ipsilateral catheter dislodgement at the aortic bifurcation. Similar precautions should be observed when dealing with the other side. The catheter should also be passed down the profunda and superficial femoral arteries of both limbs to ensure patency. Operative arteriography should be employed to ensure objective evidence that the proximal and distal arterial trees are patent.

Embolism of the upper limb is a less frequent event. The collateral supply to the upper limb is better than that of the lower limb but embolectomy should be performed in the majority of cases. Embolic material lodges with approximately equal frequency in the subclavian, axillary and brachial arteries. Using local anaesthesia, an arteriotomy is made over the axillary artery which allows adequate access both proximally and distally. Operative arteriography is carried out to ensure patency of the distal arterial tree. As long as either radial or ulnar artery is patent, then viability of the limb is ensured. A close check should be kept on the pulses after restoration of the blood flow as further embolism or thrombosis may occur.

Very occasionally, systemic heparinization in dosage 2000–4000 u hourly may result in limb salvage where surgery is contraindicated. Thrombolytic agents such as streptokinase have little or no role in the management of acute arterial embolism. When intense vasoconstriction persists, judicious and cautious use of prostaglandin E_1 (PGE_1) via a central venous catheter in carefully selected patients, may potentiate limb salvage. Where signs of irreversible ischaemia exist in the limb, e.g. fixed mottling of the skin, muscle involvement or joint contractures, early amputation at the appropriate level is indicated.

Loin pain and haematuria may follow renal artery embolism and the diagnosis should be confirmed by selective arteriography. The embolectomy technique is similar to that described for a peripheral artery. Exposure of the renal arteries is gained through a midline incision. The patient is systematically heparinized and the aorta clamped above and below the renal arteries. A transverse arteriotomy is made level with the renal arteries and using a Fogarty catheter, the embolus is extracted. The arteriotomy is closed using a continuous suture of 4/0 polypropylene. The management of mesenteric arterial embolism is dealt with in Chapter 56.

Overall, the results of arterial embolectomy for acute arterial embolism are rewarding and justify an aggressive approach both in medical and surgical terms in the management of these patients.

INFLAMMATORY ANEURYSM OF THE ABDOMINAL AORTA

First described in the surgical literature in 1972, the reported incidence of inflammatory aneurysms of the abdominal aorta ranges from 2·2% to 23%. Although there is considerable conjecture as to the exact cause of such aneurysms, most authors are agreed that the aetiology and pathogenesis remain obscure. Patients with inflammatory aneurysms tend to be younger and probably present earlier because of acute abdominal pain. Indeed the presence of an acutely tender aneurysm without evidence of circulatory collapse should suggest such a diagnosis. This may be accompanied by an elevated ESR and if intravenous urography is employed, medial ureteric displacement or possibly hydronephrosis may also suggest the diagnosis. Although inflammatory aneurysms are often small, difficult to palpate and thus diagnose, a CT scan or ultrasonography will often help clinch the diagnosis. Most inflammatory aneurysms, however, are discovered only at the time of operation. It has also been reported that they have a lesser tendency to rupture than non-inflammatory atherosclerotic abdominal aortic aneurysms.

The striking appearance of an inflammatory aneurysm is due to the dense white tissue of its anterior wall. This inflammatory process may be extensive and involve such structures as the fourth part of duodenum, ureter, mesentery, small bowel, sigmoid colon, renal vessels and inferior vena cava. Of these the duodenum is perhaps most frequently involved. However, the aorta proximal and iliac vessels distal to the aneurysm may appear relatively normal. The thickness of the anterior wall of the aneurysm can range from 1 to 3 cm, although the posterolateral wall may be thin as with non-inflammatory aneurysms. The thickness of the anterior wall is mostly adventitial. In general, patients with inflammatory aneurysms often have little in the way of diffuse arterial disease.

Aetiology

This remains obscure, although possible factors suggested include:

infection
spondylitis
retroperitoneal fibrosis
rheumatoid arthritis
sclerosing lipogranulomatosis

An infective cause seems unlikely since bacteriological culture of such aneurysms is consistently negative.

Pathogenesis

Although largely unknown, it has been postulated that the aneurysm wall could be the source of a factor which, if repeatedly released from the aneurysm wall, could initiate the inflammatory reaction. The view that this reaction is secondary to the presence of the aneurysm itself is supported on two counts. First, because symptoms usually resolve after graft replacement and second, recent histopathological studies have suggested that all atherosclerotic aneurysms are associated to some degree with a fibrotic reaction. An inflammatory aneurysm therefore may represent one end of the spectrum of inflammatory change. Slow leakage of blood resulting in peri-aortic fibrosis and inflammation is unlikely as a factor because of the virtual absence of haemosiderin pigment in the aneurysm wall. Although histologically the features of retroperitoneal fibrosis are identical to those of inflammatory aneurysms, patients with the former condition seldom if ever develop inflammatory aneurysms. It has also been suggested that there may be an immunological cause with the atherosclerotic aorta as a source of the allergen.

Histological Features

Most inflammatory aneurysms exhibit a layered appearance: a layer of atheromatous abdominal aorta surrounded by a further layer of inflammatory tissue which consists of sheets of collagen fibres infiltrated mainly with plasma cells and lymphocytes.

Treatment

Very occasionally it may be deemed too hazardous by the surgeon to attempt graft replacement of the inflammatory aneurysm because of the extensive involvement of surrounding organs. In such an instance steroid therapy should be implemented, the dose adjusted according to the patient's response and ESR. The patient should thereafter be regularly assessed by CT scanning until the inflammatory response is seen to decrease when graft replacement should be undertaken. However, the patient is still at risk from rupture during this period and should the CT scan show an increase

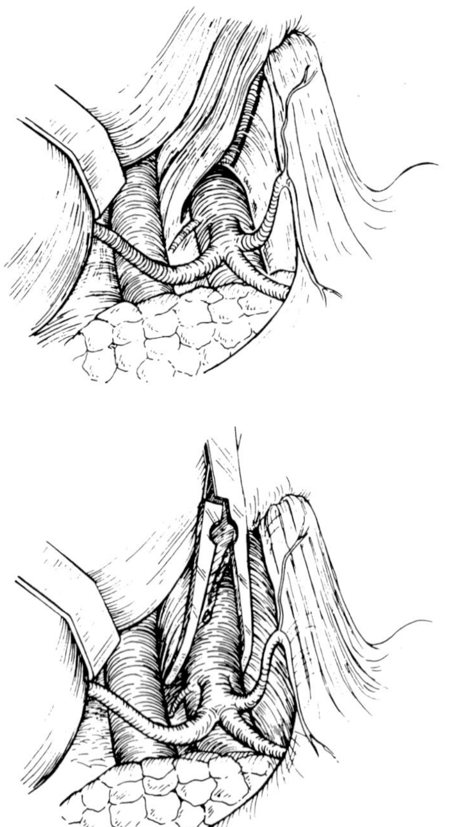

Fig. 55.2 To gain access to the supracoeliac aorta, the liver is retracted upward, the stomach downward and the posterior peritoneum incised. The muscular crus of the diaphragm is incised.

in aneurysm size or thinning of the aneurysm wall, graft replacement should be undertaken immediately. Although the hazards of operation in such cases are well documented, with an associated higher morbidity or mortality than with non-inflammatory aneurysms, an aggressive approach to primary graft replacement should be adopted. Proximal control of the aorta is easily and quickly achieved with minimal dissection of the supracoeliac aorta (*Fig.* 55.2). An alternative to this approach is to use an intra-aortic balloon which can be introduced in the midline of the aneurysm with relatively little blood loss. Dissection at all times should not stray from the midline and a plane of cleavage within the thickened aneurysmal wall can be found such that the adherent structures can be peeled off the aneurysm without injury. Unless a ureter is completely obstructed, it is probably wise to avoid ureterolysis since the inflammatory process resolves spontaneously after operation and often this will allow even a moderate hydronephrosis to resolve.

RUPTURED ABDOMINAL AORTIC ANEURYSM

Introduction

As people live longer the incidence of atherosclerotic abdominal aortic aneurysm has increased, particularly so in the Western World where it is estimated that at least 2% of the elderly population are so afflicted. Without treatment, 30% of patients with asymptomatic aneurysms survive 5 years, although the risk of rupture increases the greater the size of the aneurysm. Eighty per cent of patients with symptomatic aneurysms will die from rupture within one year if left untreated. None the less successful repair of these aneurysms whether on an elective or emergency basis is associated with an overall survival of 65% at 5 years which compares favourably with an identical population without aneurysm whose survival at five years is in the order of 76%. Although the majority of patients are male in the sixth and seventh decades of life often with a background of myocardial and/or cerebrovascular insufficiency, rupture of an abdominal aortic aneurysm has been recorded in a 7-year-old girl with a successful outcome.

Diagnosis

The diagnosis in over 90% of patients with ruptured abdominal aortic aneurysm is usually simple, the classic presentation being one of hypotension, abdominal and/or lumbar pain and a tender, pulsating, abdominal mass. Pain may be constant or intermittent with radiation to an iliac fossa, usually the left, or the groin. This is because the base of the aneurysm is usually to the left. The pain may also mimic ureteric colic and in patients over 60 years of age, such a diagnosis should take second place to a leaking or ruptured aneurysm until this is proven otherwise.

Occasionally, however, diagnosis may be difficult, especially in an obese patient where palpation of the abdomen may be unhelpful. In those patients with atypical symptoms, careful examination may reveal other signs of retroperitoneal haemorrhage such as psoas irritation, ecchymosis in the upper medial aspect of the thigh, scrotum, penis, umbilicus or flank. Rarely, perianal bruising or even anal pulsation may be noted. Less common, but equally dramatic, presentations may result from aneurysm involvement of adjacent structures. Torrential haematemesis or melaena may thus result from aorto-enteric fistula; high output cardiac failure from aortocaval fistula. Femoral and obturator neuropathy has also been observed. Although angiography is rarely necessary to establish diagnosis, on occasion it can be helpful in those difficult cases where clinical signs are sparse.

Treatment

Immediately on arrival in hospital, it is vital to establish central venous access, catheterize the bladder and cross-match the patient for 10 units of blood. A broad-spectrum prophylactic antibiotic should be administered and wherever possible Swan–Ganz catheterization employed for accurate monitoring and therapeutic purposes. A most critical period is during induction of anaesthesia where muscle relaxation may exacerbate existing hypotension, resulting in death. Successful aortic control prior to induction of anaesthesia has been reported using a Fogarty occlusion aortic balloon catheter inserted under local anaesthesia in a retrograde fashion via the common femoral artery. Using a similar technique, the brachial artery has been catheterized when the iliac segment does not permit passage of the Fogarty catheter. A simple fast and reliable method of aortic control postanaesthetic induction is to cross-clamp the supracoeliac aorta (*Fig.* 55.2). Less reliable methods of aortic control during this critical period include direct manual compression of the aorta, insertion of a thumb into the neck of the aneurysm and use of a Foley or Fogarty catheter inserted directly through the sac of the aneurysm. When control has been achieved the iliac vessels are clamped, the sac opened and the neck of the aneurysm identified. The aorta is then clamped just below the level of the renal arteries and the supracoeliac clamp removed. It may be necessary on occasion to divide the left renal vein to gain adequate access to the neck of the aneurysm. Minimal dissection is required and circumferential control of vessels unnecessary. Wherever possible a straight tube inlay graft should be used to minimize operative time. Systemic heparinization prior to cross-clamping of the vessels may be used although many surgeons prefer to instil heparin down both limbs distal to the iliac clamps. During cross-clamping, a small dose of intravenous diuretic should be given to stimulate renal function. On release of the clamps flow should be directed down both internal iliacs initially in order to avoid possible distal embolization and the possibility of the 'trash foot' syndrome. Once haemostasis has been secured, the body of the graft should be lavaged with topical antibiotic and the sac of the aneurysm tightly approximated over the graft. Prior to closure of the abdomen lower limb circulation should be checked. Where doubt exists about the viability of the left colon, the inferior mesenteric artery should be implanted into the body of the graft. Finally, the patient should be transferred to the Intensive Care Unit for critical monitoring.

Factors Influencing Mortality

Risk factors such as myocardial ischaemia, hypertension and age account for over 90% of deaths occurring within 30 days of operation. Other important factors implicated in this mortality are massive blood loss, renal failure, coagulation defects and prolonged ventilatory support. Ischaemic colitis, said to occur in 2% of patients, may in fact be more common, a figure approaching 7% being more realistic. When this does occur, a mortality of 40–75% can be expected. Approximately 85% of these ischaemic lesions follow resection of ruptured abdominal aortic aneurysms, whereas the incidence is only 15% after reconstruction for aorto-iliac occlusive disease. Rarely, paraplegia may result from ischaemic injury to the spinal cord. This is brought about by disruption of blood supply to the anterior spinal artery. Although improvements in operative technique and experience were responsible for decreasing mortality in the recent past, better anaesthesia, monitoring and supportive measures peroperatively and in the early postoperative period have mainly accounted for the success achieved today. However, prevention of rupture must surely be a better alternative and to this end, efforts should be concentrated in dealing with aneurysms before this disaster occurs.

56 *Mesenteric Vascular Disease*

Adrian Marston

The mesenteric circulation, which comprises about a quarter of the blood volume and a fifth of the cardiac output, supplies the gut almost entirely via the superior mesenteric artery (SMA) and returns blood to the liver via the portal vein. This circulatory compartment has certain behavioural characteristics which depend on its basic structure and on the way in which its haemodynamics are regulated. These have been determined largely by evolution. Clearly, the requirements of a herbivore will be very different from those of a hunting animal.

Such major species differences must be carefully borne in mind when experiments involving reduction in blood supply are studied. It is simple to occlude the SMA or its branches in the laboratory preparation and a large literature has accumulated around such studies, most of which are probably irrelevant to man.

A factor, however, which is common to all species, and which distinguishes the intestinal circulation from other vascular territories, is the potentially infective nature of the bowel contents. The gut wall lives in equilibrium with its contained population, and any reduction of viability due to ischaemia will immediately result in bacterial invasion with an inflammatory response, i.e. an 'enteritis' or 'colitis'. Whereas an infarcted kidney or myocardium can heal cleanly by fibrosis, the same does not apply to the gut, where necrosis always leads to gangrene and, unless action is taken, to the death of the patient. There appears to be a very critical margin of vascular supply after which these changes are initiated. Provided that it occurs slowly, progressive reduction in blood supply to the gut is well tolerated and at first causes no demonstrable change in structure or function. When the point is reached at which the equilibrium between bacterial challenge and mucosal defence is upset, an abrupt series of changes takes place, the consequences of which are discussed in detail below.

APPLIED ANATOMY

Of the three great vessels to the alimentary tract, the SMA is much the most important because it is functionally an end-artery which has the function of supplying blood to the entire midgut loop, i.e. from the duodenojejunal flexure to the mid-transverse colon. At the upper and lower ends of the abdomen, there are connections with extracoelomic vessels which protect against any fall in blood flow. Thus, if the coeliac axis is occluded the deficiency is quickly made up from diaphragmatic, intercostal and oesophageal vessels, supplemented by contributions from the abdominal wall, and the circulation of the liver, stomach, spleen and pancreas may hardly be affected. In the same way, because the pelvic organs have a rich supply from the internal iliac artery, the inferior mesenteric artery is, within certain limits, a dispensable vessel. Ischaemic problems in the rectum are a clinical rarity.

Generally speaking, the small bowel is supplied from the left side of the SMA and the large bowel from the right. From the left there arise from 5 to 12 'intestinal' arteries, the upper third of which supply the jejunum and the lower two-thirds the ileum, though this proportion is variable. The vessels intercommunicate in a series of arcades, which become progressively more developed from above downwards. The existence of this collateral network means that interruption of one or more of the intestinal vessels is unlikely to lead to infarction, as an effective arterial supply is maintained by its neighbours. There are, furthermore, other compensatory structures within the wall of the bowel which protect against ischaemic damage.

The rich blood supply to the small bowel, which is out of all proportion to its oxygen consumption, is in sharp contrast to the pattern of the vessels which spring from the opposite (right) side of the SMA. Here the three main arteries to the colon, i.e. (in order of their origin) the middle, right and ileocolic arteries which are comparatively slender vessels have a very simple system of anastomosis in their proximal parts. The anastomosis, such as it is, is formed by the marginal artery of the colon, which represents a condensation of the complicated arcade system of the small bowel. This marginal artery, moreover, tends to be absent or inadequate at the very point where the superior and inferior mesenteric vascular territories meet, and it is here that ischaemic damage to the colon is most often seen.

The final branches of the arcades run tangentially up to the bowel wall and penetrate alternative aspects of its circumference. A few minor vessels run backwards to supply the serosa and muscle, but the main supply passes through a number of straight vessels, arranged in roughly rectangular fashion, which penetrate through to the submucosa, where they form a vascular carpet on which the mucosa rests, extending uninterruptedly from the duodenum to the anal canal.

This provides a very efficient collateral network, which

supplements the arcade arrangement in the mesentery. The network contains both arteries and veins, but there appears to be very little if any, direct anatomical communication between them. From this submucosal plexus spring the arterioles to the villi, which are the final determinant of exchange of nutrients and oxygen. A single central arteriole runs up the villus and arborizes at its tip into a dense capillary network, draining into the venules lying beneath the basement membrane, which in turn unite to form two to three trunks running back into the submucosal plexus. The arrangement of artery and vein in the villus is of crucial importance to intestinal function.

The veins accompany the arteries in the gut wall and mesentery as periarterial plexuses, which eventually fuse to form the superior mesenteric vein. The colon is drained by the inferior mesenteric vein which runs into the splenic vein. The union of superior mesenteric and splenic veins forms the portal vein just below the hilum of the liver. Because there are no valves in this venous system it is capable of considerable expansion and variations in pressure, depending on physiological events in the liver.

CLASSIFICATION OF MESENTERIC VASCULAR DISEASE

In the past, these conditions were thought of in terms of morbid anatomy, and were classified as being due to acute or chronic arterial obstruction (embolus or thrombosis), inflammatory disease, 'non-occlusive infarction' and venous disorders. In fact the situation is much more complex.

Mesenteric embolus is now a rarity, but the condition is of scientific interest because it is the only clinical parallel of the standard laboratory model of intestinal ischaemia, i.e. the abrupt occlusion of the blood supply to the midgut loop of a healthy animal with normal vessels. Most patients who die from intestinal infarction do not in fact have emboli. Some have atheromatous lesions at the origins of their visceral arteries, but in one-third of fatal cases of gut necrosis there is no vascular occlusion detected at autopsy. Moreover, stenoses, plaques and even complete occlusions of the mesenteric vessels can be found post-mortem in individuals who have had no alimentary symptoms during life, although recent experience suggests that these lesions have been over-reported in the past.

For this reason, 'mesenteric thrombosis' can no longer be considered as a direct cause of acute intestinal ischaemia, because the relationship between the vascular lesion and what occurs in the gut is uncertain in its timing. There is circumstantial evidence, however, that persons who have atheromatous plaques on their visceral arteries may sustain an infarction if for some reason the pressure across this lesion is reduced.

A fall in central arterial pressure will lead to an increase in sympathetic drive and in the level of circulating catecholamines, which (with certain reservations) results in further vasoconstriction in the mesenteric circulatory bed.

A scientific and at the same time practical classification of mesenteric vascular disease is as follows:

Acute Intestinal Ischaemia

With arterial occlusion
Without arterial occlusion

Focal Ischaemia of the Intestine

In the small bowel
In the colon

Chronic Arterial Obstruction

Venous Obstruction

Central
Peripheral

ACUTE INTESTINAL ISCHAEMIA

By this is meant a clinical state in which the metabolic needs of the small intestine outruns its blood supply, resulting in threatened or complete necrosis of most of the alimentary tract.

The Clinical Picture

The classic description of acute ischaemia is of the sudden onset of severe abdominal colic, followed by the passage of mucus and blood per rectum, and within a few hours by peripheral circulatory failure. There is usually a history of pre-existing cardiac disease. The initial colic is later superseded by dull generalized abdominal pain, with ileus and distension, and in the absence of treatment, death occurs within 1 or 2 days.

Such striking symptomatology is easily recognized and leads to a prompt and definite diagnosis. In fact, however, few cases are diagnosed early, because the classically-described clinical picture is far from typical. For instance, it may present quite insidiously, beginning with mild cramps which are dismissed as a minor gastrointestinal upset, and the general condition of a patient with even severe degrees of intestinal damage may remain deceptively normal for hours or days. The rare embolus which lodges in the mesenteric artery of a patient recovering in hosptial from a myocardial infarction is often diagnosed early, because everyone is alerted to the possibility. But where the condition arises at home it is rarely diagnosed at all, and admission may be delayed for several days.

The situation, then, is of a patient with known rheumatic or degenerative cardiovascular disease, perhaps with a previous history of embolization, who presents with acute non-specific abdominal pain.

It is well established experimentally that the result of occluding the normal SMA is intense spasm of the small intestine (*Fig.* 56.1). This accounts for the severe colic at the onset, and for the fact that the patient seen at this stage may have no abdominal signs apart from exaggerated bowel sounds. Later the spasm relaxes and the bowel becomes immobile, though without necessarily much in the way of peritoneal reaction. At this phase, the patient presents with a moderately distended silent abdomen and slight tenderness in the right iliac fossa. As necrosis proceeds outwards to the serosa there is a peritonitic reaction and the clinical picture becomes that of a desperate illness with gross distension and ileus, exquisite tenderness and a characteristic odour on the breath. Abdominal pain and distension further interfere with respiratory movements, resulting in anxiety, restlessness, air hunger, and cyanosis. Urine output falls off as dehydration proceeds, and lowered tissue perfusion and metabolic acidosis contribute to the condition of shock.

Eventually restlessness gives place to stupor and frank coma. The clinical picture described here will obviously be modified in practice by the administration of analgesics and parenteral fluids, but it remains true that by the time that these florid physical signs have appeared, the point of recovery has probably been passed.

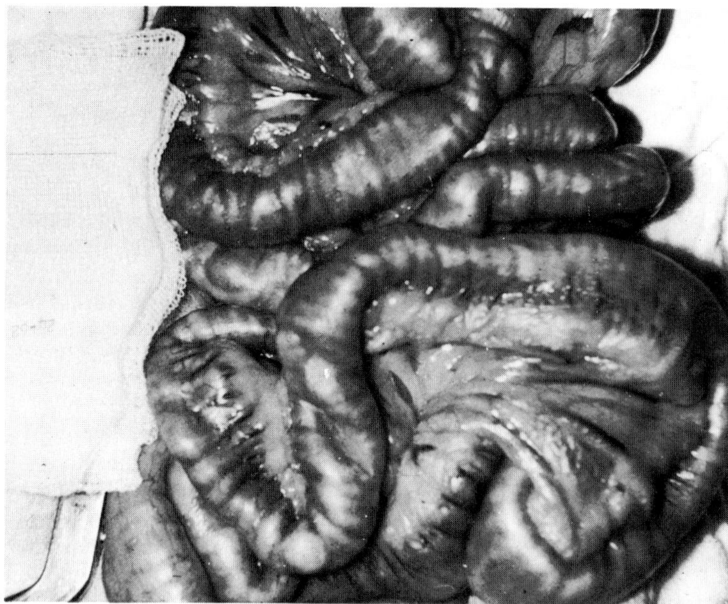

Fig. 56.1 Spasm of the bowel following experimental occlusion of the SMA.

Radiological and Laboratory Investigations

These are disappointing, and tend to confirm the clinical impression rather than to add materially to the diagnosis.

Plain films of the abdomen are described as showing gas-filled loops of small bowel, the translucent areas being separated by thickened, oedematous bowel wall. These are radiological niceties. In fact the appearances are non-specific and it is most unusual for a diagnosis to be arrived at from such radiographs. If bubbles of gas are present in the mesenteric veins, this is virtually pathognomonic of small bowel infarction. It is also, however, a sign of advanced disease.

The clinical laboratory has little help to offer in making the diagnosis. The leucocyte count is raised early in the course of the disease, so that a finding of 20 000 or 30 000 leucocytes in the peripheral blood, especially if the abdominal signs are unimpressive, should prompt the suspicion of intestinal infarction. Serum enzyme concentrations have proved surprisingly disappointing as an index to the severity of bowel necrosis. Although concentrations of alkaline phosphatase, transaminases and lactic dehydrogenase are frequently abnormal the actual pattern of enzymatic change is inconsistent and non-specific. There is some evidence that massive ischaemia is reflected by a rise in the serum levels of inorganic phosphate.

The Case for Emergency Aortography

Various authors have emphasized the importance of an immediate aortogram in the diagnosis of bowel infarction. However, the situation is not so simple.

1. As already mentioned, varying degrees of arterial occlusion are commonly found in the visceral trunks in subjects over the age of 45, without demonstrable effect on their health. It therefore follows that the presence of a blocked mesenteric artery in a patient with indeterminate abdominal pain gives little information either as to when the occlusion occurred, or whether it is the cause of the symptoms.

2. An angiographically open mesenteric vascular tree is of no diagnostic help to the surgeon and, if signs of peritonitis are present, will not and should not deter him from exploring the abdomen.

Some authors have claimed that non-occlusive intestinal failure can be diagnosed on the aortogram by the presence of a narrowed distal arterial tree with intramural spasm, and can then be treated by epidural blockade. While this is an attractive proposition, there is at present very scanty clinical evidence on which to base such a treatment policy and most experienced surgeons agree that the aortographic appearances may be misleading, and that if doubt exists, it is safer to operate. None the less, the clear demonstration of a mesenteric embolus on an aortogram certainly gives added confidence in planning the emergency operation.

Recently there have been encouraging results in cases of non-occlusive intestinal infarction, treated by injection of vasodilator drugs such as papaverine, tolazoline, glucagon and prostacyclin, directly into the SMA via the aortic catheter. This regime offers exciting possibilities of an improved success rate, but the danger of less experienced clinicians being misled by a normal aortogram into missing a surgically correctable peritonitis still exists.

Management

Threatened death of the intestine involves fluid loss and the effects of bacterial invasion. Therapy should therefore logically be directed against both these life-threatening processes.

The loss is initially of water, electrolytes and protein. This results in a rise in haematocrit and blood viscosity with a fall in circulating volume, leading to impaired tissue flow in the gut wall itself and in the rest of the body. Replacement is planned by serial measurements of the haematocrit, central venous pressure and urine output. Depending on the patient's known cardiac status and reserve, liberal quantities of balanced salt solutions (Hartmann, Ringer-lactate, PPF, or Dextran 70) are given, until the haematocrit falls to below 45 and the central venous pressure rises to 5–10 cm of saline.

Bacterial invasion and toxaemia clearly demand the use of antibiotics. While it is known from laboratory studies that pretreatment with such agents mitigates the effects of intestinal ischaemia, in the clinical context it is impossible to ensure that the antibiotic in fact reaches the site of the damage. Blood cultures are performed and the chosen drug then given intravenously. This will be either an aminoglycoside such as gentamicin, vibramycin or amikacin, or one of the recently introduced cephalosporins. The dose given will depend on the weight of the patient, the urine output and the serum concentration of the drug.

Heparin is given in order to prevent extension of thrombus in the mesenteric vessels and gut wall and, perhaps more importantly to counteract disseminated intravascular coagulation. Full heparinization is achieved by the immediate intravenous injection of 20 000 i.u. supplemented by 10 000–15 000 i.u. 6-hourly, or by continuous intravenous infusion. The only theoretical objection to heparin therapy is accentuation of the bleeding from the haemorrhagic infarct but this is rarely a major problem.

Metabolic acidosis is brought about by the combination of low-tissue perfusion, haemoconcentration, and absorption of the products of bacterial and gut necrosis. To this is added a respiratory component due to interference with chest movements and increased blood viscosity, with intrapulmonary sludging. Measurements of the base excess, P_{CO_2} and arterial pH will guide the amount of i.v. bicarbonate therapy required. Given reasonably normal pulmonary and renal function, restoration of the circulating blood volume will do much to restore correct acid–base equilibrium.

Laboratory evidence suggests that the use of α-blocking agents, such as a phenoxybenzamine, and β-stimulators, such as isoprenaline, increases flow in the mesenteric circuit and helps to preserve viability. There is little controlled clinical information and it is somewhat doubtful if, in the presence of a mesenteric vascular occlusion or massive shutdown of the minute vessels, any drug is capable of penetrating to the gut wall. Additionally, the fall in blood pressure which these agents (particularly phenoxybenzamine) bring about may be longstanding and difficult to control. By contrast, the use of vasoconstrictor agents, such as metaraminol or noradrenaline, is obviously to be condemned.

There is as yet no reported clinical experience of the use of glucagon or dopamine in this situation. Because of their reputed effect on lysosomal membrane stability, oxygen consumption, arterial resistance and complement fixation by endotoxin, the use of corticosteroids, in suprapharmacological dosage (1–2 g) has been advocated. Again, there is much experimental evidence to suggest that the precipitating event in ischaemic cell-destruction in the gut is the liberation of oxygen-free radicals, and inhibitors of the enzyme pathway such as allopurinol are effective in the laboratory preparation.

Digitalis constricts the mesenteric vessels and hence is a possible cause of intestinal ischaemia. Its cautious use may none the less be justified in the control of fast atrial fibrillation and congestive failure, as in these circumstances the effect will be to raise cardiac output and increase mesenteric blood flow.

The Operation

At the end of an assessment period of 3–4 h, or as long as is necessary to correct the fluid deficit and clarify the clinical picture, the decision regarding surgery is made. Bearing in mind that complete infarction of the midgut is for practical purposes always lethal, exploration should always be carried out if there is the remotest hope of success.

Under light general anaesthesia with intubation and muscular relaxation, the abdomen is opened through a long right paramedian incision, and the diagnosis confirmed. The situation is usually immediately obvious, because of the characteristic 'musty' smell of ischaemic small bowel: impossible to describe and unforgettable when once experienced. There is generally a small quantity of lightly blood-stained peritoneal fluid. Total, full-thickness necrosis with perforation is rare.

Arterial occlusion is usually limited to the origin of the SMA and it is fortunate that consecutive thrombosis into the distal arcades does not occur very often.

However, there is frequently some secondary occlusion of the mesenteric veins. About one-third of patients with acute midgut ischaemia have no demonstrable block in any major artery. The mortality in these circumstances is exceedingly high and we know that non-occlusive ischaemia is not susceptible to operation. If no arterial occlusion is found and the gut is still viable, the correct course is to inject liberal quantities of local anaesthetic into the coeliac and mesenteric plexuses supplemented by papaverine injected into the SMA, and to close the abdomen. Even the most recent series report a very high mortality.

If an embolus is found and the origin of the SMA is accessible, the vessel is opened and cleared with a Fogarty catheter. It may be better to carry out this manoeuvre through the ileocolic artery in the root of the caecal mesentery. A short arteriotomy is made in this vessel and a size 3 Fogarty catheter passed up into the origin of the SMA. The balloon is inflated and the embolus drawn down. This manoeuvre is repeated until as much as possible of the occluding material has been removed, the mesentery is then milked back to clear the distal vessels. The bowel is now inspected. In a reasonably early case, it begins to appear pink and healthier, with pulsation in the arcade vessels. There is a tendency at this stage for oedema and haemorrhage to occur and the loops of intestine must be handled very gently. Unless there are areas of frank gangrene, no resection should be undertaken, because it is very difficult to judge the extent of possible recovery, and suture lines are liable to break down. If the peripheral circulation to the bowel appears quite restored, the ileocolic artery can be safely ligated. If, however, as is frequently the case, there is some doubt as to patency of the origin, a side-to-side anastomosis between the ileocolic and the right common iliac arteries is carried out and the bowel thus revascularized in a retrograde fashion.

Successful revascularization is usually followed by a sharp fall in blood pressure. This is partly due to 'washout' of vaso-active material from the damaged bowel into the portal and systemic circulation, but is mainly the result of blood loss. The damaged small vessels of the bowel wall rupture and bleed when subjected to arterial pressure and replacement of 3 or 4 units of blood may be necessary at this stage, and in the postoperative period.

The postoperative course is likely to be stormy, and complicated by renal, respiratory and circulatory problems, quite apart from the prolonged period of malabsorption which follows revascularization of the ischaemic gut. None the less, the policy of routine re-operation 24 h later, virtually regardless of the state of the patient, is strongly recommended. Success or failure of revascularization can then be assessed, and any gangrenous area of bowel resected.

It has been shown by retrospective studies that it is

usually possible for a vascular rather than a gastrointestinal operation to be performed. However, a frequent finding is of massive necrosis of the midgut which quite clearly has passed the point of recovery. Under these circumstances a primary resection is carried out, and the ends exteriorized.

With the development of modern techniques of intravenous alimentation, it is possible to cope with the large fluid losses issuing from a high-level fistula. Over the next few days the patient can then be allowed to recover from all the toxic effects of massive bowel infarction, and to return to a state of metabolic normality. Continuity of the gut is then restored electively under the best possible circumstances.

The long-term effects of massive resection of the small bowel are complicated and serious, but they lie outside the scope of this chapter.

Results

It must be conceded that the results of treatment of diagnosed acute intestinal ischaemia are dismally bad. Success is virtually confined to those cases where there is a definite vascular occlusion, and there are very few recorded cases in the world literature of a fully-documented non-occlusive infarction having survived with treatment. The reasons for this enormous mortality will be apparent from *Fig.* 56.2 which illustrates the physiological disturbance engendered by massive ischaemia of the midgut. Furthermore, two other factors must be borne in mind:

1. The condition usually occurs in elderly patients, who already have established degenerative disease of the myocardium, lungs and kidneys. It is frequently a complication of central or peripheral circulatory failure, and is thus an agonal event. Under these circumstances, acute ischaemia is more a mode of dying than a cause of death.

2. Much of the study of the disease has been made in the post-mortem room. Autopsy reveals a massive infarction which was quite unsuspected during life, and the pathologist then extrapolates backwards to the clinical events leading up to it. This high preponderance of autopsy studies naturally skews the reported mortality figures. Common sense would suggest that milder forms of the illness occur, which pass unrecognized and either resolve spontaneously or else respond to incidental supportive measures.

FOCAL ISCHAEMIA OF THE INTESTINE

Infarction is a matter of degree. In the gut, a period of anoxia may be followed by total necrosis, a transient inflammatory response, or the formation of a fibrous stricture. All these processes are well recognized by the pathologist, and can be reproduced in the experimental animal.

a. Small Intestine

The following are the more important causes of focal ischaemia of the small intestine.

1. Strangulation by external hernia or adhesions.
2. Trauma to the abdomen, or surgical devascularization with partial recovery.
3. SMA occlusion.
4. Small vessel embolization.
5. Inflammatory disease of the intestinal arteries.
6. Radiation injury.
7. Action of enteric-coated potassium or other drugs on the mucosal circulation.

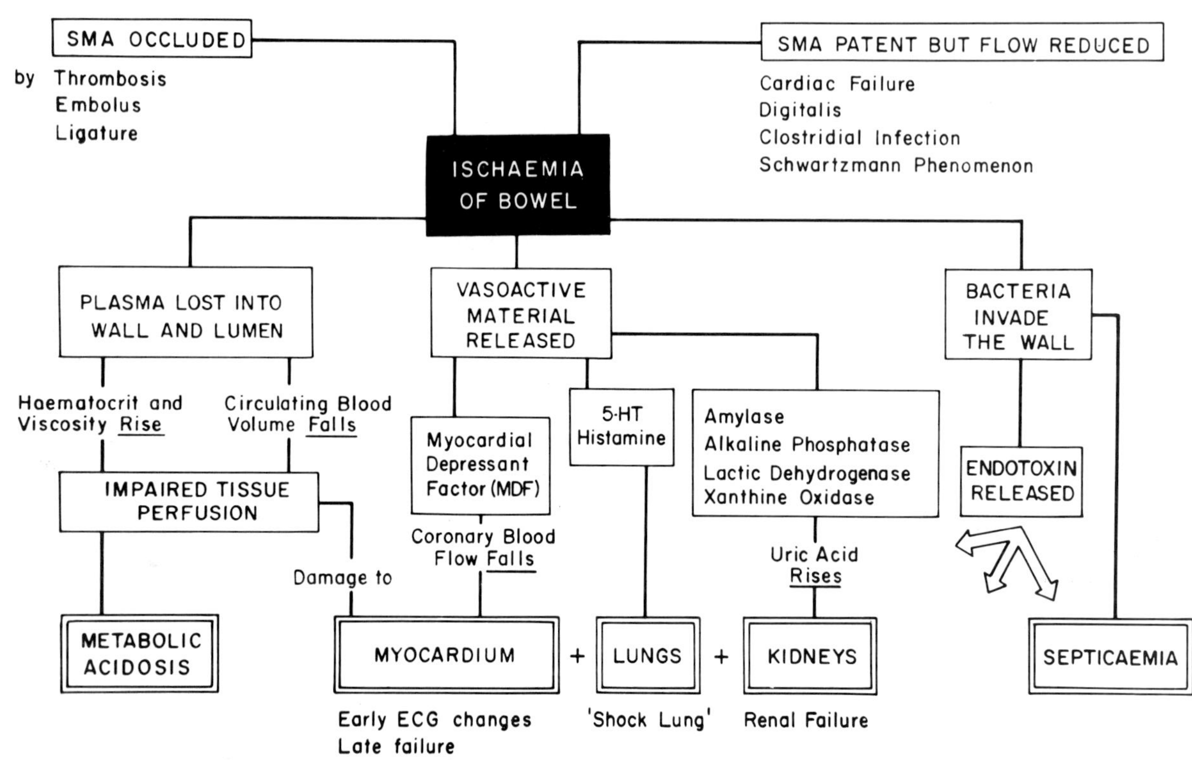

Fig. 56.2 Physiological effects of acute midgut ischaemia.

The patient presents with the typical symptoms of subacute small intestinal obstruction, i.e. colicky pain occurring after a meal, accompanied by eructations, vomiting and distension.

The symptoms usually continue for a few weeks or months and then regress, to return at a later period with rather more intensity. Untreated, the condition progresses either to frank perforation of the bowel wall or to complete intestinal obstruction, in either case the patient will be admitted as a surgical emergency. Naturally, a preceding history of strangulated hernia, ingestion of potassium tablets, episodes of ischaemia in other organs or irradiation to the pelvis, must be sought for and carefully noted.

Physical examination of the abdomen is frequently quite normal, but may on occasion show a 'ladder pattern' of distension, with visible peristalsis and exaggerated bowel sounds. Except in very advanced cases, the serum biochemistry remains normal.

Radiological examination will confirm the presence of dilated loops of jejunum with occasional fluid levels. A small bowel barium study may on occasion define the position of the stricture as well as confirm the diagnosis.

The management of one of these focal ischaemic lesions will obviously depend on the patient's symptoms, but on the whole the results of excision and primary anastomosis of such strictures are very satisfactory.

b. Large Intestine

Because of the less well-developed collateral circulation and the presence of pathogenic bacteria, focal ischaemia is more likely to occur in the colon than in the small bowel. The clinical effects vary according to the magnitude and duration of the ischaemia, but two basic types of presentation are met with. These are *gangrene* of the colon, which presents as a fulminating, undiagnosable, abdominal catastrophe, and a milder *non-gangrenous* form of the disease, which usually resolves spontaneously but may go on to the formation of a fibrous stricture, which usually affects the splenic flexure. It is this relatively common condition which is now referred to as ischaemic colitis.

Since it was originally described in 1966 ischaemic colitis has been extensively documented and the effects have been reproduced in the experimental laboratory.

Gangrene of the Colon

This may occur following a major vascular occlusion or following an episode of hypotension in a patient with atheroma of the visceral arteries.

It presents as sudden abdominal pain and collapse in an elderly patient, which is followed by diarrhoea and the passage of dark blood per rectum. On examination the patient is found to be in peripheral circulatory failure with signs of severe general peritonitis. The clinical picture is the same as in any other features of acute intestinal ischaemia (*see above*) and the management identical. Following appropriate resuscitation the abdomen is opened as soon as possible: a variable length of bowel, usually in the region of the splenic flexure, is found to be frankly necrotic and not uncommonly perforated. The safest course is immediate resection of the affected segment with a generous margin of apparently normal bowel at either end and an exteriorization of the ends. Most authors agree that primary anastomosis under these circumstances is unwise. The mortality in this group of patients is high.

Ischaemic Colitis

The majority of patients present with milder degrees of ischaemia. Typically they have acute pain in the left iliac fossa, fever and a moderate amount of dark rectal bleeding. On examination there are signs of a left-sided peritonitis and the usual provisional diagnosis is of acute diverticulitis though the degree and quality of rectal bleeding is a distinguishing feature. A polymorphonuclear leucocytosis is found in patients seen at an early stage. In those patients not operated upon, the acute illness rapidly subsides, though there may be transient episodes of bleeding over the following few weeks. From there on the disease may take one of two forms. In about one-half, the symptoms disappear completely and the radiograph returns to normal (*see below*). In the other half a stricture develops in the bowel, which leads to a permanent abnormality on the barium enema. However, most of these strictures are asymptomatic and do not require treatment.

Radiological Appearances

The changes seen on the barium enema are highly typical and it is on these that the diagnosis is made. Naturally, they depend on the timing of the examination. 'Thumb-printing' is the earliest change, and has been reported as early as 3 days after the onset of symptoms. It consists of a series of blunt semi-opaque projections into the bowel lumen. Although seen most frequently in the region of the splenic flexure, they can occur anywhere from the caecum to the rectosigmoid (*Fig.* 56.3).

The changes may disappear rapidly, persist for a few weeks or progress to the more mature changes of ulceration, narrowing of the bowel and the formation of a local stricture (*Figs.* 56.4, 56.5, 56.6). Strictures are usually permanent, but some do in fact resolve completely after surprisingly long intervals.

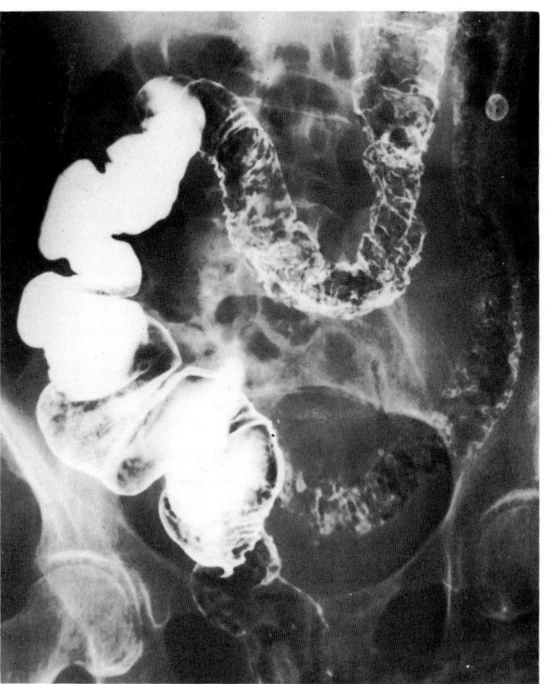

Fig. 56.3 'Thumb-printing' in the ischaemic colon.

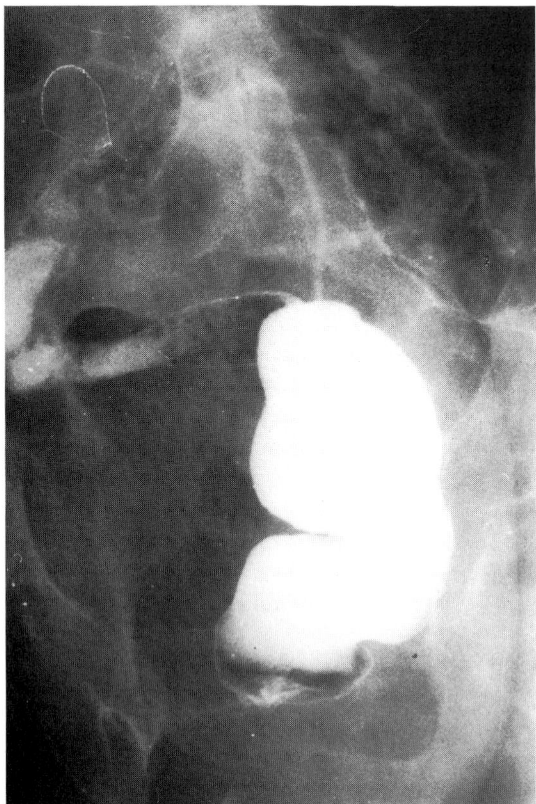

Fig. 56.4 Ischaemic colitis—barium enema showing ulceration and narrowing.

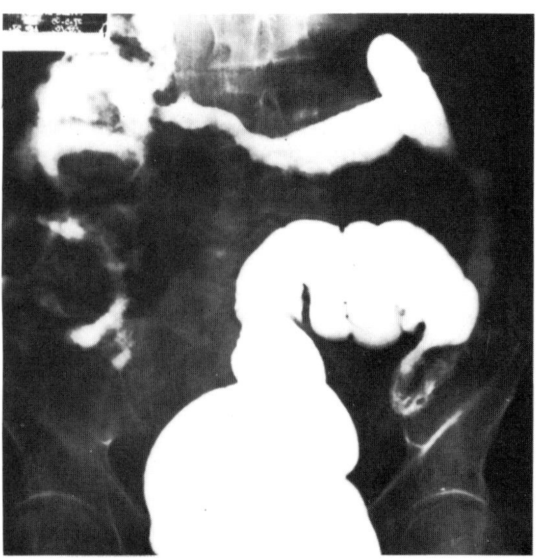

Fig. 56.5 Ischaemic colitis—a long stricture in the splenic flexure.

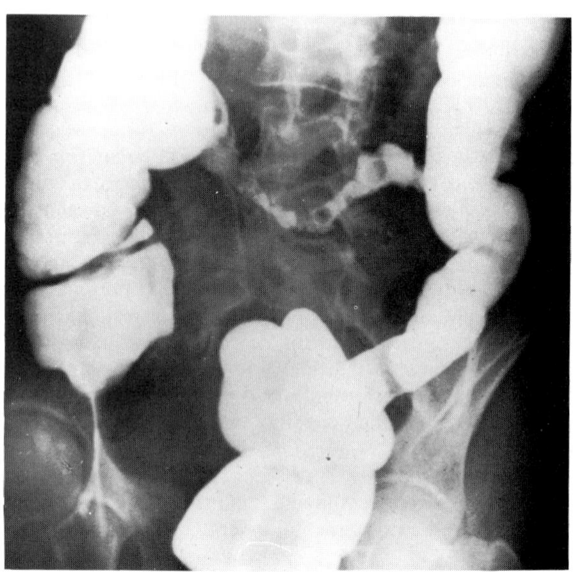

Fig. 56.6 Ischaemic colitis—a short stricture in the transverse colon

Management

This consists in the first place of making the diagnosis and ordering an early barium enema. It seems that this examination is completely safe, except of course in the presence of gangrene where the condition of the patient would obviously preclude it. Thereafter, treatment is conservative and the majority of patients will show steady spontaneous improvement. Progression from ischaemic colitis to frank gangrene is practically unknown and the only indications for surgery are persistent obstructive symptoms or the presence of a

Table 56.1 Differential diagnosis of ischaemic colitis

	Ischaemic colitis	*Ulcerative colitis*	*Crohn's disease*
Age incidence	Elderly	Young	Middle-aged
Presentation	Always acute	Acute or chronic	Chronic
Part involved	Splenic flexure (rectum rare, anus never)	Left-side or total (rectum always)	Anywhere (rectum usual, anus commonly)
Radiology	Thumbprints Stricture	Shortening Ulceration	Spicules Skip lesions
Pathology	Fibrosis Haemosiderosis	Mucosal loss Crypt abscesses	Fissures Granulomas
Associated conditions	Claudication Angina Stroke	Iritis Arthritis Pyoderma Malignant change	Enteric fistula Megaloblastic anaemia

short stricture which cannot be reliably distinguished from a neoplasm.

Differential Diagnosis

In the acute phase this is from perforated diverticular disease, and later on from inflammatory bowel disease. The main differentiating features are set out in *Table* 56.1.

CHRONIC ARTERIAL OBSTRUCTION

The concept of a muscular pain arising in the intestine in response to increased peristalsis from food, analogous to angina pectoris and stemming from obstruction to the arterial supply is attractive, particularly to the vascular surgeon. There is some evidence also that food intake 'steals' blood from the intestinal into the gastric circulation. However, the situation is not at all simple, and it has been questioned whether 'intestinal angina' is really a clinical entity. Stenosis and even complete occlusion of the main arteries is a common autopsy finding and the lesions may even be so gross as to limit resting flow. Patients with this sort of arteriographic abnormality have been investigated with great assiduity, and because the lesion is very easily reproduced in the animal laboratory, there is a thorough back-up of laboratory experience. However, no one has ever succeeded in demonstrating a structural or functional abnormality in the intestine which can be reliably correlated with diminution in blood supply, unless there is an infarction. In other words, it is an all-or-nothing situation, in that the intestine remains (to our present insensitive tests) normal, until the point is reached when its cells can no longer metabolize or resist bacterial challenge. None the less (*see below*) there are abundant case reports in the literature of severely distressed patients who have been completely relieved by arterial reconstruction. The problem is one of identification.

The Clinical Picture

The symptoms which constitute the syndrome of intestinal angina have been defined as pain coming on very shortly after eating a meal (sometimes described as 'food fear') weight loss, and disturbance of bowel habit. However, study of the literature shows that the complaints are very variable. Some patients have no pain at all, others do not lose weight, and the bowel disturbances may be in the nature of profuse diarrhoea or obstinate constipation.

Physical signs are frequently absent, and the diagnosis must be made by exclusion. The presence of an arterial bruit in the epigastrium may be a pointer, but this often arises from atheroma in the aorta itself, and is not a sure indication of trouble in the mesenteric trunks. In any event, such bruits can often be heard in fit young individuals with no symptoms. A background of cardiovascular disease, with a history of claudication, myocardial infarction or stroke, is additional circumstantial evidence that an obscure abdominal pain may be due to arterial insufficiency.

Management

Every effort is made to exclude more common and potentially treatable causes of the patient's symptoms. These include peptic ulcer, hiatus hernia, gallbladder disease, carcinoma of the stomach, pancreas or colon and, most importantly, myocardial pain referred to the abdomen. Careful history taking, complete physical examination and the standard laboratory and radiological investigations will exclude most of the alternative diagnoses.

Intense and careful investigation of intestinal function is carried out. The purpose of this is not so much to establish the diagnosis because, in the present state of knowledge this is not possible, but rather to document all available information on known cases of ischaemia, so that future sufferers can be helped. The tests employed include a small bowel barium series, and upper gastrointestinal endoscopy if the symptoms warrant this. Gastric biopsy may be included, but capsular jejunal biopsy is not performed, because of the (possibly theoretical) risk of perforation of ischaemic bowel. Laboratory tests comprise a 3-day fat balance, serum carotene, folate, vitamin B_{12} and Schilling tests, together with measurement of protein loss from the gastrointestinal tract by means of intravenously injected ^{51}Cr-labelled albumin. Xylose excretion is measured, in relation to creatinine clearance.

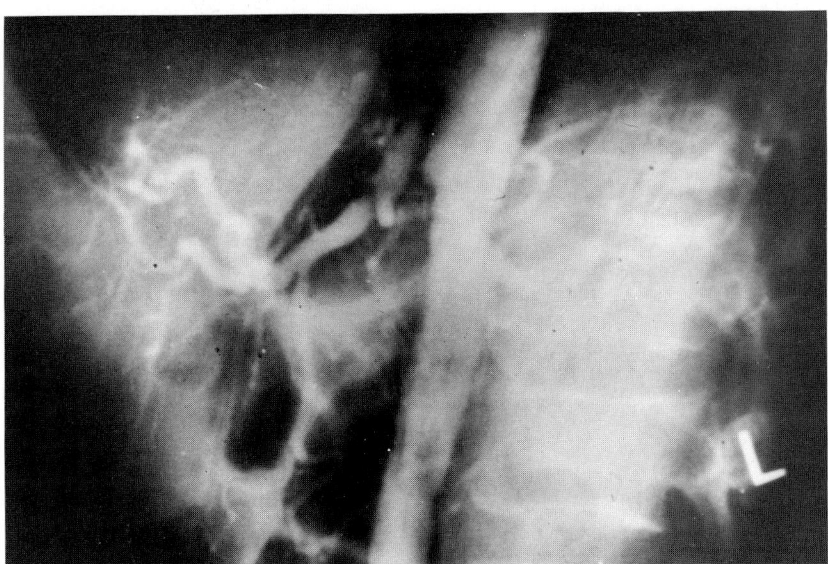

Fig. 56.7 Aortogram showing chronic occlusion of the SMA (note associated stricture of coeliac axis).

The final decision to operate must be made by aortography. In order to demonstrate the first few centimetres of the arteries, which is where the trouble is found, it is necessary to have both free and selective studies in AP and lateral views (*Fig.* 56.7). Only in this way can the extent of the arterial pathology be assessed, and most importantly, the degree to which it is compensated by cross-circulation from other vascular territories.

Treatment

When all the data are to hand and if the patient's general cardiovascular status appears to permit major surgery, reconstruction of the stenosed visceral trunk(s) must be considered. There are various ways of achieving this, which are illustrated in *Fig.* 56.8. The stenosis is almost always found at the origin of the SMA but, as in acute occlusions, it is better to operate more distally, where the artery is more accessible. A very satisfactory technique is to carry out a side-to-side anastomosis between the upper part of the SMA and the aorta.

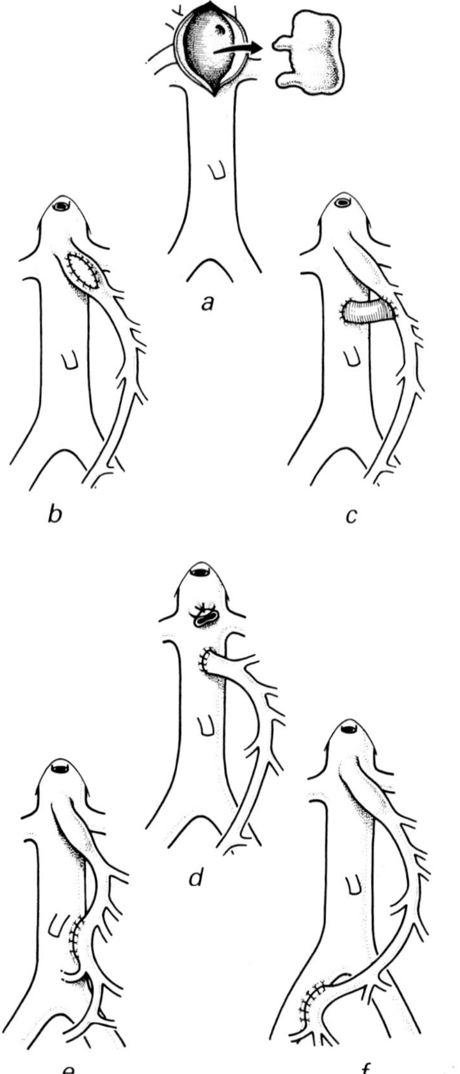

Fig. 56.8 Techniques for reconstruction of the intestinal circulation. *a*, Intra-aortic endarterectomy. *b*, External endarterectomy ± patch. *c*, Bypass. *d*, Reimplantation. *e*, Side-to-side aortic SMA anastomosis. *f*, Retrograde vascularization.

As regards the coeliac axis, this is a difficult vessel to approach, and requires a thoraco-abdominal incision. The diaphragm is divided down to the aortic hiatus and the spleen and tail of the pancreas reflected over to the right. This gives excellent access to the upper abdominal aorta, and to the origins of the visceral vessels. The most generally used and satisfactory technique for reconstruction of the coeliac axis is by patch angioplasty, with autogenous or synthetic material. Some cases have been reported in which the coeliac axis has been compressed by the fibres of the median arcuate ligament of the diaphragm, and the symptoms relieved by simple division of that structure. Little information is available, however, on the extent to which pressure and flow are influenced by this operation, and the evidence that it improves intestinal function is purely subjective. If the operation is effective, it almost certainly succeeds by some other mechanism than an increase in blood supply.

Results of Treatment

Our own experience at The Middlesex Hospital is of 100 patients investigated for suspected intestinal angina, of whom 22 were subjected to arterial reconstruction with three postoperative deaths. Fifteen of these patients have been symptomatically improved, one is unchanged and one feels rather worse. It should be pointed out that this small number represents the experience over twenty years of a unit actively interested in the problem, which illustrates the rarity of the condition.

The right patient to operate on is hard to identify, but certainly the occasional rescue of an emaciated pain-racked individual by a timely revascularization of the gut is a most satisfying surgical exercise. Additionally, though this is hard to quantify, such an operation may forestall a fatal intestinal infarction.

VENOUS OBSTRUCTION

As in other areas, the venous collateral circulation to the gut is so well developed that local obstructions and thromboses seldom have much effect. When massive venous obstruction occurs, as in the Budd–Chiari syndrome or in portal vein thrombosis, this is usually associated with a blood dyscrasia or with advanced malignancy.

It is possible to produce venous lesions in the colon which closely resemble ischaemic colitis and this may have some clinical relevance. Certainly, ischaemic (possible venous) lesions in premenopausal women seem to have a close association with the use of oral contraceptives, though the evidence is entirely circumstantial.

CONCLUSIONS

The frequency of vascular accidents in the mesenteric circulation is far less than that observed in the heart, brain or limbs. Perhaps the very lethality of such lesions has had a selective effect on the evolution of the splanchnic blood supply. Midgut necrosis is almost always fatal, and survival figures have not improved over the years in spite of advances in patient support and in operative technique. Chronic arterial stenosis which is of clinical as opposed to radiological importance is hard to find. From the practical point of view, understanding the pathophysiology of intestinal ischaemia is of most importance in relation to forms of 'enteritis' and 'colitis' whose causes have so far been unexplained.

Further Reading

Jamieson W. G., Marchuck S., Rowson J. et al. (1982) The early diagnosis of massive acute intestinal ischaemia. *Br. J. Surg.* **69**, Suppl. S52–S53.

Kazmers A., Zwolak R., Azselman H. D. et al. (1984) Pharmacologic interventions in acute ischaemia: improved survival with intravenous glucagon, methylprednisolone and prostacyclin. *J. Vasc. Surg.* **1**, 472.

Marston A. (1986) *Vascular Disease of the Gut: Pathophysiology, Recognition and Management.* London, Edward Arnold.

Marston, A., Clarke J. M. F., Garcia Garcia J. et al. (1985) Intestinal function and intestinal blood supply. *Gut* **26**, 656–666.

57 *Vein and Lymphatic Surgery*

V. V. Kakkar

DEEP VEIN THROMBOSIS

Deep vein thrombosis and pulmonary embolism have become an increasingly important cause of disability and death during the past 50 years. Fatal pulmonary embolism is a major cause of postoperative death. When no prophylaxis is given after general surgery, it has a frequency of about 1%.

Pathogenesis

The formation of venous thrombi can be explained in terms of blood coagulation and deposition in the presence of venous stasis. The three main factors postulated by Virchow in 1856 have been confirmed by subsequent work:

1. Changes in the composition of blood.
2. Damage to the blood vessels.
3. Decreased rate of blood flow.

While there is no doubt that changes in blood composition and abnormalities in the blood flow are important, there is controversy over the part played by the damage to the vessel wall or injury to the endothelial cells. Recent studies have shown that although endothelial injury is important in the development of arterial thrombi, it is probably not a prerequisite for the formation of venous thrombi. Certain groups of patients and some conditions predispose to deep vein thrombosis. The effect of age has already been mentioned. A higher incidence of leg vein thrombosis has also been reported in older patients (over 50 years), with extensive trauma, infection, congestive heart failure, blood dyscrasias, malignancy, diabetes mellitus and other metabolic disorders. Patients who have had pulmonary embolism or deep vein thrombosis in the past, are highly likely to develop these conditions again, following operation. With regard to the generally accepted danger of thrombosis in women who are using the contraceptive pill, it is good practice, whenever possible, to avoid operation for at least 6 weeks after stopping the pill.

Diagnosis of Deep Vein Thrombosis

The diagnosis of deep vein thrombosis presents two separate problems:

1. Occult and asymptomatic thrombi, common in patients confined to bed, require a quick, simple and accurate screening procedure for high-risk patients.

2. Patients presenting with suggestive clinical features require confirmatory investigations.

Clinical Features

The diagnosis is clear cut when physical examination reveals local distension, tenderness, oedema, discoloration, pain and fever, or when there is a massive thrombosis affecting the whole leg. The majority of patients have less extensive disease, and clinical diagnosis alone is unreliable; not only are there no clinical signs or symptoms in half of the patients with extensive thrombosis, but in some 30–35% of patients with a 'positive' clinical diagnosis, the deep veins are in fact normal. Considering only lower leg signs—calf tenderness, pain on dorsiflexion of the foot, and minimal ankle oedema—some 50% of positive diagnoses are false.

Venography

The introduction of modern X-ray equipment, including the image intensifier and television monitoring screen, has established venography as an effective method for demonstrating most venous thrombi of clinical interest.

All newer techniques are based on a principle of watching the filling of the deep veins of the legs with contrast medium, so that films are exposed at the correct time, allowing more precise diagnosis of the presence (or absence) of a thrombus (*Fig.* 57.1). The technique of ascending functional cinephlebography has the added advantage that it also demonstrates valvular function with the patient almost upright.

One of the complications of venography is that the large volume of contrast medium which is often employed, may initiate thrombosis by damaging the delicate intima of the deep veins; wash-out of the leg veins with heparinized solution at the end of the procedure may prevent this damage.

Radioactive Fibrinogen Uptake Test

^{125}I-labelled fibrinogen is taken up preferentially by forming thrombus, and this forms the basis of a clinical test for the detection of early thrombi. ^{125}I fibrinogen is given intravenously, and the legs are scanned at several determined points with an external scintillation counter (*Fig.* 57.2).

Because the use of labelled human fibrinogen risks transmission of viral hepatitis, the fibrinogen is taken only from accredited donors. This material has been used in over 30 000 patients, and no case of clinical serum hepatitis has occurred. There is a positive correlation of over 80% between the fibrinogen test and venography. The fibrinogen

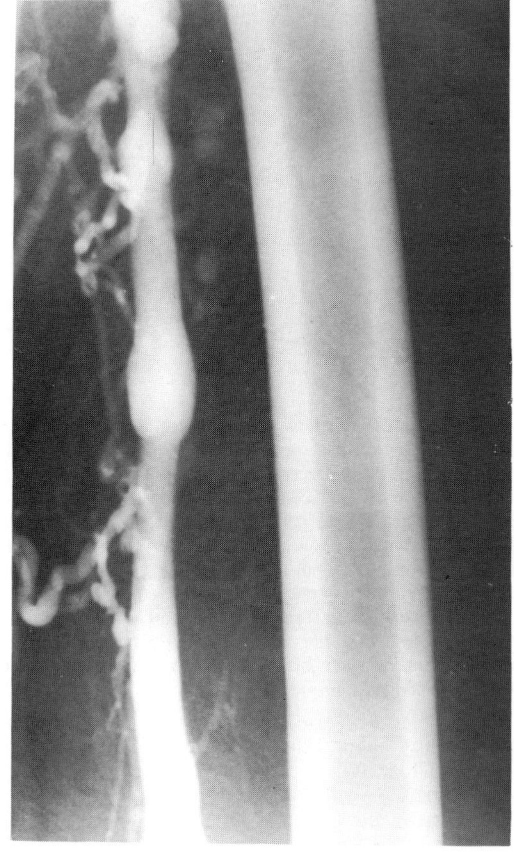

a

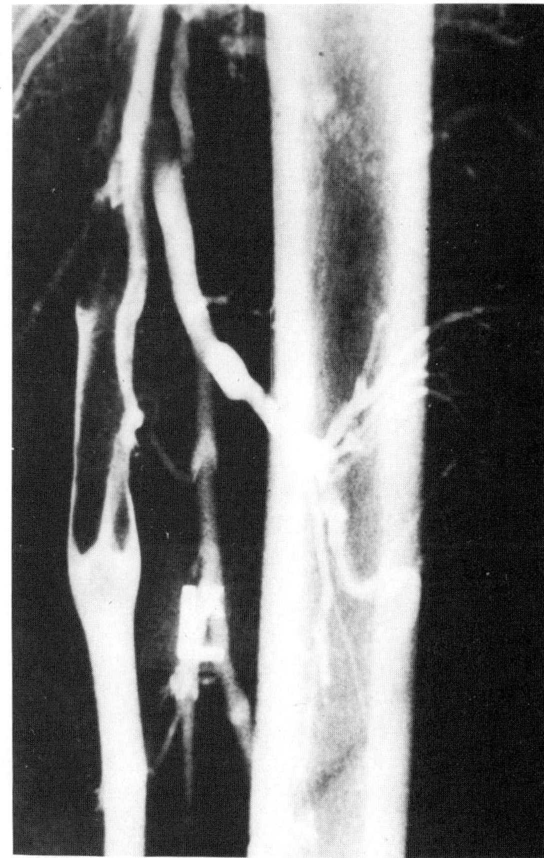

b

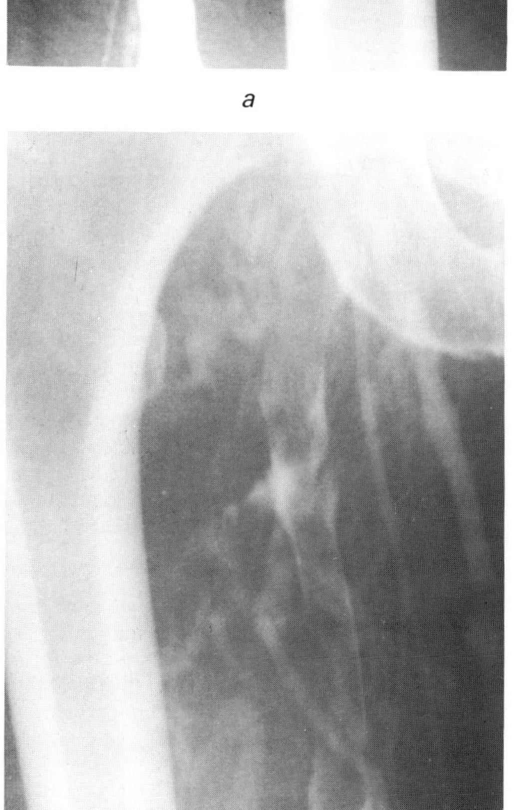

c

Fig. 57.1 *a*, Normal femoral vein. There is uniform distribution of contrast medium filling the entire lumen of the femoral vein. Both cusps of the venous valves can be seen. *b*, Partially occluding thrombi in the femoral vein. A large filling defect can be seen to be arising from a valve cusp and another proximal thrombus arising from the lateral wall. These thrombi developed following an operation of total hip replacement. *c*, Completely occluding thrombi in the femoral vein which is surrounded by a rim of contrast medium.

test shows a higher incidence of deep vein thrombosis because it detects small thrombi in the muscular veins of the calf more efficiently. However, the test is less reliable for detecting thrombosis in the common femoral and pelvic veins, because the proximity of the bladder and/or large arteries and other vascular structures gives an increased background count.

Doppler Ultrasound

The principle of this technique is shown in *Fig.* 57.3, and it depends on the detection of changes in the velocity of blood flow in the veins. The Doppler ultrasound flow velocity detector contains a crystal that directs an ultrasonic beam percutaneously to an underlying vein, where it is reflected from blood cells. If the column of blood in the vein is stationary, the frequency of the reflected beam is identical to the incident beam, and no sound is recorded. If, on the other hand, the column of blood is moving, then the beam is reflected at a changed frequency proportional to the velocity of flow. The difference between the incident and the reflected ultrasound beams is received by a second crystal

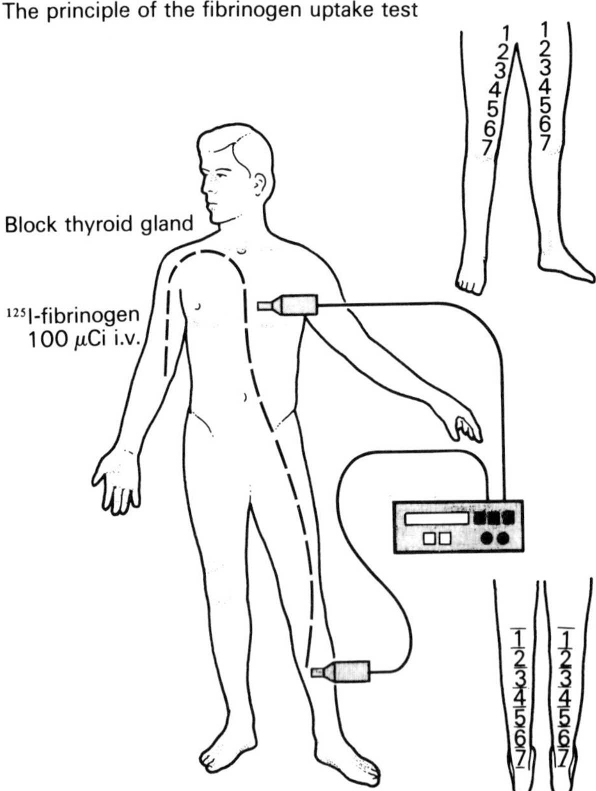

Fig. 57.2 Detection by this method depends on the incorporation into the thrombus of radio-labelled fibrinogen, which is detected by measuring the increase in surface radioactivity with an isotope detector. After blocking the thyroid gland by the oral or intravenous administration of sodium iodide, 100 μCi of ^{125}I-fibrinogen are injected into an arm vein; 4 hours later the radioactivity is recorded over the precordial region which is represented at 100%. The radioactivity from the limbs measured at fixed positions (1–7 in the thigh and calf region) is represented as a percentage of the heart counts. Venous thrombosis is diagnosed if there is an increase in radioactivity at any point, or more than 20%, which persists for at least 24 hours (i) compared with the readings over adjacent points in the same leg, or (ii) over the same point, compared with the previous day, or (iii) over a corresponding point in the opposite leg.

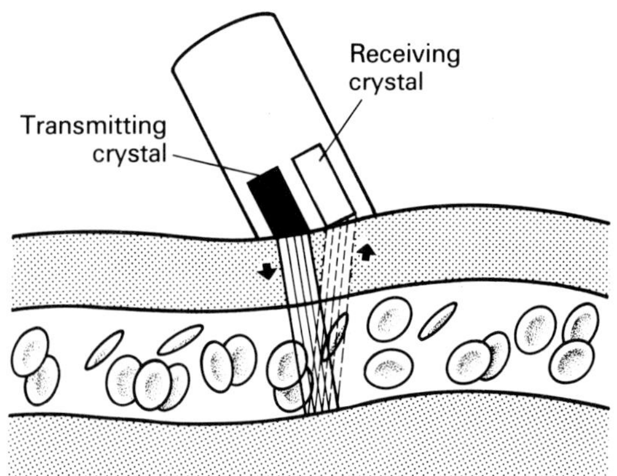

Fig. 57.3 The ultrasonic flow velocity detector is composed of two crystals, one transmits the sound, and the other receives back the scattered signal at a different frequency. The beam is passed percutaneously to an underlying vein, where it is reflected from RBCs; the reflected sound is received by the receiving crystal, and amplified into an audible sound, the magnitude of which is directly proportional to the velocity of blood flow. The velocity of blood flow in the femoral vein can be temporarily increased by compressing the thigh or calf veins. This results in the augmentation of the flow sound, called the 'A' sound. The manoeuvre fails to produce 'A' sound augmentation when blood flow is obstructed by a thrombus in the veins distal to the probe.

probe, and amplified into an audible signal or flow sound. It is an extremely simple way of detecting complete occlusion of the popliteal, femoral and iliac veins, but the test may give a false negative result when recent, non-occlusive thrombi are present. Moreover, flow in large collaterals or in a very large superficial vein may give a sound resembling flow in a patent major vein. Thrombi in the calf veins, the tributaries of the profunda, or the internal iliac veins, cannot be detected because they do not cause major vein obstruction.

Impedance Plethysmography

Thrombi of sufficient size cause obstruction of venous return from the lower leg, but usually this cannot be detected by clinical examination of the limb. Impedance plethysmography depends upon the observation that blood volume changes in the calves, produced by maximum respiratory effort or by venous occlusion by pneumatic thigh cuffs, result in changes in the electrical resistance of the calves. These changes in blood volume and electrical resistance are reduced in patients with obstruction to venous outflow due to thrombosis in the popliteal or more proximal veins (*Fig.* 57.4).

Impedance plethysmography is performed with the patient supine and the lower limbs elevated to 30° or 25°. A pneumatic cuff, 15 cm in width, is applied to the midthigh and inflated to 45 cmH_2O to occlude venous return. The pressure is maintained for 45 to 120 sec, and the cuff is then rapidly deflated. Changes in electrical resistance resulting from alterations in blood volume distal to the cuff are detected by calf electrodes, and recorded on an ECG strip. The accuracy of the test is influenced by the degree of venous filling obtained during cuff occlusion, and this can be enhanced by repeating the tests sequentially.

There have been a number of trials to evaluate the use of impedance plethysmography for the diagnosis of venous thrombosis in patients with clinically suspected venous thrombosis. These trials indicate that impedance plethysmography is highly sensitive to symptomatic proximal vein thrombosis, but is insensitive to calf vein thrombi.

Radionuclide Venography

This technique is ideal for visualizing iliac veins and the inferior vena cava. Macro-aggregated albumin particles labelled with the radio-isotope ^{99}Tc are injected through a vein on the dorsum of the foot. Images of the calf, thigh and pelvic veins are obtained by using a gamma camera.

Blood Coagulability Assays

A number of blood-assay methods have recently been developed to detect the occurrence of *in vivo* thrombosis, or changes in the blood predisposing to clot formation.

These tests measure levels of fibrinogen derivatives present in the circulation. The enzymatic action of thrombin on fibrinogen results in the formation of fibrin monomer, which then polymerizes to give fibrin. When fibrin is lysed

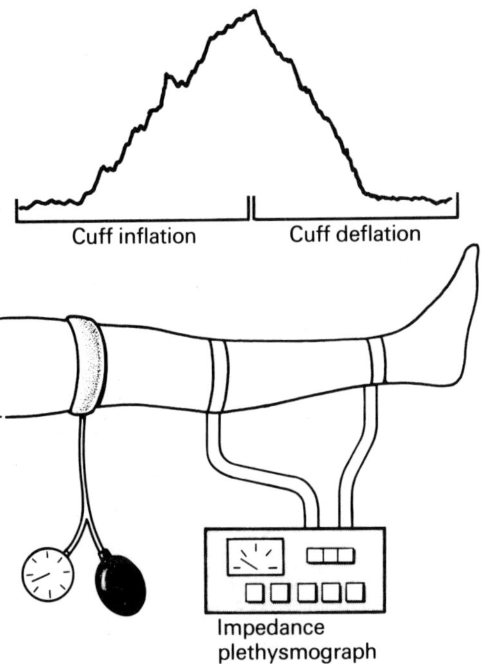

Fig. 57.4 A pressure cuff applied to the mid-thigh region produces blood volume changes in the calves, which can be detected by measuring the alteration in the electric resistance to the passage of a known current. When the calf is suddenly deflated, the venous return is resumed, and the blood volume in the calf decreases; this results in a corresponding increase in impedance or resistance, as blood conducts electric current. In the presence of venous obstruction in the popliteal or more proximal veins, the rate of venous emptying is reduced. Impedance plethysmography is undertaken with the patient supine, and the lower limbs elevated by 30–35°. A pneumatic cuff (15 cm wide) is applied to the mid-thigh region, and four electrodes to the calf region. The cuff is inflated to a pressure of 45 cmH_2O to occlude venous return; this pressure is maintained for 2 minutes, and then the cuff is rapidly deflated. Alterations in blood volume distal to the cuff are detected by calf electrodes and recorded on an ECG strip paper. The accuracy of the test is influenced by the degree of venous filling obtained during cuff occlusion.

by plasma, small fragments—fibrin-degradation products (FDP)—are released into the circulation.

Fibrin monomer complexes in the blood can be detected *in vitro* by the addition of protamine sulphate, which dissociates the complex and results in precipitation of fibrin, either as strands or gel. The serial dilution protamine sulphate (SDPS) test based on this principle is a simple, sensitive and specific haematological assay. The test is claimed to be always positive in the presence of extensive thrombosis and acute pulmonary embolism, but its value as a screening procedure for early and forming asymptomatic thrombi has yet to be established.

Large molecular weight fibrinogen complexes are known to circulate during the active thrombotic stage, but they can only be shown in highly specialized laboratories.

Selection of Test

There are two clinical situations requiring tests for detecting thrombi; screening of high-risk patients and confirming a provisional diagnosis. The strengths and weaknesses of the available tests are such that no one test is ideal for both situations.

Diagnosis of Pulmonary Embolism

Although autopsy studies indicate that pulmonary embolism occurs frequently, and is often repeated, the condition is diagnosed in relatively few patients during life. Recognition is especially difficult in patients with pre-existing cardiopulmonary disease, and even more so in those with congestive heart failure.

Clinical Diagnosis

The clinical features of pulmonary embolism depend to a large extent on the degree of vascular obstruction. Pleural pain more often reflects submassive embolism, whereas syncope indicates massive embolism; it is not possible to distinguish massive from submassive embolism from any of the other symptoms. Common physical findings such as tachypnoea, râles, loud pulmonary second sound, S_3 or S_4 gallop sounds and cyanosis may be absent in the majority of cases of submassive embolism. Though S_1, Q_3, T_3 pattern is virtually pathognomonic of pulmonary embolism if it develops suddenly, electrocardiography is usually non-specific in its diagnosis. Only about 10–20% of patients subsequently shown to have pulmonary embolism develop any ECG changes, and of these, an even smaller number show diagnostic abnormalities.

A plain chest radiograph still represents a valuable diagnostic aid, is highly desirable for comparison when a pulmonary angiogram is being interpreted, and is almost essential when interpreting isotopic lung scans.

LABORATORY TESTS. A triad of elevated serum lactic dehydrogenase (LDH), and increase in serum bilirubin concentration in association with a normal serum glutamic-oxalacetic transaminase (SGOT) activity was at one time thought to be a promising aid in distinguishing symptoms of acute chest pain. Further experience has not proved its usefulness, and these tests therefore no longer play an important role in diagnosing pulmonary embolism.

LUNG SCAN. The radio-isotope perfusion lung scan is the most valuable test for the diagnosis of pulmonary embolism. The test is carried out by injecting radio-isotope-labelled particles intravenously. These particles lodge in the precapillary arterioles, and capillaries in the lung, and their distribution reflects pulmonary blood flow. If there is pulmonary vascular obstruction, an underperfused area of lung scan can be detected by a gamma camera (*Fig.* 57.5).

The sensitivity of the lung scan to a perfusion defect depends on a number of factors: the isotope used, the sensitivity of the screening instrument, and the site of the obstruction. Multiple views of the lungs should be obtained, because defects in some of the lung segments can be seen only in certain views. A minimum of four views—anterior, posterior and right and left lateral—should be obtained. One of the limitations of perfusion lung scanning is that a number of pulmonary diseases produce abnormal perfusion (pneumonia, tuberculosis, lung tumours and chronic airway obstruction). The lung scan should therefore be interpreted only in the light of the chest radiograph findings. The perfusion lung scan findings can normally be divided into three categories: (1) A normal lung scan—if this is technically adequate, a diagnosis of pulmonary embolism is virtually excluded; (2) A high probability lung scan characterized by lobar, segmental or subsegmental perfusion defects in regions that do not show a corresponding abnormality on the chest radiograph; this indicates pulmonary embolism with

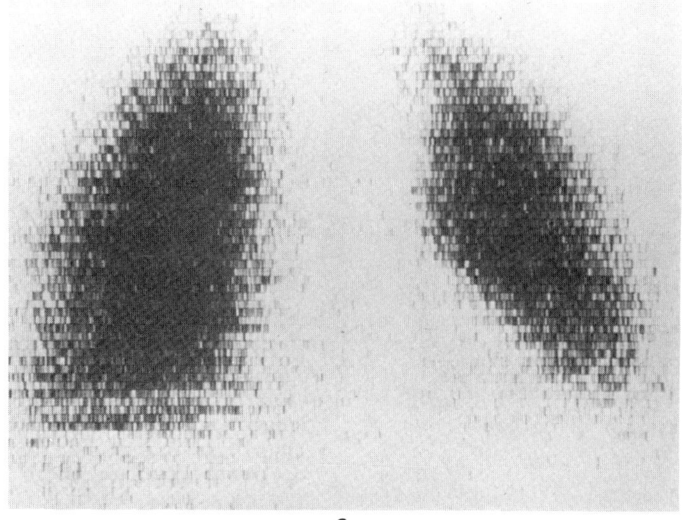

a

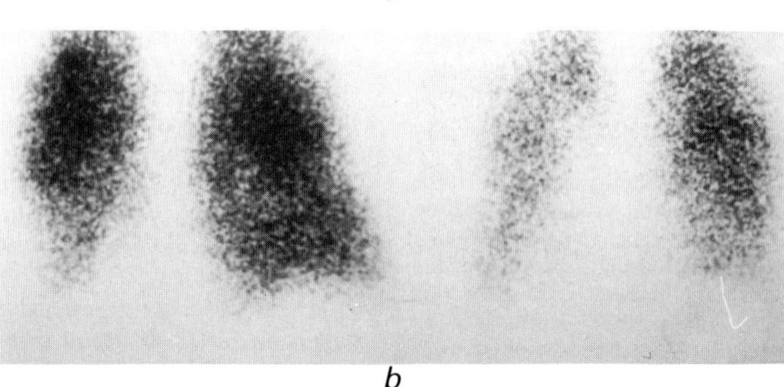

b

Fig. 57.5 *a*, Normal perfusion lung scan; there is generalized uniformity of tracer distribution. *b*, Perfusion lung scan in a patient with pulmonary embolism involving the superior and the basal segments of the right lower lobe in the anterior and posterior projections.

85% certainty; and (3) A low probability lung scan which includes non-segmental defects, and defects that correspond to chest radiograph abnormalities. In this situation, the probability of pulmonary embolism is only 10–20%.

The specificity of lung scanning for the diagnosis of pulmonary embolism can be increased by performing ventilation as well as perfusion scanning. In this technique, regional distribution of radioactive gas in the lung, after it is inhaled, is compared with pulmonary perfusion. The use of this technique is based on the assumption that a perfusion defect due to pulmonary embolism is not associated with a corresponding ventilation defect. The value of this technique may prove to be greatest in patients with low probability perfusion defects.

PULMONARY ANGIOGRAPHY. Pulmonary angiography is the definitive method for the diagnosis of pulmonary embolism. It is performed by injecting contrast medium through a catheter in the main pulmonary artery, to visualize the left and right main pulmonary arteries, lobar arteries, segmental branches and the first two subdivisions of the segmental arteries. A pulmonary angiogram is considered diagnostic for pulmonary embolism if an intraluminal filling defect can be seen, or if there is an abrupt cut-off of lobar, segmental or large subsegmental vessels. Areas of oligaemia, asymmetry of flow, and pruning of the peripheral pulmonary vessels are less specific findings (*Fig.* 57.6).

Prophylaxis

In spite of the efforts of many workers over the past 90 years or so to develop an effective prophylaxis against venous thromboembolism, the methods employed today are empirical and ineffective. This has been due to two main difficulties: first, the lack of essential knowledge concerning the nature of the 'trigger mechanism' which initiates thrombosis in the legs and, secondly, the absence of sensitive and accurate techniques for measuring with precision the effects of prophylaxis. To some extent, the second difficulty has now been overcome; by using the ^{125}I-labelled fibrinogen test, it is possible to determine the true incidence of this disease and the effectiveness of a specific regime of prevention can be judged with greater accuracy. The main attempts to prevent deep-vein thrombosis can be conveniently divided into two groups: those directed towards elimination of stasis in the deep veins and those employed to counteract changes in blood coagulability.

Elimination of Stasis

Despite general agreement that stasis plays a significant role in the pathogenesis of venous thrombosis and despite increasing wariness of the hazards of bed-rest, there is conflicting evidence as to the efficacy of early ambulation in reducing the incidence of deep vein thrombosis. More specific attempts have now been made to prevent stasis during

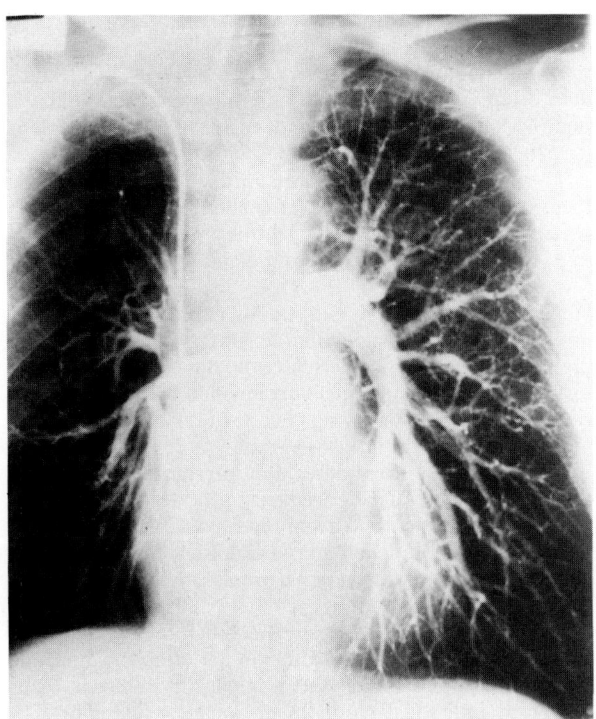

Fig. 57.6 Pulmonary angiogram in a patient with massive pulmonary embolism involving the right main pulmonary trunk. In the left pulmonary artery, there is normal distribution of the contrast medium. Lobar arteries, their primary, secondary and tertiary divisions, are visualized. In comparison, the right main pulmonary trunk is only partially filled, because of an obstructing embolus. The right lobar vessels and their divisions are inadequately visualized.

surgery, and several methods have recently been investigated for increasing venous return from the lower limbs. One of these is electrical stimulation of the calf muscles during operation: two electrodes are applied to the calf and a low-voltage current is used to contract the muscles every 2–4 sec. Another method, pneumatic compression of the calves, involves encasing the legs in an envelope of plastic material, and rhythmically altering the pressure to squeeze the calf muscles and increase venous return. In practice, an electric pump inflates each legging alternately so that compression at 40–45 mmHg for 1 min is achieved, followed by relaxation for 1 min. The advantage of this method is that it can be used not only during surgery but also in the postoperative period.

Counteracting Blood Coagulability

Many attempts have also been made to prevent thrombosis by simpler means, such as the use of chemical agents. These agents can be broadly classified into three main groups. It has been suggested that adhesion of platelets to subendothelial connective tissue at the site of presumed damaged venous endothelium and subsequent events leading to platelet aggregation may account for thrombus formation. If this platelet aggregation can be prevented, it is conceivable that the thrombus will not form. It is with this background that various drugs have been investigated which interfere with the different aspects of platelet function; these include dextran (usually dextran-70), dipyridamole, aspirin and chloroquine.

The second chemical approach has been the use of drugs which interfere with the coagulation mechanism. A vital step in the sequence of coagulation is the conversion of prothrombin to thrombin, under the influence of activated factor X. The thrombin so formed acts on fibrinogen to convert it into fibrin, which in turn forms the essential network of a venous thrombus. To block the coagulation sequence two different types of drugs have been used: oral anticoagulants, which act by reducing synthesis in the liver of various clotting factors such as prothrombin, factor X and others, and heparin which acts primarily by increasing factor X inhibitor activity. Therefore, small doses of heparin given before factor X is activated are effective in preventing thrombosis, but do not affect the clotting time.

The third group of drugs is thought to act on venous endothelium, to increase naturally occurring fibrinolytic activity in the body. Astrup (1956) has suggested that thrombosis may be due in part to a local or generalized imbalance between coagulation and fibrinolysis. A shift in the balance towards fibrinolysis could prevent thrombosis or rapidly lyse recent thrombi, while impairment of fibrinolysis would encourage the growth of the thrombus. Various investigators have shown that fibrinolytic activity in the blood and vein walls is abnormally low in the majority of patients with recent deep vein thrombosis or superficial thrombosis. The evidence that drugs such as aspirin and dipyridamole, known to interfere with platelet function, effectively reduce the incidence of deep vein thrombosis is unconvincing, and these agents should probably not be used for the prophylaxis of venous thrombosis. However, dextran infusion is effective in reducing the incidence of fatal pulmonary embolism. There is no doubt that drugs which are known to enhance naturally occurring fibrinolytic activity, such as phenformin and ethyloestranol, are totally ineffective in preventing deep vein thrombosis in surgical patients. Oral anticoagulant therapy, properly employed (starting before operation or immediately after admission to hospital), is the most effective and proved method of preventing venous thrombosis. However, in spite of strict laboratory control, the risk of haemorrhage is real and may be even greater than the dangers of thrombo-embolism if such therapy was accepted for general use.

Low-dose heparin (5000 u subcutaneously begun 2 h before operation and every 12 h thereafter for 7 days), seems to be the most promising drug for preventing deep vein thrombosis, although the optimum regimen has yet to be defined. The efficacy of this method has been assessed in a number of controlled clinical trials, and these studies have shown clearly that this form of prophylaxis is well tolerated by patients, is devoid of side-effects, requires no special monitoring, and does not result in excessive bleeding during or after surgery. Furthermore, it can be used on an extensive scale.

Treatment

There is still a great deal of argument as to which is the best form of medical treatment for patients with deep vein thrombosis. There have indeed been very few reported studies of treatment in homogeneous groups of patients where the effect of treatment has been measured by objective means such as phlebography; clinical signs are most misleading, and many examples can be found of clinical improvements despite the persisting presence of thrombus in the leg veins and, in some instances, the subsequent development of pulmonary embolus. Furthermore, none of the studies gives any indication of the efficacy of treatment so far as the long-term effects of deep vein thrombosis, the postphlebitic syndrome, are concerned.

Therapy for venous thrombosis can be broadly classified into two groups: general measures and specific drugs.

General Measures

The discomfort and pain of acute deep vein thrombosis varies considerably from case to case. All patients should be confined to bed with the foot of the bed elevated 15–22 cm, with elastic bandages applied firmly from the toe to below the inguinal region, and they should be encouraged to perform leg exercises at regular intervals in bed. At one time it was believed that this regime might provoke pulmonary emboli, but it is now generally agreed that such a risk is negligible, and these measures are of considerable value in promoting venous flow. Prolonged bed rest is unnecessary, however, and may even be harmful: it may encourage stasis and further thrombosis. The patient should only be kept in bed until the acute symptoms have disappeared. After this he should be encouraged to get up if his general condition permits. In some cases, the discomfort and pain may require analgesics. It has been suggested that local application of heat is useful and makes the patient more comfortable, but in our experience this is rarely the case.

Specific Therapy

This consists of the administration of either anticoagulants, defibrinating, or fibrinolytic agents. In understanding the action of these drugs, the whole process of thrombosis should be regarded as the final outcome of the action of two opposing reactions, one leading to the deposition and the other to the removal of fibrin. Anticoagulants restrict the further deposition of fibrin, but have no direct action on an established thrombus. Nevertheless, they may so limit its extension that they increase the possibility of spontaneous thrombolysis. In contrast, the fibrinolytic drugs have a direct thrombolytic effect, which is achieved either by activating the fibrinolytic enzyme system, or by independent proteolysis of fibrin.

ANTICOAGULANTS. Oral Anticoagulants: These act by reducing the synthesis in the liver of various clotting factors such as factor II, factor VII, factor IX and factor X. Their main action is probably as a substrate competitor with vitamin K_1 for an apoenzyme required in the synthesis of these factors.

The oral anticoagulants are of two types: the indanediones and the coumarins. Both these drugs are not effective until 48–72 h after oral administration of the initial dose; if anticoagulation is required during this period, it can be achieved by the administration of heparin, which is effective immediately after intravenous injection. The effect of oral anticoagulants lasts for 12–16 h, and when given twice daily an effective blood concentration is maintained. They are used for prolonged therapy; coumarin is commonly given. The initial dose varies between 30 and 40 mg and subsequent doses are regulated by frequent estimation of prothrombin time which is maintained at between one and a half and two times the control value.

A number of drugs may interfere with the action of oral anticoagulants. Laxatives such as liquid paraffin reduce the absorption of the fat-soluble vitamin K_1, while oral antibiotics reduce synthesis of the vitamin by intestinal flora. Many sedatives and tranquillizers increase the metabolism of coumarins by a process of 'enzyme induction'. Therefore it is essential that whenever a patient on oral anticoagulants is given any of these drugs, a strict laboratory control is maintained to regulate the dosage. Failure to do so may result in serious complications of haemorrhage. If bleeding does occur, it is controlled by the intravenous administration of vitamin K, withdrawal of the drug, and fresh blood transfusion if necessary.

The duration of oral anticoagulant therapy in the management of deep vein thrombosis remains controversial. Many people believe it should be given for a period of 3–6 weeks after the patient has become ambulant.

Heparin: As already mentioned, heparin acts by directly inhibiting various coagulation enzyme systems. Since it is rapidly metabolized in the body, the best method of administration is as a continuous infusion in saline. The dose can easily be adjusted by varying the rate of the drip; this gives a more stable effect but causes bleeding more frequently than comparable intermittent doses. For intermittent administration, a Gordh or Mitchell needle is introduced into a superficial vein on the hand to avoid repeated venepuncture. For both continuous infusion and intermittent therapy, 10 000 units of heparin given every 6 h are usually adequate for an adult of average size.

A baseline clotting time is obtained before starting heparin. Subsequent readings are made 3 h after the first and second doses, and the dosage of heparin is adjusted accordingly, as individual requirements vary considerably. The clotting time is maintained at approximately twice the control value. Deep intramuscular injections should be avoided because they can produce quite painful extensive haematomas. Heparin is usually begun in combination and is continued until the delayed effect of oral anticoagulants is established.

FIBRINOLYTIC DRUGS. These have a direct effect on the thrombus. The most widely used agent at present is streptokinase, a purified fraction from a mixture of streptococcal exotoxins, which has been shown to have a thombolytic effect. The other agent is urokinase, obtained from human urine, and claimed to induce a more predictable thrombolytic state. Both these agents act by conversion of plasminogen, an inactive plasma globulin, to plasmin, which has a specific proteolytic effect on fibrin and fibrinogen.

Streptokinase is highly antigenic in man. As a result of previous streptococcal infection, most individuals tend to have a variable level of circulating streptokinase antibody. It is essential to determine this level, because sufficient streptokinase should be given not only to neutralize these antibodies, but also to be available in excess for activation of plasminogen. It is common practice for the loading dose of 500 000 units of streptokinase to be given in 30 min, followed by a maintenance dose of 600 000 units every 6 h. The dose is dissolved in normal saline and given as a slow infusion. Although several laboratory tests have been advocated to regulate the maintenance dosage, none of them is capable of predicting the likelihood of a bleeding episode. However, thrombin-clotting time is probably the only simple and useful test which is employed frequently to monitor therapy.

Streptokinase is not always successful in producing complete lysis. Factors known to affect its action are the age and extent of the thrombus. Since the activator must reach the surface of the thrombus to produce the desired effect, thrombolysis is achieved more readily in a vessel that is not completely occluded. The age of the thrombus seems to be more important than its extent. The best results are obtained when symptoms of thrombosis have been present for less than 96 h before treatment is started.

There are, however, certain disadvantages in using streptokinase. Immediate allergic reactions and pyrexia are common and can sometimes be very troublesome. Prophylactic hydrocortisone administration may not control these effectively. The risk of haemorrhage requires very careful consideration, especially during the early postoperative period, before therapy is instituted. Another disadvantage of streptokinase is its ability to form neutralizing antibodies in high titre quite quickly which, for a time at least, would preclude a second course in the same patient.

Contraindications to Specific Therapy

Specific therapy is contraindicated when there is obvious risk of haemorrhage. The presence of recent history of a duodenal or gastric ulcer, recent gastrointestinal or cerebral haemorrhage, malignant hypertension, or any haemorrhagic diathesis are *absolute* contraindications for specific therapy. However, there are situations where the possibility of bleeding must be weighed carefully against the risk of fatal pulmonary embolism. Drugs like streptokinase and heparin should be used with caution within 72 h of major surgical operation, or even longer if there are extensive raw areas of granulation tissue present, which can act as a source of active haemorrhage.

Surgery

The availability of thrombolytic agents such as streptokinase is rapidly altering the approach to treatment of acute massive deep vein thrombosis. As a result, the indications for operative intervention have narrowed considerably. Nevertheless, the need for surgical treatment still exists in properly selected patients. Operative treatment is necessary in patients where the disease process is so extensive that the viability of the affected limb is in doubt and where anticoagulants are contraindicated or have failed to prevent pulmonary emboli.

The surgical procedures which are commonly employed in the management of deep vein thrombosis fall into two main groups: thrombectomy for acute massive thrombosis, and operations which are employed for the prevention of repeated episodes of pulmonary embolism.

Thrombectomy was first introduced in 1937; its routine use for treating patients with massive iliofemoral thrombosis has been recommended by several surgeons. These recommendations have been based upon the encouraging early results. However, in a number of studies, careful follow-up over a period of 3–10 years has shown that the operation probably does not achieve many of its objectives.

The second group of surgical procedures is employed for the prevention of repeated episodes of pulmonary embolism (*Fig.* 57.7*a*). These include ligation or plication of the inferior vena cava or the femoral vein. There is no doubt that operations performed upon the vena cava seem to be much more effective in preventing both fatal and non-fatal pulmonary embolism, when compared with the results of femoral vein ligation. Secondly, there is little to choose between total and partial interruption of the cava, though the long-term results in the majority of reported series tend to suggest that partial interruption produces a lower incidence of late stasis sequelae in the limbs. Of the various procedures we have found simple plication, as advocated by Spencer and others (1962), to be quite effective: a single row of mattress sutures is placed and tied to convert the vena cava into a series of parallel channels. The caval umbrella filter (Mobin–Uddin, Trimble and Bryant, Kimray–Greenfield) may prove to be more satisfactory if the encouraging early results are confirmed by long-term follow-up studies involving a large number of patients (*Fig.* 57.7*b*). Femoral vein ligation, to 'lock in' the thrombus, should be advocated with great caution in view of the high mortality and morbidity associated with the procedure.

Aftercare

Treatment of venous thrombosis should continue after the patient has been discharged from hosptial. It is wise to recommend the patient to sleep with the foot of the bed elevated on suitable blocks until all oedema has subsided. The patient should be advised to take regular exercise and to avoid prolonged periods in a sitting position. Elastic stockings or bandages may be of help in those cases where troublesome oedema persists in spite of adequate anticoagulant treatment. Below-knee elastic stockings are preferable to full-length ones, though the latter may be more acceptable to female patients.

VARICOSE VEINS

Varicose veins is one of the commonest conditions seen in clinical practice. It has been estimated that, in Great Britain, approximately 1 in every 15 persons over the age of 40 suffers from varicose veins. The word varicose is derived from the Latin *varix*, meaning a dilated vessel. A varicose vein is defined as one which has lost its valvular function and has undergone pathological changes, resulting in dilatation and tortuosity. Veins in the lower limb are most commonly affected.

Aetiology

Varicose veins are much more common in Europe and North America, and the cause of this preponderance is not known. Females are affected much more frequently than males, the ratio being approximately 5:1. Although no age is exempt, they commonly occur in the fourth and fifth decades.

No definite aetiology is known. Various theories have been postulated, but none seems to offer a complete and satisfactory explanation. Probably the basic abnormality is weakness of the vein wall. As a result of this, the vein dilates, and its valves become incompetent allowing retrograde flow of blood. It has also been suggested that valvular incompetence is the primary abnormality, and the changes in the vein wall are secondary in nature. Erect posture plays a definite role in the causation of varicosities since varicose veins do not occur in quadrupeds, and they are commonly seen in people engaged in occupations involving prolonged standing. Although many members of the same family may be affected, it is not known with certainty if heredity plays any significant role.

Secondary varicose veins are the result of certain known conditions. Destruction of venous valves in the deep and communicating veins by thrombosis is the commonest cause. They are also frequently seen during pregnancy; this may be due to hormonal factors causing relaxation of the smooth muscle in the vein wall, with subsequent dilatation. Direct pressure on the iliac veins by an enlarged uterus also acts as a contributory factor. They are sometimes seen with congenital arteriovenous fistulas involving the lower limb. In such cases, the skin is warm and the limb is larger than the contralateral one.

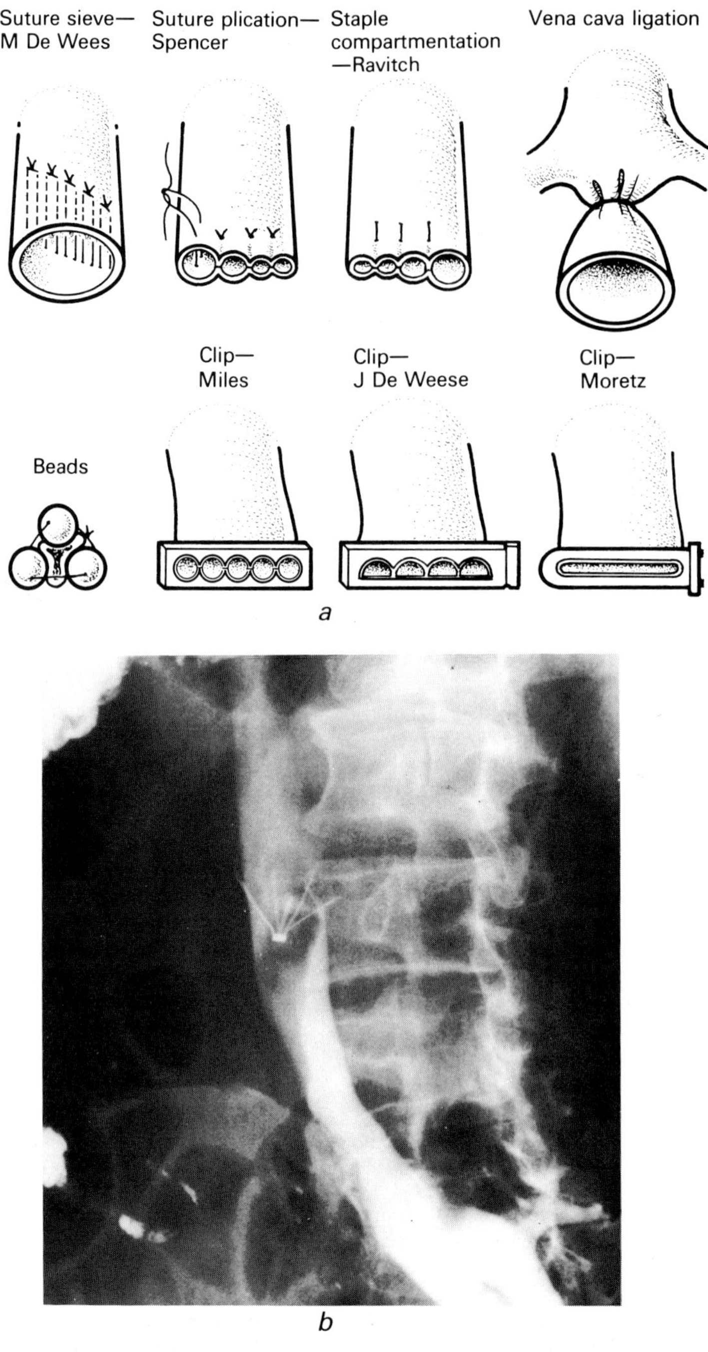

Fig. 57.7 *a*, Operative interruption of the inferior vena cava for the prevention of recurrent pulmonary embolism. Ligation of the inferior vena cava is seldom performed today. Similarly, suture sieve, suture plication and staple compartmentation are also not the procedures of choice. Application of a clip, such as that of Miles, De Wesse or Moretz, is a simple and safe procedure which is very effective in controlling recurrent pulmonary emboli, and also maintains the patency of the inferior vena cava. *b*, The umbrella filter has been passed into the infrarenal vena cava and lodged by its spikes in an inverted position.

Pathology

The veins of the lower limb are grouped into the deep, superficial and communicating systems. Normally much of the blood flows from the superficial into the deep veins through communicating veins at various levels. As the calf muscles contract, the pressure in the deep veins of the leg rises, and the blood is forced upwards. This high pressure is not transmitted to the superficial system because of the valves in the communicating veins which allow the flow of blood in one direction (*Fig.* 57.8). When these valves

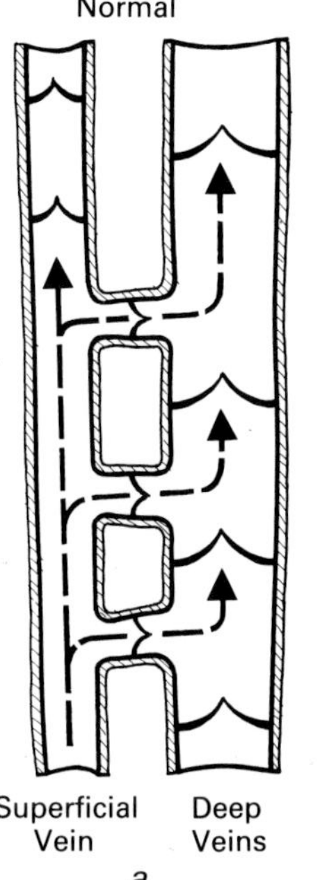

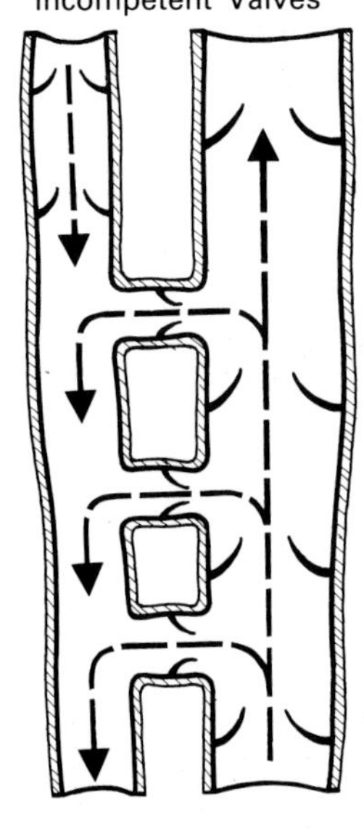

Fig. 57.8 *a*, Normal venous circulation from the superficial into the deep veins through communicating veins at the various levels. *b*, When the valves in the deep and communicating veins become incompetent or destroyed, there is reversal of flow and high pressure is also transmitted to the superficial veins.

become incompetent or are destroyed, the high pressure is transmitted to the superficial veins which subsequently dilate. This dilatation is aggravated by reversed flow of blood and stagnation. As the superficial veins become varicose, their valves also become incompetent (*Fig.* 57.8). A varicose vein may thrombose or become calcified. Microscopic examination in the advanced stages shows atrophy of the venous valves, diminution of elastic tissue and smooth muscle of the media and fibrosis. In other cases, the vein becomes so thin it ruptures easily, producing severe haemorrhage.

Clinical Features

The patient with varicose veins may have no effects other than the cosmetic appearance. Others complain of heaviness, fullness and fatigue, swelling and itching of the involved legs, especially after prolonged standing. Some patients also complain of cramps affecting the calf muscles which occur frequently during the night.

To carry out an adequate examination, the abdomen and lower limbs are exposed. All aspects of the limb are inspected and palpated in a systematic way. Inspection of the limb shows the presence of dilated veins which are localized or extend along the whole course of the long or short saphenous veins and their tributaries. Some degree of ankle oedema may be present. The skin of the involved limb may show pigmentation, induration, eczematous changes and ulceration, confined to the lower part of the leg; these features are most commonly present in cases of secondary varicose vein. The exact extent of the varicosities is detected better by palpation rather than inspection of the limb. A cough impulse is often present, and to detect this the fingers are placed distal to the saphenofemoral junction while the patient is asked to cough strongly. A positive cough impulse is detected by palpation of an expansile impulse and a course thrill; it indicates gross valvular incompetence at the saphenofemoral junction.

The incompetent communicating veins are indicated by localized blow-outs at their anatomical positions. Three communicating veins are usually present on the medial aspect of the leg, approximately at distances of 2, 4 and 6 inches from the tip of the medial malleolus. One communicating vein is often present on the lateral aspect at a distance of about 6 inches from the tip of the lateral malleolus. When incompetent, depressions are felt easily by palpating the elevated leg.

Various clinical tests have been described to determine the competence of the valves in the superficial and deep venous systems. These include the Brodie–Trendelenburg, percussion and multiple tourniquet tests. For the Brodie–Trendelenburg test, the patient lies supine on a couch and the leg is raised to empty the superficial veins. A soft rubber tourniquet is applied around the upper third of the thigh and the patient is asked to stand while the limb is examined. If the superficial veins refill quickly, and are easily palpable, it indicates incompetence of the short saphenous or communicating veins. When the tourniquet is removed and the veins fill quickly from above, it demonstrates incompetence of the saphenofemoral valve. The multiple tourniquet test is usually not performed because it is time consuming. The percussion test is used to determine the incompetence of superficial veins at all levels. A finger is placed distal to the segment to be examined, and the examiner taps proximally with the fingers of the other hand. The feeling of an impulse denotes incompetence of the intervening valves. By applying this test at all levels, the extent of valvular incompetence is determined.

General examination is undertaken to exclude other diseases, such as congestive cardiac failure, which aggravate symptoms of varicose veins. Rectal and abdominal examinations are carried out to exclude the presence of a tumour.

Investigations

Ascending phlebography is useful to demonstrate the state of the deep veins, the site of the incompetent communicating veins and superficial varicosities. It is usually undertaken in patients with a previous history of deep vein thrombosis or other causes of secondary varicosities, and recurrent varicose veins.

Diagnosis

The diagnosis of primary varicose veins is based on the presence of dilated tortuous superficial varicosities which are localized or diffuse.

With secondary varicose veins there is often a history of deep venous thrombosis and incompetent communicating veins are usually present; other features such as ankle oedema, induration, eczema and ulceration are often present. In doubtful cases, the diagnosis is confirmed by phlebography.

Management

The treatment of varicose veins is by a conservative regimen, injection of sclerosants or surgery. The aim of these procedures is to improve the venous return from the affected limb.

The conservative measures consist mainly of elastic support and avoidance of prolonged standing. They are used in patients with asymptomatic varicosities, those in whom other methods of treatment are contraindicated, and when consent for operation is refused. The length of the stocking usually extends from the base of the toes to the knee. This compresses adequately the superficial varicosities and increases the efficiency of the calf muscle pump. If the varicose veins extend to the thigh region, full-length stockings may be used, and although they are readily accepted by female patients, they are not efficient because they become loose around the knee. Elastic bandages are also used, and are more effective, but they are cumbersome, and not readily accepted because of their appearance. Venous stasis is reduced by avoiding standing for long periods, encouraging regular active exercises, periodic elevation of the limbs during the day, and sleeping with the foot of the bed elevated.

In patients with secondary varicosities due to pregnancy, it is preferable to avoid surgery or injection therapy, as in the majority of cases the varicose veins tend to regress or even disappear completely after parturition. Such cases are reviewed at the end of 4–6 months after delivery, when persistent varicosities require active treatment.

Although sclerosant therapy has been used for a long time, the technique has been recently modified by Fegan, and is being used more widely. The method is simple and safe if undertaken properly. The sites of injection are determined by localizing the points that control the varicosities effectively by digital pressure. It has been suggested that these sites represent the junction of incompetent communicating veins with the superficial venous system, and are responsible for the varicosities. A variety of sclerosants have been used; sodium tetradecyl sulphate gives good results with rare complications. An empty vein technique is used. Continuous local compression after injection is essential for the firm adherence of the localized thrombus to the vein wall with subsequent fibrosis, thus minimizing recanalization. A venepuncture is performed with the leg in a dependant position, and a fine needle is used, attached to a syringe containing 1·0 ml of sodium tetradecyl sulphate. A little blood is withdrawn and 0·1 ml of the solution is injected to clear the needle. The patient now lies down, and the limb is carefully elevated. The segment to be injected is isolated by firm digital compression (*Fig.* 57.9). An interval is allowed for emptying the vein before the sclerosant is injected. Without moving the fingers isolating the segment, the injection is made and the needle withdrawn; the site of the venepuncture is compressed with a bevelled sorbo rubber pad and a cotton crêpe bandage is applied in a criss-cross fashion, to produce immediate effective compression. The technique may be repeated at different sites on the same occasion. An elastic bandage or stocking is also applied, extending from the base of the toes to just below the knee, or proximal to the highest site of injection in the thigh. It is considered that firm elastic stockings are better than elastic bandages, as they hold the initial crêpe bandages in position. Compression is continued for 6 weeks, and during this period the patient is encouraged to walk as much as possible, and to avoid prolonged standing. After 2 weeks, the limb is inspected and further injections are given if required. The main complications of sclerosant therapy are deep vein thrombosis and ulceration. They are minimized by injecting small amounts of the solution using the empty vein technique, and local compression.

Gross varicosities are better treated by surgery unless there is some specific contraindication. The aim is to remove as many of the dilated veins as possible and, if necessary, to ligate incompetent communicating veins. High ligation of the long saphenous vein with or without retrograde injection

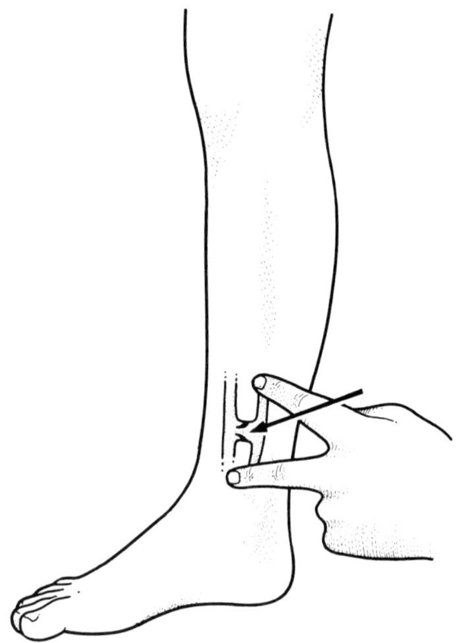

Fig. 57.9 Technique of sclerotherapy. The segment of the vein to be injected is isolated between fingers and the venepuncture is performed at the point which controls the varicosities.

of sclerosant solution has been used in the past, but is not effective. Ligation and stripping of the long and short saphenous veins is now commonly employed. To achieve satisfactory results, it is essential to carry out flush ligation of the long saphenous vein, and ligation and division of all the tributaries immediately distal to the saphenofemoral junction. Failure to do so results in the recurrence of varicosities. Incompetent tributaries of the long or short saphenous veins in the thigh or leg should be avulsed before stripping the main vein. In order to obtain good results, it requires time and patience. Before operation, it is important to mark the course of the varicose veins whilst the patient is standing erect. It is used for varicosities of both the long and short saphenous systems.

To approach the long saphenous vein, the patient is placed supine on the operating table with the leg elevated; the affected leg is externally rotated, and the feet placed apart. When operating on the short saphenous vein the patient is turned into the prone position. The long saphenous vein is approached through an incision just below and parallel to the skin crease of the groin with its midpoint one finger's breadth medial to the pulsation of the femoral artery. The subcutaneous tissues are divided and dissection reveals the long saphenous vein as it pierces the cribriform fascia to join the femoral vein. The tributaries joining the long saphenous vein in this region are dissected out in turn, and divided between ligatures. The saphenofemoral junction is clearly defined, and the long saphenous vein is ligated and divided immediately distal to the junction. A small transverse incision is made anterior to the tip of the medial malleolus, and the vein is dissected free from the surrounding tissues; particular care is taken to separate it from the saphenous nerve. The vein is ligated and a small incision is made proximal to this point. A vein stripper is introduced into the vein, and passed up to the saphenofemoral junction. Another incision is made in the vein at the groin, the stripper is advanced so that its tip may be removed, and a handle attached. The distal end of the stripper is fitted with a bullet-shaped head, and the vein is tied round it just above the distal ligature. Multiple small incisions are made over the sites of the tributaries previously marked. Each vein is grasped with two pairs of artery forceps, and by gentle traction it is pulled out of the wound; successive forceps are applied to it until the maximum length of the vein has been obtained. The extruded segment is then dealt with, and the skin incisions are closed. After the ankle wound has been sutured, the leg is elevated and dressings placed over the incisions. Crêpe bandages are applied as the stripper is withdrawn to prevent the accumulation of blood along the bed of the vein, and extensive bruising.

In difficult cases, when a short segment is very tortuous, it is necessary to make further incisions over the course of the long saphenous vein to facilitate the passage of the stripper. Sometimes retrograde passage is easier, and occasionally it is necessary to pass strippers independently from above and below. The approach to the short saphenous vein is through a small transverse incision over the popliteal fossa. It is usually easier to introduce and pass the stripper downwards, as it is difficult to identify the vein as it passes posterior to the lateral malleolus. The proximal end of the short saphenous vein is ligated deep to the deep fascia. In patients with secondary varicosities following deep vein thrombosis, ligation of incompetent communicating veins is often required; each is exposed and ligated either superficial or deep to the fascia. When venous ulceration is present, this procedure is usually avoided until the ulcer has healed.

It is difficult to localize all the incompetent communicating veins by palpation alone. Phlebography is of value in their more accurate localization, and it also demonstrates the state of the deep venous system. Ligation of incompetent communicating veins is often necessary in the treatment of persistent venous ulcers, and can be combined with excision and skin grafting.

There is some controversy as to whether it is better to carry out an extrafascial or subfascial ligation; the latter procedure entails more extensive mobilization and dissection. A vertical incision is usually made on the medial side of the leg just posterior to the border of the tibia. The incompetent communicating veins are dissected out and divided between ligatures. When a subfascial ligation is performed, the deep fascia is divided, and the anterior flap is carefully elevated to expose the communicating veins. The deep fascia is approximated with loose sutures, and the skin incision is closed.

Prognosis

Although there is considerable morbidity due to varicosities, they are hardly ever a risk to life. A number of complications sometimes occur, and are seen more frequently with secondary varicose veins. They include oedema, eczema, ulceration and haemorrhage. If bleeding occurs, the leg is elevated and local compression is applied.

VENOUS ULCERATION

Venous ulceration is a very common condition. Hippocrates first noticed the association between varicose veins and ulcers of the leg. Since then, these ulcers have been called varicose ulcers. Recently it has been observed that they occur much more frequently as the sequelae of deep vein thrombosis.

Aetiology

Venous ulceration occurs frequently in females of middle age, and a previous history of deep vein thrombosis is common. Severe and longstanding varicosities are also responsible for ulceration in a small number of cases. Local trauma, occupations involving prolonged standing, malnutrition and poor personal hygiene are all contributory factors.

Pathology

Various theories have been postulated regarding the pathogenesis of venous ulceration, but none seems to offer a complete explanation. Probably several factors play an important part in producing changes in the local circulation, and are responsible for the condition. Incompetence of valves in the deep, communicating veins and less frequently in the superficial system produces stasis of blood, and a rise in the local venous pressure. This in turn produces thickening in the wall of the capillaries and stagnation of blood in the affected area. The transport of oxygen and nutrient substances required for cellular survival is thus affected, and results in local cellular necrosis and ulceration.

There is evidence to suggest that local venous hypertension opens up the normally closed arteriovenous shunts, and arterial blood reaches the venous channels by bypassing the capillary circulation. This is supported by an increase in oxygen saturation of the blood in the tissues adjacent to the ulcer. The shunting of arterial blood produces local tissue anoxia, necrosis and ulceration.

These changes are confined to the skin and subcutaneous tissues, and are limited by the deep fascia in the earlier stages. In more advanced ulcers, the process involves the deeper structures. When the ulcer heals, the subcutaneous fat is never replaced, and there is formation of scar tissue (*Fig.* 57.10). The capillaries and venules remain dilated. In advanced stages, the skin, subcutaneous tissues and deep fascia become welded together into a firm solid mass, and this is apparent clinically as an area of induration which extends beyond that of the ulcer. Dermal lymphatics are destroyed affecting the drainage of the involved area. Contraction of the fibrous tissue may produce a tight constricting band.

Clinical Features

The ulcers are large and shallow, with an irregular sloping margin, and the base is often formed by unhealthy granulation tissue. They are usually associated with oedema of the leg, which is most marked in patients with post-thrombotic ulceration. Venous ulceration is invariably confined to the lower half of the leg in the 'gaiter area'. Before the appearance of frank ulceration, the skin in the affected area often shows eczematous changes. This is precipitated or made worse by local application of irritant substances and antibiotics. Unless these changes are controlled early and effectively, they spread rapidly to involve the whole circumference of the leg. The skin becomes pigmented due to deposition of haemosiderin in the subcutaneous tissues, derived from the breakdown of extravasated blood. The skin and subcutaneous tissues are indurated and the extent varies according to the severity and duration of the disease. In the early stages, venous ulcers are very painful, and this is made worse by infection.

Investigations

General examination of the patient is important so that conditions such as anaemia and congestive cardiac failure are

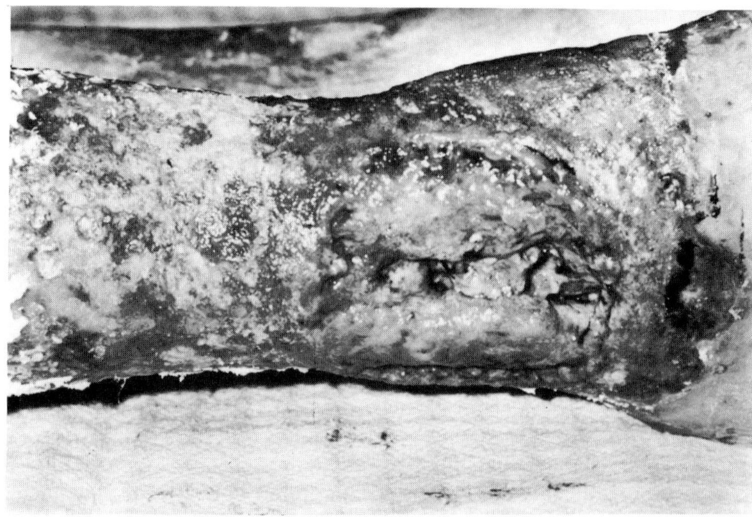

Fig. 57.10 Extensive varicose ulceration of the lower limb. Liponecrosis leads to a narrowing of the limb.

recognized and corrected. Phlebography is a useful investigation to demonstrate the state of the deep and superficial veins, and to determine the site of incompetent communicating veins.

Diagnosis

The diagnosis is based on a history of venous disease, the site of ulceration is differentiated from arterial, syphilitic and tropical ulcers. Arterial ulcers are sometimes seen in patients with severe peripheral ischaemia. They are commonly situated on the toes, heel, dorsum and lateral border of the foot. A history of trauma often precedes the onset of ulceration. These ulcers are very painful in the early stages, and examination of the leg usually reveals coldness, discoloration and the absence of peripheral pulses.

Syphilitic ulcers are usually multiple and occur in the tertiary stage of the disease. These ulcers are usually situated outside the 'gaiter area' and are painless. They have a punched-out appearance or serpiginous margin, and a wash-leather base. Other features of the disease are present elsewhere in the body. With the improved treatment of syphilis in its early stages, these ulcers are rarely seen.

Tropical ulcers seen in those living in a tropical climate occasionally present a diagnostic problem to clinicians working in temperate regions. They commonly occur in the legs or feet of malnourished individuals as a result of parasitic infestation, and are often complicated by chronic secondary infection. They are usually multiple, and are not confined to the 'gaiter area'.

Management

The aim of treatment is to heal the ulcer and prevent its recurrence. This can be achieved by local measures, elastic support and elevation. The ulcer is cleaned with normal saline, weak eusol–saline solution or cetrimide. The local application of strong cleansing agents is avoided, as they delay healing and precipitate a severe eczematous reaction. Simple non-adherent dressings are most useful as they cause minimal or no irritation to the surrounding skin, and are easily changed. When the ulcer is grossly infected, systemic antibiotics are used according to the specific sensitivity of the infecting organism.

Local venous hypertension is the main factor in the development of ulcers, and is aggravated by the erect posture. Patients with extensive ulceration infection and gross oedema are treated preferably by bed rest and elevation. They are confined to bed with the foot of the bed raised, so that the legs are above the level of the heart; this is done by using wooden blocks or bricks to a height of 6–9 inches. When combined with active calf exercises, the local venous pressure is decreased by increasing venous return and reducing the effect of gravity. Those with uncomplicated ulcers, minimal oedema and who must continue to work, are treated by the ambulant method. The use of firm elastic compression bandages also reduces effectively local venous hypertension. The bandages exert continuous pressure on the superficial and deep veins during muscular contraction, and increase the venous return by enhancing the pump-like action of the calf muscles. Although with this method healing may take longer, the patient remains ambulant and active. Many different types of bandage are available, but one-way stretch, non-adhesive, elastic webbing bandages are preferable.

The efficacy of bandaging as a method of treatment depends upon proper application. The bandages are applied working proximately from the base of the toes with full inclusion of the heel and extending to just below the knee. Each turn of the bandage overlaps the preceding one by half of its width, and the tension is greatest in the region of the ankle; it should be sufficient to afford adequate support, but not to occlude the circulation. The bandages are worn during the day only, and at night the patient is instructed to sleep with the foot of the bed elevated. The bandages are reapplied in the morning before getting out of bed. Proper understanding of this technique by the patient is essential for the success of treatment.

Elastic stockings are also used as a supporting measure, but are not as effective as bandages, although young patients accept them more readily because of their better appearance. They are less effective because they do not conform sufficiently well to the variations in oedema. Constant use and frequent laundering reduce their stretch and efficiency, and it is necessary for the patients to have several pairs, and to renew them frequently. Elastic stockings, like bandages, must include the heel, and should be made of firm material. Measurements of the patient for whom stockings are prescribed are taken in the morning, when the swelling of the limb is minimal.

If the ulcer fails to heal after a prolonged conservative regime, it is excised and a skin graft applied. Ligation of varicosities and incompetent communicating veins contributing to the ulcer is done at the same time. Recurrence of venous ulceration is prevented by the continued use of supportive measures once the ulcer has healed. In such cases, ligation of incompetent communicating veins and stripping or injection of superficial varicosities is considered. The patient is advised to avoid prolonged standing and local trauma. When at rest, the limb is elevated and regular ankle and calf exercises practised; the foot of the bed is raised at night.

Associated conditions which affect healing are treated at the same time; in particular, correction of anaemia and improvement of the general nutrition is done. If the anaemia is severe, transfusion is indicated but oral iron therapy is usually adequate.

Prognosis

Although venous ulceration is a benign condition, it has social and economic implications due to loss of work. There is a considerable morbidity due to recurrent cellulitis, phlebitis and stiffness of joints. Attacks of recurrent cellulitis cause considerable pain and discomfort; these are treated by bed rest, elevation of the limb and systemic antibiotics. In longstanding and neglected ulcers, malignant change is rarely seen. In doubtful cases, biopsy confirms the diagnosis. Wide excision of the ulcer and surrounding tissues and skin grafting is often adequate; some cases require more radical treatment by amputation.

LYMPHOEDEMA

Lymphoedema is the collection of lymph in the subcutaneous tissues due to an underlying abnormality in the lymphatic system, and the latter having an obstructive cause. Primary lymphoedema is further divided according to the age of the patient in whom it appears. The congenital type may have a hereditary background, and is then known as Milroy's disease, whereas the remaining group is divided by the arbitrary acceptance of the age of 35 into early (lymphoedema praecox) and late (lymphoedema tarda) cases. Secondary lymphoedema is classified according to the aetiological factors which are responsible for the lymphatic obstruction.

Aetiology

The basic abnormality of the lymphatics in primary lymphoedema represents a developmental anatomical variation from the normal pattern as demonstrated by lymphangiography. The most common picture is that of hypoplasia, when the lymphatic vessels are of small calibre, and reduced in number. Hyperplasia is sometimes seen when the vessels are dilated and tortuous. Total agenesis of lymphatics and lymph glands is rare. Females are much more commonly affected, and no race would seem to be exempt from the condition.

The main feature of secondary lymphoedema is obstruction to the normal lymphatic return due to a variety of causes. The blockage not only involves the regional lymph glands draining the area, but also sometimes affects the lymph vessels. Obstruction due to the dissemination of malignant tumours is a common cause of secondary lymphoedema. Direct extension of tumour growth in continuity leads to obliteration of lymphatic pathways, and this continues until there is involvement of the regional lymph glands. Once a channel has been invaded by tumour, small emboli often become detached, and lodge in the lymph glands, draining the area, causing further obstruction to lymphatic return. Although collateral pathways open up initially, it is not long before they also become involved by tumour.

With the development of modern methods in surgery, radical excision of tumours and lymph glands draining the area is practised more frequently, and this has become a common cause of secondary lymphoedema. It is particularly seen following radical mastectomy for carcinoma of the breast. It is not certain to what extent the lymphatic dissection is responsible for this, as other factors also play an important role, including trauma to the axillary vein and subsequent radiotherapy. This complication is not often of sufficient degree to cause severe disability. Radiotherapy provokes a fibrous reaction in the tissues within the field of treatment, leading to further obliteration of lymphatic channels, and thus aggravating the condition.

Chronic or recurrent inflammation leads to fibrosis and occlusion of lymph vessels. Although this is seen less commonly since the introduction of antibiotics, it still occurs in neglected cases. Minor degrees of transient lymphoedema are seen as a result of acute inflammation, but they usually resolve before irreversible changes take place. Once lymphoedema is established, chronic infection leads to progression of the condition, unless it is treated effectively. Parasitic invasion of lymphatic channels is commonly seen in the Middle and Far East, and the most common cause is filariasis. The parasites lodge in the regional lymph glands, and provoke a fibrous reaction leading to obstruction to the normal return of lymph. This type of lymphoedema not uncommonly affects the external genitalia and lower limbs, producing the grotesque appearances of elephantiasis.

Pathology

The sequence of pathological changes that occurs in lymphoedema is similar in both the primary and secondary groups. There is diminution in the return of lymph either due to a congenital abnormality, or obstruction of the lymphatic system. Transudation occurs into the surrounding tissues; this leads to accumulation and stagnation of lymph, which is followed by coagulation of the fluid because of its high protein content. Lymphoedema only affects the subcutaneous tissues as it is limited by the deep fascia, so that muscles are never involved. The accumulation and coagulation of lymph provokes a severe fibrous reaction in the adjacent tissues leading to loculation. Although initially the oedema is pitting in character, later it becomes solid, and this is typical of the advanced condition.

In the early stages, there are no apparent changes in the skin, but as the process continues, it becomes thickened. Hyperkeratosis occurs, and the skin develops a granular appearance, or there is formation of plaques or verrucae. The pathological changes are aggravated by infection. This occurs as a localized cellulitis, or as lymphangiitis and lymphadenitis. The addition of the inflammatory reaction intensifies the fibrosis occurring in the adjacent tissues, and leads to progression of the condition.

Obstruction of the main lymphatic channels and regional lymph glands acts as a stimulus to the development of collateral vessels, and the occurrence of dermal backflow, which has a characteristic pattern on lymphangiography. Recent work has suggested the appearance of lymphovenous communications following obstruction; they are of considerable importance in the dissemination of malignant tumours, and their treatment with endolymphatic radioactive isotopes.

Clinical Features

The presenting feature of primary lymphoedema is gradually increasing swelling of the affected part, although some cases do not present until complications develop. The history of swelling is sometimes related to minor trauma which is most probably coincidental. The oedema is usually unilateral, and more commonly affects the lower limb, beginning distally and gradually spreading proximally. The appearance of secondary lymphoedema is often preceded by the history of the precipitating cause, but if this remains hidden, swelling is the first sign. If it begins proximally, it is more suggestive of secondary lymphoedema, and a cause should be carefully looked for. In a small number of cases, the first features are those of infection which occurs intermittently, or becomes chronic. Malignant change occurs rarely in a limb with chronic lymphoedema. Primary lymphoedema is associated with an increased incidence of other congenital abnormalities, such as capillary haemangiomas.

Physical examination of the patient shows swelling of the affected part, and some patients with the primary type also have oedema at other sites. In the early stages, it is pitting in nature, but as the condition progresses, it becomes solid (*Fig.* 57.11). Skin changes are only found in the advanced stages of the disease, producing a granular appearance, localized plaques or verrucae. Ulceration of the skin is uncommon, although excoriation is often seen, and predisposes to infection. Lymph-filled vesicles are sometimes present, and when they rupture, produce a milky chylous discharge.

Other clinical features may be present in cases of secondary lymphoedema, and they are of value in discovering the underlying obstructive cause. Enlargement of the regional lymph glands suggests that this is due to secondary involvement by malignant disease. Surgery or radiotherapy is also responsible for this condition. Complete physical examination is of great importance, and appropriate investigations are carried out as indicated.

Investigations

Visualization of lymphatics is achieved by the intradermal injection of dyes or radio-opaque contrast media into a lymph vessel. This investigation is not indicated in every case of lymphoedema, and is undertaken when surgery is contemplated, or as a diagnostic technique to find the cause of secondary lymphoedema.

Lymphangiography shows the typical appearance in each group (*Fig.* 57.12). In primary lymphoedema, there may be hypoplasia, hyperplasia, or agenesis. Secondary lymphoedema is characterized by the presence of multiple collateral vessels, dermal back-flow and changes in the regional lymph glands. When the glands are involved by tumour, they often show filling defects, or are not visualized if there is complete

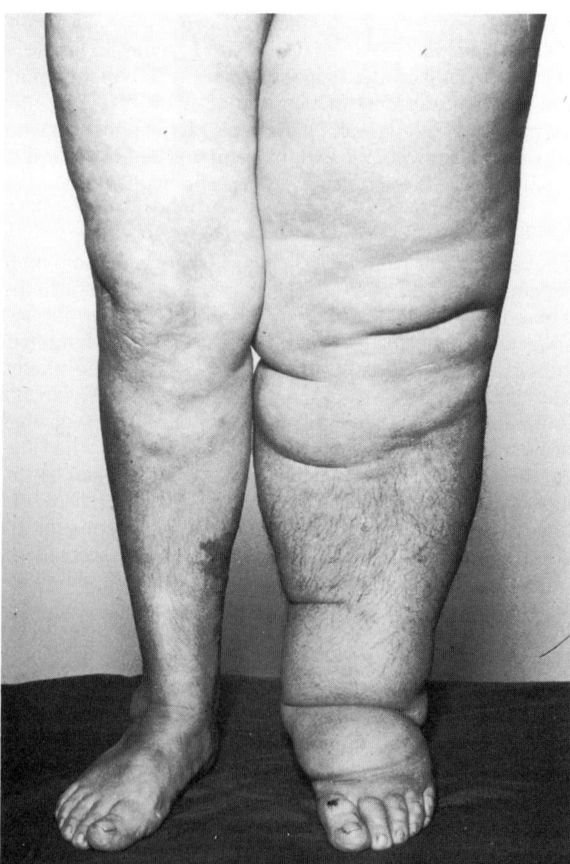

Fig. 57.11 Massive unilateral lymphoedema of the leg.

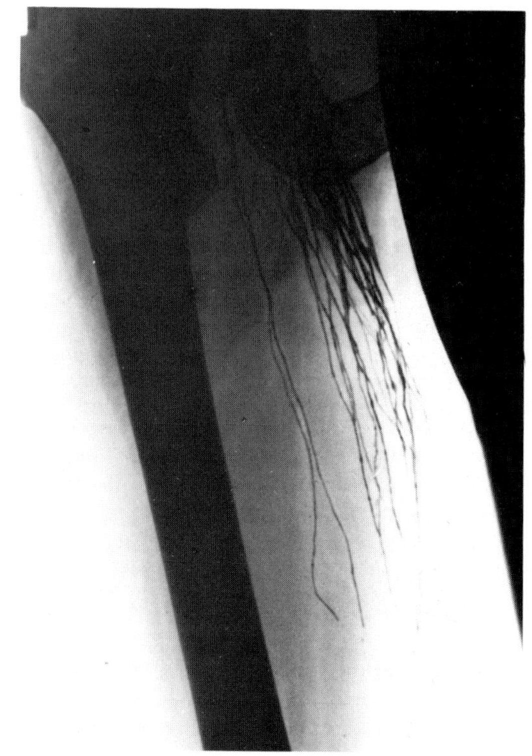

Fig. 57.12 Lymphangiogram in a patient suffering from primary lymphoedema due to hyperplasia of lymphatics. There is increase in the number of lymphatics which are dilated and the valves become incompetent.

replacement. If a chylous discharge is present, examination of the fluid shows a high protein content, and helps to distinguish it from oedema due to other causes.

Diagnosis

In the majority of cases it is based on the history and clinical assessment of the patient. Some diagnostic difficulty is encountered in the distinction between lymphoedema and the other types of oedema, such as cardiac, venous and pretibial myxoedema. Cardiac oedema usually occurs in the lower limb, but remains soft and pitting in nature; its distribution varies with posture and is also found in the sacral region. Other signs of cardiac failure are usually present, and an electrocardiogram shows evidence of ventricular strain, and a chest radiograph may show cardiac enlargement. Oedema due to venous obstruction usually has a more acute onset, and is associated with other features of deep venous insufficiency, such as incompetent communicating veins and varicose ulceration. Pretibial myxoedema is similar to the oedema of lymphatic origin, but remains localized to the anterior aspect of the leg below the knee.

Management

Most cases of lymphoedema can be controlled by conservative means using a combination of simple measures. Only patients with gross oedema will require surgical treatment, and this is not done until conservative methods have been fully tried and failed.

Elastic stockings or bandages are used to control the swelling. The technique of bandaging is carefully explained to the patient, as faulty application aggravates rather than improves the condition. Elevation of the affected part is a valuable measure, and is done whenever possible during the day, and always at night. If the lower limb is affected, the patient is encouraged to elevate the limb on a chair during the day, and to raise the foot of the bed with blocks at night. When the upper limb is involved, support in a sling or sitting for short periods with the hand on the head is recommended; during the night, the limb is elevated on pillows in a comfortable position. Frequent muscular and joint exercises are practised for short periods; they are of benefit when combined with the use of bandages, and prevent stiffness developing in the joints of the affected limb. Massage and faradic stimulation may be beneficial, and are carried out by trained physiotherapists. Ripple bags have been designed for application to the limbs, and by rhythmic variation in pressure, they help to move the lymph in a proximal direction. These simple measures help the majority of patients provided they are used energetically. The repeated short-term use of diuretics may be of value in some cases, but their use has been disappointing, especially in chronic cases when the oedema fluid is loculated.

A minority of patients need surgical treatment. Many operative procedures have been devised for the treatment of this condition, and from their variety it is apparent that none is entirely satisfactory. The procedures are extensive, and they are recommended when the possible outcome has been fully explained to the patient. The aims of surgical treatment are to reduce the weight of the affected part, and the incidence of infection, as well as to allow the wearing of normal footwear and clothing. The indications for surgery are gross swelling of the limb, and episodes of recurrent infection. The Charles operation depends on reduction en masse. The skin and affected subcutaneous tissues of the limb are excised, and the denuded area is covered by split-skin grafts taken from the removed skin. The Thompson operation combines reduction in size, with an attempt to encourage the communication of superficial and deep lymphatics. A wedge of tissue is excised, and the shaved skin flap overlying it is buried in the underlying muscles, providing an implant of dermal lymphatics so that they may communicate with the deep system.

Following the realization that lymphovenous communications may develop as a result of obstruction to the normal lymphatic return, it has been suggested recently that these could be constructed surgically in cases of secondary lymphoedema. The procedure depends on the presence of normal lymph glands within the field of drainage which are anastomosed directly into an adjacent vein. The early results of this procedure are encouraging, but it remains to be seen whether the communications remain patent as the pressure of the lymphatic flow diminishes.

Chylous reflux presents a different problem. In the surgical treatment of this condition, it is essential that lymphangiography is performed first so that all the lymphatic channels are visualized, and an attempt is then made to ligate each vessel. The results are usually good, provided that all the lymphatics are dealt with in turn.

Prognosis

It is not possible to make any generalization about the outcome of this condition. Although primary lymphoedema usually follows a mild course, it often becomes progressive, and is associated with recurrent infection of increasing severity. Gross swelling of a limb is troublesome to a patient, since it interferes with function. Excoriation of the skin and fungal infection of the interdigital clefts lead to secondary bacterial invasion, with ascending lymphangiitis and lymphadenitis. Malignant change has rarely been described in cases of longstanding lymphoedema. The outlook for secondary lymphoedema depends on the underlying cause; the prognosis is entirely different in cases due to malignant involvement of lymph glands, and those due to filariasis, which is sometimes a self-limiting condition.

58 *Reconstructive Microsurgery*

Andrew G. Batchelor

BACKGROUND

Murphy (1897) is credited with the first successful end-to-end repair of a traumatized artery. He repaired a femoral vessel injured by gunshot. Alexis Carrel won a Nobel prize for placing the techniques on a scientific basis in 1902. He described the triangulation technique (*see below*) and the use of vein grafts. Both these techniques are part of modern practice. However, we had to wait until reliable blood transfusion, antibiosis, improved instrumentation and sutures became available before these techniques could be applied. This happened in the decade 1945–1955. During this time surgeons were perplexed by their apparent inability to successfully anastomose vessels of less than 2–3 mm.

Nylen first described a microscope to improve surgical technique by raising the resolution of the surgeon's vision in 1921. It was not until the late 1950s, however, that surgeons started to experiment successfully with small-vessel anastomosis at the 1–2 mm level.

Klienert successfully revascularized a digit in 1959 but we had to wait until 1967 before a completely amputated thumb was successfully reimplanted by Tamai. From this slow beginning microvascular and microneural surgery has developed rapidly until it has become an essential part of the expertise of a reconstructive surgeon.

EQUIPMENT

Magnification

As with all specialist fields within surgery some special pieces of equipment are necessary. Some form of magnification is a prerequisite and this can be achieved in two ways. First, there are binocular loupes or magnifying glasses (*Fig.* 58.1). These are adequate for low-power work up to about ×4. This is suitable for larger blood vessels of 2–3 mm and for the exacting dissections necessary for the preparation of a vascular pedicle for higher magnification work. Higher magnification loupes are available but problems with illumination and head movement limit their usefulness. They are, however, much cheaper than a microscope, costing hundreds rather than thousands of pounds.

A modern operating microscope is a complex and elegant piece of equipment (*Fig.* 58.2). It should have integral focus and variable magnification systems remotely controlled by foot pedals. Two surgeons are provided with the same high resolution stereoscopic view while facing each other at the table. A coaxial high-intensity cold illumination system is also required. The whole must be mounted on a stable stand and supported by an articulated arm that allows precise and rigid positioning of the optical system appropriately. It can be seen that it is pointless to compromise with an old or inferior machine.

The surgeon must be completely familiar with his microscope and its various idiosyncracies so that it may be arranged to give him a perfect view of the desired field in such a way as he can still operate comfortably.

Instruments

The microsurgical instruments themselves tend to be quite personal and of a very high standard. The surgeon must be comfortable with them and not be tempted to try and 'make do' with other instruments which happen to be available. These tools are very easily damaged. If they are, and it may not be possible to see the damage without magnification, then they should be discarded as it is practically impossible to repair them to the standards necessary for trouble-free microsurgery.

The simplest set (*Fig.* 58.3) would consist of four pairs of No. 5 jeweller's forceps (two per surgeon), a pair of forceps with highly polished tips for vessel dilatation and a pair of microdissecting scissors. This may be expanded according

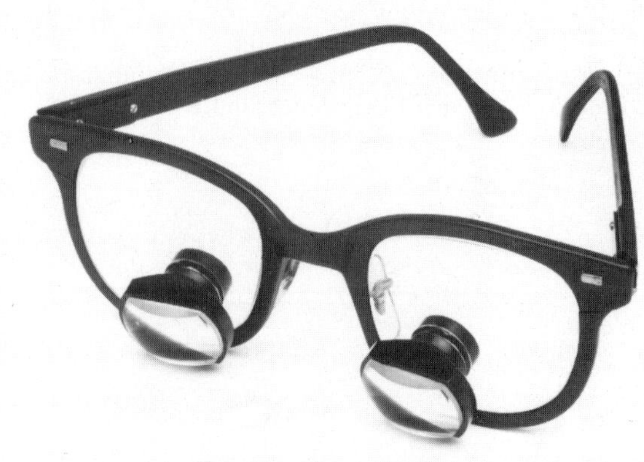

Fig. 58.1 Magnifying loupes (×2·5) suitable for low-power work.

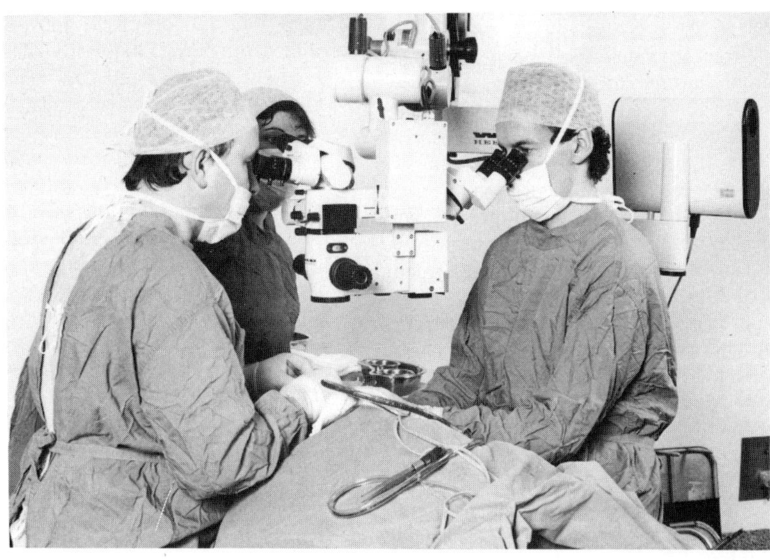

Fig. 58.2 A modern operating microscope with provision for surgeon and assistant.

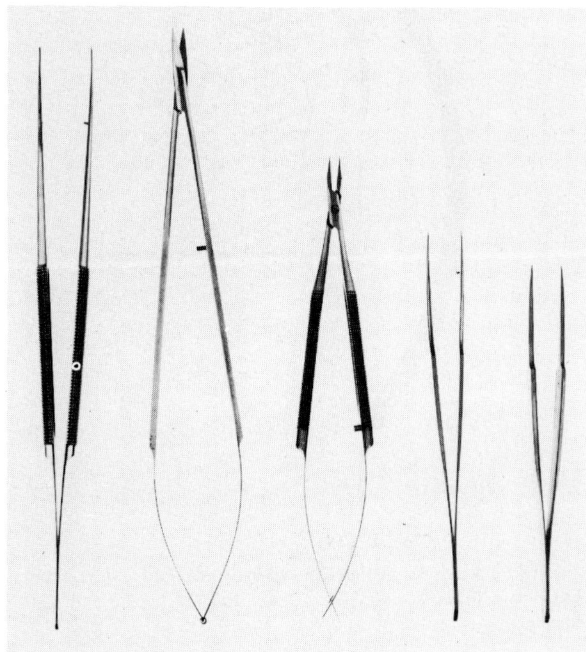

Fig. 58.3 Basic microsurgical instruments. (*Left to right*, long dissecting forceps, scissors, needleholder, vessel dilator and short forceps.)

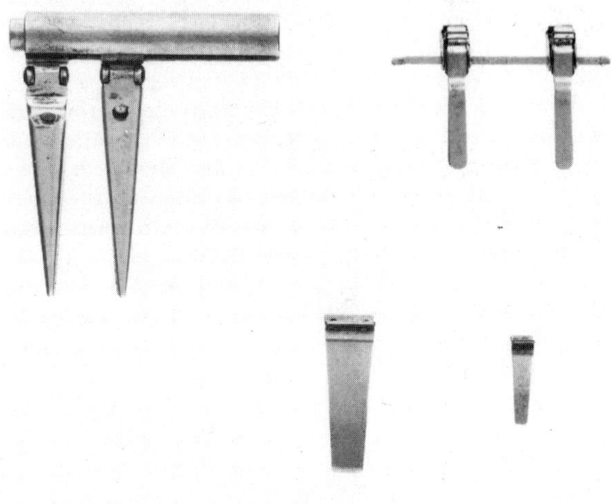

Fig. 58.4 A selection of microvascular clamps (Ackland) and double clamp approximators (*left*, Kleinert and *right*, O'Brien).

to the surgeon's preferences and pocket to include a needle-holder, longer instruments and heavier forceps.

If vascular work is being performed, then suitable vascular clamps are necessary. Most are based on neurosurgical aneurysm clips. They have, however, a very much reduced closing pressure of the order of 60–100 g to avoid crushing the vessels being anastomosed and causing thrombosis. Six clamps of varying sizes is the minimum (*Fig.* 58.4). Two arranged on a bar to approximate vessel ends are a great asset.

Appropriate atraumatic microvascular sutures are also essential. The range produced by Ethicon Laboratories is excellent.

GENERAL PRINCIPLES

Practice

The key to trouble-free microsurgery, in particular when starting, is, as with all other branches of surgery, practice. It is most valuable to have access to a microsurgical laboratory where the basic manipulative skills of handling and placing the needle and tying knots can be mastered. Unfortunately, there is no substitute for live animal work in learning the technique of microvascular anastomosis as this is necessary to assess patency, the hallmark of accurate atraumatic microvascular surgery.

Vascular Anastomosis

The keys to trouble-free microvascular anastomosis are planning, preparation and atraumatic technique.

The vessels to be anastomosed must be brought into apposition with no undue tension. Acceptable tension is always difficult to define. In this context it is safe to pull two vessel ends together if they can be held securely by a single 10/0 suture. If this is not the case then autogenous vein grafts should be used. The anastomosis should be performed in a position where it can be viewed clearly and the surgeon has comfortable access. Absolute local haemostasis is essential as only small amounts of blood will completely obscure the field. The appropriate use of tourniquets is invaluable.

The vessels must be meticulously cleared of soft tissue and mobilized so that they may be secured and controlled by vascular clamps. The inability to hold a vessel in a clamp is rarely due to the clamp pressure being inadequate, more usually either the vessel is not clean enough or the tension on the vessel too great. Once the vessels are set up then the ends should be freshened to remove any damaged tissue and adherent platelet thrombus. The lumina should be irrigated free of blood and thrombus with heparinized Hartmann's solution which should also be used to keep the operation site moist throughout the procedure. Saline is not used as it causes intimal necrosis. This is the only anticoagulation necessary as static blood does not clot in normal vessels during the time scale of surgical operations. If the vessels already have ulcerated intima, which is rare at this level even in the presence of marked atheroma, then the microvascular anastomosis is doomed to failure. Generalized anticoagulation is unhelpful. All irrigating solutions should, however, be warmed to body temperature as cold is a very potent vasospastic agent. Arrangements for delivering such warmed solutions should be a routine.

Once the vessels have been trimmed and washed then a further trimming of the adventitia under high magnification is carried out. This should be done sufficiently to ensure that no stray fronds of connective tissue are able to be trapped in the lumen during suturing as they will cause thrombosis. Too much adventitial stripping, however, will render the vessel impossible to grasp without causing damage. The vessels may now be manually dilated with an appropriate instrument. This serves two functions, first, it renders the lumen more visible as the manipulation thus far described will have caused vasospasm. Secondly, this stretching paralyses the circular muscle fibres of the media for some hours, aiding patency. It must not be overdone as the intimal damage so caused can itself lead to thrombosis.

The vessel ends can now be apposed with the clamp approximator and sutured. It cannot be stressed enough that atraumatic technique is essential. Stretching longitudinally, closing forceps across or touching the lumen of a vessel causes intimal necrosis which invites anastomotic failure. A vessel should only ever be picked up by its adventitia and never have its wall grasped directly.

To achieve this end where all movements are controlled and purposive the surgeon must work from a stable base. He should be comfortably seated if this is at all possible. His arms and hands must be firmly supported from elbow to palm so that inappropriate movements and tremor can be avoided. Inexperienced microsurgeons will frequently cut corners here and in fact lengthen the procedure by the difficulties they create.

Suture Technique

The sutures used commonly are 9, 10 and 11/0 monofilament nylon. Half-circle atraumatic needles are used and range from 50 to 130 μm in diameter (*Fig.* 58.5). All tying is done with forceps and this in itself requires some practice. The sutures are traditionally interrupted as it is suture placement that is critical and time-consuming and not knot tying. Continuous sutures may cause stenosis in such flimsy tissues. The sutures should be placed evenly around the anastomosis taking equal bites of each vessel. They should not be tied too tightly. Thus distortion of the anastomosis is minimized. The precise number and tension of the sutures depends on such factors as vessel wall thickness and discrepancy in luminal size, it can only be learned by experience. The aim should be to appose smoothly the intimal surfaces with no gaps but with the minimum number of sutures and distortion.

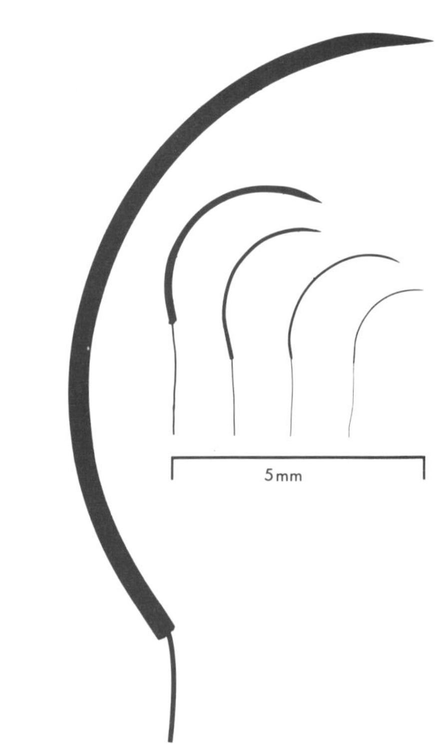

Fig. 58.5 Microsurgical needles and sutures. *Left to right*, standard 6/0, 9/0–130 needle, 10/0–75 needle, 11/0–50 needle and 12/0–30 needle.)

End-to-end Anastomosis

Initially it is best to use some variation of the triangulation technique described by Carrel and applied to microsurgery by Cobbet (*Fig.* 58.6). This reduces handling of the vessel and reduces the chance of picking up both front and back wall in the same stitch. The stay stitches may be held by an assistant or fixed to a 'cleat' on a specially modified clamp (*see Fig.* 58.4). More experienced surgeons tend to develop a more 'free hand' approach but this requires considerable practice.

The end-to-end is probably the easiest method of anastomosis but has two disadvantages. First, spasm at the site of anastomosis will cause occlusion and thrombosis, and must be avoided. A topical agent to overcome local vascular spasm engendered by handling the vessels will be helpful. Verapamil (Cordilox) in its injectable form is probably the most

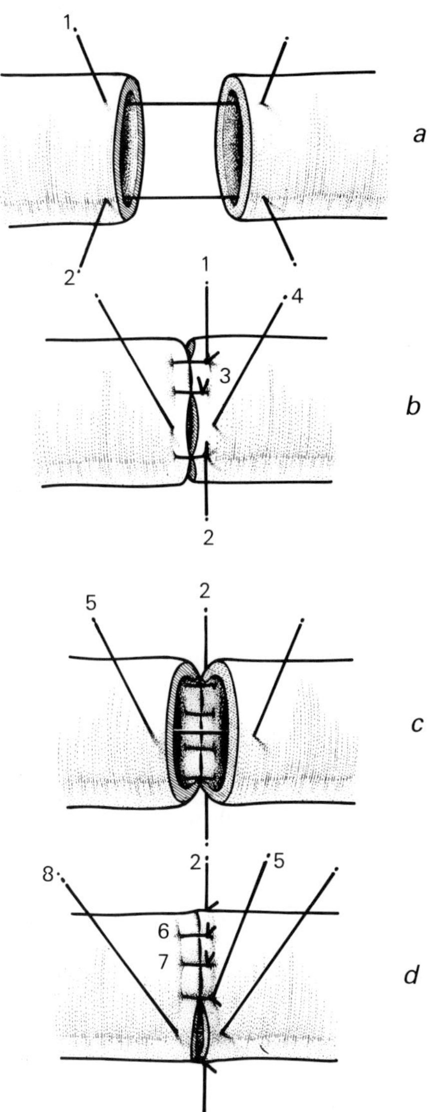

Fig. 58.6 Diagram of end-to-end anastomosis. *a*, First stay suture 1 is placed and tied, followed by 2. They are placed 120° apart on the front wall. *b*, With stays 1 and 2 held the vessel between is sutured appropriately. The anastomosis is then flipped over. *c*, The suturing is examined from the reverse side and a further stay suture is placed bisecting the back wall (5). *d*, By holding the third stay (5), it is possible to suture the gaps either side with no fear of catching the far wall. Thus the anastomosis is completed (8→).

potent substance freely available. Secondly, it requires some judgement and experience to cope with vessels of markedly different diameters.

End-to-side Anastomosis

This technique is used where a 'new branch' is to be added to a vascular tree. It is particularly useful in such procedures as free flaps (q.v.) or bypass procedures such as the intra–extracranial arterial anastomosis for cerebral ischaemia.

The arteriotomy is made transversely and as with retraction the hole produced is almost circular. There is no need to spatulate the end of the vessel to be anastomosed as the magnification allows the surgeon to see the lumen: he does not need to make it artificially bigger. The suture technique

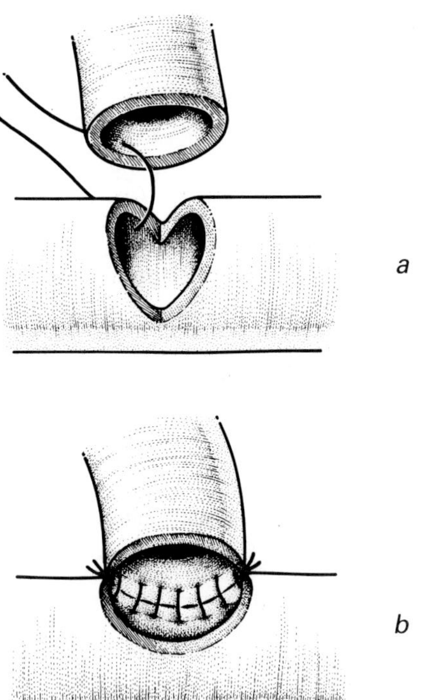

Fig. 58.7 Diagram of end-to-side anastomosis. *a*, A transverse arteriotomy is made to match the vessel to be anastomosed. The first suture is placed in the back wall (1) and then sutures are placed either side of it alternately. *b*, When the back wall is completed it is examined and the alternate suturing is continued to complete the front half. A stay suture bisecting the front wall may be used if helpful.

(*Fig.* 58.7) is a little more difficult than with end-to-end anastomosis as the inability to turn the vessels over preclude the use of triangulation as such.

There are three advantages of the technique. Vascular spasm tends to open rather than close the anastomosis; there is an analogy to the side hole in a vessel that will not stop bleeding. Next, disparity in vessel size is not a problem as one has merely to adjust the arteriotomy to match. Lastly, most importantly, this method allows the surgeon to use an important vascular pedicle without sacrificing its own function.

Nerve Repair

The aim of nerve repair is to join the nerve ends such that each proximal axon is apposed to a distal axon of the same type, i.e. motor or sensory. This is very difficult to achieve, particularly in a mixed nerve where axons of different types are mixed in each individual fascicle.

When one examines the cross-sectional morphology of a nerve (*Fig.* 58.8) it can be seen that suturing the epineurial surface alone is unlikely to ensure that each fascicle is accurately approximated to a fascicle in the distal part of the nerve, let alone the distal part of itself. Macroscopic nerve repair is a simple epineurial repair.

Microsurgeons believe that by examining the cut ends of the nerve it is possible to orientate the two surfaces accurately. The rotational orientation is the source of most discrepancy but this can be assured by examination and matching of the fascicular patterns visible on each of the cut ends. The first stitch is placed in the edge of a fascicle that can

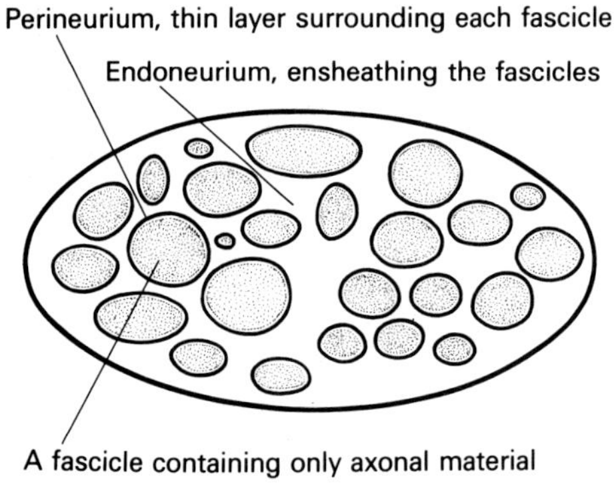

Perineurium, thin layer surrounding each fascicle

Endoneurium, ensheathing the fascicles

A fascicle containing only axonal material

Fig. 58.8 A schematic diagram of a large nerve in cross-section.

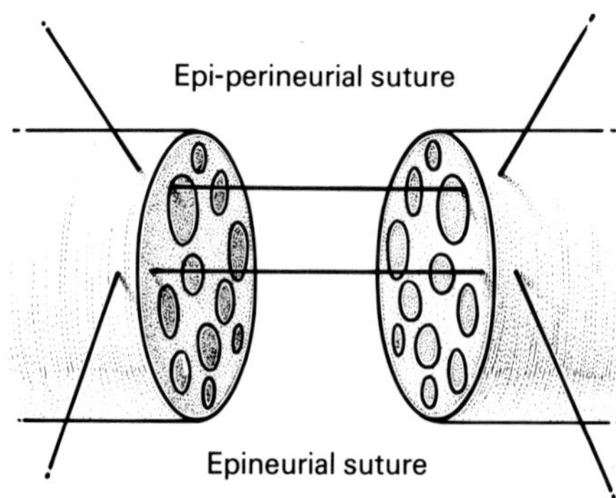

Fig. 58.9 Diagram of epineurial and epi–perineurial sutures. The epi–perineurial suture can ensure accurate rotation of the repair and matching of the fascicles.

be clearly identified on both surfaces as having been one fascicle. With careful suturing the rest should fall into place.

The accurate apposition of neural tissue alone is attempted by using epi–perineurial stitches (*Fig.* 58.9). These sutures pass through the epineurial connective tissue and include the very thin perineurium which surrounds each bundle of axons themselves. Enough of these sutures are placed to ensure apposition of the nerve without prolapsing axonal material.

CLINICAL APPLICATIONS

Broadly speaking, reconstructive microsurgery is used in three clinical settings:

Peripheral neurosurgery
Trauma—replantation and revascularization
Free flap transfer.

PERIPHERAL NEUROSURGERY

The evidence that nerves should be repaired primarily is now overwhelming. They should be repaired at the time the wound is closed. If delayed repair is employed then scarring and retraction of the cut ends will leave a gap which will require nerve grafting. The results of nerve grafts are never as good as those of primary repair.

Nerve repair should not compromise wound management. Untidy injuries must be converted into tidy injuries by wound excision. If such excision denudes a damaged nerve then it should still be repaired but protected by flap cover. Nerve repairs do badly under skin grafts as they are prone to develop painful neuromas.

If the excision includes an important nerve then primary nerve grafting may be carried out where feasible.

Performing elective nerve grafting microscopically has the advantage that the neuroma resection can be examined accurately and confirmed as complete. The grafts are then placed using epi–perineurial stitches so that they overlie accurately the cut fascicles and not the swollen and hypertrophic epineurium adjacent to the neuroma.

All nerve repairs should be splinted in a position that reduces tension on the repair for a minimum of three weeks.

Unfortunately, there is no firm evidence that micronerve repair leads to better recovery than macronerve repair. The confirmed microsurgeons believe this is because there are no accurate ways of assessing nerve recovery after such repairs.

REPLANTATION SURGERY

The initial thrust of microvascular research was aimed at replantation of traumatically amputated parts. Replantation is defined as the replacement and revascularization of a totally amputated part. Revascularization is the successful restoration of circulation to a subtotally amputated part.

Transport

In Great Britain, at least, these injuries appear to be rare. The performance of this specialized surgery is centralized in units with sufficient expertise and experience to achieve justifiable results.

The patient and the part need to be transferred to the replant centre. The patient, therefore, needs to be completely resuscitated and stable. This is rarely a problem as it only really applies to major amputations. The part requires more attention. Four hours of warm ischaemia leads to patchy failure of the microcirculation after re-establishment of vascular continuity. The amputated part should therefore be cooled to 4 °C by being placed dry in a polythene bag and the bag immersed in a mixture of ice and water. It is thus kept cool but does not get macerated. Freezing will lead to post-revascularization 'frostbite'.

Indications

Deciding whether to proceed with a potential replantation is difficult. The indications are multifactorial and contentious. They include the following considerations and each patient should be assessed on his individual merits.

The Patient

He must be fit for the procedure and well motivated. The rehabilitation is long and arduous. Total time away from work will be many times greater than for a simple amputation if the injury itself does not preclude return to work. Intelligent patients do much better than those who are less able to understand the difficulties and aims of therapy. The young do best of all. Nerve recovery and recovery from joint stiffness are so poor in the elderly that it is virtually pointless to consider a patient older than 60–65 years for replantation.

Pattern of Injury

When assessing a candidate for replant surgery the surgeon must consider the function attainable with and without the

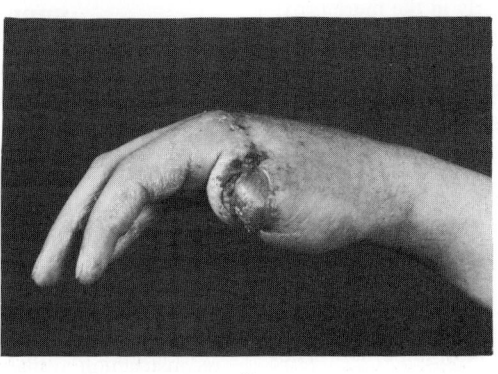

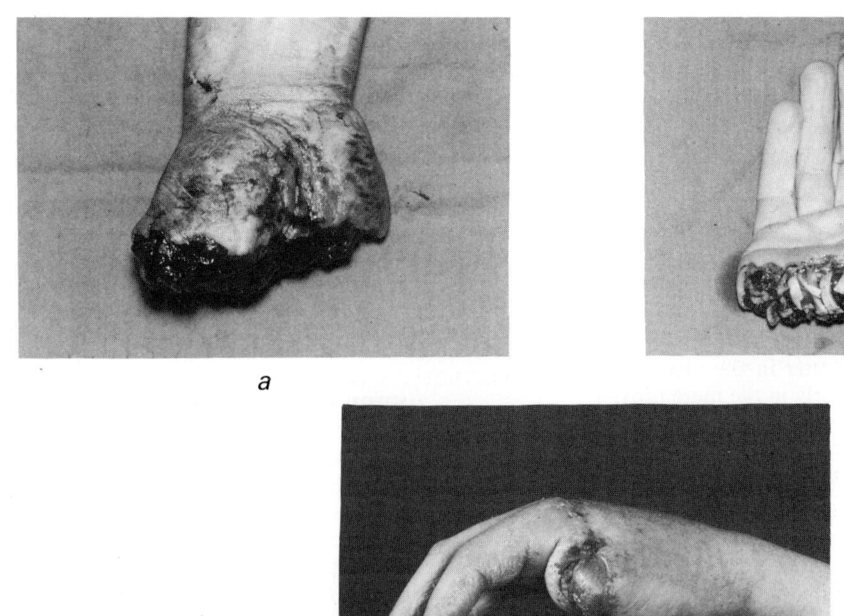

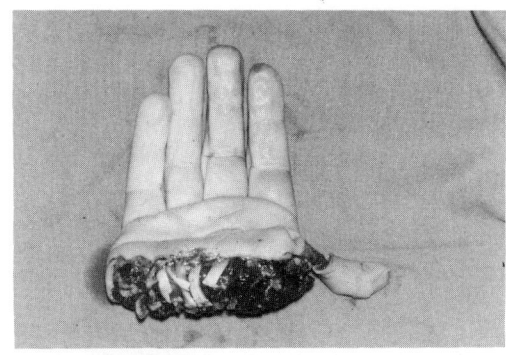

Fig. 58.10 *a*, A midpalm amputation by band saw. All hand function lost. *b*, The part—the thumb was destroyed by the machine. *c*, Two weeks following replantation. The thumb will eventually be replaced by free flap transfer of a toe.

amputated parts, bearing in mind the use of other reconstructive procedures or prostheses. That is why replantation is almost completely confined to the upper limb. Lower limb prostheses can produce functional results better than replantation.

If all the fingers or the thumb are lost the resulting hand function is poor and the indications for reimplantation are strong (*Fig.* 58.10). A single finger amputation, particularly at the border of the hand, results in little disability and a replanted finger which is stiff, insensitive and painful would not represent a therapeutic triumph.

In general, isolated thumb amputation or loss of the major part of the hand are the strongest indications for reimplant surgery.

Mechanism of Injury

Clean cutting guillotine-like injuries are the most favourable. Crush injuries may be considered if the zone of injury is narrow. Extensive crushing of the amputated part is a contraindication. Avulsion is not a contraindication in itself but the success rates are low due to unseen damage to the vascular tree, caused by stretching, long distances from the apparent site of trauma. Contamination with dirt and bacteria are not a problem as wound excision and antibiosis will overcome these problems in the successful replant.

Technique

In replantation surgery it is customary to carry out primary repair of all structures in an attempt to achieve rapid primary healing and early mobilization of the part.

The general procedure is arranged in four phases.

Preparation

The part may be examined before the patient is anaesthetized if the amount of damage it has received is uncertain. The patient may then be anaesthetized while the part is prepared. All the structures to be repaired are identified and marked while all damaged and doubtful tissue is ruthlessly excised. The vessels being used are trimmed under microscopic control as it is pointless to try to work with vessels that are in any way damaged. Considerable bone excision is usual as this can make the soft-tissue gap caused by the zone of trauma disappear. The part when prepared should be returned to the refrigerator.

The stump is prepared under tourniquet. The same sort of wound excision is performed and microvascular clamps applied to the open arteries.

The precise pattern of bone fixation and revascularization should be finalized at this stage. In multiple digit replants the order of digits to be attempted should be considered as well as which digit should be replaced on which stump. The first digit replanted is most likely to be successful so the best digit should be placed on the most appropriate stump to produce the greatest improvement in hand function. The replants should proceed in order of diminishing importance. It is not necessary to replace each finger on its original stump. Final overall hand function should be the major concern not anatomical correctness.

Musculoskeletal Stability

The bone fixation should be performed first. Rigid internal fixation is the rule. The precise technique depends on the injury and the surgeon but it must be quick, effective and not involve wide soft-tissue dissection. Adequate bone shortening must be stressed. This may allow all the soft-tissue structures to be brought together without tension after wound excision. If this is possible then the operation becomes an order of magnitude easier and therefore more likely to be successful. Damaged joints will be stiff post-operatively. They should either be arthrodesed electively or primary joint replacement performed.

Next the tendons or muscles should be repaired. Flexor tendons in 'no man's land' may be replaced by silicone rods with a view to interval tendon grafts.

If possible, the nerves should be repaired at this point. This may have to be delayed until later in the procedure because of pressure of time, particularly in the more proximal injury. It must be remembered, however, that the swelling and bleeding caused by successful revascularization may make previously easy nerve repairs difficult or impossible.

Revascularization

The arterial side should be repaired first. If necessary, vein grafts of suitable size are used to bridge any gaps or avoid tension. If vein grafts are clearly going to be needed then they can be preattached to the part during the preparation stage.

When arterialization is successful the veins of the part will fill, aiding selection of the largest and most important. They may then be repaired with or without interposition vein grafting as necessary. It is usual to repair two veins for every artery that has been anastomosed as they suffer thrombosis more frequently.

Skin Cover

The skin is closed directly. This is often feasible because of the bone shortening. Free split-skin grafts should be used if there is any doubt about viability of the skin or any suggestion of tension. Skin grafts will take perfectly on a microvascular repair.

Aftercare

The limb should be dressed in a soft, bulky dressing that allows easy observation of the part. It should be elevated. The patient must be kept warm and good analgesia provided. It may be helpful to give aspirin 75 mg/day to reduce platelet function.

The replanted part needs close observation. Anastomotic failure is not uncommon and it is certainly worthwhile to re-explore failures, if recognized early, as successful restoration of blood supply is to be expected in about half such cases.

Passive motion can be commenced on day 5 postoperatively and active motion as soon as the pattern of tendon and bone surgery will allow. If meaningful function is to be attained great attention must be paid to postoperative physiotherapy and occupational therapy. A successful replant signals the start of a 1–2 year effort on behalf of the patient, surgeon and therapists to make the initial operation justified.

Results

In the major centres success rates of over 80% are being reported for clean-cut injuries. These fall to 50–60% for severe crushing injuries. The key to high success rates is, as with other types of surgery, large numbers of patients and good patient selection. There is no real place for the occasional replant surgeon.

The individual long-term results depend very much on the original indications for the procedure. Stiffness, pain, cold intolerance and poor neurological recovery are usual sequelae. They are commoner in older patients, more proximal injuries and the more untidy injuries. Time, support and physiotherapy seem the only solutions. However, very few patients will allow a replanted part to be amputated later no matter how unsatisfactory the result appears to the surgeon.

FREE FLAP TRANSFERS

Background

Free flap transfers have become a routine part of reconstructive surgery in the last 5–10 years. As the technique has become established, the scope and power of reconstructive surgery has been extended significantly.

A flap, in plastic surgical terms, is a composite block of tissue which is moved from one site to another such that its blood supply remains intact. It is obvious that if no vascular surgery is to be performed then the donor site and defect must either be adjacent, or made so by bodily contortion and splinting. This places clear limitations on the choices of reconstruction available for a given defect. Historically the problem of distant transfer was overcome by bridging the gap with long strips of tissue containing a blood supply and formed into tubes. Many stages were required to achieve such a transfer. This led to multiple surgical procedures, entailing long hospitalization, the outcome of which was very unpredictable. It is now clear that the tube pedicle was a blind alley in the development of plastic surgery.

A free flap is a flap which has its blood supply divided and re-established during its transfer by microvascular surgery (*Fig.* 58.11). The technique frees the surgeon from many of the design constraints which previously existed, thus making available a host of reconstructive choices not hitherto possible.

As well as reliable microsurgical anastomosis much applied anatomical information was needed before free flap transfers could be developed. The knowledge that a single artery and vein might supply a specific predetermined area of skin constantly is an essential prerequisite of the donor site. McGregor and Jackson introduced the axial pattern flap and described the groin flap in 1972 and this shortly became the source of the first free skin flap. Since that time much research in applied anatomy has yielded a whole host of potential donor sites many of which are in common use.

Initially free-flap surgery had a reputation for being difficult, time consuming and unreliable. Nowadays, with improved donor sites yielding larger blood vessels in the pedicle and wider clinical experience these transfers have become routine and reliable.

Indications

The only absolute indication to use a free flap occurs when a defect defies predictable reconstruction by any other means. Such problems are rare but defects of the vertex of the scalp or lower third of the leg may fall into this group.

More usually a free flap is chosen because it is clearly advantageous to the patient. These indications are relative and may be grouped as follows.

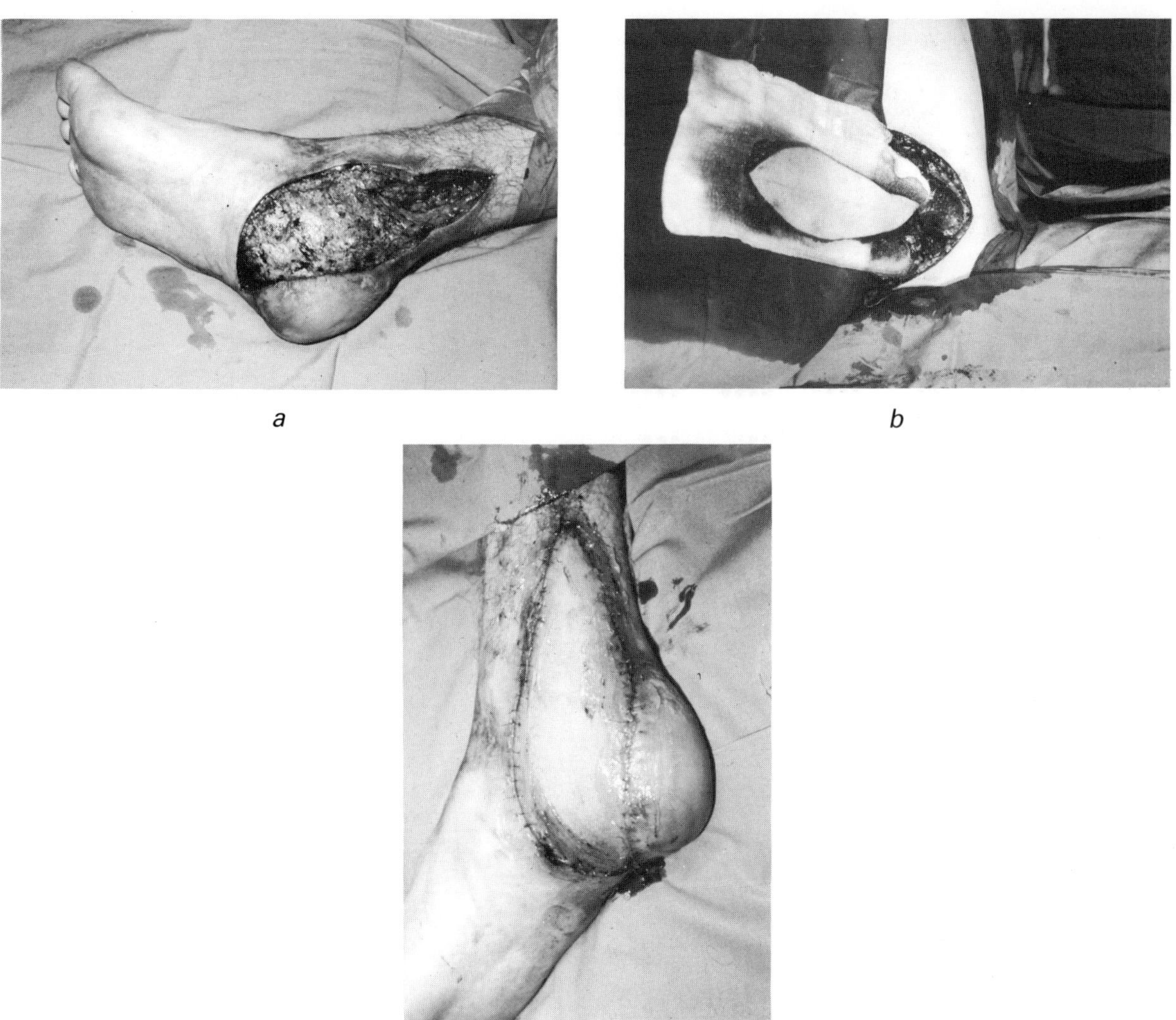

Fig. 58.11 *a*, The defect created by the excision of unstable scar from an old injury. *b*, The transverse scapular flap raised from the back. *c*, The flap after transfer, revascularization and inset.

One-stage Reconstruction

These flaps by their very nature achieve the desired result in one stage. This shortens hospital stay dramatically and avoids the multiple operations of staged procedures. The rapid time to healing and robust nature of flap allow radical surgery and radiotherapy to be used in combination. This has led to reports of improved survival in carcinoma of the oral cavity. With shorter operating times it is now feasible to consider a free flap in the acute phase of a traumatic problem as the method producing most rapid healing to allow early rehabilitation.

More Appropriate Reconstruction

When the flap closure of a major defect is being considered the surgeon, naturally enough, thinks of the surface to be covered first. This is usually in terms of matching skin quality and area. The volume of the defect must also be considered as many flaps are bulky when raised safely. This bulk can be troublesome and require thinning operations. A free flap, with the range of donor sites now available, may more nearly satisfy the requirements of a given defect and produce better functional and cosmetic results. A good example of this is the radial forearm flap in intraoral reconstruction.

The morbidity of the donor site is an important consideration and an appropriate choice of flap may make the whole operation more acceptable to the patient.

Availability of Specialized Tissues

Anatomical research into the blood supply of potential donor sites has produced a mass of information about the vascularity of a wide variety of tissues (*Table* 58.1). It is now possible to use vascularized reinnervated muscle to replace that whose action has been lost due to trauma or surgery such as in the reanimation of the paralysed face. Bone may be provided, with or without skin, so that bony defects in hostile fields may be reconstructed with some initial stability and earlier progression to bony union. The potential donor sites for bone include the pelvis, rib, radius and fibula so

Table 58.1 The 'Which' guide to free flaps. The more blobs the better, bigger, easier etc.

Flap	*Pedicle size*	*Pedicle length*	*Easy to raise*	*Skin*	*Muscle*	*Bone*	*Fascia*	*Mucosa*	*Sensation*	*Thin and flexible*	*Bulk filler*	*Donor morbidity*
Groin	•	•	•	•••	—	—	—	—	—	••	••	••••
DCIA	•••	••	••	•	•	•••	—	—	—	—	•••	••
Latissimus dorsi	•••	•••	•••	••••	••••	—	—	—	—	•	••••	•••
Serratus ınterior	•••	•••	••	••	••	••	—	—	—	—	•••	••
Scapular	••	••	••••	•••	—	—	••	—	—	••	••	••••
Intercostal	••	•	•	••	•	••	—	—	•	•	•	••
Pectoralis minor	••	•	•	—	••	—	—	—	—	•	•	••••
Rectus abdominis	•••	•••	••••	••••	••••	—	—	—	—	•	••••	•••
Gracilis	••	••	•••	••	•••	—	—	—	•	•	•••	••••
T-fascia lata	••	•	••	•••	••	—	—	—	•	•	••	••
Superior gluteal	•••	•	•	•••	•••	—	—	—	—	—	••••	•
Deltoid	•	•	•	•••	—	—	••	—	•	••	••	•
Lateral arm	••	••	•••	•••	•	••	•••	—	•	••	•	•••
Radial forearm	••••	••••	••••	•••	—	••	•••	—	•	•••	•	•••
Ulnar forearm	••••	••••	••••	•••	—	••	•••	—	•	•••	•	•••
Fibula	••••	••	••	•	—	•••	—	—	—	—	•	•
Dorsalis pedis	••••	•••	••	••	—	••	—	—	••••	•••	•	••
Temporal fascia	••	••	••	—	—	•	•••	—	—	••••	—	••••
Omentum	••••	••••	••••	–	–	–	–	–	••	••••	••••	
Jejunum	•••	••	••••	–	–	–	–	••••	–	–	–	•••

again the flap chosen can be matched to the problem presenting. The jejunum can be used as logical replacement of the hypopharynx after total pharyngolaryngectomy and decreases problems with dysphagia and stricture. One or more digits can be provided for the hand using toes on the dorsalis pedis arterial system.

Vascularity

Because of its design a free flap introduces a new axial blood supply into the region in which it is inset. This is an important consideration when the defect could be said to be 'hostile' in terms of its local blood supply and, therefore, its healing potential. A well vascularized distant flap may well heal where a local flap will fail. The powerful reconstructions available allow the generous excision of all doubtful tissue, avoiding the embarrassing situation of further local necrosis around the defect after reconstruction.

Technique

A free flap transfer is a major operative procedure only to be undertaken by those adequately trained in the technique. Once the techniques of microvascular anastomosis have been mastered then the operation becomes a straightforward organizational exercise like any other major procedure. Perhaps more so than with any other procedure in plastic surgery the ultimate success or failure depends on the smooth administration of the operation in the widest sense. Certain aspects of a free flap transfer bear further discussion as they are those which often lead to difficulties which have a habit of compounding themselves during the operation. As always, problems are far better avoided than dealt with.

Patient Preparation

It is important that specific and clear explanations be given to the patient as the aims and consequences of this type of surgery are not immediately apparent to the layman. The operation sites will be visible and painful and unexpected donor sites for flaps or vein grafts distant from the site of the original problem will cause anxiety.

Smokers must accept that they should stop completely for at least a month postoperatively as a single cigarette may produce small vessel spasm fatal to the flap.

Elective patients should be in the best possible condition for the surgery. They should be adequately nourished and have any local infection as controlled as is practical. Local oedema may lead to technical problems operatively and this should be controlled by hospitalization, elevation and intermittent compression devices.

Anaesthesia

Recent developments in anaesthesia for microvascular surgery have probably contributed as much as any surgical advance to the improved reliability of these transfers. Hypovolaemia, pain, low core and skin temperatures and low arterial $P\text{CO}_2$ values will all produce a low flow state in the flap, particularly one which is sympathetically denervated by its transfer. A low flow state through a fresh vascular anastomosis is likely to lead to thrombosis. By avoiding all these events and rendering the patient's circulation hyperdynamic the anaesthetist will be contributing as much to a successful outcome as the surgeon with painstaking technique. Some authorities also believe it is valuable to lower the blood viscosity by haemodilution. This can lead to unrecognized hypovolaemia postoperatively as the haemodilution corrects itself.

Planning

Nowadays more flaps fail because of errors in conception and planning than because of pure microsurgical problems. The planning of a case should include the following considerations.

a. Patient Selection

Radiotherapy and advanced age are no longer contraindications to a free flap. However, patients with peripheral vascular disease, longstanding diabetes, severe hypertension and heavy smokers should be assessed carefully, particularly for transfers to the leg. Atheromatous vessels are more difficult to handle and the failure rate is probably higher.

b. Flap Selection

Apart from the actual nature of the reconstruction there are purely technical considerations contributing to the choice of flap. In general one should choose the appropriate flap with the largest vessels in the pedicle. The pedicle should be long enough to make revascularization straightforward; vein grafts may be used but are best avoided. If a flap with which the surgeon is familiar is suitable then he should use it. Flaps are like friends: one should have few and know them well.

c. The Recipient Vessels

These are the blood vessels onto which the flap is to be anastomosed. They will be near the defect being filled. They should be anatomically reliable, easily approachable and in such a position that the microsurgery can be performed easily and without tension. The vessels should be normal and outside, preferably proximal to, any zone of damage associated with the defect.

Arteriograms are rarely useful as a peripheral pulse provides ample indication that a pedicle is suitable.

d. Operative Position

The patient's position during the operation should be considered in conjunction with donor site and recipient vessel selection. Access to either should not be compromised so if it cannot be avoided the patient must be repositioned during the case. A change in donor site selection may avoid this.

Postoperative Care

It is fundamental that the patient be maintained in a condition which will ensure good perfusion of the flap. Emergence from anaesthesia should be gentle. Good hydration and analgesia are also a priority. The patient must also be kept warm. Allowing him to become peripherally cold because of ambient temperature, hypovolaemia or pain invites flap failure.

Dressings must not be allowed to compress the operation site or constrict a limb proximal to an anastomosis. These flaps are prone to swell considerably postoperation and the dressings must therefore be reviewed regularly.

Flap Monitoring

If a flap should suffer either arterial or venous insufficiency it may be salvaged if this is recognized early and the intervention is swift. Observation of the flap and its colour is the mainstay of flap monitoring. The provision of experienced staff round the clock can be difficult so electromechanical monitoring systems have been investigated. At present the photoplethysmograph and muscle twitch flap monitors appear most useful.

Whichever methods of flap observation are used constant vigilance in the first 48 h will be necessary as only rapid revision of the microsurgery will be helpful.

Flap Failure

In an unselected group of patients a microsurgical failure rate of about 5% is to be expected. These failures result in total flap loss as the flap is completely dependent upon the successful restoration of its blood supply. Partial flap loss due to poor design should be rare.

When such a failure occurs it is worthwhile leaving the flap in situ while desiccation and desloughing proceeds conservatively as the resulting defect may be more easily managed than prior to the transfer. It is not unusual to be left with a defect that will support a skin graft after this chain of events even though the original defect would not have.

Rehabilitation

After 5–7 days it is usually safe to mobilize and discharge the patient from hospital. They should, however, be protected from extreme cold and direct trauma to the site of the pedicle. Flaps on the lower limb are prone to swell when the patient assumes an erect posture again. This can safely be controlled by elastic compressive bandaging, and should not be allowed to delay the patient's progress.

The Future

Free flap transfer is a new technique that has moved from the experimental stage into the realms of the routine. Doubtless some new donor sites await description. More importantly, the indications for and applications of the technique will develop rapidly in the next few years. It is already clear that the modern plastic surgeon has available a reconstructive technique of such power and flexibility that it would make his predecessors envious.

Further Reading

Beimer E. (1981) Digital replantation. In: Jackson I. T. (ed.) *Recent Advances in Plastic Surgery—2*. Edinburgh, Churchill Livingstone.

Harii K. (1981) Free flap surgery. In: Jackson I. T. (ed.) *Recent Advances in Plastic Surgery—2*. Edinburgh, Churchill Livingstone.

Millesi H. (1979) Microsurgical repair of nerves. In: Grabb W. C. and Smith J. W. (ed.) *Plastic Surgery*, 3rd ed. Boston, Little Brown.

Webster M. C. H. and Soutar D. S. (1986) *A Practical Guide to Free Tissue Transfers*. London, Butterworths.

Section 8

General Surgery

59 *Surgical Management of the Neonate*

N. V. Freeman

Paediatric surgery is a relatively young branch of general surgery. The term 'neonate' is reserved for the first 28 days after birth. Neonatal surgery is, therefore, a highly specialized branch of paediatric surgery, which in the main deals with congenital anomalies. About 14% of newborns have a single minor malformation, 3% have a single major malformation and 0·7% of newborns have multiple major malformations.

The work load of a neonatal unit is dependent on the birth rate as anomalies are fairly constant in incidence (*Table* 59.1). The table shows some interesting trends, mainly due to the recent development of screening pregnancies. Note the fall in incidence in anencephaly, spina bifida and Down's syndrome, the apparent fall in Down's syndrome in 1976 and 1985 may be due to under-reporting due to late diagnosis, as most reports suggest that the incidence has remained constant at 1 per 700 live births.

In the UK and USA, the birth rate is similar, at 11 000 live births per million people, giving an annual number of births of approximately 630 000 and 2·3 million in each country. However, in countries like India and Kuwait the birth rate is 35 000–46 000 live births per million people.

The first neonatal surgical unit to be established was in Liverpool in 1953, following a survey in 1949, which showed that of 75 neonates born and treated in 14 different hospitals in one year, there was a 72% mortality, which was reduced to 24% by concentrating the expertise of the nurses, surgeons, anaesthetists, radiologists, etc.

A working knowledge of the various congenital anomalies occurring in the neonate is essential for all doctors, obstetricians, paediatricians and nurses dealing with the newborn. This is essential as the primary diagnosis is never made by the paediatric surgeon who relies on the astute observations of those dealing with the newborn to suspect, diagnose and refer the infant, for confirmation of the diagnosis and treatment.

Aetiology of Congenital Malformations

When the baby with a congenital abnormality is born the parents often blame themselves and ask the cause of such an anomaly. In most instances it is not possible to answer this question with certainty, but several known factors should be considered. The aetiology of major congenital malformations has been found to be: idiopathic (60%), multifactorial (20%), single gene (7·5%), chromosomal (6%), (note that 60% of spontaneous abortions have a chromosomal anomaly), maternal illness (3%), congenital infection (2%), and drugs, X-ray, alcohol (1·5%).

Genetic Factors

These can be classified as *Chromosomal* (in which there is a microscopically visible chromosome anomaly); *Single gene*—either autosomal dominant, autosomal recessive or x-linked; or *Multifactorial* (more than one gene contributing to susceptibility, usually with environmental factors also contributing). Surgical examples of multifactorial disorders are, cleft

Table 59.1 Incidence of congenital anomalies per 10 000 total births 1960–1985
(Liverpool and Bootle Survey, 1960–1966, and OPCS Monitor 1986)

	Liverpool 1960–1966	*England 1976*	*Wales 1985*
Congenital heart disease	63·8	11·3	13·2
Total CNS anomalies	69·8	32·5	11·0
Spina bifida	33·5	14·5	5·5
Cleft lips and palate	15·7	14·7	12·6
Tracheo-oesophageal atresia and fistula	3·3	1·8	1·9
Rectal and anal atresia and stenosis	4·0	3·1	3·0
Exomphalos and omphalocele	3·0	3·3	2·0
Down's syndrome	14·3	6·8	6·7
Anencephaly (and spina bifida)	31·4	10·9	0·9

lip and palate, pyloric stenosis, congenital heart disease and hydrocephalus. Single gene disorders include adult polycystic disease, haemophilia, cystic fibrosis, congenital spherocytosis and intestinal polyposis.

The known teratogenic agents are:

Infections—bacterial, viral or parasitic.
Physical—heat, radiation, or mechanical factors.
Drug and chemical—including environmental chemicals such as mercury.
Maternal, metabolic and genetic.

Maternal Infection

Maternal infection by protozoal, bacterial and viral infections cause significant birth defects. The risk in rubella is 50% if the illness occurs in the first month of pregnancy and decreases to 0% after 12 weeks.

Drugs

Any drug is potentially harmful during the first three months of pregnancy and this includes alcohol, antihistamines, antibiotics, thalidomide, anticonvulsants, hydantoin, warfarin, cytotoxic and endocrine preparations, especially hormone pregnancy tests which have been known to have harmful effects. The role of tobacco is not clear.

X-rays

X-rays in early pregnancy can cause congenital anomalies, hence the '10-day rule' which used to apply in X-ray departments, i.e. that no female from 12 to 50 years of age should have an abdominal or pelvic radiograph except within the 10 days after the first day of her last menstrual period.

Mechanical Factors

Abnormal pressure either intrinsic or extrinsic exerted on the developing fetus in utero may be responsible for such anomalies as talipes and pressure dimples, congenital dislocation of the hip, plagiocephaly, torticollis, mandibular asymmetry or amniotic bands causing amputation of the digits.

Maternal Health during Pregnancy

Abnormalities are seen with vitamin-deficient diets and with folic-acid deficiency during pregnancy. Women working in such places as operating theatres with poor venting of anaesthetic waste gases are shown to have a high incidence of infertility, spontaneous abortions and birth of infants with congenital malformations.

Intrauterine Vascular Accidents

A volvulus, intussusception or strangulation for instance, at the umbilical ring, occurring in utero, often late in pregnancy is responsible for most cases of the atresia and stenosis of the bowel, excluding oesophageal, duodenal and rectal atresia. The possible mechanism is shown in *Fig.* 59.1.

THE NEONATE—SPECIFIC METABOLIC PROBLEMS

The neonate is not a 'miniature adult'.

Temperature Control

Newborn infants, especially premature infants, have difficulty in maintaining body temperature, due to a relatively large surface area, little subcutaneous fat and inability to shiver. Heat production is via the sympatheticomimetic metabolism of brown fat. The ambient temperature of the room should be maintained at 27 °C (80 °F) in order to prevent heat loss which occurs when incubator doors are opened, or when the baby is handled for any procedure such as radiography or ultrasound examination, intravenous cannulation, or during the induction of anaesthesia. In the unanaesthetized patient, cooling leads to increased metabolism by raising oxygen requirements, whereas under anaesthesia hypothermia slows metabolism and lessens oxygen demand. With cooling there is an increased demand for oxygen at tissue and cellular level. The baby vasoconstricts peripherally to maintain core temperature. The reduced peripheral circulation leads to anaerobic metabolism and a

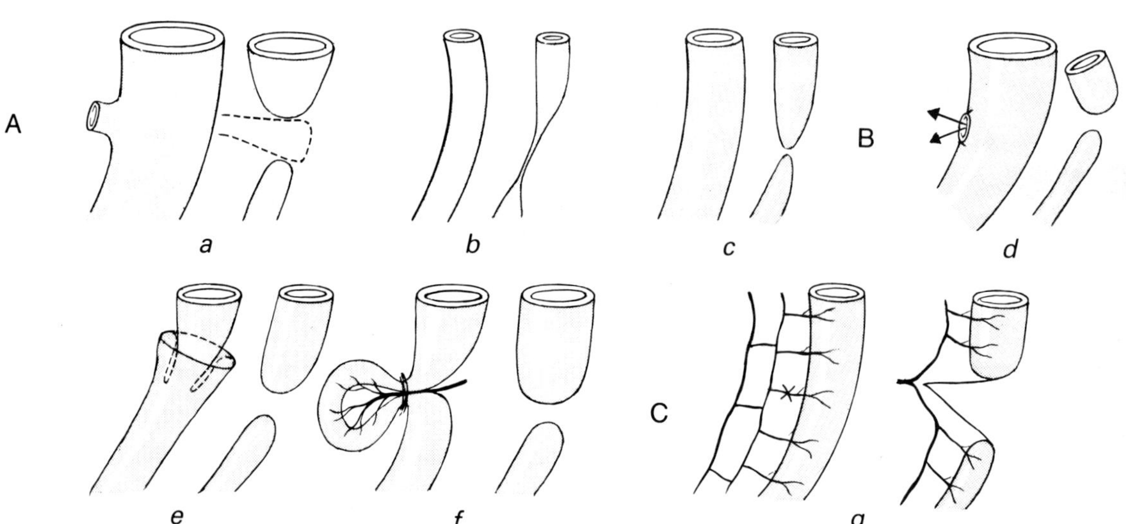

Fig. 59.1 Possible intrauterine causes of intestinal atresia. A, Embryological events: *a*, Excess reabsorption; *b*, Rapid elongation; *c*, Failure to recanalize. B, Vascular accidents: *d*, Perforation; *e*, Intussusception; *f*, Strangulation. C, Experimental: *g*, Ligation of mesenteric vessel.

build-up of acid waste products with systemic acidosis. A full-term healthy baby can respond to a brief exposure to cold by a three-fold increase in metabolic activity to maintain normal temperature. Metabolic activity is not basal as measured by the rectal temperature as this can be maintained with maximal heat production in the presence of peripheral shut down. The abdominal skin temperature should be 36·2 °C in a full-term infant and 36·5 °C in a premature infant. For minimal metabolic activity, the difference between abdominal wall and rectal temperature should be less than 1·5 °C. The temperature of the incubator should be adjusted for weight and age of the baby in order to maintain a 'neutral thermal environment' (*Fig.* 59.2).

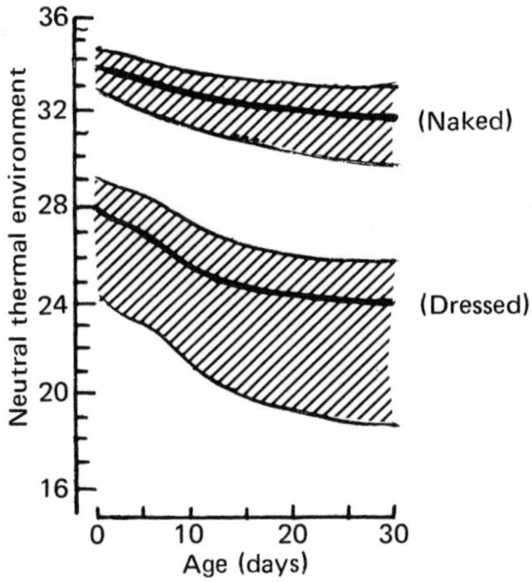

Fig. 59.2 Incubator temperature for a 2-kg baby, either naked or dressed.

Respiratory System

All medical personnel, and this includes nurses dealing with newborn babies, should be able to intubate and administer artificial ventilation. Resuscitation equipment should always be available and checked daily, to ensure working order and also to familiarize new staff.

The neonate has a reduced pulmonary reserve; is sensitive to hypoxia and acidosis; has a small calibre tracheobronchial tree which obstructs easily with thick secretions. In premature infants of 30–36 weeks' gestation there are frequent apnoeic episodes and hyaline membrane disease (respiratory distress syndrome) may aggravate the position.

The normal respiratory rate in the newborn may be up to 60/min. Note the effect of a small diaphragmatic hernia on the respiratory rate of a neonate (*Fig.* 59.3).

Cardiovascular System

The infant's cardiovascular system is unstable at birth and although the ductus arteriosus may close functionally soon after birth, any factor such as hypoxia, acidosis or increased pulmonary resistance may cause the duct to reopen and shunt the blood from right to left. The blood volume of the premature infant is 100 ml/kg reducing to 85 ml/kg body weight in the mature baby. The average haemoglobin is between 16 and 19 g/dl, with a haematocrit of 50–70%.

At operation, blood loss exceeding 10% of the blood volume needs to be replaced. In an average 3-kg baby the total blood volume is 225 ml (85×3) and losses exceeding 25 ml need replacing.

The vasomotor instability is marked by hypoxia, hypothermia and hypovolaemia with contraction of the peripheral and mesenteric circulations, depriving the tissues of oxygen to a point of actual cellular damage. A striking example of this is in the mucosal and bowel damage seen in neonatal necrotizing enterocolitis (NEC). Subsequent vasodilatation and increased permeability of the capillaries causes further loss of fluid into the tissues and further hypovolaemia. In the lungs, the capillary damage causes interstitial oedema, interfering with oxygen and carbon dioxide exchange producing hypoxia and acidosis. The normal pulse rate in a neonate is 120–160/min. Blood pressure is 70/40 mmHg in mature baby increasing to 90 mmHg systolic by the age of 3 months.

Hypoglycaemia

Definition: Less than 1·4 mmol/l (30 mEq) in full-term infants. Less than 1·1 mmol/l (20 mEq) in premature babies.

Neonatal hypoglycaemia is common, especially in preterm and 'small for dates' babies. In unrecognized or untreated hypoglycaemia, it is thought that irreversible brain damage may occur. As term approaches increasing amounts of glycogen are stored in the liver and heart muscle. At birth

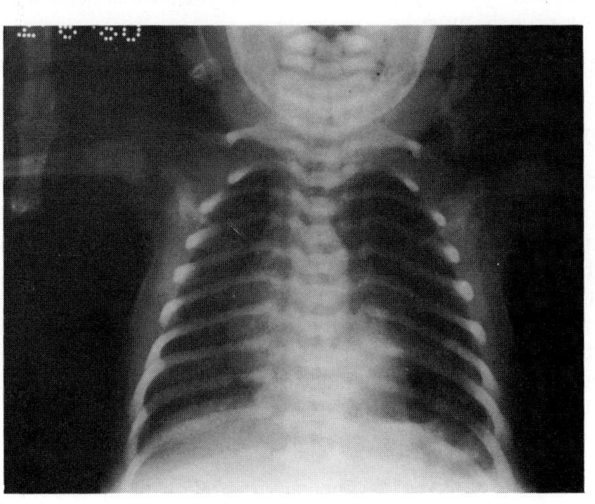

a

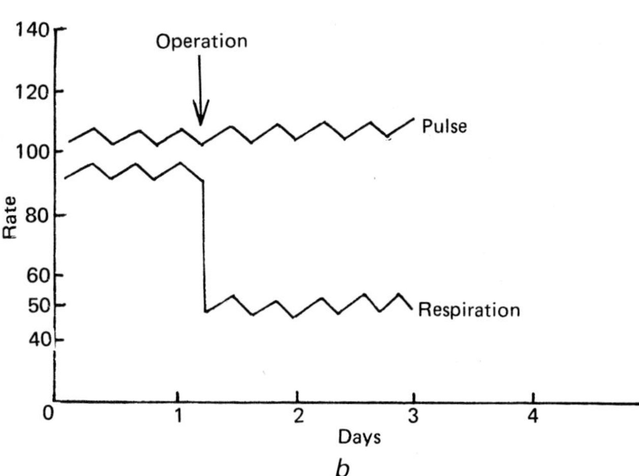

b

Fig. 59.3 *a*, Radiograph showing a small left diaphragmatic hernia; *b*, Dramatic effect of repair on the respiratory rate.

glycogenolysis occurs, depleting the glycogen stores in a few hours. As the glycogen store of energy is depleted, gluconeogenesis becomes the most important mechanism for maintaining blood sugar levels. Hypoglycaemia may also be caused by high circulating insulin levels and is seen in babies of diabetic mothers.

The symptoms of hypoglycaemia are non-specific, such as fits, jitteriness, cyanosis, apnoea, lethargy and hypotonia. All babies at risk are monitored 4-hourly by Dextrostix (Ames) estimations, from heel-prick blood.

Hypoglycaemia may be prevented at birth by an intravenous infusion of 10% dextrose infused at a rate of 2 ml 10%/kg over 1 min then 8 mg/kg/min while awaiting surgery. In symptomatic hypoglycaemia treatment with 1–2 ml/kg of 15% dextrose is indicated. This dose must not be exceeded, or given rapidly, due to the high osmolality and risk of pulmonary oedema and intraventricular haemorrhage. Intravenous infusions must be gradually reduced or rebound hypoglycaemia will occur.

Hypocalcaemia

Definition: Less than 2·13 mmol/l.

Seventy-five per cent of calcium transport across the placenta occurs after the 28th week of gestation. Full-term infants are born with calcium levels 0·25 mmol/l (1 mg/100 ml) higher than maternal levels due to placental transfer. These levels fall to about 2·3 mmol/l at 48 h. The pre-term infant produces inadequate amounts of parathormone in the first few days of life.

Administration of sodium bicarbonate decreases the ionized fraction of calcium, as does a blood transfusion using citrated blood. There are four main groups at risk: pre-term babies, infants of diabetic mothers, stressed infants, babies receiving bicarbonate or exchange transfusions.

The symptoms are similar to hypoglycaemia, namely jitteriness, twitching, fits (convulsions) and increased muscle tone. Treatment should be started on suspicion, after taking blood for analysis. While awaiting the result, infuse 10 ml of 10% calcium gluconate. This may be repeated as necessary, but is seldom required for more than 48 h. In asymptomatic cases oral calcium therapy is preferable, giving half a tablet of calcium lactate/gluconate containing 3·08 g per tablet, with four feeds per 24 h. Magnesium sulphate (0·2 ml/kg of 50% solution) by intramuscular injection on two occasions at 12-hourly intervals was found to be more effective in raising the levels of serum calcium because of the essential role of magnesium in neonatal calcium metabolism. Phenobarbitone, 7·5 mg 6-hourly, orally, may also raise the levels of serum calcium.

Hypomagnesaemia

Magnesium is the fourth most abundant cation in the body and plays a major role in cellular enzymatic activity, especially glycolysis. Sixty per cent of the magnesium is in bone, the rest, except for 1% is intracellular. Serum magnesium levels are maintained through renal regulation. Urinary excretion is increased by calcium loading. The symptoms of deficiency are increased neuromuscular irritability, tetany, severe seizures and jitteriness. Treatment is by magnesium sulphate 0·2 ml/kg of 50% solution by intramuscular injection.

Infection and Immunity

Overwhelming sepsis is one of the major causes of death in the newborn surgical patient. The diagnosis of sepsis can be quite difficult as signs and symptoms may be minimal. The temperature may be subnormal rather than elevated. Poor colour, poor feeding, abdominal distension and vomiting, bradycardia, apnoeic attacks and less activity suggest sepsis. An 'infection screen' should be carried out in all babies on suspicion. This consists of swabs of nose, throat, umbilicus and rectum, blood and urine cultures, resorting to a suprapubic aspiration if necessary. A lumbar puncture is indicated in most cases even without any signs of central nervous system involvement. A blood count, including platelets and a film, is also performed. A low platelet count and bizarre forms of red cells, such as helmet and burr cells, suggest disseminated intravascular coagulation (DIC).

The infant's immune defence mechanism appears to be deficient. Circulating B-lymphocytes and tissue plasma cells produce immunoglobulins. IgG crosses the placenta, the level is high at birth and IgG is primarily active against Gram-positive infections. IgM antibodies are effective against Gram-negative organisms, but the levels are low at birth. A high level suggests intrauterine infection with rubella, syphilis, etc. Secretory IgA and phagocytic cells are found in high concentrations in breast milk, and these may have a protective effect on the gastrointestinal tract and may prevent neonatal necrotizing enterocolitis. The cellular immune system consists of T-lymphocytes in the circulation, lymph nodes and spleen. This system is protective against viruses, fungi and protozoa and also against malignant cells. Most neonates do not appear to have a mature cellular immune system at birth. Phagocytosis is a complex process related to chemotaxis, opsonization, particle ingestion and bactericidal capacity, and all aspects are impaired in the newborn. Complement, in the globulin fraction, amplifies all the immune mechanisms; it is related to gestational age and reaches 50–60% of maternal levels at birth.

As both major defence mechanisms—cellular and humoral immunity—are immature and incompetent, prophylactic antibiotics are widely used.

As Gram-negative sepsis is the main concern to the surgeon, our current prophylactic regime uses gentamicin, penicillin and metronidazole.

Diagnosis of Congenital Anomalies

As stated previously, the diagnosis of a congenital abnormality is suspected or confirmed by the time the baby reaches the specialized neonatal unit.

In order to recognize the abnormal, the normal behaviour of a neonate must be appreciated.

Air in the Gut

Air enters the stomach with the first cry, reaches the caecum by 6 h and the rectum by about 24 h.

Passage of Urine

There is evidence of urinary secretion from the 14th week of intrauterine life. Urine is voided into the amniotic fluid from about 4 months of gestational age. An obstructive uropathy, such as posterior urethral valves, will cause gross hydroureters and hydronephrosis leading to renal failure soon after birth. This has led to the development of intrauterine decompression of the bladder or dilated renal pelvis, using ultrasound.

Passage of Meconium

During intrauterine life, the baby is swallowing up to 500 ml of amniotic fluid/24 h. Bile is secreted into the gut from 4 months of gestation. Meconium is the black, sticky, tarry material, consisting of squamous epithelial cells and hair swallowed together with mucus, bile and electrolytes, which accumulates in the colon and rectum and for reasons unknown is not passed until after birth in the normal full terms (40 weeks' gestation) baby. Delay in the passage of meconium for more than 24 h after birth is a significant observation and may suggest the diagnosis of an intestinal obstruction, such as Hirschsprung's disease.

Jaundice

So-called 'physiological jaundice' occurs in 70% of healthy newborn infants between the 2nd and 8th days after birth and is due to temporary inefficient hepatic excretion of bilirubin. The bilirubin is unconjugated and in the minority of premature infants may reach levels of 300 μmol/l at which level bile is deposited in the mid- and hind-brain (kernicterus) causing irreversible damage. Treatment is by increased fluid intake, phototherapy, phenobarbitone, and exposing the patient to artificial light, with a wavelength between 400 and 500 nm, or exchange blood transfusion.

Any degree of clinical jaundice in the first 24 h is pathological. Conjugated hyperbilirubinaemia in infancy is always pathological, arising from disorders of the hepatocyte or lesions of the biliary tree (*see* Chapter 69).

Radiology

A single, good quality plain radiograph of the abdomen in the erect and supine position, and a chest radiograph will establish the diagnosis in most cases. Occasionally injection of air or contrast medium into the stomach or rectum will be needed as supplementary procedures. More elaborate investigations including angiography, isotope scanning, etc. can be performed, but in most cases contribute little extra to the diagnosis or management of the patient.

Antenatal Ultrasound

All the known congenital defects have been diagnosed by ultrasound scan from 18 weeks of gestation. This has implications as half (69/139) the women in one series in the USA opted for termination of the pregnancy at 20 weeks regardless of the ultimate prognosis. The rapid increase in the number of babies being born with an antenatal diagnosis already established is shown in *Fig.* 59.4. Note especially the numbers of babies with dilated urinary tracts. These patients, who are completely asymptomatic, under previous circumstances may have reached adult life, prior to the diagnosis being made.

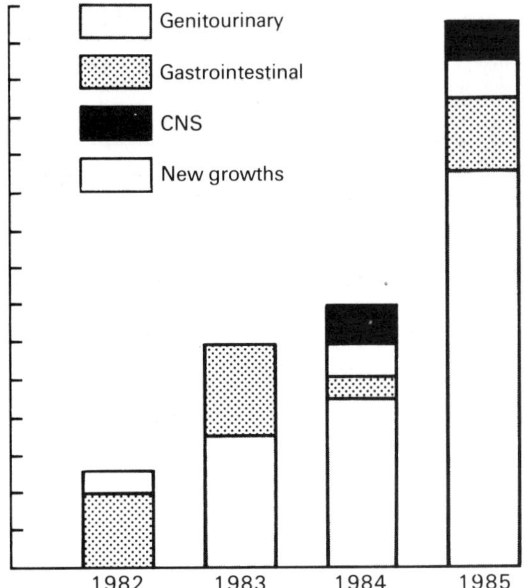

Fig. 59.4 Antenatal diagnoses, 1982–1985.

Ultrasonography

In the past 2–3 years this has become a most invaluable tool in the diagnosis and management of neonatal surgical conditions, actually changing the clinical management, e.g. in the management of neonatal hydrocephalus.

Fetal anomalies diagnosed before delivery will alert the attending doctors. Examples of the prenatal diagnosis of duodenal atresia and a choledochal cyst are shown in *Figs.* 59.5 and 59.6.

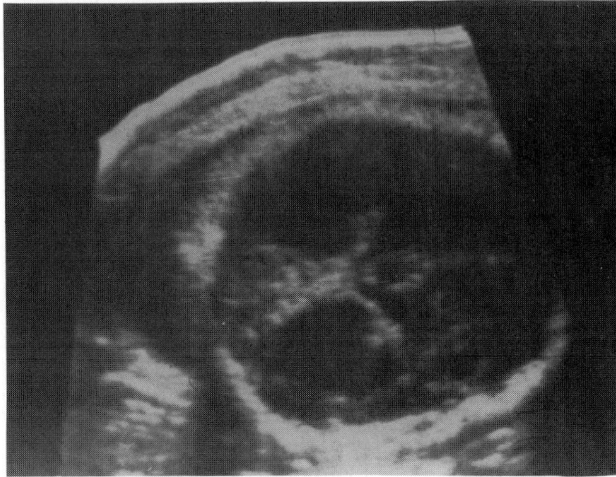

Fig. 59.5 Prenatal ultrasound scan showing a fluid level in the fetus, suggestive of duodenal atresia.

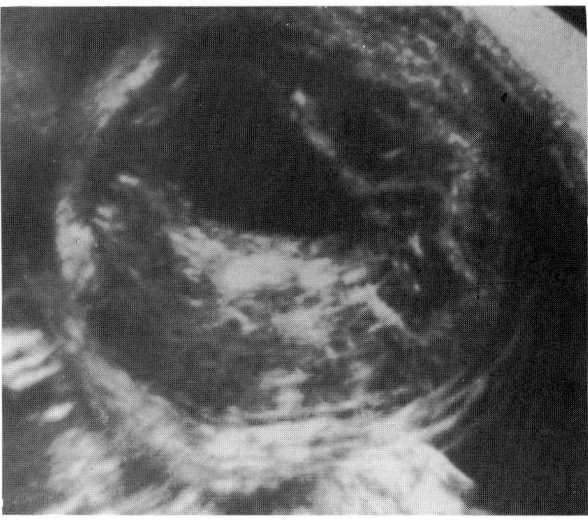

Fig. 59.6 Ultrasound scan showing choledochal cyst in the fetus at 36 weeks' gestation.

Rectal Washout

This should be regarded as an important diagnostic aid, especially in low large bowel obstruction. The washout should be performed by passing a No. 8 or 10 F Jacques catheter and syringing 10 ml normal saline gently and slowly into the rectum. The saline either leaks around the catheter or is aspirated back. The procedure can be repeated, using a total of 50–100 ml of saline. If any resistance or bleeding is noted, the procedure must be abandoned at once. In Hirschsprung's disease or the 'meconium plug syndrome' rectal washout is followed by a gush of sticky meconium and flatus, with dramatic decompression of the abdomen.

SURGICAL PROCEDURES ON NEONATES

Preoperative Preparation

Intravenous Therapy

A major difficulty in neonatal surgery is the withdrawal of blood samples and the administration of intravenous fluid and medication. Due to these conflicting interests the baby's skin overlying the antecubital fossae and feet soon looks like a pincushion!

Blood Withdrawal

In hospitals dealing with neonates the laboratories should be equipped with micromethods for biochemical estimations. This still involves the withdrawal of relatively large amounts of blood, e.g. 1·0 ml for electrolytes, 0·5 ml for bilirubin and 0·5 ml for haemoglobin estimation. The antecubital fossa is used for venepuncture, or the heel prick for capillary samples (up to 0·5 ml) and the radial artery cannulated for blood gas estimation.

Intravenous Infusion

The methods of venous access in adults (described in Chapter 6) are not usually applicable to neonates.

A 'butterfly' needle into one of the scalp veins and fixed with plaster-of-Paris is still one of the most popular methods. Various plastic i.v. cannulas (gauge 18–20) are suitable for placement in veins of the antecubital fossa, dorsum of hand, foot, external jugular and scalp veins.

Cut-down Placement of Cannulas

Open operation may be necessary in catheterization of the umbilical artery or for insertion of Silastic cannulas into central veins. Prolonged parenteral nutrition can be administered together with a second channel using a single vein with the recent development of paediatric double- or triple-lumen catheters (*Fig.* 59.7). These procedures are best performed in the operating theatre under general anaesthesia.

Intravenous Therapy

The principles of fluid and electrolyte management have already been discussed (Chapter 6). In neonates a few points need emphasis.

Water and Calorie Requirements

Many formulas exist for estimation of maintenance water requirements. None is completely accurate and all should only be used as guides. The 'meter squared method' utilizes a theoretical relationship between metabolic rate and surface area. By this method the requirements are:

Water	1200–1500 ml/m^2/24h
Sodium	40 mmol (mEq)/m^2/24h
Potassium	30 mmol (mEq)/m^2/24h

The 'caloric method' employs a formula using weight and age to calculate energy requirements, assuming 100 ml of fluid is utilized/100 calories metabolized/24 h. The average newborn requires 75 calories/kg/24 h.

For practical purposes in neonates the following simple formula is used for fluid requirements.

Day 1	20 ml
Day 2	40 ml
Day 3	60 ml
Day 4	80 ml
Day 5	100 ml/kg

Thereafter:

100 ml/kg/24 h for first 10 kg weight
50 ml/kg/24 h for next 10 kg weight
20 ml/kg/24 h thereafter

Sodium 3–4 mmol (mEq)/kg/24 h.
Potassium 3 mmol (mEq)/kg/24 h.

The most important factor to appreciate is that any formula is an initial estimate only.

Insensible water loss accounts for 40–50 ml/kg/24 h. In many units incubators are no longer humidified, as this is thought to increase the risk of *Pseudomonas* infection. If this practice is used an appropriate increase of water should be made for the extra insensible loss which occurs.

Jaundiced babies undergoing phototherapy require an extra 20 ml/kg/24 h. Losses from nasogastric aspiration, or chest drains are replaced with appropriate solutions such as

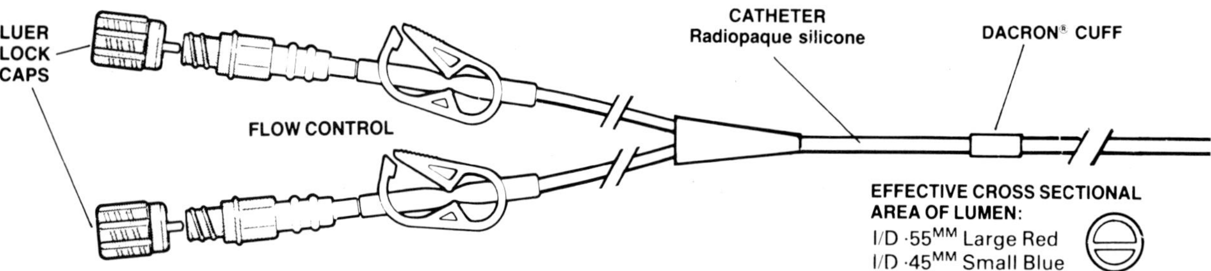

Fig. 59.7 The paediatric double-lumen chemocath provides a useful alternative to the standard adult and single-lumen paediatric sizes in case of vessel restriction in adults.

normal saline with added potassium at 36 mmol (mEq)/l for gastric aspirate and plasma or blood for pleural drainage replacement. As all regimes are guides only, clinical assessment noting the appearance of the baby's activity, skin colour, turgor and fontanelle tension should be made frequently. Weighing the baby once or twice a day is probably the most useful measure, as a loss of 1 g weight equals a loss of 1 ml of fluid. Serum electrolytes, serum and urine osmolality and haematocrit measurements are necessary daily in order to check or modify the original estimates. Not allowing a greater disparity than 2 °C between core and toe temperature is a very good guide to perfusion.

Nasogastric Feeding

The aim in any baby should be to achieve oral feeding with milk as soon as possible. This is not practical in small premature babies. These babies require large volumes of milk, usually 200 ml/kg/24 h, but this may have to be increased to 300 ml/kg/24 h as calculated on 'expected' rather than 'actual' weight. As the stomach is small and the risk of vomiting and aspiration high, the premature baby is fed via a No 6 F gauge tube at hourly intervals. In the postoperative baby even a small bolus such as this is not tolerated and a continuous milk drip infusion is necessary, injecting the same volume at a constant rate by means of an injection pump over 24 h. The 'strength' of the milk needs graduation from 'quarter' to 'half' and finally to 'full strength' before the gut will tolerate the feed. The stools should be tested, and if reducing substances are present, a lactose-free milk such as 'Galactamine' used.

Total Parenteral Nutrition

In the past 10 years this field has probably shown the biggest advances in the management of the ill surgical neonate. It has allowed one to 'buy time' while the gut is not functioning because of peritonitis, obstruction, fistulas, chronic diarrhoea, etc.

Alimentation is achieved by using either hyperosmolar solutions containing dextrose (20%), protein hydrolysate (5%), vitamins and minerals or intravenous fat solutions. The fat solutions can be administered via a peripheral or central vein, but the hyperosmolar solutions must be direct into a large vein (superior vena cava) or atrium. The central veins may be reached by cannulation of a scalp vein and threading down a fine Silastic catheter via the common facial vein and bringing out the end several centimetres away on the scalp. Meticulous care, no taps, no drugs and no withdrawal via the central line should be permitted. The entrance wound and all the junctions must be treated by strict aseptic technique with daily changing of all the solutions and infusion sets. This will go a long way in preventing most of the complications, the chief of which is sepsis, especially by *Candida albicans*. The total parenteral nutrition regime using fats or hypertonic dextrose is shown in *Tables* 59.2 and 59.3.

Table 59.2 Intravenous calories (after the 5th day of life)

DAY 1	1/5 N dextrose-saline	—4 ml	per kg 4-hourly rotation
	10% dextrose	—5 ml	
	Vamin	—4 ml	
	10% Intralipid	—3 ml	
DAY 2	10% dextrose	—5 ml	per kg 3-hourly rotation
	Vamin	—4 ml	
	10% Intralipid	—3 ml*	
DAY 3	10% dextrose	—5 ml	per kg 3-hourly rotation
	Vamin	—4 ml	
	10% Intralipid	—3 ml*	

(*suggest 5 ml for 2-kg baby, 8 ml for 3-kg baby, increase to 20% Intralipid on day 4)

ADDITIVES

1. Multibionta—add 3 ml to each 500 ml of 10% dextrose
2. 10% calcium gluconate—add 3 ml/kg to burette of 10% dextrose on days 1, 4, 7, 10, etc.
3. Dipotassium orthophosphate—add 2 ml/kg to burette of 10% dextrose on days 2, 5, 8, 11, etc.
4. 10% magnesium sulphate—add 0·2 ml/kg to burette of 10% dextrose on days 3, 6, 9, 12, etc.
5. Plasma—give once a week for 'trace elements'

INVESTIGATIONS

PBC and platelets—twice a week; U & E—three times a week; LFTs—once a week } 9 ml of blood/week
Lipidaemia—capillary check × 1/day
Urine—electrolytes and osmolality daily
Cannulas—send for culture
Sodium intake—3·0 mmol/kg/day
Potassium intake—3·0 mmol/kg/day
Calories (approx.)—100 kcal/kg/day from day 4

Table 59.3

Aminosol vitrium	10%=280 cal
Dextrose anhydrous	250 g=1000 cal
Potassium phosphate	700 mg (4 mEq/kg)
Folic acid	15 mg/ml 0·03 ml
Magnesium sulphate	50% 0·16 ml
Complete vitamin injection i.v.	1 ml
Calcium gluconate	10% 10 ml
Vitamin B_{12}	100 μg/ml 0·06 ml
Water	to 1 litre

Solution contains 25% dextrose and 70 mEq Na/1, which is equal to 1250 cal/l.

General Principles in the Operating Theatre

Operative details are beyond the scope of the book but the following points are emphasized:

Anaesthesia

1. The anaesthetic room should have extra radiant heat warmers.
2. Establish correct weight—blood volume—appropriate drug, adjusted doses.
3. Correct breathing circuits, endotracheal tubes and connectors, laryngoscopes.
4. Accurate low flow meters and vaporizers.
5. Establish i.v. line, accurate small volume-measuring i.v. sets.
6. Correct size sphygmomanometer cuff—Doppler flow detector.
7. Protection against heat loss:

Sterile cotton wool insulation;
warm water blanket;
heated humidifier in circuit;
correct ambient temperature more than 22 °C (ideally more than 26 °C);
In-line i.v. fluid warmer.

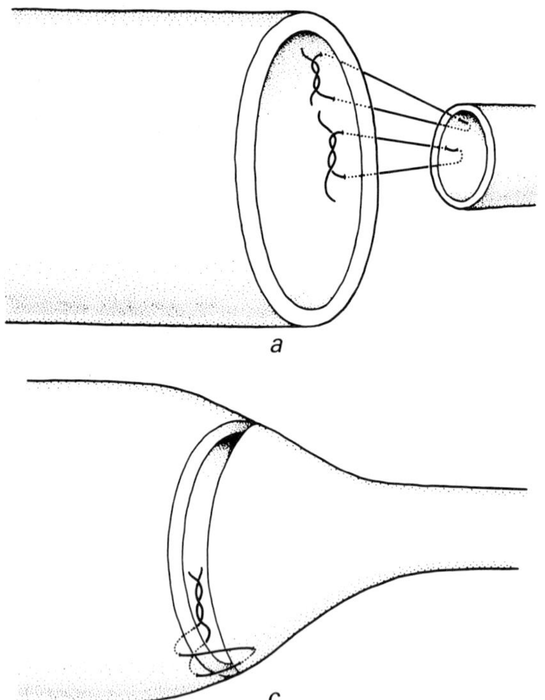

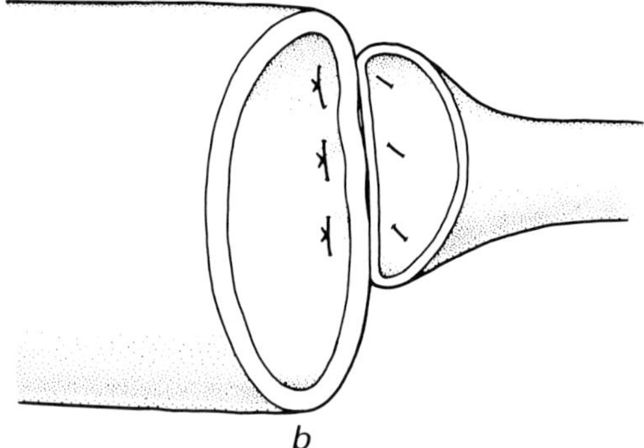

Fig. 59.8 Technique of performing an end-to-end anastomosis with a 4:1 discrepancy between proximal and distal loops.

8. Oesophageal thermometer, peripheral thermometer.
9. Oesophageal/precordial stethoscope.
10. Equipment for measuring blood loss.
11. I.V. infusion rate controller.
12. Monitors:

    Disconnection alarm
    Peripheral pulse
    ECG
    Infant capnograph
    Oximeter
    Airway pressure
    Peripheral nerve stimulator.

13. Suction equipment with small catheters, vacuum control.
14. Good assistance.
15. Prearrange for recovery and reception.

Intubation is performed either awake or under light anaesthesia and muscle relaxation with suxamethonium. Anaesthesia is maintained with nitrous oxide, oxygen, halothane and relaxants (curare or vecuronium). Awake intubation with nitrous oxide, oxygen, halothane and relaxants (curare or vecuronium) is the usual anaesthesia.

If the infant's temperature is subnormal, the operation should be postponed and the baby warmed until the temperature reaches 36–37 °C; further cooling will occur during induction of anaesthesia and surgery.

Induction of anaesthesia should be under an overhead radiant heat warmer. In the operating room the temperature of which should be 25 °C (77 °F) the baby lies on a circulating hot water blanket set at 37°C. The baby is not left exposed for any length of time. The operative field is prepared with warm solutions. Gamgee is stuck to the sides of the baby and the whole baby, including the head, covered with a large sheet of plastic Opsite or Steridrape. In spite of the precautions if the wound is large and the operation prolonged, the baby will lose heat and cool during surgery.

Operative Techniques

When resection of the bowel is necessary, the following precautions should be observed. In atresia of the intestine, the adjacent bowel may have been involved in the ischaemic process, with a subsequent reduction in motility. If possible, the grossly dilated bowel should be resected to reasonable calibre bowel which is more likely to be functionally normal. All anastomoses are performed using a single layer of 4/0 interrupted polygalactin sutures. It is not desirable to enlarge the distal small calibre bowel by cutting along the antimesenteric border and thereby ending up with an 'end-to-back' anastomosis. By careful suturing using a horizontal mattress suture on the large proximal bowel and a vertical mattress suture on the small distal bowel, discrepancies in the ratio of 4:1 or 5:1 can easily be accommodated (*Fig.* 59.8). This type of anastomosis seems to function better than the 'end-to-back' anastomosis.

Skin sutures are not often used, tape closure being preferred. Steristrip or similar material leaves a better scar and does not disturb the baby when sutures are removed.

Bleeding and Blood Replacement

Haemorrhagic disease of the newborn is a self-limiting bleeding disorder occurring on the 2nd or 3rd days of life resulting from a deficiency of coagulation factors dependent on vitamin K. All neonates undergoing surgery are given 1 mg of vitamin K_1, by intramuscular injection preoperatively. Larger doses than this produce hyperbilirubinaemia.

Disseminated Intravascular Coagulation (DIC)

DIC has been described in a large number of clinical states. A vasculitis or an endotoxin may be responsible in neonates. Depletion of the consumable coagulation factors, thrombocytopenia, haemolytic anaemia and bizarre red cell changes occur. In diseases with diffuse intravascular coagulation increased fibrinolytic activity and fibrin degradation products can be found in the circulation.

Blood Transfusion

'Top up' transfusions are frequently necessary. The fall in haemoglobin may be physiological, due to sepsis, or due to excessive blood loss from repeated venepunctures for various clinical investigations. Only small volumes need to be transfused, i.e. 25–50 ml at a time. Because the neonate is immune deficient, a satisfactory way of achieving this small blood transfusion is by using a 'walking donor'. This technique is not readily accepted as safe by some blood transfusion centres. All the staff on the unit are grouped and tested for Australia antigen, AIDS and syphilis. A copy of this list is held in the Blood Transfusion Service. Briefly the technique is as follows: the donor should be between 18 and 60 years. Their blood grouping and repeat tests for syphilis and Australia antigen are repeated in 3 months, if the donor has not been used. The infant's and maternal ABO and Rh (D) and direct antiglobulin test on the red cells are carried out. Five ml of donor serum are matched against the infant's red cells in a standard compatibility test. The donor can then be used for the next three days and aliquots of heparinized blood using 1 unit heparin per 1·0 ml blood can be withdrawn from the donor and injected directly into the neonate.

Blood Loss

The blood volume varies between 100 ml/kg in premature babies and 85 ml/kg in mature babies. All blood loss must be measured and replaced if 10% of the blood volume is exceeded. Two methods of measurement are available: weighing or colorimetric, i.e. washing the swabs and estimating the haemoglobin content of the fluid.

Monitoring

As monitoring equipment is becoming more sophisticated each year, there is a tendency to rely more and more on instrumentation. Nothing can replace the experienced nurse who spends 24 h a day at the cotside of the infant. Unless a neonatal unit can afford to have a high ratio of about 3 nurses to 1 patient, the results of neonatal surgery will be poor.

Monitoring equipment is becoming more and more sophisticated. Transcutaneous electrodes are available for both CO_2 and PO_2 measurements. The trends and figures obtained by these non-invasive methods correlate well with arterial blood sampling. The increased use of non-invasive methods of recording the babies' clinical state are becoming more common and are a welcome trend. Although these aids are available, they should never replace the clinical observations of the doctor or nurse.

Mechanical Ventilation

The trend in most hospitals is for ventilation of patients to take place in specialized intensive care untis; this is not practical for neonates. Using a simple pressure cycle ventilator such as the Vickers' Neovent, which is understood by nurses and doctors on the unit and is managed in consultation with the anaesthetist, very satisfactory results are obtained. The indications for ventilation may be:

1. Respiratory, due to raised intra-abdominal pressure from any cause pushing up the diaphragm and preventing normal excursion. Stiff lungs due to hyaline membrane disease, oedema, pneumonia, compression (i.e. diaphragmatic hernia). A baby utilizing a lot of effort to breathe with a PCO_2 approaching 55 mmHg (7·3 kPa) should be ventilated.
2. Central, due to depression of the respiratory centre by sepsis, haemorrhage, acidosis or prematurity.

RECOGNITION OF CONGENITAL ANOMALIES

The major conditions likely to be encountered are listed in *Table* 59.4 but it is not possible to discuss each condition in detail. The expected incidence of major congenital malformations is stated to be brain (10%), heart (8%), kidney (4%), limbs (2%), others (6%).

Table 59.4 Major congenital abnormalities encountered

Symptoms	*Possible anomaly*
A. *Respiratory*	Congenital heart disease
Cyanosis	Congenital diaphragmatic hernia
Breathlessness	Oesophageal atresia and tracheo-oesophageal fistula
	Neonatal lobar emphysema
B. *Intestinal Obstruction*	Atresia of small and large bowel
Vomiting (bile)	Stenosis—pylorus, small and large bowel
Distension	Malrotation
Constipation	Meconium ileus
	Meconium peritonitis
	Hirschsprung's disease
	Anorectal anomalies
	Neonatal necrotizing enterocolitis
C. *Abdominal Enlargement*	Kidney
	Poly- multi- cystic kidneys
	Hydronephrosis
	Wilms's tumour
	Liver
	Tumour or cyst
	Choledochal cyst
	Ascites
	Hydrometrocolpos
D. *Obvious Defects*	Cleft lip and palate
	Cystic hygroma
	Myelomeningocele
	Sacrococcygeal teratoma
	Exstrophy of bladder
	Hypospadias
E. *Umbilical Defects*	Exomphalos. Gastroschisis
	Vitello-intestinal duct remnants
	Urachal fistula
F. *Jaundice*	Physiological
	Neonatal hepatitis
	Biliary atresia

The number of neonates treated in Wessex, which serves a population of 2·5 million people, in a fairly typical example of a neonatal surgical unit in the UK is shown in *Table* 59.5.

The significant signs and symptoms in a neonate likely to alert the attending medical personnel to a serious underlying congenital anomaly are seen in *Table* 59.6.

Rapid Respiration may be due to:

Congenital Diaphragmatic Hernia

The defect in the diaphragm is usually posterolateral (foramen of Bochdalek) and 80% occur on the left side. The babies in whom respiratory distress is noted immediately or within the first 2–4 h of birth have a poor prognosis. Diaphragmatic hernias can be one of the most urgent neonatal conditions requiring surgery. The high mortality may be due to the following factors: (1) hypoplasia of the lung; (2) contralateral pneumothorax; (3) ischaemia of the lung which manifests itself as interstitial oedema, once the hernia is repaired, with inhibition of oxygenation; or (4) pulmonary hypertension, with re-opening of the ductus arteriosus and gross shunting. Clinical examination by means of auscultation may be grossly misleading in respiratory distress in the

Table 59.5 Congenital anomalies in neonates treated in two 3-year periods in a typical neonatal surgical unit in the UK

	Average for 1977–79	1983–85
Oesophageal atresia and tracheo-oesophageal fistula	7	6
Diaphragmatic hernia	7	7
Small bowel obstruction	14	14
Large bowel obstruction	6	3
Necrotizing enterocolitis	7	11
Anorectal anomalies	6	9
Anterior abdominal wall defect	6	4
Genito-urinary	9	13
Hydrocephalus	3	6
Spina bifida	20	10
Miscellaneous	21	36
Total per year	106	123

Note: There is a continuing decrease in the cases of spina bifida. An increase in hydrocephalus and neonatal enterocolitis, mainly in prematures. An increase in genito-urinary anomalies due to recognition by antenatal ultrasound diagnosis (*see also Fig.* 59.4).

Table 59.6 Significant signs and symptoms

Maternal hydramnios
Rapid respiration (over 50/min)
Difficult respiration (retraction, etc.)
Cyanosis (a single episode)
Excess salivation
Abdominal distension
Abdominal mass
Vomiting of bile (green)
Failure to evacuate meconium (within 24 h)
Inability to void (or inadequate or intermittent stream)
Convulsion
Lethargy (poor feeding)
Jaundice (first 24 h)

newborn and an urgent radiograph is mandatory. It is important to obtain a radiograph of the abdomen at the same time to help in the differential diagnosis. The symptoms of cyanosis, dyspnoea, apparent dextrocardia and a scaphoid abdomen are diagnostic of congenital diaphragmatic hernia. *Fig.* 59.3 is not typical due to the small size of the hernia.

The baby is transferred or transported equipped with the means of emergency intubation and insertion of bilateral underwater seal drains, or Hofnagel valves. A nasogastric tube must be passed and the stomach kept deflated. If the baby needs to be intubated and ventilated en route, it should be paralysed with pancuronium. Urgent surgery is normally required. If the baby is in a high-risk group delay with ventilation, paralysis, the use of dopamine and tolazoline may improve the prognosis. The hernia is reduced and the defect repaired via a left transverse abdominal incision.

The differential diagnosis of congenital diaphragmatic hernia includes:

Lobar emphysema, which usually involves either the upper or middle lobe of one or both lungs with over-distension causing compression of the other pulmonary lobes and gross displacement of the mediastinum. This may occur acutely in the neonatal period or more gradually later in life. Rapidly increasing dyspnoea and cyanosis result. The radiograph is characteristic although the area of translucency is occasionally mistaken for a diaphragmatic hernia or a tension pneumothorax. Emergency thoracotomy and lobectomy is the treatment of choice.

Adamantoid malformation of the lung is very rare, but it can be mistaken for a diaphragmatic hernia. The abdomen in these cases is not usually scaphoid and the radiograph shows most of the intestines within the abdomen.

Oesophageal Atresia and Tracheo-oesophageal Fistula

The incidence is approximately 1:3000 live births. The usual type is shown in *Fig.* 59.9, and accounts for approximately 85% of cases. Pure oesophageal atresia without a fistula (8%), a fistula from both upper and lower (2%) and isolated tracheo-oesophageal fistula, the so called H-type (3%), are also seen.

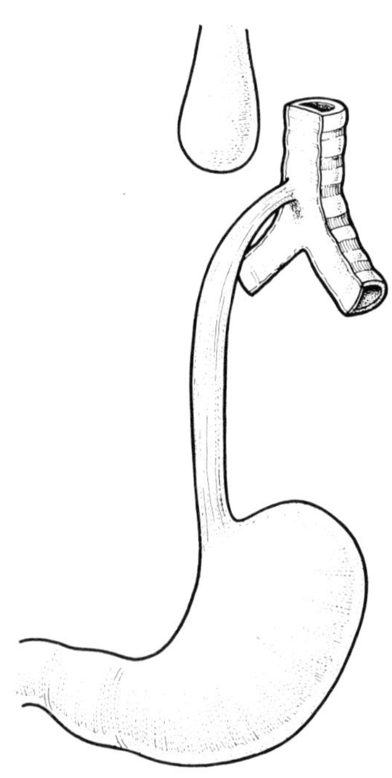

Fig. 59.9 Oesophageal atresia with tracheo-oesophageal fistula.

Untreated, the lesion is incompatible with life. Although the obvious danger to the infant appears to be inability to swallow milk or saliva with spillage into the lungs, the reflux of acid contents from the stomach into the lungs is a more serious and lethal complication.

The diagnosis should be suspected prenatally in any case of maternal hydramnios. Hydramnios is present in 85% of babies with oesophageal atresia alone, and in 35% of those with oesophageal atresia and tracheo-oesophageal fistula. The baby does not vomit but produces an abundance of frothy mucus which soon reappears after suctioning. Cyanosis, choking, coughing and dyspnoea, especially on attempting to feed or changing the baby's position is very suggestive of the diagnosis. The diagnosis is confirmed by the passage of a stiff No. 10 F radio-opaque catheter through the nose or mouth and a holding up at 7–10 cm from the alveolar margin. A single radiograph of the infant confirms the diagnosis and the presence of air in the stomach denotes the presence of an associated tracheo-oesophageal fistula. Ideally a Replogle tube should be left in the upper pouch on continuous low-grade suction. The baby should be nursed flat on its side. No pressure should be applied to the abdomen until the fistula has been ligated. Associated anomalies are recognized by the Vacterl acronym—vertebral anomalies, anal, cardiac, tracheo-oesophageal fistula, renal and limb anomalies.

Surgical treatment should be expeditious. It is not possible to predict if and when acid regurgitation into the lungs will occur. It is possible that this may have already occurred when the abdomen was squeezed in the birth canal during delivery. As the baby cries the positive pressure in the trachea, achieved by closure of the glottis, allows air to travel down the oesophagus and gross gastric distension, with splinting of the diaphragm may occur. For these two reasons, urgent gastrostomy and ligation of the tracheo-oesophageal fistula should be performed. The baby should not be intubated and ventilated unless ligation of the fistula is planned. A Stamm gastrostomy is made via a midline incision using a 14 or 16 F Malecot catheter. The upper and lower oesophagus is exposed via a retropleural approach through a Denis Browne vertical axillary incision. It is possible to achieve a primary anastomosis in about 60% of cases. In the other 40% of babies in whom a primary anastomosis is not possible, some form of staging procedure is necessary (*Fig.* 59.10). If a cervical oesophagostomy is necessary the gap between the neck and the stomach is bridged using transverse colon based on the upper left colic artery, either early at 4–6 months or later at 2 years of age (*Fig.* 59.10). More recently, neonatal colon interposition without the use of a preliminary cervical oesophagostomy has been preferred.

The overall mortality of this group is still high, in the order of 50%. However, if babies with other major anomalies, severe pneumonia or prematurity are excluded the prognosis is excellent, between 95–100% surviving. This is remarkable considering that the first baby to survive a primary transthoracic anastomosis, was at the Ann Arbor Hospital, Michigan in 1941. In a baby in whom a primary anastomosis is performed without undue tension, feeding via the gastrostomy may start after 24 h. Depending on how the baby copes with swallowing saliva, oral feeds can be introduced within 4 or 6 days and some babies are discharged home by 10 days.

Complications

Respiratory complications, either from pre- or postoperative pneumonia, pulmonary collapse or pneumothorax, need intensive physiotherapy and suction, and occasionally artificial ventilation. Disruption of the anastomosis manifests itself between the 2nd and 5th postoperative day. The great advantage of the retropleural approach has meant that the leak can be treated conservatively in many cases (*Fig.* 59.11).

If free drainage is maintained by gentle washouts or suction on the pleural drain, healing occurs in about 10 days. Anastomotic stricture may occur, even without a leak. These strictures occur: (1) early at 3–4 weeks, (2) late at 1–5 months and (3) later at 10–12 months after the original surgery. There appears to be no correlation between the clinical, radiological or endoscopic findings relating to the stricture. Dilatation with gum elastic bougies on one or more occasions usually cures the dysphagia. Any baby with persistent cough, with choking or cyanosis during feeding, following repair of a tracheo-oesophageal fistula, should be

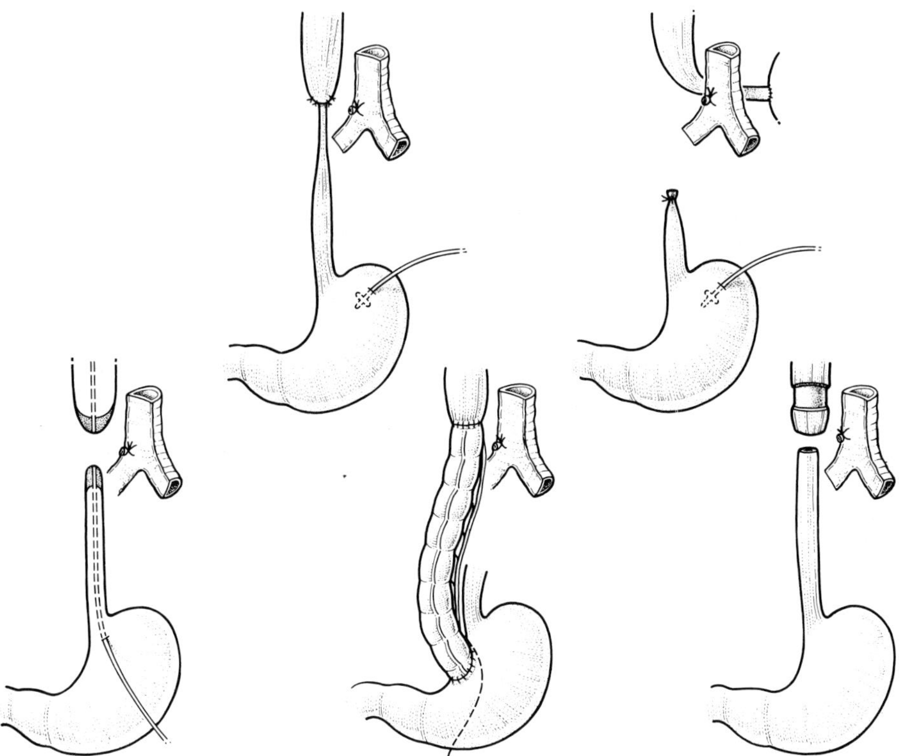

Fig. 59.10 Treatment of oesophageal atresia.

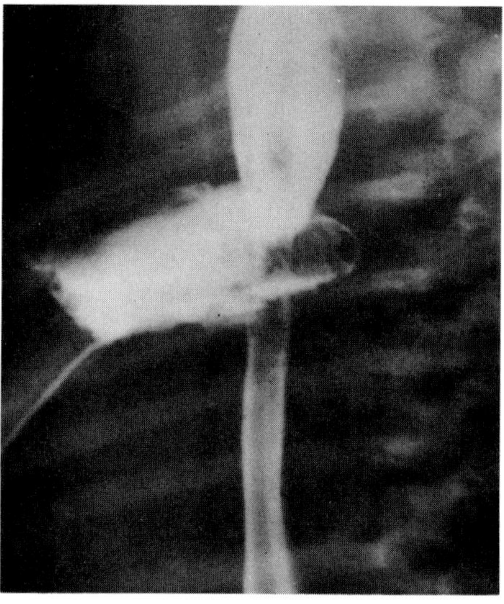

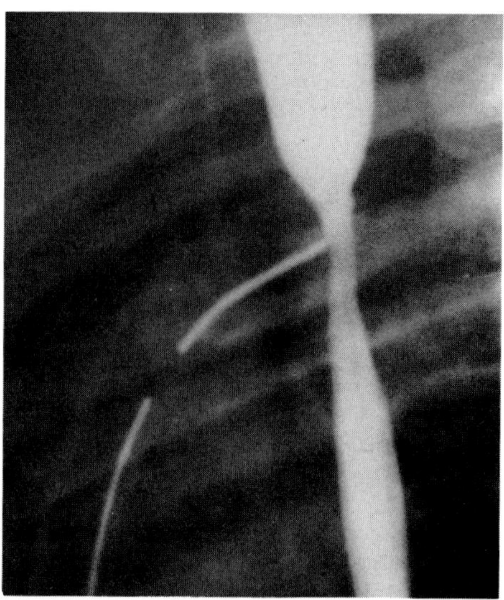

Fig. 59.11 Barium studies 14 days apart showing healing of large retropleural anastomotic leak treated conservatively.

investigated to exclude a recurrent fistula. Tracheomalacia and damage to the cords should also be excluded.

Tracheomalacia has become a more frequently recognized complication. Diagnosis is made from the history of respiratory difficulties and 'dying spells' during feeding. Diagnosis should be made on bronchoscopy with the patient breathing spontaneously. Treatment is by aortopexy, performed via a cervical incision, sternotomy or thoracotomy.

A stricture of the lower oesophagus unrelated to the anastomosis is due to gastro-oesophageal reflux and may require a Nissen fundoplication.

INTESTINAL OBSTRUCTION

Atresia and Stenosis

Atresia means 'absence or closure of normal opening'; stenosis means 'narrowing'. Atresia can occur in any part of the gastrointestinal tract from the mouth to the anus. In most cases, except possibly in the oesophagus, duodenum and rectum, the atresia is a result of an intrauterine vascular accident occurring late in pregnancy, such as volvulus, intussusception or strangulation of the bowel at the umbilical ring. As the fetus is germ free, the ischaemic portion of the bowel is absorbed and disappears almost without trace. An example of the mechanism of an intrauterine vascular accident is shown in *Fig.* 59.12.

The classic signs and symptoms of intestinal obstruction are similar to those in adults, i.e. pain, vomiting, distension and constipation.

Pain is indicated by careful observation of the baby, which reveals crying, grimacing or drawing-up of the legs coinciding with obvious visible peristaltic activity or increased obstructive bowel sounds.

After birth, babies may occasionally vomit mucus or pale yellow fluid (the carotene pigments found in colostrum). If the vomit is *green*, i.e. bile, it is likely that a significant organic cause will be found. Every baby who vomits green bile should be investigated. The cause may be a mechanical obstruction, a functional obstruction, infection, cerebral birth trauma or hypothyroidism.

The degree of abdominal distension is related to the level of obstruction. Babies with high obstructions such as duodenal atresia will have a scaphoid abdomen after a vomit, or aspiration of the stomach (*Fig.* 59.13). In complete obstruction absolute constipation is not present, if the colon is filled with bowel contents prior to the onset of obstruction. Thus, even in complete atresia of the ileum, normal meconium may be passed because the intrauterine vascular accident occurs after the formation of meconium in the colon or rectum.

Duodenal Atresia and Stenosis

In the developing embryo outpouchings occur in the area of the second part of the duodenum and from these the main bile and pancreatic ducts develop. Atresia of the duodenum occurs at the level of the ampulla of Vater, commonly duplicating the termination of the bile duct above and below the obstruction. Of babies with duodenal atresias, 30% have an associated Down's syndrome. The main feature is bile-stained vomiting, though occasionally no bile is seen as the duct enters below the atresia. The erect radiograph shows the typical 'double-bubble' appearance (*Fig.* 59.14).

Surgical treatment consists of bypassing the atresia with a duodenoduodenostomy or with a gastroenterostomy. A gastrostomy with a transanastomotic feeding tube may be added, if delay in gastric emptying is anticipated.

Jejuno-ileal Atresia

The atresia may be a single or multiple and occur at any site in the jejunum and ileum. The abdominal radiograph will usually suggest the level and possible aetiology. Except in the high jejunal atresia, near the duodenojejunal junction, it is wise to resect 10–20 cm of the dilated portion of the proximal loop as propulsion in this area is ineffective. Anastomosis should be by an end-to-end anastomosis (*see Fig.* 59.8).

Meconium Ileus

Meconium is kept fluid by the action of pancreatic enzymes. If, however, pancreatic function and mucus gland secretion

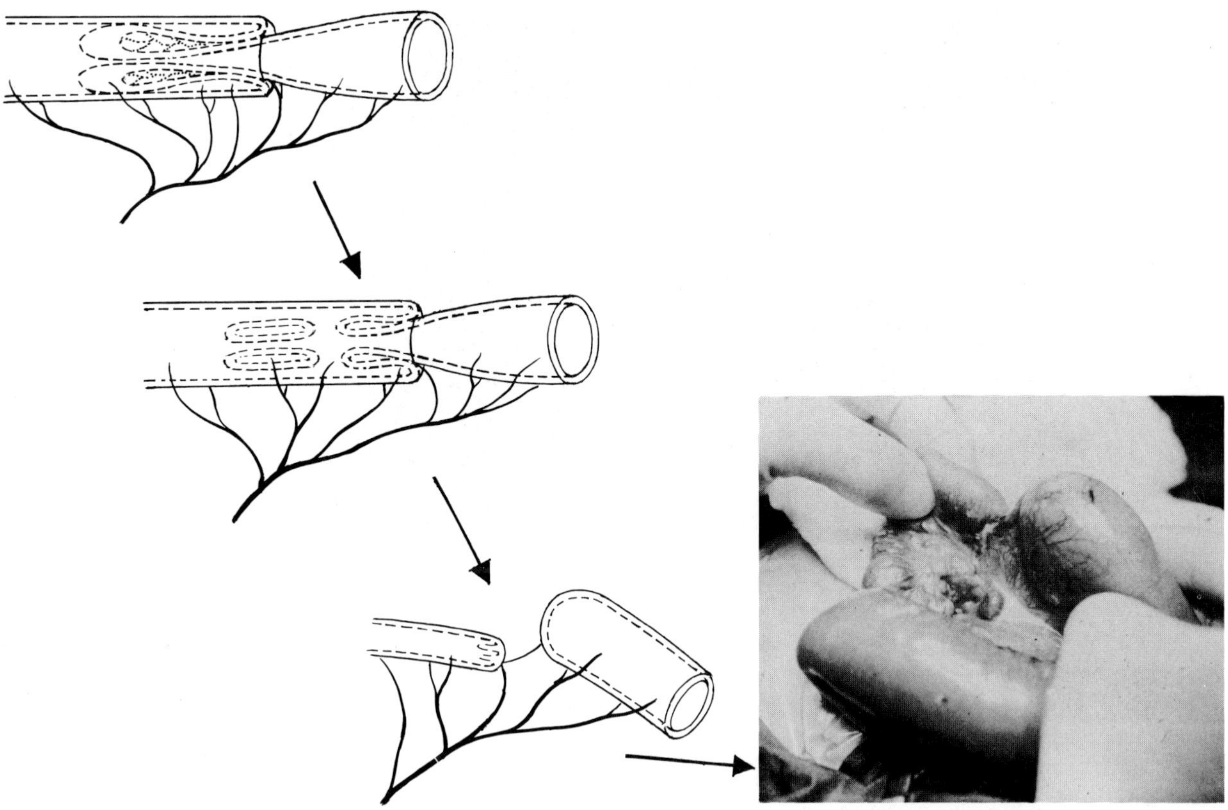

Fig. 59.12 *a*, Mechanism of intrauterine vascular accident (intussusception) resulting in *b*, an ileal atresia.

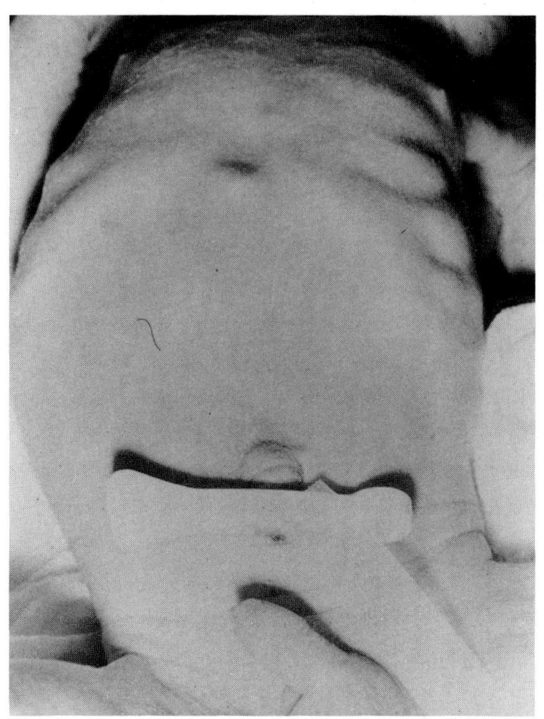

Fig. 59.13 Scaphoid abdomen without distension seen in complete duodenal obstruction (atresia).

is deficient, i.e. in fibrocystic disease of the pancreas, the meconium becomes thick and putty-like which may obstruct the terminal ileum by small pellets of inspissated meconium. This occurs prenatally and twisting (volvulus) of the grossly distended proximal bowel may lead to atresia and perforation (meconium peritonitis).

Gross abdominal distension, bile-stained vomiting, and a failure to pass meconium are the main presenting features. Large coils filled with the rubbery meconium may be palpated through the abdominal wall, and a straight abdominal radiograph shows the typical mottled granular appearance due to fat granules trapped in the sticky meconium (*Fig.* 59.15).

As the condition is due to a genetic defect (autosomal recessive) a family history of an affected sibling helps in the diagnosis. Laboratory investigations may show absence of the pancreatic enzyme, trypsin, from the stool or bile. The amount of sodium chloride in the sweat can be measured—values above 80 mmol/l are diagnostic of cystic fibrosis. In the neonate immunoreactive trypsin can be determined on a drop of blood to establish the diagnosis, as sweat tests are not easy to perform before about 6 weeks of age. In 50% of non-complicated cases the obstructed bowel may be deflated by the use of a Gastrografin enema. Gastrografin has a very high osmolarity and detergent action, which attracts fluid into the lumen of the bowel, thereby softening the inspissated meconium. In more severe cases, laparotomy, enterostomy or resection of the dilated bowel, with an end-to-side (Bishop–Koop) anastomosis is performed (*Fig.* 59.16). The

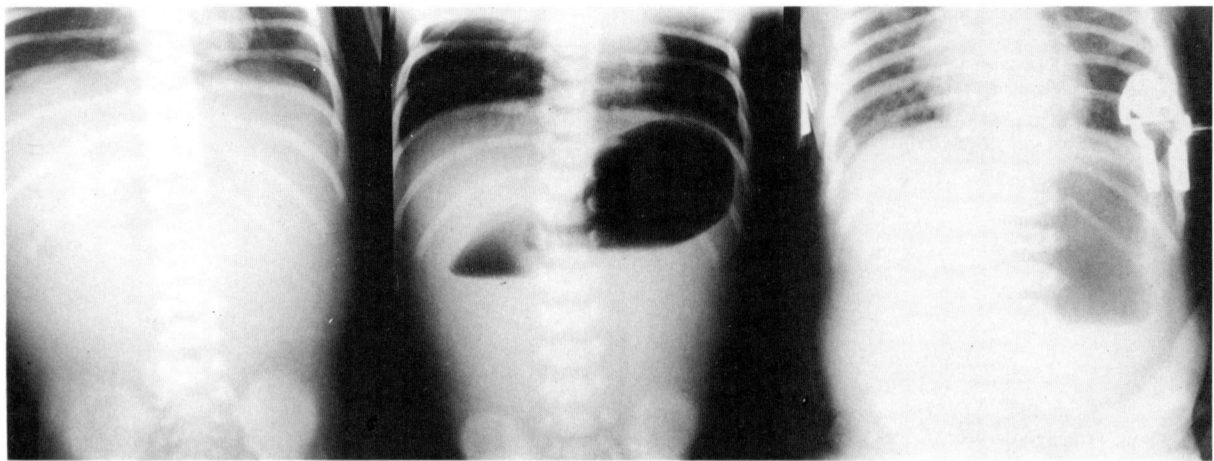

Fig. 59.14 Complete (duodenal atresia—*right* and *middle*) and partial obstruction (malrotation—*left*) of the second part of the duodenum. Note that the typical 'double bubble' is only seen on the erect films, after injection of air (*middle*), not on the supine film (*left*), and that the dilated duodenum may be easily overlooked.

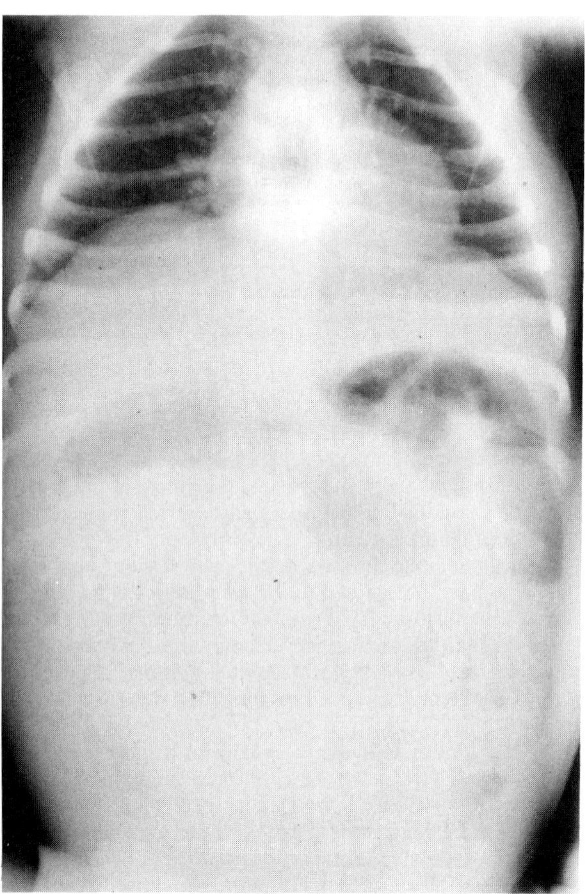

Fig. 59.15 Erect abdominal X-ray in a case of meconium ileus. Note the typical 'bubbly' appearance of meconium and air in the lower abdomen. Note the absence of fluid levels in spite of gross distension and elevation of the diaphragm, due to the abnormally viscid meconium.

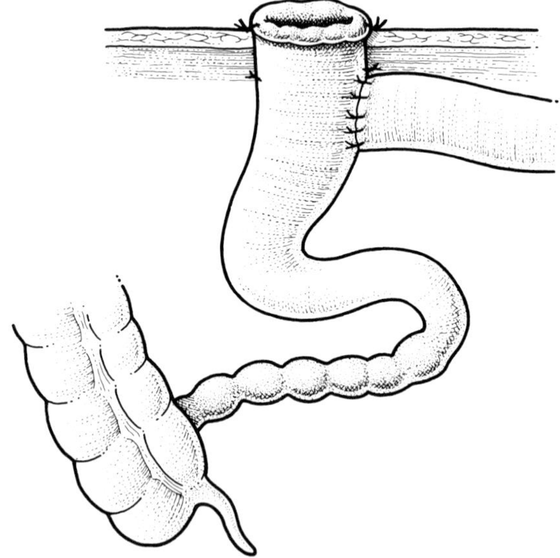

Fig. 59.16 Bishop–Koop procedure.

'chimney' opening on the abdomen allows pancreatic enzymes to be instilled into the distal bowel. Once the bowel has been cleared of the sticky meconium, oral supplementary pancreatic enzymes are given with each meal throughout life. The abnormality of mucus gland secretion remains and these patients eventually succumb from chronic respiratory failure in late teenage or early adult life.

Anomalies of Intestinal Rotation

Up to 10 weeks of gestation, the gut lies outside the abdominal cavity in a physiological hernia at the umbilicus. The gut returns in an orderly fashion to form the typical 'C' loop of the duodenum, the oblique attachment of the small bowel mesentery. The attachment of the ascending transverse and descending colon is achieved by a further rotation of 270° in an anticlockwise direction of the large bowel.

The process of rotation of the midgut (extending from the area of the bile duct papilla to the middle of the transverse colon) may be arrested at any stage and several abnormalities develop. The main effects of these abnormalities are:

1. The intestine remains free on a narrow-based mesentery and is therefore very liable to undergo volvulus with intestinal obstruction and strangulation.

2. Tight bands of peritoneum or fibrous tissue cross and obstruct the second part of the duodenum (Ladd's bands) and stretch from below the liver to the caecum, which is situated in the epigastrium, close to the origin of the superior mesenteric artery having failed to descend to the right iliac fossa. This is the commonest anomaly of rotation.

3. The intestine returns to the abdomen and rotates in a clockwise direction resulting in the third and fourth parts of the duodenum passing in front of the transverse colon and the small bowel mesentery fails to achieve a posterior attachment (reversed intestinal rotation).

4. There is a failure of rotation altogether and the small bowel lies on the right side of the abdomen with inadequate mesenteric attachment and the caecum and ascending colon are positioned in the left upper abdomen leading to the left-sided descending colon (non-rotation).

Volvulus may lead to partial obstruction of the blood vessels of the intestine, which may ultimately become gangrenous. More frequently, the symptoms that result are due to obstruction of the duodenum immediately below the entry of the bile duct into the duodenum. Vomiting usually begins very early in life and the vomitus may contain bile. Radiological examination will demonstrate that the first part of the duodenum and the stomach are distended by swallowed air ('double-bubble' sign) (*Fig.* 59.14). A valuable investigation is the injection of 20–30 ml of air through a nasogastric tube to distend the stomach and duodenum prior to the abdominal radiograph to make this feature more obvious.

Treatment is by operation. Any volvulus is corrected either by derotation in an anticlockwise direction, with division of the obstructing bands from the caecum across the duodenum. The small and large bowel cannot be returned to a normal anatomical position, therefore the duodenum is mobilized and made to lie in the right paracolic gutter, the narrow mesentery is opened up widely as an apron, and the colon is placed on the left side of the abdomen with the caecum and appendix in the left hypochondrium. No anchoring is necessary unless small bowel volvulus has been a problem. This manoeuvre effectively corrects the anomaly to one of 'non-rotation'. It is possible in some patients to convert reversed rotation to a completely normal anatomical situation.

Congenital Megacolon—Hirschsprung's Disease

The ganglion cells of the small and large bowel migrate from the neural crest along the vagi within the bowel wall in intrauterine life to reach the anus by birth. Failure of this migration to reach the anal canal will cause an aganglionic zone which extends upwards, for a varying distance, from the anal canal. The segment of bowel without ganglion cells and proper innervation by the autonomic nervous system is unable to conduct a coordinated peristaltic wave, and acts as a physiological obstruction to the onward passage of bowel contents. This results in obstruction with gross dilatation and hypertrophy of the proximal colon. Most patients (80%) present as acute large bowel obstructions in the neonatal period, with failure to pass meconium, abdominal distension and bile-stained vomiting. If the diagnosis is delayed the symptoms of vomiting, distension and diarrhoea may be due to Hirschsprung's enterocolitis. About 20% of children present less acutely, with failure to thrive or severe constipation from early infancy. They require laxatives, suppositories or enemas to achieve evacuation of the colon. The diagnosis is established by demonstrating on barium enema examination a characteristic narrow segment, a 'cone' area and dilatation of the colon above (*Fig.* 59.17). Examining histologically and with histochemistry, rectal mucosa removed through the anus, usually by a mucosal (suction) or by open biopsy, showing the absence of ganglion cells, hypertrophy of the nerve fibres and increased acetylcholine esterase activity.

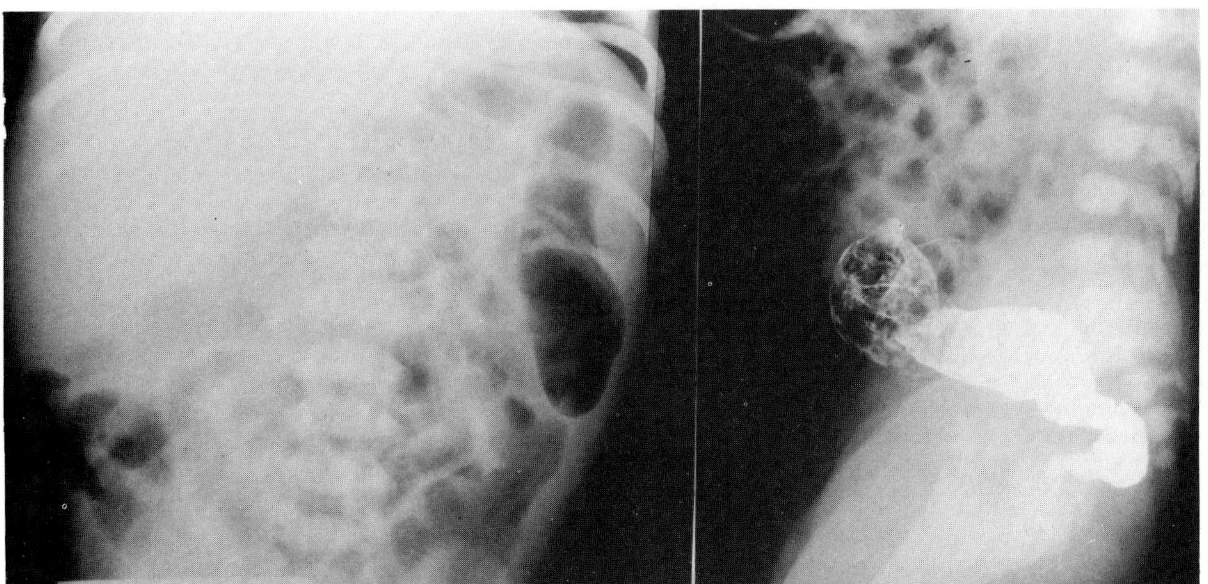

Fig. 59.17 *Left.* Note the appearance of obstruction in neonatal Hirschsprung's disease. There is a generalized distension of the whole bowel. *Right.* Note the typical 'cone' area on barium enema examination, situated at the rectosigmoid area. The cone is best demonstrated on a 24 h post-evacuation film, as above.

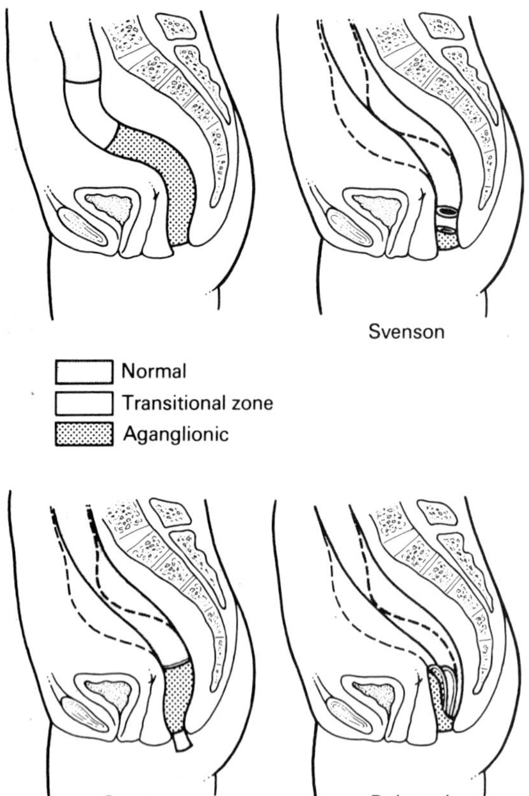

Fig. 59.18 Pull-through procedures for Hirschsprung's disease.

The normal reflex inhibition of the internal sphincter on distension of the rectum does not occur in Hirschsprung's disease and can be demonstrated on anorectal manometry.

Treatment consists of a loop colostomy, just above the cone area to relieve the obstruction, followed 6–12 months later by a definitive pull-through operation, using the Svenson, Duhamel or Soave technique. The objective being to remove most of the aganglionic segment and to restore continuity and preserve faecal continence. Surgery for this condition should only be performed by experienced surgeons. The principle of the operations is shown in *Fig.* 59.18. By not dividing about half of the internal sphincter, symptoms may persist; too low a dissection in the Duhamel operation will render the patient incontinent.

Anorectal Anomalies

The terminology in this group is confusing and there is now an international classification of anorectal anomalies describing 27 subdivisions. From a practical point, the two major subdivisions, 'high' (supralevator) and 'low' (translevator), depending on whether or not the terminal bowel (rectum) traverses the pelvic diaphragm, determine prognosis and management (*Fig.* 59.19). These two subdivisions are related either to early (6–8 weeks) or later embryological events.

Incomplete septation and migration occurs leading to 'high' anomalies. At a later stage of development incomplete migration together with overfusion result in the 'low' anomalies. The sex of the patient also influences the type of lesion as the division of the cloaca into urinary and alimentary parts in the female is modified by the development of the Müllerian system (vagina, uterus and Fallopian tubes). In the male, if separation of the cloaca does not occur, there will be a fistulous communication between the hind gut and the urinary tract, either urethra or bladder. In the female the fistulous communication is never into the urinary tract, but into the vagina (Müllerian remnant).

Diagnosis is usually made on full careful clinical examination. This includes probing any visible orifices, a plain lateral radiograph taken in the 'upside down position', centred on the greater trochanters, with the hips flexed, together with endoscopy and injection of contrast medium per urethram or via a needle in the perineum will help establish the exact anatomical abnormality, which is essential for proper management.

If no orifice is found in the perineum, a 'high' anomaly is suspected. In the female with rectal agenesis and a vaginal fistula, meconium may be seen coming from the vagina. In the male, with rectal agenesis and recto-urethral fistula, the urine may contain meconium.

The 'low' anomalies are recognized by an orifice in the perineum, which may be tiny, stenosed or in an ectopic position. In the female the orifice is usually in the fourchette just below the hymen or in any ectopic position towards the normal position. In the male the opening or fistulous tract may be recognized by meconium covered with almost transparent epithelium, in the midline, anywhere from the tip of the penis to the normal anal position.

Treatment

The 'high' anomalies present with intestinal obstruction and require a sigmoid colostomy followed by a definitive 'pull-through' operation. The timing of this operation varies. Some surgeons prefer an immediate neonatal operation, others wait until the baby is 9–12 months old. The 'pull-through' operation is performed via a sacro-perineal or posterior sagittal approach without opening the abdomen. Occasionally when the rectum is very high in the pelvis an abdominoperineal operation is necessary. The 'low' anomalies require an immediate local 'anoplasty' to widen the perineal orifice. Associated anomalies are common, especially genito-urinary (50%). The 'Vacterl' acronym of associated anomalies is as those seen in oesophageal atresia.

Prognosis

It should be made clear to the parents of babies with 'high' anomalies that, because of the missing rectum, anal sphincters and anorectal sensation, normal continence can never be achieved. It is possible, however, with careful initial surgery, and long-term regular follow-up, to achieve virtually full control in the 'low' anomalies, and 80–90% 'excellent' results in the 'high' group. 'Excellent' means that these children attend normal schools, partake in normal sporting activities, are not on regular laxatives or medication and only have the occasional 'accident'.

Neonatal Necrotizing Enterocolitis (NNEC)

The aetiology of this condition is still debated and may be multifactorial. It is primarily a mucosal ischaemic lesion due to the shunting of blood away from the terminal submucosal vessels. In the early stages the deeper layers are well vascularized, but with secondary bacterial invasion, septicaemia or endotoxic shock soon supervene. Disseminated intravascular coagulation occurs and manifests as thrombocytopenia. Hypovolaemia, and a low flow state through the splanchnic circulation, appear to be the main causative agents. Factors such as a stressful delivery, hypoxia, cold,

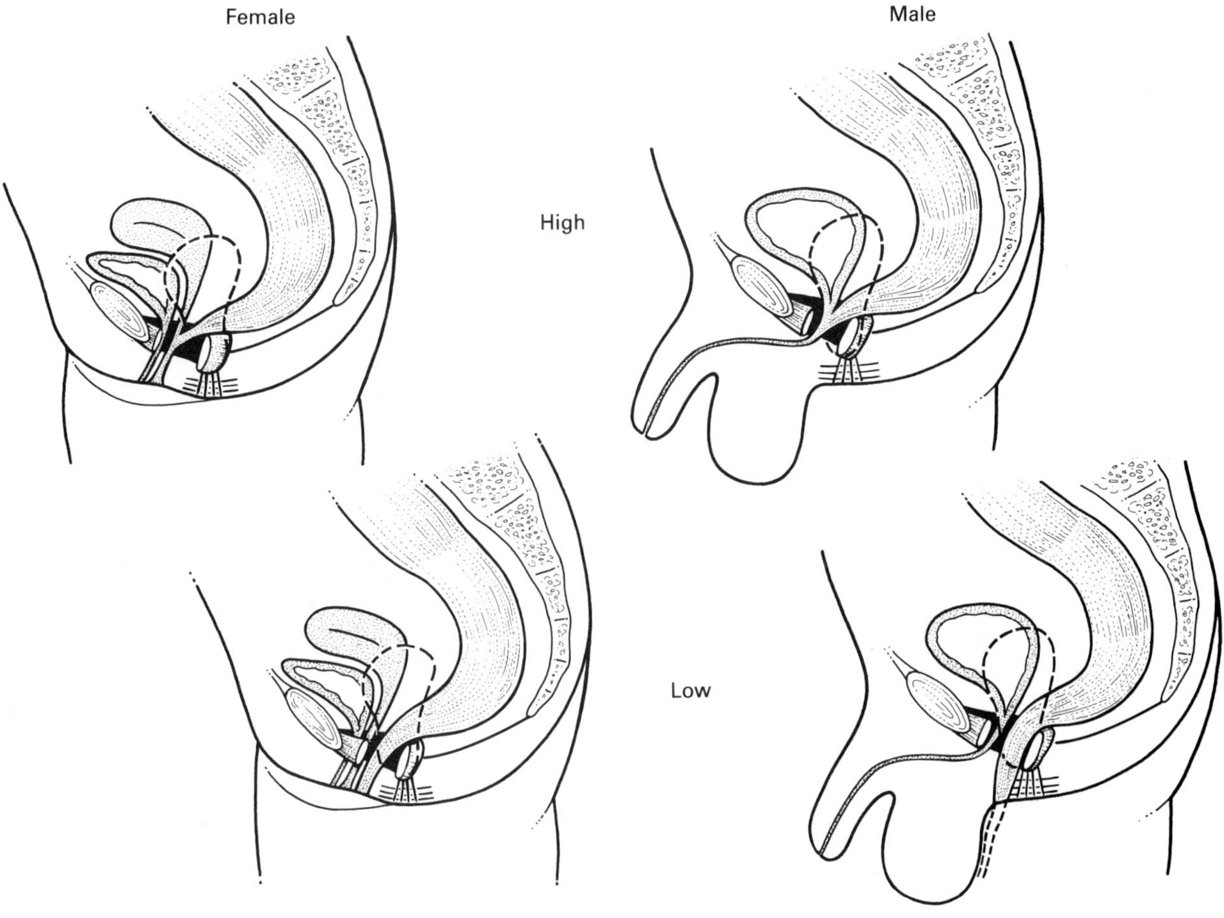

Fig. 59.19 Diagrammatic representation of 'high' and 'low' anorectal anomalies in either sex.

hyperosmolar feeds, intra-arterial and umbilical vein catheters and exchange transfusions, are recognized trigger mechanisms. The baby presents as a functional obstruction with abdominal distension, vomiting and usually passes loose stools containing blood and mucus. Radiography shows diffuse dilatation of the gut with fluid levels and in the later stages when submucosal pneumatosis occurs, the characteristic double wall shadow is seen (*Fig.* 59.20).

Treatment is mainly conservative with antibiotics (gentamicin, penicillin and metronidazole), nasogastric suction, together with intravenous feeding. Radiography is repeated 8–12-hourly and if perforation occurs, laparotomy may be indicated, with resection of the gangrenous bowel, leaving an enterostomy stoma, and a mucus fistula of the distal bowel. Continuity is later restored as the rectum is usually spared. If the baby responds to conservative management, he may develop a late stricture in the affected area at about 4–6 weeks, which requires resection. It is interesting to note that NNEC is becoming one of the more common reasons for admission to neonatal surgical units (*see Table* 59.5). It is usually encountered in premature babies and ill babies receiving intensive care.

ABDOMINAL ENLARGEMENT

Although the abdominal enlargement may be massive and obvious, the baby may be asymptomatic. A plain radiograph of the abdomen, and IVP and an ultrasound scan will usually establish the diagnosis. The renal tract, with either a multicystic kidney, hydronephrosis due to congenital pelviureteric junction obstruction, or an obstructive uropathy, or neonatal Wilms's (nephroblastoma) tumour provides the most likely diagnosis. Tumours of the liver causing enlargement are either cysts, haemangiomas, hepatoblastoma or choledochal cysts (*see* Chapters 68 and 69).

Lower abdominal distension may be due to hydrometrocolpos which occurs with or without obstruction of the uterus or vagina due to mucus retention following maternal hormone stimulation.

OBVIOUS DEFECTS

Sacrococcygeal teratoma presents as a large cystic or solid tumour arising from the tip of the coccyx and enlarging outwards or occasionally both outwards and into the pelvis as a dumb-bell. The lesion has been mistaken for a spina bifida and although excision looks formidable, it is feasible, with a good prognosis, if the coccyx is removed *en bloc* with the tumour (*Fig.* 59.21). The tumour is benign at birth, but appears to undergo malignant change with time. At Great Ormond Street Hospital, of 58 patients, 6·5% were malignant under 1 year of age and 58% of those over 1 year of age. Surprisingly little damage to the pelvic nerves, rectal or bladder sphincters occurs following excision.

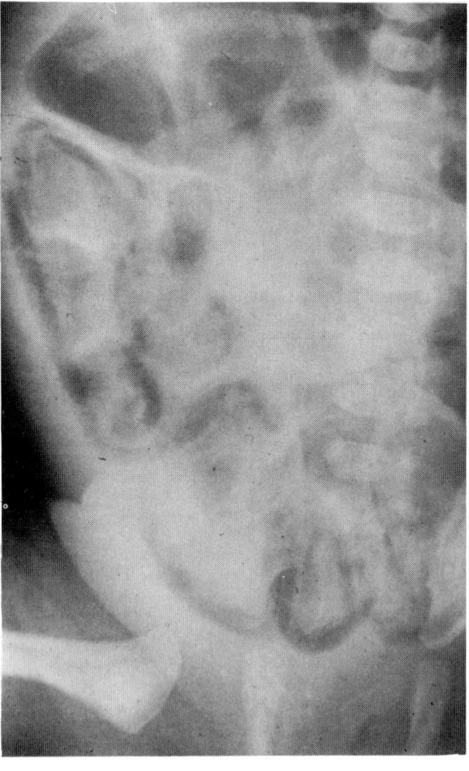

Fig. 59.20 Radiograph of a baby in a special care unit, showing typical intramural gas of neonatal necrotizing enterocolitis.

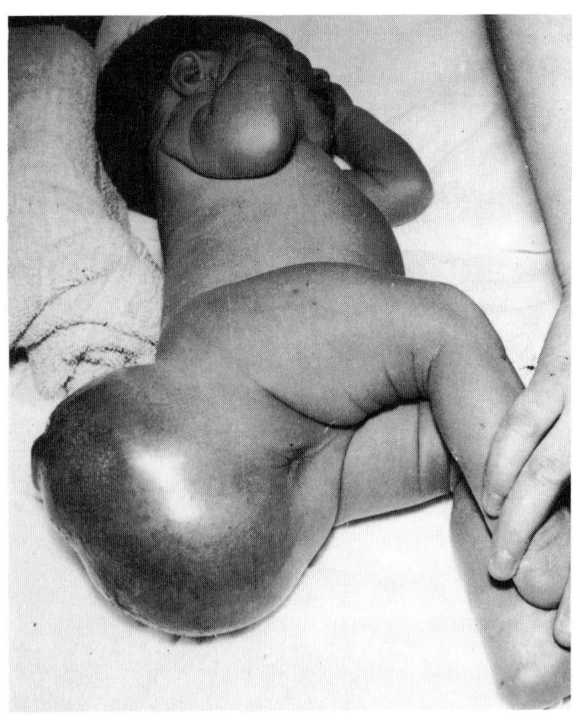

Fig. 59.21 Clinical appearance of a typical sacrococcygeal teratoma.

Other obvious defects are cleft lip and palate (*see* Chapter 25), cystic hygroma (*see* Chapter 23), myelomeningocele (*see* Chapter 33), exstrophy of the bladder (*see* Chapter 82) hypospadias (*see* Chapter 84).

UMBILICAL DEFECTS

Although these are obvious defects at birth they will be dealt with separately. The umbilical cord following ligation should shrivel, dry and separate by about 10 days. It is important that this area is looked after carefully postnatally to prevent infection, portal thrombophlebitis and septicaemia. Minor infections present as umbilical granuloma after separation of the cord. These moist, red granulations should be distinguished from the small bowel mucosa of vitello-intestinal remnants. As the granuloma has no nerve supply, treatment is simple, by cutting off with scissors and treating the base with a silver nitrate stick to stop bleeding. The granuloma should be sent for histology to exclude the presence of intestinal epithelium. If the umbilical ring fails to close completely after birth, the patient is left with an umbilical hernia. As there is a strong possibility that over the next 3 years physiological closure will occur, repair should be delayed until after this age.

Exomphalos (Omphalocele)

The physiological midgut loop hernia in the amniotic sac which is present up to 10 weeks of gestation, fails to return to the abdomen. Normal rotation and fixation of the intestines does not occur. The defect in the abdominal wall may be small, less than 5 cm (exomphalos minor) containing gut only, or larger than 5 cm (exomphalos major) containing intestines and liver. The amniotic sac covering may be intact or ruptured. The emergency treatment of both the ruptured and unruptured exomphalos should be immediate protection of the intestines with a sterile plastic bag. In the minor cases it is usually possible to return the intestines to the abdominal cavity and effect a primary closure of both muscle and skin. In the major cases it is not often possible to reduce or repair the lesion primarily. There are several alternative methods of treatment: (1) if the amniotic sac is intact, antiseptics may be applied daily until epithelization occurs from the edges; (2) the sac may be left intact and the skin only mobilized to close over the defect; (3) an artificial Silastic bag can be sewn around the defect to house the gut and liver temporarily, followed by staged reduction.

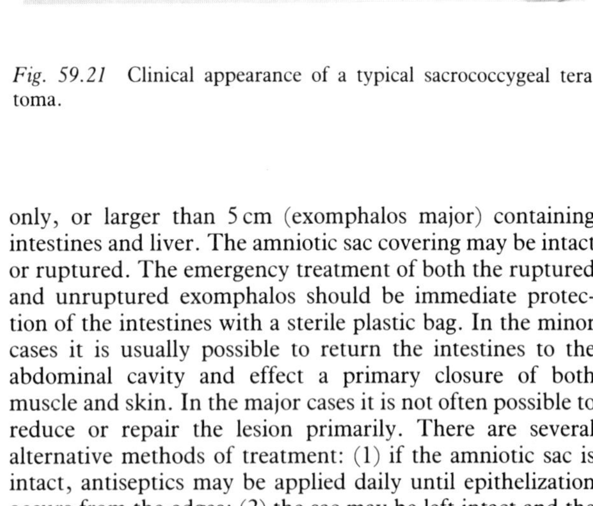

Gastroschisis

Gastroschisis is a protrusion of intestines from the abdominal cavity through a small defect to the right of the umbilicus. There is no sac visible. The gut which protrudes may vary from a normal appearance to being grossly oedematous and matted together. There is still argument as to whether gastroschisis and ruptured exomphalos are separate entities. As antenatal intrauterine rupture of an exomphalos minor will produce a similar picture to gastroschisis, and has been observed on antenatal ultrasound, this seems a more logical explanation. There are associated congenital anomalies frequently in exomphalos major but not in exomphalos minor or gastroschisis. In spite of the large amount of gut protruding and the oedematous nature of the bowel wall, primary closure is usually possible and gut function returns in 2–3 weeks. During this time intravenous feeding can be employed.

The umbilicus is also the site of urachal remnants (*see* Chapter 82) and vitello-intestinal remnants (*see* Chapter 72).

DUPLICATION OF THE ALIMENTARY TRACT

Duplications of the alimentary tract may be spherical or tubular structures and can occur anywhere from the tongue to the anus. They have three characteristics: first, attachment to at least one point of the alimentary tract, second, a well-developed coat of smooth muscle, and third the epithelial lining resembles some part of the alimentary tract. Most lie on the mesenteric aspect of the adjacent bowel or between layers of mesentery.

In the chest duplications arise as cysts in the posterior mediastinum, attached in the region of the lower cervical or upper thoracic vertebrae. Occasionally, these duplications are extensive, passing from the chest to the abdomen, through the diaphragm to reach the stomach or small bowel. Most commonly, the abdominal duplications are globular cysts, attached to the mesenteric border of the small bowel or ileal-caecal region (*Table* 59.7). Subserosal, intraluminal or tubular duplications also arise. Duplications of the colon and rectum are less common. The embryological explanation for these duplications is that the entoderm and ectoderm remain fused in the region of the notochord. Approximately 50% have anterior spina bifida or hemivertebrae in the region of the second thoracic vertebra.

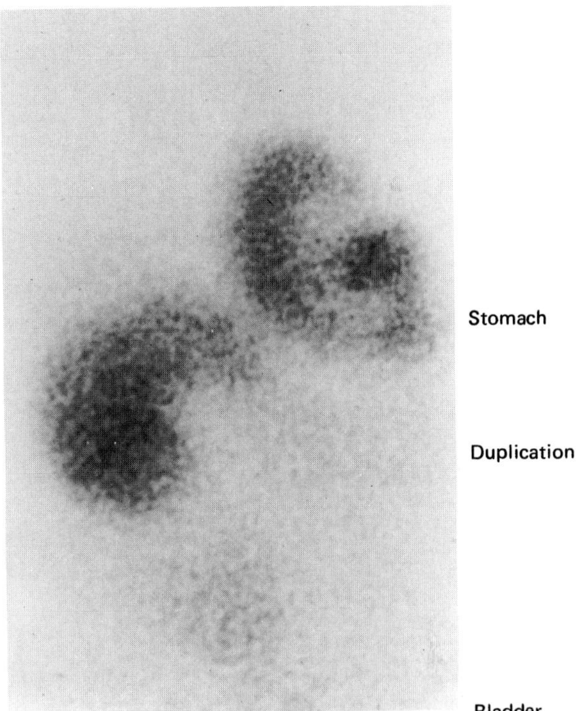

Fig. 59.22 Technetium isotope scan ($^{99}Tc^{m}$) showing stomach, bladder and large area of ectopic gastric mucosa to the right of the umbilicus.

Table 59.7 Distribution of 300 enteric duplications

Base of tongue	1
Intrathoracic	61
Related to stomach	6
Related to duodenum	22
Related to small intestine	136
Related to ileocaecal junction	26
Related to caecum	17
Related to remaining colon	9
Related to colon	9
Related to rectum	10
Intraperitoneal	8
Retroperitoneal	4
Preperitoneal	20

Symptoms

These depend on the site of the duplication and the age of the child. In the chest there may be respiratory distress as the cyst lined with mucus-secreting epithelium increases in volume. In the abdomen, the cyst may remain asymptomatic or cause obstruction by intraluminar projection, or by ribboning of the bowel across the cyst. In the tubular duplications the lining is gastric epithelium, and peptic ulcers may occur at the junction with the small bowel. Painless bleeding, in the form of melaena may be the only presenting feature. A radiograph of the chest may show the vertebral deformity in the upper thoracic spine in approximately 50% of cases. Ultrasound, computerized tomography, or the use of technetium pertechnetate ($^{99}Tc^{m}$) may confirm the presence of extrinsic gastric mucosa within the abdomen (*Fig.* 59.22).

Treatment is by surgical excision of the duplication together with adjacent bowel if necessary (*Fig.* 59.23). If an extensive resection of normal bowel appears necessary, stripping of the mucosa, but leaving the serosa, is a satisfactory alternative.

JAUNDICE

As stated previously 75% of normal newborn babies suffer from physiological jaundice. The majority of remaining cases have hyperbilirubinaemia due to unconjugated bilirubin. This group require extensive investigation to exclude haemolytic causes, ABO and Rh incompatibility, infection due to Australia antigen, rubella virus, cytomegalic virus, toxoplasmosis and syphilis, metabolic disorders, galactosaemia and alpha 1-antitrypsin deficiency.

From the practical point of view, the surgeon must exclude an obstructive cause for the jaundice. Formerly, the main differentiation was between 'neonatal hepatitis' and 'biliary atresia'. The distinction between these groups is now becoming blurred. It is now thought that this is a wide spectrum with 'neonatal hepatitis' at one end of the scale and 'biliary atresia' at the other, which may also be time related, with progression from one to the other. It is still customary to talk of intra- and extrahepatic biliary atresia. In intrahepatic atresia there may be a recognizable extrahepatic tree but no interlobular ducts. In the extrahepatic atresia the ducts are obstructed throughout or in part. A liver biopsy shows retention of bile, proliferation of bile ductules and some degree of fibrosis.

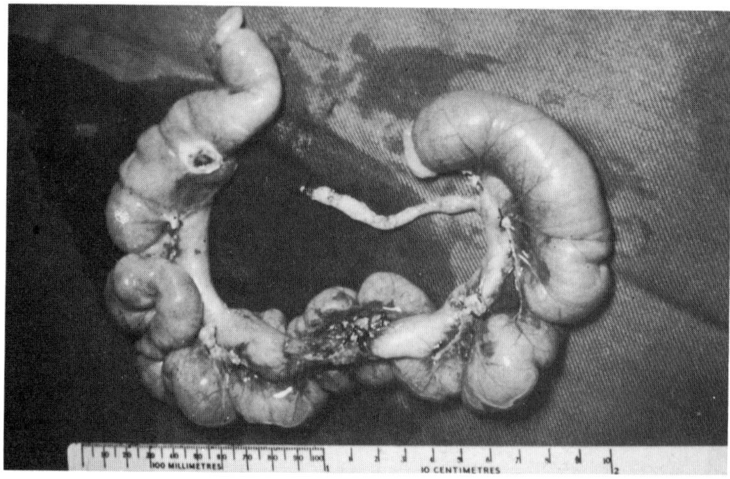

Fig. 59.23 Resected specimen of ileum together with long tubular duplication showing perforated gastric ulcer at distal end.

Diagnosis

Although several tests have been suggested as being specific, none are diagnostic. The first stool (meconium) which the infant passes in biliary atresia is always black or green and contains bile. The stools then become pale, the jaundice does not progress steadily but the level tends to plateau at about 300 µmol/l. The bilirubin is predominantly conjugated and the alkaline phosphatase is raised. Apart from the routine liver function tests, a radio-isotope scan (HIDA) may be helpful in demonstrating secretion of isotope into the duodenum, and an ultrasound scan of the liver may show dilated ducts or the presence of a choledochal cyst (*see Fig.* 59.6). If a clear-cut cause for the jaundice is not found by 4–6 weeks of age, a liver biopsy (needle) is imperative, and this should be performed within 2 months of birth. The cirrhosis is progressive, and fibrosis may become irreversible. Drainage procedures, such as the Kasai hepatic portoenterostomy, are unlikely to be successful the longer the cirrhosis is allowed to continue before surgery. If the needle biopsy indicates atresia, a limited laparotomy, with an operative cholangiogram to confirm that no suitable duct system exists, followed by a Kasai hepatic portoenterostomy or one of the many modifications may be carried out. The results of this procedure appear to be very much better in Japan than those obtained by European and American surgeons, i.e. about 30% produce bile; of these, about one-quarter survive for 5 years, but 30% of these will develop portal hypertension and oesophageal varices.

PYLORIC STENOSIS

In order to identify the specific condition found in babies, the terms 'infantile pyloric stenosis' or 'congenital pyloric stenosis' are used, these are usually shortened to 'pyloric stenosis'.

In infants, although the condition is termed congenital, the exact nature of the disease is unknown. Congenital hypertrophic pyloric stenosis has not been reported in stillborn infants. The stenosis appears to develop between 4 and 6 weeks after birth, and this holds true whether the baby is of forty weeks gestation (mature) or premature.

Although the exact cause of pyloric stenosis is uncertain, there are several interesting known facts. A definite genetic or hereditary factor is present. Mothers, who themselves have had pyloric stenosis, have a 1 in 5 chance of producing an affected child. The overall incidence of pyloric stenosis is about 1 in 400 live births (this is about equal to the incidence of spina bifida). As there is a preponderance of affected males (4:1), about 1 in every 150 male children and 1 in every 600 female children will be affected. First-born children are more often affected, and there is also a racial and social class difference. Babies of professional parents are more often affected than expected.

Experimental work in animals has not substantiated theories relating to absent or immature ganglion cells in the pyloric canal. This concept stems from the idea that pyloric stenosis is a similar disease to Hirschsprung's disease in which there is an absence of ganglion cells in the anus and rectum. This aganglionic area acts as a physiological obstruction to the passage of faeces, and the colon proximal to the aganglionic segment hypertrophies and dilates, but there is no 'tumour' as in pyloric stenosis.

In pregnant bitches receiving injections of pentagastrin or being stressed during pregnancy, there has resulted pyloric hypertrophy in newborn puppies, similar to that seen in humans.

The pathology of infantile pyloric stenosis is quite distinctive. There is gross hypertrophy and oedema of the circular sphincter muscle of the pylorus, which produces the typical 'tumour'. There is, also, oedema of the submucosa which produces narrowing of the canal (*Fig.* 59.24).

Clinical Features

Vomiting is the main presenting feature of babies with pyloric stenosis and certain features of the vomiting are characteristic.

1. The onset of the vomiting rarely occurs soon after birth, but is usually delayed for 3–4 weeks, the baby having been previously well.

2. The vomit is described as projectile. Projectile vomiting is merely an indication of forceful vomiting. The vomiting usually starts as small regurgitations and increases in

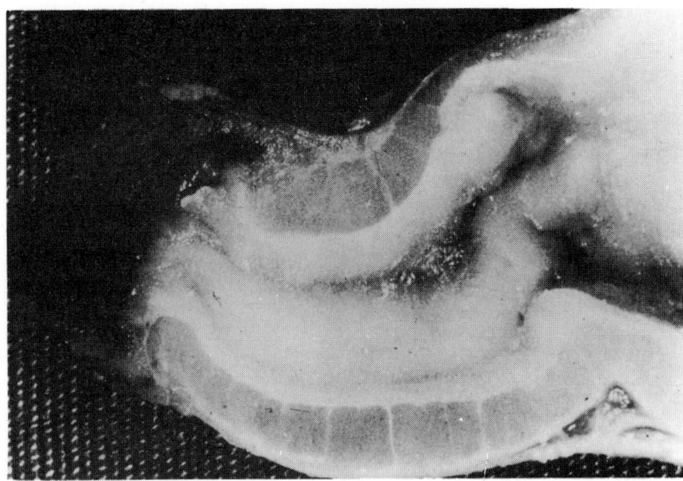

Fig. 59.24 Cross-section of pylorus showing gross oedema of the submucosa and narrowing of the pyloric canal.

volume and force as the obstruction becomes more complete. As the stomach hypertrophies, the vomiting becomes more and more forceful.

3. The vomitus is never bile stained.

4. The vomitus usually contains curdled milk, but may contain altered blood. The cause of the bleeding is due to gastritis which in turn is due to retention of the feed and gastric stasis.

5. The vomiting usually occurs during or shortly after a feed. In contradistinction to most other babies who vomit, the baby with pyloric stenosis will usually take more feed immediately after a vomit with some degree of eagerness.

The loss of the calories and water by vomiting is made worse by the excess loss of gastric juice secreted into the stomach, which contains large amounts of hydrogen, sodium, potassium and chloride ions, producing a metabolic alkalosis. Because no food, water or gastric juice reaches the bowel, the stools become more constipated or, occasionally, small frequent green stools—'hunger stools'—may be passed. Similarly, urine becomes scanty and concentrated and other signs of clinical dehydration are present; the skin turgor is reduced and the fontanelle and eyes are sunken, although the baby remains mentally alert.

The pulse and respiratory rate may be increased, and in severe advanced dehydration the baby may be lethargic or stuporose.

Diagnosis

The diagnosis is usually suspected on the history. Two physical signs are necessary to confirm the diagnosis.

1. The violent contractions of the hypertrophied obstructed stomach cause visible peristalsis. Gastric contractions, golf ball in size, appear as waves from under the left costal margin and move slowly from left to right across the epigastrium towards the umbilicus. These waves can be seen more definitely if the epigastrium is viewed with illumination from one side or from an oblique angle (*Fig.* 59.25).

2. The palpation of the pyloric 'tumour'. The tumour or swelling of the pylorus is caused by the oedema of the circular muscle and submucosa obstructing the pyloric canal. It varies in size and in hardness from moment to moment, depending on the degree of contraction of the pylorus. The tumour is best felt when the stomach is full and contracting.

For these two diagnostic physical signs to be elicited, three people need to be comfortable—the mother (or nurse), the baby, and the doctor. The examination should not be hurried and may take 20 min or more to confirm the presence of gastric peristalsis and the presence of a pyloric tumour. Eliciting these physical signs in ideal conditions forms the basis of a test feed. To carry out a test feed a warm draught-free room or corner of a ward is needed. The nurse should be seated holding the baby with the abdomen fully exposed across her knee. The doctor sits opposite the nurse so that the epigastrium can be inspected for any signs of gastric peristalsis, making sure the light falls obliquely from the side, and so that the epigastrium can be palpated with the middle finger of the left hand. The baby should be given a bottle feed of milk or may be fed from the breast. Milk should be used for the test feed rather than dextrose as it appears to induce strong contractions of the stomach and obstruction of the pylorus whereas a clear dextrose-saline feed may not. The baby usually takes the feed eagerly. As the stomach fills up with air and milk the outline of the stomach can be seen in the epigastrium, after which gastric contractions are noted towards the pylorus and becoming more and more forceful. These contractions frequently precede a large projectile vomit.

The left hand is laid across the epigastrium and an attempt is made to feel the 'tumour' against the vertebrae whilst the baby is sucking and relaxed. In spite of the anatomical position of the duodenum to the right of the midline, the tumour is more often felt in the midline between the recti muscles. Doctors or medical students feeling a tumour for the first time are often surprised at the small size of the tumour as it feels like a 'peanut under a blanket'. The tumour when palpated through the abdominal wall feels about the size of a peanut whereas when inspected at operation the pyloric thickening may measure about 2 cm × 1·5 cm × 1·5 cm.

Gastric peristalsis and a tumour should be confirmed by two observers before surgical treatment is undertaken. In about 5–10% of cases, even after more than one test feed the

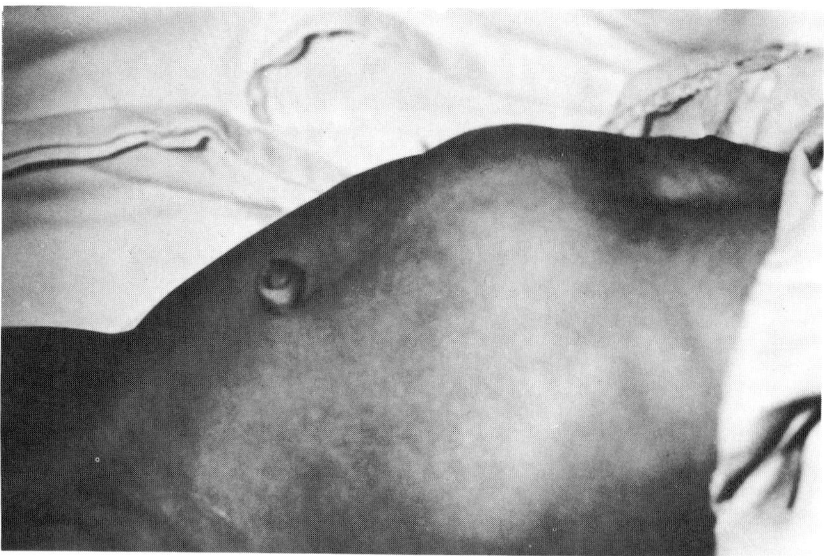

Fig. 59.25 Oblique illumination showing gastric peristalsis across the epigastrium.

examiner may still be in doubt about the diagnosis. In these cases a barium meal radiograph should be performed and this will confirm the diagnosis. Ultrasound can be used to determine the thickness of the pyloric muscle.

Differential Diagnosis

Unsatisfactory feeding technique or overfeeding is probably the commonest other condition giving rise to a suspicion of pyloric stenosis.

Hiatus hernia may give a very similar picture but the vomiting starts in the first week or two after birth, the vomitus is less copious, more frequent and effortless and may contain altered blood.

Hirschsprung's disease may be referred as pyloric stenosis, but the abdominal distension and constipation are distinguishing features. Projectile vomiting at this age is also seen in the adrenogenital syndrome with raised intracranial pressure. Rare conditions, such as enteric duplications and ectopic pancreas should also be considered.

Treatment

Once the diagnosis is confirmed the baby should be prepared for pyloromyotomy. However, in certain countries an alternative form of treatment, the so-called medical treatment is used. This consists of graduated diluted feeds, frequent stomach washouts and the use of the atropine-like drug Skopyl (methyl scopolamine nitrate) drops (2–3 drops) given before feeds to relax the pylorus. As the results of surgery are so good, this rather prolonged and uncertain form of treatment is hardly ever used today.

Operation is never an emergency, and time must be spent to make sure that the baby is in optimum condition prior to surgery. This may delay operation for 24–48 h. Sometimes the baby has been vomiting for days or even weeks before the diagnosis is established, with the result that the baby is extremely ill and grossly dehydrated, probably weighing much less than the original birthweight. In these cases especially, correction of the fluid and electrolyte status is important.

Attention must be directed to the following points:

1. Fluid and electrolyte balance: as the baby has been vomiting (and losing large amounts of water, sodium, potassium and chloride ions from the stomach) this biochemical disturbance must be corrected. The operation should be

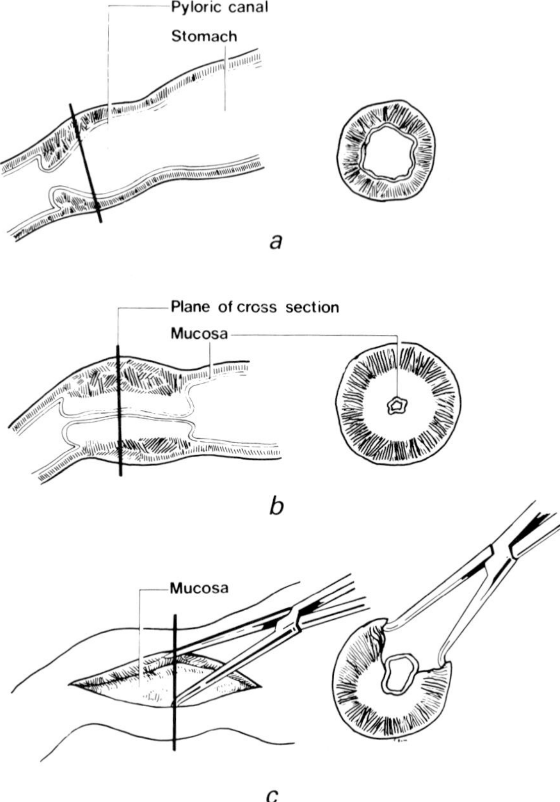

Fig. 59.26 Diagram showing: (*a*) normal pylorus; (*b*) pylorus with thickened circular fibres and oedema of submucosa; (*c*) myotomy with release of submucosa.

delayed for 24–36 h if the blood urea is raised or if the chloride is below 100 mmol/l.

The metabolic alkalosis which exists is best corrected by using intravenous normal saline and added potassium (up to 10 mmol/kg/24 h).

2. The retention of the food and fluid in the stomach leads to gastritis and an attempt should be made to reduce the inflammation before operation. This is best achieved by the passage of an 8 or 10 F gauge nasogastric tube and washing out the stomach using 50–100 ml of saline, not water, due to the osmotic effect of water on the extracellular fluid. The stomach washout should be repeated several times before operation if the gastritis is severe. The nasogastric tube should be left in situ and unspiggoted after the washout. The baby may be offered dextrose saline foods whilst awaiting operation as non-milk tends to pass through the obstructed pylorus without causing vomiting.

Operation

Pyloromyotomy is performed under general anaesthesia. There is no place today for local anaesthesia. The anaesthetic should be given by an experienced anaesthetist as the induction of anaesthesia in a baby with pyloric stenosis, inadequately prepared for operation, can be very hazardous.

A small laparotomy incision (about 2·5 cm) is made over the upper right rectus muscle. The muscle is cut with diathermy so that there is virtually no bleeding. The abdomen is entered, the stomach identified and withdrawn, first the greater curvature and then the pylorus. The appearance of the tumour is typical. The myotomy procedure consists of holding the pylorus between the thumb and index finger and splitting the thickened muscle down to the mucosa and allowing this to bulge through (*Fig.* 59.26). The anaesthetist then injects 20 ml of air down the nasogastric tube to distend the stomach and the pylorus is tested to make sure that no hole has been made in the mucosa. The abdomen is closed in layers, using adhesive strips to close the skin.

Postoperative Management

The baby is returned to the ward with the nasogastric tube in place and unspigoted. The tube is aspirated at hourly intervals for 4 h. At 4 h a small saline stomach washout (20–50 ml) is carried out after which the tube is removed and oral feeding started, according to a pyloric regimen. The aim should be to get the baby onto full strength, full volume feeds by about 48 h postoperatively, the basic principle being to alter one variable at a time, i.e. either volume or quality or time of the feed.

If the baby is breast fed, the stages of the pyloric regimen in which dextrose saline is used can be omitted. At 4 h the baby can be offered the breast for about 3 min and the length of time allowed on the breast can be increased at each hour until full feeding is achieved.

One or two vomits postoperatively are not uncommon, but if the vomiting is persistent a further stomach washout should be performed. The baby usually is well and gaining weight by 72 h and may be discharged home. The dressing may be removed from the wound in 5–6 days.

There is very rarely any additional associated anomaly with pyloric stenosis. The baby can be seen once in the outpatient department at about 2 weeks and then discharged from the clinic.

Further Reading

Connor J. M. and Ferguson-Smith M. A. (1984) *Essential Medical Genetics*. Oxford, Blackwell Scientific Publications.
Holder T. M. and Aschcraft K. W. (1980) *Pediatric Surgery*. Philadelphia, Saunders.
Mustard W. T., Ravitch M. M., Snyder W. H. et al. (1979) *Paediatric Surgery*, 3rd ed. Chicago, Year Book.
Rickham P., Lister J. and Irving I. (1978) *Neonatal Surgery*, 2nd ed. London, Butterworths.

60 The Breast

P. E. Preece

SURGICAL ANATOMICAL AND PHYSIOLOGICAL CONSIDERATIONS

The adult female breast has two components. These are the epithelial elements responsible for milk formation and transport, namely the acini and ducts, and the supporting tissues, muscle, fascia and fat. The epithelial elements consist of twenty or more lobes. Each lobe drains into a mammary duct, each of which ends separately at the nipple. The lobe consists of lobules, the number of which is very variable. Each lobule is a collection of between ten and a hundred acini grouped around, and converging on a collecting duct.

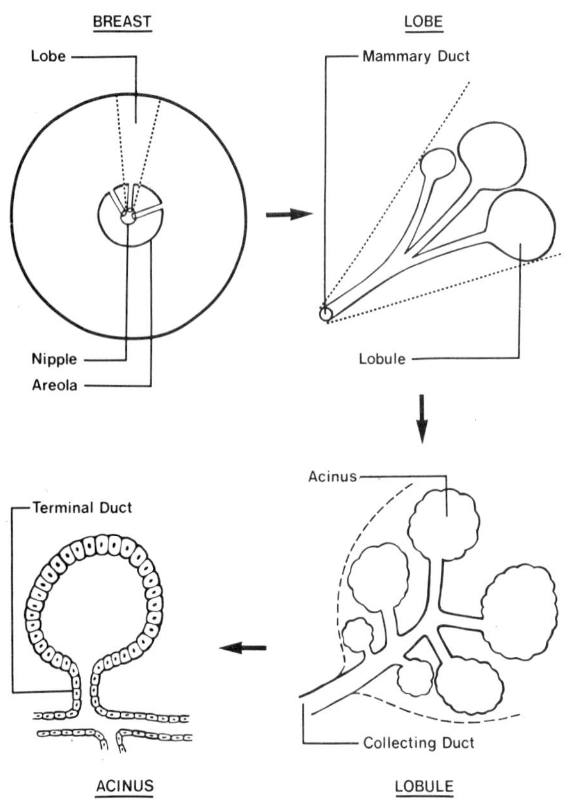

Fig. 60.1 Schematic anatomy of breast.

Each acinus is a sphere of cells capable of milk secretion, draining into a terminal duct. It is the confluence of the terminal ducts which gives rise to a collecting duct. Looking at the breast from the front, as shown in *Fig.* 60.1, the major mammary ducts lie behind the areola. The lobules occupy the more peripheral part of the breast.

The breast and axilla have surgically significant fascial planes which are usually well defined. The breast being a modified gland of the skin, it occupies a space within an envelope of superficial fascia. At operation, the plane between the small fat particles of the true subcutaneous fat (the panniculus adiposus) and the larger nodules of fat of the gland, is seen. It is loosely adherent and usually easily opened, often by strong retraction alone. In the axilla, the clavipectoral fascia, which passes from the inferior surface of the clavicle, invests pectoralis minor and ends in the skin of the floor of the axilla, is prominent as soon as the axilla is opened. Early incision of this is the key to safe and accurate exploration of the axilla.

Arterial blood to the breast comes from several sources, the lateral thoracic and acromiothoracic branches of the axillary artery, branches of the intercostal arteries, and branches of the internal mammary artery which perforate the intercostal spaces and pectoralis major muscle. Malignant tumours of the breast often induce substantial hypervascularity. The nipple and areola are the furthest away from the sources of arterial input, and their blood supply can therefore be jeopardized, especially by laterally placed incisions if these are close to the areolar margin.

The venous drainage of the breast is both superficial and deep. The superficial veins are significant because they anastomose across the midline of the anterior chest wall. The deep veins accompany the arteries. In considering the natural history of breast cancer, it is the intercostal veins which have particular significance. In addition to draining into the azygos systems, they also communicate with the vertebral veins. Such a route could explain the predilection of bone metastases from breast cancer for the axial skeleton.

Lymph vessels and nodes are even more variable than veins. Nevertheless they are highly significant in the dissemination of breast cancer. Lymph channels from the breast do not cross the midline, but they do cross the diaphragm, where they communicate with lymphatics of the liver. The regional lymph nodes of the breast are predominantly those of the axilla, but also those alongside the internal mammary artery. Many different classifications and

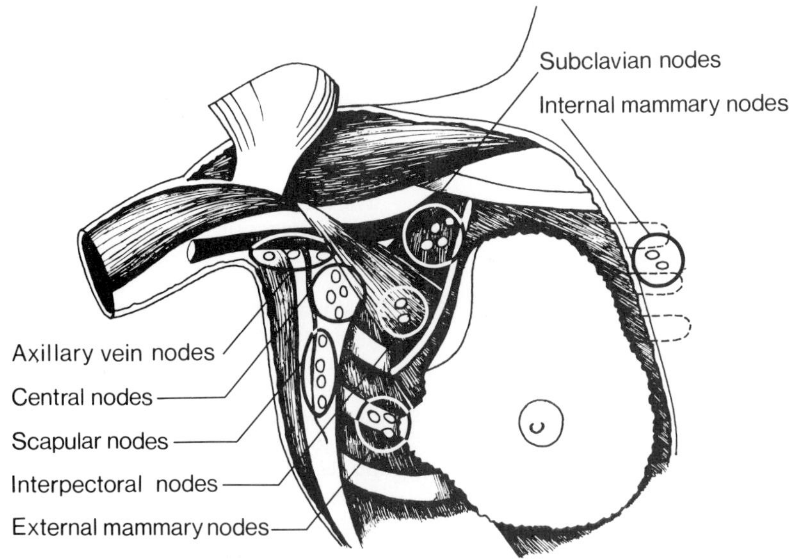

Fig. 60.2 Surgically identifiable axillary nodes.

names have been used for the axillary nodes. The accompanying *Fig.* 60.2 is a distillation of a scheme which enables ready surgical identification of axillary nodes. Internal mammary nodes are normally very small—usually only a few millimetres in diameter. They are to be found mostly behind the first three intercostal spaces, and always within 3 cm of the ipsilateral margin of the sternum. Their small size means that if not hyperplastic or neoplastic, they may well not be recognized by the naked eye, a fact which also applies, although to a lesser extent, to axillary nodes. Lymph passing through either the axillary or the internal mammary nodes reaches the jugulosubclavian venous confluence. If this is obstructed, then the lymph will pass in a retrograde way to the supraclavicular nodes.

CLINICAL INTRODUCTION

The underlying cause of complaints about the breast proves to be benign in the overwhelming majority of cases. Breast symptoms, however, induce such great anxiety in the patient that malignancy needs to be excluded as speedily as possible. The first steps in this are the classic ones of history and physical examination.

Essential points in the history include age and menstrual status, since most benign breast disease occurs during reproductive life, and family and reproductive history, as affected blood relatives and low parity are associated with mammary malignancy. So far, evidence shows no increased risks from the contraceptive pill, which may even protect against cancer. The effect of lactation is controversial, but for the individual case is unhelpful. The past medical history, particularly of previous abscess or surgery, can be helpful in interpreting both physical signs and mammograms.

In physical examination of patients with a breast complaint the patient sits, stripped to the waist. Attention is paid to:

General Appearance: Nourishment, colour, mucous membranes, palms.

Inspection from bed end
- i. Arms at side
- ii. Arms elevated

Looking for
- *a.* Symmetry of nipples and breasts
- *b.* Nipple abnormalities
- *c.* Vascularity
- *d.* Indrawing or prominence of skin
- *e.* Tethering
- *f.* Peau d'orange
- *g.* Skin nodules
- *h.* Ulceration

Palpation: with patient in the supine position
- *a.* Supraclavicular fossae
- *b.* Breasts
  - i. Lightly
  - ii. Deeply
    systematically from areola concentrically outwards including axillary tail
- *c.* Axillae
  - i. Taking weight of patient's forearm on examiner's
  - ii. Both axillae simultaneously from behind patient
- *d.* Abdomen, for ascites, hepatomegaly or abnormal masses

Chest
Inspection, percussion, auscultation

CNS
For symmetry of tone, power and reflexes

Locomotor
Percussion for tenderness over spine, straight leg raising.

Particularly valuable in practice are: (*a*) Inspection with arms firstly dependent, then elevated; (*b*) Initial light touch over the breasts prior to systematic deeper palpation in concentric circles, working outwards; (*c*) simultaneous examination of axillae performed from behind the patient.

A practical programme for the investigation of breast complaints may include one or more of the following:

Mammography — Conventional / Xeromammography — Localizing techniques for subclinical disease

Tissue diagnosis — Drill biopsy / Tru-cut needle / Fine needle aspiration / Excision with cryo or paraffin histology

Laboratory investigations
- Hb WBC Film ESR
- Liver function tests
- Calcium, phosphorus, alkaline phosphatase
- Plasma gonadotrophins
- Urinary hydroxyproline–creatinine ratio

Radiology
- Chest radiograph
- Radiographs of lumbosacral spine + pelvis
- Radiographs of sites of symptoms
- Isotope scintigraphy—bone, liver, brain
- Liver ultrasound scanning
- CT scanning

Surgery
- Laparoscopy
- Axillary dissection
- Internal mammary node biopsy
- Biopsy of suspected metastases

Mammography

Two techniques in radiology will reveal the architecture of soft tissues, without the need to use contrast media. Applied to the breast, these techniques produce respectively 'conventional mammograms' and 'xeromammograms'. Each has some advantages over the other, and the individual user tends to favour the one with which he has most experience. The basic radiological signs suspicious of malignancy are asymmetry, skin thickening, a mass (with several characteristic subtypes), distorted architecture and microcalcification.

Mammography is specially useful in supporting a clinical impression of absence of malignancy. It increases the rate of recognition of breast cancer, both in the breast of complaint and in the contralateral gland. In particular, it reveals the unsuspected, impalpable, 'subclinical' cancers.

Mammography for diagnostic purposes is done in two planes, craniocaudal and mediolateral. These enable occult lesions to be precisely localized. Combining mammography with eye, dye or needle localizing techniques ensures accurate sampling and avoids performing mutilating excision biopsies.

Mammography also has a role in the follow-up of patients who have had cancer of one breast treated. The enhanced risk of developing cancer of the second breast justifies a policy of follow-up mammography at two-yearly intervals. Careful comparison between current and previous views is essential for early recognition of a new tumour.

Mammography has an obvious place in programmes of screening for breast cancer. To be useful, the examination must be repeated at intervals over many years, the radiation dose for these purposes being kept as low as possible. Taking a single oblique view of the breast is one method used. Classification of mammographic appearances has been suggested as a means of identifying patients particularly at risk of developing cancer. A four-point scale is defined, N_1—normal, D_1—minimally prominent duct pattern, P_2—severely prominent duct pattern, and DY—the diffusely radiodense or 'dysplastic' breast (*Fig.* 60.3). P_2 and DY are the categories regarded as having an increased risk. The disadvantage of the system is that it is not easy to know how much radiodensity—which is a normal feature in the young

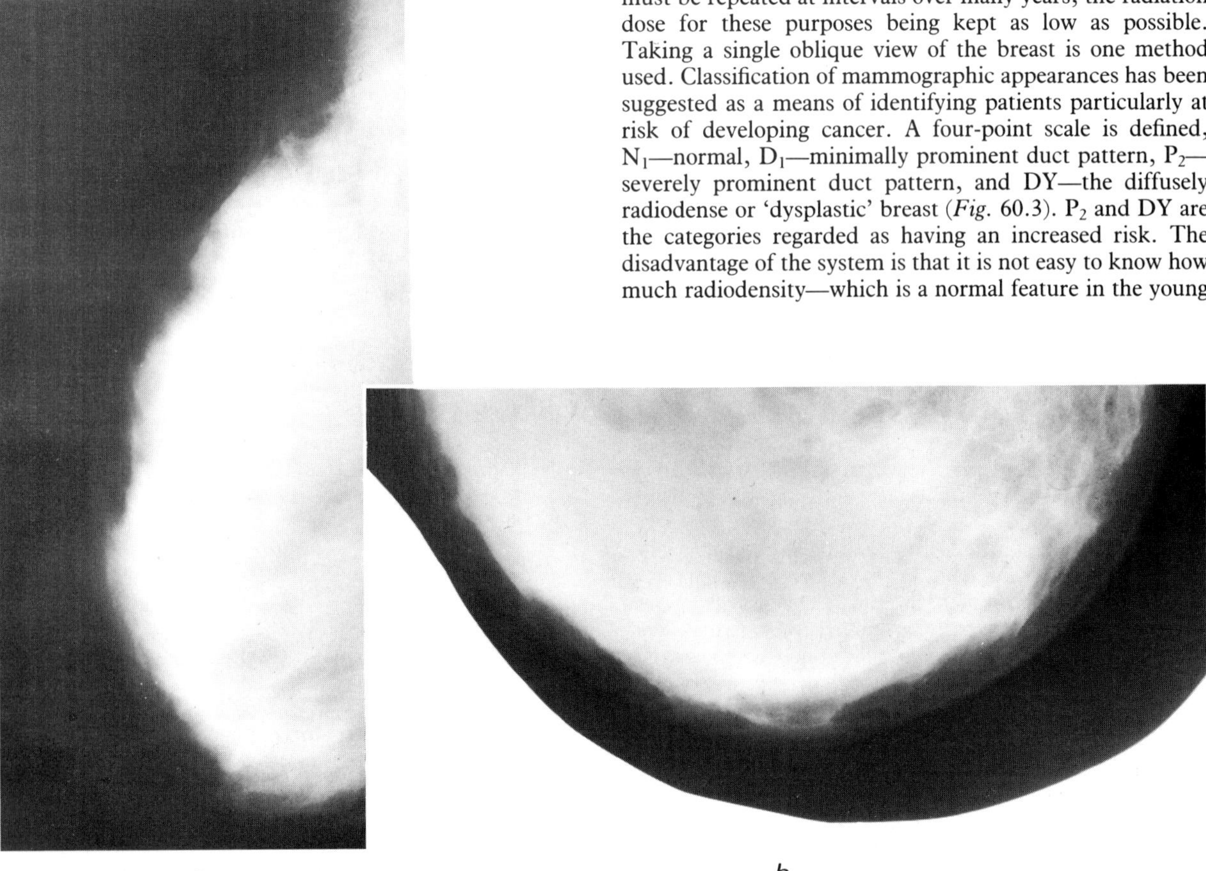

Fig. 60.3 *a*, Craniocaudal, and *b*, Mediolateral mammograms of 'dysplastic' breast in a woman aged 38 years.

breast—to allow for age. Precise complete histological correlation with radiographic images still needs to be performed.

Tissue Diagnosis

Drill biopsy, using a compressed air-driven rotary drill can be performed under local anaesthesia. The apparatus is rather cumbersome, and noisy, which increases the alarm of already apprehensive patients. Its advantage is that as long as the lesion is big enough, the material obtained is very satisfactory for histological diagnosis.

Tru-cut needle biopsy can be performed under local anaesthesia, but it is not suitable for lesions less than 1 cm in diameter. Ecchymoses and haematoma follow in a definite proportion of cases.

Fine needle aspiration for cytology rarely requires local anaesthesia. Satisfactory use of the technique requires the cooperation of a skilled cytologist. Immediate provisional results can be given. Immediate reporting has the advantage that if the first sample is inadequate, a repeat is easily obtained.

For excision biopsy, general anaesthesia is required. In these circumstances the patient is often uncertain preoperatively of what will be done. Even when frozen section is used, the answer cannot always be given immediately. For difficult proliferative lesions, an urgent paraffin histology is preferred to frozen-section histology in some centres.

Laboratory Investigations

Haematological examination rules out marrow deposits and leucoerythroblastic anaemia. A raised alkaline phosphatase and gamma glutamyl transpeptidase test will point to liver metastases in 50% of patients with hepatic deposits. Abnormal serum calcium, phosphate and alkaline phosphatase levels can give a clue that metastasis to bone has occurred. Plasma gonadotrophin levels, taken with 17-beta oestradiol will clarify menopausal status when this is in doubt, as, for example, after hysterectomy.

Twenty-four hour urinary hydroxyproline/creatinine ratio, measured in a sample collected while the patient is on a gelatin-free diet, can also point to otherwise unsuspected bone metastases.

Radiology

Radiological investigations (radiology and scintiscanning) are indicated for patients with breast cancer in an attempt at staging the extent of the disease.

Isotopic scans are not universally available. They are, in any case, of very limited value. Liver isotope scans are less discriminating than the biochemical tests of liver function mentioned above when normal but have a higher predictive value when abnormal. Ultrasound and CT liver scans are more reliable in confirming hepatic deposits. Pooled data on results of bone scanning in what can be called 'routine' use (as opposed to highly specialized research use) shows that the initial pick up rate of true occult bone metastases is poor. A high yield of suspicious lesions occurs which requires localized conventional radiology to clarify. The majority of these prove to be benign, and the diagnosis remains equivocal in some.

The best compromise currently available is *limited* radiological skeletal survey. A chest radiograph will be done in any case for most patients undergoing general anaesthesia. Plain radiographs of lumbosacral spine, pelvis, and any site where the patient complains of bone pain, complete the routine radiological investigation.

Views of thoracic inlet or cervical spine help in localizing non-neoplastic causes of breast complaints, such as cervical spondylosis and cervical rib.

Surgery

Surgical procedures have been used to stage the extent of the disease in patients with cancer of the breast. Unless there has been previous abdominal surgery or inflammation, laparoscopy allows good visualization of most of the peritoneal cavity and its contents. In particular, ovaries and liver are easily seen, and liver metastases can be biopsied percutaneously, with accurate localization via the laparoscope. Axillary and internal mammary node biopsy requires general anaesthesia, and each also necessitates approach by open operation.

Other suspected metastases may be sampled either by Tru-cut needle for histology or fine needle aspiration for cytology.

BENIGN DISEASES OF THE FEMALE BREAST

Symptoms

The symptoms of benign breast disease are the same as those of malignant disorders, but in reverse order of frequency, (i) *Pain*, (ii) *Nipple complaints*, (iii) *Lumps* and *Size/shape problems*. Benign breast disease is much the commonest reason for medical consultation relating to breast complaints.

Pain

The majority of women who see their family doctor because of a breast complaint have mastalgia amongst their symptoms. Perhaps because of the very frequency of the complaint, and its rare association with life-threatening problems, it has come to be regarded as of psychoneurotic origin. Measurement of psychoneurotic traits in women with this complaint shows them to be no more neurotic than women of similar age presenting with varicose veins. Observation of social and occupational activity of these patients gives a clear impression that most are balanced and productive members of the community—many being both housewives and mothers, as well as participating in gainful employment.

The accompanying is a classification of mastalgia, derived from close study of over four hundred cases:

Cyclical pronounced
Trigger point
Tietze's syndrome
Previous trauma
Sclerosing adenosis
Cancer
Miscellaneous and idiopathic

Numerically preponderant are the cyclical pronounced group—where the symptom has a clear relationship in time with the menstrual cycle, and the trigger point group where there is no time pattern, but a focal point within the breast from which the symptom consistently originates. The remaining types are much less common, but awareness of their existence greatly assists the management of these patients.

Cyclical pronounced mastalgia (*Fig.* 60.4) is so called since the pain has an obvious cycle-related pattern in time, and is pronounced either by virtue of its intensity or its duration or both. Intensity can be such that marital relations may be impaired, or mothers may not be able to allow their

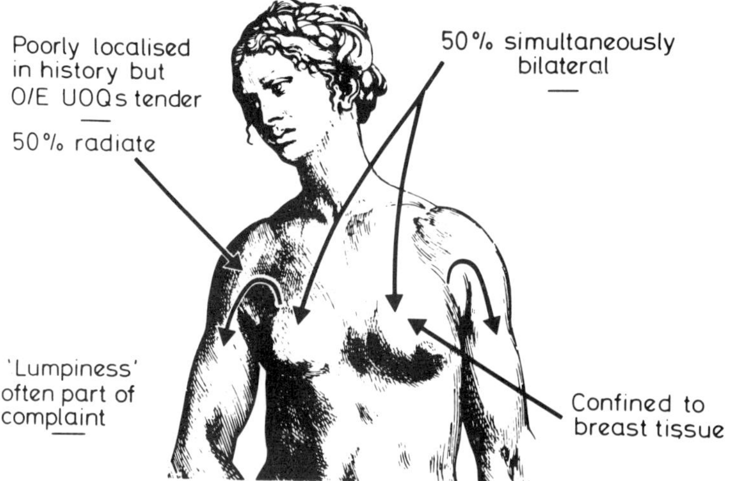

Fig. 60.4 Clinical features of cyclical pronounced mastalgia.

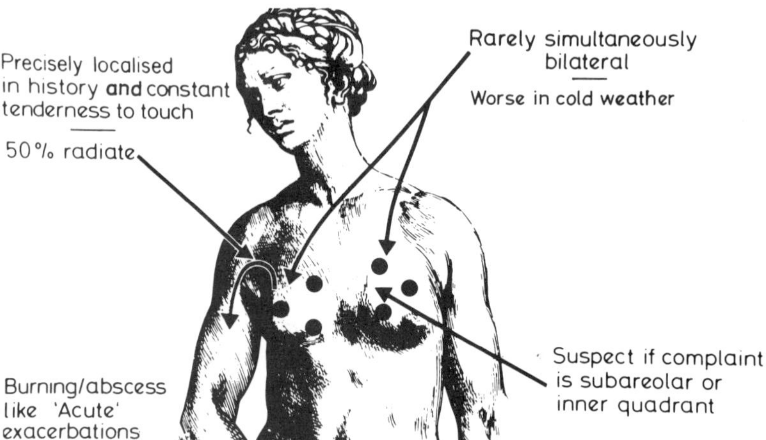

Fig. 60.5 Clinical features of trigger point pain.

children near them. Duration is often up to three-quarters of the length of each menstrual cycle. Cyclical pronounced mastalgia is often associated with palpable nodularity of the breast. This is a common clinical finding in the breasts of many women examined in the week just before menstruation is due. If biopsied it is often reported as fibroadenosis. Overall increase in total body water does not occur in these patients any more than in women with no breast symptoms.

Trigger point pain (*Fig.* 60.5) is quite distinct from cyclical pronounced, in its absence of any pattern in time, and the fact that it is consistently well localized by both the patient and the clinician. This type of pain may occur spontaneously, or may be chiefly precipitated by touch. Trigger point pain has a strong association with clinical, radiological and histopathological features of the 'duct ectasia/periductal mastitis' complex of disorders, either present or past.

The painful swollen tender costochondral junction which characterizes Tietze's syndrome is a well recognized cause of chest pain. With the female breast so closely related anatomically to the costochondral junction, this condition mimics and presents as pain in the breast.

Previous trauma to the breast may have been abscess, biopsy or injury. The scar, albeit deep in the breast and with no cutaneous component, can become a source of pain,

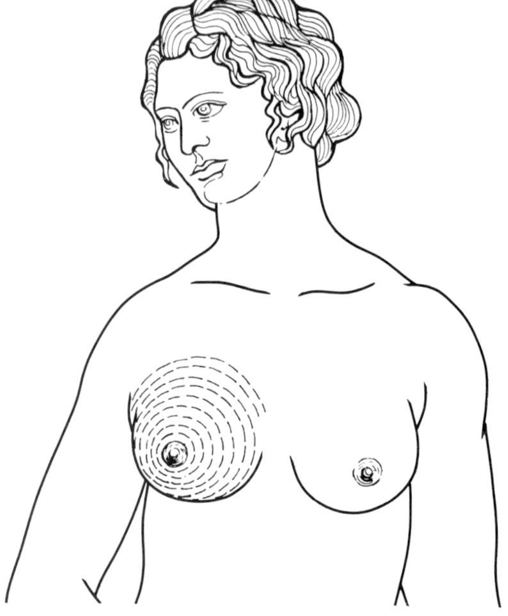

Fig. 60.6 Langer's lines on the breast.

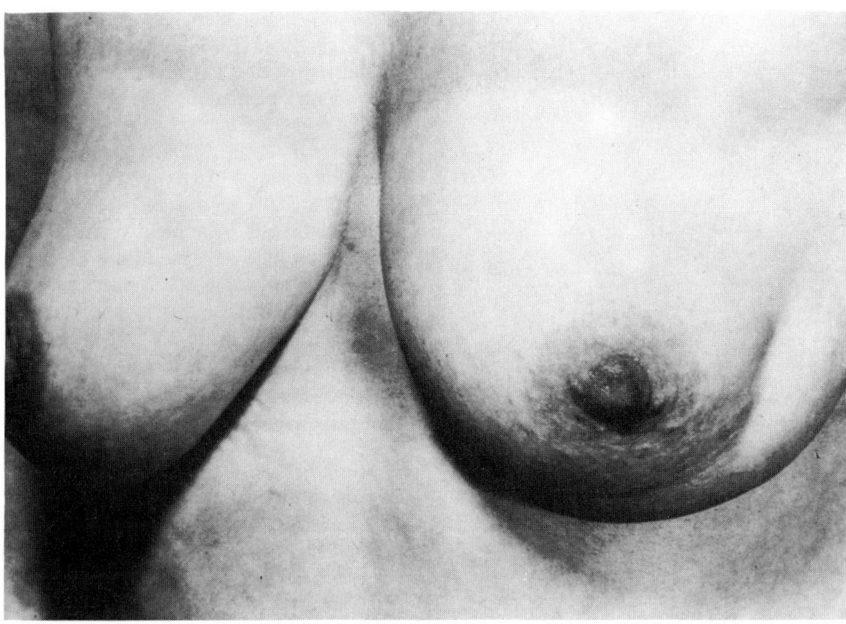

Fig. 60.7 Mondor's disease.

frequently many years after the initiating injury. Haematoma and biopsy incision made across Langer's lines (*Fig.* 60.6) predispose particularly to these painful sequelae.

Sclerosing adenosis has been a condition of importance to histopathologists rather than clinicians. Since in those cases ultimately classified as benign, it has proved to be the histopathology of the majority of biopsies done for mammographically defined suspicious lesions (usually microcalcification), it has acquired clinical significance. Many of these patients present with pain and on subsequent breast investigation a focus of suspicious microcalcification is observed on a mammogram, at the site of the pain, and can lead to the anticipation of this diagnosis. These suspicious subclinical lesions can be localized prior to excision biopsy by the techniques to be described. Urgent paraffin histology is preferable to frozen section for these mammographically defined lesions in view of difficulties with their histological interpretation.

It remains an irony, particularly to patients themselves, that pain does not commonly accompany the onset of cancer in the breast. Despite its infrequency, mastalgia can be the presenting symptom of operable breast cancer, and as such has particular potential usefulness for it can result in the diagnosis of tumours at an early stage—even subclinically—with the inherent prognostic advantages of this. Unfortunately, no particular subtypes of pain characterize these early tumours, to aid in distinguishing them from benign disease, apart from the fact that the pain is usually localized to the tumour.

Occasionally a fibroadenoma or a cyst can be painful. Discomfort in the breast is well recognized as being amongst the earliest symptoms of pregnancy, and perhaps by the same mechanism, it can follow commencement of an oral contraceptive. Fat necrosis, sclerosing periangitis of the lateral thoracic wall (Mondor's disease) and tuberculosis are causes of breast pain seen occasionally. The pathognomonic sign of Mondor's disease is guttering of the superficial veins of the breast (*Fig.* 60.7). Tuberculosis presents either as an abscess or like a malignant tumour, poorly demarcated and with skin attachment. Fat necrosis mimics cancer clinically and radiologically.

The origin of breast pain in some patients remains obscure, but the majority fall into one of the categories outlined above.

Nipple Complaints

RETRACTION. For a number of women, one or both nipples may never develop to the protruding form. This is a condition usually referred to as 'inversion'. Particularly if bilateral, the patient rarely complains, although the condition can cause difficulties with breast feeding. The drawing in or 'retraction' of a previously upstanding nipple is noticed by both patients and doctors, for both have been taught that this is associated with breast cancer. Nipple retraction accompanies benign breast disease more often than malignant. A useful distinguishing feature is that when the cause is benign, the retraction is often only partial and slit-like (*Fig.* 60.8). The inflammatory condition, periductal mastitis, associated with mammary duct ectasia, is the usual cause of benign nipple retraction.

DISCHARGE. White, cream or green nipple discharge, either thin, like milk or thick, like paste, is not sinister. Outwith a pregnancy, lactation and galactorrhoea, it is a feature of—indeed, almost pathognomonic of—mammary duct ectasia. Blood or serous nipple discharge can also be of benign origin, particularly if it consistently exudes from a single duct, as when due to a duct papilloma. Since this type of discharge can occur in cancer, investigation to exclude this possibility needs to be much more thorough than for the other types of discharge, and would usually include biopsy. A single duct can be adequately biopsied by microdochectomy. The most appropriate technique for obtaining histological material when discharge is from several ducts is subareolar duct excision (Urban's or Hadfield's operation) referred to later.

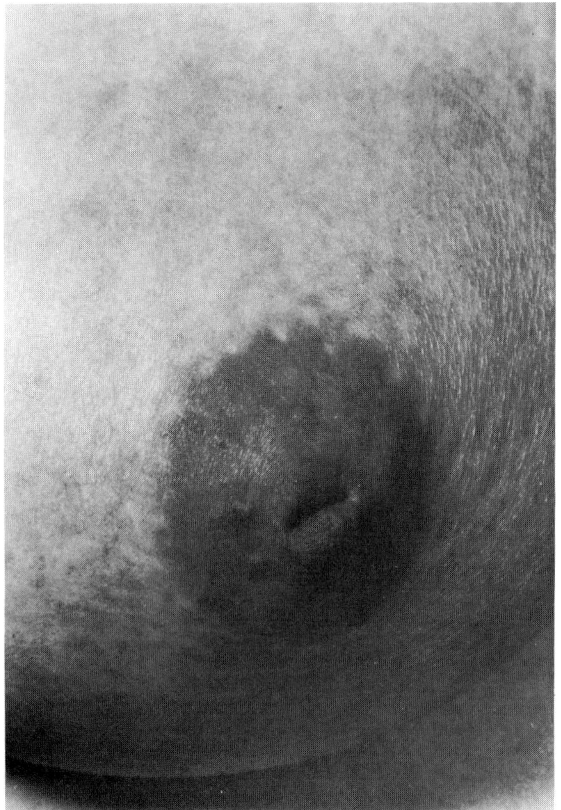

Fig. 60.8 Partial nipple retraction of duct ectasia.

SKIN CHANGE. Eczema of the nipple, usually extending on to the areola, is also a complication of mammary duct ectasia, and is usually secondary to chronic nipple discharge from this condition. In view of the difficulty of diagnosing Paget's disease of the nipple, biopsy of eczema-like lesions of the nipple is essential. In practice, the nipple and areola eczema of duct ectasia usually persists unless the ducts are excised. This provides the occasion for a histopathological diagnosis by means of which, if the skin lesion were Paget's disease, the underlying malignancy would be located in any case.

Lumps and Size/Shape Problems

These symptoms, arising from benign breast disease, present in the main during reproductive life, that is in premenopausal women. The age incidence of benign lumps can conveniently be thought of as:

teens and early twenties—fibroadenomas
twenties and thirties—fibroadenosis
forties and early fifties—cysts

Fibroadenoma ('adenofibroma') typically presents in a young woman as a usually painless lump. This lump is smooth, often spherical but may be lobulated, and highly mobile (hence 'breast mouse') without any attachment to skin or surrounding breast tissues. It feels hard, and proves to be solid on aspiration. More than one may be present. Size ranges from the smallest palpable at about 0·5 cm to huge, occupying all of and even more than the normal volume of the containing breast (*Fig.* 60.9). Giant fibroadenoma, known as cystosarcoma phylloides, is rare. With the exception of these rare giant forms, fibroadenomas, once they reach 2–3 cm diameter, do not grow further, and often remain this size for the rest of the patient's life. During pregnancy, fibroadenomas often enlarge, but usually involute again together with the rest of the breast, in the puerperium.

Fibroadenosis—stictly speaking a histopathological term—refers clinically to a very common syndrome of which the chief feature is lumpiness or multiple lumps. Many synonyms exist for this, including the pathologically imprecise terms 'chronic mastitis' and 'fibrocystic disease', and the eponyms 'Schimmelbusch disease' and the 'maladie de Reclus'. Palpable lumpiness is diffuse, as opposed to being discrete or localized. Commonly both breasts are affected similarly, and the upper outer quadrants and axillary tails tend to be most involved. The lumps have such ill-defined margins that they are difficult to measure, and they vary—tending to be most evident in the week before menstruation is due, and least evident just after a period. Pain, usually cyclical, may be associated. Cysts frequently coexist with fibroadenosis, but should not be regarded as an essential feature of the syndrome.

Cysts, or 'cystic disease', of the breasts, apart from occurring in a different age group, have very similar physical findings to fibroadenomas, i.e. they are usually painless, spherical, mobile, and often multiple. They often appear to become palpable over a very short interval of time. On aspiration fluid is obtained. This is usually watery, and either dirty brown, colourless or green. If frankly bloodstained, the possibility of intracystic carcinoma must be investigated. A residual lump after aspiration of a cyst should always be submitted to an excision biopsy.

Rare benign lumps include fat necrosis and, in women who have lactated within the past few months, the milk retention cyst known as a galactocele. As with simple cysts of the breasts, aspiration of galactoceles provides both the diagnosis as well as all the treatment that is necessary.

Gross under- or over-development of one or both female breasts is a self-evident condition which calls for surgical intervention (*see* Chapter 21). Occasionally, some women express dissatisfaction with the size and shape of breasts which appear to the clinician to be within the very wide range of normal.

A Surgeon's View of the Histopathology of Benign Breast Disease

Fibroadenomas are accurately called benign tumours of the breast. Microscopy shows that they consist of two components: (1) connective tissue stroma which has proliferated, (2) ducts and acini which appear to have multiplied in an atypical way. The epithelial lining of the ducts and acini are normal. Thus fibroadenoma would seem not to be a disorder of epithelial proliferation. There are two types of fibroadenoma: (*a*) where the connective (fibrous) tissue proliferation occurs around the breast ducts, thus called *pericanalicular*, and (*b*) where the fibrous proliferation invaginates the duct, named *intracanalicular*. Giant fibroadenoma is a variation of the intracanalicular type, subclassified as 'cellular', since the stroma contains substantially more cells than the usual fibrous tissue. Rarely these lesions, themselves misleadingly referred to as *cystosarcoma phylloides*, undergo malignant change into sarcomas.

Fibroadenosis, as the name implies, like fibroadenoma, contains two elements—connective tissue stroma and the epithelial cells of ducts and acini. Both elements undergo

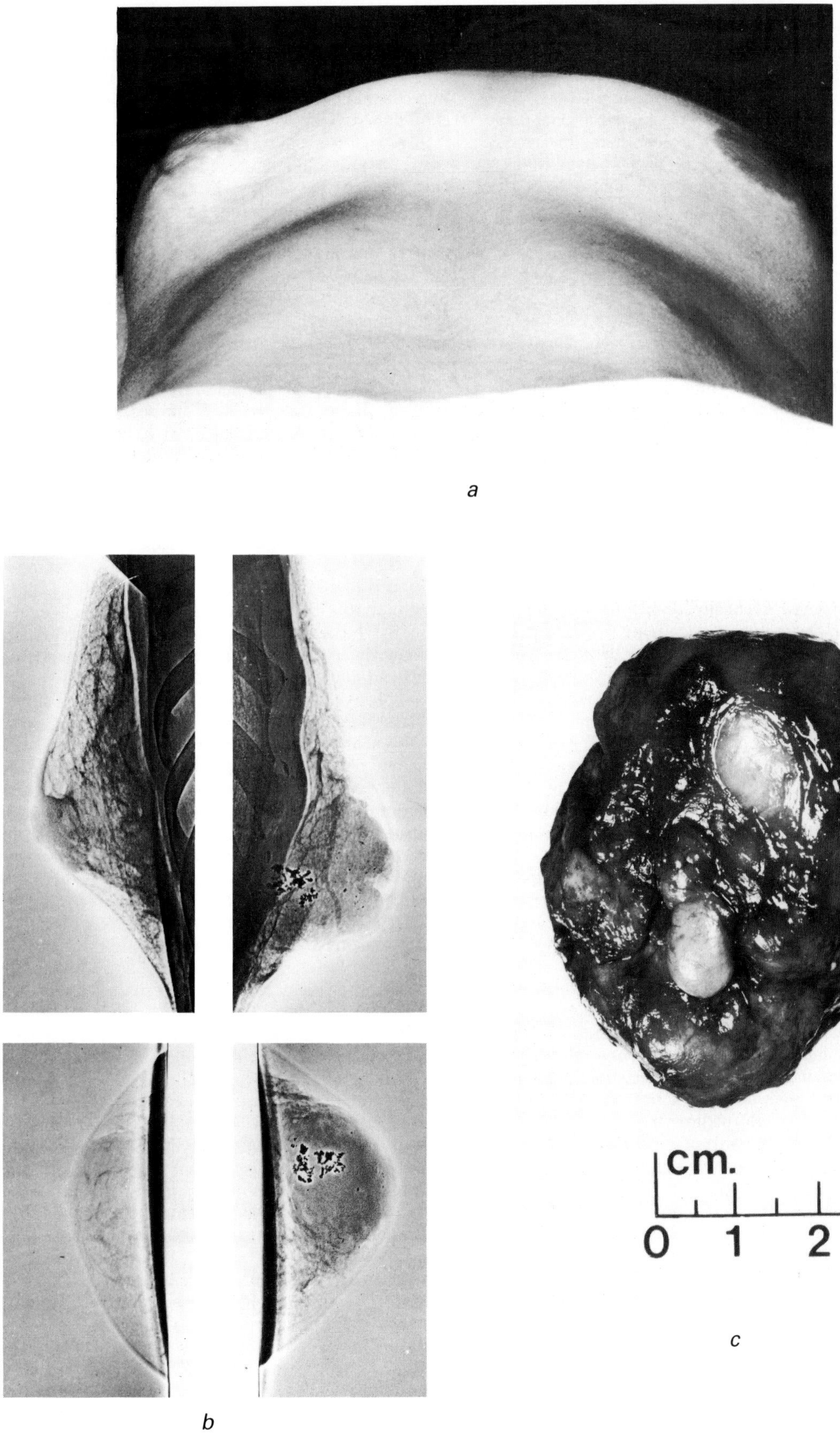

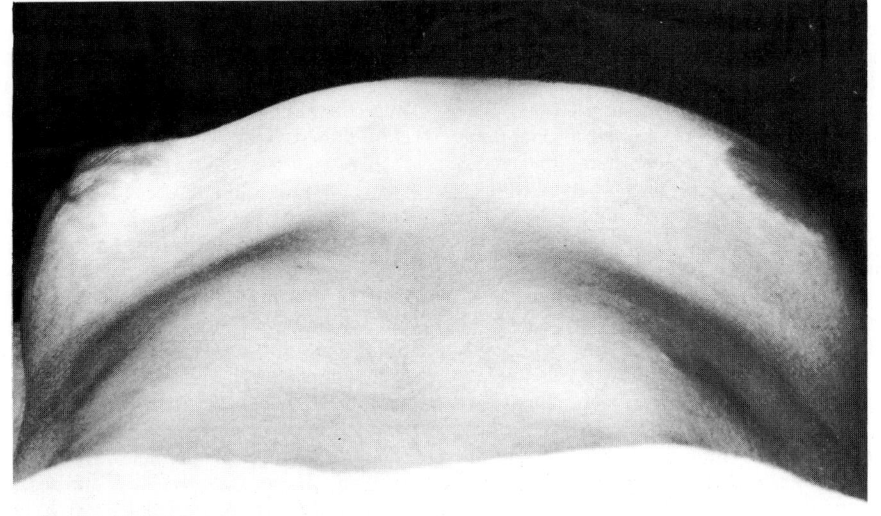

a

cm.
0 1 2

c

b

Fig. 60.9 Giant fibroadenoma. *a*, Clinical *b*, Mammographic, and *c*, Operative of right breast.

proliferation. This is most conveniently thought of separately for each element—for each may be quite independent of the other. A wide spectrum of patterns results. Chronic inflammatory cells may add to the picture, but are by no means universal. When the stroma alone proliferates, with dense sheets of fibrous tissue surrounding occasional ducts and acini, the condition is appropriately called either *fibrous disease of the breast* or *fibrosclerosis*. The other extreme is where the proliferation, which has to be regular to fit this definition, involves the breast epithelium, usually that of the terminal ducts and acini. This is *adenosis*. It can occur by itself—so-called *adenosis tumour*. *Sclerosing adenosis* is an interesting histopathological mix of fibrosis and adenosis. Both stromal and epithelial proliferation is present. Usually the stromal reaction is dominant, but if only a small area is available, as in frozen section, an epithelial component may predominate. It has now been demonstrated that these proliferating epithelial cells not only become so compressed that they appear to infiltrate the surrounding stroma, but that they can be found within both nerves and blood vessels. Such appearances, albeit by benign cells, clearly predispose to misdiagnosis. Retrospective review shows that in the past, particularly in the early days of frozen section, sclerosing adenosis was not infrequently mistaken for carcinoma.

The variant of adenosis called *blunt duct adenosis* may provide a clue to the mechanism by which cysts develop. In this variant, the terminal ductules end in small round cyst-like structures, instead of finally branching into lobules made up of acini. The epithelial cells lining these cysts may be either tall or flat, and the epithelium may be overgrown in a regular way, classified as *papillary*.

Another variant of the epithelial cells of the breast is when these become columnar in shape with a prominent pink cytoplasm. This is called *apocrine metaplasia* since the appearance is similar to that of the cells in axillary apocrine and other ordinary sweat glands, to which the breast is related developmentally. Apocrine metaplasia is frequently found as part of fibroadenosis and often forms the lining of cysts.

Cysts can be microscopic or large enough to be palpated or seen by naked eye. When microscopic, cysts are frequently multiple and aggregated as a discrete mass. *Simple cysts* are lined by a single layer of flattened epithelium. Where the epithelium has regular overgrowth without mitoses or irregularity in size or colour of nuclei, the term *papillary cyst* is used.

Three benign lesions, all of which are proliferations of the epithelium of the mammary ducts, are: *solitary duct papilloma*, *papillomatosis* and *epitheliosis*. Solitary duct papilloma is usually found in a main duct, close to the nipple. It is a regular papillary overgrowth, without hyperchromatosis or mitoses, affecting a localized area of surface of a duct. It is not premalignant, and is adequately removed by excision of the single affected duct, microdochectomy. Papillomatosis, as its name implies, is a much more extensive process, suitably regarded as a field change. The basic microscopic features are similar to those of a solitary papilloma, differing only in the extent, not only one focus of one duct being involved, but large areas of several. Epitheliosis is further classified histologically into solid and cribriform. Epitheliosis is a term which is used by different workers to mean different things. When intended for unequivocally benign epithelial proliferation, it is probably best specified as such. This proliferation means regular increase in the epithelial cells, but the tendency to formation of papillomas is not shown. When such a process contains irregular cells, with nuclear pleomorphism and increased density of staining, the term 'epitheliosis' is better not used, but instead, carcinoma-in-situ (subspecified as to whether it is lobular or ductal).

Mammary duct ectasia is a benign breast disease entity frequently encountered by clinicians and radiologists. It is a condition recognized by histopathologists, but it has to be realized that to them it is often a relative term—referring to some measure of dilatation of the ducts, without necessarily any other specific feature. Fibrotic thickening of the duct wall, atrophy of the lining epithelium, and lymphocytic infiltrate around the duct may point to this diagnosis, as does inspissation of the duct lumen with an amorphous fat-containing material. An inflammatory reaction, sometimes containing plasma cells, in the stroma surrounding ectatic ducts is a complication of duct ectasia. This process is attributed to leakage of the duct contents into the stroma where it induces a foreign body reaction called *plasma cell* or *periductal*, or *perilobular mastitis*. This condition is often bilateral. It can progress to frank abscess formation (*non-puerperal breast abscess*). If such fails to resolve completely, a chronic discharging *mammary sinus* develops, identical with the sinuses seen after infection of a buried foreign body, e.g. a silk suture.

Management of Benign Breast Disease

Pain

Lack of classification of mastalgia, and its unknown aetiology, has made rational treatment impossible. Empirical treatments have been many, including hormone supplements and diuretic therapy. The latter, probably because of its simplicity has remained the most popular, although a trial has shown it to be no more effective than placebo, and the absence of increased body water in patients with the symptom provides a theoretical reason why such therapy would not be expected to work.

A double blind trial of treatment with the dopamine agonist, bromocriptine, performed on the rationale that women with fibroadenosis are hyperprolactinaemic compared with normal controls, showed that this drug is effective in patients with cyclical symptoms, but not with non-cyclical. Bromocriptine ingestion is associated with nausea, dizziness and headache. To avoid these side-effects, it is necessary to start with 1·25 mg daily (best at night) for 3 days. Then for the next 3 days increase to 1·25 mg b.d. The nocturnal dose is then increased to 2·5 mg for the following 3 days, and after 2 weeks the maintenance dose of 2·5 mg b.d. is used. The tablets are best taken after food. Therapy is taken continuously and probably needs to be taken for a minimum of 3 menstrual cycles. No teratogenic effects have been reported, even in women taking large doses of bromocriptine over prolonged periods of time. Since the drug has indications in hyperprolactinaemic hypogonadism, adequate contraceptive methods should be used during therapy with bromocriptine when this is being used for treatment of breast pain, and administration should cease if a period is missed.

Another drug, danazol, originally developed for use as a contraceptive since it has the effect of reducing serum follicle-stimulating hormone levels and luteinizing hormone levels, has been shown to have a place in the treatment of painful lumpy breasts. Whether its benefit is confined to cyclical mastalgia is not yet clear. Amenorrhoea frequently accompanies ingestion of danazol. It is recommended that treatment should start on the first day of a period. The dosage required to be effective is variable, but ranges from

100 mg b.d. to 200 mg q.d.s., although usually the lower doses are adequate if the drug is going to relieve mastalgia. In view of the amenorrhoea induced by danazol, it is important that when this drug is being used to treat mastalgia, adequate contraceptive precautions are used, since at these doses contraceptive effects are variable.

Evening primrose oil, the richest natural source of essential fatty acids, has been shown in a placebo-controlled trial to improve cyclical mastalgia and nodularity. Like bromocriptine, it has little effect on non-cyclical symptoms, a parallel which supports the hypothesis that prolactin pathways are involved in breast disorders which have a menstrual pattern. Essential fatty acids, particularly gamma-linolenic acid, are precursors of second messengers in some prolactin-mediated mechanisms. Their deficiency is postulated in 'Western' diets, particularly when intake of polyunsaturated fatty acids is high. Dosage used has been 2 capsules of oil, together with ascorbic acid 200 mg t.d.s. To obtain full benefit from this regime, it may be necessary to ensure adequate levels of vitamins B_3 and B_6 and zinc, which are cofactors in the proposed metabolic pathways.

Trigger point pain associated with stigmas of mammary duct ectasia/periductal mastitis can be relieved by subareolar mammary duct excision. If the trigger point is distant from, but contiguous with, the main ducts, its removal with the specimen frequently reveals focal inflammation, and has been associated with relief of symptoms in a small series of patients. Perhaps explicable in terms of the microscopic appearances, local excision of foci of sclerosing adenosis and old scars frequently gives relief. Unfortunately, this is not always long lasting.

Good results have been reported of treating Tietze syndrome by perichondral injection of local anaesthetic mixed with hydrocortisone.

Nipple Complaints

Since the commonest benign histopathological cause of all the 3 nipple complaints, retraction, discharge and skin change, is mammary duct ectasia, usually with periductal mastitis—the usually effective treatment is that which eliminates the apparently causative component—namely the main mammary ducts. The operation is that devised by Urban, and popularized by Hadfield, which makes a semicircular incision in the inferior half of the areola. Nipple and areola are raised as a flap, and the circular disc of tissue beneath, which contains the larger breast ducts, is excised. To avoid recurrent problems, it is most important that no remnants of ducts are left behind attached to the nipple.

The other benign causes of nipple discharge, even though this be bloody or serous, are: (i) papillomatosis, which is adequately both investigated and treated by subareolar mammary duct excision, and (ii) solitary duct papilloma. Microdochectomy is the treatment of choice for this. Although the duct to be excised lies radially, a circumareolar incision is completely adequate.

Lumps

Fibroadenomas: Despite the established benign nature of these lesions, many women prefer them to be removed. This has the advantage that the occasional one which will grow to giant size will be prevented from so doing. In patients aged over 25 years, an apparent fibroadenoma can prove to be a circumscribed, well-differentiated carcinoma, and excision is always advisable after this age.

Fibroadenosis is best managed without surgery. Its variable and diffuse nature makes it unsuitable for local procedures, which often in the attempt to control symptoms, have to be repeated. Occasionally, either to satisfy a patient's own wishes, or to ensure the benign nature of a particular mass, open biopsy is necessary. The increasing availability of some form of needle biopsy and mammography make this less necessary.

Cysts: Simple cysts are usually rendered impalpable to both the patient and her surgeon by aspiration with a fine needle. If obvious old blood is obtained or a residual mass is palpable after aspiration or the cyst contents reaccumulate, then further investigation, usually culminating in excision biopsy, is indicated. Papillary cysts either prove solid on aspiration, or even when truly cystic, do not become impalpable when aspirated, so that biopsy is advisable.

Mammary Duct Ectasia/Periductal Mastitis

The treatment for the red inflamed manifestation of periductal mastitis is not antibiotics—since these lesions are not primarily infected. If the lesion persists for more than a few days such that symptomatic treatment is required, anti-inflammatory drugs, particularly indomethacin 25 mg t.d.s. for 5 days, taken with food (and with the standard precaution of not being used in dyspeptics), is very effective. The surgical procedures for this benign disease complex have already been outlined.

Breast Abscess

Breast abscess, either puerperal or non-puerperal, requires incision. Administration of antibiotics in puerperal cases, and anti-inflammatory drugs in non-puerperal will lead to resolution if given before a loculus of pus is present. If given in the presence of such a loculus, a hard indurated mass will persist—an *antibioma*, which will usually itself require excision. Breast abscess is best incised under general anaesthetic, so that loculi not suspected preoperatively can be opened and adequately drained. The line of incision must be parallel with the natural skin creases, Langer's lines, otherwise, ugly and often painful scarring results (*Fig.* 60.10). Drains, usually corrugated polythene or rubber, are left in place until discharge is minimal. Provided the drain is inserted in a dependent position, primary closure of the wound after evacuation of pus is followed by rapid healing and an excellent cosmetic result. Once incised, antibiotics are not necessary in the treatment of breast abscess.

Augmentation and Reduction Mammaplasties

Augmentation and reduction mammaplasties have been devised to alter the size and shape of female breasts. Before embarking on surgical augmentation, possible endocrine methods of improving obvious bilateral breast underdevelopment must be considered and ruled out for the individual patient. Where requests for augmentation or reduction do not seem justified, an attempt should be made to rule out a psychological problem which may be behind the referral. If such exists, it is unlikely to be solved by cosmetic surgery.

Three augmentation procedures are available. Grafting of dermolipomatous pads from the gluteal region was used originally; however, smooth silicone gel implants are currently the most widely used. Successful breast reconstruction using flaps of omentum has also been described. Such techniques, by themselves, only contribute to forming a mammary mound. The reconstruction of areola and nipple require even more sophisticated plastic surgical procedures, usually using transplants of labial skin or skin from the contralateral nipple (*see* Chapter 22).

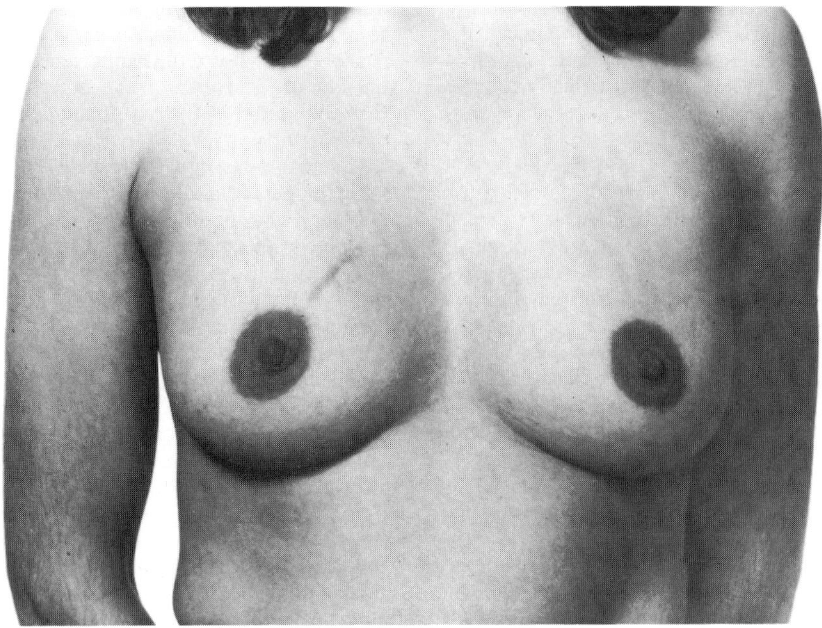

Fig. 60.10 Ugly radial scar.

Reduction mammaplasties are plastic surgical procedures which aim to reduce significantly the volume of breast tissue and yet preserve the areola and nipple. Some skin has to be removed from the breast, and this is done using an incision which will result in scars in the lower half of the reconstructed gland. The areola and nipple are usually preserved as a pedicle, but occasionally they are replaced as a free graft. The beta reduction mammaplasty is a useful and safe procedure since it leaves the vascular supply to the nipple and areola intact. The incision outlines the Greek letter beta (hence the name). Skin and breast tissue are excised from the lower half of the breast and the breast mound is restored by rotation of the medial and lateral flaps in opposite directions around the areola (*Fig.* 60.11).

BENIGN DISEASES OF THE MALE BREAST

Gynaecomastia in the Male

This is most commonly encountered as an idiopathic condition (no obvious organic cause) at puberty and old age. It is often unilateral and when bilateral may be asymmetrical in extent. In the adolescent and young adult male, it is often a source of considerable social embarrassment precluding swimming and participation in other pastimes necessitating exposure of the chest.

Gynaecomastia may, however, be secondary to a number of disorders including hypogonadism (Klinefelter's syndrome, cryptorchidism, testicular ablation by surgery or disease such as leprosy), tumours (testicular, adrenal and

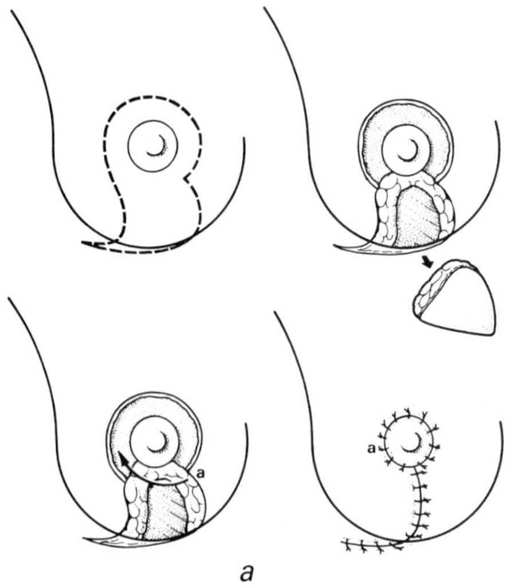

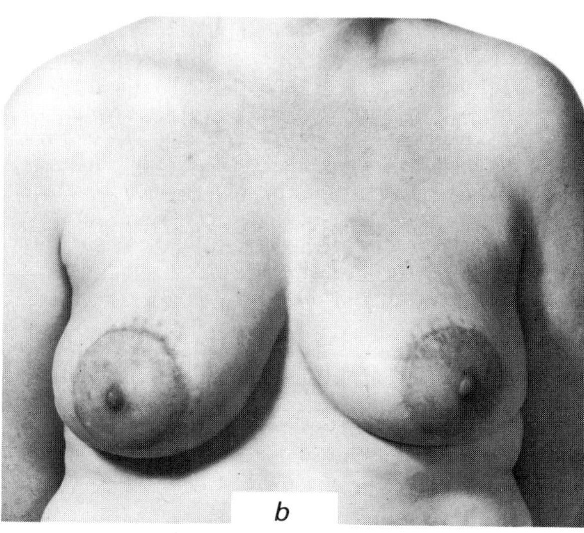

Fig. 60.11 The beta technique of reduction mammoplasty. *a*, Principle of procedure. *b*, End result.

bronchial), endocrine disorders (Addison's disease, thyrotoxicosis, and acromegaly), chronic liver disease (cirrhosis), congestive cardiac failure, end-stage renal failure, long-term dialysis and malnutrition. Drug-induced gynaecomastia is being increasingly encountered and apart from the well known effect of oestrogen and chorionic gonadotrophin therapy, drugs which are commonly associated with its development include: digoxin, spironolactone, cimetidine, isoniazid and anabolic steroids.

Surgical treatment of the idiopathic variety is often necessary in the young male and consists of a submammary excision of the breast tissue with preservation of the nipple. Treatment is not usually required for the idiopathic variety encountered in the aged. Withdrawal of the drug (if possible) is attended by a slow regression over a period of weeks to months of the gynaecomastia when this is drug-induced.

Mammary Duct Ectasia

Mammary duct ectasia is found rarely in males. It presents as in females with a pastey nipple discharge, pain, or inflammation and even on occasion as an abscess. Treatment is local excision—preserving the nipple but ensuring complete removal of all duct tissues.

MALIGNANT DISEASE OF THE FEMALE BREAST

Epidemiology

Female breast cancer is common in most Western Communities. Its incidence in the UK is 18 000 new cases per year; for the USA the figure is 72 000. About 1 in 16 women is affected at some time in her life by the disease.

Many factors in the life of an individual woman have been considered to have some effect on her chance of developing breast cancer. Clinically known as 'risk factors' these include social class, family history, height and weight, age at menarche, age at first term birth, age at menopause, prolonged breast feeding and presence of benign breast disease. Detailed studies of these factors have been performed with some conflicting results. A recent review of most available data shows a higher incidence of breast cancer in higher social class, and where there is a family history. Height certainly, and weight probably, do not affect the risk, and neither does prolonged breast feeding. Early menarche probably increases the risk. An early full-term pregnancy definitely protects against breast cancer, as does, to a lesser degree, an early menopause. Benign breast disease, considered overall, shows evidence of an increased risk. Controversy still exists as to which benign lesions predispose to subsequent cancer, although recent studies indicate that fibrocystic disease is associated with an increased risk. Most studies suggest no relationship between use of oral contraceptives and the development of breast cancer. Insufficient time has elapsed to confirm or refute an impression that these agents may be protective, although it is thought that women developing breast cancer while on the pill present at an earlier stage and so have a better prognosis.

A Surgeon's View of the Histopathology of Breast Malignancy

The majority of breast neoplasia arise from the epithelium of the mammary ducts. A minority (2–10%) appears to originate from the epithelium lining the acini and small intralobular ductules, so-called 'lobular carcinoma'. Apart from this fundamental difference, which has significant clinical implications which will be outlined, other neoplasms have relatively minor practical importance.

Invasive Neoplasia

The commonest invasive breast neoplasm, *invasive ductal carcinoma*, is referred to as 'no special type' (NST) or more recently 'not otherwise specified' (NOS). Invasive ductal carcinoma is found with a wide spectrum of differentiation. The extremely well-differentiated tumour is so characterized by recognizable duct-like structures that it is often subclassified as 'tubular'. Another subtype which by its characteristics and behaviour can be regarded as towards the better differentiated end of the spectrum of invasive ductal cancer is that aptly called 'mucinous' (also referred to as colloid, gelatinous or mucoid). The capacity of some function, albeit abnormal production of mucin by the neoplastic cells in this tumour seems consistent with the well-differentiated appearances usually observed.

In a disease such as breast cancer, where a wealth of facts is known it is mandatory to make use of all available information which might influence treatment of the individual. The preponderance of invasive breast cancers are of 'no special type' (NOS) where cellular differentiation (tubular or mucinous) cannot be recognized. A quantitative expression of differentiation in neoplasia, histological grading, was originated during the last century in Germany. Although criticized as being too subjective, good correlation between grade and outcome in breast cancer has been repeatedly demonstrated, both prospectively and in very larger series (Bloom and Richardson, 1957). The technique has fallen from regular routine use by many pathologists, probably because they did not see their efforts being used in deciding patient management. Bloom and Richardson grading has the virtues of universal application, and thus of enabling meaningful comparisons between series from different centres. The system uses the epithelial elements only. The degree of differentiation is judged by: (i) the tendency of the cells to form tubules—*tubule formation*; (ii) the size, shape and staining of the nuclei—*pleomorphism*; (iii) the frequency of hyperchromatic nuclei and mitotic figures—*mitoses* (*Fig.* 60.12).

The fact that increasingly the details of treatment of breast cancer are being based on careful selection of prognostic criteria, makes histological grading highly relevant.

Medullary carcinoma illustrates two other phenomena in breast cancer histology which correlate with prognosis, namely circumscription and lymphocytic infiltration. This type is also called *circumscribed* carcinoma, since to the naked eye it has a clearly definable margin, compared with the much more commonly seen diffuse infiltrating lesion with fronds or spicule-like extensions penetrating neighbouring tissues. Under the microscope, the most impressive feature is a dense infiltration of the stroma with lymphocytes. About 2% of breast carcinomas are medullary. Lymph node metastases tend to be less than with non-specified tumours, and the prognosis, accordingly better.

Another form of invasive mammary carcinoma with a favourable prognosis is the very rare condition *adenoidcystic carcinoma*. Histologically, these tumours are like their counterparts which occur in salivary glands, oesophagus and bronchus, consisting of mucin-containing tubules lined by small dark cells.

Invasive lobular carcinoma is characterized microscopically by a homogeneous pattern of small cells arranged in strands diffusely infiltrating the lobules. The condition is often multifocal, and frequently occurs bilaterally. Usually lobular carcinoma does not present as a lump; instead, pain is an important presenting symptom. This hystological type is not characterized by microcalcification on mammography, and so can be frequently missed at an early stage. These factors may account for the overall poorer prognosis of this subtype. Very often invasive lobular carcinoma is found together with in situ lobular neoplasia.

In situ neoplasia. About 5% of all malignant lesions of the female breast are non-invasive, or 'in situ'. These present to the surgeon as problems of management which are likely to remain unsolved for some time to come. The question is 'should a histopathological diagnosis of in situ neoplasia be followed by mastectomy, or not? *In situ lobular neoplasia* is the condition which gives greatest difficulty. First adequately described in 1941 by Foote and Stewart, the term 'lobular carcinoma-in-situ' was used to refer to non-infiltrating lobular neoplasia. By this was meant proliferation of epithelial cells lining the acini and small intralobular ductules. The cells fill up the acini and ductules so that no lumens remain. Subsequently an infiltrating form came to be recognized, and the question arose as to whether the in situ variety always progressed to the infiltrative. The evidence available points to the fact that this occurs at the most in only one-fifth of cases.

In situ lobular neoplasia was further subclassified by C. D. Haagensen in 1971 into Type A, where the cells are completely uniform, and Type B, where the cells look more

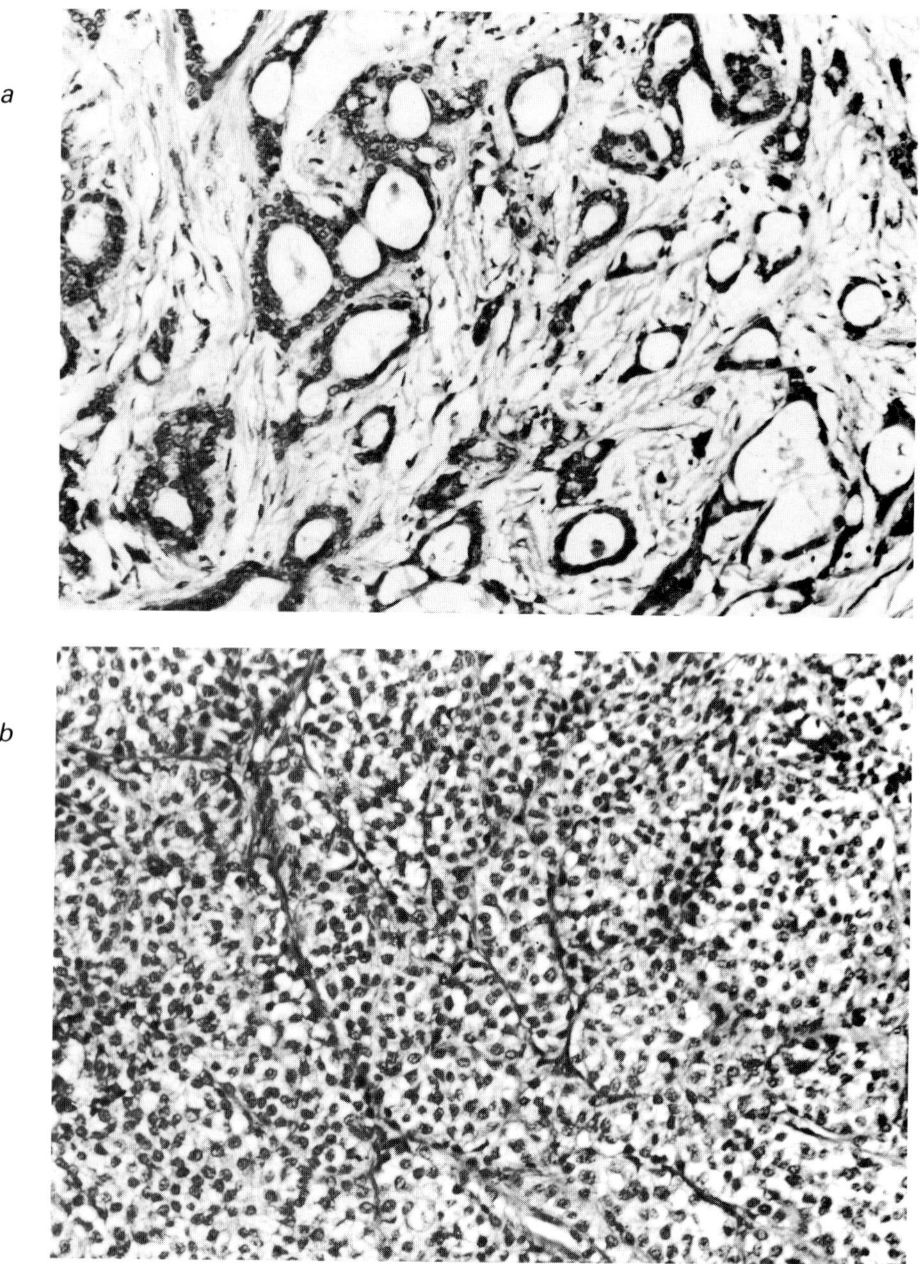

Fig. 60.12 Examples of Bloom and Richardson grading of breast cancer. *a*, C1, a high degree of differentiation means low malignancy and correlates with good survival figures. *b*, C2, medium degree of differentiation, and malignancy.

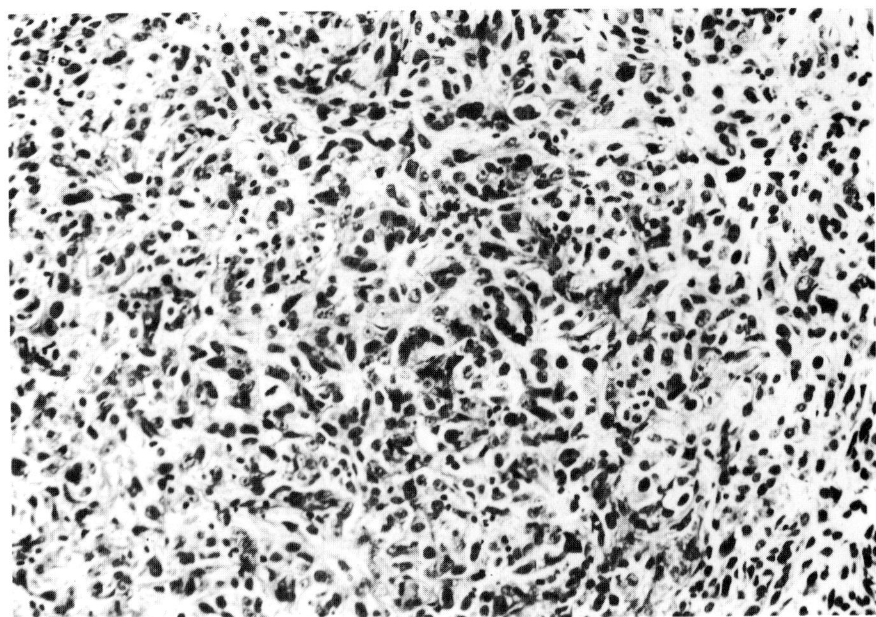

[*Fig. 60.12 continued*] *c*, C3, undifferentiated, highly malignant and correlating with short survival time. (By courtesy of Dr Margo Holley, Ninewells Hospital, Dundee.)

malignant. The two types may occur together. One feature of in situ lobular neoplasia which favours a conservative approach in its management is that it is virtually confined to premenopausal women—the implication being that it disappears at the menopause. Against this is the fact that the majority of breast biopsies for benign breast disease are done during reproductive life. Since in situ lobular neoplasia is usually an incidental finding, it is much less likely to be found after the menopause.

Such cases should be managed by close collaboration between pathologist and surgeon, who must pay close regard to what follow-up facilities are available. If cells are uniform, and follow-up good, wide biopsy and regular re-examination is acceptable. If there is wide variation in cell size, then mastectomy can reasonably be advised.

The term *'intraduct' carcinoma* causes confusion, since it is used to refer to two different conditions. First, invasive mammary carcinoma in which the predominant growth is into the lumen of the ducts. Secondly, in situ ductal carcinoma. It is the second which is relevant to discussion here, for, like in situ lobular neoplasia, it causes the surgeon problems about management. Since in situ ductal neoplasia often coexists with invasive disease, the concept arises that the invasive form is but a later manifestation of the in situ. Since only fixed sections can be examined, this hypothesis can never be directly proven or disproven. Circumstantial evidence is scanty. A working plan is to say that where the cells are markedly atypical, with any mitotic activity, the lesion should be treated as malignant.

Neoplasia requiring Special Consideration

The classification of *Paget's disease* (*Fig.* 60.13) of the breast, particularly as to whether it is an expression of invasive or in situ breast carcinoma, remains a matter of debate. Two facts are definite:

1. All Paget's cells seen in the epidermis of the nipple originate in the underlying ducts.

2. This eczematous dermatitis of the nipple (and occasionally also areola) occurs in 2% of breast cancer patients.

Age incidence is very similar to that for all breast cancer. Itching may be the earliest symptom (this needs to be distinguished from the eczema associated with the nipple discharge of mammary duct ectasia). Later follows crusting and then ulceration. Nipple biopsy will give the diagnosis. Even though Paget's disease is often an expression of only in situ ductal carcinomas, it has been convincingly demonstrated that adequate and most satisfactory treatment is total mastectomy and axillary clearance.

Intracystic Neoplasia

Occasionally carcinoma is found within cysts. Clinically this situation can be suspected if a cyst aspirate is bloodstained, or its cytology is atypical. On mammography the outline of a malignant cyst is often blurred for part of its circumference. Pneumocystography will show a ragged cavity, the same feature alerting the pathologist to the possibility of malignancy. Carcinoma in cysts tends to occur in the older age groups, are slow growing—believed not to invade for many years—and are said to occur most commonly in black women.

Inflammatory Carcinoma

This condition should be seen as a clinical entity, i.e. it is a form of breast cancer with specific clinical rather than pathological characteristics. It is rare—about 1·5% of most published series. It has no special age incidence and patients who are pregnant or lactating are not specially predisposed to it.

The first symptom is often pain. The affected breast is usually diffusely enlarged, oedematous, inflamed and indurated, and warm to the touch. The most characteristic mammographic feature is oedema. The clinical picture described can be associated with a spectrum of histopathology as wide as the whole range of invasive ductal cancer. The

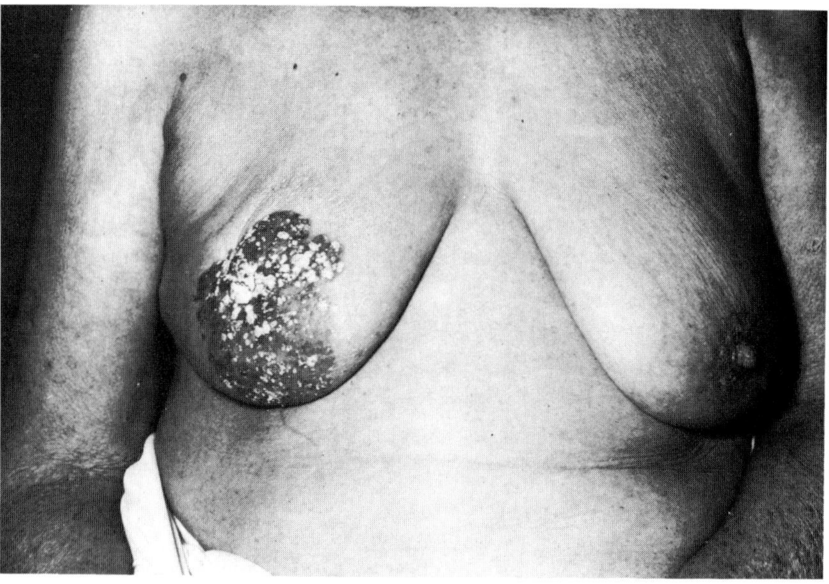

Fig. 60.13 Extensive Paget's disease of right nipple.

histopathological features associated with this condition are those which accompany highly aggressive malignancy, particularly infiltration of dilated lymphatics and blood vessels with malignant cells. Contrary to expectation, inflammatory cell infiltration is not commonly found.

This condition has a universally poor prognosis, and it is established that it should not be treated by local surgery. Control of local disease, even by radiotherapy, is difficult. Although accepting from the outset a short life expectancy, it is appropriate to use systemic therapy as part of primary treatment, in an attempt to diminish local symptoms. Endocrine and cytotoxic regimes have occasionally given remissions.

Steroid Hormone Receptors

Both the development and function of the breasts are under endocrine control. Normal breast cells contain specific binding sites for their controlling hormones. These sites are proteins known as receptors (*Fig.* 60.14). In the search for tests which would predict which breast cancers were hormone sensitive, the presence of an oestradiol-binding protein was sought. Subsequently it has been shown that the *in vivo* growth of 50% of tumours having oestrogen receptors could be inhibited by endocrine manipulations, whereas only 10% of receptor-negative tumours were so affected.

More recently it has been claimed that progesterone receptor (which itself depends on oestrogen) is a better measure of cellular synthetic function likely to be influenced by therapeutic changes in the hormonal environment. Apart from endocrine sensitivity, receptor status may be a guide to prognosis—increased receptor correlating with better prognosis. Receptor assays have an established place in advanced breast cancer. Their role in deciding management in early breast cancer has yet to emerge, although they are most

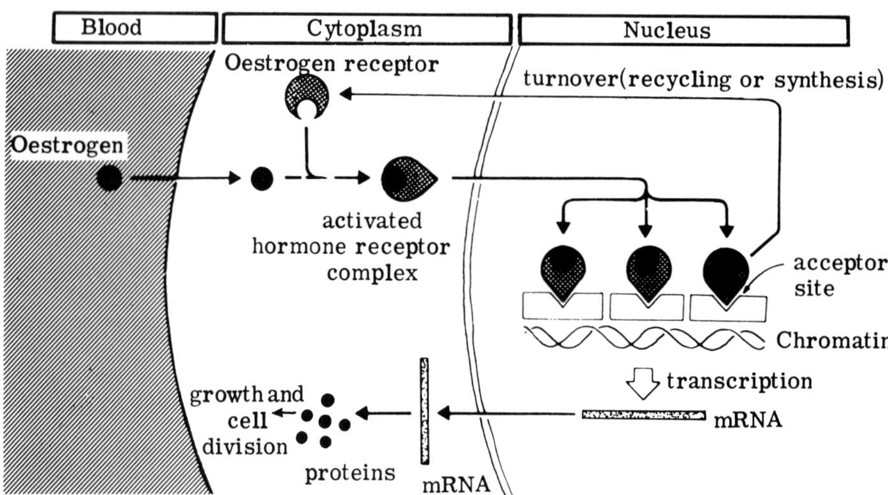

Fig. 60.14 Probable role of oestrogen receptor in breast. (By courtesy of Dr Robin Leake, Glasgow.)

satisfactorily measured on tissue which is removed initially from the primary lesion, than from metastases. Thus, in anticipation of the possibility of a patient developing recurrence, receptors may be measured at presentation.

Presenting Symptoms of Breast Cancer

The presenting symptoms are, in order of frequency: (i) lump, (ii) nipple complaint, (iii) pain, (iv) symptoms from metastases. By far the commonest of these is a lump, usually found by chance by the patient herself. There are three symptoms related to the nipple: (*a*) skin changes, (*b*) blood-stained or serous discharge, (*c*) retraction. Pain, the commonest symptom associated with benign conditions of the breast, does not, as has been popularly thought, rule out malignancy, being the first symptom in 8–10% of cases of clinically 'early' breast cancer. All of the symptoms caused by localized breast cancer can also be the symptoms of benign lesions.

Diagnosis and Pretreatment Assessment of Breast Cancer

1. *Tissue Diagnosis.* This is fundamental before any treatment. Methods available for this have already been described in the clinical introduction.
2. *Staging.* Essential and routinely used investigations are:
   Chest radiograph
   Limited skeletal survey
   Haemoglobin and blood film
   Alkaline phosphatase and gamma glutamyl transpeptidase
3. Methods of so-called 'superstaging' currently being evaulated include: (*a*) liver scans, (*b*) bone scan, (*c*) tumour markers. To date there is no evidence that results from these tests applied to treatment materially affect the outcome.

Tumour markers currently being measured include: (*a*) enzymes (e.g. gamma GTP), (*b*) acute phase reactants (e.g. C-reactive protein), (*c*) other proteins (e.g. pregnancy macroglobulin), (*d*) oncofetal antigens (e.g. CEA), (*e*) products of metabolism (e.g. hydroxyproline), (*f*) immune complexes.

It is likely in the future that serial estimations will be the most useful way of using these to indicate occult or recurrent disease activity, and the response of this to treatment. At present few give a significantly useful lead time.

Staging

Systems of staging breast cancer which have been widely accepted and used to date are: (*a*) the TNM (Tumour Nodes Metastases) System, and (*b*) the Manchester System (Stages I to IV). The Manchester System is derived directly from the TNM. Because of international agreement on the TNM staging, this system affords a means by which data from different centres can be meaningfully compared. In its application to the breast the TNM system is now sufficiently versatile to include information obtained from mammograms—namely tumour diameter, and information which results from examination of surgically removed specimens at autopsy. Mammographic measurement takes precedence over that of calliper, since it is more consistent and accurate. Where the system is used to convey information obtained after surgery the prefix 'p' is placed before the T, N and M, as appropriate. The TNM system for breast cancer is summarized as:

TIS Carcinoma-in-situ
T_0 No evidence of primary tumour
T_1 <2 cm
T_2 2–5 cm
T_3 >5 cm
(for T_1–T_3: *a*. Without fixation to fascia or muscle; *b*. With fixation to fascia or muscle)
T_4 Extension to chest wall or skin
  a. Chest wall
  b. Skin oedema or infiltration or ulceration
  c. Both chest wall and skin
N_1 Mobile axillary
  a. Not considered involved by tumour
  b. Considered involved by tumour
N_2 Fixed axillary

Considerable observer variation occurs in palpating lymph nodes. Interpretation of the pathological significance of what is felt is renowned for errors up to 40% either way. Hence when histopathological data about nodes are available, i.e. pN, they are greatly to be preferred.

Management of Malignant Breast Disease

A. *General Considerations*

Very many different trials of treatment of breast cancer have been carried out. Despite these the individual surgeon faced with treating the individual patient remains confused. All the good trials have demonstrated two facts:

1. A substantial proportion, of the order of 25% of patients who have apparently 'early' disease at presentation, take a course which proves they must have had occult dissemination when first seen.
2. A very careful assessment of the individual patient, including her domestic and emotional situation is necessary before deciding on treatment. The onus is on the surgeon to reduce to an absolute minimum the number of mastectomies, and to reduce morbidity and mutilation but not at the expense of adequate local treatment.

Two aspects of treatment should be distinguished:

1. That performed directly to the breast and its regional lymph nodes—called by Bernard Fisher of Pittsburgh 'loco-regional'.
2. That frequently called 'adjuvant'. This might be better understood if it were called prophylactic—for it is the treatment given, usually systemically, to prevent the appearance of recurrent disease, which in the nature of this condition is usually disseminated.

Two aspects of breast cancer at presentation should be distinguished:

1. Operable disease $T_1+T_2\pm T_3$ (Stage I and II)
2. Inoperable disease T_3+T_4 (Stage III and IV)

B. *Loco-regional Treatment of Primary Operable Disease*

Loco-regional treatment of operable disease means adequate treatment of: (1) primary tumour, and (2) its regional lymph nodes. This can be achieved by surgery or radiotherapy or the two combined.

1. For treatment of the primary tumour, total mastectomy, i.e. removal of the entire mammary gland (the term 'simple' referring to this is inappropriate and misleading) must still be considered preferable to local excision ('tylectomy') or segmental resection. The reasons for this are that multifocal invasive malignancy occurs in 12% of excised breasts, and the incidence of non-invasive neoplastic change can be as high as 30%. However, local excision with radiotherapy to the breast is increasingly being used, especially for Stage 1 tumours (*vide infra*).

2. Treatment of the axilla can be either axillary clearance from the level of the axillary vein downwards or by some form of axillary biopsy followed, in the presence of histological node involvement, by postoperative radiotherapy. Surgical clearance of the axilla is done by:

i. Retraction without excision of the pectoral muscles
ii. Excision of pectoralis minor (Patey)
iii. Excision of pectoralis minor and major (Halsted).

Different surgeons actually perform different axillary clearances despite naming their procedures with standard names. Whichever of these procedures is performed, and however meticulously, axillary clearance remains incomplete. Since extensive involvement of axillary nodes means that the disease is disseminated, this fact does not matter—for cure could not, in such cases, be achieved. Some surgeons refer patients for radiotherapy after doing lower axillary clearance, either because of extensive involvement of nodes by tumour or because of a high suspicion of residual disease. There is an increased incidence of lymphoedema in patients who have axillary clearance followed by radiotherapy to the axilla.

Radiotherapy to internal mammary nodes is advisable for central and medial lesions, especially if they or the axillary nodes are proved histologically to be involved.

Systemic adjuvant therapies currently being tested in trials are both endocrine and cytotoxic. For premenopausal women, ovarian ablation (with or without prednisolone) is simplest. Oral therapy with tamoxifen has been shown to benefit significantly disease-free survival in postmenopausal patients irrespective of oestrogen receptor status.

Cytotoxic therapy, both single agents (respectively thiotepa and phenylalanine mustard) and in combination (cyclophosphamide, methotrexate and 5-fluorouracil, 'CMF') have so far been shown to delay the incidence of local recurrence. CMF increases survival in premenopausal women. Cytotoxic chemotherapy, particularly combination regimes, are accompanied by serious physical and psychological sequelae. Myelodepression and alopecia occur without exception in many regimes. Induction of second cancers is being increasingly reported as more patients are followed for longer time intervals. Anxiety and depression, which are demonstrably increased when breast symptoms occur, particularly when mastectomy is performed, have been shown to persist significantly in patients receiving prophylactic cytotoxic combination chemotherapy.

C. *Treatment of 'Late' Breast Cancer*

1. Primary Inoperable Disease

Newly presenting breast cancer is unequivocally incurable by loco-regional treatment, either when it is locally advanced (i.e. Stage III) or when it is already systemic (Stage IV). Locally advanced disease often consists of a large primary tumour, frequently with direct invasion of overlying skin or frank ulceration. Skin nodules, fungation, foul odour, ipsilateral lymphadenopathy with or without lymphoedema of the arm and cancer-en-cuirasse are the causes of concern for the patient.

Overall these patients have a very poor prognosis at one year. The sole aim of treatment therefore is to palliate. Clearing infection helps. Metronidazole is particularly effective, and can be given by mouth. Local radiotherapy needs to be considered but is not always applicable or effective for a variety of reasons, including, particularly, volume of tumour, ulceration and lymphoedema. Intra-arterial combination cytotoxic therapy has been successful in a few such cases. Administration is sufficiently simple for the technique to be considered seriously for these distressing problems.

Management of disease already disseminated at presentation is as that of systemic recurrence dealt with further on.

2. Recurrent Disease

i. LOCO-REGIONAL. Locally recurrent breast cancer has two forms: (*a*) that affecting the skin flaps, (*b*) that occurring in the regional nodes—usually axillary.

a. If skin-flap recurrence is solitary and localized in or near to the scar from previous surgery, further local removal is adequate.

A wide margin of excision is essential. If necessary to achieve this a split skin graft should be used without hesitation. Applying this as a delayed procedure some 48 hours after excision gives very satisfactory healing, even when the site has been previously irradiated. If skin flap recurrence is multiple and widespread, radiotherapy is appropriate if it has not been used as part of the primary treatment. If it has, systemic treatment has to be used. This should be considered in all cases with local recurrence, albeit as an addition, even when local treatment is feasible.

b. Ipsilateral axillary node recurrence should not be seen in patients who have had a complete axillary clearance. In practice this problem is seen most frequently where initial treatment policy has been to watch the axilla, or where initial regional node treatment was by radiotherapy. Where the axilla has not been previously dealt with, the operation for excision of recrudescent disease is similar to the axillary clearance component of the radical mastectomy. Where surgery follows previous treatment, the anatomy is often very distorted, and the axillary vein particularly at risk of damage, since it seems to be drawn inferiorly towards the floor of the axilla. As with skin recurrence, if radiotherapy has not been used primarily, it is suitable for treating axillary recurrence, and is the treatment of first choice for recurrence in internal mammary nodes.

The presence of such gross disease calls for systemic measures early in the treatment. For postmenopausal women, anti-oestrogen tablets, tamoxifen 20 mg b.d., provide this, virtually free of any side-effects. Additive chemotherapy with potent agents known to induce remission in advanced breast cancer, such as adriamycin, would seem justified in this stage of disease. Alopecia always occurs, and monitoring of marrow and myocardial function is essential.

ii. SYSTEMIC. The management of patients with systemic breast cancer is not as melancholy as might at first be thought by many surgeons. It is best done in close collaboration with a radiotherapist/oncologist, ideally at an outpatient time and place which is regularly set aside for this purpose. The patient gains confidence from seeing her original medical attendant continuing to participate in her management, although this may not, by now, be necessarily uniquely surgical. She benefits by having prompt access to the most appropriate measures for symptomatic relief, during the course of her illness, whether these be a further operation, radiotherapy or drugs, or a combination of all of these. The surgeon benefits by seeing the longer term results of his early treatment policies, and by keeping in touch with medical regimes which are effective in controlling, albeit temporarily, this enigmatic disease.

The principles of treatement of disseminated breast cancer are summarized in *Table* 60.1.

Table 60.1 Principles of treatment of disseminated breast cancer

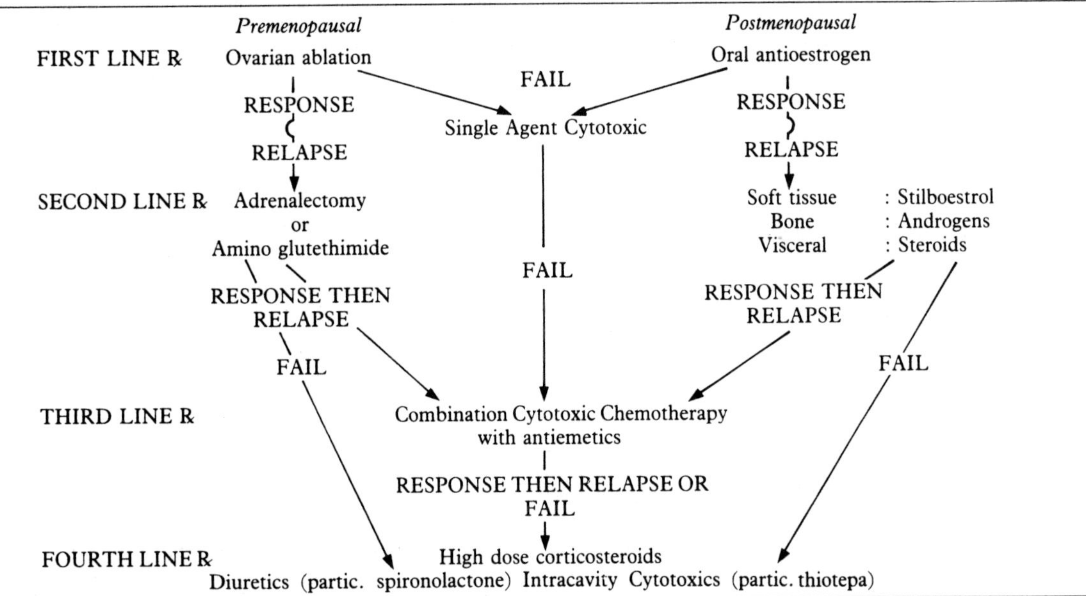

Breast Reconstruction

Female patients who require mastectomy should be offered reconstruction particularly if premenopausal and middle-aged. The reconstruction may be performed at the time of mastectomy, or more usually and preferably (for oncological reasons), delayed for some 3–6 months after the operation. The type of reconstruction used depends on local factors, e.g. amount of skin, previous radiotherapy, size of the other breast, etc. The techniques available include the insertion of a silicone implant (subcutaneously or subpectorally) and reconstruction by the latissimus dorsi myocutaneous flap over a silicone prosthesis (*Fig.* 60.15). With the first approach, a much better cosmetic appearance is obtained if a large subpectoral pouch is initially created by a temporary inflatable (expander) device which is progressively enlarged as a result of repeated injections of saline via a subcutaneous portal. Once a sufficient size is reached comparable with that of the contralateral breast, the correct size permanent silicone prosthesis is inserted after removal of the expander. This technique produces a much more aesthetically pleasing breast mound with a normal looking inframammary fold and obviates the need for reduction mammoplasty on the contralateral breast. When requested, nipple reconstruction is best achieved from a graft obtained from the opposite nipple. If this is not possible for any reason, the nipple can be reconstructed from breast skin or by a graft obtained from the ear lobe. Areolar reconstruction is done by grafting skin of the upper thigh or labia.

Breast Conservation

Although still controversial, methods of managing loco-regional cancers which conserve the affected breasts are

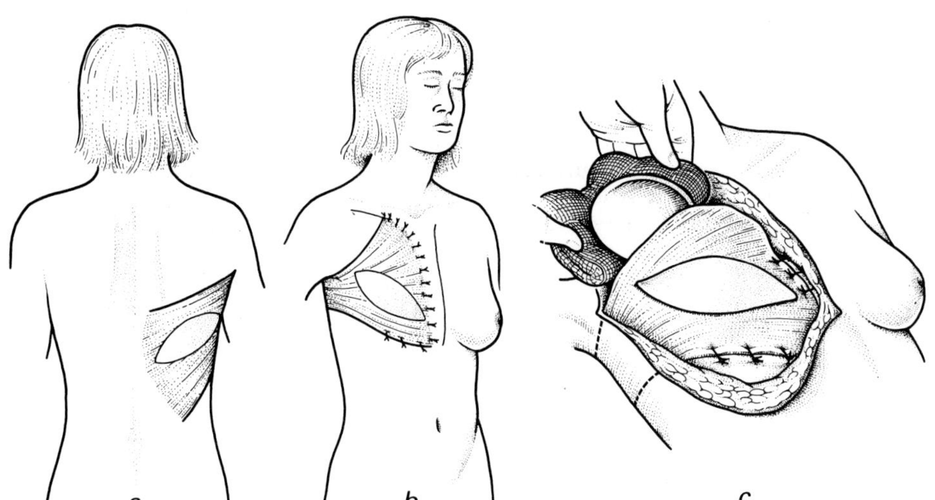

Fig. 60.15 The latissimus dorsi flap is transposed from the posterior trunk (*a*) through a tunnel in the posterior axillary fold and sutured to the anterior chest wall (*b*) over a Silastic prosthesis (*c*).

being evaluated and practised with increasing frequency. To date, long-term results of randomized trials comparing ablation with breast conservation are not available but well-validated retrospective reports are indicative of an effective control of the primary disease in selected cases. The aim of conservative treatment, in the words of one of the most experienced practitioners of this approach, Dr R. Calle, is 'to obtain survival periods of the same order as those after mastectomy, with preservation of breasts which have a good cosmetic appearance'.

Breast conservation for primary operable disease (in contradistinction to radiotherapy for locally advanced inoperable disease) is best effected by a combination of local excision and radical radiotherapy. The alternatives of radiotherapy alone or subcutaneous mastectomy are less acceptable to most surgeons and oncologists. A number of considerations are vital when breast conservation is being contemplated for 'early' breast cancer. First, a substantial proportion, i.e. about 80%, of 'early' breast cancers managed by conventional methods as described previously, will be alive and free of disease at 10 years. The medium- and long-term disease-free survival of all patients managed by conservation must therefore be monitored. Secondly, only a proportion (20–25%) of all patients presenting with 'operable' breast cancer will be suitable for conservation. Factors which determine this suitability include tumour size (up to 3·0 cm), particularly in relation to the size of the breast, and the site of the primary (excluding central lesions). Bilateral and multifocal tumours cannot be treated in this way, nor should breasts showing Paget's disease of the nipple. It is probably wise to avoid breast conservation regimens for patients with palpable homolateral axillary nodes, although it can be argued that since such patients have a poorer outlook, mastectomy is less justified. Thirdly, conservation regimens do not necessarily preclude the determination of the lymph node status. It is technically possible, without difficulty, to either sample or clear axillary nodes to obtain this important prognostic information. If clearance of the axilla is performed, the radiotherapy should not include the axilla, as otherwise an unacceptably high incidence of arm lymphoedema follows. Finally, close co-operation between the surgeon and the radiotherapist is essential during all stages of conservation, from the selection and counselling of the newly presenting patients, to the arrangements for clinical and mammographic follow-up. The radiological features of previously biopsied and irradiated breasts can be difficult to interpret and require special expertise. Often, aspiration cytology can resolve doubts as to whether recurrence is developing in these patients. This possibility of recurrence, which occurs in between 5–15% of patients so managed, needs to have been discussed with the patient and her spouse, since mastectomy then becomes inevitable. Thus patients who are suitable for breast conservation cannot be promised life-long preservation of the diseased breast. This being told to them, some patients prefer to opt for mastectomy *ab initio*.

Systemic Therapy

Systemic adjuvant therapies currently being tested in trials are both endocrine and cytotoxic. For premenopausal women, ovarian ablation (with or without prednisolone) is the simplest. Oral anti-oestrogen therapy with tamoxifen has not been completely evaluated in this situation. Cytotoxic agents in combination (cyclophosphamide, methotrexate and 5-fluorouracil—CMF) have been shown both to delay the incidence of local recurrence and increase survival in node-positive premenopausal women. Unfortunately, this treatment is often accompanied by serious physical and psychological sequelae, e.g. myelosuppression and alopecia. It may also cause second malignancies. Anxiety and depression which are demonstrably increased when breast symptoms occur particularly when mastectomy is performed, have been shown to persist significantly in patients receiving prophylactic cytotoxic combination chemotherapy. Survival has also been shown to be increased in premenopausal node-positive women by inducing a radiation menopause and administering low-dose prednisolone therapy (2·5 mg t.d.s.) to suppress production from extra-ovarian sources of oestrogens. A theoretical risk with this regimen is the development of osteoporosis if the steroid medication is continued for several years. Systemic adjuvant therapy with the anti-oestrogen Nolvadex (ICI, tamoxifen) has been proven to prolong survival significantly in postmenopausal women and results of studies of its use in premenopausal women are awaited. Tamoxifen therapy is particularly effective in the elderly and is being used as the only initial treatment in this age group with complete resolution of the tumour in 50% and reduction in size in a further 20%. In a number of centres including our own, patients aged 70 years and above are treated with tamoxifen (40 mg daily) and surgical treatment is only considered if there is no response to this initial treatment.

At present, available methods merely palliate, a fact it is essential to keep in mind when deciding which lesions to treat, and at what cost (time, travel, side-effects) to the patient.

Each method of ovarian ablation has advantages and disadvantages. Surgery is certain, complete and immediate. For the patient it means a general anaesthetic, and an abdominal operation and incision. Against this, radiotherapy is short and simple with minimal side-effects. There is always doubt about its completeness, and it can be any time up to 3 months for its effect to be complete. When relapse follows an initial response to ovarian ablation such that adrenalectomy is indicated, this can be achieved medically. In this way a further operation with its attendant risks can be avoided. Aminoglutethimide suppresses the function of the adrenal cortex. Since its effects can be severe, it is advisable for the patient to be admitted to be started and stabilized on this drug and on steroid replacement.

Anti-oestrogen therapy (tamoxifen (Nolvadex) 10–20 mg b.d.) works by competitive inhibition with oestrogen. It is probably taken up by oestrogen-binding sites. Ideally, the platelet count should be monitored (since transient falls of this have been observed), together with the serum calcium (since hypercalcaemia can develop on commencement of therapy, in the presence of bony metastases).

Stilboestrol ingestion gives nausea, vaginal bleeding and thrombo-embolism. Androgens masculinize and increase libido, occasionally sufficiently to induce suicide.

Cytotoxic agents which have been used with some benefit as single agents for established breast cancer include cyclophosphamide, 5-fluorouracil, methotrexate, doxorubicin (adriamycin) and vincristine. Adriamycin is being replaced by its epimer, epirubicin which has the same activity but is less cardiotoxic. Cyclophosphamide and vincristine used together with either 5-fluorouracil or adriamycin can produce dramatic remissions in advanced disease. Another antineoplastic drug which has been shown to be quite effective in advanced disease is mitozantrone. It is used as a single agent in a dose of 14 mg/m^2 of body surface area as a single intravenous dose which may be repeated at 21-day intervals. The dose is diluted in at least 50 ml of isotonic saline or 5% dextrose and then administered intravenously over not less than 5 minutes. Apart from myelosuppression, side-effects include nausea and vomiting, minimal alopecia, stomatitis and, rarely, gastrointestinal bleeding, acute arrhythmias and congestive cardiac failure. Regular monitoring (weekly) of full blood count and platelets is essential during treatment with all these cytotoxic agents.

After aspiration of a pleural effusion secondary to breast cancer, the cytotoxic drug bleomycin, 60 mg in 100 ml of isotonic saline, helps to delay and can often prevent the reaccumulation of the effusion. Equally good results have been reported after the intrapleural injection of *C. parvum* vaccine.

Suitable steroid regimes include prednisolone 30 mg q.d.s., reducing after a month to maintenance levels of 15–20 mg/day. Alternatively, dexamethasone or ACTH may be used. Steroids relieve pain and dyspnoea, often improve appetite, and contribute to a general sense of well-being. Occasionally a phenomenal remission occurs with these drugs.

3. Combined loco-regional and systematic disease can, in most cases, initially be regarded just as if they have systemic disease. If loco-regional elements persist while metastases improve—loco-regional radiotherapy or even surgery can have a place.

Hypercalcaemia is liable to occur in patients with breast cancer, particularly on commencing treatment, although it may occur spontaneously. It is associated with bony metastases. The symptoms are often insidious in onset, and affect several systems. They include psychological changes and sleepiness, nausea, vomiting and paralytic ileus, polyuria and dehydration. Early recognition is vital since hypercalcaemia can rapidly be fatal, particularly if a cardiac condition is also present.

Treatment consists of several facets. If hypercalcaemia was precipitated by a new treatment for the disease—this must be stopped immediately. Dehydration and electrolyte imbalance must be corrected. Since calcium is excreted with sodium, increasing salt intake helps. Oral phosphate can be given using effervescent tablets which contain 500 mg of phosphorus. Treatment is commenced starting with two tablets per day. Serum calcium levels must be watched closely—initially being checked on alternate days, and when stable, once each week. The antitumour antibiotic, mitomycin-C, is particularly effective in reducing calcium levels to normal in patients with breast cancer. A single intravenous injection of 25 μg/kg alone may work. If not, further injections after 1–4 days have been shown to produce the required effect. The mechanism of action is thought to be by temporary interference with osteoclastic function.

Corticosteroid therapy rapidly controls hypercalcaemia, and used in a short course of gradually reducing doses, is invaluable when calcium levels are found elevated at presentation of bony disease. Here, unless hypercalcaemia is first corrected, commencement of specific anticancer treatment, such as sex hormones or cytotoxics, is likely to exacerbate an already dangerous situation.

Finally the specific treatment of the causative breast cancer, by those measures most appropriate to the particular patient and the sites and stage of her disease, can control hypercalcaemia.

Prognosis

In the UK, overall corrected survival figures for breast cancer are 50% at 5 years, 35% at 10 years, and 30% at 15 years. Factors which have a bearing on survival are: (1) state of lymph nodes; (2) histological type and grading of primary; (3) some clinical variants and possibly also (4) age at presentation and (5) hormone receptor status of the primary.

1. *Nodes*. Sinus histocytosis or reactive hyperplasia of lymph nodes has been shown in some series to be associated with a good outcome. Rarely can this factor by itself be predictive. However, overall extent and the level of involvement of regional lymph nodes by tumour is consistently a good guide to prognosis. If only 3 nodes or less are involved by tumour, 5-year survival likelihood is 80%, whereas it will be 30% if 4 or more nodes are involved. Subclavian or apical node involvement is a bad sign.

2. Some *tumour types* have an especially good prognosis, particularly so-called 'medullary' carcinoma. This condition frequently shows heavy infiltration of the tumour with lymphocytes, a histological feature which, in any breast carcinoma, suggests a better prognosis. Poorly differentiated carcinoma, as anticipated, carries a poorer outlook. A quantitative guide to prognosis from histopathology is best obtained by grading, as described.

3. *Clinical variants* have a bearing on prognosis. For example, a small tumour in a large breast tends to be a good situation. Presence of oedema and inflammation, with rapid growth, as seen in inflammatory carcinoma, is a bad prognostic sign.

4. The question of *age at presentation* continues to be debated. It was popularly thought that cancer in younger women carried the worst prognosis. Other work has shown that if no account is taken of stage at presentation, cancer in older women does worse overall. The former ideas may have arisen from the impact which premature death brings. The latter figures are due to the fact that older women, at presentation, include significantly more advanced stages of the disease. Correcting for these other prognostic factors, age by itself is not a guide to outcome.

5. The presence of *hormone receptors*, in particular oestrogen receptors, in primary tumours, has been shown to correlate with both longer disease-free interval and prolonged survival time. Receptors are usually present in better differentiated 'low grade' tumours, and so may represent another expression of tumour grade.

Bilateral Breast Carcinoma

The incidence of simultaneous bilateral invasive ductal breast carcinoma is, from pooled data collected in times before mammography, about 1%. The prognosis in simultaneous bilateral disease is that of the worst of the two tumours, i.e. the presence of two simultaneous primaries does not seem to worsen the outlook significantly. From the point of view of the patients, however, the diagnosis of bilateral breast cancer is usually particularly devastating, especially when the most appropriate treatment seems to be simultaneous bilateral mastectomy. This is in practice a situation where the question of treatment has to be approached as gently as possible, and where the spouse needs to be participating in the discussions from as early a stage as possible.

A consensus of the most credible data for the same type of disease on patients observed for at least 20 years gives the metachronous incidence at 5%. This figures does not commend routine simultaneous bilateral mastectomy. The readily admitted subjective nature of the microscopy of breast lesions, and the fact that the actual biopsy site (even when called 'mirror image') is inevitably arbitrary, makes simultaneous biopsy of the contralateral breast unreliable, and even counterproductive. The increasing availability and quality of mammography now minimizes the need for any such procedure. For lobular neoplasia, different considerations need to be made. These are discussed further on under this heading.

Carcinoma of the Breast during Pregnancy

When breast cancer is discovered and treated during the first half of pregnancy, the results are as good as those for comparable stages of disease in non-pregnant women similarly treated. Thus, breast cancer in the first half of pregnancy is no more grave than otherwise. Treatment recommended for this is to allow the pregnancy to continue, and treat the cancer on its own merits. In its second half, pregnancy has a deleterious effect on breast cancer. Management advised is, depending on the circumstances and wishes of the individual patient, to treat only after term or termination.

There is no evidence that pregnancy subsequent to treatment of breast carcinoma worsens survival rate.

Despite this, with the overall mortality figures being what they are for this disease, the implications of further pregnancy in these circumstances should be given most careful consideration.

Psychological Sequelae of Mastectomy and Reconstruction

The psychological sequelae of mastectomy have now been measured. The chief problem is loss of body form, with for many women the accompanying loss of acceptability for her spouse. Restoration of a breast mound is feasible after mastectomy, either using a pedicle of omentum or a Silastic prosthesis, which may itself be placed either under the skin or under the pectoral muscles. These measures do not have universal application, even if they were advisable and appropriate in all cases. First, skin of adequate amount and thickness has to be available. Secondly, symmetry is difficult to achieve with the remaining natural breast which is usually larger and more pendulous than can be achieved by reconstruction. Thirdly, since Silastic reconstruction always diminishes blood supply to overlying skin flaps, this method would seem contraindicated where radiotherapy is also used, which itself diminishes tissue viability. Finally, it remains to be established that reconstruction will not influence adversly the natural history and follow-up of the treated disease, or that it significantly alleviates post-mastectomy psychological problems.

Follow-up Policy

Is there any benefit to the patient from regular follow-up after primary treatment for breast cancer? Most British centres see these patients quarterly for two years, half-yearly up to the end of the fifth year, and thereafter annually. The rationale for such a policy is that any recurrence will be detected fairly early, and eliminated before it overwhelms. This policy is completely justified in so far as it enables early detection, and satisfactory treatment of local recurrence or metachronous contralateral primary. Whether any benefit occurs when systemic metastasis is found is less clear. Theoretically, on the hypothesis that the smaller the tumour cell mass, the more likely it is to be successfully eliminated with minimal host damage, regular follow-up has a place. For systemic disease, the ideal would be a tumour marker in blood or urine, change in which would precede clinical manifestation of metastases. Plasma carcinoembryonic antigen, and urinary hydroxyproline–creatinine ratio offer some hope of being useful in this respect. At present, finding recurrence depends upon clinical suspicion. If suspected, a programme such as that for the initial investigation of breast complaints is necessary to refute or confirm the diagnosis.

The management of recurrent breast cancer has been outlined under the 'late breast cancer' subheading of treatment. Treatment has to be appropriate to the individual case. Particular reference must be paid to (i) the site, (ii) whether local or general, (iii) prognostic factors determined at pre- and postprimary treatment assessment, (iv) age and circumstances of individual patient.

Screening for Breast Cancer

The objective of screening for breast cancer is to detect it at a stage which is earlier than it would have been had it become symptomatic. Surgical literature has long shown that for cohorts of women, duration of survival after treatment for breast cancer is better the lower the stage of the disease at presentation.

The high incidence of the disease in the Western world and its lethal nature, make it highly desirable to prolong survival even if it cannot be detected at the pre-invasive stage as occurs with cancer of the cervix. Screening can be attempted by any one of or a combination of four techniques: self-examination, clinical examination, mammography and thermography. At least one study has shown that earlier detection than normal can be achieved in practice by women examining their own breasts at regular intervals. This apparently common sense approach is the one favoured by the majority of general practitioners who were surveyed in a large city. It leaves several questions unanswered. How small a change in the breast can women detect? Will women instructed in the ideal technique, if such exists, comply? Will there be any counterproductive effects? Preliminary results show that it is not completely harmless in that a proportion, albeit small, of subjects under instruction developed severe psychiatric sequelae.

Clinical examination requires numbers of trained personnel. By itself, clinical examination is not so effective as when combined with mammography. In addition to its costs and necessary expertise, mammography has the disadvantage that the breast is irradiated at each visit. Repeated examination is implicit in screening and the groups of women in whom repeated mammography could be of benefit rather than a hazard, have still to be defined. Thermography is completely non-invasive. However, its reliability and discrimination are much less than mammography and it is not, at present, a practical routine proposition.

Several mammographic screening programmes in different parts of the world have shown that when screening is first made available in a community, a higher yield of breast cancer is obtained than would be recognized spontaneously over the same time interval. It also looks as if the tumours found by screening are at an earlier stage and therefore carry a better prognosis than those presenting spontaneously. Furthermore, in two large studies where all the subjects screened were over 40 years of age, a 30% survival advantage has been achieved at 10 years from diagnosis. Breast screening by mammography is now being established in many Western Countries including the UK. Any method which is employed must be based on rational principles and thorough knowledge of this enigmatic disease. All programmes must be closely monitored and costed to allow their short and long term results to be evaluated. Attention must also be directed towards identifying those women who are at a higher risk than average for developing cancer of the breast.

MALIGNANT DISEASE OF THE MALE BREAST

Both compared with breast cancer in females and in terms of absolute numbers occurring, this is a small problem. Annual incidence of breast cancer in males in the UK is approximately 200 cases, i.e. about 1 per 3000 adult men. (In Klinefelter's syndrome the incidence is the same as in females.) It occurs in older age, average being 60 years (compared with the average age of 50 years for female breast cancer). Epidemiological evidence shows that it is strongly associated with chronic liver disease.

Nipple discharge, particularly serous or bloodstained is a significant symptom in males and proportionately a much more common presenting symptom of breast cancer than in females. Length of history in males is commonly expressed in years rather than the weeks or months seen in females. Partly as a consequence of this, and perhaps partly because of the relative lack of breast tissue in males, the condition is often advanced at presentation, with a predictably poor prognosis. Axillary metastases are often extensive, even when the primary is quite small.

Haagensen advocates radical mastectomy for Stage I and II male breast carcinoma, pointing out that this necessitates sacrifice of skin such that grafting is essential. Orchidectomy used for advanced male breast cancer has an excellent record, with objective remissions recorded in 70%. In the light of the fact that men with breast cancer are usually in the older age groups and that the standard loco-regional treatment when used by itself for clinically localized disease gives poor longer term results (notably poorer than such regimes in comparable disease in females) it would seem fully justified to advise orchidectomy as well as painstaking radical local treatment. When recurrence is localized, radiotherapy gives useful control. When distant recurrence occurs, particularly if disease is visceral, additive oestrogen therapy has been observed to control disease, as has the anti-oestrogen tamoxifen (Nolvadex). Chemotherapy, single or multiple agent, has a place.

Further Reading

Baum M. (1981) *Breast Cancer—The Facts.* Oxford, Oxford University Press.

Bonadonna G. and Valagussa P. (1985) Adjuvant systemic therapy for resectable breast cancer. *J. Clin. Oncol.* **3**, 259–275.

Bostwick J. (1983) *Aesthetic and Reconstructive Breast Surgery.* St Louis, Mosby.

Brinkley D. and Haybittle J. L. (1977) The curability of breast cancer. *World J. Surg.* **1**, 287–289.

Calle R., Pilleron J. P., Schlenger P. et al. (1978) Conservative management of operable breast cancer: ten years' experience at the Foundation Curie. *Cancer* **42**, 2045–2053.

Duguid H. L., Wood R. A. B., Irving A. D. et al. (1979) Needle aspiration of the breast with immediate reporting of material. *Br. Med. J.* **2**, 185–187.

Haagensen C. D. (1985) *Diseases of the Breast*, 3rd ed. Philadelphia, Saunders.

Steroid receptors in breast cancer 1980, *Cancer* (Suppl.) **46**, 2759 (whole issue).

61 The Thyroid

Andrew Gunn

EMBRYOLOGY AND ANATOMY

A detailed knowledge of gross anatomy is mandatory for the surgeon who is to operate on the thyroid gland, as is an understanding of embryology if the nature of congenital abnormalities is to be appreciated.

Embryology

The thyroid develops as an entodermal tubular structure from the posterior aspect of the fetal tongue, and grows downwards in front of the developing hyoid and larynx, bifurcating and fusing with elements from the 4th branchial pouches. The stem of the downgrowth forms the thyroglossal duct whose upper end remains as the foramen caecum of the tongue; the lower end forms the pyramidal lobe of the thyroid. The thyroglossal duct normally atrophies but may remain in whole or in part and produce abnormalities in later life. The transient ultimobranchial pouches (part of the 4th) contribute to the development of the thyroid an element which becomes the parafollicular (calcitonin secreting) cells. In lower orders, e.g. fishes, the ultimobranchial pouches form a separate endocrine gland, the ultimobranchial body, which secretes calcitonin. It is a matter of surgical importance that the 4th branchial pounches also produce the superior parathyroids which normally maintain a close relationship to the superomedial aspect of the thyroid lobes. The inferior parathyroids develop from the 3rd branchial pouch and their relationship is more to thymus than thyroid. They normally come to lie between the apex of the thymus and the lower pole of the thyroid or along the fibrous band, the thyrothymic ligament which unites them (*Fig.* 61.1).

Anatomy

The thyroid consists of two lateral lobes, pyriform in shape and united in their lower parts by an isthmus. It is applied closely to the laryngeal and cricoid cartilages and upper rings of the trachea and their uniting membranes by a dense fascia, the pretracheal fascia, and so moves with these structures on swallowing. The thyroid is covered by the strap muscles and their dense covering fascia which together form the myofascial layer of the neck. A matter of enormous importance to the surgeon is the fact that the recurrent laryngeal nerves run deep to the lobes of the thyroid in the groove between oesophagus and trachea. On the left, because of its relationship to the aortic arch, the recurrent laryngeal nerve comes to lie deeply in the groove between the oesophagus and the trachea but on the right the nerve lies more laterally. A variant, about 2% of cases, is the non-recurrent laryngeal nerve coming directly from the vagus rather than being routed round the subclavian artery.

The thyroid is richly vascular, normally accounting for 5% of the cardiac output and it derives its blood supply from four arteries. Each lateral lobe receives a superior thyroid artery at its superior pole from the external carotid and an inferior thyroid artery, indirectly from the subclavian, by way of the thyrocervical trunk, the vessel reaching the

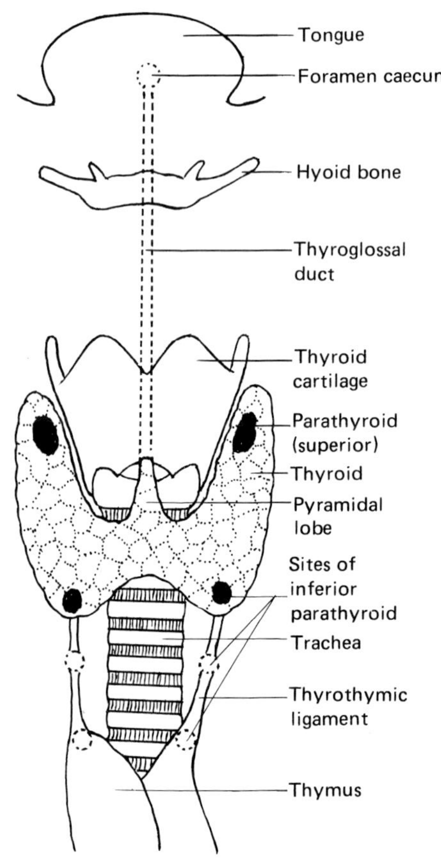

Fig. 61.1 Relationship of thyroglossal duct to thyroid, thymus and parathyroids. Anterior view.

lateral border of the thyroid lobe by piercing the fascia between the carotid sheath and the vertebral column, and having an important though variable relationship to the recurrent laryngeal nerve. An occasional fifth artery, the thyroidea ima, arising from the aorta, the brachiocephalic or internal mammary arteries, runs up the anterior border of the trachea to the thyroid.

A plexus of thin-walled veins on the surface of the gland gives rise to numerous draining veins, the principal named veins being the superior thyroid veins, running closely with the superior thyroid arteries and entering the internal jugular, the middle thyroid veins draining directly to the internal jugular and the inferior thyroid veins draining to the innominate (left brachiocephalic) vein in the superior mediastinum.

Lymphatics are numerous and drain to lymph nodes along the internal jugular vein and innominate vein. They are of great importance in the spread of thyroid carcinoma (*Figs.* 61.2, 61.3, 61.4).

PHYSIOLOGY

As will be apparent from embryological development, the thyroid is a composite of two endocrine glands. The less important element derived from the ultimobranchial pouches is that of the parafollicular cells which secrete calcitonin. Calcitonin acts on bone antagonistically to parathyroid hormone, being responsible for entry of calcium into bone, but the complete physiological action of this hormone in man awaits further research. The clinical importance of the parafollicular cells is as the source of the rare medullary carcinoma of the thyroid (*Fig.* 61.5). The follicular element of the thyroid is all important, secreting thyroxine and triiodothyronine, the principal hormones controlling the body's metabolic rate.

Thyroxine (T4) is the predominant thyroid hormone but its main action is after conversion to the more active triiodothyronine (T3). A small amount of T4 is converted to reverse T3 (rT3) in which deiodination is from the second tyrosine ring. rT3 is metabolically inactive and any biological role is as yet undefined. The importance is that this pathway may become the more significant under certain circumstances, e.g. after thyroidectomy or under the influence of certain drugs such as propranolol. Thyroid hormone is secreted by the follicular cells and stored within the follicle lumen bound to the colloid thyroglobulin from which it is dissociated to enter the circulation (*Fig.* 61.6).

Synthesis and discharge of thyroid hormone is controlled by anterior pituitary thyroid-stimulating hormone (TSH), a polypeptide, which in turn is regulated by the hypothalamic-releasing hormone, thyrotrophin-releasing hormone (TRH), a tripeptide. Ouput of TRH and TSH is regulated by many factors, chief amongst them the circulating levels of T4 and T3 feeding back to hypothalamus and pituitary (*Fig.* 61.7).

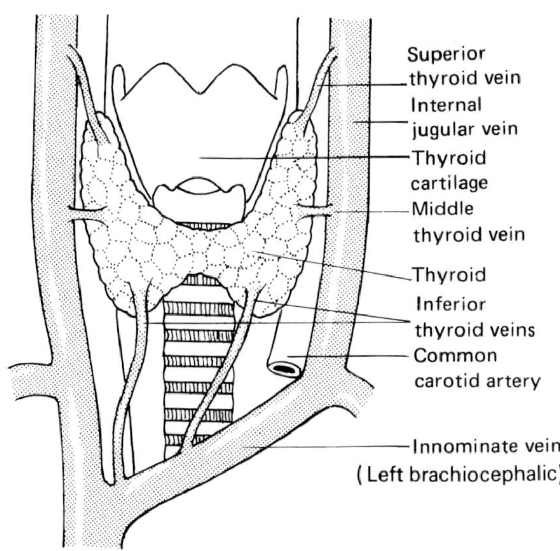

Fig. 61.2 Relations of thyroid. Anterior view.

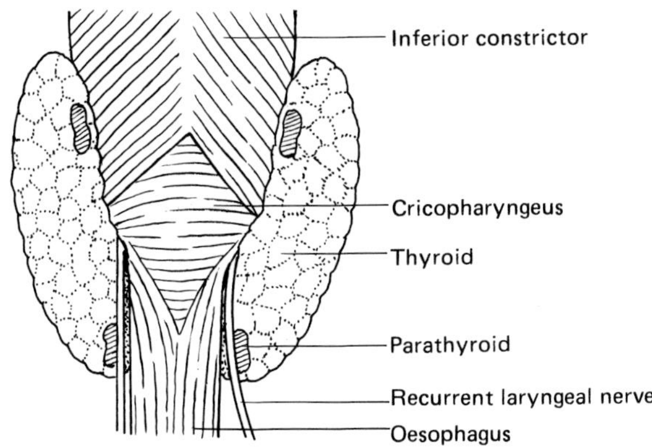

Fig. 61.3 Relations of thyroid. Posterior view.

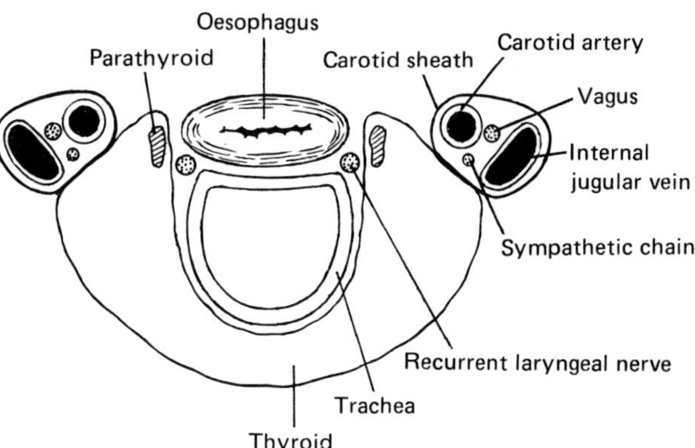

Fig. 61.4 Relations of thyroid.

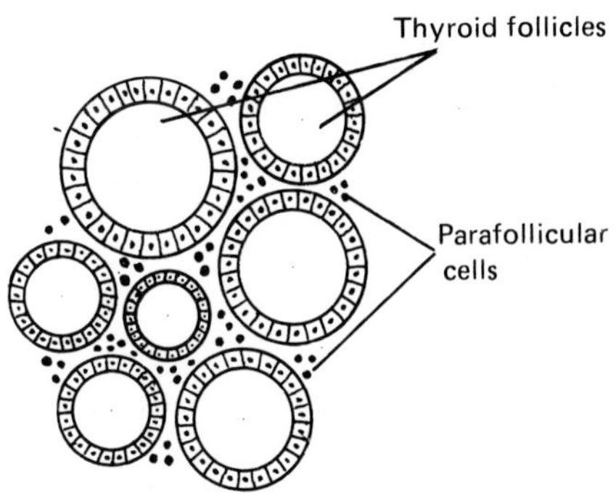

Fig. 61.5 Relationship of parafollicular cells to thyroid follicles.

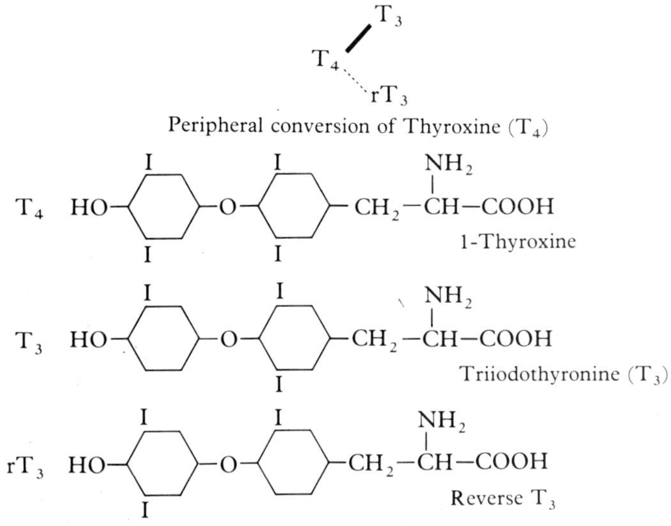

$T_4 \rightarrow T_3$ / rT_3

Peripheral conversion of Thyroxine (T_4)

T_4: HO–(ring, I, I)–O–(ring, I, I)–CH_2–CH(NH_2)–COOH — l-Thyroxine

T_3: HO–(ring, I, I)–O–(ring, I, I)–CH_2–CH(NH_2)–COOH — Triiodothyronine (T_3)

rT_3: HO–(ring, I, I)–O–(ring, I, I)–CH_2–CH(NH_2)–COOH — Reverse T_3

Fig. 61.6 Conversion of T4 to T3 and reverse T3.

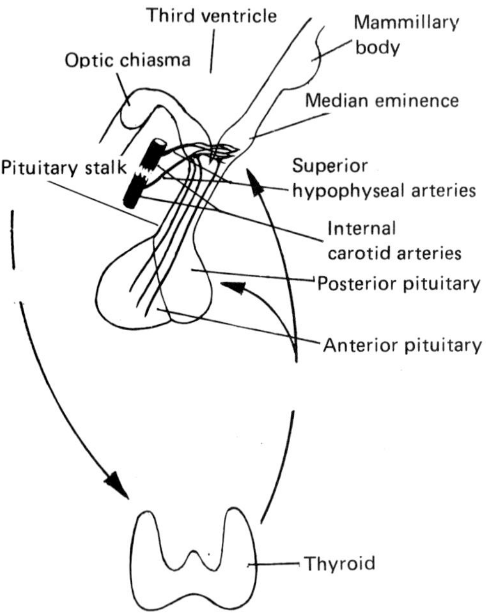

Fig. 61.7 Physiological control of the thyroid gland.

METHODS OF INVESTIGATION

Clinical

Assessment of thyroid function by a carefully elicited history and observation of clinical signs is still of fundamental importance. Symptoms and signs can be quantitated by using a diagnostic index of thyroid disease and a supply of such forms should be available in the consulting rooms (*Figs.* 61.8, 61.9).

Biochemical

It is possible to be completely objective about thyroid status because of the ready availability of sensitive assays. T3, T4 and TSH may be assayed by radioimmunoassay to give an accurate assessment of thyroid status provided account is taken of the levels of thyroid-binding globulin (TBG) which may be elevated particularly in pregnancy or as a result of oestrogen therapy, e.g. the contraceptive pill. Only a fraction of 1% of all T4 is free in the circulation and its direct measurement is difficult and expensive. Non-specific alterations in TBG can alter levels of T4 significantly. The problem can be overcome by measuring the degree of saturation of TBG using radio-iodinated T3 (the T3 index) and using this to calculate a free thyroxine index (FTI). Of increasing importance is the TRH test. Synthetic TRH is given intravenously to the patient and blood samples are taken at 0, 20 and 60 min for estimation of TSH. The degree of response to TRH can tell a great deal about the pituitary TSH reserve and hence thyroid status. The test is at its most sensitive at the lower end of the range of thyroid function and finds its greatest use in investigating incipient hypothyroidism, an important clinical problem.

Radiochemical

Radioisotopes of iodine make possible dynamic thyroid function studies. The rate of incorporation of radio-iodine into the thyroid after injection can yield a lot of information about the function of the gland. To some extent the TRH test is replacing these but they continue to have a role in difficult cases.

The isotope technetium behaves similarly to iodine, and scanning with this is important in elucidating the nature of altered function within the thyroid. Absence or ectopic situation of the thyroid can be studied by this technique. Probably its greatest use is to determine whether a lump in the thyroid is functioning ('hot') or not ('cold'). The 'hot' nodule is unlikely to be malignant (*Figs.* 61.10–61.13).

Total body scintiscanning is of great importance in certain types of carcinoma of the thyroid when, after total thyroidectomy or ablation with radio-iodine, secondary deposits can be induced to take up radio-iodine indicating which cases may benefit from therapeutic doses.

Ultrasonography

Ultrasonic scanning is of great value in determining something of the nature of swellings within the thyroid, especially those that are 'cold' on isotope scanning. Obviously it is not possible to infer a tissue diagnosis from ultrasonography, but simple fluid-filled cysts can readily be distinguished from other nodules and this has important implications for treatment. Aspiration of a simple cyst may save exploratory operation (*Figs.* 61.14, 61.15).

Biopsy

Closed biopsy techniques such as Tru-cut needle biopsy or high-speed drill biopsy have virtually ceased to have a place in histological diagnosis. They provide too small a sample and can result in complications such as bleeding or even nerve damage.

Fine needle aspiration biopsy (FNAB) using a technique similar to that used in breast disease has however come to have an important role. Interpretation is by no means easy and must be made only by a cytologist who has become specifically acquainted with thyroid FNAB cytology. There is no doubt that where thyroid FNAB cytology is available its use results in fewer thyroid explorations for 'cold' nodules.

HYPERTHYROIDISM—DIAGNOSTIC INDEX

NAME .... AGE .... DATE.................................. UNIT NO ....
HOSPITAL.. WARD/CLINIC.................................. OBSERVER ....

SYMPTOMS (of recent onset and/or increased severity)		DESCRIPTION	If PRESENT please ring numbers	
			Positive Score	Negative Score
1. Dyspnoea on effort		Age of patient taken into account	+1	0
2. Palpitations		Occurring at rest or on moderate exertion	+2	0
3. Tiredness		Unusual tiredness after usual physical effort	+2	0
4. Preference for heat (irrespective of duration)		Habit of sitting away from fire.	0	−5
Preference for cold		Preference for a cold room	+5	0
5. Sweating		Both thermal and emotional sweating	+3	0
6. Nervousness		Irritability, 'tenseness', easy loss of temper	+2	0
7. Weight	Increase	Confirm by slackness or tightness of clothing or change in weight of 7 lbs or more	0	−3
	Decrease		+3	0
8. Appetite	Increase	Less than normal, normal or excessive	+3	0
	Decrease		0	−3
SIGNS			Please ring	as indicated
			PRESENT	ABSENT
9. Palpable thyroid		Should be visible *and* palpable in females; visible *or* palpable in males	+3	−3
10. Thyroid bruit		High-pitched systolic or 'to and fro'	+2	−3
11. Exophthalmos	R. mm L. mm	Sclera seen between lower lid and iris of either eye; patient looking straight ahead	+2	0
12. Lid retraction		Sclera seen between upper lid and iris	+2	0
13. Lid lag		Sclera appears when patient's eyes moving from above downwards fixed on examiner's finger	+1	0
14. Hyperkinesis		Rapid jerky movements; wasted energy and clumsiness when removing garments	+4	−2
15. Finger tremor		Fine tremor of outstretched hands with eyes closed	+1	0
16. Hands:	Hot	Take room temperature and examiner's own hands into account	+2	−2
	Moist		+1	−1
17. Pulse rate		Counted for one minute at the end of examination		
Toxic—greater than 19		Less than 80	0	−3
Equivocal—11–19		80–90	0	0
Euthyroid—Less than 11		More than 90	+3	0
		Atrial Fibrillation	+4	0
Comments: (including any current medication)		Total Symptom and Sign Score		
		TOTAL SCORE		

Fig. 61.8 Diagnostic index of thyroid disease—hyperthyroidism.

HYPOTHYROIDISM—DIAGNOSTIC INDEX

NAME .... AGE .... SEX ....
UNIT NO .... HOSPITAL ....
OBSERVER .... DATE ....
PREVIOUS ANTITHYROID OR REPLACEMENT THERAPY: TYPE ....
DATES ....

SYMPTOMS (of recent onset)	DESCRIPTION	Score (ring appropriate value)		
		Present	*Absent*	*Doubtful*
1. Diminished sweating	Sweating in a warm room or centrally heated hall	+6	−2	0
2. Dry skin	Dryness of skin noticed spontaneously or on removing clothing, requiring skin cream	+3	−6	0
3. Cold intolerance	Preference for a warm room extra clothing or bed clothing	+4	−5	0
4. Weight increase	Recorded increase in weight; tightness of clothing	+1	−1	0
5. Constipation	Bowel habits; use of laxative	+2	−1	0
6. Hoarseness of voice	Speaking voice: singing voice	+5	−6	0
7. Paraesthesiae	Subjective sensations of numbness, tingling in *hands*	+5	−4	0
8. Deafness	Progressive impairment of hearing	+2	0	0
SIGNS				
9. Slow movements	Observe patient removing and replacing a buttoned garment	+11	−3	0
10. Coarse skin	Examine hands, forearms, elbows for roughness and thickening of skin	+7	−7	0
11. Cold skin	Compare temperature of examiner's and patient's hands	+3	−2	0
12. Periorbital puffiness	Should obscure curve of malar bone	+4	−6	0
13. Slow pulse rate	Count over 30 seconds. Slowing present if under 75/min	+4	−4	0
14. Slowing of ankle jerk	Elicit with patient kneeling on a chair, grasping its back	+15	−6	0
(−25 or less—Euthyroid) (−24 to +19—Doubtful) (+20 or over—Hypothyroid)	Positive and Negative TOTALS			
	FINAL SCORE			

COMMENTS: (Including any current medication) (overleaf)

Fig. 61.9 Diagnostic index of thyroid disease—hypothyroidism.

Immunological

Immunologically mediated disease is important in the thyroid and can be diagnosed, when taken together with the clinical and biochemical findings, by demonstrating circulating antibodies. Autoimmune thyroiditis of which Hashimoto's disease is the most severe form, can be inferred by demonstrating antibodies to thyroglobulin by agglutination of red blood cells or latex particles tanned with thyroglobulin, and antibodies to thyroid microsomes by immunofluorescence or complement fixation. Techniques for demonstration of the thyroid growth-stimulating immunoglobulin (TGSI), thyroid-stimulating immunoglobulin (TSI) and long-acting thyroid stimulator (LATS) are of importance in research but not generally available for diagnostic purposes.

CONGENITAL ABNORMALITIES (*Fig.* 61.16)

Dyshormonogenesis

There must be included abnormalities of a biochemical nature which are mostly inherited and occur in known families. The majority are due to defects at some point along the pathway of synthesis of thyroid hormone, dyshormonogenesis. Treatment is by replacement therapy. Surgical interest is in the fact that goitre may develop under the influence of TSH stimulation if treatment is suboptimal or the patient stops taking the tablets. The picture of subthyroidism in a patient with a large, perhaps pulsatile goitre should bring to mind the probability of a congenital biochemical abnormality. Treatment is to institute adequate replacement therapy. Pendred's syndrome is the association of dyshormonogenesis with congenital nerve deafness.

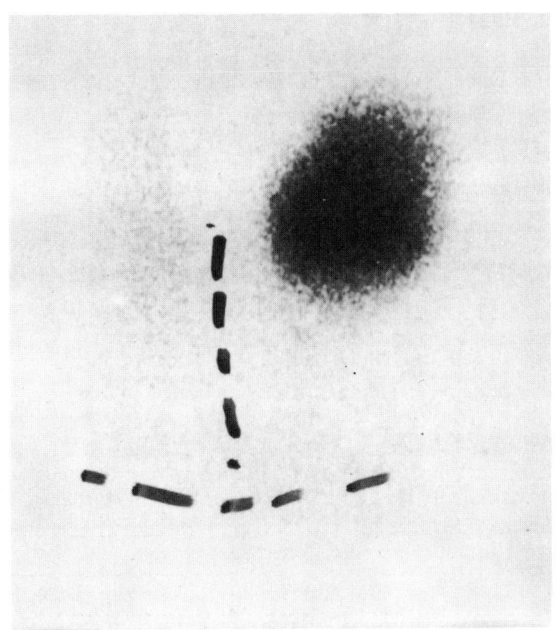

Fig. 61.10 'Hot' nodule, left lobe. Note suppression of the rest of the thyroid due to suppression of TSH.

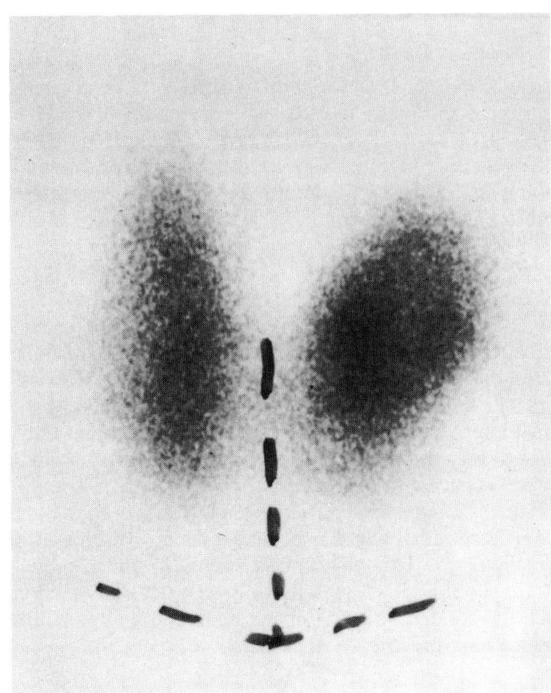

Fig. 61.11 'Hot' nodule, post TSH. Note that exogenous TSH brings up the rest of the gland.

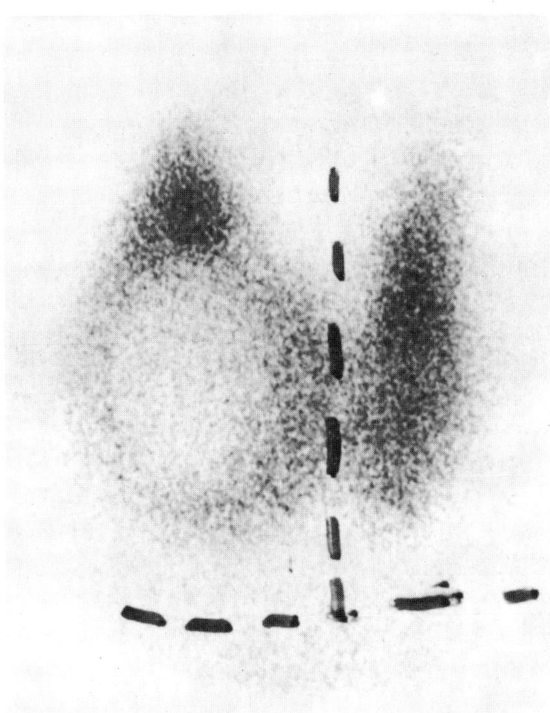

Fig. 61.12 Technetium scan. 'Cold' nodule, right lobe.

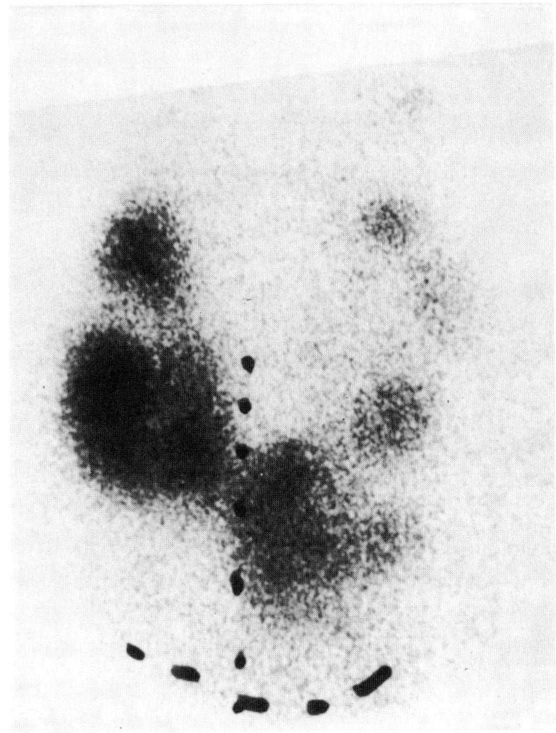

Fig. 61.13 Multinodular goitre.

Absence or Hypoplasia

Recognition of congenital absence or hypoplasia of the thyroid is one of the most critical observations that can be made in the neonate.

Treatment with adequate replacement therapy will be rewarded by normal growth and development; failure to recognize the condition must result in the severe mental and physical retardation of cretinism. Where there is a goitre at birth, as may be seen in goitrous areas, the diagnosis of goitrous cretinism should not be missed. Biochemical

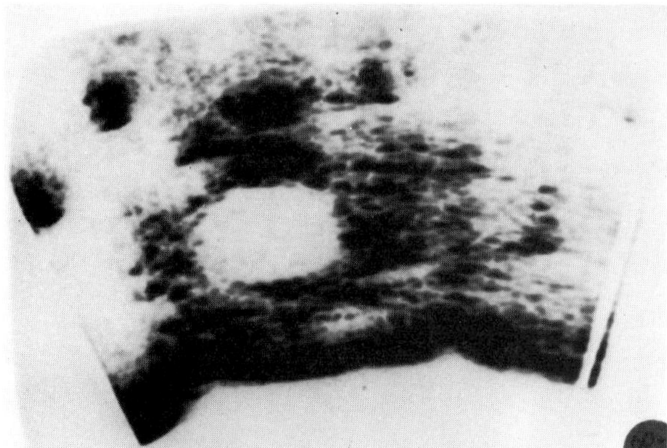

Fig. 61.14 Ultrasonic scan. Note simple cyst.

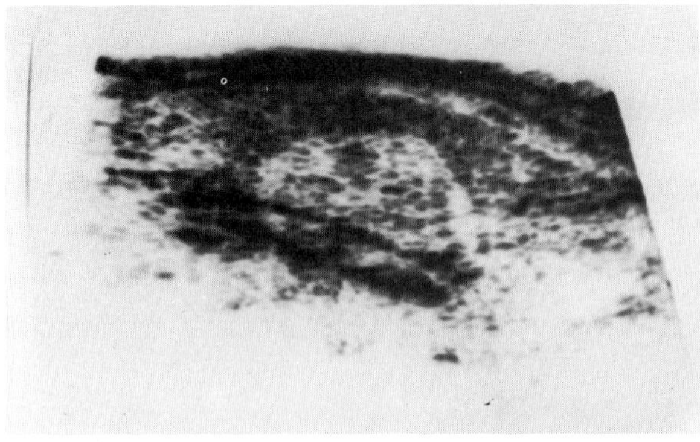

Fig. 61.15 Ultrasonic scan. Solid lesion (microfollicular adenoma).

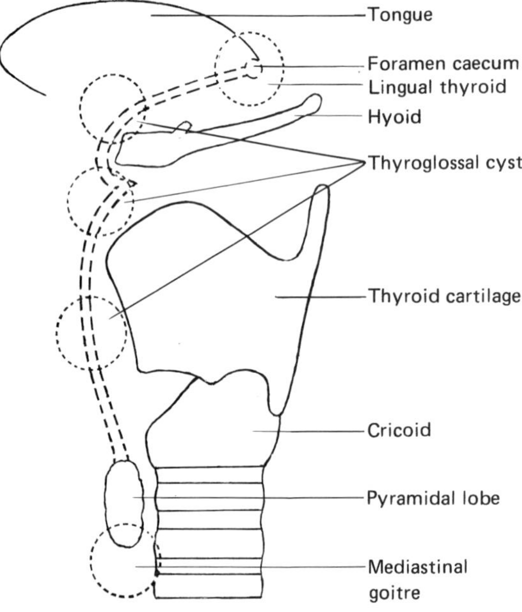

Fig. 61.16 Congenital abnormalities of thyroid development.

screening of neonates has been instituted in many centres and where this is available should make cretinism a disease of historical interest only as well as bringing to light cases where thyroid function is suboptimal.

Ectopia

Failures of migration may lead to ectopia of the thyroid gland which may lie anywhere between the base of the tongue (lingual thyroid) and the mediastinum. If masses compatible with ectopia are found then isotope scanning is desirable to determine whether there is normal thyroid tissue or whether the ectopic tissue represents all of the thyroid. Excision may be required for respiratory obstruction, other pressure symptoms, or for cosmetic reasons. Replacement therapy should probably now supplant the previous efforts at surgical reimplantation.

Thyroglossal Cyst and Fistula

These are covered in Chapter 23.

'Lateral Aberrant Thyroid'

There is no such thing as a 'lateral aberrant thyroid' and almost certainly the condition was confused with metastasis to cervical lymph nodes from an unrecognized primary thyroid tumour of well-differentiated type.

DISORDERS OF THYROID STRUCTURE

Goitre

The term 'goitre' refers only to visible or palpable enlargement of the thyroid and infers no particular alteration in thyroid function. It takes many varieties:

Physiological Goitre

Physiological goitre is the term applied to thyroid enlargement seen commonly in girls at the menarche or in women during pregnancy. The cause is unknown and normally the goitre regresses in time. No treatment is required though the patient and her family will require reassurance. It may be doubted whether the condition is truly 'physiological'.

Endemic Goitre

Goitre was once endemic in certain geographical areas, usually remote from the sea, where diet is deficient in iodine, e.g. the Himalayas, the Alps, and around the Great Lakes of North America and the Derbyshire district of England. The problem can be virtually eliminated by the iodization of salt and remains a significant problem only in those areas where this public health measure cannot be applied. Goitres may reach enormous sizes and complications may be seen as a consequence of the size of the gland alone, from metabolic consequences such as thyrotoxicosis or malignancy. The condition is essentially preventable.

Care should be taken in dealing with the individual case since the sudden addition of iodine to the diet of goitrous persons may precipitate thyrotoxicosis.

Sporadic Goitre

Goitre may occur sporadically in non-goitrous regions and in the absence of iodine deficiency. The cause is uncertain but undoubtedly some are autoimmune in nature and due to the presence of a specific growth-stimulating immunoglobulin (TGSI).

The euthyroid state is normally maintained but such patients are more prone to develop secondary thyrotoxicosis and to have a higher than average risk of thyroid cancer. The risk, however, is still small and would not *per se* justify surgical treatment. Surgery is reserved for pressure symptoms, cosmetic reasons or for the above complications.

A small number of goitres can be attributed to goitrogens in the diet, e.g. excess ingestion of vegetables of the cabbage family perhaps as part of a calorie-controlled diet, or to drugs such as PAS and lithium.

Lumps in the Thyroid

Presentation of the patient with a lump or multiple lumps in the thyroid is an important clinical problem. Where lumps are multiple the condition is usually quite benign in the pathological sense although there may be important clinical problems caused by compression of trachea or oesophagus leading to stridor or dysphagia, compression of a recurrent laryngeal nerve with voice changes, mediastinal extension, pain often from haemorrhage into an area of degeneration, or occasionally, the onset of thyrotoxicosis.

The commonest pathological change is non-toxic nodular goitre (NTNG), a disease of uncertain aetiology though some are undoubtedly autoimmune and due to the presence of TGSI. The thyroid consists of degenerating and hyperplastic areas, cystic change, fibrosis and a variable degree of lymphoid infiltration.

Investigation must include clinical and biochemical assessment of thyroid function, radiology for tracheal compression and mediastinal extension, radionuclide scanning, ultrasonography and autoantibody studies. Scanning with radio-iodine frequently gives a complex picture with areas demonstrating uptake of the isotope ('hot' or 'warm') and areas of reduced uptake ('cold') and all gradations between the widespread nature of the changes will generally help to exclude malignancy but in practice as NTNG confers no immunity to development of thyroid cancer, surgical exploration may have to be undertaken if there are suspicious areas. Complications of compression require surgical intervention and the onset of toxicity is best treated surgically. The condition is seen most often in females in the older age group.

THE CLINICALLY SOLITARY THYROID NODULE (*Fig.* 61.17)

This is more sinister than the thyroid presenting with multiple nodules and will yield a higher incidence of malignancy, between 5 and 10%. In fact, many clinically solitary

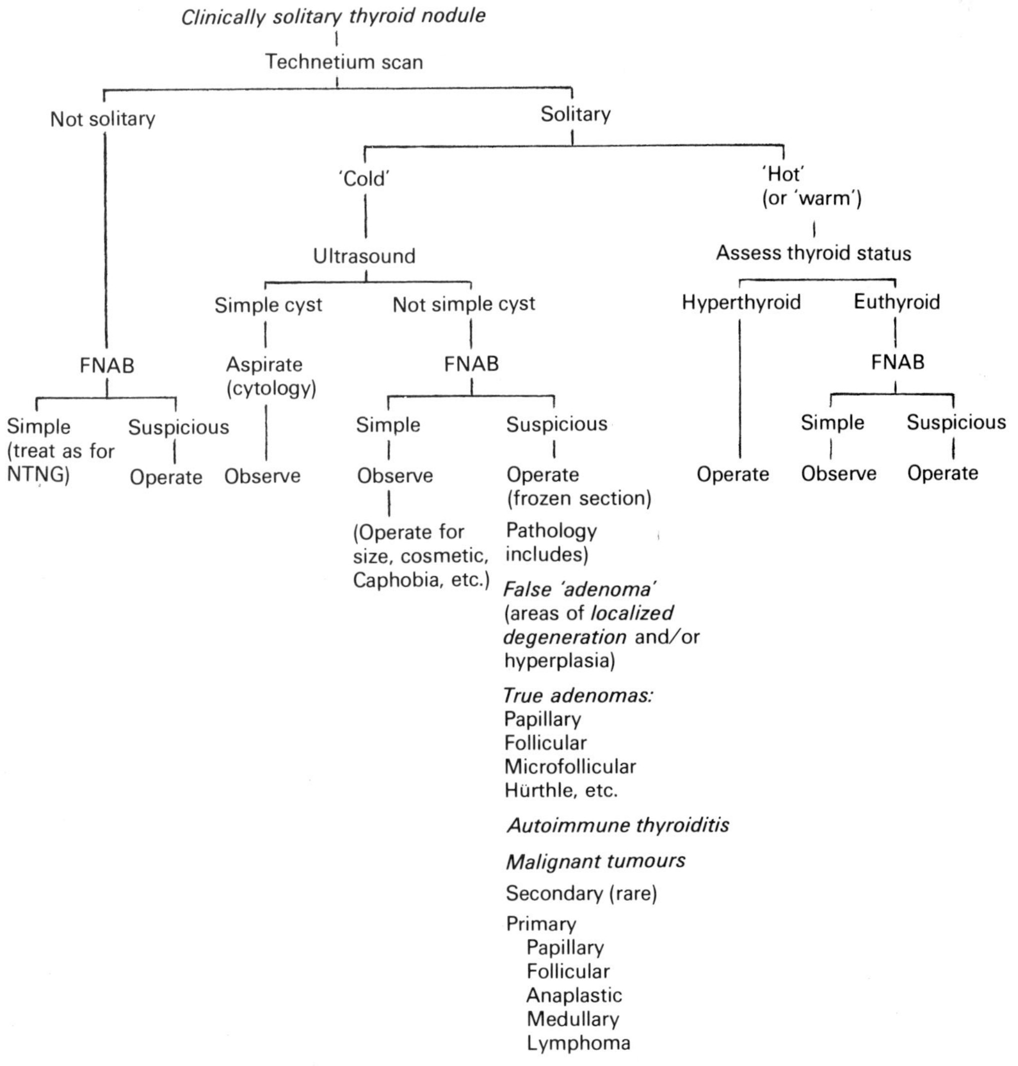

Fig. 61.17 Schema for management of the clinically solitary thyroid nodule.

nodules will be found on scanning or at thyroid exploration to be part of a more generalized change whereupon the prognosis becomes much more favourable as the lesion is then likely to be a part of a NTNG. Investigation of the clinically solitary thyroid nodule must include clinical and biochemical assessment of thyroid status, isotope scanning to assess whether it is hot or cold, ultrasonography to determine whether the lesion is cystic or not, autoantibodies and radiology of the neck and chest. Hot nodules are much less likely to be neoplastic than cold.

The changes, however, may not be absolute and all gradations between hot and cold are seen. Ultrasonography can distinguish the simple cystic lesion and the solid lesion, or the solid lesion with cystic degeneration, which is very common. The simple cystic lesion may be treated by aspiration of its contents under local anaesthesia, exploration being reserved for troublesome recurrence. The possibility of a cyst being associated with a carcinoma should be borne in mind though this is relatively uncommon. Ultrasonography cannot distinguish between pathological types of solid lesions.

The Question of Biopsy

Biopsy has been discussed above with particular reference to FNAB. With good cytology this is undoubtedly leading to reduction in the number of thyroid explorations for benign conditions. However, the operation carries an exceedingly small morbidity in experienced hands and getting rid of the lump is often of great importance to patients, many of whom have a distinct cancer phobia. Excision biopsy is the appropriate operation and should consist of total removal of the affected thyroid lobe and isthmus with careful preservation of the current laryngeal nerve and parathyroids. An experienced pathologist can give a valid opinion of frozen section but occasionally the diagnosis may have to be revised at subsequent paraffin section, though this incidence should be quite low.

BENIGN THYROID TUMOURS

Benign thyroid tumours require total lobectomy on the affected side. In practice many of the so-called adenomas are not true adenomas in a pathological sense but areas of altered function within the thyroid often with colloid retention and cystic degeneration. The true adenomas do make up a fair proportion of benign lesions and include papillary adenomas, follicular adenomas, microfollicular or 'fetal' adenomas and Hürthle cell adenomas. Hürthle cell adenoma can be difficult inasmuch as even those tumours which are histologically clearly benign do occasionally have a reputation for local recurrence. This is one of the reasons why subtotal lobectomy should be abandoned as a method of treating benign thyroid tumours.

MALIGNANT DISEASE OF THE THYROID

Secondary tumours do occur but are extremely rare.

Primary malignancies of the thyroid can be classified according to the element from which they arise:

Tumours of thyroid follicular epithelium

Papillary carcinoma
Follicular carcinoma
Anaplastic carcinoma

Tumour of parafollicular cells

Medullary carcinoma

Tumour of lymphoid element

Lymphoma

Tumours of Thyroid Follicular Epithelium

Papillary Carcinoma of Thyroid

While it may be seen at any age, papillary carcinoma has a predilection for the first three decades and may be seen in childhood. Classically it presents as a lump in the thyroid or less commonly as a solid swelling in a lymph node draining the thyroid, the primary in the thyroid being undetectable. It carries one of the most favourable prognoses of all forms of cancer with 5-year survivals of 90% scarcely reduced at 10 years and with excellent life prognosis.

There are two schools of thought on treatment.

One school favours a radical approach advising total thyroidectomy with parathyroid identification and preservation. The reason is that the disease may be multifocal and present throughout the thyroid though clinically undetectable and while the overall prognosis is excellent there is still a mortality of 10% or so and this, in a very young age group. Any involved lymph nodes are also removed. Thereafter radio-iodine total body scanning is done. If there is any uptake, therapeutic doses of radio-iodine are given. Scanning is repeated 6 monthly for 2 years and annually for 5 years.

All patients are given T3 sufficient to suppress TSH as there is evidence that TSH stimulates the tumour. A dose of 80 μg is normally sufficient for an adult. TSH should be assayed to check that it is suppressed and as a check that the patient is taking the tablets regularly. T3 is preferred to T4 since it need be stopped for only 1 week prior to scanning. T4 requires to be stopped for a month and in this time mild hypothyroidism will occur.

The recent availability of sensitive radioimmunoassays for thyroglobulin look like providing a much more efficient means of follow-up than scanning with radio-iodine. It is unnecessary to stop the thyroid hormone suppression therapy and is altogether more sensitive and much less expensive. The assay is becoming more widely available. It is a good example of a genuine 'tumour marker'.

Another school of thought feels that this rather too radical for a disease carrying such an excellent outlook and advises total thyroid lobectomy on the affected side with subtotal lobectomy on the contralateral side. Radio-iodine is not used for scanning or for therapy and reliance is placed on T3 to suppress TSH and allow regression even of established metasteses. The less experienced thyroid surgeon is advised to follow this latter course. It would take a very large controlled series over many decades to decide whether one treatment is superior to the other. A complicating factor is the difference amongst pathologists in different countries as to what constitutes papillary carcinoma of the thyroid which may have resulted in bias in some published series by inclusion of cases which would not be regarded as truly malignant by all pathologists. The field is further confused by what appears to be the real differences in incidence and in natural history of the tumour in different countries and possibly between different regions of individual countries. There is yet a third approach which advocates only local removal of the tumour and T3 suppression of TSH. This, however, cannot yet be accepted as an orthodox method of treatment. Where papillary carcinoma occurs in the older age group who tend to carry a less favourable prognosis, the radical approach is mandatory as it is in those cases of papillary carcinoma who have a history of cervical X-irradiation.

Follicular Carcinoma of Thyroid

This, too, is a tumour which may be seen in any age group but it has a predilection for the 30–50 year group. In cancer terms it carries a more favourable prognosis than most other cancers but it is much more aggressive and dangerous than papillary carcinoma, the 5-year survival being 60% and the 10-year survival 50%. Haematogenous dissemination to lung and bone is a feature of this disease.

The poorer prognosis justifies the more radical approach to follicular carcinoma. Total thyroidectomy with preservation of the parathyroids and removal of all affected lymph nodes is desirable. If total thyroidectomy is not done, then it is impossible to do total body scanning as the radio-iodine will be preferentially taken up in remaining thyroid rather than by metastases. If there is any residual thyroid tissue in the neck, it first requires to be ablated with therapeutic radio-iodine. Uptake in metastases is treated with therapeutic radio-iodine. T3 is given to suppress TSH. Scanning is done at intervals as described for the more radical approach to the treatment of papillary carcinoma of the thyroid.

Anaplastic Carcinoma of the Thyroid

This is one of the most distressing forms of cancer carrying one of the poorest prognoses. The disease affects predominantly the older age group and very few patients survive 5 years. Normally there is rapidly progressive swelling of the neck on one or both sides, voice changes due to involvement of the recurrent laryngeal nerves and stridor from tracheal compression.

Wherever possible some attempt should be made to decompress the trachea by surgery to relieve respiratory obstruction. External radiotherapy is normally used in addition though anaplastic carcinomas are rarely very sensitive. Chemotherapy has little place.

The surgeon's role is to attempt to save the patient from the great distress of death from respiratory obstruction.

Tumours of Parafollicular Tissue

Medullary Carcinoma

Medullary carcinoma of the thyroid is the most recently identified of the malignant thyroid tumours being described by Hazzard in 1959. Prior to this it was included with the anaplastic thyroid carcinomas. This may account for some unexpectedly long survivors in older series of treated anaplastic thyroid carcinomas. It arises from the parafollicular cells and has no benign variant, though a state of hyperplasia is described. The calcitonin levels in the blood are high in medullary carcinoma and this may aid diagnosis and allow progress to be monitored after surgery, another example of a 'tumour marker'. There are two sets of circumstances in which medullary carcinoma of the thyroid may be seen. It may arise sporadically or in association with other endocrine tumours. This latter is part of the pluriglandular or Sipple's syndrome but best called MEN Type II (Multiple Endocrine Neoplasia). The main association is with phaeochromocytoma but there may be other associated disorders. Medullary carcinoma arising as part of the MEN Type II syndrome is generally less aggressive than the sporadic form. This has led to suggestions of different forms of treatment. The mainstay of treatment is surgery. The tumour is not responsive to radiotherapy or chemotherapy and is not TSH stimulated.

Treatment of the sporadic form is by total thyroidectomy with parathyroid identification and preservation and prophylactic dissection of the lymph nodes of the central compartment of the neck, including those of the superior mediastinum. T3 is required for replacement therapy only. There is a school of thought that recommends for medullary carcinoma, which is part of the MEN Type II syndrome, total lobectomy on the affected side and subtotal on the contralateral side. The safer course is to advise total thyroidectomy for all cases. Five-year survivals are approximately 50%. It is of interest that there have been some cases of medullary carcinoma of thyroid associated with MEN Type II where total removal of the thyroid malignancy was not possible but where there has been nonetheless prolonged survival. This may reflect the fundamentally less aggressive nature of medullary carcinoma in MEN Type II.

Tumours of the Lymphoid Element

Primary lymphoma of the thyroid is a relatively rare tumour, and is most often seen in association with severe longstanding autoimmune thyroiditis (Hashimoto's disease). The older age group is affected. It is important to recognize the tumour for what it is because it responds extremely well to radiotherapy and where indicated to adjuvant systemic chemotherapy. Thus when operating on a suspected thyroid malignancy it is important to submit tissue early in the operation for histology. Unfortunately, the histological diagnosis can be extremely difficult between lymphoma, severe autoimmune thyroiditis and anaplastic carcinoma, but an experienced pathologist may be able to make the diagnosis from a frozen section. The importance lies in the fact that if thyroid lymphoma can be diagnosed, thyroidectomy need not be done unless it is essential for decompression, and then it should be unilateral and subtotal. Radiotherapy to the neck together with adjuvant chemotherapy, if there is evidence of spread, effects a high cure rate, though figures for 5-year survival are less meaningful because of the advanced age of many patients.

AUTOIMMUNE THYROID DISORDERS

Autoimmune Thyroiditis

Autoimmune thyroiditis is the term applied to the condition, almost certainly of autoimmune aetiology and characterized by destruction of thyroid follicles by lymphocytic infiltration, frequently organized into lymphoid follicles and with a variable degree of fibrous replacement of destroyed acini. The thyroid follicular cell has a characteristic deeply eosinophilic staining property called Askanazy cell change.

All gradations of autoimmune thyroiditis are seen from minor foci in otherwise normal glands through a spectrum to the extreme disorganization, acinar destruction and lymphoid infiltrate typical of Hashimoto's disease.

The presence in the circulation of antibodies to thyroglobulin and to the microsomes of the thyroid acinar cells is found in the vast majority of cases but there is no evidence that these have a pathogenetic role, rather they are seen as an epiphenomenon, the fundamental disorder being a cell-mediated one. Primary thyrotoxicosis fits into the spectrum of autoimmune thyroid disease and focal thyroiditis is a frequent histological component of this disorder. In the case of primary thyrotoxicosis humoral antibodies (TSI) do have a pathogenetic role, directly provoking the overactivity of the gland. Surgical interest in the autoimmune thyroiditis centres around the fact that the immunizing process is destructive to the gland, leading to ultimate thyroid failure. In severe cases autoimmune thyroiditis may lead to swelling of the gland which may be diffuse or predominantly unilateral and thus must be considered in the differential diagnosis of goitre or of a lump in the thyroid.

The typical case will be a female patient, usually post-menopausal with a thyroid swelling which is quite firm to palpation and either diffuse or affecting one side predominantly. The stigmata of mild hypothyroidism usually will be present, but the patient may be euthyroid and even hyperthyroid (Hashitoxicosis). The diagnosis depends on finding strongly positive autoantibodies, particularly to thyroid microsomes but also to thyroglobulin, but 10% of patients are antibody negative. Radionuclide scanning and ultrasonography can be suggestive but are not diagnostic. Where possible surgical intervention is to be avoided. It is rarely indicated as the disease responds well to substitution therapy to a degree that switches off TSH, which provides much of the stimulus to thyroid enlargement. Surgical intervention is called for only when possible malignancy cannot be excluded.

Riedel's Thyroiditis

It is customary to consider Riedel's thyroiditis together with autoimmune thyroiditis but there is no good evidence that the conditions are related. Riedel's thyroiditis is a very rare disease and many experienced thyroid surgeons have not personally encountered it.

There is usually painless enlargement of the thyroid gland which is extremely firm to palpation. Pressure symptoms may be present, especially tracheal compression. The thyroid is extensively replaced by fibrous tissue which may extend beyond the gland into the neck or into the mediastinum. Retroperitoneal fibrosis may also be found. None of the factors known to cause retroperitoneal fibrosis appears to be responsible for Riedel's thyroiditis. Males are affected as commonly as females and thyroid autoantibodies are negative. Surgical treatment may be required to decompress the trachea and should be as conservative as possible compatible with achieving this objective. There is no known cure. Riedel's thyroiditis has occasionally been reported in association with sclerosing cholangitis.

Acute Bacterial Thyroiditis

Specific infective thyroiditis does occur but is a rarity. Tuberculous disease is also reported but is rare.

Subacute Thyroiditis

Subacute thyroiditis (de Quervain's disease) is another rare entity. Characteristically the patient presents with or following a flu-like illness with pain and swelling of the thyroid gland. The pain radiates up into the neck to the region of the ears. The gland is tender to palpation. There is systemic upset with an elevated ESR. The condition is probably viral in nature and the mumps virus has been incriminated in some cases. Laboratory findings include reduced uptake of radio-iodine by the thyroid and transiently positive thyroid autoantibodies. There may be biochemical evidence of raised T4 in the acute phase but if the condition persists then mild hypothyroidism is the rule. The disease runs a self-limiting course with return to the euthyroid state and the disappearance of autoantibodies. Occasionally it shows a pattern of exacerbation and remission and a persistent case will require steroids before it settles. There are no permanent sequelae.

DISORDERS OF THYROID FUNCTION

Hyperthyroidism

Hyperthyroidism is a common disease and one for which surgical correction is frequently appropriate.

It occurs in three forms:

Primary thyrotoxicosis	(Graves' disease, exophthalmic goitre)
Secondary thyrotoxicosis	(thyrotoxicosis secondary to some pre-existing thyroid disorder, normally a longstanding goitre)
Tertiary thyrotoxicosis	(thyrotoxicosis due to a single functioning 'adenoma')

Primary Thyrotoxicosis

The terms 'Graves' disease' or 'exophthalmic goitre' are commonly used to describe this disease which is a complex disease affecting many body systems and of which overactivity of the thyroid is only one aspect. Nevertheless, it is this aspect which is often the most distressing to the patient and the one which can be corrected by treatment.

Primary thyrotoxicosis can now confidently be stated to be an autoimmune disease. There is a strong genetic predisposition and certain HLA types occur much more commonly than in the general population. The hyperthyroidism is due to the presence of a circulating immunoglobulin (IgG) which has the capacity to bind to and to stimulate the TSH receptors of the thyroid follicular cells. This results in increased synthesis and output of thyroid hormone which in turn feeds back to the hypothalamus and pituitary switching off TRH and TSH. This immunoglobulin is called thyroid-stimulating immunoglobulin (TSI). TSI can be assayed but the technique is complex and is essentially a research tool at present. TSI has the ability with other immunoglobulins to cross the placenta as a result of which it may produce neonatal thyrotoxicosis in the offspring of mothers who are, or who have formerly been, thyrotoxic. Neonatal thyrotoxicosis runs a self-limiting course as maternal TSI declines in the early months of life. There is growing evidence that distinct but similar autoantibodies may contribute to other manifestations of the disease, namely the ophthalmopathy and the dermatosis (pretibial myxoedema).

Greater understanding of the pathogenesis of the disease has not yet had any bearing on treatment which is directed towards making the patient euthyroid. There are three methods of treating the thyrotoxic patient:

Antithyroid drugs
Radio-iodine
Surgery.

Antithyroid Drugs

Antithyroid drugs were introduced in 1943 and act chiefly by blocking the incorporation of iodine into the tyrosine molecule, an essential step in the synthesis of T3 and T4. They are believed to work simply by preventing synthesis of thyroid hormone and so controlling hyperthyroidism until the disease remits spontaneously. There is some interest in the possibility that antithyroid drugs may effect some control over the fundamental immunological aberration but this has not been proved. Primary thyrotoxicosis is classically a disease of remissions and exacerbations. Treatment is carried on for 18 months, though some physicians stop after 6 months. Approximately half of the patients so treated will be cured but this leaves a large number who will be subjected to further attacks of the disease and for whom some form of thyroid ablation will be necessary. Unfortunately there is no way of predicting which patients will respond well to drugs and which will not. Good control on drugs depends on the patient taking the drug at 8-hourly intervals throughout the period of treatment and failure of compliance with this is a major problem. A small number of patients may suffer from drug toxicity (vomiting, skin rashes or, more severely, agranulocytosis). It is difficult to bring the symptoms of hyperthyroidism under control without producing hypothyroidism and in many clinics there is a deliberate policy to overtreat the hyperthyroidism and after the first month of treatment, when most patients will have become euthyroid, T3 is added to prevent the patient becoming hypothyroid during the drug therapy.

Radio-iodine

Radio-iodine was introduced in 1942 when it was expected to be a real advance in the treatment of thyrotoxicosis. It has undoubtedly contributed greatly to dynamic thyroid function studies and as an adjunct to surgery in some forms of thyroid cancer. In thyrotoxicosis it has proved difficult to establish a method of calculating the dose of radio-iodine appropriate to the individual thyrotoxic patient so that repeated doses may be necessary to bring the thyroid under control or alternatively for hypothyroidism to supervene. Unfortunately the tendency to hypothyroidism in the longer term is a serious drawback to the use of radio-iodine. A large percentage of treated patients (60–70%) will ultimately require replacement therapy for hypothyroidism and this figure is likely to increase with the years. Radio-iodine is still widely used in the USA for treatment of thyrotoxicosis and less widely in the UK. There is an absolute indication for the use of radio-iodine and that is where there is recurrence of thyrotoxicosis after subtotal thyroidectomy. It also has a place in the management of thyrotoxicosis in patients in the older age group or in those with a poor life prognosis.

Surgery

Subtotal thyroidectomy still presents the most certain way of rendering the majority of patients euthyroid in the shortest possible time. In experienced hands the operative morbidity is extremely small but it is universally recognized that there is no place for the 'occasional thyroidectomist'. The indications for surgery include:

RECURRENCE AFTER TREATMENT WITH ANTITHYROID DRUG. Such patients are likely always to suffer recurrence of thyrotoxicosis when drugs are stopped.

PATIENT PREFERENCE. Many patients will choose operation to the uncertainties of drug therapy.

OCCUPATIONAL OR ACADEMIC PRESSURE. Many patients require to be made euthyroid in the shortest possible time and feel that their performance at work, or their scholastic performance will suffer otherwise.

LARGE GOITRES. Patients with large goitres do less well on drugs. The goitre is likely to enlarge and they have a greater chance of recurrence on withdrawal of drug therapy.

MALES. Males seem to do even less well on antithyroid drugs than females and thyroidectomy is usually the appropriate form of treatment.

SECONDARY AND TERTIARY HYPERTHYROIDISM. Such patients tend to do less well on antithyroid drugs or radio-iodine and if there are no contraindications to operation, do well with surgery.

PREPARATION FOR SURGERY. The appropriate operation for primary thyrotoxicosis is subtotal thyroidectomy which aims to leave approximately 5 ml volume of thyroid tissue as a remnant on each side. Below this volume, the incidence of postoperative hypothyroidism becomes unacceptably high and if much more than this is left there is an increased risk of recurrence of the disease.

Classically the patient comes to surgery in the euthyroid state, controlled by a period of antithyroid drug therapy. Formerly it was the practice to stop antithyroid drugs for 10 days prior to operation and to institute iodide in the belief that this would reduce the vascularity of the gland and facilitate operation. Many surgeons now omit this step, continuing antithyroid drugs until the day before operation and not introducing iodide as they feel that this does not make sufficient difference to the operation and has possible risks, e.g. if operation has to be delayed for any reason and there is the risk of occasionally precipitating thyrotoxicosis by introducing iodine to patients who as a group are iodide deficient as a result of treatment.

Recently, there has been a lot of interest in carrying out the operation of thyroidectomy for thyrotoxicosis in patients prepared for operation by β-adrenergic blockade with propranolol. The theory is that in patients in whom thyroidectomy is contemplated there is advantage in bringing them to surgery in minimum time. Many of the severest effects of hyperthyroidism, and especially the cardiovascular manifestations, are readily controlled by β-adrenergic blockade for just a few days and it has been demonstrated in many series that surgery may be undertaken safely under the influence of propranolol alone. Large doses are needed, 40–160 mg q.d.s., depending on response, and it is important to achieve at least 25% reduction in the resting pulse rate before one can be assured that the degree of β-adrenergic blockade is sufficient.

The operation is often made easier by avoidance of antithyroid drugs which are to a degree goitrogenic. β-blockers may be tailed off after surgery and discontinued by 7 days after operation.

The principal drawback to the technique is seen in the first year after surgery when a high percentage of patients (up to 60% is quoted in some series) go through a phase of temporary biochemical hypothyroidism and a certain morbidity is seen due to weight gain. A similar proportion of patients prepared in the conventional way with antithyroid drugs also have a period of temporary hypothyroidism but it is shorter lived and so less noticeable. The problem can be overcome by putting the patient on T3 replacement (just as with antithyroid drugs) for the first year after thyroidectomy. This eliminates any morbidity due to temporary hypothyroidism and does not affect the ability of the thyroid remnant to recover, so that in the longer term the incidence of hypothyroidism is no greater than with conventional preparation.

The author's preferred method of preparing patients for thyroidectomy for thyrotoxicosis is with the long-acting non-selective β-blocker nadolol 80 mg given once daily together with potassium iodine 60 mg t.i.d. These two together are given for ten days and all patients will be rendered euthyroid in this period.

SURGICAL RISKS. In experienced hands risks are of a very low order indeed.

MORTALITY. This should be as near to zero as it is ever possible to get and there are many published series where thousands of patients have been operated upon without a death.

BLEEDING. There is always a risk of postoperative bleeding after thyroid surgery. It is rare (1% or so in many series) but dramatic and potentially fatal. The bleeding may occur in one of two sites:

1. Deep to the myofascial layer in relation to the thyroid remnant or vessels. Such occurrence is the least common but even a small amount of bleeding, because of the proximity to the larynx, is extremely serious. Evacuation must be done quickly but it will usually be possible to do this under general anaesthesia in the operating theatre rather than by dramatic opening of the neck at the bedside, known to all surgeons but probably witnessed by few.

2. Bleeding deep to the skin flaps is the more common and usually arises from veins. It can occur, for example, if anything causes the patient's blood pressure to rise in the postoperative period. Bleeding is slow but a substantial haematoma may develop and produce pressure on the airway. Evacuation is mandatory. If haematoma is seen within 12 h of operation it should probably be evacuated to prevent respiratory embarrassment developing. Little is to be gained by observation. Haematomas seen after 12 h are usually small and will mostly resolve. Where there is any degree of doubt the patient's interests are best served by evacuation. Drainage makes little difference to haematoma formation. Haematomas can accumulate even in the presence of functioning drains. It is essential that careful patient observation is exercised after thyroid surgery.

THYROTOXIC CRISIS. Thyrotoxic crisis is a serious complication but it should not be seen where there has been adequate preoperative preparation. It occurs within the first 24 h of thyroidectomy with the patient becoming confused and hyperactive, with a high temperature, profuse sweating and a rapid heart rate. Treatment must be vigorous with β-adrenergic blockade, intravenous hydrocortisone and iodide.

INFECTION. Infection after thyroidectomy should be rare but when it does occur it can be serious from the ultimate cosmetic point of view as it encourages adhesion of the scar to the trachea which is unsightly. It may ultimately require minor revision of the scar but certainly not before 12 months have elapsed as considerable improvement may be expected until then.

Because of the age group in which thyrotoxicosis most commonly occurs, occasionally acne may be found in the patient. Under these circumstances it is important not to give the patient iodide which exacerbates the acne. Antithyroid drugs are the more appropriate preparation in such a patient if surgery is contemplated. Prior to surgery the patient should wash with a cream such as Hibiscrub and apply spirit-containing hibitane such as Hibisol to the beard area and neck and upper part of the chest. Prophylaxis with antistaphylococcal antibiotics should be given in these circumstances. Where acne is severe, consideration should be given to using another form of definitive treatment such as radioactive iodine.

Recurrent Thyrotoxicosis

In UK practice this is quite unusual, about 2%, but is described as being common elsewhere and may be as much as 20%, for example, in Iceland, even though the operation carried out is similar to that which has been carried out in the UK. The reasons for this difference are not at all clear but the great variations in dietary iodide have been suggested.

Voice Changes

Some minor change in the voice is probably inevitable after thyroid surgery and this should certainly be borne in mind when considering the method of treatment appropriate to a particular patient. It does not necessarily mean that surgery must be avoided in patients to whom the quality of voice is critical since a goitre enlarging under the influence of antithyroid drugs may also affect the voice. Rarely are voice changes due to interference with recurrent laryngeal nerves since this occurs in less than 1% of cases when thyroidectomy is carried out by experienced thyroid surgeons. Probably minor changes in the muscles around the cricoid and thyroid cartilages are the most important, and it is, to some extent, inevitable that there will be some change with the mobilization of the gland.

Trauma to the external laryngeal nerve supplying the cricothyroid muscle can lead to voice changes because of difficulty in achieving vocal cord tension if the muscle is paralysed.

Damage to the internal laryngeal nerve is also serious and can occur where there is difficulty in mobilizing the superior pole. This leads to desensitization of the appropriate side of the larynx and spilling over, especially of liquids, during swallowing, or aspiration of secretions at night, may give rise to paroxysms of coughing.

Another nerve which has to be carefully preserved at thyroidectomy is the anterior cutaneous nerve of the neck (transverse cervical). This is encountered during elevation of the skin flaps and if it is damaged, desensitization of one side of the neck may create problems, especially for male patients when shaving.

Hypoparathyroidism

This is another oft-quoted but in fact rare complication of thyroidectomy. The commonly encountered hypocalcaemia of the first few days after thyroidectomy probably has little to do with hypoparathyroidism and is more likely to be a consequence of the metabolic changes taking place with re-entry of calcium into bone demineralized by hyperthyroidism ('hungry bones'). The operation of thyroidectomy is designed to leave a large amount of thyroid capsule, and with it the parathyroids, in proportion to the volume of thyroid tissue left. It is also a fact that the inferior parathyroids most usually relate to the cervical extension of the thymus than to the thyroid and are unlikely to be inadvertently removed. However, parathyroids are very small (2–8 mm in length) and are not always easy to identify at thyroidectomy for thyrotoxicosis. In addition to inadvertent removal they may suffer compromise of their blood supply. The incidence of hypoparathyroidism after surgery for thyrotoxicosis should be less than 1%. Treatment of hypoparathyroidism is with vitamin D or one of its analogues (*see* Chapter 62).

Hypothyroidism

It has been known from the earliest years of this century before definitive treatment was available for hyperthyroidism, that a third of patients would pass through the phase of hypothyroidism to ultimate thyroid failure. Surgery can do nothing to prevent this and the published incidence of hypothyroidism after surgery for thyrotoxicosis remains of this order. Surgery has the effect of bringing it on sooner, but this is no bad thing as it will appear while the patient is under clinical surveillance and treatment can be instituted. The diagnosis is much less likely to be missed or delayed in these circumstances in distinction to the situation as applies perhaps many years after treatment with radioactive iodine where the diagnosis may be delayed for some considerable time because of the insidious nature of the condition.

All forms of treatment for thyrotoxicosis will produce a population of patients prone to develop hypothyroidism, greatest after radio-iodine therapy but seen after all forms of treatment. All thyrotoxic patients should be followed for life and the institution of computer-based follow-up registers on a national basis is probably the most economical and logistically feasible method of achieving this.

THE WAY AHEAD

There are a number of interesting developments taking place in the study of thyroid disorders which hopefully will contribute to improvements in patient management.

Surgical endocrinology is establishing itself as a specialty within the field of General Surgery and is providing better opportunities for surgeons in training to become experienced in the clinical and technical aspects of disease.

In many centres close co-operation between endocrine surgeons and endocrine physicians has resulted in the establishment of joint endocrine clinics where both are involved in planning patient management from the beginning. Much of the best clinical research is coming from such joint endocrine clinics. The greater effort justifies incorporation into the clinic of other specialists such as paediatricians, gynaecologists, clinical biochemists, radiologists and nuclear medicine specialists with great overall improvement in patient care. Another excellent example of great benefits to be achieved by co-operation has come from the introduction of fine needle aspiration biopsy.

Recent work on preparation of patients for thyroidectomy for thyrotoxicosis with β-adrenergic blockade has come largely from such clinics and is an example of what can be achieved with co-operative effort. Undoubtedly the pattern has been set for the practice of surgical endocrinology for the future.

A great deal of interest centres at present on research into the fundamental nature of the immunological aberration in thyrotoxicosis. Undoubtedly, greater understanding will result. Thyrotoxicosis is a common clinical disorder and there is enormous scope for research, and it may well be that with greater understanding of the disorder that there will be important implications for the understanding and treatment of other autoimmune diseases which are so common and frequently have devastating implications for patients. This is probably the greatest expectation held by thyroidologists at present.

Finally, it is now obvious that patients with many types of thyroid disorder will require to be followed up for life if serious late sequelae are to be avoided. In a common disease this has serious implications in view of the great volume of work involved. The logistics of seeing increasing numbers of patients all requiring lifelong follow-up are critical and recourse will have to be had to more efficient methods of follow-up such as has been established now for the past 10 years in Scotland where the Scottish Automated Follow-up Register for Thyroid Disease, computer-assisted, has capacity to follow-up tens of thousands of patients in co-operation with their family physicians, leaving busy hospital specialist clinics more time to spend on patients urgently requiring their expertise. Such registers also provide a most valuable base for research.

Further Reading

Edis A. J., Ayala L. A. and Egdahl R. H. (1975) *Manual of Endocrine Surgery*. New York, Springer-Verlag.
Gunn A. (1985) *Thyroidectomy*. Videos for Surgeons. Presented jointly by Royal College of Surgeons of Edinburgh and Churchill Livingstone.
Hart I. R. and Newton R. W. (ed.) (1983) *The New Medicine*. Vol. 2. Endocrinology. Lancaster, MTP.
Montgomery D. A. D. and Welbourn R. B. (1975) *Medical and Surgical Endocrinology*. London, Arnold.
Perzik S. L. (1976) *Surgery in Thyroid Disease*. New York, Stratton International Medical Books Corporation.

62 The Parathyroids and Disorders of Calcium Metabolism

Andrew Gunn

Disorders of the parathyroid glands mostly present as disorders of calcium metabolism.

The widespread availability of autoanalysers now brings to light substantial numbers of cases, particularly of hypercalcaemia, frequently in patients without significant (or indeed any) symptoms who have blood taken for biochemistry for some unrelated condition or even just for 'screening'. It is essential to be familiar with the commoner causes of hypercalcaemia; in practice the non-parathyroid causes are fairly readily brought to light by a carefully taken history, clinical examination and a few inexpensive laboratory tests. Apart from metastatic bone disease, most general surgeons will not often be called upon to deal with bone-related disorders. This may have the effect of shielding them from contact with one of the biggest unresolved medical problems of our time, osteoporosis, particularly of the elderly female. Treatment of osteoporosis is an enormous consumer of health care resources and clearly this reflects in fewer resources being available to other fields of health care. Furthermore, it is a problem that is growing alarmingly as the demography of populations changes in favour of the aged.

History

The original description of the parathyroid glands is clearly attributable to Sir Richard Owen FRS who described them in the Indian white rhinoceros in 1850 (the specimen is conserved in the Hunterian Museum of the Royal College of Surgeons of England). The first description in man was by Ivar Sandstrom, when a senior medical student at the University of Uppsala in 1880. Their function remained something of a mystery for decades, probably because, with their close anatomical relationship to the thyroid, thyroid ablative experiments, at that time one of the few available methods for discovering the function of an organ, seemed to point to the thyroid gland itself as the source of some substance in the absence of which classic tetany occurred. Curiously, when the second calcium-regulating hormone, calcitonin, was discovered the original assumption was that it was a second parathyroid hormone, resolved by elegant perfusion experiments in sheep and goats whose thyroid and parathyroids are less intimately associated.

Embryology and Anatomy

These are considered in Chapter 61. More detailed considerations of parathyroid localization particularly in ectopic situations are given below.

Physiology

The principal hormones regulating calcium metabolism are:

Parathormone
Calcitonin

Parathormone is vastly more important and no significant sequelae are seen following total removal of the thyroid, the principal (but not exclusive) source of calcitonin, provided parathyroid function remains intact. It should be realized of course that hormones rarely work in isolation from other hormones or other metabolic processes and in the case of calcium, vitamin D, plasma magnesium, phosphate and protein metabolism are also important. Normal function of every body tissue, every cell membrane and possibly every enzyme system depends upon maintenance of a constant concentration of ionic calcium in the ECF. Disturbances of normal calcium concentrations are most readily observed in heart, muscle and nerve.

Parathormone

Parathormone (PTH) is a peptide, but because of problems of availability of human tissue for hormone extraction, most work has been carried out on bovine PTH. This shows PTH to consist of 84 amino acids of molecular weight approximately 9500; function residing in the 29 amino acid residue at the amino-terminal end. Human PTH differs in four of the amino acids in this part of the molecule which affects its immunoreactivity and hence the sensitivity of radioimmunoassays for human PTH. In essence the assay is a bovine PTH assay depending on considerable cross-reactivity with human PTH.

Secretion of PTH is principally under control of plasma ionic calcium and the fall or rise in plasma-ionized calcium is followed within minutes by the appropriate PTH response, probably necessitated by the fact that PTH has a short half-life (less than 1 hour). Plasma magnesium also affects PTH secretion, a fall in magnesium resulting in increased PTH output. Plasma phosphate appears not to affect PTH directly but administration of phosphate does cause a fall in plasma calcium and so a rise in PTH.

PTH appears to have three main sites of action:

Bone
Kidney
Intestine

Bone

The effect of PTH on bone is to increase reabsorption by osteoclasts and osteocytes. This is the basis of the classic bone changes seen in hyperparathyroidism, microcysts under the periosteum of the radial aspects of the proximal phalanges in the hands (*Figs.* 62.1 and 62.2) being diagnostic, giving way to progressively enlarging lacunae (*Figs.* 62.3 and 62.4) of longstanding disease.

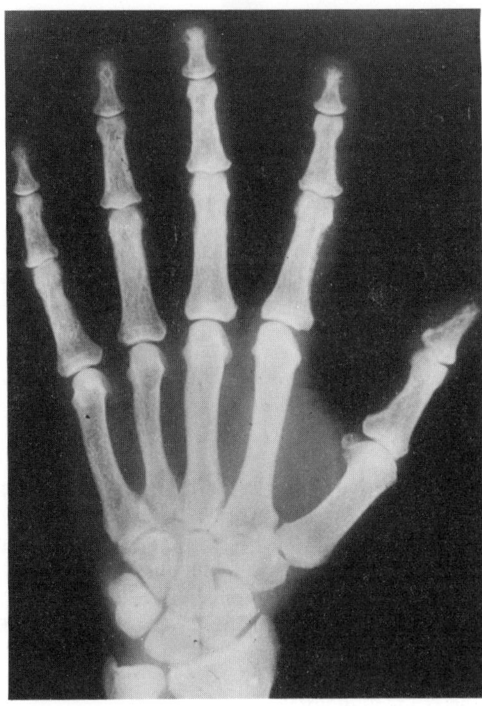

Fig. 62.1 A radiograph of the hand of a patient with primary hyperparathyroidism and early bone disease. Note the subperiosteal erosions on the radial aspect of the proximal phalanx of the index finger.

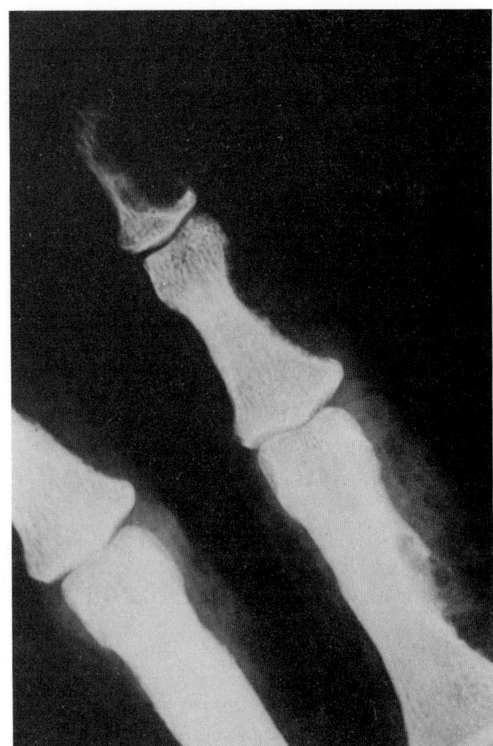

Fig. 62.2 As *Fig.* 62.1 but to an advanced degree.

Kidney

In the kidney the action of PTH has been the basis of a number of chemical tests. Administration of PTH rapidly leads to excretion of phosphate, sodium, potassium and bicarbonate, and decrease in excretion of hydrogen ion, calcium, magnesium and ammonia. As in bone, these changes are mediated through cyclic AMP. The action of PTH on phosphate has been most extensively studied and inhibition of proximal tubular reabsorption has been the basis of several tests for hyperparathyroidism. For practical clinical purposes such tests, formerly of value in the diagnosis of hyperparathyroidism, have been replaced by PTH assay.

Intestine

Active transport of calcium from the intestine is increased by PTH but evidence suggests that under normal physiological conditions passive diffusion is independent of PTH. In hyperparathyroidism, increased intestinal absorption contributes significantly to hypercalcaemia, the rationale behind the use of sodium cellulose phosphate (Calcisorb, Riker) in some mild cases of hyperparathyroidism in the elderly.

Vitamin D and PTH

There is a close interrelationship between vitamin D and PTH and it has long been known that the actions of PTH on bone and intestine are not found in cases of vitamin D deficiency. The explanation lies in the role of PTH in conversion of 25-hydroxycholecalciferol to the much more active 1,25-dihydroxycholecalciferol, a conversion which takes place in the kidney.

Calcitonin (Thyrocalcitonin)

This second calcium homeostatic hormone, acting antagonistically to PTH on bone to facilitate entry of calcium into bone, was discovered by Copp in 1960. Initially it was believed to be a second parathyroid hormone but perfusion experiments in sheep and goats showed thyroid to be the principal source. It is now established that the parafollicular ('C') cells secrete calcitonin, these being part of the APUD system of cells, containing argentaffin granules and derived from neural crest ectoderm. In fish and amphibians, reptiles and birds, this neural crest element, derived from the ultimobranchial arch, does not fuse with thyroid, remaining as a discrete endocrine gland, the ultimobranchial body. Calcitonin is a peptide of 32 amino acids and molecular weight 3400 and there is considerable species variation in the structure. Final elucidation of the role of calcitonin is awaited. In surgical practice its most important role is as a tumour marker for medullary carcinoma of the thyroid, though there is expectation that it may prove to be an effective therapy in Paget's disease (osteitis deformans).

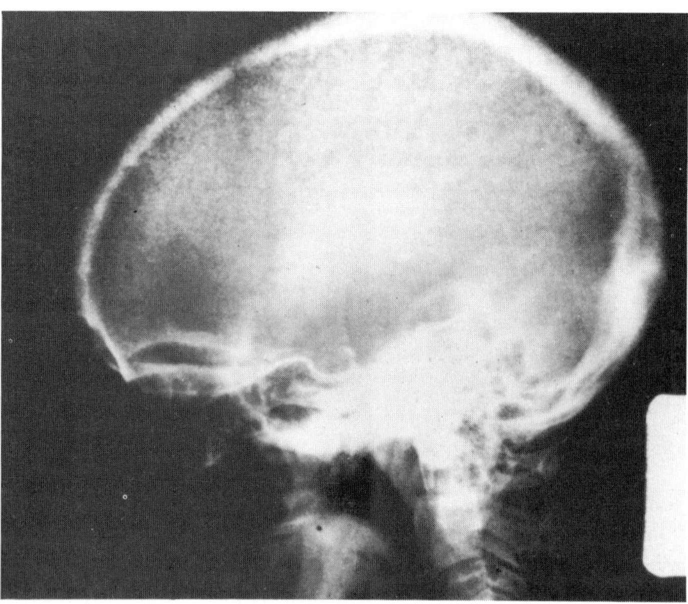

Fig. 62.3 Radiograph of skull in patient with parathyroid bone disease. Note the general fuzzy appearance of the bone and that the erosions are very irregular.

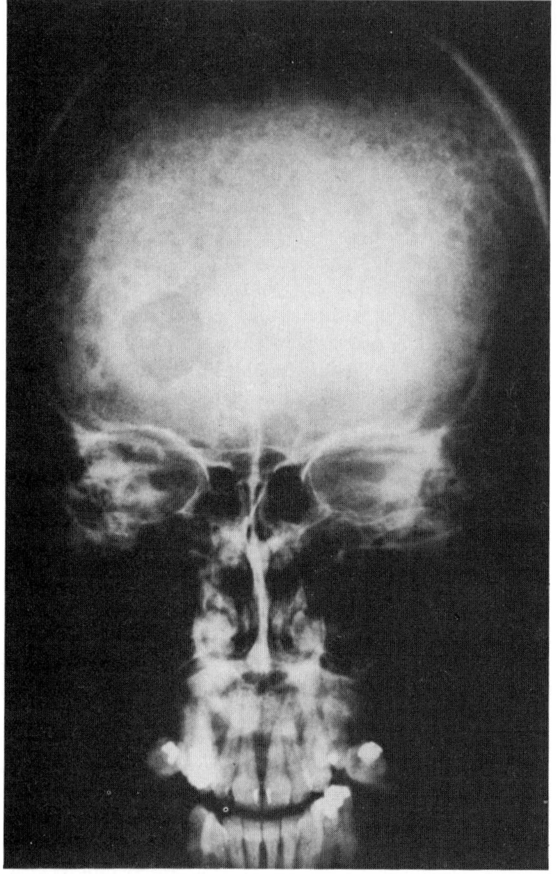

Fig. 62.4 As *Fig.* 62.3. Distinguish these from cases of metastatic bone disease where the lesions are clearly 'punched out' and there is no background of 'fuzziness' in the bones.

DISTURBANCES OF CALCIUM METABOLISM

It must be remembered that under normal circumstances 50% of calcium in blood is protein bound and is reflected in the 'serum calcium'. Mostly today laboratories will correct the figure to a plasma protein level of 4 g albumin/100 ml, the 'corrected calcium'.

Whenever calcium metabolism is disturbed, whether it be due to an inadequate intake of calcium, an excessive loss or an internal derangement of the control of its metabolism, the level of ionized calcium in the plasma will tend to move outside the limits of the normal range. An actual displacement will depend upon the response to the tendency to change by the parathyroid glands. If the parathyroid glands are normal they will initiate a homeostatic response in which the production of PTH will be appropriately modified to correct the tendency to change. For example, when calcium is lost excessively in the urine, as occurs in some forms of nephrosis, the parathyroid glands will detect the falling levels and will respond by increasing PTH production; with continuing stimulation, the glands will increase in size. Calcium levels in the blood will tend to be restored to normal, but only at the expense of the calcium stores in bone which will eventually become depleted (renal osteodystrophy). This homeostatic response with hyperplasia of the parathyroid glands is termed 'second hyperparathyroidism'. It should be noted that, although PTH is produced in excess, its purpose is only to restore plasma calcium levels to normal and that these levels do not rise above the upper limit of the normal range.

Hypocalcaemia

The theoretical list of causes of hypocalcaemia is long but for practical purposes comes down to:

Uraemic osteodystrophy
Osteomalacia

Rickets
Severe malabsorption states
Post neck surgery

Clinical Features

The most obvious result of hypocalcaemia is tetany with carpopedal spasm and (especially in infants) laryngeal spasm (laryngismus stridulus). Rarely, but again especially in infants, convulsions may result. More commonly, sensory manifestations will be complained of—paraesthesiae especially of the fingers and around the mouth. Mental change, especially depression, anxiety or feelings of impending doom, may occur and are extremely unpleasant and frightening to the patient. Longstanding, untreated hypocalcaemia may give rise to significant sequelae, of which cataract and epileptiform seizures are the most serious.

Uraemic Osteodystrophy

The pathophysiology is complicated but three elements are principally involved: hyperphosphataemia, impaired conversion of 25-hydroxycholecalciferol to the 1,25 compound and malabsorption of calcium.

Chronic Renal Failure

Chronic renal failure with phosphate retention (hyperphosphataemia) may result in osteosclerosis and soft-tissue (ectopic) calcification.

The hyperphosphataemia may induce hypocalcaemia leading to secondary hyperparathyroidism and the manifestations of osteitis fibrosa.

Since the kidney is the main source of conversion of the less active 25-hydroxycholecalciferol to the more active, 1,25-dihydroxycholecalciferol, this function may be greatly impaired in renal failure. Defective intestinal absorption of calcium may again result in the sequence of events: hypocalcaemia → secondary hyperparathyroidism → osteitis fibrosa, perhaps with superadded features of osteomalacia or in the child, rickets.

Patients with such problems may frequently be seen nowadays, a consequence of end-stage renal failure suboptimally managed by haemodialysis, CAPD or renal transplantation. In this last case the bone problems may be compounded by a need for steroids for immunosuppression.

Osteomalacia and Rickets

The two have similar pathogenesis, the end result differing in adults (osteomalacia) and in children (rickets). The causes of vitamin D deficiency are nutritional, or due to insufficient exposure to sunlight as occurs where housing conditions are poor and the atmosphere polluted, or simply from social custom as in some female immigrants from the East to Western Europe. Osteomalacia and rickets may be consequential to malabsorption in diseases such as coeliac disease, pancreatic disorders, biliary obstruction or other causes such as the osteodystrophy seen as a long-term consequence of partial gastrectomy.

Hypoparathyroidism after Surgery

Following thyroid surgery in experienced hands hypoparathyroidism should be rare, considerably less than 1% of thyroidectomies. The greatest risks attend extensive surgery for cancer (thyroid, larynx, hypopharynx) or those rare occasions where a second or subsequent thyroid operation is required. Hypoparathyroidism must be distinguished from temporary hypocalcaemia seen most frequently after thyroidectomy for thyrotoxicosis and due to great avidity of the bones for calcium which has been leeched out as a consequence of the metabolic disturbance ('hungry bones'). It is a temporary phenomenon perhaps compounded by, for example, venous congestion in the parathyroids following thyroidectomy, and resolves by the time the patient leaves hospital.

Other Causes of Hypoparathyroidism

After therapeutic use of ^{131}I
Autoimmune hypoparathyroidism
Familial hypoparathyroidism
Haemochromatosis
Third arch congenital abnormalities

All of these are rare.

Treatment

Recovery after operation is not uncommon in time and if treatment is required to relieve symptoms it must be given with caution. Acute manifestations of hypocalcaemia require intravenous injection of 10% calcium gluconate and this should be given very slowly (over several minutes). Oral calcium such as calcium lactate gluconate (Sandocal) may relieve mild symptoms which are likely to be temporary. Longer standing symptoms or chronically depressed corrected serum calcium requires the use of a vitamin D preparation such as 1α-hydroxycholecalciferol. The aim should not be to normalize the calcium level in the blood but to raise it towards the lower limit of the normal range. Regular checking of the serum calcium is essential since toxicity due to accumulation of the drug together with parathyroid recovery may occur.

Hypercalcaemia

There are many causes of hypercalcaemia but the majority are accounted for by malignant disease with skeletal metastases and hyperparathyroidism. The others are either uncommon or rare.

Differential Diagnosis

This includes:

Primary hyperparathyroidism
Malignant disease with bone metastases
Excess intake of vitamin D
The milk-alkali syndrome
Hyperthyroidism
Multiple myeloma, reticuloses and leukaemias
Sarcoidosis
Addison's disease
Paget's disease of bone
Prolonged immobilization (or weightlessness)
Thiazide diuretics
Ectopic secretion of PTH
Benign familial hypocalciuric hypercalcaemia
Renal failure

Diagnosing Hyperparathyroidism

It will be obvious from the list of principal causes of hypercalcaemia that many can be excluded on the basis of a carefully taken history, which must include drug history, specifically enquiring after vitamin D, thiazide diuretics and alkalis. After physical examination a series of simple tests including a chest radiograph, blood count and film, urea and electrolytes and serum electrophoresis will go far to exclude non-parathyroid causes of hypercalcaemia. Hyperparathyroidism, however, should not be looked upon as a diagnosis to be arrived at by exclusion. Begin by repeating the corrected serum calcium levels on a number of different occasions, looking also at the serum phosphate (is it lowish?) alkaline phosphatase and serum chloride (are they elevated?). Pay particular regard to the patient's history (has there been any change in mood (in particular, depression or confusion—in the elderly in whom the diagnosis is being increasingly recognized, it may masquerade as the beginnings of senile dementia)?) Is there any history of dyspepsia (about 30% of patients with hyperparathyroidism will admit to it and it responds satisfactorily only to the treatment of the hyperparathyroidism)? Is there polyuria, nocturia or polydipsia? Is there a history of renal stones? Is there a problem with constipation? Obviously some of these symptoms will arise in the general population but they can all be pointers to the diagnosis.

PTH Assay

It has been pointed out that the assay is not as sensitive as could be wished as it depends on antibodies to bovine PTH, which differs in the number of amino-acid residues from human PTH and hence in its immunoreactivity. Nevertheless, the assay is being improved by development of antibodies which react with different parts of the molecule and even an assay based on human PTH is not far off for clinical purposes. The presence of immunoreactive PTH in the serum in the presence of hypercalcaemia virtually clinches the diagnosis, since in other cases of hypercalcaemia PTH should be suppressed.

Steroid Suppression Test

This was formerly a common test but is now less commonly used. It depends on the fact that when corticosteroids are administered to patients with hypercalcaemia the serum calcium falls, often to normal levels, in sarcoidosis, vitamin D poisoning and in most patients with malignant disease, but does not fall in hyperparathyroidism. Hydrocortisone 40 mg t.i.d. is given orally for 10 days and the corrected serum calcium measured on alternate days. The steroids should be tailed off gradually thereafter. It should be remembered that this is a very substantial dose of steroids and the tests should not be done where contraindications are present. It is much less commonly used than formerly.

Multiple Endocrine Neoplasia (MEN)

Two syndromes of multiple endocrine neoplasia are described, both are fairly common.

In the commoner type (Type 1; MEN1), formerly known as the pluriglandular syndrome, the following abnormalities may be found:

Hyperparathyroidism (usually chief cell hyperplasia)
Pituitary tumours (acidophil or chromophobe adenomas)
Pancreatic tumours (gastrin or insulin secreting)
Adrenal cortical adenomas (rarely)
Thyroid tumours (rarely)

This disorder may be familial, inherited as an autosomal dominant.

Multiple endocrine neoplasia type 2 (MEN2), formerly known as Sipple's syndrome, may also be familial. Patients have one or more of the following:

Medullary carcinoma of the thyroid
Phaeochromocytoma
Neurofibromatosis
Hyperparathyroidism
Cushing's syndrome (rarely)

Forms of Hyperparathyroidism

Primary
Secondary } (i.e. renal disease or severe chronic
Tertiary } intestinal malabsorption)

Primary Hyperparathyroidism

The true incidence of primary hyperparathyroidism, the commonest type, is not known in the general population but of the population having hospital contact who are screened biochemically, the incidence is about one per 1000. The majority do not have symptoms clearly relating to hyperparathyroidism. About 30% on questioning will admit to having suffered from peptic ulcer or non-ulcer dyspepsia; the incidence of bone or renal symptoms or signs is not more than 10% for each. The sex incidence is two females to one male, the majority of females being postmenopausal.

This raises important principles for clinicians. There is no satisfactory medical treatment for hyperparathyroidism and no one would wish to subject the patient to major surgery simply because the serum calcium is elevated unless it can be shown that left untreated there would be a serious outcome. There is, as yet, no clear answer to this dilemma.

Probably most experienced opinions feel that it is unwise to allow the younger patient to go untreated because of the possible long-term consequences for bones and kidneys, and operation is recommended. Where there are significant symptoms—dyspepsia, polyuria, nocturia, constipation, or depression—then surgery should be advised. What of the older patient with minimal symptoms? This is the most difficult group on which to advise. Unnecessary operations must be avoided, on the other hand many of the vaguest symptoms, forgetfulness or mild confusion in the elderly, are the very symptoms likely to be helped by returning the patient to the normocalcaemic state. The author's practice, shared with his physician colleagues, is normally to recommend operation but never to pressurize the patient. The majority of patients readily submit to operation and it is gratifying how well many of them do as a result. There are few things more satisfying than returning an elderly 'presenile' patient to normal personality. Success in these terms is very difficult to evaluate but the story so often recurring amongst endocrinologists as to lead one to suppose that there is frequent and genuine improvement in these patients. If operation is declined, at least the diagnosis will have been established, and if the patient is unlucky enough to develop that most severe of complications of hyperparathyroidism, hyperparathyroid crisis, it is unlikely not to be recognized for what it is and appropriate action taken.

Preoperative Localization of the Parathyroids

Methods of localizing parathyroid glands still leave much to be desired. There is no doubt that impressive pictures can be obtained by the thallium–technetium subtraction scanning (*Figs.* 62.5–62.7) but usually in cases where parathyroid pathology could not easily be missed at exploration. It is not so easy in the case of the smaller adenoma, the ectopic adenoma or hyperplastic glands. Techniques which have been tried include:

Thallium–technetium computer subtraction scanning
Venography
Arteriography

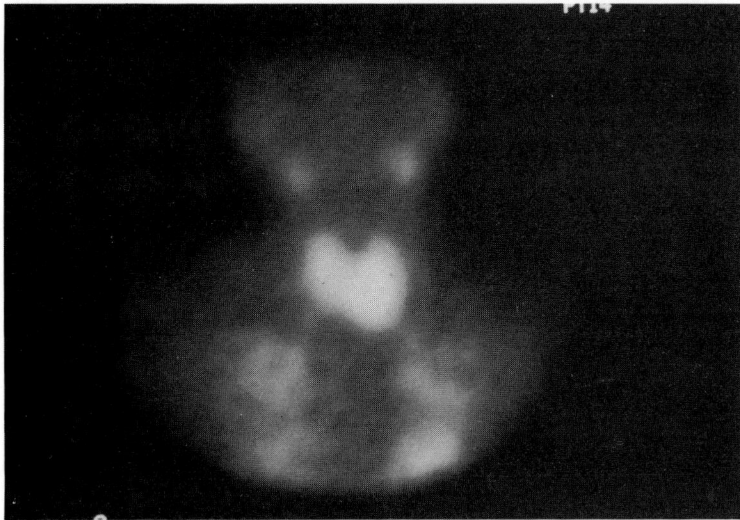

Fig. 62.5 Uptake of technetium by the thyroid.

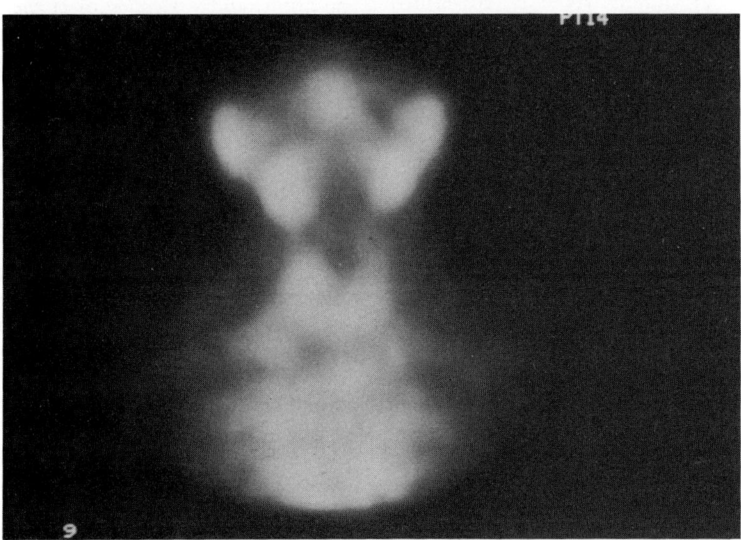

Fig. 62.6 Uptake of thallium by thyroid and parathyroid. Note also uptake by myocardium and salivary glands.

Ultrasonography
CT scanning
Selective venous catheterization

To these should be added peroperative techniques such as the use of a Geiger counter probe to detect isotope uptake in parathyroids, the peroperative infusion of methylene blue to stain parathyroids and flotation techniques to distinguish between different densities of fat, normal parathyroid and hyperplasia/adenoma.

The author's view is one which is fairly widely held amongst endocrine surgeons that localization techniques at present available should be reserved for cases in which re-exploration is to be done (not more than 2% of cases). The technique to employ will vary with availability in different centres. Probably selective venous catheterization and parathyroid hormone assay has best stood the test of time but the other non-invasive techniques are now beginning to displace it and to have an established place. More than one test may be justified when available to guide the surgeon in the highly difficult field of parathyroid re-exploration. Perhaps this is a good point at which to stress the absolute importance of accurate record keeping by parathyroid surgeons in every case. This is not a duty which should be delegated to an assistant. It is crucially important that if a second operation is required that details of findings and procedures carried out at previous exploration are completely clear and accurate.

The Pathology in Primary Hyperparathyroidism

A fairly typical series of several hundred explorations show pathology as follows:

Neoplasia
- Single adenoma 77%
- Two adenomas 4%
- Carcinoma 4%

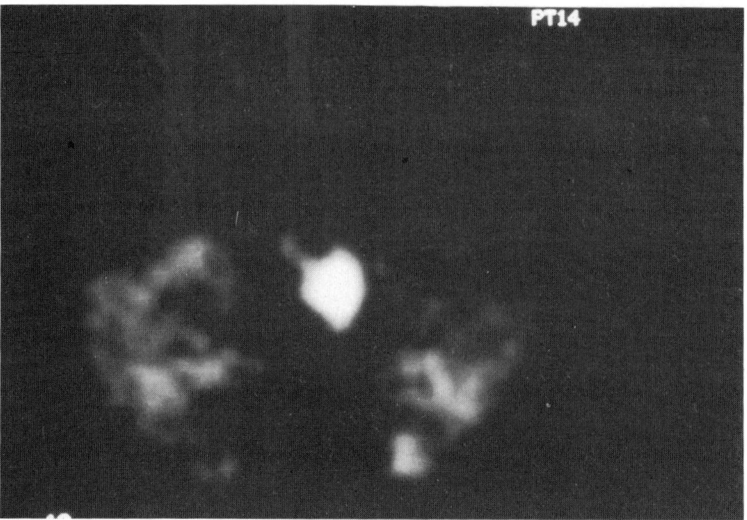

Fig. 62.7 Computer subtraction. Note that the parathyroid pathology is shown to be in the left inferior position.

Hyperplasia
  Water-clear cell 4%
  Chief cell 11%

The Surgical Objective

Straightforward operations may appear deceptively easy. This must not encourage surgeons who do not have extensive thyroid and parathyroid experience to undertake explorations. It must be concentrated in a few highly experienced hands if substantial numbers of subsequent re-explorations are to be avoided. Remember, while some cases may seem easy others can be very difficult: re-explorations are exceedingly difficult (and dangerous). The objective is to identify all parathyroid tissue, to remove any adenoma (or adenomas), and verify normal parathyroid tissue by frozen section histology. A meticulous surgical technique with absolute haemostasis is mandatory. When four-gland hyperplasia is encountered then three glands should be excised totally and a fourth divided in such a way as to leave approximately 100 mg weight of parathyroid tissue complete with its blood supply, the site being marked with a silver clip or non-absorbable sutures. Since so few patients have significant parathyroid bone disease, problems are not frequently encountered postoperatively from hypocalcaemia. If symptoms do occur—paraesthesiae or tetany—they are relieved by very slow (over five minutes) intravenous infusion of 10 ml of 10% calcium gluconate. In the rarer cases where there has been longstanding bone disease, the patient should preferably be treated for a period of three months prior to surgery with vitamin D.

Secondary Hyperparathyroidism

This is most often seen in the course of end-stage renal failure maintained by dialysis. High levels of alkaline phosphatase and a low serum calcium are encountered. Where bone demineralization is significant, parathyroidectomy may be required in preparation for renal transplantation because of the anticipated adverse effect on bone of steroids used for immunosuppression.

Tertiary Hyperparathyroidism

Some patients proceed through the phase of secondary hyperparathyroidism to a state where the parathyroid glands become autonomously functioning, hyperplastic or adenomatous, when serum calcium rises and bones rapidly soften. This is a serious state calling for parathyroidectomy. The preferred treatment is by total parathyroidectomy with reimplantation of approximately 30 mg of parathyroid tissue. The site of reimplantation is usually into the belly of the brachioradialis muscle. The parathyroid tissue must be divided into small pieces, not greater than 2 mm in any dimension and carefully implanted into the muscle in a geometric pattern, the site of each implant being marked with a non-absorbable suture (*Figs.* 62.8–62.11). The rationale behind this is that if the implanted parathyroid tissue becomes hyperplastic in the course of time it can be removed under local anaesthesia quite simply. The alternative is to do a total parathyroidectomy and maintain the patient on a vitamin D preparation.

The Negative Exploration

In experienced hands these will be few. In the event, the surgeon should seek to identify all the parathyroid tissue possible. If all four glands are found and are normal the neck should be closed and the diagnosis reconsidered. The author has encountered it only to find in time the symptoms of a liver tumour appearing, an example of the unusual situation of ectopic PTH secretion, and in cases of benign familial hypocalciuric hypercalcaemia before the syndrome was clearly recognizable. Perhaps the most worrying situation is where only three normal glands are found. Careful search must be made in all known locations for parathyroid tissue to occur including mobilization of the thymus from the neck. If no fourth gland or adenoma is encountered then total thyroid lobectomy on the side in question is justified since a proportion of parathyroids are intrathyroidal. There is no justification for mediastinal exploration at the first operation. It is important to retire to reconsider the diagnosis. In such cases, if the diagnosis cannot be revised, then

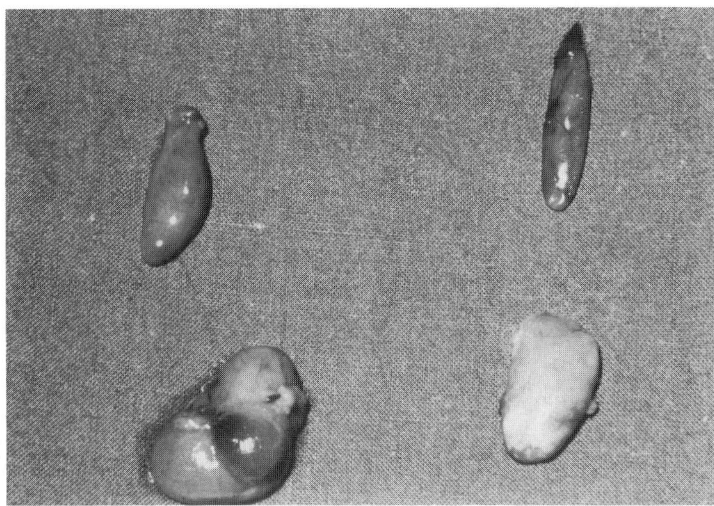

Fig. 62.8 Tertiary HPT (in a renal patient). The four hyperplastic glands are removed.

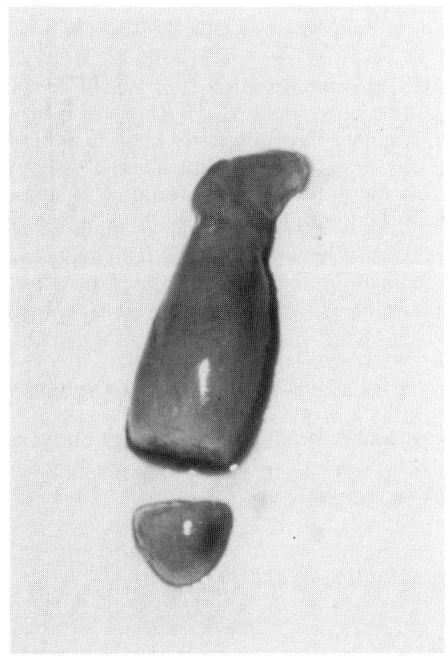

Fig. 62.9 Tertiary HPT (as *Fig.* 62.8). One parathyroid is selected and a portion approx. 30 mg removed.

some form of localization must be used to locate the adenoma before re-exploration. It has to be admitted that some locations of ectopic parathyroids defy embryological explanation. It is also a fact however, that in the vast majority of cases on re-exploration the adenoma is found in the neck! The foregoing can be no more than a guideline. Details may be found in textbooks of endocrine surgery.

Hypercalcaemic Crisis; Hyperparathyroid Crisis

These are dangerous, potentially lethal conditions in which a state of hypercalcaemia, even of mild degree, suddenly gives way to a rapid rise in plasma calcium associated with rapid deterioration of a patient's condition. This usually takes the

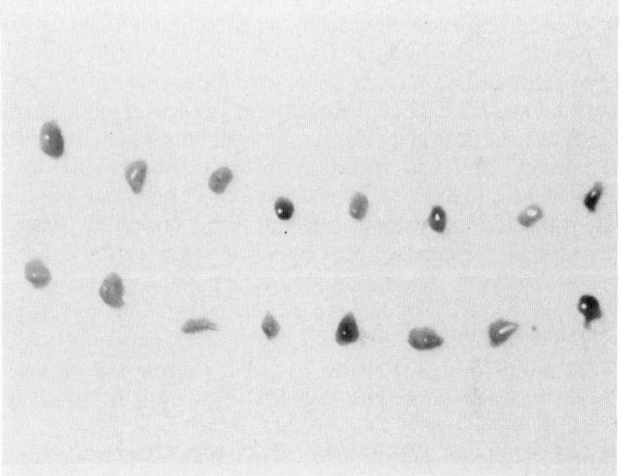

Fig. 62.10 Tertiary HPT. The 30-mg portion is divided so that no fragment is greater than 2 mm in any dimension. In this case sixteen fragments result.

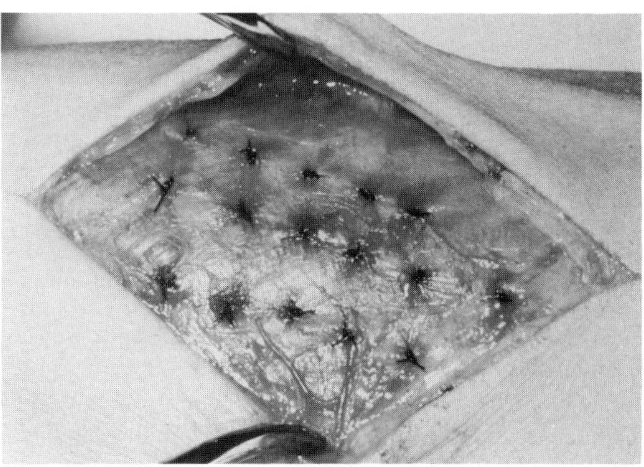

Fig. 62.11 Tertiary HPT. Each of the fragments is implanted under the fascia of the brachioradialis muscle. The arrangement should be geometric and each implant marked with a non-absorbable suture.

form of confusion, vomiting, drowsiness and dehydration, a combination which at first face may not suggest severe hypercalcaemia (levels usually upwards of 3·5 mmol/l: 7 mEq/l:14 mg/100 ml). The state may be precipitated by some intercurrent illness, infection or operation or some other condition, though on occasions no precipitating factor can be discovered. It is most important that the condition is recognized for what it is, because untreated it may prove rapidly fatal (within hours). In any confused patient, especially one who has been vomiting, hypercalcaemic crisis must be considered in the differential diagnosis. Formerly when plasma calcium estimations were a time-consuming investigation taking perhaps 48 h the outlook was serious if the condition was not diagnosed. Today, with more rapid methods of calcium estimation, there is usually time for the diagnosis to be made.

Action must be taken rapidly. Hypercalcaemic crisis not due to hyperparathyroidism usually responds rapidly to steroids, e.g. a patient who had an extensive operation for thyroid cancer was hypocalcaemic postoperatively. This required control with 1α-cholecalciferol. Recovery was complete. Weekly plasma calcium estimations were done as an outpatient and all seemed well. The time interval between estimations was therefore cautiously extended. The patient was admitted as an emergency with a clinical diagnosis of 'cerebral secondaries' (a diagnosis which looked entirely probable) and was given dexamethasone while a CT scan was being arranged. Overnight he improved and awoke normal next morning. His calcium on admission had been 4·5 mmol/l and had reverted almost to normal on dexamethasone. The diagnosis was vitamin D intoxication. Just as dramatic benefits may be seen with steroids in patients with skeletal metastases and hypercalcaemic crisis.

The hypercalcaemic crisis of hyperparathyroidism does not respond to steroids. Formerly there was no satisfactory treatment and emergency parathyroid exploration had to be undertaken as a life-saving procedure. Now it is possible to 'buy time' while the diagnosis is being confirmed by use of either calcitonin, mithramycin or intravenous phosphate. All of these must be used with great caution and preferably under the guidance of an experienced endocrine physician. Parathyroid exploration can then be done as a planned procedure. Rapid fluid replacement is, of course, mandatory in hypercalcaemic crisis.

Hyperparathyroidism together with other Conditions requiring Surgery

If faced with the situation, for example hyperparathyroidism and calculus hydronephrosis or hyperparathyroidism and severe gastric outlet obstruction due to peptic ulcer, it is important that the hyperparathyroidism be treated first otherwise operation may precipitate hyperparathyroid crisis as described above. Clearly such 'rules' are given for guidance and they have to be departed from on rare occasions; in that event it is most important that those caring for the patient are aware of the possible precipitation of crisis and understand how to manage it.

If there is a moral to be drawn from what has been written above it is to avoid the temptation to get involved in parathyroid explorations unless it is a field in which you have special expertise. As with so many surgical conditions the more straightforward cases do seem deceptively easy. Difficult cases can be very difficult and may result in considerable morbidity. Cases requiring a second exploration because of an unsatisfactory first exploration, are nothing short of a tragedy.

Further Reading

Rothmund M. and Wells S. A. (eds.) *Parathyroid surgery*. In: *Progress in Surgery*, Vol. 18. Basel, Karger.

World Journal of Surgery. Vol. 8(4) 1984. Papers presented at the International Association of Endocrine Surgeons, Sept. 1983, Hamburg.

World Journal of Surgery. Vol. 10(4) 1986. Papers presented at the International Association of Endocrine Surgeons, Sept. 1985, Paris.

63 *The Adrenal Glands*

P. Sheridan

ANATOMY OF THE ADRENAL GLANDS

Each adrenal or suprarenal gland is composed of two organs which are anatomically in close proximity but embryologically and functionally are quite different. These are the adrenal cortex and the adrenal medulla.

The adrenal cortex is derived from mesodermal cells which migrate dorsally from a site between the root of the dorsal mesentery and the developing gonad at about the fifth week of intrauterine life. The cells enlarge to form the fetal cortex. Towards the end of the second month of intrauterine life, a further proliferation of mesodermal cells takes place forming a thin layer around the fetal cortex and this becomes the definitive adult adrenal cortex. From birth the fetal cortex involutes and disappears within a few weeks and the gland which at birth is relatively large becomes smaller.

The adrenal medulla is formed from autonomic nervous tissue. Embryologically, therefore, it is derived from neural crest cells. During the seventh week of fetal life, ectodermal cells migrate from the neural crest and invade the mediodorsal aspect of the embryonic cortex which subsequently surrounds and envelops them. These neuro-ectodermal cells then develop into the adrenal medulla.

In adult life, each adrenal gland weighs about 3–5 g. They are surrounded by areolar, fatty tissue and are enclosed together with the kidneys, in the renal fascia but are separated from the kidneys by areolar fatty tissue. The right adrenal is rather pyramidal in shape. Its base lies in relation to the anteromedial aspect of the upper pole of the right kidney. Anteromedially is the inferior vena cava and anterolaterally is the right lobe of the liver. Posteriorly is the right crus of the diaphragm. The left adrenal, which is usually a little larger, is semilunar in shape, its concave aspect lying in relation to the medial aspect of the upper pole of the left kidney. The aorta is medial and anterosuperiorly is the lesser sac and below this, the pancreas and splenic vessels. Posteriorly lies the diaphragm. Accessory adrenal glands may be found in the areolar fatty tissue, in the cortex of the kidney, in the region of the coeliac plexus, in the spermatic cord and epididymis and in the broad ligament of the uterus. These are often comprised of cortical cells only.

Structurally, when cut across, the adrenal gland can be seen with the naked eye to consist of yellow cortex and a thin medulla (*Fig.* 63.1) which is red if blood is present and grey if not. There is a hilum from which the adrenal vein emerges. A thick fibrous capsule containing a plexus of arteries encloses the gland, and fibrous trabeculae with arteries pass into the cortex.

On light microscopy, the cortex is seen to be composed of three zones of cells (*Fig.* 63.2). Immediately below the capsule is the zona glomerulosa composed of columnar cells having deeply-staining nuclei and scanty basophilic cytoplasm which may contain lipid droplets. These cells are

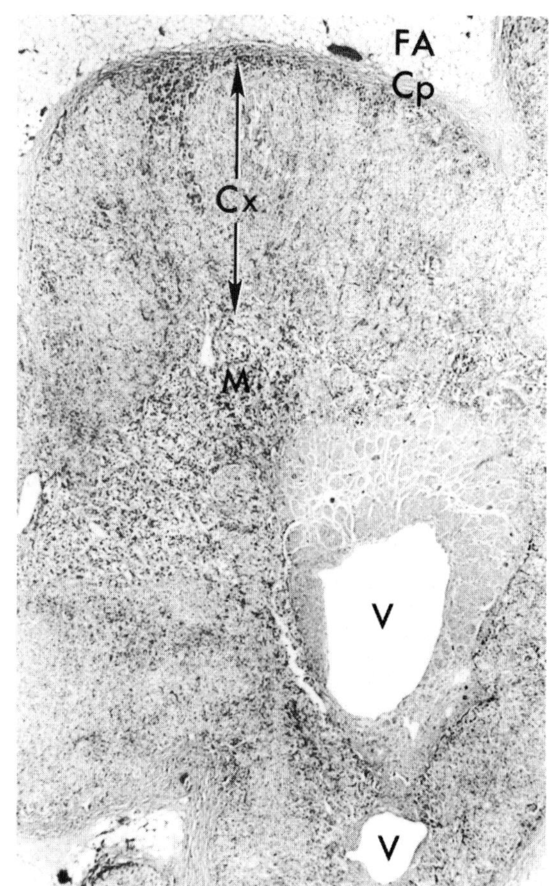

Fig. 63.1 Low-power (×25) section of normal adult adrenal gland showing fatty areolar tissue (FA), capsule (Cp), context (Cx) and medulla (M) containing large venous sinusoids (V).

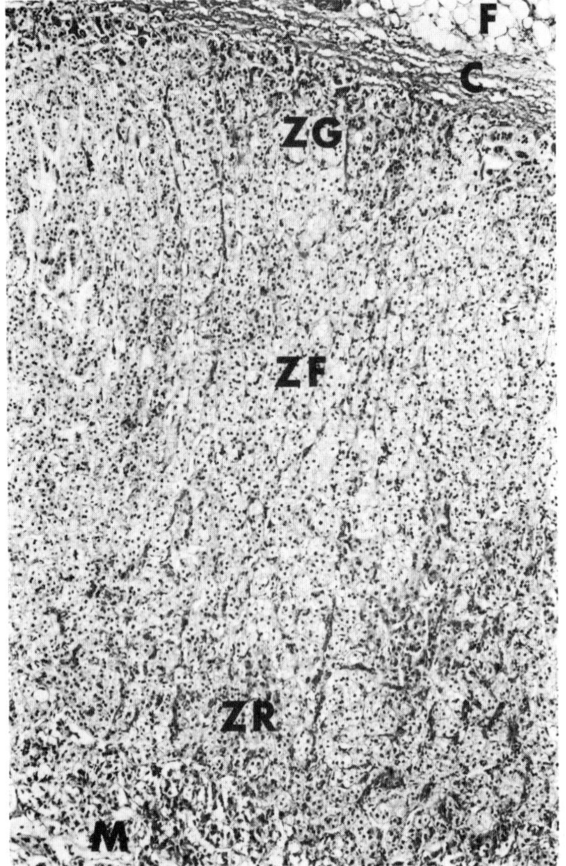

Fig. 63.2 Section (×65) of adult adrenal gland showing surrounding fat (F), capsule (C), the zones of the cortex, zona glomerulosa (ZG), zona fasciculata (ZF) and zona reticularis (ZR) and medulla (M).

arranged in rounded groups or short curved columns. The next zone is the broadest of the three layers and is called the zona fasciculata. It is composed of straight columns of polyhedral cells with basophilic cytoplasm containing many lipid droplets. The next zone which is adjacent to the medulla is called the zona reticularis. It is composed of branching columns of cells which contain a few lipid droplets.

The medulla is composed of chromaffin cells, so called because they take up the stain of chromium salts resulting in a brown pigmentation. The cells are arranged in groups and columns separated by venous sinusoids which drain into the adrenal vein at the hilum of the gland. Isolated and small groups of neurones are to be found among the chromaffin cells.

The adrenal glands are each supplied by several adrenal arteries. Superior adrenal arteries, two or three on each side, come from the right and left phrenic arteries. A middle adrenal artery on each side comes from the aorta itself and several small adrenal arteries arise from the renal arteries. These vessels give rise to the vascular plexus in the capsule described above. The adrenal glands are thus very richly supplied and are consequently very vascular. The adrenal veins emerge from the hilum of each gland. The right adrenal vein is very short and passes from the gland to the inferior vena cava. The left vein passes inferomedially to the left renal vein. Lymphatics drain to the para-aortic lymph nodes. Nerve supply is from the sympathetic system of which the adrenal medulla is part.

PHYSIOLOGY OF THE ADRENAL GLANDS

The adrenal cortex synthesizes and releases several steroid hormones into the adrenal veins and these can be grouped as follows:

Glucocorticoids: of which the most important and plentiful is hydrocortisone (cortisol).
Mineralocorticoids: of which the most important is aldosterone.
Sex hormones: including androsterone and testosterone and small amounts of oestrogen and progesterone.

Cortisol is degraded mainly in the liver to the compounds cortisone and tetrahydrocortisone which are then conjugated with glucuronic acid and excreted in the urine where they are measured as 17-oxogenic steroids. However, urinary-free cortisol measurement is now the preferred assay in studying adrenal cortical disorders.

Fig. 63.3 illustrates diagrammatically the factors controlling cortisol secretions in normal circumstances. The hypothalamic hormone, corticotrophin-releasing factor (CRF), stimulates the basophil cells of the anterior pituitary to synthesize and secrete corticotrophin (ACTH) which in turn stimulates the reticulosa cells of the adrenal cortex to synthesize and secrete cortisol (and other hormones, e.g. testosterone). The plasma level of cortisol exerts a negative feedback effect at the hypothalamus inhibiting the release of CRF when the cortisol level is high and allowing release when the level is low. A circadian rhythm regulates this system whereby release of CRF and hence ACTH and cortisol is minimal at midnight and maximal in the early

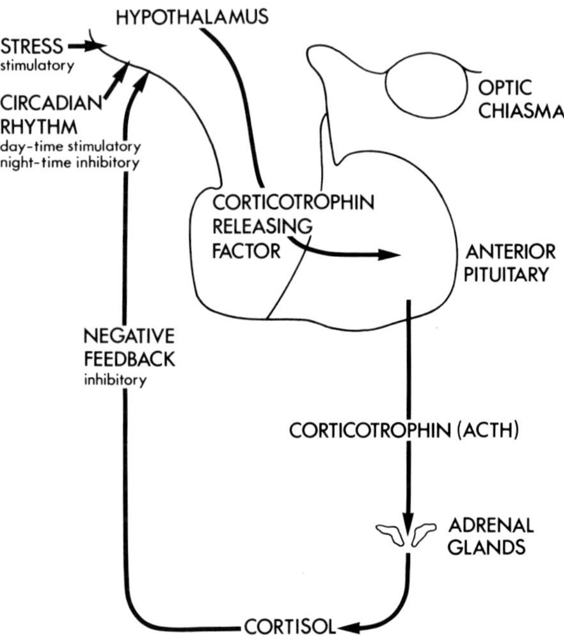

Fig. 63.3 Diagram of the hypothalamic–pituitary–adrenal axis showing the three main physiological mechanisms controlling cortisol synthesis.

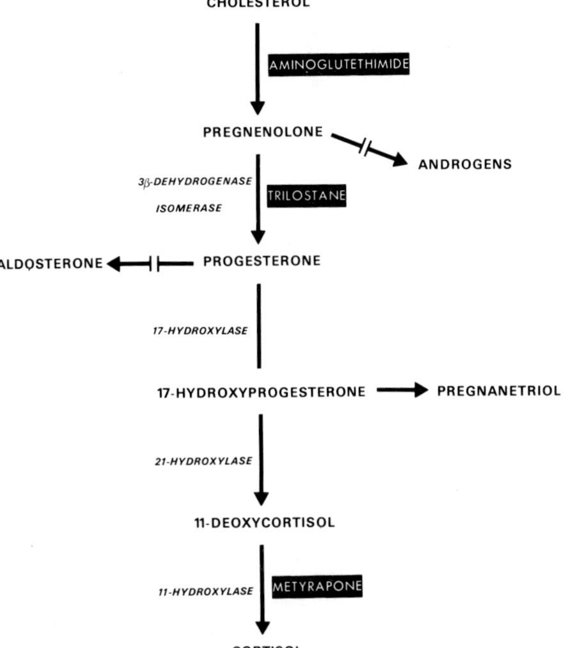

Fig. 63.4 Diagram of the major steps in the synthesis of cortisol from cholesterol in the adrenal cortex. The major intermediary metabolites are in block capitals. To the left of the main pathway in italics are the major enzymes involved and to the right in white-on-black are the drugs discussed in the text, which inhibit the enzyme at the level shown. Intermediate steps in the synthesis of androgens from pregnenolone and aldosterone from progesterone are not shown. Pregnanetriol, the urinary metabolite of 17-hydroxyprogesterone is discussed in the section on congenital adrenal hyperplasia (*see below*).

Table 63.1 Principal actions of cortisol

a. At cellular level: stimulation of synthesis of some proteins and enzymes

b. On intermediary metabolism: inhibition of glucose uptake in tissues; enhancement of gluconeogenesis

c. On water and electrolyte handling: increased free water clearance, sodium retention, potassium excretion, maintenance of extracellular fluid volume

d. On calcium metabolism: decreased intestinal absorption of calcium, increased urinary clearance of calcium

e. On growth: ill-understood role in growth and development (note: cortisol excess inhibits linear growth and skeletal maturation)

f. On inflammatory response: inhibition of classic features of inflammation

g. On immune response: inhibition of cell-mediated immunity

h. In stress: acute and chronic stress is associated with adrenocortical hyperactivity: impairment of this function may result in death

morning. Finally, stress overrides all other controlling influences resulting in secretion of large amounts of cortisol. Use is made of these three regulating mechanisms in the diagnosis of adrenal disorders. *Fig.* 63.4 illustrates the major steps involved in cortisol synthesis and shows the sites of action of drugs mentioned later in the text. The principal actions of cortisol are shown in *Table* 63.1.

Aldosterone is regulated via the renin–angiotensin–aldosterone system wherein diminution in renal bloodflow stimulates the juxtaglomerular cells of the kidney to produce renin. Renin catalyses the production of angiotensin I from

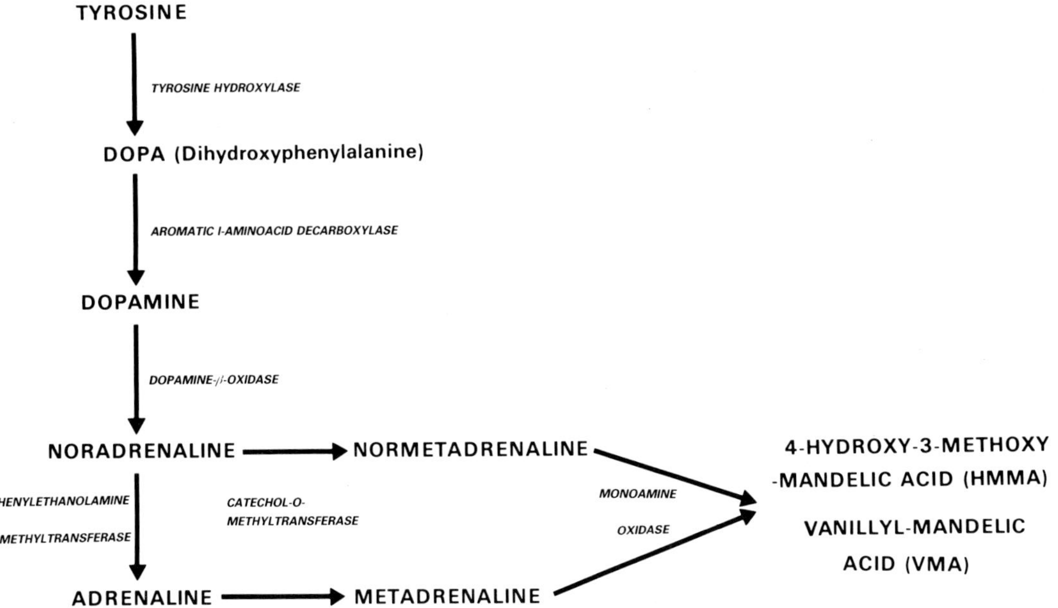

Fig. 63.5 Diagram of the major steps in the synthesis of noradrenaline (norepinephrine) and adrenaline (epinephrine) from tyrosine. Also shown are the major steps in the metabolism of noradrenaline and adrenaline to vanillyl-mandelic acid (4-hydroxy-3-methoxy-mandelic acid). The major enzymes are shown in italics.

the substrate angiotensinogen which is synthesized in the liver. The decapeptide, angiotensin I, is converted in the lungs to the more active octopeptide, angiotensin II, which stimulates aldosterone secretion from the zona glomerulosa. Aldosterone acts mainly at the distal renal tubule to promote sodium and water retention and potassium loss. Other known stimuli to aldosterone release include raised plasma potassium and reduced plasma sodium. ACTH is necessary for a complete response to these stimuli. Aldosterone is mainly degraded in the liver but some appears in the urine. Urinary levels of aldosterone may be used in diagnosis as may plasma levels.

The main source of androgens in the male is the testis and the contribution from the adrenals is not missed in its absence from whatever cause, nor do the adrenals produce sufficient androgen for virilization in gonadal deficiency syndromes. Likewise, oestrogen production from the adrenals in women is not relevant compared with the ovaries. However, in disease states of the adrenals, excessive production of either androgens or oestrogens may take place.

Fig. 63.5 illustrates the synthesis and metabolism in the adrenal medulla of the catecholamines, adrenaline (epinephrine) and noradrenaline (norepinephrine). The adrenal medulla, however, unlike the adrenal cortex, is not essential for life, for there is no deficiency of catecholamines associated with adrenal destruction or resection.

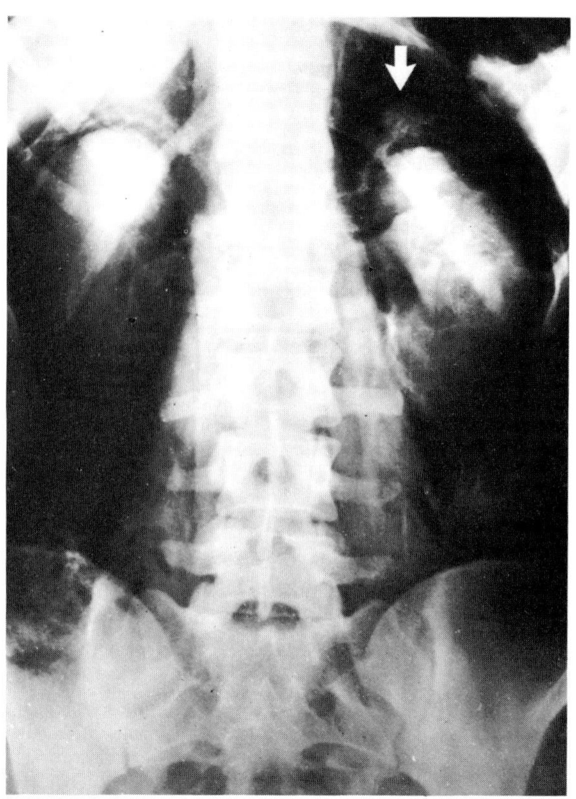

Fig. 63.6 Demonstration by retroperitoneal air insufflation of a left adrenal tumour (arrowed) which was the cause of Conn's syndrome in a young woman.

DISORDERS OF THE ADRENAL GLANDS

Introduction

Surgery of the adrenal glands is carried out for one of two reasons. First, it is carried out for a disorder of one or both adrenal glands which may be a primary disorder of the gland itself, or which may be secondary to a primary disorder elsewhere, e.g. of the pituitary gland, and which is often manifest as an endocrine syndrome. Secondly, adrenal surgery may be carried out as part of the management of advanced breast cancer. The latter is not within the scope of this chapter and is discussed in Chapter 60.

Disorders of the adrenal glands usually present to the physician or endocrinologist as endocrine syndromes before they are referred to the surgeon. The biochemical and anatomical diagnosis is usually made by the physician; nevertheless, it is important for the surgeon to appreciate the biochemical and anatomical basis of the diagnosis. In particular, two aspects of management are of especial importance to the surgeon. First, the investigation and surgery of certain adrenal disorders may be attended by serious complications unless due attention is paid to the hormonal abnormality that is present. Secondly, the abrupt change in hormonal status following surgery may itself be hazardous unless account is taken of it.

Recent years have seen the development of analytical laboratory techniques which now allow precise diagnosis of the endocrine syndrome and which have a role to play in localization of the lesion. The distinction between a bilateral and unilateral adrenal disorder and the localization of the latter has hitherto been difficult, uncomfortable and not without hazard. The insufflation of retroperitoneal air (*Fig.* 63.6) was characterized by these problems. However, the recent development of non-invasive imaging techniques such as ultrasonography, scintigraphy and computerized axial tomography (CT) has, with adrenal vein sampling for hormone assay, greatly facilitated the localization of a unilateral adrenal lesion and may indicate bilateral disease when present. CT is the best imaging method for the adrenals presently available, able to demonstrate lesions down to 5 mm diameter, smaller lesions being localized by adrenal vein sampling for hormone assay. Moreover, CT is capable of scanning the entire abdomen at one examination and this is advantageous in detecting tumour in adrenal cell rests, cortical or medullary. These rests are located at sites other than the adrenal and rarely may give rise to tumours which function exactly like tumours within the adrenal gland.

In this chapter, the pathophysiology, the clinical manifestations, the biochemical and anatomical investigations and the surgical management of adrenal disorders are discussed by considering each clinical syndrome.

Cushing's Syndrome

Introduction

In 1912, Harvey Cushing, an American neurosurgeon, described a clinical syndrome found in association with a pituitary adenoma, and adrenocortical hyperactivity. Subsequently it was shown that the condition results from the tissue effects of chronic excessive plasma concentrations of cortisol or its analogues. Moreover, a radiologically visible pituitary adenoma is now known to be a relatively uncommon cause of the disorder.

Pathology

Iatrogenic causes of Cushing's syndrome are most common and are due to treatment with cortisol or its synthetic analogues, or to treatment with ACTH or its synthetic analogues. However, the condition may arise spontaneously due to inappropriately excessive production of cortisol by the adrenal glands. This may occur as a result of excessive stimulation of the adrenal glands by ACTH from the pituitary, so-called pituitary-dependent Cushing's syndrome (sometimes referred to as Cushing's disease); whether the primary defect resides in the pituitary or in the hypothalamus or elsewhere in the brain is debated. A pituitary tumour is present in almost all patients with pituitary-dependent Cushing's syndrome but it is usually a small microadenoma and only in 20% of patients is the pituitary fossa abnormal on radiography. These adenomas may be chromophobe or basophil in cell type. The adrenal glands in this situation show cortical hyperplasia, which may be nodular. The pituitary-dependent variety accounts for about 80% of patients with non-iatrogenic Cushing's syndrome. Hyaline change (Crook's hyaline) is seen in pituitary basophil cells in all cases of Cushing's syndrome, whatever the cause.

An adrenocortical tumour, adenoma or carcinoma, which is secreting cortisol autonomously and inappropriately, outwith the normal hypothalamic–pituitary regulatory mechanism, may cause the syndrome. Adenoma accounts for 5% of patients and carcinoma for 1%. Multiple nodular adenomas are sometimes found in both adrenals and may be confused with nodular hyperplasia. Biochemical tests will distinguish (*see* below).

Finally, excessive amounts of ACTH may be produced by non-endocrine tumours, such as oat-cell carcinoma of the bronchus, giving rise to hypercortisolism, and this accounts for 15% of patients. In practice, however, this rarely gives rise to the usual clinical picture of Cushing's syndrome but manifests itself in different ways which will be discussed later in this chapter.

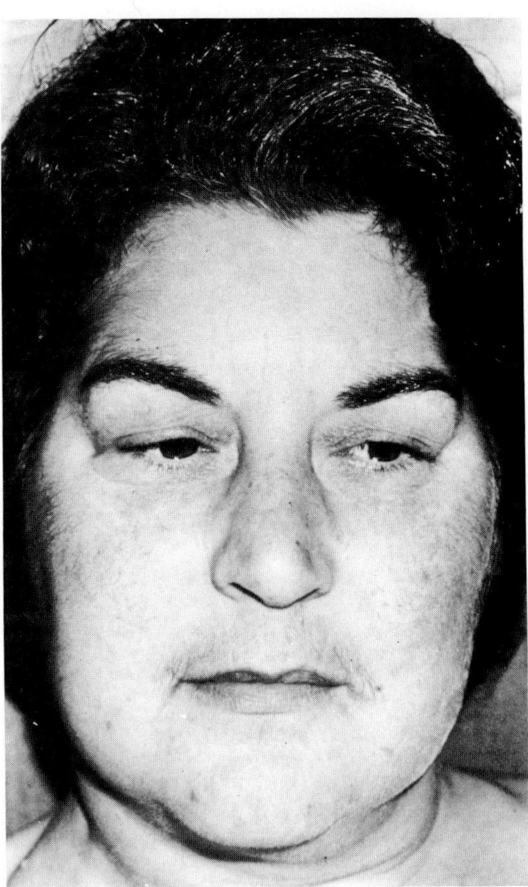

Fig. 63.7 Photograph of the face of a patient with Cushing's syndrome due to an adrenal adenoma. Note the round, plethoric facies and slight hirsutism.

Clinical

The major clinical features of Cushing's syndrome are listed in *Table* 63.2. It will be appreciated that hypercortisolism is a relatively uncommon cause for the majority of these features and in practice a patient is suspected of having Cushing's syndrome from his or her appearance, especially of the facies (*Fig.* 63.7). Since many of the features listed in *Table* 63.2 such as hypertension, diabetes mellitus and osteoporosis are very common, attempts have been made to find a simple outpatient screening procedure which would on one hand exclude Cushing's syndrome and, on the other hand, give sufficient indication of the probability of Cushing's disease to warrant further inpatient investigation. Measurement of free cortisol in an 8-hour overnight urine collection (from 11.00 p.m. to 7.00 a.m.) provides such a screening test and data from a study of this procedure are shown in *Fig.* 63.8.

Table 63.2 Clinical features of Cushing's syndrome

Obesity	: classically, of face and trunk with thin arms and legs
Moon face	: round, plethoric face (*Fig.* 63.7)
Hypertension	
Menstrual disturbances	: oligomenorrhoea, amenorrhoea (males may be impotent)
Osteoporosis	: bone pain, vertebral collapse, kyphosis, pathological fracture
Striae	: abdominal stretch marks which if purple are highly characteristic
Glucose intolerance	: glycosuria, polyuria, thirst, diabetes mellitus
Myopathy	: proximal muscle weakness and wasting
Hirsutism	: and other manifestations of androgens, e.g. acne
Depression	: also delusions and psychoses may occur
Bruising	: thin, easily traumatized skin
Oedema	
Pigmentation	

ACTH, or peptides with ACTH-like activity, may be synthesized and released from non-endocrine tumours, the commonest of which is oat-cell carcinoma of the bronchus. Less frequently, bronchial carcinoids, thymic tumours, islet-cell tumours and phaeochromocytomas secrete ACTH, and when chest radiography is negative, these sites must be considered. Usually, the clinical picture of ectopic ACTH syndrome is not that of classic Cushing's syndrome as described above, but the clinical appearance is dominated by the general effects of malignancy together with pigmentation and severe proximal myopathy, though this is not universally the case. The clue may be provided by the finding of marked hypokalaemic alkalosis. Additional clinical features may be diabetes mellitus, polyuria, hypertension and oedema. However, it occasionally happens that ACTH may

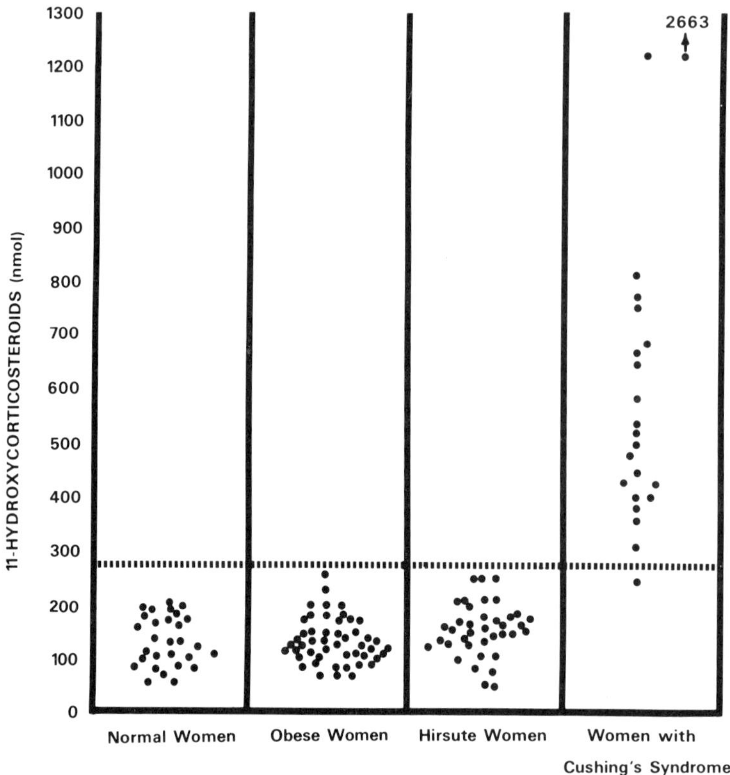

Fig. 63.8 11-Hydroxycorticosteroid content, measured by fluorimetry, of 8-hour overnight urines in women with and without Cushing's syndrome. The dotted line represents the upper limit of normal. (Reproduced by kind permission of Professor D. Mattingly and the Editors and Publishers of the *British Medical Journal.*)

be secreted by a benign tumour, such as a bronchial carcinoid or thymoma, and in this situation patients have the clinical features of classic Cushing's syndrome but in addition show the marked hypokalaemic alkalosis referred to above.

Investigations

1. Biochemical Diagnosis

If a screening test proves positive, or if the clinical suspicion is very great, the patient is admitted to hospital for more detailed investigation. The purpose of investigation is to confirm excessive secretion of cortisol and to localize the abnormality, whether pituitary or adrenal and, if the latter, to demonstrate which adrenal gland contains the tumour.

Measurement of cortisol secretion rate provides the most direct method of establishing excessive and inappropriate cortisol secretion, but this is time-consuming and involves the use of isotopes. In practice, reliable results are obtained by demonstrating increased levels of cortisol in a 24-hour urinary collection and by demonstrating disturbance of the normal circadian rhythm of cortisol secretion wherein midnight levels of plasma cortisol are elevated in contradistinction to the normal situation where low levels of plasma cortisol are obtained. It is worth emphasizing that a level of plasma cortisol at 9.00 a.m. is not necessarily elevated in Cushing's syndrome, though commonly it is so. The normal range of plasma cortisol at 10.00 a.m. is 200–650 nmol/l (6–26 μg/100 ml) and less than 250 nmol/l (8 μg/100 ml) is to be expected in normal subjects at midnight. (There are several different methods of measuring plasma and urinary cortisol and normal ranges vary according to the method and laboratory measuring them. Each laboratory should establish its own reference range.)

Once hypercortisolism has been established by demonstration of increased 24-hour urinary cortisol and disturbance of the circadian rhythm, the next step is to localize the site of the primary lesion. Pituitary-dependent Cushing's disease is the commonest variety but within this group a radiologically demonstrable pituitary tumour is uncommon, occurring in only 20% of patients. Nevertheless, radiographs to demonstrate the pituitary fossa including tomography (*Fig.* 63.9) and charting of the visual fields should be carried out; for should a pituitary tumour with or without encroachment onto the optic chiasm be demonstrated, this will have some bearing on treatment. The recently described technique of emission scintigraphy promises to be useful in identifying pituitary microadenomas undetectable by other imaging methods. In the absence of a radiologically or otherwise demonstrable pituitary tumour, biochemical methods are employed to ascertain whether the Cushing's disease is due to pituitary dysfunction or due to a primary adrenal lesion. In recent times, the development of reliable assays for plasma corticotrophin have provided a logical answer to this problem. Thus, where there is a primary adrenal lesion, plasma corticotrophin is very low or undetectable and where the hypercortisolism is due to a pituitary disorder, plasma corticotrophin levels are commonly above

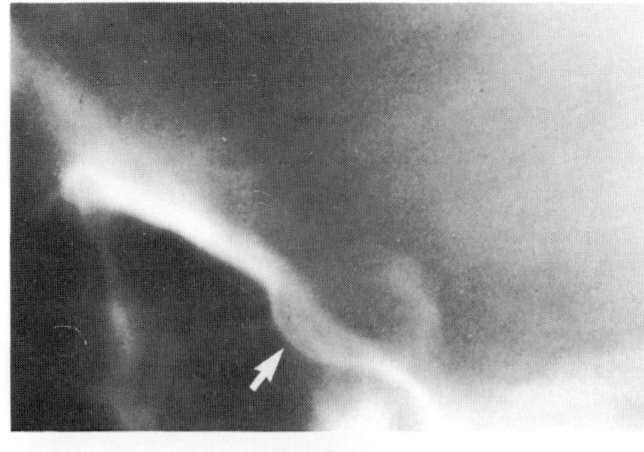

12·2cm

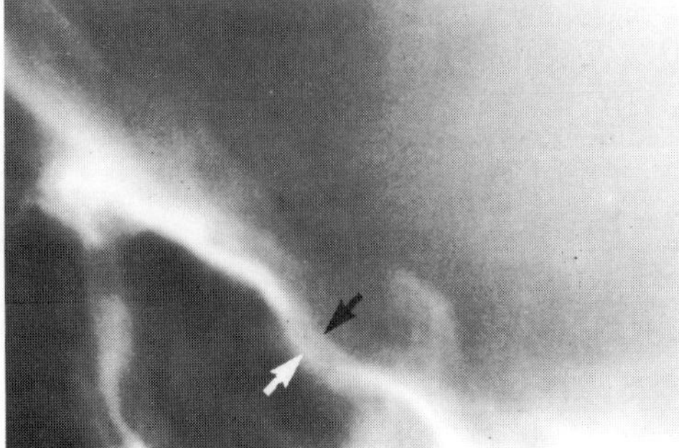

12·6cm

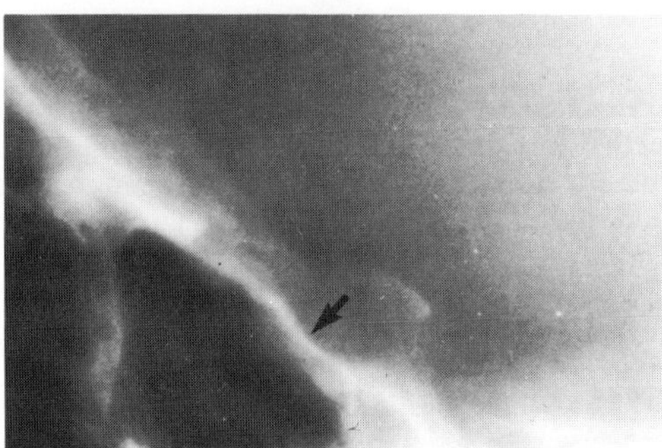

13·0cm

Fig. 63.9 Tomography of the pituitary fossa in a patient with Cushing's disease. The double floor of the fossa is clearly shown in the 12·6 cm tomograph. The 12·2 cm tomograph brings the lower floor into focus and the 13·0 cm tomograph brings the upper floor into focus.

CUSHING'S DISEASE | ADRENAL TUMOUR | ECTOPIC ACTH

PLASMA IMMUNOREACTIVE ACTH (pg/ml)

4000-12000, 2000-4000, 1000-2000, 900, 700, 500, 300, 250, 200, 150, 100, 50, 0

70 | 18 | 81

Fig. 63.10 Plasma morning N-terminal immunoreactive ACTH levels in patients with Cushing's syndrome of pituitary-dependent type (Cushing's disease), contrasted with levels in patients with Cushing's syndrome due to adrenal tumours or the ectopic ACTH syndrome. The dotted lines represent the limits of the normal range at 0900 hours. (Reproduced by kind permission of Professor L. H. Rees and Churchill Livingstone, Publishers of *Recent Advances in Endocrinology and Metabolism 1*.)

the normal range or at the upper end of the normal range. When there is ectopic ACTH production from a non-endocrine tumour, the plasma corticotrophin levels are very elevated indeed. *Fig.* 63.10 illustrates this and it will be seen that there is overlap in the plasma corticotrophin levels in patients with pituitary-dependent Cushing's syndrome and patients with ectopic ACTH production. However, because of the different clinical manifestations, this overlap rarely leads to confusion. Logically, therefore, plasma ACTH measurement is the ideal way in which to determine whether Cushing's syndrome is pituitary or adrenal in origin. Logistically, the situation is not quote so simple. In the UK at least, many hospitals do not have their own ACTH assays available and samples are sent to the Supraregional Assay Service and the delay in getting the result can be several weeks or even months. Moreover, ACTH is an unstable hormone and is adsorbed onto glass. For these reasons, samples must be taken into plastic tubes with plastic syringes and ideally the specimen tube should be ice-cold. Separation of the plasma should be undertaken within 10 minutes in a refrigerated centrifuge and the samples stored at −20°C. Samples which have to be transported for assay should be done so in tubes surrounded by carbon dioxide snow.

Because of these practical problems, the dexamethasone suppression test and metyrapone test remain useful and commonly employed procedures for determining whether Cushing's syndrome is pituitary in origin or due to primary adrenal pathology. The principle of the dexamethasone test is that dexamethasone given in high dosage (8 mg daily for 48 hours in divided dosage) will result in at least 50% reduction in plasma and urinary cortisol in pituitary-dependent Cushing's syndrome, whereas no suppression occurs in Cushing's syndrome due to primary adrenal tumour or ectopic ACTH secretion. The author's procedure

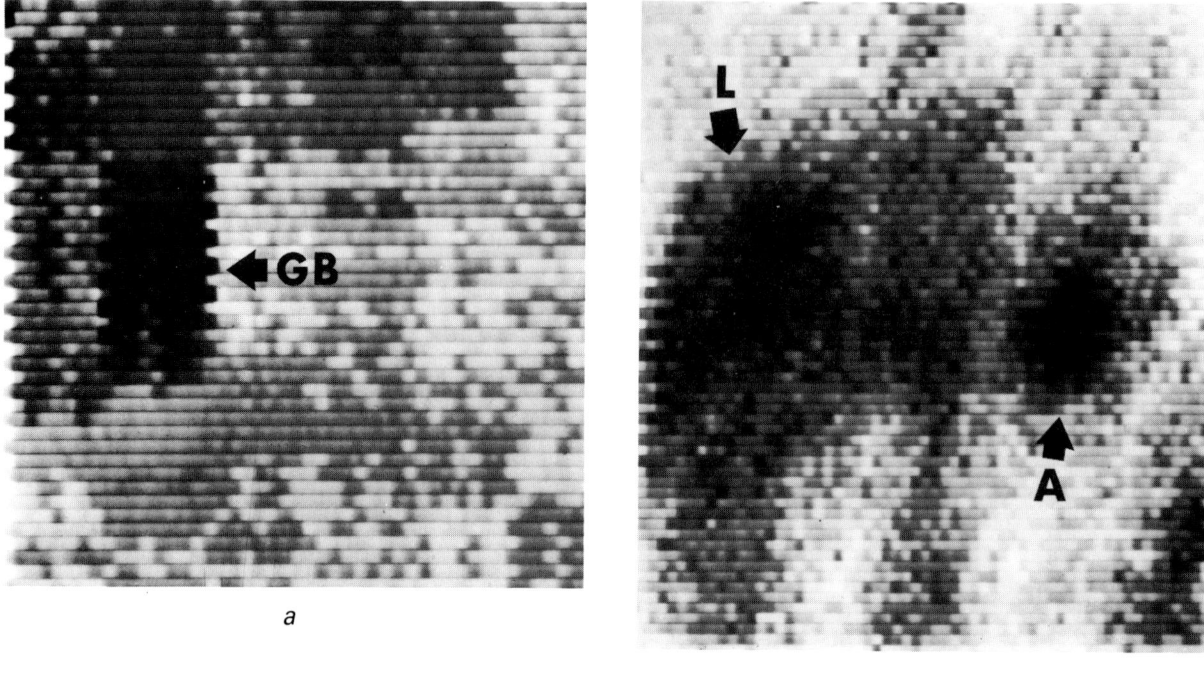

Fig. 63.11 *a*, Anterior abdominal iodocholesterol scintiscan soon after administration of the isotope in a patient suspected of having an adrenal tumour causing Cushing's syndrome. Note that the only hot spot is the gallbladder (GB), not the right adrenal. *b*, Repeat scan posteriorly in the same patient as in (*a*) 48 hours after administration of the isotope showing diffuse take up in the region of the liver (L) and a hot spot in the region of the left adrenal (A). No take up is seen in the region of the right adrenal. A left adrenal adenoma was excised from this patient.

is to administer dexamethasone 2 mg 6-hourly for 48 hours collecting a 24-hour urinary sample during the second 24-hour period and collecting a blood sample at 9.00 on the morning of completion of the 48-hour course of dexamethasone. The urine and plasma are assayed for cortisol and the results compared with the levels before administration of dexamethasone. In pituitary-dependent nodular adrenal hyperplasia, dexamethasone may fail to suppress steroid secretion. Plasma ACTH levels will distinguish between this variant and multiple nodular adenomas.

Metyrapone, which inhibits the conversion of 11-deoxycortisol to cortisol (*see Fig.* 63.4) is given at a dosage of

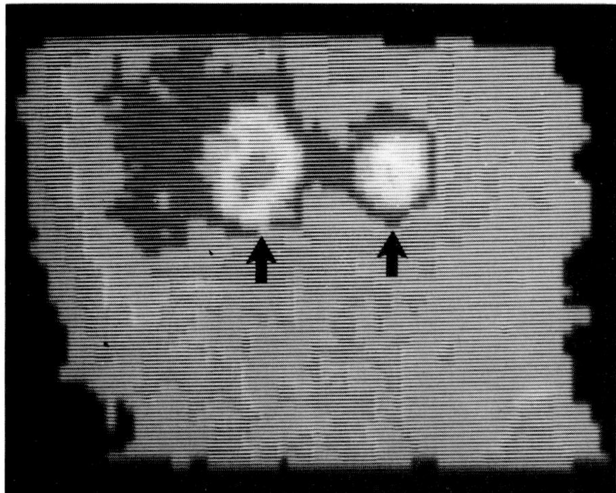

Fig. 63.12 Posterior abdominal iodocholesterol scintiscan 48 hours after administration of the isotope in a patient suspected of pituitary-dependent Cushing's disease. Note the marked take up of isotope in both adrenals (arrowed) fully compatible with the suspected diagnosis. This patient responded to the trans-sphenoidal hypophysectomy.

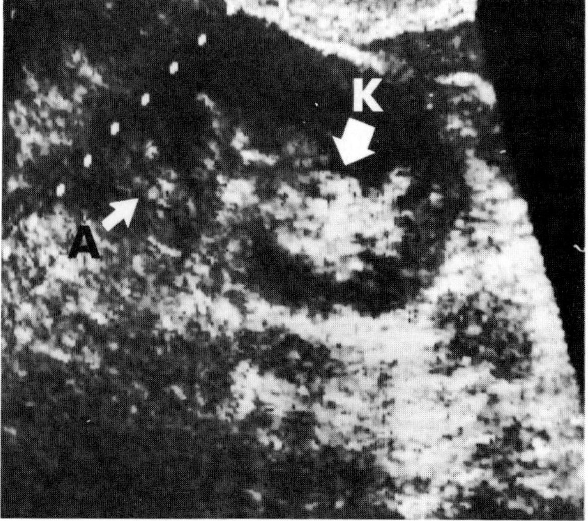

Fig. 63.13 Adrenal ultrasound study in a patient suspected of having Cushing's syndrome due to an adrenal tumour. The line of dots shows centimetre markings. The study shows a left adrenal mass (A) about 3 cm diameter in relation to the kidney (K).

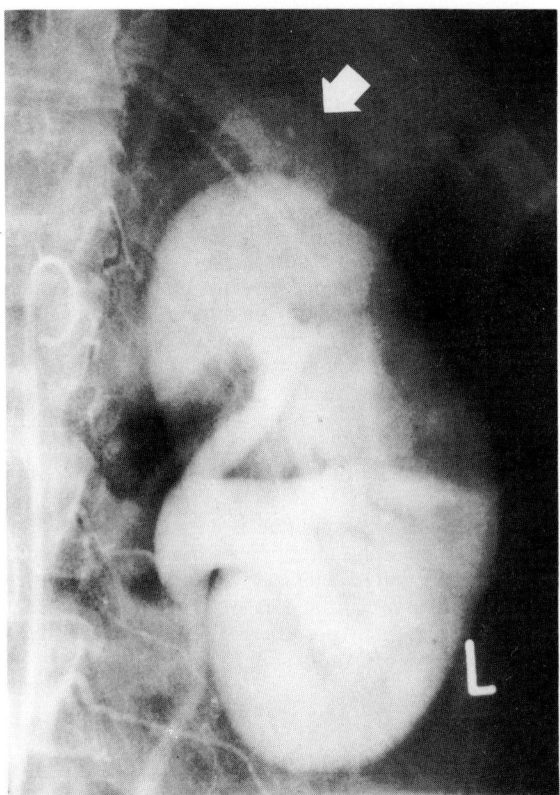

Fig. 63.14 Angiogram of left kidney and a left adrenal tumour (arrowed) in a patient suspected of Cushing's syndrome due to an adrenal tumour.

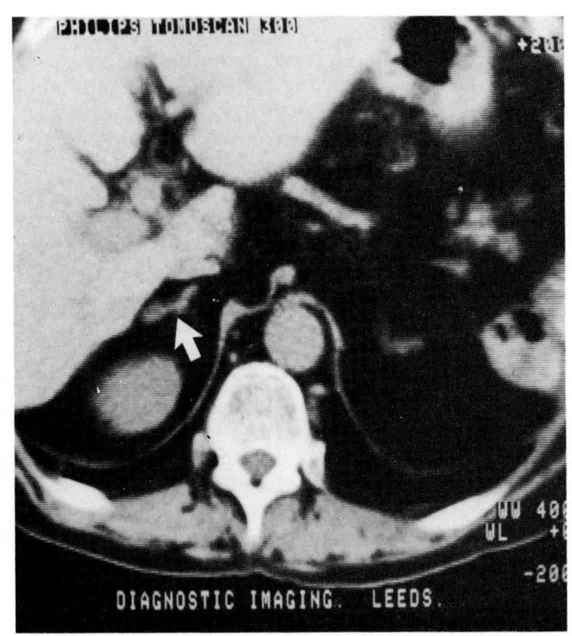

a

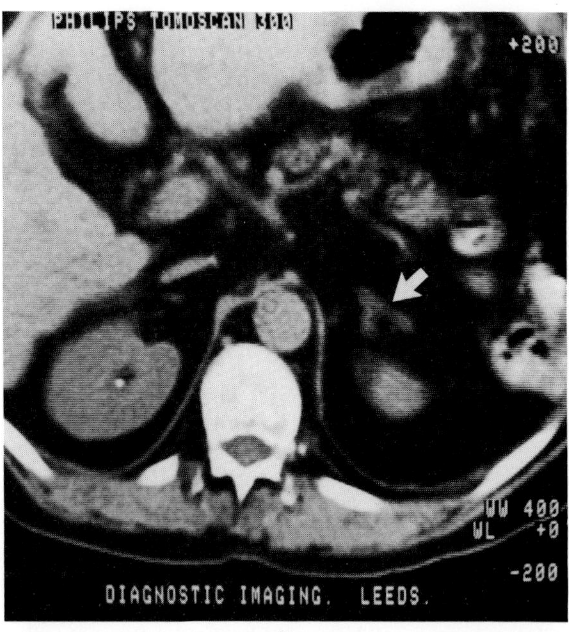

b

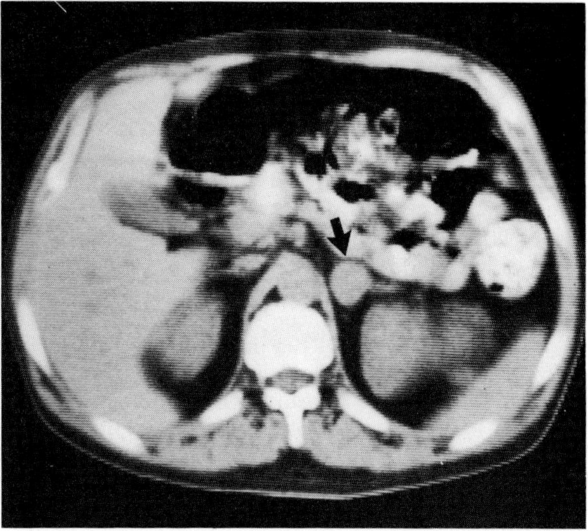

c

Fig. 63.15 *a*, *b*, Computerized axial tomographs of left adrenal (arrowed) and right adrenal (arrowed) respectively in a patient with pituitary-dependent Cushing's disease. These adrenals are of normal shape but are diffusely enlarged about 1·5 times normal compatible with bilateral hyperplasia of the adrenals due to excessive stimulation with corticotrophin. *c*, CT showing a right adrenal tumour (arrowed). (This tumour was a secondary deposit from a bronchial carcinoma.)

250 mg 4-hourly for 24 hours and urine is collected over the succeeding 24 hours and its 17-oxogenic steroid (17-OGS) content compared with basal values. In normal individuals, the 17-OGS excretion is doubled. In pituitary-dependent Cushing's disease the excretion is increased at least threefold. No response is seen with autonomous adrenal lesions. Both these tests give misleading information in a small proportion of patients.

2. Localization

If it is decided on the basis of these tests that the disorder is a primary adrenal tumour, the next step is to localize the lesion. These are several techniques currently in use to localize an adrenocortical tumour. These are ultrasonography, ^{131}I-iodocholesterol scintigraphy, adrenal arteriography, adrenal venography with sampling from adrenal veins and, more recently, CT. Examples of some of these techniques are shown in *Figs.* 63.11, 63.12, 63.13 and 63.14. Recent work has suggested that ultrasonography and scintigraphy provide high diagnostic accuracy but, as stated above, CT is now considered the investigation of choice (*Fig.* 63.15). Since angiography, especially venography, is not without serious hazard, the non-invasive procedures are to be preferred. A relative difficulty with iodocholesterol scintigraphy is that the material may accumulate in the gallbladder simulating a right adrenal hot-spot (*Fig.* 63.11*a*). Lateral scanning resolves this problem for the gallbladder is anterior whereas the adrenal is posterior. Also, adrenal take-up of isotope is still present 48–72 hours after administration, by which time the gallbladder has lost much of its isotope (*Fig.* 63.11*b*).

If the biochemistry suggests a pituitary lesion and a direct pituitary approach is contemplated by way of treatment, then further detailed radiological studies of the pituitary fossa with CT or air encephalography are desirable to determine whether suprasellar extension is present and to assess its extent for this will have some bearing on the approach to the pituitary.

Treatment

1. Choice of Surgical Procedure

Treatment of Cushing's syndrome depends on its cause. For pituitary-dependent Cushing's without obvious pituitary tumour, subtotal adrenalectomy is now no longer considered because recurrence of Cushing's syndrome is common. Bilateral total adrenalectomy is still used in many centres. The advantage of this procedure is that cortisol production is completely abolished. The disadvantages are first, the patient requires replacement therapy with hydrocortisone and fludrocortisone and, secondly, a proportion of patients, up to 30% in some series, will develop Nelson's syndrome. This condition is one of rapid expansion of a pituitary tumour, which may have been radiologically undetectable, and which may extend beyond the sella causing local neurological damage to the optic chiasma and may result in death. The syndrome may occur within months or years following adrenal surgery. The hallmark of this condition is the development of Addisonian-type skin pigmentation following bilateral adrenalectomy. For these reasons, various groups in recent years have directed their treatment to the pituitary gland itself. Such treatments have included trans-sphenoidal hypophysectomy, microsurgery in which dissection of the pituitary adenoma itself is attempted, cryosurgery and various forms of irradiation, including conventional kilovoltage external irradiation, the implantation of yttrium-90 or gold-198 and heavy particle irradiation. The choice of procedure depends very much on the expertise available locally and it is still by no means clear which of these methods of treatment will ultimately prove to be the most satisfactory. The ideal result would be abolition of the excessive ACTH production with preservation of the remaining pituitary function. Thus conventional hypophysectomy has a high remission rate with a high rate of endocrine deficit and other complications. On the other hand, external irradiation has a low incidence of endocrine deficit and complications but the remission rate is relatively low. Preliminary information would suggest that microsurgery or internal irradiation of the pituitary with radioactive yttrium or gold are capable of high remission rates with a relatively low, though not absent, incidence of endocrine deficit and other complications.

Other groups have attempted to treat pituitary-dependent Cushing's by total adrenalectomy and autotransplantation of sections of adrenal tissue into thigh muscle. This has enabled replacement therapy to be avoided and has prevented Nelson's syndrome. The possibility of recurrent Cushing's remains but is dealt with more easily.

Where there is radiological evidence of a pituitary tumour at the outset, the situation is more difficult for many of these tumours may have already spread outside the pituitary fossa. It has been suggested that a combination of surgery and irradiation should be employed in this situation and even then cortisol production may not be controlled and bilateral adrenalectomy may be required. It is evident that the best form of treatment for pituitary-dependent Cushing's is still awaited.

If the cause of the condition is an autonomous adrenal tumour, excision of the appropriate adrenal is carried out. If the condition is that of ectopic ACTH secretion, removal of the primary source will be curative. However, for oat-cell carcinoma this is rarely possible and some form of palliative therapy will have to be used (*see below*).

2. Preoperative Preparation

Because of the effects of the metabolic disorder, many patients have undergone surgery in less than ideal conditions. The obesity and poorly healing tissue present problems for the surgeon and the myopathy involving muscles of respiration may lead to postoperative respiratory problems. Cortisol excess results in impaired immune mechanisms with increased susceptibility to infections. Research has been carried out with a view to finding a satisfactory drug treatment which will suppress steroid output for a short period to enable the patient to be in much better condition for surgery. Hitherto, anti-adrenal drugs have not been satisfactory. On the one hand, the block induced by the drug has been overcome by the condition and on the other hand unacceptable side-effects have been observed. Recently, however, it has been shown that metyrapone and aminoglutethimide used in combination in doses of each insufficient to produce side-effects have been synergistic in their effect on cortisol biosynthesis. Aminoglutethimide inhibits the conversion of cholesterol to pregnenolone, a very early step in cortisol biosynthesis, and metyrapone inhibits 11-beta-hydroxylation, a late enzymatic step in cortisol biosynthesis (*see Fig.* 63.4). Aminoglutethimide, 1 or 2 g daily, together with metyrapone 2–4 g daily, adequately suppresses cortisol output as measured by urinary cortisol estimations in the majority of patients. Clinical and biochemical improvement have been reported in patients so treated. Replacement therapy is obviously necessary and dexamethasone 0·5 mg twice daily with fludrocortisone 0·1 mg daily are recommended. It is the author's practice to use this regimen in all patients who are to undergo surgery for Cushing's syndrome for 3–4 weeks before the operation. On the day of the operation this treatment is stopped and hydrocortisone hemisuccinate 400 mg over 24 hours by intravenous infusion is instituted. A very recently introduced drug, trilostane, which inhibits the conversion of pregnenolone to progesterone (*see Fig.* 63.4) may prove to be more useful than aminoglutethimide for it appears, so far, to be remarkably free from side-effects.

3. Postoperative Management

In the postoperative period hydrocortisone should be continued, given parenterally and slowly reduced to maintenance levels. It has been observed that some patients do not tolerate a speedy reduction in their steroid dosage to conventional maintenance levels, and when so treated develop features of hypoadrenalism such as vomiting and hypotension. Also seen in this situation is desquamation of the skin and hypercalcaemia. This condition responds to increasing the dose of the hydrocortisone which should then be reduced only slowly. The indication for continued replacement therapy with hydrocortisone and fludrocortisone will, of course, depend on the treatment used. Thus, following conventional trans-sphenoidal hypophysectomy or bilateral adrenalectomy, patients require steroid maintenance therapy and possibly other therapy to reverse the effects of deficiency of anterior pituitary trophic hormones. On the other hand, following the implantation of radio-yttrium, one group found that only 38% of their patients required steroid replacement therapy.

It must be borne in mind that when there is a unilateral adrenal tumour, the remaining adrenal will be completely suppressed and in the author's experience it may take very many months before this adrenal is functioning normally and therefore the patient requires steroid replacement therapy in this situation also. The therapy is slowly reduced and the function of the remaining adrenal tested periodically using adrenal stimulation tests and insulin stress tests.

4. Malignant Conditions

If the adrenal tumour is a carcinoma with metastatic spread, removal of the tumour will not cure the excessive cortisol secretion. Secondary deposits can be detected if desired by ^{131}I-iodocholesterol scintigraphy. However, the practical problem with such patients and in those with inoperable ectopic ACTH-secreting carcinomas is to suppress the excessive cortisol secretion in the hope of improving the general wellbeing of the patient. No satisfactory treatment has yet been developed but *o,p'*DDD, an adrenal cell poison which causes adrenal atrophy, has been used but itself may cause severe anorexia, nausea and depression. Metyrapone or aminoglutethimide alone are not suitable for long-term adrenal suppression, but may in combination have some effect. Trilostane (*see above*) may turn out to be a very useful drug in this situation but further evaluation is required.

Prognosis

Untreated Cushing's syndrome carries a very high mortality. The outcome for adrenal carcinoma and ectopic ACTH secretion due to carcinoma remains very poor. Removal of an autonomous adrenal adenoma is curative. The outcome in pituitary-dependent Cushing's is variable; those patients with overt pituitary tumours do less well than those without obvious tumour and this latter group generally do very well indeed.

Primary Hyperaldosteronism (Conn's Syndrome)

Introduction

In 1955, Conn described a patient with hypertension, hypokalaemia and an adrenocortical adenoma. Excision of the adenoma resulted in reduction of the blood pressure and return of the biochemical abnormalities to normal. Over the course of the next 20 years, more patients were described and studied. These studies showed that such patients have elevated levels of plasma and urinary aldosterone and reduced levels of plasma renin concentration and plasma renin activity due to autonomous hypersecretion of aldosterone. The condition was termed 'Conn's Syndrome' or primary hyperaldosteronism, to distinguish it from hyperaldosteronism associated with and caused by *high* levels of plasma renin with hypertension and often renal disease or sodium depletion, so-called secondary hyperaldosteronism. A number of subgroups of primary hyperaldosteronism have been recently described, including a variety where there is bilateral hyperplasia of the zona glomerulosa of the adrenal glands leading to the suggestion that, in these instances, the primary pathology may not reside in the adrenal glands though its precise aetiology is as yet undetermined. This has led to recent suggestions that the syndrome should be termed 'low-renin hyperaldosteronism' rather than primary hyperaldosteronism.

Pathology

The majority (about 60%) of patients with primary hyperaldosteronism have a benign adrenal adenoma. The tumours are usually small (2 cm or less in diameter; 3 g or less in weight) and about 60% are located in the left adrenal gland. The cut surface is golden yellow in colour. Histology may show various cell types in the same tumour, namely, glomerulosa-type cells, reticularis-type cells and cells with features of all adrenocortical cell types. About 40% of patients, however, will have bilateral hyperplasia with or without micronodules of the zona glomerulosa. A small subgroup cannot be classified. Very rarely an adrenocortical carcinoma is present.

Clinical

Hypertension is always present in primary hyperaldosteronism and it has been suggested that the condition may account for 1% of hypertensive patients. Other symptoms may be present, including muscle weakness, tetany, polyuria, nocturia and thirst. These are features of hypokalaemic alkalosis which is characteristically present. It is this biochemical finding that usually gives the clue that the patient is suffering from Conn's syndrome. However, the hypokalaemia may be intermittent and is less marked in those patients with bilateral hyperplasia rather than an adenoma. Plasma sodium may be elevated but may also be within the normal range. The hypertension may be asymptomatic and malignant hypertension is unusual in this condition though it may occur.

Investigations

1. Biochemical Diagnosis

When faced with a hypertensive patient with hypokalaemia, the clinician has to decide whether Conn's syndrome is likely. The effects of drugs must be eliminated, for diuretics and purgatives can cause hypokalaemia and secondary hyperaldosteronism. Carbenoxolone, liquorice and even oral contraceptives may themselves have a mineralocorticoid-like effect and other drugs used in hypertension such as methyldopa or beta-adrenergic blockers are capable of interfering with renin release. It is recommended, where possible, that the patient does not take medications for at least 4 weeks before the assessment is made. It is also recommended that during this time the patient remains on a normal dietary intake of sodium and potassium. If, under these circumstances, hypertension and hypokalaemia remain, then endogenous hyperaldosteronism may still be secondary to such conditions as renal artery stenosis, unilateral renal disease, malignant hypertension, bilateral chronic renal disease and other rarer situations such as a renin-secreting renal tumour. If hyponatraemia is present, secondary hyperaldosteronism is likely; conversely, if hypernatraemia is present, primary aldosteronism is likely. However, in both situations, the plasma sodium may be within the normal range. Studies of renin and aldosterone are therefore necessary.

Samples for plasma renin and plasma aldosterone are taken between 0900 and 1000 hours from an arm vein, the patient having remained in bed fasting from 2200 hours the previous evening. As above, the patient is off drugs and on normal salt intake for 4 weeks beforehand. The findings of a raised level of plasma aldosterone with a reduced level of plasma renin confirms the diagnosis of primary hyperaldosteronism.

2. Localization

It is important to distinguish between a unilateral adenoma and bilateral hyperplasia in this condition, for it will determine treatment. This is not always easy to do and many procedures have been described, including mathematical and statistical analysis of biochemical and clinical data, sodium loading with fludrocortisone, comparison of diurnal changes in plasma aldosterone and treatment with spironolactone. All these procedures may differentiate between hyperplasia and adenoma though overlap occurs and in individual cases their usefulness may be limited. Various techniques for imaging the adrenal glands have been used. Different centres favour different approaches to this problem and the reader is referred to the review article at the end of this chapter. At the author's centre, adrenal arteriography, venography with adrenal vein sampling, scintigraphy, ultrasonography and more recently CT have been the procedures used for differentiating between hyperplasia and adenoma, and for localizing the latter, if present. CT is now the procedure of choice. However, very small Conn's tumours (<5 mm diameter) may not be visualized and adrenal vein sampling for plasma aldosterone becomes the method of choice. In this procedure, the level of aldosterone in plasma from the side of the adenoma is at least 2·5 times that from the uninvolved side.

Treatment

1. Choice of Therapy

An adenoma is best treated by adrenalectomy and hyperplasia by medical therapy. However, recent studies have shown that in some patients, excision of an adenoma has not resulted in cure of the hypertension and such an outcome can be predicted by the response to spironolactone. Thus, if a patient's hypertension responds to spironolactone 200–400 mg daily for 4 weeks, there will be a satisfactory reduction in the blood pressure after removal of the adenoma. If the response to spironolactone is unsatisfactory, it is unlikely that surgery will further improve the blood pressure, even though the electrolyte abnormalities are normalized.

There is some debate as to whether surgery or medical therapy is the better form of treatment for the patients with bilateral hyperplasia. Such patients should be treated primarily with spironolactone or amiloride and only if they fail to respond or the drugs cannot be tolerated is surgery indicated. Preliminary evidence suggests that trilostane (*see above*) may turn out to be very useful in the medical treatment of primary hyperaldosteronism. For surgery to be effective, total or subtotal adrenalectomy is required with the attendant possibility of subsequent adrenal insufficiency on the one hand and inadequate surgery on the other. A very small group of patients appear to respond to treatment with corticosteroids and such patients will respond to dexamethasone 1–2 mg daily within a week. The mechanism for this variant of the condition is not understood. Very rarely, carcinoma of the adrenal may produce aldosterone and prompt surgery is mandatory here. Features that suggest the possibility of carcinoma include fever, abdominal pain, severe muscle weakness and a large tumour which may displace the kidney.

2. Preoperative Preparation

The patient should be normotensive and in electrolyte balance by prior treatment with spironolactone 200–400 mg daily before surgery. The side-effects of spironolactone, including gynaecomastia, impotence, irregular menses, nausea and epigastric discomfort, may prove a limiting factor in the use of this drug and amiloride is recommended as an alternative in divided doses up to 40 mg daily.

3. Postoperative Management

Selective hypoaldosteronism may be present for up to 4 weeks following resection of an aldosteronoma. This may result in hyponatraemia and hyperkalaemia and if salt is restricted in the postoperative period an acute hypoadrenal state may occur. Liberal salt intake is recommended postoperatively and it is uncommon for treatment with 9-α-fludrocortisone to be necessary. If such treatment is called for, doses of 0·05–0·1 mg daily are recommended. Preoperative treatment with spironolactone reduces the occurrence of this complication.

Prognosis

The outcome is usually very good for both adenoma and hyperplasia unless there is already renal or vascular damage due to the hypertension when the prognosis becomes that of complicated hypertension. Adrenal carcinoma carries a poor prognosis but treatment with *o*, *p*′DDD may be tried.

Phaeochromocytoma

Introduction

Phaeochromocytoma is a rare tumour derived from sympathetic nervous tissue which produces clinical syndromes due to excessive secretion of catecholamines. Hypertension is an important feature of the syndrome and Mayo in the early 1930s was the first to remove such an adrenal tumour and thus ameliorate the patient's hypertension.

Pathophysiology

Ninety per cent of phaeochromocytomas are found in the adrenal medulla; the remaining 10% may be found anywhere along the sympathetic chain from neck to pelvis. Macroscopically the tumours vary in size from small nodules to very large masses up to 4 kg in weight. They are usually well encapsulated. The cut surface is red-brown in colour and sometimes haemorrhagic. Microscopically they are composed of polygonal or spheroidal chromaffin cells and the tumour is sometimes termed 'chromaffinoma'. These cells are embedded within a markedly vascularized fibrous stroma. Malignancy is diagnosed by the finding of metastases, for many benign tumours may contain atypical bizarre cells. Recently, patients have been described with bilateral adrenal medullary hyperplasia and symptoms of catecholamine excess. Ten per cent of phaeochromocytomas are malignant and these are usually bilateral. The condition may be familial and may be associated with disorders of other tissues derived from the neuro-ectoderm. Thus, neurofibromatosis, acoustic neuroma, meningioma, glioma, astrocytoma, von Hippel's disease and other neurological tumours have been described in association with phaeochromocytoma. In addition, an association had been described with medullary cell carcinoma of the thyroid, with or without parathyroid adenoma. This variant has been termed 'multiple endocrine neoplasia (MEN), type 2' or Sipple's syndrome. It is usually familial and the phaeochromocytoma is commonly bilateral.

Fig. 63.5 illustrates the synthesis and metabolism of catecholamines and it is continuous or episodic hypersecretion of these metabolites that gives rise to the clinical features of the syndrome.

Clinical

The condition chiefly affects adults but may occur in children, with a tendency to affect boys more than girls and a tendency to be more frequently extra-adrenal than in adults. The important clinical features are shown in *Table* 63.3. It is claimed that phaeochromocytoma accounts for 0·05% of hypertensive patients. The hypertension may be sustained, though it is characteristically paroxysmal. When such paroxysms occur, there is often accompanying headache, nausea and vomiting, chest or abdominal pain, anxiety, pallor, sweating and palpitations. The attacks may last a few minutes only or may persist for several hours and may be fatal. These paroxysmal episodes can be provoked by surgery, invasive investigation such as angiography, and late pregnancy where pre-eclampsia may be simulated and mortality is high. Certain drugs may induce an attack and such drugs include histamine and glucagon. The latter is a drug that is increasingly being used in routine radiological practice as an agent for relaxing the stomach in barium meal examinations. The patient who responds to these drugs with tachycardia, pallor, sweating and hypertension should be suspected of having phaeochromocytoma. Normotensive phaeochromocytoma is an uncommon variant in which the clinical features are those of hypermetabolism, namely weight loss, sweating, tachycardia and weakness. Rarely, postural hypotension may be present. Cardiomyopathy may occur giving rise to dysrhythmias and cardiac failure. This is not mediated via adrenergic pathways but is a direct toxic effect of catecholamines on the myocardium. Mild glucose intolerance is not uncommon. It will be apparent that, though rare, phaeochromocytoma enters differential diagnosis in many situations including hypertension, hypotension, diabetes mellitus, paroxysmal tachycardia, cardiac failure, anxiety attacks, thyrotoxicosis and 'funny turns'.

Investigations

1. Biochemical Diagnosis

There are now available reliable assays for urinary (and, in some centres, plasma) catecholamines and their precursors and metabolites. These have rendered dangerous provocative tests obsolete. Thus, the precursors dopamine, metadrenaline and metnoradrenaline, the hormones adrenaline and noradrenaline and the metabolite vanillyl-mandelic acid (VMA) can be assayed. Often all these compounds are increased in the urine in patients with phaeochromocytoma but one or other may predominate. It is said that extra-adrenal and malignant phaeochromocytomas secrete largely noradrenaline and its precursors, while benign adrenal tumours tend to secrete adrenaline and its precursors.

Table 63.3 Clinical features of phaeochromocytoma

Hypertension	May be paroxysmal or sustained Hypotension or normotension may occur
Palpitations	Tachycardia, arrhythmias
Fear	Attack of unexplained apprehension with pallor, tremor and sweating. Flushing may occur
Abdominal symptoms	Pain, nausea, vomiting, diarrhoea and weight loss Chest pains and headache may also occur
Glucose intolerance	Glycosuria, hyperglycaemia
Cardiac failure	Cardiomyopathy

Table 63.4 Drugs which may give misleading information in urinary catecholamine estimation

a. Apparent increase in urinary catecholamines

Aminophylline	Tetracycline
Diazoxide	Sulphadimidine
Methyldopa	Erythromycin
Glyceryl trinitrate	Hydralazine
Phentolamine	Chloral
Levodopa	Aspirin

Phenelzine and other monoamine oxidase inhibitors
Chlorpromazine and other phenothiazines
Also cocoa, bananas and alcohol

b. Decrease in urinary catecholamines

Clonidine
Guanethidine
Reserpine

Abundant dopamine secretion is said to imply malignancy. However, these differences are by no means absolute. Many drugs are capable of giving rise to misleading results in a variety of ways. *Table* 63.4 indicates some of the drugs that produce problems in interpretation of urinary catecholamine analysis.

It is usual practice to screen all hypertensive patients with at least one 24-hour urine estimation for catecholamines though in a condition which is often episodic, the value of such screening must be limited. When clinical suspicion is strong, several urine collections must be made and preferably at the time of symptoms or signs such as elevation of blood pressure and tachycardia. At least a two-fold increase in excretion of catecholamines is found when phaeochromocytoma is present.

2. Localization

The next step is localization of the tumour or tumours. As stated above, 90% of tumours are adrenal. Of the remaining 10%, those in the thorax may be seen as a paravertebral mass on plain chest radiography with oblique and lateral views. Those in the neck may be palpable in relation to the carotid arteries, and glomus jugulare tumours which may secrete catecholamines give rise to cranial nerve lesions.

CT is unquestionably the procedure of choice in localizing phaeochromocytomas. As stated above, it can image tumours of 5-mm diameter. In addition, CT has the very marked advantage in this situation of being non-invasive and therefore, unlike angiography, does not provoke a catecholamine crisis. Moreover, at the one procedure the neck,

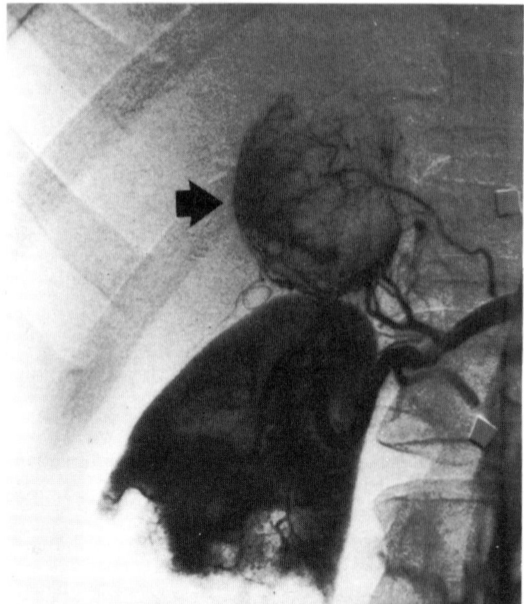

Fig. 63.16 Angiogram (subtraction study) showing a large right adrenal tumour in a patient suspected of phaeochromocytoma.

thorax, abdomen and pelvis can be scanned for ectopic tumours. If CT is not available, ultrasonography has proved useful but is not as sensitive. ^{131}I iodocholesterol scintigraphy has been used, but this isotope is better for functioning disorders of adrenal cortex and is less useful for adrenal medullary disorders. Recently, ^{131}I-meta-iodobenzylguanidine (^{131}I-mBG) has proved effective in localizing extra-adrenal phaeochromocytomas. Angiography (*Fig.* 63.16) is not as sensitive as CT and may provoke catecholamine crisis. If it is the only procedure available, meticulous care must be taken to avoid this very serious complication (*see below*).

Treatment

There are two aspects of treatment to be considered, first treatment and prevention of the effects of excess circulating catecholamines and, secondly, surgery.

1. Pharmacological Treatment

Since the effects of catecholamines are mediated by both α-adrenergic and β-adrenergic pathways, effective blockade of these pathways is essential. This is particularly so during surgery and invasive procedures such as angiography, which may cause massive and sometimes fatal hypersecretion of catecholamines. During these procedures very careful monitoring of pulse and blood pressure is mandatory. The α-blocking drug phenoxybenzamine, used with β-blocker propranolol, is favoured at many centres. To control blood pressure between investigations and surgery, phenoxybenzamine 20–80 mg daily in twice daily dosage, together with propranolol 20–40 mg daily in 6-hourly dosage are suitable. During angiography and surgery, the α-blocker phentolamine is preferred because as well as being capable of being given intravenously, it is short acting, a decided advantage in situations where blood pressure may fluctuate greatly. Recently, the drug labetalol has been found useful in some centres in the UK, both orally to control ambulant blood pressure and by infusion during invasive investigations and surgery. This drug has both α- and β-adrenergic blocking properties and in doses up to 6400 mg daily orally it has been found useful in controlling blood pressure in patients with phaeochromocytoma. Given intravenously in boluses of 50 mg it has been used to control blood pressure during angiography and surgery. However, this drug has been criticized on the grounds that the α-adrenergic blockade may be inadequate compared with β-blockade and hypertensive crisis may result from its use.

2. Operative Management

During surgery and angiography continuous recording of intra-arterial blood pressure, continuous monitoring of cardiac rate and rhythm by cardiac monitor and continuous monitoring of central venous pressure is required. Venous access for phentolamine in boluses of 1–5 mg or as continuous infusion delivering 0·5–1·0 mg/min is necessary. Propranolol in boluses up to 5 mg may be used to control tachycardia and arrhythmias. Sodium nitroprusside, a short-acting vasodilator, by continuous infusion is used in some centres instead of phentolamine. Anticholinergic drugs are not advised in preoperative preparations because of their capacity to produce tachycardia. Nitrous oxide, halothane and ethrane are acceptable anaesthetic gases. The critical stages during surgery are first when the tumour is handled at which time hypertensive crisis and arrhythmias are most likely and, secondly, after removal of the tumour when severe and sustained hypotension may occur. This is thought to be due to removal of the vasopressor stimulus of the tumour, leaving a patient with a pharmacologically paralysed autonomic system. Large volumes of blood, plasma or plasma substitute are necessary to maintain blood pressure at this stage of surgery and infusions should be commenced in anticipation of the event when the tumour blood supply is about to be severed.

3. Postoperative Care

Careful monitoring of pulse, blood pressure and central venous pressure with adjustments as appropriate are mandatory during the early postoperative period. If hypertension persists postoperatively, inadvertent renal artery or renal damage should be considered. A residual phaechromocytoma or metastases should also be considered and sought by urinary catecholamine analysis. In some patients, however, hypertension persists because either there is underlying essential hypertension or secondary renal and vascular changes have occurred before surgery. Such hypertension is treated with drugs as appropriate.

Prognosis

Removal of a benign tumour(s) with restoration of blood pressure to normal carries a good prognosis. If hypertension remains, the prognosis is that of hypertension and depends on control with drugs and existence of complications of hypertension. Malignant phaeochromocytoma with metastases is usually unresponsive to cytotoxic drugs or radiotherapy. ^{131}I-mBG has shown some initial promise in providing therapeutic internal irradiation in disseminated malignant phaeochromocytoma. The usefulness of this and other compounds taken up by a chromaffin tissue has yet to be fully evaluated. However, progression is sometimes slow and survival of 10 years or more after diagnosis has been reported. Hypertension and other manifestations are controlled by α- and β-adrenergic blockade. Some of these patients suffer from the myocarditis which cannot be controlled by adrenergic blockade but β-methyl-*p*-tyrosine may be effective in this situation.

β-Methyl-*p*-tyrosine is an agent that inhibits tyrosine hydroxylase, the rate limiting enzyme in catecholamine synthesis (*see Fig.* 63.4). Though not yet available for general use, it has been used in the UK and has been shown to diminish excretion of VMA, probably reflecting decreased synthesis of catecholamines. It also provides symptomatic relief and reduces the risks of dysrhythmia and fluctuations of blood pressure. It has been used in preparation for surgery as well as in management of patients with the malignant condition.

Neuroblastoma

This tumour of sympathetic nervous tissue is one of the commonest malignant growths of childhood. It is most frequently found in the adrenal gland though it may occur at other sites, usually associated with the sympathetic chain.

Pathophysiology

Derived from the embryonic neural crest, the cells of this tumour may be undifferentiated neuroblasts or mature ganglion cells with varying degrees of cellular differentiation, some or all of which may be seen within the same tumour.

Like phaeochromocytomas, these tumours are capable of secreting catecholamines though there is no consistency in type and quantity secreted. There are reports of neuroblastomas in fetal life secreting catecholamines which cross the placenta causing symptoms in the mother.

Local spread is common though many adrenal neuroblastomas remain encapsulated. Distant spread to lymph nodes, bone, marrow and liver frequently occurs.

Clinical

Over 80% of neuroblastomas present in children under the age of 5 and about a third of patients are under 2 years of age. Familial incidence occasionally occurs. The typical child shows a change in personality with misery and irritability, fatigue and lethargy, anorexia and weight loss. Fever, sweating and abdominal pains may occur. An abdominal mass may be palpable or visible. Commonly this mass is composed of metastases in liver or lymph nodes but it may be the primary tumour. Bone pain, skin nodules and other manifestations of metastases may be present. Particular attention should be paid to tumours in the posterior mediastinum because there is almost always a dumb-bell configuration with a protrusion within the spinal canal. Cord compression can occur and progress rapidly and signs should be carefully sought.

Investigations

Urinary catecholamines are elevated at least three-fold above normal in 90% of children with neuroblastoma. Non-invasive imaging procedures such as ultrasound and CT (*see Fig.* 63.13) are obviously preferable in children. Bone and liver scintigraphy help in detecting extent of spread. Marrow aspiration provides histological confirmation in about two-thirds of patients.

When neuroblastoma is diagnosed it is staged according to the extent of spread:

Stage I	Confined to tissue of origin
Stage II	Local spread not crossing the midline with or without ipsilateral region lymph node involvement
Stage III	Local spread across midline or involvement of regional lymph nodes on both sides
Stage IV	Distant metastases
Stage IVS	As for Stage I and II with metastases in skin, liver and bone marrow but not in any other sites

Treatment

This is determined by the stage of the disease and involves the use of surgery, cytotoxic chemotherapy and radiotherapy. Complicated regimes have been devised and the patient is best managed at a centre specialized in paediatric oncology.

Prognosis

Many factors govern prognosis, including age of patient, site and histological type of the primary tumour. The effect of chemotherapy on prognosis is controversial. Moreover, the capability (in children less than 1 year of age with Stage IVS disease) of this tumour to undergo spontaneous remission and resolution even when disseminated adds further confusion to predictability of prognosis.

Ganglioneuroma

This tumour of childhood arises from the same cell precursor as neuroblastoma and phaeochromocytoma but is always benign. They may secrete catecholamines which, however, do not usually cause symptoms. The usual clinical manifestation is a palpable abdominal mass. Resection is indicated.

Ganglioneuroblastoma

The occasional finding of foci of neuroblasts within what appears to be a ganglioneuroma has given rise to the term 'ganglioneuroblastoma'. This is best regarded as a neuroblastoma having metastatic, thus malignant, potential.

Neurofibroma

Very rarely, a neurofibroma may develop in the adrenal medulla. Clinically the features are those of a retroperitoneal mass. However, in addition, spinal cord compression may be present because of the tendency of this tumour to extend into an intervertebral canal, the so-called 'dumb-bell tumour'. Manifestations of von Recklinghausen's disease may be present. Surgical excision is indicated for this benign tumour.

Hirsutism and Virilism

Hirsutism is defined as excessive growth of hair in women outside the sites usually associated with female hair growth. The cheeks, upper lip, chin, chest, breast areolar, limbs and the linea alba may show hair growth. Virilism includes hirsutism, but, in addition, other features of marked androgen excess occur, such as male pattern of hair loss from the head, deepening of the voice, acne, male body habitus and skeletal muscle development and enlargement of the clitoris.

Pathophysiology

In the female, androgens are derived from the ovary and the adrenal cortex and disorders of these glands may result in hirsutism or virilism. Hirsutism is commonly constitutional or idiopathic but virilization usually indicates a definable cause. *Table* 63.5 lists the causes of hirsutism and virilism and, of these, adrenal causes are uncommon. Pituitary-dependent Cushing's disease is more likely to cause mild virilism than an autonomous adrenal lesion producing

Table 63.5 Causes of hirsutism and virilism

Constitutional	or idiopathic Hirsutism only
Iatrogenic	Androgens, anabolic steroids, diazoxide, phenytoin
Adrenal disorders	Cushing's syndrome, adrenal tumour, congenital adrenal hyperplasia
Ovarian disorders	Polycystic ovaries (Stein–Leventhal syndrome) Ovarian tumour

Cushing's syndrome, for ACTH stimulates adrenal androgen productions (*see Fig.* 63.4). However, adrenal tumours in childhood may produce Cushing's syndrome and virilism. Congenital adrenal hyperplasia is considered below. Adrenal adenoma or carcinoma may produce androgens only, resulting in virilization.

Clinical

In addition to the feature of hirsutism and virilism discussed above, amenorrhoea and anovulation is usual when there is a virilizing adrenal tumour.

Investigations

Plasma testosterone and urinary 17-oxosteroids are elevated where there is a virilizing adrenal tumour but may be elevated in other virilizing syndromes, such as ovarian tumour. Adrenal imaging as described above is therefore required to confirm an adrenal tumour.

Treatment

Benign adrenal tumours should be excised and this usually improves acne. Menstruation, ovulation and fertility are restored. Clitoromegaly may regress, not always completely. Regrettably, the hirsutes, a very distressing symptom, regresses only slowly and may persist if already well established. Malignant tumours may require chemotherapy as described for adrenal carcinoma causing Cushing's syndrome.

Congenital Adrenal Hyperplasia

Pathophysiology

The condition of congenital adrenal hyperplasia (adrenogenital syndrome) results from partial or complete absence of one or other of the enzymes involved in the biosynthesis of cortisol and aldosterone. The commonest variety is 21-hydroxylase deficiency (*see Fig.* 63.4). This results in deficient cortisol production (and sometimes deficient aldosterone production) which, through the negative feedback mechanism, leads to increased ACTH production and adrenocortical hyperplasia. This may be sufficient to overcome the block but at the expense of increased androgen synthesis and release. In the 'salt-losing' variety the block is not overcome and cortisol and mineralocorticoid deficiency dominate the picture.

Clinical

The clinical picture is that of ambivalent sex in infant girls due to clitoromegaly resulting from the androgen excess. In the 'salt-losing' type, acute adrenal insufficiency occurs in the first week of life. Milder cases may present as virilization in female children or rarely in female adults. Boys present with precocious puberty. Early epiphyseal fusion and ultimately short stature may occur in both sexes, though early in the condition growth is accelerated.

Investigations

Diagnosis depends on demonstration of excessive level of the steroid hormone immediately preceding the enzymatic block. Thus, for 21-hydroxylase deficiency, plasma 17-hydroxyprogesterone is present in excess. Levels of its urinary metabolite, pregnanetriol, are likewise elevated (*see Fig.* 63.4).

Treatment

The aim of treatment is to correct cortisol deficiency and suppress androgen output. This is achieved by treatment with cortisol or a synthetic steroid at 6-hourly intervals. Some centres combine this with aminoglutethimide.

The role of surgery is to correct abnormalities of the external genitalia and vagina by plastic surgery. When this should be carried out is debatable though all are agreed that surgery in infancy is unjustified. Some hold the view, however, that correction before school age is desirable.

In preparation for surgery, the patient should be considered to lack the adrenal reserve for stress. Dextrose/saline should be infused throughout the procedure and hydrocortisone 200–400 mg parenterally in divided doses on the day of the operation and for the next few days until oral feeding has been re-established.

The management of the unfortunate girl brought up as a boy is beyond the scope of this chapter and requires skilled psychiatric expertise.

Gynaecomastia

Gynaecomastia refers to development of glandular mammary tissue in men. It may be unilateral or bilateral where it may be asymmetrical. Glandular tissue must be palpable to make the diagnosis and distinguish it from adiposity. *Table* 63.6 lists the causes of gynaecomastia. Oestrogen-secreting adrenal tumours are very rare indeed. Presence of such a tumour may be suspected by the finding of high levels of plasma oestradiol in a man with gynaecomastia. Adrenal imaging is required for confirmation and localization. Treatment is surgery where possible and chemotherapy for malignancy.

Table 63.6 Causes of gynaecomastia

Puberty and old age	
Hypogonadism	e.g. Klinefelter's syndrome
Chronic liver disease	
Drugs	e.g. spironolactone, cimetidine, digoxin, oestrogens, isoniazid, chorionic gonadotrophins, anabolic steroids, etc.
Tumours	Testicular, adrenal, bronchial, breast
Testicular enzyme disorders	
Testicular feminization	
Endocrine disorders	Thyrotoxicosis, acromegaly, Addison's disease

Hypoadrenalism

Hypoadrenalism warrants mention in this chapter for two reasons. First, precautions must be taken during any form of surgery, however minor, on a patient with actual or potential adrenal insufficiency. Secondly, acute adrenal insufficiency may closely mimic an acute surgical condition.

Hypoadrenalism is the condition which results from inadequate synthesis and release of corticosteroids, principally cortisol and aldosterone. It may be due to disease of the adrenal cortex, so-called primary adrenal atrophy or, secondly, to failure of ACTH stimulation of the adrenal cortex when it is called 'secondary adrenal atrophy'.

Aetiology

The chief causes of adrenal insufficiency are listed in *Table* 63.7. Haemorrhage into the adrenal during severe infection is a rare event and all too often is only diagnosed at necropsy. Meningococcal septicaemia seems particularly likely to cause this serious condition, especially in children, but any severe infection is capable of doing so. Purpura and ecchymoses during infection should alert the clinician to the possibility of adrenal haemorrhage, especially if the patient is hypotensive. However, most septicaemic hypotensive patients are not suffering from adrenal destruction. Haemorrhage into the adrenals has been described as a complication of anticoagulant therapy and commonly is only discovered at autopsy. Adrenal vein thrombosis may rarely occur after back injury and may lead to adrenal infarction.

Addison's disease results from chronic disease destroying the adrenal cortex. At the present time, about 70% of new cases are due to autoimmune adrenalitis and antibodies to adrenal cortical cells can be demonstrated in sera from the majority of such patients. Tuberculous adrenal disease accounts for about 25% of new patients with Addison's disease and the remainder are due to a variety of conditions including metastases from carcinoma elsewhere, amyloidosis and, in the USA, to fungal disorder, such as histoplasmosis.

Adrenal cortical failure may be secondary to pituitary failure to secrete ACTH. This may be due to a variety of causes including pituitary stalk infarction during delivery (Sheehan's syndrome) or pituitary tumour. The consequent ACTH deficiency results in deficiency of cortisol and atrophy of adrenal cortical cells. Prolonged use of corticosteroid drugs leads to suppression of ACTH output via the negative feedback mechanism (*see Fig.* 63.3) and atrophy of adrenal cortex. Patients so treated lack the ability to respond to stress by increasing corticosteroid output. Moreover, should the corticosteroid drugs be discontinued, they are in a hypoadrenal state.

Clinical Features

The major clinical features of hypoadrenalism are shown in *Table* 63.8. Hypoadrenalism from any cause may present as acute adrenal insufficiency and this may be the first manifestation of hitherto unsuspected Addison's disease. Acute adrenal insufficiency presents as a severe, acute illness which may mimic the acute abdomen. Thus, the patient may present with vomiting, severe abdominal pain with rigidity, hypotension and prostration. It is not surprising that this rare situation may be mistaken for an acute surgical condition of the abdomen. However, surgery is lethal in untreated acute adrenal insufficiency.

Clues to the true nature of the condition may come from a previous history of several months of lassitude and extreme fatigue, anorexia and weight loss, giddiness and even syncope. Examination may reveal unusual pigmentation if primary adrenal disease is present or pallor and regression of secondary sexual characteristics if the hypoadrenalism is due to pituitary failure. Hyponatraemia and hyperkalaemia are usually present in acute adrenal insufficiency.

Less severe abdominal symptoms of hypoadrenalism may be mistaken for other abdominal disorders and inappropriate investigations carried out. Similarly, acute adrenal insufficiency in a patient with unsuspected hypoadrenalism may

Table 63.7 Principal causes of adrenal insufficiency

1. *Primary Adrenal Failure*
   - *a.* Addison's disease
     - autoimmune adrenalitis
     - tuberculosis
     - metastases
     - amyloidosis
     - fungal infection
   - *b.* Bilateral adrenal haemorrhage
     - septicaemia (Waterhouse–Friderichsen syndrome)
     - anticoagulant therapy
   - *c.* Bilateral adrenalectomy
   - *d.* Congenital adrenal hyperplasia
   - *e.* Bilateral adrenal vein thrombosis
   - *f.* Drugs: metyrapone, aminoglutethimide, trilostane, *o,p'*DDD
2. *Secondary Adrenal Failure*
   - *a.* Hypothalamic or pituitary disease
     - tumour—primary or secondary
     - infarction—postpartum (Sheehan's syndrome), pituitary apoplexy
     - infections—tuberculosis, syphilis, encephalitis
     - granulomatous disorders—sarcoidosis, Hand–Schüller–Christian disease
     - trauma
   - *b.* Hypophysectomy
   - *c.* Prolonged therapy with corticosteroid drugs

Table 63.8 Clinical features of hypoadrenalism

Usually Present

Weakness, tiredness, lethargy
Anorexia, weight loss
Nausea, vomiting
Pigmentation (primary adrenal failure)

Commonly Present

Hypotension (systolic BP less than 100 mmHg)
Giddiness, dizziness—often postural
—rarely syncope
Oral pigmentation (primary adrenal failure)
Abdominal pain
Muscle cramps
Diarrhoea
Other endocrine deficiency (secondary hypoadrenalism due to pituitary failure)

Occasionally Present

Active tuberculosis
Other autoimmune endocrine disease (primary hypoadrenalism)

Two-thirds of patients present with acute adrenal insufficiency be provoked by an acute surgical condition. Very careful appraisal is necessary.

Investigations

Primary adrenal insufficiency is diagnosed by demonstrating failure of plasma cortisol to rise in response to exogenous ACTH or tetracosactrin. Alternatively, the combination of subnormal plasma cortisol and elevated plasma ACTH simultaneously is diagnostic of primary adrenocortical failure. In secondary hypoadrenalism, the plasma cortisol level will increase from a low or subnormal level in response to exogenous ACTH or tetracosactrin but the response is somewhat blunted compared with that in a normal subject. Alternatively, a combination of low plasma cortisol and low or unmeasurable plasma ACTH will suggest the diagnosis.

In the situation of adrenal crisis, treatment must not be delayed pending results of investigations for the patient will die within a few hours if hydrocortisone is withheld. When acute adrenal insufficiency is suspected, a blood sample should be taken for cortisol (and ACTH) level and treatment commenced. Alternatively, treatment with prednisolone can be instituted immediately and an adrenal stimulation test carried out simultaneously.

Treatment

The patient suffering from adrenal crisis requires infusion of 4 litres of physiological saline in 24 hours. Hydrocortisone sodium succinate should be administered intravenously, 200 mg immediately and 100 mg 6-hourly thereafter. Hypoglycaemia may occur and therefore should be sought and treated with intravenous dextrose. Mineralocorticoid as deoxycorticosterone, 10 mg intramuscularly should be given also. Depending on the rate of improvement this regime is reduced over the next 4 days until oral therapy with hydrocortisone and fludrocortisone can be instituted. The procedure for simultaneous investigation and treatment is to take a blood sample for plasma cortisol. The patient is then given prednisolone phosphate, 20 mg intravenously, deoxycorticosterone acetate 10 mg intramuscularly and depot tetracosactrin 1 mg intramuscularly in addition to fluids. A second sample for plasma cortisol is taken 5 hours later. A rise in plasma cortisol of 500 nmol/l excludes adrenocortical insufficiency. A lesser increment should give rise to further study with a prolonged (3–5 day) adrenal stimulation test.

Surgery on a Patient with Hypoadrenalism

A patient with hypoadrenalism, whether due to primary adrenal disease or adrenal resection or secondary to pituitary failure, may be perfectly well on corticosteroid replacement therapy. However, such a patient has no reserve for stress and even minor procedures, such as tooth extraction, may provoke acute adrenal insufficiency with collapse, vomiting, hypotension, dehydration, hyponatraemia and death. It is recommended therefore that all surgical procedures, major and minor, are carried out with strict precautions.

On the day of surgery an infusion of saline is set up and hydrocortisone 200 mg given intravenously. The infusion is continued during and after the operation and a further two boluses of hydrocortisone, 100 mg intravenously, given during the day. Careful observation of pulse and blood pressure is mandatory and hypoadrenalism enters the differential diagnosis of postoperative collapse. Hypoglycaemia may occur and blood glucose should be checked periodically and corrected if low. Intravenous saline and hydrocortisone should be continued in the postoperative period, the duration depending on the nature and severity of the surgery until the patient's usual oral therapy can safely be reinstituted.

Further Reading

Cushing's Disease

Burke C. W. (1978) Disorders of cortisol production: diagnostic and therapeutic progress. In: O'Riordan J. L. H. (ed.) *Recent Advances in Endocrinology and Metabolism I.* Edinburgh, Churchill Livingstone, pp. 61–90.

Conn's Syndrome

Ferriss J. B. et al. (1978) Review Articles. *Am. Heart J.* **95**, 375–388, 641–658 and **96**, 97–109.

Phaeochromocytoma

Sever P. S., Roberts J. C. and Snell M. E. (1980) Phaeochromocytoma. In: Sönksen P. H. and Lowy C. (ed.) *Clinics in Endocrinology and Metabolism*, Vol. 9, No. 3. Philadelphia, Saunders, pp. 543–568.

Neuroblastoma

Jones P. G. and Campbell P. E. (ed.) (1976) Tumours of the adrenal gland and retroperitoneum. In: *Tumours of Infancy and Childhood* by the Staff of the Royal Children's Hospital, Melbourne, Ch. 18. Oxford, Blackwell, pp. 537–595.

Hypoadrenalism

Bayliss R. I. S. (1980) Adrenal cortex. In: Sönksen P. H. and Lowy C. (ed.) *Clinics in Endocrinology and Metabolism*, Vol. 9, No. 3. Philadelphia, Saunders, pp. 477–486.

64 *The Surgical Management of Morbid Obesity*

G. R. Giles and C. S. Humphrey

Throughout history there have been fat people. In certain cultures and at certain times a gross physique has been admired and sought after. However, in the richer countries, obesity threatens to be an epidemic problem with serious medical, social and economic consequences. The incidence varies but if an index of obesity is taken to be an excess of 20% over 'ideal' body weight, then approximately 15% of the male and 25% of the female population can be classified as obese.

Morbid obesity is a somewhat imprecise term applied to that subgroup of obese patients who weigh more than 200% of their 'ideal' weight, are more than 45 kg (100 lb) overweight, or who weigh more than 136 kg (300 lb). Various indices which relate weight to height or take into consideration skinfold thickness have been proposed in an attempt to add precision to the definition, but the cruder definition remains the more popular. Using data from the USA, it would seem that in men aged 21–74 years, nearly 50% weigh more than 110 kg and over 7% of women. However less than 0·1% weigh more than 136 kg.

AETIOLOGICAL FACTORS IN MORBID OBESITY

Morbid obesity is almost certainly multifactorial in aetiology, and genetic, environmental, metabolic and psychological influences have been studied intensively. Only occasionally can obesity be traced to disorders of the endocrine system.

Genetic Factors

There is an increased incidence of obesity in families where one or both of the parents are overweight, suggesting that genetic factors may be operating. Slightly more impressive evidence comes from studies which have shown a greater similarity in weight between identical twins than between fraternal twins, a difference which is still apparent, although less marked, when twins are brought up separately. Despite this, genetic influences probably play a very minor role in the genesis of morbid obesity.

Environmental and Metabolic Factors

The root cause of obesity can be traced to a positive energy balance which may be due to increased energy input, decreased energy output or a combination of these factors. In most individuals the efficiency of food absorption approaches 100% and thus it is to be expected that abnormal patterns of food intake, however, must reveal little or no difference in eating patterns between normal and obese individuals. It is not known whether obese individuals have abnormal eating patterns at some point in their lives and it is interesting that studies of obese children indicate that they may eat less than normal children.

Patients with morbid obesity exhibit grossly abnormal eating behaviour and metabolic studies have shown that a fat person may need to consume 6000 kcal/day to maintain a weight of 150 kg.

Metabolic Factors

People differ considerably in the amount of energy they appear to abstract from a meal: on a seemingly similar diet and pattern of physical activity, one person will remain lean whilst another grows fat. This being so, many people have looked for an underlying metabolic abnormality to explain the development of morbid obesity. Decreased energy output is likely in obese patients who tend to be physically less active and it has been suggested that these patients are metabolically more efficient, able to maintain body weight at a constant level despite reduced energy intake.

A number of patterns of altered metabolism can be found in the obese patient but these may be the result rather than the cause of obesity. Glucose metabolism is almost always impaired and this can be related to a reduction in insulin receptors on fat cells leading to insulin resistance. The increase in adipose tissue means an increase in size of fat cells, increased output of insulin and to hyperinsulinaemia. Despite the raised insulin, plasma glucose is frequently elevated and presumably by some form of organ fatigue a diabetic state can develop. A number of patterns of altered metabolism can be found in the obese patient. Glucose tolerance is almost always impaired and is associated with the progressive rise in fasting and stimulated insulin secretion, as weight increases. This insulin resistance is partly due to a reduction in the number of insulin receptors on fat cells. All these changes are reversed as weight is lost. The same is true for the low levels of growth hormone found in obesity. Adrenocortical activity is sometimes increased in obesity, whereas the fatty acid response to adrenaline is blunted.

All of these metabolic changes appear to be features of obesity rather than causes since they revert towards normal with weight reduction. As yet there is no evidence of the existence of any metabolic features which predate the development of obesity. One feature which deserves attention is the morphology of fatty tissue; there are two types of adipose growth associated with obesity; hyperplasia, or an increase in the number of adipocytes which are of normal volume, and hypertrophy where the fat cells are abnormally large but present in relatively normal numbers. The morbidly obese are characterized by a high percentage of hyperplastic fat. The relevance of this is that whereas the volume of fat cells can be reduced by food restriction, the number of fat cells remains constant. Thus if a morbidly obese person manages to lose weight, he is still left with an abnormally large number of fat cells, albeit relatively underfilled ones.

Fat from obese persons appears to show a decreased metabolic activity and heat production. The serum triglyceride levels are frequently elevated and the increased insulin production may lead to hepatic release of very low density lipoproteins enhancing lipogenesis and preventing triglyceride breakdown within the liver. Furthermore, cellular lipoprotein lipase activity is increased and does not show the normal response to glucose intake and an accelerated uptake of plasma triglyceride into adipose tissue results. These changes are ameliorated to some extent by weight reduction and may therefore be the result of obesity. There seems to be a self-regulating mechanism within fat which will always tend to refill adipocytes if the requisite nutrients are available. This may be why it is extremely difficult for the morbidly obese person to maintain successful weight reduction for any length of time. The other important feature of fat cellularity is the influence which overfeeding may have on the number of fat cells. Multiplication of adipocytes is believed to occur mainly during the last few weeks of uterine life and the first year, and then again towards the onset of puberty. Overfeeding during these periods in particular may result in hyperplasia of the fat cells, the numbers of which then become relatively fixed after puberty. It has been suggested that overeating during these critical periods may effectively programme the child for obesity problems in later life.

Psychological Factors

It would be surprising if the grossly obese patient did not exhibit some signs of disturbed behavioural and personality traits. Many psychological problems have been noted in the morbidly obese, including anxiety, depression and lack of self-esteem. However, as might be expected, these problems seem to be the result rather than the cause of the obesity. Morbidly obese people often show an addictive behaviour pattern which in theory would be amenable to behaviour modification therapy. In practice the amount of weight loss which can be produced by behaviour therapy alone is very small. None the less, taken in conjunction with other forms of treatment, a psychological approach to the obese personality can be quite useful. Preoperative psychological testing may indicate those patients with a greater chance of weight reduction and those likely to require psychological support afterwards. Unsuccessful surgery is more common in patients with unrealistic visions and demand and these patients tend to be younger and have a high alcohol consumption.

CONSEQUENCES OF MORBID OBESITY

Morbid obesity is associated with an earlier presentation of many commonly occurring disorders and to progress more rapidly. This increased risk is related to disturbances of endocrine pancreatic function but also with altered fat metabolism.

The only lethal condition which is directly and solely caused by extreme fatness is the Pickwickian or obesity–hypoventilation syndrome. Primary cardiopulmonary failure develops relatively rarely in the morbidly obese, but it carries a high mortality unless weight loss is achieved and maintained. It is a matter of debate whether obesity is a major risk factor for the development of coronary heart disease, independent of other factors such as hypertension, hyperlipidaemia, diabetes and physical inactivity. However, since obesity predisposes to these other risk factors, the point is academic. In practical terms, whenever obesity is found to coexist with any of these other risk factors, the need for weight reduction becomes even more urgent. Successful weight loss will often be accompanied by a reduction in blood pressure, a fall in serum cholesterol and triglycerides, an improvement in glucose tolerance and an increase in exercise tolerance.

A number of other risks to the morbidly obese are less well defined. Pulmonary embolism, pneumonia, pancreatitis and serious accidents appear to occur more commonly or to result in death more frequently than in the non-obese, although the exact relationships are not clear. The risks of surgery for coincidental problems is increased considerably, e.g. twentyfold in mortality for hysterectomy, and the incidence of problems for both mother and child is greater during pregnancy. The prevalence of gallstones is probably greater in the grossly obese, and degenerative disorders, such as arthritis, present earlier in life and are more severe.

It has been suggested that endometrial carcinoma occurs more commonly in morbidly obese women. However, it is probable that the overall incidence of neoplasm is lower because of the relatively short survival of these patients.

Thus it can be seen that the management of morbid obesity should not be thought of as extravagant, pandering to a group of patients with no willpower, but rather as an area where successful therapy can have a significant impact in terms of disease prevention.

THE MANAGEMENT OF MORBID OBESITY

Morbid obesity should be managed within the setting of a flexible yet integrated weight reduction programme which utilizes controlled dietary restriction, positive psychological support, food counselling and obesity surgery. It is a mistake to overemphasize any one of these modalities, and certainly to take surgery out of the context of a well-planned programme is to invite poor results.

Serious therapy should be commenced in patients with risk factors of the morbid obesity, e.g. angina, hypertension, arthritis. Whichever modality of therapy is used, it must be regarded as at least partly successful if the result is an alleviation of the risk factors, even though the weight reduction is modest.

Dietary Management

Dietary restriction by itself is seldom successful with the morbidly obese. This is not because weight loss cannot be achieved. On the contrary, the resting energy expenditure of a grossly overweight individual is generally greater than normal so that a severely restricted food intake may produce dramatic initial weight losses of up to 5 kg per week. Unfortunately, few patients can comply with the necessary diets for long enough to make any lasting impact upon their weight. Even the slightest lapse is liable to be followed by rapid weight gain. Despite these comments, dietary management is such an important facet of the overall treatment programme that the techniques and dangers of dieting for the morbidly obese must be mentioned.

Provided that the energy intake is less than the resting energy expenditure, weight loss is guaranteed, and the greater the energy deficit so the more weight the patient will lose. What cannot be assured from this simple approach is what the composition of that weight loss will be, and it is here that the different type of diets become important.

Weight loss during dieting can be from loss of water, fat or protein. The objective of dietary management is to produce loss of fat with conservation of lean body mass. Total starvation will produce rapid weight loss, but much of the early loss is of water and there is a substantial loss of body protein. This type of approach is rarely indicated even for short periods, and, needless to say, if used it must be supervised within hospital. 'Supplemented fasting' is a more useful technique. With this method a very low caloric intake of 400–600 kcal/day is allowed. It has been suggested that the provision of 1·5 g of protein per kg ideal weight will cause protein sparing and lead to loss of fat alone, but there is little good evidence that equal protein sparing cannot be achieved with a mixed diet. One variety of mixed but unbalanced diet which is quite popular is the ketogenic diet which utilizes protein and fat with very little carbohydrate. The idea behind these various protein-sparing diets is that if carbohydrate starvation is produced the energy requirements of the body can be met from fat stores by the production of ketones within the liver. Ketones, in patients who are starvation-adapted, can serve as alternative energy substrates to glucose and will thus prevent protein breakdown for the otherwise obligatory gluconeogenesis.

The best approach to this condition would be prevention or to stop the obese patient developing morbid obesity. There are numerous diets and pharmacological adjuvants which claim substantial benefits to the adherents; however, the morbidly obese patient is usually found to have an addictive behaviour pattern which makes it difficult to maintain the achieved weight reduction. Attempts to alter these abnormal behaviour patterns are not successful in the long term in the morbidly obese patient even in maintaining weight losses.

The Dangers of Dietary Restriction

Whichever type of diet is used, there are a number of dangers associated with weight reduction which must be appreciated. The most common of these is the production of malnutrition. In addition to protein loss, a severely restricted food intake will cause rapid depletion of electrolytes, minerals and vitamins, and supplementation will always be required with the more strict dietary programmes.

Water loss, as mentioned before, may be quite considerable in the early period of weight reduction, particularly with the ketogenic diets. This can be an advantage in lowering blood pressure and it may be psychologically good for the patient to see a rapid weight loss. However, orthostatic hypotension can be quite a problem. Acidosis and transient disturbances of renal and hepatic function have been noted, particularly with starvation regimens. Increased protein breakdown can result in hyperuricaemia and allopurinol may need to be given.

The most serious problem associated with rapid weight loss is sudden death. Sometimes this has been unexplained, but often the reason is myocardial failure. The setting in which this has occurred most frequently is with the use of the 'liquid protein' diet which was popularized extensively in the lay press. This diet comprised collagen hydrolysate as a source of very low quality protein. Many obese people used this diet with no medical supervision, and a number of sudden deaths were reported following periods of successful weight loss, sometimes within a few weeks of stopping the diet. In some patients atrophy of the myofibrils in the heart was found. It is not known whether these deaths were specifically related to the diet in question, but experimental observations suggest that too rapid weight loss from any cause may precipitate sudden death.

These observations should indicate that weight reduction in the grossly overweight must be supervised carefully. This also applies to weight loss following obesity surgery.

Selection of Patients

Intervention in the form of dental splintage or a surgical procedure is a last resort manoeuvre. Patients should have already demonstrated their ability to adhere to dietary discipline as it is easy to overcome dental splintage or gastric partitioning by consuming large quantities of high calorie/high protein meals in liquid form. A psychiatric assessment is wise for similar reasons and real psychiatric illness is unlikely to permit a patient to adhere to the rigid diet required after treatment. Alcoholism is similarly a limiting factor. Age is a significant factor as patients over 50 years with morbid obesity have a poor prognosis, being prone to deep venous thrombosis, chest infection and myocardial infarction. There may occasionally be a case in which severe angina could be alleviated by the weight reduction obtained by morbid obesity surgery and permit a coronary aortic bypass to take place. The selection of patients will inevitably be subjective but it is stressed that it is as important as the procedure itself.

Dental Splintage

The aim of this treatment is to prevent impulsive overeating which is often the result or response to psychological stress. The main requirement, other than a willingness not to imbibe high-energy liquid foods, is adequate dentition. The capping and wiring of the teeth are now fairly standard and although it is reported that complications are rare, gum sepsis does not seem uncommon. Other patients have complained of hair loss and, rarely, hypoglycaemic episodes have occurred. Patients requiring frequent attention to the splints or have broken wires are probably cheating on the prescribed diet.

Patients are expected to take a fluid diet of milk or soup base (800 kcal/day) with the addition of vitamins and iron. Patients are seen every 2–4 weeks to check the splints and every 4 weeks the splints are relaxed to permit exercise of the jaw.

Weight reduction in the correctly selected patient can be as good as a major surgical procedure. The main aim is to achieve the reduction (30 kg) over 6 months and then to maintain it after the splints are removed. Re-education of the patient is vital. The main difficulty is that many patients default once the splints are withdrawn and the long-term results of this treatment are poor in this group.

Gastric Reduction Procedures

Intragastric Balloons

From the observation that patients with gastric bezoars lose weight, gastric balloons have been designed to be passed into the stomach, inflated to 450–500 ml and then disconnected from the tube attachment. Accurate placement in the body of the stomach may be checked by endoscopy. The potential disadvantages of this system are those of a local effect on gastric mucosa and intestinal obstruction if the balloon should deflate and move distally. Experience with this procedure is limited, but adequate weight reduction has been reported in some patients, who were otherwise poor-risk candidates for surgical procedures.

Gastric Reduction

This concept arises from the universal observation that after a high Polya gastrectomy for duodenal ulcer, patients lose weight. Over the last 20 years, a group of surgeons in Iowa, led by Mason, have pioneered gastric reduction procedures initially performing a high gastric transection drained by a gastroenterostomy. It proved a difficult procedure in these morbidly obese patients with a significant mortality rate (2%) and was subsequently modified to a gastroplasty (*Fig.* 64.1) in which the stomach was partitioned into a small proximal chamber which drained into the large distal chamber by a narrow passage (*Fig.* 64.2) or by the formation of a gastroenterostomy. These procedures have now been facilitated by stapling instruments, particularly in the formation of the proximal chamber (two rows of staples). As before, the initial results were not good but certain criteria were established, namely that the proximal chamber should be no more than 50 ml and the diameter of passage about 12 mm. It now seems that the gastric partitioning is best performed in a vertical axis (*Fig.* 64.3*a*) and the stoma constructed on the lesser curvature. As the cause of failure in the early cases was a dilatation of this channel, a variety of methods are available to limit its size. The most convenient is the formation of a 12 mm linear curve channel by a circular stapler through both anterior and posterior gastric walls (*Fig.* 64.3*b*) and then the suturing of a Silastic or polyester mesh around the channel.

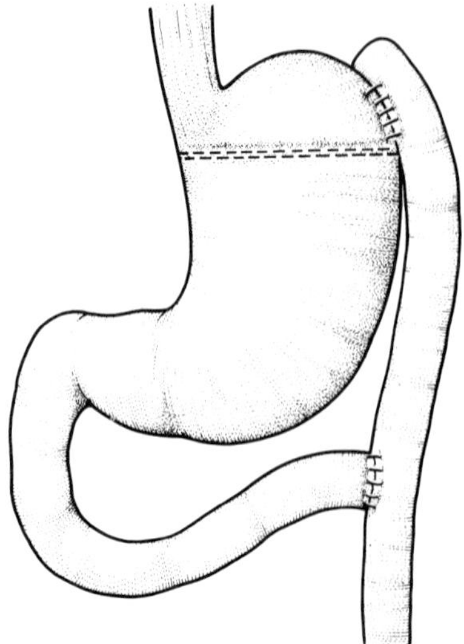

Fig. 64.1 With the introduction of stapling devices, it no longer became necessary to completely transect the stomach and a gastroenterostomy can be made to the small proximal pouch.

After gastroplasty patients are placed on a 800 kcal liquid diet for 6 weeks. An earlier introduction of solid food is likely to weaken staple lines and result in the breakdown of the partition. After six weeks, solid food with added vitamins and iron is introduced with 1000 kcal divided into three meals. Alcohol and liquid high-energy foods are forbidden.

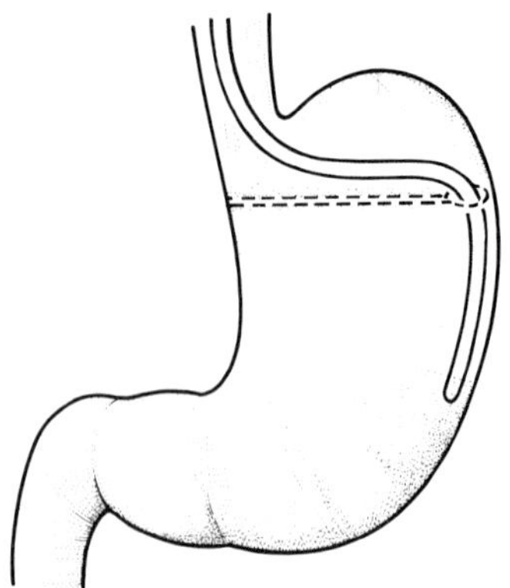

Fig. 64.2 Gastric partitioning proved to be a simpler procedure and was initially performed with a 12-mm channel on the greater curvature which was reinforced with non-absorbable sutures to prevent dilatation of the channel.

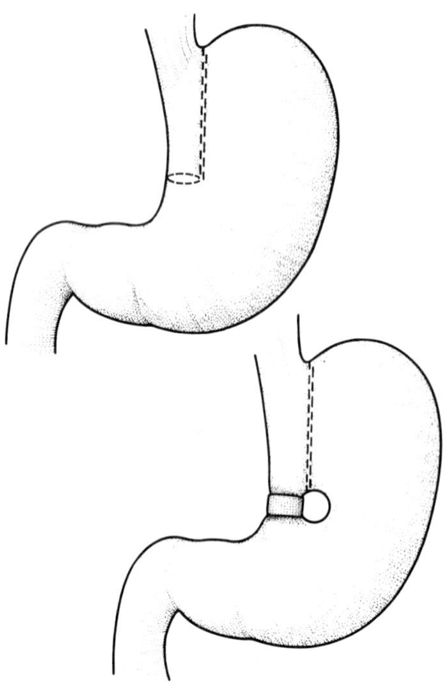

Fig. 64.3 *a*, It seems probable that vertical partitioning to produce the proximal channel gives better results and less reflux. *b*, In order to prevent dilatation of the 12-mm channel, a circular stapler is used to staple anterior and posterior gastric walls together so that the rim is 12 mm from the lesser curvature. This channel is wrapped around with a mesh to prevent dilatation.

Weight reduction after gastroplasty can be similar to that obtained after jejunal ileal bypass. Although weight reduction is initially good, the process slows down. In some cases this is due to breakdown of the gastric partition, but in others the proximal chamber dilates and permits more food to accumulate in the pouch and to trickle through slowly over several hours before the next meal is due. In other patients a poor patient compliance is the main factor.

Complications

Although much less hazardous than jejunal ileal bypass, problems can arise. Those patients with a gastroenterostomy to the proximal pouch are liable to leakage and sepsis. When solid food is introduced, patients tend to overeat and epigastric pain and vomiting are almost univeral. Occasionally the stoma may become obstructed with food particles, particularly undigested plugs of meat, or tablets. Perforation of the proximal gastric chamber has been reported as has haematemesis from erosions. Perforation requires emergency resuturing but erosions will usually cease bleeding with conservative methods.

Intestinal Bypass

This technique was described by Payne and Daniel in Los Angeles. In order to produce a sufficient degree of malabsorption all but 45–50 cm of small bowel needs to be excluded from the nutrient stream. Bypassing most of the small bowel produces a malabsorption state, but a lesser bypass does not seem to be sufficient. In fact although a rapid weight loss does occur in the first 18 months, it is associated with a reduction in intake rather than malabsorption. A variety of ways of producing this exclusion are described. Most commonly an end-to-end anastomosis is performed between the upper jejunum and terminal ileum and the excluded small bowel is drained, separated into a convenient segment of colon, usually transverse colon (*Fig.* 64.4). The end-to-side variant in which the jejunum is anastomosed to the side of the terminal ileum is less successful in terms of weight reduction. A further modification has been to anastomose the free end of jejunum to the gallbladder in order to permit absorption of bile salts in the terminal ileum.

These procedures have been carried out less frequently than previously for although the operative mortality is about 2% the morbidity commonly exceeds 20%. Nevertheless, the procedures are effective in terms of weight reduction, e.g. 35% of original body weight or 70% of excess body weight. A rebound in weight may be seen after 2 years. Other beneficial effects may be seen in the form of correction of hyperlipidaemias, reduction of insulin requirements, improved respiratory function and a social rehabilitation of many patients in domestic and professional life.

Psychological Sequelae

Generally patients undergoing morbid obesity surgery expect weight reduction to improve their psychological state. However, psychological disorders persist in some patients despite weight reduction and in the absence of significant metabolic sequelae, most preoperative studies of psychological makeup have been performed too close to the procedure when the patient may have been under 'stress' and makes it difficult to use this information to predict those patients likely to be troubled postoperatively. On a commonsense basis it might be expected that patients who did not lose weight satisfactorily would have the most severe psychological problems, however, the opposite is often the case. Improvement in self-esteem and assertiveness after weight loss may produce responses from relatives which in turn produce depression and guilt feelings. The close support of the spouse or dependants is required during weight loss and counselling of all parties is required.

It is clear that several procedures will produce weight loss in morbidly obese patients but as in other areas of surgical treatment, the technical operation is not an end to the problems faced by the patients when they are returned to their habitual environment.

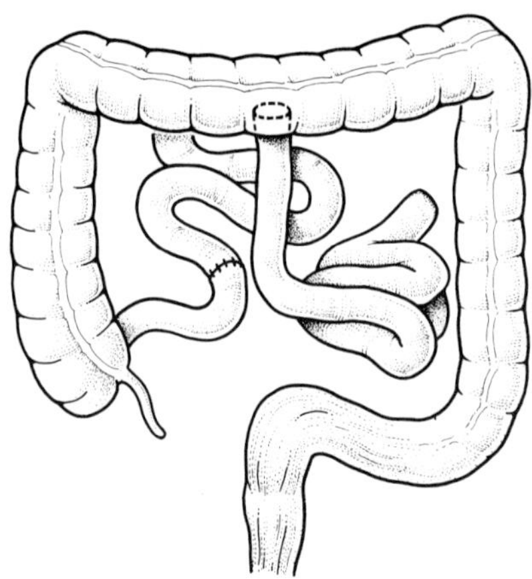

Fig. 64.4 The jejunoileal bypass keeps 50 cm of small bowel in the food stream. The remaining small bowel is drained into adjacent colon.

Metabolic Sequelae

After a successful gastric partitioning, the preoperative elevations in plasma insulin, glucose and glucagon fall. Glucose tolerance curves return to normal, plasma cholesterol, triglyceride and low-density lipoproteins fall but lipoprotein lipase levels are unchanged. There are small but significant falls in serum thyroxine and tri-iodothyronine levels. Studies of adipocytes indicate a change in metabolism at the cellular level with increasing heat production in a microcalorimeter though never quite reaching normal levels. Most of these changes are significantly correlated with the reduction in body weight and body fat and it must be concluded that these metabolic improvements are due to body fat reduction rather than being directly incriminated in the cause of the obesity.

Further Reading

Alden J. (1983) Gastric bypass for treatment of obesity. In: Delaney J. P. and Varco R. L. (ed.) *Controversies in Surgery II.* Philadelphia, Saunders. pp. 402–404.

Garrow, J. S. (1978) *Energy Balance and Obesity in Man.* Amsterdam, Elsevier Biomedical.

Gomez C. A. (1981) Gastroplasty in morbid obesity. *World J. Surg.* 5, 823–828.

Mason E. C. and Ito C. (1969) Gastric bypass. *Ann. Surg.* **170**, 329–334.

Montors W. and Doldi S. B. (1981) Jejunoileal bypass for obesity. *World J. Surg.* 5, 801–806.

65 The Oesophagus: Hiatal Hernia, Oesophagitis, Perforations and Disorders of the Diaphragm

A. Cuschieri

ANATOMICAL FEATURES

Embryology

The oesophagus starts to develop on the twentieth day after fertilization as a short tube extending from the tracheal groove to the dilatation of the foregut destined to become the stomach. This tube elongates with the ascent of the larynx and the descent of the heart, during which process the oesophageal lumen becomes temporarily obliterated by a proliferation of the endodermal columnar lining cells. Failure to recanalize is the cause of oesophageal atresia. After recanalization, the epithelial lining of the oesophagus changes to a stratified squamous type. The muscular and connective tissue coats of the oesophagues are derived from the visceral mesoderm between the sixth and twelfth weeks of life. Initially, the vagal trunks run along the side of the oesophagus, but as the stomach rotates to the right, the right vagus assumes a position posterior to the cardio-oesophageal junction and the left trunk comes to lie anterior to the gullet.

Adult Anatomy

The oesophagus is a hollow muscular tube guarded by upper and lower sphincters and extends from the lower border of the cricoid cartilage (sixth cervical vertebra) to the stomach. Its length is 25–30 cm although its measurements vary with the build and height of the individual. When viewed endoscopically, there are a number of normal constrictions, the positions of which are measured by convention from the upper incisor teeth. Thus, the beginning of the oesophagus (just distal to the cricopharyngeus) is found at 15 cm from the incisor teeth, the indentations by the aortic arch and left main bronchus occur at 22 and 27 cm respectively, and the cardio-oesophageal junction is encountered at 40 cm in the male and 37 cm in the female.

The oesophagus descends in front of the lower cervical and thoracic vertebrae but deviates to the left in the neck and then to the right of the midline in the thorax, except at the lower end when it again inclines to the left before passing through the diaphragmatic hiatus in front of the aorta. These deviations from the midline are important surgically in that the cervical oesophagus is best approached from the left side and the thoracic portion through a right thoracotomy, except the lower end which is more accessible through a left thoracotomy or left thoraco-abdominal approach.

The specialized anatomy of the lower oesophagus is shown in *Fig.* 65.1. It consists, from above downward, of:

The supradiaphragmatic portion
The inferior oesophageal constriction
The vestibule
The cardia.

Radiologically, the supradiaphragmatic portion consists of an ampulla and the 'empty' segment just distal to it. The ampulla is not an anatomical dilatation and is caused by the primary peristaltic wave (during a barium swallow) acting in conjunction with the negative intrathoracic pressure which momentarily expand this segment just before the lower oesophageal sphincter (LES) relaxes.

The inferior oesophageal constriction consists of a concentric narrowing of the oesophageal lumen present at the level of the diaphragmatic hiatus. On average, it is situated some 2 cm from the cardio-oesophageal junction. It is not synonymous with the LES although this extends to include this region. The longitudinal oesophageal mucosal folds are very prominent inside the inferior constriction but disappear readily when the oesophagus is dilated during endoscopy.

The intra-abdominal segment of the oesophagus is also known as the vestibule. It is often described as an inverted funnel or cone which inclines to the left before joining the stomach at an angle (cardiac angle or angle of His). When viewed endoscopically from within the stomach, it forms a well marked ridge at the left margin of the gastro-oesophageal junction which is referred to as the incisura.

The cardia denotes the junction between the oesophagus and the stomach. The only reliable and constant anatomical landmark of this is made by the sling or oblique fibres of the stomach but these cannot be identified endoscopically. In the clinical context, therefore, the term cardia is used to describe the junctional zone between the oesophagus and stomach. It contains the squamocolumnar junction which forms a serrated line (Z-line) marking the abrupt change from the tough, smooth, pale, squamous epithelium of the oesophagus with the epithelium of the stomach. The Z-line is situated within 1–4 cm of the anatomical gastro-oesophageal junction. A zone of junctional epithelium is interposed between the squamous lining of the oesophagus and the gastric mucosa of the rest of the stomach. It is lined by columnar cells, contains simple tubular mucous glands which are superficial to the muscularis mucosae and is resistant to acid and peptic digestion. This junctional epithelium extends upwards in patients with longstanding reflux oesophagitis when it is referred to as Barrett's epithelium.

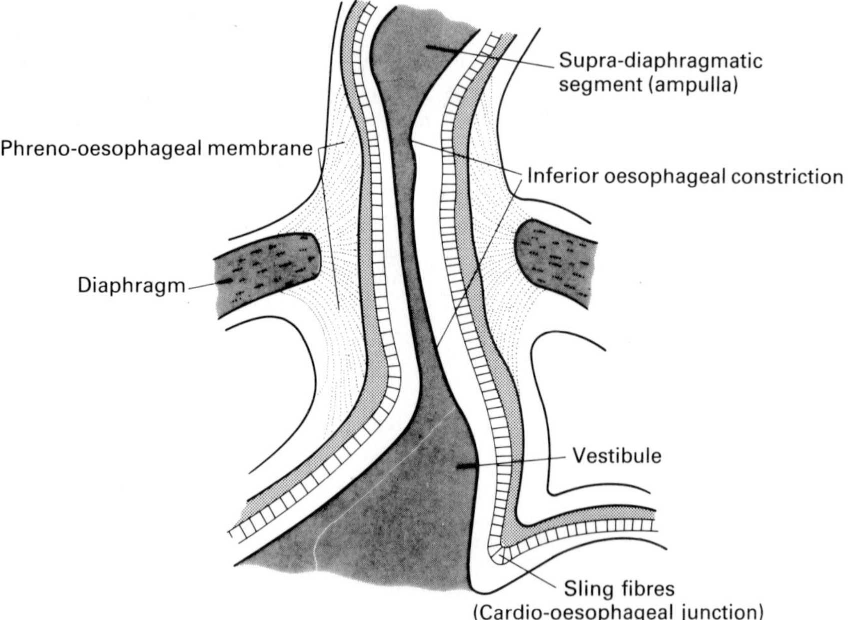

Fig. 65.1 Diagrammatic representation of the anatomy of the lower oesophagus. (Reproduced from *Surgery of the Oesophagus* (Hennessy and Cuschieri) by courtesy of Baillière, Tindall Ltd.)

Oesophageal Attachments

The oesophagus is loosely bound to adjacent structures by fibroareolar tissue throughout its course except at the upper and lower ends where fixation is more secure. Superiorly, the longitudinal muscle fibres of the oesophagus are inserted into the cricoid cartilage. The lower attachments consist of serous reflections and the phreno-oesophageal membrane (*Fig.* 65.1). The supradiaphragmatic pleural reflection is continuous with the mediastinal pleura and is separated from the lower segment of the oesophagus by a condensation of the endothoracic fascia which constitutes the phreno-oesophageal membrane. This important fibro-elastic membrane fixes the lower gullet but permits its continuous vertical displacement which occurs with respiration. The phreno-oesophageal membrane consists of a superior and an inferior limb. The latter is inserted into the cardia, and the superior limb into the lower 3·0 cm of the thoracic oesophagus. The fibres of the membrane are disposed in bundles and lamellae and are inserted deeply into the oesophageal walls, some reaching the submucous layer. As a high percentage (40–60%) of the fibres are made of elastin, the membrane has both strength and resilience which are necessary to cope with the continuous movement of the hiatus during life. The phreno-oesophageal membrane is easily identified during mobilization of the oesophagus for abdominal vagotomy. Damage to it by careless and rough mobilization predisposes to reflux disease.

Structure of the Oesophagus

Four coats are recognized: external, muscular, submucous and mucosal. The external layer is also referred to as the fibrous coat and consists of dense connective tissue containing elastin fibres. The muscle coat is composed of an outer, thicker, longitudinal and an inner circular layer. At the upper end, the longitudinal fibres separate posteriorly and sweep round to the anterior aspect of the oesophagus before their insertion into the posterior aspect of the cricoid cartilage. The resulting weak area at the back of the upper gullet below the cricopharyngeus is known as Killian's dehiscence and is the site of origin of the pharyngeal diverticulum (*Fig.* 65.2). The circular fibres are continuous with those of the cricopharyngeus superiorly and with the oblique gastric muscle fibres inferiorly. The two muscle layers of the upper quarter of the oesophagus are striated. Below this, there is a gradual replacement with smooth muscle which is the only component of the muscular coat of the lower half of the oesophagus. Although similar in appearance to skeletal muscle, the striated muscle of the oesophagus is under

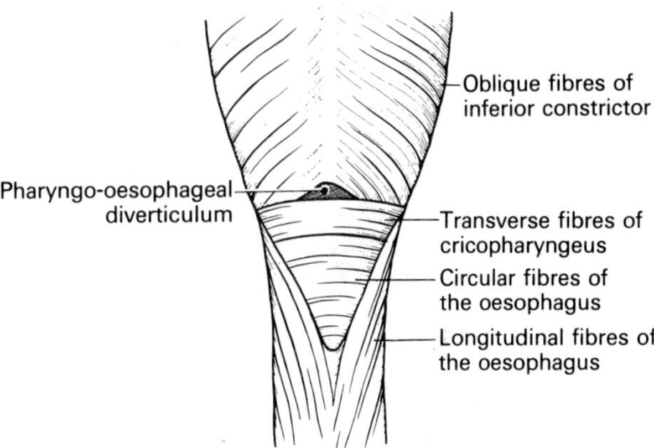

Fig. 65.2 Diagrammatic representation of the posterior aspect of the upper oesophagus and pharynx showing Killian's dehiscence as the longitudinal fibres of the oesophagus sweep anteriorly. The pharyngo-oesophageal diverticulum emerges between the oblique fibres of the inferior constrictor and the transverse fibres of the cricopharyngeus.

autonomic nervous control. At the lower end, the circular muscle layer is thickened but a definite anatomical sphincter is not present.

The submucous layer is very loose in order to permit dilatation of the gullet during swallowing. It consists of areolar–elastin tissue and contains several large vessels and the compound racemose glands of the oesophagus. The mucosal layer is made of non-keratinized squamous epithelium which is arranged in longitudinal folds especially at the lower end where the oesophageal mucosal folds form a rosette.

Vascular Supply and Lymphatic Drainage

The oesophagus receives its arterial supply from several small arterioles throughout its course: branches of the inferior thyroid, common carotid, costocervical and vertebral arteries in the neck, bronchial and direct aortic branches in the thorax, and branches of the left gastric and left inferior phrenic artery at the lower end including the abdominal portion. The venous drainage is to the inferior thyroid veins in the neck and the azygos and hemiazygos veins in the chest except at the lower end which drains into the left gastric (coronary) vein. The lower oesophagus is the most important site of communication between the portal and venous systems (*Fig.* 65.3) and is the site of occurrence of clinically significant varices in the vast majority of patients with portal hypertension. In the lower oesophagus, the veins are mainly situated within the lamina propria whereas in the more proximal oesophagus and stomach they reside in the submucous plane. This is held responsible for the propensity of the lower oesophagus to bleed in variceal portal hypertension. The lymphatics form extensive mucosal and submucosal plexuses which communicate freely and lymph flows long distances in the large submucosal plexus before passing through the muscular coat to reach the draining lymph nodes. These are grouped into three tiers: the first composed of nodes alongside the oesophagus, the second or intermediate group is made up of mediastinal lymph nodes and the third, of the deep cervical, supraclavicular, tracheobronchial and coeliac nodes from above downward.

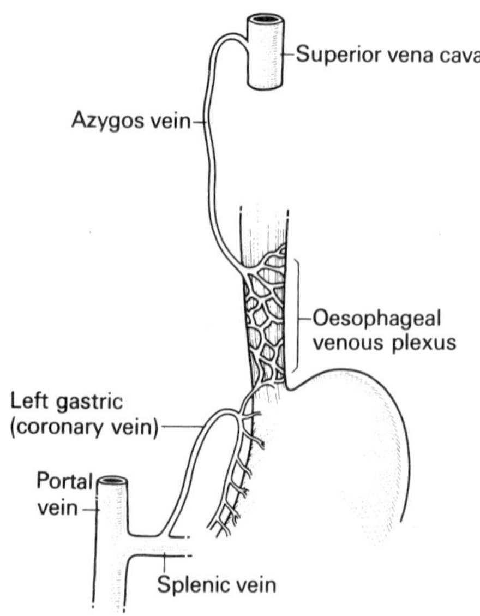

Fig. 65.3 Venous drainage of the lower oesophagus.

In general, lymph drainage from the upper two-thirds of the oesophagus occurs in a proximal direction towards the cervical region, whereas the lower third drains distally to the subdiaphragmatic region and coeliac lymph nodes.

PHYSIOLOGY AND NERVE SUPPLY

Oesophageal motility is controlled by the swallowing centre situated in the brainstem. This receives and coordinates a variety of sensory inputs from within the brainstem and from peripheral mechanoreceptors in the pharynx and oesophagus. The peripheral nerve supply of the gullet has three components:

Craniosacral (parasympathetic)
Thoracolumbar (sympathetic)
Intramural nerve plexuses.

The parasympathetic fibres which are derived from the neurones of the vagal motor nuclei travel in the glossopharyngeal, vagus and recurrent laryngeal nerves and are predominantly motor. An important sensory component is formed by the axons of the nodose ganglion, the cells of which are unipolar, their peripheral axons terminating in receptors situated in the pharynx and oesophagus. The central axons of the cells of the nodose ganglion communicate with the swallowing centre in the brainstem. The sympathetic nerve supply consists of preganglionic fibres derived from neurones situated in the intermediolateral columns of spinal cord segments T5 and T6 and terminate in the cervical, thoracic and coeliac ganglia. The postganglionic sympathetic fibres then reach the oesophagus as a periarterial plexus. The important intramural plexus is the myenteric since the submucous plexus of the oesophagus is sparse and consists of nerve fibres only.

In the fasting state, the body of the oesophagus is flaccid but both the upper and the lower sphincters are closed. The upper oesophageal sphincter (UES, cricopharyngeus) is kept closed by tonic contractions induced by a constant discharge from neurones originating in the cranial nuclei. The UES contracts reflexly in response to distension of the oesophagus, reflux of gastric contents and perfusion of the oesophagus with acid. This reflex action is essentially protective aimed at preventing aspiration. The pressure within the body of the oesophagus in the fasting state follows the intrathoracic pressure, being negative during inspiration and 0–+5 mmHg during expiration. However, at the lower 2–4 cm, a high-pressure zone (HPZ) is encountered. This is due to tonic contraction of the lower oesophageal sphincter and to mechanical factors such as the phreno-oesophageal membrane, sling fibres of the stomach, diaphragmatic crus, etc. The relative contributions of the sphincteric muscular contraction and mechanical factors in the production of the high-pressure zone remain controversial. The normal average pressure within the HPZ is 15–25 mmHg.

Only the initial step of swallowing is initiated by voluntary contractions of the tongue muscles which push the masticated bolus back towards the pharynx. This sets off an involuntary contraction in the pharyngeal musculature directed towards the cricopharyngeus. The UES relaxes momentarily to admit the bolus into the upper oesophagus and then resumes its tonically contracted state. The entry of the bolus into the upper oesophagus is accompanied by the initiation of a *primary peristaltic wave* (with amplitudes of 69–200 mmHg). This travels down the oesophagus pushing the swallowed bolus at a rate of 3–5 cm/sec. The LES relaxes when the primary peristaltic wave reaches it a few seconds after the start of the swallow.

The other contractions exhibited by the oesophagus are the *secondary peristaltic waves* and *tertiary contractions*. The former are caused by stimulation of mechanoreceptors which respond to distension of the oesophagus, as in eructation, and travel caudally from the site of distension. Tertiary contractions which occur spontaneously, are non-propulsive and usually encountered in various oesophageal motility disorders but are also observed in apparently healthy individuals, especially in old age. Tertiary contractions may be generalized (involve the whole of the oesophageal body) or localized.

ASSESSMENT OF OESOPHAGEAL DISEASE

This includes a careful history, physical examination and appropriate investigations to establish the nature of the underlying pathology.

Symptoms

The presentation of oesophageal disease is often typical with one or more of the well-known classic symptoms. Atypical presentation is not, however, infrequent and oesophageal disease may be mistaken for cardiac and pulmonary disorders. In these patients differentiation is only possible after the execution of specialized investigations. A small cohort of patients with oesophageal symptoms have no abnormality on physical examination and intensive investigations. In some, but not all of these, the symptoms reflect a psychoneurotic state.

The typical symptoms of oesophageal disease are:

Dysphagia
Regurgitation
Odynophagia
Chest pain
Waterbrash.

Dysphagia

Difficulty in swallowing may be due to organic disease (benign stricture, oesophageal carcinoma) or result from an oesophageal motility disorder (e.g. achalasia, diffuse oesophageal spasm). The patient feels the food sticking and often points to a particular site on the sternum although this does not correlate well with the exact anatomical location of the disease. Dysphagia for solids implies significant disease which may be organic or functional, whereas dysphagia for liquids only is likely to be the result of an oesophageal motility disorder. In the latter, difficulty with swallowing may be intermittent or its severity variable with exacerbations and periods of relative remission. These patients also find that food transit through the oesophagus can be facilitated by sipping fluid after each solid bolus or by repeated swallows and various postural manoeuvres such as expiration against a closed glottis (Valsalva) etc. On the other hand, persistent and progressive dysphagia indicates organic narrowing of the oesophageal lumen. This is usually associated with regurgitation and is not relieved by sipping fluids or repeated swallowing. Eventually with progression to total dysphagia, the patient is unable to swallow his saliva and exhibits constant drooling.

Globus hystericus presents as dysphagia associated with a feeling of a lump in the throat, even when fasting. It is a neurotic symptom in patients with emotional instability but requires thorough examination to exclude organic disease.

Regurgitation

This symptom results from the regurgitation of gastric or oesophageal fluid into the throat accompanied by a sour taste. It is often postural when it occurs predominantly in the supine position especially at night, the regurgitated material often staining the pillow. Postural regurgitation, which is a very common symptom of reflux disease, is precipitated by meals and activities associated with a rise in the intra-abdominal pressure, i.e. bending and straining.

Regurgitation may also occur as an overflow phenomenon due to the accumulation of food in the oesophagus proximal to a stenosing lesion. This spills back into the pharynx and mouth at night and may lead to aspiration pneumonitis. In oesophageal motility disorders, both overflow and postural regurgitation may occur, although the former is more commonly encountered in these conditions.

Odynophagia

This complaint consists of localized pain, usually in the lower sternal region, immediately the patients swallow certain foods or liquids. It always indicates organic disease, most commonly oesophagitis. Hot drinks, acid citrus beverages, coffee and heavily spiced foods are amongst the most frequent dietary items which induce odynophagia.

Pain

Oesophageal pain is of two sorts: heartburn and angina-like tightening pain which is often interpreted as evidence of coronary heart disease.

Heartburn is due to reflux of gastric juice which is injurious to the oesophageal mucosa and induces an oesophagitis. The chemical injury is accentuated by a defective clearing of the refluxate by the oesophagus consequent on an impaired motility. This increases the contact time of the acid and any other injurious substance (e.g. bile salts) with the oesophageal mucosa. Some patients complain of severe heartburn, yet on endoscopy, there is little or no evidence of inflammation. These individuals have an abnormal oesophageal mucosal sensitivity.

Oesophageal anterior chest pain described as a tightening or gripping, simulates closely angina pectoris. Thus, it may radiate to the back, jaw, arm and ear and is even relieved by sublingual nitrates. This type of pain is commonly found in patients with reflux oesophagitis or oesophageal motility disorders. It may occur in association with meals when it persists for about an hour after, but is also experienced in the fasting state and is frequently precipitated by emotion and exercise.

Waterbrash

This symptom is uncommon and restricted to patients with reflux disease. It is due to excessive salivation, the mouth becoming full of fluid which has a salty taste.

Atypical Presentation of Oesophageal Disease

Patients with oesophageal disease may present with anaemia due to chronic blood loss and, less commonly, with acute upper gastrointestinal bleeding (haematemesis, melaena). Chronic blood loss is usually due to an erosive oesophagitis and active bleeding results from the Mallory–Weiss syndrome or peptic ulceration in a hiatus hernia. Incarceration and strangulation of a para-oesophageal hiatus hernia and spontaneous perforation of the oesophagus (Boerhaave syndrome) present acutely with a severe life-threatening illness.

Reference has already been made to the frequently encountered difficulty in distinguishing oesophageal from cardiac pain. Often patients are treated for angina for a while until persistence/aggravation of symptoms indicates the need for coronary angiography. Several reports have shown that 20–40% of patients with chest pain and normal coronary angiograms are subsequently found to have oesophageal disease. Even arrhythmias may be present in some of these patients.

Presentation with pulmonary symptoms is common. These include attacks of coughing, choking and repeated chest infections due to aspiration pneumonitis in patients with overflow or postural regurgitation. The chest radiograph then shows areas of consolidation/abscess formation/pleural effusion. Furthermore, intrinsic asthma is often exacerbated by gastro-oesophageal reflux with aspiration particularly in infants and children. Effective treatment of the reflux disease is often followed by a considerable improvement in the asthmatic condition of these patients.

Physical Signs

Although the oesophagus is inaccessible to physical examination, the following signs are important and their presence should be checked for during the examination of patients with oesophageal disease:

Evidence of weight loss
Pallor due to anaemia
Neck swelling: pharyngeal pouch, enlarged lymph nodes in the left supraclavicular region
Chest signs on auscultation and percussion of the lung fields
Epigastric mass due to a carcinoma of the cardia enlarging downward
Hepatomegaly with or without clinical jaundice.

Investigations for Oesophageal Disease

These are outlined in *Table* 65.1. Some of the physiological tests require special expertise in their execution and interpretation and are, therefore, only available in major or specialist centres. In addition to these investigations, tests to exclude cardiac disease, e.g. ECG at rest and after exercise and coronary angiography may be necessary in patients who present with episodes of anterior chest pain.

Table 65.1 Investigations for oesophageal disease

Category	*Test*	*Indications*
RADIOLOGICAL	Chest radiograph	Aspiration pneumonitis, oesophageal perforation
	Barium swallow	Dysphagia, perforation, motility disorders
	Ciné-radiology	Motility disorders, reflux disease
	CT scanning	Staging of malignant disease
ULTRASOUND SCANNING	External	Diaphragmatic screening
	Endoscopic	Staging of malignant disease
RADIO-ISOTOPE STUDIES	Labelled liquid or solid bolus studies	Oesophageal transit, reflux disease
ENDOSCOPY	Fibreoptic, rigid+ biopsy, cytology	All patients with oesophageal symptoms, especially dysphagia
PHYSIOLOGICAL	Manometry	Oesophageal motility disorders, reflux disease
	Acid perfusion test (Bernstein's test)	Oesophageal sensitivity to acid
	Standard acid reflux test	Reflux disease
	Acid clearance test	Reflux disease
	24-hour pH monitoring	Reflux disease

Radiology

Chest Radiography

This investigation is necessary in all patients who have oesophageal symptoms to exclude aspiration pneumonitis, detect mediastinal widening which may suggest nodal involvement in patients with oesophageal malignancy and outline any soft tissue shadows and fluid/gas levels (intrathoracic stomach, achalasia). In patients with suspected oesophageal perforations or suture line dehiscence after an oesophagectomy, a chest radiograph to detect mediastinal emphysema and pleural effusion is an essential investigation which is performed before contrast studies.

Contrast Radiology

The standard contrast investigation for elective cases is the barium swallow which is particularly useful in the following:

Patients with dysphagia due to oesophageal motility disorders, especially achalasia and diffuse oesophageal spasm where it is often diagnostic

Oesophageal carcinoma and benign strictures: the differentiation between the two is usually possible on radiological grounds although it requires confirmation with endoscopy (*vide infra*).

Free reflux of barium into the oesophagus may be observed in the upright position and is always significant. Screening with the patient in the Trendelenburg/supine position is conventionally used to enhance and therefore better detect this reflux. However, radiological demonstration of reflux in this way is present in 20% of individuals without oesophagitis and radiological reflux is absent in 40% of patients with moderate to severe oesophagitis. The use of the barium swallow in the detection of gastro-oesophageal reflux is therefore suspect. Its main value lies in the demonstration of an associated hiatus hernia which is present in some patients and in detecting stricture formation, its extent and severity. Although oesophagitis can be detected with special radiological contrast techniques designed to obtain details of the mucosal relief, barium swallow is distinctly inferior to endoscopy in establishing this diagnosis.

A contrast swallow is an essential investigation in patients suspected of oesophageal perforation or leaking oesophageal anastomosis. Because extravasated barium can cause granuloma formation, most radiologists prefer Gastrografin (meglumine diatrizoate) in the first instance and proceed to barium studies if the diagnosis is still in doubt. Others use dilute barium for this purpose as it detects small leaks better than Gastrografin. If this practice is adopted, the surgeon must evacuate by suction any extravasated barium at operation. Although Gastrografin is rapidly absorbed following extravasation and does not exacerbate established inflammation, it is hypertonic and may lead to serious complications which include electrolyte imbalance, significant fluid shifts and pulmonary oedema. Rare instances of intestinal necrosis following its use have been reported.

Cine/Video-radiology

The use of cine fluoroscopy/videorecording is largely restricted to the investigation of patients with cricopharyngeal dysfunction and oesophageal motility disorders.

CT Scanning

Reports on the use of CT scanning have confirmed its usefulness in the preoperative assessment of oesophageal malignancy: extent of mural invasion, involvement of adjacent structures and mediastinal node enlargement although differentiation between nodal deposits and reactive lymphadenopathy is not possible. CT scanning has not, however, proved superior to contrast radiology and endoscopy in the detection of early disease.

Ultrasound Scanning

Screening for diaphragmatic respiratory movement by real-time ultrasound has largely replaced X-ray fluoroscopy for this purpose. Paralysis of a hemidiaphragm with paradoxical movement results from phrenic nerve paralysis and indicates advanced inoperable intramediastinal malignancy (oesophageal and bronchial carcinoma). Endoscopic ultrasound is a very accurate technique for the assessment of extent of intramural involvement and enlargement of the adjacent lymph nodes in both oesophageal and gastric malignancy.

Radio-isotope Studies

These are used to assess gastro-oesophageal incompetence in patients with reflux symptoms and to evaluate the oesophageal transit of liquid and solid boluses in individuals with motility disorders. The radio-isotope test for reflux entails the instillation of 300 ml of saline labelled with $^{99}Tc^{m}$ sulphur colloid inserted into the stomach via a nasogastric tube which is then removed. External scintiscanning of the lower oesophagus is used to detect reflux during a stepwise increase in the intra-abdominal pressure achieved by means of external compression of the abdomen with an inflatable binder. The pressure is increased 5 mmHg every 5 seconds. The test has a high false-positive rate and is not used extensively.

Isotope studies are more useful in the measurement of the oesophageal transit time. When a labelled liquid bolus is used, the patient is placed in the supine position and swallows on demand the labelled liquid previously held in his mouth. Normal individuals clear 90% of the liquid from the oesophagus into the stomach in 4–15 seconds. A more physiological modification employs the use of a standardized solid bolus which is swallowed by the patient in the erect position. The bolus consists of 10 ml poached egg white labelled with $^{99}Tc^{m}$ pertechnetate. External scintiscanning is started as the patient swallows the chewed bolus. The normal transit time for this test is 10 sec, s.d. 2·5 (upper limit, 15 sec). By means of computer programming, time versus activity curves can be generated outlining transit in the upper, middle and lower third in addition to the total oesophageal transit (*Fig.* 65.4). A condensed image can also be computer generated using a technique known as row summation. This outlines graphically the spatial arrangement of the labelled egg white bolus (vertical axis) with respect to time on the horizontal axis (*Fig.* 65.5). Prolonged transit times are encountered in all oesophageal motility disorders (*Fig.* 65.6) with virtually no transit in achalasia. The condensed image shows a striking sinuous outline

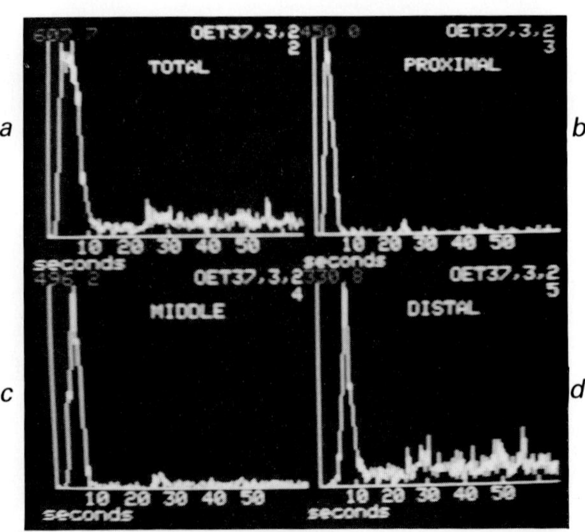

Fig. 65.4 Oesophageal isotope-labelled egg transit study. Time activity curves in a normal subject. *a*, Total transit. *b*, Transit in upper third. *c*, Transit in middle third. *d*, Transit in lower third.

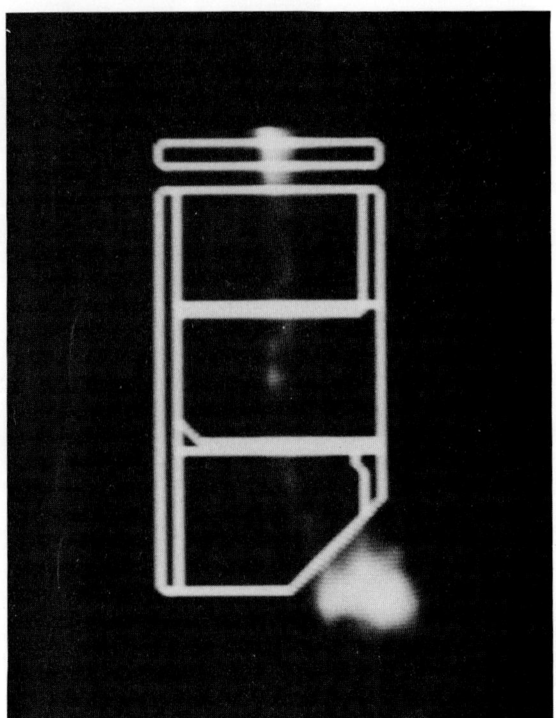

Fig. 65.5 Isotope-labelled egg transit study. Normal condensed image generated by computer using a technique known as row summation. This outlines graphically the spatial arrangement of the labelled egg white bolus (vertical axis) with respect to time on the horizontal axis.

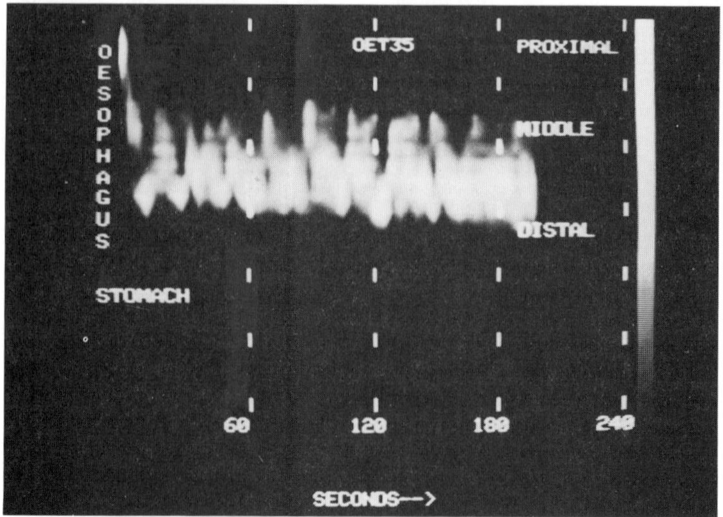

Fig. 65.6 Condensed image showing prolonged transit time in a patient with achalasia. There is virtually no movement of the labelled bolus.

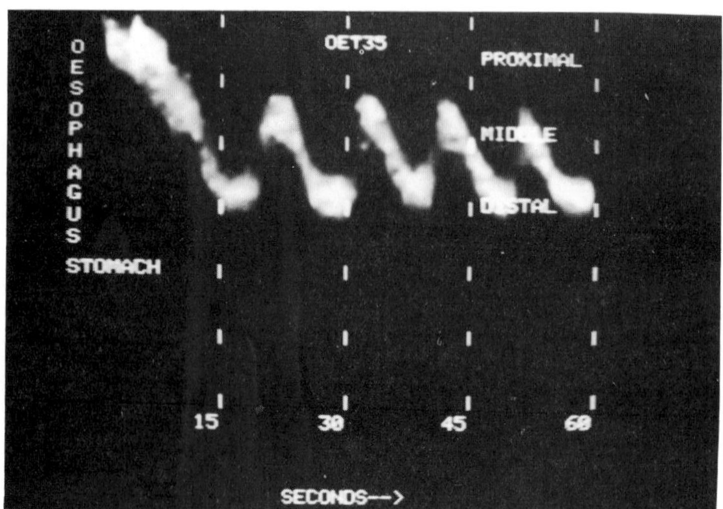

Fig. 65.7 Condensed image shows a striking sinuous outline resulting from the up and down movement of the bolus in a patient with diffuse oesophageal spasm.

resulting from the up and down movement of the bolus in patients with achalasia and diffuse oesophageal spasm (*Fig.* 65.7).

Endoscopy

Flexible endoscopy has largely replaced rigid oesophagoscopy because it provides better visualization, is safer and permits concomitant examination of the stomach. With the endoscope in the stomach and the use of the J-manoeuvre, the cardiac orifice can be inspected which is not possible with the rigid endoscope (*Fig.* 65.8). The latter is still used in the following situations:

Removal of foreign bodies

Necessity to obtain larger biopsies when a histological diagnosis cannot be established on the smaller and more superficial specimens obtained by the fibreoptic technique.

Fibreoptic endoscopy is essential in all patients with dysphagia. It gives direct visual information on the presence of oesophagitis and its severity/complications. It is the crucial test for the detection of oesophageal neoplasms. Both biopsy and brush cytology are used in the diagnosis of oesophageal malignancy and their combined accuracy rate is 96% which is better than the accuracy of either test alone (85–90%). Cytology appears to be more reliable in stenosing lesions whereas endoscopic biopsy carries a higher positive yield in exophytic tumours. Endoscopic biopsies are also necessary in the diagnosis and histological grading of reflux oesophagitis and in the detection of Barrett's epithelium in patients with longstanding reflux disease.

Physiological Tests

These include manometry, the Bernstein's or acid perfusion test, the standard acid reflux text (SART), acid clearance

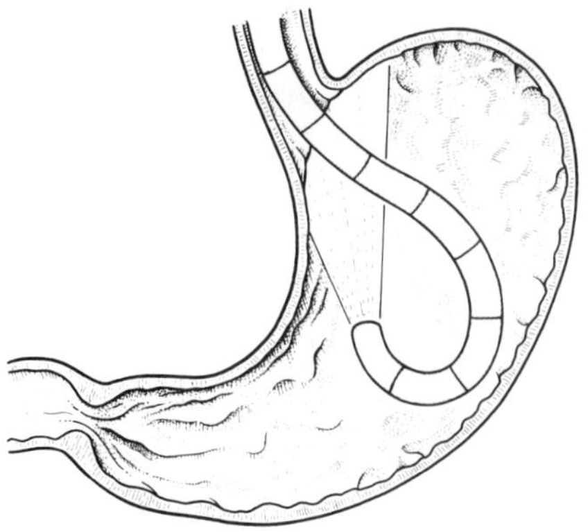

Fig. 65.8 With the endoscope in the stomach and the use of the J-manoeuvre, the cardiac orifice can be inspected which is not possible with the rigid endoscope.

test and 24-hour ambulatory pH monitoring. The latter has largely replaced SART and the acid clearance test in the assessment of patients with reflux symptoms.

Oesophageal Manometry

The techniques available for pressure recordings of the gastro-oesophageal junction use either perfused catheters connected to external transducers or catheter-mounted miniature silicone pressure transducers. The pressure profile of the stomach, cardio-oesophageal junction and proximal oesophagus is obtained by recording whilst the catheter system is withdrawn either slowly, at a rate of 6 cm/min (station pull-through technique), or more quickly (0·5–1·0 cm/sec, rapid pull-through technique). The effect of both dry and wet swallows are also observed on the manometric recording. The information obtained from these manometric studies is shown in *Table* 65.2 and *Fig.* 65.9.

Oesophageal manometry is extremely valuable in the diagnosis and characterization of the various oesophageal motility disorders. It is, however, of limited value in establishing the presence of gastro-oesophageal incompetence, since although as a group patients with reflux have a lower sphincter pressure than normal subjects, the overlap between the two groups is substantial. The specificity and predictive value of the test for the diagnosis of reflux disease is therefore low. Oesophageal manometry is, however, useful in the assessment of the results of anti-reflux surgical procedures.

Bernstein's Acid Perfusion Test

This detects the oesophageal mucosal sensitivity to acid and is very useful in the determination of the oesophageal origin of chest pain. The patient is studied in the fasting state, in the sitting-up position. A nasogastric tube is inserted and the stomach is emptied, after which the tube is pulled into the middle third of the oesophagus (30–35 cm from the incisor teeth). Perfusion is initially started with isotonic saline (100 drops/min) for 15 min and then switched, without the patient being informed, to 0·1 M HCl which reproduces the pain in patients with a sensitive oesophageal mucosa. The infusion of acid is then stopped. Thereafter, the pain should subside by 20 min.

Standard Acid Reflux Test (SART)

In this test, 300 ml of 0·1 M HCl are first instilled into the fasting stomach by means of a nasogastric tube which is then withdrawn. A pH probe is inserted and located 5·0 cm above

Table 65.2 Oesophageal manometry indices and criteria

Normal	*Abnormal*
HPZ (sphincter) pressure: 10–26 mmHg	<10·0 mmHg, >26·0 mmHg
Relaxes when reached by primary wave	No relaxation with swallowing
Primary peristaltic wave generated by wet/dry swallows: mean amplitude = 50–110 mmHg Mostly single or double peaked wave forms	Absent, increased/decreased amplitude, increased duration, abnormal wave forms multiple peaks
	Repetitive (tertiary, non-propulsive) contractions

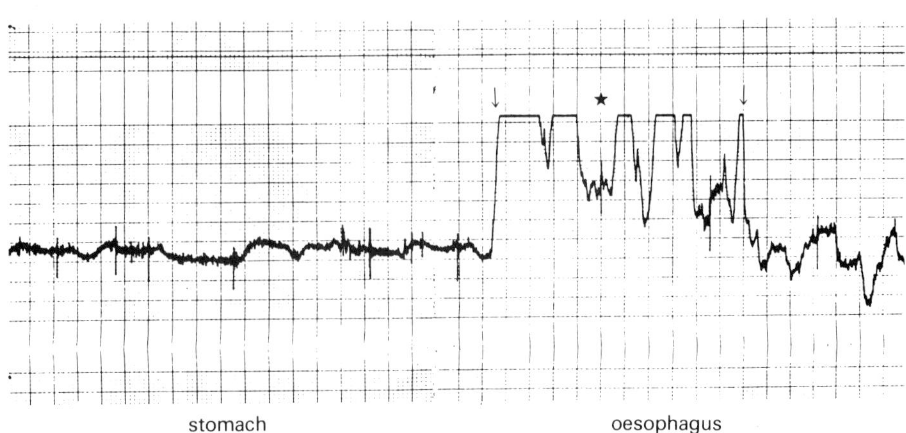

Fig. 65.9 Normal pressure tracing using the station pull-through technique. The high pressure zone extends between the two arrows. The respiratory inversion point is marked with an ★. It is due to a change from positive inspiratory to negative inspiratory deflections as the recording lumen passes from the abdominal segment into the thoracic portion.

the HPZ. The gastro-oesophageal competence is assessed after 3 coughs, 3 deep breaths, one Valsalva and Müller manoeuvres in each of the following positions: supine, right and left lateral decubitus and 20° Trendelenburg giving 20 opportunities for separate reflux episodes to occur and be detected by the pH probe. An abnormal test indicating gastro-oesophageal incompetence, is defined as the occurrence of more than 2 reflux episodes out of the 20 positions. The standard acid reflux test has 20% false negative and 20% false positive rates.

Acid Clearance Test

This test which assesses the ability of the distal oesophagus to clear an acid load by repeated swallowing, correlates well with the presence of oesophagitis. Motility of the oesophagus is impaired with the onset of oesophagitis and a vicious circle is established with prolongation of the contact time between the acid and the inflamed oesophageal epithelium. In performing the test, a pH probe is positioned 5·0 cm above the HPZ and a load of acid (15 ml of 0·1 M HCl) is then instilled above the tip of the probe. The pH drops to about 1·4. Normal individuals are able to clear the acid in 3–10 swallows. Delayed clearance is diagnosed if the patient requires more than 10 swallows to achieve return of the oesophageal pH to the pre-infusion level.

24-hour pH Monitoring

The advent of ambulatory prolonged pH monitoring, made possible with technological advances in portable solid-state data loggers and computer software for data analysis, has replaced some of the physiological tests for reflux and has allowed a better understanding of the nature of gastro-oesophageal reflux disease.

After the location of the LES is ascertained by preliminary manometry, a pH probe or telemetric pH capsule (pill) is inserted and positioned 5 cm above the HPZ (*Fig.* 65.10). If a telemetric capsule is used, it is held suspended in position by a string strapped to the cheek. A circular aerial round the patient's thorax is used to pick up the signals corresponding to the pH data in the oesophagus emitted from the capsule. The aerial is connected to a portable data logger with which the patient can interact using event buttons to store in real time pain episodes, meals, supine and erect positions (*Fig.* 65.11). Alternatively, a probe can be employed and this is connected directly to the portable pH logger. Once set up, the patient is allowed home. Monitoring is continued for 24 hours after which the pill or probe is removed and the data from the logger are transferred into a microcomputer for analysis.

The computer software analyses the data in two ways. Reflux event analysis and cumulative oesophageal exposure to acid are obtained and hard copies made. The reflux event analysis consists of the identification and characterization of all the individual reflux episodes where the oesophageal pH fell below 4·0. It gives the number of such events/hour, their mean duration, the number of long reflux events (>5 min) and the duration of the longest reflux episode throughout the 24-hour period (*Fig.* 65.12). The cumulative oesophageal exposure method depicts the frequency distribution of the oesophageal pH data points for the erect and supine periods of the run (*Fig.* 65.13). Finally, a graph of the pH against time is obtained which also depicts the time of occurrence of the special events (pain, meals, etc.). It is thus possible to determine whether a painful episode was associated with a reflux event (*Fig.* 65.14). Prolonged acid reflux episodes which occur predominantly in the supine position at night are associated with defective oesophageal clearance motility.

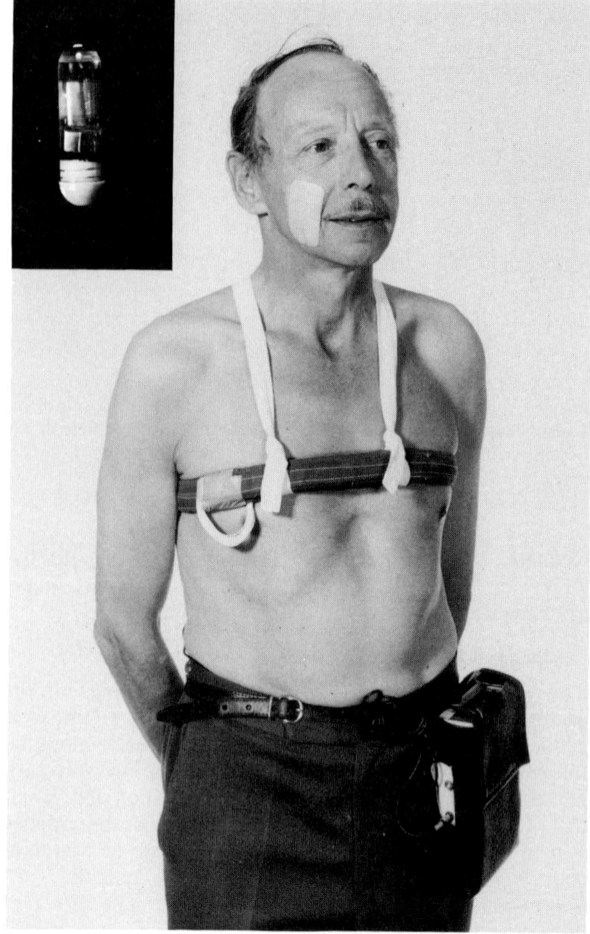

Fig. 65.10 Ambulatory oesophageal pH monitoring. The telemetric capsule (inset) has been inserted and is suspended 5 cm above the HPZ by a string taped to the patient's cheek. A circular aerial which is connected to the data logger is strapped around the patient's chest.

There is a good correlation between the results of the prolonged ambulatory pH monitoring and severity of oesophagitis at endoscopy. In addition, the results of the two investigations are complementary.

HIATAL HERNIA

Hiatal hernia is not synonymous with gastro-oesophageal reflux as evidenced by the fact that only 13% of patients with herniation of the stomach through the diaphragmatic hiatus will develop reflux oesophagitis. In addition, the prevalence of hiatus hernia has been reported to be no greater in patients with symptomatic reflux than in healthy subjects. Belsey was the first to differentiate symptoms and complications caused by reflux from those associated with hiatal hernia alone. The condition is commonly encountered from the fifth decade onwards in the West and there is a strong aetiological association with obesity. Rare instances of post-traumatic herniation of the stomach through the hiatus are well documented and must be differentiated from traumatic

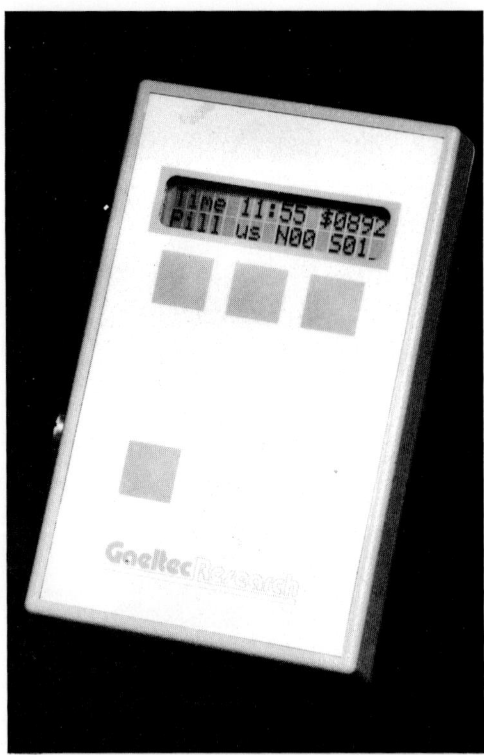

Fig. 65.11 Ninewells solid state portable data logger for pH monitoring. The patient can interact with the system through a scintillation window and by means of an event button indicate occurrence of pain and meals, position, etc. in real time. The logger can be used either with a telemetric capsule or pH probe. In the latter instance a circular aerial is not used and the probe is connected directly to the logger (instrument manufactured by Gaeltec Research, Scotland).

rupture of the diaphragm. In the vast majority of cases, however, the development of a hiatal hernia is spontaneous. Gallstones and colonic diverticular disease are commonly present in these patients (Saint's triad) and difficulty may be encountered in establishing which of the three disorders accounts for the patient's symptoms.

Pathology

Three types of hiatal hernia are recognized:

Type 1 (axial, sliding)
Type 2 (para-oesophageal)
Mixed.

Axial Hernia

This accounts for the majority (70–80%) of cases. The gastro-oesophageal junction and a variable portion of the adjacent stomach slide upwards into the mediastinum carrying with them a peritoneal sac. This results in loss of the cardiac angle of His and commonly, incompetence of the cardio-oesophageal junction (*Fig.* 65.15). The complications of this type of hernia are those which are consequent on reflux oesophagitis (chronic blood loss, stricture formation, Barrett's epithelium, etc.).

Para-oesophageal Hernia

In this type, the fundus of the stomach rotates in front of the oesophagus and herniates through the hiatus into the mediastinum. As the cardio-oesophageal junction remains in situ within the abdomen (except in large hernias), cardiac incompetence and reflux are not usually encountered (*Fig.* 65.16). This type of hernia accounts for 8–10% of cases and is found predominantly in the elderly. In large hernias, the entire stomach and pylorus may be found within the chest inside a large hernial sac which may also contain the spleen and hepatic flexure. These large hernias are prone to incarceration and strangulation with infarction and perforation of the stomach. Large hernias can also progress to complete volvulus which results in pyloric or duodenal obstruction. When a para-oesophageal hernia bleeds, this is due either to chronic gastric ulceration in the intrathoracic stomach or to an erosive gastritis in a congested/strangulated organ. The majority of uncomplicated para-oesophageal hernias can be easily reduced through the abdomen.

Mixed Hernia

This resembles a large para-oesophageal hernia but the gastro-oesophageal junction is also herniated above the diaphragm. Thus it has features and complications of both type 1 and 2 hernias. It is found in 10–15% of patients. This type of hernia is generally considered to be a late stage of the para-oesophageal variety.

PERCENTAGE OF DATA BELOW PH VALUE

RECORD:672	pH 9	8	7	6	5	4	3	2	1
ERECT	100.0	100.0	100.0	33.8	6.6	3.2	0.9	0.2	0.0
SUPINE	100.0	100.0	100.0	97.4	1.8	0.1	0.0	0.0	0.0
TOTAL	100.0	100.0	100.0	68.6	4.0	1.5	0.4	0.1	0.0

ANALYSIS BASED ON REFLUX EVENTS

RECORD NO. 672	TIME pH< 4 (min)	NO. OF EVENTS	DURATION PER EVENT (min)	REFLUX PATTERN(no. of events) <5 MINS	> 5 MINS	LONGEST EVENT (min)
ERECT	1.55	1.48	1.05	1.48	0.00	2.17
SUPINE	0.04	0.11	0.33	0.11	0.00	0.33
TOTAL	0.72	0.73	0.99	0.73	0.00	2.17

Acid reflux = pH< 4

All data standardised for one hour

Fig. 65.12 Reflux event analysis by computer of a 24-hour pH monitoring period.

OESOPHAGEAL 24 HOUR pH MONITORING

ANALYSIS BASED ON CUMULATIVE
OESOPHAGEAL ACID EXPOSURE

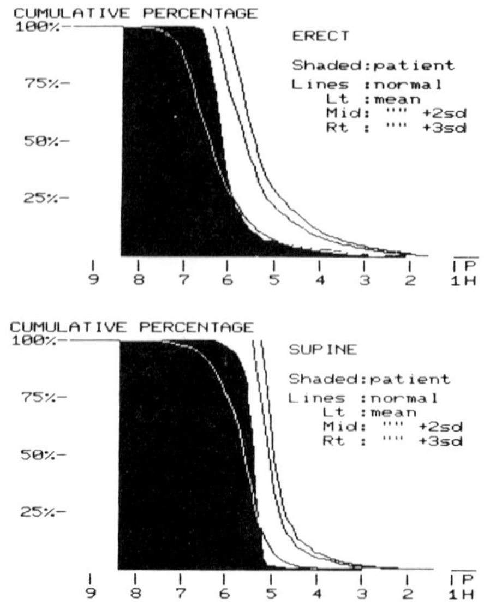

a

OESOPHAGEAL 24 HOUR pH MONITORING

ANALYSIS BASED ON CUMULATIVE
OESOPHAGEAL ACID EXPOSURE

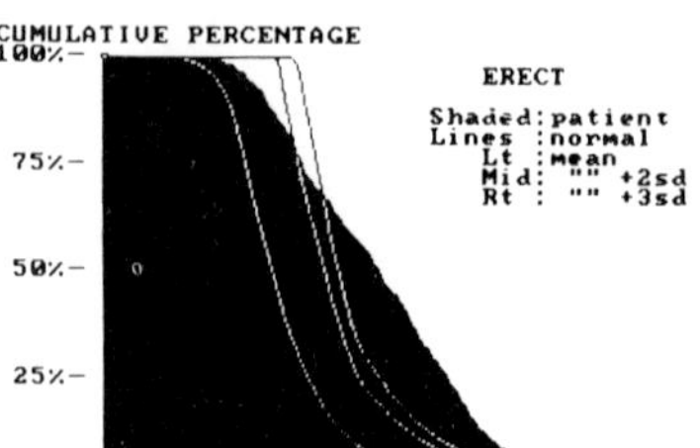

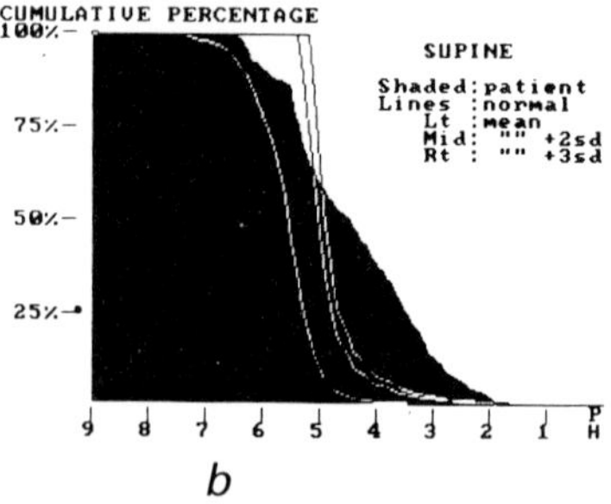

b

Fig. 65.13 Computer-generated cumulative oesophageal acid exposure of pH data from a patient during a 24-hour period. Separate graphs are shown for the erect and supine periods. The sigmoid lines represent the mean, 2 and 3 standard deviations of data obtained from normal subjects. The patient's data are superimposed as a shaded area so that abnormal acid exposure can be immediately recognized. *a*, The patient's data (shaded area) fall within the normal range both in the erect and positions. *b*, Gross reflux in both the erect and supine postures clearly shown by the shaded patient's data which exceed the normal range.

Clinical Features

These depend on the type of hernia and the onset of acute life-threatening complications which can occur with the para-oesophageal and mixed varieties.

Axial

The condition may be asymptomatic particularly in elderly patients with limited activity and a sedentary life style. When symptoms occur, they are largely due to reflux oesophagitis (*vide infra*). Chronic blood loss resulting in iron-deficiency anaemia is common but active haemorrhage is rare. Some patients may present with dysphagia due to stricture formation without a preceding symptomatic history.

Para-oesophageal and Mixed

The symptoms of para-oesophageal hernias are due to the pressure effects of the herniated stomach especially when it becomes distended with food or gas. Reflux is rare, occurring in only 3% unless the hernia is or becomes mixed. Common symptoms include pain, dyspnoea, feelings of distension and tightness which are precipitated by meals, bending and stooping. The pain is sharp, situated beneath the lower sternum and radiates to the back. It is often accompanied by a bloated sensation, anxiety, palpitations and dyspnoea. The attacks may simulate angina very closely and even cardiac arrhythmias may be present during an episode. However, the pain is often relieved by belching or vomiting. Dysphagia is found in 20% of patients with para-oesophageal hernias.

Acute Presentation

Patients with large para-oesophageal/mixed hernias may present acutely with severe upper gastrointestinal haemorrhage or strangulation/infarction/perforation of the intrathoracic stomach. In the latter instance, the patient develops severe retosternal pain and shock which are often mistaken for myocardial infarction. A chest radiograph shows a large gastric gas/fluid shadow overlying the heart. With gastric infarction and perforation, mediastinal widening and emphysema, left basal collapse and pleural effusion may be outlined by this investigation. Gastric infarction and perforation carry a high mortality from septic mediastinitis and bacteraemic shock.

Treatment

In the first instance, clinical assessment and the appropriate investigations must establish that the symptoms are due to the hiatal hernia. In elderly patients and in individuals with coexisting heart disease, case selection for surgery requires accurate clinical judgement based on the severity of the symptoms and the cardiorespiratory reserve. Middle-aged patients with significant coronary heart disease may require myocardial revascularization before surgical treatment of the hiatal hernia.

Type 1 hernia is treated with reduction and an anti-reflux procedure (*vide infra*). The majority of uncomplicated para-oesophageal hernias can be approached through the abdomen as the hernias are easily reducible via this approach. Following reduction of the hernia, the large hiatus is repaired with interrupted non-absorbable sutures and the gastro-oesophageal junction fixed beneath the diaphragm after restoring the oesophago-gastric angle (Allison's repair). Some advocate a Nissen fundoplication in addition to reduction and crural repair for these hernias.

Patients presenting with continued bleeding from a chronic gastric ulcer in an intrathoracic stomach, require emergency partial gastrectomy and repair of the hernia. An

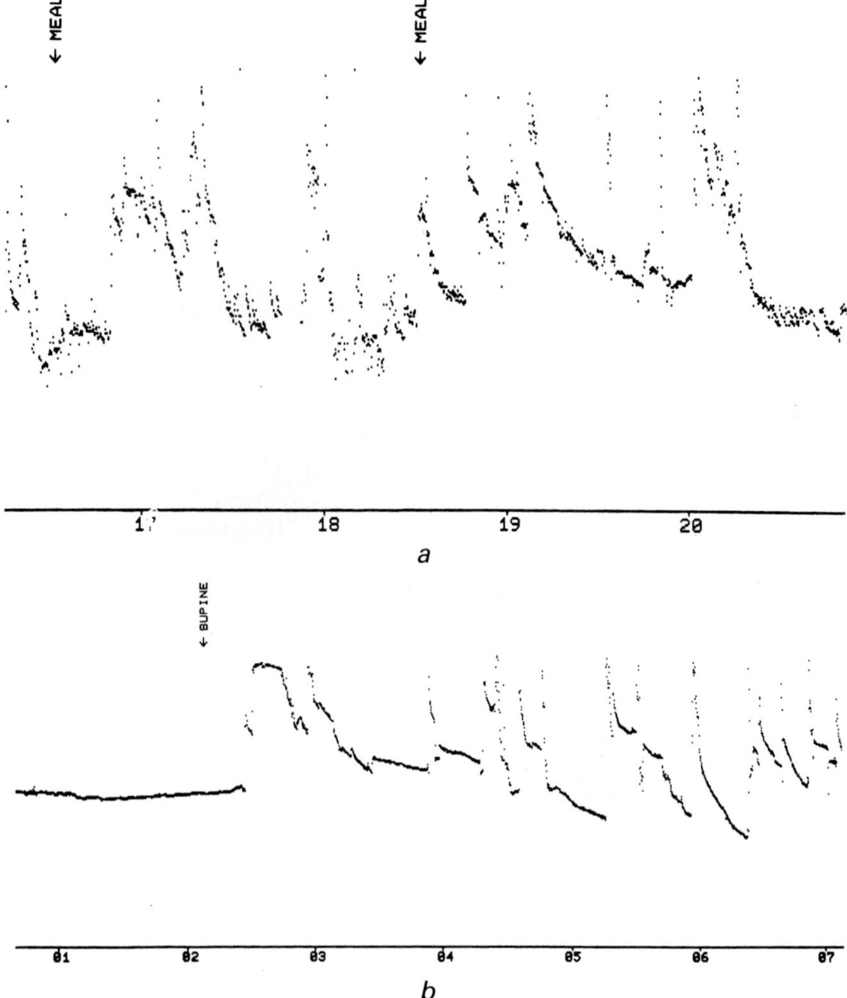

Fig. 65.14 Computer-generated graph of oesophageal pH (on the vertical axis) against time of day (horizontal axis). Special events such as pain episodes and meal times are automatically entered. *a*, Severe reflux episodes after an evening meal. *b*, Severe nocturnal reflux between 2 and 7 a.m. It is also possible to determine which painful episodes are accompanied by acid reflux into the oesophagus.

emergency thoracotomy is necessary for strangulated/infarcted para-oesophageal and mixed hernias. If the stomach is congested but viable, it is untwisted and reduced into the abdomen after which a crural repair is performed. A Belsey antireflux procedure is unwise in this situation as it may lead to gastric/oesophageal perforation. Resection of the infarcted stomach with mediastinal and pleural toilet is necessary for those patients presenting with this serious complication.

REFLUX OESOPHAGITIS

Gastro-oesophageal reflux disease is a common disorder which afflicts both sexes equally. Its prevalence is relatively constant over the age of 30 and does not seem to increase with age as does hiatal hernia. There is still some controversy regarding the exact pathophysiology of the disorder but most agree that the disease is multifactorial in origin and not simply the result of sphincter malfunction.

Normal Mechanisms of Cardio-oesophageal Competence

There is now general agreement that competence is due to the combined action of the lower oesophageal sphincter and mechanical factors which interact and function in consort. The tonic contractions of the LES are largely myogenic but neuro-endocrine influences, blood flow and hypoxia modify contractile activity of the high-pressure zone. Temporary inhibition of the LES occurs just prior to the arrival of a primary peristaltic wave induced by swallowing, to allow entry of food into the stomach, after which the sphincter resumes its contracted state. Several drugs, hormones and food substances are known to influence the contractile activity of the HPZ (*Table* 65.3). In general, the effect of the hormones on the LES have been achieved by pharmacological doses and, therefore, it is not possible to ascribe with certainty a physiological role for these peptides or hormones. In particular, it now seems unlikely that gastrin is involved in the physiological control of LES activity. Thus the resting sphincter pressure is unrelated to the basal serum gastrin levels and the observed increases in the sphincter

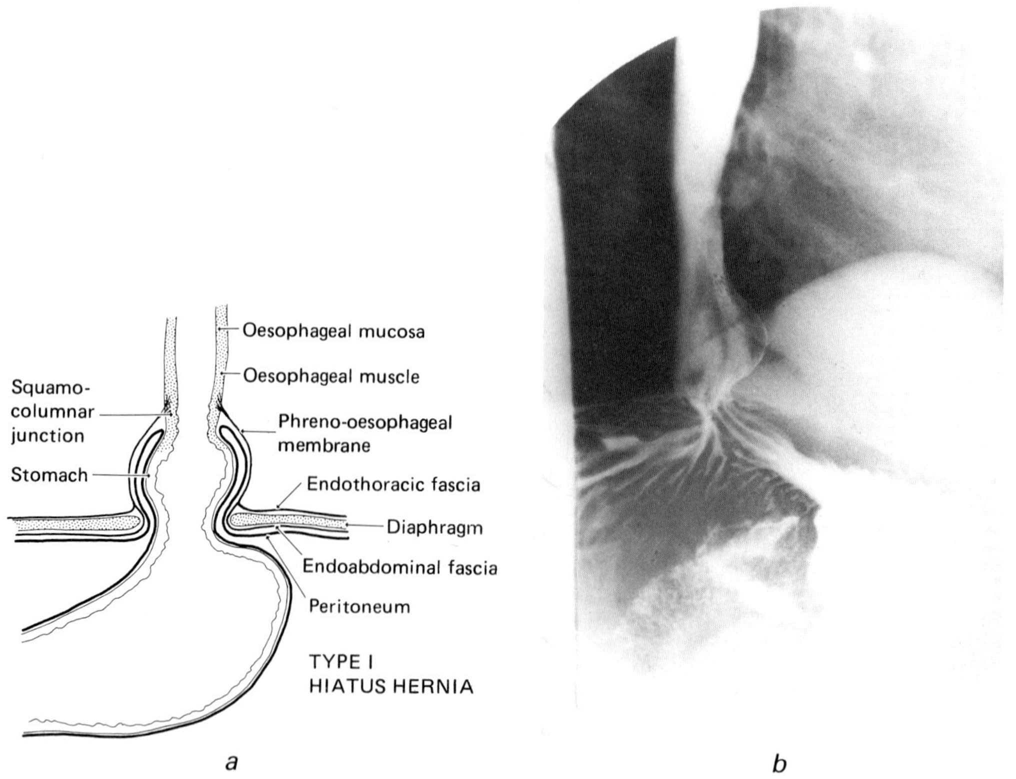

Fig. 65.15 *a*, Diagrammatic representation of Type I (axial, sliding) hiatal hernia. *b*, Barium swallow showing Type I (axial, sliding) hiatal hernia. Note displacement of the cardio-oesophageal junction into the chest.

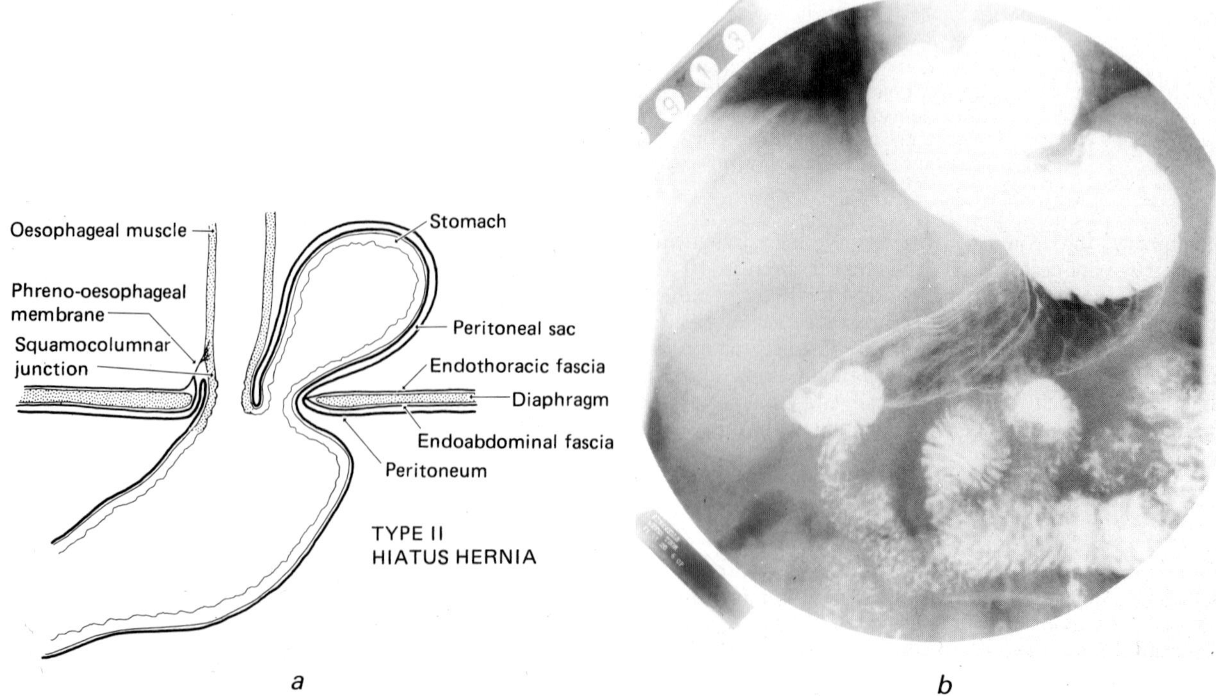

Fig. 65.16 *a*, Diagrammatic representation of Type II (para-oesophageal) hiatal hernia. *b*, Barium swallow showing large Type II (para-oesophageal) hiatal hernia. Note rotation of the fundus which rolls up in front of the cardio-oesophageal junction.

Table 65.3 Effect on the lower oesophageal sphincter pressure (high-pressure zone) by hormones, drugs and foodstuffs

	Decrease HPZ activity	*Increase HPZ activity*
HORMONES/ PEPTIDES	Glucagon Secretin Cholecystokinin VIP GIP Progesterone Oestrogens Serotonin (N-receptors) Histamine (H_2-receptors) Enkephalins	Gastrin Motilin Bombesin Histamine (H_1-receptors) Serotonin (M-receptors)
PROSTA-GLANDINS	E_1, E_2, A_2	F_2
DRUGS	Atropine Antihistamines Ca^{++}-blockers Ganglion-blockers Tricyclic antidepressants	Metoclopramide Domperidone Cisapride Cholinergic drugs Anticholinesterases
FOOD-STUFFS	Caffeine Fats Chocolate Alcohol	Protein meal
OTHERS	Smoking	

pressure after a protein meal are greater than can be expected by the measured rise in the level of the serum gastrin.

Historically, several mechanical factors have been held responsible for ensuring competence of the cardio-oesophageal junction. These include the cardiac angle with its resultant incisural fold or flap valve, the oblique fibres of the stomach, the mucosal folds at the lower end which form a rosette plugging the lumen and the pinchcock mechanism of the diaphragm. These are no longer held to be important in the prevention of gastro-oesophageal reflux.

Although the phreno-oesophageal membrane has no direct effect on closure of the lower oesophagus, it plays an important role by fixing the lower gullet and maintaining the terminal segment in the abdomen. All the experimental and clinical data indicate that competence is the result of a flutter valve, the abdominal segment being flattened anteroposteriorly against the aorta by the intra-abdominal pressure (*Fig.* 65.17). In this context, the length of the intra-abdominal segment of the oesophagus is crucial. If this exceeds 2·0 cm and the sphincter pressure is normal, pathological reflux is unlikely. Conversely, a short intra-abdominal segment together with a reduced pressure is associated with the development of pathological reflux.

Pathology of Reflux Oesophagitis

The normal baseline pH of the lower oesophagus is 5·0–6·5 with the lower value occurring at night. Prolonged ambulatory pH monitoring has shown that normal subjects have reflux episodes both in the fasting state and especially postprandially. However, these episodes are short-lived due to the efficient clearing mechanism of the oesophagus. This contrasts with the situation in reflux disease where the acid reflux episodes are more frequent and last longer resulting in a prolonged contact time between the refluxed gastric acid and the oesophageal epithelium leading to direct chemical

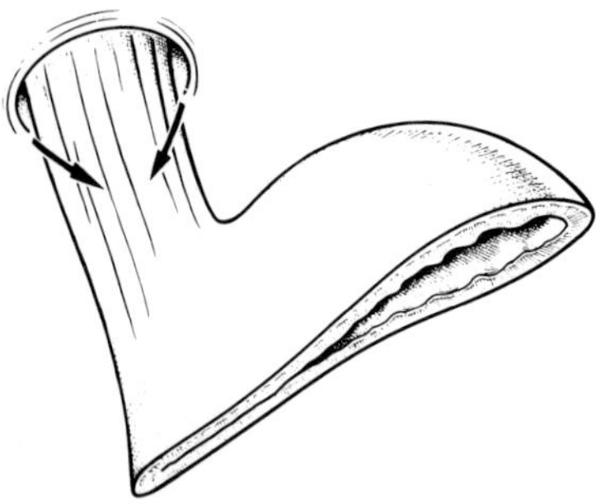

Fig. 65.17 Competence is the result of a flutter valve, the abdominal segment being flattened anteroposteriorly against the aorta by the intra-abdominal pressure. The mechanism is similar to a Heimlich valve used for chest drains instead of an underwater-seal drain.

damage when the pH falls below 4·0. It is not known whether the abnormal motility and the consequent delayed clearance is primary or secondary to the oesophagitis. Certainly the latter impairs the oesophageal contractile activity further and a vicious circle is established. However, recent studies indicate that a primary underlying motility disorder may be an essential component of reflux disease and accounts for the prolonged contact time of the refluxate with the lower oesophageal epithelium in the first instance.

Apart from acid, other substances present in the gastric juice are injurious to the oesophageal mucosa. These include pepsin, trypsin, bile salts and lysolecithin, the last three being derived from bile and duodenal juice and are the consequence of enterogastro-oesophageal reflux which is most commonly encountered after gastric surgery. Oesophagitis can therefore occur at neutral and alkaline pH (neutral, alkaline reflux) although this is much less common than acid/pepsin-induced oesophageal damage.

The histological appearances of the early stages of reflux oesophagitis are best appreciated from the examination of deep biopsies taken by the tube suction technique. The normal oesophageal epithelium consists of three layers from the lamina propria upwards: the basal (germinal layer, columnar cells), the prickle cell layer (polygonal cells with numerous bridges) and the superficial or functional layer (flattened cells with pyknotic nuclei). Inflammatory cells are few and scanty and the vascular dermal papillae project from the lamina propria to no more than half the thickness of the epithelium (*Fig.* 65.18). The histological changes of early damage include widening of the basal cell layer so as to constitute more than 15% of the total epithelial thickness and extension of the dermal papillae to more than two-thirds of the way through the epithelium to the luminal surface (*Fig.* 65.19). These changes are indicative of an increased rate of epithelial turnover and are reliable indicators of pathological reflux. With more severe damage there is an accumulation of inflammatory cells (mainly polymorphs), the total epithelial thickness is reduced and becomes entirely composed of basal cells. The papillae become widened and extend to the surface when superficial necrosis and ulceration supervene (*Fig.* 65.20). These acute ulcers are situated superficial to the muscularis mucosae. Their base consists of granulation tissue surrounded by an inflammatory infiltrate which is accompanied by submucosal oedema. Healing of these superficial ulcers does not result in fibrosis and the regenerated epithelium is of the squamous variety. However, if the ulceration and inflammation reaches the submucous layer or beyond, some fibrosis is inevitable and the

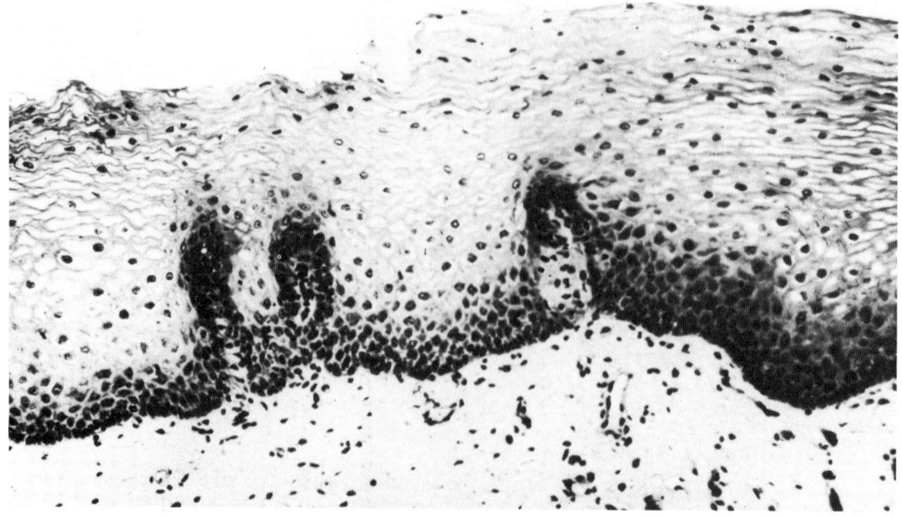

Fig. 65.18 Suction biopsy of the lower oesophageal mucosa. Normal histology: the basal layer is less than 15% of the total epithelial thickness. The papillae of the lamina propria extend less than two-thirds of the way to the luminal surface. No polymorphonuclear leucocytes are present in either lamina propria or epithelium. Mononuclear cells, normal constituents of the lamina propria, are present.

regenerated mucosa may eventually consist, entirely or in part, of columnar epithelium.

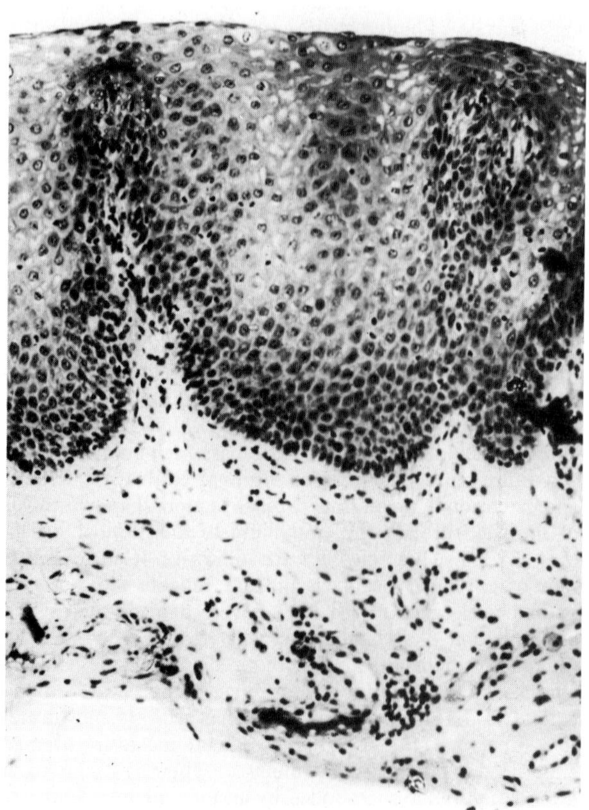

Fig. 65.19 Mild to moderate oesophagitis due to acid reflux. The basal layer occupies about 30% of the total epithelial thickness and the papillae extend nearly to the surface. No polymorphonuclear leucocytes are present.

Complications of Reflux Oesophagitis

The complications of reflux oesophagitis are:

Chronic blood loss
Deep ulceration with peri-oesophagitis
Formation of strictures and webs
Columnar-cell change.

Deep Ulceration and Peri-oesophagitis

This complication is usually found in longstanding symptomatic disease. The ulcers involve the oesophagus beyond the submucous layer and cause a peri-oesophagitis and extensive mural fibrosis which eventually leads to both stricture formation and shortening of the oesophagus. Full-thickness penetration may involve the peri-oesophageal arterial plexus and cause massive haemorrhage. However, this complication and overt perforation are rare.

Strictures and Webs

Oesophageal webs which may form at sites of ulcerative oesophagitis are the result of submucous fibrosis in a localized area of the oesophagus and are most commonly found at the lower end or at the level of the aortic arch. They may cause dysphagia with intermittent solid bolus obstruction but are easily treated by endoscopic dilatation and seldom recur thereafter.

The exact nature of the distinctive circular mucosal ridge situated at the oesophagogastric junction and known as the Schatzki's ring is still debatable. Some consider it to be a complication of reflux disease but others dispute this. Schatzki's rings tend to occur in association with hiatus hernia and are not usually associated with any evidence of oesophagitis. The majority are asymptomatic but those with a ring aperture <13 mm cause mild intermittent dysphagia with sudden episodes of total obstruction, sometimes referred to as 'the steakhouse syndrome'. In the majority of symptomatic patients, an underlying motility disorder is present in addition to the ring.

Stricture formation is the result of repeated oesophageal damage with fibrosis replacing the muscular coat of a segment of the gullet. The majority occur in patients over 60

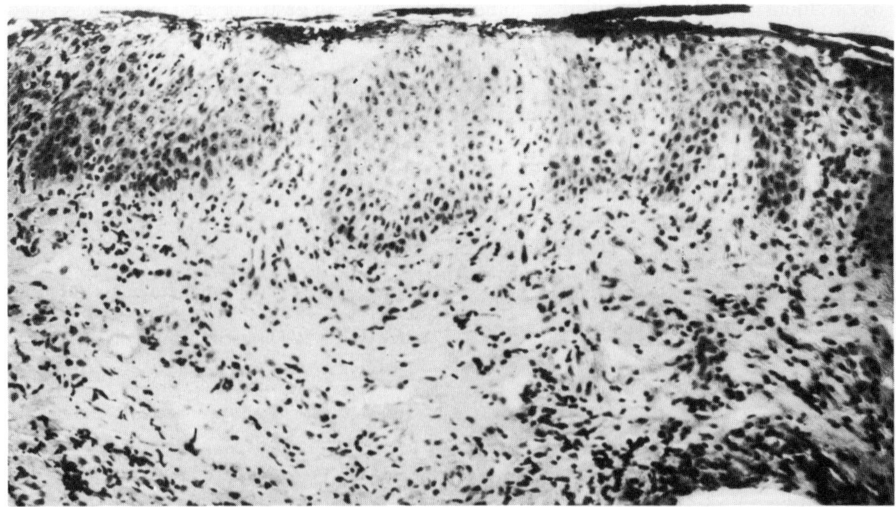

Fig. 65.20 Severe gastro-oesophageal reflux with gross erosion and exudate visible endoscopically. The total epithelial thickness is less than normal and is composed entirely of basal cells. The papillae are widened and extend all the way to the luminal surface where superficial necrosis is present. Many polymorphonuclear leucocytes are present in the lamina propria and within the epithelium.

years with longstanding symptoms, although some patients present with dysphagia due to a benign reflux (peptic) stricture without a significant history of reflux symptoms. Peptic strictures with a lumen of less than 3 mm and a length greater than 3 cm are classed as severe (*Fig.* 65.21). They account for 10% of strictures in most published series and are both difficult and dangerous to dilate. In addition, there is evidence that the initial severity of the stricture is an indicator of the propensity for recurrence after dilatation.

Columnar-cell lined (Barrett's) Oesophagus

Columnar-cell lined oesophagus was first described by Barrett as ectopic islands of gastric epithelium associated with deep ulceration and stricture formation. Initially, Barrett mistook the condition for a tubular intrathoracic stomach but later revised this opinion and suggested the term 'lower oesophagus lined by columnar epithelium'. Previously, the condition was thought to represent a congenital anomaly but this is now considered unlikely since the majority of cases are diagnosed (because of symptoms) in the sixth or seventh decade although the condition is occasionally encountered in children and young adults. The congenital theory does not explain why the columnar epithelium always occurs at the lower end as replacement of the fetal columnar epithelium, begins at the middle of the oesophagus and progresses toward each end. The acquired theory is now generally accepted. The columnar epithelium is regarded as an adaptive change which develops in response to prolonged reflux-induced damage to the oesophageal epithelium. The abnormal epithelium can extend proximally in continuity with the squamocolumnar junction or assume a patchy distribution with islands of ectopic columnar mucosa amidst squamous epithelium. It is usually confined to the lower two-thirds of the oesophagus. There is still some controversy whether the columnar epithelium is the result of change, of cephalad migration of the gastric mucosa or simply arises from the oesophageal racemose glands. The abnormal epithelium may consist of:

Junctional epithelium
Gastric epithelium of the fundic type
Intestinal change.

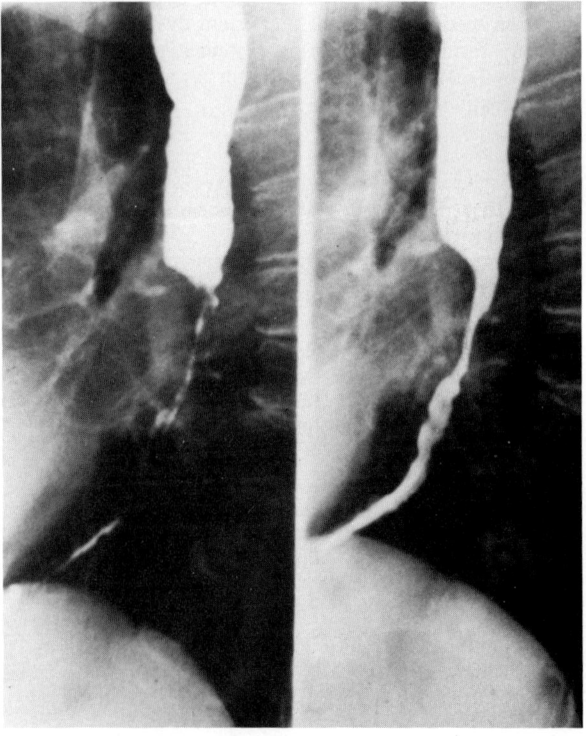

Fig. 65.21 Barium swallow showing severe reflux stricture. It exceeds 3·0 cm in length.

It seems likely, therefore, that more than one mechanism may be responsible for the actual transformation of the lower oesophageal epithelium to the columnar variety in response to prolonged reflux damage. The commonest complication of Barrett's oesophagus is stricture formation at the squamocolumnar junction. The development of large Barrett's ulcers may lead to massive haemorrhage. There is an undoubted association between Barrett's oesophagus and the development of carcinoma which is identified in some 10% of patients with this disorder. The risk is especially high in individuals with intestinal change, type IIB (incomplete) where the cells are dedifferentiated, exhibit severe dysplasia and produce an abnormal mucin (sulphomucin) instead of the normal sialomucin.

The treatment of Barrett's oesophagus depends on the pathological changes which have developed and ranges from oesophageal dilatation and antireflux procedures to oesophagectomy. The latter is indicated in patients with severe dysplasia/carcinoma-in-situ. Some reports have shown that the columnar lining may again be replaced by squamous epithelium following a successful antireflux operation.

Clinical Features

The typical reflux symptoms are heartburn, regurgitation and dysphagia. Symptoms are aggravated by posture and can be especially severe at night, after large meals and activities which increase the intra-abdominal pressure, e.g. bending, stooping, gardening, etc. Other symptoms which may occur include pain on swallowing hot or spicy foods (odynophagia) and waterbrash. Dysphagia may be due to spasm or oedema of the inflamed lower oesophagus in which case it remits with improvement of the oesophagitis consequent on medical treatment. Persistent dysphagia indicates stricture formation. A scoring system (*Table* 65.4) introduced by DeMeester is very useful for assessing the extent of symptomatic severity.

Table 65.4 DeMeester's scoring system for symptoms of gastro-oesophageal reflux

Symptoms	*Grade*	*Description*
HEARTBURN		
None	0	No heartburn
Minimal	1	Occasional episodes
Moderate	2	Reason for medical visit
Severe	3	Interference with daily activities
REGURGITATION		
None	0	No regurgitation
Minimal	1	Occasional episodes
Moderate	2	Predictable on position or straining
Severe	3	Episodes of pulmonary aspiration with chronic nocturnal cough or recurrent pneumonitis
DYSPHAGIA		
None	0	No dysphagia
Minimal	1	Occasional episodes
Moderate	2	Requires fluids to clear
Severe	3	Episode of meat impaction requiring medical treatment

Atypical presentation with chest pain which can closely mimic coronary heart disease and with pulmonary symptoms including asthma, is common and was discussed earlier in this chapter.

The important and clinically useful tests in establishing a diagnosis are barium swallow, pH monitoring and flexible endoscopy with biopsy. Oesophageal manometry is used to locate the HPZ prior to insertion of the pH probe or telemetric capsule but in itself, it is of limited use for the diagnosis of gastro-oesophageal reflux although it is valuable in assessing the efficacy of surgical treatment. The main reason for the barium swallow is to demonstrate the presence, type and size of any associated hiatal hernia. Endoscopy is mandatory in all patients with reflux symptoms and should be performed prior to commencement of therapy and must be accompanied by biopsy. The endoscopic grading of the severity of the oesophagitis is shown in *Table* 65.5.

Table 65.5 Endoscopic grading of oesophagitis

GRADE I	Distal erythema and mucosal friability
GRADE II	Superficial necrosis and linear ulcerations
GRADE III	Confluent or circumferential areas of deep ulceration
GRADE IV	Extensive mucosal necrosis and ulceration with stenosis

Treatment of Reflux Oesophagitis

Uncomplicated Disease

Management is conservative in the first instance and is designed to minimize reflux episodes, to reduce chemical damage by specific therapy and improve oesophageal motility and clearance.

The patient's co-operation is essential in achieving weight reduction and abstinence from smoking and alcohol. Large meals are to be avoided and replaced with frequent small dry snacks with fluids taken in between meals. The last meal must be taken some 3 hours before sleep. Antacids, when prescribed, are taken 1 hour after meals and at bed time. The patient is advised to sleep propped-up as near to 45° as possible by using several pillows. To avoid sliding down the bed, 20-cm blocks are placed under the foot of the bed (*Fig.* 65.22).

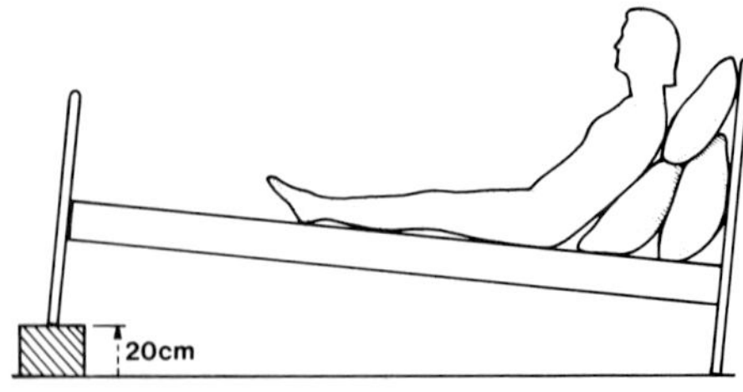

Fig. 65.22 The patient is advised to sleep propped-up as near to 45° as possible by using several pillows. To avoid sliding down the bed, 20-cm blocks are placed under the foot of the bed.

Most patients with moderate to severe symptoms from acid reflux respond well to antacid–alginate combinations such as Gaviscon. The alginic acid acts by forming a raft on the gastric juice, thereby preventing or minimizing reflux. The addition of a motility-promoting agent such as metoclopramide or domperidone is useful. These drugs may improve oesophageal clearance and sphincter tone in addition to promoting gastric emptying. Initial studies with cisapride indicate that this prokinetic drug may be very useful in patients with reflux oesophagitis by enhancing oesophageal motility and sphincter tone.

H_2-receptor blockers (cimetidine, ranitidine) which are administered in full doses for 6 weeks, can be very effective but must not be administered unless endoscopy has been performed and gastric carcinoma excluded. Initially they were reserved for resistant or severe cases when the above medications had failed. However, they are rapidly becoming the first-line treatment for established reflux oesophagitis in many centres. Recent trials have shown that combined therapy with alginate and an H_2-receptor blocker gives better results than treatment with either agent alone.

The conservative management of neutral/alkaline reflux after gastric surgery (especially total and Polya gastrectomy) is difficult and seldom effective. The administration of bile-salt-binding agents such as aluminium hydroxide gel or cholestyramine may help temporarily. However, medical treatment is usually unsuccessful in the long term and surgical intervention is required in these patients.

Surgical Treatment

The indications for surgical intervention are:

- Failure of medical therapy with persistence of severe/intractable symptoms
- Development of complications
- Patients with neutral/alkaline reflux.

The antireflux surgical procedures used nowadays share two common objectives: the restoration of a good intra-abdominal segment of the oesophagus and the creation of a valve or flap at the lower end of the oesophagus. In this respect, repair of the diaphragmatic hiatus is not essential for a good result and is considered unnecessary unless the hiatal opening is very large. Acid-reducing operations such as vagotomy are not indicated. The two most commonly used procedures are the Nissen fundoplication and the Belsey Mark IV repair. Other operations include the Hill posterior gastropexy, insertion of the Angelchick prosthesis and the Collis gastroplasty.

Nissen Fundoplication

This procedure is designed to create a circumferential 3–5 cm wrap of gastric fundus around the mobilized abdominal oesophagus. The vagal trunks are preserved but the left gastric artery is divided as it arches to form the lesser omental arcade. Mobilization of the fundus entails division of the upper short gastric vessels and any adhesions between the posterior surface of the upper stomach and the pancreas. Crural repair is performed with interrupted non-absorbable sutures but this is optional. The fundoplication sero-muscular sutures of non-absorbable material include the oesophageal wall and the uppermost one, the anterior margin of the diaphragmatic hiatus (*Fig.* 65.23). This prevents slipping of the wrap which is a serious complication as it causes an hour-glass constriction of the stomach. The wrap must be loose (floppy Nissen) to avoid dysphagia and dehiscence of the wrap. In order to ensure this, a size 35 F orogastric tube is inserted before the crural and fundoplication sutures are tied. The operation is most commonly performed through the abdomen and has the advantage of access to other upper intra-abdominal pathology which might require surgical correction at the same time, e.g. gallstones. Although an intrathoracic Nissen is performed

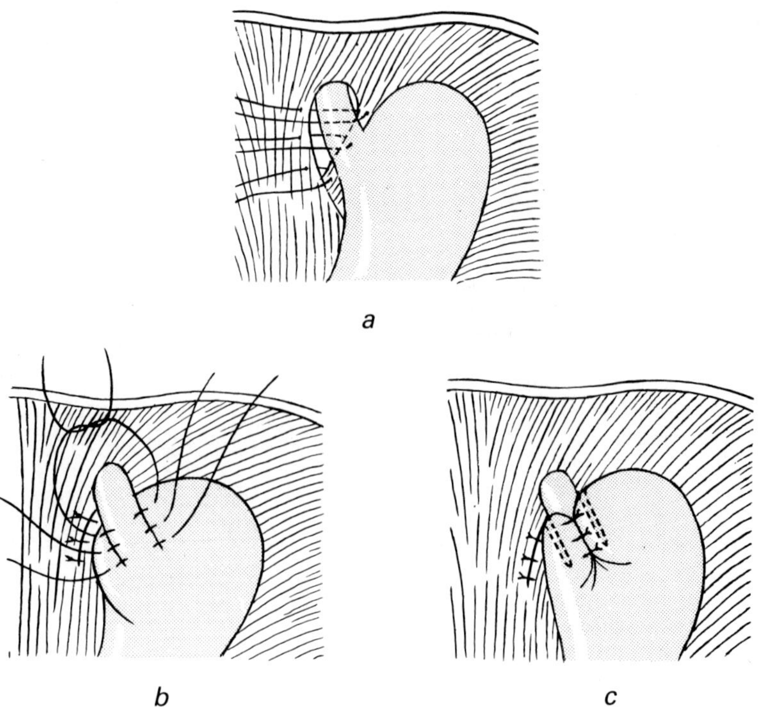

Fig. 65.23 Steps in the performance of the Nissen fundoplication: *a*, The distal oesophagus has been mobilized to restore its intra-abdominal segment and the diaphragmatic hiatus is being narrowed posteriorly. *b*, Placement of the sutures between the stomach and the oesophagus to create the 360° wrap. *c*, Fundoplication completed.

by some, this is generally regarded as less satisfactory. The main disadvantage of the classic Nissen is that it results in 'super-competence' with the development of the gas bloat syndrome in 20% of patients. This is due to gaseous distension of the stomach following the inability to belch and vomit. With a properly constructed loose Nissen, dysphagia is rarely encountered and is usually transient.

Modifications of the classic Nissen are the incomplete (270°) fundal wrap and the Rosetti–Hell procedure (*Fig.* 65.24). This creates a smaller wrap from the anterior wall of the fundus. The mobilization of the oesophagus is limited to that necessary to permit two fingers round the oesophagus. Division of the upper short gastric vessels is rarely required. The anterior fundus is brought round the oesophagus and sutured to the stomach just to the left edge of the abdominal oesophagus. The sutures do not include the oesophageal walls. Fixation of the wrap to prevent slipping is achieved by 2–3 sutures which anchor the lower edge of the wrap to the adjacent lesser curvature of the stomach. Crural repair is optional.

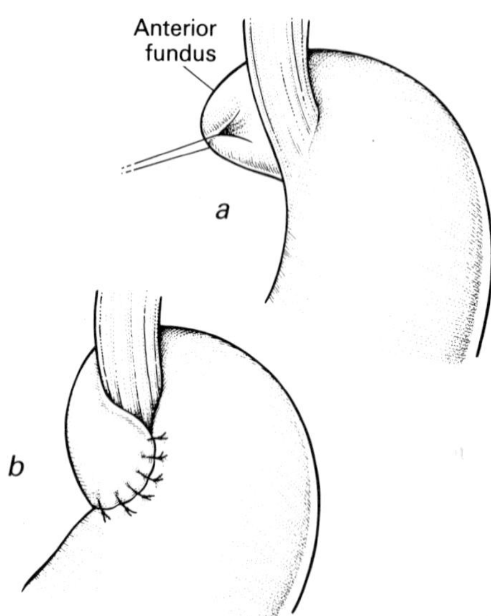

Fig. 65.24 Rosetti–Hell modification of the Nissen fundoplication. This creates a smaller wrap and consists of limited mobilization of the oesophagus and gastric fundus. The latter is then brought behind and around the right edge of the oesophagus by means of a stay suture (*a*); it is then sutured to the adjacent anterior wall of the stomach and the lower edge of the wrap is anchored tc the lesser curvature (*b*).

Belsey Mark IV Repair

The operation is performed through a left posterolateral thoracotomy through the bed of the sixth rib. The stomach is rolled around the lower 3–5 cm of the anterior two-thirds (270°) of the mobilized oesophagus by two wraps, the second burying the first and including the diaphragm. When the sutures of the second wrap are tied, the intra-abdominal segment of the oesophagus is restored (*Fig.* 65.25). With experience, this operation gives good results. Since the wrap is not circumferential, the gas bloat syndrome is not encountered. A crural repair is considered an essential component of the operation.

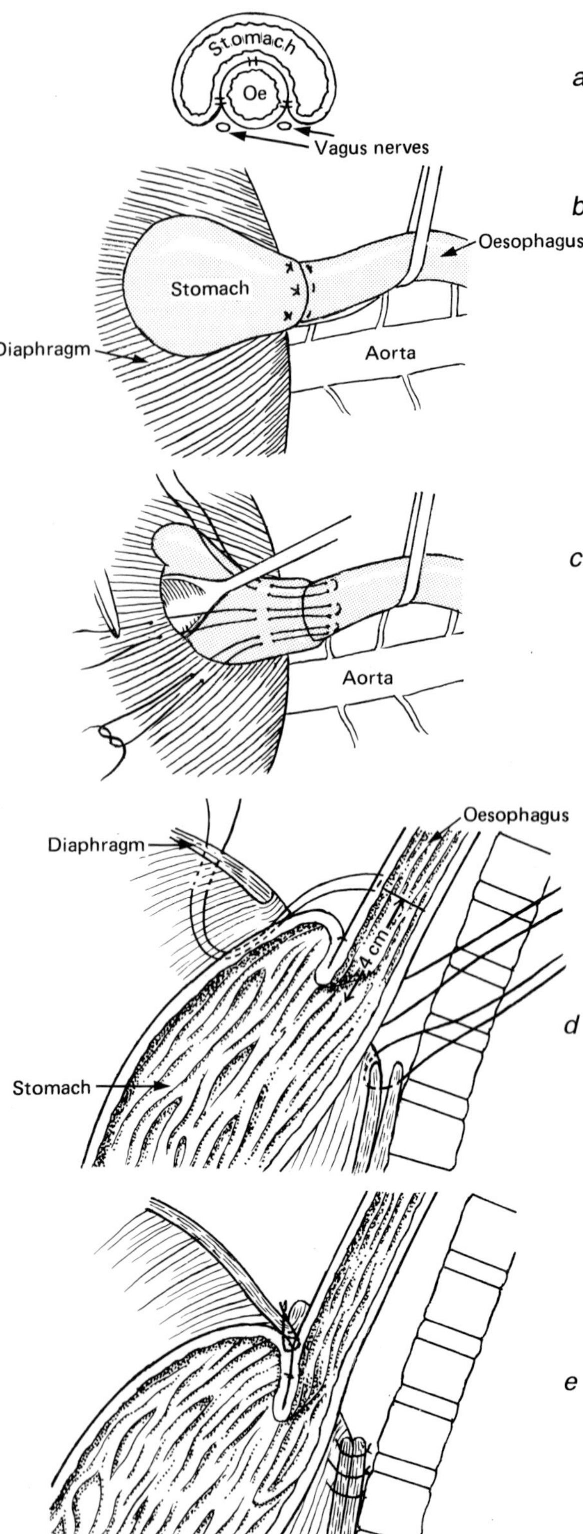

Fig. 65.25 The Belsey Mark IV repair (transthoracic). *a*, The completed 270° gastric wrap around the oesophagus (Oe). *b*, The first row of mattress sutures between the oseophagus and the stomach has been completed. *c*, Placement of the second row of mattress sutures through the diaphragm as well as stomach and oesophagus. Vertical cross-section of the repair: *d*, At time of placement of the second row of mattress sutures. *e*, At completion of the repair.

Hill Posterior Gastropexy

This procedure is always performed through the abdomen. After mobilization of the lower oesophagus, the coeliac axis is identified and the median arcuate ligament overlying the aorta is dissected. Crural repair is performed with non-absorbable sutures so that the hiatus is narrowed to an orifice which admits one finger along the oesophagus. The gastropexy is achieved by 2–3 plicating sutures which pick the cardio-oesophageal junction in front and behind the oesophagus on the medial side, in addition to the median arcuate ligament. When these sutures are tied, approximately 180° of the distal oesophagus is included in a partial gastric wrap which is fixed firmly to the arcuate ligament and pre-aortic fascia (*Fig.* 65.26). Hill employs an oesophageal manometry catheter and advocates the intraoperative monitoring of pressures during the repair to ascertain that a satisfactory narrowing of the cardia has been achieved.

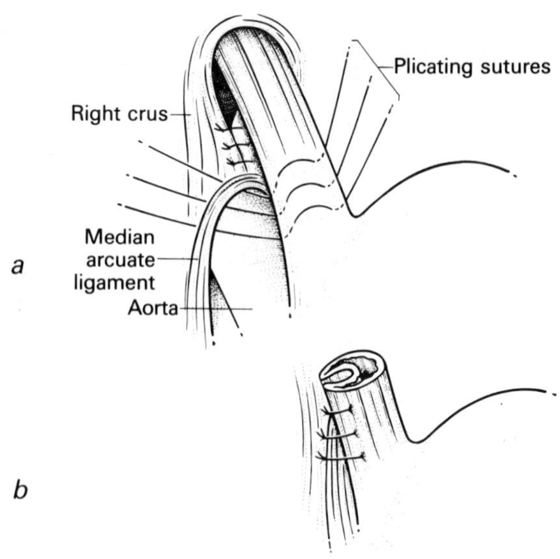

Fig. 65.26 The Hill posterior gastropexy. *a*, Crural repair has been completed. The plicating sutures in the gastro-oesophageal junction and median arcuate ligament have been inserted. *b*, The plicating sutures have been tied resulting in a 180° wrap on the medial side of the gastro-oesophageal junction which is also fixed to the median arcuate ligament.

Insertion of Angelchick Prosthesis

The prosthesis consists of an incomplete annular silicone gel-filled implant with a tape at either end. These are tied together after insertion and constitute the only anchorage (*Fig.* 65.27). It requires minimal mobilization of the oesophagus: just enough to enable insertion of the implant. Indeed, excessive mobilization favours migration of the prosthesis which weighs some 45 g. The most common displacement is distal which results in gastric obstruction. The operation is easy and quick to perform. Follow-up studies have, however, shown a high initial dysphagia rate with persistence of this distressing symptom in 8–10% of patients. This requires removal of the prosthesis as the dysphagia is unresponsive to dilatation. Erosion through the wall of the gastro-oesophageal junction is a serious complication but is fortunately rare. The risk of this eventuality is enhanced if the implant is inserted near a suture line.

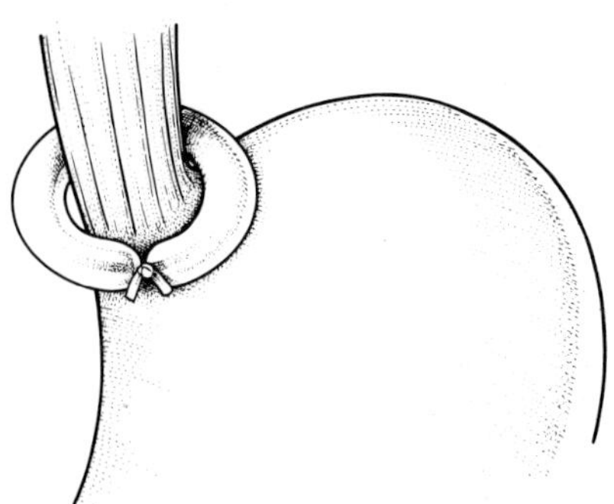

Fig. 65.27 The silicone gel Angelchick split-ring prosthesis is inserted around the gastro-oesophageal junction and the tapes tied anteriorly. Only a very limited mobilization of the oesophagus is performed.

Collis Gastroplasty

This operation was devised for patients with early strictures and shortening of the oesophagus such that its lower end cannot be replaced within the abdomen despite adequate mobilization. A tube of lesser curvature is therefore fashioned as a substitute for the intra-abdominal segment (*Fig.* 65.28). The success of the operation was initially thought to be dependent on the restoration of the cardiac angle of His. This is now known to be incorrect and experimental studies have shown that competence is due to the construction of an intra-abdominal muscular tube which is continuous with the intrathoracic oesophagus. A partial or complete gastric wrap may be added, if deemed necessary, around the neo-oesophagus.

Choice of Operation for Reflux

Aside from individual preference and experience, most general surgeons prefer the abdominal route and use the Nissen procedure or one of its modifications. Fundoplication may, however, be difficult in obese patients and those with a narrow subcostal angle and barrel-shaped chest with a deep subdiaphragmatic region. In these patients, a thoracic approach using the Belsey Mark IV is a better and safer alternative. In the author's experience, a fundoplication is difficult after a previous distal partial gastrectomy and the Hill posterior gastropexy gives better results in this situation. As a general rule, the thoracic approach is preferred in patients with severe oesophagitis, stricture formation, peri-oesophagitis and oesophageal shortening.

Treatment of Benign Strictures

The initial assessment is with radiology (barium swallow) and endoscopy. The radiological appearance may suggest malignancy but a barium swallow will misdiagnose approximately 20–25% of cancers as benign and a smaller, yet significant, number of benign lesions as malignant. Endoscopic visualization with biopsy and brush cytology is therefore essential before treatment of 'benign' oesophageal strictures. The flexible endoscope can be used not only for evaluation but also for the treatment of the stricture during the same session. If the lumen of a stricture is too narrow to permit passage of the endoscope through it, then endoscopy with biopsy must be repeated after preliminary dilatation.

Relief of dysphagia can usually be accomplished by dilatation and with the equipment available nowadays, it is unusual to encounter a stricture which cannot be dilated.

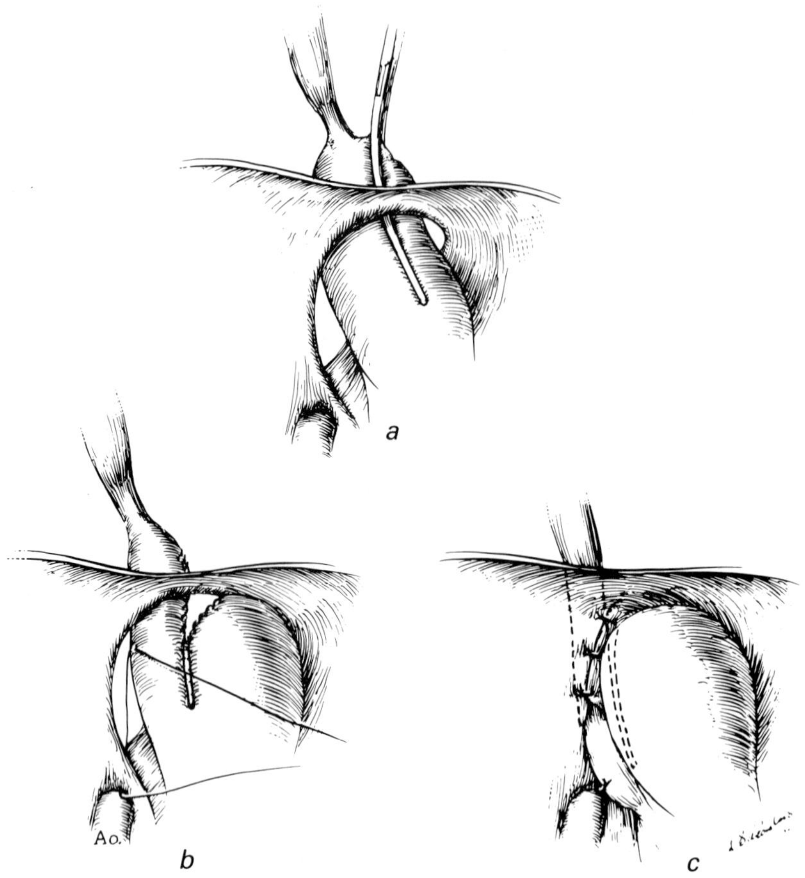

Fig. 65.28 The Collis gastroplasty. The oesophageal stricture is dilated intraoperatively. A tube is cut from the lesser curve side of the stomach. This intra-abdominal gastric tube acts as the lower oesophageal segment. It demonstrates a high-pressure zone on manometry and reflux is corrected.

However, the severe, long, tortuous strictures often pose problems, their dilatation is attended by an increased risk of perforation and they recur quickly following this treatment. The various types of dilating systems which are used are shown in *Table* 65.6. Although the mercury-tipped bougies are extremely safe and require only pharyngeal anaesthesia, they impose a burden on the patient who has to be instructed on their repeated use and many patients experience difficulty in swallowing them. The flexible endoscope systems using guidewire-guided dilators of the Puestow, Celestin or the pneumatic type have largely replaced the use of the rigid endoscope and passage of rigid dilators without guidewires (gum elastic, teflon-tipped, etc.) for the dilatation of oesophageal strictures.

Table 65.6 Dilating systems

Procedure	*Comment*
Rigid oesophagoscopy with rigid dilators without guidewire	Requires general anaesthesia, higher risk of perforation
Flexible endoscopy with guidewire-guided dilators: Puestow, Celestin, Gruntzig	Can be performed under sedation, lower risk of perforation
Non-rigid dilators: mercury-weighted rubber (e.g. Maloney)	Self-administered, lowest risk of perforation. Ineffective for severe strictures, poor patient compliance

Dilatation of a stricture should be gradual and should stop if there is discomfort or significant resistance is encountered. However, minor bleeding is not an indication to stop a dilatation session. For severe strictures, the dilatation requires to be gradual and the procedure necessitates two or more sessions with rest intervals of 1–2 weeks. During each session, dilatation should not exceed 3–4 dilator sequences corresponding to a 6–8 mm increase in diameter. This approach reduces considerably the risk of perforation.

A period of complete starvation of 6 hours is necessary after dilatation. Most also advocate a chest radiograph before oral ingestion is resumed. The complications of dilatation include haemorrhage, perforation and sèpticaemia. It is particularly important to remember that all patients with valvular heart disease should be covered with amoxycillin before endoscopy and dilatation of oesophageal strictures.

Although there is universal agreement that dilatation is the first-line treatment in patients with dysphagia due to a benign oesophageal stricture, there is considerable controversy regarding the subsequent treatment, the options for which include:

Medical and postural anti-reflux measures
Further dilatation as necessary
Anti-reflux surgery
Resection of the stricture or bypass
Long-term intubation of the stricture.

Once adequate dilatation is achieved, the results of published series with postural and medical therapy are variable: 20–50% of patients achieve a satisfactory result defined as freedom from dysphagia. A further 20% of patients will require frequent dilatations. Although some advocate anti-reflux surgery for all patients with reflux strictures if they are fit enough for surgery, this policy is debatable. Obviously clinical judgement is the important factor in case selection for surgery and management is best tailored to the individual case. There is a cohort of patients who by virtue of old age or severe cardiorespiratory disease are unfit for surgery. Medical treatment with repeated dilatation as necessary should be persisted with in these patients. If this fails either because the stricture is severe and intractable or because it requires frequent dilatations, then serious consideration should be given to intubation with an endoprosthesis which can be inserted endoscopically, such as the Atkinson system. In fit patients, the indications for surgery are:

Young patients with reflux strictures
Frequent and especially increasingly difficult dilatations
Intractable/impassable stricture
Stricture associated with Barrett's oesophagus.

Surgical Treatment of Reflux Strictures

These operations are performed through a left posterolateral or left thoraco-abdominal approach. The oesophagus is carefully mobilized from the arch of the aorta where the peri-oesophagitis is usually less severe, down to the cardia and an operative dilatation of the stricture is performed by asking the anaesthetist to pass large Maloney or gum elastic bougies starting with 35 F and progressing gradually to 60 F. The negotiation of the stricture by the bougies is guided by the surgeon's hand. Once the stricture is dilated and there is enough length of oesophagus to reduce the gastro-oesophageal junction below the diaphragm, a standard antireflux procedure such as the Belsey Mark IV or the Nissen fundoplication is performed. If there is significant oesophageal shortening which precludes restoration of the oesophageal junction below the diaphragm despite mobilization, two options are available. The first is the use of the Collis gastroplasty to create a neo-oesophagus with the stomach tube and have an intra-abdominal segment around which a wrap is formed. Alternatively, some advocate the formation of a complete Nissen fundoplication with the lower oesophagus left in the chest. The approach is not generally favoured but still has its advocates.

The *Thal fundic* patch (with or without skin cover) and a gastric wrap is shown in *Fig.* 65.29. It is reserved for severe strictures which cannot be dilated. The stricture is incised

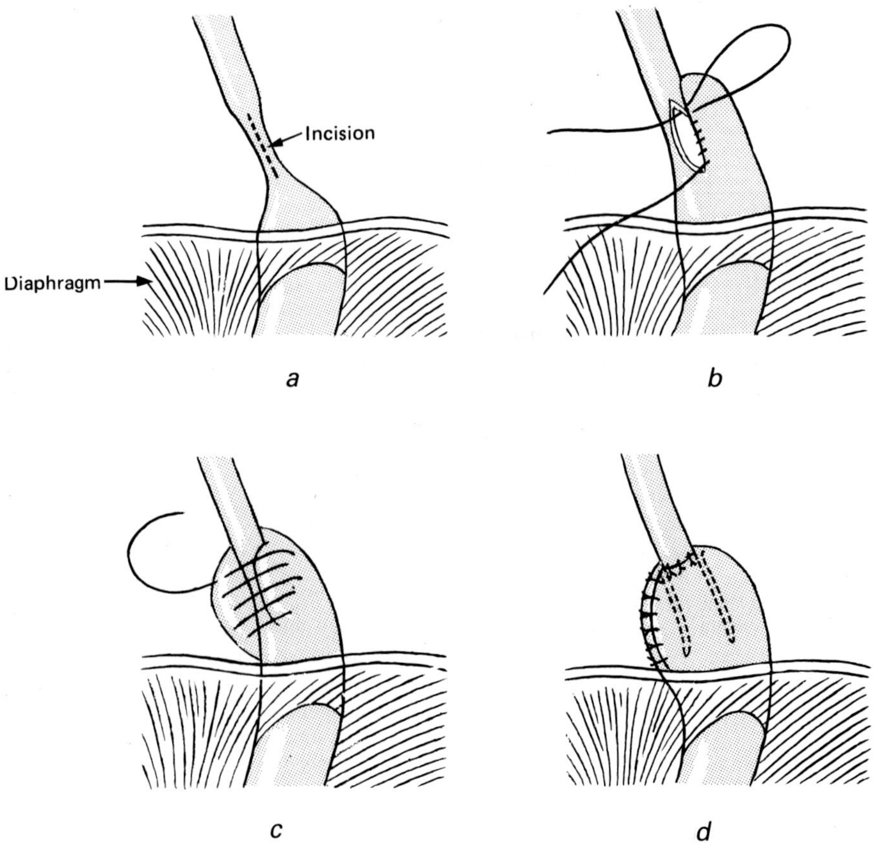

Fig. 65.29 The Thal fundic patch operation for distal oesophageal stricture. *a*, Incision and dilatation of stricture. *b*, Oesophageal defect covered by gastric serosa. *c*, Full fundoplication to prevent further reflux. *d*, Completed procedure.

longitudinally and the lumen of the oesophagus allowed to gape open. The mobilized fundus of the stomach is applied as a serosal patch to the margins of the opening in the distal oesophagus. A skin graft on the gastric serosa corresponding to the area of the oesophagus to be patched, is said to improve healing of the patch. Resection of these severe impassable strictures with replacement by interposed isoperistaltic jejunum or colon (*Fig.* 65.30) is nowadays considered preferable to the Thal fundic patch as it gives better long-term results.

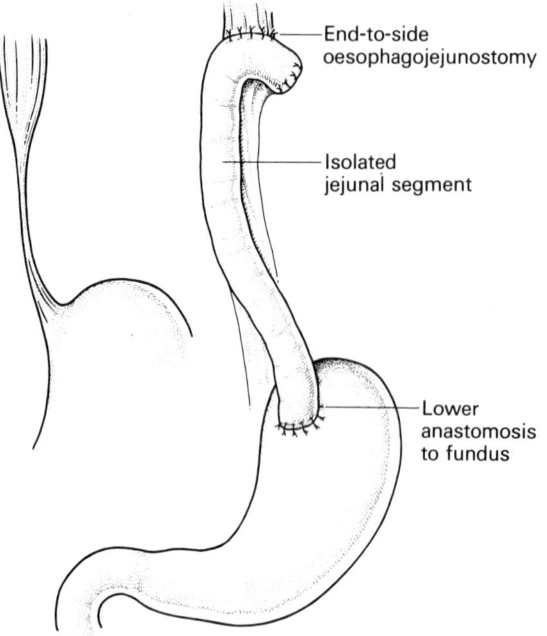

Fig. 65.30 Replacement of a severe intractable stricture with a loop of isoperistaltic jejunum isolated on a vascular pedicle. Following resection, the jejunal segment is interposed between the oesophagus and the stomach. Alternatively, a loop of colon can be used to restore continuity.

NON-REFLUX OESOPHAGITIS

The classification of non-reflux induced oesophageal damage is outlined in *Table* 65.7. Some are the result of accidental or deliberate ingestion of corrosive agents. The commonest infective oesophagitis seen nowadays is due to monilia infestation. Iatrogenic oesophageal damage may be drug induced or follow radiotherapy or insertion of a nasogastric tube. There are well documented cases of the development of severe strictures after nasogastric intubation but considering the frequency of usage of this procedure in general surgery, this complication is very rare although transient oesophagitis is very common.

Corrosive Oesophagitis

The ingestion of solid or liquid caustic agents is accidental in children, but in adults it usually represents attempted suicide in psychiatrically disturbed patients. The most common chemicals which are swallowed are alkaline caustics, acids and household bleaches. The alkaline caustics consist of sodium hydroxide (the active ingredient in household lye and drain cleaners), sodium carbonate (washing soda),

Table 65.7 Non-reflux oesophagitis

Type	*Causative agent*	*Clinical features*
CORROSIVE	Lye, acid, sodium hypochlorite, etc.	Burns, stricture, motility disorders, reflux disease
INFECTIVE	Candidosis	Occurs in chronic illnesses, immunosuppressive or antibiotic therapy, secondary to other oesophagitis
	Herpes virus	Occurs in debilitated, immunosuppressed patient particularly with lymphoproliferative disorders
DRUG INDUCED	Tetracycline, NSAIDs, doxycycline, etc	Higher incidence in patients with motility disorders and reflux disease
RADIATION	Doses greater than 20–40 Gy to the mediastinum if combined with adriamycin or actinomycin D	Ulceration and stricture formation, may simulate recurrence of neoplasm
SPECIFIC DISORDERS		Bullous dermatoses, Behçet's syndrome, Crohn's disease, aphthous oesophagitis, etc.

sodium metasalicylate (dishwashing detergent) and ammonia water (household cleaners). Oesophageal burns have also been reported following the ingestion of Clinitest tablets which contain a significant amount of anhydrous sodium hydroxide. Severe damage also results in children who swallow small alkaline batteries which consist of 45% potassium hydroxide of approximately 8 M.

These corrosive substances cause an initial burn with necrosis of the mucosa and underlying tissues, the extent of which is proportional to the concentration, amount and duration of tissue contact. In general, however, acid ingestion results in a higher incidence of stricturing and mortality which is reported to be 18% as opposed to 2% following ingestion of lye. The severity of the burn is classified as follows:

First degree: mucosal hyperaemia
Second degree: Transmucosal ulceration
Third degree: Deep ulceration, mediastinal, pleural or peritoneal perforation.

All ingested corrosives commonly affect other sites in addition to the oesophagus: oropharynx, larynx, stomach, duodenum and jejunum (rare). The oesophageal/gastric involvement may be total or segmental. In severe injuries, necrosis of the tracheal wall leads to the early development of a tracheo-oesophageal fistula which, unless recognized early and treated by prompt surgical intervention, carries a prohibitive mortality.

The burn wound progresses through acute, subacute and chronic cicatricial stages. The acute inflammatory phase occurs in the first few days following injury and is characterized by tissue coagulation, inflammatory reaction, vascular thrombosis and secondary bacterial infection. During the subacute phase which may last up to two weeks (depending on the severity of the injury), all necrotic tissues are lysed and replaced by granulation tissue. The injured oesophagus is potentially weakest during this intermediate phase (7–14 days post-injury). Symptoms of pain and dysphagia may well improve or disappear during this period. The process of epithelization is usually complete by the third to the sixth week following the injury. Maturation and contraction of the fibrous tissue results in the formation of strictures which may be multiple, short or long (tubular). At times, the fibrosis is not circumferential and on contraction, this leads to a shelf stricture. Other long-term consequences of severe corrosive oesophagitis are the development of carcinoma of the oesophagus, motility disorders of the oesophagus, hiatus hernia and gastro-oesophageal reflux. The latter is held responsible for strictures which develop years after the injury. Although there is evidence for the association between corrosive strictures and the development of oesophageal carcinoma, the risk appears small and does not justify prophylactic excision. Careful long-term follow-up of all patients with regular endoscopy is, however, necessary.

Treatment

The early management consists of assessment of the extent and severity of the injuries, supportive therapy, antibiotics and steroid administration. On admission, the whole of the oropharynx is carefully inspected. Substernal and back pain or abdominal signs may suggest mediastinal or intra-abdominal perforation. Hoarseness, stridor and dyspnoea suggest laryngeal oedema. The initial radiological investigations consist of a chest radiograph and abdominal films. Blood gases should be monitored sequentially and tracheostomy performed if airway obstruction or respiratory distress is severe or progresses. Systemic antibiotic therapy is started with a third-generation cephalosporin. In addition, some favour the oral administration of an antifungal agent (mycostatin) in severe injuries to prevent candida infestation. Shock is treated with intravenous fluids as necessary. Sedatives and analgesics are administered to relieve anxiety and pain. Fibreoptic endoscopy is performed within the first 24 hours to assess severity of the oesophageal injury. Antacids are administered for first-degree burns. Corticosteroids (methylprednisolone 1·0 mg/kg/day) are used for 21 days in patients with second-degree burns. These patients are kept on nil by mouth until they can swallow their saliva. Patients with third-degree burns require further investigation with Dionosil contrast swallow and on confirmation of necrosis/perforation are subjected to emergency oesophagogastrectomy. In less severely injured patients, a Dionosil swallow is rarely necessary in the early stages and is usually performed together with repeat endoscopy 3 weeks after the injury. Regular dilatation with Maloney mercury-tipped bougies is started for all patients with strictures. The optimal time for commencement of dilatation varies with the severity of the injury and is best delayed until re-epithelization is complete—from 10 days to several weeks, depending on the severity of the burn.

The indications for surgical reconstruction of the oesophagus after corrosive injury are:

Extensive persistent strictures
The need for frequent dilatations
Presence of high strictures or late fistula between the oesophagus and the tracheobronchial tree
Physical and psychological trauma to a child which may impair normal growth and development
Late oesophageal shortening with reflux oesophagitis
Severe dysplasia, carcinoma-in-situ, or invasive carcinoma during follow-up.

The surgical alternatives for patients with extensive oesophageal scarring are total oesophagectomy and its replacement with colon, isoperistaltic jejunum or stomach. When the mediastinum is frozen which is a common occurrence, the scarred oesophagus is left in situ and a bypass procedure is used. Colon bypass is generally preferred. This may consist of the mobilized right colon with an attached segment of terminal ileum which is tunnelled through the retrosternal space into the neck where the terminal ileum is then anastomosed to the proximal oesophagus while the colonic end of the graft is joined to the stomach. Others prefer to use the left colon based on the ascending branch of the left colic artery. Again, the colon is passed retrosternally and anastomosed end-to-end with the transected oesophagus above and to the anterior wall of the stomach as an end-to-side anastomosis below. A reversed gastric tube based proximally on the greater curvature of the stomach and receiving its blood supply from the left gastro-epiploic artery, is used when the colon proves unsuitable for oesophageal reconstruction because of anatomical abnormalities. The reversed gastric tube is also tunnelled retrosternally to the neck for anastomosis with the cervical oesophagus.

OESOPHAGEAL PERFORATIONS

The terms 'perforation' and 'rupture', although semantically different, are used synonymously with respect to oesophageal injuries. These terms do not, however, include postoperative suture line dehiscence. Perforation of the oesophagus constitutes a serious life-threatening condition which is accompanied by a high morbidity, prolonged hospital stay and an appreciable mortality. Survival depends on prompt recognition and early surgical intervention for the majority of cases, although there is a place for conservative management in selected cases.

Pathology

The categories of oesophageal perforations are outlined in *Table* 65.8, the commonest cause being endoscopy especially when associated with dilatation and/or intubation of strictures. The incidence of oesophageal perforation following

Table 65.8 Oesophageal perforations

IATROGENIC	Instrumental Postoperative
SWALLOWED FOREIGN BODIES	
EXTERNAL TRAUMA	Usually penetrating
CORROSIVE INGESTION	
SPONTANEOUS	Neonatal Intramural haematoma (incomplete perforation) Mallory–Weiss syndrome Boerhaave syndrome
PROGRESSIVE DISEASE	Peptic ulceration Hiatus hernia Tumours

insertion of a rigid endoscope is 0·5% as opposed to 0·08% after flexible endoscopy. Dilatation considerably increases the risk, the incidence of perforation varying from 0·1% with the Maloney dilators, 0·3% with the Eder–Puestow metal olives and 1–5% after pneumatic dilatation for achalasia. The pathology of oesophageal injuries caused by dilatation is shown in *Fig.* 65.31. Postoperative perforations refer to oesophageal damage sustained during 'para-oesophageal surgery', e.g. Nissen fundoplication, abdominal vagotomy, repair of hiatus hernia. The reported incidence of oesophageal perforation during abdominal vagotomy is 0·54%. The risk factors for oesophageal iatrogenic perforation during upper abdominal surgery are oesophagitis and poor surgical exposure.

Penetrating gunshot wounds of the oesophagus are common in the USA. The cervical oesophagus is the segment most commonly involved. Most cervical oesophageal injuries due to external trauma are associated with injuries to adjacent structures: spinal cord, thyroid gland, jugular vein, carotid arteries, larynx, etc.

Overall, the thoracic oesophagus (lower end) is the most commonly affected segment (*Fig.* 65.32). Thoracic injuries also carry the worst prognosis. From the clinical standpoint, oesophageal perforation is classified into early (acute) and late (chronic). An acute perforation is one which is recognized immediately or within a few hours of its occurrence. It carries a good prognosis with a reported mortality of 10% as sepsis is not established and repair is feasible since oedema of the oesophageal wall is minimal. Late perforations denote missed injuries which are diagnosed beyond 24 hours of onset. By then, there is considerable transmural oedema of the oesophagus and this precludes safe primary suture of the tear. In addition, sepsis within the mediastinum and pleural cavity is well established and the patient's cardiovascular state is unstable from septic shock. The reported mortality of late perforations ranges from 40–60%.

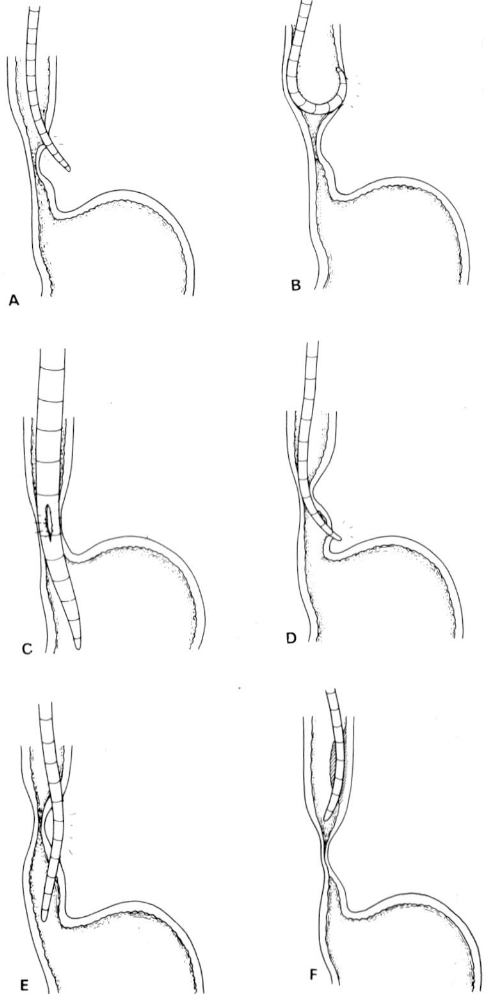

Fig. 65.31 Pathology of oesophageal injuries caused by dilatation. Injuries A and B are more prone to occur in the presence of ulceration or pseudodiverticula above the stricture or hiatal hernia. Injury C is especially likely to complicate pneumatic dilatation for achalasia and stenting of malignant strictures. Injury D occurs as a result of a sudden give, the tip of the dilator perforating the oesophagus or stomach distal to the stricture. This type of injury can also result from the use of the Eder–Puestow guidewire when an excess length of the wire is introduced and curls in the distal oesophagus and stomach. Perforation occurs as the dilator is pushed down coaxially along the curved guidewire. Injury E has a re-entry hole in the distal oesophagus and occurs in relation to strictures affecting the midoesophagus or higher, particularly malignant lesions. Injury F is an incomplete one (intramural haematoma, dissection) and usually occurs in the cervical oesophagus at, or just distal to, the cricopharyngeus; it is often caused by the endoscope, especially the rigid variety. There may or may not be a re-entry hole lower down. (Reproduced from *Surgery of the Oesophagus* (Hennessy and Cuschieri) by courtesy of Baillière, Tindall Ltd.)

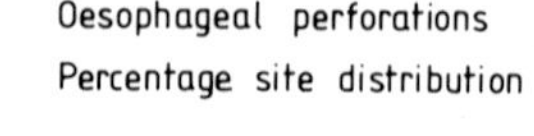

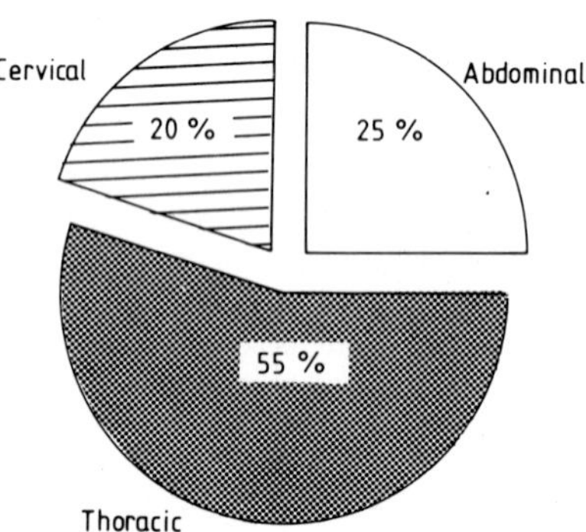

Fig. 65.32 Pie chart showing frequency distribution of the site of oesophageal perforations.

Clinical Features

The early manifestations are pain, tachycardia and fever. The site of the pain and its radiation vary with the oesophageal segment involved. The pain is, however, always severe. Patients with cervical injuries often develop a nasal voice and may have dysphagia. Haematemesis may also be found in cervical perforations. This is also a feature of incomplete injuries of the thoraco-abdominal segment. Supraclavicular swelling and crepitus (surgical emphysema) are observed in 60% of cervical and 30% of mid-oesophageal injuries. In thoracic injuries, respiratory distress is common and is accompanied by dullness on percussion and diminished air entry and breath sounds on the affected side (effusion). Upper abdominal tenderness with rebound and infrequent or absent bowel sounds indicate perforation of the abdominal segment of the oesophagus. However, these abdominal signs may be absent with small perforations (e.g. guidewire-induced, small unrecognized tears during para-oesophageal surgery) and the first intimation of this complication may be the development of a subphrenic abscess.

In late perforations, clinical evidence of established sepsis is present with fever, cardiovascular instability or fully developed septic shock. The infection is polymicrobial with aerobic and anaerobic organisms. The diagnosis is confirmed by plain and contrast radiology. Plain radiographs (neck, PA and lateral chest) are frequently diagnostic but may not accurately localize the perforation. The radiological features include presence of surgical emphysema in the mediastinum (*Fig.* 65.33) or neck, widening of the mediastinum and an increased distance between the trachea and the vertebral column. Irregularity of the mediastinal air interface is a radiological sign of mediastinitis. Free air beneath the diaphragm may be detected in patients with injuries to the abdominal oesophagus.

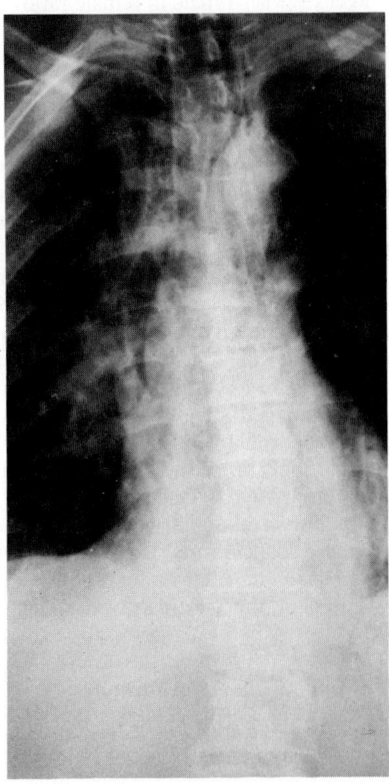

Fig. 65.33 Plain radiograph of the chest showing surgical emphysema in the mediastinum following oesophageal perforation.

A contrast swallow (*Fig.* 65.34) is always required in patients with suspected oesophageal perforation. Gastrografin is most commonly employed although Dionosil is safer. If the Gastrografin swallow is inconclusive, the investigation should be repeated with barium, in which case any extravasated barium is evacuated by suction at operation. Endoscopy is not required for complete injuries but is indicated when clinical suspicion persists despite negative contrast studies, e.g. bloodstained nasogastric aspirate or frank haematemesis. Its main indications are:

Diagnosis of incomplete (intramural) perforation and Mallory–Weiss syndrome.

Retrieval of foreign bodies and endoscopic control of bleeding.

Assessment of the burn severity after ingestion of corrosive agents.

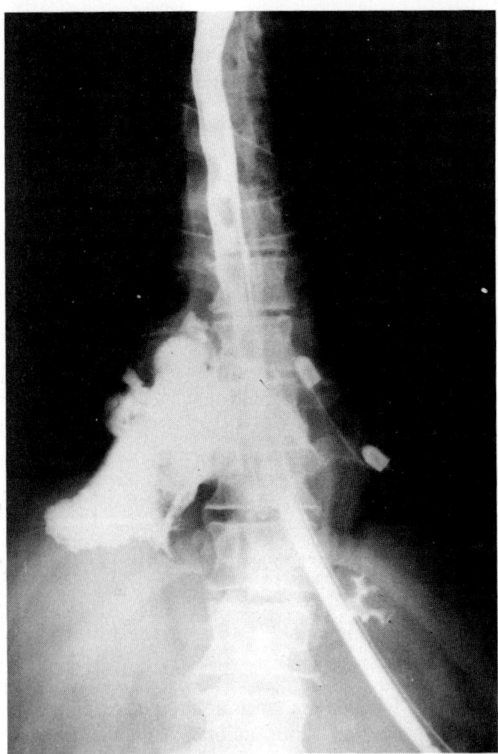

Fig. 65.34 Gastrografin swallow outlining perforation of the lower oesophagus.

Neonatal and Paediatric Oesophageal Perforations

Neonatal perforations are rare and may be traumatic or spontaneous. Both occur more commonly in premature babies and are attended with a substantial mortality, 19% for the traumatic variety and 33% for spontaneous perforation. The main distinguishing features of the two conditions are shown in *Table* 65.9.

Oesophageal injuries in children are either iatrogenic following dilatation or result from ingestion of foreign bodies and corrosive agents. The range of foreign bodies swallowed is extreme and includes coins, pins, aluminium 'pop tops', alkaline pencil batteries, etc. Unless corrosive in nature, the symptoms following ingestion of foreign bodies may be delayed several weeks to months. The swallowed object gradually burrows through the oesophageal walls and adjacent tissue often leading to the development of a tracheo-oesophageal fistula and respiratory infection. Pyrexia and persistent cough are common presenting features and paradoxically, dysphagia is rare. Endoscopy often fails to reveal the foreign body but may show an area of granulation tissue. Confirmation of the diagnosis is best achieved by radiology.

Table 65.9 Distinguishing features of traumatic and spontaneous oesophageal perforations in the neonate

	Traumatic	*Spontaneous*
SITE	Hypopharynx and cervical oesophagus	Distal oesophagus
PREMATURITY	30–35%	20%
SEX	Female preponderance	Equal
AETIOLOGY	Trauma: intubation, oral suction	Unknown, ?oesophagitis
CLINICAL FEATURES	Difficulty in passing gastric catheter, increased oral secretions/drooling	Respiratory distress
RADIOGRAPHIC FINDINGS	Non-specific changes on chest radiograph, posterior tract on contrast studies	Right-sided pneumothorax or hydropneumothorax
MORTALITY	19%	33%

Spontaneous Oesophageal Injuries in the Adult

The three conditions which come under this category are:

Intramural haematoma (incomplete perforation)
Mucosal laceration—the Mallory–Weiss syndrome
Complete spontaneous perforation—the Boerhaave syndrome.

Intramural Haematoma

This lesion which is extremely rare, arises as an oesophageal mucosal tear associated with submucosal bleeding with dissection of this plane by the expanding intramural haematoma. The clinical picture is said to be distinctive with a history of gagging or choking whilst eating, followed by sharp midepigastric/lower retrosternal pain radiating to the back and associated with haematemesis. A contrast swallow demonstrates a double-barrel oesophagogram. The condition is self-limiting and there have been no reported instances of progression to a complete perforation.

Mallory–Weiss Syndrome

This syndrome consists of painless haematemesis after vomiting, retching and straining induced by excess alcohol intake. However, there are notable and frequent exceptions to this definition. In particular, there is a high incidence of associated gastro-oesophageal disease. The Mallory–Weiss syndrome is common and accounts for 5–10% of patients undergoing endoscopy for haematemesis.

The lesion consists of a longitudinal mucosal tear involving the mucosa alone or the mucosa and submucosa on the gastric side of the oesophagogastric junction. The tear which may be single or multiple, is located on the lesser curve side in the majority of cases (85%). Associated lesions are found in 75% of patients and include hiatal hernia, oesophagitis, oesophageal varices and duodenitis/peptic ulceration. Although the bleeding stops spontaneously in the majority of patients, it may be severe and recurrent.

The condition is more often found in males (70%) and a history of alcoholism is frequently present (40–70%) but not invariable. One report showed a 20% incidence of prior aspirin ingestion. Hypovolaemia requiring blood transfusion is found in one-third of patients. The diagnosis is confirmed by upper gastrointestinal endoscopy which is delayed until resuscitation with blood transfusion is achieved in all shocked patients. The treatment is conservative with H_2-receptor blockers and antacids. Endoscopic photo- or electrocoagulation is reserved for patients with actively bleeding tears at the time of endoscopy. Surgical treatment is only indicated for those patients who continue to bleed or in whom the haemorrhage recurs after the above measures. It consists of suture ligation of the bleeding mucosal tears through a generous gastrotomy. Percutaneous embolization of the left gastric artery is used in poor-risk patients such as cirrhotic individuals.

Boerhaave Syndrome

The fatal condition of acute gastric distress, forceful vomiting, severe chest pain and collapse due to a complete tear of the lower thoracic oesophagus just above the cardia, was first described by Hermann Boerhaave in a Dutch admiral. This aristocratic gentleman succumbed in this way following a bout of overindulgence of food and drink. However, only a minority of complete spontaneous perforations of the lower thoracic oesophagus fit the classic description of Boerhaave. The condition is uncommon and occurs usually between the ages of 40–60 years with a male to female ratio of 2:1. There is frequently a long history of indigestion and chronic gastrointestinal disease such as duodenal ulcer, reflux oesophagitis and hiatal hernia. Apart from overeating, other predisposing factors include neurological disorders, tumours and gastrointestinal obstruction. The Boerhaave syndrome has also been reported during childbirth, severe convulsions and even straining during defaecation.

The manifestations consist of sudden severe epigastric pain radiating to the left chest and shoulder and upper abdomen, which develops after a violent retching episode or straining. Dyspnoea and shock rapidly supervene. The correlation between retching/vomiting and the onset of pain is only encountered in 40% of patients. Aside from the shock, physical findings include surgical emphysema in the neck, dullness and diminished air entry over the base of the left lung, tenderness and guarding in the upper abdomen and absent or infrequent bowel sounds. The condition may simulate very closely myocardial infarction, perforated peptic ulcer, pulmonary embolism, dissecting aortic aneurysm and severe acute pancreatitis with any of which it is often misdiagnosed. The chest radiograph shows a left-sided pleural effusion and the contrast swallow establishes the diagnosis.

Treatment of Oesophageal Perforations

Antibiotic therapy with a cephalosporin or aminoglycoside and metronidazole is started as soon as the diagnosis is made in addition to resuscitation with volume replacement under central venous pressure control. An underwater-seal chest drain is inserted on radiological confirmation of the presence of an effusion. A central feeding line is inserted for parenteral nutrition.

The vast majority require surgical intervention which should be carried out as soon as possible following resuscitation. There are, however, certain specific indications for adopting a conservative management. These are:

Incomplete injuries: traumatic perforation of the neonate, intramural haematoma and the Mallory–Weiss syndrome.

Complete injuries: These include minor guidewire-induced subdiaphragmatic perforation and certain thoracic perforations. The accepted criteria for a conservative

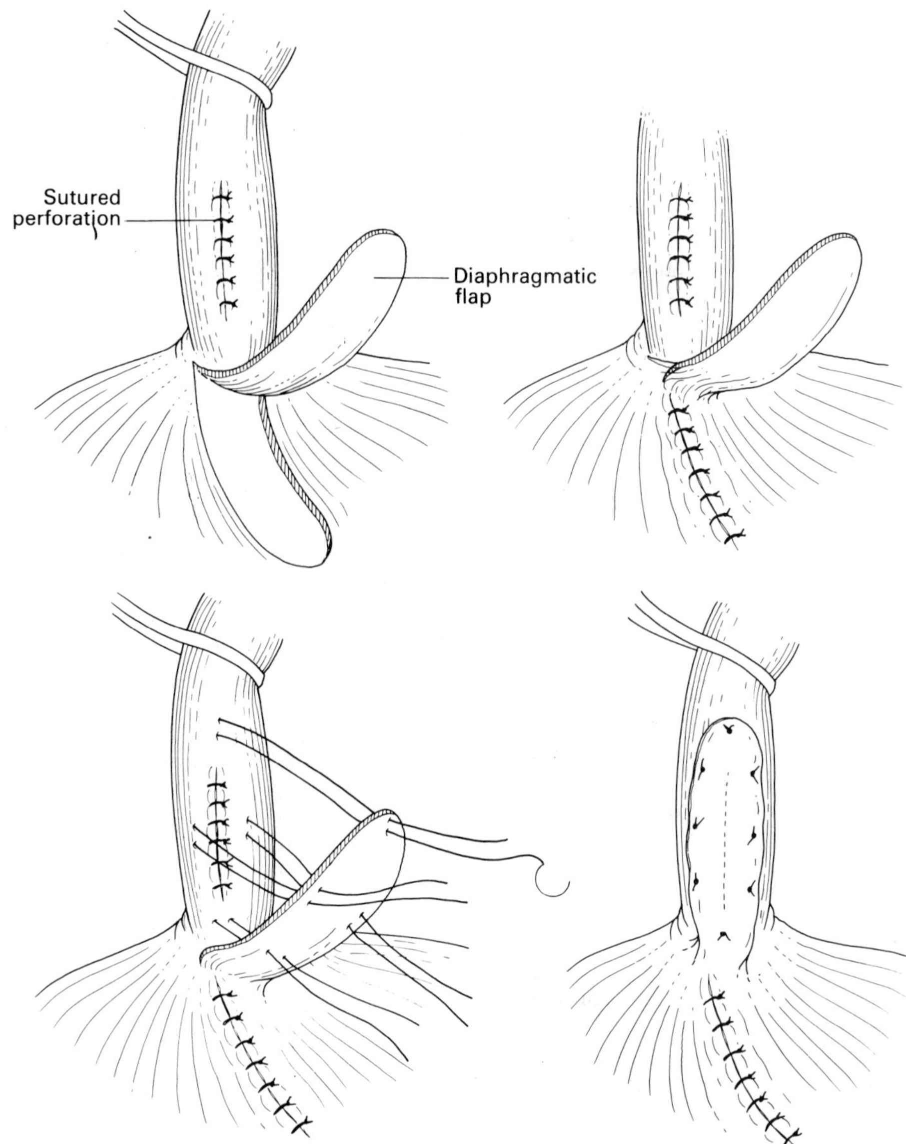

Fig. 65.35 Technique of diaphragmatic flap reinforcement of sutured oesophageal perforation. (Reproduced from *Surgery of the Oesophagus* (Hennessy and Cuschieri) by courtesy of Baillière, Tindall Ltd.)

approach in thoracic injuries are a localized perforation contained within the mediastinum or between the mediastinum and the visceral pleura, the cavity drains easily into the oesophageal lumen, minimal symptoms are present, and clinical sepsis is absent.

Conservative management entails cessation of oral food and drink, antibiotic therapy, nasogastric aspiration, parenteral nutrition and underwater-seal pleural drainage if the radiograph shows a pleural effusion. The condition of the patient is monitored closely and frequently and surgical intervention is undertaken if there is lack of progress or deterioration or the development of clinical sepsis.

Surgical Management of Oesophageal Perforations

The best results are obtained with early perforations, the mortality rising 4–5 fold if the perforation is treated surgically beyond 24 hours of onset. The approach depends on the segment of oesophagus involved: cervical injuries are approached through an incision along the anterior border of the left sternomastoid muscle, thoracic injuries through a right or left thoracotomy (depending on the exact level) and lower end/abdominal injuries through a left thoraco-abdominal approach.

Early Perforations

The surgical treatment depends on whether the perforation has occurred through an otherwise normal oesophagus or is associated with significant oesophageal disease, e.g. carcinoma, stricture. In the absence of significant oesophageal disease, the perforation is closed in layers with non-absorbable sutures and drainage established. This is sufficient for early cervical injuries but for thoracic perforations most surgeons recommend additional buttressing with pleural or intercostal flaps for high lesions and a diaphragm flap for low lesions (*Fig.* 65.35). Alternatively, the latter may be

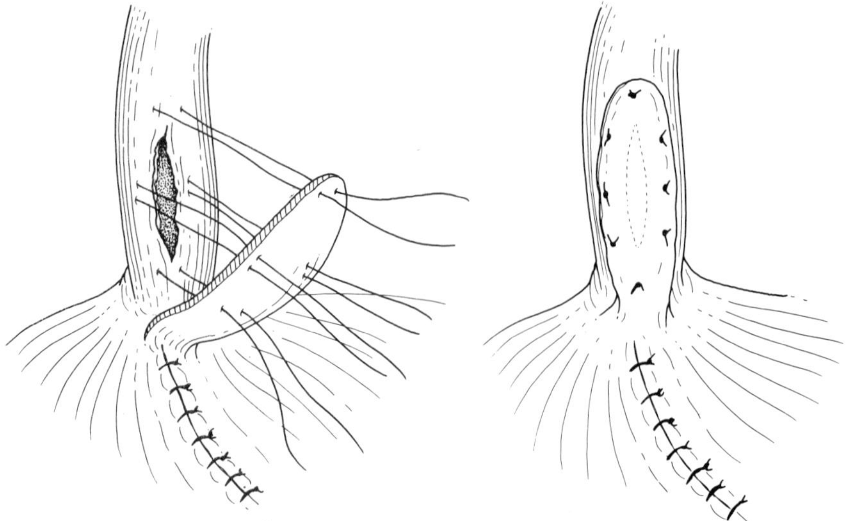

Fig. 65.36 In late perforations, the flap is used to plug the tear by sutures which are inserted from within the oesophageal lumen. (Reproduced from *Surgery of the Oesophagus* (Hennessy and Cuschieri) by courtesy of Baillière, Tindall Ltd.)

reinforced by a Thal fundal patch or a Nissen type fundoplication which is particularly useful in posteriorly placed injuries of the abdominal segment.

If the perforation is associated with significant oesophageal disease, then resection (usually oesophagogastrectomy) with primary reconstruction is performed. If the condition of the patient is precarious, the reconstruction is delayed in which case a totally diverting cervical oesophagostomy is carried out (*vide infra*) and the stomach end is closed.

Late Perforations

In late injuries direct suture of the oesophageal tear is not possible due to the severe transmural oedema. The options available are the following:

Closure of the defect with a suitable flap or gastric fundus
Oesophageal diversion with or without exclusion
Oesophageal intubation.

Closure of the defect should be attempted in lower thoracic and abdominal perforations by the use of the diaphragm flap or gastric fundus. In either event, no attempt is made to suture the perforation, the gap is either covered with a diaphragmatic flap which is sutured to healthy oesophageal wall beyond the tear (*Fig.* 65.36) or plugged with a Thal fundal patch over which a fundoplication is fashioned (*Fig.* 65.37).

Diversion is appropriate for high thoracic injuries. After pleural toilet and insertion of drains down to the perforation and in the pleural cavity, the chest is closed and a cervical oesophagostomy is performed preferably by the technique described by Ergin (*Fig.* 65.38). Some advocate diversion with exclusion for late perforations. A cervical oesophagostomy is performed and through a thoracotomy, the oesophagus is banded with Teflon distal to the perforation. Definitive treatment is carried out at a later stage if the patient survives. The disadvantage of exclusion is that a second thoracotomy is always necessary to remove the band even if the patient does not require oesophageal resection.

Oesophageal intubation is an easy alternative which is especially applicable to elderly or poor-risk patients. It entails a thoracotomy, pleural drainage and the insertion of a large T-tube (preferably silicone, size 22–24 F) into the oesophageal lumen through the perforation. Drains are also left to the mediastinum and the pleural cavity. Some surgeons advocate the repeated endoscopic application of cotton-wool pledgets soaked in 20% sodium hydroxide followed by 30% acetic acid to the edges of the perforation. Another approach consists of the insertion of a Celestin tube through the damaged oesophagus using a combined endoscopy-gastrotomy approach.

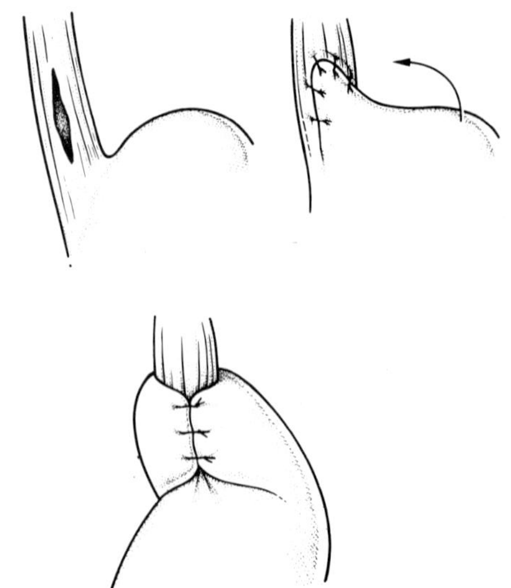

Fig. 65.37 Closure of late perforation of the lower oesophagus by a Thal fundic patch which is reinforced by a fundoplication.

THE DIAPHRAGM

The diaphragm (*Fig.* 65.39) is a dome-shaped musculotendinous structure which separates the thoracic from the abdominal cavity. It is attached anteriorly to the lower sternum, laterally to the costal margin and posteriorly (crura)

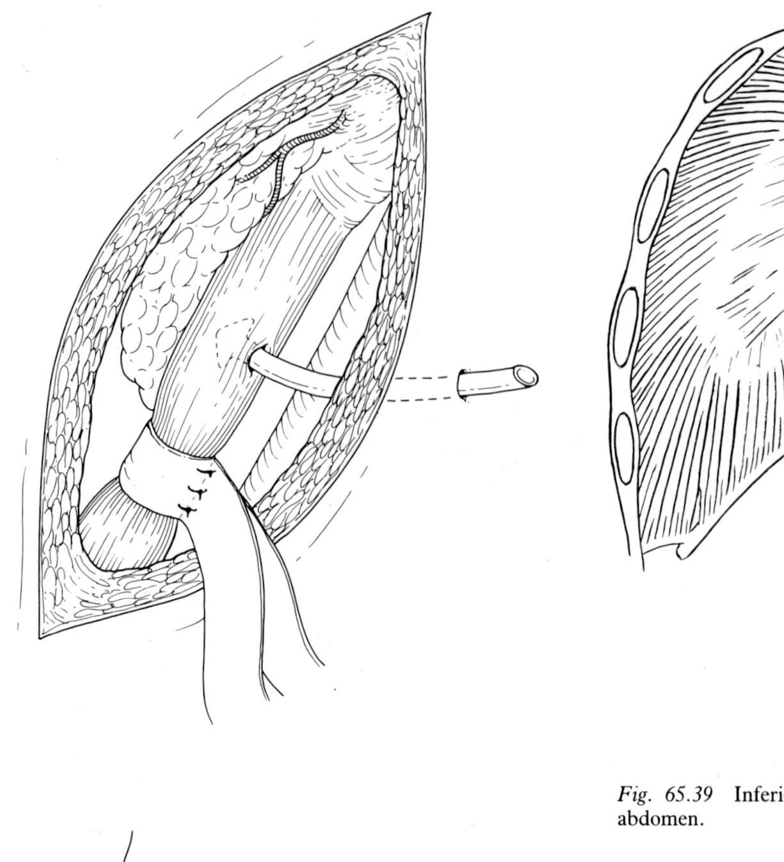

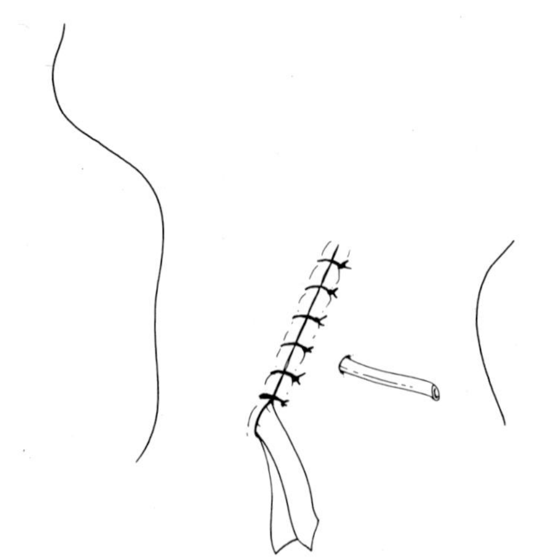

Fig. 65.38 Technique of temporary totally diverting cervical oesophagostomy. The long limbs of the band are brought out through the lower end of the incision. (Reproduced from *Surgery of the Oesophagus* (Hennessy and Cuschieri) by courtesy of Baillière, Tindall Ltd.)

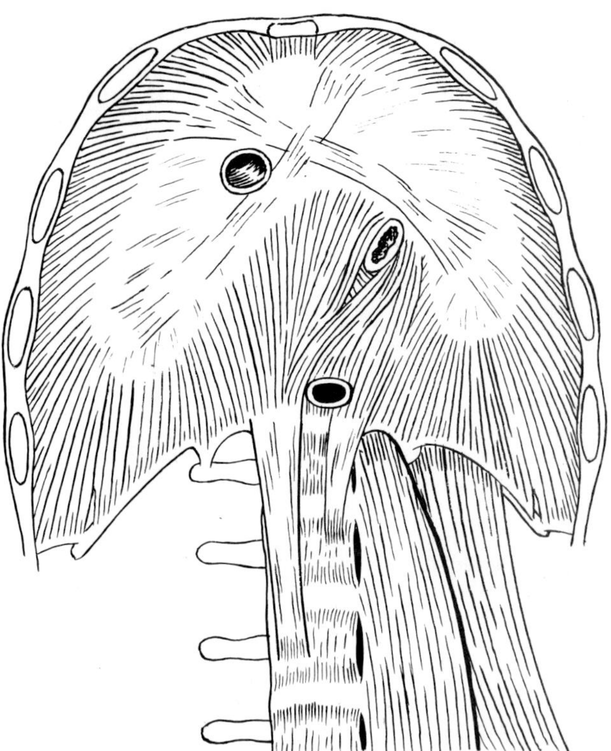

Fig. 65.39 Inferior surface of the diaphragm viewed from the abdomen.

to the first three lumbar vertebrae. The aortic hiatus (median arcuate ligament) is situated posteriorly in front of the 12th thoracic vertebra and through it pass the aorta, the thoracic duct and the azygos vein. To the left and anteriorly is situated the oesophageal hiatus at the level of the 10th thoracic vertebra (7th left costal cartilage). In the majority of individuals, the oesophageal hiatus is formed entirely by the fibres of the right crus which is more substantial than the left and arises from the bodies of the first three lumbar vertebrae and intervertebral discs. It is connected to the left crus by the median arcuate ligament after it arches over the aorta. The most common arrangement which is found in up to 60% of individuals is for the right crus to split into a large right (anterior) and a smaller left (posterior) limb. The splitting is in the ventrodorsal rather than the sagittal plane which results in a waistcoat effect and the creation of an obliquely disposed oval diaphragmatic canal rather than an orifice. The vagus nerves, oesophageal branches of the left gastric artery, veins and lymphatics accompany the oesophagus through the hiatus. Slightly to the right of the midline at the level of the 9th thoracic vertebra (6th right costal cartilage), is the vena caval foramen in the central tendon. This allows the passage of the inferior vena cava and small branches of the right phrenic nerve. The arterial blood supply to the diaphragm comes from the phrenic arteries and the lower intercostal arteries which arise directly from the aorta and the terminal branches of the internal mammary arteries.

Several other structures pass through the diaphragm. The splanchnic nerves pierce each crus, the sympathetic trunks pass behind the medial arcuate ligament, and the subcostal nerves and vessels pass behind the lateral arcuate ligament, while the left phrenic nerve pierces the left dome of the diaphragm to supply its abdominal surface. There is a rich communication between the lymphatic vessels of the posterior mediastinum and the upper abdominal lymph channels.

Congenital Diaphragmatic Hernias

The development of the diaphragm is usually complete by the 8th–10th week of intrauterine life. Congenital hernias are the result of maldevelopment of the septum transversum. The sites of congenital herniation are shown in *Fig.* 65.40.

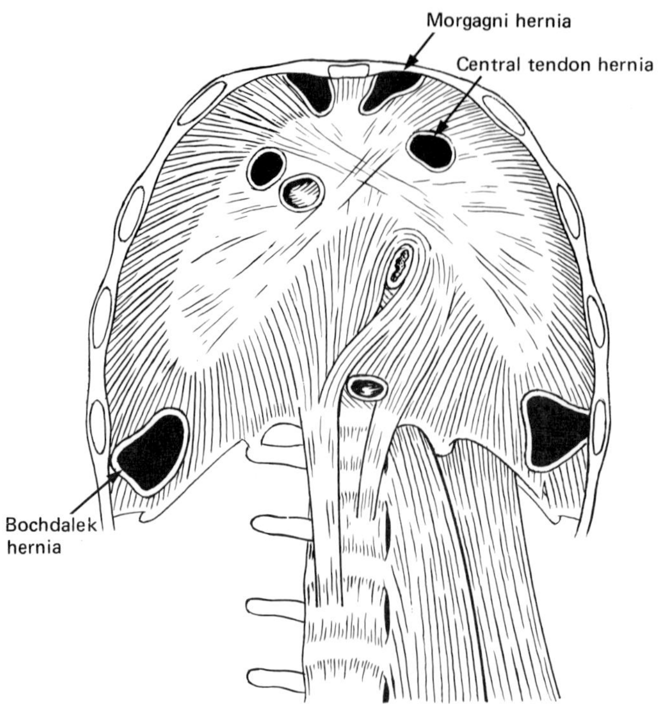

Fig. 65.40 Sites of congenital diaphragmatic hernias.

Hernia through Foramen of Bochdalek

These hernias are posteriorly situated and are due to persistence of the pleuroperitoneal canals which are the last parts of the diaphragm to close. The hernia which is usually left sided, presents acutely with respiratory distress in the neonatal period and is discussed further in Chapter 59.

Parasternal Hernia (Hernia through Foramen of Morgagni or Magendie)

This hernia is more common on the right and occurs through a triangular anterior defect lateral to the sternum between the sternal and costal attachments of the diaphragm where the superior epigastric artery, veins and lymphatics pass from the chest into the abdomen. It usually contains a loop of transverse colon but small intestine may also be found in the hernial sac. This hernia does not usually cause symptoms during infancy and childhood and presents in adult life with episodes of pain and tenderness in the right subcostal region, and intermittent obstructive symptoms. Complete intestinal obstruction may supervene. The PA chest film in these patients shows a rounded gas-containing shadow to the right of the cardiac outline. This shadow is seen to lie behind the sternum on the lateral chest film. In doubtful cases, a contrast meal is needed to confirm the diagnosis. Surgical treatment is recommended in all cases because of the risk of intestinal obstruction and strangulation. The best approach is through a midline upper abdominal incision. After reduction of the contents into the abdomen, the sac is excised and repair is performed by approximating the two diaphragmatic edges with non-absorbable interrupted sutures. Closure with a Marlex or propylene mesh is necessary for large defects.

Herniation through the Central Tendon

The deficiency in the central tendon may be situated at the apex of the right or left cupola or involve the central part in relation to the pericardium. On the right side, a hernia through the central tendon contains a mushroom-shaped portion of liver parenchyma which grows through the opening and enlarges on the thoracic surface of the diaphragm. The condition is usually diagnosed accidentally by a routine chest radiograph. It can be easily differentiated from a primary tumour of the diaphragm by ultrasound scanning. Alternatively, the induction of a pneumoperitoneum with subsequent plain radiology will demonstrate air surrounding the liver protrusion in the hernial sac. In left hernias, the fundus of the stomach usually protrudes as an air-containing 'cyst' on the top of the diaphragm. A central hernia is usually associated with a defect in the pericardium and small intestine can, therefore, herniate into the pericardial cavity.

A small defect in the central tendon on the right side does not require any treatment. However, surgical repair of the other two defects is usually recommended because of the risk of mechanical complications.

Congenital Hiatal Hernia

This is usually of the sliding type and is associated with gastro-oesophageal reflux. More rarely the hernia is of the para-oesophageal variety. Both can present in infancy and childhood.

Congenital Short Oesophagus

In the absence of congenital defects, gastro-oesophageal incompetence is often present in the neonate. The condition corrects itself spontaneously during the first few months of life probably by further development of the intra-abdominal oesophagus. True congenital shortening of the oesophagus

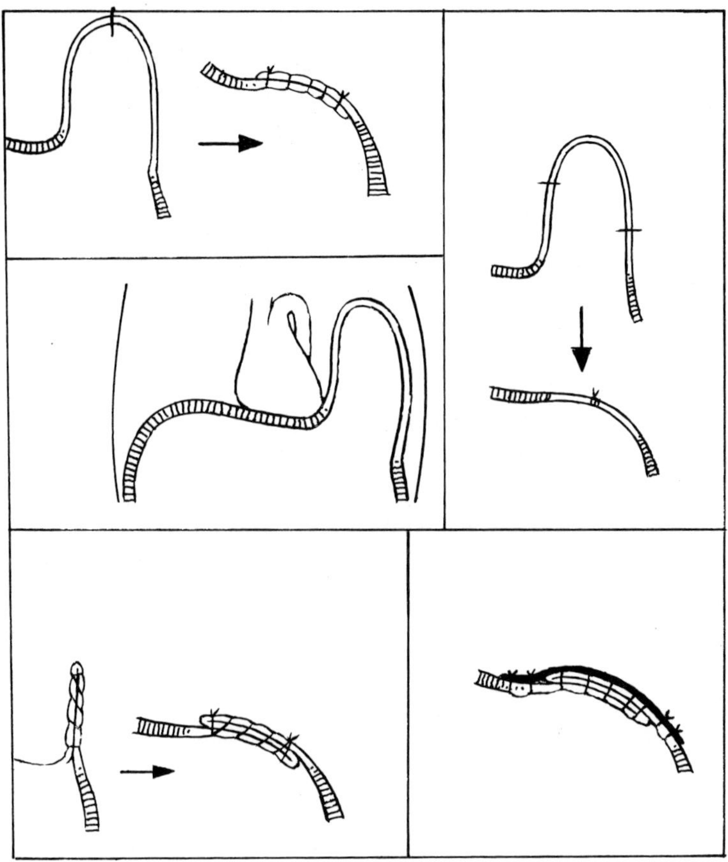

Fig. 65.41 Techniques for correction of eventration of the diaphragm.

in infancy and childhood is very rare. In this condition, the cardia and a large portion of the fundus of the stomach are situated in the mediastinum without any obvious hernial sac or sliding.

Most instances of 'congenital shortening of the oesophagus' are acquired and result from prolonged pathological reflux with fibrosis, ulceration and stricture formation. The fibrosis draws the stomach further into the chest and in extreme cases, the oesophageal stricture may be situated at the level of the aortic arch.

Whatever the aetiology, the most common symptoms are those of spontaneous regurgitation when the infant or child is in the reclining position, recurrent attacks of chest infections or asthma. Aspiration may also result in the development of a lung abscess. The condition requires treatment with an anti-reflux procedure. Most authorities favour a Collis type gastroplasty with a partial fundal wrap. Others recommend an intrathoracic Nissen.

Eventration of the Diaphragm

Anomalous congenital development of the diaphragm or its innervation may result in unilateral elevation of the diaphragm. Alternatively, phrenic nerve injury at birth or later, or injury to the diaphragm, may result in the same problem. Differentiation between eventration of the diaphragm and a large congenital hernia, especially of the Bochdalek type, may be difficult or impossible until exploration.

Eventration of the diaphragm has clinical significance only if it is associated with symptoms or when it cannot be differentiated from other serious conditions. The symptoms of eventration which are identical to those of large congenital diaphragmatic hernias may occur in the neonatal period and include respiratory distress and tachycardia with impaired cardiac function. In older children, digestive and respiratory symptoms are aggravated by obesity. In older patients, the symptoms may be minimal and management is then conservative. Surgical treatment is necessary if symptoms are severe or disabling. Approach is through a left thoracotomy. The procedures which can be used to restore the diaphragm to its normal position are illustrated in *Fig.* 65.41. They include incision or partial excision with plication of the diaphragm. In severe cases, prosthetic replacement of a very attenuated diaphragm with synthetic mesh is required.

Traumatic Diaphragmatic Hernia

Traumatic rupture of the diaphragm may result from penetrating or blunt trauma to the abdomen and chest. The tendinous portion, especially on the left side, is the usual site of laceration as the liver protects the right side of the diaphragm from most injuries except the penetrating ones. The rupture is associated with herniation of the abdominal contents and may present acutely following the injury or escape detection until several months to years later. The herniation of the abdominal viscera may occur acutely at the time of the injury or be delayed until some time after. The symptoms are related to the size of the herniated contents and to the onset of mechanical complications such as intestinal obstruction, strangulation, haemorrhage or progressive cardiorespiratory insufficiency.

The diagnosis is usually established on the plain films of the chest and abdomen when a space-occupying lesion is seen in the chest. If the omentum or spleen is the main herniated structure, the shadow appears solid. The herniated spleen is usually ruptured and accompanied by severe haemorrhage. This may result in total opacification of the left chest. Otherwise, air–fluid levels may be observed indicative of herniation of hollow viscera (colon, small intestine). Passage of a nasogastric tube identifies a herniated stomach above the diaphragm. Barium studies may be needed to confirm the diagnosis.

In acute rupture, there are often associated injuries which take precedence over the diaphragmatic injury. However, repair of the acute tear should be performed simultaneously whenever possible. The elective repair of a traumatic diaphragmatic hernia may be performed through either a left thoracotomy or an upper abdominal approach. In delayed cases, the operation may be difficult due to the presence of adhesions and/or atrophy of the damaged diaphragm. Primary repair is usually possible using interrupted non-absorbable sutures. Otherwise closure with prosthetic mesh is performed.

Further Reading

Benjamin S. B., Richter J. E., Cordova C. M. et al. (1983) Prospective manometric evaluation with pharmacological provocation of patients with suspected esophageal motility dysfunction. *Gastroenterol.* **84**, 893–901.

Campbell T. C., Andrews J. L. and Neptune W. B. (1976) Spontaneous rupture of the oesophagus (Boerhaave syndrome). Necessity of early diagnosis and treatment. *JAMA* **235**, 526–528.

Dodds W. J., Hogan W. J., Helm J. F. et al. (1981) Pathogenesis of reflux esophagitis. *Gastroenterol.* **81**, 376–394.

Ergin M. A., Wetstein L. and Giepp R. B. (1980) Temporary diverting cervical esophagostomy. *Surg. Gynecol. Obstet.* **151**, 97–98.

Goldstein L. A. and Thompson W. R. (1982) Esophageal perforations: a 15-year experience. *Am. J. Surg.* **143**, 495–503.

Hennessy T. P. J. and Cuschieri A. (ed.) (1986) *Surgery of the Oesophagus.* London, Baillière Tindall.

Ismail-Beigi F., Horton P. F. and Pope C. E. (1970) Histological consequences of gastroesophageal reflux in man. *Gastroenterol.* **58**, 163–174.

Spense R. A. J. (1984) The venous anatomy of the lower oesophagus in normal subjects and in patients with varices: an image analysis study. *Br. J. Surg.* **71**, 739–741.

Vitale G. C., Cheadle W. G., Sadek S. et al. (1984) Computerized 24-hour monitoring and esophagogastroduodenoscopy in the reflux patient: A comparative study. *Ann. Surg.* **200**, 724–728.

66 The Oesophagus: Motility Disorders, Diverticula and Tumours

A. Cuschieri

MOTILITY DISORDERS

Oesophageal motility disorders may be primary or secondary to neurological disorders (e.g. poliomyelitis, pseudobulbar palsy), myopathies (e.g. dermatomyositis), systemic disease (e.g. scleroderma) and parasitic infestations (Chagas' disease). The accepted classification of the primary oesophageal motility disorders is shown in *Table* 66.1. Controversy exists regarding the aetiology of the various primary disorders and even the separation into the various types is doubted by some since progression from one disorder to another has been documented. The differentiation of the main primary varieties is based largely on the manometric profile and on the radiological appearances of barium swallow studies. There is little doubt that primary oesophageal disorders, apart from causing distressing symptoms which affect the nutritional state and social life of the patients, carry a significant morbidity from early and late complications. The management of these patients can be difficult and surgical intervention which should not be undertaken lightly, requires careful case selection and accurate diagnosis.

Table 66.1 Classification of primary oesophageal motility disorders

SPECIFIC	Achalasia Vigorous achalasia Diffuse oesophageal spasm Nutcracker oesophagus (symptomatic oesophageal peristalsis)
NON-SPECIFIC	Hypertensive HPZ Hypo-/aperistalsis Abnormalities of peristaltic sequence

Achalasia

This is the commonest of the specific primary oesophageal motility disorders and has a reported incidence of 1:100 000 per annum. The cardinal features of the condition are:

Absence of peristaltic contractions within the oesophageal body.

Incomplete relaxation of the high-pressure zone (HPZ).

In addition, the HPZ pressure is usually elevated (>25 mmHg) and some patients exhibit an increased intra-oesophageal resting pressure relative to the gastric baseline. As both pharyngeal peristalsis and cricopharyngeal sphincter function are intact, bolus transfer into the oesophagus is normal but the oesophageal musculature lacks the ability to propel its contents down the oesophagus and into the stomach. The contractions which can be recorded manometrically are of the tertiary non-propulsive kind. The oesophageal musculature in achalasia has been shown to be hypersensitive to both cholinergic drugs (mecholyl, betanechol) and pentagastrin but this is not specific to the disease as it is also found in the majority of patients with diffuse oesophageal spasm.

Entry of food into the stomach can only occur when the hydrostatic pressure of the oesophageal contents exceeds the functional obstruction at the cardio-oesophageal junction. Passage of contents is, to limited extent, aided by intermittent intra-oesophageal pressure elevations caused by spontaneous non-peristaltic contractions. As the disease progresses, the oesophagus proximal to the constricted terminal segment, dilates and lengthens and thereby assumes a sigmoid shape in advanced cases.

This abnormal oesophageal function is the consequence of damage to the parasympathetic innervation of the oesophagus. In addition, impairment of the non-cholinergic, non-adrenergic fibres normally responsible for lower oesophageal sphincter relaxation has also been reported. Anatomical lesions have been found in the brainstem (reduction in the number and abnormalities of the cells of the dorsal motor nucleus of the vagus), the vagal fibres (Wallerian degeneration) and Auerbach's intramural plexus (mononuclear cell infiltrate, fibrosis, reduced ganglion cells and aganglionosis). However, the cause of this neuropathology and, in particular, the site of the primary lesion remain unknown.

Endoscopic examination often shows oesophagitis with mucosal ulceration. This is largely due to stasis and bacterial proliferation consequent on the retained food debris. Monilial infestation may occur spontaneously or be induced by antibiotic therapy. Leucoplakia is commonly encountered in longstanding cases of achalasia and oesophageal carcinoma is reported to develop in 3% of cases. It is not known whether this risk is influenced by effective treatment of the condition.

Clinical Features

Most reports show an equal sex incidence of the disease, the onset of which ranges from young adulthood to late middle age. However, although rare, achalasia is well documented in children. The main symptoms are dysphagia, regurgitation and chest pain. The dysphagia is common for both solids and liquids. Initially, it is intermittent, of variable severity and may be aggravated by emotional stress. Often the patients find that swallowing is improved by drinking liquids, by repeated swallowing or the adoption of certain manoeuvres such as Valsalva, eating upright, breath holding, etc. These increase the intra-oesophageal pressure and thereby help to overcome the functional resistance at the cardio-oesophageal junction.

When oesophageal dilatation is minimal, odynophagia as well as spontaneous episodes of chest pain which may be severe and simulate angina pectoris, accompany the dysphagia. With the onset of moderate dilatation of the oesophagus, both the chest pain and the dysphagia become less severe but spontaneous and postural regurgitation of foamy mucoid saliva becomes a frequent complaint. Often, the patient maintains weight and the condition may be discovered accidentally by a chest radiograph taken for some other purpose. Other patients may seek medical advice largely because of halitosis and persistent eructations of foul air. Advanced achalasia with massive dilatation of the gullet is usually accompanied by severe dysphagia, frequent regurgitation, weight loss, anaemia and prominent symptoms of respiratory complications (pneumonia, bronchiectasis, lung abscess, fibrosis and tuberculosis) with fever, sweating, cough, breathlessness and expectoration of mucopurulent material. The anaemia is nutritional in origin and may be accompanied by avitaminosis.

The essential investigations are chest radiography, barium swallow and endoscopy. Other useful investigations which may be necessary in doubtful cases are radionuclide oesophageal transit studies and manometry. The chest radiograph may reveal a soft-tissue shadow with or without a fluid level due to the dilated oesophagus. On the PA film this is observed as a convex shadow to the right of the superior vena cava and right atrium. The main reason for the chest radiograph is, however, to assess the condition of the lung fields. The barium swallow is usually diagnostic. The classic radiological features include dilatation of the oesophageal body, a beak-like tapering of the oesophagus at the gastro-oesophageal junction and absence of the gastric air bubble (*Fig.* 66.1). The latter is not, however, a constant finding and is observed in 50% of patients. A careful endoscopic examination is mandatory to exclude peptic stricture and carcinoma of the lower end of the oesophagus and cardia. The easy passage of a large bougie (50F) through the gastro-oesophageal junction should be possible in patients with achalasia and provides further reassurance that an organic stenosis is not present. In addition, a careful search

a

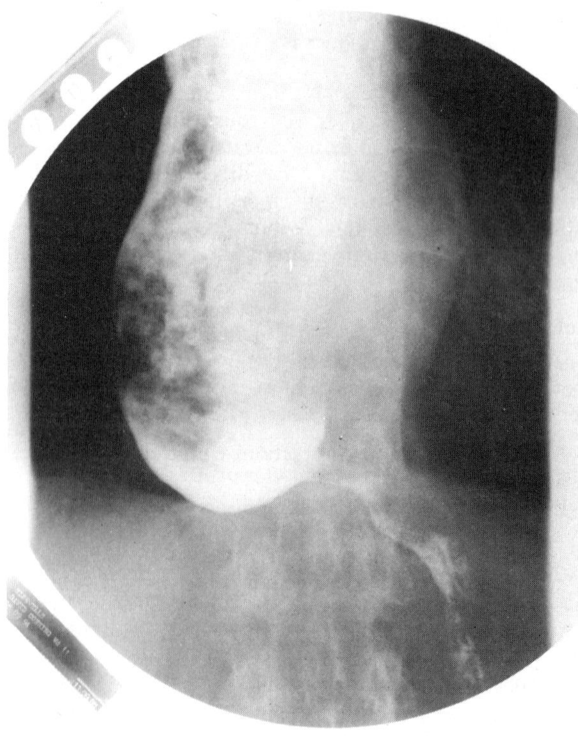

Fig. 66.1 *a*, Barium swallow in a patient with achalasia. The oesophagus is grossly dilated above an apparent narrowing at the cardia. The tapering of the oesophagus to the cardia has been likened to a bird's beak. *b*, Barium swallow showing grossly dilated sigmoid oesophagus in a patient with longstanding achalasia.

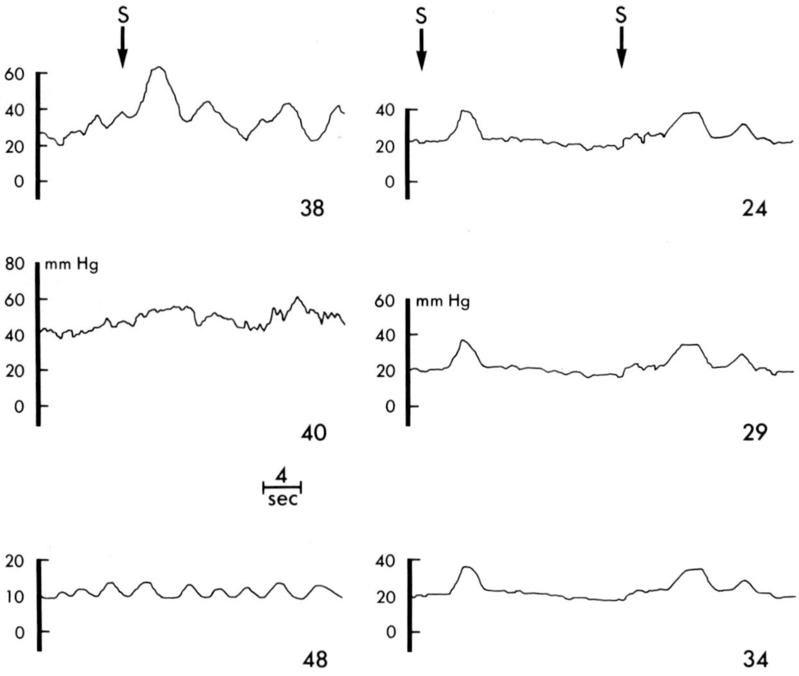

Fig. 66.2 Manometric tracing in achalasia. The panel to the left shows the body of the oesophagus (*upper tracing*), lower oesophageal sphincter high pressure zone (*middle tracing*) and stomach (*lower tracing*). No sphincteric relaxation occurs with swallowing 'S'. In the panel to the right, all three tracings are from the body of the oesophagus. In response to swallows 'S', there are low-amplitude contractions which appear simultaneously at all recording points. A peristaltic progression is never seen.

should be made to exclude cancer of the bronchus, stomach and pancreas which may cause oesophageal dilatation and exhibit radiological appearances which simulate those of achalasia.

The radionuclide oesophageal transit study (liquid or solid) shows complete retention of the isotope-labelled bolus in the upright position. Oesophageal manometry is diagnostic (*Fig.* 66.2). The provocative tests with mecholyl, betanechol and pentagastrin are no longer used as they do not reliably differentiate achalasia from diffuse oesophageal spasm.

Treatment

Some benefit may be derived from the administration of either long-acting nitrites (isosorbide) or the calcium channel blocker nifedipine. However, the long-term effect of these pharmacological agents has not been ascertained and the accepted current treatment of achalasia is either by dilatation or myotomy. Controversy exists as to whether dilatation should be the initial treatment or whether surgical intervention is the treatment of choice and should always be undertaken once the diagnosis is established. Regrettably there are no controlled clinical trials. The results of retrospective reports indicate that myotomy causes symptomatic relief in 85–100% of patients as opposed to 50–70% after dilatation. However, gastro-oesophageal reflux with the development of oesophagitis is encountered more frequently after myotomy (10–20%). Another argument for surgical intervention is that myotomy carries the best results when carried out for early disease.

In those centres where dilatation is used as the first-line treatment, surgical intervention is reserved for the following:

1. Advanced disease with severe dilatation and oesophagitis
2. Coexistent pathology requiring surgical intervention, e.g. hiatal hernia, epiphrenic diverticulum
3. Failure of dilatation or recurrence of symptoms after initial relief
4. Children.

Nowadays, the preferred method of dilatation for achalasia is by the pneumatic technique with the Hurst–Tucker or the Browne–McHardy dilators and, more recently, the Rigiflex dilator which has a pressure gauge. The latter is similar in design to the Grunzig angioplasty catheter. The balloon which is mounted on a flexible polyethylene catheter, is 10 cm long and inflates to a maximum diameter of 30 mm (90 F). Radio-opaque markers proximal and distal to the balloon help its positioning at fluoroscopy. The catheter has a soft tapered radio-opaque tip which facilitates insertion but most endoscopists prefer to use a guidewire. Following insertion, the balloon is initially partially inflated with contrast medium and its position adjusted until the constriction produced by the lower oesophageal sphincter is at the midpoint of the balloon. Inflation to the maximum diameter is then maintained for 1 min. Maximum inflation requires varying pressures depending on the resistance of the contracted sphincter. However, the inflating pressure should not exceed 1000 mmHg as this approximates to the bursting pressure of the balloon.

Although referred to as Heller's cardiomyotomy, the modern operation consists of an anteriorly-placed division of the musculature of the lower end of the oesophagus down to the mucosa which bulges out once the contracted muscle is divided (*Fig.* 66.3), whereas the procedure described by Heller consisted of an anterior and posterior cardiomyotomy. The modern anterior cardiomyotomy is performed through a left thoracotomy with careful mobilization of the lower oesophagus to preserve the vagal nerve trunks. The muscle coat of the distal oesophagus is divided longitudinally down to the oesophageal mucosa. Experts differ on the distal extent and limit of the myotomy. Some prefer to carry the incision on to the stomach only far enough to ensure complete division of the lower oesophageal musculature without incurring any damage to the phreno-oesophageal membrane and excessive dissection of the diaphragmatic hiatus. The incidence of gastro-oesophageal reflux with this technique is said to be very low. Others believe that the myotomy invariably destroys the lower oesophageal sphincter mechanism with inevitable reflux and oesophagitis unless an antireflux procedure (e.g. loose fundoplication) is added.

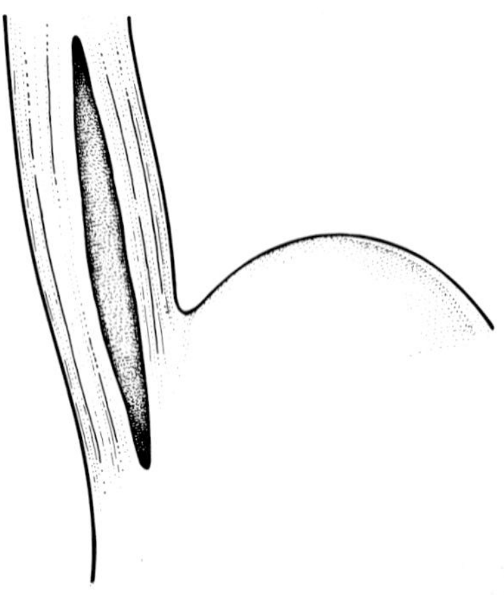

Fig. 66.3 Anterior cardiomyotomy for achalasia. The myotomy is made on the anterior surface of the lower end of the oesophagus and extends to the cardio-oesophageal junction. Some advocate the performance of a loose fundal wrap to prevent postoperative reflux.

Vigorous Achalasia

This condition was initially thought to be an early phase of achalasia but is now considered to be a separate condition. It has features of both classic achalasia and diffuse oesophageal spasm. Manometrically, it is characterized by repetitive high-amplitude non-peristaltic contractions and failure of relaxation of the lower oesophageal sphincter. Chest pain is a more prominent feature than in achalasia. In addition, the clinical manifestations include dysphagia and regurgitation. The radiological appearances are variable. There is usually segmental spasm of the lower oesophagus with dilatation of the proximal half and retention of barium within the oesophageal lumen.

Medical management with long-acting nitrates or nifedipine may give symptomatic relief but the long-term results of this treatment are not known. Dilatation is not helpful in vigorous achalasia, the surgical treatment of which consists of a longitudinal myotomy extending from the level of the aortic arch to the gastro-oesophageal junction. The results of this procedure which is performed through a left thoracotomy, are good.

Chagas' Disease

This disorder, the oesophageal component of which is known as Chagas' megaoesophagus, is the result of an infestation with *Trypanosoma cruzi*. The disease is endemic in rural parts of Latin America. The parasite invades the reticuloendothelial system, muscles and the nervous system. Destruction of the myenteric plexus of the oesophagus leads to a condition which simulates achalasia both radiologically and manometrically. Furthermore, the symptoms of the oesophageal disorder which occurs in up to 25% of patients with Chagas' disease, are similar to those of classic achalasia. In view of the usual poor general condition of patients with this chronic infestation, dilatation is the preferred method of treatment for patients with oesophageal symptoms.

Diffuse Oesophageal Spasm

This disorder is less common than achalasia and although rare instances of transition to classic achalasia have been reported, there is little evidence that the two disorders are different phases of the same pathological process. The essential features of diffuse oesophageal spasm are hypertrophy of the oesophageal muscular coats, including the muscularis mucosa of the distal oesophagus, spasm, Wallerian degeneration of the vagal fibres, hypersensitivity of the oesophageal musculature to cholinergic compounds and certain manometric findings (*Fig.* 66.4). The latter include:

The occurrence of simultaneous non-peristaltic repetitive (at least three peaks) contractions in response to swallowing. The contractions are of high amplitude and increased duration (>5·5 sec)
The occurrence of spontaneous contractions not related to swallowing
Periods of normal peristalsis
Normal relaxation of the HPZ.

The major clinical symptoms of diffuse oesophageal spasm are substernal midline chest pain, odynophagia and dysphagia. The typical sufferers tend to have an emotional personality. Pain is most commonly described as sharp, burning or constricting and is often misdiagnosed as ischaemic heart disease. Not infrequently, the diagnosis of diffuse oesophageal spasm is entertained only after normal coronary angiography has excluded a cardiac origin of the recurrent episodes of chest pain. Radiation of the pain to the back, neck and jaws is common. Although at times the pain seems to be precipitated by the ingestion of aerated beverages and hot or cold substances, it is more often spontaneous and unrelated to swallowing or other events. The suddenness and severity of some of the episodes of chest pain may closely simulate unstable angina or even myocardial infarction. Dysphagia is also common. It is of variable severity, often intermittent and may be precipitated by emotional upsets. Typically, the dysphagia is as severe for liquids as it is for solids. However, weight loss is not usually encountered and episodes of complete obstruction do not occur.

Diagnosis of diffuse oesophageal spasm requires confirmation by manometry. Other useful investigations are barium swallow, radionuclide oesophageal transit studies and the Bernstein's test which reproduces the oesophageal pain when acid is infused in the distal oesophagus. The barium swallow usually demonstrates the repetitive tertiary contractions which result in the typical 'corkscrew appearance', often also referred to as 'curling' or 'pseudodiverticulosis' (*Fig.* 66.5). The oesophageal radionuclide transit test shows an oscillatory movement of the isotope-labelled bolus

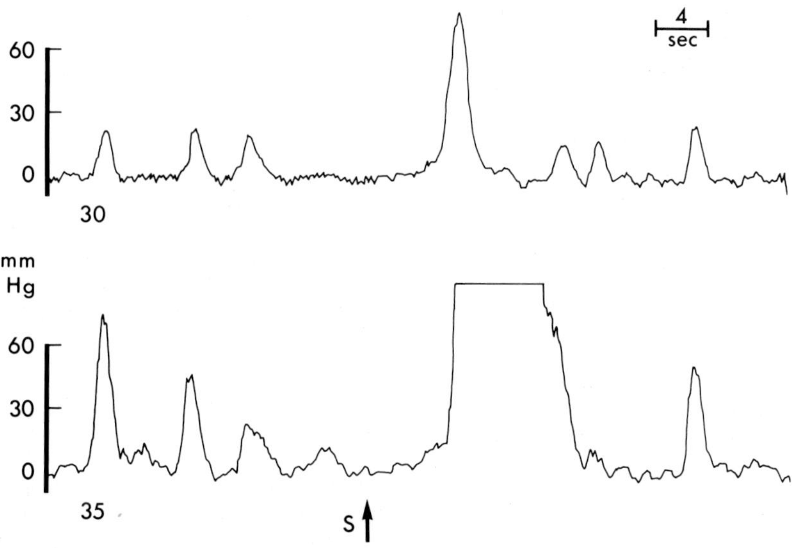

Fig. 66.4 Oesophageal motility tracing from a patient with diffuse oesophageal spasm. Tracings from two points in the body of the oesophagus, separated by 5 cm, are illustrated. There are multiple spontaneous non-peristaltic contractions. In response to a single swallow 'S', a contraction wave of unusually high amplitude and prolonged duration is recorded from the distal orifice 35 cm from the nostril. Patients with diffuse oesophageal spasm often have frequent repetitive contractions following a single swallow as well. Multi-peak contractions of long duration are also a manometric feature.

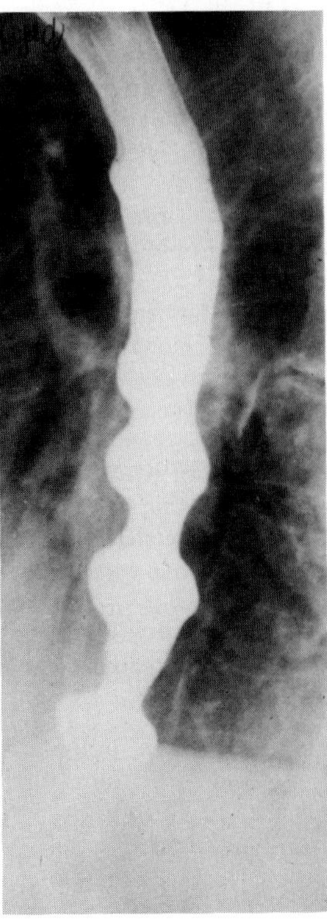

Fig. 66.5 Barium swallow in a patient with diffuse oesophageal spasm showing the typical 'corkscrew' appearance.

and marked delay in the transit time through the oesophagus. Gastro-oesophageal reflux is not a feature of the disease. Provocative tests with cholinergic compounds and edrophonium chloride (cholinesterase inhibitor) demonstrate the hypersensitivity of the oesophageal musculature to these agents but these tests do not differentiate between diffuse oesophageal spasm and achalasia. An endoscopic examination is mandatory in all cases to exclude organic disease causing partial obstruction at the cardio-oesophageal junction.

Treatment is conservative in the first instance with long-acting nitrates and tranquillizers. Good palliation of symptoms has been reported with calcium channel-blocking agents (verapamil and nifedipine) and with the drug cisapride which increases the acetylcholine concentration in the oesophageal musculature. Pneumatic dilatation also helps some patients although the results are not as consistent and dramatic as in achalasia. Surgical intervention is considered only after the above measures have failed and consists of a longitudinal myotomy from the level of the aortic arch down to the gastro-oesophageal junction. Some experts recommend the addition of a loose fundal wrap to offset the tendency to reflux after the myotomy but the wisdom of this is doubted by others since the wrap may contribute to delayed oesophageal clearance.

Nutcracker Oesophagus

Formerly this condition was considered to be a variant of diffuse oesophageal spasm. Its manometric pattern is, however, quite different and it is now regarded as a separate entity and is also referred to as *Symptomatic Oesophageal*

Peristalsis. The condition does not cause dysphagia and presents clinically with episodes of chest pain simulating angina pectoris. Some cases are associated with gastro-oesophageal reflux and treatment of the latter often results in symptomatic improvement. The manometric features of nutcracker oesophagus are:

1. Normal peristaltic waves on swallowing but the primary waves are of large amplitude (>120 mmHg in the distal oesophagus) and have an increased duration (>5·5 sec).
2. Normal peristaltic sequence.
3. No tertiary repetitive contractions.
4. Normal HPZ pressure and relaxation.

Prolonged pH monitoring should be performed in all these patients to determine whether gastro-oesophageal reflux is present or not. In addition, endoscopy should be performed to establish the presence or absence of oesophagitis. Treatment is medical. In patients with demonstrable reflux, treatment with H_2-blockers and alginate combinations often results in relief of the chest pain along with improvement of the oesophagitis. Otherwise long-acting nitrates or calcium blocking agents are prescribed.

OESOPHAGEAL DIVERTICULA

Oesophageal diverticula may be congenital or acquired. Congenital diverticula are very rare and are due to incomplete duplication of the oesophagus. Acquired diverticula are classified into *pulsion* and *traction* varieties. Pulsion diverticula arise as a consequence of a pathological elevation of the intraluminal pressure causing herniation of the mucosa through a weak area in the muscular walls. Traction diverticula are the consequence of inflammatory adhesions between the oesophagus and mediastinal structures, particularly lymph nodes, the subsequent fibrous contracture pulling the oesophageal wall (mucosa and muscle) to form a pouch.

Pseudodiverticula are the result of dilatation of the oesophageal racemose glands and are confined to the submucosal layer of the oesophagus. They are rare, usually multiple and are often associated with extensive strictures or motility disorders. Candidosis frequently complicates the clinical picture. The disorder is most commonly encountered in late middle age and a higher incidence has been reported in individuals with chronic alcoholism, immune deficiency and tuberculosis. The aetiology of oesophageal pseudodiverticulosis is obscure. The most consistent symptom of the disorder is dysphagia which becomes very painful when monilial infestation supervenes.

The clinically important oesophageal diverticula are:

1. Pharyngo-oesophageal diverticulum (Zenker's diverticulum)
2. Midthoracic diverticula
3. Epiphrenic diverticulum.

Their relative incidence is shown in *Fig.* 66.6.

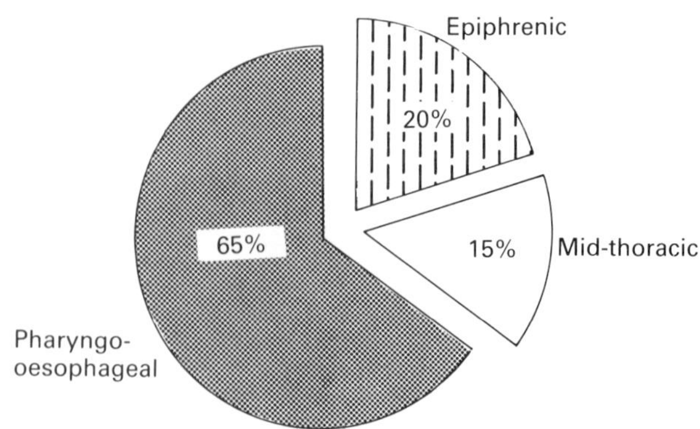

Fig. 66.6 Relative site incidence of diverticula in the oesophagus.

Pharyngo-oesophageal (Zenker's) Diverticulum

This diverticulum is of the pulsion variety and is secondary usually to cricopharyngeal dysfunction and less commonly to an oesophageal motility disorder. It develops as a midline mucosal outpouching on the posterior aspect of the pharyngo-oesophageal junction between the fibres of the inferior pharyngeal constrictor and the transverse fibres of the cricopharyngeus usually on the left side. The anatomical defect in this area, first described by Killian, is triangular in shape and is further accentuated by the absence of the longitudinal fibres of the oesophagus as they sweep anteriorly prior to their insertion into the posterior surface of the cricoid cartilage. As posterior extension is limited by the spine, the diverticulum as it enlarges, comes to lie to the side (usually left) as well as behind the oesophagus. There is evidence that more than one type of motility disturbance may be responsible for the development of a pharyngo-oesophageal diverticulum. Most commonly, cricopharyngeal dysfunction is the cause although controversy exists as to its exact nature. Some ascribe it to failure of relaxation of the cricopharyngeus with swallowing (cricopharyngeal achalasia), others to premature contraction of this upper oesophageal sphincter before the pharyngeal contraction is complete and another theory postulates a hypertonic sphincter secondary to excessive gastro-oesophageal reflux. In some patients, the diverticulum is secondary to oesophageal motility disorders such as achalasia or diffuse oesophageal spasm and some reports have documented an association between the development of pharyngo-oesophageal diverticulum and gross gastro-oesophageal reflux with or without a hiatal hernia.

The diverticulum consists mainly of mucosa and submucosa with a sparse and incomplete muscular coat. As it enlarges the pouch tends to assume a vertical lie and compresses and displaces the oesophagus such that its axis becomes in line with the pharynx (*Fig.* 66.7). Ingested food then enters the pouch more readily than the oesophagus. Symptoms such as spluttering and coughing with meals become more marked and the risks of aspiration are greatly increased. In addition, there is a great danger of iatrogenic perforation of the diverticulum at endoscopy as the scope tends to enter the diverticulum rather than the oesophagus. The complications of pharyngo-oesophageal diverticulum are:

1. Pneumonitis, lung abscess, pulmonary collapse
2. Bleeding from the diverticulum (rare)
3. Perforation (usually following endoscopy)
4. Development of carcinoma (0·3%).

Clinical Features

Pharyngo-oesophageal diverticulum is three times more common in males than females and usually occurs in late

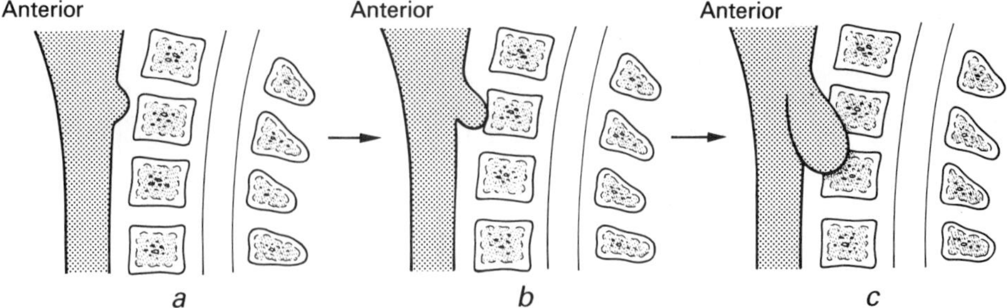

Fig. 66.7 Diagrammatic representation of the development and progress of a pharyngo-oesophageal diverticulum. The cricopharyngeal dysfunction and resultant high intraluminal pressure cause a mucosal herniation between the oblique fibres of the inferior constrictor and the transverse fibres of the cricopharyngeus. Enlargement of the pouch is limited posteriorly by the spine (*b*). It therefore becomes dependent and bulges lateral to the oesophagus usually on the left side (*c*). As it becomes dependent, food tends to enter the sac rather than the oesophageal lumen which may also be compressed by the pouch.

middle age and the elderly. Occasionally the development of the diverticulum is preceded by a period of high dysphagia characterized by difficulty in the transfer of food from the pharynx to the oesophagus. As the condition progresses, the patients complain of regurgitation, constant throat irritation, gurgling noises during swallowing, chronic cough and recurrent chest infections due to aspiration. With compression of the oesophagus, dysphagia becomes severe and attacks of coughing and spluttering are experienced with each meal. Other symptoms include halitosis, hoarseness and anorexia. These patients typically require a long period to eat even a small meal. The regurgitated material is non-acid. Rarely, the pouch enlarges sufficiently to become clinically palpable. More usually, a gurgling sound can be elicited on palpation/massage of the left side of the neck at the level of the cricoid performed after the patient is asked to swallow several gulps of air.

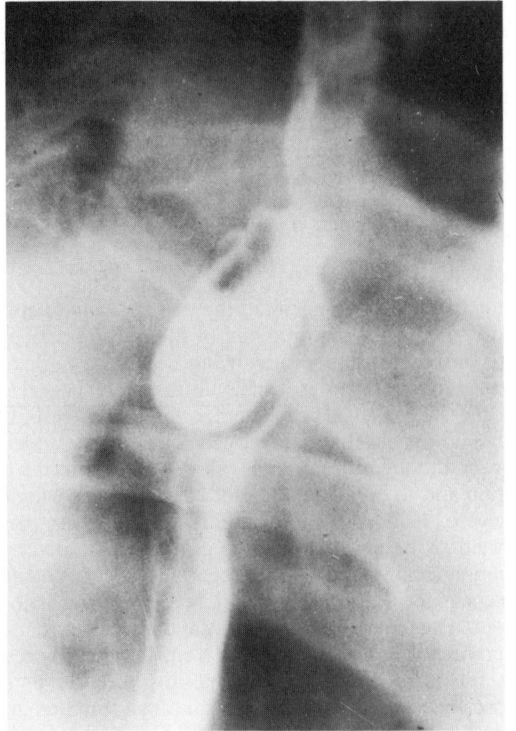

Fig. 66.8 Barium swallow demonstrating a large pharyngeal pouch. The patient had marked dysphagia and aspiration lung abscess.

The diagnosis is best confirmed by a barium swallow. The lateral films demonstrate the diverticulum better and outline its neck and any oesophageal compression (*Fig.* 66.8). It is important that a full barium swallow investigation is performed to exclude gross oesophageal motility disorders and a hiatal hernia. Endoscopy is not necessary for the diagnosis and carries a risk of perforation especially if the pouch is dependent and in line with the pharynx since the endoscope tends to enter the diverticulum rather than the oesophageal lumen. If endoscopy is considered necessary, it should be done by an experienced surgeon and the introduction of the endoscope from the level of the cricopharyngeus onwards should be performed under visual control. Oesophageal manometry, including pressure profiles of the cricopharyngeus, is done routinely in some centres but is not necessary for the diagnosis except when the contrast swallow suggests an oesophageal motility disorder. Prolonged pH monitoring is advisable in patients with hiatal hernia and those with reflux symptoms or endoscopic evidence of oesophagitis.

Treatment

The management of pharyngo-oesophageal diverticulum is usually by surgical intervention through an approach along the anterior margin of the left sternomastoid from the level of the hyoid bone to the anterior end of the clavicle. The surgical options are (*Fig.* 66.9):

1. Cricopharyngeal myotomy: this is suitable for small non-dependent diverticula.
2. Diverticulectomy: this is necessary for large dependent pouches and is sometimes combined with cricopharyngeal myotomy. It is usually carried out as a one-stage procedure although preliminary suspension to drain a grossly infected dependent pouch is still occasionally necessary before excision at a subsequent stage some weeks later.
3. Diverticulopexy: this consists of invagination and plication of the pouch. It is suitable for moderate-sized pouches which are not grossly infected or adherent to adjacent structures and is often combined with cricopharyngeal myotomy.

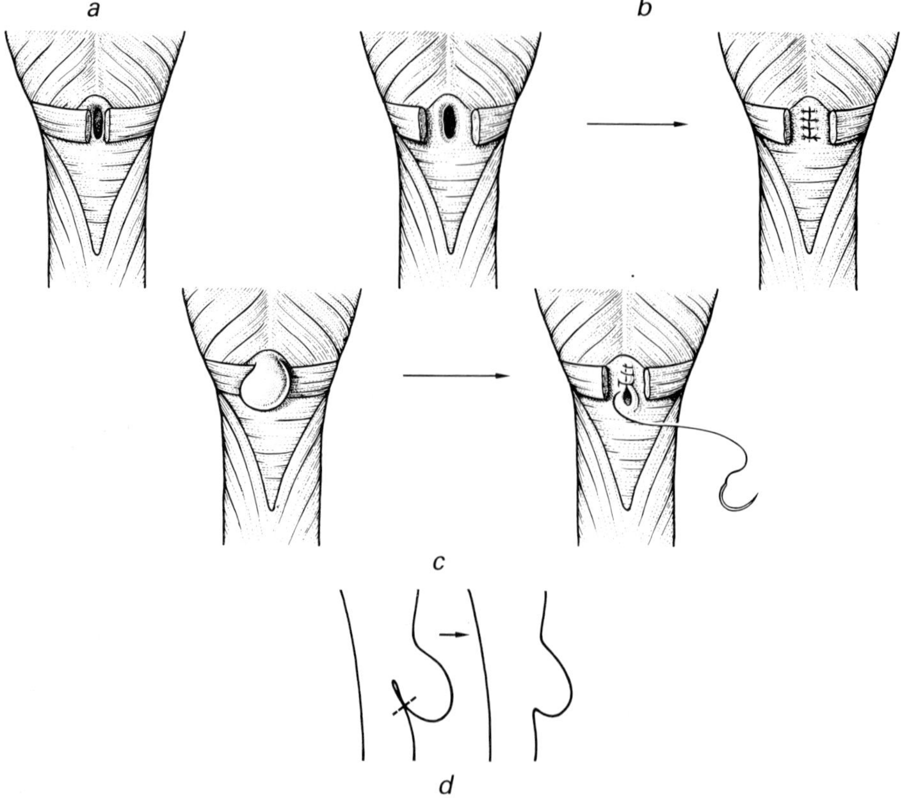

Fig. 66.9 Diagrammatic representation of procedures for pharyngo-oesophageal diverticulum. *a*, Cricopharyngeal myotomy. *b*, Cricopharyngeal myotomy with excision of the diverticulum. *c*, Cricopharyngeal myotomy with plication of the diverticulum. *d*, Endoscopic diathermy division of the septum between the pouch and the oesophageal lumen.

4. Endoscopic division of septum: in elderly poor-risk patients with large dependent diverticula, endoscopic coagulation followed by diathermy division of the septum formed by the opposed walls of the diverticulum and the oesophagus is practised in some centres. The procedure requires a special bifid endoscope. If large, the septal division is performed in stages until the cavity of the pouch communicates through its entire length with the oesophageal lumen.

Mid-thoracic Diverticula

These are of three kinds: congenital, traction and pulsion. The congenital and traction varieties have a similar radiological appearance (tented triangular shape with a wide neck) and possess a muscular coat. The congenital ones are thought to represent foregut duplications and the traction types are secondary to fibrous adhesions to healed tuberculous lymph nodes. Both the congenital and traction midoesophageal diverticula are rare and the vast majority of pouches in this region of the oesophagus are secondary to a specific (diffuse oesophageal spasm, symptomatic peristalsis) or non-specific oesophageal motility disorder which causes a persistent elevation of the oesophageal intraluminal pressure with subsequent mucosal herniation through a weak spot. These pulsion diverticula are usually narrow necked and globular in shape and do not possess a muscular coat. The complications of midoesophageal diverticula are inflammation and perforation, usually by a swallowed fish bone/foreign body leading to abscess formation and tracheo/broncho-oesophageal fistula. The surgical approach to symptomatic or complicated midthoracic diverticula is through a right thoracotomy. Excision of the sac is followed by layered closure of the oesophagus. All asymptomatic midthoracic diverticula do not require any active treatment.

Epiphrenic Diverticulum

Although a few are congenital, the vast majority of epiphrenic diverticula are acquired and of the pulsion variety, the raised intraluminal pressure being secondary either to a specific motility disorder, usually diffuse oesophageal spasm or achalasia, or to a hiatal hernia and gastro-oesophageal reflux. The symptoms are largely due to the underlying disorder although ulceration is known to occur in the diverticulum and to be a rare cause of haematemesis which may be severe. Halitosis, anorexia and obscure chest pain are reported to be specific features of epiphrenic diverticula. Although carcinoma has been reported in these pouches, it appears to be rare and a causal relationship remains unproven. The treatment of symptomatic patients is that of the underlying disorder. If the pouch is small, it usually resolves after successful therapy of the motility disorder or reflux disease. Excision of the diverticulum in addition to surgical correction of the underlying disorder is indicated if the pouch is dependent and has a narrow neck such that it cannot drain adequately, if the sac is inflamed or is compressing the oesophagus by virtue of its size.

MOTILITY DISORDERS SECONDARY TO SYSTEMIC DISORDERS

The most common condition which may lead to severe oesophageal motor dysfunction is progressive systemic sclerosis. Less commonly, patients with dermatomyositis, lupus erythematosus and rheumatoid arthritis may be similarly affected. The oesophageal motor disorder in patients with systemic sclerosis is characterized by incompetence of the lower oesophageal sphincter and weakness to the point of complete loss of peristaltic activity of the distal two-thirds of the oesophagus. The myopathy is confined to the smooth muscle portion of the oesophagus and the function of the upper striated segment and the pharynx remains normal. Histologically, marked atrophy of the smooth muscle is present together with fibrosis in the submucosa and muscularis propria. Barium swallow shows a flaccid hypotonic, slightly dilated organ with gross radiological reflux.

Nearly all patients with scleroderma and oesophageal involvement have symptoms of oesophageal reflux and these are often severe. Gross peptic oesophagitis and stricture formation are common since oesophageal clearance is grossly impaired due to the hypo-/aperistalsis. The other manifestations of the disorder such as Raynaud's phenomenon, calcinosis, tight skin, etc. are present and should point to the diagnosis in patients who present with dysphagia and severe reflux symptoms.

The management of these patients is extremely difficult. There is no specific medical therapy although motility-promoting drugs such as domperidone, metoclopramide and, more recently, cisapride are often used with variable and inconsistent results. Gastro-oesophageal reflux must be treated vigorously by standard medical regimens and any peptic strictures are dilated. Some advocate antireflux operations but these are less often successful than in ordinary gastro-oesophageal reflux because the atrophied oesophageal musculature holds sutures poorly. Furthermore, the incidence of persistent postoperative dysphagia is quite high because of the absence of effective peristalsis such that even a loose fundal wrap may lead to a hold up at the lower end of the oesophagus. The other surgical alternative is resection of the oesophagus with replacement with colon or an isoperistaltic jejunal segment. However, the reports with these procedures for this condition are few and the collective experience reported in the literature is limited such that it is not possible to comment on their overall benefit. The author's personal experience of oesophageal replacement by isoperistaltic jejunal loop in patients with scleroderma has been disappointing in terms of the relief of the dysphagia and reflux symptoms.

SIDEROPENIC DYSPHAGIA (PATERSON–KELLY, PLUMMER–VINSON SYNDROME)

This syndrome is usually associated with iron deficiency but may persist for long periods after adequate replacement therapy. It affects predominantly postmenopausal females and consists of dysphagia, microcytic hypochromic anaemia, glossitis, atrophic inflammation of the mucosa of the pharynx and upper oesophagus with areas of hyperkeratosis, ulceration and the formation of high, usually anteriorly placed, oesophageal webs. Other features include dry skin and eyes, koilonychia, splenomegaly and angular stomatitis. Cases associated with reflux oesophagitis have been described as have rare instances of the condition after gastric surgery. The oesophageal webs are flimsy and best demonstrated by a barium swallow (*Fig.* 66.10). They are easily missed and are readily ruptured at endoscopy. The dysphagia is thought to result more from oesophageal spasm associated with the inflamed atrophic mucosa than partial obstruction due to the oesophageal webs. The anaemia is usually accompanied by a low serum iron concentration. Patients with this condition require long-term follow-up because of the substantial risk of the development of upper oesophageal carcinoma, usually in the postcricoid region. The incidence of oesophageal cancer in these patients is variously reported at 10–30%.

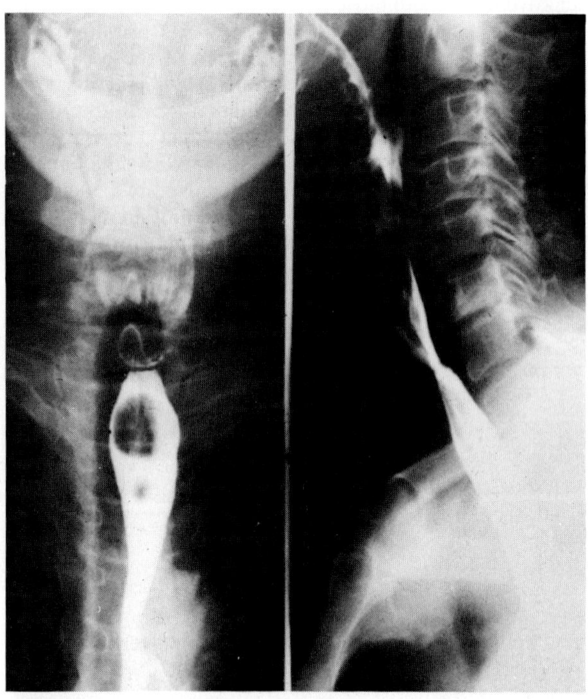

Fig. 66.10 Barium swallow showing oesophageal web in a patient with sideropenic dysphagia.

OESOPHAGEAL CYSTS AND DUPLICATIONS

Oesophageal cysts are very rare and may be acquired or congenital. The acquired variety are retention cysts of the submucous racemose glands and usually occur at the lower end of the oesophagus. They are rarely symptomatic but if large, may cause dysphagia. Removal is achieved through an oesophageal myotomy over the lesion which shells out easily and without incurring a breach of the oesophageal mucosa.

Congenital (enterogenous) cysts and reduplications share the same developmental origin and represent embryonal rests within or attached to the oesophageal walls. The cysts are most commonly lined with ciliated columnar epithelium. They usually present in infancy and childhood with pressure effects, i.e. dysphagia, and bronchial obstruction with respiratory distress as they expand within the confined space of the mediastinum. Whenever possible, enucleation of the cyst is performed without resection of the oesophagus but this is not always possible as the cyst may be densely adherent to the oesophageal mucosa as a result of previous inflammatory episodes. Reduplications are elongated structures which possess a muscular coat and are lined with squamous epithelium.

TUMOURS OF THE OESOPHAGUS

Tumours of the oesophagus are predominantly malignant. Symptomatic benign lesions are rarely encountered in clinical practice and account for less than 1% of all oesophageal neoplasms.

Benign Tumours

The commonest benign tumour of the oesophagus is leiomyoma (smooth muscle tumour). They occur most commonly in the lower oesophagus (*Fig.* 66.11) as uniform oval swellings which project into the lumen of the oesophagus and are covered by an intact mucosa. The lesions may calcify. The most common presentation is with dysphagia. Bleeding, due to ulceration is less common than with gastric leiomyomas although it is well documented. As the tumours are well encapsulated, they can be removed by enucleation without oesophageal resection. However, differentiation between benign and smooth muscle tumours can be difficult even histologically and these patients require careful follow-up.

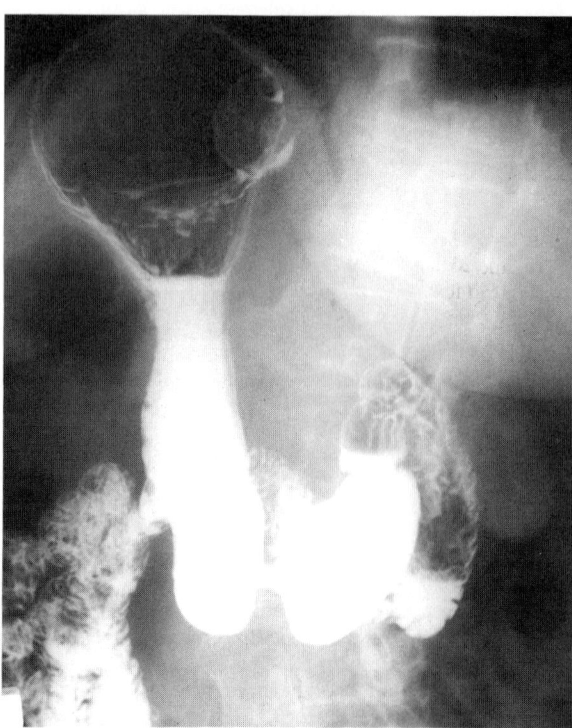

Fig. 66.11 Barium swallow showing a smooth ovoid tumour at the gastro-oesophageal junction. The lesion was a benign smooth muscle tumour (leiomyoma).

Other benign tumours include papillomas (caused by the human papilloma virus) which may occur anywhere in the oesophagus, granular-cell tumours, inflammatory polyps at the gastro-oesophageal junction, pseudotumours resulting from sclerotherapy and adenomatous polyps which are usually encountered at the lower end of the gullet and may be sessile or pedunculated. Some adenomatous oesophageal polyps arise as a consequence of reflux oesophagitis. The inflammatory polyps, also called oesophagogastric polyps or polyp–fold complexes, are covered by both gastric and oesophageal epithelium and are associated with chronic oesophagitis.

Malignant Oesophageal Neoplasms

Malignant oesophageal neoplasms are mostly carcinomas and carry a poor prognosis with an overall 5-year survival of 5%. In the West, cancer of the oesophagus is predominantly a disease of the elderly with an overall incidence of 10–20 per 100 000 per annum. The highest incidence in the Western hemisphere is found in France, followed by Scotland where the frequency of the disease has doubled in both sexes since 1970. Carcinoma of the oesophagus is some 20–30 times more common in China, Iran and the Transkei region of South Africa than in the West. The 'endemic' cancer in these high-incidence countries occurs at a younger age and the male predominance of the disease is not as marked as in Western countries.

Aetiology

The aetiology of oesophageal carcinoma remains unknown but is currently thought to be multifactorial. The important factors appear to be the following:

Excess alcohol intake
Smoking
Absence of protective substances in fruits and green vegetables
Ingestion of exogenous carcinogens and promoting factors
Infection with the human papilloma virus.

Various epidemiological surveys have shown a good correlation between excess alcohol intake and incidence of oesophageal cancer. Thus the disease is common in the whisky-distilling areas of Scotland and the red wine belt of France. Alcohol is thought to act as a promoter rather than a direct carcinogen. Certain vitamins (A, B_2, C, E) and trace elements (iron, zinc, selenium and molybdenum) are thought to be protective and deficiency of these substances either from inadequate ingestion of green vegetables and fruits or as a consequence of soil depletion (in the case of trace elements), is associated with a high incidence of oesophageal cancer. The carcinogenic compounds and promoters which have been implicated in endemic areas are nitrosamines, tannins (polyhydrophenols), alcohol and phorbol esters (present in herbal/medicinal teas).

In addition, there are certain disorders which are known to predispose to the development of cancer of the oesophagus. These are outlined in *Table* 66.2. *Tylosis Type A* is a hereditary disorder transmitted by a single autosomal gene. It is characterized by the development of hyperkeratosis of the skin of the palms and feet during the first and second decades and the subsequent development of cancer of the oesophagus in virtually all affected individuals by the seventh decade. The risk of oesophageal cancer in achalasia is not reduced by myotomy. When carcinoma develops in this condition and in patients with longstanding strictures, it is usually diagnosed late and therefore carries a poor prognosis. Despite anecdotal reports, there is no evidence that previous gastric surgery is associated with an increased risk of the development of oesophageal carcinoma. The slightly increased risk in patients with scleroderma is secondary to gastro-oesophageal reflux rather than the condition itself.

Table 66.2 Conditions which predispose to the development of oesophageal cancer

HIGH RISK
- Tylosis Type A
- Plummer–Vinson syndrome

INTERMEDIATE RISK
- Reflux disease and Barrett's oesophagus
- Achalasia
- Ectopic gastric mucosa
- Radiotherapy for Hodgkin's and non-Hodgkin's lymphomas
- Previous squamous-cell carcinoma of the head/neck

LOW RISK
- Oesophageal diverticula
- Corrosive strictures
- Coeliac disease
- Scleroderma

Pathology

The vast majority of malignant neoplasms of the oesophagus are carcinomas. The predominant histological type is squamous. Confusion has been generated by the inclusion of carcinomas of the cardia with oesophageal neoplasms. These are gastric neoplasms which invade the lower or abdominal end of the oesophagus and are considered in Chapter 67. In the West, the peak incidence of the disease is found between the age of 60 and 80 years although in the last decade there has been an increased incidence in the younger age groups (30–50 years).

Macroscopically, the disease assumes one of three forms:

Polypoid (fungating) (*Fig.* 66.12)
Stenosing (scirrhous) (*Fig.* 66.13)
Ulcerative (*Fig.* 66.14).

Early cancer of the oesophagus (confined to mucosa/submucosa) is rarely encountered because of the absence of screening programmes. The transition between severe dysplasia to carcinoma-in-situ and invasive oesophageal cancer is well documented. The results of surgical treatment for early oesophageal cancer are extremely good with a very low operative mortality and a 5-year survival of 80–85%. There is, therefore, a strong argument for screening programmes, particularly in areas of high incidence and in patients with known predisposing conditions.

Histology

The histological types of oesophageal malignancy are outlined in *Table* 66.3.

Squamous-cell Carcinoma

This accounts for 95% of oesophageal carcinomas (if cancers of the cardia are excluded). The extent of differentiation which varies from the anaplastic to the well-differentiated tumours with keratinization, does not appear to be an important factor in the prognosis. The tumour infiltrates the submucosal plane quite extensively and tends to grow longitudinally as well as circumferentially. Squamous-cell carcinomas occur throughout the length of the oesophagus and are equally common in the middle and lower thirds though they are less frequent at the upper end. The previously held statement that oesophageal cancers occur at sites of normal anatomical constrictions has not been backed by any of the large reported series of the disease. The carcinoma invades the muscle walls of the oesophagus and then adjacent mediastinal structures, particularly nerves (recurrent laryngeal and phrenic) and/or the major bronchi and trachea and pericardium. Lymph node spread from tumours of the upper third is predominantly to the supraclavicular, cervical and upper mediastinal nodes; middle third neoplasms may involve all the mediastinal nodes and those along the left gastric and coeliac artery whereas growths in the lower third usually tend to spread preferentially to the lower mediastinal and subdiaphragmatic nodes. Metastatic spread is preferentially to the liver and bones. Squamous-cell carcinoma of the oesophagus is sensitive to radiotherapy.

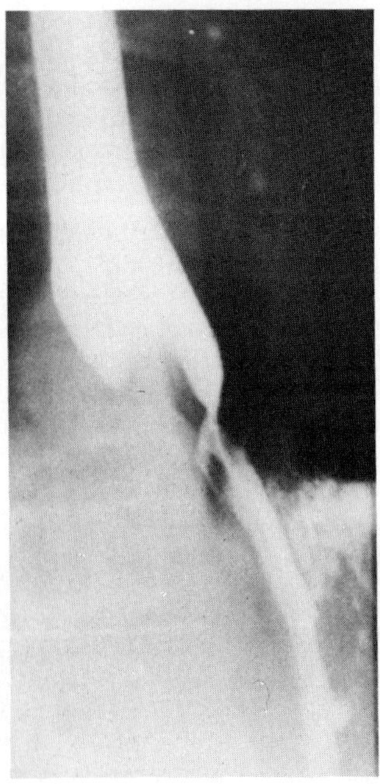

Fig. 66.12 Barium swallow showing a polypoid malignant tumour at the lower end of the oesophagus.

Adenocarcinoma

True adenocarcinomas of the oesophagus usually originate from Barrett's epithelium following longstanding reflux oesophagitis. Less commonly, they may arise from ectopic gastric epithelium or from the oesophageal submucous glands. The vast majority are found at the lower end of the oesophagus. The development of incomplete metaplasia with abnormal mucus production (sulphomucin) and de-differentation of cells and severe dysplasia precedes the onset of in situ and invasive carcinoma. The prognosis of oesophageal adenocarcinoma is poor and these tumours are relatively insensitive to radiotherapy. The mode of spread is similar to that of squamous tumours.

Sarcomas

Sarcomatous tumours of the oesophagus are rare, the commonest being leiomyosarcoma. Primary lymphomas are very uncommon and most of the reported cases have been of the non-Hodgkin's type. Secondary involvement of the oesophagus by mediastinal Hodgkin's disease is not infrequent. Oesophageal sarcomas tend to form polypoid tumours and the smooth muscle variety may present with bleeding secondary to ulceration of the neoplasm.

Mixed Tumours

These malignant tumours consist of more than one cell type. They are classified into mixed epithelial tumours (adenosquamous, muco-epidermoid) and mixed epithelial-mesenchymal neoplasms (carcinosarcomas). There are three theories concerning their origin:

1. Development from a stem cell which differentiates into more than one cell type.
2. Field hypothesis which stipulates simultaneous malignant change from mucosal and submucosal cells.
3. Mesenchymal metaplasia secondary to an undifferentiated carcinoma. This is thought to be the case with the spindle-cell type of squamous-cell carcinoma. This undifferentiated tumour often has a sarcomatous component which is thought to originate from metaplasia of the squamous neoplastic cells.

The most common mixed epithelial tumours of the oesophagus are the adenosquamous lesions. These are squamous carcinomas which also contain glandular elements. The muco-epidermoid carcinoma which is thought to arise primarily from the oesophageal glands and their ducts, is included in this group. Adenosquamous carcinomas, especially the muco-epidermoid variety, carry a poor prognosis.

Peptide-secreting Malignant Oesophageal Tumours

Although rare, these are well documented. Most, but not all, have been instances of oat-cell type tumour with secretory granules but others are histologically squamous-cell carcinomas. Inappropriate secretion of ACTH, calcitonin, parathormone and, more recently, VIP have been reported.

Diagnosis

The key investigations for establishing the diagnosis are barium swallow and endoscopy with biopsy and cytology. Both are necessary as they complement each other. Endoscopy gives precise information of the site and extent of circumferential involvement of the oesophagus by tumour. Contrast radiology gives a good assessment of the length of the lesions. Resectability and cure rates decline sharply for lesions longer than 5 cm. Both techniques are also used for

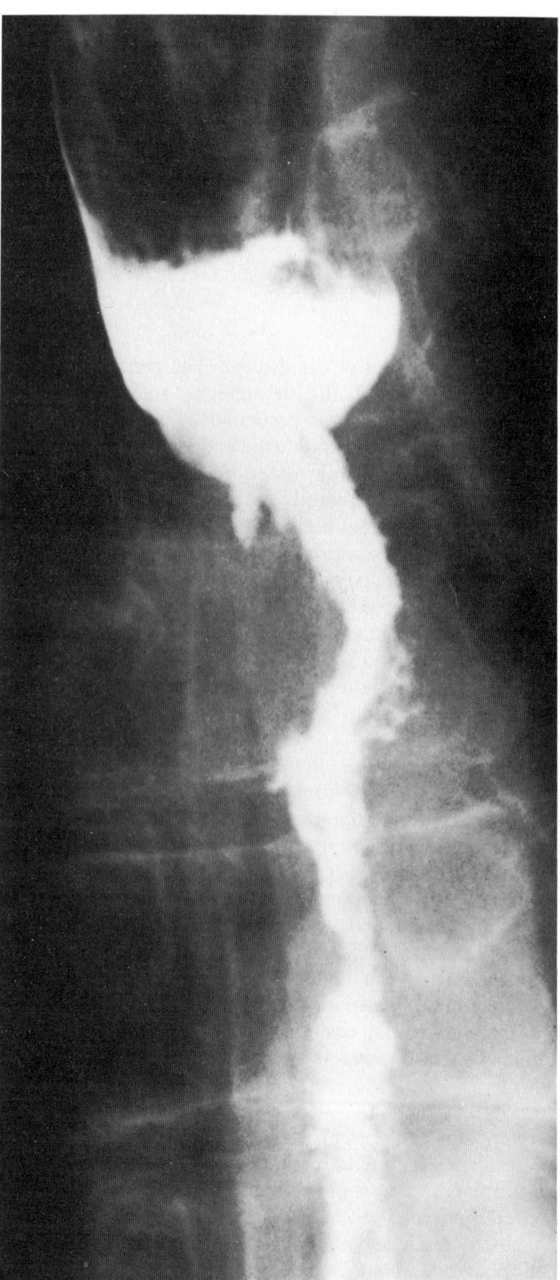

a

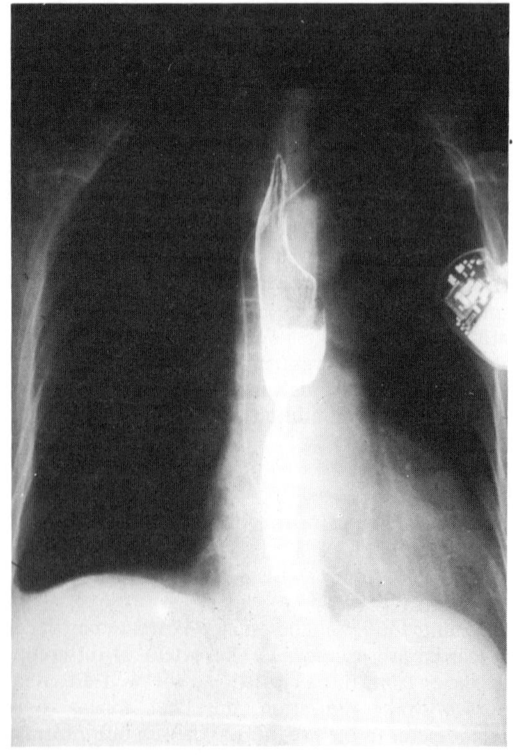

b

Fig. 66.13 *a*, Barium swallow examination demonstrating a long irregular stenosing lesion of the distal oesophagus. This neoplasm has a tendency to spread along the longitudinal axis before producing significant obstruction. *b*, Short neoplastic stricture at the midoesophageal region. The patient has a demand pacemaker.

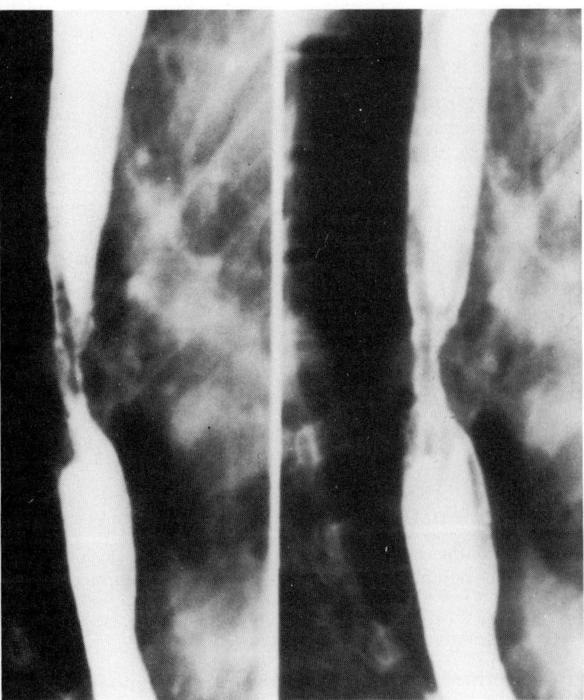

Fig. 66.14 Ulcerating type of oesophageal carcinoma situated at the lower end of the gullet.

Table 66.3 Histology of malignant oesophageal neoplasms

CARCINOMA
Squamous (95%)
Adenocarcinoma (1–2%)
Oat cell (apud tumour)
Melanoma
Adenoid cystic carcinoma
SARCOMA
Leiomyosarcoma
Rhabdomyosarcoma
Fibrosarcoma
Lymphoma
MIXED
Epithelial: adenosquamous
Epithelial+mesenchymal: carcinosarcomas

screening in high-risk areas and in individuals with known predisposing conditions. Balloon cytology whereby a rubber balloon is swallowed attached to a string and then retrieved to collect oesophageal cells, has been found to be a very effective and simple screening technique in high incidence areas such as Northern China. Serum markers have not been shown to be useful in the detection of oesophageal tumours.

Staging

Once a diagnosis of oesophageal carcinoma is made, staging of the disease is necessary to establish the appropriate method of treatment in the individual patient. The most common clinical staging system used is the TNM or the recently agreed International Staging System. The staging tests in patients with oesophageal cancer are designed to establish the presence of inoperable mediastinal disease or subdiaphragmatic involvement (hepatic and nodal). Vocal cord paralysis (ENT examination) and phrenic nerve paralysis (diaphragmatic screening by fluoroscopy or ultrasound) are indications of inoperability as is lung parenchymal involvement demonstrated on the chest radiograph. All middle and upper third neoplasms require a bronchoscopy to exclude involvement of the tracheobronchial tree. Both CT scanning and magnetic resonance imaging (MRI) have been found disappointing in the assessment of the resectability of oesophageal cancers as these techniques are unable to define individual layers of the oesophagus and do not detect early mediastinal invasion. The best and most cost-effective technique for the detection of intra-abdominal disease is laparoscopy which has been found to be superior to ultrasonography and isotope scintigraphy for this purpose.

Treatment

The treatment of patients with oesophageal cancer depends on the staging of the disease and the condition of the patients, some of whom have resectable lesions but are unfit for surgery by virtue of old age or significant intercurrent cardiorespiratory disease. The nutritional state must also be assessed by both anthropomorphic measurements (e.g. skinfold thickness, triceps girth, etc.) and biochemical and haematological tests (albumin, transferrin, Hb, serum iron, etc.). In malnourished patients, a period of parenteral or enteral nutrition for a few weeks before surgery should be undertaken.

The treatment options available are:

Surgical excision and bypass
Radiotherapy
Intubation
Laser coagulation
Combined modality treatment.

Surgical Treatment

The main objective of surgical therapy is the restoration of the ability to swallow. The procedures available are resection and bypass operations. All oesophageal surgical interventions should be covered with prophylactic antibiotic therapy (three-dose regimen) with a cephalosporin or aminoglycoside and metronidazole.

SURGICAL RESECTION. In general, some 30–40% of oesophageal tumours are resectable. At operation, a few of these are found to be inoperable and in some there is residual tumour after the resection. The mortality of oesophagectomy is dependent largely on surgical expertise and the best results are obtained from specialist or regional centres where operative mortality rates of 10–15% are obtained. The mortality is much higher overall, especially amongst those surgeons who perform an oesophagectomy from time to time and never gain sufficient experience. There is certainly a good case for the referral of these patients to centres with special experience with this procedure.

Surgical resection is the treatment of choice for tumours of the lower two-thirds of the oesophagus provided:

1. The patient is considered fit for major surgical intervention.
2. Preoperative staging tests indicate that the tumour is resectable and there is no metastatic disease.

Controversy exists regarding tumours at the upper end.

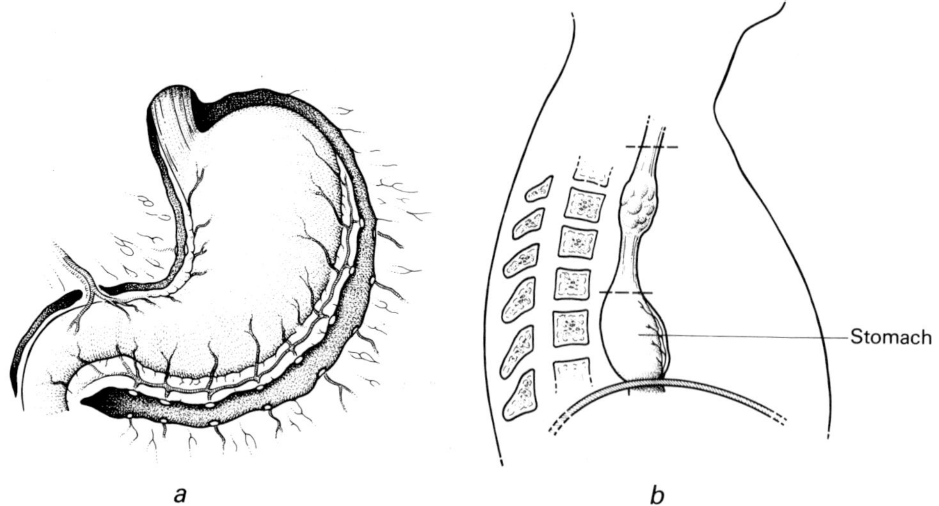

Fig. 66.15 The Lewis–Tanner two-stage oesophagectomy. *a*, Abdominal stage—the stomach and duodenum have been completely skeletonized with preservation of the right gastric and gastro-epiploic vessels. *b*, The oesophagus and tumour are mobilized through a right thoracotomy, the previously mobilized stomach is then drawn into the chest.

Some consider that these lesions are best treated by radiotherapy, others by pharyngolaryngectomy.

The two-stage Lewis–Tanner procedure (*Fig.* 66.15) has become the standard operation for resection of tumours of the lower two-thirds of the oesophagus (excluding carcinoma of the cardia). It achieves better clearance than the left thoracotomy approach which is seldom used nowadays. The abdominal or first stage of the Lewis–Tanner operation is usually performed through a midline epigastric incision. The entire stomach is mobilized and its vascular supply maintained through the right gastro-epiploic and right gastric vessels. All other arteries and veins to the stomach are ligated and divided. The short gastric vessels must be ligated individually close to the spleen to avoid bunching of the greater curvature and gastro-epiploic arcade. The left gastric artery is ligated at its origin from the coeliac axis. This prevents ischaemia of the fundus. The entire duodenum and head of the pancreas are mobilized fully to expose a long segment of the vena cava and to enable their reflection to the midline or beyond. Proximally, the peritoneum over the gastro-oesophageal junction and the phreno-oesophageal membrane are divided. The abdominal oesophagus is next mobilized, the vagal trunks are sectioned and finger dissection of the lower posterior mediastinum around the oesophagus performed. In lower third lesions, the tumour becomes palpable at this stage. Some surgeons advocate pyloromyotomy or pyloroplasty prior to closure of the abdomen but this step is unnecessary unless there is duodenal scarring or deformity since gastric retention is not usually encountered.

The thoracic or second stage is conducted through a right posterolateral thoracotomy performed through the bed of the 5th rib. The oesophagus is eminently accessible through this approach and the only overlying structure is the azygos vein. A minimum of 5 cm proximal clearance from the upper margin of the tumour is necessary because of the submucous spread of oesophageal cancer. The stomach is pulled into the chest after the oesophagus and the tumour have been mobilized. The distal resection margin is at the cardio-oesophageal junction or upper third of the stomach depending on the lower extent of the disease. The gastric end is closed and the stomach then anastomosed or stapled to the intra-thoracic oesophagus. In transecting the oesophagus, the muscle coat should be divided all the way round to expose the mucosal tube which is then transected 1·0 cm further distally (*Fig.* 66.16). This prevents retraction of the oesophageal mucosa inside the muscular layers and therefore facilitates and ensures the safety of the anastomosis. When

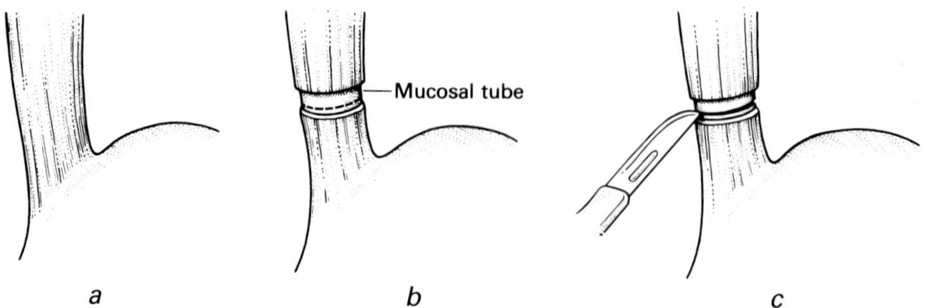

Fig. 66.16 The oesophageal muscular coat is divided all the way round down to the mucosal tube which is then transected 1·0 cm lower down. This prevents retraction of the mucosa inside the muscular layers.

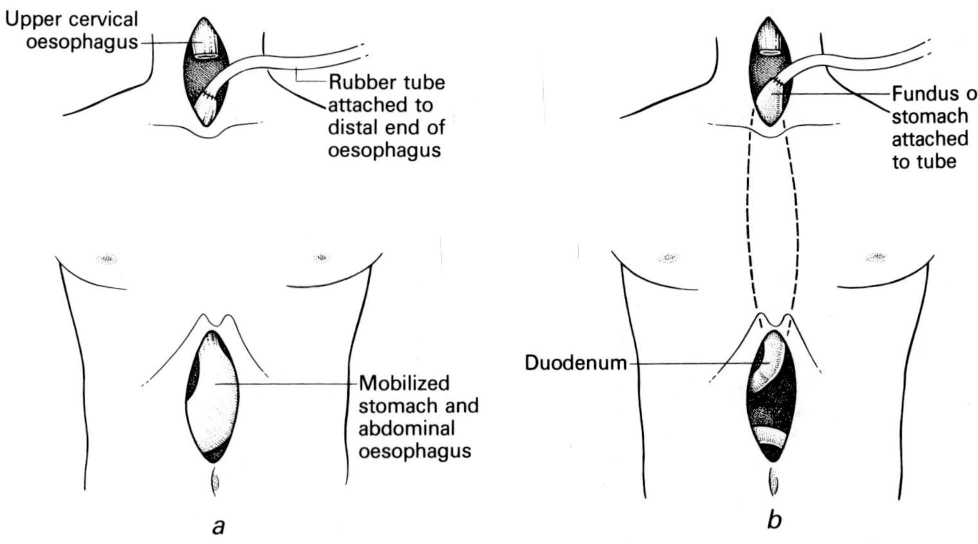

Fig. 66.17 Subtotal oesophagectomy without thoracotomy. *a*, The stomach and duodenum have been mobilized with preservation of the right gastric and epiploic vessels. The thoracic oesophagus is mobilized by hand dissection through the hiatus. The cervical and upper thoracic oesophagus are mobilized through an incision along the anterior border of the left sternomastoid muscle. The cervical oesophagus is then transected and a rubber tube attached to the distal end. The oesophagus with tumour is then withdrawn into the abdomen until the attached end of rubber tube is encountered. The oesophagus is then resected, the cardio-oesophageal junction closed and attached to the rubber tube. *b*, The stomach is brought to the neck for anastomosis to the cervical oesophagus by means of traction on the rubber tube from its cervical end.

hand sutured, the oesophageal anastomosis is carried out with a single layer technique using interrupted non-absorbable sutures. The anastomosis must not be under any tension as this will result in dehiscence.

Some surgeons have advocated subtotal oesophagectomy with anastomosis of the mobilized stomach to the cervical oesophagus. This is achieved either by means of a three-stage operation (McKeown) or by the technique of trans-hiatal oesophagectomy without thoracotomy, first described by Grey Turner and recently popularized by Orringer. The advantages of subtotal oesophagectomy are better tumour clearance and an easy anastomosis in the neck, dehiscence of which is rare and not life-threatening in this situation.

The first stage of the McKeown's procedure is identical to that of the Lewis–Tanner oesophagectomy. The second stage differs in that it entails total mobilization of the thoracic oesophagus up to and including the thoracic inlet, after which the chest is closed and the patient is repositioned in the supine posture. The cervical or third stage is conducted through an oblique incision on the left side of the neck 2·0 cm above the clavicle. After mobilization of the cervical oesophagus, the distal gullet with tumour is pulled up into the neck until the cardia appears. The gastro-oesophageal junction is then clamped, divided and closed, and the oesophagus then resected. The anastomosis is performed in the neck between the proximal cervical oesophagus and the fundus of the stomach.

In oesophagectomy without thoracotomy, the stomach is skeletonized as described previously. The thoracic oesophagus is mobilized by hand dissection through the hiatus which may be divided to facilitate the procedure. The cervical and upper thoracic oesophagus are mobilized through an approach along the anterior border of the left sternomastoid. The cervical oesophagus is then transected and a long rubber tube is attached to the distal end. The thoracic oesophagus with the tumour is then withdrawn into the abdomen, the gastro-oesophageal junction is transected and closed. The oesophagus is then detached from the rubber tube and removed. The tube is anchored to the fundus of the stomach. Traction at the cervical end of the rubber tube is used to pull up the stomach through the posterior mediastinum into the neck for anastomosis to the cervical oesophagus (*Fig.* 66.17). The advantage of this procedure is the avoidance of a thoracotomy, especially in elderly patients.

Surgeons who prefer the Lewis–Tanner operation as the routine procedure for tumours of the lower two-thirds of the oesophagus, tend to reserve subtotal oesophagectomy for high thoracic tumours. The important complication of intrathoracic oesophageal anastomosis is leakage with the development of empyema. This complication is the major

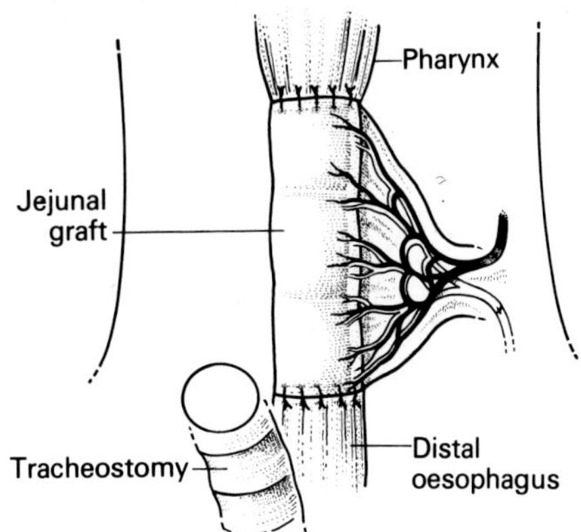

Fig. 66.18 Free revascularized jejunal graft for reconstruction after pharyngolaryngectomy. This microvascular technique gives the best results and is replacing other methods of reconstruction.

Table 66.4 Palliative bypass procedures

REVERSED GASTRIC TUBE
GASTRO-OESOPHAGOSTOMY PROXIMAL TO THE TUMOUR
COLON BYPASS, RIGHT OR LEFT
JEJUNAL BYPASS

cause of postoperative mortality after oesophageal resection. Careful attention in the performance of the anastomosis to ensure mucosa to mucosa coaptation, experience and avoidance of any tension are the most important factors in the prevention of anastomotic dehiscence.

The majority of proximal tumours arise from the hypopharyngeal area (pyriform fossa, posterior wall of the pharynx and postcricoid region) and tumours of the cervical oesophagus are rare. They carry a poor prognosis and survival beyond 1 year after treatment is uncommon. Some recommend surgical excision for all these tumours, others reserve pharyngolaryngectomy for lesions which are too extensive for radiotherapy or have recurred after this treatment. These patients have a permanent tracheostomy. Until recently, reconstruction was achieved with colon (brought up retrosternally or subcutaneously), stomach or myocutaneous flaps. However, the best results in terms of swallowing, voice production and early hospital discharge are achieved with free revascularized jejunal grafts which are interposed between the proximal pharynx and the distal oesophagus after the blood supply has been restored to the graft by anastomosis of the artery and vein of the mesenteric pedicle to the superior thyroid artery and facial vein (*Fig.* 66.18).

SURGICAL BYPASS. These are less popular than intubation procedures because they carry a high mortality which averages 30% and are major operations which do not seem justified in patients with advanced disease or poor general condition with very limited survival. When successful, however, the relief of dysphagia is better than that obtained by intubation and the patient can swallow ordinary meals.

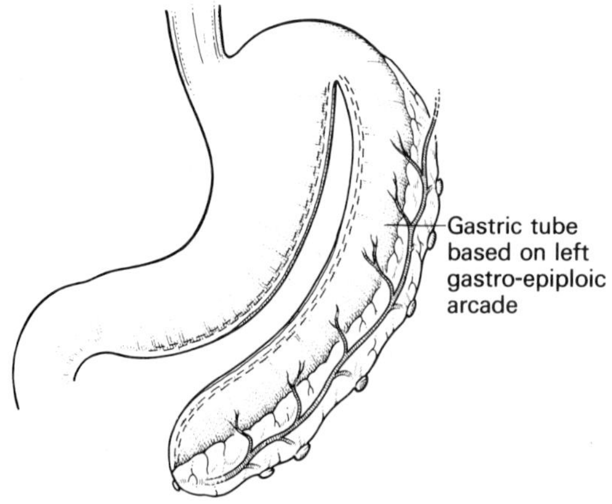

Fig. 66.19 Reversed gastric tube based on the left gastro-epiploic vessels used for bypass of inoperable oesophageal malignancy.

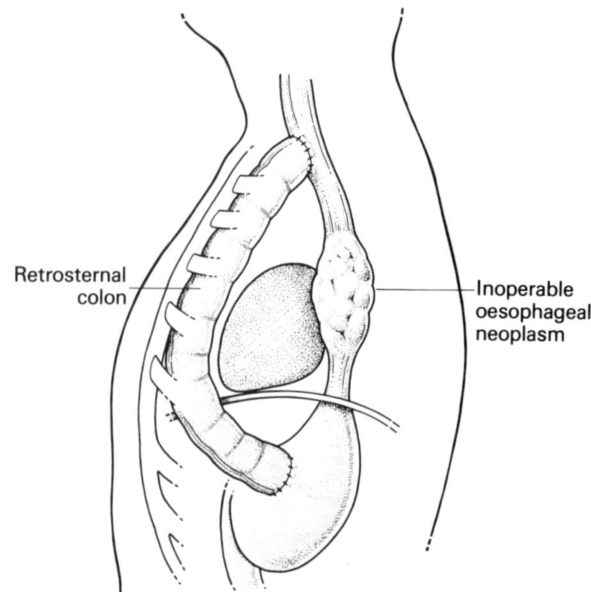

Fig. 66.20 Retrosternal colon bypass. The disadvantage of this technique is the risk of impaired venous drainage of the transposed colon with the development of necrosis which is usually fatal.

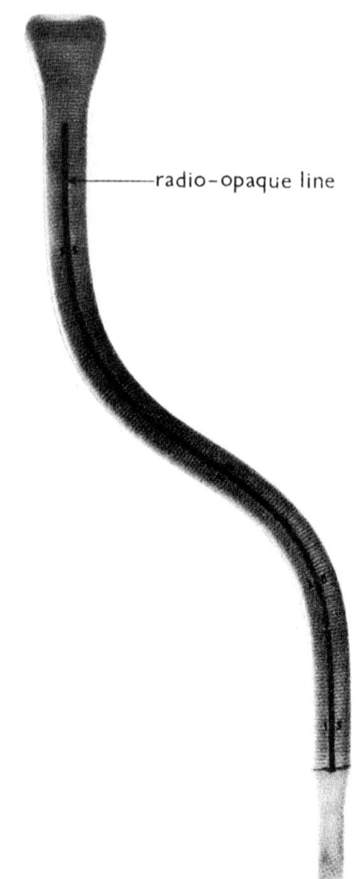

Fig. 66.21 Celestin traction tube.

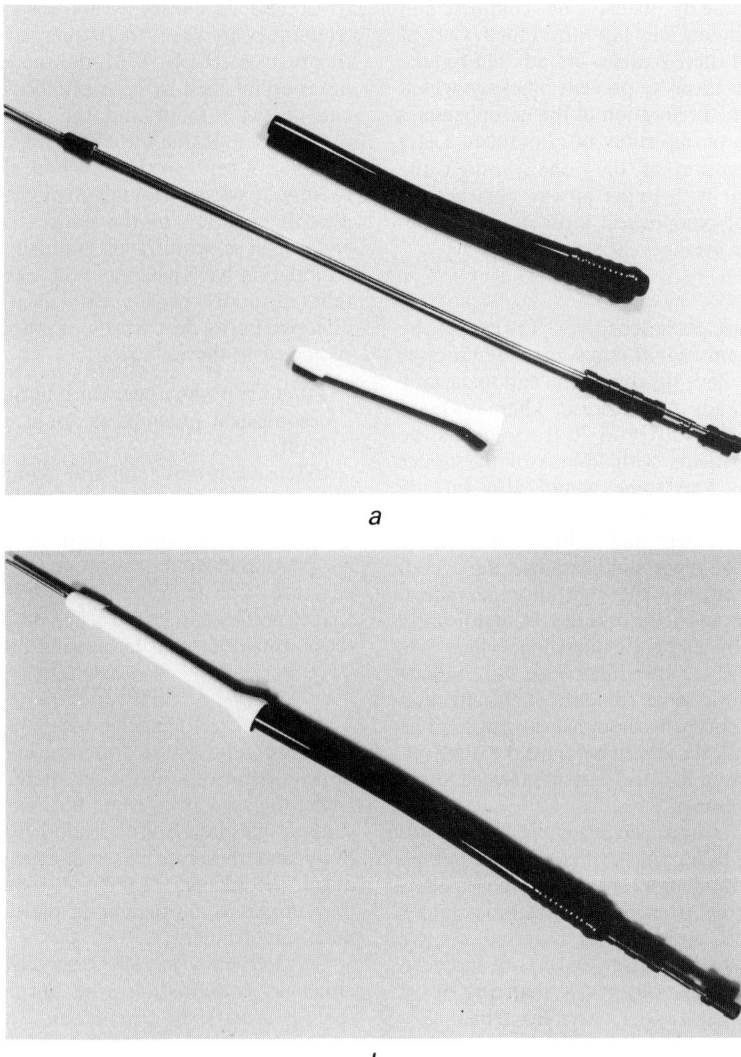

Fig. 66.22 *a*, Atkinson pulsion oesophageal tube (white) and the Nottingham introducer. The tube is made of silicone rubber and has distal shoulders to prevent upward displacement. *b*, Atkinson's tube and Nottingham oesophageal tube introducer assembled for insertion. The stricture is first dilated and then the tube-introducer assembly is guided in place over a guidewire. The introducer has a mechanism to release the tube and allow the removal of the introducer and guidewire.

Surgical bypass is the most effective method of dealing with a malignant oesophagotracheal fistula. The various procedures are outlined in *Table* 66.4.

The most commonly used bypass procedures are the reversed gastric tube and colon bypass. Gastro-oesophageal anastomosis warrants a thoracotomy and for this reason is seldom performed electively. However, it is the best option when a tumour which was deemed resectable on preoperative staging, is found to be inoperable at thoracotomy. The reversed gastric tube is fashioned along the greater curvature using staplers and is based on the left gastro-epiploic vessels (*Fig.* 66.19). It is brought up to the neck for anastomosis to the cervical oesophagus either via the subcutaneous or retrosternal route. Necrosis of the transposed colon is the main disadvantage of colon bypass for inoperable oesophageal malignancy (*Fig.* 66.20).

Intubation

This is still the most popular method of palliation of dysphagia for inoperable malignancy. *Traction* intubation entails surgical intervention to railroad the tube in position and anchor it to the stomach. The most common types of traction tube used are the Mousseau–Barbin and the Celestin tubes (*Fig.* 66.21). Increasingly, *pulsion* intubation is preferred since this avoids an operation. The initial Livingstone type was introduced over a rigid oesophagoscope and is still favoured by some surgeons. However, pulsion tubes which can be placed through the lesion by means of a flexible introducer inserted over a guidewire, are commonly used nowadays (Atkinson's and Celestin's pulsion tubes) (*Fig.* 66.22). A preliminary dilatation is usually necessary before insertion of pulsion tubes.

Intubation is more effective for distal than proximal

lesions. The palliation of the dysphagia is not complete and the patients are able to swallow only liquidized food. Care of the tube is important and these patients are advised to take aerated drinks in between meals to prevent blockage which is a common complication. Perforation of the oesophagus is a real risk at the time of insertion of the tube. Later complications include erosion of the tube through the tumour and dislodgement with upper airway obstruction. The hospital mortality of oesophageal intubation for advanced oesophageal cancer averages 20%.

Radiotherapy

Squamous carcinomas are radiosensitive. Treatment by supervoltage external beam radiotherapy may be curative (radical) or palliative to relieve the dysphagia and metastatic bone pain in patients with advanced disease. There is a good case for radical radiotherapy (50 Gy in 20 fractions) as the treatment of choice in patients with lesions of the upper third of the oesophagus and some would also include midoesophageal tumours. There are no comparative clinical trials between surgical treatment and radical radiotherapy but analysis of retrospective reports indicate that the overall results are similar except that the mortality of radical radiotherapy is negligible and its morbidity is significantly lower than that accrued by surgical extirpation. There are, however, certain definite contraindications to radical radiotherapy. These include large tumours (>9·0 cm) and the presence of a tracheo/broncho-oesophageal fistula. The main disadvantages of radical radiotherapy are the development of a fibrous stricture in half the patients treated and a high incidence of local recurrence.

Palliative treatment to relieve dysphagia is usually administered by external beam supervoltage radiotherapy although intracavitary irradiation with caesium pellets delivered by the 'Selectron After-loading Machine' into a previously inserted plastic applicator is reported to give excellent results with relief of dysphagia in 65%. It has been used as an alternative to intubation.

Laser Therapy

Laser photocoagulation is an effective method of palliation in patients with advanced oesophageal carcinoma. ND-YAG laser is used as it produces good destruction of malignant tissue and its energy is not absorbed by the blood. Two techniques are used: the sequential and the dilatation-single treatment methods. With the sequential technique, a channel is established by laser photocoagulation at the proximal end of the tumour and the 'burrowing' is progressively continued over the entire length of the tumour in several sessions. With the other method, the tumour is first dilated to allow passage through it of the flexible endoscope and photocoagulation to the entire tumour is applied as the endoscope is withdrawn gradually. The results of photocoagulation have been good in selective cases. Dysphagia is relieved in 70% of patients. Laser photocoagulation is only effective in the destruction of mucosal tumour. It is contraindicated in the following:

Tumours of the upper third of the oesophagus and gastro-oesophageal junction as application of treatment is difficult.

Extensive submucosal and extramural tumours.

The best results are obtained in short (<5 cm) tumours in the middle and lower thirds of the oesophagus. Photocoagulation of submucous tumour results in the formation of stricture. The complications of laser treatment are haemorrhage, perforation and tracheo-oesophageal fistula. The latter is usually treated by pulsion intubation.

Multi-modality Treatment

There has been considerable interest in the use of radiotherapy as adjuvant treatment to surgical excision either pre- or postoperatively. Although there are no controlled clinical trials, the data from some but not all retrospective reports suggest that preoperative radiotherapy may improve resectability and therefore survival especially in tumours of the distal oesophagus. Likewise, postoperative radiotherapy may impart some benefit in patients with extramural and nodal involvement.

Chemotherapy has also been used in the adjuvant setting either in combination with surgical excision and radiotherapy or with the latter alone. The agents used have been adriamycin, bleomycin, 5-fluorouracil, methotrexate, cisplatin and mitomycin. The results with chemotherapy alone for oesophageal carcinoma to date have been poor and do not justify their routine use.

Further Reading

Earlam R. and Cunha-Melo J. R. (1980) Oesophageal squamous cell carcinoma. A critical review of radiotherapy. *Br. J. Surg.* **67**, 457–461.

Goulbourne I. A. and Walbaum P. R. (1985) Long term results of Heller's operation for achalasia. *J. R. Coll. Surg. Edin.* **30**, 101–103.

Heimlich H. J. and Winfield J. M. (1955) The use of gastric tube to replace or bypass esophagus. *Surgery* **37**, 549–559.

Lanois B., Delarue D., Campion J. P. et al. (1981) Pre-operative radiotherapy for carcinoma of the oesophagus. *Surg. Gynecol. Obstet.* **153**, 690–692.

Lewis, I. (1946) The surgical treatment of carcinoma of the oesophagus with special reference to a new operation for growths of the middle third. *Br. J. Surg.* **34**, 18–31.

McKeown K. C. (1976) Total three-stage oesophagectomy for cancer of the oesophagus. *Br. J. Surg.* **63**, 258–262.

Orringer M. B. and Sloan H. (1978) Esophagectomy without thoracotomy. *J. Thorac. Cardiovasc. Surg.* **76**, 643–654.

Overholt B. F. (1985) Laser treatment of esophageal cancer. *Am. J. Gastroenterol.* **80**, 719–720.

Payne W. S. and King R. M. (1983) Pharyngoesophageal (Zenker's) diverticulum. *Surg. Clin. North Am.* **63**, 815–824.

Rowland C. G. and Pagliero K. M. (1985) Intracavitary irradiation in palliation of carcinoma of oesophagus and cardia. *Lancet* **2**, 981–983.

Tanner N. C. (1947) The present position of carcinoma of the oesophagus. *Postgrad. Med. J.* **23**, 109–139.

Wilson S. E., Hiatt J. R., Stabile B. E. et al. (1985) Cancer of the distal esophagus and cardia: preoperative irradiation prolongs survival. *Am. J. Surg.* **150**, 114–121.

67 The Stomach and Duodenum

C. S. Humphrey and A. Cuschieri

The functions of the stomach and duodenum are concerned with the initiation of the process of digestion. This is achieved by a combination of mechanical and acid/peptic preparation of foodstuffs together with an orderly delivery of the resulting acid chyme into the duodenum where further chemical digestion in an alkaline medium ensues. In health we are unaware of these activities, which are the result of the coordination of secretory and motor functions by neural and humoral means. Gastroduodenal disease disturbs many of these physiological mechanisms and produces symptoms related to the taking of food. Altered motility produces symptoms which vary from vomiting of food to an ill-defined feeling of epigastric fullness or distress, which, although not usually amounting to pain, can none the less influence the amount of food a patient is able to consume. Severe pain usually implies a breach in the integrity of the gastroduodenal mucosa, either chronic ulceration extending into the wall of the stomach or duodenum, or more superficial ulceration which may be discrete or widespread. The relationships between ulceration, acid and pain are not completely understood. Alterations in appetite are readily explained when the consumption of food either relieves or exacerbates symptoms, but in many cases this does not apply, and we must admit that loss of appetite sometimes occurs for no apparent reason. Likewise, loss of weight is not always explained on the basis of reduced intake.

These symptoms, together with bleeding from the gastrointestinal tract, herald the presence of disease within the stomach or duodenum.

INVESTIGATION OF THE PATIENT WITH GASTRODUODENAL DISEASE

In most cases the morphological assessment of the stomach and duodenum by contrast radiology and endoscopy gives sufficient information for further management decisions to be made. In selected cases it may be necessary to obtain a functional evaluation of the gastroduodenal region. This can be achieved by gastric secretory testing, measurement of parameters, such as gastric emptying and bile reflux, and determination of the plasma concentration of the antral hormone gastrin.

Radiology

Barium meal examination is the most commonly used diagnostic technique in investigating the stomach and duodenum. Although gross lesions are usually seen, the technique does have its limitations. Subtle mucosal changes of gastritis and of early mucosal cancer can only be detected if a meticulous double contrast technique is used in which the stomach is filled with air and the lining coated with a thin film of barium. Even with these precautions, endoscopy usually gives superior results.

A barium meal examination is notoriously unreliable in the assessment of a patient with acute upper gastrointestinal bleeding. The presence of clot within the stomach produces a variety of bizarre appearances. Even when a lesion can be identified, contrast radiology cannot demonstrate whether this has been responsible for the bleeding. For these reasons, endoscopy is the preferred investigation for the bleeding patient. Despite these criticisms, barium meal remains an extremely valuable investigation. A normal radiological appearance should not be accepted, however, in a patient with continuing dyspepsia, and supplementary endoscopy should be performed.

Endoscopy

The development of the modern flexible fibreoptic endoscopes has considerably improved the potential for accurate gastroduodenal diagnosis. With experience, the endoscopist has an accuracy rate superior to that of the radiologist.

The indications for endoscopy are numerous. Its value in the bleeding patient has already been mentioned. Precise identification of the source of bleeding may not be particularly important in many patients with haematemesis and melaena, but if bleeding is seen to be coming from varices or a diffuse haemorrhagic gastritis, important changes in management can be made with confidence. Many patients will be referred for endoscopy after a barium meal examination. This will be because the radiologist has shown a gastric ulcer or a suspicious area of mucosa, or because the appearances were normal but the patient continues to have symptoms. In the area of cancer detection, the use of multiple biopsy and brush cytology adds to the diagnostic accuracy rate. A third common indication for endoscopy is the patient with recurrent dyspepsia after gastric surgery. Demonstration of a recurrent ulcer may be quite difficult with a barium meal, and bile gastritis is seldom shown.

Upper gastrointestinal endoscopy is a safe technique. Full facilities for resuscitation should always be available. Sedation should always be kept to the minimum, particularly in any patient who may have hypovolaemia or hypoxaemia. Diazepam or midazolam in small incremental doses is usually adequate. Fortral should not be used. As with any opiate it may depress respiration significantly, and it also delays gastric emptying, thus making subsequent regurgitation and aspiration more likely. In addition, Fortral can cause pulmonary hypertension which can be significant in a patient recovering from haemorrhagic shock. Spasmolytic agents, such as Buscopan, are sometimes useful to allow visualization of the antrum, passage of the endoscope through into the duodenum and duodenoscopy.

Gastric Secretory Tests

Because of the association of duodenal ulceration with hypersecretion of acid, measurement of gastric acid output has held a fascination for many surgeons. In practice, however, measurement of acid secretion has little clinical relevance in the preoperative patient unless the Zollinger–Ellison syndrome is suspected. It is a very important investigation in the patient with a suspected recurrent ulcer.

Basal and Maximal Acid Output

Much information can be derived from measuring the unstimulated (basal) acid output in a fasting patient and then giving a 'maximal' stimulus to secretion. Basal secretion is usually measured over 1 hour. Maximal secretion is best stimulated with the synthetic gastrin analogue, 'pentagastrin', which is given by i.m. injection in a dose of 6 μg/kg (10 μg/kg in the postvagotomy patient). Secretion is then followed for 1 hour and the maximal response (peak 15 min×4) calculated. There are many pitfalls in acid secretory tests which need an experienced supervisor. The overlap between normal and disease is considerable, and the results obtained vary with body weight and sex. Typical values in preoperative patients are shown in *Table* 67.1.

Table 67.1 Typical values for basal and maximally stimulated acid secretion*

	Acid output mmol/h	
	Basal secretion	*Maximal secretion*
Normal	2	20–30
Preoperative duodenal ulcer	>5	>35
Postvagotomy	<2	10–20
Postgastrectomy	1	<10

*These values are approximations only. Secretion increases with increasing body weight and decreases progressively with age. Females secrete about two-thirds the amount of acid secreted by males.

Unless one believes in some form of selective surgery in which the type of ulcer operation is dictated by the levels of acid secretion (*see later*), the only clinical reason for acid secretory studies in a preoperative ulcer patient is to establish baseline information in the event of recurrence of dyspepsia or other symptoms after gastric surgery. Occasionally a patient with a typical ulcer history will prove to have 'duodenitis' on endoscopy and/or radiology, but no ulcer. Measurement of acid output may be of some value here, since such patients seem to get good results from ulcer surgery when they are hypersecretors. However, these patients are nowadays managed by H_2-blockers (cimetidine or ranitidine).

In the postoperative patient, maximal acid output will be reduced by 70% or more after gastrectomy and 50–70% by vagotomy. If preoperative levels of secretion are unknown, absolute levels of secretion must be judged. A postoperative maximal acid response of 20 mmol/h or greater is a fairly reliable indication of a persisting hypersecretory state (incomplete vagotomy). A response of 10 mmol/h or less effectively precludes recurrent *duodenal* ulceration, although ulcer recurrence in the stomach is still possible.

The measurement of basal acid output after gastric surgery has particular relevance to the question of ulcer recurrence due to a pancreatic gastrin producing tumour (Zollinger–Ellison syndrome—*see later*). If hypergastrinaemia exists, 'basal' secretion is already being stimulated and the characteristic findings will be of a high basal secretion which does not increase much further when a maximal stimulus is given. If basal secretion is greater than 10 mmol/h, and this represents more than 60% of the maximal response, a gastrinoma should be suspected. Proof of this requires measurement of plasma gastrin concentration (*see below*).

The Insulin Test

After complete denervation of the parietal cell mass, acid output is reduced by 50% or more. Incomplete denervation will not achieve this, and the chance of a recurrent ulcer is increased. Since many causes of recurrent ulceration exist, an assessment of the adequacy of vagotomy is important. This is achieved by the insulin test, originally described by Hollander.

The test depends upon the fact that insulin-induced hypoglycaemia stimulates hypothalamic nuclei which results in a parasympathetic response. If vagal innervation of the parietal cell mass persists, acid will be secreted in response to the hypoglycaemia. The test is performed by giving an intravenous injection of soluble insulin (0·2 u/kg) after basal secretion has been collected in four 15-min aliquots. Secretion is then followed for a further 2 hours. If the acid *concentration* in any 15-min sample after insulin is 20 mmol/l greater than in the basal period, the test is said to be positive. (If no free acid is secreted basally, then a post-insulin concentration of more than 10 mmol/l is taken as positive.) Subsequent to Hollander's original description, the interpretation of the test has been modified in many ways. The modification most commonly used is to divide a positive response into 'early' if it occurs during the first hour or 'late' if it is in the second hour.

A positive insulin test does not mean that a patient has a recurrent ulcer, merely that there is vagal innervation of the parietal cell mass. An 'early' positive response usually implies a fairly generous residual innervation and the actual *amount* of acid secreted (i.e. volume as well as concentration) is quite large. If a patient with a recurrent ulcer has an early positive response to insulin, and a maximal acid output of 20 mmol/h or more, then incomplete vagotomy is the likely cause. A 'late' positive response may not be so significant, particularly if the acid outputs to insulin and pentagastrin are small. Cephalic stimulation can also be produced by sham feeding ('chew and spit'). The gastric secretory response to sham feeding is used in some centres instead of the insulin test as it is safer and just as reliable.

One of the problems with the insulin test is that many asymptomatic patients can show a positive response. Furthermore, when serial tests have been performed after vagotomy it has been shown that negative responses in the first few months after operation can revert later. Thus, the insulin test must be interpreted with caution, and considered only in the context of all other clinical, endoscopic and secretory information. The deliberate production of hypoglycaemia is not without problems, and the test should not be carried out in patients with significant cardiac disease, cerebrovascular disease or epilepsy.

Other Gastric Function Tests

The majority of other tests are of research importance rather than clinical relevance. Measurement of gastric emptying is sometimes relevant in patients with postgastric surgery symptoms. A variety of techniques are described which use liquid, semi-solid or solid meals with or without radioisotope labelling. Rapid gastric emptying is often associated with a much shortened small bowel transit time, and useful qualitative information can be obtained using a 'physiological' food and barium meal if the more sophisticated techniques are not available.

Measurement of gastroduodenal reflux can assist in assessing patients with bile vomiting and bile gastritis. In the latter case, particularly, demonstration of increased quantities of bile acids in the stomach may suggest that reoperation for bile diversion may be profitable. Bile reflux can be quantitated by combining biliary excretion scintigraphy (Hida scan) with cholecystokinin or a milk meal.

Plasma Gastrin Concentration

The peptide hormone gastrin is elaborated in specific endocrine cells in the gastric antrum and, to a lesser extent, the duodenum. Gastrin secretion occurs in response to distension of the antrum and the presence of food, particularly protein. When the pH in the antrum falls, gastrin release is inhibited, so that a negative feedback control exists.

The concentration of gastrin in the plasma can be measured by specific radioimmunoassay. This is indicated if clinical or gastric secretory features suggest the possibility of the Zollinger–Ellison syndrome. The reported levels of plasma gastrin vary between laboratories, but values greater than 200 pg/ml are regarded as abnormally high. Values in excess of 1000 pg/ml are virtually diagnostic of a gastrinoma, provided that the patient is secreting acid. The reason for this proviso is that in an achlorhydric patient, e.g. one with pernicious anaemia, there is no fall in antral pH to shut off gastrin secretion.

Not uncommonly the plasma gastrin concentration will be found to be elevated, but not sufficiently so for the diagnosis of the Zollinger–Ellison syndrome to be made confidently. There are a number of causes of hypergastrinaemia (*Table* 67.2). Many of these can be excluded simply, but difficulty will be experienced in distinguishing a gastrinoma from antral hyperplasia, retained antrum or merely an exaggeration of the usual rise in gastrin which follows acid reduction by vagotomy. Three stimulatory tests are useful (*Fig*. 67.1):

1. *Protein meal.* Gastrin of antral origin is stimulated by protein. Provided that the antrum is present, and in continuity, gastrin levels will rise after such a meal. An exaggerated response is found in G-cell hyperplasia. Gastrin secretion from a tumour is autonomous and not affected by a meal.

2. *Calcium stimulation.* Calcium is involved in the release of many peptide hormones. Under normal circumstances an infusion of calcium causes a slight rise in gastrin concentration. If a gastrin-producing tumour is present there is a very marked release of gastrin by calcium. The usual procedure is to infuse 5 mg/kg/h for 3 hours.

Table 67.2 The cause of hypergastrinaemia

A. Primary increased secretion
- i. By tumour—Zollinger–Ellison syndrome
- ii. Antral G-cell hyperplasia

B. Increased stimulation
- Hypercalcaemia

C. Decreased inhibition
- i. Hypo- or achlorhydria, e.g. pernicious anaemia, post-vagotomy
- ii. Retained, excluded gastric antrum
- iii. Small bowel resection

D. Decreased removal
- i. Renal failure
- ii. Small bowel resection

3. *Secretin challenge.* An intravenous injection of secretin, 4 u/kg, does not affect antral gastrin, or may actually cause a slight fall in concentration. For reasons not understood, secretin causes an immediate and large release of gastrin from tumours. If this stimulus is employed it is important to use pure secretin, since many preparations of secretin contain some contaminating gastrin, or cross-reacting cholecystokinin.

THE MANAGEMENT OF GASTRODUODENAL PROBLEMS

The various surgical disorders of the stomach and duodenum are discussed later in this chapter. Many of these diseases present with varying degrees of urgency, as either perforation, bleeding or stenosis. The general management of these situations is discussed here.

Perforation

Clinical Features

Free perforation into the general peritoneal cavity is a catastrophic event, the signs and symptoms of which do not usually cause diagnostic problems. When perforation of a chronic ulcer occurs there will often have been an increase in the severity of the dyspepsia for a few days prior to the perforation. When an acute ulcer perforates there may be no premonitory symptoms, particularly in younger patients. 'Steroid-induced' perforations undoubtedly occur, but the aetiology is not straightforward. For instance, perforation is much more common in patients with rheumatoid arthritis on steroids than in patients with ulcerative colitis. This may be a reflection of the primary disease process or, alternatively may be a feature of the concomitant use of other drugs. The use of non-steroidal anti-inflammatory drugs (NSAIDs) has been shown to be associated with an increased incidence of peptic ulceration and with an increased risk of the complications of both perforation and bleeding.

Acute perforations also accompany situations of stress, such as burns, multiple injuries, sepsis and in patients receiving intensive chemotherapy and radiotherapy. Such perforations may be duodenal, pyloric or gastric. Perforation of malignant gastric ulcers is common and although most perforated gastric ulcers will be benign, biopsy is important if the ulcer is not removed.

The moment of perforation is often identified by the patient as an excruciating epigastric pain. The subsequent

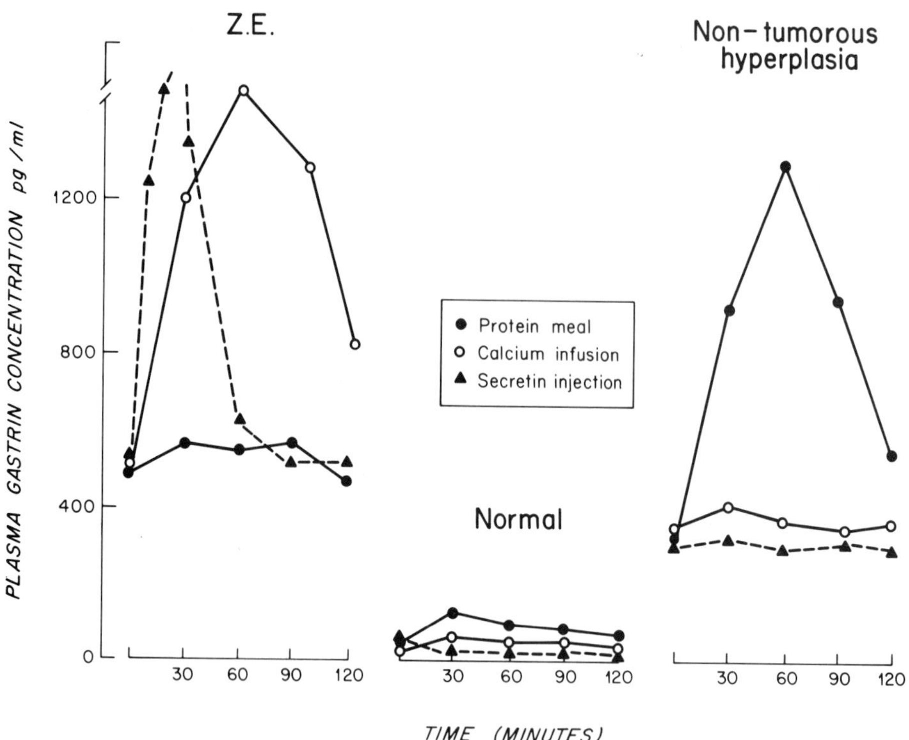

Fig. 67.1 The use of provocative gastrin stimulation tests to differentiate between the hypergastrinaemia of the Zollinger–Ellison syndrome (Z.E.) and that due to antral G-cell hyperplasia.

symptoms depend in part on the degree of peritoneal soiling and whether or not the perforation becomes sealed. The pain may become generalized. In addition, it may be felt over the shoulder if diaphragmatic irritation ensues. Sometimes the spread of gastroduodenal content is maximal along the right paracolic gutter so that pain may localize to the right iliac fossa and simulate appendicitis. Significant vomiting is uncommon unless the diagnosis is delayed and an ileus becomes established. Occasionally in the elderly or seriously ill patient, the perforation does not occur as a dramatic episode and there is a slower development of generalized peritonitis with its accompanying signs and symptoms.

The physical signs accompanying perforation will again depend upon the degree and rate of soiling. Tenderness, with guarding, may vary from being localized to the upper abdomen to being generalized. If contamination of the general peritoneal cavity has occurred there will usually be rigidity and a silent abdomen with progressive distension as a later feature. In the elderly and ill patient this may be the only significant finding. A variable degree of circulatory collapse may be present with tachycardia, hypotension, a cold periphery and a decreased urinary output. Respiration will often be shallow and grunting.

Diagnosis

The key to the diagnosis, suspected from the signs and symptoms, is the plain abdominal radiograph taken in the erect and supine positions (the lateral decubitus position may may need to be used instead of the erect in an ill patient). Although free peritoneal gas may come from any of the alimentary hollow organs, in practice the finding of subdiaphragmatic air is virtually pathognomonic of gastroduodenal perforation. Radiological features of an ileus may be present in more advanced cases.

If a pneumoperitoneum is not seen radiologically, the diagnostic problem is to differentiate between a sealed perforation with minimal localized soiling and an acute pancreatitis. In some cases of the former, differentiation may not be too important if the clinical state of the patient is improving. When it is important to differentiate between the two, contrast radiology with a water-soluble medium, such as gastrografin, may be very useful. Such studies are also helpful if a diagnosis of perforation of a gastric ulcer into the lesser sac is suspected.

In the absence of a pneumoperitoneum a serum amylase estimation should be performed. Moderate elevation of amylase concentration may be present in 10–20% of perforated ulcers, but it is uncommon to find concentrations in excess of 700 Somogyi units unless renal function is impaired as a result of hypovolaemia. If doubt persists, a diagnostic peritoneal tap or lavage may help. The amylase content will usually be very high in either condition, but it should be possible to differentiate between gastroduodenal content and the brown-coloured fluid of pancreatitis.

Management

Initial treatment should be directed toward correction of hypovolaemia and any electrolyte imbalance. Oliguria and poor peripheral perfusion are contraindications to immediate operative treatment, and their correction should take precedence even over radiological studies. If necessary, resuscitation should be monitored with measurement of central venous pressure and urine output from a urinary catheter. Colloids can be used for resuscitation, but crystalloid in the form of a balanced salt solution is equally effective. Any patient needing such aggressive therapy should also be given oxygen by mask. Pain relief should be given as soon as the physical signs have been assessed.

Pethidine is usually very effective, and a small dose can be given intravenously if absorption from a poorly perfused periphery is likely to be a problem. Nasogastric aspiration should be instituted. Antibiotics are not recommended routinely since the initial peritonitis is chemical. However, if operative cleansing of the peritoneal cavity is to be delayed much beyond 8 hours from perforation, or if the patient has chronic respiratory problems, the use of a broad-spectrum antibiotic such as Cefuroxime is justified.

Operative or Conservative Management?

There is no doubt that many patients with perforated ulcers can be managed non-operatively with initial success. A policy of nasogastric suction, intravenous fluids, antibiotics and analgesics will allow many perforations to seal spontaneously and the ileus to resolve. It is not known whether cimetidine would help. The problem with this approach to management is that there is a high incidence of residual abscess formation, particularly in the subphrenic region which will subsequently require drainage. An operative approach is therefore strongly recommended, and should be regarded as almost mandatory if free gas is seen below the diaphragm. If severe coexisting disease is regarded as precluding operation then the use of peritoneal lavage as a therapeutic measure may be considered.

Although one purpose of laparotomy is to aid in sealing the perforation, the major benefit to accrue from this approach is thorough peritoneal cleansing. Before the abdominal wound is closed the entire peritoneal cavity should be washed out with as much warm saline as is required to produce a completely clear effluent. This requires 3–4 litres of fluid. Particular attention should be paid to the subphrenic areas and the pelvis. Details of the surgical approaches to individual perforating lesions are discussed later.

Pyloric Stenosis

Pyloric stenosis is, in fact, rarely due to stenosis at the pylorus. More commonly, the site of the obstruction is on one side or the other of the pylorus—either the duodenum at the site of chronic scarring from ulceration or the antrum where a benign ulcer or a cancer is the problem. True pyloric stenosis can arise from a pyloric channel ulcer or very rarely from a congenital web or adult hypertrophic pyloric stenosis. In practical terms this distinction is pedantic since the problems are the same.

Clinical Features

Pyloric stenosis due to a duodenal ulcer usually occurs in a patient with longstanding symptoms of ulceration. A short preceding history with little in the way of characteristic ulcer pain suggests that the obstruction may be malignant. In the typical case the patient experiences yet another exacerbation of his ulcer symptoms. As obstruction develops, however, the character of the pain may change to become more of a generalized upper abdominal discomfort. Vomiting and anorexia supervene. As vomiting increases, pain may become less of a feature. The typical vomiting of pyloric stenosis is effortless and projectile and the vomitus is characterized by an absence of bile and the presence of partially digested food eaten hours or even days previously. With repeated vomiting and failure to eat, the patient often becomes constipated, although in some cases diarrhoea may develop.

Examination will usually show an underweight patient, dehydrated and often with a degree of anaemia. In such a relatively advanced case there will nearly always be evidence of gastric stasis in the form of a succussion splash. Visible peristalsis may be apparent, passing across the upper abdomen from left to right, and the dilated stomach may actually be palpable.

Metabolic Features

Prolonged vomiting of gastric contents results in a characteristic series of electrolyte disturbances. Initially the major loss is fluid rich in hydrogen and chloride ions so that a minor degree of dehydration may accompany a hypochloraemic alkalosis. At this stage the serum sodium is usually normal and hypokalaemia may not be obvious. The more marked metabolic changes which accompany unrelieved outlet obstruction result from a combination of continued losses with secondary changes in renal function. In the early stages the urine is characterized by a low chloride content and is appropriately alkaline because of enhanced bicarbonate excretion. This tends to compensate for the metabolic alkalosis, but it does so at the expense of losing sodium. If the gastric losses continue the patient thus becomes progressively more dehydrated and hyponatraemic. In an attempt to conserve circulating volume, sodium is retained by the kidneys and hydrogen ions and potassium are excreted preferentially. At this late stage, therefore, the patient with a metabolic alkalosis will have a paradoxically acid urine. Hence the alkalosis becomes more severe and hypokalaemia is more marked. As a secondary effect of the alkalosis, the concentration of plasma-ionized calcium may fall so that disturbances of conscious level and tetany may be apparent.

Management

The priority in management of the advanced case of pyloric stenosis is correction of the fluid and electrolyte disturbances. Blood transfusion may be needed: this will often become apparent as dehydration is corrected and the spuriously high haemoglobin value falls to its actual level.

Rehydration should be achieved by saline infusions with potassium supplements as indicated by electrolyte determinations. Provision of adequate sodium allows excretion of alkaline urine so that the alkalosis becomes correctable. Success is indicated by clinical improvement in the state of hydration, by an increase in urine output, a fall in blood urea and haematocrit, and restoration to normal of electrolyte concentrations.

Gastric lavage should be performed with a wide-bore tube using saline for irrigation. This should be performed twice daily initially and until the returning fluid is quite clear of particulate matter. The patient should not be allowed to eat, but fluids may be given, and milky drinks should be encouraged. One benefit of bed rest, rehydration, lavage and milk drinks is that an ulcer will begin to heal and with subsidence of the inflammatory changes the obstruction will begin to remit. Such improvement is often apparent even when the cause of the obstruction is a malignancy.

There must be no undue rush over this stage of management which will often take a week or more. The object is to get the patient into the best possible state for surgery, and it is a mistake to accept less than this ideal. During this time the patient will often benefit from chest physiotherapy. Occasionally, provision of adequate nutrition will require intravenous feeding.

It may be difficult to make a firm clinical diagnosis of the cause of the pyloric stenosis. Even when the stomach has been well prepared, radiological studies may merely confirm outlet obstruction and fail to reveal the cause. Gastroscopic examination with biopsy is appropriate once the stomach is cleansed.

Sometimes pyloric stenosis first manifests itself when active ulcer disease within the duodenum has 'burnt itself out'. A non-operative approach to the problem may then be justifiable, particularly in the elderly or medically unfit patient. Balloon dilatation of the stenosed area, via an endoscope, can sometimes relieve the obstruction. Although this may need to be repeated at intervals of a few weeks for a period, on occasions this approach can obviate the need for surgery.

A note on the more uncommon Causes of Pyloric Stenosis

Since a precise diagnosis is often not possible in pyloric stenosis, occasionally the surgeon will find himself confronted with an unexpected cause for delayed gastric emptying. A variety of benign tumours, lymphomas and granulomatous conditions can present in this way. These are discussed later.

Pyloric Hypertrophy

Thickening of the circular muscle of the pylorus to produce outlet obstruction can occur in adults. The relationship to congenital pyloric stenosis is unclear, although about 25% of such adults give a history dating back to childhood. At operation a focal or generalized thickening of the pylorus is found. There is nearly always a degree of fibrosis so that pyloroplasty rather than pyloromyotomy is the usual operation of choice.

Mucosal Diaphragm

Symptoms due to an incomplete diaphragm are often not apparent until middle age. Presumably muscular hypertrophy in the stomach is capable of overcoming the obstruction until this time. The diaphragm, consisting of mucosa and submucosa and being found in the antrum, pylorus or duodenum, represents a failure of recanalization of the embryonic gut. Gastric ulcers are sometimes found in association with this lesion. Excision of the diaphragm, with or without pyloroplasty, is all that is needed.

'Megaduodenum'

Rarely, a dilated stomach is found without an organic obstruction. The dilatation may extend into the duodenum for a variable extent. Some such cases have been well documented as being associated with degeneration of the myenteric nerve plexus. This may be as part of Chagas' disease, but in the UK the cause of the degeneration is usually unknown. Gastrojejunostomy is usually beneficial in the short term, although progression of the degeneration may occur.

Annular Pancreas

Rare instances of annular pancreas presenting in adult life as pyloric stenosis have been described. The precipitating cause is usually an attack of pancreatitis. If symptoms persist, a gastrojejunostomy is advised.

Duodenal Haematoma (*see* Chapter 75)

Arteriomesenteric Compression (Wilkie's disease)

The fourth part of the duodenum is potentially compressible between the vertebral column and the superior mesenteric vessels. Acute weight loss and immobilization in a plaster cast are cited as predisposing factors to this very rare problem.

Volvulus

Malrotation is associated with abnormal or incomplete fixation of the intestinal mesenteries so that acute twisting may occur. As commonly as volvulus, abnormal peritoneal bands associated with the malrotation (Ladd's bands) can cause duodenal obstruction.

Gastric volvulus does not really present as pyloric stenosis, but it may be reasonable to consider it here. The stomach is normally well anchored, particularly at the hiatus and pylorus. For volvulus to take place the points of tethering must be stretched and weakened. This can occur in patients with connective tissue disorders (e.g. Ehlers–Danlos syndrome), when there is extra space for the stomach to be pulled into (e.g. diaphragmatic or hiatal hernias, or anterior abdominal wall defects) or when a large tumour has caused lengthening of the connective attachments of the stomach.

Volvulus can occur around two axes—mesenterico-axial or organo-axial (*Figs.* 67.2, 67.3). In either type the presentation may be with chronic symptoms of epigastric distress and vomiting. Acute volvulus, more common with the organo-axial variety, presents as severe pain and ineffectual retching. Distension, tenderness, and signs of shock follow rapidly, and urgent surgery is indicated if strangulation and perforation are to be avoided. At operation the anatomy should be returned to normal and the stomach fixed with non-absorbable sutures. The predisposing cause may be dealt with if the patient's condition permits.

Haematemesis and Melaena

The successful treatment of acute upper gastrointestinal haemorrhage demands aggressive treatment and a policy which is flexible enough to deal with the problems peculiar to the individual patient. There are three phases in the management of the bleeding patient: resuscitation, diagnosis and definitive treatment.

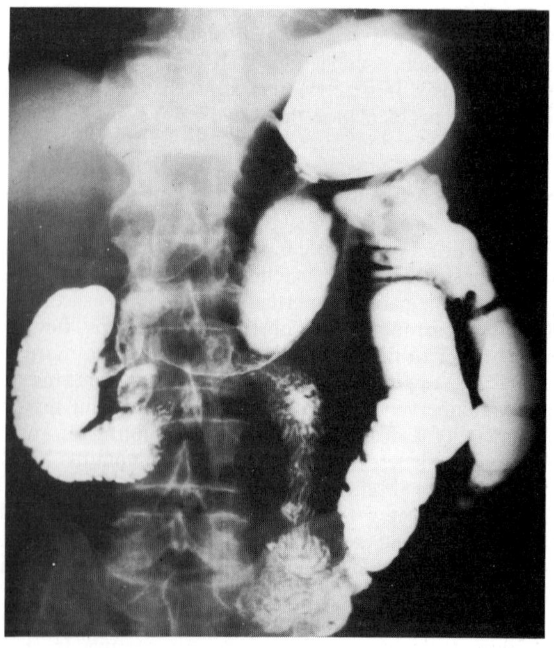

Fig. 67.2 Gastric volvulus.

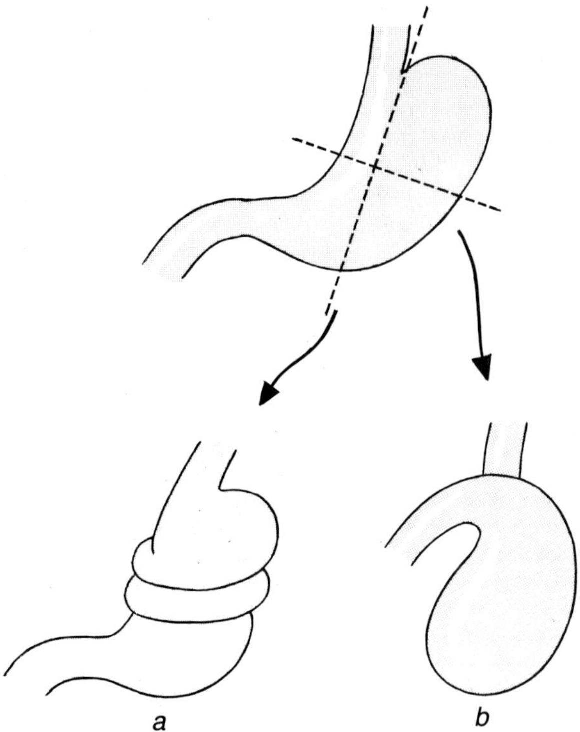

Fig. 67.3 The two types of gastric volvulus. *a*, Organo-axial. *b*, Mesenterico-axial.

Resuscitation

The general principles involved in managing haemorrhagic shock are dealt with elsewhere in this book. However, a few points merit emphasis.

Adequate resuscitation is imperative before any diagnostic measures are undertaken, and there should never be any question of sedating patients for endoscopy whilst they are still hypovolaemic from blood loss. In less severe cases it may be necessary to do no more than erect an intravenous line as a precaution against a further major bleed, but often rapid transfusion will be needed. Central venous pressure monitoring and measuring urine output are invaluable in the severely shocked patient.

All shocked patients should be given oxygen by mask, and for short periods 100% oxygen may be advisable. Confusion and restlessness demand attention for oxygenation and volume replacement, not sedation.

Diagnosis

The likely source of blood loss may be suggested by clinical features. A long dyspeptic history, stigmas of chronic liver disease, a recent high intake of alcohol and perhaps aspirin and other NSAIDs suggest a chronic ulcer, varices or erosions as the likely bleeding lesions. It must be stressed, however, that direct endoscopic visualization of the oesophagus, stomach and duodenum is the only way to make a firm decision upon which rational management can be planned.

Aside from establishing the cause of bleeding, upper gastrointestinal endoscopy is extremely valuable in predicting those patients with ulcer disease who are likely to continue to bleed or develop recurrent haemorrhage. The endoscopic stigmata which indicate this eventuality and therefore the need for early surgical intervention are:

1. Arterial spurter.
2. Identifiable vessel in base of ulcer.
3. Adherent clot.

Management

Following adequate resuscitation and diagnosis there are a number of general measures which should be carried out. The patient should be on bed rest initially and a nasogastric tube passed into the stomach. If clot is present in the stomach it is useful to remove this with cold saline lavage.

A careful watch is kept for continued or recurrent bleeding. In addition to the passage of fresh melaena or the aspiration of fresh blood from the stomach, continued blood loss is indicated by the need to give more fluid to maintain cardiovascular stability and also by increased bowel sounds on auscultation.

The role of cimetidine or ranitidine is unclear. The value of histamine H_2-receptor antagonists in bleeding from chronic duodenal ulcers, acute erosions and chronic gastric ulceration is the subject of current trials. The results to date have been disappointing and these drugs do not have an established role in the treatment of gastroduodenal haemorrhage. However, they may have a valuable contribution by preventing the development of a secondary erosive gastritis. The incidence of 'stress ulceration' during the week or so after a significant alimentary blood loss is appreciable, and on occasions this may be the source of renewed bleeding. H_2-receptor antagonists not only lower acid secretion, but also appears to have a beneficial action on the gastric mucosal barrier.

Indications for Surgery

The role of surgery is twofold: to stop bleeding which it is judged will not stop spontaneously, and to anticipate those cases in which re-bleeding is either likely or in which a rebleed would carry a significant risk to the patient. The criteria for operation thus become:

1. Continuing Bleeding

If, after the initial period of resuscitation, bleeding continues, surgery is indicated as a means of controlling haemorrhage.

2. Re-bleeding

A fresh bleed occurring some hours or days after apparent cessation of the initial haemorrhage suggests that surgery should be performed as soon as adequate transfusion has been accomplished. These patients can often be identified at the initial endoscopy.

3. The Source of Bleeding

A knowledge of the pathology responsible for the haemorrhage influences decisions on surgery and can modify other criteria. Continued or recurrent bleeding from a chronic peptic ulcer will certainly require operation, whereas there are good reasons for continuing conservative treatment in cases of bleeding erosions where surgery is less successful. If the endoscopist reports a chronic posterior wall duodenal ulcer with clot adherent to a large artery, the indications for operation are stronger than if a haemorrhagic anterior wall ulcer is all that is seen. Bleeding gastric ulcers should be operated on promptly since re-bleeding is common and carries a significant risk.

4. *Fitness of the Patient*

The presence of severe cardiorespiratory disease is a significant factor in deciding whether or not to advise surgery. It is not merely a question of deciding upon the risk of a laparotomy, but more a matter of assessing the effect that a further bleed would have on the patient. This is particularly important when cardiac disease is present, for a period of hypotension following a gastrointestinal bleed can be the cause of a myocardial infarction. In general, the older or more ill the patient, the greater is the indication for early surgery.

5. *Other Factors*

The question of the experience of the surgical and anaesthetic teams is clearly relevant, and factors such as the availability of blood need to be considered.

It should be apparent that the decision to advise laparotomy for gastrointestinal bleeding is often difficult. There are few absolute rules, and each individual patient has to be considered on his merits. The surgeon must decide what is the safest course to take for the patient in question: to operate now, or to wait?

Non-operative Management

Endoscopic treatment of bleeding lesions is feasible, although by no means always successful. The two main methods are photocoagulation with a laser, or coagulation by an electric current (electrocautery). Direct application of the latter with an electrode is not particularly effective as the coagulum is usually pulled off as the electrode is removed. Perhaps the best way of endoscopic haemostasis is by the heater probe. The exact place for this type of treatment is as yet unclear. It is asking a lot to expect an endoscopist to stop arterial bleeding from a large vessel in the base of a chronic duodenal or gastric ulcer, and indeed the results of such interventions in major upper gastrointestinal haemorrhage are disappointing. On the other hand, slower bleeding from the margins of an ulcer or discrete bleeding from an erosion can often be stopped.

Source of Bleeding Unknown

On occasions the source of an acute upper gastrointestinal bleed may be unknown. If the presenting problem is melaena alone and no blood is found in the stomach or duodenum on endoscopy then attention will turn to the lower small bowel and colon. Sometimes, however, there will be clear evidence of upper alimentary tract bleeding without any apparent source.

The problem may be one of the more unusual causes of bleeding which is merely beyond the reach of the endoscope: haemobilia, ulcerating pancreatic or duodenal tumours, aorto- or cavoduodenal fistula or a bleeding diverticulum. The decision to be made is whether to advise laparotomy, and here the most important criterion is continued bleeding. If the haemorrhage settles spontaneously, every effort should be made to secure a firm diagnosis.

In the face of continuing bleeding, the prudent surgeon will make sure that coagulation parameters are normal before embarking upon surgery, unless the rate of bleeding is such that a major vessel source is obvious and laparotomy imperative. The difficulty which may arise is that the source of bleeding is still unclear even on a full laparotomy which should include generous gastrotromy and duodenotomy incisions. Under these circumstances it is quite likely that the cause of bleeding is one of the uncommon angiodysplasias (small bowel) (*see* Chapter 72).

If it is possible to be certain that the bleeding is coming from one specific area and no other, then local suture haemostasis or resection may be feasible. If it is not possible to localize the area of bleeding, which by this time may have stopped, then it can be of great help to have an endoscope passed. The surgeon can manipulate the instrument through the bowel in a methodical manner. With the theatre lights turned down, the transillumination may show a leash of abnormal vessels. In addition, the endoscopist may see a mucosal abnormality.

Should this fail, the laparotomy should be closed. There is no place for blind resection in the hope that this will contain the source of bleeding. Emergency arteriography will need to be considered if the patient re-bleeds.

Acute Dilatation of the Stomach

Although not a specific complication of gastroduodenal surgery, acute gastric dilatation is conveniently considered at this point. The reason why the stomach should dilate to enormous dimensions so that it can contain many litres of fluid and air is unclear. Reflex inhibition of intrinsic electrical pacemaker activity has been proposed, but the variety of circumstances under which the condition may occur suggests that this explanation leaves many unanswered questions. Contrary to expectations, acute gastric dilatation rarely occurs after surgery for gastric outlet obstruction. However, this may be because appropriate nasogastric decompression is carried out routinely.

This catastrophe can follow any surgery, although upper abdominal operations, particularly splenectomy, and pelvic procedures are perhaps more common precedents. Acute dilatation of the stomach is more likely to occur in malnourished and debilitated patients, and indeed can supervene in a chronic illness without surgery having been performed. It is sometimes seen in patients who are immobilized, particularly orthopaedic patients in casts.

In addition to malnutrition, other predisposing factors include aerophagia in apprehensive patients, inadvertent distension of the stomach during ventilation or the administration of oxygen by nasal catheter, endoscopy with vigorous insufflation of gas prior to surgery and the use of opiate narcotics which can cause a significant delay in gastric emptying.

Postoperative decompression of the stomach with a nasogastric tube until such time as gastric emptying resumes may prevent some cases of acute dilatation of the stomach. There is a tendency to try to do without nasogastric tubes, or to remove them at an early stage of the postoperative course. From the point of view of patient comfort and reducing the risks of respiratory and oesophageal problems that is commendable. When nasogastric tubes are used, hourly aspiration of stomach contents should be combined with free drainage from the tube. Considerable quantities of air may accumulate especially if the tube is closed with a spigot as the patient with a nasogastric tube is continually swallowing air. On occasions it may be necessary to consider using a temporary gastrostomy or pharyngostomy for decompression if it is realized preoperatively that prolonged nasogastric intubation will be both necessary but yet undesirable.

The clinical features of acute gastric dilatation are rarely specific. Premonitory symptoms include hiccups, vague feelings of unease in the epigastric region, and small vomits which may contain altered blood. If these symptoms are heeded, a gastric splash may be elicited at this stage. The more dramatic presentation which may follow these symptoms or occur *de novo* is either as severe pain mimicking myocardial infarction or pulmonary embolus, or collapse from hypovolaemia. In either case there may be copious effortless vomiting or regurgitation of litres of foul smelling dirty fluid. Aspiration into the lungs is common.

The treatment of this emergency situation is restoration of circulating volume by crystalloid or colloid transfusion, decompression of the stomach with a large nasogastric tube, and management of any pulmonary aspiration. This may require endotracheal intubation to facilitate bronchial suction and lavage as well as antibiotics and steroids.

The mortality from such severe examples of acute gastric dilatation remains high, in part because the problem often occurs in the already debilitated patient. The need to be aware of this potential disaster, and to act promptly when early symptoms appear should be obvious.

DUODENAL ULCER DISEASE

There is no doubt that the incidence of duodenal ulcer increased considerably during the earlier part of this century and this trend now seems to be reversing. Certainly the numbers of patients coming to elective ulcer surgery are considerably fewer than they were 10 years ago. To what extent this represents a decline in the incidence of the disease is unclear. However, in the UK, the number of elective operations for duodenal ulceration has dropped significantly since the introduction of H_2-antagonists. The need for surgery for the complications of ulcer disease has changed little. In part this is due to the increasing use of non-steroidal analgesics.

Aetiological Features

Duodenal ulcer diathesis is thought to be multifactorial. Chronic duodenal ulceration is associated with hyperacidity. This general statement hides the fact that there is a considerable overlap between the ranges of acid secretion of ulcer patients and normal subjects. The primary cause of the excess acid secretion is unknown. It has been proposed that ulcer patients who have normal levels of acid secretion form a different patient group from the hypersecretors. The former are said to be predominantly of blood group O, whilst the hypersecretors are mainly of blood groups A, B and AB. In addition, the normosecretors may be more likely to develop the complications of ulcer disease.

Acid hypersecretion is usually regarded as being the result of either an increased cholinergic stimulus via the vagus nerves or an increased gastrin stimulus from the antrum. The evidence for increased vagal activity derives largely from the high levels of unstimulated overnight secretion which are typical of ulcer disease and imply overactivity of the cephalic phase of gastric secretion. Increased antral activity is sought by measuring plasma gastrin concentrations. In a very small proportion of ulcer patients fasting plasma gastrin concentrations are considerably elevated due to hyperplasia of the antral G cells. However, in the majority of patients, fasting gastrin concentrations are not elevated. Despite this, abnormalities of gastrin release can be demonstrated. The gastrin response to a meal may be exaggerated and prolonged, and the inhibition of gastrin release by acid may be defective. There is also some evidence to suggest that the local paracrine control of gastrin release may be abnormal. Despite all these uncertainties it remains true that measures which produce a sufficient reduction in acid output will allow a duodenal ulcer to heal.

Uncommonly, duodenal ulceration may be associated with other diseases. These include liver disease (particularly after shunt surgery), persistent hypercalcaemia, renal failure and after massive small bowel resection.

Campylobacter organisms (e.g. *Campylobacter pylorridis*) have been isolated from patients with duodenal ulcers. The significance of these organisms in the pathogenesis of duodenal ulcer remains uncertain, however.

Clinical Features

Duodenal ulceration is a remitting disease characterized by periods of activity and quiescence. Exacerbations may be associated with periods of stress, dietary or alcoholic indiscretions and smoking. It tends to have a seasonal variation. Early in the history of the disease, remissions may be associated with complete healing of the ulcer, but as the disease progresses there is a tendency toward fibrous scarring so that evidence of past disease may be found on investigation even when the patient is free from symptoms.

Typically the epigastric pain appears when the stomach is empty and there is nothing to buffer the acid secretions. Relief usually follows eating, milk or alkalis. Failure to produce relief, particularly if pain is felt in the back, suggests penetration of the ulcer posteriorly. Vomiting is not usually a feature of simple chronic ulceration, and its presence suggests that outlet obstruction may be developing. This may be due to fibrous pyloric stenosis (more correctly, duodenal stenosis), but may also be due to a functional delay in emptying associated with a large inflammatory ulcer mass and oedema.

Physical signs may amount to no more than diffuse epigastric tenderness, although sometimes this is well localized. Occult bleeding may produce quite marked degrees of anaemia on occasions. The presence of a succussion splash indicates delayed gastric emptying.

Investigations

Barium meal examination has been the mainstay of the investigation of dyspepsia. In patients with a chronic history this will usually demonstrate deformity in the region of the duodenal cap and will often reveal an ulcer crater. If these signs are shown and the stomach itself is seen to be normal then no further confirmation is required. If there is any doubt about the findings, or if the examination is normal despite a convincing history, endoscopy should be performed. It is bad practice to treat a patient with persisting dyspepsia but no firm diagnosis, as this invites the risk of missing an early gastric cancer.

Management

The term 'duodenal ulcer diathesis' is a useful one in so far as it emphasizes that the patient with a chronic history, i.e. two or more 'attacks', will always have the tendency to ulceration. Persuading a patient to change his life style is seldom rewarding, and treatment with alkalis alone during a relapse is often unsatisfactory. Anticholinergic drugs can sometimes reduce acid secretion sufficiently to allow an ulcer to heal, but long-term treatment is seldom practical since few patients can tolerate the dose required to reduce acid secretion.

Effective long-term reduction of acid secretion can be achieved either by a histamine H_2-receptor antagonist, such as cimetidine or ranitidine, or by an ulcer operation. It is the choice between these two modalities of treatment which confronts the surgeon faced with a patient with an uncomplicated chronic duodenal ulcer. Cimetidine or ranitidine is so effective at relieving symptoms and allowing ulcers to heal, and is without significant short-term side-effects, that there is no justification for advising operation for a patient with an uncomplicated ulcer unless they have had an adequate period of treatment with this drug. A 6–8 week course of cimetidine in full dosage (400 mg b.d. or 800 mg *nocte*) will relieve most people of ulcer symptoms, and healing can be demonstrated in 80–90% of patients. Unfortunately a relapse rate of around 80% can be expected if the drug is then stopped. However, if the full course is followed by a maintenance dose of 400 mg nightly, continuing remission occurs in 65–80% of patients. It now seems likely that maintenance treatment needs to be prolonged and in many instances, indefinite.

Duodenal ulceration is a chronic relapsing disease, and even after maintenance treatment for a year the majority of patients will experience further symptoms after stopping treatment.

Patients who fail to respond, who relapse on treatment, or who are non-compliant (do not take the tablets) should be considered as candidates for surgery. The decision to advise surgery is made on the usual criteria, namely a consideration of the amount of trouble the patient is experiencing, how much this interferes with his life and work, and how easy it is to control with simple dietary and drug therapy. In patients considered unfit for surgery—usually because of cardiorespiratory disease—it may be worth considering high long-term courses of cimetidine or ranitidine. The combination of small doses of cimetidine and an anticholinergic drug has been found to be useful in controlling the extreme hyperacidity associated with the Zollinger–Ellison syndrome, and this approach may also be considered.

Two other preparations are worth mentioning, as both have been reported as being as effective as cimetidine in inducing ulcer healing. These are Duogastrone (carbenoxolone sodium) and De Nol (tri-potassium bi-citrate bismuthate, 5 ml added to 15 ml water q.d.s.). Neither of these agents produce pain relief as rapidly as cimetidine, and the side-effects of carbenoxolone are greater. It would be unwise to contemplate long-term treatment with this latter drug, but De Nol could be used justifiably, when effective, if there were sound reasons for avoiding operation. Both of these drugs are said to have a lower relapse rate (or longer time until relapse) after stopping treatment than that after H_2-receptor antagonists. This may be due to a beneficial effect on the local tissues and, in the case of De Nol, to the local action of bismuth on campylobacter-like organisms (*see* section on gastritis).

The Choice of Operation

The aim of almost all operations for uncomplicated duodenal ulceration is to reduce acid secretion to such levels that the ulcer will heal and stay healed. The only exception to this is the operation of simple gastroenterostomy which aims at directing acid away from the area of ulceration. There is no doubt that this latter procedure is effective, but because of the high incidence of jejunal ulceration, amounting perhaps to 50% on long-term follow-up, this procedure is not often used. Advocates of gastroenterostomy alone claim that recurrent jejunal ulceration is not a problem if patients who have low levels of acid secretion are selected for the operation, or if it is used in the elderly where lower levels of secretion are more common and the life expectancy is such that recurrence over a long period is not an important consideration.

In the majority of patients, the surgeon is faced with the choice of gastric resection (to reduce the size of the parietal cell mass and to remove the antrum—the source of the gastric phase of secretion), vagal denervation (to abolish the cephalic phase of secretion and reduce the sensitivity of the parietal cells to secretory stimuli), or a combination of the two. Although the purpose of the operation is to effect permanent cure of the ulcer diathesis, this is not the only consideration, and a comparison of the various procedures demands that operative morbidity and mortality and the incidence of side-effects need to be weighed carefully against success rate in terms of recurrent ulcer risk.

The relative advantages and disadvantages of gastrectomy, vagotomy and drainage, and highly selective vagotomy are summarized in *Fig.* 67.4. Subtotal gastrectomy with gastrojejunal anastomosis is an excellent anti-ulcer operation, but its merits are seriously marred by the increased morbidity and mortality which would be expected to follow a return to the widespread use of this operation, as well as the incidence of troublesome side-effects and nutritional sequelae. The operation of truncal vagotomy and drainage is certainly safer. However, hopes that vagotomy and drainage would avoid the problems of alimentary side-effects and maintain good nutrition have not been realized, and many surgeons feel dissatisfied with this approach.

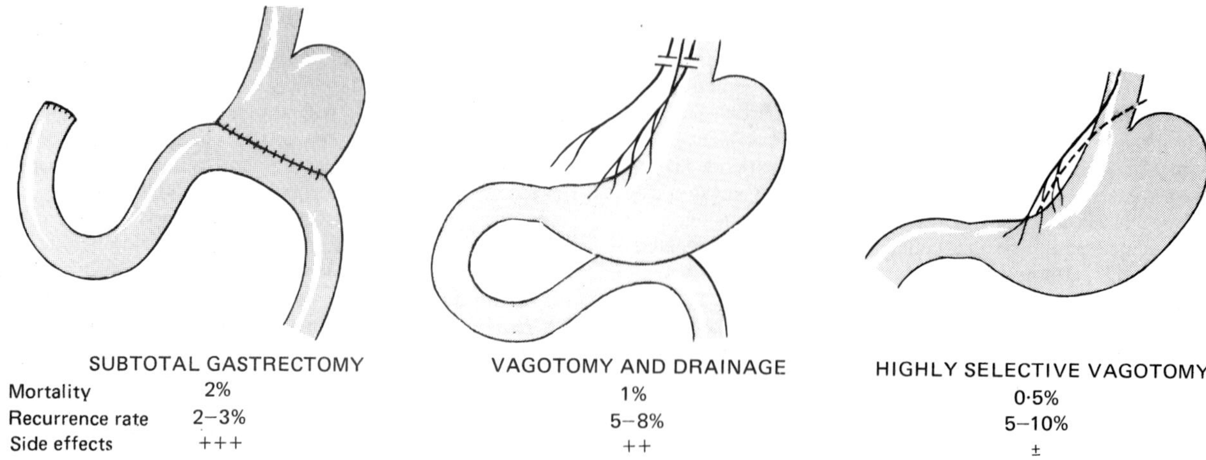

Fig. 67.4 The relative advantages and disadvantages of various operative procedures used for chronic duodenal ulceration. The figures given for mortality and recurrence rates are average values only. Choice of the 'best' operation involves a careful balance of these three factors.

Vagotomy and antrectomy possesses the advantages of a dual attack on acid secretory mechanisms, and as a result carries the lowest recurrent ulcer risk. Unfortunately, it also carries the disadvantages of both resection and vagotomy.

Vagotomy and antrectomy is probably the operation of choice for prepyloric ulcer disease which seems, for reasons not clear, to carry a much higher recurrent ulcer rate than simple duodenal ulcer.

Which Vagotomy?

Modifications of the technique of vagotomy have been introduced in an attempt to improve the results of ulcer surgery. The alternatives to truncal vagotomy are bilateral selective vagotomy, which confines the denervation to the stomach, and highly selective vagotomy (parietal cell, proximal gastric, selective proximal vagotomy) in which only the acid-producing part of the stomach is denervated.

Although selective vagotomy has been performed without gastric drainage, this is not to be recommended as many patients will experience symptoms of gastric stasis and some will develop gastric ulceration. The advantages of the selective approach are twofold. First, once the technique has been mastered it is probably easier to obtain complete gastric denervation so that the recurrent ulcer risk should be lower. Secondly, the incidence of diarrhoea is reduced. Despite these two recommendations, the overall clinical results of selective vagotomy are no better than those of truncal vagotomy, and this operation has been largely abandoned.

The major advantage of highly selective vagotomy is that a drainage procedure can be omitted as the propulsive power of the innervated antrum is retained. There is no doubt that preservation of an anatomically and physiologically intact antropyloroduodenal segment has resulted in a much lower incidence of alimentary side-effects. Particularly impressive are the low incidences of dumping, diarrhoea and bile vomiting. A second advantage of the operation is that it is extremely safe. A specific, and potentially fatal, complication of highly selective vagotomy is lesser curve necrosis, but this seems to be exceptionally rare. A possible drawback to the operation is the risk of recurrent ulceration. Some authors report recurrent ulcer rates of between 10 and 20%. On the other hand, several series report recurrence rates which are of the same order as those found after truncal vagotomy. The differences probably reflect the adequacy of the denervation. If the highly selective vagotomy achieves a complete denervation of the acid-secreting cells then the subsequent risk of recurrence is not excessive. Highly selective vagotomy is rapidly becoming the standard operation for uncomplicated duodenal ulcer disease in the UK.

Which Drainage Procedure?

Both truncal and selective vagotomy impair antral motility to such a degree that gastric stasis will supervene in a substantial number of patients if the denervated stomach is not drained. Drainage can be achieved by pyloroplasty, gastroenterostomy or antrectomy. Controlled trials have not indicated any obvious superiority of one procedure over the other. Bile vomiting may be a little more of a problem after gastroenterostomy, but this is probably offset by a slightly higher incidence of dumping after pyloroplasty. Gastroenterostomy may be a safer alternative when the ulcer area is the seat of an inflammatory mass or when there is much fibrous scarring.

If a postvagotomy patient is plagued by bile vomiting, dumping or diarrhoea, it is easy to close the gastroenterostomy. Reconstruction of the pylorus is more demanding.

Complications of Duodenal Ulceration

Perforation, bleeding and stenosis are usually complications of a chronic symptomatic ulcer, but each can occur with little or no previous history, and perforation and bleeding may present *de novo* from acute ulceration. These complications add considerably to the morbidity and mortality of duodenal ulcer disease.

Perforation

The initial management of gastroduodenal perforation has been described previously.

Simple Suture or Definitive Procedure?

Approximately 60% of patients who have had a perforated duodenal ulcer treated conservatively, or by simple suture, have further dyspepsia. One-half of these will come to operation sooner or later. These figures are probably an underestimate if one considers only those patients who have perforated an ulcer responsible for chronic symptoms. This being so, there is clearly a case for considering combining simple suture with a definitive anti-ulcer operation. In the past the criteria for deciding to perform a definitive operation were:

1. A chronic history. In this context, any patient with a history of a month or more should be regarded as having a chronic ulcer.
2. Fitness to withstand the additional operative procedure.
3. Degree of peritoneal soiling. If the perforation has resulted in widespread peritoneal contamination, and sufficient time has elapsed for the initial chemical peritonitis to become a bacterial peritonitis, then anything more than a simple suture is probably inadvisable. There is a risk of introducing infection into the mediastinal tissues during vagotomy.
4. Experience of the surgeon.

However, with the advent of H_2-receptor antagonists an emergency definitive procedure is seldom justifiable even in the presence of a long history as simple closure of the perforation followed by long-term therapy with cimetidine or ranitidine gives good results. In the presence of a duodenal perforation a pyloroplasty is best avoided unless the defect is such that closure is easier in this way. Even then a truncal vagotomy and gastroenterostomy may be prudent and if there is any evidence of stenosis it is mandatory. Highly selective vagotomy has also been used in conjunction with simple suture with good results by experienced surgeons The criteria for performing a safe definitive ulcer procedure must be present if the surgeon decides on this course of action in the individual case.

Pyloric Stenosis

Outlet obstruction of the stomach secondary to chronic duodenal ulceration is usually due to a combination of fibrosis, from repeated cycles of ulceration and healing, oedema, inflammation and pylorospasm associated with current activity of the ulcer. Although established pyloric stenosis is an almost absolute indication for surgery, much can be done by intensive medical treatment to improve the patient and make operation safer. This aspect has been discussed earlier.

Considerable hypertrophy of the stomach wall takes place

in response to outlet obstruction, so that gastric emptying may be normal despite marked fibrous stenosis. On occasions an intensive period of medical treatment may result in the resolution of the inflammatory changes around an ulcer so that less florid cases of pyloric stenosis may remit. If this happens and operation is not planned, a precise diagnosis becomes mandatory. If a malignant cause for the obstruction cannot be ruled out absolutely, with a combination of radiology and endoscopy, then operation must be advised despite the symptomatic improvement.

Surgical Treatment of Pyloric Stenosis

The twofold aim of surgery is to heal the ulcer and overcome gastric stasis. When outlet obstruction has resulted in a 'decompensated' stomach—a large flaccid bag—these objectives are best achieved by a combination of vagotomy with gastric drainage. It is true that the incidence of delayed emptying after operation is somewhat higher when pyloric stenosis existed beforehand, but there is no good evidence to support the contention that the atonic stomach is more susceptible to the effects of vagotomy. Stomal hold-up can complicate gastrectomy as well as vagotomy and drainage.

In cases where a compensated pyloric stenosis exists and the stomach still possesses good muscular tone, highly selective vagotomy has been advocated. The operation has been performed without gastric drainage, but with either dilatation of the stenosis or with a duodenoplasty. In carefully selected cases this may be a reasonable approach in the hands of surgeons well versed with the operation. There is no point in performing highly selective vagotomy *with* a drainage procedure since this negates the main advantage of the operation.

Delayed Emptying after Surgery

The incidence of delayed gastric emptying is somewhat higher when the operation is performed for pyloric stenosis, but if preoperative preparation has been adequate it should be a rare complication. There is usually no obvious cause for the problem. If excessive nasogastric aspirates continue beyond about the fifth postoperative day, and provided the abdomen is soft and bowel sounds are present, it is worth removing the tube and giving the patient something to eat.

Should stasis persist, a mechanical cause needs to be excluded by contrast radiology and endoscopy. If no cause for obstruction can be seen, non-operative treatment should be persisted with. The addition of another drainage procedure rarely solves the problem.

Pharmacological stimuli to emptying using cholinergic agents or metoclopramide and, more recently, Cisapride, may be tried, but the results are usually disappointing. It would seem more reasonable to use naturally occurring agents such as the peptide, motilin, but there is little experience with such agents. Most cases settle spontaneously, although rarely it may take many weeks. Adequate nutrition by the parenteral route will be needed in such patients.

Haematemesis and Melaena

Upper gastrointestinal haemorrhage is the single most common cause of death in patients with a chronic duodenal ulcer. It has been estimated that 25% of ulcer patients have at least one bleeding episode, and figures for the mortality from bleeding vary from 10 to 50%. The commonest causes of death in this situation are myocardial infarction and stroke, presumably resulting from hypotension in a patient with pre-existing cardiovascular disease.

The initial management of upper gastrointestinal haemorrhage centres around resuscitation and then subsequently diagnosis of the source of bleeding, preferably by endoscopy. This has been discussed previously, but it is worth emphasizing that even when the patient is known to have a particular potential bleeding lesion, the source of bleeding always remains in doubt until it has been visualized by endoscopy. Another important consideration is that it is almost never necessary to embark upon diagnostic measures until the patient has been adequately resuscitated.

Indications for Surgery

Eighty per cent of patients with a bleeding ulcer will stop bleeding spontaneously; presumably a period of hypotension from blood loss assists this. In the few patients who continue to bleed there is clearly no alternative to surgery, which should be carried out as soon as the patient is deemed fit for operation.

The majority of significant bleeds come from posterior penetrating ulcers which have eroded into the gastroduodenal artery. The presence of fibrosis in the ulcer base, the presence of an arteriosclerotic artery and clot adherent to the ulcer or an active arterial spurter at the time of endoscopy makes it unwise to assume that the patient will stop bleeding or not rebleed. Energetic medical treatment may encourage ulcer healing, but it can do nothing for the eroded vessel. There is no reason to suppose that cimetidine will improve this situation. When medical measures alone are used to deal with a chronic bleeding ulcer, the incidence of further bleeding at some time during the next five years is 50%. Some of these patients will die as a result, and another 20% or so will come to operation because of chronic symptoms. Five years after a bleed, only one-third of patients will be alive, with an intact stomach, and without further bleeding.

It is clear that a patient who has bled from a chronic posterior wall duodenal ulcer should be advised to have surgery. Furthermore, there is no justification for discharging that patient from hospital with plans for later surgery, since this merely invites a further bleed which may be fatal. If the bleed has been of a small magnitude, if the patient is young and fit, and particularly if the bleeding is seen to be coming from an anterior or superior ulcer it may be reasonable to plan for an elective operation within 7–10 days. The advantage of this approach is that at this stage the ulcer will be healing on medical treatment and may be treated as if it were an uncomplicated ulcer. Vagotomy and gastroenterostomy or highly selective vagotomy will be safe procedures under these circumstances. In most other cases the decision is whether to advise an emergency operation or whether to plan for urgent surgery within the next 24 hours. In general, older patients (60 yrs+), particularly those with coexisting cardiovascular disease, are at particular risk if re-bleeding occurs and there should be no undue delay in proceeding to operation. This also applies if the patient has been shocked, if more than 4 units of blood have been needed for resuscitation, if there is a shortage of blood, or if the patient is still bleeding during endoscopy.

Choice of Operation

The goal of surgery for bleeding ulcer is to combine an ulcer operation with reliable haemostasis. Traditionally these objectives were accomplished by partial gastrectomy, which included excision of the ulcer. There is no doubt that this is an effective operation from the standpoint of stopping haemorrhage. However, the morbidity and mortality have prompted many people to adopt the more conservative approach of underrunning the bleeding ulcer with strong non-absorbable material, pyloroplasty and truncal vagotomy. Many trials have shown that this is a favourable alternative to gastrectomy. The mortality is less, although the re-bleeding rate is somewhat higher. If the surgeon is not satisfied with the control achieved by suture he should consider gastric resection as a means of achieving better haemostasis. Under these circumstances a hemigastrectomy combined with truncal vagotomy may be preferable to subtotal gastrectomy. More recently, underrunning of the bleeding ulcer without vagotomy followed by treatment with H_2-blockers has been advocated, particularly in the elderly.

Re-bleeding after Surgery

Recurrence of bleeding within the early postoperative course may be a problem in about 5% of cases. The risk is higher after suture ligation and vagotomy than after gastrectomy. It is important to realize that the source of the bleed need not be the same as that of the initial bleed. Erosive gastritis, arising during the period of hypotension and perhaps exacerbated by postoperative gastric stasis and bile reflux, is probably more common than generally acknowledged. In addition, bleeding may occur from a suture line or from a coexisting lesion not noticed at the time of the operation. Any significant re-bleed should prompt urgent endoscopy. Fresh arterial bleeding from the original ulcer, when suture control has been used previously, needs further surgery in the form of a resection. Very few re-bleeding ulcers will settle without further intervention.

Further bleeding on long-term follow-up has been reported as occurring in up to 20% of patients, regardless of the type of surgery initially performed. This haemorrhage can occur from any site in the alimentary tract, and such cases should be treated *de novo* on their merits.

The Failures of Gastric Surgery

Unsatisfactory results follow ulcer surgery in 10–20% of cases. The reported incidence varies considerably and no doubt depends to a large extent on the thoroughness of follow-up. Poor results may be because of recurrent ulceration, alimentary side-effects or nutritional disturbances. The various operative procedures have a broadly similar incidence of unsatisfactory results, although the reasons are often different. Thus the failures of gastrectomy are usually due to severe gastrointestinal side-effects, sometimes combined with poor nutrition, rather than recurrent ulceration. After vagotomy and drainage both alimentary symptoms and recurrent ulceration are sources of poor results, whereas after highly selective vagotomy there are very few patients with gastrointestinal side-effects. In some series, however, a higher recurrent ulcer rate brings the incidence of poor results into line with the other operations.

Recurrent Ulceration

Recurrent ulceration may appear in the stomach, the duodenum, or at the site of a gastrointestinal stoma. The aetiology of gastric ulceration after previous duodenal ulcer surgery is different from recurrent ulceration in the two other sites, and usually gastric ulceration implies either delayed emptying or duodenal reflux. Recurrent duodenal or stomal ulceration suggests that the ulcer diathesis persists: in other words the hypersecretory state has not been corrected sufficiently by the previous operation. Although most cases of recurrent ulcer are the result of a failure of the previous operation, no operation will protect the stomach from drug and alcohol abuse.

The causes of recurrent ulceration are shown in *Fig.* 67.5 and discussed individually below:

1. Incomplete Vagotomy

Failure to achieve complete denervation of the parietal cell mass is the commonest cause of recurrent ulceration. The incidence of incomplete vagotomy may be as high as 20% after truncal vagotomy, as judged by the results of early postoperative insulin tests. It is true that some of these positive tests are only technically positive and may be the result of very small residual fibres only, but some are due to a major vagal trunk which has been missed, and under these circumstances a recurrent ulcer is inevitable. Peroperative tests have been described which are said to allow better visualization of the nerve fibres (leucomethylene blue) or to permit a check on the adequacy of vagotomy by observing a failure of peristalsis after electrical stimulation or an absence of acid secretion (as shown by an intragastric dye or pH probe) after pentagastrin or histamine infusion. These techniques are all time-consuming, give variable results and have not been adopted by the majority of surgeons. The most important prerequisites for successful vagotomy are the detailed knowledge of the variable anatomy of the vagus nerves and patience.

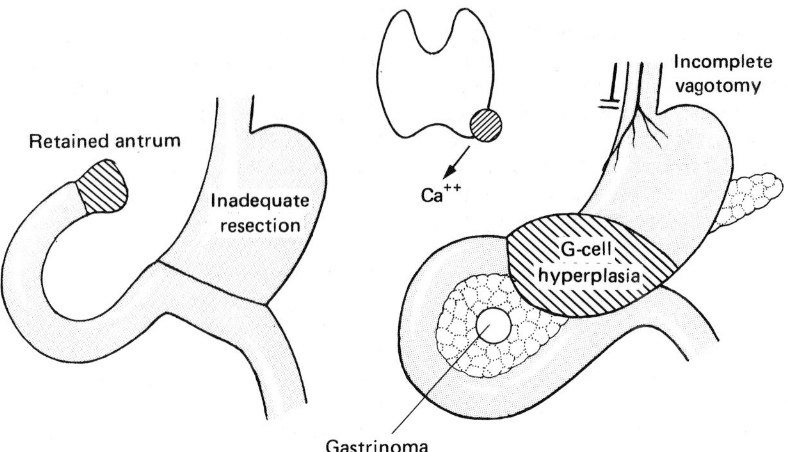

Fig. 67.5 The causes of recurrent duodenal or stomal ulceration after previous ulcer surgery.

As far as truncal vagotomy is concerned, the key is the realization that the operation can be carried out at two levels: the hiatus or above (as advocated by Dragstedt), or at the cardia. At either level it is possible to miss vagal fibres (*Fig.* 67.6), although it is less easy to miss a significant trunk if vagotomy is carried out low on the oesophagus. The solution to the problem is to divide the anterior and posterior trunks at the hiatus initially. This will enable the oesophagus to be pulled down and the region of the cardia then becomes more accessible. The lower oesophagus should then be cleared methodically until it is bared to longitudinal muscle fibres all round. The nasogastric tube should be withdrawn temporarily at this point to allow careful palpation for any remaining fibres. With this length of oesophagus cleared it is quite easy to see the region of the fundus adequately and thus prevent any vagal innervation to this area being missed.

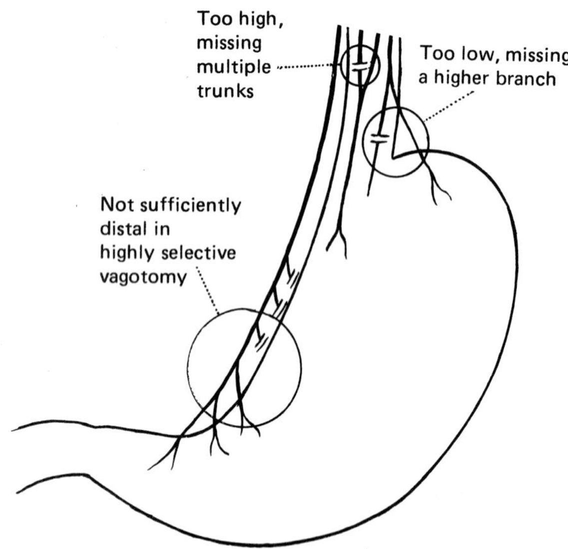

Fig. 67.6 The causes of incomplete vagotomy.

The incidence of incomplete nerve section after the selective vagotomies seems to be somewhat less than that after truncal vagotomy, once the techniques have been mastered. This is probably because the operations must be carried out on the lower oesophagus, with careful attention to clearing the oesophagus as described above. Inadequate technique will result in an alarming incidence of incomplete vagotomy and an unacceptably high recurrent ulcer rate. If complete parietal cell denervation is to be achieved by highly selective vagotomy, three aspects of technique need special attention. Clearance of at least 5 cm of distal oesophagus is needed: many studies have shown that a lesser clearance is inadequate. In addition, the lesser curve denervation must be carried distally far enough to ensure that parietal cell mass is not left innervated. The antrum/parietal cell border can be demonstrated with a pH probe or intragastric dye, but in practice it is sufficient to carry the dissection down until only the major termination of the nerve of Latarjet is left. Finally, innervation of the fundal region from the so-called criminal nerve of Grassi must be sought. This is usually not a problem if the distal oesophagus has been cleared sufficiently to allow its posterior aspect to be seen.

2. *Inadequate Resection*

If gastrectomy is to be the sole means used for reducing acid secretion, a minimum of threequarters of the stomach needs to be removed. Certainly, anything less than a 75% resection will not protect against ulcerogenesis experimentally. A related consideration is the method of restoring continuity after resection. Generally speaking, a gastrojejunal anastomosis is preferred to gastroduodenostomy. This is partly for technical reasons, and partly for the belief that the recurrent ulcer risk is less. Although this latter belief is supported by well-documeted opinion, it is difficult to substantiate. Comparisons between the two methods suffer from the defect that the extent of resection is usually ignored, and it is certainly possible that less stomach might be removed if one were striving for a gastroduodenal anastomosis. When vagotomy is combined with resection, some of the lowest recurrence rates come from centres where gastroduodenal anastomosis is the preferred method.

3. *Retained Gastric Antrum*

If residual antral tissue is left in continuity with the duodenal stump, the antral G cells, now in an alkaline environment, will secrete gastrin continuously (*see Fig.* 67.6). Under this constant stimulus the remaining parietal cells will produce sufficient acid for stomal ulceration to develop. Whenever hypergastrinaemia is found after partial gastrectomy, the retained antrum must be considered. Differentiation of this entity from autonomous tumour production of gastrin is usually possible from the results of the secretin and calcium tests, but direct confirmation of retained antral tissue may be more difficult. Radioisotope scanning with technetium may help.

4. *Zollinger–Ellison Syndrome*

This syndrome describes the association of an intractable ulcer diathesis with a gastrin-secreting tumour, usually in the pancreas. The continuous secretion of gastrin makes ulcer recurrence an inevitability, and this often occurs quite quickly after the original operation. The rapidity of the return of symptoms and their virulence, sometimes indicated by perforation or haemorrhage, should raise the suspicion of this problem. This suspicion will be heightened if gastric secretory studies are used, as they should be, to investigate the recurrent ulcer. Because the parietal cell mass is under constant stimulation, the characteristic finding is of a high level of basal secretion relative to maximal stimulated secretion. If basal secretion is greater than 60% of the response to pentagastrin or histamine, every effort must be made to exclude the Zollinger–Ellison syndrome. This is done by measuring plasma gastrin concentrations as described earlier.

5. *Hypercalcaemia*

The relationships between hypercalcaemia, gastrin, acid secretion and peptic ulceration are complex. Calcium can cause gastrin release and acid secretion, but, in addition, hyperparathyroidism may coexist with a gastrinoma. In practice, if hypercalcaemia is found in a patient with a peptic ulcer, recurrent or otherwise, parathormone levels should be measured. If hyperparathyroidism is found, and corrected surgically, plasma gastrin concentrations may fall to normal and the ulcer will often heal. There is some suggestion that this is more likely to occur if the patient has a parathyroid adenoma rather than hyperplasia. If the ulcer persists despite parathyroidectomy, and especially if gastrin concentrations remain elevated, evidence for a gastrinoma must be sought.

Management of the Patient with Recurrent 'Dyspepsia'

The persistence of indigestion, or its return after a period of freedom from symptoms suggests the possibility of recurrent ulceration. Other possibilities should not be ignored, however. These include possibly unrelated problems such as oesophageal reflux, gallstones, pancreatitis, and angina as well as complications of surgery: in particular, reflux gastritis, gastric stasis, or afferent loop problems.

It is not always an easy matter to establish a diagnosis of recurrent ulceration. On occasions the character of the indigestion may be similar to that experienced before operation, but often it is different in site or type. If vomiting is a feature, the presence of bile or food may suggest reflux gastritis or stasis as causes of the problem. Recurrent ulcers may present with bleeding or, less commonly, perforation with no accompanying dyspepsia. The rapid return of symptoms, haemorrhage or perforation, particularly in a younger patient with a strong family history should suggest the possibility of an endocrine cause for the recurrence. Coexisting diarrhoea also hints at this possibility, although post-vagotomy diarrhoea and gastrocolic fistula should be considered.

Radiological studies of the stomach and duodenum are often difficult to interpret. Scarring of the duodenum will persist even if the ulcer has healed, and the presence of a pyloroplasty may make it impossible to demonstrate an ulcer crater. Fibreoptic endoscopy is the best method for detecting ulcer recurrence, and it may also give valuable information if gastritis and/or bile reflux are present.

By no means do all recurrent ulcers need surgical treatment, and a trial of medical treatment with cimetidine or ranitidine is a reasonable approach to recurrent duodenal or stomal ulceration. Recurrent ulceration in the body of the stomach will often respond to De-Nol, and metoclopramide is a useful additional agent. Ulcer healing, under these circumstances, may be permanent and this is particularly likely if the recurrence was associated with alcohol or drugs, such as aspirin.

If the recurrence does not respond promptly to such measures, further investigation is required to establish why the ulcer has reappeared. The usual reason is that the 'hypersecretory' state persists, due either to incomplete vagotomy or inadequate resection. Gastric secretory tests should be carried out in which basal secretion and the response to a secretogogue, such as pentagastrin, are measured. If vagotomy has been performed, insulin stimulation should also be used, and this can be conveniently given after measurement of basal secretion and before the pentagastrin test.

If vagotomy has been the previous operation and investigations indicate persisting hypersecretion with incomplete vagotomy, revagotomy may be attempted by the abdominal or thoracic routes. However, it is more prudent to proceed to antrectomy with revagotomy.

When hypersecretion persists after gastrectomy, the crucial question is whether insufficient stomach was removed, or whether secretion is being driven by endogenous gastrin. In the absence of hypergastrinaemia, the addition of a truncal vagotomy to what should amount to at least a hemigastrectomy is usually adequate, and certainly safer than a re-resection.

When hypergastrinaemia is found, further investigation will be needed to differentiate retained antrum from a gastrinoma, as described earlier. Surgical removal of retained antral tissue may not be easy, and long-term cimetidine should be contemplated, particularly in the older or high risk patient.

If investigations confirm a diagnosis of the Zollinger–Ellison syndrome, selective arteriography should be used to demonstrate the blood supply of the pancreas. This may demonstrate the tumour and show whether it is multifocal. A hepatic arteriogram may reveal metastases.

SEQUELAE OF GASTRIC SURGERY

Minor postprandial complaints are commonly experienced by patients after gastric operations. These usually improve with time and dietary adjustments. In a small cohort of patients, however, variously estimated at 5–20%, the symptoms are severe, persistent and cause considerable disability and malnutrition. The various postgastric surgery syndromes arise on a background of altered anatomy and physiology of the upper gastrointestinal tract although the exact mechanisms responsible for some of the severe symptoms remain unclear. A useful classification of the sequelae of gastric surgery is shown in *Table* 67.3.

Table 67.3 Sequelae of gastric surgery

Recurrence of the disease	Recurrent ulcer or recurrence of gastric carcinoma
Nutritional consequences	Weight loss, anaemia, milk intolerance, bone disease
Dumping symptoms	
Reactive hypoglycaemia	
Bile vomiting	
Diarrhoea	
Small stomach syndrome	
Mechanical complications	Afferent/efferent loop obstruction, jejunogastric intussusception, gastro-oesophageal reflux
Other	Cholelithiasis, bezoar formation, gastric carcinoma

Disabling symptoms after gastric surgery are more often encountered in the following:

Female sex
Operations for peptic ulceration in the young (below 30 years of age)
Extensive gastrectomy with duodenal diversion (Polya).

Severe and persistent symptoms are rarely encountered after highly selective vagotomy but occur with the same frequency as that reported after gastrectomy in patients who undergo truncal vagotomy with drainage or truncal vagotomy and antrectomy. The type of drainage procedure (pyloroplasty or gastrojejunostomy) does not affect the incidence of the postprandial symptoms and other sequelae.

Nutritional Consequences of Gastric Surgery

These consist of weight loss, anaemia and bone disease.

Weight Loss

Loss or failure to gain weight is very common after gastric surgery and tends to be more marked after extensive gastrectomy, particularly of the Polya type. Significant weight loss is usually encountered in patients who obtain a bad result and experience severe postcibal symptoms. The resulting diminished calorie intake is the major factor although malabsorption of fat and nitrogen and decreased small bowel transit time may be operative at least in some patients. Although mild steatorrhoea is common, severe fat malabsorption is rare unless there is a coexisting subclinical small intestinal disease (e.g. gluten enteropathy) or gross bacterial overgrowth.

Anaemia

Iron-deficiency Anaemia

Very common after vagotomy and drainage and gastric resections, especially in females. The incidence of this complication increases with time and approximates to 60% and 80% at 10–20 years in males and females respectively. The exact pathogenesis of the iron-deficiency anaemia is unclear but is probably multifactorial. The mechanisms thought to be important include: shift to trivalent ferric iron at high pH followed by polymerization, loss of a gastric juice factor which normally facilitates the absorption of iron, diminished splitting of iron–protein complexes by the reduced peptic activity of the gastric juice and enhanced binding of dietary iron to specific proteins (e.g. gastroferrin).

In view of the high incidence of iron-deficiency anaemia after gastric surgery, prophylactic treatment with oral iron (300 mg q.d.s.) is nowadays recommended in all patients after gastrectomy and truncal vagotomy and drainage. This amount of daily iron supplementation allows sufficient absorption to restore serum iron levels to normal.

Macrocytic Anaemia

This is the result of vitamin B_{12} deficiency. Malabsorption of this vitamin is invariable after total gastrectomy due to the loss of intrinsic factor. However, megaloblastic anaemia takes several years to develop due to the large body stores of vitamin B_{12}. These patients have an abnormal Schilling test and require 3-monthly injections of cyanocobalamin indefinitely.

Subclinical deficiency of this vitamin is also encountered in some patients after partial gastrectomy or truncal vagotomy and drainage, although frank megaloblastic anaemia is rare in these groups. The main factor responsible for the impaired absorption of dietary vitamin B_{12} in patients after partial gastrectomy and truncal vagotomy is the lack of acid environment which normally facilitates the release of vitamin B_{12} bound to the ingested food. The reduced secretion of intrinsic factor reported in some of these patients is considered to be less important in this group of patients in whom the Schilling test is normal. Treatment is with oral cystalline vitamin B_{12} which is administered between meals.

Malabsorption of vitamin B_{12} may also be the consequence of bacterial overgrowth and steatorrhoea. Folate deficiency is rare and is only encountered in patients after extensive or total gastrectomy. It results from an inadequate dietary intake.

Bone Disease

This complication develops several years after gastric resection with duodenal exclusion (Polya) as the duodenum is the major site of calcium absorption. The majority of patients are females who develop osteomalacia 10–20 years after gastrectomy. However, cases with features of both osteomalacia (bone demineralization) and osteoporosis (loss of bone substance) are well documented. The biochemical features (raised alkaline phosphatase and serum calcium) and radiological changes (rarefaction) usually predate the clinical symptoms by several months to years. The clinical features of postgastrectomy bone disease include generalized bone pains, weakness due to an associated myopathy and the development of stress fractures. Treatment is with oral calcium and vitamin D supplements.

Dumping

Considerable confusion has been generated by the inclusion of patients with reactive hypoglycaemia in this group under the heading 'late dumping' to differentiate them from patients with vasomotor symptoms which occur soon after eating and in this terminology are referred to as 'early dumpers'. There is now general agreement that patients with symptoms due to reactive hypoglycaemia which occur 2–3 hours after a meal should be considered outwith the dumping category.

Although the term 'dumping' was introduced by Mix in 1922, the first description of the dumping syndrome was reported by Hertz in 1913. The syndrome which is one of the commonest sequelae of gastric surgery consists of postprandial vasomotor (systemic) and gastrointestinal symptoms (*Table* 67.4).

Table 67.4 Manifestations of the dumping syndrome

Vasomotor (Systemic)	*Gastro–intestinal*
Weakness	Fullness
Tiredness	Epigastric discomfort/heaviness
Dizziness	Nausea
Headache	Vomiting
Fainting	Distension
Warmth	Excessive borborygmi/distension
Palpitations	Diarrhoea
Dyspnoea	
Sweating	

The dumping syndrome is associated with rapid gastric emptying (*Fig.* 67.7) although some have postulated that enterogastric reflux of bile is responsible for some of the symptoms. The vasomotor symptoms occur within minutes of eating and are due to hypovolaemia which is accompanied by diminished cardiac output and peripheral resistance. The attacks are typically precipitated by high carbohydrate meals. The hypovolaemia is secondary to a massive outpouring of fluid from the vascular compartment into the bowel lumen as a consequence of the hyperosmolar nature of the intestinal contents resulting from the precipitous gastric emptying. Several vasoactive peptides have been held responsible for the vascular and gastrointestinal manifestations of the dumping syndrome. These include kinins, substance P, enteroglucagon, GIP and neurotensin. The gastrointestinal symptoms occur later during the course of a dumping attack and are often absent.

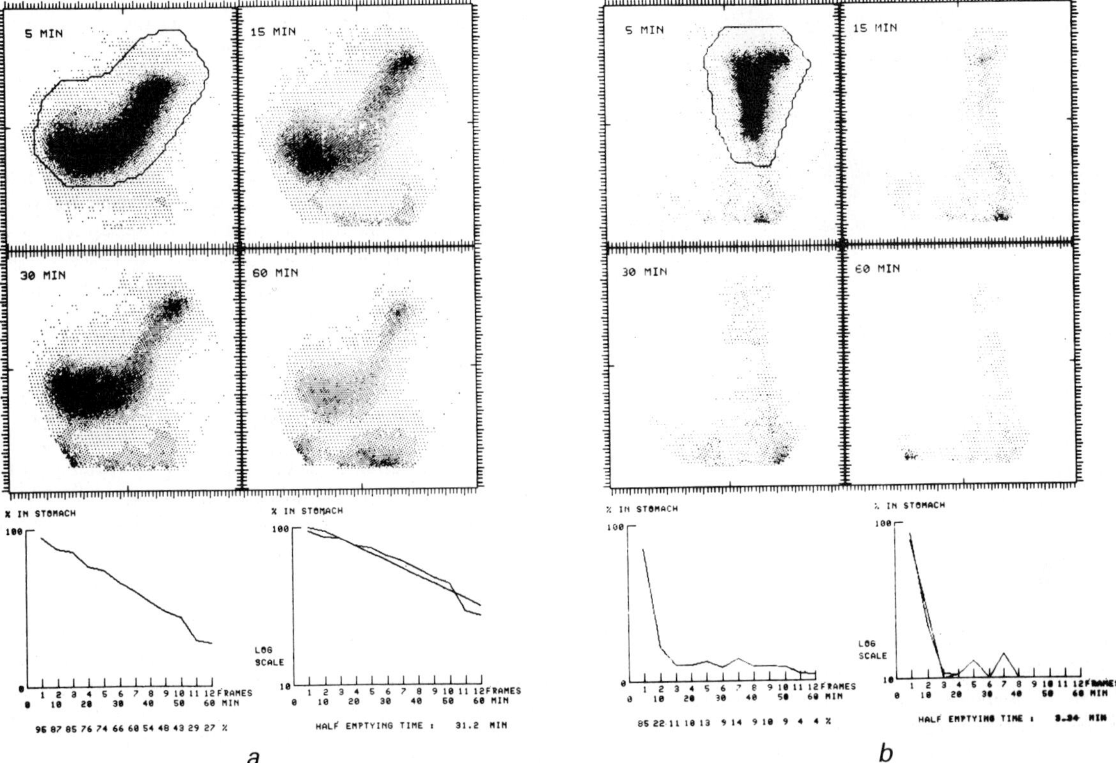

Fig. 67.7 Gastric emptying of an isotope-labelled meal: *a*, Normal single exponential emptying. *b*, Rapid initial gastric emptying in a patient with severe dumping symptoms.

Patients with mild to moderate dumping symptoms are managed satisfactorily with dietary manipulations. These patients are advised to eat small dry meals rich in protein and fat but low in carbohydrate. Additives which slow gastric emptying, such as methoxy-pectin or bran, are beneficial. However, remedial gastric surgery is required for patients with severe and persistent dumping symptoms (*vide infra*).

Reactive Hypoglycaemia

This complication is relatively uncommon and has a reported incidence of 1–6% of patients after gastric surgery. Reactive hypoglycaemia often coexists with other symptoms including vasomotor dumping and diarrhoea. The symptoms which occur 2–3 hours after a meal are due to hypoglycaemia and include sweating, tremor, difficulty in concentration and, rarely, fainting. The diagnosis is best confirmed by an extended oral glucose tolerance test which demonstrates an initial hyperglycaemia. This is accompanied by an exaggerated insulin release with elevated plasma insulin and enteroglucagon which are followed by the hypoglycaemia.

Reactive hypoglycaemia usually responds to dietary measures including low-carbohydrate, high-protein meals.

Bile Vomiting

Vomiting of bile or bile-stained fluid before or after meals is a common complaint after gastric surgery. It may be a manifestation of the following disorders:

Recurrent ulceration
Enterogastric reflux
Intermittent obstruction of the afferent or efferent loop of a gastroenterostomy
Cardio-oesophageal incompetence.

Enterogastric Reflux/Reflux Gastritis

Reflux of upper intestinal secretions (bile/pancreatic juice/succus entericus) into the stomach causes a reflux erosive gastritis and bile vomiting. The symptoms include epigastric pain, nausea and vomiting in the early postprandial period. The pain is usually of a burning nature, is aggravated by food and not relieved by antacids. The attack usually culminates in the vomiting of bile-stained fluid 1–2 hours after a meal. Less commonly, the vomiting occurs in the early morning and is preceded by nocturnal burning pain. The erosive gastritis leads to chronic blood loss with the development of an iron-deficiency anaemia and, occasionally, to severe acute gastric haemorrhage. The diagnosis is established by upper gastrointestinal endoscopy which shows a diffuse gastritis with an oedematous friable mucosa and superficial gastritis, in addition to pooling of bile-stained fluid. Quantitation of the enterogastric reflux is obtained by the modified EHIDA-test. In this investigation, EHIDA is injected intravenously and is followed by external scintiscanning of the upper abdomen with a gamma-camera. When the gallbladder is imaged by the isotope, contraction of the organ is achieved either with a milk meal or by intravenous

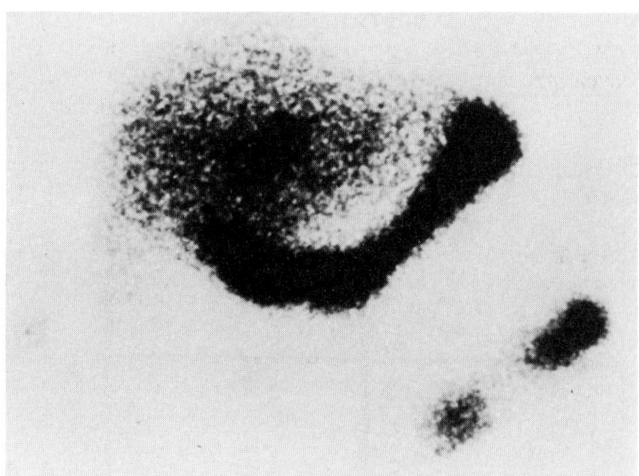

Fig. 67.8 The milk-EHIDA test for enterogastric reflux. Patient with severe bile vomiting after vagotomy and pyloroplasty—reflux of isotope (bile) into the stomach occurs in the fasting state and is enhanced after the administration of milk.

cholecystokinin. The amount of enterogastric reflux is calculated as a percentage of the total abdominal radioactivity (*Fig.* 67.8).

The symptoms of reflux gastritis and bilious vomiting may be improved by the administration of bile salt-binding agents. Often, however, conservative management along these lines fails when remedial surgical intervention becomes necessary.

Prolonged enterogastric reflux can result in atrophic gastritis and intestinal metaplasia. It has been incriminated as a factor in the development of carcinoma of the stomach after gastric surgery.

Extrinsic Loop Obstruction

This rare complication occurs after truncal vagotomy and gastroenterostomy and usually affects the afferent loop. The predisposing factors to the development of afferent loop obstruction include an antecolic anastomosis and long loops (exceeding 20 cm). The causes of extrinsic loop obstruction are:

Internal herniation
Kinking of the anastomosis
Adhesions
Volvulus
Stenosis
Jejunogastric intussusception
Development of carcinoma of the gastric remnant.

Obstruction of afferent or efferent loops is usually chronic and intermittent but may be acute. The symptoms of chronic afferent loop obstruction include fullness, cramp-like pain and nausea within 1 hour of eating. The attack culminates in vomiting of copious amounts of bile-stained fluid which relieves the symptoms. The presentation of acute afferent loop obstruction is with severe colicky abdominal pain, nausea and vomiting which is characteristically free of bile. Abdominal tenderness is present. The condition may be complicated by the development of acute pancreatitis, jaundice and necrosis with perforation.

Acute jejunogastric intussusception is a serious condition characterized by severe epigastric pain, vomiting, haematemesis, a palpable abdominal mass and high small bowel obstruction. Urgent surgical intervention is required because of the risk of strangulation and gangrene. The condition may be diagnosed preoperatively by a plain abdominal film which show a soft-tissue epigastric mass surrounded by gastric air. Alternatively, emergency barium meal or endoscopy will establish the diagnosis.

Gastro-oesophageal Reflux/Oesophagitis

The situation regarding gastro-oesophageal reflux and surgery for duodenal ulcer is both confusing and controversial. In the first instance, gastro-oesophageal reflux often accompanies duodenal ulceration and oesophagitis may, therefore, be present preoperatively. Transient dysphagia may occur after any type of vagotomy and has been attributed to oedema of the abdominal oesophagus. It is now established that vagotomy itself does not affect the oesophageal high pressure zone but damage to the oesophageal attachments, particularly the phreno-oesophageal membrane, during the mobilization of the oesophagus may cause cardio-oesophageal incompetence. If this is associated with enterogastric reflux, a severe form of oesophagitis due to reflux of bile and pancreatic juice (neutral or alkaline) may ensue and lead to stricture formation of the lower oesophagus.

Diarrhoea

The reported incidence of this complication varies widely, largely due to varying definitions. Three patterns of diarrhoea are encountered after gastric surgery: frequent loose motions, intermittent episodes of short-lived diarrhoea and severe intractable explosive diarrhoea. The latter is a serious but rare disability, being encountered in 2% of patients after truncal vagotomy. It is often accompanied by dumping symptoms and is precipitated by food. Severe intractable diarrhoea is characterized by extreme urgency and often causes incontinence during an acute attack. Although often associated with rapid gastric emptying, the exact mechanism of intractable explosive diarrhoea is unknown. Malabsorption of bile salts and/or fatty acids consequent on the intestinal denervation has been implicated. The small bowel transit is markedly accelerated.

A full malabsorption survey is necessary in all patients with severe diarrhoea as in a few patients this disability is secondary to a previously undiagnosed gastrointestinal disease (e.g. adult coeliac) or bacterial overgrowth consequent on a blind loop.

Medical management is with a low animal fat diet, intestinal sedatives (codeine phosphate, lomotil) and bile-salt binding agents such as cholestyramine. Although temporary improvement can be obtained in this way, long-term benefit is rarely obtained with conservative management, particularly in severe cases.

Small Stomach Syndrome

This term is sometimes used for the early satiety complained of by some patients after vagotomy which causes loss of receptive relaxation of the stomach during eating. It is best reserved, however, for the inability to eat experienced by some unfortunate patients, usually females, after extensive gastrectomy. The patients usually complain of a multiplicity of symptoms which preclude an adequate oral intake. The condition leads to gross malnutrition and is refractory to conservative management. Some patients can be managed by elemental diets administered via a clinifeed tube and an IVAC pump. Although many can be trained to use this in their homes and maintain an adequate nutritional state in this way, the quality of life is poor. Thus, if the patient's age and general condition are satisfactory, surgical intervention designed to reconstruct a gastric reservoir and restore duodenal continuity is indicated.

Other Complications

These include the formation of gallstones and bezoars and the development of gastric carcinoma.

Vagotomy causes dilatation of the gallbladder. However, although there are a number of reports indicating an increased risk of gallstone formation after both vagotomy and partial gastrectomy, there is no firm evidence that gastric surgery predisposes to cholelithiasis.

The factors implicated in the formation of bezoars after gastric surgery include hypoacidity, impaired proteolytic activity, inadequate mastication and loss of the antral pump. The majority of bezoars which develop after gastric surgery consist of undigested vegetable/fruit matter (notably orange pith). Bezoars can cause chronic symptoms such as nausea, vomiting, abdominal discomfort, halitosis and early satiety. They can also lead to serious complications, e.g. small bowel obstruction, severe gastritis and ulceration, bleeding, perforation and malnutrition. Treatment is initially conservative by enzymic (cellulase) digestion. Surgical intervention is undertaken if medical therapy fails or because of the development of a complication.

There is now good evidence that previous gastric surgery (partial gastrectomy, gastro-enterostomy) predisposes to the development of gastric carcinoma in the stomach remnant. Vagotomy does not appear to be implicated in this condition. Although reflux gastritis with the development of intestinal metaplasia, particularly of the type III variety, bacterial overgrowth with formation of nitrosamines in the hypochlorhydric gastric stump have been implicated, the exact mechanism for the development of invasive carcinoma remains unknown. There is a long latent period of 15–20 years and the risk, though definite, is small.

REMEDIAL SURGICAL INTERVENTION FOR POSTGASTRIC SURGERY SEQUELAE

General Considerations

As the majority of symptoms improve with time, initial management is always conservative and surgical treatment should not be undertaken before 18 months have elapsed since the gastric operation. Only patients with severe symptoms which persist beyond this time despite conservative management, should be considered as candidates for remedial surgery. All these patients ought to be investigated and assessed thoroughly to establish the dominant symptom and

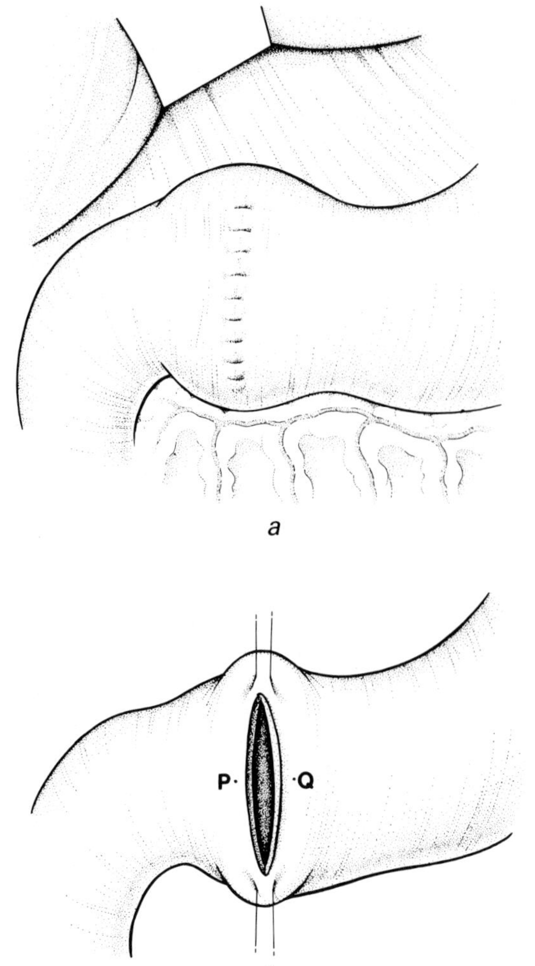

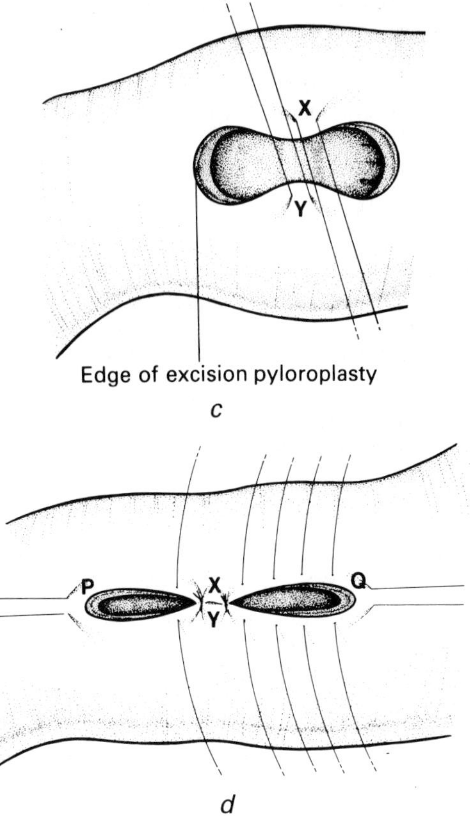

Fig. 67.9 Pyloric reconstruction for dumping after Heinicke–Mikulicz pyloroplasty: *a*, Exposure of the pyloroplasty. *b*, Insertion of stay sutures beyond both ends of the pyloroplasty scar which is incised. *c*, Restoration of the alignment of the pyloric muscular ring. *d*, The realigned antro-pyloric segment is closed with fine interrupted non-absorbable sutures.

the underlying altered gastric physiology. Although remedial surgery may impart considerable benefit to these patients, a totally symptom-free outcome is rarely obtained.

Dumping

The easiest patients to manage are those who experience severe dumping after truncal vagotomy and drainage. In these patients, the remedial surgery consists of either take down of the gastroenterostomy or pyloric reconstruction (*Fig.* 67.9) depending on the type of drainage used. Surprisingly, gastric retention is rarely encountered, although postprandial fullness is common after these remedial operations. For dumping after partial gastrectomy, an isoperistaltic jejunal interposition (10–15 cm) between the gastric remnant and the duodenum acts as an effective brake to slow down the gastric emptying.

Bile Vomiting

The commonest cause of this is enterogastric reflux. Excellent results are obtained in patients with vagotomy and gastroenterostomy by take down of the latter. Pyloric reconstruction for bilious vomiting due to enterogastric reflux in patients after vagotomy and pyloroplasty does not give satisfactory results. Severe enterogastric reflux after partial gastrectomy is usually treated by Roux-en-Y diversion. Although very effective in abolishing the bile vomiting, this procedure may lead to bacterial overgrowth. An alternative approach is the construction of an isoperistaltic jejunal segment between the gastric remnant and the duodenum.

Small Stomach Syndrome

This is the most difficult condition to treat. The patients are usually grossly malnourished and require a period of parenteral nutrition before surgical treatment. The best procedure consists of the creation of a jejunal reservoir with an isoperistaltic conduit between the gastric stump and the duodenum (*see Fig.* 67.22*c*).

Severe Explosive Diarrhoea

Although the use of reversed jejunal segments have been advocated, the outcome of these operations is poor, due to the development of episodes of postprandial colic, intestinal

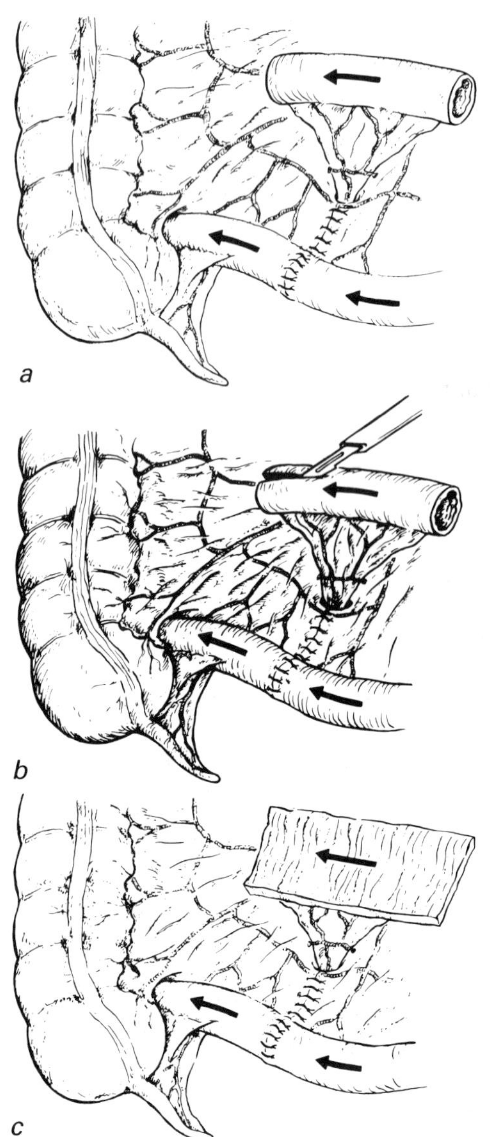

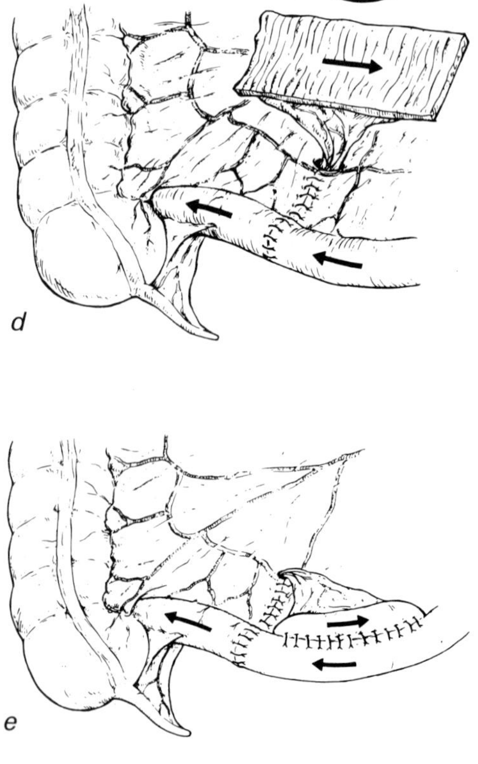

Fig. 67.10 Reversed ileal onlay graft for severe explosive diarrhoea: *a*, A 10-cm segment of ileum is isolated on an intact pedicle some 30 cm proximal to the caecum. *b*, Continuity of the small bowel is restored by an entero-enteric anastomosis. *c*, The isolated segment is split longitudinally along its antimesenteric border. *d*, Reversal of the flap. *e*, Suture of the reversed graft as an onlay to the adjacent ileum, thereby creating a passive non-propulsive segment. (Reproduced by permission from Cuschieri A. 1986. *British Journal of Surgery* **73**, 981–984.)

obstruction, distension and bacterial overgrowth. The best results are obtained by the distal onlay graft procedure which is designed to create a passive non-propulsive segment of the small intestine some 30–60 cm proximal to the ileocaecal junction (*Fig.* 67.10).

CHRONIC GASTRIC ULCER

In this section chronic gastric ulceration is discussed. The related topic of acute gastric ulcer and gastritis is considered in the next section.

Chronic ulceration in the stomach is less common than that in the duodenum in most countries, the ratio of gastric to duodenal ulcer varying from 1:4 to 1:20. There is slight male preponderance and the disease is more common in later years.

Aetiological Factors

Gastric ulceration is associated with low levels of acid secretion, although the overlap with normal subjects is considerable. Peptic ulceration cannot occur in the absence of acid. The level of secretion depends upon the site of the ulcer: the more proximal the ulcer, the lower the level of secretion. Thus, ulcers in the pyloric channel and distal antrum may be associated with normal or even high levels of gastric secretion.

Three main theories have been advanced to explain the development of chronic gastric ulcer:

1. *Antral stasis* (Harper and Dragstedt). According to this theory, delayed gastric emptying results in antral stasis, stimulation of antral gastrin and hence hypersecretion of acid.
2. *Bile reflux* (Capper). This theory again centres on the pyloric region, but differs in suggesting that the abnormality is one of abnormal reflux of bile into the stomach. Bile within the stomach is particularly irritating, but more than that it has the ability to damage the mucosa in such a way that the normal barrier to hydrogen ions is broken. Back diffusion of acid occurs from the lumen, with resulting tissue damage.
3. *Junctional theory* (Oi). There are two junctional areas on the gastric lesser curve: where antral and parietal cells meet, and where the longitudinal muscle fibres meet the oblique fibres. Oi suggested that gastric ulcers occur where the mucosal and muscular junctional zones coincide.

None of these theories satisfactorily explain all cases of gastric ulcer. It is true that some patients with a gastric ulcer have delayed emptying, perhaps resulting from the proximity of the ulcer to the antral nerves. Equally it can be argued that the hypergastrinaemia which is often present in gastric ulcer patients is the result of reduced feedback inhibition by the hypoacidity, rather than the cause of the ulcer. Certainly, when acid secretion is high in gastric ulcer patients, gastrin concentrations are low. Increased bile reflux can often be shown in the presence of a gastric ulcer, but this is not invariable. When it is present it is possible to suggest that the disordered motility is the result rather than the cause of the ulcer. Gastric ulcers do occur at the junction of antral and parietal cell mucosa. When a high lesser curve ulcer is present, a tongue of antral mucosa is found running up the lesser curve to the ulcer. This is the reason for the inverse relationship between the height of the ulcer and gastric secretion: the higher the ulcer, the larger the antrum and hence the smaller the parietal cells mass. However, the junctional theory only explains the site of the ulcer and not why it formed in the first place.

There are two quite distinct types of ulcer both clinically and in terms of therapeutic response. Gastric ulcers occurring in the body of the stomach (Type I) are associated with hypoacidity and often considerable gastritis. Type II ulcers, present in the antrum or pyloric canal have higher levels of secretion and tend to have the clinical and therapeutic features of a duodenal ulcer.

Clinical Features

Gastric ulceration is more common in the older male, but this is by no means an invariable feature. The association with chronic ill health and lower socio-economic classes is not so obvious as earlier this century.

The main clinical feature is pain, or perhaps more commonly a feeling of acute discomfort and fullness in the epigastrium. Unlike duodenal ulcer, the pain of gastic ulceration does not occur with an empty stomach: indeed, the converse is true, for eating usually produces or exacerbates the pain. Hence gastric ulcer patients tend to fear eating and are often underweight. Nausea and vomiting are more common than in duodenal ulcer, even in the absence of outlet obstruction. Periodicity of symptoms exists, but perhaps not so obviously as with duodenal ulcer.

Physical examination is not usually particularly rewarding, with epigastric tenderness being the only fairly consistent finding. Gastric ulcers may obstruct, perforate or bleed producing similar symptomatology and signs as duodenal ulcers. Occasionally a large inflammatory mass around an ulcer will be palpable, particularly if the patient has lost weight.

Management

The diagnosis of gastric ulceration will often be suspected from the patient's history. In other cases persistent indigestion will be the reason for the further investigation, usually by barium meal examination and endoscopy. Once the diagnosis of ulceration within the stomach has been confirmed, all subsequent decisions must be influenced by the overriding necessity of distinguishing between a simple chronic gastric ulcer and ulcerating cancer.

Certain radiological features may help in distinguishing the malignant gastric ulcer. The size of crater is no help, but an irregular ulcer crater is suspicious, particularly if it is impossible to demonstrate linear mucosal folds running into the crater. The area around the ulcer may be immobile, suggesting infiltration. The presence of a mass around the ulcer can sometimes be distinguished from inflammatory oedema as barium tends not to adhere to the latter.

If endoscopy is available it is wise to insist upon this as a supplement to radiology in all cases of gastric ulcer. Visualization of the ulcer should be combined with multiple biopsies and brush cytology.

A trial of medical therapy with H_2-blockers is worthwhile in most patients with uncomplicated gastric ulcer. Ulcer recurrence is high on stopping treatment and may amount to 50% more. Thus, if a patient presents with a long recurring history, surgery should be considered. If medical treatment is used, it is essential to insist that symptomatic improvement is accompanied by documented complete ulcer healing. If a gastric ulcer has shown no signs of healing within 2 months of starting adequate medical treatment, malignancy must be suspected and surgery should be advised. If partial healing is seen, it is reasonable to persist with drug therapy, but complete healing is still the objective, regardless of symptomatic success. Surgery is indicated if this is not achieved by 6 months at the outside (less if endoscopic biopsy has not been available) or if recurrence occurs after stopping treatment.

In the past the mainstays of medical treatment were bed rest, a bland diet, and advice to stop smoking. Antacids had little effect upon ulcer healing, although they might relieve symptoms. The most useful treatment is with H_2-blockers, carbenoxolone sodium (Biogastrone) and Caved S. These drugs have a proven effect on ulcer healing. Care must be exercised with Biogastrone in elderly patients or those with cardiovascular disease since this compound possesses an aldosterone-like action and can cause fluid retention. Treatment should be monitored carefully by examination for heart failure, weight gain and repeated blood electrolyte determinations. H_2-blockers have now been shown to be as effective as carbenoxolone sodium and are preferable in view of absence of serious side-effects.

Surgery for Chronic Gastric Ulcer

The objectives of gastric ulcer surgery are removal of the ulcer, thus dealing with the problem of possible malignancy—and prevention of further recurrence. Ideally the ulcer should be removed as part of a gastrectomy: on occasions local removal may be combined with some lesser procedure. Confusion over the best procedure for gastric ulcer exists partly because the aetiology is uncertain, and partly because of the existence of two types of gastric ulcer, which respond differently to acid-reducing operations.

The standard treatment is the Billroth-I type of gastrectomy, including the ulcer within the resected specimen. Restoration of continuity by gastroduodenal anastomosis is seldom a problem as the duodenum is normal. The operation is theoretically attractive since any outlet obstruction will have been dealt with, the gastric antrum is removed, and the resection includes the gastric lesser curve, the usual site of benign ulceration. This operation has a long history of success against which any alternative procedure must be weighed. The mortality is around 2% and the recurrent ulcer rate is about the same. Postoperative alimentary side-effects are produced following gastric ulcer surgery, but not with the frequency and severity as seen after Polya gastrectomy or vagotomy and drainage. Long-term nutritional problems are not usually so severe.

The main alternative to gastrectomy is vagotomy and drainage, an operation with a lower mortality. If this operation is used it must be combined with local excision of the ulcer, or at least a full-thickness biopsy. Local diathermy excision through a gastrotomy incision is usually relatively easy. This will often result in a full-thickness perforation which needs meticulous suturing. Adequate tissue for histology is essential even when the ulcer is of the pyloric canal type. Local excision alone, or local excision with a drainage procedure gives recurrence rates approaching 100%.

Vagotomy and drainage with local excision is a safe alternative to gastrectomy, with a mortality of around 1%. The recurrence rate is disturbing at around 10%. With longer follow-up this figure may be as high as 20%. Furthermore, the symptomatic results, in terms of alimentary problems, are no better than those achieved by gastrectomy.

There is, then, little justification in using vagotomy and drainage for the elective treatment of chronic gastric ulcer. The risk of missing a cancer, the high recurrence rate, and the poor symptomatic results all argue strongly in favour of gastrectomy. There may be a place for an even more conservative approach: highly selective vagotomy. A combination of careful preoperative evaluation and ulcer excision may minimize the risk of missing a cancer.

Surgery for the Complicated Gastric Ulcer

Gastric ulcers may present as an emergency with either perforation or bleeding. In both cases the mortality is higher than that of complicated duodenal ulcer: in part this is due to the average older age of the gastric ulcer patient. Early surgery is recommended in both instances. Bleeding from gastric ulcers tends to be severe and persistent.

The ideal treatment for a perforated gastric ulcer is gastrectomy. A surprisingly high percentage of seemingly benign perforated gastric ulcers prove to be malignant, perhaps 10%, so that if the ulcer is to be left in situ a biopsy is mandatory. It is often easier to resect than to try to suture a perforated ulcer after an adequate biopsy has been taken. On occasions the general condition of the patient may dictate that this simpler procedure is more advisable. There may be a place for excision of the perforated ulcer (allows histological examination) and vagotomy and drainage in the acute situation.

The bleeding gastric ulcer is best dealt with by gastrectomy. Simple suture haemostasis alone is inadequate treatment and recurrent bleeding is very common. Local excision with vagotomy and drainage may be a reasonable alternative to gastrectomy in selected patients.

Other Problems with Gastric Ulcer

1. Unsuspected Malignancy

Occasionally, postoperative histology will reveal that the apparently benign ulcer was malignant. If this report comes from biopsy or local excision, there is no alternative but to recommend further surgery in the form of an adequate gastrectomy—total if indicated. It is more difficult to be dogmatic if the previous operation was a gastrectomy which included the ulcer. The possible prognostic advantages of a greater margin of clearance from the ulcer and removal of the lymphatic drainage needs to be weighed carefully against the risk of a second resection which will usually be a near-total, if not total gastrectomy.

2. The High Lesser Curve Ulcer

Gastric ulcers around the cardio-oesophageal junction pose technical problems. The alternatives are to perform a resection distal to the ulcer, leaving it in situ (Kelling–Madlener procedure), or to excise all the lesser curve. This usually means that a Pauchet type of gastrectomy is needed in which the new lesser curve is reconstituted without the use of clamps. Unfortunately, very high lesser curve ulcers are often found in the elderly where the questions of malignancy and operative mortality are even more important. Proximal gastrectomy or total gastrectomy should not be undertaken lightly in these patients and medical therapy persisted with if the biopsy is benign. A highly selective vagotomy with local excision of the ulcer should be considered in patients who do not respond to medical treatment.

3. Combined Gastric and Duodenal Ulcer

Between 30 and 50% of patients with lesser curve gastric ulceration are said to have evidence of past or present duodenal ulceration (such gastric ulcers have been designated Type III). It is usually assumed that the duodenal ulcer precedes that in the stomach, but the precise relationship is not always clear. In theory, both delayed gastric emptying from pyloric stenosis or bile reflux through an incompetent diseased duodenal ulcer area could be responsible for the gastric ulcer. In practice, the evidence for these theories is not impressive.

Gastric ulcers occurring with duodenal ulcer disease tend to be situated fairly distally in the stomach, usually at or beyond the incisura. Levels of gastric secretion are normal or high, but not as high on average as in patients with duodenal ulcer alone. These ulcers usually respond to acid-reducing operations in a similar way to duodenal ulcers.

Surgical treatment of combined ulcer disease is by the operation the surgeon favours for duodenal ulcer. The risk of a gastric ulcer being malignant, when it is associated with a duodenal ulcer, is small but none the less present. In one large series gastric carcinoma was present in 6% of patients with gastric ulcer alone and 1·2% of patients with coexisting duodenal ulceration. All forms of gastric ulcer must be biopsied.

GASTRITIS

Under the heading of gastritis come a number of conditions characterized by inflammatory damage to the gastric mucosa. Of particular interest to the surgeon are acute erosive gastritis and the more chronic alkaline reflux gastritis.

Erosive Gastritis

Acute gastritis describes the conditions which result in the acute development of mucosal lesions of erythema, focal mucosal haemorrhage, erosions and ulcerations. Stress ulceration is an alternative term which recognizes the fact that these mucosal lesions may be precipitated by a variety of stress situations such as haemorrhagic or septic shock, head injury or severe thermal burns. Drug-induced acute gastritis is possibly of different aetiology. The drugs implicated in this problem include steroids, aspirin, phenylbutazone, indomethacin (NSAIDs) and possibly alcohol.

The precise sequence of events which link stress to ulceration are unknown. Increased acid secretion is almost certainly not a factor in most cases, although it may be of some relevance in head injury patients where increased gastrin and gastric acid secretion have been found. Acute mucosal ischaemia is probably an important factor in producing the initial mucosal injury. The subsequent development of haemorrhagic gastritis may then be related to the fact that the damaged mucosa becomes unable to maintain the normal barrier to hydrogen ions which then leak into the mucosal cells causing more damage. Bile salts are found in the stomach in increased concentration in experimental animals subjected to shock, and this may be another factor producing increased permeability to hydrogen ions. A third factor is an acute depletion of mucosal energy stores (ATP) which develops rapidly in the shock situation.

Clinical Features

The importance of stress ulceration is mainly the potential for severe bleeding from the haemorrhagic mucosa. This can arise in the context of any serious illness, although haemorrhagic shock, sepsis and trauma are the main precipitating conditions. Endoscopy has shown that acute gastritis is very common in these situations and that the earliest signs of mucosal damage can appear within a few hours of the insult. Only a small percentage of patients have overt gastrointestinal haemorrhage and this is usually not apparent for 3–8 days after the precipitating illness.

The diagnosis of gastritis as the source of acute gastrointestinal bleeding is usually made endoscopically. Once the diagnosis has been made, treatment should be conservative, whenever possible. Resuscitative measures, as discussed previously, are continued and treatment with H_2-blockers is started. These drugs have a beneficial effect in two ways: first they reduce acid secretion and so limit the amount of hydrogen ion available for back diffusion; secondly histamine H_2-receptor antagonists reduce the permeability of the gastric mucosal barrier to hydrogen ions. This form of treatment may be used as an alternative to the regular instillation of antacid into the stomach to maintain the pH above 7. If endoscopy has shown a lot of blood clot in the stomach, iced saline lavage should be used until the nasogastric aspirate is clear of old blood.

Vasopressin has been advocated for the emergency control of gastric mucosal bleeding. The best reported results come from selective arterial infusions, but even then the failure rate approaches 50%. It seems illogical to produce deliberate mucosal ischaemia when this was probably the cause of the problem initially. Somatostatin, one of the peptides normally present in gastrointestinal tissue, has a more predictable effect on mesenteric blood flow, and does not have the disadvantages of the cardiovascular problems often encountered with vasopressin. Experience with long-acting synthetic analogue of stomatostatin is limited, but it may prove more useful than vasopressin.

Surgery is not often needed for erosive gastritis. Relentless bleeding requires radical surgery. The major problem facing the surgeon is that the entire gastric mucosa is a source of bleeding. All operations short of total gastrectomy have a re-bleeding rate of 50% or more, and the mortality from such re-bleeds is extremely high. If the patient is a poor risk and the risk of death from re-bleeding is judged high, then total gastrectomy, preserving a small fundal cuff to allow a safer anastomosis, is justified. On the other hand, if the patient's condition is good enough for him to be able to tolerate reoperation, if necessary, then subtotal gastrectomy with vagotomy is indicated. The value of vagotomy is probably that it reduces mucosal blood flow by opening up arteriovenous anastomoses.

Drug-induced Gastritis

The clinical problems posed by drug-induced gastritis are similar to those of stress ulceration, although haemorrhage is not usually so severe. Perforation of acute ulcers—duodenal, pyloric or gastric—is more common.

The mechanism of drug injury is not well understood. Aspirin probably exerts a dual effect of direct mucosal damage coupled with its tendency to prolong bleeding time. Both effects can occur after a small dose regardless of whether the drug is given by mouth or parenterally. Bleeding is usually mild, even occult. The question of alcohol-induced gastritis is a little debatable. An acute overindulgence of alcohol can undoubtedly injure the gastric mucosa directly, but whether or not it can produce erosive gastritis is questionable.

It has been suggested that the mucosal damage caused by non-steroidal analgesics might be prevented by the prophylactic use of drugs which exert a 'cytoprotective' effect. Acute mucosal damage is associated with depletion of mucosal prostaglandins, and experimentally the prior administration of prostaglandins can minimize the adverse effects of drugs, including alcohol, on the gastric mucosa. Clinically the position is less clear. Prostaglandins (such as Enprostil) have been shown to exert an effect when used by patients on

NSAIDs—for example to reduce occult faecal blood loss—but the same is true for H_2-receptor antagonists. Whether cytoprotection will prove to be a clinically useful concept remains to be seen. In practice it would seem reasonable to suggest that any patient with previous dyspepsia who requires a non-steroidal drug, or one who develops dyspepsia whilst on such a drug, should be given an H_2-receptor antagonist as well.

Chronic Gastritis

The histological features of chronic gastritis are broadly similar despite a variety of different aetiologies. Two main groups are recognized: type A which is associated with a marked reduction in acid output, impaired vitamin B_{12} absorption and the presence of parietal cell antibodies in the serum; and type B in which acid secretion is not greatly affected and vitamin B_{12} absorption is rarely impaired. The distribution of the gastritis also differs. In pernicious anaemia (type A) there is a relative sparing of the gastric antrum: hence gastrin levels are grossly elevated because of the permanently high antral pH. In the more common type B gastritis the changes always begin distally in the pyloric region and spread into the antrum and body to a variable extent. Because acid secretion is not grossly reduced and because the gastritis is maximal in the antrum, gastrin levels may be normal.

The aetiology of chronic (type B) gastritis is poorly understood. Gastritis increases in frequency and severity with age and is found in association with a number of other conditions. These include duodenal ulceration (where a degree of antral gastritis is almost universal), uraemia, cirrhosis and after gastric surgery. In this latter case, reflux of duodenal contents is believed to be the causative factor. There is no good evidence to suggest that the factors responsible for acute erosive gastritis produce chronic gastritis, nor that acute gastritis progresses to the chronic condition.

Recently, a relatively distinct type of chronic gastritis has been recognized. Endoscopically the mucosal changes are perhaps best described as a 'humpy' gastritis. The gastric mucosa presents the picture of multiple small humps, on the summit of which some will bear erosions. Geographically the gastritis may be widespread or may be confined to part of the mucosa only. If these lesions are biopsied the report will usually be of 'chronic erosive gastritis'. There is no clinical correlate to these endoscopic and histological findings; sometimes the most florid of appearances can be present in an asymptomatic patient. The importance of chronic erosive gastritis is that the mucosa is usually found to contain spirochaete-like organisms similar to campylobacter—the so-called 'campylobacter-like organisms' (CLOs). These micro-organisms are readily seen in the mucus layer of the mucosa. Their presence can also be shown by demonstrating raised titres of antibody to the organisms within the bloodstream.

Whether these bacteria are truly pathogenic and responsible for the gastric lesions is unclear. The lesions are not usually responsive to H_2-receptor blockers, nor to erythromycin which is commonly effective against campylobacter. The organisms do seem to respond to topical bismuth salts (such as De Nol) and at present this is probably the most effective treatment available.

The significance of chronic gastritis is difficult to assess, and in many patients it is asymptomatic. Chronic iron-deficiency anaemia is fairly common, probably due to occult blood loss. In atrophic gastritis increased concentrations of albumin may be found in gastric juice, and it has been suggested that hypoalbuminaemia in the elderly may be produced in this way. The relationship between gastritis and dyspepsia is not clear cut. In some instances non-ulcer dyspepsia and gastritis coexist, but many people have gastritis without indigestion, and many patients with non-ulcer dyspepsia do not have gastritis.

From the surgical standpoint, two aspects of chronic gastritis are important. The first of these—alkaline reflux gastritis in the postgastric surgery patient—has already been discussed. It should be added that although symptomatic improvement follows Roux-en-Y diversion of bile away from the stomach, the gastritis often persists and may appear even more severe endoscopically. The second point is that of cancer risk; both pernicious anaemia and type B gastritis (*vide infra*) carry an increased risk for cancer of the stomach. In pernicious anaemia the risk is increased by three or fourfold. Twenty-five years after gastric resection the incidence of cancer is said to be six times the expected rate.

Rare Types of Gastritis

The gastric mucosa may become involved in a variety of rare conditions which merit brief mention.

Ménétrier's Disease

This describes the association of giant hypertrophic mucosal folds with a protein-losing gastropathy. There is gastric hypersecretion in terms of volume, but acid content is low. Often polyps form in this condition and the patient develops acute, or more commonly, chronic gastrointestinal blood loss. Severe hypoproteinaemia can result, and occasionally gastrectomy has been necessary. The condition appears to be premalignant.

Suppurative (Phlegmonous) Gastritis

This is a rare and often fatal bacterial infection producing a spreading cellulitis of the stomach wall. Haemolytic streptococcus is the commonest infecting organism. The condition usually complicates a pre-existing gastric lesion and is more common in elderly and alcoholic patients. The presentation is usually one of progressive peritonitis. The stomach appears discoloured and may be covered with exudate. Resection may be feasible if only part of the stomach is involved. Otherwise drainage is instituted and systemic antibiotics given.

Necrotizing Gastritis

This is a rare variant caused by the fusiform and spirochaete bacteria of the mouth. Primary necrosis and gangrene result.

Corrosive Gastritis

Accidental or suicidal ingestion of strong acid or alkali can produce severe mucosal inflammation. Caustic agents rarely burn the stomach seriously since the gastric acid produces rapid neutralization. Strong acids destroy the mucosa by coagulation, as do other agents such as phenol and formalin.

The acute management is by removal, dilution and neutralization. Removal should be by a soft tube and vomiting avoided. Systemic antibiotics and steroids should be used, and cimetidine might be useful to prevent further injury by endogenous acid. Laparotomy should be avoided if possible and resection is not advisable. If the patient survives, late surgery may be needed to deal with the complications of scarring.

Granulomatous Gastritis

Tuberculous infection of the stomach is almost always secondary to active pulmonary disease. It produces multiple ragged ulcers, and discrete tubercles may be seen. Serosal inflammation is common and local lymphadenopathy prominent. Antituberculous therapy is used, and surgery reserved for any late cicatricial complications.

Crohn's disease of the stomach is rare and is always accompanied by signs of disease elsewhere. Because it is part of a widespread Crohn's problem, surgery is seldom indicated.

Emphysematous Gastritis

Gas in the stomach wall may be part of pneumatosis cystoides, usually considered in relation to the colon. Associations with pyloric obstruction and with emphysematous bullae have been described. Gas-forming organisms can produce the picture, and air can be introduced by a tear during endoscopy.

GASTRIC TUMOURS

Gastric tumours may be benign or malignant. The benign group includes non-neoplastic gastric polyps which are usually of the regenerative (hyperplastic type). Carcinoma is the predominant malignant gastric tumour, lymphoma being much less common and may occur as a primary lesion or as secondary involvement from lymphomas arising elsewhere. The most common connective-tissue neoplasms are the smooth muscle tumours. Although most of these are benign (leiomyoma), some are malignant (leiomyosarcoma). The differentiation between benign and malignant smooth muscle tumours may be difficult to determine even by histological assessment in the individual case.

Adenomas and other Benign Tumours

True adenomas of the stomach are rare and account for only 5% of benign gastric polyps. Thus although progression to a carcinoma is possible as in cancer of the colon, this sequence is a very rare event in the development of invasive gastric carcinomas. The majority of gastric adenomas are found in the antrum and may be single or multiple (*Fig.* 67.11). They may form sessile, villous, pedunculated or lobulated growths. Treatment is advisable and may be achieved endoscopically but if the tumour is large or multiple, surgical local excision or partial gastrectomy is necessary.

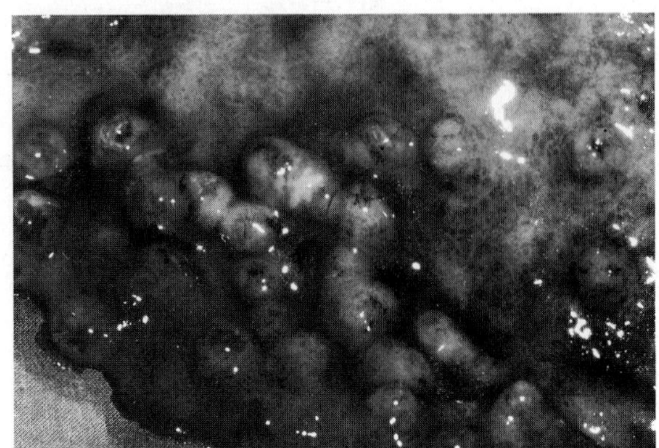

Fig. 67.11 Multiple adenomatous polyps treated by partial gastrectomy.

Other benign tumours include lipomas, neurofibromas, neurilemmomas and glomus tumours.

Non-neoplastic Gastric Polyps

The commonest site of non-neoplastic polyps of the stomach is the antropyloric region. Various types of gastric polyps are recognized (*Table* 67.5), the commonest being the regenerative (hyperplastic) variety. *Regenerative polyps* have an inflammatory origin. They often occur in association with gastritis and peptic ulceration, form smooth nodules of variable size and consist of proliferating glands with no cellular atypia. The *inflammatory fibroid polyp* is a rare lesion which is most commonly found in the gastric antrum and can be sessile or pedunculated. Histologically, it is composed of a vascular stroma containing numerous capillaries and arterioles, fibroblasts and an inflammatory cell infiltrate with an abundance of eosinophils. However, the lesion is not associated with a systemic eosinophilia or allergic conditions. In this respect it contrasts with *eosinophilic gastroenteritis* which affects the pyloric antrum and the first part of the duodenum and arises on a background of gastrointestinal allergy. The pyloric region and adjacent duodenum become diffusely thickened due to oedema of the submucosal and the muscle layers which are also infiltrated with eosinophils and occasional giant cells. Patients with eosinophilic gastroenteritis give a history of allergy and exhibit a marked eosinophilia in their peripheral blood. *Myoepithelial hamartomas* are composed of glands surrounded by smooth muscle and arise from the submucosal layer of the antrum and pylorus where they form smooth sessile masses. The hamartomatous *polyps of Peutz–Jeghers syndrome* may occur in the stomach. They very rarely become malignant. *Heterotopic pancreatic tissue* is again most commonly found in the antropyloric region.

Table 67.5 Non-neoplastic gastric polyps

Non-neoplastic gastric polyps
Regenerative (hyperplastic)
Inflammatory (fibroid)
Myoepithelial hamartomas
Peutz–Jeghers
Heterotopic pancreatic tissue

Carcinoma of the Stomach

This disease continues to carry a dismal prognosis especially in Western countries where the overall 5-year survival ranges from 5 to 10%. A better outcome is obtained in Japan which has the highest age-standardized incidence in the world (100/100 000 for males). The improved survival in Japan is due to an active screening programme resulting in earlier diagnosis and an aggressive surgical approach designed to reduce loco-regional recurrence in the gastric bed.

Epidemiology

There has been a decline in the incidence of gastric cancer during the past 30 years throughout the world. The exact reason for this is unknown but the increased consumption of refrigerated in preference to spiced and pickled foods has been postulated as a possible factor. The sharpest decline has been observed in Finland where the incidence of gastric cancer is now one-third of the rate which prevailed in the early 1950s. Within the United Kingdom, the disease is commoner in Scotland and Wales. In Scotland, the current age-standardized rate for gastric cancer is 20 and 10/100 000 for males and females respectively. This male preponderance (2:1) is encountered worldwide. The disease is rarely seen before 40 years of age and the incidence rises sharply with age to reach a maximum between 70 and 80 years. Cancer of the stomach is three times more common in social classes IV and V (semi-skilled and unskilled labourers) than in social classes I and II (professional, executive and higher management).

Aetiology

Although the results of several epidemiological studies have failed to demonstrate specific causative factors, the following have been implicated:

Highly spiced salted or pickled foods.
Polycyclic hydrocarbons, especially those generated by high temperature pyrolysis of animal fat and aromatic amino acids in grilled and barbecued meats.
Inorganic dusts (miners and potters).
High consumption of animal fat.
High salt consumption (osmotic damage to gastric mucosa).
Protein malnutrition (may lead to achlorhydria).
Viral infections (which may damage the gastric mucosa and cause temporary achlorhydria).
Excess alcohol consumption.
Tobacco smoking.
Dietary nitrates (drinking water and vegetables).
Refluxed bile acids (as tumour promoters).

Nitrates are thought to be important as they can be converted to N-nitroso compounds in the stomach. However, although these compounds are extremely potent carcinogens in animals there is no definite evidence that they are carcinogenic to humans. Both the reduction of nitrates to nitrites and the nitrosination of the nitrites with amines (with the formation of N-nitrosamines) are known to be catalysed by bacteria such as *E. coli*. Bacterial overgrowth which is commonly encountered in the human stomach in conditions of hypo- or anacidity is associated with a high concentration of nitrites and N-nitrosamines. Although plausible, the hypothesis postulating the sequence: increased dietary nitrates—bacterial proliferation in an achlorhydric stomach—excess N-nitrosamine production—cancer of the stomach, has not been confirmed in the human.

The recognized risk factors in the development of gastric carcinoma are:

Atrophic gastritis and pernicious anaemia
Previous partial gastrectomy
Hypogammaglobulinaemia
Adenomatous polyps
Blood group A.

The most researched risk factor has been atrophic gastritis in view of the high incidence (3–6 fold increase) in patients with pernicious anaemia. However, in the absence of the latter condition, gastric atrophy occurs as an inevitable consequence of ageing and is frequently encountered in patients above the age of 60 years in the Western Hemisphere. Several of the factors listed previously in the presumed aetiology are thought to act by causing a primary damage of the gastric mucosa with the development of atrophic gastritis. There is now increasing evidence for the progression of gastric atrophy to intestinal metaplasia, dysplasia and carcinoma-in-situ.

Although there is a higher incidence of intestinal metaplasia in gastric carcinoma than in benign conditions, the lesion is too common to be useful for screening purposes. However, the recognition of the various types of intestinal metaplasia by detailed histology and mucin histochemistry has clarified the picture considerably. There are three types of intestinal metaplasia depending on the degree of cell differentiation and abnormal mucus production (*Table* 67.6).

Table 67.6 Types of intestinal metaplasia

Type I (complete)	Mature absorptive and goblet cells. The latter secrete sialomucin (normal)
Type II (incomplete)	Absorptive cells are few or absent. Columnar 'intermediate' cells in various stages of de-differentiation are present and secrete sialomucin. The goblet cells secrete sialomucins and occasionally sulphomucins (abnormal mucins)
Type III (incomplete)	The cell de-differentiation is more marked than in type II. The 'intermediate' cells secrete predominantly sulphomucins (abnormal mucins). The goblet cells secrete both sialo- and sulphomucins. A variable degree of disorganized glandular architecture is present.

Various studies have now shown a strong association between type III intestinal metaplasia and gastric carcinoma of the intestinal type (*vide infra*). This type of intestinal metaplasia (*Fig.* 67.12) is also found in gastric adenomas but

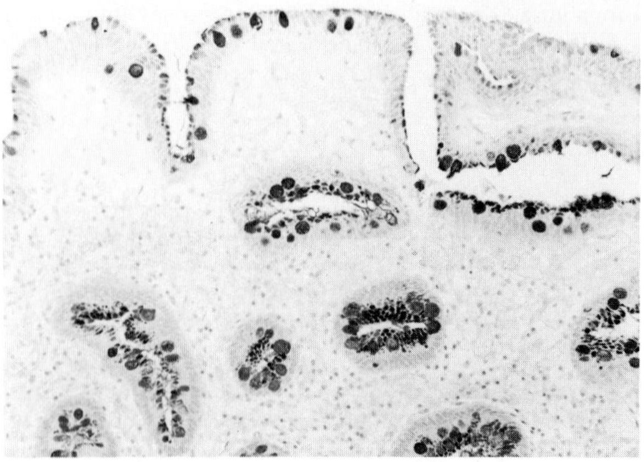

Fig. 67.12 Histochemical appearance of type IIB incomplete-intestinal metaplasia using high iron diamine alcian blue stain (HID-AB) for mucins. The normal absorptive cells are scanty and have been replaced by dedifferentiated 'intermediate' cells which secrete sulphomucin (black). The goblet cells secrete a mixture of sialo–(grey) and sulphomucin. The glandular architecture is disorganized. (By courtesy of Dr M. P. Holley, Ninewells Hospital, Dundee.)

not in regenerative polyps. Furthermore, a high incidence of type III intestinal metaplasia has been reported in relatives of patients with gastric carcinoma and in patients with pernicious anaemia.

Whereas genetic factors are important in relation to diffuse gastric carcinoma, there is no evidence for familial predisposition in the development of the intestinal type of gastric cancer. Diffuse gastric carcinoma is significantly more common in patients with blood group A, in relatives of patients with diffuse gastric cancer and in *familial hypogammaglobulinaemia*. This is a genetically determined disorder which is characterized by the defective production of IgG antibodies and is usually accompanied by pernicious anaemia. Patients with familial hypogammaglobulinaemia have a 50-fold excess risk of developing gastric carcinoma.

Pathology

There are several classifications of gastric carcinomas. The most useful to the clinician and epidemiologist is the Lauren (or Finnish or DIO) classification. This recognizes two main groups with different histogenesis and (probably) aetiology. The first group is known as the *intestinal gastric cancer* (I) as the gastric carcinoma cells exhibit a striated (brush) border and generally resemble intestinal cells. They tend to form localized expanding or ulcerated lesions and are frequently surrounded by intestinal metaplasia especially of the type III variety. The second group is known as the *diffuse gastric cancer* as the lesion infiltrates the gastric wall without forming large discrete masses. The diffuse cancer carries a worse prognosis than the intestinal variety and arises from apparently normal gastric mucosa usually over a wide field. These cancers are not usually associated with intestinal metaplasia or other precancerous conditions except pernicious anaemia and familial hypogammaglobulinaemia.

The intestinal and diffuse cancers account for 90% of all gastric carcinomas. The remainder have a mixed morphology and are referred to as *other* (O), hence the alternative name, DIO classification. However, the majority of the tumours in the 'other' category behave like the intestinal gastric cancers. Within each category (intestinal or diffuse), the tumours are graded pathologically into well differentiated, poorly differentiated and undifferentiated.

The intestinal type of gastric cancer is made up of cohesive neoplastic cells (which stick together) and when the tumour is well differentiated, these neoplastic cells form glandular tubules with a central lumen (*Fig.* 67.13). The various subtypes of the well-differentiated intestinal gastric cancer are: large gland carcinoma, small gland carcinoma and a type of colloid carcinoma in which mucus lakes are found surrounded by well-differentiated glands. The growth of intestinal cancer is mainly by expansion and macroscopically they form polypoid or fungating masses which may ulcerate centrally.

The diffuse gastric carcinomas are made of neoplastic cells which lack cohesion and therefore tend to stream out in Indian file fashion and invade the stomach wall with no tendency to organization into tubular or glandular structures (*Fig.* 67.14). They are therefore highly invasive tumours and carry a worse prognosis than the intestinal variety. The well-known linitis plastica (leather-bottle stomach) is a classic example of the diffuse type of gastric cancer. Some diffuse gastric cancers show little tendency to mucin production. Others consist of mucin-laden signet ring cells (signet-cell carcinoma) or large lakes of mucus surrounding isolated clusters of signet cells (diffuse colloid carcinoma). The

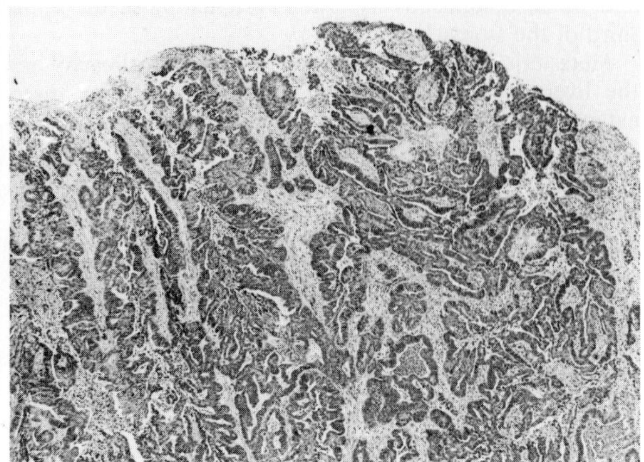

Fig. 67.13 Photomicrograph of a well-differentiated gastric cancer of the intestinal type. The cells form well-defined glandular acini.

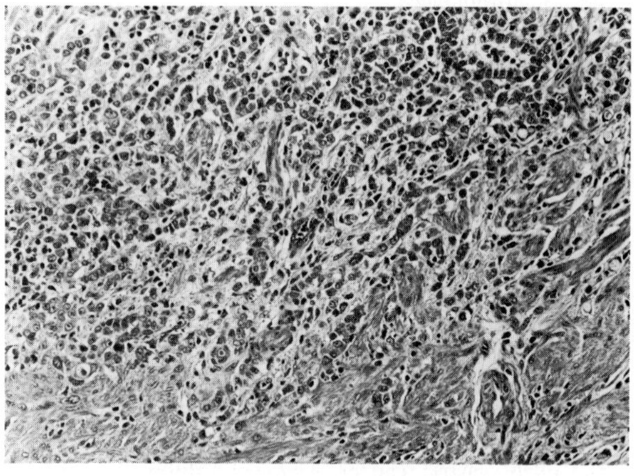

a

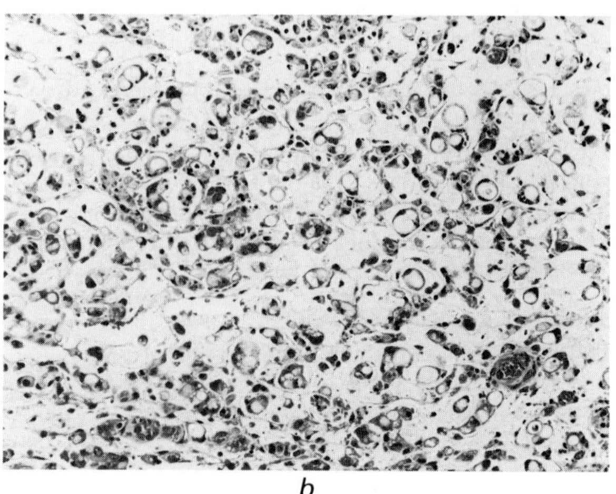

b

Fig. 67.14 *a*, Low-power view of the histological appearance of a diffuse type of gastric cancer. The cells have lost all cohesion and stream out into the surrounding stroma. *b*, High-power field showing the streaming of the malignant cells which are loaded with mucus resulting in eccentric position of the nucleus, i.e. signet-cell appearance. (By courtesy of Dr M. P. Holley, Ninewells Hospital, Dundee.)

clinicopathological differences between the intestinal and diffuse gastric carcinomas are outlined in *Table* 67.7.

Table 67.7 Contrasting features of intestinal and diffuse gastric cancers

	Intestinal	*Diffuse*
Histogenesis	Areas of intestinal metaplasia type II/III	Normal gastric mucosa
Early cancer	Protruding type	Flat, depressed or excavated
Infiltration	Localized	Diffuse
Peritoneal dissemination	Infrequent	Frequent
Hepatic metastases	Nodular	Diffuse
Sex incidence	More common in males	More frequent in females
Age incidence	More common in the elderly	More common in the young
Association with blood Group A	No	Yes
Association with pernicious anaemia	No	Yes
Genetic predisposition	No	Yes
Prognosis	Survival better than the diffuse	Dismal

Early Gastric Cancer

This is defined as cancer limited to the mucosa and submucosa and is rarely encountered in the West but accounts for up to 30% of newly diagnosed tumours in Japan as a result of screening for the disease. The prognosis with adequate resection is excellent with 5-year survival rates which exceed 80%. Early gastric cancer assumes different endoscopic appearances which have been classified as follows (*Fig.* 67.15):

Protruding
Superficial: this may be elevated, flat or depressed
Excavated.

Some 10–15% of gastric carcinomas confined histologically to the mucosal and submucosal layers have metastasized to the regional lymph nodes and have a poor prognosis. This subgroup is sometimes referred to as *early-simulating advanced gastric carcinoma.*

Advanced Gastric Carcinoma

This is defined as a tumour which has involved the muscularis propria of the stomach wall and accounts for 95% of gastric carcinomas diagnosed in the UK. In the vast majority of cases spread to the regional lymph nodes is present alone or in association with peritoneal and hepatic deposits. Advanced gastric carcinoma is further classified into macroscopic types first described by Borrmann (*Fig.* 67.16). Types 1 and 2 carry a better prognosis than types 3 and 4 which are always incurable despite attempts at radical resection.

Staging of Gastric Cancer

Until recently there were several rival staging systems for gastric carcinoma. Recently, however, an International

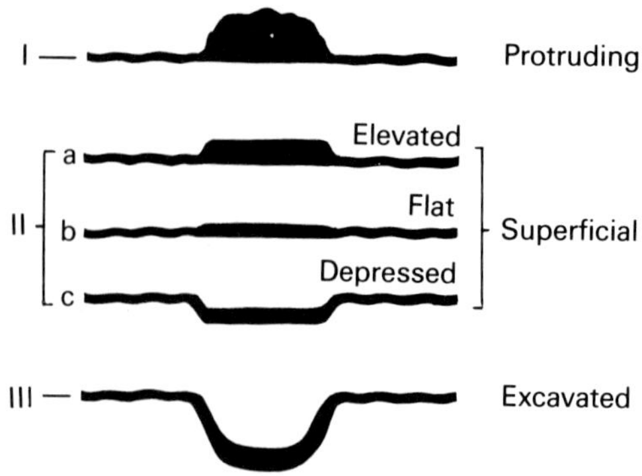

Fig. 67.15 Diagrammatic representation of the morphological types of early gastric cancer.

Staging System has been agreed. The new TNM categories are shown in *Table* 67.8. The important prognostic factors in patients without detectable distant metastases are depth of invasion of the stomach wall by the tumour and lymph node spread. Other significant but lesser prognostic variables are the type of cancer (intestinal or diffuse), location of the tumour (growths of the cardia having a poorer prognosis than lesions of the middle and lower third) and the histological type (degree of differentiation).

Spread of Gastric Carcinoma

The diffuse type of gastric cancer spreads rapidly through the submucosal and subserosal lymphatic plexuses and penetrates the gastric wall at an early stage. The intestinal variety remains localized for a while and has less tendency to disseminate. With both cancers, spread to the lymph nodes along the greater and lesser curvatures tends to occur once the muscular coat of the stomach is invaded by the neoplasm. Thereafter, spread occurs to the nodes along the coeliac axis and its trifurcation (left gastric, splenic and common hepatic arteries), to the nodes in the splenic hilum, the root of the mesentery, the retropancreatic nodes and the hepatoduodenal nodes. Involvement of the para-aortic nodes above and below the transverse colon then ensues. The exact nodal groups which are involved depend on the anatomical site of the primary tumour (upper, middle, lower third). Contrary to popular belief, involvement of the duodenum by an antral carcinoma is not unusual as is extension to the abdominal oesophagus by lesions originating in the upper third of the stomach.

Metastatic spread is usually to the peritoneal cavity and the liver. The most common organs involved by direct extension are the omentum, the transverse colon and mesocolon and the left lobe of the liver.

Clinical Features

Early gastric cancer of the intestinal type is asymptomatic but early diffuse cancer may present with dyspepsia simulating peptic ulceration. The symptoms may respond to treatment with antacids and H_2-receptor blockers and the ulcer may show evidence of healing at follow-up endoscopy. In any event, the early symptoms are often vague and include indigestion, malaise, early satiety, postprandial fullness and loss of appetite. Weight loss is a significant feature of the disease but usually signifies an advanced lesion which has involved the muscular coat of the stomach or beyond. Lesions of the cardia may present with dysphagia and

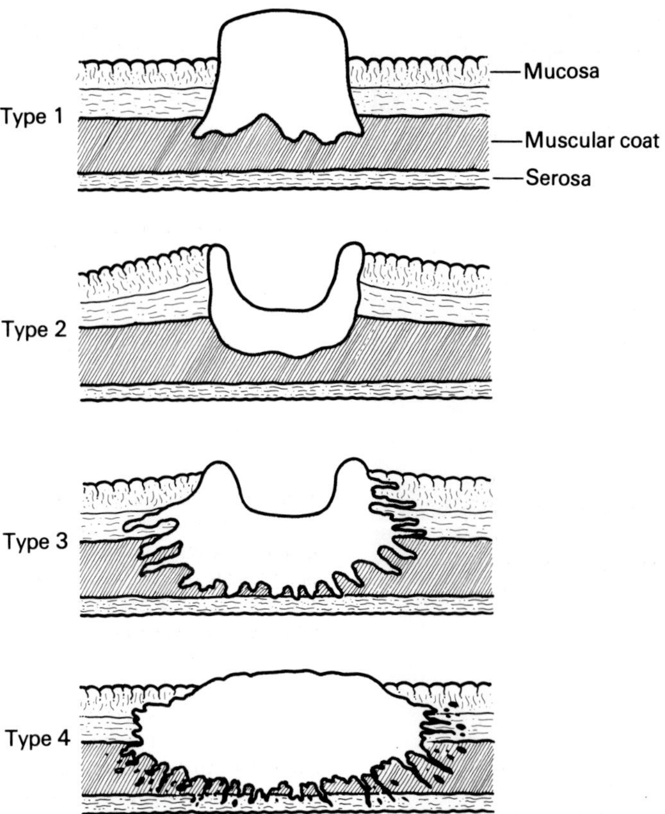

Fig. 67.16 Diagrammatic representation of the Borrmann classification of advanced gastric cancer.

Table 67.8 Staging of gastric cancer (Joint UICC, AJC and JJC*)

T—Primary Tumour
- T_1 Tumour limited to the mucosa or mucosa and submucosa
- T_2 Tumour involves the muscularis propria or subserosa
- T_3 Tumour penetrates the serosa
- T_4 Tumour involves contiguous structures

N—Regional Lymph Nodes
- N_0 No metastases to the regional lymph nodes
- N_1 Involvement of the perigastric lymph nodes within 3 cm of the primary tumour
- N_2 Involvement of the regional lymph nodes more than 3 cm from the primary including those located along the left gastric, common hepatic, splenic and coeliac arteries

M—Distant Metastases
- M_0 No evidence of distant metastases
- M_1 Evidence of distant metastases

N.B.—Involvement of lymph nodes beyond level N_2, i.e. all other intra-abdominal nodes, is regarded as distant metastases according to the new classification.

*UICC, Union International Contre le Cancer
AJC, American Joint Committee
JJC, Japanese Joint Committee

circumferential growths of the middle third and the pyloric antrum cause obstructive symptoms with vomiting after meals. Acute presentation with haematemesis or melaena is encountered more often with advanced than early lesions.

The most common presentation is that of recent dyspepsia in a patient above the age of 50 years. There are no specific features to the cancer dyspepsia. Thus, all patients who present with indigestion require full investigation including endoscopy to establish the diagnosis before treatment is started. The most frequent reason for the delay in the diagnosis of cancer of the stomach is a period of symptomatic therapy with antacids or H_2-receptor blockers often lasting several months before referral for endoscopy is undertaken. Irrespective of sex and age, the exact diagnosis of the underlying gastroduodenal disease must be established in all patients with indigestion before treatment of any sort is initiated.

Anaemia which is often present at the time of diagnosis, is usually of the iron-deficiency type due to chronic blood loss. Evidence of weight loss is usually present on examination and hypoalbuminaemia is frequent. Although often stressed, enlarged left supraclavicular lymph nodes are a rare physical finding in gastric cancer. A palpable epigastric mass usually signifies incurable, though not necessarily a nonresectable, tumour. Jaundice, hepatomegaly or ascites indicate advanced incurable disease and limited survival. Evidence of spread beyond the peritoneal cavity is unusual at the time of diagnosis of gastric carcinoma.

The key investigations are upper gastrointestinal endoscopy with multiple biopsy and brush cytology and air-contrast barium meal (*Fig.* 67.17). Other tests are used to detect extragastric disease. These include chest radiography,

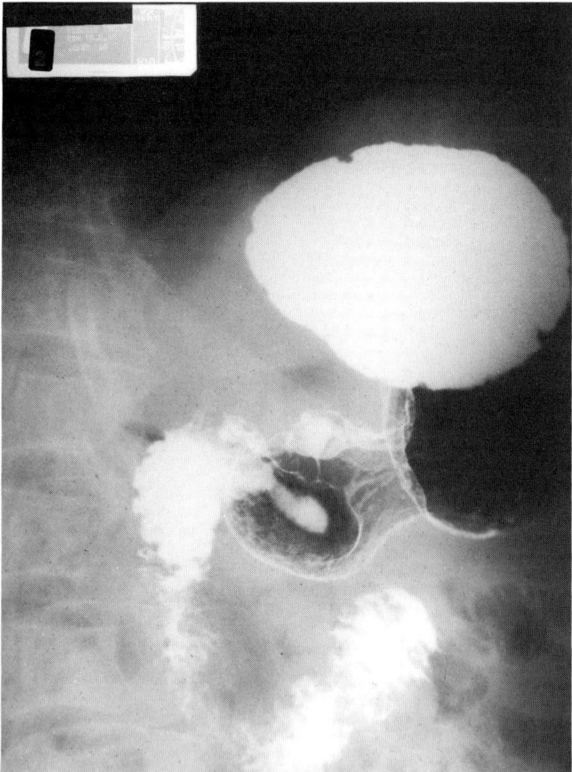

Fig. 67.17 Air-contrast (barium) meal showing an antral carcinoma.

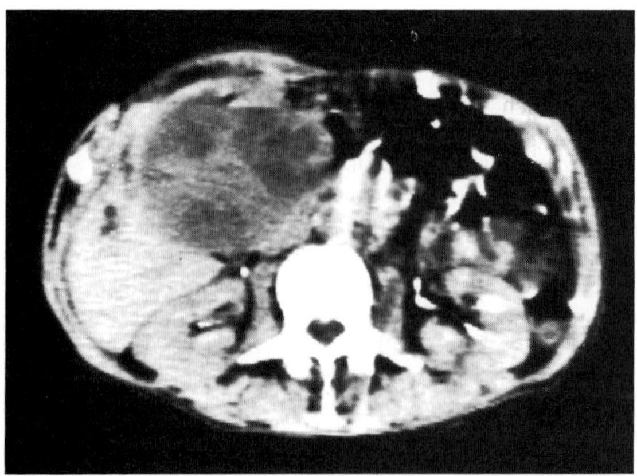

Fig. 67.18 CT scan of the liver in a patient with gastric carcinoma of the diffuse type showing multiple hepatic deposits.

liver function tests, CT or ultrasound scanning of the liver (*Fig.* 67.18) and CT scanning of the para-aortic nodes and endoscopic ultrasound examination of the stomach to determine the depth of involvement of the gastric wall by the neoplasm. Laparoscopy has also been found valuable in the assessment of the stage and curability of the disease.

Treatment of Gastric Carcinoma

An adequate surgical resection remains the only effective treatment which offers a chance of cure or long-term survival. Furthermore, a palliative resection whenever feasible is more effective in relieving symptoms than bypass or intubation procedures. With the currently available drugs, chemotherapy is ineffective as is radiotherapy.

The principles underlying a potentially curative resection of a gastric carcinoma are:

An appropriate resection with adequate tumour-free margins.
A regional lymph node clearance corresponding to the location of the primary tumour in the stomach.
Safe and well functioning reconstruction.

The Japanese Research Society for Gastric Cancer has issued a classification of gastric resections for cancer based on the radicality (R) of the procedure: R_1, R_2 and R_3. In R_1 resections, the lymph node clearance is confined to the primary group of nodes, i.e. those around the cardia, along the greater and lesser curvatures and the juxtapyloric ones (*Fig.* 67.19). In practice, this is achieved by removal of the greater and lesser omenta with the excised stomach. This is the type of resection most frequently carried out in the West and does not achieve adequate control of the disease, resulting in a high incidence of local recurrence in the gastric bed. The R_2 resection necessitates an additional clearance of the lymph nodes around the main arteries: the left gastric, coeliac, common hepatic and splenic arteries, besides the retropancreatic and splenic hilar lymph nodes. In addition to lymph node clearance of the named arteries, a splenectomy and resection of the body and tail of the pancreas are necessary to achieve this (*Fig.* 67.20). The R_3 resection extends the lymph node clearance even further to include the nodes present in the porta hepatis, behind the head of the pancreas, in the root of the mesentery, around the middle colic vessels and the para-aortic lymph nodes

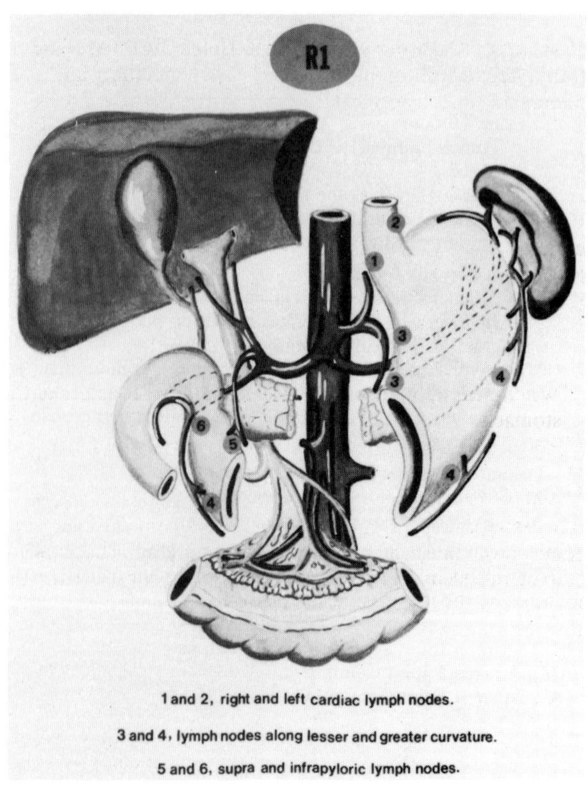

R1
1 and 2, right and left cardiac lymph nodes.
3 and 4, lymph nodes along lesser and greater curvature.
5 and 6, supra and infrapyloric lymph nodes.

Fig. 67.19 Extent of lymph node clearance in R_1 resection.

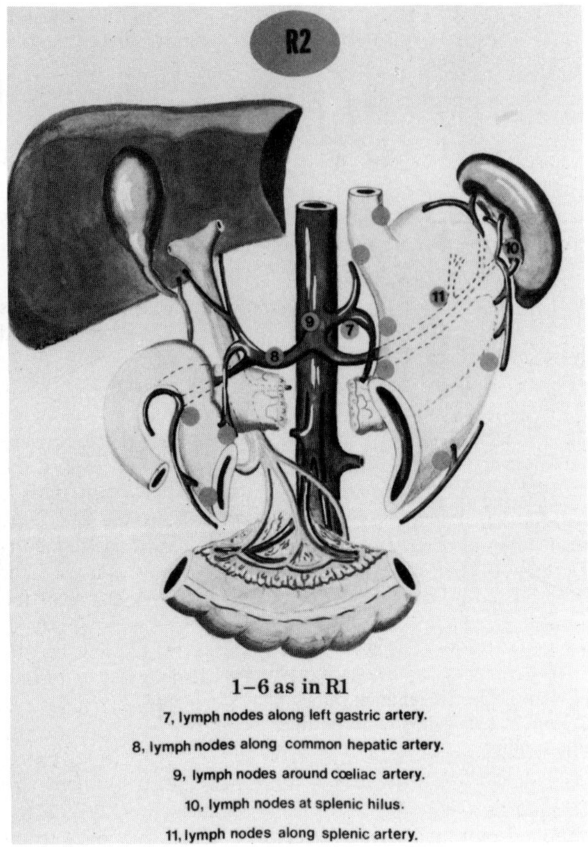

R2
1–6 as in R1
7, lymph nodes along left gastric artery.
8, lymph nodes along common hepatic artery.
9, lymph nodes around cœliac artery.
10, lymph nodes at splenic hilus.
11, lymph nodes along splenic artery.

Fig. 67.20 Extent of lymph node clearance in R_2 resection.

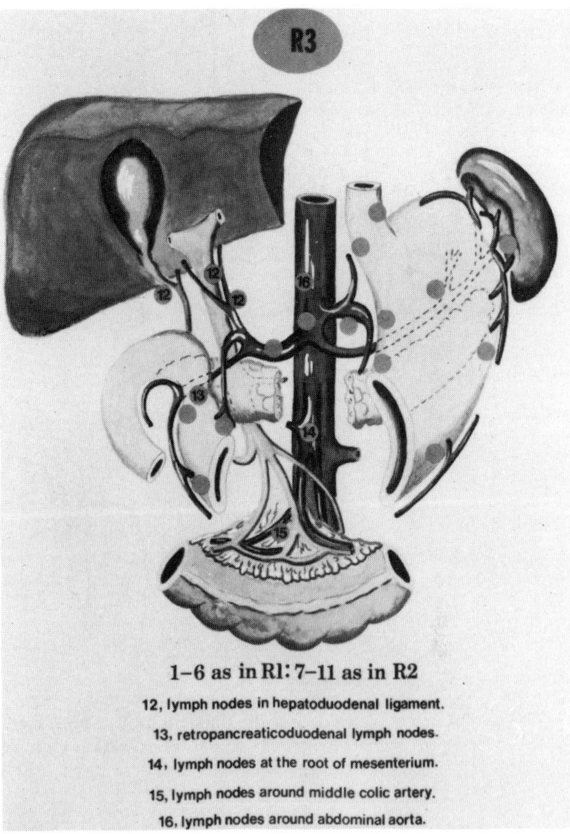

R3
1–6 as in R1: 7–11 as in R2
12, lymph nodes in hepatoduodenal ligament.
13, retropancreaticoduodenal lymph nodes.
14, lymph nodes at the root of mesenterium.
15, lymph nodes around middle colic artery.
16, lymph nodes around abdominal aorta.

Fig. 67.21 Extent of lymph node clearance in R_3 resection.

(*Fig.* 67.21). On occasions, this will involve partial colectomy, hepatic lobectomy, subtotal pancreatectomy and even pancreaticoduodenectomy.

Extent of Gastric Resection

A gastrectomy does not need to be total to be curative. Resection which provides a 2·0 cm margin for early or well circumscribed tumours and 5·0 cm for infiltrative advanced lesions is adequate. A total gastrectomy is necessary for the following:

When the proximal distance from the cardia is less than the required length to achieve a safe tumour free margin.
When the neoplasm involves two or all three sectors of the stomach.
Diffuse carcinoma (Borrmann 4) irrespective of size.

Omentectomy

The lesser omentum should be detached from the liver. The removal of the greater omentum must include the anterior leaf of the transverse mesocolon (bursectomy) to bare the colic arteries and veins and ensure the removal of the lymph nodes accompanying these vessels.

Lymph Node Clearance

This must be adequate and appropriate to the site of the primary neoplasm. Some advocate intra-operative lymph node mapping which is achieved by the peritumoural injection of dyes such as Evans Blue to outline the draining lymph nodes. The principle of an adequate node clearance is that this should encompass the tier of lymph nodes beyond those which are macroscopically involved. Thus for a tumour which is accompanied by involvement of N_1 nodes, an R_2 type of resection is necessary.

Definition of a Curative Resection

An absolute curative resection for gastric cancer may be deemed to have been performed when:

There is no peritoneal or hepatic disease.
The serosa is not involved by the tumour.
The resection margins are free of tumour by histological examination.
The R (resection) level exceeds the level of nodal involvement (N).

When the R level equals the N value, the resection is classified as relative curative.

Reconstruction

There is still considerable controversy regarding the optimum method of reconstruction after gastric resection and the various procedures may be grouped into duodenal bypass procedures and reconstructions which restore duodenal continuity. The important consideration in reconstruction after resection of gastric cancer is whether the surgeon considers that the excision performed is likely to be curative or not. In patients who are considered to have had complete excision (curative resection), the reconstruction should attempt to restore duodenal continuity since these procedures result in the best nutritional outcome in the

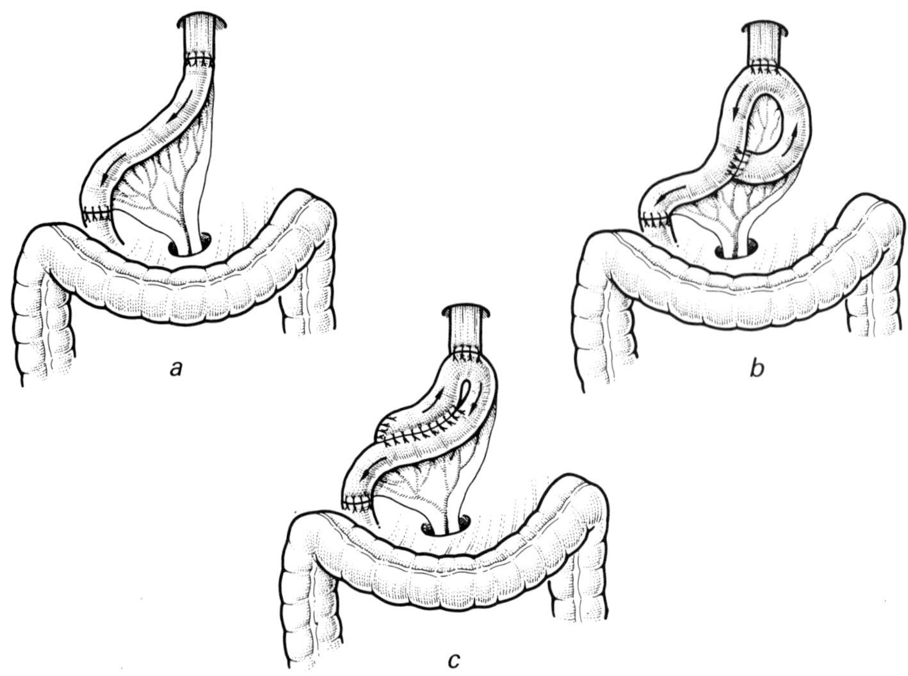

Fig. 67.22 Types of jejunal interpositions between the gastric remnant or oesophagus and the duodenum: *a*, Single isoperistaltic loop. *b*, Omega loop interposition. *c*, Reservoir jejunal interposition with isoperistaltic conduit.

long-term. Thus for patients who have had a curative distal gastrectomy, a Billroth-I procedure is the preferred method. A jejunal interposition type reconstruction (*Fig.* 67.22) is the ideal for patients who have undergone curative subtotal/total gastrectomy.

Duodenal bypass procedures (Polya for distal gastrectomy and Roux-en-Y or loop jejunostomy with entero-enteric anastomosis for more extensive resections) are performed in patients in whom the resection is considered to be non-curative (*Fig.* 67.23) as these reconstructions are less likely to be obstructed by recurrent disease.

Adjuvant Treatment

The cytotoxic agents which have some activity against gastric cancer are 5-fluorouracil, mitomycin C, adriamycin (doxorubicin) and methyl-CCNU and the most effective combination regimen is FAM (5-FU+adriamycin+mitomycin C). Although some benefit has been reported with single agent and combination treatment in some retrospective reports, there is no evidence from prospective clinical trials to date that adjuvant chemotherapy improves survival over surgical resection alone.

Adjuvant radiotherapy (preoperatively, intraoperatively and postoperatively) is also used in some centres. Postoperative radiotherapy is attractive since in 30% of patients the disease recurs in the gastric bed without any evidence of systemic spread and at least 50% of these recurrent lesions can be encompassed within a conventional radiotherapy field using external beam radiation. However, there is no firm evidence that adjuvant radiotherapy improves survival or reduces the incidence of loco-regional recurrence.

Palliative Surgical Treatment

The symptoms which require palliation are pain, vomiting, dysphagia, bleeding and malaise. The best results are obtained by a palliative gastrectomy which may have to be total if the patient's general condition permits. An antecolic gastrojejunostomy is performed for non-resectable antral neoplasms. The jejunum is anastomosed to the greater curvature after ligature and division of the lower short gastric vessels (*Fig.* 67.24). The posterior short loop gastroenterostomy favoured for benign disease is inappropriate as a palliative procedure for gastric carcinoma. The Devine's exclusion-bypass operation (*Fig.* 67.25), previously popular for inoperable antral neoplasms, is seldom performed nowadays in view of the poor results. Dysphagia due to inoperable lesions of the cardia is best treated by intubation (e.g. Celestin tube) which is preferable to the more difficult and major procedure of jejuno-oesophageal bypass.

Other Malignant Epithelial Tumours of the Stomach

These include adenosquamous, squamous and anaplastic tumours. Adenosquamous carcinomas are rare tumours which are usually found at the cardia. They are mixed tumours and both components (squamous and glandular) are histologically and biologically malignant. Until recently, anaplastic malignant tumours caused considerable difficulties with the histological diagnosis and especially the differentiation between an anaplastic carcinoma and a high-grade undifferentiated malignant lymphoma. This problem has been overcome with the advent of specific monoclonal antisera to the common leucocyte antigen (CLA) which is specific for lymphomas. Monoclonal antibodies to the epithelial membrane antigen (EMA) and cytokeratin (CAM 5.2) are used to identify the epithelial origin of anaplastic carcinomas.

Non-epithelial Tumours

The stomach is one of the common sites of smooth muscle tumours. Although they are often classified into benign

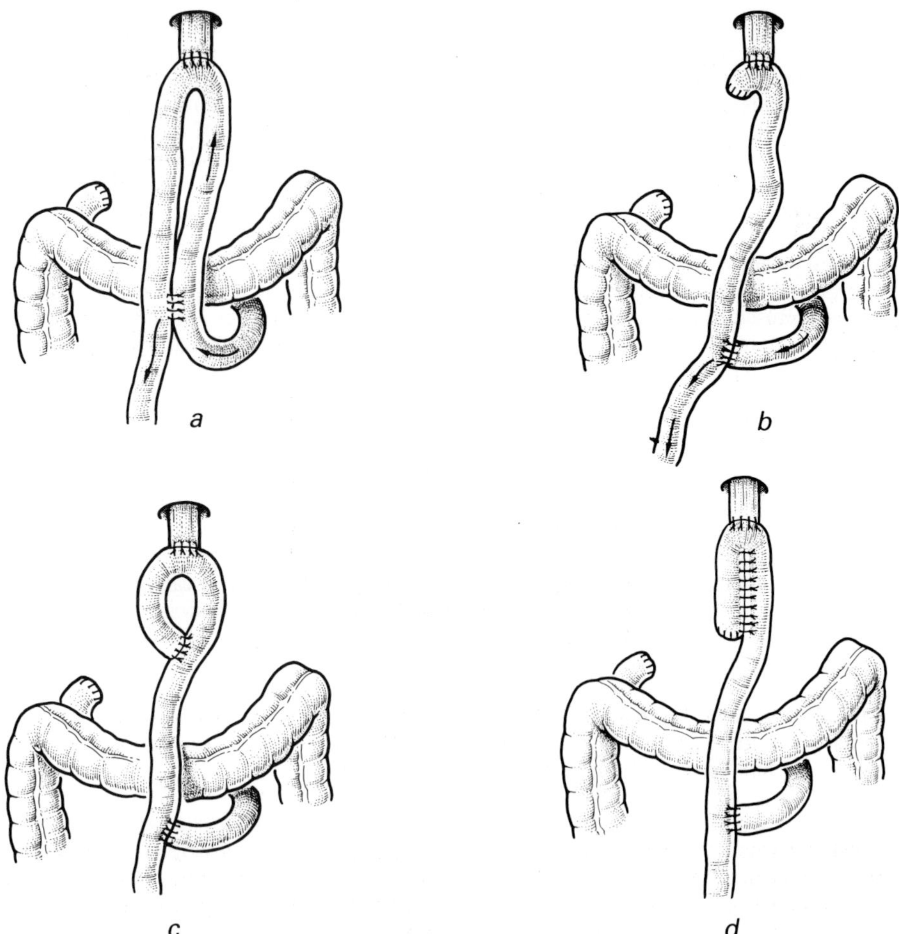

Fig. 67.23 Types of reconstructions with closure (bypass) of the duodenum: *a*, Loop oesophagojejunostomy with distal (40–60 cm) entero-enteric anastomosis. *b*, Simple Roux-en-Y reconstruction. *c*, Omega Roux-en-Y. *d*, Hunt–Lawrence Roux-en-Y pouch.

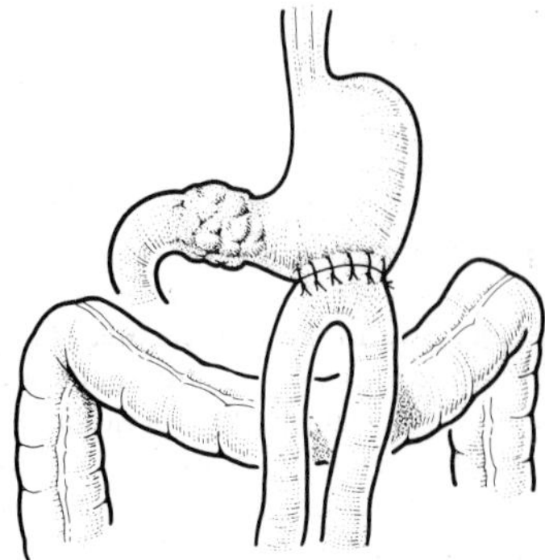

Fig. 67.24 An antecolic gastroenterostomy to the greater curvature of the stomach is an effective palliative procedure for inoperable carcinoma of the stomach.

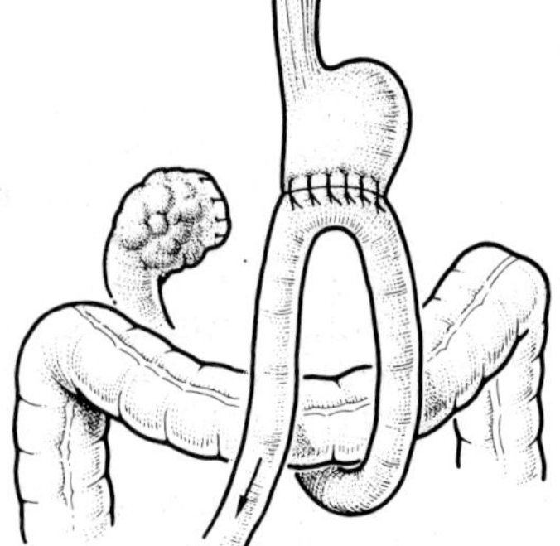

Fig. 67.25 Diagrammatic representation of Devine's antral exclusion bypass operation for inoperable carcinoma of the antrum. This operation is seldom performed nowadays. It is difficult to perform in the presence of large antral tumours and the results have been poor. It has largely been replaced by the Tanner's antecolic anastomosis to the greater curvature.

(leiomyoma) and malignant (leiomyosarcoma), the histological differentiation between the two may be difficult. However, the majority of gastric smooth muscle tumours are benign. Malignant tumours tend to be larger, show necrotic and haemorrhagic change and have a mitotic rate which exceeds 10 per 50 high power fields.

Gastric smooth muscle neoplasms form intramural tumours (submucosal or combined submucosal and intramuscular). They are encountered in the upper and middle thirds and rarely in the antrum of the stomach. When large, they may form dumb-bell swellings, the extramural portion projecting extraserosally or inside the gastric lumen. Central ulceration of the tumour is common and can result in bleeding which is a common acute presentation of gastric smooth muscle tumours. Treatment is by wedge resection if the lesion is small. Partial gastrectomy is reserved for large tumours and those considered to be malignant.

Metastatic spread from leiomyosarcomas occurs to the peritoneal surfaces, liver and lungs, nodal deposits being quite rare. Some smooth muscle tumours show areas of epithelioid differentiation and are referred to as *epithelioid smooth muscle tumours* or *epithelioid myomas* or *leiomyoblastomas*. Other non-epithelial tumours encountered in the stomach include haemangiopericytoma and Kaposi's sarcomas.

Lymphomas

In contrast to Middle Eastern countries where the small intestine is the commonest site of gastrointestinal lymphomas, in the West, the stomach is the most common site of these neoplasms and accounts for more than 50% of reported cases. However, primary gastric lymphoma is much less common than secondary involvement of the stomach by systemic lymphomas. The vast majority are non-Hodgkin's lymphomas. The classification used nowadays is that outlined in Chapter 72 (small intestine). The commonest low-grade gastric lymphomas are of the centrocytic type and the most frequently encountered high-grade tumour is the immunoblastic variety.

Although the majority of gastric lymphomas form a single lesion, a few consist of multiple polypoid masses. The tumours tend to infiltrate the wall of the stomach in a diffuse fashion causing mucosal hypertrophy and have a tendency to ulceration.

The symptoms include dyspepsia, upper abdominal pain, anorexia, nausea and vomiting, weight loss and diarrhoea. Acute presentation may occur with upper gastrointestinal bleeding (from an ulcerated tumour) or with frank perforation which occurs in 4% of cases.

The best results are obtained with resection which often entails a total gastrectomy followed by postoperative radiotherapy. Non-resectable lesions should be marked with metal clips to facilitate external beam supervoltage radiotherapy which is followed by combination chemotherapy using the CHOP regimen. The prognosis, especially for resectable lesions, is considerably better than that for gastric carcinoma with a reported 5-year survival of 50% or more.

Carcinoid and Endocrine Tumours

Carcinoid Tumour of the Stomach

Carcinoid tumours of the stomach are rare and account for only 2% of the reported gastrointestinal carcinoids. There is a known association between pernicious anaemia and the development of gastric carcinoids which may be multiple and usually arise in association with G-cell or enterochromaffin cell hyperplasia. The gastric carcinoids developing in patients with pernicious anaemia often contain gastrin and can metastasize. Gastric carcinoids arising in a previously normal gastric mucosa do not produce 5-HT but may contain histamine.

Endocrine Tumours

The endocrine tumours of the stomach either arise from normally resident endocrine cells within the gastric mucosa or from islands of ectopic pancreatic tissue. They may be single or multiple. Although rare, gastrinomas are well documented in the stomach.

Further Reading

Carter D. C. (ed.) (1983) *Peptic Ulcer*. Edinburgh, Churchill Livingstone.

Cuschieri A. (1983) Long-term sequelae of ulcer surgery. In: Carter D. C. (ed.) *Peptic Ulcer*. Edinburgh, Churchill Livingstone, pp. 149–171.

Cuschieri A. (1986) Gastrectomy for gastric cancer: definitions and objectives. *Br. J. Surg.* **73**, 513–514.

Cuschieri A. (1986) Surgical management of severe intractable postvagotomy diarrhoea. *Br. J. Surg.* **73**, 981–984.

Fielding J. W. L., Fagg S. L., Jones B. G. et al. (1983) An interim report of a prospective randomized controlled study of adjuvant chemotherapy in operable gastric cancer: British Stomach Group. *World J. Surg.* May **7** (3), 390–399.

Filipe M. I., Potet F., Bogomoletz W. V. et al. (1985) Incomplete sulphomucin-secreting intestinal metaplasia for gastric cancer. Preliminary data from a prospective study from three centres. *Gut* **26**, 1319–1326.

Gastrointestinal Tumour Study Group (1982) Controlled trial of adjuvant chemotherapy following curative resection for gastric cancer. *Cancer* **49**, 1116–1122.

Gunderson L. L. and Sosin H. (1982) Adenocarcinoma of the stomach: areas of failure in a reoperation series. *Int. J. Rad. Oncol. Biol. Phys.* **8**, 1–11.

Mackie C. R., Wisbey M. L. and Cuschieri A. (1982) Milk $^{99}Tc^{m}$-EHIDA test for enterogastric bile reflux. *Br. J. Surg.* **69**, 101–104.

Preece P. E., Cuschieri A. and Wellwood J. M. (ed.) (1986) *Cancer of the Stomach*. London, Grune & Stratton.

Reed P., Haines R., Smith P. L. et al. (1981) Gastric juice N-nitrosamines in health and gastroduodenal disease. *Lancet* **ii**, 550–552.

Regan J. F., Smutzer K. F. and Stemmer E. A. (1972) Procedures of value for the prevention and cure of dumping after vagotomy and pyloroplasty. *Am. J. Surg.* **124**, 279–286.

Tepper J. E. (1984) Intraoperative radiation therapy of gastric cancer. *Clin. Oncol.* **3**, 343–349.

68 *The Liver*

G. R. Giles

The liver is the largest organ in the body, with a weight varying from 1200 to 1600 g. It arises from the foregut endoderm as a diverticulum which extends into septum transversum and connects with the vitelline veins of the yolk sac. The caudal section of the hepatic anlage ultimately forms the biliary tract and gallbladder while the cephalic section forms the hepatic parenchyma. Ultimately the vitelline veins form the portal and hepatic veins. The left umbilical vein persists as the ductus venosum and diverts oxygenated blood from the placenta around the liver directly into the inferior vena cava. After birth the vestigial ligamentum venosum runs in the free edge of the falciform ligament. It may recanalize in patients with portal venous hypertension or can be used after dilatation for exchange blood transfusion or to permit radiological investigation of the portal venous system.

SURGICAL ANATOMY OF THE LIVER

The special nature of the hepatic vasculature has dominated thinking about this organ. Conceptually it should be regarded as a paired organ which is fused along a line which can be drawn between the gallbladder fossa and the inferior vena cava. Each lobe receives a full branch of the portal vein, hepatic artery and bile duct and the unpaired structures are the main portal vein, common hepatic artery and common hepatic bile duct. By further division of the vascular supply it will be seen that each liver is composed of 4 segments which are numbered 1–4 for the left liver and 5–8 in the right liver (*Fig.* 68.1). Recognition of the segmental nature of the livers can be ascribed to the French liver surgeon, Couinaud. It can also be seen that each numbered segment contributes hepatic veins which coalesce to form the main venous drainage of the livers and lie between the segments. There are three veins of surgical importance: the right hepatic vein drains segments 6–8 by a short vessel directly into the suprahepatic vena cava; the middle hepatic vein which drains from both livers and empties either directly into the vena cava or the left hepatic vein. The latter vein drains segments 2, 3 and 4. Segment 1, the caudate lobe, drains by several small hepatic veins directly into the infrahepatic cava.

With the demonstration of the segmental nature of the liver anatomy, it is possible to approach the question of resection of single or several segments with some confidence even in the liver which has been distorted by chronic disease. A careful identification of the vessels and ducts supplying each segment can be achieved by dissection above the portal hilum and each set may be ligated separately prior to an attempt at resection.

In the portal hilum, the portal vein which has formed behind the head of the pancreas by the junction of splenic and superior mesenteric veins, passes along the edge of the lesser omentum for 7–8 cm. It receives branches from the pylorus and the important left coronary vein from the cardio-oesophageal region (*Fig.* 68.2). In front of and to the right the common bile duct drains both livers and receives the cystic duct at a variable point of its course and on either side. To the left of the common bile duct runs the common hepatic artery giving off the main cystic artery and branches to the common bile duct prior to division into right and left branches.

An understanding of the point of the division of the structures in the portal hilum is essential for the surgeon. The main vessels and ducts, particularly the left branches,

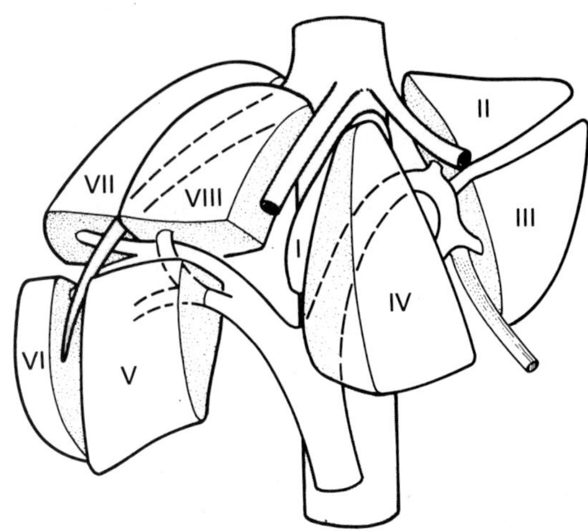

Fig. 68.1 Segmentation according to Couinaud. The liver is considered to be a paired organ, each with 4 segments. The right liver has segments numbered 5 to 8 but the left liver is somewhat more complicated. Segment 1 is the caudate lobe and segment 4 the quadrate lobe.

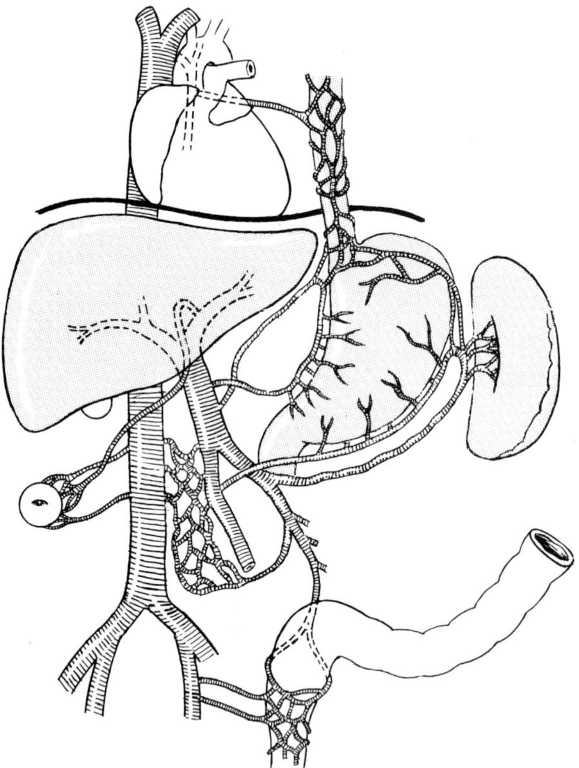

Fig. 68.2 Shows the portal venous drainage from the gastrointestinal tract and demonstrates the major anastomotic sites between the portal and systemic systems: the cardio-oesophageal junction leading up to the azygos system, the retroperitoneum, the umbilicus and in the inferior rectal plexus.

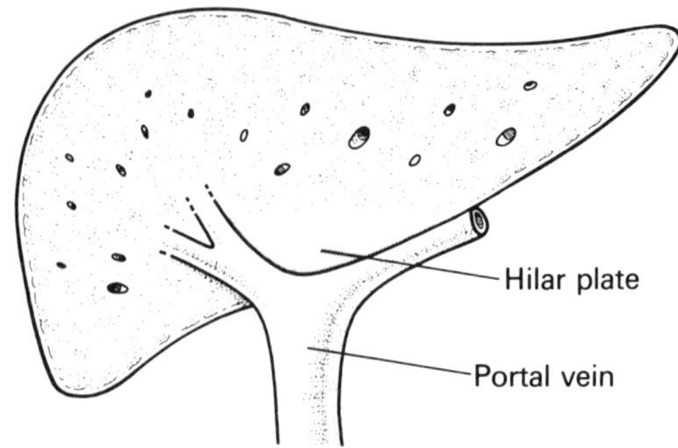

Fig. 68.3 To the undersurface of the liver, the bifurcation of the major hilar structures is secured by a dense fibrous sheath termed the hilar plate. After incising this structure the vessels to the left liver segments run for 1·5 cm before dividing into segmental branches.

are surrounded by the vasculobiliary sheath described originally by Walaeus in 1640. While the portal vein is loosely enclosed, the bile duct and hepatic artery are firmly adherent. The upper surface of the sheath which is in contact with the liver parenchyma thickens to become the hilar plate. This structure can be released from the liver surface because there are no branches along it and permits the surgeon to isolate the vessels to the left lobe and proceed to liver resection more safely (*Fig.* 68.3). The right-sided vessels are shorter and not so conveniently enclosed in a hilar plate, thus great care is required in handling.

In terms of anatomical relations, the dome of the liver can be found to reach the level of the 4th interspace and the upper surface of the left side crosses the junction of the xiphisternum and sternum. Inferiorly the tip of the right liver reaches the costal margin, though Riedel's extension commonly reaches the iliac crest. Suspending the liver from the diaphragm is the right coronary and left triangular ligament. The anterior extension of these ligaments forms the falciform ligament, which is connected to the fissure for the ligamentum venosum. The gallbladder lies in the cystic fossa on the undersurface of the liver on the line of fusion of the two sides of liver.

Conventional morphology considers that the liver is composed of pyramidal lobules based on a central vein and surrounded on the periphery by portal trunks with terminal radicles of bile duct, portal vein and hepatic artery (*Fig.* 68.4). The two vascular systems of central vein and portal tract lie on planes at right angles to one another and never interdigitate. Thus the sinusoids are arranged perpendicular to the planes of the central veins and portal blood passes to the central vein along a pressure gradient. The walls of the sinusoids are composed of endothelial and phagocytic cells termed Kupffer cells. Between the hepatocytes and Kupffer cells is the space of Disse. Bile canaliculi are shown to be channels or grooves in the hepatocyte surface, lined by microvilli. The network of canaliculi drains the liver lobules into the terminal bile ducts.

It may help in the understanding of liver injury and its consequences to view the liver morphology somewhat differently. The concept of Rappaport is to view the liver as a series of acini supplied by a portal triad of structures (*Fig.* 68.5). Three zones of sinusoids are envisaged in which the peripheral zone of the acini (Zone 3) is damaged more severely in any form of injury. Adjacent forms of injury may coalesce to form areas of bridging necrosis and later to fibrosis, producing the common pattern of post-sinusoidal block. Zones 1 and 2 may form the nidus of surviving cells which then regenerate in nodular form.

LIVER FUNCTION

Bile Formation and Excretion

About 500–1000 ml of bile are secreted each day. The liver synthesizes bile acids from cholesterol and this is the most effective form of cholesterol excretion. Almost all of the bile acids are ultimately reabsorbed by the terminal ileum and enter the enterohepatic circulation. Bile pigments are derived from the breakdown of haemoglobin by the reticulo-endothelial system to biliverdin-iron-globin, thence to unconjugated biliverdin. Biliverdin is bound to albumin for transport to the liver. Certain other chemicals, e.g. sulphonamides and salicylates compete for this binding. In the liver it is conjugated with glucuronic acid by the microsomal enzyme UDP-glucuronyl transferase. Conjugated bilirubin is secreted into the bile canaliculi and transported to the gastrointestinal tract. This enzyme is decreased in Gilbert's disease and Crigler–Najjer hyperbilirubinaemia but can be induced by phenobarbitone. A failure to excrete bilirubin into the bile ductules while maintaining bile salt excretion is a feature of the Dubin–Johnson syndrome. As bilirubin is excreted in the polar form it is not absorbed in the small intestine, but is hydrolysed and then reduced by colonic

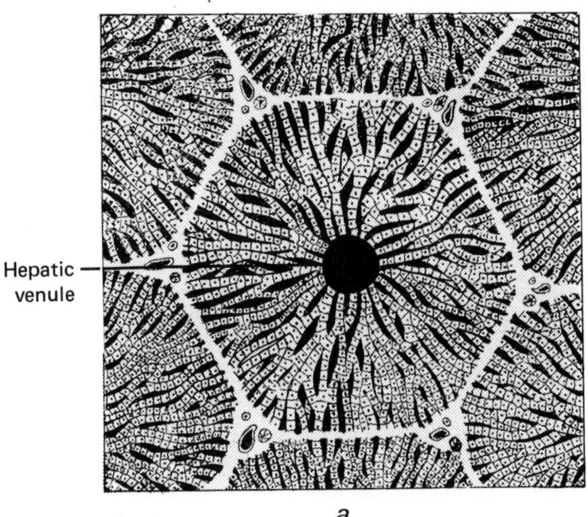

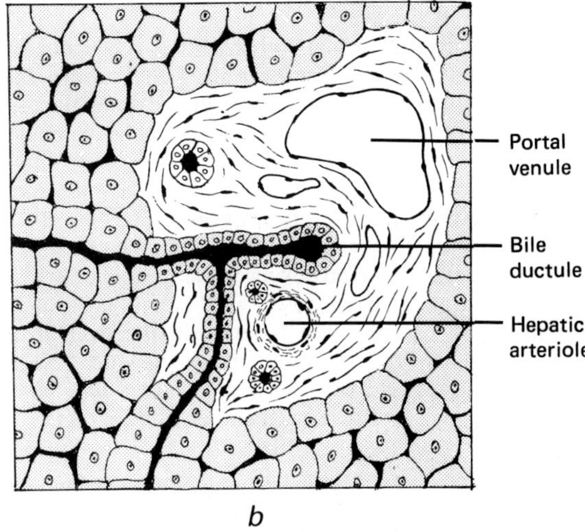

Fig. 68.4 *a*, This demonstrates the normal liver architecture in which a hepatic plate apparently surrounds a hepatic vein through which blood from the hepatic sinusoids drains. *b*, In fact it is more appropriate to centre the hepatic plate on the portal tract which contains the elements of the bile ducts into which bile can directly drain from the hepatocytes and branches of the portal vein and hepatic artery together with connective tissue stroma. Zones closest to this portal tract (Zone 1) are protected in most circumstances from liver damage. Liver cells surrounding the hepatic vein (Zone 3) are more susceptible to all forms of hepatic damage. Regenerating nodules are normally centred on a portal tract.

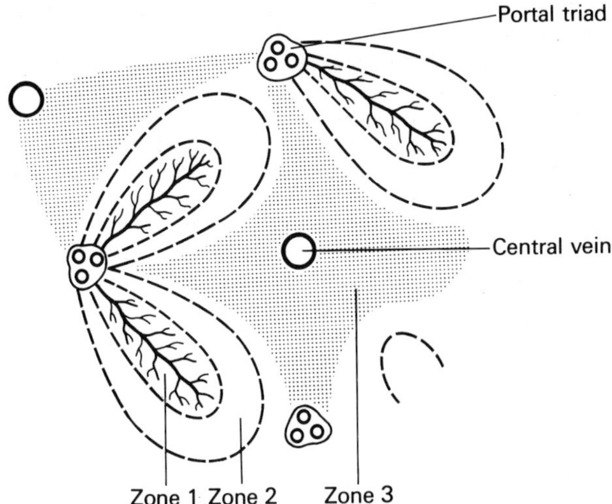

Fig. 68.5 According to Rappaport, there are three zones of liver parenchyma. Zone 1 adjacent to the portal triad is the best vascularized and least likely to injury. Zone 3 is adjacent to the central vein and most susceptible to injury.

bacteria to form urinobilinogen. Bile also contains cholesterol in micellar form, phospholipids, electrolytes, mucin and water and has an osmolality of 300 mOsm/l (*see* Chapter 69).

Jaundice due to unconjugated bilirubinaemia results from increased haemoglobin breakdown or diminished conjugation, as in Gilbert's disease. Jaundice due to conjugated bilirubinaemia is commonly associated with intrahepatic and extrahepatic bile duct obstruction and with hepatocyte damage. Bilirubin can be detected in the urine of patients with conjugated bilirubinaemia. Disturbances of the enterohepatic circulation can be shown by an absence of urinary urobilinogen. Increased urinary urobilinogen is found with increased haemoglobin breakdown and with disorders where parenchymal function is insufficient to handle the reabsorbed intestinal urobilinogen.

Protein Metabolism

The liver is a major source of beta- and gamma-globulins and the only site of production of albumin and alpha-globulins. Hepatocytes are capable of protein synthesis from amino acids and, conversely, capable of gluconeogenesis by a process of deamination of amino acids. The liver is also the major site of urea synthesis. Most of the coagulation factors are synthesized within the liver. The liver also acts to remove plasminogen activators and fibrin degradation products.

Serum albumin levels rapidly fall in hepatocellular damage and the plasma levels reflect the severity of chronic liver injury as production may be only 40% of the normal 10 g daily. However, the serum albumin level is a sensitive test only if there is no evidence of loss elsewhere, i.e. recent haemorrhage, pancreatitis, nephrotic syndrome. Globulin levels may be elevated in a wide variety of liver disorders and these disturbances are reflected in the albumin:globulin ratio. These changes are shown in the non-specific flocculation tests of liver function. Low levels of caeruloplasmin are consistent with a diagnosis of Wilson's disease, but also in terminal cirrhotic states.

Acute phase reactant proteins may be elevated in acute liver disease. The C_3 component of complement is normal in patients with chronic active hepatitis, reduced in cirrhosis and elevated with primary biliary cirrhosis. IgG shows considerable increases in patients with cryptogenic cirrhosis or chronic active hepatitis. However IgM is raised in patients with primary biliary cirrhosis and to some extent in viral hepatitis. IgA shows increases in chronic liver disease but to a lesser extent, but patterns of change are not diagnostic.

Normally, ammonia absorbed from the gut is converted to urea by the sequence demonstrated in the urea cycle. In severe hepatic dysfunction arterial blood ammonia rises. This factor may be involved in the production of portosystemic encephalopathy.

Carbohydrate Metabolism

Glycogenesis from absorbed carbohydrates is a major form of carbohydrate storage. The liver also converts the stored glycogen to glucose and it is capable of breaking glucose to pentoses via the hexose monophosphate shunt. Such compounds may be incorporated into the synthesis of nucleotides, nucleic acids and the adenosine triphosphate sequence. Furthermore, hexoses may ultimately be converted to three carbon compounds, e.g. pyruvic acid, which may form acetate and enter the tricarboxylic cycle to link protein, fat and carbohydrate metabolism.

Estimates of carbohydrate function in the liver are not generally useful, though after major hepatic resection hypoglycaemia should be guarded against. The glucose tolerance test will be flat in severe liver dysfunction.

Lipid Metabolism

Within the liver, fatty acids and glycerol are capable of conversion to acetate. Fatty acids may be converted to four carbon ketone bodies. Lipid synthesis within the liver includes glycerol, fatty acids, cholesterol, phospholipids and lipoproteins.

Cholesterol levels, particularly the esterified fraction, decrease markedly with hepatocellular failure. Conversely, a rise in cholesterol is usually seen in intra- and extrahepatic obstruction. In practice plasma levels of cholesterol or its esterified fractions are not helpful in assessing liver function.

Enzyme Secretion by the Liver

Certain enzymes of considerable metabolic importance are found in high concentration in parenchymal cells. Glutamic oxalacetic transaminase (SGOT) is found in highest levels in liver and heart muscle. Tissue injury releases the enzyme from mitochondria into the plasma. A rise to 300 units or greater (normal, 40 units), suggests hepatocellular damage. Similarly, the enzyme glutamic pyruvic transaminase (SGPT) is found in specifically high concentration in the liver compared to other organs. A rise above normal levels is usually paralleled by a rise in SGOT but may be a more specific indicator of liver injury.

The group of isoenzymes responsible for the hydrolysis of phosphate esters in an alkaline medium are termed alkaline phosphatases. These enzymes are found in liver, biliary system, bone, intestine, kidney and placenta. It is now possible to separate the isoenzymes according to the site of origin. Normally, alkaline phosphatase (AP) is excreted through the biliary tree so that biliary obstruction is accompanied by a rise in the serum alkaline phosphatase. However, most liver disorders including hepatic abscess, trauma, metastases and diffuse liver disease, e.g. hepatitis, are associated with an elevated value. There is some evidence that the elevation of serum alkaline phosphatase in these conditions may be due to overproduction, in addition to reduced biliary excretion.

A rise in the serum gamma-glutamyl transpeptidase (γ-GT) is increased in both cholestasis and hepatocellular disease. Levels tend to parallel AP in cholestasis and this can usefully confirm that the AP is of hepatobiliary origin. γ-GT is elevated in a majority of alcoholic abscesses and in patients who take regular phenobarbitone. It is often, though not invariably, elevated in patients with liver metastases.

Serum Alphafetoprotein

This protein normally circulates in fetal serum and is derived from the embryonic liver and yolk sac. The protein persists for only a few weeks after birth. It may re-appear in the plasma in adult life in patients with a variety of conditions, e.g. cirrhosis, hepatitis, liver metastasis and gastric carcinoma. More importantly, it is elevated in a proportion of patients with primary hepatocellular carcinoma (HCC). In the UK about 30% of patients are positive but in West Africa where primary liver cancer is more common the fetoprotein is elevated in 80% of patients. Serial estimations in the cirrhotic population may show small increases in the early development of HCC.

HAEMATOLOGICAL CHANGES IN LIVER DISEASE

Coagulation

As the liver manufactures most of the clotting factors, a disturbance of blood coagulation in hepatobiliary disease is common. Similarly, the liver is responsible for the clearance of activated coagulation factors including fibrin degradation products and occasionally disseminated intravascular coagulation is seen in patients with severe hepatocellular failure. The liver synthesizes fibrinogen and vitamin K-dependent factors 2, 7, 9, 10 and also factors 5, contact factors 11 and 12 and the fibrin stabilizers, factor 13. Since the half-life of these factors is short, low levels are soon found with hepatocellular disease. Rarely, abnormal coagulation factors are found, e.g. patients with hepatocellular carcinoma may produce an abnormal prothrombin (gamma carboxyprothrombin). Dysfibrinogenaemia is particularly frequent in cirrhosis, acute and chronic liver failure and is probably due to an abnormal fibrinogen molecule and is shown by prolonged thrombin time.

Vitamin K is given to all patients with a prolonged prothrombin time (10 mg intramuscularly daily × 3). Where the problem is due to bile salt deficiency the problem may be corrected as quickly as 3 hours but patients with hepatocellular disease are not so readily improved. Where the prothrombin time is prolonged greater than 3 seconds beyond the control value and some invasive procedure is absolutely required, then the coagulation defect is corrected by administering fresh frozen plasma (FFP). Platelet concentrates are used if thrombocytopenia below 60 000–80 000/mm^3 is present. Other coagulation deficiencies may be treated by administering stored blood which supplies factors 2, 7, 8 and 10. FFP and fresh blood will provide factor 5.

Peripheral Blood Changes

The bone marrow picture in chronic liver disease is one of hyperplasia and macronormoblastic. There is a relative marrow failure and the anaemia is due in part to this factor. However, as there is often a rise in the plasma volume in patients with chronic liver disease, a fall in the erythrocyte count may be due to this and the total circulating haemoglobin may be normal. Nevertheless, a picture of hypochromic anaemia is commonly seen, due to chronic blood loss associated with portal hypertension. A variety of morphological changes are seen though the erythrocytes are commonly normocytic. Macrocytes are also frequent and target cells are particularly common in cholestatic jaundice. Spur cells or thick macrocytes are found in alcoholic cirrhosis and may be associated with a poor prognosis.

Red cell distribution is increased in chronic hepatocellular disease and is due in part to hypersplenism. However, since splenectomy is not always associated with improvement this implies that many of the abnormal cells are particularly susceptible to destruction. Leucopenia and thrombocytopenia are rarely of clinical significance *per se*, thus splenectomy is rarely indicated for hypersplenism as it is followed by a high operative mortality and occasional portal venous thrombosis. Hypersplenism may suggest the need for splenectomy if the portal venous system is to be decompressed (*vide infra*). Serum folate levels and vitamin B_{12} hepatic levels are low in patients with liver disease and it is sensible to add these factors to the patient's treatment schedule.

FUNCTIONAL AND ANATOMICAL EXAMINATION OF THE LIVER

Bromsulphthalein Excretion

Sodium phenoltetrabromophthalein disulphonate (BSP) is a synthetic dye which is removed from the blood by the liver. After intravenous injection it is bound to albumin and lipoprotein and taken up by the hepatic parenchymal cells where it is conjugated and excreted into the bile. As a test of hepatic function it is given at a dose of 5 mg/kg and less than 6% should be left by 45 min. It is a very sensitive test of hepatic dysfunction and may not be of great practical value. Given by continuous infusion, it may provide a more accurate estimate of hepatic reserve in patients with cirrhosis.

It is not useful in patients with moderate jaundice, fever, severe obesity or following the recent use of radio-opaque drugs. Similar results are obtainable by the measurement of indo-cyanine green uptake of the liver.

^{131}Iodine Rose Bengal Excretion

This phthalein derivative is entirely extracted by the hepatocytes and excreted in the bile. If labelled with radioactive iodine, appropriately placed detectors will measure the rate of disappearance from the blood, hepatic uptake and excretion into the gastrointestinal tract. In practice the test does not readily distinguish between hepatocellular and *obstructive jaundice*. HIDA excretion is discussed in Chapter 69.

Anatomically, the liver parenchyma is sufficiently homogeneous for most pathological processes to be demonstrable in contrast.

Radiographic Examination of the Liver Parenchyma

A plain abdominal film may give helpful information in terms of liver size and the position of the overlying diaphragm. Rarely a small gas/fluid level may be seen within an abscess but hydatid cysts are well shown by virtue of calcification within the cyst wall. Similar findings are found in some primary liver tumours.

Ultrasonography

This mode is the investigation of choice in patients with suspected biliary tract pain, cholestasis and vague upper abdominal pain of a non-dyspeptic nature. The liver is shown as a large transonic structure in which the portal vein, hepatic veins and inferior vena cave are well shown. In patients with cholestasis, dilated intrahepatic bile ducts clearly pinpoint the presence of large duct obstruction and occasionally the cause for this obstruction may be seen distally in the biliary tree. The demonstration of gallbladder disease is particularly good and gallstones may be diagnosed with an accuracy of 95% in the best hands (Chapter 69). Visualization of the portal venous system is also possible and ultrasound is the first investigation required to demonstrate patency of the portal venous system.

It is in the screening of the liver parenchyma for focal lesions that ultrasound comes into its own and in ideal circumstances lesions as small as 1 cm can be demonstrated. Particularly well shown are liver cysts and abscesses, but also primary liver tumours and dense multifocal metastases are readily seen. Used as a screening test in patients with hepatitis B antigen positive it has proved possible to identify patients with small operable hepatocellular cancers in which prolonged survival has been reported.

Intraoperative ultrasound screening of the liver can demonstrate precisely the anatomy of vascular structures, the boundaries of palpable liver tumours and the presence of impalpable foci enabling a more appropriate resection line or preventing the performance of resection which is destined to fail. Intrahepatic gallstones are also well shown. Intraoperative probes may be side viewing and slide easily over the liver curvature and can also be used to demonstrate the anatomy and patency of hepatic veins.

Ultrasonography is of considerable help in the guidance of needles and catheters into intrahepatic collections.

Solitary echogenic areas may be haemangiomas or localized fatty infiltration and once firmly diagnosed by alternative means, e.g. CT scanning, ultrasound may be used to monitor stability of size. Liver cirrhosis is suggested by areas of increased and irregular attentuation.

CT Scanning of the Liver

This investigation is commonplace in the hepatic diagnosis and treatment planning. The principles of its application are described elsewhere in this book. Normally about 10 'slices' of the liver are performed in order to demonstrate fully the anatomical details and an imagined three-dimensional model can be constructed in which the shape, surface mass and volume can be derived. Normally the procedure is combined with contrast being swallowed to define the stomach and duodenum and intravenous contrast is administered to outline the vessels and focal lesions within the liver. The procedure is expensive and time-consuming but it is consistent and leads to relatively easy interpretation. Furthermore surrounding structures are also well shown, particularly the diaphragm, lung bases and suprahepatic vena cava.

CT scanning is particularly valuable in the diagnosis of focal disease either directly or by the direction of biopsy needles into small tumours, cysts or abscesses. After enhancement by contrast, tumours are usually more dense than the normal liver parenchyma, whereas haemangiomas are less dense centrally and commonly have lakes of contrast at the periphery. Fatty infiltration is also less dense than normal liver but hepatic adenomas and focal nodular hyperplasia may be 'invisible' because of equal density to normal liver parenchyma. Fractures in the liver substances and subcapsular haematomas are particularly well demonstrated by CT scanning.

Scintiscanning of the Liver Parenchyma

This procedure is performed less commonly than formerly and may be of two types. ^{99}Technetium^{m} (^{99}Tc^{m}) is taken up by the reticuloendothelial system and may detect focal lesions greater than 2 cm in diameter in about two-thirds of cases. Lesions in the anterior half of the liver are preferentially shown. Generalized liver disease is demonstrated as reduced or patchy uptake with increased uptake of the spleen and bone marrow. In the Budd–Chiari syndrome, reduced uptake of the liver is noted in some patients except the caudate lobe.

An alternative isotope, ^{67}gallium citrate, is concentrated in neoplastic foci and abscesses and haemangiomas concentrate the isotope ^{113}indium.

Newer Imaging Techniques

It is likely that positron emission tomography (PET) and nuclear magnetic resonance (NMR) techniques will be established as important techniques in liver disease, for certain types of cirrhosis, e.g. haemochromatosis, Wilson's disease and primary biliary cirrhosis, produce images dependent upon iron and copper deposition. Tumours are also well shown. Both techniques may indicate metabolic change within the liver parenchyma which has not yet produced structural damage and may permit monitoring of the progress of a disease and the effect of non-surgical therapy.

Examination of the Vascular Tree

The demonstration of the vascular tree is largely dependent upon invasive techniques of contrast radiology, though an increasing use of ultrasound may show the major vessels and their patency.

Hepatic Wedge Pressure and Hepatic Venography

By passing a catheter via the brachial vein, through the right atrium and directly into the hepatic veins as far as possible, the wedge pressure can be measured. It is considered to represent sinusoidal pressure and to correspond to some degree with portal vein pressure. This correlation fails in presinusoidal blocks, e.g. schistosomiasis. The technique is less commonly employed than formerly unless there is a need to demonstrate coincidentally the anatomy of hepatic veins. In patients with suspected Budd–Chiari syndrome, the technique may also demonstrate suprahepatic sources of liver congestion: congenital caval diaphragms and intraperitoneal malignant disease. By careful selective injection of contrast media, it is possible to show individual veins, the presence of thrombus and a degree of completeness of the obstruction.

Arteriography and Portography

The portal venous system may be demonstrated by splenic puncture using an intercostal route. The splenic pulse pressure is readily measured and is close to portal venous pressure. Injection of medium outlines the splenic and portal veins and often demonstrates major collaterals. Portography can also be performed via the percutaneous transhepatic route. This technique also allows selective cannulation of the left gastric vein and its embolization in poor risk patients with bleeding varices. Some centres use the left umbilical vein, after this is dilated, to inject contrast for visualization of the portal venous system.

The superior mesenteric and coeliac axis are approached by a Seldinger catheter. The arterial supply of the liver is demonstrated and the venous phase of the injection fills the superior mesenteric and portal veins or the splenic vein, according to the site of injection. The distinctive corkscrew intrahepatic arteries are characteristic of cirrhosis and a good estimate of liver size is made (*Fig.* 68.6). This technique has considerable value in planning operability of liver tumours and may be diagnostic of multifocal neoplasia when all other techniques have failed.

Needle Biopsy of the Liver

This valuable investigation is indicated in patients with undiagnosed liver disease and in some with focal abnormalities of the liver. The mortality rate should be low (less than 0·1%) provided certain precautions are taken. Normally it requires an inpatient stay and should only be performed once the prothrombin time is shown to be not more than 3 sec greater than the control and the platelet count greater than 60 000–80 000/min^3. The Menghini needle is adequate for general liver disease but is not indicated where cirrhosis is suspected. These patients require a Tru-cut needle. Normally the procedure is performed through a lateral intercostal approach but in patients with a palpable abdominal mass,

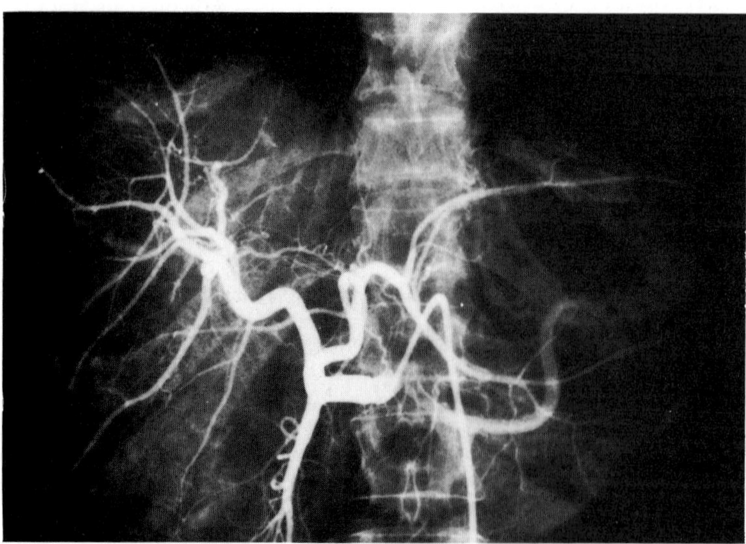

Fig. 68.6 Following selective catheterization of the common hepatic artery through the coeliac axis the hepatic arteries are well shown. In this case the terminal branches of the left hepatic artery are stretched around a large metastatic deposit within the left lateral lobe and similar metastases may be detected in the right lobe also. In certain patients the left hepatic artery will arise from the left gastric vessels and the right hepatic artery may arise, at least in part, from the superior mesenteric artery (20%).

the lesion may be approached directly. Small lesions are best biopsied by localization of the suspicious area and needle using ultrasound or CT scanning. Once the specimen is obtained, it should be placed in a container with 10% formol saline and care taken to avoid fragmentation. Biopsies taken from potential neoplastic regions may be also fixed in glutaraldehyde for electron microscopy. Complications of liver needle biopsy include pleurisy, haemorrhage from the liver and thoracic wall, intrahepatic haematoma, arteriovenous fistulas and accidental puncture of the gallbladder and large bile ducts leading to peritonitis or haemobilia. After the procedure the patient is confined to bed for 24 hours with regular and frequent pulse and blood pressure measurement.

Indications for Needle Biopsy

Investigation of acute or chronic jaundice states:

Alcoholic liver disease
Unexplained hepatomegaly
Space-occupying lesions of the liver
Drug-related liver disease

It is contraindicated in patients with coagulopathies, tense ascites and suspected haemangiomas.

CLINICAL FEATURES OF LIVER DISEASE

Many of the symptoms which can ultimately be attributed to liver disorders are non-specific, e.g. fatigue, malaise, headache, myalgia, arthralgia and fever are features commonly found with hepatitis. Confusion, forgetfulness, poor concentration and personality change are central nervous symptoms of advanced hepatic cirrhosis whereas ascites, weight loss and malnutrition and dependent oedema reflect other functional deficiencies of the same condition.

Anorexia and nausea are common in all forms of hepatic and biliary disease and it is common for pain in the right hypochondrium to be present. It is usually possible to distinguish between biliary tract colic and the dull boring pain of focal hepatic disease.

Clearly jaundice is the most obvious symptom and constitutes the greatest diagnostic problem. In many instances jaundice will be accompanied by dark urine, pale stools and pruritus. General examination may reveal early jaundice in the sclerae and palate. Pruritus may leave scratch marks and may be present earlier than other manifestations of liver disease, especially in primary biliary cirrhosis.

Chronic liver disease may show stigmata in the form of palmar erythema, finger clubbing, leuconychia, spider naevi, particularly over the upper half of the body, central nervous effects with a liver flap, peripheral neuritis and loss of consciousness ranging from confusion to full hepatic coma. A sweet musky odour may be apparent on the breath—foetor hepaticus.

On abdominal examination, there may be evidence of collateral veins in the abdominal wall, distension of the abdomen and eversion of the umbilicus from ascities, dependent oedema, gynaecomastia, testicular atrophy and loss of axillary and pubic hair. On palpation, hepatomegaly should be searched for and a decision made whether this is real or apparent, whether it is diffuse, focal or multifocal. Liver tenderness may be elicited either abdominally or by palpation or through the rib cage by percussion. Auscultation may rarely elicit a friction rub over an expanding tumour or abscess and a systolic bruit is sometimes heard. Splenomegaly may accompany hepatomegaly in patients with portal hypertension.

NON-SURGICAL DISORDERS OF THE LIVER

A full description of all liver disease is beyond the scope of this chapter. Certain conditions must be borne in mind in deciding whether a liver disorder has a surgical basis or whether it is best handled by a physician.

Drug-related Jaundice and Hepatotoxicity

Since one of the main functions of the liver is to detoxify or to metabolize many pharmaceutical agents, it is perhaps not surprising that an overdose or abnormal response to the agent may lead to problems. It is not usually the drug but a metabolite which causes the damage.

1. Directly hepatotoxic agents include carbon tetrachloride, tetracyclines, paracetamol, DDT and benzene derivatives.
2. Interference with bilirubin metabolism occurs by:

a. Haemolysis—para-aminosalicylic acid (PAS), phenacetin.
b. Abnormal bilirubin excretion—methyl testosterone and norethandrone.
c. Interference in uptake and transport of bilirubin-rifampicin, radiological agents.
d. Interference with bilirubin conjugation—novobiocin.
e. Interference with bilirubin binding—salicylates and sulphonamides.

3. Intrahepatic cholestasis: phenothiazine derivatives—chlorpromazine.
4. Hepatitis-like reaction can result from iproniazid, halothane, trichlorethylene, oxyphenisin (in laxatives) and many other drugs.
5. Hepatic fibrosis may result from the long-term use of methotrexate.

Damage is maximal in zone 3 where metabolizing enzymes are in the highest concentration and oxygen tension the lowest. The histological picture may resemble acute hepatitis and if so has a poor prognosis. In other cases the light microscopy shows only scattered fatty change and no inflammation.

A careful history of both prescribed and unprescribed medication is required for all jaundiced patients or those who have been found to have abnormal liver function tests.

Halothane Hepatitis

This useful anaesthetic agent can occasionally be incriminated as the cause of postoperative jaundice or liver failure. Although it is a rare complication, many cases only come to light if the transaminase levels are routinely monitored after surgery, particularly in patients with an unexplained pyrexia. The mechanism of hepatic injury is not certain but may have an immunological basis because of the association with pyrexia, skin rash and eosinophilia after multiple anaesthetic exposures. The clinical picture varies from a transient jaundice to fulminant hepatic failure. The surgical team should be alert to detect the minor cases in order that alternative anaesthetic agents are used for any future procedure.

Viral Hepatitis

Viral hepatitis is probably only clinically overt in one-third of patients actually affected. Type A viral hepatitis occurs in epidemic form and is largely spread via contaminated water and food (particularly shellfish), though parenteral transmission with needles can also occur. Type B viral hepatitis (serum hepatitis) is mainly spread via the parenteral route but not exclusively so and is commonly found in hospital personnel. The infection has a longer incubation period of 50–180 days compared to Type A hepatitis (15–50 days). It should also be noted that cytomegalic inclusion virus, herpesvirus, Epstein–Barr virus and yellow fever virus are all capable of producing hepatitis. Non A non B hepatitis is of four mixed types, two enterally and two parenterally acquired. The diagnosis is made after other types have been excluded. Approximately two-thirds of patients progress to chronic hepatitis.

Clinically, the disease is characterized by a prodromal pre-icteric stage lasting for up to a week with generalized malaise, skin rashes and polyarthritis. When the patient becomes jaundiced, there is a general improvement in the overall condition. Elevation of the serum transaminases may be seen before the jaundice appears, thereafter the serum bilirubin and alkaline phosphatase both rise. Normally a liver biopsy is not indicated unless the clinical diagnosis is uncertain or the disease becomes protracted.

Hepatitis B Antigen

This antigen should be looked for in *all* surgical patients who are jaundiced or have disturbed liver functions. Infection with hepatitis B virus leads to detection of several antigens in the serum: Dane particle is possibly the complete virus, both surface and core particles, hepatitis B surface antigen (HBsAg) and hepatitis B core antigen (HBcAg). There is a fourth 'e' antigen (HBeAg) which is found more frequently in patients with liver damage and those likely to progress from acute hepatitis to chronic disease and cirrhosis.

Hepatitis B virus may be transmitted by accidental inoculation or injection of HBAg-positive blood material. Blood with 'e' antigen has the highest infectivity and conversely patients with anti 'e' antibodies are less likely to transmit the disease. HBAg subtypes can be detected in the serum before the hepatitis is suspected clinically but the majority (80–90%) clear the antigen from the blood within 2 months of the disease. The remainder may have persistent antigenaemia and chronic active hepatitis and 1–2% progress to chronic aggressive hepatitis and eventually cirrhosis.

The persistent carrier rate of HBAg is about 0·2% in the UK but as high as 60% in certain areas of Polynesia. The rate is also high in drug addicts, in patients who are on immunosuppressive therapy or after cardiopulmonary bypass and in those patients suffering from polyarteritis nodosa or Down's syndrome.

Other Clinical Forms of Viral Hepatitis

1. Cholestatic Hepatitis

Some patients suffer jaundice which persists for 4–5 months. A liver biopsy will differentiate this problem from extrahepatic obstruction. A gradual reduction in the bilirubin occurs although the improvement can be accelerated by administering steroids.

2. Relapsing Hepatitis

Five to ten per cent of patients have been reported to show a relapse weeks or months after recovery from hepatitis. It may be that a premature resumption of normal physical activity is responsible.

3. Acute Liver Failure

This serious complication occurs within 10–12 days of the onset of the illness and progresses to drowsiness and coma with a bleeding tendency, hypoglycaemia, acidosis and renal failure. Once coma has developed, the mortality rate is very high.

Chronic Hepatitis

The spectrum of viral hepatitis extends from the acute fulminant form to chronic hepatitis and finally liver cirrhosis. Chronic hepatitis is divided into a number of types:

a. Chronic persistent hepatitis may be due to hepatitis B, non A non B infections, or inflammatory bowel disease. The histological picture is mild and the prognosis is excellent. No treatment is required.

b. Chronic lobular hepatitis; in this rare condition the course is characterized by remissions and relapses and often seems to be associated with patients who convert from HBeAg positive to HBe antibody positive. Steroid therapy may be indicated.

c. Chronic active hepatitis. This condition has many aetiologies including hepatitis B, non A non B, rubella, cytomegalovirus, alcohol, α_1-antitrypsin, Wilson's disease, lupoid and drugs. This diagnosis is an important one and requires thought and detailed investigation by a hepatologist. Two clinical courses are seen; mild or severe. The mild form may occasionally progress to cirrhosis; the severe form almost invariably progresses and is marked by a picture of fibrous septa extending into the liver plates with bridging between portal and central vein regions.

Chronic Carriers of Hepatitis B Virus

As a result of routine testing of patients with jaundice or liver disease, patients requiring surgery will be shown to be chronic carriers of the hepatitis B virus. In the majority there is no history of active infection but about 50% of these carriers progress to die of chronic liver disease or liver cancer.

Chronic carriers are a potential reservoir of infection for the staff, particularly in the operating room and pathology laboratory. Secondly the patient may have undetected progressive liver damage which may prejudice the outcome of operation. When a chronic carrier is detected, it is vital that a serious assessment of liver function is carried out and liver histology forms the basis of assessing the prognosis and need for treatment. The practising hepatologist will now consider active antiviral therapy for the HBe antigen positive patient in the form of adenosine arabinoside monophosphate or lymphoblastoid alpha interferons; 45–60% will respond with a disappearance of the HBV-DNA from the serum and conversion of HBe antigen to antibody. The inhibition of viral replication may lead to an improvement in the clinical liver disease and histological picture. This improvement is not seen if the patient is additionally affected by the HIV virus.

In chronic carrier patients who require elective surgery, it is necessary to take full precautions in the operative area. Ideally, elective cases should be done at the end of the working day and week and the theatre fully disinfected after use. Disposable operating clothing and drapes are sensible and additional protection by all personnel wearing gloves and the operating team protecting conjunctivae with goggles. Reverse barrier nursing is conducted at ward level.

All hospital surgical staff with a strong chance of inoculation by chronic B carriers should be vaccinated with one of the available preparations. Injections are usually repeated after one and six months. Accidental exposure or inoculation from an infected patient requires passive immunization with hyperimmune serum globulin given intramuscularly within a few hours of the injection.

Cirrhosis of the Liver

Liver cirrhosis is the end result of hepatocyte death and needs to be distinguished from hepatic fibrosis which can occur in the portal regions from chronic bile duct obstruction or congenitally, or around the central veins in chronic cardiac failure. Confluent necrosis of zones 1 and 3 leads to fibrotic bridges and the regeneration of surviving hepatocytes results in a further distortion of hepatic architecture. Three morphological types of cirrhosis can be recognized:

a. Micronodular has small regenerating nodules through the liver separated by thick fibrous septa; it is characteristically associated with alcoholism and malnutrition.

b. Macronodular has nodules of variable size and by the normal histological appearances within the larger nodules.

c. Mixed picture results from regeneration in a micronodular cirrhosis.

Clinical Presentation

Not uncommonly the condition will be unsuspected and comes to light because of a routine estimation of liver function tests or found incidentally at laparotomy. Clinical suspicion is aroused by finding palmar erythema, spider naevi, otherwise unexplained peripheral oedema or epistaxis. Alternatively, the patient may present in a later state of disease with muscle wasting and ascites, with gastrointestinal haemorrhage from varices, jaundice or hepatic encephalopathy.

In most patients, liver cirrhosis has a poor prognosis. However, it is now known that certain types, e.g. haemochromatosis and Wilson's disease can be reversed by appropriate treatment. Other diagnoses are less likely to regress but in some the prognosis may be established with appropriate management. It is of considerable importance that the risks of surgical procedures be assessed. Certain clinical criteria are worth recording:

Size of liver: large livers have better prognosis than small shrunken organs.

Jaundice: poor prognostic sign unless diagnosis is primary biliary cirrhosis.

Ascites: poor prognostic sign.

Albumin: <25 g/l is poor prognostic sign.

Hypoprothrombinaemia: if persistent, is poor prognostic sign.

Portosystemic encephalopathy: poor prognostic sign.

Alcoholic history: if abstains, prognosis better than cirrhosis of unknown origin (cryptogenic).

These prognostic factors can be combined in various mathematical models and also form the basis of the grading system devised by Child, (Grade A=good, Grade B=moderate, Grade C=poor prognosis) and modified by Pugh (*Table* 68.1).

Table 68.1 Pugh modification for assessing hepatic dysfunction

	Points awarded for abnormality 1	2	3
Encephalopathy	None	1–2	3–4
Ascites	Absent	Slight	Moderate
Albumin (g/l)	35	28–35	<28
Prothrombin time (Seconds prolonged)	1–4	4–6	6+
Bilirubin (μmol/l)	15–30	30–45	45+
Bilirubin in patients in primary biliary cirrhosis	15–60	60–150	150+

Grade A=5–6 points; Grade B=7–9 points; Grade C=10+ points.

Alcoholic Liver Disease

The liver is capable of metabolizing large quantities of alcohol via oxidation to acetaldehyde and eventually to carbon dioxide through the citric acid cycle. However, there is evidence of a direct toxic effect of alcohol on liver cells, particularly in patients who drink on a daily basis for a number of years. The earliest sign of liver damage is hepatomegaly, which may progress to a tender liver from fatty infiltration of the parenchyma. The histological picture is remarkable with the liver cells grossly distended with fat and sometimes hyaline deposits (Mallory's hyaline). This condition is reversible if the patient stops drinking.

Alcoholic hepatitis is a more serious condition and may progress to liver failure and cirrhosis. The patient may be icteric and have tender hepatomegaly. Liver function tests also show a rise in transaminase level and a leucocytosis is present. Liver histology shows a cellular infiltrate, a variable degree of fatty change and in some patients deposits of Mallory's hyaline and liver cell necrosis. The final stage of this development is a cirrhotic picture of a *micronodular* type.

Haemochromatosis

This disorder results from an excessive storage of iron in the body, up to 35 g of iron compared to a normal level of 2–4 g. The disorder is seen more frequently in middle-aged males and may be recessively linked with spontaneous causes which are equally common. Iron overload may also occur in patients receiving multiple blood transfusions and with alcoholism.

The classic clinical picture is that of a diabetic patient (75%) in whom there is a dusky brown pigmentation of the skin, buccal mucosa and conjunctiva (bronze diabetes). About half the patients have a polyarthropathy starting in the small joints. Many suffer other endocrine insufficiency as a result of iron deposition in the appropriate organ (pituitary, gonads).

A number of patients (15%) have subendocardial fibrosis due to iron deposition and right-sided heart failure is a likely result.

A liver biopsy can be stained for iron and shows excess in the hepatocytes and Kupffer cells—fibrosis is induced and eventually a macronodular cirrhosis results.

The treatment of this condition is by venesection (500 ml monthly). Each venesection removes 250 mg of iron. Chelating agents, e.g. desferrioxamine, are not effective, other than maintaining lower iron levels after venesection is complete. Untreated, most patients die within 2 years of diagnosis but with venesection over 90% will survive 5 years.

Longer term survivors have a strong tendency to develop hepatocellular carcinoma.

Primary Biliary Cirrhosis

This is a relatively rare disorder and is a cause of progressive jaundice in middle-aged, mainly female, patients. There is evidence of intrahepatic cholestasis which leads to nutritional deficiencies, including metabolic bone disease. The clinical features also include pruritus and marked deposition of cholesterol in tissues. Liver function tests shows disturbances of the levels of bilirubin, alkaline phosphatase and cholesterol. There is evidence of an immunological response with an elevation of IgM in the form of antimitochondrial and smooth muscle antibody levels. There is also evidence of a depression in lymphocyte function.

The histological picture of a liver biopsy will depend upon the stage of the disease. Typically there is a reduction in the number of small intrahepatic ducts and pericholangitis around medium-sized ducts. There is considerable overlap in the appearance on liver biopsy between primary biliary cirrhosis, chronic active hepatitis and cryptogenic cirrhosis.

Active treatment is not possible. Repletion of nutritional deficiencies by giving injections of vitamins A, D and K and calcium supplements is the only effective therapy. Medium-chain triglycerides may help prevent weight loss. Cholestyramine is given orally to control pruritus. Unfortunately a majority of patients die within 5 years.

Wilson's Disease

This inborn error of copper metabolism, which leads to a deposition of excess copper in the liver and basal ganglia of the brain, results from a decreased excretion of copper in the bile. The younger patient presents with evidence of deteriorating liver function and portal hypertension. Neurological features seem more common in the adult patient. The classic clinical feature is that of a Kayser–Fleischer ring of pigment in the cornea. Amino aciduria and phosphaturia are the result of copper deposition in the proximal tubule of the kidney.

Copper studies (serum copper and urinary copper levels and serum caeruloplasmin) should be undertaken in all young patients presenting with liver disease, and slit-lamp examination of the cornea is also carried out.

There may be some difficulty in distinguishing Wilson's liver disease from other chronic forms for in most liver disorders there is increased hepatic copper. However, the serum caeruloplasmin is low in patients with Wilson's disease.

Treatment requires the use of chelating agents, such as penicillamine, to leach the copper out of the tissues. This treatment is effective but required indefinitely.

HEPATIC ABSCESS

In temperate climates, abscesses of the liver are relatively uncommon when compared to tropical areas. This difference may be accounted for in the aetiological factors, for in warmer climates amoebic abscesses occur very frequently. Broadly there are two types—pyogenic and amoebic.

Pyogenic Abscesses

Pathogenesis

The main aetiological factor is bile-duct infection with ascending cholangitis commonly due to *E. coli* and anaerobic organisms. The suppurative process may affect both lobes of the liver or coalesce to form one large abscess. Other sources of infection include an ascending pylephlebitis with skip areas in the portal vein containing clots and bacteria which spread into the surrounding parenchyma. While any inflammatory process within the abdomen may initiate pylephlebitis, it arises particularly with complicated diverticulitis.

Some hepatic abscesses of staphylococcal and streptococcal origin arise as a complication of generalized septicaemia, others arise by direct extension from suppurating cholecystitis, penetrating peptic ulcer disease and subphrenic collections. Obviously trauma to the liver, both penetrating and non-penetrating, may devitalize liver tissue and subsequent infection produces an abscess. A significant group of patients are found in the geriatric population with symptoms of insidious and non-specific onset. Ultrasonographic examination of hepatomegaly may show surprisingly large abscesses. The microbiological basis of these abscesses is commonly the pepto-streptococcus, *Streptococcus milleri* or other microbes.

All types of abscesses are found more commonly in the right lobe.

All abscesses contain areas of liver parenchymal cell necrosis surrounded by polymorphonuclear leucocytes and lymphocyte infiltration with relatively damaged parenchyma and viable bacteria on the periphery. Ultimately a fibrous reaction is initiated which may produce a fibrous capsule containing pus. Frequently antibiotic treatment results in a solid liver abscess with a mixture of inflammatory cells, dying liver cells and fibrotic tissue—pus never forms in these areas. Since this type of abscess will not require drainage and may be confused with a neoplastic lesion, this pathological process should be considered.

Hepatic Amoebiasis (*see* Chapter 4)

This results from intestinal amoebiasis though it is not clear what proportion of infected patients are so affected. The infection spreads to the liver via the portal vein from an ulcer in the bowel wall. Most amoebae lodge in the interlobular veins and degenerate. Some act by cytolysis to invade the portal tracts and lead to cell necrosis and a coalescence of infected triads to form a larger abscess cavity. Early abscesses are solid but pus appears later, characteristically resembling anchovy paste, though in one-third of patients the pus has the usual creamy appearance. Occasionally, amoebic abscesses become secondarily infected with pyogenic bacteria.

The diagnosis is confirmed by positive serological tests, demonstration of amoebic trophozoites in abscess fluid and a rapid response to anti-amoebicides.

Amoebic abscesses tend to occur in younger patients than those with pyogenic abscess (male 3·4:female 1). Similarly, they present with a history of symptoms of shorter duration.

Clinical Features of Hepatic Abscesses

Since most pyogenic abscesses are secondary to other infective processes, the clinical features may be dominated by the primary disorder. Characteristically there is a high fever, rigors, profuse sweating, anorexia and vomiting, with pain as a relatively late symptom. These features are less striking in hepatic amoebiasis and the fever is usually low grade. However, pain is a more common feature with amoebic abscess and is aggravated by movement and coughing. An abscess may reach a very large size before causing pain if it is directed through the bare area of the liver. About half the patients with amoebic abscesses will have diarrhoea.

Hepatomegaly is common, particularly with amoebiasis. Occasionally with right lobe abscesses there is bulging and pitting oedema of the intercostal spaces. An abscess in the left lobe may present as a painful epigastric swelling. On investigation an anaemia and leucocytosis may be found, particularly with pyogenic abscess, and the ESR is markedly elevated. Disturbances of the liver function tests are not diagnostic, particularly when complicated by cholangitis, and may be absent in amoebiasis.

Stool examination is highly dependent upon the diligence of collection and the experience of the observer and it may be necessary to confirm amoebiasis by a serum complement-fixation test. Blood cultures are usually positive with pyogenic abscesses when taken during the height of pyrexia and anaerobic infection should be considered. Clinical suspicion of hepatic abscess may be confirmed by a technetium scintiscan or by ultrasonic or CT scanning of the liver which may also demonstrate the presence of pus or a multilocular defect (*Fig.* 68.7). A plain film of the abdomen and chest may rarely show an air/fluid level within the liver substance, and usually an elevated immobile diaphragm with loss of the anterior costophrenic angle is found.

Complications

Recurrent septicaemia is the most common complication of pyogenic abscesses. Extension and rupture of the abscess may occur in any direction. Peritoneal rupture results in widespread peritonitis or in the formation of a subphrenic collection. Extension through the diaphragm may lead to thoracic empyema or to a rupture into the bronchus with expectoration of large volumes of anchovy-paste-coloured pus from amoebic abscesses and bile-stained pus from cholangitic abscesses. Rarely, the abscess ruptures into the pericardium with high mortality, a feature more commonly seen with the amoebic abscess.

Treatment

Initial management is usually non-surgical with administration of antibiotics according to bacterial sensitivity. Precise microbiological identification may result from blood cultures or from aspiration of the abscess cavity with ultrasonic control. In the event of a failure to isolate organisms, the choice of antibiotic should be based on the most likely aetiological factor, i.e. cholangitic and pylophlebitic abscesses are usually infected with *E. coli* and anaerobes and may be appropriately treated with cephalosporins, gentamicin and metronidazole. Amoebic abscesses were formerly treated with emetine (65 mg daily × 10) or chloroquine phosphate (0·9 g daily × 10, 0·6 g daily × 20) but currently metronidazole can be administered with effect given in standard dosage (*see* Chapter 4). Microaerophilic streptococcal infections are sensitive to penicillin.

Emphasis is now given to drainage of the abscess cavity by repeated needle aspiration or fine-bore catheter directed under ultrasonic control. Antibiotics may be instilled into the cavity though they are not necessarily effective. Progress is monitored by repeated ultrasound examinations. Deterioration in the general condition of the patient, repeated episodes of septicaemia or a failure of the abscess to decrease in size should be treated by surgical drainage. Posteriorly placed abscesses may be approached by an extraserous dissection through the bed of the 12th rib. Larger abscesses may require abdominal drainage with wide-bore sump drains and special care being taken to avoid contamination of the peritoneal cavity. Where a pyogenic abscess is secondary to cholangitis, drainage of the bile ducts and removal of gallstones should be undertaken. Similarly, other abdominal abscesses may require drainage with appropriate treatment of the underlying disorder.

Rupture of an amoebic abscess into the lung and bronchus can usually be treated successfully by antibiotics and postural drainage. When the intrapulmonary rupture is associated with cholangitis, bile-duct drainage is essential. A persistent

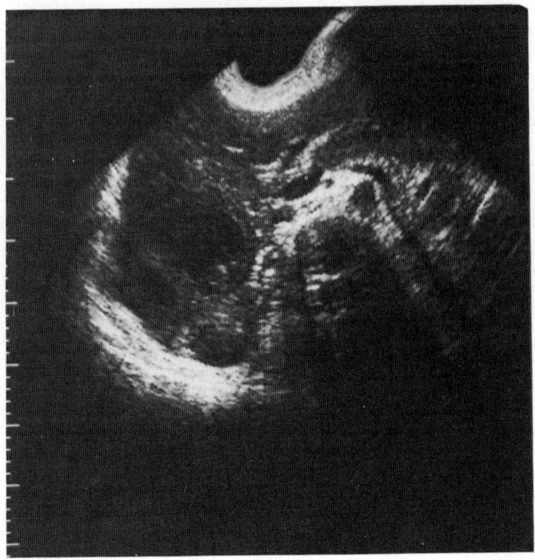

a

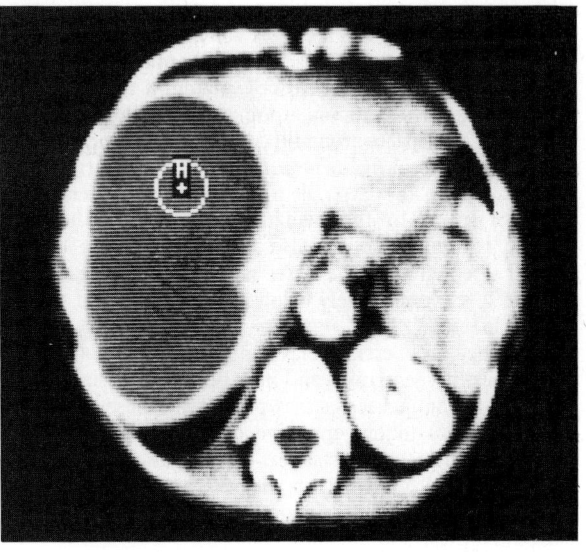

b

Fig. 68.7 *a*, An ultrasound of the liver on coronal section shows a cavity within the liver substance. *b*, CT scan demonstrates that the abscess cavity occupies most of the right lobe of the liver. Subsequent drainage of the cavity resulted in complete resolution.

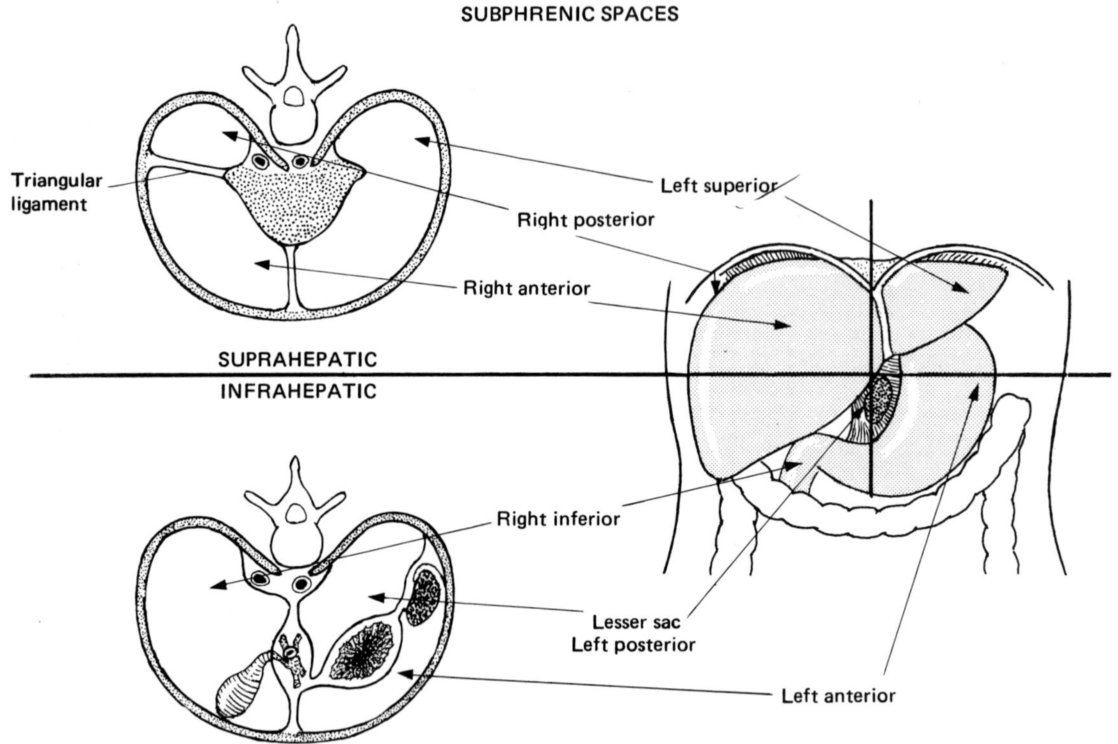

Fig. 68.8 The subphrenic spaces may be considered to be supra- and infrahepatic.

bronchopleural fistula may require formal thoracotomy, decortication of the lung and diaphragm with resection of severely damaged pulmonary tissue and diaphragmatic repair. Rupture into the pericardium requires early aspiration of the exudate and occasionally transpleural drainage.

Extrahepatic Abscess

The distribution of intra-abdominal abscesses is directly related to the precipitating lesion and to the potential peritoneal spaces. Abscesses are most common in the right and left lower quadrants as a consequence of appendicitis, diverticulitis and pelvic sepsis. Abscesses around the liver comprise the next most common group of intra-abdominal septic collections. Six spaces around the liver are described. Superiorly, the falciform ligament divides the left and right subphrenic spaces, the latter being divided into anterior and posterior spaces by the triangular ligament. In the infrahepatic region, there are also three spaces—the two on the left side including the lesser sac of the peritoneal cavity and the space immediately below the lateral lobe of the left hepatic lobe (*Fig.* 68.8).

Extrahepatic collections may contain a mixture of pus and gastrointestinal secretions and may be of major size. While any intra-abdominal sepsis may precipitate these collections most abscesses follow operative or accidental abdominal trauma. In these circumstances, extrahepatic collections of blood or serous fluid become encysted and infected (*Fig.* 68.9). Primary causes include pancreatitis, cholecystitis, perforated ulcer and appendicitis.

Clinically, suspicion of an extrahepatic collection is aroused by fever with occasional episodes of septicaemia. Non-specific abdominal symptoms and general ill-health are common, though in some patients attention is drawn to respiratory side-effects resulting from inflammatory changes induced in the lung by a subdiaphragmatic collection. When an abscess is subhepatic in site, tenderness is elicited and a mass may be palpated or percussed.

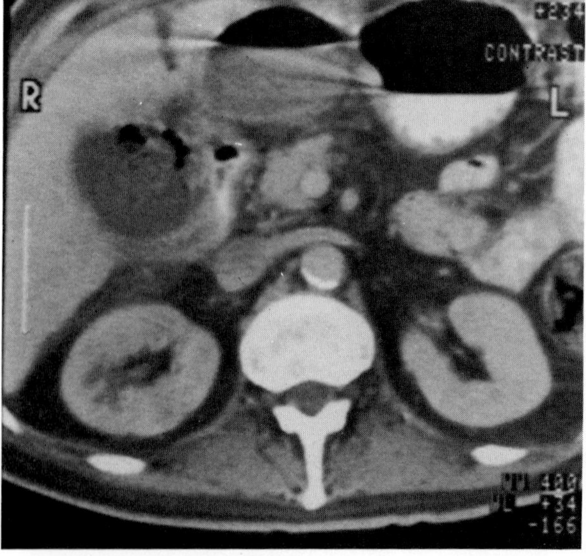

Fig. 68.9 CT scan of an infrahepatic abscess with fluid level lying between the gallbladder and gastric antrum. The abscess resulted from the infected gallbladder which contains stones seen on other sections of the CT examination.

The confirmation of an abscess may be difficult and probably many minor collections ultimately resolve and remain unproven. In the right posterior subphrenic space collections, there is typically elevation of diaphragm on chest radiography with decreased mobility of the diaphragm on screening (*Fig.* 68.10). Inflammation of the diaphragm leads to pneumonic changes in the overlying lung and a pleural effusion. For left-sided collections the combination of screening and a barium meal examination may show distortion of the gastric fundus or filled space between the fundus and dome of the diaphragm. Similarly, combined pulmonary and hepatic scintiscans may document subphrenic collections, but ultrasonic examinations are generally more helpful, particularly with reference to subhepatic collections.

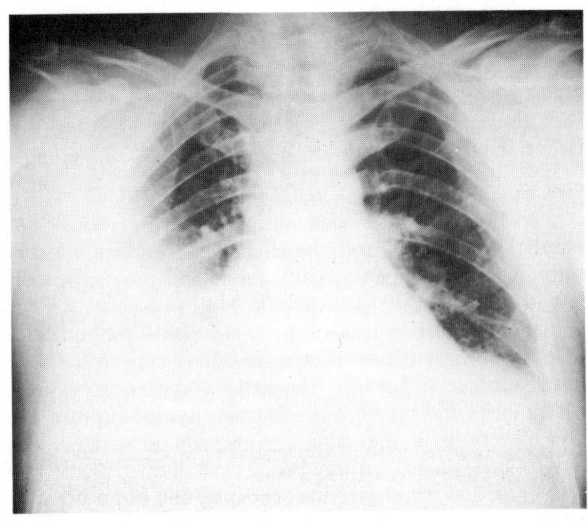

Fig. 68.10 Following cholecystectomy the patient developed a high swinging fever, together with signs at the right base and tenderness in the right hypochondrium. A chest radiograph taken at the time shows evidence of a marked pleural effusion on the right side with an underlying subphrenic collection. Drainage of the subphrenic collection led to subsequent resolution of the pleural effusion.

Management

Minor collections may resolve with antibiotics and the frequency of dense adhesions between liver and a diaphragm at elective second laparotomies suggest this is a relatively common event. However, once pus is suspected or an air fluid level is seen on radiological examination, drainage of the abscess is mandatory.

It is questionable whether subphrenic or subhepatic abscesses always require surgical drainage. With accurate localization using ultrasound or CT scanning (*Fig.* 68.9), many collections can be aspirated and a catheter left in place. In most instances the catheters are too fine to permit flow of thick pus but they do permit outlining of the cavity with opaque media to monitor progress. Some patients are best served by a surgical approach, particularly if the lesion is multilocular.

Most subhepatic abscesses may be drained surgically by an anterior approach, as may the right anterior subphrenic collection. Occasionally it is possible to enter the abscess without contamination of the peritoneal cavity. Posterior subphrenic collections are most appropriately drained by the classic extraserous approach through the bed of the 12th rib. In either approach, the abscess cavity is thoroughly explored and all loculi are broken down. Wide-calibre drains are inserted to the furthermost point of the cavity. Gradual withdrawal of the drains is indicated, with irrigation of saline and hydrogen peroxide as needed. Repeated sinograms will show loculation beyond the tip of the drain. Culture of the infected fluid is taken at the time of drainage and subsequently allows the use of appropriate antibiotics when systemic effects of infection are noted.

Abscesses occurring as a complication of surgical procedures are largely preventable. Prior to abdominal closure, a saline lavage of the peritoneal cavity with special attention to the subphrenic spaces and pelvis will reduce the incidence of postoperative abscesses to a minimum.

LIVER CYSTS AND TUMOURS

Following the widespread use of the ultrasound, echogenic foci are commonly detected in the liver and shown to be of a cystic nature. Broadly these lesions can be classified as non-parasitic or parasitic and within the non-parasitic group there are a variety of clinical conditions which reflect underlying developmental defects of the liver parenchyma or bile ducts. Some cystic lesions follow trauma in which a central rupture has resulted in a collection of bile and serum and these cysts have no epithelial lining. Others are clearly similar to dermoid cysts found in other sites. Most of the remainder have a fairly simple lining of cuboidal or endothelial epithelium and can be grouped as fibropolycystic disease. Most importantly, the lesions are associated with other well-recognized clinical entities such as congenital hepatic fibrosis, microhamartoma, Caroli's disease and choledochal cyst. With improved survival from renal failure, patients with polycystic kidneys are often found to have polycystic livers into which haemorrhage or infection develop. Clinically this condition may be mistaken for hepatic metastases. Fibropolycystic disease is also found in association with other congenital abnormalities such as cleft palate, spina bifida, cardiac defects and malrotation of the intestine.

Non-parasitic cysts are usually detected in middle life and in females. Solitary cysts are frequently tiny and discovered incidentally at laparotomy. Occasionally the cysts grow to a large size and occupy one whole hepatic lobe (*Fig.* 68.11). Characteristically the cyst contents are light brown in colour at low internal pressure in contrast to parasitic cysts. An inner lining of cuboidal epithelium is surrounded by connective stroma which is contiguous with compressed liver parenchyma. Most cysts are related to the portal tracts. Similar cysts are found in the pancreas, spleen, lungs, ovaries and kidneys in 30–50%.

Clinical Features

Most cysts are asymptomatic and only become apparent when the cysts reach sufficient size to exert pressure on adjacent viscera, producing non-specific symptoms of vomiting, upper abdominal pain and occasionally diarrhoea. Clinical examination reveals a non-tender liver tumour. Jaundice is very unusual and liver functions are rarely disturbed. Plain film of the abdomen may show displacement of the colon or stomach and the lesion may be confirmed by ultrasonography and scintiscanning. The main differential diagnosis is parasitic cysts and solid tumours. With exception of the complications of torsion, rupture and intracystic haemorrhage, the operative treatment is confined

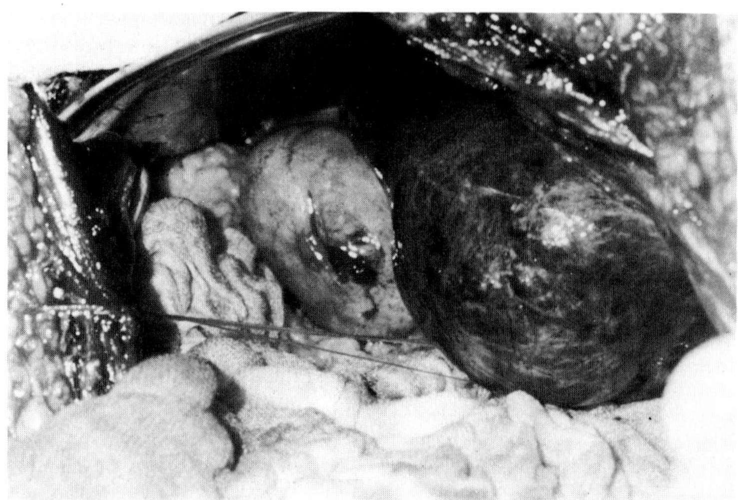

Fig. 68.11 This operative photograph shows the undersurface of the liver in which the gallbladder is seen as a whiter structure and lies adjacent to a large lymphogenous cyst of the liver. No treatment was necessary for this lesion.

to solitary cysts which are usually completely extirpated or removed by limited hepatic resection. Confirmation of polycystic liver disease may be made by ultrasonography and laparotomy—treatment is confined to patients with portal hypertension who may require portal vein decompression. Aspiration of large cysts with introduction of fibrosing agents is almost never effective. The prognosis of patients with fibropolycystic disease is generally good, though poorer in patients with Caroli's disease.

Hydatid Cysts of the Liver

This infestation is endemic in certain countries, particularly the southern half of South America, Australasia, New Zealand, France and certain areas of the USA and the UK. The life cycle and natural hosts of the organism is illustrated in *Fig.* 4.2. Man is a secondary host and becomes infected by ingesting vegetables and water fouled by dogs or more directly by handling the parasite-infested dogs as pets. After ingestion the shell of the egg is destroyed by gastric acid and hatched within the duodenum. The liberated embryos migrate through the gut wall into the mesenteric circulation and lodge within the liver. Eighty per cent of hydatid cysts are ultimately found in the liver substance. After the embryo has lodged, it is converted into a small vesicle which establishes a germinative epithelium which eventually evolves brood cysts and from these brood capsules, scolices form and invaginate themselves to protect the hooklets and suckers. Some cysts never produce brood capsules or become sterilized by secondary infection or calcification. There are two distinct pathological processes, the more common unilocular hydatid cyst, caused by *Echinococcus granulosus*, and the alveolar type, a spongy metastatic process with a poor prognosis caused by *Echinococcus multilocularis*.

Clinical Features

Since the growth of the parasite is slow, many years elapse before the cyst reaches significant size. Palpable cysts are therefore rare in children. In all ages, pain, jaundice and ascites are uncommon and in most patients, general health is good. On physical examination an anteriorly located cyst presents as a smooth rounded tense mass—the physical sign of hydatid thrill can rarely be elicited. Secondary infection results in tender hepatomegaly, rigors and pyrexia associated with a deep-seated continuous pain.

Further clinical features are the result of cyst complications. Intrabiliary rupture may give biliary colic and usually causes jaundice and fever. Associated vomitus may contain hydatid cysts and membranes. Intraperitoneal rupture produces severe pain and shock classically associated with pruritus and urticaria. Many brood cysts induce a profound fibrous reaction which sterilizes the infection but other cysts reappear in various parts of the peritoneal cavity years later. Intrathoracic rupture may be preceded by symptoms of diaphragmatic irritation and rupture into bronchus leads to a partly bloodstained sputum which frequently becomes bile stained. Hydatid allergy is manifested by urticaria or, very rarely, anaphylactic shock.

Investigational Studies

The appearance of a painless liver swelling in a patient living in an endemic area gives a high index of suspicion. An unruptured cyst may show on plain radiograph as a calcified reticulated shadow, if not calcified by displacement of the diaphragm, or a barium-filled stomach. Following intrabiliary rupture, gas may enter the cyst leading to partial collapse of the cyst wall (camellotte sign). Scintiscanning shows a large filling defect and ultrasonography reveals an echogenic cyst.

Although the cyst is isolated from the liver by an adventitial layer, there is an absorption of parasitic products which acts as an antigenic stimulus. This reflects in an eosinophilia in 25% of patients, a complement-fixation test which is accurate in 93% of patients. The Casoni test has been largely abandoned. It has been recognized that some cysts never leak and tests are never positive in these patients.

Treatment

The treatment of hydatid cysts of the liver is surgical. There is no guaranteed response to drug treatment with mebendazole or irradiation and the cyst is a potential site for serious complications. Surgical treatment involves removing the cyst without contaminating the patient. Where there are multiple cysts, several procedures may be necessary. Large cysts found on the antero-inferior and postero-inferior aspects of the liver are approached abdominally. Cysts in the dome may be reached by the posterior extraserous approach or transpleurally through the bed of the 9th rib.

The initial stage involves protection of the operative field against live cysts using multiple coloured towels soaked in hypertonic saline which isolate the main cyst from the exposed serous cavity. Since hydatid fluid is under high pressure, the cyst is decompressed by aspiration as completely as possible though daughter cysts tend to block the needle frequently. The main cyst is injected through the same needle with 20% saline and left for 5 min after which the main cyst is opened and all daughter cysts removed. In large cysts it is not feasible to remove the cyst wall and the cavity is drained for a few days and partially occluded by an omental plug which is sutured to the rim of the cyst.

Marsupialization of large cysts may be indicated when secondary infection has occurred but prolonged purulent drainage results and a secondary omentoplasty may be necessary. Cysts with extensive calcification are usually sterile and best left alone. Jaundice after intrabiliary rupture requires choledochotomy and clearance of cysts followed by T-tube drainage. Peritoneal rupture is managed by laparotomy and careful lavage. Providing the rupture has not occurred and careful surgical techniques applied, the prognosis is excellent.

Mebendazole and albendazole are two agents specifically available for hydatid. Penetration of the cyst by the drug is uncertain and although many cysts decrease in size, not all scolices are killed. Albendazole may have a role as an adjuvant to surgical treatment.

Benign Solid Tumours

Non-cystic benign tumours of the liver are commonly unsuspected and found at laparotomy for other conditions. More rarely, they reach sufficient size to be palpable or develop complications which are quite dramatic. Though the classification of these tumours is not sharply defined several types are identified:

1. Haemangioma.
2. Hamartoma.
3. Focal nodular hyperplasia.
4. Adenoma.
5. Cholangioma.
6. Biliary cystadenoma.

Haemangiomas

Haemangiomas are the commonest benign tumour but only rarely produce symptoms. They are frequently situated just beneath the liver capsule and normally of the cavernous type. Histologically the lesion is composed of blood-filled endothelial lined spaces separated by a variable degree of fibrous tissue. In the infant form of haemangioendothelioma or diffuse hepatic haemangiomatosis the lesion is multicentric and extends over a wide area.

These tumours, having grown to significant size, will eventually produce pain or dyspepsia and develop a plapable abdominal mass. Rupture is rare but leads to a major intra-abdominal haemorrhage with shock and collapse. The diffuse lesion in children may present in early life as high output cardiac failure associated with an abdominal mass and cutaneous haemangiomas (85%). A bruit is heard in about 15% of patients. CT scans are usually quite diagnostic. The lesions gradually concentrate injected contrast slowly from the periphery to the centre. This process may take 60 minutes. Where the diagnosis remains doubtful, arterioportography will demonstrate the lesion (*Fig.* 68.12). A biopsy is not indicated.

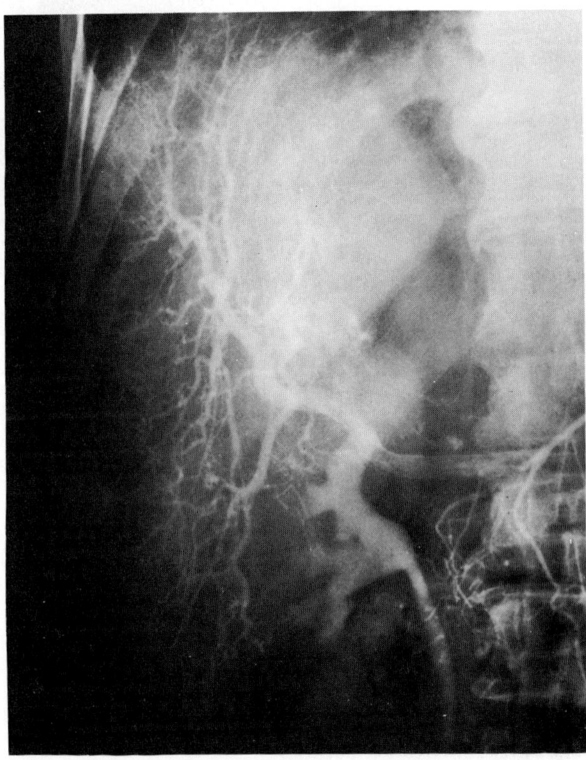

Fig. 68.12 This selective arteriogram shows an apparent tumour circulation arising from the left hepatic artery. Subsequent resection of a tumour in the left lobe showed this to be a benign cavernous haemangioma.

The preferred treatment for clinically significant haemangiomas is wedge excision where possible, with lobectomy reserved for large lesions confined to one lobe. In such cases the residual liver may contain further haemangiomas. Children presenting in the first year of life have a poor prognosis and die of cardiac failure. Scintiscanning and angiography will demonstrate the lesion and if there appears to be a major feeding vessel from the hepatic artery, it may be worthwhile ligating this vessel or the main hepatic artery. With more diffuse lesions, irradiation of the liver may result in significant shrinkage and a reduction in the volume of arteriovenous shunting. After the first year, the haemangiomatosis tends to regress as do the cutaneous lesions.

Hamartomas

Hamartomas are tumour-like malformations of congenital origin and consist of normal tissues in a disorderly arrangement. The lesions vary from minute nodules to large solid tumours and may be single or multiple. The tumours are not encapsulated, the fibrous periphery is a pseudocapsule of compressed parenchyma (*Fig.* 68.13*b*) and the histological picture demonstrates irregular distorted hepatic plates, vascular channels and extensive fibrosis. Children are commonly affected and present with an expanding abdomen with a large palpable mass. Large tumours may displace the stomach and produce vomiting and elevate the diaphragm

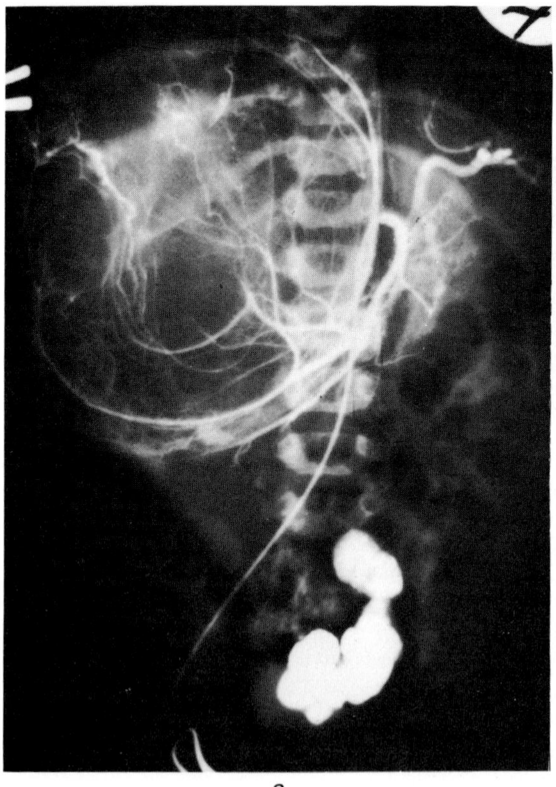

a

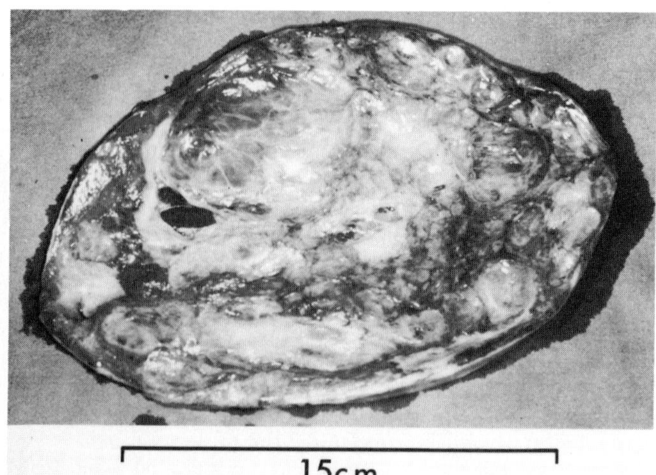

b

Fig. 68.13 *a*, A 3-year-old child presented with an expanding liver tumour. Selective arteriogram showed the hepatic vessels to be stretched around the tumour and there is little evidence of tumour circulation. *b*, The excised lesion proved to have a distinct capsule and to be multilocular. Histology showed this to be a hamartoma of the liver.

compressing the right lung. As the tumour expands inferior vena caval compression occurs.

Hamartomas show as filling defects on scintiscans and are relatively avascular tumours on angiography (*Fig.* 68.13*a*). Large tumours should be removed, usually by formal resection of a lobe, though it is sometimes possible to find a plane of cleavage. Occasionally, large tumours may show evidence of sarcomatous change and have a poor prognosis. Benign lesions have an excellent prognosis and where small and multiple may be kept under observation.

Adenomas (HA) and Focal Nodular Hyperplasia (FNH)

Adenomas are variable in size (4–30 cm) and occur uncommonly in children, postmenopausal women or males. There appears to be an increased incidence related to use of the contraceptive pill. Ten per cent appear multiple. The risk rises after 4 years of pill usage particularly in women over 30 years on pills of high hormone content.

Focal nodular hyperplasia (*Fig.* 68.14) may be distinguishable but the lesions merge in pathological terms. FNH may be a response to parenchymal injury or result from an anomalous arterial supply to a local area of liver tissue. The incidence of FNH does not appear to have increased since the introduction of the contraceptive pill. FNH is not premalignant and the natural history is such that it may be observed without serious risk. Successful management of haemorrhage from FNH appears to be ligation of the feeding hepatic artery or local resection where feasible.

In contrast, hepatic adenoma constitutes an ever-present danger with risk of rupture and haemorrhage (30%) (*Fig.* 68.15) and it may be difficult to distinguish HA from low-grade hepatomas. An adenoma, which does not regress, should be excised. However, if the diagnosis is certain, the lesions may be monitored by ultrasound for 6–12 months. If static or diminishing in size, operation may be deferred. If the patient becomes pregnant, the risk of rupture is greater. It may be appropriate to advocate sterilization.

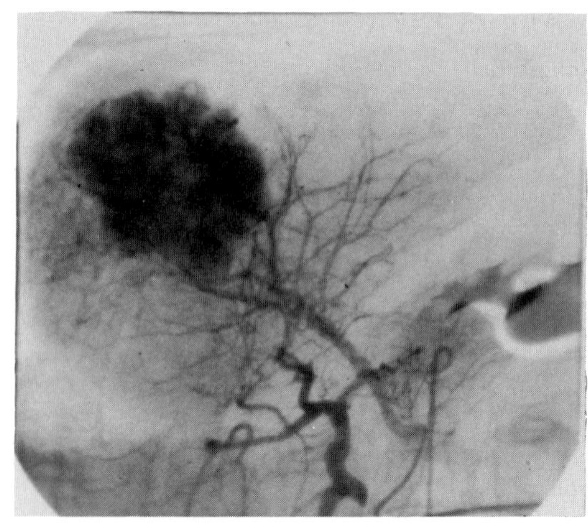

Fig. 68.14 Hepatic arteriogram demonstrates the marked nodular appearance of focal nodular hyperplasia seen during both arterial and venous phases of the study.

Diagnosis and Treatment

The lesions will appear as solid areas on scintiscans and ultrasonic examination, to have a characteristic arteriographic appearance and may be multicentric. Ruptured and bleeding tumours are excised as emergency procedures and since many of these tumours are near the surface, local excisions with a thin rim of parenchyma may be attempted. Intracapsular haemorrhage may produce an extremely large

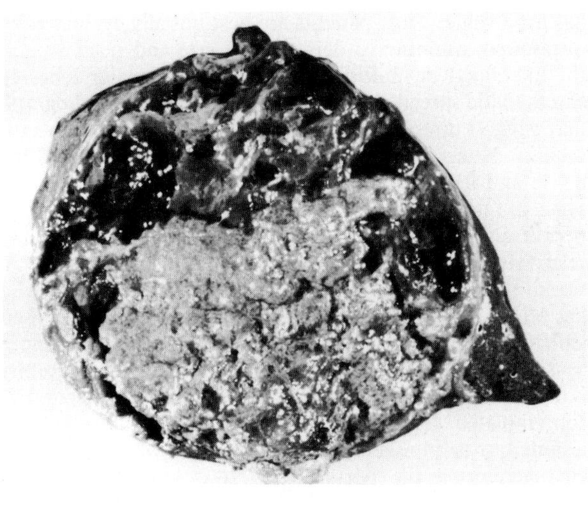

Fig. 68.15 This operative specimen of the right lobe of the liver has been cut to show the necrotic contents of a hepatic adenoma into which a major haemorrhage has occurred. The patient presented with severe upper abdominal pain and evidence of massive blood loss.

tumour demanding formal hepatic resection. Patients with multiple adenomas need prolonged careful follow-up with repeated scintigrams. Enlargement of residual adenomas requires elective excision.

Cholangioma

This rare tumour is derived from bile duct epithelium. It often has a cystic component.

Biliary Cystadenoma

This rare tumour commonly affects middle-aged women and achieves a large size usually in the right lobe; cystic degeneration is commonly found.

Primary Malignant Tumours of the Liver

Although primary malignant tumours of the liver are uncommon in European and North American populations, the condition is very common in African, Chinese and Indian communities. Considerable interest continues into the aetiological background and it has to be said that there have been definite advances in our understanding of this cancer. Significant clues can be obtained by observing the tumour incidence in the African Bantu (87% of all cancers at one end of the scale and 0·14% in Europe at the other end). Within Europe the incidence rises to 1·0% in Greece and 0·5% in Italy. In any event the incidence of liver cancer in a community is directly proportional to the incidence of viral hepatitis.

Aetiological Factors

No one factor is of overall importance and it is likely that the initiation of the tumour requires a genotoxic event followed by the action of a cocarcinogen.

a. Genetic and Racial: Although the incidence is more common in the African and Chinese there is no definite evidence of a genetic predisposition.

b. Sex: Hepatocellular cancer (HCC) is three times more common in males but this ratio parallels the chronic carrier rate of HB_sAg.

c. Alcohol: There is an increased incidence of HCC in patients with micronodular cirrhosis but this effect cannot be separated from an increased carrier rate of hepatitis B virus in this social group.

d. Chronic Liver Disease: Certain liver conditions, e.g. HB_sAg negative autoimmune chronic hepatitis and Wilson's disease are not associated with HCC but haemochromatosis has a high rate (36%). Overall the incidence of HCC in cirrhosis may reach 25% but it is greatly elevated in patients with antigen positive chronic active hepatitis (42%).

e. Mycotoxins, Aflatoxin: This agent is produced by a contaminating mould of grain and nuts particularly in West Africa. It is more likely that these toxins act as cocarcinogens rather than the initiating insult.

f. Hepatitis B virus is the most important aetiological factor in HCC development probably due to an integration of viral and host DNA, after which a cofactor becomes operative. There is no evidence that non A non B hepatitis is carcinogenic. However, not all cancers are due to this virus particularly in the European population, where 25% of tumours occur in younger patients (especially female) who are antigen negative.

Certain parasitic infestations are associated with liver cancer, e.g. *Clonorchis sinensis* but this is normally a cholangiocarcinoma. However, there is no increased incidence with schistosomiasis.

Pathological Features of HCC

Most tumours are of a large size on discovery and have necrotic centres. On cut section there may be a pale appearance with satellite projections into the surrounding liver tissue but some tumours have a homogeneous appearance and merge with the normal cut appearance. Histologically the tumour cells resemble the normal polygonal hepatocytes but develop basophilia as dedifferentiation occurs. Nevertheless it is a specialized area of pathology and some malignant tumours have a completely normal appearance on light microscopy. However, infiltration of lymphatics in the portal tracts gives an indication of malignancy.

Special features: Alphafetoprotein-secreting tumours may show PAS-positive staining. Rarer clear cell tumours may contain glycogen or lipid in the foamy cytoplasm and are sometimes associated with hypoglycaemia or hypercholesteraemia respectively.

Metastatic spread has usually occurred at the time of diagnosis. The pattern of recurrent disease after apparently successful resection suggests that direct infiltration along the hepatic veins and suprahepatic vena cava is common. Lymphatic spread to the portal tract is also common and distal lymphatic metastases are seen later in the natural history. Blood-borne metastases in the lungs are common.

Fibrolamellar carcinoma is most often found in young adults and affects both sexes equally. It is not normally associated with previous liver disease and presents with abdominal pain and a mass. Alphafetoprotein is not elevated. Although the prognosis is said to be better, few long-term cures after resection are recorded.

Rarer Tumours

Hepatocellular cholangiocarcinoma combines histological features of both types of tumour and probably represents a coincidental occurrence. Cystadenocarcinoma occurs as a large lesion usually in adults. Microscopically, cystic spaces are lined in part with cuboidal epithelium with papillary projections. Sarcoma of the liver arises from connective tissue components and results in a rapidly expanding lesion complicated by hypoglycaemia. Epithelioid haemangioendothelioma is likely to rupture and produce intraperitoneal bleeding. It has a somewhat more favourable prognosis than other angiosarcomas.

The haemangioma endothelioma or angiosarcoma is of special interest. There appears to be a definite association with vinyl chloride production or to exposure to arsenic, thorotrast or anabolic steroids. The pathological appearances are complex and include sarcomatous foci, giant cells and large cavernous sinuses lined with dedifferentiated endothelium. It is very malignant.

Hepatic Tumours in Childhood

Primary liver tumours account for about 15% of abdominal tumours in childhood. Male children develop hepatoblastoma and hepatocellular carcinoma slightly more commonly than girls. Hepatoblastomas consist of embryonic liver tissue accompanied by cartilage, osteoid, striated muscle and connective tissue in varying proportions. Hepatoblastoma tends to occur by the third year. Most tumours produce high levels of alphafetoprotein and some produce gonadotrophins which lead to sexual precocity. Where possible liver resection is indicated and about one-third of patients survive long term.

Clinical Features of Hepatic Tumours

The predominant symptom results from an abdominal mass which may have produced a dragging sensation on exercise. Other symptoms include anorexia, weight loss, abdominal or chest pain, vomiting, fever and, more rarely, changes in bowel habit and weakness. Jaundice and peripheral stigma of chronic liver disease may be present in patients with neoplastic change in a cirrhotic liver or arising in childhood biliary atresia. Physical findings include obvious abdominal distension due to hepatomegaly or the presence of a hepatic mass. A bruit is heard in about 10% of patients or a friction rub is found. Ascites is common and is sometimes bloodstained.

Additional infrequent clinical features include hypoglycaemia, hypercalcaemia, hyperlipidaemia and hyperthyroidism.

Laboratory studies frequently show abnormalities of liver function tests and may reflect underlying chronic liver disease. Haematological studies can show anaemia due to intratumour haemorrhage or polycythaemia due to anomalous erythropoietin release. Serum alphafetoprotein levels are elevated in about one-third and are a useful cancer marker after resection. However it is more commonly elevated in the USA, China and African populations. It is more likely to be elevated with undifferentiated cancers. It is a valuable marker when screening the cirrhotic population for HCC development.

Hepatitis B antigen should be looked for in all patients. For patients undergoing surgery a study of the parameters of coagulation is a sensible precaution for these may be abnormal and certainly will be affected by a major hepatic resection. Rarely there is hyperlipidaemia or hypercalcaemia with demineralization of the skeleton and spontaneous fractures.

Tumour Localization and Evaluation

Lesions greater than 2 cm in size can be detected as a filling defect on a hepatic scintiscan but this mode of investigation has little value. Most patients are best initially evaluated by ultrasound scanning to demonstrate size and position and the likelihood of multiple deposits in both major lobes or extrahepatic spread into the portal triad. A chest radiograph may suggest direct diaphragmatic involvement or show pulmonary metastases. CT scanning will also demonstrate the lesion and its relationship to major structures and the presence of satellite nodules. Both ultrasound and CT scanning permit an accurate Trucut needle biopsy to be performed relatively safely. Occasionally neither ultrasound nor CT scanning will demonstrate a lesion in a cirrhotic patient who has other indications of the presence of an HCC, e.g. raised alphafetoprotein. In these cases, arteriography is a more sensitive diagnostic technique. Normally arterioportography is reserved for those patients in whom liver resection is contemplated. Even so it is not essential for small peripheral lesions but is advisable for large tumours which appear to encroach upon the portal triad. It is essential that the technique demonstrates major and anomalous hepatic arterial supply and in the portal venous phase it should show that the main portal vein or main portal division is free from tumour encasement. Similarly with large posteriorly placed tumours, cavography is essential to exclude caval invasion but simple compression or deviation of the inferior vena cava does not preclude a successful resection. There is probably no place for a trial dissection of a hepatocellular carcinoma and the surgeon should have fully assessed the possibility of a successful procedure before embarking upon it.

Preoperative Preparation

Disturbance of liver function tests, particularly with regard to serum levels of bilirubin and albumin, may indicate the seriousness of liver damage in patients with chronic liver disease and tumour. Child's classification may be applicable to judge the operative risk prior to resection. Patients classified as Grades B or C may be thought of as having lost 50–60% of liver parenchyma. Patients with uncomplicated hepatic tumours may regenerate liver bulk but patients undergoing resection in a cirrhotic liver are not able to regenerate further liver tissue.

Fluid and electrolyte disturbances should be corrected prior to surgery and vitamin K is given routinely. Nutritional supplementation with the maximum protein load tolerable by the patient may elevate the serum albumin though albumin infusions will almost certainly be required postoperatively. It is preferred that patients receive an intravenous glucose load (1 L 10% dextrose) prior to surgery in order to ensure that hepatic glycogen is maximal.

Surgical Treatment

It is not within the scope of this chapter to detail steps in technique of liver resection. However, the object is to excise the lesion safely with a margin of healthy liver tissue of 2 cm or more (*Fig.* 68.16). This can be achieved by careful operative assessment which should include, where possible, intraoperative ultrasound to position correctly the lesion in relation to major structures and to ensure that no other foci are present. Very small liver tumours on the periphery are amenable to a careful wedge resection but this is an unusual presentation for primary liver tumours. Somewhat larger tumours occur in one segment of the liver (*Fig.* 68.17) and careful dissection of this area, based on sound anatomical detail, can resect that particular segment. This approach, i.e. segmentectomy, is most suited to patients with chronic liver disease where tumours have been detected relatively

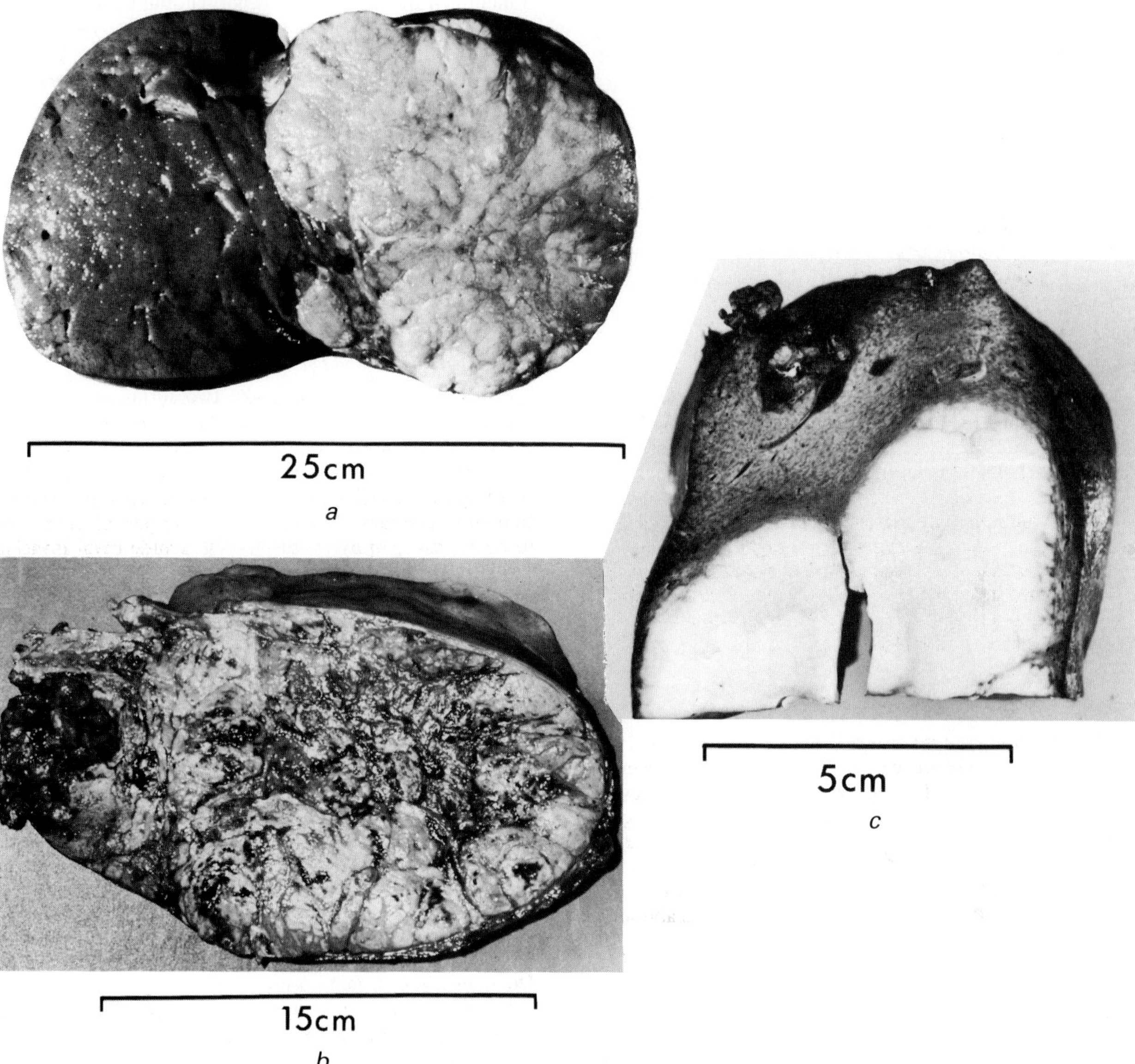

Fig. 68.16 *a*, This shows the cut surface of a right lobectomy specimen removed for a hepatoma. The large bulky tumour can be seen to be lobulated and to have necrotic areas but there is evidence of a satellite formation apart from the main tumour. *b*, This cut specimen of the right lobe contains a rare hepatic sarcoma in which the tumour arose from stromal tissue. It proved rapidly invasive. *c*, This left lateral lobe of the liver contained a reticulum-cell sarcoma. Other manifestations of the disease were responsive to standard chemotherapy for reticulosis.

early by screening. Very large tumours require a formal dissection along major planes. Where the tumour is localized to segments 5–8, a right lobectomy is preferred. A lesion in segments 2 and 3 may be excised by left lateral lobectomy but where, as is often the case, the tumour approaches the falciform ligament and segment 4, a left lobectomy is required. Some cancers extend across the plane between the two livers particularly from the right into segment 4. This lesion can be readily excised by removing segments 4–8 and, if necessary, segment 1, leaving segments 2 and 3. A careful dissection in the portal triad ensures that the remaining two segments are supplied with arterial, portal and duct branches (*Fig.* 68.17). In order to carry out these procedures it may be necessary to use a right thoraco-abdominal approach but most operations can be performed via a bilateral subcostal incision. Although hepatic transplantation was formerly practised on patients with HCC, the long-term survivors were few, no doubt the result of the preoperative dissemination and the effects of immunosuppression.

Postoperative Care after Liver Resection

Patients after liver resection require major parenteral support with diminishing daily requirements as liver adaption and regeneration take place. Following lobectomy there is transient portal hypertension and a sizeable sequestration of blood in the portal venous system. Operative blood loss may need to be supplemented by further blood transfusion to

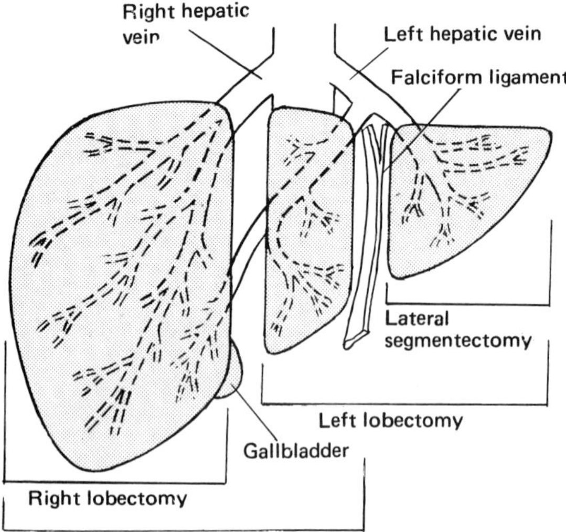

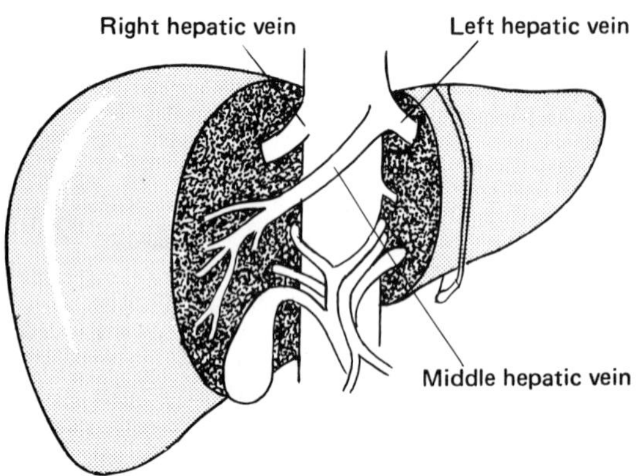

Fig. 68.17 Hepatic resection may take several forms. Resection of the liver to the left side of the falciform ligament removes half of the left lobe and is termed a lateral segmentectomy. Formal left lobectomy or formal right lobectomy requires dissection within the hilum of the liver with appropriate ligation of tributaries of the portal vein, hepatic artery and bile duct systems. It is important that the middle hepatic vein is not damaged during a formal right hepatic lobectomy. Extended right lobectomy removes segments 5–8 and sometimes segment 1.

avoid hypovolaemic shock. Arterial and venous pressure monitoring remains an excellent guide to replacement.

Jaundice is minimal and lasts about 1 week. More profound and persistent bilirubinaemia may indicate bile duct obstruction and the need for further surgery.

Hypoglycaemia can suddenly develop during surgery or in the early postoperative course. Regular monitoring of blood glucose levels is mandatory. Usually the complication can be avoided by infusing 5% glucose during and after operation. Intra- or postoperative coagulation defects can also be countered by the prophylactic use of fresh frozen plasma and vitamin K injections. Since the half-life of albumin is 8–24 hours, hypoalbuminaemia is universal after a major hepatic resection and only partly correctable by plasma infusion. Repeated plasma or albumin infusion may be necessary for at least one week postoperatively until hepatic regeneration is sufficient to maintain plasma levels.

Regeneration of liver is documented by liver scintiscans which demonstrate a fully regenerated liver volume at about 3 months if the parenchyma is normal, but a failure to fully regrow if the liver remnant is cirrhotic.

Non-surgical Management of Primary Hepatic Cancer

Chemotherapy

Primary liver cancers respond to a limited degree to systemic doxorubicin therapy given in standard dosage of 60 mg/m^2 to maximum cumulative dose of 550 mg and with reductions in dosage for jaundiced patients. About one-third of patients have an objective reduction in tumour size but 2-year survival is about 15%. Similar experiences are found with mitozantrone therapy. There are no reports of improved successes with chemotherapy given via the hepatic artery.

Intra-arterial Embolization

This form of therapy may take two forms and is quite commonly combined with chemotherapy. The hepatic artery and branches supplying the tumour are embolized with gelfoam or similar materials to produce necrosis of tumour tissue. Unfortunately, islands of tumour survive and there is little evidence that the natural history of the condition is altered. The procedure is complicated by the development of hepatic abscesses which may require drainage but it can be a useful palliative procedure. Temporary obstruction to tumour arterial blood supply may be achieved by infusing starch microgranules into the artery by the Seldinger technique or by a surgically placed catheter. The circulation is occluded for 20–30 min and if the granules are mixed with a chemotherapeutic agent, e.g. doxorubicin or mitomycin C the tumour has a prolonged exposure to the drug and may be more effective. This approach is as yet experimental.

Radiotherapy

Unfortunately, the liver parenchyma is highly sensitive to radiotherapy and doses as low as 3000 Gy are capable of producing a radiation hepatitis. Some painful HCC are palliated by this modality and hepatomegaly is reduced.

Metastatic Disease of the Liver

Direct invasion of the liver may result from locally advanced cancers of the stomach, pancreas and hepatic flexure of the colon. More commonly, hepatic metastases appear to result from embolization from the primary tumour via either the portal vein or hepatic artery. The liver would seem to be a fertile bed for such secondaries which attract a blood supply from the branches of the hepatic artery and perhaps portal venous system. Though many of the deposits appear necrotic on cut section, there is sufficient blood supply to allow multiple deposits to expand and livers weighing in excess of 10 kg at autopsy have been recorded. Although the histological picture normally reflects the primary tumour, there is a general tendency towards dedifferentiation.

Many hepatic secondaries are asymptomatic but patients with widespread involvement and expansion of the liver suffer pain in the abdomen and back. Some patients experience severe flatulence and nausea which reduces the nutritional intake of these patients. Though many patients appear physically well when liver metastases are first detectable, as the disease progresses evidence of malnutrition and cachexia becomes the rule.

By the time liver metastases become detectable clinically there is usually massive involvement. In most instances there will be no particular advantage to early detection, though some patients may wish to be kept completely informed of their prognosis. It is clear that many patients with apparently curable primary tumours have occult hepatic metastases at the time of surgery. Routine blind liver biopsy in patients with pancreatic cancer will show secondary spread in 15% of patients. Routine CT scanning has downstaged about 25% of patients with colorectal cancer. Dynamic hepatic scintigraphy will also detect a group of patients with occult metastases who develop overt liver metastases within 1 year.

^{99}Tc liver scans may detect secondary deposits over 2 cm in diameter as may ultrasonic examination of the liver. Nevertheless with both techniques, false negative examinations are high, e.g. 30–40%. Additional information may be obtained from routine liver function tests though these are not likely to show abnormalities until tumour involvement is marked. Serial monitoring of CEA will detect one-third of metastatic livers with normal liver scans, though the rise in CEA may be due to deposits elsewhere. The incidence of a false positive liver scan is about 10–15% but the incidence of false positive judgements falls to 1% if both the CEA and liver scan are positive.

Peritoneoscopy may be a helpful supplemental investigation in patients where it is important to decide whether liver involvement has occurred. The technique does not view all of the liver surface and thus the incidence of false negative tests is as high as with liver scanning but its value is that when both scans and biochemistry appear to show metastatic disease the direct vision of the liver may show an alternative liver pathology, such as cirrhosis or polycystic liver disease.

The Treatment of Liver Metastases

There would seem to be no indication for specific treatment of patients with massive liver involvement unless symptoms are not easily controlled by simple measures. However, there may be some advantage when the metastases are causing pain and nausea or when the secondary deposits are limited in extent. Three main lines of treatment may be applied to liver metastases, namely surgery, irradiation, chemotherapy or combinations of these modalities.

In patients with multifocal metastatic cancer, there is little chance of affecting survival by any form of surgical procedure unless the cancer is confined to the liver. This is rarely the case and patients usually have advanced primary tumours or locally recurrent disease. However, there are reports which suggest that patients with an apparent solitary metastasis can be treated more aggressively with benefit to the patient in terms of a more prolonged survival. In these patients surgery may be considered. Generally speaking, liver resections have not been formal lobectomies but it has been possible to locally excise the deposit with a margin of healthy liver. All successful procedures, i.e. with prolonged survival, have occurred in patients whose primary tumour was of colorectal origin. The best results were obtained when the primary tumours were small (<5 cm) and locally curable. It seems that in a small proportion of patients the ultimate prognosis must be related to the solitary metastatic deposit, for local excision can be associated with prolonged disease-free survival. Furthermore, there does not seem to be any difference in the proportion of long-term survivors after excision of the metastasis, of those who underwent synchronous excision with the primary operation compared to those who had liver resection upon the consequent development and detection of the deposit. This may suggest selection of patients with a favourable host–tumour relationship. Nevertheless, there does seem to be some advantage to resection of the solitary liver deposit in patients with colorectal cancer. Worthwhile 5-year survival (25%) has been recorded after liver resection for groups of metastases (<four) in one lobe but only after colorectal cancer. Most failures result from further metastatic disease declaring itself in the liver remnant. In order to define the role of liver resection in metastatic disease, a formal controlled trial is required.

As has already been suggested most liver metastases derive their major blood supply from the hepatic artery distal to the cystic artery. The hepatic artery ligation can be performed safely inasmuch as liver failure does not ensue and it is clear that, despite the development of some form of collateral circulation, there is massive necrosis of much of the metastatic tumour material. However, there are no reports which convincingly demonstrate that this procedure by itself significantly aids palliation or adds to survival so that its application should be combined with local chemotherapy. The exception to this rule may be in the management of patients with metastatic carcinoid tumour where hepatic artery ligation combined with as much resection of carcinoid material as possible from the liver does seem to be worthwhile.

Irradiation of the Liver

Whole organ irradiation of the liver in doses in excess of 3000R produces changes in liver function which imply serious damage to normal liver parenchyma. Since irradiation doses of this level are hardly tumoricidal, there has been little application of this therapy to the management of liver metastases. Limited clinical trials have used fractionated doses of 150 rad over 3 weeks through portals of 15 × 20 or 20 × 24 cm and there appears to be complete symptomatic relief in a majority of patients though little in the way of objective remission. It is probable that this type of treatment will be most effective against reticuloendothelial tumours though it may have a limited role in gastrointestinal cancer or in combination with other treatments.

Chemotherapy for Liver Metastases

The large bulk of most liver secondaries make systemic chemotherapy a relatively ineffective treatment when given on a systemic basis. Nevertheless, objective remissions are seen both with single agents and with combination therapy in about one-quarter of cases and the clinician may feel that this type of therapy is less likely to produce side-effects than some of the alternative treatments already discussed. Certainly for the symptomatic patient it would seem justifiable to assess the responsiveness of the tumour deposits to a complete course of appropriate chemotherapy. If there is significant palliation or some evidence of regression the treatment may be repeated or applied more locally to the liver itself.

The combination of the operation of hepatic artery ligation with placement of a catheter in the artery for consequent infusion of cytotoxic drugs has been evaluated widely but in only a few instances have untreated control patients been randomized in these trials. There is some evidence that a continuous infusion has a greater effect than intermittent therapy and this approach is now feasible by using a completely implantable pump. This system is normally primed with fluorodeoxyuridine (FUdR) which has a similar therapeutic ratio to 5-FU but requires a smaller volume. Although the system is expensive it has been implanted in large numbers of patients. There is no firm evidence that the routine gives significantly improved results over 5-FU given intermittently into the hepatic artery. Furthermore, there is some suggestion that a picture of sclerosing cholangitis can be induced by continuous therapy. Combination therapy with 5-FU, actinomycin D and methotrexate given over a 3-week cycle into the hepatic artery via an implanted chamber permits 50% to live 1 year but few longer-term survivors. Chemotherapy with yttrium microspheres selectively given into the hepatic artery is said to produce a median survival rate of 23 months.

HEPATIC TRAUMA

Liver injuries are encountered in civilian practice with regular frequency. Most are caused by blunt trauma from falls or motor vehicle accidents. More rarely in the UK, injuries are due to penetrating stab wounds and still more rarely from high-velocity missiles. Many hepatic injuries are accompanied by other intra-abdominal injury and by injuries to the head and thorax and the clinical features of these injuries may predominate.

When the injury of the liver is penetrating in nature the diagnosis is not difficult and the initial problem is to determine whether the injury extends through the diaphragm into the thoracic cavity. This requires full radiological examination of the chest and upper abdomen. Knife wounds produce a clear incised track into the liver which only rarely devitalizes liver segments and haemorrhage is easily controlled unless a major vascular structure is severed. Gunshot wounds produce much more damage and the external wounds in the body wall and liver surface may not reflect the internal damage to the liver substance where the severity of the tissue damage is directly related to the size and velocity of the missile. Similarly, the bursting type of injury may have a small laceration on the liver surface but wide cracks extend deeply into the liver parenchyma and may lead to devitalization of large segments.

The diagnosis and management of hepatic injury are considered in Chapter 19.

DISORDERS OF THE HEPATIC VASCULATURE

The unique nature of liver blood supply leads to a series of clinical problems which may be described by considering each system separately. However, there are end-points, which are common to all three systems, e.g. portal hypertension effects can follow obstruction to portal or hepatic venous systems and pathological changes in the two systems can coexist. It is advisable when evaluating a patient as hepatic vascular disorder, to demonstrate the anatomy or physiological status of all three systems.

PORTAL HYPERTENSION

Obstruction to portal venous flow leads to a rise in the pressure of the splanchnic venous circulation. While no value is absolute, portal hypertension may be assumed when the portal vein pressure exceeds 20 cm of saline. Obstruction may result from extrahepatic compression or thrombosis of the portal, mesenteric or splenic veins, from compression of portal venous radicles within the liver from a wide variety of liver diseases or from obstruction to the outflow from the liver (*Table* 68.2). Very rarely, anomalous arteriovenous communications in the portal system will result in a massive rise in portal venous flow and pressure.

Table 68.2 Pathogenesis of portal hypertension

A. Increased blood flow into portal venous system (no obstruction):
   Hepatic and splenic arteriovenous fistulas (rare)
B. Extrahepatic *outflow* obstruction:
   Hepatic vein thrombosis; Budd–Chiari syndrome
   Tricuspid incompetence, right heart failure
C. Extrahepatic *inflow* obstruction:
   Congenital malformation of portal vein
   Portal vein thrombosis
   Portal vein compression, e.g. nodes
D. Intrahepatic obstruction:
   Presinusoidal: periportal fibrosis and schistosomiasis
   Postsinusoidal: cirrhosis—alcoholic, nutritional, postnecrotic, biliary veno-occlusive diseases—senecio poisoning, haemochromatosis, Wilson's disease, congenital hepatic fibrosis.

Most commonly, portal hypertension is postsinusoidal and results from cirrhosis of the liver. While a precise diagnosis may not be relevant to the immediate management of a patient with variceal bleeding, it may ultimately indicate prognosis and further treatment. Chronic active hepatitis may improve with the use of steroids, whereas the histological features of alcoholic hepatitis should forewarn of recent liver injury which will be associated with a poor surgical risk. There is a wide spectrum of metabolic disorders of the liver (Wilson's disease, haemochromatosis) and granulomatous liver disease (toxoplasmosis, schistosomiasis), all of which have specific treatments to improve or maintain liver function if the gastrointestinal haemorrhage can be controlled.

About 25% of patients will have an extrahepatic block and a proportion of these patients will have underlying liver disease or polycythaemia. Chronic pancreaticobiliary disease or pancreatic neoplasms may be precipitating factors for portal or splenic vein thrombosis but only rarely does neonatal umbilical sepsis seem to be an aetiological factor.

Extrahepatic outflow block may result from thrombosis or occlusion of the hepatic veins. Aetiological factors may be the widespread usage of the contraceptive pill and specifically include senecio or bush tea poisoning. Other patients have congenital diaphragms in the suprahepatic vena cava or chronic congestive right heart failure. Such patients rarely present with bleeding varices but suffer with intractable ascites, painful hepatomegaly and rapidly deteriorating liver function.

Obstruction to portal venous flow is followed by enlargement of natural portosystemic communications (*see Fig.* 68.2) and by the development of new collateral channels at surgically constructed mucocutaneous junctions (colostomy, ileostomy). Rarely, portal venous blood is shunted away from the liver by an enlargement of the umbilical vein (Cruveilhier–Baumgarten syndrome) and may be detected by a venous bruit in the midline. Though there is a risk of variceal bleeding from the ileum, colon and haemorrhoidal areas, the major risk of haemorrhage is from the oesophagus and stomach. In the oesophagus the varices are large, tortuous and thin-walled with a tendency to rupture. However, in the stomach there is venous engorgement of the gastric mucosa with a tendency to erosive gastritis and a widespread diffuse haemorrhage. Most patients suffering this complication will have portal venous pressures in excess of 30 cm of saline. The predilection of the gastric cardia to develop varices is probably due to the drainage of the left coronary vein after portal hypertension has developed. Instead of draining towards the liver, blood passes along para-oesophageal veins and then via 'perforator' veins to the submucosa of the oesophagus. Three columns tend to develop and run upwards for a variable length, usually communicating into the azygos system. Blood flow from the spleen may course through the short gastric vessels to the gastric fundus and link with enlarged collaterals at the cardia. Fundal varices are well seen after inserting the fibregastroscope. Colonic varices may occasionally be seen on sigmoidoscopy though not as commonly as may be expected. Nor is the caput medusa or periumbilical plexus of veins at all common. It is most prominent in patients who develop a small para-umbilical hernia into which an omental plug provides the portal flow.

It has to be recognized that not all patients develop portal hypertension as a result of their chronic liver disease; estimates vary from 15 to 40 per cent. Furthermore only about one-half of the patients with gastro-oesophageal varices ever suffer from gastrointestinal bleeding.

Three clinical syndromes can be attributed to portal hypertension:

Hypersplenism
Ascites
Gastrointestinal bleeding.

Hypersplenism

Splenomegaly is frequently associated with portal hypertension and there may be sufficient sequestration of formed blood elements in the spleen to cause haemolytic anaemia, leucopenia and thrombocytopenia. Only rarely are these features sufficient to produce major symptoms but they do lead to general debility. After portal vein decompression, hypersplenism remains to a degree in approximately 50% of patients. Thus pancytopenia in patients requiring portal venous decompression is an indication for a splenectomy and lienorenal shunt.

Ascites

The mechanism involved in the formation of ascites by patients with portal hypertension is complex. Ascitic fluid has approximately the same composition as liver lymph and there is widespread dilatation of the lymphatics in the portal triad. Experimentally, ascites can always be produced by any procedure which blocks the outflow of the liver but not necessarily by obstruction of the portal vein and it is clinically uncommon in patients with an extrahepatic portal vein block unless the plasma albumin falls. In cirrhosis, there is a contribution from the hepatic arterial inflow in maintenance of intrahepatic communications and this augments the transudation of fluid from the venous system. It is now recognized that ascites is continually circulating and about 50% turns over each hour.

There is abnormal retention of sodium and water by the kidney; however, serum sodium may fall due to an increase in the extracellular water. It is suggested that there is reduction in the effective plasma volume which stimulates the renin–angiotensin II mechanism followed by increased aldosterone activity (*Fig.* 68.18). The reduction in the effective plasma volume is thought to result from splanchnic vasodilatations, high portal venous pressure, low plasma albumin and peripheral vasodilatation. Presumably basoceptor reflexes are invoked and result in increased levels of plasma norepinephrine and vasopressin. These mechanisms may lead to renal vasoconstriction. It is now considered that in cirrhotic patients, there is a failure of endogenous prostaglandins to inhibit the effect of increased catecholamines.

Fig. 68.18 illustrates the importance of intrahepatic outflow block, arterioportal communications, increased intrahepatic pressure and transudation of hepatic lymph, together with the relationship to the osmotic pressure and albumin levels in plasma.

Most patients with ascites can be managed successfully with salt restriction, spironolactone and other diuretics, together with adequate diet and abstinence from alcohol. For intractable ascites it may be necessary to install a

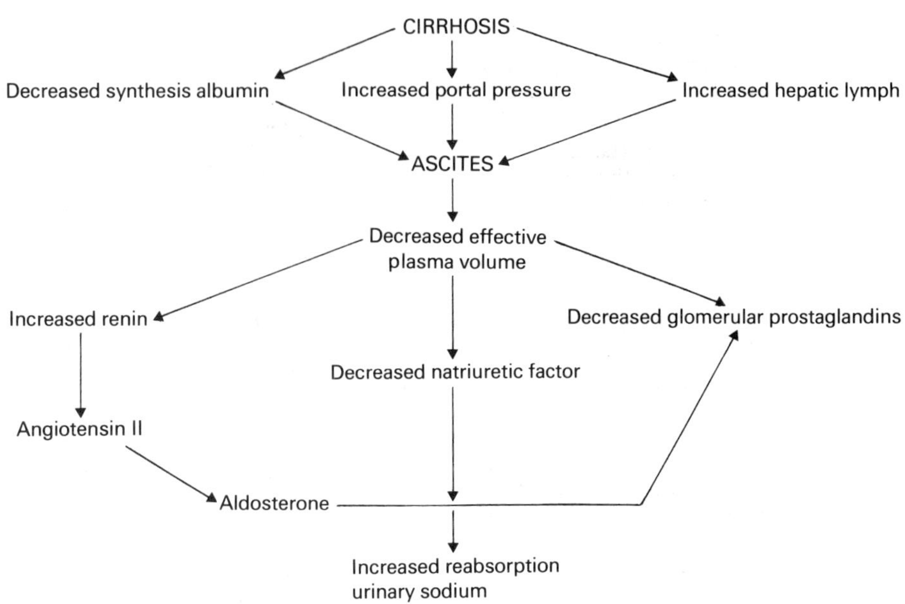

Fig. 68.18 This analogue diagram summarizes the interrelationship of factors concerned in ascites formation.

peritoneovenous shunt (Leveen shunt) or to ultrafiltrate the ascitic fluid, returning the concentrated fluid intravenously. More chronic problems may require portal decompression with a side-to-side shunt or mesentericocaval interposition graft.

Gastrointestinal Haemorrhage

About 30% of patients with varices suffer gastrointestinal haemorrhage within 2 years of diagnosis and thereafter only a smaller fraction bleed each year. Larger varices appear more likely to bleed than smaller varices and varices which are observed to increase in size over a period of one year will almost certainly bleed at some point. The pressure within the veins reaches systemic arterial pressure during coughing and straining and additional factors must initiate the haemorrhage. At endoscopy, varices with tiny cherry red spots or linear streaks are most likely to rupture. However, oesophagitis is not consistently found. Children with extrahepatic portal hypertension commonly bleed when suffering from upper respiratory tract infection.

Clinical Features

Variceal bleeding may present in the usual fashion of haematemesis of coffee-grounds material and repeated melaena. However, there is commonly a minor warning bleed of a mouthful of bright red blood followed some hours later by a major haemorrhage of fresh blood produced without retching. Such patients may be known to have or to show the peripheral stigmata of chronic liver disease. Unless bleeding is massive and continuing, every attempt is made to localize the source of bleeding by fibreoptic endoscopy.

In patients with active massive haemorrhage, a clinical diagnosis may have to suffice and resuscitation commenced, together with measures to obtain control of the haemorrhage before the patient exsanguinates. Resuscitation of variceal haemorrhage follows the general principles of management outlined in Chapter 6.

Oesophagogastroscopy should be performed as early as convenient, if possible within 8–12 hours. The source of bleeding can normally be determined, provided the stomach is not full of clot. Good visualization of the gastric mucosa is vital in order to exclude stress ulceration. Many patients will recall that they have exposed themselves to aspirin and anti-inflammatory drugs which have a similar effect on both gastric and oesophageal mucosa.

Balloon Tamponade

The major standby in the immediate control of variceal haemorrhage remains balloon tamponade. Problems arise with this technique when it is used as the only means of control over a long period and results in a mortality rate greater than if it were not used at all. However, provided the tamponade is to be applied for a limited period of 12–24 hours followed by alternative action if it fails, the balloon system can be life-saving.

Two balloon systems are commonly used: (*a*) Sengstaken tube—with a gastric balloon of about 60–100 ml capacity, which is meant to anchor the tube at the cardia and an oesophageal balloon which is inflated to 30–40 mmHg and compresses the submucosal veins of the oesophagus; (*b*) Linton tube—with a large gastric balloon of 300–700 ml capacity which is pulled against the diaphragmatic hiatus with traction and disconnects the high pressure portal venous system from the thoracic azygous veins. Both systems have disadvantages, the major one being that during use, pharyngeal and oesophageal secretions accumulate and can be aspirated into the bronchial tree. Both balloons are capable of oesophageal rupture if they are inflated when incorrectly placed. The Sengstaken gastric balloon may not anchor the tube at the cardia so that the oesophageal balloon moves headwards to obstruct the airway. It may do this anyway in a short person or in the presence of kyphosis. Polonged traction with the Linton tube leads to linear ulcers in the oesophagus which bleed profusely and are almost impossible to deal with.

Once the tube is placed, regular half-hourly or hourly aspirations of the oesophagus and stomach are performed to remove blood and secretions and determine whether variceal control has been obtained. Specimens are retained in test tubes and should show a progression from bright red blood to altered blood to clearer gastric secretions. Once control is obtained, time is spent in full resuscitation with blood transfusion, plasma and electrolyte replacement as indicated by clinical parameters and laboratory studies.

Balloon tamponade is discontinued after 12–24 hours but the tube retained initially so that gastric and oesophageal aspiration may continue. By this time, a plan of action should have been evolved to proceed further either immediately or in the event of further haemorrhage (*Fig.* 68.19). This may involve sclerotherapy or a surgical procedure on the varices or portal venous system and the decision will largely depend upon the experience and views of the attending clinicians.

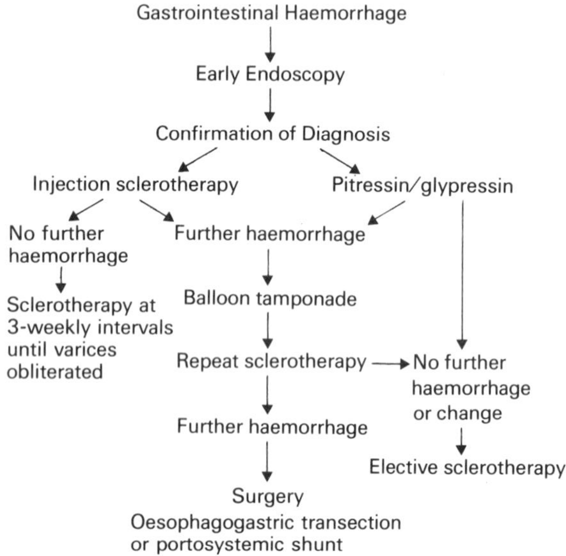

Fig. 68.19 A plan of action suggested for the management of a patient with bleeding oesophageal varices.

Vasopressin

Pitressin has been used for variceal bleeding for the past 25 years and presumably acts by constricting the smooth muscle of the splanchnic arteries, reducing mesenteric blood flow and portal vein pressure. Intramuscular injections are not effective and the agent is more effective if given intravenously as a bolus (20 u) over 20 min or continuously 0·1–0·5 u/min intravenously. The technique of selective infusion into the superior mesenteric artery has been largely abandoned. There is very little hard evidence that pitressin significantly affects the outcome of variceal bleeding and the side-effects include constriction of coronary arteries with angina, activation of plasminogen and fibrinolysis and an antidiuretic effect. However, it does seem to produce temporary control fairly readily.

It has proved more difficult to ensure supplies of pitressin, and in most units it has been replaced by the synthetic analogue, triglycyl-lysine-vasopressin (Glypressin). This drug is given as 1–2 mg doses intravenously and has a duration of 2–4 hours. Normally the agent is given at 6-hourly intervals.

An expensive alternative is the use of somatostatin (250 ug/h). The agent has a similar therapeutic effect to Glypressin.

Further Management

Once the variceal haemorrhage is under control and resuscitation is proceeding, consideration may be given to further management. The aim is to prevent further haemorrhage with its attendant risks of exsanguination and precipitation of liver failure. Currently there is an interest in the prolonged application of injection sclerotherapy, the alternative being some form of definitive surgical attempt to obliterate the varices.

Sclerotherapy for Variceal Haemorrhage

The submucosal oesophageal veins which are responsible for much variceal bleeding are accessible to injections of sclerosing agents. Though it seemed to have been effective 40 years ago the technique has not been universally adopted, no doubt due to the coincident development of portocaval shunting procedures which were unquestionably more definitive in relieving portal hypertension. It is only now that sclerotherapy is being applied more widely in the control of variceal haemorrhage, not only in the emergency situation but also as a preventive measure.

Over the past 5 years, endoscopic sclerotherapy has become a routine procedure in most gastroenterology units. Although it was not originally advocated, most clinicians proceed to variceal injection at the time of the diagnostic endoscopy. As most haemorrhage occurs at the cardia, an attempt is made to inject the varices at this point by several punctures in a circumferential fashion. Three techniques are available: (i) using the rigid oesophagoscope, the varices can be injected by a long needle usually mounted in tandem with a forward viewing telescope. After injection the instrument is passed forward to compress the injection site for a few minutes; (ii) using a fibregastroscope with a compression sheath. The object of the sheath is to isolate the varices through a small window in the distal end. A flexible needle passed through the endoscope is used for injection after which the sheath is rotated to cover the injection site (*Fig.* 68.20). Both techniques are best done with a general anaesthetic; (iii) in stable patients, it is possible to inject varices via a fibrescope without a sheath and under light intravenous anaesthesia.

It would seem that acute variceal haemorrhage will respond in 75–85% of patients although there is no firm evidence that the overall mortality is reduced when compared with other methods. There is some debate whether improved results can be obtained by injecting intravariceal or paravariceal. It is probable that the technique is particularly operator sensitive and the best results with either method are obtained by the more experienced operators. There is probably no special advantage to the use of STD (sodium tetradecyl sulphate) or ethanolamine and these are used in 2–3 ml doses in each varix to a total dose of 20–30 ml.

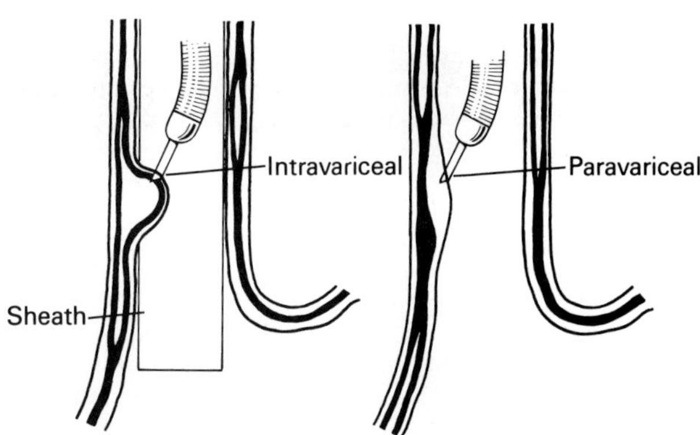

Fig. 68.20 Injection sclerotherapy can be achieved by injecting directly into the varix (intervariceal), which may be best, or immediately adjacent (paravariceal).

If haemorrhage is controlled by the initial injections, the endoscopic injection should be repeated after 7–10 days and then at 3-weekly intervals until the varices are obliterated. The varices remain visible for some time as solid cords.

The complications of sclerotherapy include oesophageal ulceration, fibrosis, stricture and perforation with mediastinitis. Many patients complain of chest pain and a number develop pleurisy with effusions. Long-term sclerotherapy appears to affect oesophageal motility leading to reflux and dysphagia.

Judged longer term, there is a reduction in the numbers of patients with recurrent variceal bleeding when compared with no active treatment. There may be an advantage in terms of survival over 3 years, though ultimately survival will be directly related to the progression of the underlying liver disease. Recurrent variceal haemorrhage may be from residual gastric fundal or colonic varices. These collaterals are not amenable to sclerotherapy and require a surgical solution.

Transhepatic Obliteration of Varices

Varices may also be thrombosed by the retrograde passage of a cannula into the portal vein and tributaries, using the transhepatic route. Injection of radio-opaque medium demonstrates the major collateral veins and these may be selectively entered and thrombosed with thrombin and Gelfoam (*Fig.* 68.21). Not all patients will be suitable but in a majority it will prove possible to control the immediate haemorrhage though recanalization seems rapid.

The technique is not effective in patients with a portal pressure >35 cm of saline. Although variceal haemorrhage is controlled in some patients, mortality is not affected.

Management of Patients with Continuing Variceal Haemorrhage

It is quite obvious that fewer patients are being offered surgical therapy than in previous years. The reasons for this change are probably twofold: first with frequent application of tamponade and Glypressin more patients are treated initially with sclerotherapy. Probably 85% of these patients stop bleeding and are then entered into a continuing sclerotherapy programme or suffer deterioriation in liver function and die. Secondly, procrastination with conservative therapy and sclerotherapy over too prolonged a period permits repeated haemorrhage with deterioration of liver function which effectively downstages the patients from Child's A/B categories to category C which is less likely to survive any

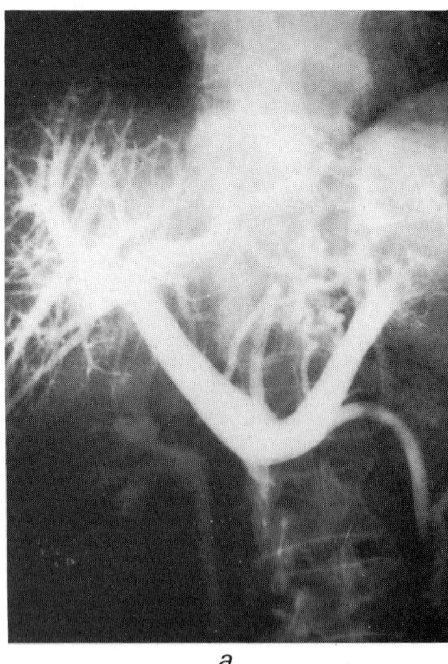

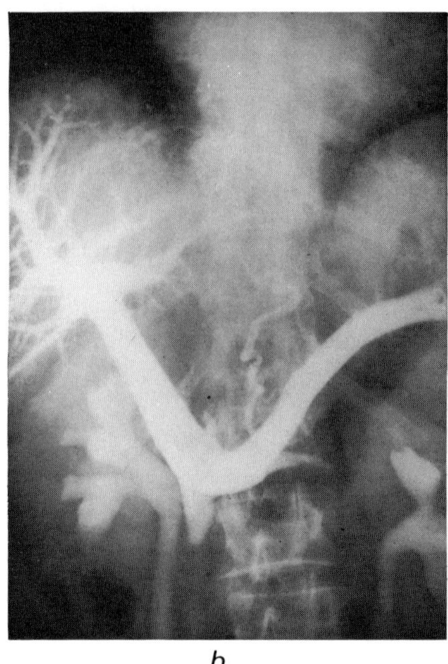

Fig. 68.21 Occasionally transhepatic embolization of bleeding varices should be attempted and can give good control of the vessels feeding the cardia, but control is only temporary.

procedure. It is important that gastroenterologists are encouraged to discuss management of individual patients at the earliest stage and that the surgical team monitor events closely. This approach is no different from that advocated in patients with gastrointestinal haemorrhage from other causes. A definite plan of action is required if the patient has further haemorrhage (*Fig.* 68.19).

Two basic surgical approaches are available: (i) either a direct surgical obliteration of bleeding varices; or (ii) some form of portal venous decompression. The timing of these procedures will be reflected in the outcome. Emergency surgery is the most hazardous particularly in the Grade C patient. Ideally the patient will have been stable for 12–24 hours if necessary with balloon tamponade and vigorous attempts will have been made to improve electrolyte and fluid balance, the blood volume and to evacuate blood from the gastrointestinal tract. However, a surgeon may be faced quite commonly with a patient in whom there is torrential haemorrhage and where tamponade no longer is effective. Active surgical intervention during bleeding cannot be avoided in this situation.

Preparation for Surgery

Careful cardiovascular and respiratory assessment prior to surgery is essential and it may be possible to detect an abnormal haemodynamic state which may determine whether patients should be subjected to emergency surgery, the time of elective surgery and postoperative care.

Careful cardiovascular investigation will also indicate the patients with the highest risk from variceal haemorrhage and operation. Three states are recognized: (i) a hyperdynamic state characterized by an increased cardiac output without evidence of peripheral vascular or pulmonary dysfunction; (ii) a balanced hyperdynamic response to stress in which a further increase in cardiac output is usually compensated for by an adequate increase in myocardial contractility and oxygen consumption; and (iii) an unbalanced hyperdynamic state in which there is evidence of severe peripheral vascular abnormality, impaired oxygen extraction and a tendency to cardiac failure. High-risk patients may require the use of inotropic drugs, such as digoxin, and prolonged ventilatory support.

Hypokalaemia needs appropriate replacement either orally or intravenously in patients with a prolonged prothrombin time; vitamin K (10–30 mg) should be given i.m. or i.v. Prolonged partial thromboplastin time indicates more serious liver dysfunction though it may be present if large amounts of stored blood have been given—fresh frozen plasma is indicated prior to and during surgery. Patients are also prepared by intestinal sterilization with 6 g of neomycin mixture orally.

If the surgical approach which is favoured is a direct attack on the varices, then there is no particular reason to visualize the portal venous system. However, if this can be done with confidence using ultrasound, then it should be done so that if circumstances change, particularly during operation, the surgeon is aware of other possibilities. Unfortunately ultrasound is often quite difficult in these critically ill patients and the vessels may be obscured by bowel gas from recent endoscopy. If necessary, arterioportography can be performed, provided that adequate care can be given to variceal control in the Radiology Department.

Direct Surgical Obliteration

This procedure is now standard in many hospitals. The original transthoracic approach, which had a 50% mortality, has been abandoned in favour of a circular stapling gun introduced via a gastrotomy. The device should transect and remove the segment of oesophagus immediately adjacent to the cardia (*Fig.* 68.22). Care is taken to avoid injury to the vagus nerves and to perform an adequate ligation of the perioesophageal veins. In practice, if the surgeons effectively devascularize the upper half of the gastric lesser curvature

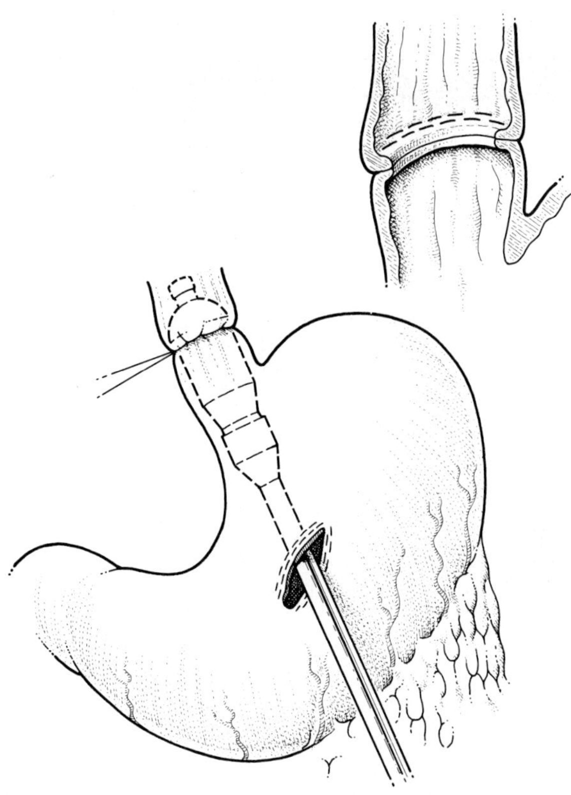

Fig. 68.22 Stapled transection of the lower oesophagus is achieved by introducing the circular stapler (28–31 mm) through a gastrotomy and by tying the oesophagus to the central axle with a strong suture before closing the gun and firing.

as in proximal gastric vagotomy, this achieves the effect of preparing the oesophagus for transection.

If it is suspected that the major source of bleeding is from gastric varices, the oesophageal stapling instrument is not effective. A double gastrotomy with separate straight staples across the anterior and posterior walls gives the same effect as the portoazygos procedure described many years ago by Tanner (*Fig.* 68.23). The procedure may be extended by adding to it a splenectomy and this is indicated if significant hypersplenism is present. Splenectomy is not without its problems, for collaterals in the lienorenal ligament are very difficult to control and the splenic vein is lost, should a decompression procedure become advisable at a future date. A staged second procedure in which the peri-oesophageal veins are ligated via a transthoracic approach constitutes the complete Sigiura procedure.

Stapling of the varices and devascularization of the oesophagogastric junction is effective in the control of haemorrhage in a large majority of patients. The operating time is short and intraoperative blood losses are minimal. However, the immediate hospital mortality is still high (35%) particularly in patients who are actively bleeding. Late rebleeding from varices also occurs fairly commonly and it is logical to carry out endoscopic examination at 3 months in survivors and if possible deal with residual varices by sclerotherapy.

Portosystemic Shunts

Whipple introduced the operation of portocaval shunt in 1945 in which the portal vein was anastomosed to the side of

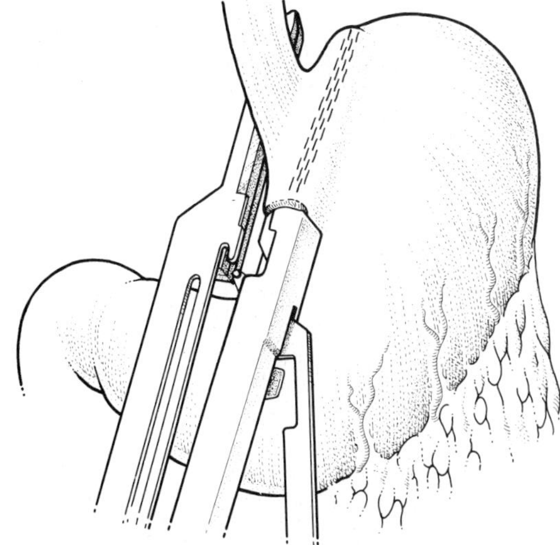

Fig. 68.23 Gastric stapling just before the cardia is performed by using two straight rows of staples on the anterior and posterior walls through a gastrotomy.

the vena cava (*Fig.* 68.24). The decompression of the portal venous system reduced the incidence of variceal bleeding and enabled ascites to be more easily controlled.

The portal pressure falls as does the hepatic venous pressure and the hepatic artery flow increases as compensation. Since these early experiences, other types of portal decompression operations have been devised but relatively few are performed in current practice because of a high incidence of post-shunt encephalopathy. This complication is higher if the patient is greater than 50 years, has previous evidence of encephalopathy or has poor liver function (Grade C). The procedures are best performed under elective conditions, i.e. where other methods have failed to prevent recurrent variceal haemorrhage but the patient can be maintained in a stable condition for some days. Patients with primary biliary cirrhosis, congenital hepatic fibrosis or high portal obstruction are most suited. Alcoholic patients, particularly if still drinking, or those who have evidence of hepatitis and patients with progressive chronic active hepatitis are least suited.

The most effective shunt for portal decompression remains the end-to-side portocaval shunt and it is easiest to perform (*Fig.* 68.24). The side-to-side shunt is thought to be nearly as effective in reducing portal pressure and appears more effective in dealing with chronic ascites possibly because decompression of the liver reduces hepatic lymph. Lienorenal or mesentericocaval shunts are also side-to-side shunts and are indicated when ascites appears to be a major complication of the portal hypertension. Significant hypersplenism suggests the need for a lienorenal shunt. These three standard shunts decompress the portal venous system and direct portal blood with its hepatotrophic factors away from the diseased liver. This fact may be responsible for the higher incidence of portosystemic encephalopathy and for the high mortality from hepatic failure in the poor-risk patients. Encephalopathy seems less of a problem with lienorenal and mesentericocaval shunts. Selective decompression of the oesophagogastric function is achieved by the distal splenorenal shunt (*Fig.* 68.24). In this operation diversion of blood from the cardia is via the short gastric

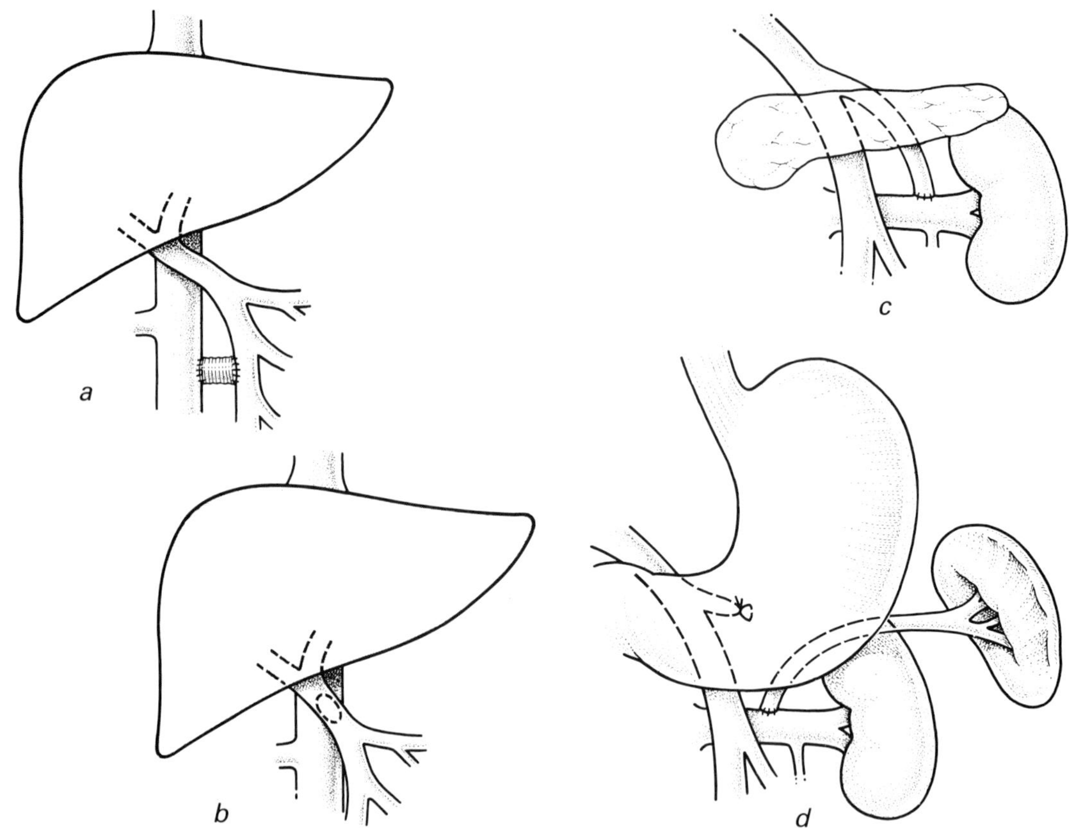

Fig. 68.24 A schematic representation of: *a*, Dacron interposition mesentericocaval shunt; *b*, side-to-side portocaval shunt; *c*, lienorenal shunt; *d*, distal splenorenal shunt.

vein into the splenic which is anastomosed to the left renal vein in a variety of ways. The object is to preserve portal venous flow to the liver and while this is achieved in the postoperative period, it does not seem that it is maintained in the long term. There is no indication for prophylactic portocaval shunt, for although bleeding is controlled, other complications ensue and there is no improvement in survival.

The operative mortality of shunt surgery performed for the emergency control of variceal bleeding varies from 20 to 70%. However, most results for emergency surgery are reported after prolonged attempts at conservative control and after massive blood transfusion. There is some evidence that if emergency shunts are performed as soon as resuscitation permits, the operative mortality is considerably lessened. Failure of conservative management should be followed by an alternative approach without procrastination.

Elective shunts can be performed with an operative mortality of about 5%. Shunt patency can be confirmed by ultrasonic examination and thrombosis would seem to occur in 10–15% of patients with lienorenal or distal splenorenal shunts. The figure may be higher in mesentericocaval shunts (40%) but very low after portocaval decompression. Late rebleeding rates reflect in the incidence of shunt obstruction.

Extrahepatic Portal Block

Infants and children with this condition will generally stop bleeding and require only blood transfusion. Recurrent haemorrhage in the early years is the rule but appears with lessened frequency in teenage and young adult life. Ideally, these patients may be managed with repeated sclerotherapy. With the failure of this approach, mesenteric angiography is performed and the larger venous tributaries can be used to construct 'make do' shunts to the vena cava or renal vein.

Adult patients should be amenable to stapling procedure and it is important that the site of bleeding between staples is accurately localized. If the spleen appears to be draining across the gastric fundus, it should be removed. Careful follow-up with endoscopy and sclerotherapy for residual varices is appropriate. Since most patients do not have liver disease, prognosis may be reasonably good and ascites or encephalopathy are rarely a problem.

Rarer Hepatic Disorders

Variceal haemorrhage from patients suffering with hepatic schistosomiasis appears to have a reasonable prognosis once the condition is recognized and treated. Both devascularization procedures and full portal decompression are reported to control variceal bleeding long term. Similarly, patients with hepatic fibrosis appear to have a favourable prognosis following portal decompression for variceal bleeding.

Certain types of storage disorders, e.g. Type 6B glycogen storage disease, familial hypercholesterolaemia, may improve following portal venous diversion.

Ascites and Fluid Retention

Most patients with chronic liver disease have a tendency to retain sodium and water and ascites increases after variceal haemorrhage or major surgery. Fluid input and output needs a careful record but daily weighing may be the only means of detecting fluid retention. Plasma electrolyte estimation may show a tendency to hyponatraemia. Increase in weight requires the use of spironolactones (up to 400 mg daily) with careful monitoring of serum electrolytes. Frusemide is effective but leads to hypokalaemia and may precipitate encephalopathy. After operation or control of haemorrhage there is a gradual rise in the serum albumin levels though dietary protein may need to be restricted to 60 g/day initially. Once the serum albumin reaches 30 g/l most patients with ascites and oedema respond to careful diuretic management.

Re-bleeding

Recurrent gastrointestinal haemorrhage is not uncommon after emergency surgery for variceal haemorrhage or even in the longer term. Recurrent variceal bleeding after shunt surgery may be controlled by injection sclerotherapy. However, it is prudent to re-endoscope the patient, for acute gastric erosion and penetrating peptic ulcers occur in about 15% of patients. In view of this complication, most surgeons prescribe cimetidine prophylactically after surgery. A note of caution should be added, for patients with hepatic and renal disease may develop CNS side-effects including coma and seizures. This should lead to prompt withdrawal of the drug before attributing the CNS symptoms to liver failure. With severe liver dysfunction, re-bleeding may be associated with a complex coagulation defect which requires investigation. Frozen plasma may correct factor deficiencies (*see* Chapter 9). As it is now known that propanolol can reduce portal pressure, this agent has been used to reduce the incidence of rebleeding. It is best given to Grade A/B patients in a dose sufficient to reduce the pulse rate by 25% 12 hours after taking the drug.

Encephalopathy. Hepatic Coma

There is a graduated scale of severity of liver dysfunction which is paralleled by CNS dysfunction and cardiorespiratory and renal failure. Clinical syndromes are seen prior to surgery or postsurgery with vagueness, lack of concentration and deterioration of intellectual function, and are worsened by gastrointestinal haemorrhage, hypokalaemia, excessive diuresis or after portal decompression. There is no specific association of preoperative encephalopathy to the severity of postshunt symptoms. About 25–30% of patients suffer progressive subcortical encephalopathy after a portocaval shunt has been performed and in about 10% the disability is crippling.

A raised blood ammonia is common in cirrhotic patients and this increases after portal decompression. It is commonly believed that this ammonia is largely derived from bacterial breakdown of protein in the gut. Blood ammonia levels do seem to correlate with the clinical state of the patient but they are sometimes normal even in patients with deep coma. Perhaps what is most important is the level of ammonia within the brain. Blood ammonia levels are therefore of limited use in assessing progress of therapy or prognosis.

There is considerable evidence of a more profound disturbance of amino acid metabolism. The high blood ammonia is associated with an increased releasing glucagon which promotes gluconeogenesis from amino acids. Plasma levels of neutral amino acids—phenylalanine, tryptophan and tyrosine increase and appear in high levels in blood and CSF. These amino acids are precursors of serotonin and catecholamines. The branched-chain amino acids—valine, leucine and isoleucine—are decreased. It has been suggested that if the ratio between the concentrations of valine plus leucine plus isoleucine and phenylalanine plus tyrosine is reduced, then encephalopathy results. Furthermore, false neurotransmitters, phenyl-ethanolamine and octopamine are produced by the action of bacteria in the colon and may replace the action of noradrenaline and dopamine in the brain. Gamma-aminobutyric acid (GABA) is an inhibiting neurotransmitter which is found in high levels in the blood of patients with hepatic failure. Although it does not normally pass through the blood–brain barrier, there is some suggestion that the barrier is ineffective in patients with encephalopathy, particularly in the presence of hypoxia and alkalosis.

The principles of management of a patient with hepatic precoma or coma are to search for and correct any precipitating cause, e.g. remove sedatives, correct electrolyte disturbances, arrest haemorrhage and treat sepsis, particularly of ascitic fluid. All dietary protein is stopped initially and when improvement occurs it is reintroduced in 10 g increments each day using, where possible, vegetable protein. The bowels are purged of magnesium sulphate orally and by enema and neomycin commenced at 2 g t.d.s. initially and gradually reduced, or by giving metronidazole 0·2 g q.d.s. Lactulose is effective (10–30 ml t.d.s.) and may act synergistically with neomycin. Lactilol is a new synthetic disaccharide and appears as effective as lactulose in reducing the ionization of ammonia in the colon.

Deep coma may be lightened at least temporarily by L-dopa but few patients seem to benefit long term. Similarly, bromocriptine can improve psychometric assessment of patients with chronic encephalopathic states but has a limited application.

Hepatorenal Syndrome

Although renal failure in cirrhotic patients may result from chronic nephritis or acute tubular necrosis due to haemorrhage, the majority of kidneys are not changed on histology and the condition is termed 'functional renal failure'. It is normally seen at the end-stage liver failure but may also complicate the postoperative period after variceal surgery. Urine volume may not be significantly decreased but sodium retention is pronounced and blood urea and creatinine rise rapidly. Hyponatraemia is usual, even reaching 110 mEq/l. The mechanism is uncertain but is certainly due to intrarenal vasoconstriction with division of blood away from the renal cortex. As evidence it is known that the thromboxane content of the urine is greatly elevated and the prostaglandin E_2 (vasodilator) is decreased.

As the functional renal failure is often precipitated by diuretics, these should be used with care and therapy with nephrotoxic drugs, e.g. aminoglycosides avoided. The best chance of reversal is the maintenance of hepatic function, and there is no improvement after renal dialysis.

Disorders of the Hepatic Artery

The anatomy of the hepatic artery is variable and in about 20% of patients additional branches to a single common hepatic trunk arising from the coeliac axis are found. The most common variants are a supply of the left lateral lobe from the left gastric artery and there is often a major trunk running from the superior mesenteric artery alongside the common bile duct which supplies the right lobe. The arterial anatomy is well shown during arterioportography.

Hepatic Artery Occlusion

This condition may develop spontaneously in an acute

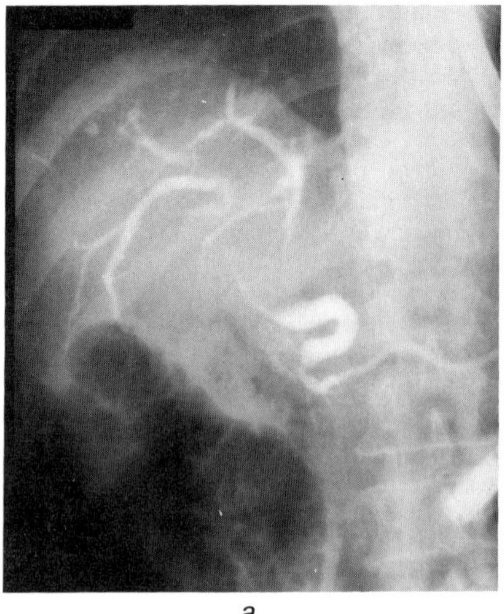

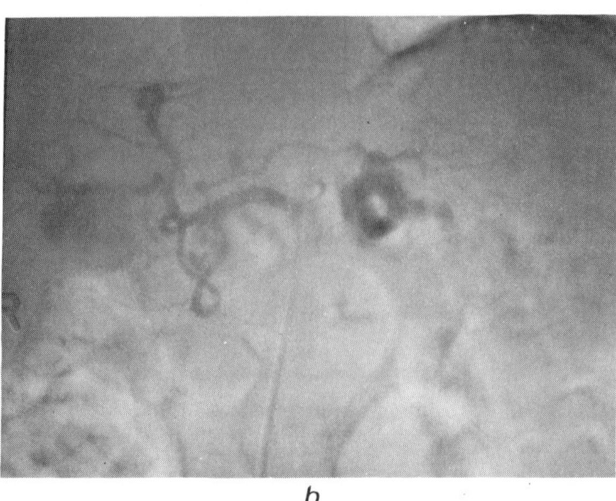

Fig. 68.25 *a*, An ERCP cholangiogram showing the distortion of the extrahepatic biliary tree of a patient with haemobilia. *b*, A hepatic arteriogram revealed a large hepatic aneurysm arising from the right hepatic artery and rupturing into the biliary tree.

fashion in patients with polyarteritis nodosa, or from an embolism or chronically from atheroma. More commonly, the occlusion is from trauma—external, surgical or radiological. Although theoretically there should be a strong chance of hepatic infarction, it is found that provided the portal vein stays patent, this complication is unlikely to occur. Hepatic artery ligation as a deliberate step has been practised for some years to devascularize tumours and appears quite safe. Hepatic artery branch embolization by radiological means does not appear to be associated with segmental infarction. This suggests that the collateral evaluation is usually quite sufficient to maintain evaluation via vessels in the subcapsular region, portal triad and phrenic regions. Where hepatic artery occlusion does occur, it is conventional to prescribe broad-spectrum antibiotics for 7 days.

Hepatic Artery Aneurysm

This interesting condition is rare but may present a diagnostic and technical challenge. The aneurysm occurs in the extra and extrahepatic arterial tree and is often mycotic in aetiology, complicating bacterial endocarditis. There is an increased incidence in patients with collagen disorders, particularly SLE and extrahepatic aneurysms may be due to atherosclerosis. Many aneurysms are the result of penetrating injuries of the liver, needle biopsy or cholecystectomy.

Two clinical syndromes are seen. The patient may present with increasing non-specific pain in the right upper quadrant which may defy diagnosis. The aneurysm may be seen on ultrasound examination and the lesion can be confirmed by arteriography. Sudden collapse with peritoneal sepsis indicates rupture (*Fig.* 68.25). The alternative presentation is similar with pain which begins to resemble biliary colic. Jaundice develops and the patient shows evidence of upper gastrointestinal haemorrhage. Both intrahepatic and extrahepatic aneurysms may rupture into the biliary tract to produce the syndrome of haemobilia.

Management

Most patients present with aneurysmal rupture though this does not necessarily produce catastrophic haemorrhage. Physical signs may not help but the endoscopic appearance of fresh blood or clot in the duodenum in the absence of an active ulcer may suggest haemobilia. Imaging by ultrasound or CT scanning may give a strong indication of both extra- and intrahepatic aneurysm.

Ideally intrahepatic aneurysms should be managed by embolization using an angiographic approach. The advantage of this approach is that all vessels feeding the aneurysm may be identified. Nevertheless, because of the tortuosity produced by atherosclerosis, it may prove impossible to position an arterial catheter. Open operation is required at which time the hepatic lobar artery is isolated and filled with Gelfoam. Aneurysms in segment 2, 3 or 4 may be dealt with by local hepatic resection (*Fig.* 68.26). Extrahepatic artery aneurysms require surgical isolation and ligation after separation from the biliary tract, which may be drained temporarily by a T-tube.

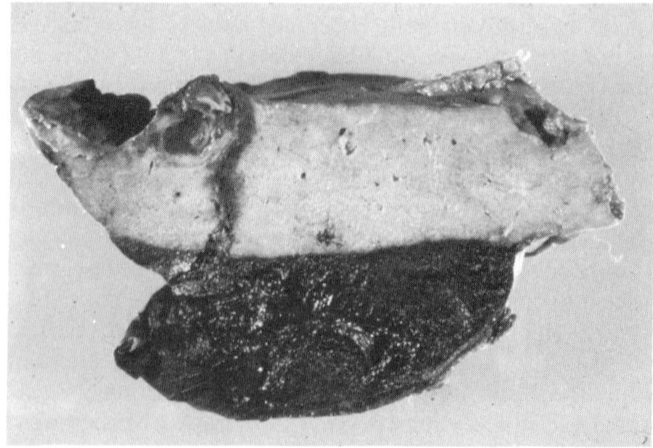

Fig. 68.26 Operative specimen of left liver lobe removed from a patient with haemoperitoneum having ruptured an intrahepatic arterial aneurysm which tracked through the liver parenchyma.

Hepatic–arteriovenous Fistula

The aetiology of this condition may follow the rupture of an aneurysm into the portal venous system or a hepatic vein.

Penetrating injuries are the commonest cause, followed by hepatic neoplasm. The lesions may occur spontaneously in hereditary telangectasia. Symptoms and signs of portal hypertension predominate. A systolic bruit may be heard over the liver. This finding indicates the need for arterioportography at which time embolization may lead to complete control.

Budd–Chiari Syndrome

The syndrome of abdominal pain with intractable ascites is diagnosed not infrequently and has considerable surgical implications. The problem arises from an obstruction to the hepatic venous system at any point from lobule to right heart. It appears more commonly in women and has been attributed to oestrogen–progesterone oral contraceptives (Chapter 79) and with haematological disorders, e.g. polycythaemia, paroxysmal nocturnal haemoglobinaemia. Collagen disorders such as lupus erythematosus may also be a factor. As the same effects are produced by suprahepatic vena caval obstruction, about one-third of cases are associated with obstruction of this organ. The aetiology may be fibrosis from previous trauma, primary or secondary tumours of the liver, adrenal, kidney or vena cava itself and a well-established condition in which a web of presumed congenital origin is found across the lumen of the vena cava. This condition is well described in Japanese patients.

Hepatic vein thrombosis may be widespread in the various radicles of the liver or distinctly patchy. In the worst cases the veins are replaced by a fibrous band but the caudate lobe which has a hepatic venous drainage survives and even enlarges enough to produce a separate caval obstruction. On histological examination the predominant feature is of centrizonal venous congestion with necrosis of the surrounding cells and areas of haemorrhage.

The condition may present fairly acutely with severe abdominal pain and vomiting and a large tender liver with ascites. Where the problem is secondary to an underlying malignancy clearly those features may predominate. The condition may progress rapidly over a few weeks to hepatic failure, coma and death. The more chronic form presents in similar fashion but at a reduced tempo and with less evidence of hepatic failure. There is usually peripheral oedema which extends on to the thighs if the vena cava becomes progressively obstructed. Serum liver function tests show disturbance but are not diagnostic. Provided that the clotting parameters will permit it, an early recourse to liver biopsy is essential. However, given the patchy nature of the condition, other diagnostic tests may also be required. Ultrasound can be very effective in the sense that hepatic veins, which are normally demonstrable, are absent and a hepatic scintiscan is grossly abnormal with poor general uptake except the caudate lobe which may show normal or greater than normal uptake. These two tests indicate the need for hepatic venography and inferior vena cavography to demonstrate the site of venous blockade. Other conditions such as cirrhosis, malignant ascites, heart failure and constrictive pericarditis clearly require to be excluded.

Treatment and Prognosis

As might be expected the prognosis is variable and dependent upon the extent of venous thrombosis. For patients with a rapid deterioration, hepatic transplantation has been effective in a small number of cases. Mild cases can be managed with low sodium diet and diuretics and spontaneous improvement appears to occur in some patients presumably as the veins recanalize and prolonged survival is recorded. The moderately severe patients present more of a problem as the time course may be relatively short (3–4 years). As anticoagulants and fibrinolysins appear of no benefit, the ascites has to be managed by portal and hepatic decompression. A side-to-side portocaval shunt can accomplish this provided the inferior vena cava is not obstructed. A more certain procedure is the meso-atrial shunt, in which a shunt is constructed from the superior mesenteric vein to right atrium using a wide-bore prosthetic material with special precautions to avoid constriction at the diaphragm. Inferior vena caval webs or diaphragms can occasionally be dealt with by balloon angioplasty but more commonly require surgical excision via the right atrial route.

69 The Biliary Tract

A. Cuschieri and I. A. D. Bouchier

SURGICAL ANATOMICAL CONSIDERATIONS

The Hepatic Ducts

The right hepatic duct is formed by the intrahepatic union of the dorsocaudal and ventrocranial branches draining the segments of the right surgical lobe of the liver (segments 5–8) (*Fig.* 69.1). The ventrocranial duct is in direct line with the right hepatic duct and crosses in front of the dorsocaudal branch as this arches downwards before reaching the confluence of the two ducts. The left hepatic duct which is formed by medial and lateral segmental branches draining segments I–IV, is longer than the right hepatic duct. It follows a partial extrahepatic course and, therefore, dilates readily in the presence of distal obstructive disease. The extrahepatic portion of the left duct can be accessed surgically at the hilus and its segment III branch by following the insertion of the round ligament (ligamentum teres) to the left branch of the portal vein in the umbilical fissure between segments III and IV of the liver (*Fig.* 69.2). This 'round ligament' approach is increasingly used as an effective method of bilo-enteric bypass for inoperable cholangiocarcinoma of the extrahepatic ducts. The majority (75–80%) of intrahepatic calculi are located in the left hepatic duct and right-sided calculi, which are far less common, are found in the ventrocranial branch of the right hepatic duct. The union of the right and left hepatic ducts is usually extrahepatic, high up in the porta hepatis and the resulting *common hepatic duct* receives the cystic duct lower down, whereupon it becomes the common bile duct. It is customary, however, in surgical anatomy to use the term 'common bile duct' or simply 'bile duct' for the entire extrahepatic conduit as it obviates difficulties in nomenclature, especially when there is a low insertion of the cystic duct. The junction of the right and left hepatic ducts is also referred to as the hilar region. It is surrounded by fibrous tissue which is condensed into a fascial plane behind (liver plate) allowing dissection of the hepatic ducts from the underlying portal vein and its two branches.

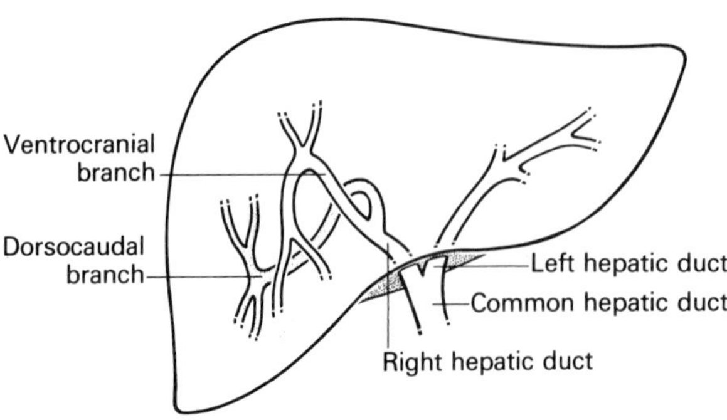

Fig. 69.1 Frontal schematic view of the liver illustrating the intrahepatic biliary tree and the ductal arrangement at the hilus. Note the left duct has a longer extrahepatic course. Within the liver, the dorsocaudal branch of the right hepatic duct curves acutely posterior to the ventrocranial branch.

The intrahepatic arrangement outlined above applies in 75% of cases. A different arrangement is encountered in the remainder when either the right dorsocaudal or ventrocranial ducts join the left hepatic duct, or the common hepatic duct forms a trifurcation (*Fig.* 69.3).

Gallbladder and Cystic Duct

The gallbladder is a pear-shaped sac about 10·0 cm in length and is situated on the inferior surface of the right lobe of the liver. It is covered with a layer of peritoneum which is reflected from the Glisson's capsule and which contains many small blood vessels which require coagulation during removal of the gallbladder. It is customarily divided into the fundus (which has the poorest blood supply, especially when the organ is distended), the body and the neck or infundibulum which leads to the cystic duct. Not infrequently, the neck has an abnormal sacculation which is referred to as Hartmann's pouch. This may become adherent to the surrounding structures of the porta hepatis, particularly the common bile duct, seriously obscuring anatomical relationships during dissection of this region.

The most common anomaly of the gallbladder encountered at laparotomy is the *phrygian cap* where the fundus is constricted and turned back on itself. The fully *intrahepatic* gallbladder is rare. The so-called *floating* gallbladder, which has a complete serosal covering and a dorsal mesentery, is relatively uncommon, as is *transposition* of the gallbladder (either between the two hepatic lobes or underneath the left lobe) and *double* gallbladder. An elongated sausage-shaped gallbladder frequently accompanies congenital cystic disease of the bile ducts. *Agenesis* (congenital absence) of the gallbladder is very rare and the condition can only be diagnosed at laparotomy in a patient who has not undergone previous

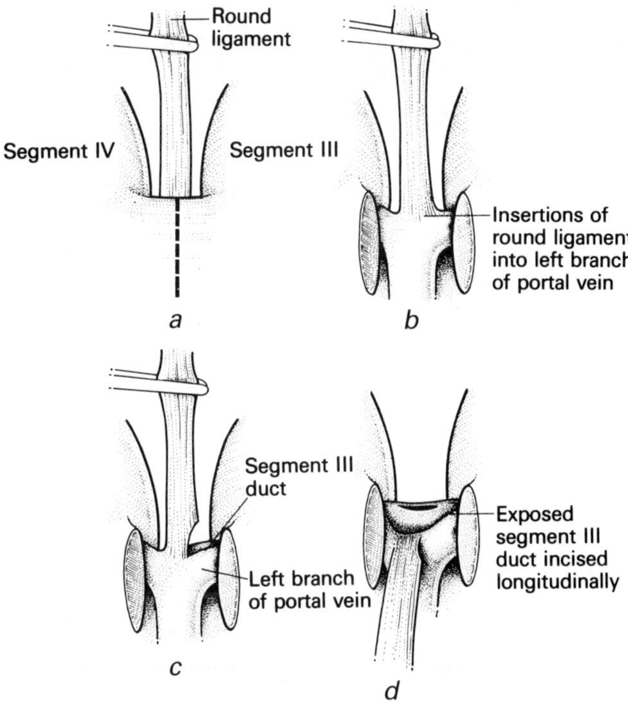

Fig. 69.2 Diagrammatic representation of the round ligament approach to segment III duct. *a*, The round ligament leads to the umbilical fissure between segment IV and segment III which are often joined by a bridge of liver tissue which overlaps the terminal insertions of the round ligament into the left branch of the portal vein. *b*, The bridge of liver tissue has been divided to expose the vascular terminations of the round ligament to the left branch of the portal vein. *c*, The terminations of the round ligament have been suture ligated and divided to expose the left branch of the portal vein. *d*, Downward traction displaces the left branch of the portal vein with exposure of segment III duct which is divided longitudinally for anastomosis to a loop of jejunum.

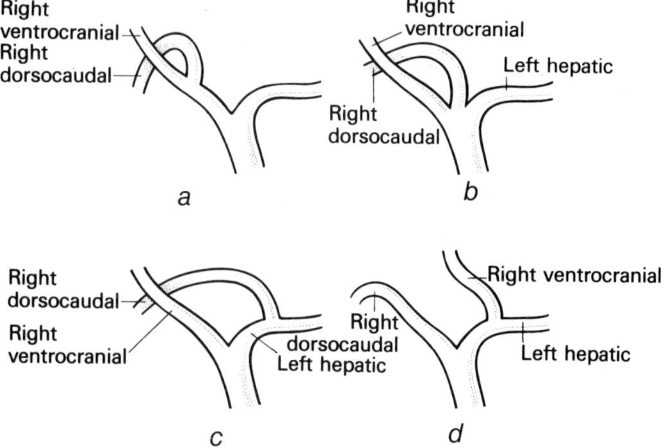

Fig. 69.3 Variations in the confluence of the major intrahepatic ducts. *a*, Normal arrangement which is found in 75% of cases. *b*, Trifurcation where the right ventrocranial, right dorsocaudal and the left hepatic ducts arise simultaneously from the common hepatic duct, there being no right hepatic duct. *c*, Termination of the right dorsocaudal branch into the left hepatic duct. *d*, Termination of the right ventrocranial duct into the left hepatic duct.

biliary tract surgery. Another rare anomaly is the *trabeculated* gallbladder, but this usually causes symptoms similar to chronic cholecystitis and is associated with abnormal gallbladder emptying.

The main arterial supply of the gallbladder is by means of the cystic artery which usually arises from the right hepatic artery. Although the cystic artery is generally considered an end-artery, blood supply also reaches the gallbladder via the vessels of the Glisson's capsule. There are several congenital anomalies of the arterial supply of the gallbladder (*Fig.* 69.4). These are important and have to be recognized during cholecystectomy before ligature of the 'cystic artery'. Careful display and verification of the anatomy is the single most important factor in the prevention of iatrogenic injuries during cholecystectomy and biliary tract surgery.

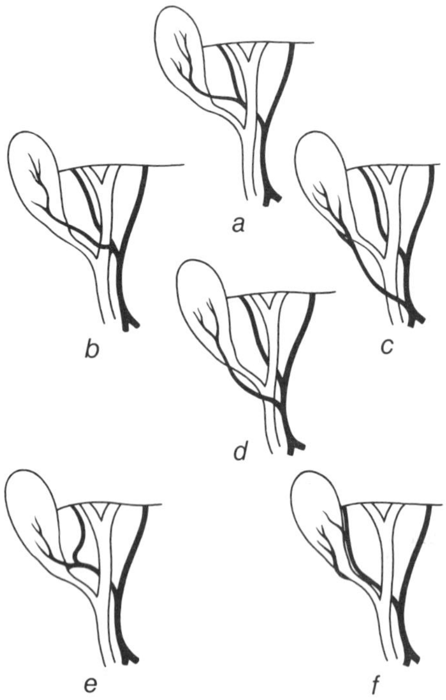

Fig. 69.4 Anomalies of the cystic artery. *a*, Normal arrangement where the cystic artery arises from the right hepatic artery soon after this emerges from behind the common hepatic duct. *b*, Origin of the cystic artery from the right hepatic to the left of the bile duct, the cystic artery then crossing in front of the common hepatic duct. *c*, Low origin of the cystic artery from the common hepatic or gastroduodenal arteries. *d*, Accessory cystic artery arising from the hepatic artery. This second artery can also arise from the left hepatic, right hepatic and gastroduodenal arteries. *e*, Looped right hepatic artery with a short cystic artery arising from the summit of the right hepatic arterial arch. *f*, The right hepatic runs close to the cystic duct and the neck of the gallbladder before giving anterior and posterior cystic branches. This anomaly is the most dangerous since the right hepatic is easily mistaken for a large cystic artery.

The *cystic duct* runs a variable course from the neck of the gallbladder to join the common hepatic duct. Its mucosa is arranged in a spiral fold or valve which often causes difficulties in cannulation during operative transcystic cholangiography. Although most anatomical textbooks indicate that the cystic duct joins the bile duct along its right margin, several large series of surgical dissections and analyses of operative cholangiograms demonstrate clearly that this arrangement is rare and is only encountered in 15–20% of cases. Much more commonly, the cystic duct enters the bile duct either posteriorly or anteriorly (40%). It may also pursue a spiral or a parallel course with the bile duct, with the two structures being enclosed in a common fibrous sheath which tends to obscure the exact location of the entry of the cystic duct into the bile duct (*Fig.* 69.5). The spiral cystic duct runs down and behind the common hepatic duct to enter on its medial aspect (35%). The parallel cystic duct runs parallel to the bile duct for a variable distance before entering it. This is the rarest arrangement and is encountered in 5–7% of patients. Rarely, the cystic duct joins the right hepatic duct and very infrequently the left duct.

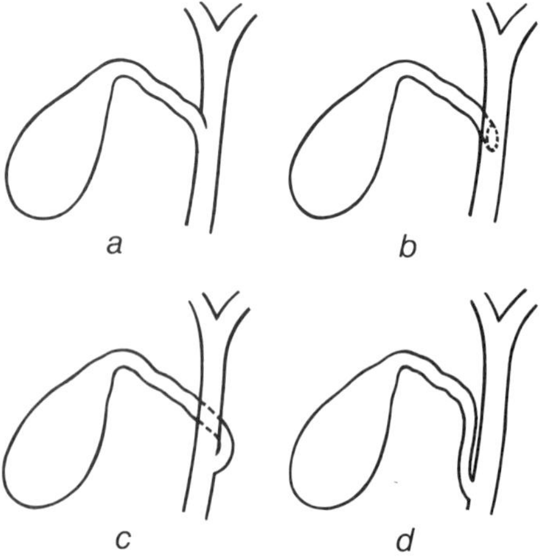

Fig. 69.5 Schematic representation of the termination of the cystic duct. *a*, Lateral insertion often depicted as the usual arrangement but which is only encountered in 15–20% of patients. *b*, Anterior or posterior termination. This is the most common type and accounts for 40% of cases. *c*, Spiral cystic duct which courses behind the bile duct to open on its medial aspect. This is fairly common and is found in 35% of patients. *d*, Parallel cystic duct. This is the rarest arrangement and is encountered in 5–7% of patients.

Common Bile Duct

The bile duct (choledochus) is formed by the union of the right and left hepatic ducts each draining the respective surgical lobes of the liver. It is joined at a variable distance along its course by the cystic duct. In strict anatomical terms, the segment between the hilar bifurcation and the cystic duct is referred to as the *common hepatic duct* and the term *common bile duct* is reserved for the portion distal to this junction. From the surgical standpoint, however, it is best to consider it as one structure which is divisible into the supraduodenal, retroduodenal, intrapancreatic and intraduodenal segments. It serves as a conduit of bile from the liver and gallbladder to the duodenal papilla, and in the adult, measures 11·0–12·0 cm in length with an average diameter of 7 mm, range 4–10 mm. The supraduodenal segment is important surgically because it is the area which is most commonly explored. It lies in the free edge of the hepatoduodenal ligament to the right of the hepatic artery and anterolateral to the portal vein. The retroduodenal segment curves to the right away from the portal vein behind the first part of the duodenum before entering the head of the pancreas—intrapancreatic segment. However, in 20% of patients the duct has a partial or complete extrapancreatic course. The transduodenal segment (also known as the infundibulum) which traverses obliquely the duodenal wall and usually joins the pancreatic duct, opens into the duodenal lumen at the summit of the *major duodenal papilla*. The lower end of the common bile duct, therefore, deviates to the right before entering the lumen of the duodenum almost at right angles. This is an important practical consideration since forcible probing through this area may perforate the bile duct and result in either a haematoma, postoperative pancreatitis, choledochoduodenal fistula or stricture of the lower end of the bile duct.

The main pancreatic duct (Wirsung) joins the posteromedial wall of the transduodenal segment of the bile duct to form a common channel in 90% of cases. A localized dilatation of the common channel to form an ampulla of Vater is uncommon (10–20%) and in 10% of patients the two ducts open separately into the duodenum (*Fig.* 69.6).

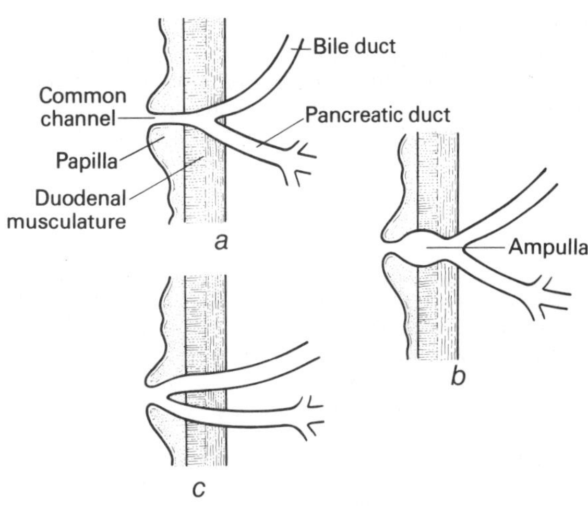

Fig. 69.6 Configuration of the lower end of the common bile and pancreatic ducts. *a*, The two ducts join to form a common channel which opens at the summit of the duodenal papilla. This is the most common arrangement. *b*, There is a localized dilatation of the common channel to form the ampulla of Vater. *c*, The two ducts open separately into the duodenum.

The *Vaterian segment* includes the lower 2·5–3·0 cm of the common bile duct, the distal part of the pancreatic duct, the ampulla or common channel and the major duodenal papilla. These structures are surrounded by a condensation of circular and longitudinal smooth muscle fibres often referred to as the sphincter of Oddi, although it was Boyden who described the detailed anatomy of the various components of this sphincteric complex. The inferior sphincter is the strongest component and is also known as the papillary muscular ball (*Fig.* 69.7). It surrounds the terminations of the bile and pancreatic ducts and the common channel. The middle sphincter is the longest and the thinnest of the components and surrounds the transduodenal and a variable portion of the transpancreatic segments of the bile duct and the duct of Wirsung. The superior sphincters consist of localized thickenings of the middle sphincters around the bile and pancreatic ducts at the proximal end of the sphincter complex.

An important variation of the anatomy of the Vaterian segment is the condition known as *pancreas divisum* which results from failure of fusion of the ventral and dorsal pancreas during embryological development. The duct of the ventral pancreas which normally forms the main pancreatic duct remains rudimentary and drains the lower portion of the pancreatic head and the uncinate process. The rest of the pancreas is drained through the duct of the dorsal anlage (duct of Santorini) which opens through the *small accessory papilla* above the major duodenal ampulla. The incidence of pancreas divisum in the general population is 5–8% but the condition is much commoner in patients with idiopathic recurrent pancreatitis (approximately 25%) and an aetiological relationship has been suggested.

The activity of the choledochal sphincteric complex is independent of the duodenal musculature but may be influenced by it. Thus, the effect of certain drugs on the choledochal sphincter differs from their action on the duodenal wall, and duodenal muscular peristaltic activity has no significant effect on the common bile duct pressure. The choledochal sphincter is an active structure and measures up to 2·5 cm in length. It consists of well-developed longitudinal and circular smooth muscle. Contraction of the longitudinal muscle tends to open the duct lumen, whereas

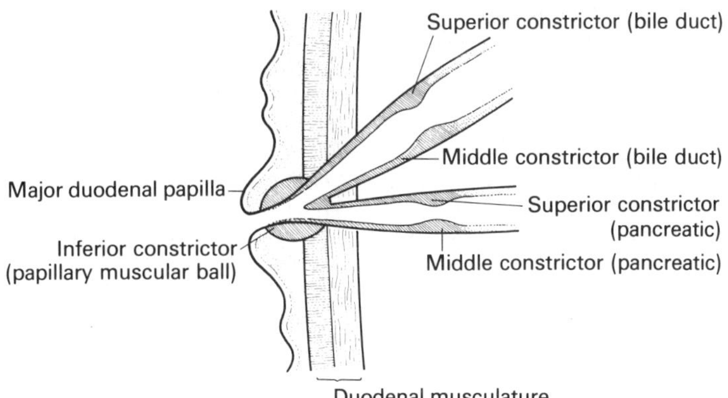

Fig. 69.7 Diagrammatic representation of the components of the sphincter complex (sphincter of Oddi) surrounding the Vaterian segment. The bile and pancreatic ducts are illustrated splayed apart to facilitate the demonstration. Normally the terminal portions of both ducts are contiguous.

the circular muscle has the opposite effect. These contracted (systolic) and relaxed (diastolic) states of the choledochal sphincter lead to quite distinct appearances of the lower end of the common bile duct at cholangiography. During contraction, contrast often forms a meniscus with the concavity facing downward simulating a stone (the pseudocalculus phenomenon) (*Fig.* 69.8).

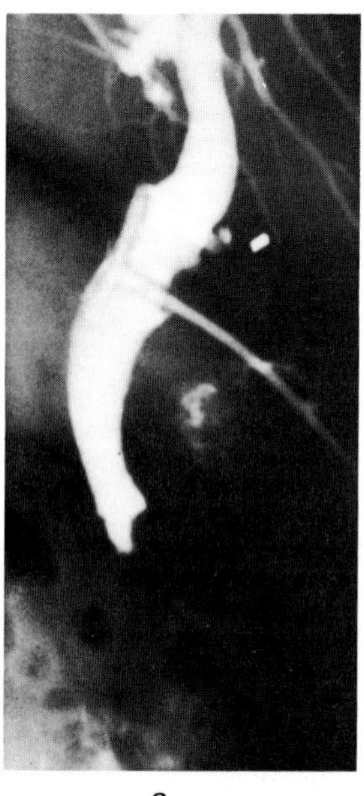

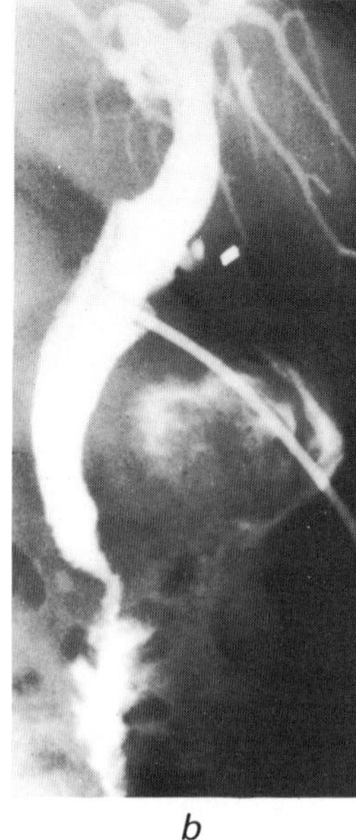

a b

Fig. 69.8 The pseudocalculus phenomenon. *a*, During the systolic phase of choledochal sphincter action, there is an apparent detachment of the lower end of the common bile duct outline from the duodenal contrast shadow with an inverted meniscus effect, the appearance simulating a stone impacted at this site. *b*, This 'filling defect' disappears when the same bile duct is visualized during diastole (relaxation) of the sphincter.

The rest of the common bile duct contains few muscle fibres. Its epithelial lining rests on a loose stroma containing elastic fibres which disappear with age or disease. Thus, stone impaction, prolonged distension or cholangitis may lead to rigidity of the common bile duct. The narrowest portion of the common bile duct occurs at its point of entrance into the duodenal wall and this area is often indicated by a notch on the cholangiogram. The diameter of the transduodenal segment is normally 5·0 mm and that of the major duodenal papilla varies from 0·5 to 1·5 mm. The commonest site for calculus arrest or impaction is just proximal to the transduodenal segment.

The major duodenal papilla is situated on the posteromedial aspect of the second part of the duodenum about 7·0–10·0 cm from the pylorus. Its appearances may vary from the usual well-defined papilla with varying degrees of projection to a flattened depression between the mucosal folds. Irrespective of its exact configuration, the major duodenal papilla frequently has a dorsal mucosal fold. The papilla is more easily located by endoscopic retrograde cholangiopancreatography (ERCP) than by direct inspection during surgical intervention. The minor (accessory) papilla is more proximally situated and assumes clinical importance only in patients with pancreas divisum.

Anomalous (Aberrant) Bile Ducts

The reported incidence of aberrant bile ducts varies widely but averages 12%. The vast majority arise from the right ductal system (especially the dorsocaudal branch of the right hepatic) and are located in the cystohepatic triangle of Calot (80%) (*Fig.* 69.9). The size of the anomalous duct and the area of hepatic parenchyma which it drains vary considerably. The anomalous duct most commonly enters the cystic or common hepatic duct and, less frequently, the gallbladder. Ligature of an aberrant hepatic duct is rarely attended by any detectable adverse effect. However, their unrecognized division may result in bile leakage and postoperative biliary peritonitis.

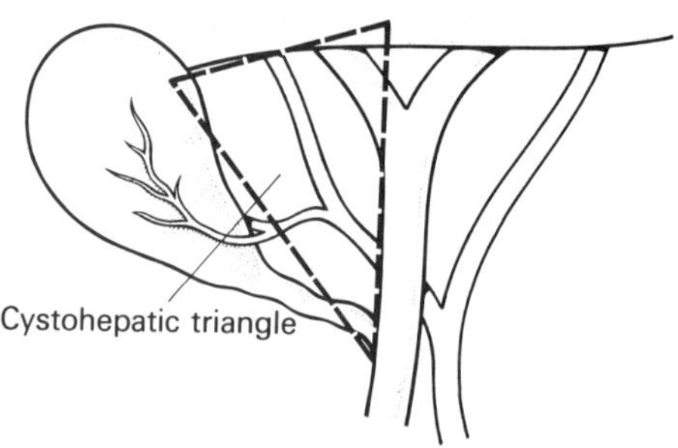

Fig. 69.9 Cystohepatic triangle of Calot formed by the cystic duct and neck of the gallbladder inferiorly, the liver edge superiorly and the common hepatic duct medially. It contains the cystic artery and lymph node and the right hepatic artery as it emerges from behind the common hepatic duct.

The cystohepatic triangle is also important surgically in the performance of cholecystectomy. It contains the right hepatic artery which usually enters the triangle behind the common hepatic duct and runs parallel to the cystic duct before it gives off the cystic artery after which it curves upwards along the right hepatic duct to the liver. The cystic lymph node is situated at the junction of the cystic with the common hepatic artery.

Anomalous Origin of the Hepatic Arteries

The usual arrangement is for the common hepatic artery to arise from the coeliac axis. After giving rise to the gastroduodenal artery behind the first part of the duodenum, it arches upwards along the left side of the bile duct and in front of the portal vein. It then bifurcates into the right and left hepatic arteries. The right hepatic artery usually crosses behind (rarely in front of) the common hepatic duct before giving rise to the cystic artery. The right gastric artery originates from the hepatic artery and soon after this gives off the gastroduodenal artery (*Fig.* 69.10*a*). The important anomalies of the hepatic arteries are origin of the right hepatic artery from the superior mesenteric, origin of the left hepatic from the left gastric artery and an accessory right hepatic artery from the superior mesenteric artery (*Fig.* 69.10*b*, *c*, *d*).

Lymphatic Drainage

Proximally, the lymphatic channels of the gallbladder communicate with those of the Glisson's capsule of the liver. The hepatic capsular lymphatics drain into the thoracic duct

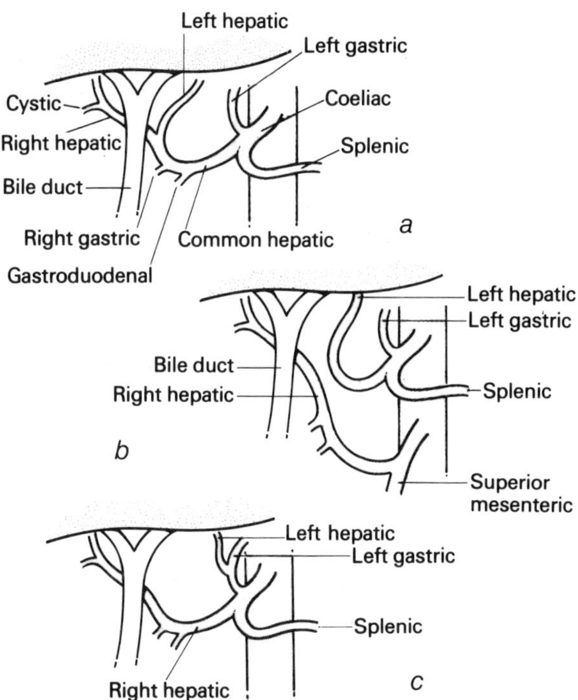

Fig. 69.10 Anomalous hepatic arteries. *a*, Usual arrangement. *b*, Origin of the right hepatic from the superior mesenteric artery. *c*, Origin of the left hepatic artery from the left gastric artery.

except those on the superior surface of the liver, flow from which reaches the retrosternal lymph nodes via several channels. Distally, the gallbladder lymphatics and those of the extrahepatic bile ducts drain into the cystic lymph node which is situated near the cystic artery close to its origin from the right hepatic artery, and to other nodes lateral to the lower end of the bile duct, particularly the retroduodenal segment.

Dilatation of the Biliary Tract

The common bile duct dilates more rapidly than the intrahepatic biliary tree. Thus, instant passive dilatation of the common bile duct demonstrated fluoroscopically, can be produced by excessive filling of the biliary tract by contrast media. Dilatation of the intrahepatic biliary tree always signifies prolonged obstruction and experimentally, it requires a minimum of 3 weeks of obstruction for the production of demonstrable intrahepatic duct dilatation.

By convention, the diameter of the common bile duct is measured just above the junction of the cystic duct. A common bile duct whose diameter exceeds 10·0 mm is considered dilated, and above 15·0 mm, the presence of significant organic disease can be safely assumed. Dilatation of the common bile duct signifies existing or recently relieved obstruction, the most common cause of which is calculous disease. There is an established positive correlation between the duct diameter and the incidence of ductal stones. On the other hand, stones may be present in a normal-sized common bile duct and in several reported series, a 5–10% incidence of ductal stones have been reported in patients with common bile ducts of 5·0 mm. Other causes of duct dilatation include pancreaticobiliary cancer, chronic pancreatitis, congenital cystic disease and parasitic infestation. Controversy persists regarding dilatation of the bile duct after truncal vagotomy. Recent studies have, however, demonstrated abnormal gallbladder emptying after this procedure but not following highly selective vagotomy.

Although there are no intrahepatic communications between the right and the left intrahepatic ductal trees in the normal state, communications between the two systems develop following the onset of extrahepatic large bile duct obstruction.

Physiology of the Extrahepatic Ductal System

The secretion of bile by the liver is largely dependent on the influx of bile acids which consists of a large component made up of bile salts which have been reabsorbed from the small intestine into the portal venous blood and a smaller component of newly synthesized bile acids. There is a small bile acid-independent fraction of bile secretion which is reduced in experimental cholestasis whereas the bile acid-dependent fraction increases under these conditions.

The basal or resting (interdigestive) common bile duct pressure which averages 6·0 mmHg ensures the continued patency of the lumen of the choledochus but is insufficient to overcome the resistance of the choledochal sphincter. The hepatic bile is stored and partitioned in the gallbladder, although the patterns of gallbladder filling and emptying are incompletely understood. Eating results in the cholecystokinetic response consisting of contraction of the gallbladder and relaxation of the sphincter of Oddi which results in the timely delivery of bile salts into the intestinal tract. This response is mediated by known hormonal mechanisms (cholecystokinin) and poorly understood neural reflexes. Recent studies have shown that gallbladder emptying occurs before the onset of gastric emptying of a meal suggesting a cephalic neural reflex. Gallbladder contractions also occur during the interdigestive period and in the human, these are coincident with phase II duodenal activity of the intestinal migratory motor complexes.

Biliary Motility

The existence of an independent choledochal sphincter is now recognized by electrophysiological criteria. It results in a high-pressure zone just within the papilla. Apart from being responsive to various hormonal influences, the choledochal sphincter has a rich nerve supply via the hepatic vagal plexus which consists predominantly of motor fibres derived from the left abdominal vagus. The sympathetic component is derived from the spinal segments T8 and 9 via the coeliac and periarterial plexuses.

In addition, the lower end of the common bile duct exhibits phasic peristaltic activity with opening (diastolic) and closing (systolic) movements that correlate with pressure waves demonstrated in man. In the fasting state these phasic contractions are cyclical and parallel the duodenal migratory motor complexes. They are considered to regulate the flow of bile and pancreatic juice into the duodenum. The sphincter is in a contracted state and offers a significant resistance to bile flow in between these phasic contractions.

Effect of Hormones

Cholecystokinin (CCK) is the main stimulus to gallbladder contraction in response to a meal and CCK administration increases gallbladder pressure, decreases the resistance through the sphincter of Oddi and enhances the bile flow in man. CCK-induced gallbladder contraction is largely inhibited by atropine. In the human, the gallbladder is less sensitive to CCK than the exocrine pancreas since the dose of exogenous CCK required to induce trypsin secretion is lower than that necessary for gallbladder contraction. CCK action on the extrahepatic biliary tract is not mediated by the nervous system although the atropine effect in reducing CCK-mediated contraction suggests that its action may be mediated by the release of acetylcholine from intrinsic cholinergic nerves. CCK administration results in the activation of intracellular phosphodiesterase activity and reduction in cyclic AMP content. CCK induces a relaxation of the sphincter of Oddi which is concomitant with contraction of the gallbladder, the response resulting in an efficient delivery of bile into the duodenum in response to a meal. CCK and motilin may be involved with the phasic activity of the choledochal sphincter which is associated with duodenal migratory myoelectrical complexes during the interdigestive stage.

The activity of CCK depends on the COOH-terminal heptapeptide, a sequence found in gastrin which has a cholecystokinetic activity 1/15 that of CCK. Thus, this effect of gastrin is a pharmacological phenomenon in both dog and man, and gastrin has no effect on the biliary pressure of cholecystectomized patients. The synthetic hepta-, octa- and decapeptides of CCK are more potent than the various molecular forms of the naturally-occurring CCK. In the human, 20 mg/kg of the COOH-terminal octapeptide of CCK (OP-CCK) reduces the gallbladder size by 40%.

Caerulein, a peptide of similar composition to CCK extracted from amphibian skin has a marked cholecystokinetic effect about 3 times that induced by CCK in the dog. Both the gallbladder contraction and the relaxation of the sphincter of Oddi are produced by a direct action on the smooth muscle. The synthetic derivative, ceruletide, has been used in the relief of biliary colic and to promote passage of retained ductal stones during saline infusion of the common bile duct through the T-tube.

Secretin does not appear to have a significant cholecystokinetic response in the human. Its effect on the gallbladder muscle vary with the species studied. Glucagon relaxes both the gallbladder musculature and the choledochal sphincter in man and the dog probably by a direct action.

VIP (vasoactive intestinal polypeptide) which has been demonstrated in nerve fibres and neurones within the gallbladder wall, induces relaxation of the gallbladder and inhibits gallbladder contraction induced by CCK. These findings suggest that VIP may act as a local neurotransmitter in the physiological neural regulation of gallbladder function.

Somatostatin-containing cells have been demonstrated in the human extrahepatic biliary tract. Somatostatin interferes with the gallbladder emptying and reduces bile flow in man.

Delivery of Bile into the Duodenum

Studies in the human have demonstrated that the bile salt output through an intact choledochal sphincter is significantly lower than that obtained from the T-tube in patients after common bile duct exploration. Whereas peak bile salt output is significantly increased after cholecystectomy, the total bile salt output is unaffected by this operation when compared to normal. The exogenous administration of CCK results in the production of a more stable bile secretion than the endogenous release of this hormone induced by the intraduodenal infusion of essential amino acids, the rhythmic release of bile following which is related to the concentration of bile salts in the duodenal lumen. The delivery of bile into the duodenum is predominantly controlled by the choledochal sphincter, the activity of which is controlled by complex neurohormonal influences that are as yet poorly understood. Alcohol ingestion induces spasm of the choledochal sphincter and intraduodenal instillation of N/10 HCl produces the same effect in the dog.

Neural Influences on Biliary Motility

In man the results of vagal stimulation by insulin-provoked hypoglycaemia suggest that the parasympathetic nervous system is involved in the maintenance of the gallbladder tone. Vagotomy causes dilatation and some delay in the gallbladder emptying when studied by cholescintigraphic techniques. Vagotomy also results in a decrease in the nerve fibres within the gallbladder wall. However, the increased prevalence of gallstones after cholecystectomy suggested by some retrospective reports remains controversial. Vagal activity appears to influence the tone of the choledochal sphincter. Electrical stimulation of the vagus nerve in the dog has been reported to result in no change or in a decreased bile flow through the sphincter and an increase in its electromyographic activity. In the human, hepatic plexus vagectomy has been reported to lower the passage pressure (the pressure head which opens the sphincter and permits bile to flow into the duodenum), indicating a lowering of the sphincteric muscular activity/contractility.

The role of the sympathetic remains undefined. An increased threshold for pain induced by biliary distension has been reported in the human following sympathetic blockade. Stimulation of the right splanchnic nerve induces a contraction of the sphincter which is abolished by an alpha-blockade, and gallbladder dilatation which is inhibited by beta-blockade.

Effect of Cholecystectomy and Sphincterotomy/Sphincteroplasty

On *a priori* grounds, removal of the gallbladder would be expected to alter the delivery of bile into the duodenum as this would then depend on the hepatic secretory pressure (maximum 25–30 cmH_2O) and the resistance of the choledochal sphincter which is expressed by the passage (yield) pressure. In practice, cholecystectomy in the human does not lead to any alterations in the total bile salt output compared to the normal situation but there is a redistribution of the pool of bile salts between the gut and the portal venous system. The effect of cholecystectomy on the cholesterol saturation of bile is uncertain, with some reports indicating a reduction and others showing no effect on the bile composition.

Although no changes in the biliary cholesterol content and gallbladder filling and response to CCK are observed after division of the sphincter (endoscopic or surgical), the concentration of lecithin and bile salts in the gallbladder are decreased as is the concentrating ability of the gallbladder. In addition, the results of animal experiments have shown an increase in the monohydroxy and dihydroxy bile salts in the gallbladder which becomes colonized by bacteria and develops histological changes of chronic inflammation. In the human, cholecystitis develops in 6% of patients with an in situ gallbladder within 6 months of an endoscopic sphincterotomy.

JAUNDICE

Bilirubin is produced in the reticuloendothelial system from the enzymic breakdown of haem which is derived from effete red blood corpuscles. As it is water-insoluble, bilirubin is carried bound to albumin in the plasma and is taken up by the hepatocytes by means of specific membrane carriers. Within the hepatocytes, the bilirubin is stored bound to specific binding proteins (ligandins Y, Z) and then conjugated by a specific enzyme (glucuronyl transferase) to the water-soluble bilirubin glucuronide (conjugated bilirubin) which is then secreted by means of specific carriers into the bile canaliculi, and finally excreted into the biliary tract and intestine. Bacterial degradation of some of the excreted conjugated bilirubin in the distal small bowel results in the formation of urobilinogen which is reabsorbed and subsequently excreted in the urine and bile. The normal upper limit of serum bilirubin is 17·0 μmol/l.

Jaundice (hyperbilirubinaemia) is a syndrome of varied aetiology which may be recognized clinically when the serum bilirubin exceeds 40·0 μmol/l. The hyperbilirubinaemia may be either *conjugated* or *unconjugated* and may result from:

- Excess bilirubin production
- Impaired uptake by the hepatocyte
- Failure of conjugation
- Impaired secretion of conjugated bilirubin into the bile canaliculi
- Impairment of bile flow subsequent to the secretion by the hepatocytes (cholestatic or obstructive jaundice).

The defect may be congenital (benign congenital hyperbilirubinaemias) but much more commonly, it is acquired as a result of haemolysis, liver disease, adverse drug reaction and biliary tract obstruction which may be intra- or extrahepatic. The early diagnosis and prompt treatment of patients with jaundice reduces both the morbidity and mortality of the underlying disease.

A useful clinical classification of jaundice is shown in *Table* 69.1. In clinical practice, the largest groups by far are the hepatocellular and cholestatic jaundice.

Table 69.1 Clinical classification of jaundice

Type	*Mechanism*
Hepatocellular	Defective secretion of conjugated bilirubin into the bile canaliculi
Cholestatic (intra/extra-hepatic)	Impairment of bile flow subsequent to the above secretory step
Haemolytic	Excess bilirubin production
Benign congenital hyperbilirubinaemias	Defective bilirubin uptake or secretory defect

N.B. A combined hepatocellular and cholestatic jaundice may be found in liver disease.
Cholestatic is synonymous with obstructive.

Hepatocellular Jaundice

This is due to parenchymatous liver disease which may be acute (viral hepatitis, liver cell necrosis, acute alcoholic hepatitis, etc.) or chronic (chronic active hepatitis, the various types of cirrhosis: alcoholic, cryptogenic, primary biliary, etc.). The principal defect is the failure of secretion of the conjugated bilirubin into the bile canaliculi. The serum transaminases are grossly elevated especially in acute disease. In patients with alcohol-related liver disease, the gamma-glutamyl transpeptidase is elevated as a result of microsomal induction rather than cholestasis. Acute hepatitis due to viral infection or drugs may also cause a cholestatic picture, in which case the alkaline phosphatase and the 5′-nucleotidase are elevated (*vide infra*). The hyperbilirubinaemia is always (predominantly) of the conjugated variety with the presence of bilirubin in the urine even in the absence of a cholestatic component.

Cholestatic Jaundice

This is the result of impaired bile flow to the duodenum subsequent to the secretion of conjugated bilirubin into the bile canaliculi. The block may be *intrahepatic* when it may be functional (e.g. drugs, hepatitis, etc.) or organic (obstruction of the intrahepatic biliary tree) or *extrahepatic*, also known as *large bile duct obstruction* which constitutes the most important surgical subgroup of cholestatic jaundice as it is always the result of organic disease, e.g. ductal calculi, pancreaticobiliary cancer, etc.

The biochemical features of cholestasis are:

- Conjugated hyperbilirubinaemia.
- Elevation of alkaline phosphatase, 5′-nucleotidase and gamma-glutamyl transpeptidase (Gamma-GT). The enzyme 5′-nucleotidase is the most reliable since its level is not influenced by bone disease and the enzyme is not induced by alcohol.
- Minimal or no elevation of the serum transaminases.
- Presence of bilirubin in the urine as the conjugated bilirubin is water soluble and is therefore filtered in the glomerulus.
- Elevation in the serum cholesterol and bile acid levels although these are not routinely measured in patients with cholestatic jaundice.

It is important to stress that the above biochemical markers of cholestasis do not distinguish between intra- and extrahepatic obstruction.

Haemolytic Jaundice

The unconjugated hyperbilirubinaemia results from excess haemolysis. Bilirubin is not present in the urine as the unconjugated pigment is water-insoluble and is carried in the plasma bound to albumin. The excess bilirubin production is accompanied by an increased secretion of the conjugated pigment in the bile and therefore increased production of urobilinogen by bacterial decomposition in the distal small intestine. The urine, therefore, contains an excess amount of urobilinogen and urobilin. A cholestatic component may develop in patients with prolonged and recurrent haemolysis (e.g. congenital haemolytic anaemias).

In some patients excess bilirubin production is present in the absence of overt haemolysis. The excess unconjugated bilirubin is thought to result from breakdown of precursor/immature red cells in the bone marrow. This form of benign non-familial congenital hyperbilirubinaemia is referred to as *shunt hyperbilirubinaemia*.

Benign Familial Congenital Hyperbilirubinaemias

This group includes Gilbert's disease, Dubin–Johnson syndrome and the Rotor syndrome. All three conditions are congenital and familial. Gilbert's disease is due to a defect in the uptake of bilirubin by the hepatocytes and results in mild unconjugated hyperbilirubinaemia. Both the Dubin–Johnson and Rotor syndromes are caused by a secretory defect of conjugated bilirubin by the hepatocytes into the bile canaliculi and therefore lead to a conjugated hyperbilirubinaemia. In addition, patients with the Dubin–Johnson syndrome are unable to excrete contrast media into the biliary tree and for this reason, the gallbladder is not visualized by oral cholecystography and intravenous cholangiography. Despite the accumulation of conjugated bilirubin in the blood and its appearance in the urine, there are no other biochemical markers of cholestasis in both conditions.

Management of the Jaundiced Patient

The investigation of the jaundiced patient has been made to appear unduly complex as a result of the introduction of a number of new investigative techniques. It is important to reiterate that a properly taken history and physical examination will allow a correct diagnosis to be made in some 80% of patients. In addition to details of the presenting symptoms, the history must always cover the following information which has to be obtained by direct questioning of the patient:

Drug intake: legal and illicit
Injections with hypodermic needles: legal and illicit
Alcohol abuse
Transfusion of blood and blood products
Contact with jaundiced individuals in the recent past
Travel to hepatitis-endemic areas
Ingestion of raw shellfish and wild mushrooms.

The investigation of jaundiced patients should proceed in a systematic manner and the sequence of tests used is designed to answer the following questions:

Is the Jaundice Cholestatic?

In cholestatic jaundice the urine is dark and frothy and the stools are often pale. Bilirubin is present in the urine and the serum alkaline phosphatase, 5′-nucleotidase of gamma-GT are elevated. A slight rise in the serum transaminases often accompanies cholestatic jaundice, but significant active hepatocellular damage is unlikely with levels below 400 iu/ml. Clinically, patients with cholestatic jaundice may complain of itching (probably due to the circulating high levels of bile salts) and often exhibit scratch marks.

Has the Patient any Evidence of Parenchymatous Liver Disease?

The stigmata of chronic liver disease are: palmar erythema, spider naevi, bruising, splenomegaly, hepatomegaly or reduced liver size, fluid retention (ascites and oedema), muscle wasting, finger clubbing, white nails, enlargement of the parotid glands and gynaecomastia/testicular atrophy in the male. Incoordination, neurological signs, such as hyperreflexia and apraxia, altered sleep rhythm, confusion, flapping tremor, stupor and foetor hepaticus are signs of impending liver failure.

Is there any Evidence of Malignancy on Clinical Examination?

The signs include recent weight loss, enlarged supraclavicular lymph nodes on the left side of the neck (Virchow's nodes, Troisier's sign), abnormal chest signs, enlarged nodular liver, palpable gallbladder (Courvoisier's sign), palpable intra-abdominal masses (epigastrium, iliac fossae), rapidly oncoming ascites and rectal neoplasm (digital examination).

Is there Dilatation of the Biliary Tree?

This is reliably demonstrated by ultrasound which allows the differentiation of large bile duct obstruction (dilated biliary tree) from intrahepatic causes of cholestasis, where the duct size is normal (*vide infra*) In addition, ultrasound will detect the majority of biliary calculi. This investigation is, however, unreliable in demonstrating the exact pathology and level of the obstructive lesion. If the ultrasound scan shows dilatation of the biliary tract and the patient is clinically jaundiced, visualization of the biliary tree is necessary by either endoscopic retrograde cholangiopancreatography (ERCP) or percutaneous transhepatic cholangiography (PTC).

Intrahepatic cholestasis requires further investigation by liver biopsy and antibody studies (anti-mitochondrial, anti-smooth muscle antibodies and immunoglobulin titres). The liver biopsy is customarily performed by the blind percutaneous technique. However, if considered necessary, either because of suspected focal disease or the possibility of bleeding, a target biopsy can be undertaken under direct laparoscopic vision. If the liver biopsy suggests bile-duct obstruction despite a non-dilated duct, visualization of the biliary tract is best achieved by ERCP.

INVESTIGATIVE TECHNIQUES IN BILIARY TRACT DISORDERS

Oral Cholecystography and Intravenous Cholangiography

Both techniques can provide adequate visualization of the gallbladder if the serum bilirubin is below 40·0–50·0 μmol/l. Oral cholecystography can also demonstrate gallbladder contractility after a fatty meal or the injection of cholecystokinin or ceruletide. Failure of the gallbladder to opacify is followed by repeated investigation using a double-dose cholecystogram. Non-visualization by this method is indicative of a diseased gallbladder if ingestion and absorption of the Telepaque tablets can be reasonably assumed (probability exceeds 90%). The sensitivity of a technically satisfactory oral cholecystogram for the detection of radiolucent stones exceeds 90%. However, visualization of the ducts is poor and is obtained in only 20% of patients after a fatty meal, although CCK- or ceruletide-cholecystography enhances the visualization of the ducts considerably (80% of patients).

Oral cholecystography is unpredictable in the ill patient who is nauseous and may vomit (e.g. acute cholecystitis). The technique is, however, useful after the acute episode has subsided and in patients with mild attacks.

The gallbladder is less well defined by the intravenous cholangiogram but the extrahepatic biliary system can be better visualized by this procedure, especially with an infusion technique used in association with tomography. Infusion cholangiography is an accurate technique for the diagnosis of cystic duct obstruction (acute cholecystitis, where the gallbladder is not opacified but the ducts are outlined). However, the technique has been largely replaced by biliary scintigraphy which appears to be more accurate.

Real-time Ultrasonography

This is now the first-line investigation for biliary tract and pancreatic disease in most hospitals. Aside from its non-invasive nature and lack of any radiation exposure, ultrasound scanning can provide simultaneous information on the following:

Presence of gallstones
Presence of gallbladder disease

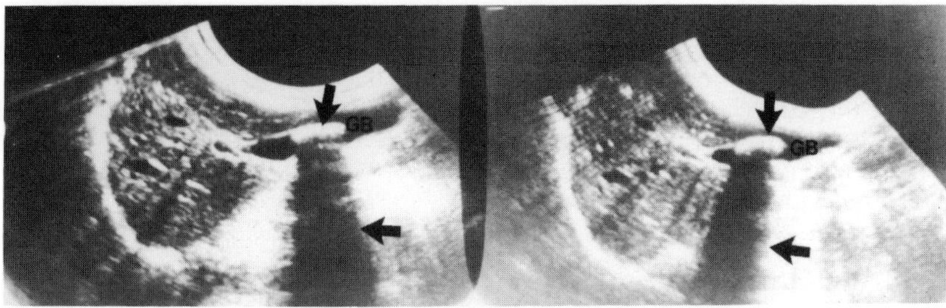

Fig. 69.11 Ultrasound examination demonstrating a large gallstone (vertical arrow) with the associated acoustic shadows (transverse arrow) which are characteristic of gallstones.

Dilatation of the biliary tract and hepatic parenchymal disease, e.g. tumour deposits
Lesions in the pancreas.

Real-time ultrasound in experienced hands can detect gallstones in over 90% of cases (*Fig.* 69.11). However, its sensitivity for ductal calculi is much less and varies considerably from centre to centre (10–80%). Gallbladder ultrasound scanning also detects gallbladder enlargement, thickening of the wall and tumours but is less sensitive in the diagnosis of adenomyomatosis than oral cholecystography. Ultrasound examination of the gallbladder has been advocated as the initial diagnostic procedure for acute cholecystitis since it enables the determination of tenderness over the sonographically identified gallbladder and is able to detect pericholecystic fluid collections and gallbladder wall oedema/thickening (ultrasonographic signs of cholecystitis), in addition to sludge and stones. However, the sensitivity and specificity of ultrasound in the diagnosis of acute cholecystitis is lower than that for gallbladder scintiscanning.

The ultrasonographic detection of a dilated biliary tract is the first step in the investigation of patients with biochemical evidence of cholestatic jaundice. In icteric patients, its accuracy in the diagnosis of extrahepatic bile duct obstruction exceeds 90% (*Fig.* 69.12). Its diagnostic yield is lower, however, in mildly jaundiced patients since it may miss minimal dilatation of the intrahepatic biliary tree. As ultrasound examination does not give accurate information on the exact site and extent of the lesion causing the extrahepatic obstruction, further investigation with ERCP or PTC is required in most patients. Percutaneous fine needle cytological aspiration of mass lesions in the liver, extrahepatic bile ducts, gallbladder and pancreas are now routinely performed in large centres under ultrasonographic guidance and often establish the definitive diagnosis regarding the benign or malignant nature of the lesion. There are no known biological hazards of ultrasound investigation.

Ultrasound examination may prove unsatisfactory for technical reasons in the following:

Obese
Following previous surgery
Ascites
Gaseous distension of the upper abdominal viscera.

In these instances CT scanning provides more reliable information.

CT Scanning and Magnetic Resonance Imaging

CT scanning can provide similar information on the biliary tree as ultrasonography but in view of cost and radiation exposure, it is usually held in reserve when ultrasound examination has failed (usually for technical reasons). Contrast enhancement (vascular or biliary) increases the diagnostic yield. CT scanning provides better detection of solid lesions in the extrahepatic bile ducts (e.g. cholangiocarcinoma), pancreas and liver.

Magnetic resonance imaging (MRI), also known as nuclear magnetic resonance, although rapidly advancing and of great potential is not used extensively for the detection of hepatobiliary disease at the present time. The technique is based on the behaviour of protons (e.g. hydrogen) of the nuclei of molecules which act as spinning magnets and align themselves in a specific direction when exposed to an external electromagnetic field. If radiofrequency (magnetic) pulses corresponding to the spinning frequency of the protons are then applied, the alignment is disturbed with each pulse and then returns or 'relaxes' to the original position. The time taken for the nuclear motion to get out of step is known as T_2 and that required for the return to the original position is known as T_1. Both these time constants vary with the proton density of the tissue and the local atomic and molecular environment of the protons (i.e. chemical state of the tissue). The movement of the nuclei resulting from the externally applied radiofrequency pulses is known as 'resonant absorption' and is accompanied by the re-emission of radiowaves which are picked up by a receiver coil placed round the patient. Different techniques of radiofrequency pulses are used to generate images of different slice thickness and in various planes. The advantages of MRI are:

Excellent soft-tissue definition, particularly of the central nervous system because of the lipid/water content.
It can image in any plane (coronal, sagittal, transverse) without movement of the patient.
It avoids radiation exposure.
It carries no known biological hazard.

Already, MRI has replaced CT scanning for the delineation of soft-tissue lesions. The future potential, including the ability to obtain information on the chemical composition of the tissue being scanned, is great and has not been fully realized (Magnetic Resonance Spectroscopy, MRS). It is likely that MRS will be able to provide the best test of liver function in the not too distant future. Already, it has been used successfully to identify specific inborn errors of metabolism due to specific enzyme deficiencies.

Percutaneous Transhepatic Cholangiography (PTC)

This is the most commonly used technique for the visualization of the biliary tract in the jaundiced patient and can be modified to allow percutaneous transhepatic drainage and insertion of endoprostheses. Its advantage over ERCP is its general availability in most radiology departments. In experienced hands, the success rate with PTC approximates to

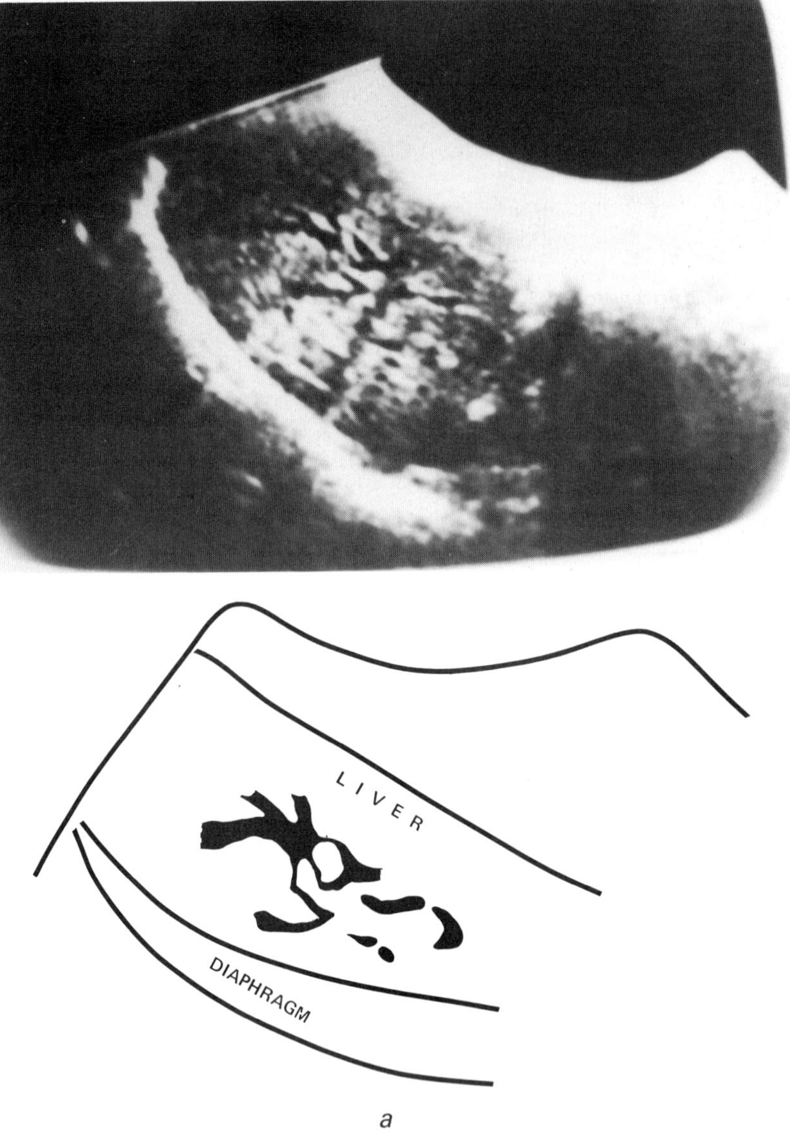

Fig. 69.12 Ultrasound examination of the liver, gallbladder and pancreas in a patient with severe cholestatic jaundice. *a*, Dilatation of the intrahepatic bile ducts.

100% in patients with dilated biliary tracts and exceeds 70% in the absence of bile duct dilatation. The reported accuracy of PTC in detecting the level and cause of the biliary obstruction averages 90% (*Fig.* 69.13). Nowadays, the procedure is carried out under sedation using the Chiba (also known as 'skinny') 22-gauge needle which has an external diameter of 0·7 mm. The use of the *Chiba* needle has largely replaced the thicker *Longdwel* trocar-cannula because of the higher success rate and a lower incidence of complications. The procedure must be covered with systemic antibiotic therapy (usually an aminoglycoside or cephalosporin or pipericillin) and any clotting abnormality must be corrected with vitamin K and/or the administration of fresh frozen plasma prior to its performance.

Preoperative percutaneous external transhepatic biliary drainage (*Fig.* 69.14) is seldom performed nowadays since several clinical trials have shown no benefit from the procedure in terms of reduced operative morbidity and mortality in severely jaundiced patients and the technique predisposes to infection of the obstructed biliary tract unless a closed collecting system which incorporates bacterial filters is used. However, the percutaneous insertion of endoprostheses (in-dwelling stents introduced over guidewires and positioned through the obstruction by means of pusher tubes) is a valuable method of palliation of patients with large bile duct obstruction due to inoperable/incurable malignancy (*Fig.* 69.15).

The complications of PTC include:

Septicaemia
Bile leakage
Haemorrhage: free bleeding into the peritoneal cavity and haemobilia
Bile embolization
Intrahepatic arterioportal fistula
Pneumothorax
Contrast reactions.

The reported incidence of major complications with the

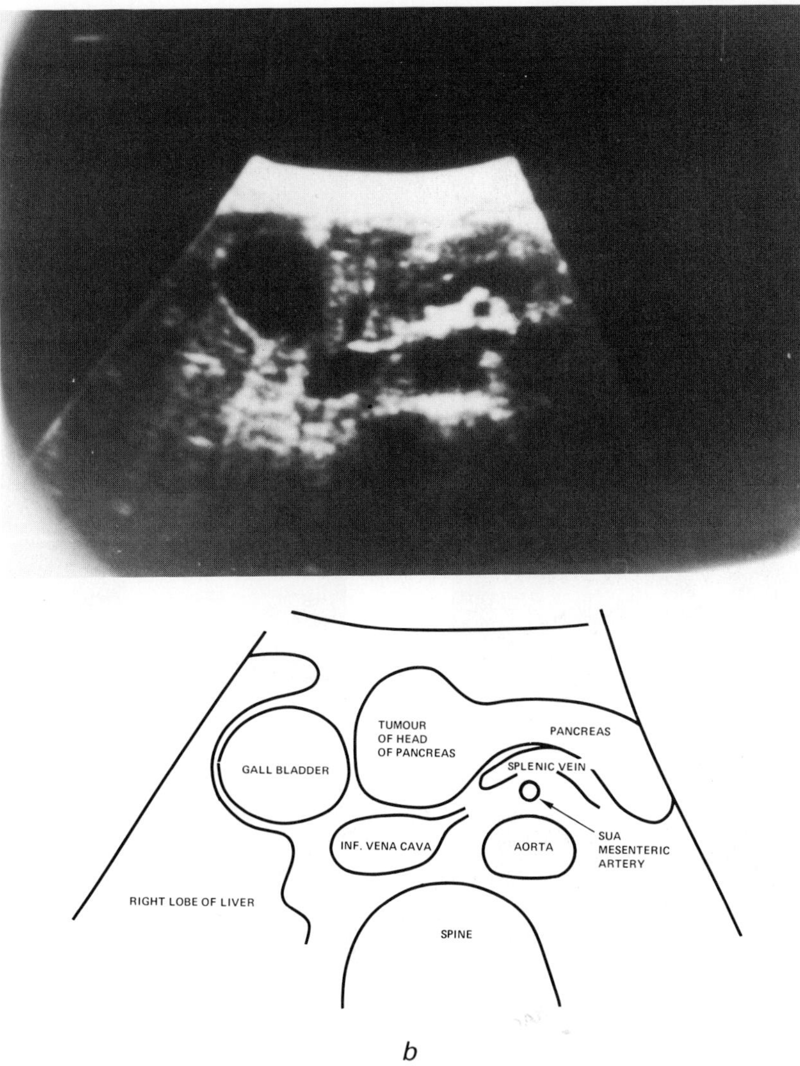

[Fig. 69.12 continued] *b*, Dilated gallbladder and mass in the head of the pancreas which on needle biopsy was shown to be an adenocarcinoma.

Chiba needle varies from 3 to 10% with a mortality of 0·1–0·3%.

Endoscopy and Endoscopic Retrograde Cholangio-pancreatography (ERCP)

Upper gastrointestinal endoscopy with a forward- or oblique-viewing panendoscope should be performed in jaundiced patients as significant gastrointestinal pathology is encountered in 25% of jaundiced patients.

ERCP, which is performed through a side-viewing endoscope, provides useful information in patients with cholestatic jaundice irrespective of whether the ductal system is dilated or not. In experienced hands, successful cholangiography is achieved by ERCP in over 90% of cases. The advantages of ERCP over PTC include:

It permits concomitant endoscopic examination and biopsy of lesions encountered during the endoscopic examination although the examination of the stomach and duodenum is more difficult and less optimal than with a forward- or oblique-viewing endoscope.

A pancreatogram can be obtained during the same investigation.

Certain lesions can be treated or palliated during the procedure, e.g. endoscopic stone removal, endoscopic nasobiliary drainage, and stent insertion for inoperable malignant large bile duct obstruction.

ERCP is, however, more difficult to perform than PTC and is not available generally. The procedure is well tolerated. Diagnostic ERCP has a very low morbidity largely due to pancreatitis (1·0%) and mortality (0·1%). The morbidity of interventional (therapeutic) ERCP, especially sphincterotomy, is, however higher (6–10%). The complications which usually follow endoscopic sphincterotomy are:

Haemorrhage
Acute pancreatitis
Cholangitis
Retroperitoneal perforation
Impacted Dormia basket
Acute cholecystitis
Gallstone ileus.

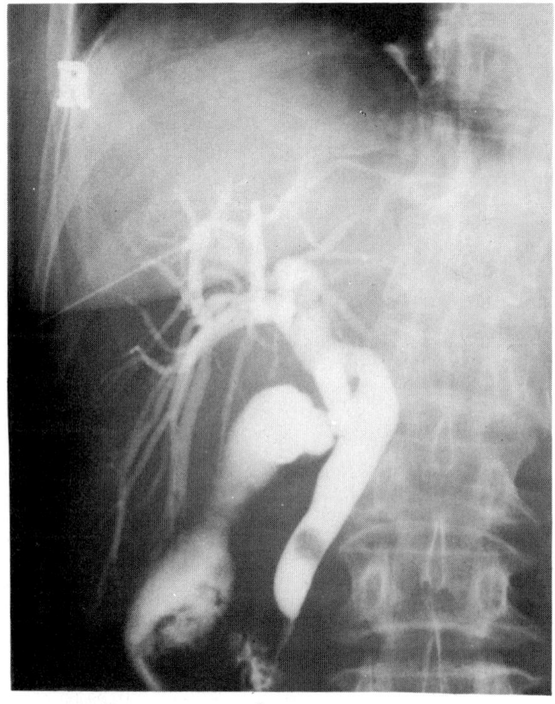

a

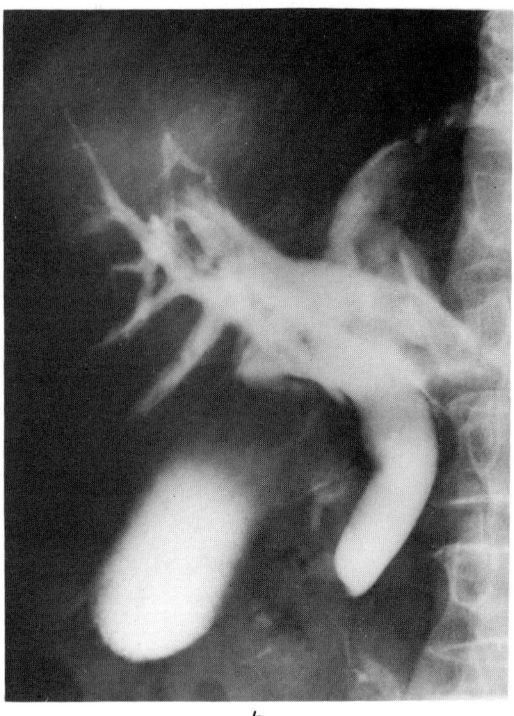

b

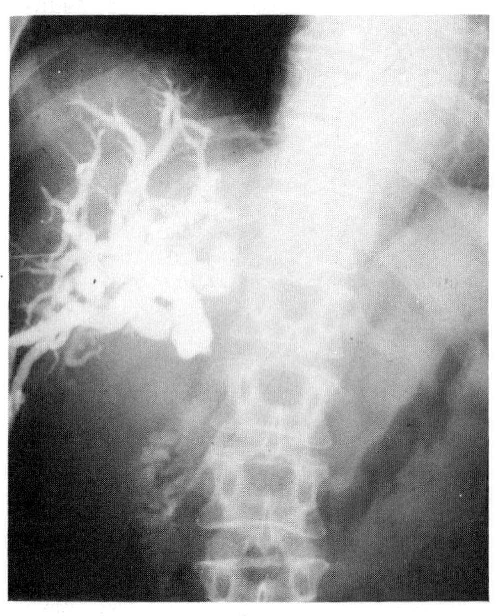

c

Fig. 69.13 Percutaneous transhepatic cholangiograms. *a*, Ductal calculi. *b*, Carcinoma of the pancreas. *c*, Bile duct stricture (iatrogenic).

The immediate mortality of endoscopic sphincterotomy averages 1·0%, although the 30-day mortality is 3%. Long-term stenosis after endoscopic sphincterotomy is rare and has not been a problem to date.

ERCP is very accurate in the diagnosis of ductal calculi (*Fig.* 69.16), tumours of the bile ducts (*Fig.* 69.17) and pancreas (*Figs.* 69.18 and 69.19) and sclerosing cholangitis. In patients with complete biliary obstructive lesions, the proximal biliary tree may not be visualized. These patients require further investigation with PTC. ERCP is less accurate than ultrasound and oral cholecystography in the diagnosis of gallbladder disease and gallstones.

Technical failure of an attempted ERCP examination may be due to:

Duodenal or pyloric stenosis
Previous Billroth II gastrectomy
Duodenal diverticulum
Uncooperative patient
Inexperience with the procedure.

Biliary Scintiscanning

The most widely used radiopharmaceutical compounds are $^{99}Tc^{m}$-labelled compounds of IDA (iminodiacetic acid) and EHIDA (diethylacetanilido-iminodiacetic acid). These agents which are powerful gamma emitters, are administered intravenously, whereupon they are selectively taken up by the hepatocytes and secreted into the bile. They are therefore ideal for the imaging of the biliary tree by a gamma camera, especially since their uptake by the liver and excretion into the biliary tract is not influenced by the presence of cholestasis.

EHIDA-cholescintiscanning is the most accurate test of acute cholecystitis irrespective of its nature (acute calculous obstructive, acalculous cholecystitis) and establishes the diagnosis within one hour of the intravenous administration of the radiopharmaceutical agent. A diagnosis of acute cholecystitis can be confidently made if the scintigram shows prompt excretion and a normal common bile duct with entry of isotope into the duodenum, *but the gallbladder is not imaged* (*Fig.* 69.20). The information is stored on magnetic tape/disc for more detailed computer analysis at a later stage. Cholescintiscanning has a sensitivity of 91–97% and a specificity of 87% for the diagnosis of acute cholecystitis. A normal gallbladder scintiscan is virtually 100% accurate in

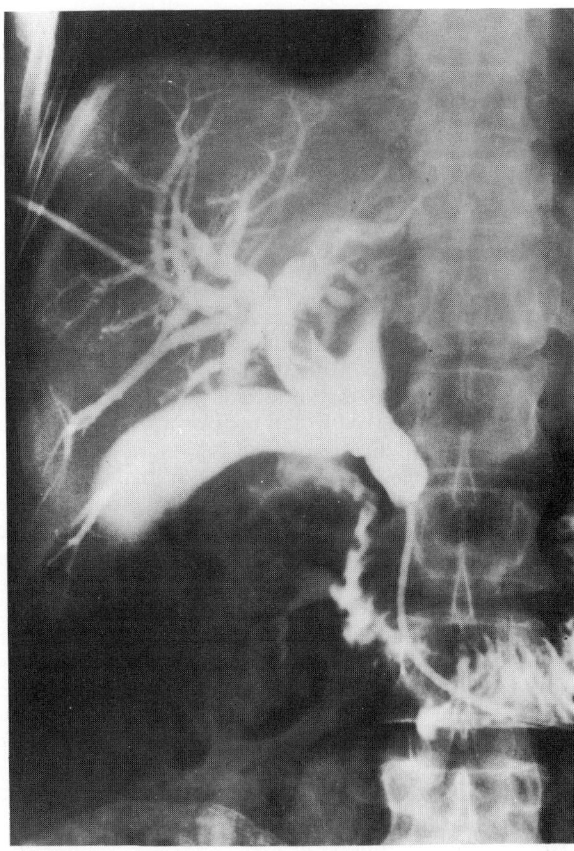

Fig. 69.14 Preoperative external biliary decompression for complete obstruction due to carcinoma of the pancreas. This technique is seldom used nowadays except as a prelude to insertion of an endoprosthesis for palliation of complete obstruction caused by inoperable pancreaticobiliary malignancy.

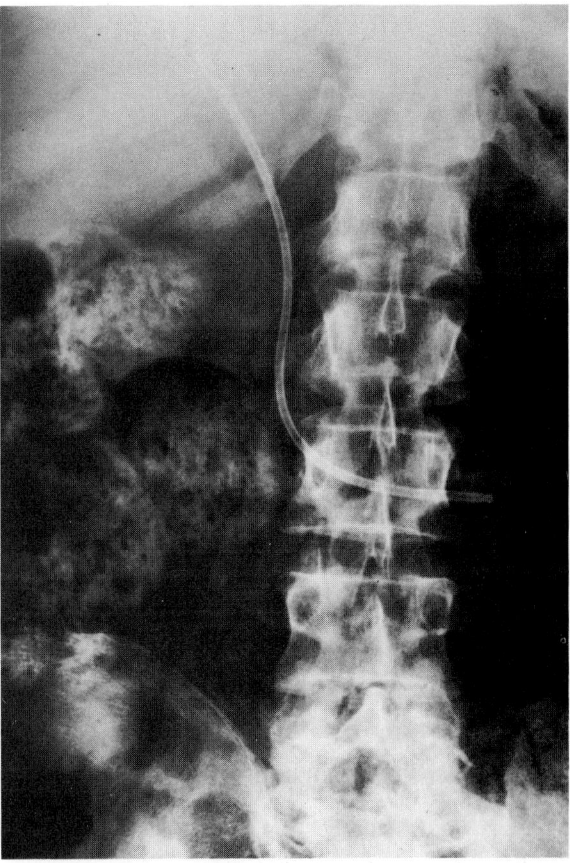

Fig. 69.15 Endoprosthesis through an incurable carcinoma of the head of the pancreas. The radio-opaque stent has side holes to drain bile from the intrahepatic biliary tree proximal to the tumour. Large stents are introduced nowadays (10–12 F) to minimize the tendency to blockage by calcium bilirubinate deposit. Replacement of the stents is often required because of blockage if the patient survives beyond 3 months.

excluding cholecystitis. False-positives are encountered in:

Chronic cholecystitis
Gallstone pancreatitis
Patients with alcoholic liver disease
Patients receiving parenteral nutrition.

Biliary scintiscanning has also been used to evaluate the jaundiced patient with a bilirubin greater than 50 μmol/l. Hepatocellular disease is diagnosed when poor liver excretion and intestinal activity are demonstrated after 18 hours of injection. Complete biliary obstruction is denoted by the absence of any intestinal activity after 18 hours, and partial obstruction by normal liver excretion, dilated ducts and delayed intestinal activity. However, biliary scintigraphy is not used routinely for the investigation of the jaundiced patient since other techniques (e.g. ultrasound and cholangiography) give more precise information of the underlying pathology. The exception to the above is provided by jaundice in the neonate where biliary scintigraphy and estimation of faecal radioactivity following the intravenous injection of the isotope is one of the routine tests used for the diagnosis of biliary atresia.

EHIDA scintigraphy is also very useful for the functional evaluation of surgically constructed bilio-enteric anastomoses (*Fig.* 69.21). EHIDA scintiscanning after gallbladder contraction induced by a milk meal or intravenous CCK is used to quantitate enterogastric reflux. Normal individuals reflux less than 5–10% of the administered dose of the radionuclide.

Peroperative Cholangiography

This is now considered to be an integral part of cholecystectomy and should be performed routinely and well. It provides a road map of the biliary tree and will indicate the need, or otherwise, for exploration of the common bile duct. It is performed by means of a variety of metal or polyethylene cannulas inserted into the common bile duct via the cystic duct. In postcholecystectomy states, operative cholangiography is usually carried out by direct puncture of the common duct using a fine intravenous type cannula or transhepatically, by means of a Chiba needle. When the gallbladder is deemed normal, cystic duct cannulation is not performed as this necessitates cholecystectomy. Instead, transcholecystic cholangiography (through the gallbladder fundus) is performed.

Nowadays, water-soluble contrast media, such as sodium diatrizoate (25–50%), are used. The volume required depends on dilatation or otherwise of the biliary tract. An initial scout film (plain) is taken prior to injection. During routine cholecystectomy small amounts (2–3 ml) are injected

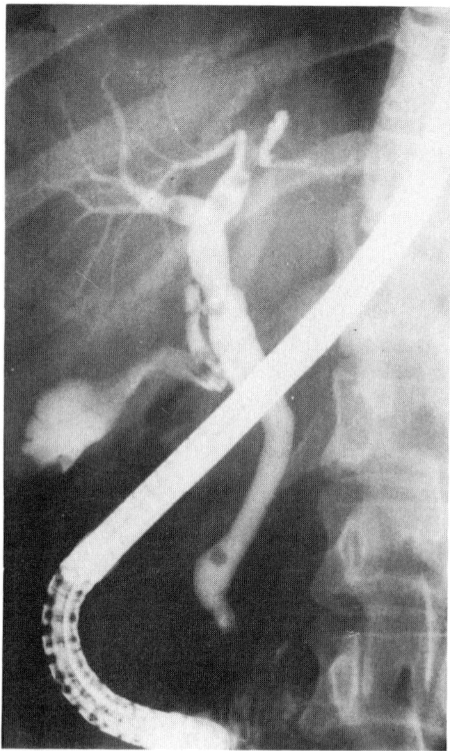

Fig. 69.16 ERCP outlining ductal calculi.

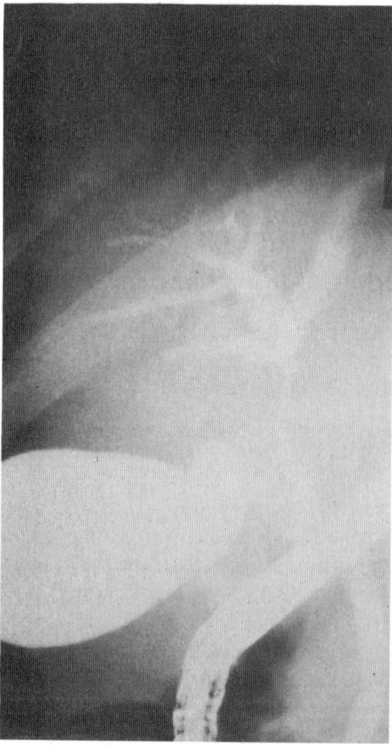

Fig. 69.17 ERCP showing a hilar cholangiocarcinoma.

before the first film if biliary fluoroscopy (image intensification) is not available, since excessive initial filling may be harmful (from cholangiovenous reflux due to the high pressure generated in the ductal system) and obscure small calculi which may therefore be overlooked. The second film is taken after the injection of a further 3 ml and the third exposure follows an additional 3 ml of contrast medium. The table should be rotated 15° to the right to obviate an intervening spinal column and the films should be taken with the operating table in a slight Trendelenburg tilt (10–20°).

With experience and meticulous technique, both false-negative and positive rates of peroperative cholangiography are low. Avoidance of haemoclips, whenever possible, is desirable as they may obscure small filling defects. The most common artefact leading to unnecessary exploration of the common bile duct, remains the air bubble which can be prevented by ensuring that the delivery system is air-free. If air bubbles are observed within the plastic cannula leading from the syringe, *aspiration should be avoided as this introduces air into the bile duct from the duodenum*. In this situation, the syringe should be disconnected from the cannula, the external end of which is held low, by the side of the drapings, such that the hydrostatic pressure of bile will slowly fill the cannula and clear any air bubbles, when the syringe is then reconnected to the system. Small blood clots, the tips of the transverse processes of the second lumbar vertebra, calcified costal cartilage, overlying gas shadows and a contracted choledochal sphincter with its meniscus effect, can also be misinterpreted as ductal calculi.

The important rules governing the performance and interpretation of peroperative cholangiography are:

Overfilling of the ductal system must be avoided.

Unequivocal flow into the duodenum must be demonstrated.

Both the intra- and extrahepatic bile ducts must be visualized. Non-filling of the intrahepatic biliary tree is always pathological and cannot be ignored. The most common cause for this during peroperative cholangiography is a hilar cholangiocarcinoma.

If doubt exists regarding the interpretation of any abnormalities, expert radiological advice should be sought (*Fig.* 69.22). Ideally, a radiologist should see and comment on the films or fluoroscopic examination routinely.

A completion T-tube cholangiogram is performed after common bile duct exploration although this is being replaced by completion choledochoscopy (*vide infra*) in many centres. Before injecting contrast, the T-tube and the extrahepatic bile duct is filled with about 60 ml of saline to remove air bubbles. Spasm of the choledochal sphincter is common after biliary manipulations during common bile duct exploration (e.g. passage of balloon catheters, etc.). This may result in a hold-up of contrast in the lower end of the bile duct. It is easily differentiated from missed organic obstruction by the intravenous administration of spasmolytic agents such as glucagon or ceruletide, etc. (*Fig.* 69.23).

The technique of *contact selective cholangiography* provides detailed anatomical information on the lower end of the common bile duct (*Fig.* 69.24). It is not used routinely but is helpful in the delineation of the pathological anatomy of the Vaterian segment of the bile duct especially during secondary biliary intervention. The technique requires mobilization of the duodenum and the head of the pancreas. This is followed by the insertion of a sterile dental film behind these mobilized structures.

Complications of peroperative cholangiography are rarely encountered and are usually due to either hypersensitivity to the contrast material or to an excessive injection pressure.

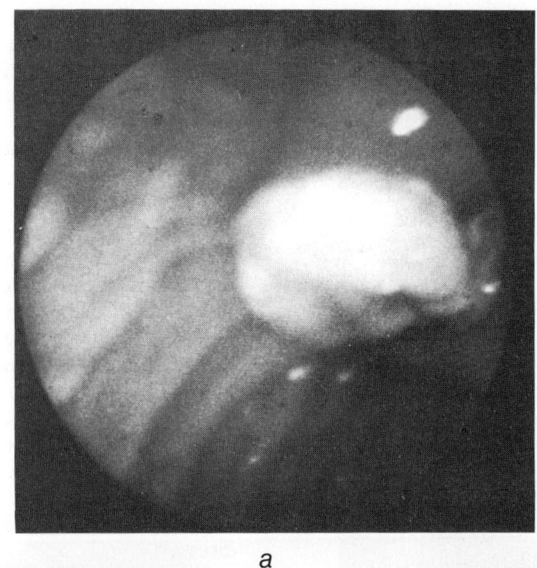

a

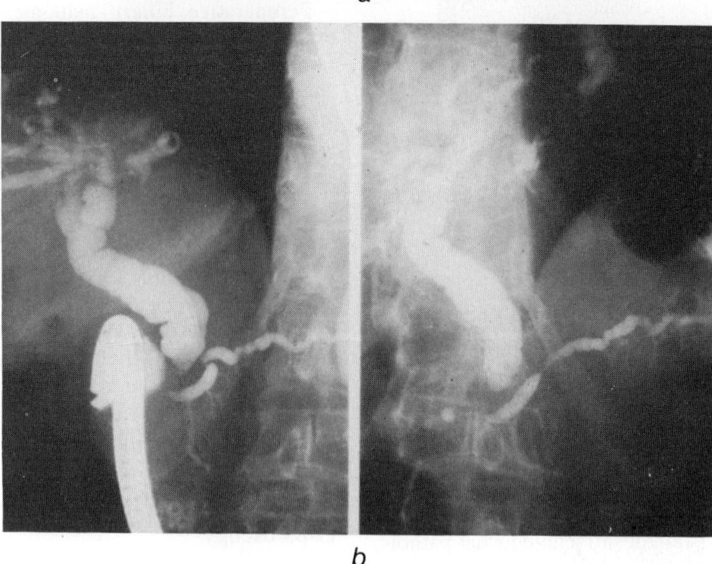

b

Fig. 69.18 *a*, Endoscopic view of a periampullary lesion of the pancreas. *b*, Cholangiopancreatogram of the same patient.

The latter can result in cholangiovenous reflux and bacteraemia especially in patients with cholangitis.

Choledochoscopy (Cholangioscopy)

Operative choledochoscopy is now well established in biliary tract surgery and is considered an integral part of common bile duct exploration. Two types of choledochoscopes are available: the flexible fibreoptic instrument and the rigid Berci–Shore choledochoscope which incorporates the Hopkin's rod lens system (*Fig.* 69.25). The rigid instrument is easier to use than the flexible endoscope and permits therapeutic manoeuvres, such as the removal under visual guidance of calculi impacted at the lower end of the common bile duct. Both instruments require saline irrigation. In most instances, gravity feed using a litre bag of saline suspended on a drip stand provides sufficient flow for adequate visualization. If not, a Fenwal pressure cuff is applied to the saline bag and insufflated to a pressure of 150–200 mmHg. However, care must be used with this system especially with the flexible endoscope (which has a wider irrigation channel) since high pressures may be generated in the biliary tract causing cholangiovenous reflux and bacteraemia. An adequate mobilization of the first and second part of the duodenum is essential for choledochoscopic inspection of the distal common bile duct. As the mobilized duodenum is put on the stretch, it straightens the lower end of the common bile duct (which normally curves acutely to the right) and this facilitates choledochoscopic inspection whether it is performed by the flexible or the rigid instrument.

The choledochoscope is introduced through a small choledochotomy in the supraduodenal part of the common bile duct. The initial inspection establishes the pathology, e.g. stones, tumour, etc. Removal of the stones can be performed under vision if the rigid instrument with the attached instrument channel is used. Either a biliary balloon catheter or a Dormia basket is introduced and the stone extracted under visual guidance. For impacted stones, the stone-grasping forceps are attached to the rigid instrument

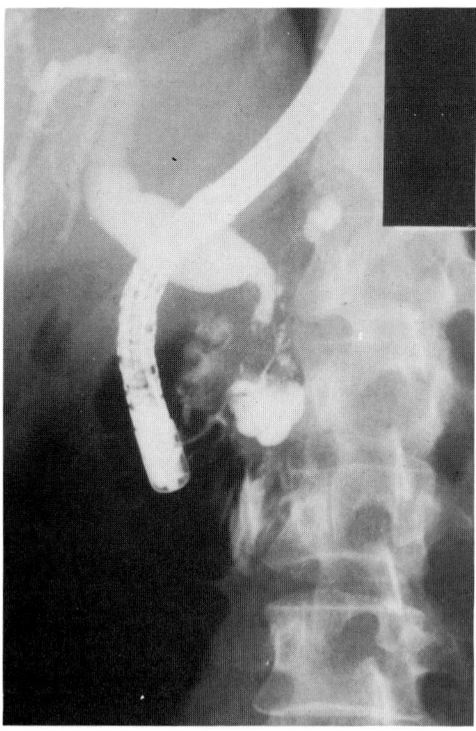

Fig. 69.19 ERCP showing a carcinoma of the head of the pancreas.

which is then re-introduced and the stone dislodged and retrieved or crushed under vision. Once all the stones have been removed (blind or under visual guidance), a completion choledochoscopic examination of the entire biliary tract is performed before the insertion of a T-tube. Completion choledochoscopy is replacing completion T-tube cholangiography in many centres.

The advantages of choledochoscopy are:

It provides a better evaluation of intracholedochal pathology.
It allows biopsy of suspicious lesions (*Fig.* 69.26).
The rigid instrument with the attached stone forceps provides an effective, safe and easy method of dealing with the problem of impacted calculi.
The routine use of completion choledochoscopy results in an almost negligible incidence of retained ductal calculi.
It reduces the incidence of trauma especially to the lower end of the bile duct caused by blind instrumentation with metal sounds and forceps.
The flexible endoscope provides an effective method of stone extraction of retained ductal calculi through the T-tube tract.

Biliary Manometry

Biliary pressure studies can be performed peroperatively or endoscopically during ERCP using a special perfusion catheter. Peroperative biliary manometry can be performed by the use of a pressure transducer connected to the cannula which is inserted into the common bile duct via the cystic duct. The transducer is attached to a channel recorder which gives an instant display of the biliary pressure. This technique is known as radiomanometry and permits the measurement of the basal (resting) pressure, and the filling pressure during the constant infusion of saline (5·0 ml/min). In addition, it demonstrates the sphincteric contractions and is used to document the effect of spasmolytic drugs on the choledochal sphincter in patients with biliary dyskinesia (*Fig.* 69.27).

The other technique used during biliary tract surgery is known as mano-debimetry. This measures the passage (yield) pressure at the choledochal sphincter and the flow rate through the common channel into the duodenum. The technique was first described by Caroli (*Fig.* 69.28). The modern modification of the Caroli instrument is known as the Tondelli mano-debitometer. After measurement of the passage pressure, the upper limit of which is 25·0 cmH_2O, the calibrated reservoir (filled with saline or contrast medium) is raised to a standard height of 30 cm above the level of the common bile duct and the flow rate through the common channel measured from the rate of emptying of the reservoir per unit time. The normal flow rate measured in this way should exceed 12·0 ml/min. A high passage pressure and a diminished flow rate are indicative of obstructive disease.

Peroperative biliary manometry is not used routinely except in specialized centres. It can provide useful information on the rare disorders of sphincter function (stenosis, spasm, hypotonia) at the lower end of the bile duct. It also enhances the diagnostic yield of peroperative cholangiography.

Endoscopic biliary manometry is still not an established routine diagnostic procedure. It is performed by the use of a special perfusion catheter attached to an external transducer and has been used in the investigation of patients with persistent symptoms and pain after cholecystectomy in an attempt to characterize abnormalities of the sphincter (stenosis, dyskinesia). The procedure measures the basal sphincter pressure, the rate and propagation of sphincteric contractions and the response to pharmacological agents such as morphine and CCK. In patients with dyskinesia increased basal pressure, altered frequency and amplitude of phasic contractions, and reversal of the normal peristaltic direction (retrograde propulsion) have been reported.

Laparoscopy

This procedure can be extremely useful in problematic cases of jaundice. Laparoscopy which can be carried out under local anaesthesia after insufflation of the peritoneal cavity with nitrous oxide, provides the same facilities as mini-laparotomy which it has largely superseded. It allows the visualization of the liver, gallbladder and peritoneal contents. Laparoscopy is often used to detect hepatic disease, secondary tumour deposits and peritoneal dissemination. The procedure allows the clinician to perform target biopsies under vision and transhepatic or transcholecystic cholangiography at the one sitting. In some patients with chronic liver disease and a bleeding tendency, laparoscopic biopsy may be undertaken in preference to the blind percutaneous procedure as bleeding from the biopsy site can be controlled by diathermy coagulation at laparoscopy.

PREOPERATIVE MANAGEMENT OF THE JAUNDICED PATIENT

Adequate timing of the surgical intervention and preparation of the patient for surgery are essential in the management of patients with obstructive lesions of the biliary tract.

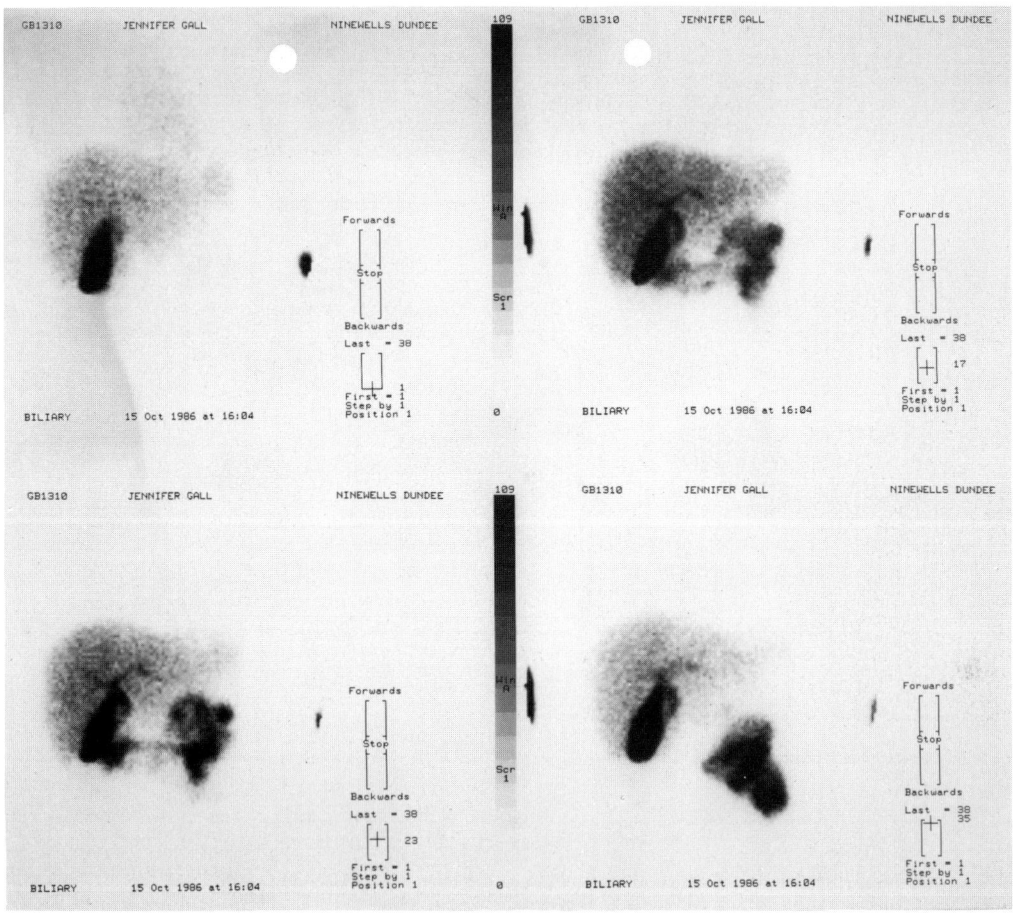

a

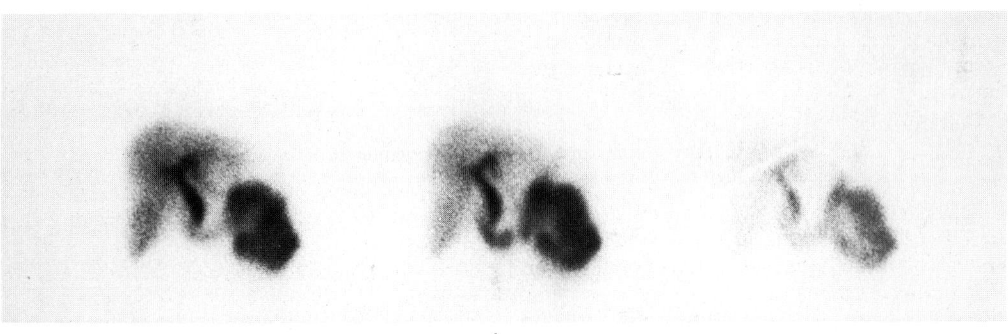

b

Fig. 69.20 Biliary scintigraphy with EHIDA. *a*, Normal cholescintigram. Both the gallbladder and the bile duct are imaged. *b*, Acute cholecystitis: a normal bile duct with prompt excretion into the duodenum is observed but the gallbladder is not outlined.

Undue delays exceeding 3–4 weeks increase both the morbidity and mortality rates following surgical intervention.

Adequate preparation entails the correction of metabolic abnormalities, improvement of the general condition and the institution of specific measures designed to minimize the incidence of complications associated with prolonged or severe cholestasis. These include:

Infections: cholangitis, septicaemia, wound infections
Disorders of the clotting mechanism
Renal failure
Liver failure
Fluid and electrolyte abnormalities.

Furthermore, the conjugation and metabolism of drugs and anaesthetic agents is impaired because of the hepatocyte malfunction. Contrary to popular belief, there is no evidence to support the view that wound healing is impaired in the presence of jaundice. Wound healing problems are largely confined to patients with malignant obstruction and are the result of the underlying disease and its association with a poor nutritional state.

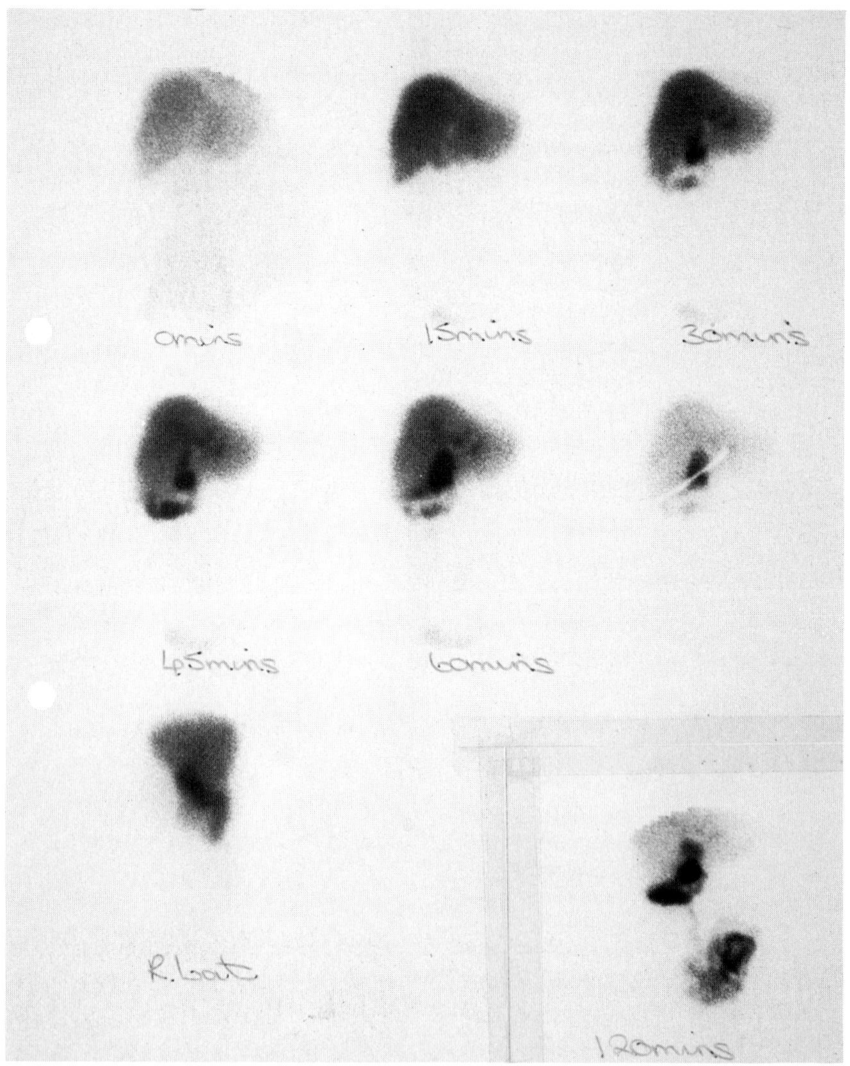

Fig. 69.21 EHIDA scintigram showing a functioning hepaticojejunostomy performed for a high bile duct stricture.

The nutritional deficits of these patients vary with the underlying pathology, age and social class of the patient. In general, parenteral nutrition should be used very selectively, and only in those patients who are grossly malnourished, because of infective risks. A high intake of carbohydrates is essential and amino acid solutions containing aromatic amino acids (phenylalanine, tyrosine and tryptophan) should be used sparingly as these may precipitate encephalopathy in susceptible patients. An oral diet is the safest and should be used whenever possible. It may be supplemented by elemental diets in nutritionally compromised patients. Some advocate the oral administration of bile salts and, more recently, lactulose to reduce the intestinal absorption of endotoxin from the intestinal microflora and thus minimize the incidence of renal failure following surgical intervention.

Hypokalaemia is frequently present and should be corrected. In general, intravenous isotonic saline administration should be restricted in the jaundiced patients and those with liver disease as the total exchangeable body sodium is elevated. The low normal values of the concentration of the serum sodium frequently encountered in these patients are due to expansion of the intra- and extravascular fluid compartments consequent on the excessive retention of water (dilutional hyponatraemia).

The hepatitis B antigen (HBsAg, HBeAg, *see* Chapter 10) status of all these patients should be ascertained at the outset and when the serology is positive, special precautions must be taken both in the ward and in the operating theatre to avoid spread of the infection to the attending medical staff. It is advisable that a strict barrier regimen should be instituted in such cases and particular attention paid at operation to avoid minor cuts amongst members of the operating team. Patients with the HBeAg antigen are especially likely to transmit the infection to the medical and nursing staff. There is now a good case for the vaccination of all surgeons and nurses against hepatitis B infection. In the event of mishap, vaccination with the hepatitis B vaccine together with the administration of high-titre anti-HBs immunoglo-

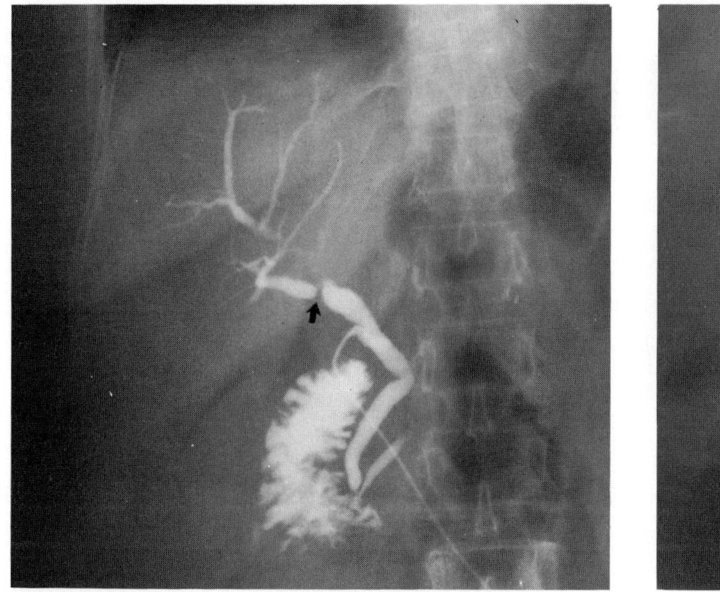

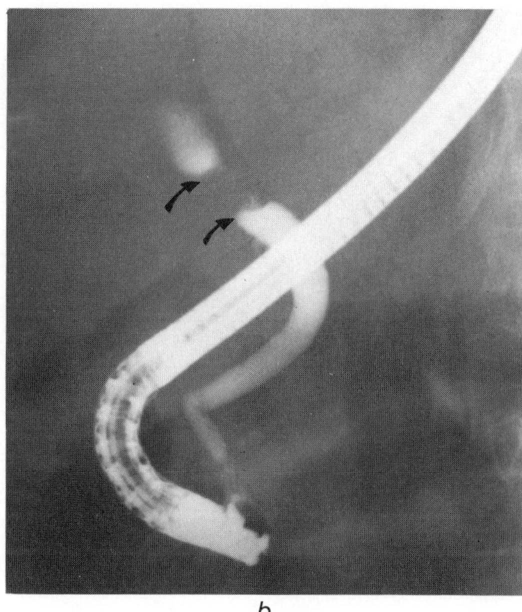

a b

Fig. 69.22 *a*, This well performed peroperative cholangiogram was interpreted as normal. The localized narrowing (arrowed) in the common hepatic duct was thought to be the result of an impression caused by the right hepatic artery. Aside from the obvious stricture, the left intrahepatic ductal system is not visualized. Regrettably, this was overlooked. *b*, The patient was referred to the author's unit 3 months later with deep jaundice. The ERCP showed an undoubted large carcinoma of the common hepatic duct (outlined between the arrows) which proved inoperable.

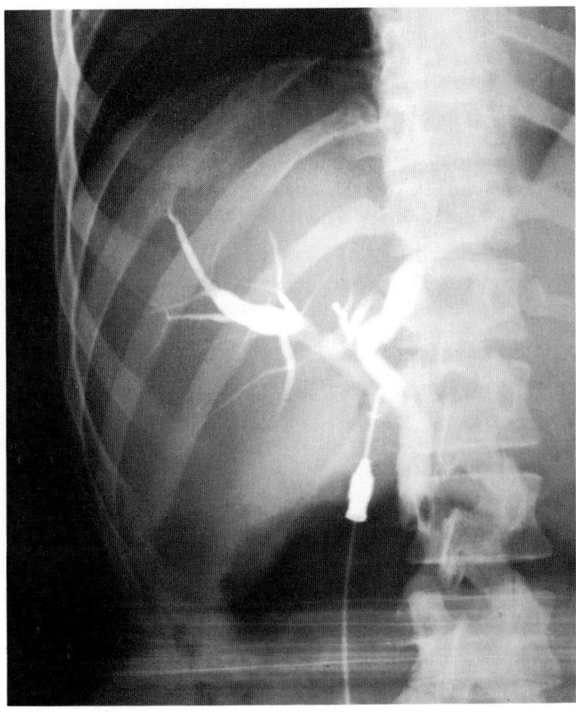

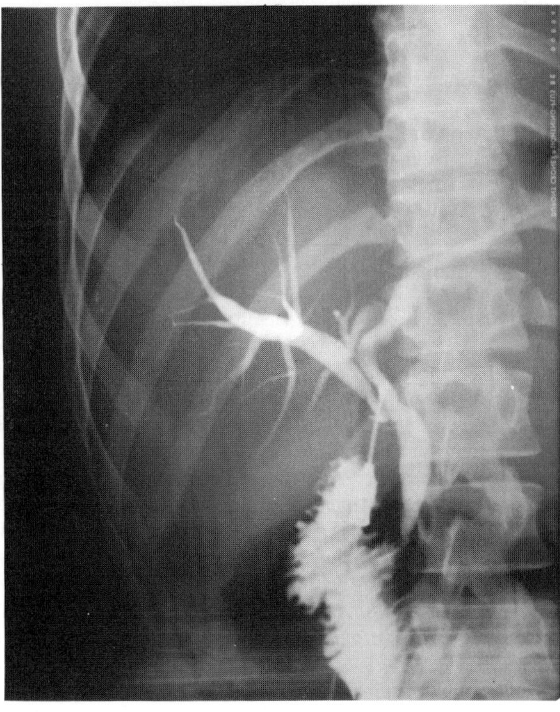

a b

Fig. 69.23 *a*, Completion peroperative T-tube cholangiogram. There is an apparent hold-up at the lower end which could be due to either spasm or a missed calculus. *b*, Repeat T-tube cholangiogram in the same patient after the administration of 1·0 μg ceruletide intravenously. There is now free flow of contrast medium into the duodenum.

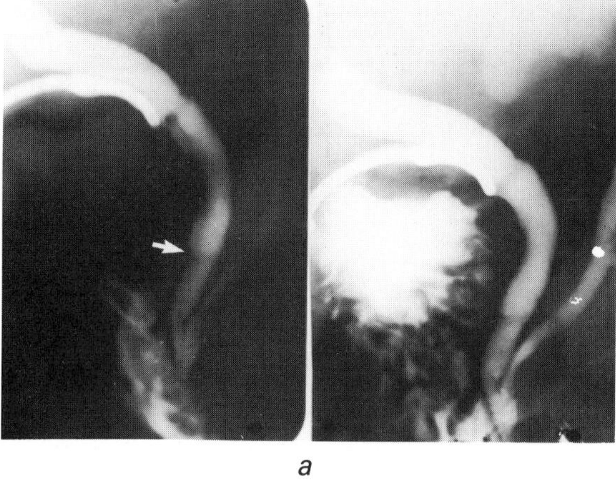

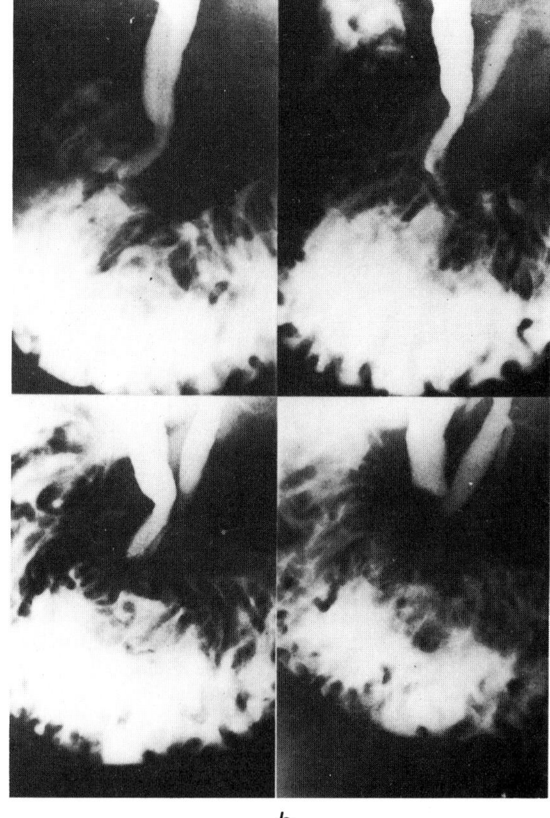

Fig. 69.24 Contact selective cholangiography. This is performed by the insertion of a sterile dental film behind the lower end of the bile duct and the head of the pancreas at operation. *a*, Details of the normal Vaterian segment of the common bile duct: the velvety fern-like pattern of the mucosal folds of the ampulla can be seen. The upper limit of the superior choledochal sphincter is depicted by a notch (arrow). *b*, Various phases of contraction of the lower sphincters surrounding the terminal segment of the common bile duct and the pancreatic duct. (By courtesy of Dr J. P. Yvergneaux.)

bulin is recommended. Normal human pooled gammaglobulin which protects against hepatitis A, is ineffective against hepatitis B infection. The general measures aimed at prevention of viral infection to the medical and nursing staff are outlined in Chapter 10.

Prevention of Infective Complications

Whereas the normal biliary tract and bile in the human is sterile, bacteria are frequently present in biliary tract disorders and may lead to septic complications, particularly cholangitis and septicaemia. Infection of the biliary tract is much more commonly present in ductal calculous disease than in patients with malignant obstructive jaundice.

Anaerobes are much less frequently found in the biliary tract and duodenum than aerobic bacteria even in the presence of pathological states. The majority of infections associated with biliary tract disorders are aerobic in origin and most commonly due to Gram-negative bacilli.

A number of clinical trials have shown that the postoperative sepsis in patients having biliary tract surgery is generally due to bacteria in the bile and the use of short-term prophylactic antibiotics (3-dose regimen perioperatively: immediately before surgery to 24 hours later) significantly lowers the incidence of sepsis only in patients who have bacteria in the bile at the time of surgery. Prophylactic antibiotics are therefore not advised in all patients undergoing surgery on the biliary tract but should be administered to those patients who are likely to have bacteria in the bile.

These higher risk groups have been identified and include:

All jaundiced patients
Patients with rigors and pyrexia
Patients undergoing emergency biliary procedures/operations
Elderly patients
Patients with common duct stones even if not jaundiced
Patients undergoing secondary biliary intervention.

Some advocate the use of Gram's staining of the bile at the time of surgery to determine both the presence and the Gram characteristics of the organisms in deciding on the appropriate antibiotic. The use of prophylactic antibiotic therapy with a cephalosporin, or aminoglycoside or pipericillin (3 doses) in the high risk groups outlined above has been shown to reduce the incidence of postoperative wound infection, cholangitis and septicaemia.

Bacterial proliferation in the bile following exploration of the common bile duct and insertion of a T-tube is extremely common and may become a source of infection or lead to the formation of calcium bilirubinate stones as a result of the deconjugation of the bilirubin–glucuronide by glucuronidase-producing bacteria, particularly *E. coli*. Thus, a closed system of T-tube drainage should always be used and a bile culture performed a few days prior to the removal of the T-tube. A course of the appropriate antibiotic should be administered if the culture is positive.

Correction of Disorders of Coagulation

The most common disorder of coagulation encountered in patients with large bile duct obstruction is a prolonged

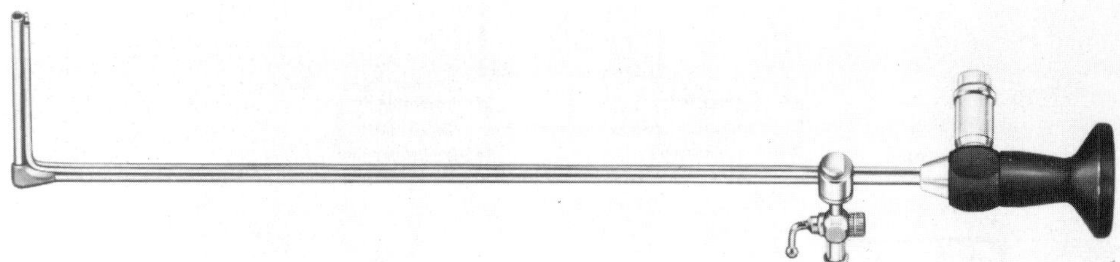

a

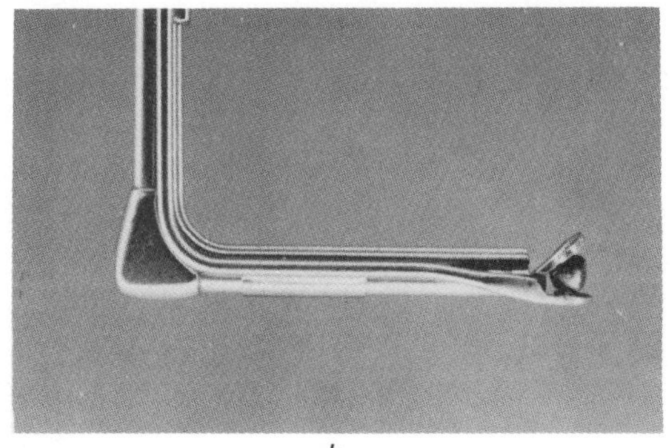

b

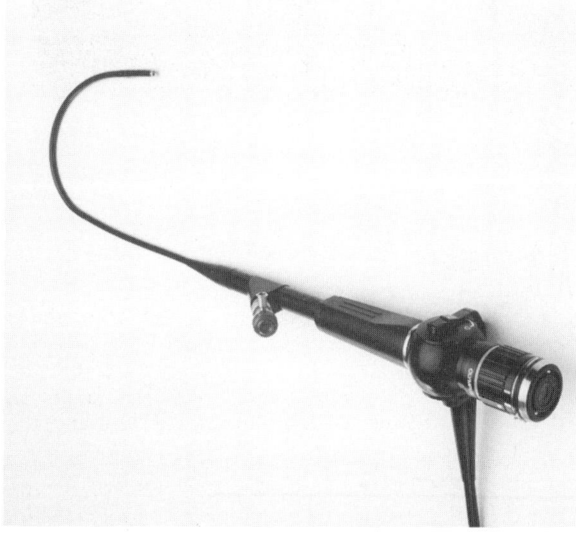

c

Fig. 69.25 *a*, The rigid choledochoscope (Berci–Shore). It has an attachable instrument channel through which biopsy forceps, biliary balloon catheters, Dormia baskets can be passed into the bile duct for visually-guided procedures such as stone extraction and biopsy of lesions. *b*, In addition, it has an attachable strong stone forceps which moves together with the instrument and is extremely useful for dealing with impacted stones at the lower end of the bile duct. The stone can be dislodged and retrieved or crushed under vision. (By courtesy of the publishers of *Common Bile Duct Exploration*, Cuschieri and Berci, 1984, Martin Nijhoff B.V.) *c*, The Olympus flexible choledochoscope.

prothrombin time resulting from a deficiency of vitamin K-dependent factors consequent on the malabsorption of this vitamin which occurs in cholestatic jaundice. The intramuscular injection of phytomenadione (10–20 mg) will reverse the multifactorial clotting deficiency within 1–3 days. Severe hepatic disease, usually with a poor prognosis, is present if the prothrombin time remains abnormally prolonged despite this treatment. If these patients require surgical intervention, administration of fresh frozen plasma is necessary to cover the perioperative period.

A more serious bleeding disorder may arise usually in the severely jaundiced patient who may develop a consumptive coagulopathy from a disseminated intravascular coagulation due to the presence of circulating endotoxin. This serious haematological complication requires careful monitoring of fibrinogen levels, fibrinogen degradation products and platelet counts. It may improve with control of the infection but often requires specific treatment with fresh frozen plasma alone or in combination with heparin. The management of this complication is outlined in Chapter 9.

Prevention of Renal Failure

The association between postoperative renal failure and severe conjugated hyperbilirubinaemia is well known but the underlying mechanism of the renal impairment is inadequately understood, although a reduced glomerular filtration is usually present. Even in the absence of infection, endotoxinaemia is frequently present in jaundiced patients when it results from absorption of endotoxin produced by the intestinal microflora. There appears to be a relationship between impaired renal function and the presence of circulating endotoxin in jaundiced patients.

Irrespective of the exact cause of the renal damage, there

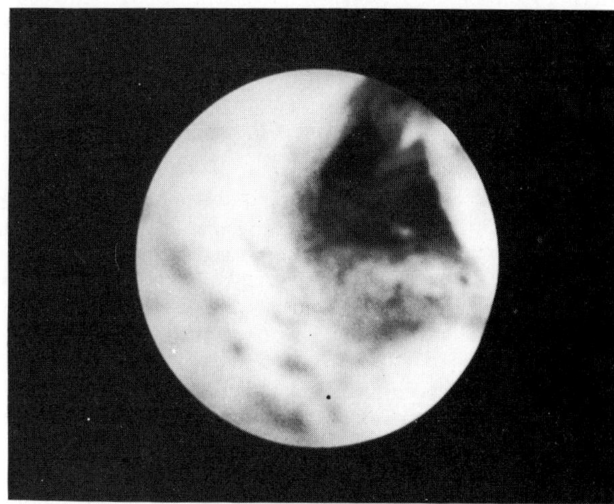

Fig. 69.26 Choledochoscopic view of a stenosing lesion of the common hepatic duct. An endoscopic biopsy confirmed the presence of a cholangiocarcinoma.

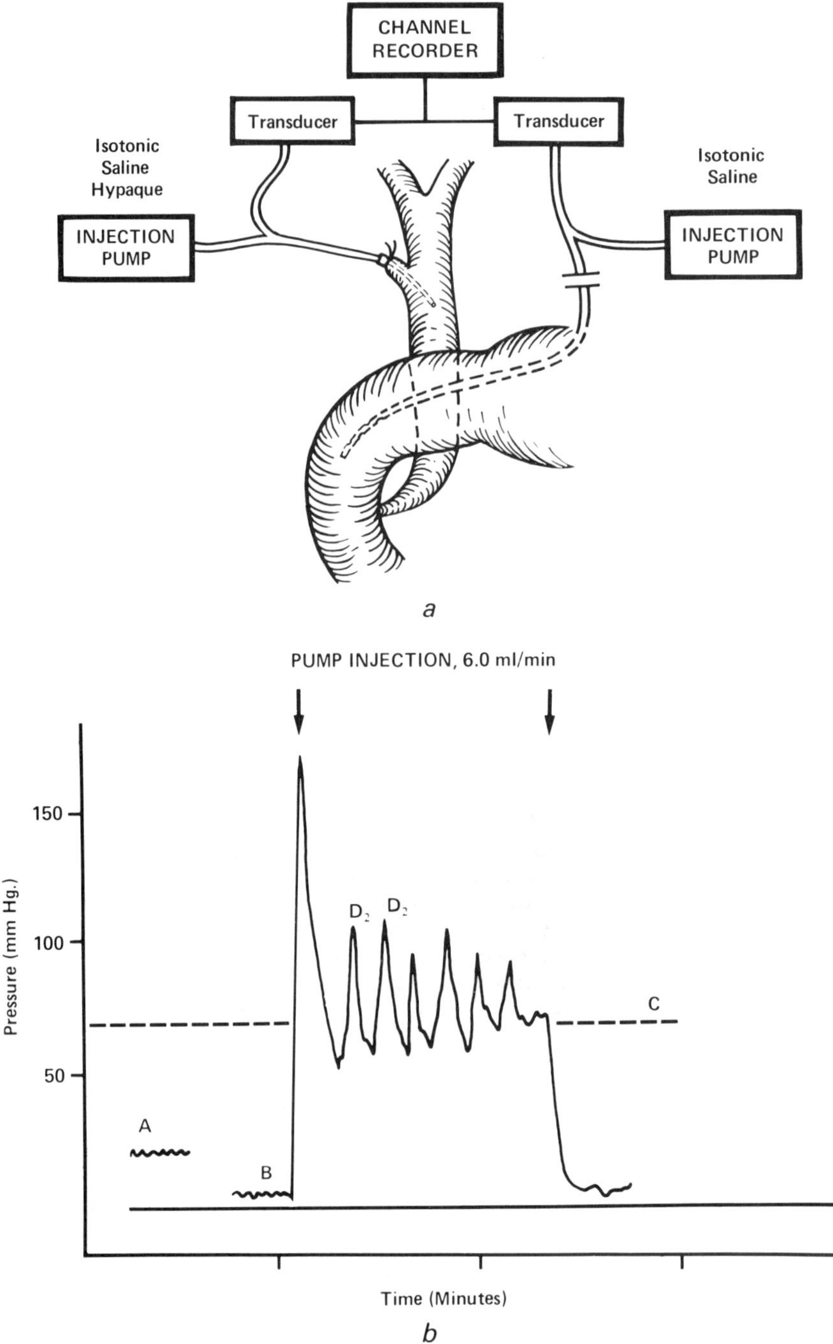

Fig. 69.27 Peroperative radiomanometry. *a*, Apparatus. *b*, Normal pressure profile of the common bile duct during constant pump infusion of isotonic saline: A, Pressure generated by the pump and intrinsic resistance of the system. B, Basal bile duct pressure. C, Filling pressure during injection. D, Contractions of the sphincter of Oddi.

is now good evidence that adequate hydration and preoperative induction of a natriuresis/diuresis reduces the incidence of renal failure after surgical intervention in jaundiced patients. It is current routine practice to administer intravenous fluids (5% dextrose) for 12–24 hours before surgery. This is followed by an osmotic diuretic (mannitol) or a loop diuretic (frusemide) administered intravenously at the time of induction of anaesthesia. All patients undergoing surgery should be catheterized and the urine output measured hourly. Further administration of diuretics (mannitol or frusemide) is indicated if the urine output falls consistently below 40 ml/hour (despite adequate hydration and normovolaemia) during operation and subsequently thereafter.

Preoperative administration of oral chenodeoxycholate commencing a few days before surgery is practised in some centres and one clinical trial has shown a reduction in the

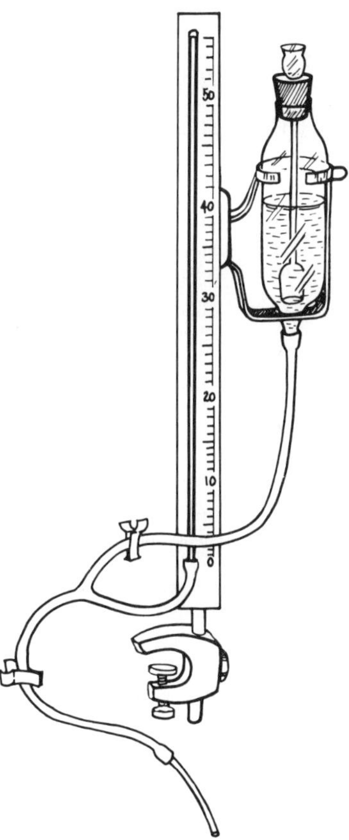

Fig. 69.28 The Caroli instrument for mano-debimetry. The technique measures the passage (yield) pressure of the choledochal sphincter and the flow rate through the common channel into the duodenum.

incidence of renal failure, although a second trial with the epimer, ursodeoxycholate, did not report any benefit. More recently, the administration of oral lactulose has been shown to reduce the incidence of renal failure in jaundiced patients undergoing surgical treatment but this requires confirmation.

Prevention of Hepatic Encephalopathy

Liver failure is usually encountered in patients with prolonged complete large bile duct obstruction or those patients with pre-existing chronic hepatocellular disease, such as cirrhosis, chronic active hepatitis, etc., who undergo surgery. If the jaundice is severe (above 150 μmol/l) or the patient shows signs of impending liver failure, a period of decompression is indicated. This is nowadays achieved by any of the following:

i. Insertion of endoprosthesis for patients with malignant obstruction. This can be performed endoscopically or percutaneously through the transhepatic route.

ii. Sphincterotomy in patients with ductal calculous disease or periampullary cancer.

External percutaneous decompression via a transhepatic tube draining into an external collecting system is no longer advocated since it predisposes to infection and leads to a loss of bile acids unless the bile is returned to the gastrointestinal tube via a nasogastric tube, but this is unpleasant and nausea provoking.

The correction of hypokalaemia, the restricted use of sedatives, hypnotics and potent analgesics, and the prompt treatment of infection cannot be overemphasized. If sedation is required, small doses of promethazine or chlorpromazine can be administered.

POSTOPERATIVE JAUNDICE

Jaundice occurring for the first time in the postoperative period may be due to a variety of causes (*Table* 69.2) and always requires detailed investigation to establish the cause and outline the necessary course of action.

Table 69.2 Causes of postoperative jaundice

SEPSIS	Leaking anastomosis, abscess formation, septicaemia, pneumonia, etc.
PRE-EXISTING LIVER DISEASE	Known or unsuspected
PRIMARY BILIARY PATHOLOGY	Residual stones, trauma and missed tumours of the biliary tract
MASSIVE BLOOD TRANSFUSION	Each unit of blood provides a bilirubin load of 250 mg/100 ml when fresh. Unconjugated hyperbilirubinaemia
HAEMOLYSIS	Unconjugated hyperbilirubinaemia, positive Coombs's test
RESIDUAL HAEMATOMAS	Unconjugated hyperbilirubinaemia
ADVERSE DRUG REACTIONS	
ANAESTHETIC AGENTS	Particularly halothane, less frequently methoxyflurane, thiopentone and cyclopropane
VIRAL HEPATITIS	Hepatitis B and non-A non-B hepatitis

A mild self-limiting conjugated hyperbilirubinaemia, sometimes referred to as *benign postoperative cholestasis* may follow prolonged operations and fever caused by chest infections. It is caused by a reactive hepatitis which is probably multifactorial in origin, resulting from a combination of reduced liver blood flow, hypoxia, hypercarbia, breakdown of transfused cells and temporary hepatocellular dysfunction. Initially, it warrants observation with repeated assessment of the patient's condition and sequential biochemical profiles, as the majority of cases with this syndrome subside within 3–4 weeks.

Severe or progressive jaundice in the postoperative period is always sinister and usually indicates a primary biliary tract problem, or significant liver disease or severe sepsis such as that resulting from an anastomotic dehiscence. Aside from the usual liver function tests, the following may be required:

Blood culture
Contrast radiological examination of recently constructed anastomoses
Ultrasound/CT scanning for the detection of abscesses
ERCP or PTC
Liver biopsy if hepatocellular disease or drug-induced jaundice is suspected.

Table 69.3 Drug-induced liver damage

Category	*Example*	*Hepatic lesion*
ANTIBIOTICS	Tetracyclines especially after i.v. use, dose related	Fatty infiltration
	Penicillins—hypersensitivity	Hepatitis
	Chloramphenicol	Hepatitis
	Sulphonamides—hypersensitivity	Granulomas, focal hepatocellular necrosis
ANALGESICS AND ANTI-INFLAMMATORY DRUGS	Paracetamol—dose dependent	Centrilobular necrosis—massive liver necrosis
	Phenylbutazone—hypersensitivity	Hepatitis with granuloma may progress to cirrhosis
	Carbamazepine	Cholestasis
	Salicylates—dose related	Focal hepatic necrosis
PSYCHOTROPIC DRUGS	Monoamine oxidase inhibitors	Hepatitis, may progress to massive hepatic necrosis
	Phenothiazines—hypersensitivity	Hepatitis and cholestasis
	Tricyclic antidepressants	Cholestatic hepatitis, more usually mild elevation of transaminases only
STEROIDS	Testosterone and anabolic steroids	Cholestasis, peliosis hepatis, hepatic tumours
	Oestrogens	Cholestasis, gallstones, hepatic tumours
ANAESTHETIC AGENTS	Halothane	Hepatitis which may progress to massive liver cirrhosis
ANTITUBERCULOUS DRUGS	PAS—hypersensitivity	Hepatitis
	INAH—occurrence related to acetylator status	Focal to severe hepatic necrosis
	Rifampicin—dose related	Defective bilirubin transport, mild hepatitis
CYTOTOXIC AND IMMUNOSUPPRESSIVE DRUGS	Azathioprine	Cholestasis and peliosis hepatis
	6-mercaptopurine—dose related	Hepatitis
	Methotrexate—long-term therapy	Fatty change, fibrosis of the portal tracts and cirrhosis
OTHERS	Benzothiazine diuretics	Cholestatic hepatitis
	Phenindione	Cholestatic hepatitis
	Chlorpropamide	Cholestatic hepatitis
	Phenytoin	Hepatocellular necrosis

Hepatitis B is rare nowadays because of better screening for the viral antigens and improved blood donor selection. Most instances of infection caused by blood and blood products are due to non-A non-B hepatitis (*see* Chapter 10). Drug-induced jaundice is common in hospital practice. Some of the important drugs which may give rise to this adverse reaction are listed in *Table* 69.3.

Severe hepatotoxicity can follow halothane anaesthesia. In the majority of patients (over 80%), this follows repeated exposure usually within 28 days (75%). The disease is usually severe and is accompanied by an overall mortality of 40%. The following recommendations have been issued by the Committee on the Safety of Medicines:

i. A careful history to determine previous exposure and reactions to halothane should be obtained from every patient.

ii. Repeated exposure to halothane within a period of at least 3 months should be avoided if at all possible.

iii. A history of unexplained jaundice or pyrexia following exposure to halothane is an absolute contraindication to further use of halothane in that individual patient.

Clinical Management of Postoperative Jaundice

In the first instance, a full examination of the patient and a careful reappraisal of the preoperative liver function tests are carried out. If liver function was normal prior to operation, the following are performed in a sequential order:

Determination of the nature of the jaundice by the liver function tests and urine testing for bilirubin.

Postoperative unconjugated hyperbilirubinaemia is most commonly due to large/massive transfusion. Each unit of blood provides a bilirubin load of 250 mg/100 ml of fresh blood. Unconjugated hyperbilirubinaemia may also result from resorption of residual haematoma/haemoperitoneum or haemolysis. Haemolytic reactions resulting from minor/major incompatibilities are accompanied by systemic signs (*see* Chapter 10). When suspected, screening tests for haemolysis should be performed.

If the jaundice is cholestatic, an assessment of all the drugs and anaesthetic agents used is followed by the withdrawal of any drug known to cause hepatotoxicity. A thorough search for sepsis by the appropriate tests (including blood cultures) is made. External leakage of bile or evidence of anastomotic dehiscence in a jaundiced patient is always serious and establishes the cause. In the absence of these, the liver function tests are repeated daily to determine the course of the biochemical profile. If the cholestasis is seen to be resolving, an expectant policy is adopted, otherwise radiological investigation with an ERCP or PTC is mandatory. If either of these two procedures excludes biliary tract pathology/trauma, a percutaneous liver biopsy is performed.

JAUNDICE IN INFANCY AND CHILDHOOD

Apart from the physiological jaundice, the aetiology of hyperbilirubinaemia in infancy may be due to haematological disorders, enzymatic defects, inborn errors of metabolism, infections and obstructive disease. The causes of jaundice in infancy and childhood are shown in *Table* 69.4. Whereas unconjugated hyperbilirubinaemia may be physiological, all causes of conjugated hyperbilirubinaemia are abnormal. Inflammatory disease of the gallbladder and cholelithiasis are rare but do occur, including acalculous cholecystitis. A higher percentage of gallstones in the paediatric age group is associated with haemolytic disorders than in the adult population. An increased incidence of gallstones is also found in patients with cystic fibrosis. Children with gallstones present with an atypical history of vague abdominal pain and distress. Classic biliary colic is rare. An ultrasound examination of the gallbladder or oral cholecystogram should be performed in all children undergoing splenectomy for haemolytic anaemia.

Table 69.4 Causes of jaundice in infancy and childhood

Physiological jaundice
Haematological disorders—inspissated bile plug
Enzymatic defects
Inborn errors of metabolism
Hepatitis and other infections
Biliary atresia
Biliary hypoplasia
Cystic disease of the bile ducts
Congenital perforation of the common bile duct

Biliary Atresia and Neonatal Hepatitis

The concept regarding the pathophysiology of these disorders proposed by Kasai has received widespread acceptance and they are now considered to be different manifestations of the same process, with atresia developing in infants who have a component of cholangitis which then progresses to fibrosis and obliteration of the extrahepatic ductal system. Experimentally, infection of mice and rhesus monkeys with retrovirus III results in congenital biliary atresia which is indistinguishable from the human disease in its pathological features and clinical course. Both biliary atresia and neonatal hepatitis present with jaundice (conjugated) at birth. Untreated biliary atresia leads to irreversible cirrhosis, often within 2–3 months of onset.

The diagnostic protocol carried out in these infants is designed to differentiate neonatal hepatitis from biliary atresia and the standard work-up, apart from liver function tests, includes screening for infectious, genetic and enzymatic disorders. Studies required include the Rose Bengal or EHIDA scan (in which there is no bile passage into the duodenum over 3–4 days in biliary atresia as assessed by faecal radioactivity), liver biopsy, and serial total bilirubin levels. A rising or flat bilirubin curve over several weeks is found in atresia whereas in neonatal hepatitis, there is a gradual fall in the serum bilirubin after an initial peak. Other congenital abnormalities, such as situs inversus and intestinal malrotation, may occur in association with biliary atresia.

The treatment of biliary atresia is surgical and must be carried out within 60 days of birth, otherwise the prognosis is poor from irreversible cirrhosis. At operation a cholecystocholangiogram (if the gallbladder is present) and a wedge liver biopsy are performed. If an extrahepatic stump of the common hepatic duct is present, a Roux-en-Y jejunal anastomosis is carried out. Hepatic portoenterostomy (the Kasai procedure) is performed if no extrahepatic ducts are discernible. The procedure consists of the progressive excision of fibrosed remnants of the ducts anterior to the portal vein at the porta hepatis together with a 1·0 cm ring of adjacent liver substance, advancing to some 2–3 cm in depth using the operating microscope until biliary structures are identified: bile ducts, collecting tubules of biliary glands or biliary glands. The excised scar tissue is subjected to histological examination to identify these structures. A modified Roux-en-Y anastomosis (Suruga II procedure) is then performed at the periphery of the saucerized area surrounding the bile ductules (*Fig.* 69.29). This has an access jejunostomy placed subcutaneously which allows irrigation, evaluation of postoperative bile flow and, if necessary, introduction of a paediatric flexible endoscope to inspect the porta hepatis. In an effort at reducing postoperative cholangitis due to reflux of intestinal contents, various valve constructions have been advocated between the portoenterostomy and the enteroenteric anastomosis. Some favour an isoperistaltic jejunal loop with a nipple valve interposed between the porta hepatis and the duodenum instead of the Roux-en-Y reconstruction.

An 80–90% successful outcome is obtained in infants in whom bile ducts communicating with the intrahepatic system have been identified at operation provided this is performed within 60 days of birth. These infants require vitamin E supplements to minimize the development of neurological sequelae. Overall, some 25% of these children

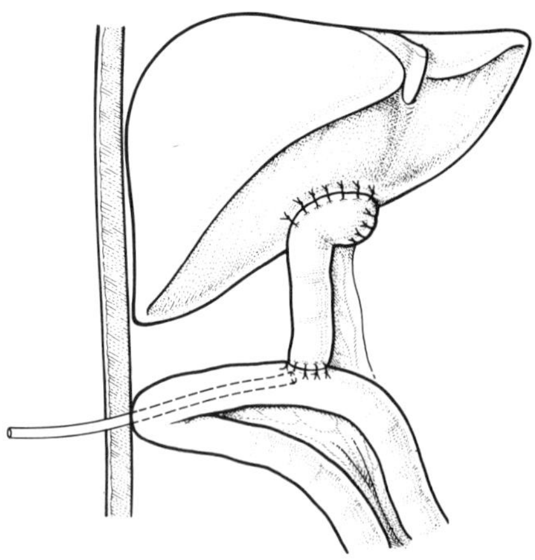

Fig. 69.29 The Suruga II procedure of intubated access jejunostomy in patients with biliary atresia.

develop cirrhosis and portal hypertension. Hepatic transplantation is now accepted as the treatment of choice in infants and children with biliary atresia in whom a portoenterostomy has failed and who develop cirrhosis.

Biliary Hypoplasia

This is usually secondary to another primary disorder, such as extrahepatic biliary atresia, choledochal cyst, neonatal hepatitis and alpha-1 antitrypsin deficiency. Early surgical treatment, when indicated, is designed to correct the primary abnormality.

Inspissated Bile Plug Syndrome

This condition is usually secondary to haemolytic disorders. The diagnosis is made by operative cholangiography and treatment, which is curative, consists of irrigation of the extrahepatic ducts.

Cystic Disease of the Biliary Tract

Cystic disease of the biliary tract is rare and in the USA accounts for 1 in 13 000 hospital admissions. The aetiology remains unknown. Most instances are thought to represent either congenital weakness of the common bile duct with distal obstruction caused by an anomalous acute or right-angle junction between the pancreatic duct and the common bile duct resulting in an abnormally long common channel (>0·6 cm). Another theory postulates an unequal proliferation of the duct epithelium. Several types are recognized (*Fig.* 69.30):

Type I Diffuse choledochal cystic dilatation commonest
Type II Localized dilatation of the supraduodenal bile duct
Type III Supraduodenal diverticulum
Type IV Intraduodenal diverticulum or choledochocele
Type V Solitary intrahepatic cyst
Type VI Multiple intrahepatic cysts (Caroli's disease)
Type VII Multiple intra- and extrahepatic cysts

Type VI (*Fig.* 69.31) which is a hereditary disorder (autosomal recessive) is known as Caroli's disease and carries a poor prognosis from recurrent cholangitis, and the development of intrahepatic stones, liver abscess formation and, eventually, cirrhosis. In some patients, multiple intrahepatic cystic disease is accompanied by congenital hepatic fibrosis. This condition is known as Grumbach's disease.

Clinical Features

There appears to be a high incidence of cystic disease in the Japanese. There is a strong female predominance worldwide (70% of reported cases in the West) and 25% of the reported cases have been diagnosed during the first year of life. Another 35% become clinically manifest over the next 10 years. The symptoms include cholestatic jaundice, abdominal mass and pain. Complications of the disease include recurrent cholangitis and pancreatitis, hepatic abscess

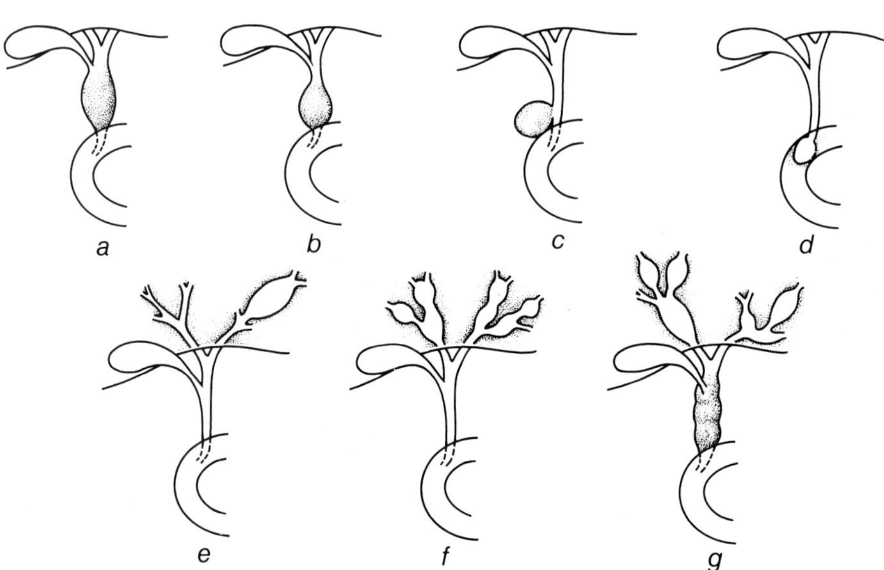

Fig. 69.30 Diagrammatic representation of the types of cystic disease of the biliary tract. *a*, Type I—Diffuse choledochal dilatation. *b*, Type II—Localized choledochal dilatation. *c*, Type III—Supraduodenal diverticulum. *d*, Type IV—Intraduodenal diverticulum (choledochocele). *e*, Type V—Solitary intrahepatic cyst. *f*, Type VI—Multiple intrahepatic cysts (Caroli's disease). *g*, Type VII—Multiple intra- and extrahepatic cysts.

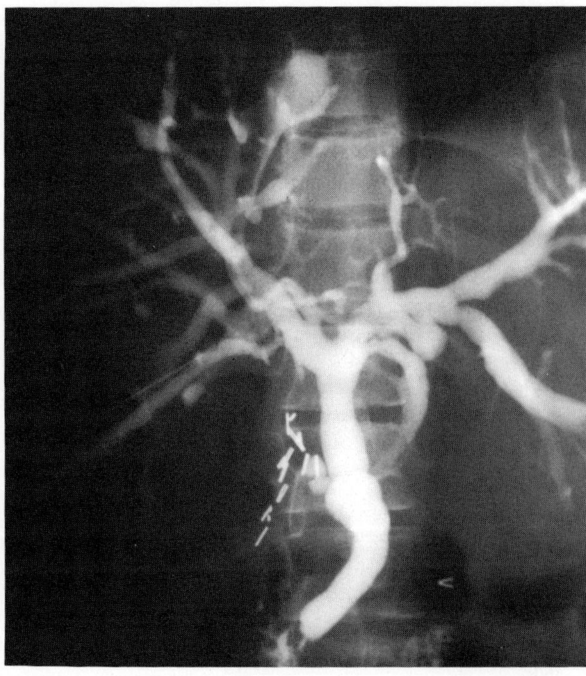

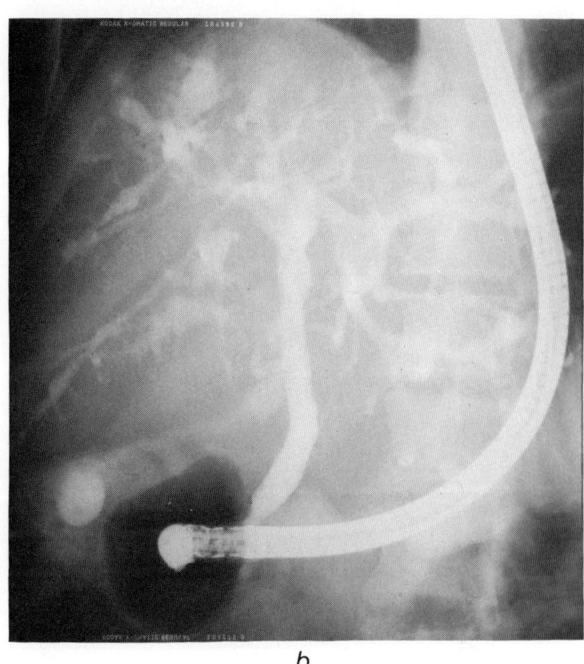

a b

Fig. 69.31 *a*, PTC showing multiple intrahepatic cysts (Caroli's disease). *b*, ERCP showing multiple intrahepatic cysts. The patient presented with bleeding from oesophageal varices. Liver biopsy showed hepatic fibrosis. The combination of diffuse intrahepatic cystic disease and hepatic fibrosis is known as Grumbach's disease.

formation, calculous disease, biliary cirrhosis, rupture of the cyst with biliary peritonitis (rare) and portal vein thrombosis. There is also an increased risk of cholangiocarcinoma which usually develops in the posteromedial wall of the cyst.

The diagnosis can be established non-invasively with ultrasound and CT scanning. Better definition of the pathological anatomy is, however, obtained with ERCP (which also demonstrates the anomalous junction of the bile and pancreatic ducts and its angle) or PTC (*Figs.* 69.32, 69.33). Type IV (intraduodenal diverticulum, choledochocele) can be recognized endoscopically as a smooth compressible elevation associated with an enlarged papilla which protrudes into the duodenum.

Treatment

The treatment of choice is surgical excision with a Roux-en-Y anastomosis. This gives much better results than drainage procedures and avoids or minimizes the risk of carcinoma. The excision is, however, difficult as the cyst is often adherent to the other structures of the porta hepatis and is best performed in centres with biliary surgical expertise. The treatment of patients with intrahepatic cystic disease is difficult. When localized, partial liver resection is advisable. It is doubtful whether distal drainage, such as choledochoduodenostomy or transduodenal/endoscopic sphincterotomy, materially influences the course of the disease of the widespread intrahepatic variety and may indeed enhance the risk of cholangitis.

Congenital Perforation of the Common Duct

This condition presents with jaundice during the first to the third month of life. The perforation which occurs at the

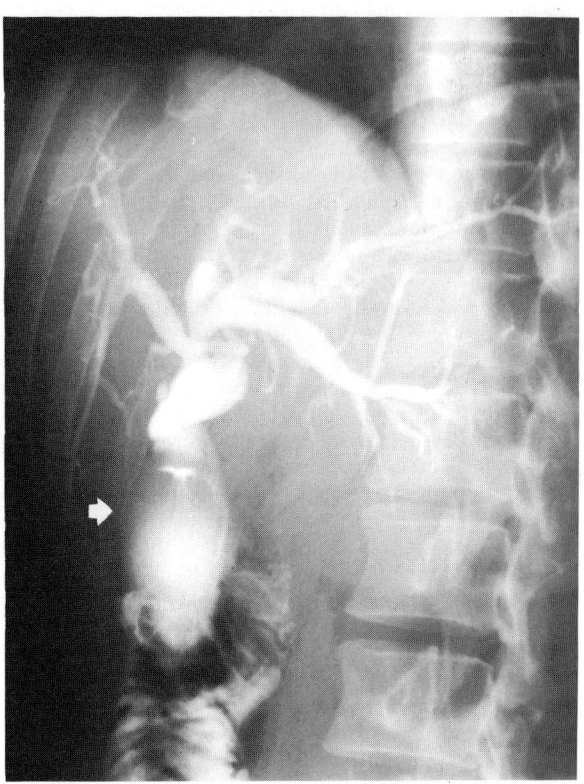

Fig. 69.32 ERCP outlining diffuse choledochal dilatation (Type I). This is the commonest variety and accounts for 80% of cases.

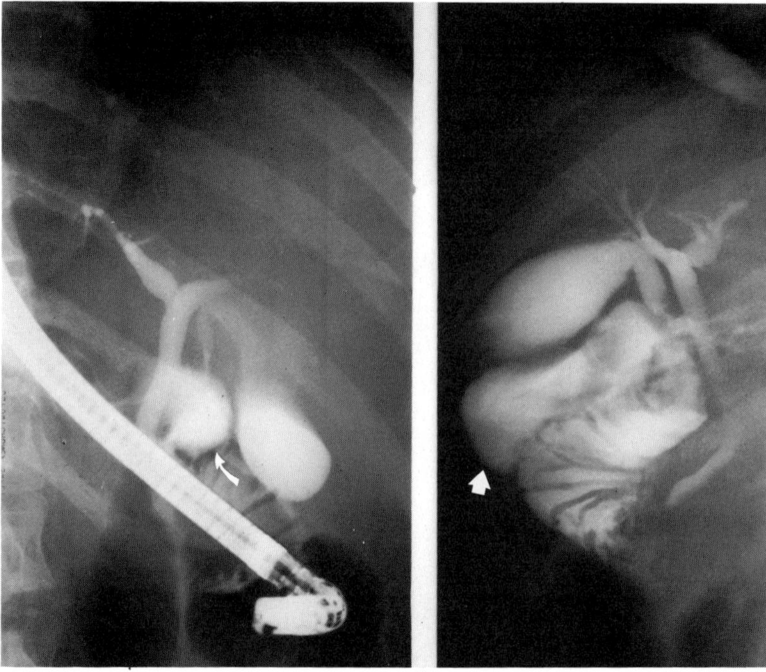

Fig. 69.33 ERCP demonstrating a supraduodenal diverticulum (Type III) beneath the gallbladder. The arrows point to the diverticulum.

junction of the cystic with the common duct, leads to the formation of a pseudocyst. Surgical treatment consists of transperitoneal drainage which is usually followed by spontaneous closure of the perforation.

GALLSTONES

There has been a marked rise in the incidence of gallstones in the Western Hemisphere during the last century. The current mean prevalence in Europe obtained from autopsy studies is 18·5% with the lowest prevalence being reported from Ireland (5%) and the highest from Sweden (38%). In UK, USA and Australia, the prevalence rates vary from 15 to 25%. In every Western country, the prevalence of gallstones in females is approximately twice that of the male population. The highest prevalence is found in the Pima Indian tribe of Arizona with a total and female prevalences of 49% and 73% respectively. A high prevalence rate is also found in S. American countries.

Gallstones are rare in Africa and most recorded rates in this continent are below 1%. The prevalence of gallstones in Japan has also risen since the early part of this century from 2 to 7%. In addition, the composition of stones in Japan has changed during the same period such that cholesterol stones now predominate over pigment stones in this country.

Classification

The old classification of Aschoff into inflammatory, metabolic, static and mixed does not correlate with the present pathophysiological information relating to the formation of gallstones and is not currently used. Likewise, the classification into 'pure' and 'mixed' stones is inaccurate as the overwhelming majority of stones are composed of more than one component. A more useful and practical classification is based on the chemical composition of gallstones:

Stones containing predominantly Cholesterol

These account for the vast majority (75%) of gallstones encountered in the Western Hemisphere. They have a protein matrix and include cholesterol, bile pigments and varying amounts of calcium salts of carbonate and palmitate which determine the radiodensity or otherwise of these yellowish-white calculi. They are usually radiolucent and cast strong acoustic shadows on ultrasonography. Cholesterol stones are often multiple and medium-sized but, when solitary, they can attain a large size and have a radiating crystalline cross-sectional appearance.

Stones containing predominantly Calcium Bilirubinate

These pigment stones may be associated with haemolytic states, biliary infections with β-glucuronidase producing bacterial infections and parasitic infestations. Pigment stones are predominant in the Asian countries. However, in Japan cholesterol stones now exceed the pigment variety. This has been attributed to the adoption of a more Western type diet in the urban population of Japan. Pigment stones account for up 25% of stones in Western countries. The cause of pigment stones in the West is not always apparent. Pigment stones are composed of calcium bilirubinate with varying amounts of cholesterol (3–25%) bound in a matrix of organic material. Most pigment stones are usually multiple, small, irregular, brown to dark green in colour. Their consistency varies from hard to soft and they have an amorphous or layered cut surface.

Stones composed predominantly of Calcium Compounds

The main components of these rare stones are calcium carbonate and calcium palmitate.

Aetiology

There is an increased prevalence of gallstones in females and the frequency of gallstones increases with age in both sexes. Although familial incidence remains unproven, a positive family history of gallstones is more often obtained from patients with symptomatic gallstone disease than in controls. The importance of genetic and ethnic factors is exemplified by the unusually high prevalence of gallstones in the American Indians, particularly the Pima tribe. The genetic disorder in this ethnic group results in the production of a supersaturated bile and a deficient secretion of bile acids by the liver. Certain risk factors are known to increase the prevalence of gallstones, others induce symptomatic disease in patients with silent gallstones without necessarily enhancing the overall frequency (*Table* 69.5).

Table 69.5 Risk factors for gallstone prevalence and symptomatic gallstone disease

Increased gallstone prevalence	*Precipitation of symptomatic disease*
Female sex*	Pregnancy
Obesity*	Clofibrate
Age*	Thiazide diuretics
Genetics and ethnic factors*	? Oral contraception
Diet: highly refined fibre depleted high animal fat*	
Diabetes mellitus*	
Ileal disease and resection	
Haemolytic states†	
Infections of the biliary tract†	
Parasitic infestations†	
Cirrhosis†	
Cystic fibrosis	

*Increased prevalence of cholesterol stones.
†Increased prevalence of pigment stones.

Although it is generally stated that the gallstones which form in patients with ileal disease or after ileal resection are of the cholesterol variety, recent studies have demonstrated that a substantial number of these stones are of the pigment variety. The enhanced lithogenicity and increased incidence of gallstones in the obese are the consequence of an increased hepatic synthesis and secretion of cholesterol. The supersaturation of bile with cholesterol is found in maturity-onset diabetes but not in the juvenile type. The exact mechanism responsible for bile lithogenicity in maturity-onset diabetes is not known. The enhanced incidence of gallstones in children with cystic fibrosis has been attributed to the abnormal mucus which impairs bile flow and favours nucleation.

Early reports demonstrated an increased incidence of symptomatic gallstones in females on the oral contraceptive pill, the relative risk being estimated at 2·5. However, more recent studies have been unable to confirm this finding. This discrepancy has been attributed to the lower oestrogen component of the modern 'mini' contraceptive pill. Studies on the prevalence of gallstones in asymptomatic populations with ultrasound scanning have shown no difference between women on the contraceptive pill and those who are not. Some reports have indicated that the modern 'mini' contraceptive pill may be associated with an increased risk of symptomatic disease in young women (aged 29 or less).

Pathogenesis of Gallstones

Despite a considerable increase in our understanding of some of the pathological mechanisms leading to the formation of gallstones, the exact sequence of events and the relative role of bile composition and gallbladder factors remain unknown. The pathogenesis of pigment and cholesterol stones is best discussed separately.

Pigment Stones

In many Eastern countries where infestation with *Ascaris lumbricoides* is endemic, the eggs of this parasite have been repeatedly identified in the nucleus of pigment stones. The precipitation of calcium bilirubinate seems to be associated in Asian countries with bacterial infections of the biliary tract particularly with *E. coli* and *B. fragilis* and bacterial β-glucuronidase has been implicated in the hydrolysis of conjugated bilirubin with the consequent precipitation of the insoluble calcium bilirubinate. In the West, however, most pigment calculi are associated with sterile bile. Either spontaneous (non-enzymatic) hydrolysis of conjugated bilirubin or the release of β-glucuronidase from the gallbladder as a result of cholestasis or damage to the gallbladder mucosa have been suggested as the responsible mechanisms in patients who develop these stones in the absence of biliary infection. The mechanism of formation of pigment stones is not clear in the majority of patients in the Western Hemisphere. The well established association of pigment stones with haemolytic states indicates that an increased bilirubin load is an important factor in these patients but the exact mechanism is not clear and the hyperbilirubinaemia does not explain the cholesterol component which is present in the majority of these calculi. Calcium bilirubinate deposition also occurs in the following:

Chronic obstructive disease of the biliary tract such as strictures.
As a deposit on indwelling latex and silicone stents/tubes/endoprosthesis.
Around non-absorbable suture material used in bile duct surgery.

Cholesterol Stones

The outstanding biochemical abnormality associated with the formation of cholesterol gallstones is the secretion of bile which is either saturated or supersaturated with cholesterol. The formation of these stones is thought to involve four processes:

Saturation
Crystallization
Nucleation
Growth

Cholesterol which is insoluble in water is held in solution in bile as a result of a molecular aggregation with bile salts and phospholipids forming micelles in which the cholesterol and phospholipid molecules form a central core surrounded by the bile salt molecules. Within the narrow range of water content of bile (80–95%), the solubility relationships of the biliary lipids can be expressed by plotting their relative

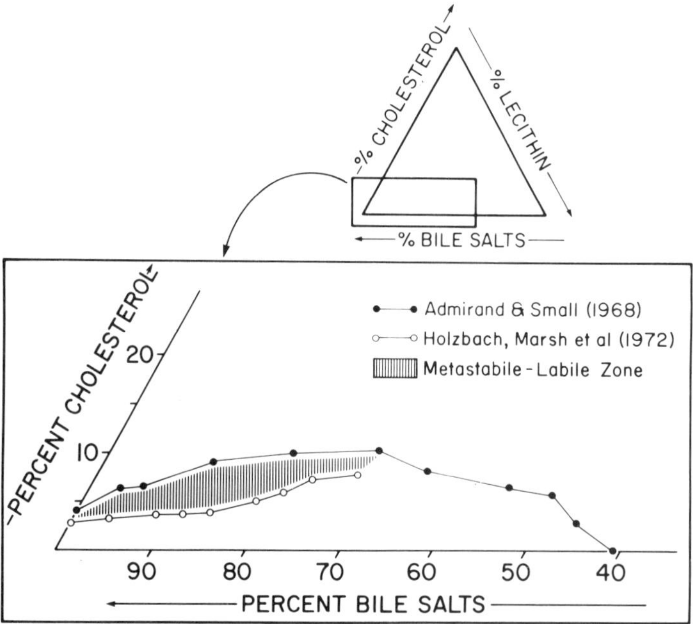

Fig. 69.34 Solubility relationships of cholesterol, bile salts and lecithin (phospholipid) expressed by plotting their relative molar concentrations on triangular coordinates. Points below the metastable-labile zone indicate unsaturated bile. (By kind permission, from Popper H. and Schaffner F. (ed.) (1976) *Progress in Liver Disease*, Vol. v, New York, Grune & Stratton.)

molar concentrations on triangular coordinates (*Fig.* 69.34). There are three main possible states regarding the physicochemical forms of cholesterol in bile. These are:

MICELLAR ZONE. Here the cholesterol is in solution within molecular complexes with bile salts and phospholipids and the bile is unsaturated with respect to cholesterol.

METASTABLE ZONE. In this intermediate zone, the bile is supersaturated with respect to cholesterol but crystal formation may or may not occur. Precipitation of cholesterol crystal is only possible around other substances, e.g. mucus calcium bilirubinate, epithelial debris, bacterial fragments, etc. (heterogeneous nucleation of cholesterol crystals).

LABILE ZONE. The concentration of cholesterol relative to the other biliary lipids is so high that spontaneous coalescence of cholesterol molecules/crystallization (cholesterol monohydrate) occurs (homogeneous nucleation). In practice, this excessive concentration of cholesterol is uncommon in human bile. The interface between the metastable and the labile concentration zones is known as the metastable–labile limit.

Other methods are used to express the solubility of cholesterol in bile. These include the percent saturation, the lithogenic index and the ratio of the concentrations of bile salts and phospholipids over the concentration of cholesterol. The lithogenic index is the ratio of the actual amount of cholesterol present to the maximum amount of cholesterol which can be dissolved in the bile sample using the triangular coordinate plots. A lithogenic index of unity or greater indicates that the bile is supersaturated with respect to cholesterol. The normal ratio: conc. bile salts + conc. phospholipids/conc. of cholesterol equals 10:1.

The relevance of saturation to gallstone formation in the human has been shown by the confirmed observation that virtually all patients with cholesterol gallstones have gallbladder bile which is supersaturated with cholesterol. However, many patients have saturated bile, in the metastable zone, and no gallstones which indicates that factors promoting or preventing nucleation are equally important in gallstone formation. There is now good evidence for a potent nucleating factor which is present in the bile of patients with gallstones but absent in patients with saturated bile but who do not have stones in the gallbladder. Chronic alcohol ingestion increases the hepatic bile acid secretion and reduces the cholesterol saturation in bile and may, therefore, have a protective action against the formation of cholesterol gallstones, although this remains unproven.

The source of the saturated bile is undoubtedly the liver and is due either to increased synthesis of cholesterol or a decreased synthesis/secretion of bile salts and phospholipids. Excess cholesterol secretion in the bile is well documented in the obese patients and is thought to result from the increased activity of the enzyme HMG CoA reductase consequent on the chronically elevated levels of insulin found in overweight individuals. Most non-obese patients with cholesterol gallstones have a reduced bile salt pool. With the exception of patients with ileal disease or after ileal resection, there is no evidence to incriminate reduced absorption as the cause of the reduction in the bile salt pool. The most likely explanation of the smaller pool in patients with gallstones (in the absence of small bowel disease) is an exaggeration of the normal feedback mechanism between the bile salt return and the hepatic synthesis of bile acids together with an increased enterohepatic cycling possibly consequent on abnormal excessive gallbladder contractility.

That the gallbladder plays an important role in gallstone

formation is evident by the fact that 85–90% of stones are encountered in this organ rather than in the bile ducts. The effect of cholecystectomy on bile saturation remains unsettled with some reports documenting a change to the unsaturated state and an increased bile salt pool and others showing no significant effect on the cholesterol saturation of bile. It has been postulated that the gallbladder may alter the physicochemical composition of bile, favouring precipitation of cholesterol crystals and growth of cholesterol microliths into stones by abnormal reabsorption of bile constituents, by stasis resulting from defective gallbladder emptying and stratification of bile or by providing essential nucleating factors such as desquamated cells, glycoprotein molecules, bile pigments, foreign bodies (suture material), bacteria or refluxed intestinal contents. It is probable that gallstones are formed at different occasions depending on the balance between hepatic and gallbladder factors (*Fig.* 69.35).

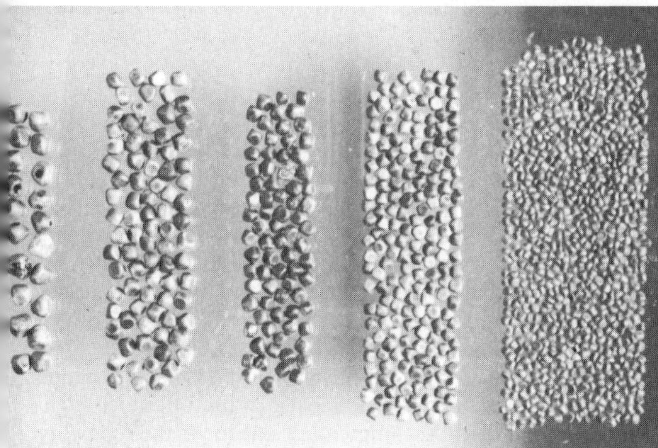

Fig. 69.35 Several generations of cholesterol stones removed from a gallbladder after cholecystectomy. The factors within the gallbladder which favour precipitation of cholesterol crystals and the growth of cholesterol microliths into discernible stones are outlined in the text.

Clinical Syndromes of Gallstone Disease

The symptomatology of gallstone disease is varied. Often non-specific, the symptoms may be acute, chronic or totally absent when gallstones are diagnosed as an incidental finding during the investigation of patients for unrelated disorders. The differentiation between silent and symptomatic gallstones is important since this affects management in the individual case.

In patients with chronic symptoms, it is important to stress that the demonstration of gallbladder disease by oral cholecystography/ultrasound scanning does not exclude other disorders being responsible for the symptoms, and a careful clinical evaluation, together with the appropriate investigative protocol, is essential in all patients with chronic symptoms and radiologically/ultrasonically confirmed gallstone disease. This is especially important in the selection of patients for elective cholecystectomy. The common coexisting diseases include:

Colonic motility disorders and diverticular disease
Gastritis and peptic ulceration
Reflux oesophagitis and hiatal hernia
Pancreatitis
Colonic cancer
Renal disease
Ischaemic heart disease

In addition to gallbladder imaging, an upper gastrointestinal endoscopy or barium series, and in certain situations, a barium enema, is advisable in all patients undergoing elective cholecystectomy for chronic symptoms.

Symptomless (Silent) Gallstones

Most surveys have shown that silent gallstones heavily outnumber the symptomatic ones. Silent gallstones are diagnosed as incidental findings most commonly by abdominal radiographs. The previous controversy regarding the management of asymptomatic gallstones has been largely resolved by prospective studies which have shown that the vast majority of silent gallstones will not cause symptoms or complications during life. Comparative evaluation of expectant versus surgical management of asymptomatic gallstones has shown that cholecystectomy reduces marginally the life expectancy in addition to being substantially more costly. Another argument for cholecystectomy in the past has been the prevention of gallbladder cancer, the development of which is known to be associated with the presence of gallstones. However, carcinoma of the gallbladder is rare and the overall operative mortality with the widespread adoption of prophylactic cholecystectomy in patients with silent gallstones would certainly exceed that due to cancer of the gallbladder by a significant margin. The evidence linking cholecystectomy with the development of colon cancer remains conflicting and cannot be used as a further argument against prophylactic cholecystectomy. The consensus of current surgical opinion is that there is no indication for cholecystectomy in the management of patients with asymptomatic gallstone disease.

Symptomatic Gallstone Disease

The clinical presentation varies and may be acute or chronic (*Table* 69.6).

Table 69.6 Spectrum of symptomatic gallstone disease

Chronic cholecystitis
Acute biliary colic/acute cholecystitis
Jaundice due to large bile duct obstruction
Cholangitis/septicaemia
Acute gallstone pancreatitis
Biliary fistulous disease
Gallstone ileus

Chronic Cholecystitis

Chronic inflammation of the gallbladder is most commonly due to stones and the term ‘chronic cholecystitis’ should be restricted to gallbladders containing gallstones with varying degrees of inflammation, from mild mucosal/submucosal changes to gross transmural fibrosis leading to a contracted fibrous encasement of the biliary calculi.

Symptoms and Signs

Most commonly, patients with chronic cholecystitis complain of recurrent attacks of epigastric or right hypochondrial pain, often radiating to the right side of the back and, less commonly, to the shoulder blade. The pain is more often persistent than intermittent. Episodes of biliary colic with severe intermittent peaks of pain lasting a few minutes to several hours, may subside spontaneously or progress to cystic duct obstruction and acute cholecystitis. Nausea and vomiting may accompany both episodes of persistent pain and the severe attacks of biliary colic. Jaundice and dark urine may follow an attack and indicate common bile duct obstruction by a calculus. The jaundice often subsides after a few days but may persist as a major presenting symptom. It is now established that indigestion, dyspepsia, flatulence, intolerance to fatty foods, abdominal distension and belching occur with the same frequency in the general population as they do in patients with chronic gallstone disease.

The only reliable sign, which is infrequently found on clinical examination, is tenderness in the right upper quadrant. More often than not, the clinical features of chronic cholecystitis are non-specific and confirmation by imaging tests (oral cholecystography, ultrasonography) is essential for diagnosis in the vast majority of cases.

Treatment

The treatment of chronic cholecystitis is surgical—cholecystectomy. There is little doubt that these patients should have their gallbladder removed as approximately 30% of them will develop complications if surgical treatment is delayed. Furthermore, the morbidity and mortality following surgical intervention are enhanced in those patients who develop complications necessitating surgical intervention. In practice, the problem concerns the selection of patients which should be based on establishing that the gallstones are the cause of the patient's symptoms since these are by no means specific and can be caused by other common gastrointestinal disorders. Poor case selection accounts for a large cohort of those patients who continue to experience symptoms after cholecystectomy (postcholecystectomy syndrome). Some of these patients are subsequently found to have disease outwith the biliary tract.

Peroperative cholangiography should be considered as an integral part of cholecystectomy. The cholangiographic findings, the presence of jaundice together with the operative appearances dictate the need for exploration of the common bile duct. Exploration of the common bile duct is usually followed by the insertion of a T-tube even in those patients who are found to have a negative exploration, although some surgeons would opt not to insert a T-tube in patients with a negative exploration and simply close the choledochotomy. Others insert a small cannula through the cystic duct remnant to enable the performance of postoperative cholangiography before discharge from hospital (*Fig.* 69.36). The T-tube should not be smaller than 14 F and its long limb should be brought out by the shortest route well laterally in the right subcostal region. These measures facilitate considerably the removal of retained ductal stones through the T-tube tract by means of the flexible choledochoscope (*vide infra*). The Whelan–Moss T-tube was specially designed to create a wide tract between the bile duct and the abdominal parieties and thus facilitate percutaneous stone extraction via the T-tube tract. Its long limb is wider than the intracholedochal portion.

Opinion on the need for drainage of the gallbladder fossa

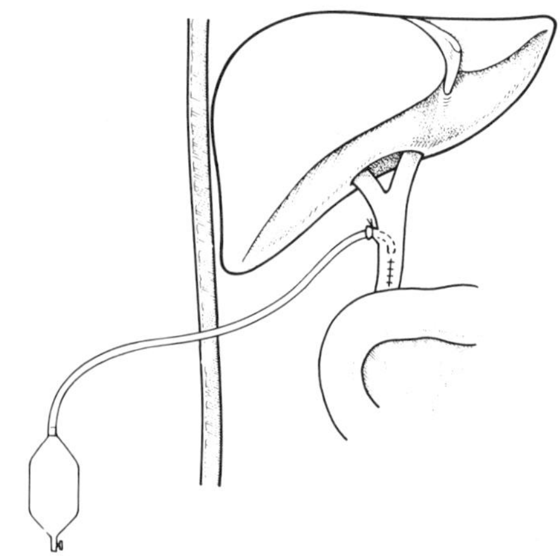

Fig. 69.36 Alternative to the use of a T-tube in patients with a negative common bile duct exploration. A fine polyethylene cannula is inserted into the common bile duct and anchored to the cystic duct by a ligature. The choledochotomy is closed. The cystic duct cannula which is exteriorized allows the performance of postoperative cholangiography.

remains divided. It would seem that the argument against drainage has been strengthened by the results of several prospective clinical trials since these have either failed to show a difference between the drained and the undrained groups, or indicated that drainage increases the postoperative sepsis and morbidity. Many of these studies have one important limitation, i.e. the small number of patients studied which may have failed to detect real differences. It seems likely that the routine uneventful cholecystectomy without exploration of the common bile duct does not require the insertion of a subhepatic drain, but most biliary surgeons would still recommend drainage for the following:

Difficult cholecystectomy
Early cholecystectomy for acute cholecystitis
In patients who require exploration of the common bile duct

The mortality of elective cholecystectomy for chronic cholecystitis is low (0·3–1·0%) but is higher in the elderly (5–6%).

GALLSTONE DISSOLUTION. The primary bile acid chenodeoxycholic acid, and its 7-β epimer, ursodeoxycholic acid, have been administered orally to dissolve gallstones but their precise place in cholesterol stone management has yet to be determined. Successful dissolution occurs if the gallbladder is functioning and the stones are not unduly large or multiple. Once dissolution has been achieved, therapy has to be maintained as otherwise the stone will reform. The results of the multicentre trial carried out in the USA have been poor. However, the protagonists of the dissolution therapy have rightly criticized this trial since the oral dose of the chenodeoxycholate used was well below the optimum required for effective dissolution of cholesterol stones. Medical dissolution is currently reserved for patients who are operative risks because of intercurrent cardiorespiratory disease and those who refuse surgery. Ursodeoxycholate is preferred to chenodeoxycholate because it causes less side-effects (especially diarrhoea) and is not hepatotoxic.

Acalculous Chronic Gallbladder Disease

Chronic inflammation of the gallbladder in the absence of

gallstones is due to adenomyomatosis or cholesterolosis of the gallbladder and these may be conveniently grouped as acalculous chronic gallbladder disease. This can give rise to vague symptoms not dissimilar to those of chronic cholecystitis. Oral cholecystography shows no abnormality of the gallbladder in 50% of these patients, or is reported as demonstrating poor function or unusual appearances. In many instances, the diagnosis is made on pathological examination of the excised gallbladder. In general, the results of cholecystectomy for these conditions have been difficult to evaluate but in the presence of persisting symptoms, most surgeons would advise operation.

Adenomyomatosis of the Gallbladder

This is variously named as adenomatous hyperplasia, diverticulosis of the gallbladder and cholecystitis glandularis proliferans. It is thought to represent a developmental defect which results in hyperplasia of the smooth muscle bundles with sacculation or diverticulum formation of the epithelial lining (Rokitansky–Aschoff sinuses). The cholecystogram may be normal or the late film taken after a fatty meal may demonstrate either the mural diverticula (*Fig.* 69.37) or a concentric narrowing of the fundus.

Cholesterolosis of the Gallbladder

In this condition, the epithelial cells and macrophages within the gallbladder mucosa become laden with cholesterol and lead to the formation of numerous lipid deposits. Chronic inflammation of the adjacent mucosa then leads to a striking appearance of the interior of the gallbladder which has been aptly described as the 'strawberry gallbladder'.

Acute Biliary Colic and Acute Cholecystitis

Acute biliary colic results in severe colicky abdominal pain usually accompanied by nausea and vomiting. The duration of the severe pain which makes the patient restless, varies from 30 min to several hours. Biliary colic often merges into acute obstructive cholecystitis. However, resolution of the severe colicky painful episode either spontaneously or as a result of analgesic medication/antispasmodic without the development of acute cholecystitis is common and many patients give a history of recurrent episodes of biliary colic before the development of acute cholecystitis.

In over 95% of cases, acute cholecystitis is *obstructive* and results from impaction of a stone in Hartmann's pouch/cystic duct. Much less commonly, acute cholecystitis is *acalculous* although the incidence of this complication in critically ill patients is diagnosed more frequently nowadays. Acute cholecystitis in the elderly may result from cystic duct obstruction due to carcinoma of the gallbladder. Whereas patients harbouring residual infection of the gallbladder with *Salmonella typhi* as typhoid carriers may cause sporadic outbursts of typhoid, acute salmonella cholecystitis is very rarely encountered in the West.

Acute Obstructive (Calculous) Cholecystitis

Following obstruction of the cystic duct/Hartmann's pouch, the gallbladder becomes hyperaemic, oedematous, tense and distended. The initial inflammation is chemically induced and is not of bacterial origin although sepsis is an important feature of the established disease and its complications. The exact cause for the initial chemical inflammation is not known but the release of mucosal phospholipase which converts the lecithin in the bile to lysolecithin is currently held responsible for the initiation of the inflammatory response although bacterial lysosomal enzymes and, more recently, prostaglandins have been implicated. In the first few days, the bile appears macroscopically normal and is sterile, but with the progress of the inflammation, absorption of pigments and bile salts takes place, and the contents then vary from a thin mucoid material to frank pus. The histological changes of the established condition involve the mucosa, fibromuscular wall and serosa and vary from mild acute inflammation with transmural oedema to severe disease with patches of necrosis usually in the fundal region of the gallbladder which becomes wrapped by the greater omentum. At the time of surgery carried out during the same admission, approximately 50% of cultures of gallbladder contents are sterile. Aerobic enteric organisms account for 94% of positive cultures and anaerobes for the remainder. The subsequent sequence of events following the acute inflammatory process may vary from:

Resolution (most common) with scarring, abnormal function or non-function of the gallbladder.

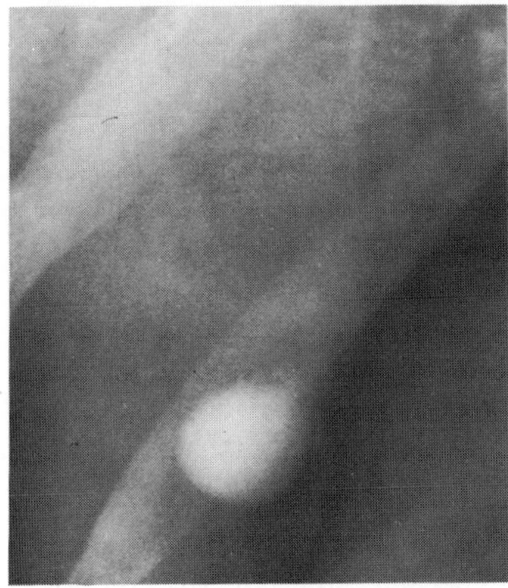

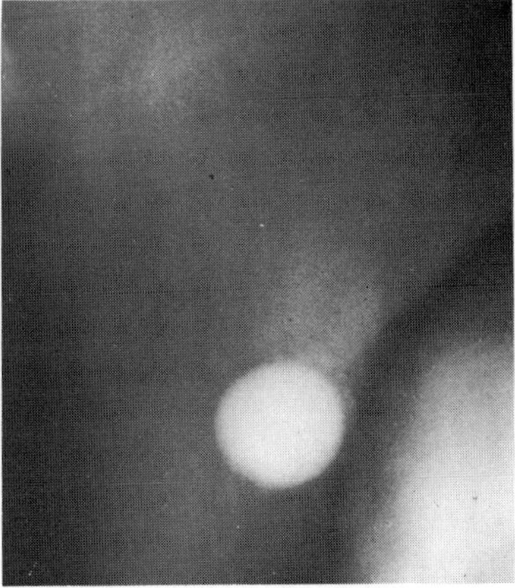

Fig. 69.37 Oral cholecystogram: a concentric narrowing of the fundus is the striking feature but on closer inspection, intramural diverticula are discernible. When encountered, these are pathognomonic of adenomyomatosis of the gallbladder. Often, however, the oral cholecystogram is normal.

Persistence of the infection: the gallbladder becomes distended with pus (empyema of the gallbladder).
Resolution of the inflammatory process within the gallbladder with persistence of the cystic duct obstruction—mucocele (hydrops) of the gallbladder.
Gangrene and acute perforation leading to localized (pericholecystic abscess or frank biliary peritonitis.
Chronic perforation with the development of bilio-enteric and bilio-bilial fistulas.

Whereas the majority of patients diagnosed as acute cholecystitis have the classic acute cystic duct obstruction and its associated inflammatory condition of the gallbladder, others are instances of chronic cholecystitis presenting with acute pain or biliary colic. Although acute cholecystitis is often suspected on clinical grounds, a definitive diagnosis can only be obtained by specific investigations (EHIDA scintiscanning, ultrasonography, intravenous cholangiography). The serum amylase should always be performed in addition to the liver function tests. Scout abdominal plain films in the supine and erect position are used to exclude perforation and the presence of gas in the biliary tract.

Symptoms and Signs

The clinical picture varies with the severity of the inflammatory process. Known pre-existing gallbladder disease may be present or chronic symptoms over several months to years may precede the acute presentation. Alternatively, acute obstructive cholecystitis may be the first intimation of gallstone disease.

In mild cases, the patient complains of right upper quadrant pain and tenderness. Pyrexia, severe pain and tenderness in the right hypochondrium with rebound reflect more severe degrees of gallbladder inflammation. In these instances, Murphy's sign (inspiratory arrest due to pain on inspiration during gentle palpation of the right subcostal region) is usually present. Nausea, vomiting, ileus, mild abdominal distension and toxicity are encountered in the severe forms of the disease. Jaundice is present in 20–25% of patients with acute obstructive cholecystitis but common duct stones are found in only 12% of these patients. In the absence of ductal calculi, jaudice has been ascribed to reactive hepatitis or oedema of the common bile duct. A tender palpable mass in the right subcostal region is found in 25% of cases and signifies one of the following:

Empyema of the gallbladder
Omental phlegmon
Abscess due to localized perforation
Carcinoma of the gallbladder, especially if the patient is elderly.

Acute cholecystitis is usually accompanied by leucocytosis and a slight elevation of the serum transaminases. The serum bilirubin and alkaline phosphatase may be elevated, either from bile duct obstruction by calculi or ductal oedema or as a result of a reactive hepatitis. The serum amylase is not infrequently elevated and may reach levels suggestive of acute pancreatitis.

Differential Diagnosis

Apart from acute pancreatitis, the important diseases which must be considered and excluded are perforation of a duodenal ulcer, right-sided pyelonephritis, lobar pneumonia and myocardial infarction. Aside from routine chest radiography and plain abdominal films, an ECG is advisable in the elderly and in those patients with a known history of ischaemic heart disease.

Acute Acalculous Cholecystitis

The incidence of this condition appears to be increasing and it now accounts for 2–8% of patients with acute cholecystitis. It is usually encountered in critically ill, elderly patients but acute acalculous cholecystitis has also been reported in children. The disorder usually occurs during the course of a prolonged serious illness, e.g. multiple trauma, following major surgical intervention, in patients with extensive burns, severe sepsis and drug overdosage. The risk factors which predispose to the development of acute acalculous cholecystitis are:

Blood volume depletion
Prolonged ileus
Morphine administration exceeding 6 days
Intravenous hyperalimentation
Multiple blood transfusions
Sepsis
Starvation.

The exact pathology is not known but the available evidence suggests that the inflammation develops as a consequence of prolonged distension of the gallbladder, bile stasis and inspissation which result in a mucosal injury and thrombosis of the blood vessels of the seromuscular layer of the gallbladder. The thrombosis is thought to be initiated by the activation of Factor XII. In the fully developed condition, the gallbladder shows marked oedema of the seromuscular layer with focal necrotic areas. Emergency cholecystectomy is necessary to prevent the onset of free perforation of the gallbladder.

Acute Emphysematous Cholecystitis

This fulminant form of acute cholecystitis is fortunately rare. It is caused by a mixed polymicrobial infection which include gas-forming bacteria (*E. coli*, *Cl. welchii*, aerobic and anaerobic streptococci). The gallbladder may or may not contain stones. Acute emphysematous cholecystitis occurs predominantly in males (70%) and has a special predilection for diabetic individuals. Thrombosis of the cystic artery has been implicated in the development of acute emphysematous cholecystitis.

The presence of air within the gallbladder lumen, its wall or the biliary tree on the plain radiograph of the abdomen is characteristic of the condition which often leads to gangrene (75%) and perforation (15%) by the time the diagnosis is made. The clinical picture is that of severe rapidly oncoming upper abdominal peritonitis with prostration and marked toxicity. Urgent surgical intervention is imperative.

Complications of Acute Cholecystitis

The important complications of all forms of acute cholecystitis are empyema, perforation and gangrene. All require urgent surgical intervention.

Empyema (Suppurative Cholecystitis)

Empyema of the gallbladder is an uncommon complication and has a reported incidence of 2–3% of all patients with gallstone disease. It presents as a tender mass in the right hypochondrium and usually affects elderly patients in whom systemic signs, including pyrexia and leucocytosis, may be minimal. Cultures of the gallbladder contents are positive in 80%.

Gangrene

Patchy gangrene of the fundus of the gallbladder is encountered in 5–7% of patients with obstructive cholecystitis. It is more commonly encountered in elderly patients, diabetics, and in patients with empyema of the gallbladder, acute acalculous cholecystitis and, especially, emphysematous cholecystitis. It may lead to localized or free perforation of the gallbladder.

Perforation

Perforation may be localized with the development of a pericholecystic abscess or free, resulting in generalized infected biliary peritonitis which carries a high mortality, variously reported as 30–50%. A localized perforation may involve the duodenum with the development of a cholecysto-duodenal fistula and resolution of the inflammatory episode. However, this bilio-enteric fistula persists and passage of a large stone through this fistula may eventually cause gallstone ileus.

Treatment of Acute Cholecystitis

Opinions still differ regarding the treatment of acute cholecystitis. The management depends on whether the inflammatory condition is progressive and life-threatening or the cholecystitis is mild and resolving.

Management of Mild or Resolving Disease

The initial treatment consists of nasogastric suction and intravenous fluid and electrolyte therapy. Antibiotic therapy is not necessary at this stage although some use it routinely. Analgesics are administered as required and the diagnosis is established by the appropriate imaging tests. Two options are available:

Interval (delayed) cholecystectomy
Early cholecystectomy.

The interval approach is the traditional one and entails conservative management of the acute episode with discharge of the patient after complete resolution of the attack. Subsequently, the patient is admitted some 2–3 months later for an elective cholecystectomy. The rationale for this treatment is that in most instances, the raised pressure within the gallbladder lumen lifts the walls of the organ off the impacted stone which then dislodges and falls into the lumen with resolution of the inflammation, the view being held that it is safer to operate several weeks after the acute inflammatory episode has subsided.

Early cholecystectomy is being increasingly performed in the management of acute cholecystitis. It must be distinguished from emergency cholecystectomy. Following initial conservative management and confirmation of the diagnosis as outlined previously, the patient is operated electively on the next available operating list or within a few days of admission. The results of several prospective clinical trials comparing early versus interval cholecystectomy have shown a clear benefit from early cholecystectomy performed during the same hospital admission. These include less time spent in hospital and lower cost of treatment. The early approach is not attended by any increase in the morbidity (including iatrogenic bile duct injury and missed stones) and mortality than interval cholecystectomy. On the other hand, the latter has several disadvantages which include:

Failure of conservative treatment in 13%
Premature re-admission with a further attack whilst waiting for elective cholecystectomy (13%)
Patient defaulting after discharge (10%).

Early cholecystectomy is best performed using the retrograde technique (fundus approach). It is customary to administer antibiotics (cephalosporins) preoperatively and 24 hours postoperatively in all patients undergoing early cholecystectomy.

Management of Progressing Disease

The indications for emergency surgical intervention are outlined in *Table* 69.7. In these patients surgical intervention is carried out under antibiotic cover active against both Gram-negative aerobes and anaerobes (cephalosporin + metronidazole or piperacillin, etc). The exact procedure depends on the operative findings. In patients with a tense empyema, preliminary decompression of the gallbladder contents using a Mayo–Ochsner suction trocar-cannula inserted through a purse-string suture in the fundus should precede the cholecystectomy which, in the acute situation, is best performed by the retrograde technique (starting at the fundus). This allows easier identification of the cystic duct and, thereby, reduces the risk of bile duct damage. At times, the precarious condition of the patient precludes a lengthy operation or the anatomy may be so obscured by the inflammatory mass as to render the cholecystectomy hazardous. In these situations, a cholecystostomy should be performed. The gallbladder contents are evacuated, any gangrenous patches of its walls are excised and a 22–24 F Malecot catheter is inserted into the organ which is closed round it by a purse-string suture. The catheter is then brought out through a separate stab wound. In these patients a cholecystectomy is advisable at a later stage unless the patient is elderly or has severe intercurrent cardiorespiratory disease because of the risk of recurrence of gallstones and symptoms. Moreover, the incidence of carcinoma of the gallbladder in patients who had previously undergone cholecystostomy is appreciable (7%).

Table 69.7 Indications for emergency surgical intervention in patients with acute cholecystitis

Progression of the disease despite conservative treatment
Failure to improve within 24 hours especially in patients >60 years
Presence of an inflammatory mass in the right hypochondrium
Detection of gas in the gallbladder/biliary tract
Established generalized peritonitis
Development of intestinal obstruction

Subtotal cholecystectomy is performed as an alternative approach to cholecystostomy in patients in whom formal cholecystectomy is considered hazardous. In this procedure, the posterior wall of the gallbladder is left in situ, attached to the liver bed, and the cystic duct is secured from within the gallbladder lumen by a purse-string suture (*Fig.* 69.38).

In all instances specimens of bile and pus are obtained for bacteriological culture. Pus is thoroughly evacuated and peritoneal lavage, preferably with an antibiotic solution, carried out when gross peritoneal sepsis is found. Adequate drainage of the gallbladder bed is still considered advisable but is no substitute for thorough peritoneal toilet. All these patients are at risk from Gram-negative septicaemia. They require a full course of antibiotic therapy for a minimum of

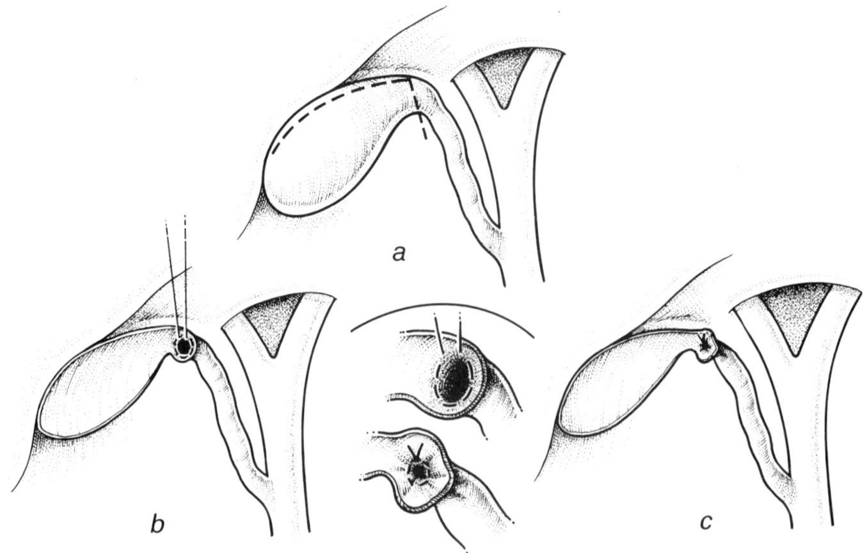

Fig. 69.38 Technique of subtotal cholecystectomy described by Borrmann and Terblanche. *a*, The broken line shows the extent of the cholecystectomy. The posterior wall of the gallbladder is left attached to the liver. *b*, A purse-string suture is inserted around the cystic duct orifice. *c*, The purse-string suture has been tied with closure of the cystic duct orifice.

7 days. The results of the culture of operative specimens of bile and pus may dictate changes in the antibiotic regimen.

Mortality of Acute Cholecystitis

The overall reported mortality of acute cholecystitis is 3%. The mortality in the elderly is higher (10%) and more than half of the deaths in patients over 65 years are secondary to cardiovascular and respiratory complications.

Ductal Calculi and Cholangitis

The majority of ductal calculi are found in the common bile duct and in the Western Hemisphere, only an estimated 5% of ductal calculi are located in the intrahepatic ducts (more commonly the left) although multiple intrahepatic calculi are common in Eastern countries, especially where parasitic infestations and recurrent pyogenic cholangitis are endemic. Ductal calculi may arise as follows:

- As secondary calculi from migration of gallstones
- As primary calculi arising *de novo* within the bile ducts.

Primary ductal calculi consist of amorphous soft concretions of cholesterol and bile pigment with a low calcium content. Not infrequently, organization into a stone has not occurred by the time of diagnosis and the appearance at operation is that of biliary mud or sludge. The factors concerned in the pathogenesis of primary ductal calculi are multiple and include:

- Stasis in the biliary ductal tree caused by obstruction, e.g. strictures, sclerosing cholangitis, etc.
- A supersaturated lithogenic hepatic bile.
- Infections with β-glucuronidase producing bacteria, e.g. *E. coli*, *B. fragilis*.
- Foreign bodies, e.g. metallic clips, non-absorbable suture material, stents, etc.
- Parasitic infestations, e.g. *Ascaris lumbricoides*, *Clonorchis sinensis*, etc.
- Recurrent pyogenic cholangitis.

Stasis due to bile duct obstruction is the most important factor and requires correction in addition to removal of the calculi and eradication of any infection.

Clinical Manifestations of Ductal Calculi

Although 15–20% of patients with stones in the common bile duct are asymptomatic, the majority present sooner or later with severe symptoms, and by and large incur a significant morbidity as the pathological potential of ductal calculi is high and may contribute to the death of the patient. Ductal calculi may present with:

- Recurrent bouts of biliary colic accompanied by intermittent jaundice
- Episodic upper abdominal pain and dyspepsia (*Fig.* 69.39)
- Stone impaction with progressive jaundice
- Cholangitis
- Gallstone pancreatitis
- Secondary biliary cirrhosis and portal hypertension.

Management of Ductal Calculi

With the development of therapeutic ERCP and its undoubted efficacy in selected cases, the management of ductal calculi varies from centre to centre depending on local facilities and expertise. The treatment of these patients is best considered in light of the clinical situation with which they present.

Patients with Ductal Calculi without Previous Cholecystectomy

The management of these patients depends on their age and general condition. A cholecystectomy and common bile duct exploration by the supraduodenal approach is the appropriate and orthodox treatment for all patients who are considered fit for surgical intervention. The stones are removed atraumatically by means of biliary balloon catheters, stone-grasping forceps or Dormia basket, preferably under visual control with the operating choledochoscope. A completion check by means of a choledochoscopic inspection virtually

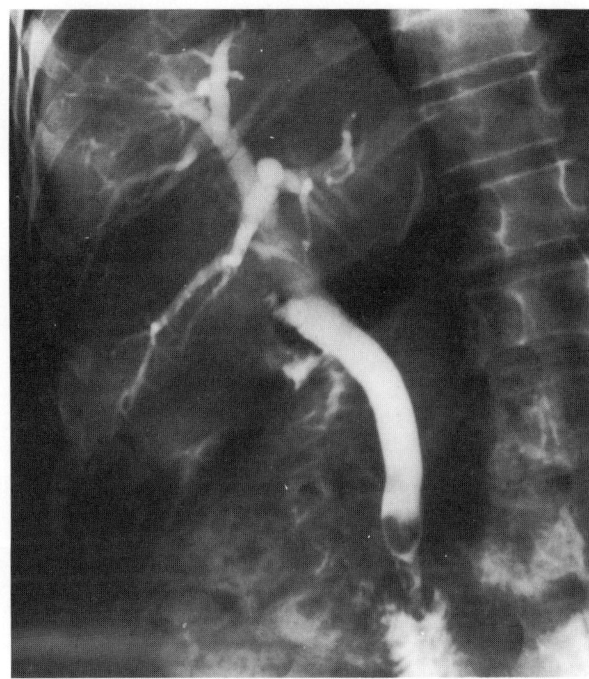

Fig. 69.39 Primary ductal calculi situated at the lower end of the bile duct 13 years after a cholecystectomy. The patient complained of dyspepsia and episodic abdominal pain. Although the patient was not jaundiced clinically, the liver function tests showed a mild elevation of the serum bilirubin and alkaline phosphatase.

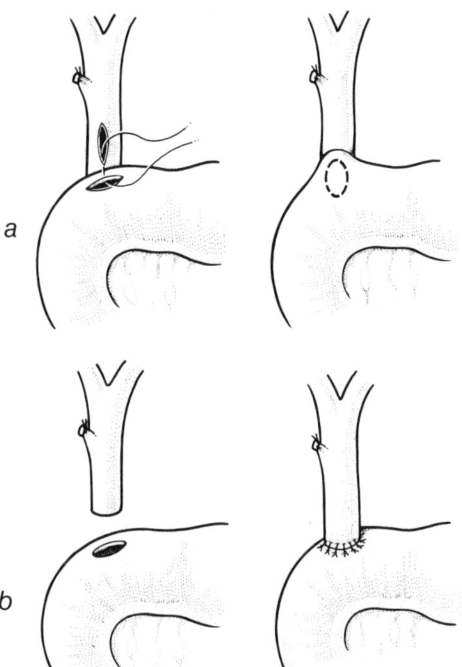

Fig. 69.40 *a*, Lateral or side-to-side choledochoduodenostomy. This may result in the passage of food debris from the duodenum through the stoma into the lower end of the bile duct (distal to the anastomosis with the development of the inspissated sump syndrome which presents with cholangitis). *b*, Diagrammatic technique of the procedure of transection choledochoduodenostomy. The bile duct is mobilized from the portal vein and hepatic artery. It is then transected as it enters the pancreas. The distal end is closed with a running suture and the proximal end is anastomosed in an end-to-side fashion to the duodenum at the junction of the first with the second part.

abolishes the incidence of residual stones. A T-tube is inserted as previously described and the choledochotomy wound is closed. In patients with multiple ductal calculi, grossly dilated bile duct (>2·0 cm) or papillary stenosis, a drainage operation is indicated: choledochoduodenostomy or transduodenal sphincteroplasty. Opinions are divided as to the relative merits of these two procedures. However, sphincteroplasty carries a significant risk of pancreatitis and involves a sizeable duodenotomy. A transection choledochoduodenostomy (*Fig.* 69.40) is preferable to the side-to-side anastomosis as it provides dependent drainage and avoids the complication of the inspissated sump syndrome.

An alternative approach has been suggested for all previously unoperated patients with ductal calculi. This consists of preoperative endoscopic sphincterotomy and stone extraction followed by cholecystectomy. However, a recent randomized trial has shown no benefit from this combined approach.

In elderly or poor-risk patients, endoscopic sphincterotomy and stone extraction is the treatment of choice if this facility is available (*Fig.* 69.41). A cholecystectomy is not performed in these patients unless they develop cholecystitis subsequently.

Patients with Ductal Calculi discovered during Elective Cholecystectomy

These account for 4–10% of cases and are discovered by routine peroperative cholangiography. The bile duct should be explored and stones are removed. In approximately 18%, the common bile duct exploration proves negative. Some advocate closure of the choledochotomy without T-tube drainage in these patients (*vide supra*).

Ductal Calculi discovered soon after Cholecystectomy and Exploration of the Common Bile Duct

These are referred to as missed, retained or residual stones. The incidence varies from 2 to 15% and averages 8%. Routine completion choledochoscopy virtually abolishes this complication. Unfortunately this is practised only in a few centres and many surgeons still rely on completion T-tube cholangiography to ascertain ductal clearance of stones.

Retained ductal calculi following biliary tract surgery are either diagnosed in the immediate postoperative period by the postoperative T-tube cholangiogram or present with recurrent symptoms usually within 2 years of cholecystectomy without exploration of the common bile duct. Ductal stones presenting beyond this interval are generally considered to be of the primary variety.

Certain general considerations apply with regard to the management of patients with residual calculi following biliary tract surgery. Urgent intervention is not indicated if the liver biochemistry is normal, the patient is asymptomatic, the T-tube cholangiogram shows no organic disease or significant dilatation. Spontaneous passage is likely if the calculi are small (less than 7 mm) and may be aided by simple measures such as T-tube clamping. If the patient tolerates

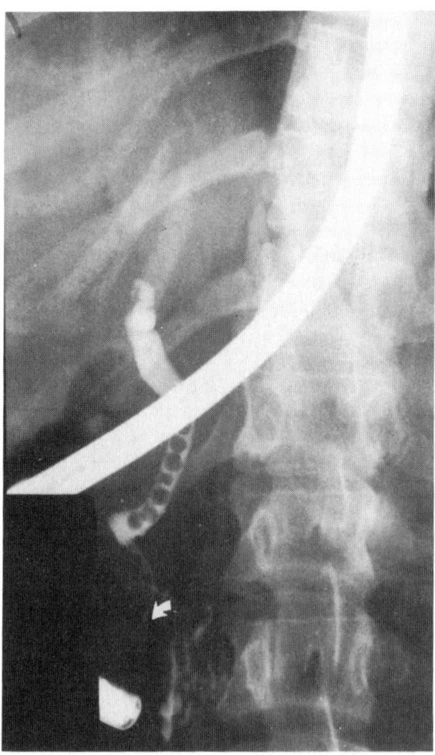

Fig. 69.41 Endoscopic papillotomy for multiple ductal calculi in an elderly patient. The wire of the sphincterotome is visible above the tip of the endoscope.

clamping and providing no untoward symptoms or complications develop, such a conservative approach can be continued for a few weeks, at the end of which time the situation is reviewed radiologically.

The various methods available for the non-surgical management of retained stones are:

Flushing
Dissolution
Percutaneous stone extraction via the T-tube tract
Endoscopic sphincterotomy and stone extraction.

The first three options are applicable only to patients with an indwelling T-tube whereas endoscopic stone extraction can be used in all patients. All the above methods are performed under antibiotic cover because of the risk of cholangitis and septicaemia.

Flushing is usually carried out with saline, heparinized saline, or lignocaine–saline solution. The technique which is simple and effective if the stones are small (<0·7 mm), is performed by infusing the solution through the T-tube under manometric control to ensure that the pressure does not exceed 30 cmH_2O as this can lead to cholangiovenous reflux and septicaemia. The efficacy of this simple method of treatment which does not require any special expertise, can be enhanced when it is accompanied by pharmacologically-induced relaxation of the sphincter of Oddi. In this respect, the results of the synthetic peptide, ceruletide, have been promising with a stone clearance of 30–50%.

Cholate infusion can dissolve cholesterol stones but its efficacy is low and it has been replaced by mono-octanoin which acts more rapidly and achieves complete stone clearance in 40%. The most effective agent for the dissolution of ductal calculi is methyl ter-butyl ether (MTBE) which is capable of achieving gallstone dissolution within hours of instillation. Early results with this agent have been very promising and it is likely that it will replace mono-octanoin.

Percutaneous stone extraction via the T-tube tract was initially performed by the Burhenne technique using a Dormia basket introduced via a specially designed steerable catheter to capture and extract the stone under fluoroscopic control. It has largely been replaced by the flexible choledochoscopic technique which is successful in 90–95% of cases. A 4–6 week period of maturation of the T-tube tract is required before the procedure can be performed safely. A guidewire is introduced into the common bile duct and the T-tube removed. Thereafter, the T-tube tract is dilated to allow the introduction of the narrow flexible choledochoscope. The retained stones are removed by means of a Dormia basket under visual control.

Endoscopic sphincterotomy with stone extraction is a very effective method of dealing with the problem of retained stones and can be performed in patients with and without T-tubes. Surgical management of missed stones is reserved for those patients in whom the above methods have failed or complications have developed during or after attempted endoscopic or percutaneous stone extraction.

Recurrent Ductal Calculi

Ductal calculi presenting 2 years or more after an operation are generally regarded to be primary. A recent study has identified suture material in 30% of cases. This finding stresses the importance of avoiding non-absorbable material during operations on the biliary tract. Recurrent ductal calculi are often multiple and are usually associated with gross dilatation of the bile duct and in some cases obvious distal ductal stenosis. This may be primary (papillary stenosis) or be secondary to trauma inflicted by metal bougies introduced through the sphincter region at the time of exploration of the common bile duct. The preferred treatment is by choledochoduodenostomy, although some favour a sphincteroplasty or endoscopic sphincterotomy and stone extraction, particularly if the patient is elderly or is considered an operative risk because of significant cardiorespiratory disease.

Multiple Intrahepatic Calculi

Although rare in the Western Hemisphere, these are common in Eastern countries and often pose serious management problems. The majority are associated with stricture formation of the hepatic ducts. If the stones are floating and located in the major intrahepatic bile ducts, removal may be possible through a standard choledochotomy with introduction of the rigid choledochoscope with an attached instrument guide channel through which either a balloon catheter or a Dormia basket is introduced. The extraction is performed under visual control.

Transhepatic lithotomy is necessary when stones are impacted above a strictured intrahepatic duct (usually left). The hepatic parenchyma of the involved liver segment is divided down to and including the involved duct. Thereafter, the stones are removed and, following irrigation, the stricture is dilated with a balloon dilator. A silicone T-tube is then inserted into the affected intrahepatic duct and the liver parenchyma is sutured around it. Resection of the involved lobe is reserved for cases with severe disease, i.e. multiple stones associated with extensive stricturing, fibrosis, gross destruction of the hepatic parenchyma and abscess formation.

CHOLANGITIS

Acute bacterial cholangitis is a serious surgical emergency which arises as a complication of large bile duct obstruction from any cause, although the most common obstructing agent is a stone impacted in the lower end of the bile duct followed by benign strictures (usually iatrogenic).

Less common causes in the Western Hemisphere include ascending cholangitis after bilioenteric anastomosis especially choledochoduodenostomy (usually the result of a narrow stoma or the inspissated sump syndrome), bile duct trauma/fistula, cystic disease of the biliary tract, duodenal diverticula, sclerosing cholangitis and malignant obstruction of the bile duct (cholangiocarcinoma, periampullary and pancreatic tumours). Malignant obstruction is less frequently complicated by cholangitis than calculous obstruction and most instances are encountered after transhepatic or endoscopic stenting for preoperative decompression or palliation. In the Far East, recurrent pyogenic cholangitis (oriental cholangiohepatitis) is a frequent cause of recurrent bacterial cholangitis.

The infection is most commonly caused by Gram-negative organisms. The classic triad of symptoms consists of pain in the right hypochondrium, intermittent fever and jaundice (Charcot's biliary fever). The patient is toxic with high intermittent pyrexia which is accompanied by rigors due to septicaemia in 50% of patients. The pain varies in intensity and can be severe. There is usually tenderness in the right hypochondrium which, if marked, suggests the presence of abscess formation (suppurative cholangitis) where the liver parenchyma becomes studded with multiple intrahepatic abscesses (honeycomb liver). The liver is often enlarged although this may be difficult to ascertain because of the abdominal tenderness. Nausea and vomiting are frequent accompaniments. Renal failure is commonly encountered at some stage during the course of the illness.

Prompt and energetic treatment is mandatory. Resuscitative measures include intravenous fluid therapy with crystalloid and colloid solutions. A blood culture is taken and systemic antibiotics commenced (cephalosporin with metronidazole or piperacillin). Active surgical intervention should be carried out if there is no improvement in the condition within 12–24 hours of active treatment. This consists of ductal clearance and insertion of a T-tube in patients with calculous disease although, increasingly, endoscopic sphincterotomy with stone extraction is being performed since this appears to be accompanied by a lower mortality in this situation. The overall reported mortality following emergency surgical intervention for cholangitis is 14%.

BILIOENTERIC FISTULAS

The various types of causation of biliary fistulas are shown in *Table* 69.8.

Spontaneous external biliary fistulas are exceeding rare and the few reported cases have been instances of neglected empyema of the gallbladder or extensive carcinoma of the gallbladder invading the abdominal wall. The vast majority of external biliary fistulas occur in the postoperative period and may result from the following:

Leakage of bile from a slipped cystic duct ligature or cut accessory bile duct.
Trauma to the extrahepatic biliary tree during cholecystectomy, gastric surgery or pancreatectomy.
Dislodged T-tube after common bile duct exploration.
Leakage from bilioenteric anastomosis.
Hepatic resections.

Leakage of bile after removal of a T-tube is short-lived and requires investigation by ERCP if it persists beyond 2–3 days. Other external biliary fistulas may follow blunt or penetrating hepatic trauma. The external biliary fistula usually occurs after the surgical treatment of the hepatic injury and is then often accompanied by sepsis.

External biliary fistulas do not result in skin excoriation but may cause significant fluid and electrolyte depletion if the output is high and prolonged. They are not usually accompanied by systemic manifestations unless sepsis is present. Abdominal tenderness and rebound indicates the concomitant presence of bile in the peritoneal cavity. Postoperative external biliary fistulas occurring in association with jaundice indicate bile duct trauma or a missed obstructive lesion of the biliary tract. These patients require urgent

Table 69.8 Biliary fistulas

Category	*Type*	*Causation*
External		Trauma and operative injuries Therapeutic (T-tube, stents, cholecystostomy)
Internal	Bilio-enteric	
	Cholecystoduodenal	Gallstones
	Cholecystocolic	Gallstones, carcinoma
	Cholecystogastric	Gallstones, carcinoma, peptic ulceration
	Choledochoduodenal	Ductal calculi, iatrogenic, duodenal ulcer, carcinoma
	Biliobilial	
	Cholecystocholedochal	Gallstones (Mirizzi's syndrome)
	Others:	
	Broncho/pleurobilial	Trauma, operative injuries, liver abscesses/hydatid, subphrenic abscess
	Cholecystorenal	Gallstones

investigation with cholangiography (ERCP or PTC) and contrast sinography. Otherwise, a conservative management is adopted as the biliary fistula usually closes spontaneously. Persistence of the fistula beyond a reasonable period (7–10 days), the development of jaundice, pyrexia or deterioration of the patient's condition are indications for urgent re-assessment and investigation.

Internal fistulas are usually spontaneous and arise from chronic or acute perforation of the gallbladder into an adjacent organ. Others are due to malignant infiltration arising from or involving the gallbladder, e.g. carcinoma of the hepatic flexure, duodenum or gallbladder. The symptoms of the non-malignant internal fistulas involving the gallbladder are similar to those of chronic cholecystitis but jaundice and cholangitis are more common and radiology of the abdomen shows gas or barium in the biliary tree. The most frequent of the internal fistulas is the cholecystoduodenal fistula followed by cholecystocolic and cholecystogastric fistulas. The Mirizzi syndrome refers to a condition characterized by obstructive jaundice caused by a stone impacted in the neck of the gallbladder which compresses the common hepatic duct and which eventually ulcerates through into the common hepatic duct causing a cholecystocholedochal fistula (*Fig.* 69.42).

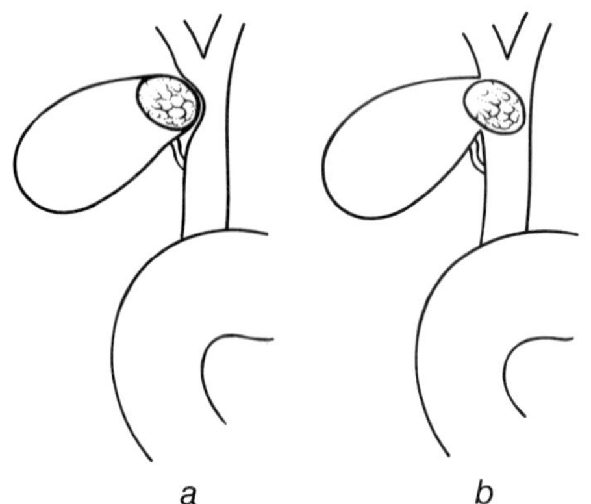

Fig. 69.42 The Mirizzi syndrome. A stone impacted in the neck/Hartmann's pouch causes extrinsic compression of the common hepatic duct followed by fistula formation between the gallbladder and the common hepatic duct.

A fistulous tract between the lower end of the bile duct and the duodenum (choledochoduodenal fistula) may arise spontaneously (secondary to ductal calculi or chronic duodenal ulcer) or be the result of iatrogenic injury from ill-advised probing of the Vaterian segment of the common bile duct during biliary surgery.

Biliopleural and bronchopleural fistulas are usually the result of hepatic abscesses and hydatid disease of the liver though some follow hepatic injuries complicated by the development of subphrenic abscesses.

The treatment of bilioenteric fistulas due to gallstone disease consists of a cholecystectomy and closure of the fistulous communication. Exploration of the common bile duct is frequently necessary and is dictated by the findings at peroperative cholangiography. Unless the Mirizzi syndrome is recognized at operation, damage to the common hepatic duct is inevitable. The surgical treatment of this condition entails leaving a small cuff of gallbladder wall which is used to close the fistulous opening. The common bile duct is explored (if necessary), through a choledochotomy lower down. The management of bronchobiliary fistulas consists of adequate drainage of the underlying hepatic/subphrenic abscess and decompression of the biliary tract when necessary.

GALLSTONE ILEUS

The condition which characteristically affects the elderly, is due to intraluminal intestinal obstruction by a large gallstone which enters the intestinal tract subsequent to the establishment of a fistula, usually between the gallbladder and the duodenum and less commonly, the gallbladder and the colon. Gallstone ileus occurs in 2% of patients with gallstone disease and in some reports, accounts for up to 20% of mechanical intestinal obstruction in the elderly.

The patient who may give a history of gallbladder disease, presents acutely with acute intestinal obstruction which in the vast majority of cases, affects the small bowel, colonic obstruction being distinctly uncommon. Characteristically, the level of the obstruction is changing until the stone becomes firmly impacted usually in the terminal ileum (70%) as this is the narrowest part of the intestinal tract and much less commonly in the duodenum. Colonic obstruction due to impaction in the colon is the result of a cholecystocolic fistula.

The condition should be suspected in the elderly patient with mechanical intestinal obstruction in the absence of the more common causes of this condition. It can be diagnosed preoperatively if gas can be demonstrated in the biliary tract or the gallstone is visualized usually in the right iliac fossa (*Fig.* 69.43).

The treatment requires emergency surgical intervention in all patients. The operative management depends on the findings and the general condition of the patient. In the elderly and frail patient with ileal obstruction, removal of the impacted calculus through a small enterotomy is performed and the cholecystoduodenal fistula is dealt with at a subsequent operation. A one-stage enterolithotomy with cholecystectomy and closure of the duodenal fistula can be performed in patients who, despite their age, are considered fit enough for this procedure. The treatment of patients with colonic obstruction and a cholecystocolic fistula consists of removal of the calculus through a colotomy, cholecystostomy (cholecystectomy if the patient is fit) and exteriorization of the colonic fistula as a proximal (diverting) colostomy.

POSTCHOLECYSTECTOMY SYNDROMES

These refer to the persistence of symptoms referable to the biliary tract after cholecystectomy. As currently defined, the syndromes exclude those patients whose symptoms are due to organic disease outwith the biliary tract. These constitute a significant percentage of patients with persistent symptoms after cholecystectomy and they are usually a reflection of failure of proper evaluation and investigation of patients prior to the cholecystectomy.

The reported incidence of postcholecystectomy syndromes vary widely and correlates with the duration of follow up. There is a female preponderance particularly in the age group 40–50 years.

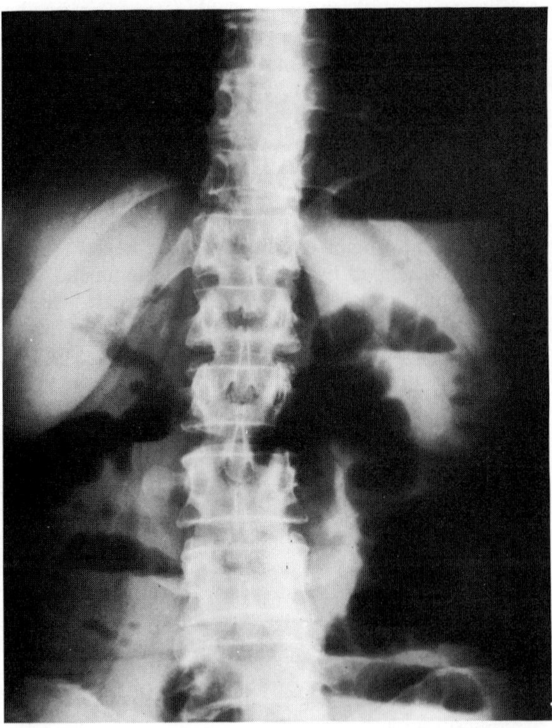

a

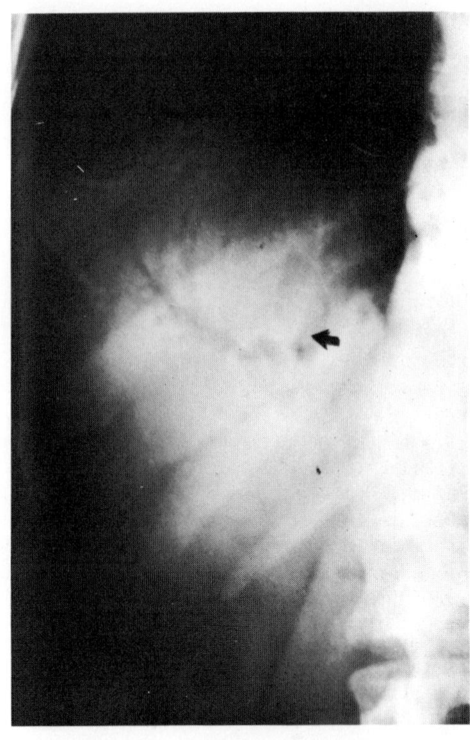

b

Fig. 69.43 *a*, Plain radiograph of the abdomen. Gas outlines the common bile duct. The patient presented with cholangitis and gallstone ileus. A spontaneous cholecystoduodenal fistula was found at operation. *b*, Gas outlining the right hepatic duct. The patient had an empyema of the gallbladder and a cholecystocolic fistula due to a carcinoma of the hepatic flexure.

A careful evaluation and a full investigation of the biliary tract including an ERCP is advisable in all patients with persistence or recurrence of symptoms after cholecystectomy. The common causes of postcholecystectomy syndromes are:

Retained or recurrent calculi
Gallbladder/cystic duct remnants
Bile duct strictures and other unrecognized iatrogenic injuries (choledochoduodenal fistula)
Papillary stenosis and biliary dyskinesia.

Persistent or recurrent symptoms after cholecystostomy are common and is one of the reasons for subsequent cholecystectomy in all patients who are considered fit for surgery. Controversy still exists regarding the role of a 'long cystic duct remnant' as a cause of persistent symptoms after cholecystectomy. There are undoubtedly patients in whom a dilated long cystic duct remnant containing stones is demonstrated on investigation and its removal together with the stones results in sustained symptomatic improvement. However, these cases are few and far between and at present there is no evidence to incriminate an otherwise normal long cystic duct remnant as one of the important causes of the postcholecystectomy syndrome.

Papillary stenosis (also known as choledochoduodenal junctional stenosis) is nowadays regarded as a rare but definite entity which results from fibrosis or fibromuscular hyperplasia of the sphincter of Oddi. An associated duodenal diverticulum is common and cannulation of the papilla is difficult. In addition to pain in the upper abdomen, the patient may exhibit slight abnormalities in the liver function tests, including mild hyperbilirubinaemia and elevated alkaline phosphatase activity. The resting sphincter pressure is elevated as is the passage pressure and there is loss of the normal phasic sphincteric activity. At operation, papillary stenosis is best demonstrated radiologically by the technique of contact selective cholangiography. In addition to duct dilatation, there is a characteristic alteration in the configuration of the infundibulum (transduodenal segment) which loses its conical shape and becomes wider than the intrapancreatic segment (*Fig.* 69.44). Biliary sludge and small ductal calculi are often present. Reflux into a dilated pancreatic duct is also observed in some cases.

The treatment of papillary stenosis is equally controversial. Endoscopic sphincterotomy or surgical transduodenal sphincteroplasty is recommended by the majority although there has not been an adequate long-term assessment of these procedures for this rare and elusive condition. In addition to the sphincteroplasty, Moody advocates the excision of the septum between the pancreatic duct and the bile duct in patients with chronic pain which he maintains is of pancreatic origin.

An alternative surgical treatment for papillary stenosis favoured by the authors is transection choledochoduodenostomy with reimplantation of the mobilized duct into the junction of the first with the second part of the duodenum (*Fig.* 69.45).

The term *biliary dyskinesia* is used to denote those patients who have persistent pain after cholecystectomy and no other abnormality on physical examination and routine testing but who exhibit the following abnormalities during ERCP manometry:

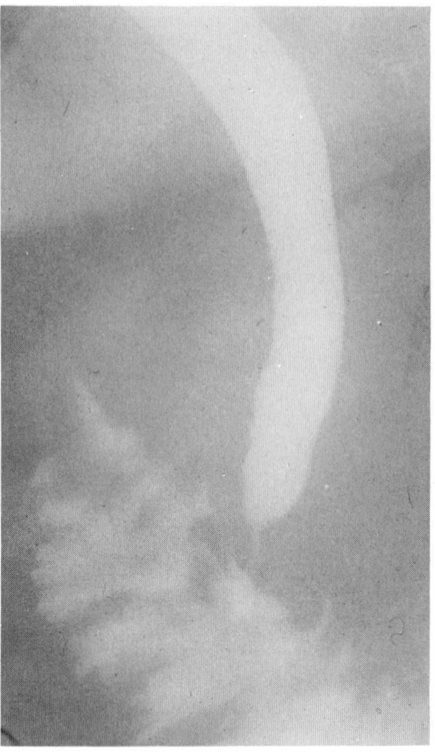

Fig. 69.44 Operative contact selective cholangiogram demonstrating papillary stenosis. There is minimal dilatation of the bile duct and the infundibulum becomes globular. Biliary sludge/small ductal calculi are often present.

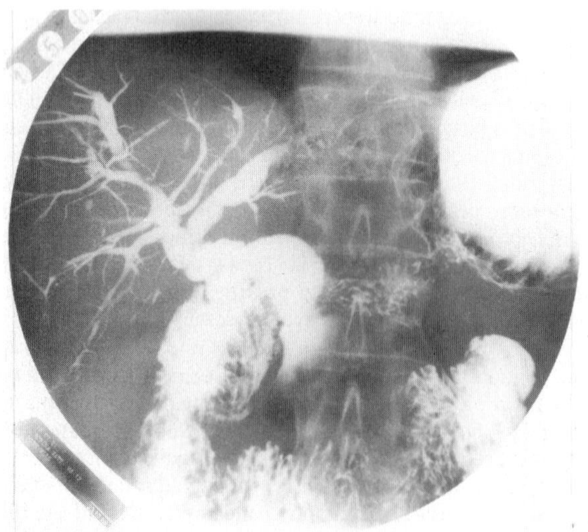

Fig. 69.45 Barium meal contrast study after transection choledochoduodenostomy performed for papillary stenosis 3 years previously.

Elevated resting pressure
Tachyarrhythmia (increased phasic activity of the sphincter)
Retrograde contractions of the sphincter
Paradoxical response to cholecystokinin.

Treatment with endoscopic sphincterotomy has been advocated for these patients but the efficacy of this in the long-term relief of symptoms remains to be ascertained.

BENIGN BILE DUCT STRICTURES

In the clinical context, benign strictures of the extrahepatic bile ducts do not exhibit a benign course since they are always attended by significant symptoms and serious complications (which are life-threatening both in the short and the long term), and carry a definite mortality. As their surgical management requires special expertise, referral to and treatment in specialized centres offers the best chance of reversal from a potentially fatal condition to long-term restoration of good health with freedom from symptoms and return to normal liver function.

The causes of benign bile duct strictures are shown in *Table* 69.9.

Table 69.9 Causes of benign bile duct strictures

Operative trauma
Penetrating and non-penetrating abdominal injuries
Chronic duodenal ulcer
Chronic pancreatitis
Recurrent pyogenic cholangitis and parasitic infestations
Sclerosing cholangitis

Pathology

In the Western Hemisphere, the vast majority of bile duct strictures are the result of preventable injuries to the extrahepatic biliary tract, usually during the operation of cholecystectomy and, less frequently, gastrectomy. The average reported incidence of operative bile duct damage is 1 in 400–500 cholecystectomies. There is little doubt that the majority of bile duct injuries sustained during operation result from failure of appreciation of the precise anatomy of the area. The situations which predispose or result in damage to the bile ducts at operation are varied and not necessarily related to the degree of technical difficulty of the operation. The more common circumstances leading to iatrogenic tragedy can be summarized as follows:

1. Bleeding from the right branch of the hepatic artery with blind hasty clamping of the area.
2. Persistence of dissection in the triangle of Calot in the presence of gross adhesions/oedema instead of performing retrograde cholecystectomy in difficult cases.
3. Excessive traction of the gallbladder and cystic duct with tenting of the common bile duct which is then inadvertently clamped.
4. Failure of appreciation of the varying anatomy of the extrahepatic biliary tract and hepatic artery and its branches. The classical described 'normal' anatomy is infrequently found at operation.
5. Inadequate display of the relevant anatomy.
6. Failure to perform and correctly interpret a peroperative cholangiogram.

7. Clamping of structures, such as the cystic artery and duct, in preference to ligation in continuity.
8. Devascularization from excessive close mobilization of the bile duct.

The lesion is most commonly a complete transection although lateral (incomplete) injuries are not infrequent. Occasionally, bile duct excision is inadvertently performed. In some instances, there is no record of any untoward mishap during the operation and the condition declares itself postoperatively or several months to years later. Most of these cases are the result of unrecognized partial injuries sustained during the cholecystectomy. A vascular element due to damage to the ascending arteries of the bile duct has been postulated by some in the pathogenesis of some of the strictures which present several months to years after cholecystectomy (*Fig.* 69.46).

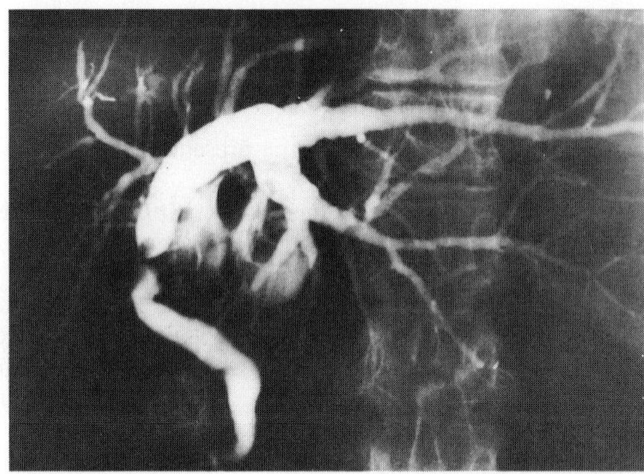

Fig. 69.46 Localized stricture of the lower hepatic duct with ductal stones 10 years after cholecystectomy and exploration of the common bile duct. The patient had been completely symptom free until then and presented acutely with cholangitis. Some have ascribed these localized late strictures to impairment of the vascular supply.

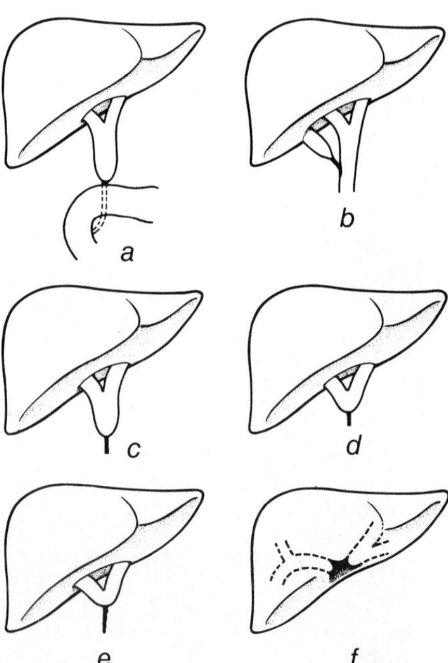

Fig. 69.47 Pathological anatomy of postoperative bile duct strictures. *a*, Distal bile duct stricture. *b*, Stricture of an anomalously inserted branch of the right hepatic. This may or may not be accompanied by stricture of the main ductal system. *c*, Low stricture of the common hepatic duct (>2·0 cm). *d*, Mid common hepatic duct stricture (<2·0 cm). *e*, High stricture with intact confluence of the right and left hepatic ducts. *f*, Obliteration of the entire hepatic duct and the confluence.

The pathological anatomy of established bile duct strictures following injuries to the extrahepatic biliary system is variable but most lesions are situated proximally and involve the hepatic duct and the bifurcation (*Fig.* 69.47). The recognized types are:

1. Stricture of the distal duct (*Fig.* 69.48). This usually follows trauma by blind metal bouginage of the lower end of the common bile duct and is often preceded by choledochoduodenal fistula and postoperative pancreatitis. It usually follows protracted attempts to dislodge an impacted stone by blind instrumentation through a supraduodenal choledochotomy.
2. Stricture of the right hepatic duct or one of its branches (ventrocranial or dorsocaudal) at the junction with the bile duct. This may or may not involve the main bile duct.
3. Low common hepatic duct stricture with a hepatic duct stump >2·0 cm (*Fig.* 69.49).
4. Mid common hepatic duct stricture with a hepatic duct stump <2·0 cm (*Fig.* 69.50).
5. High stricture with absence of the hepatic duct but an intact hilar confluence (*Fig.* 69.51).
6. Destruction of the hilar confluence. These are the most difficult strictures to repair and they often require resection of liver substance to access the right and left hepatic ducts.

Complete and partial injuries are usually accompanied by bile leakage either into the peritoneal cavity with the development of bile peritonitis or the development of an external biliary fistula in the postoperative period. The occurrence of sepsis with the formation of subphrenic and subhepatic abscesses is usual in these patients who may become septicaemic. Jaundice may be initially absent or mild, especially in patients with external biliary fistulas but cholangitis is frequent.

The late consequences, apart from frequent episodes of cholangitis, are hepatic fibrosis, secondary biliary cirrhosis and the development of portal hypertension.

A long stricture of the lower end of the common bile duct which characteristically forms an angle with the proximal dilated duct, is encountered in 15–20% of patients with chronic pancreatitis (*Fig.* 69.52). However, the differentiation between this disease and pancreatic carcinoma is often difficult in these patients. Recurrent pyogenic cholangitis and sclerosing cholangitis are considered later on in this chapter.

Clinical Features

If the lesion is not recognized at operation, the bile duct injury usually declares itself postoperatively by the development of an external biliary fistula. This is frequently associated with evidence of sepsis and the development of subphrenic/subhepatic abscesses. Peritonitis caused by leakage of bile into the peritoneal cavity may occur. The

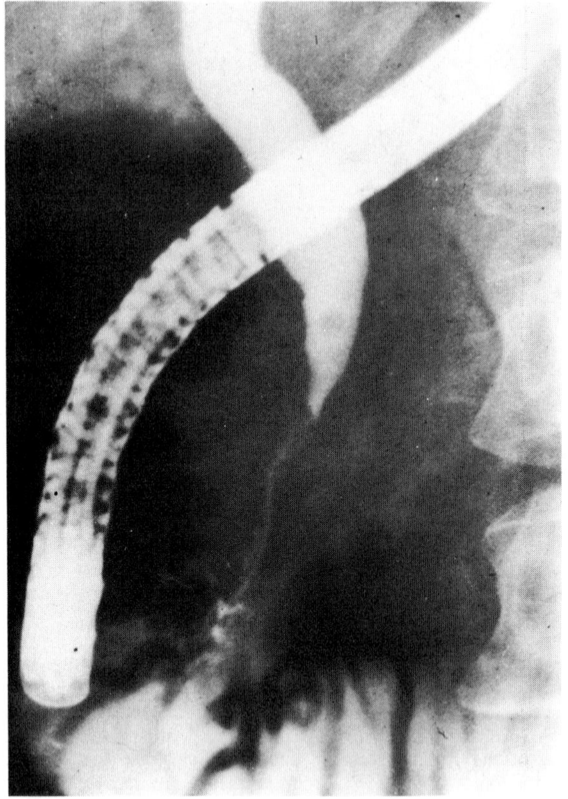

Fig. 69.48 Stricture of the lower end of the common bile duct following blind stone fragmentation of an impacted stone and forcible passage of metal bougies.

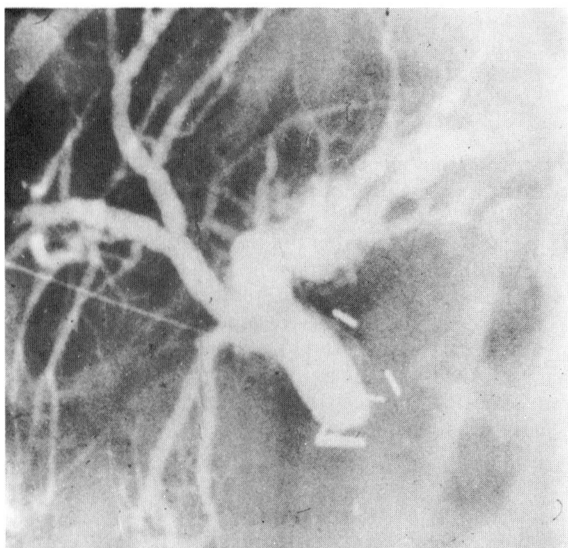

Fig. 69.49 Low common hepatic duct stricture.

patient is toxic with pyrexia and may develop rigors due to the onset of septicaemia. Jaundice is often present but may not be severe or progressive in the presence of an external biliary fistula.

Apart from liver function tests and culture of the discharge and blood, visualization of the biliary tract to ascertain the presence of bile duct damage and its severity is mandatory. A fistulogram may provide useful information on the site of the damage. Usually, however, an ERCP or PTC are required. Often both of these investigations are necessary to obtain a full picture of the state of the biliary tree and the extent of the trauma.

Treatment

This depends on whether the injury is recognized at operation or subsequently either because the patient develops

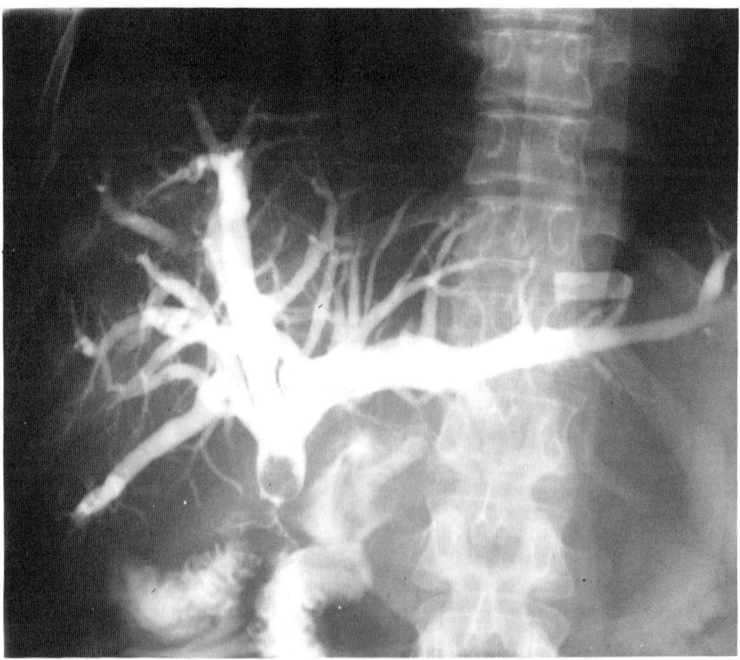

Fig. 69.50 High common hepatic duct stricture.

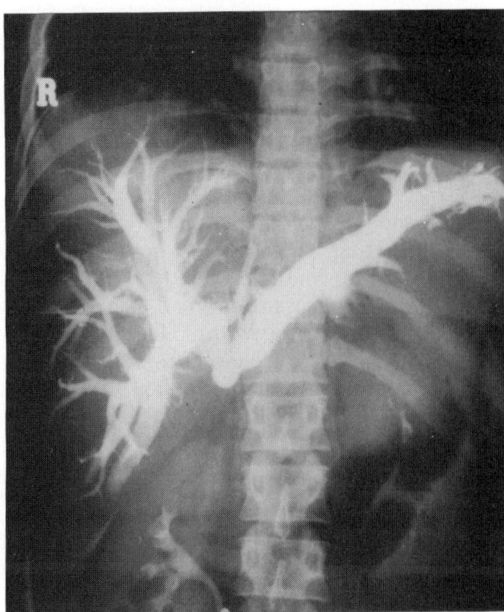

Fig. 69.51 Obliteration of the hepatic duct with an intact confluence of the right and left hepatic ducts.

serious complications postoperatively or presents after discharge from hospital with recurrent episodes of pain, fever and jaundice.

Injuries Recognized at Operation

The treatment depends on the site and extent of the damage. For high complete transections, a Roux-en-Y hepaticojejunostomy is considered preferable to a difficult direct suture repair as this usually becomes strictured in time. For lower complete injuries with a serviceable proximal duct stump, primary suture repair with fine interrupted absorbable (PDS or Vicryl) sutures over a T-tube is the treatment of choice (*Fig.* 69.53). The long limb of the T-tube must not be exteriorized through the repair site as this enhances the risks of stricture formation.

Partial (lateral) injuries are often treated by the insertion of a T-tube and a Roux-en-Y serosal patch. The long limb of the T-tube is exteriorized through the mobilized jejunum (*Fig.* 69.54). Other techniques include repair with a vein patch over a T-tube (*Fig.* 69.55).

There is an undoubted high incidence of stricture formation following primary repair of bile duct injuries (up to 60%). All these patients, therefore, require long-term follow-up with radiological assessment if they develop symptoms or abnormalities of the liver function tests.

Injuries Recognized in the Postoperative Period

The initial management is supportive. Fluid and electrolyte disorders, if present, are corrected and the patient is put on systemic antibiotics. Surgical intervention is required for the following:

Drainage of abscesses
Development of peritonitis.

Otherwise, the patient is initially managed conservatively. An ostomy bag is used to collect the bile leakage from the fistula which usually dries up. Persistence of the external biliary fistula does not constitute a serious problem since skin excoriation does not occur and the daily losses are seldom severe enough to cause significant fluid and electrolyte depletion. Surgical intervention to deal with the bile duct injury at this stage is ill-advised as the repair is difficult due to the inflammatory oedema and because the proximal ductal system is not yet dilated. Repair is, therefore, best postponed for several weeks, by which time the intra-abdominal sepsis has subsided, the stricture has matured

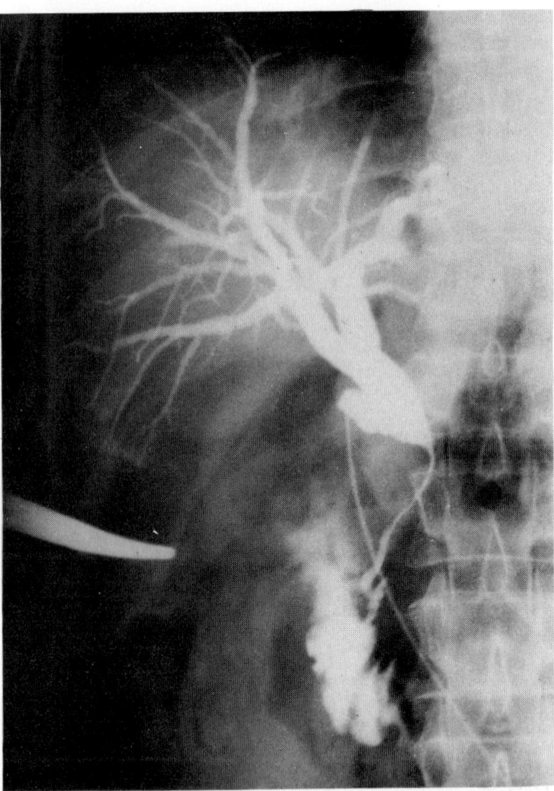

Fig. 69.52 Long stricture of the distal bile ductt in a patient with chronic alcoholic pancreatitis of 12 years' duration. There is an angle between the stricture and the proximal dilated duct. The stenosis is due to the pancreatic fibrosis which constricts the transpancreatic segment of the common bile duct.

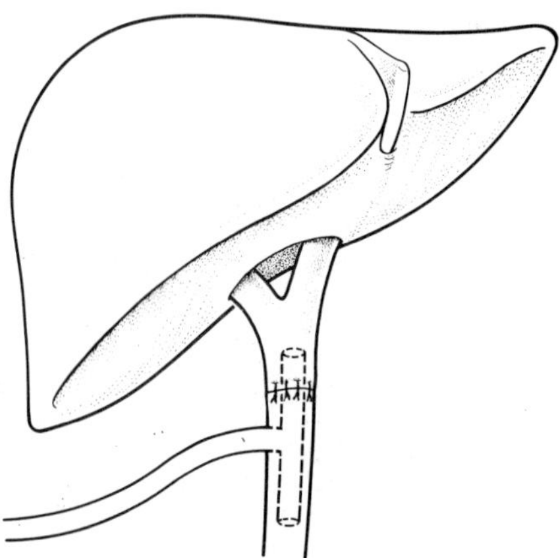

Fig. 69.53 Primary repair of a complete injury recognized at operation. The long limb of the T-tube is exteriorized below the suture repair. The risk of stenosis is considerably enhanced if the long limb of the T-tube is brought out at the site of repair.

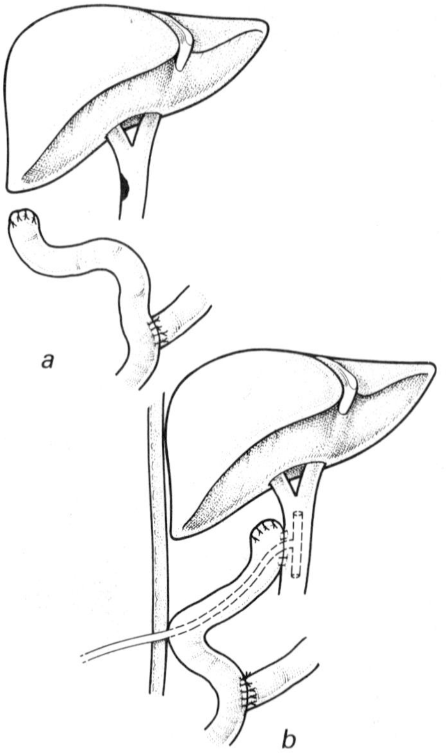

Fig. 69.54 Serosal patch Roux-en-Y technique with T-tube intubation for lateral injuries discovered at operation. *a*, Construction of a Roux-en-Y loop. *b*, The Roux loop is sutured over the defect after the insertion of a T-tube, the long limb of which is brought out through the jejunal loop.

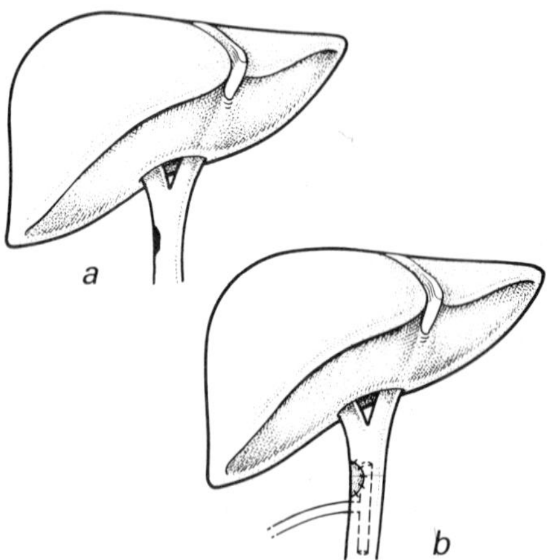

Fig. 69.55 Repair of lateral injury recognized at operation by a vein patch. The T-tube is inserted via a small choledochotomy lower down.

and the proximal ducts have dilated, thus facilitating the procedure.

Definitive Repair of Established Bile Duct Strictures

The definitive treatment of bile duct strictures is best carried out in specialized centres where the overall results, in terms of long-term freedom from jaundice and cholangitis and maintenance of good to normal liver function, are excellent (85–90%) and the operative mortality is low (1–5%). The exact treatment depends on the pathological anatomy of the stricture:

1. For lesions of the distal duct a choledochoduodenostomy (preferably of the transection type) is performed after full mobilization of the duodenum. Some would prefer a Roux-en-Y choledochojejunostomy for these strictures.

2. For common hepatic duct strictures with a serviceable extrahepatic duct stump, a Roux-en-Y hepaticojejunostomy is the treatment most commonly used (*Fig.* 69.56*a*). The establishment of a mucosa-to-mucosa anastomosis using absorbable fine sutures between the bile duct remnant and the jejunal mucosa is the single most important factor in the prevention of recurrent stricture formation. If good mucosal coaptation is achieved, there is no indication for stenting of the anastomosis and indeed this is undesirable under these circumstances. Some prefer to use an isolated jejunal isoperistaltic segment interposed between the stump of the common hepatic duct and the duodenum (*Fig.* 69.57) instead of the Roux-en-Y loop.

3. For high strictures with no residual stump but with an intact hilar confluence, dissection of the liver plate to expose the left hepatic duct as it crosses at the bottom of the quadrate lobe (anterior segment IV), enables a good anastomosis to be performed between this duct and a Roux-en-Y jejunal loop. This technique does not require any splitting or resection of the liver parenchyma (*Fig.* 69.58).

4. Destruction of the hilar confluence. These are the most difficult strictures to deal with and usually require some resection or splitting of the liver substance. An access jejunostomy is increasingly being used in addition to the repair. This allows percutaneous dilatation if the stricture recurs. All these procedures require stenting either transhepatically or through the jejunal loop. The various options are:

i. Round ligament approach with anastomosis to the segment III duct (*Fig.* 69.2). This functions well provided there is a communication between the right and the left ductal systems.

ii. Excision of the quadrate lobe to identify the right and left hepatic ducts which are then anastomosed separately to a Roux-en-Y loop (*Figs.* 69.56*b*, 69.59).

iii. The Smith's mucosal graft operation. This entails excision of scar tissue until the orifices of the right and left hepatic ducts are encountered. A Roux-en-Y loop is prepared and an ellipse of the seromuscular layer is cut on the antimesenteric border to expose the serosa. Two straight stents are introduced and anchored to the loop from the outside. The stents are inserted into the right and left ductal systems and brought out through the anterosuperior surface of the liver. When traction is applied to the stents, the jejunal mucosa is approximated to that of the hepatic ducts (*Fig.* 69.60). However, this technique and the Longmire's procedure (anastomosis of a Roux loop to the segment III duct after excision of the lateral part of the left lobe) are seldom used nowadays as their results are inferior to the above procedures.

In these high strictures, a stent is placed across the anastomosis and this is exteriorized through the jejunum which is sutured to the abdominal wall at the exit site of the tube. The site of fixation of the jejunum is marked with metal clips. This allows easy identification of this access jejunostomy, thereby permitting the introduction of fine flexible endoscopes and balloon catheters for percutaneous dilatation in the event of re-stricturing after surgical repair.

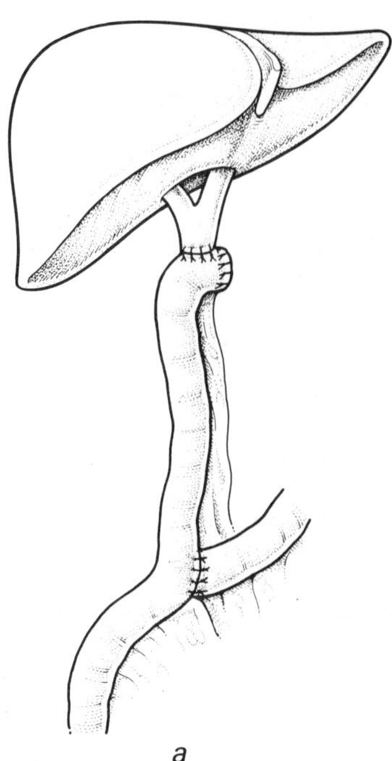

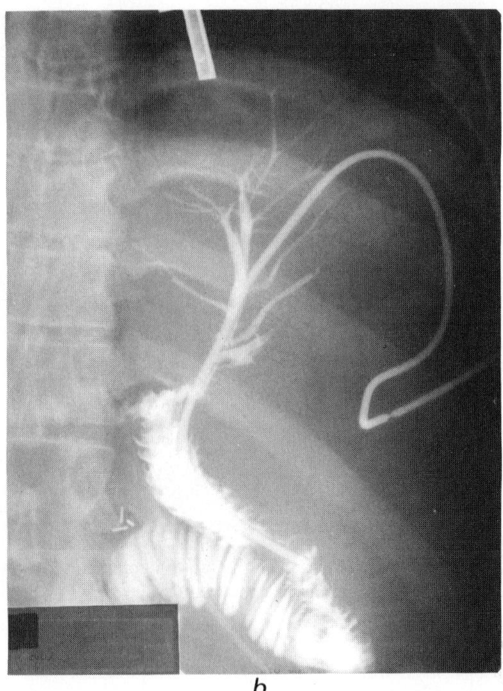

Fig. 69.56 *a*, Roux-en-Y hepaticojejunostomy for low common hepatic duct stricture. *b*, Postoperative cholangiogram after hepaticojejunostomy for high common hepatic duct stricture with destruction of hilar confluence.

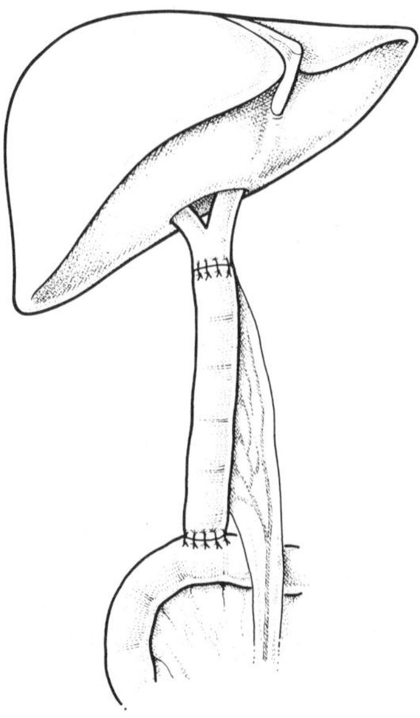

Fig. 69.57 Isoperistaltic jejunal loop interposed between the stump of the common hepatic duct and the duodenum.

SCLEROSING CHOLANGITIS

This is an obscure disorder of uncertain aetiology which results in a progressive fibrous obliteration of the biliary tract. Although sclerosing cholangitis has well-recognized histological, radiological and clinical features, there are no pathognomonic findings that reliably differentiate this disease from other hepatobiliary disorders. The distinction between primary and secondary types is no longer held to be valid. The term primary was formerly used to indicate no previous biliary surgery or biliary tract disease. Often, however, sclerosing cholangitis occurs as a secondary complication of inflammatory bowel disease, usually ulcerative colitis and, much less commonly, Crohn's disease. The condition is currently regarded as an immune-complex disorder evoked by endotoxin–antibody complexes which have been identified in the peripheral blood of patients with inflammatory bowel disease.

The classification of the disorder is based on the extent of involvement of the biliary tree by the fibrous obliterative process (*Table* 69.10).

The disease results in extensive fibrosis which extends beyond the confines of the biliary ductal walls. Histologically, the fibrosis is concentric (onion shell) with patchy, chronic inflammatory infiltrate consisting of mononuclear cells and polymorphs (*Fig.* 69.61). In addition, changes of cholestasis are seen. The gross fibrous thickening results in localized or multiple stricture formation. Although the ductal epithelium is frequently normal, it may become ulcerated and exhibit saccule formation. The disease progresses invariably to cirrhosis and the development of portal hypertension.

Sclerosing cholangitis occurs more commonly in males (3:2) and usually presents in the fifth decade. The symptoms include vague ill-health, asthenia, pain in the right hypochondrium, jaundice and itching, pyrexia and attacks of rigors. The liver is often palpable and tender. The liver function tests demonstrate a cholestatic picture and bilirubin is detected in the urine. The serum transaminases are mildly elevated. The majority of patients are HBsAg negative. The antimitochondrial, antismooth muscle and antinuclear antibodies are absent. Contrast radiological visualization shows pruning of the biliary tree (scanty ducts)

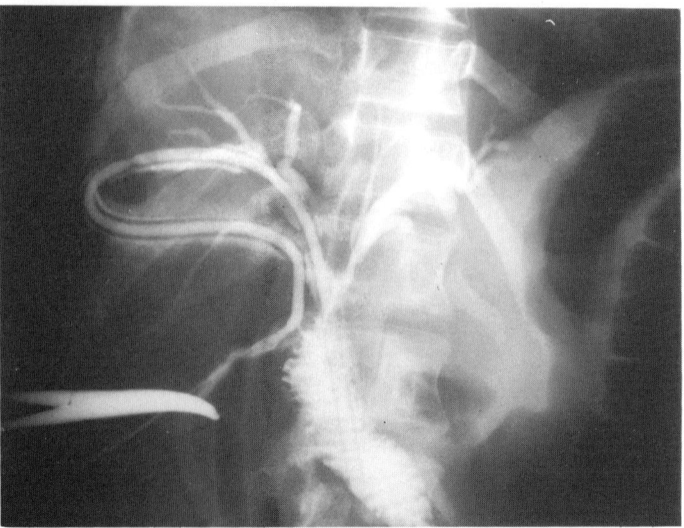

Fig. 69.58 Postoperative cholangiogram after Roux-en-Y hepaticojejunostomy for high common hepatic duct stricture.

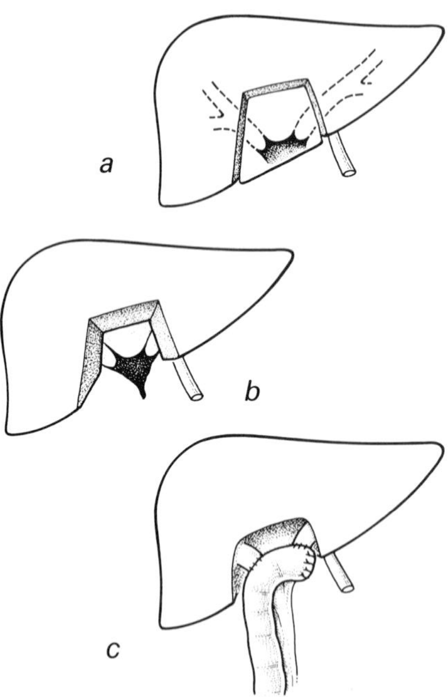

Fig. 69.59 Hepaticojejunostomy for lesions with obliteration of the hilar confluence of the right and left hepatic ducts. *a*, The quadrate lobe (segment IV) anterior to the hilus is excised (segment between the gallbladder fossa and the round ligament). *b*, Exposure of the obliterated confluence and identification of the right and left hepatic ducts. *c*, The right and left hepatic ducts are anastomosed separately to the Roux-en-Y loop.

and stricture formation which may be localized or diffuse (*Fig.* 69.62) Globular dilatations (sacculations) are often seen in patients with diffuse disease. Differentiation from hilar and diffuse cholangiocarcinoma is often difficult on radiological grounds and may not be possible even after histological examination of biopsy specimens. In these patients, only the subsequent clinical outcome can identify the true diagnosis.

Unfortunately, there is no effective medical therapy for the condition. The pruritus may be controlled by cholestyramine. Episodes of cholangitis are managed by antibiotic therapy. Surgical intervention is undertaken when adequate control of symptoms is not achieved by medical therapy, the specific indications being:

Progressive jaundice
Recurrent cholangitis.

Surgical treatment gives best results for the localized hilar disease. The hilar bifurcation is accessed through an anterior segmentectomy IV and a Roux-en-Y hepaticojejunostomy to the right and left hepatic ducts performed proximal to the stricture. For diffuse disease, intraoperative dilatation of the intrahepatic biliary tree via a choledochotomy using both metal and balloon dilators is followed by a large silicone stent introduced transhepatically down the bile duct into the duodenum (*Fig.* 69.63). Closure of the bile duct may not be possible after insertion of the stent, in which case a vein patch is used to close the defect. The stent is exteriorized through the right lowest intercostal space in the anterior axillary line. Daily irrigation with heparinized saline and prolonged antibiotic therapy are essential components of the postoperative management. The stent is left in place for at least 12 months and progress is assessed by repeat cholangiograms carried out through the stent (*Fig.* 69.64). Replacement of the stent may be necessary if it becomes blocked by encrustation with calcium bilirubinate. In recent years, hepatic transplantation has been performed for patients with diffuse disease and the early results of this treatment for severe sclerosing cholangitis have been encouraging.

RECURRENT PYOGENIC CHOLANGITIS

This condition which is prevalent in South-east Asia is characterized by recurrent attacks of bacterial cholangitis which lead to the formation of pigment stones and strictures

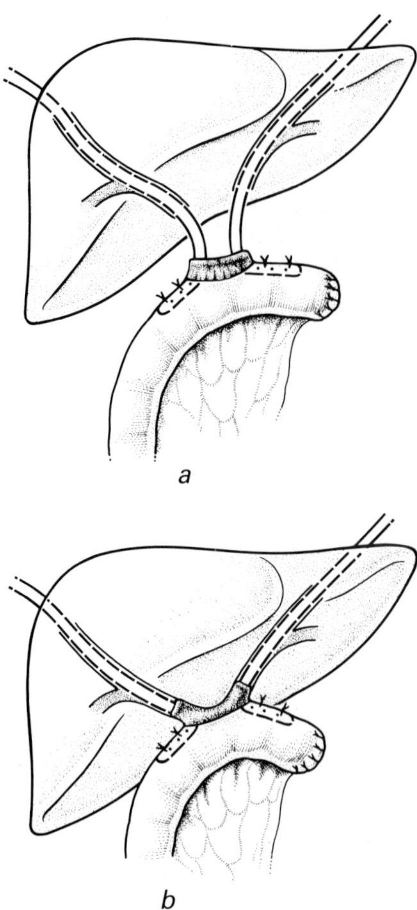

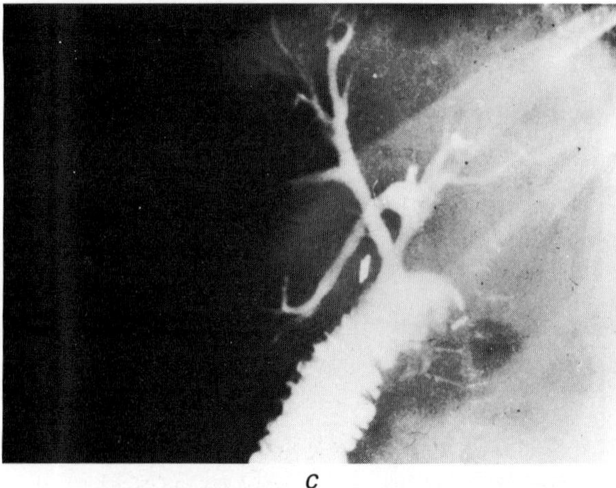

Fig. 69.60 Smith's mucosal graft operation. *a*, Stents fixed to the jejunal loop and inserted transhepatically through the right and left ductal systems before approximation. *b*, Traction on the transhepatic stents results in mucosal approximation. *c*, Cholangiogram following the mucosal graft operation.

Table 69.10 Sclerosing cholangitis: classification based on extent of involvement of the biliary tree

Type	*Incidence (%)*
Total diffuse	50
Localized hilar	25
Diffuse intrahepatic	10
Diffuse extrahepatic	10
Localized extrahepatic (distal)	5

in the biliary tract. Although the exact aetiology is unknown, infection of the biliary tract with enteric organisms (*E. coli*, *B. fragilis*, *Klebsiella* sp. and *Clostridium* sp.) in debilitated (immunocompromised) patients is regarded to be the primary event. Although parasitic infestation with *Clonorchis sinensis* and *Ascaris lumbricoides* is found in some patients, there is little evidence that these parasites play an important role in the development of recurrent pyogenic cholangitis although they may predispose to it. The disease affects both the intrahepatic and the extrahepatic bile ducts. It has a well-established predilection for the left lobe of the

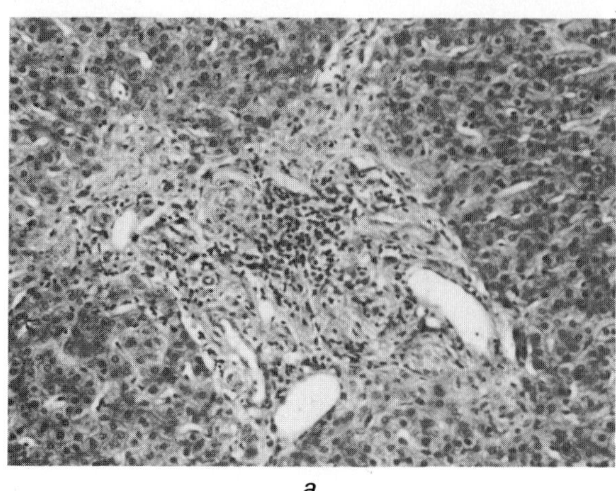

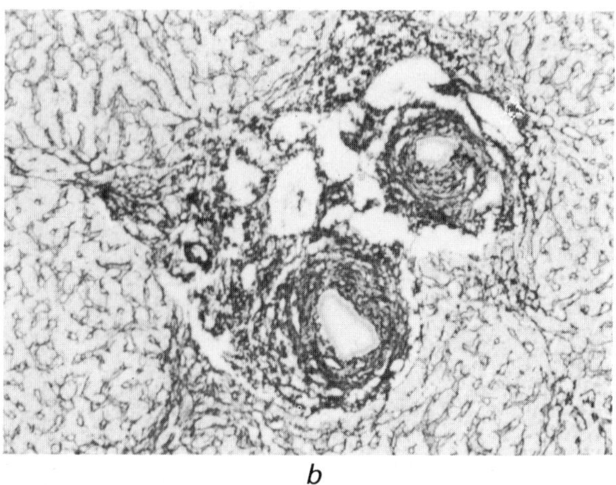

Fig. 69.61 Sclerosing cholangitis. *a*, Histology of wedge liver biopsy (H & E) showing narrowing of the intrahepatic ducts, fibrosis and cellular infiltrate. *b*, Reticulin stain of the same biopsy illustrating concentric deposition of fibrous tissue around the bile ducts.

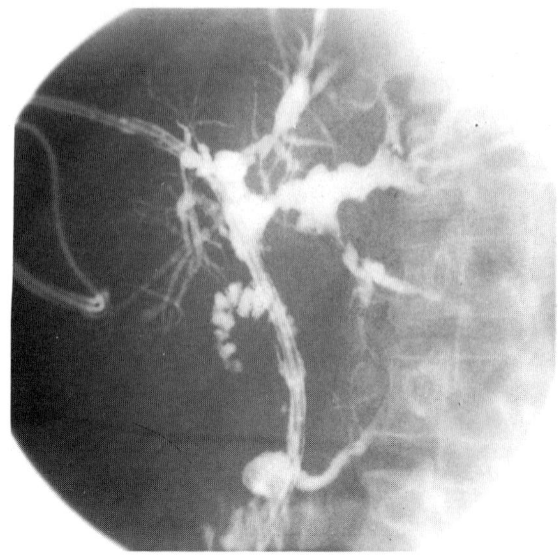

Fig. 69.62 Sclerosing cholangitis: total involvement of the biliary tract.

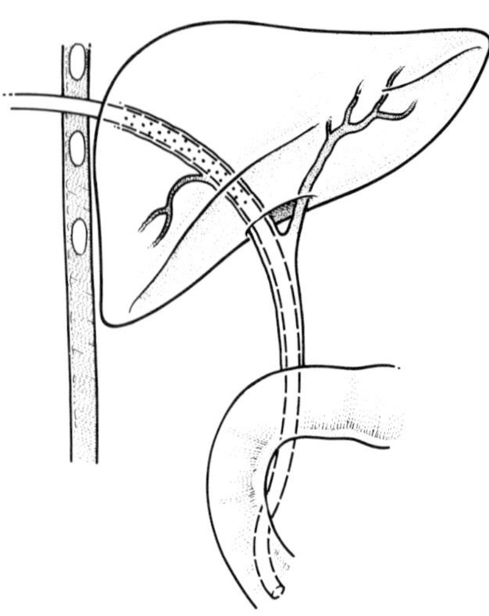

Fig. 69.63 Technique of transhepatic stenting for total diffuse sclerosing cholangitis.

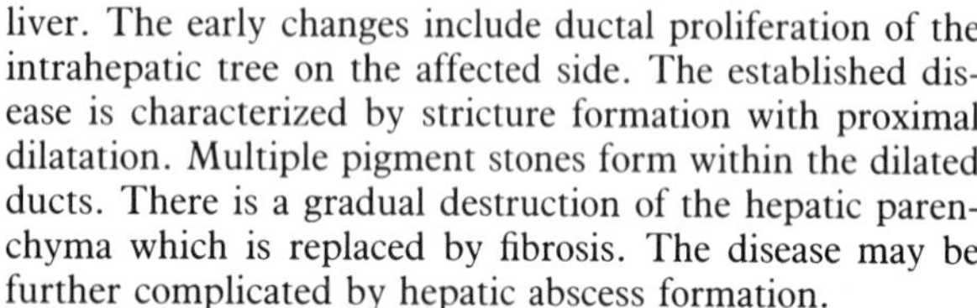

liver. The early changes include ductal proliferation of the intrahepatic tree on the affected side. The established disease is characterized by stricture formation with proximal dilatation. Multiple pigment stones form within the dilated ducts. There is a gradual destruction of the hepatic parenchyma which is replaced by fibrosis. The disease may be further complicated by hepatic abscess formation.

The condition presents with recurrent episodes of cholangitis and the diagnosis is confirmed by ERCP. The treatment depends on the site, severity and extent of the disease. It entails bile duct exploration with removal of calculi and insertion of T-tube, sphincteroplasty or bilioenteric anastomosis for strictures and hepatic resection for advanced disease of one lobe with atrophy of the liver parenchyma, multiple strictures and stones.

TUMOURS OF THE GALLBLADDER

These consist of benign lesions and carcinoma of the gallbladder.

Benign Tumours

These include adenomas and papillomas. Most are discovered in clinical practice following pathological examination of the excised gallbladder although some are identified as a fixed isolated shadow seen on the oral cholecystogram or gallbladder ultrasound scan in patients with unexplained right hypochondrium discomfort or pain. There is some evidence that adenomas may progress to carcinoma. When diagnosed, a cholecystectomy is considered advisable because of the uncertainty of the diagnosis and the possibility of malignant change.

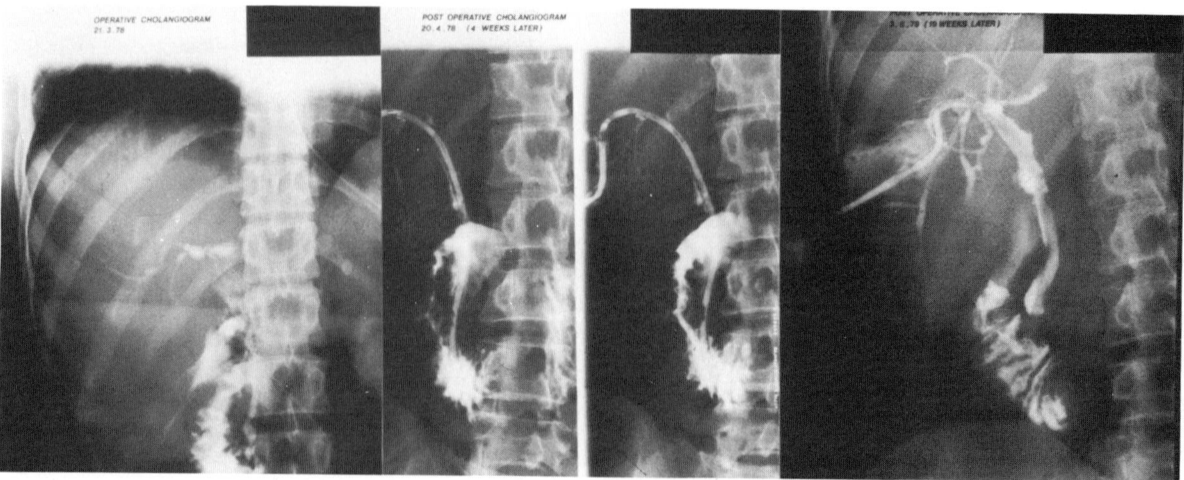

Fig. 69.64 Marked radiological improvement in a patient with sclerosing cholangitis following prolonged stenting of the intra- and extrahepatic biliary tract. The patient showed a dramatic clinical and biochemical improvement.

Carcinoma of the Gallbladder

Carcinoma of the gallbladder is the most common malignancy of the biliary tract and accounts for 3–4% of all gastrointestinal malignancies. The reported autopsy incidence is 0·6–1%. The disease is most commonly seen in elderly women (average age of 65 years) and affects females three times as commonly as males. The exact aetiology is unknown but gallstones are present in 75–90% of reported series of gallbladder cancer. An increased incidence is found in:

Chronic typhoid carriers
South American Indians
Patients with porcelain (calcified) gallbladder
Obese individuals.

The majority of tumours are adenocarcinomas, with papillary, undifferentiated, squamous and adenoacanthoma constituting a minority. Rare tumours include carcinoid, melanoma and ACTH-secreting apudomas. The staging of gallbladder cancer is based on the depth of invasion as follows:

Stage I confined to the mucosa/submucosa
Stage II involvement of the muscle layer
Stage III serosal involvement
Stage IV spread to the cystic node
Stage V invasion of the liver and adjacent organs.

Clinical Features

The disease is either discovered accidentally during cholecystectomy or presents with non-specific symptoms or acutely with an inflammatory mass in the right hypochondrium (acute cholecystitis). The non-specific symptoms include anorexia, nausea and vomiting and weight loss. The patient may be jaundiced (due to involvement of the common hepatic duct), the liver may be enlarged or the gallbladder may be palpable. Ascitis is encountered in advanced disease. Anaemia is present in 50% of patients and is due to chronic haemobilia. Even in the presence of a normal serum bilirubin, the majority of patients have an elevated alkaline phosphatase activity. Few patients with stage I or II disease are diagnosed preoperatively.

Although ultrasound examination of the gallbladder readily identifies advanced disease, it misses the early potentially curable lesions. Oral cholecystography may show a non-functioning gallbladder or a filling defect projecting into the lumen. A coeliac axis angiogram may demonstrate an enlarged cystic artery or tumour circulation in the gallbladder area.

Treatment

The treatment of the cancer of the gallbladder is surgical though opinions vary as to the exact operative procedure which should be done. For stages I and II, the best results are reported with extended cholecystectomy. Initially, the gallbladder is removed and the diagnosis is confirmed by frozen section. If this is positive, a 3–5 cm resection of surrounding hepatic parenchyma is performed together with lymph node clearance. However, some advocate simple cholecystectomy alone on the grounds that there is no firm evidence that the extended procedure improves survival. If the tumour is advanced (stages IV, V), the consensus view is that no excision should be attempted in view of the uniformly poor prognosis. In some cases with involvement of the adjacent liver parenchyma only, a right hepatic lobectomy may be considered if the patient's general condition is good. The response of gallbladder cancer to radiotherapy and chemotherapy is poor.

Survival

The overall 5-year survival is 4%. The 5-year survival for resected cases is 16·5%. The majority of long-term survivors have been patients whose tumours were confined to the mucosa or had minimal involvement of the muscularis.

TUMOURS OF THE BILE DUCTS

Benign Tumours

A variety of benign tumours of the bile duct including adenoma and papilloma have been reported but they are rare and far less common than cholangiocarcinomas. Benign bile duct tumours have a tendency to recur after excision and some have been reported to undergo malignant change. Benign bile duct tumours present with jaundice and occult chronic gastrointestinal haemorrhage (haemobilia).

Malignant Tumours

The reported autopsy incidence of malignant bile duct tumours ranges from 0·01 to 0·5%. The prevalence of carcinomas of the biliary tract and gallbladder in England and Wales is 2·8/100 000 in females and 2·0/100 000 in males. These figures underestimate the true incidence of bile duct cholangiocarcinoma since the intrahepatic ones arising from the minor bile ducts are often classified with liver tumours in many census surveys. Contrary to gallbladder cancer, there is a slight preponderance of males (1·5:1). The age at presentation varies but the peak incidence is in the sixth decade. Bile duct carcinoma is very common in Far Eastern countries where parasitic infestation is endemic (bistomiasis, *Clonorchis sinensis*, *Opisthorchis viverrini*).

The aetiology of bile duct cancer us unknown. The association with gallstones is much less marked than it is with carcinoma of the gallbladder and ductal calculiare found in 20–50% of patients who develop cholangiocarcinoma. Bacterial-induced endogenous carcinogens derived from bile salts (e.g. lithocholate) have been implicated and are supported by the findings of some epidemiological studies and the higher incidence in typhoid carriers. Cholangiocarcinoma is seen with increasing frequency in certain clinical groups (*Table* 69.11).

Table 69.11 High risk groups for the development of cholangiocarcinoma

Parasitic infestation of biliary tract
Cystic disease of the biliary tract
Chronic typhoid carriers
Ulcerative colitis
Sclerosing cholangitis

Pathology

The tumours are best classified into the anatomical site of origin:

1. Intrahepatic from the minor hepatic ducts.
2. Proximal from the right and left hepatic ducts, hilar confluence and proximal common hepatic duct (Klatskin tumours) (*Fig.* 69.65).

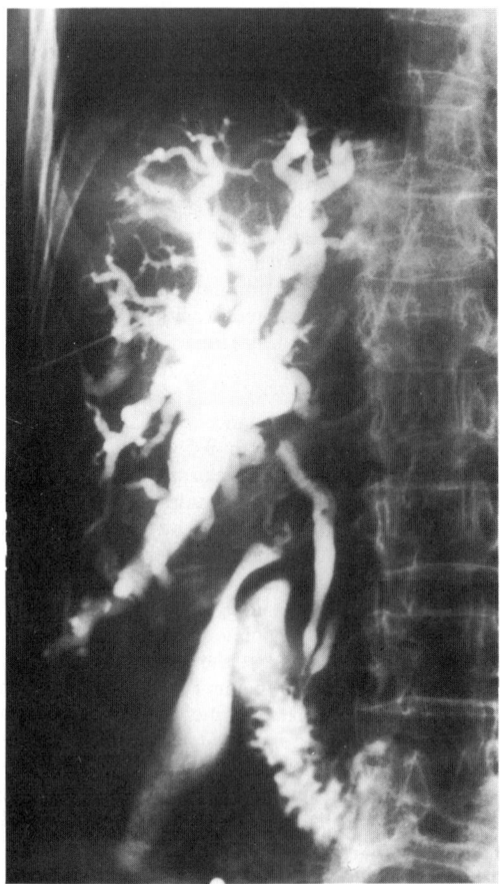

Fig. 69.65 Percutaneous transhepatic cholangiogram in a 75-year-old female who presented with marked cholestatic jaundice showing a hilar (Klatskin) tumour.

3. Middle from the distal common hepatic duct, cystic duct and its confluence with the common bile duct (*Fig.* 69.66).
4. Distal from the distal common bile duct and periampullary region (*Fig.* 69.67).

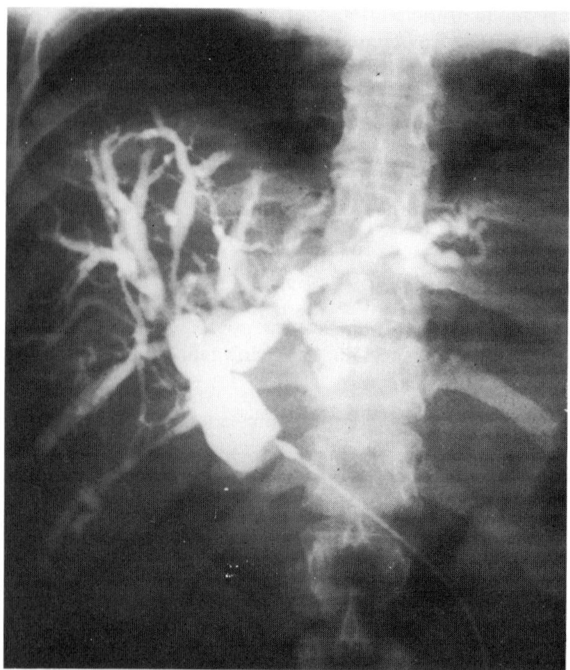

Fig. 69.66 Operative cholangiogram showing tumour at the junction of the cystic duct with the common bile duct. The patient presented with jaundice and acute cholecystitis.

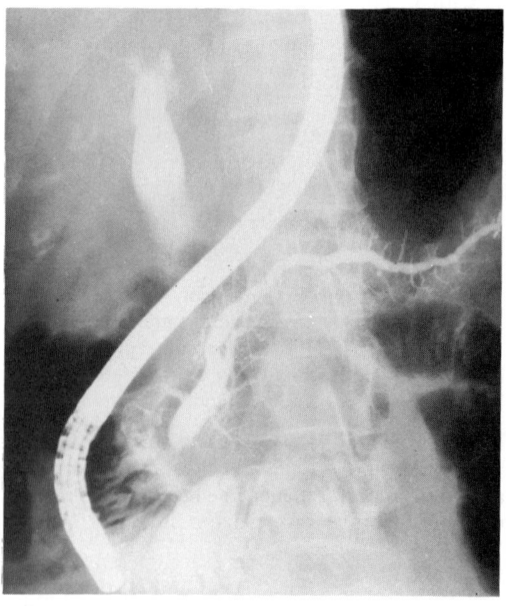

Fig. 69.67 ERCP showing a papillary tumour of the distal bile duct extending to the periampullary region.

Tumours of the minor intrahepatic ducts are often diffuse (multicentric) and difficult to differentiate from primary hepatocellular carcinomas with which they are often grouped because of similar clinical course and poor prognosis. The gross appearances of cholangiocarcinomas assume one of three forms:

Stricture (scirrhous variety)
Nodular
Papillary.

The scirrhous variety can be very difficult to distinguish from sclerosing cholangitis even on histological grounds. These tumours are generally confined to the proximal ducts (hilar) and form grey annular thickenings with clearly defined edges. The nodular tumours form extraductal nodules in addition to intraluminal projections. The papillary variety is most commonly found in the distal bile duct and periampullary region. These lesions are friable and may fill the duct lumen with vascular neoplastic tissue and tend to bleed in the ductal lumen causing haemobilia.

The majority of tumours are adenocarcinomas of varying

differentiation. The scirrhous variety are intensely fibrotic and relatively acellular, often with a few well-differentiated ductal carcinoma cells grouped as acini in a dense connective tissue stroma. Rare types include squamous-cell carcinoma, adenosquamous carcinoma, adenoacanthoma, lymphoma, carcinoid tumours and melanoma. Malignant smooth muscle tumours of the bile duct have also been reported as have two instances of primary non-secreting apudoma of the hilar region.

All cholangiocarcinomas are slow growing, locally infiltrative and metastasize late. Cholangiocarcinomas have a special predilection for perineural spread and do not metastasize beyond the liver. The best prognosis is encountered after resection especially of the distal and periampullary lesions.

Clinical Features

The main presentation (90%) is with obstructive jaundice which is progressive and accompanied by itching and anorexia. However, weight loss is not evident until the disease is advanced and is usually accompanied by evidence of hepatic involvement and ascites. Dull upper abdominal pain is a frequent symptom. Some patients present acutely with cholangitis or acute cholecystitis. The duration of symptoms is usually short and measured in months. Physical examination reveals hepatomegaly. Anaemia is present in patients with papillary tumours especially at the lower end of the bile duct and periampullary region. It is caused by chronic blood loss. The faeces of these patients have a characteristic silvery appearance due to a combination of steatorrhoea and altered blood. A palpable gallbladder is present in patients with distal tumours. A significant percentage of patients with hilar tumours have previously undergone recent cholecystectomy (within six months of diagnosis). Regrettably, these tumours are missed at operation since the small nodule in the porta hepatis is not easily palpable, the common bile duct is not dilated and there is free flow of contrast into the duodenum. Often the surgeon concerned ignores the fact that there is poor filling of the intrahepatic biliary tree or interprets a localized narrowing to extrinsic vascular compression. *An operative cholangiogram should never be passed as normal unless there is adequate and complete filling of the intrahepatic biliary tree (see Fig.* 69.22).

Although ultrasound identifies dilatation of the biliary tree, it seldom localizes the tumour. CT scanning, likewise, does not permit sufficiently precise anatomical localizaton to predict the exact site and resectability of the tumours. It can, however, demonstrate atrophy of the left lobe consequent on vascular involvement by the tumour and has been used as a guide to percutaneous fine needle cytology of these lesions. The definitive investigation is ERCP which can visualize a periampullary tumour and provide a contrast cholangiogram outlining proximal tumours. In some instances, however, proximal filling of the biliary tree is not obtained by ERCP because of tight or complete stenosis by the tumour. A PTC is needed for complete evaluation in these patients. Coeliac axis angiography is used in most specialist centres for the preoperative investigation to delineate the vascular anatomy (since anomalies are frequent) and to detect large vessel encasement which signifies inoperability.

Treatment

Resection is the best method of treatment and is indicated for all operable tumours in fit individuals. The reported resectability rate varies widely but averages 20%. The benefits of resection are:

1. The possibility of cure or long-term survival, especially for distal and periampullary tumours.
2. Resection provides the best form of palliation in terms of duration and freedom from infective complications.

The surgical procedure depends on the location of the tumours. For hilar lesions, an anterior segmentectomy IV provides good access to the confluence, allows good clearance proximal to the tumour and facilitates the hepaticojejunostomy. When the tumour extends along the right or left duct with extension to the respective lobe, the resection includes a lobectomy in continuity with the main tumour mass. However, these patients do not survive for long periods after this procedure and most would consider them to be inoperable. Middle tumours are excised from just below the confluence down to the duodenum together with the associated pericholedochal lymph nodes. The surgical treatment of periampullary tumours is with pancreaticoduodenectomy. The results of hepatic transplantation for cholangiocarcinoma (diffuse intrahepatic type) have been disappointing to date.

If at operation the tumour is found to be inoperable, a bilioenteric bypass is performed. Anastomosis of a Roux loop to the segment III duct using the round ligament approach gives the best results for inoperable hilar lesions. A cholecystojejunostomy is performed for inoperable distal tumours. A gastroenterostomy is added if duodenal obstruction is present or considered imminent in patients with periampullary tumours.

Although adjuvant postoperative radiotherapy is not routinely administered after resection of bile duct tumours, some reports indicate that recurrences may be reduced or delayed by postoperative external beam supervoltage radiotherapy.

In patients who are considered inoperable on preoperative assessment and those who are too old and frail or have serious cardiorespiratory disease, palliation of the jaundice is best achieved by percutaneous transhepatic or endoscopic stenting. The endoprosthesis has to be large (8–10 F) and may require replacement if it becomes blocked with calcium bilirubinate encrustation. The percutaneous insertion of ^{192}Ir wire has been used to provide local irradiation with good results and an average survival of 11 months. The use of intracavitary ^{192}Ir wire with supplemental external beam radiotherapy is currently being evaluated.

Cholangiocarcinomas of the bile ducts are generally regarded to be unresponsive to chemotherapy although initial reports with Mitomycin C, doxorubicin and FUDR appear to show some promise.

Survival

The best results are obtained in distal and periampullary tumours with 5-year survival rates of 30%. The outcome of diffuse intrahepatic tumours is dismal, the majority dying within 1 year of diagnosis. The reported 5-year survival of resected proximal tumours ranges from 5 to 15%.

PARASITIC INFESTATIONS OF THE BILIARY TRACT

In addition to infestations with schistosomes and the larvae of *Taenia echinococcus*, the liver and biliary tract are involved with various other parasitic disorders. Some infestations, such as toxocariasis, remain subclinical in the majority of cases. Children usually acquire infection with *Toxocara canis* from their pets. In addition to hepatic granulomas, there may be CNS and eye involvement. The latter is serious and leads to endophthalmitis and which can be mistaken for retinoblastoma in these children.

The parasitic disorders which are of significance in surgery of the biliary tract include infestation with *Ascaris lumbricoides*, *Clonorchis sinensis* and *Fasciola hepatica*.

Ascaris Lumbricoides

Infestation with this nematode is endemic and prevalent in Asia, China and Africa. It is also found in the rural areas of Europe, USA and Latin America. The adult worms live in the upper reaches of the small intestine but migrate to and from the bile duct through the ampulla of Vater, up the oesophagus and down to the appendix.

The ova are excreted in the stools of infected individuals and contaminate soil and vegetables. Following ingestion of the encysted larvae and dissolution of the cyst wall by the gastric juice, the free larvae penetrate the intestinal mucosa to reach the portal venous system and thus the liver or the lung via the intestinal lymphatics and the thoracic duct. The pulmonary larvae are carried from the alveoli to the pharynx and then swallowed to reach the upper part of the small intestine where they mature into adult worms. The larval migration may involve other organs, e.g. CNS, kidneys, etc.

The majority of adult worms migrating into the biliary tract die after a few weeks and may form a nidus for stone formation. Secondary infection of the bile with *E. coli* and other enteric organisms is common and is thought to play a role in the formation of calcium bilirubinate stones. Pyogenic liver abscess may complicate the disease. The usual hepatic lesions are granulomas surrounding the ova which are deposited in the smaller bile ducts.

Clinical Features

The stage of larval migration is accompanied by systemic symptoms: rigors, generalized aches, malaise, cough and asthmatic attacks. Eosinophilia is invariably present. Migration of the adult worms into the bile duct induces episodes of pain in the epigastric region. Jaundice is encountered in 20%. *A. lumbricoides* infestation is one of the commonest causes of jaundice in children and young adults in Africa. At this stage, the clinical picture is usually dominated by recurrent attacks of cholangitis due to calculus formation and secondary infection.

Treatment

Surgical intervention is necessary to deal with the biliary complications. An initial laparotomy is required to look for and remove (by enterotomy) adult worms which can be easily palpated through the intact bowel wall. Exploration of the bile duct, removal of stones and worms is performed next. A completion cholangiogram or, preferably, an inspection with the choledochoscope, is advisable at the end of the duct exploration. T-tube drainage is essential in all cases and should be carried out with a large tube (16–18 F) to enable subsequent percutaneous stone and parasite extraction through the T-tube tract, if necessary. Surgical intervention should be followed by antihelminthic therapy.

Clonorchis Sinensis

Man is the definitive host of this trematode which is widely distributed in China and East Asia. The adult worms live in the biliary tract and occasionally in the pancreatic duct. The eggs are excreted in the faeces and ingested by fresh water snails (e.g. *Parafossarulus manchouricus*) where they develop into cercariae. The free-swimming cercariae then penetrate fresh water fish and encyst themselves in the muscles of the host as metacercariae. Man becomes infected by eating contaminated fish, the encysted metacercariae being released in the duodenum. They then migrate into the biliary tract via the ampulla of Vater and mature into adult worms. These cause dilatation of the biliary tract with fibrosis of the ducts and adenomatous bile duct hyperplasia. Secondary infection of the biliary tract with enteric organisms is extremely common and results in death of the worm and stone formation. Recurrent episodes of cholangitis and septicaemia, and the development of bile duct carcinoma account for the appreciable mortality of this parasitic infestation. The diagnosis is confirmed by the demonstration of the typical ova in the faeces.

Treatment

Mild cases can be managed conservatively with chloroquine (300 mg for 2–6 months). Surgical intervention is needed for jaundice and cholangitis. In addition to removal of worms and calculi from the bile duct, an internal biliary drainage (choledochoduodenostomy/jejunostomy or sphincteroplasty) is performed.

Fasciola Hepatica

This is primarily an infestation of sheep and cattle. Man is an accidental host, acquiring the disease by eating wild watercress contaminated with metacercariae. The disease has a worldwide distribution and is common in Latin America and the USA. In the UK, outbreaks of the disease occur in Hampshire and the Lake District (Silverside). The ova are excreted in the faeces of infected animals, develop into miracidia in fresh water and subsequently colonize the intermediate host, a fresh water snail (*Lymnaea truncatula*). Within this host, they mature through various stages into metacercariae which become encysted on neighbouring water plants. Subsequent to ingestion, the free metacercariae are released in the upper part of the small intestine and penetrate the bowel to reach the peritoneal cavity. They then migrate across the peritoneal cavity and enter the liver parenchyma after penetration of the liver capsule. Maturation occurs in the bile ducts. Migration of the metacercariae may occur to other organs: kidneys, muscles, brain and subcutaneous tissue.

Clinical Features

The disease is often asymptomatic if the infestion is mild. Systemic symptoms signify heavy infestations and include malaise, anorexia, nausea, vomiting, fever and weight loss. An urticarial rash, jaundice or hepatosplenomegaly may develop. Diagnosis is confirmed by the demonstration of ova in the stool.

Treatment

The disease is usually treated medically with bithionol (50 mg daily for 3 weeks). Surgical intervention is indicated only in cases of biliary obstruction and cholangitis.

Further Reading

Bismuth H., Franco D. and Corlette M. B. (1978) Long term results of Roux-en-Y hepaticojejunostomy. *Surg. Gynecol. Obstet.* **146**, 161–167.

Cuschieri A. and Berci G. (1984) *Common Bile Duct Exploration.* Dordrecht, Martinus Nijhoff.

Cuschieri A. and Cheadle W. G. (1986) Tumours of the biliary tract. In: Fielding J. W. L. and Priestman T. J. (ed.) *Gastrointestinal Oncology.* Tunbridge Wells, Castle House Publications, pp. 165–195.

Escourrou J., Cordova J. A, Lazorthes F. et al. (1984) Early and late complications after endoscopic sphincterotomy for biliary lithiasis with and without the gallbladder in situ. *Gut* **25**, 589–602.

Henriksen J. H. (1985) Acute cholecystitis. Diagnostic impact of ultrasonography and cholescintigraphy. *Scand. J. Gastroenterol.* **20**, 129–132.

Ransohoff D. F., Gracie W. A., Wolfsen L. B. et al. (1983) Prophylactic cholecystectomy or expectant management for silent stones. *Ann. Intern. Med.* **99**, 199–204.

Saing H., Tam P. K. H., Lee J. M. H. et al. (1985) Surgical management of choledochal cysts: a review of 60 cases. *J. Paediatr. Surg.* **20**, 443–448.

Shukla V. K., Khandelwal C., Roy S. K. et al. (1985) Primary carcinoma of the gallbladder: review of a 16-year period at the University Hospital. *J. Surg. Oncol.* **28**, 32–35.

Suruga K., Miyano T., Arai T. et al. (1984) A study on hepatic portoenterostomy for the treatment of atresia of the biliary tract. *Surg. Gynecol. Obstet.* **159**, 53–58.

Toouli, J., Roberts-Thomson I. C., Dent J. et al. (1985) Manometric disorders in patients with suspected sphincter of Oddi dysfunction. *Gastroenterol.* **88**, 1243–1250.

70 The Pancreas

A. R. Moossa and B. E. Stabile

SURGICAL ANATOMY OF THE PANCREAS

H. Durmen has summarized the anatomical relationship of the pancreas as follows: 'The pancreas cuddles the left kidney, tickles the spleen, hugs the duodenum, cradles the aorta, opposes the inferior vena cava, dallies with the right renal pedicle, hides behind the posterior parietal peritoneum of the lesser sac and wraps itself around the superior mesenteric vessels.'

The pancreas is relatively inaccessible and, without some dissection, very little of it can be seen or palpated even at laparotomy. For this reason, it is much more difficult to manage surgically than all other abdominal viscera. Its retroperitoneal location in the upper abdomen means that it is almost completely hidden by the stomach, transverse colon and mesocolon (*Fig.* 70.1). It derives its blood supply from numerous branches arising from major branches of the coeliac and superior mesenteric arteries. A full understanding of the local vascular anatomy and its possible variations is essential for any surgeon operating on the pancreas.

In the thin patient, a part of the head of the gland may be seen directly behind the peritoneum of the supracolic and right infracolic compartments, and the inferior border of the body and tail may be visualized from the left infracolic compartment at the root of the transverse mesocolon. These views are very limited and are usually obscured by mesocolic and omental fat. The neck of the pancreas may be palpated by a finger passed through the epiploic foramen and directed inferiorly.

In order to inspect and palpate the pancreas properly, three surgical manoeuvres are necessary:

1. The hepatic flexure of the colon is mobilized downward and medially by dividing its attachments to the duode-

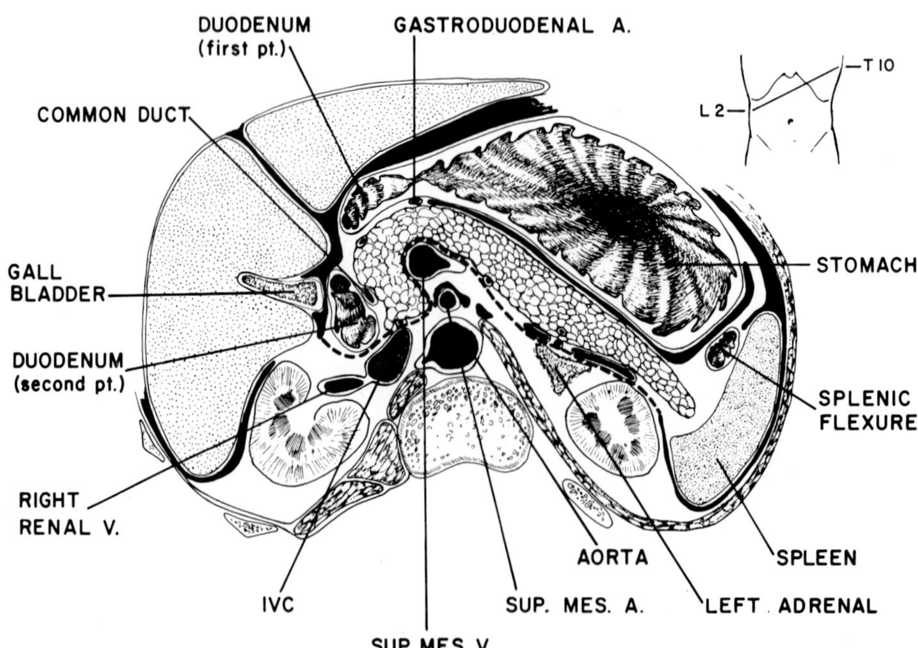

Fig. 70.1 Oblique transverse cross-section of the upper abdomen viewed from below. Section passes through the long axis of the pancreas at approximately the levels indicated in the inset figure. The disposition and relations of structures shown approximate those seen in an oblique transverse scanning.

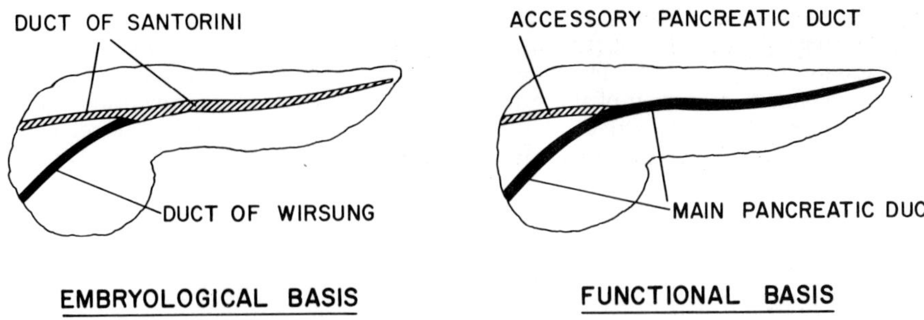

Fig. 70.2 Terminology variously applied to describe the pancreatic ductal system. An understanding of ductal embryology, particularly with regard to the development of the more unusual variations, may be served by the terms given in the left diagram. For clarity and practicality the terms given in the right diagram are preferred.

num and anterior aspects of the pancreatic head. The peritoneum lateral to the second part of the duodenum is incised and the duodenum and pancreatic head are elevated by blunt dissection (Kocher manoeuvre) from the posterior parietal structures. In this way, the right kidney, right renal vein, inferior vena cava and the root of the left renal vein are exposed. The head of the pancreas, the duodenum and the retroduodenal and pancreatic portions of the common bile duct can thus be palpated between thumb and fingers.

2. Limited visualization of the superior part of the body of the pancreas may be obtained by opening an avascular part of the lesser omentum and retracting the lesser curvature of the stomach inferiorly. This manoeuvre also brings the coeliac axis into view. The body of the pancreas can only be adequately visualized by widely opening the gastrocolic omentum, retracting the transverse colon and mesocolon inferiorly and the greater curvature of the stomach superiorly. By extending this opening to the right, into the pyloric region, the right gastro-epiploic vessels can be divided near their origins and the anterior aspect of the neck of the pancreas can be visualized. Care must be taken to avoid damage to the middle colic vessels in this region. The opening can also be extended to the left and the gastrosplenic ligament with its contained short gastric vessels can be divided to permit complete visualization of the anterior surface of the tail of the pancreas.

3. Downward and medial retraction of the dome of the spleen will tense the peritoneal leaf known as the lienorenal ligament and this can be divided to allow the spleen, splenic vessels and tail of the pancreas to be mobilized *en bloc* allowing inspection of the posterior aspect of the body and tail of the pancreas and more careful palpation of the distal portion of the gland.

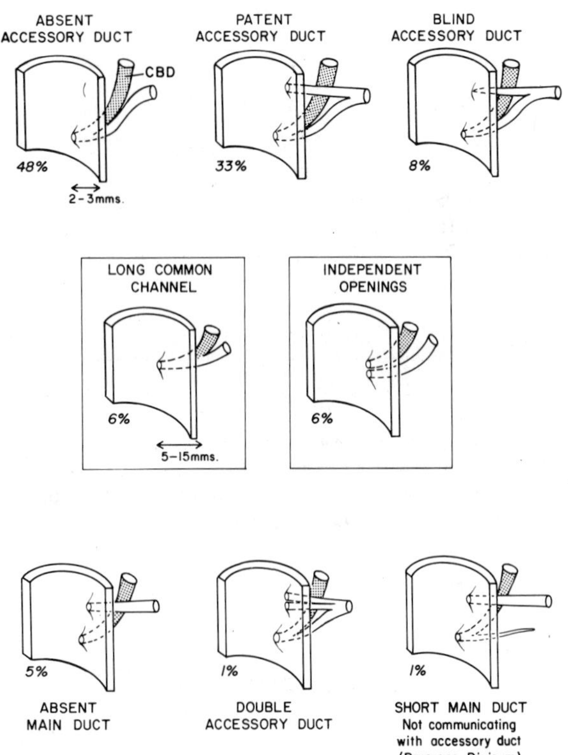

Fig. 70.3 Variations of main and accessory pancreatic ducts and their relationship to the common bile duct (CBD).

All three manoeuvres should be carried out safely, quickly and with little risk of damage to vital structures or troublesome bleeding. They will allow evaluation of all areas of the pancreas except the region of the neck and uncinate process. Further dissection and mobilization is usually necessary to assess the resectability of a pancreatic tumour. For this, a detailed knowledge of the pancreas and peripancreatic vasculature and its variations is essential.

The coeliac axis and the superior mesenteric artery and their branches vary a great deal both in their site of origin and in their direction. The same applies to the venous drainage of the foregut, its appendages, and the midgut into the portal venous trunk. The most demanding part of a pancreatic resection is dissection of the neck and head of the gland from the superior mesenteric and portal veins and the uncinate process from the superior mesenteric artery. Hence, some authorities consider it mandatory to have a coeliac and a superior mesenteric arteriogram (as well as the venous phase) prior to planning any major pancreatic resection.

As with the blood vessels, pancreatobiliary ductal anatomy is very variable and the concept of a 'normal ductal anatomy' should be abandoned. The terminology which is widely applied to describe the main pancreatic ductal system is explained in *Fig.* 70.2. The variations in termination of the main and accessory pancreatic ducts and their relationship to the lower end of the common bile duct are depicted in *Fig.* 70.3.

The pancreas occupies a central position at a complex anatomical crossroads and its lymphatic drainage is radially disposed along several major routes, namely, the splenic, hepatic and superior mesenteric nodal basins. It is thus hard to design an adequate 'cancer-operation' which, in an orderly manner, removes the primary tumour *en bloc* with primary, secondary and tertiary lymphatic nodal territories. Moreover, the intimate anatomical association of the pancreas with major vessels at once limits the extent of the procedure and dictates what must be removed. Thus, when a tumour of the pancreas spreads a short distance it involves the portal vein, superior mesenteric artery or coeliac axis, and usually becomes incurable. Similarly, if the gland is removed in radical fashion, the need to excise the vessels and lymph nodes associated with it makes removal of the spleen, duodenum, gallbladder, common bile duct, upper jejunum and most of the stomach necessary.

Where only part of the pancreas is excised or even if the gland is incised, safe management of any draining pancreatic juice becomes a matter of primary importance since the enzymes, if allowed to accumulate in the peritoneal cavity, may cause local damage. A first principle of pancreatic surgery is the provision of adequate drainage. Similarly, the collection of serum, lymph and blood following a total pancreatectomy needs to be drained. Secondly, the protein nature of catgut makes it vulnerable to digestion by trypsin. It should not, therefore, be used for ligature of major vessels, as a suture material for anastomosis, or for closure of the abdomen during pancreatic surgery. Non-absorbable material, such as silk, cotton, wire, nylon, or prolene is essential for safety

CELLULAR COMPOSITION AND PHYSIOLOGY OF THE EXOCRINE PANCREAS

The exocrine pancreas consists of acinar and ductal systems which drain its secretions into the duodenum. The exocrine tissue accounts for 98% of the pancreas by weight. Under the influence of neural and hormonal controls, the exocrine pancreas secretes water and bicarbonate from the ductal system and enzymes from the acinar cells. The parasympathetic vagal fibres have ganglia in the interlobular septa and postganglionic fibres are distributed to acinar cells and to smooth muscle cells in the ducts. The sympathetic fibres appear to be entirely distributed to the blood vessels and to be concerned solely with regulation of pancreatic blood flow rather than in the direct control of pancreatic secretion.

Fluid and electrolyte secretion from the pancreas is a ductal function and is an energy requiring process. The cationic composition of pancreatic fluid is similar to that of plasma. Sodium and potassium concentrations are identical to those in plasma and are independent of flow. During states of fluid and electrolyte secretion, calcium appears to enter the ducts passively. However, under the influence of cholecystokinin, it appears to be actively secreted in parallel with enzyme secretion. Anionic secretion consists almost entirely of bicarbonate and chloride. The sum of concentrations of these two anions remains constant—a high chloride concentration occurs at low flow rates and chloride is replaced by bicarbonate as the flow rate increases.

Pancreatic enzyme secretion originates in the acinar cell and accounts for virtually all the protein (2–8 g/day in man) in pancreatic juice. Many of the enzymes are secreted in their inactive or zymogen forms together with inhibitors. This mechanism protects the pancreas from autodigestion by its own proteolytic enzymes. It is presumed that this inhibitor is destroyed or diluted in the duodenum allowing enzyme activation to occur. The pancreas has a tremendous reserve capacity for enzyme secretion and can maintain a normal output even after 90–95% of the gland has been removed or destroyed. However, adaptive functions are probably lost in pancreatitis. The large list of enzymes which are secreted in pancreatic juice include amylase, lipase, cholesterol ester hydrolase, phospholecithinase A, trypsin, chymotrypsin A and B, elastase, carboxypeptidase A and B, collagenase, leucine aminopeptidase, ribonuclease, deoxyribonuclease and, undoubtedly, other enzymes for which a function has yet to be described.

Control of Pancreatic Exocrine Secretion

Basal pancreatic secretion results from either an intrinsic autonomy of the gland or a low level of activity of neurohormonal regulators. A complete neurohormonal control mechanism is at work and secretin, cholecystokinin (CCK-PZ) and gastrin play the dominant roles. Secretin is released in response to duodenal acidification and there is also an increase in secretin release in man in response to alcohol and, to a lesser extent, after a meal. Secretin produces a secretion of fluid and electrolytes which is initiated within 30 sec of an administered dose, the bicarbonate concentration of the fluid increasing as flow increases. It is now generally accepted that secretin is also a weak stimulant of enzyme secretion.

The stimulus for release of CCK-PZ appears to be entry of amino acids, fatty acids, hydrochloric acid and food into the duodenum. It causes an increase in the release of enzymes and a small increase in fluid and electrolyte output. In man, pancreatic secretion is initiated by CCK-PZ at a dose lower than that required for gallbladder contraction.

Gastrin has a varying effect on pancreatic secretion but, in man, it causes an increase in enzyme secretion. The actions of glucagon and vasoactive intestinal peptide (VIP) on human pancreatic secretion has yet to be defined. Chymodenin appears to selectively induce chymotrypsin secretion. Somatostatin, pancreatic polypeptide, and motilin have unidentified roles but may act as a feedback control.

Hormonal and Neural Interaction

Combinations of two or more hormones have differing effects on the acinar and ductal cells. Secretin is a strong stimulant of fluid and electrolyte secretion and a weak stimulator of enzyme secretion; acting with CCK-PZ, however, marked augmentation occurs. These hormones have different receptor sites on the acinar cell and the site of interaction is probably intracellular. Such augmentation probably has an important physiological role since only small amounts of secretin are released into the circulation in response to a meal.

The interaction between the exocrine and endocrine cells of the pancreas is currently being elucidated. Insulin is trophic to the peri-insular cells and a loss of insulin secretion in diabetes mellitus results in progressive damage to the acinar cell. The blood supply to the human pancreas first passes to the islets and then forms a capillary network around the acinar cells, allowing maximal effects of islet hormones on the acinus. Thus, insulin, glucagon, somatostatin and other islet cell secretions may affect exocrine pancreatic secretion.

In man, vagal reflexes in response to gastric distension results in a juice rich in enzymes, and this effect is abolished by truncal vagotomy. It is likely that the role of vagal stimulation is a permissive one, allowing secretin and CCK-PZ to exert their full effect. Thus, atropine, by blocking acetylcholine, depresses the responsiveness of the acinar and ductal cells to CCK-PZ in animals.

ANATOMY AND PHYSIOLOGY OF THE ENDOCRINE PANCREAS

The islets of Langerhans form the endocrine portion of the mammalian pancreas and consist of cells arranged in spherical or ovoid clusters which are well circumscribed and irregularly distributed throughout the gland. Although variable, the total number of islets in the adult human pancreas is estimated to be one million and the gland weighs 1–2 g in the adult. The islets thus form only about 2–3% of the weight of the whole gland.

Our knowledge of the cellular composition of the islets is still incomplete but the existence of four cell types has been largely accepted in mammalian islets based on ultrastructural characteristics of their secretory granules (*Fig.* 70.4). These are A, B, D and D 1 cells. A cells form approximately 20% of the normal islet cell population, B cells 75%. In the various pathological conditions affecting the islets, including diabetes mellitus, the proportion of different cell types vary. A cells (alpha cells) synthesize, store and secrete glucagon. They are concentrated in the periphery of the islets. B cells (beta cells) synthesize, store and release insulin. They are concentrated in the centre of the islets. D cells supply the tetradecapeptide somatostatin and also probably gastrin. They tend to be located in the periphery of the islets. D 1 cells are the rarest cell type encountered in normal islets and they are possibly responsible for the secretion of vasoactive intestinal polypeptide (VIP) and pancreatic polypeptide (PP). Most islets are completely devoid of D 1 cells and this explains why they have not been recognized consistently. The number of D 1 cells probably increases with age and in association with injury to pancreatic tissue. An increase in the number of D 1 cells has been documented in such conditions as diabetes, pancreatitis, mucoviscidosis, haemochromatosis and various exocrine or endocrine pancreatic tumours.

Insulin has an approximate molecular weight of 6000 and consists of two peptide chains A and B which are connected by two disulphide bridges (*Fig.* 70.5). In man, the A chain has 21 amino acids and the B chain is composed of 30 amino acids. There are structural variations from species to species. It is now known that insulin is formed in a precursor form, pro-insulin, which comprises the insulin A and B chains linked by a polypeptide segment consisting of 30–35 amino acids. This connecting peptide (C-peptide) helps in the formation of the native structure of the insulin molecule by ensuring the correct pairing of the cysteine residues during formation of the disulphide linkages between the A and B chains. Proteolytic cleavage of pro-inuslin by enzymes in the secretory granules results in the separation of insulin from the C-peptide. These two products are thus released in equimolar amounts from the B cells. Pro-insulin like components (PLC) comprise 15% of the immunoreactive insulin concentration. The kidney is an important site of pro-insulin degradation; hence levels of PLC are markedly elevated in chronic renal failure. Raised serum pro-insulin concentrations have been found in both benign and malignant insulinomas. Neither insulin nor insulin antibodies interfere in

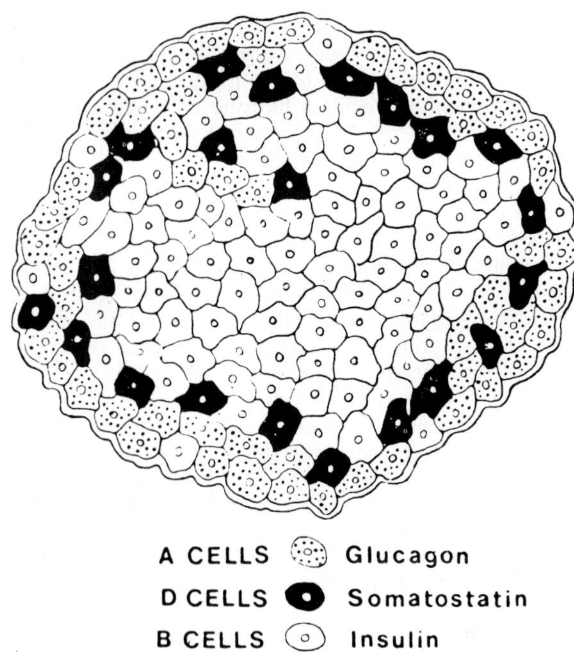

Fig. 70.4 Schematic representation of an islet of Langerhans showing distribution of the three main cell types. (Reprinted by permission from Orci L. and Unger R. H. *Lancet* 2:1243, 1975.)

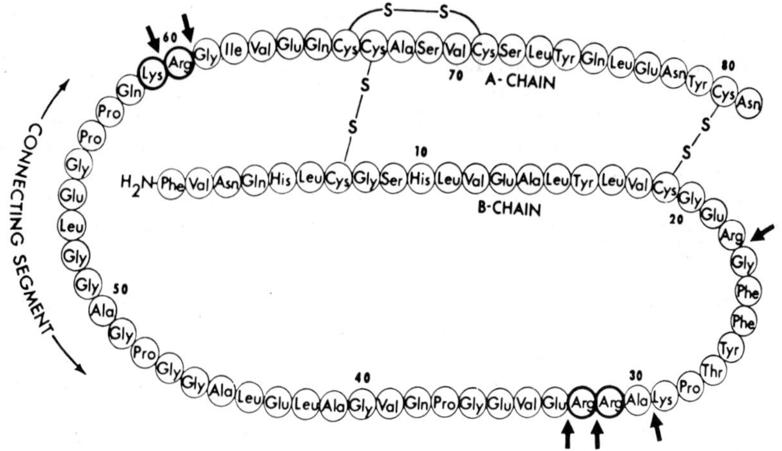

Fig. 70.5 Covalent structure of bovine pro-insulin. Arrows indicate sites of tryptic cleavage.

the immunoassay for the estimation of C-peptide concentration. Since insulin and C-peptide are formed in equimolar amounts following cleavage of pro-insulin, the circulating levels of C-peptide provide a measure of B cell secretory activity, especially in the presence of circulating insulin antibodies produced in response to exogenous insulin. Thus it gives an indication of endogenous insulin production from the beta cell. C-peptide measurement therefore has a vital role in the diagnosis of surreptitious injection of insulin and in the follow-up evaluation of patients who have undergone total or near-total pancreatectomy for nesidioblastosis or a malignant insulinoma. Following resection of the latter, significant C-peptide levels indicate residual pancreatic tissue or the presence of functioning metastases. Recurrence may be heralded by rise in C-peptide levels.

The main stimulus to insulin secretion is an increase in glucose levels. The insulin will thus cause a fall in glucose concentration and, by a negative feedback effect, this leads to a decrease in insulin release. Other stimuli for insulin release are amino acids (arginine being the most potent), glucagon, growth hormone, cortisol, placental lactogen, and the sex hormones (especially oestrogens). Glucagon releases insulin both by direct stimulatory effect on the B cells and also indirectly by mobilizing glucose from the liver. The remaining hormones mentioned above act by causing resistance to the actions of insulin and thus generate a compensatory increase in insulin secretion. A number of gastrointestinal hormones including gastrin, secretin, gut glucagon, CCK-PZ and gastric inhibitory polypeptide (GIP) may also be stimulants for insuling secretion. Insulin release is also enhanced by free fatty acids to prevent ketoacidosis which would otherwise occur during fasting in normal individuals.

Vagal stimulation is also a potent stimulus to insulin release although no impairment in the insulin release can be demonstrated following vagotomy. Adrenergic beta receptors also stimulate insulin release but adrenaline and noradrenaline, acting via alpha receptors, have an inhibitory effect on insulin secretion. The ventromedial nucleus of the hypothalamus is believed to be important in the cephalic phase of insulin release. Finally, insulin secretion is influenced by various drugs. Tolbutamide and chlorpropamide have a stimulatory effect while alloxan and streptozotocin impair insulin secretion by directly damaging the B cells.

The actions of insulin are discussed in Chapter 9.

Glucagon

Glucagon is a secretory product of the A cell and is a linear peptide composed of 29 amino acids with a molecular weight of approximately 3500. Gel filtration of acid alcohol extracts of pancreatic tissue have revealed two peaks of immunoreactivity, one with a molecular weight of in excess of 9000 (believed to represent proglucagon) and another which is a globulin-sized fraction that has been referred to as big plasma glucagon which may be a precursor of glucagon or simply glucagon bound to a larger protein.

Glucagon has catabolic actions. Hypoglycaemia produces a rise in plasma glucagon concentration and an increase in glucose concentration leads to a drop in glucagon levels. Glucagon activates adenyl cyclase which increases hepatic cyclic AMP to initiate breakdown of glycogen into glucose (glycogenolysis). It also inhibits the process of glycogenesis. It increases glucose formation from non-glucose precursors, e.g. glycerol, lactate and amino acids of the glycogenic type. Glucagon also enhances the breakdown of fat into free fatty acids and glycerol. It stimulates gluconeogenesis and thus, its infusion lowers plasma amino acids. Finally, glucagon inhibits protein synthesis. There is evidence that glucagon, through its gluconeogenic, ketogenic, and lipolytic effects, and not insulin lack alone, is responsible for the development of fulminant diabetic ketoacidosis in man.

The inter-relationship between insulin and glucagon is a complex one which is only partly understood. In general, an inverse relationship exists between insulin and glucagon levels. When glucose is needed, insulin levels fall and glucagon levels rise, producing an increased hepatic glucose production. The reverse is true in states of hyperglycaemia. Following a protein meal, a parallel change is observed in the levels of insulin and glucagon. The rise in glucagon level prevents the hypoglycaemia that would result from enhanced insulin secretion alone by amino acids. CCK-PZ, which stimulates insulin secretion, is also believed to facilitate glucagon secretion following the stimulus of a protein meal and is responsible for the buffer mechanism against hypoglycaemia arising from ingestion of protein.

Somatostatin

This tetradecapeptide is secreted by the D cell. It inhibits the release of growth hormone from the anterior pituitary and was first isolated from the hypothalamus. Its other actions include inhibition of insulin and glucagon secretion, gastrin secretion, acid and pepsin secretion from the stomach, as well as the release of pancreatic enzymes. It suppresses intestinal motility and contraction of the gallbladder. It also has a suppressive effect on glucose uptake from the gut and on appetite and may play a role in nutrient homeostasis. Infusion of somatostatin diminishes splanchnic blood flow. In view of its inhibitory effect on the exocrine pancreas, somatostatin has been tried in the treatment of patients with acute pancreatitis. Somatostatin has been isolated from a variety of tissues and organs, including the gastrointestinal tract and pancreatic islets. Its exact and full spectrum of function is as yet unknown.

Human Pancreatic Polypeptide (HPP)

HPP consists of 36 amino acids in a straight chain. The ultrastructural identification of the HPP-producing cell is not definitely settled but the D 1 cells are the prime candidates. The physiological role of HPP is unknown. It is almost totally confined to the pancreas and is thus undetectable in pancreatectomized patients. Its secretion is believed to be largely due to vagal cholinergic stimulation and, in part, by gastrointestinal humoral stimulation. It is released by ingestion of fat and protein but not by intravenous nutrients. In pharmacological doses, HPP inhibits pancreatic secretion caused by CCK-PZ and secretin, stimulates gastric emptying and intestinal transit, inhibits pentagastrin-stimulated gastric acid secretion, inhibits relaxation of the gallbladder and increases the tone of the choledochal sphincter. It has been suggested as a possible causative agent in the watery diarrhoea, hypokalaemia achlorhydria (WDHA) syndrome. Significant elevated levels of HPP are found in both maturity onset and juvenile diabetics. This observation has also been extended to patients with chronic pancreatitis. Many endocrine tumours of the pancreas and their metastases have also been found to contain numerous HPP cells and also to have a high tumour content of HPP. If this finding is substantiated, elevated circulating HPP levels in patients with these tumours may serve as an aid in diagnosis and in the monitoring of therapy in such patients.

Conclusions

The pancreatic islets consist of cell types in close topographical relationship which produce hormones with different but related actions. Gaps and tight junctions have been demonstrated between islet cells of the same as well as different types. This arrangement may play a role in coordinating the activity of the different cell types, e.g. somatostatin-containing cells are topographically closely related to B and A cells. As somatostatin inhibits insulin and glucagon release, it is possible that it serves a paracrine function by regulating the local (within the islet) release of these hormones from the appropriate cells. It is likely that the islets function as a well integrated unit and further elucidation of such mechanisms will enhance the understanding of various pathological conditions arising in this endocrine organ.

METHODS OF INVESTIGATING THE PANCREAS

Introduction

Because of its deep-seated and inaccessible location, the pancreas is a difficult organ to investigate and to visualize. A precise diagnosis of pancreatic disease is often only possible through the use of a wide battery of tests. The results of such tests should be viewed in the light of the clinical information since all the available procedures may not yield concordant data.

Procedures which are employed in the investigation of patients with suspected pancreatic disorders may be classified into five groups:

1. Procedures which outline the gland to delineate enlargement, masses, irregularities in contour, and calcification. These include:
   a. Indirect imaging of the pancreas:
   Standard radiological studies to visualize the effect of the pancreas on adjacent organs such as stomach, duodenum, small bowel, transverse colon and bile duct.
   b. Direct imaging techniques to visualize:
   The pancreatic parenchyma, e.g. ultrasonography, computerized tomography, radionuclide pancreatic scans.
   The pancreatic duct system—ERCP (endoscopic retrograde cholangiopancreatography).
   The pancreatic and peripancreatic vasculature—angiography.
2. Procedures to define pancreatic exocrine function:
   a. Faecal fat excretion.
   b. Pancreatic function tests.
3. Procedures to define pancreatic endocrine function:
   a. Measurement of fasting blood levels of glucose, and/or hormones which are secreted by the pancreatic islets under normal and/or abnormal conditions. These include serum insulin, pro-insulin, C-peptide, glucagon, somatostatin and gastrin.
   b. Provocative tests to measure the serum level of the above substances if the fasting levels are not conclusive:
   Calcium infusion test (insulinoma and gastrinoma).
   Tolbutamide tolerance test (insulinoma).
   Glucagon test (insulinoma).
   Insulin suppression test (insulinoma).
   Secretin test (gastrinoma).
4. Analysis of serum for markers of pancreatic disease:
   a. Enzymes, such as amylase, lipase, trypsin, ribonuclease.
   b. Tumour-associated antigens, such as carcinoembryonic antigen (CEA) and pancreatic oncofetal antigen (POA).
5. Pancreatic biopsy and cytology:
   a. Percutaneous fine needle aspiration cytology using ultrasonography, computerized tomography, or angiography for guidance.
   b. Endoscopic transgastric or transduodenal needle aspiration cytology or brush cytology.
   c. Laparoscopic visualization and direct vision biopsy or aspiration cytology of the pancreas.
   d. Operative visualization, palpation and biopsy of the pancreas.

Standard Radiological Investigations

Standard or routine radiological investigations rely on the detection of anatomical abnormalities by the displacement or distortion of *adjacent* viscera, such as the pancreas. Maximum information may be obtained from each type of examination if the radiologist involved is alerted to the possibility of pancreatic disease prior to the actual procedure. The main value of the various investigations to be described is that they provide important information in a clinical setting suggestive of disease in the upper abdomen. They should be employed principally to identify and/or to exclude common disorders such as peptic ulcer, gallstones, hiatus hernia, gastric cancer and colon cancer. They may, however, show a wide range of abnormalities suggestive of pancreatic disease. Two common pitfalls need to be emphasized:

1. The presence of a common benign disorder, such as hiatus hernia or gallstones does *not* preclude the simultaneous presence of pancreatic disease.
2. Normal routine radiological studies do *not* necessarily signify the absence of pancreatic disease.

A *plain radiograph of the abdomen* may show the following changes suggestive of pancreatic disease.

Pancreatic Calcification

Radiating 'sun-burst' calcification is pathognomonic of cystadenomas or cystadenocarcinomas of the pancreas. Numerous other lesions of the pancreas may also show calcifications. These include chronic pancreatitis, with or without pancreatolithiasis, lymphangiomas, haemangiomas and, occasionally, mucin-secreting adenocarcinoma or islet cell carcinoma. In hereditary pancreatitis, the incidence of pancreatic calcification is higher than in other types of pancreatitis and the incidence of pancreatic malignancy is also increased. In general, 2–4% of all patients with pancreatic calcification have a coexisting pancreatic carcinoma but, conversely, over 95% of all patients with pancreatic calcification will have benign disease.

Contrast Studies of the Gastrointestinal Tract

Pancreatic disease may reflect changes in the oesophagus, stomach, small bowel and colon.

A pancreatic pseudocyst may present in the posterior mediastinum and compress the oesophagus. Occasionally a tumour arising in the tail of the pancreas will also deform and involve the distal oesophagus. Alternatively, metastatic lymphadenopathy in the posterior mediastinum may also occlude the oesophagus. Oesophageal varices occasionally accompany pancreatitis of any type or pancreatic cancer as a result of splenic vein occlusion.

Radiological Examination of the Stomach and Duodenum

Changes produced in the stomach and duodenum can be considered under the headings of extrinsic compression and indentation, rugal and mucosal abnormalities, enlarged retrograstric space and gastric varices. If a double contrast examination is performed, some of the more subtle mucosal changes may be seen to better advantage. Motility changes of the stomach, particularly the antrum may be seen when the posterior stomach wall is invaded by an inflammatory process or a malignant disease of the pancreas.

Pancreatic disease may reflect on the duodenum in a number of different ways and these may be seen on contrast radiography as pressure defects, abnormalities of duodenal fold pattern, widening of the duodenal C-loop, displacement of the angle of Treitz, postbulbar ulceration of the duodenum (Zollinger–Ellison syndrome), disorders of duodenal motility under fluoroscopy, enlargement of the ampulla of Vater and duodenobiliary reflux.

It should be emphasized that by the time the presence of a pancreatic carcinoma is reflected by diagnosable changes on contrast radiology of the gastrointestinal tract, the lesion is advanced and incurable.

Radiological Examination of the Small Bowel

Mass lesions of the pancreas may produce displacement of the duodenojejunal area and of the small bowel. These appearances are usually seen with pancreatic pseudocysts and large tumours. Chronic pancreatic disease associated with exocrine insufficiency and steatorrhoea may show a malabsorption pattern of the small bowel with thickened, clubbed, or effaced folds. The classic appearance is seen in cystic fibrosis. Patients with the Zollinger–Ellison syndrome may show thickening of the folds in the duodenum and proximal jejunum and hypersecretion of fluid with dilution of the barium. Multiple peptic ulcerations may also be seen.

Radiological Examination of the Colon

In pancreatitis, characteristic changes have been described in the transverse colon and the region of the splenic flexure. These include ileus of the transverse colon (colon cut-off sign), displacement of the transverse colon, and, sometimes, colonic strictures, fistulas and necrosis. Some of these appearances may simulate carcinoma of the colon. Rarely, a pancreatic pseudocyst may present in an unusual location and has even been described presenting as a presacral mass indenting the rectum. Intraperitoneal seeding from metastatic pancreatic carcinoma may cause indentation of any part of the colon.

Cholangiography

Patients with pancreatic disease (cancer and/or pancreatitis) may present with biliary tract obstruction and jaundice. If the serum bilirubin exceeds 51 µmol/l (3 mg/100 ml), then oral or intravenous cholangiography no longer plays a role in the investigation. If ultrasonography or computerized tomography shows dilated biliary radicles then percutaneous transhepatic cholangiography has a place in the investigation of biliary obstruction. However, when the biliary obstruction is suspected to be in the pancreatic region, ERCP is a preferred method of visualizing the biliary tree since it can provide valuable additional information. If a patient has highly elevated serum bilirubin (greater than 200 µmol/l (12 mg/100 ml) a period of biliary decompression via the percutaneous transhepatic route may be used as an adjunct in the preparation of the patient for operation (*see* Chapter 69).

Direct Imaging of the Pancreas

Ultrasonography

Ultrasonography is probably the most important advance in pancreatic investigation of the past decade. The following features are indicators of pancreatic disease on ultrasonography:

1. Diffuse or localized enlargement of the gland may be due to inflammation, tumour or pseudocysts. Atrophy of the entire pancreas usually indicates chronic pancreatitis.
2. Alteration of the texture or 'pattern of internal echoes' within the pancreas may provide a *subjective* impression of pancreatic disease.
3. Indirect signs outside the pancreas but readily traced to the pancreatic area are dilatation of the biliary system and displacement of the vessels adjacent to the pancreas.
4. Abnormal dilatation of the pancreatic duct may be the result of cancer or chronic pancreatitis.
5. Metastases and ascites are also indirect signs of pancreatic disease which by themselves do not necessarily imply the presence of an abnormal pancreas.

The distinction between pancreatic cancer, chronic pancreatitis and a variety of other pancreatic tumours can be difficult without knowledge of the clinical situation.

Ultrasonography is relatively cheap, non-invasive, and free of radiation hazards. It can be repeated as often as necessary but it requires good equipment and enthusiastic expert staff for its performance and its interpretation. In spite of this, technical failure which prevents proper visualization of the whole pancreas occurs in about 10–15% of patients and can be attributed to obesity, gastrointestinal gas, and previous operations in the upper abdomen as well as massive ascites.

***Computerized Tomography* (*CT Scan*) (*Figs.* 70.6, 70.7)**

The CT scan is highly successful in demonstrating the pancreas and allows complete visualization of between 93 and 100% of all glands. The most valuable sign of disease shown by CT scan is the presence of localized or diffuse enlargement of the gland. As with ultrasonography, this finding is non-specific as to the type of disease. The pancreas may be abnormal without recognizable enlargement and, conversely, normal variants of size exist which may suggest abnormalities when none is present. An abnormally small pancreas may be a sign of chronic pancreatitis. The lower limit of normal is said to be one-half of a vertebral body width for the head of the pancreas and one-third for the body of the gland. Nevertheless when the size of the gland falls below these standards, the pancreas is often actually normal. Calcifications are readily identified by CT scanning. Other signs of pancreatic disease include dilatation of the hepatobiliary tree, dilatation of the pancreatic duct and liver metastases.

The accuracy of ultrasonography and CT scan in detecting abnormalities in the pancreas varies. The reported figures are dependent on the type and spectrum of diseases included in the population studied, on the nature of the equipment employed, and on the skill of the individuals involved in the study. Chronic pancreatitis produces more problems for ultrasonic detection—only about 50% of cases

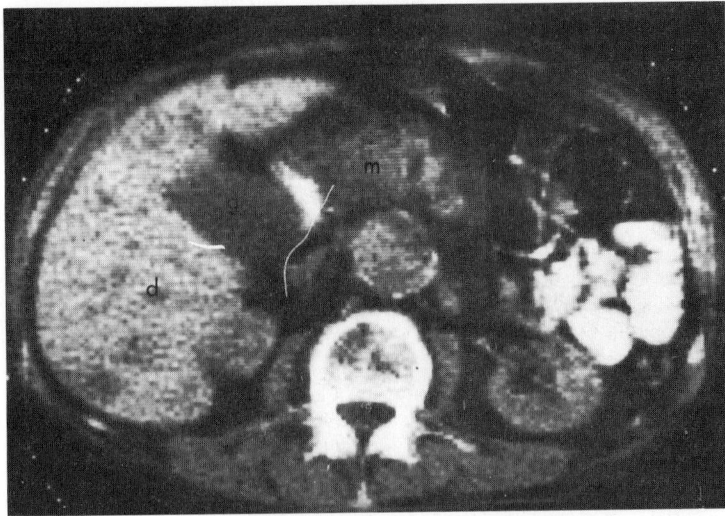

Fig. 70.6 CT scan showing typical appearance of carcinoma of the pancreas, consisting of a mass (m) in the head of the pancreas, a distended gallbladder (g) and dilated intrahepatic ducts (d). Incidental note is made of an aortic aneurysm which was better seen in more caudal sections.

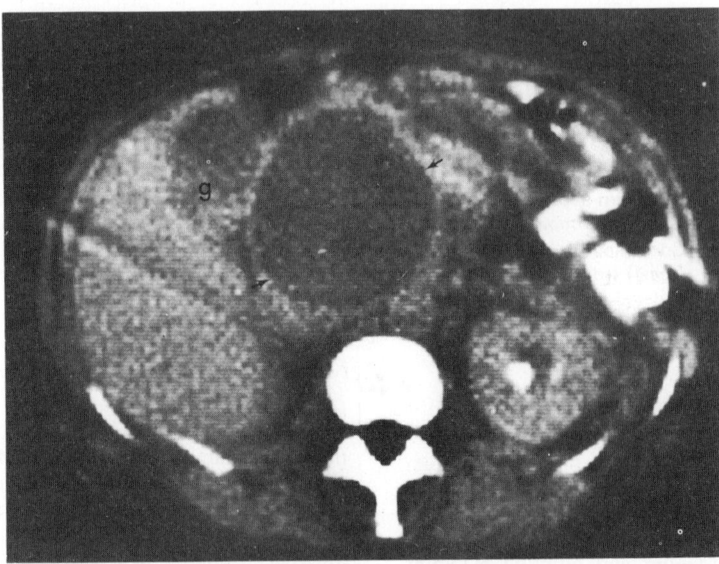

Fig. 70.7 CT scan showing typical pseudocyst (arrows) near the head of pancreas. The gallbladder (g) is also visualized.

of chronic pancreatitis may show changes detectable by ultrasound. One major difference between ultrasonography and CT scan is the frequency with which the gland can be seen. Ultrasonography has a non-visualization rate that averages 15–20% when conventional techniques are used. What is more subtle, and not known, is the frequency with which significant portions of the pancreas are hidden even though the investigator thinks the entire gland is seen. Cases of non-visualization are often excluded when an investigator tabulates his figures—the test is thus made to appear more useful than it actually is. On the other hand, failure rates for CT are significantly lower and range from 0 to 10%. CT scan has a higher chance of visualizing the gland when ascites or extreme obesity is present. On the other hand, when the patient cannot remain motionless or suspend respiration during the scanning, CT study is usually inadequate but the ultrasound examination may produce diagnostic results. Recognition of pancreatic calcification and small intrapancreatic pseudocysts is clearer with the CT scan and this facilitates diagnosis of pancreatitis. Finally, detection of gas and of the thicker walls of pancreatic abscesses is easier with a CT scan.

CT examinations are two to four times more expensive than pancreatic ultrasound. When serial or multiple studies are required, the potential risk of radiation exposure has to be taken into account with the CT scan.

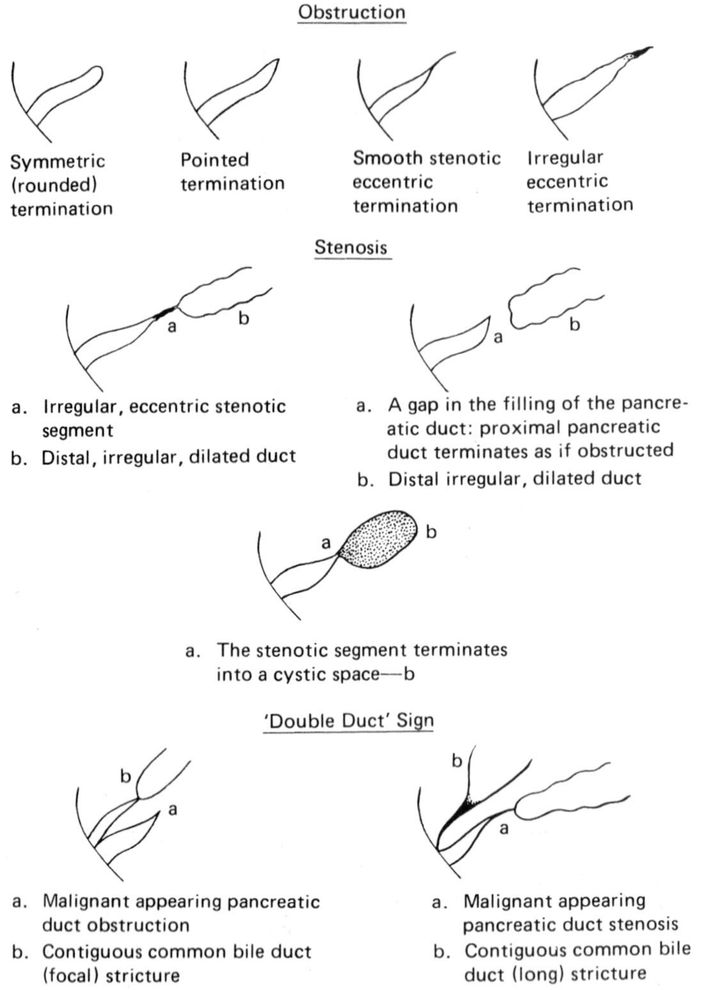

Fig. 70.8 Diagram of typical radiographic appearances of the main pancreatic duct as demonstrated by ERCP in patients with cancer of the head of pancreas.

Endoscopic Retrograde Cholangiopancreatography (ERCP)

Endoscopic Diagnosis at ERCP

ERCP endoscopy provides direct visual observation of the oesophagus, stomach, duodenum and ampulla of Vater. Inflammatory or neoplastic lesions visualized in any part of the upper gastrointestinal tract may entirely explain the clinical picture.

Tissue Diagnosis at ERCP

Conventional endoscopic biopsy with forceps, brush cytology, aspiration of pancreatic juice for cytology, or direct transduodenal needle aspiration cytology may be possible and provides valuable information if positive for malignant disease. In addition, aspirated pancreatic juice may be assayed for research into tumour markers such as CEA and POA.

Radiological Diagnosis at ERCP (Figs. 70.8, 70.9, 70.10)

Retrograde pancreatogram and/or the retrograde cholangiogram often provide information indicative of the presence of tumour, inflammatory disorders, or stone disease.

The main disadvantage of ERCP is that it requires the combined team effort of an endoscopist, an assistant who is thoroughly familiar with the equipment and technique (including disinfection procedures and the handling of specimens), a radiology technician, and, ideally, a radiologist to be present. It is time-consuming and expensive. It is an invasive procedure which carries a small risk of complications. ERCP is unsuitable for screening patients with unsuspected pancreatic disease.

Complications of ERCP

1. Injection pancreatitis—this can be prevented by careful injection of the medium into the pancreatic duct without too much pressure and without attempting to obtain an acinar phase of the pancreatogram.

2. Sepsis—pancreatic and biliary sepsis can be induced or precipitated by ERCP. Whether the sepsis is of endogenous or exogenous origin is a debatable and academic point. Suffice to say that ERCP sepsis is most frequently related to injection into an obstructed pancreatic duct, a pseudocyst or an obstructed common bile duct. ERCP sepsis can be largely prevented or abolished if the following precautions are taken:

a. Disinfection of the endoscope tip and the cannula with 2% glutaraldehyde.

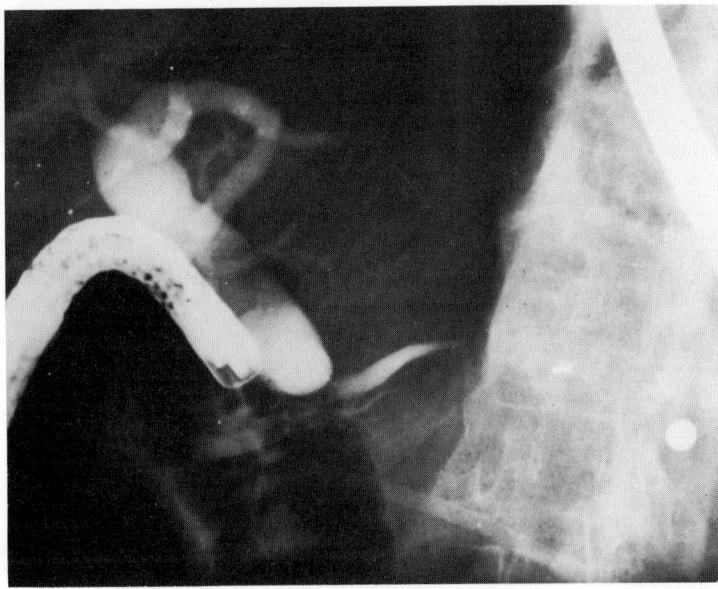

Fig. 70.9 ERCP showing 'rat tail' appearance due to obstruction of the main pancreatic duct by a carcinoma. The common bile duct is dilated. This 'double duct' sign is highly suggestive of unresectability of the cancer.

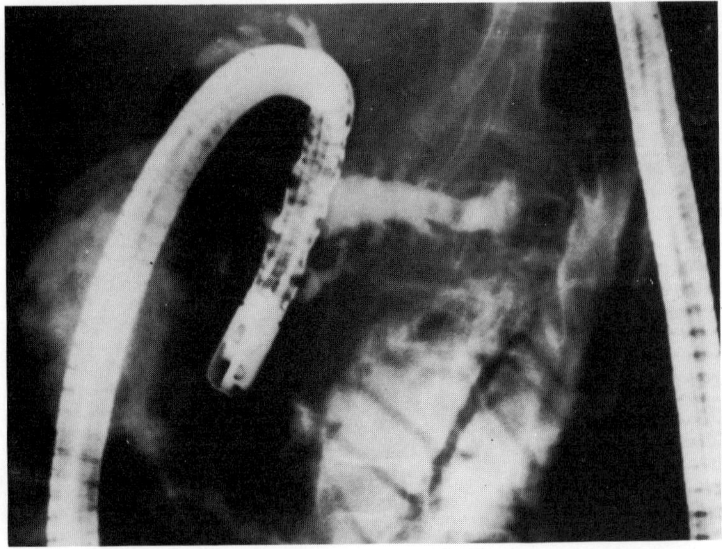

Fig. 70.10 ERCP showing grossly dilated main pancreatic duct due to chronic pancreatitis.

b. Prophylactic systemic antibiotics intravenously for 24–48 hours.

c. Addition of antibiotics (chloramphenicol or gentamicin) to the contrast material.

d. The patient should be operated on within 24 hours of ERCP if a pseudocyst or an obstructed duct is demonstrated.

3. Other rare complications of ERCP are drug reactions, instrumental injury to the upper gastrointestinal tract, and aspiration pneumonia which is associated with the amount of sedatives given to the patient.

Angiography (*Figs*. 70.11, 70.12, 70.13)

Percutaneous transfemoral catheterization for coeliac and superior mesenteric angiography is a valuable method of studying the vasculature of the pancreas. With improvement in and refinement of catheter design, various techniques of super-selective pancreatic angiography have been developed. The super-selective technique may be enhanced by magnification radiography and, in some instances, by the intra-arterial injection of various drugs which improve the visualization (pharmacoangiography) of pancreatic vessels. Vasodilators (bradykinin, tolazolin) and/or vasoconstrictors (epinepherine, norepinepherine, angiotensin) and hormones (secretin and pancreozymin) have all been tried.

The single most useful and reliable angiographic sign of a malignant tumour of the pancreas is *arterial encasement*. Encasement is seen as a narrowing and/or irregularity of a

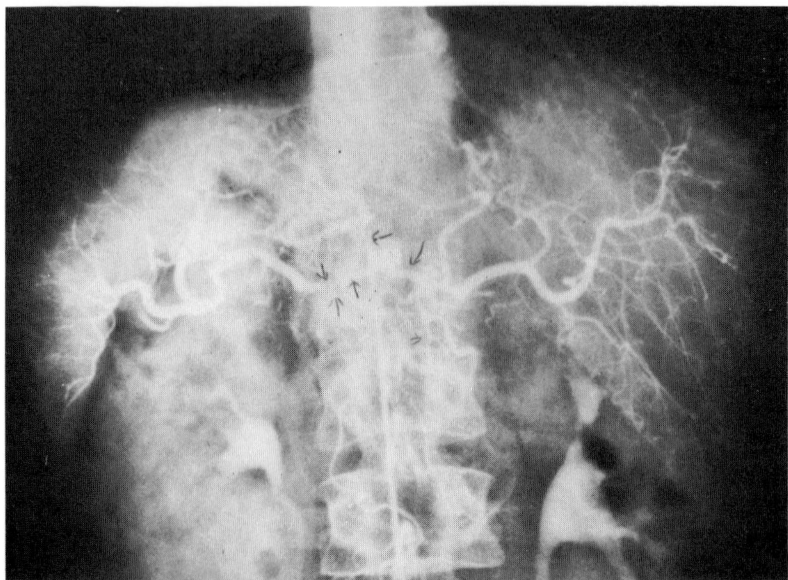

Fig. 70.11 Coeliac arteriogram showing major (hepatic, splenic, left gastric) arterial encasement, indicating unresectability of cancer of the body of the pancreas.

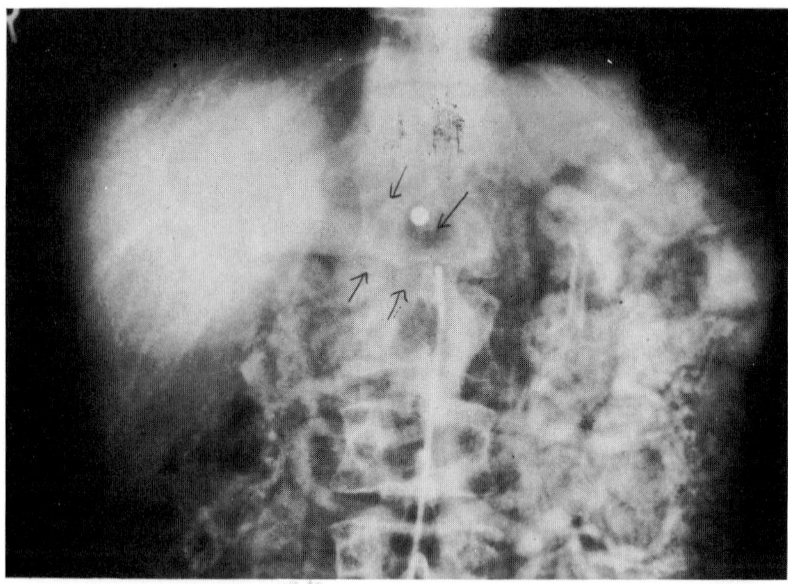

Fig. 70.12 Venous phase of coeliac and superior mesenteric angiogram showing occlusion of the portal vein. Same patient as in *Fig. 70.11* with unresectable cancer of the body of the pancreas.

vessel and is caused by invasion of the vessel by tumour or its compression by surrounding tissues. Arterial encasement may be irregular or smooth or may be serrated or serpiginous. The smooth encasement is much less specific for cancer and may be seen in pancreatitis. Large artery (splenic, hepatic, superior mesenteric, left gastric) encasement is highly suggestive of an unresectable tumour. Small artery encasement is a term applied when more distal branches supplying the pancreas are involved. In connection with the assessment of tumour resectability, the gastroduodenal artery is considered to be borderline between the two groups. A second angiographic sign of unquestionable value in the diagnosis of pancreatic cancer is the presence of *major venous involvement*. An adequate venous phase angiogram frequently reveals obstruction and narrowing or deformity of the veins. However, non-visualization of the splenic or portal vein alone, although suggestive, is not diagnostic of venous obstruction. Arterial occlusion or arterial displacement may also be caused by pancreatic tumours. Neovascularity is only *rarely* seen in pancreatic carcinoma because the cancer is typically avascular. However, hyperaemia or increased vascularity in the region of the pancreas may be seen in cases of pancreatic cancer and is usually due to secondary inflammatory changes around the tumour. Finally, an angio-

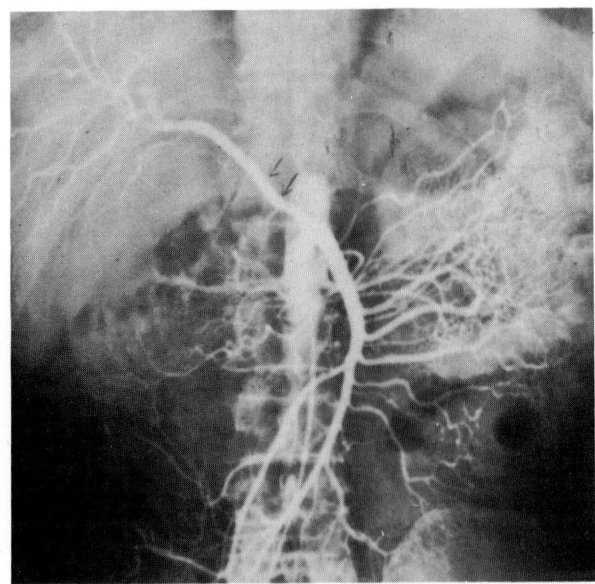

Fig. 70.13 Superior mesenteric angiogram showing a common variation of the foregut vasculature. The right hepatic artery originates from the superior mesenteric artery and can be damaged during pancreatoduodenal resections.

gram may occasionally disclose the presence of hepatic metastases, thereby suggesting the malignant nature of a pancreatic abnormality.

Islet cell tumours are typically vascular. A fine network of small vessels may be seen in the early arterial phase and, occasionally, feeding arteries and draining veins may be identified. With larger tumours, displacement of neighbouring arteries may be seen and larger, irregular 'tumour vessels' have been reported. It is difficult to correlate angiographic visualization of islet cell tumours with their malignant potential unless hepatic metastases are obviously seen or encasement (or occlusion) of arteries are striking features. When angiography does demonstrate a solitary islet cell tumour, the surgeon must be aware that there may be a second lesion not shown angiographically. When angiography shows multiple islet cell tumours, the likelihood of there being others not shown is very real. In this respect, angiography does not remove the surgeon's obligation to carry out a complete exploration of the whole pancreas.

A major value of angiography is to delineate variations in the foregut vasculature, especially the hepatic blood supply. The desirability of obtaining angiographic studies before embarking on a major pancreatic resection should be emphasized since ligation of a major hepatic arterial blood supply in a jaundiced patient may lead to fatal liver ischaemia.

Complications of Angiography

Complications at the femoral puncture site include haemorrhage, haematoma, arterial occlusion, pseudoaneurysms, and arteriovenous fistula. Embolization of thrombus formed at the puncture site, subintimal dissection of an atheromatous plaque with secondary thrombosis, distal embolization of catheter or guidewire fragments, have all been described. Postangiographic renal failure is well documented, especially in patients with pre-existing renal disease. The injected contrast media are hypertonic and may be a real hazard, especially if the patient has been dehydrated for several hours. The jaundiced patient is particularly at risk from both bleeding problems and renal failure. They should be kept well hydrated and their coagulation abnormalities should be treated prior to angiography. The spectrum of adverse sequelae is indeed very broad and this invasive procedure should not be undertaken without good indication, by inexperienced personnel or where facilities are inadequate. However, when planned and performed with care, abdominal angiography is an acceptably safe procedure and is a useful part of the diagnostic armamentarium in patients with pancreatic disorders.

Chemical Analysis of the Stool to Demonstrate Steatorrhoea

Stool examination for fat content is only useful as a screening test for *malabsorption*. Faecal fat excretion is not a valid measure of pancreatic dysfunction since about 80% of pancreatic secretory capacity may be lost without any detectable change in the test. In clinical practice, pancreatic secretory deficiency states and malabsorption syndromes coexist in about 10–20% of patients. Even with more sophisticated tolerance tests, there is an overlap of the results obtained in malabsorption states and pancreatic insufficiency.

Direct Measurement of Pancreatic Digestive and Secretory Capacity

Direct duodenal intubation and collection of pancreatic juice for analysis (duodenal drainage studies) following various stimuli is widely practised. The exact technique varies from institution to institution. In the Lundh test, a meal of fat is given and the output of pancreatic lipase in the aspirated duodenal content is determined. The pancreatic secretory response to an injection of secretin (measurement of volume of juice and bicarbonate output) or CCK-PZ (measurement of enzyme output) is often studied but data interpretation is sometimes difficult. However, they are the most reliable tests in detecting pancreatic exocrine insufficiency due to chronic pancreatitis or pancreatic carcinoma. Cytological examination of the duodenal aspirate during these maximal secretory tests often documents the presence of malignancy in cases of pancreatic cancer.

CONGENITAL ANOMALIES OF THE PANCREAS

There are three congenital anomalies of the pancreas which are of potential surgical importance. They are (1) ectopic pancreas, (2) annular pancreas and (3) pancreas divisum.

Ectopic (Heterotopic, Dystopic, Aberrant) Pancreas

Pancreatic tissue has been documented in ectopic sites in the gastrointestinal tract and even elsewhere. The most common site for nodules of aberrant pancreatic rest is on the wall of the stomach, duodenum or jejunum. The nodules may be found in submucosa (75%) and in the muscular layer or subserous coat in the remainder. The overall incidence and relative frequency with which it causes symptoms varies. Autopsy studies have found heterotopic pancreatic tissue in the duodenum in as high as 14% of individuals. Scattered pancreatic tissue has been found in Meckel's diverticulum, gallbladder, colon, spleen, liver, bile ducts, mesentery or even omentum. Enterogenous cyst of the thorax has been reported to contain typical pancreatic tissue, including islets.

With the advent of widespread upper gastrointestinal endoscopy and improvements in contrast studies of the alimentary tract, ectopic pancreas of the stomach and duodenum is being more frequently recognized. The pathognomonic radiological finding is a smooth, rounded, or negative shadow with evidence of a tiny umbilication or even a small duct which may be outlined by a line of barium. Probably most individuals with ectopic pancreas have no symptoms whatsoever. However, abdominal pain suggestive of peptic ulcer disease sometimes occurs. Interference with gastric emptying by lesions situated in the pyloric region, direct production of a peptic ulcer, gastrointestinal haemorrhage, intussusception, and development of benign or malignant neoplasm arising in the pancreatic rest, have all been documented. Even an islet cell adenoma producing bouts of hyperinsulism has been reported to be cured by resection of the ectopic pancreatic tissue from the duodenum.

Annular Pancreas

The exact embryological explanation for this malformation is debatable. The classic description of annular pancreas is almost invariably a ring of pancreatic tissue, continuous with the head of the pancreas, surrounding the second part of the duodenum proximal to the ampulla of Vater. However, the infra-ampullary location has also been documented. Eighty-five per cent of cases occur around the second portion of the duodenum and the remaining 15% are scattered around the first or third part of the duodenum. The pancreatic tissue is generally firmly attached to and embedded into the duodenal musculature; only rarely is it loosely attached and readily separable from the duodenum. There is usually a variable amount of hypertrophy of the proximal duodenal wall resulting from obstruction. Half of the reported cases have manifested themselves in the first year of life. Some believe that there is invariably an associated intrinsic atresia or stenosis of the duodenum. Other developmental anomalies are also associated in about 60–70% of cases. They include Down's syndrome, non-rotation and incomplete rotation of the mesentery, pre-duodenal portal vein, imperforate anus, oesophageal atresia with tracheo-oesophageal fistula, and congenital heart disease. There is a high frequency of polyhydramnios in the mother of those children who have a high degree of duodenal obstruction at birth.

Vomiting is the main symptom of annular pancreas. It may begin as soon as the infant starts feeding or may appear several days later. Bile may or may not be present in the vomitus. Jaundice may be present and has been explained by back pressure of the distended duodenum on the common bile duct or involvement of the ampulla of Vater by oedema at the level of the stenosis. A plain film of the abdomen may show a distended stomach and a 'double-bubble' sign at the level of the duodenum. Contrast studies may be necessary to diagnose the condition.

About one-half the cases reported present for the first time with symptoms between the ages of 21 and 70 years. The reason for such late manifestations of symptoms is generally attributed to inflammatory changes in the pancreatic ring. Duodenal ulcer, frequently reported with annular pancreas in the adult, has not been observed in infancy. The differential diagnosis in infancy rests between annular pancreas and other causes of duodenal obstruction, all of which require urgent operative relief, namely, duodenal stenosis or atresia, compression of the duodenum by Ladd's bands, pyloric stenosis, and volvulus in association with malrotation. An absolute differentiation between annular pancreas and duodenal atresia or stenosis is not possible without operation.

The operation of choice is either duodenoduodenostomy or duodenojejunostomy performed through the retrocolic route. Attempts at division of the pancreatic ring are attended with complications, including pancreatitis, pancreatic fistula, duodenal wall perforation and failures. Gastrojejunostomy is not a satisfactory operation since it inadequately decompresses the duodenum and has a high incidence of marginal ulceration. In patients with concomitant jaundice an operative cholangiogram is mandatory before a decision about the need and type of biliary diversion can be made.

Pancreas divisum and its implications are discussed in the section on pancreatitis (*see below*).

INJURIES TO THE PANCREAS

These are discussed in Chapter 75.

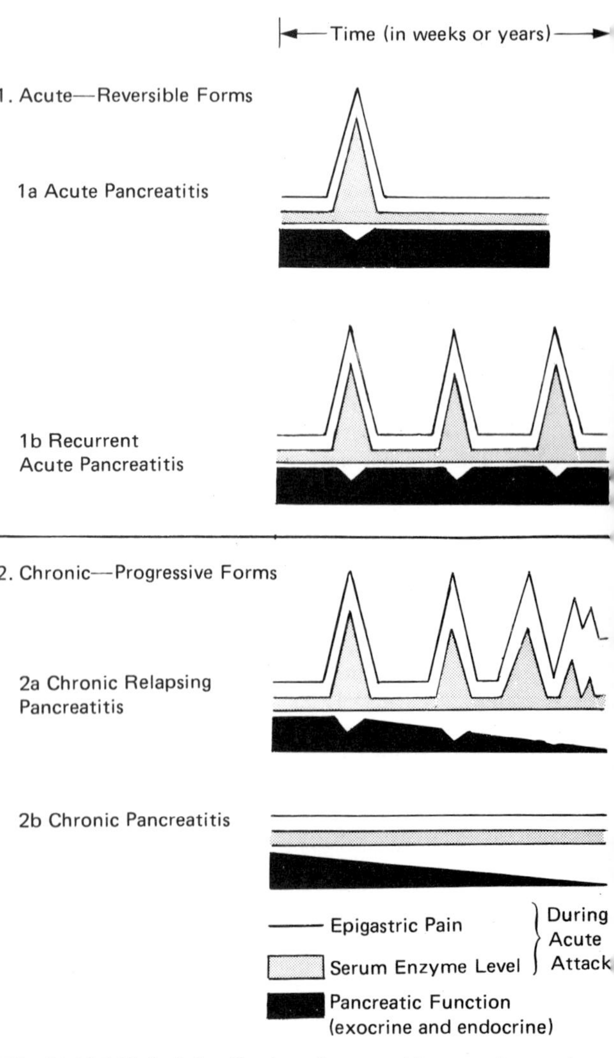

Fig. 70.14 Clinical classification of pancreatitis, according to the definition of Marseilles, as modified by Ammann and Trapnell.

PANCREATITIS

Definition and Classification

The term 'pancreatitis' implies the presence of pancreatic inflammation and autodigestion. It can be classified according to its clinical presentation (*Fig.* 70.14), according to the aetiological factors (*Table* 70.1), or according to the severity of the pathological process (*Table* 70.2). Clinically pancreatitis is referred to as *acute* or *chronic*. Restitutio ad integrum is the hallmark of the acute form whereas persistence or progression of the disease or residual damage to the pancreas indicates the chronic variety. Nevertheless, if a patient recovers from acute necrotizing pancreatitis normal recovery of pancreatic (endocrine and exocrine) function or morphology may never occur and the patient may be rightly labelled as having 'progressed' into chronic pancreatitis. Similarly, on occasion, recurrent attacks of acute pancreatitis due to any cause may merge into the chronic varieties. *Fig.* 70.14 shows a clinical classification of pancreatitis according to the definition of the Marseilles symposium as modified by Ammann and Trapnell. The emphasis on chronic pancreatitis is the absence of pain and enzyme elevation but the presence of pancreatic exocrine and endocrine insufficiency. Patients with chronic relapsing pancreatitis, in addition to the same disorders of function, experience pain which, in the overt case, is constant with relapses against the background of pain. All types of acute or chronic pancreatitis may cause complications such as biliary tract obstruction, splenic vein thrombosis, duodenal obstruction, etc.

Table 70.1 Classification of pancreatitis according to aetiological factors

1. Alcoholism
2. Biliary tract disease
3. Trauma
    - Surgical
    - Blunt
    - Penetrating
    - ERCP
    - Aortography
4. Drugs
    - Thiazides
    - Steroids
5. Metabolic disorders
    - Hyperparathyroidism
    - Hyperlipidaemia
6. Infections
    - Mumps
    - Coxsackie B Virus
    - Mycoplasma pneumoniae
    - Infectious mononucleosis
    - Septicaemia
7. Congenital mechanical obstruction of pancreatic duct, e.g.
    - Pancreas divisum
8. Periampullary cancer
9. Hereditary pancreatitis
10. Vascular disease

Table 70.2 Classification of acute pancreatitis according to severity of pathological process

1. Acute oedematous pancreatitis—mild, self-limiting
2. Acute persistent—unresolving, subacute—pancreatitis—suspect development of complications
3. Acute haemorrhagic—necrotizing, fulminant—pancreatitis

Acute Pancreatitis

Although, experimentally, acute pancreatitis has been produced in various animal models by promoting duodenopancreatic reflux, by the injection of bile salts, trypsin, etc. into the pancreatic duct, by the occlusion of pancreatic arterial blood supply, the relevance of these models to the human clinical situation is still uncertain. Acute pancreatitis has been associated with a variety of clinical disorders but the actual cause or mechanism which initiates the pancreatic autodigestion or which make it either a self-limiting disease or a progressively fatal disease remains unclear. Acute pancreatitis developing in the course of viral infection, such as mumps and Coxsackie B viruses, are usually self-limiting. So is the acute pancreatitis in association with mycoplasma pneumonia. Metabolic disorders, such as hypercalcaemia (usually associated with hyperparathyroidism) and hyperlipidaemia (usually associated with contraceptive pills) have been well documented. So is acute pancreatitis resulting from drug therapy, such as diuretics and steroids. Autopsy examination of patients dying of such conditions as fulminant liver failure, hypovolaemic shock with renal tubular necrosis, transplantation and cardiac bypass surgery have revealed fulminant pancreatitis in a significant number of these patients. From the practical point of view the two conditions most commonly associated with acute pancreatitis are alcoholism and biliary tract stone disease. The prognostic and therapeutic implications of acute pancreatitis due to these two associations are different. Gallstone pancreatitis usually occurs in patients older than 60 years old, tends to be severe and is frequently accompanied by serious complications in the acute stage. However, recurrences may be prevented by early operative intervention or, if the patient recovers quickly, by appropriately timed elective surgical treatment of the biliary tract. By contrast, alcohol-associated pancreatitis tends to be recurring. Although the first attacks are usually severe, and can be fatal, subsequent attacks are commonly mild and carry low mortality. As time passes, the recurring attacks lead to progressive destruction of the gland and eventually the clinical picture merges into that of chronic pancreatitis or chronic relapsing pancreatitis.

Acute pancreatitis may be secondary to blunt or penetrating abdominal injury or may follow some invasive clinical test, such as endoscopic retrograde cannulation of the papilla (ERCP) and translumbar aortography. Postoperative acute pancreatitis most commonly occurs after exploration of the common bile duct and is invariably due to injudicious, inexpert, forceful dilatation of the sphincter of Oddi or transduodenal sphincteroplasty. Distal pancreatitis may follow splenectomy.

Two morphological forms of acute pancreatitis are generally distinguished—the oedematous mild form and the severe, necrotizing, haemorrhagic, or suppurative type. The oedematous variety can progress to the necrotic type for reasons not well understood. Distinction between the two major forms of acute pancreatitis on the basis of the clinical features and conventional laboratory studies may be *impossible* at the *onset* of the disease. Indeed, the diagnosis itself may remain uncertain for several hours after presentation. It is not sufficiently emphasized that the diagnosis of acute pancreatitis is, at best, a shrewd guess based on clinical probabilities and backed by elevation of serum or urinary amylase levels. The renal amylase : creatinine clearance ratio, isoamylase measurements and determinations of serum lipase or trypsin have not been generally helpful in doubtful cases and are not widely available.

Clinical Features

The clinical manifestations of acute pancreatitis are protean since it can mimic any other abdominal emergency. In fact, it can coexist with some such as acute cholecystitis. It can occur at any age but is rare in children and in very young adults. In the latter group it is usually associated with infections, trauma, parasites, drugs, or is hereditary. Alcohol-related pancreatitis is usually found in the young adult less than 40 years of age, whereas the form associated with biliary tract disease manifests itself mainly in middle-aged and older persons.

The onset of symptoms may follow excess intake of food or alcohol but this is not invariable. Pain is the major initial symptom in over 90% of patients. It may vary in degree from mild to severe and is characteristically sudden in onset persisting for 12–48 hours or more. The wide spectrum of the intensity of the pain should be emphasized. Like many patients with pancreatic pain, there is a tendency for the patient to bend forward and assume various postures in order to obtain relief. Occasionally, even the severe fulminant fatal pancreatitis may be totally painless. The location of the pain is usually in the mid-epigastrium but can occur or radiate anywhere and may be diffuse or confined mainly to the back. Other common symptoms are nausea, vomiting, retching and hiccup. Less frequently, diarrhoea, dyspnoea, cyanosis, haematemesis and melaena may appear early. The bleeding may be due to erosive ulcers, bleeding diathesis, left-sided portal hypertension or erosion of the inflammatory process into the gut.

The physical findings may be minimal in striking contrast to the severity of the symptoms. Obtundation, fever, tachycardia, epigastric tenderness and muscle guarding are frequent. Shock may be the initial symptom and, in severe cases, may be profound. Mild jaundice may be observed. Abdominal distension is often present in the early phase of the disease and is the result of a diffuse or localized paralytic ileus. Several days later, a palpable epigastric mass may be felt, indicating the development of a pseudocyst or marked peripancreatic fat necrosis. Other late signs include bluish discoloration of the skin around the periumbilical area (Cullen's sign) or in the loins (Grey–Turner's sign); these indicate ecchymosis caused by seepage of blood arising from acute necrotizing pancreatitis along fascial planes. Another rare skin manifestation is nodular fat necrosis simulating erythema nodosum or Weber–Christian disease. Rarely, polyarthritis or bone pain may be observed and is also attributable to fat necrosis. Thrombophlebitis of the leg veins is only rarely seen. Abnormal physical findings on chest examination are found in less than one-third of cases but a plain chest radiograph may reveal abnormalities in a greater proportion of patients. These include elevation of the diaphragm, basal atelectasis or pneumonitis, left-sided or bilateral pleural effusion.

Diagnostic Procedures

The haematocrit is high in most patients at the onset of the disease reflecting fluid loss related to the inflammatory process and vomiting. Leucocytosis of 10 000–20 000 white blood count per mm^3 is almost invariably present.

Serum Enzyme Elevations

The key to the diagnosis of acute pancreatitis remains an elevation of pancreatic enzymes in the circulating blood or urine. Although hyperamylasaemia is a non-specific finding, the level of the serum amylase in various extrapancreatic conditions rarely attains a value five times above normal and this is commonly seen in primary acute pancreatitis. Normal serum amylase levels may be obtained if the determination is carried out 3 days or more after the onset, if previous attacks have completely destroyed the glandular tissue, or if the current attack is associated with massive destruction of the gland. Persistence of hyperamylasaemia for 10 days or longer may indicate a continuation of the acute inflammation or the development of local complications, such as pseudocyst formation, pancreatic abscess, pancreatic ascites, etc.

In view of the problems involved in the interpretation of hyperamylasaemia measurement of isoenzymes of amylase and determinations of the renal amylase : creatinine clearance ratio have recently been advocated. The P-type isoamylase cannot be detected after extirpation of the pancreas and hence is only of pancreatic origin. Its measurement is unnecessary and time-consuming for routine purposes but it is useful in establishing the cause of a persistent hyperamylasaemia.

In acute pancreatitis, the relative renal clearance of amylase increases compared to that of creatinine. It has been suggested that a clearance of amylase over the clearance of creatinine of greater than 4 is found in the first few days after an attack of acute pancreatitis and that this elevated ratio persists longer than abnormalities of blood or urinary enzyme levels. The view that the amylase : creatinine clearance is specific for acute pancreatitis has now been shown to be untrue since an elevated clearance ratio is found in numerous other conditions, such as diabetic ketoacidosis, burns, and chronic renal failure while many patients with acute pancreatitis may have normal clearance ratios.

Estimation of lipolytic activity in the blood, urine, pleural and peritoneal effusions has been advocated on the grounds that lipase is more specific for pancreatic disease than amylase and its level remains elevated for longer periods. The recent introduction of radioimmunoassay for trypsin has resulted in reports demonstrating high levels of immunoreactive trypsin in the circulation and in serous effusions in patients with acute pancreatitis. The diagnostic or prognostic value of immunoreactive trypsin assays compared with other enzymes has yet to be reported. Immunoreactive elastase levels have also been reported and are said to be elevated in patients with acute pancreatitis showing good correlation with levels of amylase.

Urinary Amylase and Lipase

Amylase clearance is increased about threefold for 1–2 weeks in patients with acute pancreatitis whose renal function is unimpaired. Thus, increased urinary output of amylase may persist for several days after normalization of the serum amylase levels. Determination of the ratio of amylase:creatinine clearance permits the diagnosis of acute pancreatitis even in the presence of renal insufficiency. Timed urinary amylase output (usually expressed in terms of total activity per hour) and amylase clearance studies are particularly of diagnostic value after serum amylase has returned to normal. Urinary lipase determination has been abandoned since it is debatable whether lipolytic activity is detectable in the urine.

Other Enzymes

Serum ribonuclease or deoxyribonuclease-I have both been advocated since elevation of the activity in serum occurs only in the presence of pancreatic necrosis. Further substantiation of this claim is needed before it can be recommended.

Hyperglycaemia and Glycosuria

Transient hyperglycaemia has been observed in a varying proportion of patients with acute pancreatitis. One of the mechanisms may be the release of glucagon from the damaged pancreatic cells. Usually the hyperglycaemia disappears with remission of the acute pancreatitis but, occasionally, following extensive parenchymal damage, diabetes mellitus may ensue.

Hypocalcaemia

The incidence, mechanism and prognostic implications of hypocalcaemia, serum calcium below 1·9 mmol/l (7·5 mg/100 ml), are still controversial. Some believe that hypoalbuminaemia accounts for most of the measured hypocalcaemia. Deposition of calcium in areas of fat necrosis, release of glucagon with secondary hypercalcitonaemia and hypomagnesaemia have all been suggested as pathogenetic factors. Impairment of parathyroid gland function has also been reported.

Whatever its mechanism, hypocalcaemia complicating acute pancreatitis is occasionally manifested by tetany and usually denotes the presence of the severe form of the disease.

Methaemalbuminaemia

The presence of this haemoglobin derivative in the serum suggests severe haemorrhagic pancreatitis rather than the oedematous variety. Elevated methaemalbumin levels, however, are not specific for necrotizing pancreatitis, because they can occur with other necrotizing intra-abdominal processes.

Blood Coagulation Tests

A rise in circulating trypsin may result in an increased antithrombin activity but this is not a reliable test for acute pancreatitis. The persistence of elevated serum fibrinogen levels, especially after the second week, is said to indicate either a severe form of acute pancreatitis or the onset of complications.

Hyperlipidaemia

Hyperlipidaemia, especially hypertriglyceridaemia, occurs in about 5–10% of patients with acute pancreatitis. The lipid rise may be primary and the cause of the acute pancreatitis or may be secondary, resulting from the pancreatitis. Long-term studies of blood lipids after subsidence of acute pancreatitis may be necessary for the differentiation of primary and secondary hyperlipidaemia. It has been suggested that many of the patients with so-called 'secondary hyperlipidaemia' may have a primary latent disorder of lipid metabolism which is unmasked by the attack of pancreatitis.

Electrocardiogram

ECG changes simulating myocardial infarction have been reported in patients with acute pancreatitis. The commonest ECG changes are S-T segment elevation or depression, inversion of T waves, and extended T wave negativity. These changes disappear rather quickly unless there is coexistent myocardial ischaemia or infarction or there are other cardiac complications of acute pancreatitis, such as pericarditis. The exact mechanisms underlying the ECG changes include several factors, such as myocardial damage due to shock, electrolyte disturbance, excessive parenteral fluid replacement, effect of severe pain on coronary circulation, particularly in patients with coronary artery disease, influence of circulating pancreatic trypsin, and vagally mediated reflexes from the pancreas to the heart.

Plain Abdominal and Chest Radiography

A plain radiograph of the abdomen and chest may show evidence of pneumoperitoneum, thus excluding the diagnosis of acute pancreatitis and indicating the need for emergency operation for a perforated viscus. It may show abnormalities suggestive of acute pancreatitis in about 50% of cases. The radiological signs include intestinal distension in the region of the pancreas (sentinel jejunal loop, colon cut-off, duodenal ileus) or a generalized paralytic ileus. Haziness in the flat plate of the abdomen is caused by retroperitoneal fluid accumulation and may be associated with obliteration of the psoas outline. Other signs are elevation of the left diaphragm, caused by basal atelectasis or subdiaphragmatic fluid collection, and pleural effusions.

Differential Diagnosis

The clinical picture of acute pancreatitis tends to change with evolution of the disease. Early (2–3 hours) after the onset, symptoms are often suggestive of acute cholecystitis—indeed, acute cholecystitis may coexist with acute pancreatitis. After 6–8 hours, a perforated duodenal ulcer or acute appendicitis may be simulated. After 2–3 days the clinical features may mimic those of an intestinal obstruction because there is marked abdominal distension and ileus. If the patient presents with profound cardiovascular collapse, myocardial infarction, acute aortic distension, ruptured aortic aneurysm, mesenteric infarction or even massive pulmonary embolism may be initially suspected. Most of these conditions may be associated with elevation of serum amylase and often of lipase. Improved diagnostic ability will result if recognition of the clinical limitations in assessment are fully appreciated. Thus, the diagnosis of acute pancreatitis is based on 'thinking about it as a possibility' and excluding other sources of abdominal pain.

Bad Prognostic Markers in Acute Pancreatitis

Ranson has postulated that the risk of death and/or developing major complications may be estimated objectively by 11 early parameters:

On admission to hospital

1. Age greater than 55 years.
2. White cell count greater than 16 000/mm^3.
3. Fasting blood glucose greater than 11·2 mmol/l (200 mg %).
4. Serum LDH greater than 350 iu/l.
5. SGOT greater than 250 S.F. Units per cent.

Within the initial 48 hours of admission

6. A haematocrit decrease greater than 10 percentage points.
7. Blood urea nitrogen increase greater than 1·8 mmol/l (5 mg %).
8. Serum calcium less than 2 mmol/l (8 mg %).
9. Arterial oxygen tension less than 7·98 kPa (60 mmHg).
10. Base deficit greater than 4 mEq/l.
11. Estimated fluid sequestration greater than 6 L.

In patients with less than 3 of these 11 signs, the mortality rate is 0·9%; with 3–4 signs, 18%; with 5–6 signs, 50%; and with more than 6 signs, 90%.

Medical Management

The mainstay of the medical treatment of acute pancreatitis entails correction of hypovolaemia by replacement of fluid, electrolytes, blood or plasma. The continuing activity of the pancreatitis and/or the development of complications may be assessed by serial clinical examination, monitoring of serum and/or urinary amylase, and by regular ultrasonography and/or CT scan of the pancreas. Current evidence suggests that anticholinergics, glucagon, or trasylol, have no place in the management of patients with acute pancreatitis.

Nasogastric suction is currently used for all patients except those with a very mild attack of pancreatitis. Oral feeding should not be instituted until 7 days (in the mild case) to 14 days (in the severe case) after the attack of pancreatitis, as measured by all parameters, has subsided. Premature feeding is probably the commonest cause of exacerbation of pancreatitis. A period of parenteral hyperalimentation may be needed.

Medical management also includes close monitoring of vital signs, hourly urine output and central venous pressure measurements. Arterial blood gases *must* be frequently measured during the first few days as clinically occult respiratory failure is common. Pulmonary arterial pressure monitoring is valuable in patients with large volume requirements and associated cardiopulmonary disease or respiratory failure.

Such careful and repeated evaluation will also permit accurate differentiation between acute pancreatitis and other acute illnesses in the majority of cases. Selected patients may need additional investigation, such as contrast studies of the alimentary tract, isotope biliary scanning, transhepatic cholangiography, or angiography to exclude with absolute certainty gastrointestinal perforation or obstruction, acute biliary tract disease, or mesenteric infarction. An even smaller group of patients will need a diagnostic laparotomy.

Early Surgical Intervention

There are three situations when early operative intervention is indicated in a patient with suspected acute pancreatitis:

1. When the diagnosis is in doubt and a perforated or a gangrenous viscus cannot be excluded.
2. Failure of the patients to improve on medical management indicates acute haemorrhagic necrotizing pancreatitis and is often an indication for operative intervention.
3. Patients with known biliary stone disease who develop an attack of acute pancreatitis which does not improve within 48–72 hours, especially if there is evidence of biliary obstruction and/or cholangitis. In this clinical setting one must suspect an inpacted stone at the ampulla and emergency ERCP with endoscopic papillotomy and stone extraction must be seriously considered. If this fails or if an experienced endoscopist is not available then early operation to relieve ampullary obstruction is mandatory. The patient who recovers following non-operative management of acute gallstone pancreatitis has a high risk of recurrence. Operative correction of the cholelithiasis should be undertaken as soon as the pancreatitis has subsided, preferably during the same hospitalization.

When laparotomy is performed early in the course of acute pancreatitis, one or more of the following procedures may be advisable:

1. Inspection only.
2. Placement of catheters for peritoneal lavage.
3. Biliary decompression via a cholecystostomy or a T-tube in the common bile duct.
4. Operative cholangiogram.
5. Cholecystectomy, common bile duct exploration, and choledocholithotomy with or without a sphincteroplasty.
6. Total or subtotal pancreatectomy.
7. Pancreatic and retroperitoneal débridement and drainage.
8. Decompressing gastrostomy and feeding jejunostomy.

Early abdominal exploration with pancreatic drainage or resection has an increased mortality in patients with *severe* pancreatitis, defined by the presence of three or more positive prognostic signs, from 18 to 67%. Peritoneal lavage by catheters placed percutaneously, coupled with adequate resuscitation, has been extremely effective in the management of early cardiovascular-respiratory-renal complications of severe pancreatitis, virtually preventing all early deaths from those causes. It should be emphasized that peritoneal lavage and laparotomy are emergency resuscitative measures for the patient who is in refractory cardiovascular collapse and respiratory embarrassment. They should not be used indiscriminately for all cases of acute pancreatitis. If laparotomy is performed, the addition of a gastrostomy and jejunostomy confers several advantages. The former allows gastric decompression and drainage which may be needed for several weeks without the discomfort of a nasogastric tube. The latter provides a route for enteral nutrition with minimal stimulation to the pancreas and obviates the use of intravenous alimentation which has the potential risk of catheter sepsis. Improvement in overall mortality following peritoneal lavage has been disappointing since lavage does not reduce the late deaths from pancreatic and peripancreatic necrosis and sepsis. It was rightly pointed out that the two surgical pitfalls in acute pancreatitis are:

1. To operate too early and do too much.
2. To operate too late and do too little.

Any patient who has persistence or reappearance of the inflammatory manifestations of acute pancreatitis must be suspected of developing a pancreatic pseudocyst or a pancreatic abscess. Clinically, fever, pain, tenderness, a palpable mass, leucocytosis and hyperamylasaemia are inconstant features. A positive blood culture is *not* usually obtained in the early development of a pancreatic abscess. If antibiotics are used the fever may be partly masked. A plain radiograph of the abdomen may demonstrate the mottled 'soap bubble' appearance suggestive of a retroperitoneal abscess in less than 20% of cases. Ultrasonography and computerized tomography are invaluable tools in these cases and obviate the need for contrast studies of the gastrointestinal tract.

Late Surgical Intervention

Apart from the eradication of biliary tract disease following an attack of acute pancreatitis which has subsided, the role of operative intervention late in the course of acute pancreatitis is for the treatment of complications. These are:

1. Pseudocyst formation.
2. Abscess formation.
3. Haemorrhage resulting from pseudoaneurysms or sectorial (left-sided) portal hypertension.

A pancreatic pseudocyst is a collection of fluid, serum and haematoma in the lesser sac and its walls have no recognizable epithelial lining. However, at some point most pseudocysts connect with the pancreatic glandular tissue or ductal system and the discharge of fluid into the cyst is maintained

Table 70.3 Pathological classification of primary malignant neoplasms of the pancreas (non-endocrine)

1. Duct (Ductular) Cell Origin	90%
Duct cell adenocarcinoma	
Giant cell carcinoma	10%
Giant cell carcinoma (epulis-osteoid)	
Adenosquamous carcinoma	
Microadenocarcinoma	
Mucinous (colloid) carcinoma	
Cystadenocarcinoma (mucinous)	
2. Acinar Cell Origin	<1%
Acinar cell carcinoma	
Cystadenocarcinoma (acinar cell)	
3. Connective Tissue Origin	<1%
'Osteogenic' sarcoma	
Leiomyosarcoma	
Haemangiopericytoma	
Malignant fibrous histocytoma	
4. Uncertain Histogenesis	8%
Pancreaticoblastoma	
Papillary and cystic neoplasm	
Mixed type: duct and islet cells	
Unclassified	
5. Miscellaneous Others	<1%
Malignant melanoma	
Oncocytoma	
Neuroblastoma	
Plasmacytoma	
Lymphoma	

via the connection. Microscopic examination of this area of a pseudocyst will reveal some epithelial lining. The majority of pancreatic epithelial cysts are neoplastic (*Table* 70.3). The differentiation between a true cyst and a pseudocyst is only histological. The epithelial lining of true cysts may atrophy due to overdistension or infection. Hence the absence of histologically recognizable epithelium in the cyst wall on biopsy may be of no significance.

Management of Pancreatic Pseudocyst

Two types of pancreatic pseudocysts can be differentiated. *Acute pseudocysts* follow an established acute attack of pancreatitis. They should be managed expectantly for 4–6 weeks. Spontaneous resolution sometimes occurs and surgical therapy is more satisfactory if the cyst wall is allowed to mature. *Chronic pseudocysts* are usually asymptomatic and no recent attack of acute pancreatitis can be identified. They should be scheduled for operation promptly following an arteriogram. Spontaneous resolution is rare and delay only invites the high risk of complications. The commonest cause of pancreatic pseudocysts in children is blunt abdominal trauma.

Other parameters which are helpful in the management of pancreatic pseudocysts are:

1. *Size.* Pseudocysts less than 5 cm in diameter may be observed and expected to resolve in many instances. Those greater than 7·5 cm in diameter will probably need surgical drainage.
2. *The development of symptoms* is indicative of an impending complication such as rupture, haemorrhage, and infection.
3. *Maturity.* As previously mentioned, an acute pseudocyst should be allowed to mature for 4–6 weeks to allow the cyst wall to mature since this facilitates internal drainage.
4. *Vascular complications.* Recent advances in visceral angiography and its widespread practice have delineated a subgroup of patients with vascular complications associated with acute pancreatitis. These include pseudo-aneurysms and left-sided portal hypertension from splenic vein thrombosis. The presence of pseudoaneurysms is an indication for pancreatic resection as opposed to internal drainage of pseudocyst. The presence of portal hypertension is an indication for splenectomy with or without gastric devascularization.
5. *The site of the pseudocyst* is another important parameter which helps the surgeon decide on the method of internal drainage. Retrogastric cysts which are enlarging anteriorly are best treated by a posterior cystogastrostomy. Cysts around the head of the pancreas close to the duodenum can easily be drained by cystoduodenostomy. Large cysts which enlarge through and bulge inferiorly into the transverse mesocolon are best drained by cystojejunostomy with Roux-en-Y. Cysts in the tail or body of the pancreas are technically more amenable to a resection (distal pancreatectomy and splenectomy) than cysts in the head and neck of the gland.

While internal drainage into the upper gastrointestinal tract is the preferred method of treating pseudocysts, there are some exceptions. Infected or ruptured cysts or the acute cysts with thin, friable walls are best drained externally with wide-bore sump suction drains. In many instances, the resulting pancreatic fistula will gradually close spontaneously. Occasionally a second procedure is needed to implant the fistulous tract into a Roux-en-Y loop of jejunum. Two additional precautionary measures should be taken whenever a pancreatic cyst is drained:

1. The cyst fluid must be routinely sent for cytological examination and a representative sample of the cyst wall must be excised for histological examination. The injudicious drainage of a cystadenoma or cystadenocarcinoma may thus be spotted and a planned re-operation for wide local excision entertained.
2. The cavity of the cyst must be explored with the index finger and septa gently divided. The cyst must be thoroughly irrigated prior to anastomosis with adjoining bowel or external drainage.

Percutaneous drainage of a pseudocyst under CT scan or ultrasound guidance is often advocated indiscriminately. It definitely has a temporizing role in some specific situations such as:

1. A patient who is unfit for or who refuses operation.
2. An acute pseudocyst which is rapidly enlarging and needs external drainage.
3. An infected pseudocyst which needs external drainage in a very sick septic patient.
4. A pseudocyst which is in an unusual location (e.g. mediastinum, pelvis) and is not readily amenable to internal drainage.

Endoscopic internal drainage of pseudocysts is too new a procedure to be evaluated. Early experience suggests that the hazards of bleeding and stenosis of the stoma are too prohibitive for the technique to be widely accepted.

Management of Pancreatic Abscess

The term 'pancreatic abscess' should *not* be used to connote a localized collection of pus in the lesser sace (infected pancreatic pseudocyst) which is easily drained externally with good results. A pancreatic abscess implies the presence of extensive pancreatic and peripancreatic necrosis with secondary infection. It has a very high mortality and morbidity and usually occurs after the second week of the onset of pancreatitis. The incidence of massive haemorrhage and injury to adjacent organs is also high. Drainage of the pancreatic bed alone is ineffective unless it is combined with wide retroperitoneal débridement to remove the pancreatic and peripancreatic slough. In most instances additional necrosis and abscess formation occur and re-operation for further débridement, lavage and drainage must be instituted.

Since pancreatic abscess formation follows an attack of acute fulminating pancreatitis and is associated with a prohibitive mortality and morbidity, some have advocated early (within a few days of onset) total pancreatectomy to control fulminating pancreatitis. The mortality for this extensive procedure in seriously ill patients is also prohibitive and all patients with the severe disease do not invariably progress to abscess formation.

Recurrent Pancreatitis

Any patient who has recovered from one or more attacks of pancreatitis must be investigated to identify and, if possible, to eliminate the aetiological factors. The need to identify surgically remediable problems, most commonly gallstones, often leads to the 'premature' performance of an oral cholecystogram or even an intravenous cholangiogram. Both these tests are unreliable for as long as 1 month after an acute attack of pancreatitis. Ultrasonography or computerized tomography are currently available and they can be used even in the acute stage. All types of cholangiography can then be reserved for doubtful or negative cases. It should also be remembered that about 5–10% of patients with an apparently normal cholecystogram have gallstones, usually small ones which are more likely to pass into the common bile duct, temporarily obstruct the papilla, and induce pancreatitis.

Stenosis of the sphincter of Oddi, often called papillitis, is without doubt a cause of recurrent pancreatitis. The stenosis is rarely of a primary nature and is probably due to a temporary impaction and later passage of a gallstone. Confidence in the diagnosis is strengthened by:

1. Documented episodes of biliary obstruction or cholangitis.
2. The endoscopic visualization of an inflamed papilla.
3. Demonstrated tightness of the ampullary orifice when it is cannulated endoscopically.
4. Documentation of delay in emptying of the common bile duct.
5. Intermittent elevations of liver enzymes, especially serum alkaline phosphatase.
6. Positive morphine-prostigmine (Nardi) test—reproduction of pain and enzyme elevation.
7. Documentation of elevated pressures in the common bile-duct by ERCP.

Treatment is sphincteroplasty which includes extensive division of the sphincter of Oddi and the septum between the common bile duct and the pancreatic duct to relieve both biliary and pancreatic outflow obstruction. The situation should be suspected in patients who have had more than one attack of pancreatitis and/or cholangitis without any other discernible cause. One word of caution—the condition of 'primary papillitis' has been overdiagnosed without adequate documentation of unexplained abdominal pain which is often not even of pancreatic or biliary origin. In such situations, the indiscriminate use of sphincteroplasty, often wrongly performed, has led the operation into disrepute. Endoscopic papillotomy may have a small place when the biliary sphincter alone needs to be divided.

Congenital malformations in the pancreas or duodenum around the ampullary region can cause recurrent pancreatitis both in children and adults. ERCP is invaluable in delineating these abnormalities some of which may be amenable to surgical correction. Probably the commonest congenital abnormality leading to recurrent pancreatitis is the pancreas divisum which is an anatomical variant occurring when there is failure of the two embryonic pancreatic ductal systems to unite. In this situation, the duct of Wirsung is very small and may measure no more than 1–2 centimetres in length while the duct of Santorini becomes the major ductal system of the pancreas and maintains its communication with the duodenum through the minor papilla. Following secretin administration, large volumes of juice can be visualized endoscopically from the minor papilla with little or none coming from the main papilla or aspirated from the duct of Wirsung during cannulation. The high incidence of recurrent pancreatic pain in patients with pancreas divisum may well be due to the very small papilla of the duct of Santorini which, in these patients, drains the majority of the pancreas, creating a marked relative stenosis of the ampulla. Surgical relief of the pain may be required for patients with recurrent pancreatitis and the choice of operation is between a distal resection with retrograde drainage into a loop of jejunum or a pancreaticoduodenectomy. Recently, endoscopic excision of the minor papilla has been advocated for this condition.

Left-sided (Sectorial) Portal Hypertension due to Pancreatitis

This occurs from thrombosis of the splenic vein and is discussed in Chapter 71.

Acute Pancreatitis in Children

In recent years, acute pancreatitis is being recognized with greater frequency in infancy and childhood. Although the treatment is not substantially different from that of adults, the aetiological factors are totally different. Biliary tract disease is not usually an aetiological factor; nor is alcoholism. A large number of mild acute pancreatitis cases result from viral infections, such as mumps. Blunt abdominal trauma, resulting from relatively minimal injury, is probably the commonest cause. Unlike the situation in adults, isolated pancreatic injury is commonly reported. A trifling fall upon a toy, such as a tricycle handlebar, may result in pancreatic trauma sufficient to induce a traumatic pancreatitis. Two clinical pictures emerge: (1) an acute abdominal emergency necessitating exploratory laparotomy when the pancreas is found to be inflamed. In such situations, care must be taken to exclude a complete pancreatic transection or major ductal injury. (2) The initial symptoms are mild and often the child is not even taken to hospital for several days or weeks when a pancreatic pseudocyst or pancreatic ascites has developed.

Drug-induced pancreatitis, familial pancreatitis (usually associated with hyperlipidaemia or amino aciduria), calculous disease of the biliary tree are all uncommon in children although occasional cases with pigment stones due to congenital spherocytosis have been described. Obstruction of the ampulla of Vater due to a congenital anomaly of the pancreatic ductual ampulla has also been documented and has been corrected by an adequate sphincteroplasty. Round worms entering into the pancreatic duct and causing pancreatitis has also been reported from time to time. Duodenal obstruction due to an annular pancreas may lead to recurrent acute pancreatitis which responds to duodenal decompression.

The management of acute or recurrent acute pancreatitis in children is essentially the same as in adults. The prognosis is much better even in the presence of complications. If the aetiological factors are removed, recovery is complete. Acute or recurrent acute pancreatitis does not progress into the chronic or chronic relapsing form in the vast majority of children.

Surgical Treatment of Chronic Pancreatitis and Chronic Relapsing Pancreatitis

Chronic pancreatitis or chronic relapsing pancreatitis is not generally considered a surgical disease. Maintenance of adequate nutrition, enzyme replacement and/or insulin supplements may be necessary in the management of exocrine and/or endocrine insufficiencies. The input of social services and of an interested psychiatric team is essential to manage the drug addiction and alcoholic problems which are often present. Direct operative procedures on the parenchyma of the gland and/or its ductal system are indicated almost exclusively for the relief of pain. The limits and hazards of surgical treatment of these patients must be emphasized.

1. No surgical procedure can restore either the endocrine or exocrine function of the pancreas. Nor is it likely to prevent further loss of glandular function.
2. The conversion of a non-reformed alcoholic or drug addict into an insulin-dependent diabetic by major pancreatic resection is likely to be lethal and must be avoided.
3. Rehabilitation of the patient must be planned well in advance otherwise surgical intervention for pain is doomed to failure. The life expectancy of the non-reformed alcoholic drug addict is extremely limited and is often shortened by the complications and late sequelae of operations.
4. Avoidance of alcohol is a more important determinant of outcome after operation than the type of procedure performed.

The indications for surgical treatment are two in number.

1. Intractable Pain

It is crucial to delineate the frequency, persistence and degree of pain. The decision to advise operation is influenced by several factors including the degree of disruption of the patient's life, the narcotic need, the control of alcoholism, the age and general condition of the patient, and, often, the surgeon's personal preferences.

2. The Development of Complications

These include (*a*) lower bile duct obstruction; (*b*) duodenal obstruction; (*c*) vascular involvement; (*d*) pancreatic cysts, pseudocysts, pancreatic ascites and pleural effusions; (*e*) the presence of a dominant mass leading to the fear or suspicion of cancer.

It is important to emphasize that correction of a complication does not invariably relieve any associated pain.

a. Lower Bile Duct Obstruction

The lower portion of the common bile duct passes through the head of the pancreas and is at risk of being narrowed by inflammation and fibrosis in this region. If frank obstructive jaudice is present, the onus is on the surgeon to exclude preoperatively and operatively the presence of an underlying cancer. On occasions this may only be possible after a total pancreatectomy. More commonly, the patient has low grade cholangitis and pain indistinguishable from pancreatic pain. Frank suppurative cholangitis and secondary biliary cirrhosis have also been described. In the mild case, serum alkaline phosphatase elevation is the most consistent although non-specific effect of biliary obstruction. As a rule, investigation of the biliary tree (by endoscopic retrograde cholangiogram) is mandatory whenever surgical treatment of chronic pancreatitis is being considered. Relief of the partial common bile duct obstruction is, in some instances, all that is needed to relieve the pain.

b. Duodenal Obstruction

This rarely occurs in patients with severe chronic pancreatitis and enlargement of the head of the pancreas. Here again a concomitant pancreatic cancer must be excluded by appropriate biopsies (in the young patient) or by total pancreatectomy (in the older patient). Vagotomy and gastrojejunostomy will adequately relieve the duodenal obstruction.

c. Development of vascular complications, such as multiple pseudo-aneurysms and sectorial portal hypertension. These have been discussed in the section on acute pancreatitis.

Once a decision for surgical treatment has been made, two most important preoperative investigations are ERCP and angiography. ERCP will delineate the state of the main pancreatic duct and common bile duct and helps in the planning of surgical therapy. However, the findings on ERCP often do not correlate with the patient's symptoms. ERCP does not indicate the state of the parenchyma; nor does it indicate the need for operative intervention except if cytological examination of the pancreatic duct aspirate is positive for cancer. However, ERCP provides a good indication of the choice of operation. Similarly, angiography delineates the anatomy of the foregut vasculature as well as vascular complications which may necessitate an alteration in surgical strategy.

As a general rule, surgery should be conservative when:

1. There is no endocrine or exocrine insufficiency.
2. A dilated duct of Wirsung is present. Dilatation (diameter >3 mm) of the main pancreatic duct, with or without partial stenosis of the duct at a number of points producing a chain of lakes appearance, may be associated with pancreatic stones in the duct. In this situation, longitudinal filleting of the main pancreatic duct and side-to-side anastomosis to a Roux-en-Y loop of jejunum (modified Puestow operation) is highly appropriate after removing any stone if present. Relief of pain is accomplished in about 70% of patients who stop consuming alcohol although recurrence of pain is common after variable intervals.

Surgery should be radical when:

1. Pancreatic cancer is suspected and/or cannot be excluded.
2. There is established endocrine or exocrine insufficiency.
3. There is extensive pancreatic destruction by ductal sclerosis, glandular fibrosis, calcification and multiple pseudocysts. A single pseudocyst may be drained internally as a preliminary step to see if the patient's pain is relieved. The presence of multiple cysts or the reformation of cysts is

an indication for pancreatic resection. The 95% distal pancreatectomy (Child's procedure) is not uniformly successful and recurrent pain associated with pancreatitis in the region of the head and the uncinate process then necessitates a second-stage pancreatoduodenectomy which can be technically difficult and hazardous. When pancreatic cancer is not suspected, total pancreatectomy can be performed in one stage with preservation of the whole stomach, pylorus and first part of the duodenum by careful preservation of the blood supply to the pyloroduodenal area. This diminishes postoperative problems associated with reduced gastric reservoir capacity and dumping syndrome.

A less radical approach which has been reported to be occasionally successful is the performance of a truncal vagotomy, antrectomy and gastrojejunal (Billroth II or Polya) anastomosis. The rationale of this operation is the elimination of neural and hormonal stimuli to pancreatic secretion, especially those normally triggered by eating. No convincing data are available to support these contentions.

Two other indirect operations, namely, cholecystectomy (for established gallbladder disease) and parathyroidectomy (for proven hyperparathyroidism) are sometimes advocated to reduce the severity of chronic pancreatitis. The incidence of gallstones in patients with chronic pancreatitis is the same as that in the general population. Cholecystectomy should be advised based on symptoms of gallbladder disease and on the risk of complications. It will not affect the natural history of chronic pancreatitis. Similarly, hyperparathyroidism should be treated to avoid the sequelae of severe hypercalcaemia without influencing the course of any incidental chronic pancreatitis.

Splanchnic neurectomies and coeliac ganglion block have generally been disappointing in the control of chronic pancreatic pain.

NEOPLASMS OF THE NON-ENDOCRINE PANCREAS

Benign neoplasms of the non-endocrine pancreas are exceedingly rare and are of no clinical significance unless they become large enough to be palpable or to impinge on adjacent structures (common bile duct, duodenum, stomach, or main pancreatic duct) and cause symptoms. Both solid and cystic benign tumours are not found, either at laparotomy or at necropsy, with sufficient frequency to suggest that they represent an early phase in the development of the more common malignant neoplasms. The reported benign tumours of the non-endocrine pancreas include adenoma, cystadenoma, lipoma, fibroma, leiomyofibroma, myoma, haemangioma, lymphangioma, haemangioendothelioma, and neuroma. These diagnoses should only be made after exclusion of the more frequent malignant tumours by some form of representative (preferably excision) biopsy.

Pancreatic Cancer

The term 'pancreatic cancer' is sometimes used to include all types of malignant neoplasms of the non-endocrine pancreas (which are classified in *Table* 70.3) as well as malignant islet cell tumours (*Table* 70.4). In clinical practice, pancreatic cancer is synonymous with pancreatic ductal adenocarcino-

Table 70.4 Cell tumours and associated clinical syndromes

Cell type	*Peptide product*	*Tumour*	*Clinical picture*
A Cell	Glucagon	Glucagonoma	Diabetes, necrolytic migratory erythema, stomatitis, glossitis Weight loss, weakness
B Cell	Insulin	Insulinoma	Neuroglycopenia Clouded sensorium Behaviour disturbance Seizures Transient neurological deficit Adrenaline discharge Sweating Tremulousness Palpitation Hunger
D Cell?	Gastrin	Gastrinoma	Fulminant peptic ulceration Diarrhoea Malabsorption
D Cell	Somatostatin	Somatostatinoma	Diabetes, pancreatic malabsorption with streatorrhoea, gallstones Weight loss
D_1 Cell?	Vasoactive intestinal polypeptide (VIP)	VIPoma	Fulminant diarrhoea, hypokalaemia, hypercalcaemia, diabetes, flushing
D_1 Cell?	Human pancreatic polypeptide	HPPoma	Uncertain
?	ACTH	?	Cushing's syndrome
?	Hydroxyindole	Carcinoid	Carcinoid syndrome?
?	Prostaglandin	?	Same as VIPoma?
?	ADH	?	?
?	None	Non-functioning islet cell tumour	Same as exocrine tumour but slow growing

ma which constitutes 90% of all primary malignant tumours arising from the gland. When the cancer originates in the head of the pancreas (in about 70% of cases) it must also be differentiated from cancer arising from the ampulla, duodenum or lower common bile duct which has a much better prognosis than true pancreatic adenocarcinoma. The incidence of pancreatic cancer has tripled over the last 40 years throughout the western world. It is highly fatal and has one of the lowest 5-year survival rates (1–2%) of all cancers. About 23 000 new pancreatic cancers are diagnosed each year in the USA and the disease now accounts for 10% of all the cancers of the digestive tract (second behind colorectal cancer) and it is the fourth most common cancer of all sites as a cause of death (behind lung, colorectal and breast). In England and Wales pancreatic cancer accounts for about 6000 deaths each year.

Cancer of the pancreas is distinctly more common in older people and is relatively uncommon, but not altogether rare below the age of 55 years. It is commoner in men than in women but the male : female ratio has decreased in recent years, suggesting that more women are now being diagnosed with this cancer.

The exact causative factors responsible for the increase in incidence of pancreatic cancer are unknown. A high protein and high fat diet, characteristic of the western population, has been implicated epidemiologically as a possible aetiological factor. The strongest association is between pancreatic cancer and cigarette smoking. Exposure to industrial carcinogens, especially betanaphthylamine and benzidine, has been documented in pancreatic cancer patients. A higher than normal incidence rate of the neoplasm has also been reported in chemists, workers in metal industries, and coke and gas plant employees. In interpreting these retrospective epidemiological data, it must be remembered that the general class of 'labourer' has, both in the USA and in Great Britain, an extensively high incidence of pancreatic cancer so that occupational risk is mixed with social class risk.

Industrial causes of pancreatic cancer are probably less important than is believed or the causative exposures are far more widespread in most occupations than is generally accepted.

Pancreatic Cancer and Diabetes Mellitus

There is no doubt that there is an association between pancreatic cancer and diabetes mellitus. Two hypotheses have been put forward—First, diabetes mellitus is an aetiological factor in the development of pancreatic cancer. The evidence for this theory is rather confusing. When recent diabetes was eliminated, some studies have found as high as a sixfold risk for pancreatic cancer in diabetic women but not in diabetic men. Several of the uncertainties result from the fact that there has been no strict delineation of the type of diabetic who is prone to develop pancreatic cancer and no sorting out of the genetic aspects of the disease in the population studied. In addition, there have been varying definitions of diabetes in all reported studies. We therefore do not know if all diabetics or a special subset are at risk from pancreatic cancer. It may well be that diabetics have so many other complications that few actually live long enough to develop pancreatic cancer.

The second hypothesis is that the presence of pancreatic cancer in some way induces glucose intolerance. This is supported by the fact that in many cases the diabetes is diagnosed within 2 years before the cancer is discovered. Thus, there may be two types of diabetes mellitus in pancreatic cancer patients: (1) in a group of individuals in whom the hereditary type is present with its possible increased risk of pancreatic cancer, and (2) another set of patients in whom the hyperglycaemia is of shorter duration and is a result of the pancreatic cancer. There is a definite suggestion of a bimodality of duration of clinical diabetes mellitus in several series of pancreatic cancer patients (40% of patients with a duration of greater than 2 years, and 50% with a duration of less than 1 year).

Alcoholism and Chronic Pancreatitis

Retrospective epidemiological data regarding an association between alcoholism and pancreatic cancer are inconclusive. As with diabetics, alcoholics have so many other problems that pancreatic cancer is one of their lesser worries. The main reason for considering an alcohol-pancreatic cancer association is that pancreatitis (which can be induced by alcohol) has been associated with pancreatic cancer. However, it must be emphasized that 'pancreatitis' may have three different meanings: (1) histological pancreatitis invariably coexists with pancreatic cancer, presumably due to ductal obstruction and/or direct destruction of parenchymatous tissues, (2) the acquired variety of chronic pancreatitis (clinical entity) does not seem to be related to pancreatic cancer, and (3) the hereditary type of chronic pancreatitis seems to have a higher predisposition to pancreatic cancer than the general population.

Clinical Features of Pancreatic Cancer

The diagnosis of pancreatic cancer varies from the simple and clinically obvious to the most difficult and almost impossible. The initial symptoms and signs depend on the site and extent of the pancreatic cancer.

Cancer of the Head of the Pancreas

As previously mentioned, this has to be differentiated from cancer of the ampulla, lower common bile duct and/or duodenum since these latter tumours may present with similar features. The term 'peri-ampullary carcinoma' is often used to denote tumours in this region irrespective of the exact site of origin. Progressive jaundice occurs in over 75% of patients with carcinoma of the head of the pancreas and the incidence of jaundice decreases as the location of the lesion progresses to the left towards the tail of the pancreas. Occasionally a tumour may invade and compress the second or third parts of the duodenum without actually obstructing the common bile duct. Pain is extremely frequent and the classic description of painless jaundice is rarely encountered. Weight loss and anorexia are also common symptoms even in the early stages. Nausea, epigastric bloating, change in bowel habits, and vomiting are occasionally present. Haematemesis and melaena occasionally occur in late cases as a result of direct invasion of the duodenal or gastric mucosa by tumour or portal hypertension secondary to splenic or portal vein compression by the tumour. Chills and fever due to ascending cholangitis can occur in longstanding biliary obstruction. A palpable gallbladder (Courvoisier's sign) is noted in only about a quarter of patients with resectable tumours. The liver is usually enlarged on palpation.

Cancer of the Body and Tail of the Pancreas

Pain and weight loss are the two main consistent symptoms. The pain may initially be dull and vague, localized to the epigastrium or to the back, or it may move to either upper quadrant. It may be episodic and related to meals or it may become constant and severe. In late cases, the patient learns to obtain partial relief by flexing the trunk forward. Severe pain invariably indicates extension of tumour into the perineural lymphatics and the posterior parietes. Weight loss is rapid and severe by the time the patient presents to hospital. Again, haematemesis and melaena may be late features due to mucosal invasion or portal hypertension. Migratory thrombophlebitis (Trousseau's sign) can be present in any patient with advanced cancer, is not specifically indicative of pancreatic carcinoma, and, by itself, does not merit diagnostic laparotomy.

Physical examination in the early stages may reveal surprisingly few abnormal physical signs. In late cases, abdominal masses or liver metastases may be palpable. A rectal shelf may be evident on rectal examination in the rectovesical or rectovaginal pouch, there may be evidence of ascites, and distant metastases may be present in the supraclavicular fossa (Troisier's sign).

Delay in Diagnosis

Over 90% of patients with pancreatic cancer present in the late stage of their disease at a time when there is no chance of cure and, often, even meaningful palliation cannot be achieved. The factors responsible for the late diagnosis are:

1. The tumour is asymptomatic in the early stages. There is some evidence that the preclinical phase of pancreatic cancer may be present for months or even years before the tumour 'appears'.
2. 'Patient delay'—the early symptoms are often vague and non-specific and the patient tolerates the discomfort.
3. 'Physician delay'—the physician often does not have a high index of suspicion and fails to properly 'evaluate' the patient in the face of a vague history and a normal physical examination, especially if these are backed by a normal barium meal, barium enema and cholecystogram.
4. The patient may not have ready and easy access to competent diagnostic centres. Centralization or regionalization of the management of difficult pancreatic problems is long overdue because of the dependence on sophisticated diagnostic and therapeutic methods.

Positive physical signs in a patient with pancreatic cancer often reflect incurability. The diagnosis therefore needs to be made before the appearance of abnormal physical signs. The clinician should always consider the diagnosis of pancreatic cancer in any patient presenting with seemingly genuine recent symptoms, absent physical signs and negative routine radiological investigations. These are the very patients in whom maximum benefit may be gained by applying the more sophisticated investigative techniques.

The Evaluation of Diagnostic Tests

It is no great triumph to diagnose incurable advanced pancreatic cancer. Any particular technique must be assessed on its ability to diagnose potentially curable lesions of the pancreas. A rational sequence of testing is as follows: Ultrasonography, with or without CT scan, is the best initial test. Patients with a demonstrable pancreatic abnormality on either of these two non-invasive tests should be subjected to endoscopic retrograde cholangiopancreatography (ERCP) combined with cytology. Angiography is not useful for diagnosing early pancreatic cancers. It should, however, be performed prior to laparotomy in any patient suspected of having a resectable pancreatic cancer for reasons previously outlined. Duodenal drainage studies are recommended to obtain material for cytological examination only when ERCP has failed for technical reasons.

It has become obvious that the diagnosis of *advanced* pancreatic cancer can be made after a careful history and routine physical examination. If obvious metastases are present such as seedlings in the retrovesical pouch or the pouch of Douglas on rectal or pelvic examination or large left supraclavicular lymph nodes (Troisier's sign) and/or obvious nodular hepatomegaly, careful consideration should be given in avoiding prolonged and unnecessary investigations and even a diagnostic laparotomy. This logic pertains especially to cancer of the body and tail of the pancreas which is rarely, if ever, curable in a symptomatic patient. Percutaneous needle biopsy of any accessible lesion, including the pancreatic mass, can achieve the diagnosis in many cases and the duration of hospitalization can be appreciably shortened. The frail elderly patient with clinically obvious cancer of the body or tail of the pancreas should be spared the mortality and morbidity of a diagnostic laparotomy. Direct percutaneous needle aspiration of the mass with ultrasonography or CT scan for guidance should be attempted (*Figs.* 70.15 and 70.16). Another way of obviating laparotomy in these seriously ill people is to perform laparoscopy and direct vision biopsy. Both these procedures are currently free from reported complications but more experience is necessary before final judgement is passed. On the other hand, the jaundiced patient, unless he is in a moribund state, should be explored with a view to internal biliary drainage as described later.

Surgical Treatment of Pancreatic Cancer

Emphasis must be placed on preoperative evaluation and adequate preparation of these patients. As mentioned previously, the newer diagnostic tests such as ERCP, cytology and arteriography, provide the surgeon with valuable preoperative information and obviate the need for time-consuming manoeuvres on the operating table. It cannot be overemphasized that pancreatic exploration with a view to resection should not be performed by the occasional surgeon or the resident-registrar in training or in institutions where there is not all the back-up expertise (endoscopy, radiology, cytology, endocrinology) necessary for the care and management of these difficult problems.

Preoperative Preparation

1. All jaundiced patients must be kept in a good state of nutrition and hydration with supplemental intravenous fluids, elemental diet and multivitamins as deemed necessary. Renal failure due to hypovolaemia is a tremendous hazard postoperatively and a continuous diuresis must be maintained at all times. If the patient is grossly malnourished, a period of parenteral hyperalimentation both before and after operation may be of additional benefit.
2. Blood clotting deficiencies must be corrected. Anaemia is corrected by blood transfusion. Daily injections of vitamin K are administered, preferably for 4–5 days prior to operation. Six units of fresh frozen plasma, six units of platelets and at least six units of blood should be made available in the operating room.
3. Cardiopulmonary function should be carefully assessed by pulmonary function tests, chest X-ray and electrocardiogram. Smoking is prohibited. Intensive pulmonary physiotherapy, active mobilization and leg exercises are strongly encouraged preoperatively. The question of prophylactic digitalization and diuretic therapy is considered in individual patients to achieve maximum cardio-vascular compensation.

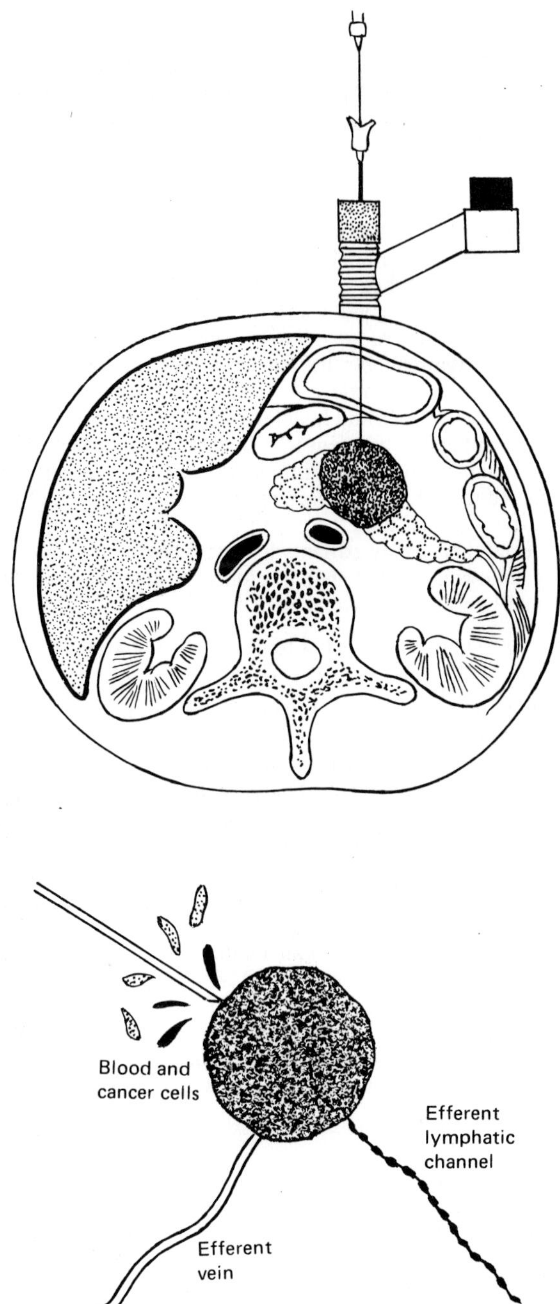

Fig. 70.15 Schematic representation of percutaneous fine needle aspiration technique of a pancreatic mass under ultrasound or CT scan control. The aspirated material is smeared on glass slides and fixed and stained by the Papanicolaou or Giemsa method for microscopic examination.

Fig. 70.16 Aspiration 'biopsy' and tumour seeding. Seeding of tumour cells occurs experimentally but is probably of no clinical significance in the vast majority of cases.

4. If a patient is critically ill with one or more of the following parameters, (*a*) a highly elevated serum bilirubin (greater than 200 µmol/l (12 mg %); (*b*) sepsis; (*c*) hepatorenal failure; (*d*) severe cardiopulmonary disease which is expected to respond to medical management; (*e*) severe malnutrition, a percutaneous transhepatic biliary decompression should be attempted to tide over the patient for 2 or 3 weeks until his general condition improves adequately for him to be considered for a major pancreatic resection. If the technique of percutaneous biliary drainage is not available, a simple cholecystostomy or T-tube drainage of the common bile duct may be undertaken under local anaesthesia.

Selection of Patients for Pancreatic Resection

Except under unusual circumstances, a major pancreatic resection should not be performed in the elderly (older than 70 years), in frail patients with multiple systemic disorders, or in those with an estimated life expectancy of less than 3 years. The operation should be reserved for the relatively fit patient under the most favourable circumstances. The surgeon must use his clinical judgement in the determination of the relative indications and contraindications for each procedure. The operative mortality should not exceed 10% and, under ideal circumstances, should be nearer 5%. A frank discussion must take place between the surgeon, the patient and his relatives prior to embarking on a potentially hazardous operation.

Surgical Options

For curative surgical treatment of a cancer in the head of the pancreas, three options are available:

1. The Whipple operation (pancreaticoduodenectomy) in which the head and neck of the pancreas together with the duodenum, the distal half of the stomach, lower common bile duct and gallbladder and upper jejunum are removed with as much of the regional lymph nodes as possible.
2. Total pancreatectomy (total pancreatoduodenectomy) includes, along with the contents of the Whipple operation, excision of the spleen, body and tail of pancreas, and a more thorough regional lymphadenectomy.
3. Regional pancreatectomy as proposed by Fortner entails extirpation of the transpancreatic portion of the portal vein, the coeliac axis, the superior mesenteric artery and the middle colic vessels, together with the structures included in a total pancreatoduodenectomy.

Of these three alternatives, total pancreatectomy with regional lymphadenectomy is recommended for the following reasons:

1. Cancer of the exocrine pancreas is potentially multifocal in origin. Papillary hyperplasia, carcinoma-in-situ, and invasive carcinoma are often found in the same gland.

Multicentricity of the malignant lesions in the gland has also been reported.

2. Gross and histological tumour spread have been documented at the line of resection after a partial pancreatectomy of the Whipple type.

3. Malignant viable cells are often present in the obstructed pancreatic ductal system and, if the gland is divided, this may be a source of seeding for local recurrence.

4. The existence of lymphatic exchange between the head and the body of the pancreas has been amply demonstrated. An adequate regional lymphadenectomy can only be performed as part of a total (as opposed to a partial) pancreatoduodenectomy.

5. Excision of the whole pancreas eliminates the risk of postoperative pancreatitis. It also obviates the need for a pancreatojejunostomy, which, even in the best of hands, has a small risk of leakage.

6. Preservation of endocrine or exocrine tissue is not sufficient justification for leaving part of the pancreas in situ. Over 80% of all pancreatic cancer patients are diabetic at the time of presentation. Late postoperative stenosis of the pancreatojejunostomy leading to insufficiency of enzyme secretion often occurs after a variable period of time.

The concept of extended resection for pancreatic cancer with resections of one or more of the major vessels (regional pancreatectomy) is uniformly attended by an increased morbidity and mortality without a concomitant improvement in cure rate. When such extensive procedures are needed to resect the local tumour, occult disease metastases are present and the disease is incurable. It must also be stated that no statistically increased survival has been documented for total pancreatectomy as compared to a Whipple operation.

The Operative Diagnosis of Pancreatic Cancer and its Differentiation from Chronic Pancreatitis

The jaundiced patient nowadays is well investigated preoperatively and usually a diagnosis is made prior to laparotomy. A general rule is as follows: hard, non-cystic masses in the head of the pancreas which are associated with obstructive jaundice and dilatation of the common bile duct are usually carcinoma, especially if acute inflammation and/or gallstones are absent. Conversely, hard, non-cystic masses involving a major part of the retroampullary part of the gland and unassociated with jaundice or dilatation of the biliary tree are usually pancreatitis.

It is important to remember that pancreatitis of varying degree invariably coexists with all carcinomas and that patients with gallstones may have a concomitant pancreatic cancer. In doubtful situations, the surgeon must decide whether to try to establish a tissue diagnosis by frozen section histology of biopsies prior to assessing resectability of any pancreatic mass. Every surgeon is influenced by his own philosophy, his experience and expertise, his pathologist's experience, and by the clinical situation. Hence, any decision in such a clinical setting can easily lead to controversy when discussed retrospectively or hypothetically. The author's *general* policy about pancreatic biopsy can be summed up as follows:

1. Since over 75% of all cancers in the head of the pancreas are identified preoperatively by a positive cytology (at ERCP or duodenal drainage), it is preferable to assess the resectability of all such masses in the first instance. If conditions are favourable, they are resected without a preliminary biopsy.

2. A suspected cancer of the body and tail of the pancreas is 'biopsied' by a distal pancreatectomy and splenectomy provided that the lesion is localized and resectable. If frozen section histological examination reveals a cancer, the 'excision biopsy' is converted into a total pancreatectomy with regional lymphadenectomy.

3. On the other hand, all unresectable and/or metastatic tumours of the pancreas are diagnosed before the surgeon leaves the operating room even if the job is time-consuming. This takes the matter out of the realm of doubt, an especially important point when a palliative procedure restores the patient to relatively good health for a long period and doubt is raised as to the true diagnosis. A known positive biopsy for adenocarcinoma of the pancreas will then prevent a fruitless second laparotomy.

4. Frozen sections and histological examination of lymph nodes peripheral or adjacent to delineated pancreatic masses are acceptable if unresectability and/or the presence of disseminated metastases has been established. The presence of a positive regional node *per se* is not an absolute criteria of unresectability. Many patients have survived longer than 3 years following total pancreatectomy in the presence of regional lymph node involvement.

These policies are supported by the following arguments:

1. Truly representative needle biopsies of the pancreas are often hard to obtain because of sampling error and confusion between tumour and associated pancreatitis (*Fig. 70.17*).

2. The establishment of diagnosis by means of biopsies for frozen section histology is sometimes time-consuming and traumatic. Factors which influence the biopsy policy of surgeons include personal experience of complications, interpretative histological errors and traditional teaching. Many senior surgeons still regard pancreatic biopsy as inaccurate and dangerous. Pancreatitis, fistula formation, haemorrhage and infection have all been reported following all biopsy techniques. However, it is often difficult to decide whether such complications are directly attributable to the biopsy itself or to the concomitant surgical manoeuvres and manipulations. The consensus of opinion is that all surgeons

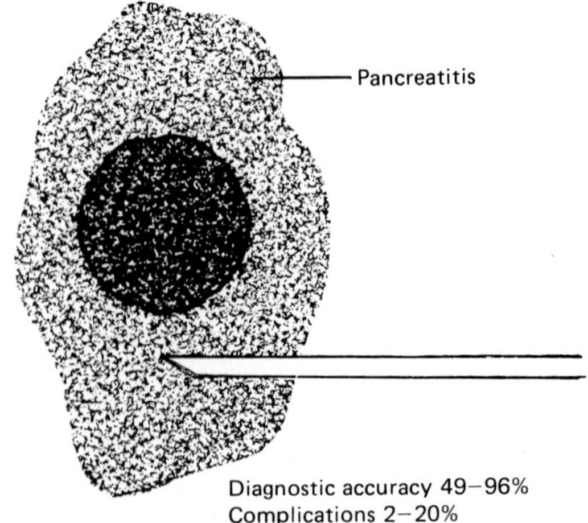

Fig. 70.17 Peroperative pancreatic biopsy. A variable degree of pancreatitis surrounds any pancreatic cancer leading to a 'sampling error' with needle biopsies. The number of biopsies taken is limited because of potential morbidity and even mortality and the biopsies may miss the cancer altogether.

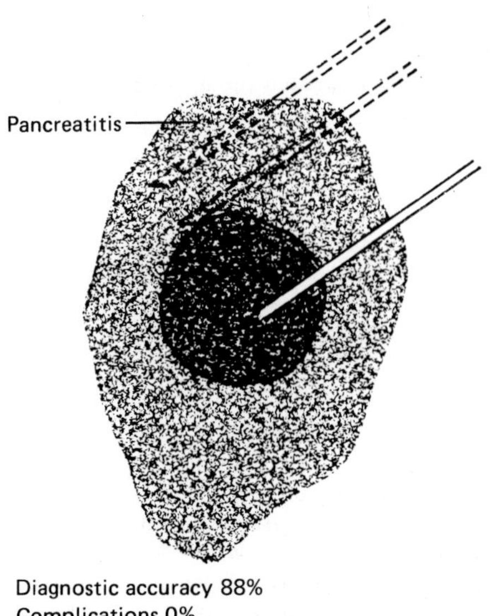

Fig. 70.18 Fine needle aspiration 'biopsy' for cytological examination. Multiple punctures may be performed with minimal risks and increase the chance of obtaining material from the cancer.

involved in the practice of pancreatic surgery should be willing and able to perform pancreatic biopsy safely if it is indicated. When this is done, the surgeon should make great efforts to avoid major pancreatic ducts and vessels, the typical anatomy of which must be well fixed in his mind. A good Kocher manoeuvre enables the surgeon to palpate the head of the pancreas between his fingers and thumb of the left hand to guide the biopsy needle through the duodenum into the appropriate suspicious area of the pancreas. The disposable Travenol 'Tru-Cut' needle is very suitable for this purpose. A less traumatic alternative is to employ a long No. 21 needle, pushing it in a similar fashion through the duodenum, and attaching a 10-ml syringe for aspiration in order to provide a smear for cytology. This is gaining in popularity with the more widespread availability of and co-operation with skilled cytopathologists (*Fig.* 70.18). Haemorrhage, when encountered, can be controlled by finger pressure. Occasionally, silk mattress sutures are needed for haemostasis of the pancreatic capsule following direct pancreatic puncture.

3. Errors in interpretation of frozen section biopsy specimens of the pancreas are sometimes made by the inexperienced histopathologist because some desmoplastic carcinomas closely resemble chronic pancreatitis.

Assessment of Resectability

A cancer of the pancreas is considered unresectable if there are distant (liver or peritoneal) metastases, invasion of major vessels (portal vein, hepatic artery, superior mesenteric vessels or coeliac axis) or any extension beyond the area of the usual total pancreatectomy specimen. Puckering of the transverse mesocolon *per se* does not always indicate unresectability since the transverse mesocolon and, if necessary, the transverse colon can be excised in a total pancreatectomy specimen if there are no contraindications to a resection.

Immediate Postoperative Care and Complications

Following a major pancreatic resection, the patient should be transferred to an intensive care unit where experienced nursing care and sophisticated monitoring techniques are readily available. They may require respiratory assistance for the first 12–24 hours. For the first 3–4 postoperative days, the patient's blood sugar is checked every 3–4 hours and small doses of regular insulin (2–5 units) are given intravenously as boluses. Alternatively, a continuous intravenous infusion of insulin can be given. It is important to maintain the blood sugar between 150 and 250 mg % (8–13 μmol/l).

Haemorrhage is the commonest intraoperative and postoperative complication encountered with total pancreatectomy. Meticulous preoperative preparation and adequate replacement of blood and clotting factors during the operation are essential. In spite of these precautions, the patient may continue to bleed at a fairly alarming rate from all raw areas in the abdominal cavity during the first 24 hours. The indications for reoperation are:

1. If there is reason to suspect a major bleeding site.
2. When clot accumulation in the abdomen causes distension and tamponade.
3. When a consumption coagulopathy is recognized.

In most cases, a discrete bleeding point is never found at reoperation. The clots are gently evacuated and the whole abdomen irrigated prior to closure with drainage.

Haemobilia following biliary decompression is not unusual. It invariably stops spontaneously.

Whenever haemorrhage is suspected, the patient must be kept normovolaemic by adequate blood and fluid replacement and by maintaining a continuous diuresis. Intermittent doses of diuretics may be given as necessary. Hepatorenal failure is the commonest sequence of events leading to postoperative death in this group of patients.

Other complications which may also be fatal include sepsis, mesenteric thrombosis, uraemia, liver insufficiency, myocardial infarction, cerebrovascular accident, congestive heart failure, and pulmonary embolism. Leakage from the biliary-enteric anastomosis or from the gastrojejunostomy are largely preventable by careful and proper construction of both anastomoses. Complications which are usually non-fatal include pneumonitis, gastric retention, paralytic ileus, bowel obstruction, wound infection, wound dehiscence, atrial fibrillation, faecal fistula and gastrojejunal fistula.

Recurrence of Jaundice after Pancreatectomy for Cancer of the Pancreas

Recurrence of jaundice and/or cholangitis may be seen after pancreatectomy and may be due to small bowel obstruction. Nausea and vomiting are usually prominent features. The obstruction may be due to recurrent tumour or simply to adhesions. Laparotomy may be indicated to establish the diagnosis and to relieve the obstruction.

Monitoring of Recurrence

There is no currently efficacious chemotherapy regimen for patients with metastatic pancreatic cancer. There is, however, a distinct clinical impression that some patients with minimal regional disease (capsular invasion and/or regional nodal spread) seem to benefit from a combination of radiation therapy and chemotherapy following total pancreatectomy. A small number of patients with resectable pancreatic cancer have elevated levels of a tumour marker such as pancreatic oncofetal antigen (POA) or carcinoembryonic antigen (CEA) levels preoperatively. When this is the case, serial monitoring of either marker may be useful in confirming the completeness of surgical excision and in the detection of recurrent pancreatic cancer.

Management of Pancreatic Endocrine Insufficiency

This is discussed in Chapter 9.

Replacement of Pancreatic Exocrine Function

Adequate pancreatin tablets (Viokase, Pancrease, Creon) must be taken with each meal. The number of tablets must be increased if steatorrhoea develops. The patient is advised to take a low fat diet in the form of frequent regular small meals.

Survival and Mortality Following Total Pancreatectomy

The mortality for major pancreatic resection is between 5 and 10% in specialized centres. Death as a result of operative complications usually occurs within the first 2 months of operation. After 2 months and up to 2 years, death is usually due to metastatic pancreatic cancer although a few individuals can present as late as the end of the third year with metastatic disease. If the patient has survived 3 years, the cause of death is usually unrelated to pancreatic cancer.

The Place of the Whipple Operation

Malignant tumours that are confined to the duodenum, ampulla of Vater or lower common bile duct are adequately treated by a pancreaticoduodenectomy of the extended Whipple type. The neck of the gland is divided to the left of the superior mesenteric vein and the body and tail of the pancreas and spleen are left undisturbed. *En bloc* excision of the regional lymph nodes from the porta hepatis, aortocaval and superior mesenteric regions again forms part of the operation. If the surgeon cannot be sure of the exact site of origin of the tumour at operation, we recommend a standard Whipple operation and immediate careful examination of the specimen by the pathologist and surgeon. If the tumour is not originating from the pancreas, the operation is adequate. On the other hand, if one cannot be sure of the exact origin of the tumour we prefer to complete the total pancreatectomy as previously stated. Another circumstance which may dictate conversion of the Whipple operation to a total pancreatectomy is when the surgeon finds that the body and tail of the pancreas is severely involved with recent pancreatitis and a pancreatojejunal anastomosis cannot be safely performed. In such a situation it is better to complete the pancreatectomy rather than risk a potentially fatal leakage from a poor pancreatojejunal anastomosis.

Palliation of Pancreatic Cancer

The surgeon can palliate incurable pancreatic cancer in several ways.

1. *Relief of jaundice, pruritus, and impending cholangitis.* The biliary tract decompression can be done either by cholecystojejunostomy or by hepaticojejunostomy (each with a diverting enterostomy), depending on whether the cystic duct is widely patent and is in full communication with the biliary tree proximal to obstructing cancer.

2. *Relief of duodenal obstruction.* If the patient lives for more than a few months, duodenal obstruction invariably occurs. It is therefore advisable to perform a gastrojejunostomy at the primary operation.

3. *Relief of pain.* The coeliac plexus can be infiltrated with 50 ml of 50% alcohol or with 20 ml of 6% phenol. This may be helpful in patients with cancer of the body of the pancreas when the pain is a prominent feature. Cordotomy, extensive sympathectomy and stereotactic thalamotomy have all been tried with minimal or no objective response. If the duct of Wirsung is dilated by a cancer in the head of the pancreas, a pancreatogastrostomy over a T-tube (as advised by Rodney Smith) may be helpful and will also permit the exocrine secretions to reach the upper alimentary tract.

All locally unresectable or metastatic masses must be biopsied until a definite histological diagnosis is made on frozen section histology. The main tumour mass must be outlined with silver clips to provide a possible radiation port. Surgical implantation of radionuclides such as ^{125}I and intraoperative radiation with electron beams are being tried in several centres but data showing objective responses have yet to be presented.

LESIONS OF THE ENDOCRINE PANCREAS

Pancreatic islet cells are components of the gastroenteropancreatic part of the diffuse neuroendocrine system. Cells belonging to this system are commonly referred to as APUD cells because they share the following cytochemical characteristics: a high amine content (A); the capacity for amine precursor uptake (PU); and the property of decarboxylation (D) of these precursors to form amines. Tumours arising from the APUD series of cells are called APUDomas. Although Pearse originally suggested that all APUD cells were probably derived from neural crest cells, it is now generally recognized that the gastroenteropancreatic APUD cells (including pancreatic islet cells) probably arise from endoderm (dedifferentiation theory). Regardless of their origin, the APUD cells share similarities in structure, properties and potential. All have characteristic histological, histochemical, immunocytochemical and electron microscopic appearances and all contain the enzyme neurone-specific enolase that is the universal marker for such cells and their hyperplastic and neoplastic lesions.

APUD cells are capable of synthesizing and secreting a great variety of peptides which exert regulatory effects by four main modes of action: (1) endocrine, i.e. involving secretion into the circulation to affect distant target sites; (2) paracrine, i.e. involving local secretion to act on adjacent cells; (3) neurocrine, i.e. involving secretion at neuronal synapses to act as a neurotransmitter; and (4) neuroendocrine, i.e. involving release of a peptide product of the neurone into the circulation to act on other tissues. Clinical syndromes may develop as a result of either inadequate or excessive production and release of the potent chemical messengers (e.g. inadequate insulin causes diabetes mellitus and excessive insulin leads to hypoglycaemia). The development of radioimmunoassays for a number of the gastroenteropancreatic peptide hormones has led to the understanding that hyperplastic as well as neoplastic pancreatic islet cells are capable of producing recognizable syndromes of hormone excess. Pancreatic tumours of the islet cell type may in fact secrete two or more identifiable peptide hormones although the threshold for the appearance of their respective clinical symptoms varies greatly and elevated levels of one hormone may be compensated by regulatory hypersecretion of other hormones. Endocrine tumours of the pancreas can be referred to as entopic if they produce hormones normally secreted by the pancreas (e.g. insulinoma, glucagonoma) and ectopic if they produce non-pancreatic hormones (e.g. gastrinoma, VIPoma). There is little correlation between tumour size and plasma hormone concentration or severity of clinical symptoms. Some 10–25% of patients harbouring pancreatic APUD tumours will have the multiple endocrine neoplasia type (MEN I) syndrome. The clinical syndromes associated with overproduction of identified pancreatic islet cell peptides is shown in *Table* 70.4.

Hyperinsulinism

Hyperinsulinism in its primary form embraces several different varieties of pancreatic islet cell disease which include B-cell hyperplasia/microadenomatosis and B-cell neoplasia (insulinoma). These conditions manifest as symptomatic hypoglycaemia. Insulinomas are the most common of pancreatic APUDomas (75% of symptomatic cases) and the most frequent cause of organic primary hyperinsulinism. In the adult, approximately 80% of insulinomas are benign solitary tumours. There is an even distribution of tumours in the head, body and tail of the pancreas. Multiple tumours are usually present in patients with MEN I syndrome and are found in about 10% of cases. B-cell carcinoma occurs in 5–10% and is characterized by local invasion and metastatic spread to regional lymph nodes and liver. Primary hyperinsulinism is rare in infants and children but, when encountered, a form of B-cell hyperplasia (nesidioblastosis) is seen much more frequently than neoplasia. In contrast, microadenomatosis or islet cell hyperplasia is only very rarely found in adults.

Clinical Features and Diagnosis of Hyperinsulinism

Hypoglycaemia induces a constellation of symptoms reflecting activation of the autonomic nervous system and release of epinephrine together with cerebral dysfunction related to insufficient glucose oxidation to meet energy needs. The symptoms of adrenergic hyperactivity are more apt to occur with rapid falls of plasma glucose and include weakness, sweating, hunger, palpitations and tremulousness. Neuroglycopenia manifests as headache, visual disturbance, dizziness and confusion and may progress to abnormal behaviour, seizures and coma. Hypoglycaemic episodes are often misinterpreted as suggesting brain tumour, epilepsy, alcoholism or drug abuse, psychosis, or even hysteria. Delays in diagnosis and treatment of hypoglycaemia are common and contribute to the morbidity and mortality of the condition. The most important clue to early correct diagnosis is the relationship of the symptoms to periods of food deprivation or physical exercise and the relief of symptoms following food ingestion. In cases where diagnosis is long delayed, patients often develop obesity from increased carbohydrate intake as a behavioural adaptation to repeated episodes of symptomatic hypoglycaemia.

Differential Diagnosis of Hypoglycaemia

Hypoglycaemia may occur in the fasting state or may be postprandial (reactive) in nature. In the latter condition, low plasma glucose concentrations occur only in response to meals. In fasting hypoglycaemia a period of hours to a few days is required to precipitate hypoglycaemia. While patients with fasting hypoglycaemia (particularly insulinomas) may also exhibit a reactive component, patients with reactive hypoglycaemia never have symptoms when food is withdrawn. Fasting hypoglycaemia usually indicates a specific underlying disease process while symptoms suggestive of postprandial hypoglycaemia are often found in the absence of an identifiable organic lesion.

Postprandial Hypoglycaemia

The more common causes of postprandial hypoglycaemia are shown in *Table* 70.5. Alimentary hypoglycaemia is the most common type seen clinically and is usually found in

Table 70.5 Causes of postprandial (reactive) hypoglycaemia

1. Alimentary hyperinsulinism
2. Hereditary fructose intolerance
3. Galactosaemia
4. Leucine sensitivity
5. Idiopathic
   True hypoglycaemia
   Non-hypoglycaemia

patients who have undergone gastrectomy, pyloroplasty, gastrojejunostomy or, rarely, proximal gastric vagotomy. Symptoms occur within a few hours postprandially and are particularly prominent after meals of high carbohydrate content in the form of mono- and disaccharides. Although the exact pathophysiological mechanisms remain to be defined, it is clear that rapid gastrin emptyimg of simple sugars by the postoperative stomach with brisk absorption of glucose and excessive insulin release are of central importance. The attacks can be provoked in affected individuals by oral ingestion of 100 g of glucose in water. A rapid abnormal rise in plasma glucose together with a parallel, and often exaggerated, plasma insulin response occur following glucose challenge. Hypoglycaemic symptoms appear within 1–2 hours as the insulin response and/or effect exceeds the requirement of euglycaemia. True alimentary hypoglycaemia may occur in the absence of gastrointestinal surgery but is rare.

Reactive hypoglycaemia is often misused as a diagnostic label in patients suffering from anxiety states rather than true idiopathic reactive hypoglycaemia. Although some of these individuals manifest a very mild and asymptomatic depression in plasma glucose during the 5-hour glucose tolerance test, hypoglycaemia cannot be documented after normal meals not containing 100 g of rapidly absorbable carbohydrate. This is in contrast to the occasional case of true idiopathic reactive hypoglycaemia where spontaneous symptomatic episodes are reproducible and accompanied by demonstrably low plasma glucose levels. Most patients without true hypoglycaemia have postprandial adrenergic discharge as a result of underlying anxiety and stress. The epinephrine-mediated symptoms suggest hypoglycaemia but occur in its absence and are presumably psychogenic in origin.

Fasting Hypoglycaemia

The major causes of fasting hypoglycaemia are shown in *Table* 70.6. In this condition one or both of the following mechanisms may be operative: (1) hepatic glucose production is not adequate to meet ordinary tissue demands; (2) peripheral glucose utilization is increased to such a degree that maximal hepatic production is insufficient to match glucose egress from the plasma component. Since hepatic glucose output in normal fasting man is between 100 g and 200 g per day, a requirement for greater than 200 g of intravenous glucose over a 24-hour period to prevent hypoglycaemia can be taken as evidence for over-utilization of glucose.

From the practical standpoint, fasting hypoglycaemia in an otherwise healthy individual is almost always due to hyperinsulinism that is attributable to an insulinoma in the adult or islet cell hyperplasia in the neonate or infant. Although patients with hyperinsulinism classically describe or manifest symptoms under fasting conditions in the early

Table 70.6 Major causes of fasting hypoglycaemia

Conditions primarily due to underproduction of glucose
1. Hormone deficiencies
   Hypopituitarism
   Adrenal insufficiency
   Catecholamine deficiency
   Glucagon deficiency
2. Enzyme defects
   Glucose-6-phosphatase
   Liver phosphorylase
   Pyruvate carboxylase
   PEP-carboxykinase
   Fructose-1 -6 diphosphatase
   Glycogen synthetase
3. Substrate deficiency
   Ketotic hypoglycaemia of infancy
   Severe malnutrition, muscle wasting
   Late pregnancy
4. Acquired liver disease
   Hepatic congestion
   Severe hepatitis
   Cirrhosis
5. Drugs
   Alcohol
   Propranolol
   Salicylates

Conditions primarily due to overutilization of glucose
1. Hyperinsulinism
   Insulinoma
   Exogenous insulin
   Sulfonylureas
   Immune disease with insulin antibodies
2. Appropriate insulin levels
   Extrapancreatic tumours
   Cachexia with fat depletion
   Carnitine deficiency
   Carnitine acyltransferase deficiency

morning hours before breakfast or in the late afternoon following exertion, attacks may be highly unpredictable and distributed randomly throughout the day. While it is obvious that the development of fasting hypoglycaemia in insuloma patients is due to excessive insulin secretion, the hypoglycaemia may result from insulin-mediated suppression of hepatic glucose production as well as augmentation of glucose utilization. Most patients learn quickly that symptoms can be relieved by intake of food or sweetened drink. Accordingly, a proportion of patients gain substantial amounts of weight.

In 1935, Whipple and Franz reviewed 35 cases of insulinoma and enunciated the primary diagnostic criteria which became known as Whipple's triad:

1. Hypoglycaemic symptoms are produced by fasting.
2. Hypoglycaemia is documented during symptomatic episodes.
3. Symptoms are relieved by glucose intake.

While the presence of Whipple's triad strongly suggests the presence of an insulinoma, differentiation from other causes of fasting hypoglycaemia is crucial. Factitious hypoglycaemia due to surreptitious self-administration of insulin must always be considered in cases posing diagnostic difficulty. Currently, the diagnosis of insulinoma is based upon three elements:

1. Recognition of the probable nature of the patient's symptoms.
2. Presence of Whipple's triad.
3. Demonstration that the plasma insulin concentration is inappropriately high for the existing level of plasma glucose.

Thus, it is not the absolute level of insulin but its concentration relative to the plasma glucose that is diagnostic. Although absolute elevations of the insulin level are present in many insulinoma patients, rapid degradation of insulin by the liver is probably responsible for the normal absolute levels seen in others with functioning islet cell tumours. For this reason, the ratio of plasma immunoreactive insulin to plasma glucose is considered of greater diagnostic accuracy than absolute levels of insulin and glucose. An insulin (μu/ml) to glucose (mg/dl) ratio of greater than 0·3 indicates insulinoma. It is therefore essential in the investigation of suspected or documented hypoglycaemia to measure simultaneous insulin and glucose levels from the same plasma sample obtained at the time of hypoglycaemia.

Virtually all insulinoma patients will develop symptomatic hypoglycaemia during a diagnostic 72-hour fast. About 90% will manifest symptoms within 48 hours, 80% within 24 hours and 40% within 2 hours of fasting. The plasma glucose level at the time of symptoms is almost invariably less than 40 mg/dl (2·2 mmol/l). In normal individuals the level of immunoreactive insulin during fasting is very low to almost undetectable. At the time of fasting hypoglycaemia almost all insulinoma patients have basal insulin levels greater than 5 μu/ml. Other causes of fasting hypoglycaemia such as fibrosarcoma and other non-pancreatic tumours, glucocorticoid deficiency or diffuse liver disease may exhibit a positive Whipple's triad but in none will the associated immunoreactive insulin level be increased.

Plasma pro-insulin levels are also helpful in the diagnosis of insulinoma. Pro-insulin is the single chain precursor of insulin and is normally present to an extent of 20% or less of the total immunoreactive insulin. Under ordinary circumstances, pro-insulin is split into C-peptide (connecting chain) and insulin prior to storage in B-cell granules, with only a small percentage being secreted into the portal venous circulation (*Fig.* 70.19). Because insulinoma tumour cells are usually less differentiated than normal B cells, they secrete more pro-insulin. Simple determination of pro-insulin in overnight fasted plasma provides good separation of patients with islet cell tumour from normal individuals in 90% of cases. Pro-insulin can be expressed as the absolute level or as a percent relative to total insulin concentration in plasma. Occasionally, some well-differentiated insulinomas may have normal pro-insulin secretion. Greatly elevated values (greater than 50% of total immunoreactive insulin) are often associated with malignant tumours.

Provocative Tests in the Diagnosis of Insulinoma

While no other test is as simple, safe and accurate as prolonged fasting with measurement of glucose and insulin, on rare occasions provocative testing may be needed. A variety of such tests have been advocated and all can be misleading and some potentially dangerous. The glucose tolerance test and the leucine infusion test are mentioned only to be condemned because of their inaccuracy. None of the others are diagnostic in more than 70% of cases. Their further disadvantage is the provocation of occasionally severe hypoglycaemic reactions resulting from release of substantial amounts of insulin from the tumour.

The calcium infusion test has been used as a provocative test for a number of APUDomas including gastrinoma,

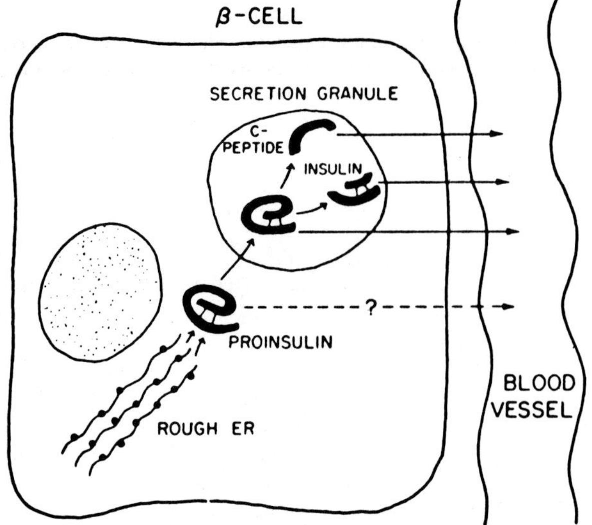

Fig. 70.19 Conversion of pro-insulin to insulin and C-peptide within the pancreatic B cell. Equimolar amounts of insulin and C-peptide are liberated during exocytosis. ER signifies endoplasmic reticulum. In normal circumstances only small amounts of the precursor, pro-insulin, are released into the bloodstream, while insulinomas release pro-insulin into the circulation in larger amounts.

medullary thyroid carcinoma and carcinoid tumours as well as insulinomas. Patients with insulinomas release insulin and pro-insulin with resultant hypoglycaemia after calcium infusion. In order to avert the hypoglycaemic attack attending calcium-stimulated insulin release, a combined glucose-calcium infusion has been devised in which insulin releases after glucose alone and after glucose plus calcium are compared. This, like all stimulation tests, suffers from a relatively low diagnostic accuracy and is indicated only when diagnostic difficulties arise.

The tolbutamide and glucagon tolerance tests are performed by intravenous administration of the respective drug followed by plasma collections for glucose and insulin determinations over a one-hour period. In the tolbutamide test, a plasma insulin level of 195 μu/ml or greater is considered diagnostic. The critical insulin value in the glucagon test is 160 μu/ml.

A useful suppression test involves infusion of fish insulin to produce hypoglycaemia. While normal subjects respond with suppression of endogenous insulin secretion, patients with insulinoma fail to suppress because of the autonomous nature of hormone release by the tumour cells. Porcine insulin may be used instead of fish insulin but C-peptide must then be measured as a marker of endogenous insulin release. While the non-suppressibility of endocrine tumours is often interpreted as a sign of malignancy, caution in this regard should be exercised with respect to insulinomas where a different degree of suppressibility reflects a different degree of functional dedifferentiation but not necessarily malignancy.

Newer tests for insulinoma which may have good diagnostic accuracy without danger of hypoglycaemia are the sequential suppression tests using somatostatin followed by diazoxide with measurement of insulin levels and glucose consumption and the computer-controlled glucose infusion system which measures the glucose infusion rate required to maintain plasma glucose constant at 80 mg/dl (4·4 μmol/l).

Factitious hypoglycaemia must always be considered and this is especially true in individuals having access to insulin or oral hypoglycaemic agents. Concomitant measurement of plasma levels of C-peptide is critical in such circumstances as insulin and C-peptide are secreted in equimolar amounts by both the normal B-cell and the insulinoma cell. C-peptide level thus serves as a direct marker of endogenous insulin release. Since all of the diagnostic tests presented can be positive following administration of exogenous insulin, the finding of an inappropriately depressed level of C-peptide can readily identify the surreptitious insulin user.

Preoperative Tumour Localization

Most insulinomas are small benign adenomas with over 75% being less than 1·5 cm in diameter. They may be wholly embedded in the pancreas and not visible on its exposed surface. Moreover, they may be difficult to distinguish by palpation from a normal lobule of pancreas or a peripancreatic lymph node. Since intraoperative definition of the lesion is often problematic and occasionally impossible, preoperative localization studies are mandatory once the definite diagnosis of hyperinsulinism has been made.

Angiography remains the most readily available and reliable method of delineating insulinomas. The use of superselective injection of contrast with subtraction technique and magnification allows confident identification of tumour in about 75% of cases. Most insulinomas are moderately hypervascular and vasoconstrictive pharmacoangiography with vasopressin or angiotensin occasionally is helpful in defining small tumours. Care must be exercised to avoid false positive localization related to presence of accessory spleens, large peripancreatic lymph nodes and hypervascular segments of normal pancreas.

Pancreatic ultrasonography and computed tomography are less efficient than angiography at localizing insulinomas but recently detection rates as high as 60% and greater have been realized. Rapid sequence CT scanning after a bolus of intravenous contrast has allowed improved definition of small slightly hypervascular tumours relative to normal pancreas. In general, however, lesions less than about 7–8 mm are poorly detected by currently available scans. Magnetic resonance imaging may prove to be very sensitive in islet cell tumour localization as the tumours appear to produce unusually intense signals.

In spite of their great utility in the localization of these small tumours, the results of imaging techniques cannot be interpreted as definitive information. When a solitary adenoma is defined, the surgeon must remember that a second tumour not seen may still be present. Likewise, when several tumours are defined, the probability of additional lesions not seen is very real. Hence, positive preoperative localization studies in no way removes the surgeon's obligation to carry out a complete exploration of the entire pancreas. Intraoperative real-time ultrasonography of the gland appears to hold considerable promise for facilitating the search.

When imaging techniques fail to identify any pancreatic or peripancreatic tumour mass, measurement of immunoreactive insulin in blood sampled from selective catheterization of small pancreatic veins via the percutaneous transhepatic route is indicated. In a few small series of insulinoma patients, this modality has correctly localized tumours with impressive regularity. At the time of portal sampling, samples are also drawn from the hepatic veins to detect metastatic or rare primary sources from within the liver. In addition, arterial samples are also drawn periodically to detect any potentially confusing variations in systemic concentrations.

Surgical Management

Without positive preoperative localization of a suspected insulinoma, the surgeon must have a high degree of conviction that the diagnosis is correct before embarking on an operative search. However, with sufficiently strong biochemical evidence supporting the presence of an insulinoma, exploratory surgery is always indicated unless the patient cannot withstand the procedure. The entire pancreas and peripancreatic area must be examined visually and by palpation at operation. This requires access, exposure, assistance and gentle technique. Full mobilization of the gland should always be performed so that careful palpation between thumb and fingers is possible. Intraoperative ultrasonography has proven to be of some use in finding small, deeply situated tumours. To palpation, insulinomas characteristically are slightly firmer than normal pancreas. Enlarged lymph nodes in the peripancreatic region and any liver lesions found should be submitted for frozen section histological evaluation to exclude metastatic disease. Histological examination of primary endocrine lesions in the pancreas is unreliable in the detection of malignancy unless obvious perineural or vascular invasion is present.

Solitary insulinomas should be enucleated whenever possible as a good cleavage plane is usually easily established between tumour and adjacent normal pancreas. Care must be taken to avoid injury to the pancreatic duct. Since the great majority of insulinomas are solitary and benign, distal pancreatectomy or, very occasionally, a Whipple type pancreaticoduodenectomy with pyloric preservation is justified for deeply situated tumours that cannot be safely enucleated. Very rarely is a Whipple operation justified for multiple tumours in the head of the pancreas since the likelihood of occult additional tumours being present in the body and tail of the gland is very substantial. Subtotal distal resection for multiple tumours throughout the gland, as seen in MEN I patients, is appropriate.

When malignant disease is encountered which can be extirpated by total pancreatectomy and regional lymphadenectomy, this should be done. Even if the tumour is inoperable, as much tumour mass is removed as is safely possible since debulking may provide good palliation with resolution of hypoglycaemic symptoms and increased efficiency of chemotherapy.

With a negative exploration, management options depend upon the clinical situation and the informed consent obtained preoperatively. If not contraindicated by these considerations, it is appropriate to perform pancreatectomy distal to the superior mesenteric vessels. If immediate examination of the thinly sliced resected specimen reveals no tumour and the patient's blood glucose exhibits no rise within 1 hour, it may be elected to perform 90% or even total pancreatectomy. Arguments in favour of the lesser procedure include: (i) a small tumour may be overlooked and subsequently found in the resected specimen; (ii) symptoms of hypoglycaemia can be controlled by this procedure alone (in the absence of tumour resection) in 20% of cases; (iii) diazoxide therapy is often successful in controlling symptoms in those uncontrolled by the operation; and (iv) the procedure usually does not cause permanent diabetes mellitus. The benefits of blind total pancreatectomy include: (i) removal of an occult lesion that could be an early malignancy; (ii) elimination of the possible need for re-exploration that is difficult and hazardous; and (iii) omission of drug therapy for prolonged periods with its undesirable side-effects. It should be mentioned that patients not evaluated preoperatively with percutaneous transhepatic portal venous sampling for insulin levels perhaps should be referred to a specialized centre for this test and then a second, more directed operation. This may be a better option than undertaking blind subtotal or total pancreatectomy at initial operation. Blind Whipple operations are likewise not recommended.

The results of surgical treatment of insulinoma suggest that about 75% of patients are cured with some 10% developing diabetes following extensive pancreatic resection. About 10–15% of patients have persistent or recurrent hypoglycaemia requiring reoperation at some time. The overall surgical mortality is between 5 and 10% and is related to the extent of resection and expertise of the surgeon. The major operative complications are pancreatitis, fistula and pseudocyst formation.

Neonatal and Infantile Hyperinsulinism

Excessive insulin secretion accounts for 20–30% of all cases of unremitting hypoglycaemia in neonates and infants. Such hypoglycaemia can lead to irreversible CNS damage and thus requires early recognition, thorough investigation and expeditious treatment. A high intravenous and/or oral glucose intake is mandatory. Additional treatment with diazoxide, somatostatin or a variety of other agents (epinephrine, diphenylhydantoin, glucocorticoids, glucagon, growth hormone) is often required. When hypoglycaemia due to documented hyperinsulinaemia cannot be adequately controlled with medical therapy, urgent operation must be undertaken. Since the overwhelming majority of neonates and infants with hyperinsulinism have nesidioblastosis, B-cell adenomatosis or islet cell hyperplasia as the cause, imaging techniques such as arteriography, ultrasonography and computed tomography have no place in the evaluation of these cases. Likewise, palpation of the pancreas at operation and biopsies for frozen section histological examination are non-contributory. The appropriate procedure is 80–90% extended distal pancreatectomy with splenic preservation. If careful postoperative monitoring of glucose levels indicates inadequacy of the resection, medical therapy should be reinstituted and consideration given to reoperation in cases of further unremitting hypoglycaemia. Reoperation consists of near total (95%) pancreatectomy with preservation of the distal bile duct and duodenum. Permanent exocrine or endocrine insufficiency is unusual in infants less than 3 months of age. This relates to the considerable regenerative capacity of the infantile pancreas.

Medical Treatment

Antisecretory therapy with diazoxide is indicated for persistent hypoglycaemia in the preoperative phase and when operation is unsuccessful or contraindicated because of the poor condition of the patient. Diazoxide is a non-diuretic benzothiadiazine which inhibits the release of secretory granules from normal islet B-cells and from insulinoma cells. Dosage is individualized based on effectiveness. Because of side-effects such as oedema, bone marrow depression, hyperuricaemia, cardiomyopathy and hirsutism in females, patients on diazoxide require close medical supervision. Long-acting analogues of somatostatin may hold considerable promise in the treatment of hyperinsulinism in inoperable patients with insulinoma. Streptozotocin, an antibiotic which selectively destroys pancreatic islet cells by inhibiting DNA synthesis, is the chemotherapeutic agent of choice for metastatic insulinoma. Objective tumour regression occurs in about 60% of patients and longevity is doubled in those who respond to the drug. Streptozotocin is highly nephrotoxic and hepatotoxic and is thus not used as routine adjunctive therapy. Combinations of streptozotocin and diazoxide are often useful in treating functioning malignant insulinoma.

Gastrinoma (Zollinger–Ellison Syndrome; ZE Syndrome)

In 1955 Zollinger and Ellison described two patients, each having a syndrome consisting of fulminant intractable peptic ulcer disease, massive gastric acid hypersecretion, and a non-beta islet cell tumour of the pancreas. Although the same clinical triad had been reported previously, Zollinger and Ellison postulated that the gastric acid excess was caused by a humoral factor released from the tumour. While their original supposition had been that glucagon was the responsible factor, the peptide hormone gastrin was subsequently extracted from such tumours which were found to be of the non-beta and non-alpha cell type. A radioimmunoassay was developed for gastrin and the hormone was found to be markedly elevated in the plasma of patients with Zollinger–Ellison syndrome.

Clinical Features and Diagnosis of Gastrinoma

By best estimate, the incidence of ZE syndrome is approximately 1 in 500 000, although the exact incidence is impossible to determine since no large population has been screened for the disease. More than 1500 cases have been reported in the literature since the original description in 1955. The disease is more common in men than women with the male-to-female ratio being 3 to 2. The ZE syndrome has been reported in patients ranging in age from 7 to 90 years but the majority of patients have been diagnosed between the third and fifth decades. Only approximately 1 in 750 patients with peptic ulcer disease will have gastrinoma as the aetiology.

About one-quarter of ZE syndrome patients have their gastrinoma as part of the MEN I syndrome. MEN I is inherited as an autosomal dominant syndrome and the lesions most commonly associated with gastrinoma are parathyroid hyperplasia and pituitary prolactinoma. Gastrinomas in MEN I patients are less likely to be malignant but are almost always multifocal. This is in contrast to patients with sporadic gastrinoma in whom the disease is more often malignant but somewhat less frequently multifocal in origin. Overall, the gastrinoma is malignant in about one-half of patients and arises in the pancreas in about 75%. Even when benign, gastrinomas are more often multiple than solitary. The most common extrapancreatic primary tumour site is the duodenum. Tumours in this location are solitary in about one-half of cases. Much less commonly, primary gastrinomas are found in the omenta, lymph nodes, liver, and gastric antrum. Malignant gastrinomas metastasize to regional lymph nodes and liver.

Peptic ulcer disease is present in over 90% of gastrinoma patients. Almost all patients with ulcers have typical dyspeptic pain which is more severe and less responsive to medical treatment than in routine peptic ulcer disease.

Coexisting diarrhoea is a significant complaint in about one-third of gastrinoma patients. About 5–7% of patients have diarrhoea as their sole presenting complaint. Large volumes of watery stools may result in dehydration, potassium loss, weakness, and wasting. The diarrhoea is of the secretory variety and frequently accompanied by steatorrhoea. A multifactoral aetiology has been elucidated but the basic underlying abnormality is acid hypersecretion. With the accompanying rapid gastric emptying, the large acid load in the duodenum and upper jejunum lowers the pH to cause inactivation of pancreatic lipase and other enzymes. This, in addition to the mucosal injury imparted by the large acid load, leads to malabsorption and steatorrhoea. There is also increased intestinal motility and inhibition of salt and water absorption from the jejunum due to the hypergastrinaemia. When severe, the mucosal injury of the distal duodenum and proximal jejunum manifests as frank peptic ulceration at these atypical sites.

The majority of patients with ZE syndrome are diagnosed only after several years of symptoms although increasing awareness of the disease is lowering the time between symptom onset and diagnosis. In the past, the majority of patients were diagnosed only after one or more failed operations for presumed routine peptic ulcer disease. Currently, many patients are being diagnosed prior to being subjected to ill-fated standard ulcer operations.

All of the complications of peptic ulcer disease are encountered in ZE syndrome patients and acute haemorrhage and perforation are each noted in approximately 20%. Vomiting and other symptoms of gastric outlet obstruction are distinctly less common as the fulminant nature of the ulcer diathesis more often precipitates acute complications.

Patients with gastrinoma most often have no abnormal physical findings. However, signs of weight loss, epigastric tenderness, and intestinal hypermotility are relatively common. Intra-abdominal tumour masses are rarely palpable but hepatic enlargement secondary to massive metastatic deposits is occasionally seen at initial presentation.

The diagnosis of ZE syndrome should be considered in any patient having: (i) severe peptic ulcer disease refractory to histamine H_2-receptor antagonists (cimetidine, ranitidine); (ii) multiple peptic ulcers or ulcers in unusual locations such as the distal duodenum or jejunum; (iii) peptic ulcer disease associated with diarrhoea; (iv) recurrent peptic ulcer disease following an acid-reducing operation; (v) peptic ulcer disease in association with a strong family history of ulcer disease or MEN I syndrome; or (vi) peptic ulcer disease without prior diagnosis of MEN I syndrome but in association with any other component of MEN I syndrome (e.g., hypercalcaemia). In addition, findings of large gastric mucosal folds and diffuse inflammation or frank ulceration distal to the duodenal bulb on endoscopic or radiological examination of the upper gastrointestinal tract are suggestive of the ZE syndrome.

In the presence of peptic ulceration and/or a secretory diarrhoea, radioimmunoassay of plasma gastrin level remains the key to diagnosis of ZE syndrome. A basal gastrin level greater than 100 pg/ml strongly supports the diagnosis of gastrinoma. The majority of patients have fasting levels greater than 200 pg/ml and not infrequently 1000 pg/ml or greater. It must be remembered that hypergastrinaemia can occur in association with gastric hypochlorhydria or achlorhydria from a variety of conditions not associated with gastrinoma. Patients with pernicious anaemia, chronic atrophic gastritis, gastric cancer, prior vagotomy or histamine H_2-receptor antagonist therapy may manifest hypergastrinaemia as a physiological response to an elevated antral pH. Thus, it is important to measure basal gastric acid output in all patients suspected to have gastrinoma based on clinical presentation and an elevated plasma gastrin level.

The principal circulating form of gastrin in patients with gastrinoma is G-34 or 'big gastrin', a situation analogous to insulinomas and other peptide-producing endocrine

Table 70.7 Differential diagnosis of hypergastrinaemia

With Acid Hypersecretion
Zollinger–Ellison syndrome
Retained gastric antrum after Billroth II gastrectomy
Antral G-cell hyperplasia
Gastric outlet obstruction
With Acid Hyposecretion
Pernicious anaemia
Atrophic gastritis
Gastric cancer

tumours where elevated levels of precursor forms of the respective hormones are often found. The measured circulating gastrin level does not reflect the degree of gastric acid stimulation by the tumour nor is there good correlation between gastrin level and tumour mass. Plasma gastrin levels normally rise following a meal and thus measurements must be made in the fasting state. Gastric outlet obstruction secondary to ordinary duodenal ulcer disease, antral G-cell hyperfunction or hyperplasia, and retained gastric antrum after Billroth II gastrectomy are other conditions associated with peptic ulcer in which elevated basal plasma gastrin levels may be found (*Table* 70.7). In order to differentiate these entities from gastrinoma and also to establish the diagnosis of gastrinoma in ulcer patients with borderline elevated basal gastrin levels, a number of provocative tests have been devised. The best of these is the secretin stimulation test. Following intravenous injection of secretin (2 u/kg), the plasma gastrin level rises within 5–10 minutes to a level 200 pg/ml greater than the basal level in patients with gastrinoma, but not in those with other conditions. The calcium stimulation test has also been used to differentiate gastrinoma from ordinary peptic ulcer disease. In this test calcium is infused at 5 mg/kg/h for 3 hours and a positive test requires that the stimulated gastrin increases by 100% over basal level. Because of untoward side-effects of hypercalcaemia, long duration and slightly lower accuracy, the calcium infusion test has been almost entirely supplanted by the secretin injection test. The meal provocation test may be used to differentiate gastrinoma from antral G-cell hyperfunction. In this test, a standard meal is ingested by the patient and causes a marked rise in plasma gastrin levels in those with G-cell hyperfunction but no rise or only a minimal one in gastrinoma patients.

In order to secure the diagnosis of gastrinoma in patients demonstrated to have hypergastrinaemia, gastric acid secretory testing is necessary. A basal level output greater than 15 mmol/h strongly supports the diagnosis as does a value greater than 5 mmol/h in the patient who has had previous acid reducing gastric surgery for peptic ulcer disease. A ratio of basal acid output to maximal acid output following stimulation with pentagastrin, histamine or betazole of greater than 0·6 has also been used as a discriminatory criterion for gastrinoma. However, this ratio is no more sensitive or specific than is the basal acid output alone. Upper gastrointestinal endoscopy and a standard barium upper gastrointestinal radiological series should be performed in all patients thought to harbour a gastrinoma. In addition to the mucosal abnormalities often found with these studies, on rare occasion a duodenal or antral polypoid lesion has proven to be a gastrinoma on biopsy.

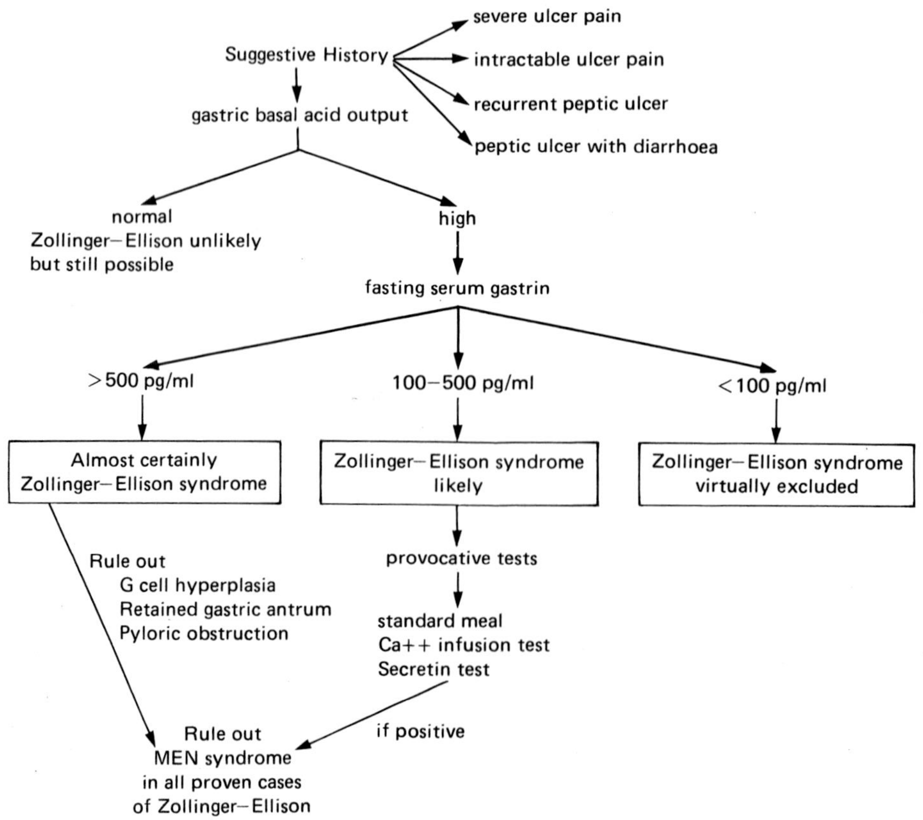

Fig. 70.20 An approach to the investigation of patients with suspected ZE syndrome.

All patients diagnosed as having ZE syndrome should be further investigated for the presence of MEN I syndrome. In addition to the plasma gastrin determinations, several serum calcium and phosphate measurements and a plasma prolactin level constitute the absolute minimal workup for the most commonly associated endocrine lesions. A family history of refractory ulcer disease, hyperparathyroidism, or other endocrine lesions warrants endocrinological screening of the immediate family as well as the patient. The diagnostic approach to the patient with suspected gastrinoma is summarized in *Fig.* 70.20.

Tumour Localization Techniques

Preoperative techniques to localize gastrinomas have not been particularly successful. Since gastrinomas may be small and deeply embedded in the pancreas, ultrasonography and computed tomography have not been very sensitive. Recent information, however, would suggest that up to two-thirds of gastrinomas can be identified with the state-of-the-art CT scanners. However, tumours smaller than 7 mm are virtually never identified. Magnetic resonance imaging has not had wide application to gastrinoma patients but since islet cell tumours in general produce an unusually intense signal, this modality may prove particularly sensitive in their detection. Since most gastrinomas are hypovascular, visceral angiography has been much less useful in localizing gastrinomas as compared to insulinomas. There has been some anecdotal suggestion that simultaneous secretin injection enhances the angiographic tumour blush and may allow detection of otherwise non-hypervascular gastrinomas. Percutaneous transhepatic selective sampling of the portal venous system for gastrin levels has been of value in a number of gastrinoma patients. This technique allows precise localization of the source or sources of hypergastrinaemia and when combined with hepatic venous gastrin level sampling, it is possible to predict the location of pancreatic tumours and the presence or absence of hepatic metastases. In general, however, presently available preoperative tests do not appear capable of localizing the tumour any more reliably than careful intraoperative exploration by the experienced surgeon. Intraoperative ultrasound examination of the pancreas may prove of ultility in the localization of small tumours within the pancreatic gland. The experience with this technique remains limited at present.

Medical Treatment

Current medical therapy for control of the acid hypersecretion in patients with ZE syndrome consists primarily of the histamine H_2-receptor antagonists cimetidine and ranitidine. Unfortunately, these drugs have proved more effective in symptom control than in ulcer healing. Approximately one-third of patients have been found to fail cimetidine treatment even when large doses are prescribed. Ranitidine may prove to be more effective but data remain inadequate. A number of newer histamine H_2-receptor antagonists are currently under evaluation. The dose of H_2-receptor antagonists must be individually titrated to ensure that basal acid output immediately prior to the next dose does not exceed 10 mmol/h. Many patients with gastrinoma require H_2-receptor antagonist drug doses two to four times that normally recommended for duodenal ulcer disease. The acid-reducing effect of the drugs may be augmented and prolonged by concomitant administration of anticholinergics. The antimuscarinic drug, pirenzipine, has been shown to be effective in this role and does not have the untoward anticholinergic side-effects of earlier drugs of the same family. Antacids may be useful in treating dyspeptic symptoms but when given alone are entirely incapable of controlling the acid hypersecretion of most gastrinoma patients.

A new class of antisecretory agents, the substituted benzimidazoles, act as inhibitors of the potassium-hydrogen ATPase of the parietal cell and are important investigational drugs which will likely have future application. Recent experience with one of these new agents (omeprazole) suggests that a major impact on the acid hypersecretion of gastrinoma patients may be in store. In a small group of patients treated with omeprazole a profound and lasting suppression of acid secretion was noted with once-a-day administration. The data thus far indicates that this drug is by far the most powerful and specific gastric antisecretory agent yet developed.

Surgical Treatment

Prior to the advent of effective antisecretory therapy, total gastrectomy was required in virtually all gastrinoma patients in order to prevent mortality from the acute complications of peptic ulceration. With current medical therapy, satisfactory control of acid secretion and the ulcer diathesis is possible in a majority of patients. The focus of the surgeon has thus shifted somewhat from control of the ulcer diathesis to control of the tumour itself. Recent experience suggests that earlier pessimism regarding surgical curability of the tumour may have been unjustified. It may be possible, in fact, that at least 20% of patients are curable by tumour excision. For example, approximately 20% of gastrinomas are located in the duodenum and about one-half of these are solitary and therefore particularly amenable to curative excision. In addition, a number of patients with primary of the pancreas, multiple primary tumours and even tumour in lymph nodes have apparently been cured by aggressive surgical excision. The vast majority of these patients have undergone enucleation or local excision of tumours rather than radical pancreatic or pancreatoduodenal resections.

An approach to the management of newly diagnosed gastrinoma patients is summarized in *Fig.* 70.21. Patients with preoperatively demonstrated liver metastases and/or MEN I syndrome are treated medically. This is particularly true if patients with metastatic disease are found to have multiple liver deposits or if patients with MEN I are found to have multiple primary tumours. If such patients fail medical therapy total gastrectomy should be performed. Whenever possible, confirmation of the multifocal nature of the disease is obtained by thorough biopsy of suspected tumours. Young and middle-aged patients without known liver metastases or MEN I are extensively evaluated with the variety of tumour localization techniques now available. These patients are offered elective laparotomy with the specific intent to accomplish complete tumour excision. Experience suggests that even patients with regionally metastatic disease to lymph nodes can be cured and thus an aggressive approach to lymph node excision is always undertaken. Adequate exploration requires full mobilization of the pancreatic gland and the duodenum. All identified lymph nodes and palpable masses within and around the pancreas are submitted for frozen section histological examination. Pancreatic tumour removal is accomplished by enucleation or distal pancreatectomy only and major resections are not performed. If preoperative localization techniques have been unsuccessful, and extensive operative search for tumour is unrewarding, blind distal pancreatectomy is not performed as most tumours occur in and around the head of the pancreas and there is no evidence that islet

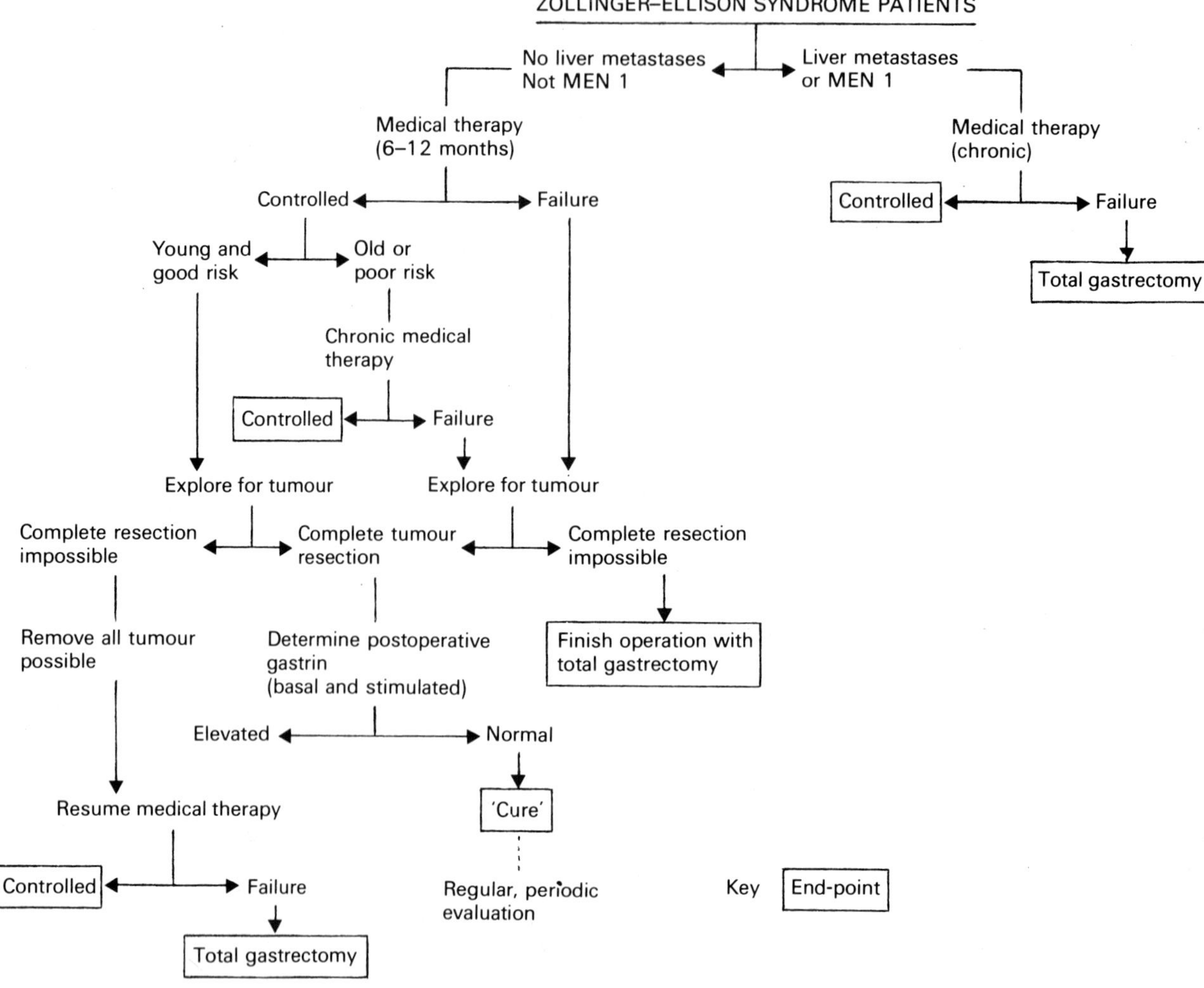

Fig. 70.21 Management of newly-diagnosed patients with ZE syndrome.

cell hyperplasia has any aetiologic role in ZE syndrome. Proximal gastric vagotomy has been advocated as an adjunctive procedure to tumour removal but its efficacy remains unproven. Patients who are well controlled on medical therapy are thus not subjected to any gastric procedure even if no tumour is found. In contrast, patients responding poorly to antisecretory drugs and at exploration are found to have either no tumour or multifocal disease are treated by total gastrectomy in order to prevent life-threatening peptic ulcer complications. Contrary to the early experience with total gastrectomy for ZE syndrome, recent reports indicate that under elective circumstances the operative mortality is below 3% and the long-term sequelae are infrequently severe.

Successful removal of all gastrin-secreting tumour is confirmed by serially negative plasma gastrin responses to secretin stimulation. Long-term surveillance is required as tumour recurrences may be late and manifest as basal hypergastrinaemia.

Results with chemotherapy for advanced hepatic metastases from gastrinoma have not been very encouraging. Streptozotocin and 5-fluorouracil have been the only drugs to have therapeutic efficacy. There may be some advantage to delivering these drugs direcly into the hepatic arterial circulation rather than intravenously but data remain sparse. Similarly, hepatic artery ligation or embolization has not been adequately evaluated.

Gastrinoma patients with MEN I syndrome and documented hyperparathyroidism should have parathyroid surgery performed prior to any attempt at gastrinoma removal. In some such patients parathyroidectomy provides marked amelioration of ulcer symptoms and concomitant decreases in gastric acid secretion and plasma gastrin levels. These salutory effects are usually transient, however, and a definitive approach to the gastrinoma is still required and should not be unduly delayed.

Vipoma (Werner–Morrison Syndrome; WDHA Syndrome; Pancreatic Cholera)

The syndrome of Watery Diarrhoea, Hypokalaemia and Achlorhydria in association with an islet cell tumour of the pancreas was initially described by Werner and Morrison in 1958. A number of hormones have been identified in these tumours (including secretin, glucagon, gastric inhibitory polypeptide, pancreatic polypeptide, and gastrin). However, vasoactive intestinal polypeptide (VIP) has been convincingly shown to be the causative agent in the majority of cases.

Patients afflicted with this condition have a secretory

diarrhoea which is profuse and causes severe dehydration and loss of potassium. Acidosis almost invariably attends the hypokalaemia and patients suffer from lethargy and weakness as a result of the dehydration and electrolyte abnormalities. Virtually all patients incur significant weight loss, a majority have abdominal colic, and a minority experience cutaneous flushing. Slightly less than half of the tumours are malignant and metastases to the liver are often found at the time of diagnosis. The primary tumour is located in the pancreas in approximately 80% of cases, is almost always solitary, and usually larger than 3 cm before causing symptoms. The extrapancreatic VIPomas include ganglioneuromas and neuroblastomas and are capable of causing the identical clinical syndrome. Unlike the 75% of pancreatic tumours which secrete pancreatic polypeptide, the extrapancreatic tumours do not.

VIP causes small intestinal secretion of water and electrolytes and is apparently responsible for the metabolic and clinical features of most cases. There are occasional patients, however, who have the identical clinical syndrome but with normal plasma VIP levels. In these cases prostaglandin E_2 is the most likely aetiological candidate.

In the setting of the proper clinical symptoms the diagnosis is made by demonstration of elevated plasma levels of VIP. Localization of the primary tumour is not difficult in view of its large size and solitary nature. Ultrasonography, computed tomography and angiography have all been effective.

Medical treatment consists of fluid and electrolyte resuscitation and support. Five or more litres of volume replacement may be required per day. Glucocorticoids or somatostatin have been helpful in antagonizing the diarrheagenic effects of the tumour.

The definitive treatment of VIPoma is surgical excision of the tumour whenever possible. Debulking of metastatic disease often provides effective palliation. Since the majority of non-metastatic cases are caused by large solitary pancreatic tumours, enucleation or distal pancreatectomy are often curative. Blind distal or subtotal pancreatectomy in the absence of tumour localization is probably unwarranted since islet cell hyperplasia is an unproven cause of the syndrome.

In patients who cannot be significantly benefited by surgical resection or who recur with multiple metastatic deposits may have symptomatic responses to long-acting somatostatin analogues. Streptozotocin has been reasonably effective in palliation but immediately following administration, diarrhoea and electrolyte losses may be exacerbated for several days, necessitating aggressive replacement. The prognosis is poor with advanced disease and thromboembolic complications due to excessive dehydration are often responsible for major morbidity and mortality. The occasional patient with pancreatic cholera secondary to prostaglandin E_2 hypersecretion may have dramatic relief with indomethacin therapy.

Glucagonoma

Glucagonomas are tumours of the A-cell of the pancreatic islet and are responsible for a characteristic syndrome consisting of severe skin rash, weight loss, diabetes mellitus, deep venous thrombosis, anaemia and hypoaminoacidaemia. This tumour is very rare and because its most salient feature, the skin rash, is frequently misdiagnosed, its true significance and the correct diagnosis are often made very late in the course. Glucagonoma is considerably more common in females and is a disease of middle age. At the time of diagnosis approximately 60% of cases have already metastasized. The typical clinical features are summarized in *Table* 70.8.

Table 70.8 The glucagonoma syndrome: clinical features and incidence

Sex	Female/Male >1
Age range (mean)	20–71 (57)
Malignancy	70–80%
Clinical diabetes (abnormal glucose tolerance test)	70% (95%)
Skin lesions	80%
Glossitis/cheilitis	90–100%
Weight loss	90–100%
Diarrhoea	50–60%
Coarse intestinal mucosal folds	50–60%
Anaemia, normocytic, normochromic	70–80%
Hypoaminoacidaemia	80%
Neurological deficit	Unusual (incidence uncertain)
Marked hyperglucagonaemia	100%
Survival	80% more than 2 years 23% more than 5½ years

The typical skin rash is termed necrolytic migratory erythema. The lesions are characteristically symmetrical and erythematous with crusted erosions involving the perineum, groins, thighs, buttocks and distal extremities. The systemic manifestations of weight loss, weakness and lethargy are due to a combination of the catabolic effects of high plasma glucagon levels and the extensive malignant disease which is often present. Hyperglycaemia results from increased hepatic glycogenolysis and gluconeogenesis. Most patients are frankly diabetic but ketonaemia rarely develops because circulating insulin levels are increased. Panhypoaminoacidaemia is a uniform finding and may be responsible for the skin rash as well as the neurological deficits that are occasionally seen. The anaemia is characteristically normocytic and normochromic and although serum iron levels may be low, the anaemia does not respond to iron and vitamin replacement.

The diagnosis is usually made upon recognition of the typical cutaneous manifestations in combination with diabetes mellitus in the setting of a chronic wasting disorder. The diagnosis is confirmed by finding an elevated plasma glucagon level. Normal values range between 50 and 150 pg/ml. Values of glucagon greater than 1000 pg/ml are often seen with glucagonoma but interpretation should be cautious in the absence of the typical skin rash or other suggestive signs. Numerous other conditions associated with hyperglucagonaemia are enumerated in *Table* 70.9. In most glucagonoma patients glucagon release from the tumour can be induced by the administration of arginine or tolbutamide. Pancreatic polypeptide levels are elevated in one-half of patients.

Since many cases are diagnosed in an advanced metastatic stage, tumour localization is not normally difficult. While topical steroids and intravenous amino acid administration have been effective in ameliorating the skin eruption in some patients, definitive treatment is surgical. Operative exploration is indicated even for advanced metastatic disease as debulking procedures may significantly alleviate the debilitating catabolic effects of the excess glucagon. When surgical resection is not an option, selective arterial embolization

Table 70.9 Conditions associated with hyperglucagonaemia

1. Diabetes
   Ketoacidosis
   Hyperosmolar syndrome
2. Chronic renal failure
3. Shock states
   Myocardial infarction
   Septicaemia
   Burns
   Hypovolaemia/haemorrhage
4. Acute pancreatitis
5. Cirrhosis
   Portosystemic shunting (natural, surgical)
6. Glucagonoma
7. Familial hyperglucagonaemia (asymptomatic)
8. Exercise
9. Antiglucagon antibodies in diabetics treated with insulin*

* These may be induced by slight glucagon impurities in commercially available insulins and manifest as hyperglucagonaemia when glucagon is measured by a double antibody immunoassay method.

and chemotherapy are indicated. Streptozotocin combined with 5-fluorouracil can produce reduction in both tumour size and glucagon levels. Dimethyltrizenoimidazole carboxamide has been effective in providing symptomatic relief and alleviation of skin rash. Somatostatin analogues may prove efficacious in suppressing glucagon production by the tumour.

Somatostatinoma

Somatostatinoma is a very rare tumour with less than two dozen cases reported to date. The patients have been mostly middle-aged and predominantly female. Over 70% of the tumours have been associated with liver metastases at the time of diagnosis. Along with somatostatin production most tumours have also elaborated other hormones such as VIP, pancreatic polypeptide, gastrin, calcitonin or cortisol.

Despite the potent inhibitory nature of somatostatin, the usual clinical syndrome is nonspecific. Abdominal pain is the most common presenting symptom and this may relate to the high prevalence of cholelithiasis in these patients. Gallbladder stasis is thought to be of aetiological importance. Other symptoms and signs commonly associated with somatostatinoma are mild diabetes mellitus, weight loss, anorexia, hypochlorhydria, steatorrhoea and anaemia. Symptoms not related to excessive somatostatin levels such as tachycardia, flushing, hypertension, hypokalaemia and hypoglycaemia are also present in some patients. The diagnosis is made by chance in most cases although a radioimmunoassay for plasma somatostatin is available. Somatostatin released by the tumour may be stimulated by tolbutamide; however, the utility of this provocative test is unknown at present.

Ideally, treatment is by surgical excision of the pancreatic or duodenal lesion. Debulking of advanced tumours may be efficacious and some patients have benefited from adjunctive therapy with streptozotocin and 5-fluorouracil.

Human Pancreatic Polypeptide Tumour (HPPoma)

A very few tumours arising from polypeptide cells and secreting this hormone exclusively have been described. They have been associated with no apparent symptom complex and the clinical and metabolic characteristics of the tumour remain to be defined.

Elevated plasma levels of pancreatic polypeptide have been found in many patients with various islet cell tumours of the pancreas (gastrinoma, glucagonoma, etc.) and carcinoid tumours. It has been suggested that elevated pancreatic polypeptide levels be used as a marker for endocrine pancreatic tumours but only approximately one-half of all patients with such tumours have abnormal elevations of the hormone. Similarly, high levels are found in approximately 50% of patients with carcinoid tumours at all sites. While plasma pancreatic polypeptide levels may be used as a screening test for tumours in patients with MEN I syndrome and their relatives, high levels must be interpreted with caution as they may be found also in elderly patients, those with renal failure, diabetes mellitus and certain inflammatory diseases. Atropine suppression of pancreatic polypeptide has been suggested as a method of determining whether the elevated hormone is the result of tumour secretion. At present it would appear that measurement of pancreatic polypeptide is of limited utility in screening for pancreatic endocrine tumours.

Non-functioning Endocrine Pancreatic Tumours

Approximately 10–15% of islet cell tumours have been diagnosed without any accompanying symptoms or signs other than those relating to a mass lesion. Such tumours are usually diagnosed late in their course, often after metastatic disease is present in the liver. A number of pancreatic tumours thought to be adenocarcinomas have, on histological examination, proven to be of the islet cell type. Some of these tumours have been found to contain pancreatic polypeptide and although this tumour is no longer regarded as biochemically silent, its clinical syndrome has yet to be defined.

Without measurable hormonal markers clinically nonfunctioning tumours will continue to be diagnosed by virtue of their large size. Thus, ultrasonography, computed tomography and angiography remain useful in their localization. As additional islet cell hormones are detected by new radioimmunoassays, other specific tumours will be described.

The best treatment currently available for nonfunctioning islet cell tumours is surgical resection of the primary tumour and of as much of the metastatic tumour as possible. Chemotherapy has been useful in a number of these cases but even without response the progression of tumour growth has, in general, been relatively slow.

Multiple Endocrine Neoplasia Type I (MEN I; MEA I; Wermer's Syndrome)

The MEN I syndrome is inherited as an autosomal dominant disorder but considerable phenotypic variability exists even within an individual family. However, recent evidence suggests that the pancreas, parathyroid glands and pituitary are involved in all patients if examined pathologically. It is also now understood that the pancreas is inevitably involved with diffuse islet cell disease consisting of micronodular and macronodular hyperplasia, and often multiple tumours secreting multiple peptide hormones.

The parathyroid glands are most frequently involved in MEN I syndrome with hyperparathyroidism being present in 85% of cases. In the vast majority of these, hyperplasia is the histological abnormality and all glands are affected. This is in contrast with the very low incidence of parathyroid hyperplasia in isolated primary hyperparathyroidism. Pancreatic abnormalities occur in over 80% of MEN I patients with non-B-cell tumours being most common. The most common pancreatic tumour found in MEN I syndrome patients is gastrinoma and in virtually all such patients, multiple pancreatic tumours are found.

Of the pituitary lesions, chromophobe adenomas and particularly prolactinomas are the most frequent lesions encountered. When small, these tumours may be without symptoms but in male patients are associated with manifestations of the antiandrogenic effect of prolactin. Tumours producing growth hormone and leading to acromegaly are the next most frequently encountered variety.

While the MEN I syndrome is classically associated with lesions of the parathyroid glands, pancreatic islets and pituitary gland, an increasing number of adrenocortical lesions have been recognized in recent years. Many of these lesions are non-functioning adenomas; however, glucocorticoid excess has been noted in some. Other occasional associations of MEN I include thyroid nodules, bronchial and intestinal carcinoids and lipomas.

All patients with endocrine pancreatic tumours should be carefully investigated for additional manifestations of MEN I syndrome. Thus, estimations of serum levels of calcium and phosphate as well as plasma assays for parathormone, insulin, gastrin, glucagon, somatostatin, pancreatic polypeptide, prolactin, growth hormone, ACTH and cortisol constitute a relatively complete though by no means exhaustive endocrine evaluation for the MEN I syndrome. Whenever a patient is diagnosed as having MEN I syndrome, screening of all available family members is indicated.

Multiple Endocrine Neoplasia Type II Syndrome (MEN II; MEA II; Sipple's Syndrome)

MEN II is another discrete endocrine syndrome which is inherited as an autosomal dominant with variable expressivity. It is not associated with pancreatic disease. It consists of hyperparathyroidism, medullary carcinoma of the thyroid gland and phaeochromocytoma. MEN IIb is a variant which is also inherited as an autosomal dominant but unlike MEN II, the incidence of parathyroid disease is extremely low. The syndrome consists of multiple mucosal neuromas, intestinal ganglioneuromatosis leading to megacolon and constipation, a Marfanoid habitus and characteristic facies with thickened lips and alae nasi, along with the medullary carcinoma of the thyroid and phaeochromocytoma.

Further Reading

Moossa A. R. (ed.) (1980) *Tumors of the Pancreas*. Baltimore, Williams & Wilkins.
Moossa A. R. (1984) Diagnostic tests and procedures in acute pancreatitis. *N. Engl. J. Med.* **311**, 639–643.
Moossa A. R., Robson M. C. and Schimpff S. C. (1986) *A Comprehensive Textbook of Oncology*. Baltimore, Williams & Wilkins.
Ranson J. H. C. (1985) Acute Pancreatitis, In: *Current Problems in Surgery*. Chicago, Year Book.
Schwartz S. I. and Ellis H. (ed.) (1985) *Maingot's Abdominal Operations*. New York, Appleton-Century-Crofts.
Warshaw A. L. (ed.) (1984) Progress Symposium on Pancreatic Cancer. *World J. Surg*. Vol. 8, No. 6.

71 *The Spleen and Lymph Nodes*

A. R. Moossa and S. R. Shackford

INTRODUCTION

The spleen and lymph nodes form part of the lymphoreticular system, a term which, if used in its broadest sense, describes all the haemopoietic and reticuloendothelial tissues. However, its use is usually confined to those circulating and fixed cellular elements which are concerned with body immune defence mechanisms, i.e. macrophages, reticuloendothelial elements and related lymphatic tissues. Because the spleen and the lymph nodes form part of this functionally related system they are often involved together in similar pathological processes. However, the spleen should not be thought of simply as a large lymph node. In addition to its extensive lymphatic tissue it has a complicated vascular system which, because of its tiny orifices and large macrophage population, acts as the optimal biological filter and constitutes a considerable hazard even for healthy red cells. Added to this, the spleen receives a disproportionate amount of the circulating blood volume for its relatively small size. Hence, it becomes involved secondarily in a wide range of haematological disorders.

Before describing the pathology and clinical aspects of disorders of the spleen and lymph nodes we shall review briefly what is known about their structure–function relationships.

STRUCTURE AND FUNCTION OF LYMPH NODES AND SPLEEN

The lymph nodes and spleen share similar immunological functions, the former processing material arriving from the tissues via lymphatics while the spleen is a haemal 'node' dealing with blood directly and without afferent lymphatics. In addition, the spleen has certain well-defined haematological functions, many of which can be carried out equally well in other organs which have a large macrophage population. Before it is possible to appreciate the haematological function of the spleen and how these are related to its immunological functions, it is necessary to consider its specialized vascular system.

It has been postulated that there are 'fast' and 'slow' passages through the red pulp which may have an anatomical basis in 'closed' and 'open' circulations (*Fig.* 71.1). The splenic artery divides to form trabecular arteries and, after several subdivisions, small radicles enter the splenic pulp

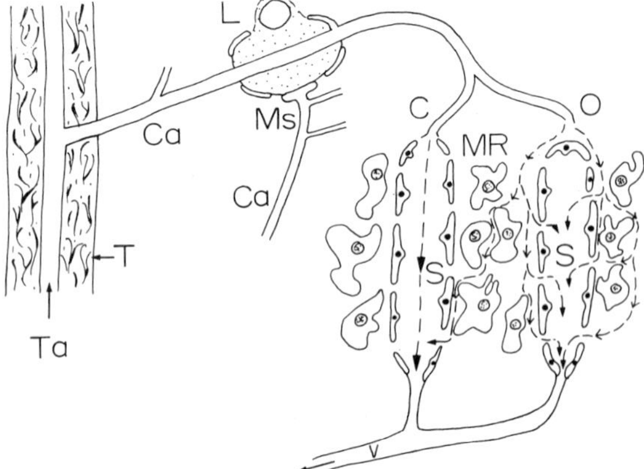

Fig. 71.1 Splenic vasculature. T=trabeculum; Ta=trabecular artery; Ca=central artery; L=lymphoid tissue; Ms=marginal sinus; C=closed circulation; O=open circulation; MR=macrophages and reticulum of red pulp; S=sinus; V=collecting vein.

where they acquire a lymphoid sheath. The arteries continue to divide and at a vessel calibre below 50 μm diameter the lymphoid modification of the adventitia is lost and the vessels enter the pulp as penicillate arteries. Lateral branches supply the marginal sinuses between the small lymphocyte sheath and a marginal zone composed of larger lymphoid cells and antigen receptive macrophages. It is at this point that lymphocytes leave the blood to enter the white pulp.

Some terminations are thought to form direct connections with the first elements of the efferent vasculature, the 'splenic sinuses', creating a closed path for red cells. Other vessels open into the meshwork, or 'cords', between the sinuses where the blood filters slowly through a grid of macrophages and reticular fibres before re-entering the vasculature through gaps in the sinus walls. This is the finest mesh through which red cells and plasma have to travel in the body.

The Haematological Functions of the Spleen

Because of the peculiar anatomical arrangement of its blood vessels, the spleen is ideally suited as a site for fine quality control of the erythrocyte population. It removes fragmented, damaged or senescent red cells from the circulating

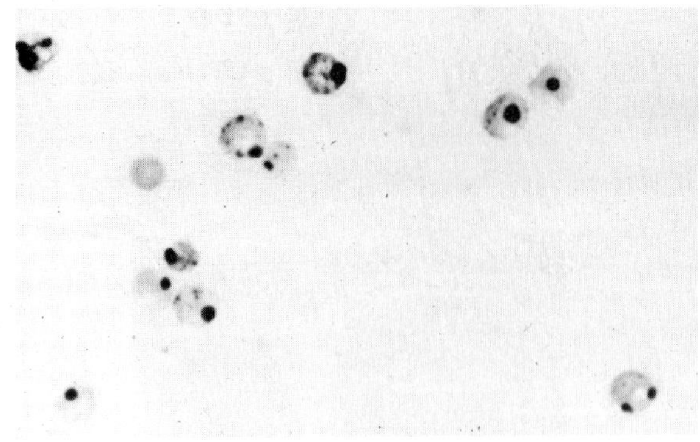

Fig. 71.2 Blood film after removal of the spleen. The red cells contain ribonucleoprotein granules (Howell–Jolly bodies) which are normally pitted out by the spleen (Giemsa stain ×680).

blood, a process known as 'culling'. It also plays a role in remodelling the surface of the maturing erythrocytes and in preserving the normal relationship between their membrane surface area and volume. Target cells, which have a relatively high ratio of membrane to intracellular content, appear in the peripheral blood soon after splenectomy. A variety of intra-erythrocyte inclusions are removed by the spleen (through a process known as 'pitting'), after which the red cells are returned to the circulation. Among the inclusions removed are Howell–Jolly bodies (*Fig.* 71.2), which are probably nuclear remnants, siderotic granules, which are haemosiderin aggregates laid down during normal erythroid maturation and Heinz bodies, which are pathological aggregates of denatured haemoglobin. Thus, after splenectomy Howell–Jolly bodies and siderotic granules may be seen in the peripheral blood and the red cells show striking changes in shape and size with the appearance of acanthocytes, irregularly crenated cells, and target forms.

The human spleen, unlike that of many animals, contains relatively little blood and hence has no important storage role. It appears to sequester a significant number of platelets, however, and after splenectomy there is nearly always a transient thrombocytosis. The spleen also clears particulate matter from the circulation, a function which may be very important in the immune response to intravenously administered antigen.

The spleen is only involved in haemopoiesis in fetal life and there is virtually no blood formation in the organ after birth. However, there may be a reversion to this fetal pattern of erythropoiesis in certain disease states and it is thought that the spleen may become an important organ of red cell production in at least some patients with progressive fibrosis of the marrow, i.e. myelosclerosis (*Fig.* 71.3). A certain amount of splenic haemopoiesis also occurs in children with congenital haemolytic anaemia.

The Immunological Functions of the Spleen

The basic arrangements of lymphoid tissue in the nodes and spleen are compared in *Fig.* 71.4. The population of lymphocytes in each is in constant motion, a substantial proportion recirculating between the two by way of the thoracic duct and bloodstream. In the case of the spleen about half the small lymphocytes recirculate fairly rapidly. Approximately a quarter of the body's total of thymus-dependent (T) cells is in the spleen at any given time.

Lymphocytes enter nodes through the walls of the post-capillary ('epithelioid') venules in the paracortex; and in the spleen through the marginal sinus bordering the Malpighian corpuscle. T-cells tend to congregate in the paracortex of lymph nodes and form a peri-arteriolar small lymphoid sheath in the spleen. B-cells pass between the T-cells to form small clusters, or primary follicles, at the periphery in the outer cortex of nodes or adjacent to the marginal sinuses in the spleen. A humoral response following antigenic stimulation involves co-operation between T- and B-cells, possibly at the site of antigen localization on the surface of large dendritic cells. Immunoglobulin-synthesizing cells appear within days in the medullary cords of nodes and in the red pulp of the spleen. Germinal centres, or secondary follicles, begin to appear within the primary follicles, and reach their maximum development at about 8 weeks. They consist of enlarged lymphocytes, with numerous mitotic figures. There appears to be an element of 'ineffective lymphopoiesis' and pyknotic nuclear remains are phagocytosed by macrophages (giving rise to so-called tingible bodies); possibly 'forbidden clones' are recognized and destroyed at this stage. In fact, the spleen may be a source of suppressor T-cells. It is thought that each secondary follicle produces polyclonal 'memory' B-cells and may be responding to more than one antigen.

A cellular immune response is recognized by enlargement of T-cells within the paracortex, cytoplasmic RNA synthesis and cell division. Some cells leave nodes by way of the efferent lymphatics, travelling up the thoracic duct to repopulate other lymphoid areas via the bloodstream. Efferent

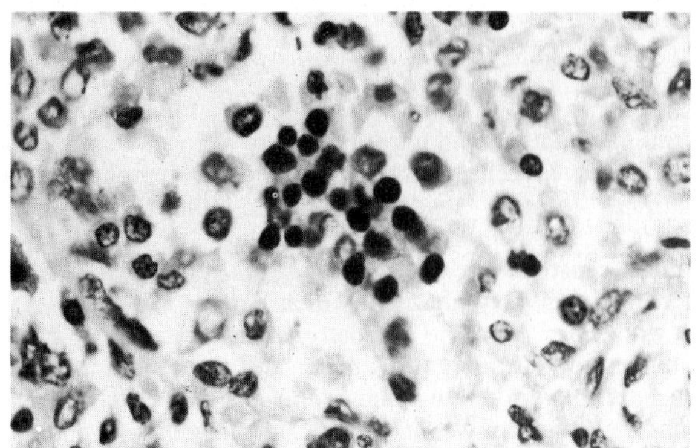

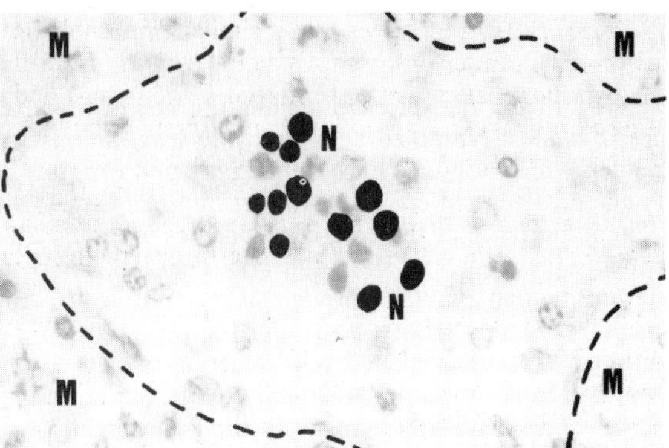

Fig. 71.3 An erythropoietic island within a sinusoid in the red pulp of the spleen from a patient with myelosclerosis. N = normoblast; --- Wall of sinus; M = red pulp meshwork surrounding the sinusoid.

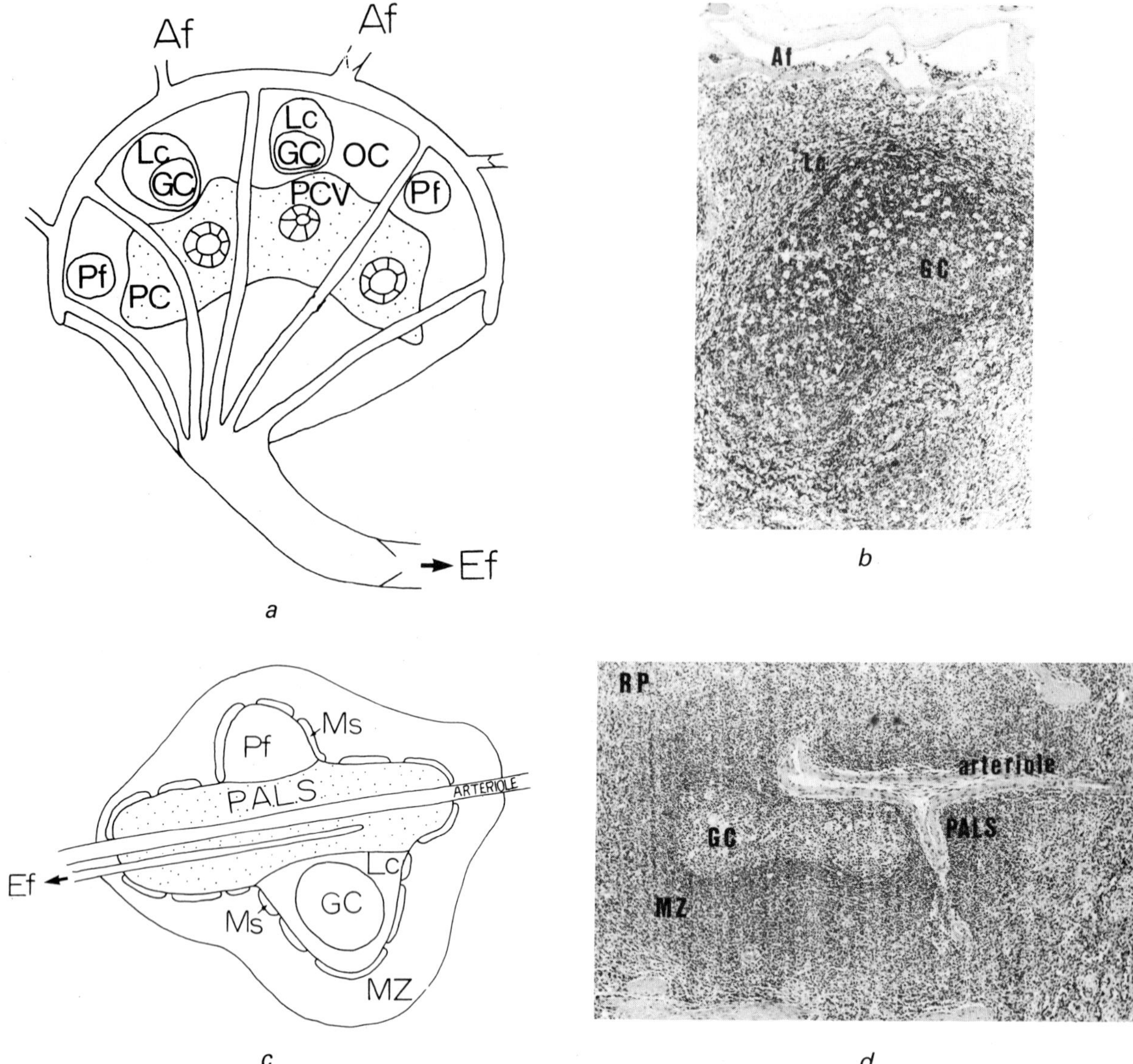

Fig. 71.4 Basic arrangement of lymphoid tissue in lymph node and spleen. *a*, Diagram of lymphatic arrangement in lymph node. *b*, Photomicrograph of a section of the spleen showing some of the features illustrated in (*a*) (H and E, ×20). *c*, Lymphatic arrangement in the splenic Malpighian body. *d*, Photomicrograph of a section of spleen illustrating some of the features shown in (*c*) (H and E, ×20). Af=afferent lymphatic; OC=outer cortex; Pf=primary follicle; GC=germinal centre; Lc=small lymphocyte corona; PC=paracortex; PCV=postcapillary venule; Ef=efferent lymphatic; MZ=marginal zone of large lymphocytes; Ms=marginal sinus; PALS=periarteriolar small lymphocyte sheath; RP=red pulp.

lymphatics from the spleen run along the line of the arterioles, but most lymphoid cells probably leave in vascular channels which originate in the white pulp and run through the marginal zone to open into the red pulp sinuses.

The importance of these observations lies in the fact that lymphoid tissues are not static collections of cells. There is a constant motion of cells through a reticulin scaffolding. Specific reactions affect particular components. When clones of 'well-differentiated cells' emerge, e.g. in chronic lymphatic leukaemia, they frequently retain the capacity to migrate and to infiltrate selectively the appropriate traffic areas. They may migrate, differentiate and form deposits in other sites, e.g. in the bone marrow in multiple myeloma. However, structural tumours analogous to follicle centres can arise in a node or group of nodes (the follicle centre cell tumours of Luke) and may give rise to a clone of circulating small cleaved cells which infiltrate other lymphoid areas without forming evident tumour follicles. Together, tumours of small, round, recirculating lymphocytes and follicle centre cleaved cells account for about 80% of acute non-Hodgkin's lymphoma in Great Britain.

Monocytes from the bloodstream are sequestered in the white pulp, the marginal sinuses and the red pulp where they are converted to fixed macrophages. Such macrophages endow the spleen with its significant phagocytic capability. There is evidence to suggest that the spleen, in certain disease states such as malaria, releases a humoral substance which acts on the bone marrow causing it to produce and

Table 71.1 Main functions of spleen

Immunological:
1. Antibody production and cell-mediated responses
2. Phagocytosis
   ? Maturation of lymphoid cells
   ? Significant lymphopoiesis
   ? Source of suppressor T-cells

Haematological:
1. Filtration of particles from blood: non-specific or antibody coated
2. Removal of red cell inclusions
3. Destruction of senescent or abnormal red cells
4. Compensatory haemopoiesis, e.g. in myelofibrosis
5. Storage of platelets, iron and Factor VIII

Table 71.2 Hyposplenism

1. CAUSES
   - Splenectomy
   - Splenic agenesis
   - Atrophy
     - Coeliac disease
     - Dermatitis herpetiformis
     - Sickle-cell anaemia
     - Thrombocytopenia
     - SLE
2. HAEMATOLOGICAL CHANGES
   - Abnormal red cells
     - Burr cells
     - Target cells
     - Pitted cells
   - Red cell inclusions
     - Howell–Jolly bodies
     - Siderotic granules
   - Abnormal platelet morphology
   - Thrombocytosis
   - Leucocytosis
     - Neutrophilia
     - Lymphocytosis
     - Monocytosis

release additional monocytes. They eventually circulate to the spleen and undergo conversion to macrophages in order to further augment phagocytic capability.

After splenectomy the primary antibody response is decreased and the secondary response is abnormal in that there is an impairment of the normal switching from IgM to IgG antibody production. In addition to specific antibody synthesis, the spleen also produces non-specific effectors of the immune response. For example, the activity of the phagocytosis-promoting tetrapeptide, tuftsin, is decreased in splenectomized patients. The spleen also influences opsonization of pneumococci in non-immune individuals and is involved in the function of the alternative pathway of complement activation.

The known functions of the spleen are summarized in *Table* 71.1.

HYPOSPLENISM

The causes and haematological features of the hyposplenic state are summarized in *Table* 71.2. Hyposplenism is suggested by the morphological appearance of the red cells and can be confirmed by technetium-sulphur colloid scanning. The qualitative and quantitative changes in the peripheral blood invariably occur regardless of the cause.

The most frequent cause of hyposplenism is surgical splenectomy.

Congenital asplenia (Ivemark syndrome) is a rare anomaly often associated with complex cardiac, gastrointestinal, genito-urinary and neuromuscular abnormalities. Advances in cardiac surgery have now permitted survival in a number of patients with congenital asplenia and complex cyanotic heart disease. The most frequently associated gastrointestinal anomalies are malrotation and situs inversus. Currently, the most frequent cause of death in these infants is overwhelming sepsis. Splenic hypoplasia may be part of the syndrome of Fanconi's anaemia (congenital hypoplastic anaemia).

Acquired hyposplenism is found in up to 76% of untreated patients with coeliac disease. The cause is unknown, but may be due to increased absorption of dietary antigen causing an increase in circulating immune complexes which overwhelm splenic filtration. Splenic function improves after withdrawal of gluten from the diet. In fact, relationship has been noted between splenic function and the morphology of the epithelium of the small intestine. Hyposplenism has also been described in association with other disorders of the gut including ulcerative colitis, Crohn's disease and intestinal lymphangiectasia.

Autoantibodies and clinical autoimmune disease, such as systemic lupus erythematosus, are noted frequently in patients with functional hyposplenism. The cause of this association is unknown, but may be due to a lack of suppressor T-cells of splenic origin.

The hyposplenism of sickle-cell anaemia is due to repeated splenic infarction.

POSTSPLENECTOMY SEPSIS

The literature on infection after splenectomy is extremely difficult to assess. There is now good evidence that asplenic patients are prone to overwhelming infection. The risk of developing serious infection appears to be dependent upon the underlying disease for which splenectomy is undertaken and the age at which it is performed. Overwhelming postsplenectomy sepsis is relatively common when the spleen is removed for thalassaemia and relatively uncommon after splenectomy for trauma (*Table* 71.3). It appears that the relative risk of postsplenectomy infection is related to the

Table 71.3 Incidence of postsplenectomy sepsis*

Splenectomy due to	*Incidence of sepsis (%)*
Trauma	1·4
Idiopathic thrombocytopenia	2·0
Incidental	2·1
Congenital spherocytosis	3·5
Acquired haemolytic anaemia	7·5
Portal hypertension	8·2
Primary anaemia	8·5
Reticuloendothelial disease	11·5
Thalassaemia	24·8

* Modified from Singer D. B. (1973) Postsplenectomy sepsis. *Perspect. Pediatr. Pathol.* **1**, 285–311.

reason for splenectomy. Thus, it is relatively common in patients with disorders such as thalassaemia which are only partially improved by the operation but rare if the spleen has been removed for trauma or for hereditary spherocytosis. Nevertheless, the risk of sepsis in otherwise healthy asplenic trauma patients is still sixty times that expected in the general population. The age at the time of splenectomy also influences risk, being greatest when the spleen is removed during the first five years of life.

Streptococcus pneumoniae has been implicated as the causative organism in over 55% of the septic episodes. Other organisms commonly cultured include *Escherichia coli*, *Haemophilus influenzae* and *Neisseria meningitidis*.

The exact nature of the susceptibility to overwhelming infection in splenectomized individuals is unknown, but it is probably related to a loss of both the filtration and the immunological properties of the spleen. The loss of splenic filtration and phagocytic functions, which decrease the size of any blood-borne inoculum, coupled with the loss of splenic IgM, tuftsin and opsonic protein severely depress the 'first line' of host immune defence.

Overwhelming postsplenectomy infection usually begins insidiously. The course, however, is fulminant and is characterized by fever, obtundation, nausea, vomiting, dehydration and hypotension, often progressing to death within 24–36 hours. Bacteraemia is often so intense that organisms can be visualized on a Gram stain of the peripheral blood. The overall mortality rate is 50–80%. Postmortem examination may fail to reveal a locus of infection, but may demonstrate bilateral adrenal haemorrhage—a common finding in patients with the syndrome. Treatment should be very aggressive with correction of fluid and electrolyte disorders, correction of coagulopathy and administration of intravenous antibiotics.

Vaccines and prophylactic antibiotics have been administered to asplenic patients to prevent postsplenectomy sepsis. Prophylactic antibiotics have met with limited success because of poor patient compliance, drug reactions and

Table 71.4 Pathological changes caused by diseases of lymph nodes and spleen

Reactive	*Lymph nodes*	*Spleen*
A. *Non-specific*: Variable emphasis on:		
i. Sinus histiocytosis	Expansion of medullary cords by histiocytes. Removal of non-antigenic material, e.g. carbon, haemoglobin or fat in dermatopathic lymphadenopathy, Gaucher's	Increased numbers of macrophages in red pulp
ii. Follicle centre reactivity	Expanded reactive follicle centres. Numerous mitoses and tingible body macrophages	Development of reactive secondary follicles in Malpighian bodies
iii. Paracortical	Expansion of paracortex, or periarterial lymphoid sheath by transforming T-cells, e.g. as in viral infection, postvaccination	
iv. Plasma cell	Large numbers of polyclonal immunoglobulin-containing plasma cells in the medullary cords	Large numbers of plasma cells, usually in red pulp
B. *Granulomatous:*		
v. Non-caseating	Compact cortical epithelioid granulomas with Langerhans giant cells, reticulin production and no necrosis in sarcoid, sarcoid reaction, e.g. draining tumours, beryllium poisoning	Similar granulomas, usually appearing first in marginal zones
vi. Caseating	Central caseous necrosis, often surrounding fibrosis, e.g. as in tuberculosis	(May show amyloid deposition)
vii. Necrotizing	Stellate micro-abscesses with polymorphs and peripheral pallisading of histiocytes, often with multinucleated giant cells in cat scratch fever, lymphogranuloma venereum	
C. *Epithelioid congeries*	Collections of small numbers of epithelioid histiocytes, without caseation or giant cells, in paracortex with active secondary centres, e.g. toxoplasmosis, occasionally pseudocysts may be seen within histiocytes. Visceral leishmaniasis, basophilic Leishman–Donovan bodies within histiocytes	Red pulp greatly expanded by histiocytes, e.g. containing parasites (L–D bodies)
D. *Angioimmunoblastic lymphadenopathy*	Debatable reactive hyperimmune state with proliferation of epithelioid venules, interstices filled with transforming lymphoid cells, polyclonal immunoblasts and mature plasma cells. May 'burn out' leaving sclerotic nodes or progress to highly malignant immunoblastic sarcoma	

inadequate drug sensitivities. A recently developed pneumococcal vaccine contains capsular polysaccharides of 23 pneumococcal types responsible for approximately 90% of the most frequently reported isolates. If possible, it is recommended that the vaccination be given 10–14 days prior to elective splenectomy. The duration of protection after vaccination is unknown. However, elevated titres of capsular type-specific antibodies have been demonstrated to persist for up to 42 months. Since no form of prophylaxis has been demonstrated to be completely effective, asplenic patients require close and frequent follow-up. They should be carefully instructed as to their potential for developing life-threatening infection and they should be advised to seek medical attention at the first sign of infection. Such a programme of follow-up may decrease the incidence and the mortality of overwhelming postsplenectomy sepsis.

Table 71.4 *continued*

Non-Hodgkin's lymphoma	*Lymph nodes*	*Spleen*
1. *Low grade*		
A. i. Small lymphocytic	Usually monoclonal B-cells, as in CLL. Expansion of usual traffic areas compressing remaining structures	Initially expands the periarteriolar lymphoid sheaths, later spilling into the red pulp. Hairy cell leukaemia involves red pulp sinusoids
ii. Plasmacytoid cells	Similar, with a spectrum of cells from small lymphocytes to those with basophilic cytoplasm and monoclonal immunoglobulin secretion (usually an IgM as in Waldenström's disease)	
B. Predominantly small cleaved cell, follicular	Pseudofollicles with fewer mitoses than a reactive follicle and very few tingible body macrophages.	Pseudofollicles initially in association with Malpighian bodies. Later in disease pseudofollicles appear in red pulp often accompanied by clone of malignant small cleaved cells in the blood/bone marrow
C. Mixed small cleaved and larger cells, follicular	Splenic follicles throughout node substance	
2. *Intermediate grade*		
D. Predominantly large cell, follicular	—	—
E. Small cleaved cells, follicular	Effacement of architecture by small cleaved cells, often with peri-adenoidal spread	Usually leukaemic with small cleaved cells in B-cell traffic areas and sinusoids
F. Mixed small and large cells, diffuse	—	—
G. Large cell, diffuse	—	—
3. *High grade*		
H. Immunoblastic	Sarcomatous, invasive and destructive proliferation. Intracytoplasmic monoclonal immunoglobulin demonstrable in B-immunoblasts and there may be some maturation to plasma cells	
I. Lymphoblastic	Sarcomatous, invasive and destructive proliferation. Similar appearance in tissue deposits of acute lymphoblastic leukaemia	
J. Small non-cleaved cell	e.g. Burkitt's lymphoma, a diffuse proliferation of non-cleaved cells with a 'starry-sky' appearance given by (non-malignant) macrophages	
4. *Miscellaneous*		
Mycosis fungoides, Sezary	Expansion of T-cell area in paracortex by lymphocytes with convoluted nuclei in Sezary syndrome	Leukaemic Sezary cells present en passage
True histiocytic	Early disease may be confined to non-selective phagocytosis by medullary and red pulp histiocytes Sometimes terminates as monocytic leukaemia	
Extramedullary plasmacytoma	Plasma cells with monoclonal intracellular immunoglobulin ± amyloid	
Unclassifiable	—	—

Hodgkin's disease	*Lymph nodes*	*Spleen*
Any of the cell types, e.g. lymphocyte predominant, nodular sclerosing, mixed cellular, or lymphocyte depleted	Usually spreads to involve next group of nodes in the downstream lymphatic drainage. Earliest involvement is seen as a reactive node with a focus of architectural destruction in the T-cell, paracortical region and with a proliferation of characteristic cells and Reed–Sternberg cells	Significance of an enlarged 'reactive' spleen at laparotomy uncertain. Debatable whether marginal zone epithelioid granulomas alone in a known case of disease elsewhere should be considered involved. Earliest involvement with recognizable Reed–Sternberg cells is usually at periphery of Malpighian body. Later architectural destruction
	In Hodgkin's disease a portion only of a node may be involved, and typically the spleen shows scattered foci, unlike non-Hodgkin's lymphoma where the whole relative structure is involved in the affected node or spleen	

PATHOLOGY OF ENLARGED LYMPH NODES AND SPLEEN

The specific pathological changes caused by diseases of the lymph nodes and spleen are summarized in *Table* 71.4; they can be described under the broad headings of immunological reactivity, neoplasia (non-Hodgkin's and Hodgkin's lymphoma) and alterations due to primary haematological disorders.

Immunological Reactivity

In reactive stages there is expansion predominantly of those compartments of the mononuclear-macrophage/lymphoid system appropriate to the immune response. Antigens eliciting an antibody response will result in increased numbers of immunoglobulin-secreting cells in the medullary cords of nodes, of red pulp of spleen, followed by the development of secondary, reactive follicle centres. Antibody response, and follicle centre reactivity, are undoubtedly beneficial in infections. Bacteria coated with specific antibody are rapidly cleared by the mononuclear-macrophage (reticulo-endothelial) cells throughout the body. Follicle centre reactivity in nodes draining tumours has been reported to have an adverse prognosis, however. Possibly tumour cells coated by antibody are less easily recognized as 'foreign' by cytotoxic T-cells.

Where cytotoxic T-cells are generated in response to a stimulus, e.g. following vaccination or in infectious mononucleosis, large dividing cells expand the paracortex around the epitheloid venules. Although the appearances may simulate neoplasia, even to the extent of showing binucleate Reed–Sternberg-like cells, there is always preservation of architecture with some reactivity evident in secondary follicles, sinuses and medullary plasma cells.

Non-antigenic material reaching nodes by way of lymphatics is removed by sinus histiocytes or, in the case of blood-borne material, by splenic red pulp macrophages. Thus, carbon pigment may be trapped in the medullary sinuses or pulmonary hilar nodes or haemosiderin in the splenic red pulp following haemolysis. Gross enlargement of lymph nodes may be seen in areas of excoriated or eczematous skin: in dermatopathic lymphadenopathy (lipomelanotic reticulosis), the sinus histiocytes become filled with fat from dead cell membranes and melanin pigment lost from the epithelial basal cells. Similarly, cells filled with lipid appear in the lymph node sinuses, or splenic pulp, in hyperlipidaemia, lipid storage disease (e.g. Gaucher's disease), or where cell membrane lipid turnover is high as in the haemolysis of thalassaemia.

Gross enlargement of the organs by expansion of the histiocytic component occurs in parasitaemia, e.g. in visceral leishmaniasis, where the histiocytes contain intracytoplasmic organisms (Leishman–Donovan bodies); and to a lesser extent in toxoplasmosis and systemic leprosy. The enlargement in malaria is more complex and involves, in addition, a major immunoresponsive component.

Neoplasia

The non-Hodgkin's tumours of the lymphoid system appear to arise in cells, the physiological counterparts of which have the capacity to migrate. Thus, the more 'differentiated' a tumour is, that is to say composed of cells morphologically closely resembling those encountered in reactive conditions, the more likely it is that sensitive methods of detecting clones of cells will demonstrate malignant cells within the appropriate traffic areas before gross destruction of architecture is evident. A good example is the overproduction of small B-lymphocytes which, if they retain their circulating capacity and appear in the blood, is called chronic lymphocytic leukaemia; or, if they become held up in nodes, with a small circulating component, lymphocytic lymphoma. Similarly in the follicular lymphomas, small cleaved cells frequently can be seen in the bone marrow (as the 'haematogones' of Rosenthal) or blood, and can be demonstrated infiltrating the B-cell areas in spleen and other lymph nodes, the architecture of which appears grossly to be preserved (*Fig.* 71.5*a*).

Demonstration of a clone of abnormal cells even within a 'normal' total white cell count, is diagnostic. Peripheral blood often proves an excellent source of such cells for immunological characterization of the tumour which often is not possible from node extracts. It is of prognostic importance since it implies that 'well-differentiated' lymphocytic lymphoma, or follicular lymphoma, detected in surgically removed nodes or spleen, is a systemic process although involvement at other sites may not be evident at the time of diagnosis.

Intermediate and high-grade lymphomas show an increasing component of large dividing cells, the tendency of which is to invade and destroy locally rather than to migrate. These tumours are often highly sensitive to radiotherapy or chemotherapy. Because they grow quickly and are soon noticed by the patient, and disseminate late, local therapy may be highly effective. Thus, it is important to stage high-grade lymphomas which, paradoxically, may have a better prognosis if locally ablated than cytologically lower-grade tumours which have spread widely by the time of diagnosis.

Hodgkin's disease differs in its tendency to spread along contiguous groups of lymph nodes, and initially to appear as a small focus within an otherwise reactive lymph node (*Fig.* 71.5*b*). In this it behaves like an epithelial tumour (cancer), although invasion of lymphatics can only rarely be demonstrated. The natural history of Hodgkin's disease has a decreasingly favourable prognosis if its composition at presentation is in the order lymphocyte predominant, nodular sclerosing, mixed cellular or lymphocyte depleted (all but nodular sclerosing tending to evolve into the lymphocyte depleted Hodgkin's 'sarcoma'). Unlike non-Hodgkin's lymphoma, Hodgkin's disease probably does not reappear at sites given adequate ablative radiotherapy. Cellular classification appears to be less important with modern radiotherapy and combination chemotherapy, but there is a real risk of the emergence of a second neoplasm, e.g. myeloid leukaemia, particularly where radiotherapy and alkylating agents have been combined.

The pathology of the non-Hodgkin's lymphomas is summarized in *Table* 71.4.

Much less is known about the nature of the true histiocytic neoplasms of lymph nodes and spleen. In the familial erythrophagocytosis (of Claireaux and Farquahar) node sinus histiocytes and splenic macrophages engulf red cells leading to profound anaemia, but there is little architectural distortion. Terminally a true monocytic leukaemia may supervene. In histiocytic medullary reticulosis a similar non-selective phagocytosis is seen. The histiocytosis-X group of diseases (eosinophilic granuloma, Hand–Schüller–Christian disease, Letterer–Siwe disease), while it may affect lymph nodes and spleen, probably is not a primary disease of these organs.

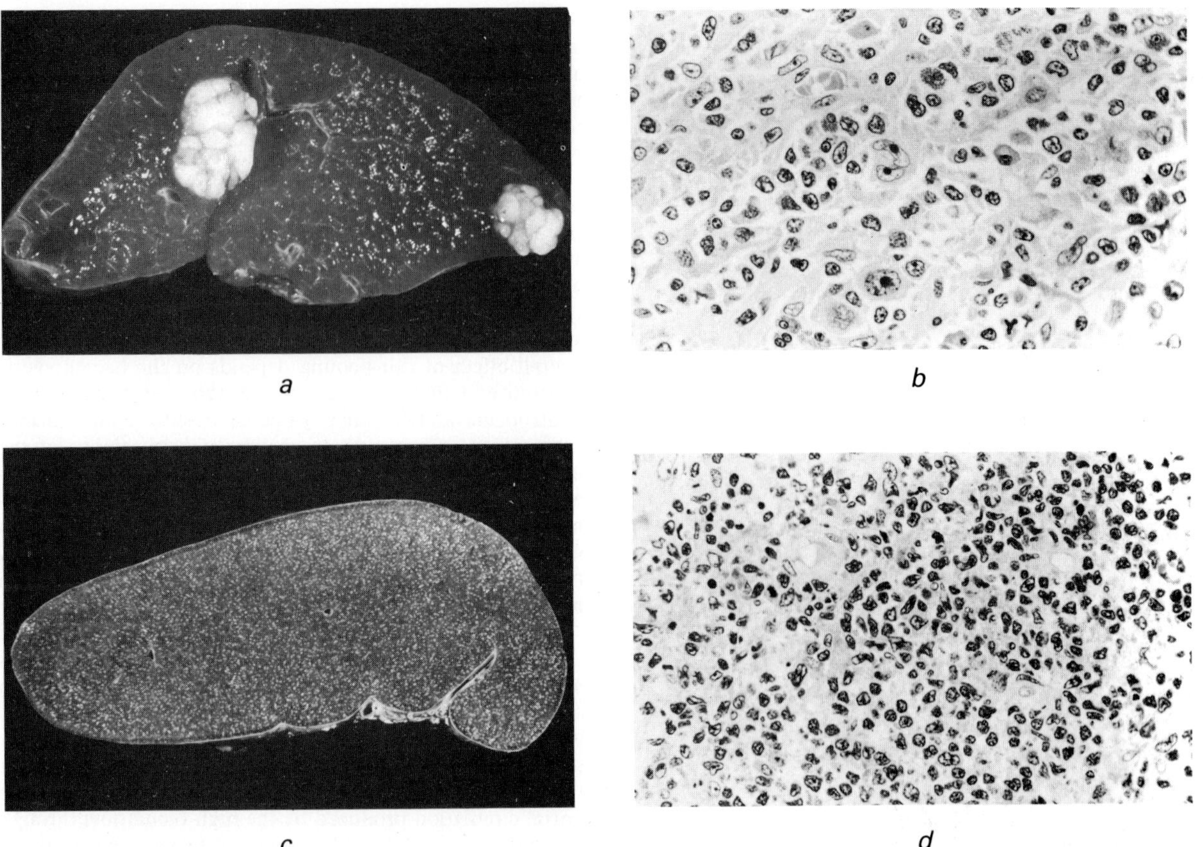

Fig. 71.5 The spleen in Hodgkin's disease and non-Hodgkin's lymphoma. *a*, Transverse section of a 200-g spleen removed at laparotomy for staging Hodgkin's disease. Two discrete tumour foci are present and histology of the intervening tissue showed only non-specific reactive features. *b*, Histology of one of the tumour nodules showing mixed cellular Hodgkin's disease. Note the central, diagnostic 'mirror image' binucleated Reed–Sternberg cell, eosinophils (with bilobed nuclei and granules in the cytoplasm, e.g. three cells from the R–S cell at one o'clock) and plasma cells (e.g. three cells away at three o'clock). The large cells with stippled nuclei are histiocytes (H and E, ×500). *c*, Transverse section of a 400-g spleen from a patient with non-Hodgkin's lymphoma. Note involvement of every Malpighian body: histologically there was minimal disturbance of architecture. *d*, Tumour cells from the white pulp of the same spleen. This is the appearance of small cleaved follicle centre cells in section: this patient had a small number of similar cleaved cells circulating with his peripheral lymphocytes in the blood (H and E, ×500).

Haematological Disorders

'Haemic reticuloses' are not often seen in biopsies of enlarged nodes since diagnosis has usually been achieved by other methods. Myeloid leukaemias may be associated with medullary lymph node proliferation, or splenic red pulp enlargement, and are readily detected by stains which bring out eosinophil granules (e.g. azo-eosin), or use of a histochemical method to demonstrate the chloracetate esterase in myelocytes. In myelosclerosis the same areas show a myeloid transformation with a high proportion of multinucleated giant cells, some resembling megakaryocytes and others the giant cells present in the bone marrow. Erythroid cells can be differentiated from lymphocytes on account of their characteristically dense nucleus, 'empty' cytoplasm and fine spherical PAS-positive cell membrane. In both genetic and acquired haemolytic anaemias there may be myeloid metaplasia in the spleen and lymph nodes.

The relative frequency of the foregoing conditions can be judged approximately from the surgical/pathological records of an average district hospital (*Tables* 71.5 and 71.6).

Table 71.5 Diagnoses in 276 surgical node biopsies

	%
Non-specific reactive	24·0
Tuberculosis	4·0
Sarcoid	1·5
Toxoplasmosis	1·4
Cat scratch fever	1·4
Miscellaneous	11·3
Secondary cancer	21·4
Non-Hodgkin's lymphoma	22·0
Hodgkin's disease	13·0

PATHOPHYSIOLOGY OF THE SPLEEN

The most important result of disordered function of the spleen is the destruction or pooling of blood cells. This may happen in two ways. First, if the spleen enlarges for any

Table 71.6 Conditions for which splenectomy was performed (655 in a 30-year period)

		%
Adjunct to other surgery		21
Traumatic rupture		18
Portal hypertension		10
Thrombocytopenic purpura		15
Hereditary spherocytosis		10
Acquired haemolytic anaemia		10
Myelofibrosis		2
'Splenic neutropenia'		1
'Splenomegaly'		13
Non-Hodgkin's lymphoma	6%	
Hodgkin's disease*	1%	
Granulocytic leukaemia	1%	
Sarcoid	1·5%	
Ill-defined	1%	
Others	2·5%	

*In the period covered splenectomy was not routinely performed in the staging of Hodgkin's disease.

reason it may trap and/or destroy cells even if they are normal. Secondly, because of its peculiar vasculature and rich macrophage population, it is well designed to destroy red cells, white cells or platelets which are in any way abnormal.

Hypersplenism

Hypersplenism is a syndrome which consists of splenomegaly associated with anaemia, leukopenia, particularly neutropenia, and thrombocytopenia. The term causes considerable confusion! Early in this century it was used to describe the role of the spleen in destroying the red cells in hereditary spherocytosis. Damashek revived it to encompass a broad spectrum of conditions in which splenomegaly is associated with depression of one or more of the formed elements of the blood. He suggested that the spleen is involved in the control of haemopoiesis, possibly through a humoral mechanism. This possibility has been examined extensively over the years but there is no experimental evidence in its favour.

The spleen can produce anaemia, neutropenia or thrombocytopenia in two ways. First, because of its peculiar vascular and phagocytic properties, it may be the site of destruction of abnormal cells. The constant exposure of the spleen to the latter, particularly red cells, produces splenic enlargement, a phenomenon which is called 'work hypertrophy'. Secondly, splenic enlargement due to primary disease of the lymphoreticular system or other pathology may result in reduction in number of one or more of the formed elements of the blood even when the latter are normal in structure and function. It is to this second group of disorders that the term 'hypersplenism' is usually applied.

Hypersplenism can be defined, therefore, as a state characterized by splenomegaly due to a wide variety of causes, associated with the following: anaemia, leucopenia, thrombocytopenia, or any combination of the three, a bone marrow which is capable of maintaining a higher output of blood cells than is apparent from their numbers in the circulation, and in which the cytopenia is corrected by splenectomy.

How does an enlarged spleen produce pancytopenia? Probably the most important mechanism is pooling of blood cells. Red cells accumulate in a splenic erythrocyte pool which increases significantly with increasing splenomegally and which may constitute up to 50% of the total red cell mass. In effect a significant number of red cells are sequestered 'outside' the circulation. This leads to a discrepancy between the peripheral venous haematocrit and the 'total body' haematocrit as obtained by isotope dilution techniques. Similarly, there may be a significant pooling of platelets in an enlarged spleen. In health, approximately 10% of the circulating platelets are in the spleen at any time; with significant splenomegaly pooling increases progressively and may involve up to 90% of the platelets. There is also significant trapping of granulocytes in enlarged spleens. The overall effect of cell pooling depends on the haemopoietic capability of the bone marrow, i.e. the degree of anaemia, neutropenia and thrombocytopenia reflects a fine balance between the magnitude of pooling and the ability of the marrow to compensate. In disorders such as myelosclerosis or chronic myeloid leukaemia, where there may be a diminished bone marrow reserve, splenic pooling may cause a severe degree of anaemia, thrombocytopenia or neutropenia; this may occur to a lesser extent or not at all if the marrow is healthy.

Hypervolaemia is another feature of splenomegaly. In diseases which limit red cell production the expanded blood volume is provided mainly by plasma and if there is a significant splenomegaly the plasma volume may be markedly increased. The result is a dilutional anaemia which tends to add to the effect of splenic pooling of red cells. The favoured mechanism is the development of a hyperkinetic portal circulation produced by the high blood flow through the enlarged spleen with expansion of the splanchnic vasculature upstream from the portal vein. How this actually produces an increased plasma volume is far from clear, however. As well as causing some degree of haemodilution the high plasma volume renders patients with hypersplenism particularly difficult to transfuse without circulatory overloading.

In addition to the trapping of a large proportion of the red cell mass in large spleens there is good evidence that the survival of normal red cells may be reduced. This may result from various 'metabolic stresses' applied to the red cells as they are packed together in the enlarged spleen. These include glucose deprivation, lactate accumulation and a fall in pH. The haemolytic component of this type of hypersplenism is mild, however. Evidence for thrombocytopenia and neutropenia due to a similar mechanism is less solid.

Specific Destruction of Blood Cells by the Spleen

Abnormal red cells may be destroyed in the spleen. Those of patients with hereditary spherocytosis are particularly prone, presumably due to their inherent metabolic abnormalities. Heinz bodies, produced by haemoglobin precipitation due to genetic defects of the molecule or the action of oxidant drugs, are 'pitted' out of cells with subsequent membrane damage. Similarly, in the warm antibody autoimmune haemolytic anaemias red cells coated with IgG, because of the peculiar anatomy of the spleen, come into close proximity to macrophages with specific receptors for these molecules. It seems likely that a similar mechanism is responsible for the destruction of platelets in some forms of idiopathic or drug-induced thrombocytopenic purpura. Similarly, there is increasing evidence that the neutropenia of Felty's syndrome (rheumatoid arthritis with splenomegaly) has an immune basis. Leucocyte-specific antinuclear factor has been demonstrated in the blood of patients with this disorder and others associated with neutropenia and splenomegaly.

Splenic Infarction

Due to the peculiar vasculature of the spleen infarction of an enlarged spleen is not uncommon. It occurs particularly in patients with myelosclerosis or chronic myeloid leukaemia but can occur with almost any cause of splenomegaly. It results in an inflammatory reaction on the serous surface and if this occurs over the area of contact with the left dome of the diaphragm it may be responsible for left basal pleurisy and pain referred to the left shoulder. It is easily recognized if accompanied by a friction rub. It requires no therapy but mild analgesia, but repeated infarction may be an indication for surgery.

Causes of Splenomegaly

The causes of splenomegaly are summarized in *Tables* 71.6 and 71.7. The spleen may enlarge transiently in a variety of acute infections, particularly those due to viruses, in chronic infections, such as brucellosis and tuberculosis, and in subacute bacterial endocarditis. Massive splenomegaly may result from several tropical disorders including malaria, leishmaniasis and schistosomiasis. Moderate enlargement may accompany any cause of portal hypertension.

Splenomegaly is a feature of a variety of disorders of the red cell. The fact that it occurs in most chronic haemolytic anaemias suggests that spleen growth may be stimulated by an increase in its workload, i.e. that when the spleen is being constantly bombarded with abnormal red cells it increases in size, allowing a larger area for red cell–macrophage interaction and therefore a vicious circle of increasing red cell destruction and increasing splenomegaly. The spleen enlarges in about one-third of patients with megaloblastic anaemia but less commonly in iron-deficiency anaemia. Similarly, splenomegaly is unusual in the acquired aplastic anaemias although for some unexplained reason it occurs in a significant number of children with the various congenital hypoplastic anaemias. It also occurs quite frequently in patients with dyserythropoietic anaemias, such as sideroblastic anaemia, some of which are preleukaemic states.

Splenomegaly is a regular finding in the myeloproliferative disorders. Although this has been explained by the process of myeloid metaplasia in myelosclerosis, histological examination of the spleen in polycythaemia vera does not show extramedullary erythropoiesis, certainly in the early stages of the illness. The spleen may also enlarge in any form of leukaemia or lymphoma; the mechanism was described earlier. However, the enlarged spleens found in association with Hodgkin's disease or non-Hodgkin's lymphoma do not always show histological evidence of the tumour. An extreme example of this phenomenon is the condition called idiopathic non-tropical splenomegaly in which massive splenomegaly with relatively normal histology may precede the clinical appearance of a lymphoma by months or even years.

Rarer causes of splenomegaly are summarized in *Table* 71.7.

Table 71.7 Causes of enlargement of the spleen

Acute bacterial, viral and other infections
Subacute bacterial endocarditis
Chronic bacterial infections; TB and brucellosis
Chronic parasitic infections.* Malaria,* kala-azar,* schistosomiasis
Idiopathic non-tropical splenomegaly*†
Tropical splenomegaly*
'Congestive'; portal hypertension
Hereditary spherocytosis (HS)†
Symptomatic elliptocytosis†
Structural haemoglobinopathy, e.g. HbC disease
Thalassaemia†
Red cell enzyme defects
Acquired haemolytic anaemia
Warm antibody haemolytic anaemia†
Cryopathic haemolytic syndrome
Primary blood dyscrasia
Acute leukaemia
Chronic myeloid leukaemia
Chronic lymphatic leukaemia
Polycythaemia vera
Myelosclerosis*†
Trauma
Perisplenic haematoma
Reticulosis
Hodgkin's disease
Non-Hodgkin's lymphoma
True histiocytic tumours
Miscellaneous
Amyloid, sarcoidosis, tumour of the spleen†
Connective tissue disorders
SLE
Felty's syndrome†

*Sometimes cause massive splenomegaly.
†Splenectomy indicated in some cases.

THE CLINICAL ASSESSMENT OF SPLENOMEGALY

The clinical significance of splenomegaly can be assessed by answering three questions: is a mass in the left upper quadrant really an enlarged spleen; if so, why it is enlarged; and will splenectomy benefit the patient?

The Differential Diagnosis of Left Upper Quadrant Masses

A mass in the left upper quadrant which moves downwards and slightly medially on respiration is usually an enlarged spleen. It is very important to start the examination with the right hand well down in the right iliac fossa and the left hand round the lower left costal margin with the patient taking moderately deep breaths with a relaxed abdomen. As the right hand moves upwards towards the left upper quadrant it will meet the edge of the spleen coming downwards and medially. If the mass is a spleen it is usually impossible to get above it and it is sometimes possible to feel a genuine edge and notch (the latter not so often!). Because the spleen is quite superficially placed it is usually dull to percussion anteriorly. If the patient has experienced pain in that region it is sometimes possible to hear a rub. The soft, enlarged spleens which accompany systemic infections are sometimes easier to feel with the patient lying on the right side.

The most common difficulty experienced with masses in the left upper quadrant is mistaking an enlarged spleen for an enlarged left kidney or a neoplasm of the splenic flexure of the colon or stomach. Renal enlargement is usually fairly obvious because the mass feels like a kidney, tends to move directly downwards on respiration rather than downwards and medially, and often has a band of resonance in front of it because of its relationship to the descending colon. Colonic and gastric masses do not move well on respiration, usually have an irregular shape and it is often possible to get above them.

In a very obese patient in whom splenomegaly is suspected it is sometimes useful to carry out a straight radiograph of the abdomen to assess the size and location of the splenic shadow. The distinction from the left kidney can be confirmed by an intravenous pyelogram and if there is still doubt a splenic scan will confirm the diagnosis. We shall consider the various ways of visualizing the spleen later in the chapter.

Investigation of the Cause of Splenomegaly

A palpable spleen is enlarged two to three times normal. A normal-sized spleen is never palpable. Splenomegaly should always be carefully investigated.

We considered the causes of splenomegaly in the previous section. With the aid of a good history and clinical examination together with a few simple laboratory and radiological investigations it is possible to determine the cause of splenomegaly in the majority of patients. However, a small group of patients will remain in whom, after all these investigations have been carried out, the cause of the splenomegaly still remains uncertain. We will consider the further management of this problem later.

In taking a history from a patient with splenomegaly it is particularly important to find out whether they have any symptoms suggestive of infection or malignant disease and where they have travelled over the preceding years. A history of previous liver disease and/or jaundice should be sought and the level of alcohol consumption should be very carefully determined from the patient or relatives (or both). It should be remembered that pruritus, particularly related to bathing or a warm bed, is a very common symptom in the myeloproliferative disorders, particularly polycythaemia vera and myelosclerosis. Clinical examination must include a very careful study of the superficial lymph nodes and the tonsillar and adenoidal tissues, a search for stigmas of liver disease, a full examination of the skin for evidence of purpura or bruising, and a complete survey of all the systems.

A few simple laboratory investigations will provide the cause for most cases of splenomegaly. Almost all the splenomegalies associated with haematological disorders can be diagnosed by a complete blood examination together with a bone marrow aspiration or biopsy. Liver disease is often associated with abnormal liver function tests or oesophageal varices on a barium swallow examination. Liver biopsy may be necessary to determine the type of liver pathology. The diagnosis of lymphoma or other RE malignancies may be accomplished by biopsy of a suitable node, the liver or another involved organ, lymphangiography or bone marrow biopsy; in some cases it may be necessary to go to a diagnostic splenectomy (*see below*). The various infections which produce splenomegaly may be identified from appropriate haematological or serological studies. In UK practice infectious mononucleosis is the commonest infective cause; it is diagnosed by the finding of atypical lymphocytes in the blood, a positive Paul–Bunnell test (or related screening procedures) and a rising anti-Epstein–Barr virus titre. In those who have travelled to the tropics, malarial parasites should be looked for and the marrow examined for Leishman–Donovan bodies. Particularly in immigrant populations the possibility of disseminated tuberculosis should always be considered; this is probably best diagnosed by liver biopsy or (rarely in the experience of the authors) by culture of the bone marrow.

Assessment of Hypersplenism

In assessing whether the removal of an enlarged spleen will benefit the patient there are two main factors to be considered; the cause of the splenomegaly and whether there is a significant degree of hypersplenism. There are some conditions in which splenectomy is almost always associated with an improvement of the patient's clinical condition; these are considered in the next section. However, there are many disorders including haemolytic anaemias, the myeloproliferative states, Felty's syndrome and some malignancies in which there may be a significant degree of splenomegaly and hypersplenism may be suspected, but it is not clear to what degree the spleen is contributing to the clinical disability. How does one proceed to determine whether splenectomy is indicated?

As mentioned earlier hypersplenism is usually associated with anaemia, neutropenia or thrombocytopenia. The neutropenia may be so severe as to cause recurrent infection and the thrombocytopenia may be associated with purpura. It is vitally important to obtain a good bone marrow sample as part of the routine work-up of patients with suspected hypersplenism. If the spleen is playing a major role in pooling or destruction of the formed elements of the blood, and if splenectomy is to be helpful, the bone marrow must be relatively cellular with adequate numbers of healthy red cell, white cell and platelet precursors. It is often necessary to carry out a trephine biopsy to assess the overall cellularity of the bone marrow. In severe hypersplenism the marrow is often hypercellular and the red and white cell precursors may be described as showing a 'maturation arrest'. This is a confusing term which simply means that there are more early precursors present than usual. This does not necessarily mean that they are 'arrested' in their maturation pathway. Rather, because of the rapid consumption of white cells in the large spleen, there is a paucity of late forms in the marrow. However, sometimes simple morphological analysis of this kind is insufficient and more sophisticated isotope techniques are required to determine the degree of hypersplenism.

In the further assessment of splenic function three questions can be asked: (1) What is the state of bone marrow function? (2) Is there pooling or destruction of formed elements of the blood in the spleen? (3) Is the spleen contributing significantly to red cell production? For assessing bone marrow function a small dose of transferrin-bound radioactive iron is administered and its rate of disappearance from the blood and its reappearance in the red cells is measured. In normal individuals about 90% of the dose of iron is incorporated into red cells in about 10–14 days, whereas if there is severe haemolysis or marrow dysfunction this figure may be altered. Rapid disappearance of iron with a reduced rate of reappearance occurs in haemolytic or dyserythropoietic disorders; slow clearance occurs in hypoplastic anaemias. The sites of erythropoiesis can be assessed by external counting over the spine, sacrum, spleen, etc. A large accumulation of iron over the spleen suggests that this is a site of significant erythropoiesis. In assessing splenic pooling it is useful to compare the circulating red cell mass with the peripheral blood haematocrit; if there is a gross discrepancy and the haematocrit is much lower than might be expected from the circulating red cell mass, this suggests that part of the latter is being held in the enlarged spleen. A plasma volume estimation is also very useful because it is often markedly elevated in patients with hypersplenism. Finally, red cell survival is measured by ^{51}Cr labelling and the major sites of destruction assessed by external scanning.

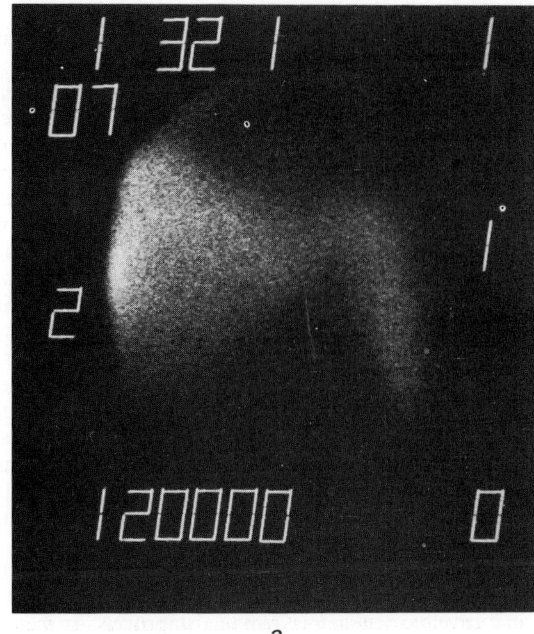

a

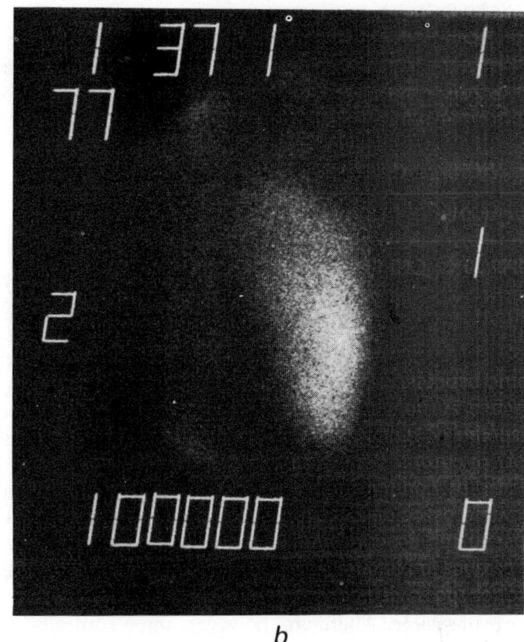

b

Fig. 71.6 Spleen scans ($^{99}Tc^{m}$). *a*, A scan showing a normal-sized spleen and liver. *b*, A much enlarged spleen with no uptake of the colloid by the liver. This is from a case of portal hypertension with cirrhosis of the liver. (By courtesy of Dr Basil Shepstone.)

A rising level of radioactivity over the spleen as compared with the liver suggests that red cell destruction is occurring mainly in the spleen. These rather crude tests give some indication of the degree of hypersplenism and the role of the spleen in haemolysis but until recently their value was strictly limited and it was very difficult to assess whether a patient with myelosclerosis, for example, was producing a significant amount of blood in the spleen.

Recently, several better techniques have been developed for analysing splenic function. It is now possible to estimate the size of the spleen, to measure phagocytic function, to identify the major sites of red cell destruction, to quantify the amount of splenic red cell destruction, to measure the size of the splenic red cell pool, and to identify and quantitate the degree of extramedullary erythropoiesis in the spleen.

The spleen can be visualized by scintillation counting following injection of labelled red cells after they have been heated at 49·5 °C for 20 min which causes them to be sequestered preferentially in the organ (*Fig.* 71.6). If, after heating they are labelled with ^{51}Cr or $^{99}Tc^{m}$ it is possible to obtain an accurate estimation of splenic size. In assessing the major sites of red cell destruction the cells are labelled with ^{51}Cr and, using a carefully calibrated external scanning system, it is possible to observe four major patterns of surface counting: (1) accumulation in the spleen alone; (2) accumulation in the liver alone; (3) no accumulation in either organ; or (4) accumulation in both organs. Recently developed techniques of quantitative scanning using ^{51}Cr or ^{81}Rb red cell labelling with a dual detector system allow the amount of red cell destruction to be quantified fairly accurately. This type of approach can be modified using red cells labelled with ^{11}C-carbon monoxide, $^{99}Tc^{m}$ or ^{51}Cr to measure the actual size of the splenic red cell pool. A normal spleen contains less than 5 per cent of the circulating red cell mass while in some disorders associated with splenomegaly and pooling as much as 40–60% of the circulating red cell mass, i.e. approximately a litre of blood, may be held in the spleen. Recently-developed techniques for producing the short-lived isotope ^{52}Fe in the cyclotron have made it possible, using a quantitative scanning technique, to determine the major sites of erythropoiesis. Interestingly, in some cases of myelosclerosis a significant amount of red cell production may occur in the spleen.

Some of the techniques mentioned above are still in the stage of development and are rarely required in clinical practice. Their major place is in the assessment of patients with myeloproliferative disorders, Felty's syndrome or other disorders in which it is difficult to predict the outcome of surgery. In the majority of other conditions the decision as to whether to remove the spleen can be made on more simple clinical grounds together with a blood count, plasma volume determination, measurement of the red cell mass and survival, and external counting over the spleen and liver to determine the major sites of red cell destruction.

INDICATIONS FOR SPLENECTOMY

The indications for splenectomy can be classified into three groups (3Ds) namely; (1) Definite or absolute, when splenectomy is essential; (2) Desirable, when splenectomy is usually beneficial; and (3) Debatable, when splenectomy may or may not help the patient.

1. Definite Indications for Splenectomy

These include the following:

a. Primary, benign or malignant, neoplasms of the spleen
b. Splenic abscess
c. Splenic echinococcal cyst
d. Splenic vein thrombosis causing left-sided hypertension and gastric varices

e. Splenic artery aneurysm
f. Radical operations for malignant lesions originating in the stomach, distal pancreas or hepatic flexure of the colon.
g. Staging for Hodgkin's lymphoma
h. Splenic injury that is not amenable to salvage.

Rupture of the Spleen

Rupture of the spleen usually occurs after severe trauma to the abdomen or chest in previously healthy patients. There are certain pathological states in which rupture is more likely to occur. It is an occasional complication of an acute viral illness such as infectious mononucleosis. The large spleens associated with tropical disorders or myelosclerosis are particularly prone to rupture after minor trauma. Rarely, a rapidly enlarging spleen in the aggressive forms of non-Hodgkin's lymphoma may rupture spontaneously. A hilar pancreatic pseudocyst associated with splenic vein thrombosis may also rupture into the spleen causing massive exsanguination.

Because of the fear of postsplenectomy sepsis discussed previously, the tendency is to preserve normal splenic tissue whenever possible. There are, however, some contraindications to splenic preservation in the trauma patient. These include the following:

1. The spleen is not amenable to salvage because of any of the following:
a. Hilar avulsion injuries
b. Blast injuries to the left upper quadrant
c. Multiple associated injuries
d. Gross intra-abdominal contamination
e. Rupture of a pathological spleen
2. The patient is unstable and/or elderly and the operative emphasis has to be shifted to quick haemostasis as opposed to splenic salvage.

The high incidence of complications after splenectomy in patients with myelosclerosis has led several centres to adopt a conservative (non-operative) approach to the presence of a small perisplenic haematoma in these patients. Such patients are then treated by strict bedrest and careful observation of the size of the splenic mass by ultrasonography or computed tomography. In many cases these lesions resolve on such conservative treatment but if the mass is enlarging or if there are signs of continuous bleeding, laparotomy is clearly indicated.

2. Desirable Indications for Splenectomy

There are certain haematological disorders which are nearly always improved or cured by splenectomy. These include symptomatic hereditary spherocytosis, chronic idiopathic thrombocytopenic purpura, warm antibody autoimmune haemolytic anaemia which has failed to respond to corticosteroid therapy, and some cases of genetic red cell enzymopathy such as pyruvate kinase deficiency.

3. Debatable Indications for Splenectomy

These include disorders in which splenectomy may be beneficial in some cases. Clinical judgement is paramount in these situations. The risk/benefit ratio must be carefully analysed in each case.

A simple cyst or pseudocyst of the spleen may be observed if it is small (under 5 cm in diameter). If operation is dictated, simple drainage and unroofing of the cyst may be all that is necessary. One must be very sure in these situations that the cyst is non-parasitic in nature.

Splenectomy may reduce blood transfusion requirements in some of the genetic disorders of haemoglobin synthesis, such as the thalassaemia syndromes. It may also be indicated in some cases of tropical splenomegaly and in patients with lymphomas in which severe neutropenia prevents the administration of adequate chemotherapy. It is also useful in the storage diseases. It may be indicated occasionally in fulminating thrombocytopenic purpura or immune haemolysis in which corticosteroid therapy has failed and there is life-threatening bleeding or anaemia.

Splenectomy as the sole treatment for patients with portal hypertension is fraught with difficulty and is best avoided. However, the operation is definitely of value in documented cases of splenic vein thrombosis with left-sided portal hypertension. Splenectomy has also a definite place as part and parcel of a gastro-oesophageal devascularization procedure such as the Siugura operation which is sometimes advocated for variceal haemorrhage.

The place of splenectomy in the myeloproliferative disorders is more controversial. Its value in the management of chronic myeloid leukaemia remains unproven. It may be occasionally indicated in myelosclerosis where it is reserved for those patients in whom there is massive splenomegaly and where isotope analysis indicates that there is a very large splenic pool of sequestered red cells but that there is an insignificant amount of erythropoiesis in the spleen as compared with the bone marrow. Splenectomy in patients with this disorder is fraught with all sorts of postoperative problems, particularly thrombocytosis which may result in postoperative thromboembolic disease. Current interest centres on the notion that the spleen should be removed early in the natural history of myelosclerosis to prevent the late complications due to massive splenomegaly, but because the disease has such a variable course and prognosis, this remains a debatable issue.

Undiagnosed Splenomegaly and Symptomatic Splenomegaly

The place of a diagnostic splenectomy in the staging of lymphoma is discussed later.

Patients are encountered occasionally in whom all diagnostic tests to determine the cause of splenomegaly are unhelpful. It is very difficult to know how to manage an otherwise healthy patient with an enlarged spleen. If the patient is symptom-free and the organ is only slightly enlarged, it is reasonable to watch him carefully for a while. If the organ is continuing to enlarge or if it is already significantly enlarged at the first examination, it is probably wiser to perform a diagnostic splenectomy. If the histology is completely normal, these patients should be followed carefully since a lymphoma may develop months or years later. In many patients with unexplained splenomegaly the histology of the spleen will provide a diagnosis, usually that of one or other form of lymphoma.

Some patients with an enlarged spleen from whatever cause develop recurrent symptoms of pain and tenderness in the left upper quadrant as a result of splenic congestion and/or infarction. If these symptoms are genuinely troublesome, splenectomy may be indicated to alleviate the problem, provided that the risks of the operation and its potential deleterious effects on the underlying disease process are carefully weighed against the benefit of pain relief.

PREOPERATIVE ASSESSMENT AND PREPARATION OF PATIENTS FOR SPLENECTOMY

Apart from the usual preoperative assessment of patients for any major operation those who are about to undergo splenectomy require particular attention to the haematological findings and liver function tests. Patients with relative bone marrow failure or with immune platelet destruction as part of chronic idiopathic thrombocytopenic purpura may be markedly thrombocytopenic before surgery. If the thrombocytopenia results from bone marrow failure it is perfectly reasonable to tide them over the period of the operation with platelet infusions. These are less successful in idiopathic thrombocytopenic purpura but if a patient is going to surgery with a platelet count of less than 50 000 it is reasonable to give platelets if there is any excess bleeding during surgery and certainly for the first 24–48 hours after the operation. The object is to keep the splenic bed dry until the platelet count is rising after the operation. Patients who are going for splenectomy with a prolonged prothrombin time or other evidence of liver failure require replacement therapy with fresh frozen plasma or concentrates. It is useful to ask the Blood Transfusion Service for blood which is as fresh as possible in patients of this type.

THE COMPLICATIONS OF SPLENECTOMY

It is convenient to consider the complications of splenectomy under the headings of early complications, and the undoubted increased proneness to infection which is usually a later complication of the operation.

Early Complications

The commonest complication at or just after surgery is bleeding. Apart from major vessel bleeding this usually is characterized by a continuous ooze from the splenic bed. It is particularly common after removal of very large spleens in which there have been one or more preceding episodes of splenic infarction as these spleens are often adherent to the peritoneal surface of the diaphragm. This type of generalized oozing may produce a large collection within several hours of surgery necessitating re-exploration of the abdomen. In addition, small collections may become infected and lead to a subphrenic abscess. This complication seems to be particularly common in patients who remain relatively thrombocytopenic after splenectomy and if the platelets remain below 50 000/µl in the days following the operation, the period should be covered with platelet infusions. It also occurs in patients with myeloproliferative diseases who have abnormal platelet function, and in those with liver disease whose coagulation abnormalities have not been adequately corrected preoperatively with fresh frozen plasma or similar concentrates. Damage to the fundus of the stomach is a well-recognized cause of subphrenic abscess after splenectomy.

Provided scrupulous care is taken to ensure complete haemostasis and early mobilization and breathing exercises are started, subphrenic abscess should be a relatively rare complication. Other surgical complications include damage to the tail of the pancreas resulting in abscess, fistula or pancreatitis.

Many patients develop a transient thrombocytosis after splenectomy. Fortunately with early mobilization serious superficial or deep vein thrombosis is rare. In that small number of patients who develop persistent thrombocytosis in excess of 1 000 000/µl, but commonly seen in individuals who have undergone splenectomy for myeloproliferative disorders, it may be necessary to use antiplatelet agents, such as aspirin or persantin, or even anticoagulants.

Infection

This has been fully discussed previously.

Late Thromboembolic Complications

A small number of patients develop migrating thrombophlebitis or more serious deep vein thrombosis and thromboembolic complications after splenectomy. This particular complication seems to occur particularly in two settings. It is seen in patients with haemolytic anaemia in whom there has been a poor response to the operation. There seems to be an inverse relationship between the postoperative haemoglobin level and the platelet count, those patients who remain anaemic having dangerously high platelet counts. The other

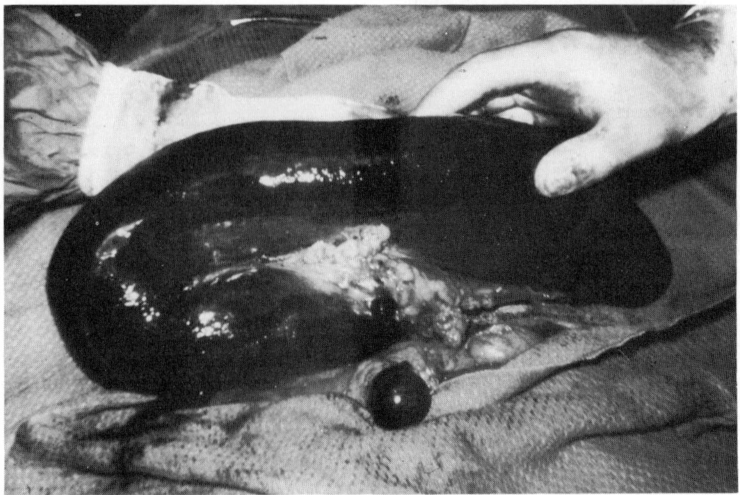

Fig. 71.7 Large spleen and accessory splenunculus in a patient with congenital spherocytosis.

group in which this complication occurs is made up of patients with myeloproliferative disorders where again the platelet count may reach extremely high values after splenectomy. These patients may require long-term anti-platelet agents or anticoagulant therapy.

Accessory Spleens

The hypertrophy of an accessory spleen is a rare but well-documented cause of a reappearance of symptoms of haemolysis or thrombocytopenia in patients with congenital spherocytosis or thrombocytopenic purpura. The accessory spleen can be visualized by one of the imaging techniques mentioned in an earlier section and, at least in the case of hereditary spherocytosis, the haemolysis can be stopped by removing the accessory spleen (*Fig.* 71.7).

There has been considerable interest recently in the possibility that splenic tissue is seeded into the peritoneum in patients who have had a ruptured spleen followed by a splenectomy. This idea arose when it was noted that the changes of hyposplenism tend to be less marked in children who have had a splenectomy following trauma than in those who have had an elective splenectomy for a haematological disorder. Since the former group seem to have less infections it is seriously suggested that when splenectomy is performed early in life some splenic tissue should be left behind in the peritoneal cavity. Indeed, successful splenic autotransplantation using splenic slices implanted into omental pouch has been reported and is desirable whenever splenic preservation is impossible, as in traumatic hilar disruption of the spleen.

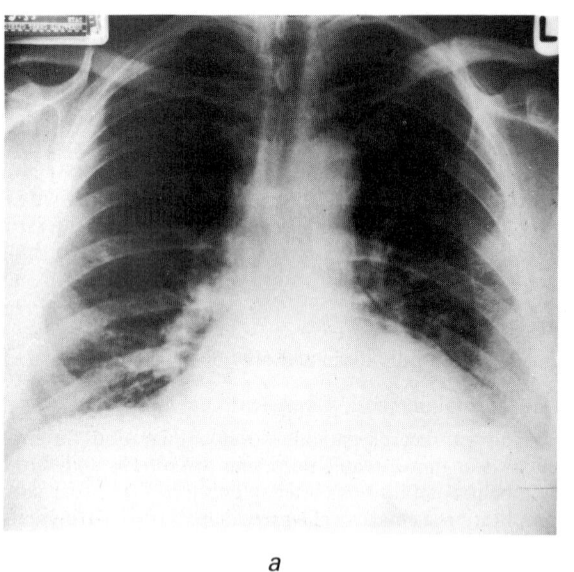

a

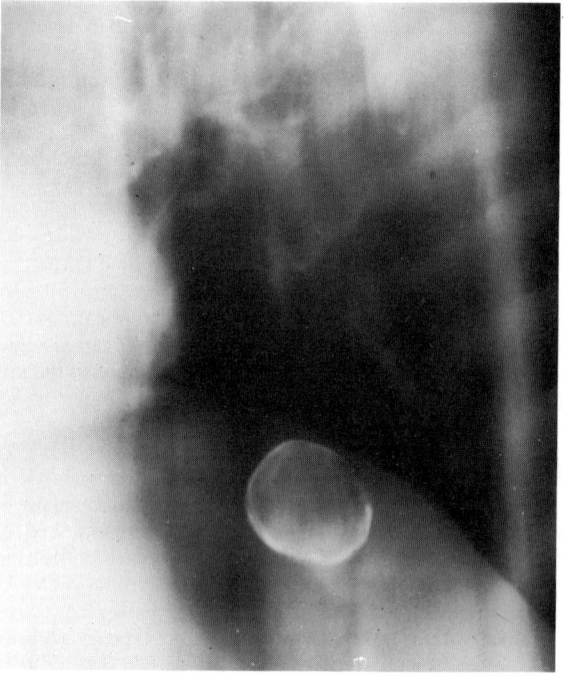

b

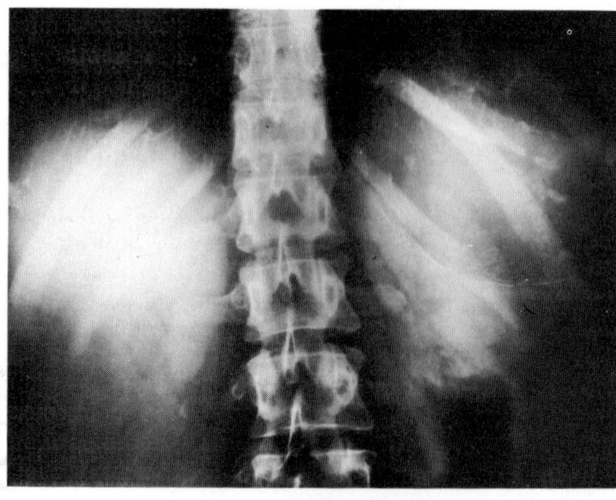

c

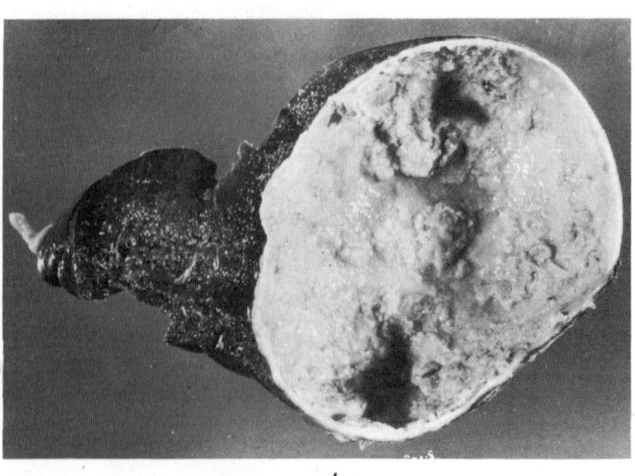

d

Fig. 71.8 *a*, Postero-anterior projection of chest showing a round opacity below the left diaphragm. This is well demonstrated in the lateral tomogram. (*b*) showing a cystic shadow with a calcified rim in the region of the spleen representing a hydatid cyst. *c*, Large, uninfected, partially calcified cyst in the spleen. The patient complained of an ache in the left hypochondrium. *d*, Resected specimen. Histological examination confirmed it as a dermoid cyst.

MISCELLANEOUS CONDITIONS

Splenic Abscess

Abscesses in the spleen may be multiple or solitary. Multiple splenic abscess formation is usually fatal and occurs as an end-stage manifestation of uncontrolled sepsis often associated with endocarditis, leukaemia, diabetes and prematurity. Solitary splenic abscess is rare. It may result from metastatic or contiguous spread of infection or follow trauma (infection of a splenic haematoma).

Presentation is usually delayed. Symptoms and signs include fever, pain and tenderness in the left upper quadrant. Splenomegaly is found in 40%. The chest radiograph often shows a left-sided effusion and the diaphragm is immobile on X-ray screening. Splenic scans (isotope/ultrasound) or arteriography have been used to confirm the diagnosis preoperatively. Untreated, the condition carries a high mortality because of the tendency for the abscess to rupture. Splenectomy performed before the onset of this complication is curative.

Splenic Cysts (*Fig.* 71.8)

The majority of cystic lesions of the spleen are post-traumatic pseudocysts. True cysts are rare and include haemangioma, lymphangioma, parasitic, epidermoid and dermoid cysts.

The symptoms of benign non-parasitic cysts are non-specific and size-related. They include a palpable mass and ache in the left upper quadrant. They may, however, rupture and present acutely with peritonitis or internal haemorrhage. Infection results in abscess formation. The diagnosis of a splenic cyst is made either by ultrasound scanning or by computed tomography. Splenectomy is recommended to relieve the symptoms and to avoid complications.

Splenic Vein Thrombosis

Thrombosis of the splenic vein not infrequently arises as a complication of chronic alcoholic pancreatitis. Splenic vein thrombosis has also been reported in infants after umbilical vein catheterization and infusion. It can also arise from involvement by pancreatic cancer.

Splenic vein thrombosis results in splenomegaly and sectorial hypertension with varices limited to the gastro-epiploic veins (*Fig.* 71.9). Often the gastric varices result in severe bleeding. The liver is normal and the pressure in the portal vein is not elevated. The condition is diagnosed either by splenoportography or by the venous phase of coeliac or superior mesenteric arteriography. Splenectomy is curative. Shunt procedures are contraindicated for bleeding varices due to sectorial hypertension consequent on splenic vein thrombosis.

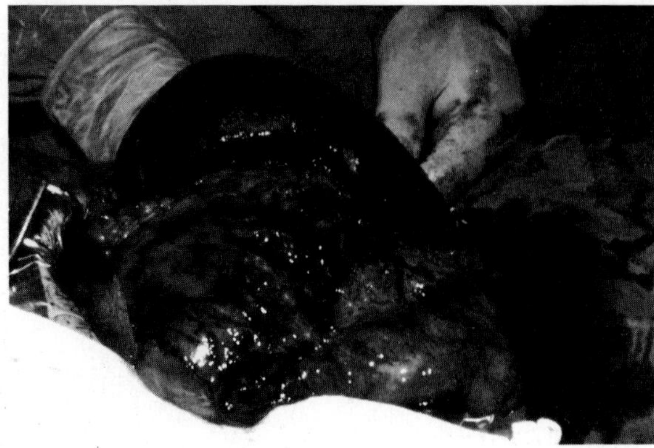

Fig. 71.9 Sectorial hypertension caused by chronic pancreatitis with splenic vein thrombosis. The patient presented with severe haematemesis. The spleen was enlarged. Endoscopy showed bleeding gastric varices. Note the distended veins along the greater curvature and in the fundal region of the stomach, together with the splenomegaly.

Gaucher's Disease

This hereditary disorder is due to a specific enzyme defect (β-glucocerebrosidase) and results in the accumulation of lipid (lipodystrophy). There are three types: Type I, the adult form (commonest), Type II, the infantile form which is neuropathic and universally fatal in early life, and Type III, the intermediate form. The adult form results in splenomegaly, thrombocytopenia, brownish discoloration of the limbs and pinqueculae. Characteristic changes are encountered in the long bones in 50% of patients and fat-laden cells (Gaucher's cells) are seen in bone marrow aspirates. Splenectomy is indicated for hypersplenism and uncomfortable massive enlargement of the spleen.

ENLARGEMENT OF THE LYMPH NODES; LYMPHADENOPATHY

The majority of important disorders of the lymphorecticular system are associated with either localized or generalized lymph node enlargement. Some of the commoner groups of causes of lymphadenopathy are summarized in *Table* 71.4.

Local Infection

Localized lymph node enlargement is a common accompaniment of many acute bacterial infections, particularly those due to the streptococcus or staphylococcus. The overlying skin and tissues may become reddened and oedematous but with appropriate antibiotic treatment it is now extremely uncommon for the lymphadenitis to progress to abscess or sinus formation. The persistence of localized lymphadenopathy in association with constitutional symptoms suggests an unusual cause. Cat scratch fever usually presents with a single tender node and is not often associated with splenomegaly. Chronic infections may produce considerable lymphadenopathy without signs of inflammation. A chronically enlarged group of cervical nodes which are matted together and firm and which show calcification and sinus formation is commonly associated with primary *bovine* tuberculosis. Syphilis, leprosy, fungus infection and lymphogranuloma venereum can produce a chronic, indolent lymphadenopathy.

The site of enlarged lymph nodes may be of some diagnostic help. Enlarged occipital nodes usually indicate chronic scalp infection; malignant lymphoreticular disease almost never begins in this site. Posterior auricular node enlargement is very frequently seen in rubella. Again, the anterior auricular nodes are not usually involved early in lymphoma and are usually associated with infections of the eyelids or conjunctivae. The commonest cause of axillary node enlargement is infection and this is a much less frequent site for presentation of lymphoma and Hodgkin's disease than the neck. Painless epitrochlear lymph node enlargement is seen commonly in many of the childhood viral diseases or in generalized tuberculosis or secondary syphilis but is very rare in sarcoidosis. Inguinal lymph nodes are easily palpable in most adults, particularly in athletes. Mediastinal or hilar nodes do not usually become enlarged with bacterial pneumonias but tuberculosis, primary or haematogenous, can produce unilateral hilar lymphadenopathy. The commonest causes of hilar adenopathy are sarcoidosis and malignant disease though infectious mononucleosis may cause mediastinal lymphadenopathy which may last for several months. Intra-abdominal or retroperitoneal lymphadenopathy is rarely of inflammatory origin, tuberculosis being the exception.

Generalized Infective Lymphadenopathy

By far the commonest cause of generalized lymphadenopathy is acute viral illness, particularly infectious mononucleosis, viral hepatitis, influenza, cytomegalovirus infection, rubella and infectious lymphocytosis. Fever and lymph node enlargement can occur in patients with secondary syphilis and acute leptospirosis, salmonellosis, typhoid and paratyphoid and generalized haematogenous tuberculosis. Protozoan infections, such as toxoplasmosis, are also relatively common causes of an illness resembling infectious mononucleosis.

Other Non-neoplastic Causes of Generalized Lymphadenopathy

Generalized lymphadenopathy may occur in association with autoimmune haemolytic anaemias, collagen vascular disorders, hypersensitivity reactions, hyperthyroidism, and with skin disorders, such as exfoliative dermatitis.

Malignant Lymphadenopathy: Secondary Carcinoma

Secondary carcinoma usually produces a hard, painless lymphadenopathy at the site of drainage of the primary tumour.

Malignant Lymphoma: Hodgkin's Disease and Non-Hodgkin's Lymphoma

A classification of Hodgkin's disease and non-Hodgkin's lymphoma is shown in *Table* 71.4. These conditions present commonly with superficial lymph node enlargement.

A historical classification of the different forms of Hodgkin's disease is shown in *Table* 71.4. It is a disorder which affects young to middle-aged adults, with a predilection for males. The most common presentation is painless lymphadenopathy and the neck is the apparent site of origin of the disease in 60–80% of patients, the left side being involved rather more often than the right. The axillary nodes are the first to appear in 6–20% of patients and the mediastinal nodes in 6–11% with the inguinal nodes being the primary site in about the same proportion of cases. Once they have appeared the nodes may grow slowly over a long period or much more rapidly, producing local pain. The size of the nodes may fluctuate considerably but they rarely disappear completely. Sooner or later systemic manifestations develop which include general malaise, lack of energy, anorexia, weight loss, sweating, intermittent bouts of fever and pruritus. As the disease progresses hepatosplenomegaly commonly develops and almost any organ system may be involved. There may be widespread lymph node involvement in the retroperitoneal, paraspinal, iliac and inguinal groups and the disease may involve the bone marrow. Ultimately it may spread to the meninges, pleura, thyroid, breast, kidneys, urinary tract and gonads. Local node masses or organ involvement may produce a variety of complications including mediastinal obstruction, neurological syndromes, intestinal obstruction and renal failure.

Over 50% of patients with non-Hodgkin's lymphomas also present with painless enlargement of one or more

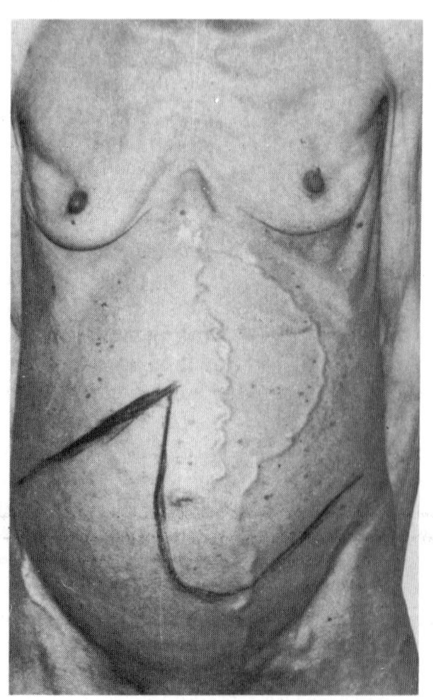

a

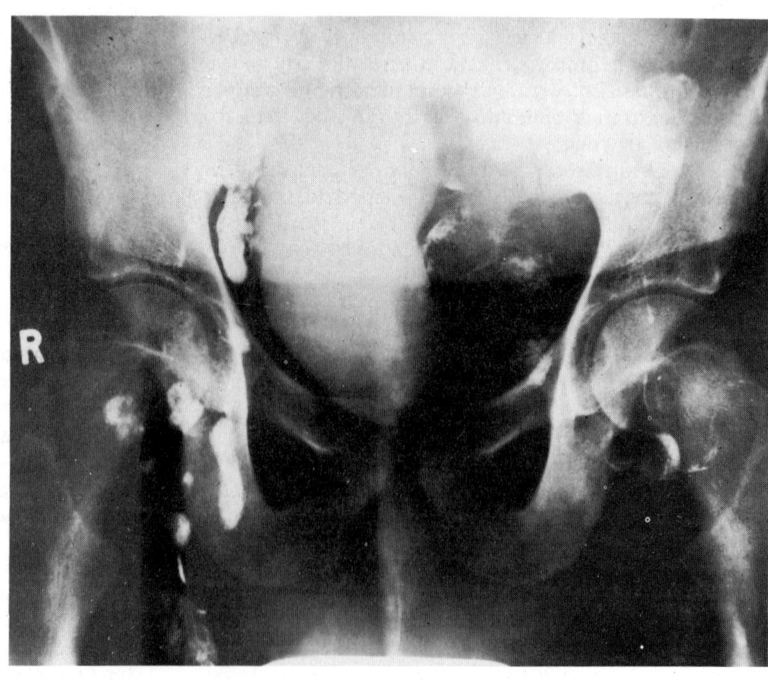

b

Fig. 71.10 Non-Hodgkin's lymphoma. *a*, Patient with a low-grade malignant non-Hodgkin's lymphoma. Note enlargement of the left groin nodes and hepatosplenomegaly. Clinically there is obstruction of the left iliac vein, with dilatation of anastomoses on the anterior abdominal wall. *b*, Lymphangiogram and intravenous pyelogram in the same patient. The very large lymph nodes on the left have filled poorly, but are demonstrated as large masses indenting the bladder.

superficial lymph node groups. The abnormal nodes may appear in any of the superficial lymph node sites but in about a quarter of patients enlargement of the retroperitoneal or mesenteric lymph nodes produces abdominal symptoms as the presenting feature. The remainder of patients with lymphomas present with involvement outside the major node areas, e.g. skin, orbit, pituitary, thyroid, tracheobronchial tree, gastrointestinal tract or involving the central or peripheral nervous system. About half of patients with lymphomas have no systemic upset at presentation but as the disease progresses similar systemic symptoms develop as those which occur in Hodgkin's disease.

Generally speaking patients with histiocytic tumours develop systemic symptoms early. Usually there is general malaise with weight loss associated with enlargement of the superficial lymph nodes and hepatosplenomegaly occurs early in the development of the illness. In some cases there may be an acute fulminating onset with fever, wasting, massive and progressive lymph node enlargement and marked hepatosplenomegaly (*Fig.* 71.10). In histiocytic medullary reticulosis the systemic features are particularly marked and the illness may be very acute with widespread lymphadenopathy, hepatosplenomegaly and osteolytic bone lesions, soft-tissue tumours resembling sarcomas and a variety of extranodal disorders. There is a significant danger of spontaneous rupture of the spleen.

In the lymphomas which involve the skin, such as mycosis fungoides and the Sezary syndrome, the cutaneous manifestations usually start early and as the disease progresses there may be marked generalized lymphadenopathy associated with systemic symptoms.

A DIAGNOSTIC APPROACH TO ENLARGED LYMPH NODES

It is usually easy to recognize lymph node enlargement secondary to local infection. There is nearly always a primary site of inflammation and provided an accurate history is taken, not forgetting such apparent trivia as cat scratches, the cause is usually obvious. If there is no local cause and if the nodes fail to regress in 2–3 weeks serious consideration should be given to carrying out a biopsy. Tuberculous adenitis is usually recognizable by its site, the texture of the nodes and, if they have been there for some time, by the presence of calcification on radiography. It may be necessary to do an excision biopsy in some cases.

Generalized Lymphadenopathy in Infection

Since by far the commonest cause is viral infection a full blood count should be carried out, particular note being taken of the differential white cell count and the presence of atypical lymphocytes on the film which would suggest a diagnosis of infectious mononucleosis. Over 95% of cases have a positive heterophil antibody response as measured by the Paul–Bunnell reaction or screening modifications of this test. A rising titre of antibody to Epstein–Barr (EB) virus occurs in about 80% of cases and may be found even when the heterophil antibody tests are negative. The antibody is usually present when patients first present and hence it is often difficult to demonstrate a rising titre; in some cases there may be a delayed rise. It should be remembered that cytomegalovirus and other viruses can produce an identical clinical picture as can toxoplasmosis. Since hepatitis is a common complication of infectious mononucleosis it is sometimes quite difficult to distinguish A or B virus hepatitis from this disorder without the appropriate serological tests.

When to Biopsy a Lymph Node

It is better to delay for a while than to rush into an early lymph node biopsy. Particularly in patients who have had a general systemic illness which suggests an infective basis for the lymphadenopathy it is always reasonable to wait for a week or two for the glands to subside. There is nothing worse than to present a pathologist with a lymph node from a patient with a viral infection. The histology may be extremely bizarre and it may be impossible to say for certain that the patient does not have a lymphoma. Hence considerable anxiety and diagnostic difficulties can be caused by a premature biopsy.

Any painless and progressive lymph node enlargement requires biopsy; unexplained lymphadenopathy lasting for more than 2 or 3 weeks should always be subjected to histology. On the whole it is best to avoid the groin as a site for biopsy. We have not been impressed with the results of lymph node aspiration and feel that a proper histological specimen must always be obtained. In extremely ill patients, e.g. those with mediastinal obstruction, it is reasonable to attempt to obtain a node under local anaesthetic but in all other cases the biopsy should be performed under general anaesthetic.

The Diagnosis of Hodgkin's Disease and Non-Hodgkin's Lymphoma

The diagnosis of the lymphomas is carried out in two stages. First, an accurate diagnosis must be made by an adequate biopsy. Having made a histological diagnosis the extent of the illness must be assessed, i.e. the lymphoma must be accurately staged.

The establishment of an accurate histological diagnosis before treating lymphomas is absolutely vital. Even in severely ill patients an adequate node biopsy must be obtained. If no superficial nodes are available it is occasionally possible to obtain a histological diagnosis from biopsy of bone marrow, liver or any particular organ that is enlarged or infiltrated. In some cases it may be necessary to go to a diagnostic laparotomy with splenectomy but where abdominal lymphoma is suspected this should always be preceded by radiological analysis of the small bowel, an intravenous pyelogram and an abdominal lymphangiogram so that the best site for biopsy can be sought (*Fig.* 71.10).

Staging Laparotomy for Lymphoma

Staging laparotomy for lymphoma is indicated whenever the findings at operation will either alter the extent of radiation therapy to be administered or make chemotherapy rather than radiotherapy the primary treatment modality. In general, staging laparotomy for lymphoma is *often* indicated in Hodgkin's disease and is *rarely* indicated in non-Hodgkin's lymphoma.

Hodgkin's Lymphoma

Extensive experience with diagnostic exploratory laparotomy over the past two decades has firmly established the role of the procedure in Hodgkin's disease and has provided a clear understanding of patterns of intra-abdominal involvement in these patients. It has also permitted a more accurate correlation of treatment approaches and outcome.

Staging laparotomy is based on the concept that Hodgkin's disease is unicentric in origin, particularly in young patients, in that it spreads in an orderly fashion via lymph channels to contiguous lymph nodes and to related lymphoreticular organs. The accepted clinical stages of Hodgkin's disease are summarized in *Table* 71.8. The clinical stage is first determined by the history which places it either into a symptomless form, i.e. grade A, or into those with systemic symptoms, i.e. grade B. This is followed by detailed clinical examination, radiological studies including a chest radiograph, straight radiograph of the abdomen, CT scan of the abdomen, and abdominal lymphangiogram. It also includes urinalysis, full blood count and a marrow aspiration and biopsy. Isotope scanning of the liver, spleen and bones by appropriate techniques are often included but they have been largely superseded by the advent of ultrasonography and computed tomography. Clinical evidence of liver involvement is based on hepatomegaly, and abnormal serum alkaline phosphatase value, two different liver function tests abnormalities, or a clear-cut abnormality on liver scan with one abnormal liver function test. Splenic involvement is accepted if there is palpable enlargement of the spleen confirmed by radiographic or radioisotopic studies or if an isotopic scan of the spleen shows filling defects.

The investigations outlined above cover the non-invasive techniques for staging the disease. It is now generally agreed that patients with clinical Stage I and Stage IIA disease should have a laparotomy although this is more controversial for those patients who have mediastinal tumours with a nodular sclerosis histology, particularly if there is no hilar, cervical or supraclavicular node involvement and the abdominal lymphangiograms are negative. There is also some controversy as to whether patients with Stage IA disease with only upper cervical or inguinal node involvement should be subjected to laparotomy as they have an excellent chance of having no abdominal foci of disease in contrast to an incidence of 40% involvement in patients who present with supraclavicular node involvement. In making these decisions, it is important to weigh the benefit of a staging laparotomy against the operative risk in terms of mortality and morbidity in each individual patient.

Table 71.8 Clinical stages of Hodgkin's disease

Stage I
Involvement of a single lymph node region, or a single extra-lymphoid organ or site (IE)

Stage II
Involvement of two or more lymph node groups on the same side of the diaphragm; or localized involvement of an extra-lymphoid organ or site and of one or more lymph node groups on the same side of the diaphragm (IIE)

Stage III
Involvement of lymph node groups on both side of the diaphragm, which may be accompanied by localized involvement of an extra-lymphoid organ (IIIE), spleen (IIIS) or both (IIISE)

Stage IV
Diffuse involvement of one or more extra-lymphoid organs with or without associated lymph node involvement: Sites denoted:

N	Lymph nodes	S	Spleen
H	Liver	L	Lung
M	Marrow	O	Bone
P	Pleura	D	Skin

A Asymptomatic.
B Weight loss greater than 10% body weight in 6 months, unexplained fever above 38°C, or night sweats.

The Stanford Group has reported the largest experience with staging laparotomy with Hodgkin's disease. Out of 814 Stage I to Stage IV patients subjected to staging abdominal exploration, 257 (31·6%) emerged from laparotomy evaluation with a pathological stage different from their initial clinical stage. 21·2% Stage IA patients and 26·6% Stage IIA patients were upstaged to Stage IIIA. Most of the upstaging occurs because of occult splenic disease or involvement of nodes not reached by the lymphangiographic dye. Downstaging of Stage II patients is very rare with laparotomy but does occur in a meaningful fraction of clinical Stage III and Stage IV cases. 30·2% of patients with clinical Stage III were demonstrated to have extranodal involvement at staging exploration.

Staging laparotomy provides a number of small benefits for subsequent management of Hodgkin's patients apart from an accurate determination of disease extent. Adequate radiation of the spleen requires a radiation port covering the left upper quadrant which overlaps with the left lung base and the upper pole of the left kidney. Removal of the spleen obviates the need to radiate this area and eliminates the possibility of radiation injury to these particular structures. Movement of the ovaries towards the midline can be accomplished during laparotomy. Such placement allows effective shielding during subsequent radiation and lessens the risk of sterility following radiation therapy. Whether or not splenectomy is associated with less white and platelet toxicity during subsequent radiation therapy and chemotherapy remains controversial. However, episodes of overwhelming sepsis from encapsulated organisms are well recognized in the splenectomized patient, especially in children and teenagers. The increased risk of this postsplenectomy syndrome has led to a rethinking of routine splenectomy and staging for Hodgkin's disease. In most institutions, splenectomy has been retained. There are currently no definitive data as to whether long-term postsurgical prophylactic antibiotics or pneumococcal vaccine would be of value in controlling this infrequent but potentially lethal complication of splenectomy.

The actual staging operation to be performed in Hodgkin's disease has been thoroughly established. Preoperative review of the lymphangiogram and CT scan directs attention to suspicious or equivocal areas of nodal involvement. The surgeon must plan his operative strategy and discuss it with the oncologist and the pathologist in advance. At laparotomy all nodal groups are carefully evaluated from the coeliac axis to the pelvis. Particular scrutiny for tumour spread to mesenteric or porta hepatis nodes is required since these areas would be missed or underdosed in standard Hodgkin's disease radiation ports. Wedge biopsies of the liver are taken from both lobes. The spleen is removed along with the splenic hilar node and clips are placed on the splenic pedicle. The amount of nodal dissection required during staging laparotomy depends to some degree on the presence or absence of splenic involvement. Therefore, once the spleen is removed, it should be immediately sectioned by the pathologist using the technique of 'bread-loafing'—making multiple sections for the entire spleen at intervals of just a few millimetres to define gross pathological involvement with Hodgkin's disease. If splenic involvement is noted, careful exploration of the lower abdomen with biopsy of nodal tissue is sufficient. If the spleen is grossly negative, several of the most suspicious nodes from different nodal groups in both upper and lower abdomen should be removed. In all cases, clips should be placed at all biopsy sites as well as around all masses of involved nodal tissue. The clips aid in radiation treatment planning and may mark changes in tumour bulk during and after therapy. This may be particularly useful in following large nodal masses not opacified adequately by the lymphangiographic contrast. After closure of the abdominal incision, a generous open bone marrow biopsy is taken from the anterior iliac crest through a separate incision. This specimen is substantially larger than that obtained through core needle biopsies and will occasionally demonstrate previously unrecognized bone marrow involvement.

With the recent trend towards combined modality treatment in a greater percentage of patients with Hodgkin's disease, the need for staging laparotomy to define possible sites of occult intra-abdominal disease may become more limited.

Non-Hodgkin's Lymphoma (NHL)

The non-Hodgkin's lymphomas (NHLs) are a heterogeneous group of tumours of the immune system with different natural histories, cellular origins, and prognosis, requiring different treatment strategies. Prior to 1956 the popular classification into giant follicular lymphoma, lymphosarcoma, and retriculum-cell sarcoma had none of the attributes of a good classification system. In 1956, Rappaport devised and reported a classification that was reproducible for pathologists and that had demonstrated clinical relevance in predicting natural history, response to treatment, and prognosis. Although Rappaport's classification has the greatest clinical data to support it, it is not perfect. In the 1970s at least five groups reported classification schemes attempting to improve the situation. Thus, there are several classifications including one from the World Health Organization and one from the British National Lymphoma Investigation group (*Table* 71.4). Because of the diverse terminology in each classification, it is difficult, certainly for surgeons, to interpret the reports and studies of the NHLs.

Rappaport's classification is basically simple to comprehend. There are two histological patterns of the NHLs in this scheme. One is a nodular (or follicular) pattern of growth and the other is a diffuse pattern of growth. Within the two patterns are described the morphological structure of the predominant cells, i.e. well-differentiated lymphocytic, poorly differentiated lymphocytic, histiocytic, mixed lymphocytic-histiocytic, undifferentiated, or lymphoblastic.

In 1982, the National Cancer Institute reported a study in which several reference pathologists and originators of each classification scheme reviewed over a thousand cases of NHL. It was agreed that no one classification was better than another scientifically or clinically. There emerged a new working formulation of NHL for clinical usage as a means of unifying the different pathological classifications with the hope that it will facilitate comparisons of clinical trials. For a more complete discussion of the classification of non-Hodgkin's lymphoma the surgeon is referred to the references at the end of this chapter.

Staging laparotomy has provided valuable information in the past concerning presentation, sites of involvement, and natural history of NHL. It appears now that, unlike Hodgkin's disease, the place for this procedure on a routine basis should be discontinued for NHL. In the Stanford experience, only 15 of 423 patients were downstaged by laparotomy while most patients were upstaged from Stage III to IV. After bone marrow biopsy alone, 43% of patients were Stage IV and after laparotomy, only an additional 12% were added that could not be detected by bone marrow examination. Following careful clinical staging including lymphangiography, bilateral bone marrow biopsies, and percutaneous liver biopsies, fully 80% of all NHL patients will have Stage III or IV disease. Approximately 20% of all NHL patients on the other hand, will have more limited disease in Stage I and II. In this situation, a laparotomy could be justified if the patient is to be given local treatment only. Anywhere from 17 to 28% of Stage I and II patients will be upstaged by laparotomy. If, on the other hand, the Stage I and II patients are to receive systemic chemotherapy, then subjecting those individuals to a relatively morbid procedure such as a laparotomy, the results of which will not alter treatment, is unjustified. Because of the advanced age of many patients with NHL, a laparotomy has a relatively high morbidity rate. In good surgical hands, the mortality rate is approximately 0·5%, but the morbidity ranges from 11 to 40% depending on the surgical series. The most common problems arising after laparotomy include pneumonia, pulmonary embolism, pancreatitis, subdiaphragmatic abscess, and gastrointestinal bleeding.

If a laparotomy is performed, it should be done in the usual systematic fashion as described for Hodgkin's lymphoma. Splenectomy, however, should not be routinely performed since it is almost always possible to identify intra-abdominal disease elsewhere, and the splenectomized patients are more susceptible to overwhelming Gram-positive sepsis, especially from the pneumococcus.

Staging Laparotomy in Children

Hodgkin's Disease

The role of surgical staging with splenectomy in the paediatric population remains controversial although it has been shown to be of value in the accurate staging of children as well as adults. Approximately one-third of children with Hodgkin's disease will have the clinical stage altered by the findings of staging laparotomy with splenectomy. Thus, there is little doubt of the value of this surgical procedure in improving the accuracy of staging in order to develop a therapy programme based upon the extent of disease. A major value of surgical staging is to define the extent of subdiaphragmatic disease so that abdominal-pelvic radiation can be carefully planned and administered on the basis of stage, thus avoiding the necessity of total lymphoid irradiation in children. Surgical staging with splenectomy has been withheld for children under the age of 5 by some investigators because of concern of overwhelming infection in an asplenic child. The suggestion of a partial splenectomy or splenic biopsy as an alternative procedure has been considered. However, there is no evidence to suggest that the age of 5 is a critical point below which the risk of septicaemia is greater. Furthermore, the false negative rate associated with partial splenectomy could be as high as 11·6%, an unacceptable level. Thus, accurate staging of the spleen requires total splenectomy with serial 'bread-loafing' of the spleen at close intervals.

Surgical staging has been documented to result in improved, relapse free survival compared to clinically staged children. In the Stanford series, the actuarial 5-year disease-free survival rate of 82% was achieved among children undergoing initial staging laparotomy, as compared with 55% of those clinically staged only. Furthermore, the relapse rate plateaued at 2 years among the surgically staged patients, while those who were clinically staged only continued to relapse greater than 5 years following diagnosis.

Non-Hodgkin's Lymphoma

Although the extent of disease is prognostically important, occult disseminated disease exists in most children with non-Hodgkin's lymphoma and meticulous surgical staging (i.e. staging laparotomy and splenectomy) is therefore not indicated. All diagnostic studies which delay the institution of specific therapy should be avoided.

THE PRINCIPLES OF TREATMENT OF HODGKIN'S DISEASE AND NON-HODGKIN'S LYMPHOMA

It is beyond the scope of this short chapter to describe the modern management of these diseases except in broad outline. The reader is referred to the sources quoted at the end of the chapter for detailed discussion.

All patients with Hodgkin's disease should be submitted to most meticulous staging before treatment is embarked on. In general, patients with Stages I and II Hodgkin's disease are treated initially with wide-field megavoltage radiotherapy. This is given in the form of the 'mantle' and inverted Y-fields after re-siting the ovaries at laparotomy. Patients with Stage IIIA disease are usually treated with wide-field radiotherapy although this is still controversial and probably multi-agent chemotherapy is equally effective. Patients with Stages IIIB and IV disease and those with severe B symptoms with little localized disease are treated with multi-agent chemotherapy. The regime of choice is the MOPP protocol which is shown in detail in *Table* 71.9. In patients who fail to respond to this regime, or who have late relapses, short remissions can be obtained by the use of other agents, such as bleomycin and the nitroso-urea compound BCNU.

The prognosis for properly staged IA and IIA Hodgkin's disease treated with adequate radiotherapy is good with up to an 80–90% 5-year survival. Patients with IB and IIB disease have a high relapse rate in the first 3 years of being treated in this way.

The approach to the management of non-Hodgkin's lymphomas is rather similar to that for Hodgkin's disease. Local radiotherapy may be the most effective treatment in Stage IA disease, Stages I and II extranodal disease, bone lesions, some lymphomas of the gastrointestinal tract and possibly the mediastinal lymphoma of children and adolescents. Usually about 3000–4000 R is given to the involved nodes and to a generous margin of the surrounding tissue over a period of about 4 weeks. If there is no relapse within the first 2 years the prognosis is relatively good. For more widespread disease combination chemotherapy is used. It is far from clear what the ideal regime is for these lymphomas but it is standard practice to use a combination of cyclophosphamide, vincristine and prednisone in pulses over several months. The response rate is much higher in the nodular and diffuse lymphocytic varieties as compared with the histiocytic malignancies.

A similar approach is used for the histiocytic tumours. Although patients with Stage I disease can sometimes be effectively treated with local radiotherapy the results in Stage II disease are much less satisfactory. Multi-agent chemotherapy such as the MOPP regime, one in which cyclophosphamide is substituted for nitrogen mustard, or more intensive regimes produce complete remissions in about 40% of patients with Stages III and IV diffuse histiocytic tumours. If complete remission is obtained these tend to persist without maintenance therapy but in those who achieve only partial remission there is usually a rapid relapse with a median interval of only about 6 months. Practically all die from the disease within a year. Central nervous system complications, particularly meningeal tumours, occur quite frequently in this group and require symptomatic CNS irradiation or intrathecal methotrexate for control.

Supportive therapy is essential for patients receiving multi-agent chemotherapy. It should be remembered that vincristine causes some degree of peripheral neuropathy and associated autonomic dysfunction may result in severe constipation going on in some cases to intestinal obstruction. Any regime which includes cyclophosphamide in large doses may be associated with a haemorrhagic cystitis. All these regimes produce a variable degree of neutropenia and thrombocytopenia. Severe infection is extremely common during the pulses of these agents and is usually treated with a broad-spectrum antibiotic regime, such as the combined use of gentamicin and carbenicillin. Any bleeding due to thrombocytopenia should be treated energetically with a platelet transfusion. There is often a severe degree of anaemia either as part of the underlying disease or secondary to bone marrow depression following chemotherapy and this should be treated by regular blood transfusion.

All patients who are neutropenic require very careful attention to the mouth and bowels. Rectal examination should be avoided. They should receive regular oral toilet and a prophylactic fungicide as part of a regular mouthwash.

Table 71.9 Some therapeutic regimes for Hodgkin's disease and non-Hodgkin's lymphoma

1. MOPP combination chemotherapy.
   Nitrogen mustard 6 mg/m^2 intravenously daily on days 1 and 8.
   Vincristine (Oncovin) 1·4 mg/m^2 intravenously daily on days 1 and 8.
   Procarbazine 100 mg/m^2 orally daily from days 1–14 inclusive.
   Prednisone (with first and fourth courses) 40 mg/m^2 orally daily from day 1 to 14 inclusive.
   It is usual to give six courses with 2 weeks' rest between completion of one course and commencement of the next. Modification of dosage may be necessary depending on the blood count.
2. CVP therapy for non-Hodgkin's lymphoma
   Cyclophosphamide 400 mg/m^2 orally days 1 to 5.
   Vincristine 1·5 mg/m^2 intravenously day 1.
   Prednisone 100 mg/m^2 orally daily days 1 to 5.
   Cycles of treatment are given every 3 weeks in the dosage stated. A reduced dose of cyclophosphamide may be used according to the blood count.

Mediastinal Obstruction

Mediastinal lymph node enlargement with the syndrome of mediastinal obstruction occurs not infrequently in Hodgkin's disease and with diffuse histiocytic tumours or undifferentiated lymphomas in childhood. Children with highly differentiated mediastinal tumours (Sternberg's sarcoma) frequently develop acute lymphoblastic leukaemia after initial periods of treatment.

Patients who present with mediastinal obstruction offer a particular therapeutic challenge. Where possible, it is most important to obtain histiological material before starting chemotherapy. This may necessitate an anterior mediastinotomy with resection of the 2nd and 3rd costal cartilages. This is particularly important in young patients because other tumours, notably teratomas, may present with an identical clinical picture. Where patients are suffering respiratory distress it may be necessary to give emergency treatment with corticosteroids and radiotherapy or vincoid alkaloids and to stage the disease accurately when the acute respiratory obstruction is overcome. Hodgkin's disease presenting in this way often carries quite a good prognosis. The malignant lymphomas of early life which are associated with acute lymphoblastic leukaemia carry a particularly poor prognosis.

Further Reading

Bowdler A. J. (1981) Disorders of the spleen. In: Hardisty R. M. and Weatherall D. J. (ed.) *Blood and its Disorders*, 3rd ed. Oxford, Blackwell.

Crosby W. H. (1963) Hyposplenism: an inquiry into normal functions of the spleen. *Annu. Rev. Med.* **14**, 349.

Donalson S. S. and Link M. P. (1986) Childhood lymphomas. In: Moossa A. R., Robson M. C. and Schimpff S. C. (ed.) *Comprehensive Textbook of Oncology*. Baltimore, Williams & Wilkins.

Green M. L. (1986) Hodgkin's disease. In: Moossa A. R., Robson M. C. and Schimpff S. C. (ed.) *Comprehensive Textbook of Oncology*. Baltimore, Williams & Wilkins.

Horning S. and Rosenberg S. (1984) The natural history of initially untreated low grade non-Hodgkin's lymphomas. *N Engl. J. Med.* **311**, 1471.

Jandl J. H. and Aster R. H. (1967) Increased splenic pooling and pathogenesis of hypersplenism. *Am. J. Med. Sci.* **253**, 383.

Kaplan H. S. (1980) *Hodgkin's Disease.* Cambridge, Mass., Harvard University Press.

Little C. and Longo D. L. (1986) Non-Hodgkin's lymphoma. In: Moossa A. R., Robson M. C. and Schimpff S. C. (ed.) *Comprehensive Textbook of Oncology*. Baltimore, Williams & Wilkins.

Moossa A. R. and Gadd M. (1985) Isolated splenic vein thrombosis. *World J. Surg.* **9**, 384–390.

O'Grady J. G., Stevens F. M., Harding B. et al. (1984) Hyposplenism and glutensensitive enteropathy. *Gastroenterol.* **87**, 1326.

Pitney W. R. (1968) The tropical splenomegaly syndrome. *Trans. R. Soc. Trop. Med. Hyg.* **62**, 717.

Robb-Smith A. H. T. (1970) Pathological lesions in surgically removed spleens. *Br. J. Hosp. Med.* **3**, 19.

Schloesser L. L. (1963) The diagnostic significance of splenomegaly. *Am. J. Med. Sci.* **245**, 84.

Szur L., Marsh G. W. and Pettit J. E. (1972) Studies of splenic function by means of radioisotope-labelled red cells. *Br. J. Haematol.* **23**, Suppl., 183.

Weiss L. (1983) The spleen. In: Weiss L. (ed.) *Histology*, 5th ed. New York, Elsevier Biomedical.

West K. W. and Grosfeld J. L. (1985) Postsplenectomy sepsis: historical background and current concepts. *World J. Surg.* **9**, 477.

72 The Small Intestine and Vermiform Appendix

A. Cuschieri

SURGICAL ANATOMICAL CONSIDERATIONS

The small intestinal loops provide a maximum possible absorptive area which is available for the assimilation of foodstuffs within the confines of the peritoneal cavity. The proximal two-fifths constitute the jejunum which is normally situated in the upper part of the infracolic compartment, mainly to the left side of the midline; whereas the ileal loops are found in the right iliac fossa and pelvis. There is no clear demarcation zone between the jejunum and the ileum. Nevertheless, the proximal jejunum is easily distinguishable from the distal ileum at operation: its walls are thicker with prominent plicae circulares, the overall diameter is twice that of the distal ileum, the mesentery contains less fat and the mesenteric vasculature consists of prominent arteries and veins which run close together and join to form 1–2 arcades in the mesentery before giving rise to the terminal intestinal branches which pursue a straight course to the jejunum. The mesenteric vasculature of the ileum is more complex, the vessels forming 4–5 levels of arcades before the origin of the terminal intestinal branches. There is a special distribution of the latter vessels to the entire length of the small intestine. Each arteriole and accompanying venule supply and drain one-half of the circumference of the small intestine, and the vessels are distributed to alternate sides of the small intestine in regular sequence (*Fig.* 72.1). This peculiar arrangement forms the basis of the intestinal lengthening operation in infants and children with the short gut syndrome, since the residual bowel can be split longitudinally with each half retaining an adequate blood supply. An understanding of the anatomy of the mesenteric vascular arcades of the small intestine is essential for the safe execution of reconstructive procedures on the gastrointestinal tract involving small bowel segments.

As a result of the pleating of the small intestine and its mesentery, certain loops of the small intestine lie normally in an antiperistaltic position with respect to the ligament of Treitz. This is an important consideration which must be kept in mind during the execution of gastrojejunal anastomoses, small bowel bypass procedures and interpositions. In general, any anastomotic procedure involving the small intestine should be constructed in an isoperistaltic fashion since this is less likely to be complicated by intestinal stasis and bacterial overgrowth.

An appreciation of the small bowel length after excisional surgery is important. Estimates are commonly based on the amount resected as a percentage of the total length of the small bowel. This practice is misleading and imparts no useful information on the long-term outcome of the patient after the small intestine resection. The reported measurements of the length of the human small intestine stripped of its mesentery at postmortem vary from 3·5 to 9 m with an average of 5 m. However, the tone of the smooth musculature reduces the small bowel length considerably during life. Accurate assessment of the intestinal length at operation is difficult owing to the changing state of the intestinal loops consequent on peristaltic activity, handling and exposure. In the adult the small bowel length, measured along its antimesenteric border and in the unstretched state after a preliminary laparotomy averages 3·5 m. An assessment of the residual small bowel length after resection is more important than accurate measurements of the resected specimen.

The basic unit of the small bowel mucosa is the *villus*, a finger-like projection measuring 0·5–1·5 mm in length. It is covered by tall columnar absorptive cells (enterocytes) which have microvilli at their luminal surfaces (brush border). The enterocytes rest on a thin basal membrane (lamina propria) and their microvilli are kept lubricated by a surface mucus known as the glycocalyx which separates the brush border from the unstirred layer of the intestinal contents. Goblet cells are found interspersed among the enterocytes. They synthesize the mucous glycoprotein and secrete it at the surface of the villus, thereby maintaining the glycocalyx. The villi are surrounded at their bases by the intestinal *crypts*

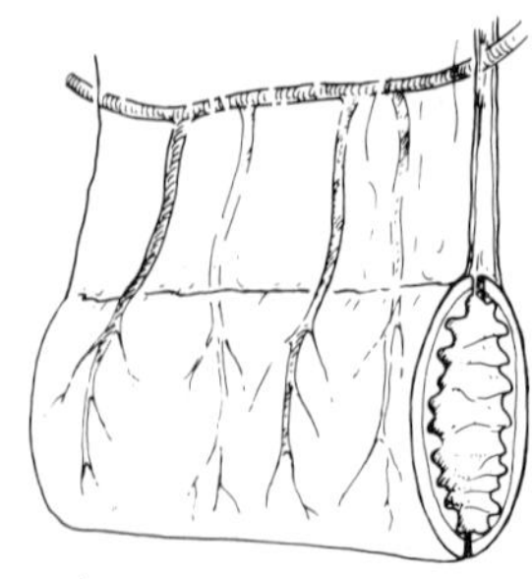

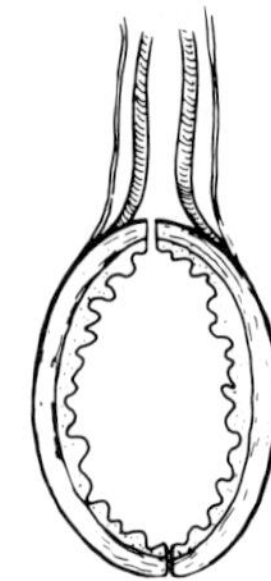

Fig. 72.1 Diagrammatic representation of the distribution of the terminal branches of the mesenteric vessels to the small intestine. These are distributed to alternate sides of the gut.

which contain the proliferative area of stem cells from which the surface epithelium is constantly replaced by a process of cell division and migration. The other cells found in the crypts are goblet cells in the upper half, Paneth cells at the base and endocrine cells. The Paneth cells are pyramidal in shape, have abundant RNA-rich cytoplasm and refractile granules containing lysosomes. Although their exact function remains uncertain, it is thought that Paneth cells are capable of phagocytosing bacteria from the crypt lumen. The endocrine cells are also known as entero-endocrine and APUD cells. The term APUD is derived from a basic characteristic of these entero-endocrine cells: the *u*ptake and *d*ecarboxylation of *a*mine *p*recursors. Although there is still considerable debate concerning the origin of the gut endocrine cells, they are no longer held to be of ectodermal origin but are thought to arise from the undifferentiated crypt stem cells. A separate group of gut endocrine cells stain with potassium chromate and silver dyes and are known as enterochromaffin cells or argentaffin cells. They elaborate and secrete 5-hydroxytryptophan and 5-hydroxytryptamine, in addition to a variety of peptide hormones, e.g. motilin, substance P etc. The other important cellular components of the villus are lymphocytes which are subdivided into those in the basal lamina (lamina propria lymphocytes, LPP) and those interspersed amongst the epithelial cells covering the villus (intra-epithelial lymphocytes, IEL).

INTRALUMINAL MICROFLORA

The alimentary tract is sterile at birth but becomes colonized by bacteria from the oral route, so that within 3–4 weeks of birth, the enteric microflora encountered in the adult is established. The contents of the stomach, duodenum and proximal jejunum in the normal adult subject are either sterile or harbour transient Gram-positive aerobes, such as lactobacilli and enterococci, in concentrations of less than 10^4 colony-forming units (CFU) per ml of contents. Coliform organisms may be found transiently in the jejunum. The bacterial flora of the terminal ileum is different, higher bacterial counts (10^5–10^8 CFU) are encountered and the flora resembles that of the large bowel. The organisms that can be cultured regularly from the ileal contents include coliforms and strict anaerobes, e.g. bacteroides. Substantially higher bacterial counts (10^9–10^{11} CFU) are found in the colon, the microflora of which is dominated by bacteroides, anaerobic lactobacilli and clostridia.

It is generally held that the enteric microflora plays an important protective role against bacterial overgrowth and infection. The postulated mechanisms for this barrier function include prevention of colonization of the surface epithelium by pathogenic bacteria, production of bacteriocins (antibiotics) by some species (*Streptococcus viridans*), and lowering of the oxidation-reduction potential by anaerobic metabolism which also results in the production of substances which are toxic to some bacteria, e.g. fatty acids and deconjugated bile acids.

Although the enteric bacteria synthesize vitamins (K and B group) in excess of their metabolic needs, these are not available to the host. In addition, the intraluminal microflora produce endotoxin which is, however, not absorbed into the bloodstream in the presence of an intact enterohepatic circulation of bile salts. Absorption of endotoxin into the bloodstream occurs whenever bile salts are prevented from reaching the small intestine as in obstructive jaundice. This endotoxinaemia is held to be responsible for the development of renal failure after surgical intervention in jaundiced patients. The enteric microflora play an important but incompletely understood role in the intraluminal metabolism of a variety of substances. Thus, some bacterial species deconjugate the taurine and glycine conjugates of the primary bile salts which then undergo hydroxylation. Intestinal organisms also metabolize proteins and other nitrogenous compounds with the production of nitroles, skatols and ammonia which is absorbed and used for the synthesis of amino acids. The excess ammonia produced by bacterial metabolism after an episode of gastrointestinal haemorrhage often precipitates encephalopathy in patients with chronic liver disease and portal hypertension. The intestinal microflora are involved in the production of other organic compounds from both exogenous (ingested food) and endogenous precursors, e.g. bile salts. Some of these are toxic and carcinogenic. The intestinal microflora, in association with other factors such as diet and its fibre content, may therefore be involved with the development of gastrointestinal cancer. There is also evidence that the enteric bacteria may be involved in the degradation of some biologically active peptides, such as gastrin.

In health a symbiotic relationship seems to exist between the gut and the intestinal organisms, and indeed the normal villus architecture and rate of regeneration of the intestinal mucosa are both dependent on the presence of a normal resident microflora. It is in pathological states which lead to bacterial overgrowth—stasis and diminished or absent gastric secretory activity—that the adverse effects become manifest clinically as maldigestion and malabsorption.

FUNCTIONS OF THE SMALL INTESTINE

The prime function of the small intestine is the digestion and assimilation of foodstuffs. Details of the mechanisms of digestion and absorption of ingested food are outside the scope of this book. It should, perhaps, be emphasized that the intraluminal digestion of carbohydrates and proteins by the pancreatic enzymes is incomplete and that intestinal surface digestion by the brush border enzymes is essential for the final hydrolysis to tri- and dipeptides and monosaccharides. Di- and tripeptides which have a high affinity for the brush border peptidases are hydrolysed to constituent amino acids before absorption; those with a low affinity for the surface enzymes are absorbed intact by the enterocytes. Triglyceride digestion and absorption is a more complex process and requires the presence of colipase and lipase which convert the triglycerides to a mixture of free fatty acids and monoglycerides, which are rendered water soluble by entering into molecular aggregation with bile acids to form micelles. At the intestinal surface, the monoglycerides and free fatty acids separate from the micelles, leaving the bile acids within the intestinal lumen. Following absorption, the fatty acids are bound to special proteins, known as the fatty acid binding proteins (FABP) and then transported to the smooth endoplasmic reticulum where they are re-esterified. Within the Golgi apparatus, the triglycerides are converted to chylomicrons which consist of a core of cholesterol and triglyceride esters covered with phospholipids, free cholesterol and apoproteins. The chylomicrons together with the lipoproteins (*vide infra*) are then transferred via the lacteals and lymph channels to the venous blood. Cholesterol follows a similar pathway to the long-chain triglycerides except that it does not bind to FABP and is released slowly from the enterocyte. The absorption of medium-chain triglycerides (MCT, 8–12 C) is different and has important therapeutic applications. In the first instance, a significant percentage of ingested MCT can be absorbed intact into the portal blood. The rest is completely broken down by pancreatic lipase to medium-chain fatty acids, and subsequent to micellar aggregation with bile acids, they are readily absorbed by the intestinal cell and transferred as free acids into the portal venous blood without chylomicron formation.

In health, the digestion and absorption of fluid, electrolytes, iron, folate, carbohydrates, fats and proteins is completed in the jejunum. The effective absorption of bile salts and vitamin B_{12} can only occur in the terminal ileum as these substances require specific transport sites which are located in this region. The reports from human studies indicate that in the absence of an ileum, the critical length of jejunum required for the absorption of water-soluble substances such as glucose, amino acids and water-soluble vitamins ranges from 30 to 120 cm. The ileum is able to perform all the jejunal absorptive functions after excision of the proximal small bowel; whereas ileal resections exceeding 150 cm will invariably produce malabsorption of fat (from a diminished bile salt pool) and vitamin B_{12}. Despite the passive absorption of bile acids which occurs in the jejunum, the loss of active transport sites in the ileum results in a loss of bile acids into the colon.

Another function of the small intestine is the synthesis of alpha (high density, HDL) and beta (low density, LDL and very low density, VLDL) lipoproteins which are closely related to the chylomicrons and contain the same apoproteins. The intestinal lipoproteins reach the plasma via the thoracic duct. Although there are other tissues which synthesize these lipoproteins, e.g. liver, the gastrointestinal tract is a major site of production. It therefore plays an important part in the metabolism of plasma lipoproteins. The synthesis of lipoproteins by the small intestine is impaired in kwashiorkor.

The various peptide and amine intestinal hormones are located within the entero-endocrine cells and in the neurones of the myenteric plexus. They modulate intestinal activity in 3 ways: some function as classic endocrine hormones, others as neurotransmitters and a further group have a paracrine action. They influence intestinal secretion and transport (neurotensin, motilin, serotonin, secretin, somatostatin), growth and differentiation (enteroglucagon), splanchnic haemodynamic state (vasoactive intestinal polypeptide, neurotensin and glucagon which enhance intestinal blood flow, and vasopressin which reduces it). Gastric inhibitory polypeptide (GIP) has been renamed as the glucose-dependent insulin-releasing hormone. Its release is inhibited by a carbohydrate meal and reduced by dietary fibre. The complex hormonal interactions within the small intestine are closely linked with the activity of the enteric nervous system which is nowadays thought to act as an independent integrative system regulating reflex activity within the gut. Within the myenteric plexus, neurones containing opioid peptides (enkephalins), substance P, VIP, serotonin, and somatostatin have been identified, in addition to the well-known adrenergic (noradrenaline) and cholinergic fibres (acetylcholine).

There is little doubt that the small intestine is involved in the immune response. It contains both lymphocytes and plasma cells, and is the major site of production of IgA. The intra-epithelial lymphocytes are thymus-dependent (T-cells) and consist of both helper and suppressor populations. The lamina propria lymphocytes are B-cells, most of which are activated to produce immunoglobulins (IgA, IgG). Primary immunological deficiency disorders, such as acquired hypogammaglobulinaemia and nodular lymphoid hyperplasia, are often accompanied by diarrhoea, malabsorption and infection with *Giardia lamblia*. Selective IgA deficiency may occur and is also associated with diarrhoea. In addition, immunological changes are found in a variety of common gastro-enterological disorders such as atrophic gastritis, Crohn's disease and coeliac disease.

INVESTIGATION OF SMALL BOWEL DISORDERS

Investigative procedures are performed on the small intestine in patients whose symptoms indicate the presence of organic small bowel disease or because of suspected malabsorption. The term 'malabsorption' can be used to describe the failure to absorb specific substances, e.g. carbohydrates, fats, proteins, minerals, etc. but when used unqualified, it is generally taken to imply fat malabsorption. It is frequently encountered in surgical practice, as it invariably follows certain excisional and bypass procedures on the gastrointestinal tract. More rarely, the balance is upset by a surgical procedure which is not usually followed by gross malabsorption in a patient with subclinical and previously undetected medical disorder, such as coeliac disease. Thus, severe steatorrhoea may develop for the first time in these patients after a truncal vagotomy and drainage procedure.

The assessment of the nature and extent of the malabsorptive defect in all these patients is crucial to their long-term management. Apart from the serum biochemistry (e.g. albumin, transferrin, electrolytes including calcium, iron), haemoglobin level and blood film, special investigations are necessary (*Table* 72.1). Tests for iron and calcium absorption are available but are not in general use.

Radiology

Plain erect and supine abdominal films, whilst invaluable in the diagnosis of acute surgical disorders such as intestinal obstructions and perforations, are of limited practical use in the investigation of chronic symptoms referable to the small intestine. Barium sulphate small bowel follow-through (SBFT) or a small bowel enema (SBE) where the contrast medium is instilled via a Bilbao–Dotter tube directly into the upper jejunum, are the established routine investigations designed to outline the small intestine in patients with chronic symptoms. Although the SBFT is easy to perform as part of a barium meal study, the small bowel enema carries a higher diagnostic yield especially for small bowel tumours, Crohn's disease and in patients with occult gastrointestinal bleeding and clinically suspected malabsorption. Lesions such as discrete or fissure ulcers, longitudinal ulceration, sinuses, fistulas, thickening and distortion of the mucosal folds, polyps, etc., are visualized more often by SBE and a more accurate prediction of the extent of the disease can be made.

The radiological criteria of malabsorption are: flocculation and segmentation of barium, thickening of the mucosal folds and dilatation of intestinal loops. However, these changes are non-specific and are frequently encountered in individuals who have no evidence of malabsorption. This diagnosis must therefore be confirmed by other more specific tests of malabsorption (*vide infra*).

Selective splanchnic angiography is the most reliable method for the detection of angiodysplastic lesions (vascular

Table 72.1 Investigations of the small intestine

Radiology	Plain abdominal films	Acute conditions
	Small bowel follow-through	
	Small bowel enema	More useful than SBFT
	Arteriography	Occult GI bleeding
	CT scanning	Detection of fistulas and pre-op. staging of GI malignancy
	Ultrasound	Diagnosis of cystic lesions
Isotope scintigraphy		Localization of GI bleeding
		Estimation of intestinal transit
		Detection of inflammatory bowel disease
Faecal fat estimation		Diagnosis of steatorrhoea
Jejunal mucosal biopsy		In patients with malabsorption
Tests of terminal ileal function	Schilling	Absorption of vitamin B_{12}
	SeHCAT	Absorption of bile salts
Breath tests	^{14}C-glycocholate/-d-xylose	Bacterial overgrowth
	^{14}C-lactose	Lactose malabsorption
	Lactulose H_2	Small bowel transit and bacterial overgrowth

malformations) which present with episodes of occult bleeding from the gastrointestinal tract. The bleeding site can be located by this radiological investigation if the patient is bleeding actively at the time of investigation. In addition, the abnormal vasculature can be demonstrated by the use of subtraction techniques.

Computed tomography (CT) of the small intestine entails the use of a special barium sulphate suspension (E–Z–CAT) to opacify the intestine. It is useful in detecting thickening of the bowel wall by disease and in demonstrating the presence of enterocolic and enterovesical fistulas. However, the indications for its use in small bowel disorders are currently limited since the information can often be obtained by ordinary contrast radiological studies. The role of CT in the preoperative staging of gastrointestinal malignancy is currently being evaluated but the initial results are encouraging. Ultrasound scanning has been used in patients with intestinal obstruction and is capable of differentiating fluid-filled dilated intestinal loops from other cystic structures in the abdomen.

Isotope Scintigraphy

External scintigraphy following the intravenous administration of radiolabelled compounds or isotope-labelled autologous cells, is useful in the investigation of patients with occult gastrointestinal bleeding or suspected intra-abdominal localized inflammation/abscess formation. It is also used to detect inflamed intestine, e.g. Crohn's disease, to estimate the intestinal transit time and to evaluate the function of bilio-enteric anastomoses.

Intestinal Bleeding

Haemorrhage of small intestinal origin may be due to a Meckel's diverticulum, polyps, tumours, especially smooth muscle neoplasms, and vascular malformations. Upper gastrointestinal endoscopy is negative in these patients and a small bowel enema may not reveal any abnormality. Radionuclide methods may help to solve these difficult problems. The tendency in recent years has been to use these isotope tests before arteriography which is then used to define the lesion, and in some cases, to control the bleeding by embolization of the bleeding vessels or by the use of vasoconstrictor drugs. Three isotope methods are available. The first involves the injection of technetium pertechnetate. This is the method of choice for the detection of a bleeding Meckel's diverticulum, and carries an accuracy rate of 90%. The technetium is excreted by the ectopic gastric mucosa into the diverticulum and shows as a hot spot (*Fig.* 72.2). For the rapid detection of bleeding sites, as in an emergency situation with active haemorrhage, ^{99m}sulphur-colloid (Tc Sc) is used. Following intravenous bolus injection, Tc Sc is cleared from the circulation by the macrophage system within 15 min, at which point the blood radioactivity declines but the extravascular radioactivity at the bleeding site increases, thereby allowing its detection as a hot spot by external scintigraphy. Technetium-labelled autologous red cells (obtained from the patient) are cleared much more slowly from the vascular compartment following their intravenous injection. This technique is preferable to the Tc Sc method in patients with intermittent gastrointestinal bleeding, since it allows repeated examination over a 24 h period (*Fig.* 72.3). Its main disadvantage concerns the long time required to label the patient's red blood cells. It is therefore clearly unsuitable for the actively bleeding patient, when Tc Sc which is readily available, should be used.

Estimation of Small Bowel Transit Time

In addition to radiological contrast studies, intestinal transit studies have been performed with radio-opaque solid and non-absorbable chemical markers. These methods are generally regarded as unphysiological and unsuitable for routine clinical practice. Estimation of the small bowel transit is best performed either by external scintigraphy after the administration of isotope-labelled meals or by

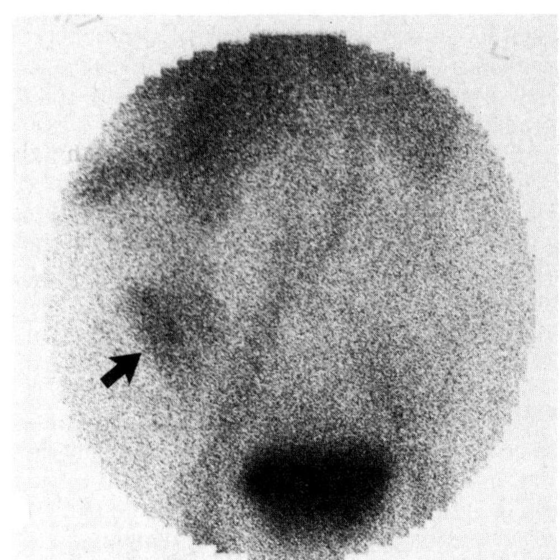

Fig. 72.2 Ectopic gastric mucosa in a bleeding Meckel's diverticulum outlined by external scintiscanning after the intravenous administration of $^{99}Tc^{m}$.

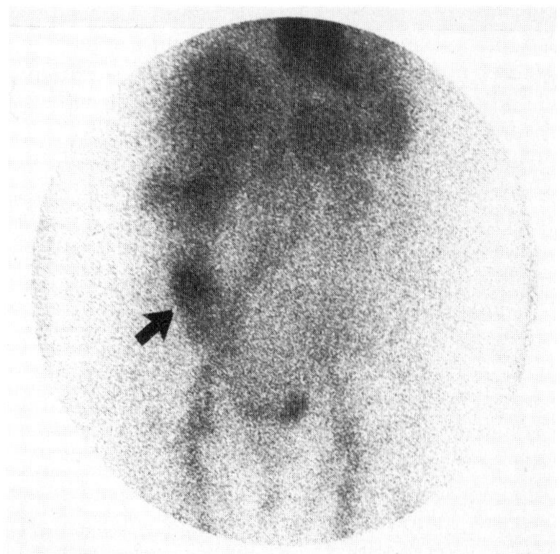

Fig. 72.3 Occult bleeding site in the ascending colon located by the $^{99}Tc^{m}$-labelled autologous red cell technique. Selective arteriography was unhelpful in this elderly patient. The lesion proved to be an angiodysplasia.

breath tests (*vide infra*). Both liquid and solid meals labelled with $^{99}Tc^{m}$ Sc or DTPA are used to estimate simultaneously gastric emptying and small bowel transit time. The detection of caecal radioactivity is used as the end point for the estimation of the small bowel transit time.

Detection of Small Bowel Inflammatory Disease

Indium^{111}-labelled autologous leucocytes, when injected intravenously, settle in areas of inflammation/abscess formation. The technique can be used to detect the extent of inflammatory bowel disease and to assess its severity. It has, however, several disadvantages when used in patients with inflammatory bowel disease, the most important being the difficulty with interpretation because of increased background radioactivity secondary to the uptake of the radiolabelled leucocytes by the bone marrow, liver and spleen. Sucralfate is an aluminium salt of polysulphated sucrose which is used in the treatment of peptic ulceration. It has a unique property of binding selectively to areas of mucosal ulceration within the gastrointestinal tract. The ^{99m}Sucralfate scanning test has proved to be a useful technique for the detection of inflammatory bowel disease and its extent in both the small and large intestine. In view of its lower radiation dosage compared to barium studies, it is being increasingly used as a screening test and in the serial assessment of disease activity. A labelled suspension of Sucralfate is administered by mouth and serial isotope scans of the abdomen are obtained between 2 and 6 h after, at 20 and 24 h later.

Estimation of Faecal Fat

The quantitative estimation of faecal fat remains the most sensitive and reliable test of disorders of digestion and absorption. The faecal fat output per day is estimated on a 3- or 5-day collection on a standard diet containing 80–100 g of fat. The normal is less than 6·0 g/day (18 mmol triglyceride). Other tests, such as the ^{14}C-triolein breath test and the oxalate loading test, are less reliable but are used in some centres as screening tests for steatorrhoea.

Jejunal Mucosal Biopsy

This is performed using the suction Crosby capsule or the Rubin multiple biopsy tube. Apart from abnormalities of villus architecture, e.g. subtotal villus atrophy in coeliac disease (*Fig.* 72.4), abnormal mucosal pathogens may be detected as in Whipple's disease, in addition to parasites, e.g. *Giardia lamblia* (*Fig.* 72.5). Special stains are used to demonstrate the presence of amyloid. A portion of the small bowel biopsy may be used to assay disaccharidase activity.

Specific Tests for Ileal Malabsorption

These consist of the Schilling test which tests the ability of the ileum to absorb vitamin B_{12} and the SeHCAT test which assesses the ileal absorptive capacity for bile salts.

Schilling Test

The absorption of vitamin B_{12} by the terminal ileum requires the presence of intrinsic factor and, to a lesser extent, the R-protein in the gastric juice. In the Schilling test, radiolabelled vitamin B_{12} (1·0 μg) is administered orally immediately after a large parenteral injection of the unlabelled vitamin (1000 μg) to ensure saturation of the body stores. Under these conditions, normal subjects will excrete 10% or more of the radiolabelled vitamin in their urine. If an abnormally low excretion is obtained in a patient, the test is repeated but the labelled vitamin B_{12} is given together with intrinsic factor. In the presence of ileal disease, the abnormally low excretion of the labelled vitamin in the urine is not altered by the addition of the intrinsic factor. On the other hand, in patients with pernicious anaemia or total gastrectomy, the administration of intrinsic factor restores the urinary excretion of the labelled vitamin to normal. Both stages of the test are invalidated by dehydration and renal disease. Bacterial overgrowth may cause malabsorption of the vitamin and an abnormal Schilling test but this will revert to normal after a course of antibiotic therapy.

SeHCAT Bile Acid Absorption Test

This is an accurate test of the ability of the terminal ileum to absorb bile acids. A synthetic selenium bile acid is used, known as SeHCAT. A dose of ^{75}Se-labelled compound is administered orally or intravenously. Initially, a whole body counter was required to perform this test and this limited its availability. More recently, the procedure has been modified to enable the use of collimated gamma-counters. Several studies have shown a very good correlation between the results of the SeHCAT test and the faecal excretion of bile acids.

Breath Tests

These simple and easily executed investigations are used for the detection of bacterial overgrowth, the demonstration of carbohydrate malabsorption and in the assessment of the small bowel transit time.

^{14}C-Glycocholate and ^{14}C-D-Xylose Breath Tests

The ^{14}C-glycocholate breath test is used to detect bacterial overgrowth in the small intestine and has replaced the urinary estimation of indican for the diagnosis of this condition. The glycine moiety of the conjugated bile salt is labelled with ^{14}C and ingested to mix with the endogenous bile salts in the intestine. Under normal conditions, the bile salts are largely reabsorbed intact in the terminal ileum to enter the enterohepatic circulation, and only a small amount reaches the colon where it is deconjugated by the colonic

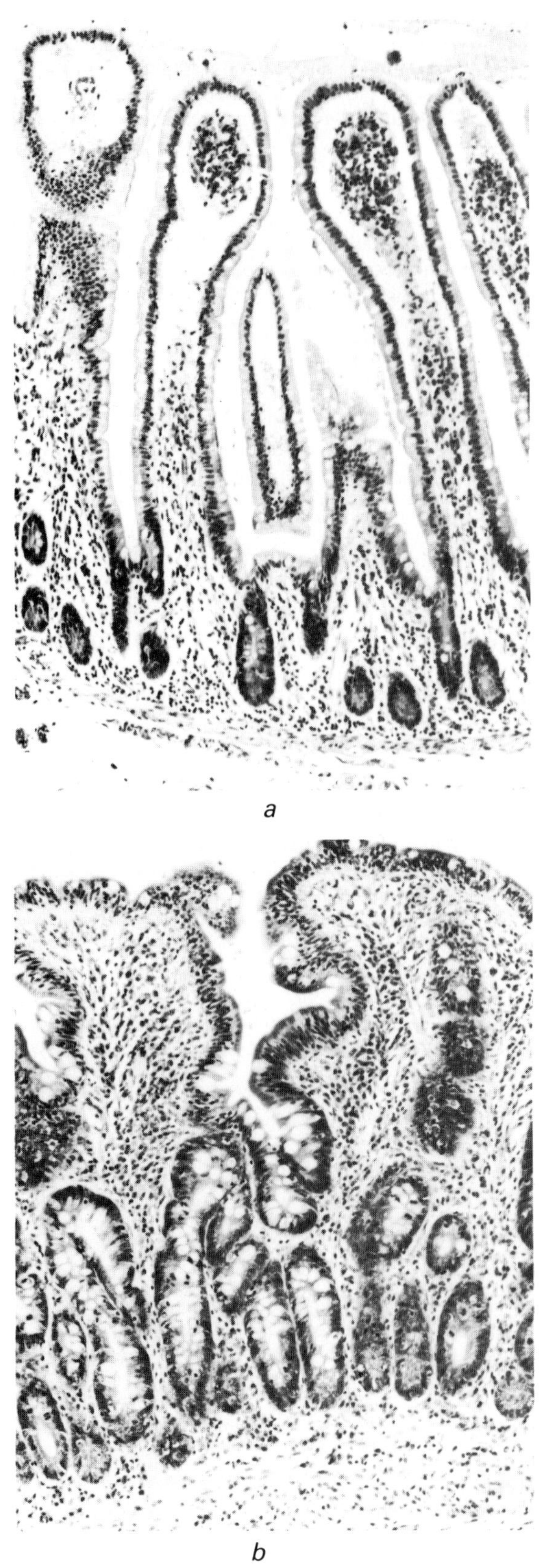

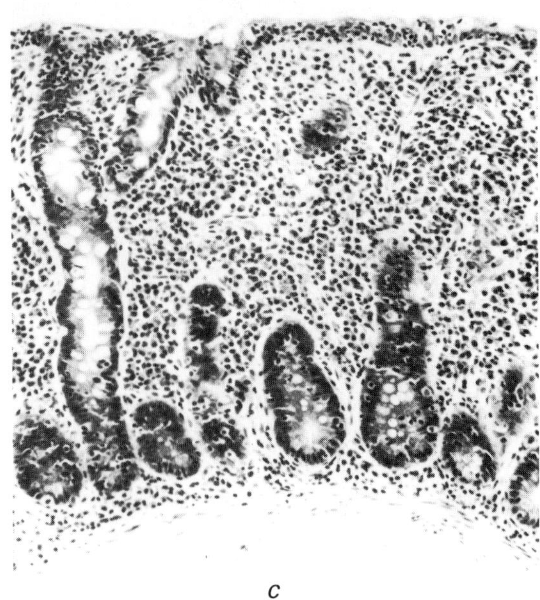

Fig. 72.4 *a*, Mucosal biopsy—normal jejunum. *b*, Mucosal biopsy—crypt hyperplasia with partial villus atrophy. *c*, Mucosal biopsy—flat mucosa due to total villus atrophy in a patient with untreated coeliac disease.

bacteria and the glycine moiety metabolized to yield $^{14}CO_2$. This is absorbed and eliminated in the expired air. However, in the presence of bacterial overgrowth, most of the ingested labelled bile salt is deconjugated by the small bowel bacteria and excess $^{14}CO_2$ is produced and eliminated in the expired air (*Fig.* 72.6). False positive results are obtained with this test in the presence of ileal disease. The ^{14}C-d-xylose test is more reliable in this respect. D-xylose is a pentose which is normally absorbed intact by the same transport mechanism as the hexoses.

Breath Tests for Carbohydrate Malabsorption

The analysis of breath $^{14}CO_2$ following the ingestion of ^{14}C-lactose is a convenient test for lactose intolerance resulting from a deficiency of the brush border enzyme lactase. The test is easy to perform, is as accurate as the lactose tolerance test, and agrees reasonably well with mucosal disaccharidase activity.

Hydrogen is evolved when carbohydrate is fermented by some bacteria. When there is lactose malabsorption, the sugar reaches the colon where it is fermented with the production of H_2. A proportion of this gas is absorbed and excreted in the expired air. Modern instruments are available which are capable of measuring very low concentrations of H_2 in a sample of end-expiratory air which has a similar composition to that of alveolar air. There is evidence that the breath H_2 concentration is more accurate than $^{14}CO_2$ excretion in the diagnosis of lactase deficiency. Both tests give false positive results in patients with bacterial overgrowth.

Hydrogen Breath Tests for Measurement of Small Bowel Transit Time and Bacterial Overgrowth

The H_2 breath test is a useful and reliable method for the determination of the small bowel transit time, and is rapidly supplanting other techniques used for this purpose in clinical practice. Repeated measurements of the H_2 in the end-expiratory air are taken every few minutes after the ingestion of a meal. The latter may be liquid in nature (drink of the

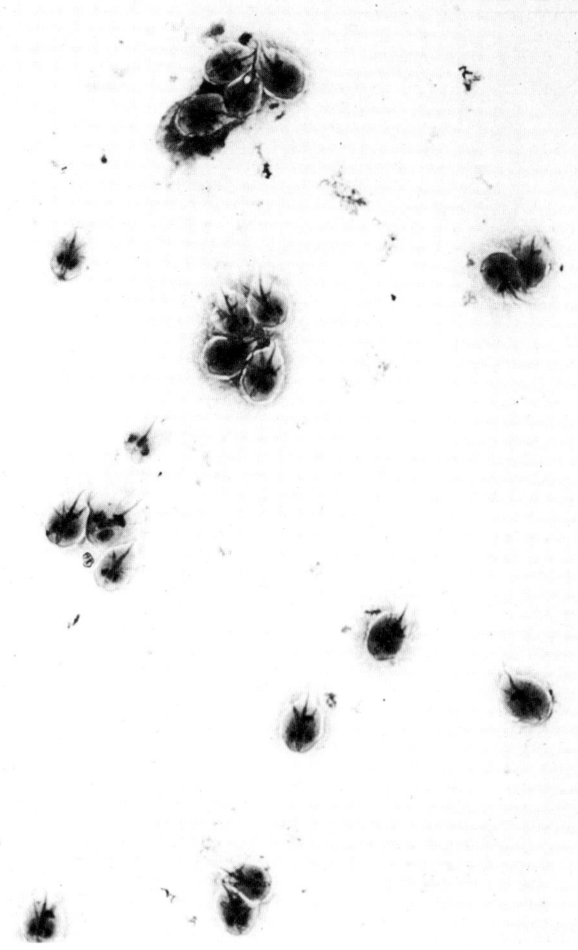

Fig. 72.5 *Giardia lamblia* obtained from a jejunal mucosal biopsy.

non-absorbable sugar lactulose) or solid, usually mashed potatoes and baked beans which contain non-absorbable oligosaccharides. When the head of the meal reaches the caecum, the resulting bacterial fermentation induces a sustained rise in the breath H_2 concentration (*Fig.* 72.7). Strictly speaking the test measures the oral–caecal transit time which includes the gastric emptying time. However, if the meal is radiolabelled with $^{99}Tc^{m}$, both gastric emptying and small bowel transit times can be calculated from the one investigation.

In patients with bacterial overgrowth, the fasting H_2 level in the expired breath is elevated. In addition, there is an early rise in the H_2 in the expired air following the administration of the lactulose solution (*Fig.* 72.8).

The investigation of a patient with suspected malabsorption should commence with estimation of the faecal fat. Once steatorrhoea is confirmed in this way, further tests are required to establish the nature of the underlying pathology. The order in which these tests are carried out is shown in *Table* 72.2. In the end malabsorption will be found to be either of small bowel origin, e.g. small intestinal disease, bacterial overgrowth, or the result of pancreatic exocrine insufficiency.

SYNDROMES RESULTING FROM DISEASE OR SURGERY ON THE GASTROINTESTINAL TRACT

These include bacterial overgrowth (stagnant loop syndrome), the short-gut syndrome and protein-losing enteropathy.

Bacterial Overgrowth

In this syndrome, the small intestine becomes colonized by bacteria. There is an increase in the concentration of organisms which are normally confined to the lower small bowel and colon. The affected intestine becomes inflamed, oedematous and dilated. The syndrome may result from surgery or disease which results in excess bacteria entering the small intestine or from delayed clearance of bacteria from the small intestine due to stasis (stagnant/blind loop syndrome)—*Table* 72.3. In some cases, the bacterial overgrowth develops in the absence of a readily demonstrable

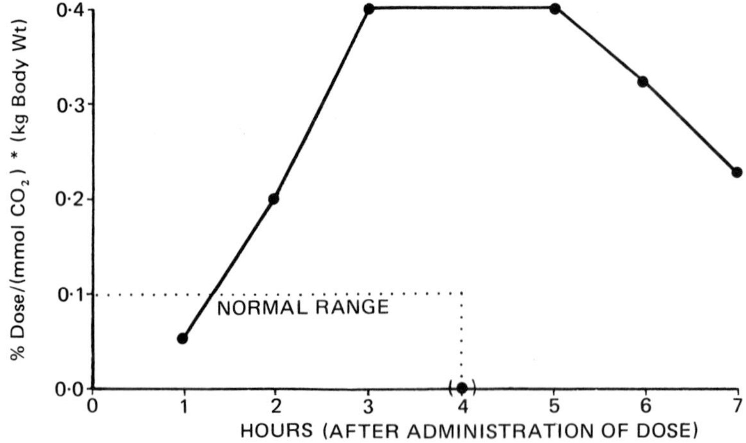

Fig. 72.6 ^{14}C-glycocholate breath test in a female patient with weight loss, hypoproteinaemia and moderate steatorrhoea. The investigation is clearly abnormal with an increased amount of labelled CO_2 being detected in the expired breath. Normally, less than 0·1% of the administered dose is recovered in the expired breath. The patient had had an ileotransverse anastomosis for Crohn's disease. The bacterial overgrowth subsided when the excluded diseased bowel was resected.

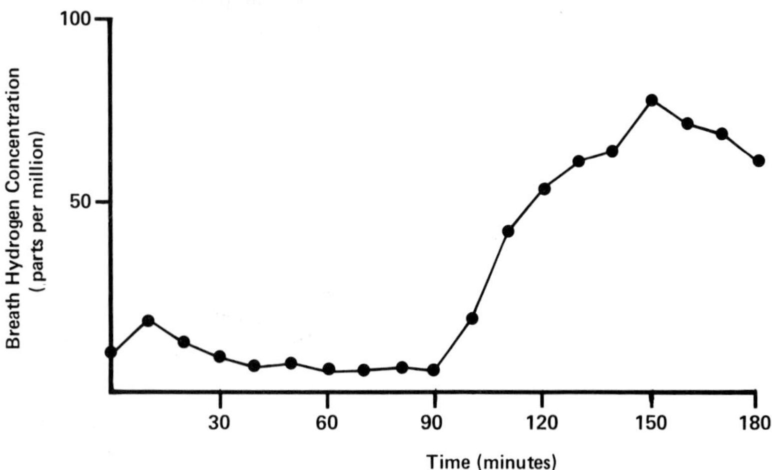

Fig. 72.7 Determination of the oral–caecal transit time by the hydrogen breath test. Following the administration of lactulose solution, serial H_2 estimations are performed on samples of the end-expiratory air. A sustained rise in the H_2 in the expired air indicates that the head of the meal has reached the caecum where bacterial fermentation of the non-absorbable carbohydrate occurs.

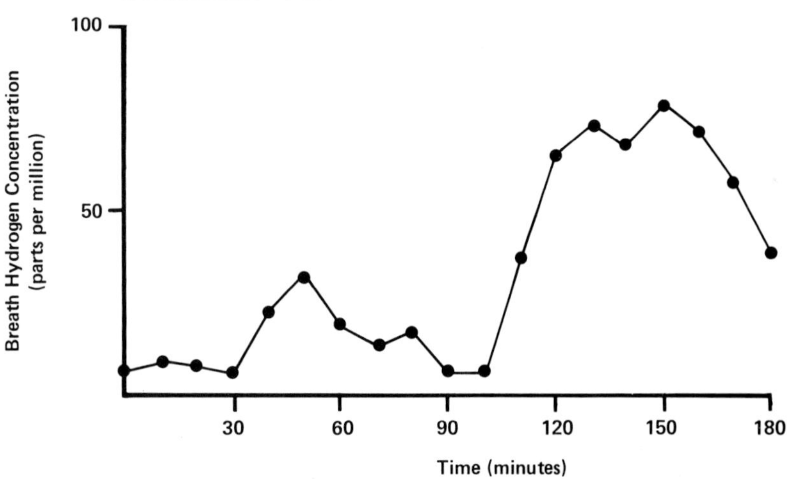

Fig. 72.8 H_2 lactulose breath test in a patient with bacterial overgrowth. The fasting level of H_2 in the expired air is high and there is an early rise in the breath H_2 after the ingestion of the lactulose solution.

local cause. This may occur in patients with malnutrition or immune deficiency.

Pathophysiology

The bacterial overgrowth in the small intestine is usually of the order of 10^7–10^9 colony-forming units per ml of intestinal contents. The bacterial colonization results in intestinal mucosal injury which is characterized by patchy inflammatory changes in the lamina propria and is accompanied by alterations in the concentrations of the brush border enzymes. The increased bacterial population deconjugates the intraluminal bile salts by removing the glycine or taurine moiety. In addition, the bacteria dehydroxylate the steroid nucleus at the C7 position with the formation of deoxycholate and lithocholate which have a tendency to precipitate at the intraluminal pH levels of the small intestine. These bile salts participate poorly in the emulsification of fat; furthermore, they are passively absorbed to a certain extent by non-ionic diffusion throughout the small intestine. There obtains, therefore, a net reduction of the concentration of the effective bile salts in the lumen of the small bowel, at times to levels below the critical micellar concentration, when malabsorption of fats and fat-soluble vitamins ensues. The bacteria also bind vitamin B_{12} and convert it to inactive derivatives (cobamides) which block the ileal receptors for the vitamin as well as the intrinsic factor. The resulting

Table 72.2 Investigation of a patient with suspected malabsorption

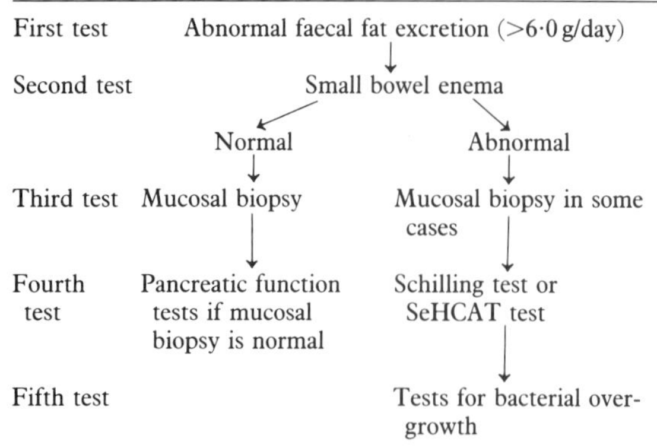

First test	Abnormal faecal fat excretion (>6·0 g/day)	
Second test	Small bowel enema	
	Normal	Abnormal
Third test	Mucosal biopsy	Mucosal biopsy in some cases
Fourth test	Pancreatic function tests if mucosal biopsy is normal	Schilling test or SeHCAT test
Fifth test		Tests for bacterial overgrowth

Table 72.3 Causes of bacterial overgrowth

Excessive entry of bacteria into the small intestine
Achlorhydria—absence of bactericidal gastric acid
Gastrojejunostomy
Partial/total gastrectomy
Enterocolic fistulas
Cholangitis
Loss of the ileocaecal valve following right hemicolectomy
Intestinal stasis
Crohn's disease—stenosis
Tuberculosis—stenosis
Small bowel diverticulosis—stasis
Afferent loop stasis
Entero-enteric anastomosis and other intestinal bypass procedures
Subacute obstruction—adhesions, strictured anastomosis
Blind loops
Diabetes mellitus—autonomic neuropathy
Radiation enteritis—stenosis, impaired intestinal motility
Scleroderma—impaired intestinal motility
Amyloidosis

malabsorption of vitamin B_{12} may lead to megaloblastic anaemia. Often, however, the anaemia has a dimorphic picture because of an iron-deficiency component due to chronic blood loss from the primary lesion itself or from malabsorption of iron. Folate deficiency is rare. The bacteria synthesize folate in substantial amounts and some patients may exhibit a high serum folate.

There is some malabsorption of carbohydrates and proteins, although this is rarely severe. The main reason for the malnutrition in patients with bacterial overgrowth is a diminished dietary intake which also accounts for the growth retardation in children. The bacteria also metabolize the triglycerides to free fatty acids which they hydroxylate to form hydroxy fatty acids which are known to impair the absorption of water and sodium by the intestinal mucosa of both small and large intestine, acting like laxatives. This, together with the action of the dehydroxylated bile salts, enterotoxin, and the osmotic load generated by the fermentation of the major dietary components, all add up to a multifactorial and potent cause for the diarrhoea in these patients.

Clinical Features

The symptomatology is varied. In the first instance, the patient may exhibit symptoms referable to the underlying pathology: postgastrectomy symptoms, recurrent intestinal colic due to subacute obstructing lesions, etc. Patients with jejunal diverticulosis (*Fig.* 72.9) are symptomless until the onset of malabsorption, but may occasionally develop complications, such as gastrointestinal bleeding or perforation of one of the diverticula which results in generalized peritonitis.

The symptoms and signs of bacterial overgrowth itself may be non-specific, and include asthenia, nausea and vomiting, excessive borborygmi and weight loss. Diarrhoea is a frequent symptom and is usually watery. Frank steatorrhoea with bulky, pale, offensive stools which are difficult to flush, is less common. Other clinical features include glossitis and stomatitis, anaemia, hypoproteinaemia with peripheral oedema, tetany, osteomalacia and rickets, and retardation of growth in children. Although rare, neurological manifestations, such as paraesthesiae and peripheral

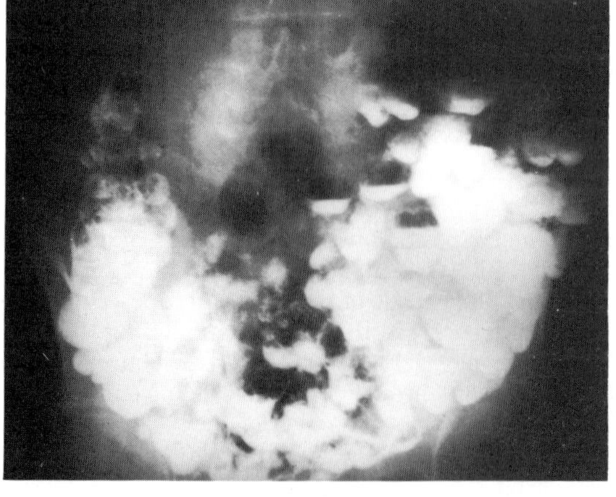

a

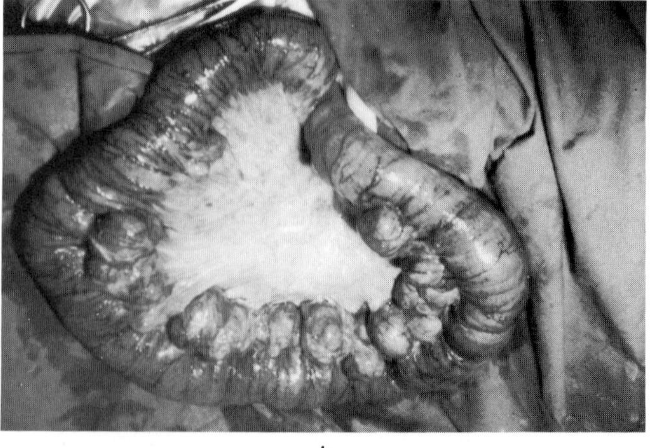

b

Fig. 72.9 a, Small bowel barium study showing extensive and multiple small intestinal diverticula in a 65-year-old female with severe malabsorption. The steatorrhoea improved considerably with oral tetracycline therapy. *b*, Multiple jejunal diverticula localized to a segment of the upper small intestine. The patient's bacterial overgrowth syndrome resolved after excision of the affected bowel.

neuropathy, may be found in association with vitamin B_{12} deficiency.

Treatment

Surgical treatment of the underlying condition, whenever possible, is the definitive and curative treatment. Situations are frequently encountered, however, where surgical treatment is not advisable because of the extensive or systemic nature of the underlying disease, e.g. extensive jejunal diverticulosis, scleroderma. In these cases, intermittent therapy with oral antibiotics is often beneficial. The two most commonly used antibiotics are tetracycline and metronidazole. As control of the anaerobic organisms seems to be the most helpful objective, the latter is generally preferred nowadays, although tetracycline is of undoubted value. The antibiotic course is usually administered for 10–14 days at a time. Although repopulation of the intestine by bacteria recurs soon after the antibiotic is stopped, symptomatic improvement may last for several months. Therefore intermittent therapy is generally preferred to long-term treatment.

Short-gut Syndrome

This is the most serious form of intestinal decompensation and is encountered after massive resection of the small bowel and in some patients subjected to jejuno-ileal bypass for morbid obesity. The lesions which may necessitate extensive resection of the small intestine in order of frequency are:

Crohn's disease
Mesenteric infarction
Radiation enteritis
Mid-gut volvulus
Multiple fistulas
Small bowel tumours.

Crohn's disease is by far the commonest cause. This disease often necessitates repeated resections over a number of years culminating in the short-gut syndrome. Hence the reason for a conservative approach in these patients with limited resections of the symptomatic disease and the judicious use of stricturoplasty for patients with short fibrous strictures without any evidence of active inflammation.

It is often stated that resections of more than half of the small bowel length are invariably accompanied by serious malabsorption. Whilst this may be true, there is some debate as to the extent of the small bowel resection which results in the short-gut syndrome. An assessment of the length of the residual small bowel after resection is the important factor as there is a critical length below which intestinal decompensation of varying degrees takes place. Thus patients with a residual small bowel length of less than 2 m have a diminished work capacity, and those with less than 100 cm require home parenteral nutrition on an indefinite basis.

The critical length of residual bowel necessary to prevent serious maldigestion and malabsorption depends on the site of resection and the retention or otherwise of the ileocaecal valve. Thus, ileal resections are less well tolerated than jejunal resections, largely because the active transport sites for bile salts and vitamin B_{12} are localized in the ileum. The importance of retaining a terminal segment of ileum and ileocaecal valve whenever possible, is documented by several clinical reports. An intact ileocaecal valve slows the transit time and limits the degree of colonization of the residual intestine by an overgrowth of colonic bacteria.

Pathophysiology

The clinical outcome following intestinal resection is dependent on the following:

Extent and site of resection
Age of the patient
Physical state and mental condition.

In cases of mesenteric infarction, varying amounts of colon are frequently resected with the small intestine. It is not known whether the extent of the associated colonic resection influences the clinical outcome. The colonic mucosa absorbs water and salt and, to a lesser extent, glucose and amino acids. Some reports indicate that it minimizes the severity of the diarrhoea and may assume some of the absorptive functions of the small intestine. Infants and neonates seem to tolerate extensive small bowel resections better than adults. A minimum of 30 cm of small intestine can support both nutrition and growth.

The intestinal decompensation that follows massive resection of the small intestine is due to a sudden reduction of the absorptive area and a greatly enhanced transit time which further aggravates the malabsorption and, in extreme cases, limits the extent of digestion. More usually, the digestion of carbohydrates, proteins and fats remains unimpaired.

Malabsorption of fats and proteins is invariably present but its severity varies with the length and site of the residual bowel. Carbohydrate absorption is less severely affected and is the first to return to normal in 4–6 weeks. The improvement in the absorptive capacity for proteins is more gradual and the absorption of fats remains impaired at a fixed percentage of the amount ingested. It is the result of interruption of the enterohepatic circulation of bile salts after ileal resection and a diminished bile salt pool, as the increased hepatic synthesis is unable to compensate for the large daily faecal losses. The spill-over into the colon where bacterial action will convert the primary bile salt conjugates into deconjugated and dehydroxylated derivatives, contributes to the diarrhoea since some of these secondary bile salts block the absorption of water and electrolytes by the colonic mucosa. The hydroxylation of the unabsorbed fatty acids by colonic bacteria has also been implicated in the pathogenesis of the diarrhoea of the short-gut syndrome. The malabsorption of fats and fat-soluble vitamins is accompanied by the malabsorption of calcium and magnesium which are precipitated as soaps with the unabsorbed fatty acids. The severe watery diarrhoea, which can amount to several litres in the first few weeks after resection, is further aggravated by the low pH of the stools and often causes severe perianal irritation.

Lactose intolerance may occur in some patients after extensive small bowel resection. It has been attributed to a rapid transit time allowing insufficient time for lactase to act, and to a reduction of the total intestinal lactase activity. The consumption of fresh milk in these patients is followed by attacks of abdominal pain and an increase in the severity of the diarrhoea. In addition to the malabsorptive defects and resultant malnutrition, other sequelae may follow massive resection or extensive bypass of the small intestine. These include:

Gastric hypersecretion
Cholesterol gallstones
Hepatic disease
Impaired renal function
Urinary stone formation
Metabolic bone disease.

Gastric Hypersecretion

In man the syndrome of gastric hypersecretion is transient and bears no relation to the extent of the intestinal excision although it appears to be more common after proximal resections. It is due to an increased rate of basal gastric acid secretion consequent on delayed clearance of gastrin. It affects some 50% of patients after extensive intestinal resection.

Gallstone Formation

There is a documented increase in the incidence of gallstones after extensive ileal resections and jejuno-ileal bypass for morbid obesity. Cholesterol stones are the result of a reduced bile salt pool. The bile therefore becomes lithogenic, i.e. supersaturated with cholesterol which precipitates as cholesterol crystals. However, pigmented gallstones also form after ileal resections.

Hepatic Disease

Mild hyperbilirubinaemia, elevation of the serum transaminases and impaired excretion of BSP are not uncommon after both massive intestinal resections and jejuno-ileal bypass. They are associated with fatty infiltration of the liver, with or without hepatic atrophy which has been documented in both conditions. The increased deposition of fat in the liver after jejuno-ileal bypass occurs in patients actively losing weight but not when the weight is stationary. Acute fulminant liver failure has been reported most commonly after jejuno-ileal bypass. The onset of the liver failure usually occurs within the first 6 months after operation and the clinical symptoms are those of a flu-like illness with anorexia, nausea, vomiting, rapid weight loss and a fall in the serum albumin. The onset of these manifestations is an indication for active intervention with restoration of intestinal continuity. Cirrhosis may develop after jejuno-ileal bypass. Initially it causes no symptoms, and therefore its onset can only be detected by serial liver biopsies.

Impaired Renal Function and Stone Formation

The severe diarrhoea may lead to fluid and electrolyte losses and to a decrease in the glomerular filtration rate with a tendency to a low urine output and a concentrated urine. The constant loss of electrolyte-rich intestinal fluid causes hyponatraemia and hypokalaemia. A metabolic acidosis ensues from the fixed base losses into the gastrointestinal tract with the excretion of a persistently acid urine. The urinary calcium excretion is low but the oxalate concentration and excretion is high especially in patients with an intact colon. Urinary calculi of all types (urate and oxalate) are very common in patients after enterectomy and the vast majority of patients will develop this complication during their lifetime.

The water and salt depletion results in an increased secretion of aldosterone in an attempt at maximal renal salt conservation but at the expense of increased potassium loss. This chronic hypokalaemia, apart from causing muscle weakness, anorexia and cardiac arrhythmias, may limit protein synthesis and impair transport and utilization of carbohydrates. In addition, it may lead to the development of a type of renal tubular nephropathy consisting of a characteristic patchy vacuolar change in the cells of the proximal convoluted tubules. This syndrome of hypokalaemic vacuolar nephropathy can complicate other disorders associated with diarrhoea, such as ulcerative colitis and coeliac disease.

Metabolic Bone Disease

Hypocalcaemia and hypomagnesaemia are common and are often associated with neuromuscular symptoms, dehydration and other electrolyte abnormalities. Both hypocalcaemia and hypomagnesaemia, if persistent or recurrent, can be effectively treated with oral 1-alpha-hydroxylated metabolites of vitamin D. Osteomalacia is common but difficult to confirm without a bone biopsy. The patients complain of bone pains and have an elevated serum alkaline phosphatase activity.

Adaptation

With time, structural and functional changes occur in the residual bowel as part of the process of adaptation to the reduced absorptive area. In the human, the structural changes consist of dilatation of the remaining intestine and villous enlargement. An increase in the length of the bowel has been reported in the human neonate. These structural changes are accompanied by a gradual improvement in the absorption of water, electrolytes, carbohydrates and protein. The enhanced absorption of water-soluble substances per unit length of intestine is not the result of greater absorption by individual cells, but rather from a normal rate of absorption by an increased cell population in the intestinal villi. Both luminal and humoral factors are involved in this adaptive villous hyperplasia. The luminal factors include alimentary secretions (pancreatico-biliary and gastroduodenal) and ingested nutrients. Duodenal juice may be particularly important as a source of epidermal growth factor. The maintenance of an adequate intraluminal nutrition by the oral ingestion of appropriate food is essential for the adaptive response. Enteroglucagon is regarded as the most important humoral agent influencing the adaptive response. The stimulus for its release is thought to result from increased exposure of the residual bowel to luminal nutrition. The enteroglucagon then acts on the mucosal cells and stimulates an increased turnover of intracellular polyamines and cell growth. There is evidence, however, that the effect of intraluminal nutrition is also mediated through direct contact of the nutrients with the epithelial cells.

The other factors with suggested involvement in the functional compensation by the residual intestine include changes in the motility pattern leading to a gradual slowing of the transit time, and increased absorption of water-soluble substances by the colon.

Treatment

The treatment is designed to support the patient during the initial stage of decompensation and through the critical stage of adaptation which may last up to 3 months until the stage of equilibrium is reached, when with adequate dietary care and oral supplements, the patient with some residual small intestine enters the final phase of rehabilitation. In patients with massive small bowel resection, indefinite total parenteral nutrition via a permanent tunnelled silicone feeding line (Broviac or Hickman) is the only option available for survival. In these patients a programme of training with regard to the management of their intravenous feeds and care of the feeding lines is started, so that they can eventually carry out the parenteral nutrition themselves in their own homes, usually at night (home parenteral nutrition).

In the immediate postoperative period, the treatment is by total parenteral nutrition. The regimen must provide 40 kcal/kg body weight and 300 mg of nitrogen/kg body weight, in addition to electrolyte, vitamin and trace metal requirements usually in a 3-litre single bag system administered daily over a period of 12 h. Accurate fluid balance must be maintained by daily charting of the input versus output which should include all measured losses. H_2-receptor blockade therapy (cimetidine 200 mg) is administered 6-hourly by the intravenous route to suppress gastric secretion. This avoids the necessity for nasogastric intubation and suction which should only be used in these patients if ileus is prolonged. Initially nothing other than weak hypotonic electrolyte solutions are tolerated orally. Small amounts should be administered (15–30 ml hourly) to avoid a dry mouth and its consequences.

When the patient's condition becomes stable (usually 3–6 weeks after the enterectomy), the transition to an oral diet is commenced in those patients with an adequate residual length of small intestine. When this exceeds one metre, ultimate resumption of a normal or near-normal oral diet is usual, whereas patients with 100 cm of residual small intestine or less will usually require long-term enteral feeding with artificial defined-formula diets (elemental/polymeric) with or without supplemental parenteral feeding. In any event, oral feeding is started gradually in all patients, initially with isotonic carbohydrate-electrolyte solutions. Thereafter, elemental diets are used. These are semi-synthetic fibre-free liquid diets containing all the basic nutrient components (protein hydrolysates, simple carbohydrates, essential lipids, vitamins and trace elements). The nitrogen component is available either as free amino acids (elemental) or as peptides (polymeric). There is some evidence that the peptide-based polymeric diets have a better nitrogen utilization than the elemental ones, although this remains controversial. The fats which contribute only a small amount of the calorie content of these artificial diets, are necessary particularly as a supply of essential fatty acids. They usually consist of a mixture of monoglycerides, diglycerides and medium-chain triglycerides. The latter have a distinct advantage in that they are absorbed directly into the portal system.

The diet is administered via a nasogastric feeding tube (Clinfeed, Dobhof, etc.) initially in a dilute form (1 in 4) and instilled by an infusion pump (Ivac, etc.) at a rate of 25 ml/h. The rate and concentration are gradually increased until the patient receives 100–120 ml of the full strength diet/hour. Great care must be taken to ensure against gastric retention as instances of gastric dilatation and pulmonary aspiration with a fatal outcome are well documented during nasogastric enteral feeding. The use of a percutaneous cervical pharyngostomy with a size 12–14 Ryle's tube is preferred by some surgeons during the first few weeks of enteral nutrition. It is less likely to block and allows intermittent aspiration of the stomach as a check for gastric retention (*Fig.* 72.10). Those patients who require long-term maintenance with chemically-defined diets can either take these as frequent small drinks throughout the day or be instructed to swallow the feeding tube and infuse the feed themselves.

One of the most common early problems is diarrhoea which is often accentuated with the start of enteral feeding. The most effective drugs which are used to control this are loperamide hydrochloride, diphenoxylate hydrochloride and codeine phosphate. In patients with an intact colon after ileal resections, cholestyramine is administered as a bile salt binding agent to limit the colonic cathartic effect of the unabsorbed bile salts. In some patients, the diarrhoea proves intractable and life threatening and requires control with an infusion of the long-acting analogue of somatostatin (SMS 201–995).

Steatorrhoea is very common in these patients and results from excess fat in the diet. Whenever possible, dietary fat should be administered as medium-chain triglycerides which do not require the presence of bile salts for their absorption into the portal venous blood. Dietary supplements of calcium, magnesium, vitamins C, D (as the 1-alpha-hydroxylated derivatives) and K, and iron are necessary. In all patients in whom the ileum has been resected,

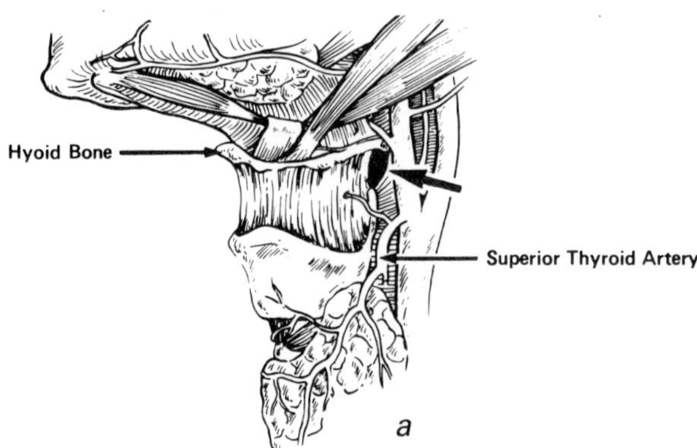

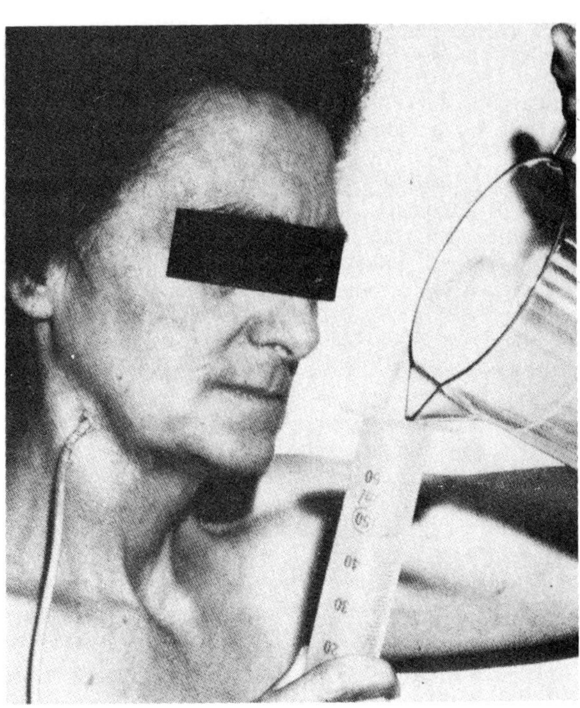

Fig. 72.10 *a*, Percutaneous cervical pharyngostomy. The position of the pyriform recess is shown by the arrow. At this site, the pharyngeal wall is close to the skin. This position is located by passing a finger through the mouth and down the lateral pharyngeal wall until the greater cornu of the hyoid can be felt. The pyriform recess lies below and medial to this point. A pair of fine right-angled forceps is guided along the finger and its tip is then pressed laterally to tent up the skin of the neck which is then incised over the tip of the forceps. A size 14 Ryle's tube is then grasped by the jaws of the forceps. (Reproduced by kind permission of the editor, Meehan et al. *Am. J. Surg.* 1984, **148**, 325–330.) *b*, Pharyngostomy tube in place and being used by the patient to feed herself. (Reproduced by kind permission of the editor, Meehan et al. *Am. J. Surg.* 1984, **148**, 325–330.)

Table 72.4 Sequential management of patients after massive resection of the small intestine

Stage of decompensation	Total parenteral nutrition, replacement of fluid and electrolyte losses, sips of oral hypotonic solutions
Transition to enteral feeding	(i) Parenteral nutrition+gradually increasing supplements of enteral feeds. (ii) Full enteral feeding by chemically defined diets (elemental, polymeric).
Final stage	(i) Home parenteral nutrition (patients with no effective residual small bowel). (ii) Enteral feeding: intermittent parenteral feeding in patients with 100 cm or less of residual small intestine. (iii) Normal low fat (medium-chain triglyceride) diet+supplements in patients with >1 m of residual small bowel.

vitamin B_{12} is administered parenterally at 3-monthly intervals on an indefinite basis. The sequential medical management of patients after massive resection of the small intestine is summarized in *Table* 72.4.

Remedial Surgical Procedures

These are rarely indicated in adult patients and should only be entertained after medical treatment, including the use of the long-acting somatostatin analogue, has failed to control the diarrhoea and malnutrition. They are designed to delay transit. Reversed (antiperistaltic) segments have been employed. Although they do delay transit, they can lead to intestinal obstruction and favour the development of bacterial overgrowth. In order to avoid risks of strangulation, the antiperistaltic segment should be constructed without reversal (*Fig.* 72.11). In neonates and infants, the procedure of intestinal lengthening has given promising results and is likely to be used more often in the future (*Fig.* 72.12). Truncal vagotomy and pyloroplasty, although often used and advocated in the past, is not indicated and in those few patients who devleop persistent gastric acid hypersecretion, cimetidine or ranitidine should be used on a long-term basis.

Protein-losing Enteropathy

In health less than 10% of the total amount of albumin catabolized daily can be accounted for enteric losses. A greatly increased bulk loss of plasma proteins (irrespective of molecular size) is found in the syndrome of protein-losing enteropathy. When severe, it leads to hypoproteinaemia and secondary hyperaldosteronism with water and salt retention. Although the fraction of the intravascular pool lost into the gut per day is the same for all the serum proteins, albumin and IgA, because of their low fractional catabolic rates, are depleted more than the other serum proteins. The syndrome of protein-losing enteropathy may be the presenting feature of the illness causing it. More usually, the clinical picture is dominated by the manifestations of the underlying disease and the hypoproteinaemia is found during the investigation of the patient. The disorders associated with protein-losing enteropathy fall into three categories:

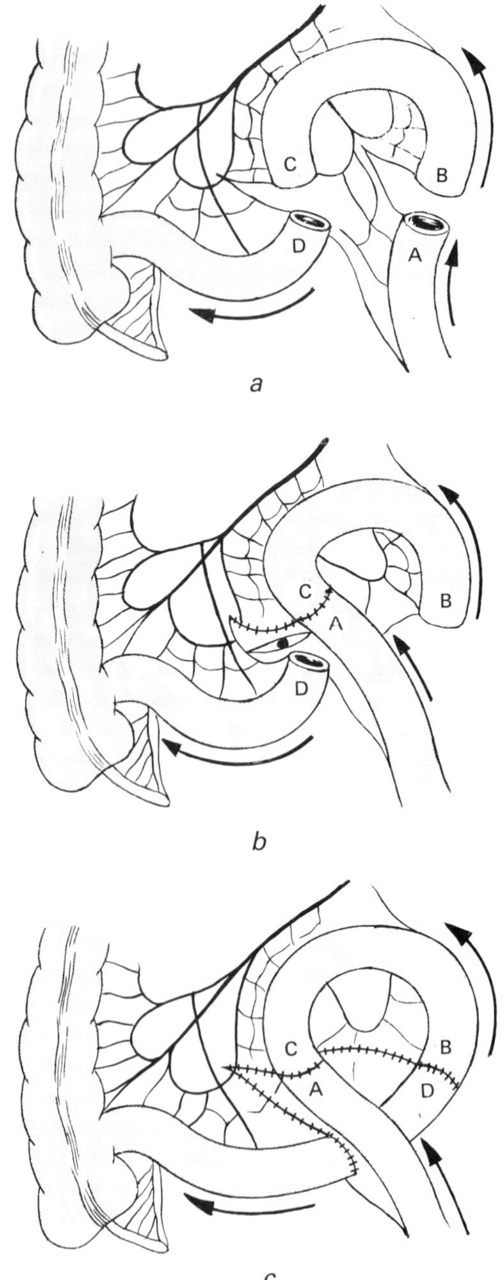

Fig. 72.11 Technique of creating an antiperistaltic segment without reversal of the mesenteric pedicle.

1. *Mucosal disease*
   Coeliac disease
   Giant rugal hypertrophy of the stomach (Ménétrier's disease)
   Whipple's disease
   Bacterial infections and parasitic infestations of the gastrointestinal tract
   Bacterial overgrowth
2. *Ulcerating lesions and tumours*
   Multiple gastric ulcers
   Malignant gastric tumours
   Colonic cancer and villous tumours
   Haemangiomas
   Inflammatory bowel disease
   Gastrojejunocolic fistula
   Radiation enteritis

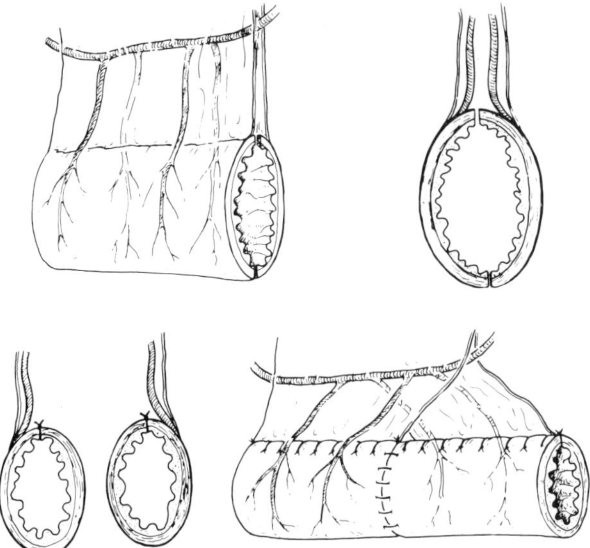

Fig. 72.12 Diagrammatic representation of the intestinal lengthening operation developed by Bianchi. The bowel is split longitudinally into two halves, each retaining its blood supply. A tube is constructed from each half. The two tubes are then joined together.

3. *Lymphatic obstruction*
   Primary lymphangiectasia
   Intestinal lymphoma
   Congestive cardiac failure

A variety of radioactive agents has been used to document protein loss in the gut but the one most frequently used in clinical practice is albumin labelled with ^{131}I or ^{51}Cr. The radionuclide is injected intravenously and its concentration in the serum followed for 2 weeks. The plasma die away curve is thus obtained. By compartmental analysis of this together with estimation of the faecal radioactivity, the extent of the enteric losses per day can be calculated. The treatment of protein-losing enteropathy is that of the underlying pathology which may necessitate surgical intervention. If the plasma albumin is very low (<3·0 g/L), this must be restored to near normal by protein infusions (Purified Protein derivative, or Albumin Solution) before surgery. These patients must be kept on a high calorie, high protein diet.

VASCULAR ANOMALIES, HAMARTOMATOUS LESIONS AND VASCULITIC/CONNECTIVE TISSUE DISORDERS OF THE GASTROINTESTINAL TRACT

Aside from the common causes of gastrointestinal haemorrhage, such as peptic ulceration and tumours, a wide spectrum of disorders may lead to recurrent and, at times, life-threatening gastrointestinal bleeding (*Table* 72.5). Prior to the advent of selective angiography, radionuclide scanning and colonoscopy, the exact cause and site of the bleeding in some of these difficult cases remained undiagnosed. Treatment then consisted of emergency laparotomy and resection of that part of the gastrointestinal tract which the surgeon considered to be responsible, based on the presence of an identifiable lesion, distribution of blood within the intestines and the application of non-crushing clamps to identify the segment which distended between two such clamps since this contained the bleeding site. The investigative modalities referred to above have largely obviated these problems. The small intestine may be involved by systemic vasculitic and connective tissue disorders. The conditions in which intestinal involvement is common are polyarteritis, Henoch–Schönlein purpura, pseudoxanthoma elasticum and Ehlers–Danlos syndrome.

Table 72.5 Vascular abnormalities and disorders

Small vessel anomalies	Angiodysplasia Phlebectasia Haemangiomas Telangiectasia
Hereditary syndromes	Osler–Weber–Rendu disease Peutz–Jeghers syndrome Blue rubber bleb naevus syndrome
Systemic vasculitic disorders	Polyarteritis Henoch–Schönlein purpura
Connective tissue disorders	Pseudoxanthoma elasticum Ehlers–Danlos syndrome

Small Vessel Anomalies

These comprise angiodysplasia, multiple phlebectasia, telangiectasis and haemangiomas.

Angiodysplasias

Angiodysplasias are referred to by a variety of names, e.g. arteriovenous malformations, vascular dysplasias, vascular ectasias. They are a common cause of recurrent occult gastrointestinal bleeding and their true incidence was not appreciated prior to the introduction of splanchnic angiography and colonoscopy. The lesions occupy the mucosa and submucosa of the gastrointestinal tract and consist of a cluster of arteriolar, venular and capillary vessels. They are, therefore, not visible or palpable from the outer aspect of the gut. Rupture of the mucosal component is the cause of the bleeding. The most common site is undoubtedly the right colon; however, they can occur in other parts of the gut, such as the stomach and the small intestine. They are considered to be acquired lesions but the exact cause remains conjectural. The various theories concerning their aetiology include chronic mucosal ischaemia secondary to arteriovenous shunting, decreased perfusion pressure and lowered oxygen tension in the terminal branches of the superior mesenteric arteries, and chronic intermittent obstruction of the submucosal veins by the muscular coat of the gut, particularly the right colon where the tension in the muscular layer is greater than elsewhere in the colon.

Clinical Features

An increased incidence of angiodysplastic lesions has been reported in patients with aortic valve disease and in patients with chronic respiratory disease. The colonic lesions have been invariably diagnosed in patients over 50–55 years of age, whereas the small bowel lesions are usually encountered in a younger age group with a mean age of 30–35 years. Patients with these arteriovenous lesions experience episodic or chronic occult gastrointestinal bleeding over a number of years and most commonly present with iron-deficiency anaemia. The majority will eventually develop attacks of overt melaena, and in some, the acute haemorrhage is severe, causing hypovolaemic shock.

The initial investigation in these patients is fibreoptic upper GI endoscopy followed by colonoscopy. Colonic angiodysplasias are well visualized by colonoscopy. The lesions are cherry-red in colour, each consisting of a central large vessel from which radiate multiple peripheral branches reminiscent of a spider naevus. If endoscopy proves negative, localization of the bleeding site can be achieved by radionuclide scintiscanning ($^{99}Tc^{m}$ Sc, $^{99}Tc^{m}$-labelled autologous red cells) or by selective angiography which can identify the vascular abnormality especially when subtraction film techniques are used. The typical angiographic finding consists of a tortuous feeding artery and dilated veins with an intervening cluster of fine vessels (*Fig.* 72.13). If the angiogram is performed during a bleeding episode, extravasation of contrast into the bowel lumen may be observed depending on the rate of bleeding. Some authors have reported extravasation with bleeding rates as low as 0·5 ml/min; others maintain that the blood loss needs to be much heavier (>6·0/min).

Treatment

Initially the patient is treated conservatively with blood volume replacement. Endoscopically defined lesions are treated with electrocoagulation using the coagulation forceps. This is particularly effective for colonic lesions. Laparotomy is reserved for lesions beyond endoscopic view, when endoscopic treatment is not practicable because of the extent of the lesions, and for continued or recurrent life-threatening haemorrhage. Peroperative endoscopy is used to transilluminate the bowel and can be very useful in identifying these vascular anomalies. The object of surgical treatment is excision of the segment of gut containing the vascular ectasia.

Phlebectasia

These lesions consist of meshwork of dilated veins having a normal endothelial lining and situated in the submucosal plane of the gut. They may be multiple and extensive. The

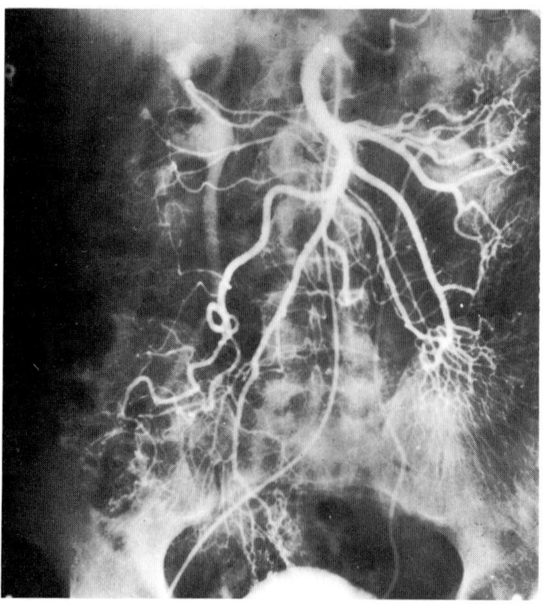

a

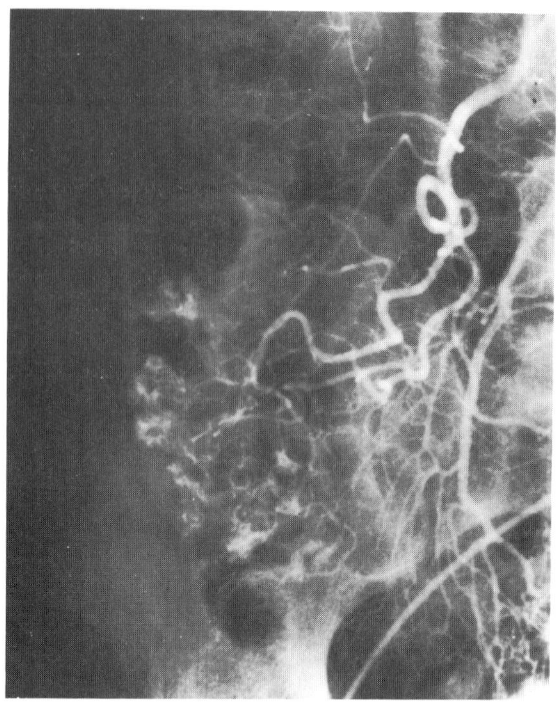

b

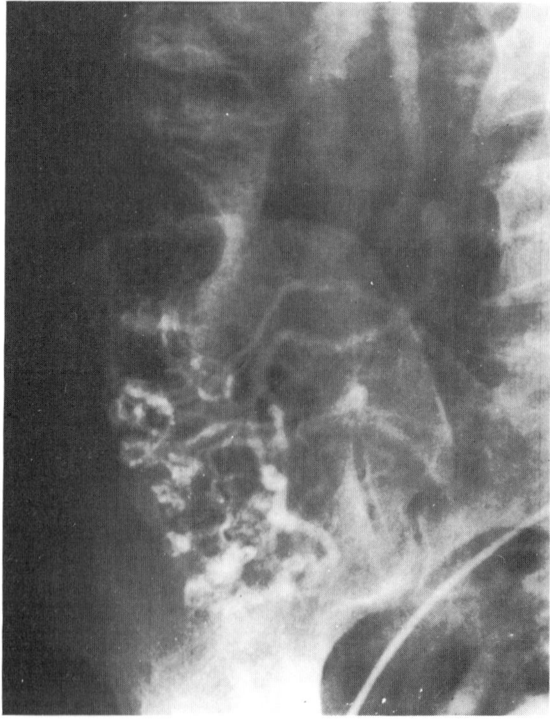

c

Fig. 72.13 Selective superior mesenteric angiogram showing extensive changes of angiodysplasia in the caecum. The angiographic features are: *a*, Prominent and early filling of clusters of irregularly dilated small vessels within the wall of the caecum supplied by enlarged branches of the ileocolic artery. *b*, Persistence of contrast within the clusters of small vessels. *c*, Early and profuse filling of enlarged draining veins from the affected area.

more frequent documented sites are the oesophagus, mid-small bowel and rectum. Blood loss is usually mild but severe haemorrhage has been reported requiring resection of the affected segment.

Haemangiomas

These are rare, congenital, non-hereditary malformations of blood vessels (vascular hamartomas). They are classified into three types: capillary, cavernous and mixed. Most of the reported cases have been in the small and large intestine. The cavernous varieties carry a poor prognosis with an overall reported mortality of 30% usually from massive haemorrhage. Haemangiomas can also present with perforation (following an intramural bleed), recurrent abdominal pain, intussusception, ulceration and intraluminal obstruction. The optimal treatment is surgical excision. Some diffuse cavernous lesions have been successfully treated by percutaneous selective arteriographic embolization.

Hereditary Haemorrhagic Telangiectasia

Also known as the Osler–Weber–Rendu disease, this rare inherited disorder is clinically recognized by repeated attacks of bleeding from multiple telangiectasias of lips, mouth, nasopharynx and gut. The lesions consist of arteriolar dilatations due to a congenital weakness of the arterial muscle and absence of elastin in the medial coat. The associated gastrointestinal telangiectasias tend to cause melaena in middle age, but the gastrointestinal bleeding is rarely severe and surgical intervention is not usually necessary.

Peutz–Jeghers Syndrome

This is an inherited autosomal dominant disorder characterized by jejunal or ileal polyps and mucocutaneous pigmentation. The polyps are hamartomatous in nature and consist of a fibromuscular stroma covered with well-differentiated epithelium. They have a tendency to ulceration and bleeding. Rarely, the polyps may be localized in the stomach, duodenum or colorectal region. The pigmentation which is due to deposits of melanin, is characteristically found in the lips and buccal mucosa. This abnormal pigmentation usually appears in infancy but the polyps are diagnosed, because of the development of symptoms or complications, in the second decade. Although malignant transformation may occur, the risk is small and has been estimated at 2–3%. Cases of Peutz–Jeghers syndrome have been documented where the mucocutaneous pigmentation is associated with intestinal haemangiomas instead of the hamartomatous polyps.

Clinical Features

Attacks of intestinal colic may predate acute intestinal obstruction from intussusception or intraluminal obstruction by a large polyp. Bleeding from the polyps is common and is usually chronic, presenting with iron-deficiency anaemia, although acute gastrointestinal haemorrhage may complicate the clinical picture.

Treatment

In view of the small but definite risk of malignancy, all polyps greater than 2·0 cm should be removed. Surgical treatment is also indicated for intestinal obstruction and haemorrhage.

Blue Rubber Bleb Naevus Syndrome

This is a hereditary autosomal disorder consisting of cavernous angiomas involving the skin, gastrointestinal tract and other organs including lungs and joints. The skin lesions appear as blue compressible swellings. The small intestine is the most commonly affected segment of the gut. The gastrointestinal lesions may give rise to profuse haemorrhage at any time between childhood and middle age. Angiographic demonstration of the bleeding site is essential before surgical intervention in those patients with continued bleeding.

Polyarteritis

This condition which is thought to be an immune-complex mediated disorder, is characterized by a systemic necrotizing vasculitis with fibrinoid necrosis and an inflammatory cell infiltrate which affect the blood vessels (arteries and veins) of several organs including the gut. The weakened vessels lead to aneurysm formation which may rupture and bleed or thrombose causing multiple organ infarcts. There are several categories of polyarteritis: classical *polyarteritis nodosa* (PAN), the *Churg–Strauss syndrome* (CSS) also known as *allergic granulomatous angiitis* (because of the eosinophilic infiltration and granuloma formation in the connective tissue in addition to the vasculitis), *microscopic polyarteritis* (MPA) and mixed forms. The first two commonly affect the gut. In addition to the systemic manifestations (fever, weight loss, malaise, hypertension) of the disorder, the usual gastrointestinal symptoms include nausea, vomiting, steatorrhoea and diarrhoea. Medical treatment is with corticosteroids and either cyclophosphamide or azathioprine. PAN, CSS and, to a lesser extent, MPA may lead to acute life-threatening complications such as intestinal infarction, perforation and massive gastrointestinal haemorrhage. The latter is caused by rupture of the inflamed aneurysmal mesenteric blood vessels. Surgical treatment is only undertaken for the above major complications. It entails resection of the affected segment. In cases of infarction, the ends are exteriorized and bowel continuity restored at a later stage.

Henoch–Schönlein Purpura

This affects children and young adults predominantly of the male sex and usually follows an upper respiratory infection and is characterized by the deposition of IgA-immune complexes in the tissues, particularly of the skin and the kidneys. The skin involvement gives rise to a characteristic purpuric rash and the renal lesions result in a glomerulonephritis. Joint and gastrointestinal tract involvement are common. The gut lesions cause submucosal oedema and mucosal haemorrhage, the former presenting as subacute intestinal obstruction with severe colicky abdominal pain, nausea and vomiting. Both severe gastrointestinal bleeding and intestinal infarction with perforation are rare. Surgical intervention is rarely necessary. The disease usually runs a benign and self-limiting course.

Connective-tissue Disorders

The two disorders which may be complicated by intestinal bleeding are the Ehlers–Danlos syndrome (EDS) and pseudoxanthoma elasticum (PE). Both are rare hereditary disorders. The basic abnormality of the EDS is a defect in the synthesis of collagen, the disease being characterized by thin, easily damaged skin which bruises easily, hyperextension and episodes of dislocation of joints, incompetence of cardiac valves due to stretching of the chordae tendineae and spontaneous rupture of arteries and viscera. The gastrointestinal manifestions include dilatation of the hollow viscera, intramural and intraluminal haemorrhage, formation of intestinal diverticula and colonic perforation.

In PE there is a defect in the metabolism of elastic tissue. The disease affects the skin, mucous membranes, blood vessels and the eyeball. The affected skin becomes lax and redundant and the eye changes lead to progressive loss of visual acuity and eventually blindness. The arteries become prematurely calcified and have a tendency to rupture spontaneously or with minimal trauma. The most common site of gastrointestinal haemorrhage is the stomach, the mucosa of which has a yellowish cobblestone appearance at endoscopy.

TUMOURS OF THE SMALL INTESTINE

Tumours of the small intestine are rare and all the benign and malignant types collectively account for less than 10% of all gastrointestinal neoplasms. The aetiology of small bowel tumours is unknown but a number of gastrointestinal disorders are associated with an increased risk. These include Crohn's disease, coeliac disease, dermatitis herpetiformis, Peutz–Jeghers syndrome, radiation enteritis and adenomas.

Benign Small Bowel Tumours

Although benign tumours constitute 60% of small bowel neoplasms, their clinical importance is limited by their usual asymptomatic course so that most are encountered as accidental findings at operation and post-mortem. They include epithelial tumours (tubular and villous adenomas), lipomas, haemangiomas and neurogenic tumours. The latter are subdivided into nerve sheath tumours (neurofibromas and neurilemmomas) and nerve cell tumours (ganglioneuromas, paraganglionomas and sympathicoblastomas). The neurofibromas may be solitary or multiple and associated with systemic neurofibromatosis and café-au-lait skin patches (Von Recklinghausen's disease).

Intestinal adenomas may occur in association with familial polyposis which includes polyposis coli, Gardner's syndrome (familial polyposis and epidermoid cysts) and Turcot's syndrome (familial polyposis and brain tumours). In addition to the well-known risk of colonic carcinoma, these patients are also liable to develop carcinoma of the duodenum and the biliary tract. Within the non-familial group of small intestinal adenomas, the villous variety is especially prone to malignant change.

The commonest presentation of benign small bowel tumours is with intestinal obstruction due to intussusception most commonly in children over the age of 2 years. Tumour-induced intussusception thus occurs later than the idiopathic variety and does not usually reduce by hydrostatic therapy. The tumour is therefore usually discovered after operative reduction and resection of the bowel segment. Chronic blood loss from a benign small bowel tumour may cause an iron-deficiency anaemia, and occasionally vascular tumours may give rise to overt gastrointestinal bleeding. Most benign small bowel tumours are, however, asymptomatic and even in the presence of chronic symptoms, there are usually no significant findings on physical examination. Treatment of the symptomatic cases is by local excision.

Malignant Small Bowel Tumours

Malignant small bowel tumours are rare and account for less than 5% of all malignant gastrointestinal neoplasms. Symptoms occur late and the tumour has usually spread beyond the confines of the bowel wall by the time of diagnosis. The important malignant small bowel tumours are:

Adenocarcinoma (40%)
Carcinoid tumours (30%)
Lymphoma (25%)
Smooth muscle tumours (5%).

The best 5-year survival rates are found in the carcinoid and lymphoma groups. The prognosis for adenocarcinoma and smooth muscle tumours is less favourable with overall 5-year survival rates of 15% and 20% respectively.

Adenocarcinoma

These are usually well-differentiated mucus-secreting tumours which are more common in the proximal part of the small intestine (duodenal 40%, jejunal 40%, ileal 20%). The majority of duodenal carcinomas are found in the periampullary region and in the third part of the duodenum. Intestinal adenocarcinomas spread primarily to the regional lymph nodes, liver and peritoneal cavity.

Clinical Features

The median age at diagnosis is 60 years with an equal sex incidence. The symptoms include epigastric or periumbilical discomfort or pain which is usually postprandial and colicky in nature, nausea and vomiting particularly in patients with duodenal carcinomas, weight loss and gastrointestinal bleeding which is usually occult and results in an iron-deficiency anaemia but may be overt, e.g. melaena and rarely frank haemorrhage. Intestinal obstruction is indicative of advanced disease, although intussusception of polypoid tumours is well documented. Patients with duodenal carcinomas may present with obstructive jaundice. The carcinoma which develops in patients with Crohn's disease has a particularly bad prognosis and differs in a number of ways from that arising *de novo*. It occurs in a younger age group (40–50 years), predominantly in males (3:1) and affects the ileum in 75% of cases. The diagnosis of duodenal carcinoma is established by fibreoptic endoscopy and hypotonic duodenography. Jejunal and ileal tumours are best identified by a small bowel contrast enema.

Treatment

Surgical resection is the mainstay of therapy since small intestinal adenocarcinoma does not respond to either chemotherapy or radiotherapy. Duodenal tumours are best treated with pancreaticoduodenectomy, although good results have been reported with segmental resection particularly for lesions situated in the third part of the duodenum. A gastroenterostomy is performed for advanced duodenal tumours. Jejunal and ileal tumours are resected with a minimum of 5 cm healthy margin on either side of the lesion together with the associated mesentery and regional lymph nodes. Carcinomas of the terminal ileum require a formal right hemicolectomy. The prognosis following resection depends on the stage of the disease in terms of extent of mural involvement, lymph-node metastases and presence of hepatic and peritoneal secondaries. The reported 5-year survival following curative resection varies from 20 to 45% and is better for the duodenal tumours.

Carcinoid Tumours

These tumour arise from the Kulchitsky cells of the crypts of Lieberkuhn. They are nowadays referred to as the enterochromaffin cells (stain with potassium chromate). Carcinoid tumours occur predominantly in the gastrointestinal tract and are classified into three groups:

1. *Foregut* tumours arise in the stomach, duodenum, pancreas, biliary tract and bronchus. These tumours consist of regularly shaped cells which assume a trabecular arrangement and contain round granules. They exhibit the argyrophilic reaction (the cells can only be stained with metallic silver in the presence of a reducing agent).
2. *Midgut* tumours. These are found in the jejunum, ileum and right colon. The cells are pleomorphic, variable in size and are arranged in nests separated by delicate connective tissue. The cells have both argentaffin (can be stained directly with metallic silver in the absence of a reducing agent) and argyrophilic staining properties.
3. *Hindgut* tumours occur in the left colon and rectum. The cells are arranged in a trabecular pattern, contain round granules but do not stain with silver.

Foregut tumours produce 5-hydroxytryptophan, 5-hydroxytryptamine (serotonin), histamine and substance P; midgut tumours 5-hydroxytryptamine, glandular kallikrein (kinin-forming enzyme) and possibly prostaglandins; but tumours of the hindgut do not usually secrete active peptides. In addition, midgut and especially foregut tumours may contain and secrete a variety of hormones: insulin, somatostatin, ACTH, gastrin, ADH, parathormone, glucagon, VIP, calcitonin, beta-MSH, cholecystokinin, growth hormone, etc. The cellular morphology does not differentiate benign from malignant carcinoids. In general, tumours smaller than 1·0 cm are rarely malignant, lesions between 1·0 and 1·9 cm may be malignant, and tumours larger than 2·0 cm are invariably invasive and usually exhibit metastatic spread. These aggressive lesions invade the bowel wall, mesentery, parietal peritoneum and adjacent organs. Metastatic spread invariably involves the regional lymph nodes and liver, and less frequently, other sites such as the lung and bones. The commonest sites of carcinoids of the gastrointestinal tract are the appendix, jejuno-ileum and rectum in that order. Carcinoid tumour of the appendix is discussed separately later in this chapter.

Duodenal Carcinoids

Carcinoid tumours of the duodenum are rare. One type is similar in nature and behaviour to the other gastrointestinal carcinoids. There is, however, an unusual type of duodenal carcinoid known as the *carcinoid-islet cell* tumour which comprises functional, morphological and histochemical features of both foregut carcinoids and pancreatic islet cell tumours (apudomas). In addition to serotinin, the tumour may elaborate and secrete a variety of peptide hormones, such as gastrin, insulin, parathyroid hormone, catecholamines, etc., causing bizarre clinical manifestations. This tumour exemplifies the similarity between carcinoid tumours of the foregut and islet cell tumours.

Jejuno-ileal Carcinoids

Carcinoid tumours of the small intestine are most commonly encountered in the ileum. The majority are malignant, 40% are multiple and in 30–35%, there is an associated malignant neoplasm, usually an adenocarcinoma.

Colorectal Carcinoids

These non-secreting tumours form polypoid lesions with identical clinical features to adenocarcinomas. Carcinoid tumours of the colon are more likely to be malignant than those of the rectum.

Clinical Features

The average age of the reported cases of small intestinal carcinoids has been 45–55 years. Duodenal carcinoids may present with vomiting due to obstruction or as a bizarre endocrine syndrome. The manifestations of jejuno-ileal carcinoids include diarrhoea, intestinal obstruction, palpable abdominal mass and, much less commonly, massive gastrointestinal haemorrhage or infarction of the small intestine. Carcinoid of the appendix usually presents as acute appendicitis (*vide infra*). The presence of symptoms of the carcinoid syndrome indicates advanced disease with extensive hepatic involvement.

Treatment

Resection of the tumour with wide margins of healthy tissue, regional lymph nodes and associated mesentery is the standard treatment. External beam supervoltage radiotherapy has been used for inoperable tumours and for residual unresectable disease but the results have been disappointing. Resectable hepatic deposits are best dealt with surgically, by segmental resection, enucleation or lobectomy, depending on the site and extent of the disease. This reduction of the tumour burden is particularly beneficial in patients with distressing symptoms due to release of pharmacologically active substances by the tumour. The overall 5-year survival of small bowel carcinoids is 60%. Many patients survive long periods despite the presence of residual or metastatic disease.

Carcinoid Syndrome

The carcinoid syndrome is very rare, is produced by less than 10% of all carcinoid tumours and in the majority of cases, the primary tumour originates in the small intestine. The carcinoid syndrome is invariably associated with extensive hepatic involvement by tumour and the manifestations are the result of inappropriate secretion of the following: 5-hydroxytryptamine (5-HT), 5-hydroxytryptophan (5-HTP), kallikrein, histamine, prostaglandins and ACTH. Biochemical confirmation of the diagnosis is usually by the determination of the urinary metabolite of 5-HT and 5-HTP, 5-hydroxyindole acetic acid (5-HIAA). The intravenous administration of 2 μg of adrenaline results in a typical attack of flushing within 2 min of injection, but this test is rarely used nowadays.

Clinical Features

These include several types of flushing syndromes, intestinal colic and diarrhoea, bronchospasm, hypoproteinaemia and oedema, cardiac lesions (tricuspid insufficiency or pulmonary stenosis), pellagra-like skin lesions (photosensitive dermatitis) and neurological signs as tryptophan is diverted to serotonin production and very little niacin is synthesized, peptic ulceration and arthralgia. The cutaneous flushing episodes affect the upper part of the body and are accompanied by sweating, itching, oedema, palpitations and hypotension.

Treatment

Considerable palliation can be obtained from reduction of the hepatic tumour burden by surgical extirpation or hepatic arterial embolization. Both procedures should be covered with antiserotonin therapy (cyproheptadine and parachlorophenylalanine). Hepatic arterial embolization is performed percutaneously using a selective angiographic technique whereby the arteries feeding the metastases are blocked by gelatin sponge (Sterispon) or human dura mater (Lyodura) delivered in an antibiotic-containing solution and followed by steel coils. In addition to antiserotonin therapy, these patients must be covered with systemic antibiotics and methylprednisolone.

Lesser degrees of palliation can be produced by chemotherapy. The drugs which have been shown to be useful are cyclophosphamide, adriamycin, 5-fluorouracil and 5-fluorodesoxyuridine and streptozotocin, used singly or in combination. Better results are obtained by prolonged infusion chemotherapy either through the hepatic artery or a tributary of the portal vein. Prolonged access to the hepatic arterial tree is now possible with the use of implantable subcutaneous stainless-steel chambers which have a silicone diaphragm which allows intermittent and prolonged infusions (*Fig.* 72.14). Totally implantable infusion pumps (Infusaid) are available but these are very expensive and do not have any special advantage over the implantable access systems which are connected to small portable battery-powered infusion pumps. Pretreatment with antiserotonin therapy is necessary to prevent a carcinoid crisis during chemotherapy. Antiserotonin therapy can be undertaken with agents that either reduce the production of 5-HT or antagonize its effects. A combination of drugs tends to be more effective than single agent therapy.

Antiserotonin Drugs

These are:

1. Parachlorophenylalanine	Relieves diarrhoea.
2. Phenoxybenzamine	Administered to achieve alpha blockade. It may relieve attacks precipitated by emotion, diet, exercise and alcohol.
3. Chlorpromazine	Has antikinin effects and may control flushing.
4. Methysergide maleate	Most potent antagonist of 5-HT. May relieve flushing diarrhoea and bronchospasm.
5. Cyproheptadine	Less potent antiserotonin agent. May relieve diarrhoea and less frequently reduce intensity of flushing.
6. Prednisolone	May relieve facial oedema, diarrhoea and the flushing symptoms of bronchial carcinoids but not when the symptoms are caused by gastrointestinal tumours.
7. Long-acting somatostatin analogue	Abolishes flushing due to gastrointestinal carcinoids and diarrhoea.
8. Ketanserin	May reduce diarrhoea.
9. Calcitonin	Same effects as somatostatin.

Primary Small Bowel Lymphoma

The important differentiation is between *primary* (arising within the small intestine) and *secondary* (small bowel involvement secondary to disease elsewhere in the body).

The criteria for the diagnosis of primary gastrointestinal lymphoma are: there are no enlargements of the peripheral lymph nodes, the WBC count is normal, the patients present with gastrointestinal symptoms, the lesions involve predominantly the gastrointestinal tract and the disease does not follow a previously diagnosed extra-abdominal lymphoma. The vast majority of gastrointestinal lymphomas are of the non-Hodgkin's variety.

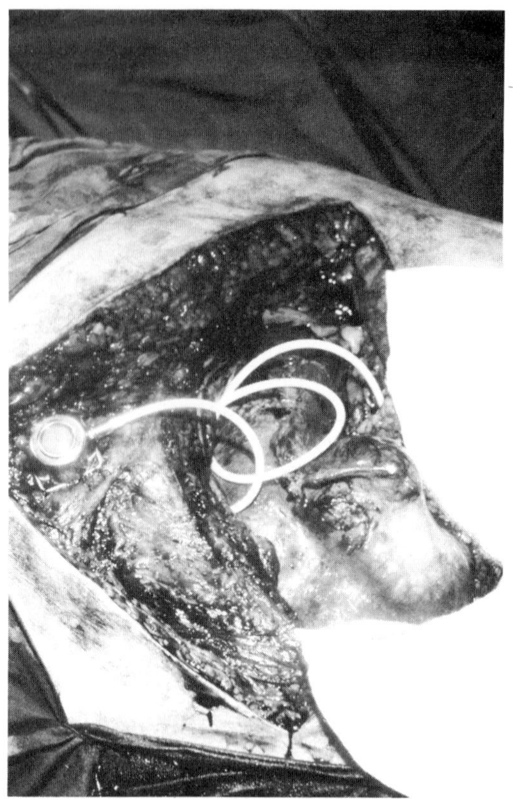

Fig. 72.14 Port-A-Cath implantable venous/arterial access system. In this particular patient, the technique has been used for prolonged hepatic arterial infusion chemotherapy for hepatic secondary deposits. In between treatments, the system is left primed with heparinized saline.

The previous terminology of non-Hodgkin's lymphomas (lymphosarcoma, reticulum-cell sarcoma, etc.) and Rappaport's classification have been abandoned in favour of newer ones based on histogenesis (cell origin of a given tumour) and monocolonal antibody markers to distinguish between T-cells, B-cells and U- (undefined) cells. There are now several different classifications which are constantly being modified and updated, such that the situation is rather confusing. However, two classifications appear to be favoured increasingly: the *modified Kiel classification* and the *Lukes and Collins functional classification*. The former arranges the non-Hodgkin's lymphomas in increasing order of malignancy into two main subdivisions: low-grade malignancy and high-grade malignancy, but takes into consideration the histogenesis, whereas the latter subdivides the tumours according to type of precursor cell origin (T-cell, B-cell, U-cell). To some extent, these two classifications are complementary. They are shown in *Tables* 72.6, 72.7.

Aetiology

The aetiology in the majority of cases remains unknown. In the West, lymphomas may arise in patients with coeliac disease. This tumour was previously considered to be a malignant histiocytosis but is now regarded as a T-cell lymphoma. Other predisposing conditions include *chronic non-specific ulcerative ileojejunitis* (a rare condition characterized by multiple small bowel ulceration, diarrhoea and malabsorption), nodular lymphoid hyperplasia with or with-

Table 72.6 Modified Kiel Classification

I. LOW-GRADE MALIGNANCY
1. ML lymphocytic
   B-chronic lymphocytic lymphoma (B-CLL)
   T-chronic lymphocytic lymphoma (T-CLL)
   Hairy-cell leukaemia
   Mycosis fungoides (T-cell cutaneous lymphoma)
   Sezary syndrome (T-cell cutaneous lymphoma + leukaemia)
   T-zone lymphomas (arise from the T-zone in between the germinal follicles)
2. ML lymphoplasmacytic/lymphoplasmacytoid or LP immunocytoma (B-cells with features of lymphocytes and plasma cells)
3. ML plasmacytic (plasmacytoma)
4. ML centrocytic (B-cells from the centre of the germinal follicle, 'centrocytes' or 'cleaved cells'
5. ML centroblastic/centrocytic (B-follicle centre non-cleaved cells or 'centroblasts')
   Follicular (tumour cells arranged in follicles)
   Follicular and diffuse
   Diffuse
   With or without sclerosis

II. HIGH-GRADE MALIGNANCY
6. ML centroblastic
   Primary
   Secondary
7. ML lymphoblastic
   B-lymphoblastic, Burkitt type and others
   T-lymphoblastic, convoluted cell types and others
   Unclassified
8. ML immunoblastic
   With plasmablastic/plasmacytic differentiation (B)
   Without plasmablastic/plasmacytic differentiation (B or T)

ML=Malignant Lymphoma

Table 72.7 Lukes and Collins functional classification of malignant lymphoma

1. U-CELL
   (Undefined)
2. T-CELL
   Small lymphocyte
   Convoluted lymphocyte
   Sezary cell—mycosis fungoides
   Immunoblastic sarcoma
3. B-CELL
   Small lymphocyte
   Plasmacytoid lymphocyte
   Follicle centre lymphoma
   Follicular or diffuse with or without sclerosis:
   - Small cleaved (centrocytes)
   - Large cleaved (centrocytes)
   - Small non-cleaved (centroblasts)
   - Large non-cleaved (centroblasts)

   Immunoblastic sarcoma
   Hairy-cell leukaemia

out hypogammaglobulinaemia and long-term cyclophosphamide therapy for carcinoma of the breast. In the Middle East, immunoproliferative small intestinal disease (IPSID) has been associated with repeated attacks of gastroenteritis, malnutrition and an abnormal immune response.

Types

Though Hodgkin's disease may involve the gastrointestinal tract late in its course, it rarely occurs as a primary GI tumour, the majority of which arise from follicle centre cells (centrocytic, centroblastic/centrocytic and centroblastic) both in the West and Middle East. The types of small bowel lymphoma, common site of origin and geographical distribution are shown in *Table* 72.8. The distinction between Western and Middle Eastern lymphoma is inappropriate as some are encountered in both areas.

Table 72.8 Classification of small bowel lymphomas

PRIMARY	LOCALIZED FOLLICLE CENTRE CELL LYMPHOMA—affects stomach and small intestine in both West and Middle East
	IMMUNOPROLIFERATIVE SMALL INTESTINAL DISEASE—affects the small intestine in the Middle East
	UNDIFFERENTIATED (BURKITT TYPE)—predominantly tumour of childhood in the West and Middle East, affecting the small intestine and ileocaecal region
	MALIGNANT HISTIOCYTOSIS OF THE SMALL INTESTINE*—arises in patients with coeliac disease in Western countries
SECONDARY	Gastrointestinal involvement secondary to extra-abdominal Hodgkin's and non-Hodgkin's lymphoma. Gastrointestinal lymphoma developing in patients with AIDS and proven Kaposi's sarcoma

*Now regarded as a T-cell lymphoma

Immunoproliferative Disease of the Small Intestine

This term was introduced by the World Health Organization to describe a spectrum of disorders which are nowadays considered to be different phases of a single disease entity occurring in Mediterranean and Middle Eastern countries and formerly referred to as alpha-chain Disease, Mediterranean lymphoma and Middle Eastern lymphoma. The condition arises from the IgA-secreting B cells of the small intestine. The benign variant (alpha-chain disease) is considered to be an early stage of the disease and progression to lymphoma has been documented. It is characterized by diffuse plasma cell infiltration of the small intestine. These abnormal plasma cells secrete a fragment of IgA (alpha or heavy chain) which can be detected in the plasma and duodenal juice of the affected patients. When it develops, the lymphoma is of the follicle centre cell (FFC) type with extreme plasmacytic differentiation. In the early stages the non-invasive plasma cells dominate the histological picture but with time, the invasive picture of FCC emerges and constitutes the bulk of the tumour. Only about one-third of patients with lymphoma have detectable alpha chain in their body fluids.

Staging of Small Bowel Lymphoma

The staging of gastrointestinal lymphoma is a good guide to prognosis in the individual case and affects the surgical management. It is shown in *Table* 72.9.

Table 72.9 Modified Ann Arbor clinical staging of lymphoma

STAGE I	Disease confined to a single extralymphatic organ
STAGE II	Localized involvement of one organ or site + involvement of one or more lymph node groups on one side of the diaphragm:
II_1	Regional adjacent lymph node involvement
II_2	Regional but non-confluent lymph node involvement
STAGE III	Localized involvement of organ or site + involvement of lymph node groups on both sides of the diaphragm
STAGE IV	Diffuse disseminated disease with involvement of more than one organ + lymph node enlargement

Clinical Features of Small Bowel Lymphoma

The presentation may be acute or insidious. In both the Middle East and the West, the disease often presents as a surgical emergency with intestinal obstruction or perforation and peritonitis. The intestinal obstruction may be due to intramural obstruction by a circumferential lesion or intussusception. The latter is particularly likely to occur with ileocaecal tumours in childhood. The chronic manifestations include malaise, abdominal pain, weight loss, diarrhoea/steatorrhoea, anaemia which may be normochromic (chronic disease) or hypochromic microcytic (chronic occult bleeding). The ESR is elevated and hypoproteinaemia is frequently present and results from a protein-losing enteropathy.

In the Middle East, IPSID is associated with gross malabsorption, bacterial overgrowth, hypoproteinaemia with oedema and ascites, and parasitic infestations, particularly giardiasis, in addition to the above chronic symptoms. It can also present acutely with intestinal obstruction, perforation and massive haemorrhage. In both regions, the commonest physical finding is a mobile abdominal mass. Diagnosis is often established with a small bowel contrast enema. More recently, abdominal ultrasound, CT scanning and laparoscopy have been used as diagnostic tests. In IPSID, the abnormal alpha chain is detected by immunocytochemistry of the tumour sections and by immunoelectrophoresis with monospecific IgA antibody of serum and duodenal juice.

Treatment

The treatment of gastrointestinal lymphomas has not been standardized and there have been few clinical trials. All patients presenting with acute abdominal disease require surgical intervention, and whenever possible the disease is resected. Further therapy is then administered soon after recovery from the operation. This may consist of combination chemotherapy with drug regimens which are commonly used in Hodgkin's disease (CHOP, CMOPP, etc.) or radiotherapy. The latter is used less frequently nowadays since it is no more effective than chemotherapy and carries a high early (bleeding, perforation) and late (radiation enteritis) morbidity.

In uncomplicated lymphoma, surgery followed by chemotherapy or radiotherapy is used for stage I and stage II of the disease. Chemotherapy alone is used for more advanced disease, but the prognosis in these cases is extremely poor. Complete remissions have been reported in patients with IPSID whose biopsy shows plasmacytic infiltration after treatment with tetracycline or cytotoxic drugs, but patients with established lymphomas are generally treated as outlined above.

Smooth Muscle Tumours

As suggested by Morson, this term or the alternative, leiomyomatous tumours, is preferable to the use of leiomyoma/leiomyosarcoma, as the distinction between the benign and malignant forms is often impossible on histological grounds alone. This includes electron microscopic appearances. Often the issue can only be settled by the subsequent clinical course. A tumour can be confidently labelled as benign only if the patient is disease-free for at least two years after surgical excision. In general, however, malignant tumours are larger, more often ulcerated and exhibit marked cellularity and necrosis. Smooth muscle tumours may occur anywhere in the small intestine but are more commonly found in the jejunum and ileum (80%).

Clinical Features

The majority of tumours present at middle age (50–60 years) with a long history, usually exceeding 12 months. The symptoms and signs include bleeding, abdominal pain, weakness and, rarely, weight loss. Acute presentation with intestinal obstruction or perforation is well documented. The most common clinical picture consists of repeated episodes of melaena when the tumour is situated in the jejuno-ileum and frank haematemesis when it originates in the duodenum. A palpable abdominal mass is present in one-third of patients. Selective angiography carries the best diagnostic yield in patients with gastrointestinal bleeding. The other useful investigation is small bowel enema.

Treatment

Smooth muscle tumours do not respond to either radio- or chemotherapy. The treatment is surgical excision with a wide healthy margin together with the regional lymph nodes and the associated mesentery.

INFECTIVE INFLAMMATORY CONDITIONS

In general, acute bacterial infections (shigellosis, cholera) and viral (small round viruses and rotavirus) infections are of limited surgical interest. Other infections which are endemic in certain tropical and underprivileged countries, can cause serious life-threatening complications which require urgent surgical intervention.

Campylobacter Infections

Infection with *Campylobacter fetus* is becoming increasingly common in the UK. It usually causes a self-limiting gastroenteritis. The diarrhoea is accompanied by abdominal pain which may be severe and mistaken for an acute abdomen when laparotomy is undertaken, usually with negative findings; although rare instances of *campylobacter* appendicitis, cholecystitis and pancreatitis have been reported.

Yersinia Infections

These Gram-negative coccobacillary rods belong to the family Enterobacteriaceae and include the organism responsible for plague, *Yersinia pestis*. The two species which cause gastrointestinal infections, particularly of the terminal ileum, appendix, ascending colon and mesenteric lymph nodes are *Y. enterocolitica* and *Y. pseudotuberculosis*. The infection is of a granulomatous nature with microabscess formation and may simulate chronic inflammatory bowel disease. The more usual clinical syndrome produced by these invasive organisms is an acute febrile gastroenteritis which is self-limiting and does not require any treatment. However, some of these patients, usually children, develop chronic symptoms (diarrhoea, rectal bleeding) that are associated with persistent inflammation of the ileum and ascending colon. These become swollen, ulcerated and exhibit radiological contrast appearances, such as nodular filling defects and cobblestone change which simulate Crohn's disease. The diagnosis is established by recovery of the organism from the stool. The *pseudoappendicitis syndrome* is also caused by *Yersinia* infection and is usually encountered in older children and adults. The clinical picture simulates acute appendicitis and at operation, the terminal ileum and the mesenteric lymph nodes are found to be inflamed and oedematous. Culture of the lymph nodes for *Yersinia* should always be performed in these patients. The terminal ileitis invariably resolves and there is no evidence that it ever progresses to Crohn's disease.

Neonatal Necrotizing Enterocolitis

This serious condition affects neonates with a mean age of onset at 10 days and consists of ischaemia and gangrene of the intestine. It carries an overall mortality of 30%. The aetiology of the condition remains unknown but is probably related to superinfection/bacterial colonization and mucosal ischaemia. The manifestations include abdominal distension and tenderness, bilious vomiting, acidosis, bloody diarrhoea, abdominal wall erythema and oliguria. The plain abdominal films may show pneumatosis intestinalis, fixed dilated intestinal loops, thickening of the bowel wall due to oedema, air/fluid levels, free fluid, gas in the portal vein and pneumoperitoneum. Medical treatment consists of gastric decompression with nasogastric suction, systemic antibiotics (gentamicin and ampicillin), fluid and electrolyte replacement and parenteral nutrition. The indications for surgical intervention are the development of a pneumoperitoneum and a positive abdominal tap (withdrawal of more than 0·5 ml of yellow-brown fluid or bacteria seen on the Gram stain). At operation, the ischaemic bowel is resected. This may involve several segmental resections. The residual bowel ends are exteriorized and restoration of continuity of the gastrointestinal tract is performed at a subsequent stage.

Enteritis Necroticans

This is a closely allied condition to the above but affects older children and adults. In Papua New Guinea it occurs in children after pig-feasting festivals and has been associated with infection by *Clostridium perfringens* although clostridial organisms have not been isolated in other series. The course of the disease varies from a self-limiting gastroenteritis to acute intestinal obstruction and perforation with peritonitis, and chronic recurrent subacute obstruction due to the development of intestinal strictures. The condition affects the small intestine, particularly the jejunum and consists of areas of necrotizing suppuration predominantly of the mucosal and submucosal layers with abscess formation. Involvement of the muscularis propria can lead to perforation. The regional lymph nodes are also involved in the inflammatory process and contain areas of suppurative necrosis. The affected bowel feels rigid and is oedematous. On the serosal aspect, the lesions appear as dark bluish patches, disposed transversely across the bowel and covered with fibrin. Necrotic and perforated bowel requires resection. Surgical treatment may also be necessary for recurrent small bowel subacute obstruction due to stricture formation.

Typhoid Fever

Typhoid fever remains endemic in tropical and subtropical countries. It is caused by *Salmonella typhi* and is characterized by an early septicaemic phase with colonization of several organs such as liver, spleen, bones and small intestine. The terminal ileum in the region of the Peyers patches bears the brunt of the intestinal infection with the formation of a longitudinal ulcerating lesion on the antimesenteric border, situated within 45 cm of the ileocaecal valve in the vast majority of patients. This intestinal typhoid ulceration may give rise to frank perforation and severe bleeding. Typhoid perforation is solitary in 85% of cases and is accompanied by peritonitis with little tendency to localization by adjacent loops of small intestine and greater omentum. The incidence of perforation varies considerably from one endemic area to another, being especially high in West Africa (15–33%) and low in Cairo and Iran (1–3%). The high incidence of perforation in West Africa has been attributed to late diagnosis of typhoid and a particularly virulent strain of *Salmonella typhi*, since intestinal perforation has been reported in this area when the disease was still septicaemic (positive blood culture and negative Widal reaction). The differential diagnosis includes perforated appendicitis and perforation associated with ascariasis.

The treatment of typhoid perforation necessitates surgical intervention under antibiotic therapy with chloramphenicol and gentamicin. Peritoneal toilet, suture of the perforation and drainage is the standard treatment. The edges of the perforation are trimmed before closure in two layers. Intestinal resection is contraindicated and carries a high mortality. This averages 15% for typhoid perforation treated by the suture closure technique. Surgical intervention may also be indicated in typhoid fever for the following complications:

Abscess formation which may occur in the septicaemic stage of the disease
Gangrenous typhoid cholecystitis
Chronic carrier state, where cholecystectomy is indicated.

Abdominal Tuberculosis

This includes tuberculous peritonitis and intestinal tuberculosis. The primary variety of gastrointestinal tuberculosis results from the ingestion of milk contaminated by *Mycobacterium bovis*. The secondary type of intestinal TB is due to swallowing of infected sputum from an active cavitating primary focus in the lungs (*Mycobacterium tuberculosis*). As a result of tuberculin testing of herds, pasteurization of milk, effective chemotherapy for pulmonary tuberculosis and general improvement in living conditions and nutrition, abdominal tuberculosis is nowadays rarely encountered in the Western countries and most cases are confined either to TB sanatoria or to the immigrant population. On the other hand, abdominal tuberculosis is very common in the underprivileged countries such as the Indian subcontinent and parts of Africa where tuberculous intestinal obstruction accounts for a significant proportion of emergency hospital admissions.

Tuberculous Peritonitis

In the majority of cases chronic tuberculous peritonitis results from reactivation of a latent primary peritoneal focus and is therefore haematogenous in origin. It causes malaise, ill health, weight loss, fever and ascites. It is not usually accompanied by active intestinal infection but is often associated with infection of other serous cavities, e.g. pleural and pericardial effusions. The latter may progress to constrictive pericarditis. The dry, plastic (fibrotic), chronic tuberculous peritonitis which gives rise to a dough-like abdomen is rare.

Acute tuberculous peritonitis occurs infrequently as part of the miliary disease or follows perforation of an intestinal lesion or rupture of tuberculous mesenteric lymph nodes.

Intestinal Tuberculosis

Pathology

Intestinal tuberculosis can assume one of four macroscopic forms: hypertrophic, ulcerative, fibrotic and ulcero-fibrotic, the first two accounting for the majority of cases.

Clinical Features

The disease usually affects children and young adults and is more common in females. In 75% of cases there are no other detectable tuberculous lesions elsewhere in the body but 25% have coexisting pulmonary disease. The systemic manifestations include chronic ill health, anorexia, fever and night sweats, dyspepsia and weight loss. The *hypertrophic type* affects predominantly the ileocaecal region and is characterized by the absence of gross caseation with marked thickening of the submucous and subserosal layers. It can also involve the ascending and transverse colon and is generally regarded as a low-virulence infection in an individual who has a high degree of immunological resistance from previous exposure to tuberculous infection. The affected patients are not usually very ill, although they exhibit the systemic manifestation of TB. The intestinal infection declares itself either because of recurrent episodes of subacute intestinal obstruction with colicky abdominal pain and vomiting, or with a mass in the right iliac fossa.

The *ulcerative type* affects predominantly the terminal ileum where multiple transverse deep ulcers develop and extend deeply to reach the serosa and may indeed lead to perforation. The serosal surface is thickened and studded with tubercles. Healing may result in multiple strictures with intervening dilated segments of ileum which often contain faecoliths. Bacterial overgrowth may develop at this stage and cause diarrhoea and malabsorption. However, the intestinal manifestations are usually those of subacute intestinal obstruction with pain, vomiting and constipation.

The *fibrotic variety* affects the terminal ileum, caecum and ascending colon. It leads to shortening and considerable narrowing of long segments of the bowel and may be accompanied by a generalized plastic tuberculous peritonitis. Presentation is again with acute or subacute intestinal obstruction.

The diagnosis of abdominal tuberculosis can pose difficulties even in endemic areas. The Mantoux test may be negative. Attempts should be made to culture the mycobacterium from gastric washings, faeces, peritoneal fluid and tissue biopsy including enlarged peripheral lymph nodes. It is important to realize, however, that certain atypical mycobacteria (not responsible for TB) may be demonstrated in certain chronic inflammatory conditions including Crohn's disease. Plain radiographs of the abdomen may show extensive calcifications. Barium studies show features of altered motility and stenotic radiological changes which may be indistinguishable from Crohn's disease. There is little doubt that the best procedure for establishing the diagnosis is laparoscopy with peritoneal biopsy and sampling of the ascitic fluid when present. Not infrequently, the diagnosis is only made at laparotomy with subsequent culture and histology of the excised specimen.

Treatment

In the absence of intestinal obstruction or perforation, the treatment is conservative with rest, adequate nutritional intake and antituberculous chemotherapy which is continued for 12 months. The most favoured first-line combination at the present time is rifampicin, isoniazid and ethambutol.

Surgical treatment is indicated usually for the onset of complications (intestinal obstruction, perforation, bleeding) and failure of medical therapy. The advent of effective chemotherapy has led to significant changes in the surgical treatment of the disease. Ileocaecal resection and right hemicolectomy are now the standard operations for ileocaecal disease and the results are excellent, provided chemotherapy is maintained for long periods after surgery. For disease in regions other than the terminal ileum and caecum, segmental resection with end-to-end anastomosis is performed. More recently stricturoplasty has been introduced to deal with fibrotic strictures causing subacute obstruction and bacterial overgrowth. Once again, this procedure must be performed under antituberculous drug therapy which has to be continued for some time after.

Actinomycosis

Abdominal (ileocaecal) actinomycosis is rare and usually follows infection with *Actinomycosis israelii* following perforated appendicitis. The patient usually presents some weeks later with a fixed indurated mass in the right iliac fossa with abscess and sinus formation. The infection spreads mainly by contiguity to the psoas muscle, abdominal wall and adjacent organs with the development of fistulas and multiple discharging sinuses. Spread of the infection by the portal venous system results in multiple intercommunicating loculated abscesses—the honeycomb liver. The treatment is conservative with prolonged penicillin and lincomycin therapy.

PARASITIC INFESTATIONS OF THE SMALL INTESTINE

The small intestine is parasitized by worms. The general features of helminthic infestations of the small intestine are dyspepsia, malabsorption, protein-losing enteropathy and anaemia (chiefly from chronic blood loss). The two common and important infestations are Ascariasis (roundworms) and Ancylostomiasis (hookworms).

Ascariasis

The infection is direct from person to person without an intermediate host. The responsible parasite is *Ascaris lumbricoides* which enters the body by the oral route. The infestation causes dyspepsia, episodes of intestinal colic with nausea and vomiting, malabsorption and an iron-deficiency anaemia due to chronic blood loss. Diagnosis is established by microscopy of fresh stool specimens for ova. Treatment is with piperazine.

The complications of the infestation are intestinal obstruction and perforation. Frank intestinal obstruction from a tangled mass of worms is far less common than subacute obstruction due to intestinal spasm. The features of ascardial intestinal obstruction include history of vomiting of worms, visible or palpable mass (worm bolus), pyrexia (usually 38 °C) and a characteristic toxaemia. Surgical treatment is necessary if the condition does not resolve. An attempt should be made to manipulate the mass of tangled worms into the caecum. If this fails, the worm bolus is extracted via an enterotomy. Occasionally, resection of a segment of bowel is necessary if its viability is considered to be compromised.

Perforation is rare and usually occurs at the site of pre-existing disease, e.g. ulcer, amoebiasis, typhoid, suture line, etc. It results in generalized peritonitis. Less commonly the infection is localized with abscess formation, the drainage of which leads to recovery of worms in the pus. In cases with frank perforation and generalized peritonitis, closure of the defect often poses technical problems. In the first instance, the bowel wall around the perforation is friable and oedematous. Therefore an adequate débridement is necessary before closure. In some cases, a localized resection of the bowel is necessary. Excision with exteriorization is advisable in patients with bowel of doubtful viability.

Ancylostomiasis

This is endemic in most tropical countries. It is caused by two filarial worms: *Ancylostoma duodenale* and *Necator americanus*. The filarial larvae enter the body by penetrating the intact skin and reach the lungs through the bloodstream. They then ascend to the pharynx where they are swallowed. The adult worm lives attached by its hooks to the mucosa of the jejunum. The female shed large numbers of ova which are excreted in the faeces. These develop into filarial larvae which repeat the cycle.

Hookworm infestation is associated with severe dyspepsia and gastrointestinal bleeding causing a microcytic anaemia and frank gastrointestinal haemorrhage especially in children. The dyspepsia is indistinguishable from that caused by duodenal ulcers and the two conditions often coexist in the tropics. A haemorrhagic duodenitis is seen endoscopically in these patients and worms may be identified in endoscopic biopsies. The diagnosis of hookworm infestation is made by stool microscopy. The treatment is with biphenium hydroxynaphthoate.

RADIATION-INDUCED BOWEL DISEASE (RADIATION ENTEROPATHY)

Although the figure of 5·0% is often quoted for the incidence of enterocolic radiation-induced bowel disease in patients who receive radiotherapy to the abdominal and pelvic regions, individual estimates vary from 3 to 25%. There is little doubt that such disorders carry a high morbidity and often contribute to the death of the patient. Most of the reported cases have received a radiation dose exceeding 40 Gy (4000 rad), usually during the course of external beam supervoltage radiotherapy, although damage, particularly to the rectum, has followed intracavitary implant treatment. The small intestine, colon and rectum are the usual affected segments, and in a substantial number of cases coexisting small and large bowel disease is present. Apart from radiation overdosage, an enhanced risk of radiation damage to the intestinal tract is encountered in:

Previous surgery
Pelvic sepsis
Old age
Cardiovascular disease
Hypertension
Diabetes.

Pathology

The immediate effect of radiation on the gastrointestinal tract is arrest of cell division in the intestinal crypts. This effect is largely restricted to the cells in the G-1 phase. With larger radiation exposure, oedema and ulceration of the mucosa ensue. As a result of the diminished cell turnover, the mucosa becomes thinner with stunted villi. If this injury is extensive and involves the small intestine, malabsorption of varying degrees will occur.

The long-term effects are due to transmural fibrosis following the appearance of atypical fibroblasts in the submucosa, and ischaemia from a proliferative endarteritis and vasculitis. Obliteration of the intestinal lymphatics with lymphatic ectasia complicates the pathological picture. The oedema is most marked in the submucosal layer. The fibrosis which affects all the coats is progressive and accompanied by hyalinization. The muscle layers, exhibit areas of myofibrillar degeneration with atrophy of the muscle fibres, patchy hyalinization and disturbed motility. The serosa becomes thickened, opaque and greyish-white and dense adhesions develop between adjacent intestinal loops. Bleeding, infarction, perforation, stricture, abscess and fistula formation are the consequences of these microscopic changes (*Fig.* 72.15). Bacterial overgrowth is invariable and contributes to the malabsorption and diarrhoea. There is also an increased risk of malignancy in radiation enteropathy, the risk factor for colon cancer being 2–8 times that of the general population.

Clinical Features

Symptoms are encountered in the majority of patients during the first few weeks of radiotherapy. The anorexia, nausea and vomiting are central nervous system effects as these are often encountered in patients receiving radiotherapy to extra-abdominal regions. These early symptoms usually subside rapidly and do not necessarily indicate the development of late sequelae which characterize radiation-induced bowel disease.

The commonest symptoms referable to bowel damage are vague abdominal discomfort, diarrhoea, mild rectal bleeding and the passage of mucus. The interval between the time of radiation and the onset of symptoms varies considerably from 2 months to 2 years. Intestinal obstruction may be acute or subacute and recurrent. Haemorrhage usually occurs as a bloody diarrhoea and massive bleeding is rare. Acute presentation with infarction and perforation carries a high mortality. Most of the serious late complications tend to occur within 2 years of the initial treatment.

The investigative procedures used in the assessment of patients must include contrast radiology of the small and large intestine, malabsorption studies, sigmoidoscopy and colonoscopy.

Treatment

Whenever possible, management should be conservative as surgical therapy has a high morbidity (50–60%) and an average reported mortality of 25%. Medical treatment involves the correction of nutritional deficiencies and the use of intestinal sedatives such as codeine phosphate, lomotil and diphenoxylate hydrochloride. Although there is no evidence that salazopyrine and steroids have a specific beneficial effect, they are commonly prescribed particularly where bleeding is a prominent symptom. Predsol enemas

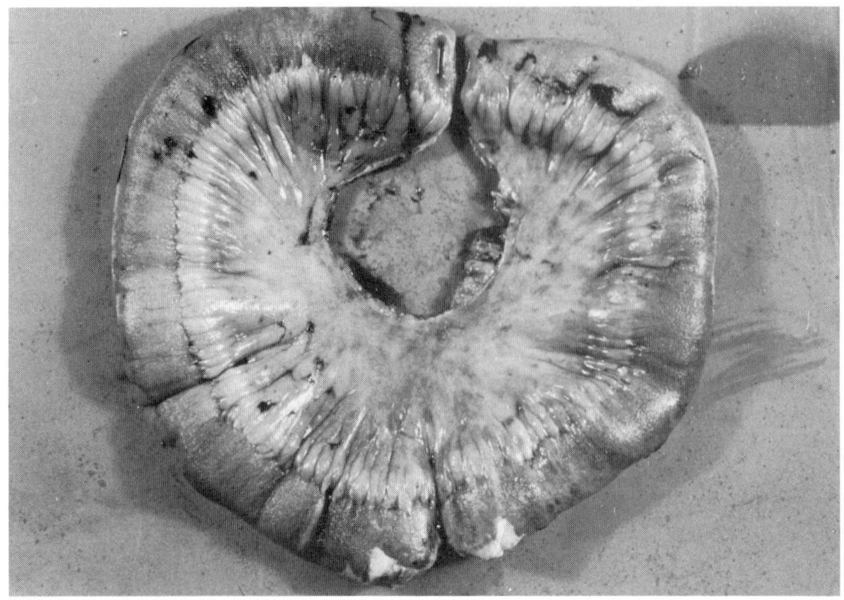

a

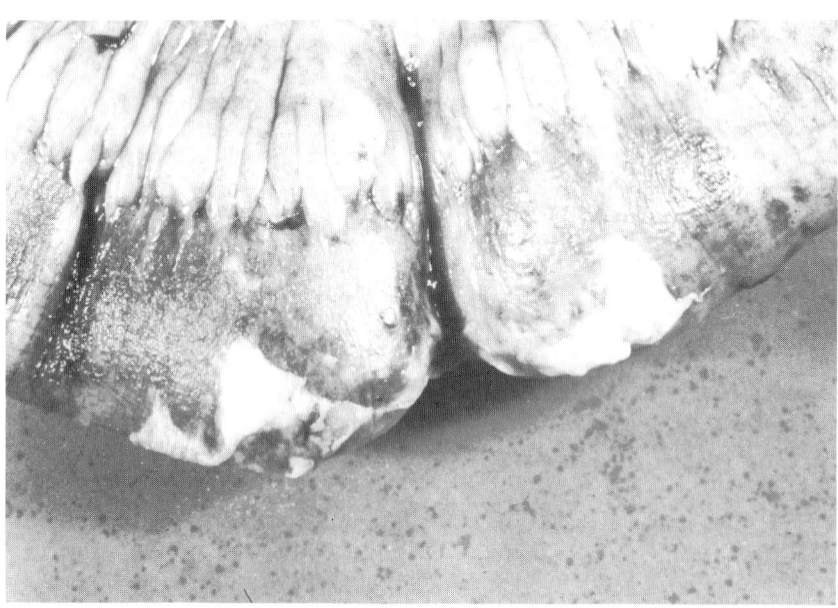

b

Fig. 72.15 *a*, Operative specimen of radiation enteropathy (chronic stage) which resulted in perforation of the affected segment. The bowel is rigid and fibrotic. The serosa is thickened with a rough granular appearance due to extensive hyalinization. There are widespread haemorrhagic areas in the bowel and its mesentery. *b*, Close-up of the bowel in the region of the perforation. (By courtesy of Mr R. A. B. Wood, Ninewells Hospital and Medical School, Dundee.)

often provide symptomatic benefit in patients with radiation proctitis and should be accompanied by the prescription of hydrophilic stool softeners in these patients. The presence of malabsorption will necessitate further measures, such as antibiotics for bacterial overgrowth or bile salt binding agents (cholestyramine) for ileal disease, together with careful dietary management, the use of elemental diets and oral supplements. Some patients with extensive small bowel disease and severe malabsorption require parenteral nutrition intermittently or indefinitely.

Emergency surgery is undertaken for infarction and perforation. The radionecrotic bowel is excised with exteriorization of the bowel ends and restoration of continuity is effected at a later stage. Elective surgery is undertaken for chronic severe symptoms due to stricture, internal fistula and unremitting severe bloody diarrhoea. A period of preoperative parenteral nutrition is advisable in these patients. Surgical management varies with the nature and extent of the disease. Some surgeons still favour bypass of the diseased segment as this carries a lower reported mortality than resection. The argument against bypass procedure concerns the outcome of the excluded segment which may bleed, ulcerate or infarct. Resection can be performed with an acceptable morbidity and mortality in patients who have localized disease provided they are prepared adequately before their elective surgical intervention. A right hemicolectomy with anastomosis of healthy mid-ileum to the transverse colon is recommended for distal ileal disease. Resection with anastomosis of the splenic flexure to a short rectal stump is the treatment of choice for rectosigmoid stenosis or bleeding. Most surgeons would advise a proximal (transverse) colostomy to protect this low anastomosis. In patients with extensive disease and enteric fistulas, the best results are obtained with complete bypass and exclusion of the diseased segment. This procedure is safer and preferable to resection in these difficult cases. In the performance of these elective operations, only those adhesions which are in the operative field are divided. Extensive enterolysis should not be performed as this is hazardous and may be followed by perforation.

DISEASES OF THE VERMIFORM APPENDIX AND MECKEL'S DIVERTICULUM

Acute Appendicitis

This is undoubtedly the most common surgical emergency in Western countries with an incidence of 1·5 and 1·9 per 1000 population in males and females respectively. It is rarely encountered before the age of 2 years, reaches its peak incidence in the 2nd and 3rd decades but may occur at any age. Although the overall incidence of perforation at the time of surgery has fallen in recent years to 15–20%, it remains high in children and the elderly, and forms the single most important factor in the high morbidity and appreciable mortality in these age groups.

Pathology

The high incidence of the disease in the Western Hemisphere has been attributed to the high-protein, low-residue diet. The incidence of the disease has increased in parts of Africa in recent years, particularly in urban districts. Acute appendicitis is thought to arise from infection superimposed on luminal obstruction by faecoliths, kinks, parasites and lymphoid hyperplasia. However, appendiceal obstruction is by no means invariable and mucosal ulceration is frequently present. This has led to the alternative hypothesis that acute appendicitis is secondary to viral infections which cause lymphoid hyperplasia and ulceration of the mucosa. The bacteria responsible for the inflammation are *Bacteroides fragilis*, *Escherichia coli*, *Streptococcus faecalis* and *Clostridium perfringens*. The intensity of the transmural inflammation varies. Often the disease progresses rapidly with thrombosis of the appendicular vessels, gangrene and perforation with either localized or generalized peritonitis. The inflammation usually stops short of the caecum.

Clinical Features

The typical history follows a sequential pattern with the development of colicky abdominal pain, vaguely distributed in the periumbilical region which is followed by nausea and vomiting. Within a few hours, the pain becomes localized in the right iliac fossa. The intensity of this constant localized pain varies with individual patients, severity of the inflammation and site of the appendix; but when severe, it indicates imminent perforation. In the absence of complications, a mild pyrexia is often present on admission to hospital.

Although frequently flushed, the patient is not usually ill. Apart from the pyrexia and tachycardia, the tongue is furred and a faecal halitosis is commonly present. Tenderness in the right iliac fossa maximal over McBurney's point (junction between upper two-thirds and lower one-third of a line joining the umbilicus to the anterior superior iliac spine) is found on light palpation. The intensity of the rebound tenderness and rigidity reflects the severity of the peritoneal irritation. A most useful indication of peritonism is pain in the right iliac fossa on coughing. Right-sided rectal tenderness is noted in a third of the patients on rectal examination. In the absence of generalized peritonitis due to perforation of a gangrenous appendix, the bowel sounds are present and initially may be hyperactive.

The diagnosis may be difficult in young children where vomiting is usually excessive and occurs before the parents become aware of any abdominal discomfort. Furthermore, the tenderness is more generalized, and fever and toxicity are invariably present. Inflammation of a pelvic appendix may simulate closely gastroenteritis with nausea, vomiting and diarrhoea and poorly localized abdominal pain. Rectal tenderness is, however, always present in these patients.

A number of classic signs of acute appendicitis, such as hyperaesthesia in Sherren's triangle, the psoas sign, etc. have a historical rather than practical importance except in the difficult diagnostic case, in which safety lies in urgent surgical intervention. Late presentation with an appendix mass/abscess may cause diagnostic problems, especially in the adult and elderly patient where it may be virtually impossible to distinguish between this condition and Crohn's disease or a perforated caecal carcinoma. Indeed, neoplasms of the caecum may obstruct the appendix and present with acute appendicitis.

Diagnosis

The typical case is readily diagnosed. The emphasis in recent years has been to err on the side of early surgical intervention, and this has contributed to the improved results. Inevitably, this policy has resulted in an appreciable incidence of normal appendicectomies which has averaged 20% of all cases undergoing this procedure. Undoubtedly, this imposes a heavy financial burden on the hospital. For this reason, some surgeons are beginning to laparoscope those patients in whom the diagnosis of acute appendicitis is in doubt prior to proceeding with appendicectomy.

A polymorphonuclear leucocytosis is present in the vast majority, and degrees of proteinuria and pyrexia are found in 10–20%. A plain abdominal film may show isolated dilated loops of small intestine.

Extensive accounts have been written on the differential diagnosis of acute appendicitis. Although many an experienced clinician has, from time to time, been caught out by a variety of disorders masquerading as acute appendicitis, the diagnostic problems commonly encountered vary with the age and sex of the patient. In children, the common diseases which must be considered are viral gastroenteritis and mesenteric lymphadenitis. The diagnosis of the latter is often made at operation when inflamed fleshy mesenteric nodes are found in the presence of a normal looking appendix. In retrospect, however, there is often a history of gastroenteritis in the family with vague abdominal pain. In addition, shifting tenderness may be present. Surgery is advisable in doubtful cases if the facility for laparoscopy is not available because of the risk of perforation which still averages 50–65% by the time of surgery in children below the age of 6 years.

In adolescent girls and premenopausal women, urinary tract infections and acute gynaecological conditions (acute salpingitis, ruptured Graafian follicle, twisted ovarian cyst, ectopic pregnancy) may resemble acute appendicitis. An increasing use is being made of diagnostic laparoscopy in acute lower abdominal pain in the child-bearing female.

In adults of both sexes, an inflammatory mass in the right iliac fossa always poses diagnostic problems and lesions such as Crohn's disease, *Yersinia* infections and other granulomatous conditions (ileocaecal TB, amoebic granuloma, etc.) or neoplasm of the caecum/ascending colon may require exclusion. Another not infrequent misdiagnosis in this age group, especially in the male, is perforated duodenal ulcer with tracking down the right paracolic gutter and tenderness in the right iliac fossa. Conversely, a high retrocaecal appendicitis may be difficult to differentiate from a perforated peptic ulcer or acute cholecystitis. The condition is most often missed or diagnosis delayed in the elderly and many of these patients undergo exploratory emergency surgery for an acute abdomen with signs of generalized peritonitis. The incidence of perforation in patients above the age of 60 years is 70%.

Complications

The complications of acute appendicitis are largely consequent on perforation of a gangrenous appendicitis. The important ones are:

- Wound infections and septicaemia
- Localized peritonitis—abscess/mass in the right iliac fossa
- Generalized peritonitis—particularly in the very young and the elderly
- Intraperitoneal abscess formation—solitary (pelvic, subphrenic) or multiple small intra-loop abscesses
- Faecal fistula—usually follows drainage of abscesses
- Recurrent intestinal obstruction—late complication from adhesions
- Pylephlebitis (portal pyaemia)

The bacteriology of the septic complications consists of Gram-negative organisms with a preponderance of bacteroides.

Treatment

Early appendicectomy is the only acceptable treatment in the majority. The base of the appendix is tied and the stump invaginated by a purse string suture in the adjacent caecal wall, although a recent trial showed that leaving the appendiceal stump unburied is not attended by an increased morbidity when compared to the standard invagination technique. In cases of perforation, abdominal lavage with an antibiotic–saline solution (tetracycline or cephalosporin) reduces the subsequent morbidity. The skin wound is best left unsutured in these patients. In addition, systemic antibiotics are administered preoperatively to all patients. In view of the importance of bacteroides and other Gram-negative anaerobes, metronidazole as suppositories is the antibiotic of choice. In patients with perforated appendicitis, systemic metronidazole together with a cephalosporin or gentamicin is continued for 5 days or more postoperatively. Clinical trials have shown that drains do not impart any benefit and increase the incidence of wound infection.

The traditional treatment of cases presenting late with appendix mass/abscess formation has been conservative with interval appendicectomy. The argument against active surgical intervention in the presence of a localized mass has been based on concern over dissemination of the infection. However, this has not been substantiated and there has been an increasing practice of early appendicectomy under appropriate antibiotic cover for this condition. Certainly the appendicectomy does not pose any great technical problems in these cases. Provided there are no indications of spreading peritoneal infection, the decision on the early or interval appendicectomy reflects individual preference and experience.

Morbidity and Mortality

The overall wound infection rate is 10–12%. Higher wound infection rates (35–75%) are found in the perforated group. The overall mortality is low and that of the unruptured disease equals that of general anaesthesia alone. The mortality in patients over the age of 60 years remains appreciable, varies from 6 to 14% and is related to the high incidence of perforation in this age group.

Controversial Issues

Chronic Appendicitis

Divergence of opinion exists regarding the entity of chronic appendicitis as a cause of recurrent pain in the right iliac fossa. This always requires full investigation to exclude inflammatory bowel disease and gynaecological disorders in the females. Some of these patients will continue to have pain despite negative investigations. The barium enema is normal but the appendix does not fill with contrast medium. Relief of pain follows appendicectomy in a proportion of these patients. The appendix is usually long, fibrotic and contains faecoliths. Histological examination shows chronic inflammation.

Incidental Appendicectomy

The incidental removal of a normal or fibrotic appendix during the course of an abdominal operation is another controversial issue. Statistical studies have shown that the risk of developing appendicitis in adults aged 40 years or more is 0·0431 for men and 0·0369 for females respectively, and the risk of death from acute appendicitis approximates to 1 in 800. These figures hardly justify incidental appendicectomy during abdominal surgery unless there is a specific indication. A stronger case can be made in children and young adolescents.

A number of retrospective reports have suggested an increased risk of cancer of the colon, breast and ovary, and lymphoma in appendicectomized individuals. However, a large prospective study involving a control group of patients having dental extractions or treatment of fractures, failed to show a higher incidence of neoplasia in the appendicectomy group.

Tumours of the Appendix

These are rare and include carcinoids, adenocarcinoma, mucinous neoplasms and lymphoma.

Carcinoid Tumours

The appendix is the most common site of carcinoid tumours, and carcinoid tumour of the appendix is the most common appendiceal tumour, accounting for 70% of tumours of this vestigeal organ. The vast majority of appendiceal carcinoids are found incidentally at the time of appendicectomy, usually at the tip of the organ. On rare occasions they arise from the base of the appendix and may then obstruct the lumen and cause acute appendicitis. Invasion of the muscularis has been reported to occur in 30%, but nodal involvement and more distant metastases are rare. Appendicectomy is curative and death from carcinoid tumour of the appendix is very rare. The carcinoid syndrome from a primary tumour of the appendix has never been reported.

Adenocarcinoma

This is a rare tumour and accounts for 17% of malignant tumours of the appendix. Most of the reported cases have presented as acute appendicitis or intestinal obstruction. The treatment is right hemicolectomy.

Mucinous Neoplasms

A simple mucocele of the appendix is a rare condition which is thought to arise as a sequel to obstruction of the appendix without the onset of infection. The appendix becomes distended by mucoid secretion and the normal mucosa becomes replaced by a single layer of mucus-secreting cells. Eventually the lesion may calcify.

Malignant mucocele, on the other hand, is a rare papilliferous cystadenoma or cystadenocarcinoma consisting of mucus-secreting cells. It rarely metastasizes but may lead to pseudomyxoma peritonei following rupture and spilling of the mucus-secreting cells.

Meckel's Diverticulum

This persistent remains of the vitello-intestinal tract has a reported incidence of 0·3–0·4%. The diverticulum was described by Heldamus more than 150 years before the comprehensive review by Meckel in 1808. It varies in length from 1 to 56 cm and arises from the antimesenteric border of the ileum within 90 cm of the ileocaecal valve. It is a true diverticulum and therefore contains all the intestinal coats. Ectopic tissue (gastric, pancreatic, duodenal, colonic) is found in 50–70% of reported cases. In infants under the age of 2 years, ulceration of the ectopic gastric mucosa in a Meckel's diverticulum is the most frequent cause of copious rectal bleeding. The presence of ectopic gastric mucosa in these patients can often be demonstrated by external scintiscanning following the intravenous administration of $^{99}Tc^{m}$ as this radionuclide is taken up by the ectopic gastric tissue. A bleeding Meckel's diverticulum can also be a cause of occult rectal bleeding in adults. Perforation of a peptic ulcer in a Meckel's diverticulum may also occur. Acute obstructive diverticulitis is clinically indistinguishable from acute appendicitis. Other acute complications include intestinal obstruction due to volvulus or compression by an adherent diverticulum.

Not infrequently an uninflamed Meckel's diverticulum is found incidentally during surgery. Removal is not necessary if the diverticulum has a wide base and feels normal on palpation. However, if the neck is narrow, or nodules are palpable in the diverticular walls, the diverticulum is chronically inflamed or contains faecoliths, removal is advisable. The treatment of complicated cases is by excision of the diverticulum together with a wedge resection of the adjacent ileum.

Further Reading

Archampong E. Q. (1985) Tropical diseases of the small bowel. *World J. Surg.* **9**, 887–896.

Bouchier I. A. D., Allan R. N., Hodgson H. J. F. et al. (ed.) (1984) *Textbook of Gastroenterology.* London, Baillière Tindall.

Camilleri M., Chadwick V. S. and Hodgson H. J. F. (1984) Vascular anomalies of the gastrointestinal tract. *Hepatogastroenterol.* **31**, 149–153.

Johnson A. M., Harman P. K. and Hanks J. B. (1985) Primary small bowel malignancies. *Am. Surg.* **51**, 31–36.

Lillemoe K. D., Brigham R. A., Harmon J. W. et al. (1983) Surgical management of small bowel radiation enteritis. *Arch. Surg.* **118**, 905–907.

Meehan S. E., Wood R. A. B. and Cuschieri A. (1984) Percutaneous cervical pharyngostomy: a comfortable and convenient alternative to protracted nasogastric intubation. *Am. J. Surg.* **148**, 325–330.

Nyhlin H., Brydon G., Danielsson A. et al. (1984) Clinical application of a selenium (^{75}Se)-labelled bile acid for the investigation of terminal ileal function. *Hepatogastroenterol.* **31**, 187–191.

Ouriel K. and Adams J. T. (1984) Adenocarcinoma of the small intestine. *Am. J. Surg.* **47**, 66–71.

Smith D. H. and DeCosse J. J. (1986) Radiation damage to the small intestine. *World J. Surg.* **10**, 189–194.

Wright D. H. and Issacson P. G. (1983) *Biopsy Pathology of the Lymphoreticular System.* London, Chapman and Hall.

73 *Inflammatory Bowel Disease*

A. Cuschieri

The term chronic inflammatory bowel disease is customarily used in a restrictive sense to cover ulcerative proctocolitis and Crohn's disease. A number of other inflammatory disorders, although excluded from this category, share some of the pathological features and must be considered in the differential diagnosis of inflammatory bowel disease. Indeed some may be misdiagnosed as inflammatory bowel disease and the diagnosis subsequently reversed or vice versa. *Tuberculous infections*, *amoebic dysentery* and *bilharzial infestations of the colon* may present as chronic inflammatory bowel disease and in certain geographical areas (Indo-Asian and African Continents), heavily outnumber the cases of both ulcerative colitis and Crohn's disease. *Salmonella enteritis and colitis* (*S. typhi*, *S. typhimurium*) and *Campylobacter infections* may mimic the full spectrum of acute severe inflammatory bowel disease, including toxic megacolon. Indeed there is evidence to support the view that at least some patients with 'ulcerative colitis' who never relapse are instances of Campylobacter infections. *Antibiotic-associated pseudomembranous* colitis due to *Clostridium difficile* which still carries a significant morbidity, is commonly encountered in hospital clinical practice nowadays. *Necrotizing enterocolitis* is usually easily differentiated from inflammatory bowel disease. A history of radiation therapy is obtained in instances of *radiation-induced colitis and enteritis*. *Ischaemic colitis* often presents with bloody diarrhoea but is rare in patients under 50 years of age. *Complicated diverticular disease of the colon*, especially with internal fistula formation, may cause diagnostic problems but the differentiation from Crohn's disease is usually possible by appropriate investigations. The symptoms of *pneumatoides cystoides intestinalis* are those of the commonly encountered irritable bowel syndrome which is often mistaken at an early stage for inflammatory bowel disease.

DIFFERENTIATION BETWEEN ULCERATIVE COLITIS AND CROHN'S DISEASE

Whereas Crohn's disease may affect both the small and large intestine singly or in combination, ulcerative colitis is a disease of the colon and rectum and does not involve the small intestine except for the development of a secondary backwash ileitis in patients with diffuse and severe disease who have an incompetent ileocaecal valve.

Although the classic cases of ulcerative proctocolitis and colonic Crohn's disease are easily differentiated on clinical, radiological and histological grounds (*Table* 73.1), patients are often encountered in whom the differentiation is impossible despite thorough and repeated investigation. From a clinical standpoint, it is becoming increasingly common practice to consider these patients as having inflammatory colonic disease and desist from futile attempts at distinction between the two entities as this can only be arbitrary in these circumstances. Some clinicians use the term *indeterminate colitis* for these patients. Indeed, the results of a computer-based analysis of a large clinical data base obtained from cases of inflammatory bowel disease, showed that patients with small bowel Crohn's disease could be easily separated from the rest and clearly formed a distinct group. However, the clinical features of Crohn's colitis could not be differentiated from those of ulcerative colitis and distinction between the two cohorts of patients was not possible.

EPIDEMIOLOGY OF INFLAMMATORY BOWEL DISEASE

Inflammatory bowel disease is common in Western Europe and North America. The incidence of ulcerative colitis in these areas varies in the different countries and regions from 2·5 to 15/100 000 per annum. In some of the European countries there has been a marginal rise in incidence of ulcerative colitis during the last decade attributable largely to improved diagnosis.

The incidence of Crohn's disease in the Western hemisphere is lower than that of ulcerative colitis and varies from country to country and often in different regions of the same country with incidence rates of 0·8–6·6/100 000 per annum. A definite true rise in the incidence of Crohn's disease (particularly of the colon) was observed in several European countries including the UK between 1960 and 1970. Since then, the incidence has remained static in most of these countries and declined in some regions (e.g. Aberdeen, Copenhagen).

Ulcerative colitis is slightly commoner in females than males but the sex incidence of Crohn's disease is equal. The peak incidence of both disorders is in early adult life (18–25 years). A smaller secondary peak for both Crohn's disease and ulcerative colitis is encountered in the elderly.

The important epidemiological factors which may have a bearing on the prevalence of inflammatory bowel disease are

Table 73.1 Differentiation between ulcerative colitis and Crohn's disease

	Ulcerative colitis	*Crohn's disease*
CLINICAL FEATURES		
Rectal bleeding	Very common	Unusual
Abdominal pain	Infrequent	Common
Abdominal mass	Rare	Sometimes
Spontaneous fistula	Very rare/never	Sometimes
Perianal infections	15%	30–40%
Rectal involvement	95%	50%
Carcinoma	Yes	Yes
RADIOLOGY		
Distribution	Continuous with rectum	Often discontinuous, along and around colon
Rectum	Usually involved	Often normal
Strictures	Rare, usually Ca	Often present
Mucosa	Granular, shallow ulcers, pseudopolyps	Fissuring, deep undermining ulcers, cobblestone appearance
Small bowel	Backwash ileitis only	Discontinuous involvement by skip lesions
HISTOPATHOLOGY		
Inflammation	Mucosal	Transmural
Vascularity	Often intense	Seldom prominent
Focal lymphoid hyperplasia	Restricted to mucosa/ submucosa	Transmural
Mucus secretion	Grossly impaired	Less severe impairment
Paneth cell metaplasia	Common	Rare
Sarcoid granuloma	Absent	50–70%
Fissuring	Rare	Very common
Precancerous dysplasia	Yes	Yes
Lymph nodes	Reactive hyperplasia	Often sarcoid foci
Anal lesions	Non-specific	Often sarcoid foci

genetic factors, race and diet. Several epidemiological studies have shown that both Crohn's disease and ulcerative colitis are more common in relatives of patients with these disorders than in the general population. However, inheritance has never been established and the higher incidence of inflammatory bowel disease in relatives may be the result of exposure to the same causative factors. Despite intensive investigations, an association between inflammatory bowel disease and HLA phenotypes has not been demonstrated although individuals with the HLA–B27 who develop inflammatory bowel disease have a substantially higher risk of developing ankylosing spondylitis.

In countries with more than one ethnic race, inflammatory bowel disease is less frequent in black or coloured races than caucasians (e.g. North America, New Zealand, South Africa). Also, inflammatory bowel disease is more common in Jewish individuals particularly those born and living in Europe and the USA.

Long-term consumption of a diet poor in fibre and high in refined sugars has been observed in several studies of patients with Crohn's disease but not ulcerative colitis. Early reports that breast feeding protects against ulcerative colitis have not been confirmed by subsequent studies. Likewise the reported association between non-smoking and ulcerative colitis and smoking with Crohn's disease remain unproven.

IMMUNOLOGICAL ABNORMALITIES IN INFLAMMATORY BOWEL DISEASE

There is no evidence that inflammatory bowel disease is caused by a primary abnormality of the immune response which is intrinsically normal in these patients. Immunological changes, humoral and cellular do, however, develop in patients with inflammatory bowel disease although their exact pathogenetic role remains unclear. Some appear to be useful indices of disease activity. The documented immunological findings in inflammatory bowel disease are:

1. Presence of subsets of T-lymphocytes in the blood which are cytotoxic to colon epithelial cells in patients with Crohn's disease and ulcerative colitis. This cytotoxicity is antibody-dependent.
2. Presence of T-lymphocytes in the lamina propria of resected bowel segments of Crohn's disease (small and large intestine) and ulcerative colitis which are cytotoxic to colon epithelial cells and red cells coated with colon epithelial antigens. This cytotoxicity is antibody-independent.
3. Presence of activation antigens (4F2, OKT9, Tac antigen) on peripheral T-lymphocytes in patients with active Crohn's disease. A very good correlation has been reported between OKT9 lymphocyte positivity and Crohn's disease activity index.

4. Presence of anticolon antibodies in patients with ulcerative colitis.

5. Defect in complement activation in patients with Crohn's disease and their relatives.

6. Presence of smooth muscle and anticytoskeletal antibodies in Crohn's disease and, to a lesser extent, ulcerative colitis.

INVESTIGATION OF PATIENTS WITH INFLAMMATORY BOWEL DISEASE

In addition to history and physical examination, certain key investigations are necessary to differentiate inflammatory bowel disease from functional or infective colonic disorders. The key initial investigations which usually establish the diagnosis are estimation of C-reactive protein, rectal biopsy and stool culture. Patients with ulcerative colitis frequently have hypochromic microcytic anaemia of moderate severity due to chronic blood loss. In cases of Crohn's disease with involvement of the distal ileum, a macrocytic anaemia may result from impaired absorption of vitamin B_{12} but iron-deficiency anaemia is distinctly less common than in ulcerative colitis. In addition to a full blood count, an ESR should be performed at regular intervals as it is a good index of activity of the disease in both Crohn's disease and ulcerative colitis. Hypoproteinaemia and a low serum albumin are often encountered and are due largely to excessive enteric losses. Stool culture and examination for parasites is always advisable at the time of first presentation of patients with diarrhoea and rectal bleeding.

Endoscopy

Sigmoidoscopy

As rectal involvement is present in 90–95% of patients with ulcerative colitis, the diagnosis of this condition is usually established by sigmoidoscopy and rectal biopsy. The flexible sigmoidoscope is being increasingly used, although for the purpose of establishing the initial diagnosis, it does not carry any special advantage over the rigid endoscope. The sigmoidoscopic appearances in ulcerative colitis include loss of the normal vascular pattern, petechial haemorrhages and an oedematous, friable, granular mucosa which bleeds spontaneously or on contact. Pseudopolyps and discrete ulceration may be seen in the more severe and chronic forms of the disease although obvious ulceration is rarely apparent in the rectosigmoid region.

Sigmoidoscope appearances are normal in 40–50% of patients with Crohn's disease but anal and perianal lesions are common—fissures, sinuses, abscesses and fistulas—and often point to the diagnosis. In those patients with Crohn's colitis and rectal involvement, the sigmoidoscopic appearances may be indistinguishable from those of ulcerative colitis or exhibit marked differences. The earliest ulcers seen in Crohn's disease are of the discrete aphthoid type. With established rectal disease, deep ulcers, mucosal thickening with considerable oedema and cobblestone change, stenosis and induration of the rectum and perineum often with multiple sinuses/fistula formation, may be encountered.

Colonoscopy

This endoscopic procedure is not required for the diagnosis of ulcerative colitis except in those rare instances with minimal rectal involvement and a normal barium enema. Colonoscopy is contraindicated in patients with severe/acute ulcerative colitis because of the risk of perforation. The indications for colonoscopy in patients with ulcerative colitis are:

1. In defining the extent of the disease in those patients whose symptoms are more severe than is expected by the barium enema findings. In some of these patients colonoscopy demonstrates that the disease is more extensive than initially suspected on the radiological findings (*Fig.* 73.1).

2. For the endoscopic visualization and biopsy of all patients who develop a stricture.

3. In the differentiation of ulcerative from Crohn's colitis when the clinical findings, histology and radiological findings are inconclusive. Multiple biopsies are taken. Despite this procedure, differentiation may not be possible when the term 'indeterminate colitis' is used to describe these patients.

4. In the long-term surveillance of patients with ulcerative colitis with regard to the possible development of colonic cancer. The current recommendation is for annual colonoscopy with multiple biopsies for all patients with total/extensive disease of 8 years' duration or more. In addition, a sigmoidoscopy with multiple biopsies is performed at 6-monthly intervals in between the colonoscopic assessments. Patients with left-sided colitis are recruited into the screening programme when the duration of the disease exceeds 15 years. A prophylactic proctocolectomy is undertaken if high-grade dysplasia or dysplasia of any grade in areas of localized macroscopic abnormality is found.

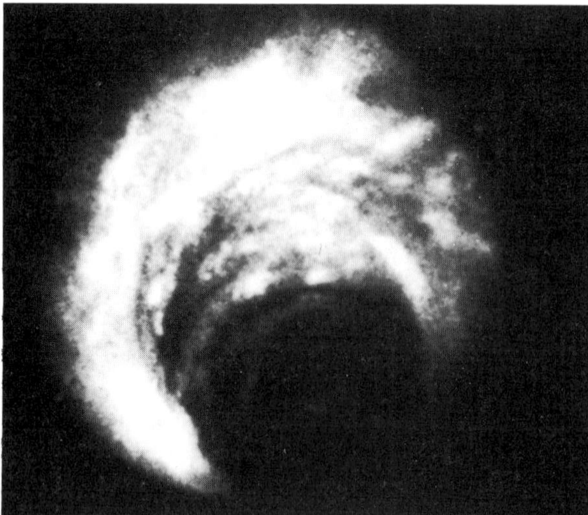

Fig. 73.1 Colonoscopic appearance of the descending colon showing extensive mucosal inflammation in a patient with a history of diarrhoea and rectal bleeding in whom the barium enema was normal.

The rigidity and foreshortening of the colon in the presence of colonic Crohn's disease eases the performance of colonoscopy in patients with this disorder. Although colonoscopy is not necessary for the diagnosis of Crohn's colitis, it is often advisable especially in the following:

1. When the rectal biopsies are equivocal. Multiple biopsies taken at colonoscopy are more likely to yield specific

histological features of the disease, particularly if taken from the margins of aphthous ulcers.

2. In patients with established small-bowel disease and suspected colonic involvement but equivocal radiological appearances of the caecum/ascending colon.

3. Assessment of strictures demonstrated by barium enema.

4. When contrast radiology is unsatisfactory or does not clearly outline the full extent of the disease.

Colonoscopy is contraindicated in patients with severe exacerbation of Crohn's colitis and in patients with deep ulceration because of the risk of colonic perforation.

Radiology

Plain Abdominal Radiographs

These are useful and necessary investigations in patients with acute inflammatory bowel disease. In general, the supine views give more reliable information than the erect exposures although both are usually performed. The main value of plain abdominal films in the acute situation lies in the diagnosis of the following complications:

1. Presence of small-bowel obstruction in patients with Crohn's disease.

2. Detection of toxic megacolon. Dilatation of the transverse colon (>5·5 cm) in the supine film is present in this condition (*Fig.* 73.2). Other radiological features include loss of haustral pattern, an irregular outline of the colonic wall, and multiple pseudopolyps visible as broad-based, soft-tissue, nodular projections into the lumen of the dilated colon.

3. Detection of colonic perforation. The best views for demonstrating free air in this condition are the midinspiratory upright chest film and the expiratory left lateral (right side up) decubitus view of the abdomen.

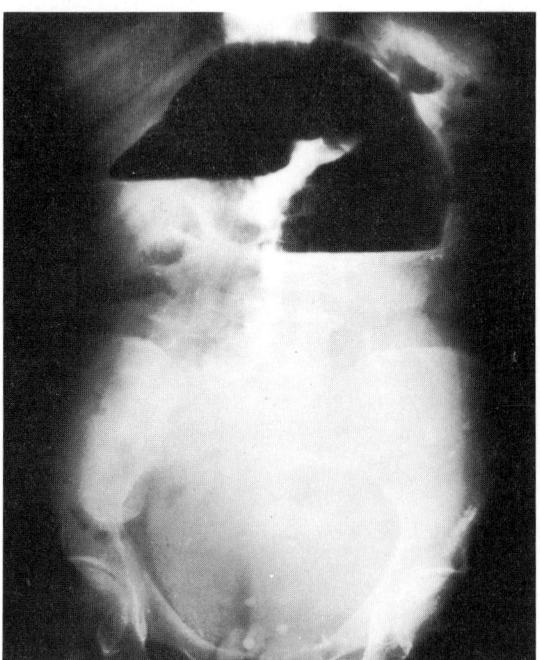

Fig. 73.2 Plain supine radiograph of the abdomen in a patient with toxic megacolon. The transverse colon is dilated with gas and is empty of any faecal residue.

4. Assessment of the extent of colonic involvement. As areas of active severe inflammation are free of faecal matter, the extent of the disease can often be surmised in the acute situation from the distribution/amount of faecal residue. 'Mucosal islands' are encountered in severe disease.

Contrast Radiology

A small-bowel enema is now the standard technique used for the detection of small-bowel Crohn's disease and has a significantly higher diagnostic yield than the small-bowel follow-through studies.

Double contrast barium enema is used in preference to the single contrast technique in colonic inflammatory bowel disease because of its superiority in defining mucosal inflammation/ulceration, in assessing the severity and extent of the disease and in the detection of carcinoma. The contraindications to a barium enema examination are toxic megacolon, suspected perforation and a rectal biopsy performed within the previous 7 days. In patients with severe disease, the 'instant enema' (without colonic preparation) is used in some centres. This consists of the gentle instillation of barium until either faeces or the caecum are reached. The following single contrast views are then obtained: whole colon, lateral rectum and oblique sigmoid. A double contrast 'instant enema' is performed in some centres in some of these patients.

As patients with severe or recurrent Crohn's disease may develop obstructive uropathy due to ureteric involvement by fibrosis, an IVP is necessary in these patients. Sinography using water-soluble contrast media, is required for the evaluation of fistulas, sinuses and abscesses in patients with Crohn's disease. CT scanning following the injection of the dye outlines in great detail the full pathological anatomy of these complications and is used in preference to conventional contrast radiology for the evaluation of these complications in centres where this facility is available.

Labelled Sucralfate Enema

Isotope-labelled ($^{99}Tc^{m}$) sucralfate which adheres to areas of mucosal ulceration has been used to define the presence and extent of inflammatory bowel disease by external scanning with a gamma camera. However, it is not, as yet, an accepted routine investigation and its advantages, apart from the much reduced radiation exposure, over contrast radiology have yet to be outlined.

Tests of Small Bowel Function

These are frequently necessary in patients with small bowel Crohn's disease, particularly the Schilling test, SeHCAT test and tests for bacterial overgrowth (*see* Chapter 72).

Liver Function Tests

All patients with inflammatory bowel disease should have periodic estimations of the liver function tests (bilirubin, protein, transaminases, alkaline phosphatase and gamma-glutamyl transpeptidase).

ULCERATIVE PROCTOCOLITIS

Despite a considerable research effort, the aetiology of ulcerative proctocolitis remains unknown. There is no evidence for the direct role of a transmissible infective agent and the immunological changes encountered in the disorder are of a secondary nature. There is some evidence that a gastrointestinal allergic diathesis may be involved in the development of the inflammatory change in the colon as evidenced by the higher incidence of atopic disease in affected patients and by the finding that some patients with ulcerative colitis benefit from a milk-free diet.

Specific mucosal abnormalities have been identified in ulcerative colitis. These consist of significant reduction in the production of type IV mucin and a decreased hydrolase activity. These abnormalities are found irrespective of the disease activity. It seems likely that the reduced mucin IV production represents loss of an important mucosal protective mechanism which enhances the susceptibility to accesss or injury by intraluminal factors. One report has shown a correlation with non-smoking and ulcerative colitis but this has not been confirmed by subsequent studies.

Pathology

The disease is largely confined to the mucosa and, to a lesser extent, the submucosa. Involvement of the muscle coats and serosa is rare and lymph node enlargement is not a significant feature of the disease. The rectum is involved in 90–95% of cases. Ulcerative colitis usually starts in the rectum as a granular proctitis and extends in continuity to involve varying extents of the colon: proctosigmoiditis, left-sided colitis, subtotal colitis and total colitis.

Macroscopic Appearances

Early disease is manifest as a haemorrhagic inflammation with loss of the normal vascular pattern, petechial haemorrhages and bleeding. Ulceration of the mucosa is seen in more advanced disease. Large areas may become denuded of mucosa and there is undermining of the mucosa which often results in the formation of mucosal bridges (*Fig.* 73.3). The mucosal destruction and undermining is accompanied by the formation of excess granulation tissue and the development of inflammatory polyps (pseudopolyps). As the mucosa heals, these polyps become totally epithelialized and persist within either a normal looking or an atrophic mucosa (*Fig.* 73.4). Relapse of the disease is accompanied by recrudescence of the inflammatory changes which can be visualized through the sigmoidoscope.

Microscopic Changes

The disease appears to start with inflammation of the crypts of Lieberkühn and the development of crypt abscesses which result in necrosis of the crypt epithelium and the appearance of a more chronic inflammatory cell infiltrate consisting of lymphocytes, plasma cells, eosinophils and mast cells in the adjacent submucosa (*Fig.* 73.5). The inflammation and crypt abscess formation is accompanied by discharge of mucus from the goblet cells which become reduced in number as the disease progresses. Ulceration and mucosal undermining are the consequences of enlargement and rupture of the micro-abscesses into the intestinal lumen. The ulcerated areas become rapidly covered by a vascular granulation tissue but excessive fibrosis is not a feature of the disease. The undermining of the inflamed mucosa and the excess granulation tissue result in the formation of polypoid mucosal excrescences, i.e. inflammatory polyps or pseudopolyps. These do not have any sinister prognostic influence in terms of the development of carcinoma which develops from areas of dysplastic mucosa (*vide infra*). Unless toxic megacolon/perforation develops, the disease remains confined to the mucosa and submucosa.

Restoration to normal histological appearance may occur with remission. However, evidence of mucosa atrophy is often observed with a reduction in the number of colonic glands which are short (fail to reach the muscularis mucosae) and branched. Hypertrophy of the muscularis mucosae and Paneth cell hyperplasia may be encountered in longstanding ulcerative colitis. However, the important long-term change is dysplasia which is thought to precede the development of carcinoma of the colon in this condition. The dysplastic areas are often widespread and may be accompanied by endoscopically or radiologically identifiable elevated plaques.

Complications

The complications of ulcerative colitis are traditionally classified into local and systemic. In general, they reflect the severity, activity, extent or duration of the disease. The

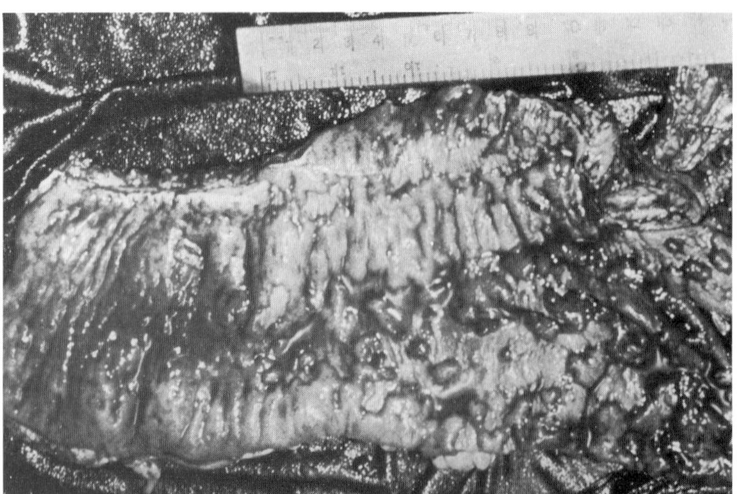

Fig. 73.3 Close-up appearances of the mucosa in fulminating ulcerative colitis—there is extensive ulceration with denuded areas covered with granulation tissue and undermining of the residual inflamed mucosa which leads to the formation of mucosal bridges.

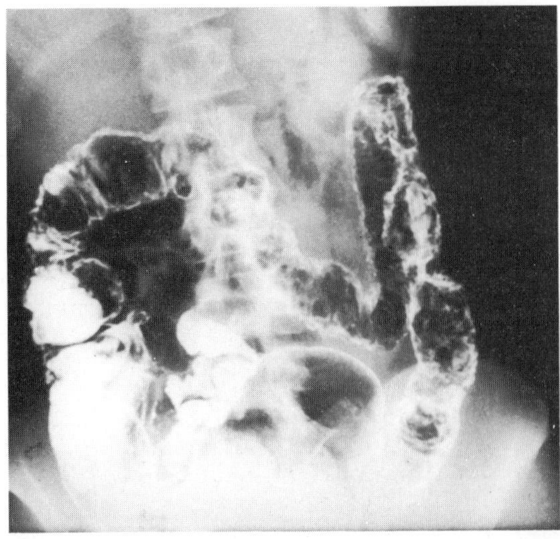

a

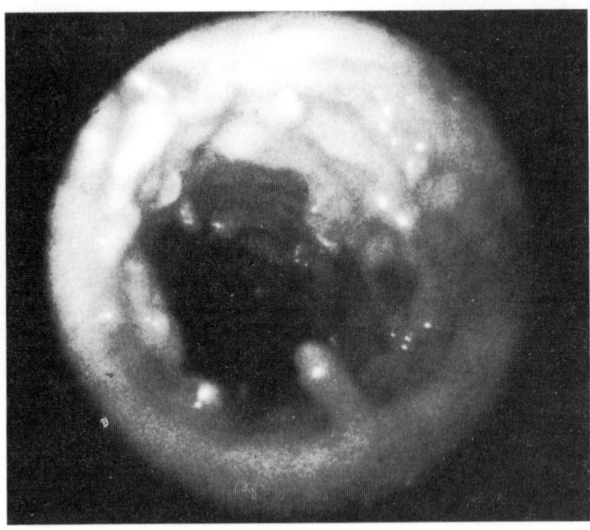

b

Fig. 73.4 *a*, Barium enema showing extensive pseudopolyp formation in a patient with total colonic involvement by ulcerative colitis. *b*, Colonoscopic appearances of pseudopolyp formation in ulcerative colitis.

systemic complications are common to both ulcerative colitis and Crohn's disease and are shown in *Table* 73.3. The local complications of ulcerative colitis are:

Toxic megacolon (acute dilatation)
Colonic perforation
Massive haemorrhage
Colonic stricture
Colonic carcinoma
Perianal suppuration/disease

The relative incidence of the local complications are shown in *Fig.* 73.6.

Toxic Megacolon

This serious complication which occurs in 2–10% carries a high reported mortality. It is not unique to idiopathic ulcerative colitis and can occur in Crohn's disease, in pseudomembranous colitis associated with antibiotic therapy, bacterial colitis (Campylobacter, Salmonella) and parasitic colitis (amoebic dysentery). It is more common in patients with extensive ulcerative colitis (total/subtotal) and is particularly prone to occur during first attacks of the disease. Certain precipitating factors may be involved in some cases. These include metabolic alkalosis, hypokalaemia and the administration of drugs which affect intestinal motility, e.g. opiates, anticholinergic agents etc. The entire colon may be affected but, more commonly, the transverse colon is predominantly involved.

Pathologically, there is a transmural extension of the inflammatory process with deep ulcers reaching the serosa, vasculitis and inflammation of the myenteric and submucous nerve plexuses. In addition, there is thinning of the bowel wall.

Toxic dilatation is heralded by a marked deterioriation in the general condition of the patient accompanied by abdominal distension, absent bowel sounds, severe systemic toxicity, fever, tachycardia, leucocytosis and marked fluid and electrolyte depletion (especially hypokalaemia), anaemia and hypovolaemia. A plain supine radiograph of the abdomen (*Fig.* 73.2) shows the gaseously distended colon which is empty of faecal residue and exhibits loss of haustration, mucosal projections (pseudopolyps), irregularities of the colonic wall and, in some instances, intramural air (tramlining). All patients suspected of developing this condition require frequent measurement of the abdominal girth throughout the day and frequent (daily, if necessary) plain abdominal films. If the condition does not respond to intensive medical therapy with high-dose systemic corticosteroid therapy within 72 hours, surgical intervention is mandatory because of the risk of colonic perforation which then approximates to 50–60% in most series. In practice, the majority of patients are nowadays treated by emergency colectomy soon after resuscitation and correction of fluid and electrolyte deficits.

Colonic Perforation

This complication carries a 50% mortality and accounts for 30% of all deaths from ulcerative colitis. It may occur in the absence of toxic megacolon and in this respect, the risk of perforation appears to be highest during the first severe attack of the disease. Although there is no evidence that corticosteroid therapy enhances the risk of perforation, steroid therapy may mask the essential physical signs and delay the diagnosis of this complication. Perforation may be precipitated by the injudicious use of barium enema or colonoscopy during an acute attack of the disease. Colonic perforation is marked by a sudden severe deterioriation in the patient's general condition and evidence of a septic shock due to the faecal peritonitis. However, the physical signs in the abdomen are often equivocal and the classic findings of peritonitis (rigidity, rebound tenderness) may be absent. The condition is best diagnosed by plain radiology (mid-inspiratory upright chest and left lateral abdominal decubitus view). Sealed perforation of the colon is found in 20% of patients undergoing emergency colectomy for toxic megacolon.

Massive Haemorrhage

This is a rare complication and usually affects patients with severe and total colonic involvement by ulcerative colitis. It usually settles with conservative management and blood transfusions, and does not contribute significantly to the mortality from the disease. Severe colonic bleeding may be associated with diffuse intravascular coagulation.

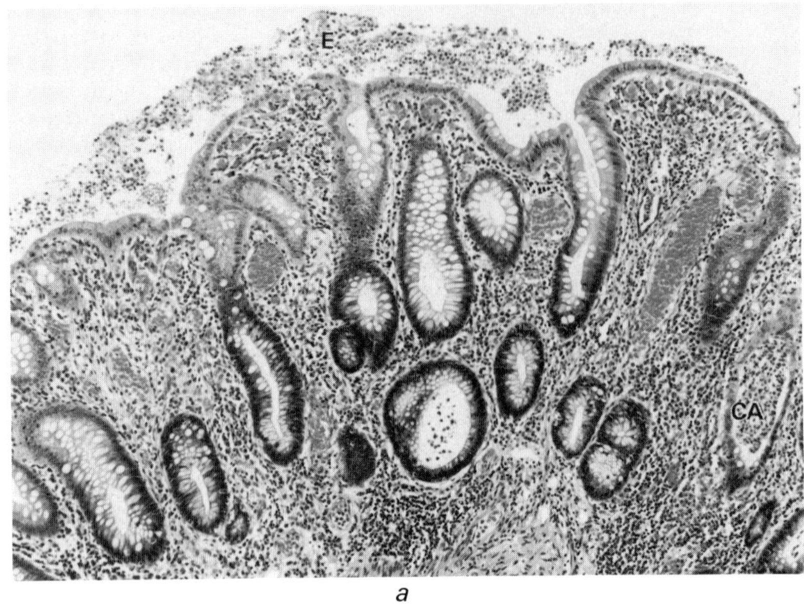

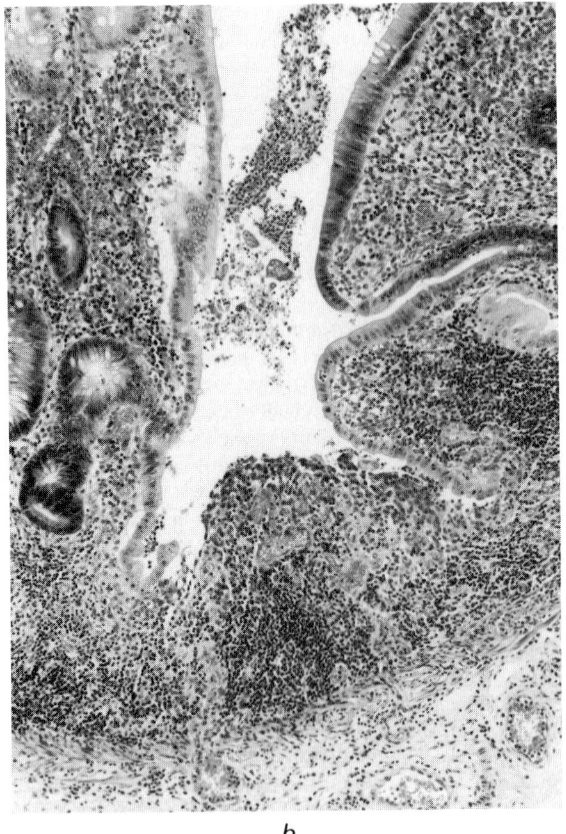

Fig. 73.5 *a*, Histological appearances of ulcerative colitis showing mucosal inflammation with surface exudate (E), cellular infiltration with lymphocytes and neutrophils, oedema, ulceration, crypt abscess (CA) formation and goblet cell depletion. *b*, Ulcerative colitis showing severe mucosal inflammation and ulceration at the bottom of a crypt where there is a total absence of epithelial cells. (By courtesy of Dr M. P. Holley, Ninewells Hospital, Dundee.)

Colonic Stricture

Radiologically demonstrable narrowing of the colon may arise from submucosal fibrosis, thickening of the muscularis mucosae or from hyperplastic mucosa and granulation tissue and may, therefore, be reversible with medical treatment. Benign fibrous strictures (*Fig.* 73.7) which occur most commonly in the rectum and transverse colon are encountered in 5–10% of cases of ulcerative colitis usually with total colonic involvement. The radiological demonstration of a stricture in these patients is an absolute indication for colonoscopy with multiple biopsies because of the real risk of carcinoma since radiological differentiation between benign stricture and carcinoma is not possible with any degree of certainty.

Colonic Cancer

The increased risk of carcinoma of the colon is well established. However, the high incidence of this complication

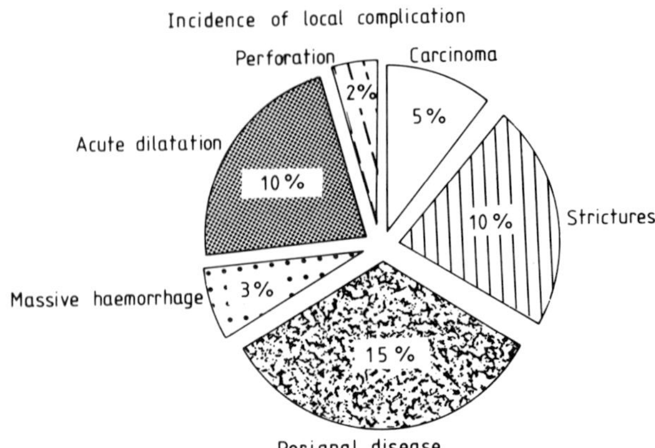

Fig. 73.6 Pie-chart showing the maximum reported overall incidence of the local complications of ulcerative colitis.

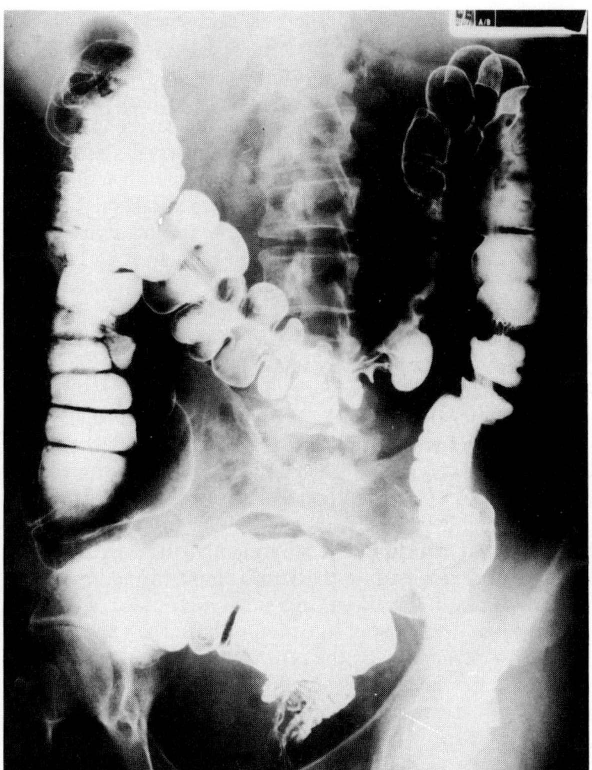

Fig. 73.7 Barium enema showing benign fibrous stricture of the transverse colon in a patient with inflammatory bowel disease. The lesion was shown to be benign by colonoscopic biopsy and required resection because of episodes of subacute obstruction.

which was reported earlier has not been substantiated by subsequent surveys of the disease. The reason for this discrepancy is that the initial estimates were based on the long-term outcome from tertiary referral centres which included a disproportionate number of patients with extensive colonic disease. Incidence rates for colon cancer in all patients with ulcerative colitis irrespective of extent of the disease average 1% at 10 years and 5% between 10 and 20 years of onset.

The risk of development of cancer in ulcerative colitis depends on:

1. Extent of the disease: Carcinoma occurs largely in patients with total and subtotal colonic involvement. It is much less common in patients with left-sided colitis and is virtually unknown in patients with rectosigmoiditis.
2. Duration of the disease: Carcinoma is rare before 7 years and its incidence then increases with the duration beyond 10 years (*Fig.* 73.8).
3. Onset of the disease in childhood: This is largely the result of long duration of the disease but some studies indicate that early onset of ulcerative colitis is a separate risk factor.

Cancer in ulcerative colitis patients occurs at a younger age than the disease in non-colitic patients. The tumours tend to be less well differentiated and are more often multiple than in ordinary colonic cancer. However, the previously held view that colitis cancer carries a worse prognosis is no longer tenable. The bad prognosis overall is due to the advanced Duke's stage of the disease and indicates the need for an effective surveillance programme in patients with ulcerative colitis. The site incidence of cancer associated with ulcerative colitis is shown in *Fig.* 73.9. The majority of tumours are found in the rectosigmoid region and the transverse colon (*Fig.* 73.10).

There is now good evidence that cancer in ulcerative colitis develops in areas of:

Dysplasia which may be mild, moderate and severe
Villous adenomatous change
Ectopic colonic mucosa in the submucosa or muscularis propria.

Dysplasia is now regarded as indicative of neoplastic transformation (*Fig.* 73.11). The affected areas may be visible at barium contrast studies and colonoscopy as flat plaques, but often the mucosa looks macroscopically normal. Repeated follow-up multiple biopsies with detailed histological and cytochemical studies are therefore necessary. The problem lies in the differentiation between dysplasia and epithelial regenerative changes. For this reason, several 'mucosal markers' have been suggested to detect dysplasia. These include enzyme activity (G6-PDH, LDH), antigen expression by the epithelial cells (CEA, second trimester fetal antigen), special staining (peanut agglutinin which binds to the T-blood antigen, and isothiocyanate-conjugated lectin which binds to abnormal mucins) etc. However, no marker has as yet proved reliable enough for

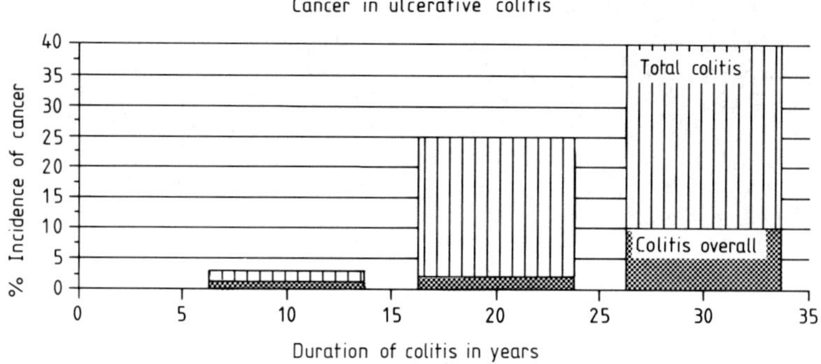

Fig. 73.8 The incidence of colonic cancer in patients with ulcerative colitis with duration of the disease in years. The solid bars represent all cases of ulcerative colitis irrespective of extent of the disease and the hatched bars denote the incidence in patients with total colitis.

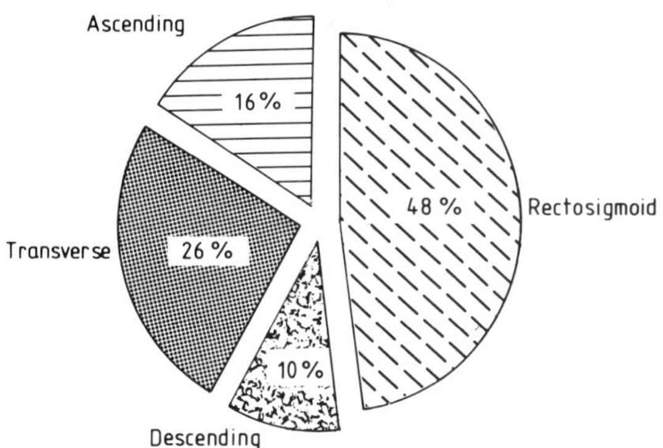

Fig. 73.9 The most common site of colitis cancer is the rectosigmoid, followed by the transverse colon, ascending and descending colon in that order.

adoption in routine surveillance. Prophylactic proctocolectomy is nowadays advised for patients with moderate to high dysplasia and in all patients with a visible lesion irrespective of the grade of dysplasia. Villous adenomatous change and ectopic colonic mucosa are associated with cancer in 70% of cases and constitute definite indications for proctocolectomy.

There is an established association between ulcerative colitis and the development of cholangiocarcinoma. These tumours tend to be of the multiple peripheral (intrahepatic type) and are not usually associated with gallstones. They occur at a younger age group than the usual bile duct tumours and because of their diffuse nature, carry a very poor prognosis. It has been estimated that patients with ulcerative colitis have a 21-fold relative risk for liver and bile duct carcinoma above the general population.

Primary colonic lymphoma has been reported in patients with ulcerative colitis and Crohn's disease. There is, as yet, insufficient information to establish inflammatory bowel disease as a definite cause for these tumours. The reported lymphomas have included both the non-Hodgkin's histiocytic types and Hodgkin's disease.

Perianal Disease

Apart from haemorrhoids which are frequently present, perianal disease (abscesses, fissures and sinuses) are encountered in patients with ulcerative colitis but much less frequently than in Crohn's disease. The highest reported incidence of perianal disease in patients with ulcerative colitis is 15%.

Clinical Features

Ulcerative colitis most commonly affects individuals in their second to fourth decades but the disease can occur both in children and the elderly where it often assumes a severe and active form. The disease is largely confined to Caucasians and is more common in females. The effect of pregnancy on the course of the disease is variable. The relapse rate in pregnant women afflicted by ulcerative colitis is 40–50% which is probably not higher than the average relapse rate for the disease. The majority of the exacerbations occur either during the first trimester or within the first 12 months following delivery. Attacks occurring for the first time during pregnancy or the puerperium are generally mild and respond to medical treatment.

The clinical course of ulcerative colitis is extremely variable and does not accurately reflect the extent of colonic involvement by the disease, although the severe intractable form which is attended by a reduced survival and a significant mortality is encountered in patients with total colitis (*Fig.* 73.12). The severity of the disease is reflected closely by the intensity of the physical symptoms and signs.

Mild ulcerative colitis is generally defined as the disease which is associated with less than four bowel motions per day and the absence of systemic symptoms and signs. It is the most common form of the disease and in the majority of patients the mucosal inflammation is limited to the rectosigmoid region, although a few patients will be found to have total colonic involvement. Apart from mild diarrhoea, mucus and some rectal bleeding, the patients often develop haemorrhoids and perianal irritation although perianal disease (abscesses, sinuses, fistulas) is uncommon. They are also subject to uveitis, erythema nodosum and other skin changes, and arthritis. Not infrequently, these extracolonic manifestations constitute the main complaints and may predate the onset of diarrhoea. In a small percentage of patients (10%), there is a slow progression of both the extent of the colonic involvement and the severity of the disease. Usually, however, the long-term prognosis of the mild disease is good, the patients rarely requiring hospitalization and the overall life expectancy is not affected by the disease.

The disease is of an intermediate severity *(moderate colitis)* in a quarter of the patients affected by the disorder. Colonic involvement varies but is usually extensive or total. Diarrhoea is more marked (4–6 times per day) and invariably contains blood. Abdominal pain (either mild colicky pain or

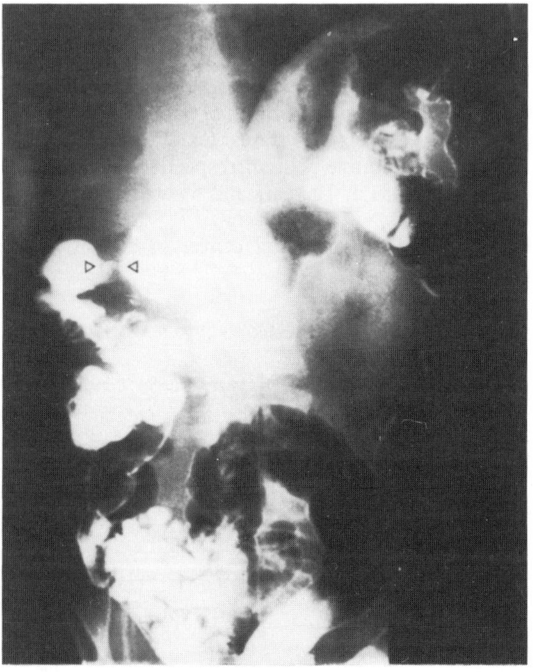

a

Fig. 73.10 *a*, Barium enema showing a neoplastic stricture at the proximal end of the transverse colon in a patient with total colitis of 12 years' duration.

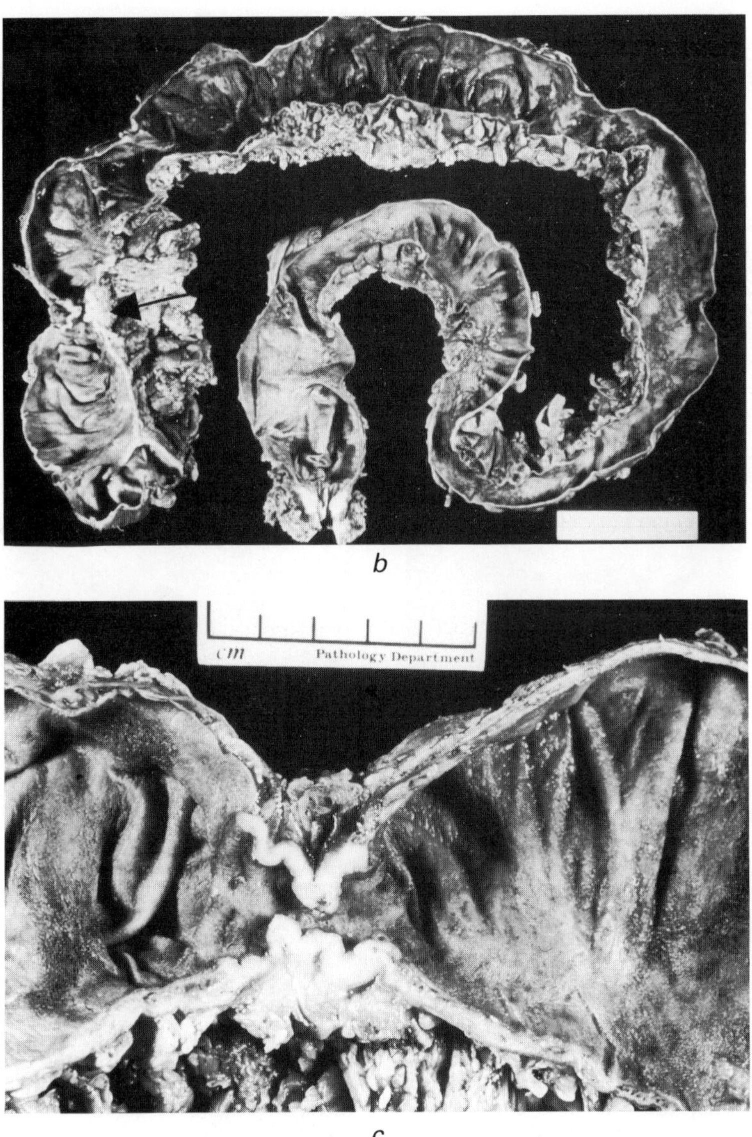

[*Fig. 73.10 continued*] *b*, The resected proctocolectomy specimen. *c*, Close-up view of the carcinoma. (By courtesy of Mr R. A. B. Wood, University of Dundee.)

lower abdominal discomfort) may be present and each attack is accompanied by low-grade pyrexia. The patients often develop iron-deficiency anaemia and may exhibit loss of appetite and weight. The disease responds well to corticosteroid therapy. However, the long-term prognosis is not good and rapid deterioriation with the development of acute local complications (toxic megacolon, massive bleeding, colonic perforation) may occur at some stage or another during the course of the disease.

Severe ulcerative colitis which occurs in 15% of patients, accounts for the vast majority of deaths from the disease. It may result from a progression of mild or moderate disease but, more usually, it starts *de novo* with a severe attack with marked colonic symptoms and systemic manifestations. The diarrhoea is marked with tenesmus and profuse rectal bleeding and is accompanied by a severe water and electrolyte depletion (Na^+ and K^+). The patient becomes dehydrated, acidotic and anaemic. Hypovolaemic shock often develops. Pyrexia is present and is accompanied by a leucocytosis. Hypoproteinaemia and hypoalbuminaemia are invariable features of severe ulcerative colitis and are due to diminished protein intake, impaired synthesis and a constant colonic loss of protein. The patient complains of severe abdominal pain. There is generalized tenderness and varying degrees of abdominal distension. Often, the response to medical treatment is poor and some of these patients require urgent or emergency colectomy for progressing disease or the onset of a serious life-threatening complication. The mortality of a severe attack of ulcerative colitis has been considerably reduced from 30% to under 5% with modern medical therapy and selective surgical intervention for those patients who do not respond to medical treatment.

Medical Treatment

The management of patients with severe disease should be a joint one between gastroenterologists and general surgeons.

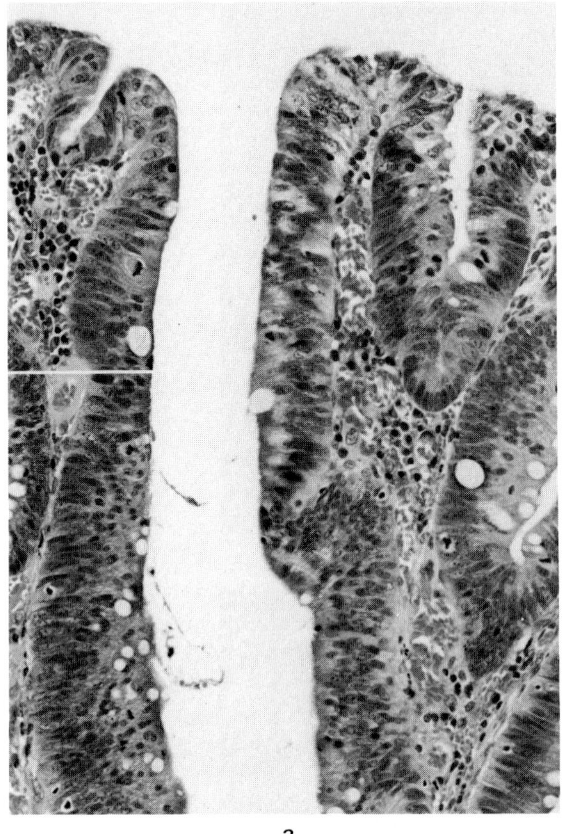

a

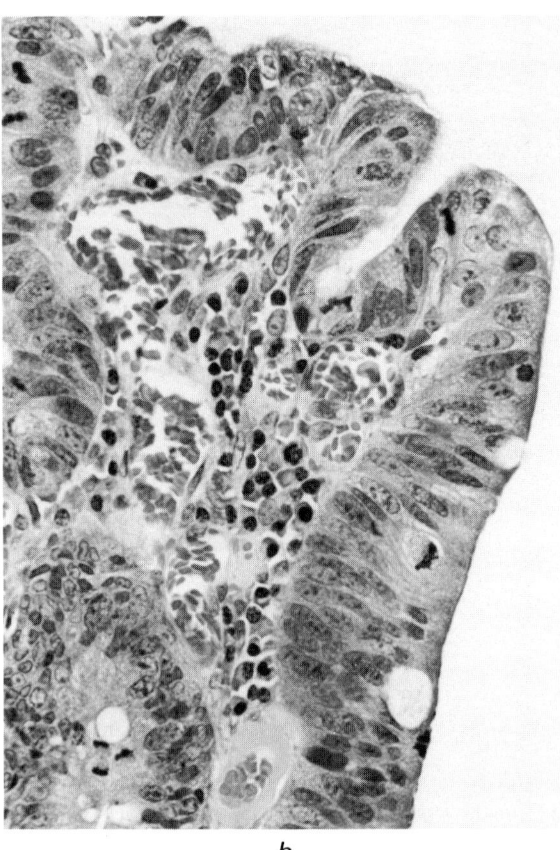

b

Fig. 73.11 Histological appearance showing severe dysplasia in a biopsy from a patient with total colitis during surveillance 9 years after onset of the disease which was well controlled by medical therapy. *a*, Low-power view. *b*, High-power view of the top portion of the left section (above white line) showing multilayering of cells with some loss of polarity, coarse nuclear chromatin and several mitotic figures. The changes amount to severe dysplasia which is an indication for colectomy. (By courtesy of Dr M. P. Holley, Ninewells Hospital, Dundee.)

As a result of better understanding of the behaviour of the disease and the outcome of controlled clinical trials on medical treatment regimens, there is now considerable agreement regarding the details of standard medical therapy and the indications for surgical intervention.

General Measures

Dietary management is important, particularly in patients with moderate to severe disease. A high fibre, calorie and protein intake must be assured. Some patients with ulcerative colitis are allergic to cow's milk proteins and a larger percentage have intestinal lactase deficiency although the exact role of the latter in the aggravation of diarrhoea has not been established. None the less, a small cohort of patients appear to benefit from a milk-free diet.

Correction of the iron-deficiency anaemia is usually achieved by oral iron therapy. The use of opiates and their synthetic derivatives or anticholinergic compounds for the symptomatic relief of the diarrhoea is not recommended because they are usually ineffective and may contribute to the development of toxic megacolon.

Treatment of Severe Attacks

These patients require hospitalization, intensive medical therapy and close and repeated monitoring. General supportive measures are essential to the survival of patients with severe colitis and include the correction of fluid and electrolyte losses, acidosis and hypovolaemia. Blood transfusions are frequently required and help to restore the haemoglobin level, the blood volume and the serum albumin. Often, transfusion of plasma protein derivative or human albumin solution are required in the presence of a marked reduction in the serum albumin level. In addition, patients with severe ulcerative colitis should receive parenteral nutrition via a central feeding line (Broviac or Hickman) until a remission is achieved.

The essential components of medical therapy for severe ulcerative colitis are:

1. Intravenous prednisolone 21-phosphate, 64 mg/day in divided doses.
2. Hydrocortisone drip enema (100 g in 100 ml of water) twice daily.
3. Repeated daily clinical assessment including abdominal girth measurements.
4. Daily radiographic monitoring with erect midinspiratory chest films and lateral decubitus abdominal view.
5. Some clinicians use systemic antibiotics (usually tetracycline and, more recently, metronidazole) in addition to the above regimen.

Sudden deterioriation of the general condition of the patient, increasing abdominal distension and absent bowel sounds indicate failure of medical therapy and the need for an emergency colectomy. In any event, a definite clinical

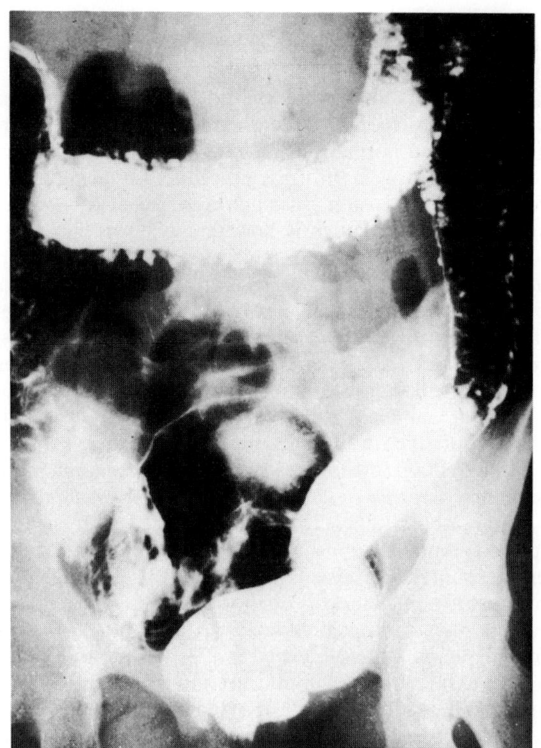

Fig. 73.12 Barium enema showing total colonic involvement with inflammatory bowel disease. There are globular or collar-stud ulcers with overhanging edges. These appearances are found in both ulcerative colitis and Crohn's disease.

improvement with medical therapy must be obtained by the 5th day. If this is not achieved, surgical treatment is required. The risk factors indicative of a likely poor response to medical therapy are:

Pyrexia >38 °C within 24 hours of admission.
Tachycardia >100/min within 24 hours of admission.
Bowel frequency >12 times/day.
Serum albumin of 30 g/litre or less during the first 4 days of treatment.

Some 70% of patients respond favourably to medical treatment in the short term. These patients are started on oral prednisolone (40 mg daily) on the 6th day together with sulphasalazine 1 g twice daily (or delayed release equivalent such as Asacol). The long-term outlook of these patients is, however, not good and 50% of them will eventually require proctocolectomy.

Treatment of Moderate Disease

These patients do not require hospitalization and are treated with oral prednisolone (40 mg daily) and sulphasalazine 1 g daily and steroid enemas. If a remission is not achieved in 2 weeks, they are admitted to hospital and treated as severe attacks.

Mild Attacks

Patients in this category are treated with sulphasalazine (or substitute, *vide infra*) and steroid enemas although some consider that small-dose oral steroid therapy (20 mg daily) should be added as this achieves a remission quicker. The prednisolone is then tailed off.

Maintenance of a Remission

Low-dose steroid therapy is ineffective in maintaining a remission and steroids are not warranted for this purpose as the doses required are too high and accompanied by significant side-effects. Sulphasalazine (or one of its derivatives) is the most effective agent in the prevention of relapse of the disease.

Steroid Enemas

These act largely by a topical action. There are three types:

1. Predsol enema which contain 20 mg prednisolone 21-phosphate: although effective, these are accompanied by absorption of about 40% of the steroid content.
2. Predenema: these contain 20 mg prednisolone metasulphobenzoate. This large steroid molecule is not absorbed by the colonic epithelium. It is as effective as the Predsol enema.
3. Colifoam enema (hydrocortisone acetate 10%, foam in aerosol): these are more acceptable to patients than the above as they lead to less disturbance in the social life and working capacity. They are as effective as the conventional varieties despite the theoretical objection than a shorter length of the colon is exposed to the steroid compound.

Sulphasalazine (salicylazosulphapyridine)

This agent which is degraded to 5-aminosalicylic acid (5-ASA) and sulphapyridine (SP) by bacterial action in the colon, may induce a remission especially in mild and left-sided colitis but is less effective than moderate doses of systemic steroids in this respect. SP and its metabolites are absorbed and largely excreted in the urine, whereas most of the 5-ASA is recovered in the faeces. It is the 5-ASA which is the effective agent against the colitis. The main use of sulphasalazine is in the maintenance therapy where it has been shown to reduce the incidence of relapse when administered in a dose of 2 g daily. Side-effects of sulphasalazine are common and some 30% of patients are intolerant of the drug because of complications which include headache, nausea, vomiting, diarrhoea, erythema nodosum and other hypersensitivity skin rashes. In addition, haematological complications, e.g. haemolytic anaemia, aplastic anaemia and agranulocytosis, may be encountered albeit rarely. Sulphasalazine also causes infertility in males from reduction of sperm counts and abnormal forms. The side-effects are usually associated with high serum levels of SP which tend to occur in slow acetylators on doses greater than 3 g daily. The acetylator status determines the ratio of free SP to total SP.

Two pharmaceutical approaches have been used to decrease sulphasalazine toxicity which is largely due to its SP moiety. One compound which is undergoing clinical testing is disodium azodisalicylate (olsalazine) which does not contain SP and consists of two 5-ASA molecules linked together by a diazo bond. This compound releases twice as much 5-ASA as sulphasalazine for a given dose. It appears, however, that the intact compound is absorbed and has a long half-life. A clinical trial with olsalazine showed it to be effective in achieving a remission when administered orally for patients with mild colitis. Another approach has been to coat 5-ASA to delay its release until the capsule reaches the colon. Two such formulations are available: Pentasa which consists of 5-ASA packaged in ethyl cellulose and Asacol where the 5-ASA tablets are coated with an acrylic-based resin. Clinical trials comparing the efficacy of these 5-ASA compounds versus sulphasalazine especially for long-term use in maintaining remission are currently in progress. The early reports indicate that tolerance for these new formulations is good.

Other Drugs

Although azathioprine has no effect on active colitis it is occasionally used to reduce the dose of steroids in those rare instances where continued steroid therapy is necessary to prevent relapse. The steroid-sparing effect of this immunosuppressive drug appears to be beneficial in reducing steriod side-effects in these selected patients. The results with disodium cromoglycate in ulcerative colitis have been disappointing and this agent does not have an established place in the treatment of this disorder although some gastroenterologists still use it for some patients with proctitis.

Surgical Treatment

Surgical intervention in patients with ulcerative colitis may be undertaken as a planned exercise under elective conditions or as an urgent measure because of failure to improve with medical therapy during an attack and finally as an emergency procedure necessitated by the onset of a life-threatening complication. There is little doubt from the results of published series that the best outcome in terms of survival and morbidity is obtained after elective surgery and the highest reported mortality is accrued when colectomy is performed as an emergency procedure. One of the important factors, apart from effective systemic steroid therapy, in reducing the overall mortality from severe ulcerative colitis during the past two decades has been the decision for earlier operation in those patients not responding adequately to standard in-hospital medical therapy and the imposition of a time limit (5 days) by which definite clinical improvement is obtained by conservative measures. These changes have resulted from an increased awareness of the natural history of the disease and the joint management of these severely ill patients.

Indications for Colectomy

These are best considered under elective, urgent and emergency procedures (*Table* 73.2).

Surgical Procedures

Until fairly recently, the accepted standard operation for ulcerative colitis has been *panproctocolectomy* with a permanent spout ileostomy. The construction of a continent ileostomy (*Fig.* 73.13) at the time of the colectomy or at a subsequent stage is still practised in some Scandinavian centres with good results. This procedure, however, requires considerable experience and has been accompanied by a tendency to pouch ileitis and bacterial overgrowth although the author has several long-term patients who have done extremely well with this procedure. In general, however, continent ileostomy has not been accepted widely and is not performed frequently nowadays.

In some instances where rectal disease is not severe *colectomy with ileorectal anastomosis* is an acknowledged alternative to be used in selected cases but with careful long-term follow-up as the risk of carcinoma though reduced is still present (10–13% at 25 years). In very ill patients undergoing emergency colectomy for toxic megacolon or colonic perforation, a *colectomy with a distal mucous fistula* is still a sensible option with proctectomy at a later stage.

In the elective situation, *colectomy with submucosal proctectomy and the creation of an anal pouch with ileo-anal anastomosis* is an established procedure in specialized centres and the reported results are constantly improving in terms of continence, spontaneous evacuation of the pouch and reduced postoperative pelvic sepsis due to separation of the ileo-anal anastomosis. Controversy, however, still exists as to the optimal pouch construction (*Fig.* 73.14) but the J-pouch appears to be the least complicated and to date has given the best overall results. Mesenteric extension is essential for the creation of a tension free ileo-anal anastomosis. The technique of mesenteric extension with preservation of the ileocolic vessels is shown in *Fig.* 73.15. The terminal trunks of the superior mesenteric vessels are ligated and divided while preserving the ileocolic arcade. This technique of mesenteric lengthening is particularly suitable for the construction of the J-pouch and ensures bilateral blood supply to each limb of the reservoir. The alternative method of mesenteric extension which is suitable for other pouches (S, W, H types) is shown in *Fig.* 73.16. Both the terminal trunks of the superior mesenteric vessels and the ileocolic vessels are divided but an arcade is preserved along the length of the distal ileum. All ileo-anal pouch procedures are covered by a temporary loop ileostomy which is subsequently closed once the anastomoses have healed. A period of training is necessary and the patients notice improvement especially in the bowel frequency over a period of several months. The complications of this procedure are:

- Dehiscence of the ileo-anal anastomosis
- Stenosis of the ileo-anal anastomosis
- Need for catheter evacuation particularly with S pouches and a long efferent limb
- Incontinence
- Inflammation of the pouch.

Although the need for re-intervention to deal with complications is high, total failure necessitating removal of the pouch with reversion to a permanent ileostomy is rare and is encountered in about 5–10%.

Table 73.2 Indications for colectomy

ELECTIVE	Failure of medical therapy—inadequate control, frequent hospitalization, need for continuous or repeated courses of steroid therapy.
	Prophylactic during cancer surveillance—dysplasia, villous adenomatous change and ectopic colonic mucosa
URGENT	Failure of medical therapy to achieve improvement within 5 days of intensive treatment for a severe attack
EMERGENCY	Toxic megacolon which does not improve within 48–72 hours with intensive medical treatment
	Colonic perforation
	Massive haemorrhage (very rare indication)

CROHN'S DISEASE

Crohn's disease is a chronic transmural inflammatory disorder of the alimentary tract manifested by marked ill-health, gastrointestinal symptoms and sometimes life-threatening complications. The disease is frequently associated with systemic manifestations (*Table* 73.3), and the clinical symptoms and signs may show considerable variation

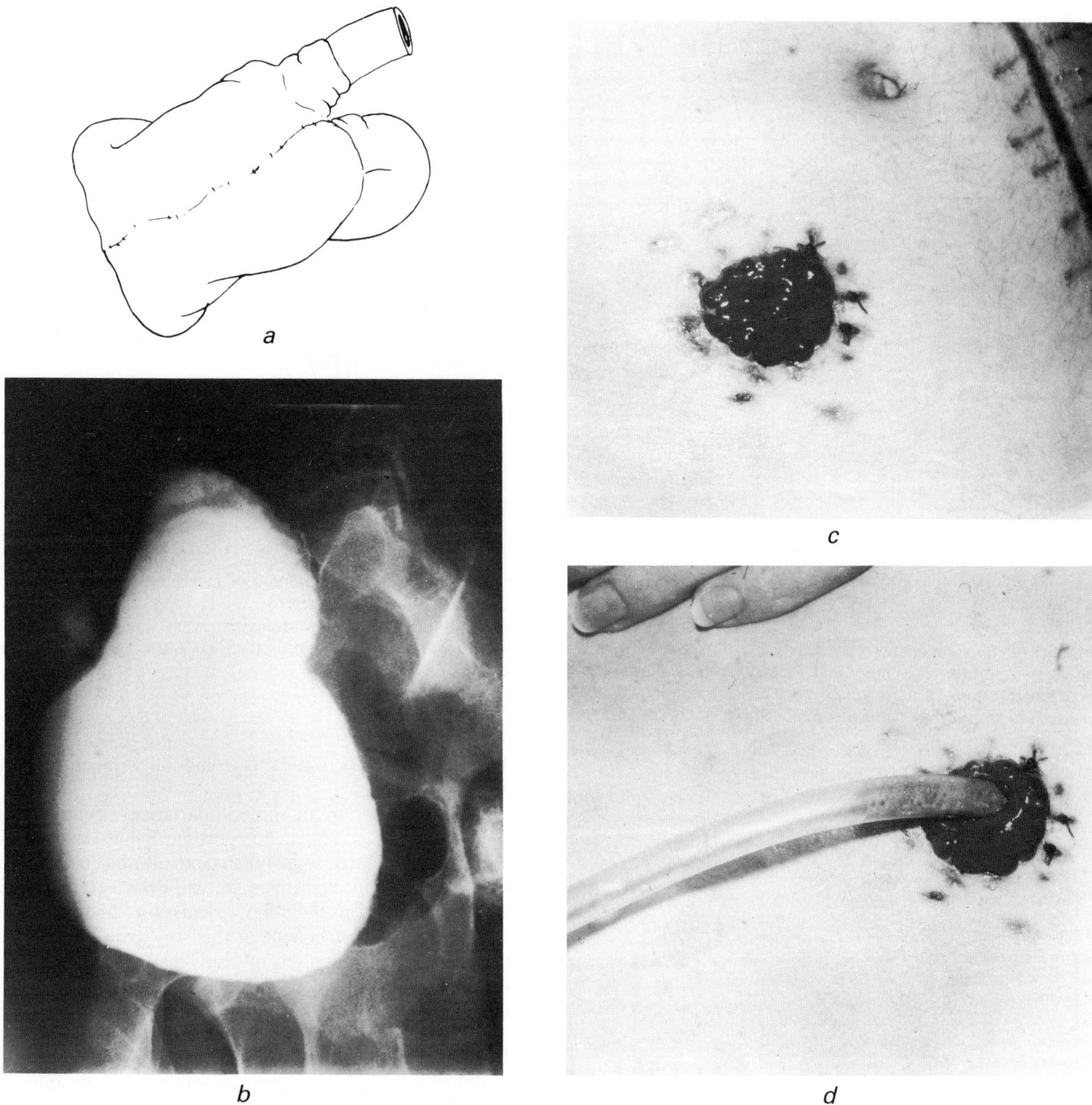

Fig. 73.13 *a*, Diagrammatic representation of Koch's continent reservoir. The nipple valve is produced by intussusception of part of the efferent limb of the reservoir. *b*, The reservoir enlarges to a capacity of 400–600 ml. Radiograph after instillation of contrast medium. *c*, Continent ileostomy in a young female after proctocolectomy for severe ulcerative colitis. *d*, The valve is opened by the insertion of a silicone catheter. Emptying of the reservoir is achieved by straining and compression of the lower abdomen. With the advent of the ileo-anal pouch, this operation although still practised in some Scandinavian centres, is less commonly performed nowadays.

from individual to individual. Crohn's disease may affect any part of the gastrointestinal tract. The most frequent site of involvement is the terminal ileum/caecum followed by the colorectal region, gastroduodenal area and the oesophagus in that order.

Aetiology

The aetiology of the disorder remains unknown. Recent work, however, suggests a possible role for both dietary antigens and certain bacteria (variant, atypical mycobacteria). Although Yersinia can cause an acute ileitis, there is no evidence for the association of the organism with the development of Crohn's disease. The immunological changes previously described in this chapter are not concerned with the development of the disorder, although some such as the lymphocyte OKT9 positivity seem to reflect the activity of the disease. One of the well-known hypotheses for the development of Crohn's disease concerns obstruction of the intestinal lymphatics either from the absorption of particulate matter (talcum powder, sand, toothpaste) or following a lymphangitis. However, although animal models simulating some of the pathological features of the human disease have been produced in this way, there has never been any firm evidence to substantiate lymphatic obstruction as the primary cause of Crohn's disease.

Several reports have demonstrated a certain personality

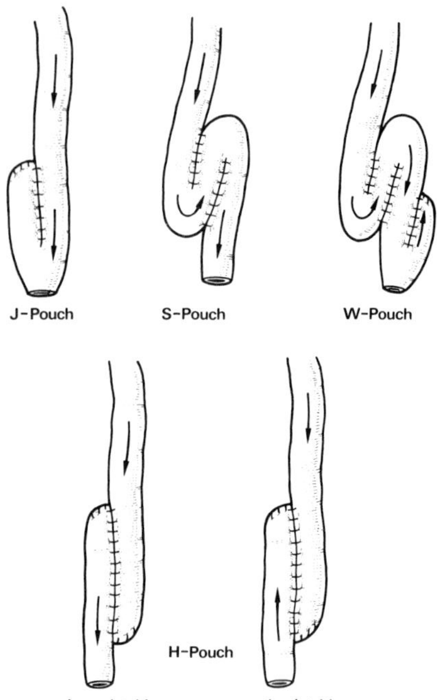

Fig. 73.14 Diagrammatic representation of the various forms of pouches used after colectomy and mucosal proctectomy. The J-pouch is the most extensively used since it is the simplest to create, is attended with the lowest incidence of complications and functions best in the long-term.

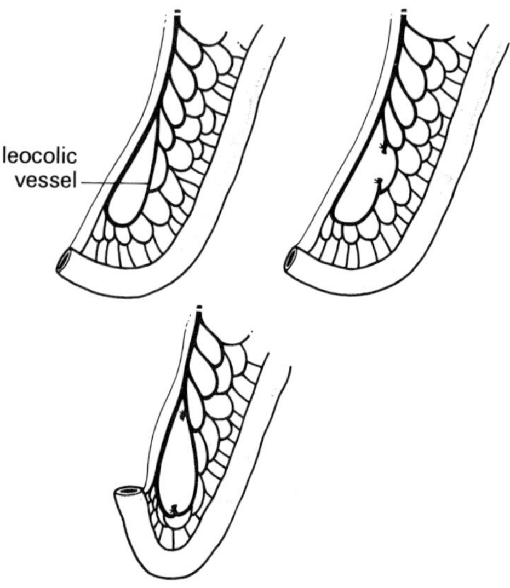

Fig. 73.15 Technique of mesenteric extension. The terminal trunks of the superior mesenteric vessels are ligated and divided while preserving the ileocolic arcade. This technique is particularly suitable for the construction of the J-pouch and ensures bilateral blood supply to each limb of the reservoir.

type with a tendency to depressive illness in patients with Crohn's disease but a causal relation between attacks of depression and the disorder has not been established. The theory behind this psychosomatic theory is that abnormal gut motility induced by psychological stress and depressive illness leads to mucosal damage and subsequent inflammation.

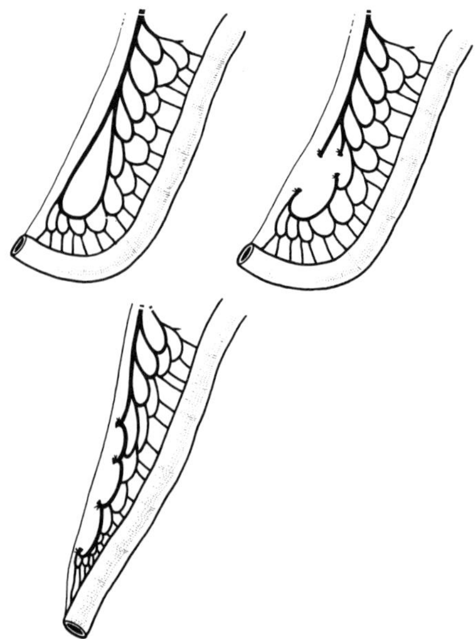

Fig. 73.16 Alternative method of mesenteric extension which is suitable for other pouches (S, W, H types). Both the terminal trunks of the superior mesenteric vessels and the ileocolic vessels are divided but an arcade is preserved along the length of the distal ileum.

Dietary factors are of some importance. Crohn's disease patients have been shown to consume a diet lower in fibre and higher in refined sugars than control subjects. Exclusion diets, whereby specific items are withdrawn from the diet, have been shown to maintain a remission. The commonest items which impart benefit in this way are dairy products and wheat. A further recent study has indicated that the administration of an elemental diet together with non-absorbable antibiotics is followed by a very high remission rate. The exact reason for the beneficial effect of elemental diets in Crohn's disease is unknown and could be the result of either a reduced luminal antigenic load or improved nutrition.

Evidence is accumulating that Crohn's disease is the result of infection by low virulence bacterial organisms. In recent years the role of two types of bacteria has been investigated:

1. Variant (or L-form) bacteria. These organisms have deficient cell walls and can develop from several bacterial species after their exposure to antibiotics. The cell-wall protein deficiency is accompanied by an alteration in virulence, antigenicity and pathogenicity. However, these variant bacteria (which can pass through filters which hold back normal bacteria), can, in time and under certain conditions, revert to their original form. *Pseudomonas maltophilia* is a variant bacterial species which has been isolated from intestinal Crohn's disease.

2. *Mycobacterium paratuberculosis* is a member of the atypical mycobacteria of the Runyon group III. It has been isolated from patients with Crohn's disease and on inoculation has been shown to produce granulomas in the terminal ileum of goats. Also, patients with Crohn's disease have IgG antibodies against this organism. However, the antibody levels bears no relation to disease activity and their level is

not altered by resection of the diseased segment of bowel. Recent studies with DNA hybridization techniques have revealed mycobacterial genomes in the tissues of patients with Crohn's disease. There is, therefore, some evidence that *M. paratuberculosis* and other closely allied atypical mycobacteria may have a causative role in this disorder although further studies are required to establish this association beyond question.

Pathology

Irrespective of the level involved, Crohn's disease is a segmental condition with areas of involvement which are sharply demarcated from the contiguous normal bowel at least on naked eye appearance (*Fig.* 73.17). The number of these skip lesions varies from none to several and widespread/continuous involvement of the small or large intestine or both.

Macroscopic Appearance

The early disease appears to start as a mucosal inflammation with small aphthoid ulcers from the edges of which granulomas can be identified on histology.

The serosal surface of the affected bowel in established Crohn's disease is granular and inflamed with a tendency for it to be encroached by the mesenteric fat, so that the intestine may at times be buried within a swollen, oedematous and foreshortened mesentery. On palpation, the involved areas feel heavy, thickened and firm (hosepipe) as a result of the transmural inflammation which is usually associated with narrowing of the bowel lumen. A close inspection of the opened bowel reveals separation of the usual anatomical layers by fibrosis which is especially marked in the submucosal and subserosal layers (*Fig.* 73.18). The mucosal oedema accounts for the characteristic cobblestone appearance of the mucosa (*Fig.* 73.19). The oedema is followed by sloughing and linear ulceration of the mucosa particularly at the mesenteric attachments (*Fig.* 73.20). Pseudopolyps and mucosal bridges may form as in ulcerative colitis. The ulcers which are typically deep, penetrate into the muscle layers (fissuring) and account for the tendency to localized perforation, adhesions and fistula formation. Regional lymphadenopathy is invariably present and is usually the result of reactive hyperplasia, although specific changes such as sarcoid granulomas are often encountered.

Fistula formation is an important frequent consequence of Crohn's disease and accounts for substantial morbidity, long periods of invalidism and a 5–10% mortality following surgical treatment. The fistulous tracts may be simple or complex and often incorporate an intervening or associated abscess. The important varieties of fistulas encountered in Crohn's disease are:

1. Enterocutaneous: some 20–30% of these may heal with drainage of the abscess and parenteral nutrition.
2. Perianal fistulas: are usually (but not always) associated with severe anorectal disease.
3. Ileosigmoid fistulas: lead to severe bacterial overgrowth of the small intestine with gross malabsorption and malnutrition.
4. Enterovesical fistulas: may involve the ileum or colon or both and usually develop in patients with longstanding disease. Enterovesical fistulas are less common than the above varieties and have a reported incidence of 5%. They usually follow a benign course and present with dysuria, pneumaturia, faecaluria and recurrent pyelonephritis. They do not respond to conservative measures and require surgical intervention, the results of which are good.

Microscopic Appearances

The histological features are characterized by a transmural inflammation consisting of chronic inflammatory cell infiltrates including eosinophils, crypt abscess formation, oedema, non-caseating epithelioid-cell granulomas containing Langhan's giant cells, dilatation and sclerosis of the intestinal lymphatics and lymphoid aggregates with or without germinal centres, in the various layers of the bowel wall, epithelial regenerative changes and angiitis. The granulomas which resemble those found in sarcoidosis, are found in the bowel wall in some 50–60% of resected specimens and, to a

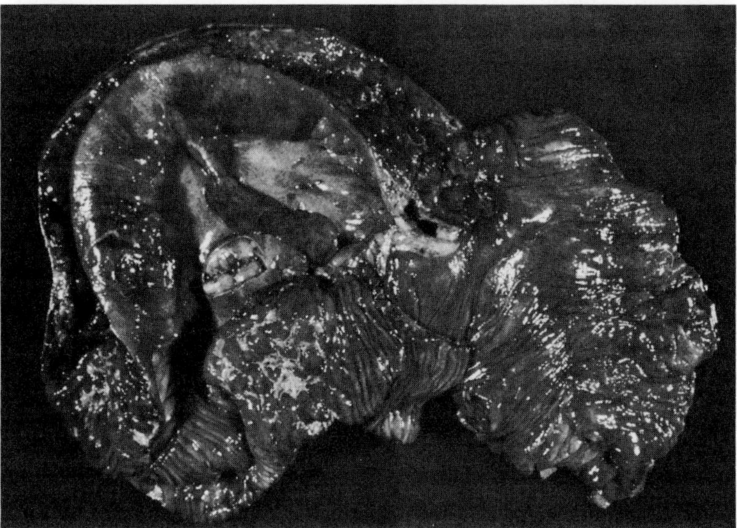

Fig. 73.17 Crohn's disease of the ileum. The affected bowel is thickened with a granular oedematous serosal surface. Note the sharp macroscopic demarcation between diseased and normal adjacent mucosa.

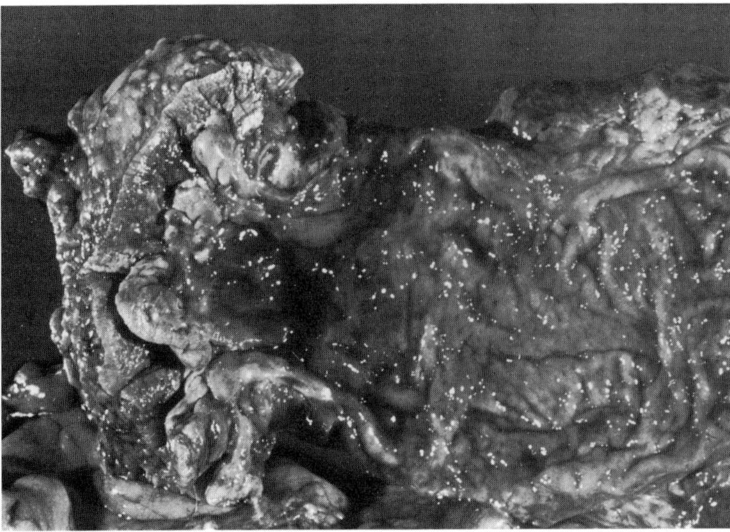

Fig. 73.18 Crohn's disease of the ileocolic region. The affected bowel has been cut longitudinally to demonstrate the transmural fibrosis which is especially marked in the subserous and submucosal layers.

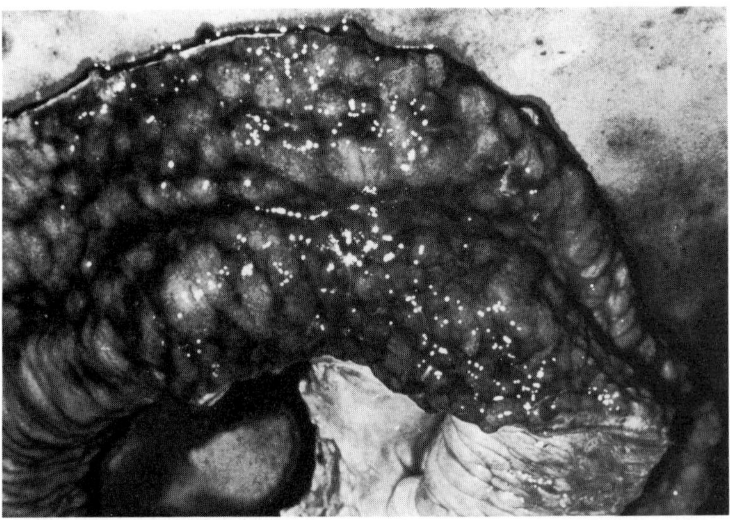

Fig. 73.19 Diffuse mucosal/submucosal oedema resulting in the characteristic cobblestone appearance of the mucosa in Crohn's disease.

lesser extent (25%), in the regional lymph nodes. The epithelial regenerative changes include the development of pseudopyloric gland metaplasia.

The distinction between ulcerative colitis and colonic Crohn's disease may be very difficult and at times impossible on histological grounds. The most important criterion for the diagnosis of Crohn's colitis is the detection of non-caseating granulomas which often require serial sectioning of multiple and often repeated biopsies.

Complications of Crohn's Disease

Some of the complications of Crohn's disease such as abscess, sinus and fistula formation, intestinal obstruction, malnutrition, etc. are so common that they are usually considered as integral clinical features of the disease. Repeated and prolonged sepsis may lead to the development of amyloid disease.

Crohn's disease may be accompanied by the *systemic manifestations* of inflammatory bowel disease (*Table* 73.3) and, like ulcerative colitis, colonic Crohn's may be complicated by the development of toxic megacolon and perforation. However, the latter may occur without acute dilatation. Massive life-threatening haemorrhage from erosion of a major vessel in a deep ulcer is a rare but well-recognized complication.

In addition to enterovesical fistulas, the urological complications of Crohn's disease include an obstructive uropathy and an increased incidence of renal calculi. The obstructive uropathy is consequent on retroperitonitis and fibrosis leading to obstruction of the ureter (usually the right) and is more frequent than is generally realized (*Fig.* 73.21). Patients with obstructive uropathy are usually totally asymptomatic although occasionally pyuria, bacteriuria and pain in the flanks are observed. If untreated, an obstructive

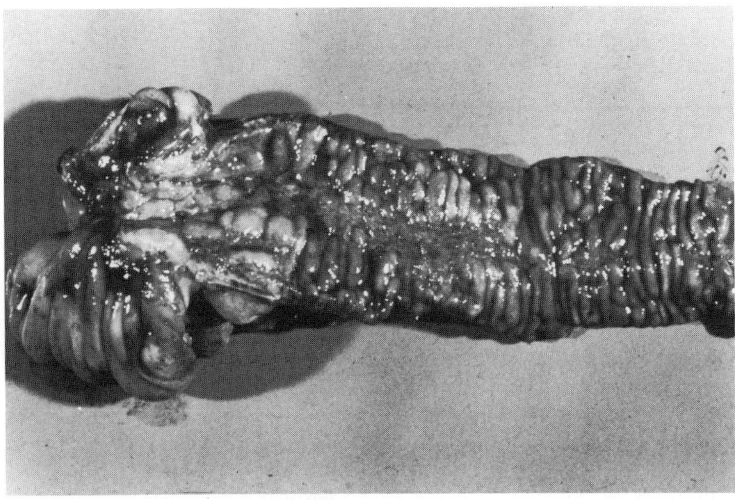

Fig. 73.20 Extensive ulceration with stricture formation in Crohn's disease of the distal ileum. The longitudinal ulceration is more prominent along the mesenteric attachment.

uropathy will lead to severe hydronephrosis, recurrent pyonephrosis and loss of functional renal tissue. Intravenous urography must be a routine part of the investigation of all patients with Crohn's disease.

Renal calculi have been reported in 7% of adults with inflammatory bowel disease with a higher incidence in Crohn's disease (10%) than in ulcerative colitis. In most of these patients, the duration of the intestinal disease is over 8–11 years. Calcium oxalate or phosphate stones account for 72% of cases and uric acid stones for 18%. Some 10% of the renal calculi cannot be classified. Only 36% of patients with renal stones have a predisposing urinary tract abnormality such as sponge kidney, obstructive uropathy or a metabolic disorder (e.g. hypercalcaemia). Increased absorption of oxalate, an increased cell turnover in the gut and a concentrated urine appear to be important factors in the formation of

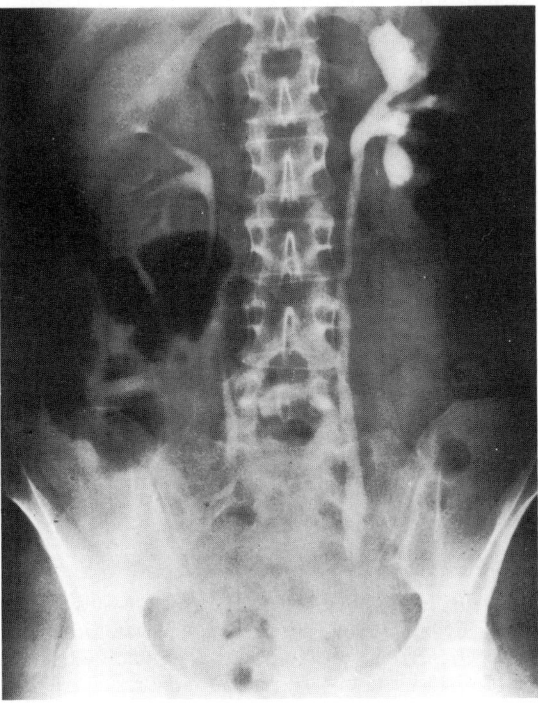

a

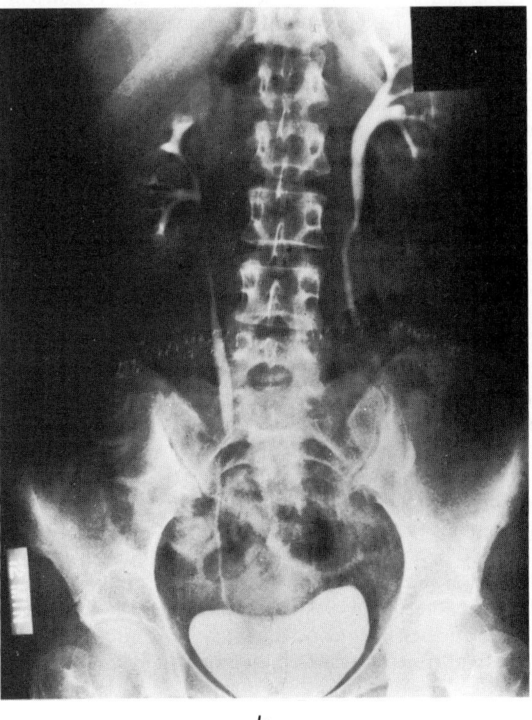

b

Fig. 73.21 *a*, Intravenous urogram demonstrating an obstructive uropathy on the left side. The patient had Crohn's disease of the ileum with fistula formation involving the sigmoid colon and resulting severe inflammation of the retroperitoneal tissue on the left side. *b*, Same patient one month following bowel resection and ureterolysis. There is complete resolution of the left hydronephrosis and hydroureter.

renal calculi in patients with inflammatory bowel disease. The prevalence of nephrolithiasis in children with Crohn's disease is said to be as high as 25%.

There is an increased incidence of gallstone formation in patients with severe ileal Crohn's disease or following ileal resections for this disorder. This is attributable to malabsorption of bile salts with interruption of the enterohepatic circulation and a consequent reduction of the bile salt pool. *Cancer of the colon* is four times more common in patients with Crohn's disease than in the general population. In addition, there is now a well-established association between Crohn's disease and *small bowel adenocarcinoma* and some 75 cases have been reported in the literature. These tumours occur at a younger age, are located predominantly in the distal ileum and carry a poor prognosis. Cases of small-bowel lymphomas and carcinoid tumours have also been reported in patients with Crohn's disease.

Clinical Features

The peak incidence of the disease is in the third decade and it occurs with the same frequency in females as in males. Crohn's disease may also affect children and the elderly. In the latter age group, it is frequently colonic and accompanied by diverticular disease. The differentiation between the two disorders in the elderly may be difficult. The clinical manifestations of Crohn's disease are protean and depend on the location and extent of the disease and the onset of specific complications which are often the presenting features.

The disease is localized in the ileocolic region in 60% of patients, to the small bowel alone in 20% and to the colon in a further 20%. Some of the clinical manifestations correlate with the site of involvement. Thus, whilst abdominal pain occurs with equal frequency in all groups (60–80%), rectal bleeding is a feature of colorectal disease and is not usually encountered in patients with small-bowel involvement. The severity of the abdominal pain varies from discomfort to severe colicky pain exacerbated by meals. The pain may be felt in the periumbilical region, the right lower quadrant or may be generalized. Some patients with small-bowel Crohn's disease complain of early satiety or a sense of fullness. The patients may also complain of abdominal distension during bouts of abdominal pain.

Pseudo-appendicitis syndrome: Some patients with Crohn's disease of the terminal ileum develop acute abdominal pain, the severity and location of which simulates closely acute appendicitis and as many as 14% of children and young adults with Crohn's disease are said to present in this manner. This clinical presentation is worthy of special consideration since acute terminal ileitis often due to *Yersinia* infection is often encountered in many such instances and has a different natural history from that of Crohn's disease. It has been estimated that only 1 in 8 acute terminal ileitis are due to Crohn's disease. Accordingly, treatment in the emergency situation should be conservative. The appendix should be removed if the caecum appears normal and swabs taken from the luminal contents for bacteriological culture. The appendicectomy which can be performed safely will prevent further diagnostic dilemmas at a later date should the patient develop recurrent symptoms.

Small Bowel Obstruction

Not infrequently, the abdominal pain and distension in Crohn's disease of the small bowel evolves into a clinical picture or partial (subacute) or intermittent obstruction (*Fig.* 73.22). Complete small bowel obstruction is, however, rare. The obstruction is more commonly due to adhesions than stenosis, although differentiation is impossible on clinical grounds. Early operation for patients with partial obstruction is advisable to avoid the risk of strangulation and the increased morbidity and mortality associated with emergency enterectomy. Patients with intermittent self-limiting obstructive episodes invariably have gross bacterial overgrowth which may cause further malabsorption, hypoproteinaemia and malnutrition.

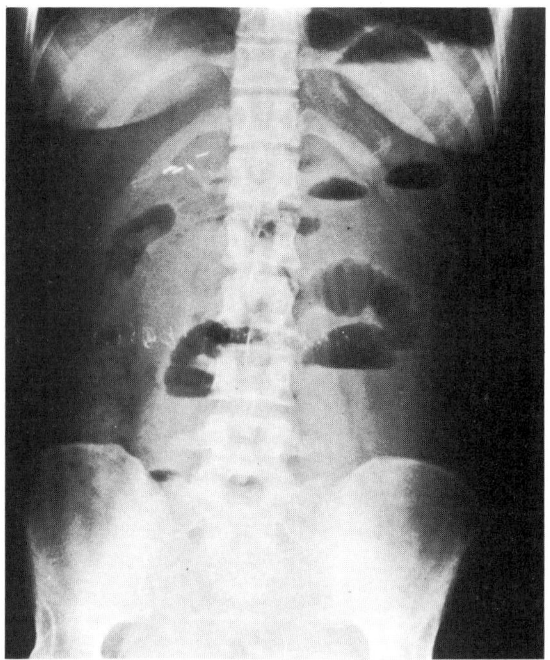

Fig. 73.22 Plain erect abdominal film showing air/fluid levels in a step ladder pattern due to mechanical bowel obstruction. The patient had had a right hemicolectomy for Crohn's disease. Such an obstructive picture may be due to adhesions or recurrence which is most commonly situated at the level of the previous anastomosis.

Abscess Formation

This is a common presentation. The abscess may result either from bowel perforation which may occur at the site of a deep fissure ulcer or proximal to a stricture. It can also arise in a mass of inflamed regional lymph nodes without a perforation of the bowel. Apart from the local signs and symptoms, abscess formation leads to malaise, increased catabolism with weight loss, fever and anorexia. The commonest site of abscess formation is in the right iliac fossa. The abscess may track into the pelvis and underneath the inguinal ligament to reach the anterior compartment of the thigh. Free perforation of Crohn's disease into the peritoneal cavity with widespread peritonitis is rare.

Fistula Formation

The most common type is perianal which usually occurs in association with perianal abscesses and sinuses (*Fig.* 73.23). These perianal complications are a significant feature of Crohn's disease and may be present months or years before intestinal symptoms are noticed. Enterocutaneous fistulas usually become evident following drainage of abdominal abscesses and are classified as high- or low-output variety in terms of the amount of faecal discharge per day. Spontaneous closure with parenteral nutrition is more likely with

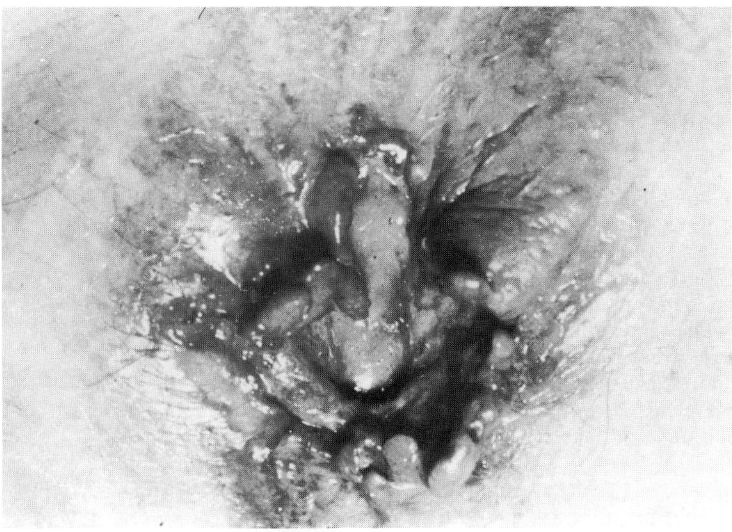

Fig. 73.23 Extensive anal and perianal disease in a patient with Crohn's colitis. The patient had a high fistula-in-ano.

the low output variety. Enterocolic fistulas are associated with bacterial overgrowth, malabsorption and diarrhoea (*Fig.* 73.24). Enterovesical fistulas due to Crohn's disease do not usually cause severe systemic disturbances and present with urinary symptoms (dysuria pneumaturia/faecaluria), and recurrent attacks of pyelonephritis.

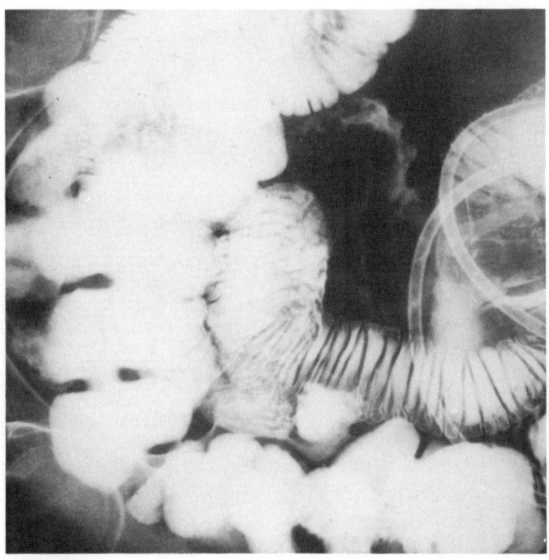

Fig. 73.24 Barium study demonstrating a fistula between the small bowel and the colon in a patient with Crohn's disease.

Diarrhoea

Diarrhoea occurs in about 70–80% of patients with Crohn's disease. However, it must be emphasized that 5–10% of patients may have constipation. The latter is found particularly in patients with isolated terminal ileal involvement. Diarrhoea tends to be most severe in patients with colonic disease and is then accompanied by the passage of mucus and blood per rectum. The diarrhoea of Crohn's disease is often accompanied by a protein-losing enteropathy and/or steatorrhoea due to bacterial overgrowth or bile salt malabsorption.

Growth Retardation

This is said to occur in approximately 20% of all children with Crohn's disease. Failure to thrive in children with Crohn's disease can have several connotations which include four basic components:

Impairment of linear growth
Weight loss or failure to gain weight
Delayed sexual maturation and closure of epiphyses
Normal endocrinological parameters.

Thyroid function in these children is consistently normal and so is growth hormone secretion when several provocative tests are employed. The major factor in growth retardation is malnutrition which is due to failure to eat because of high-grade partial intermittent small-bowel obstruction, protein and blood loss from the ulcerated inflamed areas of the small bowel, and malabsorption due to bacterial overgrowth.

When assessing the potential growth of these children, it is crucial to evaluate their bone age and to note the stature of their parents. In this way, it is possible to predict which children would be capable of responding to a therapeutic intervention (including parenteral nutrition) with linear growth. Following an appropriate bowel resection, growth resumes the normal pattern but compensatory (catch-up) growth does not occur. It is, therefore, essential to treat these children while their bones are still capable of growth. Fortunately in many of these teenagers closure of the epiphyses is delayed because of the associated malnutrition.

Diagnosis

The diagnosis of Crohn's disease rests on the evaluation of the clinical signs and symptoms which are correlated with proctosigmoidoscopic/colonoscopic, radiological and histological findings.

Sigmoidoscopic examination is best performed without bowel preparation so that an assessment of the degree of erythema, oedema and vascularity of the mucosa can be made prior to irritation by catheters and enemas. It must always be preceded by a careful inspection of the perianal and perineal regions for fissures, fleshy skin tags, sinuses, etc. If the rectum is grossly involved, the mucosa shows a patchy or diffuse erythema and, possibly, ulceration. Multiple biopsies are necessary and serial sections of these must be taken by the pathologists in their search for non-caseating sarcoid-like granulomas which constitute the histological hallmark of Crohn's disease. However, in some patients with colonic disease and no small bowel involvement differentiation from ulcerative colitis is not possible and the terms 'inflammatory bowel disease' or 'indeterminate colitis' are used.

Certain laboratory tests are important to establish the nutritional state of the patients and as an index of disease activity. A full blood count, ESR, serum electrolytes, serum proteins and, in particular, serum albumin are always necessary. Decreased serum albumin, hypochromic microcytic anaemia and low serum iron, may be found in as many as 50% of untreated patients. Occasionally, megaloblastic anaemia may be observed resulting from folic-acid deficiency or impaired vitamin B_{12} absorption. Hypocalcaemia and hypomagnesaemia resulting in paraesthesias may occasionally occur. Low serum levels of zinc and vitamin A may also be present and usually reflect impaired absorption and/or decreased ingestion. Frank malabsorption with steatorrhoea may be present in patients with extensive small-bowel disease or bacterial overgrowth. In these patients the Schilling test or the SeHCAT test may provide useful information in defining the presence of malabsorption of vitamin B_{12} and bile salts respectively. Bacterial overgrowth is documented by hydrogen breath tests and the oral ^{14}C-glycocholate test or equivalent.

The important indices of disease activity are:

ESR
Serum alpha$_1$ glycoprotein level
C-reactive protein
OKT9 lymphocyte positivity.

Demonstration of the diseased segments is most commonly achieved by contrast radiology, endoscopy and, less commonly, by external isotope scintiscanning following the intravenous administration of ^{111}In-labelled autologous leucocytes.

Radiological Appearances

The small-bowel enema is the standard investigation for the detection of small-bowel Crohn's disease. In most series, distal small-bowel or localized ileocolic involvement predominates. Narrowing of the lumen, nodularity of the mucosal pattern, thickening of the ileocaecal valve, mucosal irregularity and deep ulcerations perpendicular to the intestinal lumen and fistula formation are all characteristic features of small-bowel Crohn's disease. Long, narrow strictures result in the well-known 'string sign' of Kantor (*Fig.* 73.25). Skip lesions are characteristic with normal bowel in between strictured/diseased areas.

Large-bowel disease is evaluated by means of a barium enema. The involvement may be segmental (*Fig.* 73.26), localized (*Fig.* 73.27) or total (*Fig.* 73.28). At times differentiation of the latter from ulcerative colitis is impossible

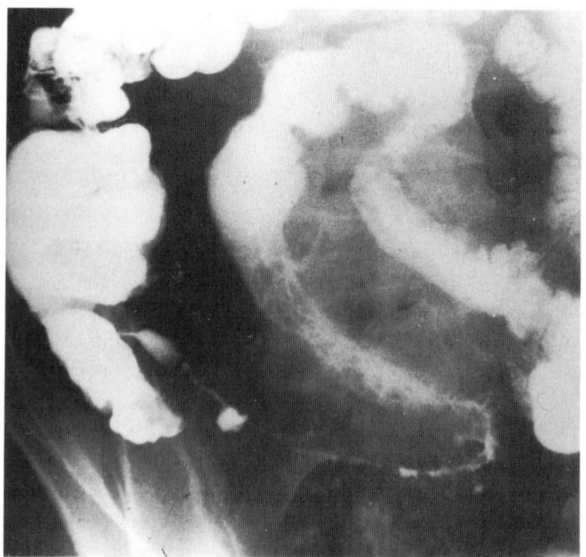

Fig. 73.25 Small-bowel enema showing several features of Crohn's disease of the distal ileum: stenosis (Kantor's string sign), cobblestoning of the mucosa, deep globular ulcer (pseudodiverticulum), deep penetrating fissure ulcers, wide separation of the intestinal loops due to thickening of the bowel walls and thickening of the ileocaecal valve due to lymphatic blockage and oedema. The patient presented with intermittent cramp-like abdominal pain after meals.

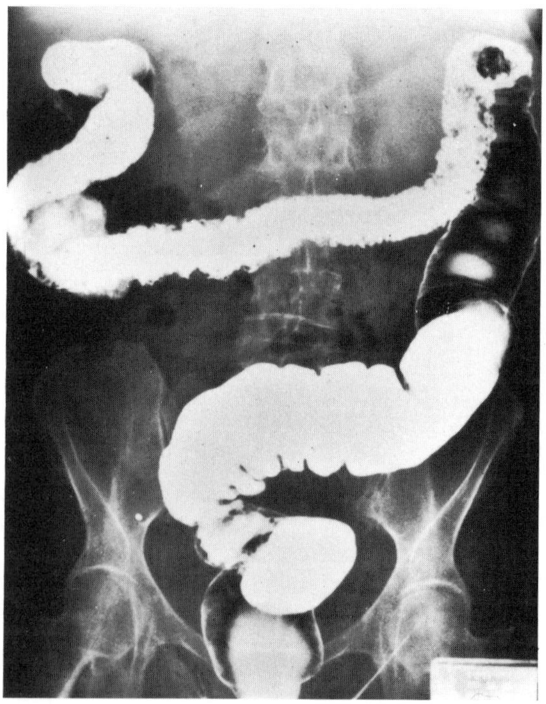

Fig. 73.26 Barium enema showing acute Crohn's colitis affecting the transverse colon in a 73-year-old diabetic woman. The segmental nature of the disease is also compatible with the diagnosis of ischaemic colitis in this age group. In addition, coexisting diverticular disease is often present in the elderly patients and differentiation between this disorder and Crohn's colitis may be difficult.

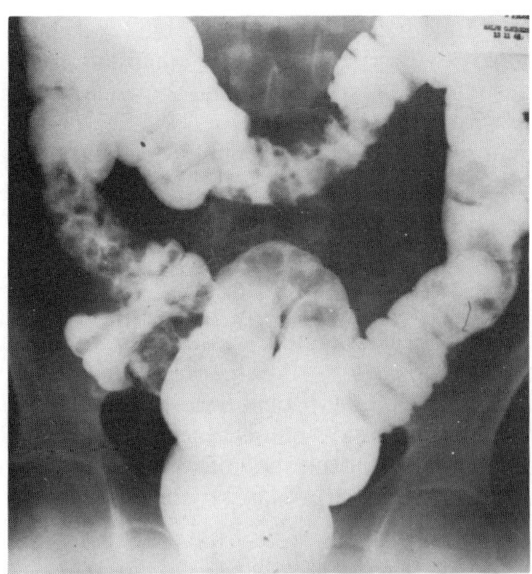

Fig. 73.27 Barium enema showing localized Crohn's disease of the colon.

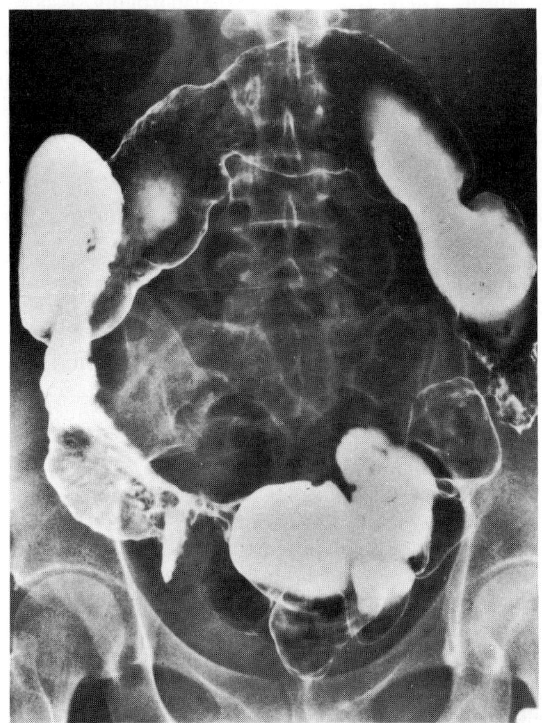

Fig. 73.28 Barium enema showing the end-stage changes of long-standing Crohn's colitis with gross architectural destruction of the colon and rectum. Similar changes may be observed in ulcerative colitis.

and remains so even after colonoscopy and multiple biopsies.

Fistulas/sinuses are evaluated by injection of contrast media following insertion of rubber catheters of the appropriate size to ensure close fitting (*Fig.* 73.29). More recently, the use of CT scanning after the injection of contrast into the fistulous tract has provided detailed appreciation of the pathological anatomy of the fistula and is

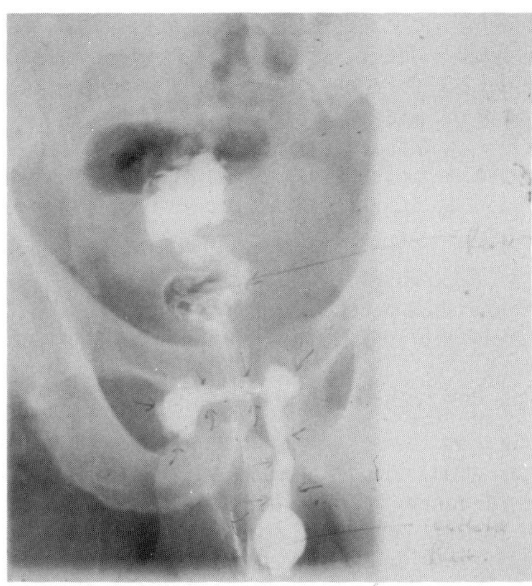

Fig. 73.29 Sinogram showing rectal fistula in a patient with Crohn's disease.

especially useful in complex types with multiple branched tracts.

Treatment

The treatment of Crohn's disease is difficult, often unsatisfactory and frequently followed by recurrence after an initial successful outcome. Management of these patients therefore lacks standardization and still generates considerable controversy.

Medical Therapy

There is no uniformly successful medical therapy for Crohn's disease. To a large extent treatment has to be tailored to the requirements of the individual patient. The important aspects of conservative management include:

- Dietary manipulations
- Parenteral nutrition
- Anti-inflammatory drugs: steroids and sulphasalazine
- Antibiotics
- Immunosuppressive drugs: azathioprine, 6-mercaptopurine, cyclosporin
- Symptomatic drug treatment.

DIETARY MANIPULATIONS. In the first instance, deficiencies including vitamins (especially A), magnesium and zinc must be corrected. Iron-deficiency anaemia is treated with oral supplements, preferably in the glutamate form. Some advocate a high-fibre low refined-sugar diet. Benefit has been reported by the use of exclusion diets where the patients are started on spring water and then items of food introduced and maintained or withdrawn according to whether or not they aggravate the condition. The most common dietary components which require exclusion are dairy products and wheat. There is some evidence for the direct benefit of elemental diet (e.g. Vivonex, Flexical, Ensure, etc.) alone or in combination with non-absorbable antibiotics, in suppressing the mucosal inflammation. The specific effect of elemental diets is thought to result from a reduction of the antigen load presented to the inflamed mucosa. However, the benefit may simply be the result of an enhanced nutritional intake. The practical snag to the long-term use of elemental diets is their unpalatability which reduces compliance in the long term.

PARENTERAL NUTRITION. This is of undoubted value in selected cases. Its indications include:

Intestinal failure with gross nutritional deficiencies and severe hypoalbuminaemia
Malnourished patients prior to surgery
In an attempt to obtain a remission in patients with active disease
In patients with enterocutaneous fistulas.

Long-term home hyperalimentation is reserved for patients with extensive small-bowel disease/resection and intestinal failure. It allows a reasonable quality of life in these patients who are taught to self-administer the parenteral feeds and look after their central lines. Long-term good health can be maintained in this way. Some patients require only intermittent or supplemental intravenous feeding and manage reasonably well with modified or elemental diets in the intervening periods. Home hyperalimentation is supervised by the medical and nursing staff of specialized Nutrition Units with facilities and staff to run the home parenteral hyperalimentation programme. Abnormalities of liver function (e.g. elevation of the transaminases) and selenium deficiency may occur as a result of the parenteral nutrition. Supplements of trace elements including selenium are necessary in patients on long-term parenteral nutrition.

Intravenous feeding is necessary on a short-term basis for patients with complications requiring elective surgical intervention but who are malnourished and hypoalbuminaemic. Improvement of the nutritional status and elevation of the serum albumin above 3·0 g/l is essential for the safe healing of intestinal anastomosis. Some 30% of enterocutaneous fistulas due to Crohn's disease may heal spontaneously by parenteral nutrition avoiding the need for surgical intervention. However, persistence of the fistula beyond 6 weeks indicates failure of the conservative regimen and the need for surgical intervention.

Some advocate cessation of oral feeding and total parenteral nutrition for several weeks to achieve a remission in patients with active Crohn's disease. Although the immediate results of this treatment are good, relapse is almost invariable within 3 months of resumption of oral food.

DRUG THERAPY. The recent large European trial on the medical therapy for Crohn's disease has shown that oral 6-methylprednisolone is the most effective treatment for small-bowel active disease and combined steroid and sulphasalazine therapy gives the best results for colonic disease. Even so, the overall response to these agents is disappointing and only 30% of patients achieve and maintain a remission for two years.

There is no evidence that sulphasalazine or steroids prevent relapse after surgical excision for Crohn's disease. The effect of 5-ASA agents in Crohn's disease has not been established but is currently being evaluated. Parenteral steroids using the same regimen as in ulcerative colitis are used in patients with severe colitis and toxic dilatation due to Crohn's. Topical steroid enemas may impart some benefit in patients with rectosigmoid disease. Metronidazole is effective for perianal disease but its long-term use is limited by its side-effects which include nausea, metallic taste and peripheral neuropathy. Various other antibiotics (sulphadioxine, pyrimethamine, co-trimoxazole) and antituberculous therapy with rifampicin and ethambutol have been tested in controlled clinical trials and shown to be ineffective in active Crohn's disease.

Azathioprine and its metabolite 6-mercaptopurine are used for their steroid-sparing effect in selected patients with active Crohn's disease and some reports indicate that their use is beneficial in the healing of fistulas due to Crohn's disease. The early reports with cyclosporin look promising but no definite conclusions can be reached owing to the small number of cases treated with this immunosuppressive agent to date.

Symptomatic treatment for diarrhoea includes the administration of loperamide or codeine phosphate and non-addictive analgesics for the abdominal pain. Cholestyramine may improve the steatorrhoea in patients with extensive ileal disease or resection.

Surgical Treatment

The results of surgical treatment for Crohn's disease are not spectacular. Surgical intervention is indicated for the complications of the disease and to resect active disease which has not responded to medical therapy and is causing severe invalidism. There is a considerable morbidity associated with surgical treatment for this disease and more than half the deaths of patients with Crohn's disease are associated with operative intervention. On the other hand, these patients constitute the hard core of severe complicated disease, the progression of which has been unchecked with repeated attempts at medical management.

INDICATIONS FOR SURGICAL INTERVENTION. Surgical treatment is necessary for the following:

1. Onset of complications:
   Small bowel obstruction
   Development of abscesses and fistulas
   Acute fulminating colitis/toxic dilatation/perforation
   Massive haemorrhage (infrequent)
   Development of obstructive uropathy
   Growth retardation in children
   Development of carcinoma of colon or ileum
   Amyloidosis complicating reasonably localized disease.
2. Failure of medical management with persistence of severe symptoms and chronic invalidism.
3. Complications of medical management: steroid side-effects in patients requiring large doses to control the disease.

Factors which also influence the decision to operate and the type of operative procedure include the anatomical site of the disease, the surgeon's preference, and whether the operation is being performed as an emergency or an elective basis.

The extra-gastrointestinal manifestations of Crohn's disease are rarely, if ever, an indication for operative intervention. Liver disease, if mild, may occasionally be arrested by surgical intervention of Crohn's colitis but this is by no means certain and remains a controversial issue.

SURGICAL TREATMENT IN CROHN'S DISEASE. The abdominal incision should be planned with attention paid to previous incisions and to the siting of a stoma which is an ever-present possibility in patients with Crohn's disease. An initial exploration to determine the extent and severity of the disease from the stomach to the rectum and to establish the state of the liver and presence or otherwise of gallstones is made on entering the peritoneum. Adhesions which are often present are taken down and the anatomy and the length of the small intestine is ascertained (especially if there has been previous surgical intervention). The previous controversy between the relative merits of resection and bypass has been settled. Localized resection of the diseased segment(s) is now the standard treatment in view of the better results. Bypass (gastroenterostomy) is reserved for gastroduodenal Crohn's (*vide infra*).

Whenever possible, abscess cavities related to diseased segments are removed together with the diseased bowel. Removal of enlarged lymph nodes is only undertaken if this does not jeopardize the mesenteric circulation.

OPERATIONS FOR SMALL-BOWEL DISEASE. In deciding the extent of small-bowel resection, a balance must be struck between removing all grossly diseased bowel and retaining sufficient for adequate absorption and nutritional support. Macroscopic assessment of the disease, by the thickening of the bowel wall and mesentery, hyperaemia and oedema, fat encroachment and the presence of ulcers at the resection line is used to determine the extent of the resection. *Areas of minimal disease may be safely left in situ.* There is no evidence that selection of the resection margins based on frozen section histology reduces the recurrence rate and this procedure is therefore unwarranted. Skip lesions in the immediate vicinity of the main disease process, should be excised *en bloc;* those at a distance are resected separately if considered significant or ignored if they are uncomplicated by significant stenosis. Currently the procedure of stricturoplasty is being evaluated (*Fig.* 73.30). This is not as yet an established procedure. It appears to be beneficial in patients with short fibrous strictures who have had previous resections provided cancer can be excluded (by frozen section histology) and the disease is not active.

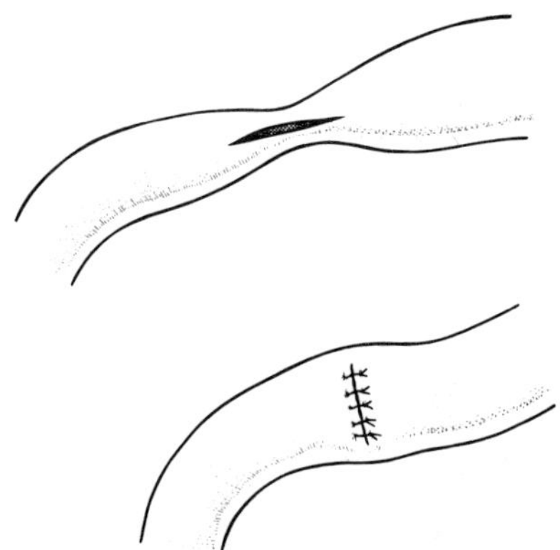

Fig. 73.30 Diagrammatic representation of the technique of stricturoplasty. This operation which is still being evaluated in specialist centres, is suitable for patients with short strictures in the absence of active inflammation. An operative biopsy of the stricture with frozen section histology is advisable to exclude carcinoma.

The recommended treatment is a conservative resection of the diseased bowel giving rise to the complication with primary anastomosis whenever appropriate. For the common ileocaecal Crohn's the resection involves the affected small bowel and the lower pole of the caecum with anastomosis of the proximal ileum to the right colon. Adhesions and fistulas between diseased bowel and adjacent hollow viscus are dealt with by careful separation of the diseased segment from the adjacent structure with débridement and primary closure of the latter. External fistulas are managed by similar excision with débridement and closure of the abdominal wall but not of the skin and subcutaneous tissues. Secondary wound closure is performed several days later. If there is a phlegmonous mass involving several loops of bowel, the surgeon must carefully identify and dissect healthy from diseased bowel. Provided that the length involved is not great, a resection 'en masse' may be performed. After all small-bowel resections the length of the residual small intestine is measured along the antimesenteric border and recorded.

Free perforation into the peritoneal cavity is rare in Crohn's disease and the commonest site is the ileum. Resection of the diseased segment, with peritoneal lavage and débridement is the treatment of choice. Primary anastomosis or exteriorization is performed, depending on the duration and the severity of the peritoneal inflammation. Again, delayed closure of the skin wound is practised. Simple drainage of an abscess invariably results in a fistula. Some 30% of enterocutaneous fistulas may heal with total parenteral nutrition. Persistence of the fistula beyond 6 weeks is an indication for surgical intervention with excision of the diseased segment. Enterocolic and enterovesical fistulas never heal by conservative management and always require surgical intervention. Perforation of the diseased bowel into the retroperitoneal tissues causes intense fibrosis and retroperitoneal inflammation resulting in an obstructive uropathy. This cannot be distinguished from pelviureteric fibrosis due to other causes. As previously stated, the obstructed ureter is most frequently asymptomatic and the resultant renal impairment may be progressive and permanent. An obstructive uropathy is an absolute indication for operation and is best relieved by appropriate bowel resection and ureterolysis.

PSEUDO-APPENDICITIS SYNDROME AND ACUTE ILEITIS. Some patients suspected of suffering from acute appendicitis are found at operation to have an acute ileitis. This may be due to Crohn's but far more commonly is the result of *Yersinia* infection, in which case spontaneous recovery occurs without the development of Crohn's disease. Unnecessary bypass or resection should thus be avoided at this stage. Contrary to previous opinion, it is perfectly safe to remove the appendix, provided the caecum is soft at its base and is non-involved. Appendicectomy will facilitate future assessment of recurrent abdominal symptoms and eliminate the risk of pyogenic appendicitis. The much feared faecal fistula following appendicectomy in such patients, rarely occurs and almost always originates from the diseased small intestine, a hazard which presumably exists whether or not the appendix is removed.

HAEMORRHAGE. Acute haemorrhage occurs in only 1% of patients with Crohn's disease and the commonest site of bleeding is in the small bowel (65%). Since arteriography often fails to delineate the bleeding site in these patients, intraoperative examination and excision of all diseased small bowel is often necessary to stop the life-threatening haemorrhage.

OPERATIONS FOR CROHN'S COLITIS. The indications for emergency operation in Crohn's colitis are perforation, acute fulminating colitis with or without toxic dilatation and, rarely, massive haemorrhage. Most centres advocate an initial period of intensive medical therapy identical to that used for severe ulcerative colitis. Failure to respond within 2–4 days, or any deterioriation are an indication for emergency surgical intervention. This consists of a total abdominal colectomy with construction of an ileostomy and a distal mucous fistula. This procedure is quick, safe and resolves the life-threatening situation. Proctocolectomy is a more extensive procedure with a higher mortality and morbidity and confers no advantage to the acutely ill patient unless there is massive bleeding from the rectum.

Elective operation for intractable colitis entails either an abdominal colectomy with primary ileorectal anastomosis or proctocolectomy with terminal ileostomy. If the distal ileum is involved with Crohn's disease, it is excised and an ileostomy is constructed in macroscopically normal ileum. Colectomy with ileorectal anastomosis is indicated if:

The rectum is minimally diseased
Perianal disease if present, is manageable
The anal sphincter is functioning.

The procedure may be performed in one or two stages. The addition of a proximal defunctioning loop ileostomy is sometimes recommended but probably does not protect the primary ileorectal anastomosis, although this is debatable.

Total proctocolectomy for Crohn's disease or ulcerative colitis does not entail a radical dissection or a regional lymphadenectomy either in the abdomen or the pelvis. The risk of impotence and other sexual difficulties in the male can thus be reduced especially if the dissection is kept close to the bowel. Koch's continent ileostomy is not an option in Crohn's disease because of the high complication rate and the risk of recurrence. Likewise, mucosal proctectomy and ileoanal reservoir reconstruction is similarly contraindicated in patients undergoing proctolectomy for Crohn's disease.

Faecal diversion with a split or loop ileostomy (*Fig.* 73.31) is sometimes used in patients with acute colonic disease which has not responded to medical therapy in an attempt to obtain a remission in young adults and in children with growth retardation. On average some 30% of patients benefit from this temporary diversion and in these a resection is avoided or postponed for some years.

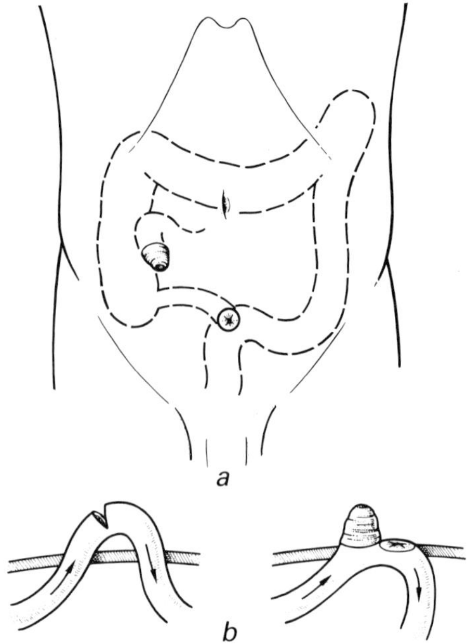

Fig. 73.31 *a*, Split ileostomy. The ileum is transected near the caecum. The proximal end is exteriorized as a spout ileostomy and the distal end as a mucous fistula. This achieves total defunctioning of the colon. *b*, Loop ileostomy for temporary diversion. The continuity of the ileum is maintained. A loop is exteriorized and opened partially to enable eversion of the proximal ileum as a spout leaving the distal small bowel as an attached mucous fistula. This technique probably achieves total defunctioning of the large bowel (although this is debatable) and is preferable to the above as the patient can manage it better since both the spout and the adjacent fistula are contained in the ileostomy bag. Furthermore, closure is possible without a further laparotomy.

TREATMENT OF PERIANAL DISEASE. The perianal complications of Crohn's disease are skin tags, abscesses, fissures, fistulas and haemorrhoids. Minor conditions such as skin tags and haemorrhoids should not be treated surgically in the presence of active rectal disease. Many patients cope well with minor fissures and skin tags with simple measures and daily baths. Adequate drainage of abscesses is obviously necessary. Further management depends on the condition of the perineum and the severity of the rectal disease and is best considered under three categories:

In patients with minimal or no rectal disease on proctoscopic examination, treatment is as for non-granulomatous lesions and includes drainage of abscesses, identification and laying out of fistulous tracts, and internal sphincterotomy, as deemed necessary. Haemorrhoids are best treated by sclero- or cryotherapy if small, and rubber band ligation if larger.

Patients with active but mild to moderate rectal disease often benefit by faecal diversion (split or loop ileostomy) in addition to the above local treatment. Resection of intra-abdominal disease is considered on its merits. Fibrous strictures of the anorectum may require dilatation.

Patients with severe rectal disease and perianal complications with destruction of the anal sphincter mechanism, require a proctectomy with appropriate excision of the proximal disease and a permanent stoma. Proctocolectomy with ileostomy is often required in these patients. The totally destroyed perineum, especially with sphincter incompetence, may also be an indication for proctectomy with appropriate proximal bowel resection and permanent stoma, even if the rectal mucosa is minimally diseased or normal.

GASTRODUODENAL CROHN'S DISEASE. Primary gastroduodenal Crohn's disease is extremely rare. Most instances represent secondary involvement in patients with known small bowel or colonic disease and gastroduodenal involvement occurs in some 4% of these patients. Gastroduodenal Crohn's disease must be differentiated from peptic ulcer disease which is often present in these patients. Misdiagnosed duodenal Crohn's disease can lead to duodenal fistula formation after operation for presumed duodenal ulcer. Most surgeons agree that bypass operations for duodenal Crohn's disease is safer and probably gives better results than resection. Whether the operation is performed for bleeding or duodenal obstruction, the procedure of choice is a highly selective vagotomy and a gastroenterostomy. A truncal vagotomy should be avoided if possible as this may compound the diarrhoea.

Complications and Results of Surgical Treatment

The operations for Crohn's disease are followed by a high incidence (10–15%) of postoperative complications such as anastomotic leakage, fistula formation, intra-abdominal abscesses and haemorrhage. The overall reported postoperative mortality rate ranges from 2 to 8%. A higher mortality is often associated with emergency operations (up to 30%) and with colonic resections. Wound complications (infection and dehiscence) can be considerably reduced by the use of transverse incisions, by proper closure of the abdominal wall with non-absorbable sutures, and by employing delayed closure of the skin and subcutaneous tissues whenever there is obvious operative contamination. Late postoperative complications include short-bowel syndrome, urinary lithiasis, cholelithiasis, gastric hypersecretion and peptic ulcer disease.

One of the unresolved problems is the high incidence of recurrence following resection. The cumulative recurrence rate after resection of small-intestinal Crohn's disease is 30% at 5 years, 50% at 10 years and 60% at 15 years. Young patients and those with ileocolic disease have the highest and earliest recurrence and the worst ultimate prognosis. Medical treatment does not influence the recurrence rate. The prognosis of patients with Crohn's colitis undergoing proctocolectomy is better in this respect as the development of ileal disease occurs in 10% and 20% of these patients at 5 and 10 years respectively. After abdominal colectomy and ileorectal anastomosis, the reported recurrence rates average 50% at 5 years.

The majority of recurrences occur at or near to the anastomosis and in patients with ileorectal anastomosis, the recurrent disease often involves the ileum and further resection does not necessarily require proctectomy and ileostomy. In assessing the widely divergent reported figures for recurrence rates after surgical intervention for Crohn's disease two points must be stressed:

1. The recurrence rate rises gradually with the duration of follow-up.
2. It is essential to differentiate patients with true recurrent Crohn's disease from those requiring re-operation for other complications including ileostomy revisions.

SYSTEMIC MANIFESTATIONS OF INFLAMMATORY BOWEL DISEASE

Systemic or extra-intestinal manifestation are common to both ulcerative colitis and Crohn's disease (*Table* 73.3). They usually accompany active disease but some may predate the intestinal symptoms or develop after resection of the disease. Some of the manifestations may develop as side-effects to medical therapy. The manifestations which regress after surgical excision of the disease are:

Finger clubbing
Enteropathic arthritis
Amyloidosis

The generally held view is that some of these systemic manifestations are the result of immune complex disease together with a defective neutrophil function. The antibody response is generated by the increased permeability of the mucosa in inflammatory bowel disease to dietary/bacterial antigens which stimulate the B-lymphocytes to excess antibody production.

Table 73.3 Systemic (extra-intestinal) manifestations of inflammatory bowel disease

LIVER	Fatty change	Both Crohn's and UC
	Pericholangitis	Both Crohn's and UC
	Sclerosing cholangitis	Usually Crohn's
	Cirrhosis	Both Crohn's and UC
	Cholangiocarcinoma	UC
SKIN	Pyoderma gangrenosum	More common in UC
	Erythema nodosum	Both Crohn's and UC
	Aphthous stomatitis	Usually Crohn's
	Finger clubbing	Both Crohn's and UC
JOINTS	Enteropathic arthritis	Both Crohn's and UC
	Sacro-ileitis/ankylosing spondylitis	Both Crohn's and UC
EYES	Uveitis	Crohn's > UC
	Episcleritis	Crohn's > UC
	Corneal infiltrates	Both Crohn's and UC
KIDNEYS	Renal calculi	Both Crohn's and UC
	Pyelonephritis	Crohn's > UC
	Obstructive uropathy	Crohn's
HAEMOPOIETIC	Autoimmune haemolytic anaemia (rare)	UC
CARDIOVASCULAR	Systemic thrombosis	Both Crohn's and UC
	Vasculitis (rare)	Both Crohn's and UC
	Takayasu's disease	Crohn's
	Pericarditis	Both Crohn's and UC
BRONCHOPULMONARY	Fibrosing alveolitis	Both Crohn's and UC
	Bronchiectasis	Both Crohn's and UC
	Pleural effusions	Both Crohn's and UC
ENDOCRINE	Goitre and hyperthyroidism	UC
OTHER	Amyloid	Crohn's

N.B. UC = Ulcerative colitis.

ILEOSTOMY CARE

The advent of modern ileostomy and stoma therapists has undoubtedly improved the quality of life of patients with a terminal ileostomy so that the majority now lead a full and unrestricted existence without any serious social or personal handicaps. Nevertheless, complications do arise and vary from trivial peristomal complications to disabling ileostomy diarrhoea and impotence, failure to maintain an ejaculation and dyspareunia. In one survey, dyspareunia was observed in 33% of females and some degree of impotence was found in 50% of males after panproctocolectomy, although male sexual performance can continue to improve over a period of 1–2 years.

To a large extent, meticulous technique in the construction of the 2·5 cm everted spout ileostomy and in the pelvic dissection during the removal of the rectum (to minimize damage to the nervi erigentes) will minimize the incidence of some of the more serious complications. Regular aftercare and adequate instruction of the patient regarding the physiological consequences that follow removal of the colon are also important. The presence of an ileostomy entails a daily obligatory loss of 500–600 ml of ileostomy fluid containing 40–50 mmol of Na^+. There is, therefore, a chronic salt-losing state. To a certain extent, there is some compensation from increased renal tubular reabsorption of Na^+ and water which results in a lowering of the urinary Na^+/K^+ ratio. The altered chemical composition of the urine which becomes concentrated is thought to be responsible at least in part for the increased incidence of renal calculi in these patients. Adequate water and salt intake is essential in patients with ileostomy, particularly in hot climates and during febrile illnesses.

The dephenylisantin content of prunes increases the ileostomy effluent by a cathartic action on the small-bowel mucosa. Apart from this, no dietary restrictions are necessary although many patients modify their diet and meal times to regulate the ileostomy function. The problem of odour due to methane and hydrogen sulphide is largely overcome by the use of stoma bags which incorporate filters or the instillation of binding chemicals in the ileostomy bag (Banish, Zephiran, etc.). The flatus-filter bags also overcome the problem of acute distension and bursting of the bag resulting from sudden decompression during air travel.

The local complications of a terminal ileostomy are:

Stenosis
Prolapse
Peristomal irritation and fistulas
Para-ileostomy hernia
Ileostomy diarrhoea
Prestomal ileitis.

The modern technique of construction of the ileostomy spout with eversion and mucocutaneous anastomosis has virtually abolished the previously common complication of stomal stenosis. Problems can, however, be encountered if the ileostomy spout is too long or too short. Its ideal height is 2·5 cm. Prolapse of the ileostomy indicates inadequate or incomplete fixation of the small-bowel mesentery to the abdominal parieties and the right paracolic gutter. Peristomal irritation with excoriation is perhaps the commonest complication (20–30%). It can be minimized by regular cleaning of the surrounding skin and the use of skin barriers (Stomadhesive, Comfeel, Hollihesive). An ill-fitting appliance is often a contributory factor. It may cause pressure necrosis of the edge of the stoma with the development of an abscess or fistula. Another cause for the latter is the use of sutures to fix the spout to the anterior rectus sheath. The advice and expert management of a stoma therapist in the prevention and treatment of these peristomal complications is essential. Para-ileostomy hernia is an incisional hernia associated with the ileostomy scar. It is less common than colostomy hernia and occurs in 5% of patients. It leads to ill fitting of the appliance and leakage and may cause internal ileal strangulation.

The onset of ileostomy diarrhoea is always an indication for thorough investigation since it usually signifies underlying pathology unless ileal resection was performed at the time of colectomy. The common causes of ileostomy diarrhoea are:

Partial obstruction
Internal abscess formation
Recurrence of Crohn's disease

The essential investigations in all patients with persistent ileostomy diarrhoea include plain radiology of the abdomen, small-bowel enema (through the stoma) and endoscopic examination of the small intestine through the ileostomy.

ANTIBIOTIC-ASSOCIATED AND PSEUDOMEMBRANOUS COLITIS

Certain antibiotics, especially the cephalosporins, ampicillin and lincomycin, may result in loss of the normal bacterial colonization and subsequent infection with *Clostridium difficile* which produces a toxin-mediated inflammation of the colonic mucosa. The severity of this varies from focal areas of superficial mucosal necrosis/ulceration covered by pseudomembranes (yellowish-white plaques consisting of fibrin and leucocytes) to complete mucosal necrosis with involvement of the lamina propria and extensive pseudomembrane formation. The term 'pseudomembranous colitis' is currently reserved for the severe category of the disease which usually involves the distal colon although cases with only right colon involvement are well documented. The disease which is rare in children who often harbour *C. difficile,* is especially prone to develop during (and occasionally weeks after) antibiotic therapy in the following:

Elderly patients
After surgical intervention
In patients with intestinal neoplasms
In patients with atherosclerotic ischaemia.

Mild antibiotic-associated colitis gives rise to watery/mucoid diarrhoea with little systemic upset but the severe disease (pseudomembranous) colitis is a serious condition with systemic toxicity, abdominal signs, fluid and electrolyte depletion. It can lead to toxic dilatation and perforation and carries a definite but variable reported mortality (0–20%). The diagnosis of antibiotic-associated colitis is established by endoscopy when biopsies should be taken for histological examination and tissue culture for *C. difficile.* Stool culture for the organisms and assays of the enterotoxin can also be performed to detect the organism although the diagnosis of the condition is established in the first instance by sigmoidoscopy.

The treatment is with oral vancomycin for 1–2 weeks. Seriously ill patients require parenteral fluids and are given metronidazole intravenously until they are able to resume oral intake when oral vancomycin is commenced. Some advocate the use of systemic corticosteroids in these patients. The other antibiotic which can be used instead of vancomycin in moderately ill patients is bacitracin. Recurrence of the pseudomembranous colitis is well documented. These patients require further antibiotic treatment. Emergency colectomy may be required if the severe disease progresses to toxic megacolon or colonic perforation ensues in which case the mortality approaches 40% in some series.

PROCTITIS

Proctitis causes distressing symptoms which are often out of proportion to the severity and extent of the inflammatory disease. Proctitis may be *specific*, i.e. caused by a known infective agent, e.g. gonorrhoeal proctitis; *factitious* due to repeated trauma following insertion of fingers, vibrators and foreign bodies and *non-specific (idiopathic)*.

Non-specific Proctitis

This accounts for the majority of cases of proctitis. The disease is generally considered to be a subtype of ulcerative colitis and in a small percentage of patients (10–15%) the disorder extends proximally and assumes the usual course of ulcerative proctosigmoiditis or left-sided colitis. However, in the majority of patients, the inflammatory condition remains localized to the rectum and the disease follows a benign but indolent course without extension or the development of systemic complications or carcinoma. However, rectal stricture may complicate longstanding non-specific proctitis.

The disease is most commonly encountered in young adults with a peak incidence in the third decade. The symptoms are seldom severe but include rectal bleeding, diarrhoea, tenesmus with the passage of mucus or mucosanguineous discharge. Systemic symptoms are usually absent. Diagnosis is made at sigmoidoscopy. The mucosa is oedematous and hyperaemic with easy contact bleeding. Macroscopic ulceration is, however, extremely rare. The histological appearances are those of a non-specific proctitis with chronic inflammatory infiltrate and mucosal/submucosal oedema. Colonic involvement is excluded by a barium enema.

Treatment is directed at the relief of the local symptoms. Often sedatives and stool softeners will be sufficient. More severe symptoms may require prednisolone suppositories/enemas, preferably of the non-absorbable steroid type (Predenema) and, rarely, oral salazopyrine or one of the newer delayed release 5-ASA compounds. Anaemia is rare and when it occurs, it is treated with oral iron. Any coexistent perianal disease (fissure, abscess, fistula, haemorrhoids) is treated by the appropriate surgical procedure.

Specific Proctitis

This is most commonly encountered in homosexual males who are subject to a variety of specific colorectal infections even when they are not immunosuppressed. The spectrum of these infections in homosexuals who do not have AIDS is collectively known as the *Gay Bowel Syndrome*. The infections may be bacterial *(Syphilis, Gonorrhoea, Chlamydia, Shigellae, Salmonella, Campylobacter, E. coli, etc.)*, viral (CMV, herpes simplex) and parasitic *(G. lamblia, E. histolytica)*. There is also a high incidence of hepatitis A and B infections in these individuals.

In addition, opportunistic rectal infections are found in patients with congenital immune deficiency (e.g. congenital hypogammaglobulinaemia, Wiskott–Aldrich syndrome, etc.) and in homosexual individuals who develop AIDS or AIDS-associated syndrome. The most common opportunistic infections encountered in this group are: *Cryptosporidium, CMV, Candida, Pneumocystis carinii, Isospora belli, Microsporidia and Mycobacterium avium intracellulare.* Some of these patients have developed Kaposi's sarcoma involving the colorectal region and bizarre invasive small-cell rectal cancers. All these tumours are rapidly fatal.

Neutropenic Anorectal Infections

A high incidence of anorectal bacterial infections *(E. coli, P. aeruginosa, S. aureus and Klebsiella)* in patients with acute leukaemia particularly of the myelocytic and myelomonocytic types. All patients who develop these infections are neutropenic. As there is little tendency to localization of these perianal infections, the induration often extends to involve the perineum, buttocks and genital region, and may progress to large areas of soft-tissue necrosis. These infections are difficult to treat. In addition to systemic antibiotics and drainage of pus, limited débridement of slough and necrotic areas is usually necessary.

IRRITABLE BOWEL SYNDROME

This loosely defined condition is the most commonly diagnosed gastroenterological disorder and denotes a variable combination of symptoms and signs of a chronic or recurrent nature precipitated by stress and emotional upsets in neurotic individuals. Unfortunately, there is no pathophysiological marker which can specifically identify this disorder. The irritable bowel syndrome is thought by some to progress to diverticular disease in the long term.

The symptoms include lower abdominal griping pain, anorexia, epigastric fullness, excessive belching, abdominal distension and constipation with passage of small hard faecal pellets. Less commonly, the patients complain of intermittent episodes of diarrhoea with the passage of mucus. The diarrhoea may be persistent or alternating with intervening episodes of constipation.

Rectal bleeding is never a feature of the irritable bowel syndrome. The majority of severely affected individuals have obvious psychoneurotic tendencies and hysterical traits are not uncommon. Colonic motility studies have shown a marked increase in both amplitude and frequency of distal colonic contractions in patients with a spastic colon and a reduced motility in patients with diarrhoea. Others have demonstrated a slow-wave frequency of 2–4 cycles/min which is quite different from that found in diverticular disease.

The diagnosis of the irritable bowel syndrome is made by exclusion and only after a thorough physical examination and the following investigations: full blood count, ESR, stool culture and examination of fresh specimens for parasites, sigmoidoscopy and barium enema. All the results should be normal except that the barium enema may reveal diffuse narrowing, increased segmentation, corrugation of the distal colon or, alternatively, absent haustration. However, these colonic radiological signs are often absent and when present, are significant only if the colonic preparation is performed with saline enemas and the use of colonic irritants avoided.

Some of these patients, especially those who complain of diarrhoea, have been shown to be intolerant to certain foods (e.g. wheat) and the exclusion of these items from the diet results in the amelioration of symptoms. There is also evidence that psychotherapy may be beneficial. The drug most commonly used for symptomatic relief is loperamide. More recently, calcium-blocking agents (nifedipine) have been introduced in the management of these patients.

SOLITARY RECTAL ULCER SYNDROME

This is a condition of unknown aetiology which is characterized by persistent rectal symptoms due to rectal ulceration which is commonly solitary but may be multiple. The lower margin of the lesion is situated at 7–10 cm from the anal verge and usually consists of a solitary well-circumscribed ulcer (70%), most commonly on the anterior or anterolateral aspect of the rectal wall (50%), although multiple ulcers and even a nodular thickening without ulceration are well described and the lesions may be found in any of the quadrants of the rectum. The ulcers vary in size and shape but have well-defined indurated margins and are usually superficial with a greyish fibrotic base. The surrounding mucosa may be normal or thickened with some oedema and nodular elevations.

The histological hallmark is fibromuscular hypertrophy of the lamina propria beneath and around the ulcerated area. In addition, ectopic mucosal elements are often found in the submucosa at the edges of the ulcer. These may undergo cystic dilatation. The lesion does not have a significant infiltration with chronic inflammatory cells. Fibromuscular hypertrophy is also encountered in rectal prolapse and is used as evidence for the association between these two conditions.

The aetiology of the solitary rectal ulcer syndrome is unknown and is presumed to be multifactorial. The following theories have been suggested:

1. Repeated trauma due to rectal prolapse. There is no doubt that the two conditions can coexist although widely different figures have been quoted (13–90% of cases). The prolapse may be complete or mucosal. Repair of the prolapse is, however, followed by healing of the ulcer in only 40–50% of cases.

2. Failure of relaxation of the puborectalis sling during defaecation. According to this hypothesis which would account for the common anterior distribution of the lesion, repeated trauma is sustained during forceful defaecation by the anterior rectal wall as it is compressed against the puborectalis bar at the top of the anal canal.

3. Rectal trauma from insertion of foreign bodies and self-digitation. This may reflect peculiar sexual preferences or habitual constipation/difficulty in rectal evacuation. A history of self-digitation/insertion of objects including vibrators into the rectum is certainly not infrequent in patients with the solitary rectal ulcer syndrome but is only obtained on direct questioning.

The disease is most commonly encountered in young adults who complain of rectal bleeding and passage of mucus during and in between defaecation. Rectal soreness and lower abdominal discomfort is another frequent complaint. Rarely, the rectal bleeding may be profuse. A history of constipation or difficult strenuous defaecation is often present. The ulcer is usually felt digitally and the diagnosis is confirmed by sigmoidoscopy and biopsy. In the assessment of these patients, the presence or absence of a rectal prolapse (partial or complete) must be ascertained.

The treatment of solitary rectal ulcer syndrome is difficult. There is no effective medical therapy. Most agree that in patients with rectal prolapse, surgical correction of the latter is indicated. This may be followed by healing of the ulcer. Persistent severely symptomatic cases are sometimes treated by low anterior resection but recurrence has been reported after this procedure. Some have advocated division of the puborectalis sling, although this is not generally accepted and may result in rectal incontinence. Persistent intractable cases may come to rectal excision with an end colostomy.

Further Reading

Chiodini R. J., van Kruiningen H. J., Thayer W. R. et al. (1984) Possible role of mycobacteria in inflammatory bowel disease. I. An unclassified mycobacterium species isolated from patients with Crohn's disease. *Dig. Dis. Sci.* **29**, 1073–1079.

Holdstock G., Savage D., Harman M. et al. (1985) An investigation into the validity of the present classification of inflammatory bowel disease. *Q. J. Med.* **54**, 183–190.

Malchow H., Ewe K., Brandes J. W. et al. (1984) European Cooperative Crohn's Disease Study (ECCDS): Results of drug treatment. *Gastroenterol.* **86**, 249–266.

Metcalf A. M., Dozois R. R., Kelly K. A. et al. (1985) Ileal J-pouch–anal anastomosis: clinical outcome. *Ann. Surg.* **202**, 735–739.

Nicholls R. J. and Pezim M. E. (1985) Restorative proctocolectomy with ileal reservoir for ulcerative colitis and familial adenomatous polyposis: comparison of three reservoir designs. *Br. J. Surg.* **72**, 470–474.

O'Morain C., Segal A. W. and Levi A. J. (1984) Elemental diet as primary treatment of acute Crohn's disease: a controlled trial. *Br. Med. J.* **288**, 1859–1862.

Ransohoff D. F., Riddell R. H. and Levin B. (1985) Ulcerative colitis and colonic cancer—problems in assessing the diagnostic usefulness of mucosal dysplasia. *Dis. Colon Rectum* **28**, 383–388.

Ren E., Marche C., Régnier B. et al. (1985) Digestive manifestations in AIDS: study of 26 patients. *Gastroenterol. Clin. Biol.* **9**, 327–335.

Rutter K. R. P. and Riddell R. H. (1975) The solitary ulcer syndrome of the rectum. *Clin. Gastroenterol.* **4**, 505.

Selby W. S., Barr G. D., Ireland A. et al. (1985) Olsalazine in active ulcerative colitis. *Br. Med. J.* **291**, 1373–1375.

74 The Colon, Rectum and Anal Canal

G. R. Giles

SURGICAL ANATOMY OF THE COLORECTUM AND ANAL CANAL

The colon arches around the abdominal cavity and surrounds the small bowel. The average length is about 140 cm and the diameter varies, being maximal in the caecum and in the rectal ampulla (7–9 cm). Elsewhere it is more constricted, particularly in the sigmoid colon (2–3 cm). The distinguishing feature of the colon is the concentration of the longitudinal muscle into three bands or taeniae coli which, being relatively short, produce sacculations or haustrations of the colon. Between the taeniae, the thin colonic wall is capable of great dilatation when obstructed, especially the right colon and caecum.

The caecum lies in the right iliac fossa with the appendix projecting from the apex. The ileum joins the posterior and medial aspect and the junction is guarded by a valve, the lips of which may prevent reflux of the caecal contents. The ascending colon is 15 cm long and fixed posteriorly. At the hepatic flexure the colon bends forwards and medially below the right lobe of the liver. The transverse colon is 40–50 cm long and lies in front of the duodenum and head of pancreas initially, before becoming completely invested in peritoneum by the attachment of the gastrocolic ligament and greater omentum. Between the left end of the transverse colon and the descending colon, the colon bends sharply at the splenic flexure. Here the colon is attached by a firm band (phrenocolic ligament) containing blood vessels which need ligating during the mobilization of the flexure. The descending colon is about 20 cm in length and is fixed to the posterior wall and where it crosses the iliac vessels, it becomes the sigmoid colon. This forms a loop 20–60 cm in length with its own mesentery which has an inverted sigma-shaped attachment on the posterior abdominal wall. The lower limb of the mesocolon extends down the front of the sacrum and ultimately joins the mesorectum. The loop of sigmoid colon commonly falls forward onto the bladder, uterus and adnexae and loops of small intestine lie against the upper surface of the sigmoid colon.

The rectum lies in the concavity of the sacrum for about 15 cm and passes through the pelvic levator muscles to angle sharply backwards to form the anal canal of 3–4 cm in length. The mesorectum is formed from the sigmoid mesocolon but is broader and thicker. The upper portion of the rectum has a complete peritoneal covering but the mid rectum has only peritoneum on the anterior and lateral aspects and lower still, only on the anterior aspect. In the male pelvis the peritoneum is reflected forwards onto the back of the seminal vesicles and bladder. In the female, the pouch of Douglas is deeper and the peritoneum reflects forwards onto the vault of the vagina, uterus and broad ligaments. These peritoneal coverings are important in ensuring safety of colorectal anastomoses. The rectum is supported in the pelvis by the adipose tissue of the mesorectum and the attachment of the levator muscles (*Fig.* 74.1). There are fibrous condensations of the fatty tissues which can be found by dissection into the lateral ligaments of the rectum; structures which need division during rectal mobilization.

The Anal Canal

Normally closed by the tonic contraction of its intrinsic musculature, the 3-cm canal is bound anteriorly by the bulbous urethra in the male, posteriorly by the anococcygeal raphe and coccyx and laterally by the fatty and vascular tissue of the ischiorectal fossae. Two cm inside the canal lies the pectinate line which marks the junction of the postallantoic gut and proctodeum. The line of the anal valves (*Fig.* 74.2) are remnants of the proctodeal membrane. At the base of each valve are small anal sinuses into which open 4–8 anal glands. Some of these glands are racemose and reach the intersphincteric layer. The function of these glands is obscure and their importance lies in the fact that they may be the route of infections into the submucous and intersphincteric spaces and lead to abscess formation. Above the pectinate line are the columns of Morgagni with a change in the mucosa from the modified skin of the lower anal canal through a graduation of several layers of cuboidal cells to a single cuboidal cell layer of the lower rectal mucosa above.

The musculature of the sphincteric area is a highly complex organ. The circular muscle layer of the rectum expands to form the internal sphincter and terminates about 0·5 cm below the pectinate line. Surrounding the lower part of the canal, the external sphincter is formed of striated muscle and is split by the interdigitating fibres of the longitudinal muscle of the rectum passing through it to attain perianal skin attachment. The levator and puborectalis muscles form an attachment to the internal sphincter (*see Fig.* 74.1).

Blood Supply and Lymphatic Drainage of the Colorectum

The patterns of arterial supply and venous drainage are well known and the main vessels are depicted in *Fig.* 74.19,

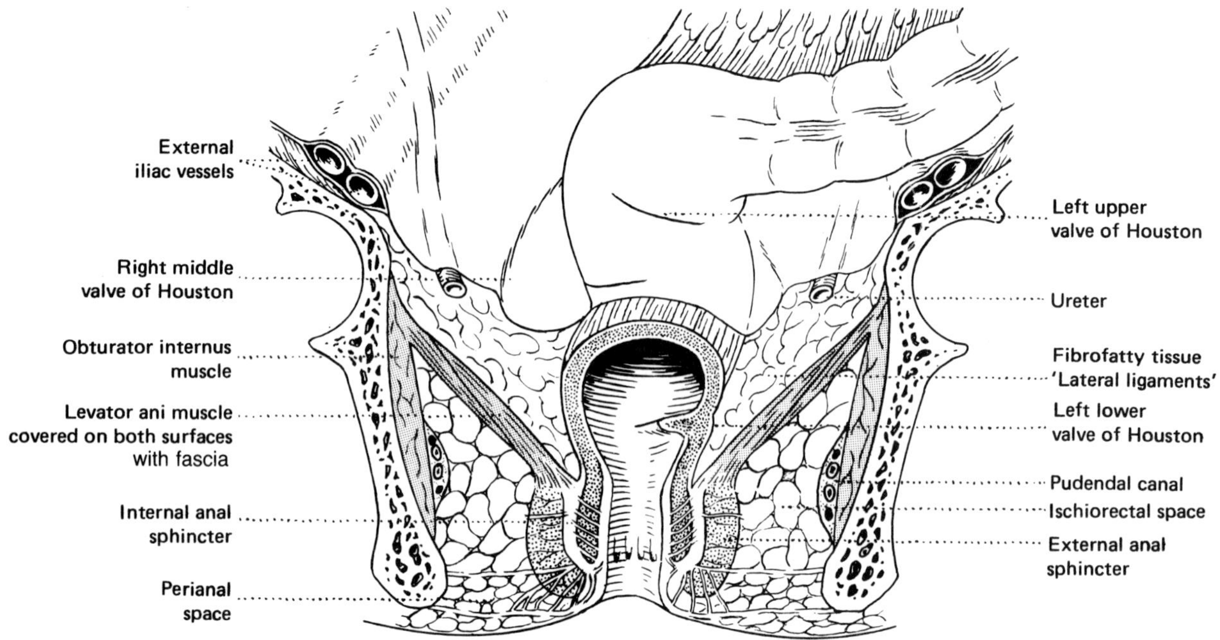

Fig. 74.1 Anatomical relationships of the rectum and sigmoid colon.

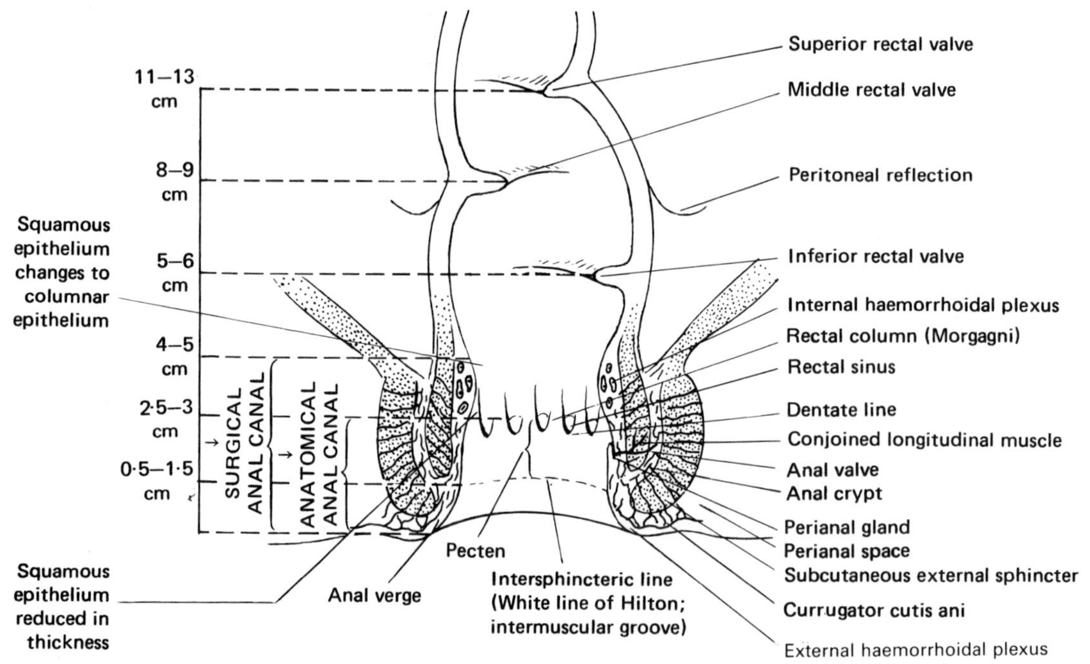

Fig. 74.2 Anatomical relationships of the anal canal and the position of the valves of Houston.

together with the arcades which permit ligation of the main vessels supplying a colonic segment without necessarily devitalizing the bowel. The marginal artery provides the ultimate blood supply of the colon via the vasa recti and provides the communication between branches of superior and inferior mesenteric arteries, by way of the long anastomotic artery of Riordan. There appear to be two critical points: namely at the splenic flexure and between the lowest branches of the sigmoid artery and the superior haemorrhoidal vessels. However, ligation of the inferior mesenteric artery flush on the aorta does not impair blood supply to the left colon nor is the viability of colerectal anastomosis impaired by a high inferior mesenteric artery tie. The veins of the colon and rectum accompany the main supplying arteries.

Lymphatic drainage is both intramural, draining the submucosal and subperitoneal spaces, and extramural, consisting of lymph vessels and nodes lying alongside the colic vessels. Four groups of lymph nodes are described: (1) epicolic nodes alongside the colonic wall, (2) paracolic nodes which lie on the marginal vessels, (3) intermediate nodes situated against the main colonic vessels, and (4) principal nodes situated along the root of the superior and inferior mesenteric vessels. Normally, lymph drainage from the gut would pass through each group but drainage from the rectum and anal canal has some special features, namely that besides an upward progression to the para-aortic glands, lymph may drain laterally to the nodes around the internal iliac vessels and more rarely in a retrograde fashion to the perianal plexuses and thence to the inguinal lymph nodes.

The nerve supply of the colon and rectum, like the lymphatics, follows the course of the main vessels. The right colon receives sympathetic nerve fibres from the lower six dorsal ganglia and parasympathetic fibres probably from the coeliac branch of the posterior vagus nerve. The left colon and rectum are supplied through the upper three lumbar ganglia and from the pre-aortic, inferior mesenteric and presacral plexus. These plexuses also receive branches from the sacral parasympathetic nerves (nervi erigentes). These nerves remain outside the parietal pelvic fascia and are sometimes injured by division of the lateral ligaments during rectal excision.

The innervation of the anal canal deserves special mention. The motor supply of the internal sphincter is via the presacral plexus whereas the external sphincter receives branches from the inferior haemorrhoidal branch of the internal pudendal nerves and the perineal branch of the 4th sacral nerve, which also supply the levator ani muscles. The sensory component below the anal canal runs with the inferior haemorrhoidal nerve whereas sensation above this level is via the autonomic system.

Physiology of the Colon and Rectum

About 1000 ml of ileal content, containing 90% water, are discharged into the caecum each day in the normal adult. Water absorption takes place during transit through the colon and only 100–200 ml of water are excreted in the faeces. The absorptive capacity of the colon depends on the rate at which faeces enter the caecum and is greater in the right colon than in the left. Normal faeces are composed of 70% water and 30% solids; about 50% of the solids are bacteria and the remainder is composed of food waste and desquamated epithelium.

Nutrients, such as glucose, amino acids, fatty acids and vitamins can be absorbed slowly through the colonic wall although only negligible amounts of such digestible matter normally reach the caecum. Sodium absorption is very efficient and is maintained by an active transport mechanism which is enhanced by mineralocorticoids and glucocorticoids. A normal person can remain in balance on as little as 5 mmol of sodium in his daily diet but following colectomy, the minimum daily requirement increases to 80–100 mmol to offset losses from the ileostomy. Chloride and water absorption is passive and follows electrical and osmotic gradients established by the sodium pump.

Potassium is actively excreted into the faeces against a concentration gradient and by secretion in mucus. Excessive mucus production in patients with colitis or with some tumours, such as villous adenomas, may lead to enormous losses of potassium in the faeces. Only a small amount of bicarbonate is secreted into the colonic lumen in exchange for chloride.

A normal bowel habit is hard to define since it is influenced by social and dietary customs. The frequency of a bowel movement in Western countries ranges from every 8 h to once every 2–3 days. Any change in bowel habits is an indication for investigation to exclude organic disease.

Diarrhoea may be defined as stools containing more than 300 ml of fluid daily. When excessive, it may be debilitating and even fatal if associated with large losses of fluid and electrolytes which are not replaced. Saline laxatives act by causing osmotic retention of water in the colonic lumen. Castor oil (ricinoleic acid), hydroxy fatty acids, and bile salts stimulate secretion of fluid by the colonic mucosa by increasing mucosal cyclic AMP. This effect can be counteracted by propranolol which inhibits adenyl cyclase. Inflammatory disease of the colonic or small bowel mucosa can cause excessive exudation of fluid and also leads to diarrhoea, as does anything that decreases intestinal transit time and decreases absorptive surface area.

The symptom of constipation has different meaning for different individuals. Some people imply infrequency of bowel movements, others hard consistency of the stools and finally others may use the term to indicate difficult expulsion of stools. In some individuals, a failure to pass a regular stool is associated with symptoms of mental depression, headache, restlessness, anorexia, nausea, coated tongue, abdominal distension and heaviness. These symptoms are aggravated by a fear of the consequences of constipation. There is no evidence that the symptoms are the result of the absorption of ill-defined toxins from the colon. Fear of constipation leads to the habitual and unnecessary use of laxatives on a daily basis. The action of laxatives is to artificially empty the colon. If the laxative is omitted, colonic activity subsides and no bowel movement occurs for 1–2 days which confirms the patient's belief that laxatives are constantly needed to avoid the dangers of constipation.

Colonic Motility

There are three patterns of motor activity in the colon.

1. *Segmentation* is the most common type of motor activity seen in the transverse and descending colon and consists of annular contractions which divide the lumen into segments, propelling faeces over short distances in both directions. Segmental contractions form, relax and reform in different locations, in a random fashion, 3–8 times per minute.
2. *Mass movement* consists of a strong contraction moving distally over relatively long distances, 30–45 cm, in the transverse and descending colon. It is infrequent and probably occurs only a few times each day, often in response to a meal.
3. *Retrograde peristalsis*, consisting of annular contractions moving proximally in the right colon and in the sigmoid and descending colon. It is more frequently seen in experimental animals than man. The retrograde movement can be shown by observing the spontaneous movement of a radio-opaque marker from the left to right colon.

A complex neurohormonal mechanism is involved in the colonic response to eating which has been inaccurately called the gastrocolic reflex. There is increased ileal emptying, increased mass movements and an urge to defaecate. Other factors influencing colonic motility are physical activity, emotional states and faecal bulk.

Thus, normal colonic emptying is slow, complex and exceedingly variable. It is difficult to define altered motility in disease states. There is no orderly laminar flow. Some of the material entering the caecum flows past faeces which has remained from earlier periods. In general, residue from a meal reaches the caecum after 4 h and the rectosigmoid by 24 h. Since there is a large amount of mixing of bowel contents in the colon, residue from a single meal may be passed in movements for 3–4 days afterwards.

Intraluminal pressure studies of the colon may be performed by use of small balloons, fine open-ended tubes or telemetring capsules. It appears that faecal transport can take place without a rise in intraluminal pressure nor can specific patterns be correlated with defined disease states. Rhythmic changes in electrical potential occur normally in colonic muscle at two frequencies—3 and 9 per minute respectively. The frequency appears to be approximately 16 per minute in the sigmoid colon with diverticular disease.

Mechanism of Anal Continence

It is generally stressed that continence is a relative phenomenon, with individuals varying greatly in their ability to control flatus and faeces. Most individuals are sometimes incontinent to liquid faecal matter and slight contamination of the anal margin is common. Normally, rectal sensation records the arrival of faeces into the rectum, whereas the sensory endings in the anal canal seem able to discriminate between flatus and faecal material. There are three patterns of response to the entrance of material into the rectum: (1) accommodation, where the rectum slowly expands but the external sphincter retains its tone until the time for defaecation; (2) sampling, where rectal contents come into contact with the sensory lining of the anal canal after temporary relaxation of the internal sphincter; and (3) defaecation, when the volume of rectal contents reaches a certain critical point, the urge to defaecate becomes overpowering and the action of the external sphincter is completely inhibited.

It is clear that the sensory component of continence is highly complex and that most individuals are able to distinguish between flatus, liquid and solid faeces. Specialized nerve endings are found within the anal canal together with free nerve endings. It is also highly likely that sensory endings in the puborectalis muscles record and control the urge to defaecate. The combination of anal mucosal and puborectalis muscular nerve endings may permit normal continence even after rectal excision has removed the reservoir function of the rectum itself. The anal mucosa above the pectinate line is relatively insensitive to tactile stimuli though not completely so, whereas the skin of the perianal region and anal canal below the pectinate line has normal cutaneous sensibility.

Motor control of continence is exhibited by a high pressure zone in the anal canal (25–120 mmHg) presumably produced by the tone of internal and external sphincters. The angle of the anal canal and rectum is about 80° and is maintained by the action of the puborectalis muscle. During defaecation in the squatting position, the thighs are flexed which straightens out this angle and permits the passage of rectal contents. It is also suggested that during raised intra-abdominal pressure, the rectum is compressed as an antero-posterior slit and acts as a flutter valve, though this mechanism will not act against raised intrarectal pressure.

Defaecation

The initial stimulus is distension of the rectum. Presumably this acts reflexly through a centre in the lumbosacral region of the spinal cord which is able to maintain reflex defaecation after spinal cord injury. Above all, man is able to exert a cerebral control if circumstances are not convenient. This cerebral conditioning leads to a degree of training or habit so that defaecation takes place once a day, even though the rectum contains faeces for much of the rest of the day.

During the act of defaecation and in the squatting position the rectum and anal canal form a straight line. The abdominal pressure is raised, the external sphincter is inhibited and the pelvic floor is lowered allowing the mass of faeces to pass through the anal canal. In some individuals, the evacuation of rectum is accompanied by mass peristalsis and emptying of the whole distal colon. In others, repeated acts of straining may produce several smaller segments of stool.

Microbiology of the Colon

The normal faecal flora survives in symbiosis with the human host and supports several physiological processes. Bile pigments are degraded by colonic bacteria to give the stool its brown colour. Characteristic faecal odour is due to the amines, indole and skatole, which are produced by bacterial action. Colon bacteria also supply vitamin K to the host, alter colonic motility and absorption and may be important in the defence against potentially more pathogenic organisms. Faecal bacteria deconjugate bile salts to produce free bile acids and also alter the steroid nucleus. These bacteria have been implicated in the pathophysiology of a variety of disease processes including the pathogenesis of carcinoma of the large bowel.

The colon of the fetus is sterile and bacterial colonization occurs soon after birth. The bacterial flora present in the colon varies with dietetic and environmental factors.

Over 99% of the normal faecal flora is anaerobic. *Bacteroides fragilis* is the most prevalent. *Lactobacillus bifidus*, clostridia of various types, and cocci of various types form the other common anaerobes. Aerobic bacteria can be divided into two groups—coliforms and enterococci. *Escherichia coli* is the predominant coliform and is present in counts of 10^7/gramme of wet faeces. *Streptococcus faecalis* is the principal enterococcus and is present in similar numbers.

The bacterial flora of the colon is readily altered by antibiotic administration. Oral neomycin and tetracycline result in resistant R factor enterococci and resistant staphylococci and bacteroides. Outbreaks of staphylococcal enterocolitis and more commonly pseudomembranous colitis from *Clostridium difficile* (Chapter 3) are frequently seen in surgical units.

CHRONIC CONSTIPATION AND MEGACOLON

Mention has already been made of the wide range of bowel habit in an apparently normal population. However, some people do seem to suffer symptoms from chronic constipation, mainly abdominal pains and distension, and in some of these patients there will be an underlying cause worthy of diagnosis and treatment. In a small proportion of individuals the colon and rectum are found to be dilated over a variable extent (megacolon and megarectum) and these patients require detailed study.

Rectal Inertia

This condition is largely but not exclusively diagnosed in children where chronic constipation is found in apparently healthy individuals with only mild abdominal distension and only occasional perianal soiling. Examination of the patient reveals an abdomen which is flat, but palpation reveals large faecal masses, largely on the left side but rarely reaching round to the right side of the colon also. On rectal examination there may be evidence of soiling and poor sphincteric tone and the rectum may contain a large hard faecal mass. In children the important differential diagnosis is from Hirschsprung's disease (*see* Chapter 59), a condition which should have given rise to some symptoms immediately after birth. Children with rectal inertia are not thought to have a problem until toilet training might be expected to be complete. As the syndrome persists, the bowel becomes overstretched with each incomplete evacuation and more faeces build up in the rectum and overflow incontinence occurs. Once this has happened, it is less likely that mere correction of bowel habit by the correct use of laxatives or rectal washouts will be effective, particularly in the older child or adult (*see below*). Bulk formers are contraindicated.

The vast majority of children have had inadequate toilet training by over-anxious parents, and in a few there has been holding back from fear of pain due to a painful anal fissure or an undetected or mismanaged anorectal anomaly such as congenital anal stenosis. Older children and adults may have a more serious psychological maladjustment and the condition appears more common in the mentally retarded or chronic epileptic population.

The condition is treated by emptying the bowel by saline rectal washouts, if necessary as an inpatient, and keeping it as empty as possible for up to 2–3 weeks. Manual evacuation of the rectum is commonly required during the initial stages. This may allow the rectum to recover its tone. After 2–3 weeks young children can recommence toilet training twice a day after a warm drink at a regular time. Waiting for a normal call to stool is not worthwhile. Adult patients may require the continued use of phosphate enemas or suppositories but children may respond to single large doses of aperients such as Senokot or Ducolax. It is important in all patients not to stimulate the proximal colon to empty its contents into the rectum as the patient will not recognize faecal contents and rectal impaction and distension can occur if aperients are given without thought.

Chronic Constipation

It is increasingly recognized that a group of patients exist with severe chronic constipation and abdominal pain. These patients have a history extending back into childhood and have often undergone series of gastrointestinal investigations over the years usually with negative results. The majority are women aged 25 to 40 years and many have undergone a hysterectomy for abdominal pain. It is probable that diagnosis is a variant of irritable bowel syndrome. However, there are reports that a total colectomy with a low ileorectal anastomosis in selected cases can be effective in dealing with the pain and constipation. It has to be emphasized that a thorough examination to exclude adult Hirschsprung's disease is required. Anorectal myomectomy is not usually effective.

Megacolon

Dilatation of the colon and rectum may occur as an acute or chronic condition.

Acute megacolon (toxic megacolon) has been described in the following conditions:

Acute phase of ulcerative colitis (*Fig.* 74.3).
Granulomatous colitis.
Severe dysentery.
Electrolyte deficiency—particularly potassium losses from diuretics, leading to colonic pseudo-obstruction.
Excessive use of anticholinergic drugs.
Ischaemia of the colon—particularly in the elderly patient.

Associated with the colonic dilatation is abdominal pain, distension and hypovolaemic collapse. Plain films of the abdominal cavity may show a whole or part of the colon dilated to a diameter of 10 cm or greater (*Fig.* 74.3) and there may also be evidence of distal small bowel distension. Barium enema examination is contraindicated and in some patients with colitis, the condition seems precipitated by this investigation.

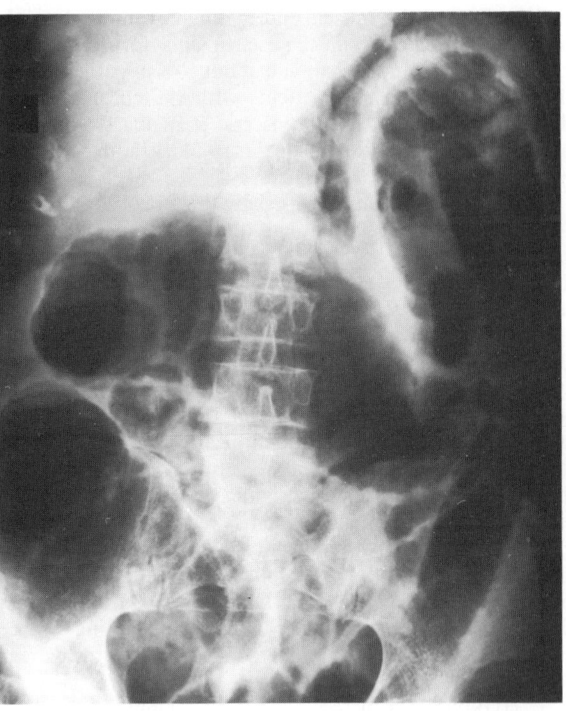

Fig. 74.3 A plain radiograph of the abdomen showing dilatation of the whole colon in a patient with ulcerative colitis. At operation the patient was found to show a sealed perforation in the sigmoid colon.

Management of this condition will be dictated by the underlying cause (*see* Chapter 73), but the prognosis is frequently grave. Early recognition and documentation of increasing dilatation can be achieved by daily or twice daily radiographs of the abdomen, sigmoidoscopy with biopsy and rectal culture. Medical treatment may avert a crisis in patients with ulcerative colitis, granulomatous colitis, dysentery and severe electrolyte disturbance. Unless a rapid resolution takes place and in patients with ischaemic colitis, there is an indication for surgical intervention. Depending upon circumstances, the safest approach would appear to be the establishment of an ileostomy and a transverse and sigmoid 'blow-hole' colostomy. When colonic gangrene or perforation has occurred a total colectomy with ileostomy or ileorectal anastomosis is required. Acute megacolon due to colonic pseudo-obstruction can be decompressed by fibreoptic colonoscopy. Repeated examinations are sometimes required.

Chronic megacolon or megarectum may also affect the bowel totally or only segmentally. The condition may be congenital as in Hirschsprung's disease (*see* Chapter 59) or may be acquired.

The acquired megacolorectum can result from a variety of causes:

1. Obstruction: chronic anal stenosis, strictures—commonly on an ischaemic basis with dilatation of the transverse colon; annular neoplasms, particularly on the left side of the colon. The muscle coat of the colon in such patients is grossly hypertrophied; a feature which is also seen in Hirschsprung's disease or Chagas' disease.

2. Chagas' disease: this disease is caused by *Trypanosoma cruzi* which enters the bloodstream via an insect bite and invades the smooth muscle and the myocardium where the organism proliferates in the Leishmania form. Repeated cycles of proliferation occur and about 10% of patients die in the acute phase. Those patients with the chronic disease develop dilatation of hollow viscera, particularly colon and oesophagus, and also develop heart block and congestive heart failure.

The disease is found especially in Brazil but also in Argentina and Chile. About half the patients, usually young adults, will suffer both mega-oesophagus and megacolon. The basic problem would appear to be a reduction in the number of myenteric ganglion cells to 4–6% of normal. Initially there is hypertonicity and hypercontractibility of the colon which eventually hypertrophies. Ultimately, stagnation leads to mucosal ulceration and in some patients to volvulus. Many patients present with chronic constipation, abdominal distension and ill-health. Eradication of this disease is largely a public health measure aimed at the insect vector and medical treatment is not effective.

For severely disabled patients rectosigmoidectomy is currently practised, leaving only 4–5 cm of rectal stump. Intestinal continuity is re-established by an abdomino-anal pull-through procedure or a Duhammel technique. It is likely, however, that the newer circular stapling devices could find a distinct role in the management of this dangerous condition.

3. Hypothyroidism: patients, who remain undiagnosed until the full clinical picture of myxoedema or cretinism develops, may be found to be suffering from chronic constipation and megarectum. Treatment is directed to the underlying endocrine abnormality.

4. Neurological disorders: are occasionally complicated by the development of a megacolon. In a child, a spina bifida condition may be apparent; in the adult the association has been reported with cauda equina lesions, paraplegia and Parkinsonism.

5. Psychological disturbances: it has previously been mentioned that irrational attention to the normal bowel habit may lead to chronic constipation and/or megacolon in the adult patient. Similarly, mentally retarded patients in long-term institutional care may be affected. When the condition arises in the psychiatrically disturbed patient on treatment it should be remembered that some psychotrophic drugs, particularly chlorpromazine, can induce megacolon in the experimental animal, acting in an unknown toxic fashion.

6. Idiopathic: some patients appear to have symptomatic megacolon without obvious cause. These patients are ultimately labelled adynamic bowel syndrome; others may prove to have previously undetected Hirschsprung's disease which has presented since early life. This may be due to an 'ultrashort aganglionic segment' just above the anal canal. In a small group of patients (whose average age is about 18 years) the clinical presentation of constipation, overflow incontinence, abdominal pain and distension has resulted in extensive investigation without demonstrating an underlying cause. The colon alone may be affected and a normal rectum present; others have a megarectum with a variable extent of dilated colon in continuity. Rectal capacity and sensation are diminished but sphincteric responses and rectal biopsy are normal. Failure of medical therapy occurs in about one-half of patients and surgical excision of the floppy, dilated, atonic colon may be indicated in the severely symptomatic patients.

VOLVULUS

Volvulus of the colon may be divided into cases in which the caecum is involved and those in which the sigmoid colon is affected. In either event, torsion is the result of poor fixation of the caecum or sigmoid colon in the respective ilial fossae. Volvulus of the transverse colon is also described.

Caecal volvulus occurs most commonly in a clockwise direction and may cause: (1) sudden strangulation leading to early gangrene with peritonitis and emergency admission, (2) closed loop obstruction with gross distension of the caecum which is no longer in the right lower quadrant but is seen to be in the upper abdomen on plain abdominal radiograph. Gangrene or perforation of the bowel results unless the volvulus untwists spontaneously or is dealt with at laparotomy (*Fig.* 74.4).

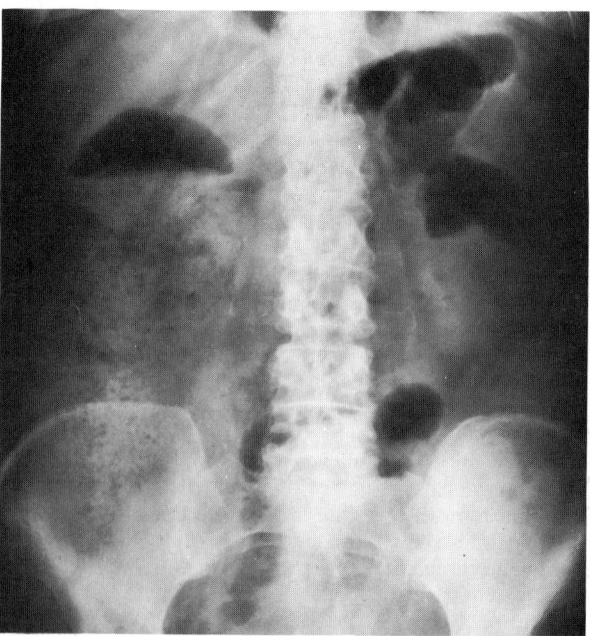

Fig. 74.4 A plain film of the abdomen in a patient with chronic ileocaecal volvulus. At laparotomy the colon was found to have failed to make its usual attachment to the right paracolic gutter and to have torted around the axis of the superior mesenteric vessels.

Sigmoid volvulus is more common and has an odd type of incidence, being rare in Europe and the USA but more common in Eastern Europe and Africa. Whether these communities have more individuals with a thick-walled, dilated, relatively long sigmoid colon is not established but it is more likely that a high residue diet overloads the sigmoid colon and leads to volvulus. It is also apparent that a higher proportion of cases arise in patients in mental institutions where chronic constipation and dilatation of the sigmoid colon predispose to volvulus. The condition appears also related to the narrowness of the base of the sigmoid mesentery and the loop of sigmoid colon is redundant. Under these circumstances the sigmoid loop can begin to twist about its base when the upper loop falls in front of the lower loop.

The symptoms of sigmoid volvulus are those of large bowel obstruction but vary in severity or acuteness. Younger patients appear to develop a more acute form of obstruction characterized by marked distension of the abdomen and collapse. The sigmoid colon may be markedly tender and a radiograph shows a dilated loop of bowel (*Fig.* 74.5) running diagonally across the abdomen from right to left and two fluid levels may be seen, one within each loop of bowel. In some elderly patients, chronic symptoms may have been present for some months highly suggestive of an obstructing carcinoma. Nevertheless, sigmoid dilatation does occur and strangulation with gangrene is the final result as it is with the acute form.

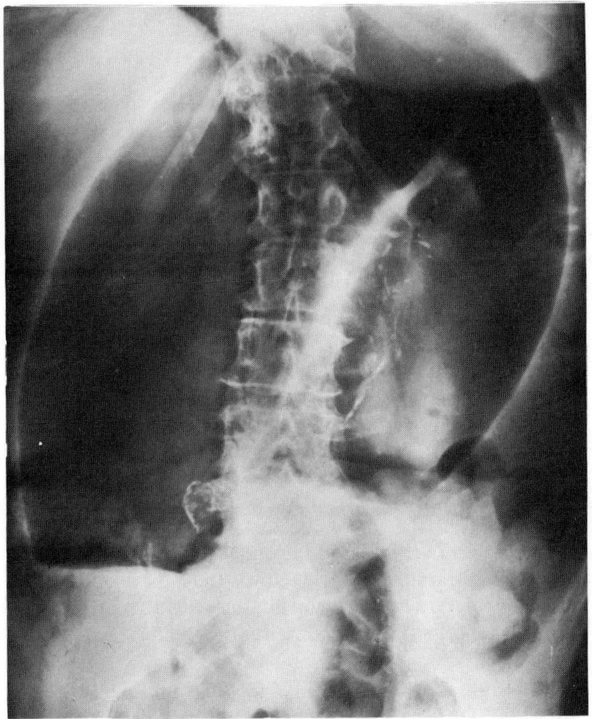

Fig. 74.5 A plain film of the abdomen showing characteristic gross distension of the sigmoid colon after a sigmoid volvulus.

Management

Early recognition of the condition and its serious consequences, in the form of intestinal gangrene, is vital and not difficult given the characteristic radiological appearance. After energetic resuscitation with intravenous fluids, early laparotomy allows untwisting of the ileocaecal volvulus and assessment of the bowel's viability. Where patches of gangrene are seen, a right hemicolectomy is required. In cases with viable bowel, fixation of the caecum behind a leaf of peritoneum is attempted but recurrence is possible. Fixation of the caecum by constructing a temporary caecostomy has some attractions in terms of simplicity.

Similarly in patients with sigmoid volvulus immediate unravelling of the volvulus is necessary. This may be possible by the gentle passage of a sigmoidoscope or flatus tube. This is more likely to be successful if performed with the patient in the knee–chest position, though many patients are too ill for this position to be adopted. When successful, there is an immediate release of large amounts of flatus and fluid and the patient's condition improves quickly. The problem is whether the volvulus has been completely reduced and whether the bowel is completely viable or not. Where there is doubt about either feature, urgent laparotomy is undertaken. Where the bowel is viable, fixation of the sigmoid colon to the posterior abdominal wall may be a safer manoeuvre for the relatively inexperienced surgeon, but resection of the large, floppy, sigmoid colon is a more satisfactory procedure provided it can be accomplished safely. Though theoretically a Paul–Mikulicz procedure should be a useful compromise, the areas of torsion are often of doubtful viability and cannot be safeguarded by being brought out of the peritoneal cavity. Where it is necessary to perform a sigmoidectomy and re-anastomosis is considered unwise, then a Hartmann's procedure may be safer, particularly now that reconstruction of the rectum is easier with stapling devices.

Following successful decompression with a flatus tube, elective resection of the sigmoid colon should take place about 7 days later.

DIVERTICULAR DISEASE OF THE COLON

Diverticula of the colon occur as congenital or acquired lesions and the latter occur commonly.

Acquired Diverticular Disease

This disorder normally develops in the latter half of life and remains asymptomatic in 90% of patients. The diverticula represent a herniation of the colonic mucosa through a defect in the circular muscle of the colon at a point where there is a weakness created by the entry of a segmental vessel and two rows are usually present (*Fig.* 74.6). Normally the sigmoid colon is primarily and most severely affected, but in many instances the disorder spreads proximally. During the early stages, the diverticula may be reducible and it has been known for sequential barium enemas to show different diverticula at different times. In obese patients the diverticula are enclosed in the fatty capsules of the appendices epiploicae.

Aetiology

Normal motility of the colon leads to segmentation of the large bowel with the intervening sections subjected to varying levels of intraluminal pressure. Under the stimulus of emotion, feeding and drugs, such as opiates, intracolonic pressures may reach as high as 90 mmHg. Persistent contraction rings may result in functional obstruction and ultimately to thickening of the circular muscle by a process which may be compared with trabeculation of the bladder. Ultimately the high pressures within the 'bladder' surrounded by the contraction rings will lead to herniation of the mucosa as diverticula.

Given that the origin of the condition results from disordered colonic motility the pathogenesis of this disease is less easy to pinpoint although it is one of the commoner colonic

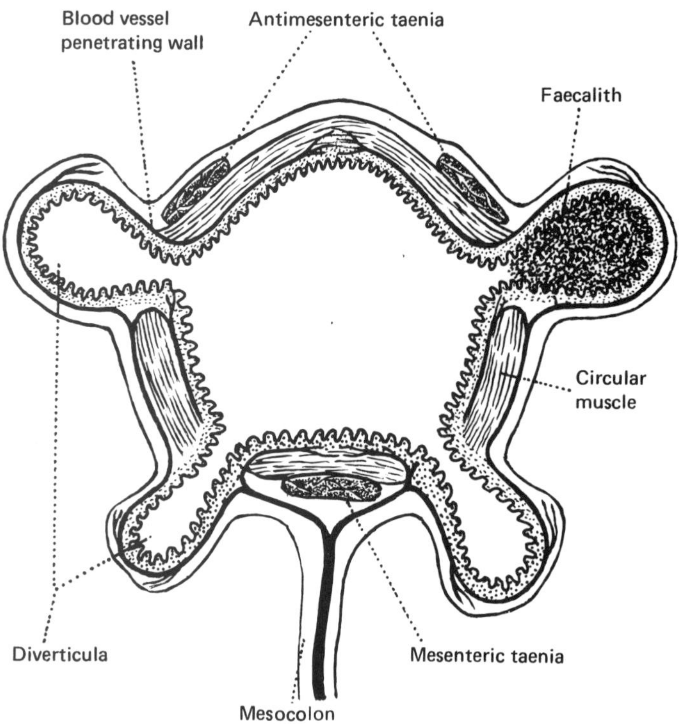

Fig. 74.6 An anatomical representation of the formation of diverticula between the taenia coli indicating the points of herniation at the entry of arterial tributaries.

diseases in Western communities. It is clearly not racial in predisposition for all races living in the same cultural environment appear to have an identical prevalence. Conventionally it is considered that the widespread use of refined sugar and flour from which all cereal fibre has been removed in the milling is the main cause of altered colonic motility. The colon is forced to propel contents of hard consistency and high segmentation pressures result.

It has been documented that the average daily stool weight of a rural African is 400 g with a transit time of 35 hours which compares with values in studies on Europeans of 150 g and 3–6 days respectively. This difference is considered to be the result of increased dietary fibre and to account for the low incidence of diverticular disease in the African community. Nevertheless, diverticulosis is appearing in African and Indian communities despite adherence to a high residue diet.

Incidence

Diverticular disease is somewhat more common in females (3:2). It is rarely found below the age of 30 years and the incidence increases with age to be maximal in the 6th and 8th decades, as judged by autopsy studies. The sigmoid colon alone is involved in about two-thirds and in combination with the rest of the colon in 96%. About 7% of colons show total involvement. Careful dissection of colons exhibiting diverticula suggest about 30% show thickening of the muscle coat but only about 15% have any pathological evidence of inflammation. There is no evidence that the disease is progressive and it seems more likely that the diverticula establish themselves early within the segments that are going to become affected.

Pathology

Diverticula never penetrate the taenia coli and usually prolapse between the antimesenteric and mesenteric taenia (*Fig.* 74.7). Formally, attention is focused upon the full saccular prolapse of mucosa with its serosal covering but small intramural and ridge diverticula are also seen within specimens. It is generally considered that the diverticula occur at the point of entry of segmental blood vessels from serosal to submucosal layer. In obese patients the diverticula are covered by the fat of the appendices epiploica but in thinner patients there are only serosal and mucosal layers. However, intramural and ridge diverticula have an attenuated layer of circular muscle in the wall as may saccular diverticula occurring through the antimesenteric intertaenial area.

On cutting open the bowel the openings of the diverticula may be seen as round or slit-like openings. The other feature is muscle thickening which affects both circular and longitudinal muscle layers, the latter leading to a degree of shortening of the bowel. There is genuine hypertrophy of the muscle fibres which may precede the development of diverticula but not necessarily so. The circular muscle and mucosa are projected as transverse folds into the lumen as interdigitating valves (*Fig.* 74.8). When marked, these folds may lead to partial obstruction of the colon.

Detailed pathological examination of specimens removed for diverticular disease reveals inflammatory changes in about 15%. When it does occur, the effects are most marked, not in the diverticula, but in the extramural pericolonic tissue and leads to peritonitis and pericolonic abscess formation. The mucosal aspect of a segment of colon affected by diverticular disease is usually intact.

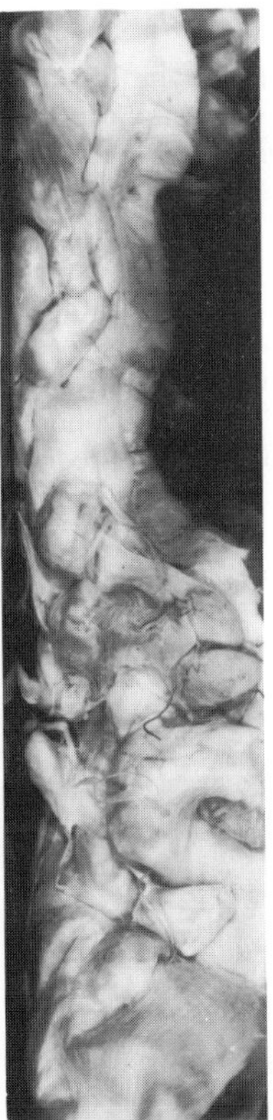

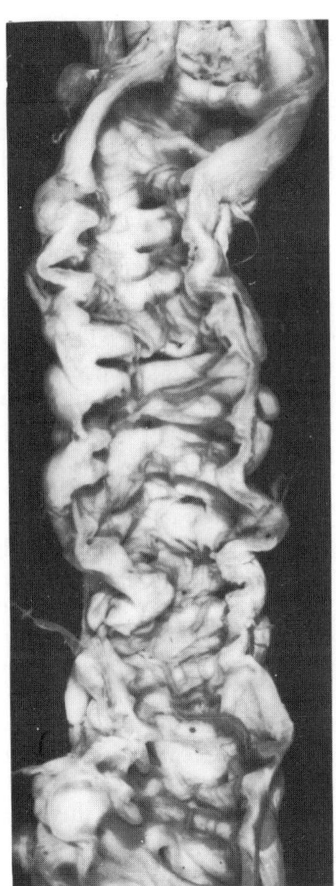

Fig. 74.7 (left) The external appearances of a resected sigmoid colon showing the dome-shaped diverticula just outside the line of the taenia coli.

Fig. 74.8 (right) The open specimen of a sigmoid colon with diverticular disease showing hypertrophy of muscle with the development of muscular bars. The internal openings of the diverticula can be seen arising between the muscular bars.

Clinical Features

In about 90% of individuals, the presence of colonic diverticula has no clinical importance. In the remainder several types of presentation are common.

Patients with diverticular pain: this is the most frequent presentation with a mild to severe pain felt in the lower abdomen, particularly the left iliac fossa. The duration of the pain may be short-lived or persist for hours or even 1–2 days. Pain may be precipitated by diet or stress but often there is no absolute relationship to food. A feeling of distension is common, only relieved by passing flatus. Bowel action in these patients may produce a stool of small hard pieces (sheep droppings) or be inconsistent with diarrhoea with mucus and constipation alternating. Normally these patients, though troubled by these symptoms, show little evidence of systemic illness.

Pain is also the most frequent symptom of acute diverticulitis. It is usually in the left lower quadrant but may occur in the midline or even on the right side of the lower abdomen. The pain is usually dull and constant. While anorexia is common, vomiting is not. Urgency or dysuria may be noted when the inflamed colon lies on the bladder or ureter. Pneumaturia is a prominent symptom in patients who have developed a colovesical fistula (*see below*).

On physical examination, low-grade fever is usually present. Tenderness, rigidity and, at times, a mass may be appreciated in the left lower quadrant. The signs and symptoms of diverticular disease may resemble those of appendicitis and the disease has been referred to as 'left-sided appendicitis'. In patients with redundant sigmoid, an area of inflammation may be present in the right lower quadrant. It is often impossible to differentiate diverticulitis from appendicitis on the basis of history and physical findings. Sigmoidoscopy in patients with acute diverticulitis may show some mucosal oedema and erythema. Occasionally a 'sentinel loop' of the small bowel may be seen on plain radiography due to proximity to the inflamed area, but barium enema is not recommended in the acute stage of diverticulitis, as it may exacerbate the disease or lead to rupture.

Barium enema performed for diagnostic reasons often shows segmental areas of spasm with resultant serrations of the bowel wall. Mucosal oedema, fixation and narrowing of the lumen are also frequently seen. A narrowed segment of sigmoid colon may be difficult to differentiate on radiography from a sigmoid carcinoma but diverticular disease usually has associated spasm and involves a longer segment of bowel than is characteristic for obstructing carcinoma (*Fig.* 74.9). The presence of other diverticula elsewhere in the colon is not helpful in differentiating a sigmoid cancer from diverticular disease because diverticula in the remainder of the colon are common in both entities. Despite the difficulties sometimes encountered, a fibreoptic examination of the affected segment is strongly recommended in all doubtful cases.

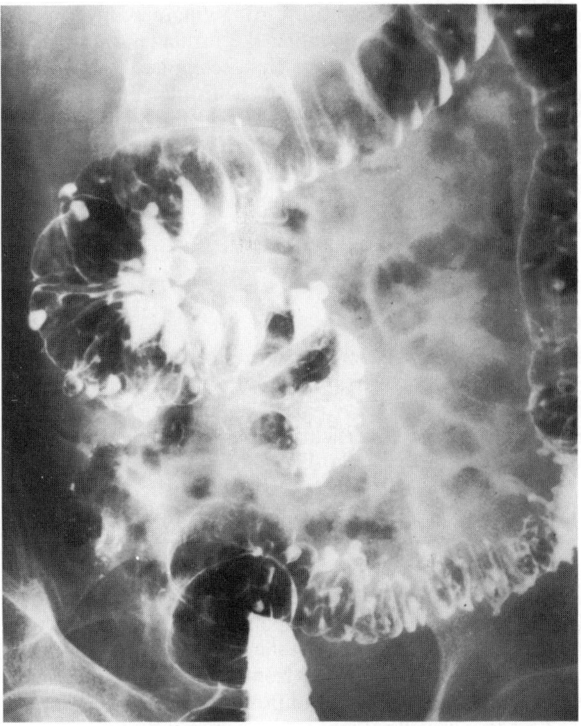

Fig. 74.9 A barium enema examination showing widespread diverticular disease, maximal in the sigmoid colon but also present in the right colon.

Secondary Complications of Inflammation

Perforation with generalized peritonitis or local abscess formation, fistula formation and obstruction of the colon are all secondary complications of diverticular inflammation.

1. Perforation

The patient has signs of left-sided peritonitis and if the suppurative area becomes walled off, a fluctuant tender mass may be palpable. If the perforation is not walled off the patient shows rapid deterioration and the signs and symptoms of generalized peritonitis develop. Ultrasound examination of the inflammatory mass will often indicate abscess formation. Barium examination may show a leak of contrast into the cavity but is not routinely recommended.

2. Intestinal Obstruction

Subacute or chronic inflammation of the colon secondary to diverticular disease causes a narrowing of the lumen due to fibrous stricture. Patients often complain of recurring attacks of left lower quadrant pain and a gradual increase in constipation. Acute large bowel obstruction may occur secondary to acute inflammation and abscess formation which obstructs the lumen of the colon. Small bowel obstruction may occur due to fixation of a loop of small bowel to the inflamed colon.

3. Fistula

As a result of the inflammation of the colon and adherence to adjacent viscera, abscesses may lead to fistula formation between the colon and the small intestine, uterus, vagina, abdominal wall and bladder. Fistula formation accounts for about 5% of the complications of diverticulitis.

Colovesical fistula is heralded by urgency and dysuria. Once the fistula has formed, pneumaturia and faecaluria make the diagnosis straightforward. Sigmoidoscopy is usually not helpful in demonstrating the fistula. Barium enema often demonstrates the tract. Cystoscopy and a cystogram may demonstrate the entrance of the fistulous tract into the bladder but not necessarily. The less common fistula formation between the colon and uterus or vagina usually produces symptoms of passage of air and faeces per vaginam.

The association of fistula-in-ano with diverticular disease is well established. If a fistula-in-ano is not responding to the usual treatment, a barium enema examination may reveal diverticulitis as the cause.

4. Haemorrhage

It is more common for this symptom to be present in patients without diverticulitis and it is now generally agreed that patients who have massive lower gastrointestinal haemorrhage and diverticular disease are bleeding from vessels in the base of the diverticula which are not themselves inflamed. Diverticular disease only accounts for a proportion of cases of massive lower gastrointestinal bleeding. This occurs most frequently in elderly individuals with associated atherosclerotic and hypertensive cardiovascular diseases. However it is now recognized that vascular ectatic lesions in the colon are responsible for major colonic haemorrhage more commonly than previously thought.

Patients with haemorrhage from diverticulosis characteristically report sudden onset of profuse bleeding per rectum. The blood is usually bright red in colour. Often the patient has had no previous history suggestive of diverticular disease. Initial investigation of the patient by proctoscopy reveals blood descending from above. Once the patient's circulatory volume has been restored, arteriography is the most efficient method of making the correct diagnosis.

Treatment of Colonic Diverticular Disease

The rationale of treatment depends in part upon the symptoms presenting in the individual patient.

Patients with Diverticular Pain

The assumption with these patients is that the symptoms are largely due to colonic spasm or excessive segmental contractions rather than an inflammatory complication of the disorder. Though a low residue diet was prescribed in the past, it is generally considered that symptoms are more likely to be relieved by faecal bulk-forming agents. The patient should be assured that there is no serious organic disease at present and that the radiological findings merely reflect an underlying disordered bowel motility. The administration of unprocessed bran (1 tablespoonful t.d.s.), and hydrophilic colloids, such as Isogel or Normacol, will generally reduce pain. The patient should be warned to expect a feeling of abdominal distension over a period of 3 weeks, which will then subside. Failure to respond to this simple measure can be managed by adding antispasmodics to the regimen. There is little to be gained by adding alimentary antiseptics to patients with this type of disease.

A few patients will remain severely symptomatic with these conservative measures and there may be a role for the operation of sigmoid myotomy to aid in management. In this procedure the circular muscle of the sigmoid colon is incised down to the submucosa of the affected bowel. Extreme care is needed not to cut through into the lumen of the bowel otherwise faecal peritonitis results. Subsequent manometric examination of these patients apparently shows a considerable reduction of the high preoperative intraluminal pressures. The original proponents of this operation report that it has proved to be 90% effective in relieving the left iliac fossa pain for which it was performed. Most surgeons prefer to perform a sigmoid colectomy in severely troubled patients.

Patients with Uncomplicated Diverticulitis

Patients with an acute attack of uncomplicated diverticulitis are normally treated expectantly in the initial stages. Bed rest, intravenous fluids in severe cases, antibiotics and analgesics (not morphine) will allow most cases to settle over 4–5 days. Subsequent progress of these patients is variable. On treatment with bran about half will remain symptom-free in the long-term and 30% will continue with mild symptoms. Only 5–10% of patients will have recurrent, severe symptoms and these will require surgical resection of the affected segment. This is best performed under elective conditions and the procedure follows the general technical outlines laid down for a high anterior resection of the rectum with carcinoma. It is preferable to preserve the supraperitoneal stump, usually 2 cm below the level of the hypertrophied circular muscle. Proximally, the line of resection is taken just above the level of inflammatory disease and more proximal diverticula in the descending colon are left in situ. The chance of getting further attacks of diverticulitis in the remaining colon is reported to be lower than 5%; where there is doubt as to the true nature of the disease, i.e. where an underlying carcinoma is suspected in the diverticular segment, the specimen should be opened at the time of surgery so that a more extensive lymph gland clearance can be attempted if this appears indicated. The long-term results of resection appear good and the morbidity is acceptably low.

Patients with Complicated Diverticular Disease
Peritonitis

Where the peritonitis appears localized, most patients respond to bed rest, intravenous fluids and broad-spectrum antibiotics. Close observation is necessary, for although most patients have signs which diminish over a few days, a few will develop an abscess in the lower abdomen or pelvis and others develop rapidly spreading peritonitis. In these patients a laparotomy is indicated urgently.

Other patients present with widespread peritonitis where the diagnosis of diverticulitis remains in doubt. Urgent resuscitation is needed to correct fluid and electrolyte depletion and to counteract septic shock (*see* Chapter 7). When the patient is fit enough, a laparotomy is undertaken. The degree of peritonitis may be purulent or frankly faecal. The condition of the diverticular segment varies from severe inflammation throughout the affected segment or associated with a periocolic abscess.

Where the affected segment appears to be only inflamed, no local treatment is necessary. Although there is evidence that a right transverse colostomy is effective in resting the left colon and inducing the inflammation to subside more quickly, it should not be performed routinely. Local collections of pus are drained and the peritoneal cavity is lavaged with saline and noxythiolin. Where the peritonitis is faecal, a perforation invariably exists. Formerly such cases were treated by a transverse colostomy, but the mortality was high and in the order of 10–30%. The left colon beyond the colostomy commonly contains bulky faeces which presumably continue to leak through the perforation. More recently, radical surgical management of this situation has been advocated. Resection of the affected segment can be accomplished in all but the most severely shocked patient. Primary anastomosis has been successfully performed but is not recommended routinely, for the incidence of anastomotic dehiscence is high. In thin patients it may be possible to exteriorize the affected segment as a left iliac colostomy. This technique depends upon the perforation being near the apex of the sigmoid loop. More commonly the patient is obese and the mesentery of the sigmoid colon sufficiently thickened so as to prevent the bowel reaching the exterior. In such patients, the safest procedure is to excise the affected segment containing the perforation, bringing the proximal end as a left iliac colostomy and closing the lower end (Hartmann's procedure). Providing the patient survives the peritonitis, it is generally possible to re-anastomose the colon after 3–6 months.

Fistulation

Contact of the sigmoid colon with the bladder, vault of vagina or other loops of bowel may lead to the establishment of a faecal fistula. Symptomatically, such patients present with chronic ill-health, lower abdominal tenderness, intermittent diarrhoea, pneumaturia and faecal vaginal discharge. These fistulas are unlikely to close spontaneously even though a covering colostomy is performed. Most patients are best treated by elective sigmoid resection with primary anastomosis and repair of the fistulous opening in the affected organ.

Haemorrhage

Occasionally severe and dramatic rectal haemorrhage can occur from an area of diverticular disease. Though frank shock is rare, profound anaemia requiring transfusion is common. Abdominal examination is usually negative but rectal examination reveals either fresh or dark, recently clotted blood. Early sigmoidoscopy is indicated and often shows fresh blood coming down from the sigmoid colon or above. Fibresigmoidoscopy may indicate the precise point of the haemorrhage but this proves to be difficult when haemorrhage is actually occurring and little is seen when the haemorrhage has ceased. Usually it is possible to determine whether the bleeding is coming from the sigmoid colon or above. Arteriography should be reserved for patients in whom the source of bleeding remains unidentified and in order to demonstrate angiodysplastic lesions.

Fortunately even with severe haemorrhage requiring transfusion the complication is frequently self-limiting and rarely recurrent. Continuing life-threatening haemorrhage requires excision of the bleeding segment, nearly always the sigmoid colon, and primary colonic anastomosis can usually be established.

Obstruction

It is clear that some patients with painful diverticular disease experience partial and temporary colonic obstruction with abdominal distension relieved by the passage of large quantities of flatus. Presumably this type of obstruction is based upon excessive segmentation in the sigmoid colon rather than a permanent narrowing of the colon.

Occasionally, patients present with more obvious mechanical obstruction to the colon or small bowel. In the latter instance, laparotomy will show the adhesion of loops of small bowel to an inflamed sigmoid colon and an adhesiotomy is probably all that is required. Where there is sufficient fibrosis or peridiverticulitis in the colon to have produced an obstruction, it would seem logical to manage these patients by sigmoid resection and primary anastomosis. The need for a covering right transverse colostomy will depend upon individual circumstances.

Caecal or Right-sided Diverticula

Careful examination of the colon with left-sided diverticulosis reveals that about 30% of patients have single or multiple diverticula on the right side. Diverticulosis of the right colon is normally asymptomatic, though the main complication of this condition is haemorrhage, melaena being the presenting symptom. Solitary diverticulum of the caecum may also be an incidental finding on barium enema or laparotomy but may on occasions become inflamed and closely mimic acute appendicitis or cholecystitis. Almost all patients will be diagnosed as appendicitis and the condition only becomes apparent at operation. Some patients develop an inflammatory mass in the right iliac fossa and this may be mistaken for carcinoma of caecum or ascending colon. Where an abscess is present, it should be drained and an interval diverticulectomy performed. If the diverticulum is discovered incidentally at operation it may be invaginated by a purse-string suture.

VASCULAR LESIONS OF THE COLON

Vascular lesions of the colon may be categorized into three groups:

1. Ischaemic disease of the large bowel.
2. Aneurysms in vessels supplying the colon.
3. Angiodysplastic lesions of the colon.

1. Ischaemic Diseases of the Large Bowel

Ischaemic disorders of the colon represent the most common of the vascular abnormalities of the large intestine. The multiple causes of colonic ischaemia are listed in *Table* 74.1. In general, ischaemia of the colon is caused by insufficient

Table 74.1 Causes of ischaemic colitis

Thrombosis—arterial or venous
Arteriosclerosis
Polycythaemia vera
Portal hypertension
Malignant disease of the colon
Hyperviscosity syndrome due to—
platelet abnormalities
high molecular weight dextran infusion
Emboli from
Left atrium (atrial fibrillation)
Left ventricle (myocardial infarction)
Atheromatous plaque in aorta
Vasculitis
Polyarteritis nodosa
Lupus erythematosus
Giant-cell arteritis (Takayasu's arteritis)
Buerger's disease
Henoch–Schönlein disease
Surgical trauma to vessels
Aortic reconstruction
Resection of adjacent intestine
Non-occlusive ischaemia
Shock—hypovolaemic or septic
Congestive heart failure
'Spontaneous' ischaemic colitis

flow through splanchnic vessels due to thrombosis or embolus. Thrombosis of arteries to the colon is usually due to progressive narrowing of the vessel by atherosclerosis and may be accompanied by the development of significant collateral blood flow. In contrast, embolic occlusion of colonic vessels is usually sudden and not associated with adequate collateral flow. In some cases ischaemia occurs in the absence of occlusive disease, but in the presence of associated conditions, such as cardiac arrhythmia, shock or congestive heart failure. Various vasculitides may be responsible for the interruption of sufficient flow to regional areas of the colon. Blood flow to the colon may be interrupted during the course of an operation on an adjacent organ, notably during aortic reconstruction, it is very rare that ligation of the inferior mesenteric artery at the aorta will lead to colonic ischaemia.

Considering the several possible aetiological factors responsible for ischaemic disease of the large bowel, it is not surprising that the ischaemia may vary in severity and there may be a wide spectrum of clinical presentations. Three distinct clinical patterns have been identified in patients with colonic ischaemia—the gangrenous, the transient and the stricturing forms. The gangrenous form is the most dramatic and the colonic infarction is usually caused by sudden occlusion of the major colic arteries in the presence of poor collateral circulation. However, no mechanical obstruction of the vascular tree is found on arteriography in a significant proportion of patients. It may also be a terminal event in patients with generalized circulatory collapse. The patient is almost always elderly and gives a history of the acute onset of intense abdominal pain (usually on the left side) accompanied by haematochezia or bloody diarrhoea. On physical examination the patient is obviously ill and the abdomen is usually extremely tender. The differential diagnosis includes diverticulitis, toxic megacolon, volvulus or perforation of the colon. Abdominal radiographs in patients with colonic infarction may show a blending of the mucosal folds, pneumatosis coli and, occasionally, air in the portal venous system. Appropriate management consists of fluid resuscitation, broad-spectrum antibiotic coverage and an early operation with resection of the infarcted segment. The mortality from this disease is usually high because of the patient's advanced age, debilitated state and gross contamination of the peritoneal cavity.

A second, less dramatic, form of the disease is more common and is characterized by ischaemic damage which is confined to mucosa and submucosa. These patients often have progressive occlusive disease of the major blood vessels supplying the colon and have developed sufficient collateral blood supply to maintain viability of the colon. The patients are middle-aged and they may have evidence of peripheral vascular disease. A history of abdominal pain of several days' duration is usually obtained and bleeding per rectum, either obvious or occult, is almost invariable. Physical examination reveals mild to moderate abdominal tenderness and proctoscopy demonstrates bleeding from above the level of the proctoscope. The disease occurs most commonly in the splenic flexure. Some patients with vasculitis or small emboli to the vascular arcades of the colon will develop a similar ischaemic pattern. Diagnosis of this type of ischaemia is often made radiographically. The common radiographic findings in ischaemic colitis are 'thumb printing', picket fence thickening of folds, and sacculation. Thumb printing consists of multiple impressions of air or barium column on the colon or ileum (*Fig.* 74.10). This can take the appearance of multiple polypoid defects if seen on end. Thumb printing is due to submucosal oedema and haemorrhage. Arteriography seldom reveals complete occlusion of a major vessel. Therapy consists of general support measures, including bowel rest and provision for adequate parenteral nutrition. In most patients the symptoms and prominent radiographic findings will resolve with time; however, these patients warrant close monitoring, as infarction of the colon may ensue.

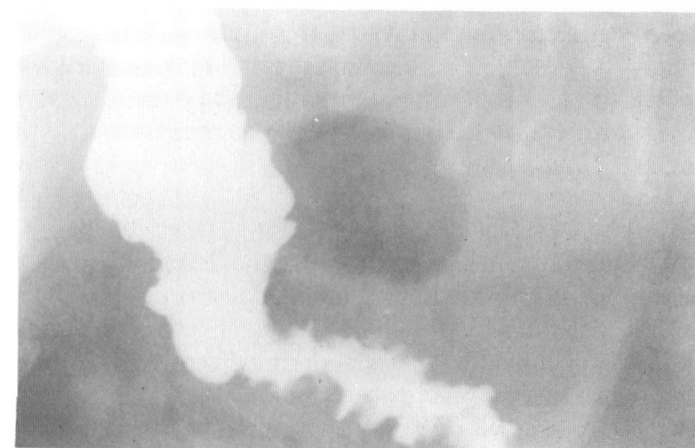

Fig. 74.10 A barium enema examination of the sigmoid colon affected by ischaemic colitis with the characteristic thumb printing pattern.

A third clinical presentation represents an entity intermediate in severity between these two extremes. Histologically, there is damage to the underlying muscularis propria of the bowel in addition to mucosal and submucosal lesions. The colon is not infarcted but sufficient interruption of blood flow results in moderately severe changes in the bowel wall. Patients usually present with severe abdominal pain and haematochezia. On physical examination, they have moderate tenderness. This group of patients also warrant close monitoring as infarction may develop. If this does occur, these patients often develop late stricture of the bowel which ultimately requires resection and can be confused, radiologically and at laparotomy, with a stenosing carcinoma.

2. Aneurysms in Vessels Supplying the Colon

Aneurysms of the visceral arteries are being detected with increasing frequency due to the more frequent use of abdominal angiography. Recent series have shown that nearly half the visceral artery aneurysms detected involve the splenic artery. Less commonly, aneurysms occur in decreasing order of frequency in the renal, hepatic and cystic arteries. In a large series of over 1000 visceral artery aneurysms the superior mesenteric artery and its branches were involved in less than 10%. Aneurysms of the colic arteries *per se* are even less common. The various factors responsible for visceral artery arterial aneurysms include: congenital, arteriosclerotic, mycotic, traumatic, luetic, medial degeneration and forms of arteritis. Aneurysms of the splenic artery are most often caused by medial degeneration whereas those of the superior mesenteric artery are most frequently mycotic. There has not been a sufficient number of colic artery aneurysms identified to make a definitive statement about a common aetiology. Although aneurysms of the colic arteries are infrequently detected, they may rupture. Rupture of visceral artery aneurysms was originally termed 'abdominal apoplexy'. The diagnosis is suggested by severe abdominal pain and signs of internal haemorrhage, especially in the presence of predisposing factors such as arteriosclerosis, hypertension or, in the case of splenic artery aneurysms, pregnancy. Arteriography is helpful in these patients and successful treatment of ruptured visceral artery aneurysms is dependent upon prompt operative intervention.

3. Vascular Ectasias of the Colon

Since angiomatous lesions of the bowel were first identified by operative angiography in 1960, the number of reported cases of such lesions in the colon has grown rapidly. Vascular lesions of the large bowel characteristically occur in patients over the age of 60 and are not associated with other angiomatous lesions of other viscera or of the skin, produce anaemia from chronic blood loss or rapid lower gastrointestinal bleeding, and can usually be diagnosed only by arteriography. The lesions are commonly small, are rarely identifiable at operation, and they almost always occur in the caecum or proximal right colon. These lesions have been called angiodysplasias, angiomas, haemangiomas, arteriovenous malformations, or vascular ectasias. The possible causes frequently cited for these lesions include congenital, neoplastic or acquired. In patients in whom the diagnosis of vascular ectasia of the colon is entertained, a careful search must be made for the stigmata of familial syndromes such as Rendu–Osler–Weber disease. Some authorities believe that vascular ectasias of the colon are acquired and are the result of chronic, partial, intermittent, low-grade obstruction of the submucosal veins. The disease is most common in the right colon, according to these authors, because the diameter of the colon is largest at that point where the Laplace relationship would dictate that the tension in the bowel wall would be greatest. Twenty per cent correlation is found with aortic stenosis in patients who were known to have vascular ectasias of the right colon.

Microaneurysms in the colonic submucosa, which result in intraluminal bleeding, are seen in patients with collagen disorders, particularly those patients who are surviving on renal failure programmes.

Detection of these lesions is largely dependent upon angiography and colonoscopy. As mentioned, the lesions are rarely demonstrable at time of operation. Magnification by visceral angiography has increased the reliability of preoperative localization. Characteristically, an early draining vein is identified parallel to the feeding artery. In the patient with chronic gastrointestinal haemorrhage in whom conventional radiographic procedures have not yielded a diagnosis, mesenteric angiography should be considered. When sophisticated equipment and expert angiographers are available selective vasopressin infusion or transcatheter embolization with Gelfoam may stop major haemorrhage. A limited right hemicolectomy or colonoscopic electrocoagulation are alternative methods of curing the disease. Although there are no reliable estimates of the frequency of this disease, it is possible that many cases of so-called right-sided diverticulosis leading to haemorrhage are vascular ectasias of the colon rather than diverticular disease. At laparotomy, the use of intraoperative transillumination of the bowel (with all other operating room lights switched off), or of the Doppler may help in localizing a vascular malformation and thus confine the bowel resection to a limited area. However, as the lesions are often multiple, it seems safer to perform a formal hemicolectomy.

POLYPS IN THE COLON AND RECTUM

The colonic mucosa is now recognized to be a highly active epithelial lining which is subjected to a prolonged exposure to a wide variety of environmental stimuli. Constant replenishment of the epithelial surface by cell division in the colonic crypts can be demonstrated in a number of ways including thymidine labelling. There are marked differences between the ascending colon and transverse colon when compared with the sigmoid colon and rectum which are consistent with a greater incidence of neoplasia on the left side of the colon. Mucosa adjacent to polyps shows a highly significant increase in thymidine labelling and in a broadening of the proliferative compartments within the crypts with an extension of proliferation towards the luminal surface. These widespread mucosal changes go some way to explain the occurrence of synchronous and metachronous neoplasms. Similar changes in the crypt cellular kinetics are found in patients with chronic ulcerative colitis.

By definition a polyp can be described as a swelling arising from the colonic mucosa on a single pedicle or stalk. This single anatomical definition covers a wide spectrum of pathological conditions, some of which may be important in the aetiology of malignant disease of the colon and rectum.

1. Inflammatory polyps occur in patients suffering from ulcerative colitis, Crohn's disease of the colon, diverticulitis, chronic dysentery and, rarely, benign lymphomatous lesions of the colon. Somewhat inaccurately this type of polyp is labelled a pseudopolyp, for it commonly exists as an island of hypertrophied mucosa in an area of inflammation and ulceration. The lesions are small, rarely exceeding 0·5 mm in diameter, and consist of inflamed congested mucosa with similar oedematous changes in the submucosa.

2. Hamartomatous polyps are found in two forms: as juvenile polyps and a familial condition, the Peutz–Jeghers syndrome. The juvenile polyps are found in infants or children and are often multiple, being round or oval with a

smooth surface. At the time of diagnosis most lesions are pedunculated with a transition from normal colonic mucosa to a type of glandular tissue at the junction of stalk and polyp. The polypoidal substance consists of vascular tissue infiltrated with inflammatory cells and contains cystic spaces maintained by mucus-secreting columnar cells.

There is a familial tendency in juvenile polyposis with the majority of patients presenting before 10 years, male children predominating over female. Fortunately they are single in 70% and since most occur in the rectum and lower sigmoid, 70% are within reach of the rigid sigmoidoscope.

The polyps occurring in the Peutz–Jeghers syndrome are associated with pigmented lesions (a bluish-brown discoloration) on the face and on the lingual and buccal mucosa. The familial tendency is very strong. The polyps are almost always multiple and are found more commonly in the small bowel than in the colon or stomach. On histological examination the basic malformation lies in the muscularis mucosae. Unlike juvenile polyposis, there is a significant malignant potential and there are many reports of carcinoma arising in these young patients.

3. Metaplastic polyps are generally plaque-like excrescences which vary in size from 1 to 2 mm but are rarely above 5 mm. Though most commonly found in the rectum, the whole colon is susceptible. There is no specific age pattern. On histological examination there appears to be lengthening of the mucosal glands with dilatation of the goblet cells and evidence of inflammatory infiltration in the lamina propria. It is not clear why these lesions arise but they rarely produce symptoms and are not premalignant. Normally biopsy will allow the diagnosis to be made and all that is required is observation.

4. Adenoma and villous papillomas are important because of their premalignant potential and their possible role in the pathogenesis of colorectal cancer. Adenomatous polyps vary in size from a split pea to 7 cm in diameter. Small lesions appear to be the same colour as colonic mucosa but as the lesion enlarges the colour tends to darken and appears more vascular. There is always a tendency to acquire a stalk, presumably as a result of the passage of faecal material; the stalk consists of normal colonic mucosa (*Fig.* 74.11).

Villous papillomas are usually sessile, 3–7 cm in diameter and may expand in a carpet-like fashion around the lumen of the bowel and both proximally and distally (*Fig.* 74.12). Whereas adenomatous polyps appear smooth and lobulated, villous papillomas demonstrate a coarse granularity.

Histologically, adenomatous polyps consist of closely-packed gland tubules with varying degrees of differentiation. The closer the lesion is to the anal canal, the more dedifferentiated the polyp is likely to be. Similarly male patients are more likely to show disturbing histology than females. Villous papillomas, on the other hand, seem to be covered by a single layer of colonic mucosa which may also show changes of carcinomatous degeneration. Careful and full examination often shows both types of histological picture. Such polyps should be described as tubulo-villous or villo-tubular depending upon predominant type.

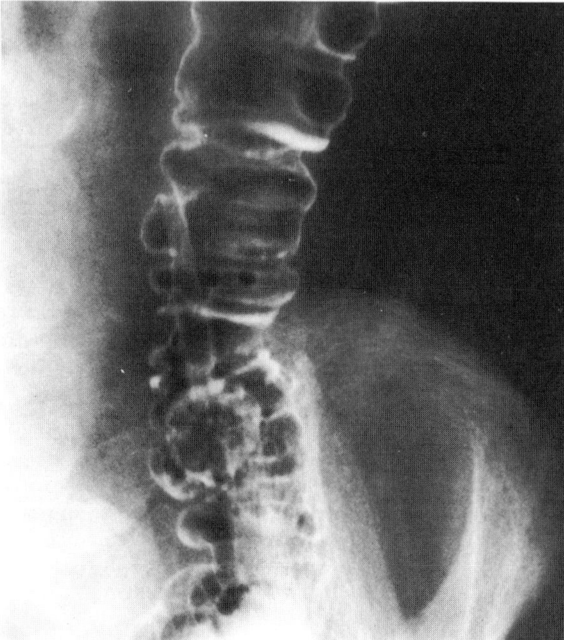

Fig. 74.11 This double contrast barium enema shows a polyp 2 cm in diameter on an extended stalk. It was treated by diathermy snaring through a colonoscope.

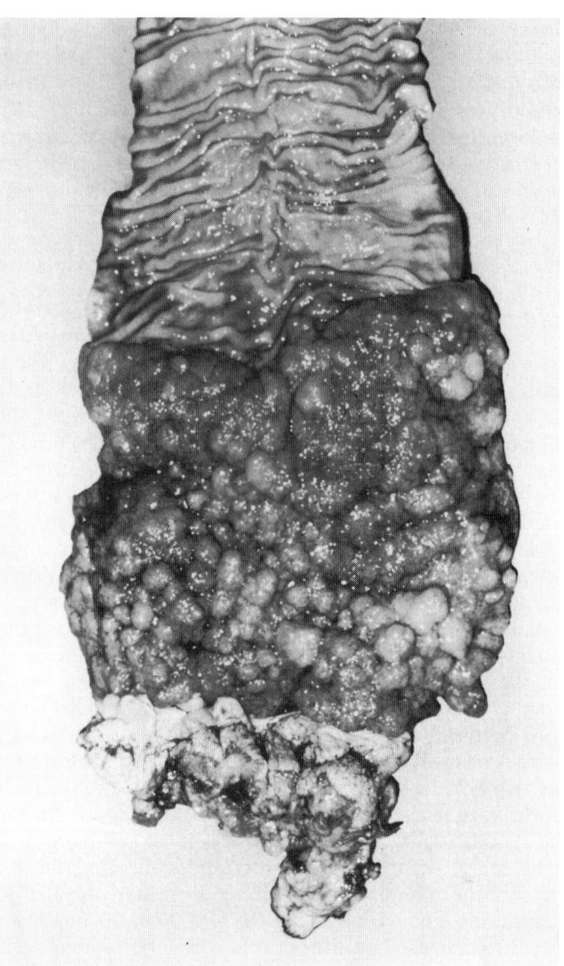

Fig. 74.12 Extensive carpet villous papilloma of the rectum. This patient presented in acute renal failure due to the severe fluid and electrolyte loss.

Incidence

About 85% of these lesions are adenomatous and 15% villous. Whereas nearly 70% of adenomas are pedunculated, 90% of villous lesions are sessile. The frequency of distribution in the colon is similar to that for cancer (*Fig.* 74.13). Villous papillomas are almost always single whereas adenomatous polyps are multiple in 17% of patients. If they coexist with colorectal carcinoma, over 30% are multiple. Although no age is excluded, the average age of diagnosis is about 60 years, with adenomatous polyps slightly predominating in males and villous papillomas in females.

Clinical Features

Most polypoidal lesions are asymptomatic and the diagnosis may be made on routine examination (2–6% of individuals). Nevertheless, occult bleeding does occur and the frequency of diagnosis of these lesions may increase with the development of haemoccult screening programmes. Frank bleeding also occurs, particularly with the larger adenomatous polyps. Occasionally, such polyps are extruded from the anal canal and may be misdiagnosed by patient and doctor as prolapsing haemorrhoids. The retrograde propulsion of larger pedunculated polyps may produce abdominal pain through spasm and colic and lead to the development of colocolic intussusception. Rectal lesions are often accompanied by tenesmus and a change in bowel habit to diarrhoea. This may be the result of mucoid discharge from the surface of the polyps. This feature is particularly common with villous papilloma where spurious diarrhoea from the abundance of mucus leads to a failure of general health, dehydration and electrolyte disturbance. In the mucus, sodium and chloride concentrations are similar to plasma but potassium concentrations are between 3 and 20 times greater. In larger papillomas, hypokalaemia and metabolic acidosis may result in lethargy, muscle weakness, mental confusion and, exceptionally, in renal failure. These metabolic disturbances require full compensation prior to any attempt at surgical treatment.

Diagnosis

Most polyps arising in the rectum and lower sigmoid colon are diagnosed on rectal and sigmoidoscopic examinations. Biopsy is not difficult and should be multiple on the more extensive villous lesions. With the increasing use of double-contrast barium enema the diagnosis of polypoidal lesions will increase. This examination should probably precede full colonoscopic examination for safety reasons. In appearance the softer, shaggy or coarsely granular polyps are likely to be villous papillomas. In the older patient, induration, increased vascularity, ulceration and an altered histological picture should warn of malignant change.

Relationship to Carcinoma of Colon and Rectum

The hypothesis is widely held that the pathogenesis of colorectal carcinoma is closely linked to the development of polyps. It is proposed that a genetic propensity to develop polyps is combined with an environmental carcinogenic factor to result in a higher incidence of colorectal cancer. There is considerable epidemiological evidence to support this view. Furthermore, once a polyp has been treated, about 40% of patients go on and develop further polyps. At routine autopsies colorectal polyps have been found in 4–10% of individuals. However, where the patient has had a colorectal cancer, the incidence rises to 30%. The distribution and frequency of polyps and cancer are similar and they commonly are associated. Patients with colonic polyps are more prone to develop colorectal cancer and patients with coexisting polyps and cancer are more likely to develop metachronous cancers. The condition of familial polyposis clearly illustrates this point (*vide infra*).

On histological examination there may be a transitional change from benign to a malignant mucosa, though it is difficult to evaluate the importance of this finding unless the muscularis mucosa is invaded. Overall about 3% of adenomatous polyps are malignant but this figure rises to 31% for villous papillomas. Presumed prolonged contact with the

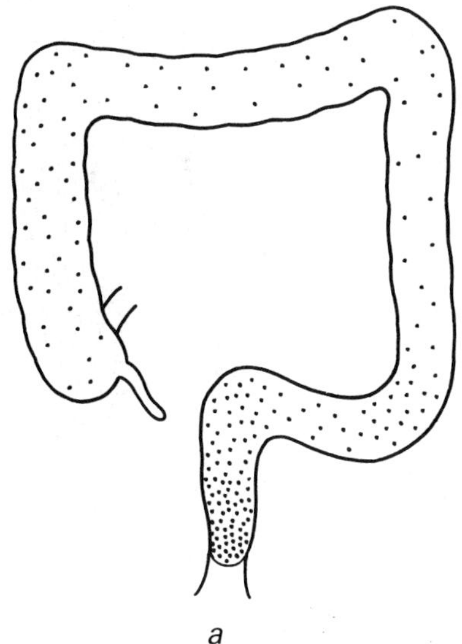

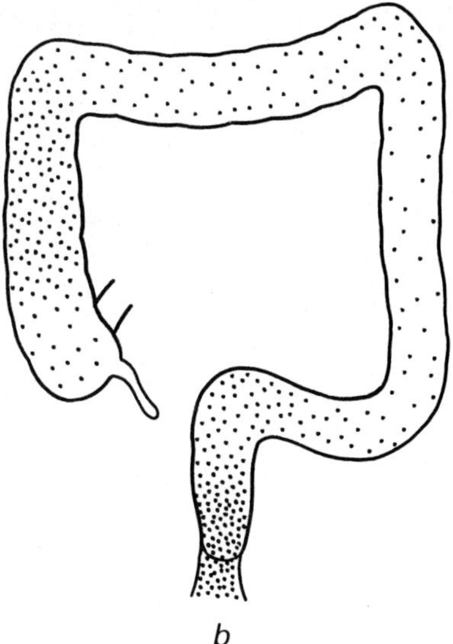

Fig. 74.13 *a*, Demonstrates the distribution of colorectal polyps within the organ, showing a high preponderance in the rectum and sigmoid colon which account for 80% of the total. *b*, Shows the distribution of colorectal cancer within the organ, again showing a higher preponderance within the retrosigmoid region but it should be noted that 22% of colorectal cancers can be found in the right colon.

carcinogen is illustrated by the increased frequency of malignant change in relation to the polyp size.

Size (mm)	*Malignant change (%)*
<0·5	<1·0
10–19	5·0
20–24	9·0
>25	14

In presenting a specimen to the pathologist it is important that it should be complete so that the full malignant potential can be estimated. This is particularly important in specimens which show features of both villous and adenomatous polyps. As much as possible of the stalk should be examined, for much store is laid by the feature of infiltration of this structure.

Familial Polyposis

This condition, first described a century ago by Cripps, is a hereditary disorder in which multiple adenomatous polyps develop in the colon (rarely elsewhere in the gastrointestinal tract). The polyps may be small sessile lesions or pedunculated and may number hundreds. All the polyps are at first non-malignant but after a variable period carcinomatous change will develop either in the polyp itself or in the adjacent mucosa.

The natural history of this condition and its hereditary nature has been well described by Dukes and appears to be transmitted in accordance with the inheritance of a dominant gene. It follows that the condition affects half the offspring and it will be transmitted only by the sufferers of this condition. The tendency is not sex-linked and both male and females are equally affected. Examination of the colorectum at birth shows the bowel to be free of polyposis and it appears that the condition develops at puberty. Certainly this is the time when symptoms are likely to develop. Carcinomatous change is diagnosed on average about 15 years after the development of the polyps and commonly occurs therefore from the age of 30 years onwards.

Coexistent with colonic polyposis, a number of patients have multiple epidermoid cysts or dermoids, connective tissue tumours or bony exostoses. This association is described as Gardner's syndrome and occurs in about 10% of polyposis patients. Normally these lesions are not premalignant though rarely sarcomas have been found. The osteomas are found commonly in the flat bones of the skull and mandible. Interestingly the soft-tissue lesions may precede the development of polyposis, and the occurrence of an epidermoid cyst in a child should raise the suspicion of colonic polyposis. It is now recognized that familial polyposis is associated with polyps in the stomach, duodenum and small bowel and more rarely with periampullary carcinoma and malignant tumours of the CNS.

Symptoms

Initially there are no symptoms from the polyps. Thereafter there may be a slight looseness of bowels and frequency increases but eventually this increases in severity and is accompanied by the passage of blood and mucus.

The diagnosis is made by rectal and sigmoidoscopic examination which differentiates between non-specific proctocolitis and colonic polyposis. On sigmoidoscopy, multiple adenomatous polyps can be seen with a normal intervening mucosa. Barium enema with double-contrast technique and colonoscopy may confirm the widespread extent of the condition (*Fig.* 74.14).

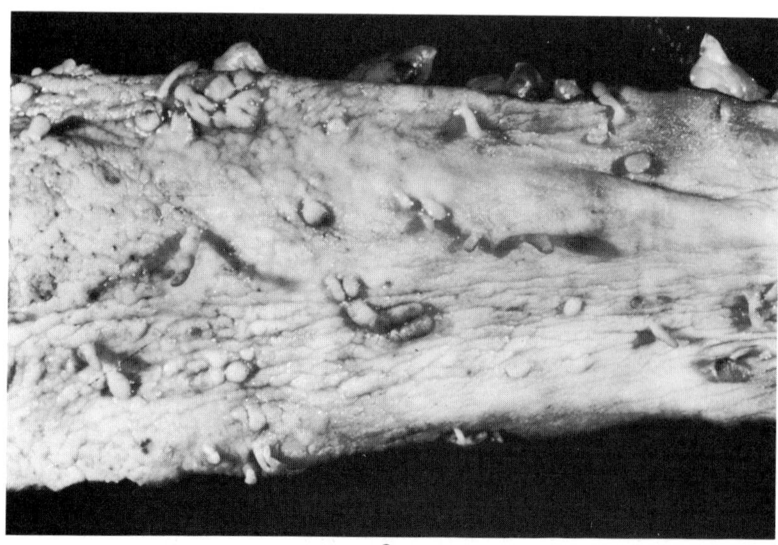

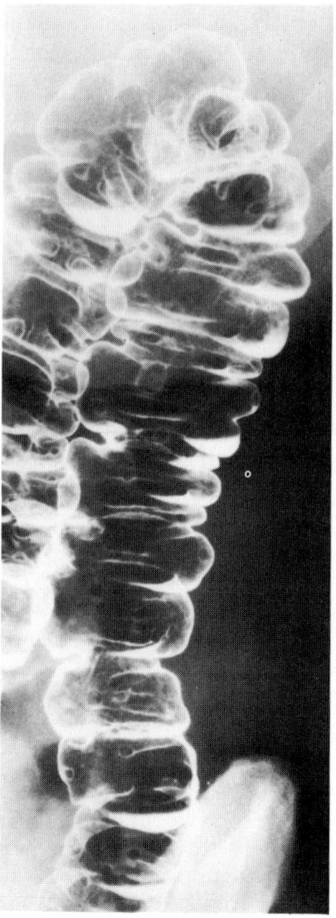

Fig. 74.14 *a,* The excised specimen of a patient with multiple polyps with familial polyposis. *b,* The barium enema examination from the same patient demonstrates the widespread nature of the sessile polyps. The colon was removed from a 17-year-old patient. None of the polyps had undergone malignant change.

Treatment of Colorectal Polyps and Villous Papillomas

Since there appears to be a definite malignant potential to colorectal polyps, there is a strong indication for removal of all lesions. The exception will be poor risk patients with small polyps, the progression of which may be documented by barium enema examination every 6–12 months or by repeated colonoscopy.

Pedunculated polyps in the lower rectum may be delivered through the anal canal and transfixed using Goodsall's sutures (*Fig.* 74.15). Rectal polyps up to 12–15 cm from the anal verge may be safely removed by diathermy snaring or coagulation using a wide bore rigid sigmoidoscope. Above this level, a safer instrument is the fibreoptic sigmoidoscope using carbon dioxide insufflation and insulated snares. By these means, most adenomas can be safely removed by snaring the pedicle or by piecemeal snaring of large sessile polyps (*Fig.* 74.16). This technique has reduced the need for polypectomy by open colotomy provided, of course, that an expert colonoscopist is available. Open colotomy is usually made with a sterile rigid sigmoidoscope and enables the polyps to be localized and removed by suture of the stalks. Frozen section is recommended in case malignant change has already occurred. In such an event a segmental colectomy is indicated, removing 12–15 cm. This operation is also indicated for large or clusters of small sessile polyps.

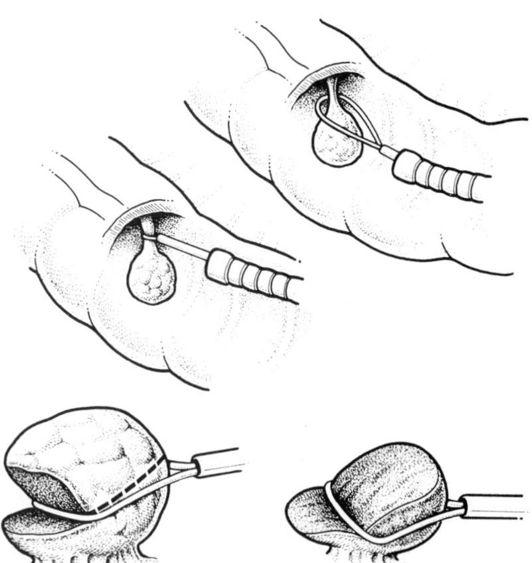

Fig. 74.16 Removal of colonic polyps by endoscopy is relatively simple when the polyp is pedunculated and can be snared. When the polyp is sessile the electrocautery may cut the lesion down to its base by taking several pieces.

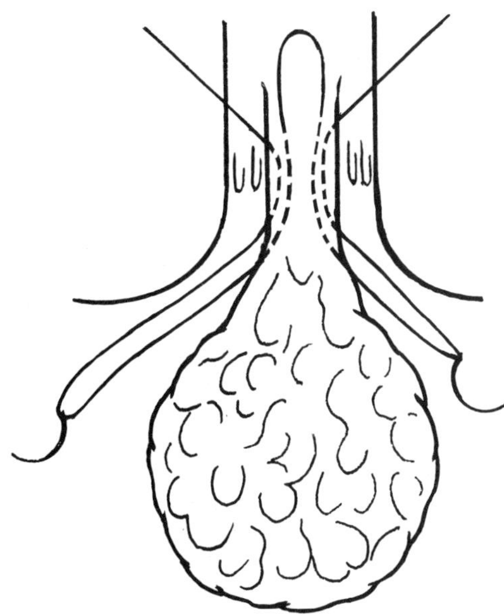

Fig. 74.15 Showing Goodsall's ligature for controlling haemorrhage from the stalk of a polyp in the lower rectum.

Patients with familial polyposis present a different problem and the polyps are far too numerous to be removed by colonoscopic means. In these patients, removal of the colon and rectum would seem a satisfactory solution. Since the operation has to be recommended at an age before malignant change has taken place, few patients at this age (15–25 years), often with minimal symptoms, will accept this treatment. Most patients will undergo a subtotal colectomy with an ileorectal anastomosis at the sacral promontory. The coexisting rectal polyps are dealt with by repeated diathermy at 6-monthly intervals. In the subsequent follow-up the development of rectal cancer has been reported to vary in incidence: 4% at St Mark's Hospital, London; however, there are reports of cancer incidence as high as 25% at 15 years' follow-up and 59% at 23 years' follow-up. In view of this incidence some surgeons appear to prefer proctocolectomy, although it seems more appropriate that mucosal proctectomy be performed after which an ileoanal pouch can be constructed (Chapter 73). An additional hazard in patients with Gardner's syndrome is the development of abdominal wall or intra-abdominal desmoids which may produce fatal obstruction of the intestinal and urinary tract.

Villous papillomas may require a somewhat different approach because of their broader base and tendency to have undergone malignant change in one or more areas. However, when situated in the lower rectum they may be removed by diathermy snaring or stalk ligation as in the case of adenomas. Normally the broader base of the lesion makes this difficult and coagulation with the diathermy button electrode over 2 or 3 sessions may be more appropriate. There are alternative techniques which enable surgical excision of these lesions provided that malignant change has not occurred. Either by a transanal approach using a large speculum, a combined abdomino-anal approach or the trans-sphincteric approach described by Yorke Mason, the mucosa around and beneath the papilloma is elevated using a very dilute solution of adrenaline. The lesion is excised with a cuff of 1–1·5 cm of normal mucosa. If the defect is small and occurs in less than half the circumference of the rectum it may be left to granulate. More extensive dissection requires approximation of the cut edges of mucosa or occasionally a pull-through of the colonic stump to the anal margin.

Where there is induration in the papilloma, malignancy should be expected. This finding and lesions which are very extensive may be best managed by a normal colonic or rectal resection in the form of anterior resection or abdomino-perineal excision of the rectum (*see Fig.* 74.20).

With the widespread availability of colonoscopy and polypectomy, there is potentially a chance that cancer will be detected early or even prevented by these means. It is not clear how often a patient should be examined after colonic polypectomy. A routine biannual colonoscopy will generate an enormous workload.

Management of Malignant Polyps

If after the local removal of the adenomatous polyp or villous papilloma, subsequent histological examination shows malignancy, further treatment may be necessary. If the report is of carcinoma-in-situ or cellular atypia, no further action is necessary other than follow-up. However, frank infiltrating carcinoma requires radical excision of the segment of colon and rectum together with the area of lymphatic drainage. This is particularly so when the differentiation is poor. With pedunculated polyps much stress is laid on the degree of malignant infiltration into the stalk and where this has reached the level of surrounding mucosa residual disease should be expected.

In very elderly and chronic sick patients with malignant rectal polyps, the choice may be diathermy fulguration of the polyp base followed by regular sigmoidoscopic examination, rather than risk rectal excision.

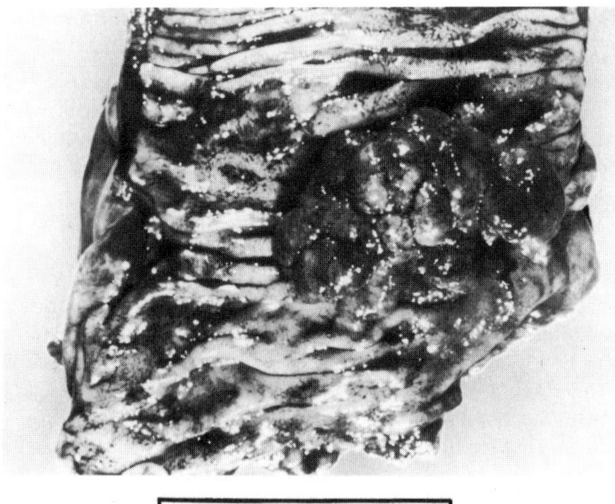

Fig. 74.17 This polypoidal cancer was situated in the sigmoid colon and presented with the passage of bright red blood per rectum.

CARCINOMA OF THE COLON AND RECTUM

There are about 17 000 deaths annually in the UK from this disease, of which about 40–45% originate in the rectum. There may be a slight decline in the prevalence of rectal cancer and a slight increase in right-sided colonic cancer; more clearly defined in the USA. Colonic cancer deaths are more frequent in women than men (11:7) but death from rectal cancer is slightly more frequent in men (6:5). No age group seems completely immune to the risk of colorectal cancer but it occurs more commonly over the age of 60 years (50% of patients) and maximally in the decade 60–69 years. About 5% of patients are under 30 years old; this may reflect familial cancer tendency or the earlier occurrence of cancer in patients with familial colonic polyposis.

The distribution of colorectal cancer is depicted in *Fig.* 74.13*b*. It will be seen that about 70% of cases occur within reach of the 50-cm flexible sigmoidoscope. By definition, rectal cancers are situated within 15 cm of the anal verge. Slightly more cancers originate in the upper and lower thirds than in the mid-rectum. Slightly more cases occur below the peritoneal reflection than above it and possibly more originate on the posterior wall of the rectum.

Pathology

At the onset the carcinoma may appear as an indurated plaque, hard nodule, or a local thickening. However, some lesions are polypoidal from the beginning. Once established the carcinomas are of five patterns:

1. Polypoidal—possibly the majority of lesions are of this form initially (*Fig.* 74.17)—As an established carcinoma, there is a tendency to infiltrate less than other forms. Carcinomas in the right colon often adopt an exaggerated cauliflower polypoidal shape.
2. Ulcerative—with the characteristic raised everted edges a variable degree of infiltration occurs into the bowel wall and a tendency to transverse extension around the bowel lumen is apparent.
3. Annular—implies that the carcinoma encompasses the whole circumference of the bowel. When situated in the colon, the cancer is fairly narrow and produces a tight constriction liable to cause complete intestinal obstruction. Similar annular carcinomas in the rectum are larger and often 5 cm or more in length.
4. Diffuse—this is the equivalent of linitis plastica of gastric cancer, the carcinoma extending widely through the muscle coats leaving the mucosal surface largely intact. Typical lesions are found in carcinoma developing in association with ulcerative colitis.
5. Colloidal—a rarer form with a gelatinous appearance due to excess mucus formation.

On histological examination there is a wide spectrum of differentiation from the original colonic mucosa. *Table* 74.2 illustrates the histological features which both Broder and Dukes were able to relate directly to pathological spread and prognosis.

Table 74.2 Classifications of grades of malignancy in colorectal cancer

Broder		*Dukes*
Grade I	Active epithelial proliferation with infiltration of muscularis mucosae—resembling an adenoma	Low-grade malignancy
Grade II	Crowded cells with regular arrangement, frequent mitoses	Average-grade malignancy
Grade III	Less differentiated with increased mitoses, crowded in irregular rings	High-grade malignancy
Grade IV	Anaplastic with no glandular arrangement; evidence of deep invasion with columns of cells	

A fifth histological type is seen in 12% of cancers with an increased amount of mucus formation and these are designated mucoid carcinoma. Permeation of the primary tumour by small cells of the lymphoid series is thought to be of prognostic significance, improvement being related to the increased numbers of lymphocytes.

Pathological spread occurs in a variety of ways with locally advanced cancers being more commonly associated with distant metastases.

1. Direct spread through the bowel wall: Spread is probably via lymphatic channels, particularly in the transverse axis and leads to annular growths. More importantly for the surgeon, spread also occurs in the longitudinal axis though this is rarely more than 15–20 mm from the edge of the growth. Anaplastic lesions are more prone to spread extensively in this direction. Direct spreading of a more penetrating nature is maximal at the midpoint of the tumour. About 85% of growths have reached the subserosal fat by the time of excision. Having reached the serosa, further extension may occur into the adjacent abdominal wall or nearby structures such as duodenum, perirenal fat, ureter or small bowel. For sigmoid lesions the uterus and ovaries in the female and the bladder in the male are commonly invaded. Lesions on the anterior rectal wall appear to be unrestricted by the thin fascia of Denonvilliers and readily penetrate the seminal vesicles, prostate and in the female the posterior wall of the vagina. Penetration of the posterior wall of rectum is partly contained to a well-defined pad of fat and lymphatic tissue by the strong fascia of Waldeyer. Careful removal of this tissue contained within its fascia constraints is a definite step in rectal excision for carcinoma.

2. Lymphatic spread: The frequency of lymph-node metastases can be directly related to the degree of penetration and the histological grade of malignancy but not to the size of the primary cancer. It is very unlikely that lymph nodes will be involved where the tumour has failed to penetrate the muscle coat. Normally, the nodes first invaded are those in the pericolic position after which nodes lying alongside the supplying colonic blood vessels become involved; eventually the para-aortic nodes are invaded. There are conflicting reports concerning the frequency of lymph-node metastases from right- and left-sided colonic cancers, thus they probably occur with equal frequency. The design of surgical procedures, with proximal ligation and excision of the blood vessels supplying the cancer, should permit the maximum lymph-node clearance. Carcinomas of the right colon are more likely to have lymph nodes involved greater than 5 cm from the tumour and require a more radical clearance. In rectal surgery this may not be possible, for lymph nodes lying alongside the internal iliac vessels are not routinely cleared, either with abdominoperineal excision or anterior resection of the rectum, and these nodes may thus account for some local recurrences. Lymph-node metastases occur in about 50% of rectal cancers compared to 35–40% of colonic cancers and in both instances more commonly in women than men. Newer techniques involving clearing of the specimen with alcohols permit a more detailed analysis of lymph nodes and indicate that the above figures considerably underestimate the incidence of lymph node involvement.

3. Bloodstream: Direct invasion of veins draining the tumour and associated bowel segment is well described, particularly in tumours with high-grade malignancy and with lymphatic metastases. There has always been an interest in the demonstration of circulating colorectal cancer cells which may reflect this invasion. Unexpectedly, most reports have not found increased numbers of circulating tumour cells induced by surgical handling of the tumour though it is sensible to keep handling at a minimum until the vessels are ligated. The practical significance of circulating cancer cells is not clear though some surgeons have used cytotoxic drugs in the operative period in an attempt to counter their metastatic potential. Presumably all distant metastases are from such cells and liver metastases ultimately occur in 35–50% of patients. Though about 12% of patients have overt hepatic metastases at the time of operation, autopsy studies of patients dying in the perioperative period indicate that probably about 25% of patients have overt or occult metastases at the time of operation. The routine use of CT scanning of the liver and dynamic hepatic scintigraphy suggests that about a quarter of apparently normal livers contain occult secondaries.

An accurate staging of the pathological extent of the tumour may be important in defining a prognosis for an individual patient. It is also important when evaluating the effect of newer surgical procedures and additional modalities such as chemotherapy and radiotherapy upon survival. Dukes' classification was originally described for rectal cancer and is now used for all colon cancers. The scheme has been modified and may be superseded by the TNM classification for clinical trials. In clinical practice, the original Dukes' scheme or its modification is most helpful.

Clinical Features

About 75% of patients with carcinoma of the colon present with vague symptoms and chronic ill-health without specific features of colonic disease. The remaining patients present either with acute-on-chronic intestinal distension (18%) or peritonitis from intestinal perforation (6·8%). Within the larger group of patients it is possible to correlate certain clinical features with the anatomical situation of the carcinoma.

1. Carcinoma of the caecum and ascending colon. The bowel habit is unchanged or slight looseness of the stool may be apparent. Abdominal pain may result from the local infiltration of advanced lesions. Other patients complain of a flatulent type of dyspepsia and are mistakenly investigated as such. Often the patient shows weight loss, weakness and anaemia due to occult blood loss.

2. Carcinoma of the transverse colon and left colon. Commonly the lesions are annular before producing symptoms. Griping abdominal pains and abdominal fullness occur, changes in bowel habit with blood and mucus in the stool are found the closer the lesion is to the rectum. A history of increasing use of laxatives is often noted.

3. Carcinoma of the rectosigmoid and rectum. Most commonly these lesions present as the passage of blood per rectum. Diarrhoea often occurs in the early morning with tenesmus or the passage of bloodstained mucus. Local pain occurs on involvement of the anal canal or by posterior infiltration into the sacral plexus. Anterior infiltration into the vagina may eventually lead to fistula formation.

The diagnosis of carcinoma of the colon or rectum should be entertained for all patients (middle-aged and above) presenting with atypical dyspepsia. Similarly a change in bowel habit for more than 2–3 weeks in patients over the age of 40 years or rectal bleeding should always be investigated.

The clinical examination should take particular note of anaemia, weight loss, abdominal and caecal distension. An abdominal mass may be detected and may represent a tumour or impacted faeces proximal to the obstructing lesion. In advanced disease it may be possible to palpate metastatic deposits in the liver, lymph nodes or omentum. Rectal examination may reveal a tumour within the rectum as a flattened indurated disc, a friable nodular mass, a malignant ulcer or a completely annular lesion. Lesions in the rectosigmoid lesion may be palpated indirectly through the anterior rectal wall and blood may be found on the examining finger. Where a carcinoma is found in the rectum the fixity of the tumour to the vagina, bladder or sacrum can be assessed. Sigmoidoscopy and biopsy of the lesion are necessary for all rectal and rectosigmoid lesions. Increasing use of the flexible fibreoptic sigmoidoscope has allowed examination and biopsy of lesions in the sigmoid and descending colon.

It is doubtful that barium enema should be performed prior to fibresigmoidoscopy but it is safer to do so if full length colonoscopy is contemplated. The use of double-contrast radiological technique will demonstrate fully annular carcinoma with the 'apple core' appearance and in most instances show earlier lesions where the carcinoma is confined to one quadrant (*Fig.* 74.18). Lesions between 1 and 2 cm may still be missed, particularly on the right side of the colon or in areas of diverticular disease. The coexistence of suspicious symptoms with positive occult blood should encourage full colonoscopic examination.

The Promotion of Early Diagnosis

There have been several studies in the UK which indicate that the time between onset of symptoms and diagnosis averages 10 months. Various approaches have been tried to combat these delays. Rapid access to diagnostic facilities for all patients presenting with appropriate symptoms will act as a case finding survey but does not usually yield up significant numbers of patients with pathologically early cancers, nor does the use of symptom questionnaires returned by members of the general public. In fact taken at face value, over 15% of the general public over 40 years admit to symptoms which normally weigh heavily in the clinical diagnosis of colorectal cancer. Cancer detection clinics are prohibitive in cost when applied to large populations and there is now a general acceptance that colorectal cancer screening will require a simple test probably based on occult blood testing of the faeces. This approach has several disadvantages not least of which relates to the sensitivity of the agent used to detect blood in the stools. An agent too insensitive will permit one-third of established cancers to remain undetected. An agent too sensitive increases the numbers of false positive tests and results in unnecessary expensive investigations. Improvements are likely to follow the introduction of immunological agents capable of detecting only human blood products. It does not appear that the use of single serum markers such as carcinoembryonic antigen are helpful in screening nor as yet has the localization of colorectal cancers with labelled antitumour monoclonal antibody added to diagnostic criteria. However, this latter approach is promising, particularly when considering specific therapy.

Treatment

Preparation for Operation

Careful assessment of the patient's cardiovascular and respiratory system are indicated with preoperative treatment as outlined in Chapter 10. It is also prudent to perform an intravenous pyelogram in situations where the carcinoma could have locally invaded the ureters or bladder if only to give an indication of the function of the unaffected side. In many instances anaemia will require preoperative blood transfusion prior to operation and where malnutrition is apparent, there is much to be gained by a period of intensive enteral or parenteral replacement.

BOWEL PREPARATION. Where possible the colon should be mechanically cleansed of faecal matter prior to resection of the cancer. If this proves possible there appears to be a reduction in most postoperative complications including anastomotic dehiscence. The long-held reliance of oral antibiotics and cathartics appears to have been superseded by fluid preparations and prophylactic antibiotics administered during surgery.

Surgical Treatment

Normally the carcinoma is approached by a paramedian incision on the side on which the carcinoma is situated.

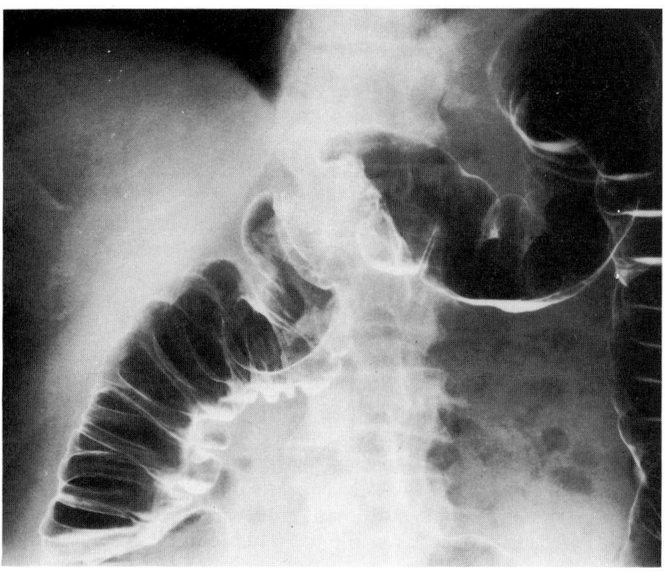

a

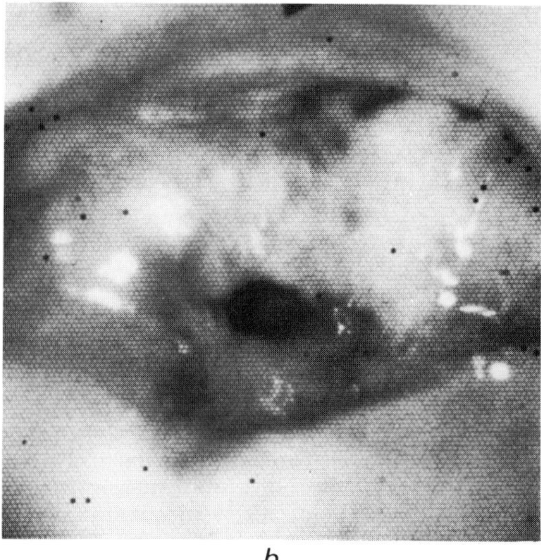

b

Fig. 74.18 *a,* A barium enema examination performed for recurrent abdominal pain shows a constricting carcinoma in the mid transverse colon with the characteristic apple-core appearance. *b,* Colonoscopic appearances of the lesion shown in the accompanying radiograph reveal an annular neoplasm with the lumen now open to only half a centimetre.

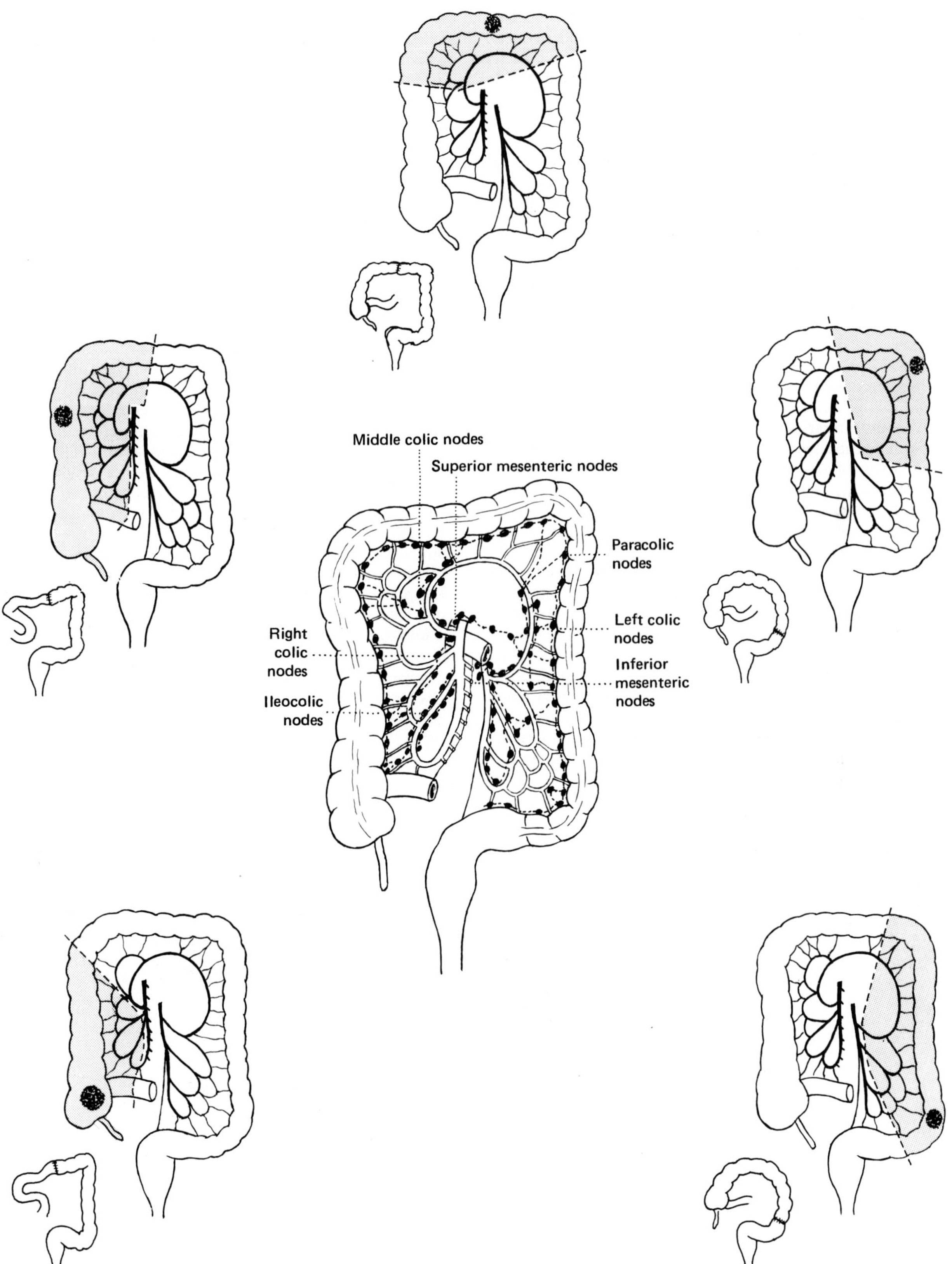

Fig. 74.19 Demonstrates the basic arterial and venous supply to the colon together with the position of the pericolic lymph nodes and lymph nodes along the major vessels. Colonic resection is based on the removal of the primary growth together with the blood supply and lymph nodes draining that particular segment of colon. End-to-end anastomosis is carried out by viable bowel which receives its blood supply from more proximal or more distal branches. The full extent of standard resection for primary cancers at the various sites are shown.

Careful laparotomy is required to detect metastatic disease and to assess resectability and operability. Whilst there is no firm evidence that the 'no touch' technique gives better survival, it is sensible not to manipulate the tumour greatly until draining vessels are ligated.

COLONIC RESECTION. The extent of colonic resection required for carcinomas at various sites is shown in *Fig.* 74.19. Normally the lines of resection follow patterns of blood vessel supply and lymphatic drainage. The divided ends of bowels are anastomosed, usually end to end, in either single or double layers of sutures or staples. End-to-side or side-to-side anastomosis has the virtue of being slightly less likely to leak but leads to the formation of intestinal blind loops in the long term.

Where there is evidence of adherent viscera, i.e. small bowel, omentum, ovaries or Fallopian tube, the lesion is removed *en bloc*, though it should be admitted that the adhesions often prove to be of an inflammatory nature rather than due to malignant infiltration. The occurrence of synchronous tumours may require more extensive colonic resection in continuity, which has the virtue of removing a large proportion of an organ which has shown the propensity for malignant field change.

The treatment of carcinoma of the rectum requires an assessment of whether the carcinoma can be removed and the anal sphincters left intact (*vide infra*).

THE SURGICAL TREATMENT OF CARCINOMA OF THE RECTUM. Carcinoma of the rectum is removed by a similar approach to that employed for colonic carcinoma. The blood supply is ligated either at the root of the inferior mesenteric artery and vein (high tie) or lower down at the origin of the superior haemorrhoidal vessels (low tie) which lie at about the aortic bifurcation (*Fig.* 74.19). In either event the object is to remove the tumour *en bloc*, with the blood vessels and accompanying lymph nodes, so that pathological staging of the specimen may be carried out. There does not appear to be any clear improvement in survival of 'high tie' operations over 'low tie'. The vessels are normally ligated above the cancer before any attempt is made to mobilize the rectum.

Carcinomas found at the level of the sacral promontory are situated at the rectosigmoid junction and are readily removed by an anterior resection (*Fig.* 74.20). Carcinomas at the pelvic peritoneal reflection lie in the midrectum. The lower edges of such lesions will lie 7–11 cm from the anal verge. Provided that an adequate margin of clearance (3 cm) can be removed below the tumour, then an attempt at a low anterior resection of the rectum is indicated. This is more readily achieved in the female patient because the pelvis permits more careful dissection and re-anastomosis. The anastomosis between the proximal cut edge of colon and lower rectum requires considerable skill and care. It should not be performed under tension and the splenic flexure of colon is usually mobilized to allow the colon to slide comfortably into the pelvis. Access to the anastomosis may be limited and formal suture in one or two layers difficult and unsatisfactory. In the past, very low resections were re-anastomosed by pull-through procedures where the top of the anal canal was everted through the anus and sutured to a colonic segment pulled through from above. The excess colon was trimmed at one week. The need for this procedure has diminished, following the reintroduction of the abdominosacral approach in which the low anastomosis is performed through an incision to the left side of the sacrum. Similarly, the use of automatic stapling devices permits the colonic segment to be drawn down onto the top of the rectal stump and by a compression device the circumferences of each are excised and stapled together (*Fig.* 74.21).

Anastomotic breakdown (10–20%) is common after anterior resection, if assessed by diodone enemas at the 10th–12th postoperative day. However, this may not show clinically. In a situation where the anastomosis at operation does not appear sound or where the colon above the anastomosis is still loaded with faecal material then a proximal transverse colostomy is safer. However, it must be stated that many experienced surgeons prefer to delay the colostomy and only perform one when an anastomotic leak develops clinically

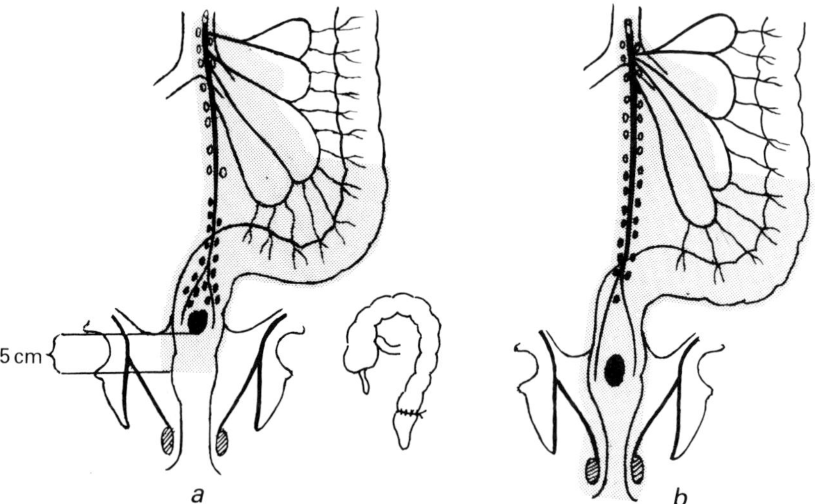

Fig. 74.20 *a*, For carcinomas above the region of about 9 cm from the anal verge (upper rectum), the neoplasm can be removed by an anterior resection with restoration of continuity via some form of end-to-end anastomotic technique. *b*, For carcinomas below the peritoneal deflection, in the mid-rectum, the ability to perform an anterior resection will be determined by the build of the patient and the degree of differentiation of the tumour. With anaplastic tumours and obese males, an abdominoperineal excision of the rectum is commonly required. The shaded area indicates the extent of resection.

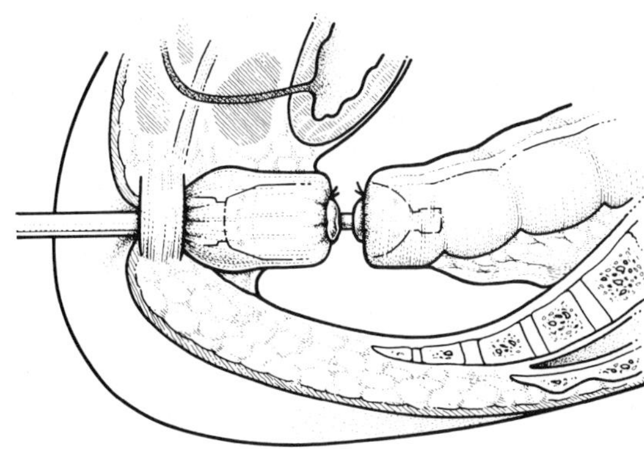

Fig. 74.21 Intestinal continuity after low anterior resection is readily achieved using a stapling device passed per anum.

and is significantly affecting a patient's progress. The decision is largely dependent upon the operator's technical experience and the particular circumstances of the case. When performed, the colostomy may be closed as soon as the anastomosis has been shown to be healed, normally 2 weeks onwards. Though this staging of procedures will delay a patient's full rehabilitation it is unquestionably safer in the hands of the trainee surgeon. On occasions a Hartmann's procedure may be performed. The indications for this procedure are found in elderly patients with advanced local and perhaps distant metastatic disease where an anastomosis will be made in an area likely to be rapidly reinfiltrated by malignant disease and where the survival time is likely to be short and thus the perineal wound of an abdominoperineal excision may be avoided.

Carcinoma of the rectum within 7 cm of the anal verge usually require an abdominoperineal excision of the rectum (*Fig.* 74.20). The anatomical dissection from the abdominal side is the same as for an anterior resection—in both instances the nodes around the internal iliac vessels are normally left intact. Given that there are now increased numbers of patients who can benefit from an anterior resection with modern approaches to a low anastomosis, the abdominal dissection is undertaken first with full rectal mobilization prior to the commencement of the perineal dissection. Very low rectal cancers can be excised by a synchronous combined procedure, provided that the pelvic cavity is not fixed from malignant infiltration. The establishment of the colostomy in the left iliac fossa requires as much care as the excisional procedure. Normally it is placed in an extraperitoneal position so as to obliterate the lateral space and mucocutaneous sutures are placed immediately. The position of the colostomy will vary slightly with the build and the sex of the patient but should not be situated too close to the iliac crest so that the colostomy appliance may sit comfortably.

Small rectal cancers in the lower rectum, particularly those which occupy less than half the circumference of the bowel and retain some polypoidal characteristics, may be excised locally. Access to these lesions may be obtained by dilatation of the anal canal and sublesional infiltration with adrenaline (1:200 000) prior to excision. For slightly higher lesions, access may be improved by the trans-sphincteric approach. Provided that the muscle wall is not totally breached and the raw area after excision does not extend around the full circumference, it is possible to leave the area to re-epithelize. More extensive lesions require that the rectal wall is pulled downwards so that a primary suture of the rectal mucosa can be accomplished. It should also be mentioned that there is considerable evidence that these small rectal cancers can be treated locally by diathermy fulguration if necessary over repeated operating sessions and by intracavitary irradiation. Local control seems at least the equivalent of more extensive procedures. Limited procedures should certainly be considered when the lesions are small and well differentiated, and when the patient is very elderly and unfit for major surgery.

Additional Treatment

The results of surgical treatment of colorectal cancer are relatively poor with failure from both distal metastases and local recurrence (*vide infra*). There is considerable interest in the use of radiotherapy and chemotherapy to counter the inadequacy of surgery alone in cancer control. The position may be summarized by stating that there is no convincing evidence to date that adjuvant radiotherapy, i.e. radiotherapy given prior to surgical excision of the rectum, materially affects long-term survival, though the Veterans Administration trial suggested that a gain of approximately 10% was achieved at 5 years in Dukes' B and C lesions. A recent study conducted under the auspices of the Medical Research Council (UK) indicates a benefit for preoperative radiotherapy (2500 R) for clinically fixed rectal cancers. Radiotherapy for colonic cancer has not been evaluated.

Similarly, the evidence that adjuvant chemotherapy effectively controls distant disease is not proven. Several control studies using single agents such as 5-FU have shown small percentage gains in 5-year survival in Dukes' C lesions but the long-term results of combination chemotherapeutic schedules are not yet available. There is no indication for the routine use of radiotherapy or chemotherapy as an adjuvant to surgery at the present time. It is probable that the future application of chemotherapy will lie in its use during the perioperative period. Portal perfusion of the liver during this period as adjuvant therapy for micrometastases is thought to improve the survival of patients with Dukes' B colonic cancer.

These treatments are, however, justifiable in dealing with painful metastatic deposits in the pelvis or liver when increased survival is not necessarily a primary aim. It is important to recognize that chemotherapy, in particular, will only be effective in a minority and failure to achieve palliation after one or two treatments is an indication to withdraw this approach.

Obstructing and Perforating Colorectal Cancer

Approximately 18% of patients with colonic cancer present with obstruction. Initial symptoms are insidious but lead to severe abdominal pain with increasing constipation. Clinical examination reveals a distended abdomen with distension and tenderness over the caecum being a disturbing feature of closed loop obstruction. Examination of the rectum may reveal ballooning and radiography of the abdomen show colonic distension and fluid levels from a point proximal to the obstructing cancer. Depending upon the completeness of the obstruction, bowel gas may be seen in the pelvic colon and rectum. Gross distension of the caecum is seen when the ileocaecal valve remains competent—closed loop obstruction.

The principles of management of colonic obstruction are considered in Chapter 75. Preoperative evaluation and correction of electrolyte and fluid disturbances are essential as is a careful assessment of cardiorespiratory and renal function in patients who are often elderly and infirm. There is some urgency in relieving the obstruction when a closed loop obstruction is present or when there is tenderness over the caecum. Laparotomy may be delayed a few hours in other patients to allow a more complete resuscitation and assessment.

At operation, it is necessary to assess the degree of infiltration of the primary tumour. Elderly patients with grossly advanced neoplasms and widespread disease may be best served by a relieving colostomy proximal to the obstruction. However, for other patients it is important that the procedure performed for cancer control should be as radical in intent whether done as an emergency or elective operation. Considerable debate remains whether left-sided colonic or rectosigmoid lesions are best dealt with by immediate resection and anastomosis or as a two-stage procedure after decompression by colostomy. There seems little doubt that in experienced hands and with selection, emergency obstruction is as successful as elective. However, in the presence of a loaded colon, some attempt to cleanse the bowel by on-table lavage seems to be required in order to minimize the incidence of anastomotic dehiscence. For the less experienced or upon finding unsatisfactory intra-abdominal conditions, there may be some advantage in performing a temporary caecostomy or transverse colostomy some 7–10 days prior to carrying out the definitive resection. Occasionally rectal cancer may produce complete obstruction, particularly in elderly patients who may be late in presenting with locally advanced lesions. An abdominoperineal resection as an emergency procedure is probably ill advised and better survival results may be found by the less radical Hartmann's procedure or delaying the major resection until the patient has stabilized after sigmoid colostomy.

Results of Treatment

It will be seen that there are many factors which affect the overall mortality of this condition. While there have been considerable improvements in the operative care offered to patients, the reported 5-year survival rate as reported by many cancer registries remains disappointingly low (20–30%). The reasons for these poor results reflect the fact that some patients with carcinoma of colon and rectum are untreated or present late with metastatic disease. It is likely that in at least 25% of patients, the carcinoma is widely disseminated by the time of diagnosis. In the remainder the prognosis can be directly related to the pathological extent of tumour spread.

The perioperative mortality has now fallen to 2–8% and is directly related to the number of palliative procedures which are included in reported series. There are few specific complications though intestinal obstruction related to adherence of the small bowel to the pelvic peritoneum and peritoneal sepsis from anastomotic breakdown should be mentioned. Patients with cancer undergoing pelvic surgery are at special risk from pulmonary embolus. Precautions to lessen the incidence of this lethal complication should be undertaken routinely, though there is as yet no strong evidence that the prophylactic use of heparin, dextrans or intermittent calf stimulation are effective in this situation.

Over the past 30 years the resectability rate of carcinoma of the colon and rectum has increased from 30% in 1949 to 95% in 1972 at specialist institutions. Clearly many of these resections will be palliative but the corrected 5-year survival rates have remained at about 40–50%.

Most reports have shown a slightly improved survival rate amongst women, about 5% greater than men. Survival rates are somewhat lower in the younger aged patient, particularly under the age of 30 years and are especially poor when the carcinoma is associated with ulcerative colitis or familial polyposis.

Certain local factors are also acting in survival statistics. Using measurement from the lower edge of the tumour to the anal verge and amalgamating published statistics, it appears that the results of curative resections (5-year survival) improve as the distance from the anal verge increases: 0–6 cm 49%; 6–10 cm 56%; 11 cm and above 66%. This is particularly relevant when the lymph nodes are found to contain metastases. There are conflicting reports concerning the influence of the site of a primary colonic neoplasm upon survival though right colonic carcinoma has an undeserved reputation for having poorer survival rates. Perhaps the only consistent feature of the collected reports in the literature is that lesions in the transverse colon, particularly at the flexures, have a poor prognosis.

Clearly the degree of fixation and local infiltration can adversely affect prognosis. The classic work of Dukes has shown that the degree of penetration of the carcinoma through the muscularis mucosa, bowel wall, serosa and spread to the lymph glands have a direct bearing upon prognosis.

Colorectal Cancer	*Corrected 5-year survival (%) following radical resection and excluding operative deaths*	
	Men	*Women*
Cancer confined to mucosa	99	94
Cancer invading muscle	76	82
Cancer with lymph-node metastases	32	33

Attempts are currently being made to improve the prognostic accuracy of Dukes' classification by creating newer categories which take account of the level of muscle invasion and the precise location of the most proximal invaded node. It is also clear that the more carefully the specimen is examined the more positive lymph nodes will be detected.

Provided that the basic tenets of cancer surgery are applied and a healthy margin of tissue is resected with the tumour, patients undergoing anterior resection have as good, if not better, prognosis than those patients required to undergo abdominoperineal excision of rectum. It is not recommended that anterior resection be performed for growths in the middle third of rectum where biopsy has shown a high-grade malignancy.

Patients undergoing low anterior resection of the rectum, by the abdomino-anal pull-through technique or the abdomino-anal approach appear to give as good results as other methods.

Where local control of rectal cancer has been attempted with diathermy fulguration or local excision, the long-term results are inevitably affected by the accuracy of selection for the procedure. It is clear that provided the lesion can be adequately removed the corrected 5-year survival rates compare with radical excision. It must be said that the selection must favour early pathological stage lesions. The same point arises in connection with survival statistics after radical radiotherapy for rectal cancer either by endocavitary contact or interstitial radium implantation where 5-year disease-free states have been reported in 70% of patients with low level, small, well-differentiated, polypoidal lesions. However, where conventional radiotherapy is employed, the local area can rarely achieve dosages of comparable radiation without producing severe radiation sickness or damage to adjacent structures.

Diagnosis and Management of Recurrent Colorectal Cancer

The failure of surgery to eradicate cancer from many patients in whom the neoplasm has invaded the muscle wall or lymph nodes implies that residual cancer exists as occult micrometastases. The rate of subsequent growth is presumably dependent upon the particular cell kinetics of the individual tumour, the suitability of the tumour bed, its vascularity and the host response to the tumour. The time scale varies but most recurrent cancer becomes clinically apparent by the third postoperative year and the mortality from colorectal cancer is nearly complete by 5 years.

The symptoms of recurrent cancer are rarely attributable to the colon or rectum unless anastomotic recurrence occurs. More frequently, there is an insidious failure of general health, anorexia, weight loss and lack of energy. In the later stages local pain or chest pain may occur. Recurrent cancer may become palpable locally or as hepatomegaly with ascites.

Though there is an emphasis on the role of distant micrometastases it is also clear that there is a local failure also. In rectal cancer, low primary lesions have a higher incidence of local recurrence ($\simeq$15%). Similarly the more advanced Dukes' stage of the primary lesion, the higher the local recurrence rate, e.g. 16% for C cases. There has always been a concern that the use of anterior resection of the rectum would lead to a higher local recurrence rate than combined rectal excision; however, this does not seem to be the case.

The commonest sites for recurrence are the anterior abdominal wall and intraperitoneally close to the anastomosis. With rectal cancer, the posterior vaginal wall, the back of the prostate and base of the bladder and the front of the sacrum are common sites. Some patients with local recurrence can benefit considerably from reoperation and a variety of approaches have been employed to deal with this problem. Before considering reoperation, a careful evaluation of the affected area, liver and lungs is advised using CT or MRI scanning.

The routine second-look procedure at 6-monthly intervals does not increase survival in asymptomatic individuals. There are a few reports indicating that a rise in the plasma CEA level, followed by re-laparotomy, can lead to a number of patients benefiting by the removal of recurrent tumour. This observation is currently tested in an MRC trial.

Management

The treatment of established liver metastases is discussed in Chapter 68. Patients with local recurrence involving the area of previous resection should be re-explored and further resection carried out where this is feasible. In the inoperable patient palliative radiotherapy does not seem particularly effective though it may reduce local bone pain. It may also be helpful in the perineal recurrence after combined excision of rectum.

Chemotherapy may also be used and though there are several combinations of drugs said to be effective in colorectal cancer, there is no convincing evidence that the results are better than single agents given alone. Currently, 5-FU delivered intravenously at 15 mg/kg for 5 days every 3–6 weeks would seem most appropriate. Lower rectal recurrences may be symptomatically improved by diathermy or cryoprobe application. In the event of the treatment failing to control pain, local nerve blocks with phenol or alcohol may be effective (*see* Chapter 13).

INVOLVEMENT OF THE COLON BY GYNAECOLOGICAL PATHOLOGY

Secondary Carcinoma

Discrete secondary deposits on the sigmoid colon are not uncommon from any primary intra-abdominal cancer but the deposits do not cause symptoms. However, direct invasion of the sigmoid colon or, more rarely, the caecum by infiltration of ovarian cancer can lead to constipation or complete colonic obstruction. Though remissions are seen with chemotherapy (*see* Chapter 79), some patients may need a relieving colostomy. In selected patients a pelvic clearance may have a role.

Endometriosis

Endometrial tissue may occasionally implant on to the serosa of the sigmoid colon and rectum. The condition frequently mimics advanced colorectal carcinoma. It is estimated that about 1 in 10 women have endometriosis during an active menstrual life and about one-quarter of these will have involvement of the rectosigmoid. Small cysts filled with dark material are seen on the surface of the bowel, usually inducing dense adhesions involving small bowel, omentum and Fallopian tubes. The involvement is almost always confined to the serosa and muscle layers and the mucosa is not usually affected. Microscopically, nests of endometrial glands are found reaching as far as the submucosa.

Clinically, the symptoms of dysmenorrhoea, dyspareunia and defaecation which is painful just before menstruation, are characteristic. These symptoms should lessen as soon as menstrual flow develops. More rarely, constipation or full colonic obstruction have been described and this has also been found in postmenopausal patients where a late stricture has developed. Full clinical examination including extended sigmoidoscopy will reveal an intact rectal and sigmoid mucosa and close questioning of previous menstrual history will support the diagnosis. However, histological diagnosis is mandatory.

When endometriosis of the bowel is severe or is found in the older woman, a hysterectomy and unilateral oophorectomy is advisable with rectosigmoidectomy to relieve obstruction, where necessary. However, in the younger patient it is preferable to attempt to excise and cauterize the endometrial implants and where possible preserve ovarian function.

PNEUMATOSIS COLI

This rare condition more commonly affects the small intestine than colon. It is usually accidentally discovered at a radiological procedure being undertaken for other reasons. Gas-filled cysts are found in the subserosal and submucosal planes and these are seen on plain films of the abdomen or as filling defects on barium examination. The condition probably results from lymphatic stasis with subsequent filling of the lymph spaces with gas, including nitrogen, carbon dioxide and hydrogen. There appears to be a definite association in patients with obstructive airways disease. No active treatment is necessary but the cysts can be induced to disappear with oxygen therapy extended over 3–4 days.

RECTAL AND ANORECTAL DISORDERS

Irradiation Proctitis

Within the therapeutic range of 4000–6000 rad, serious irradiation injury to the colorectum arises in 5–10% of patients. The injury occurs by a direct action on the mucosa about the time of therapy and subsequently as a result of an obliterative vasculitis. Irradiation injury is more likely in individuals with diabetes or cardiovascular disease. Rectal injury tends to follow external beam radiation for carcinoma of the bladder and radium treatment for carcinomas involving the uterus. Symptoms may appear within 2 weeks of treatment and are those of an idiopathic proctitis with frequent calls to stool with passage of a bloody mucus and tenesmus. Occasionally symptoms are delayed and the patient is shown to have a large rectal ulcer which requires histological diagnosis. Other patients present with symptoms related to rectal fistulation into vagina or urinary tract. Patients with irradiation proctitis may also exhibit damage to the transverse colon and small bowel particularly where adhesions from a previous laparotomy have fixed the loops of bowel in the pelvis.

Although a few cases of irradiation injury are due to excess dosage, the majority occur after conventional therapy. The routine use of a rectal monitor and the more frequent application of intracavitary cobalt may reduce the incidence.

Management

Diagnosis and extent of mucosal injury can be determined by endoscopic means. Topical steroid therapy given as suppository or mini enema is appropriate though the evidence that this therapy is capable of modifying this type of inflammatory process is lacking. Severe symptoms may require the construction of a sigmoid loop colostomy for 6–12 months, though this will not always prevent haemorrhage and tenesmus. A proximal colostomy is required if fistulation occurs and there are cases in which a Hartmann's procedure is advantageous, particularly if the rectum proves to be badly strictured or if massive haemorrhage occurs. In any event, the patient will require reassurance that symptoms will be slow to settle down. Reconstruction of the rectum after fistulation is feasible using unaffected tissues as described below.

Rectovaginal Fistulas

Persistent communication between the rectum and vagina may result from trauma. Mechanical injury results from pressure necrosis of the posterior vaginal and anterior rectal walls by the fetal head during prolonged labour and from ill-advised attempts to promote successful delivery. Alternatively, fistulas may arise from third-degree perineal tears. This type of fistula seems more common in the rural communities of developing countries.

Rectal disease may ulcerate through into the vaginal canal and fistulas are not uncommon in relatively advanced cancer of the rectum or inflammatory bowel disease of the rectum—Crohn's disease, ulcerative colitis and, more rarely, lymphogranuloma venereum.

Rectovaginal fistulas may also follow irradiation proctitis—the consequence of excessive irradiation to the tissues surrounding the cervix. These patients normally present with symptoms of proctitis and a history of previous radiotherapy. Despite all local measures, including faecal diversion by colostomy, some patients necrose the vaginal and rectal walls, leading to fistulation and distressing faecal soiling.

The principles of management are dependent upon the cause—patients with anorectal carcinoma require radical excision of the rectum and posterior vaginal wall and possibly a hysterectomy as well; patients with inflammatory bowel disease require appropriate medication (*see* Chapter 73) and depending upon the extent of the disease, either a proximal colostomy while healing takes place or colorectal excision in patients with severe and extensive disease.

Rectovaginal fistulas following obstetric or gynaecological injury may be approached with the intention to repair. Fistulas very low down on to the vaginal wall may be laid open, provided the internal opening in the anal canal is below the anorectal ring. This type of case usually results from imperfect healing after repair of a third-degree perineal tear. Where the fistula is low but above the anorectal ring, the fistula is approached either through the vagina or transperineal route and after careful dissection to free the edges of the vaginal and rectal walls, a direct suture is possible. Given the likelihood of infection and further breakdown, a preoperative proximal colostomy may seem desirable but this is not always required and most gynaecologists achieve a high success rate without recourse to it. However, if a transsphincteric approach to fistulas is embarked upon, a colostomy is essential. Fistulas at a higher level in the vagina are probably best dealt with by an abdominal approach separating the rectum and vagina completely, repairing the defect and then interposing a layer of greater omentum.

Patients with rectovaginal fistulas following irradiation pose a special problem. The vascular insufficiency produced by the irradiation makes healing difficult to achieve by either method, though an omental graft or gracilis muscle transposition into the area can lead to successful healing. Recently, reports from an American group have shown that after division of the sigmoid colon near its upper end, the distal segment may be folded between the rectum and vagina and used to patch the fistula or to widen a strictured rectum (*Fig.* 74.22). Other patients with a high fistula may be treated by an anterior resection, but it must be emphasized that since it is the low rectum which seems to be maximally affected by the radiation, the viability of the rectal stump is always doubtful. Almost certainly a colostomy will be needed for a prolonged period in these patients until it is clearly shown that delayed breakdown has not occurred.

Recto-urinary Fistulas

Communication between the sigmoid colon and bladder sometimes occurs as a result of disease in the sigmoid colon, e.g. diverticulitis, Crohn's disease, carcinoma or irradiation of the bladder. Fistulation between the prostate or urethra and rectum is rarer. In certain congenital deformities of the anal canal, the rectum opens into the prostatic urethra. The management of this problem usually requires a colostomy which may be permanent unless there is some evidence of anal sphincteric mechanisms. (These matters are discussed in Chapter 59.)

Prostatic abscesses may rupture into the rectum; typically tuberculosis can lead to chronic fistulation. Alternatively, severe inflammatory ulceration of the rectum (Crohn's disease) or malignant disease of the prostate and rectum have been known to fistulate into the prostate or bulbous urethra. Most recto-urinary fistulas result from injury, mainly as a result of prostatic or urethral instrumentation or prostatectomy (especially by the perineal approach).

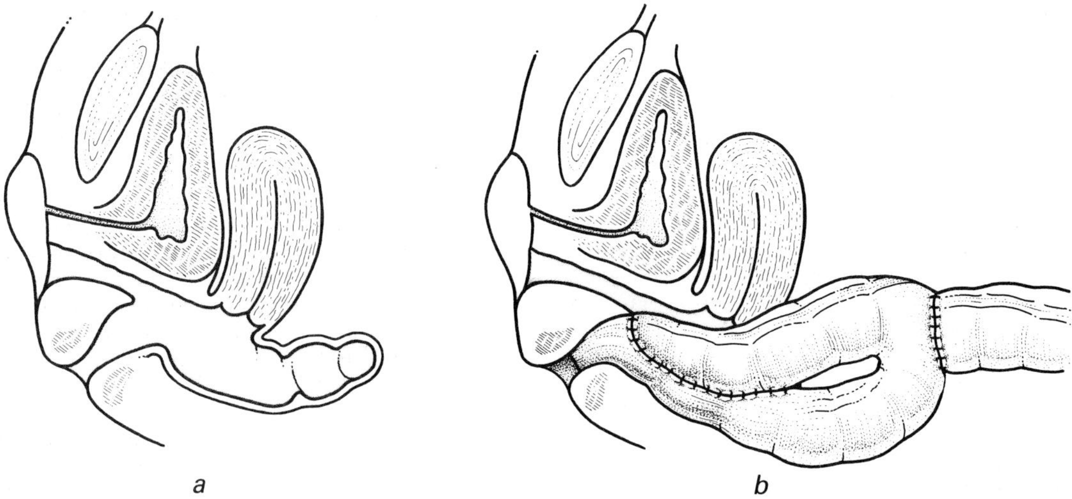

Fig. 74.22 *a*, Following trauma or radiotherapy high rectovaginal fistulas are commonly large with near-complete loss of the posterior vaginal and anterior rectal walls. *b*, This defect may be closed by mobilizing and dissecting the sigmoid colon followed by folding of the colon and suture to the margins of the defect. Both abdominal and vaginal approaches are needed.

Rectoprostatic fistulas are also a rare complication of transrectal needle biopsy of the prostate.

Management of this distressing condition includes the establishment of a suprapubic cystostomy and definitive treatment of the pathological process. Post-traumatic fistulas are amenable to direct repair either by the perineal, trans-anal or trans-sphincteric approach.

DISORDERS OF THE ANORECTAL MUSCULATURE

No doubt as a result of the interest in sphincter-saving procedures after excision of the rectum for inflammatory bowel disease or cancer, there has been a resurgence of investigation of continence and of patients with complete or partial prolapse of the rectum, slow transit constipation and solitary rectal ulcer. The evaluation of these patients largely follows the pattern of a thorough clinical and endoscopic examination to exclude specific bowel disease and careful attention during history-taking of the obstetric and perineal trauma. It is usually possible by digital examination to distinguish between damage to the anorectal ring produced by trauma and a generalized weakness of the pelvic floor (descending perineum syndrome).

In many patients, a more searching examination of the pelvic floor function is required. Radiological examination in the form of a defaecating proctogram, will delineate the rectum and anal canal in relation to the bony landmarks of the pelvis. By this means, the anorectal angle can be measured and may appear increased beyond 90° in patients with idiopathic incontinence. Similarly the distance of the anorectal line to pubococcygeal line may be lengthened. Specialized units currently use anorectal manometry and electromyography of the sphincteric and levator ani muscles to evaluate these patients. In the manometric examination, the presence of anal relaxation after rectal distension of a balloon will exclude Hirschsprung's disease. Anal canal pressures at rest reflect the activity of the internal sphincter (50–80 cmH_2O) and voluntary contraction of the external sphincter (squeeze pressure) will increase the pressure of the anal canal to 150 cmH_2O. EMG will demonstrate activity in the sphincteric and pelvic floor muscles and in its simplest form is used to demonstrate the presence of functioning muscle in patients with severe neurological deficits (cauda equina lesions) and in children with anorectal dysgenesis. A more sophisticated evaluation of pelvic floor function may be obtained by measuring the reflex latency and single fibre EMG can identify denervation because the surviving axons are required to reinnervate more muscle fibres.

Clinical Syndromes

A number of clinical states are conveniently discussed as disorders of anorectal musculature:

Rectal prolapse—complete
—partial
Solitary rectal ulcer
Anal incontinence—idiopathic
—descending perineum syndrome
—pelvic floor neuropathy.

Rectal Prolapse

The descent of the rectum through the anal canal is of two types. Prolapse involving the mucosal membrane alone is called 'incomplete' or 'partial'. Where the entire thickness of rectal wall descends, the prolapse is termed 'complete'.

Aetiology

Complete Prolapse

Cineradiographic studies appear to show that during straining at defaecation, a prolapse begins about 6–8 cm above the anal verge as a *circumferential* intussusception. When the prolapse has passed through the anal canal and is fully descended, the anterior segment may seem more prominent and can be shown to contain a sac of peritoneum from the pelvic cavity, which itself may hold loops of small bowel. It is not clear what additional factors permit this intussusception, though laxity of the pelvic floor musculature is a likely cause. This fact is borne out by the common occurrence of rectal prolapse in patients with spinal cord injuries and in the elderly patient with poor sphincteric tone. Furthermore, it has been shown that the resting activity of the sphincteric and levator ani muscles is more profoundly reduced during defaecation in patients with prolapse.

Incomplete or Partial Prolapse

Any injury to the anal sphincter reduces the fixation and support of the rectal mucosa. Thus mucosal prolapse may occur after sphincteric injury following childbirth or operation for perianal fistula. In the adult patient it would seem that the development of prolapsing haemorrhoids ultimately predisposes to a more extensive mucosal prolapse.

Prolapse in Children

In children the cause of the prolapse is less certain. Anatomically there is less curvature to the body of the sacrum so that intra-abdominal pressure may force the rectum downwards on to the anal canal in a more direct line. Children with poor toilet training who are left to strain at defaecation for a prolonged time would be at risk or children with a chronic severe cough, e.g. pertussis. While malnutrition following serious illness may weaken pelvic muscular support, this is by no means a requirement.

Clinical Features

Incidence

While prolapse can occur at any time of life, incomplete prolapse is more common in children and complete prolapse in the very elderly. Prolapse in children is a feature of the first 2 years of life being slightly more common in boys than girls which contrasts strongly with complete prolapse in adults where females are four times more susceptible. While it might be thought that this is the result of previous parturition producing lax pelvic musculature, there is little evidence to bear this out and few female patients have combined uterine and rectal prolapse. Though it is hard to explain the significance, the incidence of patients with rectal prolapse and some form of mental abnormality is rather striking.

Symptoms and Signs

In children the parents are not unnaturally concerned to see a reddened area of mucosa at the anal verge and notice also excess mucus and a trace of blood. No abnormality may be detected on preliminary examination, but the prolapse may be precipitated by inserting a suppository and putting the child on a pot. Once the prolapse has occurred (*Fig.* 74.23), careful palpation between gloved finger and thumb distinguish between two layers of mucosa and a complete prolapse. After reduction of the prolapse digital examination will probably reveal no detectable abnormality of the anal sphincter.

Adults will complain of two features, first of the prolapse itself and the soiling of underclothes from mucus, blood and faeces and secondly of a varying degree of faecal incontinence. The prolapse occurs not only at defaecation but with exertion and with coughing. Most patients resort to wearing a pad or sanitary towel, for the prolapse eventually occurs on standing and walking. On examination the anus may seem patulous and it is apparent that sphincteric tone is deficient and that active contraction of the anal sphincter on to the examining finger is weak. The patient experiences little or no discomfort and it is an obvious clinical feature that anal and rectal sensation are blunted. On bearing down the prolapse will be produced (*Fig.* 74.23) and may reach 10–12 cm from the anal verge. It is then possible to feel two complete layers of bowel wall between gloved finger and thumb and even loops of small bowel in the peritoneal sac, particularly anteriorly. A prolapse greater than 5 cm is almost certainly complete. Those less than 5 cm need careful examination to determine whether they are mucosal or complete.

The differential diagnosis in children includes a prolapsed rectal polyp or the apex of an intussusception. In adults rectal prolapse must be distinguished from large internal haemorrhoids and large polypoidal tumours of the rectum and lower sigmoid colon.

Complications

Bleeding and ulceration occur frequently with chronic complete prolapse though it is unusual for severe haemorrhage to be a problem. Rupture of the prolapse, while straining at defaecation, has been reported but is rare. While rectal prolapse is usually easily replaced, the bowel may become oedematous and the prolapse become irreducible and in some patients lead to frank gangrene of the bowel.

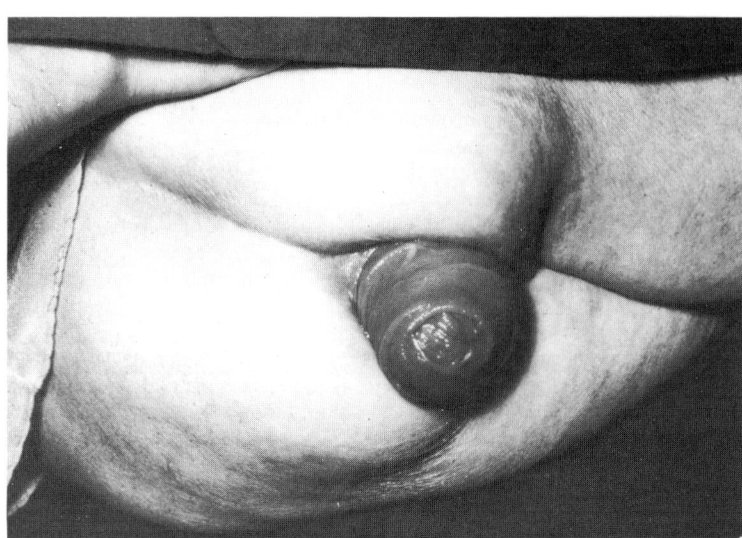

Fig. 74.23 Full rectal prolapse.

Treatment

In Children

The mucosal prolapse seen in very young children is a self-limiting disease provided that a regular habit of defaecation can be established and the straining of the constipated child alleviated. Occasionally in severe cases, constipation will require daily enemas but usually bulk-forming laxatives are adequate. Strapping the buttocks together after defaecation may be required for a short period of time.

In slightly older children, resolution of the prolapse will be hastened by injection of sclerosants, such as phenol in almond oil, or absolute alcohol, into the lower rectal mucosa. Where the prolapse seems to be complete rather than mucosal the sclerosant is given into the perirectal tissues and produces an inflammatory process which fixes the rectum to the sacrum.

Failure to respond to these conservative measures and the development of a large irreducible prolapse requires operative treatment as detailed below.

In Adults

In the initial examination of the adult patient, the rectal examination should be particularly thorough so that the tone and strength of the anal sphincter can be assessed. If the anal sphincter function appears satisfactory and the prolapse is partial or incomplete, a carefully performed 'mucosal haemorrhoidectomy' will often suffice to deal with the condition. Unfortunately, many elderly patients have poor sphincteric tone and simple excision of the prolapsing mucosa will not relieve them of all their symptoms. These patients may require training in sphincteric exercises or even operative control of their incontinence, though many patients are so frail and elderly that this may not be feasible (*see* Anal incontinence).

Complete prolapse of the rectum in adults can be successfully treated by a variety of surgical techniques but the final functional result is dependent upon the degree of continence rather than simple control of the prolapse.

In the elderly patient, a modified form of Thiersh circumanal wiring procedure is carried out, most commonly using nylon rather than wire. About half the cases are treated successfully but in many patients the nylon breaks or cuts out or the suture is too tight and leads to faecal impaction. The variant operation described by Nataras uses an implanted suture placed above the anal sphincters and levator ani muscles at a higher level in the perirectal tissues. It appears to give more support to the bowel and to control a complete prolapse more effectively. It is also less likely to cut out or produce sinuses.

A complete prolapse of major proportions and those patients with complications require more radical surgery. Partial excision of the rectum can be carried out through the anus by a rectosigmoidectomy, as described last century by Mickulicz and Miles in 1933. However, about half the patients suffer recurrent rectal prolapse and other patients are incontinent, though this may be a preoperative problem also. The operation is not in favour at the moment except for young and very elderly patients. It is, however, indicated for patients with irreducible prolapse which has developed gangrene of the bowel. An alternative approach is to excise a cuff of mucosa on the outer aspect of the prolapse and to concertina the muscle layer with sutures to approximate the cut edges of mucosa (Delorme procedure). The operation is currently practised by only a few surgeons and long-term follow-up studies are awaited. Excision of rectal prolapse by formal low anterior resection has also been advocated with apparent success in control of the full prolapse but some patients remain unsatisfactory because of prolapse of the lower rectal mucosa.

Two other principles of technique are available and often these techniques have been combined in procedures remembered by the eponymous names. Restitution of the tone of the levator ani muscles can be achieved by suturing the muscles either from a posterior or sacral approach or by the abdominal approach from above, as described by Roscoe-Graham in Toronto and Dunphy in San Francisco. Fixation of the rectum to the pelvic wall can be accomplished by direct suture to the presacral fascia or by first fixing some prosthetic material, such as polyvinyl alcohol sponge or nylon mesh, to the sacral concavity and suturing this material around the rectum after full mobilization of the rectum down to the levator ani muscles (Wells procedure). Many surgeons combine the suturing of the levator ani muscles with some form of rectal fixation.

This radical form of surgery is inappropriate for the very aged patient or young infants but where the patient is reasonably fit, it can be expected to control complete rectal prolapse in over 90% of cases. Points of failure include the occurrence in about 25% of patients of a subsequent mucosal prolapse, which can of course be treated locally. Direct complications of the procedure include damage to pelvic nerves and impotence, or sepsis around implanted materials. Sphincteric control appears to improve in about 60% of patients. Sphincteric exercises are generally encouraged in the postoperative period but there is little evidence that they are effective. Patients with severe incontinence and lax anal sphincters may benefit from a supplementary sphincteroplasty, though one cannot expect too much improvement from this procedure in these circumstances.

ANAL INCONTINENCE

There can be few symptoms more distressing to patients than the loss of anal sphincteric control with subsequent faecal soiling. It is a serious and common problem in the elderly and debilitated geriatric patient in whom a lax and disordered anal sphincteric mechanism is aggravated by a relative rectal insensibility. Digital examination reveals a patulous anus and the patient seems unaware that the examination is taking place. This lack of rectal sensation is commonly associated with faecal impaction and the trickling of liquid stool through the anus around the hard faecal masses. When this complication occurs, manual disimpaction of the rectum under a general anaesthetic is required followed by a regular use of laxatives and enemas until some form of regular bowel habit is regained.

More specific causes of anal incontinence include neurological disorders, such as spina bifida, spinal cord injuries and tumours and tabes dorsalis. Sphincteric injury may follow local trauma or obstetric injury in which the complete perineal tear includes the anal sphincter. Perhaps even more common are the sphincteric injuries which follow operations for anal fistulas, fissure or even haemorrhoidectomy, particularly when forcible manual dilatation has been added to the procedure. While a patient should be fully continent following an anterior resection of the rectum, with increasingly low procedures being performed using stapling devices or an abdominal sacral approach, a patient may not be able to fully control the passage of flatus or a liquid stool.

Similar problems may arise after correction of congenital anorectal deformities (*see* Chapter 59).

Treatment

1. Sphincteric suture is required for patients with third-degree perineal tears or those patients with operative trauma following laying open of an anal fistula. Normally the repair is carried out in two layers; an inner mucosal layer and a loosely sutured muscle layer of the divided sphincteric muscles.

2. Post-anal repair: this procedure has been popularized by the late Sir Alan Parkes. A careful reference to operative textbooks is required before embarking on this procedure which is designed for the patient with a weak pelvic floor. The principles involve a dissection posteriorly in the plane between the internal and external sphincters until the puborectalis muscles are revealed and these are buttressed with sutures to restore the anorectal angle. Finally, the external sphincter is sutured to improve its functional tone. The success of the procedure depends greatly on the experience of the surgeon but improved control for solid faeces can be obtained in the majority but it is less successful in the restoration of the control of flatus or liquid faeces.

Solitary Rectal Ulcer Syndrome

This uncommon condition is a misnomer since the lesions may be multiple and not all the cases have ulceration. No age is excluded from the complaint but it appears to be more frequent in young adults. All complain of difficulty of defaecation which involves going to the toilet several times a day but only defaecating once or twice. Usually blood and mucus are passed associated with a deep-seated perineal pain. Others have abdominal symptoms and undergo investigation resulting in the diagnosis of irritable bowel syndrome.

Investigation reveals an indurated area on digital examination and endoscopic views may show oedema or haemorrhage in the mucosa or in 50% an ulcer adjacent to a valve of Houston on the anterior surface. In most instances a neoplastic lesion will be diagnosed but repeated biopsy shows only non-specific inflammatory changes.

It is now believed that most of these patients suffer from an internal rectal prolapse or intussusception which causes trauma to the rectal wall. Many of the patients also suffer an external rectal prolapse or have some muscle abnormality or weakness. The basic abnormality can often be detected by repeating the sigmoidoscopy with the observation window removed and asking the patient to strain, when the lesion will be seen to descend into the instrument.

The management of the case may be difficult. Topical steroids may give temporary relief but once the abnormality is diagnosed with confidence, some form of abdominal rectopexy may be required.

Descending Perineum Syndrome

It is possible that this is a basic defect responsible for many cases of rectal prolapse or anal incontinence. Patients complain of an excessive need to strain at defaecation which in turn leads to a prolonged reflex inhibition of musculature with an abnormal descent of the perineum and bulging of the anterior rectal wall towards the anal canal. It is possible that the urge to strain results from a mucosal prolapse but this is not invariably present. Although the relationship of the anus to the interischial line is normal at rest (2 cm above), on straining the anus descends to greater than 1 cm below this line in patients with this syndrome.

The management is the avoidance of straining and, where needed, Bisacodyl suppositories may assist. If mucosal prolapse is present, it seems logical to excise the excess tissue in resistant cases.

ANORECTAL SUPPURATION

Anorectal Abscesses

Suppuration in the anorectal region is common, more so in men than women, a fact which may result from a less fastidious attention to hygiene. Both aerobic (staphylococcal, streptococcal, *E. coli* and pyocyaneus) and anaerobic (*Clostridium welchii*, bacteroides) organisms can be isolated and the latter group are considered to be particularly prevalent.

It is relatively unusual to find a precipitating cause and while local abrasions from hard faecal material could theoretically be a factor, it must be exceedingly rare. Some infections may be blood borne and others seem particularly to occur in patients rendered leucopenic by cytotoxic agents or adverse reactions to drugs, e.g. carbimazole. Unquestionably anorectal infections are more common in patients with a coexisting inflammatory bowel disease, such as ulcerative colitis (15%) and Crohn's colitis (25%). There is also an increased risk in patients with pulmonary tuberculosis though this is rare given modern medical treatment in the European patient.

Current views suggest that most abscesses start as an infection in the anal glands at the base of the anal crypt (*see Fig.* 74.2). The abscess develops into the plane between the internal and external sphincters and then extends to adjacent areas as the abscess expands. The classification of perianal abscess is based on the predominant area of expansion: perianal; ischiorectal; high intersphincteric or submucous; pelvirectal. The anatomical relationships of these infections are illustrated in *Fig.* 74.24.

The clinical features of perianal and ischiorectal abscess may be considered together. A severe throbbing pain develops in the perianal region which is worse on sitting and coughing. Systemic disturbance in the form of pyrexia is more common with ischiorectal abscesses. On examination a perianal abscess is shown as a red, very tender, local, rounded swelling in the perianal region with a degree of induration and sometimes fluctuation. Ischiorectal abscesses occupy a large area to one side of the anus with tender induration and some fluctuation. These abscesses are sometimes bilateral. On rectal examination, a perianal abscess will be felt as an indurated area in the anal margin with exquisite tenderness. An ischiorectal abscess is also tender but higher in the rectum. Where gas-forming organisms are involved, crepitus may be palpated in the perianal subcutaneous tissues.

A submucous abscess may present as a dull aching pain in the rectum and there is usually no external evidence of infection. Systemic disturbance is uncommon. On rectal examination it may be possible to feel a rounded smooth area of induration on one side of the upper anal canal and lower rectum. Quite often the abscess has already discharged and pus can be seen extending from an internal opening during proctoscopy.

The pelvirectal abscess is normally a complication of pelvic sepsis most usually following appendicitis, salpingitis or abdominal surgical procedures. The patient shows signs of infection with pyrexia, rigors, diarrhoea, weakness and

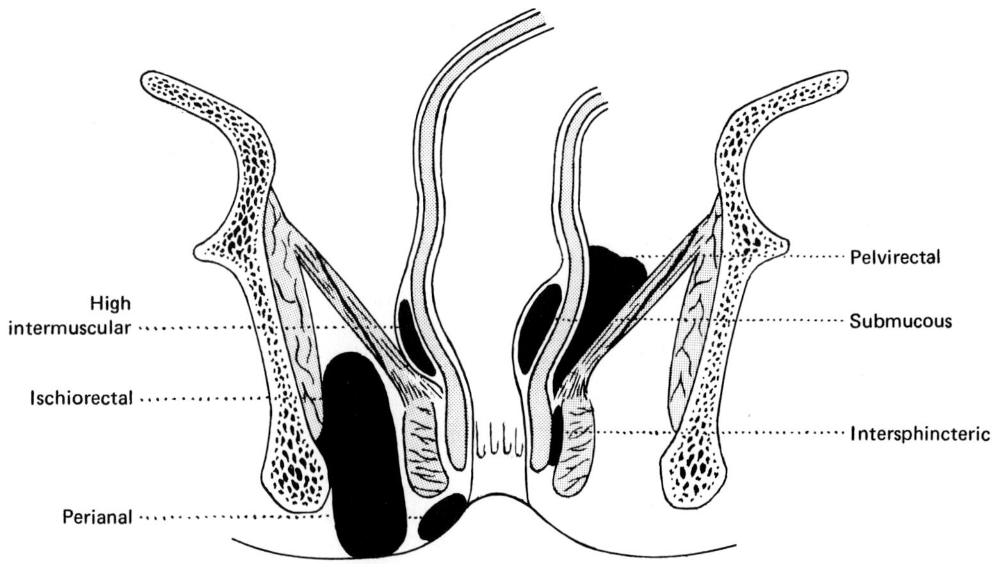

Fig. 74.24 Sites of anal abscesses.

lower abdominal tenderness or even a mass. Rectal examination is tender high on the examining finger and there is usually a firm sense to palpation which may have progressed to a characteristic boggy swelling. These patients may be extremely ill and require careful assessment and care.

Treatment

In principle the treatment of perianal abscess does not differ from the treatment of abscesses elsewhere. It is unlikely that surgeons will see patients at a stage when the infection will be contained by antibiotics, though one must suspect that a number of patients receiving antibiotics from their family practitioners do, in fact, resolve.

A careful examination under a general anaesthetic is required. Where the abscess is perianal or ischiorectal, the pus is released by a cruciate incision and the septa broken down to create one draining cavity. The examination is first extended with a blunt probe to determine whether an internal opening can be detected. If the internal opening is clearly well below the anorectal line then the track may be laid open as for a chronic anal fistula. Where there is doubt or the opening is clearly high, the abscess cavity is packed with Eusol-soaked gauze and dressings changed regularly after antiseptic baths. An alternative method, which may achieve early healing in a significant proportion of cases, involves the use of a high dose of a broad-spectrum antibiotic at the time of exploration with careful curetting of all granulations and primary closure with deep sutures which obliterate the abscess cavity. Though it is known that more patients suffer recurrent abscesses after this method, the proportion is not much greater than with the traditional method.

Most submucous abscesses will have already discharged by the time of examination but it is still appropriate to examine the abscess under anaesthetic and to ensure that adequate drainage can take place by widening the internal opening. Pelvirectal or high abscesses require more consideration, though when following acute appendicitis or salpingitis they can normally be drained with complete success into the rectum. Some seriously ill patients with complex intra-abdominal septic complications may be more adequately managed by a formal laparotomy and drainage.

Anorectal Fistulas

An opening between the skin of the perianal region and the cavity of the anal canal or rectum is termed a perianal fistula. It must be admitted that both internal and external opening will not always be demonstrated simultaneously and at times these lesions might be more appropriately termed a sinus. Not uncommonly there are multiple external openings but it is unusual for there to be other than a single internal opening. The main area of the fistulous track is lined by granulation tissue surrounded by a dense fibrous reaction. It does appear that the track in immediate continuity with the openings may be epithelized and be one factor in the chronicity of this condition.

Aetiology

It seems likely that all fistulas arise from a pyogenic abscess which has been allowed to develop to the point of spontaneously discharging or one which has not been adequately drained surgically. The point of debate thereafter is to explain why the condition has persisted. Most probably the development of an internal opening allows recurrent activation of the infection with further build-up of pus which discharges both internally and externally. In some cases faecal material may act as a foreign body but it is surprisingly rare to find such material on exploring the fistulous track. Where no internal opening can be found it may be assumed that the persistence of infection lies in the anal glands and acts as a reservoir for infection. More specific associations include ulcerative colitis, where even distal proctitis seems to be as provoking a factor as total colonic involvement; and Crohn's disease where 16–20% of patients are so affected. The striking question here is to explain why perianal disease is associated with intestinal disease elsewhere and not in continuity. While it is true that the histological features of some fistulas resemble that of Crohn's disease, this is not always the case and in any event the histological features of a Crohn's lesion are not all that specific and are seen generally with chronic infection. Active tuberculous infection may be more common than supposed and tubercle bacilli have been isolated in fistulas at rates varying from 8 to 16%. About half these patients will have evidence of healed pulmonary tuberculosis and may have acquired their perianal disease by swallowing live bacilli in sputum. The alternative sources of infection may be from infected lymphoid tissue higher in the gastrointestinal tract or the ingestion of milk infected with bovine tuberculosis. Other chronic infections include actinomycosis and lymphogranuloma venereum in endemic areas. Occasionally the extension of a carcinoma of the anal canal or low rectum particularly when this is mucus-secreting may present as a perianal fistula, and this association should be particularly excluded. Finally, some fistulas must be attributed sequelae to surgical procedures on the anal canal and perineum, e.g. haemorrhoidectomy, where infection has pocketed and subsequently discharged to produce a chronically infected track.

Classification

Most classifications can be related to the position of the underlying abscess cavity. It is, however, necessary to consider the outline of the track in two planes: horizontal and vertical. The well-known Goodsall's Rule is illustrated in *Fig.* 74.25 and demonstrates that the position of the internal opening in the circumference of the anal canal depends upon the relationship of the external opening to an imaginary line drawn between the ischial tuberosities. Fistulas with external openings anterior to Goodsall's line have their internal openings on the same radius; whereas fistulas with external openings behind this line communicate with an internal opening in the midline posteriorly. The horizontal curve of these posterior fistulas constitute one limb of the classic horseshoe shape, the constituents of which may lie on different levels as subsidiary tracks. The complex horseshoe fistulas hug the undersurface of the puborectalis muscle and the back of the anorectal junction and the outermost aspect of the external sphincter.

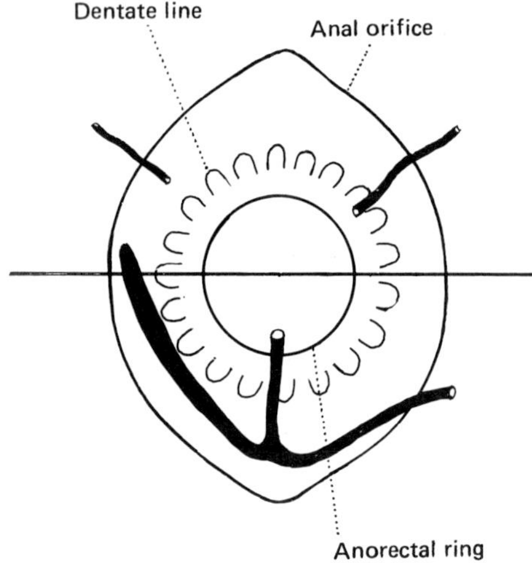

Fig. 74.25 Goodsall's Rule related to anal fistulas suggests that fistulas, with an external opening anterior to a line drawn horizontally through the anal canal, progress forwards in a radial fashion; whereas fistulas with external opening posterior to the horizontal line curve backwards and ultimately have an internal opening in the midline posteriorly. It is possible for fistulas to extend laterally on both sides leading to the characteristic horseshoe fistulas.

It is equally important to consider the course of an anorectal fistula in the vertical axis with special reference to the relationship to the external sphincter. The classic contributions to the surgical anatomy of Milligan and Morgan have more recently been added to by further contributions from Eisenhauer in the USA and Parkes in the UK.

Fig. 74.26 illustrates the vertical areas of perianal and anorectal fistulas:

1. Subcutaneous—are relatively rare and run just below the perianal skin near the pectinate line.
2. Low intersphincteric—the track runs from the region of the pectinate line in the anal canal through the lower part of the internal sphincter and skirts underneath the subcutaneous part of the external sphincter.
3. Trans-sphincteric—here the internal opening may lie higher than the pectinate line but clearly below the anorectal line. The track extends through the external sphincter to the perianal region and there is occasionally a side track extending blindly upwards between the internal and external sphincter (*Fig.* 74.26).
4. Anorectal—exceptionally there is an opening between the rectum and exterior. Much more frequently the upper part of the track is a blind sac extending upwards towards the apex of the ischiorectal fossa below the levator muscles (infralevator). Certain fistulas, originating as pelvirectal or supralevator abscesses, have a blind extension above the levator muscles and an internal opening as a side track through the pectinate line (supralevator type). Fortunately it is relatively rare for there to be a high communication with the rectum from the supralevator cavity (*Fig.* 74.26).

Differential Diagnosis

In the evaluation of patients with perianal fistulas it is important to exclude the association of colloid rectal carcinoma, proctocolitis, Crohn's disease of the small intestine, tuberculosis, actinomycosis and lymphogranuloma venereum. Strictly local conditions which may confuse the diagnosis include pilonidal sinus, suppurative hidradenitis, chronically infected Bartholin's gland and vaginal and urethral fistulas.

Clinical Features

Most patients give a history of a previous perianal abscess which discharged spontaneously, following which there occurs an intermittent or persistent discharge associated with local soreness and pruritus ani. Attacks of perianal pain occur as recurrent abscesses build up.

On examination of the perianal skin there may be redness and a brownish induration. A dorsal anal fissure is commonly present but the most striking feature is the presence of a single or multiple external opening. If the fistula is active, granulation tissue may be seen at the opening and pus can be expressed. Alternatively, the fistula may be healed temporarily.

On digital examination of the anal canal and rectum, induration is palpable and an internal opening can sometimes be felt. Where a horseshoe fistula is present, the track may be felt as a horizontally placed induration just below the anorectal ring. By continuing the examination carefully and bearing in mind the possibility of complicated anorectal fistula, it is possible to delineate extensions of tracks in the intersphincteric plane and supralevator positions.

Digital examination is followed by proctoscopy and sigmoidoscopy and, where appropriate, by full colonoscopy or radiological examination of the gastrointestinal tract. The

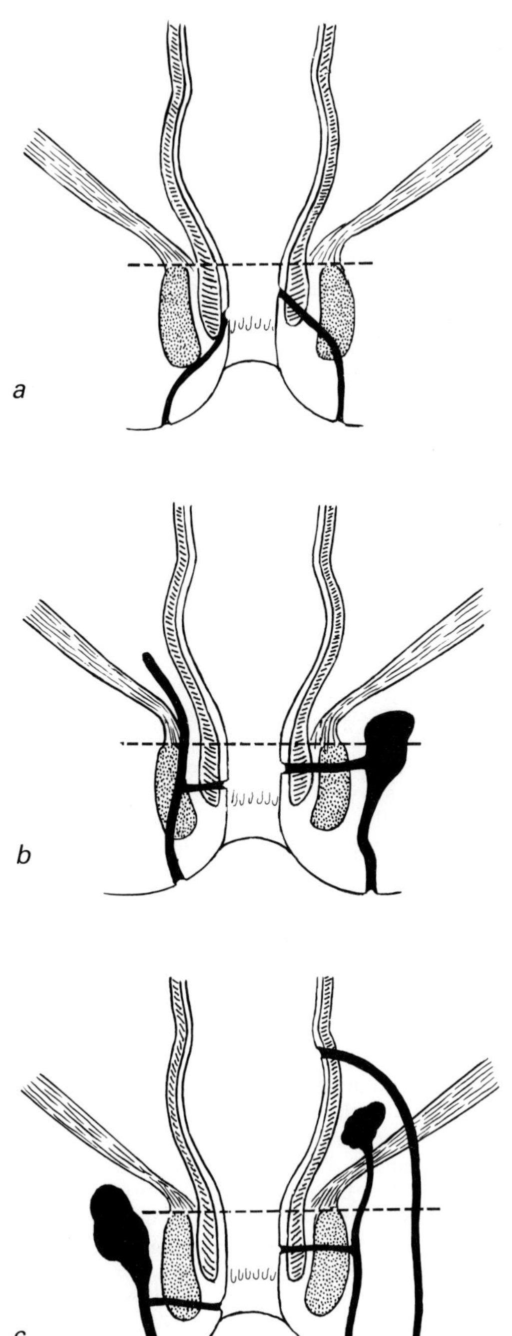

Fig. 74.26 *a*, On the left side the course of a subcutaneous fistula is shown and on the right side the course of a low intersphincteric fistula is shown. *b*, On the left side a low intersphincteric fistula has an extension between the internal and external sphincters. On the right side is depicted the commonest type of high trans-sphincteric fistula. *c*, Anorectal fistulas: On the left side the ischiorectal trans-sphincteric fistula. On the right side high pelvirectal trans-sphincteric fistulas.

most crucial local examination is to use a blunt curved probe to explore gently the fistula so that its true anatomical nature can be determined. This examination may be painful and is best carried out under a general anaesthetic.

Treatment

It is probably accurate to say no chronic fistulas will heal permanently with any form of treatment other than surgery. Local caustic agents or antibiotics are not effective. Surgical treatment is of two main types:

1. Laying open the fistulous track with healing by granulation (most commonly), primary suture or skin grafting.
2. An internal sphincterotomy draining the main abscess cavity into the anal canal and rectum and, where necessary, coring out the external point of the fistulous track.

The reader is referred to sources of operative technique for the precise details but certain principles of surgical management must be stressed. The line of the fistulous track must be defined in its relationship to the anorectal ring, where possible without anaesthetic, but if necessary under a light general anaesthetic. When it is possible to identify the type of fistula as being subcutaneous or low intersphincteric, the track may be laid open without the consequence of anal incontinence. Where the internal opening is higher and its relationship to the anorectal ring is in doubt, laying open the track may produce incontinence. Formerly a suture was threaded through the internal opening and tied tightly so that the sphincters would be held in place by fibrosis while the lower part of the track was laid open. More appropriately a suture should be loosely tied as a loop and this may be used to determine the exact position of the internal opening and the anorectal ring in the fully conscious patient subsequently.

Where there is a blind extension of the track superiorly, the cavity needs adequate drainage, if necessary by splitting the fibres of levator ani.

ANAL FISTULAS IN SPECIFIC CONDITIONS

Mention should be made of the management of perianal suppuration with a specific cause or association. Tuberculous perianal fistulas may be diagnosed on the basis of culture and histological examination of perianal tissue removed at surgery. However, where there is evidence of active tuberculosis elsewhere, e.g. pulmonary or renal, definitive surgery to the perianal disease should be delayed until after the primary foci have come under therapeutic control with appropriate agents. Often 2–3 months are needed. Once this is achieved a standard surgical approach will result in healing in 90% of cases.

Fistulas, fissures and perianal sepsis arising in combination with ulcerative colitis are slow to heal despite an apparent control of the proctocolitis by medical treatment. However, it is certainly pointless trying standard surgical procedures in the absence of energetic attempts to reduce the inflammation in the colon. Similarly with Crohn's disease both medical and surgical measures are generally required. It must be mentioned that the surgical excision of an affected segment of bowel, e.g. ileocaecal Crohn's disease, does not necessarily result in healing of indolent anal fissures or fistulas and these often require formal surgical treatment as outlined above. Perianal disease resistant to local surgical measures has been reported to be responsive to medication in the form of azathioprine, salazopyrine or, more particularly, metronidazole; but some patients never heal the perianal disease. There are patients with Crohn's disease in whom prolonged suppuration about the anus has led to amyloid deposition and death from renal and cardiac failure. Patients with severe perianal fistulation and severe proctitis may decide rectal excision and a colostomy are an acceptable alternative.

HIDRADENITIS OF THE PERIANAL SKIN

Whilst sweat (eccrine) glands are widely distributed on the body, the apocrine glands are restricted to certain zones, such as axillae, inguinoscrotal and perianal regions and the breasts. These glands are developed from hair follicles and discharge a thicker secretion than sweat into the follicle or on to adjacent skin by a rupture of cell membranes and extrusion of cytoplasm. As the glands are not active until puberty, chronic inflammation of these glands (hidradenitis) is delayed, usually into the third decade.

In clinical appearance the affected area begins as an area of induration which spreads and occasionally forms sinuses with the discharge of a little pus. Systemic disturbance is unusual, though the patient is aware of local discomfort. Histological features of the lesion confirm an acne-like disorder with leucocytes distending the affected glands and cellular infiltrate of the surrounding subcutaneous tissue. The axillae are affected predominantly in about 70% of patients and perianal region in about 30% and other areas less frequently and rarely alone. Treatment requires excision of the affected skin and subcutaneous tissue down to the deep fascia and when extensive, split skin grafts eventually give good cover.

PRURITUS ANI

This unpleasant symptom varies from a mild itching in the perianal region to an intense irritation with resultant scratching which leads to a degree of frenzy in some patients. While it is four times more common in men than women, the female incidence seems to be increasing as a result of the use of nylon underwear and hose. The condition is also exacerbated by warmth, anxiety and overwork and there is some evidence of food idiosyncrasy. It is also more common in diabetic patients and in women with a vaginal discharge.

Clinical examination may reveal only redness of the perianal skin but in more severe cases the skin is cracked, oedematous and excoriated with evidence of blood or serous discharge from scratch marks. A careful examination of the anal canal and rectum may show a precipitating cause, such as an anal fissure or fistula, haemorrhoids with a mucoid discharge, a mucus-secreting papilloma of the rectum or, more commonly, a mild to severe proctitis. In these patients appropriate management of the underlying condition will alleviate the pruritus. However, in many patients no local disease will be apparent nor will a diabetic state be detected. Some patients will be suffering from candidiasis or trichomoniasis, so culture swabs and scrapings of the excoriated skin are taken.

Idiopathic pruritus requires a careful explanation to the patient of the cycle of itching, scratching, infection and further irritation. Careful attention to anal hygiene is necessary for all patients irrespective of the underlying cause. Washing with soap and water immediately after defaecation is probably as effective as any treatment. Occasionally detergents may be an aetiological factor. Additional relief may be obtained by the twice daily application of hydrocortisone cream 0·5% or nystatin cream where candidiasis has been detected. Metronidazole is appropriately prescribed for trichomonal infection. Resistant cases may respond to the astringent lotion, Mag. Carbol., which is effective in a large proportion of cases.

There is a small group of patients who are resistant to all physical treatment and are apparently without perianal disease. Pruritus may well be a symptom of neurosis but others seem well balanced from a psychological point of view. In these patients the local injection of subcutaneous alcohol or the deliberate undercutting of the perianal skin is carried out in an attempt to diminish the sensation in the area. It is largely an act of desperation on the part of the surgeon and not without infective complications.

HAEMORRHOIDS

Haemorrhoids lying in the upper two-thirds of the anal canal are covered by columnar cell epithelium and are classified as ‘internal’. Haemorrhoids in the lower third are skin covered and termed ‘external’ (*Fig*. 74.27).

Aetiology

Haemorrhoids occur in about half the population over 50 years and men are more frequently affected than women. The submucosal haemorrhoidal plexus of the superior rectal vein is involved and the contents of the haemorrhoid also include a small branch of the superior rectal artery plus areolar tissue which becomes densely fibrotic when the haemorrhoids are longstanding. Since there are no valves in the portal venous system, internal haemorrhoids bulge into the lumen when the portal pressure is elevated particularly when the anal sphincters are relaxed during defaecation and straining. Patients with portal hypertension do not appear more likely to suffer haemorrhoids. However, in pregnancy with increased pelvic vasculature, laxity of tissues and increased venous congestion from fetal pressure, haemorrhoids are common. During defaecation the portal venous pressure is elevated by straining, the full pressure is exerted upon the anal venous plexus and distends further the haemorrhoid. Straining may be less in patients on a high residue bulk diet and this may explain the relative rareness of haemorrhoids in the native African patient. Sphincteric support of the haemorrhoids is important and when this is lacking after damage, a haemorrhoid may develop opposite the weaker point of the sphincter muscle. Congestion of the superior haemorrhoidal vein may occur as a feature of an encircling cancer of the midrectum making haemorrhoids a presenting feature of the cancer.

Anatomy

The main haemorrhoids are situated as two piles on the right side of the anal canal—anteriorly and posteriorly—and a further haemorrhoid in the left lateral position. Secondary haemorrhoids occur in between the main piles.

On straining, first-degree haemorrhoids move down to the anal margin but return spontaneously after finishing defaecation. Second-degree haemorrhoids prolapse through the anal verge on defaecation and have to be replaced manually. Third-degree haemorrhoids are those piles which prolapse repeatedly on exertion or straining and fourth-degree haemorrhoids are permanently prolapsed and irreducible.

Symptoms and Examination

Prolapse and bleeding are the cardinal symptoms of this condition. Bleeding is often slight and noticed on the toilet

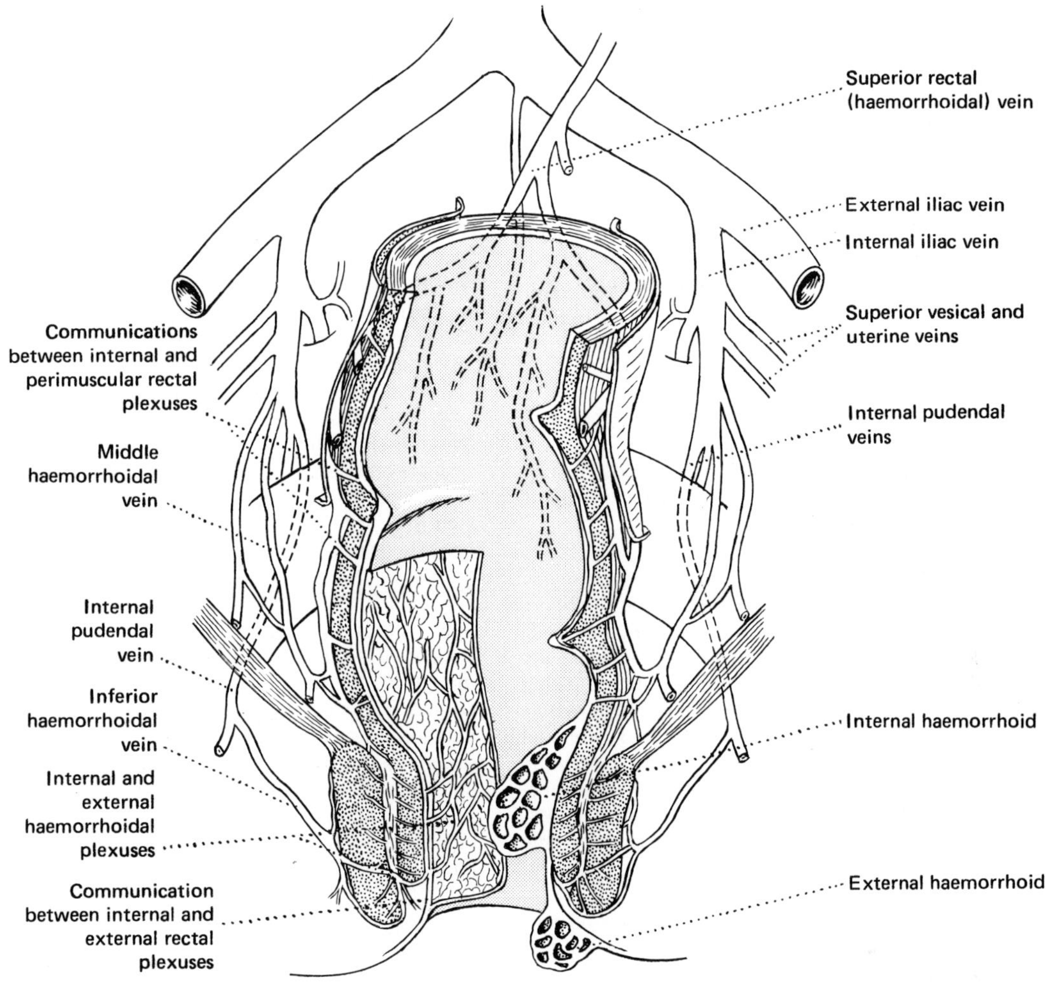

Fig. 74.27 Demonstrates the complex arterial and venous anatomy of the anal canal and the position of internal and external haemorrhoids.

paper by the patient but may be severe with prolapsed haemorrhoids and lead to marked anaemia. Pain is found in about one-fifth of patients and varies from soreness to severe pain. Prolapse is commonly associated with a mucoid discharge and with persistent wetness in the perianal region. This may lead to pruritus ani.

Large prolapsed haemorrhoids are readily seen with skin covering the lower part of pile and the darker red of the prolapsed anal mucosa forming an inner ring. Longstanding prolapse leads to a white colouring of the mucosa due to metaplasia of the anal mucosa. Less degrees of prolapsed haemorrhoids may be seen by retracting the perianal skin but first-degree haemorrhoids rarely have external changes. The piles are palpable as soft folds when longstanding; however, proctoscopy is the essential step in the examination of internal haemorrhoids, being particularly well demonstrated on withdrawal of the instrument while the patient is straining. It is imperative that all patients should proceed to a complete examination of the rectum by sigmoidoscopy.

Management

A not-insignificant group of patients have a history of anal canal bleeding from haemorrhoids but only minimal physical evidence on proctoscopy. In these patients, a trial of injection sclerotherapy is justified with a careful reappraisal at 3 weeks if this fails to control the bleeding. Additional warning symptoms of a change in bowel habit require radiological or colonoscopic examination.

Additional Measures

Advice to the patient to avoid constipation by the use of aperients or bulk-forming agents together with local antiseptic creams undoubtedly gives some patients considerable relief from pain and irritation. Such measures may be advisable during pregnancy with definitive treatment deferred for some months, though injection therapy is feasible.

Injection Therapy (Sclerotherapy)

This treatment is indicated for all first-degree haemorrhoids and for the smaller size second-degree haemorrhoids. Large piles will almost certainly return with recurrence of symptoms; however, the temporary control of symptoms may be excellent palliation in elderly patients. Injection therapy is not indicated for large haemorrhoids of third-degree severity or where the piles are complicated by thrombosis or an associated anal fissure.

The object of injection therapy is not to produce intravascular coagulation and it would be difficult to inject directly into the venous plexus. The phenol (5% in almond oil) produces a fibrotic induration after 2 or 3 weeks. The fibrosis may protect the veins during the passage of a stool and prevent further distension during straining. It may also produce a fixation of the pile to the underlying submucosa and diminish the degree of prolapse.

Injection therapy is given via proctoscopy into the submucosa at the anorectal ring and approximately 3 ml are given at the root of each major haemorrhoid. The injections may be repeated at 3–4 weeks. Only mild discomfort is felt which lasts not more than 24 h. Rarely the injections produce a localized necrosis and ulceration which may permit recurrent bleeding and irritation.

Infrared Coagulation

This recently marketed machine produces a circular burn about 2 mm in depth. Applied to the base of the haemorrhoid via a proctoscope it gives equivalent results to sclerotherapy when used on grade I and II haemorrhoids. It may be equivalent in efficiency to rubber band ligation and gives less pain and complication.

Alternative Non-operative Techniques

MANUAL DILATATION. This technique is based on the thesis that internal haemorrhoids are caused by circular constricting bands in the wall of the anorectal canal. These bands are broken down by stretching the anal canal using 4 fingers from each hand. A 4-cm anal dilator is used for some weeks afterwards. The procedure may produce cracks in the anal skin and protrusion of the rectal mucosa. The technique does not give consistent results and recurrence of haemorrhoids has been reported as occurring in 25% of patients. Furthermore, persistent anal incontinence is found in some patients and rectal prolapse has been reported in the elderly.

HAEMORRHOIDAL FREEZING. The application of cryosurgery to destroy haemorrhoids is currently under evaluation. The cryoprobe is applied to the mucosa of the haemorrhoid via access of a bivalve speculum until the surface is frosted. Usually 2 or 3 haemorrhoids can be treated at one outpatient session and it is important to give the patient adequate means of pain relief and pads to deal with the subsequent mucoid discharge. The slough produced by the technique usually takes 2–3 weeks to separate. Good control of the haemorrhoids may be expected in 80% of patients with the need for second applications or alternative treatment in the remainder.

RUBBER BAND LIGATION. This technique was designed as an outpatient procedure. Through a proctoscopy the pile is grasped in its mucosal part and one or two rubber bands are introduced over the pile to constrict the pedicle using a special instrument. In due course the pile necroses and the haemorrhoid sloughs. This appears to take 7–10 days and pain may be a severe postoperative feature for the first few days and requires potent analgesia.

Used on large second-degree haemorrhoids, the procedure is efficacious but is not advised if there are large external haemorrhoids or skin tags.

Operative Excision—Haemorrhoidectomy

As might be expected there are several described operations which aim to ligate and excise the haemorrhoid together with any external component. Very high ligation and stripping of the haemorrhoid as was practised during the early part of this century resulted in severe anal stenosis and this led to lower procedures which are currently practised widely. In this regard the report of Milligan and associates was influential, arguing that the ligated pile pedicle was tethered in the lower part of the anal canal by the fibres of the internal sphincter. The alternative to this approach is the submucosal haemorrhoidectomy described by Parkes in 1956 in which the pile pedicle was dissected from the overlying anal mucosa and ligated very high. The dissected mucosal flap covers the defect in the anal canal created by the dissection. The same effect may be obtained by various forms of closed haemorrhoidectomy (Hill–Ferguson) in which excision of the haemorrhoid is followed by primary suture of the mucosal and skin edges. Though it is clear that some of these wounds ultimately break down, there may be an advantage in terms of reduced postoperative discomfort and sepsis and the incidence of anal stenosis may be lower.

Where excision of haemorrhoids at the three primary sites leaves internal haemorrhoids in intermediate position, it is probably better to leave the mucosal bridge intact rather than attempt a complete excision and risk breakdown and stenosis. Secondary haemorrhoids often disappear subsequently or can be managed by sclerotherapy at a later date.

Postoperative Management and Complications

The rectum is normally emptied by suppositories and the patient encouraged to take a liquid diet for 1–2 days prior to operation. Normal diet may be resumed immediately after surgery and stool softeners prescribed. Though severe pain may occur during the initial postoperative defaecation, it does not disable all patients and can be controlled with analgesia. Postoperative retention of urine may occur even in young men and women but is naturally more common in older men with a degree of prostatism. Failure to respond to parasympathomimetic agents requires bladder catheterization for 2–3 days, after which normal urinary flow may establish itself. A small proportion of men may be precipitated into prostatectomy by haemorrhoidectomy.

Reactionary haemorrhage after haemorrhoidectomy occurs in a small proportion of patients and may require re-operation for haemostasis if passage of a Foley catheter and inflation of the balloon fails to control the bleeding. Secondary haemorrhage typically follows defaecation and occurs about the 7th–10th day, though it may be delayed until 2 or 3 weeks. The bleeding presumably follows separation of a slough from the base of ligated pedicle and is only rarely severe enough to require religation or suture.

Other later complications include fissure and fistula formation along the tracks of the cutaneous wounds though this is surprisingly rare. Stenosis may not be apparent on examination of the anal canal on the 7th–10th day but will often have developed by 3 weeks. Some surgeons routinely prescribe the use of an anal dilator after operation and though this is probably unnecessary for the majority of patients, it is required for those patients showing narrowing at 3 weeks. Good results from the dilator may be expected, provided that there is patient compliance. Rarely more forcible dilatation under anaesthesia is required for patients with severe stenosis.

Thrombosed Haemorrhoids

Prolapse and subsequent thrombosis of internal haemorrhoids is exceedingly painful and requires hospital admission. Conservative measures include ice packs, elevation of the foot of the bed and analgesia. While most patients will respond to these measures the alternative treatment of early excision and ligation has the attraction of immediate relief of the patient's complaint and should obviate the need for subsequent haemorrhoidal treatment. Provided that the procedure is performed carefully with preservation of mucocutaneous bridges, it appears safe and does not appear to be complicated by the theoretical complication of portal vein pyaemia.

External Haemorrhoids and Skin Tags

These result from congestion and sometimes thrombosis of the subcutaneous venous plexus of the anal margin. Pain, irritation and soreness are the predominant symptoms. External haemorrhage should not be a feature, though subcutaneous rupture of a vessel leads to the formation of a pea-sized, blue-red, perianal haematoma at the anal margin which is exquisitely painful and tender.

Many patients appear to have little or no symptoms from external piles *per se*, others find the pain and irritation sufficient to justify removal in a manner similar to the external component of a haemorrhoidectomy.

ANAL FISSURE

This minor anal complaint produces symptoms out of proportion to the pathological features of the condition. Characteristically, it is a crack in the perianal skin most commonly in the midline posteriorly. It may occasionally lie to one side of the midline or even anteriorly, particularly in women. The crack lies in the cutaneous portion of the anal canal between the anal orifice and the base of the anal valves. The fissure overlies the lower one-third of the internal sphincter and the circular muscle may sometimes be visible in the base. On the external aspect, the skin is swollen and produces a permanent skin tag to form a sentinel pile. At the upper end of the fissure there is commonly hypertrophy of an anal papilla.

Aetiology

Most fissures are of unknown aetiology. Quite often they occur in patients who are habitual laxative users who normally have a fairly liquid stool which has led to a tightly fibrosed anal canal. If these patients pass a hard mass of faeces, the skin may split. On most occasions the fissure may heal but infection and spasm of the underlying internal sphincter may prevent drainage of pus allowing the fissure to persist.

While most fissures occur posteriorly those which occur anteriorly seem quite often to follow successful childbirth. Other fissures are secondary to non-specific proctocolitis and Crohn's disease of the gastrointestinal tract or follow the operations of haemorrhoidectomy and laying open of an anal fistula.

Clinical Features

The prominent symptom is severe pain in the anal canal, especially during and for 20–30 minutes after defaecation. Bleeding is common but slight and a mucoid discharge produces perianal irritation. The patient may complain of a perianal swelling which is represented by the sentinel skin tag.

On examination, the anal orifice is seen to be contracted and pulled in, necessitating firm elevation of the buttock in order to obtain a good view. The sentinel pile may be seen as an oedematous skin tag lying at the lower edge of the fissure. Digital or proctoscopic examination will confirm the findings but in many instances is not possible because of pain and spasm of the anal sphincter.

Differential Diagnosis

Anal fissure must be distinguished from a superficial crack of the perianal skin seen with severe pruritus ani, a condition not normally associated with a sentinel pile or sphincteric spasm. Idiopathic stenosis of the anal canal is seen in the elderly and is due to submucosal fibrosis without a fissure. Atypical ulceration of the perianal margin may occur in tuberculosis and syphilis and the suspicion may be confirmed by biopsy, and culture of the tissue and by serological investigation. Gross fissures should remind one of the association with ulcerative proctocolitis and Crohn's disease and suggest the need for histological examination of the margin of the fissure. Finally, should the fissure be unduly indurated, malignancy is suspected.

Management

Most anal fissures heal spontaneously in 2 or 3 weeks. The patient should be encouraged to defaecate and mild laxatives and bulk-forming agents are prescribed. Pain may be eased by application of 5% lignocaine cream which the patient is advised to apply well within the anal canal, thus overcoming the sphincteric spasm somewhat. If this conservative management fails, then after examination under anaesthesia, two additional treatments are available: lateral cutaneous sphincterotomy divides the lower half of the internal sphincter and appears successful in about 95% of patients; less successful is forcible anal dilatation which leaves 20% of patients with symptoms and mild degrees of incontinence for flatus and liquid faeces in a similar proportion.

CARCINOMA OF THE ANAL CANAL AND ANUS

Two types of malignant neoplasm appear at the anus.

Squamous-cell Carcinoma

This is a relatively rare cancer accounting for only 3–6% of all malignant neoplasms involving the rectum and anal canal. Carcinoma of the anal margin is more common in males but carcinoma of the anal canal is more common in females. It is not clear why there should be this difference and it is not likely that anal fistulas or pruritus ani are aetiological factors. Histologically, carcinomas of the anus tend to be of low-grade malignancy whereas carcinomas of the anal canal are commonly dedifferentiated and of high-grade malignancy. Carcinomas of intermediate type may occur in the anal canal—muco-epidermoid—and are sometimes known as cloacagenic or basiloid cancers.

The appearance of the lesion is variable: a warty protuberance, flattened plaque or penetrating ulcer. Commonly the lesion is situated anteriorly and may be readily palpated through the vagina in a female patient. The patient may complain of an anal lump, of blood discharge and ultimately the growth produces painful defaecation or fistulates into the vagina.

At an early stage, anal carcinoma needs to be differentiated from an anal fissure, simple papilloma, anal condyloma, prolapsed internal haemorrhoids or the anal ulceration occurring with Crohn's disease. Commonly anal spasm makes digital examination difficult. All lesions, which appear indurated, should be examined under anaesthesia where necessary, and biopsied.

The inguinal lymph glands should also be examined carefully. There may be difficulty in distinguishing septic enlargement of the nodes from malignant infiltration though characteristically such nodes are harder.

Adenocarcinoma of the Rectum

Rectal carcinomas may spread downwards and invade the anal canal. On digital examination the lesion is usually softer than a squamous-cell carcinoma and may exude a mucoid material. A histological diagnosis by biopsy confirms the diagnosis of adenocarcinoma, which is then managed as other low-lying carcinomas of the rectum. Metastases in the inguinal nodes are rare with adenocarcinomas unless the skin of the anal orifice is invaded.

Treatment

There has been considerable controversy of the relative merits of surgery and radiotherapy. In the case of carcinomas extending above the pectinate line there is evidence that the lymph nodes around the superior haemorrhoidal vessels are readily involved and are thus less accessible to local excision and local radiotherapy. In such patients rectal excision is indicated, taking a wider margin of perianal skin and fat than is customary.

Rectal excision is not usually considered for growths of the anus and perianal region. Lymphatic spread from such lesions is exclusively to the inguinal lymph glands. Carcinomas of the anal margin may be managed by local excision of the cancer and the perianal skin taking a wide margin and if necessary sacrificing the lower part of the anal sphincters. Normally at least 2 cm of clearance around the tumour is necessary to deter local recurrence and careful follow-up is indicated.

The incidence of inguinal lymph-gland metastasis is slightly higher for carcinoma of the anal margin than for anal canal cancers but in both instances it is in the region of 40%. If the glands are clinically involved at the time of diagnosis, delayed block dissection of one or both groins is carried out 1–2 months after the primary tumour has been excised. The involvement may be confirmed by needle aspiration cytology. This delay may permit the resolution of enlarged, infected glands which appeared at first sight to be involved with metastases. Where the nodes do not appear clinically involved, two courses of action are possible. First prophylactic bilateral groin dissection may be performed but this will expose at least half the patients to an unnecessary degree of morbidity of delayed wound healing and lymphoedema of the lower limbs and external genitalia. Alternatively, the patient can be examined every month for 6 months and then every 2 months for a further 18 months followed by less frequent examination. In the event of suspicious lymphadenopathy, a superficial inguinal block dissection of the glands is carried out in that groin. Where the involved glands appear to extend above the inguinal ligament, the dissection may be deepened and extended upwards around the external iliac vessels by division of the inguinal ligament.

While treatment by irradiation from implanted radium needles or low voltage X-ray has been employed in the past, the modality was not particularly successful in cancer control, especially when the cancer arose in the anal canal. Fibrosis of the anal canal was common. Whether modern radiotherapy will prove to be better is uncertain but it is likely that improvements in technique may make radiotherapy with fast neutrons an alternative to surgery, particularly with the more superficial lesion. Combined radiotherapy and chemotherapy appear to show better results than

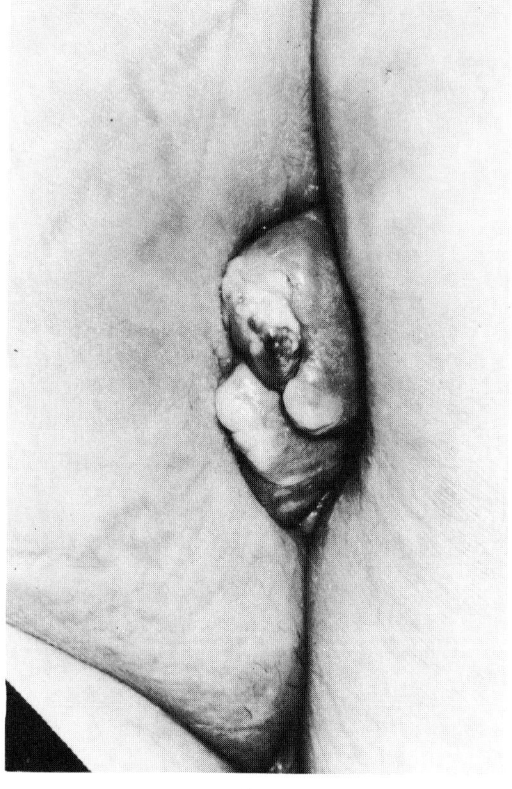

a

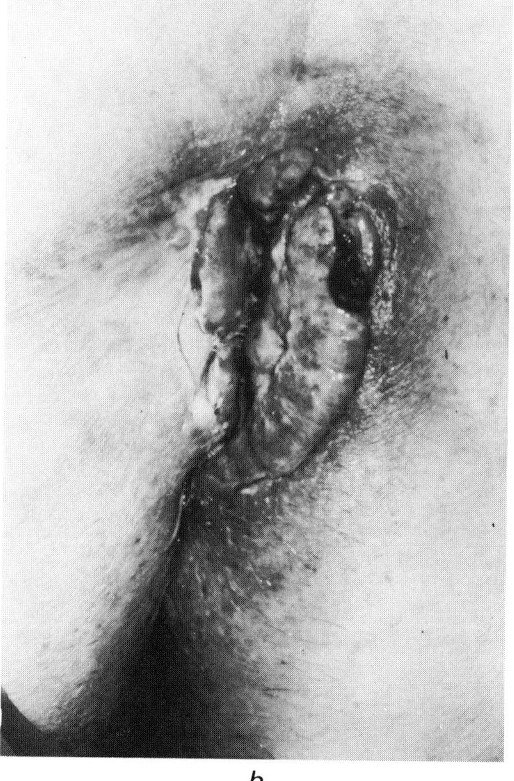

b

Fig. 74.28 *a*, Demonstrates a malignant melanoma of the anal canal which appeared as prolapsing haemorrhoids. *b*, For comparison. An advanced squamous-cell carcinoma of the anal margin is demonstrated.

radiotherapy alone. Very advanced lesions, which are unsuitable for surgery, are not often helped by radiotherapy and a colostomy may be necessary for palliation.

Results

Survival after treatment can be related directly to the pathological stage and lymph-node involvement. By using wide local excision for carcinoma of the anal margin and rectal excision for anal canal cancer, the overall 5-year survival rate for this condition is about 55%. In patients where the inguinal lymph nodes are involved at the time of diagnosis, block dissection does not improve prognosis, though occasional 5-year survivors are found. However, delayed groin dissection for involved nodes may have a prognosis of at least 60% at 5 years.

Basal Cell Carcinoma of the Anal Region

These are rare tumours of the anal region and are usually small, raised and indurated and occasionally ulcerated. Usually only 1–2 cm in diameter, they are amenable to wide surgical excision and the prognosis is excellent.

Intraepidermal cancer of the anal region (Bowen's disease) is also rare and is a diagnosis usually made after multiple biopsies of an unidentified perianal skin lesion. Wide excision and skin grafting are usually attended by good control.

Basiloid (Cloacagenic) Carcinoma

These are probably adenocarcinomas, arising from the intersphincteric anal glands, though it is fair to say that there is some debate about the origin. The lesion may be entirely submucosal and surround the anal canal and lower rectum, occasionally it may produce a deep penetrating ulcer about the level of the pectinate line with somewhat overlying edges. In most instances rectal excision is necessary.

Malignant Melanoma

Malignant melanoma of the anal canal has a poor prognosis with a highly metastasizing potential. The lesion may present as a rather protuberant but unusual looking prolapsed haemorrhoid (*Fig.* 74.28). Early spread to inguinal lymph glands seems to be the rule and both distant and local recurrences are common. After wide local excision, the patient should be followed closely and block dissection of the groins carried out upon clinical suspicion. Since the prognosis is so poor following nodal involvement, there may be an indication for adjuvant chemotherapy or immunotherapy.

75 The Acute Abdomen and Disorders of the Peritoneal Cavity

A. Cuschieri

EMERGENCY CLINICAL ASSESSMENT OF PATIENTS REFERRED FOR HOSPITAL ADMISSION

The assessment of these patients and the decision-making process regarding their management is crucial, since some will have life-threatening conditions which necessitate immediate surgical intervention or soon after resuscitation. Others require hospital admission for observation or initial conservative management. Some of these patients may well require subsequent urgent surgical intervention either because of failure of conservative management or because of the development of complications. Diagnostic errors on the initial assessment may at best lead to unnecessary surgical intervention, and at worst, to demise of the patient or a protracted clinical illness due to the development of complications which could have been avoided by earlier surgical intervention.

In the absence of obvious life-threatening intra-abdominal disorders, *the initial decision concerns the need or otherwise for hospital admission, and if so, whether the patient's underlying condition is of a surgical or medical nature.* The risk factors necessitating admission to hospital are:

1. Abdominal pain of less than 48 hours' duration.
2. Abdominal pain followed by vomiting.
3. History of recent trauma, operation or haemorrhage.
4. Abnormal physical signs—neurological, cardiovascular, respiratory, abdominal and urinary.
5. History of loss or impairment of consciousness.
6. Extremes of age.

Clinical Examination

The initial diagnosis relies heavily on a thorough clinical examination preceded by a detailed history from the patient or relatives in the case of infants and patients with mental confusion/coma from any cause. The abdominal part of the examination must be complete and should always include a rectal examination. The important abdominal findings which indicate significant intra-abdominal disease are guarding/rigidity, tenderness/rebound, distension, tender masses and external hernias, absent/tingling/hyperactive bowel sounds, and rectal tenderness/mass. Often a specific diagnosis is possible on the basis of the history and physical examination alone, e.g. acute appendicitis. At other times, the clinical evaluation establishes the presence of acute intra-abdominal pathology (acute abdomen) but only a differential diagnosis is possible and laboratory tests and other investigations are necessary to establish a definite diagnosis. Sometimes, the initial assessment is inconclusive and necessitates close observation with repeated examination of the abdomen and monitoring of the vital signs. This remains the most reliable means of establishing developing intra-abdominal pathology. It entails a constant reappraisal of the situation and an early decision for surgical intervention when conservative treatment fails. The decision to operate must not be delayed until there is definite deterioriation in the patient's general condition. *Diagnostic difficulties are most often encountered in extremes of age.*

There are certain medical disorders which may present with abdominal signs. An awareness of these is necessary since delayed recognition may prove fatal. In addition, the underlying disorder may be adversely affected by unwarranted general anaesthesia and surgical intervention. The medical conditions which may cause diagnostic problems in the emergency situation are outlined in *Table* 75.1.

Investigations

The routine investigations performed in patients with acute intra-abdominal illness include Hb, PCV, WBC, urea and electrolytes and urinalysis (microscopy, glycosuria, proteinuria). Other biochemical investigations, such as liver function tests and estimations of serum amylase, may be indicated in the individual case.

Radiology

This includes a chest radiograph and scout abdominal films (erect and supine). A chest radiograph is indicated in patients with respiratory symptoms, the elderly, patients with chronic cardiorespiratory disease and patients with acute pancreatitis. The abdominal scout films are used selectively to establish the following:

- Calculi, calcified wall of an aneurysm, etc.
- Free gas under the diaphragm (erect film).
- Dilatation of hollow organs including intestinal loops (supine film).
- Fluid levels (erect film).
- Free fluid/blood in the peritoneal cavity.
- Herniation of intra-abdominal contents through the diaphragm.
- Distortion of the stomach air bubble.

Table 75.1 Medical causes of acute abdominal pain

Myocardial infarction	The epigastrium is the sole site of the pain in 0·7% of cases and occurs at any time in 3·3%. May be misdiagnosed as peptic ulceration
Lobar pneumonia	Pain may be referred to either subcostal region depending on site of lung disease. Problem often encountered in the elderly
Diabetic ketoacidosis	May present with abdominal pain and vomiting. A diabetic history may not be obtained particularly in the young juvenile previously undiagnosed diabetic. Urine testing for sugar and ketones should be performed on all patients admitted with acute abdominal pain
Acute hepatitis	Viral or acute alcoholic hepatitis. Abdominal pain and tenderness is often present. The latter may be marked. The associated fever and jaundice may be misinterpreted as cholangitis due to ductal calculi. The diagnosis should become clear by the *marked* elevation in the serum transaminases. Often, the level of consciousness is impaired
Sickle-cell disease	The crises of this disorder which are precipitated by hypoxia, produce both abdominal pain and tenderness
Henoch–Schönlein purpura	May present with acute colicky abdominal pain, nausea and vomiting usually in children and young adults with a preponderance in males. Intestinal infarction and perforation may rarely occur in this condition which is due to the deposition of IgA-immune complexes
Congenital spherocytosis	Abdominal pain is caused by acute haemolytic episodes
Congenital erythropoietic hepatic porphyrias	Abdominal pain, vomiting, constipation. Erythropoietic type precipitated by drugs, menstruation, starvation, infection and alcohol excess
Erythrohepatic porphyria (protoporphyria)	Abdominal pain and jaundice simulating common bile duct obstruction. Cholelithiasis occurs in only 10% of these patients. Note: protoporphyrin can only be excreted in the bile. Attacks precipitated by fasting, sun exposure or iron deficiency
Herpes zoster	The pain which is most commonly in the distribution of T7–L1 may precede the blisters. The pain is of a burning nature and usually quite severe
Lead poisoning	May present with episodes of intestinal colic. A blue line may be present in the gums.
Campylobacter infections	These may cause the pseudoappendicitis syndrome, acute terminal ileitis and mesenteric lymphadenitis. However, some of these infections may cause perforation and peritonitis

N.B. Porphyrias are inherited disorders of porphyrin (haem precursor) metabolism. The main abnormalities occur either in the bone marrow (erythropoietic) or liver (hepatic). The porphyrin intermediates that accumulate are responsible for the photosensitivity.

Obliteration of the psoas outline.
Kidney outlines.
Fractures (ribs, spine, pelvis).

Contrast radiology may be necessary in the diagnosis of oesophageal perforations. Usually gastrografin is used for this purpose since it does not cause a granulomatous reaction in the event of extravasation. Gastrografin is, however, hypertonic and may lead to serious complications which include electrolyte imbalance, significant fluid shifts from the vascular compartment, pulmonary oedema, if aspirated, and rarely intestinal necrosis. Because of these potential dangers, some radiologists favour barium instead of gastrografin in these patients, in which case any extravasated barium must be removed at operation. A barium enema is required in patients with subacute large bowel obstruction. An intravenous pyelogram is necessary for all patients with haematuria and renal colic. It may also be required in theatre when the pathology found at emergency laparotomy necessitates the removal of one kidney, when the presence of an adequately functioning non-obstructed contralateral kidney can be ascertained. Selective angiography (coeliac axis/superior mesenteric/inferior mesenteric) is necessary whenever endoscopy fails to outline the cause of the bleeding. This investigation may be preceded by $^{99}Tc^{m}$ Sc scintiscanning for the localization of the bleeding site.

Endoscopy

Emergency upper gastrointestinal endoscopy has largely replaced the barium meal examination in the acute situation in view of its superior diagnostic yield. Lesions, such as oesophagitis, oesophageal ulcer, erosive gastritis are often visualized only by endoscopy. In patients with endoscopically proven varices, an alternative site of bleeding, e.g. ulcer, is found in 20–40% of cases. In cases of bleeding peptic ulcer, the endoscopic findings (fresh blood clot, black slough adherent to the ulcer, visible vessel) may indicate a high risk of rebleeding and, therefore, suggest the need for surgical intervention. In addition, endoscopy may be used to achieve haemostasis—injection sclerotherapy, laser photocoagulation and electrocoagulation of bleeding vessels at the base of a peptic ulcer.

Sigmoidoscopy and colonoscopy are extremely useful in patients with rectal bleeding and large bowel obstruction. Often they are diagnostic and in some patients they may prove therapeutic as in sigmoid volvulus, acute colonic pseudo-obstruction and colonic angiodysplasias where electrocoagulation through the colonoscope is often successful in achieving haemostasis. Sigmoidoscopy is also indicated in patients presenting with diarrhoea. The contraindications to emergency colonoscopy are the presence of active inflammation with peritoneal irritation such as toxic megacolon or acute diverticulitis, when the risk of perforation is great, and in massive haemorrhage when visualization is impossible.

Emergency Ultrasound, CT and Isotope Scintiscanning

Abdominal ultrasound has an established place in the investigation of certain patients with acute intra-abdominal disorders and is nowadays routinely used in the following situations:

Suspected cholelithiasis and acute cholecystitis.
Detection of intra-abdominal abscesses and fluid collections, e.g. pancreatic pseudocysts, ascites.
Patients admitted as an emergency with obstructive jaundice.
Examination of palpable abdominal masses.
Suspected abdominal aneurysm.

CT scanning is very accurate in the detection of intra-abdominal abscesses. It is also useful in documenting pancreatic necrosis in severe pancreatitis and in the detection of trauma to the intra-abdominal organs following blunt injury. It is not, however, generally available for emergency use except in neurosurgical units and large trauma units. Moreover, it is an expensive investigation.

Aside from its use in the diagnosis of trauma to the solid organs, isotope scintigraphy is valuable in the evaluation of patients with lower gastrointestinal bleeding ($^{99}Tc^{m}$ Sc), detection of intra-abdominal abscesses (isotope-labelled autologous WBC scan) and in patients with suspected acute cholecystitis, where the E-HIDA scanning is the most accurate test of cystic duct obstruction. A normal E-HIDA gallbladder scan excludes acute cholecystitis with a 100% reliability.

Abdominal Lavage

The four-quadrant abdominal tap using an aspiration technique with a fine needle inserted in each of the four quadrants has been replaced by peritoneal lavage because of its greater diagnostic accuracy for intra-abdominal injuries. After adequate sedation and catheterization of the bladder, a peritoneal dialysis catheter is inserted in the infra-umbilical region via a small incision. Ringer-lactate solution (15 ml/kg) is then rapidly infused and immediately collected by gravity. The test is considered positive if gross blood is returned or the RBC count is greater than 100 000/ml, the WBC > 500/ml and the amylase content of the fluid is higher than 175 u/ml. The reported diagnostic accuracy of peritoneal lavage for trauma is 80–90%. False negatives are rare and occur in relation to retroperitoneal injuries (pancreas and

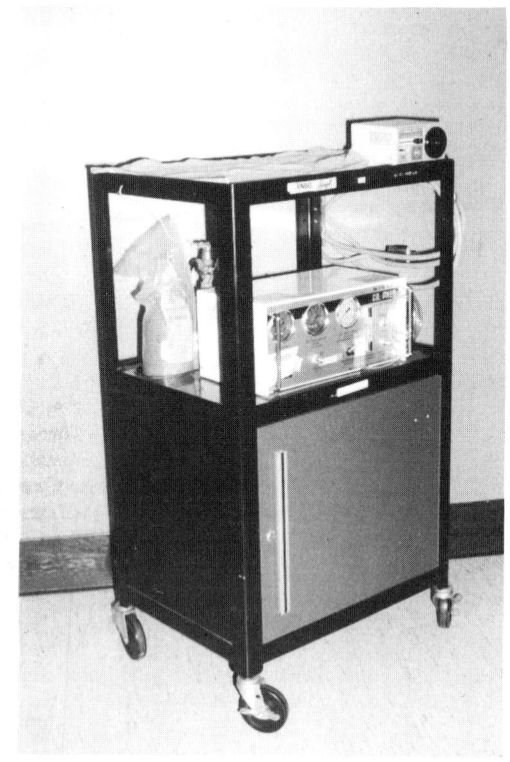

a

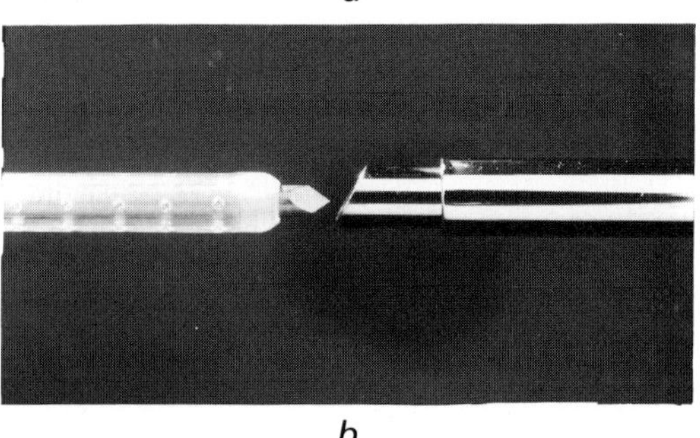

b

Fig. 75.1 *a*, Mobile trolley containing instruments, light source and nitrous oxide insufflator for minilaparoscopy. The procedure is carried out under local anaesthesia and intravenous sedation with diazepam or midazolam. (By kind permission, from Berci G. and Cuschieri A. (ed.) (1986). *Practical Laparoscopy*. London, Baillière Tindall.) *b*, Comparative sizes of the minilaparoscope and the peritoneal dialysis cannula used for peritoneal lavage.

kidneys). However, in 20% of patients with a positive lavage subjected to laparotomy, no visceral injury is encountered and the bleeding is found to have stopped at operation. The test is therefore too sensitive and results in a number of unnecessary laparotomies. Peritoneal lavage is useful in the grading of the severity of acute pancreatitis. The retrieval of bloodstained or prune-coloured fluid indicates the presence of severe haemorrhagic pancreatitis.

Emergency Laparoscopy

During the past decade, there has been an increasing use of laparoscopy in the diagnosis of acute intra-abdominal disease. There is little doubt that with modern equipment, laparoscopy is a safe and rewarding procedure which may avoid unnecessary laparotomy in the emergency situation. It, therefore, reduces morbidity incurred from unwarranted surgical intervention and saves hospital resources and expenditure. The development of minilaparoscopy has greatly facilitated this investigation. The instruments are much smaller (*Fig.* 75.1) and the external diameter of the inspecting telescope approximates to the size of a peritoneal dialysis catheter (4 mm). The procedure is carried out under local anaesthesia and intravenous sedation with diazemuls and pethidine. The peritoneal cavity is insufflated with nitrous oxide as this causes less discomfort than CO_2. Minilaparoscopy has been shown to be particularly valuable in the following conditions:

Abdominal trauma.

Acute lower abdominal and right iliac fossa pain, where it reliably differentiates acute appendicitis from gynaecological pathology.

The doubtful acute abdomen, where physical findings and the results of investigations are inconclusive. The laparoscopic findings will establish the diagnosis and the need or otherwise for surgical intervention, e.g. perforated ulcer versus acute cholecystitis or pancreatitis.

Suspicion of mesenteric ischaemia.

The contraindications to laparoscopy in the emergency situation are:

1. Established acute generalized peritonitis.
2. Obvious clinical evidence of active intra-abdominal bleeding.
3. Gross ileus and intestinal obstruction.
4. Obstructed/strangulated external hernias.
5. Extensive or multiple abdominal scars.
6. Abdominal wall sepsis.

IATROGENIC INJURIES

These consist of injuries sustained to the intra-abdominal organs during endoscopy and surgical intervention. Less commonly, complications may result from percutaneous liver biopsy (bleeding, bile peritonitis), interventional radiology involving selective angiography (arterial damage, bleeding), percutaneous transhepatic cholangiography/portography/insertion of endoprosthesis (bleeding, bile peritonitis, intrahepatic A-V fistula between portal vein and hepatic artery), peritoneal dialysis/lavage and laparoscopy (bleeding, perforation of the gastrointestinal tract or bladder).

Endoscopic Injuries

These may involve the oesophagus, stomach, colon/rectum, urethra and bladder. Iatrogenic perforations of the oesophagus account for 60–70% of all cases of oesophageal injuries. The incidence of oesophageal perforation following insertion of a rigid endoscope is 0·5% as opposed to 0·08% after flexible endoscopy. The highest incidence is encountered during oesophageal dilatation/intubation of strictures and approximates to 1 in every 400 patients undergoing this procedure. Most of these injuries involve the lower thoracic oesophagus and are described in Chapter 65. However, perforation of the abdominal oesophagus and stomach is well documented after dilatation with the Eder–Peustow system. In these instances, the injury is often caused by the guide wire. The patient develops upper abdominal pain and tenderness after the procedure and the plain radiograph may demonstrate free air under the diaphragm. As the perforation is usually small, these patients are best treated conservatively with nasogastric suction, systemic antibiotics and intravenous fluids.

Perforation of the stomach and duodenum during diagnostic upper gastrointestinal endoscopy is rare. It is distinctly more common during interventional endoscopy such as endoscopic electrocoagulation (particularly when a unipolar system is used), laser photocoagulation and endoscopic sphincterotomy. In the latter instance, the perforation occurs in the retroperitoneal aspect of the second part of the duodenum. The plain radiograph may not reveal free air underneath the diaphragm in these retroperitoneal injuries, but surgical emphysema of the retroperitoneum tracking upwards into the mediastinum and downwards along the right psoas margin, is always present. Immediate surgical intervention is required for all these injuries.

The reported incidence of colonic perforation during colonoscopy is 0·2%. Contributing factors include redundant sigmoid colon, extensive diverticular disease, pelvic surgery, inflammatory bowel disease and endoscopic polypectomy and electrocoagulation of vascular malformations. Colonic bleeding is encountered in 1–2% of cases and is usually associated with polypectomy and inadequate diathermy.

Unfortunately, not all endoscopic injuries are recognized immediately. The problem is compounded by the fact that gastrointestinal endoscopy is becoming the domain of the gastroenterologists who are less adept than their surgical colleagues in the early detection of intra-abdominal complications. Delay in surgical intervention adversely affects both the morbidity and mortality from these iatrogenic injuries.

Instrumental injuries of the urethra and bladder are usually the result of dilatation of urethral strictures and transurethral resections of the prostate and bladder tumours. They are considered in Chapters 82, 83.

Operative Injuries

Operative injuries are largely avoidable and their occurrence usually reflects inexperience, inadequate exposure of the relevant anatomy and faulty technique. The risk factors include obesity, forcible retraction and intraperitoneal adhesions. The injury may result from direct instrumental injury, e.g. laceration of liver/spleen by retractor, blind clamping to control sudden haemorrhage, scissors/scalpel division, electrocoagulation and inclusion in a ligature. Other injuries are caused by traction on peritoneal and omental attachments, e.g. laceration of the spleen during mobilization of the splenic flexure or shearing trauma in the case of adherent loops of intestine. The injury may not be recognized at operation but becomes manifest postoperatively by signs of internal bleeding, peritonitis, abscess and fistula formation. The most frequent late consequence of injury to narrow tubular organs (bile duct, ureter) is stricture formation with progressive obstruction and persistent infection. Details of the commonly injured organs and the relevant surgical procedures which are associated with these injuries are shown in *Table* 75.2.

The spleen is the most commonly injured organ at operation. The commonest type of injury is a capsular tear (65%), followed by hilar disruption (25%). Splenic repair should be attempted whenever possible, otherwise splenectomy is performed, in which case, splenic autotransplantation of small 2 mm slices in omental pouches is advocated by some in an effort at preservation of splenic function.

All injuries which are recognized at operation are repaired immediately. If performed expeditiously, this usually avoids serious immediate and late complications. These patients should receive a 5-day course of antibiotic active against Gram-negative aerobes.

PERITONITIS

Inflammation of the peritoneal cavity may be due to bacterial invasion—*septic peritonitis* or to irritation by extravasated secretions—*chemical peritonitis*, e.g. bile, urine, blood, meconium, or implanted foreign body (talc, starch, cellulose, etc.). Classification of the various forms of the disease is based on the pathogenesis. The important types are:

1. Acute secondary bacterial peritonitis.
2. Primary (spontaneous) bacterial peritonitis.
3. Acute non-bacterial peritonitis.
4. Chronic bacterial peritonitis (tuberculous).
5. Chronic non-bacterial peritonitis (granulomatous).

Acute Secondary Bacterial Peritonitis

This accounts for the majority of cases. When generalized and severe, it still carries an appreciable mortality which varies from 20 to 60%. The most common cause is perforation of the gastrointestinal tract secondary to inflammatory, ischaemic or neoplastic disease. At other times, the disruption of the gastrointestinal tract may be due to penetrating or blunt external trauma, or follow unrecognized operative injuries or dehiscence of anastomoses.

Pathology

The severity of the disease depends on the site of perforation and the underlying pathology. The peritonitis is mild in patients with perforated peptic ulcers as the escaping fluid is either sterile or has a low bacterial cell count. It is usually localized in patients with perforated appendicitis, acute salpingitis, acute diverticulitis and gangrenous cholecystitis. The severity of the disease varies from mild to moderate in these cases. Peritonitis is severe when it results from large bowel free perforations (faecal peritonitis), mesenteric infarction and following disruption of intestinal anastomoses.

The acute inflammatory response is exudative with the outpouring of large amounts of fluid rich in protein including opsonins and fibrinogen, and polymorphonuclear leucocytes. The fibrinogen polymerizes to fibrin which is involved

Table 75.2 Common operative injuries

Organ	*Operation/procedure*	*Risk factors*
Abdominal oesophagus	Para-oesophageal surgery: fundoplication, vagotomy, repair hiatus hernia,	Oesophagitis, previous surgery
Spleen	Para-oesophageal and gastric surgery, mobilization of splenic flexure	Splenomegaly, perisplenitis
Pancreas	Splenectomy	Bleeding from the mobilized spleen or hilar vessels
Bile duct	Cholecystectomy	Abnormal anatomy, inadequate display, omission of operative cholangiography, difficult cholecystectomy, bleeding
Duodenum	Right hemicolectomy	Adhesion of hepatic flexure to 3rd part of duodenum
Small intestine	Enterolysis, intestinal obstruction	Dilated, oedematous intestinal loops
Ureter	Hysterectomy, colectomy	Inadequate identification of ureter, devascularization, involvement by inflammatory mass

N.B. Operative injuries to the spleen account for 16–20% of all splenectomies. Injury to the abdominal oesophagus occurs in 0·5% of all vagotomies.

in the process of localization of the infection. The peritoneum therefore becomes oedematous, hyperaemic and is covered with a thick fibrinous exudate which coats the viscera and binds adjacent loops together and to the omentum and parietes. Concomitant with the exudative changes, there is complete cessation of peristaltic activity in the intestinal tract. This, too, favours the localization of the infection. The fibrin deposition may not be entirely advantageous to the host since it is known to impair the transport of polymorphs to the infection site. There is also some evidence that the fibrinous meshwork may be the forerunner of fibrous adhesions. The opsonins together with the complement system are necessary for phagocytosis of bacteria by the polymorphonuclear leucocytes. Toxaemia, septicaemia, endotoxinaemia and shock of varying degrees accompany all cases of acute secondary bacterial peritonitis. The massive outpouring of inflammatory exudate causes hypovolaemia. Death is usually due to the septic shock syndrome.

The infection is a mixed one with Gram-negative aerobes and anaerobes (*E. coli*, Klebsiella spp., Proteus, *Pseudomonas aeruginosa* and Bacteroides), and Gram-positive bacteria (Enterococcus, Staphylococcus, Streptococcus spp., Clostridia spp.). Usually, however, only one aerobic and one anaerobic species are recovered from the peritoneal exudate.

Clinical Features

The symptoms and signs of the causative lesion (e.g. acute appendicitis, acute diverticulitis, etc.) usually precede those of localized or spreading peritonitis. Mesenteric infarction is a notable exception to this rule. Also, perforation of a duodenal ulcer may occur without any antecedent exacerbation or, indeed, a history of dyspepsia. The patient is suddenly gripped by a severe excruciating burning epigastric pain which spreads to the entire abdomen within a few minutes to 1 h and is due to chemical irritation by the escaping gastric juice.

The pain of established bacterial peritonitis may not be severe. It has a burning quality, starts in the quadrant related to the primary lesion, and may subsequently spread to other regions or the entire abdomen. Movement and coughing exacerbate the pain. Abdominal tenderness and rebound tenderness are always marked in secondary bacterial peritonitis. The area of tenderness reflects the localized or generalized nature of the disease. Reflex spasm of the abdominal musculature with rigidity, is seen in all cases of bacterial peritonitis, and the abdominal walls cease to move with respiration. The extreme board-like rigidity with the development of the scaphoid abdomen is confined to cases of perforated peptic ulcer. The reflex spasm of the abdominal musculature is lost during the advanced stages of bacterial peritonitis.

Absence of peristaltic activity which characterizes all forms of acute generalized bacterial peritonitis, is only partly reflex in origin since bacterial toxins disrupt intestinal motility. In the absence of adequate nasogastric decompression, progressive distension of the intestine with fluid and gas ensues, and may interfere with diaphragmatic movement. The sequestration of fluid and electrolytes in the peritoneal cavity and in the dilated loops of small intestine results in hypovolaemia, dehydration and electrolyte imbalance. The tinkling sounds which can often be auscultated at this stage are due to the passive movement of fluid within distended intestinal loops.

A rising tachycardia is always present and the temperature is elevated. Hypothermia, when it ensues, is a grave prognostic sign and indicates advanced irreversible septic shock. Tachypnoea accompanies the pyrexia and is aggravated by the development of abdominal distension and diaphragmatic splinting. Fortunately, the late stages of acute bacterial peritonitis are rarely seen nowadays. The moribund patient has sunken eyeballs and drawn anxious facies (Hippocratic facies), cold clammy skin, hypotension and oliguria or anuria.

A polymorphonuclear leucocytosis is invariably present. Haematological and biochemical evidence of dehydration include a rising haematocrit and blood urea. Often there is gross electrolyte disturbance, usually a hyponatraemia. Jaundice with elevation of the transaminase enzymes, may accompany severe acute bacterial peritonitis and may be the result of a toxic (reactive) hepatitis or haemolysis consequent on septicaemia and endotoxinaemia. The latter may lead to disseminated intravascular coagulation. The plain abdominal films often demonstrate dilated small intestinal loops, free gas under the diaphragm (*Fig.* 75.2) and in some cases free fluid in the peritoneal cavity, giving a ground glass appearance.

Complications

The complications of acute secondary bacterial peritonitis are subdivided into early and late.

Early Complications

Septicaemia and septic shock.
Recurrent uncontrolled intra-abdominal sepsis with death from multi-system failure.
Residual intraperitoneal abscesses: single (e.g. subphrenic, pelvic, etc.), multiple small interloop abscesses.
Portal pyaemia (pylephlebitis, hepatic abscesses).
Wound infection and impaired wound healing.

Late Complications

Incisional hernia.
Adhesion formation and recurrent intestinal obstruction.

Differential Diagnosis

In practice, established acute secondary bacterial peritonitis is easily diagnosed by virtue of the prominent clinical signs. However, a number of medical disorders should be kept in mind since they may masquerade as an acute abdomen because of referred pain, peritonism or abdominal crises. These are summarized in *Table* 75.1. The term 'peritonism' is a clinical one and refers to any condition which produces abdominal pain and some guarding with minimal tenderness. Bowel activity is, however, present and rebound tenderness is minimal or absent.

Treatment

This is best considered under two separate headings: supportive and definitive.

SUPPORTIVE MEASURES. These include nasogastric suction, intravenous fluid to correct the hypovolaemia and electrolyte deficiencies, monitoring and prompt and adequate pain relief. Volume expansion is best carried out with crystalloid solutions such as isotonic saline/dextrose or Hartmann's solution. Specific electrolyte abnormalities are corrected as necessary. In patients who are severely shocked, colloid solutions are also administered (PPD, Haemaccel). Blood is administered if the haematocrit is low. The intravenous fluid therapy is monitored by the CVP and hourly urine output which must be kept between 30 and 50 ml/h. The relief of

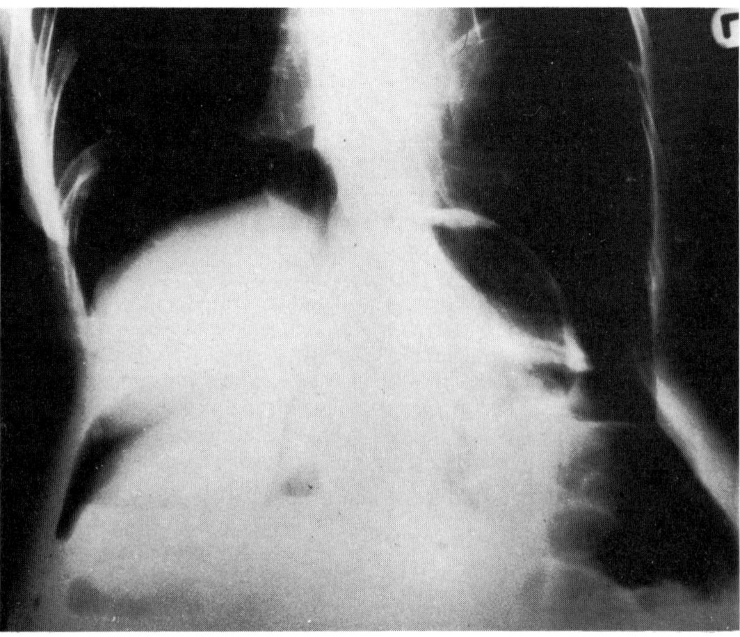

Fig. 75.2 Free air underneath the diaphragm and in the subhepatic pouch due to perforation of the caecum.

pain and neurogenic shock is an essential part of the resuscitation. It is often delayed because of an irrational fear of masking essential physical signs. In practice, the reverse is the case as a more accurate assessment of the patient and his acute abdomen is possible after adequate sedation and pain relief. The tenderness and rigidity may become localized, masses often become palpable and the patient's co-operation is assured.

DEFINITIVE MEASURES. These include:

Systemic antibiotics.
Laparotomy, surgical treatment of the primary disease and lavage.
Débridement.

Antibiotic Therapy

Secondary bacterial peritonitis is always polymicrobial in origin. Combination antibiotic therapy, usually triple, is essential against such a mixed flora. Several combinations are currently in use but the most favoured is an aminoglycoside/third-generation cephalosporin/metronidazole regimen which is maintained for 10 days. If continued beyond 2 weeks, this antibiotic combination carries a significant risk of invasive fungal infection. Blood levels of the antibiotics are essential for ensuring an adequate therapeutic level and, in the case of aminoglycosides, for the prevention of renal and eighth cranial nerve damage.

Laparotomy and Surgical Treatment

Most commonly this is performed through a midline approach. The primary lesion is located after a preliminary exploration and dealt with accordingly. Complete removal of the purulent peritoneal exudate and loose fibrinous deposits is essential. A specimen of the pus is obtained for bacteriology (aerobic and anaerobic culture). Thereafter, peritoneal lavage with saline is performed until the peritoneal cavity appears clean and free of debris. The addition of antibiotics (tetracycline, cephalosporin—0·75 g/l) is favoured by some. Drainage of the peritoneal cavity is not advisable unless continuous peritoneal lavage is contemplated in the postoperative period. Drains have been shown to increase the morbidity (wound sepsis, delayed wound healing, fistula, etc.) in these patients.

In severe cases, antibiotic lavage is extended into the postoperative period. A peritoneal silicone dialysis catheter (Tenckhoff) is introduced in the immediate subumbilical region before closure of the abdomen together with a silicone drainage catheter in the supracolic compartment, pelvis and either flank. The lavage is performed with peritoneal dialysate solution containing 1 g of cefoxitin/l infused through the Tenckhoff catheter at a rate of 250 ml/h whilst the drainage tubes are spigoted. The infusion is stopped after 1 L is administered. It is left for 30 min and then drained over the next half-hour. The continuous peritoneal lavage is maintained for 72 h after surgery. Accurate fluid balance charts should be kept and the patient must be weighed daily. Monitoring of the serum albumin and plasma potassium is essential during continuous peritoneal lavage.

Radical peritoneal débridement has been advocated recently. This entails the meticulous removal of all the fibrin membranes together with excision of abscess cavities on the premise that fibrin traps the bacteria and impairs phagocytosis by limiting leucocyte transport. However, a prospective study has not shown any benefit from this procedure which is time-consuming and accompanied by an excessive blood loss.

The abdominal wall is sutured with monofilament material but the skin wound is left open and packed with gauze soaked in acriflavine emulsion. In the absence of infection, secondary suture of the skin is performed 5–7 days later. In patients with a heavily contaminated peritoneal cavity, the entire wound is packed and then covered with Opsite. Alternatively, a Marlex mesh with a zip-fastener is sutured to the wound edges. This approach allows repeated inspection of the peritoneal cavity under intravenous sedation and is believed to reduce the recurrent sepsis rate. However, it is not, as yet, an established form of treatment and further evaluation by prospective studies is necessary before it can be recommended as a routine measure in these patients.

Primary (Spontaneous) Bacterial Peritonitis

This condition is diagnosed more frequently nowadays, although it is not clear whether this reflects an enhanced awareness of the condition or a true increased incidence of the disease. The peritonitis is primary in that there is no intra-abdominal disease or focus responsible for the bacterial invasion of the peritoneal cavity.

One type is haematogenous and occurs predominantly in children and is more common in females. It usually follows an acute febrile illness, e.g. chest and urinary tract infection, the common organisms responsible being *Strep. pneumoniae* and Group A Streptococcus. Risk factors include malnutrition, intra-abdominal malignancy, immunosuppression and splenectomy. Rare instances of primary gonococcal peritonitis in the female are well documented. Peritonitis may also follow acute gonorrhoea, septic abortion and puerperal sepsis but these are not, strictly speaking, instances of primary bacterial peritonitis.

More commonly, the disease affects patients with chronic renal and liver disease. The high risk groups are patients with the nephrotic syndrome, patients in chronic renal failure, especially those on chronic peritoneal dialysis and cirrhotic patients with ascites. The prevalence of the disease in cirrhotic patients is 8%. However, the incidence of bacterascites (positive ascitic fluid culture in an otherwise asymptomatic patient) is much higher. The majority of infections in this group of patients are caused by enteric organisms (*E. coli, S. faecalis,* Klebsiella sp., Bacteroides sp. etc.) although infections caused by *S. pneumoniae* and Haemophilus sp. are not uncommon. Most of the infections are aerobic and 50–60% of the reported cases have been caused by *E. coli.*

Clinical Features

The disease develops insidiously and localizing signs of peritonitis may be minimal. The most common manifestations include abdominal pain, fever, rebound tenderness and diminished or absent bowel sounds. In cirrhotic patients, there is an obvious deterioriation in the level of consciousness often progressing to hepatic coma. The full-blown picture is accompanied by septic shock with rigors and hypotension. A peritoneal tap with a small gauge needle attached to a 20-ml syringe should be performed in all patients suspected of having the disease. Some of the fluid which is usually turbid, is immediately Gram stained, the remainder is sent for bacteriological culture. Laparoscopy performed under local anaesthesia is also extremely helpful in establishing a definite diagnosis and in excluding primary gastrointestinal or pelvic disease. The mortality of primary bacterial peritonitis is high, varying from 20 to 80%. The highest mortality is encountered in patients with cirrhosis.

Treatment

In some patients, the differentiation of primary from secondary bacterial peritonitis proves difficult. Exploratory laparotomy is advisable in these patients, in which case, once the diagnosis is confirmed and other intra-abdominal disease is excluded at laparotomy, thorough abdominal lavage is carried out with saline containing 1 g/l of Cefoxitin. The favoured systemic antibiotic regimen in patients with renal and hepatic disease is a combination of an aminoglycoside and a third-generation cephalosporin. As systemic antibiotics may take several hours to build a sufficient concentration in the ascitic fluid, some favour the initial instillation of antibiotics into the peritoneal cavity at least in severely ill patients. Pneumococcal infections are treated with a broad-spectrum penicillin such as ampicillin, amoxycillin or augmentin (amoxycillin + clavulanic acid which inactivates bacterial penicillinases).

Acute Non-bacterial Peritonitis

In this instance, the peritoneal inflammation is due to the escape of irritant but not infected visceral contents/secretions into the peritoneal cavity, e.g. gastric juice following perforated peptic ulcer, bile after biliary surgery, urine following trauma to the urinary bladder, etc. In all these instances, the peritoneal exudate, although initially sterile, becomes infected within 6–12 h due to bacterial proliferation. Delay in treatment of these emergencies is thus accompanied by a significant rise in morbidity and mortality consequent on the development of secondary acute bacterial peritonitis.

Biliary peritonitis is most commonly encountered after biliary surgery and may arise from bile leakage from an accessory duct draining into the gallbladder. The accessory duct is avulsed during the mobilization of the gallbladder from its liver bed. Another common cause is leakage from the choledochotomy wound after removal of a T-tube following exploration of the common bile duct. In the majority of patients, a sinus tract forms around the external limb of the latex T-tube by the 7th–10th day after its insertion. However, in some patients, particularly the elderly, immunosuppressed and diabetic individuals, formation and maturation of the tract is delayed, and for this reason, bile escapes freely into the peritoneal cavity following removal of the T-tube. In these patients and whenever a silicone T-tube has been inserted instead of a latex one, a period of 4 weeks should be allowed to elapse before removal of the T-tube. Escape of bile into the peritoneal cavity is encountered after iatrogenic bile duct damage and may complicate the performance of bilio-enteric anastomosis. In all these patients the clinical signs may be minimal. The temperature is slightly elevated and the patient develops a mild tachycardia. There is tenderness with some rebound on palpation and the bowel sounds are hypoactive. Timely exploration will prevent the development of bacterial peritonitis and septic complications.

The biliary peritonitis encountered in gangrenous or emphysematous cholecystitis is a severe disease *ab initio* and differs from the above both in the prognosis and in the clinical picture. The patient is usually elderly and very ill with signs of toxaemia and established peritonitis due to the escape of infected bile. It carries a reported mortality of 30%.

Meconium peritonitis is a sterile peritonitis following perforation of the gut during late intra-uterine life. It may lead to intense fibrosis and calcification (adhesive peritonitis), meconium ascites, pseudocyst, or it may become secondarily infected. The condition is discovered in the neonatal period because of obstruction and free air under the diaphragm and is dealt with in Chapter 59.

Acute chemical peritonitis may complicate uraemia and certain collagen disorders (polyserositis).

Chronic Bacterial Peritonitis

In the majority of cases, the infection is tuberculous in origin. Tuberculous peritonitis is considered with tuberculous enteritis in Chapter 72. Abdominal actinomycosis is another example of localized chronic bacterial peritonitis.

Granulomatous Peritonitis

The formation of multiple peritoneal granulomas with the development of ascites may rarely occur as a manifestation of sarcoidosis when differentiation from tuberculous peritonitis can be difficult and is based on a positive Kveim test, negative TB cultures and a lack of response to antituberculous therapy.

Starch peritonitis (starch granuloma syndrome) is a more common cause of granulomatous peritonitis in surgical practice and can lead to a substantial early morbidity and long-term consequences. Talc (magnesium silicate) used to be the lubricant for surgical gloves and its implantation during surgery caused granuloma formation, chemical peritonitis and intra-abdominal adhesions. It was replaced by Bio-Sorb in 1949. This is the epichlorohydrinated polymer of corn starch mixed with 2% magnesium oxide and small amounts of sodium sulphate and sodium chloride. When introduced, it was claimed to be completely absorbed by the peritoneal membrane and was thus free of the disadvantages encountered with talc. Subsequent experience during the past four decades has shown that reactions to Bio-Sorb do occur and include a syndrome of starch peritonitis (starch granuloma syndrome) which has a characteristic and well-recognized clinical picture. The disease starts 2–6 weeks after abdominal surgery with low-grade fever, anorexia, nausea, vomiting, abdominal distension, cramp-like pain and tenderness. The abdominal distension is due to ileus and to the accumulation of ascitic fluid. Multiple granulomas develop on both the visceral and parietal peritoneum. The ascitic fluid is usually amber but may be serosanguineous and contains many leucocytes made up largely of lymphocytes and monocytes. The granulomatous nodules consist of collections of lymphocytes, macrophages, polymorphs and eosinophils around starch granules which have a characteristic Maltese-cross appearance on light microscopy (*Fig.* 75.3). There is still debate as to the nature of the reaction. Some ascribe its development to a state of hypersensitivity to corn starch which can be demonstrated by skin patch testing in patients who develop the condition. Others argue that it represents a foreign body reaction. This is unlikely in view of its relatively rare occurrence. The diagnosis is made on the clinical picture together with the demonstration of starch granules in the ascitic fluid obtained by an abdominal tap. The starch granules are easily identified by iodine staining or by polarized-light microscopy. Some advocate laparoscopy with biopsy to confirm the diagnosis and to exclude intra-abdominal sepsis. Surgery is avoided if the diagnosis is certain. Treatment is then conservative. Rapid resolution has been reported with systemic corticosteroid therapy. Prognosis is good and the majority of cases resolve with conservative management. The complications of starch peritonitis include sinus and fistula formation, adhesion formation and intestinal obstruction.

The prophylaxis of starch peritonitis includes the prior removal of starch from the surgical gloves. When the gloves have been put on, 10 ml of povidone-iodine (Betadine) is applied and smeared on the surface of the gloves. The black starch-iodine granules are then washed off by pouring 500 ml of sterile water from a container. More recently, gloves containing a hydrogel polymer as a lubricant only on the inner surface have been introduced (Biogel). They are totally free of starch and should eliminate the problem.

OTHER DISORDERS OF THE PERITONEAL CAVITY

A number of abnormalities other than acute inflammation are commonly encountered. Some, such as pneumoperitoneum, may accompany acute secondary bacterial peritonitis; others, e.g. adhesions and effusions, may be essential features of chronic bacterial and granulomatous peritonitis. The common non-infective disorders of the peritoneal cavity include pneumoperitoneum, haemoperitoneum, ascites, adhesions and tumours of the peritoneal lining.

Pneumoperitoneum

The introduction of as little as 1·0 ml of air into the peritoneal cavity may be demonstrated by erect films of the abdomen in the subdiaphragmatic region. Intraperitoneal air introduced at laparotomy is rapidly absorbed in infants (within 12 h), often takes longer in older children and adults (36–48 h) but may persist for 3–4 weeks in adults.

In surgical practice, pneumoperitoneum is associated with clinical evidence of peritonitis in over 90% of cases. In the absence of peritonitis, pneumoperitoneum may be due to:

Escape of air from the tracheobronchial tree in patients with chronic obstructive pulmonary disease and in patients on intermittent positive-pressure ventilation.

Pneumatosis cystoides intestinalis.

Free air after laparotomy, abdominal paracentesis and peritoneal dialysis. About 25% of patients still have demonstrable air under the diaphragm 8 days after an abdominal operation.

Gynaecological causes: tubal insufflation, pelvic examination, douching etc.

After gastrointestinal endoscopy including colonoscopy where it indicates iatrogenic perforation.

With the increasing use of CO_2 and NO_2 for peritoneal insufflation during laparoscopy, pneumoperitoneum is seldom encountered after this endoscopic procedure. Pneumoperitoneum is of clinical significance only in the presence of signs of peritoneal irritation. Otherwise a conservative approach is indicated. An overdistended viscus (e.g. hepatic flexure), adventitial gas shadows, subdiaphragmatic extraperitoneal fat and basal pulmonary collapse may produce radiological appearance simulating free air in the peritoneal cavity—*pseudopneumoperitoneum.*

Haemoperitoneum

The presence of blood in the peritoneal cavity causes acute irritation of the peritoneal lining with the development of the appropriate abdominal signs which, however, vary in intensity and can be marked, especially if the haemorrhagic exudate is due to an inflamed organ (acute pancreatitis) or contains irritant secretions (bile, urine, etc.). Haemoperitoneum is often accompanied by hypovolaemia.

Aetiology

The common causes are trauma to the intra-abdominal organs, abdominal surgery, pelvic fractures and ectopic pregnancy. The most serious life-threatening haemoperitoneum is encountered after major liver and splenic injuries where the massive intra-abdominal haemorrhage causes a

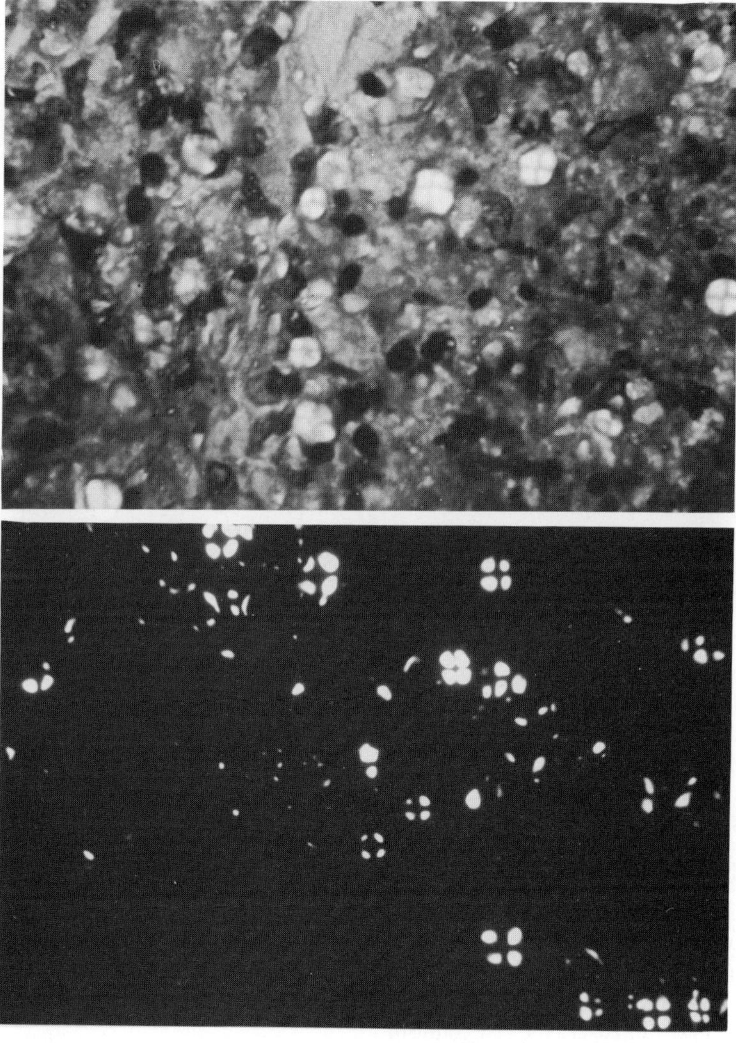

Fig. 75.3 Maltese-cross appearance of corn-starch granules visualized with polarized light. (By courtesy of Mr I. Capperauld FRCSE, Ethicon Laboratories, Edinburgh.)

tense stretched abdomen and blotchy cold lower limbs due to impairment of the blood supply and venous return consequent on the grossly elevated intra-abdominal pressure. Haemoperitoneum may follow any abdominal or pelvic operation and results from reactive or secondary haemorrhage. Spontaneous rupture of an organ may lead to a life-threatening haemoperitoneum. The organ is usually diseased, e.g. splenomegaly due to malaria or infectious mononucleosis, rupture of a primary hepatoma, ectopic pregnancy; but massive and even fatal haemoperitoneum may occur, albeit rarely, from rupture of a cyst in a physiologically normal organ such as corpus luteum cyst. A haemorrhagic effusion is commonly encountered in secondary peritoneal carcinomatosis. Rarely, bleeding into the peritoneal cavity or retroperitoneal tissues is the result of a haemorrhagic or clotting disorder (usually haemophilia). Although abdominal aneurysms predominantly rupture into the retroperitoneal tissues in the first instance, some may do so direct into the peritoneal cavity *ab initio* usually with a fatal outcome. More commonly, secondary rupture of the retroperitoneal haematoma accounts for the haemoperitoneum in these cases.

Management

The most important consideration is the state of the cardiovascular system. When the haemoperitoneum is accompanied by hypovolaemia, urgent resuscitation, volume replacement and surgical intervention are mandatory. A conservative approach is adopted in the first instance if the patient is haemodynamically stable. The diagnosis is confirmed by abdominal tap/lavage. In some centres the use of minilaparoscopy under local anaesthesia is used to establish the cause of the haemoperitoneum and the need for surgical intervention in trauma patients. In this respect, 19% of patients with a positive abdominal lavage are found at laparotomy to have no active bleeding, the blood loss usually from a minor laceration, having ceased spontaneously. In patients presenting late, the haemorrhagic exudate may track along tissue planes and result in staining and discoloration of the flanks (Grey Turner's sign in relation to haemorrhagic pancreatitis (*Fig.* 75.4), and the umbilicus (Cullen's sign observed occasionally in women with ectopic pregnancy).

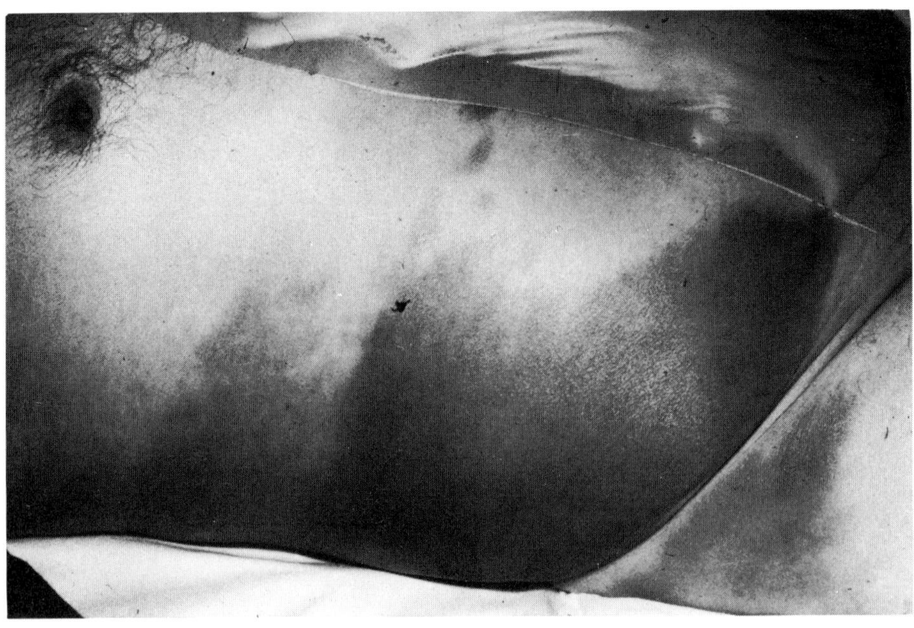

Fig. 75.4 Grey Turner's sign due to haemorrhagic pancreatitis. The discoloration in the flanks appeared on the third day of the illness.

Ascites

Ascites is clinically detected when fluid accumulation within the peritoneal cavity exceeds 1 L. Lesser amounts can be identified by ultrasonography which is the most sensitive investigation for the demonstration of both free and localized fluid collections within the peritoneal cavity. The ascitic fluid is generally regarded as a transudate and, by definition, differs from an exudate encountered in bacterial inflammation by having a low protein content (<2·0 g/l) and a low cell count. In practice, the protein content is often higher in patients with cirrhosis, tuberculous peritonitis, malignant disease and pancreatic ascites. Moreover, the cell count of the fluid may be high.

Clinical Features

The clinical detection of ascites is usually easy. With the patient in the supine position, the free fluid distends the flanks which is quite distinct from the central abdominal bulging seen in patients with intestinal obstruction. The distended flanks are dull to percussion. Furthermore, a fluid thrill and shifting dullness can be elicited. The most sensitive clinical demonstration of ascites is obtained by examining the patient in the knee–elbow position when the 'puddle sign' can be elicited and which is reputed to detect volumes of free peritoneal fluid as low as 200 ml. Difficulties in clinical differentiation from subacute obstruction can, however, be encountered in the presence of gross dilatation of the intestines with fluid and gas, where the physical findings may closely simulate those of ascites including a fluid thrill and shifting dullness. A straight erect radiograph of the abdomen will demonstrate multiple fluid levels in these patients. Other conditions which may be mistaken for ascites include large ovarian cysts, pancreatic pseudocysts, mesenteric cysts, hydramnios and acute gastric dilatation. Ultrasonography will distinguish all the cystic lesions and hydramnios. Acute gastric dilatation will become readily apparent after the insertion of a nasogastric tube.

Ascites may occur with or without evidence of generalized water and salt retention. The causes of ascites are shown in *Table* 75.3. Ascites as the sole or outstanding clinical feature is encountered in cirrhosis, tumours of the peritoneal cavity, tuberculous peritonitis and chronic pancreatitis (pancreatic ascites) due to perforation of ductal system or a pseudocyst.

Table 75.3 Mechanisms/causes of ascites

Infection	Tuberculous peritonitis, etc.
Inflammatory disease	Crohn's disease, starch peritonitis
Hypoproteinaemia	Nephrotic syndrome, liver disease, protein-losing enteropathy
Lymphatic obstruction	Tuberculosis, filariasis, lymphoma, metatastic carcinoma, Milroy's disease, rupture/damage of abdominal lymphatics
Increased lymph flow/ pressure	Congestive cardiac failure, constrictive pericarditis and cirrhosis
Portal hypertension/ congestion	Cirrhosis, congestive cardiac failure, constrictive pericarditis, Budd–Chiari syndrome
Neoplasms	Primary and secondary tumours of the peritoneal cavity
Chronic pancreatitis	Pancreatic ascites

N.B. In many instances, the ascites is multifactorial in origin.

In the investigation of all patients with ascites, a diagnostic paracentesis to obtain a sample of fluid (20–50 ml) should always be performed. The fluid is subjected to biochemical and cytological examination, and a specimen is sent for ordinary and TB culture/guinea-pig inoculation. Laparoscopy is generally reserved for those patients in whom the aetiology of the ascites cannot be ascertained by less invasive investigations.

Types of Ascites

The macroscopic appearance of the fluid often indicates the

nature of the underlying disease and is described as *serous* (yellow/green), *chylous, pseudochylous, bloodstained* or *myxomatous* (mucoid).

Ascites in Liver Disease

In cirrhosis, the ascitic fluid is usually clear, yellow to green and frothy. Stigmata of chronic liver disease are invariably present. In longstanding cirrhotic ascites, the fluid becomes opalescent and/or turbid (pseudochylous) as a result of changes in the protein constituents. It then resembles and has to be differentiated from chylous ascites which is caused by lymphatic obstruction.

Ascites in Inflammatory Disease

This is usually serous in nature and is encountered in tuberculous peritonitis and Crohn's disease. In the former, miliary tubercles are seen on laparoscopic inspection but these may be difficult to distinguish from other miliary foci such as sarcoidosis and multiple tumour deposits. Biopsies of the lesions on the parietal peritoneum are therefore essential.

Ascites in Malignant Disease

The macroscopic appearances of the fluid varies considerably. It may be clear and yellow, dark green in malignant bile duct obstruction, chylous as a result of lymphatic obstruction, frankly bloodstained and gelatinous or mucinous. Multiple tumour deposits are present on both the visceral and parietal peritoneum and on the greater omentum. When the latter is heavily involved, it becomes rolled up and forms a hard mass of malignant tissue.

Chylous Ascites

This is identified by its milky appearance. It has a high fat content on biochemical analysis. When it arises spontaneously, it indicates lymphatic obstruction by lymphoma or extensive nodal deposits from carcinoma. It is also a feature of intestinal lymphangiectasia.

Intractable Ascites

This is encountered in patients with advanced chronic liver disease, the Budd–Chiari syndrome and in patients with peritoneal carcinomatosis. Eventually some 5% of patients with chronic liver disease become refractory to medical treatment. These patients cease to respond to diuretic therapy and develop prerenal azotaemia. The ascites is gross and tense, the elevated intra-abdominal pressure causing venous congestion of the abdominal wall veins and diminished venous return from the lower limbs which aggravates the peripheral oedema. It also induces a tense uncomfortable heavy sensation frequently amounting to abdominal pain and tenderness. Respiratory distress results from splinting of the diaphragm. Mobility is considerably impaired. The umbilicus becomes everted and existing external hernias become distended. In patients with cirrhosis, prerenal azotaemia is invariably present.

The first-line treatment in patients with chronic liver disease is medical, with dietary salt restriction, spironolactone and a loop diuretic (frusemide, ethacrynic acid). The objective of medical therapy is a gradual loss of the fluid overload (3 kg fluid/week) to prevent prerenal azotaemia. When medical treatment has failed and the patient becomes oliguric, a trial of 5% albumin or fresh frozen plasma infusion (500 ml over a period of 2 h) followed by intravenous frusemide (50 mg) and 250 ml of 20% mannitol over 20–30 min is administered. If a diuresis is not established in this way, peritoneovenous shunting is indicated.

Peritoneovenous Shunting

This is now an established form of treatment which is used in patients with intractable ascites due to chronic liver disease or the Budd–Chiari syndrome. Increasingly, it is being used to palliate the tense, often painful, malignant ascites due to peritoneal carcinomatosis provided the ascitic fluid is not mucoid in consistency.

Peritoneovenous shunting is contraindicated in patients with encephalopathy, bleeding diathesis (unless corrected), renal failure due to primary renal disease, recent variceal haemorrhage, cardiac failure and active liver disease/gross jaundice.

Three types of shunt are available: LeVeen, Denver and the Cordis–Hakim varieties. The latter two have a flushing antechamber which is a distinct advantage since it substantially minimizes the risk of blockage of the valve by fibrinous deposits and cellular debris. The best results are obtained with the Cordis–Hakim shunt which is illustrated in *Fig.* 75.5. Following its insertion, the patient is instructed to compress the valve antechamber over a period of a few minutes several times daily (*Fig.* 75.6). The complications of peritoneovenous shunting include disseminated intravascular coagulation, cardiac failure and arrhythmias, infection and shunt blockage.

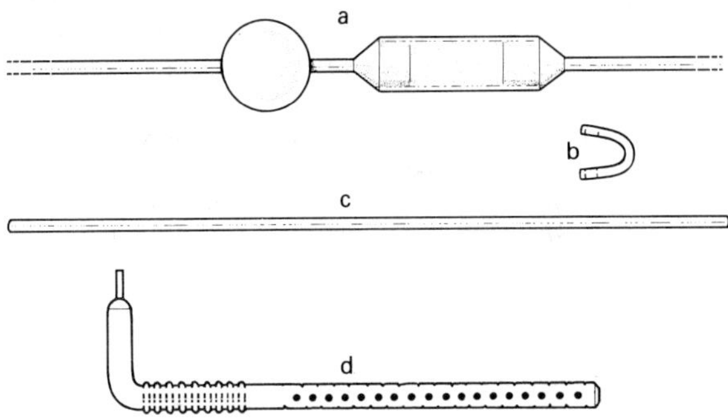

Fig. 75.5 Diagrammatic representation of the components of the Cordis–Hakim shunt: *a,* Valve unit-antechamber assembly. *b,* Metal U-shaped connector for joining the venous catheter to the valve system. *c,* Venous catheter. *d,* Peritoneal cannula with straight integral connector. (By kind permission, from Cuschieri A. and Hennessy T. P. J. (ed.) (1985). *Current Operative Surgery: General Surgery.* London, Ballière Tindall.)

TUMOURS OF THE PERITONEUM

By far the most common is secondary peritoneal carcinomatosis usually encountered in patients above the age of 40 years. The most common site of the primary is the gastrointestinal tract followed by breast, pancreas and ovary. The ascites is massive and intractable. Palliation is with simple paracentesis followed by the instillation of cytotoxic agents into the peritoneal cavity or by means of peritoneovenous shunting.

The other peritoneal neoplastic conditions are pseudomyxoma peritonei and primary mesothelioma.

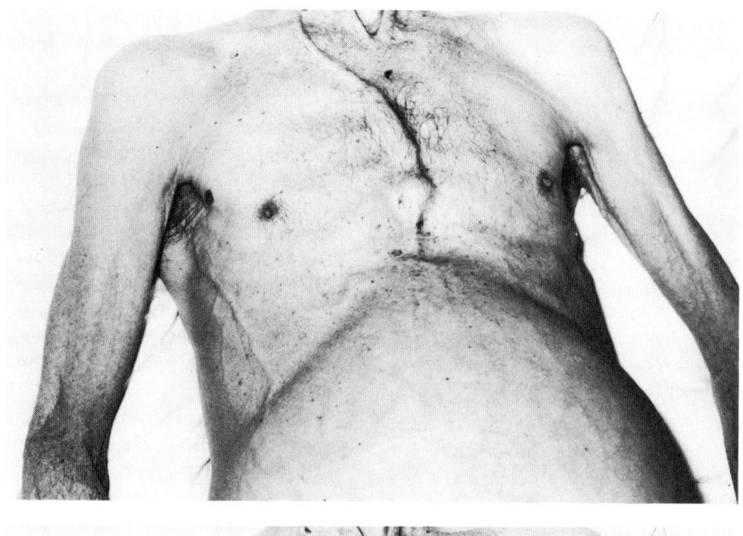

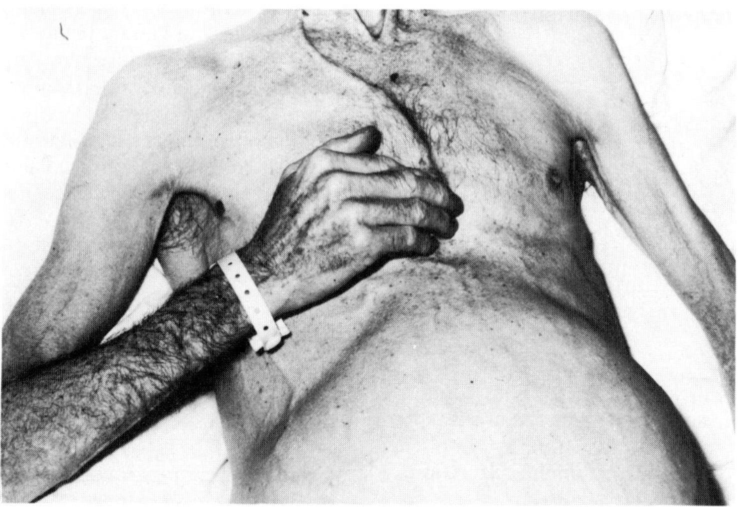

Fig. 75.6 Cordis–Hakim shunt in situ. Manual compression of the pump antechamber by the patient. This prevents blockage of the system by fibrin deposits. (By kind permission, from Cuschieri A. and Hennessy T. P. J. (ed.) (1985). *Current Operative Surgery: General Surgery*. London, Ballière Tindall.)

Pseudomyxoma Peritonei

This condition is characterized by the development of progressive abdominal distension by a yellow or brown mucoid substance which contains benign-looking cells on microscopic examination. Benign and malignant forms of the disease are recognized but the distinction is often arbitrary. The condition is caused by well-differentiated pseudomucinous cystadenoma/carcinoma. The most common primary is the ovary. Other reported sites include the appendix, uterus, bowel and urachus. The primary tumour is often slow growing and rarely metastasizes or invades adjacent viscera.

In addition to progressive abdominal distension, the condition may present as an acute abdomen or with intestinal obstruction. The treatment is aggressive by surgical evacuation, resection of the primary, systemic combination chemotherapy including cisplatin and/or intraperitoneal chemotherapy with alkylating agents. Radiotherapy is generally regarded as being ineffective in this condition. Although the prognosis is always guarded, long-term survival without recurrence of the disease is well documented. One useful prognostic factor appears to be the number of cells present in the mucus. There is a poor correlation between the histology of the primary and survival.

Peritoneal Mesothelioma

An increased incidence of peritoneal mesotheliomas has been observed since 1960, and has been attributed to asbestos exposure although several cases not associated with asbestos have been reported. In general, peritoneal mesotheliomas behave like their thoracic counterpart and carry a poor prognosis. The median survival in most series is 8–12 months after diagnosis. Two main types are recognized: the malignant mesothelioma which is diffuse and the rare benign fibrous type which is localized and usually can be cured by surgical resection. Within the malignant group, the well-differentiated papillary mesothelioma carries a reasonable prognosis with treatment and is often associated with long-term survival. The prognosis of malignant mesotheliomas is also dependent on the stage of the disease at the time of diagnosis (*Table* 75.4).

Table 75.4 Staging of malignant mesothelioma

Stage I	Tumour of one hemithorax or peritoneum
Stage II	Tumour involving mediastinum or pericardium (pleural primary only)
Stage III	Tumour invading muscle, bone, or skin of the chest/abdominal wall; involvement of lymph nodes outside the chest/abdomen; involvement of both pleural cavities
Stage IV	Abdominal and thoracic tumour with or without distant blood-borne metastases

The only treatable lesions are those confined to Stage I. The majority of cases of malignant mesotheliomas occur between the age range 40–65 years. The most common presentation is with progressive inanition, ascites and/or intestinal obstruction. Other clinical features include fever and weight loss. Diagnostic paracentesis may reveal malignant cells and laparoscopy may prove diagnostic. CT scanning is used to assess the extent and stage of the disease. In the past, diagnosis was usually made at laparotomy which is still used to stage the disease in some centres. An aggressive approach is indicated in patients with Stage I tumours, particularly if the histology demonstrates a well differentiated tumour. The treatment consists of resection of as much as is possible of the tumour followed by external beam supervoltage abdominal field radiotherapy and intraperitoneal chemotherapy or systemic combination chemotherapy. The drugs which have shown activity against the tumour in published series are cyclophosphamide, doxorubicin, cisplatin and mitomycin C. The intraperitoneal chemotherapy is administered via an indwelling Tenckhoff catheter or, more recently by means of the totally implantable Port-a-Cath (*Fig.* 75.7).

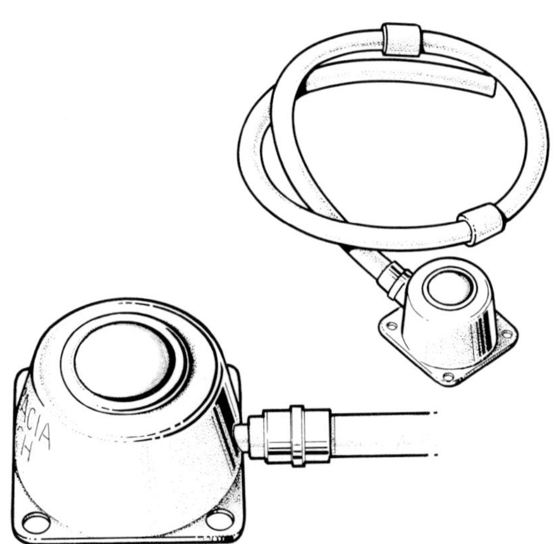

Fig. 75.7 Porta-a-Cath peritoneal access system for intraperitoneal chemotherapy.

SARCOMAS OF THE ABDOMINAL WALL

In this category are included the desmoid tumours of the anterior abdominal wall and the fully malignant soft-tissue sarcomas.

Desmoid Tumours

Desmoid tumours are sometimes grouped with other proliferative dysplastic lesions of the connective tissue under the term *musculo-aponeurotic fibromatoses* which include allied conditions such as plantar fibromatosis and nodular fasciitis. Desmoid tumours are slow growing well-circumscribed hard tumours which involve fascial and muscle layers. They have a tendency to recur after local excision (10–20%) and are found most commonly on the anterior abdominal wall but may occur elsewhere. Desmoid tumours are slightly more common in females and may become clinically obvious during or shortly after pregnancy. Some of them develop in relation to healed surgical scars. Treatment requires wide local excision. Desmoid tumours respond to radiotherapy which is used in some centres as an adjunct to surgical excision to minimize recurrence. Regression following treatment with tamoxifen which blocks oestradiol receptors has been reported in the literature.

Soft-tissue Sarcomas of the Abdominal Wall

These are rapidly growing tumours which occur in children and adults. The type depends on the tissue of origin (fibrosarcoma, rhabdomyosarcoma, Ewing's sarcoma). They are vascular tumours which may invade adjacent bone, peritoneum and intra-abdominal viscera. Treatment involves radical *en bloc* removal including a wide zone of adjacent normal tissue. Surgical treatment is usually followed by combination chemotherapy. Recurrence is common and averages 40% in reported series. The five-year survival approximates to 25%. Death is usually the result of dissemination of the disease predominantly by the bloodstream.

INTESTINAL OBSTRUCTION

The literal meaning of the word 'ileus' which is of Greek origin, is to roll or twist. It is sometimes used synonymously with obstruction which is acceptable. More often, it is incorrectly used to denote absence of peristaltic activity, a condition which is more accurately termed *paralytic* or *adynamic ileus.* The other main category of intestinal obstruction is *mechanical* where the obstruction is due to a blockage of the lumen—*intraluminal,* or results either from disease of the wall of the bowel—*intramural,* or from extrinsic compression of an otherwise normal bowel and lumen—*extramural (extrinsic* or *extra-intestinal).* Examples of intraluminal obstruction include impaction by faeces, swallowed foreign bodies, bezoars or gallstones (gallstone ileus). The commonest cause of mural obstruction is colonic cancer followed by inflammatory disease (diverticulitis and Crohn's disease). Extrinsic or extramural mechanical obstruction is most often caused by external hernias or intraperitoneal bands or adhesions. The latter is now the most frequent cause of intestinal obstruction overall.

Mechanical intestinal obstruction is designated as *simple* when the blood supply to the obstructed bowel remains intact and *strangulating/strangulated* when there is direct interference to the intestinal blood flow, most commonly by extrinsic compression by tight hernial rings or sacs and intraperitoneal adhesions/bands. Special varieties of strangulating mechanical obstructions are *intussusception* where a segment of bowel invaginates itself into an adjacent segment, *volvulus* which is a twist of a bowel loop on its mesenteric pedicle, and *closed-loop obstruction,* most commonly encountered in the colon from an obstructing mural

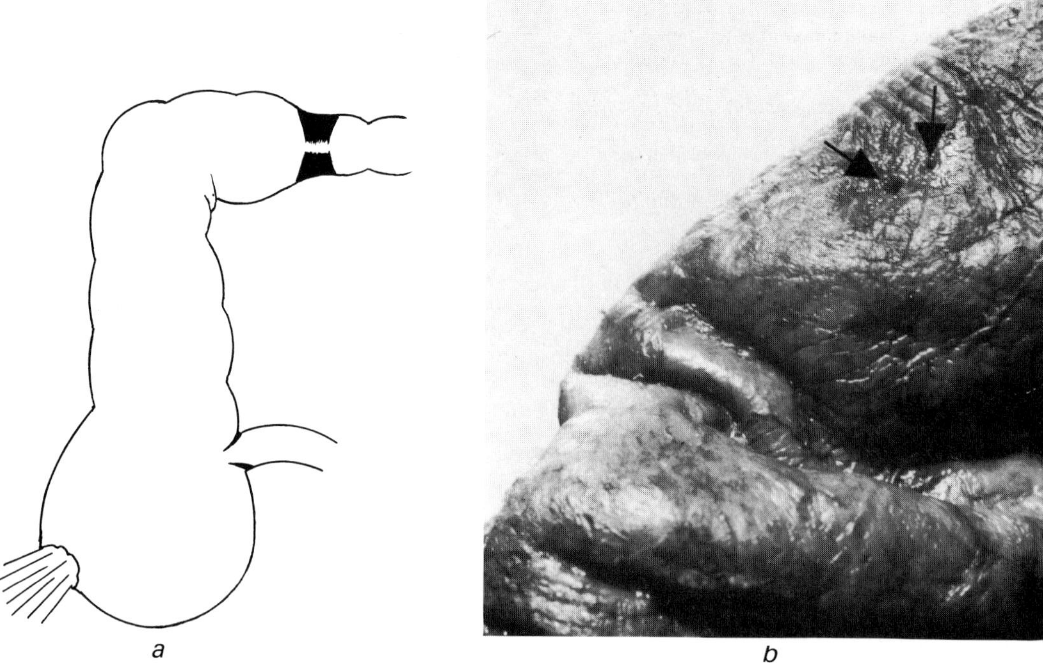

Fig. 75.8 *a*, Diagrammatic representation of a pistol-shot perforation of the caecum resulting from a closed loop obstruction due to a stenosing colonic carcinoma in the presence of a competent ileocaecal valve. *b*, Operative specimen of the same condition. The arrows point to the perforation.

lesion (e.g. annular carcinoma) in the presence of an intact ileocaecal valve (*Fig.* 75.8). This results in a rapid rise in intraluminal pressure within the closed loop and therefore an impairment of the blood supply, especially of the caecum which may undergo necrosis and perforation—'pistol-shot perforation'.

In terms of clinical presentation, mechanical intestinal obstruction is often further classified into *acute* and *chronic* obstruction. In the acute variety, the clinical course is rapid in onset with early vomiting and marked abdominal pain. The cause of the obstruction is usually in the small intestine. High small bowel acute obstructions are accompanied by severe vomiting whereas blockage of the low small intestine is characterized by marked abdominal distension. Chronic obstruction which results from colonic disease, is dominated by progressive constipation and a slower clinical course with late distension and vomiting. The term *subacute* obstruction implies an incomplete obstruction and is used for both small and large bowel disease. The manifestations consist of recurrent episodes of abdominal colicky pain and distension which are relieved by passage of a liquid or semi-formed motion. Untreated, the condition often progresses to a complete (acute) obstruction. The designation *acute-on-chronic* is confusing and rarely seen nowadays. It describes the full-blown large bowel obstruction seen in late presenting cases with dilatation of the small intestine, pain, generalized distension and vomiting.

With the improvement in the surgical services and earlier treatment of disorders which may lead to intestinal obstruction, the spectrum of disorders presenting with acute intestinal obstructions has changed dramatically in the last decade. The largest group which accounts for 35–40% of cases, is now caused by adhesions following previous intra-abdominal disease or surgical intervention (*Fig.* 75.9).

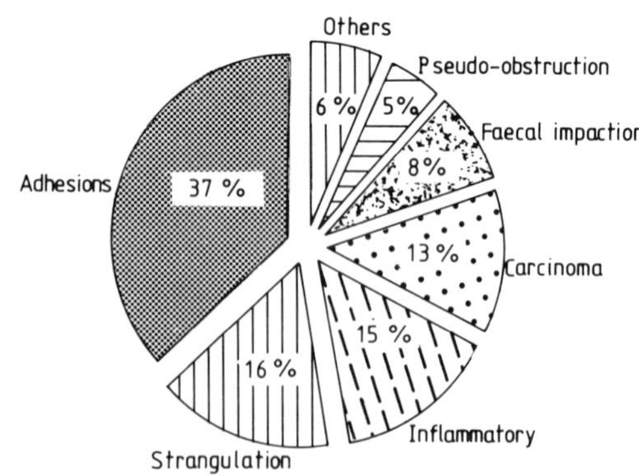

Fig. 75.9 Pie chart showing the relative frequency of the various aetiological groups of intestinal obstruction.

Although the incidence of colonic cancer remains high, this disease is presently responsible for only 13–15% of hospital admissions with acute intestinal obstruction. Similarly, obstructed external hernia is no longer a common cause of this disorder.

Pathophysiology

Simple Mechanical Obstruction

Irrespective of the aetiology and acuteness of the obstruction, the bowel proximal to the obstruction dilates and develops an altered motility. Below the point of obstruction, the intestine continues to exhibit normal peristalsis and absorption until it becomes empty when peristaltic activity diminishes and the intestine becomes contracted and pale. Consequent on the distension of the bowel proximal to the obstruction, the initial response consists of strong peristaltic contractions initiated by stimulation of the stretch reflexes. These contractions account for the severe colicky abdominal pain experienced by these patients. However, this reflex activity diminishes until a total inhibition of intestinal motility ensues, usually several hours from the onset of the obstruction. The cessation of activity has a protective action in preventing vascular damage from increasing intraluminal pressure; unless the obstruction is of the closed loop type, when ischaemic necrosis of the bowel wall ensues if surgical treatment is delayed.

The intestinal distension is caused by the excess accumulation of fluid and gas in the bowel lumen proximal to the obstruction. Soon after the onset, fluid accumulates within the walls of the obstructed intestine and excess is secreted into the lumen. The amount of fluid sequestered in the dilated intestinal loops is always substantial, and in cases of low small bowel obstruction, it may approximate to one-half of the total interstitial fluid. In health, there is a considerable daily turnover of salt and water in the gastrointestinal tract which is disrupted by intestinal obstruction. Normally, about 7–8 L of fluid enter the upper intestinal tract each day. This is made up of the following:

Food and drink	= 2000 ml
Salivary gland secretion	= 1000 ml
Gastric juice	= 1500 ml
Pancreatic juice	= 1500 ml
Bile	= 1000 ml

Most of this fluid and electrolyte load is absorbed in the small intestine (mainly jejunum) and about 1–1·5 L reaches the caecum. The colon normally absorbs most of the water and Na^+ and secretes some K^+, so that the stool water normally amounts to less than 200 ml, although the exact amount is dependent on the vegetable fibre content of the diet. In intestinal obstruction, not only is the reabsorption of the fluid and salt disrupted but, in addition, there is an increased secretion of water and electrolytes into the obstructed bowel lumen.

As the intestine dilates, its volume increases as the square of the radius. Thus the volume of a metre of intestine of 2 cm diameter approximates to 300 ml. This will increase to 1300 ml if the same segment dilates to a diameter of 4 cm. In addition to the sequestered fluid, the dilated bowel contains an excess of gas which constitutes 50% or more of the intestinal contents in simple mechanical obstruction. The normal adult has a mean intestinal gas volume of about 100 ml and excretes a variable amount ranging from 300 to 2000 ml daily. The composition which is highly variable, contains N_2 (24–80%), O_2 (0·1–2·5%), H_2 (0·6–50%), CO_2 (5–29%) and CH_4 (0–26%). Most of the N_2 is derived from swallowed air, although some may reach the bowel by diffusion from the blood. Both H_2 and CH_4 are derived exclusively from bacterial metabolism in the colon. Intestinal CO_2 arises from three sources: chemical interaction between gastric HCl with the bicarbonate of the biliary and pancreatic secretions, diffusion from the blood and bacterial metabolism. The composition of the diet affects both the quantity of intestinal gas and its composition. Inhalation of 100% O_2 for several days results in increased absorption of N_2 from the bowel by lowering the P_{N_2} of the blood to very low levels. This process of denitrogenation used to be advocated for intestinal obstruction, although it is of questionable value in this condition but it is quite effective in causing the disappearance of cysts in pneumatosis cystoides intestinalis.

The enormous increase in the intestinal gas is mainly due to the marked increase in the gut bacteria. Studies on the nature of the intestinal microflora in mechanical obstruction have shown a significant overgrowth of both aerobic and anaerobic organisms in the small intestine regardless of the level of the obstruction. In small bowel obstruction, there is a loss of the normal gradient of organisms from the jejunum to the ileum. Bacteroides organisms are recovered from 80% of cases. In large bowel obstruction, there is an increase in both aerobic and anaerobic organisms at all levels of the small intestine but the normal gradient from jejunum to ileum is retained. The increase in anaerobes is greater than that found in small bowel obstruction and bacteroides can be recovered from 100% of patients. The extreme anaerobic overgrowth seen in large bowel obstruction may explain the increased incidence of serious sepsis in these patients compared to those suffering from small intestinal obstruction.

Strangulating Mechanical Obstruction

In addition to the changes seen in simple obstruction, the viability of the bowel is threatened as a result of the impairment of its blood supply either by external compression (hernial orifices and sac, adhesions/bands) or because of interruption of the mesenteric flow (volvulus, intussusception) or from rising intraluminal pressure (closed loop obstruction) or primary obstruction of the intestinal circulation (mesenteric infarction). With the exception of the last-mentioned category, the venous return is affected before the arterial supply. The marked increase in the capillary pressure results in escape of intravascular fluid and diapedesis of red blood cells into the bowel walls, its lumen and the hernial sac or peritoneal cavity. The bowel wall therefore becomes oedematous and haemorrhagic, and both the intestinal contents and the peritoneal exudate are heavily blood-stained. Haemorrhagic infarction ensues as the arterial supply is cut off. Concomitant with the decreased or absent viability of the gut wall, transmigration of both aerobic and anaerobic organisms takes place, so that the haemorrhagic exudate in hernial sacs or peritoneal cavity in these cases, is always heavily infected with intestinal organisms. The severity of the illness and the mortality depend on the age and extent of infarction. Delay in the recognition and treatment of intestinal strangulation significantly enhances the mortality. In strangulated external hernias, the segment involved is usually short, whereas in small bowel volvulus, most of the small intestine may undergo necrosis. With long-loop strangulation, the volume of blood sequestered in the ischaemic bowel is substantial and contributes to the peripheral circulatory failure. There is a real risk of Gram-negative septicaemia in all strangulating mechanical obstructions especially when the strangulated segment is extensive and lies within the peritoneal cavity.

Paralytic or Adynamic Ileus

Loss of peristaltic activity may result from:

Reflex inhibition of intestinal motility.
Metabolic abnormalities.
Intraperitoneal sepsis.
Mesenteric vascular disease.
Drugs—tricyclic antidepressent agents.

The most common cause is inhibition ileus of the small

intestine which may follow a variety of conditions including abdominal operations, pneumonia, crush injuries, fractures of the spine, retroperitoneal haemorrhage or exudate, hyperextension of the spine (plaster jacket), etc. Reflex inhibition ileus is thought to be the result of an increased sympathetic discharge with hyperpolarization of the smooth muscle cells which become unresponsive to both neural and hormonal stimulation. The exact pathway of the reflex inhibition of small bowel motility is not known.

Absent or diminished peristaltic activity of the small intestine may accompany metabolic upsets, the most commonly encountered of which in surgical practice is hypokalaemia. Other metabolic abnormalities which may result in paralytic ileus include severe hyponatraemia, uraemia and diabetic ketoacidosis.

The paralytic ileus seen in bacterial peritonitis is due to both a reflex inhibition of intestinal motility as well as a direct effect of bacterial toxins on the myenteric nerve plexuses. The most serious form of paralytic ileus results from acute mesenteric insufficiency (*see* Chapter 56), the aetiology of which includes arterial embolism, arterial thrombosis, venous thrombosis or a low flow state secondary to a decreased cardiac output and reflex mesenteric vasoconstriction (non-occlusive vascular insufficiency).

Clinical Features

Mechanical Obstruction

The cardinal features of mechanical intestinal obstruction are abdominal pain, vomiting, distension and constipation. Other manifestations which may be encountered are dehydration from water and electrolyte losses, oliguria, hypovolaemic shock, septicaemia and respiratory embarrassment from diaphragmatic splinting consequent on abdominal distension. However, the symptomatology and physical signs vary in accordance with the exact location of the obstruction, the underlying pathology and the presence or absence of intestinal ischaemia.

PAIN. The pain of simple mechanical obstruction consists of waves of severe intestinal colic which are found to coincide with peristaltic rushes on auscultation of the abdomen. This helps to differentiate intestinal from other types of colic (e.g. ureteric). With the cessation of peristaltic activity due to increasing distension of the bowel, the colicky pain is replaced by a constant diffuse pain which is not usually severe. The development of severe constant pain whether it is preceded by intestinal colic or not, signifies the onset of strangulation. The pain caused by volvulus of the gut can be so excruciating as to precipitate irrational behaviour and mania. Simple mechanical obstruction occurring in the post-operative period may not be accompanied by colicky abdominal pain.

NAUSEA AND VOMITING. Although nausea and vomiting may accompany all forms of intestinal obstruction at some stage, the more distal the obstruction, the longer the interval between the onset of the obstruction and the appearance of these symptoms. Thus, even though total obstruction in the distal colon may have been present for several days, vomiting may not occur at all. On the other hand, nausea and vomiting are characteristic of small bowel obstruction, and in high small bowel or duodenal occlusions, vomiting is the main symptom of the disease and appears soon after the onset of the obstruction and often causes temporary relief of the intestinal colic, presumably because distension of the bowel is relieved. As the intestinal obstruction progresses, the vomitus becomes faeculent. This is due to bacterial overgrowth in the small intestine.

CONSTIPATION. This is qualified as absolute if neither faeces nor flatus can be passed and accompanies all complete intestinal obstructions. However, some patients may pass faeces or flatus or both spontaneously after the onset of intestinal obstruction. This simply reflects the natural evacuation of the intestine distal to the obstruction and has no clinical significance. Partial obstructions (faecal impaction, neoplasms of the colon), Richter's hernia, gallstone ileus and mesenteric vascular occlusion are often accompanied by diarrhoea.

DISTENSION. The degree of abdominal distension varies, as does its onset. Distension is minimal or absent in upper small bowel obstruction and mesenteric vascular occlusion. It is delayed in colonic obstructions. Severe abdominal distension is usually encountered in low small bowel obstruction, e.g. caecal neoplasm, mechanical obstruction of the left colon, volvulus of the sigmoid and Hirschsprung's disease.

PYREXIA. In patients with mechanical intestinal obstruction, fever may signify:

i. The onset of strangulation.
ii. Intestinal perforation.
iii. The presence of inflammation associated with the obstructing disease—abscess due to diverticulitis or a localized perforation of an ulcerating colonic cancer, and inflammatory bowel disease.

Hypothermia has a sinister significance and may be due to severe hyponatraemia or septic shock.

ABDOMINAL TENDERNESS. Localized tenderness in the abdomen or over an external hernia indicates strangulation. With overt infarction and/or perforation, the development of rigidity with rebound tenderness signifies the onset of peritonitis.

WATER AND SALT DEPLETION AND HAEMATOLOGICAL CHANGES. Dehydration is seen most commonly in small bowel obstructions and is due to repeated vomiting and sequestration of fluid and electrolytes in the dilated obstructed intestinal loops. The water and salt depletion results in an increase in the haematocrit, oliguria, dry skin and tongue, poor venous filling and sunken eyeballs. Hypokalaemia is not a usual feature of simple mechanical obstruction. A rise in the serum K^+ may accompany the onset of strangulation. Elevated levels of serum amylase and lactic dehydrogenase may be observed, and marked elevation of both enzymes is often encountered in strangulated bowel, but the levels of these serum enzymes do not reliably differentiate simple from strangulated obstructions. The mild leucocytosis seen in simple mechanical obstructions has been attributed to dehydration. Both marked leucocytosis and leucopenia have been described in strangulating obstructions, volvulus and mesenteric vascular occlusions.

Paralytic Ileus

This is characterized by progressive abdominal distension and effortless vomiting (in the absence of nasogastric decompression). Intestinal colic is absent but the condition is not pain free, the patients usually complain of a tight diffuse abdominal discomfort. With the recovery of intestinal motility, intestinal colic, described as 'wind pain' is often experienced by the patient.

On auscultation of the abdomen, borborygmi are not heard in paralytic ileus. Instead, high-pitched tinkling sounds are present and are due to the passive movement of fluid from one dilated intestinal loop to another.

Radiological Features

The standard radiological exposures used in intestinal obstruction are the erect and supine abdominal films, although lateral decubitus views may give useful information. The erect film demonstrates fluid levels (*Fig.* 75.10). It must be remembered, however, that the presence of fluid levels may be seen in non-obstructing conditions, e.g. inflammatory bowel disease, acute pancreatitis, intra-abdominal abscesses. They may also be observed following the administration of enemas. However, multiple fluid levels are indicative of obstruction and, if centrally placed, signify small bowel obstruction or dilatation secondary to late large bowel obstruction.

The supine film outlines the distended intestinal loops, and in general, gives more information regarding the site of intestinal obstruction. In small bowel obstructions, the dilated jejunal and ileal loops are arranged transversely in the centre of the abdomen and no gas is observed in the colon. Usually small bowel can be differentiated from the colon by the presence of circular transverse ridges due to the valvulae conniventes (plicae semilunaris). These are quite distinct from the colonic haustra which do not cross the entire distended lumen of the colon (*Fig.* 75.11).

In colonic obstruction, the dilatation of the colon, predominantly with gas, can usually be readily demonstrated in the supine film. Volvulus of the sigmoid results in a characteristic radiological appearance with a grossly dilated loop of colon with or without haustral indentations which arises from the pelvis and extends obliquely across the spine to the

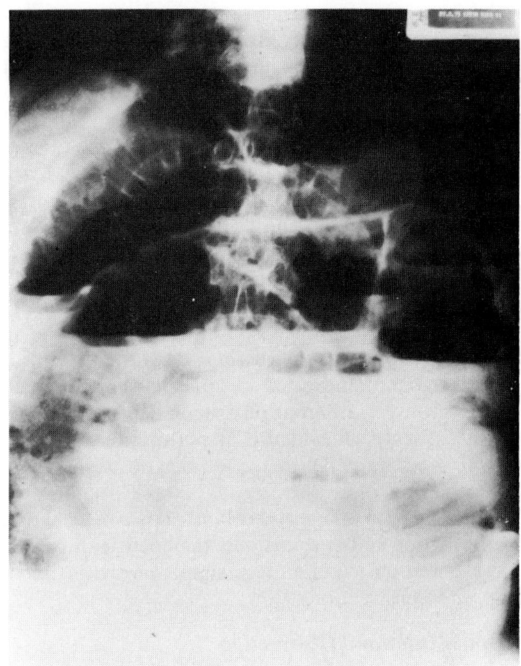

Fig. 75.10 Erect abdominal film showing multiple fluid levels in small bowel obstruction.

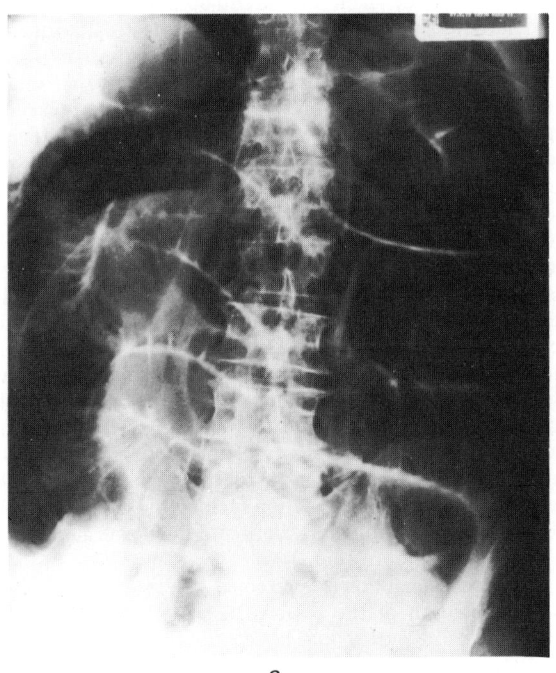

a

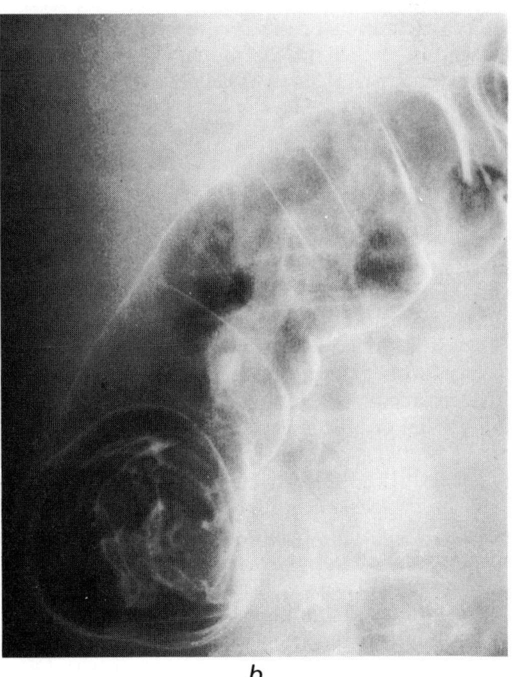

b

Fig. 75.11 *a*, Supine abdominal film demonstrating distended jejunal loops with the circular transverse ridges extending right across the width of the luminal gas shadow. *b*, Colonic haustra which do not cross the entire width of the distended bowel. Air contrast radiograph showing dilated ascending colon proximal to the carcinoma in the hepatic flexure.

upper abdomen. On close inspection, two distinct points of obstruction can usually be observed. Impacted foreign bodies may be seen on the radiographs of the abdomen. In gallstone ileus, gas is often demonstrated in the biliary tract and the offending gallstone is visualized, usually in the right iliac fossa, in about 25% of cases. It is important to stress that mechanical obstruction cannot be differentiated from paralytic ileus on the strength of the radiological findings, as both may give rise to dilatation of both the small and large intestine.

A barium meal or preferably barium instilled through the decompression-gastrointestinal tube (small bowel enema) may yield helpful if not diagnostic information on the site and nature of small bowel obstruction, e.g. intussusception. It is, however, contraindicated in large bowel obstruction since it may convert a partial obstruction into a complete one. In the absence of evidence of perforation, a barium enema will often provide the exact diagnosis in colonic obstruction.

Fibreoptic sigmoidoscopy and colonoscopy can yield diagnostic information and is sometimes therapeutic in patients with large bowel obstruction (e.g. sigmoid volvulus, acute colonic pseudo-obstruction).

Treatment of Intestinal Obstruction

Intestinal decompression by nasogastric suction and intravenous replacement and maintenance of fluid and electrolyte balance are essential components of management of all cases of intestinal obstruction. In some instances, e.g. uncomplicated paralytic ileus, these measures alone suffice. Surgical treatment is necessary for all cases of mechanical obstruction but operative intervention is often delayed in these patients until any gross fluid and electrolyte deficits have been corrected, provided there are no signs of strangulation, when early intervention is imperative. Early surgical treatment is also indicated in closed loop obstructions because of the risk of perforation. In practice, however, it is often difficult to exclude the possibility of intestinal ischaemia and the diagnosis reached in the individual case is usually a broad one: mechanical small bowel obstruction, large bowel obstruction or paralytic ileus.

Supportive Management

Nasogastric suction by a short non-vented (Ryle) or preferably vented tube (Salem) has largely replaced the use of long intestinal weighted, balloon-tipped single- or double-lumen tubes (Harris, Miller–Abbot, Levine, etc.) in most cases because of ease of introduction and increased patient comfort. Suction may be applied to the Ryle's/Salem's tube continuously or intermittently. The Salem tube is less likely to become blocked during suction than the Ryle's tube and is therefore more reliable. Whatever the exact procedure used, it is vital that the stomach is kept empty to reduce the hazard of aspiration particularly in ill patients during induction of anaesthesia and following extubation.

As the basic biochemical abnormality is water and sodium depletion, the appropriate intravenous fluid for replacement is Hartmann's solution or isotonic saline. The amount needed varies from patient to patient and is influenced by the clinical findings (skin dryness, elasticity, venous filling, urine output) and biochemical and haematological parameters (serum electrolytes, urea and haematocrit). Once the fluid and electrolyte deficit has been corrected, maintenance therapy is continued until the return of normal bowel function and motility.

There is a good case for the use of antibiotics active against both Gram-negative aerobes and anaerobes because of the inevitable bacterial overgrowth in intestinal obstruction. Antibiotic therapy is mandatory in all patients requiring resection of small or large intestine.

Surgical Treatment

Adequate exposure by the appropriate incision (most often midline if the exact cause of the obstruction is unknown) is essential. The operative assessment is directed towards the determination of the site of obstruction, the nature of the obstructing lesion and the viability of the gut. The caecum is the best guide to the site of obstruction which is often obscured by the tightly packed dilated intestinal loops. If the caecum is collapsed, the obstruction is in the small bowel and the exact site will be found if the small intestine is followed up from the ileocaecal junction. Evisceration of the dilated loops is inevitable and need not be harmful provided the loops are protected by warm saline packs. A dilated caecum indicates colonic obstruction.

Operative decompression is advisable if the dilatation of the intestinal loops is severe enough to interfere with exposure or subsequent closure. It should not, however, be undertaken lightly as it increases the risk of septic complications from spillage of the intestinal contents into the peritoneal cavity. Intestinal decompression is best performed using a Savage's intestinal decompressor introduced inside a seromuscular purse string suture which is ligated tightly around the instrument to prevent leakage of bowel contents.

The nature of the surgical procedure necessary for the relief of the obstruction will depend on the cause—division of adhesions (enterolysis), excision, bypass or proximal decompression of stenosing lesions, etc. The assessment of the viability of the intestine is often difficult, even in experienced hands. The obviously infarcted bowel with its greyish-green-black appearance and complete atony is easily distinguished. However, a heavily bruised and oedematous bowel may still be viable and careful observation is necessary for the detection of motility in these intestinal segments. The state of the mesenteric vessels and pulsations in the related mesenteric arcades is important except that infarction of the bowel may be present despite adequate pulsations in the mesenteric vessels (non-occlusive vascular insufficiency). Whilst there may be little doubt concerning the presence of a segment of infarcted bowel, it is often difficult to delineate the extent of the gangrene. A second look operation undertaken some 24 h after the first intervention may be necessary in problematic cases although this practice is usually restricted to cases with mesenteric vascular occlusion. When any doubt exists regarding the viability of the remaining bowel, the two ends of the residual intestine should be exteriorized in preference to a primary anastomosis. Apart from increased safety, this approach allows the daily inspection of the circulatory state and viability of the two exteriorized ends of the intestine. Operative methods designed to assess intestinal tissue perfusion and thus the need for and extent of resection include the Doppler probe placed on the antimesenteric border of the bowel and the use of intravenous fluorescein.

Whenever small bowel is resected, the exact site of resection, the length of the resected segment and that of the residual small bowel should be recorded. As obstructed and dilated bowel is always oedematous, only light occlusion clamps should be used on the segments of bowel to be retained. The clamps should not include the adjacent mesentery and must be clicked just enough to ensure temporary occlusion until the anastomosis is completed.

Treatment of Paralytic Ileus

Surgical treatment is necessary when the adynamic ileus is secondary to a life-threatening disorder, e.g. peritonitis, mesenteric vascular occlusion. Otherwise treatment is conservative with intestinal decompression, intravenous fluid therapy and the correction of metabolic disorders, particularly hypokalaemia which may be a major contributory factor. Rarely, paralytic ileus may be the consequence of therapy with tricyclic antidepressive drugs and withdrawal or change to a new formulation is necessary.

Elimination of the cause and adequate supportive therapy is usually successful in restoring propulsive intestinal motility. Occasionally medical therapy with an adrenergic-blocking agent in association with cholinergic stimulation, e.g. neostigmine (Catchpole regimen) is indicated for resistant cases of inhibition ileus provided an intraperitoneal cause, e.g. abscess, has been excluded as the underlying cause for the persistence of the obstruction. Recent clinical trials have demonstrated the efficacy of ceruletide over placebo and metoclopramide, especially in postoperative ileus. Ceruletide is the synthetic analogue of the naturally-occurring peptide caerulein. It has a powerful cholecystokinetic response (contraction of the gallbladder and relaxation of the sphincter of Oddi) and stimulates peristaltic contractions, especially in the small intestine. It is administered either intramuscularly or as a slow intravenous infusion.

Adhesions and Recurrent Intestinal Obstruction

The formation of intraperitoneal adhesions remains an unsolved problem in surgical practice and is attended by a significant morbidity and mortality. The important complications of intraperitoneal adhesions are repeated attacks of intestinal obstruction and strangulation of the intestines. In addition, early postoperative adhesive (mechanical) obstruction may be difficult, if not impossible, to differentiate from paralytic ileus.

Pathology of Intraperitoneal Adhesions

The causes of intraperitoneal adhesions are shown in *Table* 75.5. The most common category is postoperative adhesions. Following abdominal surgery, fibrinous adhesions always form between the intestinal loops. In the majority of cases, this fibrinous matting is absorbed. In some patients, however, the fibrinous material becomes organized with the ingrowth of both fibroblasts and capillaries to form adhesions. There is good experimental evidence that postoperative adhesions develop on a background of ischaemia in the region of surgically constructed anastomoses and following attempts at reperitonealization of raw areas. These should be left unsutured when they are rapidly filled with an inflammatory exudate and thereafter covered by a new serosa derived from the free-floating peritoneal macrophages. Adhesions are best regarded as an attempt by the body to revascularize ischaemic areas. Adhesions contain blood vessels and are least vascular at their insertion which is the optimal site for their division during adhesiolysis.

Table 75.5 Causes of intraperitoneal adhesions

Ischaemic areas	Sites of anastomoses, reperitonealization of raw areas
Foreign bodies	Talc, starch granules, gauze lint, cellulose, non-absorbable sutures
Infective disease	Peritonitis Tuberculosis
Inflammatory disease	Crohn's disease
Radiation enteritis	
Sclerosing peritonitis	Usually drug-induced (certain beta-blockers, e.g. practolol)

The implantation of foreign bodies is another important cause of adhesions. Reference has already been made to the role of talc and Bio-sorb in the formation of granulomas earlier on in this chapter. Talc is no longer used nowadays. Increasingly gloves which incorporate a hydrogel polymer (Biogel) are being worn in preference of gloves powdered with epichlorohydrinated corn starch. Gauze lint now accounts for 26% of cases of intraperitoneal granuloma formation caused by implanted foreign bodies.

Prevention of Adhesions

Aside from good surgical technique, the following measures are generally regarded as sensible precautions aimed at minimizing adhesion formation after abdominal surgery:

- Washing the peritoneal cavity with saline or dextran solutions at the end of the procedure to remove clots and implanted foreign bodies.
- Avoidance of excessive packing with gauze.
- Covering anastomoses and raw peritoneal surfaces with the greater omentum.
- Leaving raw peritoneal areas unsutured.

There have been several studies concerning drug prophylaxis of adhesions. The main agents which have been investigated are anticoagulants, dextrans of various molecular sizes, antihistamines, non-steroidal anti-inflammatory drugs, povidone and streptokinase. All the experimental studies suggest that for maximum benefit, the treatment needs to be commenced at the time of surgery. Although there have been some favourable reports with the use of these agents in clinical practice, confirmation of the benefit of such an approach has been lacking to date. Drug prophylaxis of intraperitoneal adhesions is not recommended in routine surgical practice.

Treatment of Recurrent Intestinal Obstruction due to Adhesions

The relative efficacy of the various surgical operations used in the treatment of recurrent intestinal obstruction due to adhesions has never been adequately assessed in prospective clinical trials. The operations available include adhesiolysis (enterolysis) alone, the plication operation of Noble, the Childs–Phillips procedure and intestinal intubation.

Noble's intestinal plication (*Fig.* 75.12) involves suturing the small intestinal loops with serosal sutures so that the small bowel coils become fixed in gentle curves when adhesions reform. This procedure is rarely performed nowadays because it is time-consuming and carries a high morbidity (perforation, fistula, peritonitis). Furthermore, patients complain of chronic abdominal pain and remain subject to recurrent attacks of intestinal obstruction.

In the Childs–Phillips operation of transmesenteric plication (*Fig.* 75.13) after enterolysis, the small intestine is arranged in an orderly fashion. Thereafter, the intestinal coils are fixed in position by means of transmesenteric monofilament nylon or prolene sutures passed on long needles some 3 mm from the mesenteric border of the bowel. The results of a number of retrospective reports with this procedure for recurrent small bowel obstruction due to adhesions have been good in terms of freedom from further

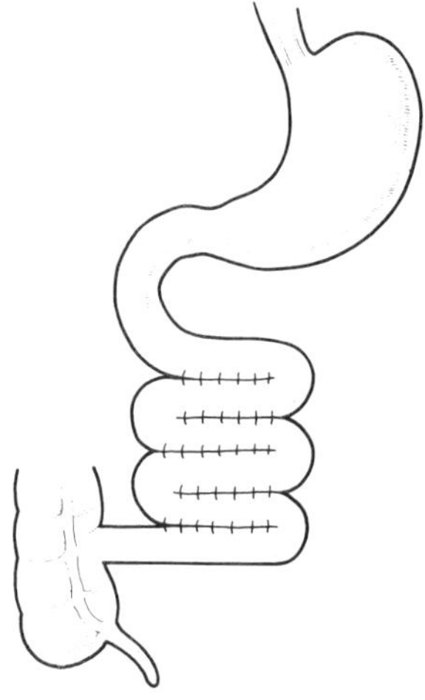

Fig. 75.12 Diagrammatic representation of Noble's plication operation. The small intestinal loops are sutured together in smooth curves by means of seromuscular sutures.

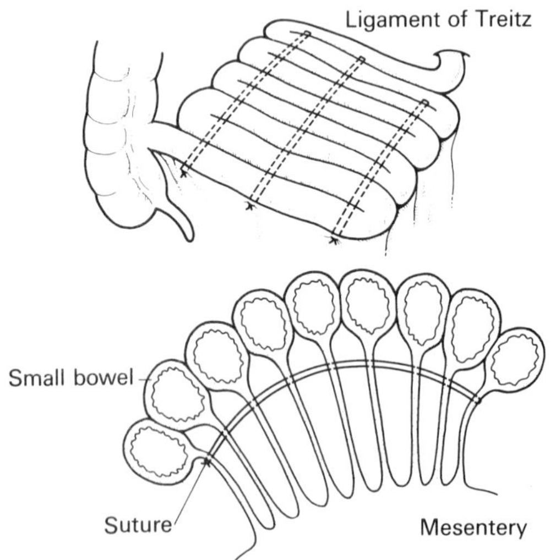

Fig. 75.13 Diagrammatic representation of the Child–Phillips operation of transmesenteric plication for recurrent small intestinal obstruction due to adhesions.

episodes of obstruction. The author's experience with this operation has been favourable.

The intraluminal tube or long intestinal tube 'stent' was proposed by White as a simple method for achieving gentle curves rather than allowing the bowel to develop acute angulations when the adhesions reform. Baker introduced the jejunostomy tube and advocated its insertion through either a purse-string suture in the upper jejunum or a Witzel jejunostomy (*Fig.* 75.14). The tube has an inflatable balloon near its tip which facilitates passage down the small intestine into the caecum. Modifications of the technique include gastrostomy stent plication with and without tube exit caecostomy (*Fig.* 75.15). The latter is unnecessary and increases the risk of infection. One of the disadvantages of intestinal intubation is the long period of ileus after the operation. The reports on the efficacy of intestinal intubation in preventing recurrent intestinal obstruction have been

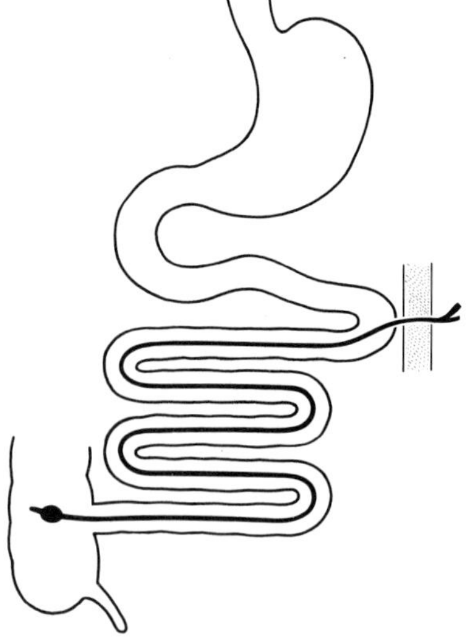

Fig. 75.14 Intestinal intubation for recurrent small bowel obstruction using a Baker's tube inserted via a Witzel jejunostomy.

conflicting. Some have found the procedure beneficial and have extended its use as a prophylactic measure in the treatment of patients with generalized peritonitis and following major abdominal surgical procedures. Other reports indicate that intestinal intubation is inferior to adhesiolysis alone.

Intestinal Pseudo-obstruction

The term 'pseudo-obstruction' is used to describe obstruction of the small or large intestine in the absence of a mechanical cause or acute intra-abdominal disease. The term covers a variety of syndromes which result from damage to the myenteric plexus (neuropathy) or smooth muscle abnormality (myopathy) or both. Small intestinal and colonic pseudo-obstruction are best discussed separately.

Small Intestinal Pseudo-obstruction

This condition may be primary (idiopathic) or secondary. Familial visceral myopathy which is included in the primary category is a particularly severe disorder which involves the smooth musculature of the oesophagus, entire gastrointestinal tract including the colon and often the urinary bladder. The secondary variety results from a neuropathy/myopathy induced by certain systemic disorders or drug abuse (excess phenothiazine administration, laxative abuse). The disorders most commonly associated with the development of secondary small intestinal pseudo-obstruction are diabetes mellitus, scleroderma, progressive systemic sclerosis, acute intermittent porphyria, hypothyroidism and Chagas' disease. More recently it has been reported as a complication of sclerotherapy for oesophageal varices. When the underlying abnormality is a neuropathy (e.g. diabetes mellitus), the pattern of intestinal motor activity is abnormal with derangements of the myoelectrical migratory complexes (MMC), absence of any normal activity or disorganized non-propulsive hypermotility. By contrast, in myopathic conditions (e.g. hypothyroidism) the pattern of motor activity is normal but the intensity of the contractile activity is reduced. The clinical picture is that of recurrent episodes of subacute intestinal obstruction with colicky abdominal pain,

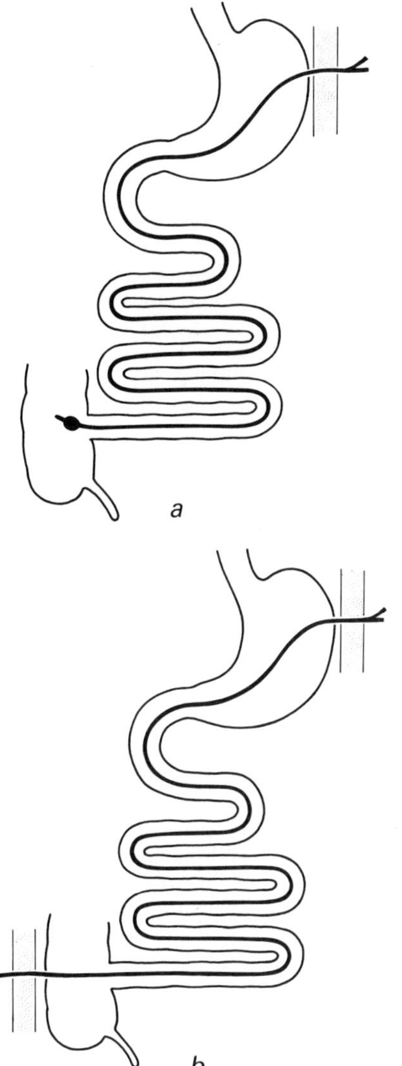

Fig. 75.15 *a*, Gastrostomy with long intestinal tube plication for recurrent small bowel obstruction. *b*, Modification of the technique with gastrostomy and tube exit-caecostomy. This technique is not generally recommended as the exit-caecostomy is considered unnecessary and increases the risk of infection.

vomiting and distension. The treatment entails the correction of any underlying disorder whenever this is possible (e.g. hypothyroidism). Metoclopramide and domperidone are sometimes beneficial. Better results have been obtained with the new drug cisapride which increases the local concentration of acetylcholine in the intestinal smooth musculature. Ceruletide which has to be administered intramuscularly or intravenously is also beneficial particularly during acute episodes. Replacement therapy is necessary in patients with hypothyroidism.

Colonic Pseudo-obstruction

Two types are recognized: acute and chronic. The acute condition was first described by Ogilvie in 1948 and is sometimes referred to as the Ogilvie's syndrome. It consists of selective dilatation of the caecum and proximal colon with a sharp cut-off usually at the splenic flexure (less frequently, hepatic flexure and sigmoid) suggestive of mechanical obstruction. It is best considered as a localized form of adynamic ileus which usually develops in patients with a major pre-existing, non-intestinal condition requiring hospitalization, e.g. major surgery, severe trauma, sepsis, myocardial infarction, severe renal and respiratory disease. The aetiology remains unknown although administration of drugs which impair colonic motility and air swallowing are thought to be contributing factors. The defect appears to be in the smooth muscle or in one of the intestinal control mechanisms and slow wave activity (electrical control activity) has been reported to be absent in these patients.

The clinical picture is dominated by abdominal distension often without vomiting. The patient complains of increasing discomfort and may develop cramp-like abdominal pain. Radiography shows features of colonic obstruction with caecal distension (7·5–22·0 cm). Caecal perforation is a well-recognized complication and is likely to occur if the radiological size of the caecum exceeds 12 cm. The standard treatment nowadays is by colonoscopic decompression which is successful in the majority of patients. Recurrence of the condition is encountered in 20% of patients. These are treated by further colonoscopy when a Baker jejunostomy tube is inserted transanally into the caecum or the colonoscope is left in situ for 2 h thereby maintaining decompression. Surgical intervention with tube caecostomy is undertaken when colonoscopy fails or is not available.

Chronic colonic pseudo-obstruction may be primary or secondary. The latter may result from a motility disorder, diabetes mellitus, hypothyroidism, malignancy, psychosis or drug and laxative abuse. Medical treatment is with cholinergic drugs including the new agent cisapride. Surgical intervention which results in good symptomatic relief, is indicated if medical treatment fails. It consists of subtotal colectomy with ileorectal anastomosis. Replacement therapy is required in patients with hypothyroidism. The prognosis of patients with chronic colonic pseudo-obstruction is thus better than that of the equivalent small bowel disease.

Special Forms of Mechanical Intestinal Obstruction

Bolus Obstruction

Intraluminal bolus obstruction, usually of the small intestine, may be caused by tricho- and phytobezoars, gallstone and a mass of worms (*Ascaris lumbricoides*). The latter is usually encountered in children and is often precipitated by antihelminthic therapy.

Phytobezoars

These are firm masses of undigested fruit or vegetable fibre which can cause gastric or small bowel obstruction. The predisposing factors include the ingestion of large amounts of high-fibre foods, inadequate mastication, previous gastric surgery producing hypo- or anacidity and loss of the antral pump mechanism. Often the phytobezoars that form after gastric surgery consist of orange pith.

Patients with gastric bezoars present with epigastric pain, loss of appetite and weight and episodes of distension and vomiting. The condition is usually diagnosed at endoscopy. Intestinal bezoars present with mechanical small bowel obstruction. Gastric phytobezoars are multiple in 17% of cases and intestinal bezoars in 4%.

Gastric phytobezoars are treated conservatively by cellulase enzymatic digestion (300 ml of 0·5% cellulase solution instilled 4-hourly via a nasogastric tube for 2 days). Laparotomy is needed for patients presenting with small bowel obstruction. Sometimes, it is possible to knead the bolus into the caecum. When this is not successful, the phytobezoar is removed by an enterotomy.

Postoperative Intestinal Obstruction

It is often incorrectly assumed that the majority of intestinal obstructions after abdominal surgery are due to protracted adynamic ileus. In practice, postoperative intestinal obstruction is more commonly of mechanical origin although the differentiation between the two is usually difficult. Early obstruction (during the first 5 days) is usually due to non-strangulating causes, e.g. anastomotic oedema, adhesive fibrinous matting with distension and kinking of the intestinal loops. As the obstruction is often incomplete, active surgical intervention is rarely necessary and the majority settle with conservative management. By contrast, later postoperative obstruction (occurring beyond 7 days of surgery) is usually caused by a band or abscess and may be strangulating in nature. Laparotomy is, therefore, advisable in these late postoperative intestinal obstructions.

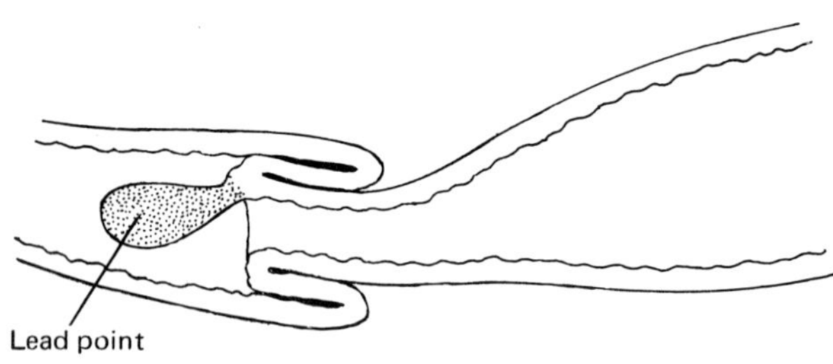

Fig. 75.16 Components of an intussusception.

Intussusception

Intussusception is a telescoping of a segment of intestine into an adjacent one (*Fig.* 75.16). The condition is encountered most commonly in childhood with a peak incidence at 4 months. Intussusception may, however, be encountered in the adult, in which case a precipitating lesion which initiates the intussusception (the lead point) is usually present, e.g. intestinal polyp, submucosal lipoma, etc. By contrast, in children some 70–95% are classed as idiopathic (no lead point) and an associated illness, such as urinary tract infection or gastroenteritis, is encountered in 30%. It is often assumed that hyperplasia of the lymphoid patches in the terminal ileum secondary to common diseases of infancy may be involved in the initiation of idiopathic intussusception in children. A definite seasonal incidence is observed in this age group with clear peaks in the spring and summer. This is suggestive of viral infections being the cause of the intestinal lymphoid hyperplasia.

Intussusception is anatomically defined as ileo-ileal, ileocaecal and ileocolic, depending on the site and extent of the telescoping observed by the time of diagnosis. The condition is a strangulating type of intestinal obstruction and if treatment is delayed, ischaemic necrosis of the involved bowel segments and peritonitis are inevitable.

The clinical features include the sudden onset of vomiting, cramp-like abdominal pain and rectal bleeding. An abdominal mass is palpable in 55–60% of cases. Children with intussusception associated with a lead point (Meckel's diverticulum, polyp, duplication, Henoch–Schönlein purpura, suture line, appendix, tumour) are usually older than the idiopathic cases.

In the absence of peritonitis and intestinal obstruction, the initial treatment is by hydrostatic barium enema which is successful in 50% and is followed by a recurrence rate of only 6%. Intussusception caused by a lead point is not likely to reduce with a hydrostatic barium enema and usually requires surgical intervention. Operative treatment is necessary when the hydrostatic reduction is incomplete, uncertain or contraindicated (peritonitis, intestinal obstruction). Operative reduction is often possible, although the viability of the bowel should be carefully checked after reduction.

Volvulus

Volvulus is a twist or rotation of a loop of intestine about its mesenteric attachments. It is, therefore, a sudden obstruction of the closed loop variety if the rotation is complete (360°) and ischaemia or total vascular occlusion may be present.

Two varieties are described: primary and secondary. Primary volvulus results from malrotation of the gut or congenital excessive mobility from loose fixation or long mesenteric attachments (volvulus of the midgut in the neonate, caecal and sigmoid volvulus in the adult). The more common secondary volvulus is due to a rotation of loop of small intestine around an adhesion, an ileostomy or colostomy.

CAECAL VOLVULUS. This is usually encountered in adult life (mean age, 50 years) and is due to undue mobility (hypofixation) of the caecum. It presents acutely with abdominal pain, nausea, vomiting and constipation, although diarrhoea is sometimes present. Dilatation of the right colon is seen on the plain abdominal film and a barium enema may demonstrate absence of barium in the caecum and a 'bird's beak' deformity. Surgical treatment consists of untwisting the caecum and fixation to the right iliac fossa (caecopexy), although some favour a caecostomy in addition. Resection is only indicated if gangrenous bowel is present.

SIGMOID VOLVULUS. This is discussed in Chapter 74.

References

Antman K. H., Klegar K. L., Pomfret E. A. et al. (1985) Early peritoneal mesotheliomas: a treatable malignancy. *Lancet* **ii**, 977–981.

Anuras S. and Shirazi S. S. (1984) Colonic pseudo-obstruction. *Am. J. Gastroenterol.* **79**, 525–532.

Berci G. and Cuschieri A. (ed.) (1986) *Practical Laparoscopy*. London, Baillière Tindall.

Childs W. A. and Phillips R. B. (1960) Experience with intestinal plication and a proposed modification. *Ann. Surg.* **152**, 258–265.

Conn H. O. (1976) Spontaneous bacterial peritonitis—multiple revisitations. *Gastroenterology* **70**, 455–457.

Ellis H. (1971) The cause and prevention of postoperative intraperitoneal adhesions. *Surg. Gynecol. Obstet.* **133**, 497–511.

Flint L. M. and Fry D. E. (1982) *Surgical Infections*. New York, Medical Examination Publishing Co., Inc.

Lykkegaard-Neilsen M., Madsen P. V. and Nielsen O. V. (1984) Ceruletide versus metoclopramide in postoperative intestinal paralysis. *Dis. Colon Rectum* **27**, 288–289.

Polk H. C. jnr. and Fry D. E. (1980) Radical peritoneal débridement for established peritonitis: a prospective, randomized, controlled trial. *Ann. Surg.* **192**, 350–355.

Seski A. and Amirikia H. (1975) Starch granuloma syndrome. *Surg. Gynecol. Obstet.* **48**, 60s–62s.

Warshaw A. L. (1972) Diagnosis of starch peritonitis by paracentesis. *Lancet* **ii**, 1054–1056.

Weinstein M. P., Iannini P. B., Stratton C. W. et al. (1978) Spontaneous bacterial peritonitis—a review of 28 cases with emphasis on improved survival and factors influencing prognosis. *Am. J. Med.* **64**, 592–598.

76 The Abdominal Wall and Hernias

G. R. Giles

ANATOMICAL FEATURES

The anterior abdominal wall is a layered muscular structure which converts to an aponeurosis as it passes towards the midline and meets its opposite partner to form the rectus sheath and linea alba. The external oblique muscle arises from the outer surface of the lower eight ribs and the anterior half of the iliac crest. Its medial attachment is to the xiphisternum, linea alba and the pubis but it has a triangular deficiency over the pubic crest, which forms the superficial inguinal ring. Between the pubic tubercle and the anterior superior iliac spine, the rolled lower edge of its aponeurosis forms the inguinal ligament.

The internal oblique muscle arises from the thoracolumbar fascia, the anterior two-thirds of the iliac crest and the lateral two-thirds of the inguinal ligament. The medial attachment is an aponeurosis which splits around the upper part of the rectus muscle to attach to the linea alba. In the lower part, all fibres pass in front of the rectus and the free posterior edge forms the arcuate ligament.

The transversus abdominis muscle arises from the lower six costal cartilages, thoracolumbar fascia, iliac crest and lateral one-third of the inguinal ligament. The medial attachment of the muscle is similar to that of the internal oblique. The lower fibres from both internal oblique and transversus muscles combine to form the conjoint tendon which passes anterior to the lower part of the rectus muscles to become attached to the pubic crest and pectineal line of the pubis (*Fig.* 76.1).

Deep to the muscle layer lies the transversalis fascia, extraperitoneal fat and peritoneum. From a firm attachment to the posterior surface of the rectus sheath, the transversalis fascia passes more loosely around the lateral abdominal wall to be continuous with the fascia of the retroperitoneum and superiorly over the diaphragm and inferiorly over the lateral wall of the pelvic cavity.

The two rectus abdominis muscles have vertically running fibres and are enclosed in the rectus sheath formed by the aponeurosis of the anterolateral muscles. The superior attachment of these muscles is to the 5th, 6th and 7th costal cartilages and xiphisternum and inferiorly to the pubic crest and pubic symphysis. The midline is composed of a strong fibrous raphe particularly between the xiphisternum and umbilicus—the linea alba.

The arterial supply of the muscles is derived from the posterior branches of the intercostal and lumbar arteries. The vessels pass forwards with the segmental nerves to form a wide anastomosis behind the rectus muscle with the superior and inferior epigastric vessels. Further anastomoses are found near the iliac crest by way of the circumflex iliac artery. The lower six intercostal nerves pass obliquely downwards between the internal oblique and transverse muscles to enter the rectus sheath. Having supplied the anterolateral muscles and skin during their course, the nerves terminate by innervating the rectus abdominis muscles and overlying skin. In the lower abdomen the iliohypogastric and ilio-inguinal vessels lie between the external and internal oblique muscle layers and are in some danger during herniorrhaphy.

Superficial lymphatic drainage is provided in each quadrant by drainage to the ipsilateral or even contralateral axillae or groin but deeper drainage may also occur through the umbilical region to the porta hepatis and para-aortic region or to the internal mammary nodes.

The function of the abdominal muscles is to contain and support the abdominal viscera and to permit movement of the viscera during respiration. By concerted action, expulsive efforts such as micturition, defaecation, vomiting and childbirth, are assisted by the abdominal muscles and movement of the trunk, particularly flexion and lateral flexion, is carried out.

ABDOMINAL WOUNDS

The average general surgeon operates upon the abdominal wall more often that any other organ system. Difficulties in

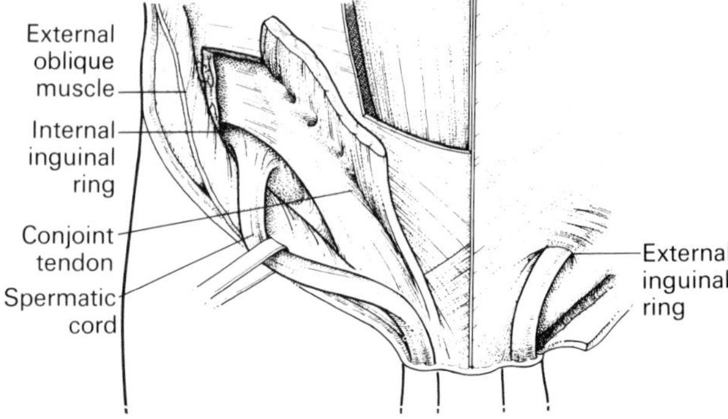

Fig. 76.1 The basic anatomical features of the inguinal region.

carrying out the definitive surgical procedure can often be attributed to an inappropriate site or size of incision and postoperative problems can be aggravated or precipitated by inadequate care in wound closure. The principles of wound management are considered in Chapter 1 but certain points are worth re-emphasizing in regard to the abdominal wound. The incision should be placed so as to give ready access to the organs requiring attention and should be capable of extension if the operation proves to be unduly difficult or additional disease is found. The incision should avoid damage to muscles and nerves where possible, as this is likely to produce a weakened closure and the development of incisional hernia. If possible the incision should not cross the main lines of tension. Thus transverse incisions may be preferable to longitudinal in terms of wound healing and cosmetic appearance. Transverse abdominal incisions, however, do not easily extend to deal with operative difficulties and often require further muscle cutting with nerve damage. Nevertheless, provided that the surgical procedure is known to be limited, e.g. hysterectomy, cholecystectomy, removal of ureteric stone, sympathectomy, etc. the transverse incision can be used with great effect and safety.

Ultimately the choice of incision depends upon a variety of factors, e.g. the diagnosis, age of the patient, degree of obesity, state of nutrition, the presence of infection or malignant disease or the multiplicity of surgical pathology. The trainee surgeon should refer to detailed texts on operative surgery for the reasoned arguments for a specific incision for a particular procedure.

However, it is pertinent to consider some of the complications of abdominal incisions and their management.

1. Wound Infection

a. Localized stitch abscess.
b. Cellulitis—usually haemolytic streptococcal organisms. *Staphylococcus aureus*, *Escherichia coli* or *Streptococcus faecalis* (*see* Chapter 3).
c. Progressive dermal gangrene—Meleney's gangrene (*see* Chapter 5).
d. Gas gangrene—usually after gastroduodenal surgery and involves *Clostridia welchii* and *Clostridia perfringens* (*see* Chapter 5).

In elective surgery, there is definite evidence that the administration of antibiotics immediately prior to surgery will reduce the incidence of wound sepsis. A heavy reliance on this approach should not be accompanied by a reduction in the discipline of aseptic surgical technique or attempts at wound protection.

In the management of obviously contaminated wounds, delayed suture of the skin and subcutaneous tissues is used too infrequently. An extension of this approach is currently being evaluated in patients who have undergone a laparotomy for severe and extensive sepsis. In such cases peritoneal débridement, irrigation or digital release of loculi of pus is required repeatedly in the postoperative period. Repeated access may be obtained by leaving the abdominal wall open, covered by soft rubber drains and moist packs or by the insertion of a Marlex mesh into which a zip fastener is sutured. The mesh is removed after 8–10 days and the wound allowed to granulate. Considerable improvement in survival of these desperately ill patients is reported.

2. Wound Dehiscence

The reported incidence of this complication varies from 0·2 to 3 per cent of abdominal wounds and it is certainly more frequent after emergency surgical procedures. Furthermore, it affects male patients much more frequently than female (4–5 : 1). The dehiscence may be partial or full but by definition it is normally considered to involve the deeper layers of the wound rather than the skin and subcutaneous tissues alone. Several patterns of clinical presentation occur:

a. The patient may have an unexpected stormy postoperative course with cardiopulmonary symptoms and a prolonged ileus, or the development of intestinal fistulas.
b. There is a serosanguineous discharge from the wound after 2 or 3 days.
c. There is a failure to develop a healing ridge over the first 10 postoperative days.
d. There is a sudden disruption of the wound on removal of the skin sutures with herniation of a knuckle of intestine through the wound.
e. There is obvious weakness and bulging on straining in the convalescent period (incisional hernia).

Wound dehiscence is more common after longitudinal than transverse incisions, though disruption is possible even with muscle-splitting, grid-iron incisions. Though midline incisions are thought to be more likely to disrupt, controlled trials of elective surgery have shown no difference in the dehiscence rate from paramedian incisions; nor with different types of anaesthesia.

Wound dehiscence results from an increased intra-abdominal pressure and poor wound healing. Factors associated with increased abdominal pressure include: prolonged postoperative ileus or adhesive obstruction, ascites, repeated retching and vomiting, persistent hiccough and coughing paroxysms. Those factors likely to be responsible for poor wound healing are many and several are present in most patients: wound infection, a drain through the wound, obesity, anaemia, hypoproteinaemia, uraemia, cachexia, the diabetic state, alcoholism, senility, vitamin deficiency, e.g. vitamin C and the use of cytotoxic agents or steroids.

Whilst most cases of dehiscence are the result of these risk factors, the use of inappropriate suture material, such as catgut, for the anterior sheath is associated with a high dehiscence rate. It does not seem critical to close the peritoneal layer of an abdominal wound, though it is certainly neater to do so. However, it is essential that suitable non-absorbable material or material with prolonged tensile strength, e.g. polydioxanone (P.D.S.), is used to repair the anterior sheath or linea alba.

The management of wound dehiscence demands urgent action. It is preferable to resuture the wound as soon as the patient's condition permits, though many of these patients have multiple problems and a period of resuscitation may be required. Normally a mass closure of all layers, except skin, with a non-absorbable monofilament suture will permit healing. Those patients with a poor healing ridge may be managed by delaying skin suture removal for several weeks and accepting an incisional hernia for repair rather than taking a risk on full disruption.

3. Wound Haematoma, Calcification and Ossification

Most wound haematomas result from an accidental penetration of a vessel in the muscle layers. It is usually self-limiting but may become infected and present as a deep abscess. When detected at an early stage, needle aspiration may allow rapid resolution. Chronic haematomas and other degenerate tissue within a wound often become impregnated with calcium salts (dystrophic calcification). In some patients, ossification of the wound may occur, probably as a result of the conversion of active wound fibroblasts into osteoblasts. The wound in both instances is hard and may appear to have metastatic disease. A radiograph of the wound will show the degenerate change and permit reassurance of the patient.

TUMOURS OF THE ABDOMINAL WALL

Benign tumours such as lipomas, fibromas, haemangiomas, keratoses and epithelial papillomas occur commonly on the abdominal wall and constitute no special problem. Neurofibromas are also common and are best excised because of the possibility of malignant change and this problem applies also to pigmented naevi.

A rare tumour arising from the muscle and aponeurotic layers is termed a 'desmoid tumour'. This may have the pathological appearance of acellular structure but the activity ranges upwards to that of a low-grade cellular fibrosarcoma. The desmoid tumour characteristically arises from the rectus abdominis muscles and the edge of the tumour can be seen to contain sequestrated muscle fibres. It is, therefore, infiltrative in nature and can enlarge to great size but it does not metastasize. Patients have local symptoms from the desmoid tumour which can be palpated easily deep to the skin and made more prominent by contraction of the rectus muscles. The cause of this tumour is unknown but it may be related to previous local trauma or childbirth and is certainly common after surgery for the variant of familial colonic polyposis known as Gardner's syndrome.

Malignant tumours of the abdominal wall are common though usually result from metastatic disease. The primary sites most frequently producing these metastases are ovary, uterus, bronchus, kidney and colon. Intra-abdominal malignancy may spread directly so as to appear at the umbilicus but others appear to result from haematogenous spread or by implantation into abdominal wounds.

Primary skin cancer of the abdominal wall is relatively rare compared with skin at other sites but does form half of all the primary malignant tumours in this region. Epidermoid cancers arising *de novo* behave as at other sites, but when arising in a scar or an area of radiation dermatitis, the prognosis is significantly worsened. Melanomas are managed by wide excision but often metastasize to more than one group of lymph glands and thus have a poorer prognosis than those on limbs.

Sarcomas (spindle-cell, rhabdomyosarcoma and neurofibrosarcoma) form the other half of primary abdominal wall tumours. These lesions readily metastasize and are best treated by wide excision and the defect repaired with prosthetic materials.

Rectal Sheath Haematoma

This condition may appear as a neoplasm of the abdominal wall and is situated almost invariably below the umbilicus. The haematoma develops from a rupture of one of the branches of the inferior epigastric artery. Usually there is a history of sudden strain or paroxysm of coughing followed by severe lower abdominal pain and the development of nausea, anorexia and vomiting. A tender swelling can be felt in the abdominal wall about 5 cm in diameter, though much larger haematomas have been seen (*Fig.* 76.2). A mild pyrexia and leucocytosis occur. If the diagnosis can be firmly established, the condition is self-limiting and resolves over 4 weeks. Where there is doubt, the haematoma is best explored and the inferior epigastric artery ligated.

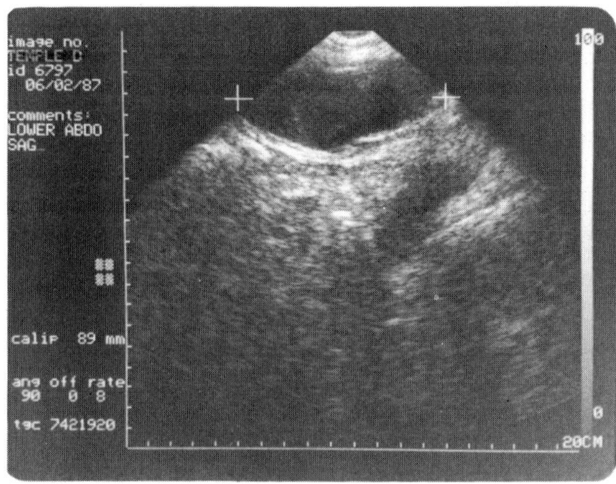

Fig. 76.2 Ultrasound of lower abdominal wall of a patient on dicoumarin therapy, who developed severe abdominal pain after a coughing spasm. The area between the '+' shows a haematoma confined by rectus sheath.

THE UMBILICUS

The umbilicus normally lies in the plane of the disc between the 3rd and 4th lumbar vertebrae, though clearly this may vary with the sex of the individual, age and degree of obesity. If examined from its deep surface, four fibrous cords are seen radiating from it and these represent structures which in fetal life traverse the umbilical cord: the umbilical vein, right and left umbilical arteries and the urachus. The additional structure to pass through the cord in embryonic development is the vitello-intestinal duct with accompanying vitelline veins.

Omphalitis

Infection of the umbilicus is fortunately a rare complication of the neonate. Faulty technique in dealing with the umbilical cord at birth leads to infection by *Staphylococcus aureus* or haemolytic streptococcus organisms with local suppuration and cellulitis. Treatment with appropriate antibiotics and local drainage is essential, for bacteraemia is common.

In the adult, infection of the umbilicus is a more chronic condition with a seropurulent, often foul-smelling, discharge and the development of granulation tissue. In the majority of patients, the fault lies in a lack of cleanliness but occasionally small foreign bodies have been 'lost' in the umbilicus and produce a persistent infection. Removal of the foreign body or sequestrated material from the depths of the umbilicus, followed by antispetic lotions, allows the condition to settle. Occasionally cautery of the granulation tissue with a silver nitrate stick is required.

Congenital Abnormalities

Patent Urachal Remnant

A persistent discharge of urine from the umbilicus results from a completely patent urachus (*see* Chapter 59). This complication may be delayed into childhood or early adult life, but in these circumstances, there is almost always an underlying urinary obstruction which has forced open the near-obliterated urachal remnant. It is important that prior to excision of the urachal remnant that the bladder should be shown to be free from any form of obstruction.

Two other urachal abnormalities may be delayed into adult life: urachal sinus and urachal cyst. In the former an intermittent umbilical discharge is the prominent symptom (*Fig*. 76.3) and in the latter the development of a very tender infected swelling in an infra-umbilical position leads to exploration and the demonstration of an infected urachal cyst. In both instances excision is indicated but repair to the dome of the bladder is not usually required.

Vitello-intestinal Duct Remnant

This condition is considered in detail in Chapter 59. The persistence of this remnant may show as a faecal fistula at the umbilicus, a bud or polyp of intestinal mucosa at the umbilicus, a cyst lying deep to the umbilicus between the

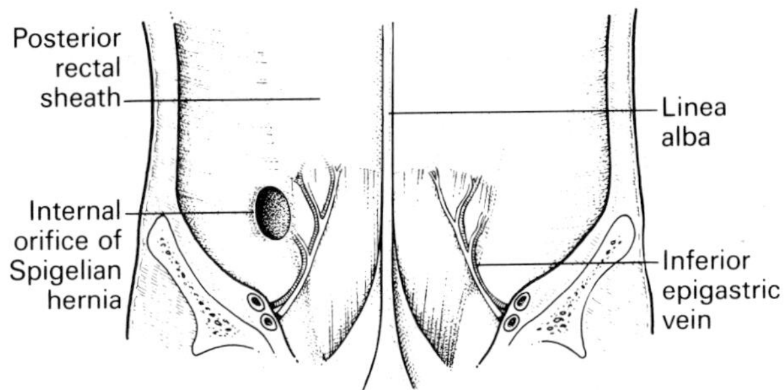

Fig. 76.3 The posterior view of the anterior abdominal wall showing the position of the sac of a Spigelian hernia.

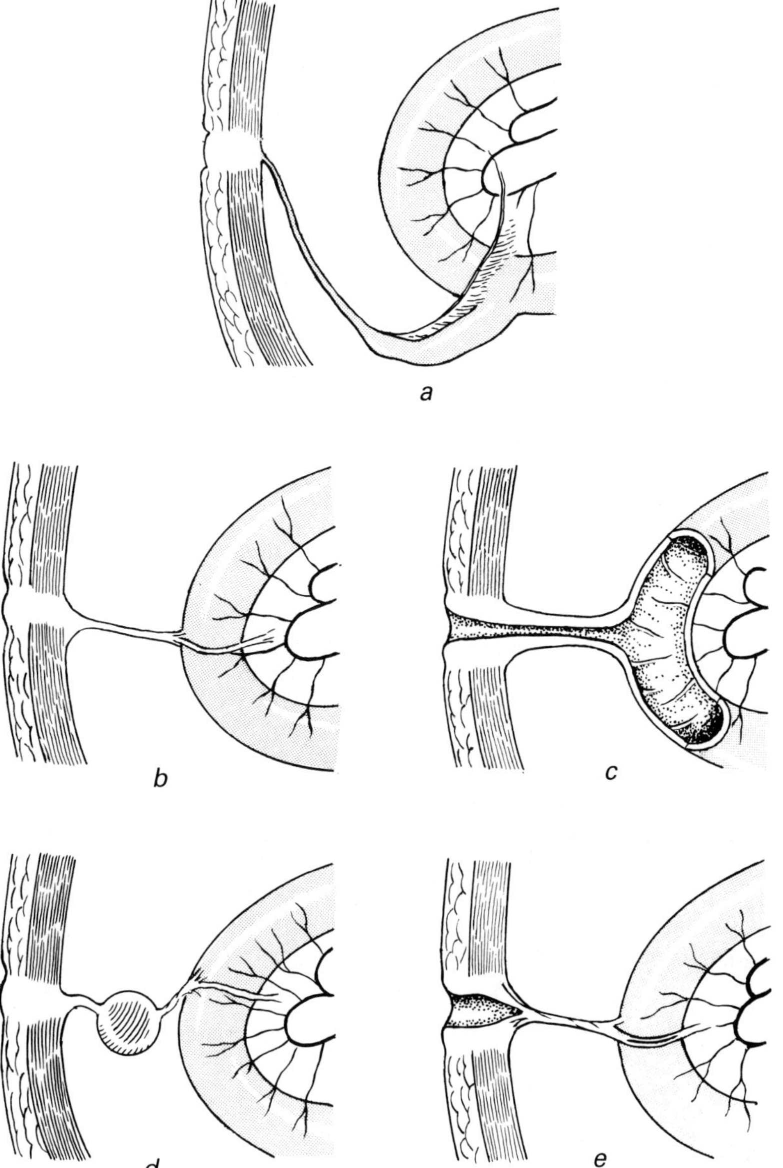

Fig. 76.4 The vitello-intestinal duct may connect with the umbilicus as: (*a*) a fibrous cord extending from a Meckel's diverticulum; (*b*) a simple fibrous cord to a loop of ileum; (*c*) an umbilical intestinal fistula; (*d*) a fibrous cord with cyst; (*e*) an umbilical sinus.

abdominal wall and ileum, a deep umbilical sinus, or a Meckel's diverticulum with or without a fibrous band attached to the posterior aspect of the umbilicus and response for intestinal obstruction by volvulus or band obstruction (*Fig.* 76.4).

The umbilical sinus, polyp or cyst usually requires excision. The completely patent vitello-intestinal duct may be complicated by partial or complete prolapse of the ileum through the umbilicus and requires early correction before this complication occurs, with excision of the umbilicus and Meckel's diverticulum.

Abdominal Wall Defects

A failure of the umbilical defect to close leads to the development of an omphalocele (*see* Chapter 59) or an umbilical hernia (*see below*). Major defects in the development of the abdominal wall are associated with exstrophy of the bladder and other forms of developmental abnormality including intestinal malrotation. The 'prune belly' baby has a gross deficiency of muscular development and the abdominal contents are covered with only skin, peritoneum and an intervening hypoplastic muscular layer.

THE POSTERIOR ABDOMINAL WALL AND RETROPERITONEUM

From both anatomical and functional points of view, this is best looked at from its ventral aspect. In the midline are the bodies, transverse processes and intervertebral discs of the 5 lumbar vertebrae. Laterally the wall extends from the 12th rib to the pelvic brim and the margin is formed by the aponeurosis of the transversus abdominis muscle. The psoas muscles take origin from the bodies and transverse process of the upper four lumbar vertebrae and are joined by the iliacus muscles on their lateral aspect. Posteriorly and laterally the quadratus lumborum muscles form the remaining support for lumbar nerves and vessels (*Fig.* 76.5).

The space between the posterior abdominal wall and peritoneal cavity is termed the retroperitoneal space. It is bounded above by the diaphragm and below by the pelvic brim. The space contains the aorta, vena cava, cysterna chyli and para-aortic glands and vessels, lumbar plexus and the chain of sympathetic ganglia. It should also be mentioned that the kidneys, ureters, adrenals and pancreas are within this retroperitoneal space.

Trauma to the space from blunt or penetrating injury is common, particularly in high-speed vehicle accidents. Damage to contained structures leads to haemorrhage and haematoma formation (*see* Chapter 75). Haemorrhage into the retroperitoneal space may also occur spontaneously, particularly in patients taking anticoagulants.

Two other retroperitoneal conditions are discussed:

Retroperitoneal Fibrosis

This relatively rare disease may be increasing in frequency. The condition results in the development of a flat grey/white plaque of tissue which is found first in the low lumbar region and then spreads laterally and upwards to encase the common iliac vessels and aorta. Rarely, it may extend upwards above the renal arteries and become contiguous with a similar process in the mediastinum, or forwards into the

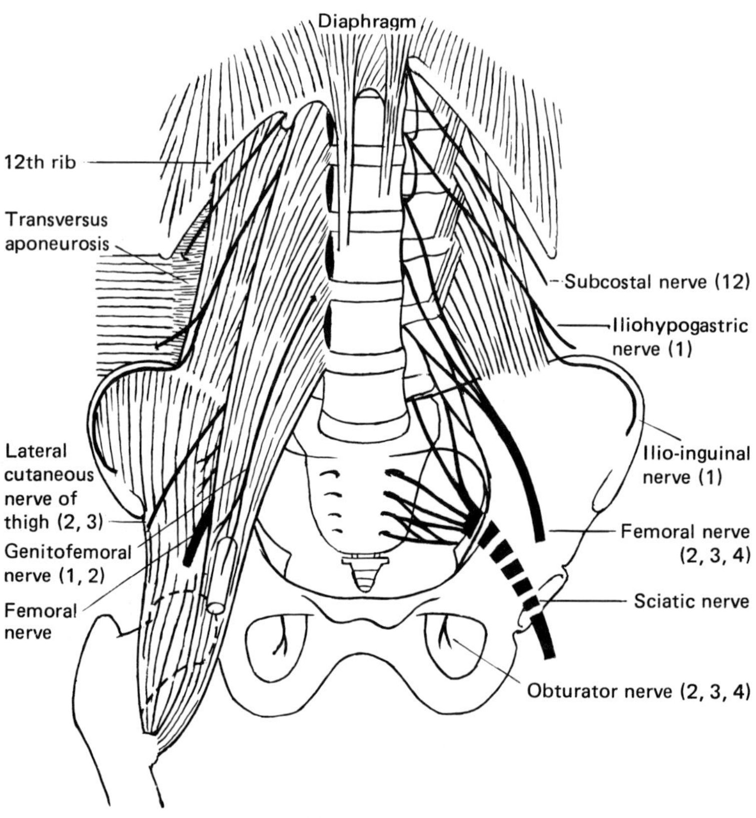

Fig. 76.5 The anatomical features of the posterior abdominal wall.

small bowel mesentery or mesocolon. The histological picture will vary from an active one which shows inflammatory cells and blood vessels surrounding bundles of collagen to a more mature picture which is relatively acellular with patches of calcification.

The aetiology is unknown and it has been attributed in the past to lymphatic and venous obstruction, lymphangitis, trauma or leakage of urine and blood. About 25% of cases seem to be associated with the administration of methysergide for migraine. The majority of the other cases would appear to be a part of a collagen disorder similar to polyarteritis nodosa.

Clinical presentation may be obtuse and result from the development of hypertension or renal failure. Many patients are middle-aged and males predominate. A nagging, ill-defined low back pain is common and there may be evidence of venous obstruction as shown by swelling of the scrotum or legs. Uncommonly, the patient may present with claudication. Examination reveals anaemia, leucocytosis and an increased sedimentation rate. Biochemical investigation may show a degree of renal failure. Where the investigation is possible, an intravenous pyelogram reveals the characteristic features of hydronephrosis, medial displacement of the ureters with gross irregularity. Patients in renal failure require cystoscopy and retrograde catheterization which produces no difficulty and permits the kidneys to drain and the renal failure to resolve.

Definitive treatment is achieved by the withdrawal of methysergide where appropriate, the administration of prednisolone and by ureterolysis. This procedure is carried out by a transabdominal approach and the freed ureters are separated from the fibrous tissue by interposing the greater omentum. A high success rate is usually possible.

Retroperitoneal Swellings

These are cystic lesions or solid tumours. Both are rare. The cysts are usually discovered incidentally and the majority are developmental remnants (Wolffian) of the urogenital tract and are situated near one of the kidneys. Teratomatous and dermoid cysts, parasitic cysts and lymphogenous cysts are all described. The lesions are readily excised to establish a true diagnosis.

Tumours in the retroperitoneum occur commonly if one includes those arising in kidneys, adrenal glands and pancreas or metastases. However, the term 'retroperitoneal tumour' is usually confined to primary tumours arising in the other tissues of these regions, e.g. muscles, fat, lymph glands and nerves. Some will be benign (20%), lipomas, leiomyomas or neurofibromas but others are malignant and include: lymphomas, sarcomas (liposarcomas, fibrosarcoma, rhabdomyosarcoma, neurofibrosarcoma) and neoplasms arising from the urogenital ridge.

Most patients present with vague symptoms including fever, abdominal discomfort, back pain, vomiting, anorexia, fatigue and weight loss and in the majority a mass is readily palpable in the abdomen. There may be evidence of tumour extension to produce vena caval compression as shown by oedematous legs, varicocele, dilated abdominal veins and ascites.

Traditionally, tumours have been demonstrated by the use of contrast radiology, intravenous pyelogram, barium examinations and angiography. There is little doubt that this is a field where computerized axial tomography is the investigation of first choice.

The treatment of these tumours will depend upon the precise pathological nature. An adequate biopsy is always required. Lymphomas are best treated by radiotherapy and/or chemotherapy once the diagnosis is established. Other malignant tumours have often extensively infiltrated the major blood vessels and other organs, e.g. kidneys, adrenal, pancreas and only 25% prove to be operable. There is some advantage to the patient to remove as much of the tumour as possible and to follow this procedure with radiotherapy and chemotherapy. If required, one kidney may be removed *en bloc* with the tumour mass, provided that an intravenous pyelogram has demonstrated that the contralateral kidney is functioning. The outlook is generally poor for these patients.

HERNIA THROUGH THE ABDOMINAL WALL

A hernia may be defined as a protrusion of a sac of peritoneum together with preperitoneal fat or an organ through a congenital or acquired defect in the muscles of the abdominal wall through which they do not normally pass (Ljungdahl). Hernias occupy a good deal of surgical time and form about 10–15% of all surgical procedures. The majority of operations (80%) are performed for inguinal hernias though this figure is even higher in the male population. The remainder are in the region of the umbilicus (8%), incisional (7%) and femoral hernias (5%). Rarer forms of hernias, though very interesting, form only a tiny proportion of the surgical problem.

Inguinal Hernias

The inguinal canal passes obliquely through the anterior abdominal wall and extends from the deep inguinal ring at the midpoint of the inguinal ligament to the superficial inguinal ring at the pubic crest. Overall the canal is about 4 cm long and contains the structures which form the spermatic cord:

Three arteries	*Three nerves*	*Three structures*
testicular	ilio-inguinal	pampiniform plexus
cremasteric	genital branch of genitofemoral	vas deferens
vas deferens	sympathetic	remnants of the processus vaginalis

The canal is formed by the descent of the testes from the posterior abdominal wall during early development and then by somatic growth in later life. The anterior wall is formed by the aponeurosis of the external oblique muscle and reinforced laterally by the internal oblique. The floor is composed of the inguinal ligament and by the expanded lacunar segment at its medial end. Fibres from the internal oblique and transversus muscles arch over the roof of the canal (conjoint tendon) and form the posterior wall medially reinforcing the strong layer of transversalis fascia which runs across the posterior wall of the canal (*Fig.* 76.6).

Indirect hernias pass through the deep inguinal ring lateral to the inferior epigastric artery; direct hernias bulge forward through the posterior inguinal wall medial to the inferior epigastric artery. Normally, two mechanisms act to prevent herniation through the inguinal canal. With increased abdominal pressure, contraction of the internal oblique and transversus muscles act upon the section of the transversus aponeurosis which arches convexly upwards over the medial half of the canal. The arch is pulled downwards and flattened so that its lower edge abuts the inguinal ligament and thus reinforces the posterior inguinal wall. The second mechanism which may in fact be more important,

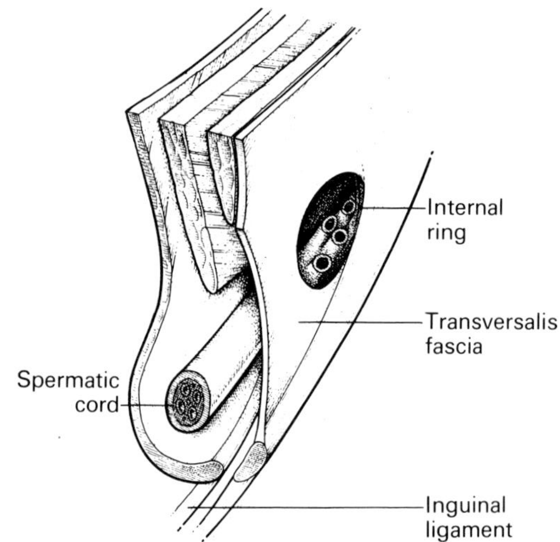

Fig. 76.6 The internal view of the deep inguinal ring and cord contents. (Derived from Nyhus L. M. and London R. E. (ed.) (1978) *Hernia* 2nd ed. Philadelphia, Lippincott.)

depends upon the attachment of the strong fascial layer forming the deep inguinal ring. This fascial ring is normally firmly adherent to the posterior surface of the transversus muscle so that contraction of the muscle pulls the ring upwards and laterally. It is important that herniorrhaphy operations should maintain or enhance these protective actions.

There is clear evidence of an increased risk of right inguinal hernia after appendicectomy, which is related to the denervation of fibres of the right transversus abdominis muscles. These fibres are responsible for the support of U-shaped deep inguinal ring of fascia.

Indirect inguinal hernias require the presence of a peritoneal sac or a potential sac passing through the deep inguinal ring. The sac is usually preformed and is thus a congenital defect of the process in which the sac is normally obliterated to form the ligament inguinale. It is quite common for the persistence of the patent processus vaginalis to be associated with other abnormalities, e.g. undescended testicle or hydroceles of the testis or cord. In the infant, the deep inguinal ring is not dilated but in the adult the ring dilates with the increasing size of hernia.

Direct hernias result from a weakening of the transversalis fascia in the posterior inguinal wall. The weakness occurs on the medial side of the inferior epigastric vessels and bulges forwards into the canal but only rarely through the external ring. Occasionally the medial wall of the sac is composed of the bladder wall. Not uncommonly, a hernia sac (indirect and direct) will be found on either side of the inferior epigastric vessels (pantaloon hernia). Studies of collagen metabolism in the fascia of patients with hernia reveal marked reduction in collagen synthesis in patients with direct hernia compared with those with indirect hernia. Other studies have, on the contrary, shown an increased rate of collagen synthesis but associated with a markedly increased rate of collagen lysis. These findings reflect in the clinical observation that direct hernias are bilateral more than twice as frequently as indirect hernias.

Inguinal Hernias in Infants and Children

Ninety per cent of inguinal hernias occur in males and the peak of incidence seems to be about 1 year when the child starts to walk. Probably about 10% of these children will develop a hernia on the other side; in about 50% this contralateral peritoneal sac will be present at operation on the presenting side. Attempts to detect these occult hernias have included the introduction of Gastrografin into the peritoneal cavity with operative radiology to demonstrate the contralateral peritoneal sac. There is no indication for routine exploration of the contralateral side. Direct inguinal hernia is excessively rare in children and the vast majority are indirect, resulting from abnormal descent of the testis and persistence of a patent processus vaginalis.

The history of a lump appearing in the groin is usually obtained from the mother who notices the hernia after a period of straining or coughing by the child. Quite frequently it is not demonstrated by the medical examiner and all that can be felt is a silky sensation on palpation of the spermatic cord as the layers of the processus vaginalis move under the examining fingers. Unfortunately many of the signs are ignored; there is a tendency for the hernia to become obstructed and to strangulate the contents. The differential diagnosis of a hydrocele, undescended testis, hydrocele of the cord, torsion of the testis or cord and a femoral hernia should be borne in mind.

This being the case, all children with a strong history should have elective exploration of the affected side. The operation consists of transection and high ligation of the patent processus (herniotomy). Repair of the inguinal canal is not required.

Inguinal Hernia in Adults

Three types of inguinal hernia may be considered:

Indirect

This hernia occurs more frequently in males in the ratio 10 males:1 female. The peritoneal sac lies lateral to the inferior epigastric vessels and accompanies the cord and its layers as it passes along the inguinal canal through the superficial inguinal ring, which it stretches, and may reach the scrotum and testicle.

Direct

The hernial sac bulges forward through the posterior inguinal wall stretching the transversalis fascia and lies behind or above the cord. The sac has a wide neck and tends to extend upwards and outwards, for the tendon of the rectus muscle and inguinal ligament are relatively strong and unyielding. It is most unusual for the sac to pass through the superficial ring into the scrotum.

Sliding (Fig. 76.7)

This type differs insomuch as there is no preformed sac but the peritoneal margins of the deep ring and the adjacent structure (e.g. caecum or sigmoid colon) slip downwards, widely stretching the fascial and muscular margins of the deep ring. The wall at the back of this hernia is extraperitoneal. These hernias may be of large size.

Recurrent

These hernias develop after an operation for hernia in the same groin regardless of whether or not the two hernias are of the same type. There is considerable doubt as to the true incidence, for the diagnosis rests completely on the interpretation of physical examination of the patient. It will be recognized that a slight bulge to one observer may be considered a recurrence by another. The approximate recurrence rates are 10% after indirect hernia repair, 20% after

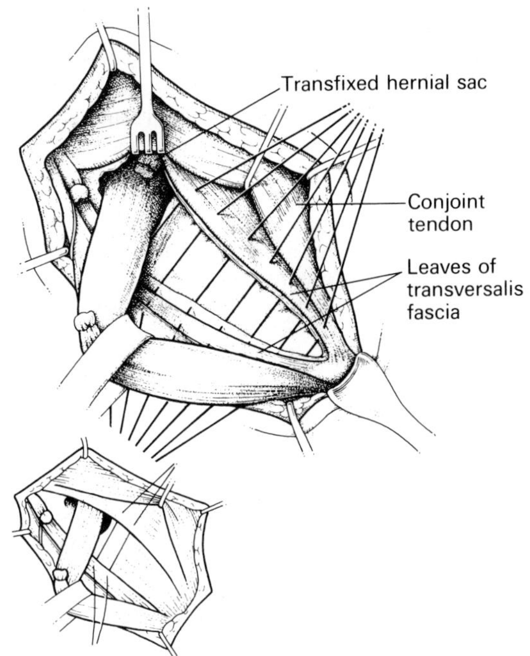

Fig. 76.7 In the repair of an inguinal hernia, the transversalis fascial layers are carefully dissected and sutured prior to any repair involving the conjoint tendon. (Derived from Nyhus L. M. and London R. E. (ed.) (1978) *Hernia* 2nd ed. Philadelphia, Lippincott.)

direct hernia repair and 30% after repair of a recurrent hernia.

Some recurrences result from obesity, persistent straining from chronic constipation, urinary obstruction or cough or premature resumption of full heavy physical activity after hernial repair. However, the majority of failures result from a failure to detect small indirect sacs within the cord at the time of repair of an apparent direct hernia or a failure to preserve and reinforce adequately the deep inguinal ring and posterior structures of the inguinal wall.

Clinical Features

The complaint common to nearly all patients is the appearance of a lump in the groin. Some patients complain of a dragging sensation or pain in the groin, particularly during the early stages, but many hernias are asymptomatic. There may be a history of a major physical strain or of heavy physical work prior to the development of the hernia. Presumably increased abdominal pressure can stretch the fascial margins of the deep inguinal ring and open up a preformed peritoneal sac.

The hernia may be best shown with the patient standing or precipitated by coughing and straining. The sac should be above and medial to the pubic tubercle. It is possible to detect a strong cough impulse in the inguinal canal and in some patients the impulse can be felt as a bulge through the external ring. In the case of a large scrotal hernia, the diagnosis is obvious and a cough impulse may be absent.

The differential diagnosis of inguinal hernia includes: femoral hernia, inguinal lymphadenopathy, ectopic testis, hydrocele of the cord, saphenous varix and psoas abscess. Endometrosis in a hernial sac may be mistaken for an incarcerated hernia as may malignant tumours in the groin. Patients with chronic groin pain constitute a difficult diagnostic problem. Most cases of chronic pain in athletes are due to soft-tissue injuries but in a number an undeclared hernia is the cause. In such instances, an investigation more detailed than clinical examination is required.

Herniography

In this technique 50–80 ml of a positive iodine contrast medium is introduced into the peritoneal cavity by fine needle puncture. The patient lies prone with a head up tilt of 25°. The contrast pools in the inguinal region and straining or moving from side to side will enhance the pooling. Three inguinal fossas are noted: suprapubic, medial and lateral. Normally the inguinal fossas do not reach beyond the rim of the pubic bone in the medial half of the posterior inguinal wall. Indirect hernias emerge from the lateral fossa whereas direct hernias may be divided into lateral direct hernias bulging from the medial fossa or medial direct hernias bulging from the suprapubic fossa. Femoral hernias are directed more caudally and curve over the pubic bone closely. Sliding hernias are not well seen by this technique but rarer forms, e.g. obturator, prevesical or sciatic are well shown. Recurrent hernias are readily demonstrable.

Ultrasonography

This technique is the method of choice for Spigelian hernias and occasionally is advocated in the differentiation of lumps in the femoral triangle.

Computerized Tomography

There can be few cases where this is justified but there are reports which have shown perineal, obturator, sciatic and Spigelian hernias which have otherwise defied diagnosis.

The Repair of Inguinal Hernias in Adults

The fundamental defect in the structure of the anterior abdominal wall which allows inguinal hernias to develop, is related to a deficiency in the fascia of the transverse abdominis muscle. If this layer remains intact, it is unlikely a hernia will develop. In a hernia repair the main object will be to restore the transverse abdominis fascia to normality. As an indirect hernia develops, it progressively stretches the internal ring of transversalis fascia and a reconstitution of this fascial ring is fundamental to the success of repair. The strength of the posterior inguinal wall is proportional to the number of transverse abdominis fibres and direct hernias are likely in those individuals found to have no aponeurotic fibres in the bulging posterior wall. In fact the bulge consists of only transversalis fascia. Unlike the situation in infants, where a herniotomy will normally suffice, adult patients require a repair to prevent recurrence of the hernia. Considerable debate ensues when the best method of repair is considered: some surgeons prefer to concentrate their attention on the deep inguinal ring and the transversalis fascia; other surgeons are more concerned to use the anterior layers of tissue (external and internal oblique aponeurosis) to reinforce the repair.

There is a general tendency to treat small indirect hernias differently from large indirect sacs and direct hernias. Small indirect hernias may be handled by high ligation and removal of the hernial sac, followed by a careful repair of the deep inguinal fascial ring medial to the spermatic cord. Where the hernia is bigger the deep ring will be stretched medially and the whole posterior inguinal wall bulges behind the conjoint tendon. In these circumstances it is appropriate to extend the repair medially by suturing the lower edge of the transversus aponeurosis to the iliopubic tract as far medially as the pubis. Variations of this technique may be described as the Bassini, Halsted or Ferguson procedures. With still larger indirect hernias, there may be some difficulty in returning the contents into the abdominal cavity, usually because of adhesions to the wall of the sac. In some of these patients, both the internal and external rings and posterior inguinal wall are grossly stretched and attenuated. In the aged patient, consideration should be given to division of the spermatic cord and orchiectomy so as to permit a complete closure of the inguinal canal. After excision of the sac, the posterior inguinal wall is repaired by a layered suture of the transversalis fascia (*Fig.* 76.8) and transversus abdominis aponeurosis to the upper fascia of the femoral sheath and Cooper's ligament, and tension avoided in the suture layer by a relieving incision in the aponeurosis of the internal oblique muscle as it forms the anterior rectus sheath. An alternative approach is to construct a mesh or darn through the layers of the posterior inguinal wall using synthetic materials (nylon, polypropylene) or fascia lata ribbon. Direct hernias do not require the sac to be excised but do require a full repair to the posterior inguinal wall. The reader is referred to detailed descriptions in textbooks of operative surgery.

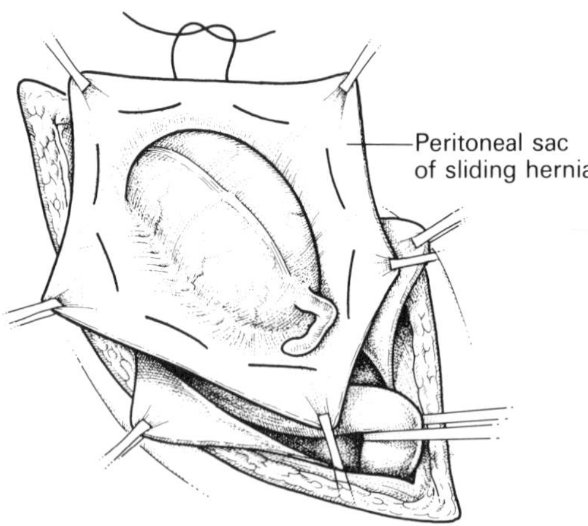

Fig. 76.8 A sliding hernia develops when the contents, usually sigmoid colon, descend into the inguinal region. The colon does not lie within the sac but the sac is applied to its surface. The bowel is liable to damage if the sac is fully dissected from the surface and is best managed by a plicating suture after which the bowel can be returned to the abdominal cavity. (Derived from Nyhus L. M. and London R. E. (ed.) (1978) *Hernia* 2nd ed. Philadelphia, Lippincott.)

Hernias in which the ileocaecal portion of the right colon and the sigmoid colon on the left side form a part of the sac wall are common and are termed the indirect sliding hernias. This variety is commonly found in the elderly and obese and tend to form large reducible hernias. A high suspicion is required and in such cases, it is necessary to open the hernial sac and to return the contents into the abdominal cavity after mobilizing colon. No attempt is made to reperitonealize the colon. The repair of the internal ring and posterior inguinal wall follow principles previously discussed.

Non-operative Treatment of Inguinal Hernia

Provided that the hernia is readily reducible, elderly patients may be content to wear a truss. Small indirect hernias are controlled by a spring truss but large indirect and direct hernias require a large pad and firm belt.

Femoral Hernia

Herniation through the femoral canal is an acquired condition and it is therefore rare in children, rising to a peak of incidence in the fifth and sixth decades. The higher incidence on the right side is inexplicable unless the right leg being in use more often than the left in severe exercise is the reason. Females are twice as prone to femoral hernias as males and this incidence is further doubled in the parous woman. This suggests that increased abdominal pressure either from pregnancy, obesity or ascites may be a factor as may the laxity of abdominal muscles and ligaments which accompany pregnancy.

There is the possibility that as a result of pressure, e.g. from a gravid uterus, the external iliac vein may at certain times stretch the coverings around the femoral canal. After the vein is decompressed, there exists a possible laxity in the tissues at this point. A final aetiological factor may be the fact that in a number of individuals, the insertion of the iliopubic tract into the pectineal line of the pubis is narrower than normal and this leads to a wide femoral canal at the upper margin.

The normal margins of the upper margin of the femoral canal ('the ostium') are: (1) laterally, the external iliac vein and a weak septum of areolar tissue; (2) anteriorly and medially, the attachments of the transversalis fascia above the inguinal ligament; and (3) posteriorly, the pubis and pectineal fascia. It appears that, contrary to previous views, the inguinal ligament and lacunar reflection normally lie about 1 cm distal to the true ostium (*Fig.* 76.9).

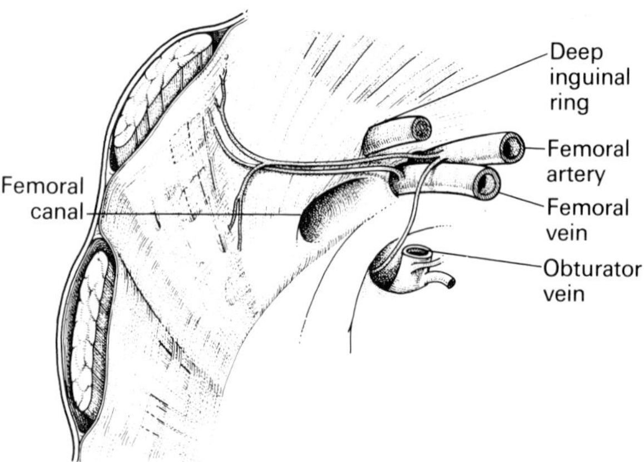

Fig. 76.9 The inner aspect of the sigmoid region which demonstrates the position of the femoral canal in relation to the femoral vessels and obturator foramen. (Derived from Nyhus L. M. and London R. E. (ed.) (1978) *Hernia* 2nd ed. Philadelphia, Lippincott.)

The femoral hernia passes downwards through the femoral canal by stretching the transversalis fascia, usually lying medial to the external iliac vein. As the hernia extends downwards, the sac eventually abuts on these ligaments and, being relatively rigid, expansion can only occur in a lateral direction. On reaching the lower end of the canal, the sac is turned forwards through the cribriform fascia and then upwards to overlie the inguinal ligament, being occasionally mistaken for an inguinal hernia. Equally the hernias may remain quite small and be invisible or scarcely palpable in the obese patient.

Most hernial sacs contain omental plugs and occasionally loops of small bowel. Since the neck of the sac is fairly rigid, it is common for the hernia to remain incarcerated and for the lump in the groin to be permanently present. Even in obese patients it is usually possible for the examiner to convince himself that the lump lies lateral and below the pubic tubercle. Normally the hernia causes only mild local discomfort, although the risk of strangulation is high (30–40%). In these circumstances, the patient has symptoms and signs of intestinal obstruction (Chapter 75) and in most instances the hernia is tender and tense and there is an absence of cough impulse.

Management

There is no effective treatment of a femoral hernia other than surgical correction and no truss should be prescribed. Femoral hernias are best dealt with as an elective procedure. Patients with a suspected strangulated hernia require emergency resuscitation as outlined in Chapter 75.

The surgical approach to a femoral hernia may be:

1. From below the inguinal ligament: The low approach is ideal for an elective procedure and requires the sac to be isolated by an incision below the inguinal ligament, and cleared up to the neck. The sac is opened and emptied with care taken to avoid injury to the bladder wall, which may bear a relationship to the medial side of the sac. The peritoneum is closed above the neck of the sac and the stump returned to the abdomen. The femoral canal is repaired by interrupted non-absorbable sutures passing from the undersurface of the inguinal ligament to Cooper's ligament behind and forming a relatively loose lattice.

In patients with strangulated hernial contents, it is important that the fluid contents are collected and cultured and that the small bowel does not return to the abdomen before its viability is assessed. This can only be done after division of the constricting ostium. Where an area of bowel wall is of doubtful viability (Richter's hernia) it may be oversewn but it is often more appropriate to proceed to a femoral local resection in these doubtful cases.

The advantages of the lower procedure is the simplicity and directness of the approach but it does have some disadvantages, notably the occasional difficulty in dealing with the constriction ring and the assessment of bowel viability. It is probably unwise to perform a bowel resection through this incision and better to carry out a formal laparotomy once the need for bowel resection has been decided upon.

2. The inguinal approach: The inguinal canal is opened anteriorly and then the neck of the femoral hernia exposed by incising the posterior inguinal canal wall. The contents of the sac can be examined by opening the sac and dealt with according to need. The repair is carried out by closing the femoral canal from above and a standard inguinal hernia repair to the posterior inguinal wall.

Though formerly advised for strangulated femoral hernia the approach holds no particular advantage.

3. The lateral rectus (McEvedy) approach: An incision just lateral to the rectus muscle permits a direct approach to the femoral ring.

4. The properitoneal approach: This is applicable to most inguinofemoral hernias. The transverse incision through the abdominal muscles above the inguinal canal allows a posterior approach to the deep inguinal ring and a superior approach to the femoral canal. It does give an improved view of the femoral canal and permits an examination of the sac and its contents, together with the ease of bowel resection should this prove necessary.

The high approach for femoral hernia allows the release of an adherent sac and contents by incision of the femoral ring of fascia. After excision of the sac, the repair is more exactly carried out by a careful repair to within a few millimetres of the femoral vein suturing the posterior inguinal wall to Cooper's ligament.

Epigastric and Umbilical Hernias

These hernias may be considered together because a para-umbilical hernia is an epigastric hernia situated just above the umbilicus. Thus the characteristic of these hernias is that they protrude through a defect in the linea alba between the xiphisternum and umbilicus.

Epigastric hernias are most commonly found in males and rarely in children. About one-quarter of cases are multiple. The defect in the linea alba allows a small pad of extraperitoneal fat to protrude and, as a result of increased intra-abdominal pressure, the defect enlarges to permit a sac of peritoneum and eventually the sac may admit omentum or even small bowel.

Most epigastric hernias are symptomless and are discovered incidentally by the patient or doctor. A small lump, which is more prominent on standing, is palpable in the midline but it is rare for a cough impulse to be present. A small number of patients present with vague upper abdominal symptoms which do not fit a dyspeptic pattern and in whom repair of the hernia gives relief. It may be that, in these patients, a degree of tension of the peritoneal sac has produced the symptoms.

Small epigastric hernias do not require treatment. Those larger than 2 cm have the potential of strangulation because of the narrow neck through the linea alba and are best treated surgically. The procedure is excision of the sac and repair of the defect by either a simple longitudinal repair or a transverse overlapping Mayo type repair. The results, except in the very obese patient, are generally very good.

Umbilical hernias require a slightly different classification:

Adult para-umbilical type
Exomphalos
Infantile umbilical type.

a. Adult Para-umbilical Hernias

These hernias are more common in females (3:1) and seem to be mainly confined to obese patients. The defect lies just above the umbilicus though deformity of the umbilical button is the earliest manifestation. The hernia may enlarge to the size of an orange but the neck of the sac remains dangerously small so that the risk of strangulation is ever present. The chronicity of the condition leads to firm adhesions forming between the peritoneal sac and its contents so that almost all large hernias are irreducible and are not treatable by the use of an abdominal support or truss. Surgical treatment is best carried out electively in all patients though it is fair to say that most patients present as emergencies with strangulation or obstruction having already taken place.

The procedure of choice is that described by W. J. Mayo in 1893. In the adult patient the umbilical cicatrix is excised to prevent infection and the sac defined and its contents removed. After excision of the sac the defect is closed by suture, the upper crescent being fixed over the front of the lower half of the defect. The recurrence rate should be no more than 2–3%.

b. Exomphalos

This rare condition occurs in about 1:5000 births. It is frequently associated with other congenital defects and not surprisingly about one-quarter of babies have malrotation of the intestine. The management of this condition is covered in Chapter 59.

c. Infantile Umbilical Hernias

These hernias occur through a persistent defect at the umbilicus and are relatively common. Indeed, umbilical hernias appear to be the rule in African infants. It must be concluded that the majority close spontaneously. Larger defects take longer and the area of the defect appears to diminish about 18% every month. The contents of the sac remain very prominent until just before the final point of closure.

It is very rare for an umbilical hernia to require surgical operation, nor is there any indication for binders or trusses. However, operation is mandatory for strangulation and incarceration. It is generally considered important to preserve the umbilical cicatrix after excising the sac and repairing the defect so that the child will not appear unusual to its fellows.

Incisional Hernias

By definition, incisional hernias develop through the area of a surgical incision. They appear to occur after 3–5% of all abdominal operations. In terms of predisposing factors, the following appear relevant and often more than one is acting in the same patient:

1. Midline or T-shaped incisions;
2. Infected wounds and wounds requiring resuture;
3. Emergency procedures are more prone;
4. Patients with poor nutritional status, e.g. hypoproteinaemia;
5. Patients with a debilitating disorder: carcinomatosis, chronic nephritis, diabetes, cirrhosis of liver, alcoholic and jaundiced patients;
6. Postoperative chest complications;
7. Obese patients;
8. Through defects left by drainage tubes.

The management of patients with incisional hernias can be difficult, not only because of the large size these hernias reach but also because the general condition may militate against aggressive surgery. Abdominal corsets are often prescribed for these patients and although such supports do control the hernia, the abdominal belt is clearly not comfortable. Every attempt should be made to persuade the patient to lose weight. Cardiorespiratory difficulties and factors liable to increase abdominal pressure, e.g. chronic constipation also require attention.

Two surgical techniques are applied:

1. The anatomical approach: For small and medium-sized incisional hernias, the ideal procedure is to excise all scar tissue until normal anatomical planes are reached. Thereafter the abdominal wall is repaired by suturing all layers individually after the clearance from the sac of adherent loops of bowel. The repair may be reinforced by overlapping of the margins of the rectus sheath, by the use of a fascia lata graft, by the inversion of the fascial margins of the sheath (Keel method) and producing a degree of relaxation in the middle of the repair by an incision through the anterior rectus sheath at the lateral margins of the rectus muscle. Provided that the abdominal exploration has not been too rigorous it should be possible to avoid a postoperative ileus and the results of repair for small and medium-sized incisional hernias should be 95% satisfactory.

2. Implantation of prosthetic materials: The larger type of incisional hernia cannot be approximated without tension and additional reinforcement is necessary. As the hernia expands the rectus muscles can no longer be brought towards one another. These sacs are sufficiently large to contain the bulk of the intestines and, as with exomphalos, there may be insufficient space within the abdominal cavity to readmit the viscera, without cardiopulmonary embarrassment. In these circumstances some surgeons resort to the use of progressive pneumoperitoneum to stretch the abdomen several weeks prior to operation. Where possible the hernial sac is kept intact. The prosthesis most commonly implanted is a polypropylene (Marlex) or polyester (Mersilene) mesh which is placed deep to the muscle layer and sutured with nylon. Redundant skin is trimmed and a satisfactory cosmetic appearance can be achieved.

Obturator Hernia

This rare hernia is found more commonly in women, possibly because the obturator foramen in the female has a greater transverse diameter. The majority of hernias pass beneath the superior ramus of the pubis to emerge under the cover of the pectineus muscle. Other hernias more rarely pass between the superior and middle fasciculi of the obturator externus muscle and still more rarely between the external and internal obturator membranes. Most commonly patients complain of referred pain at the knee due to pressure on the obturator nerve. This in combination with a vague abdominal discomfort should give the clue and careful search in the groin may give the suggestion of a lump there, though not necessarily so. The difficulty in diagnosis results in many patients only being diagnosed at laparotomy, for the sac contents are often a Richter's type hernia. By the time a diagnosis is made, gangrene in the affected segment has supervened with perforation and severe sepsis in the thigh has been reported. The surgical approach is normally through the lower abdomen though elective cases can be dealt with through the groin or inguinal canal.

Rarer Forms of Hernia

A sciatic hernia passes through the greater or lesser sciatic foramens. Pain is felt in the buttock or thigh or along the distribution of the sciatic nerve. A reducible swelling can be felt in the gluteal region with a cough impulse and radiography of the pelvis may show a gas shadow lying outside the pelvic outline. The differential diagnosis is that of a lipoma or a chronic tuberculous abscess. The hernia is normally repaired through the abdomen though a gluteal approach is also feasible.

A lumbar hernia presents in the superior or inferior lumbar triangle. Most hernias are large and reducible, with a cough impulse and pass forward to the anterior abdominal wall or over the iliac crest. Symptoms are usually local and non-specific, for the hernias have such a wide neck that obstruction and strangulation are very rare. Although some hernias appear to be of congenital origin, the majority appear to be associated with muscle weakness or related to previous incisions in the area. Many patients are satisfied with some form of abdominal support but surgical repair is not difficult and is usually successful.

Perineal hernias pass through the muscles covering the pelvic outlet and can occur in front of or behind the transverse perinei muscles. The hernias are largely confined to women, who present with soft, reducible swellings in relation to the labia or the lower margin of the gluteal muscles.

Spigelian Hernia

This hernia is a protrusion of fat and peritoneum through the semilunar line which is formed by the aponeurosis of the internal oblique muscle at its point of division to enclose the rectus muscle. In its earliest form the patient complains of a painful lump along the lateral edge of the rectus sheath and the pain is aggravated by strain or coughing (*Fig.* 76.3). Most of these lumps are fatty protrusions but eventually a full peritoneal sac develops, the contents of which are in danger of strangulation because of the narrow neck. Surgical repair is advised.

Complications of Abdominal Hernias

1. Irreducibility

Although most inguinal hernias are readily reducible by the patient, femoral and para-umbilical hernias are usually irreducible. This results from the small aperture at the neck of the sac and eventually the development of adhesions of the omentum or intestine to the hernial sac. Large inguinoscrotal hernias may also become irreducible and this is particularly the situation with sliding hernias. It is not uncommon to find patients still wearing a truss over an irreducible hernia despite its uselessness. Irreducible hernias are more likely to obstruct and strangulate and should be operated upon where possible.

2. Obstruction

A sudden increase in abdominal pressure may precipitate the intestinal obstruction. Normally only the small bowel is involved with inguinofemoral hernias but the transverse colon may obstruct in a para-umbilical hernia and the sigmoid colon in a large sliding left-sided inguinoscrotal hernia.

3. Strangulation

The contents of a hernial sac may be said to be strangulated when the blood supply is impaired—partial occlusion leads to venous congestion—complete occlusion will produce gangrene. Inguinal and femoral hernias account for 80% of cases, though the proportion of femoral and umbilical hernias which strangulate (20–30%) is greater than inguinal (2–5%).

The precipitating cause of obstruction and strangulation is usually unknown but is presumably some act which forces more abdominal viscera into the sac that can be easily returned. The contents are gripped by the neck of the sac which is usually the transversalis fascia at the deep inguinal ring or ileopectineal tract for femoral hernia. Some inguinal hernias are constricted by the inguinal canal itself (especially if the patient has worn a truss) or the external ring (children). The constricting ring in umbilical hernias is usually the fascial defect in the abdominal wall.

The contents initially become swollen and as venous congestion ensues, a bloodstained fluid is exuded. Further

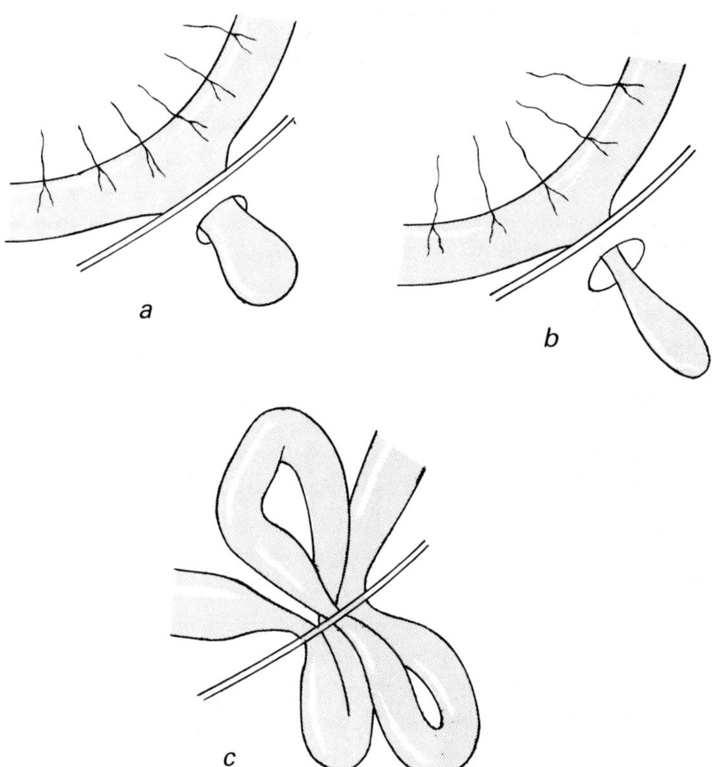

Fig. 76.10 Unusual inguinal hernias. *a*, Richter's hernia incorporates only one side of the bowel wall; *b*, Littre's hernia contains a Meckel's diverticulum; *c*, Maydl's hernia strangulates the internal loop of intestine.

swelling impairs the arterial blood supply and gangrene may follow within 4 h though it usually takes longer. Neglected cases are often complicated by peritonitis and sepsis adjacent to the hernia. The bowel tends to perforate either at the antimesenteric border, at the apex of the loop or at the site of the constricting rings.

Three additional specific types are described (*Fig.* 76.10):

Richter's hernia
Littre's hernia
Maydl's hernia

Richter's hernia is particularly important, being a small hernial protrusion involving only a part of the circumference of the bowel which is readily overlooked in clinical examination. A late diagnosis permits gangrene and perforation to occur. Operation requires clear demonstration of the ischaemic segment and repair either by inversion or excision and re-anastomosis.

Littre's hernia contains a Meckel's diverticulum and should not fully involve the ileum. Maydl's hernia involves two loops of intestine becoming incarcerated in the sac but with strangulation of the intervening intra-abdominal segment.

Clinical Features

The development of obstruction or strangulation leads to local symptoms with enlargement of the swelling over the hernial orifice. General symptoms include colicky abdominal pain, vomiting and absolute constipation. Not all of these features are present with a strangulated Richter's type hernia or when the sac contains only strangulated omentum. Examination may reveal a tender, tense swelling which is irreducible and has no cough impulse. It is not advisable to attempt a reduction of the hernia by any means other than surgical, in case the hernia is returned to the abdomen *en masse* or non-viable gut is reduced. The abdominal features may be absent initially though eventually distension will be found, with increased peristalsis. Hernias which perforate locally, lead to the development of abscesses which may produce faecal material and gas. As the condition progresses the signs of dehydration and hypovolaemia are more prominent.

The differential diagnosis of strangulated hernia depends upon its site:

Inguinal: enlarged inguinal lymph glands, hydrocele of the cord, torsion of the testis, pampiniform venous thrombosis and a strangulated femoral hernia;

Femoral: enlarged inguinal lymph nodes, saphena varix (thrombosed), lipoma, psoas abscess, obturator hernia and a strangulated inguinal hernia.

Management

Irreducible hernias should be treated by elective operation. Obstructed and strangulated hernias require emergency surgery and preoperative preparation with nasogastric aspiration and intravenous fluids according to the principles laid down in Chapter 75. Anaesthesia can be provided by either local infiltration, spinal block or inhalation anaesthesia. The surgical technique in the emergency situation requires adequate exposure through long incisions. The contents of the sac are handled gently to avoid further damage and are held in the sac while the constricting band at the neck of the sac is released. The constricted intestine is carefully assessed with regard to its viability which should improve rapidly. Non-viable bowel has lost its sheen, looks dull and oedematous and may be frankly gangrenous. Non-viable bowel requires resection and re-anastomosis. The repair of the hernia is carried out as for an elective procedure.

Postoperative care is maintained with nasogastric suction and intravenous fluids until there is a resumption of intestinal activity (*see* Chapter 75).

77 Organ Transplantation

G. R. Giles

The success of organ transplantation has been one of the most astonishing developments in medical practice over the past 20 years. Contrary to expectation, the credit for this success can be directly attributed to clinicians, particularly surgeons, with the vision to see that there is tremendous potential for this approach in end-stage organ failure of several types. A multidisciplinary approach involving clinicians, immunologists, radiologists and microbiologists is required for good results and there is little doubt that organ replacement will be used earlier and more widely over the next two decades. There is a need for increasing numbers of surgeons capable of working within a transplant team and usually leading it. Furthermore, it is likely that such teams will not be confined to the teaching centres in the future.

In this chapter, the principles and practice of organ transplantation are outlined. It will be seen that the practice does not require a detailed knowledge of immunology in order to be successful. However, many surgeons recognize that a good grounding in cell biology is advantageous and may lead to a better understanding of the control of rejection and cancer in the surgical patient.

TYPES OF GRAFT

1. Movement of tissue from one site of the body to another is termed an *autograft*, e.g. skin grafts, free nerve or tendon transplants. Microvascular techniques may extend the clinical application, e.g. free grafts of small intestine have been successfully moved to the neck in pharyngeal reconstruction.

2. Grafts between genetically identical individuals, i.e. identical twins, are termed *isografts*. There are now many patients alive and well who have received a kidney from a twin sibling. However, this will not have widespread clinical application. The importance of the isograft is in experimental work so that comparative studies of an immunological nature can be carried out.

3. Clinical grafts are usually *allografts*, i.e. between genetically dissimilar individuals of the same species. Where the graft is well vascularized, e.g. kidney, heart and liver, the immune response is strong and dependent upon the antigenic dissimilarity between the donor and recipient. Where the graft is less well vascularized and forms a structure into which host tissue ultimately grows, the immune response is weaker, e.g. bone, artery, cornea.

4. *Xenografts* are exchanged between species. This is an experimental exercise and is not likely to have a clinical application in the near future. Porcine skin has been used as a temporary dressing in patients with extensive burns but never becomes vascularized. The extracorporeal perfusion of porcine and bovine livers in patients with liver failure is effectively a temporary xenograft but it has not proven to be any more successful than more conservative methods.

Successful organ transplantation requires the facility to remove a healthy organ from the donor, to maintain the vitality of the organ for a limited period, to transplant the organ in place of the diseased structure—*orthotopically*—or to another site where it may function equally well—*heterotopically*. Finally, some means are needed to reduce the immunological response of the host against the graft. From a clinical standpoint, only kidney and corneal transplantation have made a major contribution, though it is fair to say that there are encouraging results in specialized centres in the field of cardiac, hepatic and bone marrow transplantation.

THE ORGAN DONOR

During the past decade, a change has occurred in the general public acceptance that there is a need for organ donors in most communities and consequently more cadaveric donors have become available. A second more important change in attitude has resulted by the application of brain death criteria for patients maintained on life support machines. It is not the responsibility of the transplant team to make a diagnosis of brain death (*see* Chapter 32) nor should it be. However, after the condition has been firmly diagnosed and the relatives have received the information, then in most circumstances it is appropriate for the family to be approached for permission to remove organs for donation. In some intensive care units, this request is logically introduced by a member of the medical staff responsible for care of the brain dead patient. In other hospitals, it may be appropriate for a member of the transplant team to make the request. It is also usual to inform the local coroner's office and hospital administrator that an organ donation is to take place, in the event that medicolegal matters arise, expert advice can be sought and given.

In many countries it is possible, after brain death diagnosis, to remove organs with the heart still beating and this is an absolute requirement for heart, heart–lung and liver donors. The transplant surgeon, therefore, has a responsibility to his team and the donating institution in checking that all of the criteria for the diagnosis of brain death have been adhered to and that these facts are duly recorded in the case records, together with his own note of the organs which are removed and any other abnormality noted during the donation procedure.

Most donors will be cared for in an intensive care unit, having suffered a head injury, or raised intracranial pressure from a variety of causes including intracerebral tumour, hypertension, status epilepticus, status asthmaticus and intracranial haemorrhage.

There are a number of conditions which are required for satisfactory organ donation. The organ to be removed should not have suffered adversely during the terminal illness, nor should it be the site of chronic disease, e.g. chronic nephritis, hypertensive nephropathy. Ideally the donor should be within a defined age span which will vary according to the organ to be donated. Cardiac teams prefer donors under the age of 30 years whereas kidney donation can take place quite adequately from otherwise healthy persons aged 60 years. The donor size should yield an organ compatible with transplantation into the recipient. The donor should be free from malignant disease with the proviso that certain intracerebral tumours, e.g. gliomas, astracytomas, which should not metastasize outside the CNS, can be used. Major infective complications are a barrier to transplantation, however minor infections, e.g. an adequately treated respiratory tract infection, is not a contraindication. Viral infections, e.g. herpes encephalitis, are likely to transmit the virus. However, previous cytomegalovirus infections, as shown by preoperative antibody testing, provides organs suitable for transplantation into a patient who has already been exposed to a CMV infection.

THE DONOR OPERATION

The organs which are to be donated will determine the incisions and procedural steps. It is commonplace for one, two or even three transplant teams to have an interest in one donor. It is likely that in certain localities, surgical teams will develop with a defined role for removing the organs. In any event, it is essential that the teams act in concert and that the procedure proceeds in a carefully planned way with the surgeons having agreed the technical steps before commencing the operation. It is vital that the donation goes smoothly and that the donor undergoes an operation performed with the same skill and with the same care to the tissues as though recovery was possible.

Multiple organ donation may be a lengthy procedure particularly if the liver is to be used. The donor requires full ventilatory and circulatory support during the procedure and if necessary by continuation of dopamine infusion and plasma or blood transfusion. In this way organ perfusion is optimal. It is also conventional to administer a number of agents prior to or during the donation procedure. Since a bacteraemia is possible during the donor's terminal phase, broad-spectrum antibiotics are administered intravenously if the donor is not already receiving them. Methylprednisolone and chlorpromazine are also administered to stabilize the lysosomal and cytoplasmic membranes. Renal function is supported where necessary by mannitol or dopamine infusion and a single dose of heparin will be given at an appropriate time prior to the arrest of circulation.

The procedural steps relating to heart and heart-lung transplantation are described in Chapter 49. The following account is more directed to the removal of liver and kidneys for transplantation. Although not impossible, it is not generally convenient for a donor to provide both pancreatic and hepatic grafts.

For liver/kidney donation, the abdomen and chest are cleansed and draped. The incision may be a bilateral subcostal but it is recognized that ease of access is ensured if a long midline incision with upper extension of sternal splitting is employed. After examining the abdominal contents to ensure freedom from disease, the liver is dissected by dividing the bile duct in the head of pancreas, clearing the portal vein and dissecting the hepatic artery back to the coeliac axis and aorta. Anomalies in arterial anatomy may require an alteration in technique so that a full arterial perfusion of the liver can be achieved. Similarly, the suspensory ligaments are divided, the inferior vena cava dissected free with ligation of tributaries and three phrenic veins. The liver is precooled via a catheter placed in the superior mesenteric vein and cold Hartmann's solution instilled. Overdistension of the liver is prevented by venting the venous system through the inferior vena cava. The aorta is cross-clamped above the coeliac axis after heparinization and aortic perfusion commences with an appropriate solution, e.g. hyperosmolar citrate. This perfusion cools both liver and kidneys (*Fig.* 77.1). Portal vein perfusion is continued using cold plasma protein fraction. When both liver and kidneys are washed clear of blood, the organs are rapidly removed to a side table for further

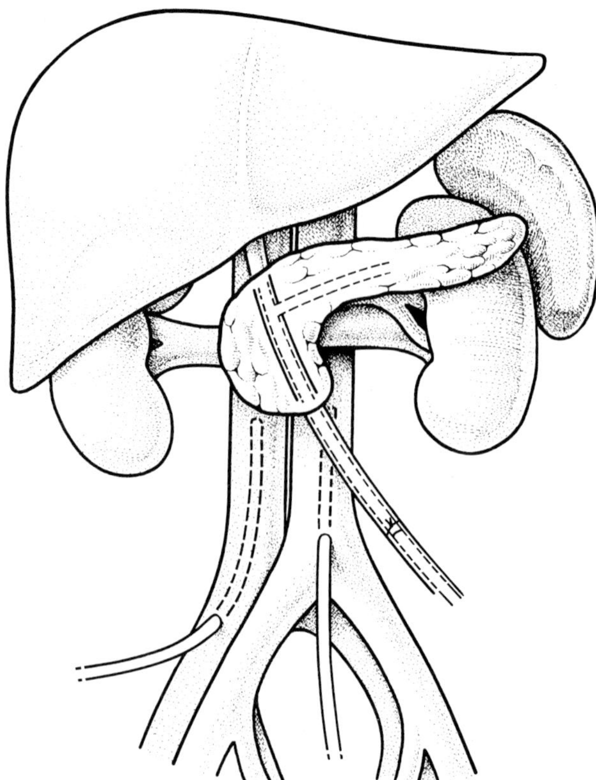

Fig. 77.1 After skeletonization of the hilar structures of the liver, cannulas are placed in the aorta and portal vein to allow in situ cooling of liver, kidneys and pancreas. A venous outflow cannula in the inferior vena cava prevents congestion of the organs.

examination. If satisfactory, the organs are placed in double plastic bags and stored in crushed ice until use.

TESTS OF COMPATIBILITY BETWEEN DONOR AND RECIPIENT

It has been known for many years that organ transplantation requires matching of ABO antigens in a similar manner which governs blood transfusion. There are occasional reports of successful transplantation across apparently incompatible ABO barriers but where this is carried out there is a higher chance that the organ would suffer hyperacute rejection. ABO red cell antigens are also expressed on most tissue cells but the Rhesus factor is only expressed on the red cell and is not taken into account normally in clinical transplantation. It is also known that in kidney transplantation there are minor differences in graft survival when O kidneys are transplanted into group A, AB or B recipients and slightly better results are obtained by absolute matching of these antigens.

THE HLA ANTIGENS

It was clear at an early stage of clinical experience that matching on the ABO antigens was not sufficient to ensure success and it was eventually discovered from work using inbred mouse strains that other histocompatibility antigens were present on tissues including leucocytes. This led to the basis of a system known as the human leucocyte antigen system (HLA). Individual tissue type is governed by a major histocompatibility complex (MHC) which appears to be present on the short arm human chromosome 6. The foci of the MHC are now determined and the HLA-A is located at a point on the chromosome which is furthest from the centromere (*Fig.* 77.2). Each short arm of the chromosome contains one HLA-A allele and 20 different A locus alleles are now known to exist. The B locus is adjacent and over 30 B alleles have been identified. Individual HLA-A and B tissue type is therefore made up of two A locus alleles and two B locus alleles, each of which has a separate coding number, e.g. A1, A11, B5, B9. The HLA-C locus exists between the

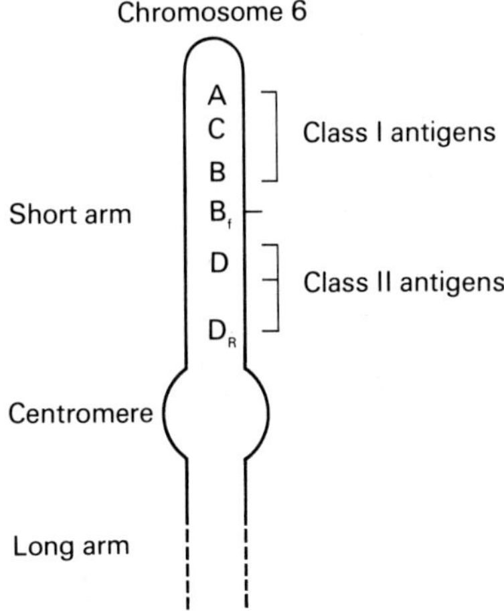

Fig. 77.2 Human chromosome 6 appears to carry the determinants of the major antigen systems. These loci are situated on the short arm and are divided into those concerned with Class I antigens (HLA-A, C, B) and Class II (D, DR).

A and B locus on chromosome 6 but appears to have an insignificant clinical role in organ matching.

There is now considerable evidence concerning the influence of matching of the HLA-A and B and antigens between the donor and recipient and although it is clear that matching on four or three antigens gives some advantage in terms of graft survival, this is not as dramatic as had originally been hoped, i.e. 1-year graft survival for matching at three and four antigens is approximately 5–10% better when compared with matching on two antigens. Since there is increasing difficulty in matching because of the large number of alleles the importance of HLA-A and B matching has declined in recent years.

The HLA-DR locus was discovered to be the closer to the centromere than the HLA-A, B and C system and appears to have two alleles but only 10 specificities have as yet been identified. This means that matching with the DR system is simpler to achieve than with the HLA-A and B and there is some evidence that matching for two DR matches gives a considerably improved survival over matches for one or no DR antigens. There is also some suggestion that failure to match on the DRW6 antigen is also associated with poorer graft survival. Matching for two DR antigens may give a kidney graft survival rate of greater than 75% compared with 60% with poorer matches. However, there are changes in immunosuppression which have coexisted with the development of DR matching and it is not completely accurate to assume that DR matching is responsible for this improved survival.

The basis of tissue typing is the separation of lymphocytes from heparinized whole blood by a Ficol–Hypaque gradient and in the case of DR testing a further separation of the B lymphocytes from the T-lymphocytes by formation of sheep red blood cell rosettes around the T-lymphocytes which are then centrifuged away from the B-cell fraction. The cells are then exposed to antibodies of known HLA-A, B and DR specificity and the cytotoxic effect of these antibodies assessed after a period of incubation and exposure to complement. The viability of the cells is measured by adding eosin dye to each mini-culture and this dye is excluded by live cells but taken up by cells killed by the cytotoxic action.

The current usage of tissue typing is particularly relevant in the investigation of a family where a live kidney donor is a possibility and it enables HLA identical siblings to be identified (*Fig.* 77.3). In organ transplantation which involves cadaveric organ donation, tissue matching is strived for, although often the clinical needs of the transplant unit or the individual patient may determine that a poorly matched organ is used rather than waiting an undefined indefinite period for a well-matched organ to appear. Following the introduction of cyclosporin and for first cadaveric kidney transplant, this is a justifiable compromise but may prejudice the long-term results in situations where a second graft is needed. A failed graft in this situation may result in the formation of circulating cytotoxic antibodies which makes the finding of a second graft much more difficult.

The influence of matching in cardiac and pancreatic transplant is not as clear-cut as in the renal transplant and there is almost no evidence for improved hepatic graft survival where matching is not normally attempted.

PREOPERATIVE DIRECT CROSSMATCH

Although matching on the HLA-A, B and DR loci gives an indication of the likely long-term outcome, it is still possible

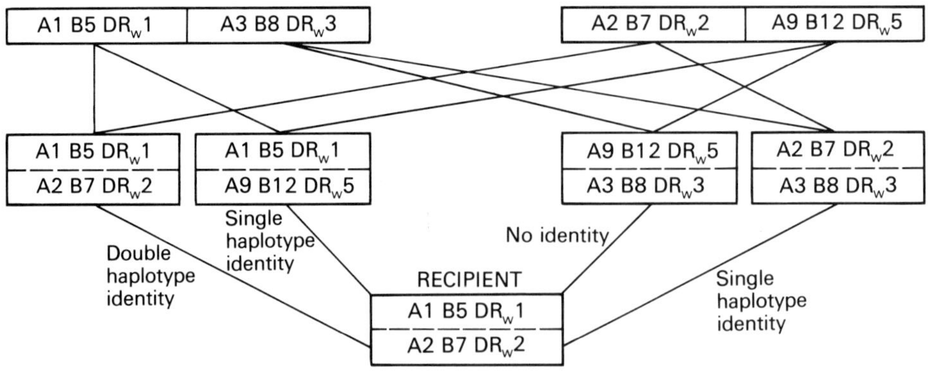

Fig. 77.3 This demonstrates the manner of transfer of Class I and II antigens in a stylized family. Ideally a recipient should receive a kidney from the sibling with double haplotype identity.

for the recipient to have preformed circulating antibodies capable of reacting against donor cells. These antibodies may be the result of prior blood transfusion, pregnancy or, more probably, viral infections and are potentially cytotoxic, normally producing an intravascular coagulation within the kidney by attaching to the endothelium and activating the complement system. Prior to transplant taking place, donor target cells are isolated, either from peripheral blood lymphocytes or from lymph node or spleen of the donor. These cells are incubated with the recipient serum in the presence of complement. Normally evidence of cytotoxicity is indication of a positive crossmatch and the transplant will not normally take place.

However, it is now known that some of these circulating antibodies, which cause a cytotoxic action against donor cells are auto-antibodies capable of giving a false positive crossmatch. These antibodies can be distinguished in the laboratory by performing parallel tests against cells from patients with chronic lymphatic leukemia. A positive reaction to both recipient and CLL cells indicate the likelihood of an immediate rejection, whereas cytotoxic antibodies to recipient cells but not to CLL cells suggests that the auto-antibodies are producing a false reaction.

Conversely, there are many instances in which a negative crossmatch is followed by an accelerated rejection following transplantation. This may represent an unrealistic response and may be detected by reviewing stored serum samples from the recipient extending back over several years. It is now routine to screen sera of patients awaiting transplantation against panels of lymphocytes. Given the large proportion of surviving patients, having had a failed renal transplant, sensitized patients may constitute one-third of the patients awaiting transplantation. Patients whose sera reacts against greater than 75% of the random panel are likely to be difficult to transplant and require detailed investigation to attempt to characterize HLA-A and B specificities. Where these monospecific antibodies are present against commonly present HLA antigens the chances of producing a negative crossmatch are exceedingly small.

KIDNEY TRANSPLANTATION

Historical Note

The earliest recorded attempts at kidney transplantation were carried out in Vienna at the turn of the century. The transplants were from goats or sheep to patients with terminal conditions and were not successful. Until the techniques of vascular surgery were developed, the basic principles of transplantation could not be tested. Once kidneys could be satisfactorily placed within the circulation, it was established experimentally that kidneys were able to function adequately on a long-term basis in heterotopic sites. However, it was found in the early 1920s that allografts would not function for more than a few days.

With the development of haemodialysis for renal failure, it became possible to maintain anuric patients for long periods of survival. The logistics of haemodialysis soon produced its own problems for the procedure is expensive and with improved patient survival, the need for haemodialysis facilities was ever expanding. Kidney transplantation began to play a serious clinical role with the development of immunosuppressive regimens in the early 1960s. Most renal failure units now function with a surgical team with special interests in providing the vascular access for haemodialysis (*see* Chapter 78) and organ transplantation. Haemodialysis, peritoneal dialysis and kidney transplantation are not competitive and these treatments should be offered in a planned integrated way to rehabilitate the patient to as full an existence as possible.

The results of clinical kidney transplantation have improved steadily over the past 25 years. In particular the improvement in patient survival has been the most impressive. In the mid 1960s patient survival at one year using cadaveric kidneys was of the order of 50%. However, in the early 1980s patient survival at one year is normally well over 90%. Several things account for this improvement in patient survival. Credit should be given to the renal physicians for the patient survival rate reflects the survival rates on dialysis. In the best centres the survival rates at 5 years on dialysis approach 75%. However, this is reduced to just under 50% when the patient suffers from diabetic nephropathy. Graft survival rates measure the true effects of transplantation. At the present time excellent results of kidney grafting are relatively short term and if the 10-year graft survival rates are considered, bearing in mind the knowledge used 10 years ago, the graft survival rates are less impressive, falling to 66% for kidneys from HLA identical siblings, 40% for parental donors and only 25% for cadaveric donors.

Indications for Transplantation

Renal transplantation should be considered for all patients

who suffer terminal renal failure and are suitable for dialysis programmes. Although the precise nature of the renal failure need not be known in order to transplant the patient, there are a number of renal disorders which may be relevant in the subsequent management of the patient. These include renal tuberculosis, diabetes, systemic lupus erythematosus, polyarteritis nodosa and congenital oxalosis. Most patients with chronic glomerulonephritis are suitable for renal transplantation, but it has to be noted that the graft survival rate of patients with dense deposit membranous glomerulonephritis is significantly worse. The acceptance of a patient onto a dialysis programme, whether it be with peritoneal dialysis or haemodialysis, implies a degree of selection and normally at that time an assessment is made of the psychiatric status of the patient and their ability to cope with the discipline required in renal failure. Patients with longstanding psychiatric disorders are generally unsuitable for both forms of treatment.

Certain other conditions preclude successful transplantation. Patients with severe cerebral vascular injury, should probably not be taken onto the renal failure programme. Patients with a history of myocardial infarction are clearly at high risk, but provided that a reasonable interval has occurred between the infarction and the transplant procedure, e.g. 6 months, then there is no reason why the operation might not go ahead. Patients with overt malignancy or within two or three years of the treatment of an invasive tumour should probably stay on the dialysis programme and not be considered for transplantation until such a time as one can be fairly certain that the malignancy has been cured by the primary treatment.

A number of patients will enter the dialysis programme with a poorly functioning lower urinary tract, either as a result of the primary disease, e.g. urogenital tuberculosis, or of congenital factors, e.g. congenital urethral valves. A complete re-evaluation of the lower urinary tract is indicated and plans can be made to deal with the urine flow from the transplanted kidney based on this evaluation.

Risk Factors

Most patients with renal failure have evidence of an arteriopathy and it is not unusual for these patients to either have angina or to have a history of myocardial infarction at some point in their lives. Patients with severe angina and marked ischaemic changes on ECG are obviously poor candidates. However, since most patients in renal failure have a low haemoglobin level, this fact must be taken into account when assessing the risk to the patient following a transplant operation. Where there is clinical evidence that angina has improved with the raising of the haemoglobin by transfusion then this may be considered to be a secondary benefit likely to accrue following a successful kidney transplant.

Patients with diabetic nephropathy are often more severely arteriopathic than expected and have a higher mortality and morbidity following renal transplantation. Nevertheless it now appears that the effect of transplantation is a beneficial one with survival patterns greater in the transplant programmes than patients confined to dialysis. Many patients have severe hypertension despite renal failure support and this is usually brought under adequate control by appropriate antihypertensive therapy (Chapter 9). There is increasing tendency to widen the age range of patients being recommended for renal transplant and, given the steroid-sparing effect of modern immunosuppressive agents, then one can justify the early application to children around the age of 5 and adults are now considered even in the 7th decade.

Blood Transfusion and Transplantation

For many years, great efforts were made to avoid blood transfusions in potential recipients before renal transplantation. Nevertheless, the present evidence suggests that recipients have a somewhat higher chance of graft survival when transfusions are given before transplantation. The mechanisms for this beneficial effect are unknown but may include:

1. Identification and exclusion of individuals with a strong immune response who form cytotoxic antibodies;
2. The induction of immunological tolerance;
3. Stimulation of anti-idiotypic antibodies;
4. Or increase in the number and function of T-suppressor cells; and
5. The depletion of immunoreactive clones.

Unfortunately it is not completely clear what are the optimal conditions in terms of the timing, number and types of blood products which produce this beneficial effect, as the reports from a wide variety of sources are conflicting.

It would appear that whole blood and frozen blood are effective as is the buffy coat (leucocyte concentrates) but platelets are probably not. Transfusion in the six months prior to transplant seems to have the greatest effect, though there is some evidence that improvements in graft survival may be obtained with blood transfusion given in the perioperative period or even postoperatively during a rejection episode. Probably the optimal effects are achieved by three separate preoperative transfusions. In patients undergoing a planned living related donor transplant, transfusion of blood from the donor (donor specific) seems to give the best results and sensitization to the donor can be minimized by the use of immunosuppression either azathioprine or cyclosporin. Normally three transfusions are given at three-week intervals in the three months preceding transplant. However, it has to be recognized that a proportion of potential recipients (10–20%) will become sensitized against the donor.

The use of cyclosporin has made more complicated the assessment of the blood transfusion effect which may not have such a beneficial effect on graft survival as when azathioprine and steroids are used as the mainstay immunosuppression.

Splenectomy and Transplantation

The importance of the spleen in the immune response of a patient to a transplant has always been controversial. The spleen is a major site of immunoglobulin-producing B-cells especially of the IgM type and appears to be the primary site of primary immune responses to antigens facilitating responses of the humoral type. Following splenectomy, a leucocytosis occurs and this may permit higher doses of azathioprine to be administered. Furthermore, humoral responses may be reduced by removal of large numbers of resident B-lymphocytes. However, splenectomy also removes large numbers of suppressor T-cells which may affect the ability of pretransplant blood transfusion to have a beneficial effect. Prospective randomized trials of splenectomy prior to renal transplantation have shown increased graft survival. Patient survival is not always safeguarded for the splenectomy effect disappears after two years and a number of patients die of post-splenectomy sepsis. Routine splenectomy is no longer practised widely.

The Technique of Kidney Transplantation

In adults an extraperitoneal approach is employed in either iliac fossa. The renal artery is anastomosed end-to-end to the internal iliac artery or end-to-side to the external iliac artery. The renal vein is sutured end-to-side to the external iliac vein (*Fig.* 77.4). After revascularization the ureter is implanted into the side wall of the bladder. Commonly an antireflux mechanism is constructed at the vesico-ureteric junction though it is not clear whether this is essential. It is safer to use as short a length of ureter as possible as the blood supply to the distal ureter is precarious. The kidney can be positioned posterior to the abdominal muscles and supported on the ilium. The organ is readily palpable in most patients. In children the kidney is often placed transperitoneally on to the common iliac vessels.

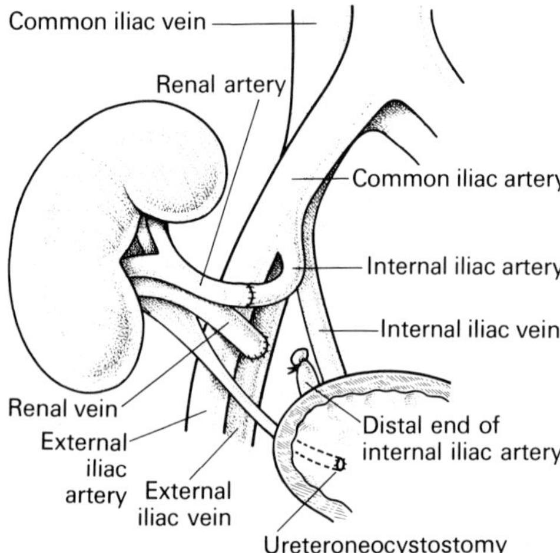

Fig. 77.4 The standard technique of renal transplantation where the arterial input is provided by the internal iliac artery (or patched to side of common or external iliac artery) and venous drainage to the external iliac vein. A ureteroneocystostomy completes the procedure. The kidney rests in an extraperitoneal position supported by the iliac crest.

Technical variations commonly have to deal with two or three renal arteries and may involve suture of an aortic button to the side of the common or external iliac artery. Multiple veins are less of a problem and only one anastomosis is needed. The kidney can be placed on the same side as a previous transplant. The kidney is readily palpable and change in size may be an indication of rejection.

Immunosuppression

Considerable changes in the immunosuppressive management of the transplant patient have taken place following the introduction of cyclosporin A (CyA). It has probably improved graft survival and has certainly slowed down the tempo of the rejection process. It is, however, an expensive drug not without complications and it should not be forgotten that very reasonable results can be achieved by the use of azathioprine and prednisone.

Azathioprine is usually commenced at high dosage (4–5 mg/kg) for 2–3 days and then reduced to 2 mg/kg for 7 days. Careful observation of the white cell and platelet count will often require that the dose be adjusted downwards in order that the white cell count does not fall below $3{\cdot}5 \times 10^3$/mm^3. A variety of prednisone doses have been administered, commencing at levels of 200 mg/day reducing by 10 mg/day to 30–60 mg. However, most transplant wards use much lower doses of 30 mg/day reducing very gradually over 3–6 months to 10–15 mg/day.

Cyclosporin A is also administered over a range of doses. Many units commence therapy at 15–17 mg/kg and reduce at set times, e.g. every 2 weeks by 2 mg/kg to 6–8 mg/kg. Alternatively, the dose may be adjusted according to trough serum or plasma levels. In this case the local method of analysis will determine the acceptable range of safe levels. As cyclosporin A is nephrotoxic, renal transplant dysfunction has to be investigated with this point in mind. When this diagnosis is made, a reduction in dosage of 30% is generally indicated. There is also uncertainty about the long-term nephrotoxicity of CyA. Many transplant units revert to azathioprine and prednisone after 6 months or perform renal biopsy in order to see whether interstitial fibrosis has developed in the graft.

The treatment of rejection normally requires the introduction or adjustment of steroid dosage as first line treatment. Methylprednisolone (250–500 mg) is given intravenously by daily × 3–5 doses. Patients treated with CyA alone may commence a regular daily dose (10–30 mg) and those already receiving prednisone with azathioprine may revert to a high dose gradually reducing again. Most transplant units set an arbitrary limit on the number of pulses of methylprednisolone they will permit the patient in order to reduce the chance of catastrophic infective complications. Additional side-effects of pulse therapy include flushing and fainting, tachycardia and tachypnoea, arthralgia and hyperglycaemia.

Antilymphocyte globulin (ALG, ATG) has few advocates at the present time. Usually raised in horses, goats or rabbit by injecting with human lymphocytes and ultimately prepared by a series of fractionation techniques from the animals' serum. There are serious problems with hypersensitivity reactions to animal protein and its use is largely confined to cardiac transplant programmes.

Currently, ALG has been superseded by the development of monoclonal antibodies which are able to destroy specific lymphocyte populations, e.g. OKT3 lymphocytes. As these products are extremely expensive, their use is currently advocated only for those patients who have a rejection which is steroid resistant. The agent is given intravenously for 7–10 days. Second courses cannot be given because of the development of hypersensitivity to mouse protein.

The place of radiation given to the graft depends upon local preference; it is doubtful whether it adds any advantage to pulses of methylprednisolone. Total lymphoid irradiation has been advocated for patients having difficulty with dialysis and having suffered an accelerated rejection of the first kidney graft. Extracorporeal irradiation of circulating blood has its advocates but shows little evidence of improved graft survival. Lymphoid depletion may also be achieved by thymectomy and by thoracic duct drainage. Neither technique has become established practice.

Investigation of Transplant Dysfunction

A deterioration in renal function may be the result of rejection or technical accident. Normally, rises are seen in the serum creatinine and urea levels and often the urine volume falls. Graft size may increase and may cause compression of the external iliac vein. Where there is doubt concerning the aetiology of the renal dysfunction an early recourse to renal imaging is justifiable and desirable.

1. Isotopic Imaging: Radionuclide procedures may be a useful test of renal perfusion and excretion. For convenience an intravenous bolus injection of technetium pertechnetate ($^{99}Tc^{m}$) is used. The result may be expressed as a percentage of the density pattern obtained from the external iliac artery. It is possible to detect accumulation of isotope in the bladder but urinary obstruction may be more accurately demonstrated by using $^{[131]}$Hippivan. A continuously rising slope may indicate ureteric obstruction and acute tubular necrosis.

2. Ultrasonic Imaging: This most valuable investigation will demonstrate renal size; calyceal and pelvic dilatation (*Fig.* 77.5). A baseline investigation early in the postoperative period permits comparison if the scan is required at a later date. Ultrasonic Doppler investigation may give an indication of total renal blood flow. Although not accurate, reductions in the diastolic phase of flow are seen in patients with cyclosporin nephrotoxicity.

3. Renal Arteriogram: This investigation is indicated in patients with deterioriating renal function, arterial bruit and hypertension.

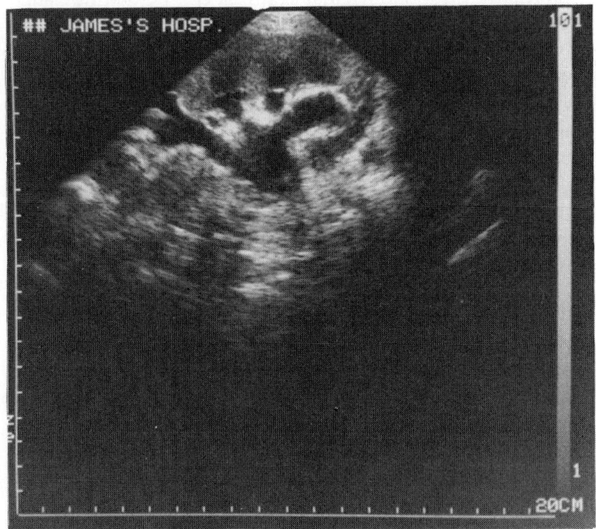

Fig. 77.5 This ultrasonic examination demonstrates renal cortex and structure. In particular the calyces and ureter are shown to be dilated and result from an obstructed ureteroneocystostomy.

Diagnosis of Rejection

The clinical features of rejection may take a number of forms:

1. *Primary non-function.* In this event, the kidney assumes a reasonable appearance on revascularization but does not produce urine. This delay is normally attributed to ischaemic damage to the organ. Unfortunately the organ may be undergoing rejection which is undetected or untreated. It is a situation not uncommon where transplantation has been performed in patients with preformed cytotoxic antibodies but with a negative crossmatch against donor cells. The kidney may be palpated as normal and minimal systemic features are found. The diagnosis may be suspected when an isotope perfusion scan(s) shows diminished or diminishing perfusion indices but, ideally, aspiration cytology, or better still, needle biopsy will confirm the rejection process. Active investigation is required for all kidneys which fail to function after 3 days and may need repeating.

2. *Hyperacute rejection.* This occurs shortly after transplantation and may be detected before the operation is complete. Preformed antibodies produce an intrarenal coagulation with cessation of blood flow and death of the organ. It should occur only very rarely and requires that the organ be removed. The kidney should be subjected to analysis in order to determine why the event was not predicted by the negative direct crossmatch between donor cells and recipient serum.

3. *Accelerated and acute rejections.* These states are related in terms of the pathological events but differ clinically by virtue of severity and timescale. The timing of an accelerated rejection is within the first few days of the transplant and is demonstrated by a reduction in renal function (all parameters) and systemic changes of pyrexia, tachycardia and some exacerbation of hypertension. Acute rejection is variable in severity and is clearly modified in part by the immunosuppression often delayed until the 3rd or 4th week. It is less dramatic in patients treated with cyclosporin. On examination the kidney may be enlarged with surrounding tenderness and there is occasional evidence of leg swelling from external iliac vein compression. Clinical diagnosis may suffice but in less obvious cases nephrotoxicity from cyclosporin or mechanical causes of malfunction should be considered. Depending upon availability, aspiration cytology, intrarenal manometry and needle biopsy are indicated. If the diagnosis remains unclear, ultrasonic examination of the kidney should be performed to exclude urinary obstruction or a lymphatic collection and if doubt persists, it is appropriate to make a clinical judgement and treat the cause as a rejection.

4. *Chronic rejection.* This process usually manifests itself by a gradual deterioration in renal function associated with increased proteinuria and exacerbated hypertension. There are few systemic features and the kidney remains small. Normally this event occurs later than 6 months and often several years after transplantation. As with other forms of rejection, it is necessary to exclude mechanical causes of malfunction such as ureter obstruction and arterial stenosis. Biopsy is required not only to confirm the extent of renal damage, but also to determine whether the transplanted kidney appears to be suffering from a recurrent glomerulonephritis, particularly of the dense deposit type of nephropathy and, more hopefully, from interstitial fibrosis consequent upon cyclosporin toxicity. This latter complication may be reversible.

The Management of Rejection

Hyperacute Rejection

If the rejection process has commenced within minutes or hours of transplantation it is likely to be mediated by antibodies. In the past, attempts have been made to modify the rejection by full heparinization. This was not successful and several patients have died despite therapy. It is more sensible to remove the kidney once the diagnosis is proven and rehabilitate the patient in the dialysis programme.

Accelerated Rejection

This process may be based on a marked cellular response or may have a humoral component. Normally methylprednisolone is given 1–2 mg/kg intravenously. Various schedules are prescribed but usually the dose is given daily for 3–5 days after which maintenance dose of oral prednisone is administered. A failure to respond is common. In a limited number of cases where humoral elements are likely to be involved in the rejection, plasmapheresis may rescue a small percentage of grafts. The role of OKT3 monoclonal antibodies is uncertain but unlikely to be effective in the absence of a marked cellular infiltration of the graft.

Acute Rejection

This process is usually treated by methylprednisolone 1–2 mg/kg intravenously daily for 3–5 days. Quite commonly, systemic features of the rejection resolve after the first treatment. A gradual improvement in renal function is expected over 3–7 days and may be monitored by normal functional parameters and repeated aspiration cytology. In patients treated with azathioprine and prednisone, an adjustment of the daily oral dose upwards is also indicated, followed by stepwise reduction as renal function improves. A 25% reduction in azathioprine dosage is advisable during the period of renal dysfunction in order to avoid unnecessary myelotoxicity. Patients treated with cyclosporin alone may require a regular daily dose of oral prednisone depending upon the recovery of renal function.

Failure to respond to methylprednisolone pulses requires additional therapy. Some centres advocate the administration of 600 Gy radiation to the graft. There may be a role for OKT3 monoclonal antibodies in this situation, though the position is not certain at this time. Similarly in some centres, antilymphocyte globulin is prescribed in this situation although its use is not universally accepted. Normally at least 60–70% of acute rejections will respond to this therapy but often the recovery is incomplete and a further set of pulses are required. Given the use of cyclosporin it should be possible to minimize graft loss from rejection to 10%.

Chronic Rejection

It is common to make this diagnosis after a biopsy in which the pathologist reports considerable destruction or obliteration of glomeruli and evidence of intrarenal vascular disease. Thus it is doubtful whether significant renal function can be obtained by administration of high-dose steroid pulses. The possibility of cyclosporin fibrosis should be considered and the possibility of conversion to azathioprine and steroids entertained. A careful review of all medication may suggest renal impairment be due in part to drug therapy. It has recently been suggested that in some patients, renal dysfunction is the result of hyperfiltration by the transplanted kidney. A carefully controlled reduction in dietary protein can result in improved renal function.

Pathological Features of Rejection

Poor renal function may result from ischaemic damage, the rejection process and cyclosporin toxicity. Pathologists may have difficulty in distinguishing absolutely between these three elements and there may be evidence that all are operative in the biopsy specimen.

It is common to find mononuclear cells in kidneys with a rejection process. However, they are invariably present in renal transplant biopsies. By themselves, they do not indicate long-term damage to the kidneys. Where the mononuclear cells are seen to be adhering to the endothelium or infiltrating into the vessel wall the prognosis is poor and the rejection process may proceed to fibrinoid necrosis. Similarly, where a large proportion of cytotoxic/suppressor T-lymphocytes and macrophages are present, then the short-term prognosis is poor.

Fibrinoid, arterial and capillary necrosis and interstitial haemorrhage is commonly seen during acute graft failure. However, it is never uniform throughout the organ. Changes predominantly affect the arcuate and interlobular vessels and although venous thromboses are commonly seen it is unlikely that these ever precipitate renal failure because of the widespread nature of the venous network. The pressence of haemorrhage is a bad prognostic sign.

Chronic rejection is characterized by obliteration of the vascular tree predominantly affecting the arterial lumens in a concentric rather than an eccentric fashion. There is progressive fibrosis and ultimately thrombosis. There may be mild infiltrates of mononuclear cells around the vessels, particularly immediately beneath the endothelium and in some vessels there are breaks in the internal elastic and lamina. The result of the obliterated process is to produce a gradual atrophy and fibrosis of the organ.

Analysis of glomerular changes in renal grafts are difficult to interpret. Severe damage in the immediate postoperative period can be attributed to rejection and is seen as increase in the mesangium, thickening of the basement membrane, fibrosis and tufts. However, some of these features may also be the result of ischaemia.

Normally these glomerular features can be distinguished from glomerulonephritis. However, this condition may develop in renal allografts or, alternatively, may have inadvertently been transplanted. It would appear that certain types of glomerulonephritis are commonly recurrent within transplanted kidneys and these include focal glomerulonephritis, dense deposit type glomerulonephritis, IgA nephropathy, oxalosis and cystinosis. Other forms of glomerulonephritis recur either rarely or are of uncertain frequency.

Alternative Causes of Renal Transplant Dysfunction

Ureteric Obstruction

It is commonly forgotten that the ureteric function is equally important as renal parenchymal function. Obstruction is most commonly the result of technical factors and occurs at several sites, of which the lower third of the ureter is the most common. Although oedema and fibrosis are responsible for some cases, the majority of problems arise because of a failed blood supply leading to necrosis of the terminal ureter often as high as the pelvic ureteric junction (*Fig.* 77.6). This problem may be detected any time during the first 6 months. Thereafter, fibrosis and kinking or even ureteric stone are more likely to be the cause.

Dilatation of the calices is readily detected by ultrasonic examination. It is sensible to perform a baseline ultrasound soon after transplantation in order that change in appearance can be assessed. If renal function has deterioriated or doubt remains a prograde pyelogram is performed by a needle inserted under ultrasonic control into an upper calix. The kidney may be drained by a percutaneous nephrostomy (*Fig.* 77.6). Ultimately, exploration of the ureter will be required. Reconstruction may occasionally be achieved by re-implantation into the dome of the bladder or, more commonly, by using the ipsilateral ureter and anastomosing this to the renal graft.

Arterial Stenosis

This complication is usually manifested by a deterioriation in renal function and increased difficulty in hypertension control. It may be suspected if an arterial bruit is heard over

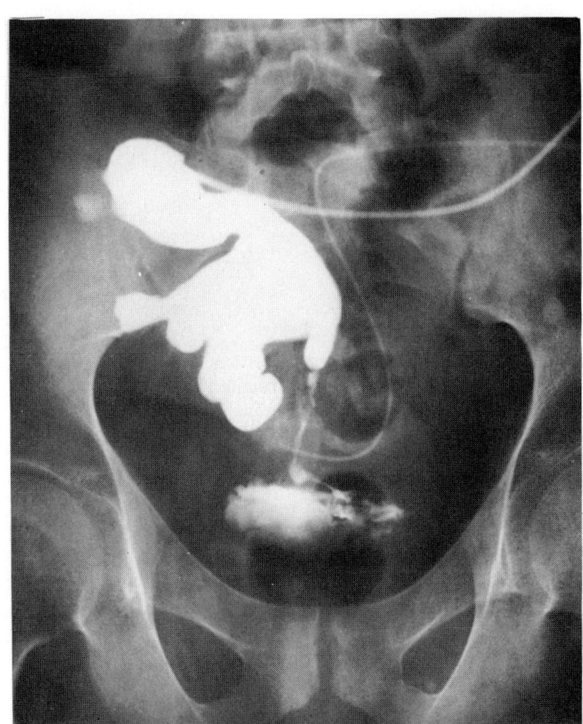

Fig. 77.6 Demonstrates necrosis of the transplanted ureter in a case 3 weeks after surgery. The kidney had to be drained percutaneously and the problem corrected after recovery of renal function by utilizing the original right ureter of the patient.

the transplant. However, confirmation is required by arteriography (*Fig.* 77.7). Ideally this examination should be performed by digital angiography with low ionic compounds. If a stenosis is detected proximal to the anastomosis, i.e. due to atheromatous disease in the recipient internal iliac artery, then a balloon angioplasty is likely to be successful, provided it is performed by an experienced operator. Stenosis of the site of anastomosis appears very difficult to dilate and it is the result of a technical failure. These cases will normally require open reconstruction of the anastomosis.

Venous Thrombosis

A sudden deterioriation of renal function associated with gross swelling of the graft and with evidence of swelling of the ipsilateral leg commonly indicates the presence of a venous thrombosis, either arising within the graft itself or within the external iliac system extending up to obstruct the venous outflow from the graft. These appearances may be occasionally mimicked by gross swelling of graft rejection with mechanical obstruction to the external iliac vein. In most instances, venous thrombosis of the graft is irrecoverable and transplant nephrectomy is required. However, where function persists, treatment with intravenous heparin should be commenced and in a proportion of cases sufficient graft function is obtained provided that the anticoagulation is continued long term.

Collections around the Renal Graft

It is a well-known fact that blood around a kidney leads to a rapid deterioration in renal function. Haematoma in the

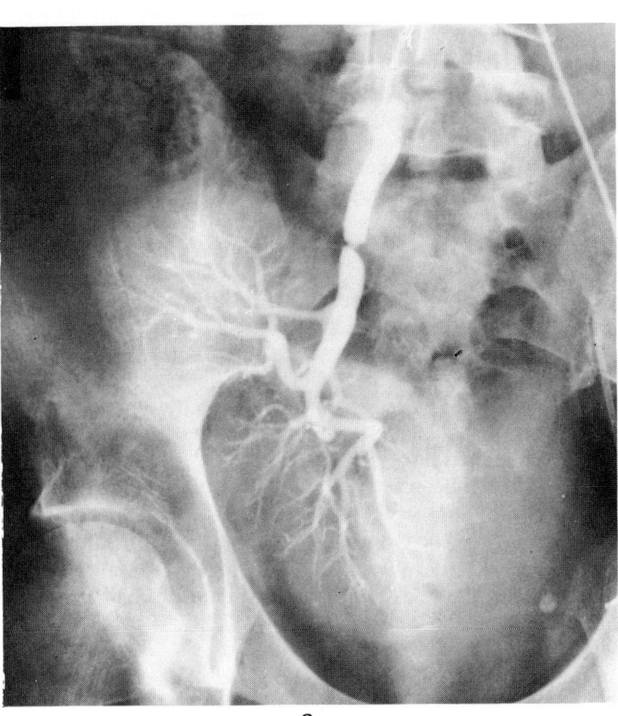

a

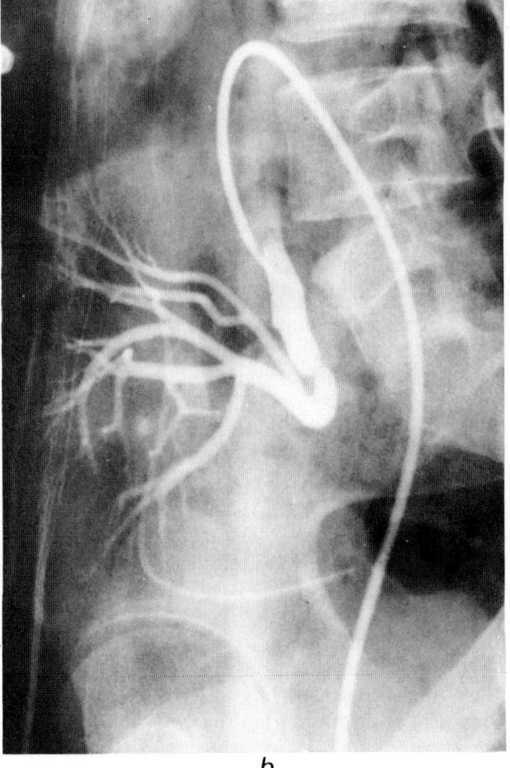

b

Fig. 77.7 *a*, Demonstrates an arteriogram of a transplanted kidney which has developed a stenosis at the mesenteric junction of internal iliac and renal arteries; *b*, Dilatation is sometimes possible by angioplasty although commonly a surgical procedure is necessary.

perirenal space may occur either immediately postoperatively and is due to technical reasons or commonly within the first month due to rupture of the graft, commonly associated with a degree of rejection. The patient complains of severe pain in the region of the graft and a swelling is normally readily apparent or can be demonstrated by ultrasonography. It may be possible to explore the graft with the intent to relieve the haematoma and to suture the defect. In the presence of severe rejection, graft nephrectomy is a wiser policy.

Occasionally a transplanted kidney becomes surrounded by an encysted collection of lymph which produces renal dysfunction. Lymphoceles may occur several months after transplantation and result from a failure to ligate the lymphatic vessels surrounding the iliac vessels. Where the collection is sufficiently large to produce renal dysfunction, it may be dealt with by draining it in through the peritoneal cavity via a laparotomy.

Although not common, large collections of pus may develop around transplanted kidneys and require drainage. Normally the wound should be left open widely and allowed to heal slowly.

Urinary Tract Complications

Urinary Tract Infection

Positive urine cultures are commonly seen during the early postoperative period, particularly when a catheter has been left in place. A persistent urinary tract infection requires treatment and if it recurs, then examination of the patient's own kidneys should be undertaken to determine whether reflux is present or not. Ideally, these kidneys should have been dealt with prior to the transplantation having taken place. Where there is recurrent infection in the absence of reflux, the patient may require antimicrobial agents for periods of up to two months.

Retention of Urine

With the advent of transplantation in the older age group both prostatic enlargement and urethral stricture have the same propensity to produce urinary obstruction or enhance urinary tract infections as in other patients. They require surgical remedies in the usual manner.

Ureteric Necrosis

Although not common, this condition may be suspected within grafts which rapidly deteriorate 7–10 days after transplant. It seems more common in kidneys with multiple arteries. It may be demonstrated by the presence of dilated calices on ultrasonic examination of the graft or by prograde pylography through the graft. Surgical exploration is indicated and the problem may be remedied by anastomosing the recipient's own ureter of that side to the pelvis of the transplanted kidney or occasionally by performing a Boari flap procedure. The condition may occasionally be mimicked by fibrotic adhesions around the ureter.

Urinary Fistula

Excess fluid in the drains or a clear fluid leaking through the wound may be due to a urinary fistula. Most commonly this results from a leak at the cystostomy suture line, ureteric implant orifice or rarely from the renal substance. An early repair is advised.

The complications of renal transplantation and immunosuppression are legion. *Table* 77.1 summarizes the commoner problems.

Table 77.1 Common complications of renal transplantation and immunosuppression

Technical
- *a.* Vascular haemorrhage: thrombosis, stenosis
- *b.* Urological: infection, fistula, obstruction
- *c.* Wound infection

Renal
- *a.* Acute tubular necrosis
- *b.* Cortical necrosis
- *c.* Lymphocele
- *d.* Graft rupture
- *e.* Recurrent glomerulonephritis

General Side-effects of Immunosuppression
- *a.* Infection: lung infections particularly protozoal, viral, fungal; meningitis all forms including Nocardia
- *b.* Septicaemia and viraemia
- *c.* Increased incidence of neoplasia particularly cutaneous lesions and reticuloses
- *d.* Aseptic necrosis of bone
- *e.* Hormonal: diabetes, hyperparathyroidism
- *f.* Peptic ulceration
- *g.* Pancreatitis
- *h.* General medical complications
  - Myocardial infarction
  - Cerebrovascular accidents
  - Hypertension
  - Thrombo-embolic phenomena
  - Colonic pseudo-obstruction/perforation

The management of infective disorders is discussed in Chapter 3. It is imperative that early signs of infection, e.g. a mild pyrexia, are pursued vigorously, repetitively and with aggression to obtain microbiological specimens, e.g. bronchial lavage. It is also required that both viral and fungal infections are constantly considered. Skin eruptions are more likely to be herpes simplex or zoster. Pulmonary infiltrations on chest radiography are often more extensive than expected from clinical examination and may result from a mixture of pulmonary oedema and infections of protozoa (*Pneumocystis carinii*), fungi (aspergillosis) or virus (CMV). The surgeon is advised that close co-operation with a renal physician trained in transplant care is required at all stages. Different skills are required at each point of care.

Patient Survival

Many factors have contributed to the improved patient survival in transplant programmes. Not least is the steady improvement in dialysis technique with more effective apparatus which has shortened both the frequency and duration of dialysis. Equally importantly, more patients are being detected at an earlier stage of renal failure and are not resuscitated under urgent conditions, having presented for the first time in terminal renal failure. In many patients it is possible to predict fairly accurately the point at which dialysis will be required so that peritoneal dialysis or arteriovenous fistula can be established well ahead of the time of first usage. General improvements in the control of hypertension, hypercalcaemia and thrombo-embolic phenomena have all played their part.

Overall, the survival of patients after renal transplantation is roughly equivalent to that achieved on dialysis. There is approximately 5% loss of patients per annum in both forms of treatment. The main causes of loss are infection, particularly chest infection from *Pneumocystis carinii*, CMV viraemia, cardiovascular failure, cerebrovascular accidents and recurrent renal failure from graft failure. Suicide rates are relatively high in both forms of treatment and the surgeon should be ready to seek expert psychiatric help.

Although the survival of young children is good, the older patient is more vulnerable, particularly if azathioprine and prednisone are the preferred immunosuppressives. One-year mortality rates of 25% are common in patients over 65 years. Similarly, diabetic patients have a significantly higher patient mortality.

Graft Survival

Survival of the renal graft is a true measure of the success of a transplant programme. For many years, graft losses have been excessive and have not matched patient survival. This was a high excusable state in programmes largely relying on cadaveric kidney usage. In the USA, where transplantation was largely based on living related organ donation, excellent results have been achieved for many years with double haplotype identical patients having 1-year graft survivals over 90% and 5-year graft survival of 75%. Kidneys from single haplotype identical donors had 1-year and 5-year graft survivals of 75% and 50% respectively. It is quite possible that these figures will be improved upon, particularly in patients receiving cyclosporin and possibly in those patients prepared for transplantation by donor specific blood transfusions.

In both living related donor and cadaveric renal transplantation, graft losses occur mainly during the first year or, more accurately, the first 3 months (*Fig.* 77.8). These losses are the result of vascular accidents, uncontrolled rejection and patient mortality. Later graft losses are at a much lower rate and largely the result of chronic rejection. It is still uncertain whether cyclosporin (short term or long term) will prevent the slow attrition over a 5–10 year period.

Prior to the introduction of cyclosporin, there was a wide disparity in the 1-year graft survival between different transplant centres (25–85%). However, with increasing experience with cyclosporin, these differences are much less marked and most centres achieve at least 75% 1-year graft survival with cadaveric graft. It is quite probable that these results can be improved on still further and that each year an increase will be seen. Controversies remain and in particular there is still disagreement on the need for preoperative blood transfusion and the impact of matching for HLA antigens. The general consensus suggests that the disadvantages of transfusion in the form of sensitization outweigh any gains in graft survival. Similarly, the general consensus suggests that organ-sharing schemes should aim to preferentially match kidneys on both DR antigens and where possible on at least one HLA-B antigen. By this policy it may be possible to raise the graft survival to 85–90%.

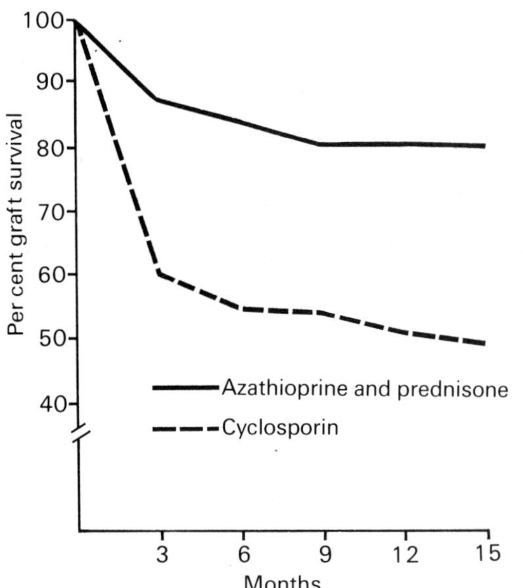

Fig. 77.8 Demonstrates the graft survival of cadaveric kidneys. The improvement seen after the introduction of cyclosporin appears dramatic but it is not possible to exclude the probability that improved organ preservation, organ matching, and patient survival all have a cumulative beneficial effect.

Second Transplants

Inevitably most renal failure programmes contain a large proportion of patients who have undergone a transplant which has failed. A large proportion of these patients will have cytotoxic antibodies which may be difficult to match against a donor. Prior to cyclosporin, the graft survival figures were significantly worse than primary transplants. However, many units are now reporting results which are only slightly inferior to first grafts and the results may be attributable to cyclosporin. This observation applies even in the presence of cytotoxic antibodies but a negative crossmatch.

Renal Transplantation in Children

Renal failure is an uncommon cause of death in children and the causes include glomerulo- and pyelonephritis but also the less common aetiologies shown in *Table* 77.2.

Table 77.2 Causes of renal failure in children

Glomerulonephritis
Pyelonephritis
Congenital hypoplasia
Hereditary nephropathy
Cystinosis
Alport's disease
Haemolytic uraemic syndrome
Bilateral nephroblastoma
Polycystic kidneys

In the most developed countries, haemodialysis and peritoneal dialysis are provided in separate children's units. Even so, long-term dialysis is not satisfactory and transplantation is the method of choice for children over 4 years. Younger children may be transplanted but constitute a relative contraindication.

Donor

There is an obvious motivation from a parent who wishes to donate a kidney, although it will normally result in only a single HLA haplotype identity. The result of cadaveric renal transplantation using cyclosporin and avoiding, where possible, regular steroids are giving equivalent results. Recipient children who are greater than 10 kg, will normally be able to accept an adult-sized kidney.

Technical consideration generally requires that the kidney is positioned on the common iliac vessels or inferior vena cava. In smaller children, the kidney may be sutured in position transperitoneally after mobilizing either right or left colon.

Postoperative Care

There are no features of adult transplantation which are not found in the child population. The control of hypertension may be a serious problem particularly in cases of chronic rejection. The stimulation of normal growth patterns is a serious aim in all children. Until recently the use of steroids was often inhibitory although alternate-day dosage does permit growth to occur. About one-half of renal recipients treated with cyclosporin do not require steroids. The best growth recovery occurs if transplantation is performed in children whose age is less than 10–12 years, with optimal graft function, male children and in children in whom levels of somatostatin are high. One other feature seen in children is that the graft is particularly susceptible to recurrence of the original disease. This event occurs particularly with the diagnoses of membranoproliferative glomerulonephritis, focal glomerulosclerosis and haemolytic uraemic syndrome.

Rehabilitation

As may be expected, there is considerable psychological stress in the child population and expert help is required from a child psychologist at all stages. About 80% of children with stable graft function are able to attend normal schools and most units have seen children who have matured and moved into post-school education programmes or into gainful employment. Provided that graft function is maintained there is no reason why these young people should not hope to enjoy a reasonable social life with an expectation of marriage and the production of normal children provided there are no underlying genetic disorders.

LIVER TRANSPLANTATION

Liver transplantation is now an accepted form of treatment for end-stage liver disease, but this position was achieved only recently after the pioneering work by Calne in the UK and Starzl in the USA. The early transplants began in 1963 but the success rates were low and there were few long-term survivors from those early attempts. The technical difficulties are much greater than those encountered in other organ replacements and there are additional difficulties as there are in heart transplantation in optimizing the timing of the procedure providing satisfactory organ support until a suitable donor is available. With an increasing confidence in the procedure and a more certain knowledge of the natural history of a number of chronic and progressive liver conditions it has been possible to offer the transplantation at a time when the patient is most likely to withstand it. Even so, the most obvious breakthrough came with the introduction of cyclosporin A which improves the immunosuppressive control, reduces the requirements for high-dose steroids and resulted in a reduction in the incidence of infective complications. It is likely now that the procedure will be more widely performed and that further technical innovation will reduce the operative mortality.

Indications for Liver Transplantation

The evaluation of a patient prior to liver transplant requires a full work-up by a fully trained gastroenterological team. The precise diagnosis will have been made with confidence and the condition of the patient brought into an optimal condition prior to the operation proceeding. In most instances the patient will have been under observation by such a team prior to the decision to advise hepatic transplantation. Both adult and paediatric age groups are likely candidates though progress in the paediatric age group is hampered by the lack of suitable donors of equivalent age and size. In the adult population primary biliary cirrhosis is a clear indication for hepatic replacement. However, since the prognosis is dependent on the time at which the diagnosis is made, the patients are selected for hepatic transplant on the basis of a progressive rise in serum bilirubin, disturbance of coagulation times and evidence of piecemeal necrosis on liver biopsy. Similar assessments are made in patients with chronic active hepatitis of the progressive type and in patients with cryptogenic cirrhosis entering the terminal phase of their illness. Patients with alcoholic hepatitis or cirrhosis require careful selection before recommending hepatic transplantation. Continuing alcoholic dependency is a contraindication. The role of liver replacement for patients with primary and secondary malignancy of the liver is uncertain at the present time. Long-term survivors have been recorded in both instances, but many failures with progressive malignant disease have been attributed to the effect of immunosuppression. Progressive liver failure in patients with inborn areas of hepatic metabolism, e.g. Wilson's disease; galactosaemia; alpha-1 antitrypsin disease; hypercholesterolaemia; Crigler–Najjar syndrome; tyrosinaemia and oxalosis, have all been conditions in which hepatic transplantation has been successfully carried out. A more recent indication for liver transplantation has been the successful replacement of livers in patients with fulminating hepatic failure from viral hepatitis.

In the paediatric age group the prime indication for liver replacement is extrahepatic biliary atresia, both in very young patients of 1–2 years and in older children who have had a period of relatively good health following a Kasai procedure (*see* Chapter 59).

Preparation for Surgery

Most patients entering a liver transplant programme show signs of impending liver failure and where possible attention is given to the correction of fluid and electrolyte disturbances, the administration of vitamin K and, where indicated, fresh frozen plasma for coagulation deficiencies. Since many patients have cardiorespiratory failure and impending renal failure, comprehensive evaluation of the patient by the medical, surgical and intensive care teams is essential in order to achieve a successful outcome. Blood specimens are taken for up-to-date haematological, electrolyte and liver function tests together with samples of urine for electrolyte and protein analysis. Microbiological swabs are taken from exposed skin sites together with urine, faeces and, where indicated, sputum. A chest radiograph and ECG are performed prior to surgery.

On the availability of a suitable donor, the patient is prepared for surgery. The donor team must acquire a suitable donor organ of sufficiently short preservation time, i.e. ideally, ischaemic time should be kept as short as possible and not more than 8–10 h. The anaesthetic team would normally be responsible for the establishment of both intravenous and arterial lines for sampling and monitoring during surgery.

The Surgical Procedure

The transplant procedure consists of two phases, first the removal of the original liver and secondly the placement of the donor organ in the orthotopic site. The initial recipient hepatectomy may be a particularly difficult and hazardous procedure made more difficult by the presence of portal hypertension with attendant haemorrhage from traumatized collaterals, or by the poor access afforded by a liver containing a large malignant tumour. Once the liver is removed, the patient is clearly in an anhepatic condition and it requires considerable skill on the part of the anaesthetic staff to maintain blood sugar, normal electrolyte patterns (particularly calcium and potassium) and to maintain the blood volume. Recently, haemodynamic difficulties have been overcome by the use of venovenous bypass using vortex pumps that do not require the use of heparin, in which blood is pumped from the lower half of the body from a cannula in the common iliac vein and joined by a similar cannula draining the portal venous system, both systems being returned to the upper half of the body via a cannula placed in the axillary vein. Flow rates as high as 3–4 L/min can be achieved by these means though lower rates are equally effective. Under these circumstances, venous congestion within the abdomen is reduced and control of bleeding points can be achieved. Furthermore, there is less pressure on the time required to perform the vascular anastomoses (*Fig.* 77.9). The new organ is anastomosed in a standard fashion to the suprahepatic vena caval stump and revascularized initially through the hepatic arterial system, after which the inferior vena cava system may be reconnected. The operation is completed with the repair of the portal vein with an end-to-end anastomosis and, finally, the biliary system is connected to the gastrointestinal tract in a number of ways (*Fig.* 77.10). The current trend in this procedure would seem to be to use both recipient and donor common bile ducts with an end-to-end anastomosis but where this is unavailable, then the technique evolved by Calne in Cambridge, UK, in which the donor gallbladder is developed into a wide conduit gives excellent results.

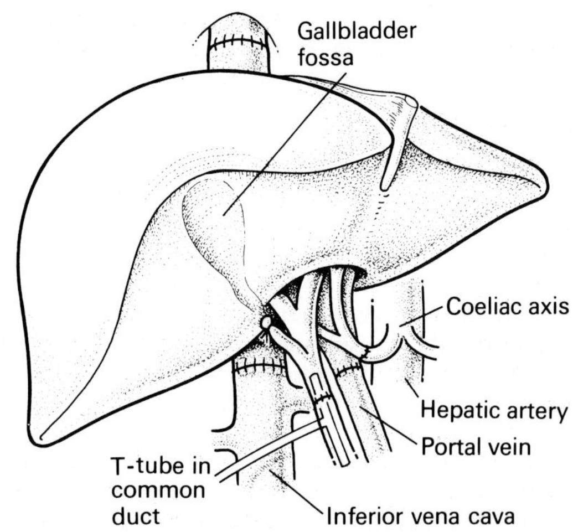

Fig. 77.10 This demonstrates the anastomoses required for orthotopic liver transplantation.

Postoperative Care

All patients undergoing liver transplantation require the fullest intensive care facility for their care in the first few days postoperatively. Ventilation is normally obligatory and the fullest monitoring system available should be used, if possible using a Swan–Ganz catheter for pulmonary artery pressures and cardiac output estimations. In most cases, inotropic drugs will be required to sustain cardiac function and to ensure that the renal function does not deteriorate.

As the reticuloendothelial system of the new liver is likely to be relatively ineffective during the early phase of transplantation, most transplant teams will use a combination of broad-spectrum antibiotics in order to reduce the chance of

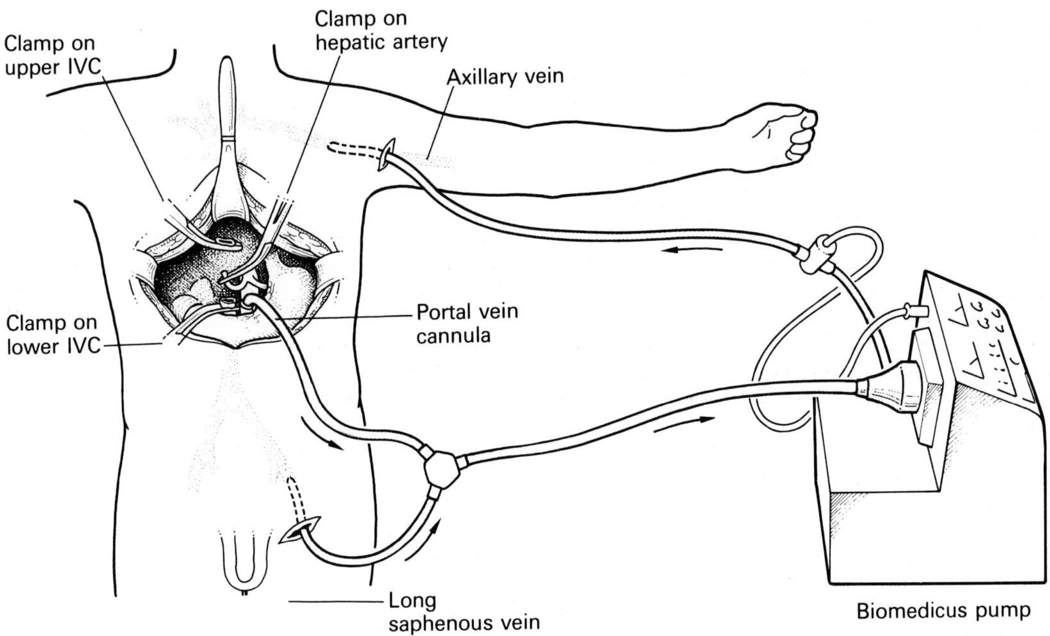

Fig. 77.9 After hepatectomy of the diseased organ, the circulatory state may be sustained by a venovenous extracorporeal circulation. The Vortex pump permits the adequate flow rates without the use of systemic heparin.

systemic infective disorders. Careful attention is also placed on oral hygiene and on the routine use of antifungal agents in the mouth. Immunosuppression is commenced as soon as the situation is haemodynamically stable. Opinion varies as to how this should be applied. The first choice is to commence immunosuppression with standard drugs of azathioprine and steroids for the first 1–2 weeks until the patient's condition is seen to be relatively stable and thereafter cyclosporin A is substituted. The advantage of this approach is that the nephrotoxicity of cyclosporin is not acting on a kidney already damaged by the events preceding transplantation and the transplantation procedure itself. Other transplant teams would argue that the dangers of an early rejection using this approach are reduced considerably by the administration of cyclosporin from the beginning and that provided care is taken in the dosage the nephrotoxicity may be minimized. The majority of patients have poor nutritional status and use of parenteral nutrition is recommended under most circumstances.

Complications of Liver Transplantation

The immediate complications relate to the surgical procedure and the failure of the new liver to function. This is commonly manifested by a haemorrhagic state which requires replacement of losses with fresh blood and fresh frozen plasma. If the organ has been taken from an unsuitable donor and suffered irreversible damage then the only hope for this patient will be the procurement of a fresh liver from a new donor. The need for cardiorespiratory support has already been alluded to.

Complications in the intermediate period include biliary fistulas, intra-abdominal sepsis arising either around the new liver or as a direct result of pigmental hepatic infarction. Rejection of the liver may occur as early as the fourth day and is manifested by disturbance in the liver function tests, pyrexia, tachycardia and a general feeling of ill-health in the patient. Normally these parameters are sufficient to give a clear indication for the use of pulsed methylprednisolone infusions but, where necessary, aspiration cytology or needle biopsy of the liver can be performed for the confirmation of the rejection process.

Of the late complications, the most serious is chronic rejection of the liver, the retransplant rate in some American units approaching 20%. Other late complications include cholangitis from biliary infections consequent on defects of biliary drainage and a recurrence of malignant disease in those patients for whom the transplant has been performed for this indication.

Results of Liver Transplantation

The results of this procedure are fast improving. Currently the major centres are able to offer a 1-year survival rate in excess of 70% and since most losses occur during this period the longer term outlook is consequently improving all the time. Patients remain at risk from the use of immunosuppression and are also at risk of chronic rejection. There are several patients now who are in excess of ten years post-transplant and are maintaining apparent good health. The next decade should see a steady improvement in the results as the technique becomes disseminated to secondary centres. It is likely that there are two new technical innovations which will make the procedure safer than currently is the case and that improved organ preservation will remove some of the difficulties consequent on the need for rapid transplant of a donor organ.

PANCREATIC TRANSPLANTATION

Insulin-dependent diabetes occurs at an incidence of 50/million population/year. The disease reduces the life expectancy by about one-third and in most Western societies it is the commonest cause of blindness. Furthermore it is responsible for one-third of the patients with renal failure and increases the susceptibility to peripheral gangrene and coronary atherosclerosis by 5 and 2 times respectively. Although insulin therapy is capable of blood sugar control, it appears that the angiopathy at the base of many diabetic complications is not prevented by adequate insulin administration.

A number of centres have commenced pancreatic transplantation to determine whether the organ can be successfully grafted and to see whether an established graft is capable of reversing or preventing vasculitic complications.

There are several problems of surgical technique which are special to pancreatic transplantation. In particular the exocrine secretion of the pancreas is troublesome and difficulties in removing these highly active proteolytic enzymes have proved to be a major stumbling block. Secondly, the vascular anastomoses are difficult and graft thrombosis is relatively common.

Initially, a full pancreaticoduodenal graft was performed but this proved bulky and prone to complication. This led to a segmental graft being employed, using body and tail vascularized by the splenic vessels. Currently, attention has returned to the whole pancreas which increases the number of active islets and gives an opportunity to use the ampullary region for the surgical drainage of exocrine secretion.

The graft is vascularized using the coeliac axis for arterial input and portal vein for venous egress. Normally the ilial system is used to provide vascular access in an extraperitoneal position (*Fig.* 77.11). However, this has the disadvantage of the pancreatic venous blood bypassing the host liver. In order that a more normal physiological state is achieved, some surgeons have anastomosed the pancreatic graft to the host splenic and mesenteric vessels in what is termed a paratopic position. It is uncertain at this stage that any overall improvement results from this approach. The segmental graft is much easier to place in the iliac fossa but suffers from the major haemodynamic disadvantage that flow from the pancreatic graft is low and thrombosis is frequent. Attempts to improve the flow by the creation of a terminal arteriovenous fistula between the splenic vessels or by transplanting the spleen in continuity have not prevented graft thrombosis.

The problem of exocrine secretion has been dealt with in two ways: (i) by the injection of a polymer into the ductal system which fills the small alveolar branches and prevents juice formation; (ii) drainage into appropriate systems of which the gastrointestinal tract seems the most ideal. This may be accomplished by constructing a Roux-en-Y loop or by anastomosing the pancreatic duct to the posterior wall of the stomach. However, both of these techniques are liable to fistulation with infection and attention has turned to drainage into the urinary tract. A number of approaches have been tried, e.g. renal pelvis and ureter, but if the iliac fossa is used, then it is most convenient to anastomose the duct directly to the bladder dome.

Normally, pancreatic transplantation is reserved for patients with diabetic complications who have already developed renal failure. In this situation the safest practice is the establishment of a successful renal graft followed by the pancreatic graft after 6 months. Some centres are now prepared to do the procedures simultaneously and a few will

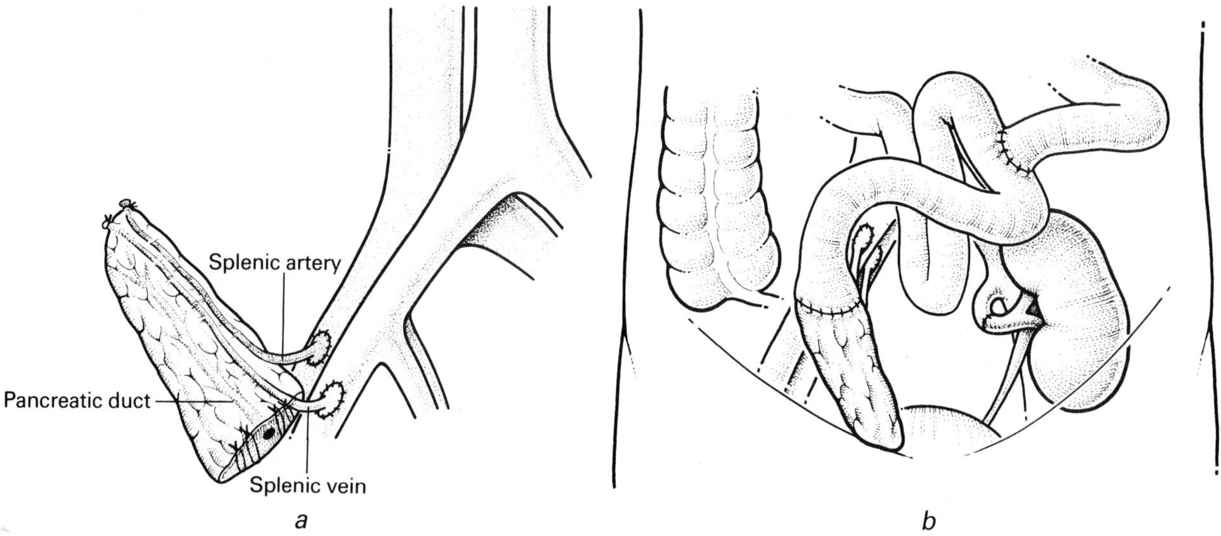

Fig. 77.11 *a*, This illustrates the placing of a partial pancreatic graft in the right iliac fossa with vascular anastomoses to the common iliac vessels. The pancreatic duct is obliterated. *b*, Alternatively, the pancreatic segment may be placed intraperitoneally and the pancreatic juice drained into a Roux-en-Y loop.

proceed to pancreatic transplantation in the absence of renal failure but on the demonstration of microalbuminuria.

Effect of Pancreatic Transplantation

Using grafts with duct drainage, the recipient becomes normoglycaemic within a few hours. Oral glucose and i.v. glucose tolerance tests become normal in about two-thirds of patients with successful grafts. When grafts with ductal obliteration are used, it may be necessary to use exogenous insulin for 2–3 weeks. However, once established there does not seem to be any major difference between the two types of graft in terms of diabetes control.

In the best hands the 1-year graft survival is about 60%. Slightly better figures have been reported following the use of segmental grafts from living related donors but it is unlikely that this method will have a wide application. As very few patients have been followed for a great length of time it is uncertain whether pancreatic grafting is capable of reversing pancreatic arteriopathy. However, it does seem that diabetic changes are not seen in transplanted kidneys and in patients who received a secondary pancreatic graft there is a reduction in the glomerular mesangium. In some patients there is an alleviation of the peripheral neuropathy. However, since this problem may also be caused by renal failure it is not clear whether it is the pancreatic or renal graft which is responsible for the improvement.

Pancreatic Graft Dysfunction

In those patients who receive a combined renal and pancreatic graft, the renal function has to serve as a marker for rejection, for the blood glucose level is slow to rise. Unfortunately the blood sugar is not elevated until 90% or more of the islets are damaged. Confirmatory evidence can be obtained by measuring the plasma insulin or C-peptide levels or by graft scanning or biopsy.

Although the fluctuations in the serum amylase are too great to be helpful it does seem that in grafts which are anastomosed to the urinary tract, the reductions in urinary amylase are diagnostic of rejection and permit early anti-rejection treatment.

78 Surgery for Vascular Access and Peritoneal Dialysis

P. J. Guillou

INTRODUCTION

Surgical procedures aimed at providing medium- or long-term access to the circulation and peritoneal cavity have become some of the most commonly performed operations undertaken in most large general hospitals, particularly those which possess a renal dialysis unit. The experience gained in performing vascular access for the haemodialysis population has become a springboard for the introduction of these procedures into other clinical disciplines. Some of the other indications for vascular access surgery are shown in *Table* 78.1 but this list is by no means exhaustive. However, subtle differences in the long-term requirements of renal as against non-renal patients do exist and the first section of this chapter describes the planning and procedures appropriate to the patient with renal failure and the second section will describe the approach in patients who require circulatory access for purposes other than haemodialysis. Finally, since many patients with chronic renal failure are now being treated by continuous ambulatory peritoneal dialysis (CAPD) this chapter concludes with a brief description of the principles and technique for the implantation of CAPD catheters into the peritoneal cavity.

Table 78.1 Indications for vascular access

1. Renal
   - Acute or chronic haemodialysis
   - Plasmapheresis
2. Poisoning
3. Burn injuries
4. Total parenteral nutrition
5. Haematological
   - Repeated transfusions (e.g. marrow aplasia)
   - Leukaemia—chemotherapy
   - Bone marrow transplantation
   - Repeated venesection
6. Chemotherapy for non-haematological malignancies
7. Frequent recurrent attacks of status asthmaticus

1. VASCULAR ACCESS SURGERY FOR RENAL FAILURE

In the provision of vascular access for the patient with renal failure, certain guiding principles have evolved which demand strict adherence if the patient is to suffer the minimum of complications and undergo optimally efficient dialysis. Central to this theme is the absolute necessity to preserve the patency of the upper limb veins. There is no more disappointing sight to the vascular access surgeon than that of a patient with chronic renal failure who is sitting in the renal unit with an intravenous infusion cannula carefully placed into the cephalic vein of the wrist of the patient's non-dominant arm. This automatically deprives the patient of any possibility of being provided with the best possible form of long-term vascular access, namely a subcutaneous arteriovenous fistula. The second important principle is that vascular access surgery must be planned and conducted by a surgeon with the appropriate training and experience in this sphere and not left to an uninterested junior member of the surgical team. With modern dialysis techniques the chronic renal failure patient has many years of dialysis life ahead of him during which a successful renal transplant may represent only a dialysis-free interlude in his chronic renal failure history and hence the importance of suitable planning of vascular access surgery can be appreciated.

The access surgeon may be called upon to provide dialysis access for patients suffering from acute reversible renal failure or an acute episode of renal failure in a patient whose renal failure is chronic and progressing inexorably down the road towards lifelong renal replacement therapy. Although these two clinical circumstances have slightly differing requirements for vascular access it should always be remembered that the apparently acute renal failure may not be reversible and the patient may ultimately have to undergo chronic dialysis. Accordingly, the absolute necessity to preserve the forearm vessels even in these patients should always be borne in mind.

A. Acute Renal Failure

Long-term haemodialysis only became a practical reality with the development of the implantable AV shunt by Quinton, Dillard and Schribner in 1960 and for many years this device was the mainstay of vascular access for both acute and chronic renal failure (*Fig.* 78.1). For the patient with acute renal failure it was a simple matter, under local anaesthesia, to insert the arterial cannula of this device into the radial artery at the wrist, the venous cannula being inserted into the adjacent cephalic vein. Both cannulas could then exit from the skin and be connected by the Teflon

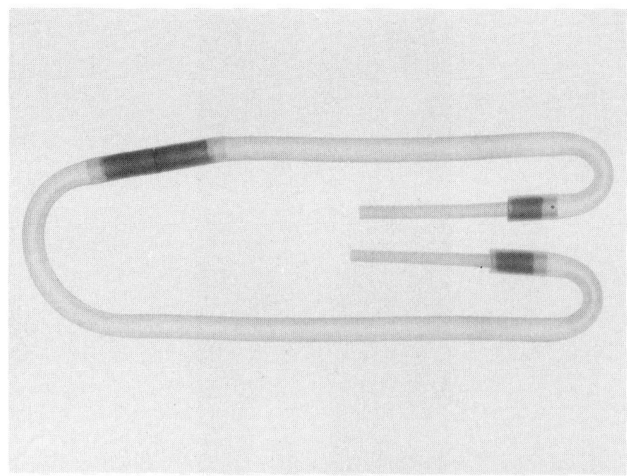

Fig. 78.1 Standard Schribner shunt: the short arm is inserted into the anterior/posterior tibial artery and long arm into the long saphenous vein.

bridging tube until required for dialysis purposes. After clamping the Silastic tubing at both ends the bridge could be disconnected prior to attaching the arterial cannula to the inflow tube to the dialysis membrane and the venous cannula to the outflow tubing from the machine, thus establishing the extracorporeal circuit for haemodialysis. It will be evident that it is now considered that this procedure transgresses one of the important principles of access surgery by destroying the cephalic vein at the wrist. Indeed, this procedure is rarely used nowadays except when alternative approaches are not feasible.

Currently the majority of patients presenting with acute renal failure are managed either by peritoneal dialysis or, if haemodialysis is mandatory, by the insertion of a subclavian venous line as described below for acute-on-chronic renal failure. If neither of these techniques is available, then haemodialysis may also be accomplished by undertaking procedures in the lower limb, consisting either of femoral vein catheterization or, as a last resort, the insertion of a Schribner AV shunt into the posterior tibial artery and long saphenous vein at the ankle. However, in the long term, the use of a Schribner shunt has been shown to have deleterious effects not only on the veins but also on the peripheral arterial supply to the foot. This may occur with particular rapidity in the patient with chronic renal failure whose arterial tree is already susceptible to the accelerated arteriopathy which results from the accompanying marked changes in plasma lipids.

B. Chronic Renal Failure

Most patients suffering from chronic renal failure present within one of two clinical scenarios each of which may play a determining role in the type of vascular access which is required at the time of presentation.

1. First, the patient may present with all the classic symptoms and signs of chronic renal failure, the diagnosis being confirmed biochemically and with renal biopsy to decide whether or not any therapeutic options exist. If not then the patient may be treated with appropriate dietary restrictions and preparations made to construct an AV fistula in the wrist of the non-dominant arm at a time convenient to both the surgeon and the patient. Thus sufficient time exists to plan the long-term management without having recourse to manoeuvres which provide temporary vascular access.

2. Acute renal failure may occur as a result of some intercurrent disorder in a patient with chronic renal failure in whom dialysis has not yet become necessary. Such a patient may already have had an AV fistula constructed in which case dialysis may commence through this, or a fistula may not yet have had time to mature or even been constructed and so an alternative form of access for urgent dialysis is required immediately. Usually this takes the form of a dialysis catheter of Uldall type (*Fig.* 78.2) inserted percutaneously into either the subclavian vein or, less desirably, into the femoral vein. Such catheters obviate the necessity to cannulate any peripheral vessels in the wrists or ankles and with modern techniques of single-needle dialysis may be utilized for up to two or three weeks to enable more permanent vascular access to be accomplished.

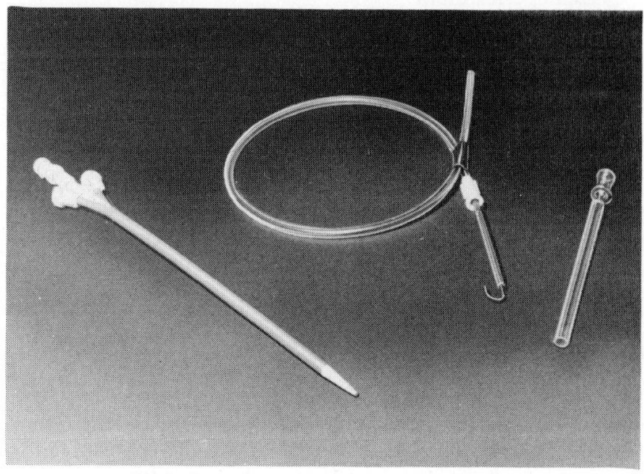

Fig. 78.2 Uldall-type double-lumen catheter and guide wire for subclavian venous catheterization for haemodialysis.

Unfortunately, percutaneously inserted central venous dialysis catheters carry a significant morbidity (*Table* 78.2) and so should be left in place for as short a time as possible whilst some form of long-term access is provided.

It can therefore be seen that by the expedient of employing some form of temporary vascular access to facilitate haemodialysis, the vast majority of chronic renal failure patients may be entered into a plan of campaign for the provision of long-term vascular access if the decision for treatment comes to lie with haemodialysis rather than continuous ambulatory peritoneal dialysis. An appropriate strategy is shown in *Table* 78.3. The absolute gold standard for the provision of vascular access for the patient with chronic renal failure is an AV fistula created at the wrist between the cephalic vein and radial artery. The principle behind this procedure is that the exposure of the venous system of the forearm to systemic arterial pressure results in the arterialization of these vessels. Because they lie subcutaneously, these vessels may be punctured repeatedly using either one double-lumen needle or two single-lumen needles to provide an extracorporeal circuit for blood to be passed through the dialysis machine and returned to the circulation.

However, the provision of vascular access in the patient with chronic renal failure is not always straightforward because of the numerous risk factors which may conspire

Table 78.2 Complications of subclavian vein catheterization for haemodialysis

A. During insertion
- Pneumothorax
- Haemothorax
- Subclavian artery injury
- Brachial plexus injury
- Caval perforation
- Guide-wire fracture

B. During or between dialyses
- Thrombus formation within the catheter or subclavian vein→Pulmonary embolus
- Sepsis
  - Exit site
  - Bloodstream
- Disconnection
  - Air embolus
  - Haemorrhage
- Migration
  - Haemopericardium
  - Intrapulmonary haemorrhage

Table 78.3 Strategy for provision of vascular access for haemodialysis

1. Chronic renal failure not yet requiring haemodialysis
   Early AV fistula formation
   Haemodialysis or CAPD
2. Acute-on-chronic renal failure with no available vascular access

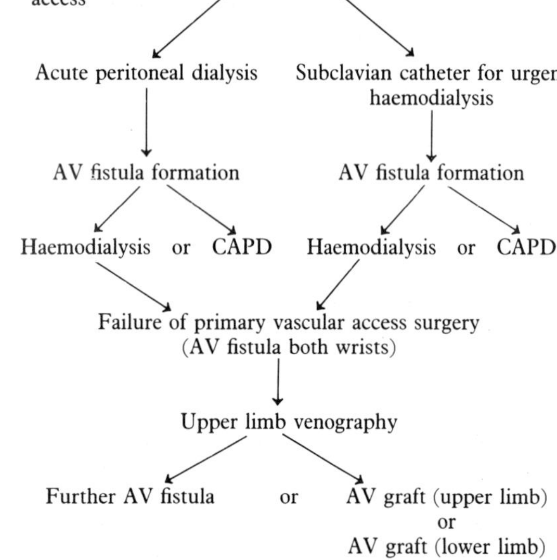

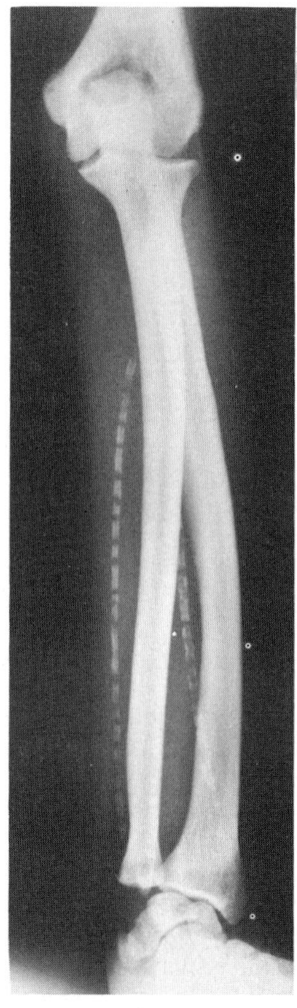

Fig. 78.3 Severe vascular calcification of radial and ulnar arteries in an 18-year-old girl with secondary hyperparathyroidism due to chronic renal failure.

against the formation of an AV fistula. Thus it is often more difficult to construct a fistula in women than in men because their veins tend to be rather less well-developed. Similarly the patient with longstanding chronic renal failure with severe aberrations of calcium metabolism may have badly calcified small vessels (*Fig.* 78.3) which may make the procedure difficult or even impossible. The development of renal failure in a patient with diabetes is a particularly notorious combination for the vascular access surgeon and, in addition, more elderly patients are being accepted onto the renal replacement therapy programmes with all their attendant vascular complications. Because of these many risk factors which may prevent successful fistula formation at the wrist and because alternative procedures are available, it has become conventional to categorize vascular access procedures into primary procedures which implies the formation of a subcutaneous AV fistula at one of a number of possible sites in the upper limbs, and secondary procedures to be employed when fistulas are either not feasible or have failed.

Primary Vascular Access Procedures for Chronic Renal Failure

Subcutaneous AV fistulas may be constructed at a number of sites in the upper limbs. Wherever possible the initial attempt should be made to perform an AV fistula between the cephalic vein and the radial artery at the wrist in the non-dominant arm so the patient may ultimately learn to cannulate the fistula himself if he is a candidate for home-based haemodialysis. If this fails or is unsuccessful then the next AV fistula should be created in the corresponding vessels of the opposite arm. The original description by Cimeno and Brescia employed a standard side-to-side configuration between the artery and vein as shown in *Fig.* 78.4. However, it has been claimed that this is associated with a higher incidence of painful hand hyperaemia than other configurations although the distended veins which develop on the dorsum of the hand may serve as useful alternative puncture sites in these patients (*Fig.* 78.5). Our own preference, based on the results of a controlled clinical trial, is for

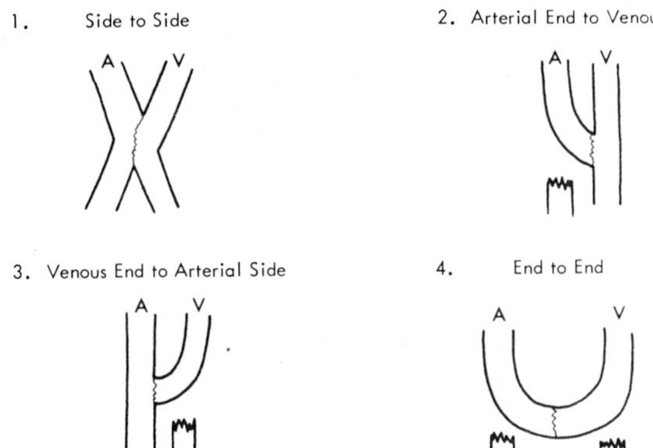

Fig. 78.4 Types of arteriovenous fistula used for haemodialysis.

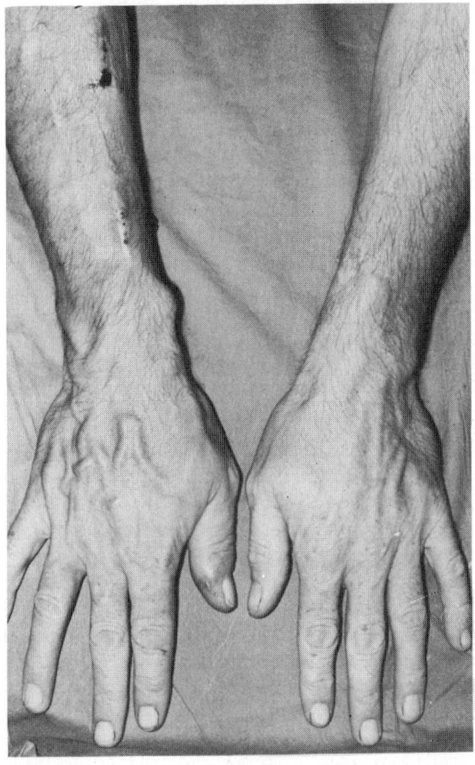

Fig. 78.5 Hyperaemia of the hand in a patient with a side-to-side arteriovenous fistula of the right wrist. Prominent veins are seen on the dorsum of the hand and the thumb is swollen with an area of skin necrosis medial to the thumb nail. A proximal venous stenosis just below the antecubital fossa was seen on venography.

an end of vein to side of artery configuration. The end-to-end configuration is occasionally used by some surgeons with good long-term results but the majority of surgeons employ one or other of the first two described above. These can easily be constructed under local anaesthesia using standard microvascular anastomotic techniques with 7/0 prolene sutures to perform the anastomosis.

If an AV fistula at these two sites is unsuccessful, then other sites may have to be considered. Fistulas created between the ulnar artery and the basilic vein tend not to be successful because of the lower flow in the ulnar artery. However, the basilic vein is always a large diameter vein (up to 4 or 5 mm) which is quite suitable for transposition across the palmar aspect of the forearm for anastomosis to the radial artery. After it has matured for two or three weeks this is usually ready for puncture for dialysis purposes and is of sufficient length to permit two-needle insertion if necessary. Alternatively, if the arteries at the wrist are inadequate to provide a sufficiently high flow then the basilic vein may be looped round subcutaneously and anastomosed to the side of the brachial artery in the antecubital fossa.

Occasionally, all the veins in the distal forearm are either thrombosed or too tenuous to be used but the veins in the antecubital fossa may have survived and under these circumstances the formation of a side-to-side AV fistula between the median cubital vein and the brachial artery may be possible. Failing this, not infrequently there is a side branch of the median cubital vein which perforates the fascia and enters the deep venous system. This may be anastomosed to the side of the brachial artery (Gracz fistula) and produces dilatation of the superficial veins for dialysis purposes.

Complications of AV Fistulas

The AV fistulas described above will provide primary vascular access for the vast majority of patients with chronic renal failure. The one-year patency rates for Cimeno–Brescia fistulas is almost 80% with some 60% subserving dialysis over a five-year period. Clearly, however, a considerable proportion of these patients suffer from one or more of the complications which may be expected when vessels are punctured two or three times per week over a protracted period of time. The potential complications to which these fistulas are prone are shown in *Table* 78.4.

Table 78.4 Complications of AV fistulas for haemodialysis

1. Primary thrombosis—fistula never used for dialysis
2. Secondary thrombosis—fistula previously used for dialysis
3. Proximal venous stenosis—hand hyperaemia
4. Puncture site infection
5. Aneurysm formation
6. Cavernous transformation
7. Left ventricular failure (very rare)

Primary thrombosis of the fistula may occur as a result of excessively tight bandaging being used to enclose the fistula wound immediately after its construction and obviously the nursing staff should be discouraged from this practice. Thrombosis early in the postoperative period will occasionally respond to re-exploration of the fistula, thrombectomy and re-anastomosis but often this is attributable to technical difficulties and flow cannot be restored. Aneurysm formation unfortunately occurs in long-lived AV fistulas and tends to occur at puncture sites which are used repeatedly. Aneurysms of alarming proportions are occasionally seen (*Fig.* 78.6) and an attempt to perform an aneurysmorrhaphy on these should be balanced against the risk of thrombosing the fistula. Hyperaemia of the hand does occur, especially with the side-to-side Cimeno–Brescia fistula. This produces intense pain in the hand, particularly the thumb, the tip of which may become necrotic as shown in *Fig.* 78.5. In this event a search should be made for a proximal stenosis in the veins higher in the forearm, again usually at the site of

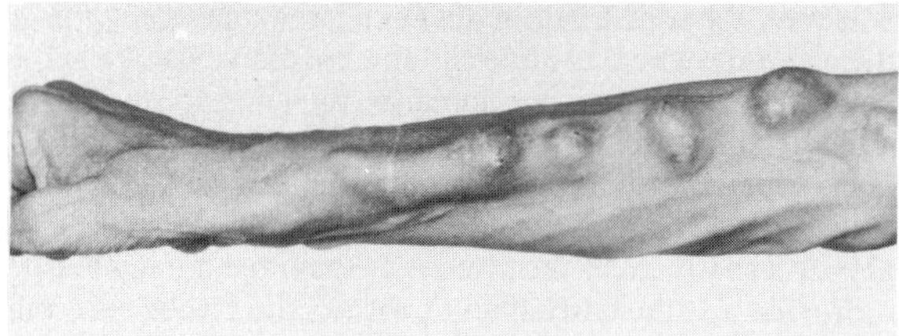

Fig. 78.6 Aneurysm formation in the proximal forearm veins of an AV fistula.

previous repeated punctures. Radiology in the form of a 'fistulogram' is essential in identifying the site of the proximal stenosis which may then be corrected surgically or, preferably, subjected to a balloon angioplasty to dilate the stricture.

Proximal stenoses of the forearm veins leading from an AV fistula may also be responsible for acute thrombosis occurring in a fistula which has previously provided satisfactory blood flow for dialysis but in which flow has gradually diminished. In all cases of sudden acute fistula thrombosis, restoration of fistula flow is dependent not just on immediate thrombectomy but also on angiography on the operating table in order to identify and correct any predisposing proximal stenosis at the time of thrombectomy. Here again, peroperative balloon angioplasty may serve the purpose very well.

A number of other complications are occasionally seen in AV fistulas. A long-term fistula may ultimately undergo cavernous transformation because of the repeated perivascular haematomas which occur at the puncture sites, thus rendering the fistula virtually unusable. Left ventricular failure as a result of distal AV fistulas is rarely seen and infection of a fistula is attributable entirely to poor asepsis and needling technique either by the patient or his nursing attendants.

Secondary Vascular Access Procedures for Chronic Renal Failure

Once the primary sites for the construction of AV fistulas have been exhausted, all the resources of ingenuity of the vascular access surgeon must be brought to bear in order to facilitate long-term access for such patients and in many instances this will involve the use of vascular grafts. The use of vascular grafts is really a last resort in vascular access surgery and should always be preceded by venography of both upper limbs. This demonstrates veins which might not be visible on ordinary physical examination and which might be suitably situated for the construction of a further AV fistula or, if not, will serve as the run-off veins for a subcutaneous AV conduit. Once the feasibility of a further upper limb AV fistula has been excluded, consideration is given to the interposition of a graft between a patent artery such as the brachial, and any appropriate upper limb vein. If no suitable veins are discerned then the insertion of a graft based on the femoral vessels may be suggested, but it should be emphasized that grafts placed in the thigh are much more subject to complications than are those at other sites.

The types of graft available for insertion for the purposes of haemodialysis have undergone considerable evolution over the past decade. A number of North American surgeons popularized the use of glutaraldehyde-preserved biological grafts such as bovine carotid artery and human umbilical cord vein allografts. However, these are subject to frequent complications, particularly those of sepsis and aneurysm formation and their use has now largely been abandoned. If the decision is made to use a biological material then autologous saphenous vein is undoubtedly the one of choice. The septic complications of autologous vein grafts are extremely low but unfortunately their poor long-term patency and susceptibility to aneurysm formation has led many surgeons to abandon even these in favour of synthetic grafts. Experience with Dacron grafts of both the knitted and double velour types was initially encouraging, the patency and blood flow achieved with such grafts being most acceptable. It soon became apparent, however, that these grafts were unable to tolerate the repeated puncturing required for haemodialysis, these sites forming false aneurysms and developing severe infective complication. Healing of tissues around the puncture sites was minimal and eventually these grafts ended by being removed as a tattered infected remnant of the original graft. This led many to examine the capacity of the newer material, expanded polytetrafluorethylene (PTFE), to withstand the repeated puncturing for haemodialysis. At present, expanded PTFE is the material of choice for forming a subcutaneous AV conduit for dialysis. Puncture sites heal readily, infective complications occur less frequently than with other synthetic grafts and can more readily be treated with antibiotics and figures from large series indicate that 60% of such grafts will be patent and subserving dialysis between 3 and 4 years after implantation.

The most frequent complication of arteriovenous grafts using PTFE are: (1) difficulty with needling due to the thickness of the PTFE graft; (2) thrombosis; (3) false aneurysm formation and sepsis.

Needling difficulties with PTFE grafts may contribute to the incidence of other complications with these grafts because of the increased amount of manipulation to which difficult grafts are subjected. However, evidence continues to accrue which suggests that thin-walled PTFE grafts are not subject to these difficulties and the consequent ease of needling is, at least in part, responsible for the greater longevity of thin-walled PTFE AV grafts compared with their standard thickness counterparts. In addition, the thin-walled PTFE graft is of a much more appropriate thickness for suturing to the thin veins which are frequently all that is available for the run-off from the graft.

Primary thrombosis of PTFE grafts within the first 24 h after operation is almost always due to technical difficulties during insertion of the graft. Although occasionally this is at the arterial end of the graft, more commonly it is the venous end where most technical complications occur. Invariably this is in association with narrow, thin-walled veins, the anastomosis narrowing the diameter of the vein at this site which is thus unable to accommodate the arterial blood flow exiting from the graft. Venous outflow obstruction is also the most common cause of secondary thrombosis of AV grafts, defined as thrombosis of a graft which has served haemodialysis for at least one month. Under these circumstances this venous outflow obstruction may be attributable either to technical error in stenosing the anastomosis with the sutures or, with longer surviving grafts, intimal hyperplasia at the venous anastomosis. This seems to be a particular complication with PTFE grafts but whether or not this will also prove to be so with thin-walled PTFE remains to be seen. However, in attempting to resurrect the graft which has undergone a secondary thrombosis it is not simply sufficient to perform thrombectomy with a balloon catheter because the complication will simply recur. At the time of thrombectomy, 'on-table' angiography should be performed to exclude the presence of venous stenosis. If such a stenosis is present this should be corrected at the time of thrombectomy, usually by means of a patch angioplasty. It seems unlikely that balloon angioplasty will have a role in this situation because of the inability to dilate the graft component of the anastomosis.

False aneurysms occurring in a PTFE AV graft may be dealt with surgically by excising the segment of the graft from which the false aneurysm arises and interposing a new segment of graft which can readily be sutured end-to-end with the old graft. However, the development of sepsis in these grafts is more ominous. If the graft is non-aneurysmal then cellulitic reactions around the graft may respond to high doses of systemic broad-spectrum antibiotics after blood cultures have been taken. If an aneurysmal graft becomes frankly infected then it is an indication for urgent removal of the graft before catastrophic haemorrhage ensues from rupture of the aneurysm. Chronic sinuses leading to exposure of the graft in the subcutaneous tissues may occasionally be covered by rotating a small local musculocutaneous flap under antibiotic cover. This may be an important manoeuvre in attempting to salvage one of the last sites for access in a haemodialysis veteran.

A number of other complications are occasionally encountered with AV grafts in the haemodialysis population. Steal syndromes resulting in either arm or leg claudication are surprisingly uncommon in such patients. Loop grafts in the forearm may achieve flows of 400–500 ml/min before symptoms occur, classically of arm claudication while shaving if the graft is in the dominant arm. This may be readily dealt with by 'banding' the graft at its arterial end whilst directly monitoring the blood flow through the distal vein with an electromagnetic flow meter. A flow of around 180–200 ml/min is sufficient to provide satisfactory flow on dialysis and still maintain the patency of the graft. Peripheral limb oedema due to venous hypertension in a limb supporting a proximal AV graft (e.g. a loop graft from common femoral artery to common femoral vein) is a much more difficult problem to contend with. Banding of the venous end of the graft in an attempt to reduce the venous pressure carries a significant risk of the graft thrombosing and graft loss. However, little else can be offered to the patient with such a complication. Cardiac decompensation resulting from a high flow arteriovenous shunt is seldom seen with primary AV fistulas but occasionally complicates arteriovenous grafts in patients whose cardiac reserve may already be compromised by anaemia and coronary artery disease.

Other secondary vascular access procedures:

1. The 'button' device. The development of implantable chamber devices which may be anastomosed to an artery and a vein, the roof of the chamber protruding from the skin, has obvious potential advantages in terms of eliminating the necessity for skin puncture in order to obtain circulatory access. One such device has been produced commercially, access to the bloodstream being achieved via a two-pronged needle which can be inserted into the chamber which has an arterial entrance tube and venous exit tube constructed of PTFE, this being anastomosed to appropriate forearm vessels. Although of potential value for haemodialysis in children, this apparatus is fraught with complications and has not been adopted for routine use.

2. Long-term central venous catheters. Satisfactory long-term circulatory access for haemodialysis using the 'single needle' technique may be obtained by the insertion of a silicone-rubber catheter of the Hickman or Broviac type into the subclavian or internal jugular veins (*Fig.* 78.7). Several techniques exist for the insertion of such catheters but all incorporate a long subcutaneous tunnel (*Fig.* 78.8) which is considered to reduce the incidence of catheter sepsis. The catheter may be inserted under local or general anaesthesia. One technique involves cutting down into the cephalic vein in the deltopectoral groove and threading the catheter along into the superior vena cava, via the subclavian vein. An alternative is to make a small incision above the medial end of the clavicle, mobilization of the internal jugular vein between the two heads of sternocleidomastoid and insertion of the catheter into a small lateral incision in the side of the internal jugular vein in the centre of a small purse-string suture of 6/0 or 7/0 prolene. This procedure may be performed under image intensification in order to position the central catheter accurately.

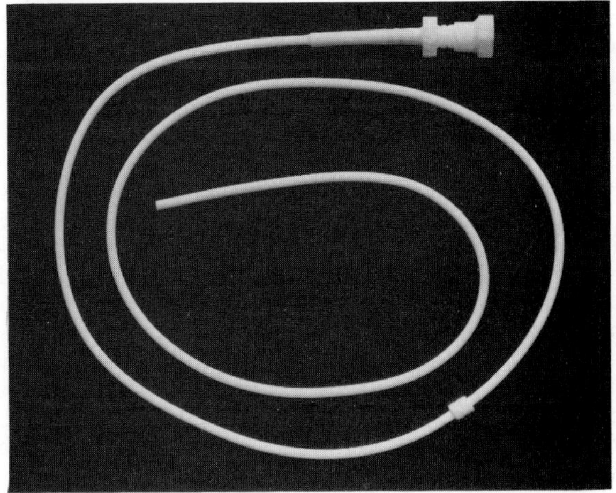

Fig. 78.7 Hickman line.

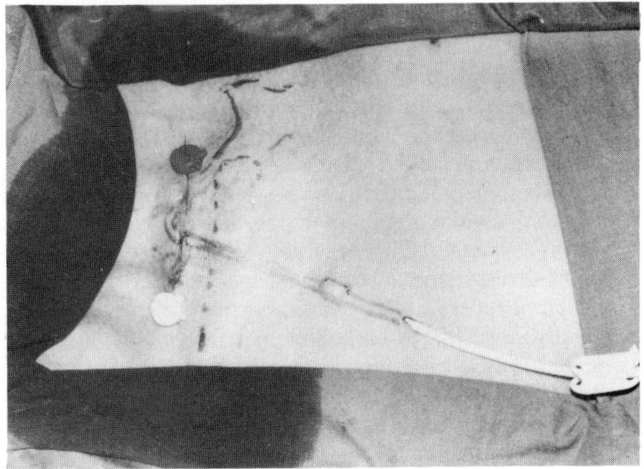

Fig. 78.8 Hickman line in subcutaneous tunnel prior to entering the internal jugular vein.

The use of such catheters is particularly valuable for the provision of dialysis access in very young children or those children who simply abhor the normal needling techniques. Unlike the percutaneously inserted Uldall catheter, these surgically implanted cathers may be relatively long-lived, providing dialysis access for up to 24 months, if cared for using strict asepsis and remembering to heparinize the catheter when it is locked off between dialyses.

Haemodialysis access in children:

The advent of chronic ambulatory peritoneal dialysis has largely superseded haemodialysis in children. However, occasionally the necessity does arise and in very small children this is best served by the insertion of a central venous Hickman or Broviac line. Small children down to the age of several weeks may be haemodialysed via this technique which may give time for the child to grow a little to a size where longer-term procedures may be performed. In bigger children (who may still remain small as a result of their uraemia) the best form of dialysis access remains a surgically created AV fistula provided this can be constructed easily using interrupted sutures which occasionally are as small as 10/0. The use of synthetic vascular grafts in children should be avoided if at all possible and in particular the use of external shunts such as the Thomas shunt (a Schribner shunt with dacron patches at the arterial and venous ends for anastomosis to the femoral vessels) has not found universal acceptance for paediatric dialysis.

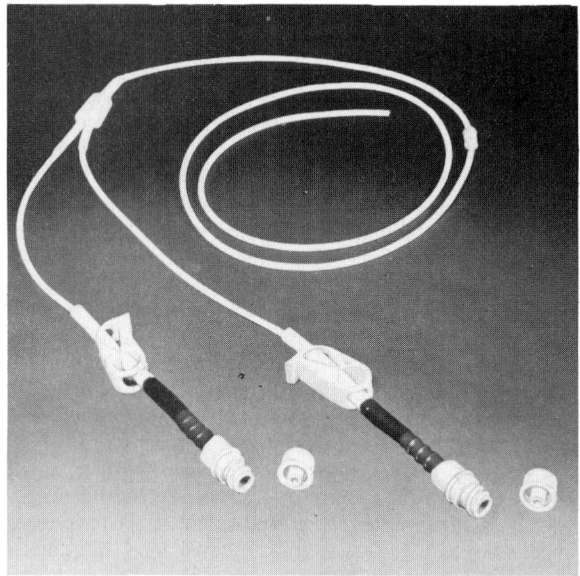

Fig. 78.9 Double-lumen Hickman line.

2. VASCULAR ACCESS FOR NON-HAEMODIALYSIS PURPOSES

It is disappointing to reflect that the principles which underly referral for access surgery in patients with chronic renal failure have not yet permeated to the referral of patients with non-renal indications. Thus, a request for circulatory access in a patient whose peripheral veins have been destroyed by prior long-term chemotherapy or repeated venepunctures and transfusion is the rule rather than the exception and thwarts any view of long-term vascular access for such patients. The lesson of early referral of these patients requires constant emphasis. In considering such patients the merits of non-permanent as against permanent circulatory access should be carefully weighed in the balance. For most purposes a Hickman line, or the smaller Broviac line in children, is satisfactory when inserted using the procedures described above. These may be inserted and removed as required. However, for the occasional patient, such as those with frequent transfusion requirements, whose life expectancy is considerable, consideration should be given to the early insertion of an AV fistula or even an AV graft if this only needs to be punctured every 4–6 weeks in order to give blood. AV fistulas tend not to be successful in patients requiring systemic chemotherapy since these appear to thrombose readily because of the drugs being administered. For such purposes a Hickman line is the preferred method, especially now that double-lumen catheters are available (*Fig.* 78.9), these providing a portal of entry for the drugs as well as a facility for the removal of blood for haematological analyses. Finally, the Hickman type line is also the procedure of choice for long-term total parenteral nutrition.

3. PERITONEAL ACCESS FOR CHRONIC AMBULATORY PERITONEAL DIALYSIS

Continuous ambulatory peritoneal dialysis (CAPD) is now an increasingly used alternative to haemodialysis with some 20% of all chronic renal failure patients in the UK being treated by this technique in 1985. The principle is that of standard intermittent peritoneal dialysis in using the peritoneum as a dialysis membrane. The rather rigid PD catheters previously available did not permit this to be used on any permanent or semipermanent basis but the development of silicone rubber catheters such as those shown in *Fig.* 78.10 together with closed system PVC bags to contain the dialysis fluid has now facilitated home-based CAPD. In practice a soft silicone rubber catheter is inserted into the pelvic sump as shown in *Fig.* 78.11. The patient is trained, using a closed system, to fill his peritoneal cavity with 2 L of peritoneal dialysis fluid for a period of 4–6 h. The fluid is then allowed to drain out and replaced, under aseptic conditions, with a new bag of dialysis fluid for a further 6 h. The bag changes take approximately 20 min to perform and all that is required is a quiet clean area in which to perform the bag change, and the necessary sterile cleaning fluids chlorhexidine and povidone–iodine. Between bag changes the patient is fully ambulant and able to work, play, eat and sleep normally without interruption other than that necessary to exchange the peritoneal dialysis fluid.

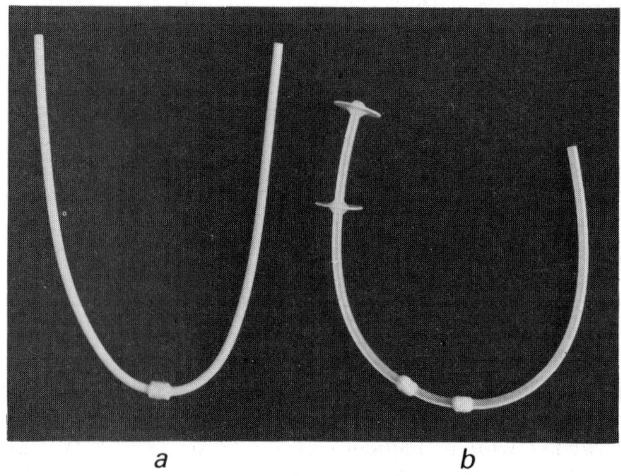

Fig. 78.10 CAPD catheters: (*a*) Tenckhoff catheter; (*b*) Oreopoulos catheter.

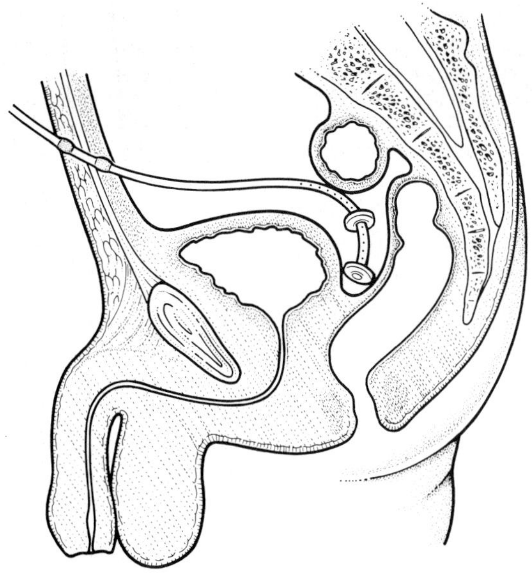

Fig. 78.11 Diagrammatic sagittal section showing idealized CAPD catheter positioning.

Table 78.5 Complications of CAPD

1. Peritonitis
   Bacterial
   Fungal
2. Tunnel infection/leakage
3. Catheter occlusion
   Omentum or fibrin
4. Catheter displacement
5. Hernia formation
   Inguinal
   Femoral
   Incisional
6. Catheter erosion
   Gastrointestinal tract
   Female genital tract
7. Membrane failure
   Sclerosing peritonitis

The most obvious and overwhelming advantage of CAPD is the freedom from haemodialysis machines and hospitalization, but, in addition, patients undergoing CAPD tend to be in a more anabolic state than their haemodialysed counterparts. This is partly because of the high glucose concentrations in the CAPD fluid and partly because of their greater biochemical stability. The commonest disadvantage and complication of CAPD is that of peritonitis but the surgeon may contribute both to its management and reducing the risk by careful implantation of the CAPD catheter.

Some centres still insert CAPD catheters under local anaesthesia without directly visualizing the pelvic sump but it is now more common practice for the catheter to be implanted surgically under general anaesthesia. This carries the additional advantage of being also able to remove the greater omentum to avoid subsequent catheter blockage by this structure. Omentectomy appears to be especially important in children because the thin omentum may initially migrate into the lumen of the catheter and occlude it. The operation may be conducted through a midline or paramedian incision, the end of the catheter being placed into the rectovesical or recto-uterine pouch so that the Dacron cuff on the catheter can be inserted into a pocket between the peritoneum and linea alba at the upper end of the wound. After closing the peritoneal and fascial layers the catheter is led through a subcutaneous tunnel to exit from the skin at a point above parallel with the umbilicus, 4–5 cm from the midline. The choice of silicone-rubber catheter is not critical but the flanges on the end of the Oreopoulos catheter may cause it to remain more readily in the pelvis than does the standard Tenckhoff catheter (*Fig.* 78.10*b*).

Complications of CAPD

The complications of CAPD are summarized in *Table* 78.5, but by far the most common complication is peritonitis, this occurring with a frequency of 1 episode per 18 patient months on average. CAPD peritonitis does not have the striking clinical features seen with a perforated intra-abdominal viscus. The symptoms, if any, are usually more insidious and CAPD peritonitis may present only with cloudy fluid noticed by the patient during bag changes. Most episodes of bacterial peritonitis may be treated with appropriate intraperitoneal and systemic antibiotics, once the bacterial species have been identified. However, occasionally fungal pathogens, especially monilia, are isolated and this represents an absolute indication for laparotomy, catheter removal and peritoneal lavage and drainage. The mortality of fungal peritonitis approaches 100% if catheter removal and peritoneal lavage is not performed.

First and second episodes of bacterial peritonitis can generally be treated successfully with antibiotics but caution is urged when a mixed bacterial flora is obtained since this may be the only indication that the catheter has eroded into a viscus. Third or subsequent episodes of peritonitis with a single contaminating organism is a relative indication for catheter removal, followed by a period of haemodialysis and replacement of the catheter at a later date.

If the catheter tip displaces from the pelvis, it may be possible to get fluid into the peritoneal cavity but this then fails to drain satisfactorily because of loss of the sump action, the catheter tip being above the pelvic fluid level. Displacement of the catheter into the subhepatic area may give rise to abdominal pain referable to the subcostal region. Both these complications require surgical removal of the catheter and simultaneous re-insertion of a new catheter in order that CAPD can be resumed.

Hernias are common in patients undergoing CAPD with an overall reported incidence between 13% and 24%. Incisional hernias appear to occur with particular readiness in female patients. All hernias which develop after the initiation of CAPD may be repaired using standard techniques without interrupting CAPD. Pre-existing groin hernias should be detected and repaired at the time of catheter insertion.

The duration for which a patient may be maintained on CAPD is determined by a number of factors including his own meticulousness in employing a scrupulously aseptic technique for bag changes. Patients who develop peritonitis episodes frequently within the first year of commencing CAPD tend not to continue with this procedure for very long. Others appear to have a trouble-free existence and some patients have now been maintained on CAPD as their sole renal replacement therapy for over 8 years. A small proportion of patients who have not previously suffered episodes of peritonitis may eventually develop failure of dialysis because of thickening of the peritoneal membrane which ceases to function as a dialysis filter. This is known as sclerosing 'peritonitis' and at laparotomy the peritoneal contents are found to be shrouded in a thick fibrous cowl, the catheter being removed of necessity. Some of these patients may ultimately be able to return to CAPD but as yet this is by no means certain. The aetiology of sclerosing peritonitis is unknown but may be related to the type of biochemical buffer (acetate rather than bicarbonate) used in some peritoneal dialysis fluids.

With care, the CAPD patient enjoys greater freedom and biochemical stability than his haemodialysed counterparts. Some patients have now dialysed by this technique for many years and with the sophisticated closed systems currently available may expect to do so for years to come.

79 Gynaecology for the General Surgeon

H. N. Macdonald

Gynaecological problems are bound to present fairly regularly in the course of general surgical practice. A surgeon must therefore be familiar with the appropriate techniques for clinical assessment and treatment of such cases. In gynaecology as in all clinical fields, careful history taking is essential; however, a patient's familiarity with her menstrual function readily results in important details being omitted or dismissed as irrelevant.

Gynaecological History

Disordered menstrual function, pain and vaginal discharge are the symptoms most likely to interest the surgeon although some heed must be paid to coitus, contraceptive habits and fertility.

Any alteration in the frequency, duration and amount of menstrual loss should be established. Frequency is calculated as the interval between onset of successive periods, not the time free of bleeding, as often quoted by patients. Periods 'twice a month' may be normal and separated by a full 28 days. Estimation of the amount of loss is very subjective and so comparison with the individual's own past experience is useful. The number of tampons used in each cycle, loss of clots (associated with abnormally rapid flow) and evidence of anaemia also assist objective evaluation.

Uterine pain is usually colicky from muscular contractions and is located diffusely over the hypogastrium with radiation down the inner thigh. Pain referred to the sacrum probably stems from the cervix. Spasmodic dysmenorrhoea is symmetrical and lasts 12–24 h from just before the onset of menstruation; when unilateral, an abnormality such as a rudimentary, even isolated, uterine horn should be suspected. Congestive dysmenorrhoea precedes menstruation often by several days, and subsides gradually after onset of the flow. As the term implies, it is due to pelvic congestion and usually secondary to pathology which is closely related to the uterus. Ovarian and tubal pain localize just above the inguinal ligament and may also be felt in the lumbosacral region. In assessing possible gynaecological pain, its site, character and duration are important, as well as any temporal relationship with menstruation. One should remember that the pain threshold is commonly reduced perimenstrually so that discomfort from a non-gynaecological cause may increase and thus mislead as to its origin.

Superficial dyspareunia arises at the vaginal introitus and is transient or continuous, the former usually indicating vaginismus. Deep dyspareunia comes from within the pelvis and is likely to be organic in origin even if intermittent. A relationship to ovulation or menstruation may be significant. Occasionally musculoskeletal disorders cause pain from unaccustomed coital posture.

Intermenstrual discharge should be qualified as to colour, odour, associated irritation or discomfort and the presence of blood. Tactful enquiry concerning recent coital experience is relevant when pregnancy, venereal infection or rupture of a cyst is suspected. Contraceptive practice must be recorded and reviewed from the standpoint of possible failure. In the case of oral contraceptives one should consider forgetfulness, gastrointestinal upset and interaction with other drugs. The past obstetrical history including involuntary infertility is also pertinent on occasion.

Gynaecological Examination

In addition to general examination the breasts should be inspected for signs of pregnancy or lactation. Abdominal examination is very much the surgeon's province and needs little elaboration except perhaps for the reminder that some highly parous women and most of those in advanced pregnancy have poor abdominal muscular tone so guarding is a less reliable sign.

The bladder is emptied before attempting pelvic examination which should be undertaken only with the permission of the patient (or her guardian if under age) and in the presence of a female chaperone. It is more easily accomplished with the patient in the dorsal position on a firm couch and embarrassment can be lessened by maintaining cover of the knees and lower legs. The vulva is inspected for signs of urethral or vaginal discharge but visualization of the upper vagina and cervix requires passage of a speculum, remembering that the vagina runs posteriorly towards the sacral promontory. A Cusco bivalve speculum is needed for examination in the dorsal position; occasional operators may prefer Sims' duckbill instrument which is inserted with the patient in the left lateral position (*Fig.* 79.1). Specimens for cytology and culture are collected before contamination with lubricants.

Vaginal examination should be performed by introducing the index and the middle finger along the posterior vaginal wall on confirmation that the introitus is of adequate calibre. Bimanual palpation is achieved by using the abdominal hand to bring the pelvic organs down onto the vaginal fingers placed in the posterior fornix. The consistency, regularity and dilatation of the cervix should be noted as well as

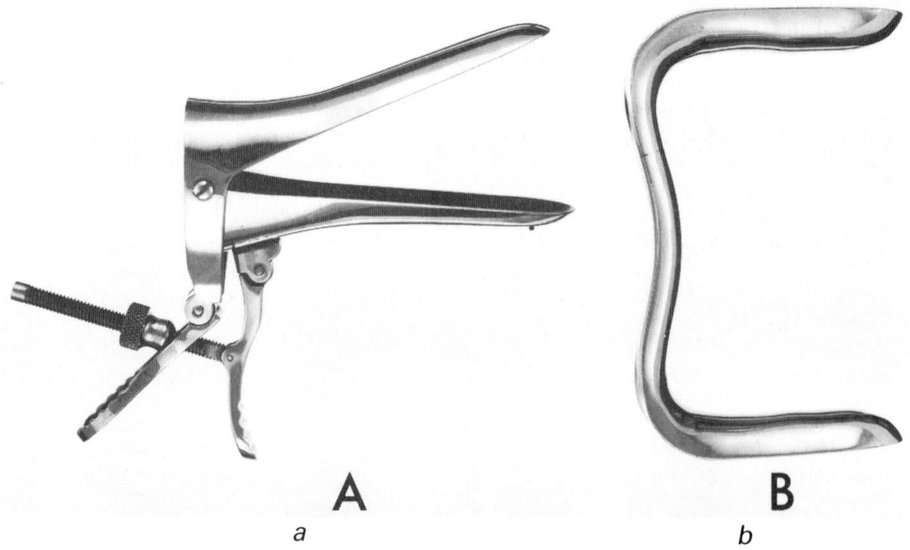

Fig. 79.1 Vaginal specula. *a*, Cusco's. *b*, Sims'.

mobility and associated tenderness. An anteverted uterus is felt easily between the two hands when its size, shape, consistency and mobility can be assessed. If retroverted, the fundus is palpable posteriorly in the pouch of Douglas and the cervix points towards the symphysis. Normal-sized ovaries are scarcely defined and are often tender on pressure. The normal fallopian tube is neither tender nor palpable. The uterosacral ligaments and pouch of Douglas should be examined for nodularity, tenderness or additional masses and a rectal examination completes assessment of the pelvis.

CONTRACEPTION

Modern contraceptive techniques are so widespread that it seems appropriate to include a brief review of those aspects which might have a bearing on surgical practice. Occlusive methods such as the sheath, cap or diaphragm and topical spermicidal agents are unlikely to present problems other than those of accidental pregnancy. In contrast, intrauterine devices and hormonal methods, whilst more reliable as contraceptives, also involve risk which can be of relevance to the surgeon.

Intrauterine Contraceptive Devices (IUCD) (*Fig.* 79.2)

These are plastic devices which prevent the implantation of a fertilized ovum by provoking a sterile inflammatory reaction in the surrounding endometrium. The contraceptive efficiency is largely dependent upon the amount of endometrial contact and can be improved by the addition of an outer coat of copper wire. The pharmacological effect of this copper appears also to be interference with implantation; its steady dissolution means that such devices must be replaced every 2–4 years. Removal of an IUCD is usually accomplished quite easily by traction on the tail which is customarily left to protrude several centimetres from the cervix. Occasionally this purpose is frustrated either by fracture or intrauterine retraction of the tail so that withdrawal necessitates invasive manipulation.

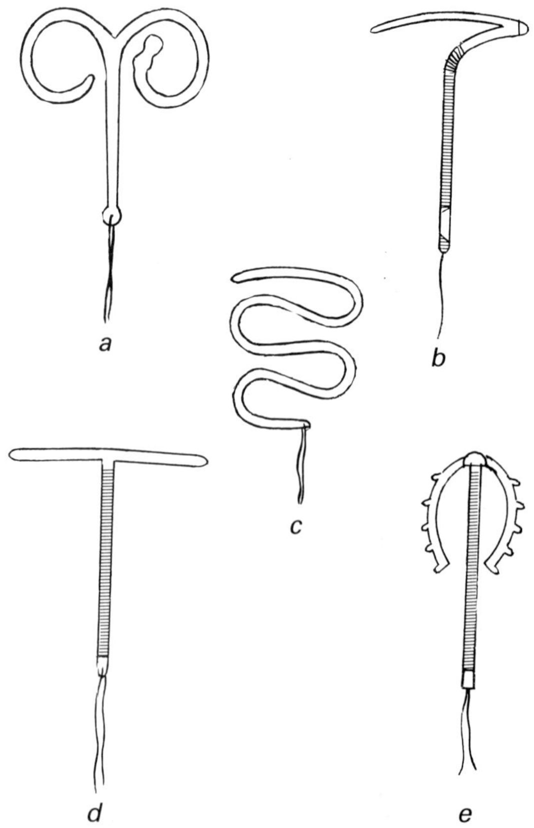

Fig. 79.2 Common types of intrauterine contraceptive devices. *a*, Saf-T-Coil. *b*, Copper-7. *c*, Lippes Loop. *d*, Copper-T. *e*, Multiload Copper 250.

The IUCD is said to prevent more than 99% of intrauterine pregnancies but only 95% of those in the fallopian tube and it offers no protection whatever against the rare chance of a primary ovarian implantation. Pregnancy complicating an IUCD is therefore tubal more often than would otherwise be expected and if intrauterine, is more prone to spontaneous abortion. Sepsis is an additional hazard in this situation, especially if the tail has retracted or the device has lodged in the myometrium so defying attempts at its removal. Where the tail has disappeared, sterile probing of the uterine cavity might be considered; a safer approach is ultrasonic scanning of the uterus which should reveal the IUCD and a pregnancy if present. Should neither be found, an abdominal radiograph is needed to exclude intraperitoneal translocation of the device as laparoscopy or laparotomy is then indicated to allow its removal. Usually an IUCD in such circumstances is found fairly harmlessly entangled within the omentum, nevertheless the bowel can be damaged or even obstructed.

Even if effective as a contraceptive, pelvic infection may complicate an IUCD and is likely to involve the uterus along with both tubes although unilateral salpingitis is said to be more frequent than usual. Infection tends to occur within the first few weeks of insertion, particularly if it has been traumatic as suggested by persistent pain or bleeding.

Hormonal Methods (*Table* 79.1)

The common hormonal regimes are intended to prevent fertilization rather than implantation and their effect is more pharmacological than that of intrauterine devices. The active agents are synthetic analogues of oestrogen and progesterone; as might be expected, neither action is reproduced

Table 79.1 Nature of oral contraceptive preparations available

Constituents		*Commercial descriptions*	
Monophasic			
Oestrogen	Progestogen	USA	UK
20 μg EE	1·0 mg NEA	Loestrin 1/20, Loestrin (Fe) 1/20	Loestrin 20
30 μg EE	0·15 mg LGL	Levlen, Nordette	Microgynon 30, Ovranette, Marvelon*
	0·25 mg NGL	—	Eugynon 30, Ovran 30
	0·3 mg NGL	Lo/Ovral	—
	1·5 mg NEA	Loestrin 1·5/30, Loestrin (Fe) 1·5/30	Loestrin 30
	2·0 mg ED	—	Conova 30
35 μg EE	0·4 mg NE	Ovcon 35	—
	0·5 mg NE	Modicon, Brevicon	Ovysmen, Brevinor
	1·0 mg NE	Norinyl 1+35, Ortho-Novum 1/35	Neocon 1/35, Norimin
	1·0 mg ED	Demulen 1/35	—
50 μg EE	0·25 mg LGL	—	Ovran
	0·5 mg NGL	Ovral	Eugynon 50
	1·0 mg ED	Demulen 1/50	—
	1·0 mg NE	Ovcon 50	—
	1·0 mg NEA	Norlestrin 1/50, Norlestrin (Fe) 1/50	Minovlar, Minovlar ED
	2·5 mg NEA	Norlestrin 2·5/50, Norlestrin (Fe) 2·5/50	Minilyn‡
	3·0 mg NEA	—	Gynovlar 21
	4·0 mg NEA	—	Anovlar 21
50 μg ME	1·0 mg NE	Norinyl 1+50, Ortho-Novum 1/50	—
80 μg ME	1·0 mg NE	Norinyl 1+80, Ortho-Novum 1/80	—
100 μg ME	1·0 mg ED	Ovulen	—
	2·0 mg NE	Norinyl 2 mg, Ortho-Novum 2 mg	—
	2·5 mg NE	Enovid-E	—
Biphasic			
35 μg EE	0·5 mg NE × 10 1·0 mg NE × 11	Ortho-Novum 10/11	× 7 × 14 Binovum
Triphasic			
35 μg EE	0·5 mg NE × 7 0·75 mg NE × 7 1·0 mg NE × 7	Ortho-Novum 7/7/7	Trinovum
	0·5 mg NE × 7 1·0 mg NE × 9 0·5 mg NE × 5	Trinorinyl	Synphase
30 μg EE 40 μg EE 30 μg EE	0·05 mg LGL × 6 0·075 mg LGL × 5 0·125 mg LGL × 10	Trilevlen, Triphasil 21	Trinordiol, Logynon, Logynon ED
Progestogen only			
	0·03 mg LGL	—	Microval, Norgeston
	0·0375 mg NGL	Ovrette	—
	0·075 mg NGL	—	Neogest
	0·35 mg NGL	Micronor, Nor-Q.D.	Micronor, Noriday
	0·5 mg ED	—	Femulen

EE—ethinyloestradiol; NE—norethisterone; ED—ethynodiol diacetate; ME—mestranol; NEA—norethisterone acetate; NGL—norgestrel; LGL—levonorgestrel.
*Desogestrel.
‡ Lynoestranol.

exactly. Mestranol and its active metabolite, ethinyloestradiol, are the usual oestrogens and as such are fairly specific in action.

Progestogens

Most of the synthetic progestogens are derivatives of 19-nortestosterone, namely norethisterone (norethindrone), norethisterone acetate (norethindrone acetate), lynoestranol, ethynodioldiacetate and norethynodrel, all of which are activated by metabolism to norethisterone *in vivo*.

Norgestrel and levonorgestrel are more recent developments which differ from other 19-norsteroids in being active without further metabolic transformation. The 19-nortestosterones have additional oestrogenic, anti-oestrogenic and even androgenic properties which depend upon their individual metabolic pathways. Medroxyprogesterone acetate, an injectable derivative of 17-alphahydroxyprogestone, is relatively free of non-progestogenic effects and norethisterone enanthate, is also available as a depot injection. These parenteral preparations give approximately 3 months protection but are preferred for relatively short-term use.

The principal progestogenic contraceptive effect is alteration of the cervical mucus to make it more viscous and impenetrable to spermatozoa. Subsidiary effects are thought to include impairment of sperm transport and fertilization, reduced tubal motility and a lower likelihood of implantation consequent upon interference with normal endometrial maturation. Higher doses may suppress ovulation but this is certain only with formulations which also include an oestrogen. For maximum contraceptive effect, therefore, progestogens must be taken at precisely the same time each day and any omission makes failure quite likely. Injectable preparations circumvent the problem of regular oral intake; their safety in long-term use is still contested. Progestogen-only contraception often results in poor cycle control with breakthrough bleeding or missed periods, but systemic side-effects, if any, seem minimal despite manufacturers' references to many of the factors cited as risks when taking the combined oestrogen-progestogen pills (*Table* 79.2). Contraceptive reliability clearly depends upon maintenance of an effective hormone level and can be as high as 99%. Theoretically there is increased likelihood of a failure being tubal but this remains to be confirmed in practice.

Combined Pills

All combined pills (oestrogen plus progestogen) are meant to suppress ovulation and to varying degrees they have supplementary progestogenic properties as outlined earlier. The range of pills (*see Table* 79.1) provides a choice both in strength and balance between oestrogen and progestogen, so that a suitable preparation can be found for most subjects. Like progestogens, the combined pill requires regular intake and absorption for full effect; however, delayed dosage is slightly less critical. Additional precautions are advisable during the first cycle on any preparation even if only changing pills, and also when absorption is doubtful because of gastrointestinal upset. Contraceptive efficacy can be reduced by interaction with other drugs which in turn may not have their otherwise expected effects (*Table* 79.3).

Assuming regular intake and none of the aforementioned complications, the combined pill is close to 100% effective as a contraceptive but has widespread systemic effects which are assuming greater importance as knowledge increases.

Side-effects of Oestrogen-progestogen Mixtures

In addition to its outstanding contraceptive reliability, the combined oral contraceptive pill is associated with a reduced incidence of troublesome gynaecological symptoms, such as premenstrual tension, dysmenorrhoea, and menorrhagia. Anaemia, acne, benign neoplasms of the breast and ovarian cysts are also less common in pill takers. Unfortunately, these benefits are largely offset by potentially more serious ill effects arising from alterations in the coagulation, cardiovascular and hepatobiliary systems.

Changes in Coagulation

The net result of oral contraception is to render the blood more coagulable. Fibrinolytic activity is increased largely by virtue of elevated plasma plasminogen but this is outweighed by complex alterations in the coagulation system. Thus increased platelet sensitivity and aggregation are accompanied by higher levels of Factors I, II, VII and X as

Table 79.2 Precautions in prescribing combined hormonal contraception

Avoid combined oral contraception where there is a history of	*Stop combined oral contraception immediately with*	*Weigh carefully need for oral contraception and monitor closely with*
Thrombotic disorders	Pregnancy	Age >35 years, obesity or smoking
Deranged lipid metabolism	Immobilization	Hypertension
Dubin–Johnson or Rotor syndromes	Surgery intended within 6 weeks	Cardiovascular disease
Acute or severe chronic liver disease	Development or aggravation of migraine	Migraine
Sickle-cell anaemia	Development or aggravation of hypertension	Depression
Mammary or uterine carcinoma	Development of pruritus or jaundice	Epilepsy
Undiagnosed abnormal vaginal bleeding	Development of visual upsets	Otosclerosis
Idiopathic jaundice or severe pruritus in pregnancy	Development of thrombotic disorder	Porphyria
Herpes or worsening of otosclerosis in pregnancy		Tetany
		Hepatic dysfunction
		Gallbladder disease
		Renal disease
		Chloasma
		Uterine fibroids
		Asthma
		Contact lenses
		Diseases prone to worsen in pregnancy

Table 79.3 Drug interaction with oral contraceptives

Probable reduction in contraceptive effect	*Possible reduction in contraceptive effect*
Absorbents—all	Analgesics and NSAIDs
Antacids—all	Aminopyrine
Anti-infectives	Antipyrine
Amoxycillin	Oxyphenbutazone
Ampicillin	Phenacetin
Cephalexin	Phenbutazone
Chloramphenicol	Salicylates
Clindamycin	Antihistamines
Co-trimoxazole	Decongestants
Dapsone	Sedatives/tranquillizers
Erithromycin	Chlordiazepoxide
Griseofulvin	Chlorpromazine
Isoniazide	Diazepam
Neomycin	Dichloralphenazone
Nitrofurantoin	Meprobamate
Penicillin V	
Rifampicin	
Sulphamethoxypyridazine	
Tetracyclines	
Tolampicillin	

Effect of oral contraceptive on interacting drug

Increased effect	*Decreased effect*	*Variable effect*
Aminocaproic acid	Anticoagulants	Anticonvulsants
Bronchodilators	Corticosteroids	
Diazepam	Hypoglycaemics	
Meperidine/pethidine	Hypotensives	
Tricyclic antidepressants		

well as decreased antithrombin III activity. The effect of these changes is amplified both by a reduction in venous flow rate secondary to increased distensibility, and loss of normal fluctuation in whole blood viscosity which remains at the upper limit of normal during treatment.

Although not necessarily all dose-dependent, these adjustments appear due to the oestrogenic component and must contribute largely to the frequency of venous thromboembolism in pill takers, which is 2–4 times that of non-users. There are also constitutional predisposing factors as blood group O is associated with a lower than average risk. The thromboembolic hazard is known to be greater when surgery, particularly abdominal, is carried out on pill takers. Elective operations should not be performed within 4 weeks of stopping the pill and emergency procedures must be covered by effective prophylaxis.

Cardiovascular Risks

Approximately 5% of pill users develop significant but reversible hypertension, possibly related to the progestogenic content. Furthermore, it seems established that oral contraception leads to alterations in carbohydrate and lipid metabolism with impaired glucose tolerance, hypercholesterolaemia and hypertriglyceridaemia. These changes may be in part responsible for the increased risk of myocardial ischaemia, coronary thrombosis and cerebrovascular accidents seen in those on the pill. Susceptibility to these conditions appears to increase with duration of use, age and, most especially, cigarette smoking. Of particular interest to the surgeon are mesenteric arterial and venous thrombosis which, although uncommon, may be more likely in pill takers. The onset of these potentially grave conditions can be insidious and so vague abdominal pain in association with oral contraception must be taken seriously. Hepatic vein thrombosis (Budd–Chiari syndrome) is another rare possible complication of the pill.

Hepatobiliary Complications

Plasma protein concentrations are altered by the pill with a decrease in albumin and increases in the binding globulins. Liver function as judged by bromsulphthalein excretion is impaired in 10–15% of users and this may progress to jaundice in a small number, especially if there is a history of pruritus, cholestasis or jaundice in pregnancy. Women on oral contraception show a twofold increase in gallbladder disease.

Liver tumours are said to be more common in pill takers. Most of the neoplasms reported have been benign and variously designated as hepatic adenoma, hamartoma and focal nodular hyperplasia. The presentation is usually with pain from intratumour or intraperitoneal haemorrhage. Hepatocellular carcinoma is also recorded in pill users although there is no real evidence of increased susceptibility and survival times appear to be significantly longer than those observed in non-users.

ECTOPIC PREGNANCY

By definition ectopic pregnancies are situated outwith the normal uterine cavity. Ninety-five per cent of all cases affect the ampullary or isthmial portions of the fallopian tube; less usual sites are the tubal extremities, ovary, abdominal cavity, cervix or a rudimentary uterine horn.

Frequency and Mortality

Reported frequencies vary from 0·1 to 0·5% of all deliveries in the UK or North America to 3·6% in the West Indies, and the higher rates are characteristic of predominantly black populations. The incidence of ectopic pregnancy appears to have increased over the past two decades as contraception has become more widespread with a possible change in sexual behaviour and a greater risk of pelvic infection. The freer use of antibiotics to retain fertility in damaged fallopian tubes may have contributed as well.

Around 10% of all maternal deaths in the UK are from ectopic pregnancy and a similar proportion of fatalities in the USA are from this cause. Individual series of cases record mortality rates from 0·5% to as high as 7% and delayed surgical intervention is the main cause of poor results. Improvement will require a high index of diagnostic suspicion, especially in view of British experience which suggests that half of the deaths occur before medical assistance can be reached.

Aetiology

The ovum is normally fertilized in the tubal ampulla and takes 4 days to reach the uterine cavity. This transfer is effected by the combined action of muscular peristalsis and endothelial ciliary activity in the fallopian tube. Any delay in transport will result in further growth of the zygote and possibly more important, differentiation with an increasing tendency to implant. Tubal motility may be reduced hormonally, especially by progesterone but the likeliest cause of delay is structural abnormality of the tubal lumen. Thus, congenital diverticula or obstructions secondary to infection, endometriosis, fibromyomas or tubal surgery will encourage ectopic pregnancy. It has been suggested that a shortened luteal phase with premature menstruation might result in retrograde flow carrying an as yet unimplanted zygote from the uterine cavity back into the fallopian tube where it lodges. Transmigration of an ovum to the contralateral tube is another possible cause of delayed transport and ectopic nidation.

Primary ovarian and abdominal pregnancies must be distinguished from those secondary to tubal implantation where the placenta has by growth spread gradually though a tubal rupture or from the fimbria to implant on neighbouring structures. Primary occurrence in these sites is extremely rare and must be the consequence of fertilization of an ovum which is either trapped within the ovary or free in the peritoneal cavity. Cervical pregnancy is a disorder of implantation which presents an entirely different clinical picture and is unlikely to involve the general surgeon.

One would therefore expect an increased risk of ectopic pregnancy in those with a history of previous appendicitis (tubal pregnancies are more often right- than left-sided), abdominal surgery, particularly tubal, involuntary infertility and gonococcal, tuberculous or other salpingitis. Recently, it has been noted that ectopic pregnancy quite frequently complicates contraception with an intrauterine device. Most probably the foreign body is more efficient at preventing intrauterine than tubal implantation and the increased risk of ectopic pregnancy is only apparent relative to the likelihood of an intrauterine pregnancy. Use of hormonal contraceptives, especially progestogens, has also been implicated as a causative factor. Alteration in tubal transport function would seem a plausible explanation of such a connection but to date the evidence is scarcely more than anecdotal.

Pathogenesis

Poor decidual reaction of the endothelium allows the implanting zygote to penetrate the muscular wall of the fallopian tube and form vascular attachments. The enlarging embryo then elevates a thin pseudocapsularis which is liable to burst, especially if situated in the relatively capacious ampulla. This results in death of the embryo followed by deterioration and detachment of the placenta. In this circumstance bleeding may be slight and ultimately absorbed along with the products of conception. Heavier bleeding will provoke tubal peristalsis causing explusion of its contents into the peritoneal cavity (tubal abortion) and muscular contraction may arrest the haemorrhage. An incomplete tubal abortion will almost certainly ensure persistent recurrent bleeding requiring intervention.

Where implantation occurs in a narrower segment, such as the tubal isthmus, the muscular wall is likely to rupture before the capsularis. Blood then escapes freely into the peritoneal cavity or rarely between the layers of the broad ligament. The conceptus perishes but bleeding from the ruptured tube may be profuse. Implantation near the fimbrial end of the tube can result in trophoblastic attachments spreading to the ovary and surrounding structures, giving rise to a secondary ovarian or abdominal pregnancy that may continue to grow and even result in a surviving infant.

Production of chorionic gonadotrophin from the abnormally and insecurely situated trophoblast is often inadequate and thus standard pregnancy tests may be negative and corpus luteal function poorly supported. The uterus undergoes some decidual change and the subject may exhibit symptoms of pregnancy but these effects are unpredictable and often breakthrough uterine bleeding or even expulsion of a decidual cast is noted.

Clinical Features

The usual presentation is lower abdominal pain, secondary amenorrhoea and vaginal bleeding in a woman of childbearing age. There may be a history of infertility, abdominal surgery, pelvic infection or even ectopic pregnancy. Neither surgical sterilization nor employment of contraception excludes the diagnosis; indeed an intrauterine device in situ might heighten the suspicion. Most cases present chronic or subacute symptoms whilst a minority progress to tubal rupture with intraperitoneal haemorrhage. Profound collapse is fortunately uncommon and best avoided by constant clinical vigilance for early pointers to the diagnosis.

Chronic or Subacute Presentation

Lower abdominal pain is the most consistent symptom, usually asymmetric and aching or colicky, resulting from progressive tubal distension and small choriodecidual haemorrhages. Syncope may accompany episodes of pain especially when due to leakage of blood from the fimbria. Epigastric or shoulder tip pain is noticed on lying flat when blood irritates the diaphragm. Amenorrhoea, which occurs in about 80% of cases, is likely to be brief and followed by continuous vaginal blood loss. Occasionally such bleeding can be heavy and even accompanied by passage of an intact or fragmented decidual cast which is easily mistaken for a blood clot. Nausea, vomiting and breast discomfort may not be particularly evident but local peritoneal irritation can cause frequency and dysuria. Accumulation of blood in the pouch of Douglas (pelvic haematocèle) often provokes urinary retention, painful defaecation and occasionally diarrhoea.

Even without circulatory embarrassment, some pallor and tachycardia is likely. An intermittent low-grade pyrexia may follow degradation and absorption of intraperitoneal blood. Breast signs of pregnancy are poorly established. Lower abdominal tenderness with guarding, maximal on the affected side, is almost invariable and there may be peritonism with some bowel distension. Shifting dullness is uncommon but periumbilical bruising (Cullen's sign) sometimes follows longstanding intraperitoneal haemorrhage.

Pelvic examination can precipitate further haemorrhage and so must be gentle; possibly it is better left until after hospital admission which is essential for all suspected cases. Marked tenderness, worse on cervical manipulation, may be the only abnormality noted on vaginal examination. Tender, often ill-defined, adnexal swelling, possibly pulsatile, or fullness in the pouch of Douglas can be found but neither their absence nor palpation of a soft, bulky uterus should be taken to exclude the diagnosis.

Acute Presentation

This dramatic, if uncommon, picture may overtake less acute symptoms or arise unheralded. Typically there is rapid onset of severe abdominal pain and hypovolaemic circulatory shock with marked pallor, poor peripheral circulatory filling, and a rapid thready pulse. The flanks may be dull but guarding can be minimal or even absent. Vaginal examination can cause further blood loss and is better omitted as it provides little additional diagnostic information and delays definitive treatment.

Table 79.4 Flow chart of diagnostic process in ectopic pregnancy

CLINICAL SUSPICION OF ECTOPIC PREGNANCY → OBVIOUS INTRAPERITONEAL HAEMORRHAGE → LAPAROTOMY

CLINICAL SUSPICION OF ECTOPIC PREGNANCY → NO OBVIOUS INTRAPERITONEAL HAEMORRHAGE → CULDOCENTESIS AND/OR PERITONEAL ASPIRATION

CULDOCENTESIS AND/OR PERITONEAL ASPIRATION → INCOAGULABLE BLOOD → LAPAROTOMY

CULDOCENTESIS AND/OR PERITONEAL ASPIRATION → NO INCOAGULABLE BLOOD → LAPAROSCOPY

Confirmation of Diagnosis (*Table* 79.4)

Only chronic or subacute cases are likely to present any problems in this regard. Haematological investigation may reveal anaemia and even leucocytosis if the haemoperitoneum has been longstanding. Pregnancy tests do not discriminate between ectopic and normally sited pregnancies and conventional immunological methods are positive in only about 50% of tubal gestations. Highly specific kits for the detection of the beta subunit of chorionic gonadotrophin are increasingly available and should be positive in virtually all cases of ectopic pregnancy.

Expert ultrasonography may show an intrauterine or ectopic gestation but can be misleading and is more useful in alerting one to the possibility of tubal pregnancy rather than in confirmation of the diagnosis (*Fig.* 79.3).

Culdocentesis

Needling of the pouch of Douglas through the posterior vaginal fornix is easily accomplished even in the conscious patient. Aspiration of non-clotting blood suggests intraperitoneal bleeding; however, a negative test is unreliable.

Examination under Anaesthesia

Although a frequent recourse in doubtful cases, vaginal examination in this situation is little better than in the conscious patient, and if less gentle is even more likely to precipitate haemorrhage. It should be followed by unequivocal diagnosis from pelvic visualization rather than risk overlooking further bleeding with an unexpected crisis later. Examination under anaesthesia has been justified by the need for uterine curettage but this is of dubious value. The histological report is inevitably delayed and there is risk of disturbing an intrauterine pregnancy. Uterine curettings reported as showing definite decidual reaction without accompanying chorionic tissue, strongly suggest an ectopic gestation. Not infrequently, however, the decidua has already been shed and the pathologist's report is unhelpful or even misleading.

Laparoscopy

Most probably it is prudent to inspect the pelvis in all cases where unconfirmed suspicion of ectopic pregnancy remains. Positive culdocentesis would indicate laparotomy and laparoscopy will clarify the remainder. Laparotomy should be substituted for laparoscopy if blood is aspirated from the Verre's needle prior to induction of pneumoperitoneum. Intra-abdominal gas pressure should be kept as low as possible to avoid gas embolism and it should be remembered that ectopic pregnancy is only reliably excluded when the entire length of both Fallopian tubes, ovaries, the uterus and pouch of Douglas have been inspected, assisted if necessary by manipulation of the uterus *per vaginam.*

Culdoscopy/Posterior Colpotomy

Culdoscopy is potentially dangerous because of the need for the knee–chest position and risk of the trocar penetrating the uterus or other structures involved with a pelvic haematocele. Posterior colpotomy offers little more than culdocentesis as visualization of the pelvis is incomplete but could be considered in those few cases where laparoscopy proves contraindicated or impossible.

Differential Diagnosis

Ectopic pregnancy often mimics other gynaecological or surgical conditions and history is the most important consideration in reaching a correct conclusion as physical signs are often rather non-specific. The important conditions to be distinguished are those that would not normally call for surgical treatment.

Dysmenorrhoea

Symptoms of pregnancy, unilateral pain, syncope and an abnormal pattern of bleeding would not be expected in this case.

Abortion of an Intrauterine Pregnancy

Bleeding almost always precedes the pain, which is symmetrical, whilst fainting or dizziness are unlikely. Abdominal

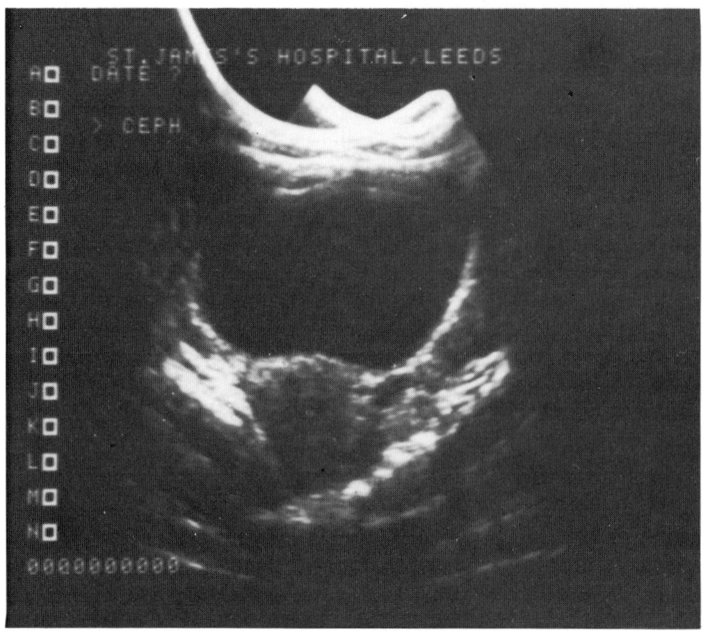

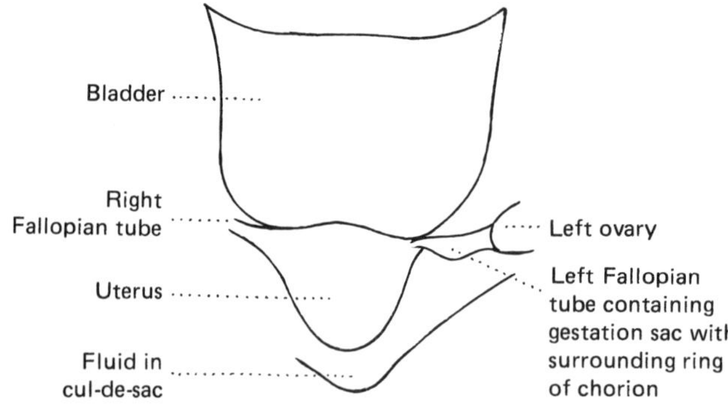

Fig. 79.3 Transverse ultrasound scan of abdomen showing left tubal pregnancy.

signs should be minimal and intrauterine products of conception may be confirmed ultrasonically or even digitally if cervical dilatation has begun. The problem becomes more complex if there is an additional pelvic mass, such as fibroids or an ovarian cyst, especially if painful because of degeneration, torsion, haemorrhage or rupture. Laparoscopy will often be required for a correct diagnosis.

Salpingitis

This is another situation where surgery should be avoided if possible. Slight irregularity of the menses can occur and pain may be somewhat asymmetric. However, syncope is most unlikely and there should not be diaphragmatic irritation. The signs are usually bilateral, possibly with swollen, tender, uterine appendages and often a purulent urethral or cervical discharge. Both pyrexia and leucocytosis would be expected. Exacerbation of a chronic pelvic infection presents particular difficulty as ectopic pregnancy is a potential complication. Culdocentesis may be inappropriate in many such cases and laparoscopy could be required.

Degeneration of a Fibroid

Whether accompanied by pregnancy or not, vaginal bleeding is unlikely and the pain is usually central. A tender, uterine irregularity may be palpated and careful ultrasonography often confirms the clinical impression.

Other Gynaecological Accidents

Torsion, rupture or haemorrhage involving ovarian cysts, tumours or pedunculated fibroids almost all require surgery and so differential diagnosis is less important. All these situations can resemble ectopic pregnancy so closely that laparotomy is indicated, irrespective of the precise cause of symptoms. Where minor haemorrhage has come from a follicular, corpus luteal or endometriotic cyst, the timing at midcycle or onset of menstruation is suggestive and might encourage conservatism, which will be rewarded by swift resolution of the symptoms and signs. More severe and persistent cases require laparoscopy if one is to avoid overlooking an early tubal pregnancy.

Surgical Conditions

Severe haemorrhage from ruptured aneurysm or intra-abdominal organs requires early surgery as do acute appendicitis and gastrointestinal perforation. It would be undesirable to approach an ectopic pregnancy through a grid-iron incision but this diagnosis should not be confused as acute appendicitis is usually accompanied by vomiting rather than by amenorrhoea, faintness or menstrual disturbance and the patient is flushed with localized rigidity of the abdominal wall. Renal colic is easily excluded by examination of the urine and radiography, if an early pregnancy can be ruled out.

Treatment

All suspected cases should be transferred to hospital with as little delay as possible. If shocked the patient must be kept flat and undisturbed. Vaginal examination should be avoided. An intravenous infusion is required and preliminary blood samples for haemoglobin, grouping and cross-matching are saved, especially if plasma expanders, such as dextrans, are to be used. Blood or plasma is the ideal replacement fluid. Morphine or pethidine, in careful dosage to avoid further hypotension, may be given for pain. This resuscitation can be accomplished in the patient's home by a flying squad but fine judgement is necessary if by summoning such aid, there will be prolonged, possibly fatal, delay in transfer of the patient to hospital.

Once decided upon, laparotomy should not be delayed. Resuscitation will proceed as swiftly as possible but in severely shocked cases improvement is unlikely until the bleeding vessels are secured. The abdomen is opened through a paramedian or low transverse incision, when the damaged tube is identified usually by palpation, and a hand used to control bleeding. If necessary, autotransfusion can be employed by removing and sieving the intraperitoneal blood which is citrated (20 ml sodium citrate to 100 ml blood) before replacement.

Choice of Operation

Unless limited by the gravity of the patient's condition, the opposite tube and ovary should be inspected before deciding upon an appropriate surgical procedure. Where preservation of reproductive capacity is desirable and especially if the opposite tube is significantly abnormal, every effort should be made to conserve function on the affected side. In some cases tubal damage and haemorrhage are slight so that the pregnancy can be milked from the fimbrial opening or through a small longitudinal incision in the antimesosalpingeal border of the tube. Provided haemostasis can be secured, a future pregnancy may be achieved. In other cases partial salpingectomy, leaving the tubal lumen unoccluded or everted as a cuff salpingostomy, may be employed. When salpingectomy is inevitable, salpingo-oophorectomy should be considered as an alternative which will ensure that all subsequent ovulation is from the opposite undamaged side. This option would of course be inappropriate if the opposite ovary was absent or functionless.

In cases where the placenta has gained attachment to neighbouring structures it should be removed or trimmed so far as is compatible with control of the resulting bleeding surface. Any retained tissue is normally absorbed in time. Hysterectomy may occasionally be considered in older women with additional pelvic pathology provided they are in good condition.

Surgery should be concluded by the covering of raw surface as completely as possible and peritoneal lavage. The specimens removed should be examined histologically and cultured for tuberculosis. The patient should be warned of the 10–15% chance of recurrence and advised to present for care early in future pregnancy.

Almost certainly some undiagnosed cases of ectopic pregnancy subside spontaneously. However, in general, surgical treatment is to be preferred to conservative management with its unpredictable risks.

ACUTE PELVIC INFECTION

The uterus, fallopian tubes, ovaries and pelvic connective tissues are all affected to some extent in most cases of pelvic infection. Excluding infection following pregnancy, involvement of the uterus is less frequent and clinically less striking than disease in the adnexae. Primary infection results from organisms ascending through the cervix which is more likely when host resistance is impaired. The risk of infection thus increases in association with intrauterine foreign bodies, haemorrhagic collections or necrotic tissue; abortion or childbirth; surgical, radiation or accidental trauma and post-menopausal atrophy. Secondary infection of the pelvis may follow appendicitis, diverticulitis or peritonitis from any cause, malignant disease of bowel or bladder and haematogenous spread from a more distant site. The general surgeon is more likely to encounter this problem in its acute form, possibly superimposed on a chronic condition, and would hope to recognize it so avoiding inappropriate surgery. This section is therefore restricted to consideration of acute pelvic sepsis.

Severe puerperal and postabortal pelvic infection is now rather uncommon; however, an increasing number of cases are seen in association with intrauterine contraceptive devices. Although sometimes secondary to other abdominal pathology, much the commonest cause of salpingitis is recent or recurrent venereal infection. There has been a marked increase in the prevalence of gonorrhoea and even more in so-called non-specific genital infection over the past two decades. Negroes appear to be particularly at risk and overall the distribution has shifted to the younger age groups. This may reflect changes in contraceptive and sexual practice. Barrier methods which can be protective, have become less acceptable and concern has been expressed about the safety of oral contraception. Wider use of intrauterine devices, even in nulliparae, may in itself have contributed to the problem. Salpingitis is said to follow 10–15% of gonorrhoeal infection of the lower genital tract but this could be an underestimate as the condition is often barely symptomatic and easily overlooked in the female.

Pathology

The changes are those of acute infection anywhere with modifications depending upon the infecting organism and its anatomical site.

Endometritis

Cyclic shedding of the endometrium and free drainage through the cervix make it difficult for bacteria to gain a hold in the uterus. Foreign bodies, necrotic tissue or trauma, especially if there has been a recent pregnancy, encourage infection which results in typical inflammatory infiltration of the endometrium and to a lesser extent, the myometrium. Obstruction of the cervical canal encourages the formation of a pyometra with uterine enlargement from distension of the cavity and inflammatory oedema of the myometrium. The uterotubal junctions may be blocked but spread to the tubes via pelvic connective tissues is common if the causative organism is at all invasive.

Salpingo-oophoritis

Salpingitis is the commonest form of pelvic infection and is usually contracted primarily from sexual transmission but may follow spread from a uterine, gastrointestinal or more distant primary focus. The pathological changes differ with the site of infection, either endosalpingeal or exosalpingeal.

Endosalpingeal infection is typically gonococcal and if progressive causes a pyosalpinx with distal and proximal tubal blockage. The fimbriae fuse and the endothelial lining is extensively damaged. A sterile hydrosalpinx may be the end result with impaired fertility.

The exosalpingeal variant follows direct intraperitoneal, blood or lymphatic-borne infection and the inflammatory process establishes in the muscular wall so that the lumen is narrowed, even closed by numerous adhesions. The fimbriae are less likely to be extensively destroyed. This picture is seen in the puerperal or postabortal infection.

Whichever form salpingitis takes, the ovary is almost certainly involved to the extent of adhering to the tubal fimbriae. The combined inflammatory mass lies in the pouch of Douglas forming a characteristic retort-shaped swelling. Bowel and omentum seal the area and a pelvic abscess if it forms, may point through the bladder, posterior vaginal fornix or rectum. Rarely, an intraligamentary abscess follows the round ligament to present in the groin. Occasionally an abscess ruptures intraperitoneally causing profound shock from the release of infected pus. Such a calamity can be spontaneous but rough manipulation might also be responsible.

Suppurative thrombophlebitis may complicate severe pelvic infection, especially when the connective tissues are significantly involved. Pyaemic abscesses can follow circulatory spread of infected clots whilst major thromboembolic catastrophes are an ever present danger.

Microbiology

Precise definition of the microbiology of pelvic inflammatory disease has been hampered by inaccessibility as cervical cultures need not reflect the pelvic pathogens. Culture of specimens obtained by culdocentesis, laparoscopy and laparotomy is now helping to clarify matters. Either *Neisseria gonorrhoeae* or *Chlamydia trachomatis* are the primary invaders in 2 out of 3 cases but secondary infection soon follows. *Neisseria gonorrhoeae* disappears early in tubal infections but may persist in urethral, vaginal and cervical secretions. Chlamydia which would appear to be the most important cause of 'non-specific genital infection', is hardier and has been isolated from the pelvis in more than 50% of patients with acute pelvic infection. In many areas chlamydia may be the commonest cause of this disease. *Mycoplasma hominis* has been reported as a primary invader much less frequently, judging from published figures.

Secondary spread from vaginal flora may replace the primary invaders or initiate infection complicating intrauterine manipulation, foreign bodies or necrotic tissue. Anaerobes which may be isolated include bacteroides, streptococci, and even *Clostridium welchii* or *tetani*. The likely aerobes are streptococci, staphylococci, *Escherichia coli* and *Haemophilus influenzae*. Other enterobacteria, such as proteus, pyocyaneus or even salmonella species, may become involved. *Mycobacterium tuberculosis* and actinomyces can cause chronic pelvic infection but acute disease is unlikely unless there is secondary invasion.

Thus the predominant infective agent may be difficult to isolate and identify. Cervical cultures are more reliable in the early stages whilst later it is necessary to examine blood and samples collected at culdocentesis, laparoscopy and laparotomy. Direct inoculation of specimens into specific transport media is desirable, indeed essential for *N. gonorrhoeae*, and culture techniques must be chosen in light of the probable pathogens. Beta-lactamase-producing variants of *N. gonorrhoeae* which are particularly prevalent on the West coasts of America and Africa, have been the subject of recent concern because of their insensitivity to the common antibiotics. Europe so far is relatively free of this problem.

Viruses such as human papillomavirus and herpes simplex are causing increasing concern as possible carcinogens involving the lower genital tract and there seems no doubt that human immunovirus infection can be acquired through coitus. As yet there is no clear evidence of viral involvement in infection of the upper genital tract; however this may only reflect difficulties in obtaining suitable material for culture and change with wider use of diagnostic laparoscopy in such cases.

Clinical Presentation

There may be a history of involuntary infertility, ectopic pregnancy or earlier acute attacks. Menorrhagia, dysmenorrhoea and dyspareunia could point to chronic pelvic infection. Recent sexual contact may be admitted and the presence of an intrauterine device is suggestive, particularly if newly inserted. Unilateral disease and septic abortions are associated with intrauterine devices but salpingitis complicating a progressing pregnancy is extremely rare.

Symptoms include malaise, fatigue, pyrexia and rigors with pain as the single most common complaint. The pain is lower abdominal, constant, bilateral, often severe but not excruciating, and may radiate to the lumbosacral area. The acute episode often arises around the time of menstruation which may be a little early or late and even prolonged. Purulent urethral or cervicovaginal discharge is quite common although easily overlooked. Frequency and dysuria are seen in a minority of cases whilst retention of urine suggests a pelvic abscess. Nausea and vomiting are infrequent complaints and lower bowel symptoms such as constipation, tenesmus and diarrhoea even less so.

Signs of general toxicity vary, with fever (>38 °C) and tachycardia present only in the more severe cases. Lower abdominal tenderness is usually bilateral with guarding rather than rigidity, and rebound is unlikely. Distension, if present, is slight and bowel sounds are usually normal. A palpable abdominal mass develops late if at all, unless the acute process has complicated fibroids, an ovarian swelling or a recent pregnancy.

Urethral discharge is best demonstrated and cultured after milking the urethra to express pus from Skene's glands and ducts. Bartholinitis and cervicovaginitis should be sought and culture specimens taken. Bimanually the vagina may feel hot and cervical movement causes pain. Adnexal tenderness is bilateral as a rule and may mask tubal swelling which tends to be minimal or even absent in early cases. Tubo-ovarian masses form a retort shape with the wider extremity curling back to adhere in the pouch of Douglas and onto the posterior leaf of the broad ligament. On rectal examination it may be fluctuant and lies mainly anterior to the examining finger.

Confirmation of Diagnosis

Accurate diagnosis is important in avoidance of inappropriate surgery but the difficulties are well exemplified by the experience of a gynaecological unit in which over 800 cases of suspected acute pelvic infection were subjected to confirmatory laparoscopy or laparotomy. Abdominopelvic visualization revealed no macroscopic pathology in 23% and a different aetiology in a further 12% of cases. Conversely, 10% of those ultimately shown to have acute pelvic infection were unsuspected prior to visual inspection undertaken with a different preoperative diagnosis.

Haematological assessment can provide some help, as both a polymorphonuclear leucocytosis and an elevated erythrocyte sedimentation rate are to be expected with pelvic infection. Excepting menorrhagia from pre-existent chronic disease, the haemoglobin should be normal. Urethral and especially cervical cultures may grow chlamydia, *N. gonorrhoeae* or almost any other organism, although not necessarily representing the predominant organism within the pelvis.

Radiography can exclude intestinal obstruction and indicate a pelvic mass which ultrasonography will confirm as structurally complex without determining its precise nature. Aspiration of pus through a wide-bore needle from the pouch of Douglas, establishes a diagnosis and provides culture material; however, there is at least a theoretical risk of injury to the bowel.

Laparoscopy has proved safe in such cases and will usually provide both pathological and bacteriological diagnosis. There is, therefore, an argument for the procedure in all cases where either the need for laparotomy cannot be confidently excluded or poor response to therapy dictates confirmation of the diagnosis and more accurate bacteriological guidance.

The conditions likely to cause diagnostic confusion are mainly gynaecological, although acute appendicitis can present problems. In the latter case, upper gastrointestinal symptoms are much commoner and there is typical localization of the signs with less pyrexia and leucocytosis.

Ectopic pregnancy may be difficult to exclude and has been considered already. Haemorrhage from pelvic endometriosis or a corpus luteum usually subsides with time and is not accompanied by general toxicity, pyrexia and leucocytosis. Ovarian tumours when painful because of infection, torsion, haemorrhage or slow leakage differ in that the swelling presents at the onset of symptoms and is usually better defined, unilateral and cystic. Ultrasound examination may assist and occasionally radiography demonstrates calcification of a cyst wall or even a tooth. Similar considerations apply to fibroids whether infected, twisted or undergoing degeneration.

Treatment (*Table* 79.5)

With a few exceptions the treatment of acute pelvic infection is medical, comprising bed rest, general supportive measures and appropriate antibiotics in adequate dosage. Thromboembolic complications of immobilization can be countered by use of a cradle to encourage free movement of the lower limbs and compression stockings; low dose heparin or dextran may be considered advisable on occasions. Good urinary output must be maintained by a high fluid intake supplemented intravenously, if necessary. Persistent vomiting or severe diarrhoea requires serum electrolyte estimations with correction if indicated; central venous pressure monitoring should be instituted if there is circulatory insufficiency. Chronic anaemia secondary to menorrhagia may be reversed by transfusion but excessive replacement is undesirable as regional blood flow is better when haemoglobin and blood viscosity are on the low side of normal.

Choice of an antibiotic regime must be made blindly

Table 79.5 Action flow chart in acute pelvic infection

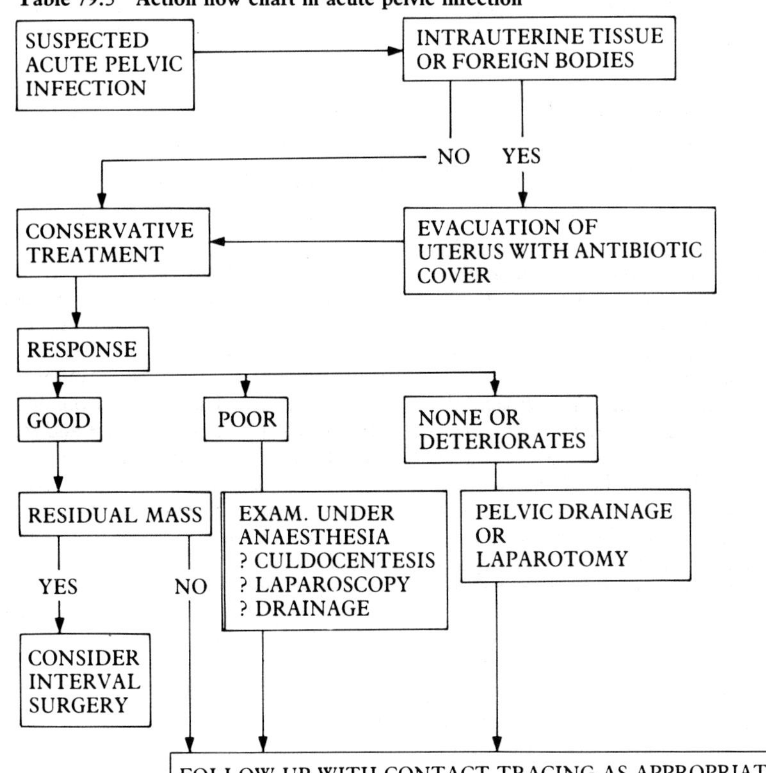

whilst awaiting bacterial sensitivities. Where previous local study has identified the usual causative pathogens, choice of treatment is easier. However, a combination of two drugs will usually be required to be effective against the likely invaders both aerobic and anaerobic. In mild to moderate cases, oral erythromycin stearate or oxytetracycline along with metronidazole would be a suitable selection. More severe cases would be better treated with an intravenous infusion of metronidazole and bolus injections of cephradine or erythromycin lactobionate (the latter is preferred when chlamydia is involved). The antibiotic regime should be reviewed according to clinical response and the laboratory culture sensitivities.

Antibiotics are continued until symptoms and pyrexia have subsided for several days which can take 2 weeks in severe cases. Poor response to treatment suggests incorrect diagnosis, inappropriate choice of antibiotics or abscess formation, possibly with intraperitoneal leakage.

Intraperitoneal Rupture

Although sometimes gradual and fortunately uncommon, intraperitoneal rupture of the pelvic abscess can be sudden with severe shock to a degree in keeping with the amount of purulent spillage. The temperature may rise or more ominously fall and tachycardia increases. Endotoxic shock can develop with circulatory failure despite a warm vasodilated periphery. General peritonitis with ileus and increasing distension of the bowel soon follows. Renal or coagulation failure are additional potential complications. Circulatory and metabolic support with corticosteroid supplementation will be required urgently. Detailed management of the condition is described in Chapter 3. Immediate laparotomy is mandatory with, at minimum, peritoneal lavage.

Surgical Measures

When response to conservative treatment is unsatisfactory a useful first step is examination under anaesthesia. This permits reassessment unhampered by tenderness but manipulation must be gentle with the risk of intraperitoneal rupture in mind. One may then proceed to whatever appears the most appropriate surgical response.

Uterine Curettage

This is indicated when infection has complicated an abortion which may be incomplete. Evacuation of the necrotic, infected remnants of choriodecidual tissue by gentle blunt curettage, should be carried out 24 h after establishing adequate antibiotic cover. An intrauterine device, if present, is removed. Cautious intrauterine manipulation is essential as the infected myometrium is soft and perforation can occur without the surgeon being aware of anything untoward.

Culdocentesis (*Fig.* 79.4)

At least fresh specimens for bacteriological assessment should be obtained by aspiration of the abscess via the posterior vaginal fornix with a large-bore needle. Thick pus may nevertheless defy aspiration and effective drainage is undoubtedly to be preferred especially if it can be accomplished through the posterior vaginal fornix.

Posterior Colpotomy (*Fig.* 79.5)

An abscess in the pouch of Douglas, particularly if dissecting the rectovaginal septum, should be amenable to drainage through the posterior vaginal fornix. After drawing the cervix downwards and anteriorly, a transverse incision is made in the posterior fornix and the abscess cavity is laid open with scissors or forceps. Loculations or a contralateral abscess should be sought and treated similarly to achieve complete drainage.

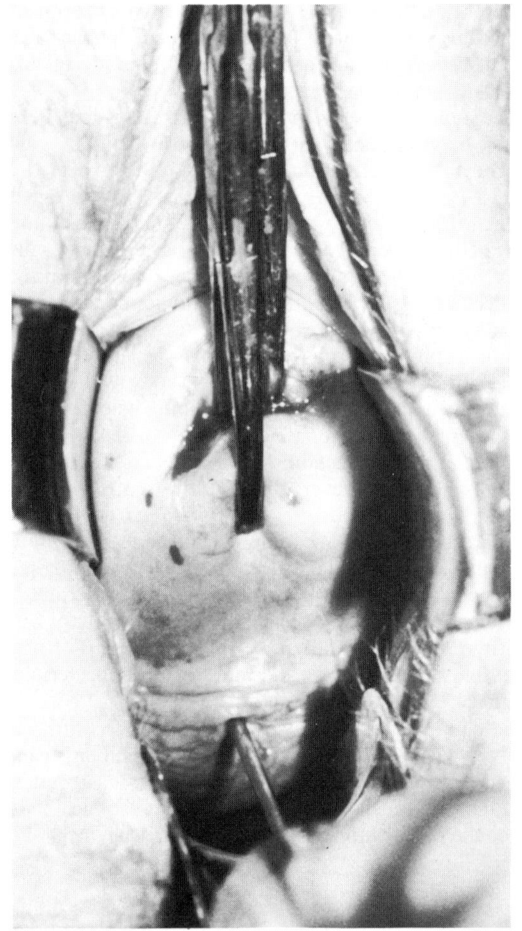

Fig. 79.4 Culdocentesis. Aspiration of the cul-de-sac using syringe and large-bore needle.

Extraperitoneal Drainage

Pelvic cellulitis may progress to a broad ligament abscess which can be drained extraperitoneally from an incision just above the inguinal ligament.

Laparoscopy

This is an appropriate course of action for confirmation of an uncertain diagnosis and collection of intraperitoneal bacteriological specimens. It would be contraindicated in the presence of general peritonitis or bowel distension, both of which make laparotomy a safer and more useful alternative.

Laparotomy

An abdominal approach must be chosen for drainage of a tubo-ovarian abscess which is not accessible vaginally. Laparotomy is also required when there is suspicion that a pelvic abscess may have ruptured intraperitoneally. Collection of culture specimens, thorough drainage and peritoneal lavage are obvious first steps. Additional measures are more controversial. In managing spontaneous intraperitoneal rupture of a pelvic abscess, some authorities advocate proceeding, where possible, to subtotal hysterectomy with bilateral

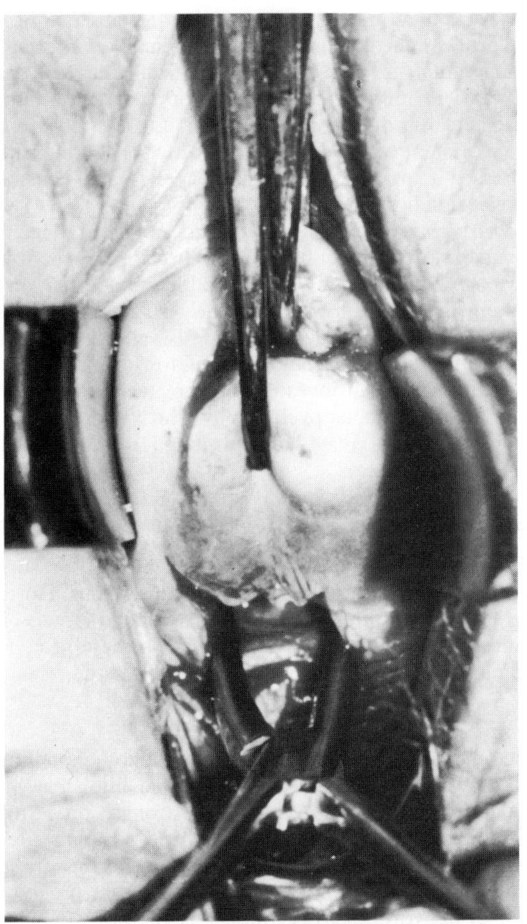

Fig. 79.5 Posterior colpotomy. Exploration of cul-de-sac with sinus forceps after transverse incision in posterior vaginal fornix.

salpingo-oophorectomy. Preservation of ovarian tissue is almost certainly impossible in this situation. Others would consider removal of a closed pyosalpinx the maximum justifiable. Yet another approach which appears to be winning growing support, is the strategic placement of suitably atraumatic Portex or similar tubing, so as to permit postoperative circulation of isotonic antiseptic or antibiotic solutions within the peritoneal cavity. It is difficult to assess these rather different philosophies. Complete or nearly complete removal of a septic focus has clear advantages as well as potential dangers. Certainly prolonged or difficult surgical procedures in a gravely ill patient might be fatal. Neither approach has been shown superior to the other nor are they mutually exclusive, but at present choice must be left to individual surgeons and made on the basis of specific circumstances.

Whichever surgical approach is employed the abdomen should be closed without conventional drainage and intensive parenteral antibiotic therapy is continued, modified as necessary by new culture data. The use of Fowler's position may reduce the risk of subphrenic collections of pus. Renal and hepatic function must be carefully monitored as impairment can have significant effects on drug metabolism with implications for dosage. Active measures to discourage thromboembolic sequelae are necessary but mobilization should be delayed until the pyrexia and toxaemia are clearly waning, if not resolved. Active encouragement of respiratory excursion and circulation in the lower limbs, as suggested earlier, would seem prudent but the use of anticoagulants might be better avoided in the postoperative situation.

Intra-abdominal rupture of a pelvic abscess with general peritonitis and septic shock is the most serious complication of pelvic infection and mortality with conventional treatment can exceed 30% if treatment is not swift and sure. In other cases future fertility is the main hostage to fortune. Follow-up should be close and coitus forbidden until pelvic examination suggests that the condition is quiescent. Chronic inflammatory disease with menstrual and coital problems is a likely outcome which may dictate pelvic clearance after a suitable interval. Where hopes of future fertility still flicker, prolonged treatment with antibiotics and short-wave diathermy can be tried. Prospects are certainly poor and attempts to demonstrate tubal patency may only serve to reinfect or aggravate dormant septic foci. Early effective antibiotic treatment which prevents abscess formation affords the best prospect of preserving fertility but at the cost of increasing susceptibility to ectopic pregnancy. In proven cases of infection with gonococcus or chlamydia, contact tracing should be arranged. One must also consider whether concomitant syphilitic infection may have been masked by antibiotics and if so undertake serological testing and follow-up.

ENDOMETRIOSIS

Endometriosis is characterized by ectopically situated, endometrial-like tissue which bleeds in response to ovarian stimulation. Repeated haemorrhage with incomplete reabsorption leads to collections of viscous fluid resembling melted tar or chocolate, and provokes marked fibrous reaction in the surrounding tissues. The continuing process can cause extensive structural damage and considerable pain which is exacerbated during menstruation.

The ovaries, pelvic peritoneum, fallopian tubes and uterine serosa are the sites most commonly affected; however, skin, bowel and bladder may be involved and there are reports of endometriosis in the kidneys, stomach, lungs and pleura. Such diversity has stimulated much ingenuity in establishing the likely aetiology. Suggestions have included implantation, transplantation, direct or metastatic spread of uterine endometrium, as well as various types of tissue metamorphosis. Some or several combinations of these possibilities would seem essential to account satisfactorily for all forms of the condition.

Endometriosis is found between the menarche and the menopause, most often in the third and fourth decades; however, developmental abnormality with haematocolpos, haematometra and haematosalpinges, encourages earlier onset. Infertility, subfertility and low parity are frequent associations which may explain an apparent predilection for the Caucasian and well-to-do. Equally it is possible that the better-off present their problems for treatment more readily. Evidence of endometriosis has been found in 5–25% of women subjected to laparotomy although such a population is necessarily selected. Wider application of more accurate diagnostic methods may establish similar rates in groups previously thought to be less susceptible.

The macroscopic appearances range from discrete patches on the ovaries or pouch of Douglas to sizeable chocolate cysts which seal the pelvis, fixing the uterus in retroposition. Surrounding fibrous reaction tends to be dense and healing may cause considerable scarring. Surprisingly intraluminal blockage of the tubes is unlikely despite peritubal adhesions which may be extensive involving the ovary and other adjacent structures. The rectosigmoid colon is often affected by widespread pelvic endometriosis and on occasions small bowel as well. Induration and nodularity of the uterosacral ligaments is common and spread to the rectovaginal septum can progress to emerge in the rectum or posterior vaginal fornix.

Clinical Features

Typically the picture is of painful, heavy periods with deep dyspareunia in women of 25–35 years who have few, if any, children. Occasionally the onset is acute, requiring emergency hospitalization because an endometriotic cyst has ruptured intraperitoneally, around the time of menstruation. More commonly symptoms are chronic with constant lower abdominal or sacral pain which is initially synchronous with menstruation, anticipating it progressively thereafter. Defaecation may be an aggravating factor and pain can be referred to the rectum, perineum or thighs.

Menorrhagia with passage of clots is likely and periodicity can be altered when there is ovarian involvement or other associated endocrine disturbance. Mucosal foci in the bladder or rectum cause cyclical haematuria or rectal bleeding. Deep dyspareunia suggests fixation of adnexal lesions in the pouch of Douglas, implants in the uterosacral ligaments or infiltration of the rectovaginal septum. Fear of painful coitus may invoke protective vaginismus and superficial dyspareunia. Surgeons must bear in mind that fibrous healing of lesions involving the lower bowel can continue following castration or the menopause causing distortion or even obstruction.

Curiously the physical signs do not always match the symptoms, and gross pathology, with little if any discomfort, is encountered almost as frequently as the converse. Sensitivity to the ovarian cycle means that physical findings are exaggerated around menstruation. Endometriotic cysts are usually fixed within the pelvis to some extent and so are palpable abdominally only if unusually large. Nevertheless, tenderness may be elicited on deep palpation of the lower abdomen superior to the inguinal ligaments.

Speculum examination of the vagina exposes lesions in the posterior fornix when present, and suggests uterine retroversion if the cervic points towards the symphysis pubis. Bimanual palpation of the pelvis vaginally or rectovaginally, reveals any tenderness or abdominal swellings as well as uterine size, position and mobility. Nodular thickening of the uterosacral ligaments with tenderness on stretching them, may be the only positive finding in less severe cases. Involvement of the ovaries causes tender enlargement and fixation to the pelvic side wall or posterior broad ligament. When extensive, endometriosis may result in retroversion of the uterus which, along with tubes and ovaries, forms a tender irregular fixed mass within the pelvis. Rupture of an endometriotic cyst presents as an acute abdomen, the severity depending upon the amount of peritoneal contamination and free bleeding.

Confirmation of Diagnosis

Despite a confident clinical diagnosis, visualization is needed for accurate assessment of the extent of the disease. This will be at laparotomy where the presentation has been acute; otherwise laparoscopy should be preferred to culdoscopy. Diagnostic curettage of the uterus is performed to exclude other causes of abnormal uterine bleeding.

Uterine fibroids frequently coexist with endometriosis; however, they are distinguished by the absence of pain, tenderness and fixation unless additionally complicated by degeneration, torsion, infection or haemorrhage.

Transient mild pyrexia and leucocytosis can occur with endometriosis during menstruation but are more marked and persistent with *pelvic infection* which is also indicated by increased temperature within the pelvis and evidence of lower genital infection.

Ovarian malignancy usually occurs in an older age group and the features do not fluctuate cyclically. The possibility is obvious when ascites is demonstrable but the risk of overlooking ovarian cancer in the early stages underlines the value of laparoscopy. *Diverticulitis* also affects an older age group and radiological studies should resolve the situation.

Additional useful investigations are testing of tubal patency and intravenous pyelography which is desirable when extensive disease may have displaced or obstructed the ureters.

Treatment

The management of endometriosis is medical or surgical, depending upon age and reproductive intentions. Hormonal therapy, often supplemented by conservative surgery, is the choice when enhancement of fertility is the object. Pelvic clearance is the most effective approach for the remainder.

Hormonal Therapy

The object of medical treatment is reduction or abolition of withdrawal bleeding in the endometrial implants. Simple ovulation suppression even with a strongly progestogenic combined contraceptive pill, has little atrophic effect as periods persist. Menstruation which may become irregular, also occurs during continuous dosage with a progestogen, such as dehydrogesterone; however, therapeutic benefit is seen quite often.

The most potent medical regimes are pseudopregnancy and pseudomenopause, so called because of the way they suspend menstrual loss. Oestrogen-progestogen mixtures in which the progestogen effect is predominant, imitate pregnancy if taken continuously for 6–9 months. Although the initial effects are proliferative and heavy bleeding can follow premature interruption of treatment, the ultimate result is atrophy with improvement of the endometriosis. Even more attractive is the use of danazol, an antigonadotrophic agent which produces a menopause-like state. There is considerable clinical as well as theoretical support for regarding this as the best available option despite its expense. The drug is given in divided doses to a total of 400–800 mg daily for 6 months or longer in severe cases. Prospects of a lasting cure are inversely proportional to the extent of the disease and as no medical regime can be expected to reverse widespread structural damage, additional surgical measures may be needed.

Surgical Treatment

Conservative

This is essentially a matter of tidying up the pelvis. Adhesions are broken down, endometriotic deposits are excised or cauterized as appropriate and the maximum possible amount of healthy ovarian tissue is preserved. The procedure is completed by ventrosuspension of the uterus and peritoneal lavage. Simultaneous presacral neurectomy for pain relief is a more controversial practice. Should the diagnosis be first made at operation it is wise to follow-up with a course of hormonal therapy unless surgical cure is complete.

Radical

Removal of uterus, tubes and ovaries is the surgical equivalent of the menopause provided all ovarian tissue is excised. This is often technically demanding when the pelvis is frozen, requiring judicious use of sharp and blunt dissection. Medial displacement of the ureters in the vicinity of the uterosacral ligaments is a potential hazard which should be borne in mind.

OVARIAN TUMOURS

Most adnexal swellings are ovarian although the broad ligament, fallopian tubes or even uterus can be sites of origin. Any enlargement of the ovary constitutes a tumour and thus the term embraces a spectrum ranging from physiological enlargement through functional disorders to benign and malignant neoplasms. Separation of the physiological from pathological and benign from malignant is of particular concern when considering the preservation or sacrifice of an organ with the functional importance of the ovary. Distinction is frequently difficult but a decision for removal should be based on better grounds than the mere fact that the other ovary will remain.

Table 79.6 lists the causes of ovarian enlargement. *Simple hypertrophy* is rare and only confirmed by exclusion following surgical or pathological section. *Cystic change* in an ovary is synonymous with active function and fluctuates through the menstrual cycle. The Graafian follicle and luteal phase corpus luteum usually measure no more than 2–3 cm, rarely if ever exceeding 5 cm.

Table 79.6 Causes of ovarian enlargement

Hypertrophy

Distension cysts
- Follicular
- Corpus luteal
- Granulosa or theca lutein

Endometriotic cysts

Infection

Ovarian pregnancy

Primary neoplasms
- Benign
- Malignant

Secondary neoplasms

A *follicular cyst* is an overdistended Graafian follicle due to haemorrhage or excess clear fluid. It is unilocular with a smooth thin wall and measures no more than 10 cm. The cyst usually reflects a failure of ovulation, appearing around mid-cycle and shrinking over the next few weeks. The subsequent menstrual loss can be delayed. A *corpus luteal cyst* arises later in the cycle, and is more prone to haemorrhage either internal or external. In size it is similar to a follicular cyst but the walls tend to be yellow tinged and thicker. Typical convolutions are usually lost with distension. The menstrual cycle is more likely to be regular and a corpus luteal cyst may persist into the third month of pregnancy. *Granulosa/theca lutein cysts* are multiple and arise from excessive ovarian stimulation or periovarian fibrosis, with less striking enlargement in the latter case. Excessive endogenous stimulation is seen with metropathia haemorrhagica, hydatidiform mole or choriocarcinoma, whilst ovulation induction is the obvious exogenous cause. The ovary can swell to a considerable size causing symptoms from distension, torsion or rupture, but withdrawal of the stimulus is followed by regression.

Endometriotic cysts of the ovary often coexist with deposits of the same disease elsewhere in the pelvis. Typically, enlargement takes place at the onset of menstruation causing discomfort which decreases gradually until the cycle repeats itself. As with other cysts, rupture may occur spontaneously or following direct trauma. Localized *oophoritis* is an uncommon complication of bloodborne infection, either bacterial or viral. Mumps is the most common cause but clinical effects are usually less than in the male with orchitis. *Ovarian pregnancy* is particularly uncommon and has been considered elsewhere.

Ovarian Neoplasms

Classification of ovarian neoplasms is a complicated exercise, both in histology and tabulation, as can be seen from *Table* 79.7. For detailed description of the various histological species the reader is referred to specialized works. Serous and mucinous cystadenomas along with cystic teratomas (dermoid cysts) account for 95% of all benign ovarian neoplasms which in turn represent 75% of the total. Interestingly, there may be inherited susceptibility to such tumours which (excepting teratomas) are more common in association with blood Group A than Group O.

Table 79.7 Classification of ovarian neoplasms

A. *Epithelial tumours*
   - i. Serous cystadenoma—carcinoma
   - ii. Mucinous cystadenoma—carcinoma
   - iii. Endometrioid tumours
   - iv. Clear cell (mesonephroid) tumours
   - v. Brenner tumour
   - vi. Mixed epithelial tumours
   - vii. Undifferentiated carcinoma

B. *Sex cord stromal tumours*
   - i. Granulosa cell tumour
   - ii. Thecoma/fibroma
   - iii. Androblastoma
   - iv. Gynandroblastoma

C. *Lipid cell tumours*

D. *Germ cell tumours*
   - i. Dysgerminoma, pure and mixed
   - ii. Endodermal sinus tumour
   - iii. Embryonal carcinoma
   - iv. Teratoma, benign and malignant
   - v. Choriocarcinoma

E. *Gonadoblastoma*

F. *Metastatic tumours*

G. *Non-specific and unclassified tumours*

Serous Cystadenoma

Around a quarter of all ovarian neoplasms are serous cystadenomas which are seen most commonly during the reproductive years. Individual cysts vary in size from a few to 20 cm in diameter and are often multiple, although confined to one ovary in about 80% of cases. The cyst is thin walled and contains clear serous fluid unless discoloured by haemorrhage. Warty plaques may be noted internally or externally and very occasionally in seeding to neighbouring structures they mimic malignancy.

Mucinous Cystadenoma

This tumour is almost as common as the serous variety and is found at all ages but especially in the fourth and fifth decades. The cysts are usually multiple and unilateral (95% of cases). Blood vessels are prominent on the thin cyst wall and condensations of fibrous tissue form between adjoining cysts. Internal papillary projections are frequent but external structures are not likely.

Benign Teratoma

Almost all teratomas are cystic and account for 15–20% of benign ovarian neoplasms. Although usually found in women of 15–45 years, it is the commonest tumour in children. Both ovaries are affected in 10–15% of cases. The tumour has a thick fibrous capsule and varies from 2 to 10 cm in size. Intracystic solid areas may be seen or felt and often include radio-opacities, such as teeth. Malignant change is fortunately uncommon as the prognosis is very poor.

Malignant Neoplasms

Ovarian carcinoma is the fourth commonest cause of death from cancer in women. It causes more fatalities than cancer of the cervix and uterus combined and is increasing in frequency. The incidence which rises with age, is higher in Western Europe and America than in Asia and Africa. Japan provides a curious statistic having a frequency one-fifth that of the disease in America, yet American-born offspring of Japanese immigrants experience the same risk as the native population, suggesting an environmental influence. High parity and long-term oral contraception appear to reduce the risk of ovarian carcinoma possibly by decreasing the frequency of ovulation.

Ninety per cent of ovarian malignancies are of epithelial origin. Almost half are serous cystadenocarcinomas which outnumber the mucinous type by 3 to 1. Endometrioid, mesonephroid, anaplastic and metastatic carcinomas also comprise an appreciable number of the total. Malignant tumours of ovary are most often both cystic and solid.

The tumour spreads directly to uterus and fallopian tubes but peritoneum and omentum are also involved at a fairly early stage so that ascites is common. Within the peritoneal cavity tumour growth is usually exophytic. Nevertheless, deeper invasion does sometimes occur affecting bowel and ureter. Lymphatic drainage leads to metastatic invasion of aortic and even supraclavicular nodes whilst haematogenous spread can involve liver, lungs and more distant sites.

Staging ovarian carcinoma requires laparotomy and is an important guide in planning treatment and assessing prognosis. The system most widely used by gynaecologists is that recommended by the International Federation of Gynaecology and Obstetrics (FIGO) (*Table* 79.8).

Table 79.8 Staging of ovarian carcinoma (FIGO)

STAGE 1	GROWTH LIMITED TO OVARIES
IA	Limited to one ovary: no ascites i. No tumour on external surface and capsule intact ii. Tumour on external surface and/or capsule ruptured
IB	Limited to both ovaries: no ascites i. As for Stage IA ii. As for Stage IA
IC	Stage IA or IB but ascites present or cytologically positive peritoneal washings
STAGE II	GROWTH INVOLVING ONE OR BOTH OVARIES WITH PELVIC EXTENSION
IIA	Extension and/or metastases to uterus and/or tubes
IIB	Extension to other pelvic tissues
IIC	Stage IIA or IIB with ascites or cytologically positive peritoneal washings
STAGE III	GROWTH OF ONE OR BOTH OVARIES WITH EXTRAPELVIC INTRAPERITONEAL SPREAD This stage also includes Stage II with histologically proven extension to small bowel or omentum and positive retroperitoneal nodes
STAGE IV	GROWTH OF ONE OR BOTH OVARIES WITH EXTRA-ABDOMINAL SPREAD Cases with pleural effusions to be included only if cytology positive. All cases with parenchymal liver metastases are Stage IV

Note: Staging is based on clinical examination and surgical exploration. Postoperative histological and cytological findings are also to be considered.

Clinical Features

Abdominal pain and enlargement are the symptoms most frequently noted with ovarian tumours, whether benign or malignant. The pain is often poorly localized and as there may also be anorexia, nausea or even vomiting, the symptoms are liable to be dismissed as gastrointestinal upset. Likewise a gradual increase in abdominal girth is readily overlooked or ascribed to fat deposition. When larger, ovarian masses may induce a sensation of heaviness and by sheer bulk impair gastrointestinal function with loss of weight, fatigue, anaemia and constipation. Dyspareunia, urinary frequency and retention suggest a mass situated deep in the pelvis.

Abnormal vaginal bleeding may arise secondary to direct infiltration of the endometrium but stimulation by abnormal hormonal production from a functioning tumour or its ovarian stromal bed is seen occasionally. Oedema of the lower limbs reflects protein deficiency, vena caval compression or venous thrombosis. More advanced disease can cause symptoms by involvement of bowel, bladder and ureter.

General examination should include a search for anaemia, oedema and lymphadenopathy, especially supraclavicular. Hydrothorax should be excluded. Percussion is valuable in confirming an abdominal mass, with central dullness and resonant flanks, assuming that there is no ascites. Cystic tumours may feel quite solid and local tenderness could indicate leakage, twisting or even malignant change. Auscultation of a friction rub suggests inflammatory reaction in the cyst wall and, rarely, detection of a fetal heart or uterine souffle leads to a revised diagnosis. Hepatomegaly or additional nodularity are ominous signs.

Bimanual examination, often more easily achieved as a combined rectovaginal palpation, is needed to differentiate ovarian from other possible pelvic masses. The bladder should first be emptied, by catheter if necessary. An ovarian mass unencumbered by adhesions should move separately from the uterus and even if closely related, a sulcus can usually be distinguished between the two. Adherent ovarian swellings, pedunculated and subserous fibroids, however, can be very confusing. Nodular peritoneal metastases are sometimes felt in the pouch of Douglas but should not be confused with the tender uterosacral nodules found in endometriosis.

Ruptured Ovarian Cyst

Spontaneous rupture of an ovarian cyst can occur but more often the accident complicates coitus, labour, or pelvic examination. Pain is sudden and quite severe. The patient may have 'felt something give'. The degree of circulatory shock and peritoneal reaction depend upon the nature and amount of the leakage. Dermoid cysts, although thicker walled, have particularly irritant contents and significant bleeding magnifies the effects. Shoulder tip pain on lying flat suggests diaphragmatic irritation and free fluid may be demonstrable in the abdomen. The ovarian cyst becomes difficult or impossible to define and so can be unsuspected unless there is a prior record. It has been suggested that salpingography is useful in subacute cases of this nature as typical displacement is found.

Torsion of an Ovarian Cyst

This is more likely to befall a modest sized cyst as larger ones are relatively immobile. Hyperactive intestinal function and recent childbirth encourage and accelerate the twisting process which causes venous and then arterial obstruction. Symptoms may wax and wane for several days before severe continuous pain indicates infarction. The ovarian mass often increases in size and becomes very tender with guarding and peritonism.

Occasionally, repeated episodes of non-fulminating torsion lead to revascularization by way of adhesion to neighbouring structures and so the cyst becomes parasitic and resistant to further torsion.

Haemorrhage or Infection of a Cyst

Serous cystadenomas and malignant cysts are prone to intracystic haemorrhage. The blood loss is usually modest and self-limiting but there is transient pain with local tenderness. Alteration of the blood with time imparts a chocolate or even tarry appearance to the cyst contents and differentiation from an endometriotic cyst can be difficult.

Intraperitoneal haemorrhage is more likely with rupture of a cyst but can occur from the surface of a malignant growth. The extent of local reaction and shock depends on the amount and persistence of the bleeding. Infection of a cyst is theoretically possible although uncommon in practice, and provided it has not been introduced by needle from the exterior, the bloodstream is almost certainly the source. The clinical picture resembles that of acute pelvic infection except that adjoining pelvic structures are less likely to be affected and consequently the ovarian swelling is more easily defined as separate.

Confirmation of Diagnosis

Physical examination is the most important diagnostic procedure in the early detection of ovarian tumours. Careful unhurried bimanual examination, vaginally in mature women, rectally or combined rectovaginally in the physically immature and some postmenopausal women, will usually permit a confident anatomical diagnosis. Anaesthesia may be required when pelvic assessment has been unsatisfactory. Provided there are no additional suspicious circumstances, ovarian swellings up to 5 cm in size found in women with reasonably normal menstrual cycles are very likely to be functional. Spontaneous regression of such tumours should become obvious within a few weeks and so justify an expectant policy. Larger swellings must be fully investigated as at least 20% will prove to be malignant.

Blood investigations are of limited value beyond demonstrating anaemia or an elevated sedimentation rate. When there is associated primary amenorrhoea, particularly if nuclear chromatin is absent in a buccal smear, chromosomal studies are indicated. Collection of blood for grouping and crossmatching prior to surgery may usefully include saving an aliquot against the unusual possibility that the tumour proves productive of some marker substance. Blood chemistry will be required when renal or bowel disturbance is present.

Pulmonary opacities or effusions and calcification within fibroids or ovarian cysts may be found on radiography of the chest and abdomen. Ultrasonic scanning should confirm the physical findings and may demonstrate intracystic solid structures, ascites, peritoneal or even hepatic metastases (*Fig.* 79.6). Computerized tomography (*Fig.* 79.7) and magnetic resonance imaging, if available, give similar useful information.

The possibility that gastrointestinal pathology has metastasized to the ovary (Krukenburg tumour) or is mimicking an ovarian tumour (e.g. sigmoid carcinoma, diverticulitis) will require full investigation in many cases. Examination of the stools for occult blood, upper and lower gastrointestinal barium studies and endoscopic techniques should resolve any doubt. Similarly, urinary cytology, cystoscopy and pyelography may be necessary where involvement of the urinary tract is suspected.

Abdominal paracentesis confirms ascites and provides fluid for bacteriological and cytological examination. Puncture of an ovarian cyst is undesirable and more easily avoided if ultrasonic guidance is employed. Examination under anaesthesia is a useful preliminary to further surgical measures. Histological assessment and thus laparotomy will usually be required; in some cases laparoscopy may be preferred if the need for open exploration is still not clear. Where laparoscopy is employed the whole abdomen including the under surfaces of the diaphragm should be inspected.

Characteristics Suggestive of Malignancy

The histology of an ovarian tumour is not always a reliable guide to its subsequent clinical course and careful assessment of the clinical characteristics can be at least as important. The features listed in *Table* 79.9 suggest malignant potential and thus justify a radical approach to treatment. Rapid increase in size, loss of weight and oedema of the lower limbs are more likely with malignant lesions but not unknown in benign ones. Ascites, if bloodstained, is ominous; however, non-malignant tumours, such as fibroma, thecoma and serous or mucinous cystadenoma can be associated with ascites and even hydrothorax (Meigs' syndrome). Cytological examination of paracentesis fluid may reveal malignant cells but a negative result has little exclusive

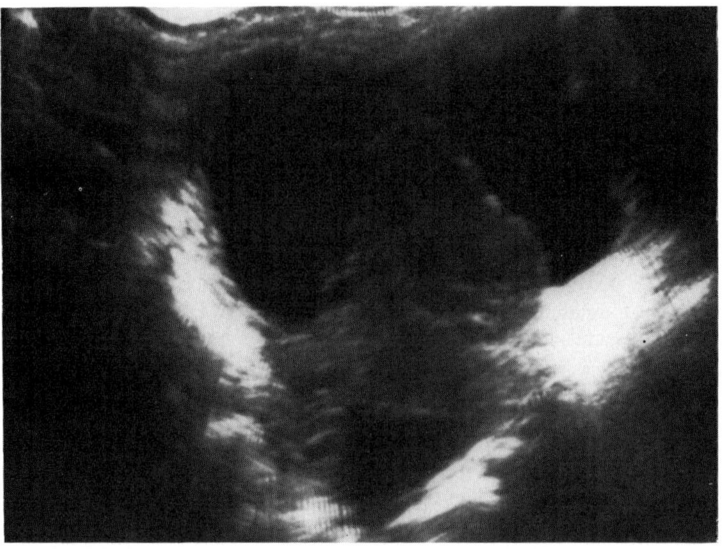

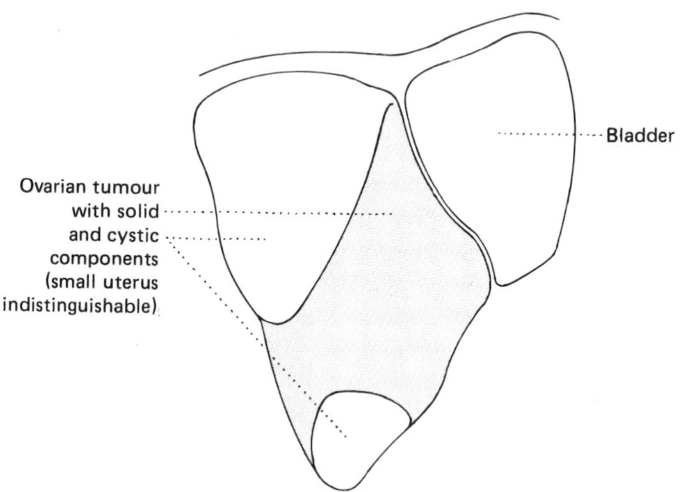

Fig. 79.6 Sagittal ultrasound scan of abdomen showing cystic/solid ovarian tumour.

value. Venous thrombosis is very suggestive of malignancy and on occasion causes the presenting symptoms. Although often useful, caution is needed in the interpretation of radiological and ultrasonic investigations which should be looked to for confirmation rather than as the sole basis upon which management is to be decided. Laparoscopy at least, should be undertaken whenever there is serious suspicion of an ovarian tumour. *Laparotomy* is required to settle any question as to operability.

Treatment

Surgery is the primary treatment of all ovarian tumours other than infective or simple transient functional ones. Laparotomy should be conducted through a paramedian incision unless the disease is confidently known to be localized in the pelvis when a low transverse approach might suffice. The size of incision presents a problem with large cysts as generally it is better to remove the swellings intact. Rupture of an ovarian cyst directly into the peritoneal cavity must be avoided; however, deliberate drainage should be possible without any risk of spilling the contents. A case can be made for eschewing near full-length abdominal incision in favour of closed drainage for very large ovarian cysts which are in any case less likely to be malignant. It should also be kept in mind that peritoneal contamination with the contents of a benign mucinous cyst can lead to pseudomyxoma peritonei, a condition which is often ultimately fatal. A wide-bore trocar with attached suction can be introduced through a thick portion of the cyst wall which has earlier been anchored by placement of a purse-string suture. Shrinkage of the cyst permits full assessment of its attachments and easy delivery through an incision of acceptable size. If present, ascitic fluid is sent for cytology, otherwise saline washings of the peritoneal cavity should be collected.

After full exploration of the abdomen, one must try to answer the question 'Is this malignant?' The suspicious features have already been discussed but frozen section may be considered. In view of the difficulties inherent in ovarian histology, however, this technique may not give a reliable answer. A superior alternative in cases where for reproductive or physiological reasons one is tempted to conserve the

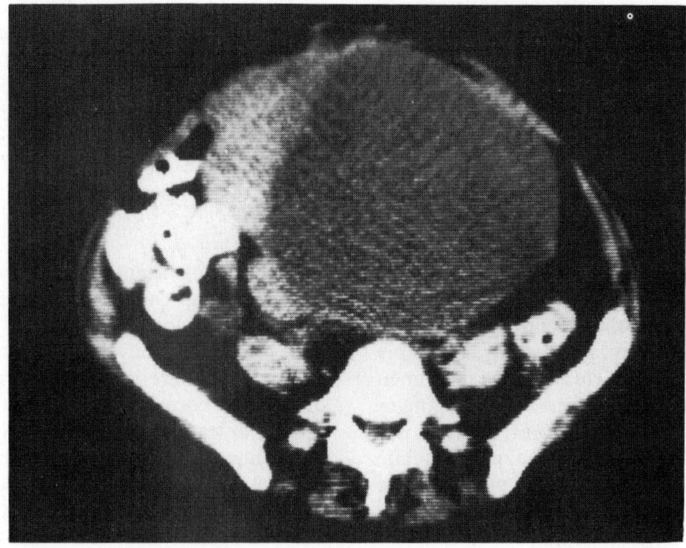

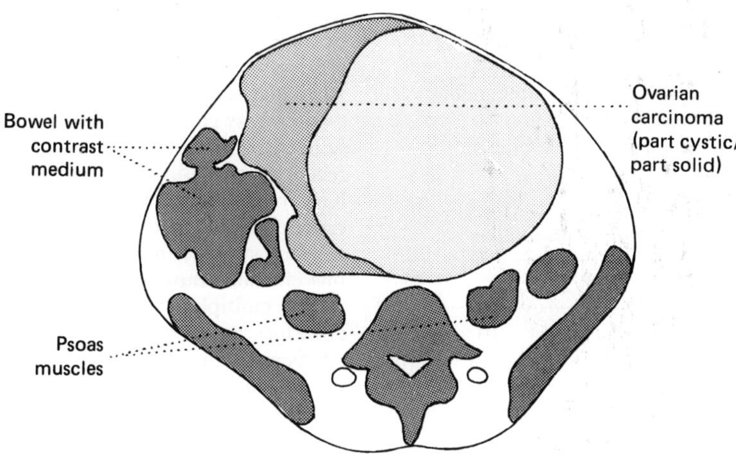

Fig. 79.7 CT transverse scan of abdomen showing ovarian carcinoma.

contralateral ovary, is to bisect it and collect a generous biopsy for more leisured histological examination.

Benign Tumours

With a tumour confidently regarded as benign and viable after unwinding any torsion, the next question is 'Should I remove the ovary or just the cyst?' The possible operations are suture of a bleeding functional cyst, ovarian cystectomy (excision of the cyst alone), and salpingo-oophorectomy with or without total hysterectomy or ovariotomy (excision of the cyst along with the ovary). One might suggest as a general rule, preservation of at least some ovarian function in all those under 45 years of age and as much as possible if less than 35 years or still desirous of further family. In making a decision the state of the contralateral ovary and both tubes must be taken into account. Ovarian cystectomy will be the usual choice when the object is retention of maximum ovarian function. Should the homolateral tube be useless and the opposite adnexae normal in a patient with hopes of future pregnancy, salpingo-oophorectomy may have advantages. In the over-45 age group, the best course is removal of both adnexae and a total hysterectomy, assuming that the

Table 79.9 Characteristics suggesting ovarian malignancy

A. *Symptomatic*
  Rapidly increasing abdominal distension
  Loss of weight
  Leg swelling especially unilateral

B. *Signs*
  Ascites, especially if bloody or positive cytology
  Bilateral and/or immobile tumours
  Additional intra-abdominal masses
  Venous thrombosis

C. *Investigations*
  Cystic and solid tumour ultrasonically
  Ultrasonic or radiological evidence of metastases

D. *Operative*
  Solid areas in tumour especially externally
  Unusual vascularity of tumour
  Areas of necrosis in the tumour wall
  Adhesion to surrounding tissues
  Omental, hepatic or peritoneal deposits
  (check undersurface of diaphragm)

patient is fit and the surgeon is equal to the technical demands.

Malignant Tumours

The fundamental concept in treatment of malignant ovarian disease is maximum surgical effort even if total clearance is not possible, as prospects for postoperative chemotherapeutic or radiotherapeutic response are inversely proportional to the residual tumour load. Total hysterectomy and bilateral salpingo-oophorectomy with excision of all other removable intra-abdominal metastases is the object. At the very least every endeavour should be made to remove both ovaries. Omentectomy is widely recommended and although not proven to alter survival significantly, it is technically simple and probably worthwhile. Before closure, the abdomen should be carefully re-examined to confirm FIGO staging of the disease. The intraperitoneal instillation of cytotoxic agents is not advised as it offers no advantage over systemic administration. Placement of tubes to allow postoperative intraperitoneal introduction of radioisotopes is favoured in some centres, especially for Stages I and II.

Adjuvant Therapy

The survival from ovarian cancer is greatly influenced both by the histological nature and extent of the disease (*Table* 79.10). Five-year salvage of only 60% in Stage Ia forces consideration of adjuvant therapy. The available modalities are radiotherapy and chemotherapy but the precise place of each is still under study.

Table 79.10 Five-year survival (%) in ovarian carcinoma

Histology	*FIGO Stage*					
	Ia	Ib + c	IIa	IIb + c	III	IV
Serous (2128)	62·1	48·8	48·8	37·5	12·0	6·0
Mucinous (609)	79·4	60·2	55·6	45·8	12·3	5·3
Endometrioid, Mesonephric (706)	67·1	60·0	54·9	43·5	5·2	4·2
Low potential malignancy	93·2	89·5	95·8	72·7	38·3	16·7

15th Annual Report FIGO—collected reports from 32 institutions (number of cases)

Radiotherapy

Postoperative external irradiation of the pelvis and lower abdomen is generally accepted as improving the prognosis in Stage II ovarian carcinoma. Irradiation of more advanced disease must include the entire abdomen and even if used with the 'moving strip' technique is associated with significant morbidity from enteritis, proctitis, nephritis and rarely hepatitis. Thus, external therapy of Stage III disease remains controversial with the exception of unusually radiosensitive tumours, such as dysgerminomas. There is some evidence that operability in Stage III tumours can be increased by irradiation 3 weeks prior to surgery. Thus an inexperienced operator might consider simple biopsy followed by radiotherapy and referral for more expert surgical exploration in such cases. External radiotherapy may also be used to palliate symptoms from specific tumour metastases.

Some groups advocate the intraperitoneal instillation of radioisotopes, gold (^{198}Au) or preferably chromic phosphate (^{32}P) which is pure beta emitter, as superior to external irradiation for management of cases in Stages I and II. Care must be taken to ensure even distribution of the solution throughout the peritoneal cavity if damage is to be avoided.

Chemotherapy

The alkylating agents have been used extensively in advanced ovarian carcinoma (Stages III and IV) and are undoubtedly capable of producing response in up to 60% of cases. Unfortunately the remission rarely exceeds 6–12 months and there is no clear evidence of improved 5-year survival. Theoretically cytotoxic therapy would be of greater benefit in early ovarian cancer when the tumour load is small; however, this remains to be substantiated by clinical trial. Meanwhile the use of cytotoxic agents is justified in most cases provided that the pospective benefit is carefully weighed against side-effects and the quality of survival.

One of the common alkylating agents such as melphalan, thiotepa, cyclophosphamide or chlorambucil has been the usual first choice as a single agent in chemotherapy of ovarian carcinoma. This combines acceptable toxicity with efficacy close to that of the various combined regimes. In particular, chlorambucil has the advantage of oral administration, easy control and few side-effects so it is a particularly useful adjuvant in the treatment of Stages I or II. More recently, cisplatin and the related compound carboplatin have been shown to have useful activity against ovarian cancer. Although toxic to bone marrow, kidneys and the nervous system, these are being used increasingly as first-line chemotherapy with promising results.

The multiplicity of chemotherapeutic agents now available for cancer makes it important that treatment is by protocol as much as possible to enable proper evaluation and the earliest possible identification of the most effective least toxic combinations for specific diseases.

There are scattered reports of benefit from treatment with various progestogens in fairly high dosage. One might expect some response in endometrioid tumours as a corollary of the atrophic effect progestogens exert on endometrial carcinoma, but as yet there is no conclusive evidence. Certainly the treatment is free from serious side-effects although cost is a drawback.

The ideal duration of cytotoxic therapy is still not established. Suggestions range from a few weeks in Stage I disease, to 5 years and even indefinitely for more advanced cases. Second look laparotomy has been advocated to confirm the safety of discontinuing drugs or to allow more definitive surgery in other cases which may have become operable following a good chemotherapeutic response. Progress may be more easily assessed in some rare germ cell tumours, such as choriocarcinoma and endodermal sinus tumours which produce markers, respectively chorionic gonadotrophin and alpha-fetoprotein, so allowing biochemical surveillance. Unlike the common epithelial carcinomas, these tumours are usually very susceptible to aggressive combination chemotherapy and genuine cures are possible. This especially is a field in which specialist advice should always be sought.

Ovarian Tumours associated with Pregnancy

Taking account of the age group, a similar range of ovarian tumours is seen both in the pregnant and non-pregnant.

Exceptions are the greater frequency of corpus luteal cysts and the absence of tumours which interfere with fertility. Radiographic investigation is obviously to be avoided. Ovarian cystectomy is possible where indicated and sacrifice of the corpus luteum at ovariotomy is not necessarily followed by abortion provided the eighth week has been reached. The uterus should be handled as little and as gently as possible. Progestogens are better avoided in view of the possible teratogenic effects. Threatened premature labour postoperatively in more advanced pregnancies, usually responds to a beta-sympathomimetic drug, such as ritodrine or salbutamol.

Suspicion of malignancy in an ovarian tumour during pregnancy raises very difficult problems if stumbled upon unsuspected. The best plan is removal of the offending ovary or ovaries where bilateral involvement is obvious, a careful search of the abdomen to establish the full extent of the disease and closure. Further management will depend upon the histology, prognosis, stage of pregnancy and the family's wishes.

Further Reading

Gaya H. and Hawkins D. F. (1981) *Gynaecological Therapeutics*. London, Baillière Tindall. Chapter 5.
Hudson C. N. (1985) *Ovarian Cancer*. Oxford, Oxford University Press.
Jones H. W. and Jones G. S. (1981) *Novak's Textbook of Gynecology*, 10th ed. Baltimore, Williams & Wilkins.
Di Saia P. J. and Creasman W. T. (1981) *Clinical Gynecologic Oncology*. St Louis, Mosby.
Tindal V. R. (1986) *Jeffcoate's Principles of Gynaecology*, 5th ed. Guildford, Butterworths.

Section 9

Genito-urinary Surgery

80 Urological Surgery

J. E. Newsam

Urological surgeons are concerned with the kidneys, ureters, bladder, urethra and the male genital system. The separation of urological surgery from general surgery has accelerated over the past few years not only because of the increasing use of resectoscopes for the treatment and assessment of benign and malignant prostatic disease and bladder tumours and the rapid development of percutaneous renal surgery and ureteroscopy, but also because of the need to assess urological patients and their diseases much more accurately than formerly.

The study of the structure, function and pathology of the kidneys, together and separately, has always taxed the ingenuities of physiologists, surgeons, pathologists, physicians and others, and renal function can be affected not only by diseases in the urinary tract and elsewhere but also by many of the drugs used for treating infections and malignant disease. In recent years the methods of studying the structure, function and pathology of the bladder, urethra and testes have also improved. The accurate assessment of all tumours is more necessary now than ever, because many of the treatments, especially chemotherapeutic agents, are expensive, unpleasant and dangerous, and it behoves us to do all we can to ensure that such treatment is eventually beneficial.

As urology separates from general surgery it becomes more dependent upon such other specialties as radiology, nuclear medicine, pathology, biochemistry, medical and radiation oncology, and bacteriology, not to mention physicists like Professor Hopkins whose invention and development of fibreoptics and rod lens telescopes have so improved endoscopy. Nevertheless, it is the urological surgeon the patient consults and his responsibility to determine what investigations, if any, the patient should have and to integrate the results of these tests with what he already knows about the patient, before he agrees what treatment is appropriate.

This chapter describes the various methods available for investigating urological patients, but it must be remembered that the use of sophisticated and often non-invasive methods of investigation does not replace the need to take an adequate history of the patient, and of his family, his work and his past medical history, and to carry out a meticulous physical examination.

HISTORY

The first thing we listen to is the history of the presenting complaint. Although we should not ask leading questions, we must remember what difficulty many patients have in describing accurately what is the matter with them. The past may throw light upon the patient's present disorder and obviously previous cardiovascular, respiratory, metabolic or neurological problems may render treatment more difficult. Many urological diseases, including polycystic disease, cystinuria and possibly medullary cystic disease, are hereditary, and the taking of a family history is essential. It is also essential to know any medicines the patient is taking, or has taken, because some, including anticholinergics, tranquillizers and hypotensive agents can cause or aggravate urinary or sexual problems. To know the patient's present and previous work is necessary, especially in patients with transitional-cell carcinoma of the kidneys, ureters and bladder, which is a prescribed industrial disease, remembering that the latent period between exposure to a carcinogen and the clinical development of a tumour averages 20 years and can exceed 45 years.

SYMPTOMATOLOGY

Haematuria

In patients with urological disease, haematuria is usually sufficient to colour the urine red or dark brown and be recognized as blood, by the patient. Clots may also be passed. Haemoglobin is a very strong pigment and even small amounts produce a red colour. Haematuria, which cannot be recognized with the naked eye and is detected only by the stick test or microscope, sometimes occurs in diseases of the collecting system of the kidney, the ureter, the bladder or the urethra, but is most often from diffuse parenchymatous disease of the kidneys.

Urine may be stained red by drugs like phenytoin, phenolphthalein, rifampicin and adriamycin or the pigment anthrocyanin (found in beet and blackberries) or reddish-brown by porphyrins, urobilinogen, bilirubin or the drugs nitrofurantoin, metronidazole, or chloroquine. Nevertheless, patients who complain of haematuria are usually correct and investigation should proceed accordingly, even if it is not possible to confirm the symptom directly.

Total haematuria in which the blood is evenly mixed with urine, suggests a source in the kidney or ureter; initial or terminal haematuria suggests a source in the bladder neck or prostate. Urethral bleeding, in which blood leaks from the urethra and stains the patient's clothes must come from the apex of the prostate or the urethra beyond the sphincters.

Haemospermia

If seminal fluid contains blood it appears red or brown. In young men haemospermia is usually caused by congestion or infection in the prostate or seminal vesicles, but in older men it may indicate unsuspected cancer of the prostate or systemic disease like hypertension. For all patients with haemospermia a good history must be taken and a full physical examination done. If the urine also contains blood, even in microscopic amounts, then cystoscopy and the other investigations appropriate to haematuria are essential.

Haemoglobinuria

The haemoglobin normally released by the breakdown of red cells is bound to large haptoglobulins and does not appear in the urine. With excessive haemolysis the haptoglobulin becomes saturated and unbound haemoglobin occurs in the urine, which appears red but as it does not contain red blood cells it is not turbid.

Pain

Acute obstruction of a calix, the pelvi-ureteric junction or the ureter produces renal or ureteric colic, which is a severe persistent pain with exacerbations in the 1st lumbar distribution. Chronic obstruction causes no pain, or pain is induced by the diuresis of a water load or diuretic. Fixed renal pain may occur in acute infections, malignant disease, infarction, haemorrhage and occasionally from vesico-ureteric reflux. Renal pain is usually unilateral, and it is questionable to ascribe bilateral loin pain to kidney disease unless there is unequivocal evidence of it although sometimes specific tests are needed to demonstrate obstruction.

Bladder pain is often referred down the urethra, even as far down as the external meatus, and may be caused by acute over-distension with urine or blood clots, by spasm from stones or infection, or by the treatment of bladder and prostatic tumours with radiotherapy. The pain of interstitial cystitis, nowadays an uncommon disease, occurs immediately before micturition and disappears as soon as it starts.

Urethral pain is usually described as dysuria. It occurs whilst passing urine and may persist for a short time afterwards. It results from infections of the prostate, bladder or urethra and by instrumentation. Mild urethral pain is perhaps better described as urethral irritation, and often gives the patient the feeling that he needs to pass urine, although he may already have done so. Prostatic disease can cause urethral pain, or pain in the perineum, the lower part of the back and the inside of the thighs. Testicular disease often causes pain in the iliac fossa, and may be mistaken for an acute abdominal disease.

Frequency

Patients who complain of increased frequency of micturition have either polyuria or 'true' frequency. However, those with polyuria usually complain of excessive thirst rather than frequency. Patients with 'true' frequency pass small volumes of urine each time they micturate, but normal volumes over 24-h periods. Urinary frequency also occurs if the bladder is irritated by infections, stones or foreign bodies; if the bladder is contracted by tumour or fibrosis; if the bladder is compressed by a pelvic tumour or pregnant uterus; if the nerves supplying the bladder are damaged by disease or injury; if the outflow of urine from the bladder is obstructed, or if the bladder is unstable for psychological reasons. Frequency is usually less during the night than during the day, but for it not to occur at all at night, suggests a psychosomatic cause.

Incontinence

Incontinence is the involuntary escape of urine. If it occurs only during sleep, it is called enuresis. There are many kinds of incontinence including overflow, stress, urge and terminal dribbling. A very careful history must be taken to try and find out exactly what kind of incontinence the patient suffers, but sometimes only urodynamics will tell us.

Outflow Obstruction from the Bladder

Many diseases of the urinary tract interfere with the free flow of urine out of the bladder, and they are discussed in more detail in later chapters. The symptoms range from slight difficulty to acute or chronic retention. In the early stages the patient complains that micturition is frequent, especially at night, is sometimes urgent, is difficult to start and difficult to finish (terminal dribbling) and produces a thin urinary stream which later deteriorates from a flow to a dribble. Later, acute or chronic urinary retention may follow, together with such complications as infection, stones or chronic renal failure.

Pneumaturia

Air or gas is lighter than water and appears at the end of micturition after all the urine has been passed. Pneumaturia can occur after cystoscopy or catheterization, particularly when the lower abdomen has been compressed to empty the bladder quickly. Otherwise it indicates a fistula between the bladder and bowel or an infection with gas-producing organisms.

RENAL FAILURE

Acute Renal Failure

Acute renal failure is the sudden severe reduction of renal function; it causes retention of urea, creatinine and other products of protein catabolism, oliguria or even anuria and results in a derangement of the internal environment, especially its content of sodium, potassium, hydrogen ions and water. The causes may be prerenal, renal or postrenal. Prerenal and renal acute renal failure are discussed in Chapter 6.

Chronic Renal Failure

Parenchymatous disease of the kidney, particularly malignant hypertension, glomerulonephritis and analgesic nephropathy account for 50%; congenital disorders, particularly polycystic disease, for 20% and obstruction for 30% of patients with chronic renal failure. The clinical features of chronic renal failure depend very much upon whether or not severe hypertension is a complicating feature, but they can include polyuria, skin pigmentation, pruritus, petechiae, osteodystrophies, potassium intoxication, water intoxication, anaemia, neuropathy, mental changes, pericarditis, tetany, sodium disturbances, acidosis and hypertension.

PHYSICAL EXAMINATION

Physical examination must be thorough and complete because urinary disease may involve any part of the body although special attention must be paid to the genito-urinary tract itself. Attempts must be made to palpate the kidneys which may be felt easily in infants, but in adults only if they are enlarged or occupy a low position. In infants the kidneys constitute about 1% of the body weight, but only 0·4% in adults. The external genitalia should be examined and a rectal examination carried out, not only to examine the prostate, the seminal vesicles and the rectum, but also to assess the tone of the anal sphincters. The lymph glands in the pelvis are impalpable, no matter how much they are involved and the abdominal ones are palpable only if they are extensively involved by tumour. The cervical lymph glands, particularly those in the lower part of the neck, must be palpated because they may be involved in patients with testicular tumours.

THE ASSESSMENT OF RENAL FUNCTION

Disease of the kidney may obviously affect the function of one or both kidneys, but diseases of the ureter, the bladder, the urethra and the prostate may all interfere with renal function by back pressure, ascending infection and vesico-ureteric reflux. The assessment of renal function is also important in patients given antibiotics for infections, or chemotherapeutic drugs for tumours, because of nephrotoxic side-effects.

Microscopic Examination of the Urine

Cells

Epithelial cells are continuously shed from the urinary tract and 3 or 4 per high power field are found together with 3 or 4 leucocytes and often 1 or 2 red blood cells. More red blood cells than this constitute haematuria. Red blood cells that originate in a glomerulus tend to be irregular in size and shape and include Burr cells and helmet cells, whereas those from the collecting system tend to be uniform in size and shape, though some may be ghost cells.

Casts

A few haline casts, which consist of Tamm–Horsfall mucoprotein, are excreted by normal people, especially after strenuous sustained exercise and with febrile diseases. Excessive quantities are excreted in most forms of chronic renal failure. Granular casts are hyaline casts with granules of albumin, lipoprotein or immunoglobin, and are found in much the same circumstances as hyaline casts. Dense granular casts, however, are always pathological, and frequently found in chronic renal failure, amyloid disease and diabetic nephropathy. Cellular casts are basically hyaline or granular casts coated with tubular epithelial cells. A few are found in any renal disease, but large numbers are seen in acute tubular necrosis. Red cell casts are made completely of red cells which have come from a glomerulus.

Crystals

The urine contains many crystals but only those of the amino acids, particularly cystine, are significant. However, amino aciduria is more readily diagnosed by chemical than microscopic techniques.

Proteinuria

The stick test consists of a paper impregnated with a buffer and the indicator bromophenol blue, which turns green with protein. It is unreliable if the urine is strongly acid or strongly alkaline or the protein is Bence Jones protein. Salicylic-sulphonic acid (25%) produces turbidity if added to urine containing more than 20 mg % of protein. The 24-h excretion of protein should be measured by the Esbach or Biuret test. Less than 0·2 g/day is normal, but this may be increased by cold, exercise or changes in posture. If these are suspected to be the cause of a significant proteinuria, short urine collections can be made with the patient erect and supine. In patients with nephrosis as much as 4–5 g/day may be found. Electrophoresis detects abnormal paraproteins, e.g. those found in myeloma.

Glomerular Filtration Rate (GFR)

The normal renal blood flow is about 1300 ml/min and the GFR is 120 ml/min. So great is the reserve capacity of the kidney, however, that GFR has to fall by 50% before nitrogenous substances are retained. The GFR is a valuable guide to renal function and depends upon the functional ability and the number of functional glomeruli. It equals the clearance value of any substance that is excreted by glomerular filtration and neither excreted nor reabsorbed by the renal tubules. Such substances include inulin, vitamin B_{12}, and endogenous creatinine. To measure the inulin clearance value is difficult, and the GFR is usually estimated by measuring the creatinine clearance value. The production of endogenous creatinine is proportional to muscle mass and obviously varies from one individual to another. It is 10% less in women than in men and falls with age. A rise or a fall means a rise or a fall in renal function so that the serial measurement of creatinine is a convenient means of assessing renal function, even though an isolated figure may not necessarily be significant. To measure the GFR with creatinine, it is necessary to know the volume and creatinine concentration of a 24-h urine specimen and the plasma creatinine concentration. ^{51}Cr-labelled ethylenediamine tetra-acetic acid (EDTA), ^{125}I- or ^{131}I-labelled diatrizoate or iothalamate, or ^{99}Tc^{m} DTPA can also be used to measure GFR. They are injected intravenously as a bolus, and blood levels are measured by a detector placed over the heart. Concentrations fall rapidly at first consequent on distribution throughout the extracellular fluid but thereafter there is an exponential decline determined by GFR.

Urea

The normal serum level is 3–7 mmol/l but it depends not only on renal function but also on protein intake, catabolic activity and the state of hydration, and it is not, therefore, a reliable test of renal function. A better test is the serum creatinine (normal level = 0·07–0·11 mmol/l).

Blood Flow

The renal plasma flow equals the clearance value of any substance excreted by both glomerular filtration and tubular excretion to the extent that it disappears completely from the circulation after one passage through the kidney. Diodrast is such a substance. More commonly orthohippurate labelled with ^{131}I is used and measured by detectors placed separately over each kidney (*see Fig.* 80.17).

Tubular Function

Concentrating Ability

The concentration of urine can be assessed by measuring its specific gravity. However, large solutes like glucose and protein increase the specific gravity disproportionately. It is better to measure the osmolality of urine which depends upon the number of particles in solution irrespective of their size. The osmotic pressure of plasma is 285–293 mmol/l and if the osmolality of any one specimen of urine passed during a 24-h period is greater than 800 mmol/l the concentrating ability of the kidney can be considered normal. Alternatively, the patient can be given, by injection, 10 units of vasopressin after which urine osmolality should exceed 800 mmol/l, and may reach as much as 1400 mmol/l. To measure the diluting ability of the kidney by water load tests is not very satisfactory and is dangerous in patients suffering from chronic renal failure and Addison's disease.

Electrolytes

In some renal diseases, failure of the renal tubules to reabsorb sodium, potassium and calcium in the normal way may be reflected by abnormal plasma levels.

Acidifying Ability

The urine is usually acid and should certainly become acid with a pH of less than 5·3 2–3 h after the ingestion of ammonium chloride (100 mg/kg body weight).

Hormonal Function

Erythropoietin in the humoral factor produced by the kidney that helps to regulate red cell mass. It is an unstable protein and has recently been quantitated by radioimmunoassay. Production is, however, normally assessed by measuring the levels of haemoglobin and the red cell mass; too little causes anaemia, too much polycythaemia.

Renin is a protein with a molecular weight of about 45 000 produced in the juxtamedullary apparatus of the kidney and released by a fall in hydrostatic pressure in the afferent arteriole. It helps control blood pressure by stimulating aldosterone production and vasoconstriction. It can be assayed in blood but levels in peripheral blood are of little value and it should be assayed in blood obtained from both renal veins by inferior veno-cavography.

Bacteriological Examination of the Urine

Apart from perinephric abscess, renal abscess and pyonephrosis, the diagnosis of urinary tract infection is based upon the demonstration of bacteriuria, though some patients with urinary tract infection may be temporarily abacteriuric, particularly after a course of antibacterial therapy. Bacteriuria means that the urine contains a significant number of organisms. If the specimen is obtained by suprapubic puncture, often used in children, any number of bacteria, apart from skin contaminants, is significant, but midstream specimens of urine or clean catch specimens are often contaminated, and therefore, significant only if they contain more than 10^5 organisms/ml. However, smaller numbers may be significant if the patient has an indwelling catheter or the organisms are proteus or pseudomonas species. The problems of collecting and preserving specimens may be overcome by using dip slides, dip spoons, or filter strips, all of which involve the inoculation of culture media with a measured amount of freshly voided urine. They provide a ready means for examining urine in domiciliary practice. Chemical tests which involve the reduction of nitrates to nitrites by bacteria are not commonly used. Microscopy may reveal pus cells, but the correlation between pyuria and bacteriuria is poor. However, persistent pyuria without bacteriuria suggests renal tuberculosis.

In urinary tract infections host factors usually overshadow the virulence characteristics of the micro-organisms. *E. coli* is the commonest pathogen and the species found are similar to those in the gut. *Proteus mirabilis* is also found in the gut; its ability to split urea into ammonia predisposes to stone formation and interferes with the activity of complement and some drugs, including nitrofurantoin. Other species of proteus like vulgaris are usually associated with catheterization or other transurethral procedures. Several staphylococci form part of the normal perineal flora and may cause infections especially in women.

In hospitalized patients *Pseudomonas aeruginosa*, species of Klebsiella and *Streptococcus faecalis* are the commonest Gram-positive organisms that infect the urinary tract.

Anaerobic organisms are rarely found in urinary tract infections but may be associated with postoperative infection. The intracellular organism Chlamydia frequently causes non-specific urethritis in men but in women it infects the cervix and causes pelvic infections.

Seriously ill patients, particularly those with bacteraemia following closed renal infections, acute pyelonephritis, or instrumentation, should have blood cultures taken because they may provide more information than urinary cultures. If renal tuberculosis is suspected at least 3 and preferably 6 or more early morning urines should be submitted to the bacteriologist for examination by the Ziehl–Neelsen stain and by culture, and in some laboratories by guinea-pig inoculation.

RADIOLOGY

Plain Radiograph of Renal Tract (*Fig.* 80.1)

The shadows in a plain radiograph reflect the differences in X-ray absorption and thickness of the tissues traversed by the beam. The atomic number of the elements making up the tissue determine its X-ray absorption. Calcium and iodine with atomic weights of 40 and 127 respectively are radio-opaque, whereas gas and fat are radiolucent. However, the fat around the kidney outlines the borders of the kidney which can usually be seen in a plain film. The plain

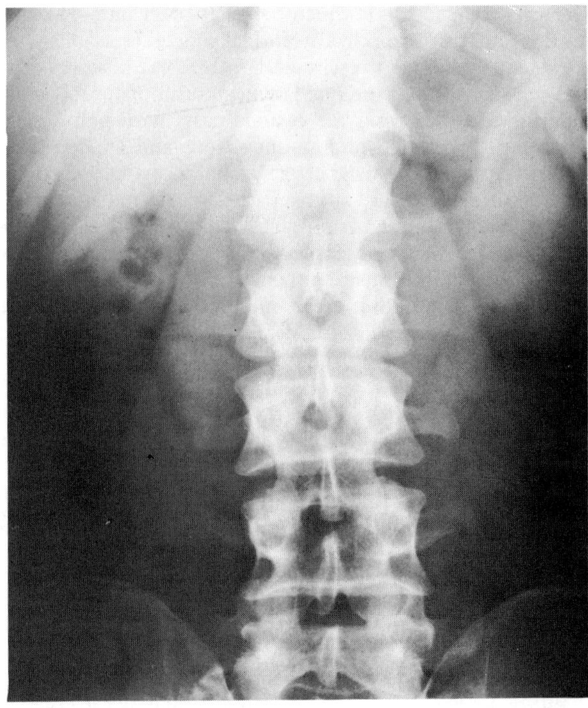

Fig. 80.1 Plain radiograph of renal tract. Note lateral borders of psoas muscles and renal outlines.

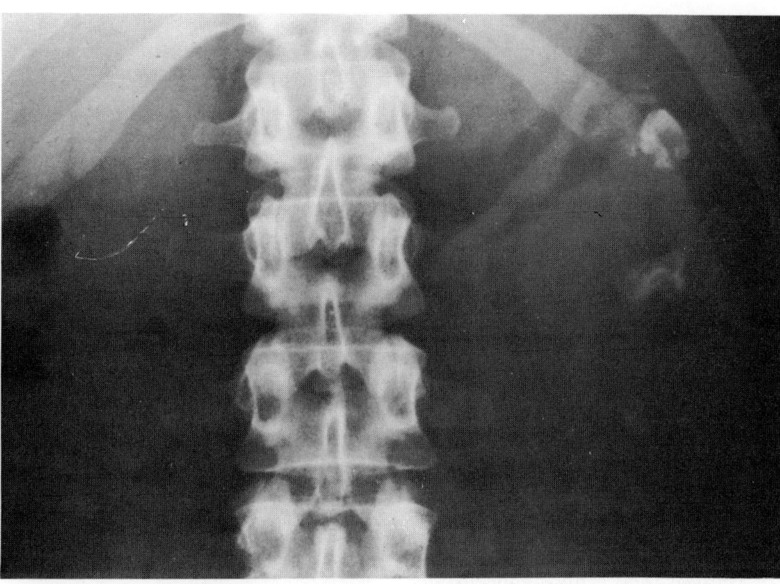

Fig. 80.2 Plain radiograph of renal tract. Shows calcification in parenchyma of left kidney (nephrocalcinosis).

radiograph is therefore examined for the renal outlines, the lateral borders of the psoas, abnormal opacities in the region of the kidneys (*Fig.* 80.2), the ureters, the bladder and the prostate. The radiograph will also give relevant information concerning skeletal structures: hips, upper femora, the ribs and the diaphragm. The value of plain films of the renal tract may be enhanced by right and left oblique films, which are particularly useful for showing whether calcification is posterior and in the kidney or ureter, or anterior and in the gallbladder or the costal cartilages. Tomograms may also be of value.

Excretion Urography

First introduced in the 1920s, excretion urography has improved enormously with the advances in contrast media and technique. Despite the rapid development of the other methods of imaging the kidneys and urinary tract it still remains the most important imaging examination. Contrast media are tri-iodinated water-soluble sodium or meglumine salts of benzoic acid derivatives, such as diatrizoates or iotholomates. The osmolality of these solutions is high compared with plasma (around 1800 mmol/l). The new generation of contrast media, such as the ioxaglates and the metrizamides have as much iodine in 2 particles as the others do in 4 and therefore exert much less osmotic pressure, but they are expensive. The kidney treats all these contrast media like inulin excreting 98% by glomerular filtration. The recommended dose of contrast amounts to 300 mg I_2/kg body weight. Better images are obtained with higher doses of contrast and do not appear to have more side-effects than smaller doses. The injection can be repeated if the films made after the first injection are unsatisfactory. The amount of contrast media excreted depends upon its plasma concentration and upon the GFR; the speed with which it passes through the kidney depends upon the pressure difference at the glomerulus. If the patient passes urine before the radiographs are taken, the bladder will be empty and the quality of the cystogram obtained some 25–30 min after injection is better. A plain radiograph of the renal tract is obtained before the injections as the interpretation of films after injection is otherwise impossible.

Nephrographic Phase (*Fig.* 80.3)

This is obtained by taking a film immediately the injection of contrast media is completed. In the proximal tubules of the kidney 80% of the water but none of the dye is reabsorbed. The contrast is rapidly concentrated and diffusely opacifies the kidney outlining functional renal tissue. It provides a picture of the size, position and contours of the kidneys and is also a test of proximal tubular function because the intensity of opacification depends on the plasma concentration of the contrast, the GFR and the ability of the proximal tubules to reabsorb water. In some patients with

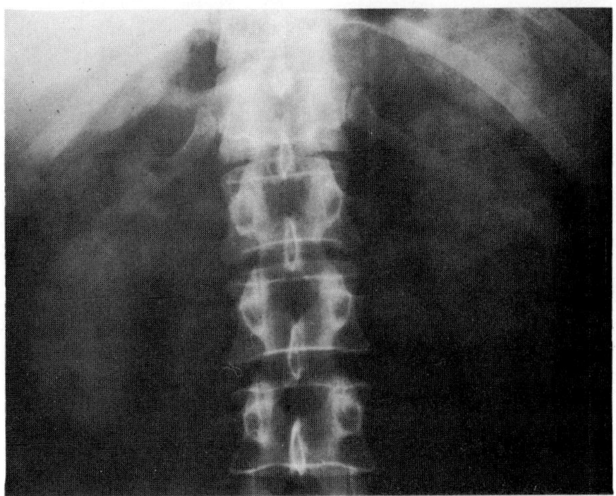

Fig. 80.3 Intravenous urogram. Film taken immediately after the injection of contrast medium was completed. Note the renal outlines. (The ovoid opacity above the left kidney is the fundus of the stomach.)

chronic renal failure, the nephrographic phase is the only contrast seen during the whole of excretion urography, yet often provides sufficient information to exclude obstruction, even though the pelvis and the calices of the kidney do not appear. In acute renal failure, too, it is of value because the nephrogram indicates the functional glomeruli. The quality of the nephrographic phase can be enhanced by taking tomograms (nephrotomography) and for this purpose a second injection may be necessary.

Pyelogram (*Fig.* 80.4)

Whereas the nephrogram depends on the proximal tubular reabsorption of water, the opacification of the calices, the pelvis and the ureters depend upon the amount of water reabsorbed in both proximal and distal tubules. In the distal tubule the amount of water reabsorbed is determined by the degree of hydration and the activity of antidiuretic hormone. The more dehydrated the patient, therefore, the more concentrated the dye becomes in the distal tubule, and the better the pyelogram. However, patients with severe chronic renal failure should not be dehydrated as the collecting systems will not opacify because they cannot concentrate urine.

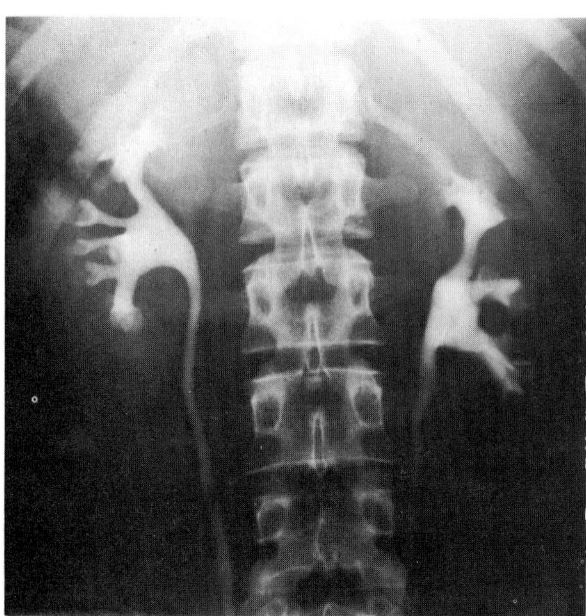

Fig. 80.4 Intravenous urogram. Film taken 10 min after injection of contrast medium.

Ureters (*Fig.* 80.5)

The ureters are rarely seen in their full lengths in excretion urograms. Better films of the pelvis, calices and ureters may be obtained by applying abdominal compression or by taking prone views.

Cystogram (*Fig.* 80.6)

The quality of the cystogram is improved if the patient voids urine before the examination. Another film of the bladder can be taken after micturition (*Fig.* 80.7). This postmicturition view may be of some value in assessing the amount of residual urine, but many patients find difficulty passing urine when asked to do so by the radiologist, and may

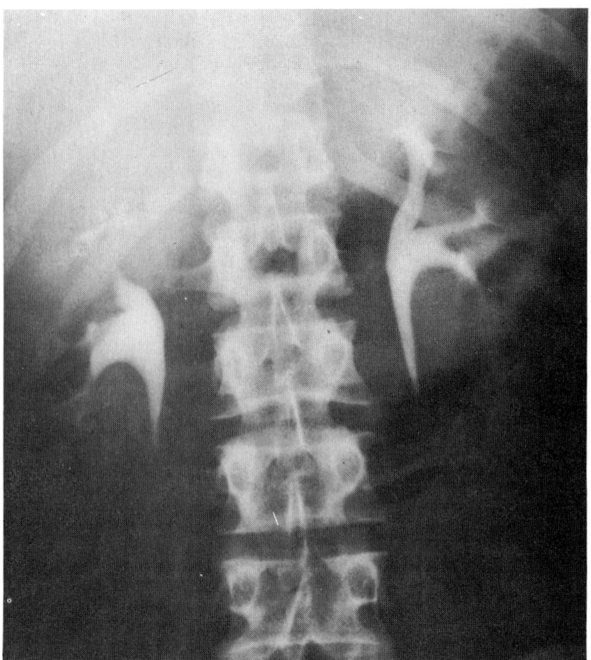

Fig. 80.5 Intravenous urogram. Film taken 15 min after injection. Good opacification of the pelvicaliceal system, but only parts of the ureter can be seen.

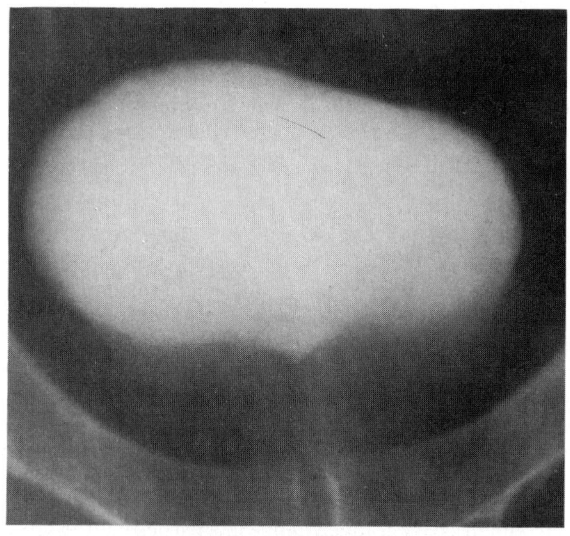

Fig. 80.6 Cystogram, premicturition.

micturate much better than the amount of dye remaining in the bladder in postmicturition films suggests.

The radiologist should look at the early films and decide if oblique films, tomograms, prone films or late films are needed. Late films are of special value in the diagnosis and assessment of obstructed kidneys (*Fig.* 80.8). If obstruction is suspected, but not obviously confirmed, further films can be made after the injection of frusemide.

Toxic Reactions

Ninety-five per cent of patients having excretion urography have no toxic reactions; minor reactions consisting of

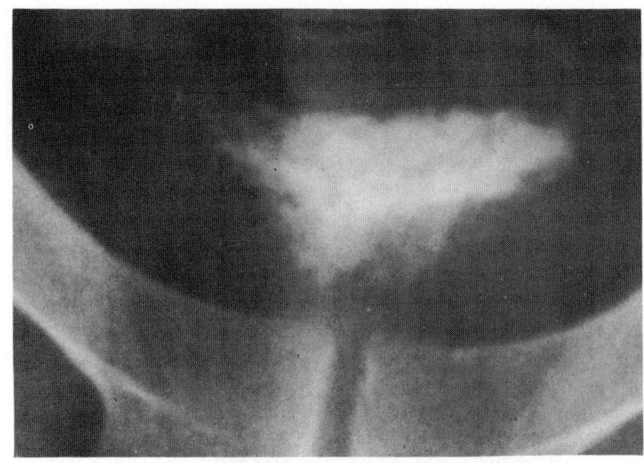

Fig. 80.7 Postmicturition cystogram.

nausea, faintness, minor skin rashes and sometimes urticaria occur in less than 4%. More severe reactions occur in about 1·5% and consist of hypotension, cardiac arrhythmias, bronchospasm and rarely airway obstruction, fits and coma. Obviously one should carry out the examination with caution in patients who complain of previous reactions to the injection of iodine compounds or who have other allergies including asthma.

Angiography

Renal angiography, main stream or selective, is carried out by the Seldinger technique. The main stream aortogram (*Fig.* 80.9) shows the number, the size, the levels and the distribution of arteries to both kidneys and, thereafter, selective angiography of the arteries of one or both kidneys can be carried out. Selective angiography can be divided into three phases:

1. The arterial phase which occurs some 3–4 sec after the injection (*Fig.* 80.10).
2. A nephrographic phase some 6–8 sec after injection, when the contrast media is in the capillaries and the tubules.
3. The venous phase some 12 sec after injection (*Fig.* 80.11).

To show the renal veins adequately requires venography. With the developments in ultrasound and digital subtraction angiography, the increasing availability and use of CT scans and the disenchantment with the preoperative embolization of renal-cell carcinomas, the use of angiography in urology has declined in the past few years. Its use now is more or less restricted to the assessment of live donors for renal transplantation, the elucidation of vascular anomalies, the investigation of some space-occupying lesions, especially bilateral ones, and as a means of angioplasty in patients with renal artery stenosis.

Digital Subtraction Angiography

This procedure uses high-quality image intensifiers and video camera recorders to visualize large arteries after the rapid injection of contrast media into a peripheral or central vein. The images obtained before injection are subtracted from those obtained after injection so enhancing the contrast between the blood vessels containing dye and other structures.

Venography (*Fig.* 80.12)

Pictures of the inferior vena cava and its branches can be obtained by using the Seldinger technique through the femoral vein. It is used less now than it was since invasion of the renal vein or vena cava in patients with renal-cell carcinoma can now be detected by ultrasound.

The procedure can, however, be extended to carry out testicular venography for the identification of undescended testes or the treatment of varicoceles by embolization.

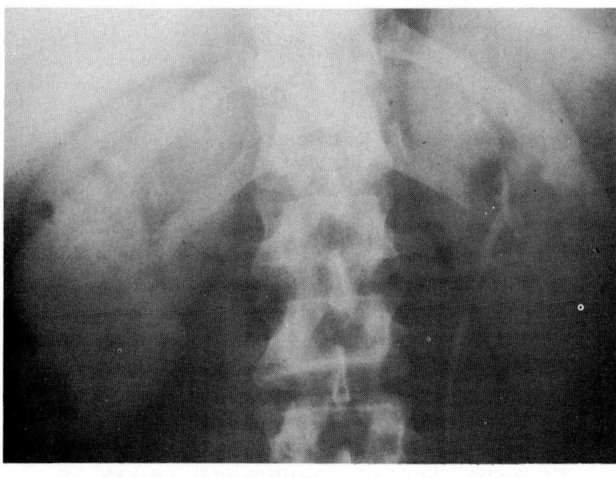

a

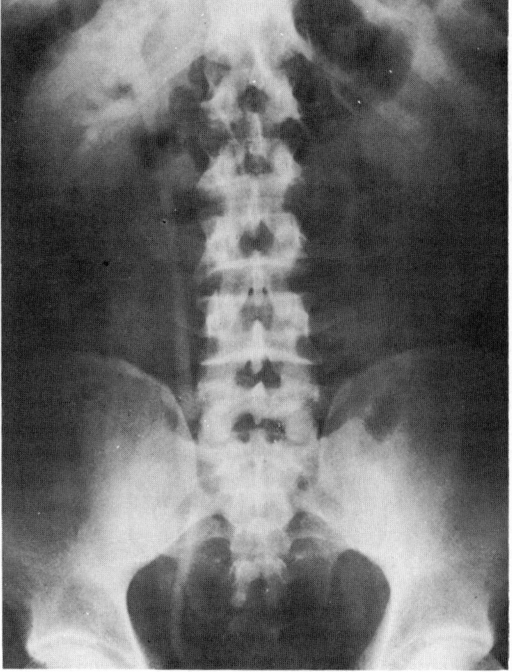

b

Fig. 80.8 *a*, Intravenous urogram 20 min after injection showing normal left kidney, nephrogram on right. *b*, Intravenous urogram 24 h after injection showing diseased right ureter.

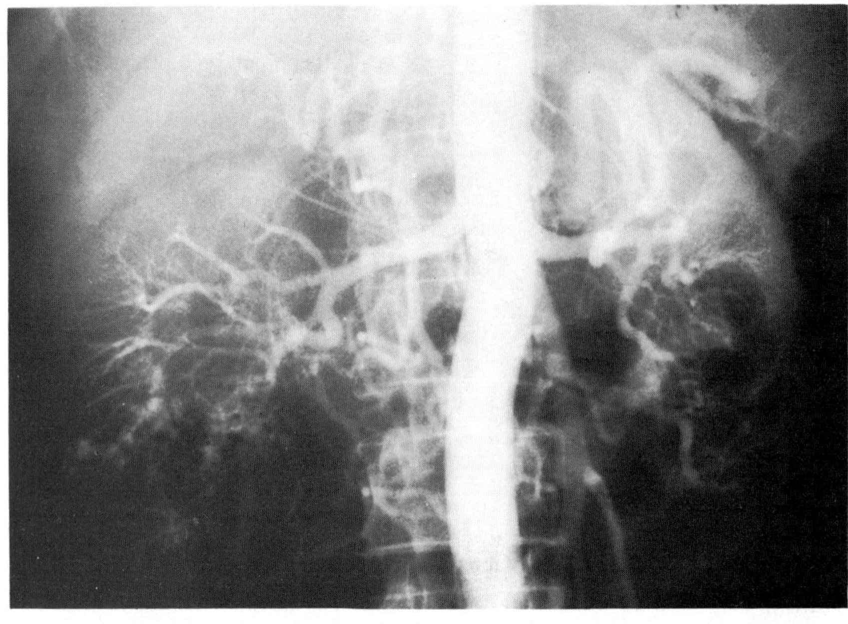

a

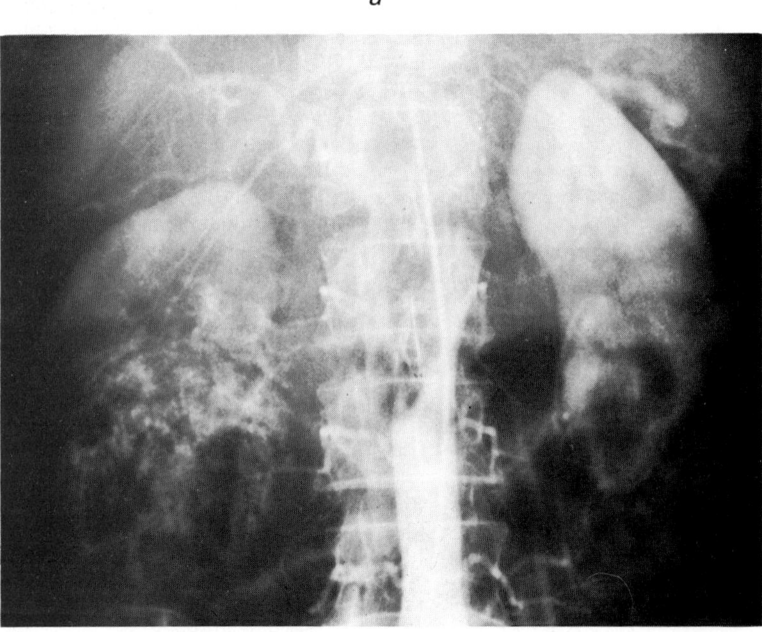

b

Fig. 80.9 Main stream aortogram; showing tumour circulation lower pole of right kidney. *a*, Arterial phase. *b*, Venous phase.

Retrograde Pyelo-ureterogram (*Fig.* 80.13)

Retrograde pyelograms are obtained much less frequently now than they were some years ago, because of the high quality of excretion urograms and the rapidly advancing non-invasive techniques of ultrasound and renal scanning. However, ureteric catheterization through a cystoscope may be necessary to clarify or obtain pictures of the renal pelvis and calices in patients with poorly functioning or non-functioning kidneys. The ureters are rarely seen in their entirety in intravenous pyelography, although late films and prone films often help and retrograde pyelo-ureterograms may be essential where ureteric lesions, particularly tumours, are suspected. Pictures of the ureters and even of the pelvis and calices are often best obtained by using bulb ureteric catheters like the Braasch and Chevassu. They are inserted no more than 2 cm into the ureteric orifice so that the bulb, which is just proximal to the tip of the catheter, plugs the orifice and thus prevents the contrast medium flowing back into the bladder as it is being injected. The technique also permits the collection of specimens from either kidney for split renal function tests, for exfoliation cytology and bacteriology. In iodine-sensitive patients caution must be exercised because if interstitial backflow occurs (12·5% of patients with obstructed kidneys), significant

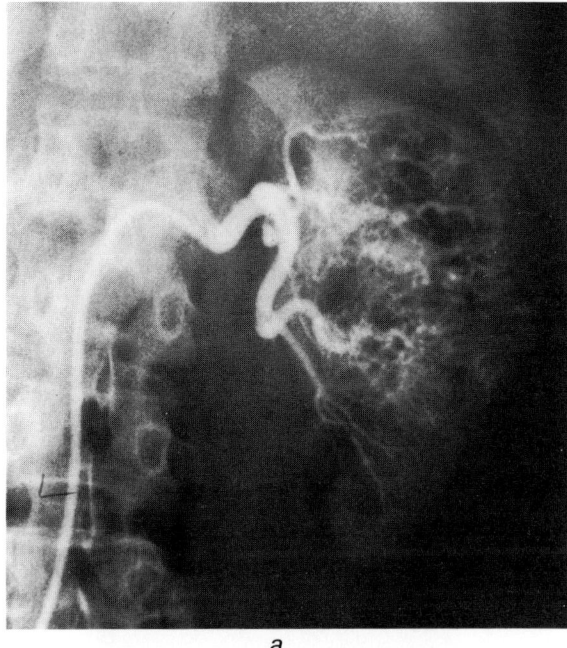

a

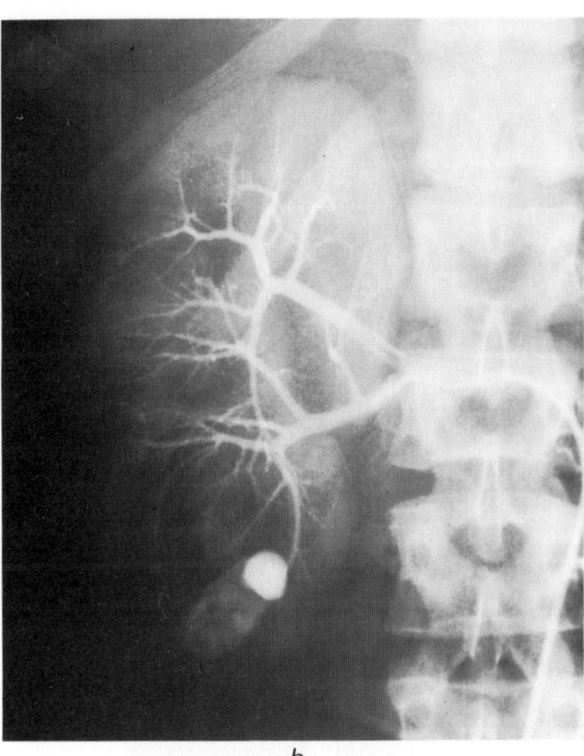

b

Fig. 80.10 Selective renal arteriogram. Arterial phase. *a*, Left kidney showing tumour. *b*, Right kidney showing false aneurysm of lower pole after nephrolithotomy.

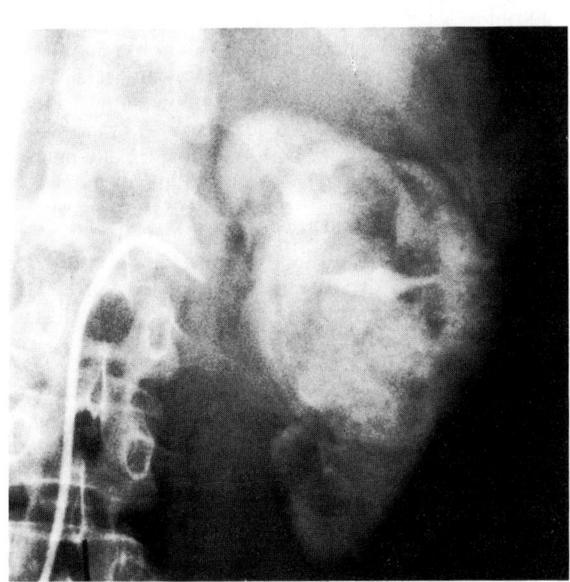

Fig. 80.11 Selective left renal angiogram. Venous phase showing tumour (same patient as in *Fig. 80.10a*).

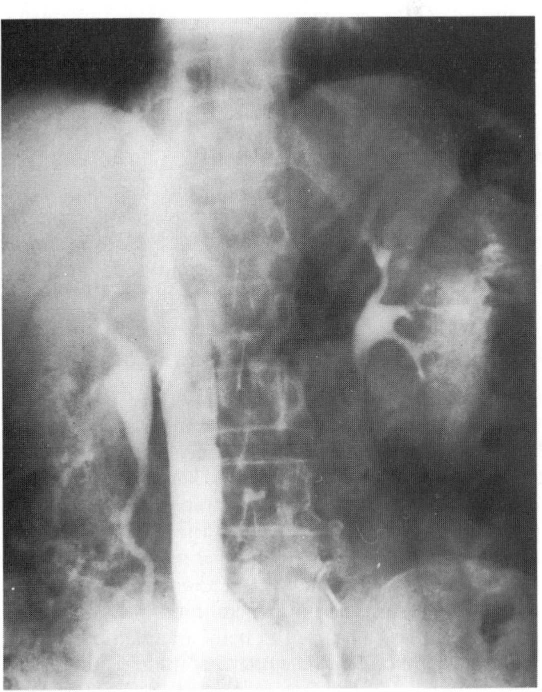

Fig. 80.12 Inferior vena cavogram. Note streaming from renal veins and kidneys.

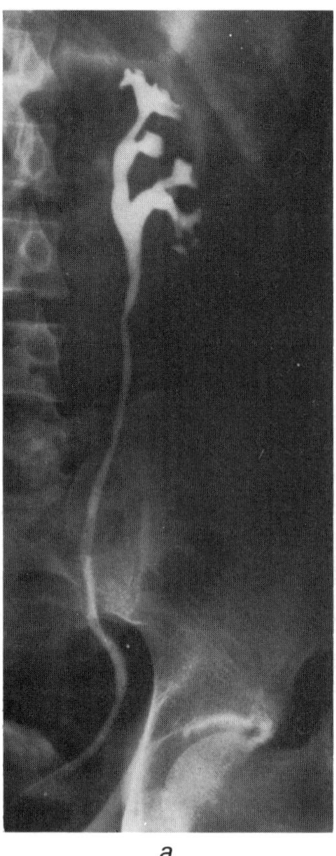

a

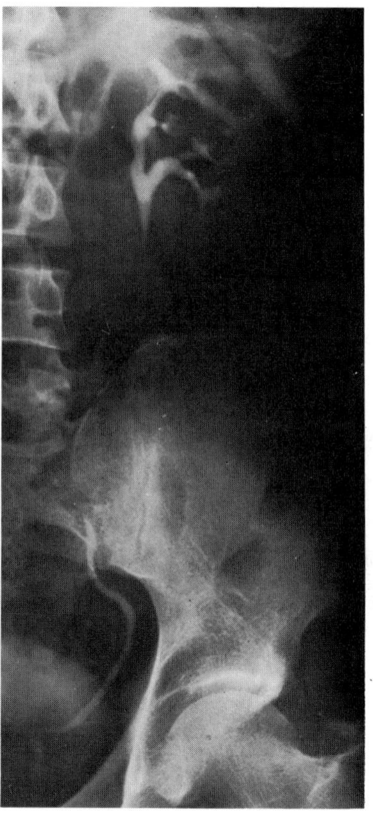

b

Fig. 80.13 Retrograde pyelogram. *a*, Retrograde pyelo-ureterogram showing full length of left ureter only the lower part of which was seen in the intravenous urogram (*b*).

amounts of iodine may be absorbed. If backflow does not occur, less than 1% of the iodine is absorbed. Pictures of the pelvis, the calices and ureters may be obtained by injecting air.

Antegrade Pyelography

If views of the pelvicaliceal system and ureter cannot be obtained by intravenous or retrograde pyelography, an antegrade pyelogram may be useful. A needle is inserted into the calices or pelvis of the kidney under radiographic or ultrasound control, urine is aspirated and contrast injected.

Retrograde Urethro-cystography

This procedure is carried out by inserting a 14 F Foley catheter into the external urethral meatus and inflating the balloon with 2–3 ml water. A 10–25% solution of one of the usual water-soluble contrast media is then slowly injected. It is very important that the small volume of dilute contrast is injected slowly, otherwise oedema of the urethral or bladder mucosa occurs or the contrast extravasates into the corpora. This procedure should demonstrate the anterior part of the urethra as far as the perineal membrane but considerable pressure often has to be used to make the media go beyond the external sphincter into the prostatic urethra and bladder. Anteroposterior and right lateral views are usually taken. Filling defects have to be interpreted with caution as they may only be air bubbles (*Fig.* 80.14).

Cystogram

A cystogram may be obtained with an intravenous pyelogram or by the procedure just described, but is best made by inserting a small catheter into the bladder and injecting 150 or 200 ml of a 10–30% solution of one of the water-soluble contrast media. Anteroposterior, left and right oblique films are obtained. A voiding view, preferably under a screen, should demonstrate whether or not vesico-ureteric reflux occurs (*Fig.* 80.15) and also provides a picture of the bladder neck and prostatic urethra, both of which usually open up widely during micturition. If adequate filling of the bladder occurs during retrograde urethrocystography a voiding view can also be made, and a picture of the whole length of the urethra obtained on one film. Postmicturition cystograms give us some idea of the amount of residual urine that remains in the bladder after micturition and confirm that it results from inadequate bladder emptying and not from vesico-ureteric reflux or diverticula.

Lymphangiography (*Fig.* 80.16)

This procedure is carried out by injecting indigo-carmine with 1% xylocaine into the skin and subcutaneous tissues in the webbed space on the dorsum of the foot. A 27 g needle can be inserted into the lymphatic channel which should become visible in 5–10 min and 5–6 ml of ethiodized oil (37% of iodine by weight) is then injected. The water-soluble contrast media are of no use because they leak out of the lymphatics. Radiographs taken 1 h after the injection

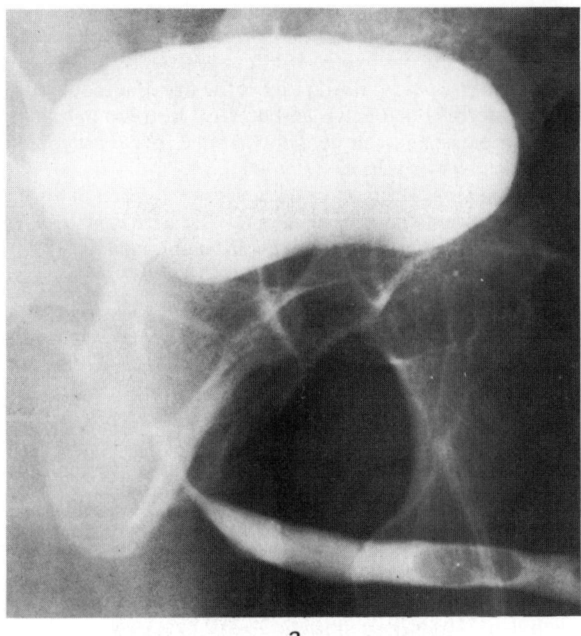

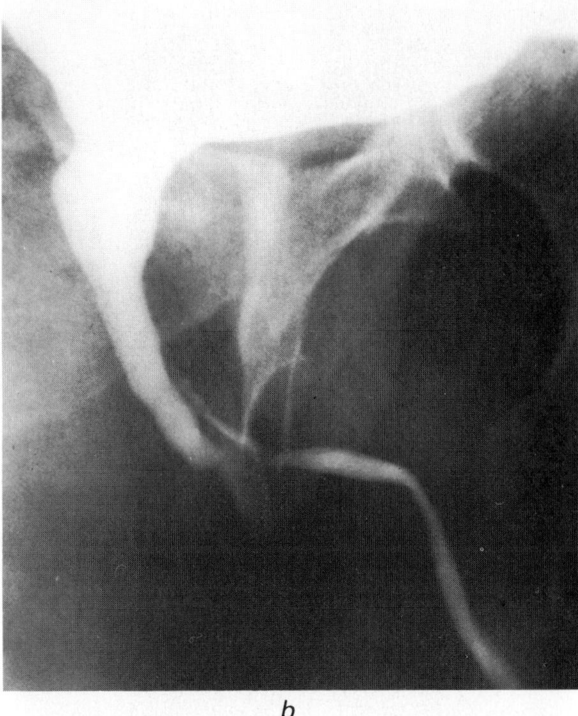

Fig. 80.14 Urethrogram. *a*, Ascending. *b*, Descending (voiding cystogram). Note that the spongy urethra is shown, but the prostatic urethra only as a thin line. Only in the descending (made same day) does dilated posterior urethra open and a false passage seen.

show the lymph vessels and 12–24 h after the injection show the lymph nodes. Some contrast leaks from the lymphatics into the veins, particularly if the lymphatics are obstructed, and this may cause pulmonary embolism. The procedure is particularly dangerous in patients who already have pulmonary disease and it is essential to have chest radiographs before the procedure starts. Lymphangiography shows the vessels in the lower limbs and the inguinal, external and common iliac and aortic lymph glands. It is of value in assessing nodal spread from tumours of the testes but of little value in carcinoma of the bladder and prostate which spread to the internal iliac glands.

NUCLEAR MEDICINE

The procedures of nuclear medicine are non-invasive, use less radiation than X-rays, require no preparation of the patient, are unaffected by gas or bowel shadows, and produce few if any reactions.

Renogram (*Fig.* 80.17*a*)

This is carried out using either *o*-iodohippurate, labelled with ^{131}I or ^{125}I, which is filtered at the glomerulus and secreted by the proximal tubules or ^{99}Tc^{m}-labelled DTPA. Concentration-time curves are recorded by scintillation counters placed over each kidney and over the heart after the intravenous injection of the labelled compound. The radiation dose from a single renogram is only one-tenth that of a straight radiograph. The curve produced has three components.

The vascular phase is the steep rise as the labelled compound arrives at the kidney. It depends on the arterial supply to the kidney and usually lasts about 20 sec.

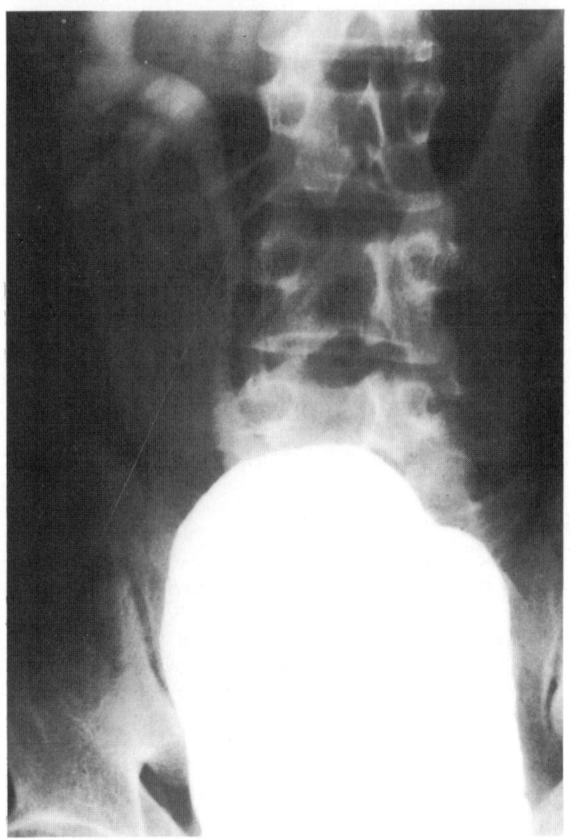

Fig. 80.15 Cystogram which shows vesico-ureteric reflux on the right side.

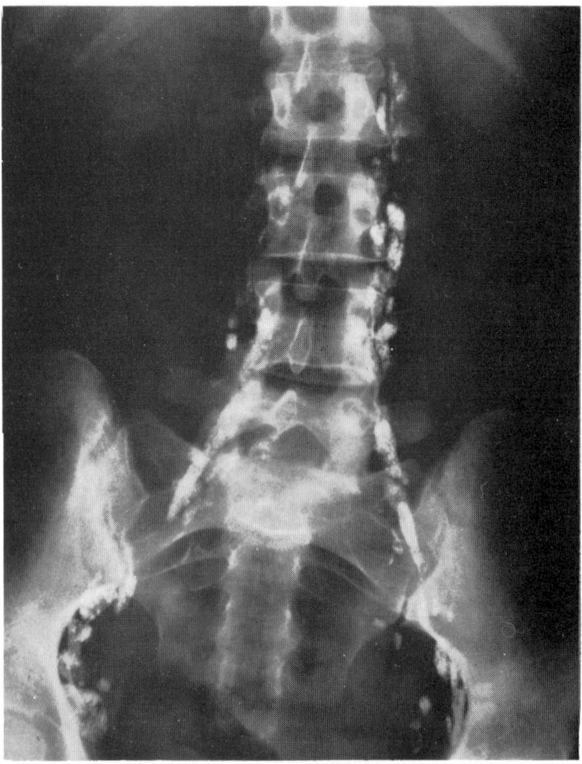

a

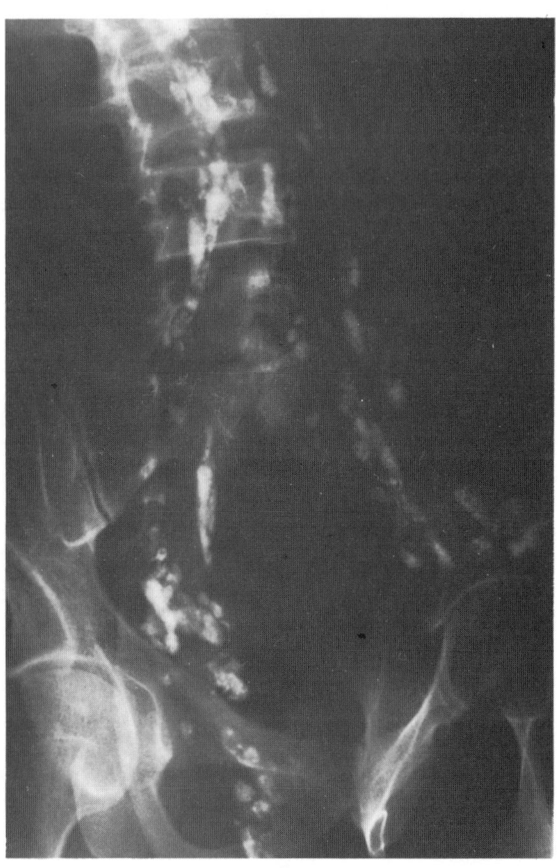

b

Fig. 80.16 Lymphangiogram. Normal. *a*, Anteroposterior. *b*, Oblique.

The secretory phase is proportional to the concentration of the dye excreted by glomerular filtration and tubular secretion, and lasts up to 5 min.

The excretory phase falls rapidly as the dye drains out of the kidney into the renal pelvis and ureter. Obstruction hinders the third phase and can be demonstrated more easily if the patient is given frusemide (*Fig.* 80.17*b*).

If the patient feels faint or has a vasovagal reaction during the examination the arterial flow to the kidney will be so much reduced that false results will be obtained.

Renal Scan

A linear scan takes 45 min so that rapidly-excreted substances like hippuran are unsuitable for routine use and chlormerodrin labelled with ^{203}Hg (half-life 47·9 days) or ^{197}Hg (half-life 2–7 days) have been substituted. Currently the ^{99}Tc^{m}-labelled chelates DTPA or DMSA are used and the image recorded by gamma-camera and computer readout. ^{99}Tc^{m} has a half-life of 6 h and is derived from the decay of the longer lived molybdenum. Hippuran labelled with ^{123}I is also useful, but is expensive and not yet freely available. Imaging can be dynamic or static.

Dynamic imaging is best carried out with ^{99}Tc^{m} DTPA (diethylene tetramine pentacetic acid) which is excreted only by glomerular filtration and can be used to assess the glomerular function of each kidney. A fifteen millicurie bolus is injected intravenously. Images at 30 sec depend upon the perfusion of the kidneys; later studies are made as the substance is excreted into the collecting system.

Static imaging (*Fig.* 80.18). For static imaging ^{99}Tc^{m} DMSA (dimercaptosuccinic acid) is used. Five millicuries are injected and after 3 h more than 50% is taken up by the parenchyma and less than 10% excreted. It images the functioning renal parenchyma of each kidney and also shows which parts of each are functioning.

For the assessment of obstruction DTPA is used and its rate of drainage from the kidney measured by a routine 30-min study. Increase in its concentration at 30 min may be caused by obstruction or by the slow emptying of a large volume collecting system. A frusemide diuresis aggravates obstruction, but rapidly washes out tracer if there is no obstruction. A DMSA scan with multiple views may demonstrate a space-occupying lesion, and can be a useful test in patients who are iodine sensitive, but is less satisfactory than ultrasound.

In acute renal failure the changes are functional rather than structural and scans using DTPA are useful, particularly in children with acute renal failure and they avoid the high osmotic loads needed for nephrotomography. In acute tubular necrosis perfusion is normal but there is neither function nor excretion; during recovery glomerular filtration increases and transit times at first slow, gradually revert to normal.

Renal scanning is now routine in the assessment of renal transplants and DTPA scans provide a measure of perfusion, function and outflow from transplanted kidneys. The onset of rejection can be recognized early by detecting a deterioration in renal perfusion.

Bone Scan

Radioisotope bone scanning using ^{99}Tc^{m}-labelled phosphate and particularly diphosphonate compounds produces an image of the whole skeleton. The substances have a half-life of about 6·2 h and the radiation dose compares favourably with that of skeletal X-rays. Radiographs show skeletal

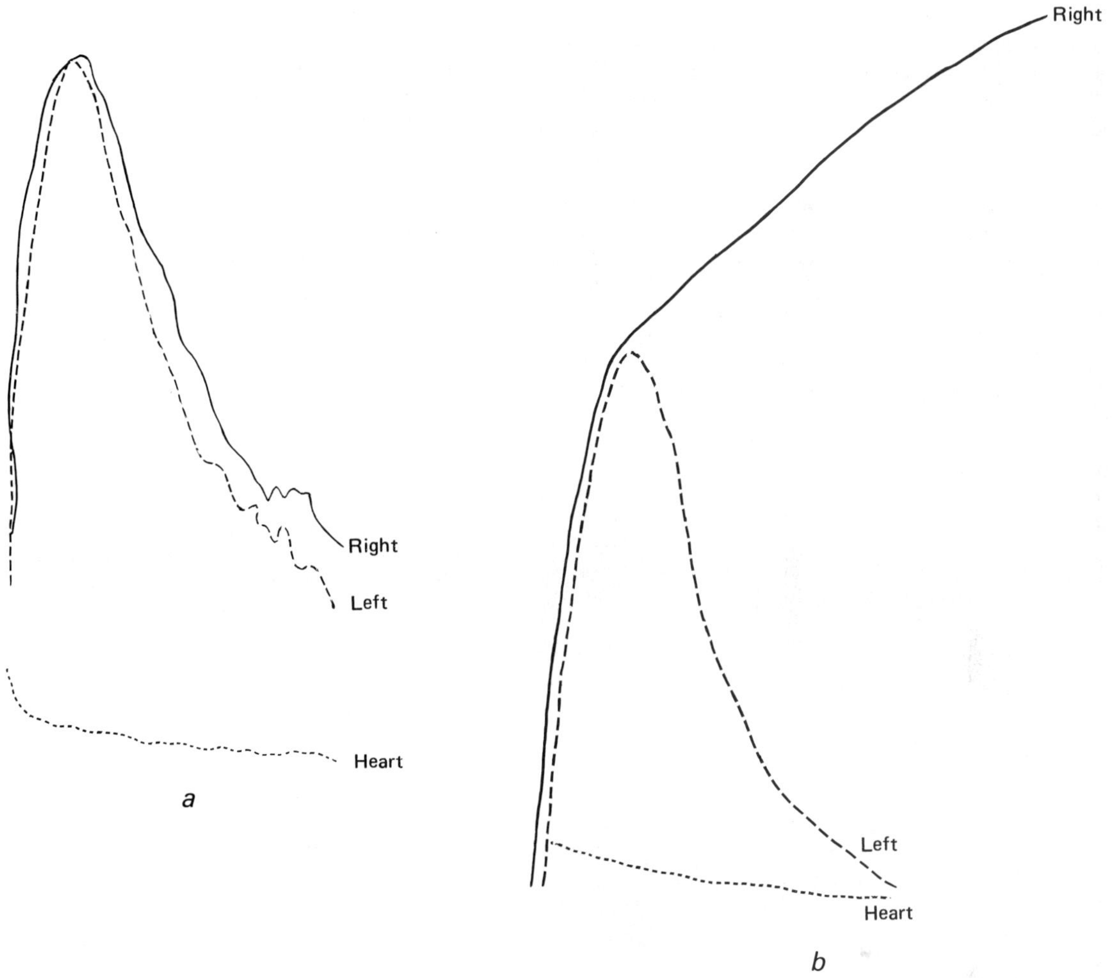

Right

Right
Left

Heart

a

Left

Heart

b

Fig. 80.17 Renogram. The upper two lines represent left and right kidneys. The lower line represents the background. *a*, Normal. *b*, Obstructed.

changes which are caused by bone reabsorption and repair, and destructive lesions have to be larger than 1·5 cm in diameter with a loss of at least 50% of bone material before they can be seen. Bone scans, on the other hand, represent skeletal metabolic activity (the mechanism by which the radioactive substances are taken up in bone are not fully understood but they are probably adsorbed on to calcium) and are affected by osteoblastic activity and bone vascularity. A scan represents the reaction of bone to neoplastic, degenerative, inflammatory or traumatic diseases and in the early stages of bone resorption radiographs may be normal but the scan abnormal. By detecting functional rather than structural changes scans show metastases, particularly from prostatic carcinoma, at an earlier stage than radiographs. However, bone scans are non-specific and it is essential to compare abnormal bone scans with the appropriate radiographs. Metastases are the most likely cause, if the scan is positive and the radiograph negative.

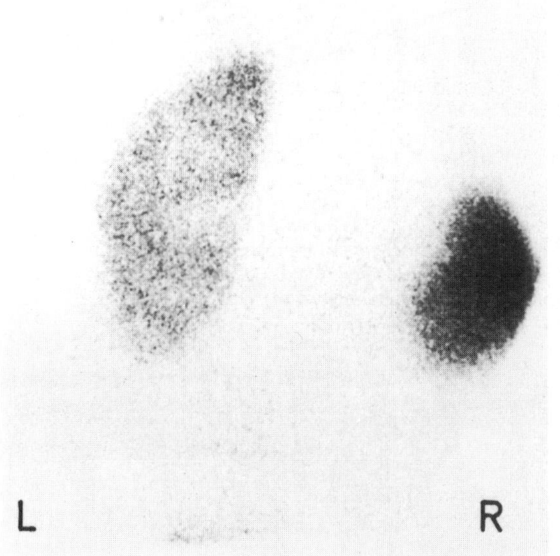

Fig. 80.18 Renal scan. Showing obstructed left kidney and a small right kidney.

ENDOSCOPY

Endoscopes have improved considerably over the past two decades, for the following three reasons:

1. The invention of fibreoptics by Hopkins and Kapany in 1954 led to the development of flexible endoscopes for gastroenterology and other specialties. In urology which uses rigid telescopes it has replaced the small distal incandescent bulb with a large external quartz iodine lamp, the light from which is transmitted through the endoscope by a large number of glass fibres.

2. The rod lens telescope was also invented by Professor Hopkins in 1960. In the old system, the telescope consisted of a tube of air with a thin glass lens; in the rod lens system it consists of a tube of glass with a thin lens of air. The advantages are twofold: first, more than twice as much light is transmitted through the rod lens system and secondly, lenses of greater diameter for a given outer diameter can be fitted, increasing the amount of light that is transmitted and the field of vision.

3. The development of a multilayer anti-reflective coating of the lens prevents the loss of light by reflection increasing the light transmitted from the object to the observer. In all, the amount of light transmitted is increased eightyfold.

CYSTO-URETHROGRAPHY

The endoscopic examination system (*Fig.* 80.19) consists of a sheath which is a straight hollow tube; 21 or 22 F is the usual size for adults, but they can be as small as 11 F for children. It is passed into the bladder with an obturator which prevents damage to the urethra. If a hollow obturator is used the urethra can be examined using a 30° or 0° telescope and constant irrigation as the sheath is passed. Once the instrument is in the bladder, the bladder is emptied and then filled with 300 ml of sterile saline 0·9% or water, and examined with both the 70° and 30° telescopes. Using an Albarran bridge, electrodes can be passed into the bladder or catheters and stone dislodgers into the ureters. Punch biopsy forceps can be used for taking biopsies from suspicious areas in the bladder and urethra and from adjacent mucosa which looks apparently normal, because in situ changes may not be obvious. Resectoscope sheaths (*Fig.* 80.20) also vary in size, but a 26 F one is probably best, using either a 30° or a 0° telescope. Saline can be used for inspection purposes, but if diathermy is required for the resection or coagulation of tumours, it must be replaced by either water or a non-electrolytic isotonic substance like glycine (1·5% amino-acetic acid). Water is best when resecting bladder tumours because it destroys any loose cells and prevents implantation.

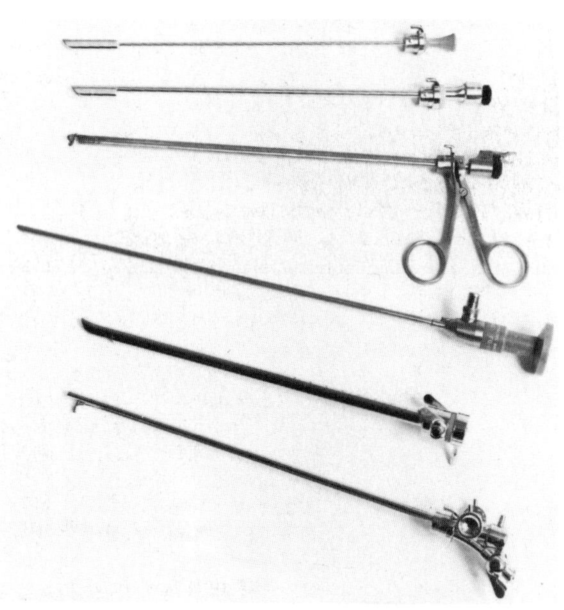

Fig. 80.19 Endoscopes. From top downwards: obturator, hollow obturator, biopsy forceps, telescope, sheath, Albarran bridge (by courtesy of ACM Endoscopy Ltd).

PERCUTANEOUS RENAL SURGERY

The procedure can be done under local or general anaesthesia and either ultrasound or intravenous urography can be used to facilitate the introduction of a needle into the kidney. Through this needle can be aspirated cysts or dye injected to obtain antegrade pyeloureterograms, or the needle can be replaced with a small tube to drain the kidney or to carry out pressure studies (Whitaker test).

For endoscopic diagnosis or treatment the needle track is dilated until a 20 or 26 F nephroscope sheath can be inserted. The appropriate telescope or working element can then be passed through the sheath into the kidney. Stones, filling defects and strictures of the pelvi-ureteric junction or caliceal necks can be evaluated. Thereafter, stones can be removed or debulked, tumours biopsied (even resected) and strictures incised.

For these procedures patients must be carefully selected and those with untreatable bleeding disorders, uncontrolled infection and marked hepato- or splenomegaly excluded.

URETERORENOSCOPY

The ureterorenoscope consists of rigid or semi-rigid examining and operating sheaths 10 and 12·5 F in diameter respectively and each long enough to extend from the external urinary meatus to the renal pelvis; the appropriate 0° telescope and a variety of instruments that can be passed visually through the sheaths to remove stones, insert stents

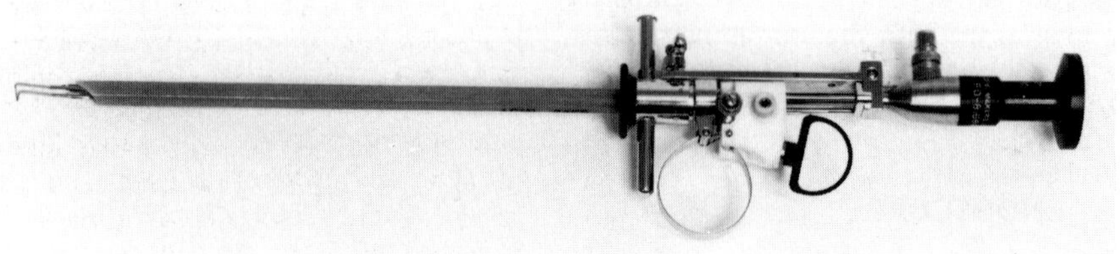

Fig. 80.20 Iglesias resectoscope (by courtesy of ACM Endoscopy Ltd).

and biopsy tumours (*Fig.* 80.21). To manipulate the instrument down the urethra into the ureteric orifice (which must first be dilated with acorn bougies or a balloon ureteric catheter) and up the ureter is not easy. It can be tedious and time-consuming and in patients with strictures, large prostates, fixed hips or angled ureters impossible.

A flexible fibreoptic cystoscope has been introduced. It can be used more easily under local anaesthesia than the rigid instruments but is presently only suitable for inspecting the bladder and urethra.

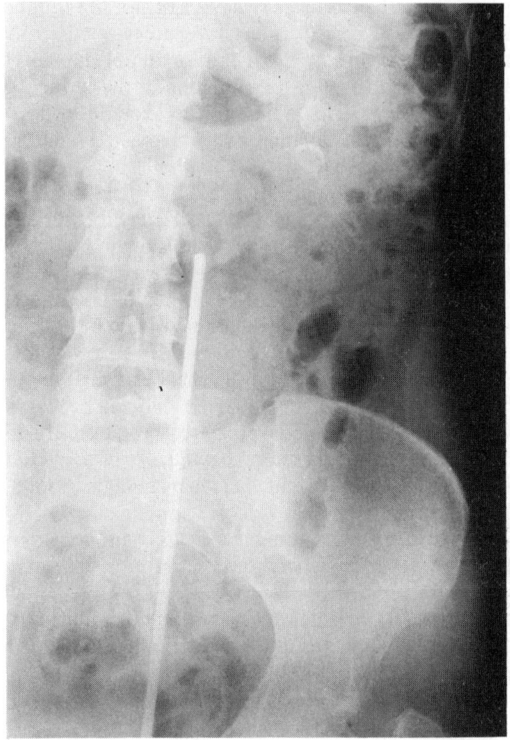

Fig. 80.21 Plain radiograph showing the Storz ureteroscope introduced, after dilatation of the ureteric orifice, up the ureter into the pelvis of the left kidney.

BIOPSY

Kidney

Needles may be passed percutaneously into the kidney for the aspiration of cysts or the performance of antegrade pyelography. Percutaneous biopsy rarely provides a sample of more than 20 glomeruli out of the total number of some 2 million and is therefore of little value in patchy diseases like pyelonephritis. It is of value in patients with asymptomatic proteinuria if more than 1 g of protein is excreted per day, especially if it is associated with microscopic haematuria or impaired renal function. Biopsy is also of value in patients with recurrent haematuria when both intravenous urography and cystoscopy are normal and proteinuria is present; with acute renal failure when there is no predisposing cause and when obstruction has been excluded; with chronic renal failure when radiologically normal size kidneys are found and in some patients with the nephrotic syndrome. The procedure is contraindicated if the opposite kidney functions inadequately or is absent, if the patient has a haemorrhagic tendency; if the platelet count is less than 10 000 per ml; if the prothrombin time is more than 16 sec and if both kidneys are shrunken.

Bladder

Biopsies can be easily and safely taken from bladder mucosa using the punch biopsy forceps passed through an endoscopic sheath and using a 30° or 0° telescope. In patients with bladder tumours, bopsies should be taken from it and from other parts of the bladder, because dysplasia or even carcinoma-in-situ may be found in areas that look normal. Biopsies are best taken from bladder tumours with a resectoscope when underlying muscle can be obtained and the tumour put into its correct T-stage.

Urine cytology may be of value in the diagnosis of transitional-cell tumours of bladder ureter and kidney.

Prostate

Biopsies can be taken from the prostate by transurethral, rectal or, less often, perineal routes. A transurethral biopsy is taken when the tumour is resected to relieve obstruction. For transrectal biopsy a Tru-cut needle is used and it can be inserted accurately into quite small nodules.

Testes

A biopsy can be taken from the testes through a small incision for subfertility investigations, but if tumour is suspected, the spermatic cord is first exposed at the deep inguinal ring. There is a high incidence of carcinoma-in-situ in the contralateral testis of those suffering from testicular tumours, and some surgeons take a biopsy from the opposite testis too.

URODYNAMICS (*Fig.* 80.22)

For many years cystoscopy, cystography, urethrography and urethroscopy have provided a satisfactory means of studying the structure of the bladder and urethra. Urodynamics provides a means of studying their function, but does not replace the need to take a careful history, which tells us much on its own account and helps us interpret the results of urodynamics. The basic study consists of measuring the urinary flow rate, the bladder pressures, the bladder filling volume and the amount of residual urine, if any. With more expensive equipment the electrical activity of the pelvic muscle and the urethral closing pressures can also be assessed.

A two-way catheter is passed into the bladder which is emptied, the residual urine is measured and examined bacteriologically; one limb of the catheter is connected to a reservoir, the other to a recording manometer which measures the bladder pressure. The bladder pressure has two components, the detrusor pressure and the intra-abdominal pressure. A pressure recorder in the rectum measures the rectal pressure which is the same as the intra-abdominal pressure, and if subtracted from the bladder pressure gives the detrusor pressure. The urinary flow rate can be measured using a urine flow meter of one kind or another and is normally 20 ml or more. The flow curve is a steep parabolic curve with a sharp ascent and sharp descent, i.e. urine is passed rapidly and completely. However, flow rates vary with the volume passed and are reduced with volumes below 250 ml or above 600 ml. It is therefore important that flow rates are measured when the patient feels he wants to pass

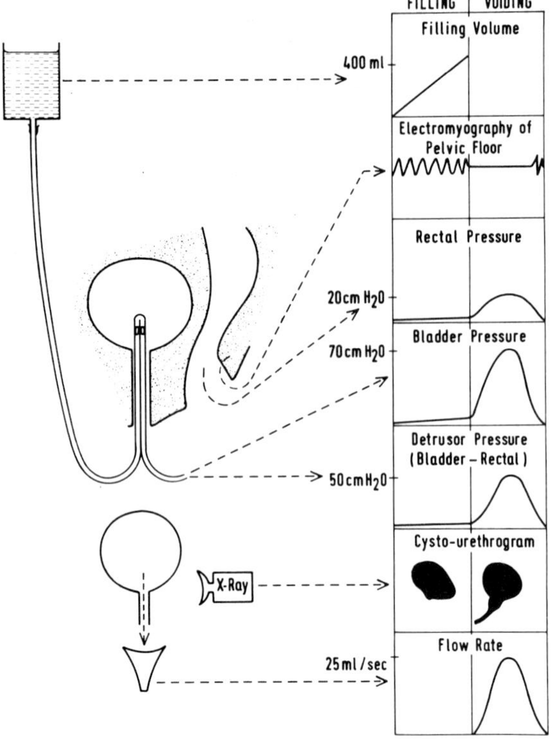

Fig. 80.22 Urodynamics.

urine. Urodynamics can be of considerable value in distinguishing stress incontinence from urge incontinence in obstruction because outflow obstruction is likely if the flow rate is less than 17 ml and the detrusor pressures more than 50 cmH_2O in women, and more than 60 cmH_2O in men. The amount of residual urine should be measured only after the patient has passed an adequate volume of urine. In patients with bladder diverticula or vesico-ureteric reflux the volume of residual urine seems higher than it is.

ULTRASOUND

Ultrasound waves are a mechanical form of energy in the form of vibrations with frequencies above those that can be appreciated by the human ear, i.e. greater than 20 000 cycles per second (20 000 Hz). In practice frequencies of 1–5 million cycles per second (1–5 MHz) are used. The higher the frequency the better the resolution but the poorer the penetration. They are produced by an ultrasound transducer which consists of a quartz crystal placed in an electrical field and directed as a narrow beam on to the object under study. When they strike interfaces between tissues of different densities and of different sound velocities, some of the beam is reflected back as echoes which are received and converted back to electrical impulses by the transducer. The echoes are then amplified by an oscilloscope, and using a scan converter can be stored, reproduced and displayed. The time delay between transmission of the wave and return of the echo indicates the depth of the interface and the amplitude of the echo, its nature. Modern instruments enable us to grade accurately the amplitude of the echo and give us a 'grey scale' image so that the contour, size and the internal architecture of the object being studied is demonstrated.

The kidneys are readily examined by contact scanning, i.e. the probe is in contact with the skin, and the quality of the images obtained is independent of the renal function (*Fig.* 80.23).

Ultrasound pictures of the kidney reveal its size, position and mobility and the size of the calices and pelvis; cystic lesions can be distinguished from solid ones and sometimes stones can be visualized. Ultrasound is of value in the investigation of hydronephrosis, trauma, space-occupying lesions, acute and chronic renal failure, and in transplanted kidneys it assists in the recognition of acute and chronic rejection. In renal-cell carcinoma it not only assists in the diagnosis but can also reveal whether or not the tumour has invaded the renal vein or inferior vena cava.

Many doctors, although the author is not among them, consider that an ultrasonic examination of the kidneys complemented by a straight radiograph to exclude stones, is as good a screening test in patients with suspected renal disease as excretion urography.

The ureter can only be imaged by ultrasound if it is dilated and filled with urine, but it may be difficult to distinguish a dilated upper ureter from a dilated renal pelvis.

Contact scanning of the bladder will reveal whether or not it is distended and some estimate of the volume of residual urine, if any. Transurethral probes have been developed and can be used to assess the size of bladder tumours and the extent to which they infiltrate the bladder wall.

The prostate can be examined by contact probes if the bladder is distended but is probably best examined with transrectal probes which can reveal the size of the gland and distinguish to some extent between benign glands and malignant ones.

The testis can be examined by contact probes or by the water bath method in which both the scrotum and probe are immersed in the same bath of water but are not in contact with each other. Solid lesions can be distinguished from cystic ones and their origin from testis or epididymis often determined.

COMPUTERIZED AXIAL TOMOGRAPHY (CT SCAN)

A CT scan is equivalent to taking many radiographs from a stationary X-ray tube while rotating the patient a little between each one, and ending up with a large number of films each taken from a different angle. The method is a useful means of demonstrating the size and the contours of the kidneys, and the presence within them of stones, haemorrhage and tumours, and lesions as small as 1 cm in diameter, have been demonstrated. However, it often contributes little more than ultrasound.

NUCLEAR MAGNETIC RESONANCE (NMR)

This is a technique that generates high-quality images of soft tissues within the body, without the harmful effects of radiation and it is non-invasive.

Unlike ultrasound it penetrates bony structures without attenuation, and unlike CT scans it can provide not only transverse scans but also coronal or sagittal ones.

It involves placing the patient in a large magnetic field which causes the hydrogen nuclei, abundant in soft tissues, to orientate themselves in the direction of the field, i.e. they behave like bar magnets. The nuclei are then excited by

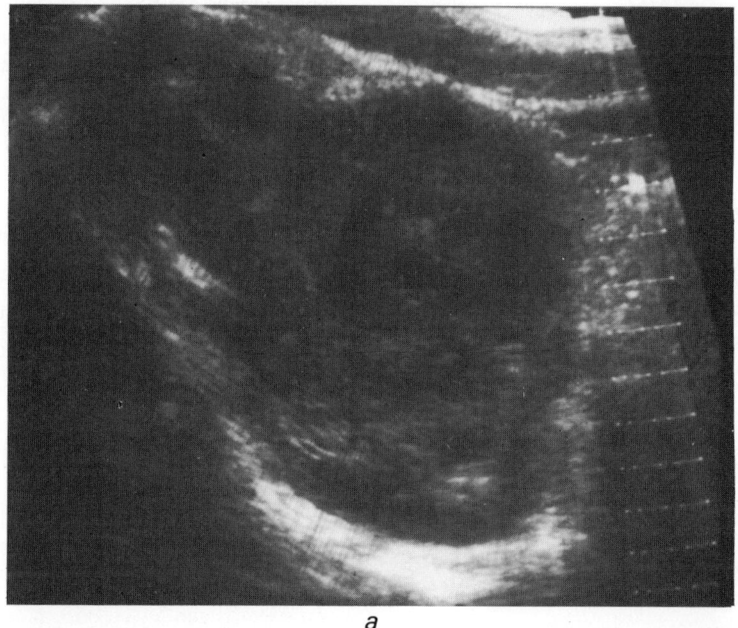

a

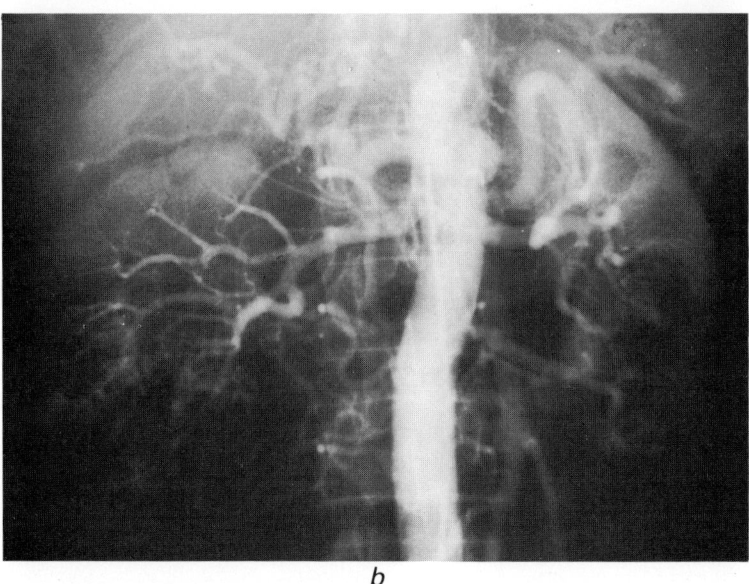

b

Fig. 80.23 *a*, Ultrasound showing large tumour of right kidney. *b*, Main stream aortogram of the same patient.

radiofrequency waves generated by a transmitter coil that is wrapped around the patient. The returning signals are detected by a receiver coil and when analysed enable the soft tissues to be differentiated from each other to produce the scan.

CONCLUSIONS AND THE WAY AHEAD

Investigations other than those described in this chapter have to be done in some patients, for instance the estimation of risk factors in the serum and urine of stone formers, of markers in the serum of patients suffering with tumours and of antibodies in the serum and seminal plasma of infertile patients. These and other special tests are described along with the relevant diseases.

Urological surgeons have always prided themselves on possessing investigative resources that enable them to diagnose and assess most diseases accurately before deciding what treatment, if any, was needed. In the last few years the old resources of intravenous urography, endoscopy and angiography have been much improved and new resources, ultrasonography, nuclear medicine, NMR, CT scanning, nephroscopy and ureteroscopy added. Now, disease can not only be diagnosed and assessed better (and often with much less discomfort and stress for the patient) but its progress and the effect upon it of treatment can be followed more easily.

But what is the value of being able to diagnose carcinoma of the kidney in more than 99% of patients who have it, if 50% have such advanced disease when they first present and of those suitable for operation less than 50% survive 5 years. The detection of disease before it causes symptoms or better, but less likely, the prevention of disease must remain the aim.

Further Reading

British Medical Bulletin. (Endoscopic Surgery) (1986) **42**, 274–284.
Hricak H. (ed.) (1986) *Genito-urinary Ultrasound*. Edinburgh, Churchill Livingstone.
Lang E. K. (ed.) (1986) *Percutaneous and Interventional Urology and Radiology*. Berlin, Springer-Verlag.
Marsh F. P. (ed.) (1985) *Postgraduate Nephrology*. London, Heinemann.
Mundy A. R. (ed.) (1986) *Scientific Basis of Urology*. Edinburgh, Churchill Livingstone.
Rintoul F. (ed.) (1986) *Farquharson's Textbook of Operative Surgery*. Edinburgh, Churchill Livingstone. pp. 504–527.
UICC (1978) *TNM Classification of Malignant Tumours.* 3rd ed. Geneva.
Whitfield H. N. and Hendry W. F. (ed.) (1985) *Textbook of Genito-urinary Surgery*. Vols. 1 and 2. Edinburgh, Churchill Livingstone.

81 *The Kidney and Ureter*

T. B. Hargreave

CONGENITAL ABNORMALITIES

Renal Development, Renal Agenesis, Hypoplasia, Dysplasia, Hypertrophy

During the 5th week of fetal development cells of the coelomic lining and underlying *mesenchyme* proliferate to form urogenital folds on either side of the midline of the posterior abdominal wall. The kidney and testes arise from this fold. Three separate excretory organs develop sequentially: the pronephros, the mesonephros and the metanephros. The first two consist of excretory tubules arranged segmentally and emptying into the mesonephric duct (Wolffian duct). The pronephros is well developed only in embryo fish and the mesonephros persists as the excretory organ of all fish and amphibians but in humans the only surviving remnants of these systems are some mesonephric tubules which form the efferent tubules of the testes and the mesonephric duct which becomes the vas deferens. The differentiation of the metanephros into renal tissue depends on the stimulus from the developing ureter and pelvis. Thus, true congenital absence of one kidney is usually associated with an absent ureter, a hemitrigone and often with absent vas deferens on that side. The incidence of congenital absence of one kidney is 1 in 2500 and it is often a chance finding following urological examination for an unrelated symptom. The diagnosis is made by the finding of a hemitrigone and absent ureter on cystoscopy, the absence of excretion on one side during intravenous urography and by the absence of the renal mass on ultrasound examination. Usually the single kidney on the other side exhibits a marked degree of hyperplasia and hypertrophy. Hypertrophy normally occurs following removal of one kidney or in the presence of unilateral renal disease and the lack of hypertrophy may indicate unsuspected bilateral renal disease. The distinction between renal hypoplasia (congenitally small kidney) and acquired shrinkage (e.g. chronic pyelonephritis) is often academic as both tend to result in renal hypertension. Dysplasia of the kidney is where the tissues show abnormal differentiation. Cases either have an abnormally structured kidney or an irregular mass of cysts.

Polycystic Disease

This is an important congenital abnormality of renal development. In the infantile type both kidneys are enormously enlarged at birth and there may be cysts in several other organs, including the liver. Babies with this disorder usually die of respiratory failure. The condition is probably inherited as a recessive characteristic and thus may affect siblings.

Adult polycystic disease is a different disorder inherited as a Mendelian dominant or arising by mutation. The disease takes a slower course, symptoms appearing for the first time in the 30s. The usual presenting features are loin pain, secondary to haemorrhage into a cyst, headache, lassitude, vomiting secondary to renal failure, cardiac failure or cerebral haemorrhage. Treatment aims at controlling hypertension and renal failure by, in some cases, renal dialysis and transplantation. Operations to deroof the cysts do not affect renal function unless the cyst is causing ureteric obstruction when a decompression operation may be justified. Pressure from a cyst can also be relieved by ultrasound guided cyst puncture.

Solitary Cysts (*Fig.* 81.1)

These are common and usually arise from the lower pole. They are usually diagnosed incidentally. Their main importance lies in distinguishing these harmless cysts from renal tumours. Ultrasound examination has revolutionized the approach to this problem. If ultrasound reveals a cyst and aspiration of the cyst fluid under ultrasound control yields clear fluid with no malignant cells, no further follow-up of the patient is required.

Medullary Cystic Disease

This is discussed in the section on stones.

Ectopic Kidneys

The kidneys arise from the lower pole of the urogenital ridge and in contradistinction to the testes migrate upwards during fetal development. Failure of migration results in a pelvic kidney (*Fig.* 81.2). Abnormal migration may result in a thoracic kidney or one kidney may cross the midline (crossed renal ectopia) (*Fig.* 81.3). The kidneys may be fused at their lower poles to give a horseshoe kidney. Most of these abnormalities are of interest only because of their rarity but it should be remembered, however, that an unsuspected mass palpated at laparotomy could be an ectopic kidney.

Fused Kidneys—Horseshoe Kidney (*Fig.* 81.4)

The commonest type of fused kidney is the horseshoe kidney joined at the lower pole. The fused lower poles of the

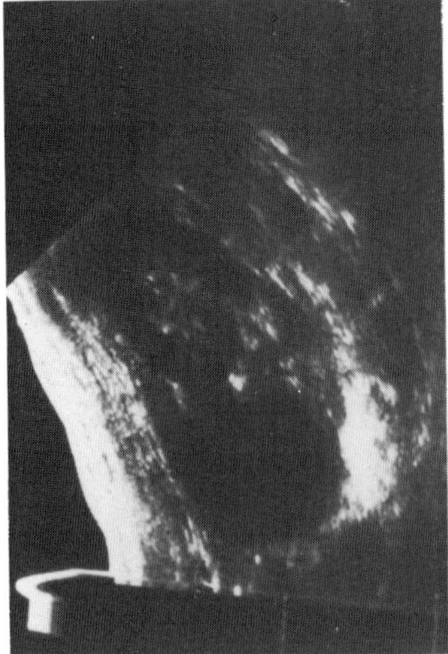
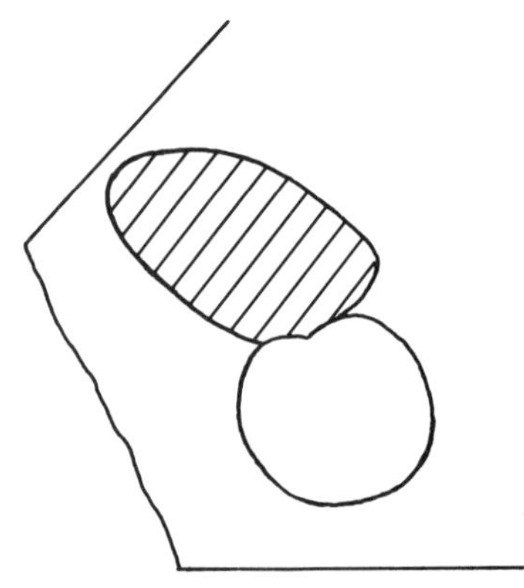

Fig. 81.1 Ultrasound showing a large lower pole renal cyst.

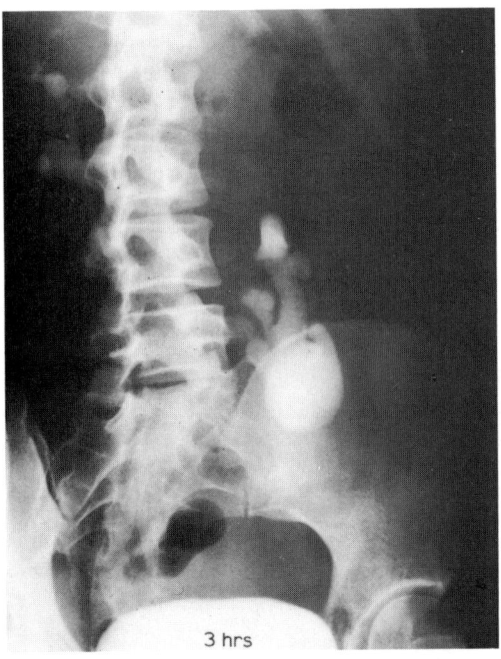

Fig. 81.2 Intravenous urogram showing a pelvic kidney.

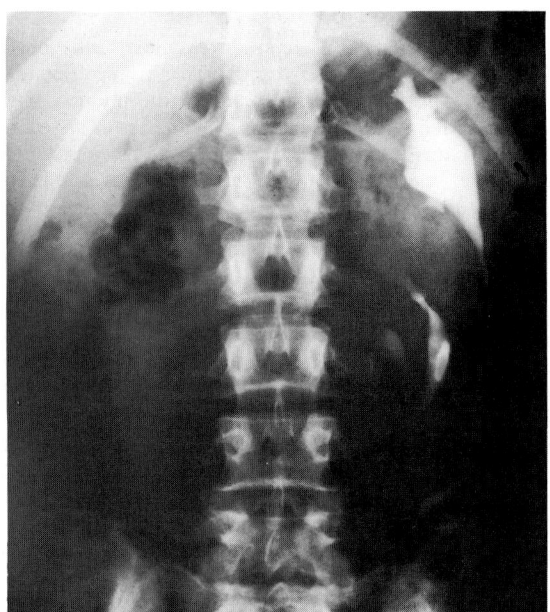

Fig. 81.3 Intravenous urogram showing crossed renal ectopia.

kidneys usually lie in front of the aorta in the region of the 4th or 5th lumbar vertebra and the ureters descend in front of the fusion. The main complication is ureteric obstruction which may require surgical correction. Presenting symptoms are pain secondary to ureteric obstruction or attacks of urinary tract infection, and a firm mass may be felt in the pelvis. An intravenous urogram shows low kidneys with non-rotated renal pelves with the ureters near the midline.

Fusion may occur in cases of crossed renal ectopia and sometimes the upper or both upper and lower poles are fused.

Duplex Kidney

A common anomaly is the duplex kidney, which has two pelves but one mass of parenchyma (which is usually longer than normal). The ureter may also be completely duplicated and both open separately into the bladder. If so the ureter from the upper moiety always opens below that from the lower. Hydronephrosis, infection, stone, or reflux may affect only one moiety, usually the lower. If the ureters are only partly duplicated urine may reflux from one into the other.

Ectopic Ureter

The upper ureter from a duplex system or the ureter from a single system may open in an ectopic position. This may be anywhere between the lateral angle of the trigone and the opening of the ejaculatory ducts in males; and anywhere between the lateral angle of the trigone and the external urethral meatus in females. Females with an ectopic ureter

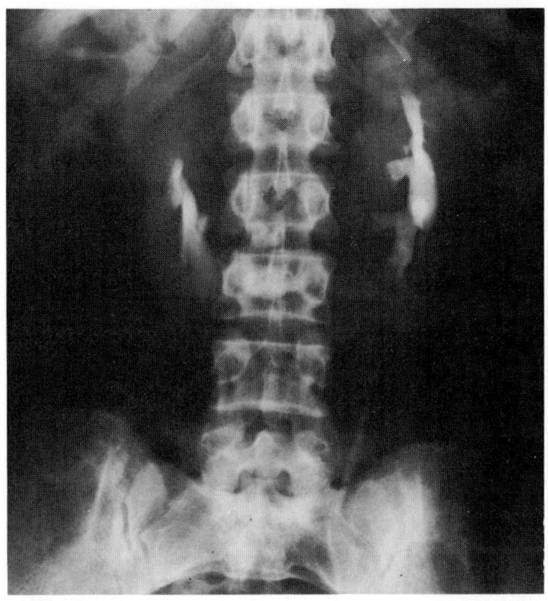

a

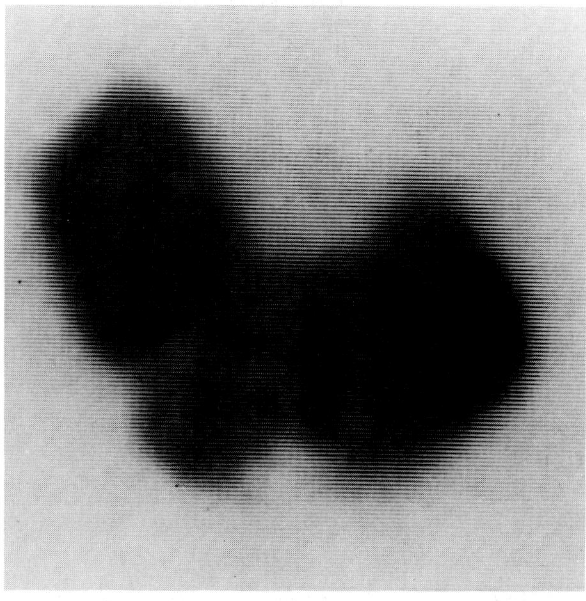

b

Fig. 81.4 *a*, Intravenous urogram of a horseshoe kidney. *b*, DMSA scan of the horseshoe kidney. Note the fusion of renal tissue across the midline shown more clearly on the scan than the urogram.

may be incontinent. The classic presentation in a female child is with dripping incontinence between normal voids.

RENAL INJURY

The kidney or its pedicle may be damaged by blunt or by penetrating injuries.

Blunt Injuries

With blunt injury the renal damage may be associated with damage to other viscera or to the skeleton, particularly the ribs, transverse processes or vertebrae. The injury can be classified as a subcapsular contusion; a laceration (which usually involves the collecting system and capsule); as fragmentation (when the kidney is split into a number of fragments) or as injury of the renal pedicle which is usually an intimal tear of the artery. Deceleration injuries involve the pedicle more often than the kidney.

Penetrating Injuries

These are uncommon in the UK but when they do occur usually involve other viscera, such as the spleen, liver, colon, mesentery or vena cava.

Clinical Features

Haematuria is the classic sign and usually obvious; however, lesions of the renal pedicle, even severe ones, may cause only transient microscopic haematuria. Lacerations cause haematuria and may form a loin mass. The first consideration is resuscitation by securing the airway and restoring the blood volume, then the extent of the renal injury can be assessed unless other visceral injuries require urgent treatment.

A plain radiograph may reveal injuries of the ribs, transverse processes or vertebrae, a soft-tissue mass obliterating the psoas shadow or an elevated diaphragm. An excretion urogram is essential; it shows the severity of the injury and confirms if the other kidney is normal. With a subcapsular bruise the kidney appears more or less normal; with a laceration the kidney continues to function but usually less well than normal and dye extravasates (*Fig.* 81.5); with fragmented kidneys and major pedicle injuries the kidney appears non-functioning. If no function is seen in the urogram an aortogram and selective renal angiogram should be done to distinguish between fragmented kidneys and injuries of the pedicle (*Fig.* 81.6). Ultrasonography reveals haematoma and renal scans show function but are of more value in following-up the patient than in the initial assessment.

Treatment

Subcapsular bruises and lacerations usually heal and can be treated conservatively. Fragmented kidneys may heal, but must be explored if the patient deteriorates. If the patient has two kidneys and one is badly damaged, nephrectomy is safe treatment. However, it is vital not to overlook the possibility of a solitary kidney. The experienced renal trauma surgeon may decide to save the kidney by draining any haematoma, stopping bleeding and reconstituting the kidney. This approach has the advantage that the patient is left with two kidneys but the disadvantage that in some cases renovascular hypertension develops later because of excess renin secretion from relatively ischaemic areas of the damaged kidney. These cases thus require further follow-up and if hypertension occurs a secondary nephrectomy may become necessary (*Fig.* 81.7).

Injuries of the pedicle are intimal tears usually with thrombosis if the lesion is closed, partial or complete tears if it is open. The kidney is usually irreversibly ischaemic by the time of diagnosis but exploration is worthwhile if the patient is seen within 12 h of injury; and essential even after that time if the patient deteriorates from continued blood loss. Sometimes the renal injury is recognized only when a

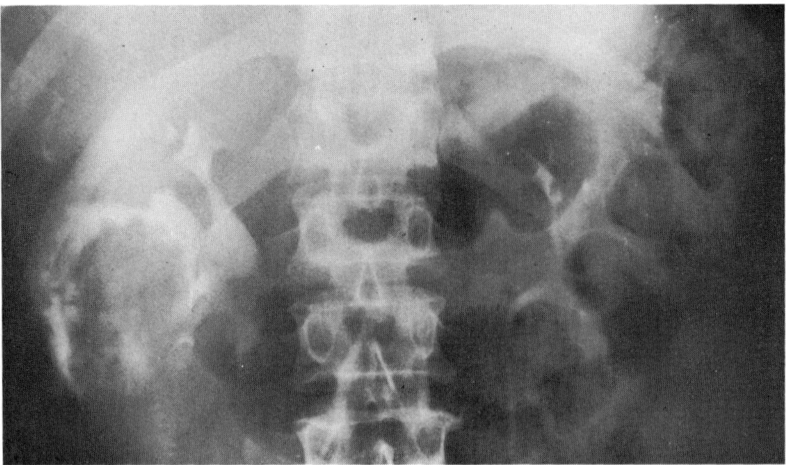

Fig. 81.5 Intravenous urogram showing an intrarenal haematoma following trauma and extravasation of the dye into the perinephric tissues.

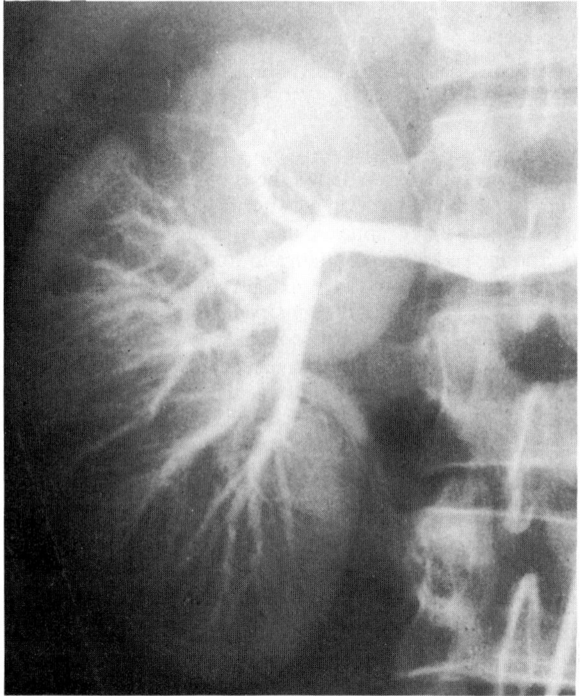

Fig. 81.6 Arteriogram showing rupture of the kidney following trauma.

retroperitoneal haematoma is found during laparotomy to control intra-abdominal bleeding. An excretion urogram should be done on the table as the function of the other kidney cannot be assessed by sight or palpation.

URETERIC TRAUMA

Ureteric injuries following external trauma are rare. Iatrogenic ureteric trauma may follow hysterectomy when the ureter can be accidentally caught as it crosses the base of the broad ligament. The ureter can also be injured by too ambitious an attempt at endoscopic ureteric stone extraction and by examination with the rigid ureteroscope. Ureteric stones should not be removed using the ureteric basket if they are too large (greater than 1 cm), more than 5 cm from the bladder or have been impacted for too long (longer than 6 weeks). Occasionally the passage of the stone may result in a spontaneous ureteric tear and extravasation. Injury to the ureter usually results in stricture or fistula or extravasation of urine. The presence of iatrogenic ureteric injury may be indicated by unexpected loin pain following an abdominal operation or by postoperative collapse because of extravasation of urine. The extent and location of the injury is assessed by intravenous urography and retrograde, ascending or antegrade urography.

Ureteric Fistula

Ureteric fistulas are rare. They may follow trauma or be associated with pelvic tumours or diverticular disease, but the commonest are ureterovaginal fistulas following hysterectomy or a perineal fistula following abdominoperineal resection of the rectum. It is sometimes difficult to decide if a fistula rises from the lower end of the ureter or from the bladder and instillation of methylene blue into the bladder may resolve the problem. The diagnosis of the site of the fistula is made by intravenous urography and, if necessary, by ascending urography with screening. These fistulas are sometimes difficult to repair because of surrounding scar tissue and are best treated by reimplanting the ureter into the bladder. A flap of greater omentum is useful to buttress the surgical repair and provide a good blood supply to the area.

RENAL OBSTRUCTION

Obstruction may occur within the kidney at the caliceal neck, at the junction of the pelvis and ureter or at some point along the length of the ureter.

Caliceal Obstruction

The usual cause is fibrosis following tuberculosis or a caliceal stone. Occasionally the distended calix may cause pain and warrant surgical exploration although it is always

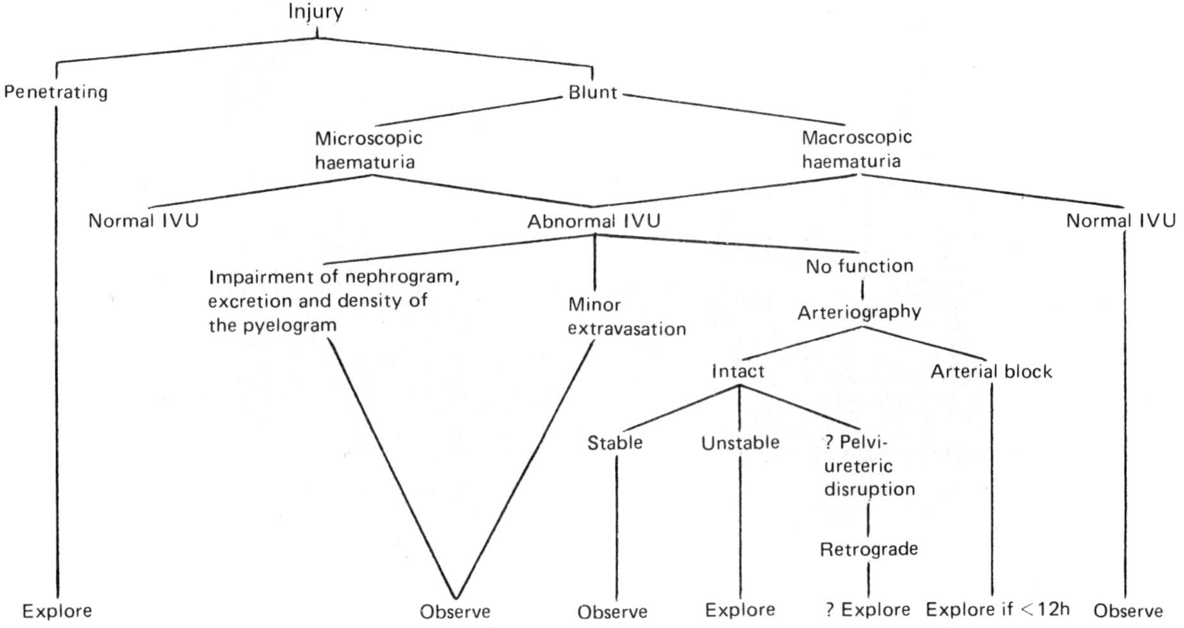

Fig. 81.7 Flow diagram showing investigation and treatment of renal injury.

very difficult to be sure that the distended calix is the cause of pain. A congenital diverticulum of the calix is usually symptomless. The upper calices sometimes become distended and cause pain secondary to crossing vessels, the superior infundibular syndrome. This syndrome is difficult to diagnose and the benefits from surgical exploration are doubtful. Hydrocalicosis, a general dilatation of all the calices is usually associated with obstruction to the renal pelvis of ureter, but may not be very marked in those cases where the renal pelvis is intrarenal or fibrosed.

Pelvi-ureteric Junction Obstruction (*Fig.* 81.8*a*)

This is a congenital abnormality, usually bilateral, where there is a functional obstruction to the passage of urine at the junction of the renal pelvis and ureter. The condition may arise either from a muscular deficiency in the last part of the renal pelvis and first part of the ureter or because of crossing vessels (*Fig.* 81.8*b*). The exact nature of the muscular deficiency is not yet understood; it has been shown that there is a disorganization of the propagation of the contraction of the muscle wall. Normally, contractions of the renal pelvis start in the calices from specialized cells adjacent to the renal papillae. The contractions start simultaneously spreading as a wave down the calices, renal pelvis and ureter, but in pelvi-ureteric junction obstruction this coordinated wave of contraction is lost. How the calices coordinate with each other is mysterious because there are no demonstrable nerve fibres.

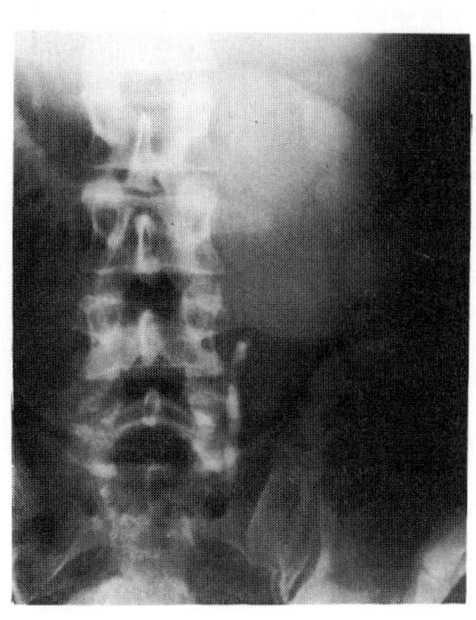

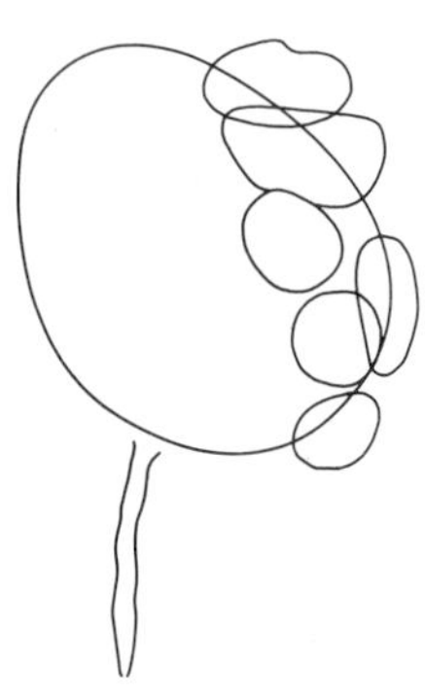

a

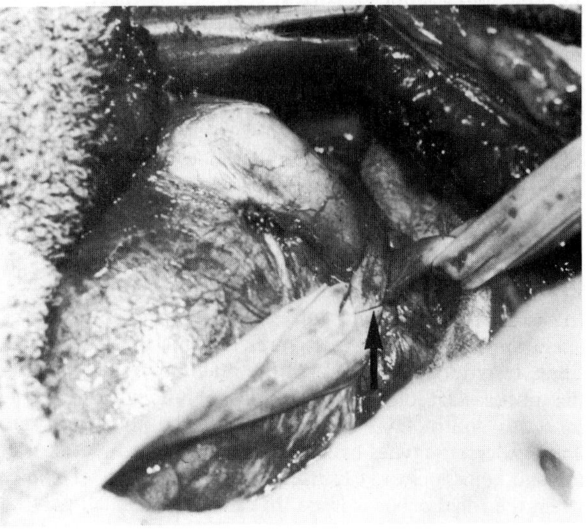

b

Fig. 81.8 *a*, Hydronephrosis and hydrocalicosis secondary to pelvi-ureteric junction obstruction. *b*, Operative photograph from the same case as shown in *a*. In this case the ureteric obstruction is secondary to crossing lower polar vessels (arrowed).

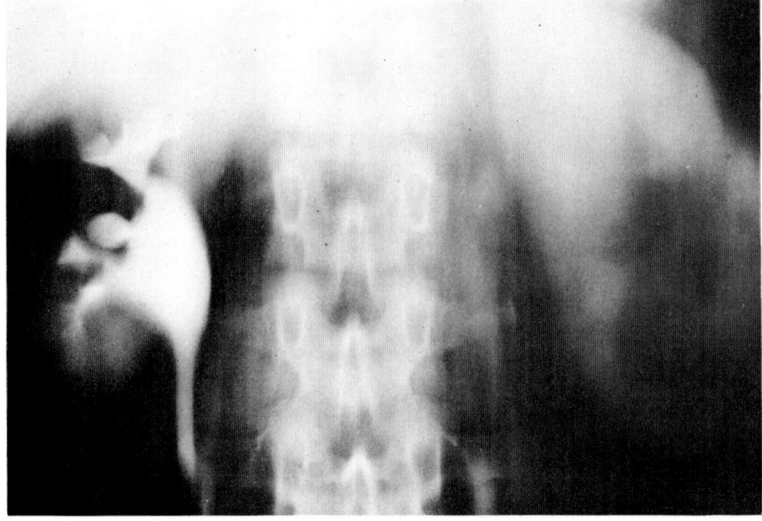

Fig. 81.9 Five-minute film in an intravenous urogram series showing unilateral renal obstruction. On the obstructed side the calices have not yet filled with contrast and show as radiolucent areas.

Clinical Features

The condition may be diagnosed in utero if an ultrasound scan is performed or it may present in babies as a failure to thrive because of renal failure and sometimes there is also a prominent abdominal mass. In older children there may be loin pain associated with symptoms of urinary infection. Adults usually present with loin pain particularly after a fluid load but in some cases, the first manifestation is renal failure. It should be remembered that the condition is often bilateral and the opposite kidney should always be carefully assessed.

Diagnosis

The diagnosis is made by intravenous urography (*Fig.* 81.9). Usually the dilated renal pelvis appears only on the late films and the ureter is not visualized. It is wise to check that the rest of the ureter is normal by retrograde urography before committing the patient to operation. Radionuclide scans may also help with the diagnosis. It is sometimes difficult to distinguish an obstructed dilated system from a dilated system with no obstruction but poor renal function and the renogram curve after the administration of frusemide may resolve this difficulty because a rising curve indicates obstruction.

Operative Treatment

In cases secondary to muscular deficiency, the object of the operation is to free the pelvi-ureteric junction from adhesions, to reduce the volume of the renal pelvis and to form the upper part of the ureter into a funnel so that the muscular contractions can better 'grip' the bolus of urine. The Anderson–Hynes pyeloplasty, where a segment of ureter and renal pelvis is excised, is the operation of choice when the renal pelvis is large. In cases with a small pelvis a flap of pelvis can be rotated to widen the upper part of the ureter—the Culp pyeloplasty. When a crossing vessel (*see Fig.* 81.8*b*) is the problem it is sometimes sufficient to move the vessels relative to the pelvi-ureteric junction but a pyeloplasty is often the best procedure even in these patients.

Ureteric Obstruction

Some causes of ureteric obstruction are listed in *Table* 81.1. Symptoms from obstruction depend on how rapidly it has developed. Rapid obstruction from a stone or blood clot usually results in classic ureteric colic radiating from loin to groin. More insidious obstruction from tumour or fibrosis

Table 81.1 Causes of ureteric obstruction

Within the lumen
Stone
Transitional-cell carcinoma of the urothelium
Blood clot
Within the wall
Congenital pelvi-ureteric junction obstruction
Vessels crossing to the lower pole of the kidney
Congenital obstruction of the ureterovesical junction
Tumour—primary sarcoma
—secondary infiltration from prostatic, cervical, rectal or bladder cancer
Infection—tuberculosis
—inflammation, xanthogranuloma
Outside the ureter
Congenital (cysts arising from the lower pole of the kidney, mesenteric or urachal cysts may obstruct the lower ureter)
Diverticulum of the bladder
Pregnancy
Tumour—Retroperitoneal glands or any tumour arising from abdominal organs
Benign prostatic hypertrophy
Inflammation of surrounding tissues secondary to diverticulitis, Crohn's disease, appendicitis
Fibrosis—idiopathic retroperitoneal fibrosis
—fibrosis secondary to diffusely infiltrating carcinoma or an aneurysm
Iatrogenic—Accidental tying of the ureter during hysterectomy, lower segment Caesarean section or colectomy

may simply be associated with a dull loin ache. The diagnosis of obstruction is confirmed by finding poorly functioning kidneys on one or both sides during intravenous urography, and the site of obstruction by ascending, retrograde or antegrade urography. Radionuclide scans will confirm renal obstruction and are particularly useful for following-up cases after treatment.

The vexed question of whether to relieve bilateral malignant ureteric obstruction is difficult. It is tempting now that we have many new modalities of anticancer treatment to relieve ureteric obstruction and to try tumour treatment. In general, most cases do very badly and the relief of obstruction is not a kindness to the patient; the exception to this is prostatic cancer infiltration involving the lower ends of both ureters where long and symptom-free survival has followed surgical relief of obstruction and treatment of the tumour. Temporary relief of obstruction can be achieved by placing Silastic ureteric stents: this is a useful treatment while waiting to see if there will be a response to chemotherapy.

Retroperitoneal Fibrosis

This may be primary idiopathic fibrosis or fibrosis secondary to diffusely infiltrating cancer or previous leakage from an aortic aneurysm. Drug-induced retroperitoneal fibrosis (e.g. methysergide) may regress if the administration of the drug ceases. It may also arise as a complication of Crohn's disease. Very often the clinical picture is difficult to distinguish and it is important in each case to ensure that abdominal malignancy is not overlooked.

Idiopathic Retroperitoneal Fibrosis

This usually occurs in men between the ages of 40 and 60. The presenting symptoms are those of renal failure: anorexia, nausea, vomiting and weight loss. There may also be a history of loin pain or backache. The typical appearance in the intravenous urogram is deviation of one or both ureters to the midline from the region of the 2nd, 3rd, or 4th lumbar vertebrae with distension of the ureter and hydronephrosis above. The erythrocyte sedimentation rate is usually raised. Retrograde urography is useful to delineate the ureter and to exclude other causes of bilateral obstruction, e.g. bilateral calculi. Characteristically the ureteric catheter will pass easily through the obstructed area and failure to do so may indicate another cause, e.g. bilateral infiltrating tumour from prostate or cervix. Treatment is to relieve the ureteric obstruction by mobilizing the ureter from its sheath of fibrous tissue. Further obstruction by extending fibrosis may be prevented by displacing the ureter laterally or into the abdominal cavity and it helps to wrap the ureter with a pedicle flap of greater omentum.

Megaureter

A wide ureter may be the result of obstruction (*see above*), ureteric reflux or may neither be obstructed nor refluxing but a congenital disorder. This latter condition may be associated with failure of development of the abdominal wall and a large bladder ('prune belly' syndrome). The distinction between refluxing and non-refluxing megaureter is made by a micturating cystogram. Obstruction is diagnosed by renography or a ureteric pressure flow study. The ureteric pressure flow study is performed by percutaneous introduction of a catheter into the renal pelvis and by placing a catheter in the bladder. The renal pelvis catheter is perfused at 10 ml/min and the pressure to produce this flow is measured. If the pressure exceeds 22 cmH_2O there is definite obstruction. Ureteric reflux is described below.

RENAL VASCULAR PROBLEMS

Renal Artery Stenosis

This may be congenital or acquired. Congenital renal artery stenosis secondary to fibromuscular dysplasia usually affects young adult women. Acquired obstruction is usually the result of atheroma and thus commoner in older men. Usually the atheroma is associated with atheroma elsewhere. The main clinical problem is the onset of hypertension at an earlier age than that of essential hypertension. Occasionally a bruit can be heard on auscultation over either the aorta or the renal area. A clue to the diagnosis may be gained from the intravenous urogram in which the affected kidney is seen to be smaller and may have slightly delayed excretion on the early films. The diagnosis can be confirmed by arteriography where a narrowed segment may be visualized. The radionuclide scan may help with the diagnosis as the delayed blood flow may be particularly marked on the early frames (*see* Chapter 80).

RENAL STONES

Patients with renal tract stones usually present to the surgeon as an emergency because of pain. Whereas effective treatment to overcome the mechanical problem is not difficult, often investigations to try to determine the aetiology of the stone are incomplete and unsatisfactory.

Symptoms

The predominant symptom is pain (*Fig.* 81.10). If the stone is lying in the renal pelvis there may only be a dull loin ache. A small stone in the pelvis may cause intermittent obstruction with colicky loin pain. Once the stone passes into the ureter the patient experiences ureteric colic—a colicky pain radiating from loin to groin. Stones in the bladder are often silent. The severe dysuria experienced as a stone passes down the urethra is called strangury.

In those parts of the world where bladder stones are endemic in children, a pathognomonic sign of bladder stone is that to initiate micturition the male child pulls at the penis and the female child presses the perineum.

The passage of a stone may also result in haematuria. Staghorn calculi are usually associated with urinary infection; thus the classic picture is a female with loin ache, dysuria, frequency and nocturia. Bilateral stones may result in renal damage and symptoms of renal failure.

The Surgical Problem

If the stone is greater than 0·5 cm in diameter it is unlikely to pass spontaneously. Consideration must be given to removing the stone and to any anatomical abnormalities predisposing to stone formation. Such factors are: (i) deformed lower calices with a nest of stones requiring partial nephrectomy; (ii) an obstructed moiety in a duplex system; (iii) a bladder stone formed in residual urine secondary to neurogenic bladders or bladder outflow obstruction; (iv) stones forming around a foreign body, e.g. an indwelling catheter.

Treatment for Stone

The last five years have seen a revolution in the treatment of renal stones and it has been said that open operation should no longer be performed. Nevertheless the standard open operative procedures described below will remain the best treatment that can be offered in places where the new technology is not yet available or too costly.

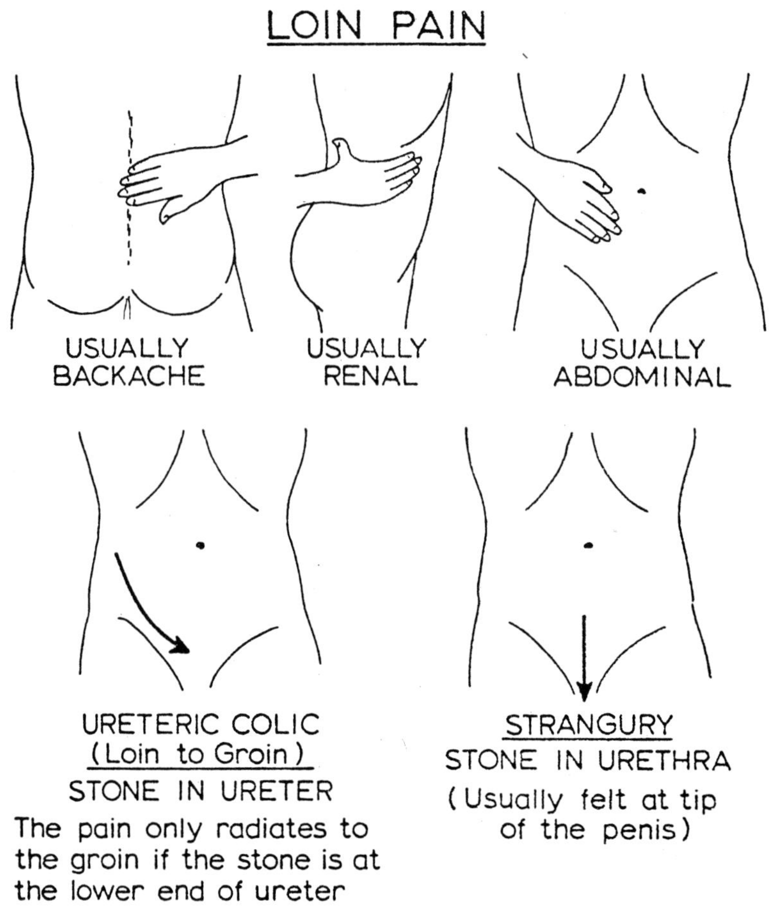

Fig. 81.10 Diagram showing types of renal and ureteric pain.

Treatment of Stone by Extracorporeal Lithotripsy (*Fig.* 81.11)

This may be the ideal treatment for nearly all renal stones but the expense of the equipment means that it is only available in a few countries. The patient is lightly anaesthetized and placed in a water bath. Shock waves are generated in the water bath by a spark and these waves are focused on the stone and cause it to disintegrate. The focusing is achieved by accurate positioning of the patient. Several hundred shock waves may be needed before the stone breaks up. The stone is then passed as small particles in the urine although in some cases larger fragments may have to be extracted using the percutaneous approach (*see below*) or a further session on the lithotripter may be necessary.

Percutaneous Stone Extraction (*Fig.* 81.12)

The second new approach to renal stone is using a direct puncture into the renal pelvis and then by introducing a specially designed nephroscope through the tract small stones can be extracted directly using grasping forceps. Larger stones can be broken up with an ultrasound probe or an electrohydraulic shock wave and then the stone pieces extracted. Stones in the upper ureter can be pushed back into the renal pelvis and extracted in a similar manner (push pull technique).

Operation for Stone

If there is any chance of the stone moving it is wise to take a plain radiograph to check the position of the stone immediately before operation, thus avoiding unnecessary surgery.

Renal Stones

The approaches to stones within the kidney are shown in *Fig.* 81.13. There are two main types of problem: (*a*) simple stones within the renal pelvis; and (*b*) complex staghorn calculi. Complex stones will often necessitate an approach through the renal pelvis combined with nephrotomy incisions. This type of surgery is made easier if the renal vessels are temporarily clamped to prevent blood loss. If this is done ischaemic renal damage must be prevented either by cooling the kidney with iced saline or by injecting inosine into the renal artery. Inosine protects tissue from ischaemic damage by repleting ATP stores.

Ureteric Stones

The approach to stones in the middle part of the ureter is shown in *Fig.* 81.14. Ideally the ureter is approached using a gridiron incision and extraperitoneal dissection. Once the stone has been removed it is important to check that there are no other stones present by passing a ureteric catheter up to the kidney and down to the bladder. Stones in the lower part of the ureter may be removed with a ureteric basket if the stone is not too large or by extraperitoneal dissection using either a modified gridiron or Pfannenstiel incision (*Fig.* 81.15).

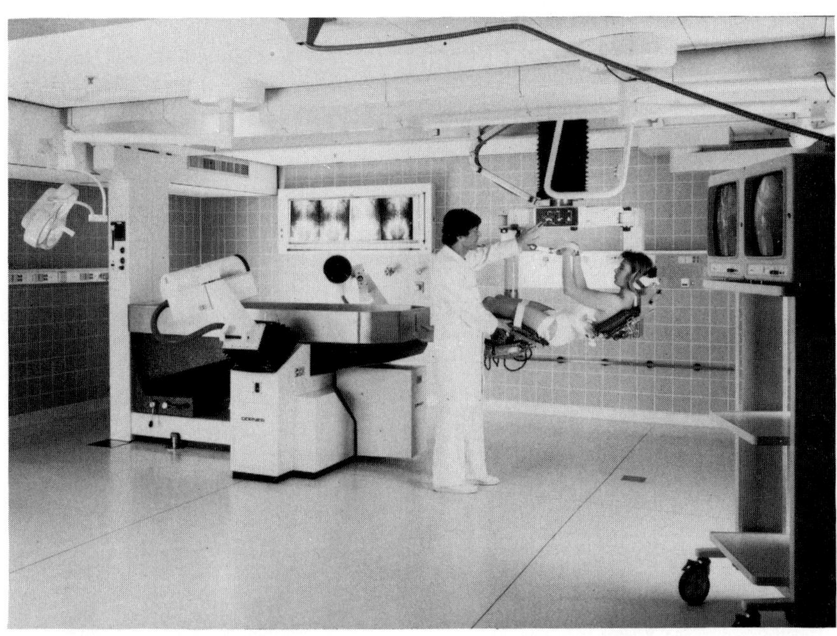

Fig. 81.11 The Dornier apparatus for extracorporeal shock wave lithotripsy (ECSWL).

Bladder Stones (*Fig.* 81.16)

In most cases in the UK bladder stones can be removed endoscopically using the lithotrite. First the stone is crushed into tiny fragments and these are then washed out through the cystoscope. For large bladder stones a small cystotomy may be necessary.

Renal Stones—The Medical Problem

Stones within the renal pelvis or ureter eventually cause deterioration in renal function and even in the absence of symptoms should be removed if there is no chance that the stone will pass spontaneously. Bilateral staghorn calculi or calculi obstructing the urinary tract of a patient with only one kidney may cause uraemia, dictating urgent relief of obstruction. Thus, patients with stone usually require renal function to be assessed by creatinine clearance. Differential renal function can be determined by renal scanning which gives good preoperative indication as to whether the kidney containing many stones can be saved or not. It is worth warning, however, that differential renal function from renal scanning does not give information about the recovery potential of a kidney following stone removal and often the final decision must be made at operation when the thickness of renal tissue can be assessed.

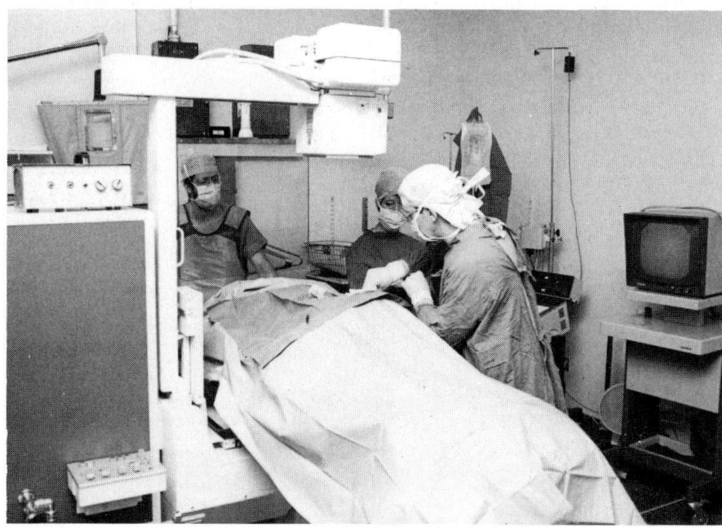

a

Fig. 81.12 Percutaneous renal surgery. *a*, Under radiological/ultrasound control, a guide-wire is initially introduced in the renal pelvis. [*continued over*]

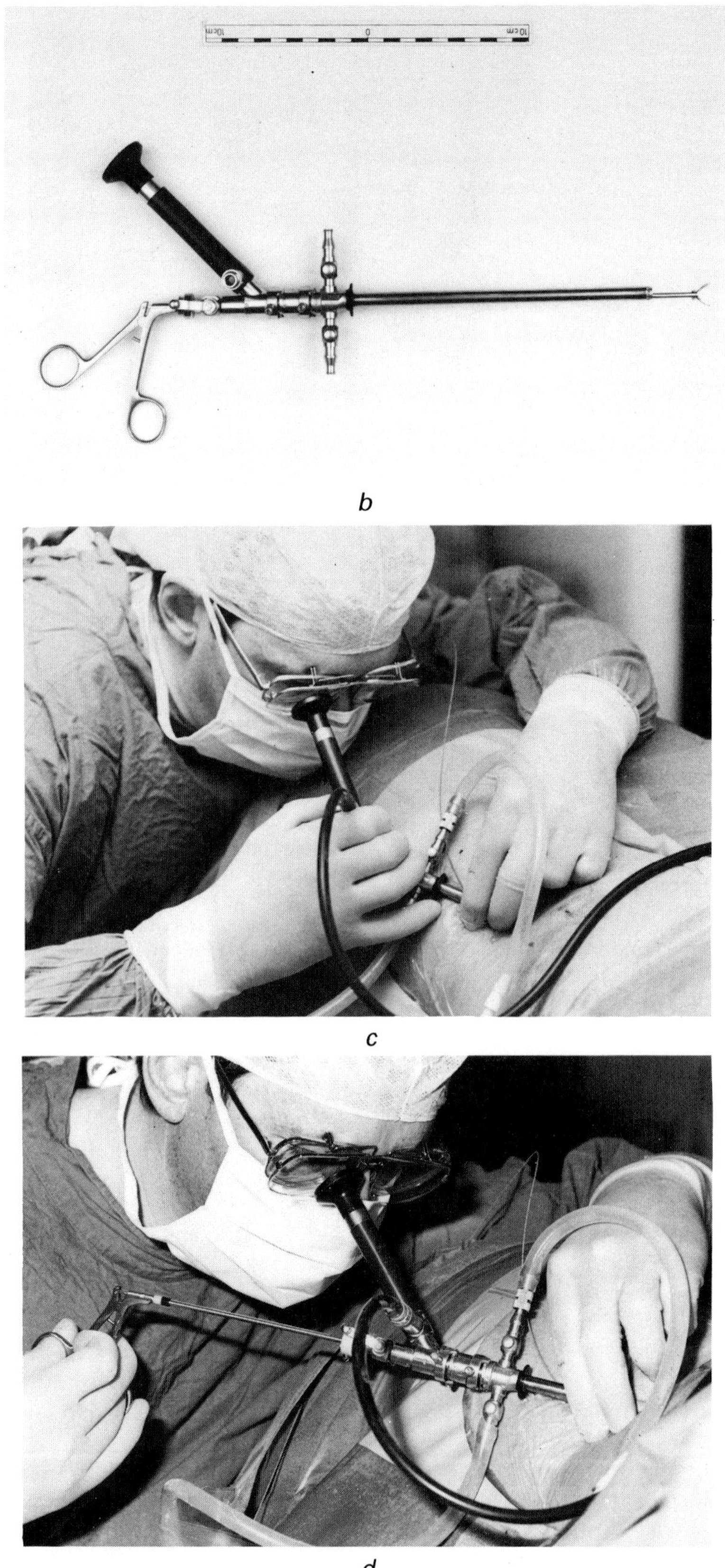

[*Fig. 81.12 continued*] (*b*) Dilators are then passed over the guide-wire to enable the sheath and the operating nephroscope to be introduced. *c*, This allows visualization of the renal pelvis, and (*d*) the introduction of instruments for biopsy and stone retrieval through the instrument guide channel.

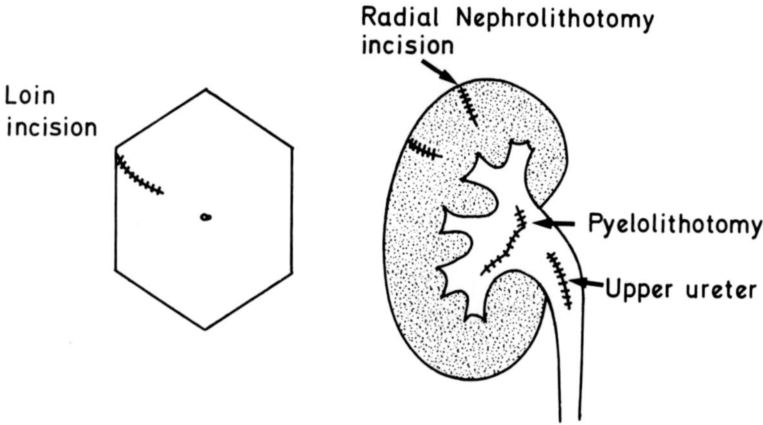

Fig. 81.13 Surgical approaches to a renal stone. Stones in the ureter at the level of the renal lower pole or above are best approached through a loin incision.

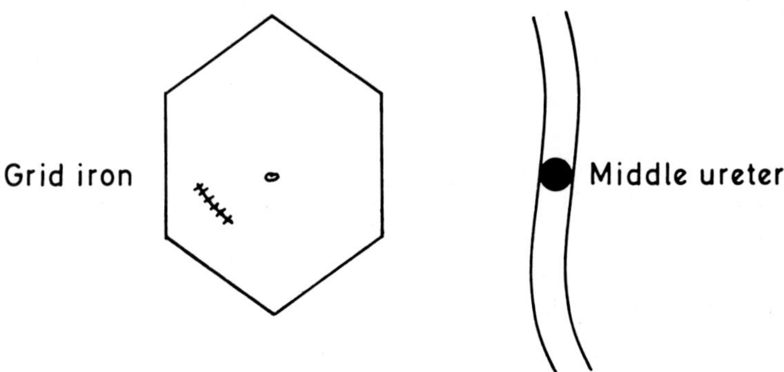

Fig. 81.14 Surgical approach to a stone in the middle ureter.

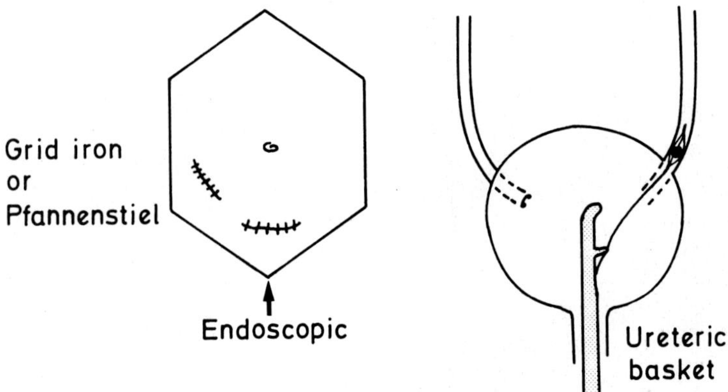

Fig. 81.15 Surgical approach to a stone in the lower ureter.

Types of Stone

Once the mechanical problem has been solved, the patient relieved of symptoms and renal function returned to normal it is appropriate to investigate the patient to try to discover the cause of stone formation. There are three main groups of stones: (i) stones associated with infection or anatomical damage, (ii) stones composed of calcium oxalate (often called idiopathic) and (iii) specific metabolic stones.

1. Staghorn Calculi (*Fig.* 81.17)

These stones are formed of magnesium ammonium phosphate hexahydrate and are nearly always associated with infection. They are often bilateral and are more common in women. Left untreated they cause progressive renal damage. The associated infection and caliceal obstruction often result in intrarenal or perinephric abscess. Treatment is to completely remove the stone, using a combination of

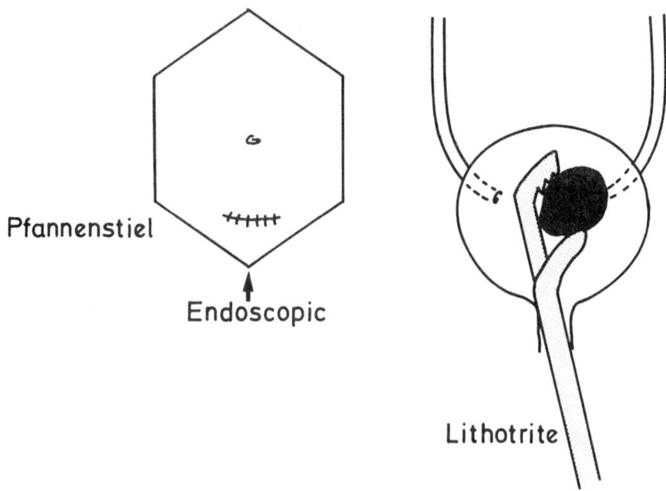

Fig. 81.16 Surgical approach to a bladder stone.

approaches through the renal pelvis and through the renal substance. It is usually necessary to secure a bloodless field using renal cooling or inosine to achieve complete stone clearance. If all of the stone is removed and the urine is kept sterile with long-term antibiotics less than 5% recur. The commonest causes of recurrence are inadequate stone clearance at operation and a failure to keep the urine sterile postoperatively.

2. *Calcium Oxalate Stones* (*Fig.* 81.18)
These so-called 'idiopathic' stones account for the majority of stones. This type of stone is commoner in the developed countries and probably related to overeating; there is a male predominance. The Medical Research Council Mineral Metabolism Unit at Leeds has investigated the genesis of these stones over a number of years and found five main risk factors: calcium concentration, oxalate concentration, urate

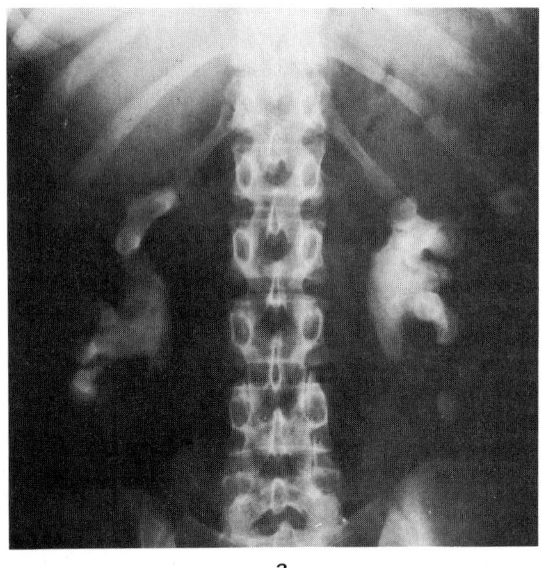

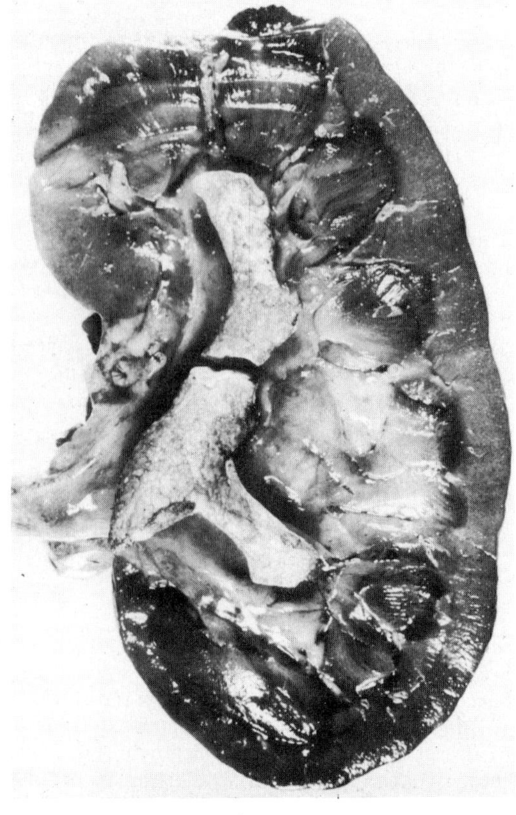

Fig. 81.17 *a*, Plain abdominal radiograph showing bilateral staghorn calculi. *b*, Staghorn calculus in situ.

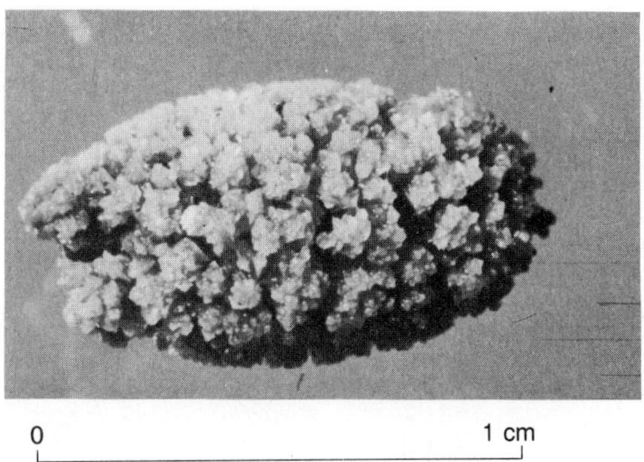

Fig. 81.18 Calcium oxalate calculus.

concentration, urinary pH and the amount of glycoaminoglycosans (e.g. heparin and chondroitin). It is interesting to note that all of these substances may remain within normal laboratory limits but the combination of a series of 'high normal' levels may put the patient at high risk of further stone formation. This finding accounts for the fact that most 24-h urine samples from stone formers show no obvious abnormality. The influence of the five factors is shown in *Fig.* 81.19.

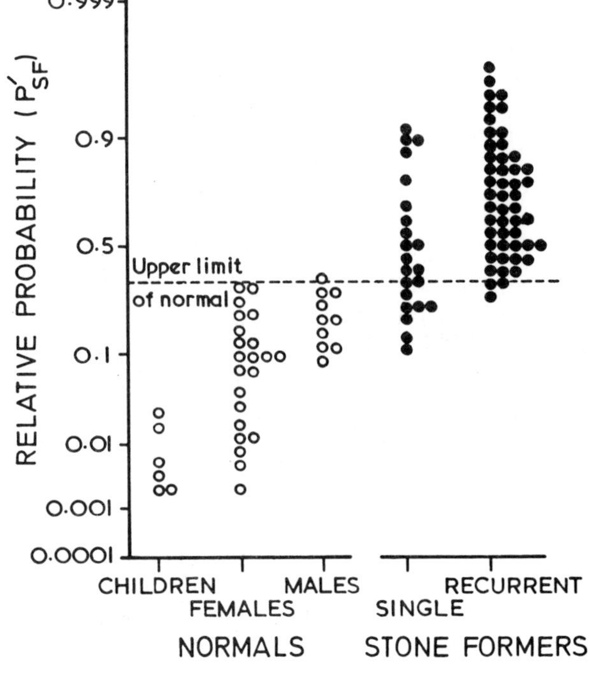

Fig. 81.19 The relative probability of stone formation judged by analysing the urinary levels of calcium, oxalate, urate, glycoaminoglycosans, and urinary pH. In many cases the individual levels fall within the normal laboratory range but when the 5 factors are analysed together the recurrent stone formers are strikingly different from non-stone formers (from Robertson et al. (1972). *Br. J. Urol.* **50**(7), 449, by kind permission of the Editor).

Once the stone has been removed, what to advise the patient? For a single stone episode there is no proven anti-stone therapy but the patient should be warned that there is an increased chance that another stone will form. When more than one stone has formed the patient should be thoroughly investigated. Obvious dietary risks, such as high milk intake, should be avoided. Fluid intake should be adequate, particularly in hot working conditions or hot climates. Good advice is to tell the patient never to eat a meal without also taking a half pint of fluid; vague advice to drink plenty does not usually work. It may also be appropriate to treat the predominant risk factor. If this is calcium then treatment with phosphate may reduce urine calcium and stone recurrence. If on the other hand the predominant risk is high uric acid, allopurinol therapy may reduce the recurrence of calcium oxalate stones. Recurrent stone formers should be followed-up regularly and renal scans are useful in this respect to check function and the absence of obstruction; the dose of radiation from a scan being less than that of an intravenous urogram.

3. *Specific Metabolic Stones*

a. STONES ASSOCIATED WITH HYPERCALCAEMIA AND HYPERCALCIURIA. The important cause to eliminate in all cases with stone is hyperparathyroidism through parathyroid adenoma accounts for only 0·5–1·0% of cases of calcium stone disease. The most reliable indicator is an elevated serum calcium. Blood should be taken with the patient fasting and the calcium value should be corrected to allow for serum protein levels. It is also unwise to rely on a single estimation (*see* Chapter 62). Any other cause of hypercalciuria may also result in calcium stone disease (*Table* 81.2), e.g. steroid therapy and prolonged immobilization.

Table 81.2 Causes of hypercalciuria

1. Plasma Calcium Elevated
Primary hyperparathyroidism
Tertiary hyperparathyroidism
2. Plasma Calcium may be Elevated
Vitamin D overdose
Sarcoidosis
Hyperthyroidism
Cushing's syndrome or steroid treatment
Immobilization
Carcinomatosis
Myelomatosis
3. Plasma Calcium Normal
Idiopathic hypercalciuria
Medullary sponge kidney
Renal tubular acidosis

b. URIC ACID STONES. As elevated urinary uric acid puts the patient at risk for calcium stone disease as described above (*Fig.* 81.19). In addition, uric acid stones may occur in gout and these account for 3·5% of cases with stones. These stones are often radiolucent, making radiological diagnosis difficult.

c. OTHER RARE METABOLIC STONES. Cystine, xanthine and pure oxalate stones occur in association with rare inborn errors of metabolism. All these stones may be radiolucent depending on their calcium content. It is worth screening for these stones in all cases of recurrent stone by a urinary amino acid chromatogram. This is particularly true for any cases of stones in children which are more likely to be due to an inborn error of metabolism as stone disease in children in this country is generally rare.

4. Medullary Sponge Kidney (Fig. 81.20)

This congenital abnormality may affect a part of or the whole of one or both kidneys. The condition is not familial. There are multiple small cysts affecting the renal medulla. These may remain symptomless but often present in middle age with infection, pyelonephritis or multiple small calculi. This condition is sometimes diagnosed when the intravenous urogram films are examined carefully from a patient with recurrent renal calculi. Treatment is symptomatic. When the abnormality involves only one or part of the kidney, nephrectomy or partial nephrectomy may be appropriate.

Investigations

Stone analysis is often neglected but provides a useful guide to aetiology. All stone formers (single or recurrent) should have a blood sample check for calcium and uric acid. It is worth checking two 24-h urine samples from all recurrent stone cases for calcium, oxalate, urate, pH and glycoaminoglycosans. Unfortunately, assays of oxalate and glycoaminoglycosans are not universally available and thus often hypercalciuria is the only risk factor that can be identified.

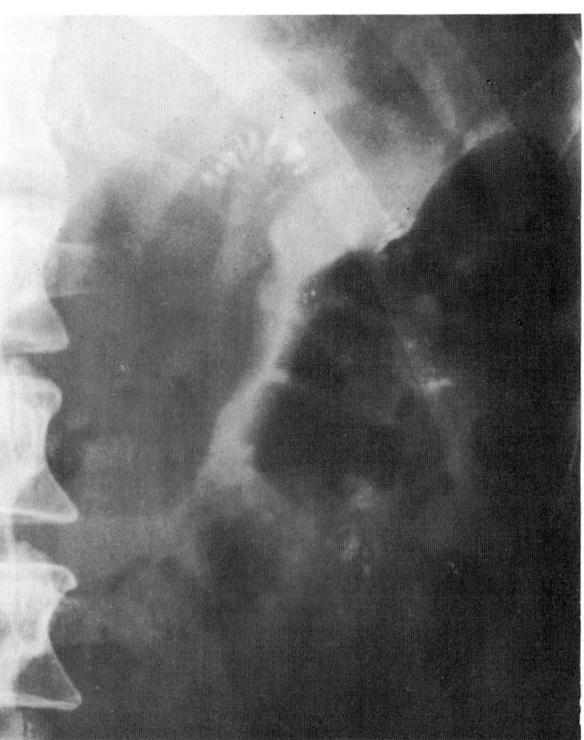

Fig. 81.20 Plain abdominal radiograph in a case of medullary sponge kidney. Note calcification in the renal medulla.

INFECTIONS

Acute Pyelonephritis

In Children

There is evidence that renal scarring secondary to pyelonephritis occurs mainly before the age of 5 years. Three factors are thought to make a child liable to this condition: (1) urinary infection; (2) reflux of urine up the ureter; (3) reflux of urine back through the renal papillae (intrarenal reflux).

1. Urinary Infection

Urinary infection is more common in girls than boys and so it is not surprising that females are more commonly affected with pyelonephritis. Boys with urinary infection should be suspected of having an abnormality of bladder outflow, such as urethral valves.

2. Ureteric Reflux

Reflux of urine up the ureter tends to disappear with age. It should also be remembered that reflux may be intermittent, thus a normal micturating cystogram does not exclude reflux which may be present only during an attack of acute cystitis. Because of the tendency to spontaneous cure as the child grows up it is not advisable to reimplant the ureter surgically unless the reflux is gross or adequate conservative treatment fails. Thus, surgical treatment is required when infection persists despite supervised long-term chemotherapy, or when reflux cannot be treated conservatively with long-term antibiotics to prevent pyelonephritis.

Reflux may be secondary to bladder outflow problems, e.g. neurogenic bladder or urethral valves; it is also associated with megacystis and megaureter, in which one or both ureters and the bladder are grossly dilated with thin walls. The exact aetiology is not understood but sometimes the ureter requires reimplantation after reduction of its width.

3. Intrarenal Reflux

There is recent evidence that abnormal renal papillae may allow intrarenal reflux. If there is also infection and ureteric reflux, pyelonephritis can occur. Normal renal papillae are cone-shaped whereas abnormal papillae are flat. Postmortem studies show that these abnormal papillae occur more frequently in the middle and lower calices which coincides with the distribution of pyelonephritic scars.

Pyelonephritis in Young Women

Approximately 30% of women have asymptomatic bacteriuria and provided the anatomy of the urinary tract is normal this usually resolves. In pregnancy, however, there is a tendency for the ureter to dilate and transient reflux to occur and women with bacteriuria are at risk from pyelonephritis. In antenatal clinics urine samples are carefully screened and patients with bacteriuria are treated even if asymptomatic.

Pyelonephritis in Older Persons

This is usually secondary to some other disease process. An example is staghorn calculi which may cause caliceal obstruction and abscess formation and later a perinephric abscess may result from rupture of the caliceal abscess. Pyelonephritis often follows a urinary diversion operation whether the ureters are diverted into the sigmoid colon or into an isolated loop of ileum. In both any degree of stenosis or obstruction at the site of ureteric implantation almost certainly guarantees pyelonephritis.

Urinary Tract Tuberculosis

The classic presentation of urinary tuberculosis is with frequency and sterile pyuria. Usually the disease starts in the kidneys and the ureters and bladder are involved secondarily. The usual presentations of urinary tract tuberculosis are listed in *Table* 81.3. It is important to prove the diagnosis by obtaining positive cultures before treatment is commenced. The plan of investigation is shown in *Table* 81.4; these investigations are intended: (i) to prove the diagnosis; and (ii) to assess the extent of disease.

Table 81.3 Clinical presentations of renal tuberculosis

Symptoms of bladder inflammation—
 frequency, dysuria, haematuria
A solitary episode of frank haematuria
Renal colic
 Loin pain
Cold abscess in loin
Genital disease
 MALE—epididymitis, orchitis
 FEMALE—infertility, tubo-ovarian abscess
Chronic renal failure
Routine investigation of:
 Tuberculosis in other organs, including miliary tuberculosis
 Apparently non-tuberculous disease, e.g. hypertension
Constitutional symptoms
 Fatigue, anorexia, weight loss

Table 81.4 Plan of investigation of renal tuberculosis

Examination of urine
 Bacteriology
 Urinalysis
Radiological examination of renal tract
Cystoscopy and retrograde pyelo-ureterography
Estimation of renal function
Radiographic examination of chest
Haematological examination
 Haemoglobin, total white blood cells and differential count, ESR, serum folate
Tuberculin test
Examination of genital tract
Identification of previous concomitant tuberculous disease and of family history of tuberculosis

Treatment depends on the extent of urinary tract damage and it has been found helpful to stage the disease according to the SEMB classification (*Fig.* 81.21). In general, SEMB Stages I and II disease can be arrested by antimicrobial therapy, sometimes with the addition of reconstructive surgery, whereas SEMB Stage III disease will often necessitate excisional surgery. Treatment of choice is chemotherapy for twelve months (*Table* 81.5). Any reconstructive surgery is carried out within the first two months of treatment.

The main surgical problems are: (1) ureteric stricture; and (2) contracture of the bladder and in recent years there has been a tendency towards more reconstructive surgery.

1. *Tuberculous Ureteric Stricture*

Stricture usually occurs at the lower end of the ureter. If the renal function deteriorates in spite of adequate antibacterial chemotherapy, reimplantation of the ureter into the bladder at an early stage is indicated because fibrosis may continue for some time after the urine has been sterilized.

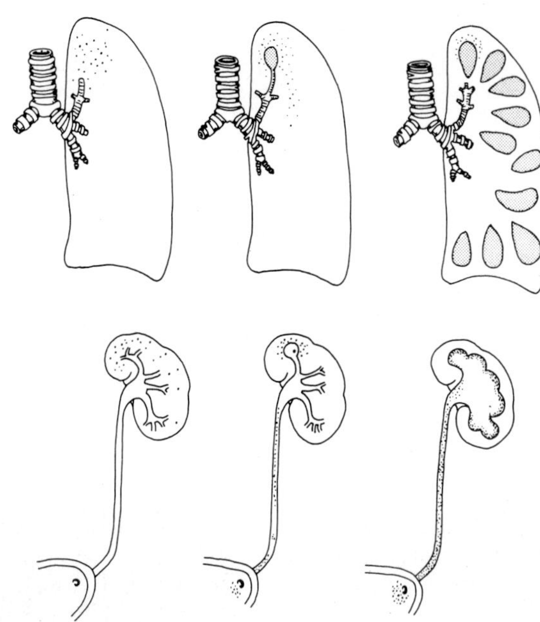

Fig. 81.21 Diagram of SEMB classification of renal tuberculosis. SEMB I—Tuberculous bacilluria or small caliceal deformity with or without genital lesion. SEMB II—Ulcerocavernous lesion affecting one or more calix. SEMB III—Extensive renal tuberculosis involving the major part of one or more calices.

Table 81.5 Nine/twelve month chemotherapy for TB

Rifampicin	450 mg daily if body weight <50 kg
	600 mg daily if body weight >50 kg
Isoniazid	300 mg daily
Ethambutal	15 mg/kg body weight daily

(care needed with ethambutal if renal function is not normal)

These three drugs are taken for 3 months or until sensitivities are obtained, thereafter rifampicin and isoniazid are given daily for a further 6 or 9 months.
Pyrazinamide can replace ethambutal.
Efforts are being made to reduce the period of treatment and the following scheme has been suggested by Gow (1979)

SHORT COURSE CHEMOTHERAPY FOR TB

Rifampicin 450 mg Pyrazinamide 1 g Isoniazid 300 mg	Taken together last thing at night for 2 months

followed by:

Rifampicin 600 mg Isoniazid 600 mg	Taken together last thing at night 3 times a week for a further 4 months

2. *Contracted Bladder*

Fibrosis following a tuberculous cystitis will often reduce the bladder capacity to an unacceptably small volume. The patient suffers from extreme urinary frequency day and night and requires surgical enlargement of the bladder (cystoplasty) or urinary diversion. Cystoplasty may be achieved either by using an isolated loop of small intestine (ileocystoplasty) or by mobilizing the caecum and replacing the excised bladder with the caecum (caecocystoplasty).

Follow-up

After treatment follow-up is carried out for 1 year but if the plain radiograph shows calcified areas longer follow-up is necessary.

RENAL TUMOUR

Types of Renal Tumour

Children—Nephroblastoma

The developmental tumour of children is the nephroblastoma or Wilms's tumour. The classic presentation is with haematuria, an abdominal mass and failure to thrive. In general, the younger the child in whom the diagnosis is made the better the prognosis. Treatment is to excise the primary tumour and to give radiotherapy to the regional nodes. Adjuvant chemotherapy is also given. This multimodality treatment has dramatically altered prognosis and there is now an 80% chance of 5-year survival (*see* Chapter 59).

Renal-cell Carcinoma (*Fig.* 81.22)

The most frequent renal tumour of adults is renal-cell carcinoma (adenocarcinoma of the kidney, hypernephroma or Grawitz tumour). The classic presentation is with haematuria, loin pain and a palpable abdominal mass. In 60% of cases haematuria is one of the presenting symptoms but this tumour is remarkable because of the various syndromes

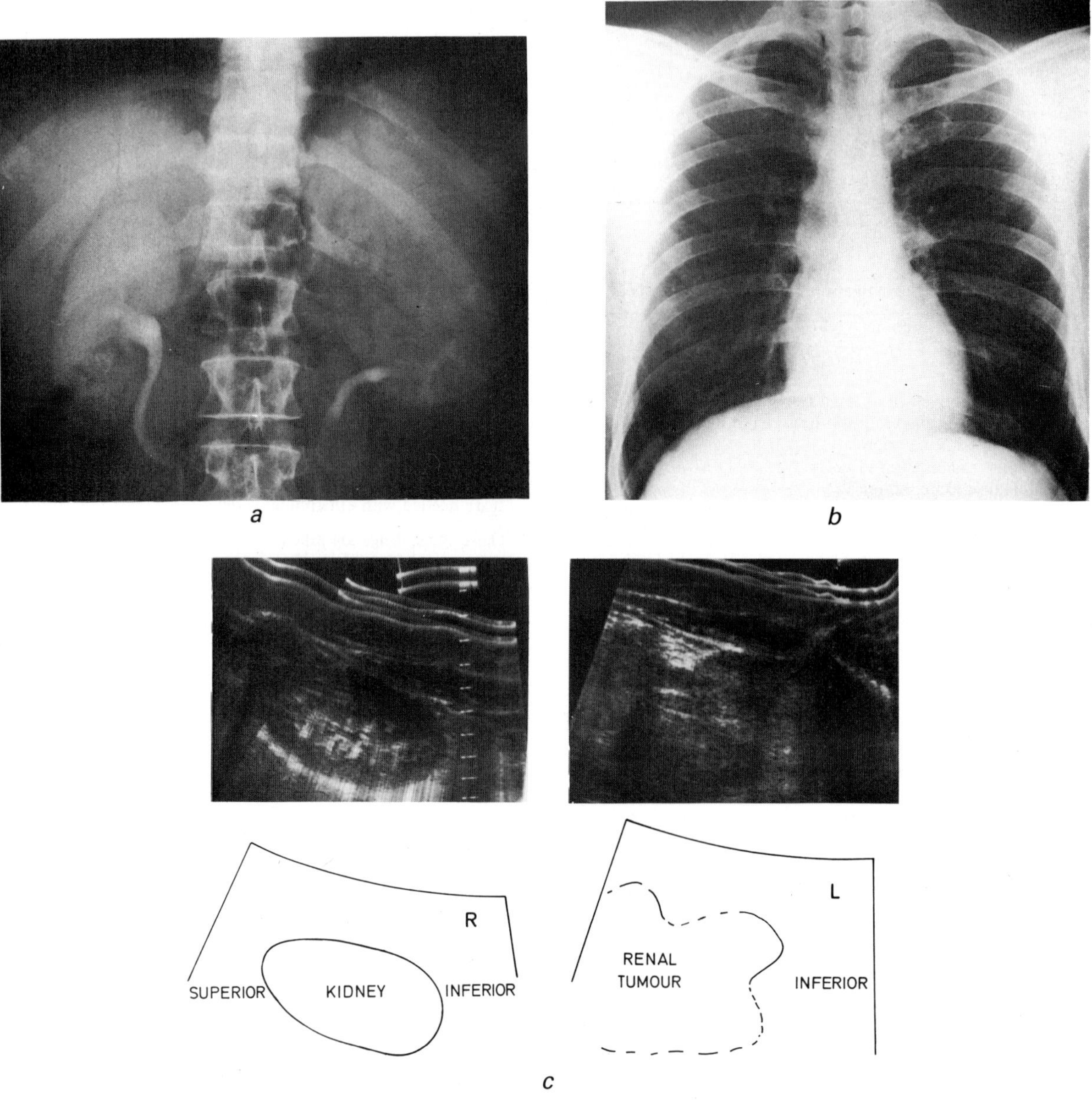

Fig. 81.22 Investigations all taken from the same case of renal-cell carcinoma. This patient presented with haematuria. *a*, Intravenous urogram shows a suspicious area at the upper pole of the left kidney. *b*, Chest radiograph reveals no obvious metastases making it reasonable to proceed with further investigation. *c*, Ultrasound reveals that the mass at the upper pole of the left kidney is solid making it likely to be a tumour. [*continued over*]

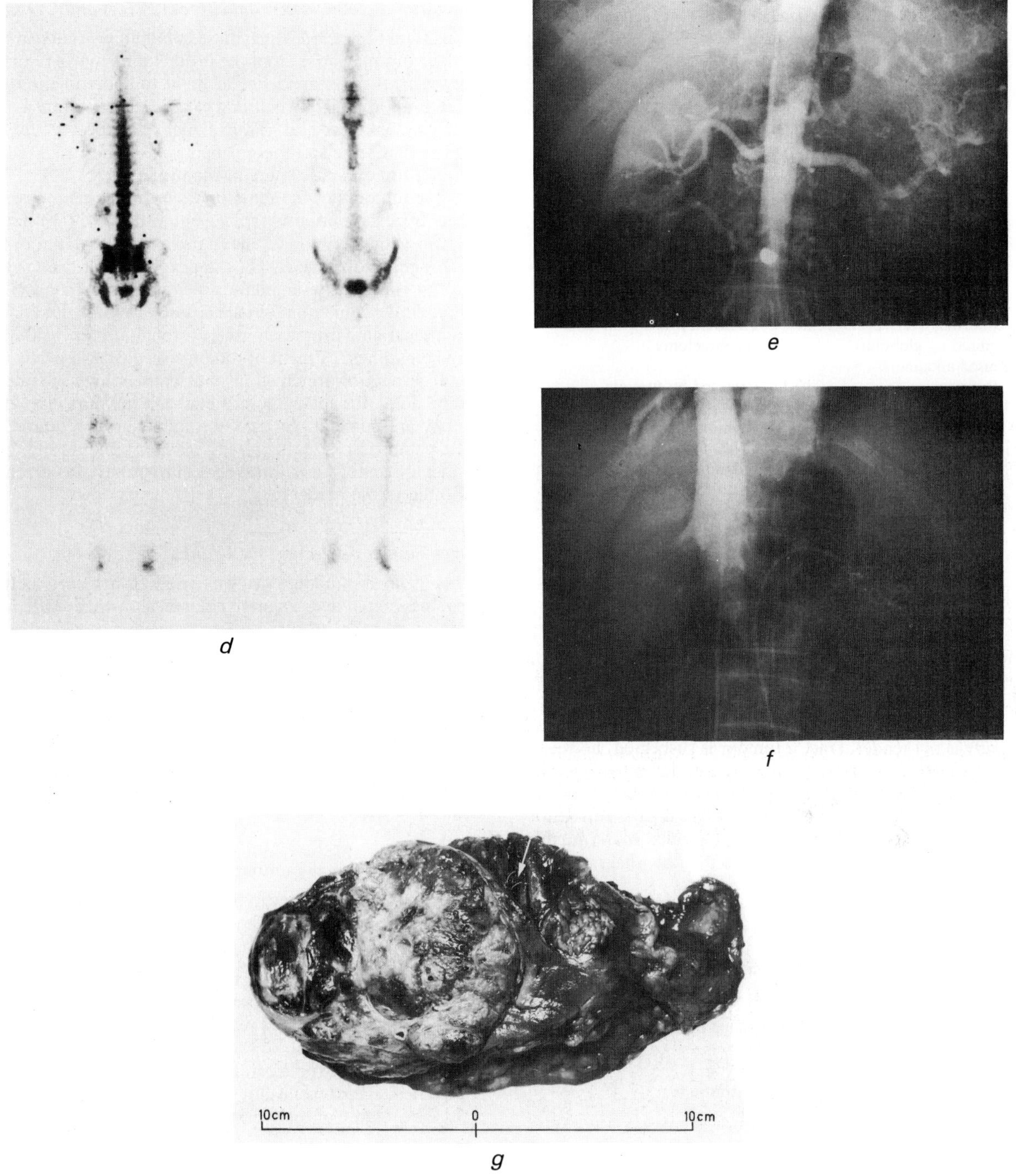

[*Fig. 81.22 continued*] *d*, Bone scan reveals no obvious bony metastases making it reasonable to proceed with further investigation and treatment. *e*, Arteriogram shows typical tumour circulation in the upper pole of the left kidney. *f*, The circulation to the kidney has been blocked by placing a coil in the left renal artery. This allows for easier operative removal of a highly vascular tumour. A catheter introduced into the inferior vena cava shows no obvious spread of tumour from the renal vein. *g*, The nephrectomy specimen shows a typical renal-cell carcinoma of the upper two-thirds of the left kidney. The arrow points to the embolectomy coils lodged in the renal artery at the time of arteriogram.

which can occur (*Table* 81.6). It is important to realize that these syndromes do not indicate metastatic disease and that they may completely regress when the primary is removed. These syndromes are often misdiagnosed because of their sporadic occurrence. Metastatic spread may result in the patient presenting with symptoms and signs unrelated to the urinary tract. Almost any organ of the body may be affected, resulting in such diverse presenting signs as pathological fracture, paraplegia, finger clubbing or melaena. The second unusual feature of renal-cell carcinoma is spontaneous regression of metastases. There are many well documented cases involving regression of lung metastases but not of

Table 81.6 Syndromes associated with renal-cell carcinoma

Findings	*% of renal tumour patients with this finding*	*Explanation*
Raised ESR	55	Changes in serum proteins associated with many tumours
Hypertension	37	Secretion of renin by tumour
Anaemia	36	Depression of erythopoiesis plus or minus haematuria
Weight loss	34	Tumour metabolites depress appetite
Pyrexia	17	Circulating pyrogèns
Abnormal liver function (raised α_2 globulin)	14	These may disappear after nephrectomy
Raised alkaline phosphatase	10·1	?secreted by tumour
Hypercalcaemia	4·9	Parathormone secretion by tumour
Polycythaemia	3·5	Erythropoietin secretion
Neuromyopathy	3·2	Tumour-associated antibodies as to the brain
Amyloidosis	2	Possibly associated with immunological reactions to the tumour

metastases in other sites. Some surgeons will perform nephrectomy in the presence of lung metastases in the hope that regression will occur but it usually does not.

On examination the enlarged kidney may be felt and usually is not tender. Once a tumour is suspected, however, palpation should be restricted because of the risk of dislodging a tumour embolus; this is particularly relevant with this tumour as it frequently grows into the renal vein. Intravenous urography will show a possible renal mass; further diagnostic investigation is shown in the flow diagram (*Fig.* 81.23).

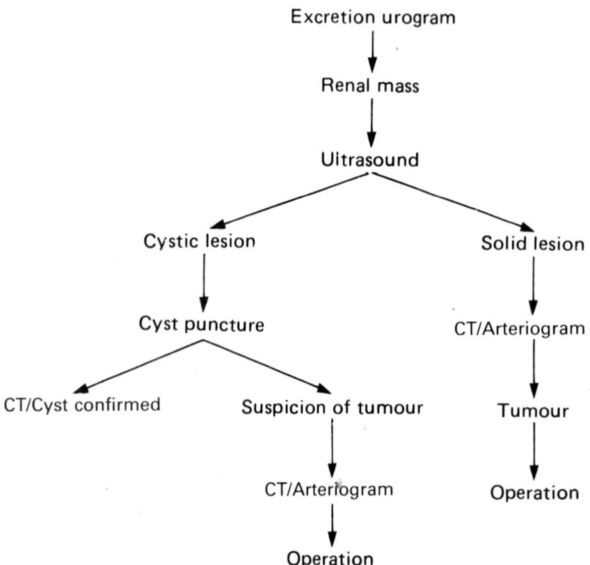

Fig. 81.23 Investigation of a renal space-occupying lesion detected in intravenous urogram.

Transitional-cell Cancer of the Renal Pelvis and Ureter

Transitional-cell carcinoma most commonly occurs in the bladder but may arise from the urothelium anywhere in the urinary tract. The incidence of these tumours in the renal pelvis is approximately half that of renal-cell carcinoma, and in the ureter rarer still. Transitional-cell cancer is often a multifocal disease and these patients are at increased risk of forming tumours elsewhere in the urinary tract.

Some tumours of the renal pelvis or ureter can be recognized by excretion urography, but others will be found only if good retrograde or sometimes antegrade pyelo-urethrograms are made. They appear as filling defects and may be confused with non-opaque stones or blood clots. Cytological examination of urine passed from the bladder or taken separately from each ureter through ureteric catheters may help. The treatment of tumours of the renal pelvis and ureter is nephro-ureterectomy but conservative operations can be done if there are transitional-cell tumours elsewhere or they are bilateral. As careful a follow-up is required for these patients as for patients with bladder tumours and must include cystoscopy and intravenous urography. Recurrences are often in the bladder.

Other Tumours affecting the Kidney

Other primary tumours are rare. Benign tumours include renal adenoma and angiomyelolipoma. Other malignant tumours include sarcomas, haemangiopericytoma and renal oncocytoma. Sarcomas and renal oncocytoma may reach a very large size before they metastasize and in the latter case operative removal may be curative despite an enormous local lesion. Secondary deposits can occur and are often bilateral and it is for this reason that it is unwise to transplant a donor kidney from a patient with malignancy outside the central nervous system. The commonest secondaries are from lung, breast and uterus.

Treatment of Renal Tumours

Before logical treatment can be recommended it is important to assess the tumour and the patient.

1. The general condition of the patient.
2. The age and wishes of the patient.
3. The degree of symptoms from the tumour.
4. The stage of local spread from the tumour (T category).
5. The stage of spread to regional gland (N category).
6. The stage of metastatic spread (M category).
7. The degree of malignancy of the tumour.

Advances in the treatment of renal tumours are hampered by the fact that the extent of assessment varies from hospital to hospital and because no single centre has sufficient cases to evaluate treatment properly.

1, 2, 3. The General Condition, Age and Symptoms State of the Patient

It is inappropriate to carry out radical surgery in a very elderly patient, especially if there are minimal symptoms; on the other hand, a nephrectomy can sometimes relieve elderly persons of severe dragging loin pain and haematuria and may be justified on these grounds even in the presence of metastases. Each case must be judged individually. In general the more aggressive therapy is reserved for younger patients.

4. *The Stage of Local Spread (T Category)* (*Fig.* 81.24)

This can often only be determined at operation. Intravenous urography will usually indicate the site of the tumour, e.g., upper or lower pole. Arteriography may give information as to the extent the tumour has invaded the capsule (parasitic circulation). The late films of the arteriogram series may show growth of tumour down the renal vein but this common form of spread is best detected by venocavography or ultrasonography. Grey scale ultrasonography and computerized tomography give good indication of invasion through the capsule. These investigations may modify the surgical approach to the tumour. If capsular invasion is likely a radical nephrectomy taking the perirenal tissue *en bloc* is the operation of choice. If the tumour is present in the renal vein it is usually wise to approach the tumour from an anterior approach and to remove the tumour from the vein before the main bulk is handled because of the very real possibility of a tumour embolus.

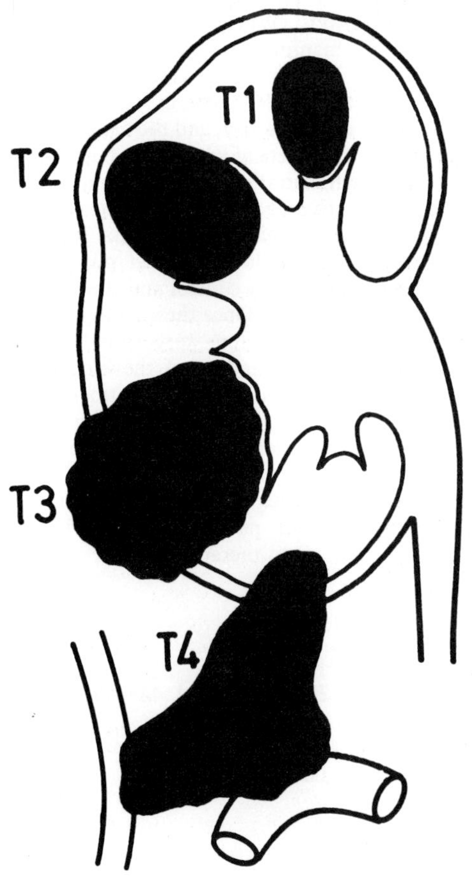

Fig. 81.24 T—Primary tumour classification.

5. *The Stage of Lymphatic Spread (N Category)* (*Fig.* 81.25)

This is determined at operation by examination of the para-aortic nodes. Some idea may be gained by preoperative computerized tomography and ultrasonography. The presence or absence of involved glands will in many cases determine whether additional radiotherapy or chemotherapy needs to be given.

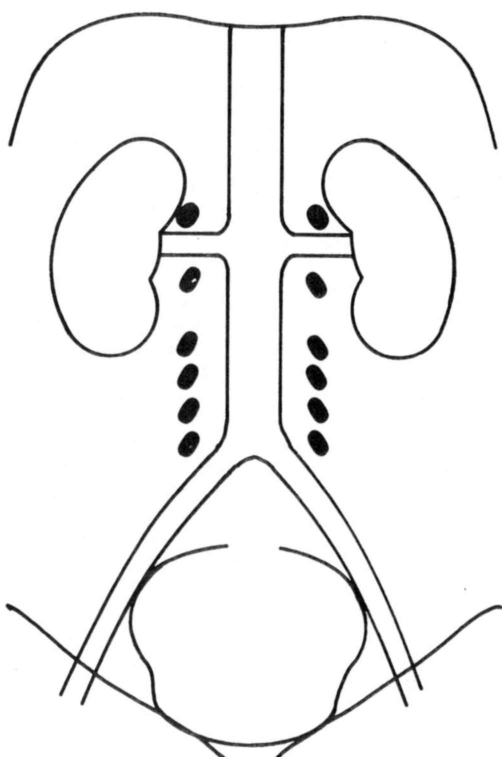

Fig. 81.25 N—Regional nodes draining kidneys: hilar and para-aortic.

6. *The Stage of Metastatic Spread (M Category)*

Renal-cell carcinoma may metastasize to any organ of the body. Commonly seen are pulmonary metastases or bony metastases. There are three particular points of note: (*a*) there have been a few well-documented cases of secondaries regressing following excision of the primary. This situation is extremely rare and only occasionally should be used as justification for a nephrectomy; (*b*) metastases may appear many months or years following removal of the primary renal-cell carcinoma. It is unwise to rely on published figures for survival unless long-term follow-up has been undertaken; (*c*) a solitary metastasis may occur following removal of the primary and operative removal of the solitary metastasis can sometimes result in cure.

In most cases treatment of metastases is attempted using chemotherapy or cytotoxic agents, however, there is no proven effective regime for these tumours.

7. *The Degree of Malignancy*

The degree of malignancy affects the prognosis. Anaplastic or poorly differentiated tumours are associated with a worse prognosis. The 5-year survival following excision of the primary tumour varies from 40% with well-differentiated lesions to 17% with high-grade anaplastic tumours. As soon as effective chemotherapy is discovered for metastases it will be tempting to offer this to patients with poor histology even when metastatic spread has not been demonstrated.

Treatment

Treatment for renal tumour is operative removal of the kidney with adjuvant radiotherapy or chemotherapy depending on the above criteria.

1. Operative removal. If possible the kidney should be removed complete with the envelope of perinephric fat intact. An anterior operative approach allows the renal artery and vein to be ligated prior to handling of the kidney and may lessen the chance of embolization. In those cases where preoperative venocavography has demonstrated a tongue of tumour invading the inferior vena cava the anterior approach is the technique of choice. If the tumour is at the upper pole a thoraco-abdominal approach is often the best option.

2. Radiotherapy. In those cases where the tumour has breached the capsule or where there is evidence of lymphatic spread it is usual to irradiate the regional glands.

3. Chemotherapy. The treatment of metastatic renal cancer with cytotoxic agents has been disappointing. In general, single-agent therapy has shown no useful response except perhaps with the nitroso-urea CCNU which has been reported as having an 11% response rate. Multiple-agent chemotherapy in theory is more attractive but the results to date have been poor. A 16% objective response rate has been reported following treatment of patients with metastatic renal cancer using Provera (medroxyprogesterone acetate).

4. Embolization of the renal artery at the time of arteriography can be used: (*a*) to reduce blood loss during the operation: this is particularly appropriate for a large vascular upper pole tumour; (*b*) as definitive treatment for a polar renal tumour in a solitary kidney; (*c*) to palliate haematuria where a nephrectomy may be of questionable value, e.g. in the presence of diffuse metastases. Following embolization there is usually a 48-h period of severe pain requiring narcotic analgesics and sometimes it may be necessary to carry out nephrectomy to relieve pain.

BENCH SURGERY AND AUTOTRANSPLANTATION

Transplantation techniques have led to the realization that the kidney can be removed from the loin to allow detailed bench surgery or transplantation into the iliac fossa. Some indications of these techniques are listed in *Table* 81.7.

Table 81.7 Indications for bench surgery and autotransplantation

Possible indications for Bench Surgery
1. Intrarenal vascular abnormalities, e.g. arteriovenous aneurysms
2. Renal tumour within a single kidney

Possible indications for Autotransplantation
1. Long length of ureter missing
2. Transitional-cell cancer within the renal pelvis of a solitary kidney. By transplanting the kidney into the iliac fossa the renal pelvis can be anastomosed directly to the bladder allowing endoscopic follow-up

THE WAY AHEAD

The accurate imaging of internal organs using new techniques has already transformed diagnosis with respect to space-occupying lesions. When these techniques are extended to involve manipulation of the kidneys exciting possibilities arise. The ability to embolize renal arteries selectively has already altered some cases of renal trauma, e.g. bleeding after a renal biopsy, and the need for operation can be avoided. This technique could be extended to perhaps the local administration of cytotoxics to a tumour or cells-specific destructive agents to a kidney secreting too much renin. Another exciting development is endoscopic removal of renal stones following direct puncture of the renal pelvis under ultrasound control and the development of extracorporeal lithotripsy. Once these techniques become more widely available open stone surgery is likely to be a rare event. Clearer understanding of the biochemistry of upper tract stones may result in specific treatment to prevent stones altogether, although it is extremely unlikely that all patients at risk will be identified before stone formation. Effective chemotherapy for renal-cell cancer is long overdue. It is strange that this tumour with so many systemic manifestations and hence possible areas of biochemical attack is still so resistant to therapy.

Further Reading

Chisholm G. D. (ed.) (1980) *Tutorial in Post Graduate Medicine—Urology*. London, Heinemann.
Robertson W. G. et al. (1978) Risk factors in calcium stone disease of urinary tract. *Br. J. Urol.* **50**, 449–454.
UICC (1978) *TNM Classification of Malignant Tumours*, 3rd ed. Geneva.
Wickham J. E. A. (ed.) (1979) *Urinary Calculus Disease*. London, Churchill Livingstone.
Williams D. I. and Chisholm G. D. (ed.) (1976) *Scientific Foundations in Urology*. London, Heinemann.

82 *The Bladder*

R. Fletcher Deane

ANATOMY

Development

The separation of the entodermal cloaca by the urorectal septum into a posterior rectal part and an anterior vesico-urethral part is complete by the 6th week of intra-uterine life when the embryo is some 16 mm in size. The vesico-urethral part of the cloaca has three sections: the upper section is the allantois and becomes the urachus and later the median umbilical ligament; the lower section is called the urogenital sinus and forms part of the urethra in men and the vaginal introitus in women; and the middle section forms the body of the bladder. The trigone of the bladder is formed from the caudal ends of the mesonephric ducts. In infancy the bladder lies in the abdomen but gradually settles down into the pelvis as the pelvis grows.

The bladder is supported in the pelvis by the puboprostatic or pubovesical ligaments. In men the posterior surface is separated from the rectum below, by the seminal vesicles and above, by the rectovesical pouch. In women it is separated above from the uterus by the uterovesical pouch, and below from the cervix and upper vagina by areolar tissue.

The bladder receives blood from the superior and inferior vesical arteries and the obturator artery, and in women from the uterine arteries by vessels which anastomose freely in the bladder walls. The veins from the bladder form a plexus on its inferolateral surfaces and drain into the internal iliac veins. Lymph drains to the internal iliac, the obturator and sacral nodes, thence to the common iliac nodes.

BLADDER FUNCTION

The bladder is an organ which stores and at intervals expels urine. Its lining is transitional cell epithelium which flattens as the bladder fills. The trigone is relatively fixed and doesn't expand or contract like the rest of the bladder. The smooth muscle fibres of the bladder are arranged in a complex way: in the body of the bladder they are reticulate and collectively called the detrusor muscle; at the bladder neck they become longitudinal or spiral and extend down the posterior urethra as far as the external sphincter. When the smooth muscle of the bladder contracts in response to parasympathetic stimulation, the detrusor muscle increases the pressure within the bladder and expels urine, whereas the muscle fibres at the bladder outlet pull open the bladder neck and the posterior urethra (*Fig.* 82.1). The bladder neck and urethra are kept closed when their muscle fibres are relaxed by elastic fibres in their walls and by tonic contraction of the external sphincter and levator ani. The function of the bladder can be assessed by history, physical examination, cystourethrography and urodynamics.

The commonest disorder of the bladder is its failure to empty properly, due either to lack of expulsive power or

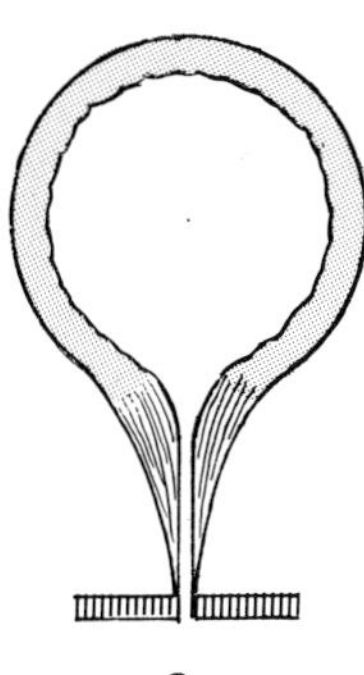

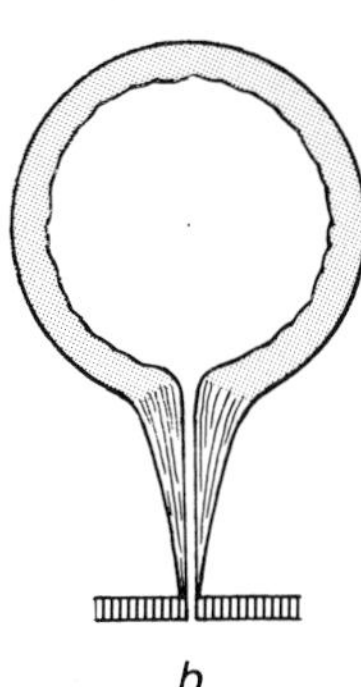

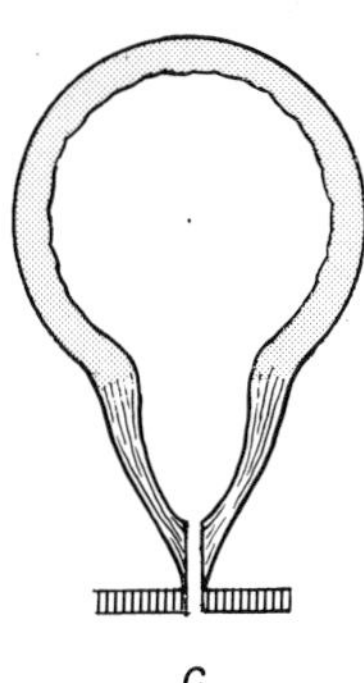

Fig. 82.1 *a*, The musculature of the bladder and the urethra. *b*, The relaxed bladder and urethra. *c*, The contracting bladder.

obstruction. If the obstruction is not relieved the detrusor muscle hypertrophies. This change can be recognized cystoscopically and sometimes radiologically, and is called trabeculation and may compensate for minor degrees of obstruction. If obstruction progressively increases, however, the bladder gradually distends to with increasing amounts of residual urine, and eventually distends to an extent that overstretches the muscle fibres and makes them atonic. The increase pressure in the distended bladder may be transmitted up into the ureters and pelves of the kidneys causing first, hydroureter and hydronephrosis and later reduces glomerular filtration and renal function. The thin layer of mucosa between bands of hypertrophied muscle may give way and diverticulum of almost any size can form. Stasis within diverticula provides a good environment for the precipitation of solutes and bacterial multiplication, causig cystitis, stones and neoplasia.

CONGENITAL ABNORMALITIES

Many abnormalities are described, but some are very rare.

A. Ectopia Vesicae

In this condition the anterior wall of the bladder, the rectus muscle and the skin of the lower abdominal wall fail to develop. The pubic bones are widely separated and the penis often split dorsally (epispadias). Varying degrees of the condition exist, but in all, the exposed bladder is liable to infection. The condition is usually obvious: there is a reddish mass on the lower abdomen which is always wet and the ureters can frequently be seen spurting out urine. Radiographs confirm diastasis of the pubic bones.

Treatment

Treatment aims at avoiding ascending infection and kidney damage and restoring function.

A formal reconstruction of the bladder, bladder neck and proximal urethra can be attempted in the neonatal period before infection and ureteric obstruction develop. Unfortunately few children achieve continence with this operation, and vesico-ureteric reflux, severe hydronephrosis and pyelonephritis can all easily develop.

Although many paediatric surgeons feel that it is worthwhile to attempt reconstruction, many children with ectopia vesicae ultimately require permanent urinary diversion.

B. Bladder Neck Obstruction

There is doubt whether or not this exists as a primary condition in infants in whom most cases of detrusor hypertrophy and unstable bladder function are caused by obstructive lesions in the urethra or by neurological disease.

Treatment

If the diagnosis is made, treatment aims at widening the bladder neck. Endoscopic resection is effective, but may render the child incontinent and later infertile and the operation of anterior vesico-urethroplasty by Y–V plasty which may be reversed later should the need arise is preferred by many surgeons.

C. Congenital Bladder Diverticulum

Bladder diverticulum in the newborn may be secondary to congenital lower urinary tract obstruction or be truly congenital and occur in the para-ureteric areas where the mesonephric ducts fuse with the entodermal cloaca. If this diverticulum enlarges it may incorporate or compress the ureteric orifice and cause vesico-ureteric reflux. It may appear small radiologically and cystoscopically and usually empties with the bladder because its wall contains muscle, unlike acquired diverticula which consist of mucosa alone or mucosa and a thin layer of muscle.

Persistence of the proximal portion of the urachus produces a vesico-urachal diverticulum in the vault of the bladder.

Treatment

Excision of the diverticulum is necessary only if it is causing infection or vesico-ureteric reflux.

Prune Belly Syndrome

This condition is typified by: deficiency of the anterior abdominal wall musculature (giving a wrinkled prune-like appearance to the overlying skin), bilateral undescended testes, and urinary tract abnormalities which include a distended thick walled bladder, a patent urachus or urachal diverticulum, dilated ureters, varying degrees of renal dysplasia and vesico-ureteric reflux.

Treatment

No specific treatment for the bladder is required so long as the child is emptying it efficiently and there is no infection. When infection and residual urine are a problem urethrotomy may improve bladder emptying and ureteroneocystostomy may be done if reflux proves to be a significant cause of infection.

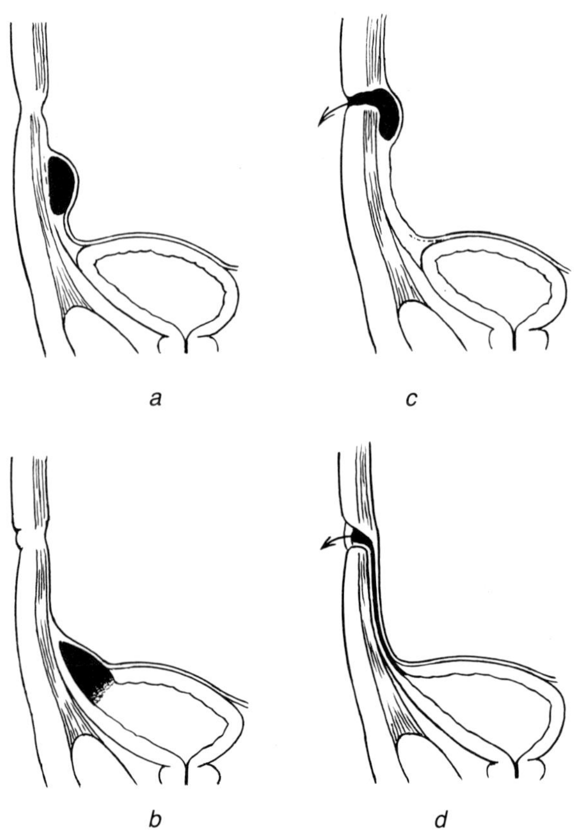

Fig. 82.2 Abnormalities of the urachus. *a*, Urachal cyst. *b*, Urachal diverticulum. *c*, External urachal sinus. *d*, Patent urachus.

Abnormalities of the Urachus

The urachus is formed from the allantois, which extends from the apex of the bladder to the umbilicus in intrauterine life, as the bladder descends into the pelvis. It usually degenerates into a fibrous cord but all or part may retain a lumen forming a fistula, a diverticulum or a cyst (*Fig.* 82.2).

CYSTITIS

Bacterial

Inflammatory conditions of the bladder are among the commonest diseases today; acute infections are particularly common and almost every woman will have at least one attack of acute cystitis at some time during her life. Acute infections of the bladder are uncommon in men unless there is some predisposing cause like obstruction or stone, and most acute lower urinary tract infections in men involve the prostate rather than the bladder.

Aetiology

Escherichia coli is the predominant organism and causes the infection in 85% of non-hospital patients, in 55% of hospital outpatients and in 45% of hospital inpatients. *Klebsiella* and *Proteus mirabilis* account for infection in about 12% of hospital patients and in 6% of non-hospital patients. Other proteus species, pseudomonas, *Streptococcuss faecalis* and enterobacter are usually found only in hospital patients, pseudomonas accounting for about 10%; each of the others for less than 10%. In hospital patients infections often follow or are associated with endoscopic or open operations like prostatectomy and are therefore commoner in men, whereas non-hospital bladder infections are 30 times commoner in women.

The *E. coli* found in urinary tract infections are identical with those recoverable from faeces and often recoverable from the vaginal introitus between infections. They can easily pass through the straight, short, wide female urethra into the bladder. There they are diluted by sterile urine from the ureters and expelled when urine is passed. But in some women they are not so easily expelled, even when there is neither anatomical abnormality nor residual urine, and infection ensues.

Diagnosis

Except for perinephric and renal abscesses, prostatic infections and infection in completely obstructed kidneys, the diagnosis of urinary tract infection depends upon the identification of organisms in significant numbers in urine, although there may be a temporary abacteriuria. If the specimen is obtained by suprapubic puncture any number is significant; if the specimen is a midstream urine more than 10^5/ml is regarded significant. The number of white blood cells in urine correlates poorly with the number of organisms; they are frequently absent in infected urine and present in sterile urines, even when the patient does not have tuberculosis.

Clinical Features

The symptoms of acute cystitis are frequent, urgent, painful micturition; suprapubic discomfort and occasionally haematuria and fever. Many patients have infection without symptoms (asymptomatic bacteriuria). Others have symptoms without infection (symptomatic abacteriuria) and provided the abacteriuria is not temporary, this group should be included with those suffering from the urethral syndrome, who will be discussed separately later.

Treatment

Asymptomatic Bacteriuria

In children infection is more likely, some say only likely, to damage the kidneys before the age of 5 years. In children, therefore, asymptomatic bacteriuria must be treated and, if it recurs, investigated by excretion urography and cysto-urethrography to exclude obstructive lesions and vesico-ureteric reflux.

In Pregnancy. Thirty per cent of women who are or become bacteriuriac during pregnancy develop pyelitis of pregnancy. Bacteriological examination of urine is an essential part of antenatal care and bacteriuria, even if asymptomatic, should be treated.

In Non-pregnant Women. There is now conclusive evidence that asymptomatic bacteriuria does no harm to non-pregnant adult women with normal urinary tracts and to treat it confers no other benefit than the relief of symptoms.

Acute Cystitis

Acute cystitis usually occurs in women after sexual activity and is treated by the family doctor. An antibiotic should be given orally for 7 days, though even 3 days may be sufficient. The choice of antibiotic is probably not important but tetracycline should be avoided especially in children, pregnant women and patients with chronic renal failure. Co-trimoxazole is as good as any. The urine can be checked some weeks later or the return of symptoms awaited as asymptomatic bacteriuria need only be treated in pregnant women and children.

Recurrent or Chronic Infections

In these groups some predisposition to bladder infection, such as obstruction, residual urine, stones or gynaecological abnormality must be excluded by excretion urography, pelvic examination and in some by cysto-urethroscopy. If the infection involves also the kidneys, diabetes, analgesic nephropathy and vesico-ureteric reflux must be excluded. If no predisposition is found, and one is not usually found, the infections can only be attributed to sexual activity and the patient must be advised to maintain a high fluid intake, to empty the bladder after intercourse, to avoid chemical douches or deodorants that might irritate the urethra and to be scrupulously hygienic so as to remove organisms from the introitus. What of antibiotics? Whether long-term low-dose maintenance therapy is used or each attack is treated when it occurs depends on the patient and doctor. There is no evidence that recurrent symptomatic infections damage the kidneys unless the organisms are of the proteus species, though the symptoms caused can obviously make the patient miserable.

Tuberculosis of the Bladder

Tuberculous cystitis is always secondary to and associated with renal tuberculosis. The changes may be confined to the area of the bladder around the ureteric orifice on the side of the affected kidney and consist of tubercles, bullous oedema or shallow ulcers. Sometimes there is a patchy non-specific looking generalized cystitis without obvious tubercles or caseation. In untreated, and even in some treated patients, considerable fibrosis occurs, reducing the bladder capacity. The patient complains of the usual symptoms of cystitis, but haematuria occurs more often than it does with non-specific infections. The diagnosis is suggested by changes in the excretion urogram suggesting tuberculosis of kidney or ureter, and confirmed by culturing the tubercle bacillus from early morning urine, and at least 3 and preferably 6 or even 12 specimens should be submitted. As soon as the diagnosis is confirmed triple therapy is commenced, as for the treatment of renal tuberculosis.

Complications

Although tuberculosis may be cured bacteriologically, the patient may be left with a fibrosed contracted bladder of low capacity. In such cases augmentation cystoplasty may be necessary and the ileum, the caecum or the colon can be used. Anti-reflux implantation of the ureters should be done in each case and, when the caecum is used, the terminal segment of ileum with its anti-reflux ileocaecal valve may be further defence against ascending renal damage. The accumulation of mucus is a problem and the function of the augmented bladder is not nearly so good as normal detrusor muscle, although in males bladder neck resection or transurethral prostatectomy may improve emptying. There is little place now for urinary diversion in the treatment of contracted tuberculous bladders.

Parasitic Cystitis

This is considered in Chapter 4.

Post-irradiation Cystitis

Radiotherapy is an established method of treating many patients with cancer of the bladder and other pelvic organs and as the bladder is sensitive to X-rays certain changes can occur. Early ones include vasodilatation with oedema, causing frequency and dysuria. Delayed changes are more serious and develop 1–10 years after exposure to radiotherapy. The principal late effect is an obliterative endarteritis causing ischaemia of the bladder wall with sloughing and ulceration of the mucosa. The muscle fibroses and diminishes the bladder capacity. Secondary bacterial invasion is common and aggravates the symptoms. Cystoscopically considerable debris may be seen with leashes of blood vessels appearing as telangiectasia in the submucosa. Bleeding from these vessels may be severe and require transfusion. Diathermy may suffice but haemorrhage may be so severe as to require the use of Helmstein's distension balloon or cystectomy. The bladder wall may necrose and cause a fistula between bladder and vagina or rectum.

Chemical Cystitis

A cystitis similar to that found after radiation can be produced by the cancericidal drug, cyclophosphamide. This drug is widely used in many forms of cancer and can cause severe haemorrhage from the bladder.

SYMPTOMATIC ABACTERIURIA

There are many patients who complain of symptoms of frequency, urgency and dysuria, indistinguishable from those of cystitis, but who show no evidence of infection and have sterile urine. However, in some patients, infection may occur secondarily to aggravate the symptoms and confuse the diagnosis. These conditions can be divided into two groups. In the first, there are physical changes in the bladder or urethra recognizable by cystoscopy; in the second, the bladder appears normal.

Group 1

Interstitial Cystitis

This condition is sometimes called Hunner's ulcer. It causes a dramatic increase in the frequency of micturition, with urgency and a characteristic suprapubic pain which occurs before and is relieved by micturition. The urine is sterile and the disease is ten times as common in women as men. At cystoscopy the bladder capacity is reduced and efforts to run more fluid into the bladder will often rouse the patient from general anaesthesia. The changes in the bladder consist of stellate ulcers in the vault of the bladder, but at cystoscopy they often appear as hyperaemic areas, which exude streams of blood as the bladder empties. This feature is regarded by many as diagnostic of interstitial cystitis. Biopsy shows a non-specific pan-cystitis with mast cells which gives some credence to a possible autoimmune aetiology and there is a loose association between patients with interstitial cystitis and those with autoimmune based diseases, such as systemic lupus erythematosus, autoimmune thyroiditis and rheumatoid arthritis.

Treatment

Distension of the bladder under general anaesthesia or cauterization of the ulcerated areas or both usually relieves symptoms for a time. If these methods fail, steroids or non-steroidal anti-inflammatory agents given parenterally or by the installation into the bladder of dimethyl sulphoxide (DMSO) or sodium oxychlorosene (Clorpactin) may be of benefit. If conservative methods fail, operations to augment the bladder capacity or even to divert urine should be considered.

Carcinoma of the Bladder

Most patients with carcinoma of the bladder present with painless haematuria. However, patients with carcinoma-in-situ and squamous carcinoma of the bladder often present with frequency, urgency and dysuria, and may have no haematuria.

Influence of the Menopause

During the menstrual cycle changes take place in the vaginal epithelium and affect the epithelium of the distal third of the female urethra which is almost an extension of the vaginal epithelium. Many patients in the postmenopausal age group have atrophic vaginitis associated with increased frequency of micturition, urgency and dysuria and atrophic changes can be observed in the distal third of the urethra by cytological examination. These changes may predispose to bacterial invasion. Urethral dilatation may provide temporary relief but the administration of oestrogens, orally or locally, often produces a dramatic improvement.

Group 2

Patients in this group have frequency and urgency without evidence of infection and without significant physical abnormality of the bladder or urethra, and are said to have the urethral syndrome, or the frequency/dysuria syndrome.

Fifty per cent of women with lower urinary tract symptoms fall into this group. Among the causes are irritation from bubble bath preparations, vaginal deodorants, nylon underwear or contraceptive creams and devices; vaginal infections or other gynaecological disorders; urethral narrowing; the trauma of intercourse; and viral or parasitic infections of the urethra or the effects of organisms in the vaginal introitus, the evidence for which, however, is unconvincing. In many women the urethral syndrome is a psychosomatic disorder and often helped by psychological treatment.

BLADDER CALCULI (*Figs.* 82.3, 82.4)

Some bladder calculi come down the ureter from the kidney but once in the bladder they are usually quickly passed because the urethra is much wider than the ureter. Such calculi, however, can remain in the bladder if it is obstructed or atonic. Stones that form in the bladder are either primary, i.e. form in a bladder that is otherwise normal, or secondary, i.e. originate in a bladder which is obstructed, infected or otherwise abnormal.

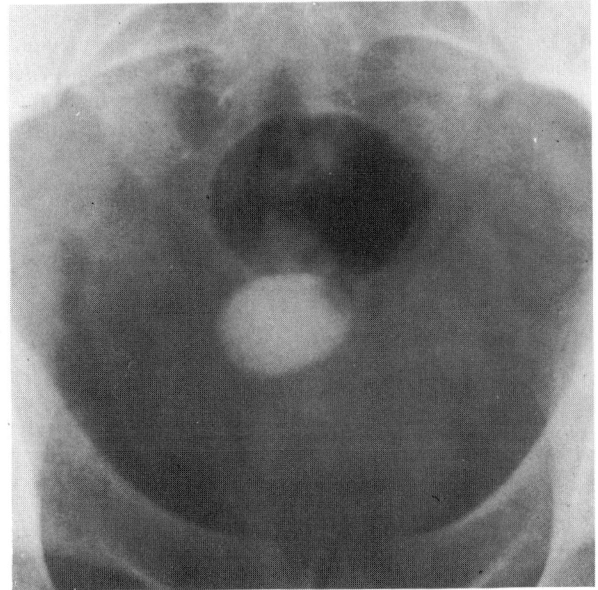

Fig. 82.3 Bladder stone.

Aetiology

Primary Stones

Endemic stone disease persists in many parts of the world including India, Pakistan, Turkey, Thailand, China, Iran, Egypt, Indonesia. Endemic stones are formed almost exclusively in male children less than 5 years old. Perhaps they do form in girls but are soon passed down the short, straight, wide female urethra. These stones are composed of ammonium acid urate and calcium oxalate, coated with phosphate if there has been much infection.

Secondary Stones

Bladder stones are not common in developed countries and when they do occur they are invariably secondary to some other disease such as obstruction to the outflow of urine from the bladder by prostatic or urethral disease; foreign bodies, particularly the inflated balloon of an indwelling Foley catheter; chronic infections, especially bilharziasis and cancer. Some bladder stones lie inside a diverticulum rather than the bladder. Metabolic diseases like gout and hyperparathyroidism rarely cause bladder stones. That many secondary bladder stones are associated with infection

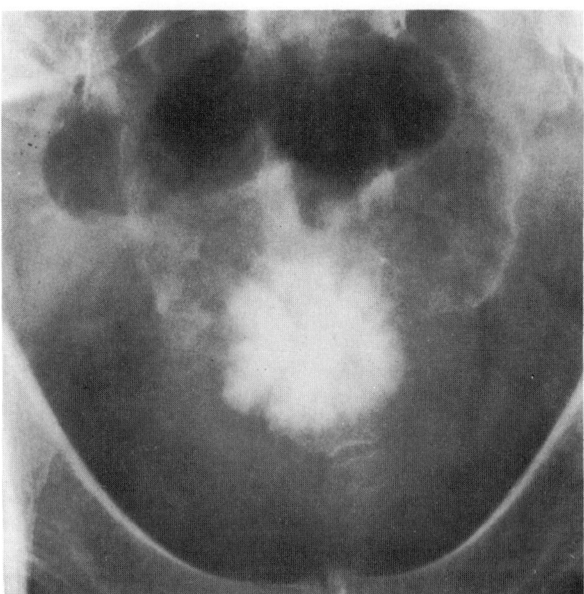

Fig. 82.4 Bladder stone.

is reflected in their composition—about 60% consist of calcium phosphate and calcium magnesium phosphate, about 25% of a calcium oxalate/calcium phosphate and 15% of pure oxalate.

Clinical Features

The patient usually has symptoms of lower urinary tract infection and haematuria as well as those of the predisposing disease. Pain characteristically occurs towards the end of micturition, is referred into the perineum and penis and associated with a sudden interruption of urinary flow.

Treatment

Most stones can be crushed endoscopically using a lithotrite which affords the operator a view of the calculus, although some urologists still favour the use of the traditional 'blind' lithotrite. The fragments of stone are evacuated and the bladder checked again with the cystoscope lest any fragments are left behind to form the nidus for further stone formation. A new method for removing bladder calculi employs ultrasonic waves to shatter the stone within the bladder. The waves are transmitted through a probe which is passed into the bladder through a cystoscope. An open operation should be done if there is a urethral stricture which renders instrumentation difficult; if the stone is lodged in a diverticulum; if the stone has developed around a foreign body which also has to be removed, and when open prostatectomy is also necessary, although usually a transurethral prostatectomy can be done and the stone crushed after the resection is completed.

DIVERTICULUM

Congenital diverticula of the bladder have already been described (p. 1356).

Acquired diverticula occur in obstructed bladders and complicate prostatic disease, urethral strictures, congenital obstructive lesions and neurogenic bladders obstructed at the bladder neck or external sphincter. They develop when increasing intravesical pressure blows out a weak spot in the bladder. These weak spots lie between the bundles of hypertrophied muscle fibres especially around the ureteric orifices where the spaces between muscle fibres are greater than elsewhere in the bladder. The neck of the diverticulum is usually narrow and the wall consists only of mucosa or of mucosa with a thin layer of muscle. They possess little if any contractility and therefore fill as the bladder empties; they become easily infected, may contain tumours or stone, lie close enough to distort the ureteric orifice and often cause reflux. The ureter is often plastered onto the wall of the diverticulum and the ureteric orifice may lie inside its neck.

Clinical Features

Diverticula are not often big enough to be palpated but they may be suspected if the urine is very infected and the patient complains of double micturition (i.e. the need and ability to pass urine some minutes after they already have done so). Large diverticula invalidate measurements of residual urine made by catheterization because some, if not all, the urine found in the bladder after micturition may have emerged from the diverticulum.

Bladder diverticula are often seen in the cystogram of excretion urograms (*Fig.* 82.5) or one made after dye is introduced into the bladder through a catheter. As acquired diverticula fill when the bladder empties they are best seen in postmicturition or voiding cystograms.

Treatment

Small diverticula require no treatment other than the relief of the obstruction causing them. Large ones can be excised at the same time as the obstruction is relieved.

INJURIES TO THE BLADDER

Aetiology

The bladder may be ruptured by direct blunt injuries of the lower abdomen or pelvis; by penetrating wounds of the pelvis or perineum, or by endoscopic or surgical procedures. Occasionally a diseased bladder ruptures spontaneously.

Intraperitoneal Rupture

Direct blunt injury to the lower abdomen can rupture a distended bladder without damaging anything else. The rupture usually involves the superior surface and the peritoneum covering it so that urine extravasates into the peritoneal cavity.

Extraperitoneal Rupture

Most injuries of the bladder occur when it is not distended and urine extravasates into the extraperitoneal tissues of the pelvis. The non-distended bladder is well protected by the bony pelvis and rarely damaged by blunt trauma unless the bony pelvis, especially the pubic bone, is fractured. Perforating injuries of the bladder by knives, gunshot wounds and impalement on fences are rarely found in this country. When they do occur other pelvic viscera are also involved. Perforating injuries and fractured pelvis may also injure the posterior urethra and sometimes both the bladder and urethra are damaged.

Surgical and Endoscopic Injuries

It is important to protect the bladder during all pelvic operations and operations on femoral and some inguinal hernias. The bladder can be damaged during endoscopic procedures, especially when resecting bladder tumours. The healthy bladder is not very likely to be damaged by catheters, bougies or cystoscopes, but malignant, tuberculous or post-radiotherapy bladders are sometimes friable and can be damaged and even perforated by these instruments; such bladders may also rupture spontaneously.

Clinical Features

With intraperitoneal rupture of the bladder the patient has peritonism and develops all the signs of an acute abdomen soon after receiving a lower abdominal injury. The features of extraperitoneal rupture are lower abdominal pain, ileus and sometimes haematuria, but they may be overshadowed by the other effects of a fractured pelvis or perforating pelvic or perineal wound, and the possibility of bladder or urethral damage should always be entertained in patients with these types of injuries, even if it is not obvious.

Diagnosis

A straight radiograph may reveal the fractured pelvis; a cystogram reveals an empty bladder and extravasation of the

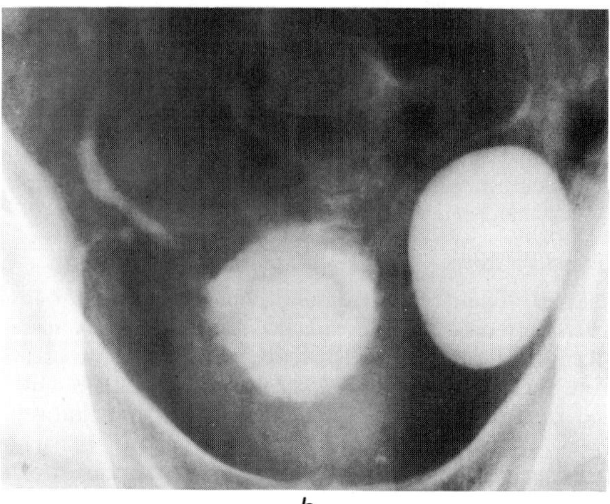

a *b*

Fig. 82.5 Cystogram showing diverticulum: *a*, Premicturition; *b*, Postmicturition.

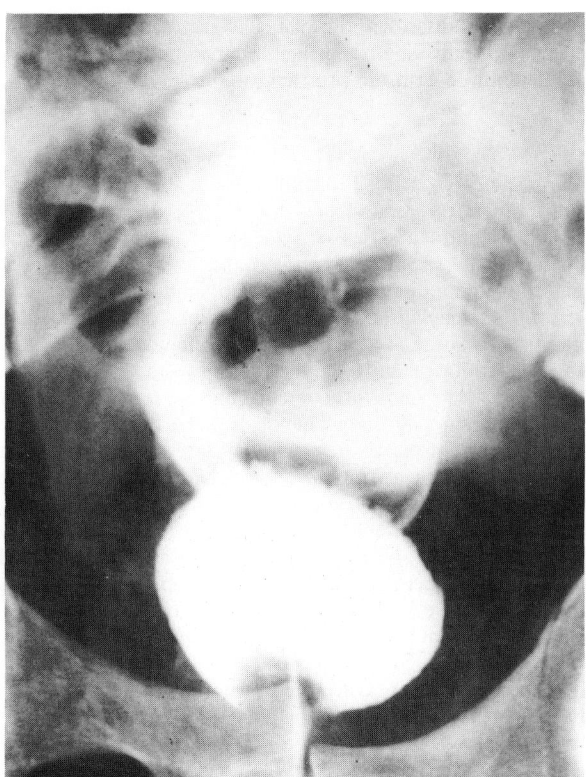

Fig. 82.6 Cystogram of a ruptured bladder with intraperitoneal extravasation of the contrast medium.

contrast medium into the peritoneal cavity (*Fig.* 82.6) or extraperitoneal tissues.

The possibility of bladder injury during pelvic surgery should be constantly borne in mind. Failure to recognize and treat it at the time may lead to the formation of a vesicovaginal, vesicocolic or vesicoperineal fistula.

A slightly different clinical picture presents when the bladder is perforated during an endoscopic procedure when the first sign is usually that the irrigating fluid fails to return and there is difficulty in seeing the lesion because the bladder does not distend. The patient, if anaesthetized by a spinal or epidural, may complain of symptoms of peritoneal irritation with rebound tenderness and shoulder-tip pain and of diffuse coldness spreading over the lower abdominal wall. The diagnosis is again confirmed by cystography.

Treatment

Much depends on the patient's general condition, particularly when the bladder rupture is part of multiple trauma. Once resuscitation has been completed the bladder should be explored surgically by the suprapubic approach. The bladder is opened, the defect identified and repaired. The bladder must be kept empty for 6 or 7 days with a catheter and the peritoneum or extraperitoneal space drained. If the bladder has been damaged during the resection of the prostate of a bladder tumour, catheter drainage alone may be all that is required.

FISTULAS

A bladder fistula is an abnormal communication between the bladder and an adjacent viscus, such as the vagina, uterus, bowel, or the skin.

Vesicovaginal Fistula

This is an abnormal communication between the bladder and the vagina.

Causes

Obstetric

The pressure of the fetal head on the anterior vaginal wall may produce a fistula if the second stage of labour is excessively prolonged. Good antenatal care enables us to anticipate such problems and fistulas caused in this way are excessively rare in developed countries. What sometimes happens, however, even in developed countries is a vesicovaginal fistula caused by a lower segment Caesarean section.

Gynaecological

The operation of hysterectomy either by the vaginal or the abdominal approach is probably the commonest cause of this fistula.

Malignant

The extension of malignant disease of the bladder into the vagina or of the cervix into the bladder produces a fistula, and sometimes a fistula is a late complication of treating either of these tumours by radiotherapy.

Traumatic

Perforating injuries of perineum may result in fistula formation, but they are rare.

Diagnosis

If the fistula is small the patient may only be incontinent when the bladder is full and urinary function is otherwise normal. With larger fistulas the patient is usually continuously wet and passes no urine in the usual way. Methylene blue can be instilled in the bladder through a catheter and leakage of dye will colour the upper of two swabs previously inserted into the vagina. An intravenous urogram reveals a normal upper urinary tract, thus distinguishing small vesicovaginal fistulas from ureterovaginal fistulas in which the affected kidney is usually hydronephrotic. The bladder opening of the fistula may be seen at cystoscopy but is often small or obscured by oedema and, furthermore, it is usually impossible to distend the bladder because the irrigating fluid leaks through the fistula into and out of the vagina. On bimanual examination the vaginal opening of the fistula may be seen or felt and is usually in or near the anterior fornix.

Treatment

Unless the fistula is malignant or postradiation it can be repaired vaginally or transvesically. Most gynaecologists prefer the vaginal route while the urologist may be more at home approaching the fistula through the bladder. At operation non-viable tissue around the edges of the fistula must be excised. The bladder and the vagina should be separated and repaired in layers and an omental graft may be interposed between them. Care must be taken to avoid damaging the ureters, and the bladder should be drained for 7–10 days.

The most common complication is recurrence of the fistula and secondary and tertiary repairs of vesicovaginal fistulas are less successful than primary repairs. Should repair be impossible or unsuccessful, urinary diversion may need to be considered.

Vesico-uterine Fistula

These are rare but may be caused by neoplasia, radiation or operations on the uterus, e.g. myomectomy. The clinical features are similar to those of vesicovaginal fistula. The site of the fistula can usually be recognized by cystoscopy or cystography.

Treatment

The fistula can be repaired if the bladder and uterus are separated, and the defects closed in separate layers. Omentum may be interposed. However, hysterectomy is often the best way of dealing with this condition.

Vesico-intestinal Fistula

A fistula may develop between bladder and bowel if a part of the bowel adheres to the bladder as a result of inflammation or neoplasia. It is possible for almost any segment of the bowel to become adherent, but the common sites are: the descending or sigmoid colon, due to diverticulitis or cancer; the terminal ileum due to Crohn's disease or tuberculosis; the appendix due to appendicitis; or Meckel's diverticulum due to infection. Perforating injuries may also cause fistulas.

Clinical Features

In nearly all cases pressure differences dictate that bowel contents enter the bladder. The bladder is irritated and micturition becomes frequent, painful and urgent. But the principal symptom which should clinch the diagnosis is pneumaturia, and if the fistula is large, the urine may contain faeces or partially digested food.

Diagnosis

A straight pelvic film in the erect posture may reveal gas in the bladder. The fistula may be demonstrated by barium enema or barium meal with follow-through visualization of the small bowel. Where the distal bowel is involved, sigmoidoscopy and perhaps biopsy should be undertaken. Alternatively, the fistula may be identified by cystography. Cystoscopy will confirm the site of the fistula, which may be obscured by oedema or phosphatic encrustations.

Treatment

Laparotomy will decide the nature and cause of the fistula. The viscus must be carefully dissected from the bladder wall. If there is severe inflammatory disease or neoplasia then the affected portion of the bowel should be excised if possible and bowel continuity restored but if there is a large abscess, drainage and colostomy may be necessary. Many surgeons prefer to treat fistulas involving the descending colon by preliminary transverse colostomy; the bowel is excised at a second operation and the colostomy closed at a third. However, if possible, it is best to repair the fistula in a one-stage procedure.

Vesicocutaneous Fistula

These are either deliberately made as suprapubic cystostomies to drain the bladder before or after operations or persist after bladder operations.

NEOPLASIA OF THE BLADDER

Carcinoma of the bladder is the commonest tumour encountered by the urologist and can cause patients more distress than almost any other tumour. Distant metastases usually occur late with this tumour and the major clinical problems are concerned with the primary tumour.

Aetiology

Primary neoplasms of the epithelium of the bladder and of the urethra, the renal pelves and ureters are regarded as a prescribed industrial disease in occupations in which certain chemicals are produced, handled and used, namely alpha-naphthylamine, beta-naphthylamine, and benzidine, and less often xenylamine, dichlorbenzidine, orthodianisidine and orthotolidine. These occupations include chemical factories; manufacturers of paints and pigments, rubber goods, coated cables; gas workers and rodent control officers. Although none of these chemicals have been used since 1967, the latent period between exposure to the carcinogen and development of tumour averages 20 years, but can be delayed as long as 45 years.

The bladder is much more frequently involved than any other urothelium, perhaps because it acts as a reservoir and urinary carcinogens can operate for a longer period; patients with obstructive lesions are more liable to the disease.

The treatment of bladder tumour is complex owing to the many variables which are encountered during the assessment of the tumour. Once the diagnosis of bladder tumour has been made the notion that this is a 'benign' condition must never be entertained because all tumours of the bladder, with rare exceptions, must be regarded as malignant.

Pathology of Bladder Tumours

1. Benign tumours do occur and include leiomyoma, fibroma, and myxoma but it is unlikely that a practising urologist would see more than one of these during his career.
2. The most common tumour is the transitional-cell carcinoma and it accounts for over 95% of all bladder tumours. All are regarded as malignant.
3. Squamous carcinoma of the bladder is rare in the Western World accounting for only 2% of all bladder tumours. They are often associated with bilharzia, vesical calculus and squamous metaplasia of the bladder.
4. Adenocarcinoma is very rare. It constitutes less than 0·5% of all bladder tumours. It is often related to ectopia vesicae, the persistence of urachal tissue in the vault of the bladder or secondary to ovarian or bowel cancer.
5. The appearance of the tumour may give an idea of its subsequent clinical behaviour. Different types are described:

   a. Papillary which tend to grow into the lumen. They tend to be well differentiated and pedunculated.

   b. Infiltrating which often appear sessile and solid with ulceration, necrosis and calcification. These growths extend through the lamina propria and muscle of the bladder wall and histologically are less well differentiated.

   c. Papillary and infiltrating: Not surprisingly there are bladder tumours which show both types of growth. The treatment and prognosis depend on the worst part of the tumour.

   d. In situ carcinoma. These lesions are flat, reddish patches on the mucosa, often indistinguishable from infection.
6. *Tumour site.* About 70% of bladder tumours arise on the lateral and posterior walls, 20% on the vault. Occasionally tumours arise within a diverticulum (*Fig.* 82.7) and they infiltrate more easily because there is little if any muscle in the wall of an acquired diverticulum.

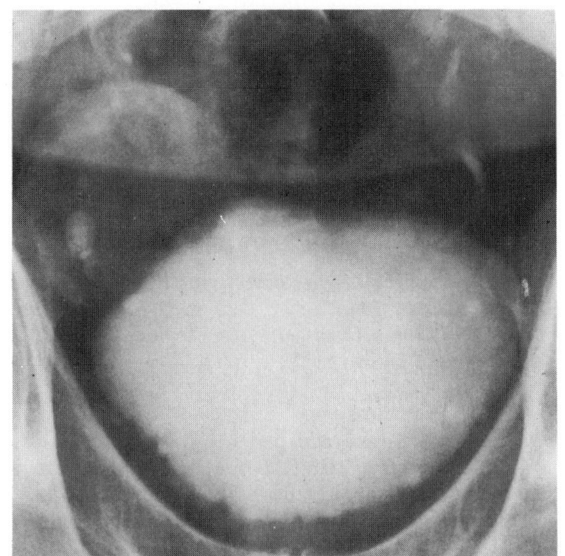

Fig. 82.7 Cystogram showing tumour in a diverticulum of the bladder.

Diagnosis

1. History

The most frequent presenting symptom is painless haematuria which is usually obvious to the patient. About 10% of tumours do not cause haematuria and may be found incidentally at cystoscopy during the investigation of some other urinary complaint. Growths near a ureteric orifice may obstruct the ureter and cause loin pain.

2. Physical Examination

This is unlikely to reveal much evidence of local disease but hepatomegaly from metastatic disease may be encountered.

3. Urinary Culture

Urinary culture with microscopy should be performed. Treatment of any secondary infection may afford the patient some relief of symptoms but the need for further investigations should not be neglected in the face of a positive urine culture.

4. Blood Examination

The serum urea and creatinine levels give an overall assessment of renal function. Haemoglobin levels should be checked as haematuria may have made the patient anaemic.

5. Urinary Cytology

The patient who presents with haematuria requires endoscopy, biopsy and radiology, but cytology does have a place in the regular screening of those exposed to possible carcinogens and as a follow-up screening test for some known cases of urothelial cancer, but it is valueless after X-ray therapy.

6. Intravenous Urography

Attention should be paid to filling defects in the cystogram, dilatation of either ureter, bladder calcification, reduced renal function and other tumours in the kidneys or ureters.

7. Cystoscopy and Biopsy

This is the most valuable single investigation and delay should be minimized between the initial presentation of symptoms and this examination. The tumour will be identified and its size, growth type, position and number of growths noted. Biopsies should be taken of the tumour and underlying muscle, of mucosa adjacent to the growth and of mucosa in other parts of the bladder.

8. Bimanual Examination of the Bladder Tumour

This should be performed at the time of the cystoscopy under general anaesthetic. The patient's abdominal wall should be completely relaxed and the bladder empty. A papillary type of growth may be palpable on the bimanual examination and slide easily between the examining fingers. When the growth begins to infiltrate the superficial layers of the muscle it may just be felt as an area of irregularity in a mobile bladder but when it infiltrates the deeper layers of muscle it is much more obvious and can be palpated even when the exophytic part of the growth has been resected. The bladder at this stage is still quite mobile. Fixation of the growth suggests spread to adjacent organs or the pelvic wall.

9. Ultrasonic Examination of the Bladder

Sometimes bladder tumours can be identified ultrasonically in the full bladder and an assessment of their degree of infiltration made to an accuracy of about 80% and is particularly useful in patients in whom a bimanual examination is unsatisfactory due to obesity, coughing, abdominal scarring or poor anaesthesia.

10. Isotope Scanning

Blood spread is uncommon, but isotope scanning of the liver and bones may identify distant metastases.

11. Chest Radiography and Skeletal Survey

The chest must be radiographed; and so must any part of the skeleton that appears abnormal in the bone scan.

12. Lymphography

Lymph nodes replaced completely with tumour may not fill with contrast and pelvic nodes are never demonstrated. Many have abandoned this procedure in the assessment of bladder tumours.

13. *Computerized Tomography*

Scanning (CT) may reveal the primary tumour, particularly if it is an infiltrating one or enlarged lymph nodes but is not usually done as a routine procedure.

After these investigations have been carried out we can attribute the tumour to its appropriate TNMG category.

T—Primary Tumour (*Fig.* 82.8).

- Tis Carcinoma-in-situ.
- T1 On bimanual examination a freely mobile mass may be felt: this should not be felt after complete transurethral resection of the lesion and/or microscopically, the tumour does not invade beyond the lamina propria. T1 tumours can be subdivided into Ta which do not invade the lamina propria and T1 which do.
- T2 On bimanual examination there is induration of the bladder wall which is mobile. There is no residual induration after complete transurethral resection of the lesion and/or there is microscopic invasion of superficial muscle.

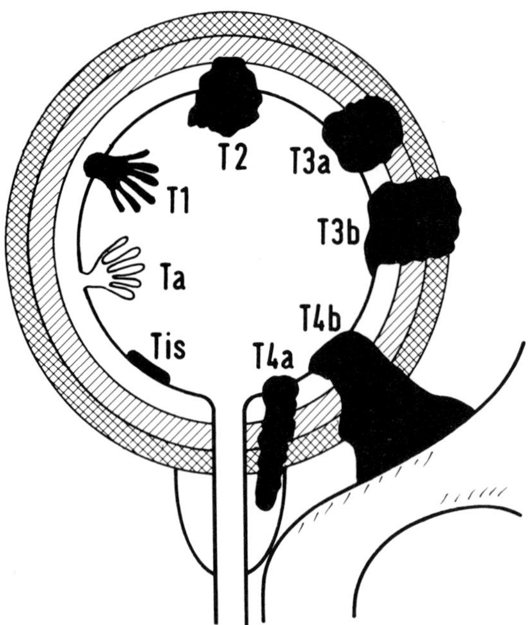

Fig. 82.8 Staging of bladder tumours (T).

T3 On bimanual examination induration or a nodular mobile mass is palpable in the bladder wall which persists after transurethral resection of the exophytic portion of the lesion and/or there is microscopic invasion of deep muscle or of extension through the bladder wall.

T3a Invasion of deep muscle.

T3b Invasion through the bladder wall.

T4 Tumour fixed or extending to neighbouring structures and/or there is microscopic evidence of such involvement.

T4a Tumour infiltrating the prostate, uterus or vagina.

T4b Tumour fixed to the pelvic wall and/or abdominal wall.

TX The minimum requirements to assess the primary tumour cannot be met.

N—Regional and Juxta-regional Lymph Nodes.

The regional lymph nodes are the pelvic nodes below the bifurcation of the common iliac arteries. The juxta-regional lymph nodes are the inguinal nodes, the common iliac nodes and the para-aortic nodes.

N0 No evidence of regional lymph node involvement.

N1 Evidence of involvement of a single homolateral regional lymph node.

N2 Evidence of involvement of contralateral or bilateral or multiple lymph nodes.

N3 Evidence of involvement of fixed regional lymph nodes (there is a fixed mass on the pelvic wall with a free space between this and the tumour).

N4 Evidence of involvement of juxta-regional lymph nodes.

NX The minimum requirements to assess the regional and/or juxta-regional lymph nodes cannot be met.

M—Distant Metastases.

M0 No evidence of distant metastases.

M1 Evidence of distant metastases.

MX The minimum requirements to assess the presence of distant metastases cannot be met.

G—Histological Grading

'G0' Papilloma, i.e. no evidence of anaplasia.

G1 High degree of differentiation.

G2 Medium degree of differentiation.

G3 Low degree of differentiation or undifferentiated.

GX Grade cannot be assessed.

Treatment of Bladder Tumours (*Fig.* 82.9)

A full assessment should be made with all speed from the first appearance of haematuria. Many methods of treatment are available to the urologist, the use of which is dependent on the degree of spread of the tumour.

Carcinoma-in-situ

At cystoscopy there are reddened areas which may be raised and mistaken for areas of infection or of interstitial cystitis. Many of these patients present without haematuria but with frequency and dysuria. Biopsy of these reddened mossy areas reveals the histological changes of carcinoma-in-situ. Other areas of the bladder should also be biopsied, because mucosa that looks normal through a cystoscope may be dysplastic. In some cases the growth can be controlled by endoscopic diathermy or resection but the recurrence rate is high, and later biopsy may show that the previous carcinoma-in-situ has become invasive. If the disease is not controlled by endoscopic means, instillations into the bladder of substances such as ethoglucid (Epodyl), mitomycin C, adriamycin, epirubicin or Bacillus Calmette-Guérin (BCG) can be tried. BCG has proved to be particularly useful in the treatment of carcinoma-in-situ despite side-effects that might have to be controlled with antituberculous therapy. In many patients the bladder can be kept free of tumour by resection or instillation, but in others the tumour becomes invasive and more radical treatment is necessary, and as these patients usually have reduced bladder capacity cystectomy is generally preferred to X-ray therapy. Provided the carcinoma-in-situ does not become invasive the bladder can be kept free of tumour in many patients, but in others more radical treatment is required and the prognosis is poor.

Treatment of T1 Tumours

These growths tend to be papillary and well differentiated and by definition do not infiltrate beyond the lamina propria of the bladder. Many are confined to the mucosa (Ta).

Endoscopic resection is the treatment of choice but more than one session may be required to deal with a big growth. However, even when the initial growth has been eradicated there is a recurrence rate of about 50%. As it is impossible to predict which cases will recur, and after what time interval, all patients need careful supervision for many years if not for life.

Although recurrences tend to be of the same histological type as the original, this is not always so and they should always be examined histologically after resection. Recurrences can usually be dealt with in the same manner as the original growth. It is interesting to note that primary growths are most commonly found on the posterior and lateral walls but recurrences are commoner on the posterior and superior walls, particularly around the air bubble region. Implantation of tumour cells at resection and diathermy via air bubbles is suggested as a possible cause.

If the tumour is too large for endoscopic resection, the size can often be reduced to manageable proportions by suction or Helmstein's technique. This involves inserting a

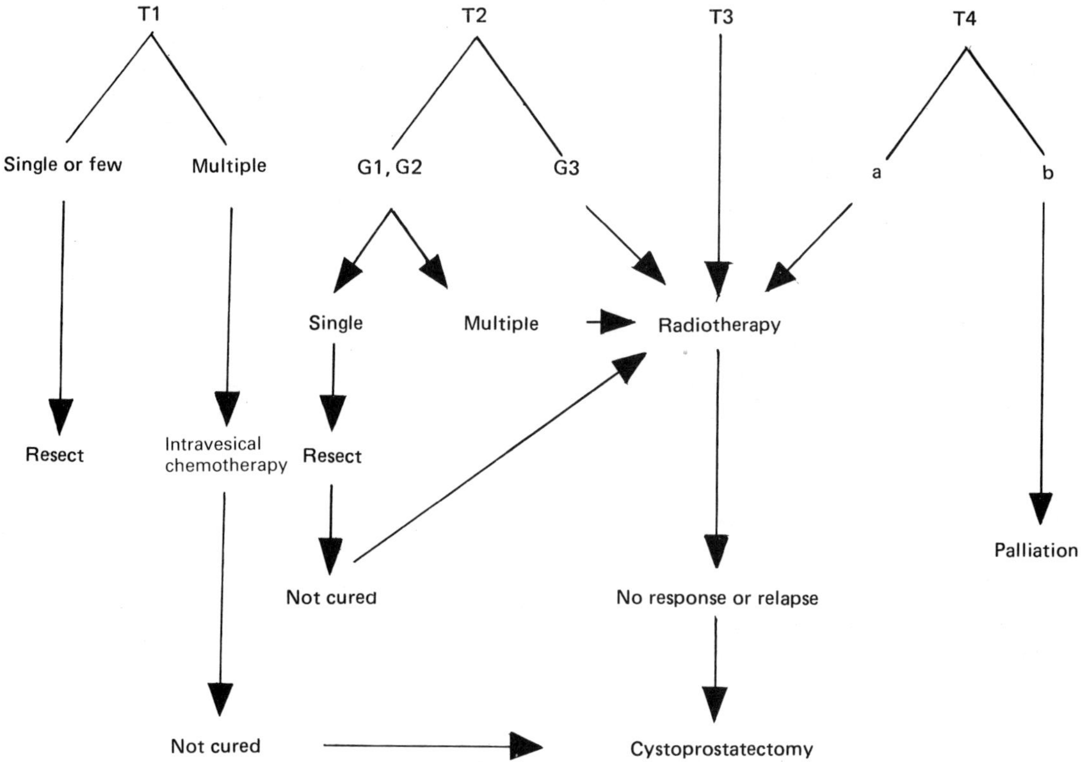

Fig. 82.9 A scheme of treatment for carcinoma of the bladder.

large balloon into the bladder on the end of a catheter and inflating it to a pressure midway between systolic and diastolic arterial pressure for several hours. Open diathermy resection should be avoided because tumour invariably implants in the bladder and wound. Multiple T1 tumours may be resected in several sessions but if they are too widespread, they can be treated by the installation into the bladder of the same substances used in the treatment of carcinoma-in-situ. These substances can also be used after a successful resection in the hope of preventing recurrence.

Occasionally if growths cannot be controlled by those methods cysto-urethrectomy may be required, especially if there are also tumours in the urethra.

The survival rate for all growths in the T1 category is over 80% at 3 years and just over 70% at 5 years, and obviously depends on the depth of spread from mucosa into lamina propria and on the degree of differentiation. G3 tumours have a poor prognosis even when detected as Tis.

Treatment of T2 Tumours

T2 tumours have penetrated the lamina propria and invaded superficial muscle. They pose a much greater problem than T1 tumours. Characteristically these growths are less often well differentiated, frequently solid rather than papillary and 'understaged' (many are probably T3).

Some can be treated by endoscopic resection, taking the muscle layer down to the deepest layers. A check cystoscopy at 12 weeks is required, when the treated and adjacent areas should be biopsied. Simple excision alone is inadequate for many and gives a 5-year survival rate of only 37%. This is due to a number of reasons: understaging, inadequate excision, the formation of new growths, or bloodborne extension, particularly if the growth is anaplastic (G3). Because of the difficulty of staging T2 growths many urological surgeons adopt a more aggressive attitude to their treatment and treat most of them as if they were T3 by radiotherapy or surgery or a combination of both, which raises the 5-year survival rate of T2 tumours to around 50%.

Treatment of T3 Tumours

By definition these tumours have spread into the deeper layers of the bladder muscle or through the bladder wall.

The 5-year survival rate for patients treated by radiotherapy or radical cystectomy or a combination of both are only in the order of 20%.

High-energy radiotherapy equipment (linear accelerators and cobalt 60 machines) was introduced some 30 years ago. Its introduction enabled the treatment of tumours in almost any part of the body with far fewer complications than occurred with machines producing only low-energy radiations. More recently cyclotrons, which produce neutrons, have been used but it is still too early to say whether they are more effective than the machines that deliver electrons.

T3 bladder tumours are treated with megavoltage radiation therapy delivered by a linear accelerator which gives about 5500 rad (55c Gray) over a 4 or 5-week period to an area with a volume of 10 cm^3. Early complications consisting of non-specific inflammatory changes in the bladder and rectum and sometimes in the small bowel are inevitable and patients complain of frequency, dysuria, urgency, rectal irritation and diarrhoea. Late complications may only develop some years after treatment and are dose-related and consist of telangiectasia, which is common, contracted bladder and fistula which fortunately are uncommon, and bowel complications consisting of stenosis, fistula, bleeding and chronic diarrhoea.

Cystoprostatectomy with an ileal loop diversion is only considered in patients whose tumour fails to respond to, or recurs after, radiation.

Some urologists treat T3 tumours by cystoprostatectomy, others by combined radiotherapy and surgery, giving some 3000 or 4000 rad over 4 weeks and carry out a cystectomy 1 week later. There is no sound evidence that either of these gives better results than radiotherapy alone for T3 tumours.

Treatment of T4 Bladder Tumours

The prognosis for growths that have spread to adjacent organs is exceptionally poor, even more so if there are metastases. There is no hope for a cure and the aim should be to make the patient as comfortable as possible. Nevertheless T4a tumours, i.e. those that invade the prostate but not other viscera or the pelvic wall can sometimes be treated radically like T3 tumours. The T4b tumours are suitable only for palliative treatment. Palliative radiotherapy may relieve bladder symptoms and can relieve pain from bony metastases. Urinary diversion sometimes combined with the application of heat or the introduction of formalin into the bladder, may also help.

Squamous Carcinoma of the Bladder

These tumours can be assessed in the same fashion as transitional-cell carcinomas. They are usually fairly extensive when first diagnosed. The treatment of choice is radiotherapy although they are often relatively radio-resistant and some patients require total cystectomy. These tumours are highly malignant and few patients survive more than one year after diagnosis and treatment.

Adenocarcinoma of the Bladder

This is a very rare tumour of the bladder but may arise in association with remnants of a urachus or ectopia vesicae. It is also very radio-resistant and cystectomy, partial or total, is the treatment of choice. Care must be taken that the tumour is not a secondary tumour which has metastasized to the bladder from ovary or colon.

Chemotherapy

Many trials are in progress to assess the effects on bladder tumours of parenterally given cytotoxic drugs, with or without X-ray therapy. It is too early to suggest an effective regime but promising results have been reported with adriamycin, methotrexate and cisplatin.

Follow-up

All patients with urothelial tumours no matter how simple, must be followed up for many years, if not for life. Patients are reviewed at 3 months after the first treatment is completed, thereafter at 6- and 12-monthly intervals if they remain tumour free, more frequently, otherwise.

THE BLADDER AND DISEASES OF THE NERVOUS SYSTEM

The features of normal micturition are that we desire to pass urine only when the bladder contains 300 ml or more; that we can suppress this desire, for a time anyway, if it is inconvenient to pass urine; that micturition starts only when we wish it to do so, and once started continues rapidly until the bladder is empty.

The filling of the bladder and continence depend upon the compliance of the bladder and upon the resistance offered by the urethra and the contractility of the striated muscles of the pelvic floor.

The emptying of the bladder depends upon the contractility of the detrusor muscle of the bladder and upon the appropriate fall in urethral pressure and relaxation of the striated muscle of the pelvic floor. The way in which disease or injuries of the brain and spinal cord may interfere with micturition can be understood best if we first review briefly the physiology of normal micturition, which is complex and still poorly understood (*Fig.* 82.10).

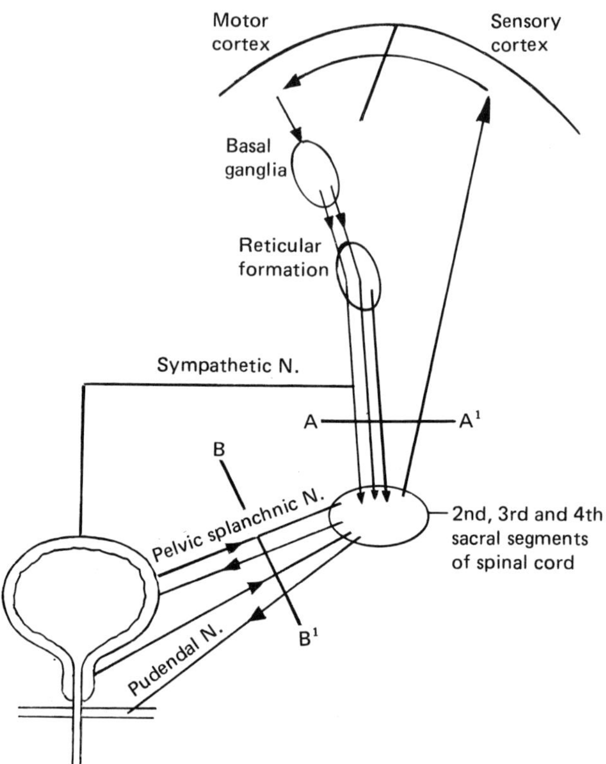

Fig. 82.10 The nerve supply of the bladder.

As the bladder fills, there is little if any change in the intravesical pressure until it is full (the normal capacity of the bladder is usually about 300 ml but can be as much as 600 ml). This is a result of the compliance of the bladder and of the inhibitory impulses from the higher motor centres (the cortex, the basal ganglia and the reticular formation) which prevent the sacral centre for micturition being excited by afferent impulses from the filling bladder until the bladder is full. Once the bladder is full the tension in its wall stimulates the receptors to such an extent that afferent impulses pass through the sacral centre and ascend to the sensory cortex and cause the desire to pass urine. If it is inconvenient to pass urine the higher motor centres increase their inhibitory influence and the desire to pass urine disappears for a time. If it is convenient to pass urine a number of things happen: the inhibitory influence of the higher motor centres is uplifted and replaced by excitatory impulses; the excited sacral centre sends impulses down the parasympathetic nerves contracting the smooth muscle of the bladder which increases the intravesical pressure and pulls open the bladder neck and the posterior urethra; as urine enters the posterior urethra, pudendal afferent nerves are stimulated; they inhibit the anterior horn cells of the pudendal efferent nerves and relax the external sphincter and levator ani; the higher motor centres continue bombarding the sacral centre with excitatory impulses until the bladder is quite emptied. It empties rapidly with a peak flow rate between 25 and 40 ml/sec; rather less in the elderly.

Sensation depends on the integrity of the afferent pathway, the bladder capacity and the ability to inhibit micturition on the inhibitory parts of the higher motor centres, and the ability to continue micturition until the bladder is empty on the excitatory parts of the higher motor centres. The filling and the emptying of the bladder involve a high degree of coordination between smooth and skeletal muscle and between autonomic and somatic reflexes. The coordinating centre is in the reticular formation in the pons: with lesions immediately above this centre micturition is coordinate but involuntary; with lesions below it is incoordinate and involuntary.

The cortex is essential for the awareness of the bladder filling and for the behavioural reflexes that put micturition under voluntary control.

Unstable or Uninhibited Bladder

Bladder activity becomes unstable or uninhibited when the higher motor centres fail to exert their usual inhibitory influences on the sacral centre. As a result this centre becomes excited and the desire to pass urine occurs when the bladder holds less, often considerably less, than 300 ml nor can the desire be inhibited. The patient complains of frequency, urgency and sometimes of urge incontinence but as excitatory activity remains normal the bladder does empty. Urodynamics reveals that the desire to pass urine occurs with a low bladder capacity and is soon followed by uninhibited bladder contractions which empty the bladder.

The causes of unstable bladder activity are many:

Physiological—the bladder often behaves in an unstable way at times of widespread excitatory activity, such as cold weather and anxiety.

Psychosomatic—bladder activity is so dominated by the inhibitory influences of the higher motor centres, including the cerebral cortex, that it is not surprising that unstable bladder activity may be a feature, even the only feature, of anxiety or depression and a frequent cause of 'symptomatic abacteriuria'.

Diseases of the nervous system—a number of diseases of the nervous system interfere with inhibitory pathways and produce unstable bladder activity. They include cerebrovascular ischaemic disease, disseminated sclerosis, Parkinsonism and some spinal injuries. Sometimes, however, although all the clinical features seem only those of unstable bladder activity, there may also be excitatory defects and the bladder may not empty completely.

Obstruction—the features of obstruction may include those of unstable bladder activity.

Treatment

Unstable bladder activity can be treated by drugs that inhibit bladder contractility. Atropine is unsuitable because of its side-effects, but propantheline bromide, flavoxate and imipramine hydrochloride are used.

Atonic Bladder

The atonic bladder possesses neither tone nor contractility and distends with urine. It evokes no sensation despite the 2 or 3 litres it may contain. No urine is passed actively, but small quantities overflow passively, incontinently and at frequent intervals from the distended bladder. Back-pressure effects and vesico-ureteric reflux (a frequent complication) cause dilatation of the ureters, renal pelves and calices and later renal failure.

Causes

Nervous Diseases

The bladder becomes atonic after acute lesions of the spinal cord or cauda equina and remains atonic during the period of spinal shock which in humans lasts several weeks. It also becomes atonic with pure sensory lesions like tabes dorsalis and some of the sacral autonomic neuropathies, like those caused by diabetes and less often by herpes zoster. In some women the bladder becomes atonic for no reason other than hysteria.

Obstruction

Chronic retention of obstructive origin overstretches the smooth muscle fibres of the bladder and as a result they lose their contractility and the bladder becomes atonic. Assessing the tone and contractility of the anal sphincter by rectal examination in patients with distended atonic bladders tells us whether the cause is obstructive or neurological. If the cause is obstructive the sphincter is usually normal, whereas if the cause is neurological it also is atonic.

Treatment

No more need be done for the obstructed atonic bladder than relieve the obstruction and drain the bladder for some days afterwards.

The others are more difficult to treat. Drugs which increase bladder contractilty, and they include distigmine bromide, bethanechol chloride and carbachol, may help patients who have difficulty passing urine after pelvic operations, but are often ineffective when used in patients with established atonic bladders. They are often best treated by intermittent catheterization which they can be taught to do themselves. For some, reducing the bladder capacity by resecting part or better by the van Werken–Hützen operation is helpful.

Automatic (Upper Motor Neurone) Bladder

The automatic bladder occurs, once the period of spinal shock if any is passed, from complete or nearly complete lesions that disconnect the sacral centres from the higher centres but leave their connection with the bladder intact. As sensation is lost the patient is incontinent, the bladder contracts in response to afferent impulses to the sacral centre from the bladder, skin or rectum, but the contractions are not sustained long enough to empty the bladder and there is residual urine.

Autonomic Bladder

The autonomic bladder occurs after lesions that destroy the sacral centre or disconnect it from the bladder. Sensation is lost and the patient is incontinent; the bladder is acontractile and can only be partially emptied by manual compression.

Modern urodynamic investigations have altered our approach to the classification of patients with bladder dysfunction and we now tend to describe them in terms of end-organ dysfunction, i.e. of dysfunction of the bladder and urethra, and it is convenient to discuss them separately.

The Detrusor (The Bladder)

The detrusor may be normal, underactive or overactive. Overactivity produces the unstable bladder and causes frequency, urgency and urge incontinence. Underactivity produces a hypotonic or acontractile bladder which is temporary in spinal shock but permanent in the pure sensory lesions and in lesions through or below the sacral centre, when voiding occurs only with manual compression or catheter drainage of one sort or another.

The Urethra

Can also be normal, overactive or underactive. In underactivity there is a loss of tone and the pelvic musculature relaxes without detrusor activity, resulting in stress incontinence.

In overactivity the urethra and pelvic muscle do not relax and may even contract during micturition and prevent the bladder emptying.

However, we describe or classify bladder dysfunction when it causes two basic problems—incontinence (failure to fill) and residual urine (failure to empty) and it is the management of these two that forms the basis of treatment although they may both produce complications that also require attention.

Complications

Residual urine predisposes to infection, stone formation, dilatation of the upper urinary tract and chronic renal failure. The more there is the more likely are these complications to occur.

Vesico-ureteric reflux is a frequent finding and more common with autonomic and atonic bladders.

Stone formation—infections and residual urine predispose to stone formation and so also do Foley catheters if left in for long periods with inflated balloons, immobility and a poor fluid intake.

Urethral diverticula and fistula—these occur in male patients usually at the penoscrotal junction and are caused by infection and the pressure of catheters, penile clamps or other incontinence appliances.

Hyper-reflexia—autonomic reflexes consisting of vasoconstriction as the bladder fills and vasodilatation as it empties occur to a subclinical level in normal people. They may be exaggerated in people with automatic bladders especially if they have cervical lesions. As the bladder fills their blood pressure increases (sometimes to seriously high levels) and they become pale and sweat; as the bladder empties the blood pressure falls and they vasodilate.

Obstruction—fibrosis and contracture of the bladder neck or spasm of the external sphincter may obstruct bladder outflow, increasing the volume of residual urine. The bladder hypertrophies and saccules and diverticula can form. The shape of the bladder often changes and it assumes a 'fir tree' appearance.

Treatment

Treatment aims at: (1) preserving the upper urinary tract and thereby renal function. This is accomplished by reducing residual urine to as low a level as possible and thus preventing infection, stones, back pressure and reflux; (2) controlling incontinence if possible without catheters.

Residual Urine

There are a number of manoeuvres which help the bladder empty better. They include contraction of abdominal wall and suprapubic compression in autonomous bladders; trigger points in the automatic, drugs that stimulate bladder contractility or inhibit the bladder neck and urethra (phenoxybenzamine, guanethidine); resection of the bladder neck or external sphincter, self-intermittent catheterization. In suitable patients, electrical devices can be used to stimulate either the conus medullaris or the anterior sacral nerve roots. Electrodes are placed on the conus or wrapped around the nerve roots and connected by subcutaneous wires to a receiver in the anterior abdominal wall. The system is activated by placing a transmitter over the receiver.

Incontinence

Many manage incontinence by careful attention to the timing of micturition; but some form of incontinence appliance is often needed.

Sexual and Reproductive Problems

In women the menstrual cycle and fertility are not usually affected and pregnancy can occur; though the effects on sexuality have not been fully studied.

In men there are problems with both sexual function and fertility, but various methods are available to help them achieve intercourse and ejaculation.

THE WAY AHEAD

Many of the bladder diseases that disabled our predecessors can now be prevented or satisfactorily treated, but incontinence and bladder tumours increasingly cause much distress and in the case of bladder tumours many premature deaths.

The science of urodynamics gives us much insight into the function and dysfunction of the bladder and urethra and is of great value in helping urologists, gynaecologists and neurologists determine the cause of incontinence and its appropriate treatment. It also enables us to study the effects of drugs on the function of bladder and urethra and although the ones presently available, and they include α agonists and blockers, parasympathetic agonists and blockers, are often ineffective or poorly tolerated because of side-effects, hopefully new ones will be developed now that we can assess their actions in humans so easily. The pharmacology of the urinary tract has lagged behind that of other parts of the body for too long.

Bladder tumours have increased in number and in malignancy, approximately one-third are now anaplastic. Many clinical trials are in progress to assess the effects upon bladder tumours of various drugs, for treatment or prophylaxis; singly or in combination, parenterally or intravesically, alone or with other treatment. Some results are promising but we have a long way to go before chemotherapy achieves the same results in bladder cancer that it does in testicular cancer.

83 *The Prostate and Urethra*

J. E. Newsam

ANATOMY

Prostate

The prostate gland is a firm, part glandular, part muscular body and surrounds the beginning of the urethra. It lies in the pelvis behind the pubis and in front of the rectum. Its base, directed upwards, is continuous with the bladder neck; its apex rests on the deep aspect of the external sphincter; its posterior surface, separated from the rectum by the two layers of the rectovesical fascia, exhibits near its upper part a depression through which the ejaculatory ducts enter. They divide the posterior surface into an upper part, called the median lobe, and a larger, lower part called the posterior lobe (*Fig.* 83.1) which lies in the shallow median furrow between the right and left lateral lobes. The lateral lobes which together form most of the 6–7 g of the normal prostate (*Fig.* 83.2) are joined together anteriorly by the anterior lobe which contains few, if any glands. The anterior surface is separated from the pubic bone by fat and veins, and partly connected to it by the puboprostatic ligaments. The prostate is supplied by arteries derived from the internal pudendal, internal iliac and middle rectal arteries. Its veins form a plexus around the gland which receives the deep vein of the penis and drains into the internal iliac veins. Its lymphatics pass to the internal iliac and sacral nodes, thence to the common iliac and para-aortic nodes, but some go first to the obturator nodes. The prostate gland consists of two sets of glands (*Fig.* 83.3), an inner zone, which surrounds the urethra and an outer zone, which surrounds the inner zone and is separated from the prostatic plexus of veins by a thick fibrous capsule.

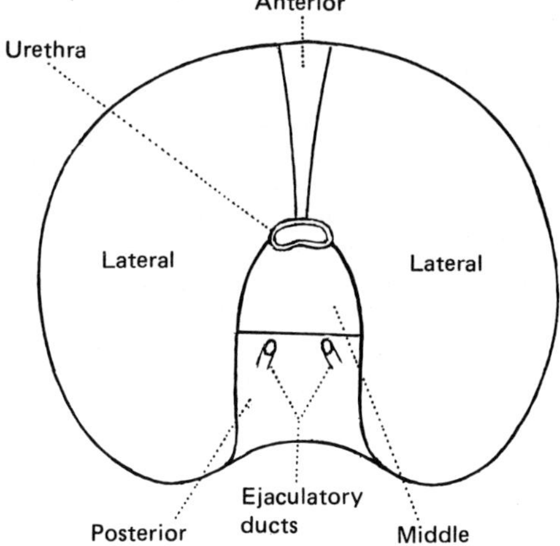

Fig. 83.1 Section of the prostate gland, showing lobes.

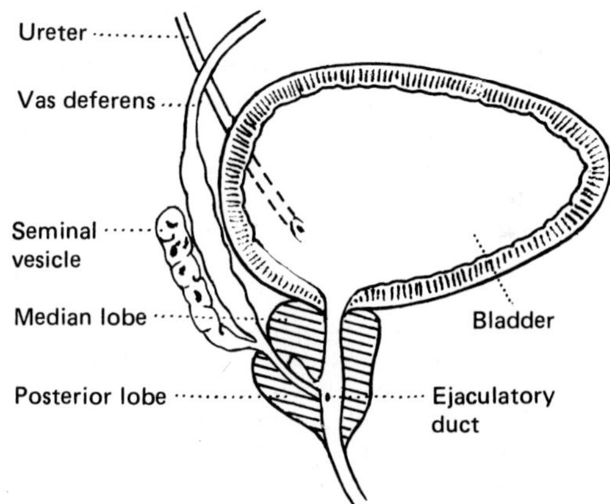

Fig. 83.2 Sagittal section of the bladder and prostate.

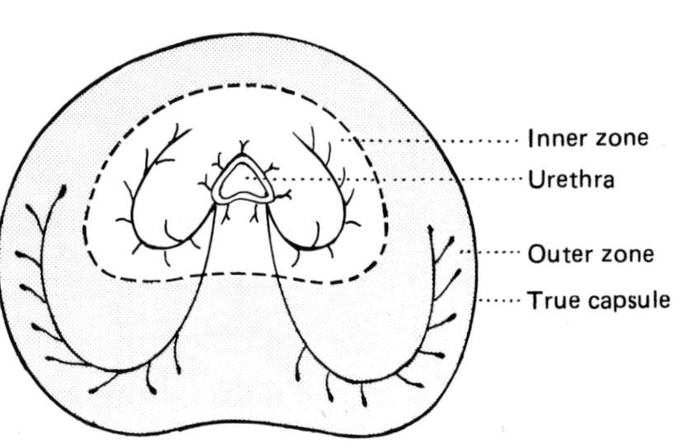

Fig. 83.3 Transverse section of the prostate.

Urethra

Male Urethra

The male urethra is about 20 cm long and can be divided into three parts. The prostatic part, which lies within the prostate gland, is the widest part and runs vertically through the prostate; on its posterior aspect is the prostatic eminence or verumontanum, on either side of which the prostatic glands and the ejaculatory ducts open (*Fig.* 83.4). The verumontanum indicates the level of the external sphincter at transurethral resections of the prostate and it must therefore be preserved.

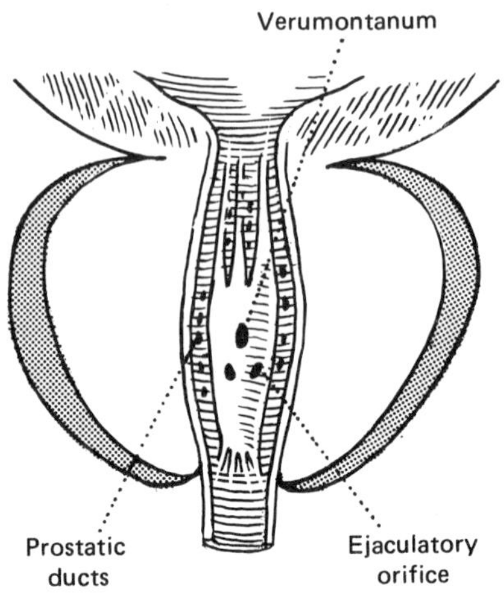

Fig. 83.4 The prostatic urethra.

The membranous part of the urethra is the shortest, and except for the external urinary meatus the narrowest part of the urethra. It is surrounded by the external sphincter.

The spongy part of the urethra extends from the membranous part to the external urethral meatus. Its beginning in the perineum is dilated forming the bulb, and it is also dilated just before it terminates, and this dilatation is called the fossa navicularis or terminalis. The urethra is lined by transitional epithelium as far as the opening of the ejaculatory ducts, then by columnar, and finally at the meatus by squamous. The urethra is distensible and a 26 F instrument can be passed through a normal urethra without difficulty.

Female Urethra

The female urethra is only 4 cm long and analogous to the posterior male urethra as far as the ejaculatory ducts. It begins at the bladder neck and runs downwards and forwards embedded in the anterior vaginal wall, ending at the external urethral meatus, directly in front of the vaginal opening. Part is lined by squamous and part by transitional epithelium, but there is considerable variation in the level at which the change occurs.

INFECTIONS

Urethritis

Urethral infections may be secondary to catheterization, urethral instrumentation or operation but most are sexually transmitted. Nevertheless, these patients may present to the urological surgeon, rather than to the genito-urinary physician with lower urinary tract infection, prostatitis or epididymitis. Sexually transmitted urethritis can be of two kinds: gonorrhoea or non-specific urethritis. Gonorrhoea is caused by the *Neisseria gonorrhoeae*, a Gram-negative diplococcus, which thrives on columnar epithelium and therefore affects the anterior urethra and sometimes the rectum in men, the endocervix in women. The commonest infective agent causing non-specific urethritis (NSU) is *Chlamydia trachomatis*. It probably accounts for about 50% of patients with NSU; *Ureaplasma urealyticum* accounts for about 25%; *Corynebacterium vaginale* for about 15% and in the remaining 5–10% the aetiological factor is a descending infection from the bladder, *Trichomonas vaginalis* or candida or *Herpes genitalis*, or the trauma from applying irritant solutions. A clinical diagnosis of gonorrhoea or non-specific urethritis cannot be made and laboratory tests consisting of smears and cultures from genital and other sites are essential. In men Gram-stained smears of the urethral discharge are accurate in more than 95% of patients; in women the diagnosis is much more difficult and swabs are taken from the urethral meatus and from the ectocervix.

Prostatitis

The prostate may be infected by organisms from the posterior urethra, especially after urethral instrumentation, from the bloodstream, from the upper urinary tract, from the bowel, possibly through lymphatic connections, or by an extension of sexually transmitted gonococcal or non-specific urethritis.

Acute infection involves the ducts and the acini of the prostate but organisms are infrequently found in the urine, nor can they usually be obtained by prostatic massage, which should probably not be done in patients with an acute prostatic infection. The usual organisms are *E. coli* and *S. faecalis*, similar to those found in the urethra and in other infections. The age group is between 30 and 50. The disease has an acute onset with fever and often rigors associated with or soon followed by frequent, difficult, painful micturition and sometimes partial or complete retention. Rectal pain, tenesmus and haematuria are often found together with pain in the perineum and over the sacrum. The prostate feels tense, swollen and tender.

In *chronic prostatitis* the organisms responsible for the infection are also rarely found and the response to antibiotics is often disappointing. The list of symptoms sometimes attributed to chronic prostatitis is daunting and includes not only urological ones like frequent, painful, urgent and difficult micturition, haematuria, perineal and urethral pains, but also weakness, lethargy, impotence, haemospermia, fever and epididymitis. On rectal examination the prostate may be tender, swollen and soft with areas of fluctuation but more often it is thickened and fibrous and these changes may extend into the seminal vesicles. Calcification may be seen on radiography and at endoscopy the prostatic urethra may be red, congested and narrowed. Organisms are rarely found in the urine, in the fluid obtained by prostatic massage or in seminal fluid, but some recommend quantitative localization cultures: organisms are counted in the first 10 ml of urine voided (VB1), the midstream urine (VB2); the secretions expressed from the prostate by massage (EPS) and the first 10 ml of urine passed afterwards (VB3). Prostatic infection is considered confirmed if the number of organisms in EPS + VB3 is greater than in VB1 + VB2. Leucocytes may be found in prostatic fluid but the numbers do not correlate with the severity of the infection or to the response to treatment. The disease tends to be relapsing and difficult to cure, but antibiotics may be given and prostatic resection carried out if there is significant obstruction.

In some 25% of the patients who present with symptoms suggesting chronic prostatitis we find neither infection nor any urological abnormality. Their symptoms are often related to stress, emotion or work and are more likely psychosomatic than organic. These patients tend to 'shop around' from one urological surgeon to another in the hope of finding treatment that might cure them, and they tend to become preoccupied with the prostate and with the symptoms they think it is causing.

Granulomatous Prostatitis

This is a rare condition and usually confused with carcinoma because the prostate feels hard and obstructs the urethra. It is called eosinophilic or allergic prostatitis if large numbers of plasma cells, eosinophils and lymphocytes are found in the gland.

CONGENITAL ANOMALIES OF THE URETHRA

The congenital urethral abnormalities of hypospadias and epispadias are discussed elsewhere (*see* Chapter 84).

Congenital Obstruction of the Urethra

This is most often found in male children and is usually caused by posterior urethral valves.

Congenital Vesical Neck Contraction

This was first described by Marion in 1933 and became a popular diagnosis in the 1950s when treatment consisted of resecting the bladder neck or reconstructing it by a VY plasty. However, it is now believed that congenital vesical neck contraction is rare and the diagnosis is not made without unequivocal evidence which should include the demonstration of a narrowed bladder outlet by voiding cysto-urethrography, bladder hypertrophy with residual urine, obstructive changes in the upper urinary tract and the absence of other causes of urethral obstruction or of neurological disease.

Posterior Urethral Valves (*Fig.* 83.5)

Posterior urethral valves are mucosal folds attached to the verumontanum and the anterior wall of the membranous urethra. They usually have two cusps which fuse anteriorly forming an oblique diaphragm. They may not be seen by retrograde injections of contrast media or at endoscopy, because they behave as one-way valves, billowing out like sails as urine passes from the bladder and causing obstruction as the free margins of the valves approximate. The posterior urethra dilates and elongates and the valves are best demonstrated by voiding cystography. Endoscopically the opening between the valves appears as a V but they gradually close like the vocal cords. They are best observed if after the bladder is filled the endoscope is kept below the verumontanum, with its tap opened so that water drains out of the bladder as the examination is made. The bladder is usually distended, hypertrophied and trabeculated, the ureters dilated and tortuous and vesico-ureteric reflux is a common accompaniment. The distended bladder and hydronephrotic kidneys can often be palpated and many patients have severe chronic renal failure with acidosis and respiratory distress. The diagnosis is made by cysto-urethrography which demonstrates the typical dilatation of the posterior urethra. The valves are treated by resection.

Other causes of congenital urethral obstruction include a hypertrophied verumontanum and phimosis which is occasionally severe enough to obstruct the outflow of urine from the bladder and meatal stricture though most meatal strictures are secondary to hypospadias, circumcision or meatal ulcers produced by a nappy rash.

Diverticula of the Urethra

These may be found in the posterior or anterior urethra. A congenital posterior urethral diverticulum represents dilatation of the prostatic utricle and usually requires no treatment. Anterior urethral diverticula are sometimes found at the penoscrotal junction. The mouth of the diverticulum is usually wide but its distal lip may be very sharp and prominent and comes into contact with the anterior urethral wall as the diverticulum fills during micturition, obstructing the flow of urine through the urethra like an anterior urethral valve.

Urethral Duplication

Two urethras are normally found in infants with two bladders or two penises. When a second one exists with a single

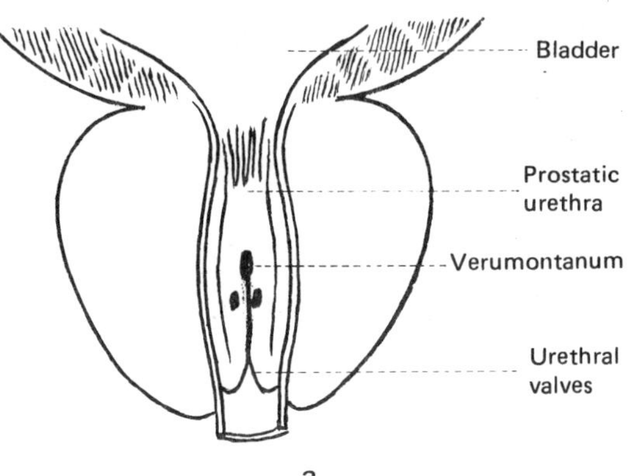

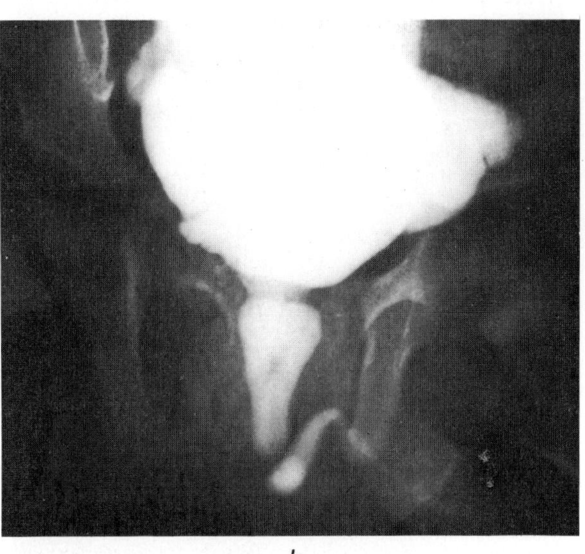

Fig. 83.5 *a*, Posterior urethral valves. *b*, Voiding cystogram showing urethral valves.

bladder and penis, it lies dorsal to the correct one and opens onto the dorsum of the glans or penile shaft. It may be a blind sinus or it may open into the bladder near the normal one and be associated with a chordee.

TRAUMA

The symptoms, the treatment and the prognosis of injuries to the bladder differ from those of injuries to the urethra but it may be difficult to distinguish one from the other except by special investigation because they are caused by similar kinds of injury, and may coexist.

Aetiology

Perforating wounds from gun shots or impalement on fences or railings are rarely seen in this country but when they do occur they often involve both bladder and urethra. The penile urethra may be damaged by blunt injuries to the erect penis and the bulb of the urethra by direct perineal injury from kicks or falls astride a plank which crush the urethra against the pubis. The non-distended bladder and the membranous and prostatic parts of the male urethra are better protected than the spongy part and damaged only by severe injury which usually fractures the pelvic bones too. Injury to the urethra or bladder should be suspected in all pubic fractures. The urethra can be damaged with bougies, cystoscopes or resectoscopes, especially when treating patients with urethral strictures, and false passages can easily be made (*Fig.* 83.6). The female urethra is not often involved in accidental trauma even with fractures of the pelvis, but may be damaged by ischaemia from a prolonged second stage of labour or by the careless use of obstetric forceps. These injuries rarely cause strictures but may cause fistulas between the vagina and urethra or damage the musculature and later cause stress incontinence. The urethra is sometimes damaged by self-inflicted injuries from instruments and other objects passed by patients to try and improve the urinary flow and in women urethral injuries may result from the attempted introduction into the vagina of deleterious agents to produce abortion.

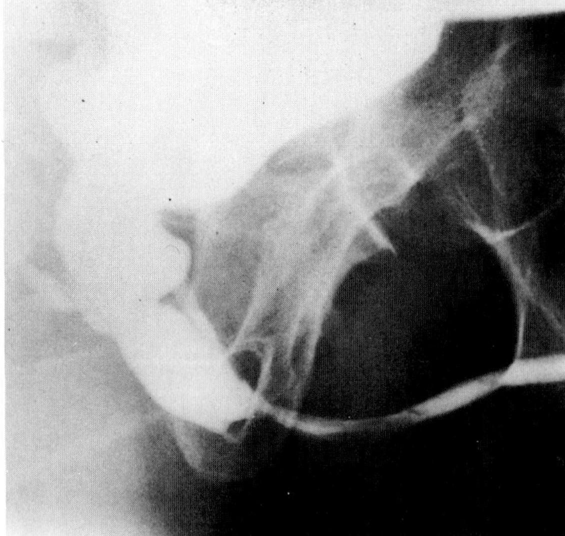

Fig. 83.6 Radiograph showing false urethral passage.

Pathology

Injuries of the anterior urethra are usually caused by direct injury and unassociated with injuries to other structures apart from the skin and the subcutaneous tissues. Injuries of the membranous and prostatic urethra are caused by severe injuries and usually associated with fractures or fracture-dislocations of the pelvis. An injury to the anterior urethra may be a contusion or a partial or complete laceration. Injuries of the posterior urethra involve the membranous part of the urethra which lies in the deep perineal pouch surrounded by the external sphincter (*Fig.* 83.7). The prostate is secured to the pubis by the puboprostatic ligaments and by the perineal membrane which are easily ruptured when the pelvis and particularly the pubic bones are fractured, allowing the gland to move upwards and backwards. The membranous urethra may only be stretched but more often is transected and the prostate dislocates upwards and backwards (*Fig.* 83.8). Sometimes the perineal membrane is also disrupted and both membranous and bulbous parts of the urethra are injured.

Clinical Features

Urethral or bladder injuries should be suspected in all patients with perineal or pelvic bone injuries. Urethral

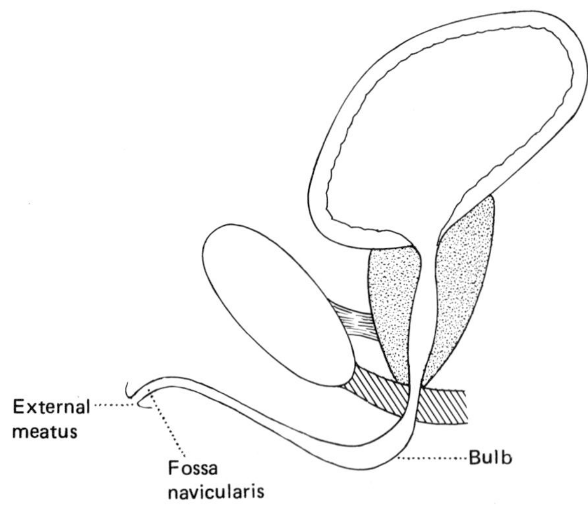

Fig. 83.7 The normal male urethra.

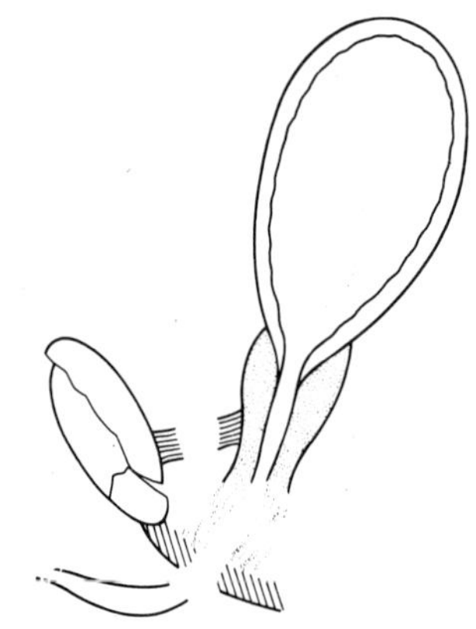

Fig. 83.8 Ruptured posterior urethra.

injuries are recognized by the nature of the accident and by urethral bleeding, perineal bruising and bladder distension. The patients rarely pass urine because the sphincters go into spasm and extravasation of urine into the pelvis or perineum is a late feature of urethral injuries, and receives too much attention in anatomical textbooks. Plain radiographs may demonstrate pelvic fractures (*Fig.* 83.9) and the soft-tissue densities of extravasated urine or blood clot which obliterate the normal soft-tissue outlines of the pelvis and displace bowel loops.

Intravenous Urography

Intravenous urography is recommended as the first investigation in all patients with suspected injury of the urinary tract. In posterior urethral injuries the bladder may look like a tear drop because it is compressed laterally by blood, blood clot and extravasated urine or it may be spherical but lie at a much higher level than usual if the prostate has dislocated upwards. Injury to the bladder may also be recognized by the extravasation of the contrast medium.

Retrograde Urethrography

Retrograde urethrography is the investigation of choice in patients with urethral injury and usually shows the site and sometimes the extent of the damage.

The water-soluble contrast medium used often extravasates into the soft tissues and veins. Twenty ml of a 20% aqueous solution of contrast medium must be slowly injected under radiographic control and the injection stopped immediately if extravasation is seen or bladder filling occurs. No force must be used, even if obstruction is encountered. Urethral injury is revealed by deformity, by contrast extravasation, or, if the injury is caused by instrumentation, by false passages or fistula. A high posterior urethral rupture with extravasation of the contrast may be difficult to distinguish from a rupture of the bladder base; however, bladder filling is never achieved with complete or extensive ruptures of the urethra, whereas some bladder filling is always seen with bladder injuries.

Treatment

There are at least three different schools of thought on the early management of urethral injuries. All three treat injuries of the bladder by early operation. All three leave the patient with suspected urethral injury, if his general condition allows, for 12–24 h after the accident. If micturition occurs no more is done; if it does not the conservative school drain the bladder suprapubically and defer further investigations like urethrography and urethroscopy for at least 3 weeks. The protagonists of this method believe that most urethral injuries are partial, and that urethroscopy and even urethrography or catheterization may damage the slender band of tissue holding the two ends of the urethra together and convert an incomplete into a complete tear. The second school carry out retrograde urethrography and cystography, but never endoscopy, to determine the site and extent of the urethral lesion and to exclude an unsuspected rupture of the bladder, but like the conservative school, they merely drain the bladder with a suprapubic catheter and defer any direct approach to the urethra for some weeks. However, if the puboprostatic ligaments, the perineal membrane and the membranous urethra have all been ruptured the prostate dislocates and there is wide separation of the cut ends of the urethra. In these circumstances many surgeons feel that the cut ends of the urethra should be approximated. This involves exposing the retropubic space, clearing it of blood and clot, passing a catheter through the external meatus and out of the distal cut end of the urethra, negotiating the catheter into the proximal cut end of the urethra and on into the bladder. Traction should not be applied by using a Foley catheter and pulling the bladder neck down with its inflated balloon but by inserting two deep sutures into the anterior prostatic capsule, passing both ends of the sutures out through the perineal skin using needles, and attaching elastic bands which can be strapped to the inside of the thighs. The third school pass a urethral catheter if the patient doesn't void urine. If clear urine is obtained the catheter is left in for some days; if bloodstained urine is obtained a cystogram is made to find out if the bladder is injured. If the

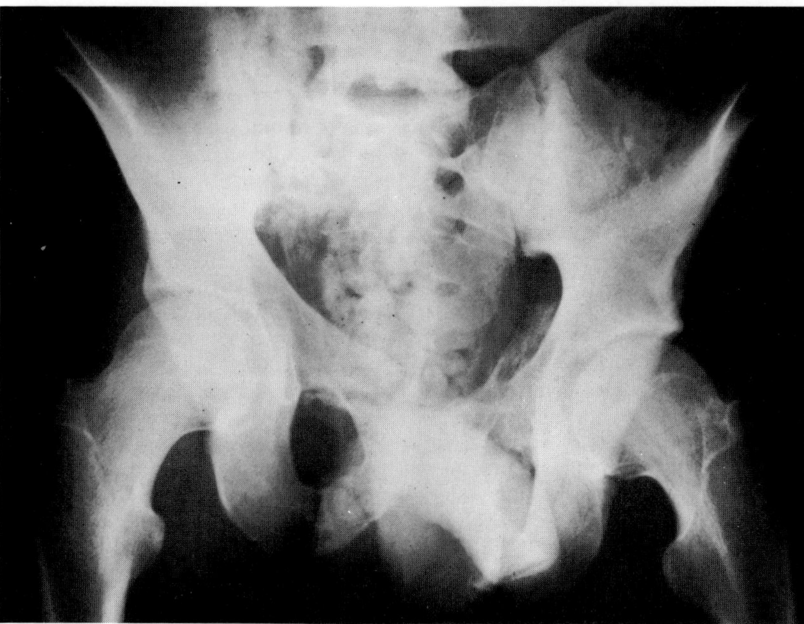

Fig. 83.9 Radiograph showing fracture dislocation of the pelvis.

catheter does not pass into the bladder, a suprapubic catheter is inserted. The second school has the best method of early management, but if it is not possible to carry out urethrography the bladder should just be drained with a suprapubic catheter and further management left for 3–6 weeks.

Prolonged follow-up is necessary in all patients who have had urethral injuries. If a stricture develops, ascending and descending urethrography and urethroscopy reveal its site and length and suggest the appropriate treatment. Apart from stricture, impotence is also a common complication of urethral injuries and may occur in as many as 50% of patients.

URETHRAL STRICTURES

Any part of the male urethra may be strictured, but the common sites are the external meatus, the bulbous part of the spongy urethra in the superficial perineal pouch and the membranous urethra (*see Fig.* 83.7). Strictures vary in length and often not only narrow but also deform and distort the urethra.

Traumatic

It is usually the bulbous and membranous parts that are involved by accidental trauma; the external meatus or membranous parts by instrumental trauma. Even a catheter, particularly if it has to be forced through a narrowed external meatus, may cause stricture of the meatus or fossa navicularis.

Infective

Of the many organisms that cause acute urethritis only the gonococcus does sufficient local damage to result in stricture formation, which is inevitable if the disease is not adequately treated. Apart from bilharziasis, chronic urethral infections are rare but it often causes dense urethral strictures as ova may be laid anywhere along the urethra and induce dense fibrosis. Tuberculosis may involve the prostate and therefore the prostatic urethra, but is rarely found elsewhere in the urethra. Balanitis xerotica obliterans involves the prepuce, causing phimosis, and sometimes the external meatus and anterior part of the urethra, causing a stricture.

Congenital

Congenital strictures of the urethra are not common but may occur at the bladder neck or external meatus. The commonest causes of congenital urethral obstruction are posterior urethral valves.

Clinical Features

Patients with urethral strictures complain of the same difficulties in passing urine as patients with prostatic disease, but tend to be younger. Because they are younger, their response to obstruction is more effective with such considerable bladder hypertrophy that their urinary stream may appear satisfactory despite marked stricture formation. They are liable to develop infections of the urethra, bladder and upper urinary tract, and if infected urine extravasates, penoscrotal abscesses. If these abscesses point at the skin a fistula results between skin and urethra and in gonococcal strictures fistulas may be multiple. Stones may develop in the bladder or in the diverticula which often arise from the urethra proximal to the stricture and, with longstanding strictures, metaplastic changes occur in the bladder and may later become malignant.

Treatment

Before deciding what treatment, if any, should be afforded the patient with a stricture, it is important to assess accurately the stricture, the bladder and the upper urinary tract and this can be done by urethroscopy, ascending and descending urethrography and excretion urography (*Fig.* 83.10).

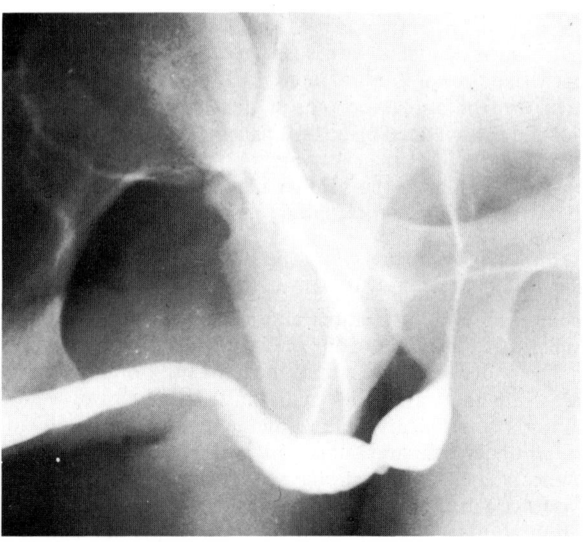

Fig. 83.10 Ascending urethrogram showing stricture of bulbous urethra.

The following methods are available for the treatment of strictures:

a. Urethral dilatation
b. Internal urethrotomy
c. External urethrotomy
d. Excision of the stricture and anastomosis
e. Urethroplasty

a. Urethral dilatation using bougies is a satisfactory means of treatment if the patient is not young and has a stricture which can be dilated easily without fever or haemorrhage and needs treatment no more often than every 6 or 12 months. Otherwise one of the other methods should be used.

b. Internal urethrotomy. This procedure can be carried out blindly with an Otis urethrotome or visually with one of the optical urethrotomes. Most endoscope manufacturers have introduced optical urethrotomes which make internal urethrotomy an accurate and easy means of dealing with strictures. After internal urethrotomy, most surgeons leave in a Silastic urethral catheter for several weeks. It is too early yet to know the long-term value of internal urethrotomy, but the results so far are promising and far fewer dilatations and urethroplasties are now done.

Strictures at the membranous urethra are perhaps better dilated than cut since it is less likely to damage the external sphincter.

c. External urethrotomy. This procedure is only used in an emergency.

d. Short strictures can be excised and the urethra reconstructed by an end-to-end anastomosis.

e. Urethroplasty. If dilatation proves unsatisfactory, and internal urethrotomy is contraindicated or ineffective, then one of the several methods of urethroplasty can be used.

PROSTATIC AND URETHRAL CALCULI

Prostatic

False prostatic calculi are calculi lodged in the prostatic urethra but derived from the kidney and bladder.

True prostatic calculi form in the acini of the gland when calcareous material deposits in the corpora amylacea which are small ovoid bodies made of desquamated epithelial cells coated with lecithin and nitrogenous substances. They vary in number, from one to several hundred, and in size, though most are very small. They are usually found only in association with chronic infection or benign prostatic hypertrophy, when they occur in the capsule rather than adenoma, and occasionally in carcinoma.

Symptoms are those of the associated disease, hypertrophy, infection or carcinoma. On rectal examination they may be confused with carcinoma unless crepitus can be elicited; and they may of course occur together with carcinoma. They can be seen in straight radiographs (*Fig*. 83.11).

Urethral calculi sometimes form in urethral diverticula or on the hair of skin used for urethroplasty. Others arrest in the fossa navicularis or proximal to a stricture en route from the bladder. They can be recognized by palpation or seen in radiographs or at urethroscopy.

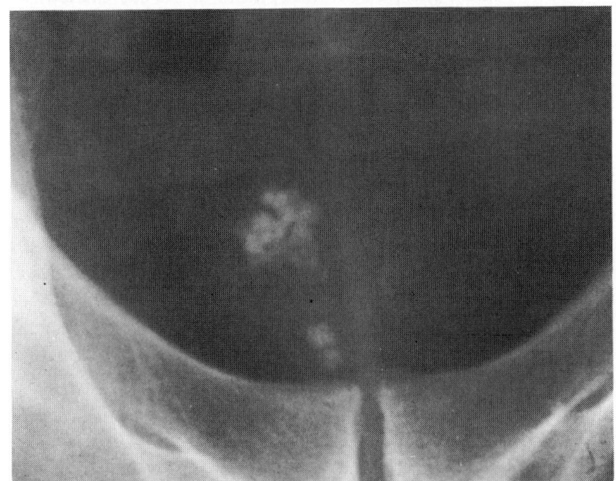

Fig. 83.11 Radiograph showing prostatic calcification.

BENIGN PROSTATIC HYPERTROPHY

Diseases of the prostate constitute much of the work load of the urological surgeon, none more so than benign prostatic hypertrophy. There are now many satisfactory ways of assessing the size of the prostate and its effects on the urethra, bladder ureters and kidneys and several safe and effective methods of dealing with it surgically, however, little progress has been made in discovering its cause nor in finding a medical means of preventing or treating it.

The disease is somehow related to the alterations in hormone activity that occur with increasing age, but the particular changes responsible have not yet been identified despite new methods of hormone assays and increasing knowledge of receptor sites and target organs.

Pathology

The prostate gland grows slowly from birth to puberty, then rapidly to the age of 30. Thereafter it remains more or less constant in size until the age of about 45, when it either hypertrophies or atrophies. The process of benign hypertrophy begins in the inner zone glands of the prostate and as it progresses it compresses, distorts, elongates and obstructs the urethra internally, interfering with the flow of urine from the bladder. Externally it compresses the outer zone glands creating a false capsule and a plane of cleavage (*Fig*. 83.12). Histologically, the changes consist of an increase in the number of glands (adenosis), an increase in the number of cells forming these new glands (epitheliosis), the formation of small cysts as some new glands distend with retained secretions and an increase in the amount of fibrous tissue. If the former changes predominate, the gland becomes large, firm and elastic. If fibrosis predominates, the gland may be no bigger than normal but can still cause severe obstruction. Hypertrophy may involve one or both lateral lobes, or the middle lobe or both middle and lateral lobes. If the middle lobe alone is involved the prostate feels normal on rectal examination (*Fig*. 83.13) because only the lateral lobes and the posterior lobe, which lies in the median furrow are palpable. Yet the middle lobe need not enlarge much to obstruct the bladder neck by the ball valve effect that occurs when it is pushed downwards as the bladder contracts. In 25% of the hypertrophied prostates removed surgically, infarction is found and in 10% an unexpected carcinoma.

Prostatic obstruction increases the resistance to the flow of urine into and along the urethra. The detrusor muscle of the bladder responds by hypertrophy, which is described as trabeculation because the muscle fibres of the detrusor are reticulate. Later, saccules and sometimes diverticula develop between the hypertrophied muscle fibres (*Fig*. 83.14). Later still there is interference with the flow of urine down the ureters and into the bladder, partly because of back pressure, partly because the intramural parts of the ureters may be elevated and obstructed by the enlarging prostate (*Fig*. 83.15) and partly because vesico-ureteric reflux often occurs with obstruction. As a result the ureters, renal pelves and calices dilate and gradually chronic renal failure ensues.

Clinical Features

There may be no symptoms if the enhanced contractility of the hypertrophied detrusor muscle compensates for the increased resistance of obstruction. Later, the patient complains that it is difficult to start passing urine and difficult to stop so that terminal dribbling occurs. The urinary stream is poor in force and calibre and may be no more than a dribble. Frequency and sometimes urgency occur and may be followed by a sensation of incomplete bladder emptying. Later still chronic retention, infection, stones or chronic renal failure may ensue. Acute retention is often the culmination of months or even years of progressively deteriorating micturition but sometimes occurs in patients who have had little if any previous trouble if the prostate suddenly enlarges with infection or congestion or oedema. Congestion and oedema of the prostate occur in patients who have congestive cardiac failure, those who suppress micturition during meals or

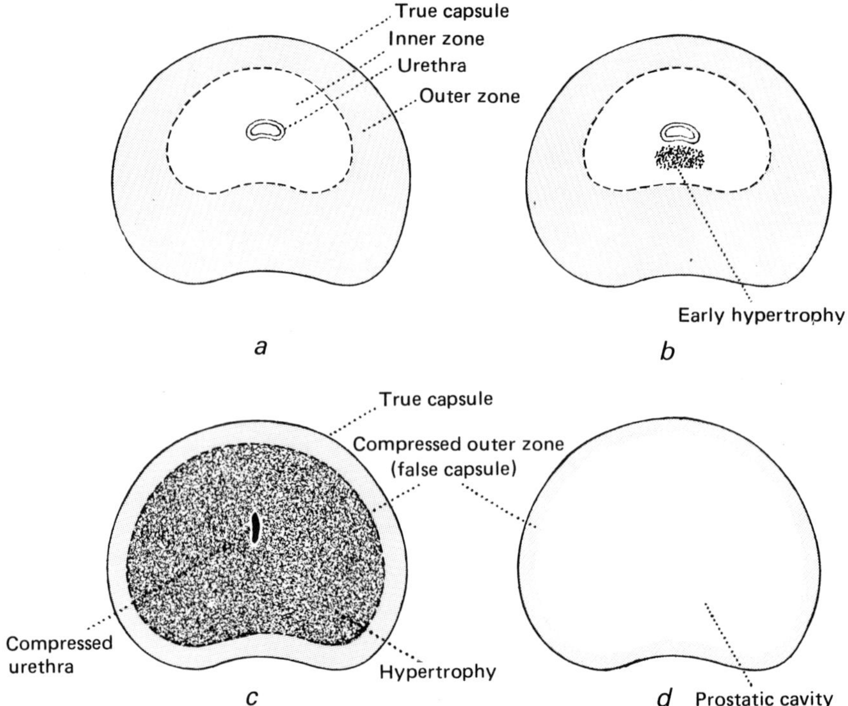

Fig. 83.12 The effects of benign prostatic hypertrophy on the prostate. *a*, Normal. *b*, Early hypertrophy. *c*, Marked hypertrophy. *d*, After prostatectomy.

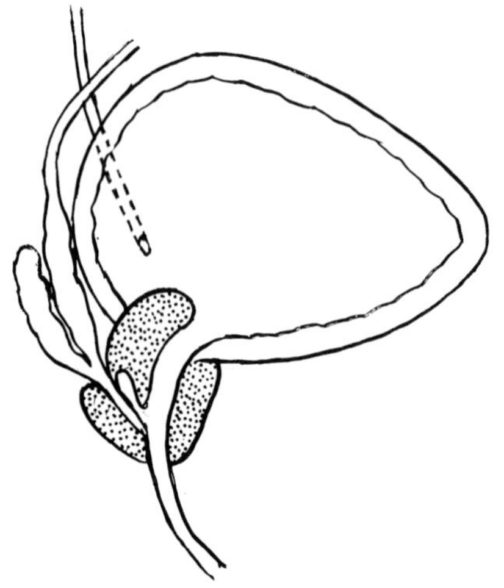

Fig. 83.13 Hypertrophy of the middle lobe of the prostate.

journeys, or patients who have had operations on structures near the prostate or endoscopic procedures like cystoscopy.

There is much evidence that unstable bladder activity also can be caused by obstruction and cured by its relief, but one must be quite certain that obstruction is present in this group before proceeding to prostatectomy, otherwise they may be worse. Benign prostatic hypertrophy is not treated because the gland is large or fibrous but because it is causing obstruction. Many large glands do not cause obstruction, whereas many small ones do. Sometimes the obstruction is obvious because the patient complains of severe difficulties with micturition or of urinary retention or of the effects of stone, infections or renal failure. Sometimes it is not obvious, especially in patients whose main complaints are of frequency and urgency, and the obstruction must be confirmed objectively.

Prostatectomy is an effective and certain way of improving and often curing the symptoms and other effects of obstruction, but it is equally certain to aggravate symptoms which are not the result of obstruction. Rectal examination is important in assessing the size of the lateral prostatic lobes and the tone and contractility of the anal sphincters (which signifies that the nerve supply to the bladder is intact). However, rectal examination does not prove that the outflow of urine from the bladder is obstructed.

Excretion urography may show dilatation of the upper urinary tract or reduced renal function. Cysto-urethroscopy will reveal trabeculation, sacculation or diverticula of the bladder and an increase in residual urine. Cysto-urethroscopy is also the most accurate way of determining the size of the prostate because the length of the prostatic urethra between verumontanum and bladder neck can be measured and the gland palpated bimanually against the instrument. Urodynamics are rarely necessary but suggest obstruction if detrusor pressures are high and flow rates poor. It must be remembered that the chronically distended bladder becomes atonic in time because its muscle fibres are overstretched.

Treatment

Medical treatment cannot alter the pathological changes in benign prostatic hypertrophy but the symptoms of the disease may be improved by treating coexistent cardiac

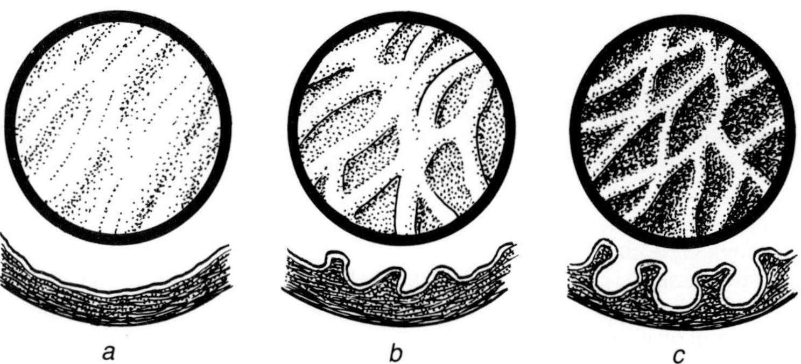

Fig. 83.14 *a*, Normal bladder. *b*, Early trabeculation. *c*. Advanced trabeculation with sacculation.

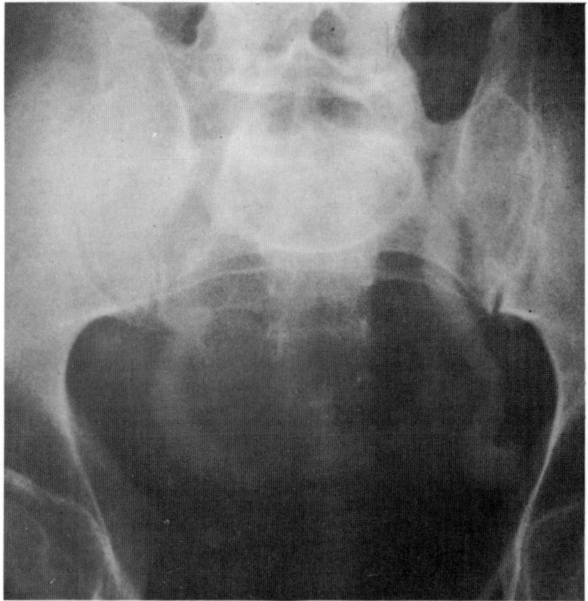

Fig. 83.15 Radiograph showing elevation of the lower ureters by an enlarged prostate.

failure (in which not only the legs and liver may become oedematous but also the prostate) or infection. α-recepter blocking agents, like phenoxybenzamine, reduce urethral resistance and have been used in patients with prostatic hypertrophy, but many patients cannot tolerate them because of side-effects. Furthermore, some drugs, particularly atropine, propantheline, flavoxate and the tricyclic antidepressants, may relax the bladder and aggravate the symptoms which often improve when the drug is stopped or its dosage reduced.

The treatment of prostatic hypertrophy is prostatectomy, which is only required if there is unequivocal subjective or objective evidence of obstruction. The surgeon should not be persuaded to carry it out prophylactically by the patient who says 'although my symptoms are few, it's surely better to do the operation now, when I'm fit, rather than in 10 years time when I may not be so fit'. The natural history of the disorder is unpredictable and it may improve or get no worse without treatment, and any form of prostatectomy may be followed by complications. The choice lies between transurethral resection or an open operation. Several distinguished urologists believe that for prostates smaller than about 25 g a bladder-neck incision, provided it is deep enough is as effective as a prostatic resection and causes fewer complications. With a transurethral resection, the hazards and complications of an incision and postoperative pain are avoided and postoperatively if the patient needs analgesia clot retention should be suspected. Normally the catheter is removed 24 or 48 h after operation and the patient discharged from hospital in half the time of open procedures. The size of each chip resected depends on the size of resectoscope, so that a 30-g prostate takes twice as long to resect as a 15 g one. The disadvantage of transurethral resection is that it requires a certain expertise which is not easily acquired and needs constant practice. Most urologists resect endoscopically prostates less than about 90 g in weight and treat by open operation (preferably retropubically) those over 90 g, but all prostates except the very small, can be effectively treated by open operation, if the surgeon responsible has not mastered the technique of endoscopic resection.

Haemorrhage remains the main immediate postoperative complication but rarely proceeds to clot retention if the bladder is irrigated through a three-way Foley catheter for the first day or two. Strictures are more of a problem after resections than open procedures, especially those at the external meatus or fossa navicularis. They can be avoided by using as small a resectoscope as possible and by dilating the urethra or incising it with an Otis urethrotome before operation.

CARCINOMA OF THE PROSTATE

For many years carcinoma of the prostate was regarded as an easy disease to diagnose and treat. Diagnosis was made by rectal examination and confirmed in some 50% of patients by finding an elevated acid phosphatase or bony metastases. Treatment in all cases, with or without metastases, involved hormonal manipulation by oestrogen therapy or orchiectomy or both. Much progress has been made in the diagnosis and the assessment but less in the treatment of the disease. In the UK carcinoma of the prostate is the fourth commonest malignant disease in men, and the second commonest site for malignant disease in the genito-urinary tract, yet only about 30% of the prostatic tumours found at post-mortem have caused symptoms during life. Geographically there is a high incidence in Norway and Sweden, and a low incidence in the Far East, especially in Japan (1·8/100 000). In the USA the disease is the second commonest malignancy in men and commoner in Black Americans (30/100 000) than White. In the UK 8000 patients present every year with prostatic carcinoma, but symptomless in situ changes are found in many more if the prostate is examined carefully pathologically.

Androgens must be involved in some way in the development of the disease, although it occurs at an age when androgen production is low because it is unknown in eunuchs and often improved by oestrogens or orchiectomy. Increasing age reduces the serum levels of testosterone, 5α-dihydrotestosterone and androsterone, but increases those of FSH, LH, sex hormone binding globulin (SHBG) and oestriol. Yet little if any differences seem to exist in these hormonal changes between normal patients and those with carcinoma or benign hypertrophy of the prostate. Whether androgens cause the disease or merely ensure that sufficient normal prostatic cells survive long enough for malignant change to develop is unknown. Senile prostatic hypertrophy seems not to be a precancerous change.

Pathology

Ninety-five per cent of prostatic carcinomas are adenocarcinomas and arise from epithelial cells of the ducts or acini of the glands in the outer zone of the prostate and many may have a multifocal origin. The tumour spreads externally into and through the capsule of the prostate and on into the trigone of the bladder, the seminal vesicles, the lower ends of the ureters, around the rectum (the rectovesical fascia tends to resist the spread of tumour into the rectum), and internally into the urethra and bladder. The tumour metastasizes along lymphatics to the nodes alongside the internal and common iliac vessels and sometimes the obturator vessels; it later spreads to the para-aortic nodes. Bony metastases are found in decreasing order of incidence: in the pelvis, the lumbosacral spine, the femora, the thoracic spine and the ribs. In 25% of the patients dying of prostatic carcinoma, pulmonary metastases are also present.

Occasionally, transitional-cell carcinomas appear in the prostate and they arise from the distal parts of the ejaculatory ducts or are secondary to bladder tumours. Tumours of the prostatic utricle are not common; they consist of tall columnar ciliated epithelium; they grow slowly and metastasize. Both these tumours and transitional-cell ones are associated with normal serum acid phosphatase levels and are unresponsive to oestrogen treatment.

Clinical Features

Patients with carcinoma of the prostate may present with symptoms or signs of obstruction to the outflow of urine from the bladder indistinguishable from those caused by benign hypertrophy, but often of shorter duration, other symptoms include bone pain from metastatic lesions, haematuria and deep venous thrombosis (carcinoma of the prostate is a not uncommon cause of a spontaneous iliofemoral venous thrombosis, and some patients present only with a swollen leg).

Diagnosis

Rectal Examination

Although some prostatic carcinomas (To) can only be diagnosed by histology, most can be recognized by rectal examination—as small nodules in the early stages and as hard, fixed, irregular masses later. In all, the diagnosis must be confirmed because stones, granulomas and even fibrosis can produce a hard gland also. Although a diagnosis can be made by the usual rectal examination in a conscious patient, the full local extent of the tumour and therefore its T category can be recognized only with a bimanual examination of the anaesthetized patient, which can be done at the same time as cysto-urethroscopy, biopsy or resection.

Cysto-urethroscopy and Transurethral Resection

This is carried out at the same time as the bimanual examination and is often combined with resection which is done to obtain a biopsy and to relieve obstruction.

Biopsy

A biopsy can be taken from the prostate through the urethra with a resectoscope, or through the rectum with a Tru-cut needle. No patient should be treated for carcinoma of the prostate without first obtaining histological proof of the disease. Most patients have obstructive problems and require a resection, which can be done at the time cystoscopy is done.

Acid Phosphatase

The prostatic acid phosphatase isoenzyme differs from that in such other tissues as red blood cells, platelets, spleen, liver and kidney because it is inhibited by L-tartrate. However, it is sometimes elevated in patients with prostatic hypertrophy, particularly after rectal examinations or resection, or if the patient has retention or the gland is infarcted. More accurate assessments of the prostatic acid phosphatase can be made by radioimmune assay techniques but these are still at an experimental stage.

Radiology

CHEST. Although pulmonary metastases are found in some 25% of patients dying of prostatic carcinoma they are rarely seen in pretreatment films, more common are sclerotic metastases in the ribs (*Fig.* 83.16).

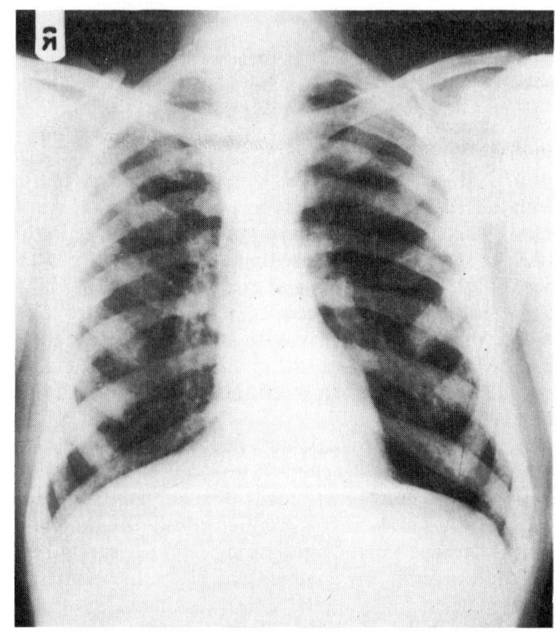

Fig. 83.16 Chest radiograph showing sclerotic metastases in the ribs.

SKELETON. Bony metastases are usually, but not always, osteosclerotic and sometimes confused with Paget's disease. Only those parts of the skeleton that appear abnormal in a bone scan are radiographed (*Fig.* 83.17).

EXCRETION UROGRAM. Obstruction of one or both ureters is a feature of locally advanced tumours and causes varying degrees of renal failure.

LYMPHANGIOGRAPHY. Pedal lymphangiography is of little value in the assessment of prostatic carcinoma because the pelvic nodes are rarely shown and the investigation has a limited place.

BONE SCAN. Prostatic bony metastases appear in bone scans before they do in radiographs. However, it is essential to radiograph those areas that are abnormal in the scan because degenerative, traumatic, infective and metabolic bone disease can produce a similar change in the scan as tumours. However, metastases can be regarded as present if the scan is abnormal and the radiographs normal (*Fig.* 83.18).

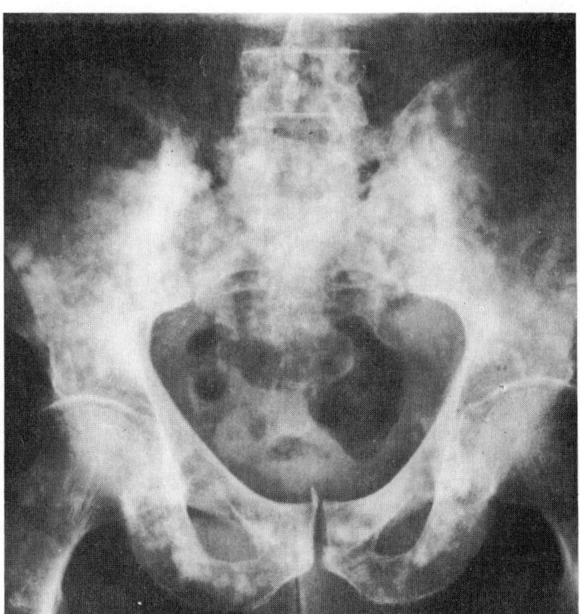

a

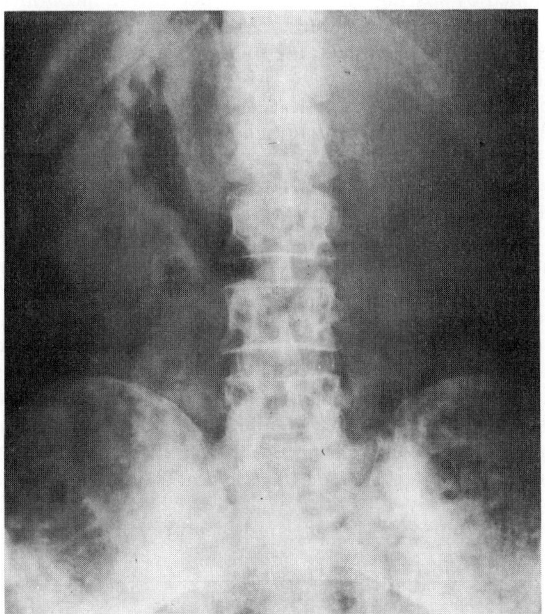

b

Fig. 83.17 Radiographs of the pelvis *a*, and lumbar spine *b*, showing osteosclerotic metastases.

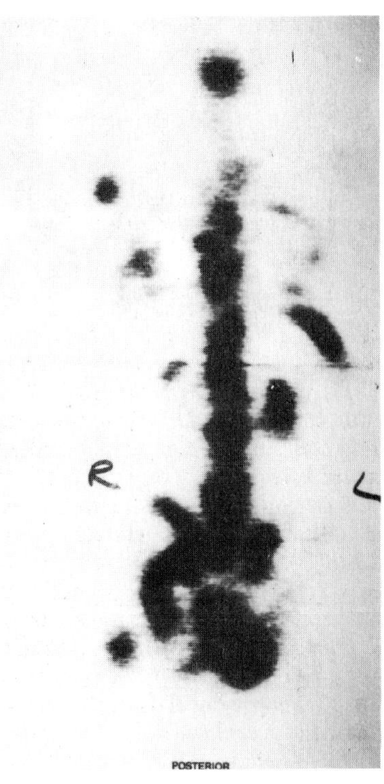

Fig. 83.18 Bone scan showing extensive deposits from a prostatic cancer.

Once these investigations have been done the tumour can be allotted its appropriate TNMG category.

The T category is determined by clinical examination, urography, endoscopy and bimanual examination.

The N category is usually impossible to assess because the regional nodes cannot be palpated nor demonstrated by lymphangiography. Pelvic node dissection is hardly justified as an investigation and most prostatic carcinomas are placed in the NX category.

The M category is determined by physical examination, bone scans, radiography and the measurement of serum acid phosphatase on at least two occasions. An elevated acid phosphatase is accepted as M1 even if bone scan and radiography are normal.

T—Primary Tumour (*Fig.* 83.19)

- Tis Pre-invasive carcinoma (carcinoma-in-situ).
- T0 No tumour palpable includes the incidental finding of carcinoma in an operative or biopsy specimen.
- T1 Tumour intracapsular surrounded by palpably normal gland.

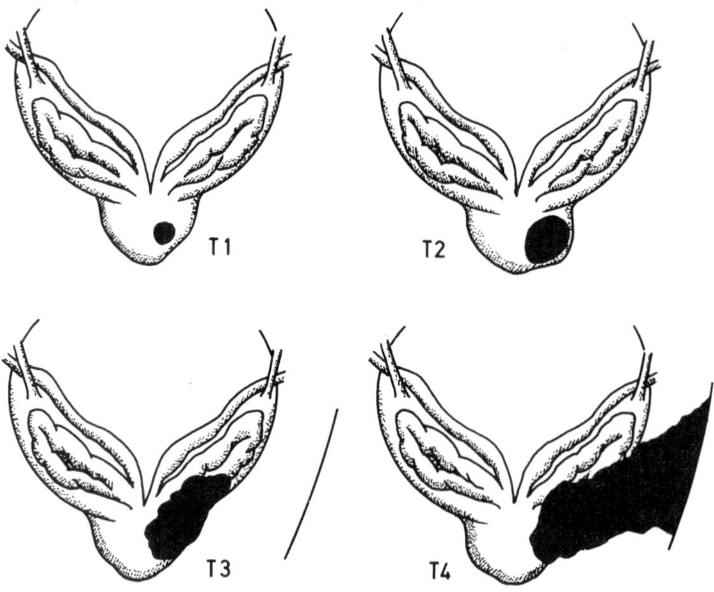

Fig. 83.19 Staging of prostatic cancer.

T2 Tumour confined to the gland. Smooth nodule deforming contour but lateral sulci and seminal vesicles not involved.
T3 Tumour extending beyond the capsule with or without involvement of the lateral sulci and/or seminal vesicles.
T4 Tumour fixed or infiltrating neighbouring structures.
TX The minimum requirements to assess the primary tumour cannot be met.

N—Regional and Juxta-regional Lymph Nodes
N0 No evidence of regional lymph node involvement.
N1 Evidence of involvement of a single homolateral regional lymph node.
N2 Evidence of involvement of contralateral or bilateral or multiple regional lymph nodes.
N3 Evidence of involvement of fixed regional lymph nodes (there is a fixed mass on the pelvic wall with a free space between this and the tumour).
N4 Evidence of involvement of juxta-regional lymph nodes.
NX The minimum requirements to assess the regional and/or juxta-regional lymph nodes cannot be met.

M—Distant Metastases
M0 No evidence of distant metastases.
M1 Evidence of distance metastases.
MX The minimum requirements to assess the presence of distant metastases cannot be met.

G—Histopathological Grading
G1 High degree of differentiation.
G2 Medium degree of differentiation.
G3 Low degree of differentiation or undifferentiated.
GX Grade cannot be assessed.

Treatment

The treatment depends upon the stage of the disease (*Fig.* 83.20) and the age and general condition of the patient. The normal prostate depends upon androgens and so also do many prostatic cancers and at one time oestrogens would be given to all, but they have side-effects, some serious, and one now reserves hormonal manipulation for patients who have metastatic disease or have failed to respond to other treatments.

In the early stages of the disease (Categories T0, T1, NX, M0) when there is no evidence of metastases there is much to be said for giving treatment only if the patient has symptoms. The alternatives are radical prostatectomy, which few if any urologists in this country would consider, or X-ray therapy. However, radical prostatectomy may become more popular now that impotence can often be avoided by sparing the appropriate nerves and incontinence can be treated by inflatable appliances. Only 10% of patients with prostatic carcinoma fall into this group (although the number is increasing), and their life history is unpredictable. An MRC trial has been devised for this group in which one half are not treated until symptoms develop and the other half are given radiotherapy, but since many patients are aged or suffer from other serious disease, not all patients are suitable for a randomized trial.

In the locally advanced tumours without metastases (Categories T2, T3, T4, N0, M0) the use of radiotherapy has been revived, in centres with megavoltage machines. It avoids the side-effects of oestrogens which include painful breasts, impotence, feminization, water and salt retention and cardiovascular problems. The risks of using them in patients who have or have had cardiovascular or thrombotic disease is unacceptable and the early results are encouraging. Many patients experience severe bladder and rectal symptoms during and after the later stages of the 4 or 5 week course of treatment, but they are usually temporary. If the tumour recurs after or does not respond to radiotherapy hormonal treatment can be given.

In the patients with metastatic disease (Categories T0 to T4, NX, M1) hormonal manipulation is used, starting with an oestrogen, or orchiectomy, or even both. Stilboestrol is used in a dose not exceeding 3 mg/day, and orchiectomy reserved for the patient who does not respond or relapses or who has cardiovascular problems. Subcapsular orchiectomy

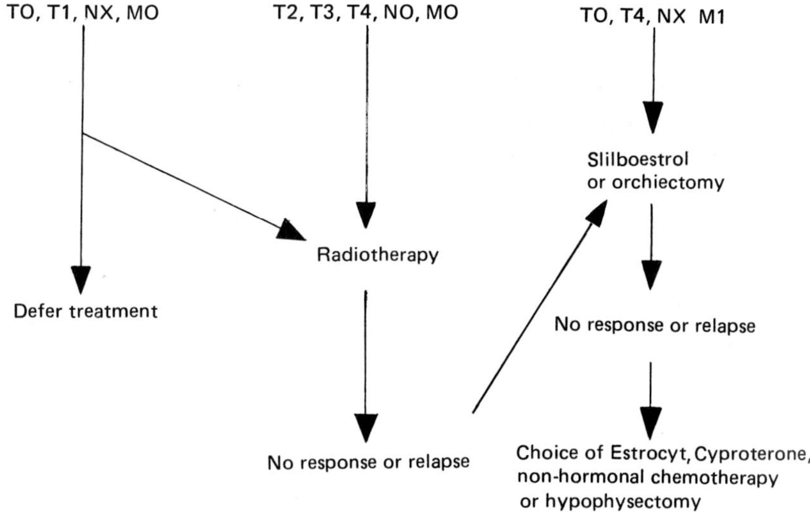

Fig. 83.20 Scheme of treatment of prostatic carcinoma.

is as effective as total orchiectomy. If one type of oestrogen fails there is little point in trying others. Few patients respond to orchiectomy if they have relapsed with stilboestrol. Alternative drugs include cyproterone acetate (which blocks androgen receptors and inhibits testosterone production), estracyt (a mixture of oestradiol and nitrogen mustard) or luteinizing hormone-releasing hormone (LHRH). The paradoxical effects of potent LHRH analogues on the hypophyseal/pituitary axis with the reduction in the production of luteinizing hormone and testosterone are well documented in animals and man. At first LHRH analogues had to be given daily but depot preparations requiring 1-mg injections each 28 days have recently been introduced. Cytotoxic chemotherapy has so far proved of little value. But for many patients, palliation is all that can be offered and includes resection for urinary problems, analgesics or local radiotherapy for bone pain. If bone pain is unrelieved by these measures a hypophysectomy should be considered.

URETHRAL TUMOURS

In the UK, urethral tumours are very rare. They may complicate strictures or be secondary to tumours of the bladder. The incidence of secondary urethral tumours in patients with bladder carcinoma is very much greater than was at one time thought; they are undoubtedly being discovered more often by the routine use of urethroscopy when reviewing these patients. The diagnosis can be made by urethroscopy and biopsy.

Condylomata acuminata (simple warts) are usually found on the glans penis, but sometimes occur within the anterior urethra and may be mistaken for more serious lesions.

CONCLUSIONS AND THE WAY AHEAD

Until some medical means arrives for treating or preventing benign prostatic hypertrophy it is unlikely that more advances will be made in the assessment and treatment of this disease. Advances, however, are to be expected in the treatment of prostatic cancer from the many clinical trials now in progress. Patients and doctors are conditioned to believe that the earlier the disease is diagnosed the easier the treatment and the better the prognosis. Obviously attitudes will change if these trials prove, as many urologists believe they will, that the asymptomatic early prostatic carcinomas (T0) should not be treated. For the late cases we look for some way of understanding and of predicting the response to treatment by manipulation of hormones and some chemotherapeutic regime for treating those who do not respond to it.

84 The Testis and External Genitalia

A. W. S. Ritchie

ANATOMY

The Testis

The testis is the central organ of male reproduction. It is an ovoid structure averaging 4–5 cm in length and 2·5–3·5 cm in width in the adult male. On the posterolateral surface of the testis the epididymis is intimately attached and connected by the efferent ductules.

Embryology

The undifferentiated gonad gives rise, during the 6th week of intrauterine life, to a group of cells (blastema) which will form the testis. The blastema is divided into a series of sex cords which become canalized to form the seminiferous tubules. The gubernaculum ('helm' in Latin) is a band of connective tissue which joins the caudal end of the developing gonad to the genital swelling. Growth in length of the fetus and the failure of the gubernaculum to elongate results in a relative caudal migration of the gonad. The testis lies behind a pouch of peritoneum (the processus vaginalis) as it traverses the inguinal canal to reach the scrotal sac by the 8th month. The lower part of the processus vaginalis becomes the tunica vaginalis and its persistence results in the infantile type of hernia.

The epididymis is formed from part of the mesonephric duct, the closed proximal portion of which remains as the appendix of the epididymis. The remainder of the mesonephric duct becomes the vas deferens and the seminal vesicles form from a diverticulum of this duct.

Blood Supply

The testis is supplied by vessels which follow the descent of the testis. The right artery usually arises from the aorta just below the origin of the renal vessels and the left arises from the left renal artery. Further blood supply follows the course of the vas deferens and may be sufficient to maintain testicular viability in instances when the testicular artery is divided.

Venous drainage of the testis is through multiple veins of the pampiniform plexus to the spermatic vein(s), usually double, emerging from the upper end of the cord before passing retroperitoneally. On the right side the testicular vein empties into the inferior vena cava and on the left into the renal vein.

The lymphatic drainage of the testis is through the spermatic cord and the inguinal canal and thence to the common iliac and periaortic nodes; the latter communicate across the midline at the level of the kidneys and also communicate with the mediastinal and supraclavicular chains.

Testicular nerves are derived from the aortic and renal plexuses, which in turn communicate with the solar plexus. Thus testicular pathology may produce abdominal and not scrotal pain. This may lead to misdiagnosis of testicular pathology, in particular testicular torsion.

Testicular Physiology

The two main functions of the testis are to produce spermatozoa and to secrete testosterone.

The seminiferous tubules and Sertoli cells are responsible for spermatogenesis and the interstitial cells of Leydig secrete androgens, predominantly testosterone. The seminiferous tubules of the testis contain germinal cells and supporting cells, the sustentacular cells of the basement membrane and the Sertoli cells. The Sertoli cell is a static, non-proliferative cell. Specialized junctional complexes between Sertoli cells are believed to form the blood–testis barrier.

Division of the germinal cells is initially mitotic to produce either stem cells to restart the process of spermatogenesis, or rapidly dividing cells, which will become spermatozoa. Meiosis occurs subsequently to produce the haploid gamete.

FSH is required to initiate spermatogenesis but its role in the control of this complex process remains controversial. The entire process of spermatogenesis takes approximately 64 days in humans. It is not until the spermatozoan has passed through further processes of maturation in the epididymis, that progressive motility and the ability to fertilize are acquired.

Between the seminiferous tubules of the testis lies the interstitial tissue containing blood vessels, lymphatic vessels, Leydig cells, macrophages and supporting cells. The Leydig cell produces androgen, mostly testosterone, under the influence of LH.

The Epididymis

This structure is composed of a single coiled epididymal tubule 12–19 feet long. The efferent ductules emerge from the rete testis to connect the testis to the epididymis. The medial surface of the epididymis attaches to the terminal portion of the spermatic cord through which blood, nerve and lymphatic supply are received. Spermatozoa undergo maturation during passage along the epididymis, which also acts as a storage reservoir.

The principal blood supply of the epididymis comes from branches of the testicular artery but it also receives some supply via branches of the inferior vesical artery. Venous drainage corresponds to the arterial supply and the lymphatic drainage is similar to the testis.

Vas Deferens

The vas deferens is a tubular structure with a thick muscle coat. The vas transports spermatozoa from the epididymis via the spermatic cord across the inguinal canal and retroperitoneally to the ampulla of the seminal vesicles.

Spermatic Cord

The spermatic cord suspends each testicle and its attached epididymis. It comprises the vas deferens, the testicular vessels, the external spermatic artery, the lymphatic drainage of the contents of the scrotum and the autonomic nerve supply to the testicle. The cord is surrounded by fibres of the cremaster muscle, which can alter the position of the testis by contraction and relaxation.

Scrotum

The scrotal sac is composed of two lateral compartments which are fused in the midline—denoted by the median raphe. Each compartment encloses the testis, epididymis and the terminal portion of the spermatic cord. Beneath the corrugated skin of the scrotum, rich in sebaceous glands, lies the dartos consisting of elastic fibres, connective tissue and smooth muscle fibres. The dartos allows for muscular contraction of the scrotum during temperature changes and sexual excitement. Together with the cremaster muscle, the dartos permits optimal temperature control of the testis. Spermatogenesis takes place at a lower temperature than that in the abdominal cavity.

The scrotum receives its blood supply from the deep pudendal branches of the femoral artery and branches of the internal pudendal arteries. The lymphatics from both sides of the scrotum anastomose freely, surround the penis and drain to the inguinal and femoral nodes. This lymphatic drainage system is separate from that of the testis and epididymis.

PENIS

The penis consists of two dorsolaterally situated parallel erectile compartments known as corpora cavernosa and the corpus spongiosum, which surrounds the urethra ventrally and terminates distally in the erectile glans penis. Each corpus cavernosum and the tubular spongy tissue are surrounded by fascial sheaths. In addition, all three corpora are surrounded by the dense fibrous Buck's fascia. The corpora cavernosa take origin from the ischial pubic rami. The suspensory ligament of the penis attaches the base of the penis to the inferior aspect of the pubis.

The principal blood supply of the penis comes from the internal pudendal arteries via the dorsal arteries.

Venous drainage is through the dorsal veins. The superficial dorsal vein drains to the saphenous vein and the deep dorsal vein enters the plexus lying anterior to the prostate.

Lymphatic drainage from the corpora cavernosa and the skin pass through the superficial and deep inguinal nodes and communicate with the iliac nodes. The lymph drainage of the glans penis parallels that of the urethra—to the subinguinal, external iliac and deep pelvic nodes.

Erection

Three basic haemodynamic changes are required for erection: (1) increased arterial flow; (2) increased intracorporeal pressure; and (3) increased venous outflow resistance. The mechanism of increased venous outflow resistance is not yet clearly established but work in the dog suggests that it may be effected by compression, by dilated sinusoids, of a venular plexus situated just beneath the fascia surrounding the corpora. Intracorporeal papaverine, used in the diagnostic assessment of impotence, has been shown to increase venous outflow resistance.

The vascular changes involved in erection are controlled by complex neural and hormonal influences.

A spinal reflex mechanism for erection is present in man and becomes obvious after spinal cord injury. The cerebral cortex clearly also has a major influence on erection without the presence of local stimulation.

The major motor nerve supply to the penis is from the sacral parasympathetic nerves. The exact anatomical course of the branches of the pelvic plexus which supply the corpora cavernosa, has only recently been described in detail. These delicate nerves run in the lateral pelvic fascia between the rectum and the prostate. At the apex of the prostate they course anteriorly to reach the lateral aspect of the membranous urethra (*Fig.* 84.1). An understanding of this anatomical pathway has allowed development of techniques to avoid their division in the course of radical pelvic surgery. The thoracolumbar sympathetic nerves form an additional nerve supply to the corpora and may be the pathway for psychologically mediated erection.

Hormonal influences on erection are not clearly understood but androgens seem necessary to maintain sexual interest and motivation. Considerable research on the

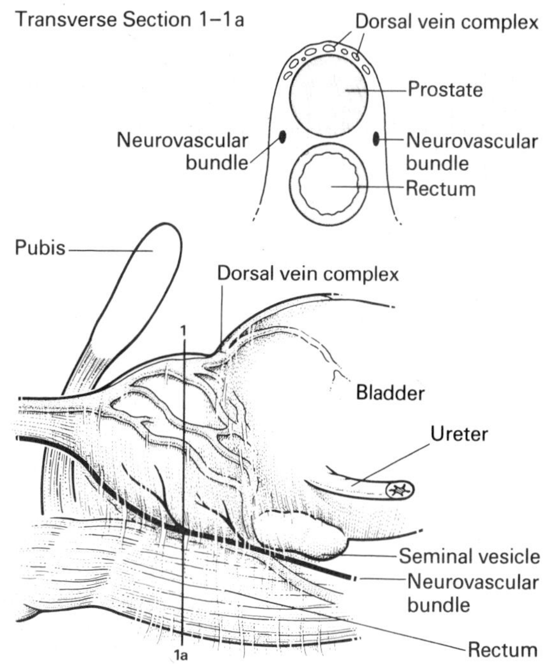

Fig. 84.1 Course of the nerve supply of the corpora cavernosa.

mechanisms of erection is in progress and a unifying hypothesis may emerge to clarify many apparently conflicting observations.

Ejaculation

The process of ejaculation has three main phases. These are seminal emission, i.e. delivery of sperm into the posterior urethra, ejaculation or propulsion of semen from the posterior urethra to the outside and bladder neck closure. This combination of events is reflex, the efferent limb for the reflex is the anterior lateral column of the spinal cord and the thoracolumbar sympathetic outflow. This latter part of the neural pathway is particularly vulnerable during surgical dissection around the distal aorta.

THE TESTIS

The Undescended Testis

Faced with a patient reported to have a problem with testicular descent there are basic questions to be answered which help to categorize the problem and thus decide upon the correct management. Is the problem uni- or bilateral? Is the testis palpable, impalpable or intermittently palpable? If the testis is palpable, is it retractile or ectopic? If the testis is not palpable, is it present at all and if so where is it located?

The Palpable Testis

Retractile Testes

The testis may be retractile due to an overactive cremasteric reflex. This condition is common and requires careful assessment by accurate examination in a relaxed atmosphere, with warm hands. Under these circumstances it should be possible to coax the testis into the scrotum where it can be held without tension. The retractile testis is usually a bilateral phenomenon and does not require surgical intervention. Demonstration of the testis in the scrotum to the parent(s) is often helpful in reassuring them that all is well.

Ectopic Testis

The ectopic testis has descended through the inguinal canal but its further descent into the scrotum is blocked by tethering misdirected gubernaculum or a fascial obstruction at the entrance to the scrotum. The ectopic positions include the superficial inguinal, femoral, perineal and pubopenile.

Some undescended testes may be intermittently palpable due to their movement into and out of the inguinal canal. Such a testis may be difficult to differentiate clinically from the ectopic testis in the superficial inguinal pouch.

The Impalpable Testis

The testis is impalpable when it is absent, atrophic, intra-abdominal or in the inguinal canal. The impalpable testis will constitute approximately 20% of all problems related to descent.

The testis should be descended in the full term infant and since the cremasteric reflex is poorly developed at birth confusion with retractile testes should not occur if early examination has been performed.

The impalpable testis is associated with a higher incidence of hernia, malignant transformation, spermatogenic failure, incomplete orchiopexy and a smaller testis. Torsion of an undescended testis is more difficult to diagnose and results in a higher incidence of ischaemic damage.

Anorchism (bilateral absence of testes) is very rare. Monorchism (absence of one testis) is more common on the left side and occurs in approximately 3% of maldescended testes.

Investigation of a child with bilateral impalpable testes is assisted by endocrine tests to identify the presence of functioning testicular tissue. These tests should be used in conjunction with a search for Müllerian structures and karyotyping. Normal basal gonadotrophins and a rise in serum testosterone after administration of human chorionic gonadotrophin (HCG) indicates the presence of functioning testicular tissue and means that surgical exploration should be undertaken. This method of investigation is unreliable in the adult male as the intra-abdominal gonad may have undergone premature failure of endocrine function.

Investigations to locate the impalpable testis prior to surgical exploration include ultrasound, laparoscopy, selective testicular arteriography and selective testicular venography. Results of such investigations allow for accurate planning of the surgical approach, although the majority of impalpable testes will be found in the inguinal canal or close to the deep ring.

Undescended testes are more common on the right side.

Endocrine Therapy

The use of HCG to induce descent of the testis is reported with varying success. Induction of descent of a true intra-abdominal testis is, however, unlikely.

Orchiopexy

The aim of this operation is to locate the testis, secure the viable organ in the scrotum without tension and remove any associated hernial sac. The purpose of orchiopexy is to improve spermatogenesis, prevent malignant change, trauma and torsion and remove any psychological ill effects of having an empty scrotum or hemi-scrotum.

Under ideal circumstances orchiopexy should be performed between 4 and 24 months and certainly before the age of 5 years. Although technically more difficult for surgeon and anaesthetist, spermatogenesis is more likely to be improved if the operation is performed before 24 months. Psychological problems can be minimized by day case surgery in suitable patients.

The operation should be performed through a skin crease incision in the groin. After identification of the testis and dissection of any associated hernial sac, careful dissection of the vas and vessels is performed to provide sufficient length for the testis to be placed in the scrotum without tension. Various methods have been described to maintain the position of the testis in the scrotum; of these the sub-dartos pouch is popular.

If sufficient length of the vessels cannot be achieved, even after extension of the dissection to the retroperitoneum there are several options. The best position obtainable can be maintained until a further dissection at a future date. Alternatively, the spermatic vessels can be divided and the testis mobilized at a future date on a pedicle of peritoneum and the artery of the vas. Auto-transplantation using microvascular anastomosis to the inferior epigastric vessels has been reported.

Testicular Tumours

Testicular tumours are uncommon but are increasing in incidence. The advent of effective chemotherapy means that early stage and low bulk disease are curable, for the most part. For this reason every effort should be directed towards early diagnosis and accurate staging so that appropriate therapy may be directed towards the entire extent of the disease.

Aetiology

The precise aetiology remains enigmatic but there are certain recognizable associated factors. Testicular maldescent is a known risk factor. The risk of malignant change in an intra-abdominal testis may be as high as 1 in 20. Intersex states have also been associated with tumours particularly of the germ cell variety.

Pathology

Tumours may arise from all the tissue types represented within the testis. The common tumours are the seminoma arising from the seminiferous tubular epithelium and the teratomas. The British Testicular Tumour Panel (BTTP) and American systems for pathological classification are shown in *Table* 84.1.

Table 84.1 Classification of testicular tumours

BTTP	*American*
Seminoma	Seminoma
Teratoma	
Teratoma differentiated	Teratoma
Malignant teratoma intermediate	Teratocarcinoma
Malignant teratoma undifferentiated	Embryonal carcinoma
Malignant teratoma trophoblastic	Choriocarcinoma
Combined tumour	
Yolk sac tumour	
Others	
Sertoli cell	
Leydig cell	
Lymphoma	

Seminoma is the commonest tumour and occurs predominantly in the 35–40 year age group. It is rare in children. Teratomas occur at an earlier age (peak age 25–30) but may also occur in childhood. The teratoma differentiated tumour of childhood can be regarded as a benign lesion but this is not so in adults. Malignant lymphoma is predominantly a disease of older men.

Presentation

The diagnosis of testicular tumours demands that every patient presenting with a testicular swelling is carefully assessed with the possibility of tumour in mind. The classical presentation is with a painless enlargement of the testicle. Up to one-third of testicular tumours are misdiagnosed on the first clinical assessment. The common errors in diagnosis result from the presence of pain, hydrocele and a history of 'trauma'. Pain may result from haemorrhage into the tumour, a hydrocele is a not uncommon accompaniment of tumour and a history of trauma should not always be taken at face value.

The differential diagnosis includes epididymo-orchitis, torsion, a syphilitic gumma, granulomatous orchitis and tuberculosis. If there is doubt about the diagnosis surgical exploration should be undertaken. Preliminary ultrasound examination of the scrotum may be helpful, especially where the testis cannot be palpated because of the presence of a large hydrocele.

Surgical Exploration

Exploration should be undertaken through an inguinal approach with early dissection and soft clamping of the cord prior to delivery of the testis. Frozen section histology is not necessary in every case and can be reserved for those in whom there is doubt about the diagnosis after visualization of the testis.

Staging

Staging investigations should not postpone the orchiectomy. The essential preoperative investigations are a chest radiograph and preferably two separate sets of the tumour markers alpha-fetoprotein (AFP) and beta-human chorionic gonadotrophin (HCG). Postoperative staging includes histological analysis of the extent of the primary tumour, with particular reference to invasion of the cord structures and the histological type.

A search for metastases should include the following: chest radiography; lymphography; IVU; ultrasound of liver and retroperitoneum; CT scan of chest and abdomen; full blood count; liver function tests; urea, electrolytes and creatine clearance; calcium; AFP; HCG; pulmonary function tests (if bleomycin is to be considered); semen analysis and semen banking, if necessary.

On the basis of information gained from the above the patient can be placed in stages I to IV (*Fig.* 84.2 and *Table* 84.2). The subgroups A, B, C of the staging system are used to indicate tumour bulk, an important concept where chemotherapy is to be considered.

Tumour Markers

The two commonly used markers are alpha-fetoprotein (AFP) and beta-human chorionic gonadotrophin (HCG). One or other marker is found in the serum of 50–90% of patients with non-seminomatous germ cell tumours. Both markers will be raised in approximately 40% of patients. The half-life of AFP in plasma is 3·5–6·2 days. HCG is a glycoprotein, consisting of two subunits, secreted by trophoblastic tissues. The alpha subunit is common to FSH, LH and HCG. The beta subunit provokes the formation of specific antibodies, under suitable conditions and the antibodies can be used for detection of the subunit in a sensitive assay. The half-life in plasma is 24–36 h. HCG levels are occasionally raised in seminomas, but AFP elevation indicates the presence of a teratomatous element, even if this has not been detected histologically.

Measurement of markers is of some prognostic guide in assessing response to orchiectomy but their main value is in patient follow-up as elevations of either marker indicate the presence of active metastases often long before disease becomes obvious on clinical or radiological examination.

Management

Since testicular tumours are relatively rare and their staging and management requires various expertise in chemotherapy, radiotherapy and surgery, in addition to active surveillance with easy access to CT scanning in follow-up, referral of these patients to a centre with a special interest may be advantageous.

Seminoma

This tumour is usually diagnosed in the early stages as it is relatively slow growing. A careful search of all pathological

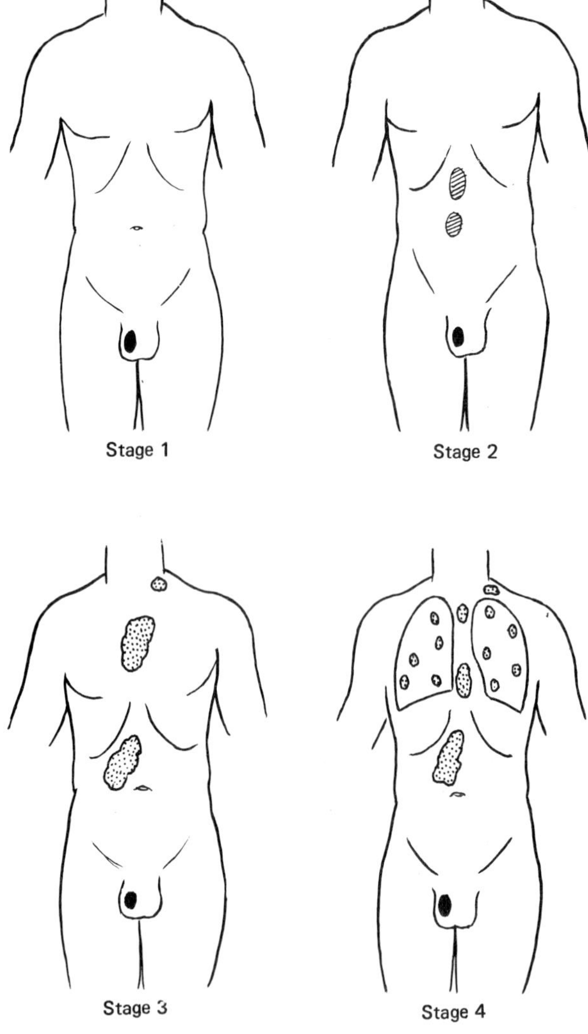

Fig. 84.2 Staging of testicular tumours.

Table 84.2 Royal Marsden Hospital staging system for testicular tumours

I	Lymphogram negative, no distant metastases, marker negative
I_M	Lymphogram negative, no distant metastases marker positive
II	Lymphogram positive, metastases confined to abdominal nodes
Subgroups:	
A	Maximum diameter of metastases <2 cm
B	Maximum diameter of metastases 2–5 cm
C	Maximum diameter of metastases >5 cm
III	Involvement of supra- and infra-diaphragmatic lymph nodes. No extra-lymphatic metastases
	Abdominal status:
	A, B, C as for II
IV	Extra-lymphatic metastases
	Lung status:
L_1	<3 small metastases
L_2	>3 metastases and <2 cm in diameter
L_3	Multiple >2 cm metastases
	Liver status:
H+	Hepatic involvement

material should be made to exclude a small teratomatous element. In addition, if the tumour markers are elevated then it can be assumed that there is a teratomatous element to the tumour. This finding has a significant bearing on the management of the patient.

Seminomas are characterized by their sensitivity to radiotherapy, which forms the main treatment of stage I and II disease.

Stage I disease is managed by radiotherapy to the para-aortic and ipsilateral pelvic nodes. The scrotum need not be irradiated unless there has been violation of the scrotal skin. In Stage I patients the relapse rate should be less than 1%.

Stage IIA and B disease are treated by a similar regime. Relapse rates are approximately 9 and 18% respectively. Stage IIC: the relapse rate for this category is unacceptably high with radiotherapy and these patients are best treated with cis-platinum based chemotherapy.

Stage III and IV disease is managed with chemotherapy.

Non-seminomatous Tumours

The management of teratomas has undergone a dramatic change in recent years. The conventional management with orchiectomy and radiotherapy or retroperitoneal node dissection has been replaced with potent chemotherapy. After adequate chemotherapy the patients are restaged and persistent bulky disease is then resected surgically.

Stage I patients with negative markers can be treated by radiotherapy, chemotherapy or no treatment with close follow-up. Patients with positive markers are treated with chemotherapy until the markers become negative.

Stage II, III and IV patients receive 4–6 cycles of chemotherapy and if the markers return to normal but a mass persists then surgical excision of the residual disease is performed. Persistent marker positive disease may require further chemotherapy.

Chemotherapy

The commonly used regime includes bleomycin, etoposide and cisplatin. These are toxic agents which demand close supervision during administration. Gastrointestinal, bone marrow, lung, skin and spermatogenic toxic effects are common.

Surgery for Residual Disease after Chemotherapy

Accurate planning with the aid of composite images made up from CT data of the site and size of residual disease is the key to success in this important facet of therapy. Although the majority of residual masses are in the retroperitoneum, combined thoraco-abdominal procedures may be required.

Mixed Tumours

Prognosis for these tumours relates to the non-seminomatous elements and they are therefore managed along the lines for teratomas.

Follow-up

There is a risk (up to 3%) of tumour developing in the opposite testis after orchiectomy for tumour. This risk is much higher (up to 45%) if the testis was originally undescended.

Surveillance for Stage I Disease

Since approximately 70% of patients with clinical stage I seminoma and 80% of clinical stage I teratoma will be cured by orchiectomy, the outcome of surveillance without primary radiotherapy or chemotherapy is being investigated. Such studies require meticulous follow-up with regular CT scan and tumour marker assessment and are helping to identify patients at high risk of relapse.

Inflammations and Infections of the Testis and Epididymis

Epididymitis

Epididymitis presents as pain, felt locally or referred along the spermatic cord, swelling and tenderness. It may occur in association with inflammation of the adjoining testis to give the clinical picture of epididymo-orchitis. For descriptive purposes epididymitis, its aetiology and treatment, will be separated from orchitis.

Patients with epididymitis can usefully be divided into three groups: children, adults up to the age of 35, and older men. In children and men over the age of 35, epididymitis is usually related to bacterial infection of the urinary tract. In the middle group of sexually active young men, epididymitis usually follows urethritis caused by sexually acquired infection. The common organisms in this group are *Neisseria gonorrhoeae* and the chlamydial organisms. Chlamydial infection is the commonest cause of non-specific urethritis (NSU) and non-gonococcal urethritis (NGU). *Chlamydia trachomatis* is one of many organisms which infect the genital tract. Fifteen serotypes of this organism have been recognized. The D-K serotypes are the common pathogens in the UK. Other causes of NGU are trauma, herpes simplex virus 1 or 2 and *Trichomonas vaginalis*.

In all age groups epididymitis may be related to a systemic infection or inflammatory disease, e.g. tuberculosis, brucella, sarcoid and cryptococcus. These latter disorders usually give rise to a clinical picture of chronic rather than acute epididymitis.

Diagnosis

The differential diagnosis of acute epididymitis includes testicular torsion and tumour. Differentiation from torsion depends on the history of preceding urinary or urethral irritation, the examination findings and the finding of pus cells and bacteria on urine microscopy. Radionuclide studies and Doppler ultrasound of the testicular vessels have been reported as helpful but none of these findings are absolute and if doubt exists, prompt surgical exploration should be undertaken.

The diagnosis of chronic epididymitis should stimulate investigation to exclude the previously noted systemic disorders.

Complications

These include abscess formation, testicular infarction, chronicity and inflammatory obstruction of sperm transport.

Abscess formation should be suspected if pain, swelling and fever fail to settle with adequate therapy. Ultrasound may be helpful in diagnosing this complication which is treated by surgical drainage. If abscess formation has produced extensive tissue destruction orchiectomy may be required.

Management

Ideally, treatment of epididymitis should be directed at a specific organism. In practice, 'best guess' therapy often has to be started in advance of bacteriological culture results.

For young men in whom the infection is likely to be associated with urethritis, a gram stain of urethral secretion should be followed by special culture. If cultures are not helpful then serological tests using immunofluorescence to type-specific IgM and IgG antibodies to the chlamydia may be helpful. Treatment is with oral oxytetracycline for 14–21 days in uncomplicated cases. Doxycycline, minocycline and erythromycin are alternative agents.

Treatment of both patient and consort should proceed simultaneously. Epididymitis in children and older men should be managed by culture of the urine, followed by administration of an antibiotic active against the common urinary pathogens. Subsequent evaluation of the urinary tract should be undertaken in these patients to exclude obstruction and other anatomical abnormalities predisposing to infection.

Non-specific measures for all patients include bed rest, analgesia and scrotal elevation to improve lymphatic drainage.

Orchitis

Infection may reach the testis by direct extension from the vas and epididymis, via the lymphatics or by blood spread. The common causes of orchitis are those associated with epididymitis, producing the clinical picture of epididymo-orchitis. Orchitis alone is relatively rare but may be caused by bacteria, viruses, chemicals, parasites and trauma.

Pyogenic Orchitis

This may occur as a focus developing after an episode of septicaemia. The patient is usually systemically unwell with a high fever and rigors. Abscess formation follows rapidly if the focus is not eradicated. Orchiectomy may be necessary if the testis is extensively destroyed by pus.

Viral Orchitis

Orchitis can occur in the course of several viral infections including the common influenza and coxsackie infections. The best known form of orchitis is that associated with mumps virus infection. This condition occurs almost exclusively in postpubertal mumps patients, approximately 18% of whom are affected. The orchitis usually starts 4–6 days after the parotitis. Testicular swelling is prominent and there is often a reactive hydrocele.

Treatment is directed to relief of symptoms. No definite benefit from ACTH or steroids has been demonstrated. Tapping of a tense hydrocele may relieve pain.

Orchitis resulting from syphilis and filariasis is rare in the UK.

Granulomatous Orchitis

Non-specific inflammation may occur in the testis, epididymis and spermatic cord following infection, trauma, exposure to chemicals and occasionally vasectomy. The testis is usually enlarged and tender. The aetiology is not always clear and biopsy may be required to exclude other specific pathology such as tuberculosis, sarcoid, malakoplakia and other rare conditions.

Testicular Torsion

Neonatal Torsion

An extravaginal torsion of the testis may occur in the neonatal period. There is often no pain or systemic upset but the testis is noted to be swollen. Commonly the testis is completely infarcted by the time of surgical exploration. If the diagnosis is not made at the time of the torsion then complete atrophy is a common sequel. Fixation of the opposite side is the remaining important task.

Torsion in Young Adults

Strictly, torsion of the testis is a misnomer, in that the pathology is a torsion of the spermatic cord. The resultant compression of the testicular veins and, later, the arterial supply, produces pain and within six hours cells within the testis begin to suffer ischaemic damage.

The underlying defect that allows an intravaginal torsion of the cord to occur is a high insertion of the tunica vaginalis, leaving a length of cord free within the tunica. This anomaly is usually bilateral and the testis may take up a horizontal lie (*Fig.* 84.3).

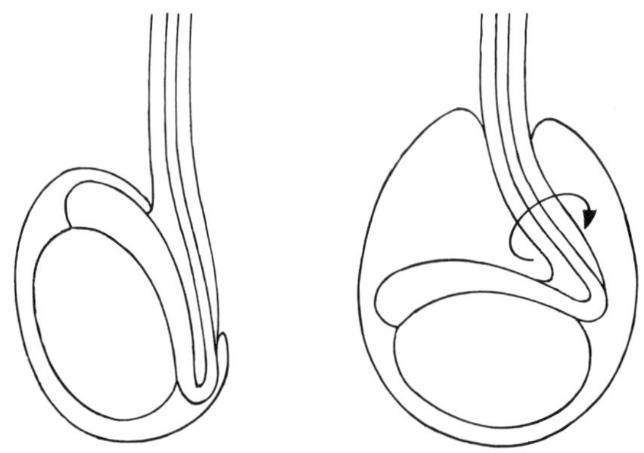

Fig. 84.3 The high insertion of the tunica vaginalis allows an intravaginal torsion to occur.

Clinical Features

Torsion of the spermatic cord is most common around the time of puberty. There are often preceding attacks of pain probably representing episodes of torsion which resolve spontaneously.

The main presenting symptom is of pain, which may be felt in the scrotum, groin or in the lower abdomen and is usually of sudden onset. There may be associated nausea and vomiting.

Examination often shows the relevant testis sitting high in the scrotum, at times with a horizontal lie. The testis and cord are tender and there may be associated swelling.

Differential Diagnosis

Infection and tumour are the main differential diagnoses. The common mistake is to treat a painful testis as infection without making a definite diagnosis. If the urine has no pus cells or bacteria on a gram stain then the diagnosis of infection should not be sustained and surgical exploration should be undertaken.

Treatment

Once a diagnosis of torsion is made it is worth trying to reduce the torsion manually. In any case prompt surgical exploration should be undertaken through a scrotal incision. The twist in the cord is reduced and the gonad inspected for viability and other congenital abnormalities. If the testis is viable it should be fixed by suturing the tunica albuginea to the dartos on at least three points using non-absorbable suture material. The opposite side should be fixed at the same time. If the testis is not viable it should be removed and the other side fixed.

Although the time limit of six hours after the onset of pain is classically associated with non-viability, it is worth performing exploration even after this time as the vascular occlusion is not always complete and the testis may be salvageable.

Torsion of Testicular Appendages

Remnants of the Müllerian duct may persist as cysts attached to the superior pole of the testis (appendix testis). These cysts may undergo torsion and produce pain and swelling out of all proportion to their size. Careful examination demonstrates localized tenderness and the rotated cyst can sometimes be visualized by transillumination of the associated small hydrocele. If the diagnosis is clear, surgical exploration is not mandatory. Usually exploration is performed to establish the diagnosis and exclude other pathology.

Testicular Trauma

The mechanism of injury may be blunt or penetrating. Penetrating wounds must be treated as for any potentially contaminated wound. Usually, however, the injury is blunt and may produce a range of damage ranging from mild bruising to complete maceration of the testis. If the tunica albuginea is split by the blunt force the testicular tissue may herniate through the split. There is usually a large haematocele in association. Surgical exploration is advised if the patient presents early and there is a suspicion of splitting of the tunica. Exploration will allow for haemostasis and repair of the split in the tunica. Untreated, the haematoma will slowly resolve and the tear in the tunica heal by fibrosis usually with resultant reduction in the volume of the testis.

Chronic Testicular Pain

Patients with chronic testicular pain require careful assessment. A thorough history should include probing to try and identify events associated with the onset of the pain and the patient's theories of the cause. Examination will identify obvious intra-scrotal pathology. If the testis and cord are normal to palpation then referred pain from intra-abdominal and musculoskeletal causes should be sought. Commonly, no physical diagnosis can be made. Psychological assessment is recommended before proceeding to regional nerve blocks and certainly before orchiectomy is considered. Orchiectomy in patients without a definitive diagnosis, commonly results in recurrence of the pain in the incision or in the opposite testis.

PENIS

Congenital Lesions

Hypospadias

Hypospadias is a developmental abnormality in which the urethra opens in an abnormal position on the underside of the penis. The abnormality can be classified according to the site of urethral opening. Thus glandular, coronal, penile and penoscrotal varieties exist. Severe hypospadias should raise the question of an intersex state and chromosome studies will be required to resolve this issue.

The hooded prepuce, often seen with hypospadias, may look unsightly but the temptation to remove it should be resisted as it may prove invaluable for plastic repair of the hypospadias.

Hypospadias is commonly associated with cordee and correction of this is an important component of any repair. The presence of cordee and its severity are best assessed by induction of an artificial erection before the start of the repair.

The choice of surgical procedure depends on the severity of the hypospadias. Not all cases require surgery. The aim of surgery is to correct the cosmetic defect and produce a meatus situated at the tip of the glans to produce a forward projected urinary stream.

The trend in surgical correction is towards one-stage procedures and these are best performed by surgeons with experience and training in this exacting area. Minor degrees may be suitable for meatal advancement and glanduloplasty (The MAGPI repair), the principles of which are illustrated in *Fig.* 84.4. The more proximally situated meatus may require preputial island flap interposition (*Fig.* 84.5).

Successful correction of the cordee can be checked by induction of erection at the end of the procedure.

Epispadias

Dorsal opening of the urethral meatus may occur alone or in conjunction with bladder exstrophy. The deformity can be subdivided into two types. In the glandular or penile variety the bladder neck is intact and continence is preserved. In the more posterior penopubic or subsymphyseal variety the bladder neck is incompetent and dribbling incontinence is present. The trigone of the bladder is often poorly developed and there is a high incidence of vesico-ureteric reflux. The corpora cavernosa are poorly developed giving rise to erectile abnormalities.

Surgical reconstruction aims to restore continence, reposition the urethral opening and correct penile deformity.

Congenital absence of the penis, duplications of the penis and true micropenis are rare congenital disorders which require specialist assessment and management.

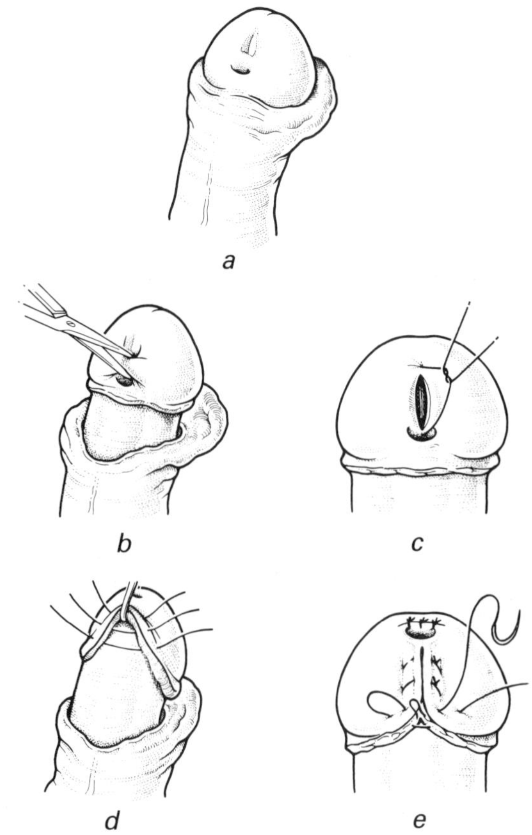

Fig. 84.4 The meatal advancement (*a–c*) and glanduloplasty (*d*, *e*) repair (MAGPI) of subcoronal hypospadias.

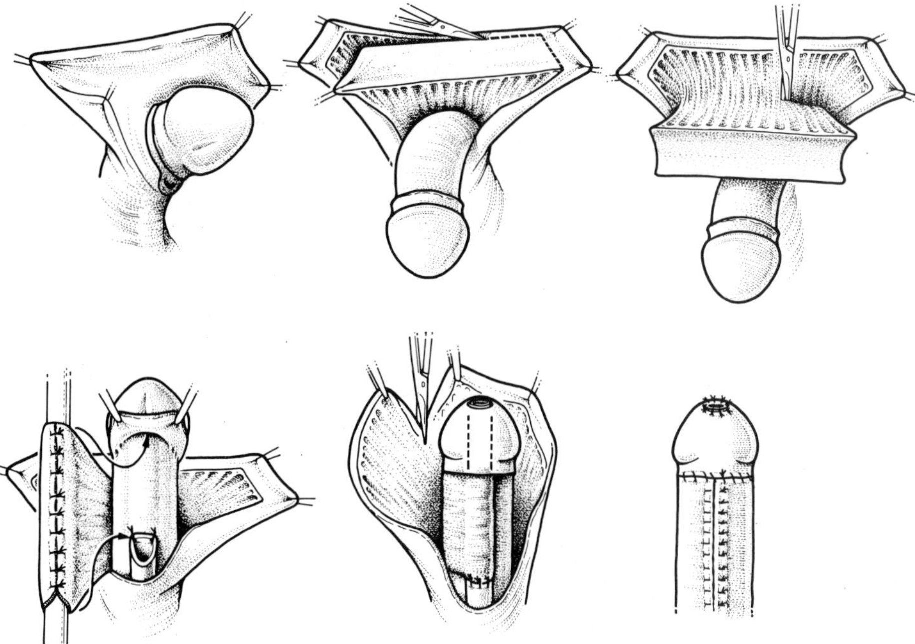

Fig. 84.5 Preputial island flap repair of penile hypospadias.

Phimosis and Paraphimosis

The prepuce is normally closely applied to the glans penis until the age of 2–3 years. Separation of the prepuce and/or circumcision before this age are not recommended as exposure of the glans to urine may result in ammoniacal dermatitis.

Phimosis describes a condition where the opening of the prepuce is narrowed and retraction is prevented. Circumcision may be indicated in the older child if the phimosis is associated with recurrent balanitis or ballooning during voiding.

Paraphimosis results from retraction of a tight phimotic ring over the glans to produce vascular congestion and oedema. A vicious cycle of increasing oedema and vascular insufficiency is created and may result in ischaemia of the glans.

The management involves anaesthesia (a ring block of plain lignocaine around the base of the penis is usually satisfactory) and gentle, persistent manual compression of the glans. This compression reduces the oedema and allows reduction of the constriction ring. Circumcision is recommended on the next suitable elective list. Emergency dorsal slit or circumcision is rarely required.

Trauma

Fracture of the penis usually occurs during athletic intercourse. The fracture affects the corpus cavernosum. The history is of an audible cracking noise with immediate detumescence of the penis. Surgical repair is recommended if the patient presents early after the injury. The resultant scarring may result in asymmetrical filling of the corpora cavernosum or impotence.

Trauma may also be caused by zipper injuries, and a variety of industrial and traffic accidents. Extensive degloving of the penile skin may require split skin grafting.

Disorders of Erection

Priapism

Named after Priapos the mythical Greek god of fertility, this condition may be defined as a painful erection of the penis without sexual stimulation or desire. The erection is confined to the corpora cavernosa. Detumescence does not occur following ejaculation. In the majority of cases there is no clear aetiology but drug therapy, alcohol abuse, perineal trauma, sickle-cell disease, leukaemia and inflammatory disorders of the urinary tract are common associated conditions.

Management

The initial management should consist of intracorporeal injection of metaraminol (Aramine), a sympathomimetic amine which effects vasoconstriction of the erectile tissue and hence detumescence. Care should be taken in administration as hypertension may occur when the agent reaches the systemic circulation. This medical treatment has taken precedence over emergency surgical decompression, which is now reserved as second-line therapy.

Embolization of the pudendal vessels is the next treatment and surgical procedures to improve the venous outflow (e.g. creation of a shunt between the corpora and the saphenous vein) have declined in popularity because of the increasing awareness that the erection is maintained by increased inflow rather than obstructed outflow.

Peyronie's Disease

This disorder is characterized by fibrotic changes in the elastic tissue of the tunica of the corpus cavernosa. This fibrosis may result in pain and/or distortion of the penis. In a minority of cases an asymptomatic lump appears in the penis. The disease may progress slowly over a period of years or may follow a rapid course producing marked angulation of the erect penis preventing intercourse.

About 10% of patients with Peyronie's disease also have Dupuytren's contracture and there are familial associations.

The aetiology is unknown although some cases undoubtedly follow trauma to the corpora.

Impotence may result from pain, psychological effects or mechanical progress of the disease.

Management

Medical management with vitamins and steroids has not stood the test of controlled trials.

Surgical intervention, if desired by the patient, is indicated for angulation interfering with satisfactory intercourse. Operative techniques are based on: (1) surgical excision of the fibrotic plaque with replacement of the defect with dermal or synthetic grafts; or (2) plication or resection of the corpus cavernosum opposite the site of maximum concavity.

Impotence in association with Peyronie's disease merits full investigation to exclude other causes but may require combined treatment of the plaque with insertion of prosthetic rods (*vide infra*).

Impotence

This can be defined as a failure to obtain an erection use for intercourse. Impotence must be separated from orders of ejaculation (*vide infra*).

Conventional classification of impotence divides the c dition into organic and psychological subgroups. In a individual patient this neat classification may be hard to sustain as there are almost always psychological elements in any patient's response to impotence. The section on the anatomy of the penis indicated that the physiology of erection is not completely understood and hence precise diagnosis of the fault within a complex phenomenon is difficult. An erection requires an increase of blood flow, reduction of venous outflow and intact parasympathetic nervi erigentes (S2, 3, (4)).

Nocturnal penile tumescence can be measured and used to separate purely organic from mixed and purely psychological cases. Intracorporeal injection of papaverine is a new technique which can be a useful aid in diagnosis. This agent will normally produce an erection lasting several hours and helps to differentiate vasculogenic impotence from psychogenic causes.

Common organic factors producing impotence are peripheral neuropathy, autonomic neuropathy commonly associated with diabetes mellitus, peripheral vascular or cardiovascular disease, drugs including antihypertensives and alcohol. Impotence may also follow pelvic fractures and other trauma including radical pelvic surgery and spinal cord injury. Local penile pathology such as priapism and Peyronie's disease may also end in impotence.

Investigations

History; examination; blood sugar; testosterone; prolactin; nocturnal penile tumescence; intra-corporeal papaverine; arteriography is rarely helpful as the pudendal vasculature is not well demonstrated except in high flow situations, e.g.

priapism; Doppler ultrasound can be used to examine blood flow and the diameter of the penile arteries.

Management

Management depends on the facts revealed by careful history taking and counselling. Anxiety is a common factor with many patients and the patient's expectations of therapy are important.

Medical treatment short of direct intracavernosal injection with such alpha-blocking agents as phentolamine or phenoxybenzamine are rarely helpful. If an organic cause has been identified or tumescence studies reveal failure of the mechanism of erection, surgery with inert prostheses may be indicated in selected patients. Such prostheses take the form of semi-rigid rods or an inflatable tube placed into the corpus cavernosa. The AMS inflatable penile prosthesis is illustrated in *Fig.* 84.6. This device includes inflatable rods which are placed in the corpora after dilatation, a reservoir placed in the retropubic space and a control mechanism and pump placed in the scrotum, where it is operated transdermally by the patient.

Disorders of Ejaculation

Complete failure of ejaculation (ejaculatory incompetence or ejaculatory impotence) is rare and usually ascribed to psychological causes. Premature ejaculation is, by contrast, common. It is also largely psychological in origin and usually responds well to sexual counselling.

Retrograde ejaculation is caused by incompetence or failure of closure of the bladder neck resulting in diversion of the ejaculate into the bladder.

Surgery to the bladder neck, diabetes, damage to the thoracolumbar outflow and drugs such as phenoxybenzamine are some common causes of retrograde ejaculation.

Carcinoma of the Penis

Aetiology

Circumcision in infancy gives complete protection from developing carcinoma of the penis. Circumcision performed after infancy but before puberty greatly decreases the risk. A non-retractile foreskin and poor hygiene are clearly associated with the development of carcinoma of the penis but there is no clear association with venereal or herpetic infection. The incidence of carcinoma of the penis shows marked geographical variations among both circumcised and uncircumcised populations.

Pathology

The lesion is usually a squamous-cell carcinoma. Very rarely a basal-cell carcinoma, malignant melanoma, sarcoma or secondary carcinoma occur in the penis. Carcinoma-in-situ of the penis shows the typical cytological features of malignancy in a thickened epidermis with a round-cell infiltrate and increased vascularity.

Clinical Features

Carcinoma-in-situ (synonyms: Bowen's disease; Paget's disease, Erythroplasia of Queyrat) may appear as a moist, red or dry, scaly patches or even as a warty lesion. The number that would go on to develop invasive cancer is probably small but they should be regarded as potentially malignant.

The invasive cancer usually presents in elderly men but may occur in patients as young as thirty years. The tumours are either proliferative growths or ulcerating and secondary infection is common. The inguinal lymph nodes are enlarged in two-thirds of cases but in half of these the lymphadenopathy is the result of secondary infection and not due to nodal metastases.

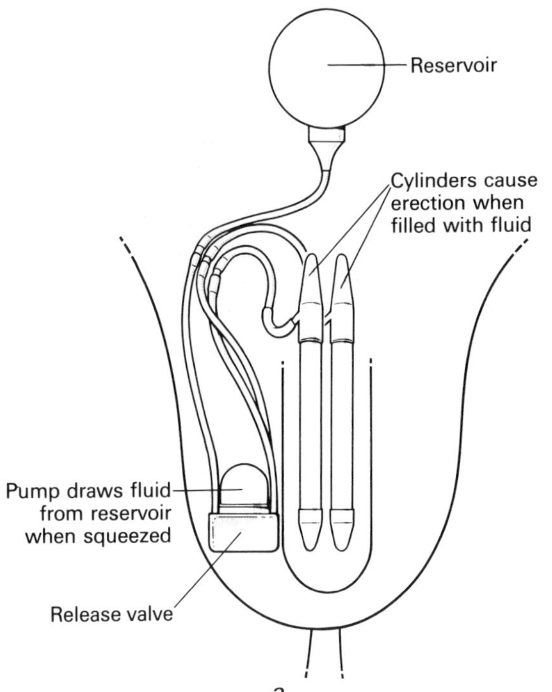

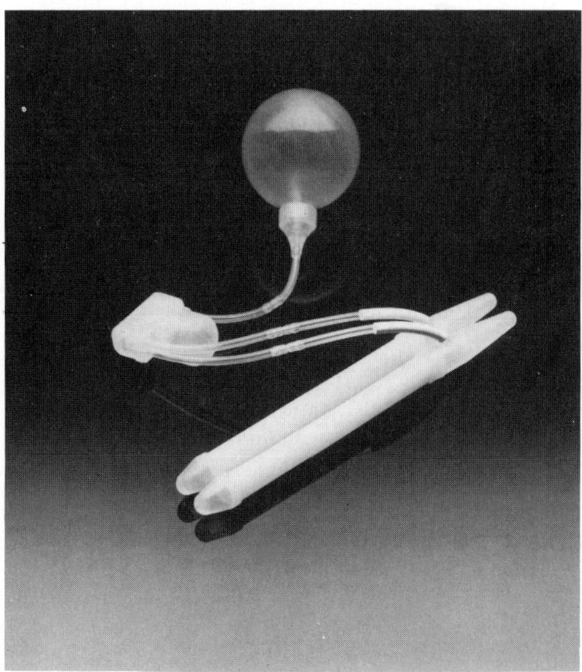

Fig. 84.6 AMS inflatable penile prosthesis.

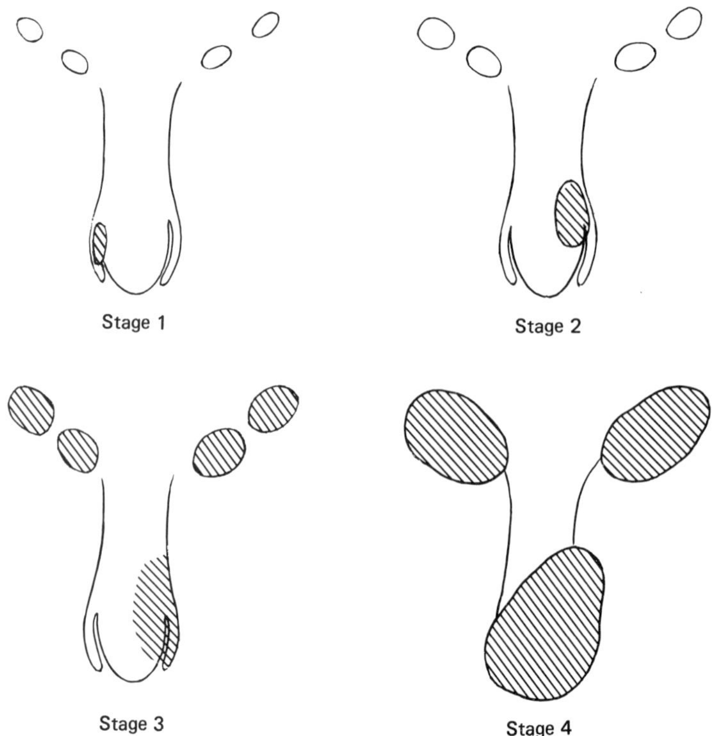

Fig. 84.7 Staging of carcinoma of the penis.

The TNM Classification and Staging

The tumours are staged according to their anatomical site (prepuce, glans penis, shaft of penis) and size (T1=<2 cm, T2=2–5 cm, T3=>5 cm or deep extension, T4=infiltrating neighbouring structures. Four stage groupings are recognized (*Fig.* 84.7).

Stage I —Confined to the glans penis and prepuce
Stage II —Invasion of the corpora cavernosa
Stage III—Inguinal lymph nodes involved but operable
Stage IV—Perineal or scotal involvement, fixed inoperable nodes, distant metastases.

Management

Diagnosis is established by biopsy which may require a dorsal slit or circumcision. The large infected and fungating tumour is best dealt with by partial or radical amputation.

The Stage I and II lesions can be treated with radiotherapy with a good cosmetic and functional result and survival at least as good as for surgery (70–90% 3-year survival).

Palpable lymph nodes should be carefully watched while the primary tumour is treated and infection cleared with a course of antibiotics. If the lymphadenopathy does not resolve a biopsy should be taken to confirm metastatic involvement. Bilateral node dissection may be complicated by lymphoedema and delayed wound healing, and may not curb the disease. An alternative, therefore, is to irradiate the nodal area. When the disease is extensive with iliac nodes involved the prognosis is dismal. So far the best chemotherapeutic agent for advanced disease is bleomycin. Carcinoma-in-situ may be treated with either radiotherapy or topical 5-fluorouracil cream.

Inflammations and Infections of the Penis and Scrotum

Balanitis and Balanoposthitis

The presence of the prepuce creates a warm moist atmosphere for the growth of organisms. Regular hygiene normally prevents abnormal growth and may be used to manage minor infections. Persistent balanitis unresponsive to local hygiene and antibiotics, guided by culture results, should be investigated to exclude other specific pathology. Not all balanitis is caused by infection and the differential diagnosis includes precancerous lesions, drug eruptions, psoriasis, scabies, dermatitis and lichen planus. If phimosis coexists then a dorsal slit may be required to expose underlying lesions of the glans penis. If doubt exists about the pathology then biopsy should be performed.

Gangrenous balanitis may result from combined infection by spirochaete and vibrio organisms and untreated may result in extensive destruction of the glans and shaft of the penis.

Balanitis xerotica obliterans is a condition similar to lichen sclerosis et atrophicus and is of uncertain aetiology. The typical white firm prepuce bleeds easily and slowly produces a dense phimosis. The atrophic sclerotic process may extend to the glans and produce meatal stenosis. The lesion is not considered premalignant and may require circumcision and meatotomy.

Genital Ulcers (*see* Chapter 5)

Ulcers of the genitalia may result from a variety of pathologies including infective, traumatic and neoplastic processes. *Table* 84.3 lists some of the more common lesions and their clinical features. Red raised lesions of the genitalia may

Table 84.3 Genital ulcers

Clinical features	*Diagnosis*
Firm, indurated, painless ulcer	Syphilis
Rolled, elevated ulcer edge	Granuloma inguinale
Punched-out ulcer	Chancroid
Group of vesicles/ ulcers on a red base	Genital herpes
Onset immediately after sexual activity	Traumatic ulcer
Specific drug ingestion	Fixed drug eruption
Raised often infected ulcer	Squamous carcinoma

cause diagnostic difficulty. Such conditions as fungal infection, erythroplasia of Queyrat, primary and metastatic tumour and balanitis circumscripta plasmacellularis will require histology, or specific culture, to confirm the diagnosis.

Genital Herpes

Herpes simplex virus (HSV) infection of the genitalia is common in sexually active adults. The condition causes considerable morbidity, is associated with cervical neoplasia in the female and remains a problem on account of the lack of curative therapy.

Infection of the genitalia is usually associated with the type II virus. The common clinical features are of urethritis, loin pain and systemic upset. Initial attack symptoms tend to be more severe than those in recurrent attacks. Proctitis may occur in homosexual men. The diagnosis is suggested by the finding of a group of vesicles on an erythematous base not corresponding to a neural distribution.

The virus can be cultured from urethral secretion and antibodies to the virus can be measured in serum. Treatment is with acyclovir which can be given orally, intravenously or topically. Treatment can shorten attacks but does not eliminate the disease.

Genital Warts

The majority of genital warts are caused by papilloma viruses and do not usually cause diagnostic difficulty. In their early stages however, they must be differentiated from benign and malignant tumours, molluscum contagiosum and condylomas of syphilis.

Warts on the genitalia outside the urethra can be treated by application of podophyllin, diathermy or cryotherapy. Warts in the urethra can be treated by local instillation of thiotepa or 5-fluorouracil.

Acquired Immune Deficiency Syndrome (AIDS)

Infection with human T-lymphotrophic viruses (specifically HTLV-III) results in abnormalities of T-cell mediated immunity with opportunistic infection and in some cases the development of tumours, e.g. Kaposi's sarcoma. The virus is spread by blood and sexual contact and the number of reported cases is increasing rapidly. There is no effective treatment for established disease which has a high fatality rate at present.

Previous exposure to the virus can be detected by serological tests.

THE SCROTUM

Acute Infective Gangrene of the Scrotum (Synonym—Fournier's Gangrene) (*see* Chapter 5)

This is usually caused by infection with more than one organism, particularly an anaerobic streptococcus. The onset is sudden and constitutional upset severe. Pain and inflammation are marked and patchy necrosis of the scrotal skin occurs which may be followed by extensive sloughing. Treatment is with antibiotics and surgical débridement when necessary. Despite the severity of its clinical signs recovery is usually complete with skin grafting rarely necessary (*see* Chapter 5).

Carcinoma of the Scrotum

An occupational aetiology has been known for this condition since it was first described in chimney sweeps and later in cotton spinners. Even today it is still likely to have resulted from occupational exposure to carcinogens so a full occupational history should be taken. Treatment is by a wide local excision with later dissection of the inguinal nodes if involved.

Genital Filariasis

Wüchereria bancrofti is the common lymphatic filarial parasite to infect the genitalia. The parasite is transmitted by mosquitoes and gains entry to the lymphatics producing inflammation and obstruction. The diagnosis can be confirmed from microscopic examination of smears of blood or hydrocele fluid. Complement-fixation and skin tests are also useful.

Management includes treatment with diethylcarbamazine. Plastic surgery may be required to remove oedematous tissue and reconstruct the scrotum.

Scrotal Swellings

Diagnosis

The diagnosis of a scrotal swelling rests with a careful history and examination and with a minimum of investigations. There are three important questions which govern the examination of a scrotal swelling:

1. Does the swelling arise in the scrotum or has it come down from above through the inguinal canal (i.e. can we get above it)?
2. Is it cystic or solid (does it transilluminate)?
3. Is the swelling in the body of the testis or not?

When examining any scrotal swelling the possibility that it is a testicular tumour must always be considered. If the swelling is found to arise from the body of the testis or if the diagnosis is in doubt then the diagnosis should be a tumour until disproved by exploration of the testis through an inguinal approach.

Hydrocele

Hydroceles presenting in childhood are due to the continued patency of the processus vaginalis and may be associated with an inguinal hernia. If the cord is explored and the processus vaginalis ligated and the hydrocele will resolve. It is not necessary to excise the hydrocele sac.

In adults the hydrocele may be primary and idiopathic or

secondary to a testicular tumour, trauma to the cord or testis, infections and filariasis. Primary hydroceles are common in the elderly and the basic defect is a delay in the absorption of fluid, presumably due to lymphatic obstruction. In all cases the body of the testis should be carefully palpated and it may be necessary to aspirate a tense hydrocele before this can be done. In 5% of cases the testis lies anteriorly in the hydrocele sac so its position should be demonstrated by transillumination before aspiration.

The management of the hydrocele is surgical (subtotal excision) unless the patient is unfit or unwilling to undergo surgery. Repeated aspirations may then keep the patient comfortable but run the risk of causing bleeding or infection.

Epididymal Cysts and Spermatoceles

Cysts arising in the region of the head of the epididymis may contain either clear fluid (epididymal cysts) or turbid fluid containing spermatozoa (spermatoceles). They may be multiple or multilocular. Aspiration is followed by recurrence and if they are large, uncomfortable or causing undue anxiety they should be excised.

Varicocele

Examination of normal adult men will reveal an abnormal dilatation of the pampiniform plexus of veins in about 8% of cases. Most varicoceles cause no symptoms but a dull ache is sometimes complained of. The left side is nearly always affected with only 2% of cases affecting the right side. A cough impulse is present and there is retrograde flow of blood down the testicular vein. Scrotal thermography reveals that there is an increase in scrotal temperature which affects both sides of the scrotum. Patients with varicoceles may have a reduction in sperm density and an increase in abnormal morphology. *See* Male Infertility.

Idiopathic Scrotal Oedema

This is a benign self-limiting condition which may be allergic and a variant of angioneurotic oedema. The oedema and erythema of the scrotum are painless and may affect both sides and extend onto the groin and penis. Spontaneous resolution occurs and will take between 2 and 4 days.

MALE INFERTILITY

Assessment of this problem must take account of two people, who should be seen together. Investigation of the male partner should only proceed as information from investigation of the female emerges. Many of the 'remedies' for infertility have proved useless when tested under controlled conditions and assessment of the couple should concentrate on accurate assessment, diagnosis and sensitive, realistic counselling. One of the most important aspects of assessment is to give the couple a realistic prognosis so that unnecessary investigation and treatment can be avoided.

Assessment

A thorough history should be obtained from both partners before investigation is considered. The history should include details of the following: previous marital history; family history; past medical history including infectious diseases (especially mumps); previous surgical history especially operations in the groin or on the genitalia; history of sexually transmitted diseases; drug history; smoking and alcohol habits; shaving habits; occupational history; gynaecological and menstrual history; sexual history including 'trying time' (duration of involuntary infertility at the time of first consultation).

Examination

Examination should include observation of anatomical abnormalities and assessment of secondary sex characteristics. Examination of the external genitalia should include estimation of testicular size, palpation of the epididymes and vasa. The presence of a varicocele should be sought by clinical examination in addition to Doppler ultrasound examination or thermography (*see below*).

Investigations

Seminal analysis: volume of ejaculate; sperm density; sperm motility; sperm morphology. Testosterone; FSH; LH; antisperm antibodies; Doppler ultrasound of the testicular veins.

Subsidiary investigations: exploratory scrototomy; testicular biopsy; vasography.

Female investigations are directed to ovulation and fallopian tubal patency.

Prognosis

Analyses of all the above factors in the assessment of a couple has shown that the trying time, the motile sperm density (millions of motile sperm/ml) and the status of the female partner are the most important predictors of the likelihood of future pregnancy. Fecundability (conception rate per month) declines rapidly with a trying time greater than 24 months and a motile sperm density less than 2 million/ml.

Management

The most common finding from investigation of male infertility is oligozoospermia. This is a description from semen analysis and is not a diagnosis as the underlying cause is not defined. Non-specific drug therapy for oligospermia has not been shown to be effective in controlled trials.

High-dose steroid treatment for selected patients with high levels of antisperm antibodies has been shown to increase the pregnancy rate. This treatment is, however, associated with significant side-effects.

Varicoceles can be ligated surgically or occluded using percutaneous transfemoral embolization techniques. The subsequent effect on sperm counts and pregnancy rates remains controversial.

Surgery for obstructive azoospermia demands an accurate diagnosis of the level of obstruction. Obstruction may be caused by congenital and acquired lesions. The common site for congenital obstruction is at the junction of the head and body of the epididymis. Inflammatory lesions and previous surgical exploration produce obstruction at various levels of the vas deferens. In general the results of surgery are better where the lesion is an acquired one.

Artificial insemination by husband, by donor and *in vitro* have an important place in the management of selected couples and have emerged as the most effective forms of therapy for infertility.

VASECTOMY AND REVERSAL OF VASECTOMY

Vasectomy

This procedure, more correctly referred to as vas sectioning and occlusion, is the most successful method of contraception in men. The operation can usually be done under local anaesthesia, is well tolerated and has few complications.

Preoperative counselling should include a detailed description of the procedure, the likely discomforts and the need for semen analysis to ensure that azoospermia occurs (two negative sperm counts). Patients should also be warned of the rare occurrence of late recanalization. Relative contraindications include local infection in the scrotal wall and systemic coagulation disorders. Consent is usually obtained from the patient and his wife although the latter is not legally necessary. The technique involves division of the vas and occlusion of the ends, either with suture or diathermy. Fascial interposition is a useful addition and reduces the incidence of late recanalization.

Histological examination of a segment of each vas is not necessary.

Complications of vasectomy are usually related to the technique. Bleeding and infection are the common early complications. Late complications include sperm granuloma, recanalization and chronic pain.

Reversal of Vasectomy

This procedure is being requested with increasing frequency. The best results (>90% vas patency) follow microsurgical vaso-vasostomy, using a two-layer technique.

Patients should understand that success is not guaranteed and that vas patency does not necessarily equate with fertility. Failure to achieve vas patency may result from technical failure or may be due to unrecognized secondary obstruction elsewhere in the vas or epididymis.

Immunological aspects of infertility following prolonged vasal obstruction require further elucidation.

THE FUTURE

Testicular Tumours

The surveillance studies now being performed should identify groups of patients at both high and low risk of relapse. Early aggressive chemotherapy for the high-risk cases and active surveillance for the low-risk cases should limit treatment toxicity for the latter and improve survival for the former.

Chemotherapy is toxic and it is hoped that less toxic analogues of cisplatin e.g. carboplatin will reduce this morbidity.

Surgical debulking will probably remain an important facet of the management of patients with heavy tumour burden at presentation.

Impotence

Improved methods of assessment should refine the diagnosis of the causes of impotence. Medical therapy with intracavernosal injection may be superseded by medication that can be absorbed transdermally. Technological improvements in inflatable penile prostheses should improve results for selected patients.

Further Reading

Hargreave T. B. (ed.) (1983) *Male Infertility*. Berlin: Springer-Verlag.

Index